Dear Ingenix Customer:

Enclosed is the 2011 pre-release draft of the International Classification of Diseases, 10th Revision, Clinical Modification (ICD-10-CM) as written by the World Health Organization (WHO) and National Center for Healthcare Statistics (NCHS). These codes will replace the current ICD-9-CM system for medical documentation and reimbursement. Our new ICD-10-CM code book will help you get a head start with training programs and system conversion.

The Department of Health and Human Services (HHS) published the final rule regarding the adoption of both ICD-10-CM and ICD-10-PCS in the January 16, 2009, *Federal Register* (45 CFR part 162 [CMS—0013—FJ]). The compliance date for implementation of ICD-10-CM and ICD-10-PCS as a replacement for ICD-9-CM is October 1, 2013.

Features and benefits include:

- **Exclusive Ingenix Edge Color Coding and Icons:**

  – check digit icons to alert coders to required 4th, 5th, 6th, and 7th characters, including a separate icon for placeholder "x" requirements

  – manifestation color coding to ensure appropriate etiology/manifestation code sequencing with no manifestation code sequenced as a first-listed or principal diagnosis

  – color-coded instructional notes that appear in red font

  – color-coded deactivated codes that appear in blue font

- **ICD-10-CM Tabular List of Diseases and Injuries 2011 Addendum:** The complete and official ICD-10-CM Tabular List of Diseases and Injuries 2011 Addendum is available on our website. Log on to www.ShopIngenix.com/productalerts then click on "ICD-9-CM News and Code Book Alerts" to review, download, and print the addendum.

- **Official Preface (2011):** Official preface provided by National Center for Health Statistics (NCHS) as guidance concerning this pre-release draft of ICD-10-CM.

- **Guidelines and Conventions (2011):** The Draft ICD-10-CM Official Guidelines for Coding and Reporting for Acute Short-term and Long-term Hospital Inpatient and Physician Office and Other Outpatient Encounters has been included to assist you with appropriate and consistent code assignment.

- **Index (2011):** Official alphabetic index to the tabular sections.

- **Neoplasm Table (2011):** The Neoplasm Table assists in the indexing and classification of neoplasms within ICD-10-CM.

- **Complete set of ICD-10-CM codes (2011):** All 21 chapters — Infectious and Parasitic Diseases through Injuries, including External Causes and Reasons for Visit.

- **Table of Drugs and Chemicals (2011):** This is a classification of drugs and other chemical substances to assist in the coding of poisoning, overdose states, underdosing, and external causes of adverse effects.

The codes in ICD-10-CM are not currently valid for coding and reporting of medical services for reimbursement purposes. However, the United States began using ICD-10 in 1999 to classify mortality data from death certificates to ensure the international comparability of health statistics.

Thank you for choosing to be an Ingenix customer. If you have any questions about your *ICD-10-CM Draft 2011* or about any Ingenix publication, please call our customer service department toll free at (800) INGENIX (464-3649).

Although this draft of ICD-10-CM is available, the codes in ICD-10-CM are not currently valid for any purpose or use. Updates to this draft are anticipated prior to implementation of ICD-10-CM.

INGENIX

ICD-10-CM

The Complete Official Draft Code Set

2011

Publisher's Notice

The *ICD-10-CM The Complete Official Draft Code Set* is designed to be an accurate and authoritative source regarding coding and every reasonable effort has been made to ensure accuracy and completeness of the content. However, Ingenix makes no guarantee, warranty, or representation that this publication is accurate, complete or without errors. It is understood that Ingenix is not rendering any legal or other professional services or advice in this publication and that Ingenix bears no liability for any results or consquences that may arise from the use of this book.

Our Commitment to Accuracy

Ingenix is committed to producing accurate and reliable materials.

To report corrections, please visit www.ingenixonline.com/accuracy or email accuracy@ingenix.com. You can also reach customer service by calling 1.800.INGENIX (464.3649), option 1.

Acknowledgments

Anita C. Hart, RHIA, CCS, CCS-P *Product Manager*
Karen Schmidt, BSN, *Technical Director*
Stacy Perry, *Manager, Desktop Publishing*
Lisa Singley, *Project Manager*
Beth Ford, RHIT, CCS, *Clinical/Technical Editor*
Melinda Stegman, MBA, CCS, *Clinical/Technical Editor*
Tracy Betzler, *Desktop Publishing Specialist*
Hope M. Dunn, *Desktop Publishing Specialist*
Toni R. Stewart, *Desktop Publishing Specialist*
Kate Holden, *Editor*

Copyright

Anita Hart, RHIA,CCS, CCS-P

Product Manager, Ingenix

Ms. Hart's experience includes conducting and publishing research in clinical medicine and human genetics for Yale University, Massachusetts General Hospital, and Massachusetts Institute of Technology. In addition, Ms. Hart has supervised medical records management, health information management, coding and reimbursement, and worker's compensation issues as the office manager for a physical therapy rehabilitation clinic. Ms. Hart is an expert in physician and facility coding, reimbursement systems, and compliance issues. Ms. Hart has developed and served as technical consultant for numerous other publications for hospital and physician practices. Currrently, Ms. Hart is the Product Manager for the ICD-9-CM and ICD-10-CM/PCS product lines.

Beth Ford, RHIT, CCS

Clinical/Technical Editor

Ms. Ford is a clinical/technical editor for Ingenix. She has extensive background in both physician and facility ICD-9-CM and CPT/HCPCS coding. Ms. Ford has served as a coding specialist, coding manager, coding trainer/educator and coding consultant, as well as a health information management director. She is an active member of the American Health Information Management Association (AHIMA).

Melinda Stegman, MBA, CCS

Clinical/Technical Editor

Ms. Stegman has more than 25 years of experience in the HIM profession and has been responsible for the update and maintenance of the ICD-9-CM, ICD-10, DRG resources and some cross coder products for Ingenix. In the past, she also managed the clinical aspects of the HSS/Ingenix HIM Consulting practice in the Washington, DC area office. Her areas of specialization include training on inpatient and DRG coding, outpatient coding, and Ambulatory Payment Classifications (APCs) for HIM professionals, software developers, and other clients; developing an outpatient billing/coding compliance tool for a major accounting firm; and managing HIM consulting practices. Ms. Stegman is a regular contributing author for *Advance for Health Information Management Professionals* and for the *Journal of Health Care Compliance*. She has performed coding assessments and educational sessions throughout the country. Ms. Stegman is credentialed by the American Health Information Management Association (AHIMA) as a Certified Coding Specialist (CCS) and holds a Master of Business Administration degree with a concentration in health care management from the University of New Mexico – Albuquerque.

Contents

ICD-10-CM Official Preface DRAFT

This 2011 pre-release draft of the International Classification of Diseases, 10th Revision, Clinical Modification (ICD-10-CM) is being published by the United States Government in recognition of its responsibility to promulgate this classification throughout the United States for morbidity coding. The International Statistical Classification of Diseases and Related Health Problems, 10th Revision (ICD-10), published by the World Health Organization (WHO), is the foundation of ICD-10-CM. ICD-10 continues to be the classification used in cause-of-death coding in the United States. The ICD-10-CM is comparable with the ICD-10. The WHO Collaborating Center for the Family of International Classifications in North America, housed at the National Center for Health Statistics (NCHS), has responsibility for the implementation of ICD and other WHO-FIC classifications and serves as a liaison with WHO, fulfilling international obligations for comparable classifications and the national health data needs of the United States. The historical background of ICD and ICD-10 can be found in the Introduction to the International Classification of Diseases and Related Health Problems (ICD-10), Second Edition, World Health Organization, Geneva, Switzerland, 2005.

ICD-10-CM is the United States' clinical modification of the World Health Organization's ICD-10. The term clinical is used to emphasize the modification's intent: to serve as a useful tool in the area of classification of morbidity data for indexing of medical records, medical care review, and ambulatory and other medical care programs, as well as for basic health statistics. To describe the clinical picture of the patient, the codes must be more precise than those needed only for statistical groupings and trend analysis.

Characteristics of ICD-10-CM

ICD-10-CM far exceeds its predecessors in the number of concepts and codes provided. The disease classification has been expanded to include health-related conditions and to provide greater specificity at the sixth digit level and with a seventh digit extension. The sixth and seventh characters are not optional; they are intended for use in recording the information documented in the clinical record.

Introduction

History and Future of ICD-10-CM

The ICD-10-CM classification system was developed by the National Center for Health Statistics (NCHS) as a clinical modification to the ICD-10 system developed by the World Health Organization (WHO), primarily as a unique system for use in the United States for morbidity and mortality reporting. Although ICD-10-CM has not yet been implemented for use in the United States, ICD-10 has been adopted for use in the coding and classification of mortality data from death certificates. ICD-10 replaced ICD-9 for this purpose as of January 1, 1999. Upon legislative approval, ICD-10-CM is planned as the replacement for ICD-9-CM, volumes 1 and 2.

ICD-10 is the copyrighted product of the World Health Organization (WHO), which has authorized the development of a clinical modification (CM) of ICD-10 for use in the United States. However, all modifications to the ICD-10 must conform to WHO conventions for ICD. The development of ICD-10-CM included comprehensive evaluation by a Technical Advisory Panel and extensive consultation with physician groups, clinical coders, and other industry experts.

The ICD-10-CM draft and crosswalk between ICD-9-CM and ICD-10-CM have been made available on the NCHS website for public comment. The initial public comment period extended from December 1997 through February 1998. A field test for ICD-10-CM was conducted in the summer of 2003 jointly by The American Hospital Association (AMA) and the American Health Information Management Association (AHIMA). Public comments and suggestions were reviewed and additional modifications to ICD-10-CM were made. Revisions were made to ICD-10-CM based on the established update process for ICD-9-CM (the ICD-9-CM Coordination and Maintenance Committee) and the World Health Organization's ICD-10 (the Update and Revision Committee).

These revisions to ICD-10-CM have included:

- information relevant to ambulatory and managed care encounters
- expanded injury codes
- creation of combination diagnosis/symptom codes to reduce the number of codes needed to fully describe a condition
- the addition of sixth and seventh character subclassifications
- incorporation of common 4th and 5th digit subclassifications
- classifications specific to laterality
- classification refinement for increased data granularity

This new structure allows for further expansion than was possible with the ICD-9-CM classification system.

This new 2011 draft update release is available for public viewing. ICD-10-CM codes are not currently valid for any purpose or use other than the reporting of mortality data for death certificates.

The Department of Health and Human Services (HHS) published the final rule regarding the adoption of both ICD-10-CM and ICD-10-PCS in the January 16, 2009 *Federal Register* (45 CFR part 162 [CMS—0013—F]). The compliance date for implementation of ICD-10-CM and ICD-10-PCS as a replacement for ICD-9-CM is October 1, 2013.

How to Use the ICD-10-CM (Draft 2011)

This draft of the International Classification of Diseases, 10th Revision, Clinical Modification (ICD-10-CM) is being published by the United States Government in recognition of its responsibility to promulgate this classification throughout the United States for morbidity coding. This code book represents an adaptation of ICD-10 which was created specifically for use in the United States. Future revisions to ICD-10-CM will be made based on the established update process for ICD-9-CM (the ICD-9-CM Coordination and Maintenance Committee) and the World Health Organization's ICD-10 (the Update and Revision Committee). Upon legislative approval, ICD-10-CM is planned as the replacement for ICD-9-CM, volumes 1 and 2.

Steps to Correct Coding

1. Before beginning to use this code book, review section 1.A., "Conventions," and section 1.B., "General Coding Guidelines of the ICD-10-CM Draft Official Guidelines for Coding and Reporting 2011."

2. Look up the main term in the Alphabetic Index and scan the subterm entries as appropriate. Review continued lines and additional subterms that may appear in the next column or on the next page.

3. Note all parenthetical terms (nonessential modifiers) that help in code selection but do not affect code assignment. Shaded guidelines in the Index are provided to help determine the indentation level for each subterm in relation to the main terms.

4. Pay close attention to the following instructions in the Index:
    - "see," "see also," and "see category" cross-references
    - "with"/"without" notes
    - "omit code" notes
    - "due to" subterms
    - other instructions found in note boxes, such as "code by site"

5. Do not code from the Alphabetic Index without verifying the accuracy of the code in the Tabular List. Locate the code in the alphanumerically arranged Tabular List.

6. To determine the appropriateness of the code selection and proper coding, read all instructional material:
    - "includes" and "excludes" notes
    - "use additional code" and "code first underlying disease" instructions
    - "code also"
    - fourth-, fifth-, and sixth-digit requirements and seventh-digit extension requirements

7. Consult the official Draft ICD-10-CM guidelines, which govern the use of specific codes. These guidelines provide both general and chapter-specific coding guidance.

8. Confirm and assign the correct code.

Organization

This book is organized in the following manner:

Introduction

The introductory material in this book includes the ICD-10-CM Official Preface, the history and future of ICD-10-CM as well as an overview of the classification system.

Draft Official ICD-10-CM Conventions and Guidelines

This section provides an explanation of the conventions and guidelines regulating the appropriate assignment and reporting of ICD-10-CM codes. This coding guidance is presented by the National Center for Health Statistics (NCHS), a governmental agency of the Centers for Disease Control and Prevention (CDC), within the United States Department of Health and Human Services (DHHS).

Alphabetic Index to Diseases

The Alphabetic Index to Diseases is arranged in alphabetic order by disease — by specific illness, injury, eponym, abbreviation, or other descriptive diagnostic term. The Index also lists diagnostic terms for other reasons for encounters with health care professionals.

Neoplasm Table

The Neoplasm Table provides the proper code based upon histology of the neoplasm and site.

Table of Drugs and Chemicals

The Table of Drugs and Chemicals is also included within the Alphabetic Index.

The Table of Drugs and Chemicals lists the drug and the specific codes that identify the drug and the intent. No additional external cause of injury and poisoning code is assigned in ICD-10-CM.

Index to External Causes

The Alphabetic Index to External Causes of injuries is arranged in alphabetic order by main term indicating the event.

Tabular List of Diseases

ICD-10-CM codes and descriptors are arranged numerically within the Tabular List of Diseases within 21 separate chapters according to body system or nature of injury and disease. Classifications which were previously considered supplemental to ICD-9-CM (e.g., V codes and E codes) are incorporated into the Tabular Listing of ICD-10-CM as individual chapters. Chapters 20 External Causes of Morbidity and 21 Factors Influencing Health Status and Contact with Health Services include chapter-specific guidelines.

ICD-1Ø-CM Draft Conventions

The ICD-1Ø-CM conventions are general rules for the use of the classification system, independent of the guidelines. These conventions are incorporated within the Index and Tabular List as instructional notes and are applicable regardless of the health care setting.

Format

ICD-1Ø-CM is divided into two main parts: the Index, an alphabetical list of terms and their corresponding code, and the Tabular List, a sequential, alphanumeric list of codes divided into chapters based on body system or condition. The Index contains the Index to Diseases and Injuries (main index) and the Index to External Causes of Injury. Also included in the main Index is the Neoplasm Table and a Table of Drugs and Chemicals.

The Tabular List contains categories, subcategories, and valid codes. ICD-1Ø-CM is an alphanumeric classification system. The first character of a three-digit category is a letter. The second and third characters may be numbers or alpha characters. A three-digit category without further subclassification is equivalent to a valid three-digit code. Subcategories are either four or five characters. Subcategory characters include either letters or numbers. Codes may be four, five, or six characters in length, in which each level of subdivision after a category is a subcategory. The final level of subdivision is a valid code. The final character in a code may be either a letter or a number.

The ICD-1Ø-CM used the letter "x" as a place-holder. A placeholder "x" is used as a fifth character place-holder at certain six-character codes to allow for future expansion, without disturbing the sixth-digit structure. For instance, an initial encounter for accidental poisoning by penicillin is coded to T36.Øx1A. The "x" in the fifth character position is a place-holder, or filler digit.

Similarly, certain categories have applicable seventh-character extensions. In these cases, the seventh-character extension is required for all codes within the category, or as otherwise instructed in the Tabular List notations. Seventh-character extensions must always be the last character in the data field. If a code is not a full six characters in length, a dummy place-holder "x" must be used to fill in the empty characters when a seventh character extension is required.

Punctuation

[ ]   In the Tabular List, brackets are used to enclose synonyms, alternative wording, or explanatory phrases. In the Index, brackets are used to identify manifestation codes.

( )   Parentheses are used in both the Index and Tabular List to enclose nonessential modifiers; supplementary words that may be present or absent in the statement of a disease or procedure without affecting the code number to which it is assigned.

:   Colons are used in the Tabular List after an incomplete term that needs one or more of the modifiers following the colon to make it assignable to a given category.

Abbreviations

NEC

The abbreviation NEC, "Not elsewhere classifiable" represents "other specified" in the ICD-1Ø-CM. An index entry that states NEC directs the coder to an "other specified" code in the Tabular List. Codes titled "Other" or "Other specified" in the Tabular List (usually a code with a fourth or sixth character 8 or z and fifth character 9) are for use when the

information in the medical record provides detail for which a specific code does not exist.

NOS

The abbreviation NOS, "Not otherwise specified," in the Tabular List may be interpreted as "unspecified." Codes in the Tabular List with "Unspecified" in the title (usually a code with a fourth or sixth character 9 and fifth character Ø) are for use when the information in the medical record is insufficient to assign a more specific code.

Typeface

Boldface

Boldface type is used for main term entries in the Alphabetic Index, and all codes and descriptions in the Tabular List.

Italicized

Italicized type is used for all exclusion notes and to identify manifestation codes, those codes that should not be reported as first-listed (principal) diagnoses.

General Notes

The following conventions and notes appear only in the Tabular List of Diseases:

Includes Notes

The word "Includes" appears immediately under certain categories to further define, clarify, or give examples of the content of a code category.

Inclusion Terms

Lists of inclusion terms are included under certain codes. These terms indicate some of the conditions for which that code number may be used. Inclusion terms may be synonyms with the code title, or, in the case of "other specified" codes, the terms may also provide a list of various conditions included within a classification code. The inclusion terms are not exhaustive. The Index may provide additional terms that may also be assigned to a given code.

Excludes Notes

ICD-1Ø-CM has two types of excludes notes. Each note has a different definition for use. However, they are similar in that they both indicate that codes excluded from each other are independent of each other.

Excludes1

An excludes1 note is a "pure" excludes. It means "NOT CODED HERE!" An excludes1 note indicates mutually exclusive codes; two conditions that cannot be reported together. For example, a congenital form of a disease may not be reported with the acquired form of the same condition. The code excluded should never be reported with the applicable codes listed above the excludes notation.

Excludes2

An excludes2 note means "NOT INCLUDED HERE." An excludes2 note indicates that although the excluded condition is not part of the condition it is excluded from, a patient may have both conditions at the same time. Therefore, when an excludes2 note appears under a code, it may be acceptable to use both the code and the excluded code together if supported by the medical documentation.

Instructional Notes in the Alphabetic Index

See/See Also
In the index, the "see" instruction following a main term or subterm refers the coder to an alternate entry to locate the correct code.

Similarly, a "see also" instruction following a main term or subterm indicates that an additional term should be referenced to provide additional information

Default Codes
In the index, the default code is the code listed next to the main term. The default code represents the condition most commonly associated with the main term. This code may be assigned when documentation does not facilitate reporting a more specific code. Alternately, it may provide an unspecified code for the condition.

Syndromes
Follow the Alphabetic Index guidance when coding syndromes. In the absence of index guidance, assign codes for the documented manifestations of the syndrome.

And
When the term "and" is used in a narrative statement it may be interpreted as "and/or."

With/Without
When "with" and "without" are the two options for the final character of a set of codes, the default is always "without." For five-character codes, a "0" as the fifth-position character represents "without", and "1" represents "with." For six-character codes, the sixth-position character "1" represents "with" and "9" represents "without."

Instructional Notes Used in the Tabular List
In the tabular section, the following instructional notes appear in red type for emphasis:

Code First/Use additional code:
These instructional notes are in red type and provide sequencing instruction. They may appear independently of each other or to designate certain etiology/manifestation paired codes. These instructions signal the coder that an additional code should be reported to provide a more complete picture of that diagnosis.

In etiology/manifestation coding, ICD-10-CM requires the underlying condition to be sequenced first, followed by the manifestation. In these situations, codes with "In diseases classified elsewhere" in the code description are never permitted as a first-listed or principal diagnosis code and must be sequenced following the underlying condition code.

Code Also:
A code also note alerts the coder that more than one code may be required to fully describe the condition. Code sequencing is discretionary. Factors that may determine sequencing include severity and reason for the encounter. These coding notes appear in red type.

Additional Conventions

Additional Digits Required
- **√4ᵗʰ** This symbol indicates that the code requires a fourth digit.
- **√5ᵗʰ** This symbol indicates that the code requires a fifth digit.
- **√6ᵗʰ** This symbol indicates that the code requires a sixth digit.
- **√7ᵗʰ** This symbol indicates that the code requires a seventh digit.
- **√x7ᵗʰ** This symbol indicates that the code requires a seventh digit following the placeholder x. Codes less than six characters that require a seventh character must contain placeholder x to fill the missing digits. The seventh character must always be a valid seventh character for that code.

Boldface

Note
The term "Note:" appears enclosed within a red icon and precedes the instructional information. These notes function as an alert, to highlight coding instruction within the text.

Color Coding

Manifestation Code
These codes appear in italic type, with a blue color bar over the title. A manifestation code cannot be reported as a first-listed or principal diagnosis. By definition, a manifestation code represents a demonstration of some aspect of an underlying disease, which is separately classifiable. In the Alphabetic Index, these codes are listed as the secondary code in brackets. The underlying disease code is listed first.

Deactivated Codes
Categories and codes that have been deactivated and are no longer in use are be displayed in blue type.

ICD-10-CM Draft Official Guidelines for Coding and Reporting 2011

Narrative changes appear in bold text

Items <u>underlined</u> have been moved within the guidelines since the 2010 version

Italics **are used to indicate revisions to heading changes**

The Centers for Medicare and Medicaid Services (CMS) and the National Center for Health Statistics (NCHS), two departments within the U.S. Federal Government's Department of Health and Human Services (DHHS) provide the following guidelines for coding and reporting using the International Classification of Diseases, 10th Revision, Clinical Modification (ICD-10-CM). These guidelines should be used as a companion document to the official version of the ICD-10-CM as published on the NCHS website. The ICD-10-CM is a morbidity classification published by the United States for classifying diagnoses and reason for visits in all health care settings. The ICD-10-CM is based on the ICD-10, the statistical classification of disease published by the World Health Organization (WHO).

These guidelines have been approved by the four organizations that make up the Cooperating Parties for the ICD-10-CM: the American Hospital Association (AHA), the American Health Information Management Association (AHIMA), CMS, and NCHS.

These guidelines are a set of rules that have been developed to accompany and complement the official conventions and instructions provided within the ICD-10-CM itself. The instructions and conventions of the classification take precedence over guidelines. These guidelines are based on the coding and sequencing instructions **in the Tabular List and Alphabetic Index** of ICD-10-CM, but provide additional instruction. Adherence to these guidelines when assigning ICD-10-CM diagnosis codes is required under the Health Insurance Portability and Accountability Act (HIPAA). The diagnosis codes (**Tabular List and Alphabetic Index**) have been adopted under HIPAA for all healthcare settings. A joint effort between the healthcare provider and the coder is essential to achieve complete and accurate documentation, code assignment, and reporting of diagnoses and procedures. These guidelines have been developed to assist both the healthcare provider and the coder in identifying those diagnoses and procedures that are to be reported. The importance of consistent, complete documentation in the medical record cannot be overemphasized. Without such documentation accurate coding cannot be achieved. The entire record should be reviewed to determine the specific reason for the encounter and the conditions treated.

The term encounter is used for all settings, including hospital admissions. In the context of these guidelines, the term provider is used throughout the guidelines to mean physician or any qualified health care practitioner who is legally accountable for establishing the patient's diagnosis. Only this set of guidelines, approved by the Cooperating Parties, is official.

The guidelines are organized into sections. Section I includes the structure and conventions of the classification and general guidelines that apply to the entire classification, and chapter-specific guidelines that correspond to the chapters as they are arranged in the classification. Section II includes guidelines for selection of principal diagnosis for non-outpatient settings. Section III includes guidelines for reporting additional diagnoses in non-outpatient settings. Section IV is for outpatient coding and reporting. It is necessary to review all sections of the guidelines to fully understand all of the rules and instructions needed to code properly.

Section I. Conventions, general coding guidelines and chapter specific guidelines

The conventions, general guidelines and chapter-specific guidelines are applicable to all health care settings unless otherwise indicated. The conventions and instructions of the classification take precedence over guidelines.

A. Conventions for the ICD-10-CM

The conventions for the ICD-10-CM are the general rules for use of the classification independent of the guidelines. These conventions are incorporated within the **Alphabetic Index and Tabular List** of the ICD-10-CM as instructional notes.

1. **The Alphabetic Index and Tabular List**

   The ICD-10-CM is divided into the **Alphabetic Index**, an alphabetical list of terms and their corresponding code, and the Tabular List, a chronological list of codes divided into chapters based on body system or condition. **The Alphabetic Index consists of the following parts: the Index of Diseases and Injury, the Index of External Causes of Injury, the Table of Neoplasms and the Table of Drugs and Chemicals.**

   See Section I.C2. General guidelines

   See Section I.C.19. Adverse effects, poisoning, underdosing and toxic effects

2. **Format and Structure:**

   The ICD-10-CM Tabular List contains categories, subcategories and codes. Characters for categories, subcategories and codes may be either a letter or a number. All categories are 3 characters. A three-character category that has no further subdivision is equivalent to a code. Subcategories are either 4 or 5 characters. Codes may be **3**, 4, 5, 6 or 7 characters. That is, each level of subdivision after a category is a subcategory. The final level of subdivision is a code. Codes that have applicable 7th characters are still referred to as codes, not subcategories. A code that has an applicable 7th character is considered invalid without the 7th character.

   The ICD-10-CM uses an indented format for ease in reference.

3. **Use of codes for reporting purposes**

   For reporting purposes only codes are permissible, not categories or subcategories, and any applicable 7th character is required.

4. **Placeholder character**

   The ICD-10-CM utilizes a placeholder character "x". The "x" is used as a placeholder at certain codes to allow for future expansion. An example of this is at the poisoning, adverse effect and underdosing codes, categories T36-T50.

   Where a placeholder exists, the x must be used in order for the code to be considered a valid code.

5. **7th Characters**

   Certain ICD-10-CM categories have applicable 7th characters. The applicable 7th character is required for all codes within the category, or as the notes in the Tabular List instruct. The 7th character must always be the 7th character in the data field. If a code that requires a 7th character is not 6 characters, a placeholder X must be used to fill in the empty characters.

6. **Abbreviations**

   a. *Alphabetic* **Index abbreviations**

      NEC "Not elsewhere classifiable"

      This abbreviation in the **Alphabetic Index** represents "other specified". When a specific code is not available for a condition, the **Alphabetic Index** directs the coder to the "other specified" code in the **Tabular List**.

      NOS "Not otherwise specified"
      This abbreviation is the equivalent of unspecified.

   b. *Tabular* **List abbreviations**

      NEC   "Not elsewhere classifiable"

      This abbreviation in the **Tabular List** represents "other specified". When a specific code is not available for a condition the **Tabular List** includes an NEC entry under a code to identify the code as the "other specified" code.

      NOS   "Not otherwise specified"

      This abbreviation is the equivalent of unspecified.

7. **Punctuation**

   [ ]   Brackets are used in the **Tabular List** to enclose synonyms, alternative wording or explanatory phrases. Brackets are used in the **Alphabetic Index** to identify manifestation codes.

   ( )   Parentheses are used in both the **Alphabetic Index** and **Tabular List** to enclose supplementary words that may be present or absent in the statement of a disease or procedure without affecting the code number to which it is assigned. The terms within the parentheses are referred to as nonessential modifiers.

   :   Colons are used in the Tabular List after an incomplete term which needs one or more of the modifiers following the colon to make it assignable to a given category.

8. **Use of "and"**

   When the term "and" is used in a narrative statement it represents and/or.

9. **Other and Unspecified codes**

   a. **"Other" codes**

      Codes titled "other" or "other specified" are for use when the information in the medical record provides detail for which a specific code does not exist. **Alphabetic Index** entries with NEC in the line designate "other" codes in the **Tabular List**. These **Alphabetic Index** entries represent specific disease entities for which no specific code exists so the term is included within an "other" code.

   b. **"Unspecified" codes**

      Codes titled "unspecified" are for use when the information in the medical record is insufficient to assign a more specific code. For those categories for which an unspecified code is not provided, the "other specified" code may represent both other and unspecified.

10. **Includes Notes**

    This note appears immediately under a three **character** code title to further define, or give examples of, the content of the category.

11. **Inclusion terms**

    List of terms is included under some codes. These terms are the conditions for which that code is to be used. The terms may be synonyms of the code title, or, in the case of "other specified" codes, the terms are a list of the various conditions assigned to that code. The inclusion terms are not necessarily exhaustive. Additional terms found only in the **Alphabetic Index** may also be assigned to a code.

12. **Excludes Notes**

    The ICD-10-CM has two types of excludes notes. Each type of note has a different definition for use but they are all similar in that they indicate that codes excluded from each other are independent of each other.

    a. **Excludes1**

       A type 1 Excludes note is a pure excludes note. It means "NOT CODED HERE!" An Excludes1 note indicates that the code excluded should never be used at the same time as the code above the Excludes1 note. An Excludes1 is used when two conditions cannot occur together, such as a congenital form versus an acquired form of the same condition.

    b. **Excludes2**

       A type 2 excludes note represents "Not included here". An excludes2 note indicates that the condition excluded is not part of the condition represented by the code, but a patient may have both conditions at the same time. When an Excludes2 note appears under a code, it is acceptable to use both the code and the excluded code together, when appropriate.

13. **Etiology/manifestation convention ("code first", "use additional code" and "in diseases classified elsewhere" notes)**

    Certain conditions have both an underlying etiology and multiple body system manifestations due to the underlying etiology. For such conditions, the ICD-10-CM has a coding convention that requires the underlying condition be sequenced first followed by the manifestation. Wherever such a combination exists, there is a "use additional code" note at the etiology code, and a "code first" note at the manifestation code. These instructional notes indicate the proper sequencing order of the codes, etiology followed by manifestation.

In most cases the manifestation codes will have in the code title, "in diseases classified elsewhere." Codes with this title are a component of the etiology/ manifestation convention. The code title indicates that it is a manifestation code. "In diseases classified elsewhere" codes are never permitted to be used as **first-listed** or principal diagnosis codes. They must be used in conjunction with an underlying condition code and they must be listed following the underlying condition. See category F02, Dementia in other diseases classified elsewhere, for an example of this convention.

There are manifestation codes that do not have "in diseases classified elsewhere" in the title. For such codes a "use additional code" note will still be present and the rules for sequencing apply.

In addition to the notes in the **Tabular List**, these conditions also have a specific **Alphabetic Index** entry structure. In the **Alphabetic Index** both conditions are listed together with the etiology code first followed by the manifestation codes in brackets. The code in brackets is always to be sequenced second.

An example of the etiology/manifestation convention is dementia in Parkinson's disease. In the **Alphabetic Index**, code G20 is listed first, followed by code F02.80 or F02.81 in brackets. Code G20 represents the underlying etiology, Parkinson's disease, and must be sequenced first, whereas codes F02.80 and F02.81 represent the manifestation of dementia in diseases classified elsewhere, with or without behavioral disturbance.

"Code first" and "Use additional code" notes are also used as sequencing rules in the classification for certain codes that are not part of an etiology/ manifestation combination.

See Section I.B.7. Multiple coding for a single condition.

14. "And"
The word "and" should be interpreted to mean either "and" or "or" when it appears in a title.

15. "With"
The word "with" should be interpreted to mean "associated with" or "due to" when it appears in a code title, the Alphabetic Index, or an instructional note in the Tabular List.

The word "with" in the Alphabetic Index is sequenced immediately following the main term, not in alphabetical order.

16. "See" and "See Also"
The "see" instruction following a main term in the **Alphabetic Index** indicates that another term should be referenced. It is necessary to go to the main term referenced with the "see" note to locate the correct code.

A "see also" instruction following a main term in the **Alphabetic Index** instructs that there is another main term that may also be referenced that may provide additional **Alphabetic Index** entries that may be useful. It is not necessary to follow the "see also" note when the original main term provides the necessary code.

17. "Code also note"
A "code also" note instructs that two codes may be required to fully describe a condition, but this note does not provide sequencing direction.

18. Default codes
A code listed next to a main term in the ICD-10-CM **Alphabetic Index** is referred to as a default code. The default code represents that condition that is most commonly associated with the main term, or is the unspecified code for the condition. If a condition is documented in a medical record (for example, appendicitis) without any additional information, such as acute or chronic, the default code should be assigned.

19. Syndromes
Follow the Alphabetic Index guidance when coding syndromes. In the absence of **Alphabetic Index** guidance, assign codes for the documented manifestations of the syndrome.

B. General Coding Guidelines

1. Locating a code in the ICD-10-CM
To select a code in the classification that corresponds to a diagnosis or reason for visit documented in a medical record, first locate the term in the **Alphabetic Index**, and then verify the code in the Tabular List. Read and be guided by instructional notations that appear in both the **Alphabetic Index** and the Tabular List.

It is essential to use both the **Alphabetic Index** and Tabular List when locating and assigning a code. The **Alphabetic Index** does not always provide the full code. Selection of the full code, including laterality and any applicable 7th character can only be done in the **Tabular List**. A dash (-) at the end of an **Alphabetic Index** entry indicates that additional characters are required. Even if a dash is not included at the **Alphabetic Index** entry, it is necessary to refer to the **Tabular List** to verify that no 7th character is required.

2. Level of Detail in Coding
Diagnosis codes are to be used and reported at their highest number of **characters** available.

ICD-10-CM diagnosis codes are composed of codes with 3, 4, 5, 6 or 7 **characters**. Codes with three **characters** are included in ICD-10-CM as the heading of a category of codes that may be further subdivided by the use of fourth and/or fifth **characters and/or sixth characters**, which provide greater detail.

A three-**character** code is to be used only if it is not further subdivided. A code is invalid if it has not been coded to the full number of characters required for that code, including the 7th character, if applicable.

3. Code or codes from A00.0 through T88.9, Z00-Z99.8
The appropriate code or codes from A00.0 through T88.9, Z00-Z99.8 must be used to identify diagnoses, symptoms, conditions, problems, complaints or other reason(s) for the encounter/visit.

4. Signs and symptoms
Codes that describe symptoms and signs, as opposed to diagnoses, are acceptable for reporting purposes when a related definitive diagnosis has not been established (confirmed) by the provider. Chapter 18 of ICD-10-CM, Symptoms, Signs, and Abnormal Clinical and Laboratory Findings, Not Elsewhere Classified (codes R00.0 - R99) contains many, but not all codes for symptoms.

5. Conditions that are an integral part of a disease process
Signs and symptoms that are associated routinely with a disease process should not be assigned as additional codes, unless otherwise instructed by the classification.

6. Conditions that are not an integral part of a disease process
Additional signs and symptoms that may not be associated routinely with a disease process should be coded when present.

7. Multiple coding for a single condition
In addition to the etiology/manifestation convention that requires two codes to fully describe a single condition that affects multiple body systems, there are other single conditions that also require more than one code. "Use additional code" notes are found in the **Tabular List** at codes that are not part of an etiology/manifestation pair where a secondary code is useful to fully describe a condition. The sequencing rule is the same as the etiology/manifestation pair, "use additional code" indicates that a secondary code should be added.

For example, for bacterial infections that are not included in chapter 1, a secondary code from category B95, Streptococcus, Staphylococcus, and Enterococcus, as the cause of diseases classified elsewhere, or B96, Other bacterial agents as the cause of diseases classified elsewhere, may be required to identify the bacterial organism causing the infection. A "use additional code" note will normally be found at the infectious disease code, indicating a need for the organism code to be added as a secondary code.

"Code first" notes are also under certain codes that are not specifically manifestation codes but may be due to an underlying cause. When there is a "code first" note and an underlying condition is present, the underlying condition should be sequenced first.

"Code, if applicable, any causal condition first", notes indicate that this code may be assigned as a principal diagnosis when the causal condition is unknown or not applicable. If a causal condition is known, then the code for that condition should be sequenced as the principal or first-listed diagnosis.

Multiple codes may be needed for late effects, complication codes and obstetric codes to more fully describe a condition. See the specific guidelines for these conditions for further instruction.

8. Acute and Chronic Conditions
If the same condition is described as both acute (subacute) and chronic, and separate subentries exist in the Alphabetic Index at the same indentation level, code both and sequence the acute (subacute) code first.

9. Combination Code
A combination code is a single code used to classify:

Two diagnoses, or

A diagnosis with an associated secondary process (manifestation)

A diagnosis with an associated complication

Combination codes are identified by referring to subterm entries in the Alphabetic Index and by reading the inclusion and exclusion notes in the Tabular List.

Assign only the combination code when that code fully identifies the diagnostic conditions involved or when the Alphabetic Index so directs. Multiple coding should not be used when the classification provides a combination code that clearly identifies all of the elements documented in the diagnosis. When the combination code lacks necessary specificity in describing the manifestation or complication, an additional code should be used as a secondary code.

10. Late Effects (Sequela)
A late effect is the residual effect (condition produced) after the acute phase of an illness or injury has terminated. There is no time limit on when a late effect code can be used. The residual may be apparent early, such as in cerebral infarction, or it may occur months or years later, such as that due to a previous injury. Coding of late effects generally requires two codes sequenced in the following order: The condition or nature of the late effect is sequenced first. The late effect code is sequenced second.

An exception to the above guidelines are those instances where the code for late effect is followed by a manifestation code identified in the Tabular List and title, or the late effect code has been expanded (at the fourth, fifth or sixth character levels) to include the manifestation(s). The code for the acute phase of an illness or injury that led to the late effect is never used with a code for the late effect.

See Section I.C.9. Sequelae of cerebrovascular disease

See Section I.C.15. Sequelae of complication of pregnancy, childbirth and the puerperium

See Section I.C.19. Code extensions

11. Impending or Threatened Condition
Code any condition described at the time of discharge as "impending" or "threatened" as follows:

If it did occur, code as confirmed diagnosis.

If it did not occur, reference the Alphabetic Index to determine if the condition has a subentry term for "impending" or "threatened" and also reference main term entries for "Impending" and for "Threatened."

If the subterms are listed, assign the given code.

If the subterms are not listed, code the existing underlying condition(s) and not the condition described as impending or threatened.

12. Reporting Same Diagnosis Code More than Once
Each unique ICD-10-CM diagnosis code may be reported only once for an encounter. This applies to bilateral conditions when there are no distinct codes identifying laterality or two different conditions classified to the same ICD-10-CM diagnosis code.

13. Laterality
For bilateral sites, the final character of the codes in the ICD-10-CM indicates laterality. An unspecified side code is also provided should the side not be identified in the medical record. If no bilateral code is provided and the condition is bilateral, assign separate codes for both the left and right side.

14. Documentation for BMI and Pressure Ulcer Stages
For the Body Mass Index (BMI) and pressure ulcer stage codes, code assignment may be based on medical record documentation from clinicians who are not the patient's provider (i.e., physician or other qualified healthcare practitioner legally accountable for establishing the patient's diagnosis), since this information is typically documented by other clinicians involved in the care of the patient (e.g., a dietitian often documents the BMI and nurses often documents the pressure ulcer stages). However, the associated diagnosis (such as overweight, obesity, or pressure ulcer) must be documented by the patient's provider. If there is conflicting medical record documentation, either from the same clinician or different clinicians, the patient's attending provider should be queried for clarification.

The BMI codes should only be reported as secondary diagnoses. As with all other secondary diagnosis codes, the BMI codes should only be assigned when they meet the definition of a reportable additional diagnosis (see Section III, Reporting Additional Diagnoses).

C. Chapter-Specific Coding Guidelines
In addition to general coding guidelines, there are guidelines for specific diagnoses and/or conditions in the classification. Unless otherwise indicated, these guidelines apply to all health care settings. Please refer to Section II for guidelines on the selection of principal diagnosis.

1. Chapter 1: Certain Infectious and Parasitic Diseases (A00-B99)
a. Human Immunodeficiency Virus (HIV) Infections
1) Code only confirmed cases
Code only confirmed cases of HIV infection/illness. This is an exception to the hospital inpatient guideline Section II, H.

In this context, "confirmation" does not require documentation of positive serology or culture for HIV; the provider's diagnostic statement that the patient is HIV positive, or has an HIV-related illness is sufficient.

2) Selection and sequencing of HIV codes
(a) Patient admitted for HIV-related condition
If a patient is admitted for an HIV-related condition, the principal diagnosis should be B20, followed by additional diagnosis codes for all reported HIV-related conditions.

(b) Patient with HIV disease admitted for unrelated condition
If a patient with HIV disease is admitted for an unrelated condition (such as a traumatic injury), the code for the unrelated condition (e.g., the nature of injury code) should be the principal diagnosis. Other diagnoses would be B20 followed by additional diagnosis codes for all reported HIV-related conditions.

(c) Whether the patient is newly diagnosed
Whether the patient is newly diagnosed or has had previous admissions/encounters for HIV conditions is irrelevant to the sequencing decision.

(d) Asymptomatic human immunodeficiency virus
Z21, Asymptomatic human immunodeficiency virus [HIV] infection status, is to be applied when the patient without any documentation of symptoms is listed as being "HIV positive," "known HIV," "HIV test positive," or similar terminology. Do not use this code if the term "AIDS" is used or if the patient is treated for any HIV-related illness

or is described as having any condition(s) resulting from his/her HIV positive status; use B20 in these cases.

(e) **Patients with inconclusive HIV serology**

Patients with inconclusive HIV serology, but no definitive diagnosis or manifestations of the illness, may be assigned code R75, Inconclusive laboratory evidence of human immunodeficiency virus [HIV].

(f) **Previously diagnosed HIV-related illness**

Patients with any known prior diagnosis of an HIV-related illness should be coded to B20. Once a patient has developed an HIV-related illness, the patient should always be assigned code B20 on every subsequent admission/encounter. Patients previously diagnosed with any HIV illness (B20) should never be assigned to R75 or Z21, Asymptomatic human immunodeficiency virus [HIV] infection status.

(g) **HIV Infection in Pregnancy, Childbirth and the Puerperium**

During pregnancy, childbirth or the puerperium, a patient admitted (or presenting for a health care encounter) because of an HIV-related illness should receive a principal diagnosis code of O98.7-, Human immunodeficiency [HIV] disease complicating pregnancy, childbirth and the puerperium, followed by B20 and the code(s) for the HIV-related illness(es). Codes from Chapter 15 always take sequencing priority.

Patients with asymptomatic HIV infection status admitted (or presenting for a health care encounter) during pregnancy, childbirth, or the puerperium should receive codes of O98.7- and Z21.

(h) **Encounters for testing for HIV**

If a patient is being seen to determine his/her HIV status, use code Z11.4, Encounter for screening for human immunodeficiency virus [HIV]. Use additional codes for any associated high risk behavior.

If a patient with signs or symptoms is being seen for HIV testing, code the signs and symptoms. An additional counseling code Z71.7, Human **immunodeficiency** virus [HIV] counseling, may be used if counseling is provided during the encounter for the test.

When a patient returns to be informed of his/her HIV test results and the test result is negative, use code Z71.7, Human immunodeficiency virus [HIV] counseling.

If the results are positive, see previous guidelines and assign codes as appropriate.

b. **Infectious agents as the cause of diseases classified to other chapters**

Certain infections are classified in chapters other than Chapter 1 and no organism is identified as part of the infection code. In these instances, it is necessary to use an additional code from Chapter 1 to identify the organism. A code from category B95, Streptococcus, Staphylococcus, and Enterococcus as the cause of diseases classified to other chapters, B96, Other bacterial agents as the cause of diseases classified to other chapters, or B97, Viral agents as the cause of diseases classified to other chapters, is to be used as an additional code to identify the organism. An instructional note will be found at the infection code advising that an additional organism code is required.

c. **Infections resistant to antibiotics**

Many bacterial infections are resistant to current antibiotics. It is necessary to identify all infections documented as antibiotic resistant. Assign code Z16, Infection with drug resistant microorganisms, following the infection code for these cases.

d. **Sepsis, Severe Sepsis, and Septic Shock**

1) **Coding of Sepsis and Severe Sepsis**

(a) **Sepsis**

For a diagnosis of sepsis, assign the appropriate code for the underlying systemic infection. If the type of infection

or causal organism is not further specified, assign code A41.9, Sepsis, unspecified.

A code from subcategory R65.2, Severe sepsis, should not be assigned unless severe sepsis or an associated acute organ dysfunction is documented.

(i) Negative or inconclusive blood cultures and sepsis
Negative or inconclusive blood cultures do not preclude a diagnosis of sepsis in patients with clinical evidence of the condition, however, the provider should be queried.

(ii) Urosepsis
The term urosepsis is a nonspecific term. It is not to be considered synonymous with sepsis. It has no default code in the Alphabetic Index. Should a provider use this term, he/she must be queried for clarification.

(iii) Sepsis with organ dysfunction
If a patient has sepsis and associated acute organ dysfunction or multiple organ dysfunction (MOD), follow the instructions for coding severe sepsis.

(iv) Acute organ dysfunction that is not clearly associated with the sepsis
If a patient has sepsis and an acute organ dysfunction, but the medical record documentation indicates that the acute organ dysfunction is related to a medical condition other than the sepsis, do not assign a code from subcategory R65.2, Severe sepsis. An acute organ dysfunction must be associated with the sepsis in order to assign the severe sepsis code. If the documentation is not clear as to whether an acute organ dysfunction is related to the sepsis or another medical condition, query the provider.

(b) **Severe sepsis**

The coding of severe sepsis requires a minimum of 2 codes: first a code for the underlying systemic infection, followed by a code from subcategory R65.2, Severe sepsis. If the causal organism is not documented, assign code A41.9, Sepsis, unspecified, for the infection. Additional code(s) for the associated acute organ dysfunction are also required.

Due to the complex nature of severe sepsis, some cases may require querying the provider prior to assignment of the codes.

2) **Septic shock**

Septic shock is circulatory failure associated with severe sepsis, and therefore, it represents a type of acute organ dysfunction. For all cases of septic shock, the code for the underlying systemic infection should be sequenced first, followed by code R65.21, Severe sepsis with septic shock. Any additional codes for the other acute organ dysfunctions should also be assigned.

Septic shock indicates the presence of severe sepsis. Code R65.21, Severe sepsis with septic shock, must be assigned if septic shock is documented in the medical record, even if the term severe sepsis is not documented.

3) **Sequencing of severe sepsis**

If severe sepsis is present on admission, and meets the definition of principal diagnosis, the underlying systemic infection should be assigned as principal diagnosis followed by the appropriate code from subcategory R65.2 as required by the sequencing rules in the Tabular List. A code from subcategory R65.2 can never be assigned as a principal diagnosis.

When severe sepsis develops during an encounter (it was not present on admission) the underlying systemic infection and the appropriate code from subcategory R65.2 should be assigned as secondary diagnoses.

Severe sepsis may be present on admission but the diagnosis may not be confirmed until sometime after admission. If the documentation is not clear whether severe sepsis was present on admission, the provider should be queried.

4) Sepsis and severe sepsis with a localized infection

If the reason for admission is both sepsis or severe sepsis and a localized infection, such as pneumonia or cellulitis, a code(s) for the underlying systemic infection should be assigned first and the code for the localized infection should be assigned as a secondary diagnosis. If the patient has severe sepsis, a code from subcategory R65.2 should also be assigned as a secondary diagnosis. If the patient is admitted with a localized infection, such as pneumonia, and sepsis/severe sepsis doesn't develop until after admission, the localized infection should be assigned first, followed by the appropriate sepsis/severe sepsis codes.

5) Sepsis due to a postprocedural infection

Sepsis resulting from a postprocedural infection is a complication of medical care. For such cases, the postprocedural infection code, such as, T80.2, Infections following infusion, transfusion, and therapeutic injection, T81.4, Infection following a procedure, T88.0, Infection following immunization, or O86.0, Infection of obstetric surgical wound, should be coded first, followed by the code for the specific infection. If the patient has severe sepsis the appropriate code from subcategory R65.2 should also be assigned with the additional code(s) for any acute organ dysfunction.

6) Sepsis and severe sepsis associated with a noninfectious process (condition)

In some cases a noninfectious process (condition), such as trauma, may lead to an infection which can result in sepsis or severe sepsis. If sepsis or severe sepsis is documented as associated with a noninfectious condition, such as a burn or serious injury, and this condition meets the definition for principal diagnosis, the code for the noninfectious condition should be sequenced first, followed by the code for the resulting infection. If severe sepsis, is present a code from subcategory R65.2 should also be assigned with any associated organ dysfunction(s) codes. It is not necessary to assign a code from subcategory R65.1, Systemic inflammatory response syndrome (SIRS) of non-infectious origin, for these cases.

If the infection meets the definition of principal diagnosis it should be sequenced before the non-infectious condition. When both the associated non-infectious condition and the infection meet the definition of principal diagnosis either may be assigned as principal diagnosis.

Only one code from category R65, Symptoms and signs specifically associated with systemic inflammation and infection, should be assigned. Therefore, when a non-infectious condition leads to an infection resulting in severe sepsis, assign the appropriate code from subcategory R65.2, Severe sepsis. Do not additionally assign a code from subcategory R65.1, Systemic inflammatory response syndrome (SIRS) of non-infectious origin.

See Section I.C.18. SIRS due to non-infectious process

7) Sepsis and septic shock complicating abortion, pregnancy, childbirth, and the puerperium

See Section I.C.15. Sepsis and septic shock complicating abortion, pregnancy, childbirth and the puerperium

8) Newborn sepsis

See Section I.C.16. Newborn sepsis

2. Chapter 2: Neoplasms (C00-D49)

General guidelines

Chapter 2 of the ICD-10-CM contains the codes for most benign and all malignant neoplasms. Certain benign neoplasms, such as prostatic adenomas, may be found in the specific body system chapters. To properly code a neoplasm it is necessary to determine from the record if the neoplasm is benign, in-situ, malignant, or of uncertain histologic

behavior. If malignant, any secondary (metastatic) sites should also be determined.

The neoplasm table in the Alphabetic Index should be referenced first. However, if the histological term is documented, that term should be referenced first, rather than going immediately to the Neoplasm Table, in order to determine which column in the Neoplasm Table is appropriate. For example, if the documentation indicates "adenoma," refer to the term in the Alphabetic Index to review the entries under this term and the instructional note to "see also neoplasm, by site, benign." The table provides the proper code based on the type of neoplasm and the site. It is important to select the proper column in the table that corresponds to the type of neoplasm. The **Tabular List** should then be referenced to verify that the correct code has been selected from the table and that a more specific site code does not exist.

See Section I.C.21. Factors influencing health status and contact with health services, Status, for information regarding Z15.0, codes for genetic susceptibility to cancer.

a. Treatment directed at the malignancy

If the treatment is directed at the malignancy, designate the malignancy as the principal diagnosis.

The only exception to this guideline is if a patient admission/encounter is solely for the administration of chemotherapy, immunotherapy or radiation therapy, assign the appropriate Z51.-- code as the first-listed or principal diagnosis, and the diagnosis or problem for which the service is being performed as a secondary diagnosis.

b. Treatment of secondary site

When a patient is admitted because of a primary neoplasm with metastasis and treatment is directed toward the secondary site only, the secondary neoplasm is designated as the principal diagnosis even though the primary malignancy is still present.

c. Coding and sequencing of complications

Coding and sequencing of complications associated with the malignancies or with the therapy thereof are subject to the following guidelines:

1) Anemia associated with malignancy

When admission/encounter is for management of an anemia associated with the malignancy, and the treatment is only for anemia, the appropriate code for the malignancy is sequenced as the principal or first-listed diagnosis followed by code D63.0, Anemia in neoplastic disease.

2) Anemia associated with chemotherapy, immunotherapy and radiation therapy

When the admission/encounter is for management of an anemia associated with an adverse effect of chemotherapy **or** immunotherapy and the only treatment is for the anemia, the appropriate adverse effect code should be sequenced first, followed by the appropriate codes for the anemia and neoplasm.

When the admission/encounter is for management of an anemia associated with an adverse effect of radiotherapy, the anemia code should be sequenced first, followed by the appropriate neoplasm code and code Y84.2, Radiological procedure and radiotherapy as the cause of abnormal reaction of the patient, or of later complication, without mention of misadventure at the time of the procedure.

3) Management of dehydration due to the malignancy

When the admission/encounter is for management of dehydration due to the malignancy and only the dehydration is being treated (intravenous rehydration), the dehydration is sequenced first, followed by the code(s) for the malignancy.

4) Treatment of a complication resulting from a surgical procedure

When the admission/encounter is for treatment of a complication resulting from a surgical procedure, designate the complication as the principal or first-listed diagnosis if treatment is directed at resolving the complication.

d. Primary malignancy previously excised

When a primary malignancy has been previously excised or eradicated from its site and there is no further treatment directed to that site and there is no evidence of any existing primary malignancy, a code from category Z85, Personal history of malignant neoplasm, should be used to indicate the former site of the malignancy. Any mention of extension, invasion, or metastasis to another site is coded as a secondary malignant neoplasm to that site. The secondary site may be the principal or first-listed with the Z85 code used as a secondary code.

e. Admissions/Encounters involving chemotherapy, immunotherapy and radiation therapy

1) Episode of care involves surgical removal of neoplasm

When an episode of care involves the surgical removal of a neoplasm, primary or secondary site, followed by adjunct chemotherapy or radiation treatment during the same episode of care, **the code for the neoplasm should be assigned as principal or first-listed diagnosis.**

2) Patient admission/encounter solely for administration of chemotherapy, immunotherapy and radiation therapy

If a patient admission/encounter is solely for the administration of chemotherapy, immunotherapy or radiation therapy assign code Z51.0, Encounter for antineoplastic radiation therapy, or Z51.11, Encounter for antineoplastic chemotherapy, or Z51.12, Encounter for antineoplastic immunotherapy as the first-listed or principal diagnosis. If a patient receives more than one of these therapies during the same admission more than one of these codes may be assigned, in any sequence.

The malignancy for which the therapy is being administered should be assigned as a secondary diagnosis.

3) Patient admitted for radiation therapy, chemotherapy or immunotherapy and develops complications

When a patient is admitted for the purpose of radiotherapy, immunotherapy or chemotherapy and develops complications such as uncontrolled nausea and vomiting or dehydration, the principal or first-listed diagnosis is Z51.0, Encounter for antineoplastic radiation therapy, or Z51.11, Encounter for antineoplastic chemotherapy, or Z51.12, Encounter for antineoplastic immunotherapy followed by any codes for the complications.

f. Admission/encounter to determine extent of malignancy

When the reason for admission/encounter is to determine the extent of the malignancy, or for a procedure such as paracentesis or thoracentesis, the primary malignancy or appropriate metastatic site is designated as the principal or first-listed diagnosis, even though chemotherapy or radiotherapy is administered.

g. Symptoms, signs, and abnormal findings listed in Chapter 18 associated with neoplasms

Symptoms, signs, and ill-defined conditions listed in Chapter 18 characteristic of, or associated with, an existing primary or secondary site malignancy cannot be used to replace the malignancy as principal or first-listed diagnosis, regardless of the number of admissions or encounters for treatment and care of the neoplasm.

See section I.C.21. Factors influencing health status and contact with health services, Encounter for prophylactic organ removal.

h. Admission/encounter for pain control/management

See Section I.C.6. for information on coding admission/encounter for pain control/management.

i. Malignancy in two or more noncontiguous sites

A patient may have more than one malignant tumor in the same organ. These tumors may represent different primaries or metastatic disease, depending on the site. Should the documentation be unclear, the provider should be queried as to the status of each tumor so that the correct codes can be assigned.

j. Disseminated malignant neoplasm, unspecified

Code C80.0, Disseminated malignant neoplasm, unspecified, is for use only in those cases where the patient has advanced metastatic disease and no known primary or secondary sites are specified. It should not be used in place of assigning codes for the primary site and all known secondary sites.

k. Malignant neoplasm without specification of site

Code C80.1, Malignant **(primary)** neoplasm, unspecified, equates to Cancer, unspecified. This code should only be used when no determination can be made as to the primary site of a malignancy. This code should rarely be used in the inpatient setting.

l. Sequencing of neoplasm codes

1) Encounter for treatment of primary malignancy

If the reason for the encounter is for treatment of a primary malignancy, assign the malignancy as the principal/**first-listed** diagnosis. The primary site is to be sequenced first, followed by any metastatic sites.

2) Encounter for treatment of secondary malignancy

When an encounter is for a primary malignancy with metastasis and treatment is directed toward the metastatic (secondary) site(s) only, the metastatic site(s) is designated as the principal/**first-listed** diagnosis. The primary malignancy is coded as an additional code.

3) Malignant neoplasm in a pregnant patient

When a pregnant woman has a malignant neoplasm, a code from subcategory **O9a.1-**, Malignant neoplasm complicating pregnancy, childbirth, and the puerperium, should be **sequenced** first, followed by the appropriate code from Chapter 2 to indicate the type of neoplasm.

4) Encounter for complication associated with a neoplasm

When an encounter is for management of a complication associated with a neoplasm, such as dehydration, and the treatment is only for the complication, the complication is coded first, followed by the appropriate code(s) for the neoplasm.

The exception to this guideline is anemia. When the admission/encounter is for management of an anemia associated with the malignancy, and the treatment is only for anemia, the appropriate code for the malignancy is sequenced as the principal or first-listed diagnosis followed by code D63.0, Anemia in neoplastic disease.

5) Complication from surgical procedure for treatment of a neoplasm

When an encounter is for treatment of a complication resulting from a surgical procedure performed for the treatment of the neoplasm, designate the complication as the principal/**first-listed** diagnosis. See guideline regarding the coding of a current malignancy versus personal history to determine if the code for the neoplasm should also be assigned.

6) Pathologic fracture due to a neoplasm

When an encounter is for a pathological fracture due to a neoplasm, if the focus of treatment is the fracture, a code from subcategory M84.5, Pathological fracture in neoplastic disease, should be sequenced first, followed by the code for the neoplasm.

If the focus of treatment is the neoplasm with an associated pathological fracture, the neoplasm code should be sequenced first, followed by a code from M84.5 for the pathological fracture.

m. Current malignancy versus personal history of malignancy

When a primary malignancy has been excised but further treatment, such as an additional surgery for the malignancy, radiation therapy or chemotherapy is directed to that site, the primary malignancy code should be used until treatment is completed.

When a primary malignancy has been previously excised or eradicated from its site, there is no further treatment (of the malignancy) directed to that site, and there is no evidence of any existing primary malignancy, a code from category Z85, Personal history of malignant neoplasm, should be used to indicate the former site of the malignancy.

See Section I.C.21. Factors influencing health status and contact with health services, History (of)

n. Leukemia, *Multiple Myeloma, and Malignant Plasma Cell Neoplasms* in remission versus personal history

The categories for leukemia, and category C90, Multiple myeloma **and malignant plasma cell neoplasms**, have codes for in remission. There are also codes Z85.6, Personal history of leukemia, and Z85.79, Personal history of other malignant neoplasms of lymphoid, hematopoietic and related tissues. If the documentation is unclear, as to whether the patient is in remission, the provider should be queried.

See Section I.C.21. Factors influencing health status and contact with health services, History (of)

o. Aftercare following surgery for neoplasm

See Section I.C.21. Factors influencing health status and contact with health services, Aftercare

p. Follow-up care for completed treatment of a malignancy

See Section I.C.21. Factors influencing health status and contact with health services, Follow-up

q. Prophylactic organ removal for prevention of malignancy

See Section I.C. 21, Factors influencing health status and contact with health services, Prophylactic organ removal

r. Malignant neoplasm associated with transplanted organ

A malignant neoplasm of a transplanted organ should be coded as a transplant complication. Assign first the appropriate code from category T86.-, Complications of transplanted **organs and tissue**, followed by code C80.2, Malignant neoplasm associated with transplanted organ. Use an additional code for the specific malignancy.

3. Chapter 3: Disease of the Blood and Blood-forming Organs and Certain Disorders Involving the Immune Mechanism (D50-D89)
Reserved for future guideline expansion

4. Chapter 4: Endocrine, Nutritional, and Metabolic Diseases (E00-E89)

a. Diabetes mellitus

The diabetes mellitus codes are combination codes that include the type of **diabetes mellitus**, the body system affected, and the complications affecting that body system. As many codes within a particular category as are necessary to describe all of the complications of the disease may be used. They should be sequenced based on the reason for a particular encounter. Assign as many codes from categories E08 – E13 as needed to identify all of the associated conditions that the patient has.

1) Type of diabetes

The age of a patient is not the sole determining factor, though most type 1 diabetics develop the condition before reaching puberty. For this reason type 1 diabetes mellitus is also referred to as juvenile diabetes.

2) Type of diabetes mellitus not documented

If the type of diabetes mellitus is not documented in the medical record the default is E11.-, Type 2 diabetes mellitus.

3) Diabetes mellitus and the use of insulin

If the documentation in a medical record does not indicate the type of diabetes but does indicate that the patient uses insulin, code E11, Type 2 diabetes mellitus, should be assigned. **Code** Z79.4, Long-term (current) use of insulin, should also be assigned to indicate that the patient uses insulin. Code Z79.4 should not be assigned if insulin is given temporarily to bring a type 2 patient's blood sugar under control during an encounter.

4) Diabetes mellitus in pregnancy and gestational diabetes

See Section I.C.15. Diabetes mellitus in pregnancy.

See Section I.C.15. Gestational (pregnancy induced) diabetes

5) Complications Due to Insulin Pump Malfunction

(a) Underdose of insulin due *to* insulin pump failure

An underdose of insulin due to an insulin pump failure should be assigned to a code from subcategory T85.6, Mechanical complication of other specified internal and external prosthetic devices, implants and grafts, that specifies the type of pump malfunction, as the principal or **first-listed** code, followed by code T38.3x6-, Underdosing of insulin and oral hypoglycemic [antidiabetic] drugs. Additional codes for the type of diabetes mellitus and any associated complications due to the underdosing should also be assigned.

(b) Overdose of insulin due to insulin pump failure

The principal or **first-listed** code for an encounter due to an insulin pump malfunction resulting in an overdose of insulin, should also be T85.6-, Mechanical complication of other specified internal and external prosthetic devices, implants and grafts, followed by code T38.3x1-, Poisoning by insulin and oral hypoglycemic [antidiabetic] drugs, accidental (unintentional).

6) Secondary Diabetes Mellitus

Codes under **categories** E08, Diabetes mellitus due to underlying condition, and E09, Drug or chemical induced diabetes mellitus, identify complications/manifestations associated with secondary diabetes mellitus. Secondary diabetes is always caused by another condition or event (e.g., cystic fibrosis, malignant neoplasm of pancreas, pancreatectomy, adverse effect of drug, or poisoning).

(a) Secondary diabetes mellitus and the use of insulin

For patients who routinely use insulin, code Z79.4, Long-term (current) use of insulin, should also be assigned. Code Z79.4 should not be assigned if insulin is given temporarily to bring a patient's blood sugar under control during an encounter.

(b) Assigning and sequencing secondary diabetes codes and its causes

The sequencing of the secondary diabetes codes in relationship to codes for the cause of the diabetes is based on the **Tabular List** instructions for categories E08 and E09. For example, for category E08, Diabetes mellitus due to underlying condition, code first the underlying condition; for category E09, Drug or chemical induced diabetes mellitus, code first the drug or chemical (T36-T65).

(i) Secondary diabetes mellitus due to pancreatectomy

For postpancreatectomy diabetes mellitus (lack of insulin due to the surgical removal of all or part of the pancreas), assign code E89.1, **Postprocedural** hypoinsulinemia. Assign a code from category **E13** and **a code from subcategory Z90.41-, Acquired absence of pancreas**, as additional codes.

(ii) Secondary diabetes due to drugs

Secondary diabetes may be caused by an adverse effect of correctly administered medications, poisoning or late effect of poisoning.

See section I.C.19.e for coding of adverse effects and poisoning, and section I.C.20 for external cause code reporting.

5. Chapter 5: Mental and behavioral disorders (F01 – F99)

a. Pain disorders related to psychological factors

Assign code F45.41, for pain that is exclusively psychological. Code F45.41, Pain disorder **exclusively** related **to** psychological factors, should be used following the appropriate code from category G89, Pain, not elsewhere classified, if there is documentation of a psychological component for a patient with acute or chronic pain.

See Section I.C.6. Pain

b. *Mental and behavioral disorders due to psychoactive substance use*

1) *In Remission*

   Selection of codes for "in remission" for categories F10-F19, Mental and behavioral disorders due to psychoactive substance use (categories F10-F19 with -.21) requires the provider's clinical judgment. The appropriate codes for "in remission" are assigned only on the basis of provider documentation (as defined in the Official Guidelines for Coding and Reporting).

2) *Psychoactive Substance Use, Abuse And Dependence*

   When the provider documentation refers to use, abuse and dependence of the same substance (e.g. alcohol, opioid, cannabis, etc.), only one code should be assigned to identify the pattern of use based on the following hierarchy:

   - If both use and abuse are documented, assign only the code for abuse
   - If both abuse and dependence are documented, assign only the code for dependence
   - If use, abuse and dependence are all documented, assign only the code for dependence
   - If both use and dependence are documented, assign only the code for dependence.

3) *Psychoactive Substance Use*

   As with all other diagnoses, the codes for psychoactive substance use (F10.9-, F11.9-, F12.9-, F13.9-, F14.9-, F15.9-, F16.9-) should only be assigned based on provider documentation and when they meet the definition of a reportable diagnosis (see Section III, Reporting Additional Diagnoses). The codes are to be used only when the psychoactive substance use is associated with a mental or behavioral disorder, and such a relationship is documented by the provider.

6. **Chapter 6: Diseases of Nervous System and Sense Organs (G00-G99)**

   a. **Dominant/nondominant side**

   Codes from category G81, Hemiplegia and hemiparesis, and subcategories, G83.1, Monoplegia of lower limb, G83.2, Monoplegia of upper limb, and G83.3, Monoplegia, unspecified, identify whether the dominant or nondominant side is affected. Should **the affected side be documented, but not specified as dominant or nondominant**, and the classification system does not indicate a default, **code selection is as follows:**

   - For ambidextrous patients, the default should be dominant.
   - **If the left side is affected, the default is non-dominant.**
   - **If the right side is affected, the default is dominant.**

   b. **Pain - Category G89**

   1) **General coding information**

      Codes in category G89, Pain, not elsewhere classified, may be used in conjunction with codes from other categories and chapters to provide more detail about acute or chronic pain and neoplasm-related pain, unless otherwise indicated below.

      If the pain is not specified as acute or chronic, post-thoracotomy, postprocedural, or neoplasm-related, do not assign codes from category G89.

      A code from category G89 should not be assigned if the underlying (definitive) diagnosis is known, unless the reason for the encounter is pain control/ management and not management of the underlying condition.

      When an admission or encounter is for a procedure aimed at treating the underlying condition (e.g., spinal fusion, kyphoplasty), a code for the underlying condition (e.g., vertebral fracture, spinal stenosis) should be assigned as the principal diagnosis. No code from category G89 should be assigned.

   (a) **Category G89 Codes as Principal or First-Listed Diagnosis**

   Category G89 codes are acceptable as principal diagnosis or the first-listed code:

   - When pain control or pain management is the reason for the admission/encounter (e.g., a patient with displaced intervertebral disc, nerve impingement and severe back pain presents for injection of steroid into the spinal canal). The underlying cause of the pain should be reported as an additional diagnosis, if known.
   - When a patient is admitted for the insertion of a neurostimulator for pain control, assign the appropriate pain code as the principal or **first-listed** diagnosis. When an admission or encounter is for a procedure aimed at treating the underlying condition and a neurostimulator is inserted for pain control during the same admission/encounter, a code for the underlying condition should be assigned as the principal diagnosis and the appropriate pain code should be assigned as a secondary diagnosis.

   (b) **Use of Category G89 Codes in Conjunction with Site Specific Pain Codes**

   (i) **Assigning Category G89 and Site-Specific Pain Codes**

      Codes from category G89 may be used in conjunction with codes that identify the site of pain (including codes from chapter 18) if the category G89 code provides additional information. For example, if the code describes the site of the pain, but does not fully describe whether the pain is acute or chronic, then both codes should be assigned.

   (ii) **Sequencing of Category G89 Codes with Site-Specific Pain Codes**

      The sequencing of category G89 codes with site-specific pain codes (including chapter 18 codes), is dependent on the circumstances of the encounter/admission as follows:

      - If the encounter is for pain control or pain management, assign the code from category G89 followed by the code identifying the specific site of pain (e.g., encounter for pain management for acute neck pain from trauma is assigned code G89.11, Acute pain due to trauma, followed by code M54.2, Cervicalgia, to identify the site of pain).
      - If the encounter is for any other reason except pain control or pain management, and a related definitive diagnosis has not been established (confirmed) by the provider, assign the code for the specific site of pain first, followed by the appropriate code from category G89.

   2) **Pain due to devices, implants and grafts**

      See Section I.C.19. Pain due to medical devices

   3) **Postoperative Pain**

      The provider's documentation should be used to guide the coding of postoperative pain, as well as *Section III. Reporting Additional Diagnoses* and *Section IV. Diagnostic Coding and Reporting in the Outpatient Setting.*

      The default for post-thoracotomy and other postoperative pain not specified as acute or chronic is the code for the acute form.

      Routine or expected postoperative pain immediately after surgery should not be coded.

   (a) **Postoperative pain not associated with specific postoperative complication**

      Postoperative pain not associated with a specific postoperative complication is assigned to the appropriate postoperative pain code in category G89.

(b) Postoperative pain associated with specific postoperative complication

Postoperative pain associated with a specific postoperative complication (such as painful wire sutures) is assigned to the appropriate code(s) found in Chapter 19, Injury, poisoning, and certain other consequences of external causes. If appropriate, use additional code(s) from category G89 to identify acute or chronic pain (G89.18 or G89.28).

4) Chronic pain

Chronic pain is classified to subcategory G89.2. There is no time frame defining when pain becomes chronic pain. The provider's documentation should be used to guide use of these codes.

5) Neoplasm Related Pain

Code G89.3 is assigned to pain documented as being related, associated or due to cancer, primary or secondary malignancy, or tumor. This code is assigned regardless of whether the pain is acute or chronic.

This code may be assigned as the principal or first-listed code when the stated reason for the admission/encounter is documented as pain control/pain management. The underlying neoplasm should be reported as an additional diagnosis.

When the reason for the admission/encounter is management of the neoplasm and the pain associated with the neoplasm is also documented, code G89.3 may be assigned as an additional diagnosis. It is not necessary to assign an additional code for the site of the pain.

See Section I.C.2 for instructions on the sequencing of neoplasms for all other stated reasons for the admission/encounter (except for pain control/pain management).

6) Chronic pain syndrome

Central pain syndrome (G89.0) and chronic pain syndrome (G89.4) are different than the term "chronic pain," and therefore codes should only be used when the provider has specifically documented this condition.

See Section I.C.5. Pain disorders related to psychological factors

7. Chapter 7: Diseases of Eye and Adnexa (H00-H59)
Reserved for future guideline expansion

8. Chapter 8: Diseases of Ear and Mastoid Process (H60-H95)
Reserved for future guideline expansion

9. Chapter 9: Diseases of Circulatory System (I00-I99)
  a. Hypertension

    1) Hypertension with Heart Disease

Heart conditions classified to I50.- or I51.4-I51.9, are assigned to, a code from category I11, Hypertensive heart disease, when a causal relationship is stated (due to hypertension) or implied (hypertensive). Use an additional code from category I50, Heart failure, to identify the type of heart failure in those patients with heart failure.

The same heart conditions (I50.-, I51.4-I51.9) with hypertension, but without a stated causal relationship, are coded separately. Sequence according to the circumstances of the admission/encounter.

    2) Hypertensive Chronic Kidney Disease

Assign codes from category I12, Hypertensive chronic kidney disease, when both hypertension and a condition classifiable to category N18, Chronic kidney disease (CKD), are present. Unlike hypertension with heart disease, ICD-10-CM presumes a cause-and-effect relationship and classifies chronic kidney disease with hypertension as hypertensive chronic kidney disease.

The appropriate code from category N18 should be used as a secondary code with a code from category I12 to identify the stage of chronic kidney disease.

See Section I.C.14. Chronic kidney disease.

If a patient has hypertensive chronic kidney disease and acute renal failure, an additional code for the acute renal failure is required.

    3) Hypertensive Heart and Chronic Kidney Disease

Assign codes from combination category I13, Hypertensive heart and chronic kidney disease, when both hypertensive kidney disease and hypertensive heart disease are stated in the diagnosis. Assume a relationship between the hypertension and the chronic kidney disease, whether or not the condition is so designated. If heart failure is present, assign an additional code from category I50 to identify the type of heart failure.

The appropriate code from category N18, Chronic kidney disease, should be used as a secondary code with a code from category I13 to identify the stage of chronic kidney disease.

See Section I.C.14. Chronic kidney disease.

The codes in category I13, Hypertensive heart and chronic kidney disease, are combination codes that include hypertension, heart disease and chronic kidney disease. The Includes note at I13 specifies that the conditions included at I11 and I12 are included together in I13. If a patient has hypertension, heart disease and chronic kidney disease then a code from I13 should be used, not individual codes for hypertension, heart disease and chronic kidney disease, or codes from I11 or I12.

For patients with both acute renal failure and chronic kidney disease an additional code for acute renal failure is required.

    4) Hypertensive Cerebrovascular Disease

For hypertensive cerebrovascular disease, first assign the appropriate code from categories I60-I69, followed by the appropriate hypertension code.

    5) Hypertensive Retinopathy

Subcategory H35.0, **Background retinopathy and retinal vascular changes**, should be used with code I10, Essential (primary) hypertension, to include the systemic hypertension. The sequencing is based on the reason for the encounter.

    6) Hypertension, Secondary

Secondary hypertension is due to an underlying condition. Two codes are required: one to identify the underlying etiology and one from category I15 to identify the hypertension. Sequencing of codes is determined by the reason for admission/encounter.

    7) Hypertension, Transient

Assign code R03.0, Elevated blood pressure reading without diagnosis of hypertension, unless patient has an established diagnosis of hypertension. Assign code O13.-, Gestational [pregnancy-induced] hypertension without significant proteinuria, or O14.-, **Pre-eclampsia**, for transient hypertension of pregnancy.

    8) Hypertension, Controlled

This diagnostic statement usually refers to an existing state of hypertension under control by therapy. Assign **the appropriate** code **from categories I10-I15, Hypertensive diseases**.

    9) Hypertension, Uncontrolled

Uncontrolled hypertension may refer to untreated hypertension or hypertension not responding to current therapeutic regimen. In either case, assign **the appropriate** code **from categories I10-I15, Hypertensive diseases.**

  b. Atherosclerotic *Coronary Artery Disease* and *Angina*

ICD-10-CM has combination codes for atherosclerotic heart disease with angina pectoris. The subcategories for these codes are I25.11, Atherosclerotic heart disease of native coronary artery with angina pectoris and I25.7, Atherosclerosis of coronary artery bypass graft(s) and coronary artery of transplanted heart with angina pectoris.

When using one of these combination codes it is not necessary to use an additional code for angina pectoris. A causal relationship can be assumed in a patient with both atherosclerosis and angina pectoris, unless the documentation indicates the angina is due to something other than the atherosclerosis.

If a patient with coronary artery disease is admitted due to an acute myocardial infarction (AMI), the AMI should be sequenced before the coronary artery disease.

See Section I.C.9. Acute myocardial infarction (AMI)

c. **Intraoperative and Postprocedural *Cerebrovascular Accident***
Medical record documentation should clearly specify the cause-and-effect relationship between the medical intervention and the cerebrovascular accident in order to assign a code for intraoperative or postprocedural cerebrovascular accident.

Proper code assignment depends on whether it was an infarction or hemorrhage and whether it occurred intraoperatively or postoperatively. If it was a cerebral hemorrhage, code assignment depends on the type of procedure performed.

d. **Sequelae of Cerebrovascular Disease**

1) **Category I69, Sequelae of Cerebrovascular disease**
Category I69 is used to indicate conditions classifiable to categories I60-I67 as the causes of late effects (neurologic deficits), themselves classified elsewhere. These "late effects" include neurologic deficits that persist after initial onset of conditions classifiable to categories I60-I67. The neurologic deficits caused by cerebrovascular disease may be present from the onset or may arise at any time after the onset of the condition classifiable to categories I60-I67.

2) **Codes from category I69 with codes from I60-I67**
Codes from category I69 may be assigned on a health care record with codes from I60-I67, if the patient has a current cerebrovascular **disease** and deficits from an old **cerebrovascular disease**.

3) **Code Z86.73**
Assign code Z86.73, Personal history of transient ischemic attack (TIA), and cerebral infarction without residual deficits (and not a code from category I69) as an additional code for history of cerebrovascular disease when no neurologic deficits are present.

e. **Acute myocardial infarction (AMI)**

1) **ST elevation myocardial infarction (STEMI) and non ST elevation myocardial infarction (NSTEMI)**
The ICD-10-CM codes for acute myocardial infarction (AMI) identify the site, such as anterolateral wall or true posterior wall. Subcategories I21.0-I21.2 and code I21.4 are used for ST elevation myocardial infarction (STEMI). Code I21.4, Non-ST elevation (NSTEMI) myocardial infarction, is used for non ST elevation myocardial infarction (NSTEMI) and nontransmural MIs.

If NSTEMI evolves to STEMI, assign the STEMI code. If STEMI converts to NSTEMI due to thrombolytic therapy, it is still coded as STEMI.

When the patient requires continued care for the myocardial infarction, codes from category I21 may continue to be reported for the duration of 4 weeks (28 days) or less from onset, regardless of the healthcare setting, including when a patient is transferred from the acute care setting to the post-acute care setting if the patient is still within the four weeks time frame. For encounters after the 4 weeks time frame and the patient requires continued care related to the myocardial infarction, the appropriate aftercare code should be assigned, rather than a code from category I21. Otherwise, code I25.2, Old myocardial infarction, may be assigned for old or healed myocardial infarction not requiring further care.

2) **Acute myocardial infarction, unspecified**
Code I21.3, ST elevation (STEMI) myocardial infarction of unspecified site, is the default for the unspecified term acute myocardial infarction. If only STEMI or transmural MI without

the site is documented, query the provider as to the site, or assign code I21.3.

3) **AMI documented as nontransmural or subendocardial but site provided**
If an AMI is documented as nontransmural or subendocardial, but the site is provided, it is still coded as a subendocardial AMI.

See Section I.C.21.3 for information on coding status post administration of tPA in a different facility within the last 24 hrs.

4) **Subsequent acute myocardial infarction**
A code from category I22, Subsequent ST elevation (STEMI) and non ST elevation (NSTEMI) myocardial infarction, is to be used when a patient who has suffered an AMI has a new AMI within the 4 week time frame of the initial AMI. A code from category I22 must be used in conjunction with a code from category I21.

The sequencing of the I22 and I21 codes depends on the circumstances of the encounter. Should a patient who is in the hospital due to an AMI have a subsequent AMI while still in the hospital code I21 would be sequenced first as the reason for admission, with code I22 sequenced as a secondary code. Should a patient have a subsequent AMI after discharge for care of an initial AMI, and the reason for admission is the subsequent AMI, the I22 code should be sequenced first followed by the I21. An I21 code must accompany an I22 code to identify the site of the initial AMI, and to indicate that the patient is still within the 4 week time frame of healing from the initial AMI.

The guidelines for assigning the correct I22 code are the same as for the initial AMI.

10. **Chapter 10: Diseases of Respiratory System (J00-J99)**

a. **Chronic Obstructive Pulmonary Disease [COPD] and Asthma**

1) **Acute exacerbation of chronic obstructive bronchitis and asthma**
The codes in categories J44 and J45 distinguish between uncomplicated cases and those in acute exacerbation. An acute exacerbation is a worsening or a decompensation of a chronic condition. An acute exacerbation is not equivalent to an infection superimposed on a chronic condition, though an exacerbation may be triggered by an infection.

b. **Acute Respiratory Failure**

1) **Acute respiratory failure as principal diagnosis**
A code from subcategory J96.0, Acute respiratory failure, or **subcategory** J96.2, Acute and chronic respiratory failure, may be assigned as a principal diagnosis when it is the condition established after study to be chiefly responsible for occasioning the admission to the hospital, and the selection is supported by the Alphabetic Index and Tabular List. However, chapter-specific coding guidelines (such as obstetrics, poisoning, HIV, newborn) that provide sequencing direction take precedence.

2) **Acute respiratory failure as secondary diagnosis**
Respiratory failure may be listed as a secondary diagnosis if it occurs after admission, or if it is present on admission, but does not meet the definition of principal diagnosis.

3) **Sequencing of acute respiratory failure and another acute condition**
When a patient is admitted with respiratory failure and another acute condition, (e.g., myocardial infarction, cerebrovascular accident, aspiration pneumonia), the principal diagnosis will not be the same in every situation. This applies whether the other acute condition is a respiratory or nonrespiratory condition. Selection of the principal diagnosis will be dependent on the circumstances of admission. If both the respiratory failure and the other acute condition are equally responsible for occasioning the admission to the hospital, and there are no chapter-specific sequencing rules, the guideline regarding two or more

diagnoses that equally meet the definition for principal diagnosis (Section II, C.) may be applied in these situations.

If the documentation is not clear as to whether acute respiratory failure and another condition are equally responsible for occasioning the admission, query the provider for clarification.

c. **Influenza due to *certain identified influenza viruses***
Code only confirmed cases of avian influenza (code J09.0-, Influenza due to identified avian influenza virus) or novel H1N1 or swine flu, code J09.1-. This is an exception to the hospital inpatient guideline Section II, H. (Uncertain Diagnosis).

In this context, "confirmation" does not require documentation of positive laboratory testing specific for avian or novel H1N1 (H1N1 or swine flu) influenza. However, coding should be based on the provider's diagnostic statement that the patient has avian influenza.

If the provider records "suspected or possible or probable avian influenza," the appropriate influenza code from category **J11**, Influenza due to **unspecified** influenza virus, should be assigned. A code from category J09, Influenza due to certain identified influenza viruses, should not be assigned.

d. **Ventilator associated Pneumonia**
1) **Documentation of Ventilator associated Pneumonia**
As with all procedural or postprocedural complications, code assignment is based on the provider's documentation of the relationship between the condition and the procedure.

Code J95.851, Ventilator associated pneumonia, should be assigned only when the provider has documented ventilator associated pneumonia (VAP). An additional code to identify the organism (e.g., Pseudomonas aeruginosa, code B96.5) should also be assigned. Do not assign an additional code from categories J12-J18 to identify the type of pneumonia.

Code J95.851 should not be assigned for cases where the patient has pneumonia and is on a mechanical ventilator but the provider has not specifically stated that the pneumonia is ventilator-associated pneumonia. If the documentation is unclear as to whether the patient has a pneumonia that is a complication attributable to the mechanical ventilator, query the provider.

2) **Ventilator associated Pneumonia Develops after Admission**
A patient may be admitted with one type of pneumonia (e.g., code J13, Pneumonia due to Streptococcus pneumonia) and subsequently develop VAP. In this instance, the principal diagnosis would be the appro- priate code from categories J12-J18 for the pneumonia diagnosed at the time of admission. Code J95.851, Ventilator assoc- iated pneumonia, would be assigned as an additional diagnosis when the provider has also documented the presence of ventilator associated pneumonia.

11. **Chapter 11: Diseases of Digestive System (K00-K94)**
Reserved for future guideline expansion

12. **Chapter 12: Diseases of Skin and Subcutaneous Tissue (L00-L99)**
a. **Pressure ulcer stage codes**
1) **Pressure ulcer stages**
Codes from category L89, Pressure ulcer, are combination codes that identify the site of the pressure ulcer as well as the stage of the ulcer.

The ICD-10-CM classifies pressure ulcer stages based on severity, which is designated by stages 1-4, unspecified stage and unstageable.

Assign as many codes from category L89 as needed to identify all the pressure ulcers the patient has, if applicable.

2) **Unstageable pressure ulcers**
Assignment of the code for unstageable pressure ulcer (L89.--0) should be based on the clinical documentation. These codes are used for pressure ulcers whose stage cannot

be clinically determined (e.g., the ulcer is covered by eschar or has been treated with a skin or muscle graft) and pressure ulcers that are documented as deep tissue injury but not documented as due to trauma. This code should not be confused with the codes for unspecified stage (L89.--9). When there is no documentation regarding the stage of the pressure ulcer, assign the appropriate code for unspecified stage (L89.--9).

3) **Documented pressure ulcer stage**
Assignment of the pressure ulcer stage code should be guided by clinical documentation of the stage or documentation of the terms found in the **Alphabetic Index**. For clinical terms describing the stage that are not found in the **Alphabetic Index**, and there is no documentation of the stage, the provider should be queried.

4) **Patients admitted with pressure ulcers documented as healed**
No code is assigned if the documentation states that the pressure ulcer is completely healed.

5) **Patients admitted with pressure ulcers documented as healing**
Pressure ulcers described as healing should be assigned the appropriate pressure ulcer stage code based on the documentation in the medical record. If the documentation does not provide information about the stage of the healing pressure ulcer, assign the appropriate code for unspecified stage.

If the documentation is unclear as to whether the patient has a current (new) pressure ulcer or if the patient is being treated for a healing pressure ulcer, query the provider.

6) **Patient admitted with pressure ulcer evolving into another stage during the admission**
If a patient is admitted with a pressure ulcer at one stage and it progresses to a higher stage, assign the code for the highest stage reported for that site.

13. **Chapter 13: Diseases of the Musculoskeletal System and Connective Tissue (M00-M99)**
a. **Site and laterality**
Most of the codes within Chapter 13 have site and laterality designations. The site represents the bone, joint or the muscle involved. For some conditions where more than one bone, joint or muscle is usually involved, such as osteoarthritis, there is a "multiple sites" code available. For categories where no multiple site code is provided and more than one bone, joint or muscle is involved, multiple codes should be used to indicate the different sites involved.

1) **Bone versus joint**
For certain conditions, the bone may be affected at the upper or lower end, (e.g., avascular necrosis of bone, M87, Osteoporosis, M80, M81). Though the portion of the bone affected may be at the joint, the site designation will be the bone, not the joint.

b. **Acute traumatic versus chronic or recurrent musculoskeletal conditions**
Many musculoskeletal conditions are a result of previous injury or trauma to a site, or are recurrent conditions. Bone, joint or muscle conditions that are the result of a healed injury are usually found in chapter 13. Recurrent bone, joint or muscle conditions are also usually found in chapter 13. Any current, acute injury should be coded to the appropriate injury code from chapter 19. Chronic or recurrent conditions should generally be coded with a code from chapter 13. If it is difficult to determine from the documentation in the record which code is best to describe a condition, query the provider.

c. **Coding of Pathologic Fractures**
7th character A is for use as long as the patient is receiving active treatment for the fracture. Examples of active treatment are: surgical treatment, emergency department encounter, evaluation and treatment by a new physician. 7th character, D is to be used

for encounters after the patient has completed active treatment. The other 7th characters, listed under each subcategory in the Tabular List, are to be used for subsequent encounters for treatment of problems associated with the healing, such as malunions, nonunions, and sequelae.

Care for complications of surgical treatment for fracture repairs during the healing or recovery phase should be coded with the appropriate complication codes.

See Section I.C.19. Coding of traumatic fractures.

d. Osteoporosis

Osteoporosis is a systemic condition, meaning that all bones of the musculoskeletal system are affected. Therefore, site is not a component of the codes under category M81, Osteoporosis without current pathological fracture. The site codes under category M80, Osteoporosis with current pathological fracture, identify the site of the fracture, not the osteoporosis.

1) **Osteoporosis without pathological fracture**
   Category M81, Osteoporosis without current pathological fracture, is for use for patients with osteoporosis who do not currently have a pathologic fracture due to the osteoporosis, even if they have had a fracture in the past. For patients with a history of osteoporosis fractures, status code **Z87.310**, Personal history of **(healed)** osteoporosis fracture, should follow the code from M81.

2) **Osteoporosis with current pathological fracture**
   Category M80, Osteoporosis with current pathological fracture, is for patients who have a current pathologic fracture at the time of an encounter. The codes under M80 identify the site of the fracture. A code from category M80, not a traumatic fracture code, should be used for any patient with known osteoporosis who suffers a fracture, even if the patient had a minor fall or trauma, if that fall or trauma would not usually break a normal, healthy bone.

14. Chapter 14: Diseases of Genitourinary System (N00-N99)

a. Chronic kidney disease

1) **Stages of chronic kidney disease (CKD)**
   The ICD-10-CM classifies CKD based on severity. The severity of CKD is designated by stages **1-5**. Stage **2**, code N18.2, equates to mild CKD; stage **3**, code N18.3, equates to moderate CKD; and stage **4**, code N18.4, equates to severe CKD. Code N18.6, End stage renal disease (ESRD), is assigned when the provider has documented end-stage-renal disease (ESRD).

   If both a stage of CKD and ESRD are documented, assign code N18.6 only.

2) **Chronic kidney disease and kidney transplant status**
   Patients who have undergone kidney transplant may still have some form of chronic kidney disease (CKD) because the kidney transplant may not fully restore kidney function. Therefore, the presence of CKD alone does not constitute a transplant complication. Assign the appropriate N18 code for the patient's stage of CKD and code Z94.0, Kidney transplant status. If a transplant complication such as failure or rejection or other transplant complication is documented, see section I.C.19.g for information on coding complications of a kidney transplant. If the documentation is unclear as to whether the patient has a complication of the transplant, query the provider.

3) **Chronic kidney disease with other conditions**
   Patients with CKD may also suffer from other serious conditions, most commonly diabetes mellitus and hypertension. The sequencing of the CKD code in relationship to codes for other contributing conditions is based on the conventions in the Tabular List.

   See I.C.9. Hypertensive chronic kidney disease.

   See I.C.19. Chronic kidney disease and kidney transplant complications.

15. Chapter 15: Pregnancy, Childbirth, and the Puerperium (O00-O9a)

a. General Rules for Obstetric Cases

1) **Codes from chapter 15 and sequencing priority**
   Obstetric cases require codes from chapter 15, codes in the range O00-O9a, Pregnancy, Childbirth, and the Puerperium. Chapter 15 codes have sequencing priority over codes from other chapters. Additional codes from other chapters may be used in conjunction with chapter 15 codes to further specify conditions. Should the provider document that the pregnancy is incidental to the encounter, then code Z33.1, Pregnant state, incidental, should be used in place of any chapter 15 codes. It is the provider's responsibility to state that the condition being treated is not affecting the pregnancy.

2) **Chapter 15 codes used only on the maternal record**
   Chapter 15 codes are to be used only on the maternal record, never on the record of the newborn.

3) **Final character for trimester**
   The majority of codes in Chapter 15 have a final character indicating the trimester of pregnancy. The timeframes for the trimesters are indicated at the beginning of the chapter. If trimester is not a component of a code it is because the condition always occurs in a specific trimester, or the concept of trimester of pregnancy is not applicable. Certain codes have characters for only certain trimesters because the condition does not occur in all trimesters, but it may occur in more than just one.

   Assignment of the final character for trimester should be based on the **provider's documentation of the** trimester (**or number of weeks**) for the current admission/encounter. This applies to the assignment of trimester for pre-existing conditions as well as those that develop during or are due to the pregnancy. **The provider's documentation of the number of weeks may be used to assign the appropriate code identifying the trimester.**

   Whenever delivery occurs during the current admission, and there is an "in childbirth" option for the obstetric complication being coded, the "in childbirth" code should be assigned.

4) **Selection of trimester for inpatient admissions that encompass more than one trimesters**
   In instances when a patient is admitted to a hospital for complications of pregnancy during one trimester and remains in the hospital into a subsequent trimester, the trimester character for the antepartum complication code should be assigned on the basis of the trimester when the complication developed, not the trimester of the discharge. If the condition developed prior to the current admission/encounter or represents a pre-existing condition, the trimester character for the trimester at the time of the admission/encounter should be assigned.

5) **Unspecified trimester**
   Each category that includes codes for trimester has a code for "unspecified trimester." The "unspecified trimester" code should rarely be used, such as when the documentation in the record is insufficient to determine the trimester and it is not possible to obtain clarification.

6) *Fetal Extensions*
   Where applicable, a 7th character is to be assigned for certain categories (O31, O32, O33.3 - O33.6, O35, O36, O40, O41, O60.1, O60.2, O64, and O69) to identify the fetus for which the complication code applies.

   Assign 7th character "0":

   - **For single gestations**
   - **When the documentation in the record is insufficient to determine the fetus affected and it is not possible to obtain clarification.**

- When it is not possible to clinically determine which fetus is affected.

b. Selection of OB Principal or First-listed Diagnosis

1) Routine outpatient prenatal visits

For routine outpatient prenatal visits when no complications are present, a code from category Z34, Encounter for supervision of normal pregnancy, should be used as the first-listed diagnosis. These codes should not be used in conjunction with chapter 15 codes.

2) Prenatal outpatient visits for high-risk patients

For routine prenatal outpatient visits for patients with high-risk pregnancies, a code from category O09, Supervision of high-risk pregnancy, should be used as the first-listed diagnosis. Secondary chapter 15 codes may be used in conjunction with these codes if appropriate.

3) Episodes when no delivery occurs

In episodes when no delivery occurs, the principal diagnosis should correspond to the principal complication of the pregnancy which necessitated the encounter. Should more than one complication exist, all of which are treated or monitored, any of the complications codes may be sequenced first.

4) When a delivery occurs

When a delivery occurs, the principal diagnosis should correspond to the main circumstances or complication of the delivery. In cases of cesarean delivery, the selection of the principal diagnosis should be the condition established after study that was responsible for the patient's admission. If the patient was admitted with a condition that resulted in the performance of a cesarean procedure, that condition should be selected as the principal diagnosis. If the reason for the admission/encounter was unrelated to the condition resulting in the cesarean delivery, the condition related to the reason for the admission/encounter should be selected as the principal diagnosis.

5) Outcome of delivery

A code from category Z37, Outcome of delivery, should be included on every maternal record when a delivery has occurred. These codes are not to be used on subsequent records or on the newborn record.

c. Pre-existing conditions versus conditions due to the pregnancy

Certain categories in Chapter 15 distinguish between conditions of the mother that existed prior to pregnancy (pre-existing) and those that are a direct result of pregnancy. When assigning codes from Chapter 15, it is important to assess if a condition was pre-existing prior to pregnancy or developed during or due to the pregnancy in order to assign the correct code.

Categories that do not distinguish between pre-existing and pregnancy-related conditions may be used for either. It is acceptable to use codes specifically for the puerperium with codes complicating pregnancy and childbirth if a condition arises postpartum during the delivery encounter.

d. Pre-existing hypertension in pregnancy

Category O10, Pre-existing hypertension complicating pregnancy, childbirth and the puerperium, includes codes for hypertensive heart and hypertensive chronic kidney disease. When assigning one of the O10 codes that includes hypertensive heart disease or hypertensive chronic kidney disease, it is necessary to add a secondary code from the appropriate hypertension category to specify the type of heart failure or chronic kidney disease.

See Section I.C.9. Hypertension.

e. Fetal Conditions Affecting the Management of the Mother

1) Codes from categories O35 and O36

Codes from categories O35, Maternal care for known or suspected fetal abnormality and damage, and O36, Maternal care for other fetal problems, are assigned only when the fetal condition is actually responsible for modifying the management of the mother, i.e., by requiring diagnostic studies, additional observation, special care, or termination of pregnancy. The fact that the fetal condition exists does not justify assigning a code from this series to the mother's record.

2) In utero surgery

In cases when surgery is performed on the fetus, a diagnosis code from category O35, Maternal care for known or suspected fetal abnormality and damage, should be assigned identifying the fetal condition. Assign the appropriate procedure code for the procedure performed.

No code from Chapter 16, the perinatal codes, should be used on the mother's record to identify fetal conditions. Surgery performed in utero on a fetus is still to be coded as an obstetric encounter.

f. HIV Infection in Pregnancy, Childbirth and the Puerperium

During pregnancy, childbirth or the puerperium, a patient admitted because of an HIV-related illness should receive a principal diagnosis from subcategory O98.7-, Human immunodeficiency [HIV] disease complicating pregnancy, childbirth and the puerperium, followed by the code(s) for the HIV-related illness(es).

Patients with asymptomatic HIV infection status admitted during pregnancy, childbirth, or the puerperium should receive codes of O98.7- and Z21, Asymptomatic human immunodeficiency virus [HIV] infection status.

g. Diabetes mellitus in pregnancy

Diabetes mellitus is a significant complicating factor in pregnancy. Pregnant women who are diabetic should be assigned a code **from category O24**, Diabetes mellitus in pregnancy, childbirth, and the puerperium, first, followed by the appropriate diabetes code(s) (E08-E13) from Chapter 4.

h. Long term use of insulin

Code Z79.4, Long-term (current) use of insulin, should also be assigned if the diabetes mellitus is being treated with insulin.

i. Gestational (pregnancy induced) diabetes

Gestational (pregnancy induced) diabetes can occur during the second and third trimester of pregnancy in women who were not diabetic prior to pregnancy. Gestational diabetes can cause complications in the pregnancy similar to those of pre-existing diabetes mellitus. It also puts the woman at greater risk of developing diabetes after the pregnancy. Codes for gestational diabetes are in subcategory O24.4, Gestational diabetes mellitus. No other code from category O24, Diabetes mellitus in pregnancy, childbirth, and the puerperium, should be used with a code from O24.4.

The codes under subcategory O24.4 include diet controlled and insulin controlled. If a patient with gestational diabetes is treated with both diet and insulin, only the code for insulin-controlled is required.

Code Z79.4, Long-term (current) use of insulin, should not be assigned with codes from subcategory O24.4.

An abnormal glucose tolerance in pregnancy is assigned a code from subcategory O99.81, Abnormal glucose complicating pregnancy, childbirth, and the puerperium.

j. Sepsis and septic shock complicating abortion, pregnancy, childbirth and the puerperium

When assigning a chapter 15 code for sepsis complicating abortion, pregnancy, childbirth, and the puerperium, a code for the specific type of infection should be assigned as an additional diagnosis. If severe sepsis is present, a code from subcategory R65.2, Severe sepsis, and code(s) for associated organ dysfunction(s) should also be assigned as additional diagnoses.

k. Puerperal sepsis

Code O85, Puerperal sepsis, should be assigned with a secondary code to identify the causal organism (e.g., for a bacterial infection, assign a code from category B95-B96, Bacterial infections in conditions classified elsewhere). A code from category A40, Streptococcal sepsis, or A41, Other sepsis, should not be used for puerperal sepsis. If applicable, use additional codes to identify severe sepsis (R65.2-) and any associated acute organ dysfunction.

l. Alcohol and tobacco use during pregnancy, childbirth and the puerperium

1) Alcohol use during pregnancy, childbirth and the puerperium
Codes under subcategory O99.31, Alcohol use complicating pregnancy, childbirth, and the puerperium, should be assigned for any pregnancy case when a mother uses alcohol during the pregnancy or postpartum. A secondary code from category F10, Alcohol related disorders, should also be assigned **to identify manifestations of the alcohol use.**

2) Tobacco use during pregnancy, childbirth and the puerperium
Codes under subcategory O99.33, Smoking (tobacco) complicating pregnancy, childbirth, and the puerperium, should be assigned for any pregnancy case when a mother uses any type of tobacco product during the pregnancy or postpartum. A secondary code from category F17, Nicotine dependence, or code Z72.0, Tobacco use, should also be assigned **to identify the type of nicotine dependence**.

m. Poisoning, toxic effects, adverse effects and underdosing in a pregnant patient
A code from subcategory O9a.2, Injury, poisoning and certain other consequences of external causes complicating pregnancy, childbirth, and the puerperium, should be sequenced first, followed by the appropriate poisoning, toxic effect, adverse effect or underdosing code, and then the additional code(s) that specifies the condition caused by the poisoning, toxic effect, adverse effect or underdosing.
See Section I.C.19. Adverse effects, poisoning, underdosing and toxic effects.

n. Normal Delivery, Code O80

1) Encounter for full term uncomplicated delivery
Code O80 should be assigned when a woman is admitted for a full-term normal delivery and delivers a single, healthy infant without any complications antepartum, during the delivery, or postpartum during the delivery episode. Code O80 is always a principal diagnosis. It is not to be used if any other code from chapter 15 is needed to describe a current complication of the antenatal, delivery, or perinatal period. Additional codes from other chapters may be used with code O80 if they are not related to or are in any way complicating the pregnancy.

2) Uncomplicated delivery with resolved antepartum complication
Code O80 may be used if the patient had a complication at some point during the pregnancy, but the complication is not present at the time of the admission for delivery.

3) Outcome of delivery for O80
Z37.0, Single live birth, is the only outcome of delivery code appropriate for use with O80.

o. The Peripartum and Postpartum Periods

1) Peripartum and Postpartum periods
The postpartum period begins immediately after delivery and continues for six weeks following delivery. The peripartum period is defined as the last month of pregnancy to five months postpartum.

2) Peripartum and postpartum complication
A postpartum complication is any complication occurring within the six-week period.

3) Pregnancy-related complications after 6 week period
Chapter 15 codes may also be used to describe pregnancy-related complications after the peripartum or postpartum period if the provider documents that a condition is pregnancy related.

4) Admission for routine postpartum care following delivery outside hospital
When the mother delivers outside the hospital prior to admission and is admitted for routine postpartum care and no complications are noted, code Z39.0, Encounter for care and

examination of mother immediately after delivery, should be assigned as the principal diagnosis.

5) Pregnancy associated cardiomyopathy
Pregnancy associated cardiomyopathy, code O90.3, is unique in that it may be diagnosed in the third trimester of pregnancy but may continue to progress months after delivery. For this reason, it is referred to as peripartum cardiomyopathy. Code O90.3 is only for use when the cardiomyopathy develops as a result of pregnancy in a woman who did not have pre-existing heart disease.

p. Code O94, Sequelae of complication of pregnancy, childbirth, and the puerperium

1) Code O94
Code O94, Sequelae of complication of pregnancy, childbirth, and the puerperium, is for use in those cases when an initial complication of a pregnancy develops a sequelae requiring care or treatment at a future date.

2) After the initial postpartum period
This code may be used at any time after the initial postpartum period.

3) Sequencing of Code O94
This code, like all late effect codes, is to be sequenced following the code describing the sequelae of the complication.

q. Abortions

1) Abortion with Liveborn Fetus
When an attempted termination of pregnancy results in a liveborn fetus, assign a code from subcategory O60.1, Preterm labor with preterm delivery, and a code from category Z37, Outcome of Delivery. The procedure code for the attempted termination of pregnancy should also be assigned.

2) Retained Products of Conception following an abortion
Subsequent encounters for retained products of conception following a spontaneous abortion or elective termination of pregnancy are assigned the appropriate code from category O03, Spontaneous abortion, or **codes O07.4, Failed attempted termination of pregnancy without complication and** Z33.2, Encounter for elective termination of pregnancy. This advice is appropriate even when the patient was discharged previously with a discharge diagnosis of complete abortion.

r. Abuse in a pregnant patient
For suspected or confirmed cases of abuse of a pregnant patient, a code(s) from subcategories O9a.3, Physical abuse complicating pregnancy, childbirth, and the puerperium, O9a.4, Sexual abuse complicating pregnancy, childbirth, and the puerperium, and O9a.5, Psychological abuse complicating pregnancy, childbirth, and the puerperium, should be sequenced first, followed by the appropriate codes (if applicable) to identify any associated current injury due to physical abuse, sexual abuse, and the perpetrator of abuse.
See Section I.C.19.f. Adult and child abuse, neglect and other maltreatment.

16. Chapter 16: Newborn (Perinatal) Guidelines (P00-P96)
For coding and reporting purposes the perinatal period is defined as before birth through the 28th day following birth. The following guidelines are provided for reporting purposes

a. General Perinatal Rules

1) Use of Chapter 16 Codes
Codes in this chapter are never for use on the maternal record. Codes from Chapter 15, the obstetric chapter, are never permitted on the newborn record. Chapter 16 **codes** may be used throughout the life of the patient if the condition is still present.

2) Principal Diagnosis for Birth Record
When coding the birth episode in a newborn record, assign a code from category Z38, Liveborn **infants** according to place of birth and type of delivery, as the principal diagnosis. A code

from category Z38 is assigned only once, to a newborn at the time of birth. If a newborn is transferred to another institution, a code from category Z38 should not be used at the receiving hospital.

A code from category Z38 is used only on the newborn record, not on the mother's record.

3) Use of Codes from other Chapters with Codes from Chapter 16

Codes from other chapters may be used with codes from chapter 16 if the codes from the other chapters provide more specific detail. Codes for signs and symptoms may be assigned when a definitive diagnosis has not been established. If the reason for the encounter is a perinatal condition, the code from chapter 16 should be sequenced first.

4) Use of Chapter 16 Codes after the Perinatal Period

Should a condition originate in the perinatal period, and continue throughout the life of the patient, the perinatal code should continue to be used regardless of the patient's age.

5) Birth process or community acquired conditions

If a newborn has a condition that may be either due to the birth process or community acquired and the documentation does not indicate which it is, the default is due to the birth process and the code from Chapter 16 should be used. If the condition is community-acquired, a code from Chapter 16 should not be assigned.

6) Code all clinically significant conditions

All clinically significant conditions noted on routine newborn examination should be coded. A condition is clinically significant if it requires:

- clinical evaluation; or
- therapeutic treatment; or
- diagnostic procedures; or
- extended length of hospital stay; or
- increased nursing care and/or monitoring; or
- has implications for future health care needs

Note: The perinatal guidelines listed above are the same as the general coding guidelines for "additional diagnoses", except for the final point regarding implications for future health care needs. Codes should be assigned for conditions that have been specified by the provider as having implications for future health care needs.

b. Observation and Evaluation of Newborns for Suspected Conditions not Found

Assign a code from categories P00-P04 to identify those instances when a healthy newborn is evaluated for a suspected condition that is determined after study not to be present. Do not use a code from categories P00-P04 when the patient has identified signs or symptoms of a suspected problem; in such cases, code the sign or symptom.

c. Coding Additional Perinatal Diagnoses

1) Assigning codes for conditions that require treatment

Assign codes for conditions that require treatment or further investigation, prolong the length of stay, or require resource utilization.

2) Codes for conditions specified as having implications for future health care needs

Assign codes for conditions that have been specified by the provider as having implications for future health care needs.

Note: This guideline should not be used for adult patients.

d. Prematurity and Fetal Growth Retardation

Providers utilize different criteria in determining prematurity. A code for prematurity should not be assigned unless it is documented. Assignment of codes in categories P05, Disorders of newborn related to slow fetal growth and fetal malnutrition, and P07, Disorders of newborn related to short gestation and low birth weight, not elsewhere classified, should be based on the recorded

birth weight and estimated gestational age. Codes from category P05 should not be assigned with codes from category P07.

When both birth weight and gestational age are available, two codes from category P07 should be assigned, with the code for birth weight sequenced before the code for gestational age.

e. Low birth weight and immaturity status

Codes from **category P07, Disorders of newborn related to short gestation and low birth weight, not elsewhere classified, are for use for a child or adult who was premature** or had a low birth weight as a newborn and this is affecting the patient's current health status.

See Section I.C.21. Factors influencing health status and contact with health services, Status.

f. Bacterial Sepsis of Newborn

Category P36, Bacterial sepsis of newborn, includes congenital sepsis. If a perinate is documented as having sepsis without documentation of congenital or community acquired, the default is congenital and a code from category P36 should be assigned. If the P36 code includes the causal organism, an additional code from category B95, Streptococcus, Staphylococcus, and Enterococcus as the cause of diseases classified elsewhere, or B96, Other bacterial agents as the cause of diseases classified elsewhere, should not be assigned. If the P36 code does not include the causal organism, assign an additional code from category B96. If applicable, use additional codes to identify severe sepsis (R65.2-) and any associated acute organ dysfunction.

g. Stillbirth

Code P95, Stillbirth, is only for use in institutions that maintain separate records for stillbirths. No other code should be used with P95. Code P95 should not be used on the mother's record.

17. Chapter 17: Congenital Malformations, Deformations, and Chromosomal Abnormalities (Q00-Q99)

Assign an appropriate code(s) from categories Q00-Q99, Congenital malformations, deformations, and chromosomal abnormalities when a malformation/deformation or chromosomal abnormality is documented. A malformation/deformation/or chromosomal abnormality may be the principal/**first-listed** diagnosis on a record or a secondary diagnosis.

When a malformation/deformation/or chromosomal abnormality does not have a unique code assignment, assign additional code(s) for any manifestations that may be present.

When the code assignment specifically identifies the malformation/deformation/or chromosomal abnormality, manifestations that are an inherent component of the anomaly should not be coded separately. Additional codes should be assigned for manifestations that are not an inherent component.

Codes from Chapter 17 may be used throughout the life of the patient. If a congenital malformation or deformity has been corrected, a personal history code should be used to identify the history of the malformation or deformity. Although present at birth, malformation/deformation/or chromosomal abnormality may not be identified until later in life. Whenever the condition is diagnosed by the physician, it is appropriate to assign a code from codes Q00-Q99.

For the birth admission, the appropriate code from category Z38, Liveborn infants, according to place of birth and type of delivery, should be sequenced as the principal diagnosis, followed by any congenital anomaly codes, Q00- **Q99**.

18. Chapter 18: Symptoms, Signs, and Abnormal Clinical and Laboratory Findings, Not Elsewhere Classified (R00-R99)

Chapter 18 includes symptoms, signs, abnormal results of clinical or other investigative procedures, and ill-defined conditions regarding which no diagnosis classifiable elsewhere is recorded. Signs and symptoms that point to a **specific** diagnosis have been assigned to a category in other chapters of the classification.

a. Use of symptom codes

Codes that describe symptoms and signs are acceptable for reporting purposes when a related definitive diagnosis has not been established (confirmed) by the provider.

b. Use of a symptom code with a definitive diagnosis code

Codes for signs and symptoms may be reported in addition to a related definitive diagnosis when the sign or symptom is not routinely associated with that diagnosis, such as the various signs and symptoms associated with complex syndromes. The definitive diagnosis code should be sequenced before the symptom code.

Signs or symptoms that are associated routinely with a disease process should not be assigned as additional codes, unless otherwise instructed by the classification.

c. Combination codes that include symptoms

ICD-10-CM contains a number of combination codes that identify both the definitive diagnosis and common symptoms of that diagnosis. When using one of these combination codes, an additional code should not be assigned for the symptom.

d. Repeated falls

Code R29.6, Repeated falls, is for use for encounters when a patient has recently fallen and the reason for the fall is being investigated.

Code Z91.81, History of falling, is for use when a patient has fallen in the past and is at risk for future falls. When appropriate, both codes R29.6 and Z91.81 may be assigned together.

e. *Coma* scale

The coma scale codes (R40.2-) can be used in conjunction with traumatic brain injury codes, **acute cerebrovascular disease** or sequelae of cerebrovascular **disease** codes. These codes are primarily for use by trauma registries, but they may be used in any setting where this information is collected. The coma scale codes should be sequenced after the diagnosis code(s).

These codes, one from each subcategory, are needed to complete the scale. The 7th character indicates when the scale was recorded. The 7th character should match for all three codes.

At a minimum, report the initial score documented on presentation at your facility. This may be a score from the emergency medicine technician (EMT) or in the emergency department. If desired, a facility may choose to capture multiple Glasgow coma scale scores.

f. Functional quadriplegia

Functional quadriplegia (code R53.2) is the lack of ability to use one's limbs or to ambulate due to extreme debility. It is not associated with neurologic deficit or injury, and code R53.2 should not be used for cases of neurologic quadriplegia. It should only be assigned if functional quadriplegia is specifically documented in the medical record.

g. SIRS due to Non-Infectious Process

The systemic inflammatory response syndrome (SIRS) can develop as a result of certain non-infectious disease processes, such as trauma, malignant neoplasm, or pancreatitis. When SIRS is documented with a noninfectious condition, and no subsequent infection is documented, the code for the underlying condition, such as an injury, should be assigned, followed by code R65.10, Systemic inflammatory response syndrome (SIRS) of non-infectious origin without acute organ dysfunction, or code R65.11, Systemic inflammatory response syndrome (SIRS) of non-infectious origin with acute organ dysfunction. If an associated acute organ dysfunction is documented, the appropriate code(s) for the specific type of organ dysfunction(s) should be assigned in addition to code R65.11. If acute organ dysfunction is documented, but it cannot be determined if the acute organ dysfunction is associated with SIRS or due to another condition (e.g., directly due to the trauma), the provider should be queried.

h. Death NOS

Code R99, Ill-defined and unknown cause of mortality, is only for use in the very limited circumstance when a patient who has already died is brought into an emergency department or other healthcare facility and is pronounced dead upon arrival. It does not represent the discharge disposition of death.

19. Chapter 19: Injury, Poisoning, and Certain Other Consequences of External Causes (S00-T88)

a. Code Extensions

Most categories in chapter 19 have 7th character extensions that are required for each applicable code. Most categories in this chapter have three extensions (with the exception of fractures): A, initial encounter, D, subsequent encounter and S, sequela.

Extension "A", initial encounter is used while the patient is receiving active treatment for the injury. Examples of active treatment are: surgical treatment, emergency department encounter, and evaluation and treatment by a new physician.

Extension "D" subsequent encounter is used for encounters after the patient has received active treatment of the injury and is receiving routine care for the injury during the healing or recovery phase. Examples of subsequent care are: cast change or removal, removal of external or internal fixation device, medication adjustment, other aftercare and follow up visits following injury treatment.

The aftercare Z codes should not be used for aftercare for injuries. For aftercare of an injury, assign the acute injury code with the 7th character "D" (subsequent encounter).

Extension "S", sequela, is for use for complications or conditions that arise as a direct result of an injury, such as scar formation after a burn. The scars are sequelae of the burn. When using extension "S", it is necessary to use both the injury code that precipitated the sequela and the code for the sequela itself. The "S" is added only to the injury code, not the sequela code. The "S" extension identifies the injury responsible for the sequela. The specific type of sequela (e.g. scar) is sequenced first, followed by the injury code.

b. Coding of Injuries

When coding injuries, assign separate codes for each injury unless a combination code is provided, in which case the combination code is assigned. **Code T07, Unspecified multiple injuries** should not be assigned unless information for a more specific code is not available. **Traumatic** injury codes (S00-T14.9) are not to be used for normal, healing surgical wounds or to identify complications of surgical wounds.

The code for the most serious injury, as determined by the provider and the focus of treatment, is sequenced first.

1) Superficial injuries

Superficial injuries such as abrasions or contusions are not coded when associated with more severe injuries of the same site.

2) Primary injury with damage to nerves/blood vessels

When a primary injury results in minor damage to peripheral nerves or blood vessels, the primary injury is sequenced first with additional code(s) for injuries to nerves and spinal cord (such as category S04), and/or injury to blood vessels (such as category S15). When the primary injury is to the blood vessels or nerves, that injury should be sequenced first.

c. Coding of Traumatic Fractures

The principles of multiple coding of injuries should be followed in coding fractures. Fractures of specified sites are coded individually by site in accordance with both the provisions within categories S02, S12, S22, S32, S42, S49, S52, S59, S62, S72, S79, S82, S89, S92 and the level of detail furnished by medical record content.

A fracture not indicated as open or closed should be coded to closed. A fracture not indicated whether displaced or not displaced should be coded to displaced.

More specific guidelines are as follows:

1) Initial vs. Subsequent Encounter for Fractures

Traumatic fractures are coded using the appropriate 7th character extension for initial encounter (A, B, C) while the patient is receiving active treatment for the fracture. Examples of active treatment are: surgical treatment, emergency department encounter, and evaluation and treatment by a new physician. **The appropriate 7th character for initial**

encounter should also be assigned for a patient who delayed seeking treatment for the fracture or nonunion.

Fractures are coded using the appropriate 7th character extension for subsequent care for encounters after the patient has completed active treatment of the fracture and is receiving routine care for the fracture during the healing or recovery phase. Examples of fracture aftercare are: cast change or removal, removal of external or internal fixation device, medication adjustment, and follow-up visits following fracture treatment.

Care for complications of surgical treatment for fracture repairs during the healing or recovery phase should be coded with the appropriate complication codes.

Care of complications of fractures, such as malunion and nonunion, should be reported with the appropriate 7th character extensions for subsequent care with nonunion (K, M, N,) or subsequent care with malunion (P, Q, R).

A code from category M80, not a traumatic fracture code, should be used for any patient with known osteoporosis who suffers a fracture, even if the patient had a minor fall or trauma, if that fall or trauma would not usually break a normal, healthy bone.

See Section I.C.13. Osteoporosis.

The aftercare Z codes should not be used for aftercare for **traumatic fractures**. For aftercare of a **traumatic fracture**, assign the acute **fracture** code with the **appropriate** 7th character.

2) **Multiple fractures sequencing**
Multiple fractures are sequenced in accordance with the severity of the fracture.

d. **Coding of Burns and Corrosions**
The ICD-10-CM **makes a distinction** between burns and corrosions. The burn codes are for thermal burns, except sunburns, that come from a heat source, such as a fire or hot appliance. The burn codes are also for burns resulting from electricity and radiation. Corrosions are burns due to chemicals. The guidelines are the same for burns and corrosions.

Current burns (T20-T25) are classified by depth, extent and by agent (X code). Burns are classified by depth as first degree (erythema), second degree (blistering), and third degree (full-thickness involvement). Burns of the eye and internal organs (T26-T28) are classified by site, but not by degree.

1) **Sequencing of burn and related condition codes**
Sequence first the code that reflects the highest degree of burn when more than one burn is present.

a. When the reason for the admission or encounter is for treatment of external multiple burns, sequence first the code that reflects the burn of the highest degree.

b. When a patient has both internal and external burns, the circumstances of admission govern the selection of the principal diagnosis or first-listed diagnosis.

c. When a patient is admitted for burn injuries and other related conditions such as smoke inhalation and/or respiratory failure, the circumstances of admission govern the selection of the principal or first-listed diagnosis.

2) **Burns of the same local site**
Classify burns of the same local site (three-**character** category level, T20-T28) but of different degrees to the subcategory identifying the highest degree recorded in the diagnosis.

3) **Non-healing burns**
Non-healing burns are coded as acute burns.

Necrosis of burned skin should be coded as a non-healed burn.

4) **Infected Burn**
For any documented infected burn site, use an additional code for the infection.

5) **Assign separate codes for each burn site**
When coding burns, assign separate codes for each burn site. Category T30, Burn and corrosion, body region unspecified is extremely vague and should rarely be used.

6) **Burns and Corrosions Classified According to Extent of Body Surface Involved**
Assign codes from category T31, Burns classified according to extent of body surface involved, or T32, Corrosions classified according to extent of body surface involved, when the site of the burn is not specified or when there is a need for additional data. It is advisable to use category T31 as additional coding when needed to provide data for evaluating burn mortality, such as that needed by burn units. It is also advisable to use category T31 as an additional code for reporting purposes when there is mention of a third-degree burn involving 20 percent or more of the body surface.

Categories T31 and T32 are based on the classic "rule of nines" in estimating body surface involved: head and neck are assigned nine percent, each arm nine percent, each leg 18 percent, the anterior trunk 18 percent, posterior trunk 18 percent, and genitalia one percent. Providers may change these percentage assignments where necessary to accommodate infants and children who have proportionately larger heads than adults, and patients who have large buttocks, thighs, or abdomen that involve burns.

7) **Encounters for treatment of late effects of burns**
Encounters for the treatment of the late effects of burns or corrosions (i.e., scars or joint contractures) should be coded with a burn or corrosion code with the 7th character "S" **for** sequela.

8) **Sequelae with a late effect code and current burn**
When appropriate, both a code for a current burn or corrosion with 7th character extension "A" or "D" and a burn or corrosion code with extension "S" may be assigned on the same record (when both a current burn and sequelae of an old burn exist). Burns and corrosions do not heal at the same rate and a current healing wound may still exist with sequela of a healed burn or corrosion.

9) **Use of an external cause code with burns and corrosions**
An external cause code should be used with burns and corrosions to identify the source and intent of the burn, as well as the place where it occurred.

e. **Adverse Effects, Poisoning , Underdosing and Toxic Effects**
Codes in categories T36-T65 are combination codes that include the substances related to adverse effects, poisonings, toxic effects and underdosing, as well as the external cause. No additional external cause code is required for poisonings, toxic effects, adverse effects and underdosing codes.

A code from categories T36-T65 is sequenced first, followed by the code(s) that specify the nature of the adverse effect, poisoning, or toxic effect. Note: This sequencing instruction does not apply to underdosing codes (fifth or sixth character "6", for example T36.0x6-).

1) **Do not code directly from the Table of Drugs**
Do not code directly from the Table of Drugs and Chemicals. Always refer back to the Tabular List.

2) **Use as many codes as necessary to describe**
Use as many codes as necessary to describe completely all drugs, medicinal or biological substances.

3) **If the same code would describe the causative agent**
If the same code would describe the causative agent for more than one adverse reaction, poisoning, toxic effect or underdosing, assign the code only once.

4) **If two or more drugs, medicinal or biological substances**
If two or more drugs, medicinal or biological substances are reported, code each individually unless **a** combination code is listed in the Table of Drugs and Chemicals.

5) **The occurrence of drug toxicity is classified in ICD-10-CM as follows:**

(a) **Adverse Effect**

Assign the appropriate code for adverse effect (for example, T36.0x5-) when the drug was correctly prescribed and properly administered. Use additional code(s) for all manifestations of adverse effects. Examples of manifestations are tachycardia, delirium, gastrointestinal hemorrhaging, vomiting, hypokalemia, hepatitis, renal failure, or respiratory failure.

(b) **Poisoning**

When coding a poisoning or reaction to the improper use of a medication (e.g., overdose, wrong substance given or taken in error, wrong route of administration), assign the appropriate code from categories T36-T50. Poisoning codes have an associated intent: accidental, intentional self-harm, assault and undetermined. Use additional code(s) for all manifestations of poisonings.

If there is also a diagnosis of abuse or dependence on the substance, the abuse or dependence is coded as an additional code.

Examples of poisoning include:

(i) Error was made in drug prescription

Errors made in drug prescription or in the administration of the drug by provider, nurse, patient, or other person.

(ii) Overdose of a drug intentionally taken

If an overdose of a drug was intentionally taken or administered and resulted in drug toxicity, it would be coded as a poisoning.

(iii) Nonprescribed drug taken with correctly prescribed and properly administered drug

If a nonprescribed drug or medicinal agent was taken in combination with a correctly prescribed and properly administered drug, any drug toxicity or other reaction resulting from the interaction of the two drugs would be classified as a poisoning.

(iv) Interaction of drug(s) and alcohol

When a reaction results from the interaction of a drug(s) and alcohol, this would be classified as poisoning.

See Section I.C.4. if poisoning is the result of insulin pump malfunctions.

(c) **Underdosing**

Underdosing refers to taking less of a medication than is prescribed by a provider or a manufacturer's instruction. For underdosing, assign the code from categories T36-T50 (fifth or sixth character "6").

Codes for underdosing should never be assigned as principal or first-listed codes. If a patient has a relapse or exacerbation of the medical condition for which the drug is prescribed because of the reduction in dose, then the medical condition itself should be coded.

Noncompliance (Z91.12-, Z91.13-) or complication of care (Y63.61, Y63.8-Y63.9) codes are to be used with an underdosing code to indicate intent, if known.

(d) **Toxic Effects**

When a harmful substance is ingested or comes in contact with a person, this is classified as a toxic effect. The toxic effect codes are in categories T51-T65.

Toxic effect codes have an associated intent: accidental, intentional self-harm, assault and undetermined.

f. **Adult and child abuse, neglect and other maltreatment**

Sequence first the appropriate code from categories T74.- **(Adult and child abuse, neglect and other maltreatment, confirmed)** or T76.- **(Adult and child abuse, neglect and other maltreatment, suspected)** for abuse, neglect and other maltreatment, followed by any accompanying mental health or injury code(s).

If the documentation in the medical record states abuse or neglect it is coded as confirmed **(T74.-).** It is coded as suspected if it is documented as suspected **(T76.-).**

For cases of confirmed abuse or neglect an external cause code from the assault section (X92-Y08) should be added to identify the cause of any physical injuries. A perpetrator code (Y07) should be added when the perpetrator of the abuse is known. For suspected cases of abuse or neglect, do not report external cause or perpetrator code.

If a suspected case of abuse, neglect or mistreatment is ruled out during an encounter code Z04.71, Suspected adult physical and sexual abuse, ruled out, or code Z04.72, Suspected child physical and sexual abuse, ruled out, should be used, not a code from T76.

See Section I.C.15.r Abuse in a pregnant patient.

g. **Complications of care**

1) **Complications of care**

(a) **Documentation of complications of care**

As with all procedural or postprocedural complications, code assignment is based on the provider's documentation of the relationship between the condition and the procedure.

2) **Pain due to medical devices**

Pain associated with devices, implants or grafts left in a surgical site (for example painful hip prosthesis) is assigned to the appropriate code(s) found in Chapter 19, Injury, poisoning, and certain other consequences of external causes. Specific codes for pain due to medical devices are found in the T code section of the ICD-10-CM. Use additional code(s) from category G89 to identify acute or chronic pain due to presence of the device, implant or graft (G89.18 or G89.28).

3) **Transplant complications**

(a) **Transplant complications other than kidney**

Codes under category T86, Complications of transplanted organs and tissues, are for use for both complications and rejection of transplanted organs. A transplant complication code is only assigned if the complication affects the function of the transplanted organ. Two codes are required to fully describe a transplant complication: the appropriate code from category T86 and a secondary code that identifies the complication.

Pre-existing conditions or conditions that develop after the transplant are not coded as complications unless they affect the function of the transplanted organs.

See I.C.21.c.3 for transplant organ removal status

See I.C.2.r for malignant neoplasm associated with transplanted organ.

(b) **Chronic kidney disease and kidney transplant complications**

Patients who have undergone kidney transplant may still have some form of chronic kidney disease (CKD) because the kidney transplant may not fully restore kidney function. Code T86.1- should be assigned for documented complications of a kidney transplant, such as transplant failure or rejection or other transplant complication. Code T86.1- should not be assigned for post kidney transplant patients who have chronic kidney (CKD) unless a transplant complication such as transplant failure or rejection is documented. If the documentation is unclear as to whether the patient has a complication of the transplant, query the provider.

For patients with CKD following a kidney transplant, but who do not have a complication such as failure or rejection, *see section I.C.14. Chronic kidney disease and kidney transplant status.*

4) Complication codes that include the external cause
As with certain other T codes, some of the complications of care codes have the external cause included in the code. The code includes the nature of the complication as well as the type of procedure that caused the complication. No external cause code indicating the type of procedure is necessary for these codes.

5) Complications of care codes within the body system chapters
Intraoperative and postprocedural complication codes are found within the body system chapters with codes specific to the organs and structures of that body system. These codes should be sequenced first, followed by a code(s) for the specific complication, if applicable.

20. Chapter 20: External Causes of Morbidity (V01-Y99)
Introduction: These guidelines are provided for the reporting of external causes of morbidity codes in order that there will be standardization in the process. These codes are secondary codes for use in any health care setting.

External cause codes are intended to provide data for injury research and evaluation of injury prevention strategies. These codes capture how the injury or health condition happened (cause), the intent (unintentional or accidental; or intentional, such as suicide or assault), the place where the event occurred the activity of the patient at the time of the event, and the person's status (e.g., civilian, military).

a. General External Cause Coding Guidelines

1) Used with any code in the range of A00.0-T88.9, Z00-Z99
An external cause code may be used with any code in the range of A00.0-T88.9, Z00-Z99, classification that is a health condition due to an external cause. Though they are most applicable to injuries, they are also valid for use with such

things as infections or diseases due to an external source, and other health conditions, such as a heart attack that occurs during strenuous physical activity.

2) External cause code used for length of treatment
Assign the external cause code, with the appropriate 7th character (initial encounter, subsequent encounter or sequela) for each encounter for which the injury or condition is being treated.

3) Use the full range of external cause codes
Use the full range of external cause codes to completely describe the cause, the intent, the place of occurrence, and if applicable, the activity of the patient at the time of the event, and the patient's status, for all injuries, and other health conditions due to an external cause.

4) Assign as many external cause codes as necessary
Assign as many external cause codes as necessary to fully explain each cause. If only one external code can be recorded, assign the code most related to the principal diagnosis.

5) The selection of the appropriate external cause code
The selection of the appropriate external cause code is guided by the **Alphabetic Index** of External Causes and by Inclusion and Exclusion notes in the Tabular List.

6) External cause code can never be a principal diagnosis
An external cause code can never be a principal **(first-listed)** diagnosis.

7) Combination external cause codes
Certain of the external cause codes are combination codes that identify sequential events that result in an injury, such as a fall which results in striking against an object. The injury may be due to either event or both. The combination external cause code used should correspond to the sequence of events regardless of which caused the most serious injury.

8) No external cause code needed in certain circumstances
No external cause code from Chapter 20 is needed if the external cause and intent are included in a code from another chapter (e.g. **T36.0x1-** Poisoning by penicillins, accidental (unintentional)).

b. Place of Occurrence Guideline
Codes from category Y92, Place of occurrence of the external cause, are secondary codes for use after other external cause codes to identify the location of the patient at the time of injury or other condition.

A place of occurrence code is used only once, at the initial encounter for treatment. No 7th characters are used for Y92. Only one code from Y92 should be recorded on a medical record. A place of occurrence code should be used in conjunction with an activity code, Y93.

Do not use place of occurrence code Y92.9 if the place is not stated or is not applicable.

c. Activity Code
Assign a code from category Y93, Activity code, to describe the activity of the patient at the time the injury or other health condition occurred.

An activity code is used only once, at the initial encounter for treatment. Only one code from Y93 should be recorded on a medical record. An activity code should be used in conjunction with a place of occurrence code, Y92.

The activity codes are not applicable to poisonings, adverse effects, misadventures or late effects.

Do not assign Y93.9, Unspecified activity, if the activity is not stated.

A code from category Y93 is appropriate for use with external cause and intent codes if identifying the activity provides additional information about the event.

d. Place of Occurrence, Activity, *and Status* Codes Used with other External Cause Code
When applicable, place of occurrence, activity, and external cause status codes are sequenced after the main external cause code(s). Regardless of the number of external cause codes assigned, there should be only one place of occurrence code, one activity code, and one external cause status code assigned to an encounter.

e. If the Reporting Format Limits the Number of External Cause Codes
If the reporting format limits the number of external cause codes that can be used in reporting clinical data, report the code for the cause/intent most related to the principal diagnosis. If the format permits capture of additional external cause codes, the cause/intent, including medical misadventures, of the additional events should be reported rather than the codes for place, activity, or external status.

f. Multiple External Cause Coding Guidelines
More than one external cause code is required to fully describe the external cause of an illness **or** injury. The assignment of external cause codes should be sequenced in the following priority:

If two or more events cause separate injuries, an external cause code should be assigned for each cause. The **first-listed** external cause code will be selected in the following order:

External cause codes for child and adult abuse take priority over all other external cause codes.

See Section I.C.19., Child and Adult abuse guidelines.

External cause codes for terrorism events take priority over all other external cause codes except child and adult abuse.

External cause codes for cataclysmic events take priority over all other external cause codes except child and adult abuse and terrorism.

External cause codes for transport accidents take priority over all other external cause codes except cataclysmic events, child and adult abuse and terrorism.

Activity and external cause status codes are assigned following all causal (intent) external cause codes.

The first-listed external cause code should correspond to the cause of the most serious diagnosis due to an assault, accident, or self-harm, following the order of hierarchy listed above.

g. **Child and Adult Abuse Guideline**

Adult and child abuse, neglect and maltreatment are classified as assault. Any of the assault codes may be used to indicate the external cause of any injury resulting from the confirmed abuse.

For confirmed cases of abuse, neglect and maltreatment, when the perpetrator is known, a code from Y07, Perpetrator of maltreatment and neglect, should accompany any other assault codes.

See Section I.C.19. Adult and child abuse, neglect and other maltreatment

h. **Unknown or Undetermined Intent Guideline**

If the intent (accident, self-harm, assault) of the cause of an injury or other condition is unknown or unspecified, code the intent as accidental intent. All transport accident categories assume accidental intent.

1) **Use of undetermined intent**

External cause codes for events of undetermined intent are only for use if the documentation in the record specifies that the intent cannot be **determined**.

i. **Late Effects of External Cause Guidelines**

1) **Late effect external cause codes**

Late effects are reported using the external cause code with the 7th character extension "S" for sequela. These codes should be used with any report of a late effect or sequela resulting from a previous injury.

2) **Late effect external cause code with a related current injury**

A late effect external cause code should never be used with a related current nature of injury code.

3) **Use of late effect external cause codes for subsequent visits**

Use a late effect external cause code for subsequent visits when a late effect of the initial injury is being treated. Do not use a late effect external cause code for subsequent visits for follow-up care (e.g., to assess healing, to receive rehabilitative therapy) of the injury when no late effect of the injury has been documented.

j. **Terrorism Guidelines**

1) **Cause of injury identified by the Federal Government (FBI) as terrorism**

When the cause of an injury is identified by the Federal Government (FBI) as terrorism, the first-listed external cause code should be a code from category Y38, Terrorism. The definition of terrorism employed by the FBI is found at the inclusion note at the beginning of category Y38. Use additional code for place of occurrence (Y92.-). More than one Y38 code may be assigned if the injury is the result of more than one mechanism of terrorism.

2) **Cause of an injury is suspected to be the result of terrorism**

When the cause of an injury is suspected to be the result of terrorism a code from category Y38 should not be assigned. Suspected cases should be classified as assault.

3) **Code Y38.9, Terrorism, secondary effects**

Assign code Y38.9, Terrorism, secondary effects, for conditions occurring subsequent to the terrorist event. This code should not be assigned for conditions that are due to the initial terrorist act.

It is acceptable to assign code Y38.9 with another code from Y38 if there is an injury due to the initial terrorist event and an injury that is a subsequent result of the terrorist event.

k. **External cause status**

A code from category Y99, External cause status, should be assigned whenever any other external cause code is assigned for an encounter, including an Activity code, except for the events noted below. Assign a code from category Y99, External cause status, to indicate the work status of the person at the time the event occurred. The status code indicates whether the event occurred during military activity, whether a non-military person was at work, whether an individual including a student or volunteer was involved in a non-work activity at the time of the causal event.

A code from Y99, External cause status, should be assigned, when applicable, with other external cause codes, such as transport accidents and falls. The external cause status codes are not applicable to poisonings, adverse effects, misadventures or late effects.

Do not assign a code from category Y99 if no other external cause codes (cause, activity) are applicable for the encounter.

An external cause status code is used only once, at the initial encounter for treatment. Only one code from Y99 should be recorded on a medical record.

Do not assign code Y99.9, Unspecified external cause status, if the status is not stated.

21. **Chapter 21: Factors Influencing Health Status and Contact with Health Services (Z00-Z99)**

Note: The chapter specific guidelines provide additional information about the use of Z codes for specified encounters.

a. **Use of Z codes in any healthcare setting**

Z codes are for use in any healthcare setting. Z codes may be used as either a **first-listed** (principal diagnosis code in the inpatient setting) or secondary code, depending on the circumstances of the encounter. Certain Z codes may only be used as **first-listed** or principal diagnosis.

b. **Z Codes indicate a reason for an encounter**

Z codes are not procedure codes. A corresponding procedure code must accompany a Z code to describe **any** procedure performed.

c. **Categories of Z Codes**

1) **Contact/Exposure**

Category Z20 indicates contact with, and suspected exposure to, communicable diseases. These codes are for patients who do not show any sign or symptom of a disease but are suspected to have been exposed to it by close personal contact with an infected individual or are in an area where a disease is epidemic.

Category Z77, indicates contact with and suspected exposures hazardous to health.

Contact/exposure codes may be used as a **first-listed** code to explain an encounter for testing, or, more commonly, as a secondary code to identify a potential risk.

2) **Inoculations and vaccinations**

Code Z23 is for encounters for inoculations and vaccinations. It indicates that a patient is being seen to receive a prophylactic inoculation against a disease. Procedure codes are required to identify the actual administration of the injection and the type(s) of immunizations given. Code Z23 may be used as a secondary code if the inoculation is given as a routine part of preventive health care, such as a well-baby visit.

3) **Status**

Status codes indicate that a patient is either a carrier of a disease or has the sequelae or residual of a past disease or condition. This includes such things as the presence of prosthetic or mechanical devices resulting from past treatment. A status code is informative, because the status may affect the course of treatment and its outcome. A status code is distinct from a history code. The history code indicates that the patient no longer has the condition.

A status code should not be used with a diagnosis code from one of the body system chapters, if the diagnosis code includes the information provided by the status code. For example, code Z94.1, Heart transplant status, should not be used with a code from subcategory T86.2, Complications of heart transplant. The status code does not provide additional information. The complication code indicates that the patient is a heart transplant patient.

For encounters for weaning from a mechanical ventilator, assign **a** code **from subcategory** J96.1, Chronic respiratory failure, followed by code Z99.11, Dependence on respirator [ventilator] status.

The status Z codes/categories are:

Z14   Genetic carrier

Genetic carrier status indicates that a person carries a gene, associated with a particular disease, which may be passed to offspring who may develop that disease. The person does not have the disease and is not at risk of developing the disease.

Z15   Genetic susceptibility to disease

Genetic susceptibility indicates that a person has a gene that increases the risk of that person developing the disease.

Codes from category Z15 should not be used as principal or first-listed codes. If the patient has the condition to which he/she is susceptible, and that condition is the reason for the encounter, the code for the current condition should be sequenced first. If the patient is being seen for follow-up after completed treatment for this condition, and the condition no longer exists, a follow-up code should be sequenced first, followed by the appropriate personal history and genetic susceptibility codes. If the purpose of the encounter is genetic counseling associated with procreative management, code Z31.5, Encounter for genetic counseling, should be assigned as the first-listed code, followed by a code from category Z15. Additional codes should be assigned for any applicable family or personal history.

Z16   Infection with drug-resistant microorganisms

This code indicates that a patient has an infection that is resistant to drug treatment. Sequence the infection code first.

Z17   Estrogen receptor status

Z18   Retained foreign body fragments

Z21   Asymptomatic HIV infection status

This code indicates that a patient has tested positive for HIV but has manifested no signs or symptoms of the disease.

Z22   Carrier of infectious disease

Carrier status indicates that a person harbors the specific organisms of a disease without manifest symptoms and is capable of transmitting the infection.

Z28.3   Underimmunization status

Z33.1   Pregnant state, incidental

This code is a secondary code only for use when the pregnancy is in no way complicating the reason for visit. Otherwise, a code from the obstetric chapter is required.

Z66   Do not resuscitate

This code may be used when it is documented by the provider that a patient is on do not resuscitate status at any time during the stay.

Z67   Blood type

Z68   Body mass index (BMI)

Z74.01 Bed confinement status

Z76.82 Awaiting organ transplant status

Z78   Other specified health status

Code Z78.1, Physical restraint status, may be used when it is documented by the provider that a patient has been put in restraints during the current encounter. Please note that this code should not be reported when it is documented by the provider that a patient is temporarily restrained during a procedure.

Z79   Long-term (current) drug therapy

Codes from this category indicate a patient's continuous use of a prescribed drug (including such things as aspirin therapy) for the long-term treatment of a condition or for prophylactic use. It is not for use for patients who have addictions to drugs. This subcategory is not for use of medications for detoxification or maintenance programs to prevent withdrawal symptoms in patients with drug dependence (e.g., methadone maintenance for opiate dependence). Assign the appropriate code for the drug dependence instead.

Assign a code from Z79 if the patient is receiving a medication for an extended period as a prophylactic measure (such as for the prevention of deep vein thrombosis) or as treatment of a chronic condition (such as arthritis) or a disease requiring a lengthy course of treatment (such as cancer). Do not assign a code from category Z79 for medication being administered for a brief period of time to treat an acute illness or injury (such as a course of antibiotics to treat acute bronchitis).

Z88   Allergy status to drugs, medicaments and biological substances

Except: Z88.9, Allergy status to unspecified drugs, medicaments and biological substances status

Z89   Acquired absence of limb

Z90   Acquired absence of organs, not elsewhere classified

Z91.0- Allergy status, other than to drugs and biological substances

Z92.82 Status post administration of tPA (rtPA) in a different facility within the last 24 hours prior to admission to a current facility

Assign code Z92.82, Status post administration of tPA (rtPA) in a different facility within the last 24 hours prior to admission to current facility, as a secondary diagnosis when a patient is received by transfer into a facility and documentation indicates they were administered tissue plasminogen activator (tPA) within the last 24 hours prior to admission to the current facility.

This guideline applies even if the patient is still receiving the tPA at the time they are received into the current facility.

The appropriate code for the condition for which the tPA was administered (such as cerebrovascular disease or myocardial infarction) should be assigned first.

Code Z92.82 is only applicable to the receiving facility record and not to the transferring facility record.

Z93   Artificial opening status

Z94   Transplanted organ and tissue status

Z95   Presence of cardiac and vascular implants and grafts

Z96   Presence of other functional implants

Z97   Presence of other devices

Z98   Other postprocedural states

Assign code Z98.85, Transplanted organ removal status, to indicate that a transplanted organ has been previously removed. This code should not be assigned for the encounter in which the transplanted organ is removed. The complication necessitating removal of the transplant organ should be assigned for that encounter.

See section I.C19.g.3. for information on the coding of organ transplant complications.

Z99   Dependence on enabling machines and devices, not elsewhere classified

Note: Categories Z89-Z90 and Z93-Z99 are for use only if there are no complications or malfunctions of the organ or tissue replaced, the amputation site or the equipment on which the patient is dependent.

4)   **History (of)**

There are two types of history Z codes, personal and family. Personal history codes explain a patient's past medical condition that no longer exists and is not receiving any treatment, but that has the potential for recurrence, and therefore may require continued monitoring.

Family history codes are for use when a patient has a family member(s) who has had a particular disease that causes the patient to be at higher risk of also contracting the disease.

Personal history codes may be used in conjunction with follow-up codes and family history codes may be used in conjunction with screening codes to explain the need for a test or procedure. History codes are also acceptable on any medical record regardless of the reason for visit. A history of an illness, even if no longer present, is important information that may alter the type of treatment ordered.

The history Z code categories are:

Z80	Family history of primary malignant neoplasm
Z81	Family history of mental and behavioral disorders
Z82	Family history of certain disabilities and chronic diseases (leading to disablement)
Z83	Family history of other specific disorders
Z84	Family history of other conditions
Z85	Personal history of malignant neoplasm
Z86	Personal history of certain other diseases
Z87	Personal history of other diseases and conditions
Z91.4-	Personal history of psychological trauma, not elsewhere classified
Z91.5	Personal history of self-harm
Z91.8-	Other specified personal risk factors, not elsewhere classified
Z92	Personal history of medical treatment

         Except: Z92.0, Personal history of contraception

         Except: Z92.82, Status post administration of tPA (rtPA) in a different facility within the last 24 hours prior to admission to a current facility

5)   **Screening**

Screening is the testing for disease or disease precursors in seemingly well individuals so that early detection and treatment can be provided for those who test positive for the disease (e.g., screening mammogram).

The testing of a person to rule out or confirm a suspected diagnosis because the patient has some sign or symptom is a diagnostic examination, not a screening. In these cases, the sign or symptom is used to explain the reason for the test.

A screening code may be a **first-listed** code if the reason for the visit is specifically the screening exam. It may also be used as an additional code if the screening is done during an office visit for other health problems. A screening code is not necessary if the screening is inherent to a routine examination, such as a pap smear done during a routine pelvic examination.

Should a condition be discovered during the screening then the code for the condition may be assigned as an additional diagnosis.

The Z code indicates that a screening exam is planned. A procedure code is required to confirm that the screening was performed.

The screening Z codes/categories:

Z11	Encounter for screening for infectious and parasitic diseases
Z12	Encounter for screening for malignant neoplasms
Z13	Encounter for screening for other diseases and disorders

         Except: Z13.9, Encounter for screening, unspecified

Z36	Encounter for antenatal screening for mother

6)   **Observation**

There are two observation Z code categories. They are for use in very limited circumstances when a person is being observed for a suspected condition that is ruled out. The observation codes are not for use if an injury or illness or any signs or symptoms related to the suspected condition are present. In such cases the diagnosis/symptom code is used with the corresponding external cause code.

The observation codes are to be used as principal diagnosis only. Additional codes may be used in addition to the observation code but only if they are unrelated to the suspected condition being observed.

Codes from subcategory Z03.7, Encounter for suspected maternal and fetal conditions ruled out, may either be used as a **first-listed** or as an additional code assignment depending on the case. They are for use in very limited circumstances on a maternal record when an encounter is for a suspected maternal or fetal condition that is ruled out during that encounter (for example, a maternal or fetal condition may be suspected due to an abnormal test result). These codes should not be used when the condition is confirmed. In those cases, the confirmed condition should be coded. In addition, these codes are not for use if an illness or any signs or symptoms related to the suspected condition or problem are present. In such cases the diagnosis/symptom code is used.

Additional codes may be used in addition to the code from subcategory Z03.7, but only if they are unrelated to the suspected condition being evaluated.

Codes from subcategory Z03.7 may not be used for encounters for antenatal screening of mother. *See Section I.C.21.c.5, Screening.*

For encounters for suspected fetal condition that are inconclusive following testing and evaluation, assign the appropriate code from category O35, O36, O40 or O41.

The observation Z code categories:

Z03	Encounter for medical observation for suspected diseases and conditions ruled out
Z04	Encounter for examination and observation for other reasons

         Except: Z04.9, Encounter for examination and observation for unspecified reason

7)   **Aftercare**

Aftercare visit codes cover situations when the initial treatment of a disease has been performed and the patient requires continued care during the healing or recovery phase, or for the long-term consequences of the disease. The aftercare Z code should not be used if treatment is directed at a current, acute disease. The diagnosis code is to be used in these cases. Exceptions to this rule are codes Z51.0, Encounter for antineoplastic radiation therapy, and codes from subcategory Z51.1, Encounter for antineoplastic chemotherapy and immunotherapy. These codes are to be **first-listed**, followed by the diagnosis code when a patient's encounter is solely to receive radiation therapy, chemotherapy, or immunotherapy for the treatment of a neoplasm. If the reason for the encounter is more than one type of antineoplastic therapy, code Z51.0 and a code from subcategory Z51.1 may be assigned together, in which case one of these codes would be reported as a secondary diagnosis.

The aftercare Z codes should also not be used for aftercare for injuries. For aftercare of an injury, assign the acute injury code with the **appropriate** 7th character (**for** subsequent encounter).

The aftercare codes are generally **first-listed** to explain the specific reason for the encounter. An aftercare code may be used as an additional code when some type of aftercare is provided in addition to the reason for admission and no diagnosis code is applicable. An example of this would be the closure of a colostomy during an encounter for treatment of another condition.

Aftercare codes should be used in conjunction with other aftercare codes or diagnosis codes to provide better detail on the specifics of an aftercare encounter visit, unless otherwise directed by the classification. Should a patient receive multiple types of antineoplastic therapy during the same encounter, code Z51.0, Encounter for antineoplastic radiation therapy, and codes from subcategory Z51.1, Encounter for antineoplastic chemotherapy and immunotherapy, may be used together on a record. The sequencing of multiple aftercare codes depends on the circumstances of the encounter.

Certain aftercare Z code categories need a secondary diagnosis code to describe the resolving condition or sequelae. For others, the condition is included in the code title.

Additional Z code aftercare category terms include fitting and adjustment, and attention to artificial openings.

Status Z codes may be used with aftercare Z codes to indicate the nature of the aftercare. For example code Z95.1, Presence of aortocoronary bypass graft, may be used with code Z48.812, Encounter for surgical aftercare following surgery on the circulatory system, to indicate the surgery for which the aftercare is being performed. A status code should not be used when the aftercare code indicates the type of status, such as using Z43.0, Encounter for attention to tracheostomy, with Z93.0, Tracheostomy status.

The aftercare Z category/codes:

Z42 Encounter for plastic and reconstructive surgery following medical procedure or healed injury
Z43 Encounter for attention to artificial openings
Z44 Encounter for fitting and adjustment of external prosthetic device
Z45 Encounter for adjustment and management of implanted device
Z46 Encounter for fitting and adjustment of other devices
Z47 Orthopedic aftercare
Z48 Encounter for other postprocedural aftercare
Z49 Encounter for care involving renal dialysis
Z51 Encounter for other aftercare

8) **Follow-up**
The follow-up codes are used to explain continuing surveillance following completed treatment of a disease, condition, or injury. They imply that the condition has been fully treated and no longer exists. They should not be confused with aftercare codes, or injury codes with **a** 7th character **for subsequent encounter**, that explain ongoing care of a healing condition or its sequelae. Follow-up codes may be used in conjunction with history codes to provide the full picture of the healed condition and its treatment. The follow-up code is sequenced first, followed by the history code.

A follow-up code may be used to explain multiple visits. Should a condition be found to have recurred on the follow-up visit, then the **diagnosis** code for the condition should be assigned **in place of the follow-up code**.

The follow-up Z code categories:

Z08 Encounter for follow-up examination after completed treatment for malignant neoplasm
Z09 Encounter for follow-up examination after completed treatment for conditions other than malignant neoplasm
Z39 Encounter for maternal postpartum care and examination

9) **Donor**
Codes in category Z52, Donors of organs and tissues, are used for living individuals who are donating blood or other body tissue. These codes are only for individuals donating for others, not for self-donations. They are not used to identify cadaveric donations.

10) **Counseling**
Counseling Z codes are used when a patient or family member receives assistance in the aftermath of an illness or injury, or when support is required in coping with family or social problems. They are not used in conjunction with a diagnosis code when the counseling component of care is considered integral to standard treatment.

The counseling Z codes/categories:

Z30.0- Encounter for general counseling and advice on contraception
Z31.5 Encounter for genetic counseling
Z31.6- Encounter for general counseling and advice on procreation
Z32.2 Encounter for childbirth instruction
Z32.3 Encounter for childcare instruction
Z69 Encounter for mental health services for victim and perpetrator of abuse
Z70 Counseling related to sexual attitude, behavior and orientation
Z71 Persons encountering health services for other counseling and medical advice, not elsewhere classified
Z76.81 Expectant mother prebirth pediatrician visit

11) **Encounters for Obstetrical and Reproductive Services**
See Section I.C.15. *Pregnancy, Childbirth, and the Puerperium, for further instruction on the use of these codes.*

Z codes for pregnancy are for use in those circumstances when none of the problems or complications included in the codes from the Obstetrics chapter exist (a routine prenatal visit or postpartum care). Codes in category Z34, Encounter for supervision of normal pregnancy, are always **first-listed** and are not to be used with any other code from the OB chapter.

The outcome of delivery, category Z37, should be included on all maternal delivery records. It is always a secondary code. Codes in category Z37 should not be used on the newborn record.

Z codes for family planning (contraceptive) or procreative management and counseling should be included on an obstetric record either during the pregnancy or the postpartum stage, if applicable.

Z codes/categories for obstetrical and reproductive services:

Z30 Encounter for contraceptive management
Z31 Encounter for procreative management
Z32.2 Encounter for childbirth instruction
Z32.3 Encounter for childcare instruction
Z33 Pregnant state
Z34 Encounter for supervision of normal pregnancy
Z36 Encounter for antenatal screening of mother
Z37 Outcome of delivery
Z39 Encounter for maternal postpartum care and examination
Z76.81 Expectant mother prebirth pediatrician visit

12) **Newborns and Infants**
See Section I.C.16. *Newborn (Perinatal) Guidelines, for further instruction on the use of these codes.*

Newborn Z codes/categories:

Z76.1 Encounter for health supervision and care of foundling
Z00.1- Encounter for routine child health examination
Z38 Liveborn infants according to place of birth and type of delivery

13) **Routine and administrative examinations**

The Z codes allow for the description of encounters for routine examinations, such as, a general check-up, or, examinations for administrative purposes, such as, a pre-employment physical. The codes are not to be used if the examination is for diagnosis of a suspected condition or for treatment purposes. In such cases the diagnosis code is used. During a routine exam, should a diagnosis or condition be discovered, it should be coded as an additional code. Pre-existing and chronic conditions and history codes may also be included as additional codes as long as the examination is for administrative purposes and not focused on any particular condition.

Some of the codes for routine health examinations distinguish between "with" and "without" abnormal findings. Code assignment depends on the information that is known at the time the encounter is being coded. For example, if no abnormal findings were found during the examination, but the encounter is being coded before test results are back, it is acceptable to assign the code for "without abnormal findings." When assigning a code for "with abnormal findings," additional code(s) should be assigned to identify the specific abnormal finding(s).

Pre-operative examination and pre-procedural laboratory examination Z codes are for use only in those situations when a patient is being cleared for a procedure or surgery and no treatment is given.

The Z codes/categories for routine and administrative examinations:

Z00   Encounter for general examination without complaint, suspected or reported diagnosis

Z01   Encounter for other special examination without complaint, suspected or reported diagnosis

Z02   Encounter for administrative examination
       Except: Z02.9, Encounter for administrative examinations, unspecified

Z32.0- Encounter for pregnancy test

14) **Miscellaneous Z codes**

The miscellaneous Z codes capture a number of other health care encounters that do not fall into one of the other categories. Certain of these codes identify the reason for the encounter; others are for use as additional codes that provide useful information on circumstances that may affect a patient's care and treatment.

Prophylactic Organ Removal

For encounters specifically for prophylactic removal of an organ (such as prophylactic removal of breasts due to a genetic susceptibility to cancer or a family history of cancer), the principal or **first-listed** code should be a code from category Z40, Encounter for prophylactic surgery, followed by the appropriate codes to identify the associated risk factor (such as genetic susceptibility or family history).

If the patient has a malignancy of one site and is having prophylactic removal at another site to prevent either a new primary malignancy or metastatic disease, a code for the malignancy should also be assigned in addition to a code from subcategory Z40.0, Encounter for prophylactic surgery for risk factors related to malignant neoplasms. A Z40.0 code should not be assigned if the patient is having organ removal for treatment of a malignancy, such as the removal of the testes for the treatment of prostate cancer.

Miscellaneous Z codes/categories:

Z28   Immunization not carried out
       Except: Z28.3, Underimmunization status

Z40   Encounter for prophylactic surgery

Z41   Encounter for procedures for purposes other than remedying health state
       Except: Z41.9, Encounter for procedure for purposes other than remedying health state, unspecified

Z53   Persons encountering health services for specific procedures and treatment, not carried out

Z55   Problems related to education and literacy

Z56   Problems related to employment and unemployment

Z57   Occupational exposure to risk factors

Z58   Problems related to physical environment

Z59   Problems related to housing and economic circumstances

Z60   Problems related to social environment

Z62   Problems related to upbringing

Z63   Other problems related to primary support group, including family circumstances

Z64   Problems related to certain psychosocial circumstances

Z65   Problems related to other psychosocial circumstances

Z72   Problems related to lifestyle

Z73   Problems related to life management difficulty

Z74   Problems related to care provider dependency
       Except: Z74.01, Bed confinement status

Z75   Problems related to medical facilities and other health care

Z76.0 Encounter for issue of repeat prescription

Z76.3 Healthy person accompanying sick person

Z76.4 Other boarder to healthcare facility

Z76.5 Malingerer [conscious simulation]

Z91.1- Patient's noncompliance with medical treatment and regimen

Z91.89 Other specified personal risk factors, not elsewhere classified

15) **Nonspecific Z codes**

Certain Z codes are so non-specific, or potentially redundant with other codes in the classification, that there can be little justification for their use in the inpatient setting. Their use in the outpatient setting should be limited to those instances when there is no further documentation to permit more precise coding. Otherwise, any sign or symptom or any other reason for visit that is captured in another code should be used.

Nonspecific Z codes/categories:

Z02.9 Encounter for administrative examinations, unspecified

Z04.9 Encounter for examination and observation for unspecified reason

Z13.9 Encounter for screening, unspecified

Z41.9 Encounter for procedure for purposes other than remedying health state, unspecified

Z52.9 Donor of unspecified organ or tissue

Z86.59 Personal history of other mental and behavioral disorders

Z88.9 Allergy status to unspecified drugs, medicaments and biological substances status

Z92.0 Personal history of contraception

16) **Z Codes That May Only be Principal/First-Listed Diagnosis**

The following Z codes/categories may only be reported as the principal/first-listed diagnosis, except when there are multiple encounters on the same day and the medical records for the encounters are combined:

Z00   Encounter for general examination without complaint, suspected or reported diagnosis

Z01   Encounter for other special examination without complaint, suspected or reported diagnosis

Z02   Encounter for administrative examination

Z03   Encounter for medical observation for suspected diseases and conditions ruled out

Z04   Encounter for examination and observation for other reasons

Z31.81 Encounter for male factor infertility in female patient

Z31.82   Encounter for Rh incompatibility status

Z31.83   Encounter for assisted reproductive fertility procedure cycle

Z31.84   Encounter for fertility preservation procedure

Z33.2   Encounter for elective termination of pregnancy

Z34   Encounter for supervision of normal pregnancy

Z39   Encounter for maternal postpartum care and examination

Z38   Liveborn infants according to place of birth and type of delivery

Z42   Encounter for plastic and reconstructive surgery following medical procedure or healed injury

Z51.Ø   Encounter for antineoplastic radiation therapy

Z51.1-   Encounter for antineoplastic chemotherapy and immunotherapy

Z52   Donors of organs and tissues
         Except: Z52.9, Donor of unspecified organ or tissue

Z76.1   Encounter for health supervision and care of foundling

Z76.2   Encounter for health supervision and care of other healthy infant and child

Z99.12   Encounter for respirator [ventilator] dependence during power failure

Section II. Selection of Principal Diagnosis

The circumstances of inpatient admission always govern the selection of principal diagnosis. The principal diagnosis is defined in the Uniform Hospital Discharge Data Set (UHDDS) as "that condition established after study to be chiefly responsible for occasioning the admission of the patient to the hospital for care."

The UHDDS definitions are used by hospitals to report inpatient data elements in a standardized manner. These data elements and their definitions can be found in the July 31, 1985, Federal Register (Vol. 5Ø, No, 147), pp. 31Ø38-4Ø.

Since that time the application of the UHDDS definitions has been expanded to include all non-outpatient settings (acute care, short term, long term care and psychiatric hospitals; home health agencies; rehab facilities; nursing homes, etc).

In determining principal diagnosis the coding conventions in the ICD-1Ø-CM, the **Tabular List and Alphabetic Index** take precedence over these official coding guidelines.

(See Section I.A., Conventions for the ICD-1Ø-CM)

The importance of consistent, complete documentation in the medical record cannot be overemphasized. Without such documentation the application of all coding guidelines is a difficult, if not impossible, task.

A. Codes for symptoms, signs, and ill-defined conditions

Codes for symptoms, signs, and ill-defined conditions from Chapter 18 are not to be used as principal diagnosis when a related definitive diagnosis has been established.

B. Two or more interrelated conditions, each potentially meeting the definition for principal diagnosis.

When there are two or more interrelated conditions (such as diseases in the same ICD-1Ø-CM chapter or manifestations characteristically associated with a certain disease) potentially meeting the definition of principal diagnosis, either condition may be sequenced first, unless the circumstances of the admission, the therapy provided, the Tabular List, or the Alphabetic Index indicate otherwise.

C. Two or more diagnoses that equally meet the definition for principal diagnosis

In the unusual instance when two or more diagnoses equally meet the criteria for principal diagnosis as determined by the circumstances of admission, diagnostic workup and/or therapy provided, and the Alphabetic Index, Tabular List, or another coding guidelines does not provide sequencing direction, any one of the diagnoses may be sequenced first.

D. Two or more comparative or contrasting conditions.

In those rare instances when two or more contrasting or comparative diagnoses are documented as "either/or" (or similar terminology), they are coded as if the diagnoses were confirmed and the diagnoses are sequenced according to the circumstances of the admission. If no further determination can be made as to which diagnosis should be principal, either diagnosis may be sequenced first.

E. A symptom(s) followed by contrasting/comparative diagnoses

When a symptom(s) is followed by contrasting/comparative diagnoses, the symptom code is sequenced first. All the contrasting/comparative diagnoses should be coded as additional diagnoses.

F. Original treatment plan not carried out

Sequence as the principal diagnosis the condition, which after study occasioned the admission to the hospital, even though treatment may not have been carried out due to unforeseen circumstances.

G. Complications of surgery and other medical care

When the admission is for treatment of a complication resulting from surgery or other medical care, the complication code is sequenced as the principal diagnosis. If the complication is classified to the T8Ø-T88 series and the code lacks the necessary specificity in describing the complication, an additional code for the specific complication should be assigned.

H. Uncertain Diagnosis

If the diagnosis documented at the time of discharge is qualified as "probable", "suspected", "likely", "questionable", "possible", or "still to be ruled out", or other similar terms indicating uncertainty, code the condition as if it existed or was established. The bases for these guidelines are the diagnostic workup, arrangements for further workup or observation, and initial therapeutic approach that correspond most closely with the established diagnosis.

Note: This guideline is applicable only to inpatient admissions to short-term, acute, long-term care and psychiatric hospitals.

I. Admission from Observation Unit

1.   **Admission Following Medical Observation**
     When a patient is admitted to an observation unit for a medical condition, which either worsens or does not improve, and is subsequently admitted as an inpatient of the same hospital for this same medical condition, the principal diagnosis would be the medical condition which led to the hospital admission.

2.   **Admission Following Post-Operative Observation**
     When a patient is admitted to an observation unit to monitor a condition (or complication) that develops following outpatient surgery, and then is subsequently admitted as an inpatient of the same hospital, hospitals should apply the Uniform Hospital Discharge Data Set (UHDDS) definition of principal diagnosis as "that condition established after study to be chiefly responsible for occasioning the admission of the patient to the hospital for care."

J. Admission from Outpatient Surgery

When a patient receives surgery in the hospital's outpatient surgery department and is subsequently admitted for continuing inpatient care at the same hospital, the following guidelines should be followed in selecting the principal diagnosis for the inpatient admission:

- If the reason for the inpatient admission is a complication, assign the complication as the principal diagnosis.
- If no complication, or other condition, is documented as the reason for the inpatient admission, assign the reason for the outpatient surgery as the principal diagnosis.
- If the reason for the inpatient admission is another condition unrelated to the surgery, assign the unrelated condition as the principal diagnosis.

Section III. Reporting Additional Diagnoses

GENERAL RULES FOR OTHER (ADDITIONAL) DIAGNOSES

For reporting purposes the definition for "other diagnoses" is interpreted as additional conditions that affect patient care in terms of requiring:

clinical evaluation; or

therapeutic treatment; or

diagnostic procedures; or

extended length of hospital stay; or

increased nursing care and/or monitoring.

The UHDDS item #11-b defines Other Diagnoses as "all conditions that coexist at the time of admission, that develop subsequently, or that affect the treatment received and/or the length of stay. Diagnoses that relate to an earlier episode which have no bearing on the current hospital stay are to be excluded." UHDDS definitions apply to inpatients in acute care, short-term, long term care and psychiatric hospital setting. The UHDDS definitions are used by acute care short-term hospitals to report inpatient data elements in a standardized manner. These data elements and their definitions can be found in the July 31, 1985, Federal Register (Vol. 50, No, 147), pp. 31038-40.

Since that time the application of the UHDDS definitions has been expanded to include all non-outpatient settings (acute care, short term, long term care and psychiatric hospitals; home health agencies; rehab facilities; nursing homes, etc).

The following guidelines are to be applied in designating "other diagnoses" when neither the Alphabetic Index nor the Tabular List in ICD-10-CM provide direction. The listing of the diagnoses in the patient record is the responsibility of the attending provider.

A. Previous conditions

If the provider has included a diagnosis in the final diagnostic statement, such as the discharge summary or the face sheet, it should ordinarily be coded. Some providers include in the diagnostic statement resolved conditions or diagnoses and status-post procedures from previous admission that have no bearing on the current stay. Such conditions are not to be reported and are coded only if required by hospital policy.

However, history codes (categories Z80-Z87) may be used as secondary codes if the historical condition or family history has an impact on current care or influences treatment.

B. Abnormal findings

Abnormal findings (laboratory, x-ray, pathologic, and other diagnostic results) are not coded and reported unless the provider indicates their clinical significance. If the findings are outside the normal range and the attending provider has ordered other tests to evaluate the condition or prescribed treatment, it is appropriate to ask the provider whether the abnormal finding should be added.

Please note: This differs from the coding practices in the outpatient setting for coding encounters for diagnostic tests that have been interpreted by a provider.

C. Uncertain Diagnosis

If the diagnosis documented at the time of discharge is qualified as "probable", "suspected", "likely", "questionable", "possible", or "still to be ruled out" or other similar terms indicating uncertainty, code the condition as if it existed or was established. The bases for these

guidelines are the diagnostic workup, arrangements for further workup or observation, and initial therapeutic approach that correspond most closely with the established diagnosis.

Note: This guideline is applicable only to inpatient admissions to short-term, acute, long-term care and psychiatric hospitals.

Section IV. Diagnostic Coding and Reporting Guidelines for Outpatient Services

These coding guidelines for outpatient diagnoses have been approved for use by hospitals/ providers in coding and reporting hospital-based outpatient services and provider-based office visits.

Information about the use of certain abbreviations, punctuation, symbols, and other conventions used in the ICD-10-CM Tabular List (code numbers and titles), can be found in Section IA of these guidelines, under "Conventions Used in the Tabular List." Information about the correct sequence to use in finding a code is also described in Section I.

The terms encounter and visit are often used interchangeably in describing outpatient service contacts and, therefore, appear together in these guidelines without distinguishing one from the other.

Though the conventions and general guidelines apply to all settings, coding guidelines for outpatient and provider reporting of diagnoses will vary in a number of instances from those for inpatient diagnoses, recognizing that:

The Uniform Hospital Discharge Data Set (UHDDS) definition of principal diagnosis applies only to inpatients in acute, short-term, long-term care and psychiatric hospitals.

Coding guidelines for inconclusive diagnoses (probable, suspected, rule out, etc.) were developed for inpatient reporting and do not apply to outpatients.

A. Selection of first-listed condition

In the outpatient setting, the term first-listed diagnosis is used in lieu of principal diagnosis.

In determining the first-listed diagnosis the coding conventions of ICD-10-CM, as well as the general and disease specific guidelines take precedence over the outpatient guidelines.

Diagnoses often are not established at the time of the initial encounter/visit. It may take two or more visits before the diagnosis is confirmed.

The most critical rule involves beginning the search for the correct code assignment through the Alphabetic Index. Never begin searching initially in the Tabular List as this will lead to coding errors.

1. Outpatient Surgery

When a patient presents for outpatient surgery (same day surgery), code the reason for the surgery as the first-listed diagnosis (reason for the encounter), even if the surgery is not performed due to a contraindication.

2. Observation Stay

When a patient is admitted for observation for a medical condition, assign a code for the medical condition as the first-listed diagnosis.

When a patient presents for outpatient surgery and develops complications requiring admission to observation, code the reason for the surgery as the first reported diagnosis (reason for the encounter), followed by codes for the complications as secondary diagnoses.

B. Codes from A00.0 through T88.9, Z00-Z99

The appropriate code(s) from A00.0 through T88.9, Z00-Z99 must be used to identify diagnoses, symptoms, conditions, problems, complaints, or other reason(s) for the encounter/visit.

C. Accurate reporting of ICD-10-CM diagnosis codes

For accurate reporting of ICD-10-CM diagnosis codes, the documentation should describe the patient's condition, using terminology which includes specific diagnoses as well as symptoms, problems, or reasons for the encounter. There are ICD-10-CM codes to describe all of these.

D. Codes that describe symptoms and signs

Codes that describe symptoms and signs, as opposed to diagnoses, are acceptable for reporting purposes when a diagnosis has not been established (confirmed) by the provider. Chapter 18 of ICD-10-CM, Symptoms, Signs, and Abnormal Clinical and Laboratory Findings Not Elsewhere Classified (codes R00-R99) contain many, but not all codes for symptoms.

E. Encounters for circumstances other than a disease or injury

ICD-10-CM provides codes to deal with encounters for circumstances other than a disease or injury. The Factors Influencing Health Status and Contact with Health Services codes (Z00-**Z99**) **are** provided to deal with occasions when circumstances other than a disease or injury are recorded as diagnosis or problems.

See Section I.C.21. Factors influencing health status and contact with health services.

F. Level of Detail in Coding

1. **ICD-10-CM codes with *3, 4, 5, 6 or 7 characters***

   ICD-10-CM is composed of codes with 3, 4, 5, 6 or 7 **characters**. Codes with three **characters** are included in ICD-10-CM as the heading of a category of codes that may be further subdivided by the use of **fourth**, fifth, sixth or seventh **characters to** provide greater specificity.

2. **Use of full number of characters required for a code**

   A three-**character** code is to be used only if it is not further subdivided. A code is invalid if it has not been coded to the full number of characters required for that code, including the 7th character extension, if applicable.

G. ICD-10-CM code for the diagnosis, condition, problem, or other reason for encounter/visit

List first the ICD-10-CM code for the diagnosis, condition, problem, or other reason for encounter/visit shown in the medical record to be chiefly responsible for the services provided. List additional codes that describe any coexisting conditions. In some cases the first-listed diagnosis may be a symptom when a diagnosis has not been established (confirmed) by the physician.

H. Uncertain diagnosis

Do not code diagnoses documented as "probable", "suspected," "questionable," "rule out," or "working diagnosis" or other similar terms indicating uncertainty. Rather, code the condition(s) to the highest degree of certainty for that encounter/visit, such as symptoms, signs, abnormal test results, or other reason for the visit.

Please note: This differs from the coding practices used by short-term, acute care, long-term care and psychiatric hospitals.

I. Chronic diseases

Chronic diseases treated on an ongoing basis may be coded and reported as many times as the patient receives treatment and care for the condition(s)

J. Code all documented conditions that coexist

Code all documented conditions that coexist at the time of the encounter/visit, and require or affect patient care treatment or management. Do not code conditions that were previously treated and no longer exist. However, history codes (categories Z80-Z87) may be used as secondary codes if the historical condition or family history has an impact on current care or influences treatment.

K. Patients receiving diagnostic services only

For patients receiving diagnostic services only during an encounter/visit, sequence first the diagnosis, condition, problem, or other reason for encounter/visit shown in the medical record to be chiefly responsible for the outpatient services provided during the encounter/visit. Codes for other diagnoses (e.g., chronic conditions) may be sequenced as additional diagnoses.

For encounters for routine laboratory/radiology testing in the absence of any signs, symptoms, or associated diagnosis, assign Z01.89, Encounter for other specified special examinations. If routine testing is performed during the same encounter as a test to evaluate a sign,

symptom, or diagnosis, it is appropriate to assign both the V code and the code describing the reason for the non-routine test.

For outpatient encounters for diagnostic tests that have been interpreted by a physician, and the final report is available at the time of coding, code any confirmed or definitive diagnosis(es) documented in the interpretation. Do not code related signs and symptoms as additional diagnoses.

Please note: This differs from the coding practice in the hospital inpatient setting regarding abnormal findings on test results.

L. Patients receiving therapeutic services only

For patients receiving therapeutic services only during an encounter/visit, sequence first the diagnosis, condition, problem, or other reason for encounter/visit shown in the medical record to be chiefly responsible for the outpatient services provided during the encounter/visit. Codes for other diagnoses (e.g., chronic conditions) may be sequenced as additional diagnoses.

The only exception to this rule is that when the primary reason for the admission/encounter is chemotherapy or radiation therapy, the appropriate Z code for the service is listed first, and the diagnosis or problem for which the service is being performed listed second.

M. Patients receiving preoperative evaluations only

For patients receiving preoperative evaluations only, sequence first a code from subcategory Z01.81, Encounter for pre-procedural examinations, to describe the pre-op consultations. Assign a code for the condition to describe the reason for the surgery as an additional diagnosis. Code also any findings related to the pre-op evaluation.

N. Ambulatory surgery

For ambulatory surgery, code the diagnosis for which the surgery was performed. If the postoperative diagnosis is known to be different from the preoperative diagnosis at the time the diagnosis is confirmed, select the postoperative diagnosis for coding, since it is the most definitive.

O. Routine outpatient prenatal visits

See Section I.C.15. Routine outpatient prenatal visits.

P. Encounters for general medical examinations with abnormal findings

The subcategories for encounters for general medical examinations, Z00.0-, provide codes for with and without abnormal findings. Should a general medical examination result in an abnormal finding, the code for general medical examination with abnormal finding should be assigned as the **first-listed** diagnosis. A secondary code for the abnormal finding should also be coded.

Q. Encounters for routine health screenings

See Section I.C.21. Factors influencing health status and contact with health services, Screening

Appendix I. Present on Admission Reporting Guidelines

(Effective with 2011 update)

Introduction

These guidelines are to be used as a supplement to the *ICD-10-CM Official Guidelines for Coding and Reporting* to facilitate the assignment of the Present on Admission (POA) indicator for each diagnosis and external cause of injury code reported on claim forms (UB-04 and 837 Institutional).

These guidelines are not intended to replace any guidelines in the main body of the *ICD-10-CM Official Guidelines for Coding and Reporting*. The POA guidelines are not intended to provide guidance on when a condition should be coded, but rather, how to apply the POA indicator to the final set of diagnosis codes that have been assigned in accordance with Sections I, II, and III of the official coding guidelines. Subsequent to the assignment of the ICD-10-CM codes, the POA indicator should then be assigned to those conditions that have been coded.

As stated in the Introduction to the *ICD-10-CM Official Guidelines for Coding and Reporting*, a joint effort between the healthcare provider and the coder is essential to achieve complete and accurate documentation, code assignment, and reporting of diagnoses and procedures. The importance of consistent, complete documentation in the medical record cannot be overemphasized. Medical record documentation from any provider involved in the care and treatment of the patient may be used to support the determination of whether a condition was present on admission or not. In the context of the official coding guidelines, the term "provider" means a physician or any qualified healthcare practitioner who is legally accountable for establishing the patient's diagnosis.

These guidelines are not a substitute for the provider's clinical judgment as to the determination of whether a condition was/was not present on admission. The provider should be queried regarding issues related to the linking of signs/symptoms, timing of test results, and the timing of findings.

General Reporting Requirements

All claims involving inpatient admissions to general acute care hospitals or other facilities that are subject to a law or regulation mandating collection of present on admission information.

Present on admission is defined as present at the time the order for inpatient admission occurs -- conditions that develop during an outpatient encounter, including emergency department, observation, or outpatient surgery, are considered as present on admission.

POA indicator is assigned to principal and secondary diagnoses (as defined in Section II of the Official Guidelines for Coding and Reporting) and the external cause of injury codes.

Issues related to inconsistent, missing, conflicting or unclear documentation must still be resolved by the provider.

If a condition would not be coded and reported based on UHDDS definitions and current official coding guidelines, then the POA indicator would not be reported.

Reporting Options

Y – Yes
N – No
U – Unknown
W – Clinically undetermined
Unreported/Not used (or "1" for Medicare usage) – (Exempt from POA reporting)

Reporting Definitions

Y – present at the time of inpatient admission
N – not present at the time of inpatient admission
U – documentation is insufficient to determine if condition is present on admission
W – provider is unable to clinically determine whether condition was present on admission or not

Timeframe for POA Identification and Documentation

There is no required timeframe as to when a provider (per the definition of "provider" used in these guidelines) must identify or document a condition to be present on admission. In some clinical situations, it may not be possible for a provider to make a definitive diagnosis (or a condition may not be recognized or reported by the patient) for a period of time after admission. In some cases it may be several days before the provider arrives at a definitive diagnosis. This does not mean that the condition was not present on admission. Determination of whether the condition was present on admission or not will be based on the applicable POA guideline as identified in this document, or on the provider's best clinical judgment.

If at the time of code assignment the documentation is unclear as to whether a condition was present on admission or not, it is appropriate to query the provider for clarification.

Assigning the POA Indicator

Condition is on the "Exempt from Reporting" list
Leave the "present on admission" field blank if the condition is on the list of ICD-10-CM codes for which this field is not applicable. This is the only circumstance in which the field may be left blank.

POA Explicitly Documented
Assign "Y" for any condition the provider explicitly documents as being present on admission.

Assign "N" for any condition the provider explicitly documents as not present at the time of admission.

Conditions diagnosed prior to inpatient admission
Assign "Y" for conditions that were diagnosed prior to admission (example: hypertension, diabetes mellitus, asthma).

Conditions diagnosed during the admission but clearly present before admission
Assign "Y" for conditions diagnosed during the admission that were clearly present but not diagnosed until after admission occurred.

Diagnoses subsequently confirmed after admission are considered present on admission if at the time of admission they are documented as suspected, possible, rule out, differential diagnosis, or constitute an underlying cause of a symptom that is present at the time of admission.

Condition develops during outpatient encounter prior to inpatient admission
Assign "Y" for any condition that develops during an outpatient encounter prior to a written order for inpatient admission.

Documentation does not indicate whether condition was present on admission
Assign "U" when the medical record documentation is unclear as to whether the condition was present on admission. "U" should not be routinely assigned and used only in very limited circumstances. Coders are encouraged to query the providers when the documentation is unclear.

Documentation states that it cannot be determined whether the condition was or was not present on admission
Assign "W" when the medical record documentation indicates that it cannot be clinically determined whether or not the condition was present on admission.

Chronic condition with acute exacerbation during the admission
If a single code identifies both the chronic condition and the acute exacerbation, see POA guidelines pertaining to combination codes.

If a single code only identifies the chronic condition and not the acute exacerbation (e.g., acute exacerbation of chronic leukemia), assign "Y."

Conditions documented as possible, probable, suspected, or rule out at the time of discharge
If the final diagnosis contains a possible, probable, suspected, or rule out diagnosis, and this diagnosis was based on signs, symptoms or clinical findings suspected at the time of inpatient admission, assign "Y."

If the final diagnosis contains a possible, probable, suspected, or rule out diagnosis, and this diagnosis was based on signs, symptoms or clinical findings that were not present on admission, assign "N".

Conditions documented as impending or threatened at the time of discharge

If the final diagnosis contains an impending or threatened diagnosis, and this diagnosis is based on symptoms or clinical findings that were present on admission, assign "Y".

If the final diagnosis contains an impending or threatened diagnosis, and this diagnosis is based on symptoms or clinical findings that were not present on admission, assign "N".

Acute and Chronic Conditions

Assign "Y" for acute conditions that are present at time of admission and N for acute conditions that are not present at time of admission.

Assign "Y" for chronic conditions, even though the condition may not be diagnosed until after admission.

If a single code identifies both an acute and chronic condition, see the POA guidelines for combination codes.

Combination Codes

Assign "N" if any part of the combination code was not present on admission (e.g., COPD with acute exacerbation and the exacerbation was not present on admission; gastric ulcer that does not start bleeding until after admission; asthma patient develops status asthmaticus after admission).

Assign "Y" if all parts of the combination code were present on admission (e.g., patient with acute prostatitis admitted with hematuria).

If the final diagnosis includes comparative or contrasting diagnoses, and both were present, or suspected, at the time of admission, assign "Y".

For infection codes that include the causal organism, assign "Y" if the infection (or signs of the infection) was present on admission, even though the culture results may not be known until after admission (e.g., patient is admitted with pneumonia and the provider documents pseudomonas as the causal organism a few days later).

Same Diagnosis Code for Two or More Conditions

When the same ICD-10-CM diagnosis code applies to two or more conditions during the same encounter (e.g. two separate conditions classified to the same ICD-10-CM diagnosis code):

> Assign "Y" if all conditions represented by the single ICD-10-CM code were present on admission (e.g. bilateral unspecified age-related cataracts).

> Assign "N" if any of the conditions represented by the single ICD-10-CM code was not present on admission (e.g. traumatic secondary and recurrent hemorrhage and seroma is assigned to a single code T79.2, but only one of the conditions was present on admission).

Obstetrical conditions

Whether or not the patient delivers during the current hospitalization does not affect assignment of the POA indicator. The determining factor for POA assignment is whether the pregnancy complication or obstetrical condition described by the code was present at the time of admission or not.

If the pregnancy complication or obstetrical condition was present on admission (e.g., patient admitted in preterm labor), assign "Y".

If the pregnancy complication or obstetrical condition was not present on admission (e.g., 2nd degree laceration during delivery, postpartum hemorrhage that occurred during current hospitalization, fetal distress develops after admission), assign "N".

If the obstetrical code includes more than one diagnosis and any of the diagnoses identified by the code were not present on admission assign "N". (e.g., Category O11, Pre-existing hypertension with pre-eclampsia).

Perinatal conditions

Newborns are not considered to be admitted until after birth. Therefore, any condition present at birth or that developed in utero is considered present at admission and should be assigned "Y". This includes conditions that occur during delivery (e.g., injury during delivery, meconium aspiration, exposure to streptococcus B in the vaginal canal).

Congenital conditions and anomalies

Assign "Y" for congenital conditions and anomalies (except for codes Q00-Q99 which are exempt). Congenital conditions are always considered present on admission.

External cause of injury codes

Assign "Y" for any external cause code representing an external cause of morbidity that occurred prior to inpatient admission (e.g., patient fell out of bed at home, patient fell out of bed in emergency room prior to admission).

Assign "N" for any external cause code representing an external cause of morbidity that occurred during inpatient hospitalization (e.g., patient fell out of hospital bed during hospital stay, patient experienced an adverse reaction to a medication administered after inpatient admission).

Categories and Codes Exempt from Diagnosis Present on Admission Requirement

Note: "Diagnosis present on admission" for these code categories are exempt because they represent circumstances regarding the healthcare encounter or factors influencing health status that do not represent a current disease or injury or are always present on admission.

B90–B94	Sequelae of infectious and parasitic diseases
E64	Sequelae of malnutrition and other nutritional deficiencies
I25.2	Old myocardial infarction
I69	Sequelae of cerebrovascular disease
O09	Supervision of high risk pregnancy
O66.5	Attempted application of vacuum extractor and forceps
O80	Encounter for full-term uncomplicated delivery
O94	Sequelae of complication of pregnancy, childbirth, and the puerperium
P00	Newborn (suspected to be) affected by maternal conditions that may be unrelated to present pregnancy
Q00 – Q99	Congenital malformations, deformations and chromosomal abnormalities
S00-T88.9	Injury, poisoning and certain other consequences of external causes with 7th character representing subsequent encounter or sequela
V00.121	Fall from non-in-line roller-skates
V00.131	Fall from skateboard
V00.141	Fall from scooter (nonmotorized)
V00.311	Fall from snowboard
V00.321	Fall from snow-skis
V40-V49	Car occupant injured in transport accident
V80-V89	Other land transport accidents
V90-V94	Water transport accidents
V95-V97	Air and space transport accidents
W03	Other fall on same level due to collision with another person
W09	Fall on and from playground equipment
W15	Fall from cliff
W17.0	Fall into well
W17.1	Fall into storm drain or manhole
W18.01	Striking against sports equipment with subsequent fall
W20.8	Other cause of strike by thrown, projected or falling object
W21	Striking against or struck by sports equipment
W30	Contact with agricultural machinery
W31	Contact with other and unspecified machinery
W32-W34	Accidental handgun discharge and malfunction

W35- W40	Exposure to inanimate mechanical forces
W52	Crushed, pushed or stepped on by crowd or human stampede
W89	Exposure to man-made visible and ultraviolet light
XØ2	Exposure to controlled fire in building or structure
XØ3	Exposure to controlled fire, not in building or structure
XØ4	Exposure to ignition of highly flammable material
X52	Prolonged stay in weightless environment
X71-X83	Intentional self-harm
Y21	Drowning and submersion, undetermined intent
Y22	Handgun discharge, undetermined intent
Y23	Rifle, shotgun and larger firearm discharge, undetermined intent
Y24	Other and unspecified firearm discharge, undetermined intent
Y3Ø	Falling, jumping or pushed from a high place, undetermined intent
Y35	Legal intervention
Y37	Military operations
Y36	Operations of war
Y38	Terrorism
Y92	Place of occurrence of the external cause
Y93	Activity code
Y99	External cause status
ZØØ	Encounter for general examination without complaint, suspected or reported diagnosis
ZØ1	Encounter for other special examination without complaint, suspected or reported diagnosis
ZØ2	Encounter for administrative examination
ZØ3	Encounter for medical observation for suspected diseases and conditions ruled out
ZØ8	Encounter for follow-up examination following completed treatment for malignant neoplasm
ZØ9	Encounter for follow-up examination after completed treatment for conditions other than malignant neoplasm
Z11	Encounter for screening for infectious and parasitic diseases
Z11.8	Encounter for screening for other infectious and parasitic diseases
Z12	Encounter for screening for malignant neoplasms
Z13	Encounter for screening for other diseases and disorders
Z13.4	Encounter for screening for certain developmental disorders in childhood
Z13.5	Encounter for screening for eye and ear disorders
Z13.6	Encounter for screening for cardiovascular disorders
Z13.83	Encounter for screening for respiratory disorder NEC
Z13.89	Encounter for screening for other disorder (inclusion term) Encounter for screening for genitourinary disorders)
Z13.89	Encounter for screening for other disorder
Z14	Genetic carrier
Z15	Genetic susceptibility to disease
Z17	Estrogen receptor status
Z18	Retained foreign body fragments
Z22	Carrier of infectious disease
Z23	Encounter for immunization
Z28	Immunization not carried out and underimmunization status
Z28.3	Underimmunization status
Z3Ø	Encounter for contraceptive management
Z31	Encounter for procreative management
Z34	Encounter for supervision of normal pregnancy
Z36	Encounter for antenatal screening of mother
Z37	Outcome of delivery
Z38	Liveborn infants according to place of birth and type of delivery

Z39	Encounter for maternal postpartum care and examination
Z41	Encounter for procedures for purposes other than remedying health state
Z42	Encounter for plastic and reconstructive surgery following medical procedure or healed injury
Z43	Encounter for attention to artificial openings
Z44	Encounter for fitting and adjustment of external prosthetic device
Z45	Encounter for adjustment and management of implanted device
Z46	Encounter for fitting and adjustment of other devices
Z47.8	Encounter for other orthopedic aftercare
Z49	Encounter for care involving renal dialysis
Z51	Encounter for other aftercare
Z51.5	Encounter for palliative care
Z51.8	Encounter for other specified aftercare
Z52	Donors of organs and tissues
Z59	Problems related to housing and economic circumstances
Z63	Other problems related to primary support groupincluding family circumstances
Z65	Problems related to other psychosocial circumstances
Z65.8	Other specified problems related to psychosocial circumstances
Z67.1-Z67.9	Blood type
Z68	Body mass index (BMI)
Z72	Problems related to lifestyle
Z74.Ø1	Bed confinement status
Z76	Persons encountering health services in other circumstances
Z77.11Ø- Z77.128	Environmental pollution and hazards in the physical environment
Z78	Other specified health status
Z79	Long term (current) drug therapy
Z8Ø	Family history of primary malignant neoplasm
Z81	Family history of mental and behavioral disorders
Z82	Family history of certain disabilities and chronic diseases (leading to disablement)
Z83	Family history of other specific disorders
Z84	Family history of other conditions
Z85	Personal history of primary malignant neoplasm
Z86	Personal history of certain other diseases
Z87	Personal history of other diseases and conditions
Z87.828	Personal history of other (healed) physical injury and trauma
Z87.891	Personal history of nicotine dependence
Z88	Allergy status to drugs, medicaments and biological substances
Z89	Acquired absence of limb
Z90.71Ø	Acquired absence of both cervix and uterus
Z91.Ø	Allergy status, other than to drugs and biological substances
Z91.4	Personal history of psychological trauma, not elsewhere classified
Z91.5	Personal history of self-harm
Z91.8	Other specified risk factors, not elsewhere classified
Z92	Personal history of medical treatment
Z93	Artificial opening status
Z94	Transplanted organ and tissue status
Z95	Presence of cardiac and vascular implants and grafts
Z97	Presence of other devices
Z98	Other postprocedural states
Z99	Dependence on enabling machines and devices, not elsewhere classified

ICD-10-CM Index to Diseases and Injuries

A

Aarskog's syndrome Q87.1
Abandonment — *see* Maltreatment, abandonment
Abasia (-astasia) (hysterical) F44.4
Abderhalden-Kaufmann-Lignac syndrome
 (cystinosis) E72.04
Abdomen, abdominal — *see also* condition
 acute R10.0
 angina K55.1
 muscle deficiency syndrome Q79.4
Abdominalgia — *see* Pain, abdominal
Abduction contracture, hip or other joint — *see*
 Contraction, joint
Aberrant (congenital) (*see also* Malposition,
 congenital)
 adrenal gland Q89.1
 artery (peripheral) Q27.8
 basilar NEC Q28.1
 cerebral Q28.3
 coronary Q24.5
 digestive system Q27.8
 eye Q15.8
 lower limb Q27.8
 precerebral Q28.1
 pulmonary Q25.7
 renal Q27.2
 retina Q14.1
 specified site NEC Q27.8
 subclavian Q27.8
 upper limb Q27.8
 vertebral Q28.1
 breast Q83.8
 endocrine gland NEC Q89.2
 hepatic duct Q44.5
 pancreas Q45.3
 parathyroid gland Q89.2
 pituitary gland Q89.2
 sebaceous glands, mucous membrane, mouth,
 congenital Q38.6
 spleen Q89.09
 subclavian artery Q27.8
 thymus (gland) Q89.2
 thyroid gland Q89.2
 vein (peripheral) NEC Q27.8
 cerebral Q28.3
 digestive system Q27.8
 lower limb Q27.8
 precerebral Q28.1
 specified site NEC Q27.8
 upper limb Q27.8
Aberration
 distantial — *see* Disturbance, visual
 mental F99
Abetalipoproteinemia E78.6
Abiotrophy R68.89
Ablatio, ablation
 retinae — *see* Detachment, retina
Ablepharia, ablepharon Q10.3
Abnormal, abnormality, abnormalities (*see also*
 Anomaly)
 acid-base balance (mixed) E87.4
 albumin R77.0
 alphafetoprotein R77.2
 alveolar ridge K08.9
 anatomical relationship Q89.9
 apertures, congenital, diaphragm Q79.1
 auditory perception H93.29-
 diplacusis — *see* Diplacusis
 hyperacusis — *see* Hyperacusis
 recruitment — *see* Recruitment, auditory
 threshold shift — *see* Shift, auditory threshold
 autosomes Q99.9
 fragile site Q95.5
 basal metabolic rate R94.8
 biosynthesis, testicular androgen E29.1
 bleeding time R79.1
 blood-gas level R79.81

Abnormal, abnormality, abnormalities— *continued*
 blood level (of)
 cobalt R79.0
 copper R79.0
 iron R79.0
 lithium R78.89
 magnesium R79.0
 mineral NEC R79.0
 zinc R79.0
 blood pressure
 elevated R03.0
 low reading (nonspecific) R03.1
 blood sugar R73.09
 bowel sounds R19.15
 absent R19.11
 hyperactive R19.12
 brain scan R94.02
 breathing R06.9
 caloric test R94.138
 cerebrospinal fluid R83.9
 cytology R83.6
 drug level R83.2
 enzyme level R83.0
 hormones R83.1
 immunology R83.4
 microbiology R83.5
 nonmedicinal level R83.3
 specified type NEC R83.8
 chemistry, blood R79.9
 C-reactive protein R79.82
 drugs — *see* Findings, abnormal, in blood
 gas level R79.81
 minerals R79.0
 pancytopenia R79.1
 specified NEC R79.89
 PTT R79.1
 toxins — *see* Findings, abnormal, in blood
 chest sounds (friction) (rales) R09.89
 chromosome, chromosomal Q99.9
 with more than three X chromosomes, female
 Q97.1
 analysis result R89.8
 bronchial washings R84.8
 cerebrospinal fluid R83.8
 cervix uteri NEC R87.89
 nasal secretions R84.8
 nipple discharge R89.8
 peritoneal fluid R85.89
 pleural fluid R84.8
 prostatic secretions R86.8
 saliva R85.89
 seminal fluid R86.8
 sputum R84.8
 synovial fluid R89.8
 throat scrapings R84.8
 vagina R87.89
 vulva R87.89
 wound secretions R89.8
 dicentric replacement Q93.2
 ring replacement Q93.2
 sex Q99.8
 female phenotype Q97.9
 specified NEC Q97.8
 male phenotype Q98.9
 specified NEC Q98.8
 structural male Q98.6
 specified NEC Q99.8
 clinical findings NEC R68.89
 coagulation D68.9
 newborn, transient P61.6
 profile R79.1
 time R79.1
 communication — *see* Fistula
 conjunctiva, vascular H11.41-
 coronary artery Q24.5
 cortisol-binding globulin E27.8
 course, eustachian tube Q17.8
 creatinine clearance R94.4

Abnormal, abnormality, abnormalities— *continued*
 cytology
 anus R85.619
 atypical squamous cells cannot exclude high
 grade squamous intraepithelial lesion
 (ASC-H) R85.611
 atypical squamous cells of undetermined
 significance (ASC-US) R85.610
 cytologic evidence of malignancy R85.614
 high grade squamous intraepithelial lesion
 (HGSIL) R85.613
 human papillomavirus (HPV) DNA test
 high risk positive R85.81
 low risk postive R85.82
 inadequate smear R85.615
 low grade squamous intraepithelial lesion
 (LGSIL) R85.612
 satisfactory cervical smear but lacking
 transformation zone R85.616
 specified NEC R85.618
 unsatisfactory smear R85.615
 female genital organs — *see* Abnormal,
 Papanicolaou (smear)
 dark adaptation curve H53.61
 dentofacial NEC — *see* Anomaly, dentofacial
 development, developmental Q89.9
 central nervous system Q07.9
 diagnostic imaging
 abdomen, abdominal region NEC R93.5
 biliary tract R93.2
 breast R92.8
 central nervous system NEC R90.89
 cerebrovascular NEC R90.89
 coronary circulation R93.1
 digestive tract NEC R93.3
 gastrointestinal (tract) R93.3
 genitourinary organs R93.8
 head R93.0
 heart R93.1
 intrathoracic organ NEC R93.8
 limbs R93.6
 liver R93.2
 lung (field) R91
 musculoskeletal system NEC R93.7
 retroperitoneum R93.5
 sites specified NEC R93.8
 skin and subcutaneous tissue R93.8
 skull R93.0
 urinary organs R93.4
 direction, teeth, fully erupted M26.30
 ear ossicles, acquired NEC H74.39-
 ankylosis — *see* Ankylosis, ear ossicles
 discontinuity — *see* Discontinuity, ossicles, ear
 partial loss — *see* Loss, ossicles, ear (partial)
 Ebstein Q22.5
 echocardiogram R93.1
 echoencephalogram R90.81
 echogram — *see* Abnormal, diagnostic imaging
 electrocardiogram [ECG] [EKG] R94.31
 electroencephalogram [EEG] R94.01
 electrolyte — *see* Imbalance, electrolyte
 electromyogram [EMG] R94.131
 electro-oculogram [EOG] R94.110
 electrophysiological intracardiac studies R94.39
 electroretinogram [ERG] R94.111
 erythrocytes
 congenital, with perinatal jaundice D58.9
 feces (color) (contents) (mucus) R19.5
 finding — *see* Findings, abnormal, without
 diagnosis
 fluid
 amniotic — *see* Abnormal, specimen, specified
 cerebrospinal — *see* Abnormal, cerebrospinal
 fluid
 peritoneal — *see* Abnormal, specimen, digestive
 organs
 pleural — *see* Abnormal, specimen, respiratory
 organs

Abnormal, abnormality, abnormalities— *continued*
- fluid— *continued*
  - synovial — *see* Abnormal, specimen, specified
  - thorax (bronchial washings) (pleural fluid) — *see* Abnormal, specimen, respiratory organs
  - vaginal — *see* Abnormal, specimen, female genital organs
- form
  - teeth K00.2
  - uterus — *see* Anomaly, uterus
- function studies
  - auditory R94.120
  - bladder R94.8
  - brain R94.09
  - cardiovascular R94.30
  - ear R94.128
  - endocrine NEC R94.7
  - eye NEC R94.118
  - kidney R94.4
  - liver R94.5
  - nervous system
    - central NEC R94.09
    - peripheral NEC R94.138
  - pancreas R94.8
  - placenta R94.8
  - pulmonary R94.2
  - special senses NEC R94.128
  - spleen R94.8
  - thyroid R94.6
  - vestibular R94.121
- gait — *see* Gait
  - hysterical F44.4
- gastrin secretion E16.4
- globulin R77.1
  - cortisol-binding E27.8
  - thyroid-binding E07.89
- glomerular, minor (*see also* N00-N07 with fourth character .0) N05.0
- glucagon secretion E16.3
- glucose tolerance (test) (non-fasting) R73.09
- gravitational (G) forces or states (effect of) T75.81
- hair (color) (shaft) L67.9
  - specified NEC L67.8
- hard tissue formation in pulp (dental) K04.3
- head movement R25.0
- heart
  - rate R00.9
    - specified NEC R00.8
  - shadow R93.1
  - sounds NEC R01.2
- hemoglobin (disease) (*see also* Disease, hemoglobin) D58.2
  - trait — *see* Trait, hemoglobin, abnormal
- histology NEC R89.7
- immunological findings R89.4
  - in serum R76.9
    - specified NEC R76.8
- increase in appetite R63.2
- involuntary movement — *see* Abnormal, movement, involuntary
- jaw closure M26.51
- karyotype R89.8
- kidney function test R94.4
- knee jerk R29.2
- leukocyte (cell) (differential) NEC D72.9
- liver
- loss of
  - height R29.890
  - weight R63.4
- mammogram NEC R92.8
  - calcification (calculus) R92.1
  - microcalcification R92.0
- Mantoux test R76.1
- movement (disorder) (*see also* Disorder, movement)
  - head R25.0
  - involuntary R25.9
    - fasciculation R25.3
      - of head R25.0
    - spasm R25.2
    - specified type NEC R25.8
    - tremor R25.1
- myoglobin (Aberdeen) (Annapolis) R89.7

Abnormal, abnormality, abnormalities— *continued*
- neonatal screening P09
- oculomotor study R94.113
- palmar creases Q82.8
- Papanicolaou (smear)
  - anus R85.619
    - atypical squamous cells cannot exclude high grade squamous intraepithelial lesion (ASC-H) R85.611
    - atypical squamous cells of undetermined significance (ASC-US) R85.610
    - cytologic evidence of malignancy R85.614
    - high grade squamous intraepithelial lesion (HGSIL) R85.613
    - human papillomavirus (HPV) DNA test
      - high risk positive R85.81
      - low risk postive R85.82
    - inadequate smear R85.615
    - low grade squamous intraepithelial lesion (LGSIL) R85.612
    - satisfactory cervical smear but lacking transformation zone R85.616
    - specified NEC R85.618
    - unsatisfactory smear R85.615
  - bronchial washings R84.6
  - cerebrospinal fluid R83.6
  - cervix R87.619
    - atypical squamous cells cannot exclude high grade squamous intraepithelial lesion (ASC-H) R87.611
    - atypical squamous cells of undetermined significance (ASC-US) R87.610
    - cytologic evidence of malignancy R87.614
    - high grade squamous intraepithelial lesion (HGSIL) R87.613
    - inadequate smear R87.615
    - low grade squamous intraepithelial lesion (LGSIL) R87.612 I
    - non-atypical endometrial cells R87.618
    - satisfactory cervical smear but lacking transformation zone R87.616
    - specified NEC R87.618
    - thin preparaton R87.619
    - unsatisfactory smear R87.615
  - nasal secretions R84.6
  - nipple discharge R89.6
  - peritoneal fluid R85.69
  - pleural fluid R84.6
  - prostatic secretions R86.6
  - saliva R85.69
  - seminal fluid R86.6
  - sites NEC R89.6
  - sputum R84.6
  - synovial fluid R89.6
  - throat scrapings R84.6
  - vagina R87.629
    - atypical squamous cells cannot exclude high grade squamous intraepithelial lesion (ASC-H) R87.621
    - atypical squamous cells of undetermined significance (ASC-US) R87.620
    - cytologic evidence of malignancy R87.624
    - high grade squamous intraepithelial lesion (HGSIL) R87.623
    - inadequate smear R87.625
    - low grade squamous intraepithelial lesion (LGSIL) R87.622
    - specified NEC R87.628
    - thin preparation R87.629
    - unsatisfactory smear R87.625
  - vulva R87.69
  - wound secretions R89.6
- partial thromboplastin time (PTT) R79.1
- plantar reflex R29.2
- pelvis (bony) — *see* Deformity, pelvis
- percussion, chest (tympany) R09.89
- periods (grossly) — *see* Menstruation
- phonocardiogram R94.39
- plasma
  - protein R77.9
    - specified NEC R77.8
  - viscosity R70.1
- pleural (folds) Q34.0

Abnormal, abnormality, abnormalities— *continued*
- posture R29.3
- product of conception O02.9
  - specified type NEC O02.8
- prothrombin time (PT) R79.1
- pulmonary
  - artery, congenital Q25.7
  - function, newborn P28.89
  - test results R94.2
- pulsations in neck R00.2
- pupillary H21.56-
  - function (reaction) (reflex) — *see* Anomaly, pupil, function
- radiological examination — *see* Abnormal, diagnostic imaging
- red blood cell(s) (morphology) (volume) R71.8
- reflex — *see* Reflex
- renal function test R94.4
- response to nerve stimulation R94.130
- retinal correspondence H53.31
- retinal function study R94.111
- rhythm, heart (*see also* Arrhythmia)
- saliva — *see* Abnormal, specimen, digestive organs
- scan
  - kidney R94.4
  - liver R93.2
  - thyroid R94.6
- secretion
  - gastrin E16.4
  - glucagon E16.3
- semen, seminal fluid — *see* Abnormal, specimen, male genital organs
- serum level (of)
  - acid phosphatase R74.8
  - alkaline phosphatase R74.8
  - amylase R74.8
  - enzymes R74.9
    - specified NEC R74.8
  - lipase R74.8
  - triacylglycerol lipase R74.8
- shape
  - gravid uterus — *see* Anomaly, uterus
- sinus venosus Q21.1
- size, tooth, teeth K00.2
- spacing, tooth, teeth, fully erupted M26.30
- specimen
  - digestive organs (peritoneal fluid) (saliva) R85.9
    - cytology R85.69
    - drug level R85.2
    - enzyme level R85.0
    - histology R85.7
    - hormones R85.1
    - immunology R85.4
    - microbiology R85.5
    - nonmedicinal level R85.3
    - specified type NEC R85.89
  - female genital organs (secretions) (smears) R87.9
    - cytology R87.619
      - cervix R87.619
        - inadequate (unsatisfactory) smear R87.615
        - human papillomavirus (HPV) DNA test
          - high risk positive R87.810
          - low risk positive R87.820
        - non-atypical endometrial cells R87.618
        - specified NEC R87.89
      - vagina R87.622
        - inadequate (unsatisfactory) smear R87.625
        - human papillomavirus (HPV) DNA test
          - high risk positive R87.811
          - low risk positive R87.821
      - vulva R87.69
    - drug level R87.2
    - enzyme level R87.0
    - histological R87.7
    - hormones R87.1
    - immunology R87.4
    - microbiology R87.5
    - nonmedicinal level R87.3
    - specified type NEC R87.89
  - male genital organs (prostatic secretions) (semen) R86.9

Abnormal, abnormality, abnormalities— *continued*
specimen— *continued*
male genital organs— *continued*
cytology R86.6
drug level R86.2
enzyme level R86.Ø
histological R86.7
hormones R86.1
immunology R86.4
microbiology R86.5
nonmedicinal level R86.3
specified type NEC R86.8
nipple discharge — *see* Abnormal, specimen, specified
respiratory organs (bronchial washings) (nasal secretions) (pleural fluid) (sputum) R84.9
cytology R84.6
drug level R84.2
enzyme level R84.Ø
histology R84.7
hormones R84.1
immunology R84.4
microbiology R84.5
nonmedicinal level R84.3
specified type NEC R84.8
specified fluid, organ, system and tissue NOS R89.9
cytology R89.6
drug level R89.2
enzyme level R89.Ø
histology R89.7
hormones R89.1
immunology R89.4
microbiology R89.5
nonmedicinal level R89.3
specified type NEC R89.8
synovial fluid — *see* Abnormal, specimen, specified
thorax (bronchial washings) (pleural fluids) — *see* Abnormal, specimen, respiratory organs
vagina (secretion) (smear) R87.629
vulva (secretion) (smear) R87.69
wound secretion — *see* Abnormal, specimen, specified
spermatozoa — *see* Abnormal, specimen, male genital organs
sputum (amount) (color) (odor) RØ9.3
stool (color) (contents) (mucus) R19.5
bloody K92.1
guaiac positive R19.5
synchondrosis Q78.8
thermography — *see* Abnormal, diagnostic imaging
thyroid-binding globulin EØ7.89
tooth, teeth (form) (size) KØØ.2
toxicology (findings) R78.9
transport protein E88.Ø9
tumor marker NEC R97.8
ultrasound results — *see* Abnormal, diagnostic imaging
umbilical cord complicating delivery O69.9
urination NEC R39.19
urine (constituents) R82.9Ø
bile R82.2
cytological examination R82.8
drugs R82.5
fat R82.Ø
glucose R81
heavy metals R82.6
hemoglobin R82.3
histological examination R82.8
ketones R82.4
microbiological examination (culture) R82.7
myoglobin R82.1
positive culture R82.7
protein — *see* Proteinuria
specified substance NEC R82.99
chromoabnormality NEC R82.91
substances nonmedical R82.6
uterine hemorrhage — *see* Hemorrhage, uterus
vectorcardiogram R94.39
visually evoked potential (VEP) R94.112

Abnormal, abnormality, abnormalities— *continued*
white blood cells D72.9
specified NEC D72.89
weight
gain R63.5
loss R63.4
X-ray examination — *see* Abnormal, diagnostic imaging
Abnormity (any organ or part) — *see* Anomaly
Abocclusion M26.29
hemolytic disease (newborn) P55.1
incompatibility reaction ABO — *see* Complication(s), transfusion, incompatibility reaction, ABO
Abolition, language R48.8
Aborter, habitual or recurrent — *see* Loss (of), pregnancy, recurrent
Abortion (complete) (spontaneous) OØ3.9
attempted (elective) (failed) OØ7.4
complicated by
afibrinogenemia OØ7.1
cardiac arrest OØ7.36
chemical damage of pelvic organ(s) OØ7.34
circulatory collapse OØ7.31
cystitis OØ7.38
defibrination syndrome OØ7.1
electrolyte imbalance OØ7.39
embolism (air) (amniotic fluid) (blood clot) (fat) (pulmonary) (septic) (soap) OØ7.2
endometritis OØ7.Ø
genital tract and pelvic infection OØ7.Ø
hemorrhage (delayed) (excessive) OØ7.1
hemolysis OØ7.1
infection
genital tract or pelvic OØ7.Ø
urinary tract tract OØ7.38
intravascular coagulation OØ7.1
laceration of pelvic organ(s) OØ7.34
metabolic disorder OØ7.33
oliguria OØ7.32
oophoritis OØ7.Ø
parametritis OØ7.Ø
pelvic peritonitis OØ7.Ø
perforation of pelvic organ(s) OØ7.34
renal failure or shutdown OØ7.32
salpingitis or salpingo-oophoritis OØ7.Ø
sepsis OØ7.37
shock OØ7.31
specified condition NEC OØ7.39
tubular necrosis (renal) OØ7.32
uremia OØ7.32
urinary tract infection OØ7.38
venous complication NEC OØ7.35
embolism (air) (amniotic fluid) (blood clot) (fat) (pulmonary) (septic) (soap) OØ7.2
complicated (by) (following) OØ3.8Ø
afibrinogenemia OØ3.6
cardiac arrest OØ3.86
chemical damage of pelvic organ(s) OØ3.84
circulatory collapse OØ3.81
cystitis OØ3.88
defibrination syndrome OØ3.6
electrolyte imbalance OØ3.89
embolism (air) (amniotic fluid) (blood clot) (fat) (pulmonary) (septic) (soap) OØ3.7
endometritis OØ3.5
genital tract and pelvic infection OØ3.5
hemolysis OØ3.6
hemorrhage (delayed) (excessive) OØ3.6
infection
genital tract or pelvic OØ3.5
urinary tract OØ3.88
intravascular coagulation OØ3.6
laceration of pelvic organ(s) OØ3.84
metabolic disorder OØ3.83
oliguria OØ3.82
oophoritis OØ3.5
parametritis OØ3.5
pelvic peritonitis OØ3.5
perforation of pelvic organ(s) OØ3.84
renal failure or shutdown OØ3.82
salpingitis or salpingo-oophoritis OØ3.5
sepsis OØ3.87

Abortion— *continued*
complicated— *continued*
shock OØ3.81
specified condition NEC OØ3.89
tubular necrosis (renal) OØ3.82
uremia OØ3.82
urinary tract infection OØ3.88
venous complication NEC OØ3.85
embolism (air) (amniotic fluid) (blood clot) (fat) (pulmonary) (septic) (soap) OØ3.7
failed — *see* Abortion, attempted
habitual or recurrent N96
with current abortion — *see* categories OØ3-OØ6
without current pregnancy N96
care in current pregnancy O26.2-
incomplete (spontaneous) OØ3.4
complicated (by) (following) OØ3.3Ø
afibrinogenemia OØ3.1
cardiac arrest OØ3.36
chemical damage of pelvic organ(s) OØ3.34
circulatory collapse OØ3.31
cystitis OØ3.38
defibrination syndrome OØ3.1
electrolyte imbalance OØ3.39
embolism (air) (amniotic fluid) (blood clot) (fat) (pulmonary) (septic) (soap) OØ3.2
endometritis OØ3.Ø
genital tract and pelvic infection OØ3.Ø
hemolysis OØ3.1
hemorrhage (delayed) (excessive) OØ3.1
infection
genital tract or pelvic OØ3.Ø
urinary tract OØ3.38
intravascular coagulation OØ3.1
laceration of pelvic organ(s) OØ3.34
metabolic disorder OØ3.33
oliguria OØ3.32
oophoritis OØ3.Ø
parametritis OØ3.Ø
pelvic peritonitis OØ3.Ø
perforation of pelvic organ(s) OØ3.34
renal failure or shutdown OØ3.32
salpingitis or salpingo-oophoritis OØ3.Ø
sepsis OØ3.37
shock OØ3.31
specified condition NEC OØ3.39
tubular necrosis (renal) OØ3.32
uremia OØ3.32
urinary infection OØ3.38
venous complication NEC OØ3.35
embolism (air) (amniotic fluid) (blood clot) (fat) (pulmonary) (septic) (soap) OØ3.2
induced (encounter for) Z33.2
complicated by OØ4.8Ø
afibrinogenemia OØ4.6
cardiac arrest OØ4.86
chemical damage of pelvic organ(s) OØ4.84
circulatory collapse OØ4.81
cystitis OØ4.88
defibrination syndrome OØ4.6
electrolyte imbalance OØ4.89
embolism (air) (amniotic fluid) (blood clot) (fat) (pulmonary) (septic) (soap) OØ4.7
endometritis OØ4.5
genital tract and pelvic infection OØ4.5
hemolysis OØ4.6
hemorrhage (delayed) (excessive) OØ4.6
infection
genital tract or pelvic OØ4.5
urinary tract OØ4.88
intravascular coagulation OØ4.6
laceration of pelvic organ(s) OØ4.84
metabolic disorder OØ4.83
oliguria OØ4.82
oophoritis OØ4.5
parametritis OØ4.5
pelvic peritonitis OØ4.5
perforation of pelvic organ(s) OØ4.84
renal failure or shutdown OØ4.82
salpingitis or salpingo-oophoritis OØ4.5
sepsis OØ4.87
shock OØ4.81

Abortion— *continued*
  induced— *continued*
    complicated by— *continued*
      specified condition NEC O04.89
      tubular necrosis (renal) O04.82
      uremia O04.82
      urinary tract infection O04.88
      venous complication NEC O04.85
        embolism (air) (amniotic fluid) (blood clot)
          (fat) (pulmonary) (septic) (soap)
          O04.7
  missed O02.1
  spontaneous — *see* Abortion (complete)
      (spontaneous)
    threatened O20.0
  threatened (spontaneous) O20.0
  tubal O00.1
  with retained products of conception — *see*
      Abortion, incomplete
Abortus fever A23.1
Aboulomania F60.7
Abrami's disease D59.8
Abramov-Fiedler myocarditis (acute isolated
    myocarditis) I40.1
Abrasion
  abdomen, abdominal (wall) S30.811
  alveolar process S00.512
  ankle S90.51-
  antecubital space — *see* Abrasion, elbow
  anus S30.817
  arm (upper) S40.81-
  auditory canal — *see* Abrasion, ear
  auricle — *see* Abrasion, ear
  axilla — *see* Abrasion, arm
  back, lower S30.810
  breast S20.11-
  brow S00.81
  buttock S30.810
  calf — *see* Abrasion, leg
  canthus — *see* Abrasion, eyelid
  cheek S00.81
    internal S00.512
  chest wall — *see* Abrasion, thorax
  chin S00.81
  clitoris S30.814
  cornea S05.0-
  costal region — *see* Abrasion, thorax
  dental K03.1
  digit(s)
    foot — *see* Abrasion, toe
    hand — *see* Abrasion, finger
  ear S00.41-
  elbow S50.31-
  epididymis S30.813
  epigastric region S30.811
  epiglottis S10.11
  esophagus (thoracic) S27.818
    cervical S10.11
  eyebrow — *see* Abrasion, eyelid
  eyelid S00.21-
  face S00.81
  finger(s) S60.41-
    index S60.41-
    little S60.41-
    middle S60.41-
    ring S60.41-
  flank S30.811
  foot (except toe(s) alone) S90.81-
    toe — *see* Abrasion, toe
  forearm S50.81-
    elbow only — *see* Abrasion, elbow
  forehead S00.81
  genital organs, external
    female S30.816
    male S30.815
  groin S30.811
  gum S00.512
  hand S60.51-
  head S00.91
    ear — *see* Abrasion, ear
    eyelid — *see* Abrasion, eyelid
    lip S00.511
    nose S00.31

Abrasion— *continued*
  head— *continued*
    oral cavity S00.512
    scalp S00.01
    specified site NEC S00.81
  heel — *see* Abrasion, foot
  hip S70.21-
  inguinal region S30.811
  interscapular region S20.419
  jaw S00.81
  knee S80.21-
  labium (majus) (minus) S30.814
  larynx S10.11
  leg (lower) S80.81-
    knee — *see* Abrasion, knee
    upper — *see* Abrasion, thigh
  lip S00.511
  lower back S30.810
  lumbar region S30.810
  malar region S00.81
  mammary — *see* Abrasion, breast
  mastoid region S00.81
  mouth S00.512
  nail
    finger — *see* Abrasion, finger
    toe — *see* Abrasion, toe
  nape S10.81
  nasal S00.31
  neck S10.91
    specified site NEC S10.81
    throat S10.11
  nose S00.31
  occipital region S00.01
  oral cavity S00.512
  orbital region — *see* Abrasion, eyelid
  palate S00.512
  palm — *see* Abrasion, hand
  parietal region S00.01
  pelvis S30.810
  penis S30.812
  perineum
    female S30.814
    male S30.810
  periocular area — *see* Abrasion, eyelid
  phalanges
    finger — *see* Abrasion, finger
    toe — *see* Abrasion, toe
  pharynx S10.11
  pinna — *see* Abrasion, ear
  popliteal space — *see* Abrasion, knee
  prepuce S30.812
  pubic region S30.810
  pudendum
    female S30.816
    male S30.815
  sacral region S30.810
  scalp S00.01
  scapular region — *see* Abrasion, shoulder
  scrotum S30.813
  shin — *see* Abrasion, leg
  shoulder S40.21-
  sternal region S20.319
  submaxillary region S00.81
  submental region S00.81
  subungual
    finger(s) — *see* Abrasion, finger
    toe(s) — *see* Abrasion, toe
  supraclavicular fossa S10.81
  supraorbital S00.81
  temple S00.81
  temporal region S00.81
  testis S30.813
  thigh S70.31-
  thorax, thoracic (wall) S20.91
    back S20.41-
    front S20.31-
  throat S10.11
  thumb S60.31-
  toe(s) (lesser) S90.416
    great S90.41-
  tongue S00.512
  tooth, teeth (dentifrice) (habitual) (hard tissues)
      (occupational) (ritual) (traditional) K03.1

Abrasion— *continued*
  trachea S10.11
  tunica vaginalis S30.813
  tympanum, tympanic membrane — *see* Abrasion,
      ear
  uvula S00.512
  vagina S30.814
  vocal cords S10.11
  vulva S30.814
  wrist S60.81-
Abrism — *see* Poisoning, food, noxious, plant
Abruptio placentae O45.9-
  with
    afibrinogenemia O45.01-
    coagulation defect O45.00-
      specified NEC O45.09-
    disseminated intravascular coagulation O45.02-
    hypofibrinogenemia O45.01-
  specified NEC O45.8-
Abruption, placenta — *see* Abruptio placentae
Abscess (connective tissue) (embolic) (fistulous)
    (infective) (metastatic) (multiple) (pernicious)
    (pyogenic) (septic) L02.91
  with
    diverticular disease (intestine) K57.80
      with bleeding K57.81
      large intestine K57.20
        with
          bleeding K57.21
          small intestine K57.40
            with bleeding K57.41
      small intestine K57.00
        with
          bleeding K57.01
          large intestine K57.40
            with bleeding K57.41
    lymphangitis—code by site under Abscess
  abdomen, abdominal
    cavity K65.1
    wall L02.211
  abdominopelvic K65.1
  accessory sinus — *see* Sinusitis
  adrenal (capsule) (gland) E27.8
  alveolar K04.7
    with sinus K04.6
  ambebic A06.4
    brain (and liver or lung abscess) A06.6
    genitourinary tract A06.82
    liver (without mention of brain or lung abscess)
        A06.4
    lung (and liver) (without mention of brain
        abscess) A06.5
    specified site NEC A06.89
    spleen A06.89
  anerobic A48.0
  ankle — *see* Abscess, lower limb
  anorectal K61.2
  antecubital space — *see* Abscess, upper limb
  antrum (chronic) (Highmore) — *see* Sinusitis,
      maxillary
  anus K61.0
  apical (tooth) K04.7
    with sinus (alveolar) K04.6
  appendix K35.3
  areola (acute) (chronic) (nonpuerperal) N61
    puerperal, postpartum or gestational — *see*
        Infection, nipple
  arm (any part) — *see* Abscess, upper limb
  artery (wall) I77.89
  atheromatous I77.2
  auricle, ear — *see* Abscess, ear, external
  axilla (region) L02.41-
    lymph gland or node L04.2
  back (any part, except buttock) L02.212
  Bartholin's gland N75.1
    with
      abortion — *see* Abortion, by type complicated
          by, sepsis
      ectopic or molar pregnancy O08.0
    following ectopic or molar pregnancy O08.0
  Bezold's — *see* Mastoiditis, acute
  bilharziasis B65.1
  bladder (wall) — *see* Cystitis, specified type NEC

Abscess— *continued*
  bone (subperiosteal) (*see also* Osteomyelitis,
    specified type NEC)
    accessory sinus (chronic) — *see* Sinusitis
    chronic or old — *see* Osteomyelitis, chronic
    jaw (lower) (upper) M27.2
    mastoid — *see* Mastoiditis, acute, subperiosteal
    petrous — *see* Petrositis
    spinal (tuberculous) A18.01
      nontuberculous — *see* Osteomyelitis, vertebra
  bowel K63.0
  brain (any part) (cystic) (otogenic) G06.0
    amebic (with abscess of any other site) A06.6
    gonococcal A54.82
    pheomycotic (chromomycotic) B43.1
    tuberculous A17.81
  breast (acute) (chronic) (nonpuerperal) N61
    newborn P39.0
    puerperal, postpartum, gestational — *see*
      Mastitis, obstetric, purulent
  broad ligament N73.2
    acute N73.0
    chronic N73.1
  Brodie's (localized) (chronic) M86.8x-
  bronchi J98.09
  buccal cavity K12.2
  bulbourethral gland N34.0
  bursa M71.00
    ankle M71.07-
    elbow M71.02-
    foot M71.07-
    hand M71.04-
    hip M71.05-
    knee M71.06-
    multiple sites M71.09
    pharyngeal J39.1
    shoulder M71.01-
    specified site NEC M71.08
    wrist M71.03-
  buttock L02.31
  canthus — *see* Blepharoconjunctivitis
  cartilage — *see* Disorder, cartilage, specified type
    NEC
  cecum K35.3
  cerebellum, cerebellar G06.0
    sequelae G09
  cerebral (embolic) G06.0
    sequelae G09
  cervical (meaning neck) L02.11
    lymph gland or node L04.0
  cervix (stump) (uteri) — *see* Cervicitis
  cheek (external) L02.01
    inner K12.2
  chest J86.9
    with fistula J86.0
    wall L02.213
  chin L02.01
  choroid — *see* Inflammation, chorioretinal
  circumtonsillar J36
  cold (lung) (tuberculous) (*see also* Tuberculosis,
    abscess, lung)
    articular — *see* Tuberculosis, joint
  colon (wall) K63.0
  colostomy K94.02
  conjunctiva — *see* Conjunctivitis, acute
  cornea H16.31-
  corpus
    cavernosum N48.21
    luteum — *see* Oophoritis
  Cowper's gland N34.0
  cranium G06.0
  cul-de-sac (Douglas') (posterior) — *see* Peritonitis,
    pelvic, female
  cutaneous — *see* Abscess, by site
  dental K04.7
    with sinus (alveolar) K04.6
  dentoalveolar K04.7
    with sinus K04.6
  diaphragm, diaphragmatic K65.1
  Douglas' cul-de-sac or pouch — *see* Peritonitis,
    pelvic, female
  Dubois A50.59

Abscess— *continued*
  ear (middle) (*see also* Otitis, media, suppurative)
    acute — *see* Otitis, media, suppurative, acute
    external H60.0-
  entamebic — *see* Abscess, amebic
  enterostomy K94.12
  epididymis N45.4
  epidural G06.2
    brain G06.0
    spinal cord G06.1
  epiglottis J38.7
  epiploon, epiploic K65.1
  erysipelatous — *see* Erysipelas
  esophagus K20.8
  ethmoid (bone) (chronic) (sinus) J32.2
  external auditory canal — *see* Abscess, ear, external
  extradural G06.2
    brain G06.0
      sequelae G09
    spinal cord G06.1
  extraperitoneal K68.19
  eye — *see* Endophthalmitis, purulent
  eyelid H00.03-
  face (any part, except ear, eye and nose) L02.01
  fallopian tube — *see* Salpingitis
  fascia M72.8
  fauces J39.1
  fecal K63.0
  femoral (region) — *see* Abscess, lower limb
  filaria, filarial — *see* Infestation, filarial
  finger (any) (*see also* Abscess, hand)
    nail — *see* Cellulitis, finger
  foot L02.61-
  forehead L02.01
  frontal sinus (chronic) J32.1
  gallbladder K81.0
  genital organ or tract
    female (external) N76.4
    male N49.9
      multiple sites N49.8
      specified NEC N49.8
  gestational mammary O91.11-
  gestational subareolar O91.11-
  gingival K05.21
  gland, glandular (lymph) (acute) — *see*
    Lymphadenitis, acute
  gluteal (region) L02.31
  gonorrheal — *see* Gonococcus
  groin L02.214
  gum K05.21
  hand L02.51-
  head NEC L02.811
    face (any part, except ear, eye and nose) L02.01
  heart — *see* Carditis
  heel — *see* Abscess, foot
  helminthic — *see* Infestation, helminth
  hepatic (cholangitic) (hematogenic) (lymphogenic)
    (pylephlebitic) K75.0
    amebic A06.4
  hip (region) — *see* Abscess, lower limb
  ileocecal K35.3
  ileostomy (bud) K94.12
  iliac (region) L02.214
    fossa K35.3
  infraclavicular (fossa) — *see* Abscess, upper limb
  inguinal (region) L02.214
    lymph gland or node L04.1
  intestine, intestinal NEC K63.0
    rectal K61.1
  intra-abdominal (*see also* Abscess, peritoneum)
    K65.1
    postoperative T81.4
      retroperitoneal K68.11
  intracranial G06.0
  intramammary — *see* Abscess, breast
  intraorbital — *see* Abscess, orbit
  intraperitoneal K65.1
  intrasphincteric (anus) K61.4
  intraspinal G06.1
  intratonsillar J36
  ischiorectal (fossa) K61.3
  jaw (bone) (lower) (upper) M27.2
  joint — *see* Arthritis, pyogenic or pyemic

Abscess— *continued*
  joint— *continued*
    spine (tuberculous) A18.01
      nontuberculous — *see* Spondylopathy,
        infective
  kidney N15.1
    with calculus N20.0
      with hydronephrosis N13.6
    puerperal (postpartum) O86.21
  knee (*see also* Abscess, lower limb)
    joint M00.9
  labium (majus) (minus) N76.4
  lacrimal
    caruncle — *see* Inflammation, lacrimal, passages,
      acute
    gland — *see* Dacryoadenitis
    passages (duct) (sac) — *see* Inflammation,
      lacrimal, passages, acute
  lacunar N34.0
  larynx J38.7
  lateral (alveolar) K04.7
    with sinus K04.6
  leg (any part) — *see* Abscess, lower limb
  lens H27.8
  lingual K14.0
    tonsil J36
  lip K13.0
  Littre's gland N34.0
  liver (cholangitic) (hematogenic) (lymphogenic)
    (pylephlebitic) (pyogenic) K75.0
    amebic (due to Entamoeba histolytica)
      (dysenteric) (tropical) A06.4
      with
        brain abscess (and liver or lung abscess)
          A06.6
        lung abscess A06.5
  loin (region) L02.211
  lower limb L02.41-
  lumbar (tuberculous) A18.01
    nontuberculous L02.212
  lung (miliary) (putrid) J85.2
    with pneumonia J85.1
      due to specified organism (see Pneumonia, in
        (due to))
    amebic (with liver abscess) A06.5
      with
        brain abscess A06.6
        pneumonia A06.5
  lymph, lymphatic, gland or node (acute) (*see also*
    Lymphadenitis, acute)
  mesentery I88.0
  malar M27.2
  mammary gland — *see* Abscess, breast
  marginal, anus K61.0
  mastoid — *see* Mastoiditis, acute
  maxilla, maxillary M27.2
    molar (tooth) K04.7
      with sinus K04.6
    premolar K04.7
    sinus (chronic) J32.0
  mediastinum J85.3
  meibomian gland — *see* Hordeolum
  meninges G06.2
  mesentery, mesenteric K65.1
  mesosalpinx — *see* Salpingitis
  mons pubis L02.215
  mouth (floor) K12.2
  muscle — *see* Myositis, infective
  myocardium I40.0
  nabothian (follicle) — *see* Cervicitis
  nasal J32.9
  nasopharyngeal J39.1
  navel L02.216
    newborn P38.9
      with mild hemorrhage P38.1
      without hemorrhage P38.9
  neck (region) L02.11
    lymph gland or node L04.0
  nephritic — *see* Abscess, kidney
  nipple N61
    associated with
      lactation — *see* Pregnancy, complicated by,
      pregnancy — *see* Pregnancy, complicated by

Abscess— *continued*

nose (external) (fossa) (septum) J34.0
  sinus (chronic) — *see* Sinusitis
omentum K65.1
operative wound T81.4
orbit, orbital — *see* Cellulitis, orbit
otogenic G06.0
ovary, ovarian (corpus luteum) — *see* Oophoritis
oviduct — *see* Oophoritis
palate (soft) K12.2
  hard M27.2
palmar (space) — *see* Abscess, hand
pancreas (duct) — *see* Pancreatitis, acute
parafrenal N48.21
parametric, parametrium N73.2
  acute N73.0
  chronic N73.1
paranephric N15.1
parapancreatic — *see* Pancreatitis, acute
parapharyngeal J39.0
pararectal K61.1
parasinus — *see* Sinusitis
parauterine (*see also* Disease, pelvis, inflammatory) N73.2
paravaginal — *see* Vaginitis
parietal region (scalp) L02.811
parodontal K05.21
parotid (duct) (gland) K11.3
  region K12.2
pectoral (region) L02.213
pelvis, pelvic
  female — *see* Disease, pelvis, inflammatory
  male, peritoneal K65.1
penis N48.21
  gonococcal (accessory gland) (periurethral) A54.1
perianal K61.0
periapical K04.7
  with sinus (alveolar) K04.6
periappendicular K35.3
pericardial I30.1
pericecal K35.3
pericemental K05.21
pericholecystic — *see* Cholecystitis, acute
pericoronal K05.21
peridental K05.21
perimetric (*see also* Disease, pelvis, inflammatory) N73.2
perinephric, perinephritic — *see* Abscess, kidney
perineum, perineal (superficial) L02.215
  urethra N34.0
periodontal (parietal) K05.21
  apical K04.7
periosteum, periosteal (*see also* Osteomyelitis, specified type NEC)
  with osteomyelitis (*see also* Osteomyelitis, specified type NEC)
    acute — *see* Osteomyelitis, acute
    chronic — *see* Osteomyelitis, chronic
peripharyngeal J39.0
peripleuritic J86.9
  with fistula J86.0
periprostatic N41.2
perirectal K61.1
perirenal (tissue) — *see* Abscess, kidney
perisinuous (nose) — *see* Sinusitis
peritoneum, peritoneal (perforated) (ruptured) K65.1
  with appendicitis K35.3
  pelvic
    female — *see* Peritonitis, pelvic, female
    male K65.1
  postoperative T81.4
  puerperal, postpartum, childbirth O85
  tuberculous A18.31
peritonsillar J36
perityphlic K35.3
periureteral N28.89
periurethral N34.0
  gonococcal (accessory gland) (periurethral) A54.1
periuterine (*see also* Disease, pelvis, inflammatory) N73.2

Abscess— *continued*

perivesical — *see* Cystitis, specified type NEC
petrous bone — *see* Petrositis
phagedenic NOS L02.91
  chancroid A57
pharynx, pharyngeal (lateral) J39.1
pilonidal L05.01
pituitary (gland) E23.6
pleura J86.9
  with fistula J86.0
popliteal — *see* Abscess, lower limb
postcecal K35.3
postlaryngeal J38.7
postnasal J34.0
postoperative (any site) T81.4
  retroperitoneal K68.11
postpharyngeal J39.0
posttonsillar J36
post-typhoid A01.09
pouch of Douglas — *see* Peritonitis, pelvic, female
premammary — *see* Abscess, breast
prepatellar — *see* Abscess, lower limb
prostate N41.2
  gonococcal (acute) (chronic) A54.22
psoas muscle K68.12
puerperal—code by site under Puerperal, abscess
pulmonary — *see* Abscess, lung
pulp, pulpal (dental) K04.0
rectovaginal septum K63.0
rectovesical — *see* Cystitis, specified type NEC
rectum K61.1
renal — *see* Abscess, kidney
retina — *see* Inflammation, chorioretinal
retrobulbar — *see* Abscess, orbit
retrocecal K65.1
retrolaryngeal J38.7
retromammary — *see* Abscess, breast
retroperitoneal NEC K68.19
  postprocedural K68.11
retropharyngeal J39.0
retrouterine — *see* Peritonitis, pelvic, female
retrovesical — *see* Cystitis, specified type NEC
root, tooth K04.7
  with sinus (alveolar) K04.6
round ligament (*see also* Disease, pelvis, inflammatory) N73.2
rupture (spontaneous) NOS L02.91
sacrum (tuberculous) A18.01
  nontuberculous M46.28
salivary (duct) (gland) K11.3
scalp (any part) L02.811
scapular — *see* Osteomyelitis, specified type NEC
sclera — *see* Scleritis
scrofulous (tuberculous) A18.2
scrotum N49.2
seminal vesicle N49.0
septal, dental K04.7
  with sinus (alveolar) K04.6
serous — *see* Periostitis
shoulder (region) — *see* Abscess, upper limb
sigmoid K63.0
sinus (accessory) (chronic) (nasal) (*see also* Sinusitis)
  intracranial venous (any) G06.0
Skene's duct or gland N34.0
skin — *see* Abscess, by site
specified site NEC L02.818
spermatic cord N49.1
sphenoidal (sinus) (chronic) J32.3
spinal cord (any part) (staphylococcal) G06.1
  tuberculous A17.81
spine (column) (tuberculous) A18.01
  epidural G06.1
  nontuberculous — *see* Osteomyelitis, vertebra
spleen D73.3
  amebic A06.89
stitch T81.4
subarachnoid G06.2
  brain G06.0
  spinal cord G06.1
subareolar — *see* Abscess, breast
subcecal K35.3

Abscess— *continued*

subcutaneous (*see also* Abscess, by site)
  pheomycotic (chromomycotic) B43.2
subdiaphragmatic K65.1
subdural G06.2
  brain G06.0
    sequelae G09
  spinal cord G06.1
subgaleal L02.811
subhepatic K65.1
sublingual K12.2
  gland K11.3
submammary — *see* Abscess, breast
submandibular (region) (space) (triangle) K12.2
  gland K11.3
submaxillary (region) L02.01
  gland K11.3
submental L02.01
  gland K11.3
subperiosteal — *see* Osteomyelitis, specified type NEC
subphrenic K65.1
  postoperative T81.4
suburethral N34.0
sudoriparous L75.8
supraclavicular (fossa) — *see* Abscess, upper limb
suprapelvic, acute N73.0
suprarenal (capsule) (gland) E27.8
sweat gland L74.8
tear duct — *see* Inflammation, lacrimal, passages, acute
temple L02.01
temporal region L02.01
temporosphenoidal G06.0
tendon (sheath) M65.00
  ankle M65.07-
  foot M65.07-
  forearm M65.03-
  hand M65.04-
  lower leg M65.06-
  pelvic region M65.05-
  shoulder region M65.01-
  specified site NEC M65.08
  thigh M65.05-
  upper arm M65.02-
testis N45.4
thigh — *see* Abscess, lower limb
thorax J86.9
  with fistula J86.0
throat J39.1
thumb (*see also* Abscess, hand)
  nail — *see* Cellulitis, finger
thymus (gland) E32.1
thyroid (gland) E06.0
toe (any) (*see also* Abscess, foot)
  nail — *see* Cellulitis, toe
tongue (staphylococcal) K14.0
tonsil(s) (lingual) J36
tonsillopharyngeal J36
tooth, teeth (root) K04.7
  with sinus (alveolar) K04.6
  supporting structures NEC K05.21
trachea J39.8
trunk L02.219
  abdominal wall L02.211
  back L02.212
  chest wall L02.213
  groin L02.214
  perineum L02.215
  umbilicus L02.216
tubal — *see* Salpingitis
tuberculous — *see* Tuberculosis, abscess
tubo-ovarian — *see* Salpingo-oophoritis
tunica vaginalis N49.1
umbilicus L02.216
upper
  limb L02.41-
  respiratory J39.8
urethral (gland) N34.0
urinary N34.0
uterus, uterine (wall) (*see also* Endometritis)
  ligament (*see also* Disease, pelvis, inflammatory) N73.2

Abscess— *continued*
　uterus, uterine (wall)—*continued*
　　neck — *see* Cervicitis
　uvula K12.2
　vagina (wall) — *see* Vaginitis
　vaginorectal — *see* Vaginitis
　vas deferens N49.1
　vermiform appendix K35.3
　vertebra (column) (tuberculous) A18.01
　　nontuberculous — *see* Osteomyelitis, vertebra
　vesical — *see* Cystitis, specified type NEC
　vesico-uterine pouch — *see* Peritonitis, pelvic, female
　vitreous (humor) — *see* Endophthalmitis, purulent
　vocal cord J38.3
　von Bezold's — *see* Mastoiditis, acute
　vulva N76.4
　vulvovaginal gland N75.1
　web space — *see* Abscess, hand
　wound T81.4
　wrist — *see* Abscess, upper limb
Absence (of) (organ or part) (complete or partial)
　adrenal (gland) (congenital) Q89.1
　　acquired E89.6
　albumin in blood E88.09
　alimentary tract (congenital) Q45.8
　　upper Q40.8
　alveolar process (acquired) — *see* Anomaly, alveolar
　ankle (acquired) Z89.44-
　anus (congenital) Q42.3
　　with fistula Q42.2
　aorta (congenital) Q25.4
　appendix, congenital Q42.8
　arm (acquired) Z89.20-
　　above elbow Z89.22-
　　　congenital (with hand present) — *see* Agenesis, arm, with hand present
　　　and hand — *see* Agenesis, forearm, and hand
　　below elbow Z89.21-
　　　congenital (with hand present) — *see* Agenesis, arm, with hand present
　　　and hand — *see* Agenesis, forearm, and hand
　　congenital — *see* Defect, reduction, upper limb
　　shoulder Z89.23-
　　　congenital (with hand present) — *see* Agenesis, arm, with hand present
　artery (congenital) (peripheral) Q27.8
　　brain Q28.3
　　coronary Q24.5
　　pulmonary Q25.7
　　specified NEC Q27.8
　　umbilical Q27.0
　atrial septum (congenital) Q21.1
　auditory canal (congenital) (external) Q16.1
　auricle (ear), congenital Q16.0
　bile, biliary duct, congenital Q44.5
　bladder (acquired) Z90.6
　　congenital Q64.5
　bowel sounds R19.11
　brain Q00.0
　　part of Q04.3
　breast(s) (and nipple(s)) (acquired) Z90.1-
　　congenital Q83.8
　broad ligament Q50.6
　bronchus (congenital) Q32.4
　canaliculus lacrimalis, congenital Q10.4
　cerebellum (vermis) Q04.3
　cervix (acquired) (with uterus) Z90.710
　　with remaining uterus Z90.712
　　congenital Q51.5
　chin, congenital Q18.8
　cilia (congenital) Q10.3
　　acquired — *see* Madarosis
　clitoris (congenital) Q52.6
　coccyx, congenital Q76.49
　cold sense R20.8
　congenital
　　lumen — *see* Atresia
　　organ or site NEC — *see* Agenesis
　　septum — *see* Imperfect, closure
　corpus callosum Q04.0

Absence— *continued*
　cricoid cartilage, congenital Q31.8
　diaphragm (with hernia), congenital Q79.1
　digestive organ(s) or tract, congenital Q45.8
　　acquired NEC Z90.49
　　upper Q40.8
　ductus arteriosus Q28.8
　duodenum (acquired) Z90.49
　　congenital Q41.0
　ear, congenital Q16.9
　　acquired H93.8-
　　auricle Q16.0
　　external Q16.0
　　inner Q16.5
　　lobe, lobule Q17.8
　　middle, except ossicles Q16.4
　　　ossicles Q16.3
　　ossicles Q16.3
　ejaculatory duct (congenital) Q55.4
　endocrine gland (congenital) NEC Q89.2
　　acquired E89.89
　epididymis (congenital) Q55.4
　　acquired Z90.79
　epiglottis, congenital Q31.8
　esophagus (congenital) Q39.8
　　acquired (partial) Z90.49
　eustachian tube (congenital) Q16.2
　extremity (acquired) Z89.9
　　congenital Q73.0
　　lower (above knee) Z89.619
　　　below knee Z89.5-
　　upper — *see* Absence, arm
　eye (acquired) Z90.01
　　congenital Q11.1
　　muscle (congenital) Q10.3
　eyeball (acquired) Z90.01
　eyelid (fold) (congenital) Q10.3
　　acquired Z90.01
　face, specified part NEC Q18.8
　fallopian tube(s) (acquired) Z90.79
　　congenital Q50.6
　family member (causing problem in home) NEC Z63.32 (*see also* Disruption, family)
　femur, congenital — *see* Defect, reduction, lower limb, longitudinal, femur
　fibrinogen (congenital) D68.2
　　acquired D65
　finger(s) (acquired) Z89.02-
　　congenital — *see* Agenesis, hand
　foot (acquired) Z89.43-
　　congenital — *see* Agenesis, foot
　forearm (acquired) — *see* Absence, arm, below elbow
　gallbladder (acquired) Z90.49
　　congenital Q44.0
　gamma globulin in blood D80.1
　　hereditary D80.0
　genital organs
　　acquired (female) (male) Z90.79
　　female, congenital Q52.8
　　　external Q52.71
　　　internal NEC Q52.8
　　male, congenital Q55.8
　genitourinary organs, congenital NEC
　　female Q52.8
　　male Q55.8
　globe (acquired) Z90.01
　　congenital Q11.1
　glottis, congenital Q31.8
　hand and wrist (acquired) Z89.11-
　　congenital — *see* Agenesis, hand
　head, part (acquired) NEC Z90.09
　heat sense R20.8
　hip Z89.62-
　hymen (congenital) Q52.4
　ileum (acquired) Z90.49
　　congenital Q41.2
　immunoglobulin, isolated NEC D80.3
　　IgA D80.2
　　IgG D80.3
　　IgM D80.4
　incus (acquired) — *see* Loss, ossicles, ear
　　congenital Q16.3

Absence— *continued*
　inner ear, congenital Q16.5
　intestine (acquired) (small) Z90.49
　　congenital Q41.9
　　　specified NEC Q41.8
　　large Z90.49
　　　congenital Q42.9
　　　　specified NEC Q42.8
　iris, congenital Q13.1
　jejunum (acquired) Z90.49
　　congenital Q41.1
　joint, congenital NEC Q74.8
　kidney(s) (acquired) Z90.5
　　congenital Q60.2
　　　bilateral Q60.1
　　　unilateral Q60.0
　labyrinth, membranous Q16.5
　larynx (congenital) Q31.8
　　acquired Z90.02
　leg (acquired) (above knee) Z89.61-
　　below knee (acquired) Z89.5-
　　congenital — *see* Defect, reduction, lower limb
　lens (acquired) (*see also* Aphakia)
　　congenital Q12.3
　　post cataract extraction Z98.4-
　limb (acquired) — *see* Absence, extremity
　lip Q38.6
　liver (congenital) Q44.7
　lung (fissure) (lobe) (bilateral) (unilateral) (congenital) Q33.3
　　acquired (any part) Z90.2
　menstruation — *see* Amenorrhea
　muscle (congenital) (pectoral) Q79.8
　　ocular Q10.3
　neck, part Q18.8
　neutrophil — *see* Agranulocytosis
　nipple(s) (with breast(s)) (acquired) Z90.1-
　　congenital Q83.2
　nose (congenital) Q30.1
　　acquired Z90.09
　organ
　　of Corti, congenital Q16.5
　　or site, congenital NEC Q89.8
　　　acquired NEC Z90.89
　osseous meatus (ear) Q16.4
　ovary (acquired)
　　bilateral Z90.722
　　congenital
　　　bilateral Q50.02
　　　unilateral Q50.01
　　unilateral Z90.721
　oviduct (acquired)
　　bilateral Z90.722
　　congenital Q50.6
　　unilateral Z90.721
　pancreas (congenital) Q45.0
　　acquired Z90.410
　　　complete Z90.410
　　　partial Z90.411
　　　total Z90.410
　parathyroid gland (acquired) E89.2
　　congenital Q89.2
　patella, congenital Q74.1
　penis (congenital) Q55.5
　　acquired Z90.79
　pericardium (congenital) Q24.8
　pituitary gland (congenital) Q89.2
　　acquired E89.3
　prostate (acquired) Z90.79
　　congenital Q55.4
　pulmonary valve Q22.0
　punctum lacrimale (congenital) Q10.4
　radius, congenital — *see* Defect, reduction, upper limb, longitudinal, radius
　rectum (congenital) Q42.1
　　with fistula Q42.0
　　acquired Z90.49
　respiratory organ NOS Q34.9
　rib (acquired) Z90.89
　　congenital Q76.6
　sacrum, congenital Q76.49
　salivary gland(s), congenital Q38.4
　scrotum, congenital Q55.29

Absence— *continued*
  seminal vesicles (congenital) Q55.4
    acquired Z90.79
  septum
    atrial (congenital) Q21.1
    between aorta and pulmonary artery Q21.4
    ventricular (congenital) Q20.4
  sex chromosome
    female phenotype Q97.8
    male phenotype Q98.8
  skull bone (congenital) Q75.8
    with
      anencephaly Q00.0
      encephalocele — *see* Encephalocele
      hydrocephalus Q03.9
        with spina bifida — *see* Spina bifida, by
          site, with hydrocephalus
      microcephaly Q02
  spermatic cord, congenital Q55.4
  spine, congenital Q76.49
  spleen (congenital) Q89.01
    acquired Z90.81
  sternum, congenital Q76.7
  stomach (acquired) (partial) Z90.3
    congenital Q40.2
  superior vena cava, congenital Q26.8
  teeth, tooth (congenital) K00.0
    acquired (complete) K08.109
      class I K08.101
      class II K08.102
      class III K08.103
      class IV K08.104
      due to
        caries K08.139
          class I K08.131
          class II K08.132
          class III K08.133
          class IV K08.134
        periodontal disease K08.129
          class I K08.121
          class II K08.122
          class III K08.123
          class IV K08.124
      specified NEC K08.199
        class I K08.191
        class II K08.192
        class III K08.193
        class IV K08.194
      trauma K08.119
        class I K08.111
        class II K08.112
        class III K08.113
        class IV K08.114
    partial K08.409
      class I K08.401
      class II K08.402
      class III K08.403
      class IV K08.404
      due to
        caries K08.439
          class I K08.431
          class II K08.432
          class III K08.433
          class IV K08.434
        periodontal disease K08.429
          class I K08.421
          class II K08.422
          class III K08.423
          class IV K08.424
      specified NEC K08.499
        class I K08.491
        class II K08.492
        class III K08.493
        class IV K08.494
      trauma K08.419
        class I K08.411
        class II K08.412
        class III K08.413
        class IV K08.414
  tendon (congenital) Q79.8
  testis (congenital) Q55.0
    acquired Z90.79

Absence— *continued*
  thumb (acquired) Z89.01-
    congenital — *see* Agenesis, hand
  thymus gland Q89.2
  thyroid (gland) (acquired) E89.0
    cartilage, congenital Q31.8
    congenital E03.1
  toe(s) (acquired) Z89.42-
    with foot — *see* Absence, foot and ankle
    congenital — *see* Agenesis, foot
    great Z89.41-
  tongue, congenital Q38.3
  trachea (cartilage), congenital Q32.1
  transverse aortic arch, congenital Q25.4
  tricuspid valve Q22.4
  umbilical artery, congenital Q27.0
  upper arm and forearm with hand present,
    congenital — *see* Agenesis, arm, with hand
    present
  ureter (congenital) Q62.4
    acquired Z90.6
  urethra, congenital Q64.5
  uterus (acquired) Z90.710
    with cervix Z90.710
    with remaining cervical stump Z90.711
    congenital Q51.0
  uvula, congenital Q38.5
  vagina, congenital Q52.0
  vas deferens (congenital) Q55.4
    acquired Z90.79
  vein (peripheral) congenital NEC Q27.8
    cerebral Q28.3
    digestive system Q27.8
    great Q26.8
    lower limb Q27.8
    portal Q26.5
    precerebral Q28.1
    specified site NEC Q27.8
    upper limb Q27.8
  vena cava (inferior) (superior), congenital Q26.8
  ventricular septum Q20.4
  vertebra, congenital Q76.49
  vulva, congenital Q52.71
  wrist (acquired) Z89.12-

Absorbent system disease I87.8
Absorption
  carbohydrate, disturbance K90.4
  chemical — *see* Table of Drugs and Chemicals
    through placenta (newborn) P04.9
      environmental substance P04.6
      nutritional substance P04.5
      obstetric anesthetic or analgesic drug P04.0
  drug NEC — *see* Table of Drugs and Chemicals
    addictive
      through placenta (newborn) P04.49
        cocaine P04.41
    medicinal
      through placenta (newborn) P04.1
    through placenta (newborn) P04.1
      obstetric anesthetic or analgesic drug P04.0
  fat, disturbance K90.4
    pancreatic K90.3
  noxious substance — *see* Table of Drugs and
    Chemicals
  protein, disturbance K90.4
  starch, disturbance K90.4
  toxic substance — *see* Table of Drugs and Chemicals
  uremic — *see* Uremia

Abstinence symptoms, syndrome
  alcohol F10.239
    with delirium F10.231
  cocaine F14.23
  neonatal P96.1
  nicotine — *see* Dependence, drug, nicotine, with,
    withdrawal
  opioid F11.93
    with dependence F11.23
  psychoactive NEC F19.939
    with
      delirium F19.931
      dependence F19.239
        with
          delirium F19.231

Abstinence symptoms, syndrome— *continued*
  psychoactive — *continued*
    with— *continued*
      dependence — *continued*
        with— *continued*
          perceptual disturbance F19.232
          uncomplicated F19.230
      perceptual disturbance F19.932
      uncomplicated F19.930
  sedative F13.939
    with
      delirium F13.931
      dependence F13.239
        with
          delirium F13.231
          perceptual disturbance F13.232
          uncomplicated F13.230
      perceptual disturbance F13.932
      uncomplicated F13.930
  stimulant NEC F15.93
    with dependence F15.23

Abulia R68.89
Abulomania F60.7
Abuse
  adult — *see* Maltreatment, adult
  as reason for
    couple seeking advice (including offender)
      Z63.0
  alcohol (non-dependent) F10.10
    with
      anxiety disorder F10.180
      intoxication F10.129
        with delirium F10.121
        uncomplicated F10.120
      mood disorder F10.14
      other specified disorder F10.188
      psychosis F10.159
        delusions F10.150
        hallucinations F10.151
      sexual dysfunction F10.181
      sleep disorder F10.182
      unspecified disorder F10.19
    counseling and surveillance Z71.41
  amphetamine (or related substance) — *see* Abuse,
    drug, stimulant NEC
  analgesics (non-prescribed) (over the counter) F55.8
  antacids F55.0
  antidepressants — *see* Abuse, drug, psychoactive
    NEC
  anxiolytic — *see* Abuse, drug, sedative
  barbiturates — *see* Abuse, drug, sedative
  caffeine — *see* Abuse, drug, stimulant NEC
  cannabis, cannabinoids — *see* Abuse, drug,
    cannabis
  child — *see* Maltreatment, child
  cocaine — *see* Abuse, drug, cocaine
  drug NEC (non-dependent) F19.10
    with sleep disorder F19.182
    amphetamine type — *see* Abuse, drug, stimulant
      NEC
    analgesics (non-prescribed) (over the counter)
      F55.8
    antacids F55.0
    antidepressants — *see* Abuse, drug, psychoactive
      NEC
    anxiolytics — *see* Abuse, drug, sedative
    barbiturates — *see* Abuse, drug, sedative
    caffeine — *see* Abuse, drug, stimulant NEC
    cannabis F12.10
      with
        anxiety disorder F12.180
        intoxication F12.129
          with
            delirium F12.121
            perceptual disturbance F12.122
          uncomplicated F12.120
        other specified disorder F12.188
        psychosis F12.159
          delusions F12.150
          hallucinations F12.151
        unspecified disorder F12.19
    cocaine F14.10

Abuse—*continued*
  drug—*continued*
    cocaine—*continued*
      with
        anxiety disorder F14.180
        intoxication F14.129
          with
            delirium F14.121
            perceptual disturbance F14.122
          uncomplicated F14.120
        mood disorder F14.14
        other specified disorder F14.188
        psychosis F14.159
          delusions F14.150
          hallucinations F14.151
        sexual dysfunction F14.181
        sleep disorder F14.182
        unspecified disorder F14.19
    counseling and surveillance Z71.51
    hallucinogen F16.10
      with
        anxiety disorder F16.180
        flashbacks F16.183
        intoxication F16.129
          with
            delirium F16.121
            perceptual disturbance F16.122
          uncomplicated F16.120
        mood disorder F16.14
        other specified disorder F16.188
        perception disorder, persisting F16.183
        psychosis F16.159
          delusions F16.150
          hallucinations F16.151
        unspecified disorder F16.19
    hashish — *see* Abuse, drug, cannabis
    herbal or folk remedies F55.1
    hormones F55.3
    hypnotics — *see* Abuse, drug, sedative
    inhalant F18.10
      with
        anxiety disorder F18.180
        dementia, persisting F18.17
        intoxication F18.129
          with delirium F18.121
          uncomplicated F18.120
        mood disorder F18.14
        other specified disorder F18.188
        psychosis F18.159
          delusions F18.150
          hallucinations F18.151
         unspecified disorder F18.19
    laxatives F55.2
    LSD — *see* Abuse, drug, hallucinogen
    marihuana — *see* Abuse, drug, cannabis
    morphine type (opioids) — *see* Abuse, drug,
      opioid
    opioid F11.10
      with
        intoxication F11.129
          with
            delirium F11.121
            perceptual disturbance F11.122
          uncomplicated F11.120
        mood disorder F11.14
        other specified disorder F11.188
        psychosis F11.159
          delusions F11.150
          hallucinations F11.151
        sexual dysfunction F11.181
        sleep disorder F11.182
        unspecified disorder F11.19
    PCP (phencyclidine) (or related substance) — *see*
      Abuse, drug, psychoactive NEC
    psychoactive NEC F19.10
      with
        amnestic disorder F19.16
        anxiety disorder F19.180
        dementia F19.17
        Intoxication F19.129
          with
            delirium F19.121
            perceptual disturbance F19.122

Abuse—*continued*
  drug—*continued*
    psychoactive—*continued*
      with—*continued*
        intoxication—*continued*
          uncomplicated F19.120
        mood disorder F19.14
        other specified disorder F19.188
        psychosis F19.159
          delusions F19.150
          hallucinations F19.151
        sexual dysfunction F19.181
        sleep disorder F19.182
        unspecified disorder F19.19
    sedative, hypnotic or anxiolytic F13.10
      with
        anxiety disorder F13.180
        intoxication F13.129
          with delirium F13.121
          uncomplicated F13.120
        mood disorder F13.14
        other specified disorder F13.188
        psychosis F13.159
          delusions F13.150
          hallucinations F13.151
        sexual dysfunction F13.181
        sleep disorder F13.182
        unspecified disorder F13.19
    solvent — *see* Abuse, drug, inhalant
    steroids F55.3
    stimulant NEC F15.10
      with
        anxiety disorder F15.180
        intoxication F15.129
          with
            delirium F15.121
            perceptual disturbance F15.122
          uncomplicated F15.120
        mood disorder F15.14
        other specified disorder F15.188
        psychosis F15.159
          delusions F15.150
          hallucinations F15.151
        sexual dysfunction F15.181
        sleep disorder F15.182
        unspecified disorder F15.19
    tranquilizers — *see* Abuse, drug, sedative
    vitamins F55.4
  hallucinogens — *see* Abuse, drug, hallucinogen
  hashish — *see* Abuse, drug, cannabis
  herbal or folk remedies F55.1
  hormones F55.3
  hypnotic — *see* Abuse, drug, sedative
  inhalant — *see* Abuse, drug, inhalant
  laxatives F55.2
  LSD — *see* Abuse, drug, hallucinogen
  marihuana — *see* Abuse, drug, cannabis
  morphine type (opioids) — *see* Abuse, drug, opioid
  non-psychoactive substance NEC F55.8
    antacids F55.0
    folk remedies F55.1
    herbal remedies F55.1
    hormones F55.3
    laxatives F55.2
    steroids F55.3
    vitamins F55.4
  opioids — *see* Abuse, drug, opioid
  PCP (phencyclidine) (or related substance) — *see*
    Abuse, drug, psychoactive NEC
  physical (adult) (child) — *see* Maltreatment, physical
    abuse
  psychoactive substance — *see* Abuse, drug,
    psychoactive NEC
  psychological (adult) (child) — *see* Maltreatment.
    psychological abuse
  sedative — *see* Abuse, drug, sedative
  sexual — *see* Maltreatment, sexual abuse
  solvent — *see* Abuse, drug, inhalant
  sterolds F55.3
  vitamins F55.4
Acalculia R48.8
  developmental F81.2

Acanthamebiasis (with) B60.10
  conjunctiva B60.12
  keratoconjunctivitis B60.13
  meningoencephalitis B60.11
  other specified B60.19
Acanthocephaliasis B83.8
Acanthocheilonemiasis B74.4
Acanthocytosis E78.6
Acantholysis L11.9
Acanthosis (acquired) (nigricans) L83
  benign Q82.8
  congenital Q82.8
  seborrheic L82.1
    inflamed L82.0
  tongue K14.3
Acapnia E87.3
Acarbia E87.2
Acardia, acardius Q89.8
Acardiacus amorphus Q89.8
Acardiotrophia I51.4
Acariasis B88.0
  scabies B86
Acarodermatitis (urticarioides) B88.0
Acarophobia F40.218
Acatalasemia, acatalasia E80.3
Acathisia (drug induced) G25.71
Accelerated atrioventricular conduction I45.6
Accentuation of personality traits (type A) Z73.1
Accessory (congenital)
  adrenal gland Q89.1
  anus Q43.4
  appendix Q43.4
  atrioventricular conduction I45.6
  auditory ossicles Q16.3
  auricle (ear) Q17.0
  biliary duct or passage Q44.5
  bladder Q64.79
  blood vessels NEC Q27.9
    coronary Q24.5
  bone NEC Q79.8
  breast tissue, axilla Q83.1
  carpal bones Q74.0
  cecum Q43.4
  chromosome(s) NEC (nonsex) Q92.9
    with complex rearrangements NEC Q92.5
      seen only at prometaphase Q92.8
    partial Q92.9
    sex
      female phenotype Q97.8
    13 — *see* Trisomy, 13
    18 — *see* Trisomy, 18
    21 — *see* Trisomy, 21
  coronary artery Q24.5
  cusp(s), heart valve NEC Q24.8
    pulmonary Q22.3
  cystic duct Q44.5
  digit(s) Q69.9
  ear (auricle) (lobe) Q17.0
  endocrine gland NEC Q89.2
  eye muscle Q10.3
  eyelid Q10.3
  face bone(s) Q75.8
  fallopian tube (fimbria) (ostium) Q50.6
  finger(s) Q69.0
  foreskin N47.8
  frontonasal process Q75.8
  gallbladder Q44.1
  genital organ(s)
    female Q52.8
      external Q52.79
      internal NEC Q52.8
    male Q55.8
  genitourinary organs NEC Q89.8
    female Q52.8
    male Q55.8
  hallux Q69.2
  heart Q24.8
    valve NEC Q24.8
      pulmonary Q22.3
  hepatic ducts Q44.5
  hymen Q52.4
  intestine (large) (small) Q43.4
  kidney Q63.0

Accessory— *continued*
　lacrimal canal Q10.6
　leaflet, heart valve NEC Q24.8
　ligament, broad Q50.6
　liver Q44.7
　　duct Q44.5
　lobule (ear) Q17.0
　lung (lobe) Q33.1
　muscle Q79.8
　navicular of carpus Q74.0
　nervous system, part NEC Q07.8
　nipple Q83.3
　nose Q30.8
　organ or site not listed — *see* Anomaly, by site
　ovary Q50.31
　oviduct Q50.6
　pancreas Q45.3
　parathyroid gland Q89.2
　parotid gland (and duct) Q38.4
　pituitary gland Q89.2
　preauricular appendage Q17.0
　prepuce N47.8
　renal arteries (multiple) Q27.2
　rib Q76.6
　　cervical Q76.5
　roots (teeth) K00.2
　salivary gland Q38.4
　sesamoid bones Q74.8
　　foot Q74.2
　　hand Q74.0
　skin tags Q82.8
　spleen Q89.09
　sternum Q76.7
　submaxillary gland Q38.4
　tarsal bones Q74.2
　teeth, tooth K00.1
　tendon Q79.8
　thumb Q69.1
　thymus gland Q89.2
　thyroid gland Q89.2
　toes Q69.2
　tongue Q38.3
　tooth, teeth K00.1
　tragus Q17.0
　ureter Q62.5
　urethra Q64.79
　urinary organ or tract NEC Q64.8
　uterus Q51.2
　vagina Q52.10
　valve, heart NEC Q24.8
　　pulmonary Q22.2
　vertebra Q76.49
　vocal cords Q31.8
　vulva Q52.79
Accident
　birth — *see* Birth, injury
　cardiac — *see* Infarct, myocardium
　cerebral I63.9
　cerebrovascular (embolic) (ischemic) (thrombotic)
　　　I63.9
　　aborted I63.9
　　hemorrhagic — *see* Hemorrhage, intracranial,
　　　intracerebral
　　old (without sequelae) Z86.73
　　　with sequelae (of) — *see* Sequelae, disease,
　　　　cerebrovascular disease
　　coronary — *see* Infarct, myocardium
　craniovascular I63.9
　vascular, brain I63.9
Accidental — *see* condition
Accommodation (disorder) (*see also* condition)
　hysterical paralysis of F44.89
　insufficiency of H52.4
　paresis — *see* Paresis, of accommodation
　spasm — *see* Spasm, of accommodation
Accouchement — *see* Delivery
Accreta placenta O43.21-
Accretio cordis (nonrheumatic) I31.0
Accretions, tooth, teeth K03.6
Acculturation difficulty Z60.3
Accumulation secretion, prostate N42.89
Acephalia, acephalism, acephalus, acephaly Q00.0
Acephalobrachia monster Q89.8

Acephalochirus monster Q89.8
Acephalogaster Q89.8
Acephalostomus monster Q89.8
Acephalothorax Q89.8
Acerophobia F40.298
Acetonemia R79.89
　in Type 1 diabetes E10.10
　　with coma E10.11
Acetonuria R82.4
Achalasia (cardia) (esophagus) K22.0
　congenital Q39.5
　pylorus Q40.0
　sphincteral NEC K59.8
Ache(s) — *see* Pain
Acheilia Q38.6
Achillobursitis — *see* Tendinitis, Achilles
Achillodynia — *see* Tendinitis, Achilles
Achlorhydria, achlorhydric (neurogenic) K31.83
　anemia D50.8
　diarrhea K31.83
　psychogenic F45.8
　secondary to vagotomy K91.1
Achluophobia F40.228
Acholia K82.8
Acholuric jaundice (familial) (splenomegalic) (*see also*
　　Spherocytosis)
　acquired D59.8
Achondrogenesis Q77.0
Achondroplasia (osteosclerosis congenita) Q77.4
Achroma, cutis L80
Achromat(ism), achromatopsia (acquired)
　　(congenital) H53.51
Achromia, congenital — *see* Albinism
Achromia parasitica B36.0
Achylia gastrica K31.89
　psychogenic F45.8
Acid
　burn — *see* Corrosion
　deficiency
　　amide nicotinic E52
　　ascorbic E54
　　folic E53.8
　　nicotinic E52
　　pantothenic E53.8
　intoxication E87.2
　peptic disease K30
　phosphatase deficiency E83.39
　stomach K30
　　psychogenic F45.8
Acidemia E87.2
　argininosuccinic E72.22
　isovaleric E71.110
　metabolic (newborn) P19.9
　　first noted before onset of labor P19.0
　　first noted during labor P19.1
　　noted at birth P19.2
　methylmalonic E71.120
　pipecolic E72.3
　propionic E71.121
Acidity, gastric (high) K30
　psychogenic F45.8
Acidocytopenia — *see* Agranulocytosis
Acidocytosis D72.1
Acidopenia — *see* Agranulocytosis
Acidosis (lactic) (respiratory) E87.2
　in Type 1 diabetes E10.10
　　with coma E10.11
　kidney, tubular N25.89
　lactic E87.2
　metabolic NEC E87.2
　　with respiratory acidosis E87.4
　　late, of newborn P74.0
　mixed metabolic and respiratory, newborn P84
　newborn P84
　renal (hyperchloremic) (tubular) N25.89
　respiratory E87.2
　　complicated by
　　　metabolic
　　　　acidosis E87.4
　　　　alkalosis E87.4
Aciduria
　argininosuccinic E72.22

Aciduria— *continued*
　glutaric (type I) E72.3
　　type II E71.313
　　type III E71.5-
　orotic (congenital) (hereditary) (pyrimidine
　　deficiency) E79.8
　　anemia D53.0
Acladiosis (skin) B36.0
Aclasis, diaphyseal Q78.6
Acleistocardia Q21.1
Aclusion — *see* Anomaly, dentofacial, malocclusion
Acne L70.9
　artificialis L70.8
　atrophica L70.2
　cachecticorum (Hebra) L70.8
　conglobata L70.1
　cystic L70.0
　decalvans L66.2
　excoriée des jeunes filles L70.5
　frontalis L70.2
　indurata L70.0
　infantile L70.4
　keloid L73.0
　lupoid L70.2
　necrotic, necrotica (miliaris) L70.2
　neonatal L70.4
　nodular L70.0
　occupational L70.8
　picker's L70.5
　pustular L70.0
　rodens L70.2
　rosacea L71.9
　specified NEC L70.8
　tropica L70.3
　varioliformis L70.2
　vulgaris L70.0
Acnitis (primary) A18.4
Acosta's disease T70.29
Acoustic — *see* condition
Acousticophobia F40.298
Acquired (*see also* condition)
　immunodeficiency syndrome (AIDS) B20
Acrania Q00.0
Acroasphyxia, chronic I73.89
Acrobystitis N47.7
Acrocephalopolysyndactyly Q87.0
Acrocephalosyndactyly Q87.0
Acrocephaly Q75.0
Acrochondrohyperplasia — *see* Syndrome, Marfan's
Acrocyanosis I73.8
　newborn P28.2
　meaning transient blue hands and feet—*omit code*
Acrodermatitis L30.8
　atrophicans (chronica) L90.4
　continua (Hallopeau) L40.2
　enteropathica (hereditary) E83.2
　Hallopeau's L40.2
　infantile papular L44.4
　perstans L40.2
　pustulosa continua L40.2
　recalcitrant pustular L40.2
Acrodynia — *see* Poisoning, mercury
Acromegaly, acromegalia E22.0
Acromelalgia I73.81
Acromicria, acromikria Q79.8
Acronyx L60.0
Acropachy, thyroid — *see* Thyrotoxicosis
Acroparesthesia (simple) (vasomotor) I73.89
Acropathy, thyroid — *see* Thyrotoxicosis
Acrophobia F40.241
Acroposthitis N47.7
Acroscleriasis, acroscleroderma, acrosclerosis —
　　see Sclerosis, systemic
Acrosphacelus I96
Acrospiroma, eccrine — *see* Neoplasm, skin, benign
Acrostealgia — *see* Osteochondropathy
Acrotrophodynia — *see* Immersion
ACTH ectopic syndrome E24.3
Actinic — *see* condition
Actinobacillosis, actinobacillus A28.8
　mallei A24.0
　muris A25.1
Actinomyces israelii (infection) — *see* Actinomycosis

Actinomycetoma (foot) B47.1
Actinomycosis, actinomycotic A42.9
  with pneumonia A42.0
  abdominal A42.1
  cervicofacial A42.2
  cutaneous A42.89
  gastrointestinal A42.1
  pulmonary A42.0
  sepsis A42.7
  specified site NEC A42.89
Actinoneuritis G62.8
Action, heart
  disorder I49.9
  irregular I49.9
    psychogenic F45.8
Active — *see* condition
Activated protein C resistance D68.51
Acute (*see also* condition)
  abdomen R10.0
  gallbladder — *see* Cholecystitis, acute
Acyanotic heart disease (congenital) Q24.9
Acystia Q64.5
Adair-Dighton syndrome (brittle bones and blue
    sclera, deafness) Q78.0
Adamantinoblastoma — *see* Ameloblastoma
Adamantinoma (*see also* Cyst, calcifying odontogenic)
  long bones C40.90
    lower limb C40.2-
    upper limb C40.0-
  malignant C41.1
    jaw (bone) (lower) C41.1
      upper C41.0
  tibial C40.2
Adamantoblastoma — *see* Ameloblastoma
Adams-Stokes (-Morgagni) disease or syndrome
  I45.9
Adaption reaction — *see* Disorder, adjustment
Addiction (*see also* Dependence) F19.20
  alcohol, alcoholic (ethyl) (methyl) (wood) (without
    remission) F10.20
    with remission F10.21
  drug — *see* Dependence, drug
  ethyl alcohol (without remission) F10.20
    with remission F10.21
  heroin — *see* Dependence, drug, opioid
  methyl alcohol (without remission) F10.20
    with remission F10.21
  methylated spirit (without remission) F10.20
    with remission F10.21
  morphine(-like substances) — *see* Dependence,
    drug, opioid
  nicotine — *see* Dependence, drug, nicotine
  opium and opioids — *see* Dependence, drug, opioid
  tobacco — *see* Dependence, drug, nicotine
Addisonian crisis E27.2
Addison's
  anemia (pernicious) D51.0
  disease (bronze) or syndrome E27.1
    tuberculous A18.7
  keloid L94.0
Addison-Biermer anemia (pernicious) D51.0
Addison-Schilder complex E71.528
Additional (*see also* Accessory)
  chromosome(s) Q99.8
    sex — *see* Abnormal, chromosome, sex
    21 — *see* Trisomy, 21
Adduction contracture, hip or other joint — *see*
  Contraction, joint
Adenitis (*see also* Lymphadenitis)
  acute, unspecified site L04.9
  axillary I88.9
    acute L04.2
    chronic or subacute I88.1
  Bartholin's gland N75.8
  bulbourethral gland — *see* Urethritis
  cervical I88.9
    acute L04.0
    chronic or subacute I88.1
  chancroid (Hemophilus ducreyi) A57
  chronic, unspecified site I88.1
  Cowper's gland — *see* Urethritis
  due to Pasteurella multocida (P. septica) A28.0

Adenitis — *continued*
  epidemic, acute B27.09
  gangrenous L04.9
  gonorrheal NEC A54.89
  groin I88.9
    acute L04.1
    chronic or subacute I88.1
  infectious (acute) (epidemic) B27.09
  inguinal I88.9
    acute L04.1
    chronic or subacute I88.1
  lymph gland or node, except mesenteric I88.9
    acute — *see* Lymphadenitis, acute
    chronic or subacute I88.1
  mesenteric (acute) (chronic) (nonspecific)
    (subacute) I88.0
  parotid gland (suppurative) — *see* Sialoadenitis
  salivary gland (any) (suppurative) — *see*
    Sialoadenitis
  scrofulous (tuberculous) A18.2
  Skene's duct or gland — *see* Urethritis
  strumous, tuberculous A18.2
  subacute, unspecified site I88.1
  sublingual gland (suppurative) — *see* Sialoadenitis
  submandibular gland (suppurative) — *see*
    Sialoadenitis
  submaxillary gland (suppurative) — *see*
    Sialoadenitis
  tuberculous — *see* Tuberculosis, lymph gland
  urethral gland — *see* Urethritis
  Wharton's duct (suppurative) — *see* Sialoadenitis
Adenoacanthoma — *see* Neoplasm, malignant, by
  site
Adenoameloblastoma — *see* Cyst, calcifying
  odontogenic
Adenocarcinoid (tumor) — *see* Neoplasm, malignant,
  by site
Adenocarcinoma (*see also* Neoplasm, malignant, by
  site)
  acidophil
    specified site — *see* Neoplasm, malignant, by site
    unspecified site C75.1
  adrenal cortical C74.0-
  alveolar — *see* Neoplasm, lung, malignant
  apocrine
    breast — *see* Neoplasm, breast, malignant
    in situ
      breast D05.8-
      specified site NEC — *see* Neoplasm, skin, in
        situ
      unspecified site D04.9
    specified site NEC — *see* Neoplasm, skin,
      malignant
    unspecified site C44.9
  basal cell
    specified site — *see* Neoplasm, skin, malignant
    unspecified site C08.9
  basophil
    specified site — *see* Neoplasm, malignant, by site
    unspecified site C75.1
  bile duct type C22.1
    liver C22.1
    specified site NEC — *see* Neoplasm, malignant,
      by site
    unspecified site C22.1
  bronchiolar — *see* Neoplasm, lung, malignant
  bronchioloalveolar — *see* Neoplasm, lung,
    malignant
  ceruminous C44.2-
  cervix, in situ D06.9 (*see also* Carcinoma, cervix uteri,
    in situ)
  chromophobe
    specified site — *see* Neoplasm, malignant, by site
    unspecified site C75.1
  diffuse type
    specified site — *see* Neoplasm, malignant, by site
    unspecified site C16.9
  duct
    infiltrating
      with Paget's disease — *see* Neoplasm, breast,
        malignant, by site

Adenocarcinoma — *continued*
  duct— *continued*
    infiltrating— *continued*
      specified site — *see* Neoplasm, malignant, by
        site
      unspecified site (female) C50.91-
        male C50.92-
    specified site — *see* Neoplasm, malignant, by site
    unspecified site
      female C56.9
      male C61
  eosinophil
    specified site — *see* Neoplasm, malignant, by site
    unspecified site C75.1
  follicular
    with papillary C73
    moderately differentiated C73
    specified site — *see* Neoplasm, malignant, by site
    trabecular C73
    unspecified site C73
    well differentiated C73
  Hurthle cell C73
  in
    adenomatous
      polyposis coli C18.9
  infiltrating duct
    with Paget's disease — *see* Neoplasm, breast,
      malignant
    specified site — *see* Neoplasm, malignant, by site
    unspecified site (female) C50.91-
      male C50.92-
  inflammatory
    specified site — *see* Neoplasm, malignant, by site
    unspecified site (female) C50.91-
      male C50.92-
  intestinal type
    specified site — *see* Neoplasm, malignant, by site
    unspecified site C16.9
  intracystic papillary
  intraductal
    breast D05.8-
    noninfiltrating
      breast D05.8-
      papillary
        with invasion
          specified site — *see* Neoplasm,
            malignant, by site
          unspecified site (female) C50.91-
            male C50.92-
        breast D05.8-
        specified site NEC — *see* Neoplasm, in situ,
          by site
        unspecified site D05.8-
      specified site NEC — *see* Neoplasm, in situ, by
        site
      unspecified site D05.8-
    papillary
      with invasion
        specified site — *see* Neoplasm, malignant,
          by site
        unspecified site (female) C50.91-
          male C50.92-
        breast D05.8-
      specified site — *see* Neoplasm, in situ, by site
      unspecified site D05.8-
    specified site NEC — *see* Neoplasm, in situ, by site
    unspecified site D05.8-
  islet cell
    with exocrine, mixed
      specified site — *see* Neoplasm, malignant, by
        site
      unspecified site C25.9
    pancreas C25.4
    specified site NEC — *see* Neoplasm, malignant,
      by site
    unspecified site C25.4
  lobular
    in situ
      breast D05.0-
      specified site NEC — *see* Neoplasm, in situ, by
        site
      unspecified site D05.0-

Adenocarcinoma— *continued*
  lobular— *continued*
    specified site — *see* Neoplasm, malignant, by site
    unspecified site (female) C50.91-
      male C50.92-
  mucoid (*see also* Neoplasm, malignant, by site)
    cell
      specified site — *see* Neoplasm, malignant, by site
      unspecified site C75.1
  nonencapsulated sclerosing C73
    with follicular C73
    follicular variant C73
    intraductal (noninfiltrating)
      with invasion
        specified site — *see* Neoplasm, malignant, by site
        unspecified site (female) C50.91-
          male C50.92-
      breast D05.8-
      specified site NEC — *see* Neoplasm, in situ, by site
      unspecified site D05.8-
  serous
    specified site — *see* Neoplasm, malignant, by site
    unspecified site C56.9
  papillocystic
    specified site — *see* Neoplasm, malignant, by site
    unspecified site C56.9
  pseudomucinous
    specified site — *see* Neoplasm, malignant, by site
    unspecified site C56.9
  renal cell C64.-
  sebaceous — *see* Neoplasm, skin, malignant
  serous (*see also* Neoplasm, malignant, by site)
    papillary
      specified site — *see* Neoplasm, malignant, by site
      unspecified site C56.9
  sweat gland — *see* Neoplasm, skin, malignant
  water-clear cell C75.0
Adenocarcinoma-in-situ (*see also* Neoplasm, in situ, by site)
  breast D05.9-
Adenofibroma
  clear cell — *see* Neoplasm, benign, by site
  endometrioid D27.9
    borderline malignancy D39.10
    malignant C56.-
  mucinous
    specified site — *see* Neoplasm, benign, by site
    unspecified site D27.9
  papillary
    specified site — *see* Neoplasm, benign, by site
    unspecified site D27.9
  prostate — *see* Enlargement, enlarged, prostate
  serous
    specified site — *see* Neoplasm, benign, by site
    unspecified site D27.9
  specified site — *see* Neoplasm, benign, by site
  unspecified site D27.9
Adenofibrosis
  breast — *see* Fibradenosis, breast
  endometrioid N80.0
Adenoiditis (chronic) J35.02
  with tonsillitis J35.03
  acute J03.90
    recurrent J03.91
    specified organism NEC J03.80
      recurrent J03.81
    staphylococcal J03.80
      recurrent J03.81
    streptococcal J03.00
      recurrent J03.01
Adenoids — *see* condition
Adenolipoma — *see* Neoplasm, benign, by site
Adenolipomatosis, Launois-Bensaude E88.89
Adenolymphoma
  specified site — *see* Neoplasm, benign, by site
  unspecified site D11.9

Adenoma (*see also* Neoplasm, benign, by site)
  acidophil
    specified site — *see* Neoplasm, benign, by site
    unspecified site D35.2
  acidophil-basophil, mixed
    specified site — *see* Neoplasm, benign, by site
    unspecified site D35.2
  adrenal (cortical) D35.00
    clear cell D35.00
    compact cell D35.00
    glomerulosa cell D35.00
    heavily pigmented variant D35.00
    mixed cell D35.00
  alpha-cell
    pancreas D13.7
    specified site NEC — *see* Neoplasm, benign, by site
    unspecified site D13.7
  alveolar D14.30
  apocrine
    breast D24.-
    specified site NEC — *see* Neoplasm, skin, benign, by site
    unspecified site D23.9
  basal cell D11.9
  basophil
    specified site — *see* Neoplasm, benign, by site
    unspecified site D35.2
  basophil-acidophil, mixed
    specified site — *see* Neoplasm, benign, by site
    unspecified site D35.2
  beta-cell
    pancreas D13.7
    specified site NEC — *see* Neoplasm, benign, by site
    unspecified site D13.7
  bile duct D13.4
    common D13.5
    extrahepatic D13.5
    intrahepatic D13.4
    specified site NEC — *see* Neoplasm, benign, by site
    unspecified site D13.4
  black D35.00
  bronchial D38.1
    cylindroid type — *see* Neoplasm, lung, malignant
  ceruminous D23.2-
  chief cell D35.1
  chromophobe
    specified site — *see* Neoplasm, benign, by site
    unspecified site D35.2
  colloid
    specified site — *see* Neoplasm, benign, by site
    unspecified site D34
  duct
  eccrine, papillary — *see* Neoplasm, skin, benign
  endocrine, multiple
    single specified site — *see* Neoplasm, uncertain behavior, by site
    two or more specified sites D44.-
    unspecified site D44.9
  endometrioid (*see also* Neoplasm, benign)
    borderline malignancy — *see* Neoplasm, uncertain behavior, by site
  eosinophil
    specified site — *see* Neoplasm, benign, by site
    unspecified site D35.2
  fetal
    specified site — *see* Neoplasm, benign, by site
    unspecified site D34
  follicular
    specified site — *see* Neoplasm, benign, by site
    unspecified site D34
  hepatocellular D13.4
  Hurthle cell D34
  islet cell
    pancreas D13.7
    specified site NEC — *see* Neoplasm, benign, by site
    unspecified site D13.7
  liver cell D13.4

Adenoma— *continued*
  macrofollicular
    specified site — *see* Neoplasm, benign, by site
    unspecified site D34
  malignant, malignum — *see* Neoplasm, malignant, by site
  microcystic
    pancreas D13.7
    specified site NEC — *see* Neoplasm, benign, by site
    unspecified site D13.7
  microfollicular
    specified site — *see* Neoplasm, benign, by site
    unspecified site D34
  mucoid cell
    specified site — *see* Neoplasm, benign, by site
    unspecified site D35.2
  multiple endocrine
    single specified site — *see* Neoplasm, uncertain behavior, by site
    two or more specified sites D44.-
    unspecified site D44.9
  nipple D24.-
  papillary (*see also* Neoplasm, benign, by site)
    eccrine — *see* Neoplasm, skin, benign, by site
  Pick's tubular
    specified site — *see* Neoplasm, benign, by site
    unspecified site
      female D27.9
      male D29.20
  pleomorphic
    carcinoma in — *see* Neoplasm, salivary gland, malignant
    specified site — *see* Neoplasm, malignant, by site
    unspecified site C08.9
  polypoid (*see also* Neoplasm, benign)
    adenocarcinoma in — *see* Neoplasm, malignant, by site
    adenocarcinoma in situ — *see* Neoplasm, in situ, by site
  prostate — *see* Neoplasm, benign, prostate
  rete cell D29.20
  sebaceous — *see* Neoplasm, skin, benign
  Sertoli cell
    specified site — *see* Neoplasm, benign, by site
    unspecified site
      female D27.9
      male D29.20
  skin appendage — *see* Neoplasm, skin, benign
  sudoriferous gland — *see* Neoplasm, skin, benign
  sweat gland — *see* Neoplasm, skin, benign
  testicular
    specified site — *see* Neoplasm, benign, by site
    unspecified site
      female D27.9
      male D29.20
  tubular (*see also* Neoplasm, benign, by site)
    adenocarcinoma in — *see* Neoplasm, malignant, by site
    adenocarcinoma in situ — *see* Neoplasm, in situ, by site
    Pick's
      specified site — *see* Neoplasm, benign, by site
      unspecified site
        female D27.9
        male D29.20
  tubulovillous (*see also* Neoplasm, benign, by site)
    adenocarcinoma in — *see* Neoplasm, malignant, by site
    adenocarcinoma in situ — *see* Neoplasm, in situ, by site
  villous — *see* Neoplasm, uncertain behavior, by site
    adenocarcinoma in — *see* Neoplasm, malignant, by site
    adenocarcinoma in situ — *see* Neoplasm, in situ, by site
  water-clear cell D35.1
Adenomatosis
  endocrine (multiple) E31.20
    single specified site — *see* Neoplasm, uncertain behavior, by site
  erosive of nipple D24.-

Adenomatosis— *continued*
  pluriendocrine — *see* Adenomatosis, endocrine
  pulmonary D38.1
    malignant — *see* Neoplasm, lung, malignant
    specified site — *see* Neoplasm, benign, by site
    unspecified site D12.6
Adenomatous
  goiter (nontoxic) E04.9
    with hyperthyroidism — *see* Hyperthyroidism, with, goiter, nodular
    toxic — *see* Hyperthyroidism, with, goiter, nodular
Adenomyoma (*see also* Neoplasm, benign, by site)
  prostate — *see* Enlarged, prostate
Adenomyometritis N80.0
Adenomyosis N80.0
Adenopathy (lymph gland) R59.9
  generalized R59.1
  inguinal R59.0
  localized R59.0
  mediastinal R59.0
  mesentery R59.0
  syphilitic (secondary) A51.49
  tracheobronchial R59.0
    tuberculous A15.4
      primary (progressive) A15.7
  tuberculous (*see also* Tuberculosis, lymph gland)
    tracheobronchial A15.4)
      primary (progressive) A15.7
Adenosalpingitis — *see* Salpingitis
Adenosarcoma — *see* Neoplasm, malignant, by site
Adenosclerosis I88.8
Adenosis (sclerosing) **breast** — *see* Fibroadenosis, breast
Adenovirus, as cause of disease classified elsewhere B97.0
Adentia (complete) (partial) — *see* Absence, teeth
Adherent (*see also* Adhesions)
  labia (minora) N90.89
  pericardium (nonrheumatic) I31.0
    rheumatic I09.2
  placenta (with hemorrhage) O72.0
    without hemorrhage O73.0
  prepuce, newborn N47.0
  scar (skin) L90.5
  tendon in scar L90.5
Adhesions, adhesive (postinfective) K66.0
  with intestinal obstruction K56.5
  abdominal (wall) — *see* Adhesions, peritoneum
  appendix K38.8
  bile duct (common) (hepatic) K83.8
  bladder (sphincter) N32.89
  bowel — *see* Adhesions, peritoneum
  cardiac I31.0
    rheumatic I09.2
  cecum — *see* Adhesions, peritoneum
  cervicovaginal N88.1
    congenital Q52.8
    postpartal O90.89
      old N88.1
  cervix N88.1
  ciliary body NEC — *see* Adhesions, iris
  clitoris N90.89
  colon — *see* Adhesions, peritoneum
  common duct K83.8
  congenital (*see also* Anomaly, by site)
    fingers — *see* Syndactylism, complex, fingers
    omental, anomalous Q43.3
    peritoneal Q43.3
    tongue (to gum or roof of mouth) Q38.3
  conjunctiva (acquired) H11.21-
    congenital Q15.8
  cystic duct K82.8
  diaphragm — *see* Adhesions, peritoneum
  due to foreign body — *see* Foreign body
  duodenum — *see* Adhesions, peritoneum
  epididymis N50.8
  epidural — *see* Adhesions, meninges
  epiglottis J38.7
  eyelid H02.59
  female pelvis N73.6
  gallbladder K82.8
  globe H44.89

Adhesions, adhesive — *continued*
  heart I31.0
    rheumatic I09.2
  ileocecal (coil) — *see* Adhesions, peritoneum
  ileum — *see* Adhesions, peritoneum
  intestine (*see also* Adhesions, peritoneum)
    with obstruction K56.5
  intra-abdominal — *see* Adhesions, peritoneum
  iris H21.50-
    anterior H21.51-
    goniosynechiae H21.52-
    posterior H21.54-
    to corneal graft T85.89
  joint — *see* Ankylosis
    knee M23.8x
    temporomandibular M26.61
  labium (majus) (minus), congenital Q52.5
  liver — *see* Adhesions, peritoneum
  lung J98.4
  mediastinum J98.5
  meninges (cerebral) (spinal) G96.12
    congenital Q07.8
    tuberculous (cerebral) (spinal) A17.0
  mesenteric — *see* Adhesions, peritoneum
  nasal (septum) (to turbinates) J34.89
  ocular muscle — *see* Strabismus, mechanical
  omentum — *see* Adhesions, peritoneum
  ovary N73.6
    congenital (to cecum, kidney or omentum) Q50.39
  paraovarian N73.6
  pelvic (peritoneal)
    female N73.6
      postprocedural N99.4
    male — *see* Adhesions, peritoneum
    postpartal (old) N73.6
    tuberculous A18.17
  penis to scrotum (congenital) Q55.8
  periappendiceal (*see also* Adhesions, peritoneum)
  pericardium (nonrheumatic) I31.0
    focal I31.8
    rheumatic I09.2
    tuberculous A18.84
  pericholecystic K82.8
  perigastric — *see* Adhesions, peritoneum
  periovarian N73.6
  periprostatic N42.89
  perirectal — *see* Adhesions, peritoneum
  perirenal N28.89
  peritoneum, peritoneal (postinfective) (postprocedural) K66.0
    with obstruction (intestinal) K56.5
    congenital Q43.3
    pelvic, female N73.6
      postprocedural N99.4
    postpartal, pelvic N73.6
    to uterus N73.6
  peritubal N73.6
  periureteral N28.89
  periuterine N73.6
  perivesical N32.89
  perivesicular (seminal vesicle) N50.8
  pleura, pleuritic J94.8
    tuberculous NEC A15.6
  pleuropericardial J94.8
  postoperative (gastrointestinal tract) K66.0
    with obstruction K91.3
    due to foreign body accidentally left in wound — *see* Foreign body, accidentally left during a procedure
    pelvic peritoneal N99.4
    urethra — *see* Stricture, urethra, postprocedural
    vagina N99.2
  postpartal, old (vulva or perineum) N90.89
  preputial, prepuce N47.5
  pulmonary J98.4
  pylorus — *see* Adhesions, peritoneum
  sciatic nerve — *see* Lesion, nerve, sciatic
  seminal vesicle N50.8
  shoulder (joint) — *see* Capsulitis, adhesive
  sigmoid flexure — *see* Adhesions, peritoneum
  spermatic cord (acquired) N50.8
    congenital Q55.4

Adhesions, adhesive — *continued*
  spinal canal G96.12
  stomach — *see* Adhesions, peritoneum
  subscapular — *see* Capsulitis, adhesive
  temporomandibular M26.61
  tendinitis (*see also* Tenosynovitis, specified type NEC)
    shoulder — *see* Capsulitis, adhesive
  testis N44.8
  tongue, congenital (to gum or roof of mouth) Q38.3
    acquired K14.8
  trachea J39.8
  tubo-ovarian N73.6
  tunica vaginalis N44.8
  uterus N73.6
    internal N85.6
    to abdominal wall N73.6
  vagina (chronic) N89.5
    postoperative N99.2
  vitreous H43.89
  vulva N90.89
Adiaspiromycosis B48.8
Adie(-Holmes) pupil or syndrome — *see* Anomaly, pupil, function, tonic pupil
Adiponecrosis neonatorum P83.8
Adiposis (*see also* Obesity)
  cerebralis E23.6
  dolorosa E88.2
Adiposity (*see also* Obesity)f
  heart — *see* Degeneration, myocardial
  localized E65
Adiposogenital dystrophy E23.6
Adjustment
  disorder — *see* Disorder, adjustment
  implanted device — *see* Encounter (for), adjustment (of)
  prosthesis, external — *see* Fitting
  reaction — *see* Disorder, adjustment
Administration of tPA (rtPA) **in a different facility within the last 24 hours prior to admission to current facility** Z92.82
Admission (for) (*see also* Encounter (for))
  adjustment (of)
    artificial
      arm Z44.00-
        complete Z44.01-
        partial Z44.02-
      eye Z44.2
      leg Z44.10-
        complete Z44.11-
        partial Z44.12-
    brain neuropacemaker Z46.2
      implanted Z45.42
    breast
      implant Z45.81
      prosthesis (external) Z44.3
    colostomy belt Z46.89
    contact lenses Z46.0
    cystostomy device Z46.6
    dental prosthesis Z46.3
    device NEC
      abdominal Z46.89
      implanted Z45.9
        cardiac Z45.09
          defibrillator (with synchronous cardiac pacemaker) Z45.02
          pacemaker Z45.018
            pulse generator Z45.010
        hearing device Z45.328
          bone conduction Z45.320
          cochlear Z45.321
        infusion pump Z45.1
        nervous system Z45.49
          CSF drainage Z45.41
          hearing device — *see* Admission, adjustment, device, implanted, hearing device
          neuropacemaker Z45.42
          visual substitution Z45.31
      specified NEC Z45.89
      vascular access Z45.2
      visual substitution Z45.31

Admission— *continued*
  adjustment—*continued*
    device—*continued*
      nervous system Z46.2
        implanted — *see* Admission, adjustment,
          device, implanted, nervous system
      orthodontic Z46.4
      prosthetic Z44.9
        arm — *see* Admission, adjustment,
          artificial, arm
        breast Z44.3
        dental Z46.3
        eye Z44.2
        leg — *see* Admission, adjustment,
          artificial, leg
        specified type NEC Z44.8
      substitution
        auditory Z46.2
          implanted — *see* Admission,
            adjustment, device, implanted,
            hearing device
        nervous system Z46.2
          implanted — *see* Admission,
            adjustment, device, implanted,
            nervous system
        visual Z46.2
          implanted Z45.31
      urinary Z46.6
    hearing aid Z46.1
      implanted — *see* Admission, adjustment,
        device, implanted, hearing device
    ileostomy device Z46.89
    intestinal appliance or device NEC Z46.89
    neuropacemaker (brain) (peripheral nerve)
      (spinal cord) Z46.2
      implanted Z45.42
    orthodontic device Z46.4
    orthopedic (brace) (cast) (device) (shoes) Z46.89
    pacemaker
      cardiac Z45.018
        pulse generator Z45.010
      nervous system Z46.2
        implanted Z45.42
    portacath (port-a-cath) Z45.2
    prosthesis Z44.9
      arm — *see* Admission, adjustment, artificial,
        arm
      breast Z44.3
      dental Z46.3
      eye Z44.2
      leg — *see* Admission, adjustment, artificial,
        leg
      specified NEC Z44.8
    spectacles Z46.0
  aftercare (*see also* Aftercare) Z51.89
    postpartum
      immediately after delivery Z39.0
      routine follow-up Z39.2
    radiation therapy (antineoplastic) Z51.0
  attention to artificial opening (of) Z43.9
    artificial vagina Z43.7
    colostomy Z43.3
    cystostomy Z43.5
    enterostomy Z43.4
    gastrostomy Z43.1
    ileostomy Z43.2
    jejunostomy Z43.4
    nephrostomy Z43.6
    specified site NEC Z43.8
      intestinal tract Z43.4
      urinary tract Z43.6
    tracheostomy Z43.0
    ureterostomy Z43.6
    urethrostomy Z43.6
  breast augmentation or reduction Z41.1
  breast reconstruction following mastectomy Z42.1
  change of
    dressing (nonsurgical) Z48.00
    neuropacemaker device (brain) (peripheral
      nerve) (spinal cord) Z46.2
      implanted Z45.42
    surgical dressing Z48.01

Admission— *continued*
  circumcision, ritual or routine (in absence of
    diagnosis) Z41.2
  clinical research investigation Z00.6
  contraceptive management Z30.9
  cosmetic surgery NEC Z41.1
  counseling (*see also* Counseling)
    dietary Z71.3
    HIV Z71.7
    human immunodeficiency virus Z71.7
    nonattending third party Z71.0
    procreative management NEC Z31.69
  delivery, full-term, uncomplicated O80
    cesarean, without indication O82
  dietary surveillance and counseling Z71.3
  ear piercing Z41.3
  examination (*see also* Examination) at health care
    facility (adult) Z00.00
    with abnormal findings Z00.01
    clinical research investigation Z00.6
    dental Z01.20
      with abnormal findings Z01.21
    donor (potential) Z00.5
    ear Z01.10
      with abnormal findings NEC Z01.118
    eye Z01.00
      with abnormal findings Z01.01
    general, specified reason NEC Z00.5
    hearing Z01.10
      with abnormal findings NEC Z01.118
    postpartum checkup Z39.2
    psychiatric (general) Z00.8
      requested by authority Z04.6
    vision Z01.00
      with abnormal findings Z01.01
  fitting (of)
    artificial
      arm — *see* Admission, adjustment, artificial,
        arm
      eye Z44.2
      leg — *see* Admission, adjustment, artificial,
        leg
    brain neuropacemaker Z46.2
      implanted Z45.42
    breast prosthesis (external) Z44.3
    colostomy belt Z46.89
    contact lenses Z46.0
    cystostomy device Z46.6
    dental prosthesis Z46.3
    dentures Z46.3
    device NEC
      abdominal Z46.89
      nervous system Z46.2
        implanted — *see* Admission, adjustment,
          device, implanted, nervous system
    orthodontic Z46.4
    prosthetic Z44.9
      breast Z44.3
      dental Z46.3
      eye Z44.2
    substitution
      auditory Z46.2
        implanted — *see* Admission,
          adjustment, device, implanted,
          hearing device
      nervous system Z46.2
        implanted — *see* Admission,
          adjustment, device, implanted,
          nervous system
      visual Z46.2
        implanted Z45.31
    hearing aid Z46.1
    ileostomy device Z46.89
    intestinal appliance or device NEC Z46.89
    neuropacemaker (brain) (peripheral nerve)
      (spinal cord) Z46.2
      implanted Z45.42
    orthodontic device Z46.4
    orthopedic device (brace) (cast) (shoes) Z46.89
    prosthesis Z44.9
      arm — *see* Admission, adjustment, artificial,
        arm
      breast Z44.3

Admission— *continued*
  fitting— *continued*
    prosthesis— *continued*
      dental Z46.3
      eye Z44.2
      leg — *see* Admission, adjustment, artificial,
        leg
      specified type NEC Z44.8
      spectacles Z46.0
  follow-up examination Z09
  intrauterine device management Z30.431
    initial prescription Z30.014
  mental health evaluation Z00.8
    requested by authority Z04.6
  observation — *see* Observation
  Papanicolaou smear, cervix Z12.4
    for suspected malignant neoplasm Z12.4
  plastic surgery, cosmetic NEC Z41.1
  postpartum observation
    immediately after delivery Z39.0
    routine follow-up Z39.2
  poststerilization (for restoration) Z31.0
    aftercare Z31.42
  plastic and reconstructive surgery following medical
    procedure or healed injury NEC Z42.8
  procreative management Z31.9
  prophylactic (measure)
    organ removal Z40.00
      breast Z40.01
      ovary Z40.02
      specified organ NEC Z40.09
      testes Z40.09
    vaccination Z23
  psychiatric examination (general) Z00.8
    requested by authority Z04.6
  radiation therapy (antineoplastic) Z51.0
  reconstructive surgery following medical procedure
    or healed injury NEC Z42.8
  removal of
    cystostomy catheter Z43.5
    drains Z48.03
    dressing (nonsurgical) Z48.00
    intrauterine contraceptive device Z30.432
    neuropacemaker (brain) (peripheral nerve)
      (spinal cord) Z46.2
      implanted Z45.42
    staples Z48.02
    surgical dressing Z48.01
    sutures Z48.02
    ureteral stent Z46.6
  respirator/ventilator use during power failure
    (Z99.12)
  restoration of organ continuity (poststerilization)
    Z31.0
    aftercare Z31.42
  sensitivity test (*see also* Test, skin)
    allergy NEC Z01.82
    Mantoux Z11.1
  tuboplasty following previous sterilization Z31.0
    aftercare Z31.42
  vasoplasty following previous sterilization Z31.0
    aftercare Z31.42
  vision examination Z01.00
    with abnormal findings Z01.01
  waiting period for admission to other facility Z75.1
Adnexitis (suppurative) — *see* Salpingo-oophoritis
Adolescent X-linked adrenoleukodystrophy
  E71.521
AIPHI R04.81
Albers-Schönberg syndrome Q78.2
Adrenal (gland) — *see* condition
Adrenalism, tuberculous A18.7
Adrenalitis, adrenitis E27.8
  autoimmune E27.1
  meningococcal, hemorrhagic A39.1
Adrenarche, premature E27.0
Adrenocortical syndrome — *see* Cushing's syndrome
Adrenogenital syndrome E25.9
  acquired E25.8
  congenital E25.0
  salt loss E25.0
Adrenogenitalism, congenital E25.0

Adrenoleukodystrophy E71.529
  neonatal E71.511
  X-linked E71.529
    Addison only phenotype E71.528
    Addison-Schilder E71.528
    adolescent E71.521
    adrenomyeloneuropathy E71.522
    childhood cerebral E71.520
    other specified E71.528
Adrenomyeloneuropathy E71.522
Adventitious bursa — *see* Bursopathy, specified type
      NEC
Adverse effect — *see* Table of Drugs and Chemicals,
      categories T36-T50, with 6th character 5
Advice — *see* Counseling
Adynamia (episodica) (hereditary) (periodic) G72.3
Aeration lung imperfect, newborn — *see* Atelectasis
Aerobullosis T70.3
Aerocele — *see* Embolism, air
Aerodermectasia
  subcutaneous (traumatic) T79.7
Aerodontalgia T70.29
Aeroembolism T70.3
Aerogenes capsulatus infection A48.0
Aero-otitis media T70.0
Aerophagy, aerophagia (psychogenic) F45.8
Aerophobia F40.228
Aerosinusitis T70.1
Aerotitis T70.0
Affection — *see* Disease
Afibrinogenemia (*see also* Defect, coagulation) D68.8
  acquired D65
  congenital D68.2
  in abortion — *see* Abortion, by type, complicated
      by, afibrinogenemia
  puerperal O72.3
African
  sleeping sickness B56.9
  tick fever A68.1
  trypanosomiasis B56.9
    gambian B56.0
    rhodesian B56.1
Aftercare (*see also* Care) Z51.89
  following surgery (for) (on)
    amputation Z47.81
    attention to
      drains Z48.03
      dressings (nonsurgical) Z48.00
        surgical Z48.01
      sutures Z48.02
    circulatory system Z48.812
    delayed (planned) wound closure Z48.1
    digestive system Z48.815
    genitourinary system Z48.816
    joint replacement Z47.1
    neoplasm Z48.3
    nervous system Z48.811
    oral cavity Z48.814
    organ transplant
      bone marrow Z48.290
      heart Z48.21
      heart-lung Z48.280
      kidney Z48.22
      liver Z48.23
      lung Z48.24
      multiple organs NEC Z48.288
      specified NEC Z48.298
    orthopedic NEC Z47.89
    planned wound closure Z48.1
    removal of internal fixation device Z47.2
    respiratory system Z48.813
    scoliosis Z47.82
    sense organs Z48.810
    skin and subcutaneous tissue Z48.817
    specified body system
      circulatory Z48.812
      digestive Z48.815
      genitourinary Z48.816
      nervous Z48.811
      oral cavity Z48.814
      respiratory Z48.813

Aftercare — *continued*
  following surgery— *continued*
    specified body system — *continued*
      sense organs Z48.810
      skin and subcutaneous tissue Z48.817
      teeth Z48.814
    specified NEC Z48.89
    spinal — *see* Aftercare, following surgery (for)
        (on), specified body system
    teeth Z48.814
  fracture—code to fracture with extension D
  involving
    removal of
      drains Z48.03
      dressings (nonsurgical) Z48.00
      staples Z48.02
      surgical dressings Z48.01
      sutures Z48.02
  neuropacemaker (brain) (peripheral nerve) (spinal
        cord) Z46.2
    implanted Z45.42
  orthopedic NEC Z47.89
  postprocedural — *see* Aftercare, following surgery
After-cataract — *see* Cataract, secondary
Agalactia (primary) O92.3
  elective, secondary or therapeutic O92.5
Agammaglobulinemia (acquired (secondary))
        (nonfamilial) D80.1
  with
    immunoglobulin-bearing B-lymphocytes D80.1
    lymphopenia D81.9
  autosomal recessive (Swiss type) D80.0
  Bruton's X-linked D80.0
  common variable (CVAgamma) D80.1
  congenital sex-linked D80.0
  hereditary D80.0
  lymphopenic D81.9
  Swiss type (autosomal recessive) D80.0
  X-linked (with growth hormone deficiency)(Bruton)
        D80.0
Aganglionosis (bowel) (colon) Q43.1
Age (old) — *see* Senility
Agenesis
  adrenal (gland) Q89.1
  alimentary tract (complete) (partial) NEC Q45.8
    upper Q40.8
  anus, anal (canal) Q42.3
    with fistula Q42.2
  aorta Q25.4
  appendix Q42.8
  arm (complete) Q71.0-
    with hand present Q71.1-
  artery (peripheral) Q27.9
    brain Q28.3
    coronary Q24.5
    pulmonary Q25.7
    specified NEC Q27.8
    umbilical Q27.0
  auditory (canal) (external) Q16.1
  auricle (ear) Q16.0
  bile duct or passage Q44.5
  bladder Q64.5
  bone Q79.9
  brain Q00.0
    part of Q04.3
  breast (with nipple present) Q83.8
    with absent nipple Q83.0
  bronchus Q32.4
  canaliculus lacrimalis Q10.4
  carpus — *see* Agenesis, hand
  cartilage Q79.9
  cecum Q42.8
  cerebellum Q04.3
  cervix Q51.5
  chin Q18.8
  cilia Q10.3
  circulatory system, part NOS Q28.9
  clavicle Q74.0
  clitoris Q52.6
  coccyx Q76.49
  colon Q42.9
    specified NEC Q42.8
  corpus callosum Q04.0

Agenesis—*continued*
  cricoid cartilage Q31.8
  diaphragm (with hernia) Q79.1
  digestive organ(s) or tract (complete) (partial) NEC
        Q45.8
    upper Q40.8
  ductus arteriosus Q28.8
  duodenum Q41.0
  ear Q16.9
    auricle Q16.0
    lobe Q17.8
  ejaculatory duct Q55.4
  endocrine (gland) NEC Q89.2
  epiglottis Q31.8
  esophagus Q39.8
  eustachian tube Q16.2
  eye Q11.1
    adnexa Q15.8
  eyelid (fold) Q10.3
  face
    bones NEC Q75.8
    specified part NEC Q18.8
  fallopian tube Q50.6
  femur — *see* Defect, reduction, lower limb,
        longitudinal, femur
  fibula — *see* Defect, reduction, lower limb,
        longitudinal, fibula
  finger (complete) (partial) — *see* Agenesis, hand
  foot (and toes) (complete) (partial) Q72.3-
  forearm (with hand present) — *see* Agenesis, arm,
        with hand present
  and hand Q71.2-
  gallbladder Q44.0
  gastric Q40.2
  genitalia, genital (organ(s))
    female Q52.8
      external Q52.71
      internal NEC Q52.8
    male Q55.8
  glottis Q31.8
  hair Q84.0
  hand (and fingers) (complete) (partial) Q71.3-
  heart Q24.8
    valve NEC Q24.8
      pulmonary Q22.0
  hepatic Q44.7
  humerus — *see* Defect, reduction, upper limb
  hymen Q52.4
  ileum Q41.2
  incus Q16.3
  intestine (small) Q41.9
    large Q42.9
      specified NEC Q42.8
  iris (dilator fibers) Q13.1
  jaw M26.09
  jejunum Q41.1
  kidney(s) (partial) Q60.2
    bilateral Q60.1
    unilateral Q60.0
  labium (majus) (minus) Q52.71
  labyrinth, membranous Q16.5
  lacrimal apparatus Q10.4
  larynx Q31.8
  leg (complete) Q72.0-
    with foot present Q72.1-
    lower leg (with foot present) — *see* Agenesis, leg,
        with foot present
    and foot Q72.2-
  lens Q12.3
  limb (complete) Q73.0
    lower — *see* Agenesis, leg
    upper — *see* Agenesis, arm
  lip Q38.0
  liver Q44.7
  lung (fissure) (lobe) (bilateral) (unilateral) Q33.3
  mandible, maxilla M26.09
  metacarpus — *see* Agenesis, hand
  metatarsus — *see* Agenesis, foot
  muscle Q79.8
    eyelid Q10.3
    ocular Q15.8
  musculoskeletal system NEC Q79.8
  nail(s) Q84.3

Agenesis— *continued*
  neck, part Q18.8
  nerve Q07.8
  nervous system, part NEC Q07.8
  nipple Q83.2
  nose Q30.1
  nuclear Q07.8
  oesophagus Q39.8
  organ
      of Corti Q16.5
      or site not listed — *see* Anomaly, by site
  osseous meatus (ear) Q16.1
  ovary
      bilateral Q50.02
      unilateral Q50.01
  oviduct Q50.6
  pancreas Q45.0
  parathyroid (gland) Q89.2
  parotid gland(s) Q38.4
  patella Q74.1
  pelvic girdle (complete) (partial) Q74.2
  penis Q55.5
  pericardium Q24.8
  pituitary (gland) Q89.2
  prostate Q55.4
  punctum lacrimale Q10.4
  radioulnar — *see* Defect, reduction, upper limb
  radius — *see* Defect, reduction, upper limb,
      longitudinal, radius
  rectum Q42.1
      with fistula Q42.0
  renal Q60.2
      bilateral Q60.1
      unilateral Q60.0
  respiratory organ NEC Q34.8
  rib Q76.6
  roof of orbit Q75.8
  round ligament Q52.8
  sacrum Q76.49
  salivary gland Q38.4
  scapula Q74.0
  scrotum Q55.29
  seminal vesicles Q55.4
  septum
      atrial Q21.1
      between aorta and pulmonary artery Q21.4
      ventricular Q20.4
  shoulder girdle (complete) (partial) Q74.0
  skull (bone) Q75.8
      with
          anencephaly Q00.0
          encephalocele — *see* Encephalocele
          hydrocephalus Q03.9
              with spina bifida — *see* Spina bifida, by
                  site, with hydrocephalus
          microcephaly Q02
  spermatic cord Q55.4
  spinal cord Q06.0
  spine Q76.49
  spleen Q89.01
  sternum Q76.7
  stomach Q40.2
  submaxillary gland(s) (congenital) Q38.4
  tarsus — *see* Agenesis, foot
  tendon Q79.8
  testicle Q55.0
  thymus (gland) Q89.2
  thyroid (gland) E03.1
      cartilage Q31.8
  tibia — *see* Defect, reduction, lower limb,
      longitudinal, tibia
  tibiofibular — *see* Defect, reduction, lower limb,
      specified type NEC
  toe (and foot) (complete) (partial) — *see* Agenesis,
      foot
  tongue Q38.3
  trachea (cartilage) Q32.1
  ulna — *see* Defect, reduction, upper limb,
      longitudinal, ulna
  upper limb — *see* Agenesis, arm
  ureter Q62.4
  urethra Q64.5
  urinary tract NEC Q64.8

Agenesis— *continued*
  uterus Q51.0
  uvula Q38.5
  vagina Q52.0
  vas deferens Q55.4
  vein(s) (peripheral) Q27.9
      brain Q28.3
      great NEC Q26.8
      portal Q26.5
  vena cava (inferior) (superior) Q26.8
  vermis of cerebellum Q04.3
  vertebra Q76.49
  vulva Q52.71
Ageusia R43.2
Agitated — *see* condition
Agitation R45.1
Aglossia (congenital) Q38.3
Aglossia-adactylia syndrome Q87.0
Aglycogenosis E74.00
Agnosia (body image) (other senses) (tactile) (visual)
      R48.1
  developmental F88
  verbal R48.1
      auditory R48.1
          developmental F80.2
      developmental F80.2
  visual object H53.16
Agoraphobia F40.00
  with panic disorder F40.01
  without panic disorder F40.02
Agrammatism R48.8
Agranulocytopenia — *see* Agranulocytosis
Agranulocytosis (chronic) (cyclical) (genetic)
      (infantile) (periodic) (pernicious) (*see also*
      Neutropenia) D70.9
  congenital D70.0
  cytoreductive cancer chemotherapy sequela D70.1
  drug-induced D70.2
      due to cytoreductive cancer chemotherapy
          D70.1
  due to infection D70.3
  secondary D70.8
      drug-induced D70.2
          due to cytoreductive cancer chemotherapy
              D70.1
Agraphia (absolute) R48.8
  with alexia R48.0
  developmental F81.81
Ague (dumb) — *see* Malaria
Agyria Q04.3
Ahumada-del Castillo syndrome E23.0
Aichomophobia F40.298
AIDS (related complex) B20
Ailment heart — *see* Disease, heart
Ailurophobia F40.218
Ainhum (disease) L94.6
AIPHI R04.81
Air
  anterior mediastinum J98.2
  compressed, disease T70.3
  conditioner lung or pneumonitis J67.7
  embolism (artery) (cerebral) (any site) T79.0
      with ectopic or molar pregnancy O08.2
      due to implanted device NEC — *see*
          Complications, by site and type, specified
          NEC
      following
          ectopic or molar pregnancy O08.2
          infusion, therapeutic injection or transfusion
              T80.0
      in pregnancy, childbirth or puerperium — *see*
          Embolism, obstetric
      traumatic T79.0
  hunger, psychogenic F45.8
  rarefied, effects of — *see* Effect, adverse, high altitude
  sickness T75.3
Airplane sickness T75.3
Akathisia (drug-induced) (treatment-induced) G25.71
  neuroleptic induced (acute) G25.71
Akinesia R29.898
Akinetic mutism R41.89
Akureyri's disease G93.3
Alactasia, congenital E73.0

Alagille's syndrome Q44.7
Alastrim B03
Albers-Schönberg syndrome Q78.2
Albert's syndrome — *see* Tendinitis, Achilles
Albinism, albino E70.30
  with hematologic abnormality E70.339
      Chédiak-Higashi syndrome E70.330
      Hermansky-Pudlak syndrome E70.331
      other specified E70.338
      I E70.320
      II E70.321
  ocular E70.319
      autosomal recessive E70.311
      other specified E70.318
      X-linked E70.310
  oculocutaneous E70.329
      other specified E70.328
      tyrosinase (ty) negative E70.320
      tyrosinase (ty) positive E70.321
  other specified E70.39
Albinismus E70.30
Albright(-McCune)(-Sternberg) **syndrome** Q78.1
Albuminous — *see* condition
Albuminuria, albuminuric (acute) (chronic)
      (subacute) (*see also* Proteinuria) R80.9
  complicating pregnancy — *see* Proteinuria,
      gestational
  with
      gestational hypertension — *see*
          Pre-eclampsia
      pre-existing hypertension — *see*
          Hypertension, complicating pregnancy,
          pre-existing, with, pre-eclampsia
  gestational — *see* Proteinuria, gestational
  with
      gestational hypertension — *see*
          Pre-eclampsia
      pre-existing hypertension — *see*
          Hypertension, complicating pregnancy,
          pre-existing, with, pre-eclampsia
  orthostatic R80.2
  postural R80.2
  pre-eclamptic — *see* Pre-eclampsia
  scarlatinal A38.8
Albuminurophobia F40.298
Alcaptonuria E70.29
Alcohol, alcoholic, alcohol-induced
  addiction (without remission) F10.20
      with remission F10.21
  amnestic disorder, persisting F10.96
      with dependence F10.26
  brain syndrome, chronic F10.97
      with dependence F10.27
  cardiopathy I42.6
  counseling and surveillance Z71.41
      family member Z71.42
  delirium (acute) (tremens) (withdrawal) F10.231
      with intoxication F10.921
          in
              abuse F10.121
              dependence F10.221
  dementia F10.97
      with dependence F10.27
  deterioration F10.97
      with dependence F10.27
  hallucinosis (acute) F10.951
      in
          abuse F10.151
          dependence F10.251
  insanity F10.959
  intoxication (acute) (without dependence) F10.129
      with
          delirium F10.121
          dependence F10.229
              with delirium F10.221
              uncomplicated F10.220
          uncomplicated F10.120
  jealousy F10.959
  Korsakoff's, Korsakov's, Korsakow's F10.26
  liver K70.9
      acute — *see* Disease, liver, alcoholic, hepatitis
  mania (acute) (chronic) F10.959
  paranoia, paranoid (type) psychosis F10.950

Alcohol, alcoholic, alcohol-induced— *continued*
  pellagra E52
  poisoning, accidental (acute) NEC — *see* Table of
    Drugs and Chemicals, alcohol, poisoning
  psychosis — *see* Psychosis, alcoholic
  withdrawal (without convulsions) F10.239
    with delirium F10.231
Alcoholism chronic) (without remission) F10.20
  with
    psychosis — *see* Psychosis, alcoholic
    remission F10.21
    Korsakov's F10.96
  with dependence F10.26
Alder (-Reilly) **anomaly or syndrome** (leukocyte
  granulation) D72.0
Aldosteronism E26.9
  familial (type I) E26.02
  glucocorticoid-remediable E26.02
  primary (due to (bilateral) adrenal hyperplasia)
    E26.09
  primary NEC E26.09
  secondary E26.1
  specified NEC E26.89
Aldosteronoma D44.10
Aldrich (-Wiskott) **syndrome**
  (eczema-thrombocytopenia) D82.0
Alektorophobia F40.218
Aleppo boil B55.1
Aleukemic — *see* condition
Aleukia
  congenital D70.0
  hemorrhagica D61.9
    congenital D61.09
  splenica D73.1
Alexia R48.0
  developmental F81.0
  secondary to organic lesion R48.0
Algoneurodystrophy M89.00
  ankle M89.07-
  foot M89.07-
  forearm M89.03-
  hand M89.04-
  lower leg M89.06-
  multiple sites M89.0-
  shoulder M89.01-
  specified site NEC M89.08
  thigh M89.05-
  upper arm M89.02-
Algophobia F40.298
Allenation, mental — *see* Psychosis
Alkalemia E87.3
Alkalosis E87.3
  metabolic E87.3
    with respiratory acidosis E87.4
  respiratory E87.3
Alkaptonuria E70.29
Allen-Masters syndrome N83.8
Allergy, allergic (reaction) (to) T78.40
  air-borne substance NEC (rhinitis) J30.89
  alveolitis (extrinsic) J67.9
    due to
      Aspergillus clavatus J67.4
      Cryptostroma corticale J67.5
      organisms (fungal, thermophilic
        actinomycete) growing in ventilation
        (air conditioning) systems J67.7
    specified type NEC J67.8
  anaphylactic shock T78.2
  angioneurotic edema T78.3
  animal (dander) (epidermal) (hair) (rhinitis) J30.81
  bee sting (anaphylactic shock) — *see* Toxicity,
    venom, arthropod, bee
  biological — *see* Allergy, drug
  colitis K52.2
  dander (animal) (rhinitis) J30.81
  dandruff (rhinitis) J30.81
  dental restorative material (existing) K08.55
  dermatitis — *see* Dermatitis, contact, allergic
  diathesis — *see* History, allergy
  drug, medicament & biological (any) (external)
    (internal) T78.40

Allergy, allergic — *continued*
  drug, medicament & biological— *continued*
    correct substance properly administered — *see*
      Table of Drugs and Chemicals, by drug,
      adverse effect
    wrong substance given or taken NEC (by
      accident) — *see* Table of Drugs and
      Chemicals, by drug, poisoning
  due to pollen J30.1
  dust (house) (stock) (rhinitis) J30.89
    with asthma — *see* Asthma, allergic extrinsic
  eczema — *see* Dermatitis, contact, allergic
  epidermal (animal) (rhinitis) J30.81
  feathers (rhinitis) J30.89
  food (any) (ingested) NEC T78.1
    anaphylactic shock — *see* Shock, anaphylactic,
      food
    dermatitis — *see* Dermatitis, due to, food
    dietary counseling and surveillance Z71.3
    in contact with skin L23.6
    rhinitis J30.5
    status (without reaction) Z91.018
      eggs Z91.012
      milk products Z91.011
      peanuts Z91.010
      seafood Z91.013
      specified NEC Z91.018
  gastrointestinal K52.2
  grain J30.1
  grass (hay fever) (pollen) J30.1
    asthma — *see* Asthma, allergic extrinsic
  hair (animal) (rhinitis) J30.81
  history (of) — *see* History, allergy
  horse serum — *see* Allergy, serum
  inhalant (rhinitis) J30.89
    pollen J30.1
  kapok (rhinitis) J30.89
  medicine — *see* Allergy, drug
  milk protein K52.2
  nasal, seasonal due to pollen J30.1
  pneumonia J82
  pollen (any) (hay fever) J30.1
    asthma — *see* Asthma, allergic extrinsic
  primrose J30.1
  primula J30.1
  purpura D69.0
  ragweed (hay fever) (pollen) J30.1
    asthma — *see* Asthma, allergic extrinsic
  rose (pollen) J30.1
  seasonal NEC J30.2
  Senecio jacobae (pollen) J30.1
  serum (prophylactic) (therapeutic) T80.6
    anaphylactic shock T80.5
  shock (anaphylactic) T78.2
    due to
      adverse effect of correct medicinal substance
        properly administered T88.6
      serum or immunization T80.5
        anaphylactic T80.5
  specific NEC T78.49
  tree (any) (hay fever) (pollen) J30.1
    asthma — *see* Asthma, allergic extrinsic
  upper respiratory J30.9
  urticaria L50.0
  vaccine — *see* Allergy, serum
Allescheriasis B48.2
Alligator skin disease Q80.9
Allocheiria, allochiria R20.8
Almeida's disease — *see* Paracoccidioidomycosis
Alopecia (hereditaria) (prematura) (seborrheica) L65.9
  androgenic L64.9
    drug-induced L64.0
    specified NEC L64.8
  areata L63.9
    ophiasis L63.2
    specified NEC L63.8
    totalis L63.0
    universalis L63.1
  cicatricial L66.9
    specified NEC L66.8
  circumscripta L63.9
  congenital, congenitalis Q84.0
  due to cytotoxic drugs NEC L65.8

Alopecia — *continued*
  mucinosa L65.2
  postinfective NEC L65.8
  postpartum L65.0
  premature L64.8
  specific (syphilitic) A51.32
  specified NEC L65.8
  syphilitic (secondary) A51.32
  totalis (capitis) L63.0
  universalis (entire body) L63.1
  X-ray L58.1
Alpers' disease G31.81
Alpine sickness T70.29
Alport syndrome Q87.81
ALTE (apparent life threatening event) **in newborn
  and infant** R68.13
Alteration (of), **Altered**
  awareness, transient R40.4
  mental status R41.82
  pattern of family relationships affecting child
    Z62.898
  sensation
    following
      cerebrovascular disease I69.998
        specified NEC I69.898
        cerebral infarction I69.398
        intracerebral hemorrhage I69.198
        nontraumatic intracranial hemorrhage
          NEC I69.298
        specified disease NEC I69.898
        subarachnoid hemorrhage I69.098
Alternating — *see* condition
Altitude, high (effects) — *see* Effect, adverse, high
  altitude
Aluminosis (of lung) J63.0
Alveolitis
  allergic (extrinsic) — *see* Pneumonitis,
    hypersensitivity
  due to
    Aspergillus clavatus J67.4
    Cryptostroma corticale J67.6
  fibrosing (cryptogenic) (idiopathic) J84.1
  jaw M27.3
  sicca dolorosa M27.3
Alveolus, alveolar — *see* condition
Alymphocytosis D72.820
  thymic (with immunodeficiency) D82.1
Alymphoplasia, thymic D82.1
Alzheimer's disease or sclerosis — *see* Disease,
  Alzheimer's
Amastia (with nipple present) Q83.8
  with absent nipple Q83.0
Amathophobia F40.228
Amaurosis (acquired) (congenital) (*see also* Blindness)
  fugax G45.3
  hysterical F44.6
  Leber's congenital H35.50
  uremic — *see* Uremia
Amaurotic idiocy (infantile) (juvenile) (late) E75.4
Amaxophobia F40.248
Ambiguous genitalia Q56.4
Amblyopia (congenital) (ex anopsia) (partial)
  (suppression) H53.00-
  anisometropic — *see* Amblyopia, refractive
  deprivation H53.01-
  hysterical F44.6
  nocturnal (*see also* Blindness, night)
    vitamin A deficiency E50.5
  refractive H53.02-
  strabismic H53.03-
  tobacco H53.8
  toxic NEC H53.8
  uremic — *see* Uremia
Ameba, amebic (histolytica) (*see also* Amebiasis)
  abscess (liver) A06.4
Amebiasis A06.9
  with abscess — *see* Abscess, amebic
  acute A06.0
  chronic (intestine) A06.1
    with abscess — *see* Abscess, amebic
  cutaneous A06.7
  cutis A06.7

Amebiasis — *continued*
  cystitis A06.81
  genitourinary tract NEC A06.82
  hepatic — *see* Abscess, liver, amebic
  intestine A06.0
  nondysenteric colitis A06.2
  skin A06.7
  specified site NEC A06.89
Ameboma (of intestine) A06.3
Amelia Q73.0
  lower limb — *see* Agenesis, leg
  upper limb — *see* Agenesis, arm
Ameloblastoma (*see also* Cyst, calcifying odontogenic)
  long bones C40.9-
    lower limb C40.2-
    upper limb C40.0-
  malignant C41.1
    jaw (bone) (lower) C41.1
      upper C41.0
  tibial C40.2-
Amelogenesis imperfecta K00.5
  nonhereditaria (segmentalis) K00.4
Amenorrhea N91.2
  hyperhormonal E28.8
  primary N91.0
  secondary N91.1
Amentia (*see also* Retardation, mental)
  Meynert's (nonalcoholic) F04
American
  leishmaniasis B55.2
  mountain tick fever A93.2
Ametropia — *see* Disorder, refraction
Amianthosis J61
Amimia R48.8
Amino-acid disorder E72.9
  anemia D53.0
Aminoacidopathy E72.9
Aminoaciduria E72.9
Amnes(t)ic syndrome (post-traumatic) F04
  induced by
    alcohol F10.96
      with dependence F10.26
    psychoactive NEC F19.96
      with
        abuse F19.16
        dependence F19.26
    sedative F13.96
      with dependence F13.26
Amnesia R41.3
  anterograde R41.1
  auditory R48.8
  dissociative F44.0
  hysterical F44.0
  postictal in epilepsy — *see* Epilepsy
  psychogenic F44.0
  retrograde R41.2
  transient global G45.4
Amnion, amniotic — *see* condition
Amnionitis — *see* Pregnancy, complicated by
Amok F68.8
Amoral traits F60.89
Ampulla
  lower esophagus K22.8
  phrenic K22.8
Amputation (*see also* Absence, by site, acquired)
  neuroma (postoperative) (traumatic) — *see*
    Complications, amputation stump, neuroma
  stump (surgical)
    abnormal, painful, or with complication (late) —
      see Complications, amputation stump
    healed or old NOS Z89.9
  traumatic (complete) (partial)
    arm (upper) (complete) S48.91-
      at
        elbow S58.01-
          partial S58.02-
        shoulder joint (complete) S48.01-
          partial S48.02-
      between
        elbow and wrist (complete) S58.11-
          partial S58.12-
        shoulder and elbow (complete) S48.11-

Amputation — *continued*
  traumatic — *continued*
    arm — *continued*
      between — *continued*
        shoulder and elbow — *continued*
          partial S48.12-
        partial S48.92-
    breast (complete) S28.21-
      partial S28.22-
    clitoris (complete) S38.211
      partial S38.212
    ear (complete) S08.11-
      partial S08.12-
    finger (complete) (metacarpophalangeal)
      S68.11-
      index S68.11-
      little S68.11-
      middle S68.11-
      partial S68.12-
        index S68.12-
        little S68.12-
        middle S68.12-
        ring S68.12-
      ring S68.11-
      thumb — *see* Amputation, traumatic, thumb
      transphalangeal (complete) S68.61-
        index S68.61-
        little S68.61-
        middle S68.61-
        partial S68.62-
          index S68.62-
          little S68.62-
          middle S68.62-
          ring S68.62-
        ring S68.61-
    foot (complete) S98.91-
      at ankle level S98.01-
        partial S98.02-
      midfoot S98.31-
        partial S98.32-
      partial S98.92-
    forearm (complete) S58.91-
      at elbow level (complete) S58.01-
        partial S58.02-
      between elbow and wrist (complete) S58.11-
        partial S58.12-
      partial S58.92-
    genital organ(s) (external)
      female (complete) S38.211
        partial S38.212
      male
        penis (complete) S38.221
          partial S38.222
        scrotum (complete) S38.231
          partial S38.232
        testes (complete) S38.231
          partial S38.232
    hand (complete) (wrist level) S68.41-
      finger(s) alone — *see* Amputation, traumatic,
        finger
      partial S68.42-
      thumb alone — *see* Amputation, traumatic,
        thumb
      transmetacarpal (complete) S68.71-
        partial S68.72-
    head
      ear — *see* Amputation, traumatic, ear
      nose (partial) S08.812
        complete S08.811
      part S08.89
        scalp S08.0
    hip (and thigh) (complete) S78.91-
      at hip joint (complete) S78.01-
        partial S78.02-
      between hip and knee (complete) S78.11-
        partial S78.12-
      partial S78.92-
    labium (majus) (minus) (complete) S38.21-
      partial S38.21-
    leg (lower) S88.91-
      at knee level S88.01-
        partial S88.02-
      between knee and ankle S88.11-

Amputation — *continued*
  traumatic — *continued*
    leg — *continued*
      between knee and ankle — *continued*
        partial S88.12-
        partial S88.92-
    nose (partial) S08.812
      complete S08.811
    penis (complete) S38.221
      partial S38.222
    scrotum (complete) S38.231
      partial S38.232
    shoulder — *see* Amputation, traumatic, arm
      at shoulder joint — *see* Amputation,
        traumatic, arm, at shoulder joint
    testes (complete) S38.231
      partial S38.232
    thigh — *see* Amputation, traumatic, hip
    thorax, part of S28.1
      breast — *see* Amputation, traumatic, breast
    thumb (complete) (metacarpophalangeal)
      S68.01-
      partial S68.02-
      transphalangeal (complete) S68.51-
        partial S68.52-
    toe (lesser) S98.13-
      great S98.11-
        partial S98.12-
      more than one S98.21-
        partial S98.22-
      partial S98.14-
    vulva (complete) S38.211
      partial S38.212
Amputee (bilateral) (old) Z89.9
Amsterdam dwarfism Q87.1
Amusia R48.8
  developmental F80.89
Amyelencephalus, amyelencephaly Q00.0
Amyelia Q06.0
Amygdalitis — *see* Tonsillitis
Amygdalolith J35.8
Amyloid heart (disease) E85.4 [I43]
Amyloidosis (generalized) (primary) E85.9
  with lung involvement E85.4 [J99]
  familial E85.2
  genetic E85.2
  heart E85.4 [I43]
  hemodialysis-associated E85.3
  liver E85.4 [K77]
  localized E85.4
  neuropathic heredofamilial E85.1
  non-neuropathic heredofamilial E85.0
  organ limited E85.4
  Portuguese E85.1
  pulmonary E85.4 [J99]
  secondary systemic E85.3
  skin (lichen) (macular) E85.4 [L99]
  specified NEC E85.8
  subglottic E85.4 [J99]
Amylopectinosis (brancher enzyme deficiency)
  E74.03
Amylophagia — *see* Pica
Amyoplasia congenita Q79.8
Amyotonia M62.89
  congenita G70.2
Amyotrophia, amyotrophy, amyotrophic G71.8
  congenita Q79.8
  diabetic — *see* Diabetes, amyotrophy
  lateral sclerosis G12.21
  neuralgic G54.5
  spinal progressive G12.21
Anacidity, gastric K31.83
  psychogenic F45.8
Anaerosis of newborn P28.89
Analbuminemia E88.09
Analgesia — *see* Anesthesia
Analphalipoproteinemia E78.6
Anaphylactic
  purpura D69.0
  shock or reaction — *see* Shock, anaphylactic
Anaphylactoid shock or reaction — *see* Shock,
  anaphylactic
Anaphylactoid syndrome of pregnancy O88.01-

Anaphylaxis — *see* Shock, anaphylactic
Anaplasia cervix (*see also* **Dysplasia, cervix**) N87.9
Anarthria R47.1
Anasarca R60.1
  cardiac — *see* Failure, heart, congestive
  lung J18.2
  newborn P83.2
  nutritional E43
  pulmonary J18.2
  renal N04.9
Anastomosis
  aneurysmal — *see* Aneurysm
  arteriovenous ruptured brain I60.8
  intestinal K63.89
    complicated NEC K91.89
      involving urinary tract N99.89
  retinal and choroidal vessels (congenital) Q14.8
Anatomical narrow angle H40.0
Ancylostoma, ancylostomiasis (braziliense)
  (caninum) (ceylanicum) (duodenale) B76.0
  Necator americanus B76.1
Andersen's disease (glycogen storage) E74.09
Anderson-Fabry disease E75.21
Andes disease T70.29
Andrews' disease (bacterid) L08.0
Androblastoma
  benign
    specified site — *see* Neoplasm, benign, by site
    unspecified site
      female D27.9
      male D29.20
  malignant
    specified site — *see* Neoplasm, malignant, by site
    unspecified site
      female C56.9
      male C62.90
  specified site — *see* Neoplasm, uncertain behavior,
    by site
  tubular
    with lipid storage
      specified site — *see* Neoplasm, benign, by site
      unspecified site
        female D27.9
        male D29.20
    specified site — *see* Neoplasm, benign, by site
    unspecified site
      female D27.9
      male D29.20
  unspecified site
    female D39.10
    male D40.10
Androgen insensitivity syndrome (*see also*
  Syndrome, androgen insensitivity) E34.50
Androgen resistance syndrome (*see also* Syndrome,
  androgen insensitivity) E34.50
Android pelvis Q74.2
  with disproportion (fetopelvic) O33.3
    causing obstructed labor O65.3
Androphobia F40.290
Anectasis, pulmonary (newborn) — *see* Atelectasis
Anemia (essential) (general) (hemoglobin deficiency)
  (infantile) (primary) (profound) D64.9
  with (due to) (in)
    disorder of
      anaerobic glycolysis D55.2
      pentose phosphate pathway D55.1
    koilonychia D50.9
  achlorhydric D50.8
  achrestic D53.1
  Addison(-Biermer) (pernicious) D51.0
  agranulocytic — *see* Agranulocytosis
  amino-acid-deficiency D53.0
  aplastic D61.9
    congenital D61.09
    drug-induced D61.1
    due to
      drugs D61.1
      external agents NEC D61.2
      infection D61.2
      radiation D61.2
    idiopathic D61.3
    red cell (pure) D60.9
      chronic D60.0

Anemia— *continued*
  aplastic — *continued*
    red cell— *continued*
      congenital D61.01
      specified type NEC D60.8
      transient D60.1
    specified type NEC D61.89
    toxic D61.2
  aregenerative
    congenital D61.09
  asiderotic D50.9
  atypical (primary) D64.9
  Baghdad spring D55.0
  Balantidium coli A07.0
  Biermer's (pernicious) D51.0
  blood loss (chronic) D50.0
    acute D62
  bothriocephalus B70.0 [D63.8]
  brickmaker's B76.9 [D63.8]
  cerebral I67.8
  childhood D58.9
  chlorotic D50.8
  chronic simple D53.9
  chronica congenita aregenerativa D61.09
  combined system disease NEC D51.0 [G32.0]
    due to dietary vitamin B12 deficiency D51.3
      [G32.0]
  complicating pregnancy, childbirth or puerperium
    — *see* Pregnancy, complicated by
    (management affected by), anemia
  congenital P61.4
    aplastic D61.09
    due to isoimmunization NOS P55.9
    dyserythropoietic, dyshematopoietic D64.4
    following fetal blood loss P61.3
    Heinz body D58.2
    hereditary hemolytic NOS D58.9
    pernicious D51.0
    spherocytic D58.0
  Cooley's (erythroblastic) D56.1
  cytogenic D51.0
  deficiency D53.9
    2, 3 diphosphoglycurate mutase D55.2
    2, 3 PG D55.2
    6 phosphogluconate dehydrogenase D55.1
    6-PGD D55.1
    amino-acid D53.0
    combined B12 and folate D53.1
    enzyme D55.9
      drug-induced (hemolytic) D59.2
      glucose-6-phosphate dehydrogenase (G6PD)
        D55.0
      glycolytic D55.2
      nucleotide metabolism D55.3
      related to hexose monophosphate (HMP)
        shunt pathway NEC D55.1
      specified type NEC D55.8
    erythrocytic glutathione D55.1
    folate D52.9
      dietary D52.0
      drug-induced D52.1
    folic acid D52.9
      dietary D52.0
      drug-induced D52.1
    G SH D55.1
    GGS-R D55.1
    glucose-6-phosphate dehydrogenase D55.0
    glutathione reductase D55.1
    glyceraldehyde phosphate dehydrogenase D55.2
    G6PD D55.0
    hexokinase D55.2
    iron D50.9
      secondary to blood loss (chronic) D50.0
    nutritional D53.9
      with
        poor iron absorption D50.8
        specified deficiency NEC D53.8
    phosphofructo-aldolase D55.2
    phosphoglycerate kinase D55.2
    PK D55.2
    protein D53.0
    pyruvate kinase D55.2

Anemia— *continued*
  deficiency— *continued*
    transcobalamin II D51.2
    triose-phosphate isomerase D55.2
    vitamin B12 NOS D51.9
      dietary D51.3
      due to
        intrinsic factor deficiency D51.0
        selective vitamin B12 malabsorption with
          proteinuria D51.1
      pernicious D51.0
      specified type NEC D51.8
  Diamond-Blackfan (congenital hypoplastic) D61.01
  dibothriocephalus B70.0 [D63.8]
  dimorphic D53.1
  diphasic D53.1
  Diphyllobothrium (Dibothriocephalus) B70.0 [D63.8]
  due to (in) (with)
    antineoplastic chemotherapy D64.81
    blood loss (chronic) D50.0
      acute D62
    chemotherapy, antineoplastic D64.81
    chronic disease classified elsewhere NEC D63.8
    chronic kidney disease D63.1
    deficiency
      amino-acid D53.0
      copper D53.8
      folate (folic acid) D52.9
        dietary D52.0
        drug-induced D52.1
      molybdenum D53.8
      protein D53.0
      zinc D53.8
    dietary vitamin B12 deficiency D51.3
    disorder of
      glutathione metabolism D55.1
      nucleotide metabolism D55.3
    drug — *see* Anemia, by type (*see also* Table of
      Drugs and Chemicals)
    end stage renal disease D63.1
    enzyme disorder D55.9
    fetal blood loss P61.3
    fish tapeworm (D.latum) infestation B70.0
      [D63.8]
    hemorrhage (chronic) D50.0
      acute D62
    impaired absorption D50.9
    loss of blood (chronic) D50.0
      acute D62
    myxedema E03.9 [D63.8]
    Necator americanus B76.1 [D63.8]
    prematurity P61.2
    selective vitamin B12 malabsorption with
      proteinuria D51.1
    transcobalamin II deficiency D51.2
  Dyke-Young type (secondary) (symptomatic) D59.1
  dyserythropoietic (congenital) D64.4
  dyshematopoietic (congenital) D64.4
  Egyptian B76.9 [D63.8]
  elliptocytosis — *see* Elliptocytosis
  enzyme-deficiency, drug-induced D59.2
  epidemic (*see also* Ancylostomiasis) B76.9 [D63.8]
  erythroblastic
    familial D56.1
    newborn (*see also* Disease, hemolytic) P55.9
    of childhood D56.1
  erythrocytic glutathione deficiency D55.1
  erythropoietin-resistant anemia (EPO resistant
    anemia) D63.1
  Faber's (achlorhydric anemia) D50.9
  factitious (self-induced blood letting) D50.0
  familial erythroblastic D56.1
  Fanconi's (congenital pancytopenia) D61.09
  favism D55.0
  fish tapeworm (D. latum) infestation B70.0 [D63.8]
  folate (folic acid) deficiency D52.9
  glucose-6-phosphate dehydrogenase (G6PD)
    deficiency D55.0
  glutathione-reductase deficiency D55.1
  goat's milk D52.0
  granulocytic — *see* Agranulocytosis
  Heinz body, congenital D58.2

Anemia— *continued*
hemolytic D58.9
acquired D59.9
with hemoglobinuria NEC D59.6
autoimmune NEC D59.1
infectious D59.4
specified type NEC D59.8
toxic D59.4
acute D59.9
due to enzyme deficiency specified type NEC D55.8
Lederer's D59.1
autoimmune D59.1
drug-induced D59.0
chronic D58.9
idiopathic D59.9
cold type (secondary) (symptomatic) D59.1
congenital (spherocytic) — *see* Spherocytosis
due to
cardiac conditions D59.4
drugs (nonautoimmune) D59.2
autoimmune D59.0
enzyme disorder D55.9
drug-induced D59.2
presence of shunt or other internal prosthetic device D59.4
familial D58.9
hereditary D58.9
due to enzyme disorder D55.9
specified type NEC D55.8
specified type NEC D58.8
idiopathic (chronic) D59.9
mechanical D59.4
microangiopathic D59.4
nonautoimmune D59.4
drug-induced D59.2
nonspherocytic
congenital or hereditary NEC D55.8
glucose-6-phosphate dehydrogenase deficiency D55.0
pyruvate kinase deficiency D55.2
type
I D55.1
II D55.2
type
I D55.1
II D55.2
secondary D59.4
autoimmune D59.1
specified (hereditary) type NEC D58.8
Stransky-Regala type (*see also* Hemoglobinopathy) D58.8
symptomatic D59.4
autoimmune D59.1
toxic D59.4
warm type (secondary) (symptomatic) D59.1
hemorrhagic (chronic) D50.0
acute D62
Herrick's D57.1
hexokinase deficiency D55.2
hookworm B76.9 [D63.8]
hypochromic (idiopathic) (microcytic) (normoblastic) D50.9
due to blood loss (chronic) D50.0
acute D62
familial sex-linked D64.0
pyridoxine-responsive D64.3
sideroblastic, sex-linked D64.0
hypoplasia, red blood cells D61.9
congenital or familial D61.09
hypoplastic (idiopathic) D61.9
congenital or familial (of childhood) D61.09
hypoproliferative (refractive) D61.9
idiopathic D64.9
aplastic D61.3
hemolytic, chronic D59.9
in (due to) (with)
chronic kidney disease D63.1
end stage renal disease D63.1
failure, kidney (renal) D63.1
neoplastic disease (*see also* Neoplasm) D63.0
intertropical (*see also* Ancylostomiasis) D63.8
iron deficiency D50.9

Anemia— *continued*
iron deficiency— *continued*
secondary to blood loss (chronic) D50.0
acute D62
specified type NEC D50.8
Joseph-Diamond-Blackfan (congenital hypoplastic) D61.01
Lederer's (hemolytic) D59.1
leukoerythroblastic D61.82
macrocytic D53.9
nutritional D52.0
tropical D52.8
malarial (*see also* Malaria) B54 [D63.8]
malignant (progressive) D51.0
malnutrition D53.9
marsh (*see also* Malaria) B54 [D63.8]
Mediterranean D56.9
megaloblastic D53.1
combined B12 and folate deficiency D53.1
hereditary D51.1
nutritional D52.0
orotic aciduria D53.0
refractory D53.1
specified type NEC D53.1
megalocytic D53.1
microcytic (hypochromic) D50.9
due to blood loss (chronic) D50.0
acute D62
familial D56.8
microelliptopoikilocytic (Rietti-GreppiMicheli) D56.9
miner's B76.9 [D63.8]
myelodysplastic D46.9
myelofibrosis D75.81
myelogenous D64.89
myelopathic D64.89
myelophthisic D61.82
myeloproliferative D47.z9
newborn P61.4
due to
ABO (antibodies, isoimmunization, maternal/fetal incompatibility) P55.1
Rh (antibodies, isoimmunization, maternal/fetal incompatibility) P55.0
following fetal blood loss P61.3
posthemorrhagic (fetal) P61.3
nonspherocytic hemolytic — *see* Anemia, hemolytic, nonspherocytic
normocytic (infectional) D64.9
due to blood loss (chronic) D50.0
acute D62
myelophthisic D61.82
nutritional (deficiency) D53.9
with
poor iron absorption D50.8
specified deficiency NEC D53.8
megaloblastic D52.0
of prematurity P61.2
orotaciduric (congenital) (hereditary) D53.0
osteosclerotic D64.89
ovalocytosis (hereditary) — *see* Elliptocytosis
paludal (*see also* Malaria) B54 [D63.8]
pernicious (congenital) (malignant) (progressive) D51.0
pleochromic D64.89
of sprue D52.8
posthemorrhagic (chronic) D50.0
acute D62
newborn P61.3
postoperative (postprocedural)
due to (acute) blood loss D62
chronic blood loss D50.0
specified NEC D64.9
postpartum O90.81
pressure D64.89
progressive D64.9
malignant D51.0
pernicious D51.0
protein-deficiency D53.0
pseudoleukemica infantum D64.89
pure red cell D60.9
congenital D61.01
pyridoxine-responsive D64.3
pyruvate kinase deficiency D55.2

Anemia— *continued*
refractory D46.4
with
excess of blasts D46.20
1 (RAEB 1) D46.21
2 (RAEB 2) D46.22
in transformation (RAEB T) — *see* Leukemia, acute myeloblastic
hemochromatosis D46.1
sideroblasts (ring) (RARS) D46.1
megaloblastic D53.1
sideroblastic D46.1
sideropenic D50.8
without ring sideroblasts, so stated D46.0
without sideroblasts without excess of blasts D46.0
Rietti-Greppi-Micheli D56.9
scorbutic D53.2
secondary to
blood loss (chronic) D50.0
acute D62
hemorrhage (chronic) D50.0
acute D62
semiplastic D61.89
sickle-cellSee Disease, sickle-cell
sideroblastic D64.3
hereditary D64.0
hypochromic, sex-linked D64.0
pyridoxine-responsive NEC D64.3
refractory D46.1
secondary (due to)
disease D64.1
drugs and toxins D64.2
specified type NEC D64.3
sideropenic (refractory) D50.9
due to blood loss (chronic) D50.0
acute D62
simple chronic D53.9
specified type NEC D64.89
spherocytic (hereditary) — *see* Spherocytosis
splenic D64.89
splenomegalic D64.89
stomatocytosis D58.8
syphilitic (acquired) (late) A52.79 [D63.8]
target cell D64.89
thalassemia D56.9
thrombocytopenic — *see* Thrombocytopenia
toxic D61.2
tropical B76.9 [D63.8]
macrocytic D52.8
tuberculous A18.89 [D63.8]
vegan D51.3
vitamin
B6-responsive D64.3
B12 deficiency (dietary) pernicious D51.0
von Jaksch's D64.89
Witts' (achlorhydric anemia) D50.8
Anencephalus, anencephaly Q00.0
Anemophobia F40.228
Anergasia — *see* Psychosis, organic
Anesthesia, anesthetic (of skin) R20.0
complication or reaction NEC (*see also* Complications, anesthesia) T88.59
due to
correct substance properly administered — *see* Table of Drugs and Chemicals, by drug, adverse effect
overdose or wrong substance given — *see* Table of Drugs and Chemicals, by drug, poisoning
cornea H18.81-
dissociative F44.6
functional (hysterical) F44.6
hyperesthetic, thalamic G89.0
hysterical F44.6
local skin lesion R20.0
sexual (psychogenic) F52.1
shock (due to) T88.2
skin R20.0
testicular N50.9
Anetoderma (maculosum) (of) L90.8
Jadassohn-Pellizzari L90.2
Schweninger-Buzzi L90.1

Aneurin deficiency E51.9
Aneurysm (anastomotic) (artery) (cirsoid) (diffuse) (false) (fusiform) (multiple) (saccular) I72.9
 abdominal (aorta) I71.4
  ruptured I71.3
  syphilitic A52.01
 aorta, aortic (nonsyphilitic) I71.9
  abdominal I71.4
   ruptured I71.3
  arch I71.2
   ruptured I71.1
  arteriosclerotic I71.9
   ruptured I71.8
  ascending I71.2
   ruptured I71.1
  congenital Q25.4
  descending I71.9
   abdominal I71.4
    ruptured I71.3
   ruptured I71.8
   thoracic I71.2
    ruptured I71.1
  ruptured I71.8
  sinus, congenital Q25.4
  syphilitic A52.01
  thoracic I71.2
   ruptured I71.1
  thoracoabdominal I71.6
   ruptured I71.5
  thorax, thoracic (arch) I71.2
   ruptured I71.1
  transverse I71.2
   ruptured I71.1
  valve (heart) (see also Endocarditis, aortic) I35.8
 arteriosclerotic I72.9
  cerebral I67.1
   ruptured — see Hemorrhage, intracranial, subarachnoid
 arteriovenous (congenital) (peripheral) (see also Malformation, arteriovenous)
  acquired I77.0
   brain I67.1
   coronary I25.41
   pulmonary I28.0
  brain Q28.2
   ruptured I60.8
  peripheral — see Malformation, arteriovenous, peripheral
  precerebral vessels Q28.0
  specified site NEC (see also Malformation, arteriovenous)
   acquired I77.0
 basal — see Aneurysm, brain
 berry (congenital) (nonruptured) I67.1
  ruptured I60.7
 brain I67.1
  arteriosclerotic I67.1
   ruptured — see Hemorrhage, intracranial, subarachnoid
  arteriovenous (congenital) (nonruptured) Q28.2
   acquired I67.1
    ruptured I60.8
   ruptured I60.8
  berry (congenital) (nonruptured) I67.1
   ruptured (see also Hemorrhage, intracranial, subarachnoid) I60.7
  congenital Q28.3
   ruptured I60.7
  meninges I67.1
   ruptured I60.8
  miliary (congenital) (nonruptured) I67.1
   ruptured (see also Hemorrhage, intracranial, subarachnoid) I60.7
  mycotic I33.0
  ruptured — see Hemorrhage, intracranial, subarachnoid
  syphilitic (hemorrhage) A52.05
 cardiac (false) (see also Aneurysm, heart) I25.3
 carotid artery (common) (external) I72.0
  internal (intracranial) I67.1
   extracranial portion I72.0
  ruptured into brain I60.0-
  syphilitic A52.09

Aneurysm— continued
 carotid artery— continued
  syphilitic— continued
   intracranial A52.05
 cavernous sinus I67.1
  arteriovenous (congenital) (nonruptured) Q28.3
   ruptured I60.8
 central nervous system, syphilitic A52.05
 cerebral — see Aneurysm, brain
 chest — see Aneurysm, thorax
 circle of Willis I67.1
  congenital Q28.3
   ruptured I60.6
  ruptured I60.6
 common iliac artery I72.3
 congenital (peripheral) Q27.8
  brain Q28.3
   ruptured I60.7
  coronary Q24.5
  digestive system Q27.8
  lower limb Q27.8
  pulmonary Q25.7
  retina Q14.1
  specified site NEC Q27.8
  upper limb Q27.8
 conjunctiva — see Abnormality, conjunctiva, vascular
 conus arteriosus — see Aneurysm, heart
 coronary (arteriosclerotic) (artery) I25.41
  arteriovenous, congenital Q24.5
  congenital Q24.5
  ruptured — see Infarct, myocardium
  syphilitic A52.06
  vein I25.89
 cylindroid (aorta) I71.9
  ruptured I71.8
  syphilitic A52.01
 ductus arteriosus Q25.0
 endocardial, infective (any valve) I33.0
 femoral (artery) (ruptured) I72.4
 heart (wall) (chronic or with a stated duration of over 4 weeks) I25.3
  valve — see Endocarditis
 iliac (common) (artery) (ruptured) I72.3
 infective I72.9
  endocardial (any valve) I33.0
 innominate (nonsyphilitic) I72.8
  syphilitic A52.09
 interauricular septum — see Aneurysm, heart
 interventricular septum — see Aneurysm, heart
 intrathoracic (nonsyphilitic) I71.2
  ruptured I71.1
  syphilitic A52.01
 lower limb I72.4
 lung (pulmonary artery) I28.1
 mediastinal (nonsyphilitic) I72.8
  syphilitic A52.09
 miliary (congenital) I67.1
  ruptured — see Hemorrhage, intracerebral, subarachnoid, intracranial
 mitral (heart) (valve) I34.8
 mural — see Aneurysm, heart
 mycotic I72.9
  endocardial (any valve) I33.0
  ruptured, brain — see Hemorrhage, intracerebral, subarachnoid
 myocardium — see Aneurysm, heart
 neck I72.0
 patent ductus arteriosus Q25.0
 peripheral NEC I72.8
  congenital Q27.8
   digestive system Q27.8
   lower limb Q27.8
   specified site NEC Q27.8
   upper limb Q27.8
 popliteal (artery) (ruptured) I72.4
 precerebral, congenital (nonruptured) Q28.1
 pulmonary I28.1
  arteriovenous Q25.7
   acquired I28.0
  syphilitic A52.09
  valve (heart) — see Endocarditis, pulmonary
 racemose (peripheral) I72.9

Aneurysm— continued
 racemose— continued
  congenital — see Aneurysm, congenital
  radial I72.1
  Rasmussen NEC A15.0
  renal (artery) I72.2
  retina (see also Disorder, retina, microaneurysms)
   congenital Q14.1
   diabetic — see Diabetes, microaneurysms, retinal
  sinus of Valsalva Q25.4
  spinal (cord) I72.8
   syphilitic (hemorrhage) A52.09
  splenic I72.8
  subclavian (artery) (ruptured) I72.8
   syphilitic A52.09
  syphilitic (aorta) A52.01
   central nervous system A52.05
   congenital (late) A50.54 [I79.0]
   spine, spinal A52.09
  thoracoabdominal (aorta) I71.6
   ruptured I71.5
   syphilitic A52.01
  thorax, thoracic (aorta) (arch) (nonsyphilitic) I71.2
   ruptured I71.1
   syphilitic A52.01
  traumatic (complication) (early), specified site — see Injury, blood vessel
  tricuspid (heart) (valve) I07.8
  ulnar I72.1
  upper limb (ruptured) I72.1
  valve, valvular — see Endocarditis
  venous (see also Varix) I86.8
   congenital Q27.8
    digestive system Q27.8
    lower limb Q27.8
    specified site NEC Q27.8
    upper limb Q27.8
  ventricle — see Aneurysm, heart
Angelman syndrome Q93.5
Anger R45.4
Angiectasis, angiectopia I99.8
Angiitis I77.6
 allergic granulomatous M30.1
 hypersensitivity M31.0
 necrotizing M31.9
  specified NEC M31.8
 nervous system, granulomatous I67.7
Angina (attack) (cardiac) (chest) (heart) (pectoris) (syndrome) (vasomotor) I20.9
 with
  atherosclerotic heart disease — see Arteriosclerosis, coronary (artery), documented spasm I20.1
 abdominal K55.1
 accelerated — see Angina, unstable
 agranulocytic — see Agranulocytosis
 angiospastic — see Angina, with documented spasm
 aphthous B08.5
 crescendo — see Angina, unstable
 croupous J05.0
 cruris I73.9
 de novo effort — see Angina, unstable
 diphtheritic, membranous A36.0
 equivalent I20.8
 exudative, chronic J37.0
 following acute myocardial infarction I23.7
 gangrenous diphtheritic A36.0
 intestinal K55.1
 Ludovici K12.2
 Ludwig's K12.2
 malignant diphtheritic A36.0
 membranous J05.0
  diphtheritic A36.0
  Vincent's A69.1
 mesenteric K55.1
 monocytic — see Mononucleosis, infectious
 of effort — see Angina, specified NEC
 phlegmonous J36
  diphtheritic A36.0
 post-infarctional I23.7
 pre-infarctional — see Angina, unstable
 Prinzmetal — see Angina, with documented spasm

Angina — *continued*
  progressive — *see* Angina, unstable
  pseudomembranous A69.1
  pultaceous, diphtheritic A36.0
  spasm-induced — *see* Angina, with documented
    spasm
  specified NEC I20.8
  stable I20.9
  stenocardia — *see* Angina, specified NEC
  stridulous, diphtheritic A36.2
  tonsil J36
  trachealis J05.0
  unstable I20.0
  variant — *see* Angina, with documented spasm
  Vincent's A69.1
Angina— *continued*
  worsening effort — *see* Angina, unstable
Angioblastoma — *see* Neoplasm, connective tissue,
  uncertain behavior
Angiocholecystitis — *see* Cholecystitis, acute
Angiocholitis — *see* Cholecystitis, acute
Angiodysgenesis spinalis G95.19
Angiodysplasia (cecum) (colon) K55.20
  with bleeding K55.21
  duodenum (and stomach) K31.819
    with bleeding K31.811
  stomach (and duodenum) K31.819
    with bleeding K31.811
Angioedema (allergic) (any site) (with urticaria) T78.3
  hereditary D84.1
Angioendothelioma — *see* Neoplasm, uncertain
  behavior, by site
  benign D18.00
    intra-abdominal D18.03
    intracranial D18.02
    skin D18.01
    specified site NEC D18.09
  bone — *see* Neoplasm, bone, malignant
  Ewing's — *see* Neoplasm, bone, malignant
Angioendotheliomatosis C85.8-
Angiofibroma (*see also* Neoplasm, benign, by site)
  juvenile
    specified site — *see* Neoplasm, benign, by site
    unspecified site D10.6
Angiohemophilia (A) (B) D68.0
Angioid streaks (choroid) (macula) (retina) H35.33
Angiokeratoma — *see* Neoplasm, skin, benign
  corporis diffusum E75.21
Angioleiomyoma — *see* Neoplasm, connective tissue,
  benign
Angiolipoma (*see also* Lipoma)
  infiltrating — *see* Lipoma
Angioma (*see also* Hemangioma, by site)
  capillary I78.1
  hemorrhagicum hereditaria I78.0
  intra-abdominal D18.03
  intracranial D18.02
  malignant — *see* Neoplasm, connective tissue,
    malignant
  plexiform D18.00
    intra-abdominal D18.03
    intracranial D18.02
    skin D18.01
    specified site NEC D18.09
  senile I78.1
  serpiginosum L81.7
  skin D18.01
  specified site NEC D18.09
  spider I78.1
  stellate I78.1
Angiomatosis Q82.8
  bacillary A79.89
  encephalotrigeminal Q85.8
  hemorrhagic familial I78.0
  hereditary familial I78.0
  liver K76.4
Angiomyolipoma — *see* Lipoma
Angiomyoliposarcoma — *see* Neoplasm, connective
  tissue, malignant
Angiomyoma — *see* Neoplasm, connective tissue,
  benign
Angiomyosarcoma — *see* Neoplasm, connective
  tissue, malignant

Angiomyxoma — *see* Neoplasm, connective tissue,
  uncertain behavior
Angioneurosis F45.8
Angioneurotic edema (allergic) (any site) (with
  urticaria) T78.3
  hereditary D84.1
Angiopathia, angiopathy I99.9
  cerebral I67.9
    amyloid E85.4 [I68.0]
  diabetic (peripheral) — *see* Diabetes, angiopathy
  peripheral I73.9
    diabetic — *see* Diabetes, angiopathy
    specified type NEC I73.89
  retinae syphilitica A52.05
  retinalis (juvenilis)
    diabetic — *see* Diabetes, retinopathy
    proliferative — *see* Retinopathy, proliferative
Angiosarcoma (*see also* Neoplasm, connective tissue,
  malignant)
  liver C22.3
Angiosclerosis — *see* Arteriosclerosis
Angiospasm (peripheral) (traumatic) (vessel) I73.9
  brachial plexus G54.0
  cerebral G45.9
  cervical plexus G54.2
  nerve
    arm — *see* Mononeuropathy, upper limb
      axillary G54.0
      median — *see* Lesion, nerve, median
      ulnar — *see* Lesion, nerve, ulnar
    axillary G54.0
    leg — *see* Mononeuropathy, lower limb
    median — *see* Lesion, nerve, median
    plantar — *see* Lesion, nerve, plantar
    ulnar — *see* Lesion, nerve, ulnar
Angiospastic disease or edema I73.9
Angiostrongyliasis
  due to
    Parastrongylus
      cantonensis B83.2
      costaricensis B81.3
  intestinal B81.3
Anguillulosis — *see* Strongyloidiasis
Angulation
  cecum — *see* Obstruction, intestine
  coccyx (acquired) (*see also* subcategory) M43.8
    congenital NEC Q76.49
  femur (acquired) (*see also* Deformity, limb, specified
    type NEC, thigh)
    congenital Q74.2
  intestine (large) (small) — *see* Obstruction, intestine
  sacrum (acquired) (*see also* subcategory) M43.8
    congenital NEC Q76.49
  sigmoid (flexure) — *see* Obstruction, intestine
  spine — *see* Dorsopathy, deforming, specified NEC
  tibia (acquired) (*see also* Deformity, limb, specified
    type NEC, lower leg)
    congenital Q74.2
  ureter N13.5
    with infection N13.6
  wrist (acquired) (*see also* Deformity, limb, specified
    type NEC, forearm)
    congenital Q74.0
Angulus infectiosus (lips) K13.0
Anhedonia R45.84
Anhidrosis L74.4
Anhydration, anhydremia E86.0
  with
    hypernatremia E87.0
    hyponatremia E87.1
Anhydremia E86.0
  with
    hypernatremia E87.0
    hyponatremia E87.1
Anidrosis L74.4
Aniridia (congenital) Q13.1
Anisakiasis (infection) (infestation) B81.0
Anisakis larvae infestation B81.0
Aniseikonia H52.32
Anisocoria (pupil) H57.09
  congenital Q13.2
Anisocytosis R71.8
Anisometropia (congenital) H52.31

Ankle — *see* condition
Ankyloblepharon (eyelid) (acquired) (*see also*
  Blepharophimosis)
  filiforme (adnatum) (congenital) Q10.3
  total Q10.3
Ankyloglossia Q38.1
Ankylosis (fibrous) (osseous) (joint) M24.60
  ankle M24.67-
  arthrodesis status Z98.1
  cricoarytenoid (cartilage) (joint) (larynx) J38.7
  dental K03.5
  ear ossicles H74.31-
  elbow M24.62-
  foot M24.67-
  hand M24.64-
  hip M24.65-
  incostapedial joint (infectional) — *see* Ankylosis, ear
    ossicles
  jaw (temporomandibular) M26.61
  knee M24.66-
  lumbosacral (joint) M43.27
  postoperative (status) Z98.1
  produced by surgical fusion, status Z98.1
  sacro-iliac (joint) M43.28
  shoulder M24.61-
  spine (joint) (*see also* Fusion, spine)
    spondylitic — *see* Spondylitis, ankylosing
  surgical Z98.1
  temporomandibular M26.61
  tooth, teeth (hard tissues) K03.5
  wrist M24.63-
Ankylostoma — *see* Ancylostoma
Ankylostomiasis — *see* Ancylostomiasis
Ankylurethria — *see* Stricture, urethra
Annular (*see also* condition)
  detachment, cervix N88.8
  organ or site, congenital NEC — *see* Distortion
  pancreas (congenital) Q45.1
Anodontia (complete) (partial) (vera) K00.0
  acquired K08.10
Anomaly, anomalous (congenital) (unspecified type)
  Q89.9
  abdominal wall NEC Q79.59
  acoustic nerve Q07.8
  adrenal (gland) Q89.1
  Alder (-Reilly) (leukocyte granulation) D72.0
  alimentary tract Q45.9
    upper Q40.9
  alveolar M26.70
    hyperplasia M26.79
      mandibular M26.72
      maxillary M26.71
    hypoplasia M26.79
      mandibular M26.74
      maxillary M26.73
    ridge (process) M26.79
    specified NEC M26.79
  ankle (joint) Q74.2
  anus Q43.9
  aorta (arch) NEC Q25.4
    coarctation (preductal) (postductal) Q25.1
  aortic cusp or valve Q23.9
  appendix Q43.8
  apple peel syndrome Q41.1
  aqueduct of Sylvius Q03.0
    with spina bifida — *see* Spina bifida, with
      hydrocephalus
  arm Q74.0
  arteriovenous NEC
    coronary Q24.5
    gastrointestinal Q27.33
      acquired — *see* Angiodysplasia
  artery (peripheral) Q27.9
    basilar NEC Q28.1
    cerebral Q28.3
    coronary Q24.5
    digestive system Q27.8
    eye Q15.8
    great Q25.9
      specified NEC Q25.8
    lower limb Q27.8
    peripheral Q27.9
      specified NEC Q27.8

Anomaly, anomalous— *continued*
  artery— *continued*
    pulmonary NEC Q25.7
    renal Q27.2
    retina Q14.1
    specified site NEC Q27.8
    subclavian Q27.8
    umbilical Q27.0
    upper limb Q27.8
    vertebral NEC Q28.1
  aryteno-epiglottic folds Q31.8
  atrial
    bands or folds Q20.8
    septa Q21.1
  atrioventricular
    excitation I45.6
    septum Q21.0
  auditory canal Q17.8
  auricle
    ear Q17.8
      causing impairment of hearing Q16.9
    heart Q20.8
  Axenfeld's Q15.0
  back Q89.9
  band
    atrial Q20.8
    heart Q24.8
    ventricular Q24.8
  Bartholin's duct Q38.4
  biliary duct or passage Q44.5
  bladder Q64.70
    absence Q64.5
    diverticulum Q64.6
    exstrophy Q64.10
      cloacal Q64.12
      extroversion Q64.19
      specified type NEC Q64.19
      supravesical fissure Q64.11
    neck obstruction Q64.31
    specified type NEC Q64.79
  bone Q79.9
    arm Q74.0
    face Q75.9
    leg Q74.2
    pelvic girdle Q74.2
    shoulder girdle Q74.0
    skull Q75.9
      with
        anencephaly Q00.0
        encephalocele — *see* Encephalocele
        hydrocephalus Q03.9
          with spina bifida — *see* Spina bifida,
            by site, with hydrocephalus
        microcephaly Q02
  brain (multiple) Q04.9
    vessel Q28.3
  breast Q83.9
  broad ligament Q50.6
  bronchus Q32.4
  bulbus cordis Q21.9
  bursa Q79.9
  canal of Nuck Q52.4
  canthus Q10.3
  capillary Q27.9
  cardiac Q24.9
    chambers Q20.9
      specified NEC Q20.8
    septal closure Q21.9
      specified NEC Q21.8
    valve NEC Q24.8
      pulmonary Q22.3
  cardiovascular system Q28.8
  carpus Q74.0
  caruncle, lacrimal Q10.6
  cascade stomach Q40.2
  cauda equina Q06.3
  cecum Q43.9
  cerebral Q04.9
    vessels Q28.3
  cervix Q51.9
  Chédiak-Higashi(-Steinbrinck) (congenital
      gigantism of peroxidase granules) E70.330
  cheek Q18.9

Anomaly, anomalous— *continued*
  chest wall Q67.8
    bones Q76.9
  chin Q18.9
  chordae tendineae Q24.8
  choroid Q14.3
    plexus Q07.8
  chromosomes, chromosomal Q99.9
    D(1) — *see* condition, chromosome 13
    E(3) — *see* condition, chromosome 18
    G — *see* condition, chromosome 21
    sex
      female phenotype Q97.8
      gonadal dysgenesis (pure) Q99.1
      Klinefelter's Q98.4
      male phenotype Q98.9
      Turner's Q96.9
    specified NEC Q99.8
  cilia Q10.3
  circulatory system Q28.9
  clavicle Q74.0
  clitoris Q52.6
  coccyx Q76.49
  colon Q43.9
  common duct Q44.5
  communication
    coronary artery Q24.5
    left ventricle with right atrium Q21.0
  concha (ear) Q17.3
  connection
    portal vein Q26.5
    pulmonary venous Q26.4
      partial Q26.3
      total Q26.2
    renal artery with kidney Q27.2
  cornea (shape) Q13.4
  coronary artery or vein Q24.5
  cranium — *see* Anomaly, skull
  cricoid cartilage Q31.8
  cystic duct Q44.5
  dental
    alveolar — *see* Anomaly, alveolar
    arch relationship M26.20
      specified NEC M26.29
  dentofacial M26.9
    alveolar — *see* Anomaly, alveolar
    dental arch relationship M26.20
      specified NEC M26.29
    functional M26.50
      specified NEC M26.59
    jaw-cranial base relationship M26.10
      asymmetry M26.12
        maxillary M26.11
      specified type NEC M26.19
    jaw size M26.00
      macrogenia M26.05
      mandibular
        hyperplasia M26.03
        hypoplasia M26.04
      maxillary
        hyperplasia M26.01
        hypoplasia M26.02
      microgenia M26.06
      specified type NEC M26.09
    malocclusion M26.4
      dental arch relationship NEC M26.29
      jaw-cranial base relationship — *see* Anomaly,
          dentofacial, jaw-cranial base relationship
      jaw size — *see* Anomaly, dentofacial, jaw size
      specified type NEC M26.89
    temporomandibular joint M26.60
      adhesions M26.61
      ankylosis M26.61
      arthralgia M26.62
      articular disc M26.63
      specified type NEC M26.69
    tooth position, fully erupted M26.30
      specified NEC M26.39
  dermatoglyphic Q82.8
  diaphragm (apertures) NEC Q79.1
  digestive organ(s) or tract Q45.9
    lower Q43.9

Anomaly, anomalous— *continued*
  digestive organ(s) or tract— *continued*
    upper Q40.9
  distance, interarch (excessive) (inadequate) M26.25
  distribution, coronary artery Q24.5
  ductus
    arteriosus Q25.0
    botalli Q25.0
  duodenum Q43.9
  dura (brain) Q04.9
    spinal cord Q06.9
  ear (external) Q17.9
    causing impairment of hearing Q16.9
    inner Q16.5
    middle (causing impairment of hearing) Q16.4
    ossicles Q16.3
  Ebstein's (heart) (tricuspid valve) Q22.5
  ectodermal Q82.9
  Eisenmenger's (ventricular septal defect) Q21.8
  ejaculatory duct Q55.4
  elbow Q74.0
  endocrine gland NEC Q89.2
  epididymis Q55.4
  epiglottis Q31.8
  esophagus Q39.9
  eustachian tube Q17.8
  eye Q15.9
    anterior segment Q13.9
    posterior segment Q14.9
    ptosis (eyelid) Q10.0
    specified NEC Q15.8
  eyebrow Q18.8
  eyelid Q10.3
    ptosis Q10.0
  face Q18.9
    bone(s) Q75.9
  fallopian tube Q50.6
  fascia Q79.9
  femur NEC Q74.2
  fibula NEC Q74.2
  finger Q74.0
  fixation, intestine Q43.3
  flexion (joint) NOS Q74.9
    hip or thigh Q65.8
  foot NEC Q74.2
    varus (congenital) Q66.3
  foramen
    Botalli Q21.1
    ovale Q21.1
  forearm Q74.0
  forehead Q75.8
  form, teeth K00.2
  fovea centralis Q14.1
  frontal bone — *see* Anomaly, skull
  gallbladder (position) (shape) (size) Q44.1
  Gartner's duct Q52.4
  gastrointestinal tract Q45.9
  genitalia, genital organ(s) or system
    female Q52.9
      external Q52.70
      internal NOS Q52.9
    male Q55.9
      hydrocele P83.5
      specified NEC Q55.8
  genitourinary NEC
    female Q52.9
    male Q55.9
  Gerbode Q21.0
  glottis Q31.8
  granulation or granulocyte, genetic (constitutional)
      (leukocyte) D72.0
  gum Q38.6
  gyri Q07.9
  hair Q84.2
  hand Q74.0
  hard tissue formation in pulp K04.3
  head — *see* Anomaly, skull
  heart Q24.9
    auricle Q20.8
    bands or folds Q24.8
    fibroelastosis cordis I42.4
    obstructive NEC Q22.6
    patent ductus arteriosus (Botalli) Q25.0

Anomaly, anomalous— *continued*
  sex chromosomes NEC (*see also* Anomaly, chromosomes)
    female phenotype Q97.8
    male phenotype Q98.9
  shoulder (girdle) (joint) Q74.0
  sigmoid (flexure) Q43.9
  simian crease Q82.8
  sinus of Valsalva Q25.4
  skeleton generalized Q78.9
  skin (appendage) Q82.9
  skull Q75.9
    with
      anencephaly Q00.0
      encephalocele — *see* Encephalocele
      hydrocephalus Q03.9
        with spina bifida — *see* Spina bifida, by site, with hydrocephalus
      microcephaly Q02
  specified organ or site NEC Q89.8
  spermatic cord Q55.4
  spine, spinal NEC Q76.49
    column NEC Q76.49
      kyphosis — *see* Kyphosis, congenital
      lordosis — *see* Lordosis, congenital
    cord Q06.9
    nerve root Q07.8
  spleen Q89.09
    agenesis Q89.01
  stenonian duct Q38.4
  sternum NEC Q76.7
  stomach Q40.3
  submaxillary gland Q38.4
  tarsus NEC Q74.2
  tendon Q79.9
  testis — *see* Malformation, testis and scrotum
  thigh NEC Q74.2
  thorax (wall) Q67.8
    bony Q76.9
  throat Q38.8
  thumb Q74.0
  thymus gland Q89.2
  thyroid (gland) Q89.2
    cartilage Q31.8
  tibia NEC Q74.2
    saber A50.56
  toe Q74.2
  tongue Q38.3
  tooth, teeth K00.9
    eruption K00.6
    position, fully erupted M26.30
    spacing, fully erupted M26.30
  trachea (cartilage) Q32.1
  tragus Q17.9
  tricuspid (leaflet) (valve) Q22.9
    atresia or stenosis Q22.4
    Ebstein's Q22.5
  Uhl's (hypoplasia of myocardium, right ventricle) Q24.8
  ulna Q74.0
  umbilical artery Q27.0
  union
    cricoid cartilage and thyroid cartilage Q31.8
    thyroid cartilage and hyoid bone Q31.8
    trachea with larynx Q31.8
  upper limb Q74.0
  urachus Q64.4
  ureter Q62.8
    obstructive NEC Q62.39
      cecoureterocele Q62.32
      orthotopic ureterocele Q62.31
  urethra Q64.70
    absence Q64.5
    double Q64.74
    fistula to rectum Q64.73
    obstructive Q64.39
      stricture Q64.32
    prolapse Q64.71
    specified type NEC Q64.79
  urinary tract Q64.9
  uterus Q51.9
    with only one functioning horn Q51.4
  uvula Q38.5

Anomaly, anomalous— *continued*
  vagina Q52.4
  valleculae Q31.8
  valve (heart) NEC Q24.8
    coronary sinus Q24.5
    inferior vena cava Q24.8
    pulmonary Q22.3
    sinus coronario Q24.5
    venae cavae inferioris Q24.8
  vas deferens Q55.4
  vascular Q27.9
    brain Q28.3
    ring Q25.4
  vein(s) (peripheral) Q27.9
    brain Q28.3
    cerebral Q28.3
    coronary Q24.5
    great Q26.9
      specified NEC Q26.8
  vena cava (inferior) (superior) Q26.9
  venous — *see* Anomaly, vein(s)
  venous return Q26.8
  ventricular
    bands or folds Q24.8
    septa Q21.0
  vertebra Q76.49
    kyphosis — *see* Kyphosis, congenital
    lordosis — *see* Lordosis, congenital
  vesicourethral orifice Q64.79
  vessel(s) Q27.9
    optic papilla Q14.2
    precerebral Q28.1
  vitelline duct Q43.0
  vitreous body or humor Q14.0
  vulva Q52.70
  wrist (joint) Q74.0
Anomia R48.8
Anonychia (congenital) Q84.3
  acquired L60.8
Anophthalmos, anophthalmus (congenital) (globe) Q11.1
  acquired Z90.01
Anopia, anopsia H53.46-
  quadrant H53.46-
Anorchia, anorchism, anorchidism Q55.0
Anorexia R63.0
  hysterical F44.89
  nervosa F50.00
    atypical F50.9
    binge-eating type F50.2
      with purging F50.02
    restricting type F50.01
Anorgasmy, psychogenic (female) F52.31
  male F52.32
Anosmia R43.0
  hysterical F44.6
  postinfectional J39.8
Anosognosia R41.89
Anosteoplasia Q78.9
Anovulatory cycle N97.0
Anoxemia R09.02
  newborn P84
Anoxia (pathological) R09.01
  altitude T70.20
  cerebral G93.1
    complicating
      anesthesia (general) (local) or other sedation T88.59
        in labor and delivery O74.3
        in pregnancy O29.21-
        postpartum, puerperal O89.2
      delivery (cesarean) (instrumental) O75.4
    during a procedure G97.81
    newborn P84
    resulting from a procedure G97.82
  due to
    drowning T75.1
    high altitude T70.20
  heart — *see* Insufficiency, coronary
  intrauterine P84
  myocardial — *see* Insufficiency, coronary
  newborn P84
  spinal cord G95.11

Anoxia — *continued*
  systemic (by suffocation) (low content in atmosphere) — *see* Asphyxia, traumatic
Anteflexion — *see* Anteversion
Antenatal
  care (normal pregnancy) Z34.90
  screening (encounter for) of mother Z36
Antepartum — *see* condition
Anterior — *see* condition
Antero-occlusion M26.220
Anteversion
  cervix — *see* Anteversion, uterus
  femur (neck), congenital Q65.8
  uterus, uterine (cervix) (postinfectional) (postpartal, old) N85.4
    congenital Q51.818
    in pregnancy or childbirth — *see* Pregnancy, complicated by
Anthophobia F40.228
Anthracosilicosis J60
Anthracosis (lung) (occupational) J60
  lingua K14.3
Anthrax A22.9
  with pneumonia A22.1
  cerebral A22.8
  colitis A22.2
  cutaneous A22.0
  gastrointestinal A22.2
  inhalation A22.1
  intestinal A22.2
  meningitis A22.8
  pulmonary A22.1
  respiratory A22.1
  sepsis A22.7
  specified manifestation NEC A22.8
Anthropoid pelvis Q74.2
  with disproportion (fetopelvic) O33.0
Anthropophobia F40.10
  generalized F40.11
Antibodies, maternal (blood group) — *see* Isoimmunization, affecting management of pregnancy
  anti-D — *see* Isoimmunization, affecting management of pregnancy, Rh
  newborn P55.0
Anticardiolipin syndrome D68.61
Anticoagulant, circulating (intrinsic) D68.31
  drug-induced (extrinsic) D68.32
Antidiuretic hormone syndrome E22.2
Antimonial cholera — *see* Poisoning, antimony
Antiphospholipid syndrome D68.61
Antisocial personality F60.2
Antithrombinemia — *see* Circulating anticoagulants
Antithromboplastinemia — *see* Circulating anticoagulants
Antithromboplastinogenemia — *see* Circulating anticoagulants
Antitoxin complication or reaction — *see* Complications, vaccination
Antlophobia F40.228
Antritis J32.0
  maxilla J32.0
    acute J01.00
      recurrent J01.01
  stomach K29.60
    with bleeding K29.61
Antrum, antral — *see* condition
Anuria R34
  calculous (impacted) (recurrent) — *see* Calculus, urinary
  following ectopic or molar pregnancy O08.4
  newborn P96.0
  postprocedural N99.0
  postrenal N13.8
  traumatic (following crushing) T79.5
Anus, anal — *see* condition
Anusitis K62.8
Anxiety F41.9
  depression F41.8
  episodic paroxysmal F41.0
  generalized F41.1
  hysteria F41.8
  neurosis F41.1

Anxiety — *continued*
  panic type F41.Ø
  reaction F41.1
  separation, abnormal (of childhood) F93.Ø
  specified NEC F41.8
  state F41.1
Aorta, aortic — *see* condition
Aortectasia — *see* Ectasia, aorta
  with aneurysm — *see* Aneurysm, aorta
Aortitis (nonsyphilitic) (calcific) I77.6
  arteriosclerotic I7Ø.Ø
  Doehle-Heller A52.Ø2
  luetic A52.Ø2
  rheumatic — *see* Endocarditis, acute, rheumatic
  specific (syphilitic) A52.Ø2
  syphilitic A52.Ø2
    congenital A5Ø.54 [I79.1]
Apathetic thyroid storm — *see* Thyrotoxicosis
Apathy R45.3
Apeirophobia F4Ø.228
Apepsia K3Ø
  psychogenic F45.8
Aperistalsis, esophagus K22.Ø
Apertognathia M26.29
Apert's syndrome Q87.Ø
Aphagia R13.Ø
  psychogenic F5Ø.9
Aphakia (acquired) (postoperative) H27.Ø-
  congenital Q12.3
Aphasia (amnestic) (global) (nominal) (semantic)
    (syntactic) R47.Ø1
  acquired, with epilepsy (Landau-Kleffner syndrome)
      F8Ø.3
  auditory (developmental) F8Ø.2
  developmental (receptive type) F8Ø.2
    expressive type F8Ø.1
    Wernicke's F8Ø.2
  following
    cerebrovascular disease I69.92Ø
      cerebral infarction I69.32Ø
      intracerebral hemorrhage I69.12Ø
      nontraumatic intracranial hemorrhage NEC
          I69.22Ø
      specified disease NEC I69.82Ø
      subarachnoid hemorrhage I69.Ø2Ø
  progressive isolated G31.Ø1 [FØ2.8Ø]
    with behavioral disturbance G31.Ø1 [FØ2.81]
  sensory F8Ø.2
  syphilis, tertiary A52.19
  Wernicke's (developmental) F8Ø.2
Aphonia (organic) R49.1
  hysterical F44.4
  psychogenic F44.4
Aphthae, aphthous (*see also* condition)
  Bednar's K12.Ø
  cachectic K14.Ø
  epizootic BØ8.8
  oral K12.Ø
  stomatitis K12.Ø
  ulcer (oral) (recurrent) K12.Ø
  fever BØ8.8
  oral (recurrent) K12.Ø
  stomatitis (major) (minor) K12.Ø
  thrush B37.Ø
  ulcer (oral) (recurrent) K12.Ø
    genital organ(s) NEC
      female N76.6
      male N5Ø.8
    larynx J38.7
Apical — *see* condition
Apiphobia F4Ø.218
Aplasia (*see also* Agenesis)
  abdominal muscle syndrome Q79.4
  alveolar process (acquired) — *see* Anomaly, alveolar
    congenital Q38.6
  aorta (congenital) Q25.4
  axialis extracorticalis (congenita) E75.29
  bone marrow (myeloid) D61.9
    congenital D61.Ø1
  brain QØØ.Ø
    part of QØ4.3
  bronchus Q32.4
  cementum KØØ.4

Aplasia — *continued*
  cerebellum QØ4.3
  cervix (congenital) Q51.5
  congenital pure red cell D61.Ø1
  corpus callosum QØ4.Ø
  cutis congenita Q84.8
  erythrocyte congenital D61.Ø1
  extracortical axial E75.29
  eye Q11.1
  fovea centralis (congenital) Q14.1
  gallbladder, congenital Q44.Ø
  iris Q13.1
  labyrinth, membranous Q16.5
  limb (congenital) Q73.8
    lower — *see* Defect, reduction, lower limb
    upper — *see* Agenesis, arm
  lung, congenital (bilateral) (unilateral) Q33.3
  pancreas Q45.Ø
  parathyroid-thymic D82.1
  Pelizaeus-Merzbacher E75.29
  penis Q55.5
  prostate Q55.4
  red cell (pure) (with thymoma) D6Ø.9
    chronic D6Ø.Ø
    congenital D61.Ø1
    constitutional D61.Ø1
    hereditary D61.Ø1
    of infants D61.Ø1
    primary D61.Ø1
    specified type NEC D6Ø.8
    transient D6Ø.1
  round ligament Q52.8
  skin Q84.8
  spermatic cord Q55.4
  spleen Q89.Ø1
  testicle Q55.Ø
  thymic, with immunodeficiency D82.1
  thyroid (congenital) (with myxedema) EØ3.1
  uterus Q51.Ø
  ventral horn cell QØ6.1
Apnea, apneic (of) (spells) RØ6.81
  newborn NEC P28.4
    obstructive P28.4
    sleep (central) (obstructive) (primary) P28.3
  prematurity P28.4
  sleep G47.3Ø
    central (primary) G47.31
      in conditions classified elsewhere G47.37
    obstructive (adult) (pediatric) G47.33
    primary central G47.31
    specified NEC G47.39
Apneumatosis, newborn P28.Ø
Apocrine metaplasia (breast) — *see* Dysplasia,
    mammary, specified type NEC
Apophysitis (bone) (*see also* Osteochondropathy)
  calcaneus M92.8
  juvenile M92.9
Apoplectiform convulsions (cerebral ischemia) I67.8
Apoplexia, apoplexy, apoplectic
  adrenal A39.1
  heart (auricle) (ventricle) — *see* Infarct, myocardium
  heat T67.Ø
  hemorrhagic (stroke) — *see* Hemorrhage,
      intracranial
  meninges, hemorrhagic — *see* Hemorrhage,
      intracranial, subarachnoid
  uremic N18.9 [I68.8]
Appearance
  bizarre R46.1
  specified NEC R46.89
  very low level of personal hygiene R46.Ø
Appendage
  epididymal (organ of Morgagni) Q55.4
  intestine (epiploic) Q43.8
  preauricular Q17.Ø
  testicular (organ of Morgagni) Q55.29
Appendicitis (pneumococcal) (retrocecal) K37
  with
    perforation or rupture K35.2
    peritoneal abscess K35.3
      with peritonitis K35.2
    peritonitis K35.2
      with perforation or rupture K35.2

Appendicitis — *continued*
  with—*continued*
    peritonitis—*continued*
      localized K35.3
      generalized K35.2
    acute (catarrhal) (fulminating) (gangrenous)
        (obstructive) (retrocecal) (suppurative) K35.8Ø
      with
        perforation or rupture K35.2
        peritoneal abscess K35.3
          with peritonitis K35.2
        peritonitis K35.2
          with perforation or rupture K35.2
          localized K35.3
          generalized K35.2
      specified NEC K35.89
  amebic AØ6.89
  chronic (recurrent) K36
  exacerbation — *see* Appendicitis, acute
  gangrenous — *see* Appendicitis, acute
  healed (obliterative) K36
  interval K36
  neurogenic K36
  obstructive K36
  recurrent K36
  relapsing K36
  subacute (adhesive) K36
  subsiding K36
  suppurative — *see* Appendicitis, acute
  tuberculous A18.32
Appendix, appendicular (*see also* condition)
  epididymis Q55.4
  Morgagni
    female Q5Ø.5
    male (epididymal) Q55.4
      testicular Q55.29
  testis Q55.29
Appendicopathia oxyurica B8Ø
Appetite
  depraved — *see* Pica
  excessive R63.2
  lack or loss (*see also* Anorexia) R63.Ø
    nonorganic origin — *see* Disorder, eating
    psychogenic F5Ø.8
  perverted (hysterical) — *see* Pica
Apple peel syndrome Q41.1
Apprehension state F41.1
Apprehensiveness, abnormal F41.9
Approximal wear KØ3.Ø
Apraxia (classic) (ideational) (ideokinetic) (ideomotor)
    (motor) (verbal) R48.2
  following
    cerebrovascular disease I69.99Ø
      specified NEC I69.89Ø
      cerebral infarction I69.39Ø
      intracerebral hemorrhage I69.19Ø
      nontraumatic intracranial hemorrhage NEC
          I69.29Ø
      specified disease NEC I69.89Ø
          subarachnoid hemorrhage I69.Ø9Ø
  oculomotor, congenital H51.8
Aptyalism K11.7
Apudoma — *see* Neoplasm, uncertain behavior, by site
Aqueous misdirection H4Ø.83-
Arabicum elephantiasis — *see* Infestation, filarial
Arachnitis — *see* Meningitis
Arachnodactyly — *see* Syndrome, Marfan's
Arachnoiditis (acute) (adhesive) (basal) (brain)
    (cerebrospinal) — *see* Meningitis
Arachnophobia F4Ø.21Ø
Arboencephalitis, Australian A83.4
Arborization block (heart) I45.5
ARC (AIDS-related complex) B2Ø
Arches — *see* condition
Arcuate uterus Q51.81Ø
Arcuatus uterus Q51.81Ø
Arcus (cornea) senilis — *see* Degeneration, cornea,
    senile
Arc-welder's lung J63.4
Areflexia R29.2
Areola — *see* condition
Argentaffinoma (*see also* Neoplasm, uncertain
    behavior , by site)

Argentaffinoma —*continued*
  malignant — *see* Neoplasm, malignant, by site
  syndrome E34.Ø
Argininemia E72.21
Arginosuccinic aciduria E72.22
Argyll Robertson phenomenon, pupil or syndrome
    (syphilitic) A52.19
  atypical H57.Ø9
  nonsyphilitic H57.Ø9
Argyria, argyriasis
  conjunctival — *see* Deposit, conjunctiva
  from drug or medicament — *see* Table of Drugs and
    Chemicals, by substance
Argyrosis, conjunctival — *see* Deposit, conjunctiva
Arhinencephaly QØ4.1
Ariboflavinosis E53.Ø
Arm — *see* condition
Arnold-Chiari disease, obstruction or syndrome
    (type II) QØ7.ØØ
  with
    hydrocephalus QØ7.Ø2
      with spina bifida QØ7.Ø3
    spina bifida QØ7.Ø1
      with hydrocephalus QØ7.Ø3
  type III — *see* Encephalocele
  type IV QØ4.8
Aromatic amino-acid metabolism disorder E7Ø.9
  specified NEC E7Ø.8
Arousals, confusional G47.51
Arrest, arrested
  cardiac I46.9
    complicating
      abortion — *see* Abortion, by type,
        complicated by, cardiac arrest
      anesthesia (general) (local) or other sedation
        — *see* Table of Drugs and Chemicals, by
        drug,
      in labor and delivery O74.2
      in pregnancy O29.11-
      postpartum, puerperal O89.1
      delivery (cesarean) (instrumental) O75.4
    due to
      cardiac condition I46.2
      specified condition NEC I46.8
    intraoperative I97.71-
    newborn P29.81
    postprocedural I97.12-
      obstetric procedure O75.4
  cardiorespiratory — *see* Arrest, cardiac
  circulatory — *see* Arrest, cardiac
  deep transverse O64.Ø
  development or growth
    bone — *see* Disorder, bone, development or
      growth
    child R62.5Ø
    tracheal rings Q32.1
  epiphyseal
    complete
      femur M89.15-
      humerus M89.12-
      tibia M89.16-
      ulna M89.13-
      forearm M89.13-
        specified NEC M89.13-
        ulna — *see* Arrest, epiphyseal, by type, ulna
      lower leg M89.16-
        specified NEC M89.168
        tibia — *see* Arrest, epiphyseal, by type, tibia
    partial
      femur M89.15-
      humerus M89.12-
      tibia M89.16-
      ulna M89.13-
      specified NEC M89.18
  granulopoiesis — *see* Agranulocytosis
  growth plate — *see* Arrest, epiphyseal
  heart — *see* Arrest, cardiac
  legal, anxiety concerning Z65.3
  physeal — *see* Arrest, epiphyseal
  respiratory RØ9.2
    newborn P28.81
  sinus I45.5

Arrest, arrested— *continued*
  spermatogenesis (complete) — *see* Azoospermia
    incomplete — *see* Oligospermia
  transverse (deep) O64.Ø
Arrhenoblastoma
  benign
    specified site — *see* Neoplasm, benign, by site
    unspecified site
      female D27.9
      male D29.2Ø
  malignant
    specified site — *see* Neoplasm, malignant, by site
    unspecified site
      female C56.9
      male C62.9Ø
  specified site — *see* Neoplasm, uncertain behavior,
    by site
  unspecified site
    female D39.1Ø
    male D4Ø.1Ø
Arrhythmia (auricle)(cardiac)(juvenile)(nodal)
    (reflex)(sinus)(supraventricular)(transitory)
    (ventricle) I49.9
  block I45.9
  extrasystolic I49.49
  newborn
    bradycardia P29.12
    tachycardia P29.11
    occurring before birth PØ3.819
      before onset of labor PØ3.81Ø
      during labor PØ3.811
  psychogenic F45.8
  specified NEC I49.8
  vagal R55
  ventricular re-entry I47.Ø
Arrillaga-Ayerza syndrome (pulmonary sclerosis with
    pulmonary hypertension) I27.Ø
Arsenical pigmentation L81.8
  from drug or medicament — *see* Table of drugs and
    medicaments
Arsenism — *see* Poisoning, arsenic
Arterial — *see* condition
Arteriofibrosis — *see* Arteriosclerosis
Arteriolar sclerosis — *see* Arteriosclerosis
Arteriolith — *see* Arteriosclerosis
Arteriolitis I77.6
  necrotizing, kidney I77.5
  renal — *see* Hypertension, kidney
Arteriolosclerosis — *see* Arteriosclerosis
Arterionephrosclerosis — *see* Hypertension, kidney
Arteriopathy I77.9
Arteriosclerosis, arteriosclerotic (diffuse)
    (obliterans) (of) (senile) (with calcification) I7Ø.9Ø
  aorta I7Ø.Ø
  arteries of extremities — *see* Arteriosclerosis,
    extremities
  brain I67.2
    extremities — *see* Arteriosclerosis,
      extremities, bypass graft
  cardiac — *see* Disease, heart, ischemic,
    atherosclerotic
  cardiopathy — *see* Disease, heart, ischemic,
    atherosclerotic
  cardiorenal — *see* Hypertension, cardiorenal
  cardiovascular — *see* Disease, heart, ischemic,
    atherosclerotic
  central nervous system I67.2
  cerebral I67.2
  cerebrovascular I67.2
  coronary (artery) I25.1Ø
    due to lipid rich plaque I25.83
    native vessel
      with
        angina pectoris I25.119
          specified type NEC I25.118
          unstable I25.11Ø
          with documented spasm I25.111
        ischemic chest pain I25.119
    bypass graft I25.81Ø
      with
        angina pectoris I25.7Ø9
          specified type NEC I25.7Ø8
          unstable I25.7ØØ

Arteriosclerosis, arteriosclerotic — *continued*
  coronary— *continued*
    bypass graft— *continued*
      with— *continued*
        angina pectoris— *continued*
          with documented spasm I25.7Ø1
        ischemic chest pain I25.7Ø9
    autologous artery I25.81Ø
      with
        angina pectoris I25.729
          specified type I25.728
          unstable I25.72Ø
          with documented spasm I25.721
        ischemic chest pain I25.729
    autologous vein I25.81Ø
      with
        angina pectoris I25.719
          specified type I25.718
          unstable I25.71Ø
          with documented spasm I25.711
        ischemic chest pain I25.719
    nonautologous biological I25.81Ø
      with
        angina pectoris I25.739
          specified type I25.738
          unstable I25.73Ø
          with documented spasm I25.731
        ischemic chest pain I25.739
    specified type NEC I25.81Ø
      with
        angina pectoris I25.799
          specified type I25.798
          unstable I25.79Ø
          with documented spasm I25.791
        ischemic chest pain I25.799
    transplanted heart I25.811
    native coronary artery I25.811
      with
        angina pectoris I25.759
          specified type I25.758
          unstable I25.75Ø
          with documented spasm I25.751
        ischemic chest pain I25.759
    bypass graft I25.812
      with
        angina pectoris I25.769
          specified type I25.768
          unstable I25.76Ø
          with documented spasm I25.761
        ischemic chest pain I25.769
  extremities (native arteries) I7Ø.2Ø9
    bypass graft I7Ø.3Ø9
      autologous vein graft I7Ø.4Ø9
        leg I7Ø.4Ø9
          with
            gangrene (and intermittent
              claudication, rest pain and
              ulcer) I7Ø.469
            intermittent claudication I7Ø.419
            rest pain (and intermittent
              claudication) I7Ø.429
          bilateral I7Ø.4Ø3
            with
              gangrene (and intermittent
                claudication, rest pain and
                ulcer) I7Ø.463
              intermittent claudication
                I7Ø.413
              rest pain (and intermittent
                claudication) I7Ø.423
            specified type NEC I7Ø.493
          left I7Ø.4Ø2
            with
              gangrene (and intermittent
                claudication, rest pain and
                ulcer) I7Ø.462
              intermittent claudication
                I7Ø.412
              rest pain (and intermittent
                claudication) I7Ø.422
              ulceration (and intermittent
                claudication and rest pain)
                I7Ø.449

Arteriosclerosis, arteriosclerotic— *continued*
  extremities— *continued*
    bypass graft— *continued*
      autologous vein graft— *continued*
        leg— *continued*
          left— *continued*
            with— *continued*
              ulceration— *continued*
                ankle I70.443
                calf I70.442
                foot site NEC I70.445
                heel I70.444
                lower leg NEC I70.448
                midfoot I70.444
                thigh I70.441
              specified type NEC I70.492
          right I70.401
            with
              gangrene (and intermittent claudication, rest pain and ulcer) I70.461
              intermittent claudication I70.411
              rest pain (and intermittent claudication) I70.421
              ulceration (and intermittent claudication and rest pain) I70.439
                ankle I70.433
                calf I70.432
                foot site NEC I70.435
                heel I70.434
                lower leg NEC I70.438
                midfoot I70.434
                thigh I70.431
              specified type NEC I70.491
          specified type NEC I70.499
        specified NEC I70.408
          with
            gangrene (and intermittent claudication, rest pain and ulcer) I70.468
            intermittent claudication I70.418
            rest pain (and intermittent claudication) I70.428
            ulceration (and intermittent claudication and rest pain) I70.45
            specified type NEC I70.498
        leg I70.309
          with
            gangrene (and intermittent claudication, rest pain and ulcer) I70.369
            intermittent claudication I70.319
            rest pain (and intermittent claudication) I70.329
          bilateral I70.303
            with
               gangrene (and intermittent claudication, rest pain and ulcer) I70.363
              intermittent claudication I70.313
              rest pain (and intermittent claudication) I70.323
            specified type NEC I70.393
          left I70.302
            with
               gangrene (and intermittent claudication, rest pain and ulcer) I70.362
              intermittent claudication I70.312
              rest pain (and intermittent claudication) I70.322
              ulceration (and intermittent claudication and rest pain) I70.349
                ankle I70.343
                calf I70.342
                foot site NEC I70.345
                heel I70.344
                lower leg NEC I70.348
                midfoot I70.344

Arteriosclerosis, arteriosclerotic— *continued*
  extremities— *continued*
    bypass graft— *continued*
      leg— *continued*
        left— *continued*
          with— *continued*
            ulceration— *continued*
              thigh I70.341
            specified type NEC I70.392
        right I70.301
          with
            gangrene (and intermittent claudication, rest pain and ulcer) I70.361
            intermittent claudication I70.311
            rest pain (and intermittent claudication) I70.321
            ulceration (and intermittent claudication and rest pain) I70.339
              ankle I70.333
              calf I70.332
              foot site NEC I70.335
              heel I70.334
              lower leg NEC I70.338
              midfoot I70.334
              thigh I70.331
            specified type NEC I70.391
        specified type NEC I70.399
        nonautologous biological graft I70.509
          leg I70.509
            with
              gangrene (and intermittent claudication, rest pain and ulcer) I70.569
              intermittent claudication I70.519
              rest pain (and intermittent claudication) I70.529
            bilateral I70.503
              with
                gangrene (and intermittent claudication, rest pain and ulcer) I70.563
                intermittent claudication I70.513
                rest pain (and intermittent claudication) I70.523
              specified type NEC I70.593
            left I70.502
              with
                gangrene (and intermittent claudication, rest pain and ulcer) I70.562
                intermittent claudication I70.512
                rest pain (and intermittent claudication) I70.522
                ulceration (and intermittent claudication and rest pain) I70.549
                  ankle I70.543
                  calf I70.542
                  foot site NEC I70.545
                  heel I70.544
                  lower leg NEC I70.548
                  midfoot I70.544
                  thigh I70.541
              specified type NEC I70.592
            right I70.501
              with
                gangrene (and intermittent claudication, rest pain and ulcer) I70.561
                intermittent claudication I70.511
                rest pain (and intermittent claudication) I70.521
                ulceration (and intermittent claudication and rest pain) I70.539
                  ankle I70.533
                  calf I70.532
                  foot site NEC I70.535

Arteriosclerosis, arteriosclerotic— *continued*
  extremities— *continued*
    bypass graft— *continued*
      nonautologous biological graft— *continued*
        leg— *continued*
          right— *continued*
            with— *continued*
              ulceration— *continued*
                heel I70.534
                lower leg NEC I70.538
                midfoot I70.534
                thigh I70.531
              specified type NEC I70.591
          specified type NEC I70.599
        specified NEC I70.508
          with
            gangrene (and intermittent claudication, rest pain and ulcer) I70.568
            intermittent claudication I70.518
            rest pain (and intermittent claudication) I70.528
            ulceration (and intermittent claudication and rest pain) I70.55
            specified type NEC I70.598
        nonbiological graft I70.609
          leg I70.609
            with
              gangrene (and intermittent claudication, rest pain and ulcer) I70.669
              intermittent claudication I70.619
              rest pain (and intermittent claudication) I70.629
            bilateral I70.603
              with
                gangrene (and intermittent claudication, rest pain and ulcer) I70.663
                intermittent claudication I70.613
                rest pain (and intermittent claudication) I70.623
              specified type NEC I70.693
            left I70.602
              with
                gangrene (and intermittent claudication, rest pain and ulcer) I70.662
                intermittent claudication I70.612
                rest pain (and intermittent claudication) I70.622
                ulceration (and intermittent claudication and rest pain) I70.649
                  ankle I70.643
                  calf I70.642
                  foot site NEC I70.645
                  heel I70.644
                  lower leg NEC I70.648
                  midfoot I70.644
                  thigh I70.641
              specified type NEC I70.692
            right I70.601
              with
                gangrene (and intermittent claudication, rest pain and ulcer) I70.661
                intermittent claudication I70.611
                rest pain (and intermittent claudication) I70.621
                ulceration (and intermittent claudication and rest pain) I70.639
                  ankle I70.633
                  calf I70.632
                  foot site NEC I70.635
                  heel I70.634
                  lower leg NEC I70.638
                  midfoot I70.634

Arteriosclerosis, arteriosclerotic— *continued*
  extremities— *continued*
    bypass graft— *continued*
      nonbiological graft— *continued*
        leg—*continued*
          right—*continued*
            with—*continued*
              ulceration—*continued*
                thigh I70.631
              specified type NEC I70.691
            specified type NEC I70.699
        specified NEC I70.608
          with
            gangrene (and intermittent
              claudication, rest pain and
              ulcer) I70.668
            intermittent claudication I70.618
            rest pain (and intermittent
              claudication) I70.628
            ulceration (and intermittent
              claudication and rest pain)
              I70.65
            specified type NEC I70.698
      specified graft NEC I70.709
        leg I70.709
          with
            gangrene (and intermittent
              claudication, rest pain and
              ulcer) I70.769
            intermittent claudication I70.719
            rest pain (and intermittent
              claudication) I70.729
          bilateral I70.703
            with
              gangrene (and intermittent
                claudication, rest pain and
                ulcer) I70.763
              intermittent claudication
                I70.713
              rest pain (and intermittent
                claudication) I70.723
            specified type NEC I70.793
          left I70.702
            with
              gangrene (and intermittent
                claudication, rest pain and
                ulcer) I70.762
              intermittent claudication
                I70.712
              rest pain (and intermittent
                claudication) I70.722
              ulceration (and intermittent
                claudication and rest pain)
                I70.749
                ankle I70.743
                calf I70.742
                foot site NEC I70.745
                heel I70.744
                lower leg NEC I70.748
                midfoot I70.744
                thigh I70.741
            specified type NEC I70.792
          right I70.701
            with
              gangrene (and intermittent
                claudication, rest pain and
                ulcer) I70.761
              intermittent claudication
                I70.711
              rest pain (and intermittent
                claudication) I70.721
              ulceration (and intermittent
                claudication and rest pain)
                I70.739
                ankle I70.733
                calf I70.732
                foot site NEC I70.735
                heel I70.734
                lower leg NEC I70.738
                midfoot I70.734
                thigh I70.731
            specified type NEC I70.791
      specified type NEC I70.799

Arteriosclerosis, arteriosclerotic— *continued*
  extremities— *continued*
    bypass graft— *continued*
      specified graft— *continued*
        specified NEC I70.708
          with
            gangrene (and intermittent
              claudication, rest pain and
              ulcer) I70.768
            intermittent claudication I70.718
            rest pain (and intermittent
              claudication) I70.728
            ulceration (and intermittent
              claudication and rest pain)
              I70.75
          specified type NEC I70.798
      specified NEC I70.308
        with
          gangrene (and intermittent
            claudication, rest pain and ulcer)
            I70.368
          intermittent claudication I70.318
          rest pain (and intermittent
            claudication) I70.328
          ulceration (and intermittent
            claudication and rest pain)
            I70.35
        specified type NEC I70.398
      leg I70.209
        with
          gangrene (and intermittent claudication,
            rest pain and ulcer) I70.269
          intermittent claudication I70.219
          rest pain (and intermittent claudication)
            I70.229
        bilateral I70.203
          with
            gangrene (and intermittent
              claudication, rest pain and ulcer)
              I70.263
            intermittent claudication I70.213
            rest pain (and intermittent
              claudication) I70.223
          specified type NEC I70.293
        left I70.202
          with
            gangrene (and intermittent
              claudication, rest pain and ulcer)
              I70.262
            intermittent claudication I70.212
            rest pain (and intermittent
              claudication) I70.222
            ulceration (and intermittent
              claudication and rest pain)
              I70.249
              ankle I70.243
              calf I70.242
              foot site NEC I70.245
              heel I70.244
              lower leg NEC I70.248
              midfoot I70.244
              thigh I70.241
          specified type NEC I70.292
        right I70.201
          with
            gangrene (and intermittent
              claudication, rest pain and ulcer)
              I70.261
            intermittent claudication I70.211
            rest pain (and intermittent
              claudication) I70.221
            ulceration (and intermittent
              claudication and rest pain)
              I70.239
              ankle I70.233
              calf I70.232
              foot site NEC I70.235
              heel I70.234
              lower leg NEC I70.238
              midfoot I70.234
              thigh I70.231
          specified type NEC I70.291
      specified type NEC I70.299

Arteriosclerosis, arteriosclerotic— *continued*
  extremities— *continued*
    specified site NEC I70.208
      with
        gangrene (and intermittent claudication,
          rest pain and ulcer) I70.268
        intermittent claudication I70.218
        rest pain (and intermittent claudication)
          I70.228
        ulceration (and intermittent claudication
          and rest pain) I70.25
      specified type NEC I70.298
  generalized I70.91
  heart (disease) — *see* Arteriosclerosis, coronary
    (artery),
  kidney — *see* Hypertension, kidney
  medial — *see* Arteriosclerosis, extremities
  mesenteric (artery) K55.1
  Mönckeberg's — *see* Arteriosclerosis, extremities
  myocarditis I51.4
  peripheral (of extremities) — *see* Arteriosclerosis,
    extremities
  pulmonary (idiopathic) I27.0
  renal (arterioles) (*see also* Hypertension, kidney
    artery I70.1)
  retina (vascular) I70.8
  specified artery NEC I70.8
  spinal (cord) G95.19
  vertebral (artery) I67.2
Arteriospasm I73.9
Arteriovenous — *see* condition
Arteritis I77.6
  allergic M31.0
  aorta (nonsyphilitic) I77.6
    syphilitic A52.02
  aortic arch M31.4
  brachiocephalic M31.4
  brain I67.7
    syphilitic A52.04
  cerebral I67.7
    in systemic lupus erythematosus M32.19
    listerial A32.89
    syphilitic A52.04
    tuberculous A18.89
  coronary (artery) I25.89
    rheumatic I01.8
      chronic I09.89
    syphilitic A52.06
  cranial (left) (right), giant cell M31.6
  deformans — *see* Arteriosclerosis
  giant cell NEC M31.6
    with polymyalgia rheumatica M31.5
  necrosing or necrotizing M31.9
    specified NEC M31.8
  nodosa M30.0
  obliterans — *see* Arteriosclerosis
  pulmonary I28.8
  rheumatic — *see* Fever, rheumatic
  senile — *see* Arteriosclerosis
  suppurative I77.2
  syphilitic (general) A52.09
    brain A52.04
    coronary A52.06
    spinal A52.09
  temporal, giant cell M31.6
  young female aortic arch syndrome M31.4
Artery, arterial (*see also* condition)
  abscess I77.89
  single umbilical Q27.0
Arthralgia (allergic) (*see also* Pain, joint)
  in caisson disease T70.3
  temporomandibular M26.62
Arthritis, arthritic (acute) (chronic) (nonpyogenic)
    (subacute) M19.90
  meaning osteoarthritis — *see* Osteoarthritis
  allergic — *see* Arthritis, specified form NEC
  ankylosing (crippling) (spine) (*see also* Spondylitis,
    ankylosing)
    sites other than spine — *see* Arthritis, specified
      form NEC
  atrophic — *see* Osteoarthritis
    spine — *see* Spondylitis, ankylosing
  back — *see* Spondylopathy, inflammatory

Index

Arthritis, arthritic—Arthritis, arthritic

Arthritis, arthritic— *continued*
  blennorrhagic (gonococcal) A54.42
  Charcot's — *see* Arthropathy, neuropathic
  Charcot's— *continued*
    diabetic — *see* Diabetes, arthropathy,
      neuropathic
    syringomyelic G95.0
  chylous (filarial) B74.9 (*see also* category M01)
  climacteric (any site) NEC — *see* Arthritis, specified
    form NEC
  crystal(-induced) — *see* Arthritis, in, crystals
  deformans — *see* Osteoarthritis
  degenerative — *see* Osteoarthritis
  due to or associated with
    acromegaly E22.0
    brucellosis — *see* Brucellosis
    caisson disease T70.3
    diabetes — *see* Diabetes, arthropathy
    dracontiasis B72 (*see also* category M01)
    enteritis NEC
      regional — *see* Enteritis, regional
    erysipelas A46
    erythema
      epidemic A25.1
      nodosum L52
    filariasis NOS B74.9
    glanders A24.0
    helminthiasis (*see also* category M01) B83.9
    hemophilia D66
    Henoch (-Schönlein) purpura D69.0
    human parvovirus (*see also* category M01) B97.6
    infectious disease NEC — *see* category M01
    leprosy (*see also* Leprosy) A30.9
    Lyme disease A69.23
    mycobacteria A31.8
    parasitic disease NEC B89 (*see also* category M01)
    paratyphoid fever (*see also* Fever, paratyphoid)
      A01.4 (*see also* category M01)
    rat bite fever A25.1
    regional enteritis — *see* Enteritis, regional
    respiratory disorder NOS J98.9
    serum sickness T80.6
    syringomyelia G95.0
    typhoid fever A01.04
  epidemic erythema A25.1
  febrile — *see* Fever, rheumatic
  gonococcal A54.42
  gouty (acute) — *see* Gout, idiopathic
  in (due to)
    acromegaly (*see also* subcategory M14.8-) E22.0
    amyloidosis (*see also* subcategory M14.8-) E85.4
    bacterial disease (*see also* subcategory M01)
      A49.9
    Behçet's syndrome M35.2
    caisson disease (*see also* subcategory M14.8-)
      T70.3
    coliform bacilli (Escherichia coli) — *see* Arthritis,
      in, pyogenic organism NEC
    crystals M11.9
      dicalcium phosphate — *see* Arthritis, in,
        crystals, specified type NEC
      hydroxyapatite M11.0-
      pyrophosphate — *see* Arthritis, in, crystals,
        specified type NEC
      specified type NEC M11.80
        ankle M11.87-
        elbow M11.82-
        foot joint M11.87-
        hand joint M11.84-
        hip M11.85-
        knee M11.86-
        multiple site M11.8-
        shoulder M11.81-
        specified joint NEC M11.88
        wrist M11.83-
    dermatoarthritis, lipoid E78.81
    dracontiasis (dracunculiasis) B72 (*see also*
      category M01)
    endocrine disorder NEC (*see also* subcategory
      M14.8-) E34.9

Arthritis, arthritic— *continued*
  in (due to)— *continued*
    enteritis, infectious NEC A09 (*see also* category
      M01)
      specified organism NEC A08.8 (*see also*
        category M01)
    erythema
      multiforme (*see also* subcategory M14.8-)
        L51.9
      nodosum (*see also* subcategory M14.8-) L52
    gout — *see* Gout, idiopathic
    Hemophilus influenzae B96.3 [M00.80]
    helminthiasis NEC B83.9 (*see also* category M01)
    hemochromatosis (*see also* subcategory M14.8-)
      E83.118
    hemoglobinopathy NEC D58.2 [M36.3]
    hemophilia NEC D66 [M36.2]
    Henoch(-Schönlein) purpura D69.0 [M36.4]
    hyperparathyroidism NEC (*see also* subcategory
      M14.8-) E21.3
    hypersensitivity reaction NEC T78.49 [M36.4]
    hypogammaglobulinemia (*see also* subcategory
      M14.8-) D80.1
    hypothyroidism NEC (*see also* subcategory
      M14.8-) E03.9
    infection — *see* Arthritis, pyogenic or pyemic
      spine — *see* Spondylopathy, infective
    infectious disease NEC (*see also* category M01)
      B99
    leprosy A30.9 (*see also* category M01)
    leukemia NEC C95.9- [M36.1]
    lipoid dermatoarthritis E78.81
    Lyme disease A69.23
    Mediterranean fever, familial (*see also*
      subcategory M14.8-) E85.0
    Meningococcus A39.83
    metabolic disorder NEC (*see also* subcategory
      M14.8-) E88.9
    multiple myelomatosis C90.0- [M36.1]
    mumps B26.85
    mycosis NEC B49 (*see also* category M01)
    myelomatosis (multiple) C90.0- [M36.1]
    neurological disorder NEC G98.0
    ochronosis (*see also* subcategory M14.8-) E70.29
    O'nyong-nyong A92.1 (*see also* category M01)
    parasitic disease NEC B89 (*see also* category M01)
    paratyphoid fever A01.4 (*see also* category M01)
    Pseudomonas — *see* Arthritis, pyogenic,
      bacterial NEC
    psoriasis L40.50
    pyogenic organism NEC — *see* Arthritis,
      pyogenic, bacterial NEC
    Reiter's disease — *see* Reiter's disease
    respiratory disorder NEC (*see also* subcategory
      M14.8-) J98.9
    reticulosis, malignant (*see also* subcategory
      M14.8-) C85.8-
    rubella B06.82
    Salmonella (arizonae) (cholerae-suis) (enteritidis)
      (typhimurium) A02.23
    sarcoidosis D86.86
    specified bacteria NEC — *see* Arthritis, pyogenic,
      bacterial NEC
    sporotrichosis B42.82
    syringomyelia G95.0
    thalassemia NEC D56.9 [M36.3]
    tuberculosis — *see* Tuberculosis, arthritis
    typhoid fever A01.04
    urethritis, Reiter's — *see* Reiter's disease
    viral disease NEC B34.9 (*see also* category M01)
  infectious or infective (*see also* Arthritis, pyogenic or
    pyemic)
    spine — *see* Spondylopathy, infective
  juvenile M08.90
    with systemic onset — *see* Still's disease
    ankle M08.97-
    elbow M08.92-
    foot joint M08.97-
    hand joint M08.94-
    hip M08.95-
    knee M08.96-
    multiple site M08.99

Arthritis, arthritic— *continued*
  juvenile— *continued*
    pauciarticular M08.40
      ankle M08.47-
      elbow M08.42-
      foot joint M08.47-
      hand joint M08.44-
      hip M08.45-
      knee M08.46-
      shoulder M08.41-
      specified joint NEC M08.48
      wrist M08.43-
    psoriatic L40.54
    rheumatoid — *see* Arthritis, rheumatoid, juvenile
    shoulder M08.91-
    vertebra M08.98
    specified type NEC M08.80
      ankle M08.87-
      elbow M08.82-
      foot joint M08.87-
      hand joint M08.84-
      hip M08.85-
      knee M08.86-
      multiple site M08.89
      shoulder M08.81-
      specified joint NEC M08.88
      wrist M08.83-
    wrist M08.93-
  meningococcal A39.83
  menopausal (any site) NEC — *see* Arthritis, specified
    form NEC
  mutilans (psoriatic) L40.52
  mycotic NEC B49 (*see also* category M01)
  neuropathic (Charcot) — *see* Arthropathy,
    neuropathic
    diabetic — *see* Diabetes, arthropathy,
      neuropathic
    nonsyphilitic NEC G98.0
    syringomyelic G95.0
  ochronotic (*see also* subcategory M14.8-) E70.29
  palindromic (any site) *see* Rheumatism, palindromic
  pneumococcal M00.10
    ankle M00.17-
    elbow M00.12-
    foot joint — *see* Arthritis, pneumococcal, ankle
    hand joint M00.14-
    hip M00.15-
    knee M00.16-
    multiple site M00.19
    shoulder M00.11-
    vertebra M00.18
    wrist M00.13-
  postdysenteric — *see* Arthropathy, postdysenteric
  postmeningococcal A39.84
  postrheumatic, chronic — *see* Arthropathy,
    postrheumatic, chronic
  primary progressive (*see also* Arthritis, specified
    form NEC)
    spine — *see* Spondylitis, ankylosing
  psoriatic L40.50
  purulent (any site except spine) — *see* Arthritis,
    pyogenic or pyemic
    spine — *see* Spondylopathy, infective
  pyogenic or pyemic (any site except spine) M00.9
    spine — *see* Spondylopathy, infective
    bacterial NEC M00.80
      ankle M00.87-
      elbow M00.82-
      foot joint — *see* Arthritis, bacterial NEC, ankle
      hand joint M00.84-
      hip M00.85-
      knee M00.86-
      multiple site M00.89
      shoulder M00.81-
      vertebra M00.88
      wrist M00.83-
    pneumococcal — *see* Arthritis, pneumococcal
    staphylococcal — *see* Arthritis, staphylococcal
    streptococcal — *see* Arthritis, streptococcal NEC
      pneumococcal — *see* Arthritis, pneumococcal
  rheumatic (*see also* Arthritis, rheumatoid)
    acute or subacute — *see* Fever, rheumatic

Arthritis, arthritic— *continued*
  rheumatoid M06.9
    with
      carditis — *see* Rheumatoid, carditis
      endocarditis — *see* Rheumatoid, carditis
      heart involvement NEC — *see* Rheumatoid, carditis
      lung involvement — *see* Rheumatoid, lung
      myocarditis — *see* Rheumatoid, carditis
      myopathy — *see* Rheumatoid, myopathy
      pericarditis — *see* Rheumatoid, carditis
      polyneuropathy — *see* Rheumatoid, polyneuropathy
      rheumatoid factor — *see* Arthritis, rheumatoid, seropositive
      splenoadenomegaly and leukopenia — *see* Felty's syndrome
      vasculitis — *see* Rheumatoid, vasculitis
      visceral involvement NEC — *see* Rheumatoid, arthritis, with involvement of organs NEC
    juvenile (with or without rheumatoid factor) M08.00
      ankle M08.07-
      elbow M08.02-
      foot joint M08.07-
      hand joint M08.04-
      hip M08.05-
      knee M08.06-
      multiple site M08.09
      shoulder M08.01-
      vertebra M08.08
      wrist M08.03-
    seronegative M06.00
      ankle M06.07-
      elbow M06.02-
      foot joint M06.07-
      hand joint M06.04-
      hip M06.05-
      knee M06.06-
      multiple site M06.09
      shoulder M06.01-
      vertebra M06.08
      wrist M06.03-
    seropositive M05.9
      specified NEC M05.80
        ankle M05.87-
        elbow M05.82-
        foot joint M05.87-
        hand joint M05.84
        hip M05.85-
        knee M05.86-
        multiple sites M05.89
        shoulder M05.81-
        wrist M05.83-
      without organ involvement M05.70
        ankle M05.77-
        elbow M05.72-
        foot joint M05.77-
        hand joint M05.74-
        hip M05.75-
        knee M05.76-
        multiple sites M05.79
        shoulder M05.71-
        vertebra — *see* Spondylitis, ankylosing
        wrist M05.73-
    specified type NEC M06.80
      ankle M06.87-
      elbow M06.82-
      foot joint M06.87-
      hand joint M06.84-
      hip M06.85-
      knee M06.86-
      multiple site M06.89
      shoulder M06.81-
      vertebra M06.88
      wrist M06.83-
    spine — *see* Spondylitis, ankylosing
  rubella B06.82
  scorbutic (*see also* subcategory M14.8-) E54
  senile or senescent — *see* Osteoarthritis

Arthritis, arthritic— *continued*
  septic (any site except spine) — *see* Arthritis, pyogenic or pyemic
    spine — *see* Spondylopathy, infective
  serum (nontherapeutic) (therapeutic) — *see* Arthropathy, postimmunization
  specified form NEC M13.80
    ankle M13.87-
    elbow M13.82-
    foot joint M13.87-
    hand joint M13.84-
    hip M13.85-
    knee M13.86-
    multiple site M13.89
    shoulder M13.81-
    specified joint NEC M13.88
    wrist M13.83-
  spine (*see also* Spondylopathy, inflammatory)
    infectious or infective NEC — *see* Spondylopathy, infective
    Marie-Strümpell — *see* Spondylitis, ankylosing
    pyogenic — *see* Spondylopathy, infective
    rheumatoid — *see* Spondylitis, ankylosing
    traumatic (old) — *see* Spondylopathy, traumatic
    tuberculous A18.01
  staphylococcal M00.00
    ankle M00.07-
    elbow M00.02-
    foot joint — *see* Arthritis, staphylococcal, ankle
    hand joint M00.04-
    hip M00.05-
    knee M00.06-
    multiple site M00.09
    shoulder M00.01-
    vertebra M00.08
    wrist M00.03-
  streptococcal NEC M00.20
    ankle M00.27-
    elbow M00.22-
    foot joint — *see* Arthritis, streptococcal, ankle
    hand joint M00.24-
    hip M00.25-
    knee M00.26-
    multiple site M00.29
    shoulder M00.21-
    vertebra M00.28
    wrist M00.23-
  suppurative — *see* Arthritis, pyogenic or pyemic
  syphilitic (late) A52.16
    congenital A50.55 [M12.80]
  syphilitica deformans (Charcot) A52.16
  temporomandibular M26.69
  toxic of menopause (any site) — *see* Arthritis, specified form NEC
  transient — *see* Arthropathy, specified form NEC
  traumatic (chronic) — *see* Arthropathy, traumatic
  tuberculous A18.02
    spine A18.01
  uratic — *see* Gout, idiopathic
  urethritica (Reiter's) — *see* Reiter's disease
  vertebral — *see* Spondylopathy, inflammatory
  villous (any site) — *see* Arthropathy, specified form NEC

Arthrocele — *see* Effusion, joint
Arthrodesis status Z98.1
Arthrodynia (*see also* Pain, joint)
Arthrofibrosis, joint — *see* Ankylosis
Arthrodysplasia Q74.9
Arthrogryposis (congenital) Q68.8
  multiplex congenita Q74.3
Arthrokatadysis M24.7
Arthropathy (*see also* Arthritis) M12.9
  Charcot's — *see* Arthropathy, neuropathic
    diabetic — *see* Diabetes, arthropathy, neuropathic
    syringomyelic G95.0
  cricoarytenoid J38.7
  crystal(-induced) — *see* Arthritis, in, crystals
  diabetic NEC — *see* Diabetes, arthropathy
  distal interphalangeal, psoriatic L40.51
  enteropathic M07.60
    ankle M07.67-
    elbow M07.62-

Arthropathy— *continued*
  enteropathic— *continued*
    foot joint M07.67-
    hand joint M07.64-
    hip M07.65-
    knee M07.66-
    multiple site M07.69
    shoulder M07.61-
    vertebra M07.68
    wrist M07.63-
  following intestinal bypass M02.00
    ankle M02.07-
    elbow M02.02-
    foot joint M02.07-
    hand joint M02.04-
    hip M02.05-
    knee M02.06-
    multiple site M02.09
    shoulder M02.01-
    vertebra M02.08
    wrist M02.03-
  gouty (*see also* Gout, idiopathic)
    in (due to)
      Lesch-Nyhan syndrome E79.1 [M14.8-]
      sickle-cell disorders D57.[M14.8-]
  hemophilic NEC D66 [M36.2]
    in (due to)
      hyperparathyroidism NEC E21.3 [M14.8-]
      metabolic disease NOS E88.9 [M14.8-]
  in (due to)
    acromegaly E22.0 [M14.8-]
    amyloidosis E85.4 [M14.8-]
    blood disorder NOS D75.9 [M36.3]
    diabetes — *see* Diabetes, arthropathy
    endocrine disease NOS E34.9 [M14.8-]
    erythema
      multiforme L51.9 [M14.8-]
      nodosum L52 [M14.8-]
    hemochromatosis E83.118 [M14.8-]
    hemoglobinopathy NEC D58.2 [M36.3]
    hemophilia NEC D66 [M36.2]
    Henoch-Schönlein purpura D69.0 [M36.4]
    hyperthyroidism E05.90 [M14.8-]
    hypothyroidism E03.9 [M14.8-]
    infective endocarditis I33.0 [M12.80]
    leukemia NEC C95.9- [M36.1]
    malignant histiocytosis C96.a [M36.1]
    metabolic disease NOS E88.9 [M14.8-]
    multiple myeloma C90.0- [M36.1]
    neoplastic disease NOS (*see also* Neoplasm) D49.9 [M36.1]
    nutritional deficiency (*see also* subcategory M14.8-) E63.9
    psoriasis NOS L40.50
    sarcoidosis D86.86
    syphilis (late) A52.77
      congenital A50.55 [M12.80]
    thyrotoxicosis (*see also* subcategory M14.8-)E05.90
    ulcerative colitis K51.90 [M07.60]
    viral hepatitis (postinfectious) NEC B19.9 [M12.80]
    Whipple's disease (*see also* subcategory M14.8-) K90.81
  Jaccoud — *see* Arthropathy, postrheumatic, chronic
  juvenile — *see* Arthritis, juvenile
  psoriatic L40.54
  mutilans (psoriatic) L40.52
  neuropathic (Charcot) M14.60
    ankle M14.67-
    diabetic — *see* Diabetes, arthropathy, neuropathic
    elbow M14.62-
    foot joint M14.67-
    hand joint M14.64-
    hip M14.65-
    knee M14.66-
    multiple site M14.69
    nonsyphilitic NEC G98.0
    shoulder M14.61-
    syringomyelic G95.0
    vertebra M14.68
    wrist M14.63-

Arthropathy— *continued*
osteopulmonary — *see* Osteoarthropathy,
   hypertrophic, specified NEC
postdysenteric M02.10
   ankle M02.17-
   elbow M02.12-
   foot joint M02.17-
   hand joint M02.14-
   hip M02.15-
   knee M02.16-
   multiple site M02.19
   shoulder M02.11-
   vertebra M02.18
   wrist M02.13-
postimmunization M02.20
   ankle M02.27-
   elbow M02.22-
   foot joint M02.27-
   hand joint M02.24-
   hip M02.25-
   knee M02.26-
   multiple site M02.29
   shoulder M02.21-
   vertebra M02.28
   wrist M02.23-
postinfectious NEC B99 [M12.80]
   in (due to)
      enteritis due to Yersinia enterocolitica A04.6
        [M12.80]
      syphilis A52.77
      viral hepatitis NEC B19.9 [M12.80]
postrheumatic, chronic (Jaccoud) M12.00
   ankle M12.07-
   elbow M12.02-
   foot joint M12.07-
   hand joint M12.04-
   hip M12.05-
   knee M12.06-
   multiple site M12.09
   shoulder M12.01-
   specified joint NEC M12.08
   wrist M12.03-
psoriatic NEC L40.59
   interphalangeal, distal L40.51
reactive M02.9
   in (due to)
      infective endocarditis I33.0 [M02.9]
   specified type NEC M02.80
      ankle M02.87-
      elbow M02.82-
      foot joint M02.87-
      hand joint M02.84-
      hip M02.85-
      knee M02.86-
      multiple site M02.89
      shoulder M02.81-
      vertebra M02.88
      wrist M02.83-
specified form NEC M12.80
   ankle M12.87-
   elbow M12.82-
   foot joint M12.87-
   hand joint M12.84-
   hip M12.85-
   knee M12.86-
   multiple site M12.89
   shoulder M12.81-
   specified joint NEC M12.88
   wrist M12.83-
syringomyelic G95.0
tabes dorsalis A52.16
tabetic A52.16
transient — *see* Arthropathy, specified form NEC
traumatic M12.50
   ankle M12.57-
   elbow M12.52-
   foot joint M12.57-
   hand joint M12.54-
   hip M12.55-
   knee M12.56-
   multiple site M12.59
   shoulder M12.51-
   specified joint NEC M12.58

Arthropathy— *continued*
traumatic—*continued*
   wrist M12.53-
Arthropyosis — *see* Arthritis, pyogenic or pyemic
Arthrosis (deformans) (degenerative) (localized)
   M19.90 (*see also* Osteoarthritis)
spine — *see* Spondylosis
Arthus' phenomenon or reaction T78.41
due to
   drug — *see* Table of Drugs and Chemicals, by
      drug
Articular — *see* condition
Articulation, reverse (teeth) M26.24
Artificial
insemination complication — *see* Complications,
   artificial, fertilization
opening status (functioning) (without complication)
   Z43.9
   anus (colostomy) Z93.3
   colostomy Z93.3
   cystostomy Z93.50
      appendico-vesicostomy Z93.52
      cutaneous Z93.51
      specified NEC Z93.59
   enterostomy Z93.4
   gastrostomy Z93.1
   ileostomy Z93.2
   intestinal tract NEC Z93.4
   jejunostomy Z93.4
   nephrostomy Z93.6
   specified site NEC Z93.8
   tracheostomy Z93.0
   ureterostomy Z93.6
   urethrostomy Z93.6
   urinary tract NEC Z93.6
   vagina Z93.8
vagina status Z93.8
Arytenoid — *see* condition
Asbestosis (occupational) J61
ASC-H (atypical squamous cells cannot exclude high
   grade squamous intraepithelial lesion on
   cytologic smear)
anus R85.611
cervix R87.611
vagina R87.621
ASC-US (atypical squamous cells of undetermined
   significance on cytologic smear)
anus R85.610
cervix R87.610
vagina R87.620
Ascariasis B77.9
with
   complications NEC B77.89
   intestinal complications B77.0
   pneumonia, pneumonitis B77.81
Ascaridosis, ascaridiasis — *see* Ascariasis
Ascaris (infection) (infestation) (lumbricoides) — *see*
   Ascariasis
Ascending — *see* condition
Aschoff's bodies — *see* Myocarditis, rheumatic
Ascites (abdominal) R18.8
cardiac I50.9
chylous (nonfilarial) I89.8
   filarial — *see* Infestation, filarial
due to
   cirrhosis, alcoholic K70.31
   hepatitis
      alcoholic K70.11
      chronic active K71.51
   S. japonicum B65.2
heart I50.9
malignant R18.0
pseudochylous R18.8
syphilitic A52.74
tuberculous A18.31
Aseptic — *see* condition
Asherman's syndrome N85.6
Asialia K11.7
Asiatic cholera — *see* Cholera
Askin's tumor — *see* Neoplasm, connective tissue,
   malignant
Asocial personality F60.2
Asomatognosia R41.4

Aspartylglucosaminuria E77.1
Asperger's disease or syndrome F84.5
Aspergilloma — *see* Aspergillosis
Aspergillosis (with pneumonia) B44.9
bronchopulmonary, allergic B44.81
disseminated B44.7
generalized B44.7
pulmonary NEC B44.1
   allergic B44.81
   invasive B44.0
specified NEC B44.89
tonsillar B44.2
Aspergillus (flavus) (fumigatus) (infection) (terreus) —
   see Aspergillosis
Aspermatogenesis — *see* Azoospermia
Aspermia (testis) — *see* Azoospermia
Asphyxia, asphyxiation (by) R09.01
antenatal P84
birth P84
bunny bag — *see* Asphyxia, due to, mechanical
   threat to breathing, trapped in bed clothes
crushing S28.0
drowning T75.1
gas, fumes, or vapor — *see* Table of Drugs and
   Chemicals
inhalation — *see* Inhalation
intrauterine P84
local I73.00
   with gangrene I73.01
mucus (*see also* Foreign body, respiratory tract,
   causing asphyxia)
newborn P84
pathological R09.01
postnatal P84
   mechanical — *see* Asphyxia, due to, mechanical
      threat to breathing
prenatal P84
reticularis R23.1
strangulation — *see* Asphyxia, due to, mechanical
   threat to breathing
submersion T75.1
traumatic T71.9
   due to
      crushed chest S28.0
      foreign body (in) — *see* Foreign body,
        respiratory tract, causing asphyxia
      low oxygen content of ambient air T71.20
      due to
        being trapped in
          low oxygen environment T71.29
          in car trunk T71.221
            circumstances undetermined
              T71.224
            done with intent to harm by
              another person T71.223
            self T71.222
          in refrigerator T71.231
            circumstances undetermined
              T71.234
            done with intent to harm by
              another person T71.233
            self T71.232
        cave-in T71.21
      mechanical threat to breathing (accidental)
        T71.191
        circumstances undetermined T71.194
        done with intent to harm by
          another person T71.193
          self T71.192
        hanging T71.161
          circumstances undetermined T71.164
          done with intent to harm by
            another person T71.163
          self T71.162
        plastic bag T71.121
          circumstances undetermined T71.124
          done with intent to harm by
            another person T71.123
          self T71.122
        smothering
          in furniture T71.151
            circumstances undetermined
              T71.154

Asphyxia, asphyxiation— *continued*
  traumatic— *continued*
    due to— *continued*
      mechanical threat to breathing—*continued*
        smothering— *continued*
          in furniture—*continued*
            done with intent to harm by
              another person T71.153
              self T71.152
            under
              another person's body T71.141
                circumstances undetermined T71.144
                done with intent to harm T71.143
              pillow T71.111
                circumstances undetermined T71.114
                done with intent to harm by
                  another person T71.113
                  self T71.112
           trapped in bed clothes T71.131
            circumstances undetermined T71.134
            done with intent to harm by
              another person T71.133
              self T71.132
  vomiting, vomitus — *see* Foreign body, respiratory tract, causing asphyxia

Aspiration
  amniotic (clear) fluid (newborn) P24.10
    with
      pneumonia (pneumonitis) P24.11
      respiratory symptoms P24.11
  blood
    newborn (without respiratory symptoms) P24.20
      with
        pneumonia (pneumonitis) P24.21
        respiratory symptoms P24.21
    specified age NEC — *see* Foreign body, respiratory tract
  bronchitis J69.0
  food or foreign body (with asphyxiation) — *see* Asphyxia, food
  liquor (amnii) (newborn) P24.10
    with
      pneumonia (pneumonitis) P24.11
      respiratory symptoms P24.11
  meconium (newborn) (without respiratory symptoms) P24.00
    with
      pneumonitis (pneumonitis) P24.01
      respiratory symptoms P24.01
  milk (newborn) (without respiratory symptoms) P24.30
    with
      pneumonia (pneumonitis) P24.31
      respiratory symptoms P24.31
    specified age NEC — *see* Foreign body, respiratory tract
  mucus (*see also* Foreign body, by site, causing asphyxia)
    newborn P24.10
      with
        pneumonia (pneumonitis) P24.11
        respiratory symptoms P24.11
  neonatal P24.9
    specific NEC (without respiratory symptoms) P24.80
      with
        pneumonia (pneumonitis) P24.81
        respiratory symptoms P24.81
  newborn P24.9
    specific NEC (without respiratory symptoms) P24.80
      with
        pneumonia (pneumonitis) P24.81
        respiratory symptoms P24.81
  pneumonia J69.0
  pneumonltis J69.0
  syndrome of newborn — *see* Aspiration, by substance, with pneumonia

Aspiration— *continued*
  vernix caseosa (newborn) P24.80
    with
      pneumonia (pneumonitis) P24.81
      respiratory symptoms P24.81
  vomitus (*see also* Foreign body, respiratory tract)
    newborn (without respiratory symptoms) P24.30
      with
        pneumonia (pneumonitis) P24.31
        respiratory symptoms P24.31
Asplenia (congenital) Q89.01
  postsurgical D73.0
Assam fever B55.0
Assault, sexual — *see* Maltreatment
Assmann's focus NEC A15.0
Astasia (-abasia) (hysterical) F44.4
Asteatosis cutis L85.3
Astereognosia, astereognosis R48.1
Asterixis R27.8
  in liver disease K71.3
Asteroid hyalitis — *see* Deposit, crystalline
Asthenia, asthenic R53.1
  cardiac (*see also* Failure, heart) I50.9
    psychogenic F45.8
  cardiovascular (*see also* Failure, heart) I50.9
    psychogenic F45.8
  heart (*see also* Failure, heart) I50.9
    psychogenic F45.8
  hysterical F44.4
  myocardial (*see also* Failure, heart) I50.9
    psychogenic F45.8
  nervous F48.8
  neurocirculatory F45.8
  neurotic F48.8
  psychogenic F48.8
  psychoneurotic F48.8
  psychophysiologic F48.8
  reaction (psychophysiologic) F48.8
  senile R54
Asthenopia (*see also* Discomfort, visual)
  hysterical F44.6
  psychogenic F44.6
Asthenospermia — *see* Abnormal, specimen, male genital organs
Asthma, asthmatic (bronchial) (catarrh) (spasmodic) J45.909
  with
    chronic obstructive bronchitis J44.9
      with
        acute lower respiratory infection J44.0
        exacerbation (acute) J44.1
    chronic obstructive pulmonary disease J44.9
      with
        acute lower respiratory infection J44.0
        exacerbation (acute) J44.1
    exacerbation (acute) J45.901
    hay fever — *see* Asthma, allergic extrinsic
    rhinitis, allergic — *see* Asthma, allergic extrinsic
    status asthmaticus J45.902
  allergic extrinsic J45.909
    with
      exacerbation (acute) J45.901
      status asthmaticus J45.902
  atopic — *see* Asthma, allergic extrinsic
  cardiac — *see* Failure, ventricular, left
  cardiobronchial I50.1
  childhood J45.909
    with
      exacerbation (acute) J45.901
      status asthmaticus J45.902
  chronic obstructive J44.9
    with
      acute lower respiratory infection J44.0
      exacerbation (acute) J44.1
  collier's J60
  cough variant J45.991
  detergent J69.8
  due to
    detergent J69.8
    inhalation of fumes J68.3
  eosinophilic J82

Asthma, asthmatic— *continued*
  extrinsic, allergic — *see* Asthma, allergic extrinsic
  grinder's J62.8
  hay — *see* Asthma, allergic extrinsic
  heart I50.1
  idiosyncratic — *see* Asthma, nonallergic
  intermittent (mild) J45.20
    with
      exacerbation (acute) J45.21
      status asthmaticus J45.22
  intrinsic, nonallergic — *see* Asthma, nonallergic
  Kopp's E32.8
  late-onset — *see* Asthma, by type
  mild intermittent J45.20
    with
      exacerbation (acute) J45.21
      status asthmaticus J45.22
  mild persistent J45.30
    with
      exacerbation (acute) J45.31
      status asthmaticus J45.32
  Millar's (laryngismus stridulus) J38.5
  miner's J60
  mixed J45.909
    with
      exacerbation (acute) J45.901
      status asthmaticus J45.902
  moderate persistent J45.40
    with
      exacerbation (acute) J45.41
      status asthmaticus J45.42
  nervous — *see* Asthma, nonallergic
  nonallergic (intrinsic) J45.909
    with
      exacerbation (acute) J45.901
      status asthmaticus J45.902
  persistent
    mild J45.30
      with
        exacerbation (acute) J45.31
        status asthmaticus J45.32
    moderate J45.40
      with
        exacerbation (acute) J45.41
        status asthmaticus J45.42
    severe J45.50
      with
        exacerbation (acute) J45.51
        status asthmaticus J45.52
  platinum J45.998
  pneumoconiotic NEC J64
  potter's J62.8
  predominantly allergic J45.909
  psychogenic F54
  pulmonary eosinophilic J82
  red cedar J67.8
  Rostan's I50.1
  sandblaster's J62.8
  sequoiosis J67.8
  severe persistent J45.50
    with
      exacerbation (acute) J45.51
      status asthmaticus J45.52
  specified NEC J45.998
  stonemason's J62.8
  thymic E32.8
  tuberculous — *see* Tuberculosis, pulmonary
  Wichmann's (laryngismus stridulus) J38.5
  wood J67.8
Astigmatism (compound) (congenital) H52.20-
  irregular H52.21-
  regular H52.22-
Astraphobia F40.220
Astroblastoma
  specified site — *see* Neoplasm, malignant, by site
  unspecified site C71.9
Astrocytoma (cystic)
  anaplastic
    specified site — *see* Neoplasm, malignant, by site
    unspecified site C71.9
  fibrillary
    specified site — *see* Neoplasm, malignant, by site
    unspecified site C71.9

Astrocytoma — *continued*
  fibrous
    specified site — *see* Neoplasm, malignant, by site
    unspecified site C71.9
  gemistocytic
    specified site — *see* Neoplasm, malignant, by site
    unspecified site C71.9
  juvenile
    specified site — *see* Neoplasm, malignant, by site
    unspecified site C71.9
  pilocytic
    specified site — *see* Neoplasm, malignant, by site
    unspecified site C71.9
  piloid
    specified site — *see* Neoplasm, malignant, by site
    unspecified site C71.9
  protoplasmic
    specified site — *see* Neoplasm, malignant, by site
    unspecified site C71.9
  specified site NEC — *see* Neoplasm, malignant, by site
  subependymal D43.2
    giant cell
      specified site — *see* Neoplasm, uncertain behavior, by site
      unspecified site D43.2
    specified site — *see* Neoplasm, uncertain behavior, by site
    unspecified site D43.2
  unspecified site C71.9
Astroglioma
  specified site — *see* Neoplasm, malignant, by site
  unspecified site C71.9
Asymbolia R48.8
Asymmetry (*see also* Distortion)
  between native and reconstructed breast N65.1
  face Q67.0
  jaw (lower) — *see* Anomaly, dentofacial, jaw-cranial base relationship, asymmetry
Asynergia, asynergy R27.8
  ventricular I51.89
Asystole (heart) — *see* Arrest, cardiac
At risk
  for falling Z91.81
Ataxia, ataxy, ataxic R27.0
  acute R27.8
  brain (hereditary) G11.9
  cerebellar (hereditary) G11.9
    with defective DNA repair G11.3
    alcoholic G31.2
    early-onset G11.1
    in
      alcoholism G31.2
      myxedema E03.9 [G13.8]
      neoplastic disease (*see also* Neoplasm) D49.9 [G13.1]
    late-onset (Marie's) G11.2
  cerebral (hereditary) G11.9
  congenital nonprogressive G11.0
  family, familial — *see* Ataxia, hereditary
  following
    cerebrovascular disease I69.993
      specified NEC I69.893
      cerebral infarction I69.393
      intracerebral hemorrhage I69.193
      nontraumatic intracranial hemorrhage NEC I69.293
      specified disease NEC I69.893
        subarachnoid hemorrhage I69.093
  Friedreich's (heredofamilial) (cerebellar) (spinal) G11.1
  gait R26.0
    hysterical F44.4
  general R27.8
  hereditary G11.9
    with neuropathy G60.2
    cerebellar — *see* Ataxia, cerebellar
    spastic G11.4
    specified NEC G11.8
    spinal (Friedreich's) G11.1
  heredofamilial — *see* Ataxia, hereditary
  Hunt's G11.1

Ataxia, ataxy, ataxic — *continued*
  hysterical F44.4
  locomotor (progressive) (syphilitic) (partial) (spastic) A52.11
    diabetic — *see* Diabetes, ataxia
  Marie's (cerebellar) (heredofamilial) (lateonset) G11.2
  nonorganic origin F44.4
  nonprogressive, congenital G11.0
  psychogenic F44.4
  Roussy-Lévy G60.0
  Sanger-Brown's (hereditary) G11.2
  spastic hereditary G11.4
  spinal
    hereditary (Friedreich's) G11.1
    progressive (syphilitic) A52.11
  spinocerebellar, X-linked recessive G11.1
  telangiectasia (Louis-Bar) G11.3
Ataxia-telangiectasia (Louis-Bar) G11.3
Atelectasis (massive) (partial) (pressure) (pulmonary) J98.11
  newborn P28.10
    due to resorption P28.11
    partial P28.19
    primary P28.0
    secondary P28.19
  primary (newborn) P28.0
  tuberculous — *see* Tuberculosis, pulmonary
Atelocardia Q24.9
Atelomyelia Q06.1
Atheroembolism
  of
    extremities
      lower I75.02-
      upper I75.01-
    kidney I75.81
    specified NEC I75.89
Atheroma, atheromatous (*see also* Arteriosclerosis) I70.90
  aorta, aortic I70.0
    valve (*see also* Endocarditis, aortic) I35.8
  aorto-iliac I70.0
  artery — *see* Arteriosclerosis
  basilar (artery) I67.2
  carotid (artery) (common) (internal) I67.2
  cerebral (arteries) I67.2
Atheroma, atheromatous
  coronary (artery) I25.10
    with angina pectoris — *see* Arteriosclerosis, coronary (artery),
  degeneration — *see* Arteriosclerosis
  heart, cardiac — *see* Disease, heart, ischemic, atherosclerotic
  mitral (valve) I34.8
  myocardium, myocardial — *see* Disease, heart, ischemic, atherosclerotic
  pulmonary valve (heart) (*see also* Endocarditis, pulmonary) I37.8
  tricuspid (heart) (valve) I36.8
  valve, valvular — *see* Endocarditis
  vertebral (artery) I67.2
Atheromatosis — *see* Arteriosclerosis
Atherosclerosis (*see also* Arteriosclerosis)
  coronary artery I25.10
    with angina pectoris — *see* Arteriosclerosis, coronary (artery),
    coronary, due to lipid rich plaque I25.83
  transplanted heart I25.811
    native coronary artery I25.811
      with angina pectoris — *see* Arteriosclerosis, coronary (artery),
      bypass graft I25.812
      with angina pectoris — *see* Arteriosclerosis, coronary (artery),
Athetosis (acquired) R25.8
  bilateral (congenital) G80.3
  congenital (bilateral) (double) G80.3
  double (congenital) G80.3
  unilateral R25.8
Athlete's
  foot B35.3
  heart I51.7
Athrepsia E41

Athyrea (acquired) (*see also* Hypothyroidism)
  congenital E03.1
Atonia, atony, atonic
  bladder (sphincter) (neurogenic) N31.2
  capillary I78.8
  cecum K59.8
    psychogenic F45.8
  colon — *see* Atony, intestine
  congenital P94.2
  esophagus K22.8
  intestine K59.8
    psychogenic F45.8
  stomach K31.89
    neurotic or psychogenic F45.8
  uterus (during labor) O62.2
    with hemorrhage (postpartum) O72.1
    postpartum (with hemorrhage) O72.1
      without hemorrhage O75.89
Atopy — *see* History, allergy
Atransferrinemia, congenital E88.09
Atresia, atretic
  alimentary organ or tract NEC Q45.8
    upper Q40.8
  ani, anus, anal (canal) Q42.3
    with fistula Q42.2
  aorta (arch) (ring) Q25.2
  aortic (orifice) (valve) Q23.0
    arch Q25.2
    congenital with hypoplasia of ascending aorta and defective development of left ventricle (with mitral stenosis) Q23.4
    in hypoplastic left heart syndrome Q23.4
  aqueduct of Sylvius Q03.0
    with spina bifida — *see* Spina bifida, with hydrocephalus
  artery NEC Q27.8
    cerebral Q28.3
    coronary Q24.5
    digestive system Q27.8
    eye Q15.8
    lower limb Q27.8
    pulmonary Q25.5
    specified site NEC Q27.8
    umbilical Q27.0
    upper limb Q27.8
  auditory canal (external) Q16.1
  bile duct (common) (congenital) (hepatic) Q44.2
    acquired — *see* Obstruction, bile duct
  bladder (neck) Q64.39
    obstruction Q64.31
  bronchus Q32.4
  cecum Q42.8
  cervix (acquired) N88.2
    congenital Q51.828
    in pregnancy or childbirth — *see* Anomaly, cervix, in pregnancy or childbirth
      causing obstructed labor O65.5
  choana Q30.0
  colon Q42.9
    specified NEC Q42.8
  common duct Q44.2
  cricoid cartilage Q31.8
  cystic duct Q44.2
    acquired K82.8
      with obstruction K82.0
  digestive organs NEC Q45.8
  duodenum Q41.0
  ear canal Q16.1
  ejaculatory duct Q55.4
  epiglottis Q31.8
  esophagus Q39.0
    with tracheoesophageal fistula Q39.1
  eustachian tube Q17.8
  fallopian tube (congenital) Q50.6
    acquired N97.1
  follicular cyst N83.0
  foramen of
    Luschka Q03.1
      with spina bifida — *see* Spina bifida, with hydrocephalus
    Magendie Q03.1
      with spina bifida — *see* Spina bifida, with hydrocephalus

Atrophy, atrophic— *continued*
  muscle, muscular— *continued*
    spinal— *continued*
      distal G12.1
      hereditary NEC G12.1
      infantile, type I (Werdnig-Hoffmann) G12.0
      juvenile form, type III (KugelbergWelander) G12.1
      progressive G12.21
      scapuloperoneal form G12.1
      specified NEC G12.8
    syphilitic A52.78
    thigh M62.55-
    upper arm M62.52-
  myocardium — *see* Degeneration, myocardial
  myometrium (senile) N85.8
    cervix N88.8
  myopathic NEC — *see* Atrophy, muscle
  myotonia G71.11
  nail L60.3
  nasopharynx J31.1
  nerve (*see also* Disorder, nerve)
    abducens — *see* Strabismus, paralytic, sixth nerve
    accessory G52.8
    acoustic or auditory — *see* subcategory H93.3
    cranial G52.9
      eighth (auditory) — *see* subcategory H93.3
      eleventh (accessory) G52.8
      fifth (trigeminal) G50.8
      first (olfactory) G52.0
      fourth (trochlear) — *see* Strabismus, paralytic, fourth nerve
      second (optic) H47.20
      sixth (abducens) — *see* Strabismus, paralytic, sixth nerve
      tenth (pneumogastric) (vagus) G52.2
      third (oculomotor) — *see* Strabismus, paralytic, third nerve
      twelfth (hypoglossal) G52.3
    hypoglossal G52.3
    oculomotor — *see* Strabismus, paralytic, third nerve
    olfactory G52.0
    optic (papillomacular bundle)
      syphilitic (late) A52.15
        congenital A50.44
    pneumogastric G52.2
    trigeminal G50.8
    trochlear — *see* Strabismus, paralytic, fourth nerve
    vagus (pneumogastric) G52.2
  neurogenic, bone, tabetic A52.11
  nutritional E41
  old age R54
  olivopontocerebellar G23.8
  optic (nerve) H47.20
    glaucomatous H47.23-
    hereditary H47.22
    syphilitic (late) A52.15
      congenital A50.44
    primary H47.21-
    specified type NEC H47.29-
  orbit H05.31-
  ovary (senile) N83.31
    with fallopian tube N83.33
  oviduct (senile) — *see* Atrophy, fallopian tube
  palsy, diffuse (progressive) G12.22
  pancreas (duct) (senile) K86.8
  parotid gland K11.0
  pelvic muscle N81.84
  penis N48.89
  pharynx J39.2
  pluriglandular E31.8
    autoimmune E31.0
  polyarthritis M15.9
  prostate N42.89
  pseudohypertrophic (muscle) G71.0
  renal (*see also* Sclerosis, renal) N26.1
  retina, retinal (postinfectional) H35.89
  rhinitis J31.0
  salivary gland K11.0
  scar L90.5

Atrophy, atrophic— *continued*
  sclerosis, lobar (of brain) G31.09 [F02.80]
    with behavioral disturbance G31.09 [F02.81]
  scrotum N50.8
  seminal vesicle N50.8
  senile R54
    due to radiation (nonionizing) (solar) L57.8
  skin (patches) (spots) L90.9
    degenerative (senile) L90.8
    due to radiation (nonionizing) (solar) L57.8
    senile L90.8
  spermatic cord N50.8
  spinal (acute) (cord) G95.89
    muscular — *see* Atrophy, muscle, spinal
    paralysis G12.20
      acute — *see* Poliomyelitis, paralytic
      meaning progressive muscular atrophy G12.21
  spine (column) — *see* Spondylopathy, specified NEC
  spleen (senile) D73.0
  stomach K29.40
    with bleeding K29.41
  striate (skin) L90.6
    syphilitic A52.79
  subcutaneous L90.9
  sublingual gland K11.0
  submandibular gland K11.0
  submaxillary gland K11.0
  Sudeck's — *see* Algoneurodystrophy
  suprarenal (capsule) (gland) E27.49
    primary E27.1
  systemic affecting central nervous system in
      myxedema E03.9 [G13.8]
      neoplastic disease (*see also* Neoplasm) D49.9 [G13.1]
  tarso-orbital fascia, congenital Q10.3
  testis N50.0
  thenar, partial — *see* Syndrome, carpal tunnel
  thymus (fatty) E32.8
  thyroid (gland) (acquired) E03.4
    with cretinism E03.1
    congenital (with myxedema) E03.1
  tongue (senile) K14.8
    papillae K14.4
  trachea J39.8
  tunica vaginalis N50.8
  turbinate J34.89
  tympanic membrane (nonflaccid) H73.82-
    flaccid H73.81-
  upper respiratory tract J39.8
  uterus, uterine (senile) N85.8
    cervix N88.8
    due to radiation (intended effect) N85.8
      adverse effect or misadventure N99.89
  vagina (senile) N95.2
  vas deferens N50.8
  vascular I99.8
  vertebra (senile) — *see* Spondylopathy, specified NEC
  vulva (senile) N90.5
  Werdnig-Hoffmann G12.0
  yellow — *see* Failure, hepatic

Attack, attacks
  with alteration of consciousness (with automatisms) — *see* Epilepsy, localization-related, symptomatic, with complex partial seizures
  Adams-Stokes I45.9
  akinetic — *see* Epilepsy, generalized, idiopathic
  angina — *see* Angina
  atonic — *see* Epilepsy, generalized, idiopathic
  cataleptic — *see* Catalepsy
  coronary — *see* Infarct, myocardium
  cyanotic, newborn P28.2
  drop NEC R55
  epileptic — *see* Epilepsy
  heart — *see* infarct, myocardium
  hysterical F44.9
  jacksonian — *see* Epilepsy, localization-related, symptomatic, with simple partial seizures
  myocardium, myocardial — *see* Infarct, myocardium
  myoclonic — *see* Epilepsy, generalized, idiopathic
  panic F41.0

Attack, attacks— *continued*
  psychomotor — *see* Epilepsy, localization-related, symptomatic, with complex partial seizures
  salaam — *see* Epilepsy, generalized, specified NEC
  schizophreniform, brief F23
  Stokes-Adams I45.9
  syncope R55
  transient ischemic (TIA) G45.9
    specified NEC G45.8
  unconsciousness R55
    hysterical F44.89
  vasomotor R55
  vasovagal (paroxysmal) (idiopathic) R55
  without alteration of consciousness — *see* Epilepsy, localization-related, symptomatic, with simple partial seizures

Attention (to)
  artificial
    opening (of) Z43.9
      digestive tract NEC Z43.4
        colon Z43.3
        ilium Z43.2
        stomach Z43.1
      specified NEC Z43.8
      trachea Z43.0
      urinary tract NEC Z43.6
        cystostomy Z43.5
        nephrostomy Z43.6
        ureterostomy Z43.6
        urethrostomy Z43.6
      vagina Z43.7
  colostomy Z43.3
  cystostomy Z43.5
  deficit disorder or syndrome F98.8
    with hyperactivity — *see* Disorder, attention-deficit hyperactivity
  gastrostomy Z43.1
  ileostomy Z43.2
  jejunostomy Z43.4
  nephrostomy Z43.6
  surgical dressings Z48.01
  sutures Z48.02
  tracheostomy Z43.0
  ureterostomy Z43.6
  urethrostomy Z43.6

Attrition
  gum K06.0
  tooth, teeth (excessive) (hard tissues) K03.0

Atypical, atypism (*see also* condition)
  cells (on cytolgocial smear) (endocervical) (endometrial) (glandular)
    cervix R87.619
    vagina R87.629
  cervical N87.9
  endometrium N85.9
    hyperplasia N85.00
  parenting situation Z62.9

Auditory — *see* condition
Aujeszky's disease B33.8
Aurantiasis, cutis E67.1
Auricle, auricular (*see also* condition)
  cervical Q18.2
Auriculotemporal syndrome G50.8
Austin Flint murmur (aortic insufficiency) I35.1
Australian
  Q fever A78
  X disease A83.4
Autism, autistic (childhood) (infantile) F84.0
  atypical F84.9
Autodigestion R68.89
Autoerythrocyte sensitization (syndrome) D69.2
Autographism L50.3
Autoimmune
  disease (systemic) M35.9
  lymphoproliferative syndrome [ALPS] D89.82
  thyroiditis E06.3
Autointoxication R68.89
Automatism G93.89
  epileptic — *see* Epilepsy, localization-related, symptomatic, with complex partial seizures
  paroxysmal, idiopathic — *see* Epilepsy, localization-related, symptomatic, with complex partial seizures

Autonomic, autonomous
  bladder (neurogenic) N31.2
  hysteria seizure F44.5
Autosensitivity, erythrocyte D69.2
Autosensitization, cutaneous L30.2
Autosome — *see* condition by chromosome involved
Autotopagnosia R48.1
Autotoxemia R68.89
Autumn — *see* condition
Avellis' syndrome G46.8
Aversion, sexual F52.1
Aviator's
  disease or sickness — *see* Effect, adverse, high
    altitude
  ear T70.0
Avitaminosis (multiple) (*see also* Deficiency, vitamin)
    E56.9
  B E53.9
    with
      beriberi E51.11
      pellagra E52
  B2 E53.0
  B6 E53.1
  B12 E53.8
  D E55.9
    with rickets E55.0
  G E53.0
  K E56.1
  nicotinic acid E52
Avulsion (traumatic)
  blood vessel — *see* Injury, blood vessel
  bone — *see* Fracture, by site
  cartilage (*see also* Dislocation, by site)
    symphyseal (inner), complicating delivery O71.6
  external site other than limb — *see* Wound, open, by
    site
  eye S05.7-
  head (intracranial)
    external site NEC S08.89
    scalp S08.0
  internal organ or site — *see* Injury, by site
  joint (*see also* Dislocation, by site)
    capsule — *see* Sprain, by site
  kidney S37.06-
  ligament — *see* Sprain, by site
  limb (*see also* Amputation, traumatic, by site)
    skin and subcutaneous tissue — *see* Wound,
      open, by site
  muscle — *see* Injury, muscle
  nerve (root) — *see* Injury, nerve
  scalp S08.0
  skin and subcutaneous tissue — *see* Wound, open,
    by site
  spleen S36.032
  symphyseal cartilage (inner), complicating delivery
    O71.6
  tendon — *see* Injury, muscle
  tooth S03.2
Awareness of heart beat R00.2
Axenfeld's
  anomaly or syndrome Q15.0
  degeneration (calcareous) Q13.4
Axilla, axillary (*see also* condition)
  breast Q83.1
Axonotmesis — *see* Injury, nerve
Ayerza's disease or syndrome (pulmonary artery
    sclerosis with pulmonary hypertension) I27.0
Azoospermia (organic) N46.01
  due to
    drug therapy N46.021
    efferent duct obstruction N46.023
    infection N46.022
    radiation N46.024
    specified cause NEC N46.029
    systemic disease N46.025
Azotemia R79.89
  meaning uremia N19
Aztec ear Q17.3
Azygos
  continuation inferior vena cava Q26.8
  lobe (lung) Q33.1

B

Baastrup's disease — *see* Kissing spine
Babesiosis B60.0
Babington's disease (familial hemorrhagic
    telangiectasia) I78.0
Babinski's syndrome A52.79
Baby
  crying constantly R68.11
  floppy (syndrome) P94.2
Bacillary — *see* condition
Bacilluria N39.0
Bacillus (*see also* Infection, bacillus)
  abortus infection A23.1
  anthracis infection A22.9
  coli infection B96.2
  Flexner's A03.1
  mallei infection A24.0
  Shiga's A03.0
  suipestifer infection — *see* Infection, salmonella
Back — *see* condition
Backache (postural) M54.9
  sacroiliac M53.3
  specified NEC M54.89
Backflow — *see* Reflux
Backward reading (dyslexia) F81.0
Bacteremia R78.81
  with sepsis — *see* Sepsis
Bactericholia — *see* Cholecystitis, acute
Bacterid, bacteride (pustular) L40.3
Bacterium, bacteria, bacterial
  agent NEC, as cause of disease classified elsewhere
    B96.89
  in blood — *see* Bacteremia
  in urine — *see* Bacteriuria
Bacteriuria, bacteruria N39.0
  asymptomatic N39.0
Bacteroides
  fragilis, as cause of disease classified elsewhere
    B96.6
Bad
  heart — *see* Disease, heart
  trip
    due to drug abuse — *see* Abuse, drug,
      hallucinogen
    due to drug dependence — *see* Dependence,
      drug, hallucinogen
Baelz's disease (cheilitis glandularis apostematosa)
    K13.0
Baerensprung's disease (eczema marginatum) B35.6
Bagasse disease or pneumonitis J67.1
Bagassosis J67.1
Baker's cyst — *see* Cyst, Baker's
Bakwin-Krida syndrome (craniometaphyseal
    dysplasia) Q78.5
Balancing side interference M26.56
Balanitis (circinata) (erosiva) (gangrenosa)
    (phagedenic) (vulgaris) N48.1
  amebic A06.82
  candidal B37.42
  due to Haemophilus ducreyi A57
  gonococcal (acute) (chronic) A54.09
  xerotica obliterans N48.0
Balanoposthitis N47.6
  gonococcal (acute) (chronic) A54.09
  ulcerative (specific) A63.8
Balanorrhagia — *see* Balanitis
Balantidiasis, balantidiosis A07.0
Bald tongue K14.4
Baldness (*see also* Alopecia)
  male-pattern — *see* Alopecia, androgenic
Balkan grippe A78
Balloon disease — *see* Effect, adverse, high altitude
Balo's disease (concentric sclerosis) G37.5
Bamberger-Marie disease — *see* Osteoarthropathy,
    hypertrophic, specified type NEC
Bancroft's filariasis B74.0
Band(s)
  adhesive — *see* Adhesions, peritoneum
  anomalous or congenital (*see also* Anomaly, by site)
    heart (atrial) (ventricular) Q24.8

Band(s)— *continued*
  anomalous or congenital— *continued*
    intestine Q43.3
    omentum Q43.3
  cervix N88.1
  constricting, congenital Q79.8
  gallbladder (congenital) Q44.1
  intestinal (adhesive) — *see* Adhesions, peritoneum
  obstructive
    intestine K56.5
    peritoneum K56.5
  periappendiceal, congenital Q43.3
  peritoneal (adhesive) — *see* Adhesions, peritoneum
  uterus N73.6
    internal N85.6
  vagina N89.5
Bandemia D72.825
Bandl's ring (contraction), **complicating delivery**
    O62.4
Bangkok hemorrhagic fever A91
Bang's disease (brucella abortus) A23.1
Bankruptcy, anxiety concerning Z59.8
Bannister's disease T78.3
  hereditary D84.1
Banti's disease or syndrome (with cirrhosis) (with
    portal hypertension) K76.6
Bar, median, prostate — *see* Enlargement, enlarged,
    prostate
Barcoo disease or rot — *see* Ulcer, skin
Barlow's disease E54
Barodontalgia T70.29
Baron Münchausen syndrome — *see* Disorder,
    factitious
Barosinusitis T70.1
Barotitis T70.0
Barotrauma T70.29
  odontalgia T70.29
  otitic T70.0
  sinus T70.1
Barraquer(-Simons) **disease or syndrome**
    (progressive lipodystrophy) E88.1
Barré-Guillain disease or syndrome G61.0
Barré-Liéou syndrome (posterior cervical
    sympathetic) M53.0
Barrel chest M95.4
Barrett's
  disease — *see* Barrett's, esophagus
  esophagus K22.70
    with dysplasia K22.719
      high grade K22.711
      low grade K22.710
    without dysplasia K22.70
  syndrome — *see* Barrett's, esophagus
  ulcer K22.10
    with bleeding K22.11
    without bleeding K22.10
Bársony (-Polgár) (-Teschendorf) **syndrome**
    (corkscrew esophagus) K22.4
Bartholinitis (suppurating) N75.8
  gonococcal (acute) (chronic) (with abscess) A54.1
Barth syndrome E78.71
Bartonellosis A44.9
  cutaneous A44.1
  mucocutaneous A44.1
  specified NEC A44.8
  systemic A44.0
Barton's fracture S52.56-
Bartter's syndrome E26.81
Basal — *see* condition
Basan's (hidrotic) **ectodermal dysplasia** Q82.4
Baseball finger — *see* Dislocation, finger
Basedow's disease (exophthalmic goiter) — *see*
    Hyperthyroidism, with, goiter
Basic — *see* condition
Basilar — *see* condition
Bason's (hidrotic) **ectodermal dysplasia** Q82.4
Basopenia — *see* Agranulocytosis
Basophilia D72.824
Basophilism (cortico-adrenal) (Cushing's) (pituitary)
    E24.0
Bassen-Kornzweig disease or syndrome E78.6
Bat ear Q17.5

Bateman's
disease B08.1
purpura (senile) D69.2
Bathing cramp T75.1
Bathophobia F40.248
Batten(-Mayou) **disease** E75.4
retina E75.4 [H36]
Batten-Steinert syndrome G71.11
Battered — see Maltreatment
Battey Mycobacterium infection A31.0
Battle exhaustion F43.0
Battledore placenta O43.19-
**Baumgarten-Cruveilhier cirrhosis, disease or
syndrome** K74.69
Bauxite fibrosis (of lung) J63.1
Bayle's disease (general paresis) A52.17
Bazin's disease (primary) (tuberculous) A18.4
Beach ear — see Swimmer's, ear
Beaded hair (congenital) Q84.1
Béal conjunctivitis or syndrome B30.2
Beard's disease (neurasthenia) F48.8
Beat(s)
atrial, premature I49.1
ectopic I49.49
elbow — see Bursitis, elbow
escaped, heart I49.49
hand — see Bursitis, hand
knee — see Bursitis, knee
premature I49.40
atrial I49.1
auricular I49.1
supraventricular I49.1
Beau's
disease or syndrome — see Degeneration,
myocardial
lines (transverse furrows on fingernails) L60.4
Bechterev's syndrome — see Spondylitis, ankylosing
Beck's syndrome (anterior spinal artery occlusion)
I65.8
Becker's
cardiomyopathy I42.8
disease
idiopathic mural endomyocardial disease I42.3
myotonia congenita, recessive form G71.12
dystrophy G71.0
pigmented hairy nevus D22.5
Beckwith-Wiedemann syndrome Q87.3
Bed confinement status Z74.01
Bed sore — see Ulcer, pressure, by site
Bedbug bite(s) — see Bite(s), by site, superficial, insect
Bedclothes, asphyxiation or suffocation by — see
Asphyxia, traumatic, due to, mechanical, trapped
Bednar's
aphthae K12.0
tumor — see Neoplasm, malignant, by site
Bedridden Z74.01
Bedsore — see Ulcer, pressure, by site
Bedwetting — see Enuresis
Bee sting (with allergic or anaphylactic shock) — see
Toxicity, venom, arthropod, bee
Begbie's disease (exophthalmic goiter) — see
Hyperthyroidism, with, goiter
Beer drinker's heart (disease) I42.6
Behavior
antisocial
adult Z72.811
child or adolescent Z72.810
disorder, disturbance — see Disorder, conduct
disruptive — see Disorder, conduct
drug seeking Z72.89
inexplicable R46.2
marked evasiveness R46.5
obsessive-compulsive R46.81
overactivity R46.3
poor responsiveness R46.4
self-damaging (life-style) Z72.89
sleep-incompatible Z72.821
slowness R46.4
specified NEC R46.89
strange (and inexplicable) R46.2
suspiciousness R46.5
type A pattern Z73.1

Behavior— continued
undue concern or preoccupation with stressful
events R46.6
verbosity and circumstantial detail obscuring reason
for contact R46.7
Behçet's disease or syndrome M35.2
Behr's disease — see Degeneration, macula
Beigel's disease or morbus (white piedra) B36.2
Bejel A65
Bekhterev's syndrome — see Spondylitis, ankylosing
Belching — see Eructation
Bell's
mania F30.8
palsy, paralysis G51.0
infant or newborn P11.3
spasm G51.3
Bence Jones albuminuria or proteinuria NEC R80.3
Bends T70.3
Benedikt's paralysis or syndrome G46.3
Benign (see also condition)
prostatic hyperplasia — see Hyperplasia, prostate
Bennett's fracture (displaced) S62.21-
Benson's disease — see Deposit, crystalline
Bent
back (hysterical) F44.4
nose M95.0
congenital Q67.4
Bereavement (uncomplicated) Z63.4
Bergeron's disease (hysterical chorea) F44.4
Berger's disease — see Nephropathy, IgA
Beriberi (dry) E51.11
heart (disease) E51.12
polyneuropathy E51.11
wet E51.12
involving circulatory system E51.11
Berlin's disease or edema (traumatic) S05.8x-
Berlock (berloque) **dermatitis** L56.2
Bernard-Horner syndrome G90.2
Bernard-Soulier disease or thrombopathia D69.1
Bernhardt (-Roth) **disease** — see Mononeuropathy,
lower limb, meralgia paresthetica
Bernheim's syndrome — see Failure, heart,
congestive
Bertielliasis B71.8
Berylliosis (lung) J63.2
Besnier-Boeck (-Schaumann) **disease** — see
Sarcoidosis
Besnier's
lupus pernio D86.3
prurigo L20.0
Bestiality F65.89
Best's disease H35.50
Beta-mercaptolactate-cysteine disulfiduria E72.09
Betalipoproteinemia, broad or floating E78.2
Betting and gambling Z72.6
pathological (compulsive) F63.0
Bezoar T18.9
intestine T18.3
stomach T18.2
Bezold's abscess — see Mastoiditis, acute
Bianchi's syndrome R48.8
Bicornate or bicornis uterus Q51.3
in pregnancy or childbirth O34.59-
causing obstructed labor O65.5
Bicuspid aortic valve Q23.1
Biedl-Bardet syndrome Q87.89
Bielschowsky (-Jansky) **disease** E75.4
Biermer's (pernicious) **anemia or disease** D51.0
Biett's disease L93.0
Bifid (congenital)
apex, heart Q24.8
clitoris Q52.6
kidney Q63.8
nose Q30.2
patella Q74.1
scrotum Q55.29
toe NEC Q74.2
tongue Q38.3
ureter Q62.8
uterus Q51.3
uvula Q35.7
Biforis uterus (suprasimplex) Q51.3

Bifurcation (congenital)
gallbladder Q44.1
kidney pelvis Q63.8
renal pelvis Q63.8
rib Q76.6
tongue, congenital Q38.3
trachea Q32.1
ureter Q62.8
urethra Q64.74
vertebra Q76.49
Big spleen syndrome D73.1
Bigeminal pulse R00.8
Bilateral — see condition
Bile
duct — see condition
pigments in urine R82.2
Bilharziasis (see also Schistosomiasis)
chyluria B65.0
cutaneous B65.3
galacturia B65.0
hematochyluria B65.0
intestinal B65.1
lipemia B65.9
lipuria B65.0
oriental B65.2
piarhemia B65.9
pulmonary NOS B65.9 [J99]
pneumonia B65.9 [J17]
tropical hematuria B65.0
vesical B65.0
Biliary — see condition
Bilirubin metabolism disorder E80.7
specified NEC E80.6
Bilirubinemia, familial nonhemolytic E80.4
Bilirubinuria R82.2
Biliuria R82.2
Bilocular stomach K31.2
Binswanger's disease I67.3
Biparta, bipartite
carpal scaphoid Q74.0
patella Q74.1
vagina Q52.10
Bird
face Q75.8
fancier's disease or lung J67.2
Birt-Hogg-Dube syndrome Q87.89
Birth
complications in mother — see Delivery,
complicated
compression during NOS P15.9
defect — see Anomaly
immature (less than 37 completed weeks) — see
Preterm infant, newborn
extremely (less than 28 completed weeks) — see
Immaturity, extreme
inattention, at or after — see Maltreatment, child,
neglect
injury NOS P15.9
basal ganglia P11.1
brachial plexus NEC P14.3
brain (compression) (pressure) P11.2
central nervous system NOS P11.9
cerebellum P11.1
cerebral hemorrhage P10.1
external genitalia P15.5
eye P15.3
face P15.4
fracture
bone P13.9
specified NEC P13.8
clavicle P13.4
femur P13.2
humerus P13.3
long bone, except femur P13.3
radius and ulna P13.3
skull P13.0
spine P11.5
tibia and fibula P13.3
intracranial P11.2
laceration or hemorrhage P10.9
specified NEC P10.8
intraventricular hemorrhage P10.2

Birth— *continued*
  injury— *continued*
    laceration
      brain P10.1
      by scalpel P15.8
      peripheral nerve P14.9
    liver P15.0
    meninges
      brain P11.1
      spinal cord P11.5
    nerve
      brachial plexus P14.3
      cranial NEC (except facial) P11.4
      facial P11.3
      peripheral P14.9
      phrenic (paralysis) P14.2
    paralysis
      facial nerve P11.3
      spinal P11.5
    penis P15.5
    rupture
      spinal cord P11.5
    scalp P12.9
    scalpel wound P15.8
    scrotum P15.5
    skull NEC P13.1
      fracture P13.0
    specified type NEC P15.8
    spinal cord P11.5
    spine P11.5
    spleen P15.1
    sternomastoid (hematoma) P15.2
    subarachnoid hemorrhage P10.3
    subcutaneous fat necrosis P15.6
    subdural hemorrhage P10.0
    tentorial tear P10.4
    testes P15.5
    vulva P15.5
  lack of care, at or after — *see* Maltreatment, child, neglect
  neglect, at or after — *see* Maltreatment, child, neglect
  palsy or paralysis, newborn, NOS (birth injury) P14.9
  premature (infant) — *see* Preterm infant, newborn
  shock, newborn P96.89
  trauma — *see* Birth, injury
  weight
    low (2499 grams or less) — *see* Low, birthweight
      extremely (999 grams or less) — *see* Low, birthweight, extreme
    4000 grams to 4499 grams P08.1
    4500 grams or more P08.0
Birthmark Q82.5
Bisalbuminemia E88.09
Biskra's button B55.1
Bite(s) (animal) (human)
  abdomen, abdominal
    wall S31.159
      with penetration into peritoneal cavity S31.659
      epigastric region S31.152
        with penetration into peritoneal cavity S31.652
      left
        lower quadrant S31.154
          with penetration into peritoneal cavity S31.654
        upper quadrant S31.151
          with penetration into peritoneal cavity S31.651
      periumbilic region S31.155
        with penetration into peritoneal cavity S31.655
      right
        lower quadrant S31.153
          with penetration into peritoneal cavity S31.653
        upper quadrant S31.150
          with penetration into peritoneal cavity S31.650
      superficial NEC S30.871
        insect S30.861
  alveolar (process) — *see* Bite, oral cavity

Bite(s) — *continued*
  amphibian (venomous) — *see* Venom, bite, amphibian
  animal (*see also* Bite, by site)
    venomous — *see* Venom
  ankle S91.05-
    superficial NEC S90.57-
      insect S90.56-
  antecubital space — *see* Bite, elbow
  anus S31.835
    superficial NEC S30.877
      insect S30.867
  arm (upper) S41.15-
    lower — *see* Bite, forearm
    superficial NEC S40.87-
      insect S40.86-
  arthropod NEC — *see* Venom, bite, arthropod
  auditory canal (external) (meatus) — *see* Bite, ear
  auricle, ear — *see* Bite, ear
  axilla — *see* Bite, arm
  back (*see also* Bite, thorax, back)
    lower S31.050
      with penetration into retroperitoneal space S31.051
      superficial NEC S30.870
        insect S30.860
  bedbug — *see* Bite(s), by site, superficial, insect
  breast S21.05-
    superficial NEC S20.17-
      insect S20.16-
  brow — *see* Bite, head, specified site NEC
  buttock S31.805
    left S31.825
    right S31.815
    superficial NEC S30.870
      insect S30.860
  calf — *see* Bite, leg
  canaliculus lacrimalis — *see* Bite, eyelid
  canthus, eye — *see* Bite, eyelid
  centipede — *see* Toxicity, venom, arthropod, centipede
  cheek (external) S01.45-
    superficial NEC S00.87
      insect S00.86
    internal — *see* Bite, oral cavity
  chest wall — *see* Bite, thorax
  chigger B88.0
  chin — *see* Bite, head, specified site NEC
  clitoris — *see* Bite, vulva
  costal region — *see* Bite, thorax
  digit(s)
    hand — *see* Bite, finger
    toe — *see* Bite, toe
  ear (canal) (external) S01.35-
    superficial NEC S00.47-
      insect S00.46-
  elbow S51.05-
    superficial NEC S50.37-
      insect S50.36-
  epididymis — *see* Bite, testis
  epigastric region — *see* Bite, abdomen
  epiglottis — *see* Bite, neck, specified site NEC
  esophagus, cervical S11.25
    superficial NEC S10.17
      insect S10.16
  eyebrow — *see* Bite, eyelid
  eyelid S01.15-
    superficial NEC S00.27-
      insect S00.26-
  face NEC — *see* Bite, head, specified site NEC
  finger(s) S61.259
    with
      damage to nail S61.359
    index S61.258
      with
        damage to nail S61.358
      left S61.251
        with
          damage to nail S61.351
      right S61.250
        with
          damage to nail S61.350
    superficial NEC S60.478

Bite(s)— *continued*
  finger(s)— *continued*
    index— *continued*
      superficial— *continued*
        insect S60.46-
    little S61.25-
      with
        damage to nail S61.35-
      superficial NEC S60.47-
        insect S60.46-
    middle S61.25-
      with
        damage to nail S61.35-
      superficial NEC S60.47-
        insect S60.46-
    ring S61.25-
      with
        damage to nail S61.35-
      superficial NEC S60.47-
        insect S60.46-
    superficial NEC S60.479
      insect S60.469
    thumb — *see* Bite, thumb
  flank — *see* Bite, abdomen, wall
  flea — *see* Bite, insect, by site
  foot (except toe(s) alone) S91.35-
    superficial NEC S90.87-
      insect S90.86-
    toe — *see* Bite, toe
  forearm S51.85-
    elbow only — *see* Bite, elbow
    superficial NEC S50.87-
      insect S50.86-
  forehead — *see* Bite, head, specified site NEC
  genital organs, external
    female S31.552
      superficial NEC S30.876
        insect S30.866
      vagina and vulva — *see* Bite, vulva
    male S31.551
      penis — *see* Bite, penis
      scrotum — *see* Bite, scrotum
      superficial NEC S30.875
        insect S30.865
      testes — *see* Bite, testis
  groin — *see* Bite, abdomen, wall
  gum — *see* Bite, oral cavity
  hand S61.45-
    finger — *see* Bite, finger
    superficial NEC S60.57-
      insect S60.56-
    thumb — *see* Bite, thumb
  head S01.95
    cheek — *see* Bite, cheek
    ear — *see* Bite, ear
    eyelid — *see* Bite, eyelid
    lip — *see* Bite, lip
    nose — *see* Bite, nose
    oral cavity — *see* Bite, oral cavity
    scalp — *see* Bite, scalp
    specified site NEC S01.85
      superficial NEC S00.87
        insect S00.86
    superficial NEC S00.97
      insect S00.96
    temporomandibular area — *see* Bite, cheek
  heel — *see* Bite, foot
  hip S71.05-
    superficial NEC S70.27-
      insect S70.26-
  hymen S31.45
  hypochondrium — *see* Bite, abdomen, wall
  hypogastric region — *see* Bite, abdomen, wall
  inguinal region — *see* Bite, abdomen, wall
  insect — *see* Bite, insect, by site
  instep — *see* Bite, foot
  interscapular region — *see* Bite, thorax, back
  jaw — *see* Bite, head, specified site NEC
  knee S81.05-
    superficial NEC S80.27-
      insect S80.26-
  labium (majus) (minus) — *see* Bite, vulva
  lacrimal duct — *see* Bite, eyelid

Bite(s)— *continued*
  larynx S11.015
    superficial NEC S10.17
      insect S10.16
  leg (lower) S81.85-
    ankle — *see* Bite, ankle
    foot — *see* Bite, foot
    knee — *see* Bite, knee
    superficial NEC S80.87-
      insect S80.86-
    toe — *see* Bite, toe
    upper — *see* Bite, thigh
  lip S01.551
    superficial NEC S00.571
      insect S00.561
  lizard (venomous) — *see* Venom, bite, reptile
  loin — *see* Bite, abdomen, wall
  lower back — *see* Bite, back, lower
  lumbar region — *see* Bite, back, lower
  malar region — *see* Bite, head, specified site NEC
  mammary — *see* Bite, breast
  marine animals (venomous) — *see* Toxicity, venom,
      marine animal
  mastoid region — *see* Bite, head, specified site NEC
  mouth — *see* Bite, oral cavity
  nail
    finger — *see* Bite, finger
    toe — *see* Bite, toe
  nape — *see* Bite, neck, specified site NEC
  nasal (septum) (sinus) — *see* Bite, nose
  nasopharynx — *see* Bite, head, specified site NEC
  neck S11.95
    involving
        cervical esophagus — *see* Bite, esophagus,
            cervical
        larynx — *see* Bite, larynx
        pharynx — *see* Bite, pharynx
        thyroid gland S11.15
        trachea — *see* Bite, trachea
    specified site NEC S11.85
      superficial NEC S10.87
        insect S10.86
    superficial NEC S10.97
      insect S10.96
    throat S11.85
      superficial NEC S10.17
        insect S10.16
  nose (septum) (sinus) S01.25
    superficial NEC S00.37
      insect S00.36
  occipital region — *see* Bite, scalp
  oral cavity S01.552
    superficial NEC S00.572
      insect S00.562
  orbital region — *see* Bite, eyelid
  palate — *see* Bite, oral cavity
  palm — *see* Bite, hand
  parietal region — *see* Bite, scalp
  pelvis S31.050
    with penetration into retroperitoneal space
        S31.051
    superficial NEC S30.870
      insect S30.860
  penis S31.25
    superficial NEC S30.872
      insect S30.862
  perineum
    female — *see* Bite, vulva
    male — *see* Bite, pelvis
  periocular area (with or without lacrimal passages)
      — *see* Bite, eyelid
  phalanges
    finger — *see* Bite, finger
    toe — *see* Bite, toe
  pharynx S11.25
    superficial NEC S10.17
      insect S10.16
  pinna — *see* Bite, ear
  poisonous — *see* Venom
  popliteal space — *see* Bite, knee
  prepuce — *see* Bite, penis
  pubic region — *see* Bite, abdomen, wall

Bite(s)— *continued*
  pudendum
    female — *see* Bite, vulva
    male — *see* Bite, pelvis
  rectovaginal septum — *see* Bite, vulva
  red bug B88.0
  reptile NEC (*see also* Venom, bite, reptile)
    nonvenomous — *see* Bite, by site
    snake — *see* Venom, bite, snake
  sacral region — *see* Bite, back, lower
  sacroiliac region — *see* Bite, back, lower
  salivary gland — *see* Bite, oral cavity
  scalp S01.05
    superficial NEC S00.07
      insect S00.06
  scapular region — *see* Bite, shoulder
  scrotum S31.35
    superficial NEC S30.873
      insect S30.863
  sea-snake (venomous) — *see* Toxicity, venom, snake,
      sea snake
  shin — *see* Bite, leg
  shoulder S41.05-
    superficial NEC S40.27-
      insect S40.26-
  snake (*see also* Venom, bite, snake)
    nonvenomous — *see* Bite, by site
  spermatic cord — *see* Bite, testis
  spider (venomous) — *see* Toxicity, venom, spider
    nonvenomous — *see* Bite, insect, by site
  sternal region — *see* Bite, thorax, front
  submaxillary region — *see* Bite, head, specified site
      NEC
  submental region — *see* Bite, head, specified site
      NEC
  subungual
    finger(s) — *see* Bite, finger
    toe — *see* Bite, toe
  superficial — *see* Bite, superficial, by site
  supraclavicular fossa S11.85
  supraorbital — *see* Bite, head, specified site NEC
  temple, temporal region — *see* Bite, head, specified
      site NEC
  temporomandibular area — *see* Bite, cheek
  testis S31.35
    superficial NEC S30.873
      insect S30.863
  thigh S71.15-
    superficial NEC S70.37-
      insect S70.36-
  thorax, thoracic (wall) S21.95
    back S21.25-
      with penetration into thoracic cavity S21.45-
    breast — *see* Bite, breast
    front S21.15-
      with penetration into thoracic cavity S21.35-
    superficial NEC S20.97
      back S20.47-
      front S20.37-
      insect S20.96
        back S20.46-
        front S20.36-
  throat — *see* Bite, neck, throat
  thumb S61.05-
    with
      damage to nail S61.15-
    superficial NEC S60.37-
      insect S60.36-
  thyroid S11.15
    superficial NEC S10.87
      insect S10.86
  toe(s) S91.15-
    with
      damage to nail S91.25-
    great S91.15-
      with
        damage to nail S91.25-
    lesser S91.15-
      with
        damage to nail S91.25-
    superficial NEC S90.47-
      great S90.47-
      insect S90.46-

Bite(s)— *continued*
  toe(s)— *continued*
    superficial— *continued*
      insect— *continued*
        great S90.46-
  tongue S01.552
  trachea S11.025
    superficial NEC S10.17
      insect S10.16
  tunica vaginalis — *see* Bite, testis
  tympanum, tympanic membrane — *see* Bite, ear
  umbilical region S31.155
  uvula — *see* Bite, oral cavity
  vagina — *see* Bite, vulva
  venomous — *see* Venom
  vocal cords S11.035
    superficial NEC S10.17
      insect S10.16
  vulva S31.45
    superficial NEC S30.874
      insect S30.864
  wrist S61.55-
    superficial NEC S60.87-
      insect S60.86-
Biting, cheek or lip K13.1
Biventricular failure (heart) I50.9
Björck (-Thorson) **syndrome** (malignant carcinoid)
    E34.0
Black
  death A20.9
  eye S00.1-
  hairy tongue K14.3
  heel (foot) S90.3-
  lung (disease) J60
  palm (hand) S60.22-
Blackfan-Diamond (congenital hypoplastic) **anemia
    or syndrome** D61.01
Blackhead L70.0
Blackout R55
Bladder — *see* condition
Blast (air) (hydraulic) (immersion) (underwater)
  blindness S05.8x-
  injury
    abdomen or thorax — *see* Injury, by site
    ear (acoustic nerve trauma) — *see* Injury, nerve,
        acoustic, specified type NEC
    syndrome NEC T70.8
Blastoma — *see* Neoplasm, malignant, by site
  pulmonary — *see* Neoplasm, lung, malignant
Blastomycosis, blastomycotic B40.9
  Brazilian — *see* Paracoccidioidomycosis
  cutaneous B40.3
  disseminated B40.7
  European — *see* Cryptococcosis
  generalized B40.7
  keloidal B48.0
  North American B40.9
  primary pulmonary B40.0
  pulmonary B40.2
    acute B40.0
    chronic B40.1
  skin B40.3
  South American — *see* Paracoccidioidomycosis
  specified NEC B40.89
Bleb(s) R23.8
  emphysematous (lung) (solitary) J43.9
  endophthalmitis H59.43
  filtering (vitreous), after glaucoma surgery Z98.83
  inflamed (infected), postprocedural H59.40
    stage 1 H59.41
    stage 2 H59.42
    stage 3 H59.43
  lung (ruptured) J43.9
    congenital — *see* Atelectasis
    newborn P25.8
  subpleural (emphysematous) J43.9
Blebitis, postprocedural H59.40
  stage 1 H59.41
  stage 2 H59.42
  stage 3 H59.43
Bleeder (familial) (hereditary) — *see* Hemophilia

Bleeding (*see also* Hemorrhage)
  anal K62.5
  anovulatory N97.0
  atonic, following delivery O72.1
  capillary I78.8
    puerperal O72.2
  contact (postcoital) N93.0
  due to uterine subinvolution N85.3
  ear — *see* Otorrhagia
  excessive, associated with menopausal onset N92.4
  familial — *see* Defect, coagulation
  following intercourse N93.0
  gastrointestinal K92.2
  hemorrhoids NEC — *see* Hemorrhoids, by type,
    bleeding
  intermenstrual (regular) N92.3
    irregular N92.1
  intraoperative — *see* Complication, intraoperative,
    hemorrhage
  irregular N92.6
  menopausal N92.4
  newborn, intraventricular — *see* Newborn, affected
    by, hemorrhage, intraventricular
  nipple N64.59
  nose R04.0
  ovulation N92.3
  postclimacteric N95.0
  postcoital N93.0
  postmenopausal N95.0
  postoperative — *see* Hemorrhage, postoperative
  preclimacteric N92.4
  puberty (excessive, with onset of menstrual periods)
    N92.2
  rectum, rectal K62.5
    newborn P54.2
  tendencies — *see* Defect, coagulation
  throat R04.1
  tooth socket (post-extraction) K91.840
  umbilical stump P51.9
  uterus, uterine NEC N93.9
    climacteric N92.4
    dysfunctional of functional N93.8
    menopausal N92.4
    preclimacteric or premenopausal N92.4
    unrelated to menstrual cycle N93.9
  vagina, vaginal (abnormal) N93.9
    dysfunctional or functional N93.8
    newborn P54.6
  vicarious N94.89
Blennorrhagia, blennorrhagic — *see* Gonorrhea
Blennorrhea (acute) (chronic) (*see also* Gonorrhea)
  inclusion (neonatal) (newborn) P39.1
  lower genitourinary tract (gonococcal) A54.00
  neonatorum (gonococcal ophthalmia) A54.31
Blepharelosis — *see* Entropion
Blepharitis (angularis) (ciliaris) (eyelid) (marginal)
  (nonulcerative) H01.009
  herpes zoster B02.39
  left H01.006
    lower H01.005
    upper H01.004
  right H01.003
    lower H01.002
    upper H01.001
  squamous H01.029
    left H01.026
      lower H01.025
      upper H01.024
    right H01.023
      lower H01.022
      upper H01.021
  ulcerative H01.019
    left H01.016
      lower H01.015
      upper H01.014
    right H01.013
      lower H01.012
      upper H01.011
Blepharochalasis H02.30
  congenital Q10.0
  left H02.36
    lower H02.35
    upper H02.34

Blepharochalasis — *continued*
  right H02.33
    lower H02.32
    upper H02.31
Blepharoclonus H02.59
Blepharoconjunctivitis H10.50-
  angular H10.52-
  contact H10.53-
  ligneous H10.51-
Blepharophimosis (eyelid) H02.529
  congenital Q10.3
  left H02.526
    lower H02.525
    upper H02.524
  right H02.523
    lower H02.522
    upper H02.521
Blepharoptosis H02.40-
  congenital Q10.0
  mechanical H02.41-
  myogenic H02.42-
  neurogenic H02.43-
  paralytic H02.43-
Blepharopyorrhea, gonococcal A54.39
Blepharospasm G24.5
  drug induced G24.01
Blighted ovum O02.0
Blind (*see also* Blindness)
  bronchus (congenital) Q32.4
  loop syndrome K90.2
    congenital Q43.8
  sac, fallopian tube (congenital) Q50.6
  spot, enlarged — *see* Defect, visual field, localized,
    scotoma, blind spot area
  tract or tube, congenital NEC — *see* Atresia, by site
Blindness (acquired) (congenital) (both eyes) H54.0
  blast S05.8x-
  color — *see* Deficiency, color vision
  concussion S05.8x-
  cortical H47.619
    left brain H47.612
    right brain H47.611
  day H53.11
  due to injury (current episode) S05.9-
    sequelae — code to injury with extension S
  eclipse (total) — *see* Retinopathy, solar
  emotional (hysterical) F44.6
  face H53.16
  hysterical F44.6
  legal (both eyes) (USA definition) H54.8
  mind R48.8
  night H53.60
    abnormal dark adaptation curve H53.61
    acquired H53.62
    congenital H53.63
    specified type NEC H53.69
    vitamin A deficiency E50.5
  one eye (other eye normal) H54.40
    left (normal vision on right) H54.42
      low vision on right H54.12
    low vision, other eye H54.10
    right (normal vision on left) H54.41
      low vision on left H54.11
  psychic R48.8
  river B73.01
  snow — *see* Photokeratitis
  sun, solar — *see* Retinopathy, solar
  transient — *see* Disturbance, vision, subjective, loss,
    transient
  traumatic (current episode) S05.9-
  word (developmental) F81.0
    acquired R48.0
    secondary to organic lesion R48.0
Blister (nonthermal)
  abdominal wall S30.821
  alveolar process S00.522
  ankle S90.52-
  antecubital space — *see* Blister, elbow
  anus S30.827
  arm (upper) S40.82-
  auditory canal — *see* Blister, ear
  auricle — *see* Blister, ear
  axilla — *see* Blister, arm

Blister — *continued*
  back, lower S30.820
  beetle dermatitis L24.89
  breast S20.12-
  brow S00.82
  calf — *see* Blister, leg
  canthus — *see* Blister, eyelid
  cheek S00.82
    internal S00.522
  chest wall — *see* Blister, thorax
  chin S00.82
  costal region — *see* Blister, thorax
  digit(s)
    foot — *see* Blister, toe
    hand — *see* Blister, finger
  due to burn — *see* Burn, by site, second degree
  ear S00.42-
  elbow S50.32-
  epiglottis S10.12
  esophagus, cervical S10.12
  eyebrow — *see* Blister, eyelid
  eyelid S00.22-
  face S00.82
  fever B00.1
  finger(s) S60.429
    index S60.42-
    little S60.42-
    middle S60.42-
    ring S60.42-
  foot (except toe(s) alone) S90.82-
    toe — *see* Blister, toe
  forearm S50.82-
    elbow only — *see* Blister, elbow
  forehead S00.82
  fracture — *omit code*
  genital organ
    female S30.826
    male S30.825
  gum S00.522
  hand S60.52-
  head S00.92
    ear — *see* Blister, ear
    eyelid — *see* Blister, eyelid
    lip S00.521
    nose S00.32
    oral cavity S00.522
    scalp S00.02
    specified site NEC S00.82
  heel — *see* Blister, foot
  hip S70.22-
  interscapular region S20.429
  jaw S00.82
  knee S80.22-
  larynx S10.12
  leg (lower) S80.82-
    knee — *see* Blister, knee
    upper — *see* Blister, thigh
  lip S00.521
  malar region S00.82
  mammary — *see* Blister, breast
  mastoid region S00.82
  mouth S00.522
  multiple, skin, nontraumatic R23.8
  nail
    finger — *see* Blister, finger
    toe — *see* Blister, toe
  nasal S00.32
  neck S10.92
    specified site NEC S10.82
    throat S10.12
  nose S00.32
  occipital region S00.02
  oral cavity S00.522
  orbital region — *see* Blister, eyelid
  palate S00.522
  palm — *see* Blister, hand
  parietal region S00.02
  pelvis S30.820
  penis S30.822
  periocular area — *see* Blister, eyelid
  phalanges
    finger — *see* Blister, finger
    toe — *see* Blister, toe

Blister—*continued*
  pharynx S10.12
  pinna — *see* Blister, ear
  popliteal space — *see* Blister, knee
  scalp S00.02
  scapular region — *see* Blister, shoulder
  scrotum S30.823
  shin — *see* Blister, leg
  shoulder S40.22-
  sternal region S20.329
  submaxillary region S00.82
  submental region S00.82
  subungual
    finger(s) — *see* Blister, finger
    toe(s) — *see* Blister, toe
  supraclavicular fossa S10.82
  supraorbital S00.82
  temple S00.82
  temporal region S00.82
  testis S30.823
  thermal — *see* Burn, second degree, by site
  thigh S70.32-
  thorax, thoracic (wall) S20.92
    back S20.42-
    front S20.32-
  throat S10.12
  thumb S60.32-
  toe(s) S90.42-
    great S90.42-
  tongue S00.522
  trachea S10.12
  tympanum, tympanic membrane — *see* Blister, ear
  upper arm — *see* Blister, arm (upper)
  uvula S00.522
  vagina S30.824
  vocal cords S10.12
  vulva S30.824
  wrist S60.82-
Bloating R14.0
Bloch-Sulzberger disease or syndrome Q82.3
Block(ed)
  alveolocapillary J84.1
  arborization (heart) I45.5
  arrhythmic I45.9
  atrioventricular (incomplete) (partial) I44.30
    with atrioventricular dissociation I44.2
    complete I44.2
      congenital Q24.6
    congenital Q24.6
    first degree I44.0
    second degree (types I and II) I44.1
    specified NEC I44.39
    third degree I44.2
    types I and II I44.1
  auriculoventricular — *see* Block, atrioventricular
  bifascicular (cardiac) I45.2
  bundle-branch (complete) (false) (incomplete) I45.4
    bilateral I45.2
    left I44.7
      with right bundle branch block I45.2
      hemiblock I44.60
        anterior I44.4
        posterior I44.5
      incomplete I44.7
        with right bundle branch block I45.2
    right I45.10
      with
        left bundle branch block I45.2
        left fascicular block I45.2
      specified NEC I45.19
    Wilson's type I45.19
  cardiac I45.9
  conduction I45.9
    complete I44.2
  fascicular (left) I44.60
    anterior I44.4
    posterior I44.5
    right I45.0
    specified NEC I44.69
  foramen Magendie (acquired) G91.1
    congenital Q03.1
      with spina bifida — *see* Spina bifida, by site, with hydrocephalus

Block(ed)— *continued*
  heart I45.9
    bundle branch I45.4
      bilateral I45.2
    complete (atrioventricular) I44.2
    congenital Q24.6
    first degree (atrioventricular) I44.0
    second degree (atrioventricular) I44.1
    specified type NEC I45.5
    third degree (atrioventricular) I44.2
  hepatic vein I82.0
  intraventricular (nonspecific) I45.4
    bundle branch
      bilateral I45.2
  kidney N28.9
    postcystoscopic or postprocedural N99.0
  Mobitz (types I and II) I44.1
  myocardial — *see* Block, heart
  nodal I45.5
  organ or site, congenital NEC — *see* Atresia, by site
  portal (vein) I81
  second degree (types I and II) I44.1
  sinoatrial I45.5
  sinoauricular I45.5
  third degree I44.2
  trifascicular I45.3
  tubal N97.1
  vein NOS I82.90
  Wenckebach (types I and II) I44.1
Blockage — *see* Obstruction
Blocq's disease F44.4
Blood
  constituents, abnormal R78.9
  disease D75.9
  donor — *see* Donor, blood
  dyscrasia D75.9
    with
      abortion — *see* Abortion, by type with excessive hemorrhage
      ectopic pregnancy O08.1
      molar pregnancy O08.1
    following ectopic or molar pregnancy O08.1
    newborn P61.9
    puerperal, postpartum O72.3
  flukes NEC — *See* Schistosomiasis
  in
    feces K92.1
      occult R19.5
    urine — *see* Hematuria
  mole O02.0
  occult in feces R19.5
  pressure
    decreased, due to shock following injury T79.4
    examination only Z01.30
    fluctuating I99.8
    high — *see* Hypertension
      incidental reading, without diagnosis of hypertension R03.0
    low (*see also* Hypotension)
      incidental reading, without diagnosis of hypotension R03.1
  spitting — *see* Hemoptysis
  staining cornea — *see* Pigmentation, cornea, stromal
  transfusion
    reaction or complication — *see* Complications, transfusion
  type
    A (Rh positive) Z67.10
      Rh negative Z67.11
    AB (Rh positive) Z67.30
      Rh negative Z67.31
    B (Rh positive) Z67.20
      Rh negative Z67.21
    O (Rh positive) Z67.40
      Rh negative Z67.41
    Rh (positive) Z67.90
      negative Z67.91
  vessel rupture — *see* Hemorrhage
  vomiting — *see* Hematemesis
Blood-forming organs, disease D75.9
Bloodgood's disease — *see* Mastopathy, cystic
Bloom (-Machacek)(-Torre) **syndrome** Q82.8

Blount's disease or osteochondrosis — *see* Osteochondrosis, juvenile, tibia
Blue
  baby Q24.9
  diaper syndrome E72.09
  dome cyst (breast) — *see* Cyst, breast
  dot cataract Q12.0
  nevus D22.9
  sclera Q13.5
    with fragility of bone and deafness Q78.0
  toe syndrome I75.02-
Blueness — *see* Cyanosis
Blues, postpartal O90.6
  baby O90.6
Blurring, visual H53.8
Blushing (abnormal) (excessive) R23.2
BMI — *see* Body, mass index
Boarder, hospital NEC Z76.4
  accompanying sick person Z76.3
  healthy infant or child Z76.2
    foundling Z76.1
Bockhart's impetigo L01.02
Bodechtel-Guttman disease (subacute sclerosing panencephalitis) A81.1
Boder-Sedgwick syndrome (ataxia-telangiectasia) G11.3
Body, bodies
  Aschoff's — *see* Myocarditis, rheumatic
  asteroid, vitreous — *see* Deposit, crystalline
  cytoid (retina) — *see* Occlusion, artery, retina
  drusen (degenerative) (macula) (retinal) (*see also* Degeneration, macula, drusen)
    optic disc — *see* Drusen, optic disc
  foreign — *see* Foreign body
  loose
    joint, except knee — *see* Loose, body, joint
      knee M23.4-
    sheath, tendon — *see* Disorder, tendon, specified type NEC
  mass index (BMI)
    adult
      19 or less Z68.1
      20.0-20.9 Z68.20
      21.0-21.9 Z68.21
      22.0-22.9 Z68.22
      23.0-23.9 Z68.23
      24.0-24.9 Z68.24
      25.0-25.9 Z68.25
      26.0-26.9 Z68.26
      27.0-27.9 Z68.27
      28.0-28.9 Z68.28
      29.0-29.9 Z68.29
      30.0-30.9 Z68.30
      31.0-31.9 Z68.31
      32.0-32.9 Z68.32
      33.0-33.9 Z68.33
      34.0-34.9 Z68.34
      35.0-35.9 Z68.35
      36.0-36.9 Z68.36
      37.0-37.9 Z68.37
      38.0-38.9 Z68.38
      39.0-39.9 Z68.39
      40.0-44.9 Z68.41
      45.0-49.9 Z68.42
      50.0-59.9 Z68.43
      60.0-69.9 Z68.44
      70 and over Z68.45
    pediatric
      5th percentile to less than 85th percentile for age Z68.52
      85th percentile to less than 95th percentile for age Z68.53
      greater than or equal to ninety-fifth percentile for age Z68.54
      less than fifth percentile for age Z68.51
  Mooser's A75.2
  rice (*see also* Loose, body, joint)
    knee M23.4-
  rocking F98.4
Boeck's
  disease or sarcoid — *see* Sarcoidosis
  lupoid (miliary) D86.3

Boerhaave's syndrome (spontaneous esophageal rupture) K22.3
Boggy
  cervix N88.8
  uterus N85.8
Boil (*see also* Furuncle, by site)
  Aleppo B55.1
  Baghdad B55.1
  Delhi B55.1
  lacrimal
    gland — *see* Dacryoadenitis
    passages (duct) (sac) — *see* Inflammation, lacrimal, passages, acute
  Natal B55.1
  orbit, orbital — *see* Abscess, orbit
  tropical B55.1
Bold hives — *see* Urticaria
Bombé, iris — *see* Membrane, pupillary
Bone — *see* condition
Bonnevie-Ullrich syndrome Q87.1
Bonnier's syndrome — *see* subcategory H81.8
Bonvale dam fever T73.3
Bony block of joint — *see* Ankylosis
BOOP (bronchiolitis obliterans organized pneumonia) J84.8
Borderline
  osteopenia M85.8-
  pelvis, with obstruction during labor O65.1
  personality F60.3
Borna disease A83.9
Bornholm disease B33.0
Boston exanthem A88.0
Botalli, ductus (patent) (persistent) Q25.0
Bothriocephalus latus infestation B70.0
Botulism (foodborne intoxication) A05.1
  infant A48.51
  non-foodborne A48.52
  wound A48.52
Bouba — *see* Yaws
Bouchard's nodes (with arthropathy) M15.2
Bouffée délirante F23
Bouillaud's disease or syndrome (rheumatic heart disease) I01.9
Bourneville's disease Q85.1
Boutonniere deformity (finger) — *see* Deformity, finger, boutonniere
Bouveret (-Hoffmann) **syndrome** (paroxysmal tachycardia) I47.9
Bovine heart — *see* Hypertrophy, cardiac
Bowel — *see* condition
Bowen's
  dermatosis (precancerous) — *see* Neoplasm, skin, in situ
  disease — *see* Neoplasm, skin, in situ
  epithelloma — *see* Neoplasm, skin, in situ
  type
    epidermoid carcinoma-in-situ — *see* Neoplasm, skin, in situ
    intraepidermal squamous cell carcinoma — *see* Neoplasm, skin, in situ
Bowing
  femur (*see also* Deformity, limb, specified type NEC, thigh)
    congenital Q68.3
  fibula (*see also* Deformity, limb, specified type NEC, lower leg)
    congenital Q68.4
  forearm — *see* Deformity, limb, specified type NEC, forearm
  leg(s), long bones, congenital Q68.5
  radius — *see* Deformity, limb, specified type NEC, forearm
  tibia (*see also* Deformity, limb, specified type NEC, lower leg)
    congenital Q68.4
Bowleg(s) (acquired) M21.16-
  congenital Q68.5
  rachitic E64.3
Boyd's dysentery A03.2
Brachial — *see* condition
Brachycardia R00.1
Brachycephaly Q75.0
Bradley's disease A08.19

Bradyarrhythmia, cardiac I49.8
Bradycardia (sinoatrial) (sinus) (vagal) R00.1
  neonatal P29.12
  reflex G90.09
  tachycardia syndrome I49.5
Bradykinesia R25.8
Bradypnea R06.89
Bradytachycardia I49.5
Brailsford's disease or osteochondrosis — *see* Osteochondrosis, juvenile, radius
Brain (*see also* condition)
  death G93.89
  syndrome — *see* Syndrome, brain
Branched-chain amino-acid disorder E71.2
Branchial — *see* condition
  cartilage, congenital Q18.2
Branchiogenic remnant (in neck) Q18.0
Brash (water) R12
Bravais-jacksonian epilepsy — *see* Epilepsy, localization-related, symptomatic, with simple partial seizures
Braxton Hicks contractions — *see* False, labor
Brazilian leishmaniasis B55.2
Break, retina (without detachment) H33.30-
  with retinal detachment — *see* Detachment, retina
  horseshoe tear H33.31-
  multiple H33.33-
  round hole H33.32-
Breakage, prosthetic join — *see* Complications, joint prosthesis, mechanical, by site
Breakdown
  device, graft or implant (*see also* Complications, by site and type, mechanical) T85.618
    arterial graft NEC — *see* Complication, cardiovascular device, mechanical, vascular
    breast (implant) T85.41
    catheter NEC T85.618
      cystostomy T83.010
      dialysis (renal) T82.41
        intraperitoneal T85.611
      infusion NEC T82.514
        spinal (epidural) (subdural) T85.610
      urinary (indwelling) T83.018
    electronic (electrode) (pulse generator) (stimulator)
      bone T84.310
      cardiac T82.119
        electrode T82.110
        pulse generator T82.111
        specified type NEC T82.118
      nervous system — *see* Complication, prosthetic device, mechanical, electronic nervous system stimulator
    urinary — *see* Complication, genitourinary, device, urinary, mechanical
    fixation, internal (orthopedic) NEC — *see* Complication, fixation device, mechanical
    gastrointestinal — *see* Complications, prosthetic device, mechanical, gastrointestinal device
    genital NEC T83.418
      intrauterine contraceptive device T83.31
      penile prosthesis T83.410
    heart NEC — *see* Complication, cardiovascular device, mechanical
    joint prosthesis — *see* Complications, joint prosthesis, internal, mechanical, by site
    ocular NEC — *see* Complications, prosthetic device, mechanical, ocular device
    orthopedic NEC — *see* Complication, orthopedic, device, mechanical
    specified NEC T85.618
    sutures, permanent T85.612
      used in bone repair — *see* Complications, fixation device, internal (orthopedic), mechanical
    urinary NEC (*see also* Complication, genitourinary, device, urinary, mechanical)
      graft T83.21
    vascular NEC — *see* Complication, cardiovascular device, mechanical
    ventricular intracranial shunt T85.01
  nervous F48.8
  perineum O90.1

Breakdown— *continued*
  respirator J95.850
    specified NEC J95.859
  ventilator J95.850
    specified NEC J95.859
Breast (*see also* condition)
  buds E30.1
    in newborn P96.89
  dense R92.2
  nodule N63
Breath
  foul R19.6
  holder, child R06.89
  holding spell R06.89
  shortness R06.02
Breathing
  labored — *see* Hyperventilation
  mouth R06.5
    causing malocclusion M26.5
  periodic R06.3
    high altitude G47.32
Breathlessness R06.81
Breda's disease — *see* Yaws
Breech presentation (mother) O32.1
  causing obstructed labor O64.1
  footling O32.8
    causing obstructed labor O64.8
  incomplete O32.8
    causing obstructed labor O64.8
Breisky's disease N90.4
Brennemann's syndrome I88.0
Brenner
  tumor (benign) D27.9
    borderline malignancy D39.1-
    malignant C56
    proliferating D39.1-
Bretonneau's disease or angina A36.0
Breus' mole O02.0
Brevicollis Q76.49
Brickmakers' anemia B76.9
Bridge, myocardial Q24.5
BRBPR K62.5
Bright red blood per rectum (BRBPR) K62.5
Bright's disease (*see also* Nephritis)
  arteriosclerotic — *see* Hypertension, kidney
Brill(-Zinsser) **disease** (recrudescent typhus) A75.1
  flea-borne A75.2
  louse-borne A75.1
Brill-Symmers' disease C82.90
Brion-Kayser disease — *see* Fever, parathyroid
Briquet's disorder or syndrome F45.0
Brissaud's
  infantilism or dwarfism E23.0
  motor-verbal tic F95.2
Brittle
  bones disease Q78.0
  nails L60.3
    congenital Q84.6
Broad (*see also* condition)
  beta disease E78.2
  ligament laceration syndrome N83.8
  Broador floating-betalipoproteinemia E78.2
Brock's syndrome (atelectasis due to enlarged lymph nodes) J98.19
Brocq-Duhring disease (dermatitis herpetiformis) L13.0
Brodie's abscess or disease M86.8x-
Broken
  arches (*see also* Deformity, limb, flat foot)
  arm (meaning upper limb) — *see* Fracture, arm
  back — *see* Fracture, vertebra
  bone — *see* Fracture
  implant or internal device — *see* Complications, by site and type, mechanical
  leg (meaning lower limb) — *see* Fracture, leg
  nose S02.2
  tooth, teeth — *see* Fracture, tooth
Bromhidrosis, bromidrosis L75.0
Bromidism, bromism G92
  due to
    correct substance properly administered — *see* Table of Drugs and Chemicals, by drug, adverse effect

Bromidism, bromism — *continued*
　due to— *continued*
　　overdose or wrong substance given or taken —
　　　see Table of Drugs and Chemicals, by drug,
　　　poisoning
　　chronic (dependence) F13.2Ø
Bromidrosiphobia F4Ø.298
Bronchi, bronchial — *see* condition
Bronchiectasis (cylindrical) (diffuse) (fusiform)
　(localized) (saccular) J47.9
　with
　　acute lower respiratory infection J47.Ø
　　exacerbation (acute) J47.1
　congenital Q33.4
　tuberculous NEC — *see* Tuberculosis, pulmonary
Bronchiolectasis — *see* Bronchiectasis
Bronchiolitis (acute) (infective) (subacute) J21.9
　with
　　bronchospasm or obstruction J21.9
　　influenza, flu or grippe — *see* Influenza, with,
　　　respiratory manifestations NEC
　chemical (chronic) J68.4
　　acute J68.Ø
　chronic (fibrosing) (obliterative) J44.9
　due to
　　external agent — *see* Bronchitis, acute, due to
　　human metapneumovirus J21.1
　　respiratory syncytial virus J21.Ø
　　specified organism NEC J21.8
　fibrosa obliterans J44.9
　influenzal — *see* Influenza, with, respiratory
　　manifestations NEC
　obliterans J42
　　with organizing pneumonia (BOOP) J84.8
　obliterative (chronic) (subacute) J44.9
　　due to fumes or vapors J68.4
　　due to chemicals, gases, fumes or vapors
　　　(inhalation) J68.4
Bronchitis (diffuse) (fibrinous) (hypostatic) (infective)
　(membranous) (with tracheitis) J4Ø
　with
　　influenza, flu or grippe — *see* Influenza, with,
　　　respiratory manifestations NEC
　　obstruction (airway) (lung) J44.9
　　tracheitis (I5 years of age and above) J4Ø
　　　acute or subacute J2Ø.9
　　　chronic J42
　　　under I5 years of age J2Ø.9
　acute or subacute (with bronchospasm or
　　obstruction) J2Ø.9
　　with
　　　bronchiectasis J47.1
　　　chronic obstructive pulmonary disease J44.Ø
　　chemical (due to gases or vapors) J68.Ø
　　due to
　　　fumes or vapors J68.Ø
　　　Haemophilus influenzae J2Ø.1
　　　Mycoplasma pneumoniae J2Ø.Ø
　　　radiation J7Ø.Ø
　　　specified organism NEC J2Ø.8
　　　Streptococcus J2Ø.2
　　　virus
　　　　coxsackie J2Ø.3
　　　　echovirus J2Ø.7
　　　　parainfluenzae J2Ø.4
　　　　respiratory syncytial J2Ø.5
　　　　rhinovirus J2Ø.6
　　viral NEC J2Ø.8
　allergic (acute) J45.9Ø9
　　with
　　　exacerbation (acute) J45.9Ø1
　　　status asthmaticus J45.9Ø2
　arachidic T17.528
　aspiration (due to fumes or vapors) J68.Ø
　asthmatic J45.9
　　chronic J44.9
　　　with
　　　　acute lower respiratory infection J44.Ø
　　　　exacerbation (acute) J44.1
　capillary — *see* Pneumonia, broncho
　caseous (tuberculous) A15.5

Bronchitis— *continued*
　Castellani's A69.8
　catarrhal (I5 years of age and above) J4Ø
　　acute — *see* Bronchitis, acute
　　chronic J41.Ø
　　under I5 years of age J2Ø.9
　chemical (acute) (subacute) J68.Ø
　　chronic J68.4
　　due to fumes or vapors J68.Ø
　　　chronic J68.4
　chronic J42
　　with
　　　airways obstruction J44.9
　　　tracheitis (chronic) J42
　　asthmatic (obstructive) J44.9
　　catarrhal J41.Ø
　　chemical (due to fumes or vapors) J68.4
　　due to
　　　chemicals, gases, fumes or vapors (inhalation)
　　　　J68.4
　　　radiation J7Ø.1
　　　tobacco smoking J41.Ø
　　emphysematous J44.9
　　mucopurulent J41.1
　　non-obstructive J41.Ø
　　obliterans J44.9
　　obstructive J44.9
　　purulent J41.1
　　simple J41.Ø
　croupous — *see* Bronchitis, acute
　due to gases, fumes or vapors (chemical) J68.Ø
　emphysematous (obstructive) J44.9
　exudative — *see* Bronchitis, acute
　fetid J41.1
　grippal — *see* Influenza, with, respiratory
　　manifestations NEC
　in those under I5 years age — *see* Bronchitis, acute
　　chronic — *see* Bronchitis, chronic
　influenzal — *see* Influenza, with, respiratory
　　manifestations NEC
　mixed simple and mucopurulent J41.8
　moulder's J62.8
　mucopurulent (chronic) (recurrent) J41.1
　　acute or subacute J2Ø.9
　　simple (mixed) J41.8
　obliterans (chronic) J44.9
　obstructive (chronic) (diffuse) J44.9
　pituitous J41.1
　pneumococcal, acute or subacute J2Ø.2
　pseudomembranous, acute or subacute — *see*
　　Bronchitis, acute
　purulent (chronic) (recurrent) J41.1
　　acute or subacute — *see* Bronchitis, acute
　putrid J41.1
　senile (chronic) J42
　simple and mucopurulent (mixed) J41.8
　smokers' J41.Ø
　spirochetal NEC A69.8
　subacute — *see* Bronchitis, acute
　suppurative (chronic) J41.1
　　acute or subacute — *see* Bronchitis, acute
　tuberculous A15.5
　under I5 years of age — *see* Bronchitis, acute
　　chronic — *see* Bronchitis, chronic
　viral NEC, acute or subacute (*see also* Bronchitis,
　　acute) J2Ø.8
Bronchoalveolitis J18.Ø
Bronchoaspergillosis B44.1
Bronchocele meaning goiter EØ4.Ø
Broncholithiasis J98.Ø9
　tuberculous NEC A15.5
Bronchomalacia J98.Ø9
　congenital Q32.2
Bronchomycosis NOS B49 [J99]
　candidal B37.1
Bronchopleuropneumonia — *see* Pneumonia,
　broncho
Bronchopneumonia — *see* Pneumonia, broncho
Bronchopneumonitis — *see* Pneumonia, broncho
Bronchopulmonary — *see* condition
Bronchopulmonitis — *see* Pneumonia, broncho
Bronchorrhagia (see Hemoptysis)

Bronchorrhea J98.Ø9
　acute J2Ø.9
　chronic (infective) (purulent) J42
Bronchospasm (acute) J98.Ø1
　with
　　bronchiolitis, acute J21.9
　　bronchitis, acute (conditions in J2Ø) — *see*
　　　Bronchitis, acute
　due to external agent — *see* condition, respiratory,
　　acute, due to
　exercise induced J45.99Ø
Bronchospirochetosis A69.8
　Castellani A69.8
Bronchostenosis J98.Ø9
Bronchus — *see* condition
Brontophobia F4Ø.22Ø
Bronze baby syndrome P83.8
Brooke's tumor — *see* Neoplasm, skin, benign
Brown enamel of teeth (hereditary) KØØ.5
Brown's sheath syndrome H5Ø.61-
Brown-Séquard disease, paralysis or
　syndrome G83.81
Bruce sepsis A23.Ø
Brucellosis (infection) A23.9
　abortus A23.1
　canis A23.3
　dermatitis A23.9
　melitensis A23.Ø
　mixed A23.8
　sepsis A23.9
　　melitensis A23.Ø
　　specified NEC A23.8
　suis A23.2
Bruck-de Lange disease Q87.1
Bruck's disease — *see* Deformity, limb
Brugsch's syndrome Q82.8
Bruise (skin surface intact) (*see also* Contusion)
　with
　　open wound — *see* Wound, open
　internal organ — *see* Injury, by site
　newborn P54.5
　scalp, due to birth injury, newborn P12.3
　umbilical cord O69.5
Bruit (arterial) RØ9.89
　cardiac RØ1.1
Brush burn — *see* Abrasion, by site
Bruton's X-linked agammaglobulinemia D8Ø.Ø
Bruxism
　psychogenic F45.8
　sleep related G47.63
Bubbly lung syndrome P27.Ø
Bubo I88.8
　blennorrhagic (gonococcal) A54.89
　chancroidal A57
　climatic A55
　due to Haemophilus ducreyi A57
　gonococcal A54.89
　indolent (nonspecific) I88.8
　inguinal (nonspecific) I88.8
　　chancroidal A57
　　climatic A55
　　due to H. ducreyi A57
　　infective I88.8
　scrofulous (tuberculous) A18.2
　soft chancre A57
　suppurating — *see* Lymphadenitis, acute
　syphilitic (primary) A51.Ø
　　congenital A5Ø.Ø7
　tropical A55
　virulent (chancroidal) A57
Bubonic plague A2Ø.Ø
Bubonocele — *see* Hernia, inguinal
Buccal — *see* condition
Buchanan's disease or osteochondrosis M91.Ø
Buchem's syndrome (hyperostosis corticalis) M85.2
Bucket-handle fracture or tear (semilunar cartilage)
　— *see* Tear, meniscus
Budd-Chiari syndrome (hepatic vein thrombosis)
　I82.Ø
Budgerigar fancier's disease or lung J67.2
Buds
　breast E3Ø.1
　　in newborn P96.89

Buerger's disease (thromboangiitis obliterans) I73.1
Bulbar — *see* condition
Bulbus cordis (left ventricle) (persistent) Q21.8
Bulimia (nervosa) F50.2
 atypical F50.9
 normal weight F50.9
Bulky
 stools R19.5
 uterus N85.2
Bulla(e) R23.8
 lung (emphysematous) (solitary) J43.9
  newborn P25.8
Bullet wound (*see also* Wound, open)
 fracture—code as Fracture, by site
 internal organ — *see* Injury, by site
Bundle
 branch block (complete) (false) (incomplete) — *see*
  Block, bundle-branch
 of His — *see* condition
Bunion — *see* Deformity, toe, hallux valgus
Buphthalmia, buphthalmos (congenital) Q15.0
Burdwan fever B55.0
Bürger-Grütz disease or syndrome E78.3
Buried roots K08.3
Burke's syndrome K86.8
Burkitt
 cell leukemia C91.0-
 lymphoma (malignant) C83.7-
  small noncleaved, diffuse C83.7-
  spleen C83.77
  undifferentiated C83.7-
 tumor C83.7-
 type
  acute lymphoblastic leukemia C91.0-
  undifferentiated C83.7-
Burn (electricity) (flame) (hot gas, liquid or hot object)
  (radiation) (steam) (thermal) T30.0
 abdomen, abdominal (muscle) (wall) T21.02
  first degree T21.12
  second degree T21.22
  third degree T21.32
 above elbow T22.039
  first degree T22.139
  left T22.032
   first degree T22.132
   second degree T22.232
   third degree T22.332
  right T22.031
   first degree T22.131
   second degree T22.231
   third degree T22.331
  second degree T22.239
  third degree T22.339
 acid (caustic) (external) (internal) — *see* Corrosion,
  by site
 alimentary tract NEC T28.2
  esophagus T28.1
  mouth T28.0
  pharynx T28.0
 alkaline (caustic) (external) (internal) — *see*
  Corrosion, by site
 ankle T25.019
  first degree T25.119
  left T25.012
   first degree T25.112
   second degree T25.212
   third degree T25.312
  multiple with foot — *see* Burn, lower, limb,
   multiple, ankle and foot
  right T25.011
   first degree T25.111
   second degree T25.211
   third degree T25.311
  second degree T25.219
  third degree T25.319
 anus — *see* Burn, buttock
 arm (lower) (upper) — *see* Burn, upper, limb
 axilla T22.049
  first degree T22.149
  left T22.042
   first degree T22.142
   second degree T22.242
   third degree T22.342

Burn— *continued*
 axilla— *continued*
  right T22.041
   first degree T22.141
   second degree T22.241
   third degree T22.341
  second degree T22.249
  third degree T22.349
 back (lower) T21.04
  first degree T21.14
  second degree T21.24
  third degree T21.34
  upper T21.03
   first degree T21.13
   second degree T21.23
   third degree T21.33
 blisters—code as Burn, second degree, by site
 breast(s) — *see* Burn, chest wall
 buttock(s) T21.05
  first degree T21.15
  second degree T21.25
  third degree T21.35
 calf T24.039
  first degree T24.139
  left T24.032
   first degree T24.132
   second degree T24.232
   third degree T24.332
  right T24.031
   first degree T24.131
   second degree T24.231
   third degree T24.331
  second degree T24.239
  third degree T24.339
 canthus (eye) — *see* Burn, eyelid
 caustic acid or alkaline — *see* Corrosion, by site
 cervix T28.3
 cheek T20.06
  first degree T20.16
  second degree T20.26
  third degree T20.36
 chemical (acids) (alkalines) (caustics) (external)
  (internal) — *see* Corrosion, by site
 chest wall T21.01
  first degree T21.11
  second degree T21.21
  third degree T21.31
 chin T20.03
  first degree T20.13
  second degree T20.23
  third degree T20.33
 colon T28.2
 conjunctiva (and cornea) — *see* Burn, cornea
 cornea (and conjunctiva) T26.1-
  chemical — *see* Corrosion, cornea
 corrosion (external) (internal) — *see* Corrosion, by
  site
 deep necrosis of underlying tissue — code as Burn,
  third degree, by site
 dorsum of hand T23.069
  first degree T23.169
  left T23.062
   first degree T23.162
   second degree T23.262
   third degree T23.362
  right T23.061
   first degree T23.161
   second degree T23.261
   third degree T23.361
  second degree T23.269
  third degree T23.369
 due to ingested chemical agent — *see* Corrosion, by
  site
 ear (auricle) (external) (canal) T20.01
  first degree T20.11
  second degree T20.21
  third degree T20.31
 elbow T22.029
  first degree T22.129
  left T22.022
   first degree T22.122
   second degree T22.222
   third degree T22.322

Burn— *continued*
 elbow— *continued*
  right T22.021
   first degree T22.121
   second degree T22.221
   third degree T22.321
  second degree T22.229
  third degree T22.329
 epidermal loss—code as Burn, second degree, by
  site
 erythema, erythematous—code as Burn, first
  degree, by site
 esophagus T28.1
 extent (percentage of body surface)
  less than 10 percent T31.0
  10-19 percent T31.10
   with 0-9 percent third degree burns T31.10
   with 10-19 percent third degree burns T31.11
  20-29 percent T31.20
   with 0-9 percent third degree burns T31.20
   with 10-19 percent third degree burns T31.21
   with 20-29 percent third degree burns T31.22
  30-39 percent T31.30
   with 0-9 percent third degree burns T31.30
   with 10-19 percent third degree burns T31.31
   with 20-29 percent third degree burns T31.32
   with 30-39 percent third degree burns T31.33
  40-49 percent T31.40
   with 0-9 percent third degree burns T31.40
   with 10-19 percent third degree burns T31.41
   with 20-29 percent third degree burns T31.42
   with 30-39 percent third degree burns T31.43
   with 40-49 percent third degree burns T31.44
  50-59 percent T31.50
   with 0-9 percent third degree burns T31.50
   with 10-19 percent third degree burns T31.51
   with 20-29 percent third degree burns T31.52
   with 30-39 percent third degree burns T31.53
   with 40-49 percent third degree burns T31.54
   with 50-59 percent third degree burns T31.55
  60-69 percent T31.60
   with 0-9 percent third degree burns T31.60
   with 10-19 percent third degree burns T31.61
   with 20-29 percent third degree burns T31.62
   with 30-39 percent third degree burns T31.63
   with 40-49 percent third degree burns T31.64
   with 50-59 percent third degree burns T31.65
   with 60-69 percent third degree burns T31.66
  70-79 percent T31.70
   with 0-9 percent third degree burns T31.70
   with 10-19 percent third degree burns T31.71
   with 20-29 percent third degree burns T31.72
   with 30-39 percent third degree burns T31.73
   with 40-49 percent third degree burns T31.74
   with 50-59 percent third degree burns T31.75
   with 60-69 percent third degree burns T31.76
   with 70-79 percent third degree burns T31.77
  80-89 percent T31.80
   with 0-9 percent third degree burns T31.80
   with 10-19 percent third degree burns T31.81
   with 20-29 percent third degree burns T31.82
   with 30-39 percent third degree burns T31.83
   with 40-49 percent third degree burns T31.84
   with 50-59 percent third degree burns T31.85
   with 60-69 percent third degree burns T31.86
   with 70-79 percent third degree burns T31.87
   with 80-89 percent third degree burns T31.88
  90 percent or more T31.90
   with 0-9 percent third degree burns T31.90
   with 10-19 percent third degree burns T31.91
   with 20-29 percent third degree burns T31.92
   with 30-39 percent third degree burns T31.93
   with 40-49 percent third degree burns T31.94
   with 50-59 percent third degree burns T31.95
   with 60-69 percent third degree burns T31.96
   with 70-79 percent third degree burns T31.97
   with 80-89 percent third degree burns T31.98
   with 90 percent or more third degree burns
    T31.99
 extremity — *see* Burn, limb
 eye(s) and adnexa T26.4-
  with resulting rupture and destruction of eyeball
   T26.2-

Burn— *continued*
  upper limb— *continued*
    third degree T22.3Ø
    wrist — *see* Burn, wrist
  uterus T28.3
  vagina T28.3
  vulva — *see* Burn, genital organs, external, female
  wrist T23.Ø79
    first degree T23.179
    left T23.Ø72
      first degree T23.172
      second degree T23.272
      third degree T23.372
    multiple sites with hand T23.Ø99
      first degree T23.199
      left T23.Ø92
        first degree T23.192
        second degree T23.292
        third degree T23.392
      right T23.Ø91
        first degree T23.191
        second degree T23.291
        third degree T23.391
      second degree T23.299
      third degree T23.399
    right T23.Ø71
      first degree T23.171
      second degree T23.271
      third degree T23.371
    second degree T23.279
    third degree T23.379
Burnett's syndrome E83.52
Burning
  feet syndrome E53.9
  sensation R2Ø.8
  tongue K14.6
Burn-out (state) Z73.Ø
Burns' disease or osteochondrosis — *see* Osteochondrosis, juvenile, ulna
Bursa — *see* condition
Bursitis M71.9
  Achilles — *see* Tendinitis, Achilles
  adhesive — *see* Bursitis, specified NEC
  ankle — *see* Enthesopathy, lower limb, ankle, specified type NEC
  calcaneal — *see* Enthesopathy, foot, specified type NEC
  collateral ligament, tibial — *see* Bursitis, tibial collateral
  due to use, overuse, pressure (*see also* Disorder, soft tissue, due to use, specified type NEC)
    specified NEC — *see* Disorder, soft tissue, due to use, specified NEC
  Duplay's M75.Ø
  elbow NEC M7Ø.3-
    olecranon M7Ø.2-
  finger — *see* Disorder, soft tissue, due to use, specified type NEC, hand
  foot — *see* Enthesopathy, foot, specified type NEC
  gonococcal A54.49
  gouty — *see* Gout, idiopathic
  hand M7Ø.1-
  hip NEC M7Ø.7-
    trochanteric M7Ø.6-
  infective NEC M71.1Ø
    abscess — *see* Abscess, bursa
    ankle M71.17-
    elbow M71.12-
    foot M71.17-
    hand M71.14-
    hip M71.15-
    knee M71.16-
    multiple sites M71.19
    shoulder M71.11-
    specified site NEC M71.18
    wrist M71.13-
  ischial — *see* Bursitis, hip
  knee NEC M7Ø.5-
    prepatellar M7Ø.4-
  occupational NEC (*see also* Disorder, soft tissue, due to, use)
  olecranon — *see* Bursitis, elbow, olecranon
  pharyngeal J39.1

Bursitis— *continued*
  popliteal — *see* Bursitis, knee
  prepatellar M7Ø.4-
  radiohumeral M77.8
  rheumatoid MØ6.2Ø
    ankle MØ6.27-
    elbow MØ6.22-
    foot joint MØ6.27-
    hand joint MØ6.24-
    hip MØ6.25-
    knee MØ6.26-
    multiple site MØ6.29
    shoulder MØ6.21-
    vertebra MØ6.28
    wrist MØ6.23-
  scapulohumeral — *see* Bursitis, shoulder
  semimembranous muscle (knee) — *see* Bursitis, knee
  shoulder M75.5-
    adhesive — *see* Capsulitis, adhesive
  specified NEC M71.5Ø
    ankle M71.57-
    due to use, overuse or pressure — *see* Disorder, soft tissue, due to, use
    elbow M71.52-
    foot M71.57-
    hand M71.54-
    hip M71.55-
    knee M71.56-
    shoulder — *see* Bursitis, shoulder
    specified site NEC M71.58
    tibial collateral M76.4-
    wrist M71.53-
  subacromial — *see* Bursitis, shoulder
  subcoracoid — *see* Bursitis, shoulder
  subdeltoid — *see* Bursitis, shoulder
  syphilitic A52.78
  Thornwaldt, Tornwaldt J39.2
  tibial collateral — *see* Bursitis, tibial collateral
  toe — *see* Enthesopathy, foot, specified type NEC
  trochanteric (area) — *see* Bursitis, hip, trochanteric
  wrist — *see* Bursitis, hand
Bursopathy M71.9
  specified type NEC M71.8Ø
    ankle M71.87-
    elbow M71.82-
    foot M71.87-
    hand M71.84-
    hip M71.85-
    knee M71.86-
    multiple sites M71.89
    shoulder M71.81-
    specified site NEC M71.88
    wrist M71.83-
Burst stitches or sutures (complication of surgery) T81.31
  external operation wound T81.31
  internal operation wound T81.32
Buruli ulcer A31.1
Bury's disease L95.1
Buschke's
  disease B45.3
  scleredema — *see* Sclerosis, systemic
Busse-Buschke disease B45.3
Buttock — *see* condition
Button
  Biskra B55.1
  Delhi B55.1
  oriental B55.1
Buttonhole deformity (finger) — *see* Deformity, finger, boutonniere
Bwamba fever A92.8
Byssinosis J66.Ø
Bywaters' syndrome T79.5

C

Cachexia R64
  cancerous R64
  cardiac — *see* Disease, heart
  dehydration E86.Ø

Cachexia— *continued*
  dehydration— *continued*
    with
      hypernatremia E87.Ø
      hyponatremia E87.1
  due to malnutrition R64
  exophthalmic — *see* Hyperthyroidism
  heart — *see* Disease, heart
  hypophyseal E23.Ø
  hypopituitary E23.Ø
  lead — *see* Poisoning, lead
  malignant R64
  marsh — *see* Malaria
  nervous F48.8
  old age R54
  paludal — *see* Malaria
  pituitary E23.Ø
  renal N28.9
  saturnine — *see* Poisoning, lead
  senile R54
  Simmonds' E23.Ø
  splenica D73.Ø
  strumipriva EØ3.4
  tuberculous NEC — *see* Tuberculosis
Café, au lait spots L81.3
Caffey's syndrome Q78.8
Caisson disease T7Ø.3
Cake kidney Q63.1
Caked breast (puerperal, postpartum) O92.79
Calabar swelling B74.3
Calcaneal spur — *see* Spur, bone, calcaneal
Calcaneo-apophysitis M92.8
Calcareous — *see* condition
Calcicosis J62.8
Calciferol (vitamin D) **deficiency** E55.9
  with rickets E55.Ø
Calcification
  adrenal (capsule) (gland) E27.1
    tuberculous B9Ø.8 [E35]
  aorta I7Ø.Ø
  artery (annular) — *see* Arteriosclerosis
  auricle (ear) — *see* Disorder, pinna, specified type NEC
  basal ganglia G23.8
  bladder N32.89
    due to Schistosoma hematobium B65.Ø
  brain (cortex) — *see* Calcification, cerebral
  bronchus J98.Ø9
  bursa M71.4Ø
    ankle M71.47-
    elbow M71.42-
    foot M71.47-
    hand M71.44-
    hip M71.45-
    knee M71.46-
    multiple sites M71.49
    shoulder M75.3-
    specified site NEC M71.48
    wrist M71.43-
  cardiac — *see* Degeneration, myocardial
  cerebral (cortex) G93.89
    artery I67.2
  cervix (uteri) N88.8
  choroid plexus G93.89
  conjunctiva — *see* Concretion, conjunctiva
  corpora cavernosa (penis) N48.89
  cortex (brain) — *see* Calcification, cerebral
  dental pulp (nodular) KØ4.2
  dentinal papilla KØØ.4
  fallopian tube N83.8
  falx cerebri G96.19
  gallbladder K82.8
  general E83.59
  heart (*see also* Degeneration, myocardial)
    valve — *see* Endocarditis
  intervertebral cartilage or disc (postinfective) — *see* Disorder, disc, specified NEC
  intracranial — *see* Calcification, cerebral
  joint — *see* Disorder, joint, specified type NEC
  kidney N28.89
    tuberculous B9Ø.1 [N29]
  larynx (senile) J38.7
  lens — *see* Cataract, specified NEC

Calcification— *continued*
  lung (active) (postinfectional) J98.4
    tuberculous B90.9
  lymph gland or node (postinfectional) I89.8
    tuberculous (*see also* Tuberculosis, lymph gland)
      B90.8
  mammographic R92.1
  massive (paraplegic) — *see* Myositis, ossificans, in,
    quadriplegia
  medial — *see* Arteriosclerosis, extremities
  meninges (cerebral) (spinal) G96.19
  metastatic E83.59
  Mönckeberg's — *see* Arteriosclerosis, extremities
  muscle M61.9
    due to burns — *see* Myositis, ossificans, in, burns
    paralytic — *see* Myositis, ossificans, in,
      quadriplegia
    specified type NEC M61.40
      ankle M61.47-
      foot M61.47-
      forearm M61.43-
      hand M61.44-
      lower leg M61.46-
      multiple sites M61.49
      pelvic region M61.45-
      shoulder region M61.41-
      specified site NEC M61.48
      thigh M61.45-
      upper arm M61.42-
  myocardium, myocardial — *see* Degeneration,
    myocardial
  ovary N83.8
  pancreas K86.8
  penis N48.89
  periarticular — *see* Disorder, joint, specified type
    NEC
  pericardium (*see also* Pericarditis) I31.1
  pineal gland E34.8
  pleura J94.8
    postinfectional J94.8
    tuberculous NEC B90.9
  pulpal (dental) (nodular) K04.2
  sclera H15.89
  spleen D73.89
  subcutaneous L94.2
  suprarenal (capsule) (gland) E27.49
  tendon (sheath) (*see also* Tenosynovitis, specified
    type NEC)
    with bursitis, synovitis or tenosynovitis—*see*
      Tendinitis, calcific
  uterus N85.8
  trachea J39.8
  ureter N28.89
  uterus N85.8
  vitreous — *see* Deposit, crystalline
Calcified — *see* Calcification
Calcinosis (interstitial) (tumoral) (universalis) E83.59
  with Raynaud's phenomenon, esophageal
    dysfunction, sclerodactyly, telangiectasia
    (CREST syndrome) M34.1
  circumscripta (skin) L94.2
  cutis L94.2
Calciphylaxis (*see also* Calcification, by site) E83.59
Calcium
  deposits — *see* Calcification, by site
  metabolism disorder E83.50
  salts or soaps in vitreous — *see* Deposit, crystalline
Calciuria R82.99
Calculi — *see* Calculus
Calculosis, intrahepatic — *see* Calculus, bile duct
Calculus, calculi, calculous
  ampulla of Vater — *see* Calculus, bile duct
  anuria (impacted) (recurrent) N20.0
  appendix K38.1
  bile duct (common) (hepatic) K80.50
    with
      calculus of gallbladder — *see* Calculus,
        gallbladder and bile duct
      cholangitis K80.30
        with
          cholecystitis — *see* Calculus, bile duct,
            with cholecystitis
          obstruction K80.31

Calculus, calculi, calculous— *continued*
  bile duct (common) (hepatic)— *continued*
    with— *continued*
      cholangitis— *continued*
        acute K80.32
          with
            chronic cholangitis K80.36
              with obstruction K80.37
            obstruction K80.33
        chronic K80.34
          with
            acute cholangitis K80.36
              with obstruction K80.37
            obstruction K80.35
      cholecystitis (with cholangitis) K80.40
        with obstruction K80.41
        acute K80.42
          with
            chronic cholecystitis K80.46
              with obstruction K80.47
            obstruction K80.43
        chronic K80.44
          with
            acute cholecystitis K80.46
              with obstruction K80.47
            obstruction K80.45
      obstruction K80.51
    biliary (*see also* Calculus, gallbladder)
      specified NEC K80.80
        with obstruction K80.81
    bilirubin, multiple — *see* Calculus, gallbladder
    bladder (encysted) (impacted) (urinary)
      (diverticulum) N21.0
    bronchus J98.09
    calyx (kidney) (renal) — *see* Calculus, kidney
    cholesterol (pure) (solitary) — *see* Calculus,
      gallbladder
    common duct (bile) — *see* Calculus, bile duct
    conjunctiva — *see* Concretion, conjunctiva
    cystic N21.0
      duct — *see* Calculus, gallbladder
    dental (subgingival) (supragingival) K03.6
    diverticulum
      bladder N21.0
      kidney N20.0
    epididymis N50.8
    gallbladder K80.20
      with
        bile duct calculus — *see* Calculus, gallbladder
          and bile duct
        cholecystitis K80.10
          with obstruction K80.11
          acute K80.00
            with
              chronic cholecystitis K80.12
                with obstruction K80.13
              obstruction K80.01
          chronic K80.10
            with
              acute cholecystitis K80.12
                with obstruction K80.13
              obstruction K80.11
        specified NEC K80.18
          with obstruction K80.19
      obstruction K80.21
    gallbladder and bile duct K80.70
      with
        cholecystitis K80.60
          with obstruction K80.61
          acute K80.62
            with
              chronic cholecystitis K80.66
                with obstruction K80.67
              obstruction K80.63
          chronic K80.64
            with
              acute cholecystitis K80.66
                with obstruction K80.67
              obstruction K80.65
        obstruction K80.71
    hepatic (duct) — *see* Calculus, bile duct
    ileal conduit N21.8
    intestinal (impaction) (obstruction) K56.49

Calculus, calculi, calculous— *continued*
  kidney (impacted) (multiple) (pelvis) (recurrent)
    (staghorn) N20.0
    with calculus, ureter N20.2
    congenital Q63.8
  lacrimal passages — *see* Dacryolith
  liver (impacted) — *see* Calculus, bile duct
  lung J98.4
  mammographic R92.1
  nephritic (impacted) (recurrent) — *see* Calculus,
    kidney
  nose J34.89
  pancreas (duct) K86.8
  parotid duct or gland K11.5
  pelvis, encysted — *see* Calculus, kidney
  prostate N42.0
  pulmonary J98.4
  pyelitis (impacted) (recurrent) N20.0
    with hydronephrosis N13.2
  pyelonephritis (impacted) (recurrent) — *see*
    category N20
    with hydronephrosis N13.2
  renal (impacted) (recurrent) — *see* Calculus, kidney
  salivary (duct) (gland) K11.5
  seminal vesicle N50.8
  staghorn — *see* Calculus, kidney
  Stensen's duct K11.5
  stomach K31.89
  sublingual duct or gland K11.5
    congenital Q38.4
  submandibular duct, gland or region K11.5
  submaxillary duct, gland or region K11.5
  suburethral N21.8
  tonsil J35.8
  tooth, teeth (subgingival) (supragingival) K03.6
  tunica vaginalis N50.8
  ureter (impacted) (recurrent) N20.1
    with calculus, kidney N20.2
      with hydronephrosis N13.2
        with infection N13.6
  urethra (impacted) N21.1
  urinary (duct) (impacted) (passage) (tract) N20.9
    with hydronephrosis N13.2
      with infection N13.6
    in (due to)
      lower N21.9
        specified NEC N21.8
  vagina N89.8
  vesical (impacted) N21.0
  Wharton's duct K11.5
  xanthine E79.8 [N22]
Calicectasis N28.89
Caliectasis N28.89
California
  disease B38.9
  encephalitis A83.5
Caligo cornea — *see* Opacity, cornea, central
Callositas, callosity (infected) L84
Callus (infected) L84
  bone — *see* Osteophyte
  excessive, following fracture—code as Sequelae of
    fracture
Calorie deficiency or malnutrition (*see also*
  Malnutrition) E46
Calvé-Perthes disease — *see* Legg-Calvé-Perthes
  disease
Calvé's disease — *see* Osteochondrosis, juvenile, spine
Calvities — *see* Alopecia, androgenic
Cameroon fever — *see* Malaria
Camptocormia (hysterical) F44.4
Camurati-Engelmann syndrome Q78.3
Canal (*see also* condition)
  atrioventricular common Q21.2
Canaliculitis (lacrimal) (acute) (subacute) H04.33-
  Actinomyces A42.89
  chronic H04.42-
Canavan's disease E75.29
Canceled procedure (surgical) Z53.9
  because of
    contraindication Z53.09
      smoking Z53.01
    left against medical advice (AMA) Z53.21
    patient's decision Z53.20

Canceled procedure— *continued*
  because of— *continued*
    patient's decision— *continued*
      for reasons of belief or group pressure Z53.1
      specified reason NEC Z53.29
     specified reason NEC Z53.8
Cancer (*see also* Neoplasm, malignant, by site)
  bile duct type liver C22.1
  blood — *see* Leukemia
  breast C50.91 (*see also* Neoplam, breast, malignant)
  hepatocellular C22.0
  lung C34.90 (*see also* Neoplasm, lung, malignant)
  ovarian C56.9 (*see also* Neoplasm, ovary, malignant)
  unspecified site (primary) C80.1
Cancer(o)phobia F45.29
Cancerous — *see* Neoplasm, malignant, by site
Cancrum oris A69.0
Candidiasis, candidal B37.9
  balanitis B37.42
  bronchitis B37.1
  cheilitis B37.83
  congenital P37.5
  cystitis B37.41
  disseminated B37.7
  endocarditis B37.6
  enteritis B37.82
  esophagitis B37.81
  intertrigo B37.2
  lung B37.1
  meningitis B37.5
  mouth B37.0
  nails B37.2
  neonatal P37.5
  onychia B37.2
  oral B37.0
  osteomyelitis B37.89
  otitis externa B37.84
  paronychia B37.2
  perionyxis B37.2
  pneumonia B37.1
  proctitis B37.82
  pulmonary B37.1
  pyelonephritis B37.49
  sepsis B37.7
  skin B37.2
  specified site NEC B37.89
  stomatitis B37.0
  systemic B37.7
  urethritis B37.41
  urogenital site NEC B37.49
  vagina B37.3
  vulva B37.3
  vulvovaginitis B37.3
Candidid L30.2
Candidosis — *see* Candidiasis
Candiru infection or infestation B88.8
Canities (premature) L67.1
  congenital Q84.2
Canker (mouth) (sore) K12.0
  rash A38.9
Cannabinosis J66.2
Canton fever A75.9
Cantrell's syndrome Q87.89
Capillariasis (intestinal) B81.1
  hepatic B83.8
Capillary — *see* condition
Caplan's syndrome — *see* Rheumatoid, lung
Capsule — *see* condition
Capsulitis (joint) (*see also* Enthesopathy)
  adhesive (shoulder) M75.0-
  hepatic K65.8
  labyrinthine — *see* Otosclerosis, specified NEC
  thyroid E06.9
Caput
  crepitus Q75.8
  medusae I86.8
  succedaneum P12.81
Car sickness T75.3
Carapata (disease) A68.0
Carate — *see* Pinta
Carbon lung J60

Carbuncle L02.93
  abdominal wall L02.231
  anus K61.0
  auditory canal, external — *see* Abscess, ear, external
  auricle ear — *see* Abscess, ear, external
  axilla L02.43-
  back (any part) L02.232
  breast N61
  buttock L02.33
  cheek (external) L02.03
  chest wall L02.233
  chin L02.03
  corpus cavernosum N48.21
  ear (any part) (external) (middle) — *see* Abscess, ear, external
  external auditory canal — *see* Abscess, ear, external
  eyelid — *see* Abscess, eyelid
  face NEC L02.03
  femoral (region) — *see* Carbuncle, lower limb
  finger — *see* Carbuncle, hand
  flank L02.231
  foot L02.63-
  forehead L02.03
  genital — *see* Abscess, genital
  gluteal (region) L02.33
  groin L02.234
  hand L02.53-
  head NEC L02.831
  heel — *see* Carbuncle, foot
  hip — *see* Carbuncle, lower limb
  kidney — *see* Abscess, kidney
  knee — *see* Carbuncle, lower limb
  labium (majus) (minus) N76.4
  lacrimal
    gland — *see* Dacryoadenitis
    passages (duct) (sac) — *see* Inflammation, lacrimal, passages, acute
  leg — *see* Carbuncle, lower limb
  lower limb L02.43-
  malignant A22.0
  multiple sites L02.93
  navel L02.236
  neck L02.13
  nose (external) (septum) J34.0
  orbit, orbital — *see* Abscess, orbit
  palmar (space) — *see* Carbuncle, hand
  partes posteriores L02.33
  pectoral region L02.233
  penis N48.21
  perineum L02.235
  pinna — *see* Abscess, ear, external
  popliteal — *see* Carbuncle, lower limb
  scalp L02.831
  seminal vesicle N49.0
  shoulder — *see* Carbuncle, upper limb
  specified site NEC L02.838
  temple (region) L02.03
  thumb — *see* Carbuncle, hand
  toe — *see* Carbuncle, foot
  trunk L02.239
    abdominal wall L02.231
    back L02.232
    chest wall L02.233
    groin L02.234
    perineum L02.235
    umbilicus L02.236
  umbilicus L02.236
  upper limb L02.43-
  urethra N34.0
  vulva N76.4
Carbunculus — *see* Carbuncle
Carcinoid (tumor) — *see* Tumor, carcinoid
Carcinoidosis E34.0
Carcinoma (malignant) (*see also* Neoplasm, malignant, by site)
  acidophil
    specified site — *see* Neoplasm, malignant, by site
    unspecified site C75.1
  acidophil-basophil, mixed
    specified site — *see* Neoplasm, malignant, by site
    unspecified site C75.1
  adnexal (skin) — *see* Neoplasm, skin, malignant
  adrenal cortical C74.0-

Carcinoma— *continued*
  alveolar — *see* Neoplasm, lung, malignant
    cell — *see* Neoplasm, lung, malignant
  ameloblastic C41.1
    upper jaw (bone) C41.0
  apocrine
    breast — *see* Neoplasm, breast, malignant
    specified site NEC — *see* Neoplasm, skin, malignant
    unspecified site C44.9
  basal cell (pigmented) (*see also* Neoplasm, skin, malignant)
    fibro-epithelial — *see* Neoplasm, skin, malignant
    morphea — *see* Neoplasm, skin, malignant
    multicentric — *see* Neoplasm, skin, malignant
  basaloid
  basal-squamous cell, mixed — *see* Neoplasm, skin, malignant
  basophil
    specified site — *see* Neoplasm, malignant, by site
    unspecified site C75.1
  basophil-acidophil, mixed
    specified site — *see* Neoplasm, malignant, by site
    unspecified site C75.1
  basosquamous — *see* Neoplasm, skin, malignant
  bile duct
    with hepatocellular, mixed C22.0
    liver C22.1
    specified site NEC — *see* Neoplasm, malignant, by site
    unspecified site C22.1
  branchial or branchiogenic C10.4
  bronchial or bronchogenic — *see* Neoplasm, lung, malignant
  bronchiolar — *see* Neoplasm, lung, malignant
  bronchioloalveolar — *see* Neoplasm, lung, malignant
  C cell
    specified site — *see* Neoplasm, malignant, by site
    unspecified site C73
  ceruminous C44.2-
  cervix uteri
    in situ D06.9
      endocervix D06.0
      exocervix D06.1
      specified site NEC D06.7
  chorionic
    specified site — *see* Neoplasm, malignant, by site
    unspecified site
      female C58
      male C62.90
  chromophobe
    specified site — *see* Neoplasm, malignant, by site
    unspecified site C75.1
  cloacogenic
    specified site — *see* Neoplasm, malignant, by site
    unspecified site C21.2
  diffuse type
    specified site — *see* Neoplasm, malignant, by site
    unspecified site C16.9
  duct (cell)
    with Paget's disease — *see* Neoplasm, breast, malignant
    infiltrating
      with lobular carcinoma (in situ)
        specified site — *see* Neoplasm, malignant, by site
        unspecified site (female) C50.91-
          male C50.92-
      specified site — *see* Neoplasm, malignant, by site
      unspecified site (female) C50.91-
        male C50.92-
  ductal
    with lobular
      specified site — *see* Neoplasm, malignant, by site
      unspecified site (female) C50.91-
        male C50.92-
  ductular, infiltrating
    specified site — *see* Neoplasm, malignant, by site
    unspecified site (female) C50.91-
      male C50.92-

Carcinoma— *continued*
  embryonal
    liver C22.7
  endometrioid
    specified site — *see* Neoplasm, malignant, by site
    unspecified site
      female C56.9
      male C61
  eosinophil
    specified site — *see* Neoplasm, malignant, by site
    unspecified site C75.1
  epidermoid (*see also* Carcinoma, squamous cell)
    in situ, Bowen's type — *see* Neoplasm, skin, in situ
  fibroepithelial, basal cell — *see* Neoplasm, skin,
      malignant
  follicular
    with papillary (mixed) C73
    moderately differentiated C73
    pure follicle C73
    specified site — *see* Neoplasm, malignant, by site
    trabecular C73
    unspecified site C73
    well differentiated C73
  generalized, with unspecified primary site C80.0
  glycogen-rich — *see* Neoplasm, breast, malignant
  granulosa cell C56.-
  hepatic cell C22.0
  hepatocellular C22.0
    with bile duct, mixed C22.0
    fibrolamellar C22.0
  hepatocholangiolitic C22.0
  Hurthle cell C73
  in
    adenomatous
      polyposis coli C18.9
    pleomorphic adenoma — *see* Neoplasm, salivary
        glands, malignant
    situ — *see* Carcinoma-in-situ
  infiltrating
    duct
      with lobular
        specified site — *see* Neoplasm, malignant,
            by site
        unspecified site (female) C50.91-
          male C50.92-
      with Paget's disease — *see* Neoplasm, breast,
          malignant
      specified site — *see* Neoplasm, malignant
      unspecified site (female) C50.91-
        male C50.92-
    ductural
      specified site — *see* Neoplasm, malignant
      unspecified site (female) C50.91-
        male C50.92-
    lobular
      unspecified site (female) C50.91-
        male C50.92-
  inflammatory
    specified site — *see* Neoplasm, malignant
    unspecified site (female) C50.91-
      male C50.92-
  intestinal type
    specified site — *see* Neoplasm, malignant, by site
    unspecified site C16.9
  intracystic
    noninfiltrating — *see* Neoplasm, in situ, by site
  intraductal (noninfiltrating)
    with Paget's disease — *see* Neoplasm, breast,
        malignant
    breast D05.8-
    papillary
      with invasion
        specified site — *see* Neoplasm, malignant,
            by site
        unspecified site (female) C50.91-
          male C50.92-
      breast D05.1-
      specified site NEC — *see* Neoplasm, in situ, by
          site
      unspecified site (female) D05.1-
    specified site NEC — *see* Neoplasm, in situ, by site
    unspecified site (female) D05.1-

Carcinoma— *continued*
  intraepidermal — *see* Neoplasm, in situ
    squamous cell, Bowen's type — *see* Neoplasm,
        skin, in situ
  intraepithelial — *see* Neoplasm, in situ, by site
    squamous cell — *see* Neoplasm, in situ, by site
  intraosseous C41.1
    upper jaw (bone) C41.0
  islet cell
    with exocrine, mixed
      specified site — *see* Neoplasm, malignant, by
          site
      unspecified site C25.9
    pancreas C25.4
    specified site NEC — *see* Neoplasm, malignant,
        by site
    unspecified site C25.4
  juvenile, breast — *see* Neoplasm, breast, malignant
  large cell
    small cell
      specified site — *see* Neoplasm, malignant, by
          site
      unspecified site C34.90
  Leydig cell (testis)
    specified site — *see* Neoplasm, malignant, by site
    unspecified site
      female C56.9
      male C62.90
  lipid-rich (female) C50.91-
    male C50.92-
  liver cell C22.0
  liver NEC C22.7
  lobular (infiltrating)
    with intraductal
      specified site — *see* Neoplasm, malignant, by
          site
      unspecified site (female) C50.91-
        male C50.92-
    noninfiltrating
      breast D05.0-
      specified site NEC — *see* Neoplasm, in situ, by
          site
      unspecified site D05.0-
    specified site — *see* Neoplasm, malignant, by site
    unspecified site (female) C50.91-
      male C50.92-
  medullary
    with
      amyloid stroma
        specified site — *see* Neoplasm, malignant,
            by site
        unspecified site C73
      lymphoid stroma
        specified site — *see* Neoplasm, malignant,
            by site
        unspecified site (female) C50.91-
          male C50.92-
  Merkel cell C4a.9
    anal margin C4a.51
    anal skin C4a.51
    canthus C4a.1-
    ear and external auricular canal C4a.2-
    external auricular canal C4a.2-
    eyelid, including canthus C4a.1-
    face C4a.30
    hip C4a.7-
    lip C4a.0
    lower limb, including hip C4a.7-
    neck C4a.4
    nodal presentation C7b.1
    nose C4a.31
      specified NEC C4a.39
    overlapping sites C4a.8
    perianal skin C4a.51
    scalp C4a.4
    secondary C7b.1
    shoulder C4a.6-
    skin of breast C4a.52
    trunk NEC C4a.59
    upper limb, including shoulder C4a.6-
    visceral metastatic C7b.1
  metastatic — *see* Neoplasm, secondary, by site

Carcinoma— *continued*
  metatypical — *see* Neoplasm, skin, malignant
  morphea, basal cell — *see* Neoplasm, skin,
      malignant
  mucoid
    cell
      specified site — *see* Neoplasm, malignant, by
          site
      unspecified site C75.1
  neuroendocrine (*see also* Tumor, neuroendocrine)
    high grade, any site C7a.1
    poorly differentiated, any site C7a.1
  nonencapsulated sclerosing C73
  noninfiltrating
    intracystic — *see* Neoplasm, in situ, by site
    intraductal
      breast D05.1-
      papillary
        breast D05.1-
        specified site NEC — *see* Neoplasm, in situ,
            by site
        unspecified site D05.1-
      specified site — *see* Neoplasm, in situ, by site
      unspecified site D05.1-
    lobular
      breast D05.0-
      specified site NEC — *see* Neoplasm, in situ, by
          site
      unspecified site (female) D05.0-
  oat cell
    specified site — *see* Neoplasm, malignant, by site
    unspecified site C34.90
  odontogenic C41.1
    upper jaw (bone) C41.0
  papillary
    with follicular (mixed) C73
    follicular variant C73
    intraductal (noninfiltrating)
      with invasion
        specified site — *see* Neoplasm, malignant,
            by site
        unspecified site (female) C50.91-
          male C50.92-
      breast D05.1-
      specified site NEC — *see* Neoplasm, in situ, by
          site
      unspecified site D05.1-
    serous
      specified site — *see* Neoplasm, malignant, by
          site
      surface
        specified site — *see* Neoplasm, malignant,
            by site
        unspecified site C56.9
      unspecified site C56.9
  papillocystic
    specified site — *see* Neoplasm, malignant, by site
    unspecified site C56.9
  parafollicular cell
    specified site — *see* Neoplasm, malignant, by site
    unspecified site C73
  pilomatrix — *see* Neoplasm, skin, malignant
  pseudomucinous
    specified site — *see* Neoplasm, malignant, by site
    unspecified site C56.9
  renal cell C64.-
  Schmincke — *see* Neoplasm, nasopharynx,
      malignant
  Schneiderian
    specified site — *see* Neoplasm, malignant, by site
    unspecified site C30.0
  sebaceous — *see* Neoplasm, skin, malignant
  secondary (*see also* Neoplasm, secondary, by site)
    Merkel cell C7b.1
    specified site NEC — *see* Neoplasm, in situ
  secretory, breast — *see* Neoplasm, breast, malignant
  serous
    papillary
      specified site — *see* Neoplasm, malignant, by
          site
      unspecified site C56.9

Carcinoma— *continued*
  serous— *continued*
    surface, papillary
      specified site — *see* Neoplasm, malignant, by site
      unspecified site C56.9
    Sertoli cell
      specified site — *see* Neoplasm, malignant, by site
      unspecified site C62.90
        female C56.9
        male C62.90
    skin appendage — *see* Neoplasm, skin, malignant
    small cell
      fusiform cell
        specified site — *see* Neoplasm, malignant, by site
        unspecified site C34.90
      intermediate cell
        specified site — *see* Neoplasm, malignant, by site
        unspecified site C34.90
      large cell
        specified site — *see* Neoplasm, malignant, by site
        unspecified site C34.90
    solid
      with amyloid stroma
        specified site — *see* Neoplasm, malignant, by site
        unspecified site C73
      microinvasive
        specified site — *see* Neoplasm, malignant, by site
        unspecified site C53.9
    sweat gland — *see* Neoplasm, skin, malignant
    theca cell C56.-
    thymic C37
    unspecified site (primary) C80.1
Carcinoma-in-situ (*see also* Neoplasm, in situ, by site)
  breast NOS D05.9-
    specified type NEC D05.8-
  epidermoid (*see also* Neoplasm, in situ, by site)
    with questionable stromal invasion
      cervix D06.9
      specified site NEC — *see* Neoplasm, in situ, by site
      unspecified site D06.9
    Bowen's type — *see* Neoplasm, skin, in situ, by site
  intraductal
    breast D05.1-
    specified site NEC — *see* Neoplasm, in situ, by site
    unspecified site D05.1-
  lobular
    with
      infiltrating duct
        breast (female) C50.91-
          male C50.92-
        specified site NEC — *see* Neoplasm, malignant
        unspecified site (female) C50.91-
          male C50.92-
      intraductal
        breast D05.8-
        specified site NEC — *see* Neoplasm, in situ, by site
        unspecified site (female) D05.8-
    breast D05.0-
    specified site NEC — *see* Neoplasm, in situ, by site
    unspecified site D05.0-
  squamous cell (*see also* Neoplasm, in situ, by site)
    with questionable stromal invasion
      cervix D06.9
      specified site NEC — *see* Neoplasm, in situ, by site
      unspecified site D06.9
Carcinomaphobia F45.29
Carcinomatosis C80.0
  peritonei C78.6
  unspecified site (primary) (secondary) C80.0
Carcinosarcoma — *see* Neoplasm, malignant, by site
  embryonal — *see* Neoplasm, malignant, by site
Cardia, cardial — *see* condition

Cardiac (*see also* condition)
  death, sudden — *see* Arrest, cardiac
  pacemaker
    in situ Z95.0
    management or adjustment Z45.018
  tamponade I31.4
Cardialgia — *see* Pain, precordial
Cardiectasis — *see* Hypertrophy, cardiac
Cardiochalasia K21.9
Cardiomalacia I51.5
Cardiomegalia glycogenica diffusa E74.02 [I43]
Cardiomegaly (*see also* Hypertrophy, cardiac)
  congenital Q24.8
  glycogen E74.02 [I43]
  idiopathic I51.7
Cardiomyoliposis I51.5
Cardiomyopathy (familial) (idiopathic) I42.9
  alcoholic I42.6
  amyloid E85.4 [I43]
  arteriosclerotic — *see* Disease, heart, ischemic, atherosclerotic
  beriberi E51.12
  cobalt-beer I42.6
  congenital I42.4
  congestive I42.0
  constrictive NOS I42.5
  dilated I42.0
  due to
    alcohol I42.6
    beriberi E51.12
    cardiac glycogenosis E74.02 [I43]
    drugs I42.7
    Friedreich's ataxia G11.1
    external agents NEC I42.7
    myotonia atrophica G71.19 [I43]
    progressive muscular dystrophy G71.0
  glycogen storage E74.02 [I43]
  hypertensive — *see* Hypertension, heart
  hypertrophic (nonobstructive) I42.2
    obstructive I42.1
      congenital Q24.8
  in
    Chagas' disease (chronic) B57.2
      acute B57.0
    sarcoidosis D86.85
  ischemic I25.5
  metabolic E88.9 [I43]
    thyrotoxic E05.90 [I43]
      with thyroid storm E05.91 [I43]
  newborn I42.8
    congenital I42.4
  nutritional E63.9 [I43]
    beriberi E51.12
  obscure of Africa I42.8
  peripartum O90.3
  postpartum O90.3
  restrictive NEC I42.5
  rheumatic I09.0
  secondary I42.9
  stress induced I51.81
  takotsubo I51.81
  thyrotoxic E05.90 [I43]
    with thyroid storm E05.91 [I43]
  toxic NEC I42.7
  tuberculous A18.84
  viral B33.24
Cardionephritis — *see* Hypertension, cardiorenal
Cardionephropathy — *see* Hypertension, cardiorenal
Cardionephrosis — *see* Hypertension, cardiorenal
Cardiopathia nigra I27.0
Cardiopathy (*see also* Disease, heart) I51.9
  idiopathic I42.9
  mucopolysaccharidosis E76.3 [I52]
Cardiopericarditis — *see* Pericarditis
Cardiophobia F45.29
Cardiorenal — *see* condition
Cardiorrhexis — *see* Infarct, myocardium
Cardiosclerosis — *see* Disease, heart, ischemic, atherosclerotic
Cardiosis — *see* Disease, heart
Cardiospasm (esophagus) (reflex) (stomach) K22.0
  congenital Q39.5
    with megaesophagus Q39.5

Cardiostenosis — *see* Disease, heart
Cardiosymphysis I31.0
Cardiovascular — *see* condition
Carditis (acute) (bacterial) (chronic) (subacute) I51.89
  meningococcal A39.50
  rheumatic — *see* Disease, heart, rheumatic
  rheumatoid — *see* Rheumatoid, carditis
  viral B33.20
Care (of) (for) (following)
  child (routine) Z76.2
  family member (handicapped) (sick)
    creating problem for family Z63.6
    provided away from home for holiday relief Z75.5
    unavailable, due to
      absence (person rendering care) (sufferer) Z74.2
      inability (any reason) of person rendering care Z74.2
  foundling Z76.1
  holiday relief Z75.5
  improper — *see* Maltreatment
  lack of (at or after birth) (infant) — *see* Maltreatment, child, neglect
  lactating mother Z39.1
  palliative Z51.5
  postpartum
    immediately after delivery Z39.0
    routine follow-up Z39.2
  respite Z75.5
  unavailable, due to
    absence of person rendering care Z74.2
    inability (any reason) of person rendering care Z74.2
  well-baby Z76.2
Caries
  bone NEC A18.03
  dental K02.9
    arrested (coronal) (root) K02.3
    chewing surface
      limited to enamel K02.51
      penetrating into dentin K02.52
      penetrating into pulp K02.53
    coronal surface
      chewing surface
        limited to enamel K02.51
        penetrating into dentin K02.52
        penetrating into pulp K02.53
      pit and fissure surface
        limited to enamel K02.51
        penetrating into dentin K02.52
        penetrating into pulp K02.53
      smooth surface
        limited to enamel K02.61
        penetrating into dentin K02.62
        penetrating into pulp K02.63
    pit and fissure surface
      limited to enamel K02.51
      penetrating into dentin K02.52
      penetrating into pulp K02.53
    smooth surface
      limited to enamel K02.61
      penetrating into dentin K02.62
      penetrating into pulp K02.63
    root K02.7
  external meatus — *see* Disorder, ear, external, specified type NEC
  hip (tuberculous) A18.02
  initial (tooth)
    chewing surface K02.51
    pit and fissure surface K02.51
    smooth surface K02.61
  knee (tuberculous) A18.02
  labyrinth — *see* subcategory H83.8
  limb NEC (tuberculous) A18.03
  mastoid process (chronic) — *see* Mastoiditis, chronic
    tuberculous A18.03
  middle ear — *see* subcategory H74.8
  nose (tuberculous) A18.03
  orbit (tuberculous) A18.03
  ossicles, ear — *see* Abnormal, ear ossicles
  petrous bone — *see* Petrositis
  root (dental) (tooth) K02.7
  sacrum (tuberculous) A18.01

Caries— *continued*
  spine, spinal (column) (tuberculous) A18.01
  syphilitic A52.77
    congenital (early) A50.02 [M90.80]
  tooth, teeth — *see* Caries, dental
  tuberculous A18.03
  vertebra (column) (tuberculous) A18.01
Carious teeth — *see* Caries, dental
Carneous mole O02.0
Carnitine insufficiency E71.40
Carotid body or sinus syndrome G90.01
Carotidynia G90.01
Carotinemia (dietary) E67.1
Carotinosis (cutis) (skin) E67.1
Carpal tunnel syndrome — *see* Syndrome, carpal tunnel
Carpenter's syndrome Q87.0
Carpopedal spasm — *see* Tetany
Carr-Barr-Plunkett syndrome Q97.1
Carrier (suspected) of
  amebiasis Z22.1
  bacterial disease NEC Z22.39
    diphtheria Z22.2
    intestinal infectious NEC Z22.1
      typhoid Z22.0
    meningococcal Z22.31
    sexually transmitted Z22.4
    specified NEC Z22.39
    staphylococcal Z22.32
    streptococcal Z22.338
      group B Z22.330
    typhoid Z22.0
  cholera Z22.1
  diphtheria Z22.2
  gastrointestinal pathogens NEC Z22.1
  genetic Z14.8
    cystic fibrosis Z14.1
    hemophilia A (asymptomatic) Z14.01
      symptomatic Z14.02
  gonorrhea Z22.4
  HAA (hepatitis Australian-antigen) Z22.59
  HB(c)(s)-AG Z22.51
  hepatitis (viral) Z22.50
    Australia-antigen (HAA) Z22.59
    B surface antigen (HBsAg) Z22.51
      with acute delta-(super)infection B17.0
    C Z22.52
    specified NEC Z22.59
  human T-cell lymphotropic virus type-1 (HTLV-1)
    infection Z22.6
  infectious organism Z22.9
    specified NEC Z22.8
  meningococci Z22.31
  Salmonella typhosa Z22.0
  serum hepatitis — *see* Carrier, hepatitis
  staphylococci Z22.32
  streptococci Z22.338
    group B Z22.330
  syphilis Z22.4
  typhoid Z22.0
  venereal disease NEC Z22.4
Carrion's disease A44.0
Carter's relapsing fever (Asiatic) A68.1
Cartilage — *see* condition
Caruncle (inflamed)
  conjunctiva (acute) — *see* Conjunctivitis, acute
  labium (majus) (minus) N90.89
  lacrimal — *see* Inflammation, lacrimal, passages
  myrtiform N89.8
  urethral (benign) N36.2
Cascade stomach K31.2
Caseation lymphatic gland (tuberculous) A18.2
Cassidy (-Scholte) **syndrome** (malignant carcinoid)
  E34.0
Castellani's disease A69.8
Castration, traumatic, male S38.231
Casts in urine R82.99
Cat
  cry syndrome Q93.4
  ear Q17.3
  eye syndrome Q92.8
Catabolism, senile R54
Catalepsy (hysterical) F44.2
  schizophrenic F20.2

Cataplexy (idiopathic)—*see* Narcolepsy
Cataract (cortical) (immature) (incipient) H26.9
  with
    neovascularization — *see* Cataract, complicated
  age-related — *see* Cataract, senile
  anterior
    and posterior axial embryonal Q12.0
    pyramidal Q12.0
  associated with
    galactosemia E74.21 [H28]
    myotonic disorders G71.19 [H28]
  blue Q12.0
  central Q12.0
  cerulean Q12.0
  complicated H26.20
    with
      neovascularization H26.21-
      ocular disorder H26.22-
      glaucomatous flecks H26.23-
  congenital Q12.0
  coraliform Q12.0
  coronary Q12.0
  crystalline Q12.0
  diabetic — *see* Diabetes, cataract
  drug-induced H26.3-
  due to
    ocular disorder — *see* Cataract, complicated
    radiation H26.8
  electric H26.8
  extraction status Z98.4-
  glass-blower's H26.8
  heat ray H26.8
  heterochromic — *see* Cataract, complicated
  hypermature — *see* Cataract, senile, morgagnian
    type
  in (due to)
    chronic iridocyclitis — *see* Cataract, complicated
    diabetes — *see* Diabetes, cataract
    endocrine disease E34.9 [H28]
    eye disease — *see* Cataract, complicated
    hypoparathyroidism E20.9 [H28]
    malnutrition-dehydration E46 [H28]
    metabolic disease E88.9 [H28]
    myotonic disorders G71.19 [H28]
    nutritional disease E63.9 [H28]
  infantile — *see* Cataract, presenile
  irradiational — *see* Cataract, specified NEC
  juvenile — *see* Cataract, presenile
  malnutrition-dehydration E46 [H28]
  morgagnian — *see* Cataract, senile, morgagnian
    type
  myotonic G71.19 [H28]
  myxedema E03.9 [H28]
  nuclear
    embryonal Q12.0
    sclerosis — *see* Cataract, senile, nuclear
  presenile H26.00-
    combined forms H26.06-
    cortical H26.01-
    lamellar — *see* Cataract, presenile, cortical
    nuclear H26.03-
    specified NEC H26.09
    subcapsular polar (anterior) H26.04-
      posterior H26.05-
    zonular — *see* Cataract, presenile, cortical
  secondary H26.40
    Soemmering's ring H26.41-
    specified NEC H26.49-
    to eye disease — *see* Cataract, complicated
  senile H25.9
    brunescens — *see* Cataract, senile, nuclear
    combined forms H25.81-
    coronary — *see* Cataract, senile, incipient
    cortical H25.01-
    hypermature — *see* Cataract, senile, morgagnian
      type
    incipient (mature) (total) H25.09-
      cortical — *see* Cataract, senile, cortical
      subcapsular — *see* Cataract, senile,
        subcapsular
    morgagnian type (hypermature) H25.2-
    nuclear (sclerosis) H25.1-

Cataract— *continued*
  senile— *continued*
    polar subcapsular (anterior) (posterior) — *see*
      Cataract, senile, incipient
    punctate — *see* Cataract, senile, incipient
    specified NEC H25.89
    subcapsular polar (anterior) H25.03-
      posterior H25.04-
  snowflake — *see* Diabetes, cataract
  specified NEC H26.8
  toxic — *see* Cataract, drug-induced
  traumatic H26.10-
    localized H26.11-
    partially resolved H26.12-
    total H26.13-
  zonular (perinuclear) Q12.0
Cataracta (*see also* Cataract)
  brunescens — *see* Cataract, senile, nuclear
  centralis pulverulenta Q12.0
  cerulea Q12.0
  complicata — *see* Cataract, complicated
  congenita Q12.0
  coralliformis Q12.0
  coronaria Q12.0
  diabetic — *see* Diabetes, cataract
  membranacea
    accreta — *see* Cataract, secondary
    congenita Q12.0
  nigra — *see* Cataract, senile, nuclear
  sunflower — *see* Cataract, complicated
Catarrh, catarrhal (acute) (febrile) (infectious)
  (inflammation) (*see also* condition) J00
  bronchial — *see* Bronchitis
  chest — *see* Bronchitis
  chronic J31.0
  due to congenital syphilis A50.03
  enteric — *see* Enteritis
  eustachian H68.009
  fauces — *see* Pharyngitis
  gastrointestinal — *see* Enteritis
  gingivitis K05.00
    plaque induced K05.00
    nonplaque induced K05.01
  hay — *see* Fever, hay
  intestinal — *see* Enteritis
  larynx, chronic J37.0
  liver B15.9
    with hepatic coma B15.0
  lung — *see* Bronchitis
  middle ear, chronic — *see* Otitis, media,
    nonsuppurative, chronic, serous
  mouth K12.1
  nasal (chronic) — *see* Rhinitis
  nasobronchial J31.1
  nasopharyngeal (chronic) J31.1
    acute J00
  pulmonary — *see* Bronchitis
  spring (eye) (vernal) — *see* Conjunctivitis, acute,
    atopic
  summer (hay) — *see* Fever, hay
  throat J31.2
  tubotympanal (*see also* Otitis, media,
    nonsuppurative)
    chronic — *see* Otitis, media, nonsuppurative,
      chronic, serous
Catatonia (schizophrenic) F20.2
Catatonic
  disorder due to known physiologic condition F06.1
  schizophrenia F20.2
  stupor R40.1
Cat-scratch (*see also* Abrasion)
  disease or fever A28.1
Cauda equina — *see* condition
Cauliflower ear M95.1-
Causalgia (upper limb) G56.4-
  lower limb G57.7-
Cause
  external, general effects T75.89
Caustic burn — *see* Corrosion, by site
Cavare's disease (familial periodic paralysis) G72.3

Cave-in, injury
  crushing (severe) — *see* Crush
  suffocation — *see* Asphyxia, traumatic, due to low
      oxygen, due to cave-in
Cavernitis (penis) N48.29
Cavernositis N48.29
Cavernous — *see* condition
Cavitation of lung (*see also* Tuberculosis, pulmonary)
  nontuberculous J98.4
Cavities, dental — *see* Caries, dental
Cavity
  lung — *see* Cavitation of lung
  optic papilla Q14.2
  pulmonary — *see* Cavitation of lung
Cavovarus foot, congenital Q66.1
Cavus foot (congenital) Q66.7
  acquired — *see* Deformity, limb, foot, specified NEC
Cazenave's disease L10.2
Cecitis K52.9
  with perforation, peritonitis, or rupture K65.8
Cecum — *see* condition
Celiac
  artery compression syndrome I77.4
  disease K90.0
  infantilism K90.0
Cell(s), cellular (*see also* condition)
  in urine R82.99
Cellulitis (diffuse) (phlegmonous) (septic)
      (suppurative) L03.90
  abdominal wall L03.311
  anaerobic A48.0
  ankle — *see* Cellulitis, lower limb
  anus K61.0
  arm — *see* Cellulitis, upper limb
  auricle (ear) — *see* Cellulitis, ear
  axilla L03.11-
  back (any part) L03.312
  broad ligament
      acute N73.0
  buttock L03.317
  cervical (meaning neck) L03.221
  cervix (uteri) — *see* Cervicitis
  cheek (external) L03.211
      internal K12.2
  chest wall L03.313
  chronic L03.90
  clostridial A48.0
  corpus cavernosum N48.22
  digit
      finger — *see* Cellulitis, finger
      toe — *see* Cellulitis, toe
  Douglas' cul-de-sac or pouch
      acute N73.0
  drainage site (following operation) T81.4
  ear (external) H60.1-
  eosinophilic (granulomatous) L98.3
  erysipelatous — *see* Erysipelas
  external auditory canal — *see* Cellulitis, ear
  eyelid — *see* Abscess, eyelid
  face NEC L03.211
  finger (intrathecal) (periosteal) (subcutaneous)
      (subcuticular) L03.01-
  foot — *see* Cellulitis, lower limb
  gangrenous — *see* Gangrene
  genital organ NEC
      female (external) N76.4
      male N49.9
          multiple sites N49.8
          specified NEC N49.8
  gluteal (region) L03.317
  gonococcal A54.89
  groin L03.314
  hand — *see* Cellulitis, upper limb
  head NEC L03.811
      face (any part, except ear, eye and nose) L03.211
  heel — *see* Cellulitis, lower limb
  hip — *see* Cellulitis, lower limb
  jaw (region) L03.211
  knee — *see* Cellulitis, lower limb
  labium (majus) (minus) — *see* Vulvitis
  lacrimal passages — *see* Inflammation, lacrimal,
      passages

Cellulitis— *continued*
  larynx J38.7
  leg — *see* Cellulitis, lower limb
  lip K13.0
  lower limb L03.11-
      toe — *see* Cellulitis, toe
  mouth (floor) K12.2
  multiple sites, so stated L03.90
  nasopharynx J39.1
  navel L03.316
      newborn P38.9
          with mild hemorrhage P38.1
          without hemorrhage P38.9
  neck (region) L03.221
  nose (septum) (external) J34.0
  orbit, orbital H05.01-
  palate (soft) K12.2
  pectoral (region) L03.313
  pelvis, pelvic (chronic)
      female (*see also* Disease, pelvis, inflammatory)
          N73.2
          acute N73.0
          following ectopic or molar pregnancy O08.0
          male K65.0
  penis N48.22
  perineal, perineum L03.315
  perirectal K61.1
  peritonsillar J36
  periurethral N34.0
  periuterine (*see also* Disease, pelvis, inflammatory)
      N73.2
          acute N73.0
  pharynx J39.1
  rectum K61.1
  retroperitoneal K68.9
  round ligament
      acute N73.0
  scalp (any part) L03.811
  scrotum N49.2
  seminal vesicle N49.0
  shoulder — *see* Cellulitis, upper limb
  specified site NEC L03.818
  submandibular (region) (space) (triangle) K12.2
      gland K11.3
  submaxillary (region) K12.2
      gland K11.3
  thigh — *see* Cellulitis, lower limb
  thumb (intrathecal) (periosteal) (subcutaneous)
      (subcuticular) — *see* Cellulitis, finger
  toe (intrathecal) (periosteal) (subcutaneous)
      (subcuticular) L03.03-
  tonsil J36
  trunk L03.319
      abdominal wall L03.311
      back (any part) L03.312
      buttock L03.317
      chest wall L03.313
      groin L03.314
      perineal, perineum L03.315
      umbilicus L03.316
  tuberculous (primary) A18.4
  umbilicus L03.316
  upper limb L03.11-
      axilla — *see* Cellulitis, axilla
      finger — *see* Cellulitis, finger
      thumb — *see* Cellulitis, finger
  vaccinal T88.0
  vocal cord J38.3
  vulva — *see* Vulvitis
  wrist — *see* Cellulitis, upper limb
Cementoblastoma, benign — *see* Cyst, calcifying
      odontogenic
Cementoma — *see* Cyst, calcifying odontogenic
Cementoperiostitis — *see* Periodontitis
Cementosis K03.4
Central auditory processing disorder H93.25
Central pain syndrome G89.0
Cephalematocele, cephal(o)hematocele
  newborn P52.8
      birth injury P10.8
  traumatic — *see* Hematoma, brain
Cephalematoma, cephalhematoma (calcified)
  newborn (birth injury) P12.0

Cephalematoma, cephalhematoma— *continued*
  traumatic — *see* Hematoma, brain
Cephalgia, cephalalgia (*see also* Headache)
  histamine G44.009
      intractable G44.001
      not intractable G44.009
  trigeminal autonomic (TAC) NEC G44.099
      intractable G44.091
      not intractable G44.099
Cephalic — *see* condition
Cephalitis — *see* Encephalitis
Cephalocele — *see* Encephalocele
Cephalomenia N94.89
Cephalopelvic — *see* condition
Cerclage (with cervical incompetence) **in pregnancy**
      — *see* Incompetence, cervix, in pregnancy
Cerebellitis — *see* Encephalitis
Cerebellum, cerebellar — *see* condition
Cerebral — *see* condition
Cerebritis — *see* Encephalitis
Cerebro-hepato-renal syndrome Q87.89
Cerebromalacia — *see* Softening, brain
  sequelae of cerebrovascular disease I69.398
Cerebroside lipidosis E75.22
Cerebrospasticity (congenital) G80.1
Cerebrospinal — *see* condition
Cerebrum — *see* condition
Ceroid-lipofuscinosis, neuronal E75.4
Cerumen (accumulation) (impacted) H61.2-
Cervical (*see also* condition)
  auricle Q18.2
  dysplasia in pregnancy — *see* Abnormal, cervix, in
      pregnancy or childbirth
  erosion in pregnancy — *see* Abnormal, cervix, in
      pregnancy or childbirth
  fibrosis in pregnancy — *see* Abnormal, cervix, in
      pregnancy or childbirth
  fusion syndrome Q76.1
  rib Q76.5
  shortening (complicating pregnancy) O26.87-
Cervicalgia M54.2
Cervicitis (acute) (chronic) (nonvenereal) (senile
      (atrophic)) (subacute) (with ulceration) N72
  with
      abortion — *see* Abortion, by type complicated by
          genital tract and pelvic infection
      ectopic pregnancy O08.0
      molar pregnancy O08.0
  chlamydial A56.09
  gonococcal A54.03
  herpesviral A60.03
  puerperal (postpartum) O86.11
  syphilitic A52.76
  trichomonal A59.09
  tuberculous A18.16
Cervicocolpitis (emphysematosa) (*see also* Cervicitis) N72
Cervix — *see* condition
Cesarean delivery, previous, affecting
      management of pregnancy O34.21
Céstan(-Chenais) **paralysis or syndrome** G46.3
Céstan-Raymond syndrome I65.8
Cestode infestation B71.9
  specified type NEC B71.8
Cestodiasis B71.9
Chabert's disease A22.9
Chacaleh E53.8
Chafing L30.4
Chagas' (-Mazza) **disease** (chronic) B57.2
  with
      cardiovascular involvement NEC B57.2
      digestive system involvement B57.30
          megacolon B57.32
          megaesophagus B57.31
          other specified B57.39
      megacolon B57.32
      megaesophagus B57.31
      myocarditis B57.2
      nervous system involvement B57.40
          meningitis B57.41
          meningoencephalitis B57.42
          other specified B57.49
      specified organ involvement NEC B57.5
  acute (with) B57.1

Chagas' (-Mazza) disease— *continued*
  acute (with)— *continued*
    cardiovascular NEC B57.0
    myocarditis B57.0
Chagres fever B50.9
Chairridden Z74.09
Chalasia (cardiac sphincter) K21.9
Chalazion H00.19
  left H00.16
    lower H00.15
    upper H00.14
  right H00.13
    lower H00.12
    upper H00.11
Chalcosis (*see also* Disorder, globe, degenerative, chalcosis)
  cornea — *see* Deposit, cornea
  crystalline lens — *see* Cataract, complicated
  retina H35.89
Chalicosis (pulmonum) J62.8
Chancre (any genital site) (hard) (hunterian) (mixed) (primary) (seronegative) (seropositive) (syphilitic) A51.0
  congenital A50.07
  conjunctiva NEC A51.2
  Ducrey's A57
  extragenital A51.2
  eyelid A51.2
  lip A51.2
  nipple A51.2
  Nisbet's A57
  of
    carate A67.0
    pinta A67.0
    yaws A66.0
  palate, soft A51.2
  phagedenic A57
  simple A57
  soft A57
    bubo A57
    palate A51.2
  urethra A51.0
  yaws A66.0
Chancroid (anus) (genital) (penis) (perineum) (rectum) (urethra) (vulva) A57
Chandler's disease (osteochondritis dissecans, hip) — *see* Osteochondritis, dissecans, hip
Change(s) (in) (of) (*see also* Removal)
  arteriosclerotic — *see* Arteriosclerosis
  bone (*see also* Disorder, bone)
    diabetic — *see* Diabetes, bone change
  bowel habit R19.4
  cardiorenal (vascular) — *see* Hypertension, cardiorenal
  cardiovascular — *see* Disease, cardiovascular
  circulatory I99.9
  cognitive (mild) (organic) R41.89
  color, tooth, teeth
    during formation K00.8
    posteruptive K03.7
  contraceptive device Z30.433
  corneal membrane H18.30
    Bowman's membrane fold or rupture H18.31-
    Descemet's membrane
      fold H18.32-
      rupture H18.33-
  coronary — *see* Disease, heart, ischemic
  degenerative, spine or vertebra — *see* Spondylosis
  dental pulp, regressive K04.2
  dressing (nonsurgical) Z48.00
    surgical Z48.01
  heart — *see* Disease, heart
  hip joint — *see* Derangement, joint, hip
  hyperplastic larynx J38.7
  hypertrophic
    nasal sinus J34.89
    turbinate, nasal J34.3
    upper respiratory tract J39.8
  indwelling catheter Z46.6
  inflammatory (*see also* Inflammation)
    sacroiliac M46.1
  job, anxiety concerning Z56.1
  joint — *see* Derangement, joint

Change(s)— *continued*
  life — *see* Menopause
  mental status R41.82
  minimal (glomerular) (*see also* N00-N07 with fourth character .0) N05.0
  myocardium, myocardial — *see* Degeneration, myocardial
  of life — *see* Menopause
  pacemaker Z45.018
    pulse generator Z45.010
  personality (enduring) F68.8
    due to (secondary to)
      general medical condition F07.0
    secondary (nonspecific) F60.89
  regressive, dental pulp K04.2
  renal — *see* Disease, renal
  retina H35.9
    myopic — *see* Disorder, globe, degenerative, myopia
  sacroiliac joint M53.3
  senile (*see also* condition) R54
  sensory R20.8
  skin R23.9
    acute, due to ultraviolet radiation L56.9
      specified NEC L56.8
    chronic, due to nonionizing radiation L57.9
      specified NEC L57.8
    cyanosis R23.0
    flushing R23.2
    pallor R23.1
    petechiae R23.3
    specified change NEC R23.8
    swelling — *see* Mass, localized
    texture R23.4
  trophic
    arm — *see* Mononeuropathy, upper limb
    leg — *see* Mononeuropathy, lower limb
  vascular I99.9
  vasomotor I73.9
  voice R49.9
    psychogenic F44.4
    specified NEC R49.8
Changing sleep-work schedule, affecting sleep G47.26
Changuinola fever A93.1
Chapping skin T69.8
Charcot-Marie-Tooth disease, paralysis or syndrome G60.0
Charcot's
  arthropathy — *see* Arthropathy, neuropathic
  cirrhosis K74.3
  disease (tabetic arthropathy) A52.16
  joint (disease) (tabetic) A52.16
    diabetic — *see* Diabetes, with, arthropathy
    syringomyelic G95.0
  syndrome (intermittent claudication) I73.9
CHARGE association Q89.8
Charley-horse (quadriceps) M62.831
  traumatic (quadriceps) S76.11-
Charlouis' disease — *see* Yaws
Cheadle's disease E54
Checking (of)
  cardiac pacemaker (battery) (electrode(s)) Z45.018
    pulse generator Z45.010
  intrauterine contraceptive device Z30.431
Check-up — *see* Examination
Chédiak-Higashi (-Steinbrinck) **syndrome** (congenital gigantism of peroxidase granules) E70.330
Cheek — *see* condition
Cheese itch B88.0
Cheese-washer's lung J67.8
Cheese-worker's lung J67.8
Cheilitis (acute) (angular) (catarrhal) (chronic) (exfoliative) (gangrenous) (glandular) (infectional) (suppurative) (ulcerative) (vesicular) K13.0
  actinic (due to sun) L56.8
    other than from sun L59.8
  candidal B37.83
Cheilodynia K13.0
Cheiloschisis — *see* Cleft, lip

Cheilosis (angular) K13.0
  with pellagra E52
  due to
    vitamin B2 (riboflavin) deficiency E53.0
Cheiromegaly M79.89
Cheiropompholyx L30.1
Cheloid — *see* Keloid
Chemical burn — *see* Corrosion, by site
Chemodectoma — *see* Paraganglioma, nonchromaffin
Chemosis, conjunctiva — *see* Edema, conjunctiva
Chemotherapy (session) (for)
  cancer Z51.11
  neoplasm Z51.11
Cherubism M27.8
Chest — *see* condition
Cheyne-Stokes breathing (respiration) R06.3
Chiari's
  disease or syndrome (hepatic vein thrombosis) I82.0
  malformation
    type I G93.5
    type II — *see* Spina bifida
  net Q24.8
Chicago disease B40.9
Chickenpox — *see* Varicella
Chiclero ulcer or sore B55.1
Chigger (infestation) B88.0
Chignon (disease) B36.8
  newborn (from vacuum extraction) (birth injury) P12.1
Chilaiditi's syndrome (subphrenic displacement, colon) Q43.3
Chilblain(s) (lupus) T69.1
Child
  custody dispute Z65.3
Childbirth — *see* Delivery
Childhood
  cerebral X-linked adrenoleukodystrophy E71.520
  period of rapid growth Z00.2
Chill(s) R68.83 with fever R50.9
  congestive in malarial regions B54
  without fever R68.83
Chilomastigiasis A07.8
Chimera 46,XX/46,XY Q99.0
Chin — *see* condition
Chinese dysentery A03.9
Chionophobia F40.228
Chitral fever A93.1
Chlamydia, chlamydial A74.9
  cervicitis A56.09
  conjunctivitis A74.0
  cystitis A56.01
  endometritis A56.11
  epididymitis A56.19
  female
    pelvic inflammatory disease A56.11
    pelviperitonitis A56.11
  orchitis A56.19
  peritonitis A74.81
  pharyngitis A56.4
  proctitis A56.3
  psittaci (infection) A70
  salpingitis A56.11
  sexually-transmitted infection NEC A56.8
  specified NEC A74.89
  urethritis A56.01
  vulvovaginitis A56.02
Chlamydiosis — *see* Chlamydia
Chloasma (skin) (idiopathic) (symptomatic) L81.1
  eyelid H02.719
    hyperthyroid E05.90 [H02.719]
      with thyroid storm E05.91 [H02.719]
    left H02.716
      lower H02.715
      upper H02.714
    right H02.713
      lower H02.712
      upper H02.711
Chloroma C92.3-
Chlorosis D50.9
  Egyptian B76.9 [D63.8]
  miner's B76.9 [D63.8]

Chlorotic anemia D50.9
Chocolate cyst (ovary) N80.1
Choked
  disc or disk — *see* Papilledema
  on food, phlegm, or vomitus NOS — *see* Asphyxia,
    food
  while vomiting NOS — *see* Asphyxia, food
Chokes (resulting from bends) T70.3
Choking sensation R09.89
Cholangiectasis K83.8
Cholangiocarcinoma
  with hepatocellular carcinoma, combined C22.0
    liver C22.1
  specified site NEC — *see* Neoplasm, malignant, by
    site
  unspecified site C22.1
Cholangiohepatitis K83.8
  due to fluke infestation B66.1
Cholangiohepatoma C22.0
Cholangiolitis (acute) (chronic) (extrahepatic)
    (gangrenous) (intrahepatic) K83.0
  paratyphoidal — *see* Fever, paratyphoid
  typhoidal A01.09
Cholangioma D13.4
  malignant — *see* Cholangiocarcinoma
Cholangitis (ascending) (primary) (recurrent)
    (sclerosing) (secondary) (stenosing)
    (suppurative) K83.0
  with calculus, bile duct — *see* Calculus, bile duct,
    with cholangitis
  chronic nonsuppurative destructive K74.3
Cholecystectasia K82.8
Cholecystitis K81.9
  with
    calculus, stones in
      bile duct (common) (hepatic) — *see* Calculus,
        bile duct, with cholecystitis
      cystic duct — *see* Calculus, gallbladder, with
        cholecystitis
      gallbladder — *see* Calculus, gallbladder, with
        cholecystitis
    choledocholithiasis — *see* Calculus, bile duct,
      with cholecystitis
    cholelithiasis — *see* Calculus, gallbladder, with
      cholecystitis
  acute (emphysematous) (gangrenous) (suppurative)
    K81.0
    with
      calculus, stones in
        cystic duct — *see* Calculus, gallbladder,
          with cholecystitis, acute
        gallbladder — *see* Calculus, gallbladder,
          with cholecystitis, acute
      choledocholithiasis — *see* Calculus, bile duct,
        with cholecystitis, acute
      cholelithiasis — *see* Calculus, gallbladder,
        with cholecystitis, acute
    chronic cholecystitis K81.2
      with gallbladder calculus K80.12
        with obstruction K80.13
  chronic K81.1
    with acute cholecystitis K81.2
      with gallbladder calculus K80.12
        with obstruction K80.13
  emphysematous (acute) — *see* Cholecystitis, acute
  gangrenous — *see* Cholecystitis, acute
  paratyphoidal, current A01.4
  suppurative — *see* Cholecystitis, acute
  typhoidal A01.09
Cholecystolithiasis — *see* Calculus, gallbladder
Choledochitis (suppurative) K83.0
Choledocholith — *see* Calculus, bile duct
Choledocholithiasis (common duct) (hepatic duct) —
    see Calculus, bile duct
  cystic — *see* Calculus, gallbladder
  typhoidal A01.09
Cholelithiasis (cystic duct) (gallbladder) (impacted)
    (multiple) — *see* Calculus, gallbladder
  bile duct (common) (hepatic) — *see* Calculus, bile
    duct
  hepatic duct — *see* Calculus, bile duct
  specified NEC K80.80
    with obstruction K80.81

Cholemia (*see also* Jaundice)
  familial (simple) (congenital) E80.4
  Gilbert's E80.4
Choleperitoneum, choleperitonitis K65.3
Cholera (Asiatic) (epidemic) (malignant) A00.9
  antimonial — *see* Poisoning, antimony
  classical A00.0
  due to Vibrio cholerae 01 A00.9
    biovar cholerae A00.0
    biovar eltor A00.1
    el tor A00.1
  el tor A00.1
Cholerine — *see* Cholera
Cholestasis NEC K83.1
  due to total parenteral nutrition (TPN) K76.8
  with hepatocyte injury K71.0
  pure K71.0
Cholesteatoma (ear) (middle) (with reaction) H71.9-
  attic H71.0-
  external ear (canal) H60.4-
  mastoid H71.2-
  postmastoidectomy cavity (recurrent) — *see*
    Complications, postmastoidectomy, recurrent
    cholesteatoma
  recurrent (postmastoidectomy) — *see*
    Complications, postmastoidectomy, recurrent
    cholesteatoma
  tympanum H71.1-
Cholesteatosis, diffuse H71.3-
Cholesteremia E78.0
Cholesterin in vitreous — *see* Deposit, crystalline
Cholesterol
  deposit
    retina H35.89
    vitreous — *see* Deposit, crystalline
  elevated (high) E78.0
    with elevated (high) triglycerides E78.2
    screening for Z13.220
  imbibition of gallbladder K82.4
Cholesterolemia (essential) (familial) (hereditary)
    (pure) E78.0
Cholesterolosis, cholesterosis (gallbladder) K82.4
  cerebrotendinous E75.5
Cholocolic fistula K82.3
Choluria R82.2
Chondritis M94.8x9
  aurical H61.03-
  costal (Tietze's) M94.0
  external ear H61.03-
  patella, posttraumatic — *see* Chondromalacia,
    patella
  pinna H61.03-
  purulent M94.8x
  tuberculous NEC A18.02
    intervertebral A18.01
Chondroblastoma (*see also* Neoplasm, bone, benign)
  malignant — *see* Neoplasm, bone, malignant
Chondrocalcinosis M11.20
  ankle M11.27-
  elbow M11.22-
  familial M11.10
    ankle M11.17-
    elbow M11.12-
    foot joint M11.17-
    hand joint M11.14-
    hip M11.15-
    knee M11.16-
    multiple site M11.19
    shoulder M11.11-
    specified joint NEC M11.18
    wrist M11.13-
  foot joint M11.27-
  hand joint M11.24-
  hip M11.25-
  knee M11.26-
  multiple site M11.29
  shoulder M11.21-
  specified joint NEC M11.28
  specified type NEC M11.20
    ankle M11.27-
    elbow M11.22-
    foot joint M11.27-

Chondrocalcinosis— *continued*
  specified type— *continued*
    hand joint M11.24-
    hip M11.25-
    knee M11.26-
    multiple site M11.29
    shoulder M11.21-
    specified joint NEC M11.28
    wrist M11.23-
  wrist M11.23-
Chondrodermatitis nodularis helicis or anthelicis
    — *see* Perichondritis, ear
Chondrodysplasia Q78.9
  with hemangioma Q78.4
  calcificans congenita Q77.3
  fetalis Q77.4
  metaphyseal (Jansen's) (McKusick's) (Schmid's)
    Q78.5
  punctata Q77.3
Chondrodystrophy, chondrodystrophia (familial)
    (fetalis) (hypoplastic) Q78.9
  calcificans congenita Q77.3
  myotonic (congenital) G71.13
  punctata Q77.3
Chondroectodermal dysplasia Q77.6
Chondrogenesis imperfecta Q77.4
Chondrolysis M94.35-
Chondroma (*see also* Neoplasm, cartilage, benign)
  juxtacortical — *see* Neoplasm, bone, benign
  periosteal — *see* Neoplasm, bone, benign
Chondromalacia (systemic) M94.20
  acromioclavicular joint M94.21-
  ankle M94.27-
  elbow M94.22-
  foot joint M94.27-
  glenohumeral joint M94.21-
  hand joint M94.24-
  hip M94.25-
  knee M94.26-
    patella M22.4-
  multiple sites M94.29
  patella M22.4-
  rib M94.28
  sacroiliac joint M94.259
  shoulder M94.21-
  sternoclavicular joint M94.21-
  vertebral joint M94.28
  wrist M94.23-
Chondromatosis (*see also* Neoplasm, cartilage,
    uncertain behavior)
  internal Q78.4
Chondromyxosarcoma — *see* Neoplasm, cartilage,
    malignant
Chondro-osteodysplasia (Morquio-Brailsford type)
    E76.219
Chondro-osteodystrophy E76.29
Chondro-osteoma — *see* Neoplasm, bone, benign
Chondropathia tuberosa M94.0
Chondrosarcoma — *see* Neoplasm, cartilage,
    malignant
  juxtacortical — *see* Neoplasm, bone, malignant
  mesenchymal — *see* Neoplasm, connective tissue,
    malignant
  myxoid — *see* Neoplasm, cartilage, malignant
Chordee (nonvenereal) N48.89
  congenital Q54.4
  gonococcal A54.09
Chorditis (fibrinous) (nodosa) (tuberosa) J38.2
Chordoma — *see* Neoplasm, vertebral (column),
    malignant
Chorea (chronic) (gravis) (posthemiplegic) (senile)
    (spasmodic) G25.5
  with
    heart involvement I02.0
      active or acute (conditions in I01-) I02.0
        rheumatic I02.9
          with valvular disorder I02.0
    rheumatic heart disease (chronic)
      (inactive)(quiescent)—code to rheumatic
      heart condition involved
  drug-induced G25.4
  habit F95.8
  hereditary G10

Chorea— *continued*
  Huntington's G1Ø
  hysterical F44.4
  minor IØ2.9
    with heart involvement IØ2.Ø
  progressive G25.5
    hereditary G1Ø
  rheumatic (chronic) IØ2.9
    with heart involvement IØ2.Ø
  Sydenham's IØ2.9
    with heart involvement — *see* Chorea, with
        rheumatic heart disease
  nonrheumatic G25.5
Choreoathetosis (paroxysmal) G25.5
Chorioadenoma (destruens) D39.2
Chorioamnionitis O41.12-
Chorioangioma D26.7
Choriocarcinoma — *see* Neoplasm, malignant, by site
  combined with
    embryonal carcinoma — *see* Neoplasm,
        malignant, by site
    other germ cell elements — *see* Neoplasm,
        malignant, by site
    teratoma — *see* Neoplasm, malignant, by site
  specified site — *see* Neoplasm, malignant, by site
  unspecified site
    female C58
    male C62.9Ø
Chorioencephalitis (acute) (lymphocytic) (serous)
    A87.2
Chorioepithelioma — *see* Choriocarcinoma
Choriomeningitis (acute) (lymphocytic) (serous)
    A87.2
Chorionepithelioma — *see* Choriocarcinoma
Chorioretinitis (*see also* Inflammation, chorioretinal)
  disseminated (*see also* Inflammation, chorioretinal,
      disseminated)
    in neurosyphilis A52.19
  focal (*see also* Inflammation, chorioretinal, focal)
  Egyptian B76.9 [D63.8]
  histoplasmic B39.9 [H32]
  in (due to)
    histoplasmosis B39.9 [H32]
    syphilis (secondary) A51.43
      late A52.71
    toxoplasmosis (acquired) B58.Ø1
      congenital (active) P37.1 [H32]
    tuberculosis A18.53
  juxtapapillary, juxtapapillaris — *see* Inflammation,
      chorioretinal, focal, juxtapapillary
  leprous A3Ø.9 [H32]
  miner's B76.9 [D63.8]
  progressive myopia (degeneration) — *see* Disorder,
      globe, degenerative, myopia
  syphilitic (secondary) A51.43
    congenital (early) A5Ø.Ø1 [H32]
      late A5Ø.32
    late A52.71
  tuberculous A18.53
Chorioretinopathy, central serous H35.71-
Choroid — *see* condition
Choroideremia H31.21
Choroiditis — *see* Chorioretinitis
Choroidopathy — *see* Disorder, choroid
Choroidoretinitis — *see* Chorioretinitis
Choroidoretinopathy, central serous — *see*
    Chorioretinopathy, central serous
Christian-Weber disease M35.6
Christmas disease D67
Chromaffinoma (*see also* Neoplasm, benign, by site)
  malignant — *see* Neoplasm, malignant, by site
Chromatopsia — *see* Deficiency, color vision
Chromhidrosis, chromidrosis L75.1
Chromoblastomycosis — *see* Chromomycosis
Chromoconversion R82.91
Chromomycosis B43.9
  brain abscess B43.1
  cerebral B43.1
  cutaneous B43.Ø
  skin B43.Ø
  specified NEC B43.8
  subcutaneous abscess or cyst B43.Ø
Chromophytosis B36.Ø

Chromosome — *see* condition by chromosome
    involved
  D(1) — *see* condition, chromosome 13
  E(3) — *see* condition, chromosome 18
  G — *see* condition, chromosome 21
Chromotrichomycosis B36.8
Chronic — *see* condition
  fracture — *see* Fracture, pathological
Churg-Strauss syndrome M3Ø.1
Chyle cyst, mesentery I89.8
Chylocele (nonfilarial) I89.8
  filarial (*see also* Infestation, filarial) B74.9 [N51]
  tunica vaginalis N5Ø.8
    filarial (*see also* Infestation, filarial) B74.9 [N51]
Chylomicronemia (fasting) (with
    hyperprebetalipoproteinemia) E78.3
Chylopericardium I31.3
  acute I3Ø.9
Chylothorax (nonfilarial) I89.8
  filarial (*see also* Infestation, filarial) B74.9 [J91.8]
Chylous — *see* condition
Chyluria (nonfilarial) R82.Ø
  due to
    bilharziasis B65.Ø
    Brugia (malayi) B74.1
      timori B74.2
    schistosomiasis (bilharziasis) B65.Ø
    Wuchereria (bancrofti) B74.Ø
  filarial — *see* Infestation, filarial
Cicatricial (deformity) — *see* Cicatrix
Cicatrix (adherent) (contracted) (painful) (vicious) (*see
    also* Scar) L9Ø.5
  adenoid (and tonsil) J35.8
  alveolar process M26.79
  anus K62.8
  auricle — *see* Disorder, pinna, specified type NEC
  bile duct (common) (hepatic) K83.8
  bladder N32.89
  bone — *see* Disorder, bone, specified type NEC
  brain G93.89
  cervix (postoperative) (postpartal) N88.1
  common duct K83.8
  cornea H17.9
    tuberculous A18.59
  duodenum (bulb), obstructive K31.5
  esophagus K22.2
  eyelid — *see* Disorder, eyelid function
  hypopharynx J39.2
  lacrimal passages — *see* Obstruction, lacrimal
  larynx J38.7
  lung J98.4
  middle ear — *see* subcategory H74.8
  mouth K13.79
  muscle M62.89
    with contracture *see* Contraction, muscle NEC
  nasopharynx J39.2
  palate (soft) K13.79
  penis N48.89
  pharynx J39.2
  prostate N42.89
  rectum K62.8
  retina — *see* Scar, chorioretinal
  semilunar cartilage — *see* Derangement, meniscus
  seminal vesicle N5Ø.8
  skin L9Ø.5
    infected LØ8.89
    postinfective L9Ø.5
    tuberculous B9Ø.8
  specified site NEC L9Ø.5
  throat J39.2
  tongue K14.8
  tonsil (and adenoid) J35.8
  trachea J39.8
  tuberculous NEC B9Ø.9
  urethra N36.8
  uterus N85.8
  vagina N89.8
    postoperative N99.2
  vocal cord J38.3
  wrist, constricting (annular) L9Ø.5
CIDP (chronic inflammatory demyelinating
    polyneuropathy) G61.81
CIN — *see* Neoplasia, intraepithelial, cervix

Cinchonism — *see* Deafness, ototoxic
  correct substance properly administered — *see*
      Table of Drugs and Chemicals, by drug,
      adverse effect
  overdose or wrong substance given or taken — *see*
      Table of Drugs and Chemicals, by drug,
      poisoning
Circle of Willis — *see* condition
Circular — *see* condition
Circulating anticoagulants D68.31
  due to drugs D68.32
  following childbirth O72.3
Circulation
  collateral, any site I99.8
  defective (lower extremity) I99.8
    congenital Q28.9
  embryonic Q28.9
  failure (peripheral) R57.9
    newborn P29.89
  fetal, persistent P29.3
  heart, incomplete Q28.9
Circulatory system — *see* condition
Circulus senilis (cornea) — *see* Degeneration, cornea,
    senile
Circumcision (in absence of medical indication) (ritual)
    (routine) Z41.2
Circumscribed — *see* condition
Circumvallate placenta O43.11-
Cirrhosis, cirrhotic (hepatic) (liver) K74.6Ø
  alcoholic K7Ø.3Ø
    with ascites K7Ø.31
  atrophic — *see* Cirrhosis, liver
  Baumgarten-Cruveilhier K74.69
  biliary (cholangiolitic) (cholangitic) (hypertrophic)
      (obstructive) (pericholangiolitic) K74.5
    due to
      Clonorchiasis B66.1
      flukes B66.3
    primary K74.3
    secondary K74.4
  cardiac (of liver) K76.1
  Charcot's K74.3
  cholangiolitic, cholangitic, cholostatic (primary)
      K74.3
  congestive K76.1
  Cruveilhier-Baumgarten K74.69
  cryptogenic (liver) K74.69
  due to
    hepatolenticular degeneration E83.Ø1
    Wilson's disease E83.Ø1
    xanthomatosis E78.2
  fatty K76.Ø
    alcoholic K7Ø.Ø
  Hanot's (hypertrophic) K74.3
  hepatic — *see* Cirrhosis, liver
  hypertrophic K74.3
  Indian childhood K74.69
  kidney — *see* Sclerosis, renal
  Laennec's K7Ø.3Ø
    with ascites K7Ø.31
    alcoholic K7Ø.3Ø
      with ascites K7Ø.31
    nonalcoholic K74.69
  liver K74.6Ø
    alcoholic K7Ø.3Ø
      with ascites K7Ø.31
      fatty K7Ø.Ø
    congenital P78.81
    syphilitic A52.74
  lung (chronic) — *see* Fibrosis, lung
  macronodular K74.69
    alcoholic K7Ø.3Ø
      with ascites K7Ø.31
  micronodular K74.69
    alcoholic K7Ø.3Ø
      with ascites K7Ø.31
  mixed type K74.69
  monolobular K74.3
  nephritis — *see* Sclerosis, renal
  nutritional K74.69
    alcoholic K7Ø.3Ø
      with ascites K7Ø.31
  obstructive — *see* Cirrhosis, biliary

Cirrhosis, cirrhotic— *continued*
  ovarian N83.8
  pancreas (duct) K86.8
  pigmentary E83.110
  portal K74.69
    alcoholic K70.30
      with ascites K70.31
    postnecrotic K74.69
    alcoholic K70.30
      with ascites K70.31
  pulmonary — *see* Fibrosis, lung
  renal — *see* Sclerosis, renal
  spleen D73.2
  stasis K76.1
  Todd's K74.3
  unilobar K74.3
  xanthomatous (biliary) K74.5
    due to xanthomatosis (familial) (metabolic)
      (primary) E78.2
Cistern, subarachnoid R93.0
Citrullinemia E72.23
Citrullinuria E72.23
Civatte's disease or poikiloderma L57.3
Clam diggers' itch B65.3
Clammy skin R23.1
Clap — *see* Gonorrhea
Clarke-Hadfield syndrome (pancreatic infantilism)
  K86.8
Clark's paralysis G80.9
Clastothrix L67.8
Claude Bernard-Horner syndrome G90.2
  traumatic — *see* Injury, nerve, cervical sympathetic
Claude's disease or syndrome G46.3
Claudication, intermittent I73.9
  cerebral (artery) G45.9
  spinal cord (arteriosclerotic) G95.19
    syphilitic A52.09
  venous (axillary) I87.8
Claudicatio venosa intermittens I87.8
Claustrophobia F40.240
Clavus (infected) L84
Clawfoot (congenital) Q66.8
  acquired — *see* Deformity, limb, clawfoot
Clawhand (acquired) (*see also* Deformity, limb,
  clawhand)
  congenital Q68.1
Clawtoe (congenital) Q66.8
  acquired — *see* Deformity, toe, specified NEC
Clay eating — *see* Pica
Cleansing of artificial opening — *see* Attention to,
  artificial, opening
Cleft (congenital) (*see also* Imperfect, closure)
  alveolar process M26.79
  branchial (cyst) (persistent) Q18.2
  cricoid cartilage, posterior Q31.8
  lip (unilateral) Q36.9
    with cleft palate Q37.9
      hard Q37.1
        with soft Q37.5
      soft Q37.3
        with hard Q37.5
    bilateral Q36.0
      with cleft palate Q37.8
        hard Q37.0
          with soft Q37.4
        soft Q37.2
          with hard Q37.4
    median Q36.1
  nose Q30.2
  palate Q35.9
    with cleft lip (unilateral) Q37.9
      bilateral Q37.8
    hard Q35.1
      with
        cleft lip (unilateral) Q37.1
          bilateral Q37.0
        soft Q35.5
          with cleft lip (unilateral) Q37.5
            bilateral Q37.4
    medial Q35.5
    soft Q35.3
      with
        cleft lip (unilateral) Q37.3

Cleft— *continued*
  palate— *continued*
    soft— *continued*
      with— *continued*
        cleft lip (unilateral)— *continued*
          bilateral Q37.2
          with cleft lip (unilateral) Q37.5
            bilateral Q37.4
  penis Q55.69
  scrotum Q55.29
  thyroid cartilage Q31.8
  uvula Q35.7
Cleidocranial dysostosis Q74.0
Cleptomania F63.2
Clicking hip (newborn) R29.4
Climacteric (female) (*see also* Menopause)
  arthritis (any site) NEC — *see* Arthritis, specified
    form NEC
  depression (single episode) F32.8
  male (symptoms) (syndrome) NEC N50.8
  paranoid state F22
  polyarthritis NEC — *see* Arthritis, specified form NEC
  symptoms (female) N95.1
Clinical research investigation (clinical trial) (control
  subject) Z00.6
Clitoris — *see* condition
Cloaca (persistent) Q43.7
Clonorchiasis, clonorchis infection (liver) B66.1
Clonus R25.8
Closed bite M26.29
**Clostridium (C.) perfringens, as cause of disease
  classified elsewhere** B96.7
Closure
  congenital, nose Q30.0
  cranial sutures, premature Q75.0
  defective or imperfect NEC — *see* Imperfect, closure
  fistula, delayed — *see* Fistula
  foramen ovale, imperfect Q21.1
  hymen N89.6
  interauricular septum, defective Q21.1
  interventricular septum, defective Q21.0
  lacrimal duct (*see also* Stenosis, lacrimal, duct)
    congenital Q10.5
  nose (congenital) Q30.0
    acquired M95.0
  of artificial opening — *see* Attention to, artificial,
    opening
  vagina N89.5
  valve — *see* Endocarditis
  vulva N90.5
Clot (blood) (*see also* Embolism)
  artery (obstruction) (occlusion) — *see* Embolism
  bladder N32.89
  brain (intradural or extradural) — *see* Occlusion,
    artery, cerebral
  circulation I74.9
  heart (*see also* Infarct, myocardium)
    not resulting in infarction I24.0
  vein — *see* Thrombosis
Clouded state R40.1
  epileptic — *see* Epilepsy, specified NEC
  paroxysmal — *see* Epilepsy, specified NEC
Cloudy antrum, antra J32.0
Clouston's (hidrotic) **ectodermal dysplasia** Q82.4
Clubbed nail pachydermoperiostosis M89.40 [L62]
Clubbing of finger(s) (nails) R68.3
Clubfinger R68.3
  congenital Q68.1
Clubfoot (congenital) Q66.8
  acquired — *see* Deformity, limb, clubfoot
  equinovarus Q66.0
  paralytic — *see* Deformity, limb, clubfoot
Clubhand (congenital) (radial) Q71.4-
  acquired — *see* Deformity, limb, clubhand
Clubnail R68.3
  congenital Q84.6
Clump, kidney Q63.1
Clumsiness, clumsy child syndrome F82
Cluttering F80.81
Clutton's joints A50.51 [M12.80]

Coagulation, intravascular (diffuse) (disseminated)
  (*see also* Defibrination syndrome)
  complicating abortion — *see* Abortion, by type,
    complicated by, intravascular coagulation
Coagulopathy (*see also* Defect, coagulation)
  consumption D65
  intravascular D65
  newborn P60
Coalminer's
  elbow — *see* Bursitis, elbow, olecranon
  lung or pneumoconiosis J60
Coalition
  calcaneo-scaphoid Q66.8
  tarsal Q66.8
Coalworker's lung or pneumoconiosis J60
Coarctation of aorta (preductal) (postductal) Q25.1
Coated tongue K14.3
Coats' disease (exudative retinopathy) — *see*
  Retinopathy, exudative
Cocainism — *see* Dependence, drug, cocaine
Coccidioidomycosis B38.9
  cutaneous B38.3
  disseminated B38.7
  generalized B38.7
  meninges B38.4
  prostate B38.81
  pulmonary B38.2
    acute B38.0
    chronic B38.1
  skin B38.3
  specified NEC B38.89
Coccidioidosis — *see* Coccidioidomycosis
Coccidiosis (intestinal) A07.3
Coccydynia, coccygodynia M53.3
Coccyx — *see* condition
Cochin-China diarrhea K90.1
Cockayne's syndrome Q87.1
Cocked up toe — *see* Deformity, toe, specified NEC
Cock's peculiar tumor L72.1
Codman's tumor — *see* Neoplasm, bone, benign
Coenurosis B71.8
Coffee-worker's lung J67.8
Cogan's syndrome (*see also* Keratitis, interstitial,
  specified type NEC)
  oculomotor apraxia H51.8
Coitus, painful (female) N94.1
  male N53.12
  psychogenic F52.6
Cold J00
  with influenza, flu, or grippe — *see* Influenza, with,
    respiratory manifestations NEC
  agglutinin disease or hemoglobinuria (chronic)
    D59.1
  bronchial — *see* Bronchitis
  chest — *see* Bronchitis
  common (head) J00
  effects of T69.9
    specified effect NEC T69.8
  excessive, effects of T69.9
    specified effect NEC T69.8
  exhaustion from T69.8
  exposure to T69.9
    specified effect NEC T69.8
  head J00
  injury syndrome (newborn) P80.0
  on lung — *see* Bronchitis
  rose J30.1
  sensitivity, auto-immune D59.1
  virus J00
Coldsore B00.1
Colibacillosis A49.8
  as the cause of other disease B96.2
  generalized A41.50
Colic (bilious) (infantile) (intestinal) (recurrent)
  (spasmodic) R10.83
  abdomen R10.83
    psychogenic F45.8
  appendix, appendicular K38.8
  bile duct — *see* Calculus, bile duct
  biliary — *see* Calculus, bile duct
  common duct — *see* Calculus, bile duct
  cystic duct — *see* Calculus, gallbladder
  Devonshire NEC — *see* Poisoning, lead

Colic— *continued*
  gallbladder — *see* Calculus, gallbladder
  gallstone — *see* Calculus, gallbladder
    gallbladder or cystic duct — *see* Calculus,
      gallbladder
  hepatic (duct) — *see* Calculus, bile duct
  hysterical F45.8
  kidney N23
  lead NEC — *see* Poisoning, lead
  mucous K58.9
    with diarrhea K58.0
    psychogenic F54
  nephritic N23
  painter's NEC — *see* Poisoning, lead
  pancreas K86.8
  psychogenic F45.8
  renal N23
  saturnine NEC — *see* Poisoning, lead
  ureter N23
  urethral N36.8
    due to calculus N21.1
  uterus NEC N94.89
    menstrual — *see* Dysmenorrhea
  worm NOS B83.9
Colicystitis — *see* Cystitis
Colitis (acute) (catarrhal) (chronic) (noninfective)
  (hemorrhagic) (*see also* Enteritis) K52.9
  allergic K52.2
  amebic (acute) (*see also* Amebiasis) A06.0
    nondysenteric A06.2
  anthrax A22.2
  bacillary — *see* Infection, Shigella
  balantidial A07.0
  Clostridium difficile A04.7
  coccidial A07.3
  collagenous K52.89
  cystica superficialis K52.89
  dietary counseling and surveillance (for) Z71.3
  dietetic K52.2
  due to radiation K52.0
  eosinophilic K52.82
  food hypersensitivity K52.2
  giardial A07.1
  granulomatous — *see* Enteritis, regional, large
    intestine
  infectious — *see* Enteritis, infectious
  ischemic K55.9
    acute (fulminant) (subacute) K55.0
    chronic K55.1
    due to mesenteric artery insufficiency K55.1
    fulminant (acute) K55.0
  left sided K51.50
    with
      complication K51.519
        specified NEC K51.518
      abscess K51.514
      fistula K51.513
      obstruction K51.512
      rectal bleeding K51.511
  lymphocytic K52.89
  membranous
    psychogenic F54
  microscopic (collagenous) (lymphocytic) K52.89
  mucous — *see* Syndrome, irritable, bowel
    psychogenic F54
  noninfective K52.9
    specified NEC K52.89
  polyposa — *see* Polyps, colon, inflammatory
  protozoal A07.9
  pseudomembranous A04.7
  pseudomucinous — *see* Syndrome, irritable, bowel
  regional — *see* Enteritis, regional, large intestine
  segmental — *see* Enteritis, regional, large intestine
  septic — *see* Enteritis, infectious
  spastic K58.9
    with diarrhea K58.0
    psychogenic F54
  staphylococcal A04.8
    foodborne A05.0
  subacute ischemic K55.0
  thromboulcerative K55.0
  toxic K52.1
  transmural — *see* Enteritis, regional, large intestine

Colitis— *continued*
  trichomonal A07.8
  tuberculous (ulcerative) A18.32
  ulcerative (chronic) K51.90
    with
      complication K51.919
        abscess K51.914
        fistula K51.913
        obstruction K51.912
        rectal bleeding K51.911
        specified complication NEC K51.918
    enterocolitis — *see* Enterocolitis, ulcerative
    ileocolitis — *see* Ileocolitis, ulcerative
    mucosal proctocolitis — *see* Proctocolitis,
      mucosal
    proctitis — *see* Proctitis, ulcerative
    pseudopolyposis — *see* Polyps, colon,
      inflammatory
    psychogenic F54
    rectosigmoiditis — *see* Rectosigmoiditis,
      ulcerative
    specified type NEC K51.80
      with
        complication K51.819
          abscess K51.814
          fistula K51.813
          obstruction K51.812
          rectal bleeding K51.811
          specified complication NEC K51.818
Collagenosis, collagen disease (nonvascular)
  (vascular) M35.9
  cardiovascular I42.8
  reactive perforating L87.1
  specified NEC M35.8
Collapse R55
  adrenal E27.2
  cardiorespiratory R57.0
  cardiovascular R57.0
    newborn P29.89
  circulatory (peripheral) R57.9
    during or after labor and delivery O75.1
    following ectopic or molar pregnancy O08.3
    newborn P29.89
  during or after labor and delivery O75.1
  external ear canal — *see* Stenosis, external ear canal
  general R55
  heart — *see* Disease, heart
  heat T67.1
  hysterical F44.89
  labyrinth, membranous (congenital) Q16.5
  lung (massive) (*see also* Atelectasis) J98.19
    pressure due to anesthesia (general) (local) or
        other sedation T88.2
      during labor and delivery O74.1
      in pregnancy O29.02-
      postpartum, puerperal O89.09
  myocardial — *see* Disease, heart
  nervous F48.8
  neurocirculatory F45.8
  nose M95.0
  postoperative (cardiovascular) T81.1
  pulmonary (*see also* Atelectasis) J98.19
    newborn — *see* Atelectasis
  trachea J39.8
  tracheobronchial J98.09
  valvular — *see* Endocarditis
  vascular (peripheral) R57.9
    during or after labor and delivery O75.1
    following ectopic or molar pregnancy O08.3
    newborn P29.89
  vertebra M48.50-
    cervical region M48.52-
    cervicothoracic region M48.53-
    in (due to)
      metastasis — *see* Collapse, vertebra, in,
        specified disease NEC
      osteoporosis (*see also* Osteoporosis) M80.88
        cervical region M80.88
        cervicothoracic region M80.88
        lumbar region M80.88
        lumbosacral region M80.88
        multiple sites M80.88
        occipito-atlanto-axial region M80.88

Collapse— *continued*
  vertebra— *continued*
    in (due to)— *continued*
      osteoporosis— *continued*
        sacrococcygeal region M80.88
        thoracic region M80.88
        thoracolumbar region M80.88
      specified disease NEC M48.50-
        cervical region M48.52-
        cervicothoracic region M48.53-
        lumbar region M48.56-
        lumbosacral region M48.57-
        occipito-atlanto-axial region M48.51-
        sacrococcygeal region M48.58-
        thoracic region M48.54-
        thoracolumbar region M48.55-
    lumbar region M48.56-
    lumbosacral region M48.57-
    occipito-atlanto-axial region M48.51-
    sacrococcygeal region M48.58-
    thoracic region M48.54-
    thoracolumbar region M48.55-
Collateral (*see also* condition)
  circulation (venous) I87.8
  dilation, veins I87.8
Colles' fracture S52.53-
Collet (-Sicard) **syndrome** G52.7
Collier's asthma or lung J60
Collodion baby Q80.2
Colloid nodule (of thyroid) (cystic) E04.1
Coloboma (iris) Q13.0
  eyelid Q10.3
  fundus Q14.8
  lens Q12.2
  optic disc (congenital) Q14.2
    acquired H47.31-
Coloenteritis — *see* Enteritis
Colon — *see* condition
Colonization status — *see* Carrier (suspected) of
Coloptosis K63.4
Color blindness — *see* Deficiency, color vision
Colostomy
  attention to Z43.3
  fitting or adjustment Z46.89
  malfunctioning K94.03
  status Z93.3
Colpitis (acute) — *see* Vaginitis
Colpocele N81.5
Colpocystitis — *see* Vaginitis
Colpospasm N94.2
Column, spinal, vertebral — *see* condition
Coma R40.20
  with
    motor response (none) R40.231
      abnormal R40.233
      extension R40.232
      flexion withdrawal R40.234
      localizes pain R40.235
      obeys commands R40.236
    opening of eyes (never) R40.211
      in response to
        pain R40.212
        sound R40.213
      spontaneous R40.214
    verbal response (none) R40.221
      confused conversation R40.224
      inappropriate words R40.223
      incomprehensible words R40.222
      oriented R40.225
  eclamptic — *see* Eclampsia
  epileptic — *see* Epilepsy
  hepatic — *see* Failure, hepatic, by type, with coma
  hyperglycemic (diabetic) — *see* Diabetes, coma
  hyperosmolar (diabetic) — *see* Diabetes, coma
  hypoglycemic (diabetic) — *see* Diabetes, coma,
    hypoglycemic
    nondiabetic E15
  in diabetes — *see* Diabetes, coma
  insulin-induced — *see* Coma, hypoglycemic
  myxedematous E03.5
  newborn P91.5
  persistent vegetative state R40.3

Comatose — *see* Coma
Combat fatigue F43.Ø
Combined — *see* condition
Comedo, comedones (giant) L7Ø.Ø
Comedocarcinoma (*see also* Neoplasm, breast, malignant)
  noninfiltrating
    breast DØ5.8-
    specified site — *see* Neoplasm, in situ, by site
    unspecified site DØ5.8-
Comedomastitis — *see* Ectasia, mammary duct
Comminuted fracture—code as Fracture, closed
Common
  arterial trunk Q2Ø.Ø
  atrioventricular canal Q21.2
  atrium Q21.1
  cold (head) JØØ
  truncus (arteriosus) Q2Ø.Ø
  variable immunodeficiency — *see* Immunodeficiency, common variable
  ventricle Q2Ø.4
Commotio, commotion (current)
  brain — *see* Injury, intracranial, concussion
  cerebri — *see* Injury, intracranial, concussion
  retinae SØ5.8x-
  spinal cord — *see* Injury, spinal cord, by region
  spinalis — *see* Injury, spinal cord, by region
Communication
  between
    base of aorta and pulmonary artery Q21.4
    left ventricle and right atrium Q2Ø.5
    pericardial sac and pleural sac Q34.8
    pulmonary artery and pulmonary vein, congenital Q25.7
  congenital between uterus and digestive or urinary tract Q51.7
Compartment syndrome (deep) (posterior) (traumatic) T79.aØ
  abdomen T79.a3
  lower extremity (hip, buttock, thigh, leg, foot, toes) T79.a2
  nontraumatic
    abdomen M79.a3
    lower extremity (hip, buttock, thigh, leg, foot, toes) M79.a2-
    specified site NEC M79.a9
    upper extremity (shoulder, arm, forearm, wrist, hand, fingers) M79.a1 -
  specified site NEC T79.a9
  upper extremity (shoulder, arm, forearm, wrist, hand, fingers) T79.a1
Compensation
  failure — *see* Disease, heart
  neurosis, psychoneurosis — *see* Disorder, factitious
Complaint (*see also* Disease)
  bowel, functional K59.9
    psychogenic F45.8
  intestine, functional K59.9
    psychogenic F45.8
  kidney — *see* Disease, renal
  miners' J6Ø
Complete — *see* condition
Complex
  Addison-Schilder E71.528
  cardiorenal — *see* Hypertension, cardiorenal
  Costen's M26.69
  disseminated mycobacterium aviumintracellulare (DMAC) A31.2
  Eisenmenger's (ventricular septal defect) I27.89
  hypersexual F52.8
  jumped process, spine — *see* Dislocation, vertebra
  primary, tuberculous A15.7
  Schilder-Addison E71.528
  subluxation (vertebral) M99.19
    abdomen M99.19
    acromioclavicular M99.17
    cervical region M99.11
    cervicothoracic M99.11
    costochondral M99.18
    costovertebral M99.18
    head region M99.1Ø
    hip M99.15
    lower extremity M99.16

Complex— *continued*
  subluxation— *continued*
    lumbar region M99.13
    lumbosacral M99.13
    occipitocervical M99.1Ø
    pelvic region M99.15
    pubic M99.15
    rib cage M99.18
    sacral region M99.14
    sacrococcygeal M99.14
    sacroiliac M99.14
    specified NEC M99.19
    sternochondral M99.18
    sternoclavicular M99.17
    thoracic region M99.12
    thoracolumbar M99.12
    upper extremity M99.17
  Taussig-Bing (transposition, aorta and overriding pulmonary artery) Q2Ø.1
Complication(s) (from) (of)
  accidental puncture or laceration during a procedure (of) — *see* Complications, intraoperative (intraprocedural), puncture or laceration
  amputation stump (surgical) (late) NEC T87.9
    infection or inflammation T87.4Ø
      lower limb T87.4-
      upper limb T87.2-
    necrosis T87.5Ø
      lower limb T87.5-
      upper limb T87.5-
    neuroma T87.3Ø
      lower limb T87.3-
      upper limb T87.3-
    specified type NEC T87.8
  anastomosis (and bypass) (*see also* Complications, prosthetic device or implant)
    intestinal (internal) NEC K91.89
      involving urinary tract N99.89
    urinary tract (involving intestinal tract) N99.89
    vascular — *see* Complications, cardiovascular device or implant
  anesthesia, anesthetic (*see also* Anesthesia, complication) T88.59
    brain, postpartum, puerperal O89.2
    cardiac
      in
        labor and delivery O74.2
        pregnancy O29.19-
      postpartum, puerperal O89.1
    central nervous system
      in
        labor and delivery O74.3
        pregnancy O29.29-
      postpartum, puerperal O89.2
    difficult or failed intubation T88.4
      in pregnancy O29.6-
    failed sedation (conscious) (moderate) during procedure T88.52
    hyperthermia, malignant T88.3
    hypothermia T88.51
    intubation failure T88.4
    malignant hyperthermia T88.3
    pulmonary
      in
        labor and delivery O74.1
        pregnancy NEC O29.Ø9-
      postpartum, puerperal O89.Ø9
    shock T88.2
    spinal and epidural
      in
        labor and delivery NEC O74.6
          headache O74.5
        pregnancy NEC O29.5x-
      postpartum, puerperal NEC O89.5
        headache O89.4
  anti-reflux device — *see* Complications, esophageal anti-reflux device
  aortic (bifurcation) graft — *see* Complications, graft, vascular
  aortocoronary (bypass) graft — *see* Complications, coronary artery (bypass) graft

Complication— *continued*
  aortofemoral (bypass) graft — *see* Complications, extremity artery (bypass) graft
  arteriovenous
    fistula, surgically created T82.9
      embolism T82.818
      fibrosis T82.828
      hemorrhage T82.838
      infection or inflammation T82.7
      mechanical
        breakdown T82.51Ø
        displacement T82.52Ø
        leakage T82.53Ø
        malposition T82.52Ø
        obstruction T82.59Ø
        perforation T82.59Ø
        protrusion T82.59Ø
      pain T82.848
      specified type NEC T82.898
      stenosis T82.858
      thrombosis T82.868
    shunt, surgically created T82.9
      embolism T82.818
      fibrosis T82.828
      hemorrhage T82.838
      infection or inflammation T82.7
      mechanical
        breakdown T82.511
        displacement T82.521
        leakage T82.531
        malposition T82.521
        obstruction T82.591
        perforation T82.591
        protrusion T82.591
      pain T82.848
      specified type NEC T82.898
      stenosis T82.858
      thrombosis T82.868
  arthroplasty — *see* Complications, joint prosthesis
  artificial
    fertilization or insemination N98.9
      attempted introduction (of)
        embryo in embryo transfer N98.3
        ovum following in vitro fertilization N98.2
      hyperstimulation of ovaries N98.1
      infection N98.Ø
      specified NEC N98.8
  heart T82.9
    embolism T82.817
    fibrosis T82.827
    hemorrhage T82.837
    infection or inflammation T82.7
    mechanical
      breakdown T82.512
      displacement T82.522
      leakage T82.532
      malposition T82.522
      obstruction T82.592
      perforation T82.592
      protrusion T82.592
    pain T82.847
    specified type NEC T82.897
    stenosis T82.857
    thrombosis T82.867
  opening
    cecostomy — *see* Complications, colostomy
    colostomy — *see* Complications, colostomy
    cystostomy — *see* Complications, cystostomy
    enterostomy — *see* Complications, enterostomy
    gastrostomy — *see* Complications, gastrostomy
    ileostomy — *see* Complications, enterostomy
    jejunostomy — *see* Complications, enterostomy
    nephrostomy — *see* Complications, stoma, urinary tract
    tracheostomy — *see* Complications, tracheostomy
    ureterostomy — *see* Complications, stoma, urinary tract
    urethrostomy — *see* Complications, stoma, urinary tract

Complication— *continued*
  balloon implant or device
    gastrointestinal T85.89
      embolism T85.81
      fibrosis T85.82
      hemorrhage T85.83
      infection and inflammation T85.79
      pain T85.84
      specified type NEC T85.89
      stenosis T85.85
      thrombosis T85.86
    vascular (counterpulsation) T82.9
      embolism T82.818
      fibrosis T82.828
      hemorrhage T82.838
      infection or inflammation T82.7
      mechanical
        breakdown T82.513
        displacement T82.523
        leakage T82.533
        malposition T82.523
        obstruction T82.593
        perforation T82.593
        protrusion T82.593
      pain T82.848
      specified type NEC T82.898
      stenosis T82.858
      thrombosis T82.868
  bile duct implant (prosthetic) T85.89
    embolism T85.81
    fibrosis T85.82
    hemorrhage T85.83
    infection and inflammation T85.79
    mechanical
      breakdown T85.510
      displacement T85.520
      malfunction T85.510
      malposition T85.520
      obstruction T85.590
      perforation T85.590
      protrusion T85.590
      specified NEC T85.590
    pain T85.84
    specified type NEC T85.89
    stenosis T85.85
    thrombosis T85.86
  bladder device (auxiliary) — see Complications,
      genitourinary, device or implant, urinary
      system
  bleeding (postoperative) — see Complication,
      postoperative, hemorrhage
    intraoperative — see Complication,
      intraoperative, hemorrhage
  blood vessel graft — see Complications, graft,
      vascular
  bone
    device NEC T84.9
      embolism T84.81
      fibrosis T84.82
      hemorrhage T84.83
      infection or inflammation T84.7
      mechanical
        breakdown T84.318
        displacement T84.328
        malposition T84.328
        obstruction T84.398
        perforation T84.398
        protrusion T84.398
      pain T84.84
      specified type NEC T84.89
      stenosis T84.85
      thrombosis T84.86
    graft — see Complications, graft, bone
    growth stimulator (electrode) — see
      Complications, electronic stimulator
      device, bone
    marrow transplant — see Complications,
      transplant, bone, marrow
  brain neurostimulator (electrode) — see
      Complications, electronic stimulator device,
      brain
  breast implant (prosthetic) T85.89
    capsular contracture T85.44

Complication— *continued*
  breast implant— *continued*
    embolism T85.81
    fibrosis T85.82
    hemorrhage T85.83
    infection and inflammation T85.79
    mechanical
      breakdown T85.41
      displacement T85.42
      leakage T85.43
      malposition T85.42
      obstruction T85.49
      perforation T85.49
      protrusion T85.49
      specified NEC T85.49
    pain T85.84
    specified type NEC T85.89
    stenosis T85.85
    thrombosis T85.86
  bypass (see also Complications, prosthetic device or
      implant)
    aortocoronary — see Complications, coronary
      artery (bypass) graft
    arterial (see also Complications, graft, vascular)
      extremity — see Complications, extremity
        artery (bypass) graft
  cardiac (see also Disease, heart)
    device, implant or graft T82.9
      embolism T82.817
      fibrosis T82.827
      hemorrhage T82.837
      infection or inflammation T82.7
        valve prosthesis T82.6
      mechanical
        breakdown T82.519
          specified device NEC T82.518
        displacement T82.529
          specified device NEC T82.528
        leakage T82.539
          specified device NEC T82.538
        malposition T82.529
          specified device NEC T82.528
        obstruction T82.599
          specified device NEC T82.598
        perforation T82.599
          specified device NEC T82.598
        protrusion T82.599
          specified device NEC T82.598
      pain T82.847
      specified type NEC T82.897
      stenosis T82.857
      thrombosis T82.867
  cardiovascular device, graft or implant T82.9
    arteriovenous
      fistula, artificial — see Complication,
        arteriovenous, fistula, surgically created
      shunt — see Complication, arteriovenous,
        shunt, surgically created
    aortic graft — see Complications, graft, vascular
    artificial heart — see Complication, artificial,
      heart
    balloon (counterpulsation) device — see
      Complication, balloon implant, vascular
    carotid artery graft — see Complications, graft,
      vascular
    coronary bypass graft — see Complication,
      coronary artery (bypass) graft
    dialysis catheter (vascular) — see Complication,
      catheter, dialysis
    electronic T82.9
      electrode T82.9
        embolism T82.817
        fibrosis T82.827
        hemorrhage T82.837
        infection T82.7
        mechanical
          breakdown T82.110
          displacement T82.120
          leakage T82.190
          obstruction T82.190
          perforation T82.190
          protrusion T82.190
          specified type NEC T82.190

Complication— *continued*
  cardiovascular device, graft or implant— *continued*
    electronic— *continued*
      electrode— *continued*
        pain T82.847
        specified NEC T82.897
        stenosis T82.857
        thrombosis T82.867
      embolism T82.817
      fibrosis T82.827
      hemorrhage T82.837
      infection T82.7
      mechanical
        breakdown T82.119
        displacement T82.129
        leakage T82.199
        obstruction T82.199
        perforation T82.199
        protrusion T82.199
        specified type NEC T82.199
      pain T82.847
      pulse generator T82.9
        embolism T82.817
        fibrosis T82.827
        hemorrhage T82.837
        infection T82.7
        mechanical
          breakdown T82.111
          displacement T82.121
          leakage T82.191
          obstruction T82.191
          perforation T82.191
          protrusion T82.191
          specified type NEC T82.191
        pain T82.847
        specified NEC T82.897
        stenosis T82.857
        thrombosis T82.867
      specified condition NEC T82.897
      specified device NEC T82.9
        embolism T82.817
        fibrosis T82.827
        hemorrhage T82.837
        infection T82.7
        mechanical
          breakdown T82.118
          displacement T82.128
          leakage T82.198
          obstruction T82.198
          perforation T82.198
          protrusion T82.198
          specified type NEC T82.198
        pain T82.847
        specified NEC T82.897
        stenosis T82.857
        thrombosis T82.867
      stenosis T82.857
      thrombosis T82.867
    extremity artery graft — see Complication,
      extremity artery (bypass) graft
    femoral artery graft — see Complication,
      extremity artery (bypass) graft
    heart-lung transplant — see Complication,
      transplant, heart, with lung
    heart
      transplant — see Complication, transplant,
        heart
      valve — see Complication, prosthetic device,
        heart valve
        graft — see Complication, heart, valve,
          graft
    infection or inflammation T82.7
    umbrella device — see Complication, umbrella
      device, vascular
    vascular graft (or anastomosis) — see
      Complication, graft, vascular
  carotid artery (bypass) graft — see Complications,
      graft, vascular
  catheter (device) NEC (see also Complications,
      prosthetic device or implant)
    cystostomy T83.89
      embolism T83.81
      fibrosis T83.82

Complication— *continued*
  catheter— *continued*
    cystostomy— *continued*
      hemorrhage T83.83
      infection and inflammation T83.59
      mechanical
        breakdown T83.010
        displacement T83.020
        leakage T83.030
        malposition T83.020
        obstruction T83.090
        perforation T83.090
        protrusion T83.090
        specified NEC T83.090
      pain T83.84
      specified type NEC T83.89
      stenosis T83.85
      thrombosis T83.86
    dialysis (vascular) T82.9
      embolism T82.818
      fibrosis T82.828
      hemorrhage T82.838
      infection and inflammation T82.7
      intraperitoneal — *see* Complications, catheter,
        intraperitoneal
      mechanical
        breakdown T82.41
        displacement T82.42
        leakage T82.43
        malposition T82.42
        obstruction T82.49
        perforation T82.49
        protrusion T82.49
      pain T82.848
      specified type NEC T82.898
      stenosis T82.858
      thrombosis T82.868
    epidural infusion T85.89
      embolism T85.81
      fibrosis T85.82
      hemorrhage T85.83
      infection and inflammation T85.79
      mechanical
        breakdown T85.610
        displacement T85.620
        leakage T85.630
        malfunction T85.610
        malposition T85.620
        obstruction T85.690
        perforation T85.690
        protrusion T85.690
        specified NEC T85.690
      pain T85.84
      specified type NEC T85.89
      stenosis T85.85
      thrombosis T85.86
    intraperitoneal dialysis T85.89
      embolism T85.81
      fibrosis T85.82
      hemorrhage T85.83
      infection and inflammation T85.71
      mechanical
        breakdown T85.611
        displacement T85.621
        leakage T85.631
        malfunction T85.611
        malposition T85.621
        obstruction T85.691
        perforation T85.691
        protrusion T85.691
        specified NEC T85.691
      pain T85.84
      specified type NEC T85.89
      stenosis T85.85
      thrombosis T85.86
    intravenous infusion T82.9
      embolism T82.818
      fibrosis T82.828
      hemorrhage T82.838
      infection or inflammation T82.7
      mechanical
        breakdown T82.514
        displacement T82.524

Complication— *continued*
  catheter— *continued*
    intravenous infusion— *continued*
      mechanical— *continued*
        leakage T82.534
        malposition T82.524
        obstruction T82.594
        perforation T82.594
        protrusion T82.594
      pain T82.848
      specified type NEC T82.898
      stenosis T82.858
      thrombosis T82.868
    subdural infusion T85.89
      embolism T85.81
      fibrosis T85.82
      hemorrhage T85.83
      infection and inflammation T85.79
      mechanical
        breakdown T85.610
        displacement T85.620
        leakage T85.630
        malfunction T85.610
        malposition T85.620
        obstruction T85.690
        perforation T85.690
        protrusion T85.690
        specified NEC T85.690
      pain T85.84
      specified type NEC T85.89
      stenosis T85.85
      thrombosis T85.86
    urethral, indwelling T83.89
      displacement T83.028
      embolism T83.81
      fibrosis T83.82
      hemorrhage T83.83
      infection and inflammation T83.51
      leakage T83.028
      malposition T83.028
      mechanical
        breakdown T83.018
      obstruction (mechanical) T83.098
      pain T83.84
      perforation T83.098
      protrusion T83.098
      specified type NEC T83.098
      stenosis T83.85
      thrombosis T83.86
    urinary (indwelling) — *see* Complications,
      catheter, urethral, indwelling
  cecostomy (stoma) — *see* Complications, colostomy
  cesarean delivery wound NEC O90.89
    disruption O90.0
    hematoma O90.2
    infection (following delivery) O86.0
  chemotherapy (antineoplastic) NEC T88.7—This
    code not for use in the inpatient setting
  chin implant (prosthetic) — *see* Complication,
    prosthetic device or implant, specified NEC
  circulatory system I99.8
    intraoperative I97.88
    postprocedural I97.89
      following cardiac surgery I97.19-
        postcardiotomy syndrome I97.0
      lymphedema after mastectomy I97.2
      hypertension I97.3
      specified NEC I97.89
  colostomy (stoma) K94.00
    hemorrhage K94.01
    infection K94.02
    malfunction K94.03
    mechanical K94.03
    specified complication NEC K94.09
  contraceptive device, intrauterine — *see*
    Complications, intrauterine, contraceptive
    device
  cord (umbilical) — *see* Complications, umbilical cord
  corneal graft — *see* Complications, graft, cornea
  coronary artery (bypass) graft T82.9
    atherosclerosis — *see* Arteriosclerosis, coronary
      (artery),

Complication— *continued*
  coronary artery— *continued*
    embolism T82.818
    fibrosis T82.828
    hemorrhage T82.838
    infection and inflammation T82.7
    mechanical
      breakdown T82.211
      displacement T82.212
      leakage T82.213
      malposition T82.212
      obstruction T82.218
      perforation T82.218
      protrusion T82.218
      specified NEC T82.218
    pain T82.848
    specified type NEC T82.897
    stenosis T82.858
    thrombosis T82.868
  counterpulsation device (balloon), intraaortic — *see*
    Complications, balloon implant, vascular
  cystostomy (stoma) N99.518
    catheter — *see* Complications, catheter,
      cystostomy
    hemorrhage N99.510
    infection N99.511
    malfunction N99.512
    specified type NEC N99.518
  delivery (*see also* Complications, obstetric) O75.9
    procedure (instrumental) (manual) (surgical)
      O75.4
    specified NEC O75.89
  dialysis (peritoneal) (renal) (*see also* Complications,
    infusion)
    catheter (vascular) — *see* Complication, catheter,
      dialysis
      peritoneal, intraperitoneal — *see*
        Complications, catheter, intraperitoneal
  dorsal column (spinal) neurostimulator — *see*
    Complications, electronic stimulator device,
    spinal cord
  drug NEC T88.7—This code not for use in the
    inpatient setting
  ear procedure (*see also* Disorder, ear)
    intraoperative H95.88-
      hematoma — *see* Complications,
        intraoperative, hemorrhage
        (hematoma) (of), ear
      hemorrhage — *see* Complications,
        intraoperative, hemorrhage
        (hematoma) (of), ear
      laceration — *see* Complications,
        intraoperative, puncture or laceration,
        ear
      specified NEC H95.88-
    postoperative H95.89-
      external ear canal stenosis H95.81-
      hematoma — *see* Complications,
        postprocedural, hemorrhage
        (hematoma) (of), ear
      hemorrhage — *see* Complications,
        postprocedural, hemorrhage
        (hematoma) (of), ear
      postmastoidectomy — *see* Complications,
        postmastoidectomy
      specified NEC H95.89-
  ectopic pregnancy O08.9
    damage to pelvic organs O08.6
    embolism O08.2
    genital infection O08.0
    hemorrhage (delayed) (excessive) O08.1
    metabolic disorder O08.5
    renal failure O08.4
    shock O08.3
    specified type NEC O08.0
    venous complication NEC O08.7
  electronic stimulator device
    bladder (urinary) — *see* Complications, electronic
      stimulator device, urinary
    bone T84.89
      breakdown T84.310
      displacement T84.320
      embolism T84.81

Complication— *continued*
  electronic stimulator device — *continued*
    bone— *continued*
      fibrosis T84.82
      hemorrhage T84.83
      infection or inflammation T84.7
      malfunction T84.31Ø
      malposition T84.32Ø
      mechanical NEC T84.39Ø
      obstruction T84.39Ø
      pain T84.84
      perforation T84.39Ø
      protrusion T84.39Ø
      specified type NEC T84.89
      stenosis T84.85
      thrombosis T84.86
    brain T85.89
      embolism T85.81
      fibrosis T85.82
      hemorrhage T85.83
      infection and inflammation T85.79
      mechanical
        breakdown T85.11Ø
        displacement T85.12Ø
        leakage T85.19Ø
        malposition T85.12Ø
        obstruction T85.19Ø
        perforation T85.19Ø
        protrusion T85.19Ø
        specified NEC T85.19Ø
      pain T85.84
      specified type NEC T85.89
      stenosis T85.85
      thrombosis T85.86
    cardiac (defibrillator) (pacemaker) — *see*
      Complications, cardiovascular device or
      implant, electronic
    muscle T84.89
      breakdown T84.418
      displacement T84.428
      embolism T84.81
      fibrosis T84.82
      hemorrhage T84.83
      infection or inflammation T84.7
      mechanical NEC T84.498
      pain T84.84
      specified type NEC T84.89
      stenosis T84.85
      thrombosis T84.86
    nervous system T85.9
      brain — *see* Complications, electronic
        stimulator device, brain
      embolism T85.81
      fibrosis T85.82
      hemorrhage T85.83
      infection and inflammation T85.79
      mechanical
        breakdown T85.118
        displacement T85.128
        leakage T85.199
        malposition T85.128
        obstruction T85.199
        perforation T85.199
        protrusion T85.199
        specified NEC T85.199
      pain T85.84
      peripheral nerve — *see* Complications,
        electronic stimulator device, peripheral
        nerve
      specified type NEC T85.89
      spinal cord — *see* Complications, electronic
        stimulator device, spinal cord
      stenosis T85.85
      thrombosis T85.86
    peripheral nerve T85.89
      embolism T85.81
      fibrosis T85.82
      hemorrhage T85.83
      infection and inflammation T85.79
      mechanical
        breakdown T85.111
        displacement T85.121
        leakage T85.191

Complication— *continued*
  electronic stimulator device — *continued*
    peripheral nerve — *continued*
      mechanical— *continued*
        malposition T85.121
        obstruction T85.191
        perforation T85.191
        protrusion T85.191
        specified NEC T85.191
      pain T85.84
      specified type NEC T85.89
      stenosis T85.85
      thrombosis T85.86
    spinal cord T85.89
      embolism T85.81
      fibrosis T85.82
      hemorrhage T85.83
      infection and inflammation T85.79
      mechanical
        breakdown T85.112
        displacement T85.122
        leakage T85.192
        malposition T85.122
        obstruction T85.192
        perforation T85.192
        protrusion T85.192
        specified NEC T85.192
      pain T85.84
      specified type NEC T85.89
      stenosis T85.85
      thrombosis T85.86
    urinary T83.9
      embolism T83.81
      fibrosis T83.82
      hemorrhage T83.83
      infection and inflammation T83.59
      mechanical
        breakdown T83.11Ø
        displacement T83.12Ø
        malposition T83.12Ø
        perforation T83.19Ø
        protrusion T83.19Ø
        specified NEC T83.19Ø
      pain T83.84
      specified type NEC T83.89
      stenosis T83.85
      thrombosis T83.86
  electroshock therapy T88.9
    specified NEC T88.8
  endocrine E34.9
    postprocedural
      adrenal hypofunction E89.6
      hypoinsulinemia E89.1
      hypoparathyroidism E89.2
      hypopituitarism E89.3
      hypothyroidism E89.Ø
      ovarian failure E89.4Ø
        asymptomatic E89.4Ø
        symptomatic E89.41
      specified NEC E89.89
      testicular hypofunction E89.5
  endodontic treatment NEC M27.59
  enterostomy (stoma) K94.1Ø
    hemorrhage K94.11
    infection K94.12
    malfunction K94.13
    mechanical K94.13
    specified complication NEC K94.19
  episiotomy, disruption O9Ø.1
  esophageal anti-reflux device T85.89
    embolism T85.81
    fibrosis T85.82
    hemorrhage T85.83
    infection and inflammation T85.79
    mechanical
      breakdown T85.511
      displacement T85.521
      malfunction T85.511
      malposition T85.521
      obstruction T85.591
      perforation T85.591
      protrusion T85.591
      specified NEC T85.591

Complication— *continued*
  esophageal anti-reflux device— *continued*
    pain T85.84
    specified type NEC T85.89
    stenosis T85.85
    thrombosis T85.86
  esophagostomy K94.3Ø
    hemorrhage K94.31
    infection K94.32
    malfunction K94.33
    mechanical K94.33
    specified complication NEC K94.39
  extracorporeal circulation T8Ø.9Ø
  extremity artery (bypass) graft T82.9
    arteriosclerosis — *see* Arteriosclerosis,
      extremities, bypass graft
    embolism T82.818
    fibrosis T82.828
    hemorrhage T82.838
    infection and inflammation T82.7
    mechanical
      breakdown T82.318
        femoral artery T82.312
      displacement T82.328
        femoral artery T82.322
      leakage T82.338
        femoral artery T82.332
      malposition T82.328
        femoral artery T82.322
      obstruction T82.398
        femoral artery T82.392
      perforation T82.398
        femoral artery T82.392
      protrusion T82.398
        femoral artery T82.392
    pain T82.848
    specified type NEC T82.898
    stenosis T82.858
    thrombosis T82.868
  eye H57.9
    corneal graft — *see* Complications, graft, cornea
    implant (prosthetic) T85.89
      embolism T85.81
      fibrosis T85.82
      hemorrhage T85.83
      infection and inflammation T85.79
      mechanical
        breakdown T85.318
        displacement T85.328
        leakage T85.398
        malposition T85.328
        obstruction T85.398
        perforation T85.398
        protrusion T85.398
        specified NEC T85.398
      pain T85.84
      specified type NEC T85.89
      stenosis T85.85
      thrombosis T85.86
    intraocular lens — *see* Complications, intraocular
      lens
    orbital prosthesis — *see* Complications, orbital
      prosthesis
  female genital N94.9
    device, implant or graft NEC — *see*
      Complications, genitourinary, device or
      implant, genital tract
  femoral artery (bypass) graft — *see* Complication,
    extremity artery (bypass) graft
  fixation device, internal (orthopedic) T84.9
    infection and inflammation T84.6Ø
      arm T84.61-
        humerus T84.61-
        radius T84.61-
        ulna T84.61-
      leg T84.629
        femur T84.62-
        fibula T84.62-
        tibia T84.62-
      specified site NEC T84.69
      spine T84.63

Complication— *continued*
  fixation device, internal (orthopedic)— *continued*
    mechanical
      breakdown
        limb T84.119
          carpal T84.210
          femur T84.11-
          fibula T84.11-
          humerus T84.11-
          metacarpal T84.210
          metatarsal T84.213
          phalanx
            foot T84.213
            hand T84.210
          radius T84.11-
          tarsal T84.213
          ulna T84.11-
          tibia T84.11-
        specified bone NEC T84.218
        spine T84.216
      displacement
        limb T84.129
          carpal T84.220
          femur T84.12-
          fibula T84.12-
          humerus T84.12-
          metacarpal T84.220
          metatarsal T84.223
          phalanx
            foot T84.223
            hand T84.220
          radius T84.12-
          tarsal T84.223
          ulna T84.12-
          tibia T84.12-
        specified bone NEC T84.228
        spine T84.226
      malposition — *see* Complications, fixation
          device, internal, mechanical,
          displacement
      obstruction — *see* Complications, fixation
          device, internal, mechanical, specified
          type NEC
      perforation — *see* Complications, fixation
          device, internal, mechanical, specified
          type NEC
      protrusion — *see* Complications, fixation
          device, internal, mechanical, specified
          type NEC
      specified type NEC
        limb T84.199
          carpal T84.290
          femur T84.19-
          fibula T84.19-
          humerus T84.19-
          metacarpal T84.290
          metatarsal T84.293
          phalanx
            foot T84.293
            hand T84.290
          radius T84.19-
          tarsal T84.293
          tibia T84.19-
          ulna T84.19-
        specified bone NEC T84.298
        vertebra T84.296
    specified type NEC T84.89
      embolism T84.81
      fibrosis T84.82
      hemorrhage T84.83
      pain T84.84
      specified complication NEC T84.89
      stenosis T84.85
      thrombosis T84.86
  following
    acute myocardial infarction NEC I23.8
      aneurysm (false) (of cardiac wall) (of heart
          wall) (ruptured) I23.3
      angina I23.7
      atrial
        septal defect I23.1
        thrombosis I23.6
      cardiac wall rupture I23.3

Complication— *continued*
  following— *continued*
    acute myocardial infarction— *continued*
      chordae tendinae rupture I23.4
      defect
        septal
          atrial (heart) I23.1
          ventricular (heart) I23.2
      hemopericardium I23.0
      papillary muscle rupture I23.5
      rupture
        cardiac wall I23.3
          with hemopericardium I23.0
        chordae tendineae I23.4
        papillary muscle I23.5
      specified NEC I23.8
      thrombosis
        atrium I23.6
        auricular appendage I23.6
        ventricle (heart) I23.6
      ventricular
        septal defect I23.2
        thrombosis I23.6
    ectopic or molar pregnancy O08.9
      cardiac arrest O08.81
      sepsis O08.82
      specified type NEC O08.89
      urinary tract infection O08.83
  gastrointestinal K92.9
    bile duct prosthesis — *see* Complications, bile
        duct implant
    esophageal anti-reflux device — *see*
        Complications, esophageal anti-reflux
        device
    postoperative
      colostomy — *see* Complications, colostomy
      dumping syndrome K91.1
      enterostomy — *see* Complications,
          enterostomy
      gastrostomy — *see* Complications,
          gastrostomy
      malabsorption NEC K91.2
      obstruction K91.3
      postcholecystectomy syndrome K91.5
      specified NEC K91.89
      vomiting after GI surgery K91.0
    prosthetic device or implant
      bile duct prosthesis — *see* Complications, bile
          duct implant
      esophageal anti-reflux device — *see*
          Complications, esophageal anti-reflux
          device
      specified type NEC
        embolism T85.81
        fibrosis T85.82
        hemorrhage T85.83
        mechanical
          breakdown T85.518
          displacement T85.528
          malfunction T85.518
          malposition T85.528
          obstruction T85.598
          perforation T85.598
          protrusion T85.598
          specified NEC T85.598
        pain T85.84
        specified complication NEC T85.89
        stenosis T85.85
        thrombosis T85.86
  gastrostomy (stoma) K94.20
    hemorrhage K94.21
    infection K94.22
    malfunction K94.23
    mechanical K94.23
    specified complication NEC K94.29
  genitourinary
    device or implant T83.9
      genital tract T83.9
        infection or inflammation T83.6
        intrauterine contraceptive device — *see*
            Complications, intrauterine,
            contraceptive device

Complication— *continued*
  genitourinary— *continued*
    device or implant— *continued*
      genital tract— *continued*
        mechanical — *see* Complications, by
            device, mechanical
        penile prosthesis — *see* Complications,
            prosthetic device, penile
        specified type NEC T83.89
          embolism T83.81
          fibrosis T83.82
          hemorrhage T83.83
          pain T83.84
          specified complication NEC T83.89
          stenosis T83.85
          thrombosis T83.86
      urinary system T83.9
        cystostomy catheter — *see* Complication,
            catheter, cystostomy
        electronic stimulator — *see*
            Complications, electronic stimulator
            device, urinary
        indwelling urethral catheter — *see*
            Complications, catheter, urethral,
            indwelling
        infection or inflammation T83.59
          indwelling urinary catheter T83.51
        kidney transplant — *see* Complication,
            transplant, kidney
        organ graft — *see* Complication, graft,
            urinary organ
        specified type NEC T83.89
          embolism T83.81
          fibrosis T83.82
          hemorrhage T83.83
          mechanical T83.198
            breakdown T83.118
            displacement T83.128
            malfunction T83.118
            malposition T83.128
            obstruction T83.198
            perforation T83.198
            protrusion T83.198
            specified NEC T83.198
          pain T83.84
          specified complication NEC T83.89
          stenosis T83.85
          thrombosis T83.86
        sphincter implant — *see* Complications,
            implant, urinary sphincter
    postprocedural
      pelvic peritoneal adhesions N99.4
      renal failure N99.0
      specified NEC N99.89
      stoma — *see* Complications, stoma, urinary
          tract
      urethral stricture — *see* Stricture, urethra,
          postprocedural
      vaginal
        adhesions N99.2
        vault prolapse N99.3
  graft (bypass) (patch) (*see also* Complications,
      prosthetic device or implant)
    aorta — *see* Complications, graft, vascular
    arterial — *see* Complication, graft, vascular
    bone T86.839
      failure T86.831
      infection T86.832
      mechanical T84.318
        breakdown T84.318
        displacement T84.328
        protrusion T84.398
        specified type NEC T84.398
      rejection T86.830
      specified type NEC T86.838
    carotid artery — *see* Complications, graft,
        vascular
    cornea T86.849
      failure T86.841
      infection T86.842
      mechanical T85.318
        breakdown T85.318
        displacement T85.328

Complication— *continued*
  graft— *continued*
    cornea— *continued*
      mechanical— *continued*
        protrusion T85.398
        specified type NEC T85.398
      rejection T86.840
      specified type NEC T86.848
    femoral artery (bypass) — *see* Complication,
      extremity artery (bypass) graft
    genital organ or tract — *see* Complications,
      genitourinary, device or implant, genital
      tract
    muscle T84.9
      breakdown T84.410
      displacement T84.420
      embolism T84.81
      fibrosis T84.82
      hemorrhage T84.83
      infection and inflammation T84.7
      mechanical NEC T84.490
      pain T84.84
      specified type NEC T84.89
      stenosis T84.85
      thrombosis T84.86
    nerve — *see* Complication, prosthetic device or
      implant, specified NEC
    skin — *see* Complications, prosthetic device or
      implant, skin graft
    tendon T84.89
      breakdown T84.410
      displacement T84.420
      embolism T84.81
      fibrosis T84.82
      hemorrhage T84.83
      infection and inflammation T84.7
      mechanical NEC T84.490
      pain T84.84
      specified type NEC T84.89
      stenosis T84.85
      thrombosis T84.86
    urinary organ T83.89
      embolism T83.81
      fibrosis T83.82
      hemorrhage T83.83
      infection and inflammation T83.59
        indwelling urinary catheter T83.51
      mechanical
        breakdown T83.21
        displacement T83.22
        leakage T83.23
        malposition T83.22
        obstruction T83.29
        perforation T83.29
        protrusion T83.29
        specified NEC T83.29
      pain T83.84
      specified type NEC T83.89
      stenosis T83.85
      thrombosis T83.86
    vascular T82.9
      embolism T82.818
      femoral artery — *see* Complication, extremity
        artery (bypass) graft
      fibrosis T82.828
      hemorrhage T82.838
      mechanical
        breakdown T82.319
          aorta (bifurcation) T82.310
          carotid artery T82.311
          specified vessel NEC T82.318
        displacement T82.329
          aorta (bifurcation) T82.320
          carotid artery T82.321
          specified vessel NEC T82.328
        leakage T82.339
          aorta (bifurcation) T82.330
          carotid artery T82.331
          specified vessel NEC T82.338
        malposition T82.329
          aorta (bifurcation) T82.320
          carotid artery T82.321
          specified vessel NEC T82.328

Complication— *continued*
  graft— *continued*
    vascular— *continued*
      mechanical— *continued*
        obstruction T82.399
          aorta (bifurcation) T82.390
          carotid artery T82.391
          specified vessel NEC T82.398
        perforation T82.399
          aorta (bifurcation) T82.390
          carotid artery T82.391
          specified vessel NEC T82.398
        protrusion T82.399
          aorta (bifurcation) T82.390
          carotid artery T82.391
          specified vessel NEC T82.398
      pain T82.848
      specified complication NEC T82.898
      stenosis T82.858
      thrombosis T82.868
  heart I51.9
    assist device
      infection and inflammation T82.7
    following acute myocardial infarction — *see*
      Complications, following, acute myocardial
      infarction
    postoperative — *see* Complications, circulatory
      system
    transplant — *see* Complication, transplant, heart
      and lung(s) — *see* Complications, transplant,
      heart, with lung
    valve
      graft (biological) T82.9
        embolism T82.817
        fibrosis T82.827
        hemorrhage T82.837
        infection and inflammation T82.7
        mechanical T82.228
          breakdown T82.221
          displacement T82.222
          leakage T82.223
          malposition T82.222
          obstruction T82.218
          perforation T82.228
          protrusion T82.228
        pain T82.847
        specified type NEC T82.897
        stenosis T82.857
        thrombosis T82.867
      prosthesis T82.09
        embolism T82.817
        fibrosis T82.827
        hemorrhage T82.837
        infection or inflammation T82.6
        mechanical T82.01
          breakdown T82.01
          displacement T82.02
          leakage T82.03
          malposition T82.02
          obstruction T82.09
          perforation T82.09
          protrusion T82.09
        pain T82.847
        specified type NEC T82.897
          mechanical T82.09
        stenosis T82.857
        thrombosis T82.867
  hematoma — *see* Complication
  hemodialysis — *see* Complications, dialysis
  ileostomy (stoma) — *see* Complications,
    enterostomy
  immunization (procedure) — *see* Complications,
    vaccination
  implant (*see also* Complications, by site and type)
    urinary sphincter T83.9
      embolism T83.81
      fibrosis T83.82
      hemorrhage T83.83
      infection and inflammation T83.59
      mechanical
        breakdown T83.111
        displacement T83.121
        leakage T83.191

Complication— *continued*
  implant— *continued*
    urinary sphincter— *continued*
      mechanical— *continued*
        malposition T83.121
        obstruction T83.191
        perforation T83.191
        protrusion T83.191
        specified NEC T83.191
      pain T83.84
      specified type NEC T83.89
      stenosis T83.85
      thrombosis T83.86
  infusion (procedure) T80.90
    air embolism T80.0
    blood — *see* Complications, transfusion
    catheter — *see* Complications, catheter
    infection T80.29
    pump — *see* Complications, cardiovascular,
      device or implant
    sepsis T80.29
    serum reaction T80.6
      anaphylactic shock T80.5
    specified type NEC T80.89
  inhalation therapy NEC T81.81
  injection (procedure) T80.90
    drug reaction — *see* Reaction, drug
    infection T80.29
    sepsis T80.29
    serum (prophylactic) (therapeutic) — *see*
      Complications, vaccination
    specified type NEC T80.89
    vaccine (any) — *see* Complications, vaccination
  inoculation (any) — *see* Complications, vaccination
  insulin pump
    infection and inflammation T85.72
    mechanical
      breakdown T85.614
      displacement T85.624
      leakage T85.633
      malposition T85.624
      obstruction T85.694
      perforation T85.694
      protrusion T85.694
      specified NEC T85.694
  intestinal pouch NEC K91.858
  intraocular lens (prosthetic) T85.89
    embolism T85.81
    fibrosis T85.82
    hemorrhage T85.83
    infection and inflammation T85.79
    mechanical
      breakdown T85.21
      displacement T85.22
      malposition T85.22
      obstruction T85.29
      perforation T85.29
      protrusion T85.29
      specified NEC T85.29
    pain T85.84
    specified type NEC T85.89
    stenosis T85.85
    thrombosis T85.86
  intraoperative (intraprocedural)
    cardiac arrest
      during cardiac surgery I97.710
      during other surgery I97.711
    cardiac functional disturbance NEC
      during cardiac surgery I97.790
      during other surgery I97.791
    hemorrhage (hematoma) (of)
      circulatory system organ or structure
        during cardiac bypass I97.411
        during cardiac catheterization I97.410
        during other circulatory system procedure
          I97.418
        during other procedure I97.42
      digestive system organ
        during procedure on digestive system
          K91.61
        during procedure on other organ K91.62

Complication— *continued*
  intraoperative — *continued*
    hemorrhage— *continued*
      ear
        during procedure on ear and mastoid
          process H95.21
        during procedure on other organ H95.22
      endocrine system organ or structure
        during procedure on endocrine system
          organ or structure E36.01
        during procedure on other organ E36.02
      eye and adnexa
        during ophthalmic procedure H59.11-
        during other procedure H59.12-
      genitourinary organ or structure
        during procedure on genitourinary organ
          or structure N99.61
        during procedure on other organ N99.62
      mastoid process
        during procedure on ear and mastoid
          process H95.21
        during procedure on other organ H95.22
      musculoskeletal structure
        during musculoskeletal surgery M96.810
        during non-orthopedic surgery M96.811
        during orthopedic surgery M96.810
      nervous system
        during a nervous system procedure
          G97.31
        during other procedure G97.32
      respiratory system
        during procedure on respiratory system
          organ or structure J95.61
        during other procedure J95.62
      skin and subcutaneous tissue
        during a dermatologic procedure L76.01
        during a procedure on other organ L76.02
      spleen
        during a procedure on the spleen D78.01
        during a procedure on other organ D78.02
    puncture or laceration (accidental)
      (unintentional) (of)
      brain
        during a nervous system procedure
          G97.48
        during other procedure G97.49
      circulatory system organ or structure
        during circulatory system procedure
          I97.51
        during other procedure I97.52
      digestive system
        during procedure on digestive system
          K91.71
        during procedure on other organ K91.72
      ear
        during procedure on ear and mastoid
          process H95.31
        during procedure on other organ H95.32
      endocrine system organ or structure
        during procedure on endocrine system
          organ or structure E36.11
        during procedure on other organ E36.12
      eye and adnexa
        during ophthalmic procedure H59.21-
        during other procedure H59.22-
      genitourinary organ or structure
        during procedure on genitourinary organ
          or structure N99.71
        during procedure on other organ N99.72
      mastoid process
        during procedure on ear and mastoid
          process H95.31
        during procedure on other organ H95.32
      musculoskeletal structure
        during musculoskeletal surgery M96.820
        during non-orthopedic surgery M96.821
        during orthopedic surgery M96.820
      nervous system
        during a nervous system procedure
          G97.48
        during other procedure G97.49

Complication— *continued*
  intraoperative — *continued*
    puncture or laceration— *continued*
      respiratory system
        during procedure on respiratory system
          organ or structure J95.71
        during other procedure J95.72
      skin and subcutaneous tissue
        during a dermatologic procedure L76.11
        during a procedure on other organ L76.12
      spleen
        during a procedure on the spleen D78.11
        during a procedure on other organ D78.12
    specified NEC
      circulatory system I97.88
      digestive system K91.81
      ear H95.88
      endocrine system E36.8
      eye and adnexa H59.88
      genitourinary system N99.81
      mastoid process H95.88
      nervous system G97.81
      respiratory system J95.88
      skin and subcutaneous tissue L76.81
      spleen D78.81
  intraperitoneal catheter (dialysis) (infusion) — *see*
    Complications, catheter, intraperitoneal
  intrauterine
    contraceptive device
      embolism T83.81
      fibrosis T83.82
      hemorrhage T83.83
      infection and inflammation T83.6
      mechanical
        breakdown T83.31
        displacement T83.32
        malposition T83.32
        obstruction T83.39
        perforation T83.39
        protrusion T83.39
        specified NEC T83.39
      pain T83.84
      specified type NEC T83.89
      stenosis T83.85
      thrombosis T83.86
    procedure (fetal), to newborn P96.5
  jejunostomy (stoma) — *see* Complications,
    enterostomy
  joint prosthesis, internal T84.9
    breakage (fracture) T84.01-
    dislocation T84.02-
    fracture T84.01-
    instability T84.02-
    subluxation T84.02-
    infection or inflammation T84.50
      hip T84.5-
      knee T84.5-
      specified joint NEC T84.59
    malposition — *see* Complications, joint
      prosthesis, mechanical, displacement
    mechanical
      breakage, broken T84.01-
      dislocation T84.02-
      fracture T84.01-
      instability T84.02-
      subluxation T84.02-
      leakage — *see* Complications, joint prosthesis,
        mechanical, specified NEC
      loosening T84.039
        hip T84.03-
        knee T84.03-
        specified joint NEC T84.038
      obstruction — *see* Complications, joint
        prosthesis, mechanical, specified NEC
      perforation — *see* Complications, joint
        prosthesis, mechanical, specified NEC
      periprosthetic
        osteolysis T84.059
          hip T84.05-
          knee T84.05-
          other specified joint T84.058
        fracture T84.049

Complication— *continued*
  joint prosthesis, internal— *continued*
    mechanical— *continued*
      periprosthetic— *continued*
        fracture— *continued*
          hip T84.04-
          knee T84.04-
          other specified joint T84.048
        protrusion — *see* Complications, joint
          prosthesis, mechanical, specified NEC
        specified complication NEC T84.099
          hip T84.09-
          knee T84.09-
          other specified joint T84.098
        wear of articular bearing surface T84.069
          hip T84.06-
          knee T84.069
          other specified joint T84.068
      specified joint NEC T84.89
      embolism T84.81
      fibrosis T84.82
      hemorrhage T84.83
      pain T84.84
      specified complication NEC T84.89
      stenosis T84.85
      thrombosis T84.86
  kidney transplant — *see* Complications, transplant,
    kidney
  labor O75.9
    specified NEC O75.89
  liver transplant (immune or nonimmune) — *see*
    Complications, transplant, liver
  lumbar puncture G97.1
    cerebrospinal fluid leak G97.0
    headache or reaction G97.1
  lung transplant — *see* Complications, transplant,
    lung
    and heart — *see* Complications, transplant, lung,
      with heart
  male genital N50.9
    device, implant or graft — *see* Complications,
      genitourinary, device or implant, genital
      tract
    postprocedural or postoperative — *see*
      Complications, genitourinary,
      postprocedural
    specified NEC N99.89
  mastoid (process) procedure
    intraoperative H95.88-
      hematoma — *see* Complications,
        intraoperative, hemorrhage
        (hematoma) (of), mastoid process
      hemorrhage — *see* Complications,
        intraoperative, hemorrhage
        (hematoma) (of), mastoid process
      laceration — *see* Complications,
        intraoperative, puncture or laceration,
        mastoid process
      specified NEC H95.88-
    postmastoidectomy — *see* Complications,
      postmastoidectomy
    postoperative H95.89-
      external ear canal stenosis H95.81-
      hematoma — *see* Complications,
        postprocedural, hemorrhage
        (hematoma) (of), mastoid process
      hemorrhage — *see* Complications,
        postprocedural, hemorrhage
        (hematoma) (of), mastoid process
      postmastoidectomy — *see* Complications,
        postmastoidectomy
      specified NEC H95.89-
  mastoidectomy cavity — *see* Complications,
    postmastoidectomy
  mechanical — *see* Complications, by site and type,
    mechanical
  medical procedures T88.9 (*see also* Complication,
    intraoperative)
  metabolic E88.9
    postoperative E89.89
      specified NEC E89.89

Complication— *continued*
- molar pregnancy NOS O08.9
  - damage to pelvic organs O08.6
  - embolism O08.2
  - genital infection O08.0
  - hemorrhage (delayed) (excessive) O08.1
  - metabolic disorder O08.5
  - renal failure O08.4
  - shock O08.3
  - specified type NEC O08.0
  - venous complication NEC O08.7
- musculoskeletal system (*see also* Complication, intraoperative (intraprocedural), by site)
  - device, implant or graft NEC — *see* Complications, orthopedic, device or implant
  - internal fixation (nail) (plate) (rod) — *see* Complications, fixation device, internal
  - joint prosthesis — *see* Complications, joint prosthesis
  - postoperative (postprocedural) M96.89
    - with osteoporosis — *see* Osteoporosis
    - fracture following insertion of device — *see* Fracture, following insertion of orthopedic implant, joint prosthesis or bone plate
    - joint instability after prosthesis removal M96.89
    - lordosis M96.4
    - postlaminectomy syndrome NEC M96.1
      - kyphosis M96.3
    - pseudarthrosis M96.0
    - specified complication NEC M96.89
  - post radiation M96.89
    - kyphosis M96.3
    - scoliosis M96.5
    - specified complication NEC M96.89
- nephrostomy (stoma) — *see* Complications, stoma, urinary tract, external NEC
- nervous system G98.8
  - central G96.9
  - device, implant or graft (*see also* Complication, prosthetic device or implant, specified NEC)
    - electronic stimulator (electrode(s)) — *see* Complications, electronic stimulator device
    - ventricular shunt — *see* Complications, ventricular shunt
  - electronic stimulator (electrode(s)) — *see* Complications, electronic stimulator device
  - postprocedural G97.82
    - intracranial hypotension G97.2
    - specified NEC G97.82
    - spinal fluid leak G97.0
- newborn, due to intrauterine (fetal) procedure P96.5
- nonabsorbable (permanent) sutures — *see* Complication, sutures, permanent
- obstetric O75.9
  - procedure (instrumental) (manual) (surgical) specified NEC O75.4
  - specified NEC O75.89
  - surgical wound NEC O90.89
    - hematoma O90.2
    - infection O86.0
- ocular lens implant — *see* Complications, intraocular lens
- ophthalmologic
  - postprocedural bleb — *see* Blebitis
- orbital prosthesis T85.89
  - embolism T85.81
  - fibrosis T85.82
  - hemorrhage T85.83
  - infection and inflammation T85.79
  - mechanical
    - breakdown T85.31-
    - displacement T85.32-
    - malposition T85.32-
    - obstruction T85.39-
    - perforation T85.39-
    - protrusion T85.39-
    - specified NEC T85.39-
  - pain T85.84
  - specified type NEC T85.89

Complication— *continued*
- orbital prosthesis— *continued*
  - stenosis T85.85
  - thrombosis T85.86
- organ or tissue transplant (partial) (total) — *see* Complications, transplant
- orthopedic (*see also* Disorder, soft tissue)
  - device or implant T84.9
    - bone
      - device or implant — *see* Complication, bone, device NEC
      - graft — *see* Complication, graft, bone
    - breakdown T84.418
    - displacement T84.428
    - electronic bone stimulator — *see* Complications, electronic stimulator device, bone
    - embolism T84.81
    - fibrosis T84.82
    - fixation device — *see* Complication, fixation device, internal
    - hemorrhage T84.83
    - infection or inflammation T84.7
    - joint prosthesis — *see* Complication, joint prosthesis, internal
    - malfunction T84.418
    - malposition T84.428
    - mechanical NEC T84.498
    - muscle graft — *see* Complications, graft, muscle
    - obstruction T84.498
    - pain T84.84
    - perforation T84.498
    - protrusion T84.498
    - specified complication NEC T84.89
    - stenosis T84.85
    - tendon graft — *see* Complications, graft, tendon
    - thrombosis T84.86
  - fracture (following insertion of device) — *see* Fracture, following insertion of orthopedic implant, joint prosthesis or bone plate
  - postprocedural M96.89
    - fracture — *see* Fracture, following insertion of orthopedic implant, joint prosthesis or bone plate
    - postlaminectomy syndrome NEC M96.1
      - kyphosis M96.3
      - lordosis M96.4
    - postradiation
      - kyphosis M96.2
      - scoliosis M96.5
    - pseudarthrosis post-fusion M96.0
    - specified type NEC M96.89
- pacemaker (cardiac) — *see* Complications, cardiovascular device or implant, electronic
- pancreas transplant — *see* Complications, transplant, pancreas
- penile prosthesis (implant) — *see* Complications, prosthetic device, penile
- perfusion NEC T80.90
- perineal repair (obstetrical) NEC O90.89
  - disruption O90.1
  - hematoma O90.2
  - infection (following delivery) O86.0
- phototherapy T88.9
  - specified NEC T88.8
- postmastoidectomy NEC H95.19-
  - cyst, mucosal H95.13-
  - granulation H95.12-
  - inflammation, chronic H95.11-
  - recurrent cholesteatoma H95.0-
- postoperative — *see* Complications, postprocedural
  - circulatory — *see* Complications, circulatory system
  - ear — *see* Complications, ear
  - endocrine — *see* Complications, endocrine
  - eye — *see* Complications, eye
  - lumbar puncture G97.1
    - cerebrospinal fluid leak G97.0
  - nervous system (central) (peripheral) — *see* Complications, nervous system

Complication— *continued*
- postoperative — *continued*
  - respiratory system — *see* Complications, respiratory system
- postprocedural (*see also* Complications, surgical procedure)
  - cardiac arrest
    - following cardiac surgery I97.120
    - following other surgery I97.121
  - cardiac functional disturbance NEC
    - following cardiac surgery I97.190
    - following other surgery I97.191
  - cardiac insufficiency
    - following cardiac surgery I97.110
    - following other surgery I97.111
  - chorioretinal scars following retinal surgery H59.81-
  - following cataract surgery
    - cataract (lens) fragments H59.02-
    - cystoid macular edema H59.03-
    - specified NEC H59.09-
    - vitreous (touch) syndrome H59.01-
  - heart failure
    - following cardiac surgery I97.130
    - following other surgery I97.131
  - hemorrhage (hematoma) (of)
    - circulatory system organ or structure
      - following a cardiac bypass I97.611
      - following a cardiac catheterization I97.610
      - following other circulatory system procedure I97.618
      - following other procedure I97.62
    - digestive system
      - following procedure on digestive system K91.840
      - following procedure on other organ K91.841
    - ear
      - following procedure on ear and mastoid process H95.41
      - following other procedure H95.42
    - endocrine system
      - following endocrine system procedure E89.810
      - following other procedure E89.811
    - eye and adnexa
      - following ophthalmic procedure H59.31-
      - following other procedure H59.32-
    - genitourinary organ or structure
      - following procedure on genitourinary organ or structure N99.820
      - following procedure on other organ N99.821
    - mastoid process
      - following procedure on ear and mastoid process H95.41
      - following other procedure H95.42
    - musculoskeletal structure
      - following musculoskeletal surgery M96.830
      - following non-orthopedic surgery M96.831
      - following orthopedic surgery M96.830
    - nervous system
      - during a nervous system procedure G97.51
      - during other procedure G97.52
    - respiratory system
      - during procedure on respiratory system organ or structure J95.830
      - during other procedure J95.831
    - skin and subcutaneous tissue
      - following a dermatologic procedure L76.21
      - following a procedure on other organ L76.22
    - spleen
      - following procedure on the spleen D78.21
      - following procedure on other organ D78.22
  - specified NEC
    - circulatory system I97.89
    - digestive K91.89

Complication— *continued*
  postprocedural— *continued*
    specified NEC— *continued*
      ear H95.89
      endocrine E89.89
      eye and adnexa H59.89
      genitourinary N99.89
      mastoid process H95.89
      metabolic E89.89
      musculoskeletal structure M96.89
      nervous system G97.82
      respiratory system J95.89
      skin and subcutaneous tissue L76.82
      spleen D78.89
  pregnancy NEC — *see* Pregnancy, complicated by
  prosthetic device or implant T85.9
    bile duct — *see* Complications, bile duct implant
    breast — *see* Complications, breast implant
    cardiac and vascular NEC — *see* Complications, cardiovascular device or implant
    corneal transplant — *see* Complications, graft, cornea
    electronic nervous system stimulator — *see* Complications, electronic stimulator device
    epidural infusion catheter — *see* Complications, catheter, epidural
    esophageal anti-reflux device — *see* Complications, esophageal anti-reflux device
    genital organ or tract — *see* Complications, genitourinary, device or implant, genital tract
    heart valve — *see* Complications, heart, valve, prosthesis
    infection or inflammation T85.79
      intestine transplant T86.892
      liver transplant T86.43
      lung transplant T86.812
      pancreas transplant T86.892
      skin graft T86.822
    intraocular lens — *see* Complications, intraocular lens
    intraperitoneal (dialysis) catheter — *see* Complications, catheter, intraperitoneal
    joint — *see* Complications, joint prosthesis, internal
    mechanical NEC T85.698
      dialysis catheter (vascular) (*see also* Complication, catheter, dialysis, mechanical)
        peritoneal — *see* Complication, catheter, intraperitoneal, mechanical
      gastrointestinal device T85.598
      ocular device T85.398
      subdural (infusion) catheter T85.690
      suture, permanent T85.692
        that for bone repair — *see* Complications, fixation device, internal (orthopedic), mechanical
      ventricular shunt
        breakdown T85.01
        displacement T85.02
        leakage T85.03
        malposition T85.02
        obstruction T85.09
        perforation T85.09
        protrusion T85.09
        specified NEC T85.09
    orbital — *see* Complications, orbital prosthesis
    penile T83.89
      embolism T83.81
      fibrosis T83.82
      hemorrhage T83.83
      infection and inflammation T83.6
      mechanical
        breakdown T83.410
        displacement T83.420
        leakage T83.490
        malposition T83.420
        obstruction T83.490
        perforation T83.490
        protrusion T83.490
        specified NEC T83.490

Complication— *continued*
  prosthetic device or implant— *continued*
    penile— *continued*
      pain T83.84
      specified type NEC T83.89
      stenosis T83.85
      thrombosis T83.86
    skin graft T86.829
      artificial skin or decellularized allodermis
        embolism T85.81
        fibrosis T85.82
        hemorrhage T85.83
        infection and inflammation T85.79
        mechanical
          breakdown T85.613
          displacement T85.623
          malfunction T85.613
          malposition T85.623
          obstruction T85.693
          perforation T85.693
          protrusion T85.693
          specified NEC T85.693
        pain T85.84
        specified type NEC T85.89
        stenosis T85.85
        thrombosis T85.86
      failure T86.821
      infection T86.822
      rejection T86.820
      specified NEC T86.828
    specified NEC T85.89
      embolism T85.81
      fibrosis T85.82
      hemorrhage T85.83
      infection and inflammation T85.79
      mechanical
        breakdown T85.618
        displacement T85.628
        leakage T85.638
        malfunction T85.618
        malposition T85.628
        obstruction T85.698
        perforation T85.698
        protrusion T85.698
        specified NEC T85.698
      pain T85.84
      specified type NEC T85.89
      stenosis T85.85
      thrombosis T85.86
    subdural infusion catheter — *see* Complications, catheter, subdural
    sutures — *see* Complications, sutures
    urinary organ or tract NEC — *see* Complications, genitourinary, device or implant, urinary system
    vascular — *see* Complications, cardiovascular device or implant
    ventricular shunt — *see* Complications, ventricular shunt (device)
  puerperium — *see* Puerperal
  puncture, spinal G97.1
    cerebrospinal fluid leak G97.0
    headache or reaction G97.1
  pyelogram N99.89
  radiation
    kyphosis M96.2
    scoliosis M96.5
  reattached
    extremity (infection) (rejection)
      lower T87.1x-
      upper T87.0x-
    specified body part NEC T87.2
  reconstructed breast
    asymmetry between native and reconstructed breast N65.1
    deformity N65.0
    disproportion between native and reconstructed breast N65.1
    excess tissue N65.0
    misshappen N65.0
  reimplant NEC (*see also* Complications, prosthetic device or implant)

Complication— *continued*
  reimplant NEC — *continued*
    limb (infection) (rejection) — *see* Complications, reattached, extremity
    organ (partial) (total) — *see* Complications, transplant
    prosthetic device NEC — *see* Complications, prosthetic device
  renal N28.9
    allograft — *see* Complications, transplant, kidney
    dialysis — *see* Complications, dialysis
  respirator
    mechanical J95.850
    specified NEC J95.859
  respiratory system J98.9
    device, implant or graft — *see* Complication, prosthetic device or implant, specified NEC
    lung transplant — *see* Complications, prosthetic device or implant, lung transplant
    postoperative J95.89
      Mendelson's syndrome (chemical pneumonitis) J95.4
      pneumothorax J95.81
      pulmonary insufficiency (acute) (after nonthoracic surgery) J95.2
        chronic J95.3
        following thoracic surgery J95.1
      respiratory failure J95.82
      specified NEC J95.89
      subglottic stenosis J95.5
      tracheostomy complication — *see* Complications, tracheostomy
    therapy T81.89
  sedation during labor and delivery O74.9
    cardiac O74.2
    central nervous system O74.3
    pulmonary NEC O74.1
  shunt (*see also* Complications, prosthetic device or implant)
    arteriovenous — *see* Complications, arteriovenous, shunt
    ventricular (communicating) — *see* Complications, ventricular shunt
  skin
    graft T86.829
      failure T86.821
      infection T86.822
      rejection T86.820
      specified type NEC T86.828
  spinal
    anesthesia — *see* Complications, anesthesia, spinal
    catheter (epidural) (subdural) — *see* Complications, catheter
    puncture or tap G97.1
      cerebrospinal fluid leak G97.0
      headache or reaction G97.1
  stent
    bile duct — *see* Complications, bile duct prosthesis
    urinary T83.89
      embolism T83.81
      fibrosis T83.82
      hemorrhage T83.83
      infection and inflammation T83.59
      mechanical
        breakdown T83.112
        displacement T83.122
        leakage T83.192
        malposition T83.122
        obstruction T83.192
        perforation T83.192
        protrusion T83.192
        specified NEC T83.192
      pain T83.84
      specified type NEC T83.89
      stenosis T83.85
      thrombosis T83.86
  stoma
    digestive tract
      colostomy — *see* Complications, colostomy
      enterostomy — *see* Complications, enterostomy

Complication— *continued*
  stoma— *continued*
    digestive tract— *continued*
      esophagostomy — *see* Complications,
        esophagostomy
      gastrostomy — *see* Complications,
        gastrostomy
    urinary tract N99.538
      cystostomy — *see* Complications, cystostomy
      external NOS N99.528
        hemorrhage N99.520
        infection N99.521
        malfunction N99.522
        specified type NEC N99.528
      hemorrhage N99.530
      infection N99.531
      malfunction N99.532
      specified type NEC N99.538
  surgical material, nonabsorbable — *see*
    Complication, suture, permanent
  surgical procedure (on) T81.9
    amputation stump (late) — *see* Complications,
      amputation stump
    cardiac — *see* Complications, circulatory system
    cholesteatoma, recurrent — *see* Complications,
      postmastoidectomy, recurrent
      cholesteatoma
    circulatory (early) — *see* Complications,
      circulatory system
    digestive system — *see* Complications,
      gastrointestinal
    dumping syndrome (postgastrectomy) K91.1
    ear — *see* Complications, ear
    elephantiasis or lymphedema I97.89
      postmastectomy I97.2
    emphysema (surgical) T81.82
    endocrine — *see* Complications, endocrine
    eye — *see* Complications, eye
    fistula (persistent postoperative) T81.83
    foreign body inadvertently left in wound
      (sponge) (suture) (swab) — *see* Foreign
      body, accidentally left during a procedure
    gastrointestinal — *see* Complications,
      gastrointestinal
    genitourinary NEC N99.89
    hematoma — *see* Complications, hematoma
    hemorrhage — *see* Complications, hemorrhage
      associated with procedure
    hepatic failure K91.82
    hyperglycemia (postpancreatectomy) E89.1
    hypoinsulinemia (postpancreatectomy) E89.1
    hypoparathyroidism (postparathyroidectomy)
      E89.2
    hypopituitarism (posthypophysectomy) E89.3
    hypothyroidism (post-thyroidectomy) E89.0
    intestinal obstruction K91.3
    intracranial hypotension following ventricular
      shunting (ventriculostomy) G97.2
    lymphedema I97.89
      postmastectomy I97.2
    malabsorption (postsurgical) NEC K91.2
      osteoporosis — *see* Osteoporosis, postsurgical
      malabsorption
    mastoidectomy cavity NEC — *see* Complications,
      postmastoidectomy
    metabolic E89.89
      specified NEC E89.89
    musculoskeletal — *see* Complications,
      musculoskeletal system
    nervous system (central) (peripheral) — *see*
      Complications, nervous system
    ovarian failure E89.40
      asymptomatic E89.40
      symptomatic E89.41
    peripheral vascular — *see* Complications, surgical
      procedure, vascular
    postcardiotomy syndrome I97.0
    postcholecystectomy syndrome K91.5
    postcommissurotomy syndrome I97.0
    postgastrectomy dumping syndrome K91.1
    postlaminectomy syndrome NEC M96.1
      kyphosis M96.3
    postmastectomy lymphedema syndrome I97.2

Complication— *continued*
  surgical procedure (on)— *continued*
    postmastoidectomy cholesteatoma — *see*
      Complications, postmastoidectomy,
      recurrent cholesteatoma
    postvagotomy syndrome K91.1
    postvalvulotomy syndrome I97.0
    pulmonary insufficiency (acute) J95.2
      chronic J95.3
      following thoracic surgery J95.1
    reattached body part — *see* Complications,
      reattached
    respiratory — *see* Complications, respiratory
      system
    shock (hypovolemic) T81.1
    spleen (postoperative) D78.89
      intraoperative D78.81
    stitch abscess T81.4
    subglottic stenosis (postsurgical) J95.5
    testicular hypofunction E89.5
    transplant — *see* Complications, organ or tissue
      transplant
    urinary NEC N99.89
    vaginal vault prolapse (posthysterectomy) N99.3
    vascular (peripheral)
      artery T81.719
        mesenteric T81.710
        renal T81.711
        specified NEC T81.718
      vein T81.72
    wound infection T81.4
  suture, permanent (wire) NEC T85.89
    with repair of bone — *see* Complications, fixation
      device, internal
    embolism T85.81
    fibrosis T85.82
    hemorrhage T85.83
    infection and inflammation T85.79
    mechanical
      breakdown T85.612
      displacement T85.622
      malfunction T85.612
      malposition T85.622
      obstruction T85.692
      perforation T85.692
      protrusion T85.692
      specified NEC T85.692
    pain T85.84
    specified type NEC T85.89
    stenosis T85.85
    thrombosis T85.86
  tracheostomy J95.00
    granuloma J95.09
    hemorrhage J95.01
    infection J95.02
    malfunction J95.03
    mechanical J95.03
    obstruction J95.03
    specified type NEC J95.09
    tracheo-esophageal fistula J95.04
  transfusion (blood) (lymphocytes) (plasma) T80.92
    air embolism T80.0
    circulatory overload E87.71
    febrile nonhemolytic transfusion reaction R50.84
    hemochromatosis E83.111
    hemolysis T80.89
    hemolytic reaction (antigen unspecified) T80.919
    incompatibility reaction (antigen unspecified)
      T80.919
      ABO T80.30
        delayed serologic (DSTR) T80.39
        hemolytic transfusion reaction (HTR)
          (unspecified time after transfusion)
          T80.319
          acute (AHTR) (less than 24 hours after
            transfusion) T80.310
          delayed (DHTR) (24 hours or more after
            transfusion) T80.311
        specified NEC T80.39
      acute (antigen unspecified) T80.910
      delayed (antigen unspecified) T80.911
      delayed serologic (DSTR) T80.89

Complication— *continued*
  transfusion— *continued*
    incompatibility reaction— *continued*
      Non-ABO (minor antigens (Duffy) (Kell) (Kidd)
        (Lewis) (M) (N) (P) (S)) T80.a0
        delayed serologic (DSTR) T80.a9
        hemolytic transfusion reaction (HTR)
          (unspecified time after transfusion)
          T80.a19
          acute (AHTR) (less than 24 hours after
            transfusion) T80.a10
          delayed (DHTR) (24 hours or more after
            transfusion) T80.a11
        specified NEC T80.a9
      Rh (antigens (C) (c) (D) (E) (e)) (factor) T80.40
        delayed serologic (DSTR) T80.49
        hemolytic transfusion reaction (HTR)
          (unspecified time after transfusion)
          T80.419
          acute (AHTR) (less than 24 hours after
            transfusion) T80.410
          delayed (DHTR) (24 hours or more after
            transfusion) T80.411
        specified NEC T80.49
    infection T80.29
    reaction NEC T80.89
    sepsis T80.29
    shock T80.89
  transplant T86.90
    bone T86.839
      failure T86.831
      infection T86.832
      rejection T86.830
      specified type NEC T86.839
    bone marrow T86.00
      failure T86.02
      infection T86.03
      rejection T86.01
      specified type NEC T86.09
    cornea T86.849
      failure T86.841
      infection T86.842
      rejection T86.840
      specified type NEC T86.848
    failure T86.92
    heart T86.20
      with lung T86.30
      cardiac allograft vasculopathy T86.290
        failure T86.32
        infection T86.33
        rejection T86.31
        specified type NEC T86.39
      failure T86.22
      infection T86.23
      rejection T86.21
      specified type NEC T86.298
    infection T86.93
    intestine T86.859
      failure T86.851
      infection T86.852
      rejection T86.850
      specified type NEC T86.858
    kidney T86.10
      failure T86.12
      infection T86.13
      rejection T86.11
      specified type NEC T86.19
    liver T86.40
      failure T86.42
      infection T86.43
      rejection T86.41
      specified type NEC T86.49
    lung T86.819
      with heart T86.30
        failure T86.32
        infection T86.33
        rejection T86.31
        specified type NEC T86.39
      failure T86.811
      infection T86.812
      rejection T86.810
      specified type NEC T86.818

Complication— *continued*
transplant— *continued*
  malignant neoplasm C80.2
  pancreas T86.899
    failure T86.891
    infection T86.892
    rejection T86.890
    specified type NEC T86.898
  post-transplant lymphoproliferative disorder
    (PTLD) D47.z1
  rejection T86.91
  skin T86.829
    failure T86.821
    infection T86.822
    rejection T86.820
    specified type NEC T86.828
  specified
    tissue T86.899
      failure T86.891
      infection T86.892
      rejection T86.890
      specified type NEC T86.898
    type NEC T86.99
trauma (early) T79.9
  specified NEC T79.8
ultrasound therapy NEC T88.9
umbilical cord NEC
  complicating delivery O69.9
  specified NEC O69.89
umbrella device, vascular T82.9
  embolism T82.818
  fibrosis T82.828
  hemorrhage T82.838
  infection or inflammation T82.7
  mechanical
    breakdown T82.515
    displacement T82.525
    leakage T82.535
    malposition T82.525
    obstruction T82.595
    perforation T82.595
    protrusion T82.595
  pain T82.848
  specified type NEC T82.898
  stenosis T82.858
  thrombosis T82.868
urethral catheter — *see* Complications, catheter,
  urethral, indwelling
vaccination T88.1
  anaphylaxis NEC T80.5
  arthropathy — *see* Arthropathy,
    postimmunization
  cellulitis T88.0
  encephalitis or encephalomyelitis G04.01
  infection (general) (local) NEC T88.0
  meningitis G03.8
  myelitis G04.89
  protein sickness T80.6
  rash T88.1
  reaction (allergic) T88.1
    Herxheimer's T88.6
    serum T80.6
  sepsis T88.0
  serum intoxication, sickness, rash, or other serum
    reaction NEC T80.6
    anaphylactic shock T80.5
  shock (allergic) (anaphylactic) T80.5
  vaccinia (generalized) (localized) T88.1
vas deferens device or implant — *see* Complications,
  genitourinary, device or implant, genital tract
vascular I99.9
  device or implant T82.9
    embolism T82.818
    fibrosis T82.828
    hemorrhage T82.838
    infection or inflammation T82.7
    mechanical
      breakdown T82.519
        specified device NEC T82.518
      displacement T82.529
        specified device NEC T82.528
      leakage T82.539
        specified device NEC T82.538

Complication— *continued*
vascular— *continued*
  device or implant— *continued*
    mechanical— *continued*
      malposition T82.529
        specified device NEC T82.528
      obstruction T82.599
        specified device NEC T82.598
      perforation T82.599
        specified device NEC T82.598
      protrusion T82.599
        specified device NEC T82.598
    pain T82.848
    specified type NEC T82.898
    stenosis T82.858
    thrombosis T82.868
  dialysis catheter — *see* Complication, catheter,
    dialysis
  graft T82.9
    embolism T82.818
    fibrosis T82.828
    hemorrhage T82.838
    mechanical
      breakdown T82.319
        aorta (bifurcation) T82.310
        carotid artery T82.311
        specified vessel NEC T82.318
      displacement T82.329
        aorta (bifurcation) T82.320
        carotid artery T82.321
        specified vessel NEC T82.328
      leakage T82.339
        aorta (bifurcation) T82.330
        carotid artery T82.331
        specified vessel NEC T82.338
      malposition T82.329
        aorta (bifurcation) T82.320
        carotid artery T82.321
        specified vessel NEC T82.328
      obstruction T82.399
        aorta (bifurcation) T82.390
        carotid artery T82.391
        specified vessel NEC T82.398
      perforation T82.399
        aorta (bifurcation) T82.390
        carotid artery T82.391
        specified vessel NEC T82.398
      protrusion T82.399
        aorta (bifurcation) T82.390
        carotid artery T82.391
        specified vessel NEC T82.398
    pain T82.848
    specified complication NEC T82.898
    stenosis T82.858
    thrombosis T82.868
  following infusion, therapeutic injection or
    transfusion T80.1
  postoperative — *see* Complications,
    postoperative, circulatory
  vena cava device (filter) (sieve) (umbrella) — *see*
    Complications, umbrella device, vascular
ventilation therapy NEC T81.81
ventilator
  mechanical J95.850
    specified NEC J95.859
ventricular (communicating) shunt (device) T85.89
  embolism T85.81
  fibrosis T85.82
  hemorrhage T85.83
  infection and inflammation T85.79
  mechanical
    breakdown T85.01
    displacement T85.02
    leakage T85.03
    malposition T85.02
    obstruction T85.09
    perforation T85.09
    protrusion T85.09
    specified NEC T85.09
  pain T85.84
  specified type NEC T85.89
  stenosis T85.85
  thrombosis T85.86

Complication— *continued*
  wire suture, permanent (implanted) — *see*
    Complications, suture, permanent
Compressed air disease T70.3
Compression
  with injury—code by Nature of injury
  artery I77.1
    celiac, syndrome I77.4
  brachial plexus G54.0
  brain (stem) G93.5
    due to
      contusion (diffuse) — *see* Injury, intracranial,
        diffuse
        focal — *see* Injury, intracranial, focal
      injury NEC — *see* Injury, intracranial, diffuse
      traumatic — *see* Injury, intracranial, diffuse
  bronchus J98.09
  cauda equina G83.4
  celiac (artery) (axis) I77.4
  cerebral — *see* Compression, brain
  cervical plexus G54.2
  cord
    spinal — *see* Compression, spinal
    umbilical — *see* Compression, umbilical cord
  cranial nerve G52.9
    eighth — *see* subcategory H93.3
    eleventh G52.8
    fifth G50.8
    first G52.0
    fourth — *see* Strabismus, paralytic, fourth nerve
    ninth G52.1
    second — *see* Disorder, nerve, optic
    seventh G52.8
    sixth — *see* Strabismus, paralytic, sixth nerve
    tenth G52.2
    third G52.8
    twelfth G52.3
  diver's squeeze T70.3
  during birth (newborn) P15.9
  esophagus K22.2
  eustachian tube — *see* Obstruction, eustachian
    tube, cartilaginous
  facies Q67.1
  fracture — *see* Fracture
  heart — *see* Disease, heart
  intestine — *see* Obstruction, intestine
  laryngeal nerve, recurrent G52.2
    with paralysis of vocal cords and larynx J38.00
      bilateral J38.02
      unilateral J38.01
  lumbosacral plexus G54.1
  lung J98.4
  lymphatic vessel I89.0
  medulla — *see* Compression, brain
  nerve (*see also* Disorder, nerve) G58.9
    arm NEC — *see* Mononeuropathy, upper limb
    axillary G54.0
    cranial — *see* Compression, cranial nerve
    leg NEC — *see* Mononeuropathy, lower limb
    median (in carpal tunnel) — *see* Syndrome,
      carpal tunnel
    optic — *see* Disorder, nerve, optic
    plantar — *see* Lesion, nerve, plantar
    posterior tibial (in tarsal tunnel) — *see*
      Syndrome, tarsal tunnel
    root or plexus NOS (in) G54.9
      intervertebral disc disorder NEC — *see*
        Disorder, disc, with, radiculopathy
        with myelopathy — *see* Disorder, disc,
          with, myelopathy
      neoplastic disease (*see also* Neoplasm) D49.9
        [G55]
      spondylosis — *see* Spondylosis, with
        radiculopathy
    sciatic (acute) — *see* Lesion, nerve, sciatic
    sympathetic G90.8
    traumatic — *see* Injury, nerve
    ulnar — *see* Lesion, nerve, ulnar
    upper extremity NEC — *see* Mononeuropathy,
      upper limb
  spinal (cord) G95.20
    by displacement of intervertebral disc NEC (*see
      also* Disorder, disc, with, myelopathy)

Compression— *continued*
  spinal (cord)— *continued*
    nerve root NOS G54.9
      due to displacement of intervertebral disc
        NEC — *see* Disorder, disc, with,
        radiculopathy
        with myelopathy — *see* Disorder, disc,
        with, myelopathy
    specified NEC G95.29
    spondylogenic (cervical) (lumbar, lumbosacral)
      (thoracic) — *see* Spondylosis, with
      myelopathy NEC
    anterior — *see* Syndrome, anterior, spinal
      artery, compression
    traumatic — *see* Injury, spinal cord, by region
  subcostal nerve (syndrome) — *see*
    Mononeuropathy, upper limb, specified NEC
  sympathetic nerve NEC G90.8
  syndrome T79.5
  trachea J39.8
  ulnar nerve (by scar tissue) — *see* Lesion, nerve,
    ulnar
  umbilical cord
    complicating delivery O69.2
      cord around neck O69.1
      prolapse O69.0
      specified NEC O69.2
  ureter N13.5
  vein I87.1
  vena cava (inferior) (superior) I87.1
Compulsion, compulsive
  gambling F63.0
  neurosis F42
  personality F60.5
  states F42
  swearing F42
    in Gilles de la Tourette's syndrome F95.2
  tics and spasms F95.9
Concato's disease (pericardial polyserositis) A19.9
  nontubercular I31.1
  pleural — *see* Pleurisy, with effusion
Concavity chest wall M95.4
Concealed penis Q55.69
Concern (normal) **about sick person in family** Z63.6
Concrescence (teeth) K00.2
Concretio cordis I31.1
  rheumatic I09.2
Concretion (*see also* Calculus)
  appendicular K38.1
  canaliculus — *see* Dacryolith
  clitoris N90.89
  conjunctiva H11.12-
  eyelid — *see* Disorder, eyelid, specified type NEC
  lacrimal passages — *see* Dacryolith
  prepuce (male) N47.8
  salivary gland (any) K11.5
  seminal vesicle N50.8
  tonsil J35.8
Concussion (brain) (cerebral) (current) S06.0x-
  blast (air) (hydraulic) (immersion) (underwater)
    abdomen or thorax — *see* Injury, blast, by site
    ear with acoustic nerve injury — *see* Injury,
      nerve, acoustic, specified type NEC
  cauda equina S34.3
  conus medullaris S34.139
  ocular S05.8x-
  spinal (cord)
    cervical S14.0
    lumbar S34.01
    sacral S34.02
    thoracic S24.0
  syndrome F07.81
Condition — *see* Disease
Conditions arising in the perinatal period — *see*
  Newborn, affected by
Conduct disorder — *see* Disorder, conduct
Condyloma A63.0
  acuminatum A63.0
  gonorrheal A54.09
  latum A51.31
  syphilitic A51.31
    congenital A50.07
  venereal, syphilitic A51.31

Conflagration (*see also* Burn)
  asphyxia (by inhalation of smoke, gases, fumes or
    vapors) — *see* Table of Drugs and Chemicals
Conflict (with) — *see also* Discord
  family Z73.9
  marital Z63.0
    involving divorce or estrangement Z63.5
Conflict — *continued*
  parent-child Z62.820
    parent-adopted child Z62.821
    parent-biological child Z62.820
    parent-foster child Z62.822
  social role NEC Z73.5
Confluent — *see* condition
Confusion, confused R41.0
  epileptic F05
  mental state (psychogenic) F44.89
  psychogenic F44.89
  reactive (from emotional stress, psychological
    trauma) F44.89
Confusional arousals G47.51
Congelation T69.9
Congenital (*see also* condition)
  aortic septum Q25.4
  intrinsic factor deficiency D51.0
  malformation — *see* Anomaly
Congestion, congestive
  bladder N32.89
  bowel K63.89
  brain G93.89
  breast N64.59
  bronchial J98.09
  catarrhal J31.0
  chest R09.89
  chill, malarial — *see* Malaria
  circulatory NEC I99.8
  duodenum K31.89
  eye — *see* Hyperemia, conjunctiva
  facial, due to birth injury P15.4
  general R68.89
  glottis J37.0
  heart — *see* Failure, heart, congestive
  hepatic K76.1
  hypostatic (lung) — *see* Edema, lung
  intestine K63.89
  kidney N28.89
  labyrinth — *see* subcategory H83.8
  larynx J37.0
  liver K76.1
  lung R09.89
    active or acute — *see* Pneumonia
  malaria, malarial — *see* Malaria
  nasal R09.81
  nose R09.81
  orbit, orbital (*see also* Exophthalmos)
    inflammatory (chronic) — *see* Inflammation, orbit
  ovary N83.8
  pancreas K86.8
  pelvic, female N94.89
  pleural J94.8
  prostate (active) N42.1
  pulmonary — *see* Congestion, lung
  renal N28.89
  retina H35.81
  seminal vesicle N50.1
  spinal cord G95.19
  spleen (chronic) D73.2
  stomach K31.89
  trachea — *see* Tracheitis
  urethra N36.8
  uterus N85.8
    with subinvolution N85.3
  venous (passive) I87.8
  viscera R68.89
Congestive — *see* Congestion
Conical
  cervix (hypertrophic elongation) N88.4
  cornea — *see* Keratoconus
  teeth K00.2
Conjoined twins Q89.4
Conjugal maladjustment Z63.0
  involving divorce or estrangement Z63.5
Conjunctiva — *see* condition

Conjunctivitis (staphylococcal) (streptococcal) NOS
  H10.9
  Acanthamoeba B60.12
  acute H10.3-
    chemical H10.21 (*see also* Corrosion, cornea)
    atopic H10.1-
    mucopurulent H10.02-
      follicular H10.01-
    pseudomembranous H10.22-
    serous except viral H10.23-
      viral — *see* Conjunctivitis, viral
    toxic H10.21-
  adenoviral (acute) (follicular) B30.1
  allergic (acute) — *see* Conjunctivitis, acute, atopic
    chronic H10.45
      vernal H10.44
  anaphylactic — *see* Conjunctivitis, acute, atopic
  Apollo B30.3
  atopic (acute) — *see* Conjunctivitis, acute, atopic
  Béal's B30.2
  blennorrhagic (gonococcal) (neonatorum) A54.31
  chemical (acute) H10.21 (*see also* Corrosion, cornea)
  chlamydial A74.0
    due to trachoma A07.0
    neonatal P39.1
  chronic (nodosa) (petrificans) (phlyctenular) H10.40-
    allergic H10.45
      vernal H10.44
    follicular H10.43-
    giant papillary H10.41-
    simple H10.42-
    vernal H10.44
  coxsackievirus 24 B30.3
  diphtheritic A36.86
  due to
    dust — *see* Conjunctivitis, acute, atopic
    filariasis B74.3
    mucocutaneous leishmaniasis B55.2
  enterovirus type 70 (hemorrhagic) B30.3
  epidemic (viral) B30.9
    hemorrhagic B30.3
  gonococcal (neonatorum) A54.31
  granular (trachomatous) A71.1
    sequelae (late effect) B94.0
  hemorrhagic (acute) (epidemic) B30.3
  herpes zoster B02.31
  in (due to)
    Acanthamoeba B60.12
    adenovirus (acute) (follicular) B30.1
    Chlamydia A74.0
    coxsackievirus 24 B30.3
    diphtheria A36.86
    enterovirus type 70 (hemorrhagic) B30.3
    filariasis B74.9
    gonococci A54.31
    herpes (simplex) virus B00.53
      zoster B02.31
    infectious disease NEC B99
    meningococci A39.89
    mucocutaneous leishmaniasis B55.2
    rosacea L71.9
    syphilis (late) A52.71
    zoster B02.31
  inclusion A74.0
  infantile P39.1
    gonococcal A54.31
  Koch-Weeks' — *see* Conjunctivitis, acute,
    mucopurulent
  light — *see* Conjunctivitis, acute, atopic
  ligneous — *see* Blepharoconjunctivitis, ligneous
  meningococcal A39.89
  mucopurulent — *see* Conjunctivitis, acute,
    mucopurulent
  neonatal P39.1
    gonococcal A54.31
  Newcastle B30.8
  of Beal B30.2
  parasitic
    filariasis B74.9
    mucocutaneous leishmaniasis B55.2
  Parinaud's H10.89
  petrificans H10.89

Conjunctivitis— *continued*
 rosacea L71.9
 specified NEC H10.89
 swimming-pool B30.1
 trachomatous A71.1
  acute A71.0
  sequelae (late effect) B94.0
 traumatic NEC H10.89
 tuberculous A18.59
 tularemic A21.1
 tularensis A21.1
 viral B30.9
  due to
   adenovirus B30.1
   enterovirus B30.3
  specified NEC B30.8
Conjunctivochalasis H11.82-
Connective tissue — *see* condition
Conn's syndrome E26.01
Conradi(-Hunermann) **disease** Q77.3
Consanguinity Z84.3
 counseling Z71.89
Conscious simulation (of illness) Z76.5
Consecutive — *see* condition
Consolidation lung (base) — *see* Pneumonia, lobar
Constipation (atonic) (neurogenic) (simple) (spastic) K59.00
 drug-induced — *see* Table of Drugs and Chemicals
 outlet dysfunction K59.02
 psychogenic F45.8
 slow transit K59.01
 specified NEC K59.09
Constitutional (*see also* condition)
 substandard F60.7
Constitutionally substandard F60.7
Constriction (*see also* Stricture)
 auditory canal — *see* Stenosis, external ear canal
 bronchial J98.09
 duodenum K31.5
 esophagus K22.2
 external
  abdomen, abdominal (wall) S30.841
  alveolar process S00.542
  ankle S90.54-
  antecubital space — *see* Constriction, external, forearm
  arm (upper) S40.84-
  auricle — *see* Constriction, external, ear
  axilla — *see* Constriction, external, arm
  back, lower S30.840
  breast S20.14-
  brow S00.84
  buttock S30.840
  calf — *see* Constriction, external, leg
  canthus — *see* Constriction, external, eyelid
  cheek S00.84
   internal S00.542
  chest wall — *see* Constriction, external, thorax
  chin S00.84
  clitoris S30.844
  costal region — *see* Constriction, external, thorax
  digit(s)
   hand — *see* Constriction, external, finger
   foot — *see* Constriction, external, toe
  ear S00.44-
  elbow S50.34-
  epididymis S30.843
  epigastric region S30.841
  esophagus, cervical S10.14
  eyebrow — *see* Constriction, external, eyelid
  eyelid S00.24-
  face S00.84
  finger(s) S60.44-
   index S60.44-
   little S60.44-
   middle S60.44-
   ring S60.44-
  flank S30.841
  foot (except toe(s) alone) S90.84-
   toe — *see* Constriction, external, toe
  forearm S50.84-
   elbow only — *see* Constriction, external, elbow

Constriction— *continued*
 external— *continued*
  forehead S00.84
  genital organs, external
   female S30.846
   male S30.845
  groin S30.841
  gum S00.542
  hand S60.54-
  head S00.94
   ear — *see* Constriction, external, ear
   eyelid — *see* Constriction, external, eyelid
   lip S00.541
   nose S00.34
   oral cavity S00.542
   scalp S00.04
   specified site NEC S00.84
  heel — *see* Constriction, external, foot
  hip S70.24-
  inguinal region S30.841
  interscapular region S20.449
  jaw S00.84
  knee S80.24-
  labium (majus) (minus) S30.844
  larynx S10.14
  leg (lower) S80.84-
   knee — *see* Constriction, external, knee
   upper — *see* Constriction, external, thigh
  lip S00.541
  lower back S30.840
  lumbar region S30.840
  malar region S00.84
  mammary — *see* Constriction, external, breast
  mastoid region S00.84
  mouth S00.542
  nail
   finger — *see* Constriction, external, finger
   toe — *see* Constriction, external, toe
  nasal S00.34
  neck S10.94
   specified site NEC S10.84
   throat S10.14
  nose S00.34
  occipital region S00.04
  oral cavity S00.542
  orbital region — *see* Constriction, external, eyelid
  palate S00.542
  palm — *see* Constriction, external, hand
  parietal region S00.04
  pelvis S30.840
  penis S30.842
  perineum
   female S30.844
   male S30.840
  periocular area — *see* Constriction, external, eyelid
  phalanges
   finger — *see* Constriction, external, finger
   toe — *see* Constriction, external, toe
  pharynx S10.14
  pinna — *see* Constriction, external, ear
  popliteal space — *see* Constriction, external, knee
  prepuce S30.842
  pubic region S30.840
  pudendum
   female S30.846
   male S30.845
  sacral region S30.840
  scalp S00.04
  scapular region — *see* Constriction, external, shoulder
  scrotum S30.843
  shin — *see* Constriction, external, leg
  shoulder S40.24-
  sternal region S20.349
  submaxillary region S00.84
  submental region S00.84
  subungual
   finger(s) — *see* Constriction, external, finger
   toe(s) — *see* Constriction, external, toe
  supraclavicular fossa S10.84
  supraorbital S00.84
  temple S00.84
  temporal region S00.84

Constriction— *continued*
 external— *continued*
  testis S30.843
  thigh S70.34-
  thorax, thoracic (wall) S20.94
   back S20.44-
   front S20.34-
  throat S10.14
  thumb S60.34-
  toe(s) (lesser) S90.44-
   great S90.44-
  tongue S00.542
  trachea S10.14
  tunica vaginalis S30.843
  uvula S00.542
  vagina S30.844
  vulva S30.844
  wrist S60.84-
 gallbladder — *see* Obstruction, gallbladder
 intestine — *see* Obstruction, intestine
 larynx J38.6
  congenital Q31.8
   specified NEC Q31.8
   subglottic Q31.1
 organ or site, congenital NEC — *see* Atresia, by site
 prepuce (acquired) (congenital) N47.1
 pylorus (adult hypertrophic) K31.1
  congenital or infantile Q40.0
  newborn Q40.0
 ring dystocia (uterus) O62.4
 spastic (*see also* Spasm)
  ureter N13.5
 ureter N13.5
  with infection N13.6
 urethra — *see* Stricture, urethra
 visual field (peripheral) (functional) — *see* Defect, visual field
Constrictive — *see* condition
Consultation
 medical — *see* Counseling, medical
 religious Z71.81
 specified reason NEC Z71.89
 spiritual Z71.81
 without complaint or sickness Z71.9
  feared complaint unfounded Z71.1
  specified reason NEC Z71.89
Consumption — *see* Tuberculosis
Contact (with) (*see also* Exposure (to))
 acariasis Z20.7
 AIDS virus Z20.6
 air pollution Z77.110
 algae and algae toxins Z77.121
 algae bloom Z77.121
 anthrax Z20.810
 aromatic amines Z77.020
 aromatic (hazardous) compounds NEC Z77.028
 aromatic dyes NOS Z77.028
 arsenic Z77.010
 asbestos Z77.090
 bacterial disease NEC Z20.818
 benzene Z77.021
 blue-green algae bloom Z77.121
 body fluids (potentially hazardous) Z77.21
 brown tide Z77.121
 chemicals (chiefly nonmedicinal) (hazardous) NEC Z77.098
 chromium compounds Z77.018
 cholera Z20.09
 communicable disease Z20.9
  bacterial NEC Z20.818
  specified NEC Z20.89
  viral NEC Z20.828
 cyanobacteria bloom Z77.121
 dyes Z77.098
 Escherichia coli (E. coli) Z20.01
 fiberglass — *see* Table of Drugs and Chemicals, fiberglass
 German measles Z20.4
 gonorrhea Z20.2
 hazardous metals NEC Z77.018
 hazardous substances NEC Z77.29
 hazards in the physical environment NEC Z77.128
 hazards to health NEC Z77.9

Contact — *continued*
  HIV Z20.6
  HTLV-III/LAV Z20.6
  human immunodeficiency virus (HIV) Z20.6
  infection Z20.9
    specified NEC Z20.89
  infestation (parasitic) NEC Z20.7
  intestinal infectious disease NEC Z20.09
    Escherichia coli (E. coli) Z20.01
  lead Z77.011
  meningococcus Z20.811
  mold (toxic) Z77.120
  nickel dust Z77.018
  noise Z77.122
  parasitic disease Z20.7
  pediculosis Z20.7
  pfiesteria piscicida Z77.121
  poliomyelitis Z20.89
  pollution
    air Z77.110
    environmental NEC Z77.118
    soil Z77.112
    water Z77.111
  polycyclic aromatic hydrocarbons Z77.028
  rabies Z20.3
  radiation, naturally occurring NEC Z77.123
  radon Z77.123
  red tide (Florida) Z77.121
  rubella Z20.4
  sexually-transmitted disease Z20.2
  smallpox (laboratory) Z20.89
  syphilis Z20.2
  tuberculosis Z20.1
  varicella Z20.820
  venereal disease Z20.2
  viral disease NEC Z20.828
  viral hepatitis Z20.5
  water pollution Z77.111
Contamination, food — *see* Intoxication, foodborne
Contraception, contraceptive
  advice Z30.09
  counseling Z30.09
  device (intrauterine) (in situ) Z97.5
    causing menorrhagia T83.83
    checking Z30.431
    complications — *see* Complications, intrauterine, contraceptive device
    in place Z97.5
    initial prescription Z30.014
    reinsertion Z30.433
    removal Z30.432
    replacement Z30.433
  emergency (postcoital) Z30.012
  initial prescription Z30.019
    injectable Z30.013
    intrauterine device Z30.014
    pills Z30.011
    postcoital (emergency) Z30.012
    specified type NEC Z30.018
    subdermal implantable Z30.019
  maintenance Z30.40
    examination Z30.8
    injectable Z30.42
    intrauterine device Z30.431
    pills Z30.41
    specified type NEC Z30.49
    subdermal implantable Z30.49
  management Z30.9
    specified NEC Z30.8
  postcoital (emergency) Z30.012
  prescription Z30.019
    repeat Z30.40
  sterilization Z30.2
  surveillance (drug) — *see* Contraception, maintenance
Contraction(s), contracture, contracted
  Achilles tendon (*see also* Short, tendon, Achilles)
    congenital Q66.8
  amputation stump (surgical) (flexion) (late) T87.8
  anus K59.8
  bile duct (common) (hepatic) K83.8
  bladder N32.89
    neck or sphincter N32.0

Contraction(s), contracture, contracted— *continued*
  bowel, cecum, colon or intestine, any part — *see* Obstruction, intestine
  Braxton Hicks — *see* False, labor
  breast implant, capsular T85.44
  bronchial J98.09
  burn (old) — *see* Cicatrix
  cervix — *see* Stricture, cervix
  cicatricial — *see* Cicatrix
  conjunctiva, trachomatous, active A71.1
    sequelae (late effect) B94.0
  Dupuytren's M72.0
  eyelid — *see* Disorder, eyelid function
  fascia (lata) (postural) M72.8
    Dupuytren's M72.0
    palmar M72.0
    plantar M72.2
  finger NEC (*see also* Deformity, finger)
    congenital Q68.1
    joint — *see* Contraction, joint, hand
  flaccid — *see* Contraction, paralytic
  gallbladder K82.0
  heart valve — *see* Endocarditis
  hip — *see* Contraction, joint, hip
  hourglass
    bladder N32.89
      congenital Q64.79
    gallbladder K82.0
      congenital Q44.1
    stomach K31.89
      congenital Q40.2
      psychogenic F45.8
    uterus (complicating delivery) O62.4
  hysterical F44.4
  internal os — *see* Stricture, cervix
  joint (abduction) (acquired) (adduction) (flexion) (rotation) M24.50
    ankle M24.57-
    congenital NEC Q68.8
      hip Q65.8
    elbow M24.52-
    foot joint M24.57-
    hand joint M24.54-
    hip M24.55-
      congenital Q65.8
    hysterical F44.4
    knee M24.56-
    shoulder M24.51-
    wrist M24.53-
  kidney (granular) (secondary) N26.9
    congenital Q63.8
    hydronephritic — *see* Hydronephrosis
    Page N26.2
    pyelonephritic — *see* Pyelitis, chronic
    tuberculous A18.11
  ligament (*see also* Disorder, ligament)
    congenital Q79.8
  muscle (postinfective) (postural) NEC M62.40
    with contracture of joint — *see* Contraction, joint
    ankle M62.47-
    congenital Q79.8
      sternocleidomastoid Q68.0
    extraocular — *see* Strabismus
    eye (extrinsic) — *see* Strabismus
    foot M62.47-
    forearm M62.43-
    hand M62.44-
    hysterical F44.4
    ischemic (Volkmann's) T79.6
    lower leg M62.46-
    multiple sites M62.49
    pelvic region M62.45-
    posttraumatic — *see* Strabismus, paralytic
    psychogenic F45.8
      conversion reaction F44.4
    shoulder region M62.41-
    specified site NEC M62.48
    thigh M62.45-
    upper arm M62.42-
  neck — *see* Torticollis
  ocular muscle — *see* Strabismus
  organ or site, congenital NEC — *see* Atresia, by site
  outlet (pelvis) — *see* Contraction, pelvis

Contraction(s), contracture, contracted— *continued*
  palmar fascia M72.0
  paralytic
    joint — *see* Contraction, joint
    muscle (*see also* Contraction, muscle NEC)
    ocular — *see* Strabismus, paralytic
  pelvis (acquired) (general) M95.5
    with disproportion (fetopelvic) O33.1
      causing obstructed labor O65.1
    inlet O33.2
    mid-cavity O33.3
    outlet O33.3
  plantar fascia M72.2
  premature
    atrium I49.1
    auriculoventricular I49.49
    heart I49.49
    junctional I49.2
    supraventricular I49.1
    ventricular I49.3
  prostate N42.89
  pylorus NEC (*see also* Pylorospasm)
    psychogenic F45.8
  rectum, rectal (sphincter) K59.8
  ring (Bandl's) (complicating delivery) O62.4
  scar — *see* Cicatrix
  spine — *see* Dorsopathy, deforming
  sternocleidomastoid (muscle), congenital Q68.0
  stomach K31.89
    hourglass K31.89
      congenital Q40.2
      psychogenic F45.8
    psychogenic F45.8
  tendon (sheath) M62.40
    with contracture of joint — *see* Contraction, joint
    Achilles — *see* Short, tendon, Achilles
    ankle M62.47-
      Achilles — *see* Short, tendon, Achilles
    foot M62.47-
    forearm M62.43-
    hand M62.44-
    lower leg M62.46-
    multiple sites M62.49
    neck M62.48
    pelvic region M62.45-
    shoulder region M62.41-
    specified site NEC M62.48
    thigh M62.45-
    thorax M62.48
    trunk M62.48
    upper arm M62.42-
  toe — *see* Deformity, toe, specified NEC
  ureterovesical orifice (postinfectional) N13.5
    with infection N13.6
  urethra (*see also* Stricture, urethra)
    orifice N32.0
  uterus N85.8
    abnormal NEC O62.9
    clonic (complicating delivery) O62.4
    dyscoordinate (complicating delivery) O62.4
    hourglass (complicating delivery) O62.4
    hypertonic O62.4
    hypotonic NEC O62.2
    inadequate
      primary O62.0
      secondary O62.1
    incoordinate (complicating delivery) O62.4
    poor O62.2
    tetanic (complicating delivery) O62.4
  vagina (outlet) N89.5
  vesical N32.89
    neck or urethral orifice N32.0
  visual field — *see* Defect, visual field, generalized
  Volkmann's (ischemic) T79.6
Contusion (skin surface intact)
  abdomen, abdominal (muscle) (wall) S30.1
  adnexa, eye NEC S05.8x-
  adrenal gland S37.812
  alveolar process S00.532
  ankle S90.0-
  antecubital space — *see* Contusion, forearm
  anus S30.3
  arm (upper) S40.02-

Contusion— *continued*
- thumb S60.01-
  - with damage to nail S60.11-
- toe(s) (lesser) S90.12-
  - with damage to nail S90.22-
  - great S90.11-
    - with damage to nail S90.21-
    - specified type NEC S90.221
- tongue S00.532
- trachea (cervical) S10.0
  - thoracic S27.52
- tunica vaginalis S30.22
- tympanum, tympanic membrane — *see* Contusion, ear
- ureter S37.12
- urethra S37.32
- urinary organ NEC S37.892
- uterus S37.62
- uvula S00.532
- vagina S30.23
- vas deferens S37.892
- vesical S37.22
- vocal cord(s) S10.0
- vulva S30.23
- wrist S60.21-

Conus (congenital) (any type) Q14.8
- cornea — *see* Keratoconus
- medullaris syndrome G95.81

Conversion hysteria, neurosis or reaction F44.9
Converter, tuberculosis (test reaction) R76.1
Conviction (legal)**, anxiety concerning** Z65.0
- with imprisonment Z65.1

Convulsions (idiopathic) (*see also* Seizure(s)) R56.9
- apoplectiform (cerebral ischemia) I67.8
- benign neonatal (familial) — *see* Epilepsy, generalized, idiopathic
- dissociative F44.5
- epileptic — *see* Epilepsy
- epileptiform, epileptoid — *see* Seizure, epileptiform
- ether (anesthetic) — *see* Table of Drugs and Chemicals, by drug
- febrile R56.00
  - with status epilepticus G40.901
  - complex R56.01
    - with status epilepticus G40.901
  - simple R56.00
- hysterical F44.5
- infantile P90
  - epilepsy — *see* Epilepsy
- jacksonian — *see* Epilepsy, localization-related, symptomatic, with simple partial seizures
- myoclonic G25.3
- neonatal, benign (familial) — *see* Epilepsy, generalized, idiopathic
- newborn P90
- obstetrical (nephritic) (uremic) — *see* Eclampsia
- paretic A52.17
- post traumatic R56.1
- psychomotor — *see* Epilepsy, localization-related, symptomatic, with complex partial seizures
- recurrent R56.9
- reflex R25.8
- scarlatinal A38.8
- tetanus, tetanic — *see* Tetanus
- thymic E32.8

Convulsive (*see also* Convulsions)
Cooley's anemia D56.1
Coolie itch B76.9
Cooper's
- disease — *see* Mastopathy, cystic
- hernia — *see* Hernia, abdomen, specified site NEC

Copra itch B88.0
Coprophagy F50.8
Coprophobia F40.298
Coproporphyria, hereditary E80.29
Cor
- biloculare Q20.8
- bovis, bovinum — *see* Hypertrophy, cardiac
- pulmonale (chronic) I27.81
  - acute I26.09
- triatriatum, triatrium Q24.2
- triloculare Q20.8
  - biatrium Q20.4

Cor— *continued*
- triloculare— *continued*
  - biventriculare Q21.1
Corbus' disease (gangrenous balanitis) N48.1
Cord (*see also* condition)
- around neck (tightly) (with compression)
  - complicating delivery O69.1
- bladder G95.89
  - tabetic A52.19
Cordis ectopia Q24.8
Corditis (spermatic) N49.1
Corectopia Q13.2
Cori's disease (glycogen storage) E74.03
Corkhandler's disease or lung J67.3
Corkscrew esophagus K22.4
Corkworker's disease or lung J67.3
Corn (infected) L84
Cornea (*see also* condition)
- donor Z52.5
- plana Q13.4
Cornelia de Lange syndrome Q87.1
Cornu cutaneum L85.8
Cornual gestation or pregnancy O00.8
Coronary (artery) — *see* condition
Coronavirus, as cause of disease classified elsewhere B97.29
- SARS-associated B97.21
Corpora (*see also* condition)
- amylacea, prostate N42.89
- cavernosa — *see* condition
Corpulence — *see* Obesity
Corpus — *see* condition
Corrected transposition Q20.5
Corrosion (injury) (acid) (caustic) (chemical) (lime) (external) (internal) T30.4
- abdomen, abdominal (muscle) (wall) T21.42
  - first degree T21.52
  - second degree T21.62
  - third degree T21.72
- above elbow T22.439
  - first degree T22.539
  - left T22.432
    - first degree T22.532
    - second degree T22.632
    - third degree T22.732
  - right T22.431
    - first degree T22.531
    - second degree T22.631
    - third degree T22.731
  - second degree T22.639
  - third degree T22.739
- alimentary tract NEC T28.7
- ankle T25.419
  - first degree T25.519
  - left T25.412
    - first degree T25.512
    - second degree T25.612
    - third degree T25.712
  - multiple with foot — *see* Corrosion, lower, limb, multiple, ankle and foot
  - right T25.411
    - first degree T25.511
    - second degree T25.611
    - third degree T25.711
  - second degree T25.619
  - third degree T25.719
- anus — *see* Corrosion, buttock
- arm(s) (meaning upper limb(s)) — *see* Corrosion, upper limb
- axilla T22.449
  - first degree T22.549
  - left T22.442
    - first degree T22.542
    - second degree T22.642
    - third degree T22.742
  - right T22.441
    - first degree T22.541
    - second degree T22.641
    - third degree T22.741
  - second degree T22.649
  - third degree T22.749
- back (lower) T21.44
  - first degree T21.54

Corrosion— *continued*
- back (lower)— *continued*
  - second degree T21.64
  - third degree T21.74
  - upper T21.43
    - first degree T21.53
    - second degree T21.63
    - third degree T21.73
- blisters—code as Corrosion, second degree, by site
- breast(s) — *see* Corrosion, chest wall
- buttock(s) T21.45
  - first degree T21.55
  - second degree T21.65
  - third degree T21.75
- calf T24.439
  - first degree T24.539
  - left T24.432
    - first degree T24.532
    - second degree T24.632
    - third degree T24.732
  - right T24.431
    - first degree T24.531
    - second degree T24.631
    - third degree T24.731
  - second degree T24.639
  - third degree T24.739
- canthus (eye) — *see* Corrosion, eyelid
- cervix T28.8
- cheek T20.46
  - first degree T20.56
  - second degree T20.66
  - third degree T20.76
- chest wall T21.41
  - first degree T21.51
  - second degree T21.61
  - third degree T21.71
- chin T20.43
  - first degree T20.53
  - second degree T20.63
  - third degree T20.73
- colon T28.7
- conjunctiva (and cornea) — *see* Corrosion, cornea
- cornea (and conjunctiva) T26.6-
- deep necrosis of underlying tissue—code as Corrosion, third degree, by site
- dorsum of hand T23.469
  - first degree T23.569
  - left T23.462
    - first degree T23.562
    - second degree T23.662
    - third degree T23.762
  - right T23.461
    - first degree T23.561
    - second degree T23.661
    - third degree T23.761
  - second degree T23.669
  - third degree T23.769
- ear (auricle) (external) (canal) T20.41
  - drum T28.91
  - first degree T20.51
  - second degree T20.61
  - third degree T20.71
- elbow T22.429
  - first degree T22.529
  - left T22.422
    - first degree T22.522
    - second degree T22.622
    - third degree T22.722
  - right T22.421
    - first degree T22.521
    - second degree T22.621
    - third degree T22.721
  - second degree T22.629
  - third degree T22.729
- entire body — *see* Corrosion, multiple body regions
- epidermal loss—code as Corrosion, second degree, by site
- epiglottis T27.4
- erythema, erythematous—code as Corrosion, first degree, by site
- esophagus T28.6
- extent (percentage of body surface)
  - less than 10 per cent T32.0

Corrosion— *continued*
  extent— *continued*
    10-19 per cent (0-9 percent third degree) T32.10
      with 10-19 percent third degree T32.11
    20-29 per cent (0-9 percent third degree) T32.20
      with
        10-19 percent third degree T32.21
        20-29 percent third degree T32.22
    30-39 per cent (0-9 percent third degree) T32.30
      with
        10-19 percent third degree T32.31
        20-29 percent third degree T32.32
        30-39 percent third degree T32.33
    40-49 per cent (0-9 percent third degree) T32.40
      with
        10-19 percent third degree T32.41
        20-29 percent third degree T32.42
        30-39 percent third degree T32.43
        40-49 percent third degree T32.44
    50-59 per cent (0-9 percent third degree) T32.50
      with
        10-19 percent third degree T32.51
        20-29 percent third degree T32.52
        30-39 percent third degree T32.53
        40-49 percent third degree T32.54
        50-59 percent third degree T32.55
    60-69 per cent (0-9 percent third degree) T32.60
      with
        10-19 percent third degree T32.61
        20-29 percent third degree T32.62
        30-39 percent third degree T32.63
        40-49 percent third degree T32.64
        50-59 percent third degree T32.65
        60-69 percent third degree T32.66
    70-79 per cent (0-9 percent third degree) T32.70
      with
        10-19 percent third degree T32.71
        20-29 percent third degree T32.72
        30-39 percent third degree T32.73
        40-49 percent third degree T32.74
        50-59 percent third degree T32.75
        60-69 percent third degree T32.76
        70-79 percent third degree T32.77
    80-89 per cent (0-9 percent third degree) T32.80
      with
        10-19 percent third degree T32.81
        20-29 percent third degree T32.82
        30-39 percent third degree T32.83
        40-49 percent third degree T32.84
        50-59 percent third degree T32.85
        60-69 percent third degree T32.86
        70-79 percent third degree T32.87
        80-89 percent third degree T32.88
    90 per cent or more (0-9 percent third degree)
      T32.90
      with
        10-19 percent third degree T32.91
        20-29 percent third degree T32.92
        30-39 percent third degree T32.93
        40-49 percent third degree T32.94
        50-59 percent third degree T32.95
        60-69 percent third degree T32.96
        70-79 percent third degree T32.97
        80-89 percent third degree T32.98
        90-99 percent third degree T32.99
  extremity — *see* Corrosion, limb
  eye(s) and adnexa T26.9-
    with resulting rupture and destruction of eyeball
      T26.7-
    conjunctival sac — *see* Corrosion, cornea
    cornea — *see* Corrosion, cornea
    lid — *see* Corrosion, eyelid
    periocular area — *see* Corrosion eyelid
    specified site NEC T26.8-
  eyeball — *see* Corrosion, eye
  eyelid(s) T26.5-
  face — *see* Corrosion, head
  finger T23.429
    first degree T23.529
    left T23.422
      first degree T23.522
      second degree T23.622
      third degree T23.722

Corrosion— *continued*
  finger— *continued*
    multiple sites (without thumb) T23.439
      with thumb T23.449
        first degree T23.549
        left T23.442
          first degree T23.542
          second degree T23.642
          third degree T23.742
        right T23.441
          first degree T23.541
          second degree T23.641
          third degree T23.741
      second degree T23.649
      third degree T23.749
    first degree T23.539
    left T23.432
      first degree T23.532
      second degree T23.632
      third degree T23.732
    right T23.431
      first degree T23.531
      second degree T23.631
      third degree T23.731
    second degree T23.639
    third degree T23.739
    right T23.421
      first degree T23.521
      second degree T23.621
      third degree T23.721
    second degree T23.629
    third degree T23.729
  flank — *see* Corrosion, abdomen
  foot T25.429
    first degree T25.529
    left T25.422
      first degree T25.522
      second degree T25.622
      third degree T25.722
    multiple with ankle — *see* Corrosion, lower, limb,
      multiple, ankle and foot
    right T25.421
      first degree T25.521
      second degree T25.621
      third degree T25.721
    second degree T25.629
    third degree T25.729
  forearm T22.419
    first degree T22.519
    left T22.412
      first degree T22.512
      second degree T22.612
      third degree T22.712
    right T22.411
      first degree T22.511
      second degree T22.611
      third degree T22.711
    second degree T22.619
    third degree T22.719
  forehead T20.46
    first degree T20.56
    second degree T20.66
    third degree T20.76
  fourth degree—code as Corrosion, third degree, by
    site
  full thickness skin loss—code as Corrosion, third
    degree, by site
  gastrointestinal tract NEC T28.7
  genital organs
    external
      female T21.47
        first degree T21.57
        second degree T21.67
        third degree T21.77
      male T21.46
        first degree T21.56
        second degree T21.66
        third degree T21.76
    internal T28.7
      from caustic or corrosive substance T28.8
  groin — *see* Corrosion, abdominal wall
  hand(s) T23.409
    back — *see* Corrosion, dorsum of hand

Corrosion— *continued*
  hand(s)— *continued*
    finger — *see* Corrosion, finger
    first degree T23.509
    left T23.402
      first degree T23.502
      second degree T23.602
      third degree T23.702
    multiple sites with wrist T23.499
      first degree T23.599
      left T23.492
        first degree T23.592
        second degree T23.692
        third degree T23.792
      right T23.491
        first degree T23.591
        second degree T23.691
        third degree T23.791
      second degree T23.699
      third degree T23.799
    palm — *see* Corrosion, palm
    right T23.401
      first degree T23.501
      second degree T23.601
      third degree T23.701
    second degree T23.609
    third degree T23.709
    thumb — *see* Corrosion, thumb
  head (and face) (and neck) T20.40
    cheek — *see* Corrosion, cheek
    chin — *see* Corrosion, chin
    ear — *see* Corrosion, ear
    eye(s) only — *see* Corrosion, eye
    first degree T20.50
    forehead — *see* Corrosion, forehead
    lip — *see* Corrosion, lip
    multiple sites T20.49
      first degree T20.59
      second degree T20.69
      third degree T20.79
    neck — *see* Corrosion, neck
    nose — *see* Corrosion, nose
    scalp — *see* Corrosion, scalp
    second degree T20.60
    third degree T20.70
  hip(s) — *see* Corrosion, lower, limb
  inhalation — *see* Corrosion, respiratory tract
  internal organ(s) T28.90
    alimentary tract T28.7
      esophagus T28.6
    esophagus T28.6
    from caustic or corrosive substance (swallowing)
      NEC — *see* Corrosion, by site
    genitourinary T28.8
    mouth T28.5
    pharynx T28.5
    specified organ NEC T28.99
  interscapular region — *see* Corrosion, back, upper
  intestine (large) (small) T28.7
  knee T24.429
    first degree T24.529
    left T24.422
      first degree T24.522
      second degree T24.622
      third degree T24.722
    right T24.421
      first degree T24.521
      second degree T24.621
      third degree T24.721
    second degree T24.629
    third degree T24.729
  labium (majus) (minus) — *see* Corrosion, genital
    organs, external, female
  lacrimal apparatus, duct, gland or sac — *see*
    Corrosion, eye, specified site NEC
  larynx T27.4
    with lung T27.5
  leg(s) (meaning lower limb(s)) — *see* Corrosion,
    lower limb
  limb(s)
    lower — *see* Corrosion, lower, limb
    upper — *see* Corrosion, upper limb

Corrosion— *continued*
- lip(s) T20.42
  - first degree T20.52
  - second degree T20.62
  - third degree T20.72
- lower
  - back — *see* Corrosion, back
  - limb T24.409
    - ankle — *see* Corrosion, ankle
    - calf — *see* Corrosion, calf
    - first degree T24.509
    - foot — *see* Corrosion, foot
    - knee — *see* Corrosion, knee
    - left T24.402
      - first degree T24.502
      - second degree T24.602
      - third degree T24.702
    - multiple sites, except ankle and foot T24.499
      - ankle and foot T25.499
        - first degree T25.599
        - left T25.492
          - first degree T25.592
          - second degree T25.692
          - third degree T25.792
        - right T25.491
          - first degree T25.591
          - second degree T25.691
          - third degree T25.791
        - second degree T25.699
        - third degree T25.799
      - first degree T24.599
      - left T24.492
        - first degree T24.592
        - second degree T24.692
        - third degree T24.792
      - right T24.491
        - first degree T24.591
        - second degree T24.691
        - third degree T24.791
      - second degree T24.699
      - third degree T24.799
    - right T24.401
      - first degree T24.501
      - second degree T24.601
      - third degree T24.701
    - second degree T24.609
    - hip — *see* Corrosion, thigh
    - thigh — *see* Corrosion, thigh
    - third degree T24.709
- lung (with larynx and trachea) T27.5
- mouth T28.5
- neck T20.47
  - first degree T20.57
  - second degree T20.67
  - third degree T20.77
- nose (septum) T20.44
  - first degree T20.54
  - second degree T20.64
  - third degree T20.74
- ocular adnexa — *see* Corrosion, eye
- orbit region — *see* Corrosion, eyelid
- palm T23.459
  - first degree T23.559
  - left T23.452
    - first degree T23.552
    - second degree T23.652
    - third degree T23.752
  - right T23.451
    - first degree T23.551
    - second degree T23.651
    - third degree T23.751
  - second degree T23.659
  - third degree T23.759
- partial thickness—code as Corrosion, unspecified degree, by site
- pelvis — *see* Corrosion, trunk
- penis — *see* Corrosion, genital organs, external, male
- perineum
  - female — *see* Corrosion, genital organs, external, female
  - male — *see* Corrosion, genital organs, external, male

Corrosion— *continued*
- periocular area — *see* Corrosion, eyelid
- pharynx T28.5
- rectum T28.7
- respiratory tract T27.7
  - larynx — *see* Corrosion, larynx
  - specified part NEC T27.6
  - trachea — *see* Corrosion, larynx
- sac, lacrimal — *see* Corrosion, eye, specified site NEC
- scalp T20.45
  - first degree T20.55
  - second degree T20.65
  - third degree T20.75
- scapular region T22.469
  - first degree T22.569
  - left T22.462
    - first degree T22.562
    - second degree T22.662
    - third degree T22.762
  - right T22.461
    - first degree T22.561
    - second degree T22.661
    - third degree T22.761
  - second degree T22.669
  - third degree T22.769
- sclera — *see* Corrosion, eye, specified site NEC
- scrotum — *see* Corrosion, genital organs, external, male
- shoulder T22.459
  - first degree T22.559
  - left T22.452
    - first degree T22.552
    - second degree T22.652
    - third degree T22.752
  - right T22.451
    - first degree T22.551
    - second degree T22.651
    - third degree T22.751
  - second degree T22.659
  - third degree T22.759
- stomach T28.7
- temple — *see* Corrosion, head
- testis — *see* Corrosion, genital organs, external, male
- thigh T24.419
  - first degree T24.519
  - left T24.412
    - first degree T24.512
    - second degree T24.612
    - third degree T24.712
  - right T24.411
    - first degree T24.511
    - second degree T24.611
    - third degree T24.711
  - second degree T24.619
  - third degree T24.719
- thorax (external) — *see* Corrosion, trunk
- throat (meaning pharynx) T28.5
- thumb(s) T23.419
  - first degree T23.519
  - left T23.412
    - first degree T23.512
    - second degree T23.612
    - third degree T23.712
  - multiple sites with fingers T23.449
    - first degree T23.549
    - left T23.442
      - first degree T23.542
      - second degree T23.642
      - third degree T23.742
    - right T23.441
      - first degree T23.541
      - second degree T23.641
      - third degree T23.741
    - second degree T23.649
    - third degree T23.749
  - right T23.411
    - first degree T23.511
    - second degree T23.611
    - third degree T23.711
  - second degree T23.619
  - third degree T23.719

Corrosion— *continued*
- toe T25.439
  - first degree T25.539
  - left T25.432
    - first degree T25.532
    - second degree T25.632
    - third degree T25.732
  - right T25.431
    - first degree T25.531
    - second degree T25.631
    - third degree T25.731
  - second degree T25.639
  - third degree T25.739
- tongue T28.5
- tonsil(s) T28.5
- total body — *see* Corrosion, multiple body regions
- trachea T27.4
  - with lung T27.5
- trunk T21.40
  - abdominal wall — *see* Corrosion, abdominal wall
  - anus — *see* Corrosion, buttock
  - axilla — *see* Corrosion, upper limb
  - back — *see* Corrosion, back
  - breast — *see* Corrosion, chest wall
  - buttock — *see* Corrosion, buttock
  - chest wall — *see* Corrosion, chest wall
  - first degree T21.50
  - flank — *see* Corrosion, abdominal wall
  - genital
    - female — *see* Corrosion, genital organs, external, female
    - male — *see* Corrosion, genital organs, external, male
  - groin — *see* Corrosion, abdominal wall
  - interscapular region — *see* Corrosion, back, upper
  - labia — *see* Corrosion, genital organs, external, female
  - lower back — *see* Corrosion, back
  - penis — *see* Corrosion, genital organs, external, male
  - perineum
    - female — *see* Corrosion, genital organs, external, female
    - male — *see* Corrosion, genital organs, external, male
  - scapular region — *see* Corrosion, upper limb
  - scrotum — *see* Corrosion, genital organs, external, male
  - shoulder — *see* Corrosion, upper limb
  - second degree T21.60
  - specified site NEC T21.49
    - first degree T21.59
    - second degree T21.69
    - third degree T21.79
  - testes — *see* Corrosion, genital organs, external, male
  - third degree T21.70
  - upper back — *see* Corrosion, back, upper
  - vagina T28.8
  - vulva — *see* Corrosion, genital organs, external, female
- unspecified site with extent of body surface involved specified
  - less than 10 per cent T32.0
  - 10-19 per cent (0-9 percent third degree) T32.10
    - with 10-19 percent third degree T32.11
  - 20-29 per cent (0-9 percent third degree) T32.20
    - with
      - 10-19 percent third degree T32.21
      - 20-29 percent third degree T32.22
  - 30-39 per cent (0-9 percent third degree) T32.30
    - with
      - 10-19 percent third degree T32.31
      - 20-29 percent third degree T32.32
      - 30-39 percent third degree T32.33
  - 40-49 per cent (0-9 percent third degree) T32.40
    - with
      - 10-19 percent third degree T32.41
      - 20-29 percent third degree T32.42
      - 30-39 percent third degree T32.43
      - 40-49 percent third degree T32.44

Coxsackie— *continued*
　specific disease NEC B33.8
Crabs, meaning pubic lice B85.3
Crack baby P04.41
Cracked nipple N64.0
　associated with
　　lactation O92.13
　　pregnancy O92.11-
Cracked tooth K03.81
Cradle cap L21.0
Craft neurosis F48.8
Cramp(s) R25.2
　abdominal — *see* Pain, abdominal
　bathing T75.1
　colic R10.83
　　psychogenic F45.8
　due to immersion T75.1
　fireman T67.2
　heat T67.2
　immersion T75.1
　intestinal — *see* Pain, abdominal
　　psychogenic F45.8
　leg, sleep related G47.62
　limb (lower) (upper) NEC R25.2
　　sleep related G47.62
　linotypist's F48.8
　　organic G25.89
　muscle (limb) (general) R25.2
　　due to immersion T75.1
　　psychogenic F45.8
　occupational (hand) F48.8
　　organic G25.89
　salt-depletion E87.1
　sleep related, leg G47.62
　stoker's T67.2
　swimmer's T75.1
　telegrapher's F48.8
　　organic G25.89
　typist's F48.8
　　organic G25.89
　uterus N94.89
　　menstrual — *see* Dysmenorrhea
Cramp— *continued*
　writer's F48.8
　　organic G25.89
Cranial — *see* condition
Craniocleidodysostosis Q74.0
Craniofenestria (skull) Q75.8
Craniolacunia (skull) Q75.8
Craniopagus Q89.4
Craniopathy, metabolic M85.2
Craniopharyngeal — *see* condition
Craniopharyngioma D44.4
Craniorachischisis (totalis) Q00.1
Cranioschisis Q75.8
Craniostenosis Q75.0
Craniosynostosis Q75.0
Craniotabes (cause unknown) M83.8
　neonatal P96.3
　rachitic E64.3
　syphilitic A50.56
Cranium — *see* condition
Craw-craw — *see* Onchocerciasis
Creaking joint — *see* Derangement, joint, specified
　　type NEC
Creeping
　eruption B76.9
　palsy or paralysis G12.22
Crenated tongue K14.8
Creotoxism A05.9
Crepitus
　caput Q75.8
　joint — *see* Derangement, joint, specified type NEC
Crescent or conus choroid, congenital Q14.3
CREST syndrome M34.1
Cretin, cretinism (congenital) (endemic)
　　(nongoitrous) (sporadic) E00.9
　pelvis
　　with disproportion (fetopelvic) O33.0
　　　causing obstructed labor O65.0
　type
　　hypothyroid E00.1
　　mixed E00.2

Cretin, cretinism — *continued*
　type— *continued*
　　myxedematous E00.1
　　neurological E00.0
Creutzfeldt-Jakob disease or syndrome (with
　　dementia) A81.00
　familial A81.09
　iatrogenic A81.09
　specified NEC A81.09
　sporadic A81.09
　variant (vCJD) A81.01
Crib death R99
Cribriform hymen Q52.3
Cri-du-chat syndrome Q93.4
Crigler-Najjar disease or syndrome E80.5
Crime, victim of Z65.4
Crimean hemorrhagic fever A98.0
Criminalism F60.2
Crisis
　abdomen R10.0
　acute reaction F43.0
　addisonian E27.2
　adrenal (cortical) E27.2
　celiac K90.0
　Dietl's N13.8
　emotional (*see also* Disorder, adjustment)
　　acute reaction to stress F43.0
　　specific to childhood and adolescence F93.8
　glaucomatocyclitic — *see* Glaucoma, secondary,
　　inflammation
　heart — *see* Failure, heart
　nitritoid I95.2
　　correct substance properly administered — *see*
　　　Table of Drugs and Chemicals, by drug,
　　　adverse effect
　　overdose or wrong substance given or taken —
　　　see Table of Drugs and Chemicals, by drug,
　　　poisoning
　oculogyric H51.8
　　psychogenic F45.8
　Pel's (tabetic) A52.11
　psychosexual identity F64.2
　renal N28.0
　sickle-cell D57.00
　　with
　　　acute chest syndrome D57.01
　　　splenic sequestration D57.02
　state (acute reaction) F43.0
　tabetic A52.11
　thyroid — *see* Thyrotoxicosis with thyroid storm
　thyrotoxic — *see* Thyrotoxicosis with thyroid storm
Crocq's disease (acrocyanosis) I73.89
Crohn's disease — *see* Enteritis, regional
Crooked septum, nasal J34.2
Cross syndrome E70.328
Crossbite (anterior) (posterior) M26.24
Cross-eye — *see* Strabismus
Croup, croupous (catarrhal) (infectious)
　　(inflammatory) (nondiphtheritic) J05.0
　bronchial J20.9
　diphtheritic A36.2
　false J38.5
　spasmodic J38.5
　　diphtheritic A36.2
　stridulous J38.5
　　diphtheritic A36.2
Crouzon's disease Q75.1
Crowding, tooth, teeth, fully erupted M26.31
CRST syndrome M34.1
Cruchet's disease A85.8
Cruelty in children — *see* Disorder, conduct
Crural ulcer — *see* Ulcer, lower limb
Crush, crushed, crushing
　abdomen S38.1
　ankle S97.0-
　arm (upper) (and shoulder) S47.-
　axilla — *see* Crush, arm
　back, lower S38.1
　buttock S38.1
　cheek S07.0
　chest S28.0
　cranium S07.1
　ear S07.0

Crush, crushed, crushing— *continued*
　elbow S57.0-
　extremity
　　lower
　　　ankle — *see* Crush, ankle
　　　below knee — *see* Crush, leg
　　　foot — *see* Crush, foot
　　　hip — *see* Crush, hip
　　　knee — *see* Crush, knee
　　　thigh — *see* Crush, thigh
　　　toe — *see* Crush, toe
　　upper
　　　below elbow S67.9-
　　　elbow — *see* Crush, elbow
　　　finger — *see* Crush, finger
　　　forearm — *see* Crush, forearm
　　　hand — *see* Crush, hand
　　　thumb — *see* Crush, thumb
　　　upper arm — *see* Crush, arm
　　　wrist — *see* Crush, wrist
　face S07.0
　finger(s) S67.1-
　　with hand (and wrist) — *see* Crush, hand,
　　　specified site NEC
　　index S67.19-
　　little S67.19-
　　middle S67.19-
　　ring S67.19-
　　thumb — *see* Crush, thumb
　foot S97.8-
　　toe — *see* Crush, toe
　forearm S57.8-
　genitalia, external
　　female S38.002
　　　vagina S38.03
　　　vulva S38.03
　　male S38.001
　　　penis S38.01
　　　scrotum S38.02
　　　testis S38.02
　hand (except fingers alone) S67.2-
　　with wrist S67.4-
　head
　　specified NEC S07.8
　heel — *see* Crush, foot
　hip S77.0-
　　with thigh S77.2-
　internal organ (abdomen, chest, or pelvis) NEC T14.8
　knee S87.0-
　labium (majus) (minus) S38.03
　larynx S17.0
　leg (lower) S87.8-
　　knee — *see* Crush, knee
　lip S07.0
　lower
　　back S38.1
　　leg — *see* Crush, leg
　neck S17.9
　nerve — *see* Injury, nerve
　nose S07.0
　pelvis S38.1
　penis S38.01
　scalp S07.8
　scapular region — *see* Crush, arm
　scrotum S38.02
　severe, unspecified site T14.8
　shoulder (and upper arm) — *see* Crush, arm
　skull S07.1
　syndrome (complication of trauma) T79.5
　testis S38.02
　thigh S77.1-
　　with hip S77.2-
　throat S17.8
　thumb S67.0-
　　with hand (and wrist) — *see* Crush, hand,
　　　specified site NEC
　toe(s) S97.10-
　　great S97.11-
　　lesser S97.12-
　trachea S17.0
　vagina S38.03
　vulva S38.03

Crush, crushed, crushing— *continued*
  wrist S67.3-
    with hand S67.4-
Crusta lactea L21.0
Crusts R23.4
Crutch paralysis — *see* Injury, brachial plexus
Cruveilhier-Baumgarten cirrhosis, disease or
  syndrome K74.69
Cruveilhier's atrophy or disease G12.8
Crying (constant) (continuous) (excessive)
  child, adolescent, or adult R45.83
  infant (baby) (newborn) R68.11
Cryofibrinogenemia D89.2
Cryoglobulinemia(essential) (idiopathic) (mixed)
  (primary) (purpura) (secondary) (vasculitis) D89.1
  with lung involvement D89.1 [J99]
Cryptitis (anal) (rectal) K62.8
Cryptococcosis, cryptococcus (infection)
  (neoformans) B45.9
  bone B45.3
  cerebral B45.1
  cutaneous B45.2
  disseminated B45.7
  generalized B45.7
  meningitis B45.1
  meningocerebralis B45.1
  osseous B45.3
  pulmonary B45.0
  skin B45.2
  specified NEC B45.8
Cryptopapillitis (anus) K62.8
Cryptophthalmos Q11.2
  syndrome Q87.0
Cryptorchid, cryptorchism, cryptorchidism Q53.9
  bilateral Q53.20
    abdominal Q53.21
    perineal Q53.22
  unilateral Q53.10
    abdominal Q53.11
    perineal Q53.12
Cryptosporidiosis A07.2
  hepatobiliary B88.8
  respiratory B88.8
Cryptostromosis J67.6
Crystalluria R82.99
Cubitus
  congenital Q68.8
  valgus (acquired) M21.0-
    congenital Q68.8
    sequelae (late effect) of rickets E64.3
  varus (acquired) M21.1-
    congenital Q68.8
    sequelae (late effect) of rickets E64.3
Cultural deprivation or shock Z60.3
Curling esophagus K22.4
Curling's ulcer — *see* Ulcer, peptic, acute
Curschmann (-Batten) (-Steinert) **disease or**
  syndrome G71.11
Curse, Ondine's — *see* Apnea, sleep
Curvature
  organ or site, congenital NEC — *see* Distortion
  penis (lateral) Q55.61
  Pott's (spinal) A18.01
  radius, idiopathic, progressive (congenital) Q74.0
  spine (acquired) (angular) (idiopathic) (incorrect)
    (postural) — *see* Dorsopathy, deforming
    congenital Q67.5
    due to or associated with
      Charcot-Marie-Tooth disease (*see also*
        subcategory M49.8) G60.0
      osteitis
        deformans M88.88
        fibrosa cystica (*see also* subcategory
          M49.8) E21.0
      tuberculosis (Pott's curvature) A18.01
    sequelae (late effect) of rickets E64.3
    tuberculous A18.01
Cushingoid due to steroid therapy E24.2
  correct substance properly administered — *see*
    Table of Drugs and Chemicals, by drug,
    adverse effect

Cushingoid due to steroid therapy— *continued*
  overdose or wrong substance given or taken — *see*
    Table of Drugs and Chemicals, by drug,
    poisoning
Cushing's
  syndrome or disease E24.9
    drug-induced E24.2
    iatrogenic E24.2
    pituitary-dependent E24.0
    specified NEC E24.8
  ulcer — *see* Ulcer, peptic, acute
Cusp, Carabelli —*omit code*
Cut (external) (*see also* Laceration)
  muscle — *see* Injury, muscle
Cutaneous (*see also* condition)
  hemorrhage R23.3
  larva migrans B76.9
Cutis (*see also* condition)
  hyperelastica Q82.8
    acquired L57.4
  laxa (hyperelastica) — *see* Dermatolysis
  marmorata R23.8
  osteosis L94.2
  pendula — *see* Dermatolysis
  rhomboidalis nuchae L57.2
  verticis gyrata Q82.8
    acquired L91.8
Cyanosis R23.0
  due to
    patent foramen botalli Q21.1
    persistent foramen ovale Q21.1
  enterogenous D74.8
  paroxysmal digital — *see* Raynaud's disease
    with gangrene I73.01
  retina, retinal H35.89
Cyanotic heart disease I24.9
  congenital Q24.9
Cycle
  anovulatory N97.0
  menstrual, irregular N92.6
Cyclencephaly Q04.9
Cyclical vomiting G43.a09 (*see also* Vomiting, cyclical)
  psychogenic F50.8
Cyclitis (*see also* Iridocyclitis) H20.9
  chronic — *see* Iridocyclitis, chronic
Cyclitis— *continued*
  Fuchs' heterochromic H20.81-
  granulomatous — *see* Iridocyclitis, chronic
  lens-induced — *see* Iridocyclitis, lens-induced
  posterior H30.2-
Cycloid personality F34.0
Cyclophoria H50.54
Cyclopia, cyclops Q87.0
Cyclopism Q87.0
Cyclosporiasis A07.4
Cyclothymia F34.0
Cyclothymic personality F34.0
Cyclotropia H50.41-
Cylindroma (*see also* Neoplasm, malignant, by site)
  eccrine dermal — *see* Neoplasm, skin, benign
  skin — *see* Neoplasm, skin, benign
Cylindruria R82.99
Cynanche
  diphtheritic A36.2
  tonsillaris J36
Cynophobia F40.218
Cynorexia R63.2
Cyphosis — *see* Kyphosis
Cyprus fever — *see* Brucellosis
Cyst (colloid) (mucous) (simple) (retention)
  adenoid (infected) J35.8
  adrenal gland E27.8
    congenital Q89.1
  air, lung J98.4
  allantoic Q64.4
  alveolar process (jaw bone) M27.40
  amnion, amniotic O41.8x-
  anterior
    chamber (eye) — *see* Cyst, iris
    nasopalatine K09.1
  antrum J34.1
  anus K62.8

Cyst— *continued*
  apical (tooth) (periodontal) K04.8
  appendix K38.8
  arachnoid, brain (acquired) G93.0
    congenital Q04.6
  arytenoid J38.7
  Baker's M71.2-
    ruptured M66.0
    tuberculous A18.02
  Bartholin's gland N75.0
  bile duct (common) (hepatic) K83.5
  bladder (multiple) (trigone) N32.89
  blue dome (breast) — *see* Cyst, breast
  bone (local) NEC M85.60
    aneurysmal M85.50
      ankle M85.57-
      foot M85.57-
      forearm M85.53-
      hand M85.54-
      jaw M27.49
      lower leg M85.56-
      multiple site M85.59
      neck M85.58
      rib M85.58
      shoulder M85.51-
      skull M85.58
      specified site NEC M85.58
      thigh M85.55-
      toe M85.57-
      upper arm M85.52-
      vertebra M85.58
    solitary M85.40
      ankle M85.47-
      fibula M85.46-
      foot M85.47-
      hand M85.44-
      humerus M85.42-
      jaw M27.49
      neck M85.48
      pelvis M85.45-
      radius M85.43-
      rib M85.48
      shoulder M85.41-
      skull M85.48
      specified site NEC M85.48
      tibia M85.46-
      toe M85.47-
      ulna M85.43-
      vertebra M85.48
    specified type NEC M85.60
      ankle M85.67-
      foot M85.67-
      forearm M85.63-
      hand M85.64-
      jaw M27.40
        developmental (nonodontogenic) K09.1
          odontogenic K09.0
        latent M27.0
      lower leg M85.66-
      multiple site M85.69
      neck M85.68
      rib M85.68
      shoulder M85.61-
      skull M85.68
      specified site NEC M85.68
      thigh M85.65-
      toe M85.67-
      upper arm M85.62-
      vertebra M85.68
  brain (acquired) G93.0
    congenital Q04.6
    hydatid B67.99 [G94]
    third ventricle (colloid), congenital Q04.6
  branchial (cleft) Q18.0
  branchiogenic Q18.0
  breast (benign) (blue dome) (pedunculated)
    (solitary) N60.0-
    involution — *see* Dysplasia, mammary, specified
      type NEC
    sebaceous — *see* Dysplasia, mammary, specified
      type NEC
  broad ligament (benign) N83.8

Cyst— *continued*
  bronchogenic (mediastinal) (sequestration) J98.4
    congenital Q33.0
  buccal K09.8
  bulbourethral gland N36.8
  bursa, bursal NEC M71.30
    with rupture — *see* Rupture, synovium
    ankle M71.37-
    elbow M71.32-
    foot M71.37-
    hand M71.34-
    hip M71.35-
    multiple sites M71.39
    pharyngeal J39.2
    popliteal space — *see* Cyst, Baker's
    shoulder M71.31-
    specified site NEC M71.38
    wrist M71.33-
  calcifying odontogenic D16.5
    upper jaw (bone) (maxilla) D16.4
  canal of Nuck (female) N94.89
    congenital Q52.4
  canthus — *see* Cyst, conjunctiva
  carcinomatous — *see* Neoplasm, malignant, by site
  cauda equina G95.89
  cavum septi pellucidi — *see* Cyst, brain
  celomic (pericardium) Q24.8
  cerebellopontine (angle) — *see* Cyst, brain
  cerebellum — *see* Cyst, brain
  cerebral — *see* Cyst, brain
  cervical lateral Q18.1
  cervix NEC N88.8
    embryonic Q51.6
    nabothian N88.8
  chiasmal optic NEC — *see* Disorder, optic, chiasm
  chocolate (ovary) N80.1
  choledochus, congenital Q44.4
  chorion O41.8x-
  choroid plexus G93.0
  ciliary body — *see* Cyst, iris
  clitoris N90.7
  colon K63.89
  common (bile) duct K83.5
  congenital NEC Q89.8
    adrenal gland Q89.1
    epiglottis Q31.8
    esophagus Q39.8
    fallopian tube Q50.4
    kidney Q61.00
      more than one (multiple) Q61.02
        specified as polycystic Q61.3
          adult type Q61.2
          infantile type NEC Q61.19
            collecting duct dilation Q61.11
      solitary Q61.01
    larynx Q31.8
    liver Q44.6
    lung Q33.0
    mediastinum Q34.1
    ovary Q50.1
    oviduct Q50.4
    periurethral (tissue) Q64.79
    prepuce Q55.69
    salivary gland (any) Q38.4
    sublingual Q38.6
    submaxillary gland Q38.6
    thymus (gland) Q89.2
    tongue Q38.3
    ureterovesical orifice Q62.8
    vulva Q52.79
  conjunctiva H11.44-
  cornea H18.89-
  corpora quadrigemina G93.0
  corpus
    albicans N83.29
    luteum (hemorrhagic) (ruptured) N83.1
  Cowper's gland (benign) (infected) N36.8
  cranial meninges G93.0
  craniobuccal pouch E23.6
  craniopharyngeal pouch E23.6
  cystic duct K82.8
  Cysticercus — *see* Cysticercosis

Cyst— *continued*
  Dandy-Walker Q03.1
    with spina bifida — *see* Spina bifida
  dental (root) K04.8
    developmental K09.0
    eruption K09.0
    primordial K09.0
  dentigerous (mandible) (maxilla) K09.0
  dermoid — *see* Neoplasm, benign, by site
    with malignant transformation C56.-
    implantation
      external area or site (skin) NEC L72.0
      iris — *see* Cyst, iris, implantation
      vagina N89.8
      vulva N90.7
    mouth K09.8
    oral soft tissue K09.8
    sacrococcygeal — *see* Cyst, pilonidal
  developmental K09.1
    odontogenic K09.0
    oral region (nonodontogenic) K09.1
    ovary, ovarian Q50.1
  dura (cerebral) G93.0
    spinal G96.19
  ear (external) Q18.1
  echinococcal — *see* Echinococcus
  embryonic
    cervix uteri Q51.6
    fallopian tube Q50.4
    vagina Q51.6
  endometrium, endometrial (uterus) N85.8
    ectopic — *see* Endometriosis
  enterogenous Q43.8
  epidermal, epidermoid (inclusion) (*see also* Cyst, skin) L72.0
    mouth K09.8
    oral soft tissue K09.8
  epididymis N50.8
  epiglottis J38.7
  epiphysis cerebri E34.8
  epithelial (inclusion) L72.0
  epoophoron Q50.5
  eruption K09.0
  esophagus K22.8
  ethmoid sinus J34.1
  external female genital organs NEC N90.7
  eye NEC H57.8
    congenital Q15.8
  eyelid (sebaceous) H02.829
    infected — *see* Hordeolum
    left H02.826
      lower H02.825
      upper H02.824
    right H02.823
      lower H02.822
      upper H02.821
  fallopian tube N83.8
    congenital Q50.4
  fimbrial (twisted) Q50.4
  fissural (oral region) K09.1
  follicle (graafian) (hemorrhagic) N83.0
    nabothian N88.8
  follicular (atretic) (hemorrhagic) (ovarian) N83.0
    dentigerous K09.0
    odontogenic K09.0
    skin L72.9
      specified NEC L72.8
  frontal sinus J34.1
  gallbladder K82.8
  ganglion — *see* Ganglion
  Gartner's duct Q52.4
  gingiva K09.0
  gland of Moll — *see* Cyst, eyelid
  globulomaxillary K09.1
  graafian follicle (hemorrhagic) N83.0
  granulosal lutein (hemorrhagic) N83.1
  hemangiomatous D18.00
    intra-abdominal D18.03
    intracranial D18.02
    skin D18.01
    specified site NEC D18.09
  hydatid (*see also* Echinococcus) B67.90
    brain B67.99 [G94]

Cyst— *continued*
  hydatid— *continued*
    liver (*see also* Cyst, liver, hydatid) B67.8
    lung NEC B67.99 [J99]
    Morgagni
      female Q50.5
      male (epididymal) Q55.4
        testicular Q55.29
    specified site NEC B67.99
  hymen N89.8
    embryonic Q52.4
  hypopharynx J39.2
  hypophysis, hypophyseal (duct) (recurrent) E23.6
    cerebri E23.6
  implantation (dermoid)
    external area or site (skin) NEC L72.0
    iris — *see* Cyst, iris, implantation
    vagina N89.8
    vulva N90.7
  incisive canal K09.1
  inclusion (epidermal) (epithelial) (epidermoid) (squamous) L72.0
    not of skin—code under Cyst, by site
  intestine (large) (small) K63.89
  intracranial — *see* Cyst, brain
  intraligamentous (*see also* Disorder, ligament)
    knee — *see* Derangement, knee
  intrasellar E23.6
  iris H21.309
    exudative H21.31-
    idiopathic H21.30-
    implantation H21.32-
    parasitic H21.33-
    pars plana (primary) H21.34-
      exudative H21.35-
  jaw (bone) (aneurysmal) (hemorrhagic) (traumatic) M27.40
    developmental (odontogenic) K09.0
    fissural K09.1
  joint NEC — *see* Disorder, joint, specified type NEC
  kidney (acquired) N28.1
    calyceal — *see* Hydronephrosis
    congenital Q61.00
      more than one (multiple) Q61.02
        specified as polycystic Q61.3
          adult type (autosomal dominant) Q61.2
          infantile type (autosomal recessive) NEC Q61.19
            collecting duct dilation Q61.11
    pyelogenic — *see* Hydronephrosis
    simple N28.1
    solitary (single) Q61.01
      acquired N28.1
  labium (majus) (minus) N90.7
    sebaceous N90.7
  lacrimal (*see also* Disorder, lacrimal system, specified NEC)
    gland H04.13-
    passages or sac — *see* Disorder, lacrimal system, specified NEC
  larynx J38.7
  lateral periodontal K09.0
  lens H27.8
    congenital Q12.8
  lip (gland) K13.0
  liver (idiopathic) K76.8
    congenital Q44.6
    hydatid B67.8
      granulosus B67.0
      multilocularis B67.5
  lung J98.4
    congenital Q33.0
    giant bullous J43.9
  lutein N83.1
  lymphangiomatous D18.1
  lymphoepithelial, oral soft tissue K09.8
  macula — *see* Degeneration, macula, hole
  malignant — *see* Neoplasm, malignant, by site
  mammary gland — *see* Cyst, breast
  mandible M27.40
    dentigerous K09.0
    radicular K04.8

Index

Cyst—Cyst

Cyst— *continued*
maxilla M27.40
  dentigerous K09.0
  radicular K04.8
medial, face and neck Q18.8
median
  anterior maxillary K09.1
  palatal K09.1
mediastinum, congenital Q34.1
meibomian (gland) — *see* Chalazion
  infected — *see* Hordeolum
membrane, brain G93.0
meninges (cerebral) G93.0
  spinal G96.19
meniscus, knee — *see* Derangement, knee,
    meniscus, cystic
mesentery, mesenteric K66.8
  chyle I89.8
mesonephric duct
  female Q50.5
  male Q55.4
milk N64.89
Morgagni (hydatid)
  female Q50.5
  male (epididymal) Q55.4
    testicular Q55.29
mouth K09.8
Müllerian duct Q50.4
  appendix testis Q55.29
  cervix Q51.6
  fallopian tube Q50.4
  female Q50.4
  male Q55.29
  prostatic utricle Q55.4
  vagina (embryonal) Q52.4
multilocular (ovary) D39.10
  benign — *see* Neoplasm, benign, by site
myometrium N85.8
nabothian (follicle) (ruptured) N88.8
nasoalveolar K09.1
nasolabial K09.1
nasopalatine (anterior) (duct) K09.1
nasopharynx J39.2
neoplastic — *see* Neoplasm, uncertain behavior, by
    site
  benign — *see* Neoplasm, benign, by site
nervous system NEC G96.8
neuroenteric (congenital) Q06.8
nipple — *see* Cyst, breast
nose (turbinates) J34.1
  sinus J34.1
odontogenic, developmental K09.0
omentum (lesser) K66.8
  congenital Q45.8
ora serrata — *see* Cyst, retina, ora serrata
oral
  region K09.9
    developmental (nonodontogenic) K09.1
    specified NEC K09.8
  soft tissue K09.9
    specified NEC K09.8
orbit H05.81-
ovary, ovarian (twisted) N83.20
  adherent N83.20
  chocolate N80.1
  corpus
    albicans N83.29
    luteum (hemorrhagic) N83.1
  dermoid D27.9
  developmental Q50.1
  due to failure of involution NEC N83.20
  endometrial N80.1
  follicular (graafian) (hemorrhagic) N83.0
  hemorrhagic N83.20
  in pregnancy or childbirth O34.8-
    with obstructed labor O65.5
  multilocular D39.10
  pseudomucinous D27.9
  retention N83.29
  serous N83.20
  specified NEC N83.29
  theca lutein (hemorrhagic) N83.1
  tuberculous A18.18

Cyst— *continued*
oviduct N83.8
palate (median) (fissural) K09.1
palatine papilla (jaw) K09.1
pancreas, pancreatic (hemorrhagic) (true) K86.2
  congenital Q45.2
  false K86.3
paralabral
  hip M24.85-
  shoulder S43.43-
paramesonephric duct Q50.4
  female Q50.4
  male Q55.29
paranephric N28.1
paraphysis, cerebri, congenital Q04.6
parasitic B89
parathyroid (gland) E21.4
paratubal N83.8
paraurethral duct N36.8
paroophoron Q50.5
parotid gland K11.6
parovarian Q50.5
pelvis, female N94.89
  in pregnancy or childbirth O34.8-
    causing obstructed labor O65.5
penis (sebaceous) N48.89
periapical K04.8
pericardial, congenital Q24.8
  acquired (secondary) I31.8
pericoronal K09.0
periodontal K04.8
  lateral K09.0
peripelvic (lymphatic) N28.1
peritoneum K66.8
  chylous I89.8
periventricular, acquired, newborn P91.1
pharynx (wall) J39.2
pilar L72.1
pilonidal (infected) (rectum) L05.91
  with abscess L05.01
  malignant C44.59
pituitary (duct) (gland) E23.6
placenta O43.19-
pleura J94.8
popliteal — *see* Cyst, Baker's
porencephalic Q04.6
  acquired G93.0
postanal (infected) — *see* Cyst, pilonidal
postmastoidectomy cavity (mucosal) —
    see Complications, postmastoidectomy, cyst
preauricular Q18.1
prepuce N47.4
  congenital Q55.69
primordial (jaw) K09.0
prostate N42.89
pseudomucinous (ovary) D27.9
pupillary, miotic H21.27-
radicular (residual) K04.8
radiculodental K04.8
ranular K11.8
Rathke's pouch E23.6
rectum (epithelium) (mucous) K62.8
renal — *see* Cyst, kidney
residual (radicular) K04.8
retention (ovary) N83.29
  salivary gland K11.6
retina H33.19-
  ora serrata H33.11-
  parasitic H33.12-
retroperitoneal K68.9
sacrococcygeal (dermoid) — *see* Cyst, pilonidal
salivary gland or duct (mucous extravasation or
    retention) K11.6
Sampson's N80.1
sclera H15.89
scrotum L72.9
  sebaceous L72.1
sebaceous (duct) (gland) L72.1
  breast — *see* Dysplasia, mammary, specified type
    NEC
  eyelid — *see* Cyst, eyelid
  genital organ NEC
    female N94.89

Cyst— *continued*
sebaceous— *continued*
  genital organ— *continued*
    male N50.8
    scrotum L72.1
semilunar cartilage (knee) (multiple) — *see*
    Derangement, knee, meniscus, cystic
seminal vesicle N50.8
serous (ovary) N83.20
sinus (accessory) (nasal) J34.1
Skene's gland N36.8
skin L72.9
  breast — *see* Dysplasia, mammary, specified type
    NEC
  epidermal, epidermoid L72.0
  epithelial L72.0
  eyelid — *see* Cyst, eyelid
  genital organ NEC
    female N90.7
    male N50.8
  inclusion L72.0
  scrotum L72.9
  sebaceous L72.1
  sweat gland or duct L74.8
solitary
  bone — *see* Cyst, bone, solitary
  jaw M27.40
  kidney N28.1
spermatic cord N50.8
sphenoid sinus J34.1
spinal meninges G96.19
spleen NEC D73.4
  congenital Q89.09
  hydatid (*see also* Echinococcus) B67.99 [D77]
Stafne's M27.0
subarachnoid intrasellar R93.0
subcutaneous, pheomycotic (chromomycotic) B43.2
subdural (cerebral) G93.0
  spinal cord G96.19
sublingual gland K11.6
submandibular gland K11.6
submaxillary gland K11.6
suburethral N36.8
suprarenal gland E27.8
suprasellar — *see* Cyst, brain
sweat gland or duct L74.8
synovial (*see also* Cyst, bursa)
  ruptured *see* Rupture, synovium
tarsal — *see* Chalazion
tendon (sheath) — *see* Disorder, tendon, specified
    type NEC
testis N44.2
  tunica albuginea N44.1
theca lutein (ovary) N83.1
Thornwaldt's J39.2
thymus (gland) E32.8
thyroglossal duct (infected) (persistent) Q89.2
thyroid (gland) E04.1
tongue K14.8
tonsil J35.8
tooth — *see* Cyst, dental
Tornwaldt's J39.2
trichilemmal L72.1
trichodermal L72.1
tubal (fallopian) N83.8
  inflammatory — *see* Salpingitis, chronic
tubo-ovarian N83.8
  inflammatory N70.13
tunica
  albuginea testis N44.1
  vaginalis N50.8
turbinate (nose) J34.1
Tyson's gland N48.89
urachus, congenital Q64.4
ureter N28.89
ureterovesical orifice N28.89
urethra, urethral (gland) N36.8
uterine ligament N83.8
uterus (body) (corpus) (recurrent) N85.8
  embryonic Q51.818
    cervix Q51.6

Cyst— *continued*
vagina, vaginal (implantation) (inclusion)
(squamous cell) (wall) N89.8
embryonic Q52.4
vallecula, vallecular (epiglottis) J38.7
vesical (orifice) N32.89
vitreous body H43.89
vulva (implantation) (inclusion) N90.7
congenital Q52.79
sebaceous gland N90.7
vulvovaginal gland N90.7
wolffian
female Q50.5
male Q55.4
Cystadenocarcinoma — *see* Neoplasm, malignant, by
site
bile duct C22.1
endometrioid — *see* Neoplasm, malignant, by site
specified site — *see* Neoplasm, malignant, by
site
unspecified site
female C56.9
male C61
mucinous
papillary
specified site — *see* Neoplasm, malignant, by
site
unspecified site C56.9
specified site — *see* Neoplasm, malignant, by site
unspecified site C56.9
papillary
mucinous
specified site — *see* Neoplasm, malignant, by
site
unspecified site C56.9
pseudomucinous
specified site — *see* Neoplasm, malignant, by
site
unspecified site C56.9
serous
specified site — *see* Neoplasm, malignant, by
site
unspecified site C56.9
specified site — *see* Neoplasm, malignant, by site
unspecified site C56.9
pseudomucinous
papillary
specified site — *see* Neoplasm, malignant, by
site
unspecified site C56.9
specified site — *see* Neoplasm, malignant, by
site
unspecified site C56.9
serous
papillary
specified site — *see* Neoplasm, malignant, by
site
unspecified site C56.9
specified site — *see* Neoplasm, malignant, by site
unspecified site C56.9
Cystadenofibroma
clear cell — *see* Neoplasm, benign, by site
endometrioid D27.9
borderline malignancy D39.1-
malignant C56.-
mucinous
specified site — *see* Neoplasm, benign, by site
unspecified site D27.9
serous
specified site — *see* Neoplasm, benign, by site
unspecified site D27.9
specified site — *see* Neoplasm, benign, by site
unspecified site D27.9
Cystadenoma (*see also* Neoplasm, benign, by site)
bile duct D13.4
endometrioid — *see* Neoplasm, benign, by site
borderline malignancy — *see* Neoplasm,
uncertain behavior, by site
malignant — *see* Neoplasm, malignant, by site
mucinous
borderline malignancy
ovary C56.-
specified site NEC — *see* Neoplasm, uncertain
behavior, by site

Cystadenoma (*see also* Neoplasm, benign, by site)
mucinous—*continued*
borderline malignancy—*continued*
unspecified site C56.9
papillary
borderline malignancy
ovary C56.-
specified site NEC — *see* Neoplasm,
uncertain behavior, by site
unspecified site C56.9
specified site — *see* Neoplasm, benign, by site
unspecified site D27.9
specified site — *see* Neoplasm, benign, by site
unspecified site D27.9
papillary
borderline malignancy
ovary C56.-
specified site NEC — *see* Neoplasm,
uncertain behavior, by site
unspecified site C56.9
lymphomatosum
specified site — *see* Neoplasm, benign, by site
unspecified site D11.9
mucinous
borderline malignancy
ovary C56.-
specified site NEC — *see* Neoplasm,
uncertain behavior, by site
unspecified site C56.9
specified site — *see* Neoplasm, benign, by site
unspecified site D27.9
pseudomucinous
borderline malignancy
ovary C56.-
specified site NEC — *see* Neoplasm,
uncertain behavior, by site
unspecified site C56.9
specified site — *see* Neoplasm, benign, by site
unspecified site D27.9
serous
borderline malignancy
ovary C56.-
specified site NEC — *see* Neoplasm,
uncertain behavior, by site
unspecified site C56.9
specified site — *see* Neoplasm, benign, by site
unspecified site D27.9
specified site — *see* Neoplasm, benign, by site
unspecified site D27.9
pseudomucinous
borderline malignancy
ovary C56.-
specified site NEC — *see* Neoplasm, uncertain
behavior, by site
unspecified site C56.9
papillary
borderline malignancy
ovary C56.-
specified site NEC — *see* Neoplasm,
uncertain behavior, by site
unspecified site C56.9
specified site — *see* Neoplasm, benign, by site
unspecified site D27.9
specified site — *see* Neoplasm, benign, by site
unspecified site D27.9
serous
borderline malignancy
specified site NEC — *see* Neoplasm, uncertain
behavior, by site
unspecified site C56.9
papillary
borderline malignancy
ovary C56.-
specified site NEC — *see* Neoplasm,
uncertain behavior, by site
unspecified site C56.9
specified site — *see* Neoplasm, benign, by site
unspecified site D27.9
specified site — *see* Neoplasm, benign, by site
unspecified site D27.9
Cystathionine synthase deficiency E72.11
Cystathioninemia E72.19
Cystathioninuria E72.19

Cystic (*see also* condition)
breast (chronic) — *see* Mastopathy, cystic
corpora lutea (hemorrhagic) N83.1
duct — *see* condition
eyeball (congenital) Q11.0
fibrosis — *see* Fibrosis, cystic
kidney (congenital) Q61.3
adult type Q61.2
infantile type NEC Q61.19
collecting duct dilatation Q61.11
medullary Q61.5
liver, congenital Q44.6
lung disease J98.4
congenital Q33.0
mastitis, chronic — *see* Mastopathy, cystic
medullary, kidney Q61.5
meniscus — *see* Derangement, knee, meniscus,
cystic
ovary N83.20
Cysticercosis, cysticerciasis B69.9
with
epileptiform fits B69.0
myositis B69.81
brain B69.0
central nervous system B69.0
cerebral B69.0
ocular B69.1
specified NEC B69.89
Cysticercus cellulose infestation — *see* Cysticercosis
Cystinosis (malignant) E72.04
Cystinuria E72.01
Cystitis (exudative) (hemorrhagic) (septic)
(suppurative) N30.90
with
fibrosis — *see* Cystitis, chronic, interstitial
hematuria N30.91
leukoplakia — *see* Cystitis, chronic, interstitial
malakoplakia — *see* Cystitis, chronic, interstitial
metaplasia — *see* Cystitis, chronic, interstitial
prostatitis N41.3
acute N30.00
with hematuria N30.01
of trigone N30.30
with hematuria N30.31
allergic — *see* Cystitis, specified type NEC
amebic A06.81
bilharzial B65.9
blennorrhagic (gonococcal) A54.01
bullous — *see* Cystitis, specified type NEC
calculous N21.0
chlamydial A56.01
chronic N30.20
with hematuria N30.21
interstitial N30.10
with hematuria N30.11
of trigone N30.30
with hematuria N30.31
specified NEC N30.20
with hematuria N30.21
cystic(a) — *see* Cystitis, specified type NEC
diphtheritic A36.85
echinococcal
granulosus B67.2
multilocularis B67.69
emphysematous — *see* Cystitis, specified type NEC
encysted — *see* Cystitis, specified type NEC
eosinophilic — *see* Cystitis, specified type NEC
follicular — *see* Cystitis, of trigone
gangrenous — *see* Cystitis, specified type NEC
glandularis — *see* Cystitis, specified type NEC
gonococcal A54.01
incrusted — *see* Cystitis, specified type NEC
interstitial (chronic) — *see* Cystitis, chronic,
interstitial
irradiation N30.40
with hematuria N30.41
irritation — *see* Cystitis, specified type NEC
malignant — *see* Cystitis, specified type NEC
of trigone N30.30
with hematuria N30.31
panmural — *see* Cystitis, chronic, interstitial
polyposa — *see* Cystitis, specified type NEC
prostatic N41.3

Cystitis—*continued*
  puerperal (postpartum) O86.22
  radiation — *see* Cystitis, irradiation
  specified type NEC N30.80
    with hematuria N30.81
  subacute — *see* Cystitis, chronic
  submucous — *see* Cystitis, chronic, interstitial
  syphilitic (late) A52.76
  trichomonal A59.03
  tuberculous A18.12
  ulcerative — *see* Cystitis, chronic, interstitial
Cystocele(-urethrocele)
  female N81.10
    with prolapse of uterus — *see* Prolapse, uterus
    lateral N81.12
    midline N81.11
    paravaginal N81.12
  in pregnancy or childbirth O34.8-
    causing obstructed labor O65.5
  male N32.89
Cystolithiasis N21.0

Cystoma (*see also* Neoplasm, benign, by site)
  endometrial, ovary N80.1
  mucinous
    specified site — *see* Neoplasm, benign, by site
    unspecified site D27.9
  serous
    specified site — *see* Neoplasm, benign, by site
    unspecified site D27.9
  simple (ovary) N83.29
Cystoplegia N31.2
Cystoptosis N32.89
Cystopyelitis — *see* Pyelonephritis
Cystorrhagia N32.89
Cystosarcoma phyllodes D48.6-
  benign D24.-
  malignant — *see* Neoplasm, breast, malignant
Cystostomy
  attention to Z43.5
  complication — *see* Complications, cystostomy
  status Z93.50
    appendico-vesicostomy Z93.52
    cutaneous Z93.51
    specified NEC Z93.59

Cystourethritis — *see* Urethritis
Cystourethrocele (*see also* Cystocele)
  female N81.10
    with uterine prolapse — *see* Prolapse, uterus
    lateral N81.12
    midline N81.11
    paravaginal N81.12
  male N32.89
Cytomegalic inclusion disease
  congenital P35.1
Cytomegalovirus infection B25.9
Cytomycosis (reticuloendothelial) B39.4
Cytopenia D75.9
  refractory
    with multilineage dysplasia D46.a
      and ring sideroblasts (RCMD RS) D46.b
Czerny's disease (periodic hydrarthrosis of the knee)
    — *see* Effusion, joint, knee

D

Daae (-Finsen) **disease** (epidemic pleurodynia) B33.0
Da Costa's syndrome F45.8
Dabney's grip B33.0
Dacryoadenitis, dacryadenitis H04.00-
  acute H04.01-
  chronic H04.02-
Dacryocystitis H04.30-
  acute H04.32-
  chronic H04.41-
  neonatal P39.1
  phlegmonous H04.31-
  syphilitic A52.71
    congenital (early) A50.01
  trachomatous, active A71.1
    sequelae (late effect) B94.0
Dacryocystoblenorrhea — *see* Inflammation,
  lacrimal, passages, chronic
Dacryocystocele — *see* Disorder, lacrimal system,
  changes
Dacryolith, dacryolithiasis H04.51-
Dacryoma — *see* Disorder, lacrimal system, changes
Dacryopericystitis — *see* Dacryocystitis
Dacryops H04.11-
Dacryostenosis (*see also* Stenosis, lacrimal)
  congenital Q10.5
Dactylitis
  bone — *see* Osteomyelitis
  sickle cell D57.00
    Hb C D57.219
    Hb SS D57.00
    specified NEC D57.819
  skin L08.9
  syphilitic A52.77
  tuberculous A18.03
Dactylolysis spontanea (ainhum) L94.6
Dactylosymphysis Q70.9
  fingers — *see* Syndactylism, complex, fingers
  toes — *see* Syndactylism, complex, toes
Damage
  arteriosclerotic — *see* Arteriosclerosis
  brain (nontraumatic) G93.9
    anoxic, hypoxic G93.1
      resulting from a procedure G97.82
    child NOS G80.9
    due to birth injury P11.2
  cardiorenal (vascular) — *see* Hypertension,
    cardiorenal
  cerebral NEC — *see* Damage, brain
  coccyx, complicating delivery O71.6
  coronary — *see* Disease, heart, ischemic
  eye, birth injury P15.3
  liver (nontraumatic) K76.9
    alcoholic K70.9
    due to drugs — *see* Disease, liver, toxic
    toxic — *see* Disease, liver, toxic
  medication T88.7 — This code not for use in the
    inpatient setting
  pelvic
    joint or ligament, during delivery O71.6
    organ NEC
      during delivery O71.5
      following ectopic or molar pregnancy O08.6
  renal — *see* Disease, renal
  subendocardium, subendocardial — *see*
    Degeneration, myocardial
  vascular I99.9
Dana-Putnam syndrome (subacute combined
  sclerosis with pernicious anemia) — *see*
  Degeneration, combined
Danbolt (-Closs) **syndrome** (acrodermatitis
  enteropathica) L08.89
Dandruff L21.0
Dandy-Walker syndrome Q03.1
  with spina bifida — *see* Spina bifida
Danlos' syndrome Q79.6
Darier(-White) **disease** (congenital) Q82.8
  meaning erythema annulare centrifugum L53.1
Darier-Roussy sarcoid D86.3
Darling's disease or histoplasmosis B39.4
Darwin's tubercle Q17.8

Dawson's (inclusion body) **encephalitis** A81.1
De Beurmann(-Gougerot) **disease** B42.1
De la Tourette's syndrome F95.2
De Lange's syndrome Q87.1
De Morgan's spots (senile angiomas) I78.1
De Quervain's
  disease (tendon sheath) M65.4
  syndrome E34.51
  thyroiditis (subacute granulomatous thyroiditis)
    E06.1
De Toni-Fanconi(-Debré) **syndrome** E72.09
  with cystinosis E72.04
Dead
  fetus, retained (mother) O36.4
    early pregnancy O02.1
  labyrinth — *see* subcategory H83.2
  ovum, retained O02.0
Deaf nonspeaking NEC H91.3
Deafmutism (acquired) (congenital) NEC H91.3
  hysterical F44.6
  syphilitic, congenital (*see also* subcategory H94.8)
    A50.09
Deafness (acquired) (complete) (hereditary) (partial)
  H91.9-
  with blue sclera and fragility of bone Q78.0
  auditory fatigue — *see* Deafness, specified type NEC
  aviation T70.0
    nerve injury — *see* Injury, nerve, acoustic,
      specified type NEC
  boilermaker's — *see* subcategory H83.3
  central — *see* Deafness, sensorineural
  conductive H90.2
    and sensorineural, mixed H90.8
      bilateral H90.6
    bilateral H90.0
    unilateral H90.1-
  congenital H90.5
    with blue sclera and fragility of bone Q78.0
  due to toxic agents — *see* Deafness, ototoxic
  emotional (hysterical) F44.6
  functional (hysterical) F44.6
  high frequency H91.9-
  hysterical F44.6
  low frequency H91.9-
  mental R48.8
  mixed conductive and sensorineural H90.8
    bilateral H90.6
    unilateral H90.7-
  nerve — *see* Deafness, sensorineural
  neural — *see* Deafness, sensorineural
  noise-induced (*see also* subcategory) H83.3
    nerve injury — *see* Injury, nerve, acoustic,
      specified type NEC
  nonspeaking H91.3
  ototoxic — *see* subcategory H91.0
  perceptive — *see* Deafness, sensorineural
  psychogenic (hysterical) F44.6
  sensorineural H90.5
    and conductive, mixed H90.8
      bilateral H90.6
    bilateral H90.3
    unilateral H90.4-
  sensory — *see* Deafness, sensorineural
  specified type NEC — *see* subcategory H91.8
  sudden (idiopathic) H91.2-
  syphilitic A52.15
  transient ischemic H93.01-
  traumatic — *see* Injury, nerve, acoustic, specified
    type NEC
  word (developmental) H93.25
Death (cause unknown) (of) (unexplained)
  (unspecified cause) R99
  cardiac (sudden) (with successful
    resuscitation)—code to underlying disease
    family history of Z82.41
    personal history of Z86.74
  family member (assumed) Z63.4
Debility (chronic) (general) (nervous) R53.81
  congenital or neonatal NOS P96.9
  old age R54
  nervous R53.81
  senile R54
Débove's disease (splenomegaly) R16.1

Decalcification
  bone — *see* Osteoporosis
  teeth K03.89
Decapsulation, kidney N28.89
Decay
  dental — *see* Caries, dental
  senile R54
  tooth, teeth — *see* Caries, dental
Deciduitis (acute)
  following ectopic or molar pregnancy O08.0
Decline (general) — *see* Debility
  cognitive, age-associated R41.81
Decompensation
  cardiac (acute) (chronic) — *see* Disease, heart
  cardiovascular — *see* Disease, cardiovascular
  heart — *see* Disease, heart
  hepatic — *see* Failure, hepatic
  myocardial (acute) (chronic) — *see* Disease, heart
  respiratory J98.8
Decompression sickness T70.3
Decrease(d)
  absolute neutrophile count — *see* Neutropenia
  blood
    platelets — *see* Thrombocytopenia
    pressure R03.1
      due to shock following
        injury T79.4
        operation T81.1
  estrogen E28.39
    postablative E89.40
      asymptomatic E89.40
      symptomatic E89.41
  fragility of erythrocytes D58.8
  function
    lipase (pancreatic) K90.3
    ovary in hypopituitarism E23.0
    parenchyma of pancreas K86.8
    pituitary (gland) (anterior) (lobe) E23.0
      posterior (lobe) E23.0
  functional activity R68.89
  glucose R73.09
  hematocrit R71.0
  hemoglobin R71.0
  leukocytes D72.819
    specified NEC D72.818
  libido R68.82
  lymphocytes D72.810
  platelets D69.6
  respiration, due to shock following injury T79.4
  sexual desire R68.82
  tear secretion NEC — *see* Syndrome, dry eye
  tolerance
    fat K90.4
    glucose R73.09
    pancreatic K90.3
    salt and water E87.8
  vision NEC H54.7
  white blood cell count D72.819
    specified NEC D72.818
Decubitus (ulcer) — *see* Ulcer, pressure, by site
  cervix N86
Deepening acetabulum — *see* Derangement, joint,
  specified type NEC, hip
Defect, defective Q89.9
  3-(hydroxysteroid dehydrogenase) E25.0
  11 hydroxylase E25.0
  21 hydroxylase E25.0
  abdominal wall, congenital Q79.59
  antibody immunodeficiency D80.9
  aorticopulmonary septum Q21.4
  atrial septal (ostium secundum type) Q21.1
    following acute myocardial infarction (current
      complication) I23.1
    ostium primum type Q21.2
  atrioventricular
    canal Q21.2
    septum Q21.2
  auricular septal Q21.1
  bilirubin excretion NEC E80.6
  biosynthesis, androgen (testicular) E29.1

Defect, defective · ICD-10-CM Draft (2011)

Index

Defect, defective—Deficiency, deficient

Defect, defective—*continued*
- bulbar septum Q21.0
- catalase E80.3
- cell membrane receptor complex (CR3) D71
- circulation I99.9
  - congenital Q28.9
  - newborn Q28.9
- coagulation (factor) (*see also* Deficiency, factor) D68.9
  - with
    - ectopic pregnancy O08.1
    - molar pregnancy O08.1
  - acquired D68.4
  - antepartum with hemorrhage — *see* Hemorrhage, antepartum, with coagulation defect
  - due to
    - liver disease D68.4
    - vitamin K deficiency D68.4
  - hereditary NEC D68.2
  - intrapartum O67.0
  - newborn, transient P61.6
  - postpartum O72.3
  - specified type NEC D68.8
- complement system D84.1
- conduction (heart) I45.9
  - bone — *see* Deafness, conductive
- congenital, organ or site not listed — *see* Anomaly, by site
- coronary sinus Q21.1
- cushion, endocardial Q21.2
- degradation, glycoprotein E77.1
- dental bridge, crown, fillings — *see* Defect, dental restoration
- dental restoration K08.50
  - specified NEC K08.59
- dentin (hereditary) K00.5
- Descemet's membrane, congenital Q13.89
- developmental (*see also* Anomaly)
  - cauda equina Q06.3
- diaphragm
  - with elevation, eventration or hernia — *see* Hernia, diaphragm
  - congenital Q79.1
    - with hernia Q79.0
    - gross (with hernia) Q79.0
- ectodermal, congenital Q82.9
- Eisenmenger's Q21.8
- enzyme
  - catalase E80.3
  - peroxidase E80.3
- esophagus, congenital Q39.9
- extensor retinaculum M62.89
- fibrin polymerization D68.2
- filling
  - bladder R93.4
  - kidney R93.4
  - stomach R93.3
  - ureter R93.4
- Gerbode Q21.0
- glycoprotein degradation E77.1
- Hageman (factor) D68.2
- hearing — *see* Deafness
- high grade F70
- interatrial septal Q21.1
- interauricular septal Q21.1
- interventricular septal Q21.0
  - with dextroposition of aorta, pulmonary stenosis and hypertrophy of right ventricle Q21.3
  - in tetralogy of Fallot Q21.3
- learning (specific) — *see* Disorder, learning
- lymphocyte function antigen-1 (LFA-1) D84.0
- lysosomal enzyme, post-translational modification E77.0
- major osseous M89.70
  - ankle M89.77-
  - carpus M89.74-
  - clavicle M89.71-
  - femur M89.75-
  - fibula M89.76-
  - fingers M89.74-
  - foot M89.77-
  - forearm M89.73-
  - hand M89.74-

Defect, defective—*continued*
- major osseous—*continued*
  - humerus M89.72-
  - lower leg M89.76-
  - metacarpus M89.74-
  - metatarsus M89.77-
  - multiple sites M89.79
  - pelvic region M89.75-
  - pelvis M89.75-
  - radius M89.73-
  - scapula M89.71-
  - shoulder region M89.71-
  - specified NEC M89.78
  - tarsus M89.77-
  - thigh M89.75-
  - tibia M89.76-
  - toes M89.77-
  - ulna M89.73-
- mental — *see* Retardation, mental
- modification, lysosomal enzymes, post-translational E77.0
- obstructive, congenital
  - renal pelvis Q62.39
  - ureter Q62.39
    - atresia — *see* Atresia, ureter
    - cecoureterocele Q62.32
    - megaureter Q62.2
    - orthotopic ureterocele Q62.31
- osseous, major M89.70
  - ankle M89.77-
  - carpus M89.74-
  - clavicle M89.71-
  - femur M89.75-
  - fibula M89.76-
  - fingers M89.74-
  - foot M89.77-
  - forearm M89.73-
  - hand M89.74-
  - humerus M89.72-
  - lower leg M89.76-
  - metacarpus M89.74-
  - metatarsus M89.77-
  - multiple sites M89.79
  - pelvic region M89.75-
  - pelvis M89.75-
  - radius M89.73-
  - scapula M89.71-
  - shoulder region M89.71-
  - specified NEC M89.78
  - tarsus M89.77-
  - thigh M89.75-
  - tibia M89.76-
  - toes M89.77-
  - ulna M89.73-
- osteochondral NEC M95.8 (*see also* Deformity)
- ostium
  - primum Q21.2
  - secundum Q21.1
- peroxidase E80.3
- placental blood supply — *see* Insufficiency, placental
- platelets, qualitative D69.1
  - constitutional D68.0
- postural NEC, spine — *see* Dorsopathy, deforming
- reduction
  - limb Q73.8
    - lower Q72.9-
      - absence — *see* Agenesis, leg
        - foot — *see* Agenesis, foot
      - split foot Q72.7-
      - longitudinal
        - femur Q72.4-
        - fibula Q72.6-
        - tibia Q72.5-
      - specified type NEC Q72.89-
    - specified type NEC Q73.8
    - upper Q71.9-
      - absence — *see* Agenesis, arm
        - forearm — *see* Agenesis, forearm
        - hand — *see* Agenesis, hand
      - lobster-claw hand Q71.6-
      - longitudinal
        - radius Q71.4-

Defect, defective—*continued*
- reduction—*continued*
  - limb—*continued*
    - upper—*continued*
      - longitudinal—*continued*
        - ulna Q71.5-
      - specified type NEC Q71.89-
- renal pelvis Q63.8
  - obstructive Q62.39
- respiratory system, congenital Q34.9
- restoration, dental K08.50
  - specified NEC K08.59
- retinal nerve bundle fibers H35.89
- septal (heart) NOS Q21.9
  - acquired (atrial) (auricular) (ventricular) (old) I51.0
  - atrial Q21.1
    - concurrent with acute myocardial infarction — *see* Infarct, myocardium
    - following acute myocardial infarction (current complication) I23.1
    - ventricular (*see also* Defect, ventricular septal) Q21.0
- sinus venosus Q21.1
- speech R47.9
  - developmental F80.9
  - specified NEC R47.89
- Taussig-Bing (aortic transposition and overriding pulmonary artery) Q20.1
- teeth, wedge K03.1
- vascular (local) I99.9
  - congenital Q27.9
- ventricular septal Q21.0
  - concurrent with acute myocardial infarction — *see* Infarct, myocardium
  - following acute myocardial infarction (current complication) I23.2
  - in tetralogy of Fallot Q21.3
- vision NEC H54.7
- visual field H53.40
  - bilateral
    - heteronymous H53.47
    - homonymous H53.46-
  - generalized contraction H53.48-
  - localized
    - arcuate H53.43-
    - scotoma (central area) H53.41-
      - blind spot area H53.42-
    - sector H53.43-
    - specified type NEC H53.45-
- voice R49.9
  - specified NEC R49.8

Deferentitis N49.1
- gonorrheal (acute) (chronic) A54.23

Defibrination (syndrome) D65
- antepartum — *see* Hemorrhage, antepartum, with coagulation defect, disseminated intravascular coagulation
- following ectopic or molar pregnancy O08.1
- intrapartum O67.0
- newborn P60
- postpartum O72.3

Deficiency, deficient
- 3B hydroxysteroid dehydrogenase E25.0
- 5-alpha reductase (with male pseudohermaphroditism) E29.1
- 11 hydroxylase E25.0
- 21 hydroxylase E25.0
- abdominal muscle syndrome Q79.4
- accelerator globulin (Ac G) (blood) D68.2
- AC globulin (congenital) (hereditary) D68.2
  - acquired D68.4
- acid phosphatase E83.39
- activating factor (blood) D68.2
- adenosine deaminase (ADA) D81.3
- aldolase (hereditary) E74.19
- alpha-1-antitrypsin E88.01
- amino-acids E72.9
- anemia — *see* Anemia
- aneurin E51.9
- antibody with
  - hyperimmunoglobulinemia D80.6
  - near-normal immunoglobins D80.6

Deficiency, deficient —continued

antidiuretic hormone E23.2
anti-hemophilic
  factor (A) D66
    B D67
    C D68.1
  globulin (AHG) NEC D66
antithrombin (antithrombin III) D68.59
ascorbic acid E54
attention (disorder) (syndrome) F98.8
  with hyperactivity — see Disorder,
    attention-deficit hyperactivity
autoprothrombin
  I D68.2
  II D67
  C D68.2
beta-glucuronidase E76.29
biotin E53.8
biotin-dependent carboxylase D81.819
biotinidase D81.810
brancher enzyme (amylopectinosis) E74.03
calciferol E55.9
  with
    adult osteomalacia M83.8
    rickets — see Rickets
calcium (dietary) E58
calorie, severe E43
  with marasmus E41
    and kwashiorkor E42
cardiac — see Insufficiency, myocardial
carnitine E71.40
  due to
    hemodialysis E71.43
    inborn errors of metabolism E71.42
    Valproic acid therapy E71.43
  iatrogenic E71.43
  muscle palmityltransferase E71.314
  primary E71.41
  secondary E71.448
carotene E50.9
central nervous system G96.8
ceruloplasmin (Wilson) E83.01
choline E53.8
Christmas factor D67
chromium E61.4
clotting (blood) (see also Deficiency, coagulation
  factor) D68.9
clotting factor NEC (hereditary) (see also Deficiency,
  factor) D68.2
coagulation NOS D68.9
  with
    ectopic pregnancy O08.1
    molar pregnancy O08.1
  acquired (any) D68.4
  antepartum hemorrhage — see Hemorrhage,
    antepartum, with coagulation defect
  clotting factor NEC (see also Deficiency, factor)
    D68.2
  due to
    hyperprothrombinemia D68.4
    liver disease D68.4
    vitamin K deficiency D68.4
  newborn, transient P61.6
  postpartum O72.3
  specified NEC D68.8
cognitive F09
color vision H53.50
  achromatopsia H53.51
  acquired H53.52
  deuteranomaly H53.53
  protanomaly H53.54
  specified type NEC H53.59
  tritanomaly H53.55
combined glucocorticoid and mineralocorticoid
  E27.49
contact factor D68.2
copper (nutritional) E61.0
corticoadrenal E27.40
  primary E27.1
craniofacial axis Q75.0
cyanocobalamin E53.8
C1 esterase inhibitor (C1-INH) D84.1
debrancher enzyme (limit dextrinosis) E74.03

Deficiency, deficient — continued

dehydrogenase
  long chain/very long chain acyl CoA E71.310
  medium chain acyl CoA E71.311
  short chain acyl CoA E71.312
diet E63.9
disaccharidase E73.9
edema — see Malnutrition, severe
endocrine E34.9
energy-supply — see Malnutrition
enzymes, circulating NEC E88.09
ergosterol E55.9
  with
    adult osteomalacia M83.8
    rickets — see Rickets
essential fatty acid (EFA) E63.0
factor (see also Deficiency, coagulation)
  Hageman D68.2
  I (congenital) (hereditary) D68.2
  II (congenital) (hereditary) D68.2
  IX (congenital) (functional) (hereditary) (with
    functional defect) D67
  multiple (congenital) D68.8
    acquired D68.4
  V (congenital) (hereditary) D68.2
  VII (congenital) (hereditary) D68.2
  VIII (congenital) (functional) (hereditary) (with
    functional defect) D66
    with vascular defect D68.0
  X (congenital) (hereditary) D68.2
  XI (congenital) (hereditary) D68.1
  XII (congenital) (hereditary) D68.2
  XIII (congenital) (hereditary) D68.2
femoral, proximal focal (congenital) — see Defect,
  reduction, lower limb, longitudinal, femur
fibrin-stabilizing factor (congenital) (hereditary)
  D68.2
  acquired D68.4
fibrinase D68.2
fibrinogen (congenital) (hereditary) D68.2
  acquired D65
folate E53.8
folic acid E53.8
foreskin N47.3
fructokinase E74.11
fructose 1,6-diphosphatase E74.19
fructose-1-phosphate aldolase E74.19
galactokinase E74.29
galactose-1-phosphate uridyl transferase E74.29
gammaglobulin in blood D80.1
  hereditary D80.0
glass factor D68.2
glucocorticoid E27.49
  mineralocorticoid E27.49
glucose-6-phosphatase E74.01
glucose-6-phosphate dehydrogenase anemia D55.0
glucuronyl transferase E80.5
glycogen synthetase E74.09
gonadotropin (isolated) E23.0
growth hormone (idiopathic) (isolated) E23.0
Hageman factor D68.2
hemoglobin D64.9
hepatophosphorylase E74.09
homogentisate 1,2-dioxygenase E70.29
hormone
  anterior pituitary (partial) NEC E23.0
    growth E23.0
  growth (isolated) E23.0
  pituitary E23.0
  testicular E29.1
hypoxanthine-(guanine)-phosphoribosyltransferase
  (HGPRT) (total H-PRT) E79.1
immunity D84.9
  cell-mediated D84.8
    with thrombocytopenia and eczema D82.0
  combined D81.9
  humoral D80.9
  IgA (secretory) D80.2
  IgG D80.3
  IgM D80.4
immuno — see Immunodeficiency
immunoglobulin, selective
  A (IgA) D80.2

Deficiency, deficient — continued

immunoglobulin, selective—continued
  G (IgG) (subclasses) D80.3
  M (IgM) D80.4
inositol (B complex) E53.8
intrinsic
  factor (congenital) D51.0
  sphincter N36.42
    with urethral hypermobility N36.43
iodine E61.8
  congenital syndrome — see Syndrome,
    iodine-deficiency, congenital
iron E61.1
  anemia D50.9
kalium E87.6
kappa-light chain D80.8
labile factor (congenital) (hereditary) D68.2
  acquired D68.4
lacrimal fluid (acquired) (see also Syndrome, dry eye)
  congenital Q10.6
lactase
  congenital E73.0
  secondary E73.1
Laki-Lorand factor D68.2
lecithin cholesterol acyltransferase E78.6
lipocaic K86.8
lipoprotein (familial) (high density) E78.6
liver phosphorylase E74.09
lysosomal (-1, 4 glucosidase) E74.02
magnesium E61.2
major histocompatibility complex
  class I D81.6
  class II D81.7
manganese E61.3
menadione (vitamin K) E56.1
  newborn P53
mental (familial) (hereditary) — see Retardation,
  mental
methylenetetrahydrofolate reductase (MTHFR)
  E72.12
mineral NEC E61.8
mineralocorticoid E27.49
  with glucocorticoid E27.49
molybdenum (nutritional) E61.5
moral F60.2
multiple nutrient elements E61.7
muscle
  carnitine (palmityltransferase) E71.314
  phosphofructokinase E74.09
myoadenylate deaminase E79.2
myocardial — see Insufficiency, myocardial
myophosphorylase E74.04
NADH diaphorase or reductase (congenital) D74.0
NADH-methemoglobin reductase (congenital)
  D74.0
natrium E87.1
niacin (amide) (-tryptophan) E52
nicotinamide E52
nicotinic acid E52
number of teeth — see Anodontia
nutrient element E61.9
  multiple E61.7
  specified NEC E61.8
nutrition, nutritional E63.9
  sequelae — see Sequelae, nutritional deficiency
  specified NEC E63.8
ornithine transcarbamylase E72.4
ovarian E28.39
oxygen — see Anoxia
pantothenic acid E53.8
parathyroid (gland) E20.9
perineum (female) N81.89
phenylalanine hydroxylase E70.1
phosphoenolpyruvate carboxykinase E74.4
phosphofructokinase E74.19
phosphomannomutase E74.8
phosphomannose isomerase E74.8
phosphomannosyl mutase E74.8
phosphorylase kinase, liver E74.09
pituitary hormone (isolated) E23.0
plasma thromboplastin
  antecedent (PTA) D68.1
  component (PTC) D67

Deficiency, deficient — *continued*
 platelet NEC D69.1
  constitutional D68.Ø
 polyglandular E31.8
  autoimmune E31.Ø
 potassium (K) E87.6
 prepuce N47.3
 proaccelerin (congenital) (hereditary) D68.2
  acquired D68.4
 proconvertin factor (congenital) (hereditary) D68.2
  acquired D68.4
 protein (*see also* Malnutrition) E46
  anemia D53.Ø
  C D68.59
  S D68.59
 prothrombin (congenital) (hereditary) D68.2
  acquired D68.4
 Prower factor D68.2
 pseudocholinesterase E88.Ø9
 PTA (plasma thromboplastin antecedent) D68.1
 PTC (plasma thromboplastin component) D67
 purine nucleoside phosphorylase (PNP) D81.5
 pyracin (alpha) (beta) E53.1
 pyridoxal E53.1
 pyridoxamine E53.1
 pyridoxine (derivatives) E53.1
 pyruvate
  carboxylase E74.4
  dehydrogenase E74.4
 riboflavin (vitamin B2) E53.Ø
 salt E87.1
 secretion
  ovary E28.39
  salivary gland (any) K11.7
  urine R34
 selenium (dietary) E59
 serum antitrypsin, familial E88.Ø1
 short stature homeobox gene (SHOX)
  with
   dyschondrosteosis Q78.8
   short stature (idiopathic) E34.3
   Turner's syndrome Q96.9
 sodium (Na) E87.1
 SPCA (factor VII) D68.2
 sphincter, intrinsic N36.42
  with urethral hypermobility N36.43
 stable factor (congenital) (hereditary) D68.2
  acquired D68.4
 Stuart-Prower (factor X) D68.2
 sucrase E74.39
 sulfatase E75.29
 sulfite oxidase E72.19
 thiamin, thiaminic (chloride) E51.9
  beriberi (dry) E51.11
   wet E51.12
 thrombokinase D68.2
  newborn P53
 thyroid (gland) — *see* Hypothyroidism
 tocopherol E56.Ø
 tooth bud KØØ.Ø
 transcobalamine II (anemia) D51.2
 vanadium E61.6
 vascular I99.9
 vasopressin E23.2
 viosterol — *see* Deficiency, calciferol
 vitamin (multiple) NOS E56.9
  A E5Ø.9
   with
    Bitot's spot (corneal) E5Ø.1
    follicular keratosis E5Ø.8
    keratomalacia E5Ø.4
    manifestations NEC E5Ø.8
    night blindness E5Ø.5
    scar of cornea, xerophthalmic E5Ø.6
    xeroderma E5Ø.8
    xerophthalmia E5Ø.7
    xerosis
     conjunctival E5Ø.Ø
      and Bitot's spot E5Ø.1
     cornea E5Ø.2
      and ulceration E5Ø.3
   sequelae E64.1

Deficiency, deficient — *continued*
 vitamin (multiple)—*continued*
  B (complex) NOS E53.9
   with
    beriberi (dry) E51.11
     wet E51.12
    pellagra E52
  B1 NOS E51.9
   beriberi (dry) E51.11
    with circulatory system manifestations E51.11
    wet E51.12
  B12 E53.8
  B2 (riboflavin) E53.Ø
  B6 E53.1
  C E54
   sequelae E64.2
  D E55.9
   with
    adult osteomalacia M83.8
    rickets — *see* Rickets
   25-hydroxylase E83.32
  E E56.Ø
  folic acid E53.8
  G E53.Ø
  group B E53.9
   specified NEC E53.8
  H (biotin) E53.8
  K E56.1
   of newborn P53
  nicotinic E52
  P E56.8
  PP (pellagra-preventing) E52
  specified NEC E56.8
  thiamin E51.9
   beriberi — *see* Beriberi
  zinc, dietary E6Ø
Deficit (*see also* Deficiency)
 attention and concentration R41.84Ø
  disorder — *see* Attention, deficit
 cognitive communication R41.841
 cognitive NEC R41.89
  following
   cerebral infarction I69.31
   cerebrovascular disease I69.91
    specified disease NEC I69.8
   intracerebral hemorrhage I69.11
   nontraumatic intracranial hemorrhage NEC I69.21
   subarachnoid hemorrhage I69.Ø1
  cognitive communication R41.841
  concentration R41.84Ø
  executive function R41.844
  frontal lobe R41.844
  neurologic NEC R29.818
   ischemic
    reversible (RIND) I63.9
    prolonged (PRIND) I63.9
  oxygen RØ9.Ø2
  prolonged reversible ischemic neurologic (PRIND) I63.9
  psychomotor R41.843
  visuospatial R41.842
Deflection
 radius — *see* Deformity, limb, specified type NEC, forearm
 septum (acquired) (nasal) (nose) J34.2
 spine — *see* Curvature, spine
 turbinate (nose) J34.2
Defluvium
 capillorum — *see* Alopecia
 ciliorum — *see* Madarosis
 unguium L6Ø.8
Deformity Q89.9
 abdomen, congenital Q89.9
 abdominal wall
  acquired M95.8
  congenital Q79.59
 acquired (unspecified site) M95.9
 adrenal gland Q89.1
 alimentary tract, congenital Q45.9
  upper Q4Ø.9

Deformity —*continued*
 ankle (joint) (acquired) (*see also* Deformity, limb, lower leg)
  abduction — *see* Contraction, joint, ankle
  congenital Q68.8
  contraction — *see* Contraction, joint, ankle
  specified type NEC — *see* Deformity, limb, foot, specified NEC
 anus (acquired) K62.8
  congenital Q43.9
 aorta (arch) (congenital) Q25.4
  acquired I77.89
 aortic
  arch, acquired I77.89
  cusp or valve (congenital) Q23.8
   acquired (*see also* Endocarditis, aortic) I35.8
 arm (acquired) (upper) (*see also* Deformity, limb, upper arm)
  congenital Q68.8
  forearm — *see* Deformity, limb, forearm
 artery (congenital) (peripheral) NOS Q27.9
  acquired I77.89
  coronary (acquired) I25.9
   congenital Q24.5
  umbilical Q27.Ø
 atrial septal Q21.1
 auditory canal (external) (congenital) (*see also* Malformation, ear, external)
  acquired — *see* Disorder, ear, external, specified type NEC
 auricle
  ear (congenital) (*see also* Malformation, ear, external)
   acquired — *see* Disorder, pinna, deformity
 back — *see* Dorsopathy, deforming
 bile duct (common) (congenital) (hepatic) Q44.5
  acquired K83.8
 biliary duct or passage (congenital) Q44.5
  acquired K83.8
 bladder (neck) (trigone) (sphincter) (acquired) N32.89
  congenital Q64.79
 bone (acquired) M95.9
  congenital Q79.9
  turbinate M95.Ø
 brain (congenital) QØ4.9
  acquired G93.89
  reduction QØ4.3
 breast (acquired) N64.89
  congenital Q83.9
  reconstructed N65.Ø
 bronchus (congenital) Q32.4
  acquired NEC J98.Ø9
 bursa, congenital Q79.9
 canaliculi (lacrimalis) (acquired) (*see also* Disorder, lacrimal system, changes)
  congenital Q1Ø.6
 canthus, acquired — *see* Disorder, eyelid, specified type NEC
 capillary (acquired) I78.8
 cardiovascular system, congenital Q28.9
 caruncle, lacrimal (acquired) (*see also* Disorder, lacrimal system, changes)
  congenital Q1Ø.6
 cascade, stomach K31.2
 cecum (congenital) Q43.9
  acquired K63.89
 cerebral, acquired G93.89
  congenital QØ4.9
 cervix (uterus) (acquired) NEC N88.8
  congenital Q51.9
 cheek (acquired) M95.2
  congenital Q18.9
 chest (acquired) (wall) M95.4
  congenital Q67.8
  sequelae (late effect) of rickets E64.3
 chin (acquired) M95.2
  congenital Q18.9
 choroid (congenital) Q14.3
  acquired H31.8
  plexus QØ7.8
   acquired G96.19
 cicatricial — *see* Cicatrix

Deformity— *continued*
　cilia, acquired — *see* Disorder, eyelid, specified type NEC
　clavicle (acquired) M95.8
　　congenital Q68.8
　clitoris (congenital) Q52.6
　　acquired N90.89
　clubfoot — *see* Clubfoot
　coccyx (acquired) — *see* subcategory M43.8
　colon (congenital) Q43.9
　　acquired K63.89
　concha (ear), congenital (*see also* Malformation, ear, external)
　　acquired — *see* Disorder, pinna, deformity
　cornea (acquired) H18.70
　　congenital Q13.4
　　descemetocele — *see* Descemetocele
　　ectasia — *see* Ectasia, cornea
　　specified NEC H18.79-
　　staphyloma — *see* Staphyloma, cornea
　coronary artery (acquired) I25.9
　　congenital Q24.5
　cranium (acquired) — *see* Deformity, skull
　cricoid cartilage (congenital) Q31.8
　　acquired J38.7
　cystic duct (congenital) Q44.5
　　acquired K82.8
　Dandy-Walker Q03.1
　　with spina bifida — *see* Spina bifida
　diaphragm (congenital) Q79.1
　　acquired J98.6
　digestive organ NOS Q45.9
　ductus arteriosus Q25.0
　duodenal bulb K31.89
　duodenum (congenital) Q43.9
　　acquired K31.89
　dura — *see* Deformity, meninges
　ear (acquired) (*see also* Disorder, pinna, deformity)
　　congenital (external) Q17.9
　　　internal Q16.5
　　　middle Q16.4
　　　　ossicles Q16.3
　　　ossicles Q16.3
　ectodermal (congenital) NEC Q84.9
　ejaculatory duct (congenital) Q55.4
　　acquired N50.8
　elbow (joint) (acquired) (*see also* Deformity, limb, upper arm)
　　congenital Q68.8
　　contraction — *see* Contraction, joint, elbow
　endocrine gland NEC Q89.2
　epididymis (congenital) Q55.4
　　acquired N50.8
　epiglottis (congenital) Q31.8
　　acquired J38.7
　esophagus (congenital) Q39.9
　　acquired K22.8
　eustachian tube (congenital) NEC Q17.8
　eye, congenital Q15.9
　eyebrow (congenital) Q18.8
　eyelid (acquired) (*see also* Disorder, eyelid, specified type NEC)
　　congenital Q10.3
　face (acquired) M95.2
　　congenital Q18.9
　fallopian tube, acquired N83.8
　femur (acquired) — *see* Deformity, limb, specified type NEC, thigh
　fetal
　　with fetopelvic disproportion O33.7
　　　causing obstructed labor O66.3
　finger (acquired) M20.00-
　　boutonniere M20.02-
　　congenital Q68.1
　　flexion contracture — *see* Contraction, joint, hand
　　mallet finger M20.01-
　　specified NEC M20.09-
　　swan-neck M20.03-
　flexion (joint) (acquired) (*see also* Deformity, limb, flexion) M21.20
　　congenital NOS Q74.9
　　　hip Q65.8

Deformity— *continued*
　foot (acquired) (*see also* Deformity, limb, lower leg)
　　cavovarus (congenital) Q66.1
　　congenital NOS Q66.9
　　　specified type NEC Q66.8
　　specified type NEC — *see* Deformity, limb, foot, specified NEC
　　valgus (congenital) Q66.6
　　　acquired — *see* Deformity, valgus, ankle
　　varus (congenital) NEC Q66.3
　　　acquired — *see* Deformity, varus, ankle
　forearm (acquired) (*see also* Deformity, limb, forearm congenital) Q68.8
　forehead (acquired) M95.2
　　congenital Q75.8
　frontal bone (acquired) M95.2
　　congenital Q75.8
　gallbladder (congenital) Q44.1
　　acquired K82.8
　gastrointestinal tract (congenital) NOS Q45.9
　　acquired K63.89
　genitalia, genital organ(s) or system NEC
　　female (congenital) Q52.9
　　　acquired N94.89
　　　external Q52.70
　　male (congenital) Q55.9
　　　acquired N50.8
　globe (eye) (congenital) Q15.8
　　acquired H44.89
　gum, acquired NEC K06.8
　hand (acquired) — *see* Deformity, limb, forearm
　　congenital Q68.1
　head (acquired) M95.2
　　congenital Q75.8
　heart (congenital) Q24.9
　　septum Q21.9
　　　auricular Q21.1
　　　ventricular Q21.0
　　valve (congenital) NEC Q24.8
　　　acquired — *see* Endocarditis
　heel (acquired) — *see* Deformity, foot
　hepatic duct (congenital) Q44.5
　　acquired K83.8
　hip (joint) (acquired) (*see also* Deformity, limb, thigh)
　　congenital Q65.9
　　due to (previous) juvenile osteochondrosis — *see* Coxa, plana
　　flexion — *see* Contraction, joint, hip
　hourglass — *see* Contraction, hourglass
　humerus (acquired) M21.82-
　　congenital Q74.0
　hypophyseal (congenital) Q89.2
　ileocecal (coil) (valve) (acquired) K63.89
　　congenital Q43.9
　ileum (congenital) Q43.9
　　acquired K63.89
　ilium (acquired) M95.5
　　congenital Q74.2
　integument (congenital) Q84.9
　intervertebral cartilage or disc (acquired) — *see* Disorder, disc, specified NEC
　intestine (large) (small) (congenital) NOS Q43.9
　　acquired K63.89
　intrinsic minus or plus (hand) — *see* Deformity, limb, specified type NEC, forearm
　iris (acquired) H21.89
　　congenital Q13.2
　ischium (acquired) M95.5
　　congenital Q74.2
　jaw (acquired) (congenital) M26.9
　joint (acquired) NEC M21.90
　　congenital Q68.8
　　elbow M21.92-
　　hand M21.94-
　　hip M21.95-
　　knee M21.96-
　　shoulder M21.92-
　　wrist M21.93-
　kidney(s) (calyx) (pelvis) (congenital) Q63.9
　　acquired N28.89
　　artery (congenital) Q27.2

Deformity— *continued*
　kidney(s)—*continued*
　　artery—*continued*
　　　acquired I77.89
　Klippel-Feil (brevicollis) Q76.1
　knee (acquired) NEC (*see also* Deformity, limb, lower leg)
　　congenital Q68.2
　labium (majus) (minus) (congenital) Q52.79
　　acquired N90.89
　lacrimal passages or duct (congenital) NEC Q10.6
　　acquired — *see* Disorder, lacrimal system, changes
　larynx (muscle) (congenital) Q31.8
　　acquired J38.7
　　web (glottic) Q31.0
　leg (upper) (acquired) NEC (*see also* Deformity, limb, thigh)
　　congenital Q68.8
　　lower leg — *see* Deformity, limb, lower leg
　lens (acquired) H27.8
　　congenital Q12.9
　lid (fold) (acquired) (*see also* Disorder, eyelid, specified type NEC)
　　congenital Q10.3
　ligament (acquired) — *see* Disorder, ligament
　　congenital Q79.9
　limb (acquired) M21.90
　　clawfoot M21.53-
　　clawhand M21.51-
　　clubfoot M21.54-
　　clubhand M21.52-
　　congenital, except reduction deformity Q74.9
　　flat foot M21.4-
　　flexion M21.20
　　　ankle M21.27-
　　　elbow M21.22-
　　　finger M21.24-
　　　hip M21.25-
　　　knee M21.26-
　　　shoulder M21.21-
　　　toe M21.27-
　　　wrist M21.23-
　　foot
　　　claw — *see* Deformity, limb, clawfoot
　　　club — *see* Deformity, limb, clubfoot
　　　drop M21.37-
　　　flat — *see* Deformity, limb, flat foot
　　　specified NEC M21.6x-
　　forearm M21.93-
　　hand M21.94-
　　lower leg M21.96-
　　specified type NEC M21.80
　　　forearm M21.83-
　　　lower leg M21.86-
　　　thigh M21.85-
　　　upper arm M21.82-
　　thigh M21.95-
　　unequal length M21.70
　　　short site is
　　　　femur M21.75-
　　　　fibula M21.76-
　　　　humerus M21.72-
　　　　radius M21.73-
　　　　tibia M21.76-
　　　　ulna M21.73-
　　upper arm M21.92-
　　valgus — *see* Deformity, valgus
　　varus — *see* Deformity, varus
　　wrist drop M21.33-
　lip (acquired) NEC K13.0
　　congenital Q38.0
　liver (congenital) Q44.7
　　acquired K76.8
　lumbosacral (congenital) (joint) (region) Q76.49
　　acquired — *see* subcategory M43.8
　　kyphosis — *see* Kyphosis, congenital
　　lordosis — *see* Lordosis, congenital
　lung (congenital) Q33.9
　　acquired J98.4
　lymphatic system, congenital Q89.9
　Madelung's (radius) Q74.0
　mandible (acquired) (congenital) M26.9

Deformity— *continued*
  maxilla (acquired) (congenital) M26.9
  meninges or membrane (congenital) Q07.9
    cerebral Q04.8
      acquired G96.19
    spinal cord (congenital) G96.19
      acquired G96.19
  metacarpus (acquired) — *see* Deformity, limb,
      forearm
    congenital Q74.0
  metatarsus (acquired) — *see* Deformity, foot
    congenital Q66.9
  middle ear (congenital) Q16.4
    ossicles Q16.3
  mitral (leaflets) (valve) I05.8
    parachute Q23.2
    stenosis, congenital Q23.2
  mouth (acquired) K13.79
    congenital Q38.6
  multiple, congenital NEC Q89.7
  muscle (acquired) M62.89
    congenital Q79.9
      sternocleidomastoid Q68.0
  musculoskeletal system (acquired) M95.9
    congenital Q79.9
    specified NEC M95.8
  nail (acquired) L60.8
    congenital Q84.6
  nasal — *see* Deformity, nose
  neck (acquired) M95.3
    congenital Q18.9
      sternocleidomastoid Q68.0
  nervous system (congenital) Q07.9
  nipple (congenital) Q83.9
    acquired N64.89
  nose (acquired) (cartilage) M95.0
    bone (turbinate) M95.0
    congenital Q30.9
      bent or squashed Q67.4
    saddle M95.0
      syphilitic A50.57
    septum (acquired) J34.2
      congenital Q30.8
    sinus (wall) (congenital) Q30.8
      acquired M95.0
    syphilitic (congenital) A50.57
      late A52.73
  ocular muscle (congenital) Q10.3
    acquired — *see* Strabismus, mechanical
  opticociliary vessels (congenital) Q13.2
  orbit (eye) (acquired) H05.30
    atrophy — *see* Atrophy, orbit
    congenital Q10.7
    due to
      bone disease NEC H05.32-
      trauma or surgery H05.33-
    enlargement — *see* Enlargement, orbit
    exostosis — *see* Exostosis, orbit
  organ of Corti (congenital) Q16.5
  ovary (congenital) Q50.39
    acquired N83.8
  oviduct, acquired N83.8
  palate (congenital) Q38.5
    acquired M27.8
    cleft (congenital) — *see* Cleft, palate
  pancreas (congenital) Q45.3
    acquired K86.8
  parathyroid (gland) Q89.2
  parotid (gland) (congenital) Q38.4
    acquired K11.8
  patella (acquired) — *see* Disorder, patella, specified
      NEC
  pelvis, pelvic (acquired) (bony) M95.5
    with disproportion (fetopelvic) O33.0
      causing obstructed labor O65.0
    congenital Q74.2
    rachitic sequelae (late effect) E64.3
  penis (glans) (congenital) Q55.69
    acquired N48.89
  pericardium (congenital) Q24.8
    acquired — *see* Pericarditis
  pharynx (congenital) Q38.8
    acquired J39.2

Deformity— *continued*
  pinna, acquired (*see also* Disorder, pinna, deformity)
    congenital Q17.9
  pituitary (congenital) Q89.2
  posture — *see* Dorsopathy, deforming
  prepuce (congenital) Q55.69
    acquired N47.8
  prostate (congenital) Q55.4
    acquired N42.89
  pupil (congenital) Q13.2
    acquired — *see* Abnormality, pupillary
  pylorus (congenital) Q40.3
    acquired K31.89
  rachitic (acquired), old or healed E64.3
  radius (acquired) (*see also* Deformity, limb, forearm)
    congenital Q68.8
  rectum (congenital) Q43.9
    acquired K62.8
  reduction (extremity) (limb), congenital (*see also*
      condition and site) Q73.8
    brain Q04.3
    lower — *see* Defect, reduction, lower limb
    upper — *see* Defect, reduction, upper limb
  renal — *see* Deformity, kidney
  respiratory system (congenital) Q34.9
  rib (acquired) M95.4
    congenital Q76.6
      cervical Q76.5
  rotation (joint) (acquired) *see* Deformity, limb,
      specified site NEC
    congenital Q74.9
    hip — *see* Deformity, limb, specified type NEC,
        thigh
      congenital Q65.8
  sacroiliac joint (congenital) Q74.2
    acquired — *see* subcategory M43.8
  sacrum (acquired) — *see* subcategory M43.8
  saddle
    back — *see* Lordosis
    nose M95.0
      syphilitic A50.57
  salivary gland or duct (congenital) Q38.4
    acquired K11.8
  scapula (acquired) M95.8
    congenital Q68.8
  scrotum (congenital) (*see also* Malformation, testis
      and scrotum)
    acquired N50.8
  seminal vesicles (congenital) Q55.4
    acquired N50.8
  septum, nasal (acquired) J34.2
  shoulder (joint) (acquired) — *see* Deformity, limb,
      upper arm
    congenital Q74.0
    contraction — *see* Contraction, joint, shoulder
  sigmoid (flexure) (congenital) Q43.9
    acquired K63.89
  skin (congenital) Q82.9
  skull (acquired) M95.2
    congenital Q75.8
      with
        anencephaly Q00.0
        encephalocele — *see* Encephalocele
        hydrocephalus Q03.9
          with spina bifida — *see* Spina bifida,
            by site, with hydrocephalus
        microcephaly Q02
  soft parts, organs or tissues (of pelvis)
    in pregnancy or childbirth NEC O34.8-
      causing obstructed labor O65.5
  spermatic cord (congenital) Q55.4
    acquired N50.8
    torsion — *see* Torsion, spermatic cord
  spinal — *see* Dorsopathy, deforming
    column (acquired) — *see* Dorsopathy, deforming
    congenital Q67.5
    cord (congenital) Q06.9
      acquired G95.89
    nerve root (congenital) Q07.9
  spine (acquired) (*see also* Dorsopathy, deforming)
    congenital Q67.5
    rachitic E64.3

Deformity— *continued*
  spine—*continued*
    specified NEC — *see* Dorsopathy, deforming,
        specified NEC
  spleen
    acquired D73.89
    congenital Q89.09
  Sprengel's (congenital) Q74.0
  sternocleidomastoid (muscle), congenital Q68.0
  sternum (acquired) M95.4
    congenital NEC Q76.7
  stomach (congenital) Q40.3
    acquired K31.89
  submandibular gland (congenital) Q38.4
  submaxillary gland (congenital) Q38.4
    acquired K11.8
  talipes — *see* Talipes
  testis (congenital) (*see also* Malformation, testis and
      scrotum)
    acquired N44.8
      torsion — *see* Torsion, testis
  thigh (acquired) (*see also* Deformity, limb, thigh)
    congenital NEC Q68.8
  thorax (acquired) (wall) M95.4
    congenital Q67.8
    sequelae of rickets E64.3
  thumb (acquired) (*see also* Deformity, finger)
    congenital NEC Q68.1
  thymus (tissue) (congenital) Q89.2
  thyroid (gland) (congenital) Q89.2
    cartilage Q31.8
      acquired J38.7
  tibia (acquired) — *see also* Deformity, limb, specified
      type NEC, lower leg
    congenital NEC Q68.8
    saber (syphilitic) A50.56 [M90.80]
  toe (acquired) M20.6-
    congenital Q66.9
    hallux rigidus M20.2-
    hallux valgus M20.1-
    hallux varus M20.3-
    hammer toe M20.4-
    specified NEC M20.5x-
  tongue (congenital) Q38.3
    acquired K14.8
  tooth, teeth K00.2
  trachea (rings) (congenital) Q32.1
    acquired J39.8
  transverse aortic arch (congenital) Q25.4
  tricuspid (leaflets) (valve) I07.8
    atresia or stenosis Q22.4
    Ebstein's Q22.5
  trunk (acquired) M95.8
    congenital Q89.9
  ulna (acquired) (*see also* Deformity, limb, forearm)
    congenital NEC Q68.8
  urachus, congenital Q64.4
  ureter (opening) (congenital) Q62.8
    acquired N28.89
  urethra (congenital) Q64.79
    acquired N36.8
  urinary tract (congenital) Q64.9
    urachus Q64.4
  uterus (congenital) Q51.9
    acquired N85.8
  uvula (congenital) Q38.5
  vagina (acquired) N89.8
    congenital Q52.4
  valgus NEC M21.00
    ankle M21.07-
    elbow M21.02-
    knee M21.06-
  valve, valvular (congenital) (heart) Q24.8
    acquired — *see* Endocarditis
  varus NEC M21.10
    ankle M21.17-
    elbow M21.12-
    knee M21.16-
    tibia — *see* Osteochondrosis, juvenile, tibia
  vas deferens (congenital) Q55.4
    acquired N50.8
  vein (congenital) Q27.9
    great Q26.9

Deformity— *continued*
  vertebra — *see* Dorsopathy, deforming
  vesicourethral orifice (acquired) N32.89
    congenital NEC Q64.79
  vessels of optic papilla (congenital) Q14.2
  visual field (contraction) — *see* Defect, visual field
  vitreous body, acquired H43.89
  vulva (congenital) Q52.79
    acquired N90.89
  wrist (joint) (acquired) (*see also* Deformity, limb,
    forearm)
    congenital Q68.8
    contraction — *see* Contraction, joint, wrist

Degeneration, degenerative
  adrenal (capsule) (fatty) (gland) (hyaline)
    (infectional) E27.8
  amyloid (*see also* Amyloidosis) E85.9
  anterior cornua, spinal cord G12.29
  anterior labral S43.49-
  aorta, aortic I70.0
    fatty I77.89
  aortic valve (heart) — *see* Endocarditis, aortic
  arteriovascular — *see* Arteriosclerosis
  artery, arterial (atheromatous) (calcareous) (*see also*
    Arteriosclerosis)
    cerebral, amyloid E85.4 [I68.0]
    medial — *see* Arteriosclerosis, extremities
  articular cartilage NEC — *see* Derangement, joint,
    articular cartilage, by site
  atheromatous — *see* Arteriosclerosis
  basal nuclei or ganglia G23.9
    specified NEC G23.8
  bone NEC — *see* Disorder, bone, specified type NEC
  brachial plexus G54.0
  brain (cortical) (progressive) G31.9
    alcoholic G31.2
    arteriosclerotic I67.2
    childhood G31.9
      specified NEC G31.89
    cystic G31.89
      congenital Q04.6
    in
      alcoholism G31.2
      beriberi E51.2
      cerebrovascular disease I67.9
      congenital hydrocephalus Q03.9
        with spina bifida (*see also* Spina bifida)
      Fabry-Anderson disease E75.21
      Gaucher's disease E75.22
      Hunter's syndrome E76.1
      lipidosis
        cerebral E75.4
        generalized E75.6
      mucopolysaccharidosis — *see*
        Mucopolysaccharidosis
      myxedema E03.9 [G32.8]
      neoplastic disease (*see also* Neoplasm) D49.6
        [G32.8]
      Niemann-Pick disease E75.249 [G32.8]
      sphingolipidosis E75.3 [G32.8]
      vitamin B12 deficiency E53.8 [G32.8]
    senile NEC G31.1
  breast N64.89
  Bruch's membrane — *see* Degeneration, choroid
  capillaries (fatty) I78.8
    amyloid E85.8 [I79.8]
  cardiac (*see also* Degeneration, myocardial)
    valve, valvular — *see* Endocarditis
  cardiorenal — *see* Hypertension, cardiorenal
  cardiovascular (*see also* Disease, cardiovascular)
    renal — *see* Hypertension, cardiorenal
  cerebellar NOS G31.9
    alcoholic G31.2
    primary (hereditary) (sporadic) G11.9
  cerebral — *see* Degeneration, brain
  cerebrovascular I67.9
    due to hypertension I67.4
  cervical plexus G54.2
  cervix N88.8
    due to radiation (intended effect) N88.8
      adverse effect or misadventure N99.89
  chamber angle H21.21-
  changes, spine or vertebra — *see* Spondylosis

Degeneration, degenerative— *continued*
  chorioretinal (*see also* Degeneration, choroid)
    hereditary H31.20
  choroid (colloid) (drusen) H31.11-
    atrophy — *see* Atrophy, choroidal
    hereditary — *see* Dystrophy, choroidal,
      hereditary
  ciliary body H21.22-
  cochlear — *see* subcategory H83.8
  combined (spinal cord) (subacute) E53.8 [G32.0]
    with anemia (pernicious) D51.0 [G32.0]
      due to dietary vitamin B12 deficiency D51.3
        [G32.0]
    in (due to)
      vitamin B12 deficiency E53.8 [G32.0]
        anemia D51.9 [G32.0]
  conjunctiva H11.10
    concretions — *see* Concretion, conjunctiva
    deposits — *see* Deposit, conjunctiva
    pigmentations — *see* Pigmentation, conjunctiva
    pinguecula — *see* Pinguecula
    xerosis — *see* Xerosis, conjunctiva
  cornea H18.40
    calcerous H18.43
      band keratopathy H18.42-
    familial, hereditary — *see* Dystrophy, cornea
    hyaline (of old scars) H18.49
    keratomalacia — *see* Keratomalacia
    nodular H18.45-
    peripheral H18.46-
    senile H18.41-
    specified type NEC H18.49
  cortical (cerebellar) (parenchymatous) G31.89
    alcoholic G31.2
    diffuse, due to arteriopathy I67.2
  cutis L98.8
    amyloid E85.4 [L99]
  dental pulp K04.2
  disc disease — *see* Degeneration, intervertebral disc
    NEC
  dorsolateral (spinal cord) — *see* Degeneration,
    combined
  extrapyramidal G25.9
  eye, macular (*see also* Degeneration, macula)
    congenital or hereditary — *see* Dystrophy, retina
  facet joints — *see* Spondylosis
  fatty
    liver NEC K76.0
      alcoholic K70.0
  grey matter (brain) (Alpers') G31.81
  heart (*see also* Degeneration, myocardial)
    amyloid E85.4 [I43]
    atheromatous — *see* Disease, heart, ischemic,
      atherosclerotic
    ischemic — *see* Disease, heart, ischemic
  hepatolenticular (Wilson's) E83.01
  hepatorenal K76.7
  hyaline (diffuse) (generalized)
    localized — *see* Degeneration, by site
  infrapatellar fat pad M79.4
  intervertebral disc NOS
    with
      myelopathy — *see* Disorder, disc, with,
        myelopathy
      radiculitis or radiculopathy — *see* Disorder,
        disc, with, radiculopathy
    cervical, cervicothoracic — *see* Disorder, disc,
      cervical, degeneration
      with
        myelopathy — *see* Disorder, disc, cervical,
          with myelopathy
        neuritis, radiculitis or radiculopathy — *see*
          Disorder, disc, cervical, with neuritis
    lumbar region M51.36
      with
        myelopathy M51.06
        neuritis, radiculitis, radiculopathy or
          sciatica M51.16
    lumbosacral region M51.37
      with
        myelopathy M51.07
        neuritis, radiculitis, radiculopathy or
          sciatica M51.17

Degeneration, degenerative— *continued*
  intervertebral disc—*continued*
    sacrococcygeal region M53.3
    thoracic region M51.34
      with
        myelopathy M51.04
        neuritis, radiculitis, radiculopathy M51.14
    thoracolumbar region M51.35
      with
        myelopathy M51.05
        neuritis, radiculitis, radiculopathy M51.15
  intestine, amyloid E85.4
  iris (pigmentary) H21.23-
  ischemic — *see* Ischemia
  joint disease — *see* Osteoarthritis
  kidney N28.89
    amyloid E85.4 [N29]
    cystic, congenital Q61.9
    fatty N28.89
    polycystic Q61.3
      adult type (autosomal dominant) Q61.2
      infantile type (autosomal recessive) NEC
        Q61.19
      collecting duct dilatation Q61.11
  Kuhnt-Junius — *see* Degeneration, macula
  lens — *see* Cataract
  lenticular (familial) (progressive) (Wilson's) (with
    cirrhosis of liver) E83.01
  liver (diffuse) NEC K76.8
    amyloid E85.4 [K77]
    cystic K76.8
      congenital Q44.6
    fatty NEC K76.0
      alcoholic K70.0
    hypertrophic K76.8
    parenchymatous, acute or subacute K72.00
      with coma K72.01
    pigmentary K76.8
    toxic (acute) K71.9
  lung J98.4
  lymph gland I89.8
    hyaline I89.8
  macula, macular (acquired) (atrophic) (exudative)
    (senile) H35.30
    angioid streaks H35.33
    congenital or hereditary — *see* Dystrophy, retina
    cystoid H35.35-
    drusen H35.36-
    exudative H35.31
    hole H35.34-
    nonexudative H35.32
    puckering H35.37-
    toxic H35.38-
  membranous labyrinth, congenital (causing
    impairment of hearing) Q16.5
  meniscus — *see* Derangement, meniscus
  mitral — *see* Insufficiency, mitral
  Monckeberg's — *see* Arteriosclerosis, extremities
  motor centers, senile G31.1
  multi-system G90.3
  mural — *see* Degeneration, myocardial
  muscle (fatty) (fibrous) (hyaline) (progressive)
    M62.89
    heart — *see* Degeneration, myocardial
  myelin, central nervous system G37.9
  myocardial, myocardium (fatty) (hyaline) (senile)
    I51.5
    with rheumatic fever (conditions in I00) I09.0
      active, acute or subacute I01.2
        with chorea I02.0
      inactive or quiescent (with chorea) I09.0
    hypertensive — *see* Hypertension, heart
    rheumatic — *see* Degeneration, myocardial, with
      rheumatic fever
    syphilitic A52.06
  nasal sinus (mucosa) J32.9
    frontal J32.1
    maxillary J32.0
  nerve — *see* Disorder, nerve
  nervous system G31.9
    alcoholic G31.2
    amyloid E85.4 [G99.8]
    autonomic G90.9

Degeneration, degenerative— *continued*
  nervous system—*continued*
    fatty G31.89
    specified NEC G31.89
  nipple N64.89
  olivopontocerebellar (hereditary) (familial) G23.8
  osseous labyrinth — *see* subcategory H83.8
  ovary N83.8
    cystic N83.20
    microcystic N83.20
  pallidal pigmentary (progressive) G23.0
  pancreas K86.8
    tuberculous A18.83
  penis N48.89
  pigmentary (diffuse) (general)
    localized — *see* Degeneration, by site
    pallidal (progressive) G23.0
  pineal gland E34.8
  pituitary (gland) E23.6
  popliteal fat pad M79.4
  posterolateral (spinal cord) — *see* Degeneration, combined
  pulmonary valve (heart) I37.8
  pulp (tooth) K04.2
  pupillary margin H21.24-
  renal — *see* Degeneration, kidney
  retina H35.9
    hereditary (cerebroretinal) (congenital) (juvenile) (macula) (peripheral) (pigmentary) — *see* Dystrophy, retina
    Kuhnt-Junius — *see* Degeneration, macula, hole
    macula (cystic) (exudative) (hole) (nonexudative) (pseudohole) (senile) (toxic) — *see* Degeneration, macula
    peripheral H35.40
      lattice H35.41-
      microcystoid H35.42-
      paving stone H35.43-
      secondary
        pigmentary H35.45-
        vitreoretinal H35.46-
      senile reticular H35.44-
    pigmentary (primary) (*see also* Dystrophy, retina)
      secondary — *see* Degeneration, retina, peripheral, secondary
    posterior pole — *see* Degeneration, macula
  saccule, congenital (causing impairment of hearing) Q16.5
  senile R54
    brain G31.1
    cardiac, heart or myocardium — *see* Degeneration, myocardial
    motor centers G31.1
    vascular — *see* Arteriosclerosis
  sinus (cystic) (*see also* Sinusitis)
    polypoid J33.1
  skin L98.8
    amyloid E85.4 [L99]
    colloid L98.8
  spinal (cord) G31.89
    amyloid E85.4 [G32.8]
    combined (subacute) — *see* Degeneration, combined
    dorsolateral — *see* Degeneration, combined
    familial NEC G31.89
    fatty G31.89
    funicular — *see* Degeneration, combined
    posterolateral — *see* Degeneration, combined
    subacute combined — *see* Degeneration, combined
    tuberculous A17.81
  spleen D73.0
    amyloid E85.4 [D77]
  stomach K31.89
  striatonigral G23.2
  suprarenal (capsule) (gland) E27.8
  synovial membrane (pulpy) — *see* Disorder, synovium, specified type NEC
  tapetoretinal — *see* Dystrophy, retina
  thymus (gland) E32.8
    fatty E32.8
  thyroid (gland) E07.89
  tricuspid (heart) (valve) I07.9

Degeneration, degenerative— *continued*
  tuberculous NEC — *see* Tuberculosis
  turbinate J34.89
  uterus (cystic) N85.8
  vascular (senile) — *see* Arteriosclerosis
    hypertensive — *see* Hypertension
  vitreoretinal, secondary — *see* Degeneration, retina, peripheral, secondary, vitreoretinal
  vitreous (body) H43.81-
  Wallerian — *see* Disorder, nerve
  Wilson's hepatolenticular E83.01
Deglutition
  paralysis R13.0
    hysterical F44.4
  pneumonia J69.0
Degos' disease I77.89
Dehiscence (of)
  cesarean wound O90.0
  closure of
    cornea T81.31
    craniotomy T81.32
    fascia (muscular) (superficial) T81.32
    internal organ or tissue T81.32
    laceration (external) (internal) T81.33
    ligament T81.32
    mucosa T81.31
    muscle or muscle flap T81.32
    ribs or rib cage T81.32
    skin and subcutaneous tissue (full-thickness) (superficial) T81.31
    skull T81.32
    sternum (sternotomy) T81.32
    tendon T81.32
    traumatic laceration (external) (internal) T81.33
  episiotomy O90.1
  operation wound NEC T81.31
    external operation wound (superficial) T81.31
    internal operation wound (deep) T81.32
  perineal wound (postpartum) O90.1
  traumatic injury wound repair T81.33
  wound T81.30
    traumatic repair T81.33
Dehydration E86.0
  hypertonic E87.0
  hypotonic E87.1
  newborn P74.1
Déjérine-Roussy syndrome G93.89
Déjérine-Sottas disease or neuropathy (hypertrophic) G60.0
Déjérine-Thomas atrophy G23.8
Delay, delayed
  any plane in pelvis
    complicating delivery O66.9
  birth or delivery NOS O63.9
  closure, ductus arteriosus (Botalli) P29.3
  coagulation — *see* Defect, coagulation
  conduction (cardiac) (ventricular) I45.9
  delivery, second twin, triplet, etc O63.2
  development R62.50
    global F88
    intellectual (specific) F81.9
    language F80.9
      due to hearing loss F80.4
    learning F81.9
    pervasive F84.9
    physiological R62.50
      specified stage NEC R62.0
    reading F81.0
    sexual E30.0
    speech F80.9
      due to hearing loss F80.4
    spelling F81.81
  gastric emptying K30
  menarche E28.39
  menstruation (cause unknown) N91.0
  milestone R62.0
  passage of meconium (newborn) P76.0
  primary respiration P28.9
  puberty (constitutional) E30.0
  separation of umbilical cord P96.82
  sexual maturation, female E30.0
  sleep phase syndrome G47.21
  union, fracture — *see* Fracture, by site

Delay, delayed— *continued*
  vaccination Z28.9
Deletion(s)
  autosome Q93.9
    identified by fluorescence in situ hybridization (FISH) Q93.89
    identified by in situ hybridization (ISH) Q93.89
  chromosome
    with complex rearrangements NEC Q93.7
    part of NEC Q93.5
    seen only at prometaphase Q93.89
    short arm
      4 Q93.3
      5p Q93.4
      22q11.2 Q93.81
    specified NEC Q93.89
  long arm chromosome 18 or 21 Q93.89
    with complex rearrangements NEC Q93.7
  microdeletions NEC Q93.88
Delhi boil or button B55.1
Delinquency (juvenile) (neurotic) F91.8
  group Z72.810
Delinquent immunization status Z28.3
Delirium, delirious (acute or subacute) (not alcohol or drug-induced) (with dementia) R41.0
  alcoholic (acute) (tremens) (withdrawal) F10.921
    with intoxication F10.921
      in
        abuse F10.121
        dependence F10.221
  due to (secondary to)
    alcohol
      intoxication F10.921
        in
          abuse F10.121
          dependence F10.221
      withdrawal F10.231
    amphetamine intoxication F15.921
      in
        abuse F15.121
        dependence F15.221
    anxiolytic
      intoxication F13.921
        in
          abuse F13.121
          dependence F13.221
      withdrawal F13.231
    cannabis intoxication (acute) F12.921
      in
        abuse F12.121
        dependence F12.221
    cocaine intoxication (acute) F14.921
      in
        abuse F14.121
        dependence F14.221
    general medical condition F05
    hallucinogen intoxication F16.921
      in
        abuse F16.121
        dependence F16.221
    hypnotic
      intoxication F13.921
        in
          abuse F13.121
          dependence F13.221
      withdrawal F13.231
    inhalant intoxication (acute) F18.921
      in
        abuse F18.121
        dependence F18.221
    multiple etiologies F05
    opioid intoxication (acute) F11.921
      in
        abuse F11.121
        dependence F11.221
    phencyclidine intoxication (acute) F19.921
      in
        abuse F19.121
        dependence F19.221
    psychoactive substance NEC intoxication (acute) F19.921
      in
        abuse F19.121

Delirium, delirious —*continued*
  due to—*continued*
    psychoactive substance NEC
      intoxication—*continued*
      in—*continued*
        dependence F19.221
      sedative
        intoxication F13.921
          in
            abuse F13.121
            dependence F13.221
        withdrawal F13.231
      unknown etiology F05
    exhaustion F43.0
    hysterical F44.89
    postprocedural (postoperative) F05
    puerperal F05
    thyroid — *see* Thyrotoxicosis with thyroid storm
    traumatic — *see* Injury, intracranial
    tremens (alcohol-induced) F10.231
      sedative-induced F13.231
Delivery (childbirth) (labor)
  arrested active phase O62.1
  cesarean (for)
    abnormal
      pelvis (bony) (deformity) (major) NEC with
        disproportion (fetopelvic) O33.0
          with obstructed labor O65.0
        presentation or position O32.9
    abruptio placentae(*see also* Abruptio placentae)
      O45.
    acromion presentation O32.2
    atony, uterus O62.2
    breech presentation O32.1
      incomplete O32.8
    brow presentation O32.3
    cephalopelvic disproportion O33.9
    cerclage O34.3-
    chin presentation O32.3
    cicatrix of cervix O34.4-
    contracted pelvis (general)
      inlet O33.2
      outlet O33.3
    cord presentation or prolapse O69.0
    cystocele O34.8-
    deformity (acquired) (congenital)
      pelvic organs or tissues NEC O34.8-
      pelvis (bony) NEC O33.0
    disproportion NOS O33.9
    eclampsia — *see* Eclampsia
    face presentation O32.3
    failed
      forceps O66.5
      induction of labor O61.9
        instrumental O61.1
        mechanical O61.1
        medical O61.0
        specified NEC O61.8
        surgical O61.1
      trial of labor NOS O66.40
        following previous cesarean delivery O66.41
      vacuum extraction O66.5
      ventouse O66.5
    fetal-maternal hemorrhage O43.01-
    hemorrhage (intrapartum) O67.9
      with coagulation defect O67.0
      specified cause NEC O67.8
    high head at term O32.4
    hydrocephalic fetus O33.6
    incarceration of uterus O34.51-
    incoordinate uterine action O62.4
    increased size, fetus O33.5
    inertia, uterus O62.2
      primary O62.0
      secondary O62.1
    lateroversion, uterus O34.59-
    mal lie O32.9
    malposition
      fetus O32.9
      pelvic organs or tissues NEC O34.8-
      uterus NEC O34.59-
    malpresentation NOS O32.9

Delivery— *continued*
  cesarean—*continued*
    oblique presentation O32.2
    oversize fetus O33.5
    pelvic tumor NEC O34.8-
    placenta previa O44.1-
      without hemorrhage O44.0-
    placental insufficiency O36.51-
    polyp, cervix O34.4-
      causing obstructed labor O65.5
    poor dilatation, cervix O62.0
    pre-eclampsia O14.9-
      mild O14.0-
      moderate O14.0-
      severe
        with HELLP O14.2-
    previous
      cesarean delivery O34.21
      surgery (to)
        cervix O34.4-
        gynecological NEC O34.8-
        rectum O34.7-
        uterus O34.29
        vagina O34.6-
    prolapse
      arm or hand O32.2
      uterus O34.52-
    prolonged labor NOS O63.9
    rectocele O34.8-
    retroversion
      uterus O34.59-
    rigid
      cervix O34.4-
      pelvic floor O34.8-
      perineum O34.7-
      vagina O34.6-
      vulva O34.7-
    sacculation, pregnant uterus O34.59-
    scar(s)
      cervix O34.4-
      cesarean delivery O34.21
      uterus O34.29
    Shirodkar suture in situ O34.3-
    shoulder presentation O32.2
    stenosis or stricture, cervix O34.4-
    streptococcus B carrier state O99.824
    transverse presentation or lie O32.2
    tumor, pelvic organs or tissues NEC O34.8-
      cervix O34.4-
    umbilical cord presentation or prolapse O69.0
    without indication O82
  completely normal case O80
  complicated O75.9
    by
      abnormal, abnormality (of)
        forces of labor O62.9
          specified type NEC O62.8
        glucose O99.814
        uterine contractions NOS O62.9
      abruptio placentae O45.9-
      abuse
        physical O9A.32
        psychological O9A.52
        sexual O9A.42
      adherent placenta O72.0
        without hemorrhage O73.0
      alcohol use O99.314
      anemia (pre-existing) O99.02
      anesthetic death O74.8
      annular detachment of cervix O71.3
      atony, uterus O62.2
      attempted vacuum extraction and forceps
        O66.5
      Bandl's ring O62.4
      bariatric surgery status O99.844
      bleeding — *see* Delivery, complicated by,
        hemorrhage
      blood disorder NEC O99.12
      cervical dystocia (hypotonic) O62.2
        primary O62.0
        secondary O62.1
      circulatory system disorder O99.42
      compression of cord (umbilical) NEC O69.2

Delivery— *continued*
  complicated—*continued*
    by—*continued*
      condition NEC O99.89
      contraction, contracted ring O62.4
      cord (umbilical)
        around neck
          with compression O69.1
          without compression O69.81
        bruising O69.5
        complication O69.9
          specified NEC O69.89
        compression NEC O69.2
        entanglement O69.2
          without compression O69.82
        hematoma O69.5
        presentation O69.0
        prolapse O69.0
        short O69.3
        thrombosis (vessels) O69.5
        vascular lesion O69.5
      Couvelaire uterus O45.8x-
      delay following rupture of membranes
        (spontaneous) — *see* Pregnancy,
        complicated by, premature rupture of
        membranes
      damage to (injury to) NEC
        perineum O71.82
        periurethral tissue O71.82
        vulva O71.82
      depressed fetal heart tones O76
      diabetes O24.92
        gestational O24.429
          diet controlled O24.420
          insulin controlled O24.424
        pre-existing O24.32
          specified NEC O24.82
          type 1 O24.02
          type 2 O24.12
      diastasis recti (abdominis) O71.89
      dilatation
        bladder O66.8
        cervix incomplete, poor or slow O62.0
      disease NEC O99.89
      disruptio uteri — *see* Delivery, complicated by,
        rupture, uterus
      drug use O99.324
      dysfunction, uterus NOS O62.9
        hypertonic O62.4
        hypotonic O62.2
          primary O62.0
          secondary O62.1
        incoordinate O62.4
      eclampsia O15.1
      embolism (pulmonary) — *see* Embolism,
        obstetric
      endocrine, nutritional or metabolic disease
        NEC O99.284
      failed
        attempted vaginal birth after previous
          cesarean delivery O66.41
        induction of labor O61.9
          instrumental O61.1
          mechanical O61.1
          medical O61.0
          specified NEC O61.8
          surgical O61.1
        trial of labor O66.40
      female genital mutilation O65.5
      fetal
        abnormal acid-base balance O68
        acidemia O68
        acidosis O68
        alkalosis O68
        death, early O02.1
        deformity O66.3
        heart rate or rhythm (abnormal)
          (non-reassuring) O76
        hypoxia O77.8
        stress O77.9
          due to drug administration O77.1
          electrocardiographic evidence of
            O77.8

Delivery— *continued*
  complicated— *continued*
    by— *continued*
      fetal —*continued*
        stress—*continued*
          ultrasound evidence of O77.8
          specified NEC O77.8
      fever during labor O75.2
      gastric banding status O99.844
      gastric bypass status O99.844
      gastrointestinal disease NEC O99.62
      gestational diabetes O24.429
        diet controlled O24.420
        insulin (and diet) controlled O24.424
      gonorrhea O98.22
      hematoma O71.7
        ischial spine O71.7
        pelvic O71.7
        vagina O71.7
        vulva or perineum O71.7
      hemorrhage (uterine) O67.9
        associated with
          afibrinogenemia O67.0
          coagulation defect O67.0
          hyperfibrinolysis O67.0
          hypofibrinogenemia O67.0
        due to
          low-lying placenta O44.1-
            without hemorrhage O44.0-
          placenta previa O44.1-
            without hemorrhage O44.0-
          premature separation of placenta
            (normally implanted) (*see also*
            Abruptio placentae) O45.
          retained placenta O72.0
          uterine leiomyoma O67.8
        placenta NEC O67.8
        postpartum NEC (atonic) (immediate)
          O72.1
          with retained or trapped placenta
            O72.0
          delayed O72.2
          secondary O72.2
          third stage O72.0
      hourglass contraction, uterus O62.4
      hypertension, hypertensive (pre-existing) —
        see Hypertension, complicated by,
        childbirth (labor)
      hypotension O26.5-
      incomplete dilatation (cervix) O62.0
      incoordinate uterus contractions O62.4
      inertia, uterus O62.2
        during latent phase of labor O62.0
        primary O62.0
        secondary O62.1
      infection (maternal) O98.92
        carrier state NEC O99.834
        gonorrhea O98.22
        human immunodeficiency (HIV) O98.72
        sexually transmitted NEC O98.32
        specified NEC O98.82
        syphilis O98.12
        tuberculosis O98.02
        viral hepatitis O98.42
        viral NEC O98.52
      injury (to mother) (*see* also Delivery,
        complicated by, damage to) O71.9
        nonobstetric O9A.22
          caused by abuse — *see* Delivery,
            complicated by, abuse
      intrauterine fetal death, early O02.1
      inversion, uterus O71.2
      laceration (perineal) O70.9
        anus (sphincter) O70.4
          with third degree laceration O70.2
            with mucosa O70.3
          without third degree laceration O70.4
        bladder (urinary) O71.5
        bowel O71.5
        cervix (uteri) O71.3
        fourchette O70.0
        hymen O70.0
        labia O70.0

Delivery— *continued*
  complicated— *continued*
    by— *continued*
      laceration— *continued*
        pelvic
          floor O70.1
          organ NEC O71.5
        perineum, perineal O70.9
          first degree O70.0
          fourth degree O70.3
          muscles O70.1
          second degree O70.1
          skin O70.0
          slight O70.0
          third degree O70.2
        peritoneum (pelvic) O71.5
        rectovaginal (septum) (without perineal
          laceration) O71.4
          with perineum O70.2
            with anal or rectal mucosa O70.3
        specified NEC O71.89
        sphincter ani — *see* Delivery, complicated,
          by, laceration, anus (sphincter)
        urethra O71.5
        uterus O71.81
          before labor O71.81
        vagina, vaginal (deep) (high) (without
          perineal laceration) O71.4
          with perineum O70.0
          muscles, with perineum O70.1
        vulva O70.0
      liver disorder O26.62
      malignancy O9A.12
      malnutrition O25.2
      malposition, malpresentation
        placenta (with hemorrhage) O44.1-
        uterus or cervix O65.5
        without obstruction (*see also* Delivery,
          complicated by, obstruction) O32.9
          breech O32.1
          compound O32.6
          face (brow) (chin) O32.3
          footling O32.8
          high head O32.4
          oblique O32.2
          specified NEC O32.8
          transverse O32.2
          unstable lie O32.0
      meconium in amniotic fluid O77.0
      mental disorder NEC O99.344
      metrorrhexis — *see* Delivery, complicated by,
        rupture, uterus
      nervous system disorder O99.354
      obesity (pre-existing) O99.214
      obesity surgery status O99.844
      obstetric trauma O71.9
        specified NEC O71.89
      obstruction
        due to
          breech (complete) (frank) presentation
            O64.1
            incomplete O64.8
          brow presenation O64.3
          buttock presentation O64.1
          chin presentation O64.2
          compound presentation O64.5
          contracted pelvis O65.1
          deep transverse arrest O64.0
          deformed pelvis O65.0
          dystocia (fetal) O66.9
            due to
              conjoined twins O66.3
              fetal
                abnormality NEC O66.3
                ascites O66.3
                hydrops O66.3
                meningomyelocele O66.3
                sacral teratoma O66.3
                tumor O66.3
             hydrocephalic fetus O66.3
          shoulder O66.0
          face presentation O64.2
          fetopelvic disproportion O65.4

Delivery— *continued*
  complicated— *continued*
    by— *continued*
      obstruction— *continued*
        due to— *continued*
          footling presentation O64.8
          impacted shoulders O66.0
          incomplete rotation of fetal head
            O64.0
          large fetus O66.2
          locked twins O66.1
          malposition O64.9
            specified NEC O64.8
          malpresentation O64.9
            specified NEC O64.8
          multiple fetuses NEC O66.6
          pelvic
            abnormality (maternal) O65.9
              organ O65.5
              specified NEC O65.8
            contraction
              inlet O65.2
              mid-cavity O65.3
              outlet O65.3
          persistent (position)
            occipitoiliac O64.0
            occipitoposterior O64.0
            occipitosacral O64.0
            occipitotransverse O64.0
          prolapsed arm O64.4
          shoulder presentation O64.4
        specified NEC O66.8
      pathological retraction ring, uterus O62.4
      penetration, pregnant uterus by instrument
        O71.1
      perforation — *see* Delivery, complicated by,
        laceration
      placenta, placental
        ablatio O45.9-
        abnormality O43.9-
          specified NEC O43.89-
        abruptio O45.9-
        accreta O43.21-
        adherent (with hemorrhage) O72.0
          without hemorrhage O73.0
        detachment (premature) O45.9-
        disorder O43.9-
        hemorrhage NEC O67.8
        increta O43.22 -
        low (implantation) O44.1-
          without hemorrhage O44.0-
        malformation O43.10-
        malposition O44.1-
          without hemorrhage O44.0-
        percreta O43.23 -
        previa (central) (lateral) (low) (marginal)
          (partial) (total) O44.1-
        retained (with hemorrhage) O72.0
          without hemorrhage O73.0
        separation (premature) O45.9-
          specified NEC O45.8x-
        vicious insertion O44.1-
      precipitate labor O62.3
      premature rupture, membranes (*see also*
        Pregnancy, complicated by, premature
        rupture of membranes) O42.90
      prolapse
        arm or hand O32.8
        cord (umbilical) O69.0
        foot or leg O32.8
        uterus O34.52-
      prolonged labor O63.9
        first stage O63.0
        second stage O63.1
      protozoal disease (maternal) O98.62
      respiratory disease NEC O99.52
      retained membranes or portions of placenta
        O72.2
        without hemorrhage O73.1
      retarded birth O63.9
      retention of secundines (with hemorrhage)
        O72.0
        without hemorrhage O73.0

Delivery— *continued*
  complicated— *continued*
    by— *continued*
      retention of secundines—*continued*
        partial O72.2
          without hemorrhage O73.1
      rupture
        bladder (urinary) O71.5
        cervix O71.3
        pelvic organ NEC O71.5
        urethra O71.5
        uterus (during or after labor) O71.1
          before labor O71.0-
      separation, pubic bone (symphysis pubis)
        O71.6
      shock O75.1
      shoulder presentation O64.4
      skin disorder NEC O99.72
      spasm, cervix O62.4
      stenosis or stricture, cervix O65.5
      streptococcus B carrier state O99.824
      subluxation of symphysis (pubis) O26.72
      syphilis (maternal) O98.12
      tear — *see* Delivery, complicated by, laceration
      tetanic uterus O62.4
      trauma (obstetrical) (*see also* Delivery,
        complicated, by damage to) O71.9
        non-obstetric O9A.22
        periurethral O71.82
      tuberculosis (maternal) O98.02
      tumor, pelvic organs or tissues NEC O65.5
      umbilical cord around neck
        with compression O69.1
        without compression O69.81
      uterine inertia O62.2
        during latent phase of labor O62.0
        primary O62.0
        secondary O62.1
      vasa previa O69.4
      velamentous insertion of cord O43.12-
    specified complication NEC O75.89
  delayed NOS O63.9
    following rupture of membranes
      artificial O75.5
    second twin, triplet, etc. O63.2
  forceps, low following failed vacuum extraction
    O66.5
  missed (at or near term) O36.4
  normal O80
  obstructed — *see* Delivery, complicated by,
    obstruction
  precipitate O62.3
  preterm (*see also* Pregnancy, complicated by,
    preterm labor) O60.10
  spontaneous O80
  term pregnancy NOS O80
  uncomplicated O80
  vaginal, following previous cesarean delivery O34.21
Delusions (paranoid) — *see* Disorder, delusional
Dementia (degenerative (primary)) (old age)
      (persisting) F03
  with
    Lewy bodies G31.83 [F02.80]
      with behavioral disturbance G31.83 [F02.81]
    Parkinsonism G31.83 [F02.80]
      with behavioral disturbance G31.83 [F02.81]
  alcoholic F10.97
    with dependence F10.27
  Alzheimer's type — *see* Disease, Alzheimer's
  arteriosclerotic — *see* Dementia, vascular
  atypical, Alzheimer's type — *see* Disease,
      Alzheimer's, specified NEC
  congenital — *see* Retardation, mental
  frontal (lobe) G31.09 [F02.80]
    with behavioral disturbance G31.09 [F02.81]
  frontotemporal G31.09 [F02.80]
    with behavioral disturbance G31.09 [F02.81]
    specified NEC G31.09 [F02.80]
      with behavioral disturbance G31.09 [F02.81]
  in (due to)
    alcohol F10.97
      with dependence F10.27
    Alzheimer's disease — *see* Disease, Alzheimer's

Dementia —*continued*
  in (due to)— *continued*
    arteriosclerotic brain disease — *see* Dementia,
        vascular
    cerebral lipidoses E75.[F02.80]
      with behavioral disturbance E75.[F02.81]
    Creutzfeldt-Jakob disease (*see also*
        Creutzfeldt-Jakob disease or syndrome
        (with dementia)) A81.00
    epilepsy G40.[F02.80]
      with behavioral disturbance G40.[F02.81]
    hepatolenticular degeneration E83.01 [F02.80]
      with behavioral disturbance E83.01 [F02.81]
    human immunodeficiency virus (HIV) disease
        B20 [F02.80]
      with behavioral disturbance B20 [F02.81]
    Huntington's disease or chorea G10
    hypercalcemia E83.52 [F02.80]
      with behavioral disturbance E83.52 [F02.81]
    hypothyroidism, acquired E03.9 [F02.80]
      with behavioral disturbance E03.9 [F02.81]
      due to iodine deficiency E01.8 [F02.80]
        with behavioral disturbance E01.8 [F02.81]
    inhalants F18.97
      with dependence F18.27
    multiple
      etiologies F03
        sclerosis G35 [F02.80]
          with behavioral disturbance G35 [F02.81]
    neurosyphilis A52.17 [F02.80]
      with behavioral disturbance A52.17 [F02.81]
      juvenile A50.49 [F02.80]
        with behavioral disturbance A50.49
          [F02.81]
    niacin deficiency E52 [F02.80]
      with behavioral disturbance E52 [F02.81]
    paralysis agitans G20 [F02.80]
      with behavioral disturbance G20 [F02.81]
    Parkinson's disease (parkinsonism) G20 [F02.80]
      with behavioral disturbance G20 [F02.81]
    pellagra E52 [F02.80]
      with behavioral disturbance E52 [F02.81]
    Pick's G31.01 [F02.80]
      with behavioral disturbance G31.01 [F02.81]
    polyarteritis nodosa M30.0 [F02.80]
      with behavioral disturbance M30.0 [F02.81]
    psychoactive drug F19.97
      with dependence F19.27
      inhalants F18.97
        with dependence F18.27
      sedatives, hypnotics or anxiolytics F13.97
        with dependence F13.27
    sedatives, hypnotics or anxiolytics F13.97
      with dependence F13.27
    systemic lupus erythematosus M32.[F02.80]
      with behavioral disturbance M32.[F02.81]
    trypanosomiasis
      African B56.9 [F02.80]
        with behavioral disturbance B56.9
          [F02.81]
    unknown etiology F03
    vitamin B12 deficiency E53.8 [F02.80]
      with behavioral disturbance E53.8 [F02.81]
    volatile solvents F18.97
      with dependence F18.27
    with behavioral disturbance G31.83 [F02.81]
  infantile, infantilis F84.3
  Lewy body G31.83 [F02.80]
  multi-infarct — *see* Dementia, vascular
  paralytica, paralytic (syphilitic) A52.17 [F02.80]
    with behavioral disturbance A52.17 [F02.81]
    juvenilis A50.45 [F02.80]
      with behavioral disturbance A50.45 [F02.81]
  paretic A52.17
  praecox — *see* Schizophrenia
  presenile F03
    Alzheimer's type — *see* Disease, Alzheimer's,
        early onset
  primary degenerative F03
  progressive, syphilitic A52.17
  senile F03
    with acute confusional state F05

Dementia— *continued*
  senile— *continued*
    Alzheimer's type — *see* Disease, Alzheimer's, late
        onset
    depressed or paranoid type F03
  vascular (acute onset) (mixed) (multi-infarct)
      (subcortical) F01.50
    with behavioral disturbance F01.51
Demineralization, bone — *see* Osteoporosis
Demodex folliculorum (infestation) B88.0
Demophobia F40.248
Demoralization R45.3
Demyelination, demyelinization
  central nervous system G37.9
    specified NEC G37.8
  corpus callosum (central) G37.1
  disseminated, acute G36.9
    specified NEC G36.8
  global G35
  in optic neuritis G36.0
Dengue (classical) (fever) A90
  hemorrhagic A91
  sandfly A93.1
Dennie-Marfan syphilitic syndrome A50.45
Dens evaginatus, in dente or invaginatus K00.2
Dense breasts R92.2
Density
  increased, bone (disseminated) (generalized)
      (spotted) — *see* Disorder, bone, density and
      structure, specified type NEC
  lung (nodular) J98.4
Dental (*see also* condition)
  examination Z01.20
    with abnormal findings Z01.21
  restoration
    aesthetically inadequate or displeasing K08.56
    defective K08.50
      specified NEC K08.59
    failure of marginal integrity K08.51
    failure of periodontal anatomical integrity K08.54
Dentia praecox K00.6
Denticles (pulp) K04.2
Dentigerous cyst K09.0
Dentin
  irregular (in pulp) K04.3
  opalescent K00.5
  secondary (in pulp) K04.3
  sensitive K03.89
Dentinogenesis imperfecta K00.5
Dentinoma — *see* Cyst, calcifying odontogenic
Dentition (syndrome) K00.7
  delayed K00.6
  difficult K00.7
  precocious K00.6
  premature K00.6
  retarded K00.6
Dependence (on) (syndrome) F19.20
  with remission F19.21
  alcohol (ethyl) (methyl) (without remission) F10.20
    with
      amnestic disorder, persisting F10.26
      anxiety disorder F10.280
      dementia, persisting F10.27
      intoxication F10.229
        with delirium F10.221
        uncomplicated F10.220
      mood disorder F10.24
      psychotic disorder F10.259
        with
          delusions F10.250
          hallucinations F10.251
      remission F10.21
      sexual dysfunction F10.281
      sleep disorder F10.282
      specified disorder NEC F10.288
      withdrawal F10.239
        with
          delirium F10.231
          perceptual disturbance F10.232
        uncomplicated F10.230
    counseling and surveillance Z71.41
  amobarbital — *see* Dependence, drug, sedative

Dependence— *continued*
  amphetamine(s) (type) — *see* Dependence, drug, stimulant NEC
  amytal (sodium) — *see* Dependence, drug, sedative
  analgesic NEC F55.8
  anesthetic (agent) (gas) (general) (local) NEC — *see* Dependence, drug, psychoactive NEC
  anxiolytic NEC — *see* Dependence, drug, sedative
  barbital(s) — *see* Dependence, drug, sedative
  barbiturate(s) (compounds) (drugs classifiable to T42) — *see* Dependence, drug, sedative
  benzedrine — *see* Dependence, drug, stimulant NEC
  bhang — *see* Dependence, drug, cannabis
  bromide(s) NEC — *see* Dependence, drug, sedative
  caffeine — *see* Dependence, drug, stimulant NEC
  cannabis (sativa) (indica) (resin) (derivatives) (type) — *see* Dependence, drug, cannabis
  chloral (betaine) (hydrate) — *see* Dependence, drug, sedative
  chlordiazepoxide — *see* Dependence, drug, sedative
  coca (leaf) (derivatives) — *see* Dependence, drug, cocaine
  cocaine — *see* Dependence, drug, cocaine
  codeine — *see* Dependence, drug, opioid
  combinations of drugs F19.20
  dagga — *see* Dependence, drug, cannabis
  demerol — *see* Dependence, drug, opioid
  dexamphetamine — *see* Dependence, drug, stimulant NEC
  dexedrine — *see* Dependence, drug, stimulant NEC
  dextromethorphan — *see* Dependence, drug, opioid
  dextromoramide — *see* Dependence, drug, opioid
  dextro-nor-pseudo-ephedrine — *see*Dependence, drug, stimulant NEC
  dextrorphan — *see* Dependence, drug, opioid
  diazepam — *see* Dependence, drug, sedative
  dilaudid — *see* Dependence, drug, opioid
  D-lysergic acid diethylamide — *see* Dependence, drug, hallucinogen
  drug NEC F19.20
    with sleep disorder F19.282
    cannabis F12.20
      with
        anxiety disorder F12.280
        intoxication F12.229
          with
            delirium F12.221
            perceptual disturbance F12.222
          uncomplicated F12.220
        other specified disorder F12.288
        psychosis F12.259
          delusions F12.250
          hallucinations F12.251
        unspecified disorder F12.29
      in remission F12.21
    cocaine F14.20
      with
        anxiety disorder F14.280
        intoxication F14.229
          with
            delirium F14.221
            perceptual disturbance F14.222
          uncomplicated F14.220
        mood disorder F14.24
        other specified disorder F14.288
        psychosis F14.259
          delusions F14.250
          hallucinations F14.251
        sexual dysfunction F14.281
        sleep disorder F14.282
        unspecified disorder F14.29
        withdrawal F14.23
      in remission F14.21
      withdrawal symptoms in newborn P96.1
    counseling and surveillance Z71.51
    hallucinogen F16.20
      with
        anxiety disorder F16.280
        flashbacks F16.283
        intoxication F16.229
          with delirium F16.221
          uncomplicated F16.220

Dependence— *continued*
  drug— *continued*
    hallucinogen—*continued*
      with—*continued*
        mood disorder F16.24
        other specified disorder F16.288
        perception disorder, persisting F16.283
        psychosis F16.259
          delusions F16.250
          hallucinations F16.251
        unspecified disorder F16.29
      in remission F16.21
    in remission F19.21
    inhalant F18.20
      with
        amnestic disorder F13.26
        anxiety disorder F18.280
        dementia, persisting F18.27
        intoxication F18.229
          with delirium F18.221
          uncomplicated F18.220
        mood disorder F18.24
        other specified disorder F18.288
        psychosis F18.259
          delusions F18.250
          hallucinations F18.251
        sexual dysfunction F13.281
        unspecified disorder F18.29
        withdrawal F13.239
          with
            delirium F13.231
            perceptual disturbance F13.232
          uncomplicated F13.230
      in remission F18.21
    nicotine F17.200
      with disorder F17.209
        remission F17.201
        specified disorder NEC F17.208
        withdrawal F17.203
      chewing tobacco F17.220
        with disorder F17.229
          remission F17.221
          specified disorder NEC F17.228
          withdrawal F17.223
      cigarettes F17.210
        with disorder F17.219
          remission F17.211
          specified disorder NEC F17.218
          withdrawal F17.213
      specified product NEC F17.290
        with disorder F17.299
          remission F17.291
          specified disorder NEC F17.298
          withdrawal F17.293
    opioid F11.20
      with
        intoxication F11.229
          with
            delirium F11.221
            perceptual disturbance F11.222
          uncomplicated F11.220
        mood disorder F11.24
        other specified disorder F11.288
        psychosis F11.259
          delusions F11.250
          hallucinations F11.251
        sexual dysfunction F11.281
        sleep disorder F11.282
        unspecified disorder F11.29
        withdrawal F11.23
      in remission F11.21
    psychoactive NEC F19.20
      with
        amnestic disorder F19.26
        anxiety disorder F19.280
        dementia F19.27
        intoxication F19.229
          with
            delirium F19.221
            perceptual disturbance F19.222
          uncomplicated F19.220
        mood disorder F19.24
        other specified disorder F19.288

Dependence— *continued*
  drug— *continued*
    psychoactive—*continued*
      with—*continued*
        psychosis F19.259
          delusions F19.250
          hallucinations F19.251
        sexual dysfunction F19.281
        sleep disorder F19.282
        unspecified disorder F19.29
        withdrawal F19.239
          with
            delirium F19.231
            perceptual disturbance F19.232
          uncomplicated F19.230
    sedative, hypnotic or anxiolytic F13.20
      with
        amnestic disorder F13.26
        anxiety disorder F13.280
        dementia, persisting F13.27
        intoxication F13.229
          with delirium F13.221
          uncomplicated F13.220
        mood disorder F13.24
        other specified disorder F13.288
        psychosis F13.259
          delusions F13.250
          hallucinations F13.251
        sexual dysfunction F13.281
        sleep disorder F13.282
        unspecified disorder F13.29
        withdrawal F13.239
          with
            delirium F13.231
            perceptual disturbance F13.232
          uncomplicated F13.230
      in remission F13.21
    stimulant NEC F15.20
      with
        anxiety disorder F15.280
        intoxication F15.229
          with
            delirium F15.221
            perceptual disturbance F15.222
          uncomplicated F15.220
        mood disorder F15.24
        other specified disorder F15.288
        psychosis F15.259
          delusions F15.250
          hallucinations F15.251
        sexual dysfunction F15.281
        sleep disorder F15.282
        unspecified disorder F15.29
        withdrawal F15.23
      in remission F15.21
  ethyl
    alcohol (without remission) F10.20
      with remission F10.21
    bromide — *see* Dependence, drug, sedative
    carbamate F19.20
    chloride F19.20
    morphine — *see* Dependence, drug, opioid
  ganja — *see* Dependence, drug, cannabis
  glue (airplane) (sniffing) — *see* Dependence, drug, inhalant
  glutethimide — *see* Dependence, drug, sedative
  hallucinogenics — *see* Dependence, drug, hallucinogen
  hashish — *see* Dependence, drug, cannabis
  hemp — *see* Dependence, drug, cannabis
  heroin (salt) (any) — *see* Dependence, drug, opioid
  hypnotic NEC — *see* Dependence, drug, sedative
  Indian hemp — *see* Dependence, drug, cannabis
  inhalants — *see* Dependence, drug, inhalant
  khat — *see* Dependence, drug, stimulant NEC
  laudanum — *see* Dependence, drug, opioid
  LSD(-25) (derivatives) — *see* Dependence, drug, hallucinogen
  luminal — *see* Dependence, drug, sedative
  lysergic acid — *see* Dependence, drug, hallucinogen
  maconha — *see* Dependence, drug, cannabis
  marihuana — *see* Dependence, drug, cannabis
  meprobamate — *see* Dependence, drug, sedative

Dependence— *continued*
mescaline — *see* Dependence, drug, hallucinogen
methadone — *see* Dependence, drug, opioid
methamphetamine(s) — *see* Dependence, drug, stimulant NEC
methaqualone — *see* Dependence, drug, sedative
methyl
  alcohol (without remission) F10.20
    with remission F10.21
  bromide — *see* Dependence, drug, sedative
  morphine — *see* Dependence, drug, opioid
  phenidate — *see* Dependence, drug, stimulant NEC
sulfonal — *see* Dependence, drug, sedative
morphine (sulfate) (sulfite) (type) — *see* Dependence, drug, opioid
narcotic (drug) NEC — *see* Dependence, drug, opioid
nembutal — *see* Dependence, drug, sedative
neraval — *see* Dependence, drug, sedative
neravan — *see* Dependence, drug, sedative
neurobarb — *see* Dependence, drug, sedative
nicotine — *see* Dependence, drug, nicotine
nitrous oxide F19.20
nonbarbiturate sedatives and tranquilizers with similar effect — *see* Dependence, drug, sedative
on
  aspirator Z99.0
  care provider (because of) Z74.9
    impaired mobility Z74.09
    need for
      assistance with personal care Z74.1
      continuous supervision Z74.3
    no other household member able to render care Z74.2
    specified reason NEC Z74.8
  machine Z99.89
    enabling NEC Z99.89
    specified type NEC Z99.89
  renal dialysis (hemodialysis) (peritoneal) Z99.2
  respirator Z99.11
  ventilator Z99.11
  wheelchair Z99.3
opiate — *see* Dependence, drug, opioid
opioids — *see* Dependence, drug, opioid
opium (alkaloids) (derivatives) (tincture) — *see* Dependence, drug, opioid
oxygen (long-term) (supplemental) Z99.81
paraldehyde — *see* Dependence, drug, sedative
paregoric — *see* Dependence, drug, opioid
PCP (phencyclidine) F19.20
pentobarbital — *see* Dependence, drug, sedative
pentobarbitone (sodium) — *see* Dependence, drug, sedative
pentothal — *see* Dependence, drug, sedative
peyote — *see* Dependence, drug, hallucinogen
phencyclidine (PCP) (and related substances) F19.20
phenmetrazine — *see* Dependence, drug, stimulant NEC
phenobarbital — *see* Dependence, drug, sedative
polysubstance F19.20
psilocibin, psilocin, psilocyn, psilocyline — *see* Dependence, drug, hallucinogen
psychostimulant NEC — *see* Dependence, drug, stimulant NEC
secobarbital — *see* Dependence, drug, sedative
seconal — *see* Dependence, drug, sedative
sedative NEC — *see* Dependence, drug, sedative
specified drug NEC — *see* Dependence, drug
stimulant NEC — *see* Dependence, drug, stimulant NEC
substance NEC — *see* Dependence, drug
supplemental oxygen Z99.81
tobacco — *see* Dependence, drug, nicotine
  counseling and surveillance Z71.6
tranquilizer NEC — *see* Dependence, drug, sedative
vitamin B6 E53.1
volatile solvents — *see* Dependence, drug, inhalant
Dependency
care-provider Z74.9
passive F60.7
reactions (persistent) F60.7

Depersonalization (in neurotic state) (neurotic) (syndrome) F48.1
Depletion
extracellular fluid E86.9
plasma E86.1
potassium E87.6
  nephropathy N25.89
salt or sodium E87.1
  causing heat exhaustion or prostration T67.4
  nephropathy N28.9
volume NOS E86.9
Deployment (current) (military) **status** Z56.82
in theater or in support of military war, peacekeeping and humanitarian operations Z56.82
personal history of Z91.82
  military war, peacekeeping and humanitarian deployment (current or past conflict) Z91.82
returned from Z91.82
Depolarization, premature I49.40
atrial I49.1
junctional I49.2
specified NEC I49.49
ventricular I49.3
Deposit
bone in Boeck's sarcoid D86.89
calcareous, calcium — *see* Calcification
cholesterol
  retina H35.89
  vitreous (body) (humor) — *see* Deposit, crystalline
conjunctiva H11.11-
cornea H18.00-
  argentous H18.02-
  due to metabolic disorder H18.03-
  Kayser-Fleischer ring H18.04-
  pigmentation — *see* Pigmentation, cornea
crystalline, vitreous (body) (humor) H43.2-
hemosiderin in old scars of cornea — *see* Pigmentation, cornea, stromal
metallic in lens — *see* Cataract, specified NEC
skin R23.8
tooth, teeth (betel) (black) (green) (materia alba) (orange) (tobacco) K03.6
urate, kidney — *see* Calculus, kidney
Depraved appetite — *see* Pica
Depressed
HDL cholesterol E78.6
Depression (acute) (mental) F32.9
agitated (single episode) F32.2
anaclitic — *see* Disorder, adjustment
anxiety F41.8
  persistent F34.1
arches (*see also* Deformity, limb, flat foot)
atypical (single episode) F32.8
basal metabolic rate R94.8
bone marrow D75.89
central nervous system R09.2
cerebral R29.81
  newborn P91.4
cerebrovascular I67.9
chest wall M95.4
climacteric (single episode) F32.8
endogenous (without psychotic symptoms) F33.2
  with psychotic symptoms F33.3
functional activity R68.89
hysterical F44.89
involutional (single episode) F32.8
major F32.9
  with psychotic symptoms F32.3
major (recurrent) — *see* Disorder, depressive, recurrent
manic-depressive — *see* Disorder, depressive, recurrent
masked (single episode) F32.8
medullary G93.89
menopausal (single episode) F32.8
metatarsus — *see* Depression, arches
monopolar F33.9
nervous F34.1
neurotic F34.1
nose M95.0

Depression— *continued*
postnatal F53
postpartum F53
post-psychotic of schizophrenia F32.8
post-schizophrenic F32.8
psychogenic (reactive) (single episode) F32.9
psychoneurotic F34.1
psychotic (single episode) F32.3
  recurrent F33.3
reactive (psychogenic) (single episode) F32.9
  psychotic (single episode) F32.3
recurrent — *see* Disorder, depressive, recurrent
respiratory center G93.89
seasonal — *see* Disorder, depressive, recurrent
senile F03
severe, single episode F32.2
situational F43.21
skull Q67.4
specified NEC (single episode) F32.8
sternum M95.4
visual field — *see* Defect, visual field
vital (recurrent) (without psychotic symptoms) F33.2
  with psychotic symptoms F33.3
  single episode F32.2
Deprivation
cultural Z60.3
effects NOS T73.9
  specified NEC T73.8
emotional NEC Z65.8
  affecting infant or child — *see* Maltreatment, child, psychological
food T73.0
protein — *see* Malnutrition
sleep Z72.820
social Z60.4
  affecting infant or child — *see* Maltreatment, child, psychological
specified NEC T73.8
vitamins — *see* Deficiency, vitamin
water T73.1
Derangement
ankle (internal) — *see* Derangement, joint, ankle
cartilage (articular) NEC — *see* Derangement, joint, articular cartilage, by site
  recurrent — *see* Dislocation, recurrent
cruciate ligament, anterior, current injury — *see* Sprain, knee, cruciate, anterior
elbow (internal) — *see* Derangement, joint, elbow
hip (joint) (internal) (old) — *see* Derangement, joint, hip
joint (internal) M24.9
  ankylosis — *see* Ankylosis
  articular cartilage M24.10
    ankle M24.17-
    elbow M24.12-
    foot M24.17-
    hand M24.14-
    hip M24.15-
    knee NEC M23.9-
    loose body — *see* Loose, body
    shoulder M24.11-
    wrist M24.13-
  contracture — *see* Contraction, joint
  current injury (*see also* Dislocation)
    knee, meniscus or cartilage — *see* Tear, meniscus
  dislocation
    pathological — *see* Dislocation, pathological
    recurrent — *see* Dislocation, recurrent
  knee — *see* Derangement, knee
  ligament — *see* Disorder, ligament
  loose body — *see* Loose, body
  recurrent — *see* Dislocation, recurrent
  specified type NEC M24.80
    ankle M24.87-
    elbow M24.82-
    foot joint M24.87-
    hand joint M24.84-
    hip M24.85-
    shoulder M24.81-
    wrist M24.83-
    temporomandibular M26.69

Derangement—*continued*
  knee (recurrent) M23.9-
    ligament disruption, spontaneous M23.60-
      anterior cruciate M23.61-
      capsular M23.67-
      instability, chronic M23.5-
      lateral collateral M23.64-
      medial collateral M23.63-
      posterior cruciate M23.62-
    loose body M23.4-
    meniscus M23.30-
      cystic M23.00-
        lateral M23.02-
          anterior horn M23.04-
          posterior horn M23.05-
          specified NEC M23.06-
        medial M23.00-
          anterior horn M23.01-
          posterior horn M23.02-
          specified NEC M23.03-
      degenerate — *see* Derangement, knee,
        meniscus, specified NEC
      detached — *see* Derangement, knee,
        meniscus, specified NEC
      due to old tear or injury M23.20-
        lateral M23.20-
          anterior horn M23.24-
          posterior horn M23.25-
          specified NEC M23.26-
        medial M23.20-
          anterior horn M23.21-
          posterior horn M23.22-
          specified NEC M23.23-
      retained — *see* Derangement, knee,
        meniscus, specified NEC
      specified NEC M23.30-
        lateral M23.30-
          anterior horn M23.34-
          posterior horn M23.35-
          specified NEC M23.36-
        medial M23.30-
          anterior horn M23.31-
          posterior horn M23.32-
          specified NEC M23.33-
      old M23.8x-
      specified NEC — *see* subcategory M23.8
  low back NEC — *see* Dorsopathy, specified NEC
  meniscus — *see* Derangement, knee, meniscus
  mental — *see* Psychosis
  patella, specified NEC — *see* Disorder, patella,
    derangement NEC
  semilunar cartilage (knee) — *see* Derangement,
    knee, meniscus, specified NEC
  shoulder (internal) — *see* Derangement, joint,
    shoulder
Dercum's disease E88.2
Derealization (neurotic) F48.1
Dermal — *see* condition
Dermaphytid — *see* Dermatophytosis
Dermatitis (eczematous) L30.9
  ab igne L59.0
  acarine B88.0
  actinic (due to sun) L57.8
    other than from sun L59.8
  allergic — *see* Dermatitis, contact, allergic
  ambustionis, due to burn or scald — *see* Burn
  amebic A06.7
  ammonia L22
  arsenical (ingested) L27.8
  artefacta L98.1
    psychogenic F54
  atopic L20.9
    psychogenic F54
    specified NEC L20.89
  autoimmune progesterone L30.8
  berlock, berloque L56.2
  blastomycotic B40.3
  blister beetle L24.89
  bullous, bullosa L13.9
    mucosynechial, atrophic L12.1
    seasonal L30.8
    specified NEC L13.8

Dermatitis— *continued*
  calorica L59.0
    due to burn or scald — *see* Burn
  caterpillar L24.89
  cercarial B65.3
  combustionis L59.0
    due to burn or scald — *see* Burn
  congelationis T69.1
  contact (occupational) L25.9
    allergic L23.9
      due to
        adhesives L23.1
        cement L23.5
        chemical products NEC L23.5
        chromium L23.0
        cosmetics L23.2
        dander (cat) (dog) L23.81
        drugs in contact with skin L23.3
        dyes L23.4
        food in contact with skin L23.6
        hair (cat) (dog) L23.81
        insecticide L23.5
        metals L23.0
        nickel L23.0
        plants, non-food L23.7
        plastic L23.5
        rubber L23.5
        specified agent NEC L23.89
    due to
      chemical products NEC L25.3
      cosmetics L25.0
      dander (cat) (dog) L23.81
      drugs in contact with skin L25.1
      dyes L25.2
      food in contact with skin L25.4
      hair (cat) (dog) L23.81
      plants, non-food L25.5
      specified agent NEC L25.8
    irritant L24.9
      due to
        chemical products NEC L24.5
        cosmetics L24.3
        detergents L24.0
        drugs in contact with skin L24.4
        food in contact with skin L24.6
        oils and greases L24.1
        plants, non-food L24.7
        solvents L24.2
        specified agent NEC L24.89
  contusiformis L52
  diabetic — *see* E08-E13 with .63
  diaper L22
  diphtheritica A36.3
  dry skin L85.3
  due to
    acetone (contact) (irritant) L24.2
    acids (contact) (irritant) L24.5
    adhesive(s) (allergic) (contact) (plaster) L23.1
      irritant L24.5
    alcohol (irritant) (skin contact) (substances in
      T51.00-T51.93) L24.2
      taken internally L27.8
    alkalis (contact) (irritant) L24.5
    arsenic (ingested) L27.8
    carbon disulfide (contact) (irritant) L24.2
    caustics (contact) (irritant) L24.5
    cement (contact) L24.5
    cereal (ingested) L27.2
    chemical(s) NEC L24.5
      taken internally L27.8
    chlorocompounds L24.2
    chromium (contact) (irritant) L24.81
    coffee (ingested) L27.2
    cold weather L30.8
    cosmetics (contact) L25.0
      allergic L23.2
      irritant L24.3
    cyclohexanes L24.2
    dander (cat) (dog) L23.81
    Demodex species B88.0
    Dermanyssus gallinae B88.0
    detergents (contact) (irritant) L24.0
    dichromate L24.81

Dermatitis— *continued*
  due to— *continued*
    drugs and medicaments (generalized) (internal
      use) L27.0
      external — *see* Dermatitis, due to, drugs, in
        contact with skin
      in contact with skin L25.1
        allergic L23.3
        irritant L24.4
      localized skin eruption L27.1
      specified substance — *see* Table of Drugs and
        Chemicals
    dyes (contact) L25.2
      allergic L23.4
      irritant L24.89
    epidermophytosis — *see* Dermatophytosis
    esters L24.2
    external irritant NEC L24.9
    fish (ingested) L27.2
    flour (ingested) L27.2
    food (ingested) L27.2
      in contact with skin L23.6
    fruit (ingested) L27.2
    furs (allergic) (contact) L23.81
    glues — *see* Dermatitis, due to, adhesives
    glycols L24.2
    greases NEC (contact) (irritant) L24.1
    hair (cat) (dog) L23.81
    hot
      objects and materials — *see* Burn
      weather or places L59.0
    hydrocarbons L24.2
    infrared rays L59.8
    ingestion, ingested substance L27.9
      chemical NEC L27.8
      drugs and medicaments — *see* Dermatitis,
        due to, drugs
      food L27.2
      specified NEC L27.8
    insecticide in contact with skin L24.5
    internal agent L27.9
      drugs and medicaments (generalized) — *see*
        Dermatitis, due to, drugs
      food L27.2
    irradiation — *see* Dermatitis, due to, radioactive
      substance
    ketones L24.2
    lacquer tree (allergic) (contact) L23.7
    light (sun) NEC L57.8
      acute L56.8
      other L59.8
    Liponyssoides sanguineus B88.0
    low temperature L30.8
    meat (ingested) L27.2
    metals, metal salts (contact) (irritant) L24.81
    milk (ingested) L27.2
    nickel (contact) (irritant) L24.81
    nylon (contact) (irritant) L24.5
    oils NEC (contact) (irritant) L24.1
    paint solvent (contact) (irritant) L24.2
    petroleum products (contact) (irritant)
      (substances in T52.0) L24.2
    plants NEC (contact) L25.5
      allergic L23.7
      irritant L24.7
    plasters (adhesive) (any) (allergic) (contact) L23.1
      irritant L24.5
    plastic (contact) L24.5
    preservatives (contact) — *see* Dermatitis, due to,
      chemical, in contact with skin
    primrose (allergic) (contact) L23.7
    primula (allergic) (contact) L23.7
    radiation L59.8
      nonionizing (chronic exposure) L57.8
      sun NEC L57.8
        acute L56.8
    radioactive substance L58.9
      acute L58.0
      chronic L58.1
    radium L58.9
      acute L58.0
      chronic L58.1
    ragweed (allergic) (contact) L23.7

Dermatitis— *continued*
  due to— *continued*
    Rhus (allergic) (contact) (diversiloba) (radicans)
      (toxicodendron) (venenata) (verniciflua)
      L23.7
    rubber (contact) L24.5
    Senecio jacobaea (allergic) (contact) L23.7
    solvents (contact) (irritant) (substances in
      T52.00-T53.93) L24.2
    specified agent NEC (contact) L25.8
      allergic L23.89
      irritant L24.89
    sunshine NEC L57.8
      acute L56.8
    tetrachlorethylene (contact) (irritant) L24.2
    toluene (contact) (irritant) L24.2
    turpentine (contact) L24.2
    ultraviolet rays (sun NEC) (chronic exposure)
      L57.8
      acute L56.8
    vaccine or vaccination L27.0
      specified substance — *see* Table of Drugs and
        Chemicals
    varicose veins — *see* Varix, leg, with,
      inflammation
    X-rays L58.9
      acute L58.0
      chronic L58.1
  dyshydrotic L30.1
  dysmenorrheica N94.6
  escharotica — *see* Burn
  exfoliative, exfoliativa (generalized) L26
    neonatorum L00
  eyelid (*see also* Dermatosis, eyelid)
    allergic H01.119
      left H01.116
        lower H01.115
        upper H01.114
      right H01.113
        lower H01.112
        upper H01.111
    contact — *see* Dermatitis, eyelid, allergic
    due to
      Demodex species B88.0
      herpes (zoster) B02.39
        simplex B00.59
    eczematous H01.139
      left H01.136
        lower H01.135
        upper H01.134
      right H01.133
        lower H01.132
        upper H01.131
  facta, factitia, factitial L98.1
    psychogenic F54
  flexural NEC L20.82
  friction L30.4
  fungus B36.9
    specified type NEC B36.8
  gangrenosa, gangrenous infantum L08.0
  harvest mite B88.0
  heat L59.0
  herpesviral, vesicular (ear) (lip) B00.1
  herpetiformis (bullous) (erythematous) (pustular)
    (vesicular) L13.0
    juvenile L12.2
    senile L12.0
  hiemalis L30.8
  hypostatic, hypostatica — *see* Varix, leg, with,
    inflammation
  infectious eczematoid L30.3
  infective L30.3
  irritant — *see* Dermatitis, contact, irritant
  Jacquet's (diaper dermatitis) L22
  Leptus B88.0
  lichenified NEC L28.0
  medicamentosa (generalized) (internal use) — *see*
    Dermatitis, due to drugs
  mite B88.0
  multiformis L13.0
    juvenile L12.2
  napkin L22
  neurotica L13.0

Dermatitis— *continued*
  nummular L30.0
  papillaris capillitii L73.0
  pellagrous E52
  perioral L71.0
  photocontact L56.2
  polymorpha dolorosa L13.0
  pruriginosa L13.0
  pruritic NEC L30.8
  psychogenic F54
  purulent L08.0
  pustular
    contagious B08.02
    subcorneal L13.1
  pyococcal L08.0
  pyogenica L08.0
  repens L40.2
  Ritter's (exfoliativa) L00
  Schamberg's L81.7
  schistosome B65.3
  seasonal bullous L30.8
  seborrheic L21.9
    infantile L21.1
    specified NEC L21.8
  sensitization NOS L23.9
  septic L08.0
  solare L57.8
  specified NEC L30.8
  stasis I87.2
    with varicose ulcer — *see* Varix, leg, with, ulcer,
      with inflammation
    due to postthrombotic syndrome — *see*
      Syndrome, postthrombotic
  suppurative L08.0
  traumatic NEC L30.4
  trophoneurotica L13.0
  ultraviolet (sun) (chronic exposure) L57.8
    acute L56.8
  varicose — *see* Varix, leg, with, inflammation
  vegetans L10.1
  verrucosa B43.0
  vesicular, herpesviral B00.1
Dermatoarthritis, lipoid E78.81
Dermatochalasis, eyelid H02.839
  left H02.836
    lower H02.835
    upper H02.834
  right H02.833
    lower H02.832
    upper H02.831
Dermatofibroma (lenticulare) — *see* Neoplasm, skin,
  benign
  protuberans — *see* Neoplasm, skin, uncertain
    behavior
Dermatofibrosarcoma (pigmented) (protuberans) —
  see Neoplasm, skin, malignant
Dermatographia L50.3
Dermatolysis (exfoliativa) (congenital) Q82.8
  acquired L57.4
  eyelids — *see* Blepharochalasis
  palpebrarum — *see* Blepharochalasis
  senile L57.4
Dermatomegaly NEC Q82.8
Dermatomucosomyositis M33.10
  with
    myopathy M33.12
    respiratory involvement M33.11
    specified organ involvement NEC M33.19
Dermatomycosis B36.9
  furfuracea B36.0
  specified type NEC B36.8
Dermatomyositis (acute) (chronic) (*see also*
  Dermatopolymyositis)
  in (due to) neoplastic disease (*see also* Neoplasm)
    D49.9 [M36.0]
Dermatoneuritis of children — *see* Poisoning,
  mercury
Dermatophilosis A48.8
Dermatophytid L30.2
Dermatophytide — *see* Dermatophytosis

Dermatophytosis (epidermophyton) (infection)
  (Microsporum) (tinea) (Trichophyton) B35.9
  beard B35.0
  body B35.4
  capitis B35.0
  corporis B35.4
  deep-seated B35.8
  disseminated B35.8
  foot B35.3
  granulomatous B35.8
  groin B35.6
  hand B35.2
  nail B35.1
  perianal (area) B35.6
  scalp B35.0
  specified NEC B35.8
Dermatopolymyositis M33.90
  with
    myopathy M33.92
    respiratory involvement M33.91
    specified organ involvement NEC M33.99
  in neoplastic disease (*see also* Neoplasm) D49.9
    [M36.0]
  juvenile M33.00
    with
      myopathy M33.02
      respiratory involvement M33.01
      specified organ involvement NEC M33.09
  specified NEC M33.10
    myopathy M33.12
    respiratory involvement M33.11
    specified organ involvement NEC M33.19
Dermatopolyneuritis — *see* Poisoning, mercury
Dermatorrhexis Q79.6
  acquired L57.4
Dermatosclerosis (*see also* Scleroderma)
  localized L94.0
Dermatosis L98.9
  Andrews' L08.89
  Bowen's — *see* Neoplasm, skin, in situ
  bullous L13.9
    specified NEC L13.8
  exfoliativa L26
  eyelid (noninfectious)
    dermatitis — *see* Dermatitis, eyelid
    discoid lupus erythematosus — *see* Lupus,
      erythematosus, eyelid
    xeroderma — *see* Xeroderma, acquired, eyelid
  factitial L98.1
  febrile neutrophilic L98.2
  gonococcal A54.89
  herpetiformis L13.0
    juvenile L12.2
  linear IgA L13.8
  menstrual NEC L98.8
  neutrophilic, febrile L98.2
  occupational — *see* Dermatitis, contact
  papulosa nigra L82.1
  pigmentary L81.9
    progressive L81.7
    Schamberg's L81.7
  psychogenic F54
  purpuric, pigmented L81.7
  pustular, subcorneal L13.1
  transient acantholytic L11.1
Dermographia, dermographism L50.3
Dermoid (cyst) (*see also* Neoplasm, benign, by site)
  with malignant transformation C56.-
  due to radiation (nonionizing) L57.8
Dermopathy
  infiltrative with thyrotoxicosis — *see* Thyrotoxicosis
  nephrogenic fibrosing L90.8
Dermophytosis — *see* Dermatophytosis
Descemetocele H18.73-
Descemet's membrane — *see* condition
Descending — *see* condition
Descensus uteri — *see* Prolapse, uterus
Desert
  rheumatism B38.0
  sore — *see* Ulcer, skin
Desertion (newborn) — *see* Maltreatment,
  abandonment

Desmoid (extra-abdominal) (tumor) — *see* Neoplasm, connective tissue, uncertain behavior
  abdominal D48.1
Despondency F32.9
Desquamation, skin R23.4
Destruction, destructive (*see also* Damage)
  articular facet — *see also* Derangement, joint, specified type NEC
    knee M23.8x-
    vertebra — *see* Spondylosis
  bone — *see also* Disorder, bone, specified type NEC
    syphilitic A52.77
  joint (*see also* Derangement, joint, specified type NEC)
    sacroiliac M53.3
  rectal sphincter K62.8
  septum (nasal) J34.89
  tuberculous NEC — *see* Tuberculosis
  tympanum, tympanic membrane (nontraumatic) — *see* Disorder, tympanic membrane, specified NEC
  vertebral disc — *see* Degeneration, intervertebral disc
Destructiveness (*see also* Disorder, conduct)
  adjustment reaction — *see* Disorder, adjustment
Desultory labor O62.2
Detachment
  cartilage — *see* Sprain
  cervix, annular N88.8
    complicating delivery O71.3
  choroid (old) (postinfectional) (simple) (spontaneous) H31.40-
    hemorrhagic H31.41-
    serous H31.42-
  ligament — *see* Sprain
  meniscus (knee) (*see also* Derangement, knee, meniscus, specified NEC)
    current injury — *see* Tear, meniscus
    due to old tear or injury — *see* Derangement, knee, meniscus, due to old tear
  retina (without retinal break) (serous) H33.2-
    with retinal:
      break H33.00-
        giant H33.03-
        multiple H33.02-
        single H33.01-
      dialysis H33.04-
    pigment epithelium — *see* Degeneration, retina, separation of layers, pigment epithelium detachment
    rhegmatogenous — *see* Detachment, retina, with retinal, break
    specified NEC H33.8
    total H33.05-
    traction H33.4-
  vitreous (body) H43.89
Detergent asthma J69.8
Deterioration
  epileptic F06.8
  general physical R53.81
  heart, cardiac — *see* Degeneration, myocardial
  mental — *see* Psychosis
  myocardial, myocardium — *see* Degeneration, myocardial
  senile (simple) R54
Deuteranomaly (anomalous trichromat) H53.53
Deuteranopia (complete) (incomplete) H53.53
Development
  abnormal, bone Q79.9
  arrested R62.50
    bone — *see* Arrest, development or growth, bone
    child R62.50
    due to malnutrition E45
  defective, congenital (*see also* Anomaly, by site)
    cauda equina Q06.3
    left ventricle Q24.8
      in hypoplastic left heart syndrome Q23.4
    valve Q24.8
      pulmonary Q22.2
  delayed (*see also* Delay, development) R62.50
    arithmetical skills F81.2
    language (skills) (expressive) F80.1

Development— *continued*
  delayed—*continued*
    learning skill F81.9
    mixed skills F88
    motor coordination F82
    reading F81.0
    specified learning skill NEC F81.89
    speech F80.9
    spelling F81.81
    written expression F81.81
  imperfect, congenital (*see also* Anomaly, by site)
    heart Q24.9
    lungs Q33.6
  incomplete
    bronchial tree Q32.4
    organ or site not listed — *see* Hypoplasia, by site
    respiratory system Q34.9
    sexual, precocious NEC E30.1
  tardy, mental (*see also* Retardation, mental) F79
Developmental — *see* condition
  testing, child — *see* Examination, child
Devergie's disease (pityriasis rubra pilaris) L44.0
Deviation (in)
  conjugate palsy (eye) (spastic) H51.0
  esophagus (acquired) K22.8
  eye, skew H51.8
  midline (jaw) (teeth) (dental arch) M26.29
    specified site NEC — *see* Malposition
  nasal septum J34.2
    congenital Q67.4
  opening and closing of the mandible M26.53
  organ or site, congenital NEC — *see* Malposition, congenital
  septum (nasal) (acquired) J34.2
    congenital Q67.4
  sexual F65.9
    bestiality F65.89
    erotomania F52.8
    exhibitionism F65.2
    fetishism, fetishistic F65.0
      transvestism F65.1
    frotteurism F65.81
    masochism F65.51
    multiple F65.89
    necrophilia F65.89
    nymphomania F52.8
    pederosis F65.4
    pedophilia F65.4
    sadism, sadomasochism F65.52
    satyriasis F52.8
    specified type NEC F65.89
    transvestism F64.1
    voyeurism F65.3
  teeth, midline M26.29
  trachea J39.8
  ureter, congenital Q62.61
Device
  cerebral ventricle (communicating) in situ Z98.2
  contraceptive — *see* Contraceptive, device
  drainage, cerebrospinal fluid, in situ Z98.2
Devic's disease G36.0
Devil's
  grip B33.0
  pinches (purpura simplex) D69.2
Devitalized tooth K04.99
Devonshire colic — *see* Poisoning, lead
Dextraposition, aorta Q20.3
  in tetralogy of Fallot Q21.3
Dextrinosis, limit (debrancher enzyme deficiency) E74.03
Dextrocardia (true) Q24.0
  with
    complete transposition of viscera Q89.3
    situs inversus Q89.3
Dextrotransposition, aorta Q20.3
d-glycericacidemia E72.59
Dhat syndrome F48.8
Dhobi itch B35.6
Di George's syndrome D82.1
Di Guglielmo's disease C94.0-
Diabetes, diabetic (mellitus) (sugar) E11.9
  with
    amyotrophy E11.44

Diabetes, diabetic— *continued*
  with— *continued*
    arthropathy NEC E11.618
    autonomic (poly)neuropathy E11.43
    cataract E11.36
    Charcot's joints E11.610
    chronic kidney disease E11.22
    circulatory complication NEC E11.59
    complication E11.8
      specified NEC E11.69
    dermatitis E11.620
    foot ulcer E11.621
    gangrene E11.52
    gastroparesis E11.43
    glomerulonephrosis, intracapillary E11.21
    glomerulosclerosis, intercapillary E11.21
    hyperglycemia E11.65
    hyperosmolarity E11.00
      with coma E11.01
    hypoglycemia E11.649
      with coma E11.641
    kidney complications NEC E11.29
    Kimmelstiel-Wilson disease E11.21
    loss of protective sensation (LOPS) — Diabetes, by type, with neuropathy
    mononeuropathy E11.41
    myasthenia E11.44
    necrobiosis lipoidica E11.620
    nephropathy E11.21
    neuralgia E11.42
    neurologic complication NEC E11.49
    neuropathic arthropathy E11.610
    neuropathy E11.40
    ophthalmic complication NEC E11.39
    oral complication NEC E11.638
    periodontal disease E11.630
    peripheral angiopathy E11.51
      with gangrene E11.52
    polyneuropathy E11.42
    renal complication NEC E11.29
    renal tubular degeneration E11.29
    retinopathy E11.319
      with macular edema E11.311
      nonproliferative E11.329
        with macular edema E11.321
        mild E11.329
          with macular edema E11.321
        moderate E11.339
          with macular edema E11.331
        severe E11.349
          with macular edema E11.341
      proliferative E11.359
        with macular edema E11.351
    skin complication NEC E11.628
    skin ulcer NEC E11.622
  bronzed E83.110
  complicating pregnancy — *see* Pregnancy, complicated by, diabetes
  dietary counseling and surveillance Z71.3
  due to drug or chemical E09.9
    with
      amyotrophy E09.44
      arthropathy NEC E09.618
      autonomic (poly)neuropathy E09.43
      cataract E09.36
      Charcot's joints E09.610
      chronic kidney disease E09.22
      circulatory complication NEC E09.59
      complication E09.8
        specified NEC E09.69
      dermatitis E09.620
      foot ulcer E09.621
      gangrene E09.52
      gastroparesis E09.43
      glomerulonephrosis, intracapillary E09.21
      glomerulosclerosis, intercapillary E09.21
      hyperglycemia E09.65
      hyperosmolarity E09.00
        with coma E09.01
      hypoglycemia E09.649
        with coma E09.641
      ketoacidosis E09.10
        with coma E09.11

Diabetes, diabetic— *continued*
  due to drug or chemical— *continued*
    with—*continued*
      kidney complications NEC E09.29
      Kimmelsteil-Wilson disease E09.21
      mononeuropathy E09.41
      myasthenia E09.44
      necrobiosis lipoidica E09.620
      nephropathy E09.21
      neuralgia E09.42
      neurologic complication NEC E09.49
      neuropathic arthropathy E09.610
      neuropathy E09.40
      ophthalmic complication NEC E09.39
      oral complication NEC E09.638
      periodontal disease E09.630
      peripheral angiopathy E09.51
        with gangrene E09.52
      polyneuropathy E09.42
      renal complication NEC E09.29
      renal tubular degeneration E09.29
      retinopathy E09.319
        with macular edema E09.311
        nonproliferative E09.329
          with macular edema E09.321
          mild E09.329
            with macular edema E09.321
          moderate E09.339
            with macular edema E09.331
          severe E09.349
            with macular edema E09.341
        proliferative E09.359
          with macular edema E09.351
      skin complication NEC E09.628
      skin ulcer NEC E09.622
  due to underlying condition E08.9
    with
      amyotrophy E08.44
      arthropathy NEC E08.618
      autonomic (poly)neuropathy E08.43
      cataract E08.36
      Charcot's joints E08.610
      chronic kidney disease E08.22
      circulatory complication NEC E08.59
      complication E08.8
        specified NEC E08.69
      dermatitis E08.620
      foot ulcer E08.621
      gangrene E08.52
      gastroparesis E08.43
      glomerulonephrosis, intracapillary E08.21
      glomerulosclerosis, intercapillary E08.21
      hyperglycemia E08.65
      hyperosmolarity E08.00
        with coma E08.01
      hypoglycemia E08.649
        with coma E08.641
      ketoacidosis E08.10
        with coma E08.11
      kidney complications NEC E08.29
      Kimmelsteil-Wilson disease E08.21
      mononeuropathy E08.41
      myasthenia E08.44
      necrobiosis lipoidica E08.620
      nephropathy E08.21
      neuralgia E08.42
      neurologic complication NEC E08.49
      neuropathic arthropathy E08.610
      neuropathy E08.40
      ophthalmic complication NEC E08.39
      oral complication NEC E08.638
      periodontal disease E08.630
      peripheral angiopathy E08.51
        with gangrene E08.52
      polyneuropathy E08.42
      renal complication NEC E08.29
      renal tubular degeneration E08.29
      retinopathy E08.319
        with macular edema E08.311
        nonproliferative E08.329
          with macular edema E08.321
          mild E08.329
            with macular edema E08.321

Diabetes, diabetic—
  due to underlying condition— *continued*
    with—*continued*
      retinopathy—*continued*
        nonproliferative—*continued*
          moderate E08.339
            with macular edema E08.331
          severe E08.349
            with macular edema E08.341
        proliferative E08.359
          with macular edema E08.351
      skin complication NEC E08.628
      skin ulcer NEC E08.622
  gestational (in pregnancy) O24.419
    affecting newborn P70.0
    diet controlled O24.410
    in childbirth O24.429
      diet controlled O24.420
      insulin (and diet) controlled O24.424
    insulin (and diet) controlled O24.414
    puerperal O24.439
      diet controlled O24.430
      insulin (and diet) controlled O24.434
  inadequately controlled—code to Diabetes, by
      type, with hyperglycemia
  insipidus E23.2
    nephrogenic N25.1
    pituitary E23.2
    vasopressin resistant N25.1
  insulin dependent—code to type of diabetes
  juvenile-onset — *see* Diabetes, type 1
  ketosis-prone — *see* Diabetes, type 1
  latent R73.09
  neonatal (transient) P70.2
  non-insulin dependent—code to type of diabetes
  out of control—code to Diabetes, by type, with
      hyperglycemia
  phosphate E83.39
  poorly controlled—code to Diabetes, by type, with
      hyperglycemia
  postpancreatectomy — *see* Diabetes, specified type
      NEC
  postprocedural — *see* Diabetes, specified type NEC
  secondary diabetes mellitus NEC — *see* Diabetes,
      specified type NEC
  specified type NEC E13.9
    with
      amyotrophy E13.44
      arthropathy NEC E13.618
      autonomic (poly)neuropathy E13.43
      cataract E13.36
      Charcot's joints E13.610
      chronic kidney disease E13.22
      circulatory complication NEC E13.59
      complication E13.8
        specified NEC E13.69
      dermatitis E13.620
      foot ulcer E13.621
      gangrene E13.52
      gastroparesis E13.43
      glomerulonephrosis, intracapillary E13.21
      glomerulosclerosis, intercapillary E13.21
      hyperglycemia E13.65
      hyperosmolarity E13.00
        with coma E13.01
      hypoglycemia E13.649
        with coma E13.641
      ketoacidosis E13.10
        with coma E13.11
      kidney complications NEC E13.29
      Kimmelsteil-Wilson disease E13.21
      mononeuropathy E13.41
      myasthenia E13.44
      necrobiosis lipoidica E13.620
      nephropathy E13.21
      neuralgia E13.42
      neurologic complication NEC E13.49
      neuropathic arthropathy E13.610
      neuropathy E13.40
      ophthalmic complication NEC E13.39
      oral complication NEC E13.638
      periodontal disease E13.630

Diabetes, diabetic— *continued*
  specified type—*continued*
    with—*continued*
      peripheral angiopathy E13.51
        with gangrene E13.52
      polyneuropathy E13.42
      renal complication NEC E13.29
      renal tubular degeneration E13.29
      retinopathy E13.319
        with macular edema E13.311
        nonproliferative E13.329
          with macular edema E13.321
          mild E13.329
            with macular edema E13.321
          moderate E13.339
            with macular edema E13.331
          severe E13.349
            with macular edema E13.341
        proliferative E13.359
          with macular edema E13.351
      skin complication NEC E13.628
      skin ulcer NEC E13.622
  steroid-induced — *see* Diabetes, due to, drug or
      chemical
  type 1 E10.9
    with
      amyotrophy E10.44
      arthropathy NEC E10.618
      autonomic (poly)neuropathy E10.43
      cataract E10.36
      Charcot's joints E10.610
      chronic kidney disease E10.22
      circulatory complication NEC E10.59
      complication E10.8
        specified NEC E10.69
      dermatitis E10.620
      foot ulcer E10.621
      gangrene E10.52
      gastroparesis E10.43
      glomerulonephrosis, intracapillary E10.21
      glomerulosclerosis, intercapillary E10.21
      hyperglycemia E10.65
      hypoglycemia E10.649
        with coma E10.641
      ketoacidosis E10.10
        with coma E10.11
      kidney complications NEC E10.29
      Kimmelsteil-Wilson disease E10.21
      mononeuropathy E10.41
      myasthenia E10.44
      necrobiosis lipoidica E10.620
      nephropathy E10.21
      neuralgia E10.42
      neurologic complication NEC E10.49
      neuropathic arthropathy E10.610
      neuropathy E10.40
      ophthalmic complication NEC E10.39
      oral complication NEC E10.638
      periodontal disease E10.630
      peripheral angiopathy E10.51
        with gangrene E10.52
      polyneuropathy E10.42
      renal complication NEC E10.29
      renal tubular degeneration E10.29
      retinopathy E10.319
        with macular edema E10.311
        nonproliferative E10.329
          with macular edema E10.321
          mild E10.329
            with macular edema E10.321
          moderate E10.339
            with macular edema E10.331
          severe E10.349
            with macular edema E10.341
        proliferative E10.359
          with macular edema E10.351
      skin complication NEC E10.628
      skin ulcer NEC E10.622
  type 2 E11.9
    with
      amyotrophy E11.44
      arthropathy NEC E11.618
      autonomic (poly)neuropathy E11.43

Diabetes, diabetic— *continued*
  type 2— *continued*
    with— *continued*
      cataract E11.36
      Charcot's joints E11.610
      chronic kidney disease E11.22
      circulatory complication NEC E11.59
      complication E11.8
        specified NEC E11.69
      dermatitis E11.620
      foot ulcer E11.621
      gangrene E11.52
      gastroparesis E11.43
      glomerulonephrosis, intracapillary E11.21
      glomerulosclerosis, intercapillary E11.21
      hyperglycemia E11.65
      hyperosmolarity E11.00
        with coma E11.01
      hypoglycemia E11.649
        with coma E11.641
      kidney complications NEC E11.29
      Kimmelsteil-Wilson disease E11.21
      mononeuropathy E11.41
      myasthenia E11.44
      necrobiosis lipoidica E11.620
      nephropathy E11.21
      neuralgia E11.42
      neurologic complication NEC E11.49
      neuropathic arthropathy E11.610
      neuropathy E11.40
      ophthalmic complication NEC E11.39
      oral complication NEC E11.638
      periodontal disease E11.630
      peripheral angiopathy E11.51
        with gangrene E11.52
      polyneuropathy E11.42
      renal complication NEC E11.29
      renal tubular degeneration E11.29
      retinopathy E11.319
        with macular edema E11.311
        nonproliferative E11.329
          with macular edema E11.321
          mild E11.329
            with macular edema E11.321
          moderate E11.339
            with macular edema E11.331
          severe E11.349
            with macular edema E11.341
        proliferative E11.359
          with macular edema E11.351
      skin complication NEC E11.628
      skin ulcer NEC E11.622
Diacyclothrombopathia D69.1
Diagnosis deferred R69
Dialysis (intermittent) (treatment)
  noncompliance (with) Z91.15
  renal (hemodialysis) (peritoneal), status Z99.2
  retina, retinal — *see* Detachment, retina, with
    retinal, dialysis
Diamond-Blackfan anemia (congenital hypoplastic)
  D61.01
Diamond-Gardener syndrome
  (autoerythrocytesensitization) D69.2
Diaper rash L22
Diaphoresis (excessive) R61
Diaphragm — *see* condition
Diaphragmalgia R07.1
Diaphragmatitis, diaphragmitis J98.6
Diaphysial aclasis Q78.6
Diaphysitis — *see* Osteomyelitis, specified type NEC
Diarrhea, diarrheal (disease) (infantile)
  (inflammatory) R19.7
  achlorhydric K31.83
  allergic K52.2
  amebic (*see also* Amebiasis) A06.0
    with abscess — *see* Abscess, amebic
    acute A06.0
    chronic A06.1
    nondysenteric A06.2
  bacillary — *see* Dysentery, bacillary
  balantidial A07.0
  cachectic NEC K52.89
  Chilomastix A07.8

Diarrhea, diarrheal— *continued*
  choleriformis A00.1
  chronic (noninfectious) K52.9
  coccidial A07.3
  Cochin-China K90.1
    strongyloidiasis B78.0
  Dientamoeba A07.8
  dietetic K52.2
  due to
    bacteria A04.9
      specified NEC A04.8
    Campylobacter A04.5
    Capillaria philippinensis B81.1
    Clostridium difficile A04.7
    Clostridium perfringens (C) (F) A04.8
    Cryptosporidium A07.2
    Escherichia coli A04.4
      enteroaggregative A04.4
      enterohemorrhagic A04.3
      enteroinvasive A04.2
      enteropathogenic A04.0
      enterotoxigenic A04.1
      specified NEC A04.4
    food hypersensitivity K52.2
    Necator americanus B76.1
    S. japonicum B65.2
    specified organism NEC A08.8
      bacterial A04.8
      viral A08.39
    Staphylococcus A04.8
    Trichuris trichiuria B79
    virus — *see* Enteritis, viral
    Yersinia enterocolitica A04.6
  dysenteric A09
  endemic A09
  epidemic A09
  flagellate A07.9
  Flexner's (ulcerative) A03.1
  functional K59.1
    following gastrointestinal surgery K91.89
    psychogenic F45.8
  Giardia lamblia A07.1
  giardial A07.1
  hill K90.1
  infectious A09
  malarial — *see* Malaria
  mite B88.0
  mycotic NEC B49
  neonatal (noninfectious) P78.3
  nervous F45.8
  neurogenic K59.1
  noninfectious K52.9
  postgastrectomy K91.1
  postvagotomy K91.1
  protozoal A07.9
    specified NEC A07.8
  psychogenic F45.8
  specified
    bacterium NEC A04.8
    virus NEC A08.39
  strongyloidiasis B78.0
  toxic K52.1
  trichomonal A07.8
  tropical K90.1
  tuberculous A18.32
  viral — *see* Enteritis, viral
Diastasis
  cranial bones M84.88
    congenital NEC Q75.8
  joint (traumatic) — *see* Dislocation
  muscle M62.00
    ankle M62.07-
    congenital Q79.8
    foot M62.07-
    forearm M62.03-
    hand M62.04-
    lower leg M62.06-
    pelvic region M62.05-
    shoulder region M62.01-
    specified site NEC M62.08
    thigh M62.05-
    upper arm M62.02-

Diastasis —*continued*
  recti (abdomen)
    complicating delivery O71.89
    congenital Q79.59
Diastema, tooth, teeth, fully erupted M26.32
Diastematomyelia Q06.2
Diataxia, cerebral G80.4
Diathesis
  allergic — *see* History, allergy
  bleeding (familial) D69.9
  cystine (familial) E72.00
  gouty — *see* Gout
  hemorrhagic (familial) D69.9
    newborn NEC P53
  spasmophilic R29.0
Diaz's disease or osteochondrosis (juvenile) (talus)
  — *see* Osteochondrosis, juvenile, tarsus
Dibothriocephalus, dibothriocephaliasis (latus)
  (infection) (infestation) B70.0 larval B70.1
Dicephalus, dicephaly Q89.4
Dichotomy, teeth K00.2
Dichromat, dichromatopsia (congenital) — *see*
  Deficiency, color vision
Dichuchwa A65
Dicroceliasis B66.2
Didelphia, didelphys — *see* Double uterus
Didymytis N45.1
  with orchitis N45.3
Dietary
  inadequacy or deficiency E63.9
  surveillance and counseling Z71.3
Dietl's crisis N13.8
Dieulafoy lesion (hemorrhagic)
  duodenum K31.82
  esophagus K22.8
  intestine (colon) K63.81
  stomach K31.82
Difficult, difficulty (in)
  acculturation Z60.3
  feeding R63.3
    newborn P92.9
      breast P92.5
      specified NEC P92.8
    nonorganic (infant or child) F98.29
  intubation, in anesthesia T88.4
  mechanical, gastroduodenal stoma K91.89
    causing obstruction K91.3
  reading (developmental) F81.0
    secondary to emotional disorders F93.9
  spelling (specific) F81.81
    with reading disorder F81.89
    due to inadequate teaching Z55.8
  swallowing — *see* Dysphagia
  walking R26.2
  work
    conditions NEC Z56.5
    schedule Z56.3
Diffuse — *see* condition
DiGeorge's syndrome (thymic hypoplasia) D82.1
Digestive — *see* condition
Diktyoma — *see* Neoplasm, malignant, by site
Dilaceration, tooth K00.4
Dilatation
  anus K59.8
    venule — *see* Hemorrhoids
  aorta (focal) (general) — *see* Ectasia, aorta
    with aneurysm — *see* Aneurysm, aorta
  artery — *see* Aneurysm
  bladder (sphincter) N32.89
    congenital Q64.79
  blood vessel I99.8
  bronchial J47.9
    with
      exacerbation (acute) J47.1
      lower respiratory infection J47.0
  calyx (due to obstruction) — *see* Hydronephrosis
  capillaries I78.8
  cardiac (acute) (chronic) (*see also* Hypertrophy,
    cardiac)
    congenital Q24.8
      valve NEC Q24.8
        pulmonary Q22.2
    valve — *see* Endocarditis

Dilatation— *continued*
- cavum septi pellucidi Q06.8
- cervix (uteri) (*see also* Incompetency, cervix)
  - incomplete, poor, slow complicating delivery O62.0
- colon K59.3
  - congenital Q43.1
  - psychogenic F45.8
- common duct (acquired) K83.8
  - congenital Q44.5
- cystic duct (acquired) K82.8
  - congenital Q44.5
- duct, mammary — *see* Ectasia, mammary duct
- duodenum K59.8
- esophagus K22.8
  - congenital Q39.5
  - due to achalasia K22.0
- eustachian tube, congenital Q17.8
- gallbladder K82.8
- gastric — *see* Dilatation, stomach
- heart (acute) (chronic) (*see also* Hypertrophy, cardiac)
  - congenital Q24.8
  - valve — *see* Endocarditis
- ileum K59.8
  - psychogenic F45.8
- jejunum K59.8
  - psychogenic F45.8
- kidney (calyx) (collecting structures) (cystic) (parenchyma) (pelvis) (idiopathic) N28.89
- lacrimal passages or duct — *see* Disorder, lacrimal system, changes
- lymphatic vessel I89.0
- mammary duct — *see* Ectasia, mammary duct
- Meckel's diverticulum (congenital) Q43.0
  - malignant — *see* Table of Neoplasms, small intestine, malignant
- myocardium (acute) (chronic) — *see* Hypertrophy, cardiac
- organ or site, congenital NEC — *see* Distortion
- pancreatic duct K86.8
- pericardium — *see* Pericarditis
- pharynx J39.2
- prostate N42.89
- pulmonary
  - artery (idiopathic) I28.8
  - valve, congenital Q22.2
- pupil H57.04
- rectum K59.3
- saccule, congenital Q16.5
- salivary gland (duct) K11.8
- sphincter ani K62.8
- stomach K31.89
  - acute K31.0
  - psychogenic F45.8
- submaxillary duct K11.8
- trachea, congenital Q32.1
- ureter (idiopathic) N28.82
  - congenital Q62.2
  - due to obstruction N13.4
- urethra (acquired) N36.8
- vasomotor I73.9
- vein I86.8
- ventricular, ventricle (acute) (chronic) (*see also* Hypertrophy, cardiac)
  - cerebral, congenital Q04.8
- venule NEC I86.8
- vesical orifice N32.89

Dilated, dilation — *see* Dilatation

Diminished, diminution
- hearing (acuity) — *see* Deafness
- sense or sensation (cold) (heat) (tactile) (vibratory) R20.8
- vision NEC H54.7
- vital capacity R94.2

Diminuta taenia B71.0

Dimitri-Sturge-Weber disease Q85.8

Dimple
- parasacral, pilonidal or postanal — *see* Cyst, pilonidal

Dioctophyme renalis (infection) (infestation) B83.8

Dipetalonemiasis B74.4

Diphallus Q55.69

Diphtheria, diphtheritic (gangrenous) (hemorrhagic) A36.9
- carrier (suspected) Z22.2
- cutaneous A36.3
- faucial A36.0
- infection of wound A36.3
- laryngeal A36.2
- myocarditis A36.81
- nasal, anterior A36.89
- nasopharyngeal A36.1
- neurological complication A36.89
- pharyngeal A36.0
- specified site NEC A36.89
- tonsillar A36.0

Diphyllobothriasis (intestine) B70.0
- larval B70.1

Diplacusis H93.22-

Diplegia (upper limbs) G83.0
- congenital (cerebral) G80.8
- facial G51.0
- lower limbs G82.20
- spastic G80.1

Diplococcus, diplococcal — *see* condition

Diplopia H53.2

Dipsomania F10.20
- with
  - psychosis — *see* Psychosis, alcoholic
  - remission F10.21

Dipylidiasis B71.1

Direction, teeth, abnormal, fully erupted M26.30

Dirofilariasis B74.8

Dirt-eating child F98.3

Disability
- heart — *see* Disease, heart
- knowledge acquisition F81.9
- learning F81.9
- limiting activities Z73.6
- spelling, specific F81.81

Disappearance of family member Z63.4

Disarticulation — *see* Amputation
- meaning traumatic amputation — *see* Amputation, traumatic

Discharge (from)
- abnormal finding in — *see* Abnormal, specimen
- breast (female) (male) N64.52
- diencephalic autonomic idiopathic — *see* Epilepsy, specified NEC
- ear (*see also* Otorrhea)
  - blood — *see* Otorrhagia
- excessive urine R35.8
- nipple N64.52
- penile R36.9
- postnasal R09.82
- prison, anxiety concerning Z65.2
- urethral R36.9
  - without blood R36.0
  - hematospermia R36.1
- vaginal N89.8

Discitis, diskitis M46.40
- cervical region M46.42
- cervicothoracic region M46.43
- lumbar region M46.46
- lumbosacral region M46.47
- multiple sites M46.49
- occipito-atlanto-axial region M46.41
- pyogenic — *see* Infection, intervertebral disc, pyogenic
- sacrococcygeal region M46.48
- thoracic region M46.44
- thoracolumbar region M46.45

Discoid
- meniscus (congenital) Q68.6
- semilunar cartilage (congenital) — *see* Derangement, knee, meniscus, specified NEC

Discoloration
- nails L60.8
- teeth (posteruptive) K03.7
  - during formation K00.8

Discomfort
- chest R07.89
- visual H53.14-

Discontinuity, ossicles, ear H74.2-

Discord (with)
- boss Z56.4
- classmates Z55.4
- counselor Z64.4
- employer Z56.4
- family Z63.8
- fellow employees Z56.4
- in-laws Z63.1
- landlord Z59.2
- lodgers Z59.2
- neighbors Z59.2
- probation officer Z64.4
- social worker Z64.4
- teachers Z55.4
- workmates Z56.4

Discordant connection
- atrioventricular (congenital) Q20.5
- ventriculoarterial Q20.3

Discrepancy
- centric occlusion maximum intercuspation M26.55
- leg length (acquired) — *see* Deformity, limb, unequal length
  - congenital — *see* Defect, reduction, lower limb
- uterine size date O26.84-

Discrimination
- ethnic Z60.5
- political Z60.5
- racial Z60.5
- religious Z60.5
- sex Z60.5

Disease, diseased (*see also* Syndrome)
- absorbent system I87.8
- acid-peptic K30
- Acosta's T70.29
- Adams-Stokes (-Morgagni) (syncope with heart block) I45.9
- Addison's anemia (pernicious) D51.0
- adenoids (and tonsils) J35.9
- adrenal (capsule) (cortex) (gland) (medullary) E27.9
  - hyperfunction E27.0
  - specified NEC E27.8
- ainhum L94.6
- airway
  - obstructive, chronic J44.9
    - due to
      - cotton dust J66.0
      - specific organic dusts NEC J66.8
  - reactive — *see* Asthma
- akamushi (scrub typhus) A75.3
- Albers-Schönberg's (marble bones) Q78.2
- Albert's — *see* Tendinitis, Achilles
- alimentary canal K63.9
- alligator-skin Q80.9
  - acquired L85.0
- alpha heavy chain C88.3
- alpine T70.29
- altitude T70.20
- alveolar ridge
  - edentulous K06.9
    - specified NEC K06.8
- alveoli, teeth K08.9
- Alzheimer's G30.9 [F02.80]
  - with behavioral disturbance G30.9 [F02.81]
  - early onset G30.0 [F02.80]
    - with behavioral disturbance G30.0 [F02.81]
  - late onset G30.1 [F02.80]
    - with behavioral disturbance G30.1 [F02.81]
  - specified NEC G30.8 [F02.80]
    - with behavioral disturbance G30.8 [F02.81]
- amyloid — *see* Amyloidosis
- Andersen's (glycogenosis IV) E74.09
- Andes T70.29
- Andrews' (bacterid) L08.89
- angiospastic I73.9
  - cerebral G45.9
  - vein I87.8
- anterior
  - chamber H21.9
  - horn cell G12.29
- antiglomerular basement membrane (antiGBM)
  - antibody M31.0
  - tubulo-interstitial nephritis N12
- antral — *see* Sinusitis, maxillary

Disease, diseased— *continued*
anus K62.9
  specified NEC K62.8
aorta (nonsyphilitic) I77.9
  syphilitic NEC A52.02
aortic (heart) (valve) I35.9
  rheumatic I06.9
Apollo B30.3
aponeuroses — *see* Enthesopathy
appendix K38.9
  specified NEC K38.8
aqueous (chamber) H21.9
Arnold-Chiari — *see* Arnold-Chiari disease
arterial I77.9
  occlusive — *see* Occlusion, by site
    due to stricture or stenosis I77.1
arteriocardiorenal — *see* Hypertension, cardiorenal
arteriolar (generalized) (obliterative) I77.9
arteriorenal — *see* Hypertension, kidney
arteriosclerotic (*see also* Arteriosclerosis)
  cardiovascular — *see* Disease, heart, ischemic,
    atherosclerotic
  coronary (artery) — *see* Disease, heart, ischemic,
    atherosclerotic
  heart — *see* Disease, heart, ischemic,
    atherosclerotic
artery I77.9
  cerebral I67.9
  coronary I25.10
    with angina pectoris — *see* Arteriosclerosis,
      coronary (artery),
arthropod-borne NOS (viral) A94
  specified type NEC A93.8
atticoantral, chronic H66.20
  left H66.22
    with right H66.23
  right H66.21
    with left H66.23
auditory canal — *see* Disorder, ear, external
auricle, ear NEC — *see* Disorder, pinna
Australian X A83.4
autoimmune (systemic) NOS M35.9
  hemolytic (cold type) (warm type) D59.1
    drug-induced D59.0
  thyroid E06.3
aviator's — *see* Effect, adverse, high altitude
Ayala's Q78.5
Ayerza's (pulmonary artery sclerosis with pulmonary
    hypertension) I27.0
Babington's (familial hemorrhagic telangiectasia)
    I78.0
bacterial A49.9
  specified NEC A48.8
  zoonotic A28.9
    specified type NEC A28.8
Baelz's (cheilitis glandularis apostematosa) K13.0
bagasse J67.1
balloon — *see* Effect, adverse, high altitude
Bang's (brucella abortus) A23.1
Bannister's T78.3
barometer makers' — *see* Poisoning, mercury
Barraquer (-Simons') (progressive lipodystrophy)
    E88.1
Barrett's — *see* Barrett's, esophagus
Bartholin's gland N75.9
basal ganglia G25.9
  degenerative G23.9
    specified NEC G23.8
  specified NEC G25.89
Basedow's (exophthalmic goiter) — *see*
    Hyperthyroidism, with, goiter (diffuse)
Bateman's B08.1
Batten-Steinert G71.11
Battey A31.0
Beard's (neurasthenia) F48.8
Becker
  idiopathic mural endomyocardial I42.3
  myotonia congenita G71.12
Begbie's (exophthalmic goiter) — *see*
    Hyperthyroidism, with, goiter (diffuse)
Beigel's (white piedra) B36.2
behavioral, organic F07.9
Benson's — *see* Deposit, crystalline

Disease, diseased— *continued*
Bernard-Soulier (thrombopathy) D69.1
Bernhardt (-Roth) — *see* Mononeuropathy, lower
    limb, meralgia paresthetica
Biermer's (pernicious anemia) D51.0
bile duct (common) (hepatic) K83.9
  with calculus, stones — *see* Calculus, bile duct
  specified NEC K83.8
biliary (tract) K83.9
  specified NEC K83.8
Billroth's — *see* Spina bifida
bird fancier's J67.2
black lung J60
bladder N32.9
  in (due to)
    schistosomiasis (bilharziasis) B65.0 [N33]
  specified NEC N32.89
bleeder's D66
blood D75.9
  forming organs D75.9
  vessel I99.9
Bloodgood's — *see* Mastopathy, cystic
Bodechtel-Guttmann (subacute sclerosing
    panencephalitis) A81.1
bone (*see also* Disorder, bone)
  aluminum M83.4
  fibrocystic NEC
    jaw M27.49
bone-marrow D75.9
Borna A83.9
Bornholm (epidemic pleurodynia) B33.0
Bouchard's (myopathic dilatation of the stomach)
    K31.0
Bouillaud's (rheumatic heart disease) I01.9
Bourneville (-Brissaud) (tuberous sclerosis) Q85.1
Bouveret (-Hoffmann) (paroxysmal tachycardia)
    I47.9
bowel K63.9
  functional K59.9
    psychogenic F45.8
brain G93.9
  arterial, artery I67.9
  arteriosclerotic I67.2
  congenital Q04.9
  degenerative — *see* Degeneration, brain
  inflammatory — *see* Encephalitis
  organic G93.9
    arteriosclerotic I67.2
  parasitic NEC B71.9 [G94]
  senile NEC G31.1
  specified NEC G93.89
breast (*see also* Disorder, breast) N64.9
  cystic (chronic) — *see* Mastopathy, cystic
  fibrocystic — *see* Mastopathy, cystic
  Paget's
    female, unspecified side C50.91-
    male, unspecified side C50.92-
  specified NEC N64.89
Breda's — *see* Yaws
Bretonneau's (diphtheritic malignant angina) A36.0
Bright's — *see* Nephritis
  arteriosclerotic — *see* Hypertension, kidney
Brill's (recrudescent typhus) A75.1
Brill-Zinsser (recrudescent typhus) A75.1
Brion-Kayser — *see* Fever, paratyphoid
broad
  beta E78.2
  ligament (noninflammatory) N83.9
    inflammatory — *see* Disease, pelvis,
      inflammatory
    specified NEC N83.8
Brocq-Duhring (dermatitis herpetiformis) L13.0
Brocq's
  meaning
    dermatitis herpetiformis L13.0
    prurigo L28.2
bronchopulmonary J98.4
bronchus NEC J98.09
bronze Addison's E27.1
  tuberculous A18.7
budgerigar fancier's J67.2
bullous L13.9
  chronic of childhood L12.2

Disease, diseased— *continued*
bullous—*continued*
  specified NEC L13.8
Buerger's (thromboangiitis obliterans) I73.1
Bürger-Grütz (essential familial hyperlipemia) E78.3
bursa — *see* Bursopathy
caisson T70.3
California — *see* Coccidioidomycosis
capillaries I78.9
  specified NEC I78.8
Carapata A68.0
cardiac — *see* Disease, heart
cardiopulmonary, chronic I27.9
cardiorenal (hepatic) (hypertensive) (vascular) —
    see Hypertension, cardiorenal
cardiovascular (atherosclerotic) I25.10
  with angina pectoris — *see* Arteriosclerosis,
    coronary (artery),
  congenital Q28.9
  newborn P29.9
    specified NEC P29.89
  hypertensive — *see* Hypertension, heart
  renal (hypertensive) — *see* Hypertension,
    cardiorenal
  syphilitic (asymptomatic) A52.00
cartilage — *see* Disorder, cartilage
Castellani's A69.8
cat-scratch A28.1
Cavare's (familial periodic paralysis) G72.3
cecum K63.9
celiac (adult) (infantile) K90.0
cellular tissue L98.9
central core G71.2
cerebellar, cerebellum — *see* Disease, brain
cerebral (*see also* Disease, brain)
  degenerative — *see* Degeneration, brain
cerebrospinal G96.9
cerebrovascular I67.9
  acute I67.8
    embolic I63.4-
    thrombotic I63.3-
  arteriosclerotic I67.2
  specified NEC I67.8
cervix (uteri) (noninflammatory) N88.9
  inflammatory — *see* Cervicitis
  specified NEC N88.8
Chabert's A22.9
Chandler's (osteochondritis dissecans, hip) — *see*
    Osteochondritis, dissecans, hip
Charlouis — *see* Yaws
Chédiak-Steinbrinck (-Higashi) (congenital
    gigantism of peroxidase granules) D72.0
chest J98.9
Chiari's (hepatic vein thrombosis) I82.0
Chicago B40.9
Chignon B36.8
chigo, chigoe B88.1
childhood granulomatous D71
Chinese liver fluke B66.1
chlamydial A74.9
  specified NEC A74.89
cholecystic K82.9
choroid H31.9
  specified NEC H31.8
Christmas D67
chronic bullous of childhood L12.2
chylomicron retention E78.3
ciliary body H21.9
  specified NEC H21.89
circulatory (system) NEC I99.8
  newborn P29.9
  syphilitic A52.00
    congenital A50.54
coagulation factor deficiency (congenital) — *see*
    Defect, coagulation
coccidioidal — *see* Coccidioidomycosis
cold
  agglutinin or hemoglobinuria D59.1
    paroxysmal D59.6
  hemagglutinin (chronic) D59.1
collagen NOS (nonvascular) (vascular) M35.9
  specified NEC M35.8

Disease, diseased— *continued*
  colon K63.9
    functional K59.9
      congenital Q43.2
    ischemic K55.0
  combined system — *see* Degeneration, combined
  compressed air T70.3
  Concato's (pericardial polyserositis) I31.1
    pleural — *see* Pleurisy, with effusion
  conjunctiva H11.9
    chlamydial A74.0
    specified NEC H11.89
    viral B30.9
      specified NEC B30.8
  connective tissue, systemic (diffuse) M35.9
    in (due to)
      hypogammaglobulinemia D80.1 [M36.8]
      ochronosis E70.29 [M36.8]
    specified NEC M35.8
  Conor and Bruch's (boutonneuse fever) A77.1
  Cooper's — *see* Mastopathy, cystic
  Cori's (glycogenosis III) E74.03
  corkhandler's or corkworker's J67.3
  cornea H18.9
    specified NEC H18.89-
  coronary (artery) — *see* Disease, heart, ischemic,
    atherosclerotic
    congenital Q24.5
    ostial, syphilitic (aortic) (mitral) (pulmonary)
      A52.03
  corpus cavernosum N48.9
    specified NEC N48.89
  Cotugno's — *see* Sciatica
  coxsackie (virus) NEC B34.1
  cranial nerve NOS G52.9
  Creutzfeldt-Jakob — *see* Creutzfeldt-Jakob disease
    or syndrome
  Crocq's (acrocyanosis) I73.89
  Crohn's — *see* Enteritis, regional
  Curschmann's G71.19
  cystic
    breast (chronic) — *see* Mastopathy, cystic
    kidney, congenital Q61.9
    liver, congenital Q44.6
    lung J98.4
      congenital Q33.0
  cytomegalic inclusion (generalized) B25.9
    with pneumonia B25.0
    congenital P35.1
  cytomegaloviral B25.9
    specified NEC B25.8
  Czerny's (periodic hydrarthrosis of the knee) — *see*
    Effusion, joint, knee
  Daae (-Finsen) (epidemic pleurodynia) B33.0
  Darling's — *see* Histoplasmosis capsulati
  Débove's (splenomegaly) R16.1
  deer fly — *see* Tularemia
  Degos' I77.89
  demyelinating, demyelinizating (nervous system)
    G37.9
    multiple sclerosis G35
    specified NEC G37.8
  dense deposit (*see also* N00-N07 with fourth
    character .6) N05.6
  deposition, hydroxyapatite — *see* Disease,
    hydroxyapatite deposition
  de Quervain's (tendon sheath) M65.4
    thyroid (subacute granulomatous thyroiditis)
      E06.1
  Devergie's (pityriasis rubra pilaris) L44.0
  Devic's G36.0
  diaphorase deficiency D74.0
  diaphragm J98.6
  diarrheal, infectious NEC A09
  digestive system K92.9
    specified NEC K92.89
  disc, degenerative — *see* Degeneration,
    intervertebral disc
  discogenic (*see also* Displacement, intervertebral
    disc NEC)
    with myelopathy — *see* Disorder, disc, with,
      myelopathy
  diverticular — *see* Diverticula

Disease, diseased— *continued*
  Dubois (thymus) A50.59
  Duchenne-Griesinger G71.0
  Duchenne's
    muscular dystrophy G71.0
    pseudohypertrophy, muscles G71.0
  ductless glands E34.9
  duodenum K31.9
    specified NEC K31.89
  Dupré's (meningism) R29.1
  Dupuytren's (muscle contracture) M72.0
  Durand-Nicholas-Favre (climatic bubo) A55
  Duroziez's (congenital mitral stenosis) Q23.2
  ear — *see* Disorder, ear
  Eberth's — *see* Fever, typhoid
  Ebola (virus) A98.4
  Ebstein's heart Q22.5
  Echinococcus — *see* Echinococcus
  echovirus NEC B34.1
  Eddowes' (brittle bones and blue sclera) Q78.0
  edentulous (alveolar) ridge K06.9
    specified NEC K06.8
  Edsall's T67.2
  Eichstedt's (pityriasis versicolor) B36.0
  Ellis-van Creveld (chondroectodermal dysplasia)
    Q77.6
  end stage renal (ESRD) N18.6
    due to hypertension I12.0
  endocrine glands or system NEC E34.9
  endomyocardial (eosinophilic) I42.3
  English (rickets) E55.0
  enterovirus, enterovirus NEC B34.1
    central nervous system NEC A88.8
  epidemic B99.9
    specified NEC B99.8
  epididymis N50.9
  Erb (-Landouzy) G71.0
  esophagus K22.9
    functional K22.4
    psychogenic F45.8
    specified NEC K22.8
  Erdheim-Chester (ECD) E88.89
  Eulenburg's (congenital paramyotonia) G71.19
  eustachian tube — *see* Disorder, eustachian tube
  external
    auditory canal — *see* Disorder, ear, external
    ear — *see* Disorder, ear, external
  extrapyramidal G25.9
    specified NEC G25.89
  eye H57.9
    anterior chamber H21.9
    inflammatory NEC H57.8
    muscle (external) — *see* Strabismus
    specified NEC H57.8
    syphilitic — *see* Oculopathy, syphilitic
  eyeball H44.9
    specified NEC H44.89
  eyelid — *see* Disorder, eyelid
    specified NEC — *see* Disorder, eyelid, specified
      type NEC
  eyeworm of Africa B74.3
  facial nerve (seventh) G51.9
    newborn (birth injury) P11.3
  Fahr (of brain) G23.8
  Fahr Volhard (of kidney) I12.-
  fallopian tube (noninflammatory) N83.9
    inflammatory — *see* Salpingo-oophoritis
    specified NEC N83.8
  familial periodic paralysis G72.3
  Fanconi's (congenital pancytopenia) D61.09
  fascia NEC *see also* Disorder, muscle
    inflammatory — *see* Myositis
    specified NEC M62.89
  Fauchard's (periodontitis) — *see* Periodontitis
  Favre-Durand-Nicolas (climatic bubo) A55
  Fede's K14.0
  Feer's — *see* Poisoning, mercury
  female pelvic inflammatory (*see also* Disease, pelvis,
    inflammatory) N73.9
    syphilitic (secondary) A51.42
    tuberculous A18.17
  Fernels' (aortic aneurysm) I71.9

Disease, diseased— *continued*
  fibrocaseous of lung — *see* Tuberculosis, pulmonary
  fibrocystic — *see* Fibrocystic disease
  Fiedler's (leptospiral jaundice) A27.0
  fifth B08.3
  file-cutter's — *see* Poisoning, lead
  fish-skin Q80.9
    acquired L85.0
  Flajani (-Basedow) (exophthalmic goiter) — *see*
    Hyperthyroidism, with, goiter (diffuse)
  flax-dresser's J66.1
  fluke — *see* Infestation, fluke
  foot and mouth B08.8
  foot process — *see* Nephrosis
  Forbes' (glycogenosis III) E74.03
  Fordyce-Fox (apocrine miliaria) L75.2
  Fordyce's (ectopic sebaceous glands) (mouth) Q38.6
  Forestier's (rhizomelic pseudopolyarthritis) M35.3
    meaning ankylosing hyperostosis — *see*
      Hyperostosis, ankylosing
  Fothergill's
    neuralgia — *see* Neuralgia, trigeminal
    scarlatina anginosa A38.9
  Fournier's N49.3
  fourth B08.8
  Fox (-Fordyce) (apocrine miliaria) L75.2
  Francis' — *see* Tularemia
  Franklin C88.2
  Frei's (climatic bubo) A55
  Friedreich's
    combined systemic or ataxia G11.1
    myoclonia G25.3
  frontal sinus — *see* Sinusitis, frontal
  fungus NEC B49
  Gaisböck's (polycythemia hypertonica) D75.1
  gallbladder K82.9
    calculus — *see* Calculus, gallbladder
    cholecystitis — *see* Cholecystitis
    cholesterolosis K82.4
    fistula — *see* Fistula, gallbladder
    hydrops K82.1
    obstruction — *see* Obstruction, gallbladder
    perforation K82.2
    specified NEC K82.8
  gamma heavy chain C88.2
  Gamna's (siderotic splenomegaly) D73.2
  Gamstorp's (adynamia episodica hereditaria) G72.3
  Gandy-Nanta (siderotic splenomegaly) D73.2
  ganister J62.8
  gastric — *see* Disease, stomach
  gastroesophageal reflux (GERD) K21.9
    with esophagitis K21.0
  gastrointestinal (tract) K92.9
    amyloid E85.4
    functional K59.9
      psychogenic F45.8
    specified NEC K92.89
  Gee (-Herter) (-Heubner) (-Thaysen) (nontropical
    sprue) K90.0
  genital organs
    female N94.9
    male N50.9
  Gerhardt's (erythromelalgia) I73.81
  Gibert's (pityriasis rosea) L42
  Gierke's (glycogenosis I) E74.01
  Gilles de la Tourette's (motor-verbal tic) F95.2
  gingiva K06.9
    specified NEC K06.8
  gland (lymph) I89.9
  Glanzmann's (hereditary hemorrhagic
    thrombasthenia) D69.1
  glass-blower's (cataract) — *see* Cataract, specified
    NEC
    salivary gland hypertrophy K11.1
  Glisson's — *see* Rickets
  globe H44.9
    specified NEC H44.89
  glomerular (*see also* Glomerulonephritis)
    with edema — *see* Nephrosis
    acute — *see* Nephritis, acute
    chronic — *see* Nephritis, chronic
    minimal change N05.0
    rapidly progressive N01.9

Disease, diseased— *continued*
  glycogen storage E74.00
    Andersen's E74.09
    Cori's E74.03
    Forbes' E74.03
    generalized E74.00
    glucose-6-phosphatase deficiency E74.01
    heart E74.02 [I43]
    hepatorenal E74.09
    Hers' E74.09
    liver and kidney E74.01
    McArdle's E74.04
    muscle phosphofructokinase E74.09
    myocardium E74.02 [I43]
    Pompe's E74.02
    Tauri's E74.09
    type 0 E74.09
    type I E74.01
    type II E74.02
    type III E74.03
    type IV E74.09
    type V E74.04
    type VI-XI E74.09
    Von Gierke's E74.01
  Goldstein's (familial hemorrhagic telangiectasia)
      I78.0
  gonococcal NOS A54.9
  graft-versus-host (GVH) D89.813
    acute D89.810
    acute on chronic D89.812
    chronic D89.811
  grainhandler's J67.8
  granulomatous (childhood) (chronic) D71
  Graves' (exophthalmic goiter) — *see*
      Hyperthyroidism, with, goiter (diffuse)
  Griesinger's — *see* Ancylostomiasis
  Grisel's M43.6
  Gruby's (tinea tonsurans) B35.0
  Guillain-Barré G61.0
  Guinon's (motor-verbal tic) F95.2
  gum K06.9
  gynecological N94.9
  H (Hartnup's) E72.02
  Haff — *see* Poisoning, mercury
  Hageman (congenital factor XII deficiency) D68.2
  hair (color) (shaft) L67.9
    follicles L73.9
      specified NEC L73.8
  Hamman's (spontaneous mediastinal emphysema)
      J98.2
  hand, foot and mouth B08.4
  Hansen's — *see* Leprosy
  Hantavirus, with pulmonary manifestations B33.4
    with renal manifestations A98.5
  Harada's H30.81-
  Hartnup (pellagra-cerebellar ataxia-renal
      aminoaciduria) E72.02
  Hart's (pellagra-cerebellar ataxia-renal
      aminoaciduria) E72.02
  Hashimoto's (struma lymphomatosa) E06.3
  Hb — *see* Disease, hemoglobin
  heart (organic) I51.9
    with
      pulmonary edema (acute) (*see also* Failure,
          ventricular, left) I50.1
      rheumatic fever (conditions in I00)
        active I01.9
          with chorea I02.0
          specified NEC I01.8
        inactive or quiescent (with chorea) I09.9
          specified NEC I09.89
    amyloid E85.4 [I43]
    aortic (valve) I35.9
    arteriosclerotic or sclerotic (senile) — *see*
        Disease, heart, ischemic, atherosclerotic
    artery, arterial — *see* Disease, heart, ischemic,
        atherosclerotic
    beer drinkers' I42.6
    beriberi (wet) E51.12
    black I27.0
    congenital Q24.9
      cyanotic Q24.9
      specified NEC Q24.8

Disease, diseased— *continued*
  heart— *continued*
    coronary — *see* Disease, heart, ischemic
    cryptogenic I51.9
    fibroid — *see* Myocarditis
    functional I51.89
      psychogenic F45.8
    glycogen storage E74.02 [I43]
    gonococcal A54.83
    hypertensive — *see* Hypertension, heart
    hyperthyroid (*see also* Hyperthyroidism) E05.90
        [I43]
      with thyroid storm E05.91 [I43]
    ischemic (chronic or with a stated duration of
        over 4 weeks) I25.9
      atherosclerotic (of) I25.10
        with angina pectoris — *see*
            Arteriosclerosis, coronary (artery)
        coronary artery bypass graft — *see*
            Arteriosclerosis, coronary (artery),
      cardiomyopathy I25.5
      diagnosed on ECG or other special
          investigation, but currently presenting
          no symptoms I25.6
      silent I25.6
      specified form NEC I25.89
    kyphoscoliotic I27.1
    meningococcal A39.50
      endocarditis A39.51
      myocarditis A39.52
      pericarditis A39.53
    mitral I05.9
      specified NEC I05.8
    muscular — *see* Degeneration, myocardial
    psychogenic (functional) F45.8
    pulmonary (chronic) I27.9
      in schistosomiasis B65.9 [I52]
      specified NEC I27.89
    rheumatic (chronic) (inactive) (old) (quiescent)
        (with chorea) I09.9
      active or acute I01.9
        with chorea (acute) (rheumatic)
            (Sydenham's) I02.0
      specified NEC I09.89
    senile — *see* Myocarditis
    syphilitic A52.06
      aortic A52.03
        aneurysm A52.01
      congenital A50.54 [I52]
    thyrotoxic (*see also* Thyrotoxicosis) E05.90 [I43]
      with thyroid storm E05.91 [I43]
    valve, valvular (obstructive) (regurgitant) (*see
        also* Endocarditis)
      congenital NEC Q24.8
        pulmonary Q22.3
    vascular — *see* Disease, cardiovascular
  heavy chain NEC C88.2
    alpha C88.3
    gamma C88.2
    mu C88.2
  Hebra's
    pityriasis
      maculata et circinata L42
      rubra pilaris L44.0
    prurigo L28.2
  hematopoietic organs D75.9
  hemoglobin or Hb
    abnormal (mixed) NEC D58.2
      with thalassemia D56.9
    AS genotype D57.3
    Bart's D56.8
    C (Hb-C) D58.2
      with other abnormal hemoglobin NEC D58.2
      elliptocytosis D58.1
      Hb-S D57.2-
      sickle-cell D57.2-
    thalassemia D56.9
    D (Hb-D) D58.2
    E (Hb-E) D58.2
    elliptocytosis D58.1
    H (Hb-H) (thalassemia) D56.0
      with other abnormal hemoglobin NEC D56.9
    I thalassemia D56.9

Disease, diseased— *continued*
  hemoglobin or Hb—*continued*
    M D74.0
    S or SS D57.1
    SC D57.2-
    SD D57.8-
    SE D57.8-
    spherocytosis D58.0
    unstable, hemolytic D58.2
  hemolytic (newborn) P55.9
    autoimmune (cold type) (warm type) D59.1
    drug-induced D59.0
    due to or with
      incompatibility
        ABO (blood group) P55.1
        blood (group) (Duffy) (K(ell)) (Kidd) (Lewis)
            (M) (S) NEC P55.8
        Rh (blood group) (factor) P55.0
        Rh negative mother P55.0
    specified type NEC P55.8
    unstable hemoglobin D58.2
  hemorrhagic D69.9
    newborn P53
  Henoch (-Schönlein) (purpura nervosa) D69.0
  hepatic — *see* Disease, liver
  hepatolenticular E83.01
  heredodegenerative NEC
    spinal cord G95.89
  herpesviral, disseminated B00.7
  Hers' (glycogenosis VI) E74.09
  Herter (-Gee) (-Heubner) (nontropical sprue) K90.0
  Heubner-Herter (nontropical sprue) K90.0
  high fetal gene or hemoglobin thalassemia D56.9
  Hildenbrand's — *see* Typhus
  hip (joint) M25.9
    congenital Q65.8
    suppurative M00.9
    tuberculous A18.02
  His (-Werner) (trench fever) A79.0
  Hodgson's I71.9
    ruptured I71.8
  Holla — *see* Spherocytosis
  hookworm B76.9
    specified NEC B76.8
  host-versus-graft D89.813
    acute D89.810
    acute on chronic D89.812
    chronic D89.811
  human immunodeficiency virus (HIV) B20
  Huntington's G10
  Hutchinson's (cheiropompholyx) L30.1
  hyaline (diffuse) (generalized)
    membrane (lung) (newborn) P22.0
      adult J80
  hydatid — *see* Echinococcus
  hydroxyapatite deposition M11.00
    ankle M11.07-
    elbow M11.02-
    foot joint M11.07-
    hand joint M11.04-
    hip M11.05-
    knee M11.06-
    multiple site M11.09
    shoulder M11.01-
    vertebra M11.08
    wrist M11.03-
  hyperkinetic — *see* Hyperkinesia
  hypertensive — *see* Hypertension
  hypophysis E23.7
  Iceland G93.3
  I-cell E77.0
  immune D89.9
  immunoproliferative (malignant) C88.9
    small intestinal C88.3
    specified NEC C88.8
  inclusion B25.9
    salivary gland B25.9
  infectious, infective B99.9
    congenital P37.9
      specified NEC P37.8
    viral
      specified NEC B99.8

Disease, diseased— *continued*
  inflammatory
    penis N48.29
      abscess N48.21
      cellulitis N48.22
    prepuce N47.7
      balanoposthitis N47.6
    tubo-ovarian — *see* Salpingo-oophoritis
  intervertebral disc (*see also* Disorder, disc)
    with myelopathy — *see* Disorder, disc, with,
        myelopathy
    cervical, cervicothoracic — *see* Disorder, disc,
        cervical
    with
        myelopathy — *see* Disorder, disc, cervical,
            with myelopathy
        neuritis, radiculitis or radiculopathy — *see*
            Disorder, disc, cervical, with neuritis
        specified NEC — *see* Disorder, disc,
            cervical, specified type NEC
    lumbar (with)
        myelopathy M51.06
        neuritis, radiculitis, radiculopathy or sciatica
            M51.16
        specified NEC M51.86
    lumbosacral (with)
        myelopathy M51.07
        neuritis, radiculitis, radiculopathy or sciatica
            M51.17
        specified NEC M51.87
    specified NEC — *see* Disorder, disc, specified NEC
    thoracic (with)
        myelopathy M51.04
        neuritis, radiculitis or radiculopathy M51.14
        specified NEC M51.84
    thoracolumbar (with)
        myelopathy M51.05
        neuritis, radiculitis or radiculopathy M51.15
        specified NEC M51.85
  intestine K63.9
    functional K59.9
        psychogenic F45.8
        specified NEC K59.8
    organic K63.9
    protozoal A07.9
    specified NEC K63.89
  iris H21.9
    specified NEC H21.89
  iron metabolism or storage E83.10
  island (scrub typhus) A75.3
  itai-itai — *see* Poisoning, cadmium
  Jakob-Creutzfeldt — *see* Creutzfeldt-Jakob disease
        or syndrome
  jaw M27.9
    fibrocystic M27.49
    specified NEC M27.8
  jigger B88.1
  joint (*see also* Disorder, joint)
    Charcot's — *see* Arthropathy, neuropathic
        (Charcot)
    degenerative — *see* Osteoarthritis
        multiple M15.9
        spine — *see* Spondylosis
    hypertrophic — *see* Osteoarthritis
    sacroiliac M53.3
    specified NEC — *see* Disorder, joint, specified
        type NEC
    spine NEC — *see* Dorsopathy
    suppurative — *see* Arthritis, pyogenic or pyemic
  Jourdain's (acute gingivitis) K05.00
    plaque induced K05.00
    nonplaque induced K05.01
  Kaschin-Beck (endemic polyarthritis) M12.10
    ankle M12.17-
    elbow M12.12-
    foot joint M12.17-
    hand joint M12.14-
    hip M12.15-
    knee M12.16-
    multiple site M12.19
    shoulder M12.11-
    vertebra M12.18
    wrist M12.13-

Disease, diseased— *continued*
  Katayama B65.2
  Kedani (scrub typhus) A75.3
  Keshan E59
  kidney (functional) (pelvis) N28.9
    chronic N18.9
        hypertensive — *see* Hypertension, kidney
        stage 1 N18.1
        stage 2 (mild) N18.2
        stage 3 (moderate) N18.3
        stage 4 (severe) N18.4
        stage 5 N18.5
    complicating pregnancy — *see* Pregnancy,
        complicated by, renal disease
    cystic (congenital) Q61.9
    fibrocystic (congenital) Q61.8
    hypertensive — *see* Hypertension, kidney
    in (due to)
        schistosomiasis (bilharziasis) B65.9 [N29]
    multicystic Q61.4
    polycystic Q61.3
        adult type Q61.2
        childhood type NEC Q61.19
            collecting duct dilatation Q61.11
  Kimmelstiel (-Wilson) (intercapillary polycystic
        (congenital) glomerulosclerosis) — *see*
        E08-E13 with .21
  Kinnier Wilson's (hepatolenticular degeneration)
        E83.01
  kissing — *see* Mononucleosis, infectious
  Klebs' (*see also* Glomerulonephritis) N05.-
  Klippel-Feil (brevicollis) Q76.1
  Köhler-Pellegrini-Stieda (calcification, knee joint) —
        see Bursitis, tibial collateral
  Kok Q89.8
  König's (osteochondritis dissecans) — *see*
        Osteochondritis, dissecans
  Korsakoff's (nonalcoholic) F04
    alcoholic F10.96
        with dependence F10.26
  Kostmann's (infantile genetic agranulocytosis) D70.0
  kuru A81.81
  Kyasanur Forest A98.2
  labyrinth, ear — *see* Disorder, ear, inner
  lacrimal system — *see* Disorder, lacrimal system
  Lafora's G25.3
  Lancereaux-Mathieu (leptospiral jaundice) A27.0
  Landry's G61.0
  Larrey-Weil (leptospiral jaundice) A27.0
  larynx J38.7
  legionnaires' A48.1
    nonpneumonic A48.2
  Lenegre's I44.2
  lens H27.9
    specified NEC H27.8
  Lev's (acquired complete heart block) I44.2
  Lewy body (dementia) G31.83 [F02.80]
    with behavioral disturbance G31.83 [F02.81]
  Lichtheim's (subacute combined sclerosis with
        pernicious anemia) D51.0
  Lightwood's (renal tubular acidosis) N25.89
  Lignac's (cystinosis) E72.04
  lip K13.0
  lipid-storage E75.6
    specified NEC E75.5
  Lipschütz's N76.6
  liver (chronic) (organic) K76.9
    alcoholic (chronic) K70.9
        acute — *see* Disease, liver, alcoholic, hepatitis
        cirrhosis K70.30
            with ascites K70.31
        failure K70.40
            with coma K70.41
        fatty liver K70.0
        fibrosis K70.2
        hepatitis K70.10
            with ascites K70.11
        sclerosis K70.2
    cystic, congenital Q44.6
    drug-induced (idiosyncratic) (toxic) (predictable)
        (unpredictable) — *see* Disease, liver, toxic
    end stage K72.90
        due to hepatitis — *see* Hepatitis

Disease, diseased— *continued*
  liver— *continued*
    fatty, nonalcoholic (NAFLD) K76.0
        alcoholic K70.0
    fibrocystic (congenital) Q44.6
    fluke
        Chinese B66.1
        oriental B66.1
        sheep B66.3
    glycogen storage E74.09 [K77]
    in (due to)
        schistosomiasis (bilharziasis) B65.9 [K77]
    inflammatory K75.9
        alcoholic K70.1
        specified NEC K75.89
    polycystic (congenital) Q44.6
    toxic K71.9
        with
            cholestasis K71.0
            cirrhosis (liver) K71.7
            fibrosis (liver) K71.7
            focal nodular hyperplasia K71.8
            hepatic granuloma K71.8
            hepatic necrosis K71.10
                with coma K71.11
            hepatitis NEC K71.6
                acute K71.2
                chronic
                    active K71.50
                        with ascites K71.51
                    lobular K71.4
                    persistent K71.3
                lupoid K71.50
                    with ascites K71.51
            peliosis hepatis K71.8
            veno-occlusive disease (VOD) of liver
                K71.8
        veno-occlusive K76.5
  Lobo's (keloid blastomycosis) B48.0
  Lobstein's (brittle bones and blue sclera) Q78.0
  Ludwig's (submaxillary cellulitis) K12.2
  lumbosacral region M53.87
  lung J98.4
    black J60
    congenital Q33.9
    cystic J98.4
        congenital Q33.0
    fibroid (chronic) — *see* Fibrosis, lung
    fluke B66.4
        oriental B66.4
    in
        amyloidosis E85.4 [J99]
        sarcoidosis D86.0
        Sjögren's syndrome M35.02
        systemic
            lupus erythematosus M32.13
            sclerosis M34.81
    interstitial J84.9
        acute B59
        specified NEC J84.8
    obstructive (chronic) J44.9
        with
            acute
                bronchitis J44.0
                exacerbation NEC J44.1
                lower respiratory infection J44.0
            alveolitis, allergic J67.9
            asthma J44.9
            bronchiectasis J47.9
                with
                    exacerbation (acute) J47.1
                    lower respiratory infection J47.0
            bronchitis J44.9
                with
                    exacerbation (acute) J44.1
                    lower respiratory infection J44.0
            emphysema J44.9
            hypersensitivity pneumonitis J67.9
        decompensated J44.1
            with
                exacerbation (acute) J44.1
    polycystic J98.4
        congenital Q33.0

Disease, diseased— *continued*
　lung—*continued*
　　rheumatoid (diffuse) (interstitial) — *see*
　　　Rheumatoid, lung
　Lutembacher's (atrial septal defect with mitral
　　stenosis) Q21.1
　Lyme A69.2Ø
　lymphatic (gland) (system) (channel) (vessel) I89.9
　lymphoproliferative D47.9
　　specified NEC D47.z9
　　T-gamma D47.z9
　　X-linked D82.3
　Magitot's M27.2
　malarial — *see* Malaria
　malignant (*see also* Neoplasm, malignant, by site)
　Manson's B65.1
　maple bark J67.6
　maple-syrup-urine E71.Ø
　Marburg (virus) A98.3
　Marion's (bladder neck obstruction) N32.Ø
　Marsh's (exophthalmic goiter) — *see*
　　Hyperthyroidism, with, goiter (diffuse)
　mastoid (process) — *see* Disorder, ear, middle
　Mathieu's (leptospiral jaundice) A27.Ø
　Maxcy's A75.2
　McArdle (-Schmid-Pearson) (glycogenosis V) E74.Ø4
　mediastinum J98.5
　medullary center (idiopathic) (respiratory) G93.89
　Meige's (chronic hereditary edema) Q82.Ø
　meningococcal — *see* Infection, meningococcal
　mental F99
　　organic FØ9
　mesenchymal M35.9
　mesenteric embolic K55.Ø
　metabolic, metabolism E88.9
　　bilirubin E8Ø.7
　metal-polisher's J62.8
　metastatic (see also Neoplasm, secondary, by site)
　　C79.9
　microvascular code to condition
　microvillus inclusion (MVD) Q43.8
　middle ear — *see* Disorder, ear, middle
　Mikulicz' (dryness of mouth, absent or decreased
　　lacrimation) K11.8
　Milroy's (chronic hereditary edema) Q82.Ø
　Minamata — *see* Poisoning, mercury
　minicore G71.2
　Minor's G95.19
　Minot's (hemorrhagic disease, newborn) P53
　Minot-von Willebrand-Jürgens (angiohemophilia)
　　D68.Ø
　Mitchell's (erythromelalgia) I73.81
　mitral (valve) IØ5.9
　　nonrheumatic I34.9
　mixed connective tissue M35.1
　Monge's T7Ø.29
　Morgagni-Adams-Stokes (syncope with heart block)
　　I45.9
　Morgagni's (syndrome) (hyperostosis frontalis
　　interna) M85.2
　Morton's (with metatarsalgia) — *see* Lesion, nerve,
　　plantar
　Morvan's G95.Ø
　motor neuron (bulbar) (familial) (mixed type)
　　(spinal) G12.2Ø
　　amyotrophic lateral sclerosis G12.21
　　progressive bulbar palsy G12.22
　　specified NEC G12.29
　moldy hay J67.Ø
　moyamoya I67.5
　mu heavy chain disease C88.2
　multicore G71.2
　muscle *see also* Disorder, muscle
　　inflammatory — *see* Myositis
　　ocular (external) — *see* Strabismus
　musculoskeletal system, soft tissue (*see also*
　　Disorder, soft tissue)
　　specified NEC — *see* Disorder, soft tissue,
　　　specified type NEC
　mushroom workers' J67.5
　mycotic B49
　myelodysplastic, not classified C94.6

Disease, diseased— *continued*
　myeloproliferative, not classified C94.6
　　chronic D47.1
　myocardium, myocardial (*see also* Degeneration,
　　myocardial) I51.5
　　primary (idiopathic) I42.9
　myoneural G7Ø.9
　Naegeli's D69.1
　nails L6Ø.9
　　specified NEC L6Ø.8
　Nairobi (sheep virus) A93.8
　nasal J34.9
　nemaline body G71.2
　nerve — *see* Disorder, nerve
　nervous system G98.8
　　autonomic G9Ø.9
　　central G96.9
　　　specified NEC G96.8
　　congenital QØ7.9
　　parasympathetic G9Ø.9
　　specified NEC G98.8
　　sympathetic G9Ø.9
　　vegetative G9Ø.9
　neuromuscular system G7Ø.9
　Newcastle B3Ø.8
　Nicolas (-Durand)-Favre (climatic bubo) A55
　nipple N64.9
　　Paget's C5Ø.Ø1-
　　　female C5Ø.Ø1-
　　　male C5Ø.Ø2-
　Nishimoto (-Takeuchi) I67.5
　nonarthropod-borne NOS (viral) B34.9
　　enterovirus NEC B34.1
　nonautoimmune hemolytic D59.4
　　drug-induced D59.2
　Nonne-Milroy-Meige (chronic hereditary edema)
　　Q82.Ø
　nose J34.9
　nucleus pulposus — *see* Disorder, disc
　nutritional E63.9
　oast-house-urine E72.19
　　ocular
　　　herpesviral BØØ.5Ø
　　　zoster BØ2.3Ø
　obliterative vascular I77.1
　Ohara's — *see* Tularemia
　Opitz's (congestive splenomegaly) D73.2
　Oppenheim-Urbach (necrobiosis lipoidica
　　diabeticorum) — *see* EØ8-E13 with .63
　optic nerve NEC — *see* Disorder, nerve, optic
　orbit — *see* Disorder, orbit
　Oriental liver fluke B66.1
　Oriental lung fluke B66.4
　Ormond's N13.5
　Oropouche virus A93.Ø
　Osler-Rendu (familial hemorrhagic telangiectasia)
　　I78.Ø
　osteofibrocystic E21.Ø
　Otto's M24.7
　outer ear — *see* Disorder, ear, external
　ovary (noninflammatory) N83.9
　　cystic N83.2Ø
　　inflammatory — *see* Salpingo-oophoritis
　　polycystic E28.2
　　specified NEC N83.8
　Owren's (congenital) — *see* Defect, coagulation
　pancreas K86.9
　　cystic K86.2
　　fibrocystic E84.9
　　specified NEC K86.8
　panvalvular IØ8.9
　　specified NEC IØ8.8
　parametrium (noninflammatory) N83.9
　parasitic B89
　　cerebral NEC B71.9 [G94]
　　intestinal NOS B82.9
　　mouth B37.Ø
　　skin NOS B88.9
　　specified type — *see* Infestation
　　tongue B37.Ø
　parathyroid (gland) E21.5
　　specified NEC E21.4
　Parkinson's G2Ø

Disease, diseased— *continued*
　parodontal KØ5.6
　Parrot's (syphilitic osteochondritis) A5Ø.Ø2
　Parry's (exophthalmic goiter) — *see*
　　Hyperthyroidism, with, goiter (diffuse)
　Parson's (exophthalmic goiter) — *see*
　　Hyperthyroidism, with, goiter (diffuse)
　Paxton's (white piedra) B36.2
　pearl-worker's — *see* Osteomyelitis, specified type
　　NEC
　Pellegrini-Stieda (calcification, knee joint) — *see*
　　Bursitis, tibial collateral
　pelvis, pelvic
　　female NOS N94.9
　　　specified NEC N94.89
　　gonococcal (acute) (chronic) A54.24
　　inflammatory (female) N73.9
　　　acute N73.Ø
　　　chronic N73.1
　　　specified NEC N73.8
　　　syphilitic (secondary) A51.42
　　　　late A52.76
　　　tuberculous A18.17
　　organ, female N94.9
　　peritoneum, female NEC N94.89
　penis N48.9
　　inflammatory N48.29
　　　abscess N48.21
　　　cellulitis N48.22
　　specified NEC N48.89
　periapical tissues NOS KØ4.9Ø
　periodontal KØ5.6
　　specified NEC KØ5.5
　periosteum — *see* Disorder, bone, specified type
　　NEC
　peripheral
　　arterial I73.9
　　autonomic nervous system G9Ø.9
　　nerves — *see* Polyneuropathy
　　vascular NOS I73.9
　peritoneum K66.9
　　pelvic, female NEC N94.89
　　specified NEC K66.8
　persistent mucosal (middle ear) H66.2Ø
　　left H66.22
　　　with right H66.23
　　right H66.21
　　　with left H66.23
　Petit's — *see* Hernia, abdomen, specified site NEC
　pharynx J39.2
　　specified NEC J39.2
　Phocas' — *see* Mastopathy, cystic
　photochromogenic (acid-fast bacilli) (pulmonary)
　　A31.Ø
　　nonpulmonary A31.9
　Pick's G31.Ø1 [FØ2.8Ø]
　　with behavioral disturbance G31.Ø1 [FØ2.81]
　pigeon fancier's J67.2
　pineal gland E34.8
　pink — *see* Poisoning, mercury
　Pinkus' (lichen nitidus) L44.1
　pinworm B8Ø
　Piry virus A93.8
　pituitary (gland) E23.7
　pituitary-snuff-taker's J67.8
　pleura (cavity) J94.9
　　specified NEC J94.8
　pneumatic drill (hammer) T75.21
　Pollitzer's (hidradenitis suppurativa) L73.2
　polycystic
　　kidney or renal Q61.3
　　　adult type Q61.2
　　　childhood type NEC Q61.19
　　　　collecting duct dilatation Q61.11
　　liver or hepatic Q44.6
　　lung or pulmonary J98.4
　　　congenital Q33.Ø
　　ovary, ovaries E28.2
　　spleen Q89.Ø9
　Pompe's (glycogenosis II) E74.Ø2
　Posada-Wernicke B38.9
　Potain's (pulmonary edema) J18.2

Disease, diseased— *continued*
  prepuce N47.8
    inflammatory N47.7
      balanoposthitis N47.6
  Pringle's (tuberous sclerosis) Q85.1
  prion, central nervous system A81.9
    specified NEC A81.89
  prostate N42.9
    specified NEC N42.89
  protozoal B64
    acanthamebiasis — *see* Acanthamebiasis
    African trypanosomiasis — *see* African trypanosomiasis
    babesiosis B60.0
    Chagas disease — *see* Chagas disease
    intestine, intestinal A07.9
    leishmaniasis — *see* Leishmaniasis
    malaria — *see* Malaria
    naegleriasis B60.2
    pneumocystosis B59
    specified organism NEC B60.8
    toxoplasmosis — *see* Toxoplasmosis
  pseudo-Hurler's E77.0
  psychiatric F99
  psychotic — *see* Psychosis
  Puente's (simple glandular cheilitis) K13.0
  puerperal — *see* Puerperal
  pulmonary (*see also* Disease, lung)
    artery I28.9
    chronic obstructive J44.9
      with
        acute bronchitis J44.0
        exacerbation (acute) J44.1
        lower respiratory infection (acute) J44.0
      decompensated J44.1
        with
          exacerbation (acute) J44.1
    heart I27.9
      specified NEC I27.89
    hypertensive (vascular) I27.0
    valve I37.9
      rheumatic I09.89
  pulp (dental) NOS K04.90
  pulseless M31.4
  Putnam's (subacute combined sclerosis with pernicious anemia) D51.0
  Pyle (-Cohn) (craniometaphyseal dysplasia) Q78.5
  ragpicker's or ragsorter's A22.1
  Raynaud's — *see* Raynaud's disease
  reactive airway — *see* Asthma
  Reclus' (cystic) — *see* Mastopathy, cystic
  rectum K62.9
    specified NEC K62.8
  Refsum's (heredopathia atactica polyneuritiformis) G60.1
  renal (chronic) (functional) (pelvis) (*see also* Disease, kidney) N28.9
    with
      edema — *see* Nephrosis
      glomerular lesion — *see* Glomerulonephritis
        with edema — *see* Nephrosis
      interstitial nephritis N12
    acute N28.9
    cystic, congenital Q61.9
    diabetic — *see* E08-E13 with .22
    end-stage (failure) N18.6
      due to hypertension I12.0
    fibrocystic (congenital) Q61.8
    hypertensive — *see* Hypertension, kidney
    lupus M32.14
    phosphate-losing (tubular) N25.0
    polycystic (congenital) Q61.3
      adult type Q61.2
      childhood type NEC Q61.19
        collecting duct dilatation Q61.11
    rapidly progressive N01.9
    subacute N01.9
  Rendu-Osler-Weber (familial hemorrhagic telangiectasia) I78.0
  renovascular (arteriosclerotic) — *see* Hypertension, kidney

Disease, diseased— *continued*
  respiratory (tract) J98.9
    acute or subacute NOS J06.9
      due to
        chemicals, gases, fumes or vapors (inhalation) J68.3
        external agent J70.9
          specified NEC J70.8
        radiation J70.0
      noninfectious J39.8
    chronic NOS J98.9
      due to
        chemicals, gases, fumes or vapors J68.4
        external agent J70.9
          specified NEC J70.8
        radiation J70.1
      newborn P27.9
        specified NEC P27.8
    due to
      chemicals, gases, fumes or vapors J68.9
        acute or subacute NEC J68.3
        chronic J68.4
      external agent J70.9
        specified NEC J70.8
    newborn P28.9
      specified type NEC P28.89
    upper J39.9
      acute or subacute J06.9
      noninfectious NEC J39.8
      specified NEC J39.8
      streptococcal J06.9
  retina, retinal H35.9
    Batten's or Batten-Mayou E75.4 [H36]
    specified NEC H35.89
  rheumatoid — *see* Arthritis, rheumatoid
  rickettsial NOS A79.9
    specified type NEC A79.89
  Riga (-Fede) (cachectic aphthae) K14.0
  Riggs' (compound periodontitis) — *see* Periodontitis
  Ritter's L00
  Rivalta's (cervicofacial actinomycosis) A42.2
  Robles' (onchocerciasis) B73.1
  Roger's (congenital interventricular septal defect) Q21.0
  Rosenthal's (factor XI deficiency) D68.1
  Rossbach's (hyperchlorhydria) K30
  Ross River B33.1
  Rotes Quérol — *see* Hyperostosis, ankylosing
  Roth (-Bernhardt) — *see* Mononeuropathy, lower limb, meralgia paresthetica
  Runeberg's (progressive pernicious anemia) D51.0
  sacroiliac NEC M53.3
  salivary gland or duct K11.9
    inclusion B25.9
    specified NEC K11.8
    virus B25.9
  sandworm B76.9
  Schimmelbusch's — *see* Mastopathy, cystic
  Schmorl's — *see* Schmorl's disease or nodes
  Schönlein (-Henoch) (purpura rheumatica) D69.0
  Schottmüller's — *see* Fever, paratyphoid
  Schultz's (agranulocytosis) — *see* Agranulocytosis
  Schwalbe-Ziehen-Oppenheim G24.1
  Schwartz-Jampel G71.13
  sclera H15.9
    specified NEC H15.89
  scrofulous (tuberculous) A18.2
  scrotum N50.9
  sebaceous glands L73.9
  semilunar cartilage, cystic (*see also* Derangement, knee, meniscus, cystic)
  seminal vesicle N50.9
  serum NEC T80.6
  sexually transmitted A64
    anogenital
      herpesviral infection — *see* Herpes, anogenital
      warts A63.0
    chancroid A57
    chlamydial infection — *see* Chlamydia
    gonorrhea — *see* Gonorrhea
    granuloma inguinale A58
    specified organism NEC A63.8

Disease, diseased— *continued*
  sexually transmitted—*continued*
    syphilis — *see* Syphilis
    trichomoniasis — *see* Trichomoniasis
  Sézary C84.1-
  shimamushi (scrub typhus) A75.3
  shipyard B30.0
  sickle-cell D57.1
    with crisis (vasoocclusive pain) D57.00
      with
        acute chest syndrome D57.01
        splenic sequestration D57.02
    elliptocytosis D57.8-
    Hb-C D57.20
      with crisis (vasoocclusive pain) D57.219
        with
          acute chest syndrome D57.211
          splenic sequestration D57.212
      without crisis D57.20
    Hb-SD D57.80
      with crisis D57.819
        with
          acute chest syndrome D57.811
          splenic sequestration D57.812
    Hb-SE D57.80
      with crisis D57.819
        with
          acute chest syndrome D57.811
          splenic sequestration D57.812
    specified NEC D57.80
      with crisis D57.819
        with
          acute chest syndrome D57.811
          splenic sequestration D57.812
    spherocytosis D57.80
      with crisis D57.819
        with
          acute chest syndrome D57.811
          splenic sequestration D57.812
    thalassemia D57.40
      with crisis (vasoocclusive pain) D57.419
        with
          acute chest syndrome D57.411
          splenic sequestration D57.412
      without crisis D57.40
  silo-filler's J68.8
    bronchitis J68.0
    pneumonitis J68.0
    pulmonary edema J68.1
  simian B B00.4
  Simons' (progressive lipodystrophy) E88.1
  sin nombre virus B33.4
  sinus — *see* Sinusitis
  Sirkari's B55.0
  sixth B08.20
    due to human herpesvirus 6 B08.21
    due to human herpesvirus 7 B08.22
  skin L98.9
    due to metabolic disorder NEC E88.9 [L99]
    specified NEC L98.8
  slim (HIV) B20
  small vessel I73.9
  Sneddon-Wilkinson (subcorneal pustular dermatosis) L13.1
  South African creeping B88.0
  spinal (cord) G95.9
    congenital Q06.9
    specified NEC G95.89
  spine (*see also* Spondylopathy)
    joint — *see* Dorsopathy
    tuberculous A18.01
  spinocerebellar (hereditary) G11.9
    specified NEC G11.8
  spleen D73.9
    amyloid E85.4 [D77]
    organic D73.9
    polycystic Q89.09
    postinfectional D73.89
  sponge-diver's — *see* Toxicity, venom, marine animal, sea anemone
  Startle Q89.8
  Steinert's G71.11
  Sticker's (erythema infectiosum) B08.3

Disease, diseased— *continued*
- Stieda's (calcification, knee joint) — *see* Bursitis, tibial collateral
- Stokes' (exophthalmic goiter) — *see* Hyperthyroidism, with, goiter (diffuse)
- Stokes-Adams (syncope with heart block) I45.9
- stomach K31.9
  - functional, psychogenic F45.8
  - specified NEC K31.89
- stonemason's J62.8
- storage
  - glycogen — *see* Disease, glycogen storage
  - mucopolysaccharide — *see* Mucopolysaccharidosis
- striatopallidal system NEC G25.89
- Stuart-Prower (congenital factor X deficiency) D68.2
- Stuart's (congenital factor X deficiency) D68.2
- subcutaneous tissue — *see* Disease, skin
- supporting structures of teeth K08.9
  - specified NEC K08.8
- suprarenal (capsule) (gland) E27.9
  - hyperfunction E27.0
  - specified NEC E27.8
- sweat glands L74.9
  - specified NEC L74.8
- Swift (-Feer) — *see* Poisoning, mercury
- swimming-pool granuloma A31.1
- Sylvest's (epidemic pleurodynia) B33.0
- sympathetic nervous system G90.9
- synovium — *see* Disorder, synovium
- syphilitic — *see* Syphilis
- systemic tissue mast cell C96.2
- tanapox (virus) B08.71
- Tangier E78.6
- Tarral-Besnier (pityriasis rubra pilaris) L44.0
- Tauri's E74.09
- tear duct — *see* Disorder, lacrimal system
- tendon, tendinous (*see also* Disorder, tendon)
  - nodular — *see* Trigger finger
- terminal vessel I73.9
- testis N50.9
- thalassemia Hb-S — *see* Disease, sickle cell, thalassemia
- Thaysen-Gee (nontropical sprue) K90.0
- Thomsen G71.12
- throat J39.2
  - septic J02.0
- thromboembolic — *see* Embolism
- thymus (gland) E32.9
  - specified NEC E32.8
- thyroid (gland) E07.9
  - heart (*see also* Hyperthyroidism) E05.90 [I43]
    - with thyroid storm E05.91 [I43]
  - specified NEC E07.89
- Tietze's M94.0
- tongue K14.9
  - specified NEC K14.8
- tonsils, tonsillar (and adenoids) J35.9
- tooth, teeth K08.9
  - hard tissues K03.9
    - specified NEC K03.89
  - pulp NEC K04.99
  - specified NEC K08.8
- Tourette's F95.2
- trachea NEC J39.8
- tricuspid I07.9
  - nonrheumatic I36.9
- triglyceride-storage E75.5
- trophoblastic — *see* Mole, hydatidiform
- tsutsugamushi A75.3
- tube (fallopian) (noninflammatory) N83.9
  - inflammatory — *see* Salpingitis
  - specified NEC N83.8
- tuberculous NEC — *see* Tuberculosis
- tubo-ovarian (noninflammatory) N83.9
  - inflammatory — *see* Salpingo-oophoritis
  - specified NEC N83.8
- tubotympanic, chronic — *see* Otitis, media, suppurative, chronic, tubotympanic
- tubulo-interstitial N15.9
  - specified NEC N15.8
- tympanum — *see* Disorder, tympanic membrane
- Uhl's Q22.6

Disease, diseased— *continued*
- Underwood's (sclerema neonatorum) P83.0
- Unverricht (-Lundborg) — *see* Epilepsy, generalized, idiopathic
- Urbach-Oppenheim (necrobiosis lipoidica diabeticorum) — *see* E08-E13 with .63
- ureter N28.9
  - in (due to)
    - schistosomiasis (bilharziasis) B65.0 [N29]
- urethra N36.9
  - specified NEC N36.8
- urinary (tract) N39.9
  - bladder N32.9
    - specified NEC N32.89
  - specified NEC N39.8
- uterus (noninflammatory) N85.9
  - infective — *see* Endometritis
  - inflammatory — *see* Endometritis
  - specified NEC N85.8
- uveal tract (anterior) H21.9
  - posterior H31.9
- vagabond's B85.1
- vagina, vaginal (noninflammatory) N89.9
  - inflammatory NEC N76.89
  - specified NEC N89.8
- valve, valvular I38
  - multiple I08.9
    - specified NEC I08.8
- van Creveld-von Gierke (glycogenosis I) E74.01
- vas deferens N50.9
- vascular I99.9
  - arteriosclerotic — *see* Arteriosclerosis
  - ciliary body NEC — *see* Disorder, iris, vascular
  - hypertensive — *see* Hypertension
  - iris NEC — *see* Disorder, iris, vascular
  - obliterative I77.1
    - peripheral I73.9
  - occlusive I99.8
  - peripheral (occlusive) I73.9
    - in diabetes mellitus — *see* E08-E13 with .51
- vasomotor I73.9
- vasospastic I73.9
- vein I87.9
- venereal (*see also* Disease, sexually transmitted) A64
  - chlamydial NEC A56.8
    - anus A56.3
    - genitourinary NOS A56.2
    - pharynx A56.4
    - rectum A56.3
  - fifth A55
  - sixth A55
  - specified nature or type NEC A63.8
- vertebra, vertebral (*see also* Spondylopathy)
  - disc — *see* Disorder, disc
- vibration — *see* Vibration, adverse effects
- viral, virus (*see also* Disease, by type of virus) B34.9
  - arbovirus NOS A94
  - arthropod-borne NOS A94
  - congenital P35.9
    - specified NEC P35.8
  - Hanta (with renal manifestations) (Dobrava) (Puumala) (Seoul) A98.5
    - with pulmonary manifestations (Andes) (Bayou) (Bermejo) (Black Creek Canal) (Choclo) (Juquitiba) (Laguna negra) (Lechiguanas) (New York) (Oran) (Sin nombre) B33.4
  - Hantaan (Korean hemorrhagic fever) A98.5
  - human immunodeficiency (HIV) B20
  - Kunjin A83.4
  - nonarthropod-borne NOS B34.9
  - Powassan A84.8
  - Rocio (encephalitis) A83.6
  - Sin nombre (Hantavirus (cardio)-pulmonary syndrome) B33.4
  - Tahyna B33.8
  - vesicular stomatitis A93.8
- vitreous H43.9
  - specified NEC H43.89
- vocal cord J38.3
- Volkmann's, acquired T79.6
- von Eulenburg's (congenital paramyotonia) G71.19
- von Gierke's (glycogenosis I) E74.01

Disease, diseased— *continued*
- von Graefe's — *see* Strabismus, paralytic, ophthalmoplegia, progressive
- von Willebrand (-Jürgens) (angiohemophilia) D68.0
- Vrolik's (osteogenesis imperfecta) Q78.0
- vulva (noninflammatory) N90.9
  - inflammatory NEC N76.89
  - specified NEC N90.89
- Wallgren's (obstruction of splenic vein with collateral circulation) I87.8
- Wassilieff's (leptospiral jaundice) A27.0
- wasting NEC R64
  - due to malnutrition E41
- Waterhouse-Friderichsen A39.1
- Wegner's (syphilitic osteochondritis) A50.02
- Weil's (leptospiral jaundice of lung) A27.0
- Weir Mitchell's (erythromelalgia) I73.81
- Werdnig-Hoffmann G12.0
- Wermer's E31.21
- Werner-His (trench fever) A79.0
- Werner-Schultz (neutropenic splenomegaly) D73.81
- Wernicke-Posadas B38.9
- whipworm B79
- white blood cells D72.9
  - specified NEC D72.89
- white matter R90.82
- white-spot, meaning lichen sclerosus et atrophicus L90.0
  - penis N48.0
  - vulva N90.4
- Wilkie's K55.1
- Wilkinson-Sneddon (subcorneal pustular dermatosis) L13.1
- Willis' — *see* Diabetes
- Wilson's (hepatolenticular degeneration) E83.01
- woolsorter's A22.1
- yaba monkey tumor B08.72
- yaba pox (virus) B08.72
- zoonotic, bacterial A28.9
  - specified type NEC A28.8

Disfigurement (due to scar) L90.5
Disgerminoma — *see* Dysgerminoma
DISH (diffuse idiopathic skeletal hyperostosis) — *see* Hyperostosis, ankylosing
Disinsertion, retina — *see* Detachment, retina
Dislocatable hip, congenital Q65.6
Dislocation (articular)
- with fracture — *see* Fracture
- acromioclavicular (joint) S43.10-
  - with displacement
    - 100%-200% S43.12-
    - more than 200% S43.13-
  - inferior S43.14-
  - posterior S43.15-
- ankle S93.0-
- astragalus — *see* Dislocation, ankle
- atlantoaxial S13.121
- atlantooccipital S13.111
- atloidooccipital S13.111
- breast bone S23.29
- capsule, joint—code by site under Dislocation
- carpal (bone) — *see* Dislocation, wrist
- carpometacarpal (joint) NEC S63.05-
  - thumb S63.04-
- cartilage (joint)—code by site under Dislocation
- cervical spine (vertebra) — *see* Dislocation, vertebra, cervical
- chronic — *see* Dislocation, recurrent
- clavicle — *see* Dislocation, acromioclavicular joint
- coccyx S33.2
- congenital NEC Q68.8
- coracoid — *see* Dislocation, shoulder
- costal cartilage S23.29
- costochondral S23.29
- cricoarytenoid articulation S13.29
- cricothyroid articulation S13.29
- dorsal vertebra — *see* Dislocation, vertebra, thoracic
- ear ossicle — *see* Discontinuity, ossicles, ear
- elbow S53.10-
  - congenital Q68.8
  - pathological — *see* Dislocation, pathological NEC, elbow
  - radial head alone — *see* Dislocation, radial head

Dislocation — *continued*
 elbow— *continued*
  recurrent — *see* Dislocation, recurrent, elbow
  traumatic S53.10-
   anterior S53.11-
   lateral S53.14-
   medial S53.13-
   posterior S53.12-
   specified type NEC S53.19-
 eye, nontraumatic — *see* Luxation, globe
 eyeball, nontraumatic — *see* Luxation, globe
 femur
  distal end — *see* Dislocation, knee
  proximal end — *see* Dislocation, hip
 fibula
  distal end — *see* Dislocation, ankle
  proximal end — *see* Dislocation, knee
 finger S63.25-
  index S63.25-
  interphalangeal S63.27-
   distal S63.29-
    index S63.29-
    little S63.29-
    middle S63.29-
    ring S63.29-
   index S63.27-
   little S63.27-
   middle S63.27-
   proximal S63.28-
    index S63.28-
    little S63.28-
    middle S63.28-
    ring S63.28-
   ring S63.27-
  little S63.25-
  metacarpophalangeal S63.26-
   index S63.26-
   little S63.26-
   middle S63.26-
   ring S63.26-
  middle S63.25-
  recurrent — *see* Dislocation, recurrent, finger
  ring S63.25-
  thumb — *see* Dislocation, thumb
 foot S93.30-
  recurrent — *see* Dislocation, recurrent, foot
  specified site NEC S93.33-
  tarsal joint S93.31-
  tarsometatarsal joint S93.32-
  toe — *see* Dislocation, toe
 fracture — *see* Fracture
 glenohumeral (joint) — *see* Dislocation, shoulder
 glenoid — *see* Dislocation, shoulder
 habitual — *see* Dislocation, recurrent
 hip S73.00-
  anterior S73.03-
   obturator S73.02-
  central S73.04-
  congenital (total) Q65.2
   bilateral Q65.1
   partial Q65.5
    bilateral Q65.4
    unilateral Q65.3-
   unilateral Q65.0-
  developmental M24.85-
  pathological — *see* Dislocation, pathological NEC, hip
  posterior S73.01-
  recurrent — *see* Dislocation, recurrent, hip
 humerus, proximal end — *see* Dislocation, shoulder
 incomplete — *see* Subluxation, by site
 incus — *see* Discontinuity, ossicles, ear
 infracoracoid — *see* Dislocation, shoulder
 innominate (pubic junction) (sacral junction) S33.39
  acetabulum — *see* Dislocation, hip
 interphalangeal (joint(s))
  finger S63.279
   distal S63.29-
    index S63.29-
    little S63.29-
    middle S63.29-
    ring S63.29-
   index S63.27-

Dislocation — *continued*
 interphalangeal (joint(s))— *continued*
  finger— *continued*
   little S63.27-
   middle S63.27-
   proximal S63.28-
    index S63.28-
    little S63.28-
    middle S63.28-
    ring S63.28-
   ring S63.27-
  foot or toe — *see* Dislocation, toe
  thumb S63.12-
   distal joint S63.14-
   proximal joint S63.13-
 jaw (cartilage) (meniscus) S03.0
 joint prosthesis — *see* Complications, joint
  prosthesis, mechanical, displacement, by site
 knee S83.106
  cap — *see* Dislocation, patella
  congenital Q68.2
  old M23.8x-
  patella — *see* Dislocation, patella
  pathological — *see* Dislocation, pathological NEC, knee
  proximal tibia
   anteriorly S83.11-
   laterally S83.14-
   medially S83.13-
   posteriorly S83.12-
  recurrent (*see also* Derangement, knee, specified NEC)
  specified type NEC S83.19-
 lacrimal gland H04.16-
 lens (complete) H27.1-
  anterior H27.12-
  congenital Q12.1
  ocular implant — *see* Complications, intraocular lens
  partial H27.11-
  posterior H27.13-
  traumatic S05.8x-
 ligament—code by site under Dislocation
 lumbar (vertebra) — *see* Dislocation, vertebra, lumbar
 lumbosacral (vertebra) (*see also* Dislocation, vertebra, lumbar)
  congenital Q76.49
 mandible S03.0
 meniscus (knee) — *see* Tear, meniscus
 other sites—code by site under Dislocation
 metacarpal (bone)
  distal end — *see* Dislocation, finger
  proximal end S63.06-
 metacarpophalangeal (joint)
  finger S63.26-
   index S63.26-
   little S63.26-
   middle S63.26-
   ring S63.26-
  thumb S63.11-
 metatarsal (bone) — *see* Dislocation, foot
 metatarsophalangeal (joint(s)) — *see* Dislocation, toe
 midcarpal (joint) S63.03-
 midtarsal (joint) — *see* Dislocation, foot
 neck S13.20
  specified site NEC S13.29
  vertebra — *see* Dislocation, vertebra, cervical
 nose (septal cartilage) S03.1
 occipitoatloid S13.111
 old — *see* Derangement, joint, specified type NEC
 ossicles, ear — *see* Discontinuity, ossicles, ear
 partial — *see* Subluxation, by site
 patella S83.006
  congenital Q74.1
  lateral S83.01-
  recurrent (nontraumatic) M22.0-
   incomplete M22.1-
  specified type NEC S83.09-
 pathological NEC M24.30
  ankle M24.37-
  elbow M24.32-

Dislocation — *continued*
 pathological— *continued*
  foot joint M24.37-
  hand joint M24.34-
  hip M24.35-
  knee M24.36-
  lumbosacral joint — *see* subcategory M53.2
  pelvic region — *see* Dislocation, pathological, hip
  sacroiliac — *see* subcategory M53.2
  shoulder M24.31-
  wrist M24.33-
 pelvis NEC S33.30
  specified NEC S33.39
 phalanx
  finger or hand — *see* Dislocation, finger
  foot or toe — *see* Dislocation, toe
 prosthesis, internal — *see* Complications, prosthetic device, by site, mechanical
 radial head S53.006
  anterior S53.01-
  posterior S53.02-
  specified type NEC S53.09-
 radiocarpal (joint) S63.02-
 radiohumeral (joint) — *see* Dislocation, radial head
 radioulnar (joint)
  distal S63.01-
  proximal — *see* Dislocation, elbow
 radius
  distal end — *see* Dislocation, wrist
  proximal end — *see* Dislocation, radial head
 recurrent M24.40
  ankle M24.47-
  elbow M24.42-
  finger M24.44-
  foot joint M24.47-
  hand joint M24.44-
  hip M24.45-
  knee M24.46-
   patella — *see* Dislocation, patella, recurrent
  patella — *see* Dislocation, patella, recurrent
  sacroiliac — *see* subcategory M53.2
  shoulder M24.41-
  toe M24.47-
  vertebra (*see also* subcategory) M43.5
   atlantoaxial M43.4
    with myelopathy M43.3
  wrist M24.43-
 rib (cartilage) S23.29
 sacrococcygeal S33.2
 sacroiliac (joint) (ligament) S33.2
  congenital Q74.2
  recurrent — *see* subcategory M53.2
 sacrum S33.2
 scaphoid (bone) (hand) (wrist) — *see* Dislocation, wrist
  foot — *see* Dislocation, foot
 scapula — *see* Dislocation, shoulder, girdle, scapula
 semilunar cartilage, knee — *see* Tear, meniscus
 septal cartilage (nose) S03.1
 septum (nasal) (old) J34.2
 sesamoid bone—code by site under Dislocation
 shoulder (blade) (ligament) (joint) (traumatic) S43.006
  acromioclavicular — *see* Dislocation, acromioclavicular
  chronic — *see* Dislocation, recurrent, shoulder
  congenital Q68.8
  girdle S43.30-
   scapula S43.31-
   specified site NEC S43.39-
  humerus S43.00-
   anterior S43.01-
   inferior S43.03-
   posterior S43.02-
  pathological — *see* Dislocation, pathological NEC, shoulder
  recurrent — *see* Dislocation, recurrent, shoulder
  specified type NEC S43.08-
 spine
  cervical — *see* Dislocation, vertebra, cervical
  congenital Q76.49
  due to birth trauma P11.5
  lumbar — *see* Dislocation, vertebra, lumbar

Dislocation — *continued*
 spine—*continued*
  thoracic — *see* Dislocation, vertebra, thoracic
 spontaneous — *see* Dislocation, pathological
 sternoclavicular (joint) S43.206
  anterior S43.21-
  posterior S43.22-
 sternum S23.29
 subglenoid — *see* Dislocation, shoulder
 symphysis pubis S33.4
 talus — *see* Dislocation, ankle
 tarsal (bone(s)) (joint(s)) — *see* Dislocation, foot
 tarsometatarsal (joint(s)) — *see* Dislocation, foot
 temporomandibular (joint) S03.0
 thigh, proximal end — *see* Dislocation, hip
 thorax S23.20
  specified site NEC S23.29
  vertebra — *see* Dislocation, vertebra
 thumb S63.10-
  interphalangeal joint — *see* Dislocation, interphalangeal (joint), thumb
  metacarpophalangeal joint — *see* Dislocation, metacarpophalangeal (joint), thumb
 thyroid cartilage S13.29
 tibia
  distal end — *see* Dislocation, ankle
  proximal end — *see* Dislocation, knee
 tibiofibular (joint)
  distal — *see* Dislocation, ankle
  superior — *see* Dislocation, knee
 toe(s) S93.106
  great S93.10-
   interphalangeal joint S93.11-
   metatarsophalangeal joint S93.12-
  interphalangeal joint S93.119
  lesser S93.106
   interphalangeal joint S93.11-
   metatarsophalangeal joint S93.12-
  metatarsophalangeal joint S93.12-
 tooth S03.2
 trachea S23.29
 ulna
  distal end S63.07-
  proximal end — *see* Dislocation, elbow
 ulnohumeral (joint) — *see* Dislocation, elbow
 vertebra (articular process) (body) (traumatic)
  cervical S13.101
   atlantoaxial joint S13.121
   atlantooccipital joint S13.111
   atloidooccipital joint S13.111
   joint between
    C0 and C1 S13.111
    C1 and C2 S13.121
    C2 and C3 S13.131
    C3 and C4 S13.141
    C4 and C5 S13.151
    C5and C6 S13.161
    C6and C7 S13.171
    C7and T1 S13.181
   occipitoatloid joint S13.111
  congenital Q76.49
  lumbar S33.101
   joint between
    L1and L2 S33.111
    L2and L3 S33.121
    L3 and L4 S33.131
    L4and L5 S33.141
  nontraumatic — *see* Displacement, intervertebral disc
  partial — *see* Subluxation, by site
  recurrent NEC — *see* subcategory M43.5
  thoracic S23.101
   joint between
    T1 and T2 S23.111
    T2 and T3 S23.121
    T3 and T4 S23.123
    T4 and T5 S23.131
    T5 and T6 S23.133
    T6 and T7 S23.141
    T7 and T8 S23.143
    T8 and T9 S23.151
    T9 and T10 S23.153
    T10 and T11 S23.161

Dislocation — *continued*
 vertebra—*continued*
  thoracic—*continued*
   joint between—*continued*
    T11 and T12 S23.163
    T12 and L1 S23.171
 wrist (carpal bone) S63.006
  carpometacarpal joint — *see* Dislocation, carpometacarpal (joint)
  distal radioulnar joint — *see* Dislocation, radioulnar (joint), distal
  metacarpal bone, proximal — *see* Dislocation, metacarpal (bone), proximal end
  midcarpal — *see* Dislocation, midcarpal (joint)
  radiocarpal joint — *see* Dislocation, radiocarpal (joint)
  recurrent — *see* Dislocation, recurrent, wrist
  specified site NEC S63.09-
  ulna — *see* Dislocation, ulna, distal end
 xiphoid cartilage S23.29
Disorder (of) (*see also* Disease)
 acantholytic L11.9
  specified NEC L11.8
 acute
  psychotic — *see* Psychosis, acute
  stress F43.0
 adjustment (grief) F43.20
  with
   anxiety F43.22
    with depressed mood F43.23
   conduct disturbance F43.24
    with emotional disturbance F43.25
   depressed mood F43.21
    with anxiety F43.23
   other specified symptom F43.29
 adrenal (capsule) (gland) (medullary) E27.9
  specified NEC E27.8
 adrenogenital E25.9
  drug-induced E25.8
  iatrogenic E25.8
  idiopathic E25.8
 adult personality (and behavior) F69
  specified NEC F68.8
 affective (mood) — *see* Disorder, mood
 aggressive, unsocialized F91.1
 alcohol-related F10.99
  with
   amnestic disorder, persisting F10.96
   anxiety disorder F10.980
   dementia, persisting F10.97
   intoxication F10.929
    with delirium F10.921
    uncomplicated F10.920
   mood disorder F10.94
   other specified F10.988
   psychotic disorder F10.959
    with
     delusions F10.950
     hallucinations F10.951
   sexual dysfunction F10.981
   sleep disorder F10.988
 allergic — *see* Allergy
 alveolar NEC J84.0
 amino-acid
  cystathioninuria E72.19
  cystinosis E72.04
  cystinuria E72.01
  glycinuria E72.09
  homocystinuria E72.11
  metabolism — *see* Disturbance, metabolism, amino-acid
  specified NEC E72.8
  neonatal, transitory P74.8
  renal transport NEC E72.09
  transport NEC E72.09
 amnesic, amnestic
  alcohol-induced F10.96
   with dependence F10.26
  due to (secondary to) general medical condition F04
  psychoactive NEC-induced F19.96
   with
    abuse F19.16

Disorder—*continued*
 amnesic, amnestic—*continued*
  psychoactive NEC-induced—*continued*
   with—*continued*
    dependence F19.26
   sedative, hypnotic or anxiolytic-induced F13.96
    with dependence F13.26
 anaerobic glycolysis with anemia D55.2
 anxiety F41.9
  due to (secondary to)
   alcohol F10.980
   amphetamine F15.980
    in
     abuse F15.180
     dependence F15.280
   anxiolytic F13.980
    in
     abuse F13.180
     dependence F13.280
   caffeine F15.980
    in
     abuse F15.180
     dependence F15.280
   cannabis F12.980
    in
     abuse F12.180
     dependence F12.280
   cocaine F14.980
    in
     abuse F14.180
     dependence F14.180
   general medical condition F06.4
   hallucinogen F16.980
    in
     abuse F16.180
     dependence F16.280
   hypnotic F13.980
    in
     abuse F13.180
     dependence F13.280
   inhalant F18.980
    in
     abuse F18.180
     dependence F18.280
   phencyclidine F19.980
    in
     abuse F19.180
     dependence F19.280
   psychoactive substance NEC F19.980
    in
     abuse F19.180
     dependence F19.280
   sedative F13.980
    in
     abuse F13.180
     dependence F13.280
   volatile solvents F18.980
    in
     abuse F18.180
     dependence F18.280
  generalized F41.1
  mixed
   with depression (mild) F41.8
   specified NEC F41.3
  organic F06.4
  phobic F40.9
   of childhood F40.8
  specified NEC F41.8
 aortic valve — *see* Endocarditis, aortic
 aromatic amino-acid metabolism E70.9
  specified NEC E70.8
 arteriole NEC I77.89
 artery NEC I77.89
 articulation — *see* Disorder, joint
 attachment (childhood)
  disinhibited F94.2
  reactive F94.1
 attention-deficit hyperactivity (adolescent) (adult) (child) F90.9
  combined type F90.2
  hyperactive type F90.1
  inattentive type F90.0
  specified type NEC F90.8

Disorder — *continued*
  attention-deficit without hyperactivity (adolescent) (adult) (child) F90.0
  auditory processing (central) H93.25
  autistic F84.0
  autonomic nervous system G90.9
    specified NEC G90.8
  avoidant, child or adolescent F40.10
  balance
    acid-base E87.8
      mixed E87.4
    electrolyte E87.8
    fluid NEC E87.8
  behavioral (disruptive) — *see* Disorder, conduct
  beta-amino-acid metabolism E72.8
  bile acid and cholesterol metabolism E78.70
    Barth syndrome E78.71
    other specified E78.79
    Smith-Lemli-Opitz syndrome E78.72
  bilirubin excretion E80.6
  binocular
    movement H51.9
      convergence
        excess H51.12
        insufficiency H51.11
      internuclear ophthalmoplegia — *see* Ophthalmoplegia, internuclear
      palsy of conjugate gaze H51.0
      specified type NEC H51.8
    vision NEC — *see* Disorder, vision, binocular
  bipolar (I) F31.9
    current episode
      depressed F31.9
        with psychotic features F31.5
        without psychotic features F31.30
          mild F31.31
          moderate F31.32
          severe (without psychotic features) F31.4
          with psychotic features F31.5
      hypomanic F31.0
      manic F31.9
        with psychotic features F31.2
        without psychotic features F31.10
          mild F31.11
          moderate F31.12
          severe (without psychotic features) F31.13
          with psychotic features F31.2
      mixed F31.60
        mild F31.61
        moderate F31.62
        severe (without psychotic features) F31.63
          with psychotic features F31.64
      severe depression (without psychotic features) F31.4
        with psychotic features F31.5
    in remission (currently) F31.70
      in full remission
        most recent episode
          depressed F31.76
          hypomanic F31.72
          manic F31.74
          mixed F31.78
      in partial remission
        most recent episode
          depressed F31.75
          hypomanic F31.71
          manic F31.73
          mixed F31.77
    organic F06.30
    single manic episode F30.9
      mild F30.11
      moderate F30.12
      severe (without psychotic symptoms) F30.13
        with psychotic symptoms F30.2
    specified NEC F31.89
  bipolar II F31.81
  bladder N32.9
    functional NEC N31.9
    in schistosomiasis B65.0 [N33]
    specified NEC N32.89
  bleeding D68.9

Disorder — *continued*
  blood D75.9
    in congenital early syphilis A50.09 [D77]
  body dysmorphic F45.22
  bone M89.9
    continuity M84.9
      specified type NEC M84.80
        ankle M84.87-
        fibula M84.86-
        foot M84.87-
        hand M84.84-
        humerus M84.82-
        neck M84.88
        pelvis M84.859
        radius M84.83-
        rib M84.88
        shoulder M84.81-
        skull M84.88
        thigh M84.85-
        tibia M84.86-
        ulna M84.83-
        vertebra M84.88
    density and structure M85.9
      cyst (*see also* Cyst, bone, specified type NEC)
        aneurysmal — *see* Cyst, bone, aneurysmal
        solitary — *see* Cyst, bone, solitary
      diffuse idiopathic skeletal hyperostosis — *see* Hyperostosis, ankylosing
      fibrous dysplasia (monostotic) — *see* Dysplasia, fibrous, bone
      fluorosis — *see* Fluorosis, skeletal
      hyperostosis of skull M85.2
      osteitis condensans — *see* Osteitis, condensans
      specified type NEC M85.8-
        ankle M85.87-
        foot M85.87-
        forearm M85.83-
        hand M85.84-
        lower leg M85.86-
        multiple sites M85.89
        neck M85.88
        rib M85.88
        shoulder M85.81-
        skull M85.88
        thigh M85.85-
        upper arm M85.82-
        vertebra M85.88
    development and growth NEC M89.20
      carpus M89.24-
      clavicle M89.21-
      femur M89.25-
      fibula M89.26-
      finger M89.24-
      humerus M89.22-
      ilium M89.259
      ischium M89.259
      metacarpus M89.24-
      metatarsus M89.27-
      multiple sites M89.29
      neck M89.28
      radius M89.23-
      rib M89.28
      scapula M89.21-
      skull M89.28
      tarsus M89.27-
      tibia M89.26-
      toe M89.27-
      ulna M89.23-
      vertebra M89.28
      specified type NEC M89.8x-
  brachial plexus G54.0
  branched-chain amino-acid metabolism E71.2
    specified NEC E71.19
  breast N64.9
    agalactia — *see* Agalactia
    associated with
      lactation O92.70
        specified NEC O92.79
      pregnancy O92.20
        specified NEC O92.29
      puerperium O92.20
        specified NEC O92.29

Disorder — *continued*
  breast — *continued*
    cracked nipple — *see* Cracked nipple
    galactorrhea *see* Galactorrhea
    hypogalactia O92.4
    lactation disorder NEC O92.79
    mastitis — *see* Mastitis
    nipple infection — *see* Infection, nipple
    retracted nipple — *see* Retraction, nipple
    specified type NEC N64.89
  Briquet's F45.0
  bullous, in diseases classified elsewhere L14
  cannabis use
    due to drug abuse — *see* Abuse, drug, cannabis
    due to drug dependence — *see* Dependend, drug, cannabis
  carbohydrate
    absorption, intestinal NEC E74.39
    metabolism (congenital) E74.9
      specified NEC E74.8
  cardiac, functional I51.89
  carnitine metabolism E71.40
  cartilage M94.9
    articular NEC — *see* Derangement, joint, articular cartilage
    chondrocalcinosis — *see* Chondrocalcinosis
    specified type NEC M94.8x-
      articular — *see* Derangement, joint, articular cartilage
      multiple sites M94.8x0
  catatonic
    due to (secondary to) known physiological condition F06.1
    organic F06.1
  central auditory processing H93.25
  cervical
    region NEC M53.82
    root (nerve) NEC G54.2
  character NEC F68.8
  childhood disintegrative NEC F84.3
  cholesterol and bile acid metabolism E78.70
    Barth syndrome E78.71
    other specified E78.79
    Smith-Lemli-Opitz syndrome E78.72
  choroid H31.9
    atrophy — *see* Atrophy, choroid
    degeneration — *see* Degeneration, choroid
    detachment — *see* Detachment, choroid
    dystrophy — *see* Dystrophy, choroid
    hemorrhage — *see* Hemorrhage, choroid
    rupture — *see* Rupture, choroid
    scar — *see* Scar, chorioretinal
    solar retinopathy — *see* Retinopathy, solar
    specified type NEC H31.8
  ciliary body — *see* Disorder, iris
    degeneration — *see* Degeneration, ciliary body
  coagulation (factor) (*see also* Defect, coagulation) D68.9
    newborn, transient P61.6
  coccyx NEC M53.3
  cognitive F09
    due to (secondary to) general medical condition F09
    persisting R41.89
      due to
        alcohol F10.97
          with dependence F10.27
        anxiolytics F13.97
          with dependence F13.27
        hypnotics F13.97
          with dependence F13.27
        sedatives F13.97
          with dependence F13.27
        specified substance NEC F19.97
          with
            abuse F19.17
            dependence F19.27
  communication F80.9
  conduct (childhood) F91.9
    adjustment reaction — *see* Disorder, adjustment
    adolescent onset type F91.2
    childhood onset type F91.1
    compulsive F63.9

Disorder — *continued*
    conduct (childhood)— *continued*
        confined to family context F91.0
        depressive F91.8
        group type F91.2
        hyperkinetic — *see* Disorder, attention-deficit
            hyperactivity
        oppositional defiance F91.3
        socialized F91.2
        solitary aggressive type F91.1
        specified NEC F91.8
        unsocialized (aggressive) F91.1
    conduction, heart I45.9
    congenital glycosylation (CDG) E74.8
    conjunctiva H11.9
        infection — *see* Conjunctivitis
    connective tissue, localized L94.9
        specified NEC L94.8
    conversion — *see* Disorder, dissociative
    convulsive (secondary) — *see* Convulsions
    cornea H18.9
        deformity — *see* Deformity, cornea
        degeneration — *see* Degeneration, cornea
        deposits — *see* Deposit, cornea
        due to contact lens H18.82-
            specified as edema — *see* Edema, cornea
        edema — *see* Edema, cornea
        keratitis — *see* Keratitis
        keratoconjunctivitis — *see* Keratoconjunctivitis
        membrane change — *see* Change, corneal
            membrane
        neovascularization — *see* Neovascularization,
            cornea
        scar — *see* Opacity, cornea
        specified type NEC H18.89-
        ulcer — *see* Ulcer, cornea
    corpus cavernosum N48.9
    cranial nerve — *see* Disorder, nerve, cranial
    cyclothymic F34.0
    defiant oppositional F91.3
    delusional (persistent) (systematized) F22
        induced F24
    depersonalization F48.1
    depressive F32.9
        major F32.9
            with psychotic symptoms F32.3
            in remission (full) F32.5
                partial F32.4
            recurrent F33.9
            single episode F32.9
                mild F32.0
                moderate F32.1
                severe (without psychotic symptoms)
                    F32.2
                    with psychotic symptoms F32.3
        organic F06.31
        recurrent F33.9
            current episode
                mild F33.0
                moderate F33.1
                severe (without psychotic symptoms)
                    F33.2
                    with psychotic symptoms F33.3
            in remission F33.40
                full F33.42
                partial F33.41
            specified NEC F33.8
        single episode — *see* Episode, depressive
    developmental F89
        arithmetical skills F81.2
        coordination (motor) F82
        expressive writing F81.81
        language F80.9
            expressive F80.1
            receptive type F80.2
            specified NEC F80.89
        learning F81.9
            arithmetical F81.2
            reading F81.0
        mixed F88
        motor coordination or function F82
        pervasive F84.9
            specified NEC F84.8

Disorder — *continued*
    developmental— *continued*
        phonological F80.0
        reading F81.0
        scholastic skills (*see also* Disorder, learning)
            mixed F81.89
            specified NEC F88
        speech F80.9
            articulation F80.0
            specified NEC F80.89
        written expression F81.81
    diaphragm J98.6
    digestive (system) K92.9
        newborn P78.9
            specified NEC P78.89
        postprocedural — *see* Complication,
            gastrointestinal
        psychogenic F45.8
    disc (intervertebral) M51.9
        with
            myelopathy
                cervical region M50.00
                cervicothoracic region M50.03
                lumbar region M51.06
                lumbosacral region M51.07
                mid-cervical region M50.02
                occipito-atlanto-axial region M50.01
                sacrococcygeal region M53.3
                thoracic region M51.04
                thoracolumbar region M51.05
            radiculopathy
                cervical region M50.10
                cervicothoracic region M50.13
                lumbar region M51.16
                lumbosacral region M51.17
                mid-cervical region M50.12
                occipito-atlanto-axial region M50.11
                sacrococcygeal region M53.3
                thoracic region M51.14
                thoracolumbar region M51.15
        cervical M50.90
            with
                myelopathy M50.00
                    cervicothoracic region M50.03
                    mid-cervical region M50.02
                    occipito-atlanto-axial region M50.01
                neuritis, radiculitis or radiculopathy
                    M50.10
                    cervicothoracic region M50.13
                    mid-cervical region M50.12
                    occipito-atlanto-axial region M50.11
            cervicothoracic region M50.93
            degeneration M50.30
                cervicothoracic region M50.33
                mid-cervical region M50.32
                occipito-atlanto-axial region M50.31
            displacement M50.20
                cervicothoracic region M50.23
                mid-cervical region M50.22
                occipito-atlanto-axial region M50.21
            mid-cervical region M50.92
            occipito-atlanto-axial region M50.91
            specified type NEC M50.80
                cervicothoracic region M50.83
                mid-cervical region M50.82
                occipito-atlanto-axial region M50.81
        specified NEC
            lumbar region M51.86
            lumbosacral region M51.87
            sacrococcygeal region M53.3
            thoracic region M51.84
            thoracolumbar region M51.85
    disinhibited attachment (childhood) F94.2
    disintegrative, childhood NEC F84.3
    disruptive behavior F98.9
    dissocial personality F60.2
    dissociative F44.9
        affecting
            motor function F44.4
                and sensation F44.7
            sensation F44.6
                and motor function F44.7
        brief reactive F43.0

Disorder — *continued*
    dissociative— *continued*
        due to (secondary to) general medical condition
            F06.8
        mixed F44.7
        organic F06.8
        other specified NEC F44.89
    double heterozygous sickling See Disease,
        sickle-cell
    dream anxiety F51.5
    drug induced hemorrhagic D68.32
    drug related F19.99
        abuse — *see* Abuse, drug
        dependence — *see* Dependence, drug
    dysmorphic body F45.1
    dysthymic F34.1
    ear H93.9-
        bleeding — *see* Otorrhagia
        deafness — *see* Deafness
        degenerative H93.09-
        discharge — *see* Otorrhea
        external H61.9-
            auditory canal stenosis — *see* Stenosis,
                external ear canal
            exostosis — *see* Exostosis, external ear canal
            impacted cerumen — *see* Impaction, cerumen
            otitis — *see* Otitis, externa
            perichondritis — *see* Perichondritis, ear
            pinna — *see* Disorder, pinna
            specified type NEC H61.89-
        inner H83.9-
            vestibular dysfunction — *see* Disorder,
                vestibular function
        middle H74.9-
            ossicle — *see* Abnormal, ear ossicles
            polyp — *see* Polyp, ear (middle)
            specified NEC, in diseases classified elsewhere
                H75.8-
            postprocedural — *see* Complications, ear,
                procedure
            specified NEC, in diseases classified elsewhere
                H94.8
    eating (adult) (psychogenic) F50.9
        anorexia — *see* Anorexia
        bulimia F50.2
        child F98.29
            pica F98.3
            rumination disorder F98.21
        pica F50.8
            childhood F98.3
    electrolyte (balance) NEC E87.8
        with
            abortion — *see* Abortion by type complicated
                by specified condition NEC
            ectopic pregnancy O08.5
            molar pregnancy O08.5
        acidosis (metabolic) (respiratory) E87.2
        alkalosis (metabolic) (respiratory) E87.3
    elimination, transepidermal L87.9
        specified NEC L87.8
    emotional (persistent) F34.9
        of childhood F93.9
            specified NEC F93.8
    endocrine E34.9
        postprocedural E89.89
            specified NEC E89.89
    erectile (male) (organic) (*see also* Dysfunction,
        sexual, male, erectile) N52.9
        nonorganic F52.21
    erythematous — *see* Erythema
    esophagus K22.9
        functional K22.4
        psychogenic F45.8
    eustachian tube H69.9-
        infection — *see* Salpingitis, eustachian
        obstruction — *see* Obstruction, eustachian tube
        patulous — *see* Patulous, eustachian tube
        specified NEC H69.8-
    extrapyramidal G25.9
        specified type NEC G25.89
    eye H57.9
        postprocedural *see* Complication,
            postprocedural, eye

Disorder — *continued*
- eyelid H02.9
  - cyst — *see* Cyst, eyelid
  - degenerative H02.70
    - chloasma — *see* Chloasma, eyelid
    - madarosis — *see* Madarosis
    - specified type NEC H02.79
    - vitiligo — *see* Vitiligo, eyelid
    - xanthelasma — *see* Xanthelasma
  - dermatochalasis — *see* Dermatochalasis
  - edema — *see* Edema, eyelid
  - elephantiasis — *see* Elephantiasis, eyelid
  - foreign body, retained — *see* Foreign body, retained, eyelid
  - function H02.59
    - abnormal innervation syndrome — *see* Syndrome, abnormal innervation
    - blepharochalasis — *see* Blepharochalasis
    - blepharoclonus — *see* Blepharoclonus
    - blepharophimosis — *see* Blepharophimosis
    - blepharoptosis — *see* Blepharoptosis
    - lagophthalmos — *see* Lagophthalmos
    - lid retraction — *see* Retraction, lid
  - hypertrichosis — *see* Hypertrichosis, eyelid
  - specified type NEC H02.89
  - vascular H02.879
    - left H02.876
      - lower H02.875
      - upper H02.874
    - right H02.873
      - lower H02.872
      - upper H02.871
- factitious F68.10
  - with predominantly
    - psychological symptoms F68.11
      - with physical symptoms F68.13
    - physical symptoms F68.12
      - with psychological symptoms F68.13
- factor, coagulation — *see* Defect, coagulation
- fatty acid
  - metabolism E71.30
    - specified NEC E71.39
  - oxidation
    - LCAD E71.310
    - MCAD E71.311
    - SCAD E71.312
    - specified deficiency NEC E71.318
- feeding (infant or child) (*see also* Disorder, eating) R63.3
- feigned (with obvious motivation) Z76.5
  - without obvious motivation — *see* Disorder, factitious
- female
  - hypoactive sexual desire F52.0
  - orgasmic F52.31
  - sexual arousal F52.22
- fibroblastic M72.9
  - specified NEC M72.8
- fluency
  - adult onset F98.5
  - childhood onset F80.81
  - following
    - cerebral infarction I69.323
    - cerebrovascular disease I69.923
      - specified disease NEC I69.823
    - intracerebral hemorrhage I69.123
    - nontraumatic intracranial hemorrhage NEC I69.223
    - subarachnoid hemorrhage I69.023
  - in conditions classified elsewhere R47.82
- fluid balance E87.8
- follicular (skin) L73.9
  - specified NEC L73.8
- fructose metabolism E74.10
  - essential fructosuria E74.11
  - fructokinase deficiency E74.11
  - fructose-1, 6-diphosphatase deficiency E74.19
  - hereditary fructose intolerance E74.12
  - other specified E74.19
- functional polymorphonuclear neutrophils D71
- gallbladder, biliary tract and pancreas in diseases classified elsewhere K87
- gamma-glutamyl cycle E72.8

Disorder — *continued*
- gastric (functional) K31.9
  - motility K30
  - psychogenic F45.8
  - secretion K30
- gastrointestinal (functional) NOS K92.9
  - newborn P78.9
  - psychogenic F45.8
- gender-identity or -role F64.9
  - childhood F64.2
  - effect on relationship F66
  - of adolescence or adulthood (nontranssexual) F64.1
  - specified NEC F64.8
  - uncertainty F66
- genitourinary system
  - female N94.9
  - male N50.9
  - psychogenic F45.8
- globe H44.9
  - degenerated condition H44.50
    - absolute glaucoma H44.51-
    - atrophy H44.52-
    - leucocoria H44.53-
  - degenerative H44.30
    - chalcosis H44.31-
    - myopia H44.2-
    - siderosis H44.32-
    - specified type NEC H44.39-
  - endophthalmitis — *see* Endophthalmitis
  - foreign body, retained — *see* Foreign body, intraocular, old, retained
  - hemophthalmos — *see* Hemophthalmos
  - hypotony H44.40
    - due to
      - ocular fistula H44.42-
      - specified disorder NEC H44.43-
    - flat anterior chamber H44.41-
    - primary H44.44-
  - luxation — *see* Luxation, globe
  - specified type NEC H44.89
- glomerular (in) N05.9
  - amyloidosis E85.4 [N08]
  - cryoglobulinemia D89.1 [N08]
  - disseminated intravascular coagulation D65 [N08]
  - Fabry's disease E75.21 [N08]
  - familial lecithin cholesterol acyltransferase deficiency E78.6 [N08]
  - Goodpasture's syndrome M31.0
  - hemolytic-uremic syndrome D59.3
  - Henoch (-Schönlein) purpura D69.0 [N08]
  - malariae malaria B52.0
  - microscopic polyangiitis M31.7 [N08]
  - multiple myeloma C90.0- [N08]
  - mumps B26.83
  - schistosomiasis B65.9 [N08]
  - sepsis NEC A41.9 [N08]
    - streptococcal A40.9 [N08]
  - sickle-cell disorders D57.[N08]
  - strongyloidiasis B78.9 [N08]
  - subacute bacterial endocarditis I33.0 [N08]
  - syphilis A52.75
  - systemic lupus erythematosus M32.14
  - thrombotic thrombocytopenic purpura M31.1 [N08]
  - Waldenström macroglobulinemia C88.0 [N08]
  - Wegener's granulomatosis M31.31
- gluconeogenesis E74.4
- glucosaminoglycan metabolism — *see* Disorder, metabolism, glucosaminoglycan
- glycine metabolism E72.50
  - d-glycericacidemia E72.59
  - hyperhydroxyprolinemia E72.59
  - hyperoxaluria E72.53
  - hyperprolinemia E72.59
  - non-ketotic hyperglycinemia E72.51
  - oxalosis E72.53
  - oxaluria E72.53
  - sarcosinemia E72.59
  - trimethylaminuria E72.52
- glycoprotein metabolism E77.9
  - specified NEC E77.8

Disorder — *continued*
- habit (and impulse) F63.9
  - involving sexual behavior NEC F65.9
  - specified NEC F63.89
- heart action I49.9
- hematological D75.9
  - newborn (transient) P61.9
    - specified NEC P61.8
- hematopoietic organs D75.9
- hemorrhagic NEC D69.9
  - drug-induced D68.32
  - due to extrinsic circulating anticoagulants D68.32
  - due to intrinsic circulating anticoagulants D68.31
    - following childbirth O72.3
- hemostasis — *see* Defect, coagulation
- histidine metabolism E70.40
  - histidinemia E70.41
  - other specified E70.49
- hyperkinetic — *see* Disorder, attention-deficit hyperactivity
- hyperleucine-isoleucinemia E71.19
- hypervalinemia E71.19
- hypoactive sexual desire F52.0
- hypochondriacal F45.20
  - body dysmorphic F45.22
  - neurosis F45.21
  - other specified F45.29
- identity
  - dissociative F44.81
  - of childhood F93.8
- immune mechanism (immunity) D89.9
  - specified type NEC D89.8
- impaired renal tubular function N25.9
  - specified NEC N25.89
- impulse (control) F63.9
- inflammatory
  - penis N48.29
    - abscess N48.21
    - cellulitis N48.22
- integument, newborn P83.9
  - specified NEC P83.8
- intermittent explosive F63.81
- internal secretion pancreas — *see* Increased, secretion, pancreas, endocrine
- intestine, intestinal
  - carbohydrate absorption NEC E74.39
    - postoperative K91.2
  - functional NEC K59.9
    - postoperative K91.89
  - psychogenic F45.8
  - vascular K55.9
    - chronic K55.1
    - specified NEC K55.8
- intraoperative (intraprocedural) — *see* Complications, intraoperative
- involuntary emotional expression (IEED) F07.89
- iris H21.9
  - adhesions — *see* Adhesions, iris
  - atrophy — *see* Atrophy, iris
  - chamber angle recession — *see* Recession, chamber angle
  - cyst — *see* Cyst, iris
  - degeneration — *see* Degeneration, iris
  - in diseases classified elsewhere H22
  - iridodialysis — *see* Iridodialysis
  - iridoschisis — *see* Iridoschisis
  - miotic pupillary cyst — *see* Cyst, pupillary
  - pupillary
    - abnormality — *see* Abnormality, pupillary
    - membrane — *see* Membrane, pupillary
  - specified type NEC H21.89
  - vascular NEC H21.1x-
- iron metabolism E83.10
  - specified NEC E83.19
- isovaleric acidemia E71.110
- jaw, developmental M27.0
  - temporomandibular — *see* Anomaly, dentofacial, temporomandibular joint
- joint M25.9
  - derangement — *see* Derangement, joint
  - effusion — *see* Effusion, joint
  - fistula — *see* Fistula, joint

Disorder — *continued*
  joint— *continued*
    hemarthrosis — *see* Hemarthrosis
    instability — *see* Instability, joint
    osteophyte — *see* Osteophyte
    pain — *see* Pain, joint
    psychogenic F45.8
    specified type NEC M25.80
      ankle M25.87-
      elbow M25.82-
      foot joint M25.87-
      hand joint M25.84-
      hip M25.85-
      knee M25.86-
      shoulder M25.81-
      wrist M25.83-
    stiffness — *see* Stiffness, joint
  ketone metabolism E71.32
  kidney N28.9
    functional (tubular) N25.9
    in
      schistosomiasis B65.9 [N29]
    tubular function N25.9
      specified NEC N25.89
  lacrimal system H04.9
    changes H04.69
      fistula — *see* Fistula, lacrimal
    gland H04.19
      atrophy — *see* Atrophy, lacrimal gland
      cyst — *see* Cyst, lacrimal, gland
      dacryops — *see* Dacryops
      dislocation — *see* Dislocation, lacrimal gland
      dry eye syndrome — *see* Syndrome, dry eye
      infection — *see* Dacryoadenitis
      granuloma — *see* Granuloma, lacrimal
      inflammation — *see* Inflammation, lacrimal
      obstruction — *see* Obstruction, lacrimal
      specified NEC H04.89
  lactation NEC O92.79
  language (developmental) F80.9
    expressive F80.1
    mixed receptive and expressive F80.2
    receptive F80.2
  late luteal phase dysphoric N94.89
  learning (specific) F81.9
    acalculia R48.8
    alexia R48.0
    mathematics F81.2
    reading F81.0
    specified NEC F81.89
    spelling F81.81
    written expression F81.81
  lens H27.9
    aphakia — *see* Aphakia
    cataract — *see* Cataract
    dislocation — *see* Dislocation, lens
    specified type NEC H27.8
  ligament M24.20
    ankle M24.27-
    attachment, spine — *see* Enthesopathy, spinal
    elbow M24.22-
    foot joint M24.27-
    hand joint M24.24-
    hip M24.25-
    knee — *see* Derangement, knee, specified NEC
    shoulder M24.21-
    vertebra M24.28
    wrist M24.23-
  ligamentous attachments (*see also* Enthesopathy)
    spine — *see* Enthesopathy, spinal
  lipid
    metabolism, congenital E78.9
    storage E75.6
      specified NEC E75.5
  lipoprotein
    deficiency (familial) E78.6
    metabolism E78.9
      specified NEC E78.89
  liver K76.9
    malarial B54 [K77]
  low back (*see also* Dorsopathy, specified NEC)
  lumbosacral
    plexus G54.1

Disorder — *continued*
  lumbosacral— *continued*
    root (nerve) NEC G54.4
  lung, interstitial, drug-induced J70.4
    acute J70.2
    chronic J70.3
  lymphoproliferative, post-transplant (PTLD) D47.z1
  lysine and hydroxylysine metabolism E72.3
  male
    erectile (organic) (*see also* Dysfunction, sexual, male, erectile) N52.9
      nonorganic F52.21
    hypoactive sexual desire F52.0
    orgasmic F52.32
  manic F30.9
    organic F06.33
  mastoid (*see also* Disorder, ear, middle)
    postprocedural — *see* Complications, ear, procedure
  meniscus — *see* Derangement, knee, meniscus
  menopausal N95.9
    specified NEC N95.8
  menstrual N92.6
    psychogenic F45.8
    specified NEC N92.5
  mental (or behavioral) (nonpsychotic) F99
    due to (secondary to)
      amphetamine
        due to drug abuse — *see* Abuse, drug, stimulant
        due to drug dependence — *see* Dependence, drug, stimulant
      brain disease, damage and dysfunction F09
      caffeine use
        due to drug abuse — *see* Abuse, drug, stimulant
        due to drug dependence — *see* Dependence, drug, stimulant
      cannabis use
        due to drug abuse — *see* Abuse, drug, cannabis
        due to drug dependence — *see* Dependence, drug, cannabis
      general medical condition F09
      sedative or hypnotic use
        due to drug abuse — *see* Abuse, drug, sedative
        due to drug dependence — *see* Dependence, drug, sedative
      tobacco (nicotine) use — *see* Dependence, drug, nicotine
    following organic brain damage F07.9
      frontal lobe syndrome F07.0
      personality change F07.0
      postconcussional syndrome F07.81
      specified NEC F07.89
    infancy, childhood or adolescence F98.9
    neurotic — *see* Neurosis
    organic or symptomatic F09
    presenile, psychotic F03
    problem NEC
    psychoneurotic — *see* Neurosis
    psychotic — *see* Psychosis
    puerperal F53
    senile, psychotic NEC F03
  metabolic, amino acid, transitory, newborn P74.8
  metabolism NOS E88.9
    amino-acid E72.9
      aromatic E70.9
        albinism — *see* Albinism
        histidine E70.40
          histidinemia E70.41
          other specified E70.49
        hyperphenylalaninemia EE70.1
          classical phenylketonuria E70.0
        other specified E70.8
        tryptophan E70.5
        tyrosine E70.20
          hypertyrosinemia E70.21
          other specified E70.29
      branched chain E71.2
        3-methylglutaconic aciduria E71.111
        hyperleucine-isoleucinemia E71.19

Disorder — *continued*
  metabolism— *continued*
    amino-acid— *continued*
      branched chain— *continued*
        hypervalinemia E71.19
        isovaleric acidemia E71.110
        maple syrup urine disease E71.0
        methylmalonic acidemia E71.120
        organic aciduria NEC E71.118
        other specified E71.19
        propionate NEC E71.128
        propionic acidemia E71.121
      glycine E72.50
        d-glycericacidemia E72.59
        hyperhydroxyprolinemia E72.59
        hyperoxaluria E72.53
        hyperprolinemia E72.59
        non-ketotic hyperglycinemia E72.51
        other specified E72.59
        sarcosinemia E72.59
        trimethylaminuria E72.52
      hydroxylysine E72.3
      lysine E72.3
      ornithine E72.4
      other specified E72.8
        beta-amino acid E72.8
        gamma-glutamyl cycle E72.8
      straight-chain E72.8
      sulfur-bearing E72.10
        homocystinuria E72.11
        methylenetetrahydrofolate reductase deficiency E72.12
        other specified E72.19
    bile acid and cholesterol metabolism E78.70
    bilirubin E80.7
      specified NEC E80.6
    calcium E83.50
      hypercalcemia E83.52
      hypocalcemia E83.51
      other specified E83.59
    carbohydrate E74.9
      specified NEC E74.8
    cholesterol and bile acid metabolism E78.70
    congenital E88.9
    copper E83.00
      Wilson's disease E83.01
      specified type NEC E83.09
    cystinuria E72.01
    fructose E74.10
    galactose E74.20
    glucosaminoglycan E76.9
      mucopolysaccharidosis — *see* Mucopolysaccharidosis
      specified NEC E76.8
    glutamine E72.8
    glycine E72.50
    glycogen storage (hepatorenal) E74.01
    glycoprotein E77.9
      specified NEC E77.8
    glycosaminoglycan E76.9
      specified NEC E76.8
    in labor and delivery O75.89
    iron E83.10
    isoleucine E71.19
    leucine E71.19
    lipoid E78.9
    lipoprotein E78.9
      specified NEC E78.89
    magnesium E83.40
      hypermagnesemia E83.41
      hypomagnesemia E83.42
      other specified E83.49
    mineral E83.9
      specified NEC E83.89
    mitochondrial E88.40
      MELAS syndrome E88.41
      MERRF syndrome E88.42
      other specified E88.49
    ornithine E72.4
    phosphatases E83.30
    phosphorus E83.30
      acid phosphatase deficiency E83.39
      hypophosphatasia E83.39

Disorder — *continued*
  metabolism— *continued*
    phosphorus— *continued*
      hypophosphatemia E83.39
        familial E83.31
      other specified E83.39
      pseudovitamin D deficiency E83.32
    plasma protein NEC E88.09
    porphyrin — *see* Porphyria
    postprocedural E89.89
      specified NEC E89.89
    purine E79.9
      specified NEC E79.8
    pyrimidine E79.9
      specified NEC E79.8
    pyruvate E74.4
    serine E72.8
    sodium E87.8
    specified NEC E88.89
    threonine E72.8
    valine E71.19
    zinc E83.2
  methylmalonic acidemia E71.120
  micturition NEC R39.19
    feeling of incomplete emptying R39.14
    hesitancy R39.11
    poor stream R39.12
    psychogenic F45.8
    split stream R39.13
    straining R39.16
    urgency R39.15
  mitochondrial metabolism E88.40
  mitral (valve) — *see* Endocarditis, mitral
  mixed
    anxiety and depressive F41.8
    of scholastic skills (developmental) F81.89
    receptive expressive language F80.2
  mood F39
    bipolar — *see* Disorder, bipolar
    depressive — *see* Disorder, depressive
    due to (secondary to)
      alcohol F10.959
      amphetamine F15.94
        in
          abuse F15.14
          dependence F15.24
      anxiolytic F13.94
        in
          abuse F13.14
          dependence F13.24
      cocaine F14.94
        in
          abuse F14.14
          dependence F14.24
      general medical condition F06.30
      hallucinogen F16.94
        in
          abuse F16.14
          dependence F16.24
      hypnotic F13.94
        in
          abuse F13.14
          dependence F13.24
      inhalant F18.94
        in
          abuse F18.14
          dependence F18.24
      opioid F11.94
        in
          abuse F11.14
          dependence F11.24
      phencyclidine (PCP) F19.94
        in
          abuse F19.14
          dependence F19.24
      physiological condition F06.30
        with
          depressive features F06.31
          major depressive-like episode F06.32
          manic features F06.33
          mixed features F06.34

Disorder — *continued*
  mood— *continued*
    due to (secondary to)— *continued*
      psychoactive substance NEC F19.94
        in
          abuse F19.14
          dependence F19.24
      sedative F13.94
        in
          abuse F13.14
          dependence F13.24
      volatile solvents F18.94
        in
          abuse F18.14
          dependence F18.24
    manic episode F30.9
      with psychotic symptoms F30.2
      in remission (full) F30.4
        partial F30.3
      specified type NEC F30.8
      without psychotic symptoms F30.10
        mild F30.11
        moderate F30.12
        severe F30.13
    organic F06.30
      right hemisphere F07.89
    persistent F34.9
      cyclothymia F34.0
      dysthymia F34.1
      specified type NEC F34.8
    recurrent F39
    right hemisphere organic F07.89
  movement G25.9
    drug-induced G25.70
      akathisia G25.71
      specified NEC G25.79
    hysterical F44.4
    periodic limb G47.61
      sleep related G47.61
    specified NEC G25.89
    sleep related NEC G47.69
    stereotyped F98.4
    treatment-induced G25.9
  multiple personality F44.81
  muscle M62.9
    attachment, spine — *see* Enthesopathy, spinal
    in trichinellosis — *see* Trichinellosis, with muscle disorder
    psychogenic F45.8
    specified type NEC M62.89
    tone, newborn P94.9
      specified NEC P94.8
  muscular
    attachments (*see also* Enthesopathy)
      spine — *see* Enthesopathy, spinal
      urethra N36.44
  musculoskeletal system, soft tissue — *see* Disorder, soft tissue
    postprocedural M96.89
    psychogenic F45.8
  myoneural G70.9
    due to lead G70.1
    specified NEC G70.8
    toxic G70.1
  myotonic NEC G71.19
  nail, in diseases classified elsewhere L62
  neck region NEC — *see* Dorsopathy, specified NEC
  nerve G58.9
    abducent NEC — *see* Strabismus, paralytic, sixth nerve
    accessory G52.8
    acoustic — *see* subcategory H93.3
    auditory — *see* subcategory H93.3
    auriculotemporal G50.8
    axillary G54.0
    cerebral — *see* Disorder, nerve, cranial
    cranial G52.9
      eighth — *see* subcategory H93.3
      eleventh G52.8
      fifth G50.9
      first G52.0
      fourth NEC — *see* Strabismus, paralytic, fourth nerve

Disorder — *continued*
  nerve— *continued*
    cranial— *continued*
      multiple G52.7
      ninth G52.1
      second NEC — *see* Disorder, nerve, optic
      seventh NEC G51.9
      sixth NEC — *see* Strabismus, paralytic, sixth nerve
      specified NEC G52.8
      tenth G52.2
      third NEC — *see* Strabismus, paralytic, third nerve
      twelfth G52.3
    entrapment — *see* Neuropathy, entrapment
    facial G51.9
      specified NEC G51.8
    femoral — *see* Lesion, nerve, femoral
    glossopharyngeal NEC G52.1
    hypoglossal G52.3
    intercostal G58.0
    lateral
      cutaneous of thigh — *see* Mononeuropathy, lower limb, meralgia paresthetica
      popliteal — *see* Lesion, nerve, popliteal
    lower limb — *see* Mononeuropathy, lower limb
    medial popliteal — *see* Lesion, nerve, popliteal, medial
    median NEC — *see* Lesion, nerve, median
    multiple G58.7
    oculomotor NEC — *see* Strabismus, paralytic, third nerve
    olfactory G52.0
    optic NEC H47.09-
      hemorrhage into sheath — *see* Hemorrhage, optic nerve
      ischemic H47.01-
    peroneal — *see* Lesion, nerve, popliteal
    phrenic G58.8
    plantar — *see* Lesion, nerve, plantar
    pneumogastric G52.2
    posterior tibial — *see* Syndrome, tarsal tunnel
    radial — *see* Lesion, nerve, radial
    recurrent laryngeal G52.2
    root
      cervical G54.2
      lumbosacral G54.1
      specified NEC G54.8
      thoracic G54.3
    sciatic NEC — *see* Lesion, nerve, sciatic
    specified NEC G58.8
      lower limb — *see* Mononeuropathy, lower limb, specified NEC
      upper limb — *see* Mononeuropathy, upper limb, specified NEC
    sympathetic G90.9
    tibial — *see* Lesion, nerve, popliteal, medial
    trigeminal G50.9
      specified NEC G50.8
    trochlear NEC — *see* Strabismus, paralytic, fourth nerve
    ulnar — *see* Lesion, nerve, ulnar
    upper limb — *see* Mononeuropathy, upper limb
    vagus G52.2
  nervous system G98.8
    autonomic (peripheral) G90.9
      specified NEC G90.8
    central G96.9
      specified NEC G96.8
    parasympathetic G90.9
    specified NEC G98.8
    sympathetic G90.9
    vegetative G90.9
  neurohypophysis NEC E23.3
  neurological NEC R29.81
  neuromuscular G70.9
    hereditary NEC G71.9
    specified NEC G70.8
    toxic G70.1
  neurotic F48.9
    specified NEC F48.8
  neutrophil, polymorphonuclear D71
  nicotine use — *see* Dependence, drug, nicotine

Disorder — *continued*
 nightmare F51.5
 nose J34.9
  specified NEC J34.89
 obsessive-compulsive F42
 odontogenesis NOS K00.9
 oesophagus — *see* Disorder, esophagus
 opioid use
  due to drug abuse — *see* Abuse, drug, opioid
  due to drug dependence — *see* Dependence,
    drug, opioid
 oppositional defiant F91.3
 optic
  chiasm H47.49
   due to
    inflammatory disorder H47.41
    neoplasm H47.42
    vascular disorder H47.43
  disc H47.39-
   coloboma — *see* Coloboma, optic disc
   drusen — *see* Drusen, optic disc
   pseudopapilledema — *see*
      Pseudopapilledema
  radiations — *see* Disorder, visual, pathway
  tracts — *see* Disorder, visual, pathway
 orbit H05.9
  cyst — *see* Cyst, orbit
  deformity — *see* Deformity, orbit
  edema — *see* Edema, orbit
  enophthalmos — *see* Enophthalmos
  exophthalmos — *see* Exophthalmos
  hemorrhage — *see* Hemorrhage, orbit
  inflammation — *see* Inflammation, orbit
  myopathy — *see* Myopathy, extraocular muscles
  retained foreign body — *see* Foreign body, orbit,
    old
  specified type NEC H05.89
 organic
  anxiety F06.4
  catatonic F06.1
  delusional F06.2
  dissociative F06.8
  emotionally labile (asthenic) F06.8
  mood (affective) F06.30
  schizophrenia-like F06.2
 orgasmic (female) F52.31
  male F52.32
 ornithine metabolism E72.4
 overanxious F41.1
  of childhood F93.8
 pain
  with related psychological factors F45.42
  exclusively related to psychological factors F45.41
 pancreatic internal secretion E16.9
  specified NEC E16.8
 panic F41.0
  with agoraphobia F40.01
 papulosquamous L44.9
  in diseases classified elsewhere L45
  specified NEC L44.8
 paranoid F22
  induced F24
  shared F24
 parathyroid (gland) E21.5
  specified NEC E21.4
 parietoalveolar NEC J84.0
 paroxysmal, mixed R56.9
 patella M22.9-
  chondromalacia — *see* Chondromalacia, patella
  derangement NEC M22.3x-
  recurrent
   dislocation — *see* Dislocation, patella,
      recurrent
   subluxation — *see* Dislocation, patella,
      recurrent, incomplete
  specified NEC M22.8x-
 patellofemoral M22.2x-
 pentose phosphate pathway with anemia D55.1
 perception, due to hallucinogens F16.983
  in
   abuse F16.183
   dependence F16.283
 peripheral nervous system NEC G64

Disorder — *continued*
 peroxisomal E71.50
  biogenesis
   neonatal adrenoleukodystrophy E71.511
   specified disorder NEC E71.518
   Zellweger syndrome E71.510
  rhizomelic chondrodysplasia punctata E71.540
  specified form NEC E71.548
   group 1 E71.518
   group 2 E71.53
   group 3 E71.542
  X-linked adrenoleukodystrophy E71.529
   adolescent E71.521
   adrenomyeloneuropathy E71.522
   childhood E71.520
   specified form NEC E71.528
  Zellweger-like syndrome E71.541
 persistent
  (somatoform) pain F45.41
  affective (mood) F34.9
 personality (*see also* Personality) F60.9
  affective F34.0
  aggressive F60.3
  amoral F60.2
  anankastic F60.5
  antisocial F60.2
  anxious F60.6
  asocial F60.2
  asthenic F60.7
  avoidant F60.6
  borderline F60.3
  change (secondary) due to general medical
    condition F07.0
  compulsive F60.5
  cyclothymic F34.0
  dependent (passive) F60.7
  depressive F34.1
  dissocial F60.2
  emotional instability F60.3
  expansive paranoid F60.0
  explosive F60.3
  following organic brain damage F07.9
  histrionic F60.4
  hyperthymic F34.0
  hypothymic F34.1
  hysterical F60.4
  immature F60.89
  inadequate F60.7
  labile F60.3
  mixed (nonspecific) F60.89
  moral deficiency F60.2
  narcissistic F60.81
  negativistic F60.89
  obsessional F60.5
  obsessive(-compulsive) F60.5
  organic F07.9
  overconscientious F60.5
  paranoid F60.0
  passive(-dependent) F60.7
  passive-aggressive F60.89
  pathological NEC F60.9
  pseudosocial F60.2
  psychopathic F60.2
  schizoid F60.1
  schizotypal F21
  self-defeating F60.7
  specified NEC F60.89
  type A F60.5
  unstable (emotional) F60.3
 pervasive, developmental F84.9
 phobic anxiety, childhood F40.8
 phosphate-losing tubular N25.0
 pigmentation L81.9
  choroid, congenital Q14.3
  diminished melanin formation L81.6
  iron L81.8
  specified NEC L81.8
 pinna (noninfective) H61.10-
  deformity, acquired H61.11-
  hematoma H61.12-
  perichondritis — *see* Perichondritis, ear
  specified type NEC H61.19-
 pituitary gland E23.7

Disorder — *continued*
 pituitary gland— *continued*
  iatrogenic (postprocedural) E89.3
  specified NEC E23.6
 platelets D69.1
 plexus G54.9
  specified NEC G54.8
 polymorphonuclear neutrophils D71
 porphyrin metabolism — *see* Porphyria
 postconcussional F07.81
 posthallucinogen perception F16.983
  in
   abuse F16.183
   dependence F16.283
 postmenopausal N95.9
  specified NEC N95.8
 postprocedural (postoperative) — *see*
   Complications, postprocedural
 post-transplant lymphoproliferative D47.z1
 post-traumatic stress (PTSD) F43.10
  acute F43.0
  chronic F43.12
 premenstrual dysphoric (PMDD) N94.3
 prepuce N47.8
 propionic acidemia E71.121
 prostate N42.9
  specified NEC N42.89
 psychogenic NOS (*see also* condition) F45.9
  anxiety F41.8
  appetite F50.9
  asthenic F48.8
  cardiovascular (system) F45.8
  compulsive F42
  cutaneous F54
  depressive F32.9
  digestive (system) F45.8
  dysmenorrheic F45.8
  dyspneic F45.8
  endocrine (system) F54
  eye NEC F45.8
  feeding — *see* Disorder, eating
  functional NEC F45.8
  gastric F45.8
  gastrointestinal (system) F45.8
  genitourinary (system) F45.8
  heart (function) (rhythm) F45.8
  hyperventilatory F45.8
  hypochondriacal — *see* Disorder,
    hypochondriacal
  intestinal F45.8
  joint F45.8
  learning F81.9
  limb F45.8
  lymphatic (system) F45.8
  menstrual F45.8
  micturition F45.8
  monoplegic NEC F44.4
  motor F44.4
  muscle F45.8
  musculoskeletal F45.8
  neurocirculatory F45.8
  obsessive F42
  occupational F48.8
  organ or part of body NEC F45.8
  paralytic NEC F44.4
  phobic F40.9
  physical NEC F45.8
  rectal F45.8
  respiratory (system) F45.8
  rheumatic F45.8
  sexual (function) F52.9
  skin (allergic) (eczematous) F54
  sleep F51.9
  specified part of body NEC F45.8
  stomach F45.8
 psychological F99
  associated with
   disease classified elsewhere F54
   sexual
    development F66
    relationship F66
   uncertainty about gender identity F66

Disorder — *continued*
 psychomotor NEC F44.4
  hysterical F44.4
 psychoneurotic (*see also* Neurosis)
  mixed NEC F48.8
 psychophysiologic — *see* Disorder, somatoform
 psychosexual F65.9
  development F66
  identity of childhood F64.2
 psychosomatic NOS — *see* Disorder, somatoform
  multiple F45.0
  undifferentiated F45.1
 psychotic — *see* Psychosis
  transient (acute) F23
 puberty E30.9
  specified NEC E30.8
 pulmonary (valve) — *see* Endocarditis, pulmonary
 purine metabolism E79.9
 pyrimidine metabolism E79.9
 pyruvate metabolism E74.4
 reactive attachment (childhood) F94.1
 reading R48.0
  developmental (specific) F81.0
 receptive language F80.2
 receptor, hormonal, peripheral (*see also* Syndrome,
   androgen insensitivity) E34.50
 recurrent brief depressive F33.8
 reflex R29.2
 refraction H52.7
  aniseikonia H52.32
  anisometropia H52.31
  astigmatism — *see* Astigmatism
  hypermetropia — *see* Hypermetropia
  myopia — *see* Myopia
  presbyopia H52.4
  specified NEC H52.6
 relationship F68.8
  due to sexual orientation F66
 REM sleep behavior G47.52
 renal function, impaired (tubular) N25.9
 resonance R49.9
  specified NEC R49.8
 respiratory function, impaired (*see also* Failure,
   respiration)
  postprocedural — *see* Complication,
    postoperative, respiratory system
  psychogenic F45.8
 retina H35.9
  angioid streaks H35.33
  changes in vascular appearance H35.01-
  degeneration — *see* Degeneration, retina
  dystrophy (hereditary) — *see* Dystrophy, retina
  edema H35.81
  hemorrhage — *see* Hemorrhage, retina
  ischemia H35.82
  macular degeneration — *see* Degeneration,
   macula
  microaneurysms H35.04-
  microvascular abnormality NEC H35.09
  neovascularization — *see* Neovascularization,
   retina
  retinopathy — *see* Retinopathy
  separation of layers H35.70
   central serous chorioretinopathy H35.71-
   pigment epithelium detachment (serous)
    H35.72-
    hemorrhagic H35.73-
  specified type NEC H35.89
  telangiectasis — *see* Telangiectasis, retina
  vasculitis — *see* Vasculitis, retina
 retroperitoneal K68.9
 right hemisphere organic affective F07.89
 rumination (infant or child) F98.21
 sacrum, sacrococcygeal NEC M53.3
 schizoaffective F25.9
  bipolar type F25.8
  depressive type F25.1
  manic type F25.0
  mixed type F25.8
  specified NEC F25.8
 schizoid of childhood F84.5
 schizophreniform F20.81
  brief F23

Disorder — *continued*
 schizotypal (personality) F21
 secretion, thyrocalcitonin E07.0
 seizure R56.9
  intractable G40.919
   with status epilepticus G40.911
 semantic pragmatic F80.89
  with autism F84.0
 sense of smell R43.1
  psychogenic F45.8
 separation anxiety, of childhood F93.0
 sexual
  arousal, female F52.22
  aversion F52.1
  function, psychogenic F52.9
  maturation F66
  nonorganic F52.9
  preference (*see also* Deviation, sexual) F65.9
   fetishistic transvestism F65.1
  relationship F66
 shyness, of childhood and adolescence F40.10
 sibling rivalry F93.8
 sickle-cell (sickling) (homozygous) See Disease,
   sickle-cell
  heterozygous D57.3
  specified type NEC D57.8-
  trait D57.3
 sinus (nasal) J34.9
  specified NEC J34.89
 skin L98.9
  atrophic L90.9
   specified NEC L90.8
  newborn P83.9
   specified NEC P83.8
  granulomatous L92.9
   specified NEC L92.8
  hypertrophic L91.9
   specified NEC L91.8
  infiltrative NEC L98.6
  psychogenic (allergic) (eczematous) F54
 sleep G47.9
  breathing-related — *see* Apnea, sleep
  circadian rhythm G47.20
   advance sleep phase type G47.22
   delayed sleep phase type G47.21
   due to
    alcohol
     abuse F10.182
     dependence F10.282
     use F10.982
    amphetamines
     abuse F15.182
     dependence F15.282
     use F15.982
    caffeine
     abuse F15.182
     dependence F15.282
     use F15.982
    cocaine
     abuse F14.182
     dependence F14.282
     use F14.982
    drug NEC
     abuse F19.182
     dependence F19.282
     use F19.982
    opioid
     abuse F11.182
     dependence F11.282
     use F11.982
    psychoactive substance NEC
     abuse F19.182
     dependence F19.282
     use F19.982
    sedative, hypnotic, or anxiolytic
     abuse F13.182
     dependence F13.282
     use F13.982
    stimulant NEC
     abuse F15.182
     dependence F15.282
     use F15.982
   free running type G47.24

Disorder — *continued*
 sleep— *continued*
  circadian rhythm— *continued*
   in conditions classified elsewhere G47.27
   irregular sleep wake type G47.23
   jet lag type G47.25
   shift work type G47.26
   specified NEC G47.29
   due to
    alcohol
     abuse F10.182
     dependence F10.282
     use F10.982
    amphetamine
     abuse F15.182
     dependence F15.282
     use F15.982
    anxiolytic
     abuse F13.182
     dependence F13.282
     use F13.982
    caffeine
     abuse F15.182
     dependence F15.282
     use F15.982
    cocaine
     abuse F14.182
     dependence F14.282
     use F14.982
    drug NEC
     abuse F19.182
     dependence F19.282
     use F19.982
    hypnotic
     abuse F13.182
     dependence F13.282
     use F13.982
    opioid
     abuse F11.182
     dependence F11.282
     use F11.982
    psychoactive substance NEC
     abuse F19.182
     dependence F19.282
     use F19.982
    sedative
     abuse F13.182
     dependence F13.282
     use F13.982
    stimulant NEC
     abuse F15.182
     dependence F15.282
     use F15.982
  emotional F51.9
  excessive somnolence — *see* Hypersomnia
  hypersomnia type — *see* Hypersomnia
  initiating or maintaining — *see* Insomnia
  nightmares F51.5
  nonorganic F51.9
   specified NEC F51.8
  parasomnia type G47.50
  specified NEC G47.8
  terrors F51.4
  walking F51.3
 sleep-wake pattern or schedule — *see* Disorder,
   sleep, circadian rhythm
 social
  anxiety of childhood F40.10
  functioning in childhood F94.9
   specified NEC F94.8
 soft tissue M79.9
  ankle M79.9
  due to use, overuse and pressure M70.90
   ankle M70.97-
   bursitis — *see* Bursitis
   foot M70.97-
   forearm M70.93-
   hand M70.94-
   lower leg M70.96-
   multiple sites M70.99
   pelvic region M70.95-
   shoulder region M70.91-
   specified site NEC M70.98

Displacement, displaced— *continued*
canaliculus (lacrimalis), congenital Q10.6
cardia through esophageal hiatus (congenital) Q40.1
cerebellum, caudal (congenital) Q04.8
cervix — *see* Malposition, uterus
colon (congenital) Q43.3
device, implant or graft (*see also* Complications, by site and type, mechanical) T85.9
   arterial graft NEC — *see* Complication, cardio-vascular device, mechanical, vascular
   breast (implant) T85.42
   catheter NEC T85.628
    dialysis (renal) T82.42
     intraperitoneal T85.621
    infusion NEC T82.524
     spinal (epidural) (subdural) T85.620
    urinary (indwelling) T83.028
     cystostomy T83.020
   electronic (electrode) (pulse generator) (stimulator) — *see* Complication, electronic stimulator
   fixation, internal (orthopedic) NEC — *see* Complication, fixation device, mechanical
   gastrointestinal — *see* Complications, prosthetic device, mechanical, gastrointestinal device
   genital NEC T83.428
    intrauterine contraceptive device T83.32
    penile prosthesis T83.420
   heart NEC — *see* Complication, cardiovascular device, mechanical
   joint prosthesis — *see* Complications, joint prosthesis, mechanical
   ocular — *see* Complications, prosthetic device, mechanical, ocular device
   orthopedic NEC — *see* Complication, orthopedic, device or graft, mechanical
   specified NEC T85.628
   urinary NEC (*see also* Complication, genitourinary, device, urinary, mechanical)
    graft T83.22
   vascular NEC — *see* Complication, cardiovascular device, mechanical
   ventricular intracranial shunt T85.02
electronic stimulator
   bone T84.320
   cardiac — *see* Complications, cardiac device, electronic
   nervous system — *see* Complication, prosthetic device, mechanical, electronic nervous system stimulator
   urinary — *see* Complications, electronic stimulator, urinary
esophageal mucosa into cardia of stomach, congenital Q39.8
esophagus (acquired) K22.8
   congenital Q39.8
eyeball (acquired) (lateral) (old) — *see* Displacement, globe
   congenital Q15.8
   current — *see* Avulsion, eye
fallopian tube (acquired) N83.4
   congenital Q50.6
   opening (congenital) Q50.6
gallbladder (congenital) Q44.1
gastric mucosa (congenital) Q40.2
globe (acquired) (old) (lateral) H05.21-
   current — *see* Avulsion, eye
heart (congenital) Q24.8
   acquired I51.89
hymen (upward) (congenital) Q52.4
intervertebral disc NEC
   with myelopathy — *see* Disorder, disc, with, myelopathy
   cervical, cervicothoracic (with) M50.20
    myelopathy — *see* Disorder, disc, cervical, with myelopathy
    neuritis, radiculitis or radiculopathy — *see* Disorder, disc, cervical, with neuritis
   due to trauma — *see* Dislocation, vertebra
   lumbar region M51.26
    with
     myelopathy M51.06

Displacement, displaced— *continued*
intervertebral disc— *continued*
   lumbar region— *continued*
    with— *continued*
     neuritis, radiculitis, radiculopathy or sciatica M51.16
   lumbosacral region M51.27
    with
     myelopathy M51.07
     neuritis, radiculitis, radiculopathy or sciatica M51.17
   sacrococcygeal region M53.3
   thoracic region M51.24
    with
     myelopathy M51.04
     neuritis, radiculitis, radiculopathy M51.14
   thoracolumbar region M51.25
    with
     myelopathy M51.05
     neuritis, radiculitis, radiculopathy M51.15
intrauterine device T83.32
kidney (acquired) N28.83
   congenital Q63.2
lachrymal, lacrimal apparatus or duct (congenital) Q10.6
lens, congenital Q12.1
macula (congenital) Q14.1
Meckel's diverticulum Q43.0
   malignant — *see* Table of Neoplasms, small intestine, malignant
nail (congenital) Q84.6
   acquired L60.8
oesophagus (acquired) — *see* Displacement, esophagus
opening of Wharton's duct in mouth Q38.4
organ or site, congenital NEC — *see* Malposition, congenital
ovary (acquired) N83.4
   congenital Q50.39
   free in peritoneal cavity (congenital) Q50.39
   into hernial sac N83.4
oviduct (acquired) N83.4
   congenital Q50.6
parathyroid (gland) E21.4
parotid gland (congenital) Q38.4
punctum lacrimale (congenital) Q10.6
sacro-iliac (joint) (congenital) Q74.2
   current injury S33.2
   old — *see* subcategory M53.2
salivary gland (any) (congenital) Q38.4
spleen (congenital) Q89.09
stomach, congenital Q40.2
sublingual duct Q38.4
tongue (downward) (congenital) Q38.3
tooth, teeth, fully erupted M26.30
   horizontal M26.33
   vertical M26.34
trachea (congenital) Q32.1
ureter or ureteric opening or orifice (congenital) Q62.62
uterine opening of oviducts or fallopian tubes Q50.6
uterus, uterine — *see* Malposition, uterus
ventricular septum Q21.0
   with rudimentary ventricle Q20.4
Disproportion
between native and reconstructed breast N65.1
fiber-type G71.2
Disruptio uteri — *see* Rupture, uterus
Disruption (of)
ciliary body NEC H21.89
closure of
   cornea T81.31
   craniotomy T81.32
   fascia (muscular) (superficial) T81.32
   internal organ or tissue T81.32
   laceration (external) (internal) T81.33
   ligament T81.32
   mucosa T81.31
   muscle or muscle flap T81.32
   ribs or rib cage T81.32
   skin and subcutaneous tissue (full-thickness) (superficial) T81.31
   skull T81.32

Disruption — *continued*
closure of— *continued*
   sternum (sternotomy) T81.32
   tendon T81.32
   traumatic laceration (external) (internal) T81.33
family Z63.8
   due to
    absence of family member NEC Z63.32
    absence of family member due to military deployment Z63.31
    alcoholism and drug addiction in family Z63.72
    bereavement Z63.4
    death (assumed) or disappearance of family member Z63.4
    divorce or separation Z63.5
    drug addiction in family Z63.72
    return of family member from military deploy-ment (current or past conflict) Z63.71
    stressful life events NEC Z63.79
iris NEC H21.89
ligament(s) (*see also* Sprain)
   knee
    current injury — *see* Dislocation, knee
    old (chronic) — *see* Derangement, knee, instability
    spontaneous NEC — *see* Derangement, knee, disruption ligament
ossicular chain — *see* Discontinuity, ossicles, ear
pelvic ring (stable) S32.810
   unstable S32.811
wound T81.30
   episiotomy O90.1
   operation T81.31
    cesarean O90.0
    external operation wound (superficial) T81.31
    internal operation wound (deep) T81.32
   perineal (obstetric) O90.1
   traumatic injury repair T81.33
   traumatic injury wound repair T81.33
Dissatisfaction with
employment Z56.9
school environment Z55.4
Dissecting — *see* condition
Dissection
aorta I71.00
   abdominal I71.02
   thoracic I71.01
   thoracoabdominal I71.03
artery
   carotid I77.71
   cerebral (nonruptured) I67.0
    ruptured — *see* Hemorrhage, intracranial, subarachnoid
   coronary I25.42
   iliac I77.72
   renal I77.73
   specified NEC I77.79
   vertebral I77.74
traumatic — *see* Wound, open, by site
vascular I99.8
wound — *see* Wound, open
Disseminated — *see* condition
Dissociation
auriculoventricular or atrioventricular (AV) (any degree) (isorhythmic) I45.89
   with heart block I44.2
interference I45.89
Dissociative reaction, state F44.9
Dissolution, vertebra — *see* Osteoporosis
Distension, distention
abdomen R14.0
bladder N32.89
cecum K63.89
colon K63.89
gallbladder K82.8
intestine K63.89
kidney N28.89
liver K76.8
seminal vesicle N50.8
stomach K31.89
   acute K31.0
   psychogenic F45.8

Distension, distention— *continued*
  ureter — *see* Dilatation, ureter
  uterus N85.8
Distoma hepaticum infestation B66.3
Distomiasis B66.9
  bile passages B66.3
  hemic B65.9
  hepatic B66.3
    due to Clonorchis sinensis B66.1
  intestinal B66.5
  liver B66.3
    due to Clonorchis sinensis B66.1
  lung B66.4
  pulmonary B66.4
Distomolar (fourth molar) K00.1
Disto-occlusion (Division I) (Division II) M26.212
Distortion(s) (congenital)
  adrenal (gland) Q89.1
  arm NEC Q68.8
  bile duct or passage Q44.5
  bladder Q64.79
  brain Q04.9
  cervix (uteri) Q51.9
  chest (wall) Q67.8
    bones Q76.8
  clavicle Q74.0
  clitoris Q52.6
  coccyx Q76.49
  common duct Q44.5
  coronary Q24.5
  cystic duct Q44.5
  ear (auricle) (external) Q17.3
    inner Q16.5
    middle Q16.4
      ossicles Q16.3
  endocrine NEC Q89.2
  eustachian tube Q17.8
  eye (adnexa) Q15.8
  face bone(s) NEC Q75.8
  fallopian tube Q50.6
  femur NEC Q68.8
  fibula NEC Q68.8
  finger(s) Q68.1
  foot Q66.9
  genitalia, genital organ(s)
    female Q52.8
      external Q52.79
      internal NEC Q52.8
  gyri Q04.8
  hand bone(s) Q68.1
  heart (auricle) (ventricle) Q24.8
    valve (cusp) Q24.8
  hepatic duct Q44.5
  humerus NEC Q68.8
  hymen Q52.4
  intrafamilial communications Z63.8
  jaw NEC M26.89
  labium (majus) (minus) Q52.79
  leg NEC Q68.8
  lens Q12.8
  liver Q44.7
  lumbar spine Q76.49
    with disproportion O33.8
      causing obstructed labor O65.0
  lumbosacral (joint) (region) Q76.49
    kyphosis — *see* Kyphosis, congenital
    lordosis — *see* Lordosis, congenital
  nerve Q07.8
  nose Q30.8
  organ
    of Corti Q16.5
    or site not listed — *see* Anomaly, by site
  ossicles, ear Q16.3
  oviduct Q50.6
  pancreas Q45.3
  parathyroid (gland) Q89.2
  pituitary (gland) Q89.2
  radius NEC Q68.8
  sacroiliac joint Q74.2
  sacrum Q76.49
  scapula Q74.0
  shoulder girdle Q74.0

Distortion(s)— *continued*
  skull bone(s) NEC Q75.8
    with
      anencephalus Q00.0
      encephalocele — *see* Encephalocele
      hydrocephalus Q03.9
        with spina bifida — *see* Spina bifida, with
          hydrocephalus
      microcephaly Q02
  spinal cord Q06.8
  spine Q76.49
    kyphosis — *see* Kyphosis, congenital
    lordosis — *see* Lordosis, congenital
  spleen Q89.09
  sternum NEC Q76.7
  thorax (wall) Q67.8
    bony Q76.8
  thymus (gland) Q89.2
  thyroid (gland) Q89.2
  tibia NEC Q68.8
  toe(s) Q66.9
  tongue Q38.3
  trachea (cartilage) Q32.1
  ulna NEC Q68.8
  ureter Q62.8
  urethra Q64.79
    causing obstruction Q64.39
  uterus Q51.9
  vagina Q52.4
  vertebra Q76.49
    kyphosis — *see* Kyphosis, congenital
    lordosis — *see* Lordosis, congenital
  visual (*see also* Disturbance, vision)
    shape and size H53.15
  vulva Q52.79
  wrist (bones) (joint) Q68.8
Distress
  abdomen — *see* Pain, abdominal
  acute respiratory (adult) (child) J80
  epigastric R10.13
  fetal P84
    complicating pregnancy — *see* Stress, fetal
  gastrointestinal (functional) K30
    psychogenic F45.8
  intestinal (functional) NOS K59.9
    psychogenic F45.8
  maternal, during labor and delivery O75.0
  respiratory R06.00
    adult J80
    child J80
    newborn P22.9
      specified NEC P22.8
    orthopnea R06.01
    psychogenic F45.8
    shortness of breath R06.02
    specified type NEC R06.09
Distribution vessel, atypical Q27.9
  coronary artery Q24.5
  precerebral Q28.1
Districhiasis L68.8
Disturbance(s) (*see also* Disease)
  absorption K90.9
    calcium E58
    carbohydrate K90.4
    fat K90.4
      pancreatic K90.3
    protein K90.4
    starch K90.4
    vitamin — *see* Deficiency, vitamin
  acid-base equilibrium E87.8
    mixed E87.4
  activity and attention (with hyperkinesis) — *see*
    Disorder, attention-deficit hyperactivity
  amino acid transport E72.00
  assimilation, food K90.9
  auditory nerve, except deafness — *see* subcategory
    H93.3
  behavior — *see* Disorder, conduct
  blood clotting (mechanism) (*see also* Defect,
    coagulation) D68.9
  cerebral
    nerve — *see* Disorder, nerve, cranial

Disturbance(s) — *continued*
  cerebral— *continued*
    status, newborn P91.9
      specified NEC P91.8
  circulatory I99.9
  conduct (*see also* Disorder, conduct) F91.9
    adjustment reaction — *see* Disorder, adjustment
    compulsive F63.9
    disruptive F91.9
    hyperkinetic — *see* Disorder, attention-deficit
      hyperactivity
    socialized F91.2
    specified NEC F91.8
    unsocialized F91.1
  coordination R27.8
  cranial nerve — *see* Disorder, nerve, cranial
  deep sensibility — *see* Disturbance, sensation
  digestive K30
    psychogenic F45.8
  electrolyte (*see also* Imbalance, electrolyte)
    newborn, transitory P74.4
      hyperammonemia P74.6
      potassium balance P74.3
      sodium balance P74.2
      specified type NEC P74.4
  emotions specific to childhood and adolescence
    F93.9
    with
      anxiety and fearfulness NEC F93.8
      elective mutism F94.0
      oppositional disorder F91.3
      sensitivity (withdrawal) F40.10
      shyness F40.10
      social withdrawal F40.10
    involving relationship problems F93.8
    mixed F93.8
    specified NEC F93.8
  endocrine (gland) E34.9
    neonatal, transitory P72.9
      specified NEC P72.8
  equilibrium R42
  fructose metabolism E74.10
  gait — *see* Gait
    hysterical F44.4
    psychogenic F44.4
  gastrointestinal (functional) K30
    psychogenic F45.8
  habit, child F98.9
  hearing, except deafness and tinnitus — *see*
    Abnormal, auditory perception
  heart, functional (conditions in I44-I50)
    due to presence of (cardiac) prosthesis I97.19-
    postoperative I97.89
      cardiac surgery I97.19-
  hormones E34.9
  innervation uterus (parasympathetic) (sympathetic)
    N85.8
  keratinization NEC
    gingiva K05.10
      plaque induced K05.10
      nonplaque induced K05.11
    lip K13.0
    oral (mucosa) (soft tissue) K13.29
    tongue K13.29
  learning (specific) — *see* Disorder, learning
  memory — *see* Amnesia
    mild, following organic brain damage F06.8
  mental F99
    associated with diseases classified elsewhere F54
  metabolism E88.9
    with
      abortion — *see* Abortion, by type with other
        specified complication
      ectopic pregnancy O08.5
      molar pregnancy O08.5
    amino-acid E72.9
      aromatic E70.9
      branched-chain E71.2
      straight-chain E72.8
      sulfur-bearing E72.10
    ammonia E72.20
    arginine E72.21
    arginosuccinic acid E72.22

Disturbance(s) — *continued*
  metabolism— *continued*
    carbohydrate E74.9
    cholesterol E78.9
    citrulline E72.23
    cystathionine E72.19
    general E88.9
    glutamine E72.8
    histidine E70.40
    homocystine E72.19
    hydroxylysine E72.3
    in labor or delivery O75.89
    iron E83.10
    lipoid E78.9
    lysine E72.3
    methionine E72.19
    neonatal, transitory P74.9
      calcium and magnesium P71.9
        specified type NEC P71.8
      carbohydrate metabolism P70.9
        specified type NEC P70.8
      specified NEC P74.8
    ornithine E72.4
    phosphate E83.39
    sodium NEC E87.8
    threonine E72.8
    tryptophan E70.5
    tyrosine E70.20
    urea cycle E72.20
  motor R29.2
  nervous, functional R45.0
  neuromuscular mechanism (eye), due to syphilis
    A52.15
  nutritional E63.9
    nail L60.3
  ocular motion H51.9
    psychogenic F45.8
  oculogyric H51.8
    psychogenic F45.8
  oculomotor H51.9
    psychogenic F45.8
  olfactory nerve R43.1
  optic nerve NEC — *see* Disorder, nerve, optic
  oral epithelium, including tongue NEC K13.29
  perceptual due to
    alcohol withdrawal F10.232
    amphetamine intoxication F15.922
      in
        abuse F15.122
        dependence F15.222
    anxiolytic withdrawal F13.232
    cannabis intoxication (acute) F12.922
      in
        abuse F12.122
        dependence F12.222
    cocaine intoxication (acute) F14.922
      in
        abuse F14.122
        dependence F14.222
    hypnotic withdrawal F13.232
    opioid intoxication (acute) F11.922
      in
        abuse F11.122
        dependence F11.222
    phencyclidine intoxication (acute) F19.922
      in
        abuse F19.122
        dependence F19.222
    sedative withdrawal F13.232
  personality (pattern) (trait) (*see also* Disorder,
    personality) F60.9
    following organic brain damage F07.9
  polyglandular E31.9
    specified NEC E31.8
  potassium balance, newborn P74.3
  psychogenic F45.9
  psychomotor F44.4
  psychophysical visual H53.16
  pupillary — *see* Anomaly, pupil, function
  reflex R29.2
  rhythm, heart I49.9
  salivary secretion K11.7

Disturbance(s) — *continued*
  sensation (cold) (heat) (localization) (tactile
    discrimination) (texture) (vibratory) NEC R20.9
    hysterical F44.6
    skin R20.9
      anesthesia R20.0
      hyperesthesia R20.3
      hypoesthesia R20.1
      paresthesia R20.2
      specified type NEC R20.8
    smell R43.9
      and taste (mixed) R43.8
      anosmia R43.0
      parosmia R43.1
      specified NEC R43.8
    taste R43.9
      and smell (mixed) R43.8
      parageusia R43.2
      specified NEC R43.8
  sensory — *see* Disturbance, sensation
  situational (transient) (*see also* Disorder, adjustment)
    acute F43.0
  sleep G47.9
    nonorganic origin F51.9
  smell — *see* Disturbance, sensation, smell
  sociopathic F60.2
  sodium balance, newborn P74.2
  speech R47.9
    developmental F80.9
    specified NEC R47.89
  stomach (functional) K31.9
  sympathetic (nerve) G90.9
  taste — *see* Disturbance, sensation, taste
  temperature
    regulation, newborn P81.9
      specified NEC P81.8
    sense R20.8
      hysterical F44.6
  tooth
    eruption K00.6
    formation K00.4
    structure, hereditary NEC K00.5
  touch — *see* Disturbance, sensation
  vascular I99.9
    arteriosclerotic — *see* Arteriosclerosis
  vasomotor I73.9
  vasospastic I73.9
  vision, visual H53.9
    following
      cerebrovascular disease I69.998
        specified NEC I69.898
        cerebral infarction I69.398
        intracerebral hemorrhage I69.198
        nontraumatic intracranial hemorrhage
          NEC I69.298
        specified disease NEC I69.898
        subarachnoid hemorrhage I69.098
    psychophysical H53.16
    specified NEC H53.8
    subjective H53.10
      day blindness H53.11
      discomfort H53.14-
      distortions of shape and size H53.15
      loss
        sudden H53.13-
        transient H53.12-
      specified type NEC H53.19
  voice R49.9
    psychogenic F44.4
    specified NEC R49.8
Diuresis R35.8
Diver's palsy, paralysis or squeeze T70.3
Diverticulitis (acute) K57.92
  bladder — *see* Cystitis
  ileum — *see* Diverticulitis, intestine, small
  intestine K57.92
    with
      abscess, perforation or peritonitis K57.80
        with bleeding K57.81
      bleeding K57.93
    congenital Q43.8
    large K57.32

Diverticulitis — *continued*
  intestine— *continued*
    large— *continued*
      with
        abscess, perforation or peritonitis K57.20
          with bleeding K57.21
        bleeding K57.33
        small intestine K57.52
          with
            abscess, perforation or peritonitis
              K57.40
                with bleeding K57.41
              bleeding K57.53
    small K57.12
      with
        abscess, perforation or peritonitis K57.00
          with bleeding K57.01
        bleeding K57.13
        large intestine K57.52
          with
            abscess, perforation or peritonitis
              K57.40
                with bleeding K57.41
              bleeding K57.53
Diverticulosis K57.90
  with bleeding K57.91
  large intestine K57.30
    with
      bleeding K57.31
      small intestine K57.50
        with bleeding K57.51
  small intestine K57.10
    with
      bleeding K57.11
      large intestine K57.50
        with bleeding K57.51
Diverticulum, diverticula (multiple) K57.90
  appendix (noninflammatory) K38.2
  bladder (sphincter) N32.3
    congenital Q64.6
  bronchus (congenital) Q32.4
    acquired J98.09
  calyx, calyceal (kidney) N28.89
  cardia (stomach) K31.4
  cecum — *see* Diverticulosis, intestine, large
    congenital Q43.8
  colon — *see* Diverticulosis, intestine, large
    congenital Q43.8
  duodenum — *see* Diverticulosis, intestine, small
    congenital Q43.8
  epiphrenic (esophagus) K22.5
  esophagus (congenital) Q39.6
    acquired (epiphrenic) (pulsion) (traction) K22.5
  eustachian tube — *see* Disorder, eustachian tube,
    specified NEC
  fallopian tube N83.8
  gastric K31.4
  heart (congenital) Q24.8
  ileum — *see* Diverticulosis, intestine, small
  jejunum — *see* Diverticulosis, intestine, small
  kidney (pelvis) (calyces) N28.89
    with calculus — *see* Calculus, kidney
  Meckel's (displaced) (hypertrophic) Q43.0
    malignant — *see* Table of Neoplasms, small
      intestine, malignant
  midthoracic K22.5
  organ or site, congenital NEC — *see* Distortion
  pericardium (congenital) (cyst) Q24.8
    acquired I31.8
  pharyngoesophageal (congenital) Q39.6
    acquired K22.5
  pharynx (congenital) Q38.7
  rectosigmoid — *see* Diverticulosis, intestine, large
    congenital Q43.8
  rectum — *see* Diverticulosis, intestine, large
  Rokitansky's K22.5
  seminal vesicle N50.8
  sigmoid — *see* Diverticulosis, intestine, large
    congenital Q43.8
  stomach (acquired) K31.4
    congenital Q40.2
  trachea (acquired) J39.8

Diverticulum, diverticula — *continued*
  ureter (acquired) N28.89
    congenital Q62.8
  ureterovesical orifice N28.89
  urethra (acquired) N36.1
    congenital Q64.79
  ventricle, left (congenital) Q24.8
  vesical N32.3
    congenital Q64.6
  Zenker's (esophagus) K22.5
Division
  cervix uteri (acquired) N88.8
  glans penis Q55.69
  labia minora (congenital) Q52.79
  ligament (partial or complete) (current) (*see also*
      Sprain)
    with open wound — *see* Wound, open
  muscle (partial or complete) (current) (*see also*
      Injury, muscle)
    with open wound — *see* Wound, open
  nerve (traumatic) — *see* Injury, nerve
  spinal cord — *see* Injury, spinal cord, by region
  vein I87.8
Divorce, causing family disruption Z63.5
Dix-Hallpike neurolabyrinthitis — *see* Neuronitis,
    vestibular
Dizziness R42
  hysterical F44.89
  psychogenic F45.8
DMAC (disseminated mycobacterium
    aviumtracellulare complex) A31.2
DNR (do not resuscitate) Z66
Doan-Wiseman syndrome (primary splenic
    neutropenia) — *see* Agranulocytosis
Doehle-Heller aortitis A52.02
Dog bite — *see* Bite
Dohle body panmyelopathic syndrome D72.0
Dolichocephaly Q67.2
Dolichocolon Q43.8
Dolichostenomelia — *see* Syndrome, Marfan's
Donohue's syndrome E34.8
Donor (organ or tissue) Z52.9
  blood (whole) Z52.000
    autologous Z52.010
    specified donor NEC Z52.090
    specified component (lymphocytes) (platelets)
        NEC Z52.008
      autologous Z52.018
      specified donor NEC Z52.098
    stem cells Z52.001
      autologous Z52.011
      specified donor NEC Z52.091
  bone Z52.20
    autologous Z52.21
    marrow Z52.3
    specified type NEC Z52.29
  cornea Z52.5
  egg (Oocyte) Z52.819
    age 35 and over Z52.812
      anonymous recipient Z52.812
      designated recipient Z52.813
    under age 35 Z52.810
      anonymous recipient Z52.810
      designated recipient Z52.811
  kidney Z52.4
  liver Z52.6
  lung Z52.89
  lymphocyte *see* Donor, blood, specified components
      NEC
  Oocyte — *see* Donor, egg
  platelets Z52.008
  potential, examination of Z00.5
  semen Z52.89
  skin Z52.10
    autologous Z52.11
    specified type NEC Z52.19
  specified organ or tissue NEC Z52.89
  sperm Z52.89
Donovanosis A58
Dorsalgia M54.9
  psychogenic F45.41
  specified NEC M54.89

Dorsopathy M53.9
  deforming M43.9
    specified NEC — *see* subcategory M43.8
  specified NEC M53.80
    cervical region M53.82
    cervicothoracic region M53.83
    lumbar region M53.86
    lumbosacral region M53.87
    occipito-atlanto-axial region M53.81
    sacrococcygeal region M53.88
    thoracic region M53.84
    thoracolumbar region M53.85
Double
  albumin E88.09
  aortic arch Q25.4
  auditory canal Q17.8
  auricle (heart) Q20.8
  bladder Q64.79
  cervix Q51.820
    with doubling of uterus (and vagina) Q51.10
      with obstruction Q51.11
  inlet ventricle Q20.4
  kidney with double pelvis (renal) Q63.0
  meatus urinarius Q64.75
  monster Q89.4
  outlet
    left ventricle Q20.2
    right ventricle Q20.1
  pelvis (renal) with double ureter Q62.5
  tongue Q38.3
  ureter (one or both sides) Q62.5
    with double pelvis (renal) Q62.5
  urethra Q64.74
  urinary meatus Q64.75
  uterus Q51.2
    with
      doubling of cervix (and vagina) Q51.10
        with obstruction Q51.11
    in pregnancy or childbirth O34.59-
      causing obstructed labor O65.5
  vagina Q52.10
    with doubling of uterus (and cervix) Q51.10
      with obstruction Q51.11
  vision H53.2
  vulva Q52.79
Down syndrome Q90.9
  meiotic nondisjunction Q90.0
  mitotic nondisjunction Q90.1
  mosaicism Q90.1
  translocation Q90.2
Dracontiasis B72
Dracunculiasis, dracunculosis B72
Dream state, hysterical F44.89
Dreschlera (hawaiiensis) (infection) B43.8
Drepanocytic anemia — *see* Disease, sickle-cell
Dresbach's syndrome (elliptocytosis) D58.1
Dressler's syndrome I24.1
Drift, ulnar — *see* Deformity, limb, specified type NEC,
    forearm
Drinking (alcohol)
  excessive, to excess NEC (without dependence)
      F10.10
    habitual (continual) (without remission) F10.20
      with remission F10.21
Drip, postnasal (chronic) R09.82
  due to
    allergic rhinitis — *see* Rhinitis, allergic
    common cold J00
    gastroesophageal reflux — *see* Reflux,
        gastroesophageal
    nasopharyngitis — *see* Nasopharyngitis
    other know condition—code to condition
    sinusitis — *see* Sinusitis
Droop
  facial R29.810
    cerebrovascular disease I69.992
      specified NEC I69.892
      cerebral infarction I69.392
      intracerebral hemorrhage I69.192
      nontraumatic intracranial hemorrhage NEC
          I69.292
      specified disease NEC I69.892
      subarachnoid hemorrhage I69.092

Drop (in)
  attack NEC R55
  finger — *see* Deformity, finger
  foot — *see* Deformity, limb, foot, drop
  hematocrit (precipitous) R71.0
  hemoglobin R71.0
  toe — *see* Deformity, toe, specified NEC
  wrist — *see* Deformity, limb, wrist drop
Dropped heart beats I45.9
Dropsy, dropsical (*see also* Hydrops)
  abdomen R18.8
  brain — *see* Hydrocephalus
  cardiac, heart — *see* Failure, heart, congestive
  gangrenous — *see* Gangrene
  heart — *see* Failure, heart, congestive
  kidney — *see* Nephrosis
  lung — *see* Edema, lung
  newborn due to isoimmunization P56.0
  pericardium — *see* Pericarditis
Drowned, drowning (near) T75.1
Drowsiness R40.0
Drug
  abuse counseling and surveillance Z71.51
  addiction — *see* Dependence
  dependence — *see* Dependence
  habit — *see* Dependence
  harmful use — *see* Abuse, drug
  induced fever R50.2
  overdose — *see* Table of Drugs and Chemicals, by
      drug, poisoning
  poisoning — *see* Table of Drugs and Chemicals, by
      drug, poisoning
  resistant organism infection Z16
  therapy
    long term (current) (prophylactic) — *see* Therapy,
        drug long-term (current) (prophylactic)
    short term — *omit code*
  wrong substance given or taken in error — *see* Table
      of Drugs and Chemicals, by drug, poisoning
Drunkenness (without dependence) F10.129
  acute in alcoholism F10.229
  chronic (without remission) F10.20
    with remission F10.21
  pathological (without dependence) F10.129
    with dependence F10.229
  sleep F51.9
Drusen
  macula (degenerative) (retina) — *see* Degeneration,
      macula, drusen
  optic disc H47.32-
Dry, dryness (*see also* condition)
  larynx J38.7
  mouth R68.2
    due to dehydration E86.0
  nose J34.89
  socket (teeth) M27.3
  throat J39.2
DSAP L56.5
Duane's syndrome H50.81-
Dubin-Johnson disease or syndrome E80.6
Dubois' disease (thymus gland) A50.59 [E35]
Dubowitz' syndrome Q87.1
Duchenne-Aran muscular atrophy G12.21
Duchenne-Griesinger disease G71.0
Duchenne's
  disease or syndrome
    motor neuron disease G12.22
    muscular dystrophy G71.0
  locomotor ataxia (syphilitic) A52.11
  paralysis
    birth injury P14.0
    due to or associated with
      motor neuron disease G12.22
      muscular dystrophy G71.0
Ducrey's chancre A57
Duct, ductus — *see* condition
Duhring's disease (dermatitis herpetiformis) L13.0
Dullness, cardiac (decreased) (increased) R01.2
Dumb ague — *see* Malaria
Dumbness — *see* Aphasia
Dumdum fever B55.0
Dumping syndrome (postgastrectomy) K91.1

Duodenitis (nonspecific) (peptic) K29.80
  with bleeding K29.81
Duodenocholangitis — see Cholangitis
Duodenum, duodenal — see condition
Duplay's bursitis or periarthritis — see Tendinitis, calcific, shoulder
Duplication, duplex (see also Accessory)
  alimentary tract Q45.8
  anus Q43.4
  appendix (and cecum) Q43.4
  biliary duct (any) Q44.5
  bladder Q64.79
  cecum (and appendix) Q43.4
  cervix Q51.820
  chromosome NEC
    with complex rearrangements NEC Q92.5
    seen only at prometaphase Q92.8
  cystic duct Q44.5
  digestive organs Q45.8
  esophagus Q39.8
  frontonasal process Q75.8
  intestine (large) (small) Q43.4
  kidney Q63.0
  liver Q44.7
  oesophagus Q39.8
  pancreas Q45.3
  penis Q55.69
  respiratory organs NEC Q34.8
  salivary duct Q38.4
  spinal cord (incomplete) Q06.2
  stomach Q40.2
Dupré's disease (meningism) R29.1
Dupuytren's contraction or disease M72.0
Durand-Nicolas-Favre disease A55
Durotomy (inadvertent) (incidental) G97.41
Duroziez's disease (congenital mitral stenosis) Q23.2
Dutton's relapsing fever (West African) A68.1
Dwarfism E34.3
  achondroplastic Q77.4
  congenital E34.3
  constitutional E34.3
  hypochondroplastic Q77.4
  hypophyseal E23.0
  infantile E34.3
  Laron-type E34.3
  Lorain(-Levi) type E23.0
  metatropic Q77.8
  nephrotic-glycosuric (with hypophosphatemic rickets) E72.09
  nutritional E45
  pancreatic K86.8
  pituitary E23.0
  renal N25.0
  thanatophoric Q77.1
Dyke-Young anemia (secondary) (symptomatic) D59.1
Dysacusis — see Abnormal, auditory perception
Dysadrenocortism E27.9
  hyperfunction E27.0
Dysarthria R47.1
  following
    cerebral infarction I69.322
    cerebrovascular disease I69.922
      specified disease NEC I69.822
    intracerebral hemorrhage I69.122
    nontraumatic intracranial hemorrhage NEC I69.222
    subarachnoid hemorrhage I69.022
Dysautonomia (familial) G90.1
Dysbarism T70.3
Dysbasia R26.2
  angiosclerotica intermittens I73.9
  hysterical F44.4
  lordotica (progressiva) G24.1
  nonorganic origin F44.4
  psychogenic F44.4
Dysbetalipoproteinemia (familial) E78.2
Dyscalculia R48.8
  developmental F81.2
Dyschezia K59.00
Dyschondroplasia (with hemangiomata) Q78.4
Dyschromia (skin) L81.9
Dyscollagenosis M35.9

Dyscranio-pygo-phalangy Q87.0
Dyscrasia
  blood (with) D75.9
    antepartum hemorrhage — see Hemorrhage, antepartum, with coagulation defect
    newborn P61.9
      specified type NEC P61.8
    intrapartum hemorrhage O67.0
    puerperal, postpartum O72.3
  polyglandular, pluriglandular E31.9
Dysendocrinism E34.9
Dysentery, dysenteric (catarrhal) (diarrhea) (epidemic) (hemorrhagic) (infectious) (sporadic) (tropical) A09
  abscess, liver A06.4
  amebic (see also Amebiasis) A06.0
    with abscess — see Abscess, amebic
    acute A06.0
    chronic A06.1
  arthritis A09 (see also category M01)
    bacillary A03.9 (see also category M01)
  bacillary A03.9
    arthritis A03.9 (see also category M01)
    Boyd A03.2
    Flexner A03.1
    Schmitz(-Stutzer) A03.0
    Shiga(-Kruse) A03.0
    Shigella A03.9
      boydii A03.2
      dysenteriae A03.0
      flexneri A03.1
      group A A03.0
      group B A03.1
      group C A03.2
      group D A03.3
      sonnei A03.3
      specified type NEC A03.8
    Sonne A03.3
    specified type NEC A03.8
  balantidial A07.0
  Balantidium coli A07.0
  Boyd's A03.2
  candidal B37.82
  Chilomastix A07.8
  Chinese A03.9
  coccidial A07.3
  Dientamoeba (fragilis) A07.8
  Embadomonas A07.8
  Entamoeba, entamebic — see Dysentery, amebic
  Flexner-Boyd A03.2
  Flexner's A03.1
  Giardia lamblia A07.1
  Hiss-Russell A03.1
  Lamblia A07.1
  leishmanial B55.0
  malarial — see Malaria
  metazoal B82.0
  monilial B37.82
  protozoal A07.9
  Salmonella A02.0
  schistosomal B65.1
  Schmitz(-Stutzer) A03.0
  Shiga(-Kruse) A03.0
  Shigella NOS — see Dysentery, bacillary
  Sonne A03.3
  strongyloidiasis B78.0
  trichomonal A07.8
  viral (see also Enteritis, viral) A08.4
Dysequilibrium R42
Dysesthesia R20.8
  hysterical F44.6
Dysfibrinogenemia (congenital) D68.2
Dysfunction
  adrenal E27.9
    hyperfunction E27.0
  autonomic
    due to alcohol G31.2
    somatoform F45.8
  bladder N31.9
    neurogenic NOS — see Dysfunction, bladder, neuromuscular
    neuromuscular NOS N31.9
      atonic (motor) (sensory) N31.2

Dysfunction— continued
  bladder— continued
    neuromuscular— continued
      autonomous N31.2
      flaccid N31.2
      nonreflex N31.2
      reflex N31.1
      specified NEC N31.8
      uninhibited N31.0
    bleeding, uterus N93.8
  cerebral G93.89
  colon K59.9
    psychogenic F45.8
  colostomy K94.03
  cystic duct K82.8
  cystostomy (stoma) — see Complications, cystostomy
  ejaculatory N53.19
    anejaculatory orgasm N53.13
    painful N53.12
    premature F52.4
    retarded N53.11
  endocrine NOS E34.9
  endometrium N85.8
  enterostomy K94.13
  gallbladder K82.8
  gastrostomy (stoma) K94.23
  gland, glandular NOS E34.9
  heart I51.89
  hemoglobin D75.89
  hepatic K76.8
  hypophysis E23.7
  hypothalamic NEC E23.3
  ileostomy (stoma) K94.13
  jejunostomy (stoma) K94.13
  kidney — see Disease, renal
  labyrinthine — see subcategory H83.2
  left ventricular, following sudden emotional stress I51.81
  liver K76.8
  male — see Dysfunction, sexual, male
  orgasmic (female) F52.31
    male F52.32
  ovary E28.9
    specified NEC E28.8
  papillary muscle I51.89
  parathyroid E21.4
  physiological NEC R68.89
    psychogenic F59
  pineal gland E34.8
  pituitary (gland) E23.3
  platelets D69.1
  polyglandular E31.9
    specified NEC E31.8
  psychophysiologic F59
  psychosexual F52.9
    with
      dyspareunia F52.6
      premature ejaculation F52.4
      vaginismus F52.5
  pylorus K31.9
  rectum K59.9
    psychogenic F45.8
  reflex (sympathetic) — see Syndrome, pain, complex regional I
  segmental — see Dysfunction, somatic
  senile R54
  sexual (due to) R37
    alcohol F10.981
    amphetamine F15.981
      in
        abuse F15.181
        dependence F15.281
    anxiolytic F13.981
      in
        abuse F13.181
        dependence F13.281
    cocaine F14.981
      in
        abuse F14.181
        dependence F14.281
    excessive sexual drive F52.8

Dysphasia— *continued*
developmental— *continued*
receptive type F80.2
following
cerebrovascular disease I69.921
cerebral infarction I69.321
intracerebral hemorrhage I69.121
nontraumatic intracranial hemorrhage NEC I69.221
specified disease NEC I69.821
subarachnoid hemorrhage I69.021
Dysphonia R49.0
functional F44.4
hysterical F44.4
psychogenic F44.4
spastica J38.3
Dysphoria, postpartal O90.6
Dyspituitarism E23.3
Dysplasia (*see also* Anomaly)
acetabular, congenital Q65.8
anus (histologically confirmed) (mild) (moderate) K62.82
severe D01.3
arrhythmogenic right ventricular I42.8
arterial, fibromuscular I77.3
asphyxiating thoracic (congenital) Q77.2
brain Q07.9
bronchopulmonary, perinatal P27.1
cervix (uteri) N87.9
mild N87.0
moderate N87.1
severe D06.9
chondroectodermal Q77.6
colon D12.6
craniometaphyseal Q78.5
dentinal K00.5
diaphyseal, progressive Q78.3
dystrophic Q77.5
ectodermal (anhidrotic) (congenital) (hereditary) Q82.4
hydrotic Q82.8
epithelial, uterine cervix — *see* Dysplasia, cervix
eye (congenital) Q11.2
fibrous
bone NEC (monostotic) M85.00
ankle M85.07-
foot M85.07-
forearm M85.03-
hand M85.04-
lower leg M85.06-
multiple site M85.09
neck M85.08
rib M85.08
shoulder M85.01-
skull M85.08
specified site NEC M85.08
thigh M85.05-
toe M85.07-
upper arm M85.02-
vertebra M85.08
diaphyseal, progressive Q78.3
jaw M27.8
polyostotic Q78.1
florid osseous (*see also* Cyst, calcifying odontogenic)
high grade, focal D12.6
hip, congenital Q65.8
joint, congenital Q74.8
kidney Q61.4
multicystic Q61.4
leg Q74.2
lung, congenital (not associated with short gestation) Q33.6
mammary (gland) (benign) N60.9-
cyst (solitary) — *see* Cyst, breast
cystic — *see* Mastopathy, cystic
duct ectasia — *see* Ectasia, mammary duct
fibroadenosis — *see* Fibroadenosis, breast
fibrosclerosis — *see* Fibrosclerosis, breast
specified type NEC N60.8-
metaphyseal (Jansen's) (McKusick's) (Schmid's) Q78.5
muscle Q79.8

Dysplasia — *continued*
oculodentodigital Q87.0
periapical (cemental) (cemento-osseous) — *see* Cyst, calcifying odontogenic
periosteum — *see* Disorder, bone, specified type NEC
polyostotic fibrous Q78.1
prostate (*see also* Neoplasia, intraepithelial, prostate) N42.3
severe D07.5
renal Q61.4
multicystic Q61.4
retinal, congenital Q14.1
right ventricular, arrhythmogenic I42.8
septo-optic Q04.4
skin L98.8
spinal cord Q06.1
spondyloepiphyseal Q77.7
thymic, with immunodeficiency D82.1
vagina N89.3
mild N89.0
moderate N89.1
severe NEC D07.2
vulva N90.3
mild N90.0
moderate N90.1
severe NEC D07.1
Dyspnea (nocturnal) (paroxysmal) R06.00
asthmatic (bronchial) J45.909
with
exacerbation (acute) J45.901
bronchitis J45.909
with
exacerbation (acute) J45.901
status asthmaticus J45.902
chronic J44.9
status asthmaticus J45.902
cardiac — *see* Failure, ventricular, left
cardiac — *see* Failure, ventricular, left
functional F45.8
hyperventilation R06.4
hysterical F45.8
newborn
orthopnea R06.01
psychogenic F45.8
shortness of breath R06.02
specified type NEC R06.09
Dyspraxia R27.8
developmental (syndrome) F82
Dysproteinemia E88.09
Dysreflexia, autonomic G90.4
Dysrhythmia
cardiac I49.9
newborn
bradycardia P29.12
tachycardia P29.11
occurring before birth P03.819
before onset of labor P03.810
during labor P03.811
postoperative I97.89
cerebral or cortical — *see* Epilepsy
Dyssomnia — *see* Disorder, sleep
Dyssynergia
biliary K83.8
bladder sphincter N36.44
cerebellaris myoclonica (Hunt's ataxia) G11.1
Dysthymia F34.1
Dysthyroidism E07.9
Dystocia O66.9
affecting newborn P03.1
cervical (hypotonic) O62.2
affecting newborn P03.6
primary O62.0
secondary O62.1
contraction ring O62.4
fetal O66.9
abnormality NEC O66.3
conjoined twins O66.3
oversize O66.2
maternal O66.9
positional O64.9
shoulder (girdle) O66.0
causing obstructed labor O66.0

Dystocia — *continued*
uterine NEC O62.4
Dystonia G24.9
deformans progressiva G24.1
drug induced NEC G24.09
acute G24.02
specified NEC G24.09
familial G24.1
idiopathic G24.1
familial G24.1
nonfamilial G24.2
orofacial G24.4
lenticularis G24.8
musculorum deformans G24.1
neuroleptic induced (acute) G24.02
orofacial (idiopathic) G24.4
oromandibular G24.4
due to drug G24.01
specified NEC G24.8
torsion (familial) (idiopathic) G24.1
acquired G24.8
genetic G24.1
symptomatic (nonfamilial) G24.2
Dystonic movements R25.8
Dystrophy, dystrophia
adiposogenital E23.6
Becker's type G71.0
cervical sympathetic G90.2
choroid (hereditary) H31.20
central areolar H31.22
choroideremia H31.21
gyrate atrophy H31.23
specified type NEC H31.29
cornea (hereditary) H18.50
endothelial H18.51
epithelial H18.52
granular H18.53
lattice H18.54
macular H18.55
specified type NEC H18.59
myotonic (myotonica) G71.11
Duchenne's type G71.0
due to malnutrition E45
Erb's G71.0
Fuchs' H18.52
Gower's muscular G71.0
hair L67.8
infantile neuraxonal G31.89
Landouzy-Déjérine G71.0
Leyden-Möbius G71.0
muscular G71.0
benign (Becker type) G71.0
congenital (hereditary) (progressive) G71.2
myotonic G71.11
distal G71.0
Duchenne type G71.0
Emery-Dreifuss G71.0
Erb type G71.0
facioscapulohumeral G71.0
Gower's G71.0
hereditary (progressive) G71.0
Landouzy-Déjérine type G71.0
limb-girdle G71.0
myotonic G71.11
progressive (hereditary) G71.0
Charcot-Marie(-Tooth) type G60.0
pseudohypertrophic (infantile) G71.0
severe (Duchenne type) G71.0
myocardium, myocardial — *see* Degeneration, myocardial
myotonic, myotonica G71.11
nail L60.3
congenital Q84.6
nutritional E45
ocular G71.0
oculocerebrorenal E72.03
oculopharyngeal G71.0
ovarian N83.8
polyglandular E31.8
reflex (neuromuscular) (sympathetic) — *see* Syndrome, pain, complex regional I

Dystrophy, dystrophia— *continued*
  retinal (hereditary) H35.50
    in
      lipid storage disorders E75.6 [H36]
      systemic lipidoses E75.6 [H36]
    involving
      pigment epithelium H35.54
      sensory area H35.53
    pigmentary H35.52
    vitreoretinal H35.51
  Salzmann's nodular — *see* Degeneration, cornea, nodular
  scapuloperoneal G71.0
  skin NEC L98.8
  sympathetic (reflex) — *see* Syndrome, pain, complex regional I
    cervical G90.2
  tapetoretinal H35.54
  thoracic, asphyxiating Q77.2
  unguium L60.3
    congenital Q84.6
  vitreoretinal H35.51
  vulva N90.4
  yellow (liver) — *see* Failure, hepatic
Dysuria R30.0
  psychogenic F45.8

E

Eales' disease — *see* Vasculitis, retina
Ear (*see also* condition)
  piercing Z41.3
  tropical B36.8
  wax (impacted) H61.20
    left H61.22
      with right H61.23
    right H61.21
      with left H61.23
Earache — *see* subcategory H92.0
Early satiety R68.81
Eaton-Lambert syndrome G73.1
  not associated with neoplasm G70.8
Eberth's disease (typhoid fever) A01.00
Ebola virus disease A98.4
Ebstein's anomaly or syndrome (heart) Q22.5
Eccentro-osteochondrodysplasia E76.29
Ecchondroma — *see* Neoplasm, bone, benign
Ecchondrosis D48.0
Ecchymosis R58
  conjunctiva — *see* Hemorrhage, conjunctiva
  eye (traumatic) — *see* Contusion, eyeball
  eyelid (traumatic) — *see* Contusion, eyelid
  newborn P54.5
  spontaneous R23.3
  traumatic — *see* Contusion
Echinococciasis — *see* Echinococcus
Echinococcosis — *see* Echinococcus
Echinococcus (infection) B67.90
  granulosus B67.4
    bone B67.2
    liver B67.0
    lung B67.1
    multiple sites B67.32
    specified site NEC B67.39
    thyroid B67.31 [E35]
  liver NOS B67.8
    granulosus B67.0
    multilocularis B67.5
  lung NEC B67.99
    granulosus B67.1
    multilocularis B67.69
  multilocularis B67.7
    liver B67.5
    multiple sites B67.61
    specified site NEC B67.69
  specified site NEC B67.99
    granulosus B67.39
    multilocularis B67.69
  thyroid NEC B67.99
    granulosus B67.31 [E35]

Echinococcus — *continued*
  thyroid— *continued*
    multilocularis B67.69 [E35]
Echinorhynchiasis B83.8
Echinostomiasis B66.8
Echolalia R48.8
Echovirus, as cause of disease classified elsewhere B97.12
Eclampsia, eclamptic (coma) (convulsions) (delirium) (with hypertension) NEC O15.9
  during labor and delivery O15.1
  postpartum O15.2
  pregnancy O15.0-
  puerperal O15.2
Economic circumstances affecting care Z59.9
Economo's disease A85.8
Ectasia, ectasis
  annuloaortic I35.8
  aorta I77.819
    with aneurysm — *see* Aneurysm, aorta
      abdominal I77.811
      thoracic I77.810
      thoracoabdominal I77.812
  breast — *see* Ectasia, mammary duct
  capillary I78.8
  cornea H18.71-
  gastric antral vascular (GAVE) K31.819
    with hemorrhage K31.811
    without hemorrhage K31.819
  mammary duct N60.4-
  salivary gland (duct) K11.8
  sclera — *see* Sclerectasia
Ecthyma L08.0
  contagiosum B08.02
  gangrenosum L08.0
  infectiosum B08.02
Ectocardia Q24.8
Ectodermal dysplasia (anhidrotic) Q82.4
Ectodermosis erosiva pluriorificialis L51.1
Ectopic, ectopia (congenital)
  abdominal viscera Q45.8
    due to defect in anterior abdominal wall Q79.59
  ACTH syndrome E24.3
  adrenal gland Q89.1
  anus Q43.5
  atrial beats I49.1
  beats I49.49
    atrial I49.1
    ventricular I49.3
  bladder Q64.10
  bone and cartilage in lung Q33.5
  brain Q04.8
  breast tissue Q83.8
  cardiac Q24.8
  cerebral Q04.8
  cordis Q24.8
  endometrium — *see* Endometriosis
  gastric mucosa Q40.2
  gestation — *see* Pregnancy, by site
  heart Q24.8
  hormone secretion NEC E34.2
  kidney (crossed) (pelvis) Q63.2
  lens, lentis Q12.1
  mole — *see* Pregnancy, by site
  organ or site NEC — *see* Malposition, congenital
  pancreas Q45.3
  pregnancy — *see* Pregnancy, ectopic
  pupil — *see* Abnormality, pupillary
  renal Q63.2
  sebaceous glands of mouth Q38.6
  spleen Q89.09
  testis Q53.00
    bilateral Q53.02
    unilateral Q53.01
  thyroid Q89.2
  tissue in lung Q33.5
  ureter Q62.63
  ventricular beats I49.3
  vesicae Q64.10
Ectromelia Q73.8
  lower limb — *see* Defect, reduction, limb, lower, specified type NEC

Ectromelia — *continued*
  upper limb — *see* Defect, reduction, limb, upper, specified type NEC
Ectropion H02.109
  cervix N86
    with cervicitis N72
  congenital Q10.1
  eyelid (paralytic) H02.109
    cicatricial H02.119
      left H02.116
        lower H02.115
        upper H02.114
      right H02.113
        lower H02.112
        upper H02.111
    congenital Q10.1
    left H02.106
      lower H02.105
      upper H02.104
    mechanical H02.129
      left H02.126
        lower H02.125
        upper H02.124
      right H02.123
        lower H02.122
        upper H02.121
    right H02.103
      lower H02.102
      upper H02.101
    senile H02.139
      left H02.136
        lower H02.135
        upper H02.134
      right H02.133
        lower H02.132
        upper H02.131
    spastic H02.149
      left H02.146
        lower H02.145
        upper H02.144
      right H02.143
        lower H02.142
        upper H02.141
  iris H21.89
  lip (acquired) K13.0
    congenital Q38.0
  urethra N36.8
  uvea H21.89
Eczema (acute) (chronic) (erythematous) (fissum) (rubrum) (squamous) (*see also* Dermatitis) L30.9
  contact — *see* Dermatitis, contact
  dyshydrotic L30.1
  external ear — *see* Otitis, externa, acute, eczematoid
  flexural L20.82
  herpeticum B00.0
  hypertrophicum L28.0
  hypostatic — *see* Varix, leg, with, inflammation
  impetiginous L01.1
  infantile (due to any substance) L20.83
    intertriginous L21.1
    seborrheic L21.1
  intertriginous NEC L30.4
    infantile L21.1
  intrinsic (allergic) L20.84
  lichenified NEC L28.0
  marginatum (hebrae) B35.6
  pustular L30.3
  stasis — *see* Varix, leg, with, inflammation
  vaccination, vaccinatum T88.1
  varicose — *see* Varix, leg, with, inflammation
Eczematid L30.2
Eddowes(-Spurway) **syndrome** Q78.0
Edema, edematous (infectious) (pitting) (toxic) R60.9
  with nephritis — *see* Nephrosis
  allergic T78.3
  amputation stump (surgical) (sequelae (late effect)) T87.8
  angioneurotic (allergic) (any site) (with urticaria) T78.3
    hereditary D84.1
  angiospastic I73.9
  Berlin's (traumatic) S05.8x-

Edema, edematous— *continued*
　brain (cytotoxic) (vasogenic) G93.6
　　due to birth injury P11.Ø
　　newborn (anoxia or hypoxia) P52.4
　　　birth injury P11.Ø
　　traumatic — *see* Injury, intracranial, cerebral
　　　edema
　cardiac — *see* Failure, heart, congestive
　cardiovascular — *see* Failure, heart, congestive
　cerebral — *see* Edema, brain
　cerebrospinal — *see* Edema, brain
　cervix (uteri) (acute) N88.8
　　puerperal, postpartum O9Ø.89
　chronic hereditary Q82.Ø
　circumscribed, acute T78.3
　　hereditary D84.1
　conjunctiva H11.42-
　cornea H18.2-
　　idiopathic H18.22-
　　secondary H18.23-
　　　due to contact lens H18.21-
　due to
　　lymphatic obstruction I89.Ø
　　salt retention E87.Ø
　epiglottis — *see* Edema, glottis
　essential, acute T78.3
　　hereditary D84.1
　extremities, lower — *see* Edema, legs
　eyelid NEC HØ2.849
　　left HØ2.846
　　　lower HØ2.845
　　　upper HØ2.844
　　right HØ2.843
　　　lower HØ2.842
　　　upper HØ2.841
　familial, hereditary Q82.Ø
　famine — *see* Malnutrition, severe
　generalized R6Ø.1
　glottis, glottic, glottidis (obstructive) (passive) J38.4
　　allergic T78.3
　　　hereditary D84.1
　heart — *see* Failure, heart, congestive
　heat T67.7
　hereditary Q82.Ø
　inanition — *see* Malnutrition, severe
　intracranial G93.6
　iris H21.89
　joint — *see* Effusion, joint
　larynx — *see* Edema, glottis
　legs R6Ø.Ø
　　due to venous obstruction I87.1
　　　hereditary Q82.Ø
　localized R6Ø.Ø
　　due to venous obstruction I87.1
　lower limbs — *see* Edema, legs
　lung J81.1
　　with heart condition or failure — *see* Failure,
　　　ventricular, left
　　acute J81.Ø
　　chemical (acute) J68.1
　　　chronic J68.1
　　chronic J81.1
　　　due to
　　　　chemicals, gases, fumes or vapors
　　　　　(inhalation) J68.1
　　　　external agent J7Ø.9
　　　　　specified NEC J7Ø.8
　　　　radiation J7Ø.1
　　due to
　　　chemicals, fumes or vapors (inhalation) J68.1
　　　external agent J7Ø.9
　　　　specified NEC J7Ø.8
　　　high altitude T7Ø.29
　　　near drowning T75.1
　　　radiation J7Ø.Ø
　　meaning failure, left ventricle I5Ø.1
　lymphatic I89.Ø
　　due to mastectomy I97.2
　macula H35.81
　　cystoid, following cataract surgery — *see*
　　　Complications, postprocedural, following
　　　cataract surgery
　　diabetic — *see* Diabetes, macular edema

Edema, edematous— *continued*
　malignant — *see* Gangrene, gas
　Milroy's Q82.Ø
　nasopharynx J39.2
　newborn P83.3Ø
　　hydrops fetalis — *see* Hydrops, fetalis
　　specified NEC P83.39
　nutritional (*see also* Malnutrition, severe)
　　with dyspigmentation, skin and hair E4Ø
　optic disc or nerve — *see* Papilledema
　orbit HØ5.22-
　pancreas K86.8
　papilla, optic — *see* Papilledema
　penis N48.89
　periodic T78.3
　　hereditary D84.1
　pharynx J39.2
　pulmonary — *see* Edema, lung
　Quincke's T78.3
　　hereditary D84.1
　renal — *see* Nephrosis
　retina H35.81
　　diabetic — *see* Diabetes, macular edema
　salt E87.Ø
　scrotum N5Ø.8
　seminal vesicle N5Ø.8
　spermatic cord N5Ø.8
　spinal (cord) (vascular) (nontraumatic) G95.19
　starvation — *see* Malnutrition, severe
　stasis — *see* Hypertension, venous, (chronic)
　subglottic — *see* Edema, glottis
　supraglottic — *see* Edema, glottis
　testis N44.8
　tunica vaginalis N5Ø.8
　vas deferens N5Ø.8
　vulva (acute) N9Ø.89
Edentulism — *see* Absence, teeth, acquired
Edsall's disease T67.2
Educational handicap Z55.9
　specified NEC Z55.8
Edward's syndrome — *see* Trisomy, 18
Effect, adverse
　abnormal gravitational (G) forces or states T75.81
　abuse — *see* Maltreatment
　air pressure T7Ø.9
　　specified NEC T7Ø.8
　altitude (high) — *see* Effect, adverse, high altitude
　anesthesia (*see also* Anesthesia) T88.59
　　in labor and delivery O74.9
　　in pregnancy NEC O29.3-
　　local, toxic
　　　in labor and delivery O74.4
　　　postpartum, puerperal O89.3
　　postpartum, puerperal O89.9
　　specified NEC T88.59
　　　in labor and delivery O74.8
　　　postpartum, puerperal O89.8
　　spinal and epidural T88.59
　　　headache T88.59
　　　　in labor and delivery O74.5
　　　　postpartum, puerperal O89.4
　　　specified NEC
　　　　in labor and delivery O74.6
　　　　postpartum, puerperal O89.5
　antitoxin — *see* Complications, vaccination
　atmospheric pressure T7Ø.9
　　due to explosion T7Ø.8
　　high T7Ø.3
　　low — *see* Effect, adverse, high altitude
　　specified effect NEC T7Ø.8
　biological, correct substance properly administered
　　— *see* Effect, adverse, drug
　blood (derivatives) (serum) (transfusion) — *see*
　　Complications, transfusion
　chemical substance — *see* Table of Drugs and
　　Chemicals
　cold (temperature) (weather) T69.9
　　chilblains T69.1
　　frostbite — *see* Frostbite
　　specified effect NEC T69.8
　drugs and medicaments T88.7—This code not for
　　use in the inpatient setting

Effect, adverse— *continued*
　drugs and medicaments— *continued*
　　specified drug — *see* Table of Drugs and
　　　Chemicals, by drug, adverse effect
　　specified effect—code to condition
　electric current, electricity (shock) T75.4
　　burn — *see* Burn
　exertion (excessive) T73.3
　exposure — *see* Exposure
　external cause NEC T75.89
　foodstuffs T78.1
　　allergic reaction — *see* Allergy, food
　　　causing anaphylaxis — *see* Shock,
　　　　anaphylactic, food
　　noxious — *see* Poisoning, food, noxious
　gases, fumes, or vapors — *see* Table of Drugs and
　　Chemicals
　glue (airplane) sniffing
　　due to drug abuse — *see* Abuse, drug, inhalant
　　due to drug dependence — *see* Dependence,
　　　drug, inhalant
　heat — *see* Heat
　high altitude NEC T7Ø.29
　　anoxia T7Ø.2Ø
　　on
　　　ears T7Ø.Ø
　　　sinuses T7Ø.1
　　polycythemia D75.1
　high pressure fluids T7Ø.8
　hot weather — *see* Heat
　hunger T73.Ø
　immersion, foot — *see* Immersion
　immunization — *see* Complications, vaccination
　immunological agents — *see* Complications,
　　vaccination
　infrared (radiation) (rays) NOS
　　dermatitis or eczema L59.8
　infusion — *see* Complications, infusion
　lack of care of infants — *see* Maltreatment, child
　lightning — *see* Lightning
　medical care T88.9
　　specified NEC T88.8
　medicinal substance, correct, properly administered
　　— *see* Effect, adverse, drug
　motion T75.3
　noise, on inner ear — *see* subcategory H83.3
　overheated places — *see* Heat
　psychosocial, of work environment Z56.5
　radiation (diagnostic) (infrared) (natural source)
　　(therapeutic) (ultraviolet) (X-ray) NOS
　　dermatitis or eczema — *see* Dermatitis, due to,
　　　radiation
　　fibrosis of lung J7Ø.1
　　pneumonitis J7Ø.Ø
　　pulmonary manifestations
　　　acute J7Ø.Ø
　　　chronic J7Ø.1
　　skin L59.9
　radioactive substance NOS
　　dermatitis or eczema — *see* Radiodermatitis
　　dermatitis or eczema — *see* Radiodermatitis
　reduced temperature T69.9
　　immersion foot or hand — *see* Immersion
　　specified effect NEC T69.8
　serum (prophylactic) (therapeutic) NEC T8Ø.6
　specified NEC T78.8
　　external cause NEC T75.89
　strangulation — *see* Asphyxia, traumatic
　submersion T75.1
　thirst T73.1
　toxic — *see* Toxicity
　transfusion — *see* Complications, transfusion
　ultraviolet (radiation) (rays) NOS
　　burn (see Burn)
　　dermatitis or eczema — *see* Dermatitis, due to,
　　　ultraviolet rays
　　　acute L56.8
　vaccine (any) — *see* Complications, vaccination
　vibration — *see* Vibration, adverse effects
　water pressure NEC T7Ø.9
　　specified NEC T7Ø.8
　weightlessness T75.82
　whole blood — *see* Complications, transfusion

Effect, adverse— *continued*
  work environment Z56.5
Effect(s) (of) (from) — *see* Effect, adverse NEC
Effects, late — *see* Sequelae
Effluvium
  anagen L65.1
  telogen L65.0
Effort syndrome (psychogenic) F45.8
Effusion
  amniotic fluid — *see* Pregnancy, complicated by,
      prematue rupture of membranes
  brain (serous) G93.6
  bronchial — *see* Bronchitis
  cerebral G93.6
  cerebrospinal (*see also* Meningitis)
      vessel G93.6
  chest — *see* Effusion, pleura
  chylous, chyliform (pleura) J94.0
  intracranial G93.6
  joint M25.40
      ankle M25.47-
      elbow M25.42-
      foot joint M25.47-
      hand joint M25.44-
      hip M25.45-
      knee M25.46-
      shoulder M25.41-
      specified joint NEC M25.48
      wrist M25.43-
  malignant pleural J91.0
  meninges — *see* Meningitis
  pericardium, pericardial (noninflammatory) I31.3
      acute — *see* Pericarditis, acute
  peritoneal (chronic) R18.8
  pleura, pleurisy, pleuritic, pleuropericardial J90
      chylous, chyliform J94.0
      due to systemic lupus erythematosis M32.13
      influenzal — *see* Influenza, with, respiratory
          manifestations NEC
      malignant J91.0
      newborn P28.89
      tuberculous NEC A15.6
          primary (progressive) A15.7
  spinal — *see* Meningitis
  thorax, thoracic — *see* Effusion, pleura
Egg shell nails L60.3
  congenital Q84.6
Egyptian splenomegaly B65.1
Ehrlichiosis A77.40
  due to
      E. chafeensis A77.41
      E. sennetsu A79.81
      specified organism NEC A77.49
Ehlers-Danlos syndrome Q79.6
Eichstedt's disease B36.0
Eisenmenger's
  complex or syndrome I27.89
  defect Q21.8
Ejaculation
  painful N53.12
  premature F52.4
  retarded N53.11
  retrograde N53.14
  semen, painful N53.12
      psychogenic F52.6
Ekbom's syndrome (restless legs) G25.81
Ekman's syndrome (brittle bones and blue sclera)
  Q78.0
Elastic skin Q82.8
  acquired L57.4
Elastofibroma — *see* Neoplasm, connective tissue,
  benign
Elastoma (juvenile) Q82.8
  Miescher's L87.2
Elastomyofibrosis I42.4
Elastosis
  actinic, solar L57.8
  atrophicans (senile) L57.4
  perforans serpiginosa L87.2
  senilis L57.4
Elbow — *see* condition
Electric current, electricity, effects (concussion
  (fatal) (nonfatal) (shock) T75.4 burn — *see* Burn

Electric feet syndrome E53.8
Electrocution T75.4
  from electroshock gun (taser) T75.4
Electrolyte imbalance E87.8
  with
      abortion — *see* Abortion by type complicated by
          specified condition NEC
      ectopic pregnancy O08.5
      molar pregnancy O08.5
Elephantiasis (nonfilarial) I89.0
  arabicum — *see* Infestation, filarial bancroftian
      B74.0
  congenital (any site) (hereditary) Q82.0
  due to
      Brugia (malayi) B74.1
          timori B74.2
      mastectomy I97.2
      Wuchereria (bancrofti) B74.0
  eyelid H02.859
      left H02.856
          lower H02.855
          upper H02.854
      right H02.853
          lower H02.852
          upper H02.851
  filarial, filariensis — *see* Infestation, filarial
  glandular I89.0
  graecorum A30.9
  lymphangiectatic I89.0
  lymphatic vessel I89.0
      due to mastectomy I97.2
  scrotum (nonfilarial) I89.0
  streptococcal I89.0
  surgical I97.89
      postmastectomy I97.2
  telangiectodes I89.0
  vulva (nonfilarial) N90.89
Elevated, elevation
  antibody titer R76.0
  basal metabolic rate R94.8
  blood pressure (*see also* Hypertension)
      reading (incidental) (isolated) (nonspecific), no
          diagnosis of hypertension R03.0
  blood sugar R73.09
  body temperature (of unknown origin) R50.9
  C-reactive protein (CRP) R79.82
  cancer antigen 125 [CA 125] R97.1
  carcinoembryonic antigen [CEA] R97.0
  cholesterol E78.0
      with high triglycerides E78.2
  conjugate, eye H51.0
  diaphragm, congenital Q79.1
  erythrocyte sedimentation rate R70.0
  fasting glucose R73.01
  fasting triglycerides E78.1
  finding on laboratory examination — *see* Findings,
      abnormal, inconclusive, without diagnosis, by
      type of exam
  GFR (glomerular filtration rate) — *see* Findings,
      abnormal, inconclusive, without diagnosis, by
      type of exam
  glucose tolerance (oral) R73.02
  immunoglobulin level R76.8
  indolacetic acid R82.5
  lactic acid dehydrogenase (LDH) level R74.0
  leukocytes D72.829
  lipoprotein a level E78.8
  liver function
      study R94.5
      test R79.89
          alkaline phosphatase R74.8
          aminotransferase R74.0
          bilirubin R17
          hepatic enzyme R74.8
          lactate dehydrogenase R74.0
  lymphocytes D72.820
  prostate specific antigen [PSA] R97.2
  Rh titer T80.4 — *see* Complication(s), transfusion,
      incompatiblity reaction, Rh (factor)
  scapula, congenital Q74.0
  sedimentation rate R70.0
  SGOT R74.0
  SGPT R74.0

Elevated, elevation— *continued*
  transaminase level R74.0
  triglycerides E78.1
      with high cholesterol E78.2
  tumor associated antigens [TAA] NEC R97.8
  tumor specific antigens [TSA] NEC R97.8
  urine level of
      catecholamine R82.5
      indoleacetic acid R82.5
      17-ketosteroids R82.5
      steroids R82.5
      vanillylmandelic acid (VMA) R82.5
  venous pressure I87.8
  white blood cell count D72.829
      specified NEC D72.828
Elliptocytosis (congenital) (hereditary) D58.1 Hb C
  (disease) D58.1
  hemoglobin disease D58.1
  sickle-cell (disease) D57.8-
      trait D57.3
Ellison-Zollinger syndrome E16.4
Ellis-van Creveld syndrome (chondroectodermal
  dysplasia) Q77.6
Elongated, elongation (congenital) (*see also*
  Distortion)
  bone Q79.9
  cervix (uteri) Q51.828
      acquired N88.4
      hypertrophic N88.4
  colon Q43.8
  common bile duct Q44.5
  cystic duct Q44.5
  frenulum, penis Q55.69
  labia minora (acquired) N90.6
  ligamentum patellae Q74.1
  petiolus (epiglottidis) Q31.8
  tooth, teeth K00.2
  uvula Q38.6
Eltor cholera A00.1
Emaciation (due to malnutrition) E41
Embadomoniasis A07.8
Embedded tooth, teeth K01.0
  root only K08.3
Embolic — *see* condition
Embolism (multiple) (paradoxical) I74.9
  air (any site) (traumatic) T79.0
      following
          abortion — *see* Abortion by type complicated
              by embolism
          ectopic pregnancy O08.2
          infusion, therapeutic injection or transfusion
              T80.0
          molar pregnancy O08.2
          procedure NEC
              artery T81.719
                  mesenteric T81.710
                  renal T81.711
                  specified NEC T81.718
              vein T81.72
      in pregnancy, childbirth or puerperium — *see*
          Embolism, obstetric
  amniotic fluid (pulmonary) (*see also* Embolism,
      obstetric)
      following
          abortion — *see* Abortion by type complicated
              by embolism
          ectopic pregnancy O08.2
          molar pregnancy O08.2
  aorta, aortic I74.10
      abdominal I74.0
      bifurcation I74.0
      saddle I74.0
      thoracic I74.11
  artery I74.9
      auditory, internal I65.8
      basilar — *see* Occlusion, artery, basilar
      carotid (common) (internal) — *see* Occlusion,
          artery, carotid
      cerebellar (anterior inferior) (posterior inferior)
          (superior) I66.3
      cerebral — *see* Occlusion, artery, cerebral
      choroidal (anterior) I66.8
      communicating posterior I66.8

Embolism — *continued*
  artery— *continued*
    coronary (*see also* Infarct, myocardium)
      not resulting in infarction I24.Ø
    extremity I74.4
      lower I74.3
      upper I74.2
    hypophyseal I66.8
    iliac I74.5
    limb I74.4
      lower I74.3
      upper I74.2
    mesenteric (with gangrene) K55.Ø
    ophthalmic — *see* Occlusion, artery, retina
    peripheral I74.4
    pontine I66.8
    precerebral — *see* Occlusion, artery, precerebral
    pulmonary — *see* Embolism, pulmonary
    renal N28.Ø
    retinal — *see* Occlusion, artery, retina
    septic I76
    specified NEC I74.8
    vertebral — *see* Occlusion, artery, vertebral
  basilar (artery) I65.1
  blood clot
    following
      abortion — *see* Abortion by type complicated
        by embolism
      ectopic or molar pregnancy OØ8.2
    in pregnancy, childbirth or puerperium — *see*
      Embolism, obstetric
  brain (*see also* Occlusion, artery, cerebral)
    following
      abortion — *see* Abortion by type complicated
        by embolism
      ectopic or molar pregnancy OØ8.2
      puerperal, postpartum, childbirth — *see*
        Embolism, obstetric
  capillary I78.8
  cardiac (*see also* Infarct, myocardium)
    not resulting in infarction I24.Ø
  carotid (artery) (common) (internal) — *see*
    Occlusion, artery, carotid
  cavernous sinus (venous) — *see* Embolism,
    intracranial venous sinus
  cerebral — *see* Occlusion, artery, cerebral
  cholesterol — *see* Atheroembolism
  coronary (artery or vein) (systemic) — *see* Occlusion,
    coronary
  due to device, implant or graft (*see also*
    Complications, by site and type, specified
    NEC)
    arterial graft NEC T82.818
    breast (implant) T85.81
    catheter NEC T85.81
      dialysis (renal) T82.818
        intraperitoneal T85.81
      infusion NEC T82.818
        spinal (epidural) (subdural) T85.81
      urinary (indwelling) T83.81
    electronic (electrode) (pulse generator)
      (stimulator)
      bone T84.81
      cardiac T82.817
      nervous system (brain) (peripheral nerve)
        (spinal) T85.81
      urinary T83.81
    fixation, internal (orthopedic) NEC T84.81
    gastrointestinal (bile duct) (esophagus) T85.81
    genital NEC T83.81
    heart (graft) (valve) T82.817
    joint prosthesis T84.81
    ocular (corneal graft) (orbital implant) T85.81
    orthopedic (bone graft) NEC T86.838
    specified NEC T85.81
    urinary (graft) NEC T83.81
    vascular NEC T82.818
    ventricular intracranial shunt T85.81
  extremities
    lower — *see* Embolism, vein, lower extremity
      arterial I74.3
    upper I74.2
  eye H34.9

Embolism — *continued*
  fat (cerebral) (pulmonary) (systemic) T79.1
    following
      abortion — *see* Abortion by type complicated
        by embolism
      ectopic or molar pregnancy OØ8.2
    complicating delivery — *see* Embolism, obstetric
  following
    abortion — *see* Abortion by type complicated by
      embolism
    ectopic or molar pregnancy OØ8.2
    infusion, therapeutic injection or transfusion
      air T8Ø.Ø
      thrombus T8Ø.1
  heart (fatty) (*see also* Infarct, myocardium)
    not resulting in infarction I24.Ø
  hepatic (vein) I82.Ø
  in pregnancy, childbirth or puerperium — *see*
    Embolism, obstetric
  intestine (artery) (vein) (with gangrene) K55.Ø
  intracranial — *see also* Occlusion, artery, cerebral
    venous sinus (any) GØ8
      nonpyogenic I67.6
  intraspinal venous sinuses or veins GØ8
    nonpyogenic G95.19
  kidney (artery) N28.Ø
  lateral sinus (venous) — *see* Embolism, intracranial,
    venous sinus
  leg — *see* Embolism, vein, lower extremity
    arterial I74.3
  longitudinal sinus (venous) — *see* Embolism,
    intracranial, venous sinus
  lung (massive) — *see* Embolism, pulmonary
  meninges I66.8
  mesenteric (artery) (vein) (with gangrene) K55.Ø
  obstetric (in) (pulmonary)
    childbirth O88.82
      air O88.Ø2
      amniotic fluid O88.12
      blood clot O88.22
      fat O88.82
      pyemic O88.32
      septic O88.32
      specified type NEC O88.82
    pregnancy O88.81-
      air O88.Ø1-
      amniotic fluid O88.11-
      blood clot O88.21-
      fat O88.81-
      pyemic O88.31-
      septic O88.31-
      specified type NEC O88.81-
    puerperal O88.83
      air O88.Ø3
      amniotic fluid O88.13
      blood clot O88.23
      fat O88.83
      pyemic O88.33
      septic O88.33
      specified type NEC O88.83
  ophthalmic — *see* Occlusion, artery, retina
  penis N48.81
  peripheral artery NEC I74.8
  pituitary E23.6
  popliteal (artery) I74.3
  portal (vein) I81
  postoperative, postrpocedural
    artery T81.719
      mesenteric T81.71Ø
      renal T81.711
      specified NEC T81.718
    vein T81.72
  precerebral artery — *see* Occlusion, artery,
    precerebral
  puerperal — *see* Embolism, obstetric
  pulmonary (acute) (artery) (vein) I26.99
    with acute cor pulmonale I26.Ø9
    chronic I27.82
    healed or old Z86.71
    following
      abortion — *see* Abortion by type complicated
        by embolism
      ectopic or molar pregnancy OØ8.2

Embolism — *continued*
  pulmonary— *continued*
    in pregnancy, childbirth or puerperium — *see*
      Embolism, obstetric
    personal history of Z86.71
    septic I26.9Ø
      with acute cor pulmonale I26.Ø1
  pyemic (multiple) I76
    following
      abortion — *see* Abortion by type complicated
        by embolism
      ectopic or molar pregnancy OØ8.2
    Hemophilus influenzae A41.3
    pneumococcal A4Ø.3
      with pneumonia J13
    puerperal, postpartum, childbirth (any organism)
      — *see* Embolism, obstetric
    specified organism NEC A41.89
    staphylococcal A41.2
    streptococcal A4Ø.9
  renal (artery) N28.Ø
    vein I82.3
  retina, retinal — *see* Occlusion, artery, retina
  saddle (aorta) I74.Ø
  septic (arterial) I76
    complicating abortion — *see* Abortion, by type,
      complicated by, embolism
  sinus — *see* Embolism, intracranial, venous sinus
  soap complicating abortion — *see* Abortion, by
    type, complicated by, embolism
  spinal cord G95.19
    pyogenic origin GØ6.1
  spleen, splenic (artery) I74.8
  upper extremity I74.2
  vein (acute) I82.9Ø
    antecubital I82.61-
      chronic I82.71
    axillary I82.a1-
      chronic I82.a2-
    basilic I82.61-
      chronic I82.71
    brachial I82.62-
      chronic I82.72
    brachiocephalic (innominate) I82.29Ø
      chronic I82.291
    cephalic I82.61-
      chronic I82.71
    chronic I82.91
      upper extremity I82.7Ø
    deep (DVT) I82.4Ø-
      calf I82.4z-
        chronic I82.5z-
      lower leg I82.4z-
        chronic I82.5z-
      thigh I82.4y-
        chronic I82.5y-
      upper leg I82.4y-
        chronic I82.5y-
    femoral I82.41-
      chronic I82.51
    iliac (iliofemoral) I82.42-
      chronic I82.51-
    innominate I82.29Ø
      chronic I82.291
    internal jugular I82.c1-
      chronic I82.c2-
    lower extremity
      deep I82.4Ø-
        chronic I82.5Ø-
          specifed NEC I82.49-
            chronic NEC I82.59-
      distal
        deep I82.4z-
      proximal
        deep I82.4y-
          chronic I82.5y-
      superficial I82.81
    mesenteric (with gangrene) K55.Ø
    popliteal I82.43-
      chronic I82.53-
    radial I82.62-
      chronic I82.72-
    renal I82.3

Embolism — *continued*
  vein (acute)— *continued*
    saphenous (greater) (lesser) I82.81-
    specified NEC I82.890
      chronic I82.891
    subclavian I82.b1-
      chronic I82.b2-
    thoracic NEC I82.290
      chronic I82.291
    tibial I82.44-
      chronic I82.54-
    ulnar I82.62-
      chronic I82.72-
    upper extremity I82.60-
      chronic I82.70-
      deep I82.62-
        chronic I82.72-
      superficial I82.61-
        chronic I82.71
  vena cava
    inferior (acute) I82.220
      chronic I82.221
    superior (acute) I82.210
      chronic I82.211
  venous sinus G08
  vessels of brain — *see* Occlusion, artery, cerebral
Embolus — *see* Embolism
Embryoma (*see also* Neoplasm, uncertain behavior, by site)
  benign — *see* Neoplasm, benign, by site
  kidney C64.-
  liver C22.0
  malignant (*see also* Neoplasm, malignant, by site)
    kidney C64.-
    liver C22.0
    testis C62.9-
      descended (scrotal) C62.1-
      undescended C62.0-
  testis C62.9-
    descended (scrotal) C62.1-
    undescended C62.0-
Embryonic
  circulation Q28.9
  heart Q28.9
  vas deferens Q55.4
Embryopathia NOS Q89.9
Embryotoxon Q13.4
Emesis — *see* Vomiting
Emotional lability R45.86
Emotionality, pathological F60.3
Emotogenic disease — *see* Disorder, psychogenic
Emphysema (atrophic) (bullous) (chronic) (interlobular) (lung) (obstructive) (pulmonary) (senile) (vesicular) J43.9
  cellular tissue (traumatic) T79.7
    surgical T81.82
  centrilobular J43.2
  compensatory J98.3
  congenital (interstitial) P25.0
  conjunctiva H11.89
  connective tissue (traumatic) T79.7
    surgical T81.82
  due to chemicals, gases, fumes or vapors J68.4
  eyelid(s) — see Disorder, eyelid, specified type NEC
    surgical T81.82
    traumatic T79.7
  interstitial J98.2
    congenital P25.0
    perinatal period P25.0
  laminated tissue T79.7
    surgical T81.82
  mediastinal J98.2
    newborn P25.2
  orbit, orbital — see Disorder, orbit, specified type NEC
  panacinar J43.1
  panlobular J43.1
  specified NEC J43.8
  subcutaneous (traumatic) T79.7
    nontraumatic J98.2
    postprocedural T81.82
    surgical T81.82
  surgical T81.82
  thymus (gland) (congenital) E32.8

Emphysema — *continued*
  traumatic (subcutaneous) T79.7
  unilateral J43.0
Empty nest syndrome Z60.0
Empyema (acute) (chest) (double) (pleura) (supradiaphragmatic) (thorax) J86.9
  with fistula J86.0
  accessory sinus (chronic) — *see* Sinusitis
  antrum (chronic) — *see* Sinusitis, maxillary
  brain (any part) — *see* Abscess, brain
  ethmoidal (chronic) (sinus) — *see* Sinusitis, ethmoidal
  extradural — *see* Abscess, extradural
  frontal (chronic) (sinus) — *see* Sinusitis, frontal
  gallbladder K81.0
  mastoid (process) (acute) — *see* Mastoiditis, acute
  maxilla, maxillary M27.2
    sinus (chronic) — *see* Sinusitis, maxillary
  nasal sinus (chronic) — *see* Sinusitis
  sinus (accessory) (chronic) (nasal) — *see* Sinusitis
  sphenoidal (sinus) (chronic) — *see* Sinusitis, sphenoidal
  subarachnoid — *see* Abscess, extradural
  subdural — *see* Abscess, subdural
  tuberculous A15.6
  ureter — *see* Ureteritis
  ventricular — *see* Abscess, brain
En coup de sabre lesion L94.1
Enamel pearls K00.2
Enameloma K00.2
Enanthema, viral B09
Encephalitis (chronic) (hemorrhagic) (idiopathic) (nonepidemic) (spurious) (subacute) G04.90
  acute (*see also* Encephalitis, viral) A86
    disseminated G04.00
      infectious G04.00
      noninfectious G04.81
      postimmunization (postvaccination) G04.01
      postinfectious G04.00
    inclusion body A85.8
    necrotizing hemorrhagic (postinfectious) G04.30
      postimmunization G04.31
  arboviral, arbovirus NEC A85.2
  arthropod-borne NEC (viral) A85.2
  Australian A83.4
  California (virus) A83.5
  Central European (tick-borne) A84.1
  Czechoslovakian A84.1
  Dawson's (inclusion body) A81.1
  diffuse sclerosing A81.1
  disseminated, acute G04.00
  due to
    cat scratch disease A28.1
    malaria — *see* Malaria
    rickettsiosis — *see* Rickettsiosis
    smallpox inoculation G04.01
    typhus — *see* Typhus
  Eastern equine A83.2
  endemic (viral) A86
  epidemic NEC (viral) A86
  equine (acute) (infectious) (viral) A83.9
    Eastern A83.2
    Venezuelan A92.2
    Western A83.1
  Far Eastern (tick-borne) A84.0
  following vaccination or other immunization procedure G04.01
  herpes zoster B02.0
  herpesviral B00.4
    due to herpesvirus 6 B10.01
    due to herpesvirus 7 B10.09
    specified NEC B10.09
  Ilheus (virus) A83.8
  inclusion body A81.1
  in (due to)
    actinomycosis A42.82
    adenovirus A85.1
    African trypanosomiasis B56.9 [G05.3]
    Chagas' disease (chronic) B57.42
    cytomegalovirus B25.8
    enterovirus A85.0
    herpes (simplex) virus B00.4
      due to herpesvirus 6 B10.01
      due to herpesvirus 7 B10.09

Encephalitis — *continued*
  in (due to)— *continued*
    herpes (simplex) virus—*continued*
      specified NEC B10.09
    infectious disease NEC B99 [G05.3]
    influenza — *see* Influenza, with, encephalopathy
    listeriosis A32.12
    measles B05.0
    mumps B26.2
    naegleriasis B60.2
    parasitic disease NEC B89 [G05.3]
    poliovirus A80.9 [G05.3]
    rubella B06.01
    syphilis
      congenital A50.42
      late A52.14
    systemic lupus erythematosus M32.19
    toxoplasmosis (acquired) B58.2
      congenital P37.1
    tuberculosis A17.82
    zoster B02.0
  infectious (acute) (virus) NEC A86
  Japanese (B type) A83.0
  La Crosse A83.5
  lead — *see* Poisoning, lead
  lethargica (acute) (infectious) A85.8
  louping ill A84.8
  lupus erythematosus, systemic M32.19
  lymphatica A87.2
  Mengo A85.8
  meningococcal A39.81
  Murray Valley A83.4
  otitic NEC H66.40 [G05.3]
  parasitic NOS B71.9
  periaxial G37.0
  periaxialis (concentrica) (diffuse) G37.5
  postchickenpox B01.11
  postexanthematous NEC B09
  postimmunization G04.01
  postmeasles B05.0
  postvaccinal G04.01
  postvaricella B01.11
  postviral NEC A86
  Powassan A84.8
  Rasmussen G04.81
  Rio Bravo A85.8
  Russian
    autumnal A83.0
    spring-summer (taiga) A84.0
  saturnine — *see* Poisoning, lead
  specified NEC G04.81
  St. Louis A83.3
  subacute sclerosing A81.1
  summer A83.0
  suppurative G04.81
  tick-borne A84.9
  Torula, torular (cryptococcal) B45.1
  toxic NEC G92
  trichinosis B75 [G05.3]
  type
    B A83.0
    C A83.3
  van Bogaert's A81.1
  Venezuelan equine A92.2
  Vienna A85.8
  viral, virus A86
    arthropod-borne NEC A85.2
      mosquito-borne A83.9
        Australian X disease A83.4
        California virus A83.5
        Eastern equine A83.2
        Japanese (B type) A83.0
        Murray Valley A83.4
        specified NEC A83.8
        St. Louis A83.3
        type B A83.0
        type C A83.3
        Western equine A83.1
      tick-borne A84.9
        biundulant A84.1
        central European A84.1
        Czechoslovakian A84.1
        diphasic meningoencephalitis A84.1

Encephalitis — *continued*
  viral, virus— *continued*
    arthropod-borne— *continued*
      tick-borne— *continued*
        Far Eastern A84.0
        Russian spring-summer (taiga) A84.0
        specified NEC A84.8
      specified type NEC A85.8
    Western equine A83.1
Encephalocele Q01.9
  frontal Q01.0
  nasofrontal Q01.1
  occipital Q01.2
  specified NEC Q01.8
Encephalocystocele — *see* Encephalocele
Encephalomalacia (brain) (cerebellar) (cerebral) —
    see Softening, brain
Encephalomeningitis — *see* Meningoencephalitis
Encephalomeningocele — *see* Encephalocele
Encephalomeningomyelitis — *see*
    Meningoencephalitis
Encephalomyelitis (*see also* Encephalitis) G04.90
  acute disseminated (postinfectious) G04.00
    infectious G04.00
    noninfectious G04.81
    postimmunization G04.01
  acute necrotizing hemorrhagic (postinfectious) G04.30
    postimmunization G04.31
  benign myalgic G93.3
  equine A83.9
    Eastern A83.2
    Venezuelan A92.2
    Western A83.1
  in diseases classified elsewhere G05.3
  myalgic, benign G93.3
  postchickenpox B01.11
  postinfectious NEC G04.00
  postmeasles B05.0
  postvaccinal G04.01
  postvaricella B01.11
  rubella B06.01
  specified NEC G04.81
  Venezuelan equine A92.2
Encephalomyelocele — *see* Encephalocele
Encephalomyelomeningitis — *see*
    Meningoencephalitis
Encephalomyelopathy G96.9
Encephalomyeloradiculitis (acute) G61.0
Encephalomyeloradiculoneuritis (acute)
    (Guillain-Barré) G61.0
Encephalomyeloradiculopathy G96.9
Encephalopathia hyperbilirubinemica, newborn
    P57.9
  due to isoimmunization (conditions in P55) P57.0
Encephalopathy (acute) G93.40
  acute necrotizing hemorrhagic (postinfectious)
      G04.30
    postimmunization G04.31
  alcoholic G31.2
  anoxic — *see* Damage, brain, anoxic
  arteriosclerotic I67.2
  centrolobar progressive (Schilder) G37.0
  congenital Q07.9
  demyelinating callosal G37.1
  hepatic — *see* Failure, hepatic
  hyperbilirubinemic, newborn P57.9
    due to isoimmunization (conditions in P55) P57.0
  hypertensive I67.4
  hypoglycemic E16.2
  hypoxic — *see* Damage, brain, anoxic
  hypoxic ischemic P91.60
    mild P91.61
    moderate P91.62
    severe P91.63
  in (due to) (with)
    birth injury P11.1
    hyperinsulinism E16.1 [G94]
    influenza — *see* Influenza, with, encephalopathy
    lack of vitamin (*see also* Deficiency, vitamin)
        E56.9 [G32.8]
    neoplastic disease (*see also* Neoplasm) D49.9 [G13.1]
    serum (nontherapeutic) (therapeutic) T80.6
    syphilis A52.17

Encephalopathy — *continued*
  in (due to)— *continued*
    trauma (postconcussional) F07.81
      current injury — *see* Injury, intracranial
    vaccination G04.01
  lead — *see* Poisoning, lead
  metabolic G93.41
    toxic G92
  myoclonic, early, symptomatic — *see* Epilepsy,
      generalized, specified NEC
  necrotizing, subacute (Leigh) G31.82
  pellagrous E52 [G32.8]
  portosystemic — *see* Failure, hepatic
  postcontusional F07.81
    current injury — *see* Injury, intracranial, diffuse
  posthypoglycemic (coma) E16.1 [G94]
  postradiation G93.89
  saturnine — *see* Poisoning, lead
  septic G93.41
  specified NEC G93.49
  spongioform, subacute (viral) A81.09
  toxic G92
    metabolic G92
  traumatic (postconcussional) F07.81
    current injury — *see* Injury, intracranial
  vitamin B deficiency NEC E53.9 [G32.8]
    vitamin B1 E51.2
  Wernicke's E51.2
Encephalorrhagia — *see* Hemorrhage, intracranial,
    intracerebral
Encephalosis, posttraumatic F07.81
Enchondroma (*see also* Neoplasm, bone, benign)
Enchondromatosis (cartilaginous) (multiple) Q78.4
Encopresis R15.9
  functional F98.1
  nonorganic origin F98.1
  psychogenic F98.1
Encounter (with health service) (for) Z76.89
  adjustment and management (of)
    breast implant Z45.81
    implanted device NEC Z45.89
    myringotomy device (stent) (tube) Z45.82
  administrative purpose only Z02.9
    examination for
      adoption Z02.82
      armed forces Z02.3
      disability determination Z02.71
      driving license Z02.4
      employment Z02.1
      insurance Z02.6
      medical certificate NEC Z02.79
      paternity testing Z02.81
      residential institution admission Z02.2
      school admission Z02.0
      sports Z02.5
    specified reason NEC Z02.89
  aftercare — *see* Aftercare
  antenatal screening Z36
  assisted reproductive fertility procedure cycle Z31.83
  blood typing Z01.83
    Rh typing Z01.83
  breast augmentation or reduction Z41.1
  breast implant exchange (different material)
      (different size) Z45.81
  breast reconstruction following mastectomy Z42.1
  check-up — *see* Examination
  chemotherapy for neoplasm Z51.11
  colonoscopy, screening Z12.11
  counseling — *see* Counseling
  delivery, full-term, uncomplicated O80
    cesarean, without indication O82
  examination — *see* Examination
  expectant parent(s) (adoptive) pre-birth
      pediatrician visit Z76.81
  fertility preservation procedure (prior to cancer
      therapy) (prior to removal of gonads) Z31.84
  fitting (of) — *see* Fitting (and adjustment) (of)
  genetic
    counseling Z31.5
    testing — *see* Test, genetic
  hearing conservation and treatment Z01.12
  immunotherapy for neoplasm Z51.12
  in vitro fertilization cycle Z31.83

Encounter — *continued*
  instruction (in)
    childbirth Z32.2
    child care (postpartal) (prenatal) Z32.3
    natural family planning
      procreative Z31.61
      to avoid pregnancy Z30.02
  insulin pump titration Z46.81
  laboratory (as part of a general medical
      examination) Z00.00
    with abnormal findings Z00.01
  mental health services (for)
    abuse NEC
      perpetrator Z69.82
      victim Z69.81
    child abuse
      nonparental
        perpetrator Z69.021
        victim Z69.020
      parental
        perpetrator Z69.011
        victim Z69.010
    spousal or partner abuse
      perpetrator Z69.12
      victim Z69.11
  observation (for) (ruled out)
    exposure to (suspected)
      anthrax Z03.810
      biological agent NEC Z03.818
  pediatrician visit, by expectant parent(s) (adoptive)
      Z76.81
  plastic and reconstructive surgery following medical
      procedure or healed injury NEC Z42.8
  pregnancy
    supervision of — *see* Pregnancy, supervision of
    test Z32.00
      result negative Z32.02
      result positive Z32.01
  radiation therapy (antineoplastic) Z51.0
  radiological (as part of a general medical
      examination) Z00.00
    with abnormal findings Z00.01
  reconstructive surgery following medical procedure
      or healed injury NEC Z42.8
  removal (of) (*see also* Removal)
    artificial
      arm Z44.00-
        complete Z44.01-
        partial Z44.02-
      eye Z44.2-
      leg Z44.10-
        complete Z44.11-
        partial Z44.12-
    breast implant Z45.81
      tissue expander (without synchronous
          insertion of permanent implant) Z45.81
    device Z46.9
      specified NEC Z46.89
    external
      fixation device—code to fracture with extension
          D
      prosthesis, prosthetic device Z44.9
        breast Z44.3-
        specified NEC Z44.8
    implanted device NEC Z45.89
    internal fixation device Z47.2
    insulin pump Z46.81
    myringotomy device (stent) (tube) Z45.82
    nervous system device NEC Z46.2
      brain neuropacemaker Z46.2
      visual substitution device Z46.2
        implanted Z45.31
    non-vascular catheter Z46.82
    orthodontic device Z46.4
    stent
      ureteral Z46.6
    urinary device Z46.6
  repeat cervical smear to confirm findings of recent
      normal smear following initial abnormal
      smear Z01.42
  respirator/ventilator use during power failure (Z99.12)
  Rh typing Z01.83
  screening — *see* Screening

Encounter — *continued*
  specified NEC Z76.89
  sterilization Z30.2
  suspected condition, ruled out
    amniotic cavity and membrane Z03.71
    cervical shortening Z03.75
    fetal anomaly Z03.73
    fetal growth Z03.74
    maternal and fetal conditions NEC Z03.79
    oligohydramnios Z03.71
    placental problem Z03.72
    polyhydramnios Z03.71
  suspected exposure (to), ruled out
    anthrax Z03.810
    biological agents NEC Z03.818
  termination of pregnancy, elective Z33.2
  testing — *see* Test
  therapeutic drug level monitoring Z51.81
  titration, insulin pump Z46.81
  training
    insulin pump Z46.81
  X-ray of chest
    as part of a general medical examination Z00.00
    with abnormal findings Z00.01
Encystment — *see* Cyst
Endarteritis (bacterial, subacute) (infective) I77.6
  brain I67.7
  cerebral or cerebrospinal I67.7
  deformans — *see* Arteriosclerosis
  embolic — *see* Embolism
  obliterans (*see also* Arteriosclerosis)
    pulmonary I28.8
  pulmonary I28.8
  retina — *see* Vasculitis, retina
  senile — *see* Arteriosclerosis
  syphilitic A52.09
    brain or cerebral A52.04
    congenital A50.54 [I79.8]
  tuberculous A18.89
Endemic — *see* condition
Endocarditis (chronic) (marantic) (nonbacterial
    thrombotic) (valvular) I38
  with rheumatic fever (conditions in I00)
    active — *see* Endocarditis, acute, rheumatic
    inactive or quiescent (with chorea) I09.1
  acute or subacute I33.9
    infective I33.0
    rheumatic (aortic) (mitral) (pulmonary)
      (tricuspid) I01.1
      with chorea (acute) (rheumatic) (Sydenham's)
        I02.0
  aortic (heart) (nonrheumatic) (valve) I35.8
    with
      mitral disease I08.0
        with tricuspid (valve) disease I08.3
        active or acute I01.1
          with chorea (acute) (rheumatic)
            (Sydenham's) I02.0
      rheumatic fever (conditions in I00)
        active — *see* Endocarditis, acute,
          rheumatic
        inactive or quiescent (with chorea) I06.9
      tricuspid (valve) disease I08.2
        with mitral (valve) disease I08.3
    acute or subacute I33.9
    arteriosclerotic I35.8
    rheumatic I06.9
      with mitral disease I08.0
        with tricuspid (valve) disease I08.3
        active or acute I01.1
          with chorea (acute) (rheumatic)
            (Sydenham's) I02.0
      active or acute I01.1
        with chorea (acute) (rheumatic)
          (Sydenham's) I02.0
      specified NEC I06.8
    specified cause NEC I35.8
    syphilitic A52.03
  arteriosclerotic I38
  atypical verrucous (Libman-Sacks) M32.11
  bacterial (acute) (any valve) (subacute) I33.0
  candidal B37.6
  congenital Q24.8

Endocarditis — *continued*
  constrictive I33.0
  Coxiella burnetii A78 [I39]
  Coxsackie B33.21
  due to
    prosthetic cardiac valve T82.6
    Q fever A78
    Serratia marcescens I33.0
    typhoid (fever) A01.02
  gonococcal A54.83
  infectious or infective (acute) (any valve) (subacute)
    I33.0
  lenta (acute) (any valve) (subacute) I33.0
  Libman-Sacks M32.11
  listerial A32.82
  Löffler's I42.3
  malignant (acute) (any valve) (subacute) I33.0
  meningococcal A39.51
  mitral (chronic) (double) (fibroid) (heart) (inactive)
    (valve) (with chorea) I05.9
    with
      aortic (valve) disease I08.0
        with tricuspid (valve) disease I08.3
        active or acute I01.1
          with chorea (acute) (rheumatic)
            (Sydenham's) I02.0
      rheumatic fever (conditions in I00)
        active — *see* Endocarditis, acute,
          rheumatic
        inactive or quiescent (with chorea) I05.9
      tricuspid (valve) disease I08.1
        with aortic (valve) disease I08.3
    active or acute I01.1
      with chorea (acute) (rheumatic) (Sydenham's)
        I02.0
    bacterial I33.0
    arteriosclerotic I34.8
    nonrheumatic I34.8
      acute or subacute I33.9
    specified NEC I05.8
  monilial B37.6
  multiple valves I08.9
    specified disorders I08.8
  mycotic (acute) (any valve) (subacute) I33.0
  pneumococcal (acute) (any valve) (subacute) I33.0
  pulmonary (chronic) (heart) (valve) I37.8
    with rheumatic fever (conditions in I00)
      active — *see* Endocarditis, acute, rheumatic
      inactive or quiescent (with chorea) I09.89
        with aortic, mitral or tricuspid disease
          I08.8
    acute or subacute I33.9
      rheumatic I01.1
        with chorea (acute) (rheumatic)
          (Sydenham's) I02.0
    arteriosclerotic I37.8
    congenital Q22.2
    rheumatic (chronic) (inactive) (with chorea) I09.89
      active or acute I01.1
        with chorea (acute) (rheumatic)
          (Sydenham's) I02.0
    syphilitic A52.03
  purulent (acute) (any valve) (subacute) I33.0
  Q fever A78 [I39]
  rheumatic (chronic) (inactive) (with chorea) I09.1
    active or acute (aortic) (mitral) (pulmonary)
      (tricuspid) I01.1
      with chorea (acute) (rheumatic) (Sydenham's)
        I02.0
  rheumatoid — *see* Rheumatoid, carditis
  septic (acute) (any valve) (subacute) I33.0
  streptococcal (acute) (any valve) (subacute) I33.0
  subacute — *see* Endocarditis, acute
  suppurative (acute) (any valve) (subacute) I33.0
  syphilitic A52.03
  toxic I33.9
  tricuspid (chronic) (heart) (inactive) (rheumatic)
    (valve) (with chorea) I07.9
    with
      aortic (valve) disease I08.2
        mitral (valve) disease I08.3
      mitral (valve) disease I08.1
        aortic (valve) disease I08.3

Endocarditis — *continued*
  tricuspid— *continued*
    with— *continued*
      rheumatic fever (conditions in I00)
        active — *see* Endocarditis, acute,
          rheumatic
        inactive or quiescent (with chorea) I07.8
    active or acute I01.1
      with chorea (acute) (rheumatic) (Sydenham's)
        I02.0
    arteriosclerotic I36.8
    nonrheumatic I36.8
      acute or subacute I33.9
    specified cause, except rheumatic I36.8
  tuberculous — *see* Tuberculosis, endocarditis
  typhoid A01.02
  ulcerative (acute) (any valve) (subacute) I33.0
  vegetative (acute) (any valve) (subacute) I33.0
  verrucous (atypical) (nonbacterial) (nonrheumatic)
    M32.11
Endocardium, endocardial (*see also* condition)
  cushion defect Q21.2
Endocervicitis (*see also* Cervicitis)
  due to intrauterine (contraceptive) device T83.6
  hyperplastic N72
Endocrine — *see* condition
Endocrinopathy, pluriglandular E31.9
Endodontic
  overfill M27.52
  underfill M27.53
Endodontitis K04.0
Endomastoiditis — *see* Mastoiditis
Endometrioma N80.9
Endometriosis N80.9
  appendix N80.5
  bladder N80.8
  bowel N80.5
  broad ligament N80.3
  cervix N80.0
  colon N80.5
  cul-de-sac (Douglas') N80.3
  exocervix N80.0
  fallopian tube N80.2
  female genital organ NEC N80.8
  gallbladder N80.8
  in scar of skin N80.6
  internal N80.0
  intestine N80.5
  lung N80.8
  myometrium N80.0
  ovary N80.1
  parametrium N80.3
  pelvic peritoneum N80.3
  peritoneal (pelvic) N80.3
  rectovaginal septum N80.4
  rectum N80.5
  round ligament N80.3
  skin (scar) N80.6
  specified site NEC N80.8
  stromal D39.0
  umbilicus N80.8
  uterus (internal) N80.0
  vagina N80.4
  vulva N80.8
Endometritis (decidual) (nonspecific) (purulent)
    (senile) (atrophic) (suppurative) N71.9
  with ectopic pregnancy O08.0
  acute N71.0
  blenorrhagic (gonococcal) (acute) (chronic) A54.24
  cervix, cervical (with erosion or ectropion) (*see also*
    Cervicitis)
    hyperplastic N72
  chlamydial A56.11
  chronic N71.1
  following
    abortion — *see* Abortion by type complicated by
      genital infection
    ectopic or molar pregnancy O08.0
  gonococcal, gonorrheal (acute) (chronic) A54.24
  hyperplastic (*see also* Hyperplasia, endometrial)
    N85.00
    cervix N72
  puerperal, postpartum, childbirth O86.12

Endometritis — *continued*
  subacute N71.0
  tuberculous A18.17
Endometrium — *see* condition
Endomyocarditis — *see* Endocarditis
Endomyocardiopathy, South African I42.3
Endomyofibrosis I42.3
Endomyometritis — *see* Endometritis
Endopericarditis — *see* Endocarditis
Endoperineuritis — *see* Disorder, nerve
Endophlebitis — *see* Phlebitis
Endophthalmia — *see* Endophthalmitis, purulent
Endophthalmitis (acute) (infective) (metastatic)
    (subacute) H44.009
  bleb associated (*see also* Bleb, inflammed (infected),
    postprocedural) H59.4
  gonorrheal A54.39
  in (due to)
    cysticercosis B69.1
    onchocerciasis B73.01
    toxocariasis B83.0
  panuveitis — *see* Panuveitis
  parasitic H44.12-
  purulent H44.00-
    panophthalmitis — *see* Panophthalmitis
    vitreous abscess H44.02-
  specified NEC H44.19
  sympathetic — *see* Uveitis, sympathetic
Endosalpingioma D28.2
Endosalpingiosis N94.89
Endosteitis — *see* Osteomyelitis
Endothelioma, bone — *see* Neoplasm, bone,
    malignant
Endotheliosis (hemorrhagic infectional) D69.8
Endotoxemia —code to condition
Endotrachelitis — *see* Cervicitis
Engelmann(-Camurati) syndrome Q78.3
English disease — *see* Rickets
Engman's disease L30.3
Engorgement
  breast N64.59
    newborn P83.4
    puerperal, postpartum O92.79
  lung (passive) — *see* Edema, lung
  pulmonary (passive) — *see* Edema, lung
  stomach K31.89
  venous, retina — *see* Occlusion, retina, vein,
    engorgement
Enlargement, enlarged (*see also* Hypertrophy)
  adenoids J35.2
    with tonsils J35.3
  alveolar ridge K08.8
    congenital — *see* Anomaly, alveolar
  apertures of diaphragm (congenital) Q79.1
  gingival K06.1
  heart, cardiac — *see* Hypertrophy, cardiac
  lacrimal gland, chronic H04.03-
  liver — *see* Hypertrophy, liver
  lymph gland or node R59.9
    generalized R59.1
    localized R59.0
  orbit H05.34-
  organ or site, congenital NEC — *see* Anomaly, by site
  parathyroid (gland) E21.0
  pituitary fossa R93.0
  prostate N40.0
    with lower urinary tract symptoms (LUTS) N40.1
    without lower urinary tract symtpoms (LUTS)
      N40.0
  sella turcica R93.0
  spleen — *see* Splenomegaly
  thymus (gland) (congenital) E32.0
  thyroid (gland) — *see* Goiter
  tongue K14.8
  tonsils J35.1
    with adenoids J35.3
  uterus N85.2
Enophthalmos H05.40-
  due to
    orbital tissue atrophy H05.41-
    trauma or surgery H05.42-

Enostosis M27.8
Entamebic, entamebiasis — *see* Amebiasis
Entanglement
  umbilical cord(s) O69.2
    with compression O69.2
      without compression O69.82
    around neck (with compression) O69.1
      without compression O69.81
    of twins in monoamniotic sac O69.2
Enteralgia — *see* Pain, abdominal
Enteric — *see* condition
Enteritis (acute) (diarrheal) (hemorrhagic)
    (noninfective) (septic) K52.9
  aertrycke infection A02.0
  adenovirus A08.2
  allergic K52.2
  amebic (acute) A06.0
    with abscess — *see* Abscess, amebic
    chronic A06.1
      with abscess — *see* Abscess, amebic
      nondysenteric A06.2
    nondysenteric A06.2
  astrovirus A08.32
  bacillary NOS A03.9
  bacterial A04.9
    specified NEC A04.8
  calicivirus A08.31
  candidal B37.82
  Chilomastix A07.8
  choleriformis A00.1
  chronic (noninfectious) K52.9
    ulcerative — *see* Colitis, ulcerative
  cicatrizing (chronic) — *see* Enteritis, regional, small
    intestine
  Clostridium
    botulinum (food poisoning) A05.1
    difficile A04.7
  coccidial A07.3
  coxsackie virus A08.39
  dietetic K52.2
  due to
    astrovirus A08.32
    calicivirus A08.31
    coxsackie virus A08.39
    echovirus A08.39
    enterovirus NEC A08.39
    food hypersensitivity K52.2
    infectious organism (bacterial) (viral) —
      see Enteritis, infectious
    torovirus A08.39
    Yersinia enterocolitica A04.6
  echovirus A08.39
  eltor A00.1
  enterovirus NEC A08.39
  eosinophilic K52.81
  epidemic (infectious) A09
  fulminant K55.0
  gangrenous — *see* Enteritis, infectious
  giardial A07.1
  infectious NOS A09
    due to
      adenovirus A08.2
      Aerobacter aerogenes A04.8
      Arizona (bacillus) A02.0
      bacteria NOS A04.9
        specified NEC A04.8
      Campylobacter A04.5
      Clostridium perfringens A04.8
      Enterobacter aerogenes A04.8
      enterovirus A08.39
      Escherichia coli A04.4
        enteroaggregative A04.4
        enterohemorrhagic A04.3
        enteroinvasive A04.2
        enteropathogenic A04.0
        enterotoxigenic A04.1
        specified NEC A04.4
      specified
        bacteria NEC A04.8
        virus NEC A08.39
      Staphylococcus A04.8

Enteritis— *continued*
  infectious—*continued*
    due to—*continued*
      virus NEC A08.4
        specified type NEC A08.39
      Yersinia enterocolitica A04.6
    specified organism NEC A08.8
  influenzal — *see* Influenza, with, digestive
    manifestations
  ischemic K55.9
    acute K55.0
    chronic K55.1
  microsporidial A07.8
  mucomembranous, myxomembranous — *see*
    Syndrome, irritable bowel
  mucous — *see* Syndrome, irritable bowel
  necroticans A05.2
  necrotizing of newborn — *see* Enterocolitis,
    necrotizing, in newborn
  neurogenic — *see* Syndrome, irritable bowel
  newborn necrotizing — *see* Enterocolitis,
    necrotizing, in newborn
  noninfectious K52.9
  norovirus A08.11
  parasitic NEC B82.9
  paratyphoid (fever) — *see* Fever, paratyphoid
  protozoal A07.9
    specified NEC A07.8
  radiation K52.0
  regional (of) K50.90
    with
      complication K50.919
        abscess K50.914
        fistula K50.913
        intestinal obstruction K50.912
        rectal bleeding K50.911
        specified complication NEC K50.918
    colon — *see* Enteritis, regional, large intestine
    duodenum — *see* Enteritis, regional, small
      intestine
    ileum — *see* Enteritis, regional, small intestine
    jejunum — *see* Enteritis, regional, small intestine
    large bowel — *see* Enteritis, regional, large
      intestine
    large intestine (colon) (rectum) K50.10
      with
        complication K50.119
          abscess K50.114
          fistula K50.113
          intestinal obstruction K50.112
          rectal bleeding K50.111
          small intestine (duodenum) (ileum)
            (jejunum) involvement K50.80
            with
              complication K50.819
                abscess K50.814
                fistula K50.813
                intestinal obstruction
                  K50.812
                rectal bleeding K50.811
                specified complication NEC
                  K50.818
          specified complication NEC K50.118
    rectum — *see* Enteritis, regional, large intestine
    small intestine (duodenum) (ileum) (jejunum)
      K50.00
      with
        complication K50.019
          abscess K50.014
          fistula K50.013
          intestinal obstruction K50.012
          large intestine (colon) (rectum)
            involvement K50.80
            with
              complication K50.819
                abscess K50.814
                fistula K50.813
                intestinal obstruction
                  K50.812
                rectal bleeding K50.811
                specified complication NEC
                  K50.818

Enteritis— *continued*
 regional—*continued*
  small intestine—*continued*
   with—*continued*
    complication—*continued*
     rectal bleeding K50.011
     specified complication NEC K50.018
  rotaviral A08.0
  Salmonella, salmonellosis (arizonae) (cholerae-suis)
   (enteritidis) (typhimurium) A02.0
  segmental — *see* Enteritis, regional
  septic A09
  Shigella — *see* Infection, Shigella
  small round structured NEC A08.19
  spasmodic, spastic — *see* Syndrome, irritable bowel
  staphylococcal A04.8
   due to food A05.0
  torovirus A08.39
  toxic K52.1
  trichomonal A07.8
  tuberculous A18.32
  typhosa A01.00
  ulcerative (chronic) — *see* Colitis, ulcerative
  viral A08.4
   adenovirus A08.2
   enterovirus A08.39
   Rotavirus A08.0
   small round structured NEC A08.19
   specified NEC A08.39
   virus specified NEC A08.39
Enterobiasis B80
Enterobius vermicularis (infection) (infestation) B80
Enterocele (*see also* Hernia, abdomen)
 pelvic, pelvis (acquired) (congenital) N81.5
 vagina, vaginal (acquired) (congenital) NEC N81.5
Enterocolitis (*see also* Enteritis) K52.9
 due to Clostridium difficile A04.7
 fulminant ischemic K55.0
 granulomatous — *see* Enteritis, regional
 hemorrhagic (acute) K55.0
  chronic K55.1
 infectious NEC A09
 ischemic K55.9
 necrotizing
  due to Clostridium difficile A04.7
  in newborn P77.9
   stage 1 (without pneumatosis, without
    perforation) P77.1
   stage 2 (with pneumatosis, without
    perforation) P77.2
   stage 3 (with pneumatosis, with perforation)
    P77.3
 noninfectious K52.9
  newborn — *see* Enterocolitis, necrotizing, in
   newborn
 pseudomembranous (newborn) A04.7
 radiation K52.0
  newborn — *see* Enterocolitis, necrotizing, in
   newborn
 ulcerative (chronic) *see* Pancolitis, ulcerative
  (chronic)
Enterogastritis — *see* Enteritis
Enteropathy K63.9
 gluten-sensitive K90.0
 hemorrhagic, terminal K55.0
 protein-losing K90.4
Enteroperitonitis — *see* Peritonitis
Enteroptosis K63.4
Enterorrhagia K92.2
Enterospasm (*see also* Syndrome, irritable, bowel)
 psychogenic F45.8
Enterostenosis K56.69 — *see also* Obstruction,
  intestine
Enterostomy
 complication — *see* Complication, enterostomy
 status Z93.4
Enterovirus, as cause of disease classified
  elsewhere B97.10
 coxsackievirus B97.11
 echovirus B97.12
 other specified B97.19
Enthesopathy (peripheral) M77.9
 Achilles tendinitis — *see* Tendinitis, Achilles

Enthesopathy — *continued*
 ankle and tarsus M77.9
  specified type NEC — *see* Enthesopathy, foot,
   specified type NEC
 anterior tibial syndrome M76.81-
 calcaneal spur — *see* Spur, bone, calcaneal
 elbow region M77.8
  lateral epicondylitis — *see* Epicondylitis, lateral
  medial epicondylitis — *see* Epicondylitis, medial
 foot NEC M77.9
  metatarsalgia — *see* Metatarsalgia
  specified type NEC M77.5-
 forearm M77.9
 gluteal tendinitis — *see* Tendinitis, gluteal
 hand M77.9
 hip — *see* Enthesopathy, lower limb, thigh, specified
  type NEC
 iliac crest spur — *see* Spur, bone, iliac crest
 iliotibial band syndrome — *see* Syndrome, iliotibial
  band
 knee — *see* Enthesopathy, lower limb, lower leg,
  specified type NEC
 lateral epicondylitis — *see* Epicondylitis, lateral
 lower limb (excluding foot) M76.9
  Achilles tendinitis — *see* Tendinitis, Achilles
  anterior tibial syndrome M76.81-
  gluteal tendinitis — *see* Tendinitis, gluteal
  iliac crest spur — *see* Spur, bone, iliac crest
  iliotibial band syndrome — *see* Syndrome,
   iliotibial band
  patellar tendinitis — *see* Tendinitis, patellar
  pelvic region — *see* Enthesopathy, lower limb,
   thigh
  peroneal tendinitis — *see* Tendinitis, peroneal
  posterior tibial syndrome M76.82
  psoas tendinitis — *see* Tendinitis, psoas
  shoulder M77.9
  specified type NEC M76.89-
  tibial collateral bursitis — *see* Bursitis, tibial
   collateral
 medial epicondylitis — *see* Epicondylitis,
  medialmetatarsalgia — *see* Metatarsalgia
 multiple sites M77.9
 patellar tendinitis — *see* Tendinitis, patellar
 pelvis M77.9
 periarthritis of wrist — *see* Periarthritis, wrist
 peroneal tendinitis — *see* Tendinitis, peroneal
 posterior tibial syndrome M76.82-
 psoas tendinitis — *see* Tendinitis, psoas
 shoulder region — *see* Lesion, shoulder
 specified site NEC M77.9
 specified type NEC M77.8
 spinal M46.00
  cervical region M46.02
  cervicothoracic region M46.03
  lumbar region M46.06
  lumbosacral region M46.07
  multiple sites M46.09
  occipito-atlanto-axial region M46.01
  sacrococcygeal region M46.08
  thoracic region M46.04
  thoracolumbar region M46.05
 tibial collateral bursitis — *see* Bursitis, tibial
  collateral
 upper arm M77.9
 wrist and carpus NEC M77.8
  calcaneal spur — *see* Spur, bone, calcaneal
  periarthritis of wrist — *see* Periarthritis, wrist
Entomophobia F40.218
Entomophthoromycosis B46.8
Entrance, air into vein — *see* Embolism, air
Entrapment, nerve — *see* Neuropathy, entrapment
Entropion (eyelid) (paralytic) H02.009
 cicatricial H02.019
  left H02.016
   lower H02.015
   upper H02.014
  right H02.013
   lower H02.012
   upper H02.011
 congenital Q10.2

Entropion — *continued*
 left H02.006
  lower H02.005
  upper H02.004
 mechanical H02.029
  left H02.026
   lower H02.025
   upper H02.024
  right H02.023
   lower H02.022
   upper H02.021
 right H02.003
  lower H02.002
  upper H02.001
 senile H02.039
  left H02.036
   lower H02.035
   upper H02.034
  right H02.033
   lower H02.032
   upper H02.031
 spastic H02.049
  left H02.046
   lower H02.045
   upper H02.044
  right H02.043
   lower H02.042
   upper H02.041
Enucleated eye (traumatic, current) S05.7-
Enuresis R32
 functional F98.0
 habit disturbance F98.0
 nocturnal R32
  psychogenic F98.0
 nonorganic origin F98.0
 psychogenic F98.0
Eosinopenia — *see* Agranulocytosis
Eosinophilia (allergic) (hereditary) (idiopathic)
  (secondary) D72.1
 infiltrative J82
 Löffler's J82
 peritonal — *see* Peritonitis, eosinophilic
 pulmonary NEC J82
 tropical (pulmonary) J82
Eosinophilia-myalgia syndrome M35.8
Ependymitis (acute) (cerebral) (chronic) (granular) —
  see Encephalomyelitis
Ependymoblastoma
 specified site — *see* Neoplasm, malignant, by site
 unspecified site C71.9
Ependymoma (epithelial) (malignant)
 anaplastic
  specified site — *see* Neoplasm, malignant, by site
  unspecified site C71.9
 benign
  specified site — *see* Neoplasm, benign, by site
  unspecified site D33.2
 myxopapillary D43.2
  specified site — *see* Neoplasm, uncertain
   behavior, by site
  unspecified site D43.2
 papillary D43.2
  specified site — *see* Neoplasm, uncertain
   behavior, by site
  unspecified site D43.2
 specified site — *see* Neoplasm, malignant, by site
 unspecified site C71.9
Ependymopathy G93.89
Ephelis, ephelides L81.2
Epiblepharon (congenital) Q10.3
Epicanthus, epicanthic fold (eyelid) (congenital)
  Q10.3
Epicondylitis (elbow)
 lateral M77.1-
 medial M77.0-
Epicystitis — *see* Cystitis
Epidemic — *see* condition
Epidermidalization, cervix — *see* Dysplasia, cervix
Epidermis, epidermal — *see* condition
Epidermodysplasia verruciformis B07.8

Epilepsy, epileptic, epilepsia — *continued*
  uncinate (gyrus) — *see* Epilepsy,
      localization-related, symptomatic, with
      complex partial seizures
  Unverricht (-Lundborg) (familial myoclonic) — *see*
      Epilepsy, generalized, idiopathic
  visceral — *see* Epilepsy, specified NEC
  visual — *see* Epilepsy, specified NEC
Epiloia Q85.1
Epimenorrhea N92.0
Epipharyngitis — *see* Nasopharyngitis
Epiphora H04.20-
  due to
      excess lacrimation H04.21-
      insufficient drainage H04.22-
Epiphyseal arrest — *see* Arrest, epiphyseal
Epiphyseolysis, epiphysiolysis — *see*
      Osteochondropathy
Epiphysitis (*see also* Osteochondropathy)
  juvenile M92.9
  syphilitic (congenital) A50.02
Epiplocele — *see* Hernia, abdomen
Epiploitis — *see* Peritonitis
Epiplosarcomphalocele — *see* Hernia, umbilicus
Episcleritis (suppurative) H15.10-
  in (due to)
      syphilis A52.71
      tuberculosis A18.51
  nodular H15.12-
  periodica fugax H15.11-
      angioneurotic — *see* Edema, angioneurotic
  syphilitic (late) A52.71
  tuberculous A18.51
Episode
  affective, mixed F39
  depersonalization (in neurotic state) F48.1
  depressive F32.9
      major F32.9
          mild F32.0
          moderate F32.1
          severe (without psychotic symptoms) F32.2
              with psychotic symptoms F32.3
      recurrent F33.9
          brief F33.8
      specified NEC F32.8
  hypomanic F30.8
  manic F30.9
      with
          psychotic symptoms F30.2
          remission (full) F30.4
              partial F30.3
      other specified F30.8
      recurrent F31.89
      without psychotic symptoms F30.10
          mild F30.11
          moderate F30.12
          severe (without psychotic symptoms) F30.13
              with psychotic symptoms F30.2
  psychotic F23
      organic F06.8
  schizophrenic (acute) NEC, brief F23
Epispadias (female) (male) Q64.0
Episplenitis D73.89
Epistaxis (multiple) R04.0
  hereditary I78.0
  vicarious menstruation N94.89
Epithelioma (malignant) (*see also* Neoplasm,
      malignant, by site)
  adenoides cysticum — *see* Neoplasm, skin, benign
  basal cell — *see* Neoplasm, skin, malignant
  benign — *see* Neoplasm, benign, by site
  Bowen's — *see* Neoplasm, skin, in situ
  calcifying, of Malherbe — *see* Neoplasm, skin,
      benign
  external site — *see* Neoplasm, skin, malignant
  intraepidermal, Jadassohn — *see* Neoplasm, skin,
      benign
  squamous cell — *see* Neoplasm, malignant, by site
Epitheliomatosis pigmented Q82.1
Epitheliopathy, multifocal placoid pigment H30.14-
Epithelium, epithelial — *see* condition
Epituberculosis (with atelectasis) (allergic) A15.7
Eponychia Q84.6

Epstein's
  nephrosis or syndrome — *see* Nephrosis
  pearl K09.8
Epulis (gingiva) (fibrous) (giant cell) K06.8
Equinia A24.0
Equinovarus (congenital) (talipes) Q66.0
  acquired — *see* Deformity, limb, clubfoot
Equivalent
  convulsive (abdominal) — *see* Epilepsy, specified
      NEC
  epileptic (psychic) — *see* Epilepsy,
      localization-related, symptomatic, with
      complex partial seizures
Erb(-Duchenne) **paralysis** (birth injury) (newborn)
      P14.0
Erb-Goldflam disease or syndrome G70.00
  with exacerbation (acute) G70.01
  in crisis G70.01
Erb's
  disease G71.0
  palsy, paralysis (brachial) (birth) (newborn) P14.0
      spinal (spastic) syphilitic A52.17
  pseudohypertrophic muscular dystrophy G71.0
Erdheim's syndrome (acromegalic macrospondylitis)
      E22.0
Erection, painful (persistent) — *see* Priapism
Ergosterol deficiency (vitamin D) E55.9
  with
      adult osteomalacia M83.8
      rickets — *see* Rickets
Ergotism (*see also* Poisoning, food, noxious, plant)
  from ergot used as drug (migraine therapy) — *see*
      Table of Drugs and Chemicals
Erosio interdigitalis blastomycetica B37.2
Erosion
  artery I77.2
      without rupture I77.89
  bone — *see* Disorder, bone, density and structure,
      specified NEC
  bronchus J98.09
  cartilage (joint) — *see* Disorder, cartilage, specified
      type NEC
  cervix (uteri) (acquired) (chronic) (congenital) N86
      with cervicitis N72
  cornea (nontraumatic) — *see* Ulcer, cornea
      recurrent H18.83-
      traumatic — *see* Abrasion, cornea
  dental (idiopathic) (occupational) (due to diet, drugs
      or vomiting) K03.2
  duodenum, postpyloric — *see* Ulcer, duodenum
  esophagus K22.10
      with bleeding K22.11
  gastric — *see* Ulcer, stomach
  gastrojejunal — *see* Ulcer, gastrojejunal
  intestine K63.3
  lymphatic vessel I89.8
  pylorus, pyloric (ulcer) — *see* Ulcer, stomach
  spine, aneurysmal A52.09
  stomach — *see* Ulcer, stomach
  teeth (idiopathic) (occupational) (due to diet, drugs
      or vomiting) K03.2
  urethra N36.8
  uterus N85.8
Erotomania F52.8
Error
  metabolism, inborn — *see* Disorder, metabolism
  refractive — *see* Disorder, refraction
Eructation R14.2
  nervous or psychogenic F45.8
Eruption
  creeping B76.9
  drug (generalized) (taken internally) L27.0
      fixed L27.1
      in contact with skin — *see* Dermatitis, due to
          drugs
      localized L27.1
  Hutchinson, summer L56.4
  Kaposi's varicelliform B00.0
  napkin L22
  polymorphous light (sun) L56.4
  recalcitrant pustular L13.8
  ringed R23.8

Eruption—*continued*
  skin (nonspecific) R21
      creeping (meaning hookworm) B76.9
      due to inoculation/vaccination (generalized) (*see
          also* Dermatitis, due to, vaccine) L27.0
          localized L27.0
      erysipeloid A26.0
      feigned L98.1
      Kaposi's varicelliform B00.0
      lichenoid L28.0
      meaning dermatitis — *see* Dermatitis
      toxic NEC L53.0
  tooth, teeth, abnormal (incomplete) (late)
      (premature) (sequence) K00.6
  vesicular R23.8
Erysipelas (gangrenous) (infantile) (newborn)
      (phlegmonous) (suppurative) A46
  external ear A46 [H62.40]
  puerperal, postpartum O86.89
Erysipeloid A26.9
  cutaneous (Rosenbach's) A26.0
  disseminated A26.8
  sepsis A26.7
  specified NEC A26.8
Erythema, erythematous (infectional) (inflammation)
      L53.9
  ab igne L59.0
  annulare (centrifugum) (rheumaticum) L53.1
  arthriticum epidemicum A25.1
  brucellum — *see* Brucellosis
  chronic figurate NEC L53.3
  chronicum migrans (Borrelia burgdorferi) A69.20
  diaper L22
  due to
      chemical NEC L53.0
          in contact with skin L24.5
      drug (internal use) — *see* Dermatitis, due to,
          drugs
  elevatum diutinum L95.1
  endemic E52
  epidemic, arthritic A25.1
  figuratum perstans L53.3
  gluteal L22
  heat—code by site under Burn, first degree
  ichthyosiforme congenitum bullous Q80.3
  in diseases classified elsewhere L54
  induratum (nontuberculous) L52
      tuberculous A18.4
  infectiosum B08.3
  intertrigo L30.4
  iris L51.9
  marginatum L53.2
      in (due to) acute rheumatic fever I00
  medicamentosum — *see* Dermatitis, due to, drugs
  migrans A26.0
      chronicum A69.20
      tongue K14.1
  multiforme (major) (minor) L51.9
      bullous, bullosum L51.1
      conjunctiva L51.1
      nonbullous L51.0
      pemphigoides L12.0
      specified NEC L51.8
  napkin L22
  neonatorum P83.8
      toxic P83.1
  nodosum L52
      tuberculous A18.4
  palmar L53.8
  pernio T69.1
  rash, newborn P83.8
  scarlatiniform (recurrent) (exfoliative) L53.8
  solare L55.0
  specified NEC L53.8
  toxic, toxicum NEC L53.0
      newborn P83.1
  tuberculous (primary) A18.4
Erythematous, erythematosus — *see* condition
Erythermalgia (primary) I73.81
Erythralgia I73.81
Erythrasma L08.1
Erythredema (polyneuropathy) — *see* Poisoning,
      mercury

Erythremia (acute) C94.0-
   chronic D45
   secondary D75.1
Erythroblastopenia (*see also* Aplasia, red cell) D60.9
   congenital D61.01
Erythroblastophthisis D61.09
Erythroblastosis (fetalis) (newborn) P55.9
   due to
      ABO (antibodies) (incompatibility)
         (isoimmunization) P55.1
      Rh (antibodies) (incompatibility)
         (isoimmunization) P55.0
Erythrocyanosis (crurum) I73.89
Erythrocythemia — *see* Erythremia
Erythrocytosis (megalosplenic) (secondary) D75.1
   familial D75.0
   oval, hereditary — *see* Elliptocytosis
   secondary D75.1
   stress D75.1
Erythroderma (secondary) (*see also* Erythema) L53.9
   bullous ichthyosiform, congenital Q80.3
   desquamativum L21.1
   ichthyosiform, congenital (bullous) Q80.3
   neonatorum P83.8
   psoriaticum L40.8
Erythrodysesthesia, palmar plantar (PPE) L27.1
Erythrogenesis imperfecta D61.09
Erythroleukemia C94.0-
Erythromelalgia I73.81
Erythrophagocytosis D75.89
Erythrophobia F40.298
Erythroplakia, oral epithelium, and tongue K13.29
Erythroplasia (Queyrat) D07.4
   specified site — *see* Neoplasm, skin, in situ
   unspecified site D07.4
Escherichia (E.) coli, as cause of disease classified elsewhere B96.2
Esophagismus K22.4
Esophagitis (acute) (alkaline) (chemical) (chronic)
   (infectional) (necrotic) (peptic) (postoperative)
   K20.9
   candidal B37.81
   due to gastrointestinal reflux disease K21.0
   eosinophilic K20.0
   reflux K21.0
   specified NEC K20.8
   tuberculous A18.83
   ulcerative K22.10
      with bleeding K22.11
Esophagocele K22.5
Esophagomalacia K22.8
Esophagospasm K22.4
Esophagostenosis K22.2
Esophagostomiasis B81.8
Esophagotracheal — *see* condition
Esophagus — *see* condition
Esophoria H50.51
   convergence, excess H51.12
   divergence, insufficiency H51.8
Esotropia — *see* Strabismus, convergent concomitant
Espundia B55.2
Essential — *see* condition
Esthesioneuroblastoma C30.0
Esthesioneurocytoma C30.0
Esthesioneuroepithelioma C30.0
Esthiomene A55
Estivo-autumnal malaria (fever) B50.9
Estrangement (marital) Z63.5
   parent-child NEC Z62.890
Estriasis — *see* Myiasis
Ethanolism — *see* Alcoholism
Etherism — *see* Dependence, drug, inhalant
Ethmoid, ethmoidal — *see* condition
Ethmoiditis (chronic) (purulent) (nonpurulent) (*see also* Sinusitis, ethmoidal)
   influenzal — *see* Influenza, with, respiratory
      manifestations NEC
   Woakes' J33.1
Ethylism — *see* Alcoholism
Eulenburg's disease (congenital paramyotonia)
   G71.19
Eumycetoma B47.0

Eunuchoidism E29.1
   hypogonadotropic E23.0
European blastomycosis — *see* Cryptococcosis
Eustachian — *see* condition
Evaluation (for) (of)
   development state
      adolescent Z00.3
      period of
         delayed growth in childhood Z00.70
            with abnormal findings Z00.71
         rapid growth in childhood Z00.2
         puberty Z00.3
   growth and developmental state (period of rapid
      growth) Z00.2
      delayed growth Z00.70
         with abnormal findings Z00.71
   mental health (status) Z00.8
      requested by authority Z04.6
   period of
      delayed growth in childhood Z00.70
         with abnormal findings Z00.71
      rapid growth in childhood Z00.2
   suspected condition — *see* Observation
Evans syndrome D69.41
Event apparent life threatening in newborn and infant (ALTE) R68.13
Eventration (*see also* Hernia, ventral)
   colon into chest — *see* Hernia, diaphragm
   diaphragm (congenital) Q79.1
Eversion
   bladder N32.89
   cervix (uteri) N86
      with cervicitis N72
   foot NEC (*see also* Deformity, valgus, ankle)
      congenital Q66.6
   punctum lacrimale (postinfectional) (senile) H04.52-
   ureter (meatus) N28.89
   urethra (meatus) N36.8
   uterus N81.4
Evidence
   cytologic
      of malignancy on anal smear R85.614
      of malignancy on cervical smear R87.614
      of malignancy on vaginal smear R87.624
Evisceration
   birth injury P15.8
   traumatic NEC
      eye — *see* Enucleated eye
Evulsion — *see* Avulsion
Ewing's sarcoma or tumor — *see* Neoplasm, bone, malignant
Examination (for) (following) (general) (of) (routine)
   Z00.00
   with abnormal findings Z00.01
   abuse, physical (alleged), ruled out
      adult Z04.71
      child Z04.72
   adolescent (development state) Z00.3
   alleged rape or sexual assault (victim), ruled out
      adult Z04.41
      child Z04.42
   allergy Z01.82
   annual (adult) (periodic) (physical) Z00.00
      with abnormal findings Z00.01
      gynecological Z01.419
         with abnormal findings Z01.411
   antibody response Z01.84
   blood — *see* Examination, laboratory
   blood pressure Z01.30
      with abnormal findings Z01.31
   cancer staging — *see* Neoplasm, malignant, by site
   cervical Papanicolaou smear Z12.4
      as part of routine gynecological examination
         Z01.419
         with abnormal findings Z01.411
   child (over 28 days old) Z00.129
      with abnormal findings Z00.121
      under 28 days old — *see* Newborn, examination
   clinical research control or normal comparison Z00.6
   contraceptive (drug) maintenance (routine) Z30.8
      device (intrauterine) Z30.431
   developmental — *see* Examination, child

Examination — *continued*
   dental Z01.20
      with abnormal findings Z01.21
   donor (potential) Z00.5
   ear Z01.10
      with abnormal findings NEC Z01.118
   eye Z01.00
      with abnormal findings Z01.01
   following
      accident NEC Z04.3
         transport Z04.1
         work Z04.2
      assault, alleged, ruled out
         adult Z04.71
         child Z04.72
      motor vehicle accident Z04.1
      treatment (for) Z09
         combined NEC Z09
            fracture Z09
            malignant neoplasm Z08
         malignant neoplasm Z08
         mental disorder Z09
         specified condition NEC Z09
   follow-up (routine) (following) Z09
      chemotherapy NEC Z09
         malignant neoplasm Z08
      fracture Z09
      malignant neoplasm Z08
      postpartum Z39.2
      psychotherapy Z09
      radiotherapy NEC Z09
         malignant neoplasm Z08
      surgery NEC Z09
         malignant neoplasm Z08
   gynecological Z01.419
      with abnormal findings Z01.411
      for contraceptive maintenance Z30.8
   health — *see* Examination, medical
   hearing Z01.10
      with abnormal findings NEC Z01.118
      following failed hearing screening Z01.110
   immunity status testing Z01.84
   laboratory (as part of a general medical
      examination) Z00.00
      with abnormal findings Z00.01
      preprocedural Z01.812
   lactating mother Z39.1
   medical (adult) (for) (of) Z00.00
      with abnormal findings Z00.01
      administrative purpose only Z02.9
         specified NEC Z02.89
      admission to
         armed forces Z02.3
         old age home Z02.2
         prison Z02.89
         residential institution Z02.2
         school Z02.0
            following illness or medical treatment
               Z02.0
         summer camp Z02.89
      adoption Z02.82
      blood alcohol or drug level Z02.83
      camp (summer) Z02.89
      clinical research, normal subject Z00.6
      control subject in clinical research Z00.6
      donor (potential) Z00.5
      driving license Z02.4
      general (adult) Z00.00
         with abnormal findings Z00.01
      immigration Z02.89
      insurance purposes Z02.6
      marriage Z02.89
      medicolegal reasons NEC Z04.8
      naturalization Z02.89
      participation in sport Z02.5
      paternity testing Z02.81
      population survey Z00.8
      pre-employment Z02.1
      pre-operative — *see* Examination,
         pre-procedural
      pre-procedural
         cardiovascular Z01.810
         respiratory Z01.811

Examination — *continued*
  medical—*continued*
    pre-procedural—*continued*
      specified NEC Z01.818
    preschool children
      for admission to school Z02.0
    prisoners
      for entrance into prison Z02.89
    recruitment for armed forces Z02.3
    specified NEC Z00.8
    sport competition Z02.5
  medicolegal reason NEC Z04.8
  newborn — *see* Newborn, examination
  pelvic (annual) (periodic) Z01.419
    with abnormal findings Z01.411
  period of rapid growth in childhood Z00.2
  periodic (adult) (annual) (routine) Z00.00
    with abnormal findings Z00.01
  physical (adult) (*see also* Examination, medical)
      Z00.00
    sports Z02.5
  postpartum
    immediately after delivery Z39.0
    routine follow-up Z39.2
  prenatal (normal pregnancy) — *see* Category O34
  pre-chemotherapy (antineoplastic) Z01.818
  pre-procedural (pre-operative)
    cardiovascular Z01.810
    laboratory Z01.812
    respiratory Z01.811
    specified NEC Z01.818
  prior to chemotherapy (antineoplastic) Z01.818
  psychiatric NEC Z00.8
    follow-up not needing further care Z09
    requested by authority Z04.6
  radiological (as part of a general medical
      examination) Z00.00
    with abnormal findings Z00.01
  repeat cervical smear to confirm findings of recent
      normal smear following initial abnormal
      smear Z01.42
  skin (hypersensitivity) Z01.82
  special (*see also* Examination, by type) Z01.89
    specified type NEC Z01.89
  specified type or reason NEC Z04.8
  teeth Z01.20
    with abnormal findings Z01.21
  urine — *see* Examination, laboratory
  vision Z01.00
    with abnormal findings Z01.01
Exanthem, exanthema (*see also* Rash)
  with enteroviral vesicular stomatitis B08.4
  Boston A88.0
  epidemic with meningitis A88.0 [G02]
  subitum B08.20
    due to human herpesvirus 6 B08.21
    due to human herpesvirus 7 B08.22
  viral, virus B09
    specified type NEC B08.8
Excess, excessive, excessively
  alcohol level in blood R78.0
  androgen (ovarian) E28.1
  attrition, tooth, teeth K03.0
  carotene, carotin (dietary) E67.1
  cold, effects of T69.9
    specified effect NEC T69.8
  convergence H51.12
  crying
    in child, adolescent, or adult R45.83
    in infant R68.11
  development, breast N62
  divergence H51.8
  drinking (alcohol) NEC (without dependence)
      F10.10
    habitual (continual) (without remission) F10.20
  eating R63.2
  estrogen E28.0
  fat (*see also* Obesity)
    in heart — *see* Degeneration, myocardial
    localized E65
  foreskin N47.8
  gas R14.0
  glucagon E16.3

Excess, excessive, excessively— *continued*
  heat — *see* Heat
  intermaxillary vertical dimension of fully erupted
      teeth M26.37
  interocclusal distance of fully erupted teeth M26.37
  kalium E87.5
  large
    colon K59.3
      congenital Q43.8
    infant P08.0
    organ or site, congenital NEC — *see* Anomaly, by
        site
  long
    organ or site, congenital NEC — *see* Anomaly, by
        site
  menstruation (with regular cycle) N92.0
    with irregular cycle N92.1
  napping Z72.821
  natrium E87.0
  number of teeth K00.1
  nutrient (dietary) NEC R63.2
  potassium (K) E87.5
  salivation K11.7
  secretion (*see also* Hypersecretion)
    milk O92.6
    sputum R09.3
    sweat R61
  sexual drive F52.8
  short
    organ or site, congenital NEC — *see* Anomaly, by
        site
    umbilical cord in labor or delivery O69.3
  skin, eyelid (acquired) — *see* Blepharochalasis
    congenital Q10.3
  sodium (Na) E87.0
  spacing of fully erupted teeth M26.32
  sputum R09.3
  sweating R61
  thirst R63.1
    due to deprivation of water T73.1
  tuberosity of jaw M26.07
  vitamin
    A (dietary) E67.0
      administered as drug (prolonged intake) —
          see Table of Drugs and Chemicals,
          vitamins, adverse effect
      overdose or wrong substance given or taken
          — *see* Table of Drugs and Chemicals,
          vitamins, poisoning
    D (dietary) E67.3
      administered as drug (prolonged intake) —
          see Table of Drugs and Chemicals,
          vitamins, adverse effect
      overdose or wrong substance given or taken
          — *see* Table of Drugs and Chemicals,
          vitamins, poisoning
  weight
    gain R63.5
    loss R63.4
Excitability, abnormal, under minor stress
    (personality disorder) F60.3
Excitation
  anomalous atrioventricular I45.6
  psychogenic F30.8
  reactive (from emotional stress, psychological
      trauma) F30.8
Excitement
  hypomanic F30.8
  manic F30.9
  mental, reactive (from emotional stress,
      psychological trauma) F30.8
  state, reactive (from emotional stress, psychological
      trauma) F30.8
Excoriation (traumatic) (*see also* Abrasion)
  neurotic L98.1
Exfoliation
  due to erythematous conditions according to extent
      of body surface involved L49.0
    10-19 percent of body surface L49.1
    20-29 percent of body surface L49.2
    30-39 percent of body surface L49.3
    40-49 percent of body surface L49.4
    50-59 percent of body surface L49.5

Exfoliation—*continued*
  due to erythematous conditions according to
      extent of body surface involved—*continued*
    60-69 percent of body surface L49.6
    70-79 percent of body surface L49.7
    80-89 percent of body surface L49.8
    90-99 percent of body surface L49.9
    less than 10 percent of body surface L49.0
  teeth, due to systemic causes K08.0
Exfoliative — *see* condition
Exhaustion, exhaustive (physical NEC) R53.83
  battle F43.0
  cardiac — *see* Failure, heart
  delirium F43.0
  due to
    cold T69.8
    excessive exertion T73.3
    exposure T73.2
    neurasthenia F48.8
  heart — *see* Failure, heart
  heat (*see also* Heat, exhaustion) T67.5
    due to
      salt depletion T67.4
      water depletion T67.3
  maternal, complicating delivery O75.81
  mental F48.8
  myocardium, myocardial — *see* Failure, heart
  nervous F48.8
  old age R54
  psychogenic F48.8
  psychosis F43.0
  senile R54
  vital NEC Z73.0
Exhibitionism F65.2
Exocervicitis — *see* Cervicitis
Exomphalos Q79.2
  meaning hernia — *see* Hernia, umbilicus
Exophoria H50.52
  convergence, insufficiency H51.11
  divergence, excess H51.8
Exophthalmos H05.2-
  congenital Q15.8
  constant NEC H05.24-
  displacement, globe — *see* Displacement, globe
  due to thyrotoxicosis (hyperthyroidism) — *see*
      Hyperthyroidism, with, goiter (diffuse)
  dysthyroid — *see* Hyperthyroidism, with, goiter
      (diffuse)
  goiter — *see* Hyperthyroidism, with, goiter (diffuse)
  intermittent NEC H05.25-
  malignant — *see* Hyperthyroidism, with, goiter
      (diffuse)
  orbital
    edema — *see* Edema, orbit
    hemorrhage — *see* Hemorrhage, orbit
  pulsating NEC H05.26-
  thyrotoxic, thyrotropic — *see* Hyperthyroidism,
      with, goiter (diffuse)
Exostosis (*see also* Disorder, bone)
  cartilaginous — *see* Neoplasm, bone, benign
  congenital (multiple) Q78.6
  external ear canal H61.81-
  gonococcal A54.49
  jaw (bone) M27.8
  multiple, congenital Q78.6
  orbit H05.35-
  osteocartilaginous — *see* Neoplasm, bone, benign
  syphilitic A52.77
Exotropia — *see* Strabismus, divergent concomitant
Explanation of
  investigation finding Z71.2
  medication Z71.89
Exposure (to) (*see also* Contact, with) T75.89
  acariasis Z20.7
  AIDS virus Z20.6
  air pollution Z77.110
  algae and algae toxins Z77.121
  algae bloom Z77.121
  anthrax Z20.810
  aromatic amines Z77.020
  aromatic (hazardous) compounds NEC Z77.028
  aromatic dyes NOS Z77.028
  arsenic Z77.010

Exposure — *continued*
  asbestos Z77.090
  bacterial disease NEC Z20.818
  benzene Z77.021
  blue-green algae bloom Z77.121
  body fluids (potentially hazardous) Z77.21
  brown tide Z77.121
  chemicals (chiefly nonmedicinal) (hazardous) NEC Z77.098
  cholera Z20.09
  chromium compounds Z77.018
  cold, effects of T69.9
    specified effect NEC T69.8
  communicable disease Z20.9
    bacterial NEC Z20.818
    specified NEC Z20.89
    viral NEC Z20.828
  cyanobacteria bloom Z77.121
  disaster Z65.5
  discrimination Z60.5
  dyes Z77.098
  Escherichia coli (E. coli) Z20.01
  effects of T73.9
  environmental tobacco smoke (acute) (chronic) Z77.22
  exhaustion due to T73.2
  fiberglass — *see* Table of Drugs and Chemicals, fiberglass
  German measles Z20.4
  gonorrhea Z20.2
  hazardous metals NEC Z77.018
  hazardous substances NEC Z77.29
  hazards in the physical environment NEC Z77.128
  hazards to health NEC Z77.9
  human immunodeficiency virus (HIV) Z20.6
  human T-lymphotropic virus type-1 (HTLV-1) Z20.89
  infestation (parasitic) NEC Z20.7
  intestinal infectious disease NEC Z20.09
    Escherichia coli (E. coli) Z20.01
  lead Z77.011
  meningococcus Z20.811
  mold (toxic) Z77.120
  nickel dust Z77.018
  noise Z77.122
  occupational
    air contaminants NEC Z57.39
    dust Z57.2
    environmental tobacco smoke Z57.31
    extreme temperature Z57.6
    noise Z57.0
    radiation Z57.1
    risk factors Z57.9
      specified NEC Z57.8
    toxic agents (gases) (liquids) (solids) (vapors) in agriculture Z57.4
    toxic agents (gases) (liquids) (solids) (vapors) in industry NEC Z57.5
    vibration Z57.7
  parasitic disease NEC Z20.7
  pediculosis Z20.7
  persecution Z60.5
  pfiesteria piscicida Z77.121
  poliomyelitis Z20.89
  polycyclic aromatic hydrocarbons Z77.028
  pollution
    air Z77.110
    environmental NEC Z77.118
    soil Z77.112
    water Z77.111
  prenatal (drugs) (toxic chemicals) — *see* Newborn, affected by (suspected to be), noxious substances transmitted via placenta or breast milk
  rabies Z20.3
  radiation, naturally occurring NEC Z77.123
  radon Z77.123
  red tide (Florida) Z77.121
  rubella Z20.4
  second hand tobacco smoke (acute) (chronic) Z77.22
    in the perinatal period P96.81
  sexually-transmitted disease Z20.2
  smallpox (laboratory) Z20.89

Exposure — *continued*
  syphilis Z20.2
  terrorism Z65.4
  torture Z65.4
  tuberculosis Z20.1
  varicella Z20.820
  venereal disease Z20.2
  viral disease NEC Z20.828
  war Z65.5
  water pollution Z77.110
Exsanguination — *see* Hemorrhage
Exstrophy
  abdominal contents Q45.8
  bladder Q64.10
    cloacal Q64.12
    specified type NEC Q64.19
    supravesical fissure Q64.11
Extensive — *see* condition
Extra *(see also* Accessory)
  marker chromosomes (normal individual) Q92.61
    in abnormal individual Q92.62
  rib Q76.6
    cervical Q76.5
Extrasystoles (supraventricular) I49.49
  atrial I49.1
  auricular I49.1
  junctional I49.2
  ventricular I49.3
Extrauterine gestation or pregnancy — *see* Pregnancy, by site
Extravasation
  blood R58
  chyle into mesentery I89.8
  pelvicalyceal N13.8
  pyelosinus N13.8
  urine (from ureter) R39.0
  vesicant agent
    antineoplastic chemotherapy T80.810
    other agent NEC T80.818
Extremity — *see* condition, limb
Extrophy — *see* Exstrophy
Extroversion
  bladder Q64.19
  uterus N81.4
    complicating delivery O71.2
    postpartal (old) N81.4
Extruded tooth (teeth) M26.34
Extrusion
  breast implant (prosthetic) T85.42
  eye implant (globe) (ball) T85.328
  intervertebral disc — *see* Displacement, intervertebral disc
  ocular lens implant (prosthetic) — *see* Complications, intraocular lens
  vitreous — *see* Prolapse, vitreous
Exudate
  pleural — *see* Effusion, pleura
  retina H35.89
Exudative — *see* condition
Eye, eyeball, eyelid — *see* condition
Eyestrain — *see* Disturbance, vision, subjective
Eyeworm disease of Africa B74.3

F

Faber's syndrome (achlorhydric anemia) D50.9
Fabry(-Anderson) disease E75.21
Faciocephalalgia, autonomic *(see also* Neuropathy, peripheral, autonomic) G90.09
Factor(s)
  psychic, associated with diseases classified elsewhere F54
  psychological
    affecting physical conditions F54
    or behavioral
      affecting general medical condition F54
      associated with disorders or diseases classified elsewhere F54
Fahr disease (of brain) G23.8
Fahr Volhard disease (of kidney) I12.-

Failure, failed
  abortion — *see* Abortion, attempted
  aortic (valve) I35.8
    rheumatic I06.8
  attempted abortion — *see* Abortion, attempted
  biventricular I50.9
  bone marrow — *see* Anemia, aplastic
  cardiac — *see* Failure, heart
  cardiorenal (chronic) I50.9
    hypertensive I13.2
  cardiorespiratory *(see also* Failure, heart) R09.2
  cardiovascular (chronic) — *see* Failure, heart
  cerebrovascular I67.9
  cervical dilatation in labor O62.0
  circulation, circulatory (peripheral) R57.9
  compensation — *see* Disease, heart
  compliance with medical treatment or regimen — *see* Noncompliance
  congestive — *see* Failure, heart, congestive
  dental implant (endosseous) M27.69
    due to
      failure of dental prosthesis M27.63
      lack of attached gingiva M27.62
      occlusal trauma (poor prosthetic design) M27.62
      parafunctional habits M27.62
      periodontal infection (peri-implantitis) M27.62
      poor oral hygiene M27.62
    osseointegration M27.61
      due to
        complications of systemic disease M27.61
        poor bone quality M27.61
      iatrogenic M27.61
    post-osseointegration
      biological M27.62
        due to complications of systemic disease M27.62
      iatrogenic M27.62
      mechanical M27.63
    pre-integration M27.61
    pre-osseointegration M27.61
    specified NEC M27.69
  descent of head (at term) of pregnancy (mother) O32.4
  endosseous dental implant — *see* Failure, dental implant
  engagement of head (term of pregnancy) (mother) O32.4
  erection (penile) N52.9 *(see also* Dysfunction, sexual, male, nonorganic erectile)
    nonorgqanic F52.21
  examination(s), anxiety concerning Z55.2
  expansion terminal respiratory units (newborn) (primary) P28.0
  forceps NOS (with subsequent cesarean delivery) O66.5
  gain weight (child over 28 days old) R62.51
    adult R62.7
    newborn P92.6
  genital response (male) F52.21
    female F52.22
  heart (acute) (senile) (sudden) I50.9
    with
      acute pulmonary edema — *see* Failure, ventricular, left
      decompensation — *see* Failure, heart, congestive
      dilatation — *see* Disease, heart
    arteriosclerotic I70.90
    biventricular I50.9
    combined left-right sided I50.9
    compensated I50.9
    complicating
      anesthesia (general) (local) or other sedation
        in labor and delivery O74.2
        in pregnancy O29.12-
        postpartum, puerperal O89.1
      delivery (cesarean) (instrumental) O75.4

Failure, failed— *continued*
  heart— *continued*
    congestive (compensated) (decompensated)
      I50.9
      with rheumatic fever (conditions in I00)
        active I01.8
        inactive or quiescent (with chorea) I09.81
      newborn P29.0
      rheumatic (chronic) (inactive) (with chorea)
        I09.81
        active or acute I01.8
          with chorea I02.0
    decompensated I50.9
    degenerative — *see* Degeneration, myocardial
    diastolic (congestive) I50.30
      acute (congestive) I50.31
        and (on) chronic (congestive) I50.33
      chronic (congestive) I50.32
        and (on) acute (congestive) I50.33
      combined with systolic (congestive) I50.40
        acute (congestive) I50.41
          and (on) chronic (congestive) I50.43
        chronic (congestive) I50.42
          and (on) acute (congestive) I50.43
    due to presence of cardiac prosthesis I97.13-
    following cardiac surgery I97.13-
    high output NOS I50.9
    hypertensive — *see* Hypertension, heart
    left (ventricular) — *see* Failure, ventricular, left
    low output (syndrome) NOS I50.9
    newborn P29.0
    organic — *see* Disease, heart
    peripartum O90.3
    postprocedural I97.13-
    rheumatic (chronic) (inactive) I09.9
    right (ventricular) (secondary to left heart failure)
      — *see* Failure, heart, congestive
    systolic (congestive) I50.20
      acute (congestive) I50.21
        and (on) chronic (congestive) I50.23
      chronic (congestive) I50.22
        and (on) acute (congestive) I50.23
      combined with diastolic (congestive) I50.40
        acute (congestive) I50.41
          and (on) chronic (congestive) I50.43
        chronic (congestive) I50.42
          and (on) acute (congestive) I50.43
    thyrotoxic (*see also* Thyrotoxicosis) E05.90 [I43]
      with thyroid storm E05.91 [I43]
    valvular — *see* Endocarditis
  hepatic K72.90
    with coma K72.91
    acute or subacute K72.00
      with coma K72.01
      due to drugs K71.10
        with coma K71.11
    alcoholic (acute) (chronic) (subacute) K70.40
      with coma K70.41
    chronic K72.10
      with coma K72.11
      due to drugs (acute) (subacute) (chronic)
        K71.10
        with coma K71.11
    due to drugs (acute) (subacute) (chronic) K71.10
      with coma K71.11
    postprocedural K91.82
  hepatorenal K76.7
  induction (of labor) O61.9
    abortion — *see* Abortion, attempted
    by
      oxytocic drugs O61.0
      prostaglandins O61.0
    instrumental O61.1
    mechanical O61.1
    medical O61.0
    specified NEC O61.8
    surgical O61.1
  intubation during anesthesia T88.4
    in pregnancy O29.6-
    labor and delivery O74.7
    postpartum, puerperal O89.6
  involution, thymus (gland) E32.0

Failure, failed— *continued*
  kidney (*see also* Disease, kidney, chronic) N19
    acute (*see also* Failure, renal, acute) N17.9
  lactation (complete) O92.3
    partial O92.4
  Leydig's cell, adult E29.1
  liver — *see* Failure, hepatic
  menstruation at puberty N91.0
  mitral I05.8
  myocardial, myocardium (*see also* Failure, heart)
    I50.9
    chronic (*see also* Failure, heart, congestive) I50.9
    congestive (*see also* Failure, heart, congestive)
      I50.9
  orgasm (female) (psychogenic) F52.31
    male F52.32
  ovarian (primary) E28.39
    iatrogenic E89.40
      asymptomatic E89.40
      symptomatic E89.41
    postprocedural (postablative) (postirradiation)
      (postsurgical) E89.40
      asymptomatic E89.40
      symptomatic E89.41
  ovulation causing infertility N97.0
  polyglandular, autoimmune E31.0
  prosthetic joint implant — *see* Complications, joint
    prosthesis, mechanical, breakdown, by site
  renal N19
    tubular necrosis (acute) N17.0
    acute N17.9
      with
        cortical necrosis N17.1
        medullary necrosis N17.2
        tubular necrosis N17.0
      specified NEC N17.8
    chronic N18.9
      hypertensive — *see* Hypertension, kidney
    congenital P96.0
    end stage (chronic) N18.6
      due to hypertension I12.0
    following
      abortion — *see* Abortion by type complicated
        by specified condition NEC
      crushing T79.5
      ectopic or molar pregnancy O08.4
      labor and delivery (acute) O90.4
    hypertensive — *see* Hypertension, kidney
    postprocedural N99.0
  respiration, respiratory J96.90
    with
      hypercapnia J96.92
      hypoxia J96.91
    acute
      with
        hypercapnia J96.02
        hypoxia J96.01
    acute and (on) chronic J96.20
      with
        hypercapnia J96.22
        hypoxia J96.21
    center G93.89
    chronic J96.10
      with
        hypercapnia J96.12
        hypoxia J96.11
    newborn P28.5
    postprocedural J95.82
  rotation
    cecum Q43.3
    colon Q43.3
    intestine Q43.3
    kidney Q63.2
  sedation (conscious) (moderate) during procedure
    T88.52
    history of Z92.83
  segmentation (*see also* Fusion)
    fingers — *see* Syndactylism, complex, fingers
    toes Q70.2
    vertebra Q76.49
      with scoliosis Q76.3
  seminiferous tubule, adult E29.1
  senile (general) R54

Failure, failed— *continued*
  sexual arousal (male) F52.21
    female F52.22
  testicular endocrine function E29.1
  to thrive (child over 28 days old) R62.51
    adult R62.7
    female F52.22
    newborn P92.6
  transplant T86.92
    bone T86.831
      marrow T86.02
    cornea T86.841
    heart T86.22
      with lung(s) T86.32
    intestine T86.891
    kidney T86.12
    liver T86.42
    lung(s) T86.811
      with heart T86.32
    pancreas T86.891
    skin (allograft) (autograft) T86.821
    specified organ or tissue NEC T86.891
  trial of labor (with subsequent cesarean delivery) O66.40
    following previous cesarean delivery O66.41
  tubal ligation N99.89
  urinary — *see* Disease, kidney, chronic
  vacuum extraction NOS (with subsequent cesarean
    delivery) O66.5
  vasectomy N99.89
  ventouse NOS (with subsequent cesarean delivery) O66.5
  ventricular (*see also* Failure, heart) I50.9
    left I50.1
      with rheumatic fever (conditions in I00)
        active I01.8
          with chorea I02.0
        inactive or quiescent (with chorea) I09.81
      rheumatic (chronic) (inactive) (with chorea) I09.81
        active or acute I01.8
          with chorea I02.0
    right (*see also* Failure, heart, congestive) I50.9
  vital centers, newborn P91.8
Fainting (fit) R55
Fallen arches — *see* Deformity, limb, flat foot
Falling, falls (repeated) R29.6
  any organ or part — *see* Prolapse
Fallopian
  insufflation Z31.41
  tube — *see* condition
Fallot's
  pentalogy Q21.3
  tetrad or tetralogy Q21.3
  triad or trilogy Q22.2
False (*see also* condition)
  croup J38.5
  joint — *see* Nonunion, fracture
  labor (pains) O47.9
    at or after 37 completed weeks of gestation O47.1
    before 37 completed weeks of gestation O47.0-
  passage, urethra (prostatic) N36.0
  pregnancy F45.8
Family, familial (*see also* condition)
  disruption Z63.8
    involving divorce or separation Z63.5
  Li-Fraumeni (syndrome) Z15.01
  planning advice Z30.09
  problem Z63.9
    specified NEC Z63.8
  retinoblastoma C69.2-
Famine (effects of) T73.0
  edema — *see* Malnutrition, severe
Fanconi(-de Toni)(-Debré) **syndrome** E72.09
  with cystinosis E72.04
Fanconi's anemia (congenital pancytopenia) D61.09
Farber's disease or syndrome E75.29
Farcy A24.0
Farmer's
  lung J67.0
  skin L57.8
Farsightedness — *see* Hypermetropia
Fascia — *see* condition
Fasciculation R25.3
Fasciitis M72.9
  diffuse (eosinophilic) M35.4

Fasciitis—*continued*
  infective M72.8
    necrotizing M72.6
  necrotizing M72.6
  nodular M72.4
  perirenal (with ureteral obstruction) N13.5
    with infection N13.6
  plantar M72.2
  specified NEC M72.8
  traumatic (old) M72.8
    current — code by site under Sprain
Fascioliasis B66.3
Fasciolopsis, fasciolopsiasis (intestinal) B66.5
Fascioscapulohumeral myopathy G71.0
Fast pulse R00.0
Fat
  embolism — *see* Embolism, fat
  excessive (*see also* Obesity)
    in heart — *see* Degeneration, myocardial
  in stool R19.5
  localized (pad) E65
    heart — *see* Degeneration, myocardial
    knee M79.4
    retropatellar M79.4
  necrosis
    breast N64.1
    mesentery K65.4
    omentum K65.4
  pad E65
    knee M79.4
Fatigue R53.83
  auditory deafness — *see* Deafness
  chronic R53.82
  combat F43.0
  general R53.83
    psychogenic F48.8
  heat (transient) T67.6
  muscle M62.89
  myocardium — *see* Failure, heart
  neoplasm-related R53.0
  nervous, neurosis F48.8
  operational F48.8
  psychogenic (general) F48.8
  senile R54
  voice R49.8
Fatness — *see* Obesity
Fatty (*see also* condition)
  apron E65
  degeneration — *see* Degeneration, fatty
  heart (enlarged) — *see* Degeneration, myocardial
  liver NEC K76.0
    alcoholic K70.0
    nonalcoholic K76.0
  necrosis — *see* Degeneration, fatty
Fauces — *see* condition
Fauchard's disease (periodontitis) — *see* Periodontitis
Faucitis J02.9
Favism (anemia) D55.0
Favus — *see* Dermatophytosis
Fazio-Londe disease or syndrome G12.1
Fear complex or reaction F40.9
Fear of — *see* Phobia
Feared complaint unfounded Z71.1
Febris, febrile (*see also* Fever)
  flava (*see also* Fever, yellow) A95.9
  melitensis A23.0
  pestis — *see* Plague
  recurrens — *see* Fever, relapsing
  rubra A38.9
Fecal
  incontinenece R15.9
  smearing R15.1
  soiling R15.1
  urgency R15.2
Fecalith (impaction) K56.41
  appendix K38.1
  congenital P76.8
Fede's disease K14.0
Feeble rapid pulse due to shock following injury T79.4
Feeble-minded F70
Feeding
  difficulties R63.3

Feeding—*continued*
  problem R63.3
    newborn P92.9
      specified NEC P92.8
    nonorganic (adult) — *see* Disorder, eating
Feeling (of)
  foreign body in throat R09.89
Feer's disease — *see* Poisoning, mercury
Feet — *see* condition
Feigned illness Z76.5
Feil-Klippel syndrome (brevicollis) Q76.1
Feinmesser's (hidrotic) **ectodermal dysplasia** Q82.4
Felinophobia F40.218
Felon (*see also* Cellulitis, digit)
  with lymphangitis — *see* Lymphangitis, acute, digit
Felty's syndrome M05.00
  ankle M05.07-
  elbow M05.02-
  foot joint M05.07-
  hand joint M05.04-
  hip M05.05-
  knee M05.06-
  multiple site M05.09
  shoulder M05.01-
  vertebra — *see* Spondylitis, ankylosing
  wrist M05.03-
Female gential cutting status — *see* Female genital mutilation status (FGM)
Female genital mutilation status (FGM) N90.810
  specified NEC N90.818
  type I (clitorectomy status) N90.811
  type II (clitorectomy with excision of labia minora status) N90.812
  type III (infibulation status) N90.813
  type IV N90.818
Femur, femoral — *see* condition
Fenestration, fenestrated (*see also* Imperfect, closure)
  aortico-pulmonary Q21.4
  cusps, heart valve NEC Q24.8
    pulmonary Q22.2
  pulmonic cusps Q22.2
Fernell's disease (aortic aneurysm) I71.9
Fertile eunuch syndrome E23.0
Fetid
  breath R19.6
  sweat L75.0
Fetishism F65.0
  transvestic F65.1
Fetus, fetal (*see also* condition)
  alcohol syndrome (dysmorphic) Q86.0
  compressus O31.0-
  hydantoin syndrome Q86.1
  lung tissue P28.0
  papyraceous O31.0-
Fever (inanition) (of unknown origin) (persistent) (with chills) (with rigor) R50.9
  abortus A23.1
  Aden (dengue) A90
  African tick-borne A68.1
  American
    mountain (tick) A93.2
    spotted A77.0
  aphthous B08.8
  arbovirus, arboviral A94
    hemorrhagic A94
    specified NEC A93.8
  Argentinian hemorrhagic A96.0
  Assam B55.0
  Australian Q A78
  Bangkok hemorrhagic A91
  Barmah forest A92.8
  Bartonella A44.0
  bilious, hemoglobinuric B50.8
  blackwater B50.8
  blister B00.1
  Bolivian hemorrhagic A96.1
  Bonvale dam T73.3
  boutonneuse A77.1
  brain — *see* Encephalitis
  Brazilian purpuric A48.4
  breakbone A90
  Bullis A77.0

Fever— *continued*
  Bunyamwera A92.8
  Burdwan B55.0
  Bwamba A92.8
  Cameroon — *see* Malaria
  Canton A75.9
  catarrhal (acute) J00
    chronic J31.0
  cat-scratch A28.1
  Central Asian hemorrhagic A98.0
  cerebral — *see* Encephalitis
  cerebrospinal meningococcal A39.0
  Chagres B50.9
  Chandipura A92.8
  Changuinola A93.1
  Charcot's (biliary) (hepatic) (intermittent) — *see* Calculus, bile duct
  Chikungunya (viral) (hemorrhagic) A92.0
  Chitral A93.1
  Colombo — *see* Fever, paratyphoid
  Colorado tick (virus) A93.2
  congestive (remittent) — *see* Malaria
  Congo virus A98.0
  continued malarial B50.9
  Corsican — *see* Malaria
  Crimean-Congo hemorrhagic A98.0
  Cyprus — *see* Brucellosis
  dandy A90
  deer fly — *see* Tularemia
  dengue (virus) A90
    hemorrhagic A91
    sandfly A93.1
  desert B38.0
  drug induced R50.2
  due to heat T67.0
  due to conditions classified elsewhere R50.81
  enteric A01.00
  enteroviral exanthematous (Boston exanthem) A88.0
  ephemeral (of unknown origin) R50.9
  epidemic hemorrhagic A98.5
  erysipelatous — *see* Erysipelas
  estivo-autumnal (malarial) B50.9
  famine A75.0
  five day A79.0
  following delivery O86.4
  Fort Bragg A27.89
  gastroenteric A01.00
  gastromalarial — *see* Malaria
  Gibraltar — *see* Brucellosis
  glandular — *see* Mononucleosis, infectious
  Guama (viral) A92.8
  Haverhill A25.1
  hay (allergic) J30.1
    with asthma (bronchial) J45.909
      with
        exacerbation (acute) J45.901
        status asthmaticus J45.902
      due to
        allergen other than pollen J30.89
        pollen, any plant or tree J30.1
  heat (effects) T67.0
  hematuric, bilious B50.8
  hemoglobinuric (malarial) (bilious) B50.8
  hemorrhagic (arthropod-borne) NOS A94
    with renal syndrome A98.5
    arenaviral A96.9
      specified NEC A96.8
    Argentinian A96.0
    Bangkok A91
    Bolivian A96.1
    Central Asian A98.0
    Chikungunya A92.0
    Crimean-Congo A98.0
    dengue (virus) A91
    epidemic A98.5
    Junin (virus) A96.0
    Korean A98.5
    Kyasanur forest A98.2
    Machupo (virus) A96.1
    mite-borne A93.8
    mosquito-borne A92.8
    Omsk A98.1
    Philippine A91

Fever— *continued*
 hemorrhagic—*continued*
  Russian A98.5
  Singapore A91
  Southeast Asia A91
  Thailand A91
  tick-borne NEC A93.8
  viral A99
   specified NEC A98.8
 hepatic — *see* Cholecystitis
 herpetic — *see* Herpes
 icterohemorrhagic A27.0
 Indiana A93.8
 infective B99.9
  specified NEC B99.8
 intermittent (bilious) (*see also* Malaria)
  of unknown origin R50.9
  pernicious B50.9
 iodide R50.2
 Japanese river A75.3
 jungle (*see also* Malaria)
  yellow A95.0
 Junin (virus) hemorrhagic A96.0
 Katayama B65.2
 kedani A75.3
 Kenya (tick) A77.1
 Kew Garden A79.1
 Korean hemorrhagic A98.5
 Lassa A96.2
 Lone Star A77.0
 Machupo (virus) hemorrhagic A96.1
 malaria, malarial — *see* Malaria
 Malta A23.9
 Marseilles A77.1
 marsh — *see* Malaria
 Mayaro (viral) A92.8
 Mediterranean — *see* Brucellosis
  familial E85.0
  tick A77.1
 meningeal — *see* Meningitis
 Meuse A79.0
 Mexican A75.2
 mianeh A68.1
 miasmatic — *see* Malaria
 mosquito-borne (viral) A92.9
  hemorrhagic A92.8
 mountain (*see also* Brucellosis)
  meaning Rocky Mountain spotted fever A77.0
  tick (American) (Colorado) (viral) A93.2
 Mucambo (viral) A92.8
 mud A27.9
 Neapolitan — *see* Brucellosis
 neutropenic D70.9
 newborn P81.9
  environmental P81.0
 Nine-Mile A78
 non-exanthematous tick A93.2
 North Asian tick-borne A77.2
 Omsk hemorrhagic A98.1
 O'nyong-nyong (viral) A92.1
 Oropouche (viral) A93.0
 Oroya A44.0
 paludal — *see* Malaria
 Panama (malarial) B50.9
 Pappataci A93.1
 paratyphoid A01.4
  A A01.1
  B A01.2
  C A01.3
 parrot A70
 periodic (Mediterranean) E85.0
 persistent (of unknown origin) R50.9
 petechial A39.9
 pharyngoconjunctival B30.2
 Philippine hemorrhagic A91
 phlebotomus A93.1
 Piry (virus) A93.8
 Pixuna (viral) A92.8
 Plasmodium ovale B53.0
 polioviral (nonparalytic) A80.4
 Pontiac A48.2
 postimmunization R50.83

Fever— *continued*
 postoperative R50.82
  due to infection T81.4
 postoperative R50.82
 posttransfusion R50.84
 postvaccination R50.83
 presenting with conditions classified elsewhere R50.81
 pretibial A27.89
 puerperal O86.4
 Q A78
 quadrilateral A78
 quartan (malaria) B52.9
 Queensland (coastal) (tick) A77.3
 quintan A79.0
 rabbit — *see* Tularemia
 rat-bite A25.9
  due to
   Spirillum A25.0
   Streptobacillus moniliformis A25.1
 recurrent — *see* Fever, relapsing
 relapsing (Borrelia) A68.9
  Carter's (Asiatic) A68.1
  Dutton's (West African) A68.1
  Koch's A68.9
  louse-borne A68.0
  Novy's
   louse-borne A68.0
   tick-borne A68.1
  Obermeyer's (European) A68.0
  tick-borne A68.1
 remittent (bilious) (congestive) (gastric) — *see* Malaria
 rheumatic (active) (acute) (chronic) (subacute) I00
  with central nervous system involvement I02.9
  active with heart involvement — *see* category I01
  inactive or quiescent with
   cardiac hypertrophy I09.89
   carditis I09.9
   endocarditis I09.1
    aortic (valve) I06.9
     with mitral (valve) disease I08.0
    mitral (valve) I05.9
     with aortic (valve) disease I08.0
    pulmonary (valve) I09.89
    tricuspid (valve) I07.8
   heart disease NEC I09.89
   heart failure (congestive) (conditions in I50.9) I09.81
   left ventricular failure (conditions in I50.1) I09.81
   myocarditis, myocardial degeneration (conditions in I51.4) I09.0
   pancarditis I09.9
   pericarditis I09.2
 Rift Valley (viral) A92.4
 Rocky Mountain spotted A77.0
 rose J30.1
 Ross River B33.1
 Russian hemorrhagic A98.5
 San Joaquin (Valley) B38.0
 sandfly A93.1
 Sao Paulo A77.0
 scarlet A38.9
 seven day (leptospirosis) (autumnal) (Japanese) A27.89
  dengue A90
 shin-bone A79.0
 Singapore hemorrhagic A91
 solar A90
 Songo A98.5
 sore B00.1
 South African tick-bite A68.1
 Southeast Asia hemorrhagic A91
 spinal — *see* Meningitis
 spirillary A25.0
 splenic — *see* Anthrax
 spotted A77.9
  American A77.0
  Brazilian A77.0
  cerebrospinal meningitis A39.0
  Colombian A77.0

Fever— *continued*
 spotted—*continued*
  due to Rickettsia
   australis A77.3
   conorii A77.1
   rickettsii A77.0
   sibirica A77.2
   specified type NEC A77.8
  Ehrlichiosis A77.40
   due to
    E. chafeensis A77.41
    specified organism NEC A77.49
  Rocky Mountain A77.0
 steroid R50.2
 streptobacillary A25.1
 subtertian B50.9
 Sumatran mite A75.3
 sun A90
 swamp A27.9
 swine A02.8
 sylvatic, yellow A95.0
 Tahyna B33.8
 tertian — *see* Malaria, tertian
 Thailand hemorrhagic A91
 thermic T67.0
 three-day A93.1
 tick
  American mountain A93.2
  Colorado A93.2
  Kemerovo A93.8
  Mediterranean A77.1
  mountain A93.2
  nonexanthematous A93.2
  Quaranfil A93.8
 tick-bite NEC A93.8
 tick-borne (hemorrhagic) NEC A93.8
 trench A79.0
 tsutsugamushi A75.3
 typhogastric A01.00
 typhoid (abortive) (hemorrhagic) (intermittent) (malignant) A01.00
  complicated by
   arthritis A01.04
   heart involvement A01.02
   meningitis A01.01
   osteomyelitis A01.05
   pneumonia A01.03
   specified NEC A01.09
 typhomalarial — *see* Malaria
 typhus — *see* Typhus (fever)
 undulant — *see* Brucellosis
 unknown origin R50.9
 uveoparotid D86.89
 valley B38.0
 Venezuelan equine A92.2
 vesicular stomatitis A93.8
 viral hemorrhagic — *see* Fever, hemorrhagic, by type of virus
 Volhynian A79.0
 Wesselsbron (viral) A92.8
 West
  African B50.8
  Nile (viral) A92.30
   with
    complications NEC A92.39
    cranial nerve disorders A92.32
    encephalitis A92.31
    encephalomyelitis A92.31
    neurologic manifestation NEC A92.32
    optic neuritis A92.32
    polyradiculitis A92.32
 Whitmore's — *see* Melioidosis
 Wolhynian A79.0
 worm B83.9
 yellow A95.9
  jungle A95.0
  sylvatic A95.0
  urban A95.1
 Zika (viral) A92.8
Fibrillation
 atrial or auricular (established) I48.0
 cardiac I49.8
 heart I49.8

Fibrillation—*continued*
  muscular M62.89
  ventricular I49.Ø1
Fibrin
  ball or bodies, pleural (sac) J94.1
  chamber, anterior (eye) (gelatinous exudate) — *see*
    Iridocyclitis, acute
Fibrinogenolysis — *see* Fibrinolysis
Fibrinogenopenia D68.8
  acquired D65
  congenital D68.2
Fibrinolysis (hemorrhagic) (acquired) D65
  antepartum hemorrhage — *see* Hemorrhage,
    antepartum, with coagulation defect
  following
    abortion — *see* Abortion by type complicated by
      hemorrhage
    ectopic or molar pregnancy OØ8.1
  intrapartum O67.Ø
  newborn, transient P6Ø
  postpartum O72.3
Fibrinopenia (hereditary) D68.2
  acquired D68.4
Fibrinopurulent — *see* condition
Fibrinous — *see* condition
Fibroadenoma
  cellular intracanalicular D24.-
  giant D24.-
  intracanalicular
    cellular D24.-
    giant D24.-
    specified site — *see* Neoplasm, benign, by site
    unspecified site D24.-
  juvenile D24.-
  pericanalicular
    specified site — *see* Neoplasm, benign, by site
    unspecified site D24.-
  phyllodes D24.-
  prostate D29.1
  specified site NEC — *see* Neoplasm, benign, by site
  unspecified site D24.-
Fibroadenosis, breast (chronic) (cystic) (diffuse)
    (periodic) (segmental) N6Ø.2-
Fibroangioma (*see also* Neoplasm, benign, by site)
  juvenile
    specified site — *see* Neoplasm, benign, by site
    unspecified site D1Ø.6
Fibrochondrosarcoma — *see* Neoplasm, cartilage,
    malignant
Fibrocystic
  disease (*see also* Fibrosis, cystic)
    breast — *see* Mastopathy, cystic
    jaw M27.49
    kidney (congenital) Q61.8
    liver Q44.6
    pancreas E84.9
  kidney (congenital) Q61.8
Fibrodysplasia ossificans progressiva — *see*
    Myositis, ossificans, progressiva
Fibroelastosis (cordis) (endocardial) (endomyocardial)
    I42.4
Fibroid (tumor) (*see also* Neoplasm, connective tissue,
    benign)
  disease, lung (chronic) — *see* Fibrosis, lung
  heart (disease) — *see* Myocarditis
  in pregnancy or childbirth O34.1-
    causing obstructed labor O65.5
  induration, lung (chronic) — *see* Fibrosis, lung
  lung — *see* Fibrosis, lung
  pneumonia (chronic) — *see* Fibrosis, lung
  uterus D25.9
Fibrolipoma — *see* Lipoma
Fibroliposarcoma — *see* Neoplasm, connective tissue,
    malignant
Fibroma (*see also* Neoplasm, connective tissue, benign)
  ameloblastic — *see* Cyst, calcifying odontogenic
  bone (nonossifying) — *see* Disorder, bone, specified
    type NEC
    ossifying — *see* Neoplasm, bone, benign
  cementifying — *see* Neoplasm, bone, benign
  chondromyxoid — *see* Neoplasm, bone, benign
  desmoplastic — *see* Neoplasm, connective tissue,
    uncertain behavior

Fibroma—*continued*
  durum — *see* Neoplasm, connective tissue, benign
  fascial — *see* Neoplasm, connective tissue, benign
  invasive — *see* Neoplasm, connective tissue,
    uncertain behavior
  molle — *see* Lipoma
  myxoid — *see* Neoplasm, connective tissue, benign
  nasopharynx, nasopharyngeal (juvenile) D1Ø.6
  nonosteogenic (nonossifying) — *see* Dysplasia,
    fibrous
  odontogenic (central) — *see* Cyst, calcifying
    odontogenic
  ossifying — *see* Neoplasm, bone, benign
  periosteal — *see* Neoplasm, bone, benign
  soft — *see* Lipoma
Fibromatosis M72.9
  abdominal — *see* Neoplasm, connective tissue,
    uncertain behavior
  aggressive — *see* Neoplasm, connective tissue,
    uncertain behavior
  congenital generalized — *see* Neoplasm, connective
    tissue, uncertain behavior
  Dupuytren's M72.Ø
  gingival KØ6.1
  palmar (fascial) M72.Ø
  plantar (fascial) M72.2
  pseudosarcomatous (proliferative) (subcutaneous)
    M72.4
  retroperitoneal D48.3
  specified NEC M72.8
Fibromyalgia M79.7
Fibromyoma (*see also* Neoplasm, connective tissue,
    benign)
  uterus (corpus) (*see also* Leiomyoma, uterus)
    in pregnancy or childbirth — *see* Fibroid, in
      pregnancy or childbirth
    causing obstructed labor O65.5
Fibromyositis M79.7
Fibromyxolipoma D17.9
Fibromyxoma — *see* Neoplasm, connective tissue, benign
Fibromyxosarcoma — *see* Neoplasm, connective
    tissue, malignant
Fibro-odontoma, ameloblastic — *see* Cyst, calcifying
    odontogenic
Fibro-osteoma — *see* Neoplasm, bone, benign
Fibroplasia, retrolental H35.17-
Fibropurulent — *see* condition
Fibrosarcoma (*see also* Neoplasm, connective tissue,
    malignant)
  ameloblastic C41.1
    upper jaw (bone) C41.Ø
  congenital — *see* Neoplasm, connective tissue,
    malignant
  fascial — *see* Neoplasm, connective tissue,
    malignant
  infantile — *see* Neoplasm, connective tissue,
    malignant
  odontogenic C41.1
    upper jaw (bone) C41.Ø
  periosteal — *see* Neoplasm, bone, malignant
Fibrosclerosis
  breast N6Ø.3-
  multifocal M35.5
  penis (corpora cavernosa) N48.6
Fibrosis, fibrotic
  adrenal (gland) E27.8
  amnion O41.8x-
  anal papillae K62.8
  arteriocapillary — *see* Arteriosclerosis
  bladder N32.89
    interstitial — *see* Cystitis, chronic, interstitial
    localized submucosal — *see* Cystitis, chronic,
      interstitial
    panmural — *see* Cystitis, chronic, interstitial
  breast — *see* Fibrosclerosis, breast
  capillary (*see also* Arteriosclerosis) I7Ø.9Ø
    lung (chronic) — *see* Fibrosis, lung
  cardiac — *see* Myocarditis
  cervix N88.8
  chorion O41.8x-
  corpus cavernosum (sclerosing) N48.6

Fibrosis, fibrotic—*continued*
  cystic (of pancreas) E84.9
    with
      distal intestinal obstruction syndrome E84.19
      fecal impaction E84.19
      intestinal manifestations NEC E84.19
      pulmonary manifestations E84.Ø
      specified manifestations NEC E84.8
  due to device, implant or graft (*see also*
    Complications, by site and type, specified
    NEC) T85.82
    arterial graft NEC T82.828
    breast (implant) T85.82
    catheter NEC T85.82
      dialysis (renal) T82.828
        intraperitoneal T85.82
      infusion NEC T82.828
        spinal (epidural) (subdural) T85.82
      urinary (indwelling) T83.82
    electronic (electrode) (pulse generator)
      (stimulator)
      bone T84.82
      cardiac T82.827
      nervous system (brain) (peripheral nerve)
        (spinal) T85.82
      urinary T83.82
    fixation, internal (orthopedic) NEC T84.82
    gastrointestinal (bile duct) (esophagus) T85.82
    genital NEC T83.82
    heart NEC T82.827
    joint prosthesis T84.82
    ocular (corneal graft) (orbital implant) NEC
      T85.82
    orthopedic NEC T84.82
    specified NEC T85.82
    urinary NEC T83.82
    vascular NEC T82.828
    ventricular intracranial shunt T85.82
  ejaculatory duct N5Ø.8
  endocardium — *see* Endocarditis
  endomyocardial (tropical) I42.3
  epididymis N5Ø.8
  eye muscle — *see* Strabismus, mechanical
  heart — *see* Myocarditis
  hepatic — *see* Fibrosis, liver
  hepatolienal (portal hypertension) K76.6
  hepatosplenic (portal hypertension) K76.6
  infrapatellar fat pad M79.4
  intrascrotal N5Ø.8
  kidney N26.9
  liver K74.Ø
    with sclerosis K74.2
    alcoholic K7Ø.2
  lung (atrophic) (capillary) (chronic) (confluent)
    (massive) (perialveolar) (peribronchial) J84.1
    with
      anthracosilicosis J6Ø
      anthracosis J6Ø
      asbestosis J61
      bagassosis J67.1
      bauxite J63.1
      berylliosis J63.2
      byssinosis J66.Ø
      calcicosis J62.8
      chalicosis J62.8
      dust reticulation J64
      farmer's lung J67.Ø
      ganister disease J62.8
      graphite J63.3
      pneumoconiosis NOS J64
      siderosis J63.4
      silicosis J62.8
    congenital P27.8
    diffuse (idiopathic) (interstitial) J84.1
      chemicals, gases, fumes or vapors (inhalation)
        J68.4
      talc J62.Ø
    following radiation J7Ø.1
    idiopathic J84.1
    postinflammatory J84.1
    silicotic J62.8
    tuberculous — *see* Tuberculosis, pulmonary
  lymphatic gland I89.8

Fibrosis, fibrotic— continued
- median bar — see Hyperplasia, prostate
- mediastinum (idiopathic) J98.5
- meninges G96.19
- myocardium, myocardial — see Myocarditis
- ovary N83.8
- oviduct N83.8
- pancreas K86.8
- penis NEC N48.6
- pericardium I31.0
- perineum, in pregnancy or childbirth O34.7-
  - causing obstructed labor O65.5
- pleura J94.1
- popliteal fat pad M79.4
- prostate (chronic) — see Hyperplasia, prostate
- pulmonary (see also Fibrosis, lung)
  - congenital P27.8
- rectal sphincter K62.8
- retroperitoneal, idiopathic (with ureteral
  - obstruction) N13.5
  - with infection N13.6
- sclerosing mesenteric (idiopathic) K65.4
- scrotum N50.8
- seminal vesicle N50.8
- senile R54
- skin L90.5
- spermatic cord N50.8
- spleen D73.89
  - in schistosomiasis (bilharziasis) B65.9 [D77]
- subepidermal nodular — see Neoplasm, skin,
  - benign
- submucous (oral) (tongue) K13.5
- testis N44.8
  - chronic, due to syphilis A52.76
- thymus (gland) E32.8
- tongue, submucous K13.5
- tunica vaginalis N50.8
- uterus (non-neoplastic) N85.8
- vagina N89.8
- valve, heart — see Endocarditis
- vas deferens N50.8
- vein I87.8

Fibrositis (periarticular) M79.7
- nodular, chronic (Jaccoud's) (rheumatoid) — see
  - Arthropathy, postrheumatic, chronic

Fibrothorax J94.1

Fibrotic — see Fibrosis

Fibrous — see condition

Fibroxanthoma (see also Neoplasm, connective tissue,
- benign)
- atypical — see Neoplasm, connective tissue,
  - uncertain behavior
- malignant — see Neoplasm, connective tissue,
  - malignant

Fibroxanthosarcoma — see Neoplasm, connective
- tissue, malignant

Fiedler's
- disease (icterohemorrhagic leptospirosis) A27.0
- myocarditis (acute) I40.1

Fifth disease B08.3
- venereal A55

Filaria, filarial, filariasis — see Infestation, filarial

Filatov's disease — see Mononucleosis, infectious

File-cutter's disease — see Poisoning, lead

Filling defect
- biliary tract R93.2
- bladder R93.4
- duodenum R93.3
- gallbladder R93.2
- gastrointestinal tract R93.3
- intestine R93.3
- kidney R93.4
- stomach R93.3
- ureter R93.4

Fimbrial cyst Q50.4

Financial problem affecting care NOS Z59.9
- bankruptcy Z59.8
- foreclosure on loan Z59.8

**Findings, abnormal, inconclusive, without
diagnosis** (see also Abnormal)
- 17-ketosteroids, elevated R82.5
- acetonuria R82.4
- alcohol in blood R78.0

**Findings, abnormal, inconclusive, without
diagnosis** — continued
- antenatal screening of mother O28.9
  - biochemical O28.1
  - cytological O28.2
  - chromosomal O28.5
  - genetic O28.5
  - hematological O28.0
  - radiological O28.4
  - specified NEC O28.8
  - ultrasonic O28.3
- anisocytosis R71.8
- antibody titer, elevated R76.0
- bacteriuria N39.0
- bicarbonate E87.8
- bile in urine R82.2
- blood sugar (high) R73.09
  - low (transient) E16.2
- casts, urine R82.99
- catecholamines R82.5
- cells, urine R82.99
- chloride E87.8
- cholesterol E78.9
  - high E78.0
    - with high triglycerides E78.2
- chyluria R82.0
- cloudy
  - dialysis effluent R88.0
  - urine R82.90
- creatinine clearance R94.4
- crystals, urine R82.99
- culture
  - blood R78.81
  - positive — see Positive, culture
- echocardiogram R93.1
- electrolyte level, urinary R82.99
- function study NEC R94.8
  - bladder R94.8
  - endocrine NEC R94.7
    - thyroid R94.6
  - kidney R94.4
  - liver R94.5
  - pancreas R94.8
  - placenta R94.8
  - pulmonary R94.2
  - spleen R94.8
- gallbladder, nonvisualization R93.2
- glucose (tolerance test) (non-fasting) R73.09
- glycosuria R81
- heart
  - shadow R93.1
  - sounds R01.2
- hematinuria R82.3
- hematocrit drop (precipitous) R71.0
- hemoglobinuria R82.3
- human papillomavirus (HPV) DNA test positive
  - cervix
    - high risk R87.810
    - low risk R87.820
  - vagina
    - high risk R87.811
    - low risk R87.821
- in blood (of substance not normally found in blood)
  - R78.9
  - addictive drug NEC R78.4
  - alcohol (excessive level) R78.0
  - cocaine R78.2
  - hallucinogen R78.3
  - heavy metals (abnormal level) R78.79
  - lead R78.71
  - lithium (abnormal level) R78.89
  - opiate drug R78.1
  - psychotropic drug R78.5
  - specified substance NEC R78.89
  - steroid agent R78.6
- indolacetic acid, elevated R82.5
- ketonuria R82.4
- lactic acid dehydrogenase (LDH) R74.0
- liver function test R79.89
- mammogram NEC R92.8
  - calcification (calculus) R92.1
  - inconclusive result (due to dense breasts) R92.2
  - microcalcification R92.0

**Findings, abnormal, inconclusive, without
diagnosis** — continued
- mediastinal shift R93.1
- melanin, urine R82.99
- myoglobinuria R82.1
- neonatal screening P09
- nonvisualization of gallbladder R93.2
- odor of urine NOS R82.90
- Papanicolaou cervix R87.619
  - non-atypical endometrial cells R87.618
- pneumoencephalogram R93.0
- poikilocytosis R71.8
- potassium (deficiency) E87.6
  - excess E87.5
- PPD R76.1
- radiologic (X-ray) R93.8
  - abdomen R93.5
  - biliary tract R93.2
  - breast R92.8
  - gastrointestinal tract R93.3
  - genitourinary organs R93.4
  - head R93.0
  - inconclusive due to excess body fat of patient
    - R93.9
  - intrathoracic organs NEC R93.1
  - placenta R93.8
  - retroperitoneum R93.5
  - skin R93.8
  - skull R93.0
  - subcutaneous tissue R93.8
- red blood cell (count) (morphology) (sickling)
  - (volume) R71.8
- scan NEC R94.8
  - bladder R94.8
  - bone R94.8
  - kidney R94.4
  - liver R93.2
  - lung R94.2
  - pancreas R94.8
  - placental R94.8
  - spleen R94.8
  - thyroid R94.6
- sedimentation rate, elevated R70.0
- SGOT R74.0
- SGPT R74.0
- sodium (deficiency) E87.1
  - excess E87.0
- specified body fluid NEC R88.8
- stress test R94.39
- thyroid (function) (metabolic rate) (scan) (uptake)
  - R94.6
- transaminase (level) R74.0
- triglycerides E78.9
  - high E78.1
    - with high cholesterol E78.2
- tuberculin skin test (without active tuberculosis)
  - R76.1
- urine R82.90
  - acetone R82.4
  - bacteria N39.0
  - bile R82.2
  - casts or cells R82.99
  - chyle R82.0
  - culture positive R82.7
  - glucose R81
  - hemoglobin R82.3
  - ketone R82.4
  - sugar R81
- vanillylmandelic acid (VMA), elevated R82.5
- vectorcardiogram (VCG) R93.1
- ventriculogram R93.0
- white blood cell (count) (differential) (morphology)
  - D72.9
- xerography R92.8

Finger — see condition

Fire, Saint Anthony's — see Erysipelas

Fire-setting
- pathological (compulsive) F63.1

Fish hook stomach K31.89

Fishmeal-worker's lung J67.8

Fissure, fissured
anus, anal K60.2
  acute K60.0
  chronic K60.1
  congenital Q43.8
ear, lobule, congenital Q17.8
epiglottis (congenital) Q31.8
larynx J38.7
  congenital Q31.8
lip K13.0
  congenital — see Cleft, lip
nipple N64.0
  associated with
    lactation O92.13
    pregnancy O92.11-
    puerperium O92.12
nose Q30.2
palate (congenital) — see Cleft, palate
skin R23.4
spine (congenital) (see also Spina bifida)
  with hydrocephalus — see Spina bifida, by site,
    with hydrocephalus
tongue (acquired) K14.5
  congenital Q38.3

Fistula (cutaneous) L98.8
abdomen (wall) K63.2
  bladder N32.2
  intestine NEC K63.2
  ureter N28.89
  uterus N82.5
abdominorectal K63.2
abdominosigmoidal K63.2
abdominothoracic J86.0
abdominouterine N82.5
  congenital Q51.7
abdominovesical N32.2
accessory sinuses — see Sinusitis
actinomycotic — see Actinomycosis
alveolar antrum — see Sinusitis, maxillary
alveolar process K04.6
anorectal K60.5
antrobuccal — see Sinusitis, maxillary
antrum — see Sinusitis, maxillary
anus, anal (recurrent) (infectional) K60.3
  congenital Q43.6
    with absence, atresia and stenosis Q42.2
  tuberculous A18.32
aorta-duodenal I77.2
appendix, appendicular K38.3
arteriovenous (acquired) (nonruptured) I77.0
  brain I67.1
    congenital Q28.2
      ruptured I60.8
    ruptured I60.8
  cerebral — see Fistula, arteriovenous, brain
  congenital (peripheral) (see also Malformation,
    arteriovenous)
    brain Q28.2
      ruptured I60.8
    coronary Q24.5
    pulmonary Q25.7
  coronary I25.41
    congenital Q24.5
  pulmonary I28.0
    congenital Q25.7
  surgically created (for dialysis) Z99.2
    complication — see Complication,
      arteriovenous, fistula, surgically created
  traumatic — see Injury, blood vessel
artery I77.2
aural (mastoid) — see Mastoiditis, chronic
auricle (see also Disorder, pinna, specified type NEC)
  congenital Q18.1
Bartholin's gland N82.8
bile duct (common) (hepatic) K83.3
  with calculus, stones — see Calculus, bile duct
biliary (tract) — see Fistula, bile duct
bladder (sphincter) NEC (see also Fistula, vesico-)
  N32.2
  into seminal vesicle N32.2
bone (see also Disorder, bone, specified type NEC)
  with osteomyelitis, chronic — see Osteomyelitis,
    chronic, with draining sinus

Fistula — continued
brain G93.89
  arteriovenous (acquired) I67.1
    congenital Q28.2
branchial (cleft) Q18.0
branchiogenous Q18.0
breast N61
  puerperal, postpartum or gestational, due to
    mastitis (purulent) — see Mastitis,
    obstetric, purulent
bronchial J86.0
bronchocutaneous, bronchomediastinal,
  bronchopleural, bronchopleuromediastinal
  (infective) J86.0
  tuberculous NEC A15.5
bronchoesophageal J86.0
  congenital Q39.2
    with atresia of esophagus Q39.1
bronchovisceral J86.0
buccal cavity (infective) K12.2
cecosigmoidal K63.2
cecum K63.2
cerebrospinal (fluid) G96.0
cervical, lateral Q18.1
cervicoaural Q18.1
cervicosigmoidal N82.4
cervicovesical N82.1
cervix N82.8
chest (wall) J86.0
cholecystenteric — see Fistula, gallbladder
cholecystocolic — see Fistula, gallbladder
cholecystocolonic — see Fistula, gallbladder
cholecystoduodenal — see Fistula, gallbladder
cholecystogastric — see Fistula, gallbladder
cholecystointestinal — see Fistula, gallbladder
choledochoduodenal — see Fistula, bile duct
cholocolic K82.3
coccyx — see Sinus, pilonidal
colon K63.2
colostomy K94.09
common duct — see Fistula, bile duct
congenital, site not listed — see Anomaly, by site
coronary, arteriovenous I25.41
  congenital Q24.5
costal region J86.0
cul-de-sac, Douglas' N82.8
cystic duct (see also Fistula, gallbladder)
  congenital Q44.5
dental K04.6
diaphragm J86.0
duodenum K31.6
ear (external) (canal) — see Disorder, ear, external,
  specified type NEC
enterocolic K63.2
enterocutaneous K63.2
enterouterine N82.4
  congenital Q51.7
enterovaginal N82.4
  congenital Q52.2
  large intestine N82.3
  small intestine N82.2
enterovesical N32.1
epididymis N50.8
  tuberculous A18.15
esophagobronchial J86.0
  congenital Q39.2
    with atresia of esophagus Q39.1
esophagocutaneous K22.8
esophagopleural-cutaneous J86.0
esophagotracheal J86.0
  congenital Q39.2
    with atresia of esophagus Q39.1
esophagus K22.8
  congenital Q39.2
    with atresia of esophagus Q39.1
ethmoid — see Sinusitis, ethmoidal
eyeball (cornea) (sclera) — see Disorder, globe,
  hypotony
eyelid H01.8
fallopian tube, external N82.5
fecal K63.2
  congenital Q43.6
from periapical abscess K04.6

Fistula — continued
frontal sinus — see Sinusitis, frontal
gallbladder K82.3
  with calculus, cholelithiasis, stones — see
    Calculus, gallbladder
gastric K31.6
gastrocolic K31.6
  congenital Q40.2
  tuberculous A18.32
gastroenterocolic K31.6
gastroesophageal K31.6
gastrojejunal K31.6
gastrojejunocolic K31.6
genital tract (female) N82.9
  specified NEC N82.8
  to intestine NEC N82.4
  to skin N82.5
hepatic artery-portal vein, congenital Q26.6
hepatopleural J86.0
hepatopulmonary J86.0
ileorectal or ileosigmoidal K63.2
ileovaginal N82.2
ileovesical N32.1
ileum K63.2
in ano K60.3
  tuberculous A18.32
inner ear (labyrinth) — see subcategory H83.1
intestine NEC K63.2
intestinocolonic (abdominal) K63.2
intestinoureteral N28.89
intestinouterine N82.4
intestinovaginal N82.4
  large intestine N82.3
  small intestine N82.2
intestinovesical N32.1
ischiorectal (fossa) K61.3
jejunum K63.2
joint M25.10
  ankle M25.17-
  elbow M25.12-
  foot joint M25.17-
  hand joint M25.14-
  hip M25.15-
  knee M25.16-
  shoulder M25.11-
  specified joint NEC M25.18
  tuberculous — see Tuberculosis, joint
  wrist M25.13-
kidney N28.89
labium (majus) (minus) N82.8
labyrinth — see subcategory H83.1
lacrimal (gland) (sac) H04.61-
lacrimonasal duct — see Fistula, lacrimal
laryngotracheal, congenital Q34.8
larynx J38.7
lip K13.0
  congenital Q38.0
lumbar, tuberculous A18.01
lung J86.0
lymphatic I89.8
mammary (gland) N61
mastoid (process) (region) — see Mastoiditis,
  chronic
maxillary J32.0
medial, face and neck Q18.8
mediastinal J86.0
mediastinobronchial J86.0
mediastinocutaneous J86.0
middle ear — see subcategory H74.8
mouth K12.2
nasal J34.89
  sinus — see Sinusitis
nasopharynx J39.2
nipple N64.0
nose J34.89
oral (cutaneous) K12.2
  maxillary J32.0
  nasal (with cleft palate) — see Cleft, palate
orbit, orbital — see Disorder, orbit, specified type
  NEC
oroantral J32.0
oviduct, external N82.5
palate (hard) M27.8

Fistula — *continued*
  pancreatic K86.8
  pancreaticoduodenal K86.8
  parotid (gland) K11.4
    region K12.2
  penis N48.89
  perianal K60.3
  pericardium (pleura) (sac) — *see* Pericarditis
  pericecal K63.2
  perineorectal K60.4
  perineosigmoidal K63.2
  perineum, perineal (with urethral involvement) NEC N36.0
    tuberculous A18.13
    ureter N28.89
  perirectal K60.4
    tuberculous A18.32
  peritoneum K65.9
  pharyngoesophageal J39.2
  pharynx J39.2
    branchial cleft (congenital) Q18.0
  pilonidal (infected) (rectum) — *see* Sinus, pilonidal
  pleura, pleural, pleurocutaneous, pleuroperitoneal J86.0
    tuberculous NEC A15.6
  pleuropericardial I31.8
  portal vein-hepatic artery, congenital Q26.6
  postauricular H70.81-
  postoperative, persistent T81.83
    specified site — *see* Fistula, by site
  preauricular (congenital) Q18.1
  prostate N42.89
  pulmonary J86.0
    arteriovenous I28.0
      congenital Q25.7
    tuberculous — *see* Tuberculosis, pulmonary
  pulmonoperitoneal J86.0
  rectolabial N82.4
  rectosigmoid (intercommunicating) K63.2
  rectoureteral N28.89
  rectourethral N36.0
    congenital Q64.73
  rectouterine N82.4
    congenital Q51.7
  rectovaginal N82.3
    congenital Q52.2
    tuberculous A18.18
  rectovesical N32.1
    congenital Q64.79
  rectovesicovaginal N82.3
  rectovulval N82.4
    congenital Q52.79
  rectum (to skin) K60.4
    congenital Q43.6
      with absence, atresia and stenosis Q42.0
    tuberculous A18.32
  renal N28.89
  retroauricular — *see* Fistula, postauricular
  salivary duct or gland (any) K11.4
    congenital Q38.4
  scrotum (urinary) N50.8
    tuberculous A18.15
  semicircular canals — *see* subcategory H83.1
  sigmoid K63.2
    to bladder N32.1
  sinus — *see* Sinusitis
  skin L98.8
    to genital tract (female) N82.5
  splenocolic D73.89
  stercoral K63.2
  stomach K31.6
  sublingual gland K11.4
  submandibular gland K11.4
  submaxillary (gland) K11.4
    region K12.2
  thoracic J86.0
    duct I89.8
  thoracoabdominal J86.0
  thoracogastric J86.0
  thoracointestinal J86.0
  thorax J86.0
  thyroglossal duct Q89.2
  thyroid E07.89

Fistula — *continued*
  trachea, congenital (external) (internal) Q32.1
  tracheoesophageal J86.0
    congenital Q39.2
      with atresia of esophagus Q39.1
      following tracheostomy J95.04
  traumatic arteriovenous — *see* Injury, blood vessel, by site
  tuberculous—code by site under Tuberculosis
  typhoid A01.09
  umbilicourinary Q64.8
  urachus, congenital Q64.4
  ureter (persistent) N28.89
  ureteroabdominal N28.89
  ureterorectal N28.89
  ureterosigmoido-abdominal N28.89
  ureterovaginal N82.1
  ureterovesical N32.2
  urethra N36.0
    congenital Q64.79
    tuberculous A18.13
  urethroperineal N36.0
  urethroperineovesical N32.2
  urethrorectal N36.0
    congenital Q64.73
  urethroscrotal N50.8
  urethrovaginal N82.1
  urethrovesical N32.2
  urinary (tract) (persistent) (recurrent) N36.0
  uteroabdominal N82.5
    congenital Q51.7
  uteroenteric, uterointestinal N82.4
    congenital Q51.7
  uterorectal N82.4
    congenital Q51.7
  uteroureteric N82.1
  uterourethral Q51.7
  uterovaginal N82.8
  uterovesical N82.1
    congenital Q51.7
  uterus N82.8
  vagina (postpartal) (wall) N82.8
  vaginocutaneous (postpartal) N82.5
  vaginointestinal NEC N82.4
    large intestine N82.3
    small intestine N82.2
  vaginoperineal N82.5
  vasocutaneous, congenital Q55.7
  vesical NEC N32.2
  vesicoabdominal N32.2
  vesicocervicovaginal N82.1
  vesicocolic N32.1
  vesicocutaneous N32.2
  vesicoenteric N32.1
  vesicointestinal N32.1
  vesicometrorectal N82.4
  vesicoperineal N32.2
  vesicorectal N32.1
    congenital Q64.79
  vesicosigmoidal N32.1
  vesicosigmoidovaginal N82.3
  vesicoureteral N32.1
  vesicoureterovaginal N82.1
  vesicourethral N32.2
  vesicourethrorectal N32.1
  vesicouterine N82.1
    congenital Q51.7
  vesicovaginal N82.0
  vulvorectal N82.4
    congenital Q52.79

Fit R56.9
  epileptic — *see* Epilepsy
  fainting R55
  hysterical F44.5
  newborn P90
Fitting (and adjustment) (of)
  artificial
    arm — *see* Admission, adjustment, artificial, arm
    breast Z44.3
    eye Z44.2
    leg — *see* Admission, adjustment, artificial, leg
  automatic implantable cardiac defibrillator (with synchronous cardiac pacemaker) Z45.02

Fitting — *continued*
  brain neuropacemaker Z46.2
    implanted Z45.42
  cardiac defibrillator — *see* Fitting (and adjustment) (of), automatic implantable cardiac defibrillator
  catheter, non-vascular Z46.82
  colostomy belt Z46.89
  contact lenses Z46.0
  cystostomy device Z46.6
  defibrillator, cardiac — *see* Fitting (and adjustment) (of), automatic implantable cardiac defibrillator
  dentures Z46.3
  device NOS Z46.9
    abdominal Z46.89
    gastrointestinal NEC Z46.59
    implanted NEC Z45.89
    nervous system Z46.2
      implanted — *see* Admission, adjustment, device, implanted, nervous system
    orthodontic Z46.4
    orthoptic Z46.0
    orthotic Z46.89
    prosthetic (external) Z44.9
      breast Z44.3
      dental Z46.3
      eye Z44.2
      specified NEC Z44.8
    specified NEC Z46.89
    substitution
      auditory Z46.2
        implanted — *see* Admission, adjustment, device, implanted, hearing device
      nervous system Z46.2
        implanted — *see* Admission, adjustment, device, implanted, nervous system
      visual Z46.2
        implanted Z45.31
    urinary Z46.6
  gastric lap band Z46.51
  gastrointestinal appliance NEC Z46.59
  glasses (reading) Z46.0
  hearing aid Z46.1
  ileostomy device Z46.89
  insulin pump Z46.81
  intestinal appliance NEC Z46.89
  myringotomy device (stent) (tube) Z45.82
  neuropacemaker Z46.2
    implanted Z45.42
  non-vascular catheter Z46.82
  orthodontic device Z46.4
  orthopedic device (brace) (cast) (corset) (shoes) Z46.89
  pacemaker (cardiac) Z45.018
    nervous system (brain) (peripheral nerve) (spinal cord) Z46.2
      implanted Z45.42
    pulse generator Z45.010
  portacath (port-a-cath) Z45.2
  prosthesis (external) Z44.9
    arm — *see* Admission, adjustment, artificial, arm
    breast Z44.3
    dental Z46.3
    eye Z44.2
    leg — *see* Admission, adjustment, artificial, leg
    specified NEC Z44.8
  spectacles Z46.0
  wheelchair Z46.89
Fitzhugh-Curtis syndrome
  due to
    Chlamydia trachomatis A74.81
    Neisseria gonorrhorea (gonococcal peritonitis) A54.85
Fitz's syndrome (acute hemorrhagic pancreatitis) K85.8
Fixation
  joint — *see* Ankylosis
  larynx J38.7
  stapes — *see* Ankylosis, ear ossicles
    deafness — *see* Deafness, conductive
  uterus (acquired) — *see* Malposition, uterus
  vocal cord J38.3

Flabby ridge K06.8
Flaccid (*see also* condition)
  palate, congenital Q38.5
Flail
  chest S22.5-
    newborn (birth injury) P13.8
  joint (paralytic) M25.2Ø
    ankle M25.27-
    elbow M25.22-
    foot joint M25.27-
    hand joint M25.24-
    hip M25.25-
    knee M25.26-
    shoulder M25.21-
    specified joint NEC M25.28
    wrist M25.23-
Flajani's disease — *see* Hyperthyroidism, with, goiter
    (diffuse)
Flashbacks (residual to hallucinogen use) F16.283
Flap, liver K71.3
Flat
  chamber (eye) — *see* Disorder, globe, hypotony, flat
      anterior chamber
  chest, congenital Q67.8
  foot (acquired) (fixed type) (painful) (postural) (*see
      also* Deformity, limb, flat foot)
    congenital (rigid) (spastic (everted)) Q66.5
    rachitic sequelae (late effect) E64.3
  organ or site, congenital NEC — *see* Anomaly, by site
  pelvis M95.5
    with disproportion (fetopelvic) O33.Ø
      causing obstructed labor O65.Ø
    congenital Q74.2
Flatau-Schilder disease G37.0
Flatback syndrome M40.30
  lumbar region M4Ø.36
  lumbosacral region M4Ø.37
  thoracolumbar region M4Ø.35
Flattening
  head, femur M89.8x5
  hip — *see* Coxa, plana
  lip (congenital) Q18.8
  nose (congenital) Q67.4
    acquired M95.Ø
Flatulence R14.3
  psychogenic F45.8
Flatus R14.3
  vaginalis N89.8
Flax-dresser's disease J66.1
Flea bite — *see* Injury, bite, insect
Flecks, glaucomatous (subcapsular) — *see* Cataract,
    complicated
Fleischer (-Kayser) **ring** (cornea) H18.Ø4-
Fleshy mole O02.0
Flexibilitas cerea — *see* Catalepsy
Flexion
  cervix — *see* Malposition, uterus
  contracture, joint — *see* Contraction, joint
  deformity, joint (*see also* Deformity, limb, flexion)
      M21.2Ø
    hip, congenital Q65.8
  uterus (*see also* Malposition, uterus)
    lateral — *see* Lateroversion, uterus
Flexner-Boyd dysentery A03.2
Flexner's dysentery A03.1
Flexure — *see* Flexion
Flint murmur (aortic insufficiency) I35.1
Floater, vitreous — *see* Opacity, vitreous
Floating
  cartilage (joint) (*see also* Loose, body, joint)
    knee — *see* Derangement, knee, loose body
  gallbladder, congenital Q44.1
  kidney N28.89
    congenital Q63.8
  spleen D73.89
Flooding N92.0
Floor — *see* condition
Floppy
  baby syndrome (nonspecific) P94.2
  iris syndrome (intraoperative) (IFIS) H21.81
  nonrheumatic mitral valve syndrome I34.1

Flu (*see also* Influenza)
  avian — *see* Influenza, due to identified avian
      influenza virus
  bird — *see* Influenza, due to identified avian
      influenza virus
  intestinal NEC A08.4
  swine — *see* Influenza, due to identified novel H1N1
      influenza virus
Fluctuating blood pressure I99.8
Fluid
  abdomen R18.8
  chest J94.8
  heart — *see* Failure, heart, congestive
  joint — *see* Effusion, joint
  loss (acute) E86.9
    with
      hypernatremia E87.Ø
      hyponatremia E87.1
  lung — *see* Edema, lung
  overload E87.7Ø
    specified NEC E87.79
  peritoneal cavity R18.8
  pleural cavity J94.8
  retention E87.7Ø
Flukes NEC (*see also* Infestation, fluke)
  blood NEC — *see* Schistosomiasis
  liver B66.3
Fluor (vaginalis) N89.8
  trichomonal or due to Trichomonas (vaginalis)
      A59.ØØ
Fluorosis
  dental K00.3
  skeletal M85.1Ø
    ankle M85.17-
    foot M85.17-
    forearm M85.13-
    hand M85.14-
    lower leg M85.16-
    multiple site M85.19
    neck M85.18
    rib M85.18
    shoulder M85.11-
    skull M85.18
    specified site NEC M85.18
    thigh M85.15-
    toe M85.17-
    upper arm M85.12-
    vertebra M85.18
Flush syndrome E34.0
Flushing R23.2
  menopausal N95.1
Flutter
  atrial or auricular I48.1
  heart I49.8
    atrial or auricular I48.1
    ventricular I49.Ø2
  ventricular I49.Ø2
Fochier's abscess — code by site under Abscess
FNHTR (febrile nonhemolytic transfusion reaction)
    R5Ø.84
Focus, Assmann's — *see* Tuberculosis, pulmonary
Fogo selvagem L10.3
Foix-Alajouanine syndrome G95.19
Fold, folds (anomalous) (*see also* Anomaly, by site)
  Descemet's membrane — *see* Change, corneal
      membrane, Descemet's, fold
  epicanthic Q10.3
  heart Q24.8
Folie à deux F24
Follicle
  cervix (nabothian) (ruptured) N88.8
  graafian, ruptured, with hemorrhage N83.Ø
  nabothian N88.8
Follicular — *see* condition
Folliculitis (superficial) L73.9
  abscedens et suffodiens L66.3
  cyst N83.0
  decalvans L66.2
  deep — *see* Furuncle, by site
  gonococcal (acute) (chronic) A54.Ø1
  keloid, keloidalis L73.Ø
  pustular LØ1.Ø2
  ulerythematosa reticulata L66.4

Folliculome lipidique
  specified site — *see* Neoplasm, benign, by site
  unspecified site
    female D27.9
    male D29.2Ø
Folling's disease E70.0
Follow-up — *see* Examination, follow-up
Fong's syndrome (hereditary osteo-onychodysplasia)
    Q78.5
Food
  allergy L27.2
  asphyxia (from aspiration or inhalation) — *see*
      Asphyxia, food
  choked on — *see* Asphyxia, food
  deprivation T73.Ø
    specified kind of food NEC E63.8
  intoxication — *see* Poisoning, food
  lack of T73.Ø
  poisoning — *see* Poisoning, food
  rejection NEC — *see* Disorder, eating
  strangulation or suffocation — *see* Asphyxia, food
  toxemia — *see* Poisoning, food
Foot — *see* condition
Foramen ovale (nonclosure) (patent) (persistent)
    Q21.1
Forbes' glycogen storage disease E74.03
Fordyce-Fox disease L75.2
Fordyce's disease (mouth) Q38.6
Forearm — *see* condition
Foreign body
  with
    laceration — *see* Laceration, by site, with foreign
        body
    puncture wound — *see* Puncture, by site, with
        foreign body
  accidentally left following a procedure T81.5Ø9
    aspiration T81.5Ø6
      resulting in
        adhesions T81.516
        obstruction T81.526
        perforation T81.536
        specified complication NEC T81.596
    cardiac catheterization T81.5Ø5
      resulting in
        acute reaction T81.6Ø
          aseptic peritonitis T81.61
          specified NEC T81.69
        adhesions T81.515
        obstruction T81.525
        perforation T81.535
        specified complication NEC T81.595
    endoscopy T81.5Ø4
      resulting in
        adhesions T81.514
        obstruction T81.524
        perforation T81.534
        specified complication NEC T81.594
    immunization T81.5Ø3
      resulting in
        adhesions T81.513
        obstruction T81.523
        perforation T81.533
        specified complication NEC T81.593
    infusion T81.5Ø1
      resulting in
        adhesions T81.511
        obstruction T81.521
        perforation T81.531
        specified complication NEC T81.591
    injection T81.5Ø3
      resulting in
        adhesions T81.513
        obstruction T81.523
        perforation T81.533
        specified complication NEC T81.593
    kidney dialysis T81.5Ø2
      resulting in
        adhesions T81.512
        obstruction T81.522
        perforation T81.532
        specified complication NEC T81.592

Foreign body— *continued*
  larynx T17.3Ø8
    causing
      asphyxiation T17.3ØØ
        food (bone) (seed) T17.32Ø
        gastric contents (vomitus) T17.31Ø
        specified type NEC T17.39Ø
      injury NEC T17.3Ø8
        food (bone) (seed) T17.328
        gastric contents (vomitus) T17.318
        specified type NEC T17.398
  lens — *see* Foreign body, intraocular
  ocular muscle SØ5.4-
    old, retained — *see* Foreign body, orbit, old
  old or residual
    soft tissue (residual) M79.5
  operation wound, left accidentally — *see* Foreign
    body, accidentally left during a procedure
  orbit SØ5.4-
    old, retained HØ5.5-
  pharynx T17.2Ø8
    causing
      asphyxiation T17.2ØØ
        food (bone) (seed) T17.22Ø
        gastric contents (vomitus) T17.21Ø
        specified type NEC T17.29Ø
      injury NEC T17.2Ø8
        food (bone) (seed) T17.228
        gastric contents (vomitus) T17.218
        specified type NEC T17.298
  respiratory tract T17.9Ø8
    bronchioles — *see* Foreign body, respiratory
      tract, specified site NEC
    bronchus — *see* Foreign body, bronchus
    causing
      asphyxiation T17.9ØØ
        food (bone) (seed) T17.92Ø
        gastric contents (vomitus) T17.91Ø
        specified type NEC T17.99Ø
      injury NEC T17.9Ø8
        food (bone) (seed) T17.928
        gastric contents (vomitus) T17.918
        specified type NEC T17.998
    larynx — *see* Foreign body, larynx
    lung — *see* Foreign body, respiratory tract,
      specified site NEC
    multiple parts — *see* Foreign body, respiratory
      tract, specified site NEC
    nasal sinus T17.Ø
    nasopharynx — *see* Foreign body, pharynx
    nose T17.1
    nostril T17.1
    pharynx — *see* Foreign body, pharynx
    specified site NEC T17.8Ø8
      causing
        asphyxiation T17.8ØØ
          food (bone) (seed) T17.82Ø
          gastric contents (vomitus) T17.81Ø
          specified type NEC T17.89Ø
        injury NEC T17.8Ø8
          food (bone) (seed) T17.828
          gastric contents (vomitus) T17.818
          specified type NEC T17.898
    throat — *see* Foreign body, pharynx
    trachea — *see* Foreign body, trachea
  retained (old) (nonmagnetic) (in)
    anterior chamber (eye) — *see* Foreign body,
      intraocular, old, retained, anterior chamber
      magnetic — *see* Foreign body, intraocular, old,
        retained, magnetic, anterior chamber
    ciliary body — *see* Foreign body, intraocular, old,
      retained, ciliary body
      magnetic — *see* Foreign body, intraocular, old,
        retained, magnetic, ciliary body
    eyelid HØ2.819
      left HØ2.816
        lower HØ2.815
        upper HØ2.814
      right HØ2.813
        lower HØ2.812
        upper HØ2.811

Foreign body— *continued*
  retained— *continued*
    fragments — see Retained, foreign body
      fragments (type of)
    globe — *see* Foreign body, intraocular, old,
      retained
      magnetic — *see* Foreign body, intraocular, old,
        retained, magnetic
    intraocular — *see* Foreign body, intraocular, old,
      retained
      magnetic — *see* Foreign body, intraocular, old,
        retained, magnetic
    iris — *see* Foreign body, intraocular, old, retained,
      iris
      magnetic — *see* Foreign body, intraocular, old,
        retained, magnetic, iris
    lens — *see* Foreign body, intraocular, old,
      retained, lens
      magnetic — *see* Foreign body, intraocular, old,
        retained, magnetic, lens
    muscle — *see* Foreign body, retained, soft tissue
    orbit — *see* Foreign body, orbit, old
    posterior wall of globe — *see* Foreign body,
      intraocular, old, retained, posterior wall
      magnetic — *see* Foreign body, intraocular, old,
        retained, magnetic, posterior wall
    retrobulbar — *see* Foreign body, orbit, old,
      retrobulbar
    soft tissue M79.5
    vitreous — *see* Foreign body, intraocular, old,
      retained, vitreous body
      magnetic — *see* Foreign body, intraocular, old,
        retained, magnetic, vitreous body
  retina SØ5.5-
  superficial, without open wound
    abdomen, abdominal (wall) S3Ø.851
    alveolar process SØØ.552
    ankle S9Ø.55-
    antecubital space — *see* Foreign body,
      superficial, forearm
    anus S3Ø.857
    arm (upper) S4Ø.85-
    auditory canal — *see* Foreign body, superficial,
      ear
    auricle — *see* Foreign body, superficial, ear
    axilla — *see* Foreign body, superficial, arm
    back, lower S3Ø.85Ø
    breast S2Ø.15-
    brow SØØ.85
    buttock S3Ø.85Ø
    calf — *see* Foreign body, superficial, leg
    canthus — *see* Foreign body, superficial, eyelid
    cheek SØØ.85
      internal SØØ.552
    chest wall — *see* Foreign body, superficial, thorax
    chin SØØ.85
    clitoris S3Ø.854
    costal region — *see* Foreign body, superficial,
      thorax
    digit(s)
      hand — *see* Foreign body, superficial, finger
      foot — *see* Foreign body, superficial, toe
    ear SØØ.45-
    elbow S5Ø.35-
    epididymis S3Ø.853
    epigastric region S3Ø.851
    epiglottis S1Ø.15
    esophagus, cervical S1Ø.15
    eyebrow — *see* Foreign body, superficial, eyelid
    eyelid SØØ.25-
    face SØØ.85
    finger(s) S6Ø.459
      index S6Ø.45-
      little S6Ø.45-
      middle S6Ø.45-
      ring S6Ø.45-
    flank S3Ø.851
    foot (except toe(s) alone) S9Ø.85-
      toe — *see* Foreign body, superficial, toe
    forearm S5Ø.85-
      elbow only — *see* Foreign body, superficial,
        elbow
    forehead SØØ.85

Foreign body— *continued*
  superficial, without open wound—*continued*
    genital organs, external
      female S3Ø.856
      male S3Ø.855
    groin S3Ø.851
    gum SØØ.552
    hand S6Ø.55-
    head SØØ.95
      ear — *see* Foreign body, superficial, ear
      eyelid — *see* Foreign body, superficial, eyelid
      lip SØØ.551
      nose SØØ.35
      oral cavity SØØ.552
      scalp SØØ.Ø5
      specified site NEC SØØ.85
    heel — *see* Foreign body, superficial, foot
    hip S7Ø.25-
    inguinal region S3Ø.851
    interscapular region S2Ø.459
    jaw SØØ.85
    knee S8Ø.25-
    labium (majus) (minus) S3Ø.854
    larynx S1Ø.15
    leg (lower) S8Ø.85-
      knee — *see* Foreign body, superficial, knee
      upper — *see* Foreign body, superficial, thigh
    lip SØØ.551
    lower back S3Ø.85Ø
    lumbar region S3Ø.85Ø
    malar region SØØ.85
    mammary — *see* Foreign body, superficial, breast
    mastoid region SØØ.85
    mouth SØØ.552
    nail
      finger — *see* Foreign body, superficial, finger
      toe — *see* Foreign body, superficial, toe
    nape S1Ø.85
    nasal SØØ.35
    neck S1Ø.95
      specified site NEC S1Ø.85
      throat S1Ø.15
    nose SØØ.35
    occipital region SØØ.Ø5
    oral cavity SØØ.552
    orbital region — *see* Foreign body, superficial,
      eyelid
    palate SØØ.552
    palm — *see* Foreign body, superficial, hand
    parietal region SØØ.Ø5
    pelvis S3Ø.85Ø
    penis S3Ø.852
    perineum
      female S3Ø.854
      male S3Ø.85Ø
    periocular area — *see* Foreign body, superficial,
      eyelid
    phalanges
      finger — *see* Foreign body, superficial, finger
      toe — *see* Foreign body, superficial, toe
    pharynx S1Ø.15
    pinna — *see* Foreign body, superficial, ear
    popliteal space — *see* Foreign body, superficial,
      knee
    prepuce S3Ø.852
    pubic region S3Ø.85Ø
    pudendum
      female S3Ø.856
      male S3Ø.855
    sacral region S3Ø.85Ø
    scalp SØØ.Ø5
    scapular region — *see* Foreign body, superficial,
      shoulder
    scrotum S3Ø.853
    shin — *see* Foreign body, superficial, leg
    shoulder S4Ø.25-
    sternal region S2Ø.359
    submaxillary region SØØ.85
    submental region SØØ.85
    subungual
      finger(s) — *see* Foreign body, superficial,
        finger
      toe(s) — *see* Foreign body, superficial, toe

Fracture, traumatic — *continued*
- carpal bone(s) S62.109
    - capitate (displaced) S62.13-
        - nondisplaced S62.13-
    - cuneiform — *see* Fracture, carpal bone, triquetrum
    - hamate (body) (displaced) S62.143
        - hook process (displaced) S62.15-
            - nondisplaced S62.15-
        - nondisplaced S62.14-
    - larger multangular — *see* Fracture, carpal bones, trapezium
    - lunate (displaced) S62.12-
        - nondisplaced S62.12-
    - navicular S62.00-
        - distal pole (displaced) S62.01-
            - nondisplaced S62.01-
        - middle third (displaced) S62.02-
            - nondisplaced S62.02-
        - proximal third (displaced) S62.03-
            - nondisplaced S62.03-
        - volar tuberosity — *see* Fracture, carpal bones, navicular, distal pole
    - os magnum — *see* Fracture, carpal bones, capitate
    - pisiform (displaced) S62.16-
        - nondisplaced S62.16-
    - semilunar — *see* Fracture, carpal bones, lunate
    - smaller multangular — *see* Fracture, carpal bones, trapezoid
    - trapezium (displaced) S62.17-
        - nondisplaced S62.17-
    - trapezoid (displaced) S62.18-
        - nondisplaced S62.18-
    - triquetrum (displaced) S62.11-
        - nondisplaced S62.11-
    - unciform — *see* Fracture, carpal bones, hamate
- cervical — *see* Fracture, vertebra, cervical
- clavicle S42.00-
    - acromial end (displaced) S42.03-
        - nondisplaced S42.03-
    - birth injury P13.4
    - lateral end — *see* Fracture, clavicle, acromial end
    - shaft (displaced) S42.02-
        - nondisplaced S42.02-
    - sternal end (anterior) (displaced) S42.01-
        - nondisplaced S42.01-
        - posterior S42.01-
- coccyx S32.2
- collapsed — *see* Collapse, vertebra
- collar bone — *see* Fracture, clavicle
- Colles' — *see* Colles' fracture
- compression, not due to trauma — *see* Collapse, vertebra
- coronoid process — *see* Fracture, ulna, upper end, coronoid process
- corpus cavernosum penis S39.840
- costochondral cartilage S23.41
- costochondral, costosternal junction — *see* Fracture, rib
- cranium — *see* Fracture, skull
- cricoid cartilage S12.8
- cuboid (ankle) — *see* Fracture, tarsal, cuboid
- cuneiform
    - foot — *see* Fracture, tarsal, cuneiform
    - wrist — *see* Fracture, carpal, triquetrum
- delayed union — *see* Delay, union, fracture
- dental restorative material K08.539
    - with loss of material K08.531
    - without loss of material K08.530
- due to
    - birth injury — *see* Birth, injury, fracture
    - osteoporosis — *see* Osteoporosis, with fracture
- Dupuytren's — *see* Fracture, ankle, lateral malleolus
- elbow S42.40-
- ethmoid (bone) (sinus) — *see* Fracture, skull, base
- face bone S02.92
- fatigue (*see also* Fracture, stress)
    - vertebra M48.40
        - cervical region M48.42
        - cervicothoracic region M48.43
        - lumbar region M48.46
        - lumbosacral region M48.47

Fracture, traumatic — *continued*
- fatigue—*continued*
    - vertebra—*continued*
        - occipito-atlanto-axial region M48.41
        - sacrococcygeal region M48.48
        - thoracic region M48.44
        - thoracolumbar region M48.45
- femur, femoral S72.9-
    - birth injury P13.2
    - capital epiphyseal S79.01-
    - condyles, epicondyles — *see* Fracture, femur, lower end
    - distal end — *see* Fracture, femur, lower end
    - epiphysis
        - head — *see* Fracture, femur, upper end, epiphysis
        - lower — *see* Fracture, femur, lower end, epiphysis
        - upper — *see* Fracture, femur, upper end, epiphysis
    - following insertion of implant, prosthesis or plate M96.66-
    - head — *see* Fracture, femur, upper end, head
    - intertrochanteric — *see* Fracture, femur, trochanteric
    - intratrochanteric — *see* Fracture, femur, trochanteric
    - lower end S72.40-
        - condyle (displaced) S72.41-
            - lateral (displaced) S72.42-
                - nondisplaced S72.42-
            - medial (displaced) S72.43-
                - nondisplaced S72.43-
            - nondisplaced S72.41-
        - epiphysis (displaced) S72.44-
            - nondisplaced S72.44-
        - physeal S79.10-
            - Salter-Harris
                - Type I S79.11-
                - Type II S79.12-
                - Type III S79.13-
                - Type IV S79.14-
            - specified NEC S79.19-
        - specified NEC S72.49-
        - supracondylar (displaced) S72.45-
            - with intracondylar extension (displaced) S72.46-
                - nondisplaced S72.46-
            - nondisplaced S72.45-
        - torus S72.47-
    - neck — *see* Fracture, femur, upper end, neck
    - pertrochanteric — *see* Fracture, femur, trochanteric
    - shaft (lower third) (middle third) (upper third) S72.30-
        - comminuted (displaced) S72.35-
            - nondisplaced S72.35-
        - oblique (displaced) S72.33-
            - nondisplaced S72.33-
        - segmental (displaced) S72.36-
            - nondisplaced S72.36-
        - specified NEC S72.39-
        - spiral (displaced) S72.34-
            - nondisplaced S72.34-
        - transverse (displaced) S72.32-
            - nondisplaced S72.32-
    - specified site NEC — *see* subcategory S72.8
    - subcapital (displaced) S72.01-
    - subtrochanteric (region) (section) (displaced) S72.2-
        - nondisplaced S72.2-
    - transcervical — *see* Fracture, femur, upper end, neck
    - transtrochanteric — *see* Fracture, femur, trochanteric
    - trochanteric S72.10-
        - apophyseal (displaced) S72.14-
            - nondisplaced S72.14-
        - greater trochanter (displaced) S72.11-
            - nondisplaced S72.11-
        - intertrochanteric (displaced) S72.13-
            - nondisplaced S72.13-

Fracture, traumatic — *continued*
- femur, femoral— *continued*
    - trochanteric—*continued*
        - lesser trochanter (displaced) S72.12-
            - nondisplaced S72.12-
    - upper end S72.00-
        - apophyseal (displaced) S72.13-
            - nondisplaced S72.13-
        - cervicotrochanteric — *see* Fracture, femur, upper end, neck, base
        - epiphysis (displaced) S72.02-
            - nondisplaced S72.02-
        - head S72.05-
            - articular (displaced) S72.06-
                - nondisplaced S72.06-
            - specified NEC S72.09-
        - intertrochanteric (displaced) S72.14-
            - nondisplaced S72.14-
        - intracapsular S72.01-
        - midcervical (displaced) S72.03-
            - nondisplaced S72.03-
        - neck S72.00-
            - base (displaced) S72.04-
                - nondisplaced S72.04-
            - specified NEC S72.09-
        - pertrochanteric — *see* Fracture, femur, upper end, trochanteric
        - physeal S79.00-
            - Salter-Harris type I S79.01-
            - specified NEC S79.09-
        - subcapital (displaced) S72.01-
        - subtrochanteric (displaced) S72.2-
            - nondisplaced S72.2-
        - transcervical — *see* Fracture, femur, upper end, midcervical
        - trochanteric S72.10-
            - greater (displaced) S72.11-
                - nondisplaced S72.11-
            - lesser (displaced) S72.12-
                - nondisplaced S72.12-
- fibula (shaft) (styloid) S82.40-
    - comminuted (displaced) S82.45-
        - nondisplaced S82.45-
    - following insertion of implant, prosthesis or plate M96.67-
    - involving ankle or malleolus — *see* Fracture, fibula, lateral malleolus
    - lateral malleolus (displaced) S82.6-
        - nondisplaced S82.6-
    - lower end
        - physeal S89.30-
            - Salter-Harris
                - Type I S89.31-
                - Type II S89.32-
            - specified NEC S89.39-
        - specified NEC S82.83-
        - torus S82.82-
    - oblique (displaced) S82.43-
        - nondisplaced S82.43-
    - segmental (displaced) S82.46-
        - nondisplaced S82.46-
    - specified NEC S82.49-
    - spiral (displaced) S82.44-
        - nondisplaced S82.44-
    - transverse (displaced) S82.42-
        - nondisplaced S82.42-
    - upper end
        - physeal S89.20-
            - Salter-Harris
                - Type I S89.21-
                - Type II S89.22-
            - specified NEC S89.29-
        - specified NEC S82.83-
        - torus S82.81-
- finger (except thumb) S62.60-
    - distal phalanx (displaced) S62.63-
        - nondisplaced S62.66-
    - index S62.60-
        - distal phalanx (displaced) S62.63-
            - nondisplaced S62.66-
        - medial phalanx (displaced) S62.62-
            - nondisplaced S62.65-

Fracture, traumatic — *continued*
  finger (except thumb)— *continued*
    index—*continued*
      proximal phalanx (displaced) S62.61-
        nondisplaced S62.64-
      little S62.60-
        distal phalanx (displaced) S62.63-
          nondisplaced S62.66-
        medial phalanx (displaced) S62.62-
          nondisplaced S62.65-
        proximal phalanx (displaced) S62.61-
          nondisplaced S62.64-
      medial phalanx (displaced) S62.62-
        nondisplaced S62.65-
      middle S62.60-
        distal phalanx (displaced) S62.63-
          nondisplaced S62.66-
        medial phalanx (displaced) S62.62-
          nondisplaced S62.65-
        proximal phalanx (displaced) S62.61-
          nondisplaced S62.64-
      proximal phalanx (displaced) S62.61-
        nondisplaced S62.64-
      ring S62.60-
        distal phalanx (displaced) S62.63-
          nondisplaced S62.66-
        medial phalanx (displaced) S62.62-
          nondisplaced S62.65-
        proximal phalanx (displaced) S62.61-
          nondisplaced S62.64-
    thumb — *see* Fracture, thumb
  following insertion (intraoperative) (postoperative) of orthopedic implant, joint prosthesis or bone plate M96.69
    femur M96.66-
    fibula M96.67-
    humerus M96.62-
    pelvis M96.65
    radius M96.63-
    specified bone NEC M96.69
    tibia M96.67-
    ulna M96.63-
  foot S92.90-
    astragalus — *see* Fracture, tarsal, talus
    calcaneus — *see* Fracture, tarsal, calcaneus
    cuboid — *see* Fracture, tarsal, cuboid
    cuneiform — *see* Fracture, tarsal, cuneiform
    metatarsal — *see* Fracture, metatarsal
    navicular — *see* Fracture, tarsal, navicular
    talus — *see* Fracture, tarsal, talus
    tarsal — *see* Fracture, tarsal
    toe — *see* Fracture, toe
  forearm S52.9-
    radius — *see* Fracture, radius
    ulna — *see* Fracture, ulna
  fossa (anterior) (middle) (posterior) S02.19
  frontal (bone) (skull) S02.0
    sinus S02.19
  glenoid (cavity) (scapula) — *see* Fracture, scapula, glenoid cavity
  greenstick — *see* Fracture, by site
  hallux — *see* Fracture, toe, great
  hand S62.9-
    carpal — *see* Fracture, carpal bone
    finger (except thumb) — *see* Fracture, finger
    metacarpal — *see* Fracture, metacarpal
    navicular (scaphoid) (hand) — *see* Fracture, carpal bone, navicular
    thumb — *see* Fracture, thumb
  healed or old
    with complications — code by Nature of the complication
  heel bone — *see* Fracture, tarsal, calcaneus
  Hill-Sachs S42.29-
  hip — *see* Fracture, femur, neck
  humerus S42.30-
    anatomical neck — *see* Fracture, humerus, upper end
    articular process — *see* Fracture, humerus, lower end
    capitellum — *see* Fracture, humerus, lower end, condyle, lateral
    distal end — *see* Fracture, humerus, lower end

Fracture, traumatic — *continued*
  humerus— *continued*
    epiphysis
      lower — *see* Fracture, humerus, lower end, physeal
      upper — *see* Fracture, humerus, upper end, physeal
    external condyle — *see* Fracture, humerus, lower end, condyle, lateral
    following insertion of implant, prosthesis or plate M96.62-
    great tuberosity — *see* Fracture, humerus, upper end, greater tuberosity
    intercondylar — *see* Fracture, humerus, lower end
    internal epicondyle — *see* Fracture, humerus, lower end, epicondyle, medial
    lesser tuberosity — *see* Fracture, humerus, upper end, specified NEC
    lower end S42.40-
      condyle
        lateral (displaced) S42.45-
          nondisplaced S42.45-
        medial (displaced) S42.46-
          nondisplaced S42.46-
      epicondyle
        lateral (displaced) S42.43-
          nondisplaced S42.43-
        medial (displaced) S42.44-
          incarcerated S42.44-
          nondisplaced S42.44-
      physeal S49.10-
        Salter-Harris
          Type I S49.11-
          Type II S49.12-
          Type III S49.13-
          Type IV S49.14-
          specified NEC S49.19-
      specified NEC (displaced) S42.49-
        nondisplaced S42.49-
      supracondylar (simple) (displaced) S42.41-
        comminuted (displaced) S42.42-
          nondisplaced S42.42-
        nondisplaced S42.41-
      torus S42.48-
      transcondylar (displaced) S42.47-
        nondisplaced S42.47-
    proximal end — *see* Fracture, humerus, upper end
    shaft S42.30-
      comminuted (displaced) S42.35-
        nondisplaced S42.35-
      greenstick S42.31-
      oblique (displaced) S42.33-
        nondisplaced S42.33-
      segmental (displaced) S42.36-
        nondisplaced S42.36-
      specified NEC S42.39-
      spiral (displaced) S42.34-
        nondisplaced S42.34-
      transverse (displaced) S42.32-
        nondisplaced S42.32-
    supracondylar — *see* Fracture, humerus, lower end
    surgical neck — *see* Fracture, humerus, upper end, surgical neck
    trochlea — *see* Fracture, humerus, lower end, condyle, medial
    tuberosity — *see* Fracture, humerus, upper end
    upper end S42.20-
      anatomical neck — *see* Fracture, humerus, upper end, specified NEC
      articular head — *see* Fracture, humerus, upper end, specified NEC
      epiphysis — *see* Fracture, humerus, upper end, physeal
      greater tuberosity (displaced) S42.25-
        nondisplaced S42.25-
      lesser tuberosity (displaced) S42.26-
        nondisplaced S42.26-
      physeal S49.00-
        Salter-Harris
          Type I S49.01-

Fracture, traumatic — *continued*
  humerus— *continued*
    upper end—*continued*
      physeal—*continued*
        Salter-Harris—*continued*
          Type II S49.02-
          Type III S49.03-
          Type IV S49.04-
          specified NEC S49.09-
      specified NEC (displaced) S42.29-
        nondisplaced S42.29-
      surgical neck (displaced) S42.21-
        four-part S42.24-
        nondisplaced S42.21-
        three-part S42.23-
        two-part (displaced) S42.22-
          nondisplaced S42.22-
      torus S42.27-
      transepiphyseal — *see* Fracture, humerus, upper end, physeal
  hyoid bone S12.8
  ilium S32.30-
    with disruption of pelvic ring — *see* Disruption, pelvic ring
    avulsion (displaced) S32.31-
      nondisplaced S32.31-
    specified NEC S32.39-
  impaction, impacted—code as Fracture, by site
  innominate bone — *see* Fracture, ilium
  instep — *see* Fracture, foot
  ischium S32.60-
    with disruption of pelvic ring — *see* Disruption, pelvic ring
    avulsion (displaced) S32.61-
      nondisplaced S32.61-
    specified NEC S32.69-
  jaw (bone) (lower) — *see* Fracture, mandible
    upper — *see* Fracture, maxilla
  joint prosthesis — *see* Complications, joint prosthesis, mechanical, breakdown, by site
    periprosthetic — *see* Complications, joint prosthesis, mechanical, periprosthesis, fracture, by site
  knee cap — *see* Fracture, patella
  larynx S12.8
  late effects — *see* Sequelae, fracture
  leg (lower) S82.9-
    ankle — *see* Fracture, ankle
    femur — *see* Fracture, femur
    fibula — *see* Fracture, fibula
    malleolus — *see* Fracture, ankle
    patella — *see* Fracture, patella
    specified site NEC S82.89-
    tibia — *see* Fracture, tibia
  lumbar spine — *see* Fracture, vertebra, lumbar
  lumbosacral spine S32.9
  Maisonneuve's (displaced) S82.86-
    nondisplaced S82.86-
  malar bone (*see also* Fracture, maxilla) S02.400
  malleolus — *see* Fracture, ankle
  malunion — *see* Malunion, fracture
  mandible (lower jaw (bone) S02.609
    alveolous S02.67
    angle (of jaw) S02.65
    body, unspecified S02.600
    condylar process S02.61
    coronoid process S02.63
    ramus, unspecified S02.64
    specified site NEC S02.69
    subcondylar process S02.62
    symphysis S02.66
  manubrium (sterni) S22.21
    dissociation from sternum S22.23
  march — *see* Fracture, traumatic, stress, by site
  maxilla, maxillary (bone) (sinus) (superior) (upper jaw) S02.401
    alveolus S02.42
    inferior — *see* Fracture, mandible
    LeFort I S02.411
    LeFort II S02.412
    LeFort III S02.413

Fracture, traumatic — *continued*
  metacarpal S62.309
    base (displaced) S62.319
      nondisplaced S62.349
    fifth S62.30-
      base (displaced) S62.31-
        nondisplaced S62.34-
      neck (displaced) S62.33-
        nondisplaced S62.36-
      shaft (displaced) S62.32-
        nondisplaced S62.35-
      specified NEC S62.398
    first S62.20-
      base NEC (displaced) S62.23-
        nondisplaced S62.23-
      Bennett's — *see* Bennett's fracture
      neck (displaced) S62.25-
        nondisplaced S62.25-
      shaft (displaced) S62.24-
        nondisplaced S62.24-
      specified NEC S62.29-
    fourth S62.30-
      base (displaced) S62.31-
        nondisplaced S62.34-
      neck (displaced) S62.33-
        nondisplaced S62.36-
      shaft (displaced) S62.32-
        nondisplaced S62.35-
      specified NEC S62.39-
    neck (displaced) S62.33-
      nondisplaced S62.36-
    Rolando's — *see* Rolando's fracture
    second S62.30-
      base (displaced) S62.31-
        nondisplaced S62.34-
      neck (displaced) S62.33-
        nondisplaced S62.36-
      shaft (displaced) S62.32-
        nondisplaced S62.35-
      specified NEC S62.39-
    shaft (displaced) S62.32-
      nondisplaced S62.35-
    third S62.30-
      base (displaced) S62.31-
        nondisplaced S62.34-
      neck (displaced) S62.33-
        nondisplaced S62.36-
      shaft (displaced) S62.32-
        nondisplaced S62.35-
      specified NEC S62.39-
    specified NEC S62.399
  metastatic (*see also* Neoplasm) — *see* Fracture, pathological, due to, neoplastic disease
  metatarsal bone S92.30-
    fifth (displaced) S92.35-
      nondisplaced S92.35-
    first (displaced) S92.31-
      nondisplaced S92.31-
    fourth (displaced) S92.34-
      nondisplaced S92.34-
    second (displaced) S92.32-
      nondisplaced S92.32-
    third (displaced) S92.33-
      nondisplaced S92.33-
  Monteggia's — *see* Monteggia's fracture
  multiple
    hand (and wrist) NEC — *see* Fracture, by site
    ribs — *see* Fracture, rib, multiple
  nasal (bone(s)) S02.2
  navicular (scaphoid) (foot) (*see also* Fracture, tarsal, navicular)
    hand — *see* Fracture, carpal, navicular
  neck S12.9
    cervical vertebra S12.9
      fifth (displaced) S12.400
        nondisplaced S12.401
        specified type NEC (displaced) S12.490
          nondisplaced S12.491
      first (displaced) S12.000
        burst (stable) S12.01
          unstable S12.02
        lateral mass (displaced) S12.040
          nondisplaced S12.041

Fracture, traumatic — *continued*
  neck— *continued*
    cervical vertebra— *continued*
      first—*continued*
        nondisplaced S12.001
        posterior arch (displaced) S12.030
          nondisplaced S12.031
        specified type NEC (displaced) S12.090
          nondisplaced S12.091
      fourth (displaced) S12.300
        nondisplaced S12.301
        specified type NEC (displaced) S12.390
          nondisplaced S12.391
      second (displaced) S12.100
        nondisplaced S12.101
        dens (anterior) (displaced) (type II) S12.110
          nondisplaced S12.112
          posterior S12.111
          specified type NEC (displaced) S12.120
            nondisplaced S12.121
        specified type NEC (displaced) S12.190
          nondisplaced S12.191
      seventh (displaced) S12.600
        nondisplaced S12.601
        specified type NEC (displaced) S12.690
          displaced S12.691
      sixth (displaced) S12.500
        nondisplaced S12.501
        specified type NEC (displaced) S12.590
          displaced S12.591
      third (displaced) S12.200
        nondisplaced S12.201
        specified type NEC (displaced) S12.290
          displaced S12.291
    hyoid bone S12.8
    larynx S12.8
    specified site NEC S12.8
    thyroid cartilage S12.8
    trachea S12.8
  neoplastic NEC — *see* Fracture, pathological, due to, neoplastic disease
  neural arch — *see* Fracture, vertebra
  newborn — *see* Birth, injury, fracture
  nontraumatic — *see* Fracture, pathological
  nonunion — *see* Nonunion, fracture
  nose, nasal (bone) (septum) S02.2
  occiput — *see* Fracture, skull, base, occiput
  odontoid process — *see* Fracture, neck, cervical vertebra, second
  olecranon (process) (ulna) — *see* Fracture, ulna, upper end, olecranon process
  orbit, orbital (bone) (region) S02.8
    floor (blow-out) S02.3
    roof S02.19
  os
    calcis — *see* Fracture, tarsal, calcaneus
    magnum — *see* Fracture, carpal, capitate
    pubis — *see* Fracture, pubis
  palate S02.8
  parietal bone (skull) S02.0
  patella S82.00-
    comminuted (displaced) S82.04-
      nondisplaced S82.04-
    longitudinal (displaced) S82.02-
      nondisplaced S82.02-
    osteochondral (displaced) S82.01-
      nondisplaced S82.01-
    specified NEC S82.09-
    transverse (displaced) S82.03-
      nondisplaced S82.03-
  pedicle (of vertebral arch) — *see* Fracture, vertebra
  pelvis, pelvic (bone) S32.9
    acetabulum — *see* Fracture, acetabulum
    circle — *see* Disruption, pelvic ring
    following insertion of implant, prosthesis or plate M96.65
    ilium — *see* Fracture, ilium
    ischium — *see* Fracture, ischium
    multiple with disruption of pelvic ring — *see* Disruption, pelvic ring
    pubis — *see* Fracture, pubis
    specified site NEC S32.89

Fracture, traumatic — *continued*
  pelvis— *continued*
    sacrum — *see* Fracture, sacrum
  phalanx
    foot — *see* Fracture, toe
    hand — *see* Fracture, finger
  pisiform — *see* Fracture, carpal, pisiform
  pond — *see* Fracture, skull
  prosthetic device, internal — *see* Complications, prosthetic device, by site, mechanical
  pubis S32.50-
    with disruption of pelvic ring — *see* Disruption, pelvic ring
    specified site NEC S32.59-
    superior rim S32.51-
  radius S52.9-
    distal end — *see* Fracture, radius, lower end
    following insertion of implant, prosthesis or plate M96.63-
    head — *see* Fracture, radius, upper end, head
    lower end S52.50-
      Barton's — *see* Barton's fracture
      Colles' — *see* Colles' fracture
      extraarticular NEC S52.55-
      intraarticular NEC S52.57-
      physeal S59.20-
        Salter-Harris
          Type I S59.21-
          Type II S59.22-
          Type III S59.23-
          Type IV S59.24-
        specified NEC S59.29-
      Smith's — *see* Smith's fracture
      specified NEC S52.59-
      styloid process (displaced) S52.51-
        nondisplaced S52.51-
      torus S52.52-
    neck — *see* Fracture, radius, upper end
    proximal end — *see* Fracture, radius, upper end
    shaft S52.30-
      bent bone S52.38-
      comminuted (displaced) S52.35-
        nondisplaced S52.35-
      Galeazzi's — *see* Galeazzi's fracture
      greenstick S52.31-
      oblique (displaced) S52.33-
        nondisplaced S52.33-
      segmental (displaced) S52.36-
        nondisplaced S52.36-
      specified NEC S52.39-
      spiral (displaced) S52.34-
        nondisplaced S52.34-
      transverse (displaced) S52.32-
        nondisplaced S52.32-
    upper end S52.10-
      head (displaced) S52.12-
        nondisplaced S52.12-
      neck (displaced) S52.13-
        nondisplaced S52.13-
      specified NEC S52.18-
      physeal S59.10-
        Salter-Harris
          Type I S59.11-
          Type II S59.12-
          Type III S59.13-
          Type IV S59.14-
        specified NEC S59.19-
      torus S52.11-
  ramus
    inferior or superior, pubis — *see* Fracture, pubis
    mandible — *see* Fracture, mandible
  restorative material (dental) K08.539
    with loss of material K08.531
    without loss of material K08.530
  rib S22.3-
    with flail chest — *see* Flail, chest
    multiple S22.4-
      with flail chest — *see* Flail, chest
  root, tooth — *see* Fracture, tooth
  sacrum S32.10
    specified NEC S32.19
    Type
      1 S32.14

Fracture, traumatic — *continued*
  sacrum— *continued*
    Type— *continued*
      2 S32.15
      3 S32.16
      4 S32.17
      Zone
        I S32.119
          displaced (minimally) S32.111
            severely S32.112
          nondisplaced S32.110
        II S32.129
          displaced (minimally) S32.121
            severely S32.122
          nondisplaced S32.120
        III S32.139
          displaced (minimally) S32.131
            severely S32.132
          nondisplaced S32.130
  scaphoid (hand) (*see also* Fracture, carpal, navicular)
    foot — *see* Fracture, tarsal, navicular
  scapula S42.10-
    acromial process (displaced) S42.12-
      nondisplaced S42.12-
    body (displaced) S42.11-
      nondisplaced S42.11-
    coracoid process (displaced) S42.13-
      nondisplaced S42.13-
    glenoid cavity (displaced) S42.14-
      nondisplaced S42.14-
    neck (displaced) S42.15-
      nondisplaced S42.15-
    specified NEC S42.19-
  semilunar bone, wrist — *see* Fracture, carpal, lunate
  sequelae — *see* Sequelae, fracture
  sesamoid bone
    hand — *see* Fracture, carpal
    other—code by site under Fracture
  shepherd's — *see* Fracture, tarsal, talus
  shoulder (girdle) S42.9-
    blade — *see* Fracture, scapula
  sinus (ethmoid) (frontal) S02.19
  skull S02.91
    base S02.10
      occiput S02.119
        condyle S02.113
          type I S02.110
          type II S02.111
          type III S02.112
        specified NEC S02.118
      specified NEC S02.19
    birth injury P13.0
    frontal bone S02.0
    parietal bone S02.0
    specified site NEC S02.8
    temporal bone S02.19
    vault S02.0
  Smith's — *see* Smith's fracture
  sphenoid (bone) (sinus) S02.19
  spine — *see* Fracture, vertebra
  spinous process — *see* Fracture, vertebra
  spontaneous (cause unknown) — *see* Fracture, pathological
  stave (of thumb) — *see* Fracture, metacarpal, first
  sternum S22.20
    with flail chest — *see* Flail, chest
    body S22.22
    manubrium S22.21
    xiphoid (process) S22.24
  stress M84.30
    ankle M84.37-
    carpus M84.34-
    clavicle M84.31-
    femoral neck M84.359
    femur M84.35-
    fibula M84.36-
    finger M84.34-
    hip M84.359
    humerus M84.32-
    ilium M84.350
    ischium M84.350
    metacarpus M84.34-
    metatarsus M84.37-

Fracture, traumatic — *continued*
  stress— *continued*
    neck — *see* Fracture, fatigue, vertebra
    pelvis M84.350
    radius M84.33-
    rib M84.38
    scapula M84.31-
    skull M84.38
    tarsus M84.37-
    tibia M84.36-
    toe M84.37-
    ulna M84.33-
    vertebra — *see* Fracture, fatigue, vertebra
  supracondylar, elbow — *see* Fracture, humerus, lower end, supracondylar
  symphysis pubis — *see* Fracture, pubis
  talus (ankle bone) — *see* Fracture, tarsal, talus
  tarsal bone(s) S92.20-
    astragalus — *see* Fracture, tarsal, talus
    calcaneus S92.00-
      anterior process (displaced) S92.02-
        nondisplaced S92.02-
      body (displaced) S92.01-
        nondisplaced S92.01-
      extraarticular NEC (displaced) S92.05-
        nondisplaced S92.05-
      intraarticular (displaced) S92.06-
        nondisplaced S92.06-
      tuberosity (displaced) S92.04-
        avulsion (displaced) S92.03-
          nondisplaced S92.03-
        nondisplaced S92.04-
    cuboid (displaced) S92.21-
      nondisplaced S92.21-
    cuneiform
      intermediate (displaced) S92.23-
        nondisplaced S92.23-
      lateral (displaced) S92.22-
        nondisplaced S92.22-
      medial (displaced) S92.24-
        nondisplaced S92.24-
    navicular (displaced) S92.25-
      nondisplaced S92.25-
    scaphoid — *see* Fracture, tarsal, navicular
    talus S92.10-
      avulsion (displaced) S92.15-
        nondisplaced S92.15-
      body (displaced) S92.12-
        nondisplaced S92.12-
      dome (displaced) S92.14-
        nondisplaced S92.14-
      head (displaced) S92.12-
        nondisplaced S92.12-
      lateral process (displaced) S92.14-
        nondisplaced S92.14-
      neck (displaced) S92.11-
        nondisplaced S92.11-
      posterior process (displaced) S92.13-
        nondisplaced S92.13-
      specified NEC S92.19-
  temporal bone (styloid) S02.19
  thorax (bony) S22.9
    with flail chest — *see* Flail, chest
    rib S22.3-
      multiple S22.4-
        with flail chest — *see* Flail, chest
    sternum S22.20
      body S22.22
      manubrium S22.21
      xiphoid process S22.24
    vertebra (displaced) S22.009
      burst (stable) S22.001
        unstable S22.002
      eighth S22.069
        burst (stable) S22.061
          unstable S22.062
        specified type NEC S22.068
        wedge compression S22.060
      eleventh S22.089
        burst (stable) S22.081
          unstable S22.082
        specified type NEC S22.088
        wedge compression S22.080

Fracture, traumatic — *continued*
  thorax (bony)— *continued*
    vertebra (displaced)— *continued*
      fifth S22.059
        burst (stable) S22.051
          unstable S22.052
        specified type NEC S22.058
        wedge compression S22.050
      first S22.019
        burst (stable) S22.011
          unstable S22.012
        specified type NEC S22.018
        wedge compression S22.010
      fourth S22.049
        burst (stable) S22.041
          unstable S22.042
        specified type NEC S22.048
        wedge compression S22.040
      ninth S22.079
        burst (stable) S22.071
          unstable S22.072
        specified type NEC S22.078
        wedge compression S22.070
      nondisplaced S22.001
      second S22.029
        burst (stable) S22.021
          unstable S22.022
        specified type NEC S22.028
        wedge compression S22.020
      seventh S22.069
        burst (stable) S22.061
          unstable S22.062
        specified type NEC S22.068
        wedge compression S22.060
      sixth S22.059
        burst (stable) S22.051
          unstable S22.052
        specified type NEC S22.058
        wedge compression S22.050
      specified type NEC S22.008
      tenth S22.079
        burst (stable) S22.071
          unstable S22.072
        specified type NEC S22.078
        wedge compression S22.070
      third S22.039
        burst (stable) S22.031
          unstable S22.032
        specified type NEC S22.038
        wedge compression S22.030
      twelfth S22.089
        burst (stable) S22.081
          unstable S22.082
        specified type NEC S22.088
        wedge compression S22.080
      wedge compression S22.000
    thumb S62.50-
      distal phalanx (displaced) S62.52-
        nondisplaced S62.52-
      proximal phalanx (displaced) S62.51-
        nondisplaced S62.51-
    thyroid cartilage S12.8
    tibia (shaft) S82.20-
      comminuted (displaced) S82.25-
        nondisplaced S82.25-
      condyles — *see* Fracture, tibia, upper end
      distal end — *see* Fracture, tibia, lower end
      epiphysis
        lower — *see* Fracture, tibia, lower end
        upper — *see* Fracture, tibia, upper end
      following insertion of implant, prosthesis or plate M96.67-
      head (involving knee joint) — *see* Fracture, tibia, upper end
      intercondyloid eminence — *see* Fracture, tibia, upper end
      involving ankle or malleolus — *see* Fracture, ankle, medial malleolus
      lower end S82.30-
        physeal S89.10-
          Salter-Harris
            Type I S89.11-
            Type II S89.12-

Fracture, traumatic — *continued*
  tibia (shaft)— *continued*
    lower end—*continued*
      physeal—*continued*
        Salter-Harris—*continued*
          Type III S89.13-
          Type IV S89.14-
          specified NEC S89.19-
      pilon (displaced) S82.87-
        nondisplaced S82.87-
      specified NEC S82.39-
      torus S82.31-
    malleolus — *see* Fracture, ankle, medial malleolus
    oblique (displaced) S82.23-
      nondisplaced S82.23-
    pilon — *see* Fracture, tibia, lower end, pilon
    proximal end — *see* Fracture, tibia, upper end
    segmental (displaced) S82.26-
      nondisplaced S82.26-
    specified NEC S82.29-
    spine — *see* Fracture, upper end, spine
    spiral (displaced) S82.24-
      nondisplaced S82.24-
    transverse (displaced) S82.22-
      nondisplaced S82.22-
    tuberosity — *see* Fracture, tibia, upper end,
      tuberosity
    upper end S82.10-
      bicondylar (displaced) S82.14-
        nondisplaced S82.14-
      lateral condyle (displaced) S82.12-
        nondisplaced S82.12-
      medial condyle (displaced) S82.13-
        nondisplaced S82.13-
      physeal S89.00-
        Salter-Harris
          Type I S89.01-
          Type II S89.02-
          Type III S89.03-
          Type IV S89.04-
          specified NEC S89.09-
      plateau — *see* Fracture, tibia, upper end,
        bicondylar
      spine (displaced) S82.11-
        nondisplaced S82.11-
      torus S82.16-
      specified NEC S82.19-
      tuberosity (displaced) S82.15-
        nondisplaced S82.15-
  toe S92.91-
    great (displaced) S92.40-
      distal phalanx (displaced) S92.42-
        nondisplaced S92.42-
      nondisplaced S92.40-
      proximal phalanx (displaced) S92.41-
        nondisplaced S92.41-
      specified NEC S92.49-
    lesser (displaced) S92.50-
      distal phalanx (displaced) S92.53-
        nondisplaced S92.53-
      medial phalanx (displaced) S92.52-
        nondisplaced S92.52-
      nondisplaced S92.50-
      proximal phalanx (displaced) S92.51-
        nondisplaced S92.51-
      specified NEC S92.59-
  tooth (root) S02.5
  trachea (cartilage) S12.8
  transverse process — *see* Fracture, vertebra
  trapezium or trapezoid bone — *see* Fracture, carpal
  trimalleolar — *see* Fracture, ankle, trimalleolar
  triquetrum (cuneiform of carpus) — *see* Fracture,
    carpal, triquetrum
  trochanter — *see* Fracture, femur, trochanteric
  tuberosity (external)—code by site under Fracture
  ulna (shaft) S52.20-
    bent bone S52.28-
    coronoid process — *see* Fracture, ulna, upper
      end, coronoid process
    distal end — *see* Fracture, ulna, lower end
    following insertion of implant, prosthesis or plate
      M96.63-
    head S52.00-

Fracture, traumatic — *continued*
  ulna (shaft)— *continued*
    lower end S52.60-
      physeal S59.00-
        Salter-Harris
          Type I S59.01-
          Type II S59.02-
          Type III S59.03-
          Type IV S59.04-
        specified NEC S59.09-
      specified NEC S52.69-
      styloid process (displaced) S52.61-
        nondisplaced S52.61-
      torus S52.62-
    proximal end — *see* Fracture, ulna, upper end
    shaft S52.20-
      comminuted (displaced) S52.25-
        nondisplaced S52.25-
      greenstick S52.21-
      Monteggia's — *see* Monteggia's fracture
      oblique (displaced) S52.23-
        nondisplaced S52.23-
      segmental (displaced) S52.26-
        nondisplaced S52.26-
      specified NEC S52.29-
      spiral (displaced) S52.24-
        nondisplaced S52.24-
      transverse (displaced) S52.22-
        nondisplaced S52.22-
    upper end S52.00-
      coronoid process (displaced) S52.04-
        nondisplaced S52.04-
      olecranon process (displaced) S52.02-
        with intraarticular extension S52.03-
          with intraarticular extension S52.03-
        nondisplaced S52.02-
          with intraarticular extension S52.03-
            with intraarticular extension
              S52.03-
          with intraarticular extension
            S52.03-
          with intraarticular extension S52.03-
      specified NEC S52.09-
      torus S52.01-
  unciform — *see* Fracture, carpal, hamate
  vault of skull S02.0
  vertebra, vertebral (arch) (body) (column) (neural
    arch) (pedicle) (spinous process) (transverse
    process)
    atlas — *see* Fracture, neck, cervical vertebra, first
    axis — *see* Fracture, neck, cervical vertebra,
      second
    cervical (teardrop) S12.9
      axis — *see* Fracture, neck, cervical vertebra,
        second
      first (atlas) — *see* Fracture, neck, cervical
        vertebra, first
      second (axis) — *see* Fracture, neck, cervical
        vertebra, second
    chronic M84.48
    coccyx S32.2
    dorsal — *see* Fracture, thorax, vertebra
    lumbar S32.009
      burst (stable) S32.001
        unstable S32.002
      fifth S32.059
        burst (stable) S32.051
          unstable S32.052
        specified type NEC S32.058
        wedge compression S32.050
      first S32.019
        burst (stable) S32.011
          unstable S32.012
        specified type NEC S32.018
        wedge compression S32.010
      fourth S32.049
        burst (stable) S32.041
          unstable S32.042
        specified type NEC S32.048
        wedge compression S32.040
      second S32.029
        burst (stable) S32.021
          unstable S32.022

Fracture, traumatic — *continued*
  vertebra, vertebral— *continued*
    lumbar—*continued*
      specified type NEC S32.028
        wedge compression S32.020
      specified type NEC S32.008
      third S32.039
        burst (stable) S32.031
          unstable S32.032
        specified type NEC S32.038
        wedge compression S32.030
      wedge compression S32.000
    metastatic (*see also* Neoplasm) — *see* Collapse,
      vertebra, in, specified disease NEC
    newborn (birth injury) P11.5
    sacrum S32.10
      specified NEC S32.19
      Type
        1 S32.14
        2 S32.15
        3 S32.16
        4 S32.17
      Zone
        I S32.119
          displaced (minimally) S32.111
            severely S32.112
          nondisplaced S32.110
        II S32.129
          displaced (minimally) S32.121
            severely S32.122
          nondisplaced S32.120
        III S32.139
          displaced (minimally) S32.131
            severely S32.132
          nondisplaced S32.130
    thoracic — *see* Fracture, thorax, vertebra
  vertex S02.0
  vomer (bone) S02.2
  wrist S62.10-
    carpal — *see* Fracture, carpal bone
    navicular (scaphoid) (hand) — *see* Fracture,
      carpal, navicular
  xiphisternum, xiphoid (process) S22.24
  zygoma S02.402
Fragile, fragility
  autosomal site Q95.5
  bone, congenital (with blue sclera) Q78.0
  capillary (hereditary) D69.8
  hair L67.8
  nails L60.3
  non-sex chromosome site Q95.5
  X chromosome Q99.2
Fragilitas
  crinium L67.8
  ossium (with blue sclerae) (hereditary) Q78.0
  unguium L60.3
    congenital Q84.6
Fragments, cataract (lens)**, following cataract
  surgery** H59.02-
  retained foreign body — *see* Retained, foreign body
    fragments (type of)
Frailty (frail) R54
  mental R41.81
Frambesia, frambesial (tropica) (*see also* Yaws)
  initial lesion or ulcer A66.0
  primary A66.0
Frambeside
  gummatous A66.4
  of early yaws A66.2
Frambesioma A66.1
Franceschetti-Klein (-Wildervanck) **disease or
  syndrome** Q75.4
Francis' disease — *see* Tularemia
Franklin disease C88.2
Frank's essential thrombocytopenia D69.3
Fraser's syndrome Q87.0
Freckle(s) L81.2
  malignant melanoma In — *see* Melanoma
  melanotic (Hutchinson's) — *see* Melanoma, in situ
  retinal D49.81

Frederickson's hyperlipoproteinemia, type
  I and V E78.3
  IIA E78.0
  IIB and III E78.2
  IV E78.1
Freeman Sheldon syndrome Q87.0
Freezing (*see also* Effect, adverse, cold) T69.9
Freiberg's disease (infraction of metatarsal head or
  osteochondrosis) — *see* Osteochondrosis,
  juvenile, metatarsus
Frei's disease A55
Fremitus, friction, cardiac R01.2
Frenum, frenulum
  external os Q51.828
  tongue (shortening) (congenital) Q38.1
Frequency micturition (nocturnal) R35.0
  psychogenic F45.8
Frey's syndrome
  auriculotemporal G50.8
  hyperhidrosis L74.52
Friction
  burn — *see* Burn, by site
  fremitus, cardiac R01.2
  precordial R01.2
  sounds, chest R09.89
Friderichsen-Waterhouse syndrome or disease
  A39.1
Friedländer's B (bacillus) **NEC** (*see also* condition)
  A49.8
Friedreich's
  ataxia G11.1
  combined systemic disease G11.1
  facial hemihypertrophy Q67.4
  sclerosis (cerebellum) (spinal cord) G11.1
Frigidity F52.22
Fröhlich's syndrome E23.6
Frontal (*see also* condition)
  lobe syndrome F07.0
Frostbite (superficial) T33.90
  with
      partial thickness skin loss — *see* Frostbite
        (superficial), by site
      tissue necrosis T34.90
  abdominal wall T33.3
      with tissue necrosis T34.3
  ankle T33.81-
      with tissue necrosis T34.81-
  arm T33.4-
      with tissue necrosis T34.4-
      finger(s) — *see* Frostbite, finger
      hand — *see* Frostbite, hand
      wrist — *see* Frostbite, wrist
  ear T33.01-
      with tissue necrosis T34.01-
  face T33.09
      with tissue necrosis T34.09
  finger T33.53-
      with tissue necrosis T34.53-
  foot T33.82-
      with tissue necrosis T34.82-
  hand T33.52-
      with tissue necrosis T34.52-
  head T33.09
      with tissue necrosis T34.09
      ear — *see* Frostbite, ear
      nose — *see* Frostbite, nose
  hip (and thigh) T33.6-
      with tissue necrosis T34.6-
  knee T33.7-
      with tissue necrosis T34.7-
  leg T33.9-
      with tissue necrosis T34.9-
      ankle — *see* Frostbite, ankle
      foot — *see* Frostbite, foot
      knee — *see* Frostbite, knee
      lower T33.7-
          with tissue necrosis T34.7-
      thigh — *see* Frostbite, hip
      toe — *see* Frostbite, toe
  limb
      lower T33.99
          with tissue necrosis T34.99
      upper — *see* Frostbite, arm

Frostbite —*continued*
  neck T33.1
      with tissue necrosis T34.1
  nose T33.02
      with tissue necrosis T34.02
  pelvis T33.3
      with tissue necrosis T34.3
  specified site NEC T33.99
      with tissue necrosis T34.99
  thigh — *see* Frostbite, hip
  thorax T33.2
      with tissue necrosis T34.2
  toes T33.83-
      with tissue necrosis T34.83-
  trunk T33.99
      with tissue necrosis T34.99
  wrist T33.51-
      with tissue necrosis T34.51-
Frotteurism F65.81
Frozen (*see also* Effect, adverse, cold) T69.9
  pelvis (female) N94.89
      male K66.8
  shoulder — *see* Capsulitis, adhesive
Fructokinase deficiency E74.11
Fructose 1,6 diphosphatase deficiency E74.19
Fructosemia (benign) (essential) E74.19
Fructosuria (benign) (essential) E74.11
Fuchs'
  black spot (myopic) — *see* Disorder, globe,
      degenerative, myopia
  dystrophy (corneal endothelium) H18.52
  heterochromic cyclitis — *see* Cyclitis, Fuchs'
      heterochromic
Fucosidosis E77.1
Fugue R68.89
  dissociative F44.1
  hysterical (dissociative) F44.1
  postictal in epilepsy — *see* Epilepsy
  reaction to exceptional stress (transient) F43.0
Fulminant, fulminating — *see* condition
Functional (*see also* condition)
  bleeding (uterus) N93.8
Functioning, intellectual, borderline R41.83
Fundus — *see* condition
Fungemia NOS B49
Fungus, fungous
  cerebral G93.89
  disease NOS B49
  infection — *see* Infection, fungus
Funiculitis (acute) (chronic) (endemic) N49.1
  gonococcal (acute) (chronic) A54.23
  tuberculous A18.15
Funnel
  breast (acquired) M95.4
      congenital Q67.6
      sequelae (late effect) of rickets E64.3
  chest (acquired) M95.4
      congenital Q67.6
      sequelae (late effect) of rickets E64.3
  pelvis (acquired) M95.5
      with disproportion (fetopelvic) O33.3
          causing obstructed labor O65.3
      congenital Q74.2
FUO (fever of unknown origin) R50.9
Furfur L21.0
  microsporon B36.0
Furrier's lung J67.8
Furrowed K14.5
  nail(s) (transverse) L60.4
      congenital Q84.6
  tongue K14.5
      congenital Q38.3
Furuncle L02.92
  abdominal wall L02.221
  ankle — *see* Furuncle, lower limb
  anus K61.0
  antecubital space — *see* Furuncle, upper limb
  arm — *see* Furuncle, upper limb
  auditory canal, external — *see* Abscess, ear, external
  auricle (ear) — *see* Abscess, ear, external
  axilla (region) L02.42-
  back (any part) L02.222
  breast N61

Furuncle — *continued*
  buttock L02.32
  cheek (external) L02.02
  chest wall L02.223
  chin L02.02
  corpus cavernosum N48.21
  ear, external — *see* Abscess, ear, external
  external auditory canal — *see* Abscess, ear, external
  eyelid — *see* Abscess, eyelid
  face L02.02
  femoral (region) — *see* Furuncle, lower limb
  finger — *see* Furuncle, hand
  flank L02.221
  foot L02.62-
  forehead L02.02
  gluteal (region) L02.32
  groin L02.224
  hand L02.52-
  head L02.821
      face L02.02
  hip — *see* Furuncle, lower limb
  kidney — *see* Abscess, kidney
  knee — *see* Furuncle, lower limb
  labium (majus) (minus) N76.4
  lacrimal
      gland — *see* Dacryoadenitis
      passages (duct) (sac) — *see* Inflammation,
          lacrimal, passages, acute
  leg (any part) — *see* Furuncle, lower limb
  lower limb L02.42-
  malignant A22.0
  mouth K12.2
  navel L02.226
  neck L02.12
  nose J34.0
  orbit, orbital — *see* Abscess, orbit
  palmar (space) — *see* Furuncle, hand
  partes posteriores L02.32
  pectoral region L02.223
  penis N48.21
  perineum L02.225
  pinna — *see* Abscess, ear, external
  popliteal — *see* Furuncle, lower limb
  prepatellar — *see* Furuncle, lower limb
  scalp L02.821
  seminal vesicle N49.0
  shoulder — *see* Furuncle, upper limb
  specified site NEC L02.828
  submandibular K12.2
  temple (region) L02.02
  thumb — *see* Furuncle, hand
  toe — *see* Furuncle, foot
  trunk L02.229
      abdominal wall L02.221
      back L02.222
      chest wall L02.223
      groin L02.224
      perineum L02.225
      umbilicus L02.226
  umbilicus L02.226
  upper limb L02.42-
  vulva N76.4
Furunculosis — *see* Abscess, by site
Fused — *see* Fusion, fused
Fusion, fused (congenital)
  astragaloscaphoid Q74.2
  atria Q21.1
  auditory canal Q16.1
  auricles, heart Q21.1
  binocular with defective stereopsis H53.32
  bone Q79.8
  cervical spine M43.22
  choanal Q30.0
  commissure, mitral valve Q23.2
  cusps, heart valve NEC Q24.8
      mitral Q23.2
      pulmonary Q22.1
      tricuspid Q22.4
  ear ossicles Q16.3
  fingers Q70.0-
  hymen Q52.3
  joint (acquired) (*see also* Ankylosis)
      congenital Q74.8

Fusion, fused — *continued*
kidneys (incomplete) Q63.1
labium (majus) (minus) Q52.5
larynx and trachea Q34.8
limb, congenital Q74.8
lower Q74.2
upper Q74.0
lobes, lung Q33.8
lumbosacral (acquired) M43.27
arthrodesis status Z98.1
congenital Q76.49
postprocedural status Z98.1
nares, nose, nasal, nostril(s) Q30.0
organ or site not listed — *see* Anomaly, by site
ossicles Q79.9
auditory Q16.3
pulmonic cusps Q22.1
ribs Q76.6
sacroiliac (joint) (acquired) M43.25
arthrodesis status Z98.1
congenital Q74.2
postprocedural status Z98.1
spine (acquired) NEC M43.20
arthrodesis status Z98.1
cervical region M43.22
cervicothoracic region M43.23
congenital Q76.49
lumbar M43.26
lumbosacral region M43.27
occipito-atlanto-axial region M43.21
postoperative status Z98.1
sacrococcygeal region M43.28
thoracic region M43.24
thoracolumbar region M43.25
sublingual duct with submaxillary duct at opening
in mouth Q38.4
testes Q55.1
toes Q70.2-
tooth, teeth K00.2
trachea and esophagus Q39.8
twins Q89.4
vagina Q52.4
ventricles, heart Q21.0
vertebra (arch) — *see* Fusion, spine
vulva Q52.5
Fusospirillosis (mouth) (tongue) (tonsil) A69.1
Fussy baby R68.12

G

Gain in weight (abnormal) (excessive) (*see also*
Weight, gain)
Gaisböck's disease (polycythemia hypertonica) D75.1
Gait abnormality R26.9
ataxic R26.0
falling R29.6
hysterical (ataxic) (staggering) F44.4
paralytic R26.1
spastic R26.1
specified type NEC R26.89
staggering R26.0
unsteadiness R26.81
walking difficulty NEC R26.2
Galactocele (breast) N64.89
puerperal, postpartum O92.79
Galactokinase deficiency E74.29
Galactophoritis N61
gestational, puerperal, postpartum — *see* Mastitis,
obstetric, purulent
Galactorrhea O92.6
not associated with childbirth N64.3
Galactosemia (classic) (congenital) E74.21
Galactosuria E74.29
Galacturia R82.0
schistosomiasis (bilharziasis) B65.0
Galeazzi's fracture S52.37-
Galen's vein — *see* condition
Galeophobia F40.218
Gall duct — *see* condition
Gallbladder (*see also* condition)
acute K81.0

Gallop rhythm R00.8
Gallstone (colic) (cystic duct) (gallbladder) (impacted)
(multiple) (*see also* Calculus, gallbladder)
with
cholecystitis — *see* Calculus, gallbladder, with
cholecystitis
bile duct (common) (hepatic) — *see* Calculus, bile
duct
causing intestinal obstruction K56.3
specified NEC K80.80
with obstruction K80.81
Gambling Z72.6
pathological (compulsive) F63.0
Gammopathy (of undetermined significance [MGUS])
D47.2
associated with lymphoplasmacytic dyscrasia D47.2
monoclonal D47.2
polyclonal D89.0
Gamna's disease (siderotic splenomegaly) D73.1
Gamophobia F40.298
Gampsodactylia (congenital) Q66.7
Gamstorp's disease (adynamia episodica hereditaria)
G72.3
Gandy-Nanta disease (siderotic splenomegaly) D73.1
Gang
membership offenses Z72.810
Gangliocytoma D36.10
Ganglioglioma — *see* Neoplasm, uncertain behavior,
by site
Ganglion (compound) (diffuse) (joint) (tendon
(sheath)) M67.40
ankle M67.47-
foot M67.47-
forearm M67.43-
hand M67.44-
lower leg M67.46-
multiple sites M67.49
of yaws (early) (late) A66.6
pelvic region M67.45-
periosteal — *see* Periostitis
shoulder region M67.41-
specified site NEC M67.48
thigh region M67.45-
tuberculous A18.09
upper arm M67.42-
wrist M67.43-
Ganglioneuroblastoma — *see* Neoplasm, nerve,
malignant
Ganglioneuroma D36.10
malignant — *see* Neoplasm, nerve, malignant
Ganglioneuromatosis D36.10
Ganglionitis
fifth nerve — *see* Neuralgia, trigeminal
gasserian (postherpetic) (postzoster) B02.21
geniculate G51.1
newborn (birth injury) P11.3
postherpetic, postzoster B02.21
herpes zoster B02.21
postherpetic geniculate B02.21
Gangliosidosis E75.10
GM1 E75.19
GM2 E75.00
other specified E75.09
Sandhoff disease E75.01
Tay-Sachs disease E75.02
GM3 E75.19
mucolipidosis IV E75.11
Gangosa A66.5
Gangrene, gangrenous (connective tissue) (dropsical)
(dry) (moist) (skin) (ulcer) (*see also* Necrosis) I96
with diabetes (mellitus) — *see* Diabetes, gangrene
abdomen (wall) I96
alveolar M27.3
appendix K35.3
with
perforation or rupture K35.2
peritoneal abscess K35.3
peritonitis, localized K35.3
with perforation or rupture K35.2
generalized K35.2
arteriosclerotic (general) (senile) — *see*
Arteriosclerosis, extremities, with, gangrene

Gangrene, gangrenous — *continued*
auricle I96
Bacillus welchii A48.0
bladder (infectious) — *see* Cystitis, specified type
NEC
bowel, cecum, or colon — *see* Gangrene, intestine
Clostridium perfringens or welchii A48.0
cornea H18.89-
corpora cavernosa N48.29
noninfective N48.89
cutaneous, spreading I96
decubital — *see* Ulcer, pressure, by site
diabetic (any site) — *see* Diabetes, gangrene
epidemic — *see* Poisoning, food, noxious, plant
epididymis (infectional) N45.1
erysipelas — *see* Erysipelas
emphysematous — *see* Gangrene, gas
extremity (lower) (upper) I96
Fournier's N49.3
female N76.89
fusospirochetal A69.0
gallbladder — *see* Cholecystitis, acute
gas (bacillus) A48.0
following
abortion — *see* Abortion by type complicated
by infection
ectopic or molar pregnancy O08.0
glossitis K14.0
hernia — *see* Hernia, by site, with gangrene
intestine, intestinal (hemorrhagic) (massive) K55.0
with
mesenteric embolism K55.0
obstruction — *see* Obstruction, intestine
laryngitis J04.0
limb (lower) (upper) I96
lung J85.0
spirochetal A69.8
lymphangitis I89.1
Meleney's (synergistic) — *see* Ulcer, skin
mesentery K55.0
with
embolism K55.0
intestinal obstruction — *see* Obstruction,
intestine
mouth A69.0
ovary — *see* Oophoritis
pancreas K85.9
penis N48.29
noninfective N48.89
perineum I96
pharynx (*see also* Pharyngitis)
Vincent's A69.1
presenile I73.1
progressive synergistic — *see* Ulcer, skin
pulmonary J85.0
pulpal (dental) K04.1
quinsy J36
Raynaud's (symmetric gangrene) I73.01
retropharyngeal J39.2
scrotum N49.3
noninfective N50.8
senile (atherosclerotic) — *see* Arteriosclerosis,
extremities, with, gangrene
spermatic cord N49.1
noninfective N50.8
spine I96
spirochetal NEC A69.8
spreading cutaneous I96
stomatitis A69.0
symmetrical I73.01
testis (infectional) N45.2
noninfective N44.8
throat (*see also* Pharyngitis)
diphtheritic A36.0
Vincent's A69.1
thyroid (gland) E07.89
tooth (pulp) K04.1
tuberculous NEC — *see* Tuberculosis
tunica vaginalis N49.1
noninfective N50.8
umbilicus I96
uterus — *see* Endometritis
uvulitis K12.2

Gangrene, gangrenous — *continued*
  vas deferens N49.1
    noninfective N50.8
  vulva N76.89
Ganister disease J62.8
Ganser's syndrome (hysterical) F44.89
Gardner-Diamond syndrome (autoerythrocyte
    sensitization) D69.2
Gargoylism E76.01
Garré's disease, osteitis (sclerosing), **osteomyelitis**
    — *see* Osteomyelitis, specified type NEC
Garrod's pad, knuckle M72.1
Gartner's duct
  cyst Q52.4
  persistent Q50.6
Gas R14.3
  asphyxiation, inhalation, poisoning, suffocation NEC
    — *see* Table of Drugs and Chemicals
  excessive R14.0
  gangrene A48.0
    following
      abortion — *see* Abortion by type complicated
        by infection
      ectopic or molar pregnancy O08.0
  on stomach R14.0
  pains R14.1
Gastralgia (*see also* Pain, abdominal)
Gastrectasis K31.0
  psychogenic F45.8
Gastric — *see* condition
Gastrinoma
  malignant
    pancreas C25.4
    specified site NEC — *see* Neoplasm, malignant,
      by site
    unspecified site C25.4
  specified site — *see* Neoplasm, uncertain behavior
  unspecified site D37.9
Gastritis (simple) K29.70
  with bleeding K29.71
  acute (erosive) K29.00
    with bleeding K29.01
  alcoholic K29.20
    with bleeding K29.21
  allergic K29.60
    with bleeding K29.61
  atrophic (chronic) K29.40
    with bleeding K29.41
  chronic (antral) (fundal) K29.50
    with bleeding K29.51
    atrophic K29.40
      with bleeding K29.41
    superficial K29.30
      with bleeding K29.31
  dietary counseling and surveillance Z71.3
  due to diet deficiency E63.9
  eosinophilic K52.81
  giant hypertrophic K29.60
    with bleeding K29.61
  granulomatous K29.60
    with bleeding K29.61
  hypertrophic (mucosa) K29.60
    with bleeding K29.61
  nervous F54
  spastic K29.60
    with bleeding K29.61
  specified NEC K29.60
    with bleeding K29.61
  superficial chronic K29.30
    with bleeding K29.31
  tuberculous A18.83
  viral NEC A08.4
Gastrocarcinoma — *see* Neoplasm, malignant,
    stomach
Gastrocolic — *see* condition
Gastrodisciasis, gastrodiscoidiasis B66.8
Gastroduodenitis K29.90
  with bleeding K29.91
  virus, viral A08.4
    specified type NEC A08.39
Gastrodynia — *see* Pain, abdominal

Gastroenteritis (acute) (chronic) (noninfectious) (*see
    also* Enteritis) K52.9
  allergic K52.2
  dietetic K52.2
  due to
    Cryptosporidium A07.2
    food poisoning — *see* Intoxication, foodborne
    radiation K52.0
  eosinophilic K52.81
  epidemic (infectious) A09
  food hypersensitivity K52.2
  infectious — *see* Enteritis, infectious
  influenzal — *see* Influenza, with gastroenteritis
  noninfectious K52.9
    specified NEC K52.89
  rotaviral A08.0
  Salmonella A02.0
  toxic K52.1
  viral NEC A08.4
    acute infectious A08.39
      type Norwalk A08.11
    infantile (acute) A08.39
    Norwalk agent A08.11
    rotaviral A08.0
    severe of infants A08.39
    specified type NEC A08.39
Gastroenteropathy (*see also* Gastroenteritis) K52.9
  acute, due to Norwalk agent A08.11
  acute, due to Norovirus A08.11
  infectious A09
Gastroenteroptosis K63.4
**Gastroesophageal laceration hemorrhage
    syndrome** K22.6
Gastrointestinal — *see* condition
Gastrojejunal — *see* condition
Gastrojejunitis (*see also* Enteritis) K52.9
Gastrojejunocolic — *see* condition
Gastroliths K31.89
Gastromalacia K31.89
Gastroparalysis K31.89
  diabetic — *see* Diabetes, gastroparalysis
Gastroparesis K31.89
  diabetic — *see* Diabetes, by type, with gastroparesis
Gastropathy K31.9
  congestive portal K31.89
  erythematous K29.70
  exudative K90.89
  portal hypertensive K31.89
Gastroptosis K31.89
Gastrorrhagia K92.2
  psychogenic F45.8
Gastroschisis (congenital) Q79.3
Gastrospasm (neurogenic) (reflex) K31.89
  neurotic F45.8
  psychogenic F45.8
Gastrostaxis — *see* Gastritis, with bleeding
Gastrostenosis K31.89
Gastrostomy
  attention to Z43.1
  status Z93.1
Gastrosuccorrhea (continuous) (intermittent) K31.89
  neurotic F45.8
  psychogenic F45.8
Gatophobia F40.218
Gaucher's disease or splenomegaly (adult) infantile)
    E75.22
Gee (-Herter)(-Thaysen) **disease** (nontropical sprue)
    K90.0
Gélineau's syndrome G47.419
  with cataplexy G47.411
Gemination, tooth, teeth K00.2
Gemistocytoma
  specified site — *see* Neoplasm, malignant, by site
  unspecified site C71.9
General, generalized — *see* condition
Genetic
  carrier (status)
    cystic fibrosis Z14.1
    hemophilia A (asymptomatic) Z14.01
      symptomatic Z14.02
    specified NEC Z14.8

Genetic—*continued*
  susceptibility to disease NEC Z15.89
    malignant neoplasm Z15.09
      breast Z15.01
      endometrium Z15.04
      ovary Z15.02
      prostate Z15.03
      specified NEC Z15.09
    multiple endocrine neoplasia Z15.81
Genital — *see* condition
Genito-anorectal syndrome A55
Genitourinary system — *see* condition
Genu
  congenital Q74.1
  extrorsum (acquired) (*see also* Deformity, varus,
      knee)
    congenital Q74.1
    sequelae (late effect) of rickets E64.3
  introrsum (acquired) (*see also* Deformity, valgus,
      knee)
    congenital Q74.1
    sequelae (late effect) of rickets E64.3
  rachitic (old) E64.3
  recurvatum (acquired) (*see also* Deformity, limb,
      specified type NEC, lower leg)
    congenital Q68.2
    sequelae (late effect) of rickets E64.3
  valgum (acquired) (knock-knee) M21.06-
    congenital Q74.1
    sequelae (late effect) of rickets E64.3
  varum (acquired) (bowleg) M21.16-
    congenital Q74.1
    sequelae (late effect) of rickets E64.3
Geographic tongue K14.1
Geophagia — *see* Pica
Geotrichosis B48.3
  stomatitis B48.3
Gephyrophobia F40.242
Gerbode defect Q21.0
GERD (gastroesophageal reflux disease) K21.9
Gerhardt's
  disease (erythromelalgia) I73.81
  syndrome (vocal cord paralysis) J38.00
    bilateral J38.02
    unilateral J38.01
German measles (*see also* Rubella)
  exposure to Z20.4
Germinoblastoma (diffuse) C85.9-
  follicular C82.9-
Germinoma — *see* Neoplasm, malignant, by site
Gerontoxon — *see* Degeneration, cornea, senile
Gerstmann-Sträussler-Scheinker syndrome (GSS)
    A81.82
Gerstmann's syndrome (developmental) F81.2
Gestation (period) (*see also* Pregnancy)
  ectopic — *see* Pregnancy
  multiple O30.9-
    greater than quadruplets — *see* Pregnancy,
        multiple (gestation), specified NEC
    specified NEC — *see* Pregnancy, multiple
        (gestation), specified NEC
Gestational
  mammary abscess O91.11-
  purulent mastitis O91.11-
  subareolar abscess O91.11-
Ghon tubercle, primary infection A15.7
Ghost
  teeth K00.4
  vessels (cornea) H16.41-
Ghoul hand A66.3
Gianotti-Crosti disease L44.4
Giant
  cell
    epulis K06.8
    peripheral granuloma K06.8
  esophagus, congenital Q39.5
  kidney, congenital Q63.3
  oesophagus, congenital Q39.5
  urticaria T78.3
    hereditary D84.1
Giardiasis A07.1
Gibert's disease or pityriasis L42

Giddiness R42
　hysterical F44.89
　psychogenic F45.8
Gierke's disease (glycogenosis I) E74.01
Gigantism (cerebral) (hypophyseal) (pituitary) E22.0
　constitutional E34.4
Gilbert's disease or syndrome E80.4
Gilchrist's disease B40.9
Gilford-Hutchinson disease E34.8
Gilles de la Tourette's disease or syndrome
　(motor-verbal tic) F95.2
Gingivitis K05.10
　acute (catarrhal) K05.00
　　necrotizing A69.1
　　plaque induced K05.00
　　nonplaque induced K05.01
　chronic (desquamative) (hyperplastic) (simple
　　marginal) (ulcerative) K05.10
　　plaque induced K05.10
　　nonplaque induced K05.11
　expulsiva — *see* Periodontitis
　necrotizing ulcerative (acute) A69.1
　pellagrous E52
　　acute necrotizing A69.1
　Vincent's A69.1
Gingivoglossitis K14.0
Gingivopericementitis — *see* Periodontitis
Gingivosis — *see* Gingivitis, chronic
Gingivostomatitis B00.2
　herpesviral B00.2
　necrotizing ulcerative (acute) A69.1
Gland, glandular — *see* condition
Glanders A24.0
Glanzmann (-Naegeli) **disease or thrombasthenia**
　D69.1
Glass-blower's disease (cataract) — *see* Cataract,
　specified NEC
Glaucoma H40.9
　with
　　increased episcleral venous pressure H40.81-
　　pseudoexfoliation of lens — *see* Glaucoma, open
　　　angle, primary, capsular
　absolute H44.51-
　angle-closure (primary) H40.20
　　acute H40.21-
　　chronic H40.22-
　　intermittent H40.23-
　　residual stage H40.24-
　borderline H40.0
　capsular (with pseudoexfoliation of lens) — *see*
　　Glaucoma, open angle, primary, capsular
　childhood Q15.0
　closed angle — *see* Glaucoma, angle-closure
　congenital Q15.0
　corticosteroid-induced — *see* Glaucoma, secondary,
　　drugs
　hypersecretion H40.82-
　in (due to)
　　amyloidosis E85.4 [H42]
　　aniridia Q13.1 [H42]
　　concussion of globe — *see* Glaucoma, secondary,
　　　trauma
　　dislocation of lens — *see* Glaucoma, secondary
　　disorder of lens NEC — *see* Glaucoma, secondary
　　drugs — *see* Glaucoma, secondary, drugs
　　endocrine disease NOS E34.9 [H42]
　　eye
　　　inflammation — *see* Glaucoma, secondary,
　　　　inflammation
　　　trauma — *see* Glaucoma, secondary, trauma
　　hypermature cataract — *see* Glaucoma,
　　　secondary
　　iridocyclitis — *see* Glaucoma, secondary,
　　　inflammation
　　lens disorder — *see* Glaucoma, secondary,
　　Lowe's syndrome E72.03 [H42]
　　metabolic disease NOS E88.9 [H42]
　　ocular disorders NEC — *see* Glaucoma, secondary
　　onchocerciasis B73.02
　　pupillary block — *see* Glaucoma, secondary
　　retinal vein occlusion — *see* Glaucoma,
　　　secondary
　　Rieger's anomaly Q13.81 [H42]

Glaucoma — *continued*
　in (due to)—*continued*
　　rubeosis of iris — *see* Glaucoma, secondary
　　tumor of globe — *see* Glaucoma, secondary
　infantile Q15.0
　low tension — *see* Glaucoma, open angle,
　　low-tension
　malignant H40.83-
　narrow angle — *see* Glaucoma, angle-closure
　newborn Q15.0
　noncongestive (chronic) — *see* Glaucoma, open
　　angle
　nonobstructive — *see* Glaucoma, open angle
　obstructive (*see also* Glaucoma, angle-closure)
　　due to lens changes — *see* Glaucoma, secondary
　open angle H40.10
　　primary H40.11
　　　capsular (with pseudoexfoliation of lens)
　　　　H40.14-
　　　low-tension H40.12-
　　　pigmentary H40.13-
　　　residual stage H40.15-
　phacolytic — *see* Glaucoma, secondary
　pigmentary — *see* Glaucoma, open angle,
　　pigmentary
　postinfectious — *see* Glaucoma, secondary,
　　inflammation
　secondary (to) H40.5-
　　drugs H40.6-
　　inflammation H40.4-
　　trauma H40.3-
　simple (chronic) — *see* Glaucoma, open angle
　simplex — *see* Glaucoma, open angle
　specified type NEC H40.89
　suspect H40.0
　syphilitic A52.71
　traumatic (*see also* Glaucoma, secondary, trauma)
　　newborn (birth injury) P15.3
　tuberculous A18.59
Glaucomatous flecks (subcapsular) — *see* Cataract,
　complicated
Glazed tongue K14.4
Gleet (gonococcal) A54.01
Glénard's disease K63.4
Glioblastoma (multiforme)
　with sarcomatous component
　　specified site — *see* Neoplasm, malignant, by site
　　unspecified site C71.9
　giant cell
　　specified site — *see* Neoplasm, malignant, by site
　　unspecified site C71.9
　specified site — *see* Neoplasm, malignant, by site
　unspecified site C71.9
Glioma (malignant)
　astrocytic
　　specified site — *see* Neoplasm, malignant, by site
　　unspecified site C71.9
　mixed
　　specified site — *see* Neoplasm, malignant, by site
　　unspecified site C71.9
　nose Q30.8
　specified site NEC — *see* Neoplasm, malignant, by
　　site
　subependymal D43.2
　　specified site — *see* Neoplasm, uncertain
　　　behavior, by site
　　unspecified site D43.2
　unspecified site C71.9
Gliomatosis cerebri C71.0
Glioneuroma — *see* Neoplasm, uncertain behavior, by
　site
Gliosarcoma
　specified site — *see* Neoplasm, malignant, by site
　unspecified site C71.9
Gliosis (cerebral) G93.89
　spinal G95.89
Glisson's disease — *see* Rickets
Globinuria R82.3
Globus (hystericus) F45.8
Glomangioma D18.00
　intra-abdominal D18.03
　intracranial D18.02
　skin D18.01

Glomangioma—*continued*
　specified site NEC D18.09
Glomangiomyoma D18.00
　intra-abdominal D18.03
　intracranial D18.02
　skin D18.01
　specified site NEC D18.09
Glomangiosarcoma — *see* Neoplasm, connective
　tissue, malignant
Glomerular
　disease in syphilis A52.75
　nephritis — *see* Glomerulonephritis
Glomerulitis — *see* Glomerulonephritis
Glomerulonephritis (*see also* Nephritis) N05.9
　with
　　edema — *see* Nephrosis
　　minimal change N05.0
　　minor glomerular abnormality N05.0
　acute N00.9
　chronic N03.9
　crescentic (diffuse) NEC (*see also* N00–N07 with
　　fourth character .7) N05.7
　dense deposit (*see also* N00–N07 with fourth
　　character .6) N05.6
　diffuse
　　crescentic (*see also* N00–N07 with fourth
　　　character .7) N05.7
　　endocapillary proliferative (*see also* N00–N07 with
　　　fourth character .4) N05.4
　　membranous (*see also* N00–N07 with fourth
　　　character .2) N05.2
　　mesangial proliferative (*see also* N00–N07 with
　　　fourth character .3) N05.3
　　mesangiocapillary (*see also* N00–N07 with fourth
　　　character .5) N05.5
　　sclerosing N05.8
　　　endocapillary proliferative (diffuse)
　　　　NEC (*see also* N00–N07 with
　　　　fourth character .4) N05.4
　extracapillary NEC (*see also* N00–N07 with fourth
　　character .7) N05.7
　focal (and segmental) (*see also* N00–N07 with fourth
　　character .1) N05.1
　hypocomplementemic — *see* Glomerulonephritis,
　　membranoproliferative
　IgA — *see* Nephropathy, IgA
　immune complex (circulating) NEC N05.8
　in (due to)
　　amyloidosis E85.4 [N08]
　　bilharziasis B65.9 [N08]
　　cryoglobulinemia D89.1 [N08]
　　defibrination syndrome D65 [N08]
　　diabetes mellitus — *see* Diabetes,
　　　glomerulosclerosis
　　disseminated intravascular coagulation D65
　　　[N08]
　　Fabry(-Anderson) disease E75.21 [N08]
　　Goodpasture's syndrome M31.0
　　hemolytic-uremic syndrome D59.3
　　Henoch(-Schönlein) purpura D69.0 [N08]
　　lecithin cholesterol acyltransferase deficiency
　　　E78.6 [N08]
　　microscopic polyangiitis M31.7 [N08]
　　multiple myeloma C90.0- [N08]
　　Plasmodium malariae B52.0
　　schistosomiasis B65.9 [N08]
　　sepsis A41.9 [N08]
　　　streptococcal A40.- [N08]
　　sickle-cell disorders D57.- [N08]
　　strongyloidiasis B78.9 [N08]
　　subacute bacterial endocarditis I33.0 [N08]
　　syphilis (late) congenital A50.59 [N08]
　　systemic lupus erythematosus M32.14
　　thrombotic thrombocytopenic purpura M31.1
　　　[N08]
　　typhoid fever A01.09
　　Waldenström macroglobulinemia C88.0 [N08]
　　Wegener's granulomatosis M31.31
　latent or quiescent N03.9
　lobular, lobulonodular — *see* Glomerulonephritis,
　　membranoproliferative

Glomerulonephritis — *continued*
  membranoproliferative (diffuse)(type 1 or 3)(*see also* N00-N07 with fourth character .5) N05.5
    dense deposit (type 2) NEC (*see also* N00-N07 with fourth character .6) N05.6
  membranous (diffuse) NEC (*see also* N00-N07 with fourth character .2) N05.2
  mesangial
    IgA/IgG — *see* Nephropathy, IgA
    proliferative (diffuse) NEC (*see also* N00-N07 with fourth character .3) N05.3
  mesangiocapillary (diffuse) NEC (*see also* N00-N07 with fourth character .5) N05.5
  necrotic, necrotizing NEC (*see also* N00N07 with fourth character .8) N05.8
  nodular — *see* Glomerulonephritis, membranoproliferative
  poststreptococcal NEC N05.9
    acute N00.9
    chronic N03.9
    rapidly progressive N01.9
  proliferative NEC (*see also* N00-N07 with fourth character .8) N05.8
    diffuse (lupus) M32.14
  rapidly progressive N01.9
  sclerosing, diffuse N05.8
  specified pathology NEC (*see also* N00N07 with fourth character .8) N05.8
  subacute N01.9
Glomerulopathy — *see* Glomerulonephritis
Glomerulosclerosis (*see also* Sclerosis, renal)
  intercapillary (nodular) (with diabetes) — *see* Diabetes, glomerulosclerosis
  intracapillary — *see* Diabetes, glomerulosclerosis
Glossagra K14.6
Glossalgia K14.6
Glossitis (chronic superficial) (gangrenous) (Moeller's) K14.0
  areata exfoliativa K14.1
  atrophic K14.4
  benign migratory K14.1
  cortical superficial, sclerotic K14.0
  Hunter's D51.0
  interstitial, sclerous K14.0
  median rhomboid K14.2
  pellagrous E52
  superficial, chronic K14.0
Glossocele K14.8
Glossodynia K14.6
  exfoliativa K14.0
Glossoncus K14.8
Glossopathy K14.9
Glossophytia K14.3
Glossoplegia K14.8
Glossoptosis K14.8
Glossopyrosis K14.6
Glossotrichia K14.3
Glossy skin L90.8
Glottis — *see* condition
Glottitis (*see also* Laryngitis) J04.0
Glucagonoma
  pancreas
    benign D13.7
    malignant C25.4
    uncertain behavior D37.8
  specified site NEC
    benign — *see* Neoplasm, benign, by site
    malignant — *see* Neoplasm, malignant, by site
    uncertain behavior — *see* Neoplasm, uncertain behavior, by site
  unspecified site
    benign D13.7
    malignant C25.4
    uncertain behavior D37.9
Glucoglycinuria E72.51
Glucose-galactose malabsorption E74.39
Glue
  ear — *see* Otitis, media, nonsuppurative, chronic, mucoid
  sniffing (airplane) — *see* Abuse, drug, inhalant
    dependence — *see* Dependence, drug, inhalant
Glutaric aciduria E72.3
Glycinemia E72.51

Glycinuria (renal) (with ketosis) E72.09
Glycogen
  infiltration — *see* Disease, glycogen storage
  storage disease — *see* Disease, glycogen storage
Glycogenosis (diffuse) (generalized) (*see also* Disease, glycogen storage)
  cardiac E74.02 [I43]
  diabetic, secondary — *see* Diabetes, glycogenosis, secondary
Glycopenia E16.2
Glycosuria R81
  renal E74.8
Gnathostoma spinigerum (infection) (infestation), **gnathostomiasis** (wandering swelling) B83.1
Goiter (plunging) (substernal) E04.9
  with
    hyperthyroidism (recurrent) — *see* Hyperthyroidism, with, goiter
    thyrotoxicosis — *see* Hyperthyroidism, with, goiter
  adenomatous — *see* Goiter, nodular
  cancerous C73
  congenital (nontoxic) E03.0
    diffuse E03.0
    parenchymatous E03.0
    transitory, with normal functioning P72.0
  cystic E04.2
    due to iodine-deficiency E01.1
  due to
    enzyme defect in synthesis of thyroid hormone E07.1
    iodine-deficiency (endemic) E01.2
  dyshormonogenetic (familial) E07.1
  endemic (iodine-deficiency) E01.2
    diffuse E01.0
    multinodular E01.1
  exophthalmic — *see* Hyperthyroidism, with, goiter
  iodine-deficiency (endemic) E01.2
    diffuse E01.0
    multinodular E01.1
    nodular E01.1
  lingual Q89.2
  lymphadenoid E06.3
  malignant C73
  multinodular (cystic) (nontoxic) E04.2
    toxic or with hyperthyroidism E05.20
      with thyroid storm E05.21
  neonatal NEC P72.0
  nodular (nontoxic) (due to) E04.9
    with
      hyperthyroidism E05.20
        with thyroid storm E05.21
      thyrotoxicosis E05.20
        with thyroid storm E05.21
    endemic E01.1
    iodine-deficiency E01.1
    sporadic E04.9
    toxic E05.20
      with thyroid storm E05.21
  nontoxic E04.9
    diffuse (colloid) E04.0
    multinodular E04.2
    simple E04.0
    specified NEC E04.8
    uninodular E04.1
  simple E04.0
  toxic — *see* Hyperthyroidism, with, goiter
  uninodular (nontoxic) E04.1
    toxic or with hyperthyroidism E05.10
      with thyroid storm E05.11
Goiter-deafness syndrome E07.1
Goldberg syndrome Q89.8
Goldberg-Maxwell syndrome E34.51
Goldblatt's hypertension or kidney I70.1
Goldenhar (-Gorlin) **syndrome** Q87.0
Goldflam-Erb disease or syndrome G70.00
  with exacerbation (acute) G70.01
  in crisis G70.01
Goldscheider's disease Q81.8
Goldstein's disease (familial hemorrhagic telangiectasia) I78.0
Golfer's elbow — *see* Epicondylitis, medial

Gonadoblastoma
  specified site — *see* Neoplasm, uncertain behavior, by site
  unspecified site
    female D39.10
    male D40.10
Gonecystitis — *see* Vesiculitis
Gongylonemiasis B83.8
Goniosynechiae — *see* Adhesions, iris, goniosynechiae
Gonococcemia A54.86
Gonococcus, gonococcal (disease) (infection) (*see also* condition) A54.9
  anus A54.6
  bursa, bursitis A54.49
  conjunctiva, conjunctivitis (neonatorum) A54.31
  endocardium A54.83
  eye A54.30
    conjunctivitis A54.31
    iridocyclitis A54.32
    keratitis A54.33
    newborn A54.31
    other specified A54.39
  fallopian tubes (acute) (chronic) A54.24
  genitourinary (organ) (system) (tract) (acute)
    lower A54.00
      with abscess (accessory gland) (periurethral) A54.1
    upper (*see also* condition) A54.29
  heart A54.83
  iridocyclitis A54.32
  joint A54.42
  lymphatic (gland) (node) A54.89
  meninges, meningitis A54.81
  musculoskeletal A54.40
    arthritis A54.42
    osteomyelitis A54.43
    other specified A54.49
    spondylopathy A54.41
  pelviperitonitis A54.24
  pelvis (acute) (chronic) A54.24
  pharynx A54.5
  proctitis A54.6
  pyosalpinx (acute) (chronic) A54.24
  rectum A54.6
  skin A54.89
  specified site NEC A54.89
  tendon sheath A54.49
  throat A54.5
  urethra (acute) (chronic) A54.01
    with abscess (accessory gland) (periurethral) A54.1
  vulva (acute) (chronic) A54.02
Gonocytoma
  specified site — *see* Neoplasm, uncertain behavior, by site
  unspecified site
    female D39.10
    male D40.10
Gonorrhea (acute) (chronic) A54.9
  Bartholin's gland (acute) (chronic) (purulent) A54.02
    with abscess (accessory gland) (periurethral) A54.1
  bladder A54.01
  cervix A54.03
  conjunctiva, conjunctivitis (neonatorum) A54.31
  contact Z20.2
  Cowper's gland (with abscess) A54.1
  exposure to Z20.2
  fallopian tube (acute) (chronic) A54.24
  kidney (acute) (chronic) A54.21
  lower genitourinary tract A54.00
    with abscess (accessory gland) (periurethral) A54.1
  ovary (acute) (chronic) A54.24
  pelvis (acute) (chronic) A54.24
    female pelvic inflammatory disease A54.24
  penis A54.09
  prostate (acute) (chronic) A54.22
  seminal vesicle (acute) (chronic) A54.23
  specified site not listed (*see also* Gonococcus) A54.89
  spermatic cord (acute) (chronic) A54.23

Gonorrhea —*continued*
  urethra A54.01
    with abscess (accessory gland) (periurethral) A54.1
  vagina A54.02
  vas deferens (acute) (chronic) A54.23
  vulva A54.02
Goodall's disease A08.19
Goodpasture's syndrome M31.0
Gopalan's syndrome (burning feet) E53.0
Gorlin-Chaudry-Moss syndrome Q87.0
Gottron's papules L94.4
Gougerot's syndrome (trisymptomatic) L81.7
Gougerot-Blum syndrome (pigmented purpuric lichenoid dermatitis) L81.7
Gougerot-Carteaud disease or syndrome (confluent reticulate papillomatosis) L83
Gouley's syndrome (constrictive pericarditis) I31.1
Goundou A66.6
Gout, gouty (acute) (attack) (flare) (*see also* Gout, chronic) M10.9
  drug-induced M10.20
    ankle M10.27-
    elbow M10.22-
    foot joint M10.27-
    hand joint M10.24-
    hip M10.25-
    knee M10.26-
    multiple site M10.29
    shoulder M10.21-
    specified joint NEC M10.28
    wrist M10.23-
  idiopathic M10.00
    ankle M10.07-
    elbow M10.02-
    foot joint M10.07-
    hand joint M10.04-
    hip M10.05-
    knee M10.06-
    multiple site M10.09
    shoulder M10.01-
    specified joint NEC M10.08
    wrist M10.03-
  in (due to) renal impairment M10.30
    ankle M10.37-
    elbow M10.32-
    foot joint M10.37-
    hand joint M10.34-
    hip M10.35-
    knee M10.36-
    multiple site M10.39
    shoulder M10.31-
    specified joint NEC M10.38
    wrist M10.33-
  lead-induced M10.10
    ankle M10.17-
    elbow M10.12-
    foot joint M10.17-
    hand joint M10.14-
    hip M10.15-
    knee M10.16-
    multiple site M10.19
    shoulder M10.11-
    specified joint NEC M10.18
    wrist M10.13-
  primary — *see* Gout, idiopathic
  saturnine — *see* Gout, lead-induced
  secondary NEC M10.40
    ankle M10.47-
    elbow M10.42-
    foot joint M10.47-
    hand joint M10.44-
    hip M10.45-
    knee M10.46-
    multiple site M10.49
    shoulder M10.41-
    specified joint NEC M10.48
    wrist M10.43-
  syphilitic (*see also* subcategory M14.8-) A52.77
  tophi — *see* Gout by type
Gout, chronic (*see also* Gout) (acute) M1a.9
  drug-induced M1a.20
    ankle M1a.27-

Gout, chronic — *continued*
  drug-induced—*continued*
    elbow M1a.22-
    foot joint M1a.27-
    hand joint M1a.24-
    hip M1a.25-
    knee M1a.26-
    multiple site M1a.29-
    shoulder M1a.21-
    specified joint NEC M1a.28 -
    wrist M1a.23-
  idiopathic M1a.00
    ankle M1a.07-
    elbow M1a.02-
    foot joint M1a.07-
    hand joint M1a.04-
    hip M1a.05-
    knee M1a.06-
    multiple site M1a.09
    shoulder M1a.01-
    specified joint NEC M1a.08
    wrist M1a.03-
  in (due to) renal impairment M1a.30
    ankle M1a.37-
    elbow M1a.32-
    foot joint M1a.37-
    hand joint M1a.34-
    hip M1a.35-
    knee M1a.36-
    multiple site M1a.39
    shoulder M1a.31-
    specified joint NEC M1a.38
    wrist M1a.33
  lead-induced M1a.10
    ankle M1a.17-
    elbow M1a.12-
    foot joint M1a.17-
    hand joint M1a.14-
    hip M1a.15-
    knee M1a.16
    multiple site M1a.19
    shoulder M1a.11-
    specified joint NEC M1a.18 -
    wrist M1a.13
  primary — *see* Gout, chronic, idiopathic
  saturnine — *see* Gout, chronic, lead-induced
  secondary NEC M1a.40
    ankle M1a.47-
    elbow M1a.42-
    foot joint M1a.47-
    hand joint M1a.44-
    hip M1a.45-
    knee M1a.46-
    multiple site M1a.49
    shoulder M1a.41-
    specified joint NEC M1a.48 -
    wrist M1a.43-
  syphilitic A52.77 (*see also* subcategory) M1a.8-
  tophi — *see* Gout by type
Gower's
  muscular dystrophy G71.0
  syndrome (vasovagal attack) R55
Gradenigo's syndrome — *see* Otitis, media, suppurative, acute
Graefe's disease — *see* Strabismus, paralytic, ophthalmoplegia, progressive
Graft-versus-host disease D89.813
  acute D89.810
  acute on chronic D89.812
  chronic D89.811
Grainhandler's disease or lung J67.8
Grain mite (itch) B88.0
Grand mal — *see* Epilepsy, generalized, idiopathic
Grand multipara status only (not pregnant) Z64.1
  pregnant — *see* Pregnancy, complicated by, grand multiparity
Granite worker's lung J62.8
Granular (*see also* condition)
  inflammation, pharynx J31.2
  kidney (contracting) — *see* Sclerosis, renal
  liver K74.69

Granulation tissue (abnormal) (excessive) L92.9
  postmastoidectomy cavity — *see* Complications, postmastoidectomy, granulation
Granulocytopenia (primary) (malignant) — *see* Aganulocytosis
Granuloma L92.9
  abdomen K66.8
    from residual foreign body L92.3
    pyogenicum L98.0
  actinic L57.5
  annulare (perforating) L92.0
  apical K04.5
  aural — *see* Otitis, externa, specified NEC
  beryllium (skin) L92.3
  bone
    eosinophilic C96.6
    from residual foreign body — *see* Osteomyelitis, specified type NEC
    lung C96.6
  brain (any site) G06.0
    schistosomiasis B65.9 [G07]
  canaliculus lacrimalis — *see* Granuloma, lacrimal
  candidal (cutaneous) B37.2
  cerebral (any site) G06.0
  coccidioidal (primary) (progressive) B38.7
    lung B38.1
    meninges B38.4
  colon K63.89
  conjunctiva H11.22-
  dental K04.5
  ear, middle — *see* Cholesteatoma
  eosinophilic C96.6
    bone C96.6
    lung C96.6
    oral mucosa K13.4
    skin L92.2
  eyelid H01.8
  facial(e) L92.2
  foreign body (in soft tissue) NEC M60.20
    ankle M60.27-
    foot M60.27-
    forearm M60.23-
    hand M60.24-
    in operation wound — *see* Foreign body, accidentally left during a procedure
    lower leg M60.26-
    pelvic region M60.25-
    shoulder region M60.21-
    skin L92.3
    specified site NEC M60.28
    subcutaneous tissue L92.3
    thigh M60.25-
    upper arm M60.22-
  gangraenescens M31.2
  genito-inguinale A58
  giant cell (central) (reparative) (jaw) M27.1
    gingiva (peripheral) K06.8
  gland (lymph) I88.8
  hepatic NEC K75.3
    in (due to)
      berylliosis J63.2 [K77]
      sarcoidosis D86.89
  Hodgkin C81.9
  ileum K63.89
  infectious B99.9
    specified NEC B99.8
  inguinale (Donovan) (venereal) A58
  intestine NEC K63.89
  intracranial (any site) G06.0
  intraspinal (any part) G06.1
  iridocyclitis — *see* Iridocyclitis, chronic
  jaw (bone) (central) M27.1
    reparative giant cell M27.1
  kidney (*see also* Infection, kidney) N15.8
  lacrimal H04.81-
  larynx J38.7
  lethal midline (faciale(e)) M31.2
  liver NEC — *see* Granuloma, hepatic
  lung (infectious) (*see also* Fibrosis, lung)
    coccidioidal B38.1 [J99]
    eosinophilic C96.6
  Majocchi's B35.8
  malignant (facial(e)) M31.2

Granuloma — *continued*
  mandible (central) M27.1
  midline (lethal) M31.2
  monilial (cutaneous) B37.2
  nasal sinus — *see* Sinusitis
  operation wound T81.89
    foreign body — *see* Foreign body, accidentally
      left during a procedure
    stitch T81.89
    talc — *see* Foreign body, accidentally left during
      a procedure
  oral mucosa K13.4
  orbit, orbital H05.11-
  paracoccidioidal B41.8
  penis, venereal A58
  periapical K04.5
  peritoneum K66.8
    due to ova of helminths NOS (*see also*
      Helminthiasis) B83.9 [K67]
  postmastoidectomy cavity — *see* Complications,
    postmastoidectomy, recurrent cholesteatoma
  prostate N42.89
  pudendi (ulcerating) A58
  pulp, internal (tooth) K03.3
  pyogenic, pyogenicum (of) (skin) L98.0
    gingiva K06.8
    maxillary alveolar ridge K04.5
    oral mucosa K13.4
  rectum K62.8
  reticulohistiocytic D76.3
  rubrum nasi L74.8
  Schistosoma — *see* Schistosomiasis
  septic (skin) L98.0
  silica (skin) L92.3
  sinus (accessory) (infective) (nasal) — *see* Sinusitis
  skin L92.9
    from residual foreign body L92.3
    pyogenicum L98.0
  spine
    syphilitic (epidural) A52.19
    tuberculous A18.01
  stitch (postoperative) T81.89
  suppurative (skin) L98.0
  swimming pool A31.1
  talc (*see also* Granuloma, foreign body)
    in operation wound — *see* Foreign body,
      accidentally left during a procedure
  telangiectaticum (skin) L98.0
  tracheostomy J95.09
  trichophyticum B35.8
  tropicum A66.4
  umbilicus L92.9
  urethra N36.8
  uveitis — *see* Iridocyclitis, chronic
  vagina A58
  venereum A58
  vocal cord J38.3
Granulomatosis L92.9
  lymphoid C83.8-
  miliary (listerial) A32.89
  necrotizing, respiratory M31.30
  progressive septic D71
  specified NEC L92.8
  Wegener's M31.30
    with renal involvement M31.31

Granulomatous tissue (abnormal) (excessive) L92.9
Granulosis rubra nasi L74.8
Graphite fibrosis (of lung) J63.3
Graphospasm F48.8
  organic G25.89
Grating scapula M89.8x1
Gravel (urinary) — *see* Calculus, urinary
Graves' disease — *see* Hyperthyroidism, with, goiter
Gravis — *see* condition
Grawitz tumor C64.-
Gray syndrome (newborn) P93.0
Grayness, hair (premature) L67.1
  congenital Q84.2
Green sickness D50.8
Greenfield's disease
  meaning
    concentric sclerosis (encephalitis periaxialis
      concentrica) G37.5
    metachromatic leukodystrophy E75.25
Greenstick fracture—code as Fracture, by site
Grey syndrome (newborn) P93.0
Grief F43.21
  prolonged F43.29
  reaction (*see also* Disorder, adjustment) F43.20
Griesinger's disease B76.9
Grinder's lung or pneumoconiosis J62.8
Grinding, teeth
  psychogenic F45.8
  sleep related G47.63
Grip
  Dabney's B33.0
  devil's B33.0
Grippe, grippal (*see also* Influenza)
  Balkan A78
  summer, of Italy A93.1
Grisel's disease M43.6
Groin — *see* condition
Grooved tongue K14.5
Ground itch B76.9
Grover's disease or syndrome L11.1
Growing pains, children R29.898
Growth (fungoid) (neoplastic) (new) (*see also*
  Neoplasm)
  adenoid (vegetative) J35.8
  benign — *see* Neoplasm, benign, by site
  malignant — *see* Neoplasm, malignant, by site
  rapid, childhood Z00.2
  secondary — *see* Neoplasm, secondary, by site
Gruby's disease B35.0
Gubler-Millard paralysis or syndrome G46.3
Guerin-Stern syndrome Q74.3
Guidance, insufficient anterior (occlusal) M26.54
Guillain-Barré disease or syndrome G61.0
  sequelae G65.0
Guinea worms (infection) (infestation) B72
Guinon's disease (motor-verbal tic) F95.2
Gull's disease E03.4
Gum — *see* condition
Gumboil K04.7
  with sinus K04.6

Gumma (syphilitic) A52.79
  artery A52.09
    cerebral A52.04
  bone A52.77
    of yaws (late) A66.6
  brain A52.19
  cauda equina A52.19
  central nervous system A52.3
  ciliary body A52.71
  congenital A50.59
  eyelid A52.71
  heart A52.06
  intracranial A52.19
  iris A52.71
  kidney A52.75
  larynx A52.73
  leptomeninges A52.19
  liver A52.74
  meninges A52.19
  myocardium A52.06
  nasopharynx A52.73
  neurosyphilitic A52.3
  nose A52.73
  orbit A52.71
  palate (soft) A52.79
  penis A52.76
  pericardium A52.06
  pharynx A52.73
  pituitary A52.79
  scrofulous (tuberculous) A18.4
  skin A52.79
  specified site NEC A52.79
  spinal cord A52.19
  tongue A52.79
  tonsil A52.73
  trachea A52.73
  tuberculous A18.4
  ulcerative due to yaws A66.4
  ureter A52.75
  yaws A66.4
    bone A66.6
Gunn's syndrome Q07.8
Gunshot wound (*see also* Wound, open)
  fracture—code as Fracture, by site
  internal organs — *see* Injury, by site
Gynandrism Q56.0
Gynandroblastoma
  specified site — *see* Neoplasm, uncertain behavior,
    by site
  unspecified site
    female D39.10
    male D40.10
Gynecological examination (periodic) (routine)
  Z01.419
  with abnormal findings Z01.411
Gynecomastia N62
Gynephobia F40.291
Gyrate scalp Q82.8

H

H (Hartnup's) disease E72.02
Haas' disease or osteochondrosis (juvenile) (head of humerus) — *see* Osteochondrosis, juvenile, humerus
Habit, habituation
  bad sleep Z72.821
  chorea F95.8
  disturbance, child F98.9
  drug — *see* Dependence, drug
  irregular Z72.821
  laxative F55.2
  spasm — *see* Tic
  tic — *see* Tic
Haemophilus (H.) **influenzae, as cause of disease classified elsewhere** B96.3
Haff disease — *see* Poisoning, mercury
Hageman's factor defect, deficiency or disease D68.2
Haglund's disease or osteochondrosis (juvenile) (os tibiale externum) — *see* Osteochondrosis, juvenile, tarsus
Hailey-Hailey disease Q82.8
Hair(*see also* condition)
  plucking F63.3
    in stereotyped movement disorder F98.4
  tourniquet syndrome (*see also* Constriction, external, by site)
    finger S60.44-
    penis S30.842
    thumb S60.34-
    toe S90.44-
Hairball in stomach T18.2
Hair-pulling, pathological (compulsive) F63.3
Hairy black tongue K14.3
Half vertebra Q76.49
Halitosis R19.6
Hallerman-Streiff syndrome Q87.0
Hallervorden-Spatz disease G23.0
Hallopeau's acrodermatitis or disease L40.2
Hallucination R44.3
  auditory R44.0
  gustatory R44.2
  olfactory R44.2
  specified NEC R44.2
  tactile R44.2
  visual R44.1
Hallucinosis (chronic) F28
  alcoholic (acute) F10.951
    in
        abuse F10.151
        dependence F10.251
  drug-induced F19.951
    cannabis F12.951
    cocaine F14.951
    hallucinogen F16.151
    in
        abuse F19.151
           cannabis F12.151
           cocaine F14.151
           hallucinogen F16.151
           inhalant F18.151
           opioid F11.151
           sedative, anxiolytic or hypnotic F13.151
           stimulant NEC F15.151
        dependence F19.251
           cannabis F12.251
           cocaine F14.251
           hallucinogen F16.251
           inhalant F18.251
           opioid F11.251
           sedative, anxiolytic or hypnotic F13.251
           stimulant NEC F15.251
    inhalant F18.951
    opioid F11.951
    sedative, anxiolytic or hypnotic F13.951
Hallucinosis (chronic) F28
  stimulant NEC F15.951
  organic F06.0

Hallux
  deformity (acquired) NEC M20.5x-
  limitus M20.5x-
  malleus (acquired) NEC M20.3-
  rigidus (acquired) M20.2-
    congenital Q74.2
    sequelae (late effect) of rickets E64.3
  valgus (acquired) M20.1-
    congenital Q66.6
  varus (acquired) M20.3-
    congenital Q66.3
Halo, visual H53.19
Hamartoma, hamartoblastoma Q85.9
  epithelial (gingival), odontogenic, central or peripheral — *see* Cyst, calcifying odontogenic
Hamartosis Q85.9
Hamman-Rich syndrome J84.1
Hammer toe (acquired) NEC (*see also* Deformity, toe, hammer toe)
  congenital Q66.8
  sequelae (late effect) of rickets E64.3
Hand — *see* condition
Hand-foot syndrome L27.1
Handicap, handicapped
  educational Z55.9
    specified NEC Z55.8
Hand-Schüller-Christian disease or syndrome C96.5
Hanging (asphyxia) (strangulation) (suffocation) — *see* Asphyxia, traumatic, due to mechanical threat
Hangnail (*see also* Cellulitis, digit)
  with lymphangitis — *see* Lymphangitis, acute, digit
Hangover (alcohol) F10.129
Hanhart's syndrome Q87.0
Hanot-Chauffard(-Troisier) **syndrome** E83.19
Hanot's cirrhosis or disease K74.3
Hansen's disease — *see* Leprosy
Hantaan virus disease (Korean hemorrhagic fever) A98.5
Hantavirus disease (with renal manifestations) (Dobrava) (Puumala) (Seoul) A98.5
  with pulmonary manifestations (Andes) (Bayou) (Bermejo) (Black Creek Canal) (Choclo) (Juquitiba) (Laguna negra) (Lechiguanas) (New York) (Oran) (Sin nombre) B33.4
Happy puppet syndrome Q93.5
Harada's disease or syndrome H30.81-
Hardening
  artery — *see* Arteriosclerosis
  brain G93.89
Harelip (complete) (incomplete) — *see* Cleft, lip
Harlequin (newborn) Q80.4
Harley's disease D59.6
Harmful use (of)
  alcohol F10.10
  anxiolytics — *see* Abuse, drug, sedative
  cannabinoids — *see* Abuse, drug, cannabis
  cocaine — *see* Abuse, drug, cocaine
  drug — *see* Abuse, drug
  hallucinogens — *see* Abuse, drug, hallucinogen
  hypnotics — *see* Abuse, drug, sedative
  opioids — *see* Abuse, drug, opioid
  PCP (phencyclidine) — *see* Abuse, drug NEC
  sedatives — *see* Abuse, drug, sedative
  stimulants NEC — *see* Abuse, drug, stimulant
Harris' lines — *see* Arrest, epiphyseal
Hartnup's disease E72.02
Harvester's lung J67.0
Harvesting ovum for in vitro fertilization Z31.83
Hashimoto's disease or thyroiditis E06.3
Hashitoxicosis (transient) E06.3
Hassal-Henle bodies or warts (cornea) H18.49
Haut mal — *see* Epilepsy, generalized, idiopathic
Haverhill fever A25.1
Hay fever J30.1
Hayem-Widal syndrome D59.8
Haygarth's nodes M15.8
Haymaker's lung J67.0
Hb (abnormal)
  Bart's disease D56.8
  disease — *see* Disease, hemoglobin
  trait — *see* Trait
Head — *see* condition

Headache R51
  allergic NEC G44.89
  associated with sexual activity G44.82
  chronic daily R51
  cluster G44.009
    chronic G44.029
      intractable G44.021
      not intractable G44.029
    episodic G44.019
      intractable G44.011
      not intractable G44.019
    intractable G44.001
    not intractable G44.009
  cough (primary) G44.83
  daily chronic R51
  drug-induced NEC G44.40
    intractable G44.41
    not intractable G44.40
  exertional (primary) G44.84
  histamine G44.009
    intractable G44.001
    not intractable G44.009
  hypnic G44.81
  lumbar puncture G97.1
  medication overuse G44.40
    intractable G44.41
    not intractable G44.40
  menstrual — *see* Migraine, menstrual
  migraine (type) (*see also* Migraine) G43.909
  nasal septum R51
  neuralgiform, short lasting unilateral, with conjunctival injection and tearing (SUNCT) G44.059
    intractable G44.051
    not intractable G44.059
  new daily persistent (NDPH) G44.52
  orgasmic G44.82
  periodic syndromes in adults and children G43.c09
    intractable G43.c19
      with status migrainosus G43.c11
      without status migrainosus G43.c19
    not intractable G43.c09
      with status migrainosus G43.c01
      without status migrainosus G43.c09
  postspinal puncture G97.1
  post-traumatic G44.309
    acute G44.319
      intractable G44.311
      not intractable G44.319
    chronic G44.329
      intractable G44.321
      not intractable G44.329
    intractable G44.301
    not intractable G44.309
  pre-menstrual — *see* Migraine, menstrual
  preorgasmic G44.82
  primary
    cough G44.83
    exertional G44.84
    stabbing G44.85
    thunderclap G44.53
  rebound G44.40
    intractable G44.41
    not intractable G44.40
  short lasting unilateral neuralgiform, with conjunctival injection and tearing (SUNCT) G44.059
    intractable G44.051
    not intractable G44.059
  specified syndrome NEC G44.89
  spinal and epidural anesthesia induced T88.59
    in labor and delivery O74.5
    in pregnancy O29.4-
    postpartum, puerperal O89.4
  spinal fluid loss (from puncture) G97.1
  stabbing (primary) G44.85
  tension(-type) G44.209
    chronic G44.229
      intractable G44.221
      not intractable G44.229

Hb—*continued*
tension(-type)—*continued*
episodic G44.219
intractable G44.211
not intractable G44.219
intractable G44.2Ø1
not intractable G44.2Ø9
thunderclap (primary) G44.53
vascular NEC G44.1Ø
intractable G44.11
not intractable G44.1Ø
Healthy
infant
accompanying sick mother Z76.3
receiving care Z76.2
person accompanying sick person Z76.3
Hearing examination ZØ1.1Ø
with abnormal findings NEC ZØ1.118
following failed hearing screening ZØ1.11Ø
for hearing conservation and treatment ZØ1.12
Heart — *see* condition
Heart beat
abnormality RØØ.9
specified NEC RØØ.8
awareness RØØ.2
rapid RØØ.Ø
slow RØØ.1
Heartburn R12
psychogenic F45.8
Heat (effects) T67.9
apoplexy T67.Ø
burn (*see also* Burn) L55.9
collapse T67.1
cramps T67.2
dermatitis or eczema L59.Ø
edema T67.7
erythema—code by site under Burn, first degree
excessive T67.9
specified effect NEC T67.8
exhaustion T67.5
anhydrotic T67.3
due to
salt (and water) depletion T67.4
water depletion T67.3
with salt depletion T67.4
fatigue (transient) T67.6
fever T67.Ø
hyperpyrexia T67.Ø
prickly L74.Ø
prostration — *see* Heat, exhaustion
pyrexia T67.Ø
rash L74.Ø
specified effect NEC T67.8
stroke T67.Ø
sunburn — *see* Sunburn
syncope T67.1
Heavy-for-dates NEC (infant) (4ØØØg to 4499g) PØ8.1
exceptionally (45ØØg or more) PØ8.Ø
Hebephrenia, hebephrenic (schizophrenia) F2Ø.1
Heberden's disease or nodes (with arthropathy) M15.1
Hebra's
pityriasis L26
prurigo L28.2
Heel — *see* condition
Heerfordt's disease D86.89
Hegglin's anomaly or syndrome D72.Ø
Heilmeyer-Schoner disease D45
Heine-Medin disease A8Ø.9
Heinz body anemia, congenital D58.2
Heliophobia F4Ø.228
Heller's disease or syndrome F84.3
HELLP syndrome O14.2-
Helminthiasis (*see also* Infestation, helminth)
Ancylostoma B76.Ø
intestinal B82.Ø
mixed types (types classifiable to more than one of the titles B65.Ø-B81.3 and B81.8) B81.4
specified type NEC B81.8
mixed types (intestinal) (types classifiable to more than one of the titles B65.Ø-B81.3 and B81.8) B81.4
Necator (americanus) B76.1

Helminthiasis —*continued*
specified type NEC B83.8
Heloma L84
Hemangioblastoma — *see* Neoplasm, connective tissue, uncertain behavior
malignant — *see* Neoplasm, connective tissue, malignant
Hemangioendothelioma (*see also* Neoplasm, uncertain behavior, by site)
benign D18.ØØ
intra-abdominal D18.Ø3
intracranial D18.Ø2
skin D18.Ø1
specified site NEC D18.Ø9
bone (diffuse) — *see* Neoplasm, bone, malignant
epithelioid (*see also* Neoplasm, uncertain behavior, by site)
malignant — *see* Neoplasm, malignant, by site
malignant — *see* Neoplasm, connective tissue, malignant
Hemangiofibroma — *see* Neoplasm, benign, by site
Hemangiolipoma — *see* Lipoma
Hemangioma D18.ØØ
arteriovenous D18.ØØ
intra-abdominal D18.Ø3
intracranial D18.Ø2
skin D18.Ø1
specified site NEC D18.Ø9
capillary D18.ØØ
intra-abdominal D18.Ø3
intracranial D18.Ø2
skin D18.Ø1
specified site NEC D18.Ø9
cavernous D18.ØØ
intra-abdominal D18.Ø3
intracranial D18.Ø2
skin D18.Ø1
specified site NEC D18.Ø9
epithelioid D18.ØØ
intra-abdominal D18.Ø3
intracranial D18.Ø2
skin D18.Ø1
specified site NEC D18.Ø9
histiocytoid D18.ØØ
intra-abdominal D18.Ø3
intracranial D18.Ø2
skin D18.Ø1
specified site NEC D18.Ø9
infantile D18.ØØ
intra-abdominal D18.Ø3
intracranial D18.Ø2
skin D18.Ø1
specified site NEC D18.Ø9
intra-abdominal D18.Ø3
intracranial D18.Ø2
intramuscular D18.ØØ
intra-abdominal D18.Ø3
intracranial D18.Ø2
skin D18.Ø1
specified site NEC D18.Ø9
juvenile D18.ØØ
malignant — *see* Neoplasm, connective tissue, malignant
plexiform D18.ØØ
intra-abdominal D18.Ø3
intracranial D18.Ø2
skin D18.Ø1
specified site NEC D18.Ø9
racemose D18.ØØ
intra-abdominal D18.Ø3
intracranial D18.Ø2
skin D18.Ø1
specified site NEC D18.Ø9
sclerosing — *see* Neoplasm, skin, benign
simplex D18.ØØ
intra-abdominal D18.Ø3
intracranial D18.Ø2
skin D18.Ø1
specified site NEC D18.Ø9
skin D18.Ø1
specified site NEC D18.Ø9
venous D18.ØØ
intra-abdominal D18.Ø3

Hemangioma —*continued*
venous—*continued*
intracranial D18.Ø2
skin D18.Ø1
specified site NEC D18.Ø9
verrucous keratotic D18.ØØ
intra-abdominal D18.Ø3
intracranial D18.Ø2
skin D18.Ø1
specified site NEC D18.Ø9
Hemangiomatosis (systemic) I78.8
involving single site — *see* Hemangioma
Hemangiopericytoma (*see also* Neoplasm, connective tissue, uncertain behavior)
benign — *see* Neoplasm, connective tissue, benign
malignant — *see* Neoplasm, connective tissue, malignant
Hemangiosarcoma — *see* Neoplasm, connective tissue, malignant
Hemarthrosis (nontraumatic) M25.ØØ
ankle M25.Ø7-
elbow M25.Ø2-
foot joint M25.Ø7-
hand joint M25.Ø4-
hip M25.Ø5-
in hemophilic arthropathy — *see* Arthropathy, hemophilic
knee M25.Ø6-
shoulder M25.Ø1-
specified joint NEC M25.Ø8
traumatic — *see* Sprain, by site
wrist M25.Ø3-
Hematemesis K92.Ø
with ulcer—code by site under Ulcer, with hemorrhage K27.4
newborn, neonatal P54.Ø
due to swallowed maternal blood P78.2
Hematidrosis L74.8
Hematinuria (*see also* Hemoglobinuria)
malarial B5Ø.8
Hematobilia K83.8
Hematocele
female NEC N94.89
with ectopic pregnancy OØØ.9
ovary N83.8
male N5Ø.1
Hematochezia (*see also* Melena) K92.1
Hematochyluria (*see also* Infestation, filarial)
schistosomiasis (bilharziasis) B65.Ø
Hematocolpos (with hematometra or hematosalpinx) N89.7
Hematocornea — *see* Pigmentation, cornea, stromal
Hematogenous — *see* condition
Hematoma (traumatic) (skin surface intact) (*see also* Contusion)
with
injury of internal organs — *see* Injury, by site
open wound — *see* Wound, open
amputation stump (surgical) (late) T87.8
aorta, dissecting I71.ØØ
abdominal I71.Ø2
thoracic I71.Ø1
thoracoabdominal I71.Ø3
arterial (complicating trauma) — *see* Injury, blood vessel, by site
auricle — *see* Contusion, ear
nontraumatic — *see* Disorder, pinna, hematoma
birth injury NEC P15.8
brain (traumatic)
with
cerebral laceration or contusion (diffuse) — *see* Injury, intracranial, diffuse
focal — *see* Injury, intracranial, focal
cerebellar, traumatic SØ6.37-
newborn NEC P52.4
birth injury P1Ø.1
intracerebral, traumatic — *see* Injury, intracranial, intracerebral hemorrhage
nontraumatic — *see* Hemorrhage, intracranial
subarachnoid, arachnoid, traumatic — *see* Injury, intracranial, subarachnoid hemorrhage
subdural, traumatic — *see* Injury, intracranial, subdural hemorrhage

Hematoma —continued
  breast (nontraumatic) N64.89
  broad ligament (nontraumatic) N83.7
    traumatic S37.892
  cerebellar, traumatic S06.37-
  cerebral — see Hematoma, brain
  cerebrum S06.36-
    left S06.35-
    right S06.34-
  cesarean delivery wound O90.2
  complicating delivery (perineal) (pelvic) (vagina) (vulva) O71.7
  corpus cavernosum (nontraumatic) N48.89
  epididymis (nontraumatic) N50.1
  epidural (traumatic) — see Injury, intracranial, epidural hemorrhage
    spinal — see Injury, spinal cord, by region
  episiotomy O90.2
  face, birth injury P15.4
  genital organ NEC (nontraumatic)
    female (nonobstetric) N94.89
      traumatic S30.202
    male N50.1
      traumatic S30.201
  internal organs — see Injury, by site
  intracerebral, traumatic — see Injury, intracranial, intracerebral hemorrhage
  intraoperative — see Complications, intraoperative, hemorrhage
  labia (nontraumatic) (nonobstetric) N90.89
  liver (subcapsular) (nontraumatic) K76.8
    birth injury P15.0
  mediastinum — see Injury, intrathoracic
  mesosalpinx (nontraumatic) N83.7
    traumatic S37.529
      bilateral S37.522
      unilateral S37.521
  muscle—code by site under Contusion
  nontraumatic
    muscle M79.81
    soft tissue M79.81
  obstetrical surgical wound O90.2
  orbit, orbital (nontraumatic) (see also Hemorrhage, orbit)
    traumatic — see Contusion, orbit
  pelvis (female) (nontraumatic) (nonobstetric) N94.89
    obstetric O71.7
    traumatic — see Injury, by site
  penis (nontraumatic) N48.89
    birth injury P15.5
  perineal S30.23
    complicating delivery O71.7
  perirenal — see Injury, kidney
  pinna — see Contusion, ear
    nontraumatic — see Disorder, pinna, hematoma
  placenta O43.89-
  postoperative (postprocedural) — see Complication, postprocedural, hemorrhage
  retroperitoneal (nontraumatic) K66.1
    traumatic S36.892
  scrotum, superficial S30.22
    birth injury P15.5
  seminal vesicle (nontraumatic) N50.1
    traumatic S37.892
  spermatic cord (traumatic) S37.892
    nontraumatic N50.1
  spinal (cord) (meninges) (see also Injury, spinal cord, by region)
    newborn (birth injury) P11.5
  spleen D73.5
    intraoperative see Complications, intraoperative, hemorrhage, spleen
    postprocedural (postoperative) see Complications, postprocedural, hemorrhage, spleen
  sternocleidomastoid, birth injury P15.2
  sternomastoid, birth injury P15.2
  subarachnoid (traumatic) — see Injury, intracranial, subarachnoid hemorrhage
    newborn (nontraumatic) P52.5
      due to birth injury P10.3

Hematoma —continued
  subarachnoid (traumatic) —continued
    nontraumatic — see Hemorrhage, intracranial, subarachnoid
  subdural (traumatic) — see Injury, intracranial, subdural hemorrhage
    newborn (localized) P52.8
      birth injury P10.0
    nontraumatic — see Hemorrhage, intracranial, subdural
  superficial, newborn P54.5
  testis (nontraumatic) N50.1
    birth injury P15.5
  tunica vaginalis (nontraumatic) N50.1
  umbilical cord, complicating delivery O69.5
  uterine ligament (broad) (nontraumatic) N83.7
    traumatic S37.62
  vagina (ruptured) (nontraumatic) N89.8
    complicating delivery O71.7
  vas deferens (nontraumatic) N50.1
    traumatic S37.892
  vitreous — see Hemorrhage, vitreous
  vulva (nontraumatic) (nonobstetric) N90.89
    complicating delivery O71.7
    newborn (birth injury) P15.5
Hematometra N85.7
  with hematocolpos N89.7
Hematomyelia (central) G95.19
  newborn (birth injury) P11.5
  traumatic T14.8
Hematomyelitis G04.90
Hematoperitoneum — see Hemoperitoneum
Hematophobia F40.230
Hematopneumothorax (see Hemothorax)
Hematopoiesis, cyclic D70.4
Hematoporphyria — see Porphyria
Hematorachis, hematorrhachis G95.19
  newborn (birth injury) P11.5
Hematosalpinx N83.6
  with
    hematocolpos N89.7
    hematometra N85.7
      with hematocolpos N89.7
  infectional — see Salpingitis
Hematospermia R36.1
Hematothorax (see Hemothorax)
Hematuria R31.9
  due to sulphonamide, sulfonamide — see Table of Drugs and Chemicals, by drug
  benign (familial) (of childhood) (see also Hematuria, idiopathic)
    essential microscopic R31.1
  endemic (see also Schistosomiasis) B65.0
  gross R31.0
  idiopathic N02.9
    with glomerular lesion
      crescentic (diffuse) glomerulonephritis N02.7
      dense deposit disease N02.6
      endocapillary proliferative glomerulonephritis N02.4
      focal and segmental hyalinosis or sclerosis N02.1
      membranoproliferative (diffuse) N02.5
      membranous (diffuse) N02.2
      mesangial proliferative (diffuse) N02.3
      mesangiocapillary (diffuse) N02.5
      minor abnormality N02.0
      proliferative NEC N02.8
      specified pathology NEC N02.8
  intermittent — see Hematuria, idiopathic
  malarial B50.8
  microscopic NEC R31.2
    benign essential R31.1
  paroxysmal (see also Hematuria, idiopathic)
    nocturnal D59.5
  persistent — see Hematuria, idiopathic
  recurrent — see Hematuria, idiopathic
  tropical (see also Schistosomiasis) B65.0
  tuberculous A18.13
Hemeralopia (day blindness) H53.11
  vitamin A deficiency E50.5
Hemi-akinesia R41.4
Hemianalgesia R20.0

Hemianencephaly Q00.0
Hemianesthesia R20.0
Hemianopia, hemianopsia (heteronymous) H53.47
  homonymous H53.46-
  syphilitic A52.71
Hemiathetosis R25.8
Hemiatrophy R68.89
  cerebellar G31.9
  face, facial, progressive (Romberg) G51.8
  tongue K14.8
Hemiballism(us) G25.5
Hemicardia Q24.8
Hemicephalus, hemicephaly Q00.0
Hemichorea G25.5
Hemicolitis, left — see Colitis, left sided
Hemicrania
  congenital malformation Q00.0
  continua G44.51
  meaning migraine (see also Migraine) G43.909
  paroxysmal G44.039
    chronic G44.049
      intractable G44.041
      not intractable G44.049
    episodic G44.039
      intractable G44.031
      not intractable G44.039
    intractable G44.031
    not intractable G44.039
Hemidystrophy — see Hemiatrophy
Hemiectromelia Q73.8
Hemihypalgesia R20.8
Hemihypesthesia R20.1
Hemi-inattention R41.4
Hemimelia Q73.8
  lower limb — see Defect, reduction, lower limb, specified type NEC
  upper limb — see Defect, reduction, upper limb, specified type NEC
Hemiparalysis — see Hemiplegia
Hemiparesis — see Hemiplegia
Hemiparesthesia R20.2
Hemiparkinsonism G20
Hemiplegia G81.9-
  alternans facialis G83.89
  ascending NEC G81.90
    spinal G95.89
  congenital (cerebral) G80.8
    spastic G80.2
  embolic (current episode) I63.4-
  flaccid G81.0-
  following
    cerebrovascular disease I69.959
      cerebral infarction I69.35-
      intracerebral hemorrhage I69.15-
      nontraumatic intracranial hemorrhage NEC I69.25-
      specified disease NEC I69.85-
      stroke NOS I69.35-
      subarachnoid hemorrhage I69.05-
  hysterical F44.4
  newborn NEC P91.8
    birth injury P11.9
  spastic G81.1-
    congenital G80.2
  thrombotic (current episode) I63.3
Hemisection, spinal cord — see Injury, spinal cord, by region
Hemispasm (facial) R25.2
Hemisporosis B48.8
Hemitremor R25.1
Hemivertebra Q76.49
  failure of segmentation with scoliosis Q76.3
  fusion with scoliosis Q76.3
Hemochromatosis E83.119
  with refractory anemia D46.1
  due to repeated red blood cell transfusion E83.111
  hereditary (primary) E83.110
  primary E83.110
  specified NEC E83.118
Hemoglobin (see also condition)
  abnormal (disease) — see Disease, hemoglobin
  AS genotype D57.3
  fetal, hereditary persistence (HPFH) D56.4

Hemoglobin —continued
    low NOS D64.9
    S (Hb S), heterozygous D57.3
Hemoglobinemia D59.9
    due to blood transfusion T80.89
    paroxysmal D59.6
        nocturnal D59.5
Hemoglobinopathy (mixed) D58.2
    with thalassemia D56.9
    sickle-cell D57.1
        with thalassemia D57.40
            with crisis (vasoocclusive pain) D57.419
                with
                    acute chest syndrome D57.411
                    splenic sequestration D57.412
            without crisis D57.40
Hemoglobinuria R82.3
    with anemia, hemolytic, acquired (chronic) NEC
        D59.6
    cold (agglutinin) (paroxysmal) (with Raynaud's
        syndrome) D59.6
    due to exertion or hemolysis NEC D59.6
    intermittent D59.6
    malarial B50.8
    march D59.6
    nocturnal (paroxysmal) D59.5
    paroxysmal (cold) D59.6
        nocturnal D59.5
Hemolymphangioma D18.1
Hemolysis
    intravascular
        with
            abortion — see Abortion, by type,
                complicated by, hemorrhage
            ectopic or molar pregnancy O08.1
            hemorrhage
                antepartum — see Hemorrhage,
                    antepartum
                intrapartum (see also Hemorrhage,
                    complicating, delivery) O67.0
            postpartum O72.3
    neonatal (excessive) P58.8
Hemolytic — see condition
Hemopericardium I31.2
    following acute myocardial infarction (current
        complication) I23.0
    newborn P54.8
    traumatic — see Injury, heart, with
        hemopericardium
Hemoperitoneum K66.1
    infectional K65.9
    traumatic S36.899
        with open wound — see Wound, open, with
            penetration into peritoneal cavity
Hemophilia (classical) (familial) (hereditary) D66
    A D66
    B D67
    C D68.1
    calcipriva (see also Defect, coagulation) D68.4
    nonfamilial (see also Defect, coagulation) D68.4
    secondary D68.31
    vascular D68.0
Hemophthalmos H44.81-
Hemopneumothorax (see also Hemothorax)
    traumatic S27.2
Hemoptysis R04.2
    newborn P26.9
    tuberculous — see Tuberculosis, pulmonary
Hemorrhage, hemorrhagic (concealed) R58
    abdomen R58
    accidental antepartum — see Hemorrhage,
        antepartum
    acute idiopathic pulmonary, in infants R04.81
    adenoid J35.8
    adrenal (capsule) (gland) E27.49
        medulla E27.8
        newborn P54.4
    after delivery — see Hemorrhage, postpartum
    alveolar
        lung, newborn P26.8
        process K08.8
    alveolus K08.8
    amputation stump (surgical) T87.8

Hemorrhage, hemorrhagic —continued
    anemia (chronic) D50.0
        acute D62
    antepartum (with) O46.90
        with coagulation defect O46.00-
            afibrinogenemia O46.01-
            disseminated intravascular coagulation
                O46.02-
            hypofibrinogenemia — see Hemorrhage,
                antepartum, with coagulation defect,
                afibrinogenemia
            specified defect NEC O46.09-
        before 20 weeks gestation O20.9
            specified type NEC O20.8
            threatened abortion O20.0
        due to
            abruptio placenta (see also Abruptio
                placentae) O45.
            leiomyoma, uterus — see Hemorrhage,
                antepartum, specified cause NEC
            placenta previa O44.1-
        specified cause NEC — see subcategory O46.8x-
    anus (sphincter) K62.5
    apoplexy (stroke) — see Hemorrhage, intracranial,
        intracerebral
    arachnoid — see Hemorrhage, intracranial,
        subarachnoid
    artery R58
        brain — see Hemorrhage, intracranial,
            intracerebral
    basilar (ganglion) I61.0
    bladder N32.89
    bowel K92.2
        newborn P54.3
    brain (miliary) (nontraumatic) — see Hemorrhage,
        intracranial, intracerebral
        due to
            birth injury P10.1
            syphilis A52.05
        epidural or extradural (traumatic) — see Injury,
            intracranial, epidural hemorrhage
        newborn P52.4
            birth injury P10.1
        subarachnoid — see Hemorrhage, intracranial,
            subarachnoid
        subdural — see Hemorrhage, intracranial,
            subdural
    brainstem (nontraumatic) I61.3
        traumatic S06.38-
    breast N64.59
    bronchial tube — see Hemorrhage, lung
    bronchopulmonary — see Hemorrhage, lung
    bronchus — see Hemorrhage, lung
    bulbar I61.5
    capillary I78.8
        primary D69.8
    cecum K92.2
    cerebellar, cerebellum (nontraumatic) I61.4
        newborn P52.6
        traumatic S06.37-
    cerebral, cerebrum (see also Hemorrhage,
        intracranial, intracerebral)
        newborn (anoxic) P52.4
            birth injury P10.1
        lobe I61.1
    cerebromeningeal I61.8
    cerebrospinal — see Hemorrhage, intracranial,
        intracerebral
    cervix (uteri) (stump) NEC N88.8
    chamber, anterior (eye) — see Hyphema
    childbirth — see Hemorrhage, complicating,
        delivery
    choroid H31.30-
        expulsive H31.31-
    ciliary body — see Hyphema
    cochlea — see subcategory H83.8
    colon K92.2
    complicating
        abortion — see Abortion, by type, complicated
            by, hemorrhage
        delivery O67.9

Hemorrhage, hemorrhagic —continued
    complicating—continued
        delivery—continued
            associated with coagulation defect
                (afibrinogenemia) (DIC)
                (hyperfibrinolysis) O67.0
            specified cause NEC O67.8
            surgical procedure — see Hemorrhage,
                intraoperative
    conjunctiva H11.3-
        newborn P54.8
    cord, newborn (stump) P51.9
    corpus luteum (ruptured) cyst N83.1
    cortical (brain) I61.1
    cranial — see Hemorrhage, intracranial
    cutaneous R23.3
        due to autosensitivity, erythrocyte D69.2
        newborn P54.5
    delayed
        following ectopic or molar pregnancy O08.1
        postpartum O72.2
    diathesis (familial) D69.9
    disease D69.9
        newborn P53
        specified type NEC D69.8
    due to or associated with
        afibrinogenemia or other coagulation defect
            (conditions in categories D65-D69)
            antepartum — see Hemorrhage, antepartum,
                with coagulation defect
            intrapartum O67.0
    dental implant M27.61
    device, implant or graft (see also Complications,
        by site and type, specified NEC) T85.83
        arterial graft NEC T82.838
        breast T85.83
        catheter NEC T85.83
            dialysis (renal) T82.838
                intraperitoneal T85.83
            infusion NEC T82.838
                spinal (epidural) (subdural) T85.83
            urinary (indwelling) T83.83
        electronic (electrode) (pulse generator)
            (stimulator)
            bone T84.83
            cardiac T82.837
            nervous system (brain) (peripheral nerve)
                (spinal) T85.83
            urinary T83.83
        fixation, internal (orthopedic) NEC T84.83
        gastrointestinal (bile duct) (esophagus)
            T85.83
        genital NEC T83.83
        heart NEC T82.837
        joint prosthesis T84.83
        ocular (corneal graft) (orbital implant) NEC
            T85.83
        orthopedic NEC T84.83
            bone graft T86.838
        specified NEC T85.83
        urinary NEC T83.83
        vascular NEC T82.838
        ventricular intracranial shunt T85.83
    duodenum, duodenal K92.2
        ulcer — see Ulcer, duodenum, with hemorrhage
    dura mater — see Hemorrhage, intracranial,
        subdural
    endotracheal — see Hemorrhage, lung
    epicranial subaponeurotic (massive), birth injury
        P12.2
    epidural (traumatic) (see also Injury, intracranial,
        epidural hemorrhage)
        nontraumatic I62.1
    esophagus K22.8
        varix I85.01
            secondary I85.11
    excessive, following ectopic gestation (subsequent
        episode) O08.1
    extradural (traumatic) — see Injury, intracranial,
        epidural hemorrhage
        birth injury P10.8
        newborn (anoxic) (nontraumatic) P52.8
        nontraumatic I62.1

Hemorrhage, hemorrhagic —*continued*
- eye NEC H57.8
  - fundus — *see* Hemorrhage, retina
  - lid — *see* Disorder, eyelid, specified type NEC
- fallopian tube N83.6
- fibrinogenolysis — *see* Fibrinolysis
- fibrinolytic (acquired) — *see* Fibrinolysis
- from
  - ear (nontraumatic) — *see* Otorrhagia
  - tracheostomy stoma J95.01
- fundus, eye — *see* Hemorrhage, retina
- funis — *see* Hemorrhage, umbilicus, cord
- gastric — *see* Hemorrhage, stomach
- gastroenteric K92.2
  - newborn P54.3
- gastrointestinal (tract) K92.2
  - newborn P54.3
- genital organ, male N50.1
- genitourinary (tract) NOS R31.9
- gingiva K06.8
- globe (eye) — *see* Hemophthalmos
- graafian follicle cyst (ruptured) N83.0
- gum K06.8
- heart I51.89
- hypopharyngeal (throat) R58
- intermenstrual (regular) N92.3
  - irregular N92.1
- internal (organs) NEC R58
  - capsule I61.0
  - ear — *see* subcategory H83.8
  - newborn P54.8
- intestine K92.2
  - newborn P54.3
- intra-abdominal R58
- intra-alveolar (lung), newborn P26.8
- intracerebral (nontraumatic) — *see* Hemorrhage, intracranial, intracerebral
- intracranial (nontraumatic) I62.9
  - birth injury P10.9
  - epidural, nontraumatic I62.1
  - extradural, nontraumatic I62.1
  - newborn P52.9
    - specified NEC P52.8
  - intracerebral (nontraumatic) (in) I61.9
    - brain stem I61.3
    - cerebellum I61.4
    - newborn P52.4
      - birth injury P10.1
    - hemisphere I61.2
      - cortical (superficial) I61.1
      - subcortical (deep) I61.0
    - intraoperative
      - during a nervous system procedure G97.31
      - during other procedure G97.32
    - intraventricular I61.5
    - multiple localized I61.6
    - postprocedural
      - during a nervous system procedure G97.51
      - during other procedure G97.52
    - specified NEC I61.8
    - superficial I61.1
    - traumatic (diffuse) — *see* Injury, intracranial, diffuse
      - focal — *see* Injury, intracranial, focal
  - subarachnoid (nontraumatic) (from) I60.9
    - newborn P52.5
      - birth injury P10.3
    - intracranial (cerebral) artery I60.7
      - anterior communicating I60.2-
      - basilar I60.4
      - carotid siphon and bifurcation I60.0-
      - communicating I60.7
        - anterior I60.2-
        - posterior I60.3-
      - middle cerebral I60.1-
      - posterior communicating I60.3-
      - specified artery NEC I60.6
      - vertebral I60.5-
    - specified NEC I60.8
    - traumatic S06.6x-

Hemorrhage, hemorrhagic —*continued*
- intracranial (nontraumatic)—*continued*
  - subdural (nontraumatic) I62.00
    - acute I62.01
    - birth injury P10.0
    - chronic I62.03
    - newborn (anoxic) (hypoxic) P52.8
      - birth injury P10.0
    - spinal G95.19
    - subacute I62.02
    - traumatic — *see* Injury, intracranial, subdural hemorrhage
  - traumatic — *see* Injury, intracranial, focal brain injury
- intramedullary NEC G95.19
- intraocular — *see* Hemophthalmos
- intraoperative, intraprocedural — *see* Complication, hemorrhage (hematoma), intraoperative (intraprocedural), by site
- intrapartum — *see* Hemorrhage, complicating, delivery
- intrapelvic
  - female N94.89
  - male K66.1
- intraperitoneal K66.1
- intrapontine I61.3
- intraprocedural — *see* Complication, hemorrhage (hematoma), intraoperative (intraprocedural), by site
- intrauterine N85.7
  - complicating delivery (see also Hemorrhage, complicating, delivery) O67.9
  - postpartum — *see* Hemorrhage, postpartum
- intraventricular I61.5
  - newborn (nontraumatic) (see also Newborn, affected by, hemorrhage) P52.3
    - due to birth injury P10.2
    - grade
      - 1 P52.0
      - 2 P52.1
      - 3 P52.21
      - 4 P52.22
- intravesical N32.89
- iris (postinfectional) (postinflammatory) (toxic) — *see* Hyphema
- joint (nontraumatic) — *see* Hemarthrosis
- kidney N28.89
- knee (joint) (nontraumatic) — *see* Hemarthrosis, knee
- labyrinth — *see* subcategory H83.8
- lenticular striate artery I61.0
- ligature, vessel — *see* Hemorrhage, postoperative
- liver K76.8
- lung R04.89
  - newborn P26.9
    - massive P26.1
    - specified NEC P26.8
  - tuberculous — *see* Tuberculosis, pulmonary
- massive umbilical, newborn P51.0
- mediastinum — *see* Hemorrhage, lung
- medulla I61.3
- membrane (brain) I60.8
  - spinal cord — *see* Hemorrhage, spinal cord
- meninges, meningeal (brain) (middle) I60.8
  - spinal cord — *see* Hemorrhage, spinal cord
- mesentery K66.1
- metritis — *see* Endometritis
- mouth K13.79
- mucous membrane NEC R58
  - newborn P54.8
- muscle M62.89
- nail (subungual) L60.8
- nasal turbinate R04.0
  - newborn P54.8
- navel, newborn P51.9
- newborn P54.9
  - specified NEC P54.8
- nipple N64.59
- nose R04.0
  - newborn P54.8
- omentum K66.1
- optic nerve (sheath) H47.02-
- orbit, orbital H05.23-

Hemorrhage, hemorrhagic —*continued*
- ovary NEC N83.8
- oviduct N83.6
- pancreas K86.8
- parathyroid (gland) (spontaneous) E21.4
- parturition — *see* Hemorrhage, complicating, delivery
- penis N48.89
- pericardium, pericarditis I31.2
- peritoneum, peritoneal K66.1
- peritonsillar tissue J35.8
  - due to infection J36
- petechial R23.3
  - due to autosensitivity, erythrocyte D69.2
- pituitary (gland) E23.6
- pleura — *see* Hemorrhage, lung
- polioencephalitis, superior E51.2
- polymyositis — *see* Polymyositis
- pons, pontine I61.3
- posterior fossa (nontraumatic) I61.8
  - newborn P52.6
- postmenopausal N95.0
- postnasal R04.0
- postoperative — *see* Complications, postprocedural, hemorrhage, by site
- postpartum NEC (following delivery of placenta) O72.1
  - delayed or secondary O72.2
  - retained placenta O72.0
  - third stage O72.0
- pregnancy — *see* Hemorrhage, antepartum
- preretinal — *see* Hemorrhage, retina
- prostate N42.1
- puerperal — *see* Hemorrhage, postpartum
  - delayed or secondary O72.2
- pulmonary R04.89
  - newborn P26.9
    - massive P26.1
    - specified NEC P26.8
  - tuberculous — *see* Tuberculosis, pulmonary
- purpura (primary) D69.3
- rectum (sphincter) K62.5
  - newborn P54.2
- recurring, following initial hemorrhage at time of injury T79.2
- renal N28.89
- respiratory passage or tract R04.9
  - specified NEC R04.89
- retina, retinal (vessels) H35.6-
  - diabetic — *see* Diabetes, retinal, hemorrhage
- retroperitoneal R58
- scalp R58
- scrotum N50.1
- secondary (nontraumatic) R58
  - following initial hemorrhage at time of injury T79.2
- seminal vesicle N50.1
- skin R23.3
  - newborn P54.5
- slipped umbilical ligature P51.8
- spermatic cord N50.1
- spinal (cord) G95.19
  - newborn (birth injury) P11.5
- spleen D73.5
  - intraoperative — *see* Complications, intraoperative, hemorrhage, spleen
  - postprocedural — *see* Complications, postprocedural, hemorrhage, spleen
- stomach K92.2
  - newborn P54.3
  - ulcer — *see* Ulcer, stomach, with hemorrhage
- subarachnoid (nontraumatic) — *see* Hemorrhage, intracranial, subarachnoid
- subconjunctival (see also Hemorrhage, conjunctiva)
  - birth injury P15.3
- subcortical (brain) I61.0
- subcutaneous R23.3
- subdiaphragmatic R58
- subdural (acute) (nontraumatic) — *see* Hemorrhage, intracranial, subarachnoid
- subependymal
  - newborn P52.0

Hemorrhage, hemorrhagic —*continued*
　subependymal —*continued*
　　newborn —*continued*
　　　with intraventricular extension P52.1
　　　　and intracerebral extension P52.22
　subhyaloid — *see* Hemorrhage, retina
　subperiosteal — *see* Disorder, bone, specified type
　　NEC
　subretinal — *see* Hemorrhage, retina
　subtentorial — *see* Hemorrhage, intracranial,
　　subarachnoid
　subungual L60.8
　suprarenal (capsule) (gland) E27.49
　　newborn P54.4
　tentorium (traumatic) NEC — *see* Hemorrhage, brain
　　newborn (birth injury) P10.4
　testis N50.1
　third stage (postpartum) O72.0
　thorax — *see* Hemorrhage, lung
　throat R04.1
　thymus (gland) E32.8
　thyroid (cyst) (gland) E07.89
　tongue K14.8
　tonsil J35.8
　trachea — *see* Hemorrhage, lung
　tracheobronchial R04.89
　　newborn P26.0
　traumatic—code to specific injury
　　cerebellar — *see* Hemorrhage, brain
　　intracranial — *see* Hemorrhage, brain
　　recurring or secondary (following initial
　　　hemorrhage at time of injury) T79.2
　tuberculous NEC (*see also* Tuberculosis, pulmonary)
　　A15.0
　tunica vaginalis N50.1
　ulcer—code by site under Ulcer, with hemorrhage
　　K27.4
　umbilicus, umbilical
　　cord
　　　after birth, newborn P51.9
　　　complicating delivery O69.5
　　newborn P51.9
　　　massive P51.0
　　　slipped ligature P51.8
　　stump P51.9
　urethra (idiopathic) N36.8
　uterus, uterine (abnormal) N93.9
　　climacteric N92.4
　　complicating delivery — *see* Hemorrhage,
　　　complicating, delivery
　　dysfunctional or functional N93.8
　　intermenstrual (regular) N92.3
　　　irregular N92.1
　　postmenopausal N95.0
　　postpartum — *see* Hemorrhage, postpartum
　　preclimacteric or premenopausal N92.4
　　prepubertal N93.8
　　pubertal N92.2
　vagina (abnormal) N93.9
　　newborn P54.6
　vas deferens N50.1
　vasa previa O69.4
　ventricular I61.5
　vesical N32.89
　viscera NEC R58
　　newborn P54.8
　vitreous (humor) (intraocular) H43.1-
　vulva N90.89
Hemorrhoids I84.20
　bleeding I84.101
　external I84.22
　　with internal I84.23
　　　bleeding I84.131
　　　prolapsed I84.132
　　　strangulated I84.133
　　　thrombosed I84.03
　　　ulcerated I84.134
　　　　bleeding I84.121
　　prolapsed I84.122
　　strangulated I84.123
　　thrombosed I84.02
　　ulcerated I84.124

Hemorrhoids —*continued*
　internal I84.21
　　with external I84.23
　　　bleeding I84.131
　　　prolapsed I84.132
　　　strangulated I84.133
　　　thrombosed I84.03
　　　ulcerated I84.134
　　　　bleeding I84.111
　　prolapsed I84.112
　　strangulated I84.113
　　thrombosed I84.01
　　ulcerated I84.114
　　prolapsed I84.102
　skin tags, residual I84.6
　strangulated I84.103
　thrombosed I84.00
　ulcerated I84.104
Hemosalpinx N83.6
　with
　　hematocolpos N89.7
　　hematometra N85.7
　　　with hematocolpos N89.7
Hemosiderosis (dietary) E83.19
　pulmonary, idiopathic E83.19 [J99]
　transfusion T80.89
Hemothorax (bacterial) (nontuberculous) J94.2
　newborn P54.8
　traumatic S27.1
　　with pneumothorax S27.2
　tuberculous NEC A15.6
Henoch(-Schönlein) disease or syndrome (purpura)
　D69.0
Henpue, henpuye A66.6
Hepar lobatum (syphilitic) A52.74
Hepatalgia K76.8
Hepatitis K75.9
　acute B17.9
　　with coma K72.01
　　with hepatic failure — *see* Failure, hepatic
　　alcoholic — *see* Hepatitis, alcoholic
　　infectious B15.9
　　　with hepatic coma B15.0
　　viral B17.9
　alcoholic (acute) (chronic) K70.10
　　with ascites K70.11
　amebic — *see* Abscess, liver, amebic
　anicteric (viral) — *see* Hepatitis, viral
　antigen-associated (HAA) — *see* Hepatitis, B
　Australia-antigen (positive) — *see* Hepatitis, B
　autoimmune K75.4
　B B19.10
　　with hepatic coma B19.11
　　acute B16.9
　　　with
　　　　delta-agent (coinfection) (without hepatic
　　　　　coma) B16.1
　　　　　with hepatic coma B16.0
　　　　hepatic coma (without delta-agent
　　　　　coinfection) B16.2
　　chronic B18.1
　　　with delta-agent B18.0
　bacterial NEC K75.89
　C (viral) B19.20
　　with hepatic coma B19.21
　　acute B17.10
　　　with hepatic coma B17.11
　　chronic B18.2
　catarrhal (acute) B15.9
　　with hepatic coma B15.0
　cholangiolitic K75.89
　cholestatic K75.89
　chronic K73.9
　　active NEC K73.2
　　lobular NEC K73.1
　　persistent NEC K73.0
　　specified NEC K73.8
　cytomegaloviral B25.1
　due to ethanol (acute) (chronic) — *see* Hepatitis,
　　alcoholic
　epidemic B15.9
　　with hepatic coma B15.0
　fulminant NEC (viral) — *see* Hepatitis, viral

Hepatitis —*continued*
　giant cell P59.29
　granulomatous NEC K75.3
　herpesviral B00.81
　history of
　　B Z86.19
　　C Z86.19
　homologous serum — *see* Hepatitis, viral, type B
　in (due to)
　　mumps B26.81
　　toxoplasmosis (acquired) B58.1
　　　congenital (active) P37.1 [K77]
　infectious, infective (acute) (chronic) (subacute)
　　B15.9
　　with hepatic coma B15.0
　inoculation — *see* Hepatitis, viral, type B
　interstitial (chronic) K74.69
　lupoid NEC K73.2
　malignant NEC (with hepatic failure) K72.90
　　with coma K72.91
　neonatal (idiopathic) (toxic) P59.29
　newborn P59.29
　postimmunization — *see* Hepatitis, viral, type B
　post-transfusion — *see* Hepatitis, viral, type B
　reactive, nonspecific K75.2
　serum — *see* Hepatitis, viral, type B
　specified type NEC
　　with hepatic failure — *see* Failure, hepatic
　syphilitic (late) A52.74
　　congenital (early) A50.08 [K77]
　　　late A50.59 [K77]
　　secondary A51.45
　toxic (*see also* Disease, liver, toxic) K71.6
　tuberculous A18.83
　viral, virus B19.9
　　with hepatic coma B19.0
　　acute B17.9
　　chronic B18.9
　　　specified NEC B18.8
　　　type
　　　　B B18.1
　　　　　with delta-agent B18.0
　　　　C B18.2
　　congenital P35.3
　　coxsackie B33.8 [K77]
　　cytomegalic inclusion B25.1
　　in remission, any type—code to Hepatitis, chronic,
　　　by type
　　non-A, non-B B17.8
　　specified type NEC (with or without coma) B17.8
　　type
　　　A B15.9
　　　　with hepatic coma B15.0
　　　B B19.10
　　　　with hepatic coma B19.11
　　　　acute B16.9
　　　　　with
　　　　　　delta-agent (coinfection) (without
　　　　　　　hepatic coma) B16.1
　　　　　　　with hepatic coma B16.0
　　　　　　hepatic coma (without delta-agent
　　　　　　　coinfection) B16.2
　　　　chronic B18.1
　　　　　with delta-agent B18.0
　　　C B19.20
　　　　with hepatic coma B19.21
　　　　acute B17.10
　　　　　with hepatic coma B17.11
　　　　chronic B18.2
　　　E B17.2
　　　non-A, non-B B17.8
Hepatization lung (acute) — *see* Pneumonia, lobar
Hepatoblastoma C22.2
Hepatocarcinoma C22.0
Hepatocholangiocarcinoma C22.0
Hepatocholangioma, benign D13.4
Hepatocholangitis K75.89
Hepatolenticular degeneration E83.01
Hepatoma (malignant) C22.0
　benign D13.4
　embryonal C22.0

Hepatomegaly (*see also* Hypertrophy, liver)
  with splenomegaly R16.2
  congenital Q44.7
  in mononucleosis
    gammaherpesviral B27.09
    infectious specified NEC B27.89
Hepatoptosis K76.8
Hepatorenal syndrome following labor and delivery O90.4
Hepatosis K76.8
Hepatosplenomegaly R16.2
  hyperlipemic (Bürger-Grütz type) E78.3 [K77]
Hereditary — *see* condition
Heredodegeneration, macular — *see* Dystrophy, retina
Heredopathia atactica polyneuritiformis G60.1
Heredosyphilis — *see* Syphilis, congenital
Herlitz' syndrome Q81.1
Hermansky-Pudlak syndrome E70.331
Hermaphrodite, hermaphroditism (true) Q56.0
  46,XX with streak gonads Q99.1
  46,XX/46,XY Q99.0
  46,XY with streak gonads Q99.1
  chimera 46,XX/46,XY Q99.0
Hernia, hernial (acquired) (recurrent) K46.9
  with
    gangrene — *see* Hernia, by site, with, gangrene
    incarceration — *see* Hernia, by site, with, obstruction
    irreducible — *see* Hernia, by site, with, obstruction
    obstruction — *see* Hernia, by site, with, obstruction
    strangulation — *see* Hernia, by site, with, obstruction
  abdomen, abdominal K46.9
    with
      gangrene (and obstruction) K46.1
      obstruction K46.0
    femoral — *see* Hernia, femoral
    incisional — *see* Hernia, incisional
    inguinal — *see* Hernia, inguinal
    specified site NEC K45.8
      with
        gangrene (and obstruction) K45.1
        obstruction K45.0
    umbilical — *see* Hernia, umbilical
    wall — *see* Hernia, ventral
  appendix — *see* Hernia, abdomen
  bladder (mucosa) (sphincter)
    congenital (female) (male) Q79.51
    female — *see* Cystocele
    male N32.89
  brain, congenital — *see* Encephalocele
  cartilage, vertebra — *see* Displacement, intervertebral disc
  cerebral, congenital (*see also* Encephalocele)
    endaural Q01.8
  ciliary body (traumatic) S05.2-
  colon — *see* Hernia, abdomen
  Cooper's — *see* Hernia, abdomen, specified site NEC
  crural — *see* Hernia, femoral
  diaphragm, diaphragmatic K44.9
    with
      gangrene (and obstruction) K44.1
      obstruction K44.0
    congenital Q79.0
  direct (inguinal) — *see* Hernia, inguinal
  diverticulum, intestine — *see* Hernia, abdomen
  double (inguinal) — *see* Hernia, inguinal, bilateral
  due to adhesions (with obstruction) K56.5
  epigastric — *see* Hernia, ventral
  esophageal hiatus — *see* Hernia, hiatal
  external (inguinal) — *see* Hernia, inguinal
  fallopian tube N83.4
  fascia M62.89
  femoral K41.90
    with
      gangrene (and obstruction) K41.40
        not specified as recurrent K41.40
        recurrent K41.41
      obstruction K41.30
        not specified as recurrent K41.30

Hernia, hernial—*continued*
  femoral—*continued*
    with—*continued*
      obstruction—*continued*
        recurrent K41.31
      bilateral K41.20
        with
          gangrene (and obstruction) K41.10
            not specified as recurrent K41.10
            recurrent K41.11
          obstruction K41.00
            not specified as recurrent K41.00
            recurrent K41.01
        not specified as recurrent K41.20
        recurrent K41.21
      unilateral K41.90
        with
          gangrene (and obstruction) K41.40
            not specified as recurrent K41.40
            recurrent K41.41
          obstruction K41.30
            not specified as recurrent K41.30
            recurrent K41.31
        not specified as recurrent K41.90
        recurrent K41.91
    not specified as recurrent K41.90
    recurrent K41.91
  foramen magnum G93.5
    congenital Q01.8
  funicular (umbilical) (*see also* Hernia, umbilicus)
    spermatic (cord) — *see* Hernia, inguinal
  gastrointestinal tract — *see* Hernia, abdomen
  Hesselbach's — *see* Hernia, femoral, specified site NEC
  hiatal (esophageal) (sliding) K44.9
    with
      gangrene (and obstruction) K44.1
      obstruction K44.0
    congenital Q40.1
  incarcerated (*see also* Hernia, by site, with obstruction)
    with gangrene — *see* Hernia, by site, with gangrene
  incisional K43.91
    with
      gangrene (and obstruction) K43.11
      obstruction K43.01
  indirect (inguinal) — *see* Hernia, inguinal
  inguinal (direct) (external) (funicular) (indirect) (internal) (oblique) (scrotal) (sliding) K40.90
    with
      gangrene (and obstruction) K40.40
        not specified as recurrent K40.40
        recurrent K40.41
      obstruction K40.30
        not specified as recurrent K40.30
        recurrent K40.31
    not specified as recurrent K40.90
    recurrent K40.91
    bilateral K40.20
      with
        gangrene (and obstruction) K40.10
          not specified as recurrent K40.10
          recurrent K40.11
        obstruction K40.00
          not specified as recurrent K40.00
          recurrent K40.01
      not specified as recurrent K40.20
      recurrent K40.21
    unilateral K40.90
      with
        gangrene (and obstruction) K40.40
          not specified as recurrent K40.40
          recurrent K40.41
        obstruction K40.30
          not specified as recurrent K40.30
          recurrent K40.31
      not specified as recurrent K40.90
      recurrent K40.91
  internal (*see also* Hernia, abdomen)
  inguinal — *see* Hernia, inguinal
  interstitial — *see* Hernia, abdomen

Hernia, hernial—*continued*
  intervertebral cartilage or disc — *see* Displacement, intervertebral disc
  intestine, intestinal — *see* Hernia, by site
  intra-abdominal — *see* Hernia, abdomen
  iris (traumatic) S05.2-
  irreducible (*see also* Hernia, by site, with obstruction)
    with gangrene — *see* Hernia, by site, with gangrene
  ischiatic — *see* Hernia, abdomen, specified site NEC
  ischiorectal — *see* Hernia, abdomen, specified site NEC
  lens (traumatic) S05.2-
  linea (alba) (semilunaris) — *see* Hernia, ventral
  Littre's — *see* Hernia, abdomen
  lumbar — *see* Hernia, abdomen, specified site NEC
  lung (subcutaneous) J98.4
  mediastinum J98.5
  mesenteric (internal) — *see* Hernia, abdomen
  muscle (sheath) M62.89
  nucleus pulposus — *see* Displacement, intervertebral disc
  oblique (inguinal) — *see* Hernia, inguinal
  obstructive (*see also* Hernia, by site, with obstruction)
    with gangrene — *see* Hernia, by site, with gangrene
  obturator — *see* Hernia, abdomen, specified site NEC
  omental — *see* Hernia, abdomen
  ovary N83.4
  oviduct N83.4
  paraesophageal (*see also* Hernia, diaphragm congenital) Q40.1
  paraumbilical — *see* Hernia, umbilicus
  perineal — *see* Hernia, abdomen, specified site NEC
  Petit's — *see* Hernia, abdomen, specified site NEC
  postoperative — *see* Hernia, incisional
  pregnant uterus — *see* Abnormal, uterus in pregnancy or childbirth
  prevesical N32.89
  properitoneal — *see* Hernia, abdomen, specified site NEC
  pudendal — *see* Hernia, abdomen, specified site NEC
  rectovaginal N81.6
  retroperitoneal — *see* Hernia, abdomen, specified site NEC
  Richter's — *see* Hernia, abdomen, with obstruction
  Rieux's, Riex's — *see* Hernia, abdomen, specified site NEC
  sac condition (adhesion) (dropsy) (inflammation) (laceration) (suppuration)—code by site under Hernia
  sciatic — *see* Hernia, abdomen, specified site NEC
  scrotum, scrotal — *see* Hernia, inguinal
  sliding (inguinal) (*see also* Hernia, inguinal)
    hiatus — *see* Hernia, hiatal
  spigelian — *see* Hernia, ventral
  spinal — *see* Spina bifida
  strangulated (*see also* Hernia, by site, with obstruction)
    with gangrene — *see* Hernia, by site, with gangrene
  supra-umbilicus — *see* Hernia, ventral
  tendon — *see* Disorder, tendon, specified type NEC
  Treitz's (fossa) — *see* Hernia, abdomen, specified site NEC
  tunica vaginalis Q55.29
  umbilicus, umbilical K42.9
    with
      gangrene (and obstruction) K42.1
      obstruction K42.0
  ureter N28.89
  urethra, congenital Q64.79
  urinary meatus, congenital Q64.79
  uterus N81.4
    pregnant — *see* Abnormal, uterus in pregnancy or childbirth
  vaginal (anterior) (wall) — *see* Cystocele
  Velpeau's — *see* Hernia, femoral

Hernia, hernial—*continued*
  ventral K43.90
    with
      gangrene (and obstruction) K43.10
      obstruction K43.00
    recurrent — *see* Hernia, incisional
    incisional K43.91
      with
        gangrene (and obstruction) K43.11
        obstruction K43.01
      specified NEC K43.99
        with
          gangrene (and obstruction) K43.19
          obstruction K43.09
  vesical
    congenital (female) (male) Q79.51
    female — *see* Cystocele
    male N32.89
  vitreous (into wound) S05.2-
    into anterior chamber — *see* Prolapse, vitreous
Herniation (*see also* Hernia)
  brain (stem) G93.5
  cerebral G93.5
  mediastinum J98.5
  nucleus pulposus — *see* Displacement,
    intervertebral disc
Herpangina B08.5
Herpes, herpesvirus, herpetic B00.9
  anogenital A60.9
    perianal skin A60.1
    rectum A60.1
    urogenital tract A60.00
      cervix A60.03
      male genital organ NEC A60.02
      penis A60.01
      specified site NEC A60.09
      vagina A60.04
      vulva A60.04
  blepharitis (zoster) B02.39
    simplex B00.59
  circinatus B35.4
    bullosus L12.0
  conjunctivitis (simplex) B00.53
    zoster B02.31
  cornea B02.33
  encephalitis B00.4
    due to herpesvirus 6 B10.01
    due to herpesvirus 7 B10.09
    specified NEC B10.09
  eye (zoster) B02.30
    simplex B00.50
  eyelid (zoster) B02.39
    simplex B00.59
  facialis B00.1
  febrilis B00.1
  geniculate ganglionitis B02.21
  genital, genitalis A60.00
    female A60.09
    male A60.02
  gestational, gestationis O26.4-
  gingivostomatitis B00.2
  human B00.9
    1 — *see* Herpes, simplex
    2 — *see* Herpes, simplex
    3 — *see* Varicella
    4 — *see* Mononucleosis, Epstein-Barr (virus)
    5 — *see* Disease, cytomegalic inclusion
      (generalized)
    6
      encephalitis B10.01
      specified NEC B10.81
    7
      encephalitis B10.09
      specified NEC B10.82
    8 B10.89
  infection NEC B10.89
    Kaposi's sarcoma associated B10.89
  iridocyclitis (simplex) B00.51
    zoster B02.32
  iris (vesicular erythema multiforme) L51.9
  iritis (simplex) B00.51
  Kaposi's sarcoma associated B10.89

Herpes, herpesvirus, herpetic —*continued*
  keratitis (simplex) (dendritic) (disciform) (interstitial)
    B00.52
    zoster (interstitial) B02.33
  keratoconjunctivitis (simplex) B00.52
    zoster B02.33
  labialis B00.1
  lip B00.1
  meningitis (simplex) B00.3
    zoster B02.1
  ophthalmicus (zoster) NEC B02.30
    simplex B00.50
  penis A60.01
  perianal skin A60.1
  pharyngitis, pharyngotonsillitis B00.2
  rectum A60.1
  scrotum A60.02
  sepsis B00.7
  simplex B00.9
    complicated NEC B00.89
    congenital P35.2
    conjunctivitis B00.53
    external ear B00.1
    eyelid B00.59
    hepatitis B00.81
    keratitis (interstitial) B00.52
    myeitis B00.82
    specified complication NEC B00.89
    visceral B00.89
  stomatitis B00.2
  tonsurans B35.0
  visceral B00.89
  vulva A60.04
  whitlow B00.89
  zoster (*see also* condition) B02.9
    auricularis B02.21
    complicated NEC B02.8
    conjunctivitis B02.31
    disseminated B02.7
    encephalitis B02.0
    eye(lid) B02.39
    geniculate ganglionitis B02.21
    keratitis (interstitial) B02.33
    meningitis B02.1
    myelitis B02.24
    neuritis, neuralgia B02.29
    ophthalmicus NEC B02.30
    oticus B02.21
    polyneuropathy B02.23
    specified complication NEC B02.8
    trigeminal neuralgia B02.22
Herpesvirus (human) — *see* Herpes
Herpetophobia F40.218
Herrick's anemia — *see* Disease, sickle-cell
Hers' disease E74.09
Herter-Gee syndrome K90.0
Herxheimer's reaction T88.6
Hesitancy
  of micturition R39.11
  urinary R39.11
Hesselbach's hernia — *see* Hernia, femoral, specified
  site NEC
Heterochromia (congenital) Q13.2
  cataract — *see* Cataract, complicated
  cyclitis (Fuchs) — *see* Cyclitis, Fuchs' heterochromic
  hair L67.1
  iritis — *see* Cyclitis, Fuchs' heterochromic
  retained metallic foreign body (nonmagnetic) — *see*
    Foreign body, intraocular, old, retained
    magnetic — *see* Foreign body, intraocular, old,
      retained, magnetic
  uveitis — *see* Cyclitis, Fuchs' heterochromic
Heterophoria — *see* Strabismus, heterophoria
Heterophyes, heterophyiasis (small intestine) B66.8
Heterotopia, heterotopic (*see also* Malposition,
  congenital)
  cerebralis Q04.8
Heterotropia — *see* Strabismus
Heubner-Herter disease K90.0
Hexadactylism Q69.9

HGSIL (cytology finding) (high grade squamous
  intraepithelial lesion on cytologic smear) (Pap
  smear finding)
  anus R85.613
  cervix R87.613
    biopsy (histology) finding—code to CIN II or CIN
      III
  vagina R87.623
    biopsy (histology) finding—code to VAIN II or
      VAIN III
Hibernoma — *see* Lipoma
Hiccup, hiccough R06.6
  epidemic B33.0
  psychogenic F45.8
Hidradenitis (axillaris) (suppurative) L73.2
Hidradenoma (nodular) (*see also* Neoplasm, skin,
  benign)
  clear cell — *see* Neoplasm, skin, benign
  papillary — *see* Neoplasm, skin, benign
Hidrocystoma — *see* Neoplasm, skin, benign
High
  altitude effects T70.20
    anoxia T70.20
    on
      ears T70.0
      sinuses T70.1
    polycythemia D75.1
  arch
    foot Q66.7
    palate, congenital Q38.5
  arterial tension — *see* Hypertension
  basal metabolic rate R94.8
  blood pressure (*see also* Hypertension)
    reading (incidental) (isolated) (nonspecific),
      without diagnosis of hypertension R03.0
  cholesterol E78.0
    with high triglycerides E78.2
  diaphragm (congenital) Q79.1
  expressed emotional level within family Z63.8
  head at term O32.4
  palate, congenital Q38.5
    infant NEC Z76.2
    sexual behavior (heterosexual) Z72.51
      bisexual Z72.53
      homosexual Z72.52
  temperature (of unknown origin) R50.9
  thoracic rib Q76.6
  triglycerides E78.1
    with high cholesterol E78.2
Hildenbrand's disease A75.0
Hilum — *see* condition
Hip — *see* condition
Hippel's disease Q85.8
Hippophobia F40.218
Hippus H57.09
Hirschsprung's disease or megacolon Q43.1
Hirsutism, hirsuties L68.0
Hirudiniasis
  external B88.3
  internal B83.4
Hiss-Russell dysentery A03.1
Histidinemia, histidinuria E70.41
Histiocytoma (*see also* Neoplasm, skin, benign)
  fibrous (*see also* Neoplasm, skin, benign)
    atypical — *see* Neoplasm, connective tissue,
      uncertain behavior
    malignant — *see* Neoplasm, connective tissue,
      malignant
Histiocytosis D76.3
  acute differentiated progressive C96.0
  Langerhans' cell NEC C96.6
    multifocal X
      multisystemic (disseminated) C96.0
      unisystemic C96.5
    unifocal (X) C96.6
  lipid, lipoid (essential) D76.3
  malignant C96.a
  mononuclear phagocytes NEC D76.1
    Langerhans' cells C96.6
  non-Langerhans cell D76.3
  polyostotic sclerosing D76.3
  sinus, with massive lymphadenopathy D76.3
  syndrome NEC D76.3

Histiocytosis —*continued*
    X NEC C96.6
        acute (progressive) C96.0
        chronic C96.6
        multifocal C96.5
        multisystemic C96.0
        unifocal C96.6
Histoplasmosis B39.9
    with pneumonia NEC B39.2 [J17]
    African B39.5
    American — *see* Histoplasmosis, capsulati
    capsulati B39.4
        disseminated B39.3
        generalized B39.3
        pulmonary B39.2
            acute B39.0
            chronic B39.1
    Darling's B39.4
    duboisii B39.5
    lung NEC B39.2
History
    family (of) — *see also* History, personal (of)
        alcohol abuse Z81.1
        allergy NEC Z84.89
        anemia Z83.2
        arthritis Z82.61
        asthma Z82.5
        blindness Z82.1
        cardiac death (sudden) Z82.41
        carrier of genetic disease Z84.81
        chromosomal anomaly Z82.79
        chronic
            disabling disease NEC Z82.8
            lower respiratory disease Z82.5
        colonic polyps Z83.71
        congenital malformations and deformations Z82.79
            polycystic kidney Z82.71
        consanguinity Z84.3
        deafness Z82.2
        diabetes mellitus Z83.3
        disability NEC Z82.8
        disease or disorder (of)
            allergic NEC Z84.89
            behavioral NEC Z81.8
            blood and blood-forming organs Z83.2
            cardiovascular NEC Z82.49
            chronic disabling NEC Z82.8
            digestive Z83.79
            ear NEC Z83.5
            endocrine NEC Z83.49
            eye NEC Z83.5
            genitourinary NEC Z84.2
            hematological Z83.2
            immune mechanism Z83.2
            infectious NEC Z83.1
            ischemic heart Z82.49
            kidney Z84.1
            mental NEC Z81.8
            metabolic Z83.49
            musculoskeletal NEC Z82.69
            neurological NEC Z82.0
            nutritional Z83.49
            parasitic NEC Z83.1
            psychiatric NEC Z81.8
            respiratory NEC Z83.6
            skin and subcutaneous tissue NEC Z84.0
            specified NEC Z84.89
        drug abuse NEC Z81.3
        epilepsy Z82.0
        genetic disease carrier Z84.81
        hearing loss Z82.2
        human immunodeficiency virus (HIV) infection Z83.0
        Huntington's chorea Z82.0
        leukemia Z80.6
        malignant neoplasm (of) NOS Z80.9
            bladder Z80.52
            breast Z80.3
            bronchus Z80.1
            digestive organ Z80.0
            gastrointestinal tract Z80.0
            genital organ Z80.49

History—*continued*
    family (of)—*continued*
        malignant neoplasm (of)—*continued*
            genital organ—*continued*
                ovary Z80.41
                prostate Z80.42
                specified organ NEC Z80.49
                testis Z80.43
            hematopoietic NEC Z80.7
            intrathoracic organ NEC Z80.2
            kidney Z80.51
            lung Z80.1
            lymphatic NEC Z80.7
            ovary Z80.41
            prostate Z80.42
            respiratory organ NEC Z80.2
            specified site NEC Z80.8
            testis Z80.43
            trachea Z80.1
            urinary organ or tract Z80.59
                bladder Z80.52
                kidney Z80.51
        mental
            disorder NEC Z81.8
            retardation Z81.0
        multiple endocrine neoplasia (MEN) syndrome Z83.41
        osteoporosis Z82.62
        polycystic kidney Z82.71
        polyps (colon) Z83.71
        psychiatric disorder Z81.8
        psychoactive substance abuse NEC Z81.3
        respiratory condition NEC Z83.6
            asthma and other lower respiratory conditions Z82.5
        self-harmful behavior Z81.8
        skin condition Z84.0
        specified condition NEC Z84.89
        stroke (cerebrovascular) Z82.3
        substance abuse NEC Z81.4
            alcohol Z81.1
            drug NEC Z81.3
            psychoactive NEC Z81.3
            tobacco Z81.2
        sudden cardiac death Z82.41
        tobacco abuse Z81.2
        violence, violent behavior Z81.8
        visual loss Z82.1
    personal (of) — *see also* History, family (of)
        abuse
            childhood Z62.819
                physical Z62.810
                psychological Z62.811
                sexual Z62.810
            adult Z91.419
                physical and sexual Z91.410
                psychological Z91.411
        alcohol dependence F10.21
        allergy (to) Z88.9
            analgesic agent NEC Z88.6
            anesthetic Z88.4
            antibiotic agent NEC Z88.1
            anti-infective agent NEC Z88.3
            contrast media Z91.041
            drugs, medicaments and biological substances Z88.9
                specified NEC Z88.8
            food Z91.018
                additives Z91.02
                eggs Z91.012
                milk products Z91.011
                peanuts Z91.010
                seafood Z91.013
                specified food NEC Z91.018
            insect Z91.038
                bee Z91.030
            latex Z91.040
            medicinal agents Z88.9
                specified NEC Z88.8
            narcotic agent NEC Z88.5
            nonmedicinal agents Z91.048
            penicillin Z88.0
            serum Z88.7

History—*continued*
    personal (of)—*continued*
        allergy—*continued*
            specified NEC Z91.09
            sulfonamides Z88.2
            vaccine Z88.7
        anaphylactic shock Z88.9
        behavioral disorders Z86.59
        benign carcinoid tumor Z86.012
        benign neoplasm Z86.018
            carcinoid Z86.012
            brain Z86.011
            colonic polyps Z86.010
        brain injury (traumatic) Z87.820
        breast implant removal Z98.86
        calculi, renal Z87.442
        cancer — *see* History, personal (of), malignant neoplasm (of)
        cardiac arrest (death), successfully resuscitated Z86.74
        cerebral infarction without residual deficit Z86.73
        cervical dysplasia Z87.410
        chemotherapy for neoplastic condition Z92.21
        childhood abuse — *see* History, personal (of), abuse
        cleft lip (corrected) Z87.730
        cleft palate (corrected) Z87.730
        collapsed vertebra (healed) Z87.311
            due to osteoporosis Z87.310
        combat and operational stress reaction Z86.51
        congenital malformation (corrected) Z87.798
            circulatory system (corrected) Z87.74
            digestive system (corrected) NEC Z87.738
            ear (corrected) Z87.720
            eye (corrected) Z87.721
            face and neck (corrected) Z87.790
            genitourinary system (corrected) NEC Z87.718
            heart (corrected) Z87.74
            integument (corrected) Z87.76
            limb(s) (corrected) Z87.76
            musculoskeletal system (corrected) Z87.76
            neck (corrected) Z87.790
            nervous system (corrected) NEC Z87.728
            respiratory system (corrected) Z87.75
            sense organs (corrected) NEC Z87.728
            specified NEC Z87.798
        contraception Z92.0
        deployment (military) Z91.82
        disease or disorder (of) Z87.898
            blood and blood-forming organs Z86.2
            circulatory system Z86.79
                specified condition NEC Z86.79
            connective tissue NEC Z87.39
            digestive system Z87.19
                colonic polyp Z86.010
                peptic ulcer disease Z87.11
                specified condition NEC Z87.19
            ear Z86.69
            endocrine Z86.39
                diabetic foot ulcer Z86.31
                specified type NEC Z86.39
            eye Z86.69
            genital system (track) system NEC
                female Z87.42
                male Z87.438
            hematological Z86.2
            Hodgkin Z85.71
            immune mechanism Z86.2
            infectious Z86.19
                malaria Z86.13
                poliomyelitis Z86.12
                specified NEC Z86.19
                tuberculosis Z86.11
            mental NEC Z86.59
            metabolic Z86.39
                diabetic foot ulcer Z86.31
                specified type NEC Z86.39
            musculoskeletal NEC Z87.39
            nervous system Z86.69
            nutritional Z86.39
            parasitic Z86.19
            respiratory system NEC Z87.09
            sense organs Z86.69

History—*continued*
  personal (of)—*continued*
    disease or disorder (of)—*continued*
      skin Z87.2
      specified site or type NEC Z87.898
      subcutaneous tissue Z87.2
      trophoblastic Z87.59
      urinary system NEC Z87.448
    drug dependence — *see* Dependence, drug, by
      type, in remission
    drug therapy
      antineoplastic chemotherapy Z92.21
      estrogen Z92.23
      immunosupression Z92.25
      inhaled steroids Z92.240
      monoclonal drug Z92.22
      specified NEC Z92.29
      steroid Z92.241
      systemic steroids Z92.241
    dysplasia
      cervical Z87.410
      prostatic Z87.430
      vaginal Z87.411
      vulvar Z87.412
    embolism (venous) Z86.71
    encephalitis Z86.61
    estrogen therapy Z92.23
    extracorporeal membrane oxygenation (ECMO)
      Z92.81
    failed moderate sedation Z92.83
    failed conscious sedation Z92.83
    fall, falling Z91.81
    fracture (healed)
      fatigue Z87.312
      fragility Z87.310
      osteoporosis Z87.310
      pathological NEC Z87.311
      stress Z87.312
      traumatic Z87.81
    hepatitis
      B Z86.19
      C Z86.19
    Hodgkin disease Z85.71
    hyperthermia, malignant Z88.4
    hypospadias (corrected) Z87.710
    hysterectomy Z90.710
    immunosupression therapy Z92.25
    in situ neoplasm
      breast Z86.000
      cervix uteri Z86.001
      specified NEC Z86.008
    infection NEC Z86.19
      central nervous system Z86.61
      urinary (recurrent) (tract) Z87.440
    injury NEC Z87.828
    in utero procedure during pregnancy Z98.870
    in utero procedure while a fetus Z98.871
    irradiation Z92.3
    kidney stones Z87.442
    leukemia Z85.6
    lymphoma (non-Hodgkin) Z85.72
    malignant melanoma (skin) Z85.820
    malignant neoplasm (of) Z85.9
      accessory sinuses Z85.22
      anus NEC Z85.048
        carcinoid Z85.040
      bladder Z85.51
      bone Z85.830
      brain Z85.841
      breast Z85.3
      bronchus NEC Z85.118
        carcinoid Z85.110
      carcinoid — *see* History, personal (of),
        malignant neoplasm, by site, carcinioid
      cervix Z85.41
      colon NEC Z85.038
        carcinoid Z85.030
      digestive organ Z85.00
        specified NEC Z85.09
      endocrine gland NEC Z85.858
      epididymis Z85.48
      esophagus Z85.01
      eye Z85.840

History—*continued*
  personal (of)—*continued*
    malignant neoplasm (of)—*continued*
      gastrointestinal tract — *see* History,
        malignant neoplasm, digestive organ
      genital organ
        female Z85.40
          specified NEC Z85.44
        male Z85.45
          specified NEC Z85.49
      hematopoietic NEC Z85.79
      intrathoracic organ Z85.20
      kidney NEC Z85.528
        carcinoid Z85.520
      large intestine NEC Z85.030
        carcinoid Z85.030
      larynx Z85.21
      liver Z85.05
      lung NEC Z85.118
        carcinoid Z85.110
      mediastinum Z85.29
      Merkel cell Z85.821
      middle ear Z85.22
      nasal cavities Z85.22
      nervous system NEC Z85.848
      oral cavity Z85.819
        specified site NEC Z85.818
      ovary Z85.43
      pancreas Z85.07
      pharynx Z85.819
        specified site NEC Z85.818
      pelvis Z85.53
      pleura Z85.29
      prostate Z85.46
      rectosigmoid junction NEC Z85.048
        carcinoid Z85.040
      rectum NEC Z85.048
        carcinoid Z85.040
      respiratory organ Z85.20
      sinuses, accessory Z85.22
      skin NEC Z85.828
        melanoma Z85.820
        Merkel cell Z85.821
      small intestine NEC Z85.068
        carcinoid Z85.060
      soft tissue Z85.831
      specified site NEC Z85.89
      stomach NEC Z85.028
        carcinoid Z85.020
      testis Z85.47
      thymus NEC Z85.238
        carcinoid Z85.230
      thyroid Z85.850
      tongue Z85.810
      trachea Z85.12
      urinary organ or tract Z85.50
        specified NEC Z85.59
      uterus Z85.42
    maltreatment Z91.89
    medical treatment NEC Z92.89
    melanoma (malignant) (skin) Z85.820
    meningitis Z86.61
    mental disorder Z86.59
    Merkel cell carcinoma (skin) Z85.821
    military deployment Z91.82
    military war, peacekeeping and humanitarian
      deployment (current or past conflict)
      Z91.82
    myocardial infarction (old) I25.2
    neglect (in)
      adult Z91.412
      childhood Z62.812
    neoplasm
      benign Z86.018
        brain Z86.011
        colon polyp Z86.010
      in situ
        breast Z86.000
        cervix uteri Z86.001
        specified NEC Z86.008
      malignant — *see* History of, malignant
        neoplasm
      uncertain behavior Z86.03

History—*continued*
  personal (of)—*continued*
    nephrotic syndrome Z87.441
    nicotine dependence Z87.891
    noncompliance with medical treatment or
      regimen — *see* Noncompliance
    nutritional deficiency Z86.39
    obstetric complications Z87.59
      childbirth Z87.59
      pregnancy Z87.59
      pre-term labor Z87.51
      puerperium Z87.59
    osteoporosis fractures Z87.31
    parasuicide (attempt) Z91.5
    physical trauma NEC Z87.828
      self-harm or suicide attempt Z91.5
    poisoning NEC Z91.89
      self-harm or suicide attempt Z91.5
    poor personal hygiene Z91.89
    pneumonia (recurrent) Z87.01
    preterm labor Z87.51
    prolonged reversible ischemic neurologic deficit
      (PRIND) Z86.73
    procedure during pregnancy Z98.870
    procedure while a fetus Z98.871
    prostatic dysplasia Z87.430
    psychological
      abuse
        adult Z91.411
        child Z62.811
      trauma, specified NEC Z91.49
    radiation therapy Z92.3
    removal
      implant
        breast Z98.86
    renal calculi Z87.442
    respiratory condition NEC Z87.09
    retained foreign body fully removed Z87.821
    risk factors NEC Z91.89
    self-harm Z91.5
    self-poisoning attempt Z91.5
    sex reassignment Z87.890
    sleep-wake cycle problem Z72.821
    specified NEC Z87.898
    steroid therapy (systemic) Z92.241
      inhaled Z92.240
    stroke without residual deficits Z86.73
    substance abuse NEC F10 F19
      with fifth character 1
    sudden cardiac arrest Z86.74
    sudden cardiac death successfully resuscitated Z86.74
    suicide attempt Z91.5
    surgery NEC Z98.89
      sex reassignment Z87.890
      transplant — *see* Transplant
    thrombophlebitis Z86.72
    thrombosis (venous) Z86.71
    tobacco dependence
    transient ischemic attack (TIA) without residual
      deficits Z86.73
    trauma (physical) NEC Z87.828
      self-harm Z91.5
    traumatic brain injury Z87.820
      psychological NEC Z91.49
    unhealthy sleep-wake cycle Z72.821
    urinary calculi Z87.442
    urinary (recurrent) (tract) infection(s) Z87.440
    vaginal dysplasia Z87.411
    venous thrombosis or embolism Z86.71
    vulvar dysplasia Z87.412
His-Werner disease A79.0
HIV B20
  laboratory evidence (nonconclusive) R75
  positive, seropositive Z21
  nonconclusive test (in infants) R75
Hives (bold) — *see* Urticaria
Hoarseness R49.0
Hobo Z59.0
Hodgkin disease — *see* Lymphoma, Hodgkin
Hodgson's disease I71.2
  ruptured I71.1
Hoffa-Kastert disease E88.89
Hoffa's disease E88.89

Hoffmann-Bouveret syndrome I47.9
Hoffmann's syndrome E03.9[G73.7]
Hole (round)
    macula H35.34-
    retina (without detachment) — see Break, retina,
        round hole
        with detachment — see Detachment, retina, with
            retinal, break
Holiday relief care Z75.5
Hollenhorst's plaque — see Occlusion, artery, retina
Hollow foot (congenital) Q66.7
    acquired — see Deformity, limb, foot, specified NEC
Holoprosencephaly Q04.2
Holt-Oram syndrome Q87.2
Homelessness Z59.0
Homesickness — see Disorder, adjustment
Homocystinemia, homocystinuria E72.11
Homogentisate 1,2-dioxygenase deficiency E70.29
Homologous serum hepatitis (prophylactic)
    (therapeutic) — see Hepatitis, viral, type B
Honeycomb lung J98.4
    congenital Q33.0
Hooded
    clitoris Q52.6
    penis Q55.69
Hookworm (anemia) (disease) (infection) (infestation)
    B76.9
    specified NEC B76.8
Hordeolum (eyelid) (externum) (recurrent) H00.019
    internum H00.029
        left H00.026
            lower H00.025
            upper H00.024
        right H00.023
            lower H00.022
            upper H00.021
    left H00.016
        lower H00.015
        upper H00.014
    right H00.013
        lower H00.012
        upper H00.011
Horn
    cutaneous L85.8
    nail L60.2
        congenital Q84.6
Horner(-Claude Bernard) **syndrome** G90.2
    traumatic — see Injury, nerve, cervical sympathetic
Horseshoe kidney (congenital) Q63.1
Horton's headache or neuralgia G44.099
    intractable G44.091
    not intractable G44.099
Hospital hopper syndrome — see Disorder, factitious
Hospitalism in children — see Disorder, adjustment
Hostility R45.5
    towards child Z62.3
Hot flashes
    menopausal N95.1
Hourglass (contracture) (see also Contraction,
        hourglass)
    stomach K31.89
        congenital Q40.2
        stricture K31.2
Household, housing circumstance affecting care
    Z59.9
    specified NEC Z59.8
Housemaid's knee — see Bursitis, prepatellar
Hudson(-Stähli) **line** (cornea) — see Pigmentation,
    cornea, anterior
Human
    bite (open wound) (see also Bite)
        intact skin surface — see Bite, superficial
    herpesvirus — see Herpes
    immunodeficiency virus (HIV) disease (infection)
        B20
        asymptomatic status Z21
        contact Z20.6
        counseling Z71.7
        dementia B20 [F02.80]
            with behavioral disturbance B20 [F02.81]
        exposure to Z20.6
        laboratory evidence R75

Human—continued
    immunodeficiency virus (HIV)—continued
        type-2 (HIV 2) as cause of disease classified
            elsewhere B97.35
    papillomavirus (HPV)
        DNA test positive
            high risk
                cervix R87.810
                vagina R87.811
            low risk
                cervix R87.820
                vagina R87.821
        screening for Z11.51
    T-cell lymphotropic virus
        type-1 (HTLV-I) infection B33.3
            as cause of disease classified elsewhere
                B97.33
            carrier Z22.6
        type-2 (HTLV-II) as cause of disease classified
            elsewhere B97.34
Humidifier lung or pneumonitis J67.7
Humiliation (experience) **in childhood** Z62.898
Humpback (acquired) — see Kyphosis
Hunchback (acquired) — see Kyphosis
Hunger T73.0
    air, psychogenic F45.8
Hungry bone syndrome E83.81
Hunner's ulcer — see Cystitis, chronic, interstitial
Hunter's
    glossitis D51.0
    syndrome E76.1
Huntington's disease or chorea G10
    with dementia G10 [F02.80]
        with behavioral disturbance G10 [F02.81]
Hunt's
    disease or syndrome (herpetic geniculate
        ganglionitis) B02.21
        dyssynergia cerebellaris myoclonica G11.1
        neuralgia B02.21
Hurler (-Scheie) **disease or syndrome** E76.02
Hurst's disease G36.1
Hurthle cell
    adenocarcinoma C73
    adenoma D34
    carcinoma C73
    tumor D34
Hutchinson-Boeck disease or syndrome — see
    Sarcoidosis
Hutchinson-Gilford disease or syndrome E34.8
Hutchinson's
    disease meaning
        angioma serpiginosum L81.7
        pompholyx L30.1
        prurigo estivalis L56.4
        summer eruption or summer prurigo L56.4
    melanotic freckle — see Melanoma, in situ
        malignant melanoma in — see Melanoma
    teeth or incisors (congenital syphilis) A50.52
    triad (congenital syphilis) A50.53
Hyalin plaque, sclera, senile H15.89
Hyaline membrane (disease) (lung) (pulmonary)
    (newborn) P22.0
Hyalinosis
    cutis (et mucosae) E78.89
    focal and segmental (glomerular) (see also N00-N07
        with fourth character .1) N05.1
Hyalitis, hyalosis, asteroid (see also Deposit,
    crystalline)
    syphilitic (late) A52.71
Hydatid
    cyst or tumor — see Echinococcus
    mole — see Hydatidiform mole
    Morgagni
        female Q50.5
        male (epididymal) Q55.4
        testicular Q55.29
Hydatidiform mole (benign) (complicating
    pregnancy) (delivered) (undelivered) O01.9
    classical O01.0
    complete O01.0
    incomplete O01.1
    invasive D39.2
    malignant D39.2

Hydatidiform mole—continued
    partial O01.1
Hydatidosis — see Echinococcus
Hydradenitis (axillaris) (suppurative) L73.2
Hydradenoma — see Hidradenoma
Hydramnios O40.-
Hydrancephaly, hydranencephaly Q04.3
    with spina bifida — see Spina bifida, with
        hydrocephalus
Hydrargyrism NEC — see Poisoning, mercury
Hydrarthrosis (see also Effusion, joint)
    gonococcal A54.42
    intermittent M12.40
        ankle M12.47-
        elbow M12.42-
        foot joint M12.47-
        hand joint M12.44-
        hip M12.45-
        knee M12.46-
        multiple site M12.49
        shoulder M12.41-
        specified joint NEC M12.48
        wrist M12.43-
    of yaws (early) (late) (see also subcategory M14.8-)
        A66.6
    syphilitic (late) A52.77
        congenital A50.55 [M12.80]
Hydremia D64.89
Hydrencephalocele (congenital) — see Encephalocele
Hydrencephalomeningocele (congenital) — see
    Encephalocele
Hydroa R23.8
    aestivale L56.4
    vacciniforme L56.4
Hydroadenitis (axillaris) (suppurative) L73.2
Hydrocalycosis — see Hydronephrosis
Hydrocele (spermatic cord) (testis) (tunica vaginalis)
    N43.3
    canal of Nuck N94.89
    communicating N43.2
        congenital P83.5
    congenital P83.5
    encysted N43.0
    female NEC N94.89
    infected N43.1
    newborn P83.5
    round ligament N94.89
    specified NEC N43.2
    spinalis — see Spina bifida
    vulva N90.89
Hydrocephalus (acquired) (external) (internal)
    (malignant) (recurrent) G91.9
    aqueduct Sylvius stricture Q03.0
    causing disproportion O33.6
        with obstructed labor O66.3
    communicating G91.0
    congenital (external) (internal) Q03.9
        with spina bifida Q05.4
            cervical Q05.0
            dorsal Q05.1
            lumbar Q05.2
            lumbosacral Q05.2
            sacral Q05.3
            thoracic Q05.1
            thoracolumbar Q05.1
        specified NEC Q03.8
    due to toxoplasmosis (congenital) P37.1
    foramen Magendie block (acquired) G91.1
        congenital (see also Hydrocephalus, congenital)
            Q03.1
    in (due to)
        infectious disease NEC G91.4
        neoplastic disease NEC (see also Neoplasm) G91.4
        parasitic disease G91.4
    newborn Q03.9
        with spina bifida — see Spina bifida, with
            hydrocephalus
    noncommunicating G91.1
    normal pressure G91.2
        secondary G91.0
    obstructive G91.1
    otitic G93.2
    post-traumatic NEC G91.3

Hydrocephalus—continued
secondary G91.4
post-traumatic G91.3
specified NEC G91.8
syphilitic, congenital A50.49
Hydrocolpos (congenital) N89.8
Hydrocystoma — see Neoplasm, skin, benign
Hydroencephalocele (congenital) — see
Encephalocele
Hydroencephalomeningocele (congenital) — see
Encephalocele
Hydrohematopneumothorax — see Hemothorax
Hydromeningitis — see Meningitis
Hydromeningocele (spinal) (see also Spina bifida)
cranial — see Encephalocele
Hydrometra N85.8
Hydrometrocolpos N89.8
Hydromicrocephaly Q02
Hydromphalos (since birth) Q45.8
Hydromyelia Q06.4
Hydromyelocele — see Spina bifida
Hydronephrosis (atrophic) (early) (functionless)
(intermittent) (primary) (secondary) NEC N13.30
with
infection N13.6
obstruction (by) (of)
renal calculus N13.2
with infection N13.6
ureteral NEC N13.1
with infection N13.6
calculus N13.2
with infection N13.6
ureteropelvic junction (congenital) Q62.0
with infection N13.6
ureteral stricture NEC N13.1
with infection N13.6
congenital Q62.0
specified type NEC N13.39
tuberculous A18.11
Hydropericarditis — see Pericarditis
Hydropericardium — see Pericarditis
Hydroperitoneum R18.8
Hydrophobia — see Rabies
Hydrophthalmos Q15.0
Hydropneumohemothorax — see Hemothorax
Hydropneumopericarditis — see Pericarditis
Hydropneumopericardium — see Pericarditis
Hydropneumothorax J94.8
traumatic — see Injury, intrathoracic, lung
tuberculous NEC A15.6
Hydrops R60.9
abdominis R18.8
articulorum intermittens — see Hydrarthrosis,
intermittent
cardiac — see Failure, heart, congestive
causing obstructed labor (mother) O66.3
endolymphatic H81.0-
gallbladder K82.1
joint — see Effusion, joint
labyrinth H81.0-
newborn (idiopathic) P83.2
due to
ABO isoimmunization P56.0
hemolytic disease P56.90
specified NEC P56.99
isoimmunization (ABO) (Rh) P56.0
Rh incompatibility P56.0
nutritional — see Malnutrition, severe
pericardium — see Pericarditis
pleura — see Hydrothorax
spermatic cord — see Hydrocele
Hydropyonephrosis N13.6
Hydrorachis Q06.4
Hydrorrhea (nasal) J34.89
pregnancy — see Rupture, membranes, premature
Hydrosadenitis (axillaris) (suppurative) L73.2
Hydrosalpinx (fallopian tube) (follicularis) N70.11
Hydrothorax (double) (pleura) J94.8
chylous (nonfilarial) I89.8
filarial (see also Infestation, filarial) B74.9 [J91.8]
traumatic — see Injury, intrathoracic
tuberculous NEC (non primary) A15.6

Hydroureter
(see also Hydronephrosis) N13.4
with infection N13.6
congenital Q62.39
Hydroureteronephrosis — see Hydronephrosis
Hydrourethra N36.8
Hydroxykynureninuria E70.8
Hydroxylysinemia E72.3
Hydroxyprolinemia E72.59
Hygiene, sleep
abuse Z72.821
inadequate Z72.821
poor Z72.821
Hygroma (congenital) (cystic) D18.1
praepatellare, prepatellar — see Bursitis, prepatellar
Hymen — see condition
Hymenolepis, hymenolepiasis (diminuta) (infection)
(infestation) (nana) B71.0
Hypalgesia R20.8
Hyperacidity (gastric) K31.89
psychogenic F45.8
Hyperactive, hyperactivity F90.9
basal cell, uterine cervix — see Dysplasia, cervix
bowel sounds R19.12
cervix epithelial (basal) — see Dysplasia, cervix
child F90.9
attention deficit — see Disorder, attention-deficit
hyperactivity
detrusor muscle N32.81
gastrointestinal K31.89
psychogenic F45.8
nasal mucous membrane J34.3
stomach K31.89
thyroid (gland) — see Hyperthyroidism
Hyperacusis H93.23-
Hyperadrenalism E27.5
Hyperadrenocorticism E24.9
congenital E25.0
iatrogenic E24.2
correct substance properly administered — see
Table of Drugs and Chemicals, by drug,
adverse effect
overdose or wrong substance given or taken —
see Table of Drugs and Chemicals, by drug,
poisoning
not associated with Cushing's syndrome E27.0
pituitary-dependent E24.0
Hyperaldosteronism E26.9
familial (type I) E26.02
glucocorticoid-remediable E26.02
primary (due to (bilateral) adrenal hyperplasia) E26.09
primary NEC E26.09
secondary E26.1
specified NEC E26.89
Hyperalgesia R20.8
Hyperalimentation R63.2
carotene, carotin E67.1
specified NEC E67.8
vitamin
A E67.0
D E67.3
Hyperaminoaciduria
arginine E72.21
cystine E72.01
lysine E72.3
ornithine E72.4
Hyperammonemia (congenital) E72.20
Hyperazotemia — see Uremia
Hyperbetalipoproteinemia (familial) E78.0
with prebetalipoproteinemia E78.2
Hyperbilirubinemia
constitutional E80.6
familial conjugated E80.6
neonatal (transient) — see Jaundice, newborn
Hypercalcemia, hypocalciuric, familial E83.52
Hypercalciuria, idiopathic E83.52
Hypercapnia R06.89
newborn P84
Hypercarotenemia, hypercarotinemia (dietary)
E67.1
Hypercementosis K03.4
Hyperchloremia E87.8

Hyperchlorhydria K31.89
neurotic F45.8
psychogenic F45.8
Hypercholesterinemia — see Hypercholesterolemia
Hypercholesterolemia (essential) (familial)
(hereditary) (primary) (pure) E78.0
with hyperglyceridemia, endogenous E78.2
dietary counseling and surveillance Z71.3
Hyperchylia gastrica, psychogenic F45.8
Hyperchylomicronemia (familial) (primary) E78.3
with hyperbetalipoproteinemia E78.3
Hypercoagulable (state) D68.59
activated protein C resistance D68.51
antithrombin (III) deficiency D68.59
factor V Leiden mutation D68.51
primary NEC D68.59
protein C deficiency D68.59
protein S deficiency D68.59
prothrombin gene mutation D68.52
secondary D68.69
specified NEC D68.69
Hypercoagulation (state) D68.59
Hypercorticalism, pituitary-dependent E24.0
Hypercorticosolism — see Cushing's syndrome
Hypercorticosteronism E24.2
correct substance properly administered — see
Table of Drugs and Chemicals, by drug,
adverse effect
overdose or wrong substance given or taken — see
Table of Drugs and Chemicals, by drug,
poisoning
Hypercortisonism E24.2
correct substance properly administered — see
Table of Drugs and Chemicals, by drug,
adverse effect
overdose or wrong substance given or taken — see
Table of Drugs and Chemicals, by drug,
poisoning
Hyperekplexia Q89.8
Hyperelectrolytemia E87.8
Hyperemesis R11.10
with nausea R11.2
gravidarum (mild) O21.0
with
carbohydrate depletion O21.1
dehydration O21.1
electrolyte imbalance O21.1
metabolic disturbance O21.1
severe (with metabolic disturbance) O21.1
projectile R11.12
psychogenic F45.8
Hyperemia (acute) (passive) R68.89
anal mucosa K62.8
bladder N32.89
cerebral I67.8
conjunctiva H11.43-
ear internal, acute — see subcategory H83.0
enteric K59.8
eye — see Hyperemia, conjunctiva
eyelid (active) (passive) — see Disorder, eyelid,
specified type NEC
intestine K59.8
iris — see Disorder, iris, vascular
kidney N28.89
labyrinth — see subcategory H83.0
liver (active) K76.8
lung (passive) — see Edema, lung
pulmonary (passive) — see Edema, lung
renal N28.89
retina H35.89
stomach K31.89
Hyperesthesia (body surface) R20.3
larynx (reflex) J38.7
hysterical F44.89
pharynx (reflex) J39.2
hysterical F44.89
Hyperestrogenism (drug-induced) (iatrogenic) E28.0
Hyperexplexia Q89.8
Hyperfibrinolysis — see Fibrinolysis
Hyperfructosemia E74.19

Hyperfunction
adrenal cortex, not associated with Cushing's
syndrome E27.Ø
medulla E27.5
adrenomedullary E27.5
virilism E25.9
congenital E25.Ø
ovarian E28.8
pancreas K86.8
parathyroid (gland) E21.3
pituitary (gland) (anterior) E22.9
specified NEC E22.8
polyglandular E31.1
testicular E29.Ø
Hypergammaglobulinemia D89.2
polyclonal D89.Ø
Waldenström D89.Ø
Hypergastrinemia E16.4
Hyperglobulinemia R77.1
Hyperglycemia, hyperglycemic (transient) R73.9
coma — *see* Diabetes, by type, with coma
postpancreatectomy E89.1
Hyperglyceridemia (endogenous) (essential) (familial)
(hereditary) (pure) E78.1
mixed E78.3
Hyperglycinemia (non-ketotic) E72.51
Hypergonadism
ovarian E28.8
testicular (primary) (infantile) E29.Ø
Hyperheparinemia — *see* Circulating anticoagulants
Hyperhidrosis, hyperidrosis R61
focal
primary L74.519
axilla L74.51Ø
face L74.511
palms L74.512
soles L74.513
secondary L74.52
generalized R61
localized
primary L74.519
axilla L74.51Ø
face L74.511
palms L74.512
soles L74.513
secondary L74.52
psychogenic F45.8
secondary R61
focal L74.52
Hyperhistidinemia E70.41
Hyperhomocysteinemia E72.11
Hyperhydroxyprolinemia E72.59
Hyperinsulinism (functional) E16.1
with
coma (hypoglycemic) E15
encephalopathy E16.1 [G94]
ectopic E16.1
therapeutic misadventure (from administration of
insulin) — *see* subcategory T38.3
Hyperkalemia E87.5
Hyperkeratosis (*see also* Keratosis) L85.9
cervix N88.Ø
due to yaws (early) (late) (palmar or plantar) A66.3
follicularis Q82.8
penetrans (in cutem) L87.Ø
palmoplantaris climacterica L85.1
pinta A67.1
senile (with pruritus) L57.Ø
universalis congenita Q80.8
vocal cord J38.3
vulva N90.4
Hyperkinesia, hyperkinetic (disease) (reaction)
(syndrome) (childhood) (adolescence) (*see also*
Disorder, attention-deficit hyperactivity)
heart I51.89
Hyperleucine-isoleucinemia E71.19
Hyperlipemia, hyperlipidemia E78.5
combined E78.2
familial E78.4
group
A E78.Ø
B E78.1

Hyperlipemia, hyperlipidemia—*continued*
group—*continued*
C E78.2
D E78.3
mixed E78.2
specified NEC E78.4
Hyperlipidosis E75.6
hereditary NEC E75.5
Hyperlipoproteinemia E78.5
Fredrickson's type
I E78.3
IIa E78.Ø
IIb E78.2
III E78.2
IV E78.1
V E78.3
low-density-lipoprotein-type (LDL) E78.Ø
very-low-density-lipoprotein-type (VLDL) E78.1
Hyperlucent lung, unilateral J43.Ø
Hyperlysinemia E72.3
Hypermagnesemia E83.41
neonatal P71.8
Hypermenorrhea N92.Ø
Hypermethioninemia E72.19
Hypermetropia (congenital) H52.Ø-
Hypermobility, hypermotility
cecum — *see* Syndrome, irritable bowel
coccyx — *see* subcategory M53.2
colon — *see* Syndrome, irritable bowel
psychogenic F45.8
ileum K58.9
intestine (*see also* Syndrome, irritable bowel) K58.9
psychogenic F45.8
meniscus (knee) — *see* Derangement, knee,
meniscus
scapula — *see* Instability, joint, shoulder
stomach K31.89
psychogenic F45.8
syndrome M35.7
urethra N36.41
with intrinsic sphincter deficiency N36.43
Hypernasality R49.21
Hypernatremia E87.Ø
Hypernephroma C64.-
Hyperopia — *see* Hypermetropia
Hyperorexia nervosa F50.2
Hyperornithinemia E72.4
Hyperosmia R43.1
Hyperosmolality E87.Ø
Hyperostosis (monomelic) (*see also* Disorder, bone,
density and structure, specified NEC)
ankylosing (spine) M48.1Ø
cervical region M48.12
cervicothoracic region M48.13
lumbar region M48.16
lumbosacral region M48.17
multiple sites M48.19
occipito-atlanto-axial region M48.11
sacrococcygeal region M48.18
thoracic region M48.14
thoracolumbar region M48.15
cortical (skull) M85.2
infantile M89.8x-
frontal, internal of skull M85.2
interna frontalis M85.2
skeletal, diffuse idiopathic — *see* Hyperostosis,
ankylosing
skull M85.2
congenital Q75.8
vertebral, ankylosing — *see* Hyperostosis,
ankylosing
Hyperovarism E28.8
Hyperoxaluria (primary) E72.53
Hyperparathyroidism E21.3
primary E21.Ø
secondary (renal) N25.81
non-renal E21.1
specified NEC E21.2
tertiary E21.2
Hyperpathia R20.8
Hyperperistalsis R19.2
psychogenic F45.8
Hyperpermeability, capillary I78.8

Hyperphagia R63.2
Hyperphenylalaninemia NEC E70.1
Hyperphoria (alternating) H50.53
Hyperphosphatemia E83.39
Hyperpiesis, hyperpiesia — *see* Hypertension
Hyperpigmentation (*see also* Pigmentation)
melanin NEC L81.4
postinflammatory L81.Ø
Hyperpinealism E34.8
Hyperpituitarism E22.9
Hyperplasia, hyperplastic adenoids J35.2
adrenal (capsule) (cortex) (gland) E27.8
with
sexual precocity (male) E25.9
congenital E25.Ø
virilism, adrenal E25.9
congenital E25.Ø
virilization (female) E25.9
congenital E25.Ø
congenital E25.Ø
salt-losing E25.Ø
adrenomedullary E27.5
appendix (lymphoid) K38.Ø
artery, fibromuscular I77.3
bone (*see also* Hypertrophy, bone)
marrow D75.89
breast (*see also* Hypertrophy, breast)
ductal (atypical) N60.9-
C-cell, thyroid E07.Ø
cementation (tooth) (teeth) K03.4
cervical gland R59.Ø
cervix (uteri) (basal cell) (endometrium) (polypoid)
(*see also* Dysplasia, cervix)
congenital Q51.828
clitoris, congenital Q52.6
denture K06.2
endocervicitis N72
endometrium, endometrial (adenomatous) (benign)
(cystic) (glandular) (glandular-cystic)
(polypoid) N85.ØØ
with atypia N85.Ø2
cervix — *see* Dysplasia, cervix
complex (without atypia) N85.Ø1
simple (without atypia) N85.Ø1
epithelial L85.9
focal, oral, including tongue K13.29
nipple N62
skin L85.9
tongue K13.29
vaginal wall N89.3
erythroid D75.89
fibromuscular of artery (carotid) (renal) I77.3
genital
female NEC N94.89
male N50.8
gingiva K06.1
glandularis cystica uteri (interstitialis) (*see also*
Hyperplasia, endometrial) N85.ØØ
gum K06.1
hymen, congenital Q52.4
irritative, edentulous (alveolar) K06.2
jaw M26.Ø9
alveolar M26.79
lower M26.Ø3
alveolar M26.72
upper M26.Ø1
alveolar M26.71
kidney (congenital) Q63.3
labia N90.6
epithelial N90.3
liver (congenital) Q44.7
nodular, focal K76.8
lymph gland or node R59.9
mandible, mandibular M26.Ø3
alveolar M26.72
unilateral condylar M27.8
maxilla, maxillary M26.Ø1
alveolar M26.71
myometrium, myometrial N85.2
nose
lymphoid J34.89
polypoid J33.9
oral mucosa (irritative) K13.6

Hyperplasia, hyperplastic—*continued*
- organ or site, congenital NEC — *see* Anomaly, by site
- ovary N83.8
- palate, papillary (irritative) K13.6
- pancreatic islet cells E16.9
  - alpha E16.8
    - with excess
      - gastrin E16.4
      - glucagon E16.3
  - beta E16.1
- parathyroid (gland) E21.0
- pharynx (lymphoid) J39.2
- prostate (adenofibromatous) (nodular) N40.0
  - with lower urinary tract symptoms (LUTS) N40.1
  - without lower urinary tract symtpoms (LUTS) N40.0
- renal artery I77.89
- reticulo-endothelial (cell) D75.89
- salivary gland (any) K11.1
- Schimmelbusch's — *see* Mastopathy, cystic
- suprarenal capsule (gland) E27.8
- thymus (gland) (persistent) E32.0
- thyroid (gland) — *see* Goiter
- tonsils (faucial) (infective) (lingual) (lymphoid) J35.1
  - with adenoids J35.3
- unilateral condylar M27.8
- uterus, uterine N85.2
  - endometrium (glandular)(*see also* Hyperplasia, endometrial) N85.00
- vulva N90.6
  - epithelial N90.3
Hyperpnea — *see* Hyperventilation
Hyperpotassemia E87.5
Hyperprebetalipoproteinemia (familial) E78.1
Hyperprolactinemia E22.1
Hyperprolinemia (type I) (type II) E72.59
Hyperproteinemia E88.09
Hyperprothrombinemia, causing coagulation factor deficiency D68.4
Hyperpyrexia R50.9
- heat (effects) T67.0
- malignant, due to anesthetic T88.3
- rheumatic — *see* Fever, rheumatic
- unknown origin R50.9
Hyper-reflexia R29.2
Hypersalivation K11.7
Hypersecretion
- ACTH (not associated with Cushing's syndrome) E27.0
  - pituitary E24.0
- adrenaline E27.5
- adrenomedullary E27.5
- androgen (testicular) E29.0
  - ovarian (drug-induced) (iatrogenic) E28.1
- calcitonin E07.0
- catecholamine E27.5
- corticoadrenal E24.9
- cortisol E24.9
- epinephrine E27.5
- estrogen E28.0
- gastric K31.89
  - psychogenic F45.8
- gastrin E16.4
- glucagon E16.3
- hormone(s)
  - ACTH (not associated with Cushing's syndrome) E27.0
    - pituitary E24.0
  - antidiuretic E22.2
  - growth E22.0
  - intestinal NEC E34.1
  - ovarian androgen E28.1
  - pituitary E22.9
  - testicular E29.0
  - thyroid stimulating E05.80
    - with thyroid storm E05.81
- insulin — *see* Hyperinsulinism
- lacrimal glands — *see* Epiphora
- medulloadrenal E27.5
- milk O92.6
- ovarian androgens E28.1
- salivary gland (any) K11.7

Hypersecretion—*continued*
- thyrocalcitonin E07.0
- upper respiratory J39.8
Hypersegmentation, leukocytic, hereditary D72.0
Hypersensitive, hypersensitiveness, hypersensitivity (*see also* Allergy)
- carotid sinus G90.01
- colon — *see* Irritable, colon
- drug T88.7 —This code not for use in the inpatient setting
- gastrointestinal K52.2
  - psychogenic F45.8
- labyrinth — *see* subcategory H83.2
- pain R20.8
- pneumonitis — *see* Pneumonitis, allergic
- reaction T78.40
  - upper respiratory tract NEC J39.3
Hypersomnia (organic) G47.10
- due to
  - alcohol
    - abuse F10.182
    - dependence F10.282
    - use F10.982
  - amphetamines
    - abuse F15.182
    - dependence F15.282
    - use F15.982
  - caffeine
    - abuse F15.182
    - dependence F15.282
    - use F15.982
  - cocaine
    - abuse F14.182
    - dependence F14.282
    - use F14.982
  - drug NEC
    - abuse F19.182
    - dependence F19.282
    - use F19.982
  - medical condition G47.14
  - mental disorder F51.13
  - opioid
    - abuse F11.182
    - dependence F11.282
    - use F11.982
  - psychoactive substance NEC
    - abuse F19.182
    - dependence F19.282
    - use F19.982
  - sedative, hypnotic, or anxiolytic
    - abuse F13.182
    - dependence F13.282
    - use F13.982
  - stimulant NEC
    - abuse F15.182
    - dependence F15.282
    - use F15.982
- idiopathic G47.11
  - with long sleep time G47.11
  - without long sleep time G47.12
- menstrual related G47.13
- nonorganic origin F51.11
  - specified NEC F51.19
- not due to a substance or known physiological condition F51.11
  - specified NEC F51.19
- primary F51.11
- recurrent G47.13
- specified NEC G47.19
Hypersplenia, hypersplenism D73.1
Hyperstimulation, ovaries (associated with induced ovulation) N98.1
Hypersusceptibility — *see* Allergy
Hypertelorism (ocular) (orbital) Q75.2
Hypertension, hypertensive (accelerated) (benign) (essential) (idiopathic) (malignant) (systemic) I10
- with
  - heart involvement (conditions in I51.4 - I51.9 due to hypertension) — *see* Hypertension, heart
  - kidney involvement — *see* Hypertension, kidney
- benign, intracranial G93.2

Hypertension, hypertensive — *continued*
- cardiorenal (disease) I13.10
  - with heart failure I13.0
    - with stage 1 through stage 4 chronic kidney disease I13.0
    - with stage 5 or end stage renal disease I13.2
  - without heart failure I13.10
    - with stage 1 through stage 4 chronic kidney disease I13.10
    - with stage 5 or end stage renal disease I13.11
  - disease (arteriosclerotic) (sclerotic) — *see* Hypertension, heart
- cardiovascular
  - renal (disease) — *see* Hypertension, cardiorenal
- chronic venous — *see* Hypertension, venous (chronic)
- complicating
  - childbirth (labor) O10.92
    - with
      - heart disease O10.12
        - with renal disease O10.32
      - renal disease O10.22
        - with heart disease O10.32
    - essential O10.02
    - secondary O10.42
  - pregnancy O16.-
    - with edema (*see also* Pre-eclampsia) O14.9-
    - gestational (pregnancy induced) (transient) (without proteinuria) O13.-
      - with proteinuria O14.9-
        - mild pre-eclampsia O14.0-
        - moderate pre-eclampsia O14.0-
        - severe pre-eclampsia O14.1-
    - pre-existing O10.91-
      - with
        - heart disease O10.11-
          - with renal disease O10.31-
        - pre-eclampsia O11.-
        - renal disease O10.21-
          - with heart disease O10.31-
      - essential O10.01-
      - secondary O10.41-
  - puerperium O10.93
    - with
      - heart disease O10.13
        - with renal disease O10.33
      - renal disease O10.23
        - with heart disease O10.33
    - essential O10.03
    - secondary O10.43
- due to
  - endocrine disorders I15.2
  - pheochromocytoma I15.2
  - renal disorders NEC I15.1
    - arterial I15.0
  - renovascular disorders I15.0
  - specified disease NEC I15.8
- encephalopathy I67.4
- gestational (without significant proteinuria) (pregnancy-induced) (transient) O13.-
  - with significant proteinuria — *see* Pre-eclampsia
- Goldblatt's I70.1
- heart (disease) (conditions in I51.4-I51.9 due to hypertension) I11.9
  - with
    - heart failure (congestive) I11.0
    - kidney disease (chronic) — *see* Hypertension, cardiorenal
- intracranial (benign) G93.2
- kidney I12.9
  - with
    - heart disease — *see* Hypertension, cardiorenal
    - stage 5 chronic kidney disease (CKD) or end stage renal disease (ESRD) I12.0
    - stage 1 through stage 4 chronic kidney disease I12.9
- lesser circulation I27.0
- newborn P29.2
  - pulmonary (persistent) P29.3
- ocular H40.0
- pancreatic duct—code to underlying condition
  - with chronic pancreatitis K86.1

© 2011 Ingenix

Hypertension, hypertensive —continued
- portal (due to chronic liver disease) (idiopathic) K76.6
  - gastropathy K31.89
  - in (due to) schistosomiasis (bilharziasis) B65.9 [K77]
- postoperative I97.3
- psychogenic F45.8
- pulmonary (artery) (secondary) NEC I27.2
  - of newborn (persistent) P29.3
  - primary (idiopathic) I27.Ø
- renal — see Hypertension, kidney
- renovascular I15.Ø
- secondary NEC I15.9
  - due to
    - endocrine disorders I15.2
    - pheochromocytoma I15.2
    - renal disorders NEC I15.1
      - arterial I15.Ø
    - renovascular disorders I15.Ø
  - specified NEC I15.8
- venous (chronic)
  - due to
    - deep vein thrombosis — see Syndrome, postthrombotic
  - idiopathic I87.3Ø9
    - with
      - inflammation I87.32-
        - with ulcer I87.33-
      - specified complication NEC I87.39-
      - ulcer I87.31-
        - with inflammation I87.33-
    - asymptomatic I87.3Ø-

Hypertensive urgency — see Hypertension

Hyperthecosis ovary E28.8

Hyperthermia (of unknown origin)(see also Hyperpyrexia)
- malignant, due to anesthesia T88.3
- newborn P81.9
  - environmental P81.Ø

Hyperthyroid (recurrent) — see Hyperthyroidism

Hyperthyroidism (latent) (pre-adult) (recurrent) EØ5.9Ø
- with
  - goiter (diffuse) EØ5.ØØ
    - with thyroid storm EØ5.Ø1
    - nodular (multinodular) EØ5.2Ø
      - with thyroid storm EØ5.21
      - uninodular EØ5.1Ø
        - with thyroid storm EØ5.11
  - storm EØ5.91
- due to ectopic thyroid tissue EØ5.3Ø
  - with thyroid storm EØ5.31
- neonatal, transitory P72.1
- specified NEC EØ5.8Ø
  - with thyroid storm EØ5.81

Hypertony, hypertonia, hypertonicity
- bladder N31.8
- congenital P94.1
- stomach K31.89
  - psychogenic F45.8
- uterus, uterine (contractions) (complicating delivery) O62.4

Hypertrichosis L68.9
- congenital Q84.2
- eyelid HØ2.869
  - left HØ2.866
    - lower HØ2.865
    - upper HØ2.864
  - right HØ2.863
    - lower HØ2.862
    - upper HØ2.861
- lanuginosa Q84.2
  - acquired L68.1
- localized L68.2
- specified NEC L68.8

Hypertriglyceridemia, essential E78.1

Hypertrophy, hypertrophic
- adenofibromatous, prostate — see Enlargement, enlarged, prostate
- adenoids (infective) J35.2
  - with tonsils J35.3
- adrenal cortex E27.8

Hypertrophy, hypertrophic—continued
- alveolar process or ridge — see Anomaly, alveolar
- anal papillae K62.8
- artery I77.89
  - congenital NEC Q27.8
    - digestive system Q27.8
    - lower limb Q27.8
    - specified site NEC Q27.8
    - upper limb Q27.8
- auricular — see Hypertrophy, cardiac
- Bartholin's gland N75.8
- bile duct (common) (hepatic) K83.8
- bladder (sphincter) (trigone) N32.89
- bone M89.3Ø
  - carpus M89.34-
  - clavicle M89.31-
  - femur M89.35-
  - fibula M89.36-
  - finger M89.34-
  - humerus M89.32-
  - ilium M89.359
  - ischium M89.359
  - metacarpus M89.34-
  - metatarsus M89.37-
  - multiple sites M89.39
  - neck M89.38
  - radius M89.33-
  - rib M89.38
  - scapula M89.31-
  - skull M89.38
  - tarsus M89.37-
  - tibia M89.36-
  - toe M89.37-
  - ulna M89.33-
  - vertebra M89.38
- brain G93.89
- breast N62
  - cystic — see Mastopathy, cystic
  - newborn P83.4
  - pubertal, massive N62
  - puerperal, postpartum — see Disorder, breast, specified type NEC
  - senile (parenchymatous) N62
- cardiac (chronic) (idiopathic) I51.7
  - with rheumatic fever (conditions in IØØ)
    - active IØ1.8
    - inactive or quiescent (with chorea) IØ9.89
  - congenital NEC Q24.8
  - fatty — see Degeneration, myocardial
  - hypertensive — see Hypertension, heart
  - rheumatic (with chorea) IØ9.89
    - active or acute IØ1.8
      - with chorea IØ2.Ø
  - valve — see Endocarditis
- cartilage — see Disorder, cartilage, specified type NEC
- cecum — see Megacolon
- cervix (uteri) N88.8
  - congenital Q51.828
  - elongation N88.4
- clitoris (cirrhotic) N9Ø.89
  - congenital Q52.6
- colon (see also Megacolon)
  - congenital Q43.2
- conjunctiva, lymphoid H11.89
- corpora cavernosa N48.89
- cystic duct K82.8
- duodenum K31.89
- endometrium (glandular) (see also Hyperplasia, endometrial) N85.ØØ
  - cervix N88.8
- epididymis N5Ø.8
- esophageal hiatus (congenital) Q79.1
  - with hernia — see Hernia, hiatal
- eyelid — see Disorder, eyelid, specified type NEC
- fat pad E65
  - knee (infrapatellar) (popliteal) (prepatellar) (retropatellar) M79.4
- foot (congenital) Q74.2
- frenulum, frenum (tongue) K14.8
  - lip K13.Ø
- gallbladder K82.8

Hypertrophy, hypertrophic—continued
- gastric mucosa K29.6Ø
  - with bleeding K29.61
- gland, glandular R59.9
  - generalized R59.1
  - localized R59.Ø
- gum (mucous membrane) KØ6.1
- heart (idiopathic) (see also Hypertrophy, cardiac)
  - valve (see also Endocarditis) I38
- hemifacial Q67.4
- hepatic — see Hypertrophy, liver
- hiatus (esophageal) Q79.1
- hilus gland R59.Ø
- hymen, congenital Q52.4
- ileum K63.89
- intestine NEC K63.89
- jejunum K63.89
- kidney (compensatory) N28.81
  - congenital Q63.3
- labium (majus) (minus) N9Ø.6
- ligament — see Disorder, ligament
- lingual tonsil (infective) J35.1
  - with adenoids J35.3
- lip K13.Ø
  - congenital Q18.6
- liver R16.Ø
  - acute K76.8
  - congenital Q44.7
  - cirrhotic — see Cirrhosis, liver
  - fatty — see Fatty, liver
- lymph, lymphatic gland R59.9
  - generalized R59.1
  - localized R59.Ø
  - tuberculous — see Tuberculosis, lymph gland
- mammary gland — see Hypertrophy, breast
- Meckel's diverticulum (congenital) Q43.Ø
  - malignant — see Table of Neoplasms, small intestine, malignant
- median bar — see Hyperplasia, prostate
- meibomian gland — see Chalazion
- meniscus, knee, congenital Q74.1
- metatarsal head — see Hypertrophy, bone, metatarsus
- metatarsus — see Hypertrophy, bone, metatarsus
- mucous membrane
  - alveolar ridge KØ6.2
  - gum KØ6.1
  - nose (turbinate) J34.3
- muscle M62.89
- muscular coat, artery I77.89
- myocardium (see also Hypertrophy, cardiac)
  - idiopathic I42.2
- myometrium N85.2
- nail L6Ø.2
  - congenital Q84.5
- nasal J34.89
  - alae J34.89
  - bone J34.89
  - cartilage J34.89
  - mucous membrane (septum) J34.3
  - sinus J34.89
  - turbinate J34.3
- nasopharynx, lymphoid (infectional) (tissue) (wall) J35.2
- nipple N62
- organ or site, congenital NEC — see Anomaly, by site
- ovary N83.8
- palate (hard) M27.8
  - soft K13.79
- pancreas, congenital Q45.3
- parathyroid (gland) E21.Ø
- parotid gland K11.1
- penis N48.89
- pharyngeal tonsil J35.2
- pharynx J39.2
  - lymphoid (infectional) (tissue) (wall) J35.2
- pituitary (anterior) (fossa) (gland) E23.6
- prepuce (congenital) N47.8
  - female N9Ø.89
- prostate — see Enlargement, enlarged, prostate
  - congenital Q55.4
- pseudomuscular G71.Ø

Hypertrophy, hypertrophic—*continued*
pylorus (adult) (muscle) (sphincter) K31.1
congenital or infantile Q40.0
rectal, rectum (sphincter) K62.8
rhinitis (turbinate) J31.0
salivary gland (any) K11.1
congenital Q38.4
scaphoid (tarsal) — *see* Hypertrophy, bone, tarsus
scar L91.0
scrotum N50.8
seminal vesicle N50.8
sigmoid — *see* Megacolon
skin L91.9
specified NEC L91.8
spermatic cord N50.8
spleen — *see* Splenomegaly
spondylitis — *see* Spondylosis
stomach K31.89
sublingual gland K11.1
submandibular gland K11.1
suprarenal cortex (gland) E27.8
synovial NEC M67.20
acromioclavicular M67.21-
ankle M67.27-
elbow M67.22-
foot M67.27-
hand M67.24-
hip M67.25-
knee M67.26-
multiple sites M67.29
specified site NEC M67.28
wrist M67.23-
tendon — *see* Disorder, tendon, specified type NEC
testis N44.8
congenital Q55.29
thymic, thymus (gland) (congenital) E32.0
thyroid (gland) — *see* Goiter
toe (congenital) Q74.2
acquired (*see also* Deformity, toe, specified NEC)
tongue K14.8
congenital Q38.2
papillae (foliate) K14.3
tonsils (faucial) (infective) (lingual) (lymphoid) J35.1
with adenoids J35.3
tunica vaginalis N50.8
ureter N28.89
urethra N36.8
uterus N85.2
neck (with elongation) N88.4
puerperal O90.89
uvula K13.79
vagina N89.8
vas deferens N50.8
vein I87.8
ventricle, ventricular (heart) (*see also* Hypertrophy, cardiac)
congenital Q24.8
in tetralogy of Fallot Q21.3
verumontanum N36.8
vocal cord J38.3
vulva N90.6
stasis (nonfilarial) N90.6
Hypertropia H50.2-
Hypertyrosinemia E70.21
Hyperuricemia (asymptomatic) E79.0
Hypervalinemia E71.19
Hyperventilation (tetany) R06.4
hysterical F45.8
psychogenic F45.8
syndrome F45.8
Hypervitaminosis (dietary) NEC E67.8
A E67.0
administered as drug (prolonged intake) — *see* Table of Drugs and Chemicals, vitamins, adverse effect
overdose or wrong substance given or taken — *see* Table of Drugs and Chemicals, vitamins, poisoning
B6 E67.2
D E67.3
administered as drug (prolonged intake) — *see* Table of Drugs and Chemicals, vitamins, adverse effect

Hypervitaminosis—*continued*
D E67.3—*continued*
overdose or wrong substance given or taken — *see* Table of Drugs and Chemicals, vitamins, poisoning
K E67.8
administered as drug (prolonged intake) — *see* Table of Drugs and Chemicals, vitamins, adverse effect
overdose or wrong substance given or taken — *see* Table of Drugs and Chemicals, vitamins, poisoning
Hypervolemia E87.70
specified NEC E87.79
Hypesthesia R20.1
cornea — *see* Anesthesia, cornea
Hyphema H21.0-
traumatic S05.1-
Hypoacidity, gastric K31.89
psychogenic F45.8
Hypoadrenalism, hypoadrenia E27.40
primary E27.1
tuberculous A18.7
Hypoadrenocorticism E27.40
pituitary E23.0
primary E27.1
Hypoalbuminemia E88.09
Hypoaldosteronism E27.40
Hypoalphalipoproteinemia E78.6
Hypobarism T70.29
Hypobaropathy T70.29
Hypobetalipoproteinemia (familial) E78.6
Hypocalcemia E83.51
dietary E58
neonatal P71.1
due to cow's milk P71.0
phosphate-loading (newborn) P71.1
Hypochloremia E87.8
Hypochlorhydria K31.89
neurotic F45.8
psychogenic F45.8
Hypochondria, hypochondriac, hypochondriasis (reaction) F45.21
sleep F51.03
Hypochondrogenesis Q77.0
Hypochondroplasia Q77.4
Hypochromasia, blood cells D50.8
Hypodontia — *see* Anodontia
Hypoeosinophilia D72.89
Hypoesthesia R20.1
Hypofibrinogenemia D68.8
acquired D65
congenital (hereditary) D68.2
Hypofunction
adrenocortical E27.40
drug-induced E27.3
postprocedural E89.6
primary E27.1
adrenomedullary, postprocedural E89.6
cerebral R29.81
corticoadrenal NEC E27.49
intestinal K59.8
labyrinth — *see* subcategory H83.2
ovary E28.39
pituitary (gland) (anterior) E23.0
testicular E29.1
postprocedural (postsurgical) (postirradiation) (iatrogenic) E89.5
Hypogalactia O92.4
Hypogammaglobulinemia (*see also* Agammaglobulinemia) D80.1
hereditary D80.0
nonfamilial D80.1
transient, of infancy D80.7
Hypogenitalism (congenital) — *see* Hypogonadism
Hypoglossia Q38.3
Hypoglycemia (spontaneous) E16.2
coma E15
diabetic — *see* Diabetes, coma
diabetic — *see* Diabetes, hypoglycemia
dietary counseling and surveillance Z71.3
drug-induced E16.0
with coma (nondiabetic) E15

Hypoglycemia—*continued*
due to insulin E16.0
with coma (nondiabetic) E15
therapeutic misadventure — *see* subcategory T38.3
functional, nonhyperinsulinemic E16.1
iatrogenic E16.0
with coma (nondiabetic) E15
in infant of diabetic mother P70.1
gestational diabetes P70.0
infantile E16.1
leucine-induced E71.19
neonatal (transitory) P70.4
iatrogenic P70.3
reactive (not drug-induced) E16.1
transitory neonatal P70.4
Hypogonadism
female E28.39
hypogonadotropic E23.0
male E29.1
ovarian (primary) E28.39
pituitary E23.0
testicular (primary) E29.1
Hypohidrosis, hypoidrosis L74.4
Hypoinsulinemia, postprocedural E89.1
Hypokalemia E87.6
Hypoleukocytosis — *see* Agranulocytosis
Hypolipoproteinemia (alpha) (beta) E78.6
Hypomagnesemia E83.42
neonatal P71.2
Hypomania, hypomanic reaction F30.8
Hypomenorrhea — *see* Oligomenorrhea
Hypometabolism R63.8
Hypomotility
gastrointestinal (tract) K31.89
psychogenic F45.8
intestine K59.8
psychogenic F45.8
stomach K31.89
psychogenic F45.8
Hyponasality R49.22
Hyponatremia E87.1
Hypo-osmolality E87.1
Hypo-ovarianism, hypo-ovarism E28.39
Hypoparathyroidism E20.9
familial E20.8
idiopathic E20.0
neonatal, transitory P71.4
postprocedural E89.2
specified NEC E20.8
Hypoperfusion (in)
newborn P96.89
Hypopharyngitis — *see* Laryngopharyngitis
Hypophoria H50.53
Hypophosphatemia, hypophosphatasia (acquired) (congenital) (renal) E83.39
familial E83.31
Hypophyseal, hypophysis (*see also* condition)
dwarfism E23.0
gigantism E22.0
Hypopiesis — *see* Hypotension
Hypopinealism E34.8
Hypopituitarism (juvenile) E23.0
drug-induced E23.1
due to
hypophysectomy E89.3
radiotherapy E89.3
iatrogenic NEC E23.1
postirradiation E89.3
postpartum E23.0
postprocedural E89.3
Hypoplasia, hypoplastic
adrenal (gland), congenital Q89.1
alimentary tract, congenital Q45.8
upper Q40.8
anus, anal (canal) Q42.3
with fistula Q42.2
aorta, aortic Q25.4
ascending, in hypoplastic left heart syndrome Q23.4
valve Q23.1
in hypoplastic left heart syndrome Q23.4
areola, congenital Q83.8

Hypoplasia, hypoplastic—*continued*
  arm (congenital) — *see* Defect, reduction, upper limb
  artery (peripheral) Q27.8
    brain (congenital) Q28.3
    coronary Q24.5
    digestive system Q27.8
    lower limb Q27.8
    pulmonary Q25.7
      functional, unilateral J43.0
    retinal (congenital) Q14.1
    specified site NEC Q27.8
    umbilical Q27.0
    upper limb Q27.8
  auditory canal Q17.8
    causing impairment of hearing Q16.9
  biliary duct or passage Q44.5
  bone NOS Q79.9
    face Q75.8
    marrow D61.9
      megakaryocytic D69.49
    skull — *see* Hypoplasia, skull
  brain Q02
    gyri Q04.3
    part of Q04.3
  breast (areola) N64.82
  bronchus Q32.4
  cardiac Q24.8
  carpus — *see* Defect, reduction, upper limb, specified type NEC
  cartilage hair Q78.5
  cecum Q42.8
  cementum K00.4
  cephalic Q02
  cerebellum Q04.3
  cervix (uteri), congenital Q51.821
  clavicle (congenital) Q74.0
  coccyx Q76.49
  colon Q42.9
    specified NEC Q42.8
  corpus callosum Q04.0
  cricoid cartilage Q31.2
  digestive organ(s) or tract NEC Q45.8
    upper (congenital) Q40.8
  ear (auricle) (lobe) Q17.2
    middle Q16.4
  enamel of teeth (neonatal) (postnatal) (prenatal) K00.4
  endocrine (gland) NEC Q89.2
  endometrium N85.8
  epididymis (congenital) Q55.4
  epiglottis Q31.2
  erythroid, congenital D61.09
  esophagus (congenital) Q39.8
  eustachian tube Q17.8
  eye Q11.2
  eyelid (congenital) Q10.3
  face Q18.8
    bone(s) Q75.8
  femur (congenital) — *see* Defect, reduction, lower limb, specified type NEC
  fibula (congenital) — *see* Defect, reduction, lower limb, specified type NEC
  finger (congenital) — *see* Defect, reduction, upper limb, specified type NEC
  focal dermal Q82.8
  foot — *see* Defect, reduction, lower limb, specified type NEC
  gallbladder Q44.0
  genitalia, genital organ(s)
    female, congenital Q52.8
      external Q52.79
      internal NEC Q52.8
    in adiposogenital dystrophy E23.6
  glottis Q31.2
  hair Q84.2
  hand (congenital) — *see* Defect, reduction, upper limb, specified type NEC
  heart Q24.8
  humerus (congenital) — *see* Defect, reduction, upper limb, specified type NEC

Hypoplasia, hypoplastic—*continued*
  intestine (small) Q41.9
    large Q42.9
      specified NEC Q42.8
  jaw M26.09
    alveolar M26.79
    lower M26.04
      alveolar M26.74
    upper M26.02
      alveolar M26.73
  kidney(s) Q60.5
    bilateral Q60.4
    unilateral Q60.3
  labium (majus) (minus), congenital Q52.79
  larynx Q31.2
  left heart syndrome Q23.4
  leg (congenital) — *see* Defect, reduction, lower limb
  limb Q73.8
    lower (congenital) — *see* Defect, reduction, lower limb
    upper (congenital) — *see* Defect, reduction, upper limb
  liver Q44.7
  lung (lobe) (not associated with short gestation) Q33.6
    associated with immaturity, low birth weight, prematurity, or short gestation P28.0
  mammary (areola), congenital Q83.8
  mandible, mandibular M26.04
    alveolar M26.74
    unilateral condylar M27.8
  maxillary M26.02
    alveolar M26.73
  medullary D61.9
  megakaryocytic D69.49
  metacarpus — *see* Defect, reduction, upper limb, specified type NEC
  metatarsus — *see* Defect, reduction, lower limb, specified type NEC
  muscle Q79.8
  nail(s) Q84.6
  nose, nasal Q30.1
  optic nerve H47.03-
  osseous meatus (ear) Q17.8
  ovary, congenital Q50.39
  pancreas Q45.0
  parathyroid (gland) Q89.2
  parotid gland Q38.4
  patella Q74.1
  pelvis, pelvic girdle Q74.2
  penis (congenital) Q55.62
  peripheral vascular system Q27.8
    digestive system Q27.8
    lower limb Q27.8
    specified site NEC Q27.8
    upper limb Q27.8
  pituitary (gland) (congenital) Q89.2
  pulmonary (not associated with short gestation) Q33.6
    artery, functional J43.0
    associated with short gestation P28.0
  radioulnar — *see* Defect, reduction, upper limb, specified type NEC
  radius — *see* Defect, reduction, upper limb
  rectum Q42.1
    with fistula Q42.0
  respiratory system NEC Q34.8
  rib Q76.6
  right heart syndrome Q22.6
  sacrum Q76.49
  scapula Q74.2
  scrotum Q55.1
  shoulder girdle Q74.0
  skin Q82.8
  skull (bone) Q75.8
    with
      anencephaly Q00.0
      encephalocele — *see* Encephalocele
      hydrocephalus Q03.9
        with spina bifida — *see* Spina bifida, by site, with hydrocephalus
      microcephaly Q02
  spinal (cord) (ventral horn cell) Q06.1

Hypoplasia, hypoplastic—*continued*
  spine Q76.49
  sternum Q76.7
  tarsus — *see* Defect, reduction, lower limb, specified type NEC
  testis Q55.1
  thymic, with immunodeficiency D82.1
  thymus (gland) Q89.2
    with immunodeficiency D82.1
  thyroid (gland) E03.1
    cartilage Q31.2
  tibiofibular (congenital) — *see* Defect, reduction, lower limb, specified type NEC
  toe — *see* Defect, reduction, lower limb, specified type NEC
  tongue Q38.3
  Turner's K00.4
  ulna (congenital) — *see* Defect, reduction, upper limb
  umbilical artery Q27.0
  unilateral condylar M27.8
  ureter Q62.8
  uterus, congenital Q51.811
  vagina Q52.4
  vascular NEC peripheral Q27.8
    brain Q28.3
    digestive system Q27.8
    lower limb Q27.8
    specified site NEC Q27.8
    upper limb Q27.8
  vein(s) (peripheral) Q27.8
    brain Q28.3
    digestive system Q27.8
    great Q26.8
    lower limb Q27.8
    specified site NEC Q27.8
    upper limb Q27.8
  vena cava (inferior) (superior) Q26.8
  vertebra Q76.49
  vulva, congenital Q52.79
  zonule (ciliary) Q12.8
Hypopotassemia E87.6
Hypoproconvertinemia, congenital (hereditary) D68.2
Hypoproteinemia E77.8
Hypoprothrombinemia (congenital) (hereditary) (idiopathic) D68.2
  acquired D68.4
  newborn, transient P61.6
Hypoptyalism K11.7
Hypopyon (eye) (anterior chamber) — *see* Iridocyclitis, acute, hypopyon
Hypopyrexia R68.0
Hyporeflexia R29.2
Hyposecretion
  ACTH E23.0
  antidiuretic hormone E23.2
  ovary E28.39
  salivary gland (any) K11.7
  vasopressin E23.2
Hyposegmentation, leukocytic, hereditary D72.0
Hyposiderinemia D50.9
Hypospadias Q54.9
  balanic Q54.0
  coronal Q54.0
  glandular Q54.0
  penile Q54.1
  penoscrotal Q54.2
  perineal Q54.3
  specified NEC Q54.8
Hypospermatogenesis — *see* Oligospermia
Hyposplenism D73.0
Hypostasis pulmonary, passive — *see* Edema, lung
Hypostatic — *see* condition
Hyposthenuria N28.89
Hypotension (arterial) (constitutional) I95.9
  chronic I95.89
  due to (of) hemodialysis I95.3
  drug-induced I95.2
  iatrogenic I95.89
  idiopathic (permanent) I95.0
  intracranial, following ventricular shunting (ventriculostomy) G97.2

Hypotension—continued
  intra-dialytic I95.3
  maternal, syndrome (following labor and delivery)
      O26.5-
  neurogenic, orthostatic G90.3
  orthostatic (chronic) I95.1
    due to drugs I95.2
    neurogenic G90.3
  postoperative I95.81
  postural I95.1
  specified NEC I95.89
Hypothermia (accidental) T68
  due to anesthesia, anesthetic T88.51
  low environmental temperature T68
  neonatal P80.9
    environmental (mild) NEC P80.8
    mild P80.8
    severe (chronic) (cold injury syndrome) P80.0
    specified NEC P80.8
  not associated with low environmental temperature
      R68.0
Hypothyroidism (acquired) E03.9
  congenital (without goiter) E03.1
    with goiter (diffuse) E03.0
  due to
    exogenous substance NEC E03.2
    iodine-deficiency, acquired E01.8
      subclinical E02
    irradiation therapy E89.0
    medicament NEC E03.2
    P-aminosalicylic acid (PAS) E03.2
    phenylbutazone E03.2
    resorcinol E03.2
    sulfonamide E03.2
    surgery E89.0
    thiourea group drugs E03.2
  iatrogenic NEC E03.2
  iodine-deficiency (acquired) E01.8
  congenital — see Syndrome, iodine deficiency,
      congenital
    subclinical E02
  neonatal, transitory P72.2
  postinfectious E03.3
  postirradiation E89.0
  postprocedural E89.0
  postsurgical E89.0
  specified NEC E03.8
  subclinical, iodine-deficiency related E02
Hypotonia, hypotonicity, hypotony
  bladder N31.2
  congenital (benign) P94.2
  eye — see Disorder, globe, hypotony
Hypotrichosis — see Alopecia
Hypotropia H50.2-
Hypoventilation R06.89
  congenital central alveolar G47.35
  sleep related
    idiopathic nonobstructive alveolar G47.34
    in conditions classified elsewhere G47.36
Hypovitaminosis — see Deficiency, vitamin
Hypovolemia E86.1
  surgical shock T81.1
  traumatic (shock) T79.4
Hypoxemia R09.02
  newborn P84
  sleep related, in conditions classified elsewhere
      G47.36
Hypoxia (see also Anoxia) R09.01
  cerebral, during a procedure NEC G97.81
    postprocedural NEC G97.82
  intrauterine P84
  myocardial — see Insufficiency, coronary
  newborn P84
  sleep-related G47.34
Hypsarhythmia — see Epilepsy, generalized, specified
      NEC
Hysteralgia, pregnant uterus O26.89-
Hysteria, hysterical (conversion) (dissociative state)
      F44.9
  anxiety F41.8
  convulsions F44.5
  psychosis, acute F44.9
Hysteroepilepsy F44.5

I

Ichthyoparasitism due to Vandellia cirrhosa B88.8
Ichthyosis (congenital) Q80.9
  acquired L85.0
  fetalis Q80.4
  hystrix Q80.8
  lamellar Q80.2
  lingual K13.29
  palmaris and plantaris Q82.8
  simplex Q80.0
  vera Q80.8
  vulgaris Q80.0
  X-linked Q80.1
Ichthyotoxism — see Poisoning, fish
  bacterial — see Intoxication, foodborne
Icteroanemia, hemolytic (acquired) D59.9
  congenital — see Spherocytosis
Icterus (see also Jaundice)
  conjunctiva R17
  newborn P59.9
  gravis, newborn P55.0
  hematogenous (acquired) D59.9
  hemolytic (acquired) D59.9
    congenital — see Spherocytosis
  hemorrhagic (acute) (leptospiral) (spirochetal) A27.0
    newborn P53
  infectious B15.9
    with hepatic coma B15.0
    leptospiral A27.0
    spirochetal A27.0
  neonatorum — see Jaundice, newborn
  spirochetal A27.0
Ictus solaris, solis T67.0
Ideation
  homicidal R45.850
  suicidal R45.851
Identity disorder (child) F64.9
  gender role F64.2
  psychosexual F64.2
Id reaction (due to bacteria) L30.2
Idioglossia F80.0
Idiopathic — see condition
Idiot, idiocy (congenital) F73
  amaurotic (Bielschowsky(-Jansky)) (family)
      (infantile) (late)) (juvenile (late))
      (Vogt-Spielmeyer) E75.4
  microcephalic Q02
IgE asthma J45.909
Ileitis (chronic) (noninfectious) (see also Enteritis) K52.9
  backwash — see Pancolitis, ulcerative (chronic)
  infectious A09
  regional (ulcerative) — see Enteritis, regional, small
      intestine
  segmental — see Enteritis, regional
  terminal (ulcerative) — see Enteritis, regional, small
      intestine
Ileocolitis (see also Enteritis) K52.9
  regional — see Enteritis, regional
  infectious A09
Ileostomy
  attention to Z43.2
  malfunctioning K94.13
  status Z93.2
    with complication — see Complications,
        enterostomy
Ileotyphus — see Typhoid
Ileum — see condition
Ileus (bowel) (colon) (inhibitory) (intestine) K56.7
  adynamic K56.0
  due to gallstone (in intestine) K56.3
  duodenal (chronic) K31.5
  gallstone K56.3
  mechanical NEC K56.69
  meconium P76.0
    in cystic fibrosis E84.11
    meaning meconium plug (without cystic fibrosis)
        P76.0
  myxedema K59.8
  neurogenic K56.0
    Hirschsprung's disease or megacolon Q43.1

Ileus—continued
  newborn
    due to meconium P76.0
      in cystic fibrosis E84.11
      meaning meconium plug (without cystic
          fibrosis) P76.0
    transitory P76.1
  obstructive K56.69
  paralytic K56.0
Iliac — see condition
Iliotibial band syndrome M76.3-
Illiteracy Z55.0
Illness (see also Disease) R69
  manic-depressive — see Disorder, bipolar
Imbalance R26.89
  autonomic G90.8
  constituents of food intake E63.1
  electrolyte E87.8
    with molar pregnancy O08.5
    due to hyperemesis gravidarum O21.1
    following ectopic or molar pregnancy O08.5
    neonatal, transitory NEC P74.4
      potassium P74.3
      sodium P74.2
  endocrine E34.9
  eye muscle NOS H50.9
  hormone E34.9
  hysterical F44.4
  labyrinth — see subcategory H83.2
  posture R29.3
  protein-energy — see Malnutrition
  sympathetic G90.8
Imbecile, imbecility (I.Q. 35-49) F71
Imbedding, intrauterine device T83.39
Imbibition, cholesterol (gallbladder) K82.4
Imbrication, teeth,, fully erupted M26.30
Imerslund (-Gräsbeck) **syndrome** D51.1
Immature (see also Immaturity)
  birth (less than 37 completed weeks) see Preterm
      infant, newborn
    extremely (less than 28 completed weeks) — see
        Immaturity, extreme
  personality F60.89
Immaturity (less than 37 completed weeks) — see
      Preterm infant, newborn
  extreme P07.20
    with gestation of:
      less than 24 weeks P07.21
      24-26 weeks P07.22
      27 weeks P07.23
  fetus or infant light-for-dates — see Light-for-dates
  lung, newborn P28.0
  organ or site NEC — see Hypoplasia
  pulmonary, newborn P28.0
  reaction F60.89
  sexual (female) (male), after puberty E30.0
Immersion T75.1
  hand T69.01-
  foot T69.02-
Immobile, immobility
  complete, due to severe physical disability or frailty
      R53.2
  intestine K59.8
  syndrome (paraplegic) M62.3
Immune reconstitution (inflammatory) syndrome
      [IRIS] D89.3
Immunization (see also Vaccination)
  ABO — see Incompatibility, ABO
    in newborn P55.1
  complication — see Complications, vaccination
  not done (not carried out) Z28.9
    because (of)
      contraindication NEC Z28.09
  encounter for Z23
    acute illness of patient Z28.01
    allergy to vaccine (or component) Z28.04
    caregiver refusal Z28.82
    chronic illness of patient Z28.02
    group pressure Z28.1
    guardian refusal Z28.82
    immune compromised state of patient Z28.03
    parent refusal Z28.82
    patient's belief Z28.1

Immunization —*continued*
  encounter for—*continued*
    patient had disease being vaccinated against
        Z28.81
    patient refusal Z28.21
    religious beliefs of patient Z28.1
    specified reason NEC Z28.89
      of patient Z28.29
    unspecified patient reason Z28.20
  Rh factor
    affecting management of pregnancy NEC
        O36.09-
      anti-D antibody O36.01-
    from transfusion — *see* Complication(s)
        transfusion, incompatibility reaction, Rh
        (factor)
Immunocytoma — *see* Lymphoma, non-Hodgkin's,
    diffuse, small cell
Immunodeficiency D84.9
  with
    adenosine-deaminase deficiency D81.3
    antibody defects D80.9
      specified type NEC D80.8
    hyperimmunoglobulinemia D80.6
    increased immunoglobulin M (IgM) D80.5
    major defect D82.9
      specified type NEC D82.8
    partial albinism D82.8
    short-limbed stature D82.2
    thrombocytopenia and eczema D82.0
  antibody with
    hyperimmunoglobulinemia D80.6
    near-normal immunoglobulins D80.6
  autosomal recessive, Swiss type D80.0
  combined D81.9
    biotin-dependent carboxylase D81.819
      biotinidase D81.810
      holocarboxylase synthetase D81.818
      specified type NEC D81.818
    severe (SCID) D81.9
      with
        low or normal B-cell numbers D81.2
        low T- and B-cell numbers D81.1
        reticular dysgenesis D81.0
      specified type NEC D81.89
  common variable D83.9
    with
      abnormalities of B-cell numbers and function
          D83.0
      autoantibodies to B- or T-cells D83.2
      immunoregulatory T-cell disorders D83.1
    specified type NEC D83.8
  following hereditary defective response to
      Epstein-Barr virus (EBV) D82.3
  selective, immunoglobulin
    A (IgA) D80.2
    G (IgG) (subclasses) D80.3
    M (IgM) D80.4
  severe combined (SCID) D81.9
  specified type NEC D84.8
  X-linked, with increased IgM D80.5
Immunotherapy (encounter for)
  antineoplastic Z51.12
Impaction, impacted
  bowel, colon, rectum (*see also* Impaction, fecal)
      K56.49
    by gallstone K56.3
  calculus — *see* Calculus
  cerumen (ear) (external) H61.2-
  cuspid — *see* Impaction, tooth
  dental (same or adjacent tooth) K01.1
  fecal, feces K56.41
  fracture — *see* Fracture, by site
  gallbladder — *see* Calculus, gallbladder
  gallstone(s) — *see* Calculus, gallbladder
    bile duct (common) (hepatic) — *see* Calculus, bile
        duct
    cystic duct — *see* Calculus, gallbladder
    in intestine, with obstruction (any part) K56.3
  intestine (calculous) NEC *see also* impaction, fecal
      K56.49
    gallstone, with ileus K56.3
  intrauterine device (IUD) T83.39

Impaction, impacted—*continued*
  molar — *see* Impaction, tooth
  shoulder, causing obstructed labor O66.0
  tooth, teeth K01.1
  turbinate J34.89
Impaired, impairment (function)
  auditory discrimination — *see* Abnormal, auditory
      perception
  cognitive, mild, so stated G31.84
  dual sensory Z73.82
  fasting glucose R73.01
  glucose tolerance (oral) R73.02
  hearing — *see* Deafness
  heart — *see* Disease, heart
  kidney N28.9
    disorder resulting from N25.9
      specified NEC N25.89
  liver K72.90
    with coma K72.91
  mastication K08.8
  mild cognitive, so stated G31.84
  mobility
    ear ossicles — *see* Ankylosis, ear ossicles
    requiring care provider Z74.09
  myocardium, myocardial — *see* Insufficiency,
      myocardial
  rectal sphincter R19.8
  renal (acute) (chronic) N28.9
    disorder resulting from N25.9
      specified NEC N25.89
  vision NEC H54.7
    both eyes H54.3
Impediment, speech R47.9
  psychogenic (childhood) F98.8
  slurring R47.81
  specified NEC R47.89
Impending
  coronary syndrome I20.0
  delirium tremens F10.239
  myocardial infarction I20.0
Imperception auditory (acquired) (*see also* Deafness)
  congenital H93.25
Imperfect
  aeration, lung (newborn) NEC — *see* Atelectasis
  closure (congenital)
    alimentary tract NEC Q45.8
      lower Q43.8
      upper Q40.8
    atrioventricular ostium Q21.2
    atrium (secundum) Q21.1
    branchial cleft or sinus Q18.0
    choroid Q14.3
    cricoid cartilage Q31.8
    cusps, heart valve NEC Q24.8
      pulmonary Q22.3
    ductus
      arteriosus Q25.0
      Botalli Q25.0
    ear drum (causing impairment of hearing) Q16.4
    esophagus with communication to bronchus or
        trachea Q39.1
    eyelid Q10.3
    foramen
      botalli Q21.1
      ovale Q21.1
    genitalia, genital organ(s) or system
      female Q52.8
        external Q52.79
        internal NEC Q52.8
      male Q55.8
    glottis Q31.8
    interatrial ostium or septum Q21.1
    interauricular ostium or septum Q21.1
    interventricular ostium or septum Q21.0
    larynx Q31.8
    lip — *see* Cleft, lip
    nasal septum Q30.3
    nose Q30.2
    omphalomesenteric duct Q43.0
    optic nerve entry Q14.2
    organ or site not listed — *see* Anomaly, by site

Imperfect—*continued*
  closure—*continued*
    ostium
      interatrial Q21.1
      interauricular Q21.1
      interventricular Q21.0
    palate — *see* Cleft, palate
    preauricular sinus Q18.1
    retina Q14.1
    roof of orbit Q75.8
    sclera Q13.5
    septum
      aorticopulmonary Q21.4
      atrial (secundum) Q21.1
      between aorta and pulmonary artery Q21.4
      heart Q21.9
      interatrial (secundum) Q21.1
      interauricular (secundum) Q21.1
      interventricular Q21.0
        in tetralogy of Fallot Q21.3
      nasal Q30.3
      ventricular Q21.0
        with pulmonary stenosis or atresia,
            dextraposition of aorta, and
            hypertrophy of right ventricle Q21.3
        in tetralogy of Fallot Q21.3
    skull Q75.0
      with
        anencephaly Q00.0
        encephalocele — *see* Encephalocele
        hydrocephalus Q03.9
          with spina bifida — *see* Spina bifida,
              by site, with hydrocephalus
        microcephaly Q02
      spine (with meningocele) — *see* Spina bifida
    trachea Q32.1
    tympanic membrane (causing impairment of
        hearing) Q16.4
    uterus Q51.818
    vitelline duct Q43.0
  erection — *see* Dysfunction, sexual, male, erectile
  fusion — *see* Imperfect, closure
  inflation, lung (newborn) — *see* Atelectasis
  posture R29.3
  rotation, intestine Q43.3
  septum, ventricular Q21.0
Imperfectly descended testis — *see* Cryptorchid
Imperforate (congenital) (*see also* Atresia)
  anus Q42.3
    with fistula Q42.2
  cervix (uteri) Q51.828
  esophagus Q39.0
    with tracheoesophageal fistula Q39.1
  hymen Q52.3
  jejunum Q41.1
  pharynx Q38.8
  rectum Q42.1
    with fistula Q42.0
  urethra Q64.39
  vagina Q52.4
Impervious (congenital) (*see also* Atresia)
  anus Q42.3
    with fistula Q42.2
  bile duct Q44.2
  esophagus Q39.0
    with tracheoesophageal fistula Q39.1
  intestine (small) Q41.9
    large Q42.9
      specified NEC Q42.8
  rectum Q42.1
    with fistula Q42.0
  ureter — *see* Atresia, ureter
  urethra Q64.39
Impetiginization of dermatoses L01.1
Impetigo (any organism) (any site) (circinate)
    (contagiosa) (simplex) (vulgaris) L01.00
  Bockhart's L01.02
  bullous, bullosa L01.03
  external ear L01.00 [H62.40]
  follicularis L01.02
  furfuracea L30.5
  herpetiformis L40.1
    nonobstetrical L40.1

Impetigo—continued
  neonatorum L01.03
  nonbullous L01.01
  specified type NEC L01.09
  ulcerative L01.09
Impingement (on teeth)
  soft tissue
    anterior M26.81
    posterior M26.82
Implant, endometrial N80.9
Implantation
  anomalous — see Anomaly, by site
    ureter Q62.63
  cyst
    external area or site (skin) NEC L72.0
    iris — see Cyst, iris, implantation
    vagina N89.8
    vulva N90.7
  dermoid (cyst) — see Implantation, cyst
Impotence (sexual) N52.9
  counseling Z70.1
  organic origin (see also Dysfunction, sexual, male,
    erectile) N52.9
  psychogenic F52.21
Impression, basilar Q75.8
Imprisonment, anxiety concerning Z65.1
Improper care (child) (newborn) — see Neglect
Improperly tied umbilical cord (causing
  hemorrhage) P51.8
Impulsiveness (impulsive) R45.87
Inability to swallow — see Aphagia
Inaccessible, inaccessibility
  health care NEC Z75.3
    due to
      waiting period Z75.2
        for admission to facility elsewhere Z75.1
    other helping agencies Z75.4
Inactive — see condition
Inadequate, inadequacy
  aesthetics of dental restoration K08.56
  biologic, constitutional, functional, or social F60.7
  development
    child R62.50
    genitalia
      after puberty NEC E30.0
      congenital
        female Q52.8
          external Q52.79
          internal Q52.8
        male Q55.8
    lungs Q33.6
      associated with short gestation P28.0
    organ or site not listed — see Anomaly, by site
  diet (causing nutritional deficiency) E63.9
  eating habits Z72.4
  environment, household Z59.1
  family support Z63.8
  food (supply) NEC Z59.4
    hunger effects T73.0
  functional F60.7
  household care, due to
    family member
      handicapped or ill Z74.2
      on vacation Z75.5
      temporarily away from home Z74.2
    technical defects in home Z59.1
    temporary absence from home of person
      rendering care Z74.2
  housing (heating) (space) Z59.1
  income (financial) Z59.6
  intrafamilial communication Z63.8
  material resources Z59.9
  mental — see Retardation, mental
  parental supervision or control of child Z62.0
  personality F60.7
  pulmonary
    function R06.89
      newborn P28.5
    ventilation, newborn P28.5
  sample of cytologic smear
    anus R85.615
    cervix R87.615
    vagina R87.625

Inadequate, inadequacy—continued
  social F60.7
    insurance Z59.7
    skills NEC Z73.4
  supervision of child by parent Z62.0
  teaching affecting education Z55.8
  welfare support Z59.7
Inanition R64
  with edema — see Malnutrition, severe
  due to
    deprivation of food T73.0
    malnutrition — see Malnutrition
  fever R50.9
Inappropriate
  diet or eating habits Z72.4
  secretion
    antidiuretic hormone (ADH) (excessive) E22.2
      deficiency E23.2
    pituitary (posterior) E22.2
Inattention at or after birth — see Neglect
Incarceration, incarcerated
  enterocele K46.0
    gangrenous K46.1
  epiplocele K46.0
    gangrenous K46.1
  exophthalmos K42.0
    gangrenous K42.1
  hernia (see also Hernia, by site, with obstruction)
    with gangrene — see Hernia, by site, with
      gangrene
  iris, in wound — see Injury, eye, laceration, with
    prolapse
  lens, in wound — see Injury, eye, laceration, with
    prolapse
  omphalocele K42.0
  prison, anxiety concerning Z65.1
  rupture — see Hernia, by site
  sarcoepiplocele K46.0
    gangrenous K46.1
  sarcoepiplomphalocele K42.0
    with gangrene K42.1
  uterus N85.8
    gravid O34.51-
      causing obstructed labor O65.5
Incised wound
  external — see Laceration
  internal organs — see Injury, by site
Incision, incisional
  hernia — see Hernia, ventral
  surgical, complication — see Complications, surgical
    procedure
  traumatic
    external — see Laceration
    internal organs — see Injury, by site
Inclusion
  azurophilic leukocytic D72.0
  blennorrhea (neonatal) (newborn) P39.1
  gallbladder in liver (congenital) Q44.1
Incompatibility
  ABO
    affecting management of pregnancy O36.11-
      anti-A sensitization O36.11-
      anti-B sensitization O36.19-
      specified NEC O36.19-
    infusion or transfusion reaction — see
      Complication(s), transfusion,
      incompatibility reaction, ABO
    newborn P55.1
  blood (group) (Duffy) (K(ell)) (Kidd) (Lewis) (M) (S)
    NEC
    affecting management of pregnancy O36.11-
      anti-A sensitization O36.11-
      anti-B sensitization O36.19-
    infusion or transfusion reaction T80.89
    newborn P55.8
  divorce or estrangement Z63.5
  Rh (blood group) (factor) Z31.82
    affecting management of pregnancy NEC
      O36.09-
      anti-D antibody O36.01-
    infusion or transfusion reaction — see
      Complication(s), transfusion,
      incompatibility reaction, Rh (factor)

Incompatibility—continued
  Rh—continued
    newborn P55.0
  rhesus — see Incompatibility, Rh
Incompetency, incompetent, incompetence
  annular
    aortic (valve) — see Insufficiency, aortic
    mitral (valve) I34.0
    pulmonary valve (heart) I37.1
  aortic (valve) — see Insufficiency, aortic
  cardiac valve — see Endocarditis
  cervix, cervical (os) N88.3
    in pregnancy O34.3-
  chronotropic I45.89
    with
      autonomic dysfunction G90.8
      ischemic heart disease I25.89
      left ventricular dysfunction I51.89
      sinus node dysfunction I49.8
  esophagogastric (junction) (sphincter) K22.0
  mitral (valve) — see Insufficiency, mitral
  pelvic fundus N81.89
  pubocervical tissue N81.82
  pulmonary valve (heart) I37.1
    congenital Q22.3
  rectovaginal tissue N81.83
  tricuspid (annular) (valve) — see Insufficiency,
    tricuspid
  valvular — see Endocarditis
    congenital Q24.8
  vein, venous (saphenous) (varicose) — see Varix, leg
Incomplete (see also condition)
  bladder, emptying R33.9
  defecation R15.0
  expansion lungs (newborn) NEC — see Atelectasis
  rotation, intestine Q43.3
Inconclusive
  diagnostic imaging due to excess body fat of patient
    R93.9
  findings on diagnostic imaging of breast NEC R92.8
  mammogram (due to dense breasts) R92.2
Incontinence R32
  anal sphincter R15.9
  feces R15.9
    nonorganic origin F98.1
  overflow N39.490
  psychogenic F45.8
  rectal R15.9
  reflex N39.498
  stress (female) (male) N39.3
    and urge N39.46
  urethral sphincter R32
  urge N39.41
    and stress (female) (male) N39.46
  urine (urinary) R32
    continuous N39.45
    due to cognitive impairment, or severe physical
      disability or immobility R39.81
    functional R39.81
    mixed (stress and urge) N39.46
    nocturnal N39.44
    nonorganic origin F98.0
    overflow N39.490
    post dribbling N39.43
    reflex N39.498
    specified NEC N39.498
    stress (female) (male) N39.3
      and urge N39.46
    total N39.498
    unaware N39.42
    urge N39.41
      and stress (female) (male) N39.46
Incontinentia pigmenti Q82.3
Incoordinate, incoordination
  esophageal-pharyngeal (newborn) — see
    Dysphagia
  muscular R27.8
  uterus (action) (contractions) (complicating
    delivery) O62.4
Increase, increased
  abnormal, in development R63.8
  androgens (ovarian) E28.1

Increase, increased—*continued*
anticoagulants (antithrombin) (anti-VIIIa) (anti-IXa)
(anti-Xa) (anti-XIa) — *see* Circulating
anticoagulants
cold sense R20.8
estrogen E28.0
function
adrenal
cortex — *see* Cushing's syndrome
medulla E27.5
pituitary (gland) (anterior) (lobe) E22.9
posterior E22.2
heat sense R20.8
intracranial pressure (benign) G93.2
permeability, capillaries I78.8
pressure, intracranial G93.2
secretion
gastrin E16.4
glucagon E16.3
pancreas, endocrine E16.9
growth hormone-releasing hormone E16.8
pancreatic polypeptide E16.8
somatostatin E16.8
vasoactive-intestinal polypeptide E16.8
sphericity, lens Q12.4
splenic activity D73.1
venous pressure I87.8
portal K76.6
Increta placenta O43.22-
Incrustation, cornea, foreign body (lead)(zinc) — *see*
Foreign body, cornea
Incyclophoria H50.54
Incyclotropia — *see* Cyclotropia
Indeterminate sex Q56.4
India rubber skin Q82.8
Indigestion (acid) (bilious) (functional) K30
catarrhal K31.89
due to decomposed food NOS A05.9
nervous F45.8
psychogenic F45.8
Indirect — *see* condition
Induratio penis plastica N48.6
Induration, indurated
brain G93.89
breast (fibrous) N64.51
puerperal, postpartum O92.29
broad ligament N83.8
chancre
anus A51.1
congenital A50.07
extragenital NEC A51.2
corpora cavernosa (penis) (plastic) N48.6
liver (chronic) K76.8
lung (black) (brown) (chronic) (fibroid) — *see*
Fibrosis, lung
penile (plastic) N48.6
phlebitic — *see* Phlebitis
skin R23.4
Inebriety (without dependence) — *see* Alcohol,
intoxication
Inefficiency, kidney N28.9
Inelasticity, skin R23.4
Inequality, leg (length) (acquired) (*see also* Deformity,
limb, unequal length)
congenital — *see* Defect, reduction, lower limb
lower leg — *see* Deformity, limb, unequal length
Inertia
bladder (neurogenic) N31.2
stomach K31.89
psychogenic F45.8
uterus, uterine during labor O62.2
during latent phase of labor O62.0
primary O62.0
secondary O62.1
vesical (neurogenic) N31.2
Infancy, infantile, infantilism (*see also* condition)
celiac K90.0
genitalia, genitals (after puberty) E30.0
Herter's (nontropical sprue) K90.0
intestinal K90.0
Lorain E23.0
pancreatic K86.8

Infancy, infantile, infantilism—*continued*
pelvis M95.5
with disproportion (fetopelvic) O33.1
causing obstructed labor O65.1
pituitary E23.0
renal N25.0
uterus — *see* Infantile, genitalia
Infant(s) (*see also* Infancy)
excessive crying R68.11
irritable child R68.12
lack of care — *see* Neglect
liveborn (singleton) Z38.2
born in hospital Z38.00
by cesarean Z38.01
born outside hospital Z38.1
multiple NEC Z38.8
born in hospital Z38.68
by cesarean Z38.69
born outside hospital Z38.7
quadruplet Z38.8
born in hospital Z38.63
by cesarean Z38.64
born outside hospital Z38.7
quintuplet Z38.8
born in hospital Z38.65
by cesarean Z38.66
born outside hospital Z38.7
triplet Z38.8
born in hospital Z38.61
by cesarean Z38.62
born outside hospital Z38.7
twin Z38.5
born in hospital Z38.30
by cesarean Z38.31
born outside hospital Z38.4
of diabetic mother (syndrome of) P70.1
gestational diabetes P70.0
Infantile (*see also* condition)
genitalia, genitals E30.0
os, uterine E30.0
penis E30.0
testis E29.1
uterus E30.0
Infantilism — *see* Infancy
Infarct, infarction
adrenal (capsule) (gland) E27.49
appendices epiploicae K55.0
bowel K55.0
brain (stem) — *see* Infarct, cerebral
breast N64.89
brewer's (kidney) N28.0
cardiac — *see* Infarct, myocardium
cerebellar — *see* Infarct, cerebral
cerebral (*see also* Occlusion, artery cerebral or
precerebral, with infarction) I63.9
aborted I63.9
cortical I63.9
due to
cerebral venous thrombosis, nonpyogenic
I63.6
embolism
cerebral arteries I63.4-
precerebral arteries I63.1-
occlusion NEC
cerebral arteries I63.5-
precerebral arteries I63.2-
stenosis NEC
cerebral arteries I63.5-
precerebral arteries I63.2-
thrombosis
cerebral artery I63.3-
precerebral artery I63.0-
intraoperative
during cardiac surgery I97.810
during other surgery I97.811
postprocedural
following cardiac surgery I97.820
following other surgery I97.821
specified NEC I63.8
colon (acute) (agnogenic) (embolic) (hemorrhagic)
(nonocclusive) (nonthrombotic) (occlusive)
(segmental) (thrombotic) (with gangrene)
K55.0

Infarct, infarction—*continued*
coronary artery — *see* Infarct, myocardium
embolic — *see* Embolism
fallopian tube N83.8
gallbladder K82.8
heart — *see* Infarct, myocardium
hepatic K76.3
hypophysis (anterior lobe) E23.6
impending (myocardium) I20.0
intestine (acute) (agnogenic) (embolic)
(hemorrhagic) (nonocclusive)
(nonthrombotic) (occlusive) (thrombotic)
(with gangrene) K55.0
kidney N28.0
liver K76.3
lung (embolic) (thrombotic) — *see* Embolism,
pulmonary
lymph node I89.8
mesentery, mesenteric (embolic) (thrombotic) (with
gangrene) K55.0
muscle (ischemic) M62.20
ankle M62.27-
foot M62.27-
forearm M62.23-
hand M62.24-
lower leg M62.26-
pelvic region M62.25-
shoulder region M62.21-
specified site NEC M62.28
thigh M62.25-
upper arm M62.22-
myocardium, myocardial (acute) (with stated
duration of 4 weeks or less) I21.3
diagnosed on ECG, but presenting no symptoms
I25.2
healed or old I25.2
intraoperative
during cardiac surgery I97.790
during other surgery I97.791
non-Q wave I21.4
non-ST elevation (NSTEMI) I21.4
subsequent I22.2
nontransmural I21.4
past (diagnosed on ECG or other investigation,
but currently presenting no symptoms)
I25.2
postprocedural
following cardiac surgery I97.190
following other surgery I97.191
Q wave (*see also*, Infarct, myocardium, by site)
I21.3
ST elevation (STEMI) I21.3
anterior (anteroapical) (anterolateral)
(anteroseptal) (Q wave) (wall) I21.09
subsequent I22.0
inferior (diaphragmatic) (inferolateral)
(inferoposterior) (wall) NEC I21.19
subsequent I22.1
inferoposterior transmural (Q wave) I21.11
involving
coronary artery of anterior wall NEC I21.09
coronary artery of inferior wall NEC I21.19
diagonal coronary artery I21.02
left anterior descending coronary artery
I21.02
left circumflex coronary artery I21.21
left main coronary artery I21.01
oblique marginal coronary artery I21.21
right coronary artery I21.11
lateral (apical-lateral) (basal-lateral) (high)
I21.29
subsequent I22.8
posterior (posterobasal) (posterolateral)
(posteroseptal) (true) I21.29
subsequent I22.8
septal I21.29
subsequent I22.8
specified NEC I21.29
subsequent I22.8
subsequent I22.9
subsequent (recurrent) (reinfarction) I22.9
anterior (anteroapical) (anterolateral)
(anteroseptal) (wall) I22.0

Infection, infected, infective —*continued*
    cholera — *see* Cholera
    Cladosporium
        bantianum (brain abscess) B43.1
        carrionii B43.0
        castellanii B36.1
        trichoides (brain abscess) B43.1
        werneckii B36.1
    Clonorchis (sinensis) (liver) B66.1
    Clostridium NEC
        bifermentans A48.0
        botulinum (food poisoning) A05.1
            infant A48.51
            wound A48.52
        difficile
            as cause of disease classified elsewhere
                B96.89
            foodborne (disease) A05.8
            gas gangrene A48.0
            necrotizing enterocolitis A05.8
            sepsis A41.4
        gas-forming NEC A48.0
        histolyticum A48.0
        novyi, causing gas gangrene A48.0
        oedematiens A48.0
        perfringens
            as cause of disease classified elsewhere B96.7
            due to food A05.2
            foodborne (disease) A05.2
            gas gangrene A48.0
            sepsis A41.4
        septicum, causing gas gangrene A48.0
        sordellii, causing gas gangrene A48.0
        welchii
            as cause of disease classified elsewhere B96.7
            foodborne (disease) A05.2
            gas gangrene A48.0
            necrotizing enteritis A05.2
            sepsis A41.4
    Coccidioides (immitis) — *see* Coccidioidomycosis
    colon — *see* Enteritis, infectious
    colostomy K94.02
    common duct — *see* Cholangitis
    congenital P39.9
        Candida (albicans) P37.5
        cytomegalovirus P35.1
        hepatitis, viral P35.3
        herpes simplex P35.2
        infectious or parasitic disease P37.9
            specified NEC P37.8
        listeriosis (disseminated) P37.2
        malaria NEC P37.4
            falciparum P37.3
        Plasmodium falciparum P37.3
        poliomyelitis P35.8
        rubella P35.0
        skin P39.4
        toxoplasmosis (acute) (subacute) (chronic) P37.1
        tuberculosis P37.0
        urinary (tract) P39.3
        vaccinia P35.8
        virus P35.9
            specified type NEC P35.8
    Conidiobolus B46.8
    coronavirus NEC B34.2
        as cause of disease classified elsewhere B97.29
        severe acute respiratory syndrome (SARS associated) B97.21
    corpus luteum — *see* Salpingo-oophoritis
    Corynebacterium diphtheriae — *see* Diphtheria
    cotia virus B08.8
    Coxiella burnetii A78
    coxsackie — *see* Coxsackie
    Cryptococcus neoformans — *see* Cryptococcosis
    Cryptosporidium A07.2
    Cunninghamella — *see* Mucormycosis
    cyst — *see* Cyst
    cystic duct (*see also* Cholecystitis) K81.9
    Cysticercus cellulosae — *see* Cysticercosis
    cytomegalovirus, cytomegaloviral B25.9
        congenital P35.1
        maternal, maternal care for (suspected) damage to fetus O35.3

Infection, infected, infective —*continued*
    cytomegalovirus, cytomegaloviral—*continued*
        mononucleosis B27.10
            with
                complication NEC B27.19
                meningitis B27.12
                polyneuropathy B27.11
    delta-agent (acute), in hepatitis B carrier B17.0
    dental (pulpal origin) K04.7
    Deuteromycetes B47.0
    Dicrocoelium dendriticum B66.2
    Dipetalonema (perstans) (streptocerca) B74.4
    diphtherial — *see* Diphtheria
    Diphyllobothrium (adult) (latum) (pacificum) B70.0
        larval B70.1
    Diplogonoporus (grandis) B71.8
    Dipylidium caninum B67.4
    Dirofilaria B74.8
    Dracunculus medinensis B72
    Drechslera (hawaiiensis) B43.8
    Ducrey Haemophilus (any location) A57
    due to or resulting from
        artificial insemination N98.0
        central venous catheter T80.21
        device, implant or graft (*see also* Complications, by site and type, infection or inflammation) T85.79
            arterial graft NEC T82.7
            breast (implant) T85.79
            catheter NEC T85.79
                dialysis (renal) T82.7
                    intraperitoneal T85.71
                infusion NEC T82.7
                    spinal (epidural) (subdural) T85.79
                urinary (indwelling) T83.51
            electronic (electrode) (pulse generator) (stimulator)
                bone T84.7
                cardiac T82.7
                nervous system (brain) (peripheral nerve) (spinal) T85.79
                urinary T83.59
            fixation, internal (orthopedic) NEC — *see* Complication, fixation device, infection
            gastrointestinal (bile duct) (esophagus) T85.79
            genital NEC T83.6
            heart NEC T82.7
                valve (prosthesis) T82.6
                    graft T82.7
            joint prosthesis — *see* Complication, joint prosthesis, infection
            ocular (corneal graft) (orbital implant) NEC T85.79
            orthopedic NEC T84.7
            specified NEC T85.79
            urinary NEC T83.59
            vascular NEC T82.7
            ventricular intracranial shunt T85.79
        immunization or vaccination T88.0
        infusion, injection or transfusion NEC T80.29
        injury NEC code by site under Wound, open
        portacath (port-a-cath) T80.21
        surgery T81.4
        umbilical venous catheter T80.21
    during labor NEC O75.3
    ear (middle) (*see also* Otitis media)
        external — *see* Otitis, externa, infective
        inner — *see* subcategory H83.0
    Eberthella typhosa A01.00
    Echinococcus — *see* Echinococcus
    echovirus
        as cause of disease classified elsewhere B97.12
        unspecified nature or site B34.1
    endocardium I33.0
    endocervix — *see* Cervicitis
    Entamoeba — *see* Amebiasis
    enteric — *see* Enteritis, infectious
    Enterobacter sakazakii B96.89
    Enterobius vermicularis B80
    enterostomy K94.12

Infection, infected, infective —*continued*
    enterovirus B34.1
        as cause of disease classified elsewhere B97.10
            coxsackievirus B97.11
            echovirus B97.12
            specified NEC B97.19
    Entomophthora B46.8
    Epidermophyton — *see* Dermatophytosis
    epididymis — *see* Epididymitis
    episiotomy (puerperal) O86.0
    Erysipelothrix (insidiosa) (rhusiopathiae) — *see* Erysipeloid
    erythema infectiosum B08.3
    Escherichia (E.) coli NEC A49.8
        as cause of disease classified elsewhere B96.2
        congenital P36.4
            sepsis P36.4
        generalized A41.51
        intestinal — *see* Enteritis, infectious, due to, Escherichia coli
    ethmoidal (chronic) (sinus) — *see* Sinusitis, ethmoidal
    eustachian tube (ear) — *see* Salpingitis, eustachian
    external auditory canal (meatus) NEC — *see* Otitis, externa, infective
    eye (purulent) — *see* Endophthalmitis, purulent
    eyelid — *see* Inflammation, eyelid
    fallopian tube — *see* Salpingo-oophoritis
    Fasciola (gigantica) (hepatica) (indica) B66.3
    Fasciolopsis (buski) B66.5
    filarial — *see* Infestation, filarial
    finger (skin) L08.9
        nail L03.01-
            fungus B35.1
    fish tapeworm B70.0
        larval B70.1
    flagellate, intestinal A07.9
    fluke — *see* Infestation, fluke
    focal
        teeth (pulpal origin) K04.7
        tonsils J35.01
    Fonsecaea (compactum) (pedrosoi) B43.0
    food — *see* Intoxication, foodborne
    foot (skin) L08.9
        dermatophytic fungus B35.3
    Francisella tularensis — *see* Tularemia
    frontal (sinus) (chronic) — *see* Sinusitis, frontal
    fungus NOS B49
        beard B35.0
        dermatophytic — *see* Dermatophytosis
        foot B35.3
        groin B35.6
        hand B35.2
        nail B35.1
        pathogenic to compromised host only B48.8
        perianal (area) B35.6
        scalp B35.0
        skin B36.9
            foot B35.3
            hand B35.2
            toenails B35.1
    Fusarium B48.8
    gallbladder — *see* Cholecystitis
    gas bacillus — *see* Gangrene, gas
    gastrointestinal — *see* Enteritis, infectious
    generalized NEC — *see* Sepsis
    genital organ or tract
        female — *see* Disease, pelvis, inflammatory
        male N49.9
            multiple sites N49.8
            specified NEC N49.8
    Ghon tubercle, primary A15.7
    Giardia lamblia A07.1
    gingiva (chronic) K05.10
        acute K05.00
            plaque induced K05.00
            nonplaque induced K05.01
        plaque induced K05.10
        nonplaque induced K05.11
    glanders A24.0
    glenosporopsis B48.0
    Gnathostoma (spinigerum) B83.1
    Gongylonema B83.8

Infection, infected, infective —*continued*
  gonococcal — *see* Gonococcus
  gram-negative bacilli NOS A49.9
  guinea worm B72
  gum (chronic) KØ5.1Ø
    acute KØ5.ØØ
      plaque induced KØ5.ØØ
      nonplaque induced KØ5.Ø1
    plaque induced KØ5.1Ø
    nonplaque induced KØ5.11
  Haemophilus — *see* Infection, Hemophilus
  heart — *see* Carditis
  Helicobacter pylori AØ4.5
    as cause of disease classified elsewhere B96.81
  helminths B83.9
    intestinal B82.Ø
      mixed (types classifiable to more than one of
        the titles B65.Ø-B81.3 and B81.8) B81.4
      specified type NEC B81.8
    specified type NEC B83.8
  Hemophilus
    aegyptius, systemic A48.4
    ducrey (any location) A57
    influenzae NEC A49.2
      as cause of disease classified elsewhere B96.3
    generalized A41.3
  herpes (simplex) (*see also* Herpes)
    congenital P35.2
    disseminated BØØ.7
    zoster BØ2.9
  herpesvirus, herpesviral — *see* Herpes
  Heterophyes (heterophyes) B66.8
  Histoplasma — *see* Histoplasmosis
    American B39.4
    capsulatum B39.4
  hookworm B76.9
  human
    papilloma virus A63.Ø
    T-cell lymphotropic virus type-1 (HTLV-1) B33.3
  hydrocele N43.Ø
  Hymenolepis B71.Ø
  hypopharynx — *see* Pharyngitis
  inguinal (lymph) glands LØ4.1
    due to soft chancre A57
  intervertebral disc, pyogenic M46.3Ø
    cervical region M46.32
    cervicothoracic region M46.33
    lumbar region M46.36
    lumbosacral region M46.37
    multiple sites M46.39
    occipito-atlanto-axial region M46.31
    sacrococcygeal region M46.38
    thoracic region M46.34
    thoracolumbar region M46.35
  intestine, intestinal — *see* Enteritis, infectious
    specified NEC AØ8.8
  intra-amniotic affecting newborn NEC P39.2
  Isospora belli or hominis AØ7.3
  Japanese B encephalitis A83.Ø
  jaw (bone) (lower) (upper) M27.2
  joint — *see* Arthritis, pyogenic or pyemic
  kidney (cortex) (hematogenous) N15.9
    with calculus N2Ø.Ø
      with hydronephrosis N13.6
    following ectopic gestation OØ8.89
    pelvis and ureter (cystic) N28.85
    puerperal (postpartum) O86.21
    specified NEC N15.8
  Klebsiella (K.) pneumoniae NEC A49.8
    as cause of disease classified elsewhere B96.1
  knee (skin) NEC LØ8.9
    joint MØØ.9
  Koch's — *see* Tuberculosis
  labia (majora) (minora) (acute) — *see* Vulvitis
  lacrimal
    gland — *see* Dacryoadenitis
    passages (duct) (sac) — *see* Inflammation,
      lacrimal, passages
  lancet fluke B66.2
  larynx NEC J38.7
  leg (skin) NOS LØ8.9
  Legionella pneumophila A48.1
    nonpneumonic A48.2

Infection, infected, infective —*continued*
  Leishmania (*see also* Leishmaniasis)
    aethiopica B55.1
    braziliensis B55.2
    chagasi B55.Ø
    donovani B55.Ø
    infantum B55.Ø
    major B55.1
    mexicana B55.1
    tropica B55.1
  lentivirus, as cause of disease classified elsewhere
    B97.31
  Leptosphaeria senegalensis B47.Ø
  Leptospira interrogans A27.9
    autumnalis A27.89
    canicola A27.89
    hebdomadis A27.89
    icterohaemorrhagiae A27.Ø
    pomona A27.89
    specified type NEC A27.89
  leptospirochetal NEC — *see* Leptospirosis
  Listeria monocytogenes (*see also* Listeriosis)
    congenital P37.2
  Loa loa B74.3
    with conjunctival infestation B74.3
    eyelid B74.3
  Loboa loboi B48.Ø
  local, skin (staphylococcal) (streptococcal) LØ8.9
    abscess code by site under Abscess
    cellulitis code by site under Cellulitis
    specified NEC LØ8.89
    ulcer — *see* Ulcer, skin
  Loefflerella mallei A24.Ø
  lung (*see also* Pneumonia) J18.9
    atypical Mycobacterium A31.Ø
    spirochetal A69.8
    tuberculous — *see* Tuberculosis, pulmonary
    virus — *see* Pneumonia, viral
  lymph gland (*see also* Lymphadenitis, acute)
    mesenteric I88.Ø
  lymphoid tissue, base of tongue or posterior
    pharynx, NEC (chronic) J35.Ø3
  Madurella (grisea) (mycetomii) B47.Ø
  major
    following ectopic or molar pregnancy OØ8.Ø
    puerperal, postpartum, childbirth O85
  Malassezia furfur B36.Ø
  Malleomyces
    mallei A24.Ø
    pseudomallei (whitmori) — *see* Melioidosis
  mammary gland N61
  Mansonella (ozzardi) (perstans) (streptocerca) B74.4
  mastoid — *see* Mastoiditis
  maxilla, maxillary M27.2
    sinus (chronic) — *see* Sinusitis, maxillary
  mediastinum J98.5
  Medina (worm) B72
  meibomian cyst or gland — *see* Hordeolum
  meninges — *see* Meningitis, bacterial
  meningococcal (*see also* condition) A39.9
    adrenals A39.1
    brain A39.81
    cerebrospinal A39.Ø
    conjunctiva A39.89
    endocardium A39.51
    heart A39.5Ø
      endocardium A39.51
      myocardium A39.52
      pericardium A39.53
    joint A39.83
    meninges A39.Ø
    meningococcemia A39.4
      acute A39.2
      chronic A39.3
    myocardium A39.52
    pericardium A39.53
    retrobulbar neuritis A39.82
    specified site NEC A39.89
  mesenteric lymph nodes or glands NEC I88.Ø
  Metagonimus B66.8
  metatarsophalangeal MØØ.9
  Microsporum, microsporic — *see* Dermatophytosis
  mixed flora (bacterial) NEC A49.8

Infection, infected, infective —*continued*
  Monilia — *see* Candidiasis
  Monosporium apiospermum B48.2
  mouth, parasitic B37.Ø
  Mucor — *see* Mucormycosis
  muscle NEC — *see* Myositis, infective
  mycelium NOS B49
  mycetoma
    actinomycotic NEC B47.1
    mycotic NEC B47.Ø
  Mycobacterium, mycobacterial — *see*
    Mycobacterium
  Mycoplasma NEC A49.3
    pneumoniae, as cause of disease classified
      elsewhere B96.Ø
  mycotic NOS B49
    pathogenic to compromised host only B48.8
    skin NOS B36.9
  myocardium NEC I4Ø.Ø
  nail (chronic)
    with lymphangitis — *see* Lymphangitis, acute,
      digit
    finger LØ3.Ø1-
      fungus B35.1
    ingrowing L6Ø.Ø
    toe LØ3.Ø3-
      fungus B35.1
  nasal sinus (chronic) — *see* Sinusitis
  nasopharynx — *see* Nasopharyngitis
  navel LØ8.82
  Necator americanus B76.1
  Neisseria — *see* Gonococcus
  Neotestudina rosatii B47.Ø
  newborn P39.9
    intra-amniotic NEC P39.2
    skin P39.4
    specified type NEC P39.8
  nipple N61
    associated with
      lactation O91.Ø3
      pregnancy O91.Ø1-
      puerperium O91.Ø2
  Nocardia — *see* Nocardiosis
  obstetrical surgical wound (puerperal) O86.Ø
  Oesophagostomum (apiostomum) B81.8
  Oestrus ovis — *see* Myiasis
  Oidium albicans B37.9
  Onchocerca (volvulus) — *see* Onchocerciasis
  oncovirus, as cause of disease classified elsewhere
    B97.32
  operation wound T81.4
  Opisthorchis (felineus) (viverrini) B66.Ø
  orbit, orbital — *see* Inflammation, orbit
  orthopoxvirus NEC BØ8.Ø9
  ovary — *see* Salpingo-oophoritis
  Oxyuris vermicularis B8Ø
  pancreas (acute) K85.9
    abscess — *see* Pancreatitis, acute
    specified NEC K85.8
  papillomavirus, as cause of disease classified
    elsewhere B97.7
  papovavirus NEC B34.4
  Paracoccidioides brasiliensis — *see*
    Paracoccidioidomycosis
  Paragonimus (westermani) B66.4
  parainfluenza virus B34.8
  parameningococcus NOS A39.9
  parapoxvirus BØ8.6Ø
    specified NEC BØ8.69
  parasitic B89
  Parastrongylus
    cantonensis B83.2
    costaricensis B81.3
    paratyphoid AØ1.4
      Type A AØ1.1
      Type B AØ1.2
      Type C AØ1.3
  paraurethral ducts N34.2
  parotid gland — *see* Sialoadenitis
  parvovirus NEC B34.3
    as cause of disease classified elsewhere B97.6

Index

Infection, infected, infective —continued

Pasteurella NEC A28.0
  multocida A28.0
  pestis — see Plague
  pseudotuberculosis A28.0
  septica (cat bite) (dog bite) A28.0
  tularensis — see Tularemia
pelvic, female — see Disease, pelvis, inflammatory
Penicillium (marneffei) B48.4
penis (glans) (retention) NEC N48.29
periapical K04.5
peridental, periodontal K05.20
  generalized K05.22
  localized K05.21
perinatal period P39.9
  specified type NEC P39.8
perineal repair (puerperal) O86.0
periorbital — see Inflammation, orbit
perirectal K62.8
perirenal — see Infection, kidney
peritoneal — see Peritonitis
periureteral N28.89
Petriellidium boydii B48.2
pharynx (see also Pharyngitis)
  coxsackievirus B08.5
  posterior, lymphoid (chronic) J35.03
Phialophora
  gougerotii (subcutaneous abscess or cyst) B43.2
  jeanselmei (subcutaneous abscess or cyst) B43.2
  verrucosa (skin) B43.0
Piedraia hortae B36.3
pinta A67.9
  intermediate A67.1
  late A67.2
  mixed A67.3
  primary A67.0
pinworm B80
pityrosporum furfur B36.0
pleuro-pneumonia-like organism (PPLO) NEC A49.3
  as cause of disease classified elsewhere B96.0
pneumococcus, pneumococcal NEC A49.1
  as cause of disease classified elsewhere B95.3
  generalized (purulent) A40.3
    with pneumonia J13
Pneumocystis carinii (pneumonia) B59
Pneumocystis jiroveci (pneumonia) B59
postoperative T81.4
postoperative wound T81.4
postprocedural T81.4
postvaccinal T88.0
prepuce NEC N47.7
  with penile inflammation N47.6
prion — see Disease, prion, central nervous system
prostate (capsule) — see Prostatitis
Proteus (mirabilis) (morganii) (vulgaris) NEC A49.8
  as cause of disease classified elsewhere B96.4
protozoal NEC B64
  intestinal A07.9
    specified NEC A07.8
  specified NEC B60.8
Pseudoallescheria boydii B48.2
Pseudomonas NEC A49.8
  as cause of disease classified elsewhere B96.5
  mallei A24.0
  pneumonia J15.1
  pseudomallei — see Melioidosis
puerperal O86.4
  genitourinary tract NEC O86.89
  major or generalized O85
  minor O86.4
  specified NEC O86.89
pulmonary — see Infection, lung
purulent — see Abscess
Pyrenochaeta romeroi B47.0
Q fever A78
rectum (sphincter) K62.8
renal (see also Infection, kidney)
  pelvis and ureter (cystic) N28.85
reovirus, as cause of disease classified elsewhere B97.5
respiratory (tract) NEC J98.8
  acute J22
  chronic J98.8

Infection, infected, infective —continued

respiratory—continued
  influenzal (upper) (acute) — see Influenza, with, respiratory manifestations NEC
  lower (acute) J22
    chronic — see Bronchitis, chronic
  rhinovirus J00
  syncytial virus, as cause of disease classified elsewhere B97.4
  upper (acute) NOS J06.9
    chronic J39.8
    streptococcal J06.9
    viral NOS J06.9
resulting from
  presence of internal prosthesis, implant, graft — see Complications, by site and type, infection
retortamoniasis A07.8
retroperitoneal NEC K68.9
retrovirus B33.3
  as cause of disease classified elsewhere B97.30
    human
      immunodeficiency, type 2 (HIV 2) B97.35
      T-cell lymphotropic
        type I (HTLV-I) B97.33
        type II (HTLV-II) B97.34
    lentivirus B97.31
    oncovirus B97.32
    specified NEC B97.39
Rhinosporidium (seeberi) B48.1
rhinovirus
  as cause of disease classified elsewhere B97.8
  unspecified nature or site B34.8
Rhizopus — see Mucormycosis
rickettsial NOS A79.9
roundworm (large) NEC B82.0
  Ascariasis (see also Ascariasis) B77.9
rubella — see Rubella
Saccharomyces — see Candidiasis
salivary duct or gland (any) — see Sialoadenitis
Salmonella (aertrycke) (arizonae) (callinarum) (cholerae-suis) (enteritidis) (suipestifer) (typhimurium) A02.9
  with
    (gastro)enteritis A02.0
    sepsis A02.1
    specified manifestation NEC A02.8
  due to food (poisoning) A02.9
  hirschfeldii A01.3
  localized A02.20
    arthritis A02.23
    meningitis A02.21
    osteomyelitis A02.24
    pneumonia A02.22
    pyelonephritis A02.25
    specified NEC A02.29
  paratyphi A01.4
    A A01.1
    B A01.2
    C A01.3
  schottmuelleri A01.2
  typhi, typhosa — see Typhoid
Sarcocystis A07.8
scabies B86
Schistosoma — see Infestation, Schistosoma
scrotum (acute) NEC N49.2
seminal vesicle — see Vesiculitis
septic
  localized, skin — see Abscess
sheep liver fluke B66.3
Shigella A03.9
  boydii A03.2
  dysenteriae A03.0
  flexneri A03.1
  group
    A A03.0
    B A03.1
    C A03.2
    D A03.3
  Schmitz (-Stutzer) A03.0
  schmitzii A03.0
  shigae A03.0
  sonnei A03.3

Infection, infected, infective —continued

Shigella—continued
  specified NEC A03.8
sinus (accessory) (chronic) (nasal) (see also Sinusitis)
  pilonidal — see Sinus, pilonidal
  skin NEC L08.89
Skene's duct or gland — see Urethritis
skin (local) (staphylococcal) (streptococcal) L08.9
  abscess code by site under Abscess
  cellulitis code by site under Cellulitis
  due to fungus B36.9
    specified type NEC B36.8
  mycotic B36.9
    specified type NEC B36.8
  newborn P39.4
  ulcer — see Ulcer, skin
slow virus A81.9
  specified NEC A81.89
Sparganum (mansoni) (proliferum) (baxteri) B70.1
specific (see also Syphilis)
  to perinatal period — see Infection, congenital
specified NEC B99.8
spermatic cord NEC N49.1
sphenoidal (sinus) — see Sinusitis, sphenoidal
spinal cord NOS (see also Myelitis) G04.91
  abscess G06.1
  meninges — see Meningitis
  streptococcal G04.89
Spirillum A25.0
spirochetal NOS A69.9
  lung A69.8
  specified NEC A69.8
Spirometra larvae B70.1
spleen D73.89
Sporotrichum, Sporothrix (schenckii) — see Sporotrichosis
staphylococcal NEC A49.0
  as cause of disease classified elsewhere B95.8
    aureus B95.6
    specified NEC B95.7
  food poisoning A05.0
  generalized (purulent) A41.2
  pneumonia — see Pneumonia, staphylococcal
Stellantchasmus falcatus B66.8
streptobacillus moniliformis A25.1
streptococcal NEC A49.1
  as cause of disease classified elsewhere B95.5
  B genitourinary complicating
    childbirth O98.82
    pregnancy O98.81-
    puerperium O98.83
  congenital
    sepsis P36.10
      group B P36.0
      specified NEC P36.19
  generalized (purulent) A40.9
Streptomyces B47.1
Strongyloides (stercoralis) — see Strongyloidiasis
stump (amputation) (surgical) — see Complication, amputation stump, infection
subcutaneous tissue, local L08.89
suipestifer — see Infection, salmonella
swimming pool bacillus A31.1
Taenia — see Infestation, Taenia
Taeniarhynchus saginatus B68.1
tapeworm — see Infestation, tapeworm
tendon (sheath) — see Tenosynovitis, infective NEC
Ternidens diminutus B81.8
testis — see Orchitis
threadworm B80
throat — see Pharyngitis
thyroglossal duct K14.8
toe (skin) L08.9
  cellulitis L03.03-
    fungus B35.1
  nail L03.03-
    fungus B35.1
tongue NEC K14.0
  parasitic B37.0
tonsil (and adenoid) (faucial) (lingual) (pharyngeal) — see Tonsillitis

Infection, infected, infective —*continued*
  tooth, teeth K04.7
    periapical K04.7
    peridental, periodontal K05.20
      generalized K05.22
      localized K05.21
    pulp K04.0
    socket M27.3
  TORCH — *see* Infection, congenital
    without active infection P00.2
  Torula histolytica — *see* Cryptococcosis
  Toxocara (canis) (cati) (felis) B83.0
  Toxoplasma gondii — *see* Toxoplasma
  trachea, chronic J42
  trematode NEC — *see* Infestation, fluke
  trench fever A79.0
  Treponema pallidum — *see* Syphilis
  Trichinella (spiralis) B75
  Trichomonas A59.9
    cervix A59.09
    intestine A07.8
    prostate A59.02
    specified site NEC A59.8
    urethra A59.03
    urogenitalis A59.00
    vagina A59.01
    vulva A59.01
  Trichophyton, trichophytic — *see* Dermatophytosis
  Trichosporon (beigelii) cutaneum B36.2
  Trichostrongylus B81.2
  Trichuris (trichiura) B79
  Trombicula (irritans) B88.0
  Trypanosoma
    brucei
      gambiense B56.0
      rhodesiense B56.1
    cruzi — *see* Chagas' disease
  tubal — *see* Salpingo-oophoritis
  tuberculous NEC — *see* Tuberculosis
  tubo-ovarian — *see* Salpingo-oophoritis
  tunica vaginalis N49.1
  tympanic membrane NEC — *see* Myringitis
  typhoid (abortive) (ambulant) (bacillus) — *see*
    Typhoid
  typhus A75.9
    flea-borne A75.2
    mite-borne A75.3
    recrudescent A75.1
    tick-borne A77.9
      African A77.1
      North Asian A77.2
  umbilicus L08.82
  ureter N28.86
  urethra — *see* Urethritis
  urinary (tract) N39.0
    bladder — *see* Cystitis
    complicating
      pregnancy O23.4-
        specified type NEC O23.3-
    kidney — *see* Infection, kidney
    newborn P39.3
    puerperal (postpartum) O86.20
    tuberculous A18.13
    urethra — *see* Urethritis
  uterus, uterine — *see* Endometritis
  vaccination T88.0
  vaccinia not from vaccination B08.011
  vagina (acute) — *see* Vaginitis
  varicella B01.9
  varicose veins — *see* Varix
  vas deferens NEC N49.1
  vesical — *see* Cystitis
  Vibrio
    cholerae A00.0
      El Tor A00.1
    parahaemolyticus (food poisoning) A05.3
    vulnificus
      as cause of disease classified elsewhere
        B96.82
      foodborne intoxication A05.5
  Vincent's (gum) (mouth) (tonsil) A69.1
  virus, viral NOS B34.9
    adenovirus

Infection, infected, infective —*continued*
  virus, viral—*continued*
    as cause of disease classified elsewhere B97.0
      unspecified nature or site B34.0
    arborvirus, arbovirus arthropod-borne A94
    as cause of disease classified elsewhere B97.8
      adenovirus B97.0
      coronavirus B97.29
        SARS-associated B97.21
      coxsackievirus B97.11
      echovirus B97.12
      enterovirus B97.10
        coxsackievirus B97.11
        echovirus B97.12
        specified NEC B97.19
      human
        immunodeficiency, type 2 (HIV 2) B97.35
        T-cell lymphotropic,
          type I (HTLV-I) B97.33
          type II (HTLV-II) B97.34
        metapneumovirus B97.8
      papillomavirus B97.7
      parvovirus B97.6
      reovirus B97.5
      respiratory syncytial B97.4
      retrovirus B97.30
        human
          immunodeficiency, type 2 (HIV 2)
            B97.35
        T-cell lymphotropic,
          type I (HTLV-I)B97.33
          type II (HTLV-II)B97.34
        lentivirus B97.31
        oncovirus B97.32
        specified NEC B97.39
      specified NEC B97.8
    central nervous system A89
      atypical A81.9
        specified NEC A81.89
      enterovirus NEC A88.8
        meningitis A87.0
      slow virus A81.9
        specified NEC A81.89
      specified NEC A88.8
    chest J98.8
    cotia B08.8
    coxsackie (*see also* Infection, coxsackie) B34.1
      as cause of disease classified elsewhere
        B97.11
    ECHO
      as cause of disease classified elsewhere
        B97.12
      unspecified nature or site B34.1
    encephalitis, tick-borne A84.9
    enterovirus, as cause of disease classified
      elsewhere B97.10
      coxsackievirus B97.11
      echovirus B97.12
      specified NEC B97.19
    exanthem NOS B09
    human papilloma as cause of disease classified
      elsewhere B97.7
    human metapneumovirus as cause of disease
      classified elsewhere B97.8
    intestine — *see* Enteritis, viral
    respiratory syncytial
      as cause of disease classified elsewhere B97.4
      bronchopneumonia J12.1
      common cold syndrome J00
      nasopharyngitis (acute) J00
    rhinovirus
      as cause of disease classified elsewhere B97.8
      unspecified nature or site B34.8
    slow A81.9
      specified NEC A81.89
    specified type NEC B33.8
      as cause of disease classified elsewhere B97.8
      unspecified nature or site B34.8
    unspecified nature or site B34.9
    West Nile — *see* Virus, West Nile
  vulva (acute) — *see* Vulvitis
  West Nile — *see* Virus, West Nile
  whipworm B79

Infection, infected, infective —*continued*
  worms B83.9
    specified type NEC B83.8
  Wuchereria (bancrofti) B74.0
    malayi B74.1
  yatapoxvirus B08.70
    specified NEC B08.79
  yeast (*see also* Candidiasis) B37.9
  yellow fever — *see* Fever, yellow
  Yersinia
    enterocolitica (intestinal) A04.6
    pestis — *see* Plague
    pseudotuberculosis A28.2
  Zeis' gland — *see* Hordeolum
  zoonotic bacterial NOS A28.9
  Zopfia senegalensis B47.0
Infective, infectious — *see* condition
Infertility
  female N97.9
    age-related N97.8
    associated with
      anovulation N97.0
      cervical (mucus) disease or anomaly N88.3
      congenital anomaly
        cervix N88.3
        fallopian tube N97.1
        uterus N97.2
        vagina N97.8
      dysmucorrhea N88.3
      fallopian tube disease or anomaly N97.1
      pituitary-hypothalamic origin E23.0
      specified origin NEC N97.8
      Stein-Leventhal syndrome E28.2
      uterine disease or anomaly N97.2
      vaginal disease or anomaly N97.8
    due to
      cervical anomaly N88.3
      fallopian tube anomaly N97.1
      ovarian failure E28.39
      Stein-Leventhal syndrome E28.2
      uterine anomaly N97.2
      vaginal anomaly N97.8
    nonimplantation N97.2
    origin
      cervical N88.3
      tubal (block) (occlusion) (stenosis) N97.1
      uterine N97.2
      vaginal N97.8
  male N46.9
    azoospermia N46.01
      extratesticular cause N46.029
        drug therapy N46.021
        efferent duct obstruction N46.023
        infection N46.022
        radiation N46.024
        specified cause NEC N46.029
        systemic disease N46.025
    oligospermia N46.11
      extratesticular cause N46.129
        drug therapy N46.121
        efferent duct obstruction N46.123
        infection N46.122
        radiation N46.124
        specified cause NEC N46.129
        systemic disease N46.125
    specified type NEC N46.8
Infestation B88.9
  Acanthocheilonema (perstans) (streptocerca) B74.4
  Acariasis B88.0
    demodex folliculorum B88.0
    sarcoptes scabiei B86
    trombiculae B88.0
  Agamofilaria streptocerca B74.4
  Ancylostoma, ankylostoma (braziliense) (caninum)
    (ceylanicum) (duodenale) B76.0
    americanum B76.1
    new world B76.1
  Anisakis larvae, anisakiasis B81.0
  arthropod NEC B88.2
  Ascaris lumbricoides — *see* Ascariasis
  Balantidium coli A07.0
  beef tapeworm B68.1

Inflammation, inflamed, inflammatory —*continued*
oculomotor (nerve) — *see* Strabismus, paralytic, third nerve
optic nerve — *see* Neuritis, optic
orbit (chronic) H05.10
acute H05.00
abscess — *see* Abscess, orbit
cellulitis — *see* Cellulitis, orbit
osteomyelitis — *see* Osteomyelitis, orbit
periostitis — *see* Periostitis, orbital
tenonitis — *see* Tenonitis, eye
granuloma — *see* Granuloma, orbit
myositis — *see* Myositis, orbital
ovary — *see* Salpingo-oophoritis
oviduct — *see* Salpingo-oophoritis
pancreas (acute) — *see* Pancreatitis
parametrium N73.0
parotid region L08.9
pelvis, female — *see* Disease, pelvis, inflammatory
penis (corpora cavernosa) N48.29
perianal K62.8
pericardium — *see* Pericarditis
perineum (female) (male) L08.9
perirectal K62.8
peritoneum — *see* Peritonitis
periuterine — *see* Disease, pelvis, inflammatory
perivesical — *see* Cystitis
petrous bone (acute) (chronic) — *see* Petrositis
pharynx (acute) — *see* Pharyngitis
pia mater — *see* Meningitis
pleura — *see* Pleurisy
polyp, colon (*see also* Polyp, colon, inflammatory) K51.40
prostate (*see also* Prostatitis)
specified type NEC N41.8
rectosigmoid — *see* Rectosigmoiditis
rectum (*see also* Proctitis) K62.8
respiratory, upper (*see also* Infection, respiratory, upper) J06.9
acute, due to radiation J70.0
chronic, due to external agent — *see* condition, respiratory, chronic, due to
due to
chemicals, gases, fumes or vapors (inhalation) J68.2
radiation J70.1
retina — *see* Chorioretinitis
retrocecal — *see* Appendicitis
retroperitoneal — *see* Peritonitis
salivary duct or gland (any) (suppurative) — *see* Sialoadenitis
scorbutic, alveoli, teeth E54
scrotum N49.2
seminal vesicle — *see* Vesiculitis
sigmoid — *see* Enteritis
sinus — *see* Sinusitis
Skene's duct or gland — *see* Urethritis
skin L08.9
spermatic cord N49.1
sphenoidal (sinus) — *see* Sinusitis, sphenoidal
spinal
cord — *see* Encephalitis
membrane — *see* Meningitis
nerve — *see* Disorder, nerve
spine — *see* Spondylopathy, inflammatory
spleen (capsule) D73.89
stomach — *see* Gastritis
subcutaneous tissue L08.9
suprarenal (gland) E27.8
synovial — *see* Tenosynovitis
tendon (sheath) NEC — *see* Tenosynovitis
testis — *see* Orchitis
throat (acute) — *see* Pharyngitis
thymus (gland) E32.8
thyroid (gland) — *see* Thyroiditis
tongue K14.0
tonsil — *see* Tonsillitis
trachea — *see* Tracheitis
trochlear (nerve) — *see* Strabismus, paralytic, fourth nerve
tubal — *see* Salpingo-oophoritis
tuberculous NEC — *see* Tuberculosis

Inflammation, inflamed, inflammatory —*continued*
tubo-ovarian — *see* Salpingo-oophoritis
tunica vaginalis N49.1
tympanic membrane — *see* Tympanitis
umbilicus, umbilical L08.82
uterine ligament — *see* Disease, pelvis, inflammatory
uterus (catarrhal) — *see* Endometritis
uveal tract (anterior) NOS (*see also* Iridocyclitis)
posterior — *see* Chorioretinitis
vagina — *see* Vaginitis
vas deferens N49.1
vein (*see also* Phlebitis)
intracranial or intraspinal (septic) G08
thrombotic I80.9
leg — *see* Phlebitis, leg
lower extremity — *see* Phlebitis, leg
vocal cord J38.3
vulva — *see* Vulvitis
Wharton's duct (suppurative) — *see* Sialoadenitis
Inflation, lung, imperfect (newborn) — *see* Atelectasis
Influenza (bronchial) (epidemic) (respiratory (upper) (unidentified influenza virus) J11.1
with
digestive manifestations J11.2
encephalopathy J11.81
enteritis J11.2
gastroenteritis J11.2
gastrointestinal manifestations J11.2
laryngitis J11.1
myocarditis J11.82
otitis media J11.83
pharyngitis J11.1
pneumonia J11.00
specified type J11.08
respiratory manifestations NEC J11.1
specified manifestation NEC J11.89
A/H5N1 — *see* Influenza, due to, identified avian influenza virus
avian — *see* Influenza, due to, identified avian influenza virus
novel (2009) H1N1 influenza — *see* Influenza, due to identified novel H1N1 influenza virus
novel influenza A/H1N1 — *see* Influenza, due to identified novel H1N1 influenza virus
due to
identified avian influenza virus J09.02
with
digestive manifestations J09.03
encephalopathy J09.090
enteritis J09.03
gastroenteritis J09.03
gastrointestinal manifestations J09.03
laryngitis J09.02
myocarditis J09.091
otitis media J09.092
pharyngitis J09.02
pneumonia (unspecified type) J09.019
due to identified avian influenza virus J09.010
specified type NEC J09.018
respiratory manifestations NEC J09.02
specified manifestation NEC J09.098
identified influenza virus NEC J10.1
with
digestive manifestations J10.2
encephalopathy J10.81
enteritis J10.2
gastroenteritis J10.2
gastrointestinal manifestations J10.2
laryngitis J10.1
myocarditis J10.82
otitis media J10.83
pharyngitis J10.1
pneumonia (unspecified type) J10.00
with same identified influenza virus J10.01
specified type NEC J10.08
respiratory manifestations NEC J10.1
specified manifestation NEC J10.89

Influenza —*continued*
due to—*continued*
identified novel H1N1 influenza virus J09.12
with
digestive manifestations J09.13
encephalopathy J09.190
enteritis J09.13
gastroenteritis J09.13
gastrointestinal manifestations J09.13
laryngitis 9.12
myocarditis J09.191
otitis media J09.192
pharyngitis J09.12
pneumonia (unspecified type) J09.119
due to identified novel H1N1 influenza virus J09.110
specified type NEC J09.118
respiratory manifestations NEC J09.12
specified manifestation NEC J09.198
Influenza-like disease — *see* Influenza
Influenzal— *see* Influenza
Infraction, Freiberg's (metatarsal head) — *see* Osteochondrosis, juvenile, metatarsus
Infraeruption of tooth (teeth) M26.34
Infusion complication, misadventure, or reaction — *see* Complications, infusion
Ingestion
chemical — *see* Table of Drugs and Chemicals, by substance, poisoning
drug or medicament
correct substance properly administered — *see* Table of Drugs and Chemicals, by drug, adverse effect
overdose or wrong substance given or taken — *see* Table of Drugs and Chemicals, by drug, poisoning
foreign body — *see* Foreign body, alimentary tract
tularemia A21.3
Ingrowing
hair (beard) L73.1
nail (finger) (toe) L60.0
Inguinal (*see also* condition)
testicle Q53.9
bilateral Q53.21
unilateral Q53.11
Inhalation
anthrax A22.1
flame T27.3
food or foreign body — *see* Asphyxia, food
gases, fumes, or vapors NEC — *see* Table of Drugs and Chemicals, by substance
liquid or vomitus — *see* Asphyxia
meconium (newborn) P24.00
with
pneumonia (pneumonitis) P24.01
with respiratory symptoms P24.01
mucus — *see* Asphyxia, mucus
oil or gasoline (causing suffocation) — *see* Asphyxia, food
smoke — *see* Toxicity, vapors
steam — *see* Toxicity, vapors
stomach contents or secretions (*see also* Asphyxia, food)
due to anesthesia (general) (local) or other sedation T88.59
in labor and delivery O74.0
in pregnancy O29.01-
postpartum, puerperal O89.01
Inhibition, orgasm
female F52.32
male F52.31
Inhibitor, systemic lupus erythematosus (presence of) D68.62
Iniencephalus, iniencephaly Q00.2
Injection, traumatic jet (air) (industrial) (water) (paint or dye) T70.4
Injury (*see also* specified injury type) T14.90
abdomen, abdominal S39.91
blood vessel — *see* Injury, blood vessel, abdomen
cavity — *see* Injury, intra-abdominal
contusion S30.1
internal — *see* Injury, intra-abdominal

Injury —*continued*
abdomen, abdominal—*continued*
  intra-abdominal organ — *see* Injury,
    intra-abdominal
  nerve — *see* Injury, nerve, abdomen
  open — *see* Wound, open, abdomen
  specified NEC S39.81
  superficial — *see* Injury, superficial, abdomen
Achilles tendon S86.00-
  laceration S86.02-
  specified type NEC S86.09-
  strain S86.01-
acoustic, resulting in deafness — *see* Injury, nerve,
  acoustic
adrenal (gland) S37.819
  contusion S37.812
  laceration S37.813
  specified type NEC S37.818
alveolar (process) S09.93
ankle S99.91-
  contusion — *see* Contusion, ankle
  dislocation — *see* Dislocation, ankle
  fracture — *see* Fracture, ankle
  nerve — *see* Injury, nerve, ankle
  open — *see* Wound, open, ankle
  specified type NEC S99.81-
  sprain — *see* Sprain, ankle
  superficial — *see* Injury, superficial, ankle
anterior chamber, eye — *see* Injury, eye, specified
  site NEC
anus — *see* Injury, abdomen
aorta (thoracic) S25.00
  abdominal S35.00
    laceration (minor) (superficial) S35.01
      major S35.02
    specified type NEC S35.09
  laceration (minor) (superficial) S25.01
    major S25.02
  specified type NEC S25.09
arm (upper) S49.9-
  blood vessel — *see* Injury, blood vessel, arm
  contusion — *see* Contusion, arm, upper
  fracture — *see* Fracture, humerus
  lower — *see* Injury, forearm
  muscle — *see* Injury, muscle, shoulder
  nerve — *see* Injury, nerve, arm
  open — *see* Wound, open, arm
  specified type NEC S49.8-
  superficial — *see* Injury, superficial, arm
artery (complicating trauma) (*see also* Injury, blood
  vessel, by site)
  cerebral or meningeal — *see* Injury, intracranial
auditory canal (external) (meatus) S09.91
auricle, auris, ear S09.91
axilla — *see* Injury, shoulder
back — *see* Injury, back, lower
bile duct — *see* Injury, gallbladder
birth (*see also* Birth, injury) P15.9
bladder (sphincter) S37.20
  at delivery O71.5
  contusion S37.22
  laceration S37.23
  obstetrical trauma O71.5
  specified type NEC S37.29
blast (air) (hydraulic) (immersion) (underwater) NEC
  T14.8
  acoustic nerve trauma — *see* Injury, nerve,
    acoustic
  bladder — *see* Injury, bladder, blast injury
  brain — *see* Concussion
  colon — *see* Injury, intestine, large, blast injury
  ear (primary) S09.31-
    secondary S09.39-
  generalized T70.8
  lung — *see* Injury, intrathoracic, lung, blast injury
  multiple body organs T70.8
  peritoneum S36.81
  rectum S36.61
  retroperitoneum S36.898
  small intestine S36.419
    duodenum S36.410
    specified site NEC S36.418

Injury —*continued*
blast—*continued*
  specified
    intra-abdominal organ NEC S36.898
    pelvic organ NEC S37.899
blood vessel NEC T14.8
  abdomen S35.90
    aorta — *see* Injury, aorta, abdominal
    celiac artery — *see* Injury, blood vessel, celiac
      artery
    iliac vessel — *see* Injury, blood vessel, iliac
    laceration S35.91
    mesenteric vessel — *see* Injury, mesenteric
    portal vein — *see* Injury, blood vessel, portal
      vein
    renal vessel — *see* Injury, blood vessel, renal
    specified T14.8
      site NEC — *see* subcategory S35.8
      type NEC S35.99
    splenic vessel — *see* Injury, blood vessel,
      splenic
    vena cava — *see* Injury, vena cava, inferior
  ankle — *see* Injury, blood vessel, foot
  aorta (abdominal) (thoracic) — *see* Injury, aorta
  arm (upper) NEC S45.90-
    forearm — *see* Injury, blood vessel, forearm
    laceration S45.91-
    specified
      site NEC S45.80-
        laceration S45.81-
        specified type NEC S45.89-
      type NEC S45.99-
    superficial vein S45.30-
      laceration S45.31-
      specified type NEC S45.39-
  axillary
    artery S45.00-
      laceration S45.01-
      specified type NEC S45.09-
    vein S45.20-
      laceration S45.21-
      specified type NEC S45.29-
  azygos vein — *see* Injury, blood vessel, thoracic,
    specified site NEC
  brachial
    artery S45.10-
      laceration S45.11-
      specified type NEC S45.19-
    vein S45.20-
      laceration S45.219
      specified type NEC S45.29-
  carotid artery (common) (external) (internal,
    extracranial) S15.00-
    internal, intracranial S06.8-
    laceration (minor) (superficial) S15.01-
      major S15.02-
    specified type NEC S15.09-
  celiac artery S35.219
    branch S35.299
      laceration (minor) (superficial) S35.291
        major S35.292
      specified NEC S35.298
    laceration (minor) (superficial) S35.211
      major S35.212
    specified type NEC S35.218
  cerebral — *see* Injury, intracranial
  deep plantar — *see* Injury, nerve, medial plantar
  digital (hand) — *see* Injury, blood vessel, finger
  dorsal
    artery (foot) S95.00-
      laceration S95.01-
      specified type NEC S95.09-
    vein (foot) S95.20-
      laceration S95.21-
      specified type NEC S95.29-
  due to accidental laceration during procedure —
    see Laceration, accidental complicating
    surgery
  extremity — *see* Injury, blood vessel, limb
  femoral
    artery (common) (superficial) S75.00-
      laceration (minor) (superficial) S75.01-
        major S75.02-

Injury —*continued*
blood vessel—*continued*
  femoral—*continued*
    artery—*continued*
      specified type NEC S75.09-
    vein (hip level) (thigh level) S75.10-
      laceration (minor) (superficial) S75.11-
        major S75.12-
      specified type NEC S75.19-
  finger S65.50-
    index S65.50-
      laceration S65.51-
      specified type NEC S65.59-
    laceration S65.51-
    little S65.50-
      laceration S65.51-
      specified type NEC S65.59-
    middle S65.50-
      laceration S65.51-
      specified type NEC S65.59-
      laceration S65.51-
      specified type NEC S65.59-
    specified type NEC S65.59-
    thumb — *see* Injury, blood vessel, thumb
  foot S95.90-
    dorsal
      artery — *see* Injury, blood vessel, dorsal,
        artery
      vein — *see* Injury, blood vessel, dorsal,
        vein
    laceration S95.91-
    plantar artery — *see* Injury, blood vessel,
      plantar artery
    specified
      site NEC S95.80-
        laceration S95.81-
        specified type NEC S95.89-
      specified type NEC S95.99-
  forearm S55.90-
    laceration S55.91-
    radial artery — *see* Injury, blood vessel, radial
      artery
    specified
      site NEC S55.80-
        laceration S55.81-
        specified type NEC S55.89-
      type NEC S55.99-
    ulnar artery — *see* Injury, blood vessel, ulnar
      artery
    vein S55.20-
      laceration S55.21-
      specified type NEC S55.29-
  gastric
    artery — *see* Injury, mesenteric, artery, branch
    vein — *see* Injury, blood vessel, abdomen
  gastroduodenal artery — *see* Injury, mesenteric,
    artery, branch
  greater saphenous vein (lower leg level) S85.30-
    hip (and thigh) level S75.20-
      laceration (minor) (superficial) S75.21-
        major S75.22-
      specified type NEC S75.29-
    laceration S85.31-
    specified type NEC S85.39-
  hand (level) S65.90-
    finger — *see* Injury, blood vessel, finger
    laceration S65.91-
    palmar arch — *see* Injury, blood vessel, palmar
      arch
    radial artery — *see* Injury, blood vessel, radial
      artery, hand
    specified
      site NEC S65.80-
        laceration S65.81-
        specified type NEC S65.89-
      type NEC S65.99-
    thumb — *see* Injury, blood vessel, thumb
    ulnar artery — *see* Injury, blood vessel, ulnar
      artery, hand
  head S09.0
    intracranial — *see* Injury, intracranial
    multiple S09.0

Injury —*continued*
  blood vessel—*continued*
    hepatic
      artery — *see* Injury, mesenteric, artery
      vein — *see* Injury, vena cava, inferior
    hip S75.90-
      femoral artery — *see* Injury, blood vessel, femoral, artery
      femoral vein — *see* Injury, blood vessel, femoral, vein
      greater saphenous vein — *see* Injury, blood vessel, greater saphenous, hip level
      laceration S75.91-
      specified
        site NEC S75.80-
          laceration S75.81-
          specified type NEC S75.89-
        type NEC S75.99-
    hypogastric (artery) (vein) — *see* Injury, blood vessel, iliac
    iliac S35.5-
      artery S35.51-
      specified vessel NEC S35.5-
      uterine vessel — *see* Injury, blood vessel, uterine
      vein S35.51-
    innominate — *see* Injury, blood vessel, thoracic, innominate
    intercostal (artery) (vein) — *see* Injury, blood vessel, thoracic, intercostal
    jugular vein (external) S15.20-
      internal S15.30-
        laceration (minor) (superficial) S15.31-
          major S15.32-
        specified type NEC S15.39-
      laceration (minor) (superficial) S15.21-
        major S15.22-
      specified type NEC S15.29-
    leg (level) (lower) S85.90-
      greater saphenous — *see* Injury, blood vessel, greater saphenous
      laceration S85.91-
      lesser saphenous — *see* Injury, blood vessel, lesser saphenous
      peroneal artery — *see* Injury, blood vessel, peroneal artery
      popliteal
        artery — *see* Injury, blood vessel, popliteal, artery
        vein — *see* Injury, blood vessel, popliteal, vein
      specified
        site NEC S85.80-
          laceration S85.81-
          specified type NEC S85.89-
        type NEC S85.99-
      thigh — *see* Injury, blood vessel, hip
      tibial artery — *see* Injury, blood vessel, tibial artery
    lesser saphenous vein (lower leg level) S85.40-
      laceration S85.41-
      specified type NEC S85.49-
    limb
      lower — *see* Injury, blood vessel, leg
      upper — *see* Injury, blood vessel, arm
    lower back — *see* Injury, blood vessel, abdomen
    specified NEC — *see* Injury, blood vessel, abdomen, specified, site NEC
    mammary (artery) (vein) — *see* Injury, blood vessel, thoracic, specified site NEC
    mesenteric (inferior) (superior)
      artery — *see* Injury, mesenteric, artery
      vein — *see* Injury, blood vessel, portal vein
    neck S15.9
      specified site NEC S15.8
    ovarian (artery) (vein) — *see* subcategory S35.8
    palmar arch (superficial) S65.20-
      deep S65.30-
        laceration S65.31-
        specified type NEC S65.39-
      laceration S65.21-
      specified type NEC S65.29-

Injury —*continued*
  blood vessel—*continued*
    pelvis — *see* Injury, blood vessel, abdomen
    specified NEC — *see* Injury, blood vessel, abdomen, specified, site NEC
    peroneal artery S85.20-
      laceration S85.21-
      specified type NEC S85.29-
    plantar artery (deep) (foot) S95.10-
      laceration S95.11-
      specified type NEC S95.19-
    popliteal
      artery S85.00-
        laceration S85.01-
        specified type NEC S85.09-
      vein S85.50-
        laceration S85.51-
        specified type NEC S85.59-
    portal vein S35.319
      laceration S35.311
      specified type NEC S35.318
    precerebral — *see* Injury, blood vessel, neck
    pulmonary (artery) (vein) — *see* Injury, blood vessel, thoracic, pulmonary
    radial artery (forearm level) S55.10-
      hand and wrist (level) S65.10-
        laceration S65.11-
        specified type NEC S65.19-
      laceration S55.11-
      specified type NEC S55.19-
    renal
      artery S35.40-
        laceration S35.41-
        specified NEC S35.49-
      vein S35.40-
        laceration S35.41-
        specified NEC S35.49-
    saphenous vein (greater) (lower leg level) — *see* Injury, blood vessel, greater saphenous
      hip and thigh level — *see* Injury, blood vessel, greater saphenous, hip level
      lesser — *see* Injury, blood vessel, lesser saphenous
    shoulder
      specified NEC — *see* Injury, blood vessel, arm, specified site NEC
      superficial vein — *see* Injury, blood vessel, arm, superficial vein
    specified NEC
    splenic
      artery — *see* Injury, blood vessel, celiac artery, branch
      vein S35.329
        laceration S35.321
        specified NEC S35.328
    subclavian — *see* Injury, blood vessel, thoracic, innominate
    thigh — *see* Injury, blood vessel, hip
    thoracic S25.90
      aorta S25.00
        laceration (minor) (superficial) S25.01
          major S25.02
        specified type NEC S25.09
      azygos vein — *see* Injury, blood vessel, thoracic, specified, site NEC
      innominate
        artery S25.10-
          laceration (minor) (superficial) S25.11-
            major S25.12-
          specified type NEC S25.19-
        vein S25.30-
          laceration (minor) (superficial) S25.31-
            major S25.32-
          specified type NEC S25.39-
      intercostal S25.50-
        laceration S25.51-
        specified type NEC S25.59-
      laceration S25.91
      mammary vessel — *see* Injury, blood vessel, thoracic, specified, site NEC
      pulmonary S25.40-
        laceration (minor) (superficial) S25.41-
          major S25.42-

Injury —*continued*
  blood vessel—*continued*
    thoracic—*continued*
      pulmonary—*continued*
        specified type NEC S25.49-
      specified
        site NEC S25.80-
          laceration S25.81-
          specified type NEC S25.89-
        type NEC S25.99
      subclavian — *see* Injury, blood vessel, thoracic, innominate
      vena cava (superior) S25.20
        laceration (minor) (superficial) S25.21
          major S25.22
        specified type NEC S25.29
    thumb S65.40-
      laceration S65.41-
      specified type NEC S65.49-
    tibial artery S85.10-
      anterior S85.13-
        laceration S85.14-
        specified injury NEC S85.15-
      laceration S85.11-
      posterior S85.16-
        laceration S85.17-
        specified injury NEC S85.18-
      specified injury NEC S85.12-
    ulnar artery (forearm level) S55.00-
      hand and wrist (level) S65.00-
        laceration S65.01-
        specified type NEC S65.09-
      laceration S55.01-
      specified type NEC S55.09-
    upper arm (level) — *see* Injury, blood vessel, arm
      superficial vein — *see* Injury, blood vessel, arm, superficial vein
    uterine S35.5-
      artery S35.53-
      vein S35.53-
    vena cava — *see* Injury, vena cava
    vertebral artery S15.10-
      laceration (minor) (superficial) S15.11-
        major S15.12-
      specified type NEC S15.19-
    wrist (level) — *see* Injury, blood vessel, hand
  brachial plexus S14.3
    newborn P14.3
  brain (traumatic) S06.9-
    diffuse (axonal) S06.2x-
    focal S06.30-
    traumatic — *see* category S06
  brainstem S06.38-
  breast NOS S29.9
  broad ligament — *see* Injury, pelvic organ, specified site NEC
  bronchus, bronchi — *see* Injury, intrathoracic, bronchus
  brow S09.90
  buttock S39.92
  canthus, eye S05.90
  cardiac plexus — *see* Injury, nerve, thorax, sympathetic
  cauda equina S34.3
  cavernous sinus — *see* Injury, intracranial
  cecum — *see* Injury, colon
  celiac ganglion or plexus — *see* Injury, nerve, lumbosacral, sympathetic
  cerebellum — *see* Injury, intracranial
  cerebral — *see* Injury, intracranial
  cervix (uteri) — *see* Injury, uterus
  cheek (wall) S09.93
  chest — *see* Injury, thorax
  childbirth (newborn) (*see also* Birth, injury)
    maternal NEC O71.9
  chin S09.93
  choroid (eye) — *see* Injury, eye, specified site NEC
  clitoris S39.94
  coccyx (*see also* Injury, back, lower)
    complicating delivery O71.6
  colon — *see* Injury, intestine, large
  common bile duct — *see* Injury, liver
  conjunctiva (superficial) — *see* Injury, eye, conjunctiva

Injury —*continued*
conus medullaris — *see* Injury, spinal, sacral
cord
  spermatic (pelvic region) S37.898
    scrotal region S39.848
  spinal — *see* Injury, spinal cord, by region
cornea — *see* Injury, eye, specified site NEC
  abrasion — *see* Injury, eye, cornea, abrasion
cortex (cerebral) (*see also* Injury, intracranial)
  visual — *see* Injury, nerve, optic
costal region NEC S29.9
costochondral NEC S29.9
cranial
  cavity — *see* Injury, intracranial
  nerve — *see* Injury, nerve, cranial
crushing — *see* Crush
cutaneous sensory nerve
cystic duct — *see* Injury, liver
deep tissue — *see* Contusion, by site
  meaning pressure ulcer — *see* Ulcer, pressure,
    unstageable, by site
delivery (newborn) P15.9
  maternal NEC O71.9
Descemet's membrane — *see* Injury, eyeball,
  penetrating
diaphragm — *see* Injury, intrathoracic, diaphragm
duodenum — *see* Injury, intestine, small, duodenum
ear (auricle) (external) (canal) S09.91
  abrasion — *see* Abrasion, ear
  bite — *see* Bite, ear
  blister — *see* Blister, ear
  bruise — *see* Contusion, ear
  contusion — *see* Contusion, ear
  external constriction — *see* Constriction,
    external, ear
  hematoma — *see* Hematoma, ear
  inner — *see* Injury, ear, middle
  laceration — *see* Laceration, ear
  middle S09.30-
    blast — *see* Injury, blast, ear
    specified NEC S09.39-
  puncture — *see* Puncture, ear
  superficial — *see* Injury, superficial, ear
eighth cranial nerve (acoustic or auditory) — *see*
  Injury, nerve, acoustic
elbow S59.90-
  contusion — *see* Contusion, elbow
  dislocation — *see* Dislocation, elbow
  fracture — *see* Fracture, ulna, upper end
  open — *see* Wound, open, elbow
  specified NEC S59.80-
  sprain — *see* Sprain, elbow
  superficial — *see* Injury, superficial, elbow
eleventh cranial nerve (accessory) — *see* Injury,
  nerve, accessory
epididymis S39.94
epigastric region S39.91
epiglottis NEC S19.89
esophageal plexus — *see* Injury, nerve, thorax,
  sympathetic
esophagus (thoracic part) (*see also* Injury,
  intrathoracic, esophagus)
  cervical NEC S19.85
eustachian tube S09.91
eye S05.9-
  avulsion S05.7-
  ball — *see* Injury, eyeball
  conjunctiva S05.0-
  cornea
    abrasion S05.0-
    laceration S05.3-
      with prolapse S05.2-
  lacrimal apparatus S05.8x-
  orbit penetration S05.4-
  specified site NEC S05.8x-
  eyeball S05.8x-
    contusion S05.1-
    penetrating S05.6-
      with
        foreign body S05.5-
        prolapse or loss of intraocular tissue S05.2-

Injury —*continued*
eyeball—*continued*
  penetrating—*continued*
    without prolapse or loss of intraocular tissue
      S05.3-
    specified type NEC S05.8-
eyebrow S09.93
eyelid S09.93
  abrasion — *see* Abrasion, eyelid
  contusion — *see* Contusion, eyelid
  open — *see* Wound, open, eyelid
face S09.93
fallopian tube S37.509
  bilateral S37.502
    blast injury S37.512
    contusion S37.522
    laceration S37.532
    specified type NEC S37.592
  blast injury (primary) S37.519
    bilateral S37.512
    secondary — *see* Injury, fallopian tube,
      specified type NEC
    unilateral S37.511
  contusion S37.529
    bilateral S37.522
    unilateral S37.521
  laceration S37.539
    bilateral S37.532
    unilateral S37.531
  specified type NEC S37.599
    bilateral S37.592
    unilateral S37.591
  unilateral S37.501
    blast injury S37.511
    contusion S37.521
    laceration S37.531
    specified type NEC S37.591
fascia — *see* Injury, muscle
fifth cranial nerve (trigeminal) — *see* Injury, nerve,
  trigeminal
finger (nail) S69.9-
  blood vessel — *see* Injury, blood vessel, finger
  contusion — *see* Contusion, finger
  dislocation — *see* Dislocation, finger
  fracture — *see* Fracture, finger
  muscle — *see* Injury, muscle, finger
  nerve — *see* Injury, nerve, digital, finger
  open — *see* Wound, open, finger
  specified NEC S69.8-
  sprain — *see* Sprain, finger
  superficial — *see* Injury, superficial, finger
first cranial nerve (olfactory) — *see* Injury, nerve,
  olfactory
flank — *see* Injury, abdomen
foot S99.92-
  blood vessel — *see* Injury, blood vessel, foot
  contusion — *see* Contusion, foot
  dislocation — *see* Dislocation, foot
  fracture — *see* Fracture, foot
  muscle — *see* Injury, muscle, foot
  open — *see* Wound, open, foot
  specified type NEC S99.82-
  sprain — *see* Sprain, foot
  superficial — *see* Injury, superficial, foot
forceps NOS P15.9
forearm S59.91-
  blood vessel — *see* Injury, blood vessel, forearm
  contusion — *see* Contusion, forearm
  fracture — *see* Fracture, forearm
  muscle — *see* Injury, muscle, forearm
  nerve — *see* Injury, nerve, forearm
  open — *see* Wound, open, forearm
  specified NEC S59.81-
  superficial — *see* Injury, superficial, forearm
forehead S09.90
fourth cranial nerve (trochlear) — *see* Injury, nerve,
  trochlear
gallbladder S36.129
  contusion S36.122
  laceration S36.123
  specified NEC S36.128

Injury —*continued*
ganglion
  celiac, coeliac — *see* Injury, nerve, lumbosacral,
    sympathetic
  gasserian — *see* Injury, nerve, trigeminal
  stellate — *see* Injury, nerve, thorax, sympathetic
  thoracic sympathetic — *see* Injury, nerve, thorax,
    sympathetic
gasserian ganglion — *see* Injury, nerve, trigeminal
gastric artery — *see* Injury, blood vessel, celiac
  artery, branch
gastroduodenal artery — *see* Injury, blood vessel,
  celiac artery, branch
gastrointestinal tract — *see* Injury, intra-abdominal
  with open wound into abdominal cavity — *see*
    Wound, open, with penetration into
    peritoneal cavity
  colon — *see* Injury, intestine, large
  rectum — *see* Injury, intestine, large, rectum
    with open wound into abdominal cavity
      S36.61
  specified site NEC — *see* Injury, intra-abdominal,
    specified, site NEC
  stomach — *see* Injury, stomach
  small intestine — *see* Injury, intestine, small
genital organ(s)
  external S39.94
    specified NEC S39.848
  internal S37.90
    fallopian tube — *see* Injury, fallopian tube
    ovary — *see* Injury, ovary
    prostate — *see* Injury, prostate
    seminal vesicle — *see* Injury, pelvis, organ,
      specified site NEC
    uterus — *see* Injury, uterus
    vas deferens — *see* Injury, pelvis, organ,
      specified site NEC
  obstetrical trauma O71.9
gland
  lacrimal laceration — *see* Injury, eye, specified
    site NEC
  salivary S09.90
  thyroid NEC S19.84
globe (eye) S05.90
  specified NEC S05.8x-
groin — *see* Injury, abdomen
gum S09.90
hand S69.9-
  blood vessel — *see* Injury, blood vessel, hand
  contusion — *see* Contusion, hand
  fracture — *see* Fracture, hand
  muscle — *see* Injury, muscle, hand
  nerve — *see* Injury, nerve, hand
  open — *see* Wound, open, hand
  specified NEC S69.8-
  sprain — *see* Sprain, hand
  superficial — *see* Injury, superficial, hand
head S09.90
  with loss of consciousness S06.9-
  specified NEC S09.8
heart S26.90
  with hemopericardium S26.00
    contusion S26.01
    laceration (mild) S26.020
      moderate S26.021
      major S26.022
    specified type NEC S26.09
  contusion S26.91
  laceration S26.92
  specified type NEC S26.99
  without hemopericardium S26.10
    contusion S26.11
    laceration S26.12
    specified type NEC S26.19
heel — *see* Injury, foot
hepatic
  artery — *see* Injury, blood vessel, celiac artery,
    branch
  duct — *see* Injury, liver
  vein — *see* Injury, vena cava, inferior
hip S79.91-
  blood vessel — *see* Injury, blood vessel, hip
  contusion — *see* Contusion, hip

Injury —*continued*
  hip—*continued*
    dislocation — *see* Dislocation, hip
    fracture — *see* Fracture, femur, neck
    muscle — *see* Injury, muscle, hip
    nerve — *see* Injury, nerve, hip
    open — *see* Wound, open, hip
    sprain — *see* Sprain, hip
    superficial — *see* Injury, superficial, hip
    specified NEC S79.81-
  hymen S39.94
  hypogastric
    blood vessel — *see* Injury, blood vessel, iliac
    plexus — *see* Injury, nerve, lumbosacral,
        sympathetic
  ileum — *see* Injury, intestine, small
  iliac region S39.91
  instrumental (during surgery) — *see* Laceration,
      accidental complicating surgery
    birth injury — *see* Birth, injury
    nonsurgical — *see* Injury, by site
    obstetrical O71.9
      bladder O71.5
      cervix O71.3
      high vaginal O71.4
      perineal NOS O70.9
      urethra O71.5
      uterus O71.5
        with rupture or perforation O71.1
  internal T14.8
    aorta — *see* Injury, aorta
    bladder (sphincter) — *see* Injury, bladder
      with
        ectopic or molar pregnancy O08.6
        following ectopic or molar pregnancy O08.6
        obstetrical trauma O71.5
    bronchus, bronchi — *see* Injury, intrathoracic,
        bronchus
    cecum — *see* Injury, intestine, large
    cervix (uteri) *(see also* Injury, uterus)
      with ectopic or molar pregnancy O08.6
      following ectopic or molar pregnancy O08.6
      obstetrical trauma O71.3
    chest — *see* Injury, intrathoracic
    gastrointestinal tract — *see* Injury,
        intra-abdominal
    heart — *see* Injury, heart
    intestine NEC — *see* Injury, intestine
    intrauterine — *see* Injury, uterus
    mesentery — *see* Injury, intra-abdominal,
        specified, site NEC
    pelvis, pelvic (organ) S37.90
      following ectopic or molar pregnancy
          (subsequent episode) O08.6
      obstetrical trauma NEC O71.5
        rupture or perforation O71.1
      specified NEC S39.83
    rectum — *see* Injury, intestine, large, rectum
    stomach — *see* Injury, stomach
    ureter — *see* Injury, ureter
    urethra (sphincter) following ectopic or molar
        pregnancy O08.6
    uterus — *see* Injury, uterus
  interscapular area — *see* Injury, thorax
  intestine
    large S36.509
      ascending (right) S36.500
        blast injury (primary) S36.510
          secondary S36.590
        contusion S36.520
        laceration S36.530
        specified type NEC S36.590
      blast injury (primary) S36.519
        ascending (right) S36.510
        descending (left) S36.512
        rectum S36.61
        sigmoid S36.513
        specified site NEC S36.518
        transverse S36.511
      contusion S36.529
        ascending (right) S36.520
        descending (left) S36.522
        rectum S36.62

Injury —*continued*
  intestine —*continued*
    large—*continued*
      contusion—*continued*
        sigmoid S36.523
        specified site NEC S36.528
        transverse S36.521
      descending (left) S36.502
        blast injury (primary) S36.512
          secondary S36.592
        contusion S36.522
        laceration S36.532
        specified type NEC S36.592
      laceration S36.539
        ascending (right) S36.530
        descending (left) S36.532
        rectum S36.63
        sigmoid S36.533
        specified site NEC S36.538
        transverse S36.531
      rectum S36.60
        blast injury (primary) S36.61
          secondary S36.69
        contusion S36.62
        laceration S36.63
        specified type NEC S36.69
      sigmoid S36.503
        blast injury (primary) S36.513
          secondary S36.593
        contusion S36.523
        laceration S36.533
        specified type NEC S36.593
      specified
        site NEC S36.508
          blast injury (primary) S36.518
            secondary S36.598
          contusion S36.528
          laceration S36.538
          specified type NEC S36.598
        type NEC S36.599
          ascending (right) S36.590
          descending (left) S36.592
          rectum S36.69
          sigmoid S36.593
          specified site NEC S36.598
          transverse S36.591
      transverse S36.501
        blast injury (primary) S36.511
          secondary S36.591
        contusion S36.521
        laceration S36.531
        specified type NEC S36.591
    small S36.409
      blast injury (primary) S36.419
        duodenum S36.410
        secondary S36.499
          duodenum S36.490
          specified site NEC S36.498
        specified site NEC S36.418
      contusion S36.429
        duodenum S36.420
        specified site NEC S36.428
      duodenum S36.400
        blast injury (primary) S36.410
          secondary S36.490
        contusion S36.420
        laceration S36.430
        specified NEC S36.490
      laceration S36.439
        duodenum S36.430
        specified site NEC S36.438
      specified
        type NEC S36.499
          duodenum S36.490
          specified site NEC S36.498
        site NEC S36.408
    intra-abdominal S36.90
      adrenal gland — *see* Injury, adrenal gland
      bladder — *see* Injury, bladder
      colon — *see* Injury, intestine, large
      contusion S36.92
      fallopian tube — *see* Injury, fallopian tube
      gallbladder — *see* Injury, gallbladder

Injury —*continued*
  intra-abdominal—*continued*
    intestine — *see* Injury, intestine
    laceration S36.93
    liver — *see* Injury, liver
    kidney — *see* Injury, kidney
    ovary — *see* Injury, ovary
    pancreas — *see* Injury, pancreas
    pelvic NOS S37.90
    peritoneum — *see* Injury, intra-abdominal,
        specified, site NEC
    prostate — *see* Injury, prostate
    rectum — *see* Injury, intestine, large, rectum
    retroperitoneum — *see* Injury, intra-abdominal,
        specified, site NEC
    seminal vesicle — *see* Injury, pelvis, organ,
        specified site NEC
    small intestine — *see* Injury, intestine, small
    specified
      site NEC S36.899
        contusion S36.892
        laceration S36.893
        specified type NEC S36.898
      type NEC S36.99
    pelvic S37.90
      specified
        site NEC S37.899
          specified type NEC S37.898
        type NEC S37.99
    spleen — *see* Injury, spleen
    stomach — *see* Injury, stomach
    ureter — *see* Injury, ureter
    urethra — *see* Injury, urethra
    uterus — *see* Injury, uterus
    vas deferens — *see* Injury, pelvis, organ, specified
        site NEC
  intracranial (traumatic) S06.9-
    cerebellar hemorrhage, traumatic — *see* Injury,
        intracranial, focal
    cerebral edema, traumatic S06.1x-
      diffuse S06.1x-
      focal S06.1x-
    diffuse (axonal) S06.2x-
    epidural hemorrhage (traumatic) S06.4x-
    focal brain injury S06.30-
      contusion — *see* Contusion, cerebral
      laceration — *see* Laceration, cerebral
    intracerebral hemorrhage, traumatic S06.36-
      left side S06.35-
      right side S06.34-
    subarachnoid hemorrhage, traumatic S06.6x-
    subdural hemorrhage, traumatic S06.5x-
  intraocular — *see* Injury, eyeball, penetrating
  intrathoracic S27.9
    bronchus S27.409
      bilateral S27.402
      blast injury (primary) S27.419
        bilateral S27.412
        secondary — *see* Injury, intrathoracic,
            bronchus, specified type NEC
        unilateral S27.411
      contusion S27.429
        bilateral S27.422
        unilateral S27.421
      laceration S27.439
        bilateral S27.432
        unilateral S27.431
      specified type NEC S27.499
        bilateral S27.492
        unilateral S27.491
      unilateral S27.401
    diaphragm S27.809
      contusion S27.802
      laceration S27.803
      specified type NEC S27.808
    esophagus (thoracic) S27.819
      contusion S27.812
      laceration S27.813
      specified type NEC S27.818
    heart — *see* Injury, heart
    hemopneumothorax S27.2
    hemothorax S27.1

Injury —continued
  muscle —continued
    finger—continued
      middle—continued
        intrinsic S66.50-
          laceration S66.52-
          specified type NEC S66.59-
          strain S66.51-
      ring
        extensor (forearm level)
          hand level S66.30-
            laceration S66.32-
            specified type NEC S66.39-
            strain S66.31-
          laceration S56.42-
          specified type NEC S56.49-
          strain S56.41-
        flexor (forearm level)
          hand level S66.10-
            laceration S66.12-
            specified type NEC S66.19-
            strain S66.11-
          laceration S56.12-
          specified type NEC S56.19-
          strain S56.11-
        intrinsic S66.50-
          laceration S66.52-
          specified type NEC S66.59-
          strain S66.51-
    flexor
      finger(s) (other than thumb) — see Injury,
        muscle, finger
      forearm level, specified NEC — see Injury,
        muscle, forearm, flexor
      thumb — see Injury, muscle, thumb, flexor
      toe (long) (ankle level) (foot level) — see
        Injury, muscle, toe, flexor
    foot S96.90-
      intrinsic S96.20-
        laceration S96.22-
        specified type NEC S96.29-
        strain S96.21-
      laceration S96.92-
      long extensor, toe — see Injury, muscle, toe,
        extensor
      long flexor, toe — see Injury, muscle, toe,
        flexor
      specified
        site NEC S96.80-
          laceration S96.82-
          specified type NEC S96.89-
          strain S96.81-
        type NEC S96.99-
      strain S96.91-
    forearm (level) S56.90-
      extensor S56.50-
        laceration S56.52-
        specified type NEC S56.59-
        strain S56.51-
      flexor S56.20-
        laceration S56.22-
        specified type NEC S56.29-
        strain S56.21-
      laceration S56.92-
      specified S56.99-
        site NEC S56.80-
          laceration S56.82-
          strain S56.81-
          type NEC S56.89-
      strain S56.91-
    hand (level) S66.90-
      laceration S66.92-
      specified
        site NEC S66.80-
          laceration S66.82-
          specified type NEC S66.89-
          strain S66.81-
          type NEC S66.99-
      strain S66.91-
    head S09.10
      laceration S09.12
      specified type NEC S09.19
      strain S09.11

Injury —continued
  muscle —continued
    hip NEC S76.00-
      laceration S76.02-
      specified type NEC S76.09-
      strain S76.01-
    intrinsic
      ankle and foot level — see Injury, muscle, foot,
        intrinsic
      finger (other than thumb) — see Injury,
        muscle, finger by site, intrinsic
      foot (level) — see Injury, muscle, foot, intrinsic
      thumb — see Injury, muscle, thumb, intrinsic
    leg (level) (lower) S86.90-
      Achilles tendon — see Injury, Achilles tendon
      anterior muscle group — see Injury, muscle,
        anterior muscle group
      laceration S86.92-
      peroneal muscle group — see Injury, muscle,
        peroneal muscle group
      posterior muscle group — see Injury, muscle,
        posterior muscle group, leg level
      specified
        site NEC S86.80-
          laceration S86.82-
          specified type NEC S86.89-
          strain S86.81-
        type NEC S86.99-
      strain S86.91-
    long
      extensor toe, at ankle and foot level — see
        Injury, muscle, toe, extensor
      flexor, toe, at ankle and foot level — see Injury,
        muscle, toe, flexor
      head, biceps — see Injury, muscle, biceps,
        long head
    lower back S39.002
      laceration S39.022
      specified type NEC S39.092
      strain S39.012
    neck (level) S16.9
      laceration S16.2
      specified type NEC S16.8
      strain S16.1
    pelvis S39.003
      laceration S39.023
      specified type NEC S39.093
      strain S39.013
    peroneal muscle group, at leg level (lower)
      S86.30-
      laceration S86.32-
      specified type NEC S86.39-
      strain S86.31-
    posterior muscle (group)
      leg level (lower) S86.10-
        laceration S86.12-
        specified type NEC S86.19-
        strain S86.11-
      thigh level S76.30-
        laceration S76.32-
        specified type NEC S76.39-
        strain S76.31-
    quadriceps (thigh) S76.10-
      laceration S76.12-
      specified type NEC S76.19-
      strain S76.11-
    shoulder S46.90-
      laceration S46.92-
      rotator cuff — see Injury, rotator cuff
      specified site NEC S46.80-
        laceration S46.82-
        strain S46.81-
        specified type NEC S46.89-
      strain S46.91-
      specified type NEC S46.99-
    thigh NEC (level) S76.90-
      adductor — see Injury, muscle, adductor,
        thigh
      laceration S76.92-
      posterior muscle (group) — see Injury, muscle,
        posterior muscle, thigh level
      quadriceps — see Injury, muscle, quadriceps

Injury —continued
  muscle —continued
    thigh NEC—continued
      specified
        site NEC S76.80-
          laceration S76.82-
          specified type NEC S76.89-
          strain S76.81-
        type NEC S76.99-
      strain S76.91-
    thorax (level) S29.009
      back wall S29.002
      front wall S29.001
      laceration S29.029
        back wall S29.022
        front wall S29.021
      specified type NEC S29.099
        back wall S29.092
        front wall S29.091
      strain S29.019
        back wall S29.012
        front wall S29.011
    thumb
      abductor (forearm level) S56.30-
        laceration S56.32-
        specified type NEC S56.39-
        strain S56.31-
      extensor (forearm level) S56.30-
        hand level S66.20-
          laceration S66.22-
          specified type NEC S66.29-
          strain S66.21-
        laceration S56.32-
        specified type NEC S56.39-
        strain S56.31-
      flexor (forearm level) S56.00-
        hand level S66.00-
          laceration S66.02-
          specified type NEC S66.09-
          strain S66.01-
        laceration S56.02-
        specified type NEC S56.09-
        strain S56.01-
        wrist level — see Injury, muscle, thumb,
          flexor, hand level
      intrinsic S66.40-
        laceration S66.42-
        specified type NEC S66.49-
        strain S66.41-
    toe (see also Injury, muscle, foot)
      extensor, long S96.10-
        laceration S96.12-
        specified type NEC S96.19-
        strain S96.11-
      flexor, long S96.00-
        laceration S96.02-
        specified type NEC S96.09-
        strain S96.01-
    triceps S46.30-
      laceration S46.32-
      specified type NEC S46.39-
      strain S46.31-
    wrist (and hand) level — see Injury, muscle, hand
  musculocutaneous nerve — see Injury, nerve,
    musculocutaneous
  myocardium — see Injury, heart
  nape — see Injury, neck
  nasal (septum) (sinus) S09.92
  nasopharynx S09.92
  neck S19.9
    specified NEC S19.80
      specified site NEC S19.89
  nerve NEC T14.8
    abdomen S34.9
      peripheral S34.6
      specified site NEC S34.8
    abducens S04.4-
      contusion S04.4-
      laceration S04.4-
      specified type NEC S04.4-
    abducent — see Injury, nerve, abducens

Injury —*continued*
  nerve —*continued*
    accessory S04.7-
      contusion S04.7-
      laceration S04.7-
      specified type NEC S04.7-
    acoustic S04.6-
      contusion S04.6-
      laceration S04.6-
      specified type NEC S04.6-
    ankle S94.9-
      cutaneous sensory S94.3-
      specified site NEC — *see* subcategory S94.8
    anterior crural, femoral — *see* Injury, nerve, femoral
    arm (upper) S44.9-
      axillary — *see* Injury, nerve, axillary
      cutaneous — *see* Injury, nerve, cutaneous, arm
      median — *see* Injury, nerve, median, upper arm
      musculocutaneous — *see* Injury, nerve, musculocutaneous
      radial — *see* Injury, nerve, radial, upper arm
      specified site NEC — *see* subcategory S44.8
      ulnar — *see* Injury, nerve, ulnar, arm
    auditory — *see* Injury, nerve, acoustic
    axillary S44.3-
    brachial plexus — *see* Injury, brachial plexus
    cervical sympathetic S14.5
    cranial S04.9
      contusion S04.9
      eighth (acoustic or auditory) — *see* Injury, nerve, acoustic
      eleventh (accessory) — *see* Injury, nerve, accessory
      fifth (trigeminal) — *see* Injury, nerve, trigeminal
      first (olfactory) — *see* Injury, nerve, olfactory
      fourth (trochlear) — *see* Injury, nerve, trochlear
      laceration S04.9
      ninth (glossopharyngeal) — *see* Injury, nerve, glossopharyngeal
      second (optic) — *see* Injury, nerve, optic
      seventh (facial) — *see* Injury, nerve, facial
      sixth (abducent) — *see* Injury, nerve, abducens
      specified
        nerve NEC S04.89-
          contusion S04.89-
          laceration S04.89-
          specified type NEC S04.89-
        type NEC S04.9
      tenth (pneumogastric or vagus) — *see* Injury, nerve, vagus
      third (oculomotor) — *see* Injury, nerve, oculomotor
      twelfth (hypoglossal) — *see* Injury, nerve, hypoglossal
    cutaneous sensory
      ankle (level) S94.3-
      arm (upper) (level) S44.5-
      foot (level) — *see* Injury, nerve, cutaneous sensory, ankle
      forearm (level) S54.3-
      hip (level) S74.2-
      leg (lower level) S84.2-
      shoulder (level) — *see* Injury, nerve, cutaneous sensory, arm
      thigh (level) — *see* Injury, nerve, cutaneous sensory, hip
    deep peroneal — *see* Injury, nerve, peroneal, foot
    digital
      finger S64.4-
        index S64.49-
        little S64.49-
        middle S64.49-
        ring S64.49-
      thumb S64.3-
      toe — *see* Injury, nerve, ankle, specified site NEC

Injury —*continued*
  nerve —*continued*
    eighth cranial (acoustic or auditory) — *see* Injury, nerve, acoustic
    eleventh cranial (accessory) — *see* Injury, nerve, accessory
    facial S04.5-
      contusion S04.5-
      laceration S04.5-
      newborn P11.3
      specified type NEC S04.5-
    femoral (hip level) (thigh level) S74.1-
    fifth cranial (trigeminal) — *see* Injury, nerve, trigeminal
    finger (digital) — *see* Injury, nerve, digital, finger
    first cranial (olfactory) — *see* Injury, nerve, olfactory
    foot S94.9-
      cutaneous sensory S94.3-
      deep peroneal S94.2-
      lateral plantar S94.0-
      medial plantar S94.1-
      specified site NEC — *see* subcategory S94.8
    forearm (level) S54.9-
      cutaneous sensory — *see* Injury, nerve, cutaneous sensory, forearm
      median — *see* Injury, nerve, median
      radial — *see* Injury, nerve, radial
      specified site NEC — *see* subcategory S54.8
      ulnar — *see* Injury, nerve, ulnar
    fourth cranial (trochlear) — *see* Injury, nerve, trochlear
    glossopharyngeal S04.89-
      specified type NEC S04.89-
    hand S64.9-
      median — *see* Injury, nerve, median, hand
      radial — *see* Injury, nerve, radial, hand
      specified NEC — *see* subcategory S64.8
      ulnar — *see* Injury, nerve, ulnar, hand
    hip (level) S74.9-
      cutaneous sensory — *see* Injury, nerve, cutaneous sensory, hip
      femoral — *see* Injury, nerve, femoral
      sciatic — *see* Injury, nerve, sciatic
      specified site NEC — *see* subcategory S74.8
    hypoglossal S04.89-
      specified type NEC S04.89-
    lateral plantar S94.0-
    leg (lower) S84.9-
      cutaneous sensory — *see* Injury, nerve, cutaneous sensory, leg
      peroneal — *see* Injury, nerve, peroneal
      specified site NEC — *see* subcategory S84.8
      tibial — *see* Injury, nerve, tibial
      upper — *see* Injury, nerve, thigh
    lower
      back — *see* Injury, nerve, abdomen, specified site NEC
      peripheral — *see* Injury, nerve, abdomen, peripheral
      limb — *see* Injury, nerve, leg
    lumbar plexus — *see* Injury, nerve, lumbosacral, sympathetic
    lumbar spinal — *see* Injury, nerve spinal, lumbar
    lumbosacral
      plexus — *see* Injury, nerve, lumbosacral, sympathetic
      sympathetic S34.5
    medial plantar S94.1-
    median (forearm level) S54.1-
      hand (level) S64.1-
      upper arm (level) S44.1-
      wrist (level) — *see* Injury, nerve, median, hand
    musculocutaneous S44.4-
    musculospiral (upper arm level) — *see* Injury, nerve, radial, upper arm
    neck S14.9
      peripheral S14.4
      specified site NEC S14.8
      sympathetic S14.5
    ninth cranial (glossopharyngeal) — *see* Injury, nerve, glossopharyngeal

Injury —*continued*
  nerve —*continued*
    oculomotor S04.1-
      contusion S04.1-
      laceration S04.1-
      specified type NEC S04.1-
    olfactory S04.81-
      specified type NEC S04.81-
    optic S04.01-
      contusion S04.01-
      laceration S04.01-
      specified type NEC S04.01-
    pelvic girdle — *see* Injury, nerve, hip
    pelvis — *see* Injury, nerve, abdomen, specified site NEC
      peripheral — *see* Injury, nerve, abdomen, peripheral
    peripheral NEC T14.8
      abdomen — *see* Injury, nerve, abdomen, peripheral
      lower back — *see* Injury, nerve, abdomen, peripheral
      neck — *see* Injury, nerve, neck, peripheral
      pelvis — *see* Injury, nerve, abdomen, peripheral
      specified NEC T14.8
    peroneal (lower leg level) S84.1-
      foot S94.2-
    plexus
      brachial — *see* Injury, brachial plexus
      celiac, coeliac — *see* Injury, nerve, lumbosacral, sympathetic
      mesenteric, inferior — *see* Injury, nerve, lumbosacral, sympathetic
      sacral — *see* Injury, lumbosacral plexus
      spinal
        brachial — *see* Injury, brachial plexus
        lumbosacral — *see* Injury, lumbosacral plexus
    pneumogastric — *see* Injury, nerve, vagus
    radial (forearm level) S54.2-
      hand (level) S64.2-
      upper arm (level) S44.2-
      wrist (level) — *see* Injury, nerve, radial, hand
    root — *see* Injury, nerve, spinal, root
    sacral plexus — *see* Injury, lumbosacral plexus
    sacral spinal — *see* Injury, nerve, spinal. sacral
    sciatic (hip level) (thigh level) S74.0-
    second cranial (optic) — *see* Injury, nerve, optic
    seventh cranial (facial) — *see* Injury, nerve, facial
    shoulder — *see* Injury, nerve, arm
    sixth cranial (abducent) — *see* Injury, nerve, abducens
    spinal
      plexus — *see* Injury, nerve, plexus, spinal
      root
        cervical S14.2
        dorsal S24.2
        lumbar S34.21
        sacral S34.22
        thoracic — *see* Injury, nerve, spinal, root, dorsal
    splanchnic — *see* Injury, nerve, lumbosacral, sympathetic
    sympathetic NEC — *see* Injury, nerve, lumbosacral, sympathetic
      cervical — *see* Injury, nerve, cervical sympathetic
    tenth cranial (pneumogastric or vagus) — *see* Injury, nerve, vagus
    thigh (level) — *see* Injury, nerve, hip
      cutaneous sensory — *see* Injury, nerve, cutaneous sensory, hip
      femoral — *see* Injury, nerve, femoral
      sciatic — *see* Injury, nerve, sciatic
      specified NEC — *see* Injury, nerve, hip
    third cranial (oculomotor) — *see* Injury, nerve, oculomotor
    thorax S24.9
      peripheral S24.3
      specified site NEC S24.8
      sympathetic S24.4
    thumb, digital — *see* Injury, nerve, digital, thumb

Injury —continued
  nerve —continued
    tibial (lower leg level) (posterior) S84.0-
    toe — see Injury, nerve, ankle
    trigeminal S04.3-
      contusion S04.3-
      laceration S04.3-
      specified type NEC S04.3-
    trochlear S04.2-
      contusion S04.2-
      laceration S04.2-
      specified type NEC S04.2-
    twelfth cranial (hypoglossal) — see Injury, nerve, hypoglossal
    ulnar (forearm level) S54.0-
      arm (upper) (level) S44.0-
      hand (level) S64.0-
      wrist (level) — see Injury, nerve, ulnar, hand
    vagus S04.89-
      specified type NEC S04.89-
    wrist (level) — see Injury, nerve, hand
  ninth cranial nerve (glossopharyngeal) — see Injury, nerve, glossopharyngeal
  nose (septum) S09.92
  obstetrical O71.9
    specified NEC O71.89
  occipital (region) (scalp) S09.90
    lobe — see Injury, intracranial
  optic chiasm S04.02
  optic radiation S04.03-
  optic tract and pathways S04.03-
  orbit, orbital (region) — see Injury, eye
    penetrating (with foreign body) — see Injury, eye, orbit, penetrating
    specified NEC — see Injury, eye, specified site NEC
  ovary, ovarian S37.409
    bilateral S37.402
      contusion S37.422
      laceration S37.432
      specified type NEC S37.492
    blood vessel — see Injury, blood vessel, ovarian
    contusion S37.429
      bilateral S37.422
      unilateral S37.421
    laceration S37.439
      bilateral S37.432
      unilateral S37.431
    specified type NEC S37.499
      bilateral S37.492
      unilateral S37.491
    unilateral S37.401
      contusion S37.421
      laceration S37.431
      specified type NEC S37.491
  palate (hard) (soft) S09.93
  pancreas S36.209
    body S36.201
      contusion S36.221
      laceration S36.231
        major S36.261
        minor S36.241
        moderate S36.251
      specified type NEC S36.291
    contusion S36.229
    head S36.200
      contusion S36.220
      laceration S36.230
        major S36.260
        minor S36.240
        moderate S36.250
      specified type NEC S36.290
    laceration S36.239
      major S36.269
      minor S36.249
      moderate S36.259
    specified type NEC S36.299
    tail S36.202
      contusion S36.222
      laceration S36.232
        major S36.262
        minor S36.242
        moderate S36.252
      specified type NEC S36.292

Injury —continued
  parietal (region) (scalp) S09.90
    lobe — see Injury, intracranial
  patellar ligament (tendon) S76.10-
    laceration S76.12-
    specified NEC S76.19-
    strain S76.11-
  pelvis, pelvic (floor) S39.93
    complicating delivery O70.1
    joint or ligament, complicating delivery O71.6
    organ S37.90
      with ectopic or molar pregnancy O08.6
      complication of abortion — see Abortion
      contusion S37.92
      following ectopic or molar pregnancy O08.6
      laceration S37.93
      obstetrical trauma NEC O71.5
      specified
        site NEC S37.899
          contusion S37.892
          laceration S37.893
          specified type NEC S37.898
        type NEC S37.99
    specified NEC S39.83
  penis S39.94
  perineum S39.94
  peritoneum — see Injury, intra-abdominal, specified site NEC
  periurethral tissue — see Injury, urethra
    complicating delivery O71.82
  phalanges
    foot — see Injury, foot
    hand — see Injury, hand
  pharynx NEC S19.85
  pleura — see Injury, intrathoracic, pleura
  plexus
    brachial — see Injury, brachial plexus
    cardiac — see Injury, nerve, thorax, sympathetic
    celiac, coeliac — see Injury, nerve, lumbosacral, sympathetic
    esophageal — see Injury, nerve, thorax, sympathetic
    hypogastric — see Injury, nerve, lumbosacral, sympathetic
    lumbar, lumbosacral — see Injury, lumbosacral plexus
    mesenteric — see Injury, nerve, lumbosacral, sympathetic
    pulmonary — see Injury, nerve, thorax, sympathetic
  postcardiac surgery (syndrome) I97.0
  prepuce S39.94
  prostate S37.829
    contusion S37.822
    laceration S37.823
    specified type NEC S37.828
  pubic region S39.94
  pudendum S39.94
  pulmonary plexus — see Injury, nerve, thorax, sympathetic
  rectovaginal septum NEC S39.83
  rectum — see Injury, intestine, large, rectum
  retina — see Injury, eye, specified site NEC
    penetrating — see Injury, eyeball, penetrating
  retroperitoneal — see Injury, intra-abdominal, specified site NEC
  rotator cuff (muscle(s)) (tendon(s)) S46.00-
    laceration S46.02-
    specified type NEC S46.09-
    strain S46.01-
  round ligament — see Injury, pelvic organ, specified site NEC
  sacral plexus — see Injury, lumbosacral plexus
  salivary duct or gland S09.93
  scalp S09.90
    newborn (birth injury) P12.9
      due to monitoring (electrode) (sampling incision) P12.4
      specified NEC P12.89
        caput succedaneum P12.81
  scapular region — see Injury, shoulder
  sclera — see Injury, eye, specified site NEC
    penetrating — see Injury, eyeball, penetrating

Injury —continued
  scrotum S39.94
  second cranial nerve (optic) — see Injury, nerve, optic
  seminal vesicle — see Injury, pelvic organ, specified site NEC
  seventh cranial nerve (facial) — see Injury, nerve, facial
    blood vessel — see Injury, blood vessel, arm
    contusion — see Contusion, shoulder
    dislocation — see Dislocation, shoulder
    fracture — see Fracture, shoulder
    muscle — see Injury, muscle, shoulder
    nerve — see Injury, nerve, shoulder
    open — see Wound, open, shoulder
    specified type NEC S49.8-
    sprain — see Sprain, shoulder girdle
    superficial — see Injury, superficial, shoulder
  sinus
    cavernous — see Injury, intracranial
    nasal S09.92
  sixth cranial nerve (abducent) — see Injury, nerve, abducens
  skeleton, birth injury P13.9
    specified part NEC P13.8
  skin NEC T14.8
    surface intact — see Injury, superficial
  skull NEC S09.90
  specified NEC T14.8
  spermatic cord (pelvic region) S37.898
    scrotal region S39.848
  spinal (cord)
    cervical (neck) S14.109
      anterior cord syndrome S14.139
        C1 level S14.131
        C2 level S14.132
        C3 level S14.133
        C4 level S14.134
        C5 level S14.135
        C6 level S14.136
        C7 level S14.137
        C8 level S14.138
      Brown-Séquard syndrome S14.149
        C1 level S14.141
        C2 level S14.142
        C3 level S14.143
        C4 level S14.144
        C5 level S14.145
        C6 level S14.146
        C7 level S14.147
        C8 level S14.148
      C1 level S14.101
      C2 level S14.102
      C3 level S14.103
      C4 level S14.104
      C5 level S14.105
      C6 level S14.106
      C7 level S14.107
      C8 level S14.108
      central cord syndrome S14.129
        C1 level S14.121
        C2 level S14.122
        C3 level S14.123
        C4 level S14.124
        C5 level S14.125
        C6 level S14.126
        C7 level S14.127
        C8 level S14.128
      complete lesion S14.119
        C1 level S14.111
        C2 level S14.112
        C3 level S14.113
        C4 level S14.114
        C5 level S14.115
        C6 level S14.116
        C7 level S14.117
        C8 level S14.118
      concussion S14.0
      edema S14.0
      incomplete lesion specified NEC S14.159
        C1 level S14.151
        C2 level S14.152
        C3 level S14.153

Injury —*continued*
  superficial—*continued*
    foot—*continued*
      external constriction — *see* Constriction, external, foot
      foreign body — *see* Foreign body, superficial, foot
    forearm S50.91-
      abrasion — *see* Abrasion, forearm
      bite — *see* Bite, forearm, superficial
      blister — *see* Blister, forearm
      contusion — *see* Contusion, forearm
      elbow only — *see* Injury, superficial, elbow
      external constriction — *see* Constriction, external, forearm
      foreign body — *see* Foreign body, superficial, forearm
    forehead — *see* Injury, superficial, head NEC
    foreign body — *see* Foreign body, superficial
    genital organs, external
      female S30.97
      male S30.96
    globe (eye) — *see* Injury, eye, specified site NEC
    groin S30.92
    gum — *see* Injury, superficial, oral cavity
    hand S60.92-
      abrasion — *see* Abrasion, hand
      bite — *see* Bite, superficial, hand
      contusion — *see* Contusion, hand
      external constriction — *see* Constriction, external, hand
      foreign body — *see* Foreign body, superficial, hand
    head S00.90
      ear — *see* Injury, superficial, ear
      eyelid — *see* Injury, superficial, eyelid
      nose S00.30
      oral cavity S00.502
      scalp S00.00
      specified site NEC S00.80
    heel — *see* Injury, superficial, foot
    hip S70.91-
      abrasion — *see* Abrasion, hip
      bite — *see* Bite, superficial, hip
      blister — *see* Blister, hip
      contusion — *see* Contusion, hip
      external constriction — *see* Constriction, external, hip
      foreign body — *see* Foreign body, superficial, hip
    iliac region — *see* Injury, superficial, abdomen
    inguinal region — *see* Injury, superficial, abdomen
    insect bite — *see* Bite, insect, by site
    interscapular region — *see* Injury, superficial, thorax, back
    jaw — *see* Injury, superficial, head, specified NEC
    knee S80.91-
      abrasion — *see* Abrasion, knee
      bite — *see* Bite, superficial, knee
      blister — *see* Blister, knee
      contusion — *see* Contusion, knee
      external constriction — *see* Constriction, external, knee
      foreign body — *see* Foreign body, superficial, knee
    labium (majus) (minus) S30.95
    lacrimal (apparatus) (gland) (sac) — *see* Injury, eye, specified site NEC
    larynx — *see* Injury, superficial, throat
    leg (lower) S80.92-
      abrasion — *see* Abrasion, leg
      bite — *see* Bite, superficial, leg
      contusion — *see* Contusion, leg
      external constriction — *see* Constriction, external, leg
      foreign body — *see* Foreign body, superficial, leg
      knee — *see* Injury, superficial, knee
    limb NEC T14.8
    lip S00.501
    lower back S30.91
    lumbar region S30.91

Injury —*continued*
  superficial—*continued*
    malar region — *see* Injury, superficial, head, specified NEC
    mammary — *see* Injury, superficial, breast
    mastoid region — *see* Injury, superficial, head, specified NEC
    mouth — *see* Injury, superficial, oral cavity
    muscle NEC T14.8
    nail NEC T14.8
      finger — *see* Injury, superficial, finger
      toe — *see* Injury, superficial, toe
    nasal (septum) — *see* Injury, superficial, nose
    neck S10.90
      specified site NEC S10.80
    nose (septum) S00.30
    occipital region — *see* Injury, superficial, scalp
    oral cavity S00.502
    orbital region — *see* Injury, superficial, periocular area
    palate — *see* Injury, superficial, oral cavity
    palm — *see* Injury, superficial, hand
    parietal region — *see* Injury, superficial, scalp
    pelvis S30.91
      girdle — *see* Injury, superficial, hip
    penis S30.93
    perineum
      female S30.95
      male S30.91
    periocular area S00.20-
      abrasion — *see* Abrasion, eyelid
      bite — *see* Bite, superficial, eyelid
      contusion — *see* Contusion, eyelid
      external constriction — *see* Constriction, external, eyelid
      foreign body — *see* Foreign body, superficial, eyelid
    phalanges
      finger — *see* Injury, superficial, finger
      toe — *see* Injury, superficial, toe
    pharynx — *see* Injury, superficial, throat
    pinna — *see* Injury, superficial, ear
    popliteal space — *see* Injury, superficial, knee
    prepuce S30.93
    pubic region S30.91
    pudendum
      female S30.97
      male S30.96
    sacral region S30.91
    scalp S00.00
    scapular region — *see* Injury, superficial, shoulder
    sclera — *see* Injury, eye, specified site NEC
    scrotum S30.94
    shin — *see* Injury, superficial, leg
    shoulder S40.91-
      abrasion — *see* Abrasion, shoulder
      bite — *see* Bite, superficial, shoulder
      blister — *see* Blister, shoulder
      contusion — *see* Contusion, shoulder
      external constriction — *see* Constriction, external, shoulder
      foreign body — *see* Foreign body, superficial, shoulder
    skin NEC T14.8
    sternal region — *see* Injury, superficial, thorax, front
    subconjunctival — *see* Injury, eye, specified site NEC
    subcutaneous NEC T14.8
    submaxillary region — *see* Injury, superficial, head, specified NEC
    submental region — *see* Injury, superficial, head, specified NEC
    subungual
      finger(s) — *see* Injury, superficial, finger
      toe(s) — *see* Injury, superficial, toe
    supraclavicular fossa — *see* Injury, superficial, neck
    supraorbital — *see* Injury, superficial, head, specified NEC
    temple — *see* Injury, superficial, head, specified NEC

Injury —*continued*
  superficial—*continued*
    temporal region — *see* Injury, superficial, head, specified NEC
    testis S30.94
    thigh S70.92-
      abrasion — *see* Abrasion, thigh
      bite — *see* Bite, superficial, thigh
      blister — *see* Blister, thigh
      contusion — *see* Contusion, thigh
      external constriction — *see* Constriction, external, thigh
      foreign body — *see* Foreign body, superficial, thigh
    thorax, thoracic (wall) S20.90
      abrasion — *see* Abrasion, thorax
      back S20.40-
      bite — *see* Bite, thorax, superficial
      blister — *see* Blister, thorax
      contusion — *see* Contusion, thorax
      external constriction — *see* Constriction, external, thorax
      foreign body — *see* Foreign body, superficial, thorax
      front S20.30-
    throat S10.10
      abrasion S10.11
      bite S10.17
        insect S10.16
      blister S10.12
      contusion S10.0
      external constriction S10.14
      foreign body S10.15
    thumb S60.93-
      abrasion — *see* Abrasion, thumb
      bite — *see* Bite, superficial, thumb
      blister — *see* Blister, thumb
      contusion — *see* Contusion, thumb
      external constriction — *see* Constriction, external, thumb
      foreign body — *see* Foreign body, superficial, thumb
      insect bite — *see* Bite, insect, thumb
        specified type NEC S60.392
        specified type NEC S60.391
      specified type NEC S60.399
    toe(s) S90.93-
      abrasion — *see* Abrasion, toe
      bite — *see* Bite, toe
      blister — *see* Blister, toe
      contusion — *see* Contusion, toe
      external constriction — *see* Constriction, external, toe
      foreign body — *see* Foreign body, superficial, toe
      great S90.93-
    tongue — *see* Injury, superficial, oral cavity
    tooth, teeth — *see* Injury, superficial, oral cavity
    trachea S10.10
    tunica vaginalis S30.94
    tympanum, tympanic membrane — *see* Injury, superficial, ear
    uvula — *see* Injury, superficial, oral cavity
    vagina S30.95
    vocal cords — *see* Injury, superficial, throat
    vulva S30.95
    wrist S60.91-
  supraclavicular region — *see* Injury, neck
  supraorbital S09.93
  suprarenal gland (multiple) — *see* Injury, adrenal
  surgical complication (external or internal site) — *see* Laceration, accidental complicating surgery
  temple S09.90
  temporal region S09.90
  tendon (*see also* Injury, muscle, by site)
    abdomen — *see* Injury, muscle, abdomen
    Achilles — *see* Injury, Achilles tendon
    lower back — *see* Injury, muscle, lower back
    pelvic organs — *see* Injury, muscle, pelvis
  tenth cranial nerve (pneumogastric or vagus) — *see* Injury, nerve, vagus
  testis S39.94

Injury —continued
  thigh S79.92-
    blood vessel — see Injury, blood vessel, hip
    contusion — see Contusion, thigh
    fracture — see Fracture, femur
    muscle — see Injury, muscle, thigh
    nerve — see Injury, nerve, thigh
    open — see Wound, open, thigh
    specified NEC S79.82-
    superficial — see Injury, superficial, thigh
  third cranial nerve (oculomotor) — see Injury, nerve, oculomotor
  thorax, thoracic S29.9
    blood vessel — see Injury, blood vessel, thorax
    cavity — see Injury, intrathoracic
    dislocation — see Dislocation, thorax
    external (wall) S29.9
      contusion — see Contusion, thorax
      nerve — see Injury, nerve, thorax
      open — see Wound, open, thorax
      specified NEC S29.8
      sprain — see Sprain, thorax
      superficial — see Injury, superficial, thorax
    fracture — see Fracture, thorax
    internal — see Injury, intrathoracic
    intrathoracic organ — see Injury, intrathoracic
    sympathetic ganglion — see Injury, nerve, thorax, sympathetic
  throat — see Injury, neck
  thumb S69.9-
    blood vessel — see Injury, blood vessel, thumb
    contusion — see Contusion, thumb
    dislocation — see Dislocation, thumb
    fracture — see Fracture, thumb
    muscle — see Injury, muscle, thumb
    nerve — see Injury, nerve, digital, thumb
    open — see Wound, open, thumb
    specified NEC S69.8-
    sprain — see Sprain, thumb
    superficial — see Injury, superficial, thumb
  thymus (gland) — see Injury, intrathoracic, specified organ NEC
  thyroid (gland) NEC S19.84
  toe S99.92-
    contusion — see Contusion, toe
    dislocation — see Dislocation, toe
    fracture — see Fracture, toe
    muscle — see Injury, muscle, toe
    open — see Wound, open, toe
    specified type NEC S99.82-
    sprain — see Sprain, toe
    superficial — see Injury, superficial, toe
  tongue S09.93
  tonsil S09.93
  tooth S09.93
  trachea (cervical) NEC S19.82
    thoracic — see Injury, intrathoracic, trachea, thoracic
  transfusion-related acute lung (TRALI) J95.84
  tunica vaginalis S39.94
  twelfth cranial nerve (hypoglossal) — see Injury, nerve, hypoglossal
  ureter S37.10
    contusion S37.12
    laceration S37.13
    specified type NEC S37.39
  urethra (sphincter) S37.30
    at delivery O71.5
    contusion S37.32
    laceration S37.33
    specified type NEC S37.39
  urinary organ S37.90
    contusion S37.92
    laceration S37.93
    specified site NEC S37.899
      contusion S37.892
      laceration S37.893
      specified type NEC S37.898
    type NEC S37.99
  uterus, uterine S37.60
    with ectopic or molar pregnancy O08.6
    blood vessel — see Injury, blood vessel, iliac
    contusion S37.62

Injury —continued
  uterus, uterine—continued
    laceration S37.63
      cervix at delivery O71.3
      rupture associated with obstetrics — see Rupture, uterus
    specified type NEC S37.69
  uvula S09.93
  vagina S39.93
    abrasion S30.814
    bite S31.45
      insect S30.864
      superficial NEC S30.874
    contusion S30.23
    crush S38.03
    during delivery — see Laceration, vagina, during delivery
    external constriction S30.844
    insect bite S30.864
    laceration S31.41
      with foreign body S31.42
    open wound S31.40
    puncture S31.43
      with foreign body S31.44
    superficial S30.95
      foreign body S30.854
  vas deferens — see Injury, pelvic organ, specified site NEC
  vascular NEC T14.8
  vein — see Injury, blood vessel
  vena cava (superior) S25.20
    inferior S35.10
      laceration (minor) (superficial) S35.11
        major S35.12
      specified type NEC S35.19
    laceration (minor) (superficial) S25.21
      major S25.22
    specified type NEC S25.29
  vesical (sphincter) — see Injury, bladder
  visual cortex S04.04-
  vitreous (humor) S05.90
    specified NEC S05.8x-
  vocal cord NEC S19.83
  vulva S39.94
    abrasion S30.814
    bite S31.45
      insect S30.864
      superficial NEC S30.874
    contusion S30.23
    crush S38.03
    during delivery — see Laceration, perineum, female, during delivery
    external constriction S30.844
    insect bite S30.864
    laceration S31.41
      with foreign body S31.42
    open wound S31.40
    puncture S31.43
      with foreign body S31.44
    superficial S30.95
      foreign body S30.854
  whiplash (cervical spine) S13.4
  wrist S69.9-
    blood vessel — see Injury, blood vessel, hand
    contusion — see Contusion, wrist
    dislocation — see Dislocation, wrist
    fracture — see Fracture, wrist
    muscle — see Injury, muscle, hand
    nerve — see Injury, nerve, hand
    open — see Wound, open, wrist
    specified NEC S69.8-
    sprain — see Sprain, wrist
    superficial — see Injury, superficial, wrist
Inoculation (see also Vaccination)
  complication or reaction — see Complications, vaccination
Insanity, insane (see also Psychosis)
  adolescent — see Schizophrenia
  confusional F28
    acute or subacute F05
  delusional F22
  senile F03

Insect
  bite — see Bite, insect, by site
  venomous, poisoning NEC (by) — see Venom, arthropod
Insensitivity
  adrenocorticotropin hormone (ACTH) E27.49
  androgen E34.50
    complete E34.51
    partial E34.52
Insertion
  cord (umbilical) lateral or velamentous O43.12-
  intrauterine contraceptive device (encounter for) — see Intrauterine contraceptive device
Insolation (sunstroke) T67.0
Insomnia (organic) G47.00
  adjustment F51.02
  adjustment disorder F51.02
  behavioral, of childhood Z73.819
    combined type Z73.812
    limit setting type Z73.811
    sleep-onset association type Z73.810
  childhood Z73.819
  chronic F51.04
    somatized tension F51.04
  conditioned F51.04
  due to
    alcohol
      abuse F10.182
      dependence F10.282
      use F10.982
    amphetamines
      abuse F15.182
      dependence F15.282
      use F15.982
    anxiety disorder F51.05
    caffeine
      abuse F15.182
      dependence F15.282
      use F15.982
    cocaine
      abuse F14.182
      dependence F14.282
      use F14.982
    depression F51.05
    drug NEC
      abuse F19.182
      dependence F19.282
      use F19.982
    medical condition G47.01
    mental disorder NEC F51.05
    opioid
      abuse F11.182
      dependence F11.282
      use F11.982
    psychoactive substance NEC
      abuse F19.182
      dependence F19.282
      use F19.982
    sedative, hypnotic, or anxiolytic
      abuse F13.182
      dependence F13.282
      use F13.982
    stimulant NEC
      abuse F15.182
      dependence F15.282
      use F15.982
  fatal familial (FFI) A81.83
  idiopathic F51.01
  learned F51.3
  nonorganic origin F51.01
  not due to a substance or known physiological condition F51.01
    specified NEC F51.09
  organic G47.00
    specified NEC G47.09
  paradoxical F51.03
  primary F51.01
  psychiatric F51.05
  psychophysiologic F51.04
  related to psychopathology F51.05
  short-term F51.02
  specified NEC G47.09
  stress-related F51.02

Insomnia—*continued*
   transient F51.02
   without objective findings F51.02
Inspiration
   food or foreign body — *see* Asphyxia, food
   mucus — *see* Asphyxia, mucus
Inspissated bile syndrome (newborn) P59.1
Instability
   emotional (excessive) F60.3
   joint (post-traumatic) M25.30
     ankle M25.37-
     due to old ligament injury — *see* Disorder,
       ligament
     elbow M25.32-
     flail — *see* Flail, joint
     foot M25.37-
     hand M25.34-
     hip M25.35-
     knee M25.36-
     lumbosacral — *see* subcategory M53.2
     prosthesis — *see* Complications, joint prosthesis,
       mechanical, displacement, by site
     sacroiliac — *see* subcategory M53.2
     secondary to
       old ligament injury — *see* Disorder, ligament
       removal of joint prosthesis M96.89
     shoulder (region) M25.31-
     spine — *see* subcategory M53.2
     wrist M25.33-
   knee (chronic) M23.5-
   lumbosacral — *see* subcategory M53.2
   nervous F48.8
   personality (emotional) F60.3
   spine — *see* Instability, joint, spine
   vasomotor R55
Institutional syndrome (childhood) F94.2
Institutionalization, affecting child Z62.22
   disinhibited attachment F94.2
Insufficiency, insufficient
   accommodation, old age H52.4
   adrenal (gland) E27.40
     primary E27.1
   adrenocortical E27.40
     drug-induced E27.3
     iatrogenic E27.3
     primary E27.1
   anterior (occlusal) guidance M26.54
   anus K62.8
   aortic (valve) I35.1
     with
       mitral (valve) disease I08.0
         with tricuspid (valve) disease I08.3
       stenosis I35.2
       tricuspid (valve) disease I08.2
         with mitral (valve) disease I08.3
     congenital Q23.1
     rheumatic I06.1
       with
         mitral (valve) disease I08.0
           with tricuspid (valve) disease I08.3
         stenosis I06.2
           with mitral (valve) disease I08.0
             with tricuspid (valve) disease I08.3
         tricuspid (valve) disease I08.2
           with mitral (valve) disease I08.3
     specified cause NEC I35.1
     syphilitic A52.03
   arterial I77.1
     basilar G45.0
     carotid (hemispheric) G45.1
     cerebral I67.8
     coronary (acute or subacute) I24.9
     mesenteric K55.1
     peripheral I73.9
     precerebral (multiple) (bilateral) G45.2
     vertebral G45.0
   arteriovenous I99.8
   biliary K83.8
   cardiac (*see also* Insufficiency, myocardial)
     due to presence of (cardiac) prosthesis I97.11-
     postprocedural I97.11-
   cardiorenal, hypertensive I13.2
   cardiovascular — *see* Disease, cardiovascular

Insufficiency, insufficient—*continued*
   cerebrovascular (acute) I67.8
     with transient focal neurological signs and
       symptoms G45.8
   circulatory NEC I99.8
     newborn P29.89
   convergence H51.11
   coronary (acute or subacute) I24.8
     chronic or with a stated duration of over 4 weeks
       I25.89
   corticoadrenal E27.40
     primary E27.1
   dietary E63.9
   divergence H51.8
   food T73.0
   gastroesophageal K22.8
   gonadal
     ovary E28.39
     testis E29.1
   heart (*see also* Insufficiency, myocardial)
     newborn P29.0
     valve — *see* Endocarditis
   hepatic — *see* Failure, hepatic
   idiopathic autonomic G90.09
   interocclusal distance of fully erupted teeth (ridge)
     M26.36
   kidney N28.9
     acute N28.9
     chronic N18.9
   lacrimal (secretion) H04.12-
     passages — *see* Stenosis, lacrimal
   liver — *see* Failure, hepatic
   lung — *see* Insufficiency, pulmonary
   mental (congenital) — *see* Retardation, mental
   mesenteric K55.1
   mitral (valve) I34.0
     with
       aortic valve disease I08.0
         with tricuspid (valve) disease I08.3
       obstruction or stenosis I05.2
         with aortic valve disease I08.0
       tricuspid (valve) disease I08.1
         with aortic (valve) disease I08.3
     congenital Q23.3
     rheumatic I05.1
       with
         aortic valve disease I08.0
           with tricuspid (valve) disease I08.3
         obstruction or stenosis I05.2
           with aortic valve disease I08.0
             with tricuspid (valve) disease I08.3
         tricuspid (valve) disease I08.1
           with aortic (valve) disease I08.3
       active or acute I01.1
         with chorea, rheumatic (Sydenham's) I02.0
     specified cause, except rheumatic I34.0
   muscle (*see also* Disease, muscle)
     heart — *see* Insufficiency, myocardial
     ocular NEC H50.9
   myocardial, myocardium (with arteriosclerosis) I50.9
     with
       rheumatic fever (conditions in I00) I09.0
         active, acute or subacute I01.2
           with chorea I02.0
         inactive or quiescent (with chorea) I09.0
     congenital Q24.8
     hypertensive — *see* Hypertension, heart
     newborn P29.0
     rheumatic I09.0
       active, acute, or subacute I01.2
     syphilitic A52.06
   nourishment T73.0
   pancreatic K86.8
   parathyroid (gland) E20.9
   peripheral vascular (arterial) I73.9
   pituitary E23.0
   placental (mother) O36.51-
   platelets D69.6
   prenatal care affecting management of pregnancy
     O09.3-
   progressive pluriglandular E31.0

Insufficiency, insufficient—*continued*
   pulmonary J98.4
     acute, following surgery (nonthoracic) J95.2
       thoracic J95.1
     chronic, following surgery J95.3
     following
       shock J80
       trauma J80
     newborn P28.5
     valve I37.1
       with stenosis I37.2
       congenital Q22.2
       rheumatic I09.89
         with aortic, mitral or tricuspid (valve)
           disease I08.8
   pyloric K31.89
   renal (acute) N28.9
     chronic N18.9
   respiratory R06.89
     newborn P28.5
   rotation — *see* Malrotation
   sleep syndrome F51.12
   social insurance Z59.7
   suprarenal E27.40
     primary E27.1
   tarso-orbital fascia, congenital Q10.3
   testis E29.1
   thyroid (gland) (acquired) E03.9
     congenital E03.1
   tricuspid (valve) (rheumatic) I07.1
     with
       aortic (valve) disease I08.2
         with mitral (valve) disease I08.3
       mitral (valve) disease I08.1
         with aortic (valve) disease I08.3
       obstruction or stenosis I07.2
         with aortic (valve) disease I08.2
           with mitral (valve) disease I08.3
     congenital Q22.8
     nonrheumatic I36.1
       with stenosis I36.2
   urethral sphincter R32
   valve, valvular (heart) — *see* Endocarditis
     congenital Q24.8
   vascular I99.8
     intestine K55.9
       acute K55.0
     mesenteric K55.1
     peripheral I73.9
     renal — *see* Hypertension, kidney
   velopharyngeal
     acquired K13.79
     congenital Q38.8
   venous (chronic) (peripheral) I87.2
   ventricular — *see* Insufficiency, myocardial
   welfare support Z59.7
Insufflation, fallopian Z31.41
Insular — *see* condition
Insulinoma
   pancreas
     benign D13.7
     malignant C25.4
     uncertain behavior D37.8
   specified site
     benign — *see* Neoplasm, by site, benign
     malignant — *see* Neoplasm, by site, malignant
     uncertain behavior — *see* Neoplasm, by site,
       uncertain behavior
   unspecified site
     benign D13.7
     malignant C25.4
     uncertain behavior D37.9
Insuloma — *see* Insulinoma
Interference
   balancing side M26.56
   non-working side M26.56
Intermenstrual — *see* condition
Intermittent — *see* condition
Internal — *see* condition
Interruption
   bundle of His I44.30
   phase-shift, sleep cycle
   sleep phase-shift, or 24 hour sleep-wake cycle

J

Jaccoud's syndrome — *see* Arthropathy, postrheumatic, chronic
Jackson's
  membrane Q43.3
  paralysis or syndrome G83.89
  veil Q43.3
Jacquet's dermatitis (diaper dermatitis) L22
Jadassohn-Pellizari's disease or anetoderma L90.2
Jadassohn's
  blue nevus — *see* Nevus
  intraepidermal epithelioma — *see* Neoplasm, skin, benign
Jaffe-Lichtenstein (-Uehlinger) **syndrome** — *see* Dysplasia, fibrous, bone NEC
Jakob-Creutzfeldt disease or syndrome — *see* Creutzfeldt-Jakob disease or syndrome
Jaksch-Luzet disease D64.89
Jamaican
  neuropathy G92
  paraplegic tropical ataxic-spastic syndrome G92
Janet's disease F48.8
Janiceps Q89.4
Jansky-Bielschowsky amaurotic idiocy E75.4
Japanese
  B-type encephalitis A83.0
  river fever A75.3
Jaundice (yellow) R17
  acholuric (familial) (splenomegalic) (*see also* Spherocytosis)
    acquired D59.8
  breast-milk (inhibitor) P59.3
  catarrhal (acute) B15.9
    with hepatic coma B15.0
  cholestatic (benign) R17
  due to or associated with
    delayed conjugation P59.8
      associated with (due to) preterm delivery P59.0
    preterm delivery P59.0
  epidemic (catarrhal)
    with hepatic coma B15.0
    leptospiral A27.0
    spirochetal A27.0
  familial nonhemolytic (congenital) (Gilbert) E80.4
    congenital E80.5
  febrile (acute) B15.9
    with hepatic coma B15.0
    due to or associated with
      ABO
        antibodies P55.1
        incompatibility, maternal/fetal P55.1
        isoimmunization P55.1
      absence or deficiency of enzyme system for bilirubin conjugation (congenital) P59.8
      bleeding P58.1
      breast milk inhibitors to conjugation P59.3
        associated with preterm delivery P59.0
      bruising P58.0
      Crigler-Najjar syndrome E80.5
      delayed conjugation P59.8
        associated with preterm delivery P59.0
      drugs or toxins
        given to newborn P58.42
        transmitted from mother P58.41
      excessive hemolysis P58.9
        due to
          bleeding P58.1
          bruising P58.0
          drugs or toxins
            given to newborn P58.42
            transmitted from mother P58.41
          infection P58.2
          polycythemia P58.3
          swallowed maternal blood P58.5
        specified type NEC P58.8
      galactosemia E74.21
      Gilbert's syndrome E80.4
      hemolytic disease P55.9
        ABO isoimmunization P55.1
        Rh isoimmunization P55.0

Jaundice—*continued*
  febrile—*continued*
    due to or associated with—*continued*
      hemolytic disease—*continued*
        specified NEC P55.8
      hepatocellular damage P59.20
        specified NEC P59.29
      hereditary hemolytic anemia P58.8
      hypothyroidism, congenital E03.1
      incompatibility, maternal/fetal NOS P55.9
      infection P58.2
      inspissated bile syndrome P59.1
      isoimmunization NOS P55.9
      mucoviscidosis E84.9
      polycythemia P58.3
      preterm delivery P59.0
      Rh
        antibodies P55.0
        incompatibility, maternal/fetal P55.0
        isoimmunization P55.0
      specified cause NEC P59.8
      swallowed maternal blood P58.5
    leptospiral A27.0
    spherocytosis (congenital) D58.0
    spirochetal A27.0
  hematogenous D59.9
  hemolytic (acquired) D59.9
    congenital — *see* Spherocytosis
  hemorrhagic (acute) (leptospiral) (spirochetal) A27.0
  infectious (acute) (subacute) B15.9
    with hepatic coma B15.0
    leptospiral A27.0
    spirochetal A27.0
  leptospiral (hemorrhagic) A27.0
  malignant (without coma) K72.90
    with coma K72.91
  newborn P59.9
    due to or associated with
      Gilbert syndrome E80.4
  neonatal — *see* Jaundice, newborn
  nonhemolytic congenital familial (Gilbert) E80.4
  nuclear, newborn (*see also* Kernicterus of newborn) K57.9
  obstructive (*see also* Obstruction, bile duct) K83.1
  post-immunization — *see* Hepatitis, viral, type, B
  post-transfusion — *see* Hepatitis, viral, type, B
  regurgitation (*see also* Obstruction, bile duct) K83.1
  serum (homologous) (prophylactic) (therapeutic) — *see* Hepatitis, viral, type, B
  spirochetal (hemorrhagic) A27.0
  symptomatic R17
    newborn P59.9
Jaw — *see* condition
Jaw-winking phenomenon or syndrome Q07.8
Jealousy
  alcoholic F10.988
  childhood F93.8
  sibling F93.8
Jejunitis — *see* Enteritis
Jejunostomy status Z93.4
Jejunum, jejunal — *see* condition
Jensen's disease — *see* Inflammation, chorioretinal, focal, juxtapapillary
Jerks, myoclonic G25.3
Jervell-Lange-Nielsen syndrome I45.81
Jeune's disease Q77.2
Jigger disease B88.1
Job's syndrome (chronic granulomatous disease) D71
Joint (*see also* condition)
  mice — *see* Loose, body, joint
    knee M23.4-
Jordan's anomaly or syndrome D72.0
Joseph-Diamond-Blackfan anemia (congenital hypoplastic) D61.09
Jungle yellow fever A95.0
Jüngling's disease — *see* Sarcoidosis
Juvenile — *see* condition

K

Kahler's disease C90.0-

Kakke E51.11
Kala-azar B55.0
Kallmann's syndrome E23.0
Kanner's syndrome (autism) — *see* Psychosis, childhood
Kaposi's
  dermatosis (xeroderma pigmentosum) Q82.1
  lichen ruber L44.0
    acuminatus L44.0
  sarcoma
    colon C46.4
    connective tissue C46.1
    gastrointestinal organ C46.4
    lung C46.5-
    lymph node (multiple) C46.3
    palate (hard) (soft) C46.2
    rectum C46.4
    skin (multiple sites) C46.0
    specified site NEC C46.7
    stomach C46.4
    unspecified site C46.9
  varicelliform eruption B00.0
  vaccinia T88.1
Kartagener's syndrome or triad (sinusitis, bronchiectasis, situs inversus) Q89.3
Karyotype
  with abnormality except iso (Xq) Q96.2
  45,X Q96.0
  46,X
    iso (Xq) Q96.1
  46,XX Q98.3
    with streak gonads Q50.32
    hermaphrodite (true) Q99.1
    male Q98.3
  46,XY
    with streak gonads Q56.1
    female Q97.3
    hermaphrodite (true) Q99.1
  47,XXX Q97.0
  47,XXY Q98.0
  47,XYY Q98.5
Kaschin-Beck disease — *see* Disease, Kaschin-Beck
Katayama's disease or fever B65.2
Kawasaki's syndrome M30.3
Kayser-Fleischer ring (cornea) (pseudosclerosis) H18.04-
Kaznelson's syndrome (congenital hypoplastic anemia) D61.01
Kearns-Sayre syndrome H49.81-
Kedani fever A75.3
Kelis L91.0
Kelly (-Patterson) **syndrome** (sideropenic dysphagia) D50.1
Keloid, cheloid L91.0
  acne L73.0
  Addison's L94.0
  cornea — *see* Opacity, cornea
  Hawkin's L91.0
  scar L91.0
Keloma L91.0
Kenya fever A77.1
Keratectasia (*see also* Ectasia, cornea)
  congenital Q13.4
Keratinization of alveolar ridge mucosa
  excessive K13.23
  minimal K13.22
Keratinized residual ridge mucosa
  excessive K13.23
  minimal K13.22
Keratitis (nodular) (nonulcerative) (simple) (zonular) H16.9
  with ulceration (central) (marginal) (perforated) (ring) — *see* Ulcer, cornea
  actinic — *see* Photokeratitis
  arborescens (herpes simplex) B00.52
  areolar — *see* Keratitis, macular
  bullosa H16.8
  deep H16.309
    specified type NEC H16.399

Keratitis —*continued*
  dendritic(a) (herpes simplex) B00.52
  disciform(is) (herpes simplex) B00.52
    varicella B01.81
  filamentary H16.12-
  gonococcal (congenital or prenatal) A54.33
  herpes, herpetic (simplex) B00.52
    zoster B02.33
  in (due to)
    acanthamebiasis B60.13
    adenovirus B30.0
    exanthema (*see also* Exanthem) B09
    herpes (simplex) virus B00.52
    measles B05.81
    syphilis A50.31
    tuberculosis A18.52
    zoster B02.33
  interstitial (nonsyphilitic) H16.30-
    diffuse H16.32-
    herpes, herpetic (simplex) B00.5-
      zoster B02.3-
    sclerosing H16.33-
    specified type NEC H16.39-
    syphilitic (congenital) (late) A50.31
    tuberculous A18.52
  macular H16.11-
  nummular — *see* Keratitis, macular
  oyster shuckers' H16.8
  parenchymatous — *see* Keratitis, interstitial
  petrificans H16.8
  postmeasles B05.81
  punctata
    leprosa A30.9
    syphilitic (profunda) A50.31
  punctate H16.14-
  purulent H16.8
  rosacea L71.8
  sclerosing — *see* Keratitis, interstitial, sclerosing
  specified type NEC H16.8
  superficial (stellate) (striate) H16.10-
    with conjunctivitis — *see* Keratoconjunctivitis
    due to light — *see* Photokeratitis
    filamentary — *see* Keratitis, filamentary
    macular — *see* Keratitis, macular
    punctate — *see* Keratitis, punctate
  suppurative H16.8
  syphilitic (congenital) (prenatal) A50.31
  trachomatous A71.1
    sequelae B94.0
  tuberculous A18.52
  vesicular H16.8
  xerotic (*see also* Keratomalacia) H16.8
    vitamin A deficiency E50.4
Keratoacanthoma L85.8
Keratocele — *see* Descemetocele
Keratoconjunctivitis H16.20-
  Acanthamoeba B60.13
  adenoviral B30.0
  epidemic B30.0
  exposure H16.21-
  herpes, herpetic (simplex) B00.52
    zoster B02.33
  in exanthema (*see also* Exanthem) B09
  infectious B30.0
  lagophthalmic — *see* Keratoconjunctivitis, specified
    type NEC
  neurotrophic H16.23-
  phlyctenular H16.25-
  postmeasles B05.81
  shipyard B30.0
  sicca (Sjogren's) M35.0-
    not Sjogren's H16.22-
  specified type NEC H16.29-
  tuberculous (phlyctenular) A18.52
  vernal H16.26-
Keratoconus H18.60-
  congenital Q13.4
  stable H18.61-
  unstable H18.62-
Keratocyst (dental) (odontogenic) — *see* Cyst,
    calcifying odontogenic

Keratoderma, keratodermia (congenital) (palmaris et
    plantaris) (symmetrical) Q82.8
  acquired L85.1
    in diseases classified elsewhere L86
  climactericum L85.1
  gonococcal A54.89
  gonorrheal A54.89
  punctata L85.2
  Reiter's — *see* Reiter's disease
Keratodermatocele — *see* Descemetocele
Keratoglobus (congenital) H18.79
  congenital Q15.8
    with glaucoma Q15.0
Keratohemia — *see* Pigmentation, cornea, stromal
Keratoiritis (*see also* Iridocyclitis)
  syphilitic A50.39
  tuberculous A18.54
Keratoma L57.0
  palmaris and plantaris hereditarium Q82.8
  senile L57.0
Keratomalacia H18.44-
  vitamin A deficiency E50.4
Keratomegaly Q13.4
Keratomycosis B49
  nigrans, nigricans (palmaris) B36.1
Keratopathy H18.9
  band H18.42-
  bullous H18.1-
  bullous (aphakic), following cataract surgery
    H59.01-
Keratoscleritis, tuberculous A18.52
Keratosis L57.0
  actinic L57.0
  arsenical L85.8
  congenital, specified NEC Q80.8
  female genital NEC N94.89
  follicularis Q82.8
    acquired L11.0
    congenita Q82.8
    et parafollicularis in cutem penetrans L87.0
    spinulosa (decalvans) Q82.8
    vitamin A deficiency E50.8
  gonococcal A54.89
  male genital (external) N50.8
  nigricans L83
  obturans, external ear (canal) — *see* Cholesteatoma,
    external ear
  palmaris et plantaris (inherited) (symmetrical) Q82.8
    acquired L85.1
  penile N48.89
  pharynx J39.2
  pilaris, acquired L85.8
  punctata (palmaris et plantaris) L85.2
  scrotal N50.8
  seborrheic L82.1
    inflamed L82.0
  senile L57.0
  solar L57.0
  tonsillaris J35.8
  vagina N89.4
  vegetans Q82.8
  vitamin A deficiency E50.8
  vocal cord J38.3
Kerato-uveitis — *see* Iridocyclitis
Kerunoparalysis T75.09
Kerion (celsi) B35.0
Kernicterus of newborn (not due to isoimmunization)
    P57.9
  due to isoimmunization (conditions in P55.0-P55.9)
    P57.0
  specified type NEC P57.8
Keshan disease E59
Ketoacidosis E87.2
  diabetic — *see* Diabetes, by type, with complication,
    ketosis
Ketonuria R82.4
Ketosis NEC E88.89
  diabetic — *see* Diabetes, by type, with complication,
    ketosis
Kew Garden fever A79.1
Kidney — *see* condition

Kienböck's disease (*see also* Osteochondrosis,
    juvenile, hand, carpal lunate)
  adult M93.1
Kimmelstiel (-Wilson) **disease** — *see* Diabetes,
    Kimmelstiel (-Wilson) disease
Kink, kinking
  artery I77.1
  hair (acquired) L67.8
  ileum or intestine — *see* Obstruction, intestine
  Lane's — *see* Obstruction, intestine
  organ or site, congenital NEC — *see* Anomaly, by site
  ureter (pelvic junction) N13.5
    with
      hydronephrosis N13.1
        with infection N13.6
      pyelonephritis (chronic) N11.1
    congenital Q62.39
  vein(s) I87.8
    caval I87.1
    peripheral I87.1
Kinnier Wilson's disease (hepatolenticular
    degeneration) E83.01
Kissing spine M48.20
  cervical region M48.22
  cervicothoracic region M48.23
  lumbar region M48.26
  lumbosacral region M48.27
  occipito-atlanto-axial region M48.21
  thoracic region M48.24
  thoracolumbar region M48.25
Klatskin's tumor C22.1
Klauder's disease A26.8
Klebs' disease (*see also* Glomerulonephritis) N05.-
**Klebsiella (K.) pneumoniae, as cause of disease
    classified elsewhere** B96.1
Klein(e)-Levin syndrome G47.13
Kleptomania F63.2
Klinefelter's syndrome Q98.4
  karyotype 47,XXY Q98.0
  male with more than two X chromosomes Q98.1
Klippel-Feil deficiency, disease, or syndrome
    (brevicollis) Q76.1
Klippel's disease I67.2
Klippel-Trenaunay (-Weber) **syndrome** Q87.2
Klumpke (-Déjerine) **palsy, paralysis** (birth)
    (newborn) P14.1
Knee — *see* condition
Knock knee (acquired) M21.06-
  congenital Q74.1
Knot(s)
  intestinal, syndrome (volvulus) K56.2
  surfer S89.8-
  umbilical cord (true) O69.2
Knotting (of)
  hair L67.8
  intestine K56.2
Knuckle pad (Garrod's) M72.1
Koch's
  infection — *see* Tuberculosis
  relapsing fever A68.9
Koch-Weeks' conjunctivitis — *see* Conjunctivitis,
    acute, mucopurulent
Köebner's syndrome Q81.8
Köenig's disease (osteochondritis dissecans) — *see*
    Osteochondritis, dissecans
Köhler-Pellegrini-Steida disease or syndrome
    (calcification, knee joint) — *see* Bursitis, tibial
    collateral
Köhler's disease
  patellar — *see* Osteochondrosis, juvenile, patella
  tarsal navicular — *see* Osteochondrosis, juvenile,
    tarsus
Koilonychia L60.3
  congenital Q84.6
Kojevnikov's, Kozhevnikof's epilepsy G40.509
  intractable G40.519
    with status epilepticus G40.511
    without status epilepticus G40.519
  not intractable G40.509
    with status epilepticus G40.501
    without status epilepticus G40.509
Koplik's spots B05.9

Kopp's asthma E32.8
Korsakoff's (Wernicke) **disease, psychosis or syndrome** (alcoholic) F10.96
   with dependence F10.26
   drug-induced
      due to drug abuse — see Abuse, drug, by type, with amnestic disorder
      due to drug dependence — see Dependence, drug, by type, with amnestic disorder
   nonalcoholic F04
Korsakov's disease, psychosis or syndrome — see Korsakoff's disease
Korsakow's disease, psychosis or syndrome — see Korsakoff's disease
Kostmann's disease or syndrome (infantile genetic agranulocytosis) — see Agranulocytosis
Krabbe's
   disease E75.23
   syndrome, congenital muscle hypoplasia Q79.8
Kraepelin-Morel disease — see Schizophrenia
Kraft-Weber-Dimitri disease Q85.8
Kraurosis
   ani K62.8
   penis N48.0
   vagina N89.8
   vulva N90.4
Kreotoxism A05.9
Krukenberg's
   spindle — see Pigmentation, cornea, posterior
   tumor C79.6-
Kufs' disease E75.4
Kugelberg-Welander disease G12.1
Kuhnt-Junius degeneration — see Degeneration, macula
Kümmell's disease or spondylitis — see Spondylopathy, traumatic
Kupffer cell sarcoma C22.3
Kuru A81.81
Kussmaul's
   disease M30.0
   respiration E87.2
      in diabetic acidosis — see Diabetes, by type, with ketoacidosis
Kwashiorkor E40
   marasmic, marasmus type E42
Kyasanur Forest disease A98.2
Kyphoscoliosis, kyphoscoliotic (acquired) (see also Scoliosis) M41.9
   congenital Q67.5
   heart (disease) I27.1
   sequelae of rickets E64.3
   tuberculous A18.01
Kyphosis, kyphotic (acquired) M40.209
   cervical region M40.202
   cervicothoracic region M40.203
   congenital Q76.419
      cervical region Q76.412
      cervicothoracic region Q76.413
      occipito-atlanto-axial region Q76.411
      thoracic region Q76.414
      thoracolumbar region Q76.415
   Morquio-Brailsford type (spinal) (see also subcategory M49.8) E76.219
   postlaminectomy M96.3
   postradiation therapy M96.2
   postural (adolescent) M40.00
      cervicothoracic region M40.03
      thoracic region M40.04
      thoracolumbar region M40.05
   secondary NEC M40.10
      cervical region M40.12
      cervicothoracic region M40.13
      thoracic region M40.14
      thoracolumbar region M40.15
   sequelae of rickets E64.3
   specified type NEC M40.299
      cervical region M40.292
      cervicothoracic region M40.293
      thoracic region M40.294
      thoracolumbar region M40.295
   syphilitic, congenital A50.56
   thoracic region M40.204
   thoracolumbar region M40.205

Kyphosis, kyphotic—continued
   tuberculous A18.01
Kyrle disease L87.0

L

Labia, labium — see condition
Labile
   blood pressure R09.89
   vasomotor system I73.9
Labioglossal paralysis G12.29
Labium leporinum — see Cleft, lip
Labor — see Delivery
Labored breathing — see Hyperventilation
Labyrinthitis (circumscribed) (destructive) (diffuse) (inner ear) (latent) (purulent) (suppurative) (see also subcategory) H83.0
   syphilitic A52.79
Laceration
   with abortion — see Abortion, by type, complicated by laceration of pelvic organs
   abdomen, abdominal
      wall S31.119
         with
            foreign body S31.129
            penetration into peritoneal cavity S31.619
               with foreign body S31.629
         epigastric region S31.112
            with
               foreign body S31.122
               penetration into peritoneal cavity S31.612
                  with foreign body S31.622
         left
            lower quadrant S31.114
               with
                  foreign body S31.124
                  penetration into peritoneal cavity S31.614
                     with foreign body S31.624
            upper quadrant S31.111
               with
                  foreign body S31.121
                  penetration into peritoneal cavity S31.611
                     with foreign body S31.621
         periumbilic region S31.115
            with
               foreign body S31.125
               penetration into peritoneal cavity S31.615
                  with foreign body S31.625
         right
            lower quadrant S31.113
               with
                  foreign body S31.123
                  penetration into peritoneal cavity S31.613
                     with foreign body S31.623
            upper quadrant S31.110
               with
                  foreign body S31.120
                  penetration into peritoneal cavity S31.610
                     with foreign body S31.620
   accidental, complicating surgery — see Complications, surgical, accidental puncture or laceration
   Achilles tendon S86.02-
   adrenal gland S37.813
   alveolar (process) — see Laceration, oral cavity
   ankle S91.01-
      with
         foreign body S91.02-
   antecubital space — see Laceration, elbow
   anus (sphincter) S31.831
      with
         ectopic or molar pregnancy O08.6
         foreign body S31.832

Laceration—continued
   anus—continued
      complicating delivery — see Delivery, complicated, by, laceration, anus (sphincter)
      following ectopic or molar pregnancy O08.6
      nontraumatic, nonpuerperal — see Fissure, anus
   arm (upper) S41.11-
      with foreign body S41.12-
      lower — see Laceration, forearm
   auditory canal (external) (meatus) — see Laceration, ear
   auricle, ear — see Laceration, ear
   axilla — see Laceration, arm
   back (see also Laceration, thorax, back)
      lower S31.010
         with
            foreign body S31.020
               with penetration into retroperitoneal space S31.021
            penetration into retroperitoneal space S31.011
   bile duct S36.13
   bladder S37.23
      with ectopic or molar pregnancy O08.6
      following ectopic or molar pregnancy O08.6
      obstetrical trauma O71.5
   blood vessel — see Injury, blood vessel
   bowel (see also Laceration, intestine)
      with ectopic or molar pregnancy O08.6
      complicating abortion — see Abortion, by type, complicated by, specified condition NEC
      following ectopic or molar pregnancy O08.6
      obstetrical trauma O71.5
   brain (any part) (cortex) (diffuse) (membrane) (see also Injury, intracranial, diffuse)
      during birth P10.8
         with hemorrhage P10.1
      focal — see Injury, intracranial, focal brain injury
   brainstem S06.38-
   breast S21.01-
      with foreign body S21.02-
   broad ligament S37.893
      with ectopic or molar pregnancy O08.6
      following ectopic or molar pregnancy O08.6
      laceration syndrome N83.8
      obstetrical trauma O71.6
      syndrome (laceration) N83.8
   buttock S31.801
      with foreign body S31.802
      left S31.821
         with foreign body S31.822
      right S31.811
         with foreign body S31.812
   calf — see Laceration, leg
   canaliculus lacrimalis — see Laceration, eyelid
   canthus, eye — see Laceration, eyelid
   capsule, joint — see Sprain
   causing eversion of cervix uteri (old) N86
   central (perineal), complicating delivery O70.9
   cerebellum, traumatic S06.37-
   cerebral S06.33-
      left side S06.32-
         during birth P10.8
            with hemorrhage P10.1
      right side S06.31-
   cervix (uteri)
      with ectopic or molar pregnancy O08.6
      following ectopic or molar pregnancy O08.6
      nonpuerperal, nontraumatic N88.1
      obstetrical trauma (current) O71.3
      old (postpartal) N88.1
      traumatic S37.63
   cheek (external) S01.41-
      with foreign body S01.42-
      internal — see Laceration, oral cavity
   chest wall — see Laceration, thorax
   chin — see Laceration, head, specified site NEC
   chordae tendinae NEC I51.1
      concurrent with acute myocardial infarction — see Infarct, myocardium
      following acute myocardial infarction (current complication) I23.4

Laceration—*continued*
- clitoris — *see* Laceration, vulva
- colon — *see* Laceration, intestine, large, colon
- common bile duct S36.13
- cortex (cerebral) — *see* Injury, intracranial, diffuse
- costal region — *see* Laceration, thorax
- cystic duct S36.13
- diaphragm S27.803
- digit(s)
  - hand — *see* Laceration, finger
  - foot — *see* Laceration, toe
- duodenum S36.430
- ear (canal) (external) S01.31-
  - with foreign body S01.32-
  - drum S09.2-
- elbow S51.01-
  - with
    - foreign body S51.02-
- epididymis — *see* Laceration, testis
- epigastric region — *see* Laceration, abdomen, wall, epigastric region
- esophagus K22.8
  - traumatic
    - cervical S11.21
      - with foreign body S11.22
    - thoracic S27.813
- eye(ball) S05.3-
  - with prolapse or loss of intraocular tissue S05.2-
  - penetrating S05.6-
- eyebrow — *see* Laceration, eyelid
- eyelid S01.11-
  - with foreign body S01.12-
- face NEC — *see* Laceration, head, specified site NEC
- fallopian tube S37.539
  - bilateral S37.532
  - unilateral S37.531
- finger(s) S61.219
  - with
    - damage to nail S61.319
      - with
        - foreign body S61.329
    - foreign body S61.229
  - index S61.218
    - with
      - damage to nail S61.318
        - with
          - foreign body S61.328
      - foreign body S61.228
    - left S61.211
      - with
        - damage to nail S61.311
          - with
            - foreign body S61.321
        - foreign body S61.221
    - right S61.210
      - with
        - damage to nail S61.310
          - with
            - foreign body S61.320
        - foreign body S61.220
  - little S61.218
    - with
      - damage to nail S61.318
        - with
          - foreign body S61.328
      - foreign body S61.228
    - left S61.217
      - with
        - damage to nail S61.317
          - with
            - foreign body S61.327
        - foreign body S61.227
    - right S61.216
      - with
        - damage to nail S61.316
          - with
            - foreign body S61.326
        - foreign body S61.226
  - middle S61.218
    - with
      - damage to nail S61.318
        - with
          - foreign body S61.328

Laceration—*continued*
- finger(s)—*continued*
  - middle—*continued*
    - with—*continued*
      - foreign body S61.228
    - left S61.213
      - with
        - damage to nail S61.313
          - with
            - foreign body S61.323
        - foreign body S61.223
    - right S61.212
      - with
        - damage to nail S61.312
          - with
            - foreign body S61.322
        - foreign body S61.222
  - ring S61.218
    - with
      - damage to nail S61.318
        - with
          - foreign body S61.328
      - foreign body S61.228
    - left S61.215
      - with
        - damage to nail S61.315
          - with
            - foreign body S61.325
        - foreign body S61.225
    - right S61.214
      - with
        - damage to nail S61.314
          - with
            - foreign body S61.324
        - foreign body S61.224
- flank S31.119
  - with foreign body S31.129
- foot (except toe(s) alone) S91.319
  - with foreign body S91.329
  - left S91.312
    - with foreign body S91.322
  - right S91.311
    - with foreign body S91.321
  - toe — *see* Laceration, toe
- forearm S51.819
  - with
    - foreign body S51.829
  - elbow only — *see* Laceration, elbow
  - left S51.812
    - with
      - foreign body S51.822
  - right S51.811
    - with
      - foreign body S51.821
- forehead S01.81
  - with foreign body S01.82
- fourchette O70.0
  - with ectopic or molar pregnancy O08.6
  - complicating delivery O70.0
  - following ectopic or molar pregnancy O08.6
- gallbladder S36.123
- genital organs, external
  - female S31.512
    - with foreign body S31.522
    - vagina — *see* Laceration, vagina
    - vulva — *see* Laceration, vulva
  - male S31.511
    - with foreign body S31.521
    - penis — *see* Laceration, penis
    - scrotum — *see* Laceration, scrotum
    - testis — *see* Laceration, testis
- groin — *see* Laceration, abdomen, wall
- gum — *see* Laceration, oral cavity
- hand S61.419
  - with
    - foreign body S61.429
  - finger — *see* Laceration, finger
  - left S61.412
    - with
      - foreign body S61.422
  - right S61.411
    - with
      - foreign body S61.421

Laceration—*continued*
- hand—*continued*
  - thumb — *see* Laceration, thumb
- head S01.91
  - with foreign body S01.92
  - cheek — *see* Laceration, cheek
  - ear — *see* Laceration, ear
  - eyelid — *see* Laceration, eyelid
  - lip — *see* Laceration, lip
  - nose — *see* Laceration, nose
  - oral cavity — *see* Laceration, oral cavity
  - scalp S01.01
    - with foreign body S01.02
  - specified site NEC S01.81
    - with foreign body S01.82
  - temporomandibular area — *see* Laceration, cheek
- heart — *see* Injury, heart, laceration
- heel — *see* Laceration, foot
- hepatic duct S36.13
- hip S71.019
  - with foreign body S71.029
  - left S71.012
    - with foreign body S71.022
  - right S71.011
    - with foreign body S71.021
- hymen — *see* Laceration, vagina
- hypochondrium — *see* Laceration, abdomen, wall
- hypogastric region — *see* Laceration, abdomen, wall
- ileum S36.438
- inguinal region — *see* Laceration, abdomen, wall
- instep — *see* Laceration, foot
- internal organ — *see* Injury, by site
- interscapular region — *see* Laceration, thorax, back
- intestine
  - large
    - colon S36.539
      - ascending S36.530
      - descending S36.532
      - sigmoid S36.533
      - specified site NEC S36.538
    - rectum S36.63
    - transverse S36.531
  - small S36.439
    - duodenum S36.430
    - specified site NEC S36.438
- intra-abdominal organ S36.93
  - intestine — *see* Laceration, intestine
  - liver — *see* Laceration, liver
  - pancreas — *see* Laceration, pancreas
  - peritoneum S36.81
  - specified site NEC S36.893
  - spleen — *see* Laceration, spleen
  - stomach — *see* Laceration, stomach
- intracranial NEC (*see also* Injury, intracranial, diffuse)
  - birth injury P10.9
- jaw — *see* Laceration, head, specified site NEC
- jejunum S36.438
- joint capsule — *see* Sprain, by site
- kidney S37.03-
  - major (greater than 3 cm) (massive) (stellate) S37.06-
  - minor (less than 1 cm) S37.04-
  - moderate (1 to 3 cm) S37.05-
  - multiple S37.06-
- knee S81.01-
  - with foreign body S81.02-
- labium (majus) (minus) — *see* Laceration, vulva
- lacrimal duct — *see* Laceration, eyelid
- large intestine — *see* Laceration, intestine, large
- larynx S11.011
  - with foreign body S11.012
- leg (lower) S81.819
  - with foreign body S81.829
  - foot — *see* Laceration, foot
  - knee — *see* Laceration, knee
  - left S81.812
    - with foreign body S81.822
  - right S81.811
    - with foreign body S81.821
  - upper — *see* Laceration, thigh
- ligament — *see* Sprain

Laceration—continued
- lip S01.511
  - with foreign body S01.521
- liver S36.113
  - major (stellate) S36.116
  - minor S36.114
  - moderate S36.115
- loin — see Laceration, abdomen, wall
- lower back — see Laceration, back, lower
- lumbar region — see Laceration, back, lower
- lung S27.339
  - bilateral S27.332
  - unilateral S27.331
- malar region — see Laceration, head, specified site NEC
- mammary — see Laceration, breast
- mastoid region — see Laceration, head, specified site NEC
- meninges — see Injury, intracranial, diffuse
- meniscus — see Tear, meniscus
- mesentery S36.893
- mesosalpinx S37.539
  - bilateral S37.532
  - unilateral S37.531
- mouth — see Laceration, oral cavity
- muscle — see Injury, muscle, by site, laceration
- nail
  - finger — see Laceration, finger, with damage to nail
  - toe — see Laceration, toe, with damage to nail
- nasal (septum) (sinus) — see Laceration, nose
- nasopharynx — see Laceration, head, specified site NEC
- neck S11.91
  - with foreign body S11.92
  - involving
    - cervical esophagus S11.21
      - with foreign body S11.22
    - larynx — see Laceration, larynx
    - pharynx — see Laceration, pharynx
    - thyroid gland — see Laceration, thyroid gland
    - trachea — see Laceration, trachea
  - specified site NEC S11.81
    - with foreign body S11.82
- nerve — see Injury, nerve
- nose (septum) (sinus) S01.21
  - with foreign body S01.22
- ocular NOS S05.3-
  - adnexa NOS S01.11-
- oral cavity S01.512
  - with foreign body S01.522
- orbit (eye) — see Wound, open, ocular, orbit
- ovary S37.439
  - bilateral S37.432
  - unilateral S37.431
- palate — see Laceration, oral cavity
- palm — see Laceration, hand
- pancreas S36.239
  - body S36.231
    - major S36.261
    - minor S36.241
    - moderate S36.251
  - head S36.230
    - major S36.260
    - minor S36.240
    - moderate S36.250
  - major S36.269
  - minor S36.249
  - moderate S36.259
  - tail S36.232
    - major S36.262
    - minor S36.242
    - moderate S36.252
- pelvic S31.010
  - with
    - foreign body S31.020
      - penetration into retroperitoneal cavity S31.021
    - penetration into retroperitoneal cavity S31.011
  - floor (see also Laceration, back, lower)
    - with ectopic or molar pregnancy O08.6
    - complicating delivery O70.1

Laceration—continued
- pelvic—continued
  - with—continued
    - following ectopic or molar pregnancy O08.6
    - old (postpartal) N81.89
  - organ S37.93
    - with ectopic or molar pregnancy O08.6
    - adrenal gland S37.813
    - bladder S37.23
    - fallopian tube — see Laceration, fallopian tube
    - following ectopic or molar pregnancy O08.6
    - kidney — see Laceration, kidney
    - obstetrical trauma O71.5
    - ovary — see Laceration, ovary
    - prostate S37.823
    - specified site NEC S37.893
    - ureter S37.13
    - urethra S37.33
    - uterus S37.63
- penis S31.21
  - with foreign body S31.22
- perineum
  - female S31.41
    - with
      - ectopic or molar pregnancy O08.6
      - foreign body S31.42
    - during delivery O70.9
      - first degree O70.0
      - fourth degree O70.3
      - second degree O70.1
      - third degree O70.2
    - old (postpartal) N81.89
    - postpartal N81.89
    - secondary (postpartal) O90.1
  - male S31.119
    - with foreign body S31.129
- periocular area (with or without lacrimal passages) — see Laceration, eyelid
- peritoneum S36.893
- periumbilic region — see Laceration, abdomen, wall, periumbilic
- periurethral tissue — see Laceration, urethra
- phalanges
  - finger — see Laceration, finger
  - toe — see Laceration, toe
- pharynx S11.21
  - with foreign body S11.22
- pinna — see Laceration, ear
- popliteal space — see Laceration, knee
- prepuce — see Laceration, penis
- prostate S37.823
- pubic region S31.119
  - with foreign body S31.129
- pudendum — see Laceration, genital organs, external
- rectovaginal septum — see Laceration, vagina
- rectum S36.63
- retroperitoneum S36.893
- round ligament S37.893
- sacral region — see Laceration, back, lower
- sacroiliac region — see Laceration, back, lower
- salivary gland — see Laceration, oral cavity
- scalp S01.01
  - with foreign body S01.02
- scapular region — see Laceration, shoulder
- scrotum S31.31
  - with foreign body S31.32
- seminal vesicle S37.893
- shin — see Laceration, leg
- shoulder S41.019
  - with foreign body S41.029
  - left S41.012
    - with foreign body S41.022
  - right S41.011
    - with foreign body S41.021
- small intestine — see Laceration, intestine, small
- spermatic cord — see Laceration, testis
- spinal cord (meninges) (see also Injury, spinal cord, by region)
  - due to injury at birth P11.5
  - newborn (birth injury) P11.5

Laceration—continued
- spleen S36.039
  - major (massive) (stellate) S36.032
  - moderate S36.031
  - superficial (minor) S36.030
- sternal region — see Laceration, thorax, front
- stomach S36.33
- submaxillary region — see Laceration, head, specified site NEC
- submental region — see Laceration, head, specified site NEC
- subungual
  - finger(s) — see Laceration, finger, with damage to nail
  - toe(s) — see Laceration, toe, with damage to nail
- suprarenal gland — see Laceration, adrenal gland
- temple, temporal region — see Laceration, head, specified site NEC
- temporomandibular area — see Laceration, cheek
- tendon — see Injury, muscle, by site, laceration
  - Achilles S86.02-
- tentorium cerebelli — see Injury, intracranial, diffuse
- testis S31.31
  - with foreign body S31.32
- thigh S71.11-
  - with foreign body S71.12-
- thorax, thoracic (wall) S21.91
  - with foreign body S21.92
    - back S21.22-
      - with penetration into thoracic cavity S21.42-
    - front S21.12-
      - with penetration into thoracic cavity S21.32-
  - back S21.21-
    - with
      - foreign body S21.22-
        - with penetration into thoracic cavity S21.42-
      - penetration into thoracic cavity S21.41-
  - breast — see Laceration, breast
  - front S21.11-
    - foreign body S21.12-
      - with penetration into thoracic cavity S21.32-
    - penetration into thoracic cavity S21.31-
- thumb S61.019
  - with
    - damage to nail S61.119
      - with
        - foreign body S61.129
    - foreign body S61.029
  - left S61.012
    - with
      - damage to nail S61.112
        - with
          - foreign body S61.122
      - foreign body S61.022
  - right S61.011
    - with
      - damage to nail S61.111
        - with
          - foreign body S61.121
      - foreign body S61.021
- thyroid gland S11.11
  - with foreign body S11.12
- toe(s) S91.119
  - with
    - damage to nail S91.219
      - with
        - foreign body S91.229
    - foreign body S91.129
  - great S91.113
    - with
      - damage to nail S91.213
        - with
          - foreign body S91.223
      - foreign body S91.123

Laceration—*continued*
  toe(s)—*continued*
    great—*continued*
      left S91.112
        with
          damage to nail S91.212
            with
              foreign body S91.222
          foreign body S91.122
      right S91.111
        with
          damage to nail S91.211
            with
              foreign body S91.221
          foreign body S91.121
     lesser S91.116
      with
        damage to nail S91.216
          with
            foreign body S91.226
        foreign body S91.126
      left S91.115
        with
          damage to nail S91.215
            with
              foreign body S91.225
          foreign body S91.125
      right S91.114
        with
          damage to nail S91.214
            with
              foreign body S91.224
          foreign body S91.124
  tongue — *see* Laceration, oral cavity
  trachea S11.021
    with foreign body S11.022
  tunica vaginalis — *see* Laceration, testis
  tympanum, tympanic membrane — *see* Laceration, ear, drum
  umbilical region S31.115
    with foreign body S31.125
  ureter S37.13
  urethra S37.33
    with or following ectopic or molar pregnancy O08.6
    obstetrical trauma O71.5
  urinary organ NEC S37.893
  uterus S37.63
    with ectopic or molar pregnancy O08.6
    following ectopic or molar pregnancy O08.6
    nonpuerperal, nontraumatic N85.8
    obstetrical trauma NEC O71.81
    old (postpartal) N85.8
  uvula — *see* Laceration, oral cavity
  vagina S31.41
    with
      ectopic or molar pregnancy O08.6
      foreign body S31.42
    during delivery O71.4
      with perineal laceration — *see* Laceration, perineum, female, during delivery
    following ectopic or molar pregnancy O08.6
    nonpuerperal, nontraumatic N89.8
    old (postpartal) N89.8
  vas deferens S37.893
  vesical — *see* Laceration, bladder
  vulva S31.41
    with
      ectopic or molar pregnancy O08.6
      foreign body S31.42
    complicating delivery O70.0
    following ectopic or molar pregnancy O08.6
    nonpuerperal, nontraumatic N90.89
    old (postpartal) N90.89
  wrist S61.519
    with
      foreign body S61.529
    left S61.512
      with
        foreign body S61.522
    right S61.511
      with
        foreign body S61.521

Lack of
  achievement in school Z55.3
  adequate
    food Z59.4
    intermaxillary vertical dimension of fully erupted teeth M26.36
    sleep Z72.820
  appetite — *see* Anorexia
  awareness R41.9
  care
    in home Z74.2
    of infant (at or after birth) T76.02
      confirmed T74.02
  cognitive functions R41.9
  coordination R27.9
    ataxia R27.0
    specified type NEC R27.8
  development (physiological) R62.50
    failure to thrive (child over 28 days old) R62.51
      adult R62.7
      newborn P92.6
    short stature R62.52
    specified type NEC R62.59
  energy R53.83
  financial resources Z59.6
  food T73.0
  growth R62.52
  heating Z59.1
  housing (permanent) (temporary) Z59.0
    adequate Z59.1
  learning experiences in childhood Z62.8
  leisure time (affecting life-style) Z73.2
  material resources Z59.9
  memory (*see also* Amnesia)
    mild, following organic brain damage F06.8
  ovulation N97.0
  parental supervision or control of child Z62.0
  person able to render necessary care Z74.2
  physical exercise Z72.3
  play experience in childhood Z62.8
  posterior occlusal support M26.57
  relaxation (affecting life-style) Z73.2
  sexual
    desire F52.0
    enjoyment F52.1
  shelter Z59.0
  sleep (adequate) Z72.820
  supervision of child by parent Z62.0
  support, posterior occlusal M26.57
  water T73.1
Lacrimal — *see* condition
Lacrimation, abnormal — *see* Epiphora
Lacrimonasal duct — *see* condition
Lactation, lactating (breast) (puerperal, postpartum)
  associated
    cracked nipple O92.13
    retracted nipple O92.03
  defective O92.4
  disorder NEC O92.79
  excessive O92.6
  failed (complete) O92.3
    partial O92.4
  mastitis NEC — *see* Mastitis, obstetric
  mother (care and/or examination) Z39.1
  nonpuerperal N64.3
Lacticemia, excessive E87.2
Lacunar skull Q75.8
Laennec's cirrhosis K74.69
  alcoholic K70.30
    with ascites K70.31
Lafora's disease — *see* Epilepsy, generalized, idiopathic
Lag, lid (nervous) — *see* Retraction, lid
Lagophthalmos (eyelid) (nervous) H02.209
  cicatricial H02.219
    left H02.216
      lower H02.215
      upper H02.214
    right H02.213
      lower H02.212
      upper H02.211
  keratoconjunctivitis — *see* Keratoconjunctivitis

Lagophthalmos—*continued*
  left H02.206
    lower H02.205
    upper H02.204
  mechanical H02.229
    left H02.226
      lower H02.225
      upper H02.224
    right H02.223
      lower H02.222
      upper H02.221
  paralytic H02.239
    left H02.236
      lower H02.235
      upper H02.234
    right H02.233
      lower H02.232
      upper H02.231
  right H02.203
    lower H02.202
    upper H02.201
Laki-Lorand factor deficiency — *see* Defect, coagulation, specified type NEC
Lalling F80.0
Lambert-Eaton syndrome G73.1
  not associated with neoplasm G70.8
Lambliasis, lambliosis A07.1
Landau-Kleffner syndrome F80.3
Landouzy-Déjérine dystrophy or facioscapulohumeral atrophy G71.0
Landouzy's disease (icterohemorrhagic leptospirosis) A27.0
Landry-Guillain-Barré, syndrome or paralysis G61.0
Landry's disease or paralysis G61.0
Lane's
  band Q43.3
  kink — *see* Obstruction, intestine
  syndrome K90.2
Langdon Down syndrome — *see* Trisomy, 21
Lapsed immunization schedule status Z28.3
Large
  baby (regardless of gestational age) (4000g to 4499g) P08.1
  ear, congenital Q17.1
  physiological cup Q14.2
  stature R68.89
Large-for-dates NEC (infant) (4000g to 4499g) P08.1
  affecting management of pregnancy O36.6-
  exceptionally (4500g or more) P08.0
Larsen-Johansson disease orosteochondrosis — *see* Osteochondrosis, juvenile, patella
Larsen's syndrome (flattened facies and multiple congenital dislocations) Q74.8
Larva migrans
  cutaneous B76.9
    Ancylostoma B76.0
  visceral B83.0
Laryngeal — *see* condition
Laryngismus (stridulus) J38.5
  congenital P28.89
  diphtheritic A36.2
Laryngitis (acute) (edematous) (fibrinous) (infective) (infiltrative) (malignant) (membranous) (phlegmonous) (pneumococcal) (pseudomembranous) (septic) (subglottic) (suppurative) (ulcerative) J04.0
  with
    influenza, flu, or grippe — *see* Influenza, with, laryngitis
    tracheitis (acute) — *see* Laryngotracheitis
  atrophic J37.0
  catarrhal J37.0
  chronic J37.0
    with tracheitis (chronic) J37.1
  diphtheritic A36.2
  due to external agent — *see* Inflammation, respiratory, upper, due to
  Hemophilus influenzae J04.0
  H. influenzae J04.0
  hypertrophic J37.0
  influenzal — *see* Influenza, with, respiratory manifestations NEC
  obstructive J05.0

Laryngitis—continued
 sicca J37.0
 spasmodic J05.0
  acute J04.0
 streptococcal J04.0
 stridulous J05.0
 syphilitic (late) A52.73
  congenital A50.59 [J99]
   early A50.03 [J99]
 tuberculous A15.5
 Vincent's A69.1
Laryngocele (congenital) (ventricular) Q31.3
Laryngofissure J38.7
 congenital Q31.8
Laryngomalacia (congenital) Q31.5
Laryngopharyngitis (acute) J06.0
 chronic J37.0
 due to external agent — see Inflammation,
  respiratory, upper, due to
Laryngoplegia J38.00
 bilateral J38.02
 unilateral J38.01
Laryngoptosis J38.7
Laryngospasm J38.5
Laryngostenosis J38.6
Laryngotracheitis (acute) (Infectional) (infective)
  (viral) J04.2
 atrophic J37.1
 catarrhal J37.1
 chronic J37.1
 diphtheritic A36.2
 due to external agent — see Inflammation,
  respiratory, upper, due to
 Hemophilus influenzae J04.2
 hypertrophic J37.1
 influenzal — see Influenza, with, respiratory
  manifestations NEC
 pachydermic J38.7
 sicca J37.1
 spasmodic J38.5
  acute J05.0
 streptococcal J04.2
 stridulous J38.5
 syphilitic (late) A52.73
  congenital A50.59 [J99]
   early A50.03 [J99]
 tuberculous A15.5
 Vincent's A69.1
Laryngotracheobronchitis — see Bronchitis
Larynx, laryngeal — see condition
Lassa fever A96.2
Lassitude — see Weakness
Late
 talker R62.0
 walker R62.0
Late effect(s) — see Sequelae
Latent — see condition
Laterocession — see Lateroversion
Lateroflexion — see Lateroversion
Lateroversion
 cervix — see Lateroversion, uterus
 uterus, uterine (cervix) (postinfectional) (postpartal,
  old) N85.4
  congenital Q51.818
  in pregnancy or childbirth — see subcategory
   O34.5
Lathyrism — see Poisoning, food, noxious, plant
Launois' syndrome (pituitary gigantism) E22.0
Launois-Bensaude adenolipomatosis E88.89
Laurence-Moon(-Bardet)-Biedl syndrome Q87.89
Lax, laxity (see also Relaxation)
 ligament(ous) (see also Disorder, ligament)
  familial M35.7
  knee — see Derangement, knee
 skin (acquired) L57.4
  congenital Q82.8
Laxative habit F55.2
Lazy leukocyte syndrome D70.8
Lead miner's lung J63.6
Leak, leakage
 amniotic fluid — see Rupture, membranes,
  premature

Leak, leakage—continued
 blood (microscopic), fetal, into maternal circulation
  affecting management of pregnancy — see
  Pregnancy, complicated by
 cerebrospinal fluid G96.0
  from spinal (lumbar) puncture G97.0
 device, implant or graft (see also Complications, by
  site and type, mechanical)
  arterial graft NEC — see Complication,
   cardiovascular device, mechanical, vascular
  breast (implant) T85.43
  catheter NEC T85.638
   dialysis (renal) T82.43
    intraperitoneal T85.631
   infusion NEC T82.534
    spinal (epidural) (subdural) T85.630
   urinary, indwelling T83.038
    cystostomy T83.030
  gastrointestinal — see Complications, prosthetic
   device, mechanical, gastrointestinal device
  genital NEC T83.498
   penile prosthesis T83.490
  heart NEC — see Complication, cardiovascular
   device, mechanical
  joint prosthesis — see Complications, joint
   prosthesis, mechanical, specified NEC, by
   site
  ocular NEC — see Complications, prosthetic
   device, mechanical, ocular device
  orthopedic NEC — see Complication, orthopedic,
   device, mechanical
  specified NEC T85.638
  urinary NEC (see also Complication,
   genitourinary, device, urinary, mechanical)
   graft T83.23
  vascular NEC — see Complication, cardiovascular
   device, mechanical
  ventricular intracranial shunt T85.03
  joint prosthesis — see Complications, joint
   prosthesis, mechanical, specified NEC, by
   site
 urine — see Incontinence
Leaky heart — see Endocarditis
Learning defect (specific) F81.9
Leather bottle stomach C16.9
Leber's
 congenital amaurosis H35.50
 optic atrophy (hereditary) H47.22
Lederer's anemia D59.1
Leeches (external) — see Hirudiniasis
Leg — see condition
Legg(-Calvé)**-Perthes disease**, syndrome or
  osteochondrosis M91.1-
Legionellosis A48.1
 nonpneumonic A48.2
Legionnaires'
 disease A48.1
  nonpneumonic A48.2
 pneumonia A48.1
Leigh's disease G31.82
Leiner's disease L21.1
Leiofibromyoma — see Leiomyoma
Leiomyoblastoma — see Neoplasm, connective
  tissue, benign
Leiomyofibroma (see also Neoplasm, connective
  tissue, benign)
 uterus (cervix) (corpus) D25.9
Leiomyoma (see also Neoplasm, connective tissue,
  benign)
 bizarre — see Neoplasm, connective tissue, benign
 cellular — see Neoplasm, connective tissue, benign
 epithelioid — see Neoplasm, connective tissue,
  benign
 uterus (cervix) (corpus) D25.9
  intramural D25.1
  submucous D25.0
  subserosal D25.2
 vascular — see Neoplasm, connective tissue, benign
Leiomyoma, leiomyomatosis (intravascular) — see
  Neoplasm, connective tissue, uncertain behavior

Leiomyosarcoma (see also Neoplasm, connective
  tissue, malignant)
 epithelioid — see Neoplasm, connective tissue,
  malignant
 myxoid — see Neoplasm, connective tissue,
  malignant
Leishmaniasis B55.9
 American (mucocutaneous) B55.2
  cutaneous B55.1
 Asian Desert B55.1
 Brazilian B55.2
 cutaneous (any type) B55.1
 dermal (see also Leishmaniasis, cutaneous)
  post-kala-azar B55.0
 eyelid B55.1
 infantile B55.0
 Mediterranean B55.0
 mucocutaneous (American) (New World) B55.2
 naso-oral B55.2
 nasopharyngeal B55.2
 old world B55.1
 tegumentaria diffusa B55.1
 visceral B55.0
Leishmanoid, dermal (see also Leishmaniasis,
  cutaneous)
 post-kala-azar B55.0
Lenegre's disease I44.2
Lengthening, leg — see Deformity, limb, unequal
  length
Lennert's lymphoma — see Lymphoma, Lennert's
Lennox-Gastaut syndrome — see Epilepsy,
  generalized, specified NEC
Lens — see condition
Lenticonus (anterior) (posterior) (congenital) Q12.8
Lenticular degeneration, progressive E83.01
Lentiglobus (posterior) (congenital) Q12.8
Lentigo (congenital) L81.4
 maligna (see also Melanoma, in situ)
  melanoma — see Melanoma
Lentivirus, as cause of disease classified elsewhere
  B97.31
Leontiasis
 ossium M85.2
 syphilitic (late) A52.78
  congenital A50.59
Lepothrix A48.8
Lepra — see Leprosy
Leprechaunism E34.8
Leprosy A30.-
 with muscle disorder A30.9 [M63.80]
  ankle A30.9 [M63.87-]
  foot A30.9 [M63.87-]
  forearm A30.9 [M63.83-]
  hand A30.9 [M63.84-]
  lower leg A30.9 [M63.86-]
  multiple sites A30.9 [M63.89]
  pelvic region A30.9 [M63.85-]
  shoulder region A30.9 [M63.81-]
  specified site NEC A30.9 [M63.88]
  thigh A30.9 [M63.85-]
  upper arm A30.9 [M63.82-]
 anesthetic A30.9
 BB A30.3
 BL A30.4
 borderline (infiltrated) (neuritic) A30.3
  lepromatous A30.4
  tuberculoid A30.2
 BT A30.2
 dimorphous (infiltrated) (neuritic) A30.3
 I A30.0
 indeterminate (macular) (neuritic) A30.0
 lepromatous (diffuse) (infiltrated) (macular)
  (neuritic) (nodular) A30.5
 LL A30.5
 macular (early) (neuritic) (simple) A30.9
 maculoanesthetic A30.9
 mixed A30.3
 neural A30.9
 nodular A30.5
 primary neuritic A30.3
 specified type NEC A30.8
 TT A30.1
 tuberculoid (major) (minor) A30.1

Leptocytosis, hereditary D56.9
Leptomeningitis (chronic) (circumscribed) (hemorrhagic) (nonsuppurative) — *see* Meningitis
Leptomeningopathy G96.19
Leptospiral — *see* condition
Leptospirochetal — *see* condition
Leptospirosis A27.9
  canicola A27.89
  due to Leptospira interrogans serovar icterohaemorrhagiae A27.Ø
  icterohemorrhagica A27.Ø
  pomona A27.89
  Weil's disease A27.Ø
Leptus dermatitis B88.Ø
Leriche's syndrome (aortic bifurcation occlusion) I74.Ø
Leri's pleonosteosis Q78.8
Leri-Weill syndrome Q77.8
Lermoyez' syndrome — *see* Vertigo, peripheral NEC
Lesch-Nyhan syndrome E79.1
Leser-Trélat disease L82.1
  inflamed L82.Ø
Lesion(s) (nontraumatic)
  abducens nerve — *see* Strabismus, paralytic, sixth nerve
  alveolar process KØ8.9
  angiocentric immunoproliferative D47.z9
  anorectal K62.9
  aortic (valve) I35.9
  auditory nerve — *see* subcategory H93.3
  basal ganglion G25.9
  bile duct — *see* Disease, bile duct
  biomechanical M99.9
    specified type NEC M99.89
      abdomen M99.89
      acromioclavicular M99.87
      cervical region M99.81
      cervicothoracic M99.81
      costochondral M99.88
      costovertebral M99.88
      head region M99.8Ø
      hip M99.85
      lower extremity M99.86
      lumbar region M99.83
      lumbosacral M99.83
      occipitocervical M99.8Ø
      pelvic region M99.85
      pubic M99.85
      rib cage M99.88
      sacral region M99.84
      sacrococcygeal M99.84
      sacroiliac M99.84
      specified NEC M99.89
      sternochondral M99.88
      sternoclavicular M99.87
      thoracic region M99.82
      thoracolumbar M99.82
      upper extremity M99.87
  bladder N32.9
  bone — *see* Disorder, bone
  brachial plexus G54.Ø
  brain G93.9
    congenital QØ4.9
    vascular I67.9
      degenerative I67.9
      hypertensive I67.4
  buccal cavity K13.79
  calcified — *see* Calcification
  canthus — *see* Disorder, eyelid
  carate — *see* Pinta, lesions
  cardia K22.9
  cardiac (*see also* Disease, heart) I51.9
    congenital Q24.9
    valvular — *see* Endocarditis
  cauda equina G83.4
  cecum K63.9
  cerebral — *see* Lesion, brain
  cerebrovascular I67.9
    degenerative I67.9
    hypertensive I67.4
  cervical (nerve) root NEC G54.2

Lesion(s)—*continued*
  chiasmal — *see* Disorder, optic, chiasm
  chorda tympani G51.8
  coin, lung R91
  colon K63.9
  congenital — *see* Anomaly, by site
  conjunctiva H11.9
  conus medullaris — *see* Injury, conus medullaris
  coronary artery — *see* Ischemia, heart
  cranial nerve G52.9
    eighth — *see* Disorder, ear
    eleventh G52.9
    fifth G5Ø.9
    first G52.Ø
    fourth — *see* Strabismus, paralytic, fourth nerve
    seventh G51.9
    sixth — *see* Strabismus, paralytic, sixth nerve
    tenth G52.2
    twelfth G52.3
  cystic — *see* Cyst
  degenerative — *see* Degeneration
  duodenum K31.9
  edentulous (alveolar) ridge, associated with trauma, due to traumatic occlusion KØ6.2
  en coup de sabre L94.1
  eyelid — *see* Disorder, eyelid
  gasserian ganglion G5Ø.8
  gastric K31.9
  gastroduodenal K31.9
  gastrointestinal K63.9
  gingiva, associated with trauma KØ6.2
  glomerular
    focal and segmental (*see also* NØØ-NØ7 with fourth character .1) NØ5.1
    minimal change (*see also* NØØ-NØ7 with fourth character .Ø) NØ5.Ø
  heart (organic) — *see* Disease, heart
  hyperchromic, due to pinta (carate) A67.1
  hyperkeratotic — *see* Hyperkeratosis
  hypothalamic E23.7
  ileocecal K63.9
  ileum K63.9
  iliohypogastric nerve G57.8-
  inflammatory — *see* Inflammation
  intestine K63.9
  intracerebral — *see* Lesion, brain
  intrachiasmal (optic) — *see* Disorder, optic, chiasm
  intracranial, space-occupying R9Ø.Ø
  joint — *see* Disorder, joint
    sacroiliac (old) M53.3
  keratotic — *see* Keratosis
  kidney — *see* Disease, renal
  laryngeal nerve (recurrent) G52.2
  lip K13.Ø
  liver K76.9
  lumbosacral
    plexus G54.1
    root (nerve) NEC G54.4
  lung (coin) R91
  maxillary sinus J32.Ø
  mitral IØ5.9
  Morel-Lavallée — *see* Hematoma, by site
  motor cortex NEC G93.89
  mouth K13.79
  nerve G58.9
    femoral G57.2-
    median G56.1-
      carpal tunnel syndrome — *see* Syndrome, carpal tunnel
    plantar G57.6-
    popliteal (lateral) G57.3-
      medial G57.4-
    radial G56.3-
    sciatic G57.Ø-
    spinal — *see* Injury, nerve, spinal
    ulnar G56.2-
  nervous system, congenital QØ7.9
  nonallopathic — *see* Lesion, biomechanical
  nose (internal) J34.89
  obstructive — *see* Obstruction
  obturator nerve G57.8-
  oral mucosa K13.7Ø
  organ or site NEC — *see* Disease, by site

Lesion(s)—*continued*
  osteolytic — *see* Osteolysis
  peptic K27.9
  periodontal, due to traumatic occlusion KØ5.5
  pharynx J39.2
  pigment, pigmented (skin) L81.9
  pinta — *see* Pinta, lesions
  polypoid — *see* Polyp
  prechiasmal (optic) — *see* Disorder, optic, chiasm
  primary (*see also* Syphilis, primary) A51.Ø
    carate A67.Ø
    pinta A67.Ø
    yaws A66.Ø
  pulmonary J98.4
    valve I37.9
  pylorus K31.9
  rectosigmoid K63.9
  retina, retinal H35.9
  sacroiliac (joint) (old) M53.3
  salivary gland K11.9
    benign lymphoepithelial K11.8
  saphenous nerve G57.8-
  sciatic nerve G57.Ø-
  secondary — *see* Syphilis, secondary
  shoulder (region) M75.9-
    specified NEC M75.8-
  sigmoid K63.9
  sinus (accessory) (nasal) J34.89
  skin L98.9
    suppurative LØ8.Ø
  SLAP S43.43-
  spinal cord G95.9
    congenital QØ6.9
  spleen D73.89
  stomach K31.9
  superior glenoid labrum S43.43-
  syphilitic — *see* Syphilis
  tertiary — *see* Syphilis, tertiary
  thoracic root (nerve) NEC G54.3
  tonsillar fossa J35.9
  tooth, teeth KØ8.9
    white spot
      chewing surface KØ2.51
      pit and fissure surface KØ2.51
      smooth surface KØ2.61
  traumatic — *see* specific type of injury by site
  tricuspid (valve) IØ7.9
    nonrheumatic I36.9
  trigeminal nerve G5Ø.9
  ulcerated or ulcerative — *see* Ulcer, skin
  uterus N85.9
  vagus nerve G52.2
  valvular — *see* Endocarditis
  vascular I99.9
    affecting central nervous system I67.9
    following trauma NEC T14.8
    umbilical cord, complicating delivery O69.5
  warty — *see* Verruca
  white spot (tooth)
    chewing surface KØ2.51
    pit and fissure surface KØ2.51
    smooth surface KØ2.61
Lethargic — *see* condition
Lethargy R53.83
Letterer-Siwe's disease C96.Ø
Leuc(o) — *see* Leuk(o)
Leukemia, leukemic C95.9-
  acute basophilic C94.8-
  acute bilineal C95.Ø-
  acute erythoid C94.Ø-
  acute lymphoblastic C91.Ø-
  acute megakaryoblastic C94.2-
  acute megakaryocytic C94.2-
  acute mixed lineage C95.Ø-
  acute monoblastic (monoblastic/monocytic) C93.Ø-
  acute monocytic (monoblastic/monocytic) C93.Ø-
  acute myeloblastic (minimal differentiation) (with maturation) C92.Ø-

Leukemia, leukemic—*continued*
  acute myeloid
    with
      11q23-abnormality C92.6-
      dysplasia of remaining hematopoesis and/or
        myelodysplastic disease in its history
        C92.a-
      multilineage dysplasia C92.a-
      variation of MLL-gene C92.6-
    M6(a)(b) C94.0-
    M7 C94.2-
  acute myelomonocytic C92.5-
  acute promyelocytic C92.4-
  adult T-cell (HTLV-1-associated) (acute variant)
    (chronic variant) (lymphomatoid variant)
    (smouldering variant) C91.5-
  aggressive NK-cell C94.8-
  AML (1/ETO) (MØ) (M1) (M2) (without a FAB
    classification) C92.0-
  AML M3 C92.4-
  AML M4 (Eo with inv(16) or t(16;16)) C92.5-
  AML M5 C93.0-
  AML M5a C93.0-
  AML M5b C93.0-
  AML Me with t(15;17) and variants C92.4-
  atypical chronic myeloid, BCR/ABL-negative C92.2-
  biphenotypic acute C95.0-
  blast cell C95.0-
  Burkitt-type, mature B-cell C91.a-
  chronic lymphocytic, of B-cell type C91.1-
  chronic monocytic C93.1-
  chronic myelogenous (Philadelphia chromosome
    (Ph1) positive) (t(9;22) (q34;q11) (with crisis of
    blast cells) C92.1-
  chronic myeloid, BCR/ABL-positive C92.1-
    atypical, BCR/ABL-negative C92.2-
  chronic myelomonocytic C93.1-
  chronic neutrophilic D47.1
  CMML (-1) (-2) (with eosinophilia) C93.1-
  granulocytic C92.9 (*see also* Category C92
  hairy cell C91.4-
  juvenile myelomonocytic C93.3-
  lymphoid C91.9-
    specified NEC C91.z-
  mast cell C94.3-
  mature B-cell, Burkitt-type C91.a-
  monocytic (subacute) C93.9-
    specified NEC C93.z-
  myelogenous C92.9— *see also* Category C92
  myeloid C92.9-
    specified NEC C92.z-
  plasma cell C90.1-
  plasmacytic C90.1-
  prolymphocytic
    of B-cell type C91.3-
    of T-cell type C91.6-
  specified NEC C94.8-
  stem cell, of unclear lineage C95.0-
  subacute lymphocytic C91.9-
  T-cell large granular lymphocytic C91.z-
  unspecified cell type C95.9-
    acute C95.0-
    chronic C95.1-
Leukemoid reaction (*see also* Reaction, leukemoid)
  D72.823
Leukoaraiosis (hypertensive) I67.8
Leukoariosis — *see* Leukoaraiosis
Leukocoria — *see* Disorder, globe, degenerated
  condition, leucocoria
Leukocytopenia D72.819
Leukocytosis D72.829
  eosinophilic D72.1
Leukoderma, leukodermia NEC L81.5
  syphilitic A51.39
    late A52.79
Leukodystrophy E75.29
Leukoedema, oral epithelium K13.29
Leukoencephalitis G04.81
  acute (subacute) hemorrhagic G36.1
    postimmunization or postvaccinal G04.01
  postinfectious G04.02
  subacute sclerosing A81.1
  van Bogaert's (sclerosing) A81.1

Leukoencephalopathy (*see also* Encephalopathy)
  G93.49
  Binswanger's F03
  heroin vapor G92
  metachromatic E75.25
  multifocal (progressive) A81.2
  postimmunization and postvaccinal G04.01
  progressive multifocal A81.2
  reversible, posterior G93.6
  van Bogaert's (sclerosing) A81.1
  vascular, progressive I67.3
Leukoerythroblastosis D75.9
Leukokeratosis (*see also* Leukoplakia)
  mouth K13.21
  nicotina palati K13.24
  oral mucosa K13.21
  tongue K13.21
  vocal cord J38.3
Leukokraurosis vulva(e) N90.4
Leukoma (cornea) (*see also* Opacity, cornea)
  adherent H17.0-
  interfering with central vision — *see* Opacity,
    cornea, central
Leukomalacia, cerebral, newborn P91.2
  periventricular P91.2
Leukomelanopathy, hereditary D72.0
Leukonychia (punctata) (striata) L60.8
  congenital Q84.4
Leukopathia unguium L60.8
  congenital Q84.4
Leukopenia D72.819
  basophilic D72.818
  chemotherapy (cancer) induced D70.1
  congenital D70.0
  cyclic D70.0
  drug induced NEC D70.2
    due to cytoreductive cancer chemotherapy
      D70.1
  eosinophilic D72.818
  familial D70.0
  infantile genetic D70.0
  malignant D70.9
  periodic D70.0
  transitory neonatal P61.5
Leukopenic — *see* condition
Leukoplakia
  anus K62.8
  bladder (postinfectional) N32.89
  buccal K13.21
  cervix (uteri) N88.0
  esophagus K22.8
  gingiva K13.21
  hairy (oral mucosa) (tongue) K13.3
  kidney (pelvis) N28.89
  larynx J38.7
  lip K13.21
  mouth K13.21
  oral epithelium, including tongue (mucosa) K13.21
  palate K13.21
  pelvis (kidney) N28.89
  penis (infectional) N48.0
  rectum K62.8
  syphilitic (late) A52.79
  tongue K13.21
  ureter (postinfectional) N28.89
  urethra (postinfectional) N36.8
  uterus N85.8
  vagina N89.4
  vocal cord J38.3
  vulva N90.4
Leukorrhea N89.8
  due to Trichomonas (vaginalis) A59.00
  trichomonal A59.00
Leukosarcoma C85.9-
Levocardia (isolated) Q24.1
  with situs inversus Q89.3
Levotransposition Q20.5
Lev's disease or syndrome (acquired complete heart
  block) I44.2
Levulosuria — *see* Fructosuria
Levurid L30.2
Lewy body(ies) (dementia) (disease) G31.83
Leyden-Moebius dystrophy G71.0

Leydig cell
  carcinoma
    specified site — *see* Neoplasm, malignant, by site
    unspecified site
      female C56.9-
      male C62.9-
  tumor
    benign
      specified site — *see* Neoplasm, benign, by site
      unspecified site
        female D27.-
        male D29.2-
    malignant
      specified site — *see* Neoplasm, malignant, by
        site
      unspecified site
        female C56.-
        male C62.9-
    specified site — *see* Neoplasm, uncertain
      behavior, by site
    unspecified site
      female D39.1-
      male D40.1-
Leydig-Sertoli cell tumor
  specified site — *see* Neoplasm, benign, by site
  unspecified site
    female D27.-
    male D29.2-
LGSIL (Low grade squamous intraepithelial lesion on
  cytologic smear of)
  anus R85.612
  cervix R87.612
  vagina R87.622
Liar, pathologic F60.2
Libido
  decreased R68.82
Libman-Sacks disease M32.11
Lice (infestation) B85.2
  body (Pediculus corporis) B85.1
  crab B85.3
  head (Pediculus capitis) B85.0
  mixed (classifiable to more than one of the titles
    B85.0-B85.3) B85.4
  pubic (Phthirus pubis) B85.3
Lichen L28.0
  albus L90.0
    penis N48.0
    vulva N90.4
  amyloidosis E85.4 [L99]
  atrophicus L90.0
    penis N48.0
    vulva N90.4
  congenital Q82.8
  myxedematosus L98.5
  nitidus L44.1
  pilaris Q82.8
    acquired L85.8
  planopilaris L66.1
  planus (chronicus) L43.9
    annularis L43.8
    bullous L43.1
    follicular L66.1
    hypertrophic L43.0
    moniliformis L44.3
    of Wilson L43.9
    specified NEC L43.8
    subacute (active) L43.3
    tropicus L43.3
  ruber
    acuminatus L44.0
    moniliformis L44.3
    planus L43.9
  sclerosus (et atrophicus) L90.0
    penis N48.0
    vulva N90.4
  scrofulosus (primary) (tuberculous) A18.4
  simplex (chronicus) (circumscriptus) L28.0
  striatus L44.2
  urticatus L28.2
Lichenification L28.0
Lichenoides tuberculosis (primary) A18.4
Lichtheim's disease or syndrome — *see*
  Degeneration, combined

Lien migrans D73.89
Ligament — *see* condition
Light
  for gestational age — *see* Light for dates
  headedness R42
Light-for-dates (infant) P05.00
  with weight of
    499 grams or less P05.01
    500-749 grams P05.02
    750-999 grams P05.03
    1000-1249 grams P05.04
    1250-1499 grams P05.05
    1500-1749 grams P05.06
    1750-1999 grams P05.07
    2000-2499 grams P05.08
  and small-for-dates — *see* Small for dates
  affecting management of pregnancy O36.59-
Lightning (effects) (stroke) (struck by) T75.00
  burn — *see* Burn
  foot E53.8
  shock T75.01
  specified effect NEC T75.09
Lightwood-Albright syndrome N25.89
Lightwood's disease or syndrome (renal tubular
    acidosis) N25.89
Lignac (-de Toni) (-Fanconi) (-Debré) **disease or
    syndrome** E72.09
  with cystinosis E72.04
Ligneous thyroiditis E06.5
Likoff's syndrome I20.8
Limb — *see* condition
Limbic epilepsy personality syndrome F07.0
Limitation, limited
  activities due to disability Z73.6
  cardiac reserve — *see* Disease, heart
  eye muscle duction, traumatic — *see* Strabismus,
    mechanical
  mandibular range of motion M26.52
Lindau (-von Hippel) **disease** Q85.8
Line(s)
  Beau's L60.4
  Harris' — *see* Arrest, epiphyseal
  Hudson's (cornea) — *see* Pigmentation, cornea,
    anterior
  Stähli's (cornea) — *see* Pigmentation, cornea,
    anterior
Linea corneae senilis — *see* Change, cornea, senile
Lingua
  geographica K14.1
  nigra (villosa) K14.3
  plicata K14.5
  tylosis K13.29
Lingual — *see* condition
Linguatulosis B88.8
Linitis (gastric) **plastica** C16.9
Lip — *see* condition
Lipedema — *see* Edema
Lipemia (*see also* Hyperlipidemia)
  retina, retinalis E78.3
Lipidosis E75.6
  cerebral (infantile) (juvenile) (late) E75.4
  cerebroretinal E75.4
  cerebroside E75.22
  cholesterol (cerebral) E75.5
  glycolipid E75.21
  hepatosplenomegalic E78.3
  sphingomyelin — *see* Niemann-Pick disease or
    syndrome
  sulfatide E75.29
Lipoadenoma — *see* Neoplasm, benign, by site
Lipoblastoma — *see* Lipoma
Lipoblastomatosis — *see* Lipoma
Lipochondrodystrophy E76.01
Lipodermatosclerosis — *see* Varix, leg, with,
    inflammation
  ulcerated — *see* Varix, leg, with, ulcer, with
    inflammation by site
Lipochrome histiocytosis (familial) D71
Lipodystrophia progressiva E88.1
Lipodystrophy (progressive) E88.1
  insulin E88.1
  intestinal K90.81
  mesenteric K65.4

Lipofibroma — *see* Lipoma
Lipofuscinosis, neuronal (with ceroidosis) E75.4
Lipogranuloma, sclerosing L92.8
Lipogranulomatosis E78.89
Lipoid (*see also* condition)
  histiocytosis D76.3
    essential E75.29
  nephrosis N04.9
  proteinosis of Urbach E78.89
Lipoidemia — *see* Hyperlipidemia
Lipoidosis — *see* Lipidosis
Lipoma D17.9
  fetal D17.9
    fat cell D17.9
  infiltrating D17.9
  intramuscular D17.9
  pleomorphic D17.9
  site classification
    arms (skin) (subcutaneous) D17.2-
    connective tissue D17.30
      intra-abdominal D17.5
      intrathoracic D17.4
      peritoneum D17.7
      retroperitoneum D17.7
      specified site NEC D17.39
      spermatic cord D17.6
    face (skin) (subcutaneous) D17.0
    head (skin) (subcutaneous) D17.0
    intra-abdominal D17.5
    intrathoracic D17.4
    legs (skin) (subcutaneous) D17.2-
    neck (skin) (subcutaneous) D17.0
    peritoneum D17.7
    retroperitoneum D17.7
    skin D17.30
      specified site NEC D17.39
    specified site NEC D17.7
    spermatic cord D17.6
    subcutaneous D17.30
      specified site NEC D17.39
    trunk (skin) (subcutaneous) D17.1
  unspecified D17.9
  spindle cell D17.9
Lipomatosis E88.2
  dolorosa (Dercum) E88.2
  fetal — *see* Lipoma
  Launois-Bensaude E88.89
Lipomyoma — *see* Lipoma
Lipomyxoma — *see* Lipoma
Lipomyxosarcoma — *see* Neoplasm, connective
    tissue, malignant
Lipoprotein metabolism disorder E78.9
Lipoproteinemia E78.5
  broad-beta E78.2
  floating-beta E78.2
  hyper-pre-beta E78.1
Liposarcoma (*see also* Neoplasm, connective tissue,
    malignant)
  dedifferentiated — *see* Neoplasm, connective tissue,
    malignant
  differentiated type — *see* Neoplasm, connective
    tissue, malignant
  embryonal — *see* Neoplasm, connective tissue,
    malignant
  mixed type — *see* Neoplasm, connective tissue,
    malignant
  myxoid — *see* Neoplasm, connective tissue,
    malignant
  pleomorphic — *see* Neoplasm, connective tissue,
    malignant
  round cell — *see* Neoplasm, connective tissue,
    malignant
  well differentiated type — *see* Neoplasm,
    connective tissue, malignant
Liposynovitis prepatellaris E88.89
Lipping, cervix N86
Lipschütz disease or ulcer N76.6
Lipuria R82.0
  schistosomiasis (bilharziasis) B65.0
Lisping F80.0
Lissauer's paralysis A52.17
Lissencephalia, lissencephaly Q04.3

Listeriosis, listerellosis A32.9
  congenital (disseminated) P37.2
  cutaneous A32.0
  neonatal, newborn (disseminated) P37.2
  oculoglandular A32.81
  specified NEC A32.89
Lithemia E79.0
Lithiasis — *see* Calculus
Lithosis J62.8
Lithuria R82.99
Litigation, anxiety concerning Z65.3
Little leaguer's elbow — *see* Epicondylitis, medial
Little's disease G80.9
Littre's
  gland — *see* condition
  hernia — *see* Hernia, abdomen
Littritis — *see* Urethritis
Livedo (annularis) (racemosa) (reticularis) R23.1
Liver — *see* condition
Living alone (problems with) Z60.2
  with handicapped person Z74.2
Lloyd's syndrome — *see* Adenomatosis, endocrine
Loa loa, loaiasis, loasis B74.3
Lobar — *see* condition
Lobomycosis B48.0
Lobo's disease B48.0
Lobotomy syndrome F07.0
Lobstein (-Ekman) **disease or syndrome** Q78.0
Lobster-claw hand Q71.6-
Lobulation (congenital) (*see also* Anomaly, by site)
  kidney, Q63.1
  liver, abnormal Q44.7
  spleen Q89.09
Lobule, lobular — *see* condition
Local, localized — *see* condition
Locked-in state G83.5
Locked twins causing obstructed labor O66.1
Locking
  joint — *see* Derangement, joint, specified type NEC
    knee — *see* Derangement, knee
Lockjaw — *see* Tetanus
Löffler's
  endocarditis I42.3
  eosinophilia J82
  pneumonia J82
  syndrome (eosinophilic pneumonitis) J82
Loiasis (with conjunctival infestation) (eyelid) B74.3
Lone Star fever A77.0
Long
  labor O63.9
    first stage O63.0
    second stage O63.1
  QT syndrome I45.81
Long-term (current) (prophylactic) **drug therapy** (use
    of)
  agents affecting estrogen receptors and estrogen
    levels NEC Z79.818
  anastrozole (Arimidex) Z79.811
  antibiotics Z79.2
    short-term use — *omit code*
  anticoagulants Z79.01
  anti-inflammatory, non-steroidal (NSAID) Z79.1
  antiplatelet Z79.02
  antithrombotics Z79.02
  aromatase inhibitors Z79.811
  aspirin Z79.82
  birth control pill or patch Z79.3
  contraceptive, oral Z79.3
  drug, specified NEC Z79.899
  estrogen receptor downregulators Z79.818
  Evista Z79.810
  exemestane (Aromasin) Z79.811
  Fareston Z79.810
  fulvestrant (Faslodex) Z79.818
  gonadotropin-releasing hormone (GnRH) agonist
    Z79.818
  goserelin acetate (Zoladex) Z79.818
  hormone replacement (postmenopausal) Z79.890
  insulin Z79.4
  letrozole (Femara) Z79.811
  leuprolide acetate (leuprorelin) (Lupron) Z79.818
  megestrol acetate (Megace) Z79.818
  methadone for pain management Z79.891

Long-term drug therapy —*continued*
  Nolvadex Z79.810
  non-steroidal anti-inflammatories (NSAID) Z79.1
  opiate analgesic Z79.891
  oral contraceptive Z79.3
  raloxifene (Evista) Z79.810
  selective estrogen receptor modulators (SERMs) Z79.810
  steroids
    inhaled Z79.51
    systemic Z79.52
  tamoxifen (Nolvadex) Z79.810
  toremifene (Fareston) Z79.810
Longitudinal stripes or grooves, nails L60.8
  congenital Q84.6
Loop
  intestine — *see* Volvulus
  vascular on papilla (optic) Q14.2
Loose (*see also* condition)
  body
    joint M24.00
      ankle M24.07-
      elbow M24.02-
      hand M24.04-
      hip M24.05-
      knee M23.4-
      shoulder (region) M24.01-
      specified site NEC M24.08
      vertebra M24.08
      toe M24.07-
      wrist M24.03-
    knee M23.4-
    sheath, tendon — *see* Disorder, tendon, specified type NEC
  cartilage — *see* Loose, body, joint
  tooth, teeth K08.8
Loosening
  aseptic
    joint prosthesis — *see* Complications, joint prosthesis, mechanical, loosening, by site
  epiphysis — *see* Osteochondropathy
  mechanical
    joint prosthesis — *see* Complications, joint prosthesis, mechanical, loosening, by site
Looser-Milkman (-Debray) **syndrome** M83.8
Lop ear (deformity) Q17.3
Lorain (-Levi) **short stature syndrome** E23.0
Lordosis M40.50
  acquired — *see* Lordosis, specified type NEC
  congenital Q76.429
    lumbar region Q76.426
    lumbosacral region Q76.427
    sacral region Q76.428
    sacrococcygeal region Q76.428
    thoracolumbar region Q76.425
  lumbar region M40.56
  lumbosacral region M40.57
  postsurgical M96.4
  postural — *see* Lordosis, specified type NEC
  rachitic (late effect) (sequelae) E64.3
  sequelae of rickets E64.3
  specified type NEC M40.40
    lumbar region M40.46
    lumbosacral region M40.47
    thoracolumbar region M40.45
  thoracolumbar region M40.55
  tuberculous A18.01
Loss (of)
  appetite R63.0
    hysterical F50.8
    nonorganic origin F50.8
    psychogenic F50.8
  blood — *see* Hemorrhage
  control, sphincter, rectum R15.9
    nonorganic origin F98.1
  consciousness, transient R55
    traumatic — *see* Injury, intracranial
  elasticity, skin R23.4
  family (member) in childhood Z62.898
  fluid (acute) E86.9
    with
      hypernatremia E87.0
      hyponatremia E87.1

Loss —*continued*
  function of labyrinth — *see* subcategory H83.2
  hair, nonscarring — *see* Alopecia
  hearing (*see also* Deafness)
    central NOS H90.5
    neural NOS H90.5
    perceptive NOS H90.5
    sensorineural NOS H90.5
    sensory NOS H90.5
  height R29.890
  limb or member, traumatic, current — *see* Amputation, traumatic
  love relationship in childhood Z62.898
  memory (*see also* Amnesia)
    mild, following organic brain damage F06.8
  mind — *see* Psychosis
  occlusal vertical dimension of fully erupted teeth M26.37
  organ or part — *see* Absence, by site, acquired
  ossicles, ear (partial) H74.32-
  parent in childhood Z63.4
  pregnancy, recurrent N46
    care in current pregnancy O26.2-
    without current pregnancy N96
  recurrent pregnancy — *see* Loss, pregnancy, recurrent
  self-esteem, in childhood Z62.898
  sense of
    smell — *see* Disturbance, sensation, smell
    taste — *see* Disturbance, sensation, taste
    touch R20.8
  sensory R44.9
    dissociative F44.6
  sexual desire F52.0
  sight (acquired) (complete) (congenital) — *see* Blindness
  substance of
    bone — *see* Disorder, bone, density and structure, specified NEC
    cartilage — *see* Disorder, cartilage, specified type NEC
      auricle (ear) — *see* Disorder, pinna, specified type NEC
    vitreous (humor) H15.89
  tooth, teeth *see* Absence, teeth, acquired
  vision, visual H54.7
    both eyes H54.3
    one eye H54.60
      left (normal vision on right) H54.62
      right (normal vision on left) H54.61
    specified as blindness — *see* Blindness
    subjective
      sudden H53.13-
      transient H53.12-
  vitreous — *see* Prolapse, vitreous
  voice — *see* Aphonia
  weight (abnormal) (cause unknown) R63.4
Louis-Bar syndrome (ataxia-telangiectasia) G11.3
Louping ill (encephalitis) A84.8
Louse, lousiness — *see* Lice
Low
  achiever, school Z55.3
  back syndrome M54.5
  basal metabolic rate R94.8
  birthweight (2499 grams or less) P07.10
    with weight of
      1000-1249 grams P07.14
      1250-1499 grams P07.15
      1500-1749 grams P07.16
      1750-1999 grams P07.17
      2000-2499 grams P07.18
    extreme (999 grams or less) P07.00
      with weight of
        499 grams or less P07.01
        500-749 grams P07.02
        750-999 grams P07.03
    for gestational age — *see* Light for dates
  blood pressure (*see also* Hypotension)
    reading (incidental) (isolated) (nonspecific) R03.1
  cardiac reserve — *see* Disease, heart
  function (*see also* Hypofunction)
    kidney N28.9
  hematocrit D64.9

Loss —*continued*
  hemoglobin D64.9
  income Z59.6
  level of literacy Z55.0
  lying
    kidney N28.89
    organ or site, congenital — *see* Malposition, congenital
  output syndrome (cardiac) — *see* Failure, heart
  platelets (blood) — *see* Thrombocytopenia
  reserve, kidney N28.89
  salt syndrome E87.1
  self esteem R45.81
  set ears Q17.4
  vision H54.2
    one eye (other eye normal) H54.50
      left (normal vision on right) H54.52
      other eye blind — *see* Blindness
      right (normal vision on left) H54.51
Low-density-lipoprotein-type (LDL) **hyperlipoproteinemia** E78.0
Lowe's syndrome E72.03
Lown-Ganong-Levine syndrome I45.6
LSD reaction (acute) (without dependence) F16.90
  with dependence F16.20
L-shaped kidney Q63.8
Ludwig's angina or disease K12.2
Lues (venerea), **luetic** — *see* Syphilis
Luetscher's syndrome (dehydration) E86.0
Lumbago, lumbalgia M54.5
  with sciatica M54.4-
    due to intervertebral disc disorder M51.17
  due to displacement, intervertebral disc M51.27
    with sciatica M51.17
Lumbar — *see* condition
Lumbarization, vertebra, congenital Q76.49
Lumbermen's itch B88.0
Lump — *see* Mass
Lunacy — *see* Psychosis
Lung — *see* condition
Lupoid (miliary) **of Boeck** D86.3
Lupus
  anticoagulant D68.62
  discoid (local) L93.0
  erythematosus (discoid) (local) L93.0
    disseminated — *see* Lupus, erythematosus, systemic
    eyelid H01.129
      left H01.126
        lower H01.125
        upper H01.124
      right H01.123
        lower H01.122
        upper H01.121
    profundus L93.2
    specified NEC L93.2
    subacute cutaneous L93.1
    systemic M32.9
      with organ or system involvement M32.10
        endocarditis M32.11
        lung M32.13
        pericarditis M32.12
        renal (glomerular) M32.14
          tubulo-interstitial M32.15
        specified organ or system NEC M32.19
      drug-induced M32.0
      inhibitor (presence of) D68.62
      specified NEC M32.8
  exedens A18.4
  hydralazine M32.0
    correct substance properly administered — *see* Table of Drugs and Chemicals, by drug, adverse effect
    overdose or wrong substance given or taken — *see* Table of Drugs and Chemicals, by drug, poisoning
  nephritis (chronic) M32.14
  nontuberculous, not disseminated L93.0
  panniculitis L93.2
  pernio (Besnier) D86.3
  systemic — *see* Lupus, erythematosus, systemic
  tuberculous A18.4
    eyelid A18.4

Lymphoma —*continued*
  BALT C88.4
  B-cell C85.1-
  B-precursor C83.5-
  blastic NK-cell C86.4
  bronchial-associated lymphoid tissue
      [BALT-lymphoma] C88.4
  Burkitt (atypical) C83.7-
  Burkitt-like C83.7-
  centrocytic C83.1-
  cutaneous follicle center C82.6-
  cutaneous T-cell C84.a-
  diffuse follicle center C82.5-
  diffuse large cell C83.3-
      anaplastic C83.3-
      B-cell C83.3-
      CD30-positive C83.3-
      centroblastic C83.3-
      immunoblastic C83.3-
      plasmablastic C83.3-
      subtype not specified C83.3-
      T-cell rich C83.3-
  enteropathy-type (associated) (intestinal) T-cell
      C86.2
  extranodal NK/T-cell, nasal type C86.0
  extranodal marginal zone B-cell lymphoma of
      mucosa-associated lymphoid tissue
      [MALT-lymphoma] C88.4
  follicular C82.9-
      grade
        I C82.0-
        II C82.1-
        III C82.2-
        IIIa C82.3-
        IIIb C82.4-
      specified NEC C82.8-
  hepatosplenic T-cell (alpha-beta) (gamma-delta)
      C86.1
  histiocytic C85.9-
      true C96.a
  Hodgkin C81.9
      classical C81.7-
        lymphocyte depleted C81.3-
        lymphocyte-rich C81.4-
        mixed cellularity C81.2-
        nodular sclerosis C81.1-
        specified NEC C81.7-
      lymphocyte depleted classical C81.3-
      lymphocyte-rich classical C81.4-
      mixed cellularity classical C81.2-
      nodular
        lymphocyte predominant C81.0-
        sclerosis classical C81.1-
  intravascular large B-cell C83.8-
  Lennert's C84.4-
  lymphoblastic B-cell C83.5-
  lymphoblastic (diffuse) C83.5-
  lymphoblastic T-cell C83.5-
  lymphoepithelioid C84.4-
  lymphoplasmacytic C83.0-
      with IgM-production C88.0
  MALT C88.4
  mantle cell C83.1-
  mature T-cell NEC C84.4-
  mature T/NK-cell C84.9-
      specified NEC C84.z-
  mediastinal (thymic) large B-cell C85.2-
  Mediterranean C88.3
  mucosa-associated lymphoid tissue
      [MALT-lymphoma] C88.4
  NK/T cell C84.9-
  nodal marginal zone C83.0-
  non-follicular C83.9-
      specified NEC C83.8-
  non-Hodgkin (*see also* Lymphoma, by type) C85.9
      specified NEC C85.8-
  non-leukemic variant of B-CLL C83.0-
  peripheral T-cell, not classified C84.4-
  primary cutaneous
      anaplastic large cell C86.6
      CD30-positive T-cell C86.6
  primary effusion B-cell C83.8-
  SALT C88.4

Lymphoma —*continued*
  skin-associated lymphoid tissue [SALT-lymphoma]
      C88.4
  small cell B-cell C83.0-
  splenic marginal zone C83.0-
  subcutaneous panniculitis-like T-cell C86.3
  T-precursor C83.5-
  true histiocytic C96.a
Lymphomatosis — *see* Lymphoma
Lymphopathia venereum, veneris A55
Lymphopenia D72.810
Lymphoplasmacytic leukemia — *see* Leukemia,
    chronic lymphocytic, B-cell type
Lymphoproliferation, X-linked disease D82.3
Lymphoreticulosis, benign (of inoculation) A28.1
Lymphorrhea I89.8
    Lymphosarcoma (diffuse) (*see also* Lymphoma) C85.9
Lymphostasis I89.8
Lypemania — *see* Melancholia
Lysine and hydroxylysine metabolism disorder
    E72.3
Lyssa — *see* Rabies

M

Macacus ear Q17.3
Maceration, wet feet, tropical (syndrome) T69.02-
MacLeod's syndrome J43.0
Macrocephalia, macrocephaly Q75.3
Macrocheilia, macrochilia (congenital) Q18.6
Macrocolon (*see also* Megacolon) Q43.1
Macrocornea Q15.8
    with glaucoma Q15.0
Macrocytic — *see* condition
Macrocytosis D75.89
Macrodactylia, macrodactylism (fingers) (thumbs)
    Q74.0
    toes Q74.2
Macrodontia K00.2
Macrogenia M26.05
Macrogenitosomia (adrenal) (male) (praecox) E25.9
    congenital E25.0
Macroglobulinemia (idiopathic) (primary) C88.0
    monoclonal (essential) D47.2
    Waldenström C88.0
Macroglossia (congenital) Q38.2
    acquired K14.8
Macrognathia, macrognathism (congenital)
    (mandibular) (maxillary) M26.09
Macrogyria (congenital) Q04.8
Macrohydrocephalus — *see* Hydrocephalus
Macromastia — *see* Hypertrophy, breast
Macrophthalmos Q11.3
    in congenital glaucoma Q15.0
Macropsia H53.15
Macrosigmoid K59.3
    congenital Q43.2
Macrospondylitis , acromegalic E22.0
Macrostomia (congenital) Q18.4
Macrotia (external ear) (congenital) Q17.1
Macula
    cornea, corneal — *see* Opacity, cornea
    degeneration (atrophic) (exudative) (senile) (*see also*
        Degeneration, macula)
      hereditary — *see* Dystrophy, retina
Maculae ceruleae — B85.1
Maculopathy, toxic — *see* Degeneration, macula,
    toxic
Madarosis (eyelid) H02.729
    left H02.726
      lower H02.725
      upper H02.724
    right H02.723
      lower H02.722
      upper H02.721
Madelung's
    deformity (radius) Q74.0
    disease
      radial deformity Q74.0
      symmetrical lipomas, neck E88.89
Madness — *see* Psychosis

Madura
    foot B47.9
      actinomycotic B47.1
      mycotic B47.0
Maduromycosis B47.0
Maffucci's syndrome Q78.4
Magnesium metabolism disorder — *see* Disorder,
    metabolism, magnesium
Main en griffe (acquired) (*see also* Deformity, limb,
    clawhand)
    congenital Q74.0
Maintenance (encounter for)
    antineoplastic chemotherapy Z51.11
    antineoplastic radiation therapy Z51.0
Majocchi's disease L81.7
    granuloma B35.8
Major — *see* condition
Malabar itch (any site) B35.5
Malabsorption K90.9
    calcium K90.89
    carbohydrate K90.4
    disaccharide E73.9
    fat K90.4
    galactose E74.20
    glucose(-galactose) E74.39
    intestinal K90.9
      specified NEC K90.89
    isomaltose E74.31
    lactose E73.9
    methionine E72.19
    monosaccharide E74.39
    postgastrectomy K91.2
    postsurgical K91.2
    protein K90.4
    starch K90.4
    sucrose E74.39
    syndrome K90.9
      postsurgical K91.2
Malacia, bone (adult) M83.9
    juvenile — *see* Rickets
Malacoplakia
    bladder N32.89
    pelvis (kidney) N28.89
    ureter N28.89
    urethra N36.8
Malacosteon, juvenile — *see* Rickets
Maladaptation — *see* Maladjustment
Maladie de Roger Q21.0
Maladjustment
    conjugal Z63.0
      involving divorce or estrangement Z63.5
    educational Z55.4
    family Z63.9
    marital Z63.0
      involving divorce or estrangement Z63.5
    occupational NEC Z56.89
    simple, adult — *see* Disorder, adjustment
    situational — *see* Disorder, adjustment
    social Z60.9
      due to
        acculturation difficulty Z60.3
        discrimination and persecution (perceived)
            Z60.5
        exclusion and isolation Z60.4
        life-cycle (phase of life) transition Z60.0
        rejection Z60.4
        specified reason NEC Z60.8
Malaise R53.81
Malakoplakia — *see* Malacoplakia
Malaria, malarial (fever) B54
    with
      blackwater fever B50.8
        hemoglobinuric (bilious) B50.8
      hemoglobinuria B50.8
    accidentally induced (therapeutically)—code by
        type under Malaria
    algid B50.9
    cerebral B50.0 [G94]
    clinically diagnosed (without parasitological
        confirmation) B54
    congenital NEC P37.4
    falciparum P37.3

Malaria, malarial—*continued*
congestion, congestive B54
continued (fever) B50.9
estivo-autumnal B50.9
falciparum B50.9
  with complications NEC B50.8
    cerebral B50.0 [G94]
  severe B50.8
hemorrhagic B54
malariae B52.9
  with
    complications NEC B52.8
    glomerular disorder B52.0
malignant (tertian) — *see* Malaria, falciparum
mixed infections—code to first listed type in
  B50-B53
ovale B53.0
parasitologically confirmed NEC B53.8
pernicious, acute — *see* Malaria, falciparum
Plasmodium (P.)
  falciparum NEC — *see* Malaria, falciparum
  malariae NEC B52.9
    with Plasmodium
      falciparum (and or vivax) — *see* Malaria,
        falciparum
      vivax (*see also* Malaria, vivax)
        and falciparum — *see* Malaria,
          falciparum
  ovale B53.0
    with Plasmodium malariae (*see also* Malaria,
      malariae)
      and vivax (*see also* Malaria, vivax)
        and falciparum — *see* Malaria,
          falciparum
  simian B53.1
    with Plasmodium malariae (*see also* Malaria,
      malariae)
      and vivax (*see also* Malaria, vivax)
        and falciparum — *see* Malaria,
          falciparum
  vivax NEC B51.9
    with Plasmodium falciparum — *see* Malaria,
      falciparum
quartan — *see* Malaria, malariae
quotidian — *see* Malaria, falciparum
recurrent B54
remittent B54
specified type NEC (parasitologically confirmed)
  B53.8
spleen B54
subtertian (fever) — *see* Malaria, falciparum
tertian (benign) (*see also* Malaria, vivax)
  malignant B50.9
tropical B50.9
typhoid B54
vivax B51.9
  with
    complications NEC B51.8
    ruptured spleen B51.0
Malassimilation K90.9
Malassez's disease (cystic) N50.8
Mal de los pintos — *see* Pinta
Mal de mer T75.3
Maldescent, testis Q53.9
bilateral Q53.20
  abdominal Q53.21
  perineal Q53.22
unilateral Q53.10
  abdominal Q53.11
  perineal Q53.12

Maldevelopment (*see also* Anomaly)
brain Q07.9
colon Q43.9
hip Q74.2
  congenital dislocation Q65.2
    bilateral Q65.1
    unilateral Q65.0-
mastoid process Q75.8
middle ear Q16.4
  except ossicles Q16.4
  ossicles Q16.3
ossicles Q16.3
spine Q76.49

Maldevelopment—*continued*
toe Q74.2
Male type pelvis Q74.2
with disproportion (fetopelvic) O33.3
  causing obstructed labor O65.3
Malformation (congenital) (*see also* Anomaly)
adrenal gland Q89.1
affecting multiple systems with skeletal changes
  NEC Q87.5
alimentary tract Q45.9
  specified type NEC Q45.8
  upper Q40.9
    specified type NEC Q40.8
aorta Q25.9
  atresia Q25.2
  coarctation (preductal) (postductal) Q25.1
  patent ductus arteriosus Q25.0
  specified type NEC Q25.4
  stenosis (supravalvular) Q25.3
aortic valve Q23.9
  specified NEC Q23.8
arteriovenous, aneurysmatic (congenital) Q27.30
  brain Q28.2
  cerebral Q28.2
  peripheral Q27.30
    digestive system Q27.33
    lower limb Q27.32
    other specified site Q27.39
    renal vessel Q27.34
    upper limb Q27.31
  precerebral vessels (nonruptured) Q28.0
auricle
  ear (congenital) Q17.3
    acquired H61.119
      left H61.112
        with right H61.113
      right H61.111
        with left H61.113
bile duct Q44.5
bladder Q64.79
  aplasia Q64.5
  diverticulum Q64.6
  exstrophy — *see* Exstrophy, bladder
  neck obstruction Q64.31
bone Q79.9
  face Q75.9
    specified type NEC Q75.8
  skull Q75.9
    specified type NEC Q75.8
brain (multiple) Q04.9
  arteriovenous Q28.2
  specified type NEC Q04.8
branchial cleft Q18.2
breast Q83.9
  specified type NEC Q83.8
broad ligament Q50.6
bronchus Q32.4
bursa Q79.9
cardiac
  chambers Q20.9
    specified type NEC Q20.8
  septum Q21.9
    specified type NEC Q21.8
cerebral Q04.9
  vessels Q28.3
cervix uteri Q51.9
  specified type NEC Q51.828
Chiari
  Type I G93.5
  Type II Q07.01
choroid (congenital) Q14.3
  plexus Q07.8
circulatory system Q28.9
cochlea Q16.5
cornea Q13.4
coronary vessels Q24.5
corpus callosum (congenital) Q04.0
diaphragm Q79.1
digestive system NEC, specified type NEC Q45.8
dura Q07.9
  brain Q04.9
  spinal Q06.9

Malformation—*continued*
ear Q17.9
  causing impairment of hearing Q16.9
  external Q17.9
    accessory auricle Q17.0
    causing impairment of hearing Q16.9
      absence of
        auditory canal Q16.1
        auricle Q16.0
    macrotia Q17.1
    microtia Q17.2
    misplacement Q17.4
    misshapen NEC Q17.3
    prominence Q17.5
    specified type NEC Q17.8
  inner Q16.5
  middle Q16.4
    absence of eustachian tube Q16.2
    ossicles (fusion) Q16.3
  ossicles Q16.3
  specified type NEC Q17.8
epididymis Q55.4
esophagus Q39.9
  specified type NEC Q39.8
eye Q15.9
  lid Q10.3
  specified NEC Q15.8
fallopian tube Q50.6
genital organ
  male Q55.9
    epididymis — *see* Malformation, epididymis
    penis — *see* Malformation, penis
    prostate — *see* Malformation, prostate
    scrotum — *see* Malformation, scrotum
    seminal vesicle — *see* Malformation, seminal
      vesicle
    specified type NEC Q55.8
    testis — *see* Malformation, testis
    vas deferens — *see* Malformation, vas
      deferens
    vasocutaneous fistula Q55.7
great
  artery Q25.9
    aorta — *see* Malformation, aorta
    pulmonary artery — *see* Malformation,
      pulmonary, artery
    specified type NEC Q25.8
  vein Q26.9
    anomalous
      portal venous connection Q26.5
      pulmonary venous connection Q26.4
        partial Q26.3
        total Q26.2
    persistent left superior vena cava Q26.1
    portal vein-hepatic artery fistula Q26.6
    specified type NEC Q26.8
    vena cava stenosis, congenital Q26.0
gum Q38.6
hair Q84.2
heart Q24.9
  specified type NEC Q24.8
integument Q84.9
  specified type NEC Q84.8
internal ear Q16.5
intestine Q43.9
  specified type NEC Q43.8
iris Q13.2
joint Q74.9
  ankle Q74.2
  lumbosacral Q76.49
  sacroiliac Q74.2
  specified type NEC Q74.8
kidney Q63.9
  accessory Q63.0
  giant Q63.3
  horseshoe Q63.1
  hydronephrosis Q62.0
  malposition Q63.2
  specified type NEC Q63.8
lacrimal apparatus Q10.6
lip Q38.0
lingual Q38.3
liver Q44.7

Malformation —*continued*
 lung Q33.9
 meninges or membrane (congenital) Q07.9
  cerebral Q04.8
  spinal (cord) Q06.9
 middle ear Q16.4
  ossicles Q16.3
 mitral valve Q23.9
  specified NEC Q23.8
 Mondini's (congenital) (malformation, cochlea)
   Q16.5
 mouth (congenital) Q38.6
 multiple types NEC Q89.7
 musculoskeletal system Q79.9
 myocardium Q24.8
 nail Q84.6
 nervous system (central) Q07.9
 nose Q30.9
  specified type NEC Q30.8
 optic disc Q14.2
 orbit Q10.7
 ovary Q50.39
 palate Q38.5
 parathyroid gland Q89.2
 pelvic organs or tissues NEC
  in pregnancy or childbirth O34.8-
   causing obstructed labor O65.5
 penis Q55.69
  aplasia Q55.5
  curvature (lateral) Q55.61
  hypoplasia Q55.62
 pericardium Q24.8
 peripheral vascular system Q27.9
  specified type NEC Q27.8
 pharynx Q38.8
 precerebral vessels Q28.1
 prostate Q55.4
 pulmonary
  artery Q25.9
   atresia Q25.5
   specified type NEC Q25.7
   stenosis Q25.6
  valve Q22.3
 renal artery Q27.2
 respiratory system Q34.9
 retina Q14.1
 scrotum — *see* Malformation, testis and scrotum
 seminal vesicles Q55.4
 sense organs NEC Q07.9
 skin Q82.9
 specified NEC Q89.8
 spinal
  cord Q06.9
  nerve root Q07.8
 spine Q76.49
  kyphosis — *see* Kyphosis, congenital
  lordosis — *see* Lordosis, congenital
 spleen Q89.09
 stomach Q40.3
  specified type NEC Q40.2
 teeth, tooth K00.9
 tendon Q79.9
 testis and scrotum Q55.20
  aplasia Q55.0
  hypoplasia Q55.1
  polyorchism Q55.21
  retractile testis Q55.22
  scrotal transposition Q55.23
  specified NEC Q55.29
 throat Q38.8
 thorax, bony Q76.9
 thyroid gland Q89.2
 tongue (congenital) Q38.3
  hypertrophy Q38.2
  tie Q38.1
 trachea Q32.1
 tricuspid valve Q22.9
  specified type NEC Q22.8
 umbilical cord NEC (complicating delivery) O69.89
 umbilicus Q89.9
 ureter Q62.8
  agenesis Q62.4
  duplication Q62.5

Malformation —*continued*
 ureter—*continued*
  malposition — *see* Malposition, congenital, ureter
  obstructive defect — *see* Defect, obstructive,
    ureter
  vesico-uretero-renal reflux Q62.7
 urethra Q64.79
  aplasia Q64.5
  duplication Q64.74
  posterior valves Q64.2
  prolapse Q64.71
  stricture Q64.32
 urinary system Q64.9
 uterus Q51.9
  specified type NEC Q51.818
 vagina Q52.4
 vascular system, peripheral Q27.9
 vas deferens Q55.4
  atresia Q55.3
 venous — *see* Anomaly, vein(s)
 vulva Q52.70
Malfunction (*see also* Dysfunction)
 cardiac electronic device T82.119
  electrode T82.110
  pulse generator T82.111
  specified type NEC T82.118
 catheter device NEC T85.618
  cystostomy T83.010
  dialysis (renal) (vascular) T82.41
   intraperitoneal T85.611
  infusion NEC T82.514
   spinal (epidural) (subdural) T85.610
  urinary, indwelling T83.018
 colostomy K94.03
  valve K94.03
 cystostomy (stoma) N99.512
  catheter T83.010
 enteric stoma K94.13
 enterostomy K94.13
 esophagostomy K94.33
 gastroenteric K31.89
 gastrostomy K94.23
 ileostomy K94.13
  valve K94.13
 jejunostomy K94.13
 pacemaker — *see* Malfunction, cardiac electronic
    device
 prosthetic device, internal — *see* Complications,
    prosthetic device, by site, mechanical
 tracheostomy J95.03
 urinary device NEC — *see* Complication,
    genitourinary, device, urinary, mechanical
 valve
  colostomy K94.03
  heart T82.09
  ileostomy K94.13
 vascular graft or shunt NEC — *see* Complication,
    cardiovascular device, mechanical, vascular
 ventricular (communicating shunt) T85.01
Malherbe's tumor — *see* Neoplasm, skin, benign
Malibu disease L98.8-
Malignancy (*see also* Neoplasm, malignant, by site)
 unspecified site (primary) C80.1
Malignant — *see* condition
Malingerer, malingering Z76.5
Mallet finger (acquired) — *see* Deformity, finger,
    mallet finger
 congenital Q74.0
 sequelae of rickets E64.3
Malleus A24.0
Mallory's bodies R89.7
Mallory-Weiss syndrome K22.6
Malnutrition E46
 degree
  first E44.1
  mild (protein) E44.1
  moderate (protein) E44.0
  second E44.0
  severe (protein-energy) E43
   intermediate form E42
    with
     kwashiorkor (and marasmus) E42
     marasmus E41

Malnutrition—*continued*
 degree—*continued*
  third E43
 following gastrointestinal surgery K91.2
 intrauterine
  light-for-dates — *see* Light for dates
  small-for-dates — *see* Small for dates
 lack of care, or neglect (child) (infant) T76.02
  confirmed T74.02
 malignant E40
 protein E46
  calorie
   mild E44.1
   moderate E44.0
   severe E43
    intermediate form E42
     with
      kwashiorkor (and marasmus) E42
      marasmus E41
  energy E46
   mild E44.1
   moderate E44.0
   severe E43
    intermediate form E42
     with
      kwashiorkor (and marasmus) E42
      marasmus E41
 severe (protein-energy) E43
  with
   kwashiorkor (and marasmus) E42
   marasmus E41
Malocclusion (teeth) M26.4
 Angle's M26.219
  class I M26.211
  class II M26.212
  class III M26.213
 due to
  abnormal swallowing M26.59
  mouth breathing M26.59
  tongue, lip or finger habits M26.59
 temporomandibular (joint) M26.69
Malposition
 cervix — *see* Malposition, uterus
 congenital
  adrenal (gland) Q89.1
  alimentary tract Q45.8
   lower Q43.8
   upper Q40.8
  aorta Q25.4
  appendix Q43.8
  arterial trunk Q20.0
  artery (peripheral) Q27.8
   coronary Q24.5
   digestive system Q27.8
   lower limb Q27.8
   pulmonary Q25.7
   specified site NEC Q27.8
   upper limb Q27.8
  auditory canal Q17.8
   causing impairment of hearing Q16.9
  auricle (ear) Q17.4
   causing impairment of hearing Q16.9
  cervical Q18.2
  biliary duct or passage Q44.5
  bladder (mucosa) — *see* Exstrophy, bladder
  brachial plexus Q07.8
  brain tissue Q04.8
  breast Q83.8
  bronchus Q32.4
  cecum Q43.8
  clavicle Q74.0
  colon Q43.8
  digestive organ or tract NEC Q45.8
   lower Q43.8
   upper Q40.8
  ear (auricle) (external) Q17.4
   ossicles Q16.3
  endocrine (gland) NEC Q89.2
  epiglottis Q31.8
  eustachian tube Q17.8
  eye Q15.8
  facial features Q18.8
  fallopian tube Q50.6

Marasmus—*continued*
  senile R54
  tuberculous NEC — *see* Tuberculosis
Marble
  bones Q78.2
  skin R23.8
Marburg virus disease A98.3
March
  fracture — *see* Fracture, traumatic, stress, by site
  hemoglobinuria D59.6
Marchesani(-Weill) **syndrome** Q87.0
Marchiafava(-Bignami) **syndrome or disease** G37.1
Marchiafava-Micheli syndrome D59.5
Marcus Gunn's syndrome Q07.8
Marfan's syndrome
  — *see* Syndrome, Marfan's
Marie-Bamberger disease — *see* Osteoarthropathy,
    hypertrophic, specified NEC
Marie-Charcot-Tooth neuropathic muscular
    atrophy G60.0
Marie's
  cerebellar ataxia (late-onset) G11.2
  disease or syndrome (acromegaly) E22.0
Marie-Strümpell arthritis, disease or spondylitis —
    see Spondylitis, ankylosing
Marion's disease (bladder neck obstruction) N32.0
Marital conflict Z63.0
Mark
  port wine Q82.5
  raspberry Q82.5
  strawberry Q82.5
  stretch L90.6
  tattoo L81.8
Marker heterochromatin — *see* Extra, marker
    chromosomes
Maroteaux-Lamy syndrome (mild) (severe) E76.29
Marrow (bone)
  arrest D61.9
  poor function D75.89
Marseilles fever A77.1
Marsh fever — *see* Malaria
Marshall's (hidrotic) **ectodermal dysplasia** Q82.4
Marsh's disease (exophthalmic goiter) E05.00
  with storm E05.01
Masculinization (female) **with adrenal hyperplasia**
    E25.9
  congenital E25.0
Masculinovoblastoma D27.-
Masochism (sexual) F65.51
Mason's lung J62.8
Mass
  abdominal R19.00
    epigastric R19.06
    generalized R19.07
    left lower quadrant R19.04
    left upper quadrant R19.02
    periumbilic R19.05
    right lower quadrant R19.03
    right upper quadrant R19.01
    specified site NEC R19.09
  breast N63
  chest R22.2
  cystic — *see* Cyst
  ear H93.8-
  head R22.0
  intra-abdominal (diffuse) (generalized) — *see* Mass,
    abdominal
  kidney N28.89
  liver R16.0
  localized (skin) R22.9
    chest R22.2
    head R22.0
    limb
      lower R22.4-
      upper R22.3-
    neck R22.1
    trunk R22.2
  lung R91
  malignant — *see* Neoplasm, malignant, by site
  neck R22.1
  pelvic (diffuse) (generalized) — *see* Mass, abdominal
  specified organ NEC — *see* Disease, by site
  splenic R16.1

Mass—*continued*
  substernal thyroid — *see* Goiter
  superficial (localized) R22.9
  umbilical (diffuse) (generalized) R19.09
Massive — *see* condition
Mast cell
  disease, systemic tissue D47.0
  leukemia C94.3-
  sarcoma C96.2
  tumor D47.0
    malignant C96.2-
Mastalgia N64.4
Masters-Allen syndrome N83.8
Mastitis (acute) (diffuse) (nonpuerperal) (subacute)
    N61
  chronic (cystic) — *see* Mastopathy, cystic
  cystic (Schimmelbusch's type) — *see* Mastopathy,
    cystic
  fibrocystic — *see* Mastopathy, cystic
  infective N61
    newborn P39.0
  interstitial, gestational or puerperal — *see* Mastitis,
    obstetric
  neonatal (noninfective) P83.4
    infective P39.0
  obstetric (interstitial) (nonpurulent)
    associated with
      lactation O91.23
      pregnancy O91.21-
      puerperium O91.22
    purulent
      associated with
        lactation O91.13
        pregnancy O91.11-
        puerperium O91.12
  periductal — *see* Ectasia, mammary duct
  phlegmonous — *see* Mastopathy, cystic
  plasma cell — *see* Ectasia, mammary duct
Mastocytoma D47.0
  malignant C96.2
Mastocytosis Q82.2
  aggressive systemic C96.2
  indolent systemic D47.0
  malignant C96.2
  systemic, associated with clonal hematopoetic
    non-mast-cell disease (SM-AHNMD) D47.0
Mastodynia N64.4
Mastoid — *see* condition
Mastoidalgia — *see* subcategory H92.0
Mastoiditis (coalescent) (hemorrhagic) (suppurative)
    H70.9-
  acute, subacute H70.00-
    complicated NEC H70.09-
    subperiosteal H70.01-
  chronic (necrotic) (recurrent) H70.1-
  in (due to)
    infectious disease NEC B99 [H75.0-]
    parasitic disease NEC B89 [H75.0-]
    tuberculosis A18.03
  petrositis — *see* Petrositis
  postauricular fistula — *see* Fistula, postauricular
  specified NEC H70.89-
  tuberculous A18.03
Mastopathy, mastopathia N64.9
  chronica cystica — *see* Mastopathy, cystic
  cystic (chronic) (diffuse) N60.1-
    with epithelial proliferation N60.3-
  diffuse cystic — *see* Mastopathy, cystic
  estrogenic, oestrogenica N64.89
  ovarian origin N64.89
Mastoplasia, mastoplastia N62
Masturbation (excessive) F98.8
Maternal care (for) — *see* Pregnancy (complicated by)
    (management affected by)
Matheiu's disease (leptospiral jaundice) A27.0
Mauclaire's disease or osteochondrosis — *see*
    Osteochondrosis, juvenile, hand, metacarpal
Maxcy's disease A75.2
Maxilla, maxillary — *see* condition
May(-Hegglin) **anomaly or syndrome** D72.0
McArdle(-Schmid)(-Pearson) **disease** (glycogen
    storage) E74.04
McCune-Albright syndrome Q78.1

McQuarrie's syndrome (idiopathic familial
    hypoglycemia) E16.2
Meadow's syndrome Q86.1
Measles (black) (hemorrhagic) (suppressed) B05.9
  with
    complications NEC B05.89
    encephalitis B05.0
    intestinal complications B05.4
    keratitis (keratoconjunctivitis) B05.81
    meningitis B05.1
    otitis media B05.3
    pneumonia B05.2
  French — *see* Rubella
  German — *see* Rubella
  Liberty — *see* Rubella
Meatitis, urethral — *see* Urethritis
Meatus, meatal — *see* condition
Meat-wrappers' asthma J68.9
Meckel-Gruber syndrome Q61.9
Meckel's diverticulitis, diverticulum (displaced)
    (hypertrophic) Q43.0
  malignant — *see* Table of Neoplasms, small
    intestine, malignant
Meconium
  ileus, newborn P76.0
    in cystic fibrosis E84.11
  obstruction, newborn P76.0
    in mucoviscidosis E84.11
  peritonitis P78.0
  plug syndrome (newborn) NEC P76.0
Median (*see also* condition)
  arcuate ligament syndrome I77.4
  bar (prostate) (vesical orifice) — *see* Hyperplasia,
    prostate
  rhomboid glossitis K14.2
Mediastinal shift R93.1
Mediastinitis (acute) (chronic) J98.5
  syphilitic A52.73
  tuberculous A15.8
Mediastinopericarditis (*see also* Pericarditis)
  acute I30.9
  adhesive I31.0
  chronic I31.8
    rheumatic I09.2
Mediastinum, mediastinal — *see* condition
Medical services provided for — *see* Health, services
    provided because of (of)
Medicine poisoning — *see* Table of Drugs and
    Chemicals, by drug, poisoning
Mediterranean
  fever — *see* Brucellosis
    familial E85.0
    tick A77.1
  kala-azar B55.0
  leishmaniasis B55.0
  tick fever A77.1
Medulla — *see* condition
Medullary cystic kidney Q61.5
Medullated fibers
  optic (nerve) Q14.8
  retina Q14.1
Medulloblastoma
  desmoplastic C71.6
  specified site — *see* Neoplasm, malignant, by site
  unspecified site C71.6
Medulloepithelioma (*see also* Neoplasm, malignant,
    by site)
  teratoid — *see* Neoplasm, malignant, by site
Medullomyoblastoma
  specified site — *see* Neoplasm, malignant, by site
  unspecified site C71.6
Meekeren-Ehlers-Danlos syndrome Q79.6
Megacolon (acquired) (functional) (not Hirschsprung's
    disease) (in) K59.3
  Chagas' disease B57.32
  congenital, congenitum (aganglionic) Q43.1
  Hirschsprung's (disease) Q43.1
  toxic K59.3
Megaesophagus (functional) K22.0
  congenital Q39.5
  in (due to) Chagas' disease B57.31
Megalencephaly Q04.5
Megalerythema (epidemic) B08.3

Melanoma—*continued*
  spindle cell
    with epithelioid, mixed — *see* Melanoma, skin,
      by site
    type A C69.4-
    type B C69.4-
  superficial spreading — *see* Melanoma, skin, by site
Melanosarcoma (*see also* Melanoma)
  epithelioid cell (*see* Melanoma)
Melanosis L81.4
  addisonian E27.1
    tuberculous A18.7
  adrenal E27.1
  colon K63.89
  conjunctiva — *see* Pigmentation, conjunctiva
    congenital Q13.89
  cornea (presenile) (senile) (*see also* Pigmentation,
    cornea)
    congenital Q13.4
  eye NEC H57.8
    congenital Q15.8
  lenticularis progressiva Q82.1
  liver K76.8
  precancerous — *see also* Melanoma, in situ
    malignant melanoma in — *see* Melanoma
  Riehl's L81.4
  sclera H15.89
    congenital Q13.89
  suprarenal E27.1
  tar L81.4
  toxic L81.4
Melanuria R82.91
MELAS syndrome E88.41
Melasma L81.1
  adrenal (gland) E27.1
  suprarenal (gland) E27.1
Melena K92.1
  with ulcer code by site under Ulcer, with
    hemorrhage K27.4
  due to swallowed maternal blood P78.2
  newborn, neonatal P54.1
    due to swallowed maternal blood P78.2
Meleney's
  gangrene (cutaneous) — *see* Ulcer, skin
  ulcer (chronic undermining) — *see* Ulcer, skin
Melioidosis A24.9
  acute A24.1
  chronic A24.2
  fulminating A24.1
  pneumonia A24.1
  pulmonary (chronic) A24.2
    acute A24.1
    subacute A24.2
  sepsis A24.1
  specified NEC A24.3
  subacute A24.2
Melitensis, febris A23.0
Melkersson(-Rosenthal) syndrome G51.2
Mellitus, diabete — *see* Diabetes
Melorheostosis (bone) — *see* Disorder, bone, density
    and structure, specified NEC
Meloschisis Q18.4
Melotia Q17.4
Membrana
  capsularis lentis posterior Q13.89
  epipapillaris Q14.2
Membranacea placenta O43.19-
Membranaceous uterus N85.8
Membrane(s), membranous — *see also* condition
  cyclitic — *see* Membrane, pupillary
  folds, congenital — *see* Web
  Jackson's Q43.3
  over face of newborn P28.9
  premature rupture — *see* Rupture, membranes,
    premature
  pupillary H21.4-
    persistent Q13.89
  retained (with hemorrhage) (complicating delivery)
    O72.2
    without hemorrhage O73.1
  secondary cataract — *see* Cataract, secondary
  unruptured (causing asphyxia) — *see* Asphyxia,
    newborn

Membrane(s), membranous—*continued*
  vitreous — *see* Opacity, vitreous, membranes and
    strands
Membranitis — *see* Chorioamnionitis
Memory disturbance, lack or loss — *see also*
    Amnesia
  mild, following organic brain damage F06.8
Menadione deficiency E56.1
Menarche
  delayed E30.0
  precocious E30.1
Mendacity, pathologic F60.2
Mendelson's syndrome (due to anesthesia) J95.4
  in labor and delivery O74.0
  in pregnancy O29.01-
  obstetric O74.0
  postpartum, puerperal O89.01
Ménétrier's disease or syndrome K29.60
  with bleeding K29.61
Ménière's disease, syndrome or vertigo H81.0-
Meninges, meningeal — *see* condition
Meningioma (*see also* Neoplasm, meninges, benign)
  angioblastic — *see* Neoplasm, meninges, benign
  angiomatous — *see* Neoplasm, meninges, benign
  endotheliomatous — *see* Neoplasm, meninges,
    benign
  fibroblastic — *see* Neoplasm, meninges, benign
  fibrous — *see* Neoplasm, meninges, benign
  hemangioblastic — *see* Neoplasm, meninges,
    benign
  hemangiopericytic — *see* Neoplasm, meninges,
    benign
  malignant — *see* Neoplasm, meninges, malignant
  meningiothelial — *see* Neoplasm, meninges, benign
  meningotheliomatous — *see* Neoplasm, meninges,
    benign
  mixed — *see* Neoplasm, meninges, benign
  multiple — *see* Neoplasm, meninges, uncertain
    behavior
  papillary — *see* Neoplasm, meninges, uncertain
    behavior
  psammomatous — *see* Neoplasm, meninges,
    benign
  syncytial — *see* Neoplasm, meninges, benign
  transitional — *see* Neoplasm, meninges, benign
Meningiomatosis (diffuse) — *see* Neoplasm,
    meninges, uncertain behavior
Meningism — *see* Meningismus
Meningismus (infectional) (pneumococcal) R29.1
  due to serum or vaccine R29.1
  influenzal — *see* Influenza, with, manifestations NEC
Meningitis (basal) (basic) (brain) (cerebral) (cervical)
    (congestive) (diffuse) (hemorrhagic) (infantile)
    (membranous) (metastatic) (nonspecific)
    (pontine) (progressive) (simple) (spinal)
    (subacute) (sympathetic) (toxic) G03.9
  abacterial G03.0
  actinomycotic A42.81
  adenoviral A87.1
  arbovirus A87.8
  aseptic (acute) G03.0
  bacterial G00.9
    Escherichia coli (E. coli) G00.8
    Friedländer (bacillus) G00.8
    gram-negative G00.9
    H. influenzae G00.0
    Klebsiella G00.8
    pneumococcal G00.1
    specified organism NEC G00.8
    staphylococcal G00.3
    streptococcal (acute) G00.2
  benign recurrent (Mollaret) G03.2
  candidal B37.5
  caseous (tuberculous) A17.0
  cerebrospinal A39.0
  chronic NEC G03.1
  clear cerebrospinal fluid NEC G03.0
  coxsackievirus A87.0
  cryptococcal B45.1
  diplococcal (gram positive) A39.0
  echovirus A87.0
  enteroviral A87.0
  eosinophilic B83.2

Meningitis—*continued*
  epidemic NEC A39.0
  Escherichia coli (E. coli) G00.8
  fibrinopurulent G00.9
    specified organism NEC G00.8
  Friedländer (bacillus) G00.8
  gonococcal A54.81
  gram-negative cocci G00.9
  gram-positive cocci G00.9
  Haemophilus (influenzae) G00.0
  H. influenzae G00.0
  in (due to)
    adenovirus A87.1
    African trypanosomiasis B56.9
    anthrax A22.8
    bacterial disease NEC A48.8 [G01]
    Chagas' disease (chronic) B57.41
    chickenpox B01.0
    coccidioidomycosis B38.4
    Diplococcus pneumoniae G00.1
    enterovirus A87.0
    herpes (simplex) virus B00.3
      zoster B02.1
    infectious mononucleosis B27.92
    leptospirosis A27.81
    Listeria monocytogenes A32.11
    Lyme disease A69.21
    measles B05.1
    mumps (virus) B26.1
    neurosyphilis (late) A52.13
    parasitic disease NEC B89 [G02]
    poliovirus A80.9 [G02]
    preventive immunization, inoculation or
      vaccination G03.8
    rubella B06.02
    Salmonella infection A02.21
    specified cause NEC G03.8
    typhoid fever A01.01
    varicella B01.0
    viral disease NEC A87.8
    whooping cough A37.90
    zoster B02.1
  infectious G00.9
  influenzal (H. influenzae) G00.0
  Klebsiella G00.8
  leptospiral (aseptic) A27.81
  lymphocytic (acute) (benign) (serous) A87.2
  meningococcal A39.0
  Mima polymorpha G00.8
  Mollaret (benign recurrent) G03.2
  monilial B37.5
  mycotic NEC B49 [G02]
  Neisseria A39.0
  nonbacterial G03.0
  nonpyogenic NEC G03.0
  ossificans G96.19
  pneumococcal G00.1
  poliovirus A80.9 [G02]
  postmeasles B05.1
  purulent G00.9
    specified organism NEC G00.8
  pyogenic G00.9
    specified organism NEC G00.8
  Salmonella (arizonae) (Cholerae-Suis) (enteritidis)
    (typhimurium) A02.21
  septic G00.9
    specified organism NEC G00.8
  serosa circumscripta NEC G03.0
  serous NEC G93.2
  specified organism NEC G00.8
  sporotrichosis B42.81
  staphylococcal G00.3
  sterile G03.0
  streptococcal (acute) G00.2
  suppurative G00.9
    specified organism NEC G00.8
  syphilitic (late) (tertiary) A52.13
    acute A51.41
    congenital A50.41
    secondary A51.41
  Torula histolytica (cryptococcal) B45.1
  traumatic (complication of injury) T79.8
  tuberculous A17.0

Meningitis—*continued*
  typhoid A0.01
  viral NEC A87.9
  Yersinia pestis A20.3
Meningocele (spinal) (*see also* Spina bifida)
  with hydrocephalus — *see* Spina bifida, by site, with
    hydrocephalus
  acquired (traumatic) G96.19
  cerebral — *see* Encephalocele
Meningocerebritis — *see* Meningoencephalitis
Meningococcemia A39.4
  acute A39.2
  chronic A39.3
Meningococcus, meningococcal (*see also* condition)
  A39.9
  adrenalitis, hemorrhagic A39.1
  carrier (suspected) of Z22.31
  meningitis (cerebrospinal) A39.0
Meningoencephalitis (*see also* Encephalitis) G04.90
  acute NEC (*see also* Encephalitis, viral) A86
  bacterial NEC G04.2
  California A83.5
  diphasic A84.1
  eosinophilic B83.2
  epidemic A39.81
  herpesviral, herpetic B00.4
    due to herpesvirus 6 B10.01
    due to herpesvirus 7 B10.09
    specified NEC B10.09
  in (due to)
    blastomycosis NEC B40.81
    diseases classified elsewhere G05.3
    free-living amebae B60.2
    Hemophilus influenzae (H. influenzae) G04.2
    herpes B00.4
      due to herpesvirus 6 B10.01
      due to herpesvirus 7 B10.09
      specified NEC B10.09
    H. influenzae G00.0
    Lyme disease A69.22
    mercury — *see* subcategory T56.1
    mumps B26.2
    Naegleria (amebae) (organisms) (fowleri) B60.2
    Parastrongylus cantonensis B83.2
    toxoplasmosis (acquired) B58.2
      congenital P37.1
  infectious (acute) (viral) A86
  influenzal (H. influenzae) G04.2
  Listeria monocytogenes A32.12
  lymphocytic (serous) A87.2
  mumps B26.2
  parasitic NEC B89 [G05.3]
  pneumococcal G00.1
  primary amebic B60.2
  specific (syphilitic) A52.14
  specified organism NEC G04.81
  staphylococcal G04.2
  streptococcal G04.2
  syphilitic A52.14
  toxic NEC G92
    due to mercury — *see* subcategory T56.1
  tuberculous A17.82
  virus NEC A86
Meningoencephalocele (*see also* Encephalocele)
  syphilitic A52.19
    congenital A50.49
Meningoencephalomyelitis (*see also*
  Meningoencephalitis)
  acute NEC (viral) A86
    disseminated G04.00
      postimmunization or postvaccination G04.01
      postinfectious G04.00
  due to
    actinomycosis A42.82
    Toxoplasma or toxoplasmosis (acquired) B58.2
      congenital P37.1
  postimmunization or postvaccination G04.01
Meningoencephalomyelopathy G96.9
Meningoencephalopathy G96.9
Meningomyelitis (*see also* Meningoencephalitis)
  bacterial NEC G04.2
  blastomycotic NEC B40.81
  cryptococcal B45.1

Meningomyelitis—*continued*
  in diseases classified elsewhere G05.4
  meningococcal A39.81
  syphilitic A52.14
  tuberculous A17.82
Meningomyelocele (*see also* Spina bifida)
  syphilitic A52.19
Meningomyeloneuritis — *see* Meningoencephalitis
Meningoradiculitis — *see* Meningitis
Meningovascular — *see* condition
Menkes' disease or syndrome E83.09
  meaning maple-syrup-urine disease E71.0
Menometrorrhagia N92.1
Menopause, menopausal (asymptomatic) (state)
  Z78.0
  arthritis (any site) NEC — *see* Arthritis, specified
    form NEC
  bleeding N92.4
  depression (single episode) F32.8
    agitated (single episode) F32.2
      recurrent episode F33.9
    psychotic (single episode) F32.8
      recurrent episode F33.9
    recurrent episode F33.9
  melancholia (single episode) F32.8
    recurrent episode F33.9
  paranoid state F22
  premature E28.319
    asymptomatic E28.319
      postirradiation E89.40
      postsurgical E89.40
    symptomatic E28.310
      postirradiation E89.41
      postsurgical E89.41
  psychosis NEC F28
  symptomatic N95.1
  toxic polyarthritis NEC — *see* Arthritis, specified
    form NEC
Menorrhagia (primary) N92.0
  climacteric N92.4
    menopausal N92.4
  menopausal N92.4
  postclimacteric N95.0
  postmenopausal N95.0
  preclimacteric or premenopausal N92.4
  pubertal (menses retained) N92.2
Menostaxis N92.0
Menses, retention N94.89
Menstrual — *see* Menstruation
Menstruation
  absent — *see* Amenorrhea
  anovulatory N97.0
  cycle, irregular N92.6
  delayed N91.0
  disorder N93.9
    psychogenic F45.8
  during pregnancy O20.8
  excessive (with regular cycle) N92.0
    with irregular cycle N92.1
    at puberty N92.2
  frequent N92.0
  infrequent — *see* Oligomenorrhea
  irregular N92.6
    specified NEC N92.5
  latent N92.5
  membranous N92.5
  painful (*see also* Dysmenorrhea) N94.6
    primary N94.4
    psychogenic F45.8
    secondary N94.5
  passage of clots N92.0
  precocious E30.1
  protracted N92.5
  rare — *see* Oligomenorrhea
  retained N94.89
  retrograde N92.5
  scanty — *see* Oligomenorrhea
  suppression N94.89
  vicarious (nasal) N94.89
Mental (*see also* condition)
  deficiency — *see* Retardation, mental
  deterioration — *see* Psychosis
  disorder — *see* Disorder, mental

Mental—*continued*
  exhaustion F48.8
  insufficiency (congenital) — *see* Retardation, mental
  observation without need for further medical care
    Z03.89
  retardation — *see* Retardation, mental
  subnormality — *see* Retardation, mental
  upset — *see* Disorder, mental
Meralgia paresthetica G57.1-
Mercurial — *see* condition
Mercurialism — *see* subcategory T56.1
MERFF syndrome E88.42
Merkel cell tumor — *see* Carcinoma, Merkel cell
Merocele — *see* Hernia, femoral
Meromelia
  lower limb — *see* Defect, reduction, lower limb
    intercalary
      femur — *see* Defect, reduction, lower limb,
        specified type NEC
        tibiofibular (complete) (incomplete) — *see*
          Defect, reduction, lower limb
  upper limb — *see* Defect, reduction, upper limb
    intercalary, humeral, radioulnar — *see* Agenesis,
      arm, with hand present
Merzbacher-Pelizaeus disease E75.29
Mesaortitis — *see* Aortitis
Mesarteritis — *see* Arteritis
Mesencephalitis — *see* Encephalitis
Mesenchymoma (*see also* Neoplasm, connective
  tissue, uncertain behavior)
  benign — *see* Neoplasm, connective tissue, benign
  malignant — *see* Neoplasm, connective tissue,
    malignant
Mesenteritis
  retractile K65.4
  sclerosing K65.4
Mesentery, mesenteric — *see* condition
Mesiodens, mesiodentes K00.1
Mesio-occlusion M26.213
Mesocolon — *see* condition
Mesonephroma (malignant) — *see* Neoplasm,
  malignant, by site
  benign — *see* Neoplasm, benign, by site
Mesophlebitis — *see* Phlebitis
Mesostromal dysgenesis Q13.89
Mesothelioma (malignant) C45.9
  benign
    mesentery D19.1
    mesocolon D19.1
    omentum D19.1
    peritoneum D19.1
    pleura D19.0
    specified site NEC D19.7
    unspecified site D19.9
  biphasic C45.9
    benign
      mesentery D19.1
      mesocolon D19.1
      omentum D19.1
      peritoneum D19.1
      pleura D19.0
      specified site NEC D19.7
      unspecified site D19.9
  cystic D48.4
  epithelioid C45.9
    benign
      mesentery D19.1
      mesocolon D19.1
      omentum D19.1
      peritoneum D19.1
      pleura D19.0
      specified site NEC D19.7
      unspecified site D19.9
  fibrous C45.9
    benign
      mesentery D19.1
      mesocolon D19.1
      omentum D19.1
      peritoneum D19.1
      pleura D19.0
      specified site NEC D19.7
      unspecified site D19.9

Mesothelioma—continued
  site classification
    liver C45.7
    lung C45.7
    mediastinum C45.7
    mesentery C45.1
    mesocolon C45.1
    omentum C45.1
    pericardium C45.2
    peritoneum C45.1
    pleura C45.0
      parietal C45.0
    retroperitoneum C45.7
    specified site NEC C45.7
    unspecified C45.9
Metabolic syndrome E88.81
Metagonimiasis B66.8
Metagonimus infestation (intestine) B66.8
Metal
  pigmentation L81.8
  polisher's disease J62.8
Metamorphopsia H53.15
Metaplasia
  apocrine (breast) — see Dysplasia, mammary,
      specified type NEC
  cervix (squamous) — see Dysplasia, cervix
  endometrium (squamous) (uterus) N85.8
  esophagus
  kidney (pelvis) (squamous) N28.89
  myelogenous D73.1
  myeloid (agnogenic) (megakaryocytic) D73.1
  spleen D73.1
  squamous cell, bladder N32.89
Metastasis, metastatic
  abscess — see Abscess
  calcification E83.59
  cancer
    from specified site — see Neoplasm, malignant,
        by site
    to specified site — see Neoplasm, secondary, by
        site
  deposits (in) — see Neoplasm, secondary, by site
  disease (see also Neoplasm, secondary, by site)C79.9
  spread (to) — see Neoplasm, secondary, by site
Metastrongyliasis B83.8
Metatarsalgia M77.4-
  anterior G57.6-
  Morton's G57.6-
Metatarsus, metatarsal (see also condition)
  valgus (abductus), congenital Q66.6
  varus (adductus) (congenital) Q66.2
Methadone use F11.20
Methemoglobinemia D74.9
  acquired (with sulfhemoglobinemia) D74.8
  congenital D74.0
  enzymatic (congenital) D74.0
  Hb M disease D74.0
  hereditary D74.0
  toxic D74.8
Methemoglobinuria — see Hemoglobinuria
Methioninemia E72.19
Methylmalonic acidemia E71.120
Metritis (catarrhal) (hemorrhagic) (septic)
    (suppurative) (see also Endometritis)
  cervical — see Cervicitis
Metropathia hemorrhagica N93.8
Metroperitonitis — see Peritonitis, pelvic, female
Metrorrhagia N92.1
  climacteric N92.4
  menopausal N92.4
  postpartum NEC (atonic) (following delivery of
      placenta) O72.1
    delayed or secondary O72.2
  preclimacteric or premenopausal N92.4
  psychogenic F45.8
Metrorrhexis — see Rupture, uterus
Metrosalpingitis N70.91
Metrostaxis N93.8
Metrovaginitis — see Endometritis
Meyer-Schwickerath and Weyers syndrome Q87.0

Meynert's amentia (nonalcoholic) F04
  alcoholic F10.96
    with dependence F10.26
Mibelli's disease (porokeratosis) Q82.8
Mice, joint — see Loose, body, joint
  knee M23.4-
Micrencephalon, micrencephaly Q02
Microalbuminuria R80.9
Microaneurysm, retinal (see also Disorder, retina,
    microaneurysms)
  diabetic — see E08-E13 with .31
Microangiopathy (peripheral) I73.9
  thrombotic M31.1
Microcalcifications, breast R92.0
Microcephalus, microcephalic, microcephaly Q02
  due to toxoplasmosis (congenital) P37.1
Microcheilia Q18.7
Microcolon (congenital) Q43.8
Microcornea (congenital) Q13.4
Microcytic — see condition
Microdeletions NEC Q93.88
Microdontia K00.2
Microdrepanocytosis D56.8
Microembolism
  atherothrombotic — see Atheroembolism
  retinal — see Occlusion, artery, retina
Microencephalon Q02
Microfilaria streptocerca infestation B73.1
Microgastria (congenital) Q40.2
Microgenia M26.06
Microgenitalia, congenital
  female Q52.8
  male Q55.8
Microglioma — see Lymphoma, non-Hodgkin,
    specified NEC
Microglossia (congenital) Q38.3
Micrognathia, micrognathism (congenital)
    (mandibular) (maxillary) M26.09
Microgyria (congenital) Q04.3
Microinfarct of heart — see Insufficiency, coronary
Microlentia (congenital) Q12.8
Microlithiasis, alveolar, pulmonary J84.0
Micromastia N64.82
Micromyelia (congenital) Q06.8
Micropenis Q55.62
Microphakia (congenital) Q12.8
Microphthalmos, microphthalmia (congenital)
    Q11.2
  due to toxoplasmosis P37.1
Micropsia H53.15
Microscopic polyangiitis (polyarteritis) M31.7
Microsporidiosis B60.8
  intestinal A07.8
Microsporon furfur infestation B36.0
Microsporosis (see also Dermatophytosis)
  nigra B36.1
Microstomia (congenital) Q18.5
Microtia (congenital) (external ear) Q17.2
Microtropia H50.40
Microvillus inclusion disease (MVD) Q43.8
Micturition
  disorder NEC R39.19
    psychogenic F45.8
  frequency R35.0
    psychogenic F45.8
  hesitancy R39.11
  incomplete emptying R39.14
  nocturnal R35.1
  painful R30.9
    dysuria R30.0
    psychogenic F45.8
    tenesmus R30.1
  poor stream R39.12
  split stream R39.13
  straining R39.16
  urgency R39.15
Mid plane — see condition
Middle
  ear — see condition
  lobe (right) syndrome J98.19
Miescher's elastoma L87.2
Mietens' syndrome Q87.2

Migraine (idiopathic) G43.909
  basilar — see Migraine, with aura
  classical — see Migraine, with aura
  common — see Migraine, without aura
  equivalents — see Migraine, with aura
  familiar — see Migraine, hemiplegic
  hemiplegic G43.409
    intractable G43.419
      with status migrainosus G43.411
      without status migrainosus G43.419
    not intractable G43.409
      with status migrainosus G43.401
      without status migrainosus G43.409
  intractable G43.919
    with status migrainosus G43.911
    without status migrainosus G43.919
  menstrual G43.d09
    intractable G43.d19
      with status migrainosus G43.d11
      without status migrainosus G43.d19
    not intractable G43.d09
      with status migrainosus G43.d01
      without status migrainosus G43.d09
  menstrually related — see Migraine, menstrual
  not intractable G43.909
    with status migrainosus G43.901
    without status migrainosus G43.919
  ophthalmoplegic G43.b09
    intractable G43.b19
      with status migrainosus G43.b11
      without status migrainosus G43.b19
    not intractable G43.b09
      with status migrainosus G43.b01
      without status migrainosus G43.b09
  persistent aura (with, without) cerebral infarction —
      see Migraine, with aura, persistent
  preceded or accompanied by transient focal
      neurological phenomena — see Migraine,
      with aura
  pre-menstrual — see Migraine, menstrual
  pure menstrual — see Migraine, menstrual
  retinal — see Migraine, with aura
  specified NEC G43.809
    intractable G43.819
      with status migrainosus G43.811
      without status migrainosus G43.819
    not intractable G43.809
      with status migrainosus G43.801
      without status migrainosus G43.809
  sporadic — see Migraine, hemiplegic
  transformed — see Migraine, without aura, chronic
  triggered seizures — see Migraine, with aura
  with aura (acute-onset) (prolonged) (typical)
      (without headache) G43.109
    intractable G43.119
      with status migrainosus G43.111
      without status migrainosus G43.119
    not intractable G43.109
      with status migrainosus G43.101
      without status migrainosus G43.109
    persistent G43.509
      with cerebral infarction G43.609
        intractable G43.619
          with status migrainosus G43.611
          without status migrainosus G43.619
        not intractable G43.609
          with status migrainosus G43.601
          without status migrainosus G43.609
      without cerebral infarction G43.509
        intractable G43.519
          with status migrainosus G43.511
          without status migrainosus G43.519
        not intractable G43.509
          with status migrainosus G43.501
          without status migrainosus G43.509
  without aura G43.009
    chronic G43.709
      intractable
        with status migrainosus G43.711
        without status migrainosus G43.719
      not intractable
        with status migrainosus G43.701
        without status migrainosus G43.709

Migraine —continued
  without aura—continued
    intractable
      with status migrainosus G43.011
      without status migrainosus G43.019
    not intractable
      with status migrainosus G43.001
      without status migrainosus G43.009
Migrant, social Z59.0
Migration, anxiety concerning Z60.3
Migratory, migrating (see also condition)
  person Z59.0
  testis Q55.29
Mikity-Wilson disease or syndrome P27.0
Mikulicz' disease or syndrome K11.8
Miliaria L74.3
  alba L74.1
  apocrine L75.2
  crystallina L74.1
  profunda L74.2
  rubra L74.0
  tropicalis L74.2
Miliary — see condition
Milium L72.0
  colloid L57.8
Milk
  crust L21.0
  excessive secretion O92.6
  poisoning — see Poisoning, food, noxious
  retention O92.79
  sickness — see Poisoning, food, noxious
  spots I31.0
Milk-alkali disease or syndrome E83.59
Milk-leg (deep vessels) (nonpuerperal) — see
  Embolism, vein, lower extremity
  complicating pregnancy O22.3-
  puerperal, postpartum, childbirth O87.1
Milkman's disease or syndrome M83.8
Milky urine — see Chyluria
Millard-Gubler(-Foville) **paralysis or syndrome** G46.3
Millar's asthma J38.5
Miller Fisher syndrome G61.0
Mills' disease — see Hemiplegia
Millstone maker's pneumoconiosis J62.8
Milroy's disease (chronic hereditary edema) Q82.0
Minamata disease T26.1-
Minkowski-Chauffard syndrome — see
  Spherocytosis
Miners' asthma or lung J60
Minkowski-Chauffard syndrome — see
  Spherocytosis
Minor — see condition
Minor's disease (hematomyelia) G95.19
Minot's disease (hemorrhagic disease), newborn P53
**Minot-von Willebrand-Jurgens disease or
  syndrome** (angiohemophilia) D68.0
Minus (and plus) **hand** (intrinsic) — see Deformity,
  limb, specified type NEC, forearm
Miosis (pupil) H57.03
Mirizzi's syndrome (hepatic duct stenosis) K83.1
Mirror writing F81.0
Misadventure (of) (prophylactic) (therapeutic) (see
  also Complications) T88.9
  administration of insulin (by accident) — see
    subcategory T38.3
  infusion — see Complications, infusion
  local applications (of fomentations, plasters, etc.)
    T88.9
    burn or scald — see Burn
    specified NEC T88.8
  medical care (early) (late) T88.9
    adverse effect of drugs or chemicals — see Table
      of Drugs and Chemicals
  medical care (early) (late)
    burn or scald — see Burn
    specified NEC T88.8
  specified NEC T88.8
  surgical procedure (early) (late) — see
    Complications, surgical procedure
  transfusion — see Complications, transfusion
  vaccination or other immunological procedure —
    see Complications, vaccination
Miscarriage O03.9

Misdirection, aqueous H40.83-
Misperception, sleep state F51.02
Misplaced, misplacement
  ear Q17.4
  kidney (acquired) N28.89
    congenital Q63.2
  organ or site, congenital NEC — see Malposition,
    congenital
Missed
  abortion O02.1
  delivery O36.4
Missing — see Absence
Misuse of drugs F19.99
Mitchell's disease (erythromelalgia) I73.81
Mite(s) (infestation) B88.9
  diarrhea B88.0
  grain (itch) B88.0
  hair follicle (itch) B88.0
  in sputum B88.0
Mitral — see condition
Mittelschmerz N94.0
Mixed — see condition
MNGIE (Mitochondrial Neurogastrointestinal
  Encephalopathy) syndrome E88.49
Mobile, mobility
  cecum Q43.3
  excessive — see Hypermobility
  gallbladder, congenital Q44.1
  kidney N28.89
  organ or site, congenital NEC — see Malposition,
    congenital
Mobitz heart block (atrioventricular) I44.30
Moebius, Möbius
  disease (ophthalmoplegic migraine) — see
    Migraine, ophthalmoplegic
  syndrome Q87.0
    congenital oculofacial paralysis (with other
      anomalies) Q87.0
    ophthalmoplegic migraine — see Migraine,
      ophthalmoplegic
Moeller's glossitis K14.0
Mohr's syndrome (Types I and II) Q87.0
Mola destruens D39.2
Molar pregnancy O02.0
Molarization of premolars K00.2
Molding, head (during birth) **omit code**
Mole (pigmented) (see also Nevus)
  blood O02.0
  Breus' O02.0
  cancerous — see Melanoma
  carneous O02.0
  destructive D39.2
  fleshy O02.0
  hydatid, hydatidiform (benign) (complicating
    pregnancy) (delivered) (undelivered) O01.9
    classical O01.0
    complete O01.0
    incomplete O01.1
    invasive D39.2
    malignant D39.2
    partial O01.1
  intrauterine O02.0
  invasive (hydatidiform) D39.2
  malignant
    meaning
      malignant hydatidiform mole D39.2
      melanoma — see Melanoma
  nonhydatidiform O02.0
  nonpigmented — see Nevus
  pregnancy NEC O02.0
  skin — see Nevus
  tubal O00.1
  vesicular — see Mole, hydatidiform
Molimen, molimina (menstrual) N94.3
Molluscum contagiosum (epitheliale) B08.1
Mönckeberg's arteriosclerosis, disease, or sclerosis
  — see Arteriosclerosis, extremities
Mondini's malformation (cochlea) Q16.5
Mondor's disease I80.8
Monge's disease T70.29
Monilethrlx (congenital) Q84.1
Moniliasis (see also Candidiasis) B37.9
  neonatal P37.5

Monitoring (encounter for)
  therapeutic drug level Z51.81
Monkey malaria B53.1
Monkeypox B04
Monoarthritis M13.10
  ankle M13.17-
  elbow M13.12-
  foot joint M13.17-
  hand joint M13.14-
  hip M13.15-
  knee M13.16-
  shoulder M13.11-
  wrist M13.13-
Monoblastic — see condition
Monochromat(ism), monochromatopsia (acquired)
  (congenital) H53.51
Monocytic — see condition
Monocytopenia D72.818
Monocytosis (symptomatic) D72.821
Monomania — see Psychosis
Mononeuritis G58.9
  cranial nerve — see Disorder, nerve, cranial
  femoral nerve G57.2-
  lateral
    cutaneous nerve of thigh G57.1-
    popliteal nerve G57.3-
  lower limb G57.9-
    specified nerve NEC G57.8-
  medial popliteal nerve G57.4-
  median nerve G56.1-
  multiplex G58.7
  plantar nerve G57.6-
  posterior tibial nerve G57.5-
  radial nerve G56.3-
  sciatic nerve G57.0-
  specified NEC G58.8
  tibial nerve G57.4-
  ulnar nerve G56.2-
  upper limb G56.9-
    specified nerve NEC G56.8-
  vestibular — see subcategory H93.3
Mononeuropathy G58.9
  carpal tunnel syndrome — see Syndrome, carpal
    tunnel
  diabetic NEC — see E08-E13 with .41
  femoral nerve — see Lesion, nerve, femoral
  ilioinguinal nerve G57.8-
  intercostal G58.0
  lower limb G57.9-
    causalgia — see Causalgia, lower limb
    femoral nerve — see Lesion, nerve, femoral
    meralgia paresthetica G57.1-
    plantar nerve — see Lesion, nerve, plantar
    popliteal nerve — see Lesion, nerve, popliteal
    sciatic nerve — see Lesion, nerve, sciatic
    specified NEC G57.8-
    tarsal tunnel syndrome — see Syndrome, tarsal
      tunnel
  median nerve — see Lesion, nerve, median
  multiplex G58.7
  obturator nerve G57.80
  popliteal nerve — see Lesion, nerve, popliteal
  radial nerve — see Lesion, nerve, radial
  saphenous nerve G57.8-
  specified NEC G58.8
  tarsal tunnel syndrome — see Syndrome, tarsal
    tunnel
  tuberculous A17.83
  ulnar nerve — see Lesion, nerve, ulnar
  upper limb G56.9-
    carpal tunnel syndrome — see Syndrome, carpal
      tunnel
    causalgia — see Causalgia
    median nerve — see Lesion, nerve, median
    radial nerve — see Lesion, nerve, radial
    specified site NEC G56.8-
    ulnar nerve — see Lesion, nerve, ulnar
Mononucleosis, infectious B27.90
  with
    complication NEC B27.99
    meningitis B27.92
    polyneuropathy B27.91

Mononucleosis, infectious—*continued*
  cytomegaloviral B27.10
    with
      complication NEC B27.19
      meningitis B27.12
      polyneuropathy B27.11
  Epstein-Barr (virus) B27.00
    with
      complication NEC B27.09
      meningitis B27.02
      polyneuropathy B27.01
  gammaherpesviral B27.00
    with
      complication NEC B27.09
      meningitis B27.02
      polyneuropathy B27.01
  specified NEC B27.80
    with
      complication NEC B27.89
      meningitis B27.82
      polyneuropathy B27.81
Monoplegia G83.3-
  congenital (cerebral) G80.8
    spastic G80.1
  embolic (current episode) I63.4
  following
    cerebrovascular disease
      cerebral infarction
        lower limb I69.34-
        upper limb I69.33-
      intracerebral hemorrhage
        lower limb I69.14-
        upper limb I69.13-
      lower limb I69.94-
      nontraumatic intracranial hemorrhage NEC
        lower limb I69.24-
        upper limb I69.23-
      specified disease NEC
        lower limb I69.84-
        upper limb I69.83-
      stroke NOS
        lower limb I69.34-
        upper limb I69.33-
      subarachnoid hemorrhage
        lower limb I69.04-
        upper limb I69.03-
      upper limb I69.93-
  hysterical (transient) F44.4
  lower limb G83.1-
  psychogenic (conversion reaction) F44.4
  thrombotic (current episode) I63.3
  transient R29.81
  upper limb G83.2-
Monorchism, monorchidism Q55.0
Monosomy (see also Deletion, chromosome) Q93.9
  specified NEC Q93.89
  whole chromosome
    meiotic nondisjunction Q93.0
    mitotic nondisjunction Q93.1
    mosaicism Q93.1
  X Q96.9
Monster, monstrosity (single) Q89.7
  acephalic Q00.0
  twin Q89.4
Monteggia's fracture (-dislocation) S52.27-
Mooren's ulcer (cornea) — *see* Ulcer, cornea, Mooren's
Moore's syndrome — *see* Epilepsy, specified NEC
Mooser-Neill reaction A75.2
Mooser's bodies A75.2
Morbidity not stated or unknown R69
Morbilli — *see* Measles
Morbus (*see also* Disease)
  angelicus, anglorum E55.0
  Beigel B36.2
  caducus — *see* Epilepsy
  celiacus K90.0
  comitialis — *see* Epilepsy
  cordis (*see also* Disease, heart) I51.9
    valvulorum — *see* Endocarditis
  coxae senilis M16.9
    tuberculous A18.02
  hemorrhagicus neonatorum P53
  maculosus neonatorum P54.5

Morel(-Stewart)(-Morgagni) **syndrome** M85.2
Morel-Kraepelin disease — *see* Schizophrenia
Morel-Moore syndrome M85.2
Morgagni's
  cyst, organ, hydatid, or appendage
    female Q50.5
    male (epididymal) Q55.4
      testicular Q55.29
  syndrome M85.2
Morgagni-Stokes-Adams syndrome I45.9
Morgagni-Stewart-Morel syndrome M85.2
Morgagni-Turner(-Albright) **syndrome** Q96.9
Moria F07.0
Moron (I.Q. 50-69) F70
Morphea L94.0
Morphinism (without remission) F11.20
  with remission F11.21
Morphinomania (without remission) F11.20
  with remission F11.21
Morquio(-Ullrich)(-Brailsford) **disease or syndrome**
  — *see* Mucopolysaccharidosis
Mortification (dry) (moist) — *see* Gangrene
Morton's metatarsalgia (neuralgia)(neuroma)
  (syndrome) G57.6-
Morvan's disease or syndrome G60.8
Mosaicism, mosaic (autosomal) (chromosomal)
  45,X/other cell lines NEC with abnormal sex
    chromosome Q96.4
  45,X/46,XX Q96.3
  sex chromosome
    female Q97.8
    lines with various numbers of X chromosomes
      Q97.2
    male Q98.7
    XY Q96.3
Moschowitz' disease M31.1
Mother yaw A66.0
Motion sickness (from travel, any vehicle) (from
  roundabouts or swings) T75.3
Mottled, mottling, teeth (enamel) (endemic)
  (nonendemic) K00.3
Mounier-Kuhn syndrome Q32.4
  with bronchiectasis J47.9
    exacerbation (acute) J47.1
    lower respiratory infection J47.0
  acquired J98.09
    with bronchiectasis J47.9
      with
        exacerbation (acute) J47.1
        lower respiratory infection J47.0
Mountain
  sickness T70.29
    with polycythemia , acquired (acute) D75.1
  tick fever A93.2
Mouse, joint — *see* Loose, body, joint
  knee M23.4-
Mouth — *see* condition
Movable
  coccyx — *see* subcategory M53.2
  kidney N28.89
    congenital Q63.8
  spleen D73.89
Movements, dystonic R25.8
Moyamoya disease I67.5
MRSA (Methacillin Resistant Staphylococcus Aureus)
  Z16
Mucha-Habermann disease L41.0
Mucinosis (cutaneous) (focal) (papular) (skin) L98.5
  oral K13.79
Mucocele
  appendix K38.8
  buccal cavity K13.79
  gallbladder K82.1
  lacrimal sac, chronic H04.43-
  nasal sinus J34.1
  nose J34.1
  salivary gland (any) K11.6
  sinus (accessory) (nasal) J34.1
  turbinate (bone) (middle) (nasal) J34.1
  uterus N85.8

Mucolipidosis
  I E77.1
  II, III E77.0
  IV E75.11
Mucopolysaccharidosis E76.3
  beta-gluduronidase deficiency E76.29
  cardiopathy E76.3 [I52]
  Hunter's syndrome E76.1
  Hurler's syndrome E76.01
  Hurler-Scheie syndrome E76.02
  Maroteaux-Lamy syndrome E76.29
  Morquio syndrome E76.219
    A E76.210
    B E76.211
    classic E76.210
  Sanfilippo syndrome E76.22
  Scheie's syndrome E76.03
  specified NEC E76.29
  type
    I
      Hurler's syndrome E76.01
      Hurler-Scheie syndrome E76.02
      Scheie's syndrome E76.03
    II E76.1
    III E76.22
    IV E76.219
    IVA E76.210
    IVB E76.211
    VI E76.29
    VII E76.29
Mucormycosis B46.5
  cutaneous B46.3
  disseminated B46.4
  gastrointestinal B46.2
  generalized B46.4
  pulmonary B46.0
  rhinocerebral B46.1
  skin B46.3
  subcutaneous B46.3
Mucositis (ulcerative) K12.30
  due to drugs NEC K12.32
  gastrointestinal K92.81
  mouth (oral) (oropharyngeal) K12.30
    due to antineoplastic therapy K12.31
    due to drugs NEC K12.32
    due to radiation K12.33
    specified NEC K12.39
    viral K12.39
  nasal J34.81
  oral cavity — *see* Mucositis, mouth
  oral soft tissues — *see* Mucositis, mouth
  vagina and vulva N76.81
Mucositis necroticans agranulocytica — *see*
  Agranulocytosis
Mucous (*see also* condition)
  patches (syphilitic) A51.39
    congenital A50.07
Mucoviscidosis E84.9
  with meconium obstruction E84.11
Mucus
  asphyxia or suffocation — *see* Asphyxia, mucus
  in stool R19.5
  plug — *see* Asphyxia, mucus
Muguet B37.0
Mulberry molars (congenital syphilis) A50.52
Müllerian mixed tumor
  specified site — *see* Neoplasm, malignant, by site
  unspecified site C54.9
Multicystic kidney (development) Q61.4
Multiparity (grand) Z64.1
  affecting management of pregnancy, labor and
    delivery (supervision only) O09.4-
  requiring contraceptive management — *see*
    Contraception
Multipartita placenta O43.19-
Multiple, multiplex (*see also* condition)
  digits (congenital) Q69.9
  endocrine neoplasia — *see* Neoplasia, endocrine,
    multiple (MEN)
  personality F44.81
Mumps B26.9
  arthritis B26.85
  complication NEC B26.89

Mumps—*continued*
encephalitis B26.2
hepatitis B26.81
meningitis (aseptic) B26.1
meningoencephalitis B26.2
myocarditis B26.82
oophoritis B26.89
orchitis B26.0
pancreatitis B26.3
polyneuropathy B26.84
Mumu (*see also* Infestation, filarial) B74.9 [N51]
Münchhausen's syndrome — *see* Disorder, factitious
Münchmeyer's syndrome — *see* Myositis, ossificans, progressiva
Mural — *see* condition
Murmur (cardiac) (heart) (organic) R01.1
abdominal R19.15
aortic (valve) — *see* Endocarditis, aortic
benign R01.0
diastolic — *see* Endocarditis
Flint I35.1
functional R01.0
Graham Steell I37.1
innocent R01.0
mitral (valve) — *see* Insufficiency, mitral
nonorganic R01.0
presystolic, mitral — *see* Insufficiency, mitral
pulmonic (valve) I37.8
systolic (valvular) — *see* Endocarditis
tricuspid (valve) I07.9
valvular — *see* Endocarditis
Murri's disease (intermittent hemoglobinuria) D59.6
Muscle, muscular (*see also* condition)
carnitine (palmityltransferase) deficiency E71.314
Musculoneuralgia — *see* Neuralgia
Mushroom-workers' (pickers') **disease or lung** J67.5
Mushrooming hip — *see* Derangement, joint, specified NEC, hip
Mutation
factor V Leiden D68.51
prothrombin gene D68.52
Mutism (*see also* Aphasia)
deaf (acquired) (congenital) NEC H91.3
elective (adjustment reaction) (childhood) F94.0
hysterical F44.4
selective (childhood) F94.0
Myalgia M79.1
epidemic (cervical) B33.0
traumatic NEC T14.8
Myasthenia G70.9
congenital G70.2
cordis — *see* Failure, heart
developmental G70.2
gravis G70.00
with exacerbation (acute)G70.01
in crisis G70.01
neonatal, transient P94.0
pseudoparalytica G70.00
with exacerbation (acute) G70.01
in crisis G70.01
stomach, psychogenic F45.8
syndrome
in
diabetes mellitus — *see* E08-E13 with .44
neoplastic disease (*see also* Neoplasm) D49.9 [G73.3]
pernicious anemia D51.0 [G73.3]
thyrotoxicosis E05.90 [G73.3]
with thyroid storm E05.91 [G73.3]
Myasthenic M62.81
Mycelium infection B49
Mycetismus — *see* Poisoning, food, noxious, mushroom
Mycetoma B47.9
actinomycotic B47.1
bone (mycotic) B47.9 [M90.80]
eumycotic B47.0
foot B47.9
actinomycotic B47.1
mycotic B47.0
madurae NEC B47.9
mycotic B47.0
maduromycotic B47.0

Mycetoma—*continued*
mycotic B47.0
nocardial B47.1
Mycobacteriosis — *see* Mycobacterium
Mycobacterium, mycobacterial (infection) A31.9
anonymous A31.9
atypical A31.9
cutaneous A31.1
pulmonary A31.0
tuberculous — *see* Tuberculosis, pulmonary
specified site NEC A31.8
avium (intracellulare complex) A31.0
balnei A31.1
Battey A31.0
chelonei A31.8
cutaneous A31.1
extrapulmonary systemic A31.8
fortuitum A31.8
intracellulare (Battey bacillus) A31.0
kansasii (yellow bacillus) A31.0
kakaferifu A31.8
kasongo A31.8
leprae (*see also* Leprosy) A30.9
luciflavum A31.1
marinum (M. balnei) A31.1
nonspecific — *see* Mycobacterium, atypical
pulmonary (atypical) A31.0
tuberculous — *see* Tuberculosis, pulmonary
scrofulaceum A31.8
simiae A31.8
systemic, extrapulmonary A31.8
szulgai A31.8
terrae A31.8
triviale A31.8
tuberculosis (human, bovine) seeTuberculosis
ulcerans A31.1
xenopi A31.8
Mycoplasma (M.) pneumoniae, as cause of disease classified elsewhere B96.0
Mycosis, mycotic B49
cutaneous NEC B36.9
ear B36.8
fungoides (extranodal) (solid organ) C84.0-
mouth B37.0
nails B35.1
opportunistic B48.8
skin NEC B36.9
specified NEC B48.8
stomatitis B37.0
vagina, vaginitis (candidal) B37.3
Mydriasis (pupil) H57.04
Myelatelia Q06.1
Myelinolysis, pontine, central G37.2
Myelitis (acute) (ascending) (childhood) (chronic) (descending) (diffuse) (disseminated) (idiopathic) (pressure) (progressive) (spinal cord) (subacute) (*see also* Encephalitis) G04.91
herpes simplex B00.82
herpes zoster B02.24
in diseases classified elsewhere G05.4
necrotizing, subacute G37.4
optic neuritis in G36.0
postchickenpox B01.12
postherpetic B02.24
postimmunization G04.89
postinfectious NEC G04.89
postvaccinal G04.89
specified NEC G04.89
syphilitic (transverse) A52.14
toxic G92
transverse (in demyelinating diseases of central nervous system) G37.3
tuberculous A17.82
varicella B01.12
Myeloblastic — *see* condition
Myeloblastoma
granular cell (*see also* Neoplasm, connective tissue)
malignant — *see* Neoplasm, connective tissue, malignant
tongue D10.1
Myelocele — *see* Spina bifida
Myelocystocele — *see* Spina bifida
Myelocytic — *see* condition

Myelodysplasia D46.9
specified NEC D46.z
spinal cord (congenital) Q06.1
Myelodysplastic syndrome D46.9
with
5q deletion D46.c
isolated del(5q) chromosomal abnormality D46.c
specified NEC D46.z
Myeloencephalitis — *see* Encephalitis
Myelofibrosis D75.81
with myeloid metaplasia D47.4
acute C94.4-
idiopathic (chronic) D47.4
primary D75.81
secondary D75.81
in myeloproliferative disease D47.4
Myelogenous — *see* condition
Myeloid — *see* condition
Myelokathexis D70.9
Myeloleukodystrophy E75.29
Myelolipoma — *see* Lipoma
Myeloma (multiple) C90.0-
plasma cell C90.0-
solitary (*see also* Plasmacytoma, solitary) C90.3
Myelomalacia G95.89
Myelomatosis C90.0-
Myelomeningitis — *see* Meningoencephalitis
Myelomeningocele (spinal cord) — *see* Spina bifida
Myelo-osteo-musculodysplasia hereditaria Q79.8
Myelopathic
anemia D64.89
muscle atrophy — *see* Atrophy, muscle, spinal
pain syndrome G89.0
Myelopathy (spinal cord) G95.9
drug-induced G95.89
in (due to)
degeneration or displacement, intervertebral disc NEC — *see* Disorder, disc, with, myelopathy
infection — *see* Encephalitis
intervertebral disc disorder (*see also* Disorder, disc, with, myelopathy)
mercury — *see* subcategory T56.1
neoplastic disease (*see also* Neoplasm) D49.9 [G99.2]
pernicious anemia D51.0 [G99.2]
spondylosis — *see* Spondylosis, with myelopathy NEC
necrotic (subacute) (vascular) G95.19
radiation-induced G95.89
spondylogenic NEC — *see* Spondylosis, with myelopathy NEC
toxic G95.89
transverse, acute G37.3
vascular G95.19
vitamin B12 E53.8 [G32.0]
Myelophthisis D61.82
Myeloradiculitis G04.91
Myeloradiculodysplasia (spinal) Q06.1
Myelosarcoma C92.3-
Myelosclerosis D75.89
with myeloid metaplasia D47.4
disseminated, of nervous system G35
megakaryocytic D47.4
with myeloid metaplasia D47.4
Myelosis
acute C92.0-
aleukemic C92.9-
chronic D47.1
erythremic (acute) C94.0-
megakaryocytic C94.2-
nonleukemic D72.828
subacute C92.9-
Myiasis (cavernous) B87.9
aural B87.4
creeping B87.0
cutaneous B87.0
dermal B87.0
ear (external) (middle) B87.4
eye B87.2
genitourinary B87.81
intestinal B87.82
laryngeal B87.3

Myiasis—continued
  nasopharyngeal B87.3
  ocular B87.2
  orbit B87.2
  skin B87.0
  specified site NEC B87.89
  traumatic B87.1
  wound B87.1
Myoadenoma, prostate — see Hyperplasia, prostate
Myoblastoma
  granular cell (see also Neoplasm, connective tissue, benign)
    malignant — see Neoplasm, connective tissue, malignant
  tongue D10.1
Myocardial — see condition
Myocardiopathy (congestive) (constrictive) (familial) (hypertrophic nonobstructive) (idiopathic) (infiltrative) (obstructive) (primary) (restrictive) (sporadic) (see also Cardiomyopathy) I42.9
  alcoholic I42.6
  cobalt-beer I42.6
  glycogen storage E74.02 [I43]
  hypertrophic obstructive I42.1
  in (due to)
    beriberi E51.12 [I43]
    cardiac glycogenosis E74.02 [I43]
    Friedreich's ataxia G11.1 [I43]
    myotonia atrophica G71.19 [I43]
    progressive muscular dystrophy G71.0 [I43]
  obscure (African) I42.8
  secondary I42.7
  thyrotoxic E05.90 [I43]
    with storm E05.91 [I43]
  toxic NEC I42.7
Myocarditis (with arteriosclerosis)(chronic)(fibroid) (interstitial) (old) (progressive) (senile) I51.4
  with
    rheumatic fever (conditions in I00) I09.0
      active — see Myocarditis, acute, rheumatic
      inactive or quiescent (with chorea) I09.0
  active I40.9
    rheumatic I01.2
      with chorea (acute) (rheumatic) (Sydenham's) I02.0
  acute or subacute (interstitial) I40.9
    due to
      streptococcus (beta-hemolytic) I01.2
    idiopathic I40.1
    rheumatic I01.2
      with chorea (acute) (rheumatic) (Sydenham's) I02.0
    specified NEC I40.8
  aseptic of newborn B33.22
  bacterial (acute) I40.0
  Coxsackie (virus) B33.22
  diphtheritic A36.81
  eosinophilic I40.1
  epidemic of newborn (Coxsackie) B33.22
  Fiedler's (acute) (isolated) I40.1
  giant cell (acute) (subacute) I40.1
  gonococcal A54.83
  granulomatous (idiopathic) (isolated) (nonspecific) I40.1
  hypertensive — see Hypertension, heart
  idiopathic (granulomatous) I40.1
  in (due to)
    diphtheria A36.81
    epidemic louse-borne typhus A75.0 [I41]
    Lyme disease A69.29
    sarcoidosis D86.85
    scarlet fever A38.1
    toxoplasmosis (acquired) B58.81
    typhoid A01.02
    typhus NEC A75.9 [I41]
  infective I40.0
  influenzal — see Influenza, with, myocarditis
  isolated (acute) I40.1
  meningococcal A39.52
  mumps B26.82
  nonrheumatic, active I40.9
  parenchymatous I40.9
  pneumococcal I40.0

Myocarditis—continued
  rheumatic (chronic) (inactive) (with chorea) I09.0
    active or acute I01.2
      with chorea (acute) (rheumatic) (Sydenham's) I02.0
  rheumatoid — see Rheumatoid, carditis
  septic I40.0
  staphylococcal I40.0
  suppurative I40.0
  syphilitic (chronic) A52.06
  toxic I40.8
    rheumatic — see Myocarditis, acute, rheumatic
  tuberculous A18.84
  typhoid A01.02
  valvular — see Endocarditis
  virus, viral I40.0
    of newborn (Coxsackie) B33.22
Myocardium, myocardial — see condition
Myocardosis — see Cardiomyopathy
Myoclonus, myoclonic, myoclonia (familial) (essential) (multifocal) (simplex) G25.3
  drug-induced G25.3
  epilepsy, familial (progressive) G25.3
  epileptica G40.309
    with status epilepticus G40.301
  facial G51.3
  familial progressive G25.3
  Friedreich's G25.3
  jerks G25.3
  massive G25.3
  palatal G25.3
  pharyngeal G25.3
Myocytolysis I51.5
Myodiastasis — see Diastasis, muscle
Myoendocarditis — see Endocarditis
Myoepithelioma — see Neoplasm, benign, by site
Myofasciitis (acute) — see Myositis
Myofibroma (see also Neoplasm, connective tissue, benign)
  uterus (cervix) (corpus) — see Leiomyoma
Myofibromatosis D48.1
  infantile Q89.8
Myofibrosis M62.89
  heart — see Myocarditis
  scapulohumeral — see Lesion, shoulder, specified NEC
Myofibrositis M79.7
  scapulohumeral — see Lesion, shoulder, specified NEC
Myoglobulinuria, myoglobinuria (primary) R82.1
Myokymia, facial G51.4
Myolipoma — see Lipoma
Myoma (see also Neoplasm, connective tissue, benign)
  malignant — see Neoplasm, connective tissue, malignant
  prostate D29.1
  uterus (cervix) (corpus) — see Leiomyoma
Myomalacia M62.89
Myometritis — see Endometritis
Myometrium — see condition
Myonecrosis, clostridial A48.0
Myopathy G72.9
  alcoholic G72.1
  benign congenital G70.9
  central core G70.9
  centronuclear G71.2
  congenital (benign) G71.2
  distal G71.0
  drug-induced G72.0
  endocrine NEC E34.9 [G73.7]
  extraocular muscles H05.82-
  facioscapulohumeral G71.0
  hereditary G71.9
    specified NEC G71.8
  immune NEC G72.49
  in (due to)
    Addison's disease E27.1 [G73.7]
    alcohol G72.1
    amyloidosis E85.0 [G73.7]
    cretinism E00.9 [G73.7]
    Cushing's syndrome E24.9 [G73.7]
    drugs G72.0
    endocrine disease NEC E34.9 [G73.7]

Myopathy—continued
  in—continued
    giant cell arteritis M31.6 [G73.7]
    glycogen storage disease E74.00 [G73.7]
    hyperadrenocorticism E24.9 [G73.7]
    hyperparathyroidism NEC E21.3 [G73.7]
    hypoparathyroidism E20.9 [G73.7]
    hypopituitarism E23.0 [G73.7]
    hypothyroidism E03.9 [G73.7]
    infectious disease NEC B99 [G73.7]
    lipid storage disease E75.6 [G73.7]
    metabolic disease NEC E88.9 [G73.7]
    myxedema E03.9 [G73.7]
    parasitic disease NEC B89 [G73.7]
    polyarteritis nodosa M30.0 [G73.7]
    rheumatoid arthritis — see Rheumatoid, myopathy
    sarcoidosis D86.87
    scleroderma M34.82
    sicca syndrome M35.03
    Sjögren's syndrome M35.03
    systemic lupus erythematosus M32.19
    thyrotoxicosis (hyperthyroidism) E05.90 [G73.7]
      with thyroid storm E05.91 [G73.7]
    toxic agent NEC G72.2
  inflammatory NEC G72.49
  limb-girdle G71.0
  mitochondrial NEC G71.3
  myotonic, proximal (PROMM) G71.11
  myotubular G71.2
  nemaline G71.2
  ocular G71.0
  oculopharyngeal G71.0
  primary G71.9
    specified NEC G71.8
  progressive NEC G72.8
  proximal myotonic (PROMM) G71.11
  rod G71.2
  scapulohumeral G71.0
  specified NEC G72.8
  toxic G72.2
Myopericarditis (see also Pericarditis)
  chronic rheumatic I09.2
Myopia (axial) (congenital) (progressive) H52.1-
  degenerative (malignant) — see Disorder, globe, degenerative, myopia
  malignant — see Disorder, globe, degenerative, myopia
  pernicious — see Disorder, globe, degenerative, myopia
  progressive high (degenerative) — see Disorder, globe, degenerative, myopia
Myosarcoma — see Neoplasm, connective tissue, malignant
Myosis (pupil) H57.03
  stromal (endolymphatic) D39.0
Myositis M60.9
  clostridial A48.0
  due to posture — see Myositis, specified type NEC
  epidemic B33.0
  fibrosa or fibrous (chronic), Volkmann's T79.6
  foreign body granuloma — see Granuloma, foreign body
  in (due to)
    bilharziasis B65.9 [M63]
    cysticercosis B69.81
    leprosy A30.9 [M63]
    mycosis B49 [M63]
    sarcoidosis D86.87
    schistosomiasis B65.9 [M63]
    syphilis
      late A52.78
      secondary A51.49
    toxoplasmosis (acquired) B58.82
    trichinellosis B75 [M63]
    tuberculosis A18.09
  inclusion body [IBM] G72.41
  infective M60.009
    arm M60.002
      left M60.001
      right M60.000

Myositis—*continued*
  infective—*continued*
    leg M60.005
      left M60.004
      right M60.003
    lower limb M60.005
      ankle M60.07-
      foot M60.07-
      lower leg M60.06-
      thigh M60.05-
      toe M60.07-
    multiple sites M60.09
    specified site NEC M60.08
    upper limb M60.002
      finger M60.04-
      forearm M60.03-
      hand M60.04-
      shoulder region M60.01-
      upper arm M60.02-
  interstitial M60.10
    ankle M60.17-
    foot M60.17-
    forearm M60.13-
    hand M60.14-
    lower leg M60.16-
    multiple sites M60.19
    shoulder region M60.11-
    specified site NEC M60.18
    thigh M60.15-
    upper arm M60.12-
  mycotic B49 [M63]
  orbital, chronic H05.12-
  ossificans or ossifying (circumscripta) (*see also*
    Ossification, muscle, specified NEC)
    in (due to)
      burns M61.30
        ankle M61.37-
        foot M61.37-
        forearm M61.33-
        hand M61.34-
        lower leg M61.36-
        multiple sites M61.39
        pelvic region M61.35-
        shoulder region M61.31-
        specified site NEC M61.38
        thigh M61.35-
        upper arm M61.32-
      quadriplegia or paraplegia M61.20
        ankle M61.27-
        foot M61.27-
        forearm M61.23-
        hand M61.24-
        lower leg M61.26-

Myositis—*continued*
  ossificans or ossifying—*continued*
    in—*continued*
      quadriplegia or paraplegia—*continued*
        multiple sites M61.29
        pelvic region M61.25-
        shoulder region M61.21-
        specified site NEC M61.28
        thigh M61.25-
        upper arm M61.22-
    progressiva M61.10
      ankle M61.17-
      finger M61.14-
      foot M61.17-
      forearm M61.13-
      hand M61.14-
      lower leg M61.16-
      multiple sites M61.19
      pelvic region M61.15-
      shoulder region M61.11-
      specified site NEC M61.18
      thigh M61.15-
      toe M61.17-
      upper arm M61.12-
    traumatica M61.00
      ankle M61.07-
      foot M61.07-
      forearm M61.03-
      hand M61.04-
      lower leg M61.06-
      multiple sites M61.09
      pelvic region M61.05-
      shoulder region M61.01-
      specified site NEC M61.08
      thigh M61.05-
      upper arm M61.02-
  purulent — *see* Myositis, infective
  specified type NEC M60.80
    ankle M60.87-
    foot M60.87-
    forearm M60.83-
    hand M60.84-
    lower leg M60.86-
    multiple sites M60.89
    pelvic region M60.85-
    shoulder region M60.81-
    specified site NEC M60.88
    thigh M60.85-
    upper arm M60.82-
  suppurative — *see* Myositis, infective
  traumatic (old) — *see* Myositis, specified type NEC

Myospasia impulsiva F95.2
Myotonia (acquisita) (intermittens) M62.89
  atrophica G71.11
  chondrodystrophic G71.13
  congenita (acetazolamide responsive) (dominant)
    (recessive) G71.12
  drug-induced G71.14
  dystrophica G71.11
  fluctuans G71.19
  levior G71.12
  permanens G71.19
  symptomatic G71.19
Myotonic pupil — *see* Anomaly, pupil, function, tonic
  pupil
Myriapodiasis B88.2
Myringitis H73.2-
  with otitis media — *see* Otitis, media
  acute H73.00-
    bullous H73.01-
    specified NEC H73.09-
  bullous — *see* Myringitis, acute, bullous
  chronic H73.1-
Mysophobia F40.228
Mytilotoxism — *see* Poisoning, fish
Myxadenitis labialis K13.0
Myxedema (adult) (idiocy) (infantile) (juvenile) (*see
  also* Hypothyroidism) E03.9
  circumscribed E05.90
    with storm E05.91
  coma E03.5
  congenital E00.1
  cutis L98.5
  localized (pretibial) E05.90
    with storm E05.91
  papular L98.5
Myxochondrosarcoma — *see* Neoplasm, cartilage,
  malignant
Myxofibroma — *see* Neoplasm, connective tissue,
  benign
  odontogenic — *see* Cyst, calcifying odontogenic
Myxofibrosarcoma — *see* Neoplasm, connective
  tissue, malignant
Myxolipoma D17.9
Myxoliposarcoma — *see* Neoplasm, connective tissue,
  malignant
Myxoma (*see also* Neoplasm, connective tissue,
  benign)
  nerve sheath — *see* Neoplasm, nerve, benign
  odontogenic — *see* Cyst, calcifying odontogenic
Myxosarcoma — *see* Neoplasm, connective tissue,
  malignant

This page was intentionally left blank

N

Naegeli's
  disease Q82.8
  leukemia, monocytic C93.1-
Naegleriasis (with meningoencephalitis) B60.2
Naffziger's syndrome G54.0
Naga sore — see Ulcer, skin
Nägele's pelvis M95.5
  with disproportion (fetopelvic) O33.0
    causing obstructed labor O65.0
Nail (see also condition)
  biting F98.8
  patella syndrome Q87.2
Nanism, nanosomia — see Dwarfism
Nanophyetiasis B66.8
Nanukayami A27.89
Napkin rash L22
Narcolepsy G47.419
  with cataplexy G47.411
  in conditions classified elsewhere G47.429
    with cataplexy G47.421
Narcosis R06.89
Narcotism — see Dependence
NARP (Neuropathy, Ataxia and Retinitis pigmentosa)
  syndrome E88.49
Narrow
  anterior chamber angle H40.0
  pelvis — see Contraction, pelvis
Narrowing (see also Stenosis)
  artery I77.1
    auditory, internal I65.8
    basilar — see Occlusion, artery, basilar
    carotid — see Occlusion, artery, carotid
    cerebellar — see Occlusion, artery, cerebellar
    cerebral — see Occlusion artery, cerebral
    choroidal — see Occlusion, artery, cerebral,
      specified NEC
    communicating posterior — see Occlusion,
      artery, cerebral, specified NEC
    coronary (see also Disease, heart, ischemic,
      atherosclerotic)
      congenital Q24.5
        syphilitic A50.54 [I52]
      due to syphilis NEC A52.06
    hypophyseal — see Occlusion, artery, cerebral,
      specified NEC
    pontine — see Occlusion, artery, cerebral,
      specified NEC
    precerebral — see Occlusion, artery, precerebral
    vertebral — see Occlusion, artery, vertebral
  auditory canal (external) — see Stenosis, external
    ear canal
  eustachian tube — see Obstruction, eustachian tube
  eyelid — see Disorder, eyelid function
  larynx J38.6
  mesenteric artery K55.0
  palate M26.89
  palpebral fissure — see Disorder, eyelid function
  ureter N13.5
    with infection N13.6
  urethra — see Stricture, urethra
Narrowness, abnormal, eyelid Q10.3
Nasal — see condition
Nasolachrymal, nasolacrimal — see condition
Nasopharyngeal (see also condition)
  pituitary gland Q89.2
  torticollis M43.6
Nasopharyngitis (acute) (infective) (streptococcal)
  (subacute) J00
  chronic (suppurative) (ulcerative) J31.1
Nasopharynx, nasopharyngeal — see condition
Natal tooth, teeth K00.6
Nausea (without vomiting) R11.0
  with vomiting R11.2
  gravidarum — see Hyperemesis, gravidarum
  marina T75.3
  navalis T75.3
Navel — see condition
Neapolitan fever — see Brucellosis
Near drowning T75.1
Nearsightedness — see Myopia

Near-syncope R55
Nebula, cornea — see Opacity, cornea
Necator americanus infestation B76.1
Necatoriasis B76.1
Neck — see condition
Necrobiosis R68.89
  lipoidica NEC L92.1
    with diabetes — see E08-E13 with .63
Necrolysis, toxic epidermal L51.2
  due to drug
    correct substance properly administered — see
      Table of Drugs and Chemicals, by drug,
      adverse effect
    overdose or wrong substance given or taken —
      see Table of Drugs and Chemicals, by drug,
      poisoning
Necrophilia F65.89
Necrosis, necrotic (ischemic) (see also Gangrene)
  adrenal (capsule) (gland) E27.49
  amputation stump (surgical) (late) T87.50
    arm T87.5-
    leg T87.5-
  antrum J32.0
  aorta (hyaline) (see also Aneurysm, aorta)
    cystic medial — see Dissection, aorta
  artery I77.5
  bladder (aseptic) (sphincter) N32.89
  bone (see also Osteonecrosis) M87.9
    aseptic or avascular — see Osteonecrosis
      idiopathic M87.00
    ethmoid J32.2
    jaw M27.2
    tuberculous — see Tuberculosis, bone
  brain I67.8
  breast (aseptic) (fat) (segmental) N64.1
  bronchus J98.09
  central nervous system NEC I67.8
  cerebellar I67.8
  cerebral I67.8
  colon K55.0
  cornea H18.40
  cortical (acute) (renal) N17.1
  cystic medial (aorta) — see Dissection, aorta
  dental pulp K04.1
  esophagus K22.8
  ethmoid (bone) J32.2
  eyelid — see Disorder, eyelid, degenerative
  fat, fatty (generalized) (see also Disorder, soft tissue,
    specified type NEC)
    abdominal wall K65.4
    breast (aseptic) (segmental) N64.1
    localized — see Degeneration, by site, fatty
    mesentery K65.4
    omentum K65.4
    pancreas K86.8
    peritoneum K65.4
    skin (subcutaneous), newborn P83.0
    subcutaneous, due to birth injury P15.6
  gallbladder — see Cholecystitis, acute
  heart — see Infarct, myocardium
  hip, aseptic or avascular — see Osteonecrosis, by
    type, femur
  intestine (acute) (hemorrhagic) (massive) K55.0
  jaw M27.2
  kidney (bilateral) N28.0
    acute N17.9
    cortical (acute) (bilateral) N17.1
      with ectopic or molar pregnancy O08.4
    medullary (bilateral) (in acute renal failure)
      (papillary) — see Pyelitis
    papillary (bilateral) (in acute renal failure) — see
      Pyelitis
    tubular N17.0
      with ectopic or molar pregnancy O08.4
      complicating
        abortion — see Abortion, by type,
          complicated by, tubular necrosis
        ectopic or molar pregnancy O08.4
        pregnancy — see Pregnancy, complicated
          by, diseases of, specified type or
          system NEC
      following ectopic or molar pregnancy O08.4
      traumatic T79.5

Necrosis, necrotic—continued
  larynx J38.7
  liver (with hepatic failure) (cell)—see Failure, hepatic
    hemorrhagic, central K76.2
  lung J85.0
  lymphatic gland — see Lymphadenitis, acute
  mammary gland (fat) (segmental) N64.1
  mastoid (chronic) — see Mastoiditis, chronic
  medullary (acute) (renal) N17.2
  mesentery K55.0
    fat K65.4
  mitral valve — see Insufficiency, mitral
  myocardium, myocardial — see Infarct, myocardium
  nose J34.0
  omentum (with mesenteric infarction) K55.0
    fat K65.4
  orbit, orbital — see Osteomyelitis, orbit
  ossicles, ear — see Abnormal, ear ossicles
  ovary N70.92
  pancreas (aseptic) (duct) (fat) K86.8
    acute (infective) — see Pancreatitis, acute
    infective — see Pancreatitis, acute
  papillary (acute) (renal) N17.2
  perineum N90.89
  peritoneum (with mesenteric infarction) K55.0
    fat K65.4
  pharynx J02.9
    in granulocytopenia — see Neutropenia
      Vincent's A69.1
  phosphorus — see subcategory T54.2
  pituitary (gland) (postpartum) (Sheehan) E23.0
  pressure — see Ulcer, pressure, by site
  pulmonary J85.0
  pulp (dental) K04.1
  radiation — see Necrosis, by site
  radium — see Necrosis, by site
  renal — see Necrosis, kidney
  sclera H15.89
  scrotum N50.8
  skin or subcutaneous tissue NEC I96
  spine, spinal (column) (see also Osteonecrosis, by
    type, vertebra)
    cord G95.19
  spleen D73.5
  stomach K31.89
  stomatitis (ulcerative) A69.0
  subcutaneous fat, newborn P83.8
  subendocardial (acute) I21.4
    chronic I25.89
  suprarenal (capsule) (gland) E27.49
  testis N50.8
  thymus (gland) E32.8
  tonsil J35.8
  trachea J39.8
  tuberculous NEC — see Tuberculosis
  tubular (acute) (anoxic) (renal) (toxic) N17.0
    postprocedural N99.0
  vagina N89.8
  vertebra (see also Osteonecrosis, by type, vertebra)
    tuberculous A18.01
  vulva N90.89
  X-ray — see Necrosis, by site
Necrospermia — see Infertility, male
Need (for)
  care provider because (of)
    assistance with personal care Z74.1
    continuous supervision required Z74.3
    impaired mobility Z74.09
    no other household member able to render care
      Z74.2
    specified reason NEC Z74.8
  immunization — see Vaccination
  vaccination — see Vaccination
Neglect
  adult
    confirmed T74.01
    history of Z91.412
    suspected T76.01
  child (childhood)
    confirmed T74.02
    history of Z62.812
    suspected T76.02

Neglect—*continued*
  emotional, in childhood Z62.8
  hemispatial R41.4
  left-sided R41.4
  sensory R41.4
  visuospatial R41.4
Neisserian infection NEC — *see* Gonococcus
Nelaton's syndrome G60.8
Nelson's syndrome E24.1
Nematodiasis (intestinal) B82.0
  Ancylostoma B76.0
Neonatal (*see also* Newborn)
  acne L70.4
  bradycardia P29.12
  tachycardia P29.11
  screening, abnormal findings on P09
  tooth, teeth K00.6
Neonatorum — *see* condition
Neoplasia
  endocrine, multiple (MEN) E31.20
    type I E31.21
    type IIA E31.22
    type IIB E31.23
  intraepithelial (histologically confirmed)
    anal (AIN)
      grade I K62.82
      grade II K62.82
      severe D01.3
    cervical glandular (histologically confirmed)
      D06.9
    cervix (uteri) (CIN) (histologically confirmed)
      N87.9
      glandular D06.9
      grade I N87.0
      grade II N87.1
      grade III (severe dysplasia) D06.9 *see also*
        Carcinoma, cervix uteri, in situ
    vagina (histologically confirmed) (VAIN) N89.3
      grade I N89.0
      grade II N89.1
      grade III (severe dysplasia) D07.2
    prostate (histologically confirmed) (PIN I) (PIN II)
      N42.3
      grade I N42.3
      grade II N42.3
      severe D07.5
    vulva (histologically confirmed) (VIN) N90.3
      grade I N90.0
      grade II N90.1
      grade III (severe dysplasia) D07.1
Neoplasm, neoplastic — *see* Table of Neoplasms
Neovascularization
  ciliary body — *see* Disorder, iris, vascular
  cornea H16.40-
    deep H16.44-
    ghost vessels — *see* Ghost, vessels
    localized H16.43-
    pannus — *see* Pannus
  iris — *see* Disorder, iris, vascular
  retina H35.05-
Nephralgia N23
Nephritis, nephritic (albuminuric) (azotemic)
    (congenital) (disseminated) (epithelial) (familial)
    (focal) (granulomatous) (hemorrhagic) (infantile)
    (nonsuppurative, excretory) (uremic) N05.9
  with
    dense deposit disease N05.6
    diffuse
      crescentic glomerulonephritis N05.7
      endocapillary proliferative
        glomerulonephritis N05.4
      membranous glomerulonephritis N05.2
      mesangial proliferative glomerulonephritis
        N05.3
      mesangiocapillary glomerulonephritis N05.5
    edema — *see* Nephrosis
    focal and segmental glomerular lesions N05.1
    foot process disease N04.9
    glomerular lesion
      diffuse sclerosing N05.8
      hypocomplementemic — *see* Nephritis,
        membranoproliferative
      IgA — *see* Nephropathy, IgA

Nephritis, nephritic—*continued*
  with—*continued*
    glomerular lesion—*continued*
      lobular, lobulonodular — *see* Nephritis,
        membranoproliferative
      nodular — *see* Nephritis,
        membranoproliferative
    lesion of
      glomerulonephritis, proliferative N05.8
      renal necrosis N05.9
    minor glomerular abnormality N05.0
    specified morphological changes NEC N05.8
  acute N00.9
  with
    dense deposit disease N00.6
    diffuse
      crescentic glomerulonephritis N00.7
      endocapillary proliferative
        glomerulonephritis N00.4
      membranous glomerulonephritis N00.2
      mesangial proliferative
        glomerulonephritis N00.3
      mesangiocapillary glomerulonephritis
        N00.5
    focal and segmental glomerular lesions N00.1
    minor glomerular abnormality N00.0
    specified morphological changes NEC N00.8
  amyloid E85.4 [N08]
  antiglomerular basement membrane (anti-GBM)
    antibody NEC
    in Goodpasture's syndrome M31.0
  antitubular basement membrane
    (tubulo-interstitial) NEC N12
    toxic — *see* Nephropathy, toxic
  arteriolar — *see* Hypertension, kidney
  arteriosclerotic — *see* Hypertension, kidney
  ascending — *see* Nephritis, tubulo-interstitial
  atrophic N03.9
  Balkan (endemic) N15.0
  calculous, calculus — *see* Calculus, kidney
  cardiac — *see* Hypertension, kidney
  cardiovascular — *see* Hypertension, kidney
  chronic N03.9
    with
      dense deposit disease N03.6
      diffuse
        crescentic glomerulonephritis N03.7
        endocapillary proliferative
          glomerulonephritis N03.4
        membranous glomerulonephritis N03.2
        mesangial proliferative
          glomerulonephritis N03.3
        mesangiocapillary glomerulonephritis
          N03.5
      focal and segmental glomerular lesions N03.1
      minor glomerular abnormality N03.0
      specified morphological changes NEC N03.8
    arteriosclerotic — *see* Hypertension, kidney
  cirrhotic N26.9
  croupous N00.9
  degenerative — *see* Nephrosis
  diffuse sclerosing N05.8
  due to
    diabetes mellitus — *see* E08-E13 with .21
    subacute bacterial endocarditis I33.0
    systemic lupus erythematosus (chronic) M32.14
    typhoid fever A01.09
  gonococcal (acute) (chronic) A54.21
  hypocomplementemic — *see* Nephritis,
    membranoproliferative
  IgA — *see* Nephropathy, IgA
  immune complex (circulating) NEC N05.8
  infective — *see* Nephritis, tubulo-interstitial
  interstitial — *see* Nephritis, tubulo-interstitial
  lead N14.3
  membranoproliferative (diffuse) (type 1 or 3) (*see
    also* N00-N07 with fourth character .5) N05.5
    type 2 (*see also* N00-N07 with fourth character .6)
      N05.6
  minimal change N05.0
  necrotic, necrotizing NEC (*see also* N00-N07 with
    fourth character .8) N05.8
  nephrotic — *see* Nephrosis

Nephritis, nephritic—*continued*
  nodular — *see* Nephritis, membranoproliferative
  polycystic Q61.3
    adult type Q61.2
    autosomal
      dominant Q61.2
      recessive NEC Q61.19
    childhood type NEC Q61.19
    infantile type NEC Q61.19
  poststreptococcal N05.9
    acute N00.9
    chronic N03.9
    rapidly progressive N01.9
  proliferative NEC (*see also* N00-N07 with fourth
    character .8) N05.8
  purulent — *see* Nephritis, tubulo-interstitial
  rapidly progressive N01.9
    with
      dense deposit disease N01.6
      diffuse
        crescentic glomerulonephritis N01.7
        endocapillary proliferative
          glomerulonephritis N01.4
        membranous glomerulonephritis N01.2
        mesangial proliferative
          glomerulonephritis N01.3
        mesangiocapillary glomerulonephritis
          N01.5
      focal and segmental glomerular lesions N01.1
      minor glomerular abnormality N01.0
      specified morphological changes NEC N01.8
  salt losing or wasting NEC N28.89
  saturnine N14.3
  sclerosing, diffuse N05.8
  septic — *see* Nephritis, tubulo-interstitial
  specified pathology NEC (*see also* N00-N07 with
    fourth character .8) N05.8
  subacute N01.9
  suppurative — *see* Nephritis, tubulo-interstitial
  syphilitic (late) A52.75
    congenital A50.59 [N08]
    early (secondary) A51.44
  toxic — *see* Nephropathy, toxic
  tubal, tubular — *see* Nephritis, tubulo-interstitial
  tuberculous A18.11
  tubulo-interstitial (in) N12
    acute (infectious) N10
    chronic (infectious) N11.9
      nonobstructive N11.8
        reflux-associated N11.0
      obstructive N11.1
      specified NEC N11.8
    due to
      brucellosis A23.9 [N16]
      cryoglobulinemia D89.1 [N16]
      glycogen storage disease E74.00 [N16]
    Sjögren's syndrome M35.04
  vascular — *see* Hypertension, kidney
  war N00.9
Nephroblastoma (epithelial) (mesenchymal) C64.-
Nephrocalcinosis E83.59 [N29]
Nephrocystitis, pustular — *see* Nephritis,
    tubulo-interstitial
Nephrolithiasis (congenital) (pelvis) (recurrent)—*see
    also* Calculus, kidney
Nephroma C64.-
  mesoblastic D41.0-
Nephronephritis — *see* Nephrosis
Nephronophthisis Q61.5
Nephropathia epidemica A98.5
Nephropathy (*see also* Nephritis) N28.9
  with
    edema — *see* Nephrosis
    glomerular lesion — *see* Glomerulonephritis
  amyloid, hereditary E85.0
  analgesic N14.0
    with medullary necrosis, acute N17.2
  Balkan (endemic) N15.0
  chemical — *see* Nephropathy, toxic
  diabetic — *see* E08-E13 with .21
  drug-induced N14.2
    specified NEC N14.1
  focal and segmental hyalinosis or sclerosis N02.1

Nephropathy —*continued*
  heavy metal-induced N14.3
  hereditary NEC N07.9
    with
      dense deposit disease N07.6
      diffuse
        crescentic glomerulonephritis N07.7
        endocapillary proliferative
          glomerulonephritis N07.4
        membranous glomerulonephritis N07.2
        mesangial proliferative
          glomerulonephritis N07.3
        mesangiocapillary glomerulonephritis
          N07.5
      focal and segmental glomerular lesions N07.1
      minor glomerular abnormality N07.0
      specified morphological changes NEC N07.8
  hypercalcemic N25.89
  hypertensive — *see* Hypertension, kidney
  hypokalemic (vacuolar) N25.89
  IgA N02.8
    with glomerular lesion N02.9
      focal and segmental hyalinosis or sclerosis N02.1
      membranoproliferative (diffuse) N02.5
      membranous (diffuse) N02.2
      mesangial proliferative (diffuse) N02.3
      mesangiocapillary (diffuse) N02.5
      proliferative NEC N02.8
      specified pathology NEC N02.8
  lead N14.3
  membranoproliferative (diffuse) N02.5
  membranous (diffuse) N02.2
  mesangial (IgA/IgG) — *see* Nephropathy, IgA
    proliferative (diffuse) N02.3
  mesangiocapillary (diffuse) N02.5
  obstructive N13.8
  phenacetin N17.2
  phosphate-losing N25.0
  potassium depletion N25.89
  pregnancy-related O26.83-
  proliferative NEC (*see also* N00-N07 with fourth
    character .8) N05.8
  protein-losing N25.89
  saturnine N14.3
  sickle-cell D57.[N08]
  toxic NEC N14.4
    due to
      drugs N14.2
        analgesic N14.0
        specified NEC N14.1
      heavy metals N14.3
  vasomotor N17.0
  water-losing N25.89
Nephroptosis N28.83
Nephropyosis — *see* Abscess, kidney
Nephrorrhagia N28.89
Nephrosclerosis (arteriolar)(arteriosclerotic) (chronic)
  (hyaline) (*see also* Hypertension, kidney)
  hyperplastic — *see* Hypertension, kidney
  senile N26.9
Nephrosis, nephrotic (Epstein's) (syndrome)
  (congenital) N04.9
  with glomerular lesion N04.1
    foot process disease N04.9
    hypocomplementemic N04.5
  acute N04.9
  anoxic — *see* Nephrosis, tubular
  chemical — *see* Nephrosis, tubular
  cholemic K76.7
  diabetic — *see* E08-E13 with .21
  Finnish type (congenital) Q89.8
  hemoglobin N10
  hemoglobinuric — *see* Nephrosis, tubular
  in
    amyloidosis E85.4 [N08]
    diabetes mellitus — *see* E08-E13 with .21
    epidemic hemorrhagic fever A98.5
    malaria (malariae) B52.0
  ischemic — *see* Nephrosis, tubular
  lipoid N04.9
  lower nephron — *see* Nephrosis, tubular
  malarial (malariae) B52.0

Nephrosis, nephrotic—*continued*
  minimal change N04.0
  myoglobin N10
  necrotizing — *see* Nephrosis, tubular
  osmotic (sucrose) N25.89
  radiation N04.9
  syphilitic (late) A52.75
  toxic — *see* Nephrosis, tubular
  tubular (acute) N17.0
    postprocedural N99.0
    radiation N04.9
Nephrosonephritis, hemorrhagic (endemic) A98.5
Nephrostomy
  attention to Z43.6
  status Z93.6
Nerve (*see also* condition)
  injury — *see* Injury, nerve, by body site
Nerves R45.0
Nervous (*see also* condition) R45.0
  heart F45.8
  stomach F45.8
  tension R45.0
Nervousness R45.0
Nesidioblastoma
  pancreas D13.7
  specified site NEC — *see* Neoplam, benign, by site
  unspecified site D13.7
Nettleship's syndrome Q82.2
Neumann's disease or syndrome L10.1
Neuralgia, neuralgic (acute) M79.2
  accessory (nerve) G52.8
  acoustic (nerve) — *see* subcategory H93.3
  auditory (nerve) — *see* subcategory H93.3
  ciliary G44.009
    intractable G44.001
    not intractable G44.009
  cranial
    nerve (*see also* Disorder, nerve, cranial)
      fifth or trigeminal — *see* Neuralgia, trigeminal
    postherpetic, postzoster B02.29
  ear — *see* subcategory H92.0
  facialis vera G51.1
  Fothergill's — *see* Neuralgia, trigeminal
  glossopharyngeal (nerve) G52.1
  Horton's G43.809
  Hunt's B02.21
  hypoglossal (nerve) G52.3
  infraorbital — *see* Neuralgia, trigeminal
  malarial — *see* Malaria
  migrainous G44.009
    intractable G44.001
    not intractable G44.009
  Morton's G57.6-
  nerve, cranial — *see* Disorder, nerve, cranial
  nose G52.0
  occipital M54.81
  olfactory G52.0
  penis N48.9
  perineum R10.2
  postherpetic NEC B02.29
    trigeminal B02.22
  pubic region R10.2
  scrotum R10.2
  Sluder's G90.09
  specified nerve NEC G58.8
  spermatic cord R10.2
  sphenopalatine (ganglion) G44.89
  trifacial — *see* Neuralgia, trigeminal
  trigeminal G50.0
    postherpetic, postzoster B02.22
  vagus (nerve) G52.2
  writer's F48.8
    organic G25.89
Neurapraxia — *see* Injury, nerve
Neurasthenia F48.8
  cardiac F45.8
  gastric F45.8
  heart F45.8
Neurilemmoma (*see also* Neoplasm, nerve, benign)
  acoustic (nerve) D33.3
  malignant (*see also* Neoplasm, nerve, malignant)
    acoustic (nerve) C72.4-

Neurilemmosarcoma — *see* Neoplasm, nerve,
  malignant
Neurinoma — *see* Neoplasm, nerve, benign
Neurinomatosis — *see* Neoplasm, nerve, uncertain
  behavior
Neuritis (rheumatoid) M79.2
  abducens (nerve) — *see* Strabismus, paralytic, sixth
    nerve
  accessory (nerve) G52.8
  acoustic (nerve) (*see also* subcategory) H93.3
    in (due to)
      infectious disease NEC B99 [H94.0-]
      parasitic disease NEC B89 [H94.0-]
    syphilitic A52.15
  alcoholic G62.1
    with psychosis — *see* Psychosis, alcoholic
  amyloid, any site E85.4 [G63]
  auditory (nerve) — *see* subcategory H93.3
  brachial — *see* Radiculopathy
    due to displacement, intervertebral disc — *see*
      Disorder, disc, cervical, with neuritis
  cranial nerve
    due to Lyme disease A69.22
    eighth or acoustic or auditory — *see* subcategory
      H93.3
    eleventh or accessory G52.8
    fifth or trigeminal G51.0
    first or olfactory G52.0
    fourth or trochlear — *see* Strabismus, paralytic,
      fourth nerve
    second or optic — *see* Neuritis, optic
    seventh or facial G51.8
      newborn (birth injury) P11.3
    sixth or abducent — *see* Strabismus, paralytic,
      sixth nerve
    tenth or vagus G52.2
    third or oculomotor — *see* Strabismus, paralytic,
      third nerve
    twelfth or hypoglossal G52.3
  Déjérine-Sottas G60.0
  diabetic (mononeuropathy) — *see* E08-E13 with .41
    polyneuropathy — *see* E08-E13 with .42
  due to
    beriberi E51.11 [G63]
    displacement, prolapse or rupture, intervertebral
      disc — *see* Disorder, disc, with,
      radiculopathy
    herniation, nucleus pulposus M51.9 [G55]
  endemic E51.11 [G63]
  facial G51.8
    newborn (birth injury) P11.3
  general — *see* Polyneuropathy
  geniculate ganglion G51.1
    due to herpes (zoster) B02.21
  gouty M10.00 [G63]
  hypoglossal (nerve) G52.3
  ilioinguinal (nerve) G57.9-
  infectious (multiple) NEC G61.0
  interstitial hypertrophic progressive G60.0
  lumbar M54.16
  lumbosacral M54.17
  multiple (*see also* Polyneuropathy)
    endemic E51.11
    infective, acute G61.0
  multiplex endemica E51.11
  nerve root — *see* Radiculopathy
  oculomotor (nerve) — *see* Strabismus, paralytic,
    third nerve
  olfactory nerve G52.0
  optic (nerve) (hereditary) (sympathetic) H46.9
    with demyelination G36.0
    in myelitis G36.0
    nutritional H46.2
    papillitis — *see* Papillitis, optic
    retrobulbar H46.1-
    specified type NEC H46.8
    toxic H46.3
  peripheral (nerve) G62.9
    multiple — *see* Polyneuropathy
    single — *see* Mononeuritis
  pneumogastric (nerve) G52.2
  postherpetic, postzoster B02.29
  progressive hypertrophic interstitial G60.0

Neuritis—*continued*
retrobulbar (*see also* Neuritis, optic, retrobulbar)
in (due to)
late syphilis A52.15
meningococcal infection A39.82
meningococcal A39.82
syphilitic A52.15
sciatic (nerve) (*see also* Sciatica)
due to displacement of intervertebral disc — *see* Disorder, disc, with, radiculopathy
serum T80.6
shoulder-girdle G54.5
specified nerve NEC G58.8
spinal (nerve) root — *see* Radiculopathy
syphilitic A52.15
thenar (median) G56.1-
thoracic M54.14
toxic NEC G62.2
trochlear (nerve) — *see* Strabismus, paralytic, fourth nerve
vagus (nerve) G52.2
Neuroastrocytoma — *see* Neoplasm, uncertain behavior, by site
Neuroavitaminosis E56.9 [G99.8]
Neuroblastoma
olfactory C30.0
specified site — *see* Neoplasm, malignant, by site
unspecified site C74.90
Neurochorioretinitis — *see* Chorioretinitis
Neurocirculatory asthenia F45.8
Neurocysticercosis B69.0
Neurocytoma — *see* Neoplasm, benign, by site
Neurodermatitis (circumscribed) (circumscripta) (local) L28.0
atopic L20.81
diffuse (Brocq) L20.81
disseminated L20.81
Neuroencephalomyelopathy, optic G36.0
Neuroepithelioma (*see also* Neoplasm, malignant, by site)
olfactory C30.0
Neurofibroma (*see also* Neoplasm, nerve, benign)
melanotic — *see* Neoplasm, nerve, benign
multiple — *see* Neurofibromatosis
plexiform — *see* Neoplasm, nerve, benign
Neurofibromatosis (multiple) (nonmalignant) Q85.00
acoustic Q85.02
malignant — *see* Neoplasm, nerve, malignant
specified NEC Q85.09
type 1 (von Recklinghausen) Q85.01
type 2 Q85.02
Neurofibrosarcoma — *see* Neoplasm, nerve, malignant
Neurogenic (*see also* condition)
bladder (*see also* Dysfunction, bladder, neuromuscular) N31.9
cauda equina syndrome G83.4
bowel NEC K59.2
heart F45.8
Neuroglioma — *see* Neoplasm, uncertain behavior, by site
Neurolabyrinthitis (of Dix and Hallpike) — *see* Neuronitis, vestibular
Neurolathyrism — *see* Poisoning, food, noxious, plant
Neuroleprosy A30.9
Neuroma (*see also* Neoplasm, nerve, benign)
acoustic (nerve) D33.3
amputation (stump) (traumatic) (surgical complication) (late) T87.3-
arm T87.3-
leg T87.3-
digital (toe) G57.6-
interdigital (toe) G58.8
lower limb G57.8-
upper limb G56.8-
intermetatarsal G57.8-
Morton's G57.6-
nonneoplastic
arm G56.9-
leg G57.9-
lower extremity G57.9-
upper extremity G56.9-
optic (nerve) D33.3

Neuroma—*continued*
plantar G57.6-
plexiform — *see* Neoplasm, nerve, benign
surgical (nonneoplastic)
arm G56.9-
leg G57.9-
lower extremity G57.9-
upper extremity G56.9-
Neuromyalgia — *see* Neuralgia
Neuromyasthenia (epidemic) (postinfectious) G93.3
Neuromyelitis G36.9
ascending G61.0
optica G36.0
Neuromyopathy G70.9
paraneoplastic D49.9 [G13.0]
Neuromyotonia (Isaacs) G71.19
Neuronevus — *see* Nevus
Neuronitis G58.9
ascending (acute) G57.2-
vestibular H81.23
left H81.21
with right H81.22
right H81.20
with left H81.22
Neuroparalytic — *see* condition
Neuropathy, neuropathic G62.9
acute motor G62.81
alcoholic G62.1
with psychosis — *see* Psychosis, alcoholic
arm G56.9-
autonomic, peripheral — *see* Neuropathy, peripheral, autonomic
axillary G56.9-
bladder N31.9
atonic (motor) (sensory) N31.2
autonomous N31.2
flaccid N31.2
nonreflex N31.2
reflex N31.1
uninhibited N31.0
brachial plexus G54.0
cervical plexus G54.2
chronic
progressive segmentally demyelinating G62.89
relapsing demyelinating G62.89
Déjérine-Sottas G60.0
diabetic — *see* E08-E13 with .40
mononeuropathy — *see* E08-E13 with .41
polyneuropathy — *see* E08-E13 with .42
entrapment G58.9
iliohypogastric nerve G57.8-
ilioinguinal nerve G57.8-
lateral cutaneous nerve of thigh G57.1-
median nerve G56.0-
obturator nerve G57.8-
peroneal nerve G57.3-
posterior tibial nerve G57.5-
saphenous nerve G57.8-
ulnar nerve G56.2-
facial nerve G51.9
hereditary G60.9
motor and sensory (types I-IV) G60.0
sensory G60.8
specified NEC G60.8
hypertrophic G60.0
Charcot-Marie-Tooth G60.0
Déjérine-Sottas G60.0
interstitial progressive G60.0
of infancy G60.0
Refsum G60.1
idiopathic G60.9
progressive G60.3
specified NEC G60.8
in association with hereditary ataxia G60.2
intercostal G58.0
ischemic — *see* Disorder, nerve
Jamaica (ginger) G62.2
leg NEC G57.9-
lower extremity G57.9-
lumbar plexus G54.1
median nerve G56.1-
motor and sensory (*see also* Polyneuropathy)
hereditary (types I-IV) G60.0

Neuropathy, neuropathic —*continued*
multiple (acute) (chronic) — *see* Polyneuropathy
optic (nerve) (*see also* Neuritis, optic)
ischemic H47.01-
paraneoplastic (sensorial) (Denny Brown) D49.9 [G13.0]
peripheral (nerve) (*see also* Polyneuropathy) G62.9
autonomic G90.9
idiopathic G90.09
in (due to)
amyloidosis E85.4 [G99.0]
diabetes mellitus — *see* E08-E13 with .43
endocrine disease NEC E34.9 [G99.0]
gout M10.00 [G99.0]
hyperthyroidism E05.90 [G99.0]
with thyroid storm E05.91 [G99.0]
metabolic disease NEC E88.9 [G99.0]
idiopathic G60.9
progressive G60.3
in (due to)
antitetanus serum G62.0
arsenic G62.2
drugs NEC G62.0
lead G62.2
organophosphate compounds G62.2
toxic agent NEC G62.2
plantar nerves G57.6-
progressive
hypertrophic interstitial G60.9
inflammatory G62.81
radicular NEC — *see* Radiculopathy
sacral plexus G54.1
sciatic G57.0-
serum G61.1
toxic NEC G62.2
trigeminal sensory G50.8
ulnar nerve G56.2-
uremic N18.9 [G63]
vitamin B12 E53.8 [G63]
with anemia (pernicious) D51.0 [G63]
due to dietary deficiency D51.3 [G63]
Neurophthisis (*see also* Disorder, nerve)
peripheral, diabetic — *see* E08-E13 with .42
Neuroretinitis — *see* Chorioretinitis
Neuroretinopathy, hereditary optic H47.22
Neurosarcoma — *see* Neoplasm, nerve, malignant
Neurosclerosis — *see* Disorder, nerve
Neurosis, neurotic F48.9
anankastic F42
anxiety (state) F41.1
panic type F41.0
asthenic F48.8
bladder F45.8
cardiac (reflex) F45.8
cardiovascular F45.8
character F60.9
colon F45.8
compensation F68.8
compulsive, compulsion F42
conversion F44.9
craft F48.8
cutaneous F45.8
depersonalization F48.1
depressive (reaction) (type) F34.1
environmental F48.8
excoriation L98.1
fatigue F48.8
functional — *see* Disorder, somatoform
gastric F45.8
gastrointestinal F45.8
heart F45.8
hypochondriacal F45.21
hysterical F44.9
incoordination F45.8
larynx F45.8
vocal cord F45.8
intestine F45.8
larynx (sensory) F45.8
hysterical F44.4
mixed NEC F48.8
musculoskeletal F45.8
obsessional F42
obsessive-compulsive F42

Neurosis, neurotic —*continued*
  occupational F48.8
  ocular NEC F45.8
  organ — *see* Disorder, somatoform
  pharynx F45.8
  phobic F40.9
  posttraumatic (acute) (situational) F43.9
  psychasthenic (type) F48.8
  railroad F48.8
  rectum F45.8
  respiratory F45.8
  rumination F45.8
  sexual F65.9
  situational F48.8
  social F40.10
    generalized F40.11
  specified type NEC F48.8
  state F48.9
    with depersonalization episode F48.1
  stomach F45.8
  traumatic F43.10
    acute F43.11
    chronic F43.12
  vasomotor F45.8
  visceral F45.8
  war F48.8
Neurospongioblastosis diffusa Q85.1
Neurosyphilis (arrested) (early) (gumma) (late) (latent)
    (recurrent) (relapse) A52.3
  with ataxia (cerebellar) (locomotor) (spastic) (spinal)
    A52.19
  aneurysm (cerebral) A52.05
  arachnoid (adhesive) A52.13
  arteritis (any artery) (cerebral) A52.04
  asymptomatic A52.2
  congenital A50.40
  dura (mater) A52.13
  general paresis A52.17
  hemorrhagic A52.05
  juvenile (asymptomatic) (meningeal) A50.40
  leptomeninges (aseptic) A52.13
  meningeal, meninges (adhesive) A52.13
  meningitis A52.13
  meningovascular (diffuse) A52.13
  optic atrophy A52.15
  parenchymatous (degenerative) A52.19
  paresis, paretic A52.17
    juvenile A50.45
  remission in (sustained) A52.3
  serological (without symptoms) A52.2
  specified nature or site NEC A52.19
  tabes, tabetic (dorsalis) A52.11
    juvenile A50.45
  taboparesis A52.17
    juvenile A50.45
  thrombosis (cerebral) A52.05
  vascular (cerebral) NEC A52.05
Neurothekeoma — *see* Neoplasm, nerve, benign
Neurotic — *see* Neurosis
Neurotoxemia — *see* Toxemia
Neutroclusion M26.211
Neutropenia, neutropenic (chronic) (genetic)
    (idiopathic) (immune) (infantile) (malignant)
    (pernicious) (splenic) D70.9
  congenital (primary) D70.0
  cyclic D70.4
  cytoreductive cancer chemotherapy sequela D70.1
  drug-induced D70.2
    due to cytoreductive cancer chemotherapy
      D70.1
  due to infection D70.3
  fever D70.9
  neonatal, transitory (isoimmune) (maternal transfer)
    P61.5
  periodic D70.4
  secondary (cyclic) (periodic) (splenic) D70.4
    drug-induced D70.2
      due to cytoreductive cancer chemotherapy
        D70.1
  toxic D70.8
Neutrophilia, hereditary giant D72.0
Nevocarcinoma — *see* Melanoma

Nevus D22.9
  achromic
  amelanotic
  angiomatous D18.00
    intra-abdominal D18.03
    intracranial D18.02
    skin D18.01
    specified site NEC D18.09
  araneus I78.1
  balloon cell
  bathing trunk D48.5
  blue
    cellular
    giant
    Jadassohn's
    malignant — *see* Melanoma
  capillary D18.00
    intra-abdominal D18.03
    intracranial D18.02
    skin D18.01
    specified site NEC D18.09
  cavernous D18.00
    intra-abdominal D18.03
    intracranial D18.02
    skin D18.01
    specified site NEC D18.09
  cellular
    blue
  choroid D31.3-
  comedonicus Q82.5
  conjunctiva D31.0-
  dermal
    with epidermal nevus
  dysplastic
  eye D31.9-
  flammeus Q82.5
  hemangiomatous D18.00
    intra-abdominal D18.03
    intracranial D18.02
    skin D18.01
    specified site NEC D18.09
  iris D31.4-
  lacrimal gland D31.5-
  lymphatic D18.1
    specified site — *see* Neoplasm, benign, by site
    unspecified site D31.40
  malignant — *see* Melanoma
  meaning hemangioma D18.00
    intra-abdominal D18.03
    intracranial D18.02
    skin D18.01
    specified site NEC D18.09
  mouth (mucosa) D10.30
    specified site NEC D10.39
    white sponge Q38.6
  multiplex Q85.1
  non-neoplastic I78.1
  oral mucosa D10.30
    specified site NEC D10.39
    white sponge Q38.6
  orbit D31.6-
    giant (*see also* Neoplasm, skin, uncertain
      behavior) D48.5
    malignant melanoma in — *see* Melanoma
  portwine Q82.5
  retina D31.2-
  retrobulbar D31.6-
  sanguineous Q82.5
  senile I78.1
  skin D22.9
    abdominal wall D22.5
    ala nasi D22.39
    ankle D22.7-
    anus, anal D22.5
    arm D22.6-
    auditory canal (external) D22.2-
    auricle (ear) D22.2-
    auricular canal (external) D22.2-
    axilla, axillary fold D22.5
    back D22.5
    breast D22.5
    brow D22.39
    buttock D22.5

Nevus —*continued*
  skin—*continued*
    canthus (eye) D22.1-
    cheek (external) D22.39
    chest wall D22.5
    chin D22.39
    ear (external) D22.2-
    external meatus (ear) D22.2-
    eyebrow D22.39
    eyelid (lower) (upper) D22.1-
    face D22.30
      specified NEC D22.39
    female genital organ (external) NEC D28.0
    finger D22.6-
    flank D22.5
    foot D22.7-
    forearm D22.6-
    forehead D22.39
    foreskin D29.0
    genital organ (external) NEC
      female D28.0
      male D29.9
    gluteal region D22.5
    groin D22.5
    hand D22.6-
    heel D22.7-
    helix D22.2-
    hip D22.7-
    interscapular region D22.5
    jaw D22.39
    knee D22.7-
    labium (majus) (minus) D28.0
    leg D22.7-
    lip (lower) (upper) D22.0
    lower limb D22.7-
    male genital organ (external) D29.9
    nail D22.9
      finger D22.6-
      toe D22.7-
    nasolabial groove D22.39
    nates D22.5
    neck D22.4
    nose (external) D22.39
    palpebra D22.1-
    penis D29.0
    perianal skin D22.5
    perineum D22.5
    pinna D22.2-
    popliteal fossa or space D22.7-
    prepuce D29.0
    pudendum D28.0
    scalp D22.4
    scrotum D29.4
    shoulder D22.6-
    skin D22.9
    specified site NEC — *see* Neoplasm, benign, by
      site
    submammary fold D22.5
    temple D22.39
    thigh D22.7-
    toe D22.7-
    trunk NEC D22.5
    umbilicus D22.5
    upper limb D22.6-
    vulva D28.0
  spider I78.1
  stellar I78.1
  strawberry Q82.5
  Sutton's
  unius lateris Q82.5
  Unna's Q82.5
  vascular Q82.5
  verrucous Q82.5
Newborn (infant) (liveborn) (singleton) Z38.2
  acne L70.4
  abstinence syndrome P96.1
  affected by (suspected to be)
    abnormalities of membranes P02.9
      specified NEC P02.8
    abruptio placenta P02.1
    amino-acid metabolic disorder, transitory P74.8
    amniocentesis (while in utero) P00.6
    amnionitis P02.7

Newborn —*continued*
  affected by—*continued*
    apparent life threatening event (ALTE) R68.13
    bleeding (into)
      cerebral cortex P52.22
      germinal matrix P52.0
      ventricles P52.1
    breech delivery P03.0
    cardiac arrest P29.81
    cardiomyopathy I42.8
    congenital I42.4
    cerebral ischemia P91.0
    Cesarean delivery P03.4
    chemotherapy agents P04.1
    chorioamnionitis P02.7
    cocaine (crack) P04.41
    complications of labor and delivery P03.9
      specified NEC P03.89
    compression of umbilical cord NEC P02.5
    contracted pelvis P03.1
    delivery P03.9
      Cesarean P03.4
      forceps P03.2
      vacuum extractor P03.3
    environmental chemicals P04.6
    entanglement (knot) in umbilical cord P02.5
    fetal (intrauterine)
      growth retardation P05.9
      malnutrition not light or small for gestational
        age P05.2
    forceps delivery P03.2
    heart rate abnormalities P29.1
      bradycardia P29.12
      intrauterine P03.819
        before onset of labor P03.810
        during labor P03.811
      tachycardia P29.11
    hemorrhage (antepartum) P02.1
      cerebellar (nontraumatic) P52.6
      intracerebral (nontraumatic) P52.4
      intracranial (nontraumatic) P52.9
        specified NEC P52.8
      intraventricular (nontraumatic) P52.3
        grade 1 P52.0
        grade 2 P52.1
        grade 3 P52.21
        grade 4 P52.22
      posterior fossa (nontraumatic) P52.6
      subarachnoid (nontraumatic) P52.5
      subependymal P52.0
        with intracerebral extension P52.22
        with intraventricular extension P52.1
          with enlargment of ventricles P52.21
        without intraventricular extension P52.0
    hypoxic ischemic encephalopathy [HIE] P91.60
      mild P91.61
      moderate P91.62
      severe P91.63
    induction of labor P03.89
    intestinal perforation P78.0
    intrauterine (fetal) blood loss P50.9
      due to (from)
        cut end of co-twin cord P50.5
        hemorrhage into
          co-twin P50.3
          maternal circulation P50.4
        placenta P50.2
        ruptured cord blood P50.1
        vasa previa P50.0
      specified NEC P50.8
    intrauterine (fetal) hemorrhage P50.9
    intrauterine (in utero) procedure P96.5
    malpresentation (malposition) NEC P03.1
    maternal (complication of) (use of)
      alcohol P04.3
      analgesia (maternal) P04.0
      anesthesia (maternal) P04.0
      blood loss P02.1
      circulatory disease P00.3
      condition P00.9
        specified NEC P00.89

Newborn —*continued*
  affected by—*continued*
    maternal—*continued*
      delivery P03.9
        Cesarean P03.4
        forceps P03.2
        vacuum extractor P03.3
      diabetes mellitus (pre-existing) P70.1
      disorder P00.9
        specified NEC P00.89
      drugs (addictive) (illegal) NEC P04.49
      ectopic pregnancy P01.4
      gestational diabetes P70.0
      hemorrhage P02.1
      hypertensive disorder P00.0
      incompetent cervix P01.0
      infectious disease P00.2
      injury P00.5
      labor and delivery P03.9
      malpresentation before labor P01.7
      maternal death P01.6
      medical procedure P00.7
      medication P04.1
      multiple pregnancy P01.5
      nutritional disorder P00.4
      oligohydramnios P01.2
      parasitic disease P00.2
      periodontal disease P00.81
      placenta previa P02.0
      polyhydramnios P01.3
      precipitate delivery P03.5
      pregnancy P01.9
        specified P01.8
      premature rupture of membranes P01.1
      renal disease P00.1
      respiratory disease P00.3
      surgical procedure P00.6
      urinary tract disease P00.1
      uterine contraction (abnormal) P03.6
    meconium peritonitis P78.0
    medication (legal) (maternal use) (prescribed)
      P04.1
    membrane abnormalities P02.9
      specified NEC P02.8
    membranitis P02.7
    methamphetamine(s) P04.49
    mixed metabolic and respiratory acidosis P84
    neonatal abstinence syndrome P96.1
    noxious substances transmitted via placenta or
      breast milk P04.9
      specified NEC P04.8
    nutritional supplements P04.5
    placenta previa P02.0
    placental
      abnormality (functional) (morphological)
        P02.20
        specified NEC P02.29
      dysfunction P02.29
      infarction P02.29
      insufficiency P02.29
      separation NEC P02.1
      transfusion syndromes P02.3
    placentitis P02.7
    precipitate delivery P03.5
    prolapsed cord P02.4
    respiratory arrest P28.81
    slow intrauterine growth P05.9
    tobacco P04.2
    twin to twin transplacental transfusion P02.3
    umbilical cord (tightly) around neck P02.5
    umbilical cord condition P02.60
      short cord P02.69
      specified NEC P02.69
    uterine contractions (abnormal) P03.6
    vasa previa P02.69
      from intrauterine blood loss P50.0
  apnea P28.3
    primary P28.3
    obstructive P28.4
    specified P28.4
  born in hospital Z38.00
    by cesarean Z38.01
  born outside hospital Z38.1

Newborn —*continued*
  breast buds P96.89
  breast engorgement P83.4
  check-up — *see* Newborn, examination
  convulsion P90
  dehydration P74.1
  examination
    8 to 28 days old Z00.111
    under 8 days old Z00.110
  fever P81.9
    environmentally-induced P81.0
  hyperbilirubinemia P59.9
    of prematurity P59.0
  hypernatremia P74.2
  hyponatremia P74.2
  infection P39.9
    candidal P37.5
    specified NEC P39.8
    urinary tract P39.3
  jaundice P59.8
    due to
      breast milk inhibitor P593.
      hepatocellular damage P59.20
        specified NEC P59.29
      preterm delivery P59.0
    of prematurity P59.0
    specified NEC P59.8
  late metabolic acidosis P74.0
  mastitis P39.0
    infective P39.0
    noninfective P83.4
  multiple born NEC Z38.8
    born in hospital Z38.68
      by cesarean Z38.69
    born outside hospital Z38.7
  omphalitis P38.9
    with mild hemorrhage P38.1
    without hemorrhage P38.9
  post-term P08.21
  prolonged gestation (over 42 completed weeks)
    P08.22
  quadruplet Z38.8
    born in hospital Z38.63
      by cesarean Z38.64
    born outside hospital Z38.7
  quintuplet Z38.8
    born in hospital Z38.65
      by cesarean Z38.66
    born outside hospital Z38.7
  seizure P90
  sepsis (congenital) P36.9
    due to
      anaerobes NEC P36.5
      Escherichia coli P36.4
      Staphylococcus P36.30
        aureus P36.2
        specified NEC P36.39
      Streptococcus P36.10
        group B P36.0
        specified NEC P36.19
      specified NEC P36.8
  triplet Z38.8
    born in hospital Z38.61
      by cesarean Z38.62
    born outside hospital Z38.7
  twin Z38.5
    born in hospital Z38.30
      by cesarean Z38.31
    born outside hospital Z38.4
  vomiting P92.09
    bilious P92.01
  weight check Z00.111
Newcastle conjunctivitis or disease B30.8
Nezelof's syndrome (pure alymphocytosis) D81.4
Niacin(amide) **deficiency** E52
Nicolas(-Durand)**-Favre disease** A55
Nicotine — *see* Tobacco
Nicotinic acid deficiency E52
Niemann-Pick disease or syndrome E75.249
  specified NEC E75.248
  type
    A E75.240
    B E75.241

Niemann-Pick disease or syndrome—*continued*
  type—*continued*
    C E75.242
    D E75.243
Night
  blindness — *see* Blindness, night
  sweats R61
  terrors (child) F51.4
Nightmares (REM sleep type) F51.5
Nipple — *see* condition
Nisbet's chancre A57
Nishimoto (-Takeuchi) **disease** I67.5
Nitritoid crisis or reaction — *see* Crisis, nitritoid
Nitrosohemoglobinemia D74.8
Njovera A65
Nocardiosis, nocardiasis A43.9
  cutaneous A43.1
  lung A43.0
  pneumonia A43.0
  pulmonary A43.0
  specified site NEC A43.8
Nocturia R35.1
  psychogenic F45.8
Nocturnal — *see* condition
Nodal rhythm I49.8
Node(s) (*see also* Nodule)
  Bouchard's (with arthropathy) M15.2
  Haygarth's M15.8
  Heberden's (with arthropathy) M15.1
  larynx J38.7
  lymph — *see* condition
  milker's B08.03
  Osler's I33.0
  Schmorl's — *see* Schmorl's disease
  singer's J38.2
  teacher's J38.2
  tuberculous — *see* Tuberculosis, lymph gland
  vocal cord J38.2
Nodule(s), nodular
  actinomycotic — *see* Actinomycosis
  breast NEC N63
  colloid (cystic), thyroid E04.1
  cutaneous — *see* Swelling, localized
  endometrial (stromal) D26.1
  Haygarth's M15.8
  inflammatory — *see* Inflammation
  juxta-articular
    syphilitic A52.77
    yaws A66.7
  larynx J38.7
  milker's B08.03
  prostate — *see* Enlargement, enlarged, prostate
  retrocardiac R09.89
  rheumatoid M06.30
    ankle M06.37-
    elbow M06.32-
    foot joint M06.37-
    hand joint M06.34-
    hip M06.35-
    knee M06.36-
    multiple site M06.39
    shoulder M06.31-
    vertebra M06.38
    wrist M06.33-
  scrotum (inflammatory) N49.2
  singer's J38.2
  solitary, lung J98.4
  subcutaneous — *see* Swelling, localized
  teacher's J38.2
  thyroid (cold) (gland) (nontoxic) E04.1
    with thyrotoxicosis E05.20
      with thyroid storm E05.21
    toxic or with hyperthyroidism E05.20
      with thyroid storm E05.21
  vocal cord J38.2
Noma (gangrenous) (hospital) (infective) A69.0
  auricle I96
  mouth A69.0
  pudendi N76.89
  vulvae N76.89
Nomad, nomadism Z59.0
Nonautoimmune hemolytic anemia D59.4
  drug-induced D59.2

Nonclosure (*see also* Imperfect, closure)
  ductus arteriosus (Botallo's) Q25.0
  foramen
    botalli Q21.1
    ovale Q21.1
Noncompliance Z91.19
  with
    dietary regimen Z91.11
    dialysis Z91.15
    medical treatment Z91.19
    medication regimen NEC Z91.14
      underdosing (*see also* Table of Drugs and
        Chemicals, categories T36-T50, with
        final character 6) Z91.14
        intentional NEC Z91.128
          due to financial hardship of patient
            Z91.120
        unintentional NEC Z91.138
          due to patient's age related debility
            Z91.130
  renal dialysis Z91.15
Nondescent (congenital) (*see also* Malposition,
  congenital)
  cecum Q43.3
  colon Q43.3
  testicle Q53.9
    bilateral Q53.20
      abdominal Q53.21
      perineal Q53.22
    unilateral Q53.10
      abdominal Q53.11
      perineal Q53.12
Nondevelopment
  brain Q02
    part of Q04.3
  heart Q24.8
  organ or site, congenital NEC — *see* Hypoplasia
Nonengagement
  head NEC O32.4
    in labor, causing obstructed labor O64.8
Nonexanthematous tick fever A93.2
Nonexpansion, lung (newborn) P28.0
Nonfunctioning
  cystic duct (*see also* Disease, gallbladder) K82.8
  gallbladder (*see also* Disease, gallbladder) K82.8
  kidney N28.9
  labyrinth — *see* subcategory H83.2
Non-Hodgkin lymphoma NEC — *see* Lymphoma,
  non-Hodgkin
Non-working side interference M26.56
Nonimplantation, ovum N97.2
Noninsufflation, fallopian tube N97.1
Non-ketotic hyperglycinemia E72.51
Nonne-Milroy syndrome Q82.0
Nonovulation N97.0
Nonpatent fallopian tube N97.1
Nonpneumatization, lung NEC P28.0
Nonrotation — *see* Malrotation
Nonsecretion, urine — *see* Anuria
Nonunion
  fracture — *see* Fracture, by site
  organ or site, congenital NEC — *see* Imperfect,
    closure
  symphysis pubis, congenital Q74.2
Nonvisualization, gallbladder R93.2
Nonvital, nonvitalized tooth K04.99
Noonan's syndrome Q87.1
Normocytic anemia (infectional) due to blood loss
  (chronic) D50.0
  acute D62
Norrie's disease (congenital) Q15.8
North American blastomycosis B40.9
Norwegian itch B86
Nose, nasal — *see* condition
Nosebleed R04.0
Nose-picking F98.8
Nosomania F45.21
Nosophobia F45.22
Nostalgia F43.20
Notch of iris Q13.2
Notching nose, congenital (tip) Q30.2

Nothnagel's
  syndrome — *see* Strabismus, paralytic, third nerve
  vasomotor acroparesthesia I73.89
Novy's relapsing fever A68.9
  louse-borne A68.0
  tick-borne A68.1
Noxious
  foodstuffs, poisoning by — *see* Poisoning, food,
    noxious, plant
  substances transmitted through placenta or breast
    milk P04.9
Nucleus pulposus — *see* condition
Numbness R20.0
Nuns' knee — *see* Bursitis, prepatellar
Nursemaid's elbow S53.03-
Nutcracker esophagus K22.4
Nutmeg liver K76.1
Nutrient element deficiency E61.9
  specified NEC E61.8
Nutrition deficient or insufficient (*see also*
  Malnutrition) E46
  due to
    insufficient food T73.0
    lack of
      care (child) T76.02
        adult T76.01
      food T73.0
Nutritional stunting E45
Nyctalopia (night blindness) — *see* Blindness, night
Nycturia R35.1
  psychogenic F45.8
Nymphomania F52.8
Nystagmus H55.00
  benign paroxysmal — *see* Vertigo, benign
    paroxysmal
  central positional — *see* subcategory H81.4
  congenital H55.01
  dissociated H55.04
  latent H55.02
  miners' H55
  positional
    benign paroxysmal — *see* subcategory H81.4
    central — *see* subcategory H81.4
  specified form NEC H55.09
  visual deprivation H55.03

O

Obermeyer's relapsing fever (European) A68.0
Obesity E66.9
  with alveolar hyperventilation E66.2
  adrenal E27.8
  complicating
    childbirth O99.214
    pregnancy O99.21-
    puerperium O99.215
  constitutional E66.8
  dietary counseling and surveillance Z71.3
  drug-induced E66.1
  due to
    drug E66.1
    excess calories E66.09
      morbid E66.01
      severe E66.01
  endocrine E66.8
  endogenous E66.8
  familial E66.8
  glandular E66.8
  hypothyroid — *see* Hypothyroidism
  morbid E66.01
    with alveolar hypoventilation E66.2
    due to excess calories E66.01
  nutritional E66.09
  pituitary E23.6
  severe E66.01
  specified type NEC E66.8
Oblique — *see* condition
Obliteration
  appendix (lumen) K38.8
  artery I77.1
  bile duct (noncalculous) K83.1

Obliteration—continued
  common duct (noncalculous) K83.1
  cystic duct — see Obstruction, gallbladder
  disease, arteriolar I77.1
  endometrium N85.8
  eye, anterior chamber — see Disorder, globe,
      hypotony
  fallopian tube N97.1
  lymphatic vessel I89.0
      due to mastectomy I97.2
  organ or site, congenital NEC — see Atresia, by site
  ureter N13.5
      with infection N13.6
  urethra — see Stricture, urethra
  vein I87.8
  vestibule (oral) K08.8
Observation (following) (for) (without need for further
      medical care) Z04.9
  accident NEC Z04.3
      at work Z04.2
      transport Z04.1
  adverse effect of drug Z03.6
  alleged rape or sexual assault (victim), ruled out
      adult Z04.41
      child Z04.42
  criminal assault Z04.8
  development state
      adolescent Z00.3
      period of rapid growth in childhood Z00.2
      puberty Z00.3
  disease, specified NEC Z03.89
  following work accident Z04.2
  growth and development state — see Observation,
      development state
  injuries (accidental) NEC (see also Observation,
      accident)
  newborn (for suspected condition, ruled out)—see
      Newborn, affected by (suspected to be),
      maternal (complication of) (use of)
  postpartum
      immediately after delivery Z39.0
      routine follow-up Z39.2
  pregnancy (normal) (without complication) Z34.9-
      high risk O09.9-
  suicide attempt, alleged NEC Z03.89
      self-poisoning Z03.6
  suspected, ruled out (see also Suspected condition,
      ruled out)
      abuse, physical
          adult Z04.71
          child Z04.72
      accident at work Z04.2
      adult battering victim Z04.71
      child battering victim Z04.72
      condition NEC Z03.89
  newborn see Newborn, affected by (suspected to
      be), maternal (complication of) (use of)
  drug poisoning or adverse effect Z03.6
  exposure (to)
      anthrax Z03.810
      biological agent NEC Z03.818
  inflicted injury NEC Z04.8
  suicide attempt, alleged Z03.89
      self-poisoning Z03.6
  toxic effects from ingested substance (drug)
      (poison) Z03.6
  toxic effects from ingested substance (drug)
      (poison) Z03.6
Obsession, obsessional state F42
Obsessive-compulsive neurosis or reaction F42
Obstetric embolism, septic — see Embolism,
      obstetric, septic
Obstetrical trauma (complicating delivery) O71.9
  with or following ectopic or molar pregnancy O08.6
  specified type NEC O71.89
Obstipation — see Constipation

Obstruction, obstructed, obstructive
  airway J98.8
      with
          allergic alveolitis J67.9
          asthma J45.909
              with
                  exacerbation (acute) J45.901
                  status asthmaticus J45.902
          bronchiectasis J47.9
              with
                  exacerbation (acute) J47.1
                  lower respiratory infection J47.0
          bronchitis (chronic) J44.9
          emphysema J43.9
      chronic J44.9
          with
              allergic alveolitis — see Pneumonitis,
                  hypersensitivity
              bronchiectasis J47.9
                  with
                      exacerbation (acute) J47.1
                      lower respiratory infection J47.0
      foreign body — see Foreign body, by site,
          causing asphyxia
      inhalation of fumes or vapors J68.9
      laryngospasm J38.5
  ampulla of Vater K83.1
  aortic (heart) (valve) — see Stenosis, aortic
  aortoiliac I74.0
  aqueduct of Sylvius G91.1
      congenital Q03.0
          with spina bifida — see Spina bifida, by site,
              with hydrocephalus
  Arnold-Chiari — see Arnold-Chiari disease
  artery (see also Embolism, artery) I74.9
      basilar (complete) (partial) — see Occlusion,
          artery, basilar
      carotid (complete) (partial) — see Occlusion,
          artery, carotid
      cerebellar — see Occlusion, artery, cerebellar
      cerebral (anterior) (middle) (posterior) — see
          Occlusion, artery, cerebral
      precerebral — see Occlusion, artery, precerebral
      renal I70.1
      retinal NEC — see Occlusion, artery, retina
      vertebral (complete) (partial) — see Occlusion,
          artery, vertebral
  band (intestinal) K56.69
  bile duct or passage (common) (hepatic)
      (noncalculous) K83.1
      with calculus K80.51
      congenital (causing jaundice) Q44.3
  biliary (duct) (tract) K83.1
      gallbladder K82.0
  bladder-neck (acquired) N32.0
      congenital Q64.31
      due to hyperplasia (hypertrophy) of prostate —
          see Hyperplasia, prostate
  bowel — see Obstruction, intestine
  bronchus J98.09
  canal, ear — see Stenosis, external ear canal
  cardia K22.2
  caval veins (inferior) (superior) I87.1
  cecum — see Obstruction, intestine
  circulatory I99.8
  colon — see Obstruction, intestine
  common duct (noncalculous) K83.1
  coronary (artery) — see Occlusion, coronary
  cystic duct (see also Obstruction, gallbladder)
      with calculus K80.21
  device, implant or graft (see also Complications, by
      site and type, mechanical) T85.628
      arterial graft NEC — see Complication,
          cardiovascular device, mechanical, vascular
      catheter NEC T85.628
          cystostomy T83.090
          dialysis (renal) T82.49
              intraperitoneal T85.691
          infusion NEC T82.594
              spinal (epidural) (subdural) T85.690
          urinary, indwelling T83.098
      due to infection T85.79

Obstruction, obstructed, obstructive—continued
  device, implant or graft—continued
      gastrointestinal — see Complications, prosthetic
          device, mechanical, gastrointestinal device
      genital NEC T83.498
          intrauterine contraceptive device T83.39
          penile prosthesis T83.490
      heart NEC — see Complication, cardiovascular
          device, mechanical
      joint prosthesis — see Complications, joint
          prosthesis, mechanical, specified NEC, by
          site
      orthopedic NEC — see Complication, orthopedic,
          device, mechanical
      specified NEC T85.628
      urinary NEC (see also Complication,
          genitourinary, device, urinary, mechanical)
          graft T83.29
      vascular NEC — see Complication, cardiovascular
          device, mechanical
      ventricular intracranial shunt T85.09
  due to foreign body accidentally left in operative
      wound T81.529
  duodenum K31.5
  ejaculatory duct N50.8
  esophagus K22.2
  eustachian tube (complete) (partial) H68.10-
      cartilagenous (extrinsic) H68.13-
          intrinsic H68.12-
      osseous H68.11-
  fallopian tube (bilateral) N97.1
  fecal K56.41
      with hernia — see Hernia, by site, with
          obstruction
  foramen of Monro (congenital) Q03.8
      with spina bifida — see Spina bifida, by site, with
          hydrocephalus
  foreign body — see Foreign body
  gallbladder K82.0
      with calculus, stones K80.21
      congenital Q44.1
  gastric outlet K31.1
  gastrointestinal — see Obstruction, intestine
  hepatic K76.8
      duct (noncalculous) K83.1
  ileum — see Obstruction, intestine
  iliofemoral (artery) I74.5
  intestine K56.60
      with
          adhesions (intestinal) (peritoneal) K56.5
          adynamic K56.0
          by gallstone K56.3
          congenital (small) Q41.9
              large Q42.9
                  specified part NEC Q42.8
          neurogenic K56.0
              Hirschsprung's disease or megacolon Q43.1
          newborn P76.9
              due to
                  fecaliths P76.8
                  inspissated milk P76.2
                  meconium (plug) P76.0
                      in mucoviscidosis E84.11
              specified NEC P76.8
          postoperative K91.3
          reflex K56.0
          specified NEC K56.69
          volvulus K56.2
  intracardiac ball valve prosthesis T82.09
  jejunum — see Obstruction, intestine
  joint prosthesis — see Complications, joint
      prosthesis, mechanical, specified NEC, by site
  kidney (calices) N28.89
  labor — see Delivery
  lacrimal (passages) (duct)
      by
          dacryolith — see Dacryolith
          stenosis — see Stenosis, lacrimal
      congenital Q10.5
      neonatal H04.53-
  lacrimonasal duct — see Obstruction, lacrimal
  lacteal, with steatorrhea K90.2
  laryngitis — see Laryngitis

Obstruction, obstructed, obstructive—*continued*
    larynx NEC J38.6
        congenital Q31.8
    lung J98.4
        disease, chronic J44.9
    lymphatic I89.0
    meconium (plug)
        newborn P76.0
            due to fecaliths P76.0
            in mucoviscidosis E84.11
    mitral — *see* Stenosis, mitral
    nasal J34.89
    nasolacrimal duct (*see also* Obstruction, lacrimal)
        congenital Q10.5
    nasopharynx J39.2
    nose J34.89
    organ or site, congenital NEC — *see* Atresia, by site
    pancreatic duct K86.8
    parotid duct or gland K11.8
    pelviureteral junction N13.5
        congenital Q62.39
    pharynx J39.2
    portal (circulation) (vein) I81
    prostate (*see also* Hyperplasia, prostate)
        valve (urinary) N32.0
    pulmonary valve (heart) I37.0
    pyelonephritis (chronic) N11.1
    pylorus
        adult K31.1
        congenital or infantile Q40.0
    rectosigmoid — *see* Obstruction, intestine
    rectum K62.4
    renal N28.89
        outflow N13.8
        pelvis, congenital Q62.39
    respiratory J98.8
        chronic J44.9
    retinal (vessels) H34.9
    salivary duct (any) K11.8
        with calculus K11.5
    sigmoid — *see* Obstruction, intestine
    sinus (accessory) (nasal) J34.89
    Stensen's duct K11.8
    stomach NEC K31.89
        acute K31.0
        congenital Q40.2
        due to pylorospasm K31.3
    submandibular duct K11.8
    submaxillary gland K11.8
        with calculus K11.5
    thoracic duct I89.0
    thrombotic — *see* Thrombosis
    trachea J39.8
    tracheostomy airway J95.03
    tricuspid (valve) — *see* Stenosis, tricuspid
    upper respiratory, congenital Q34.8
    ureter (functional) (pelvic junction) NEC N13.5
        with
            hydronephrosis N13.1
                with infection N13.6
            pyelonephritis (chronic) N11.1
        congenital Q62.39
        due to calculus — *see* Calculus, ureter
    urethra NEC N36.8
        congenital Q64.39
    urinary (moderate) N13.9
        due to hyperplasia (hypertrophy) of prostate —
            see Hyperplasia, prostate
        organ or tract (lower) N13.9
        prostatic valve N32.0
        specified NEC N13.8
    uropathy N13.9
    uterus N85.8
    vagina N89.5
    valvular — *see* Endocarditis
    vein, venous I87.1
        caval (inferior) (superior) I87.1
        thrombotic — *see* Thrombosis
    vena cava (inferior) (superior) I87.1
    vesical NEC N32.0
    vesicourethral orifice N32.0
        congenital Q64.31
    vessel NEC I99.8

Obturator — *see* condition
Occlusal wear, teeth K03.0
Occlusio pupillae — *see* Membrane, pupillary
Occlusion, occluded
    anus K62.4
        congenital Q42.3
            with fistula Q42.2
    aortoiliac (chronic) I74.0
    aqueduct of Sylvius G91.1
        congenital Q03.0
            with spina bifida — *see* Spina bifida, by site,
                with hydrocephalus
    artery (*see also* Embolism, artery) I74.9
        auditory, internal I65.8
        basilar I65.1
            with
                infarction I63.22
                    due to
                        embolism I63.12
                        thrombosis I63.02
        brain or cerebral I66.9
            with infarction (due to) I63.5
                embolism I63.4
                thrombosis I63.3
        carotid I65.2-
            with
                infarction I63.23-
                    due to
                        embolism I63.13-
                        thrombosis I63.03-
        cerebellar (anterior inferior) (posterior inferior)
                (superior) I66.3
            with infarction I63.54-
                due to
                    embolism I63.44-
                    thrombosis I63.34-
        cerebral I66.9
            with infarction I63.50
                due to
                    embolism I63.40
                        specified NEC I63.49
                    thrombosis I63.30
                        specified NEC I63.39
            anterior I66.1-
                with infarction I63.52-
                    due to
                        embolism I63.42-
                        thrombosis I63.32-
            middle I66.0-
                with infarction I63.51-
                    due to
                        embolism I63.41-
                        thrombosis I63.31-
            posterior I66.2-
                with infarction I63.53-
                    due to
                        embolism I63.43-
                        thrombosis I63.33-
            specified NEC I66.8
                with infarction I63.59
                    due to
                        embolism I63.4
                        thrombosis I63.3
        choroidal (anterior) — *see* Occlusion, artery,
            cerebral, specified NEC
        communicating posterior — *see* Occlusion,
            artery, cerebral, specified NEC
        complete
            coronary I25.82
            extremities I70.92
        coronary (acute) (thrombotic) (without
                myocardial infarction) I24.0
            with myocardial infarction — *see* Infarction,
                myocardium
            chronic total I25.82
            complete I25.82
            healed or old I25.2
            total (chronic) I25.82
        hypophyseal — *see* Occlusion, artery,
            precerebral, specified NEC
        iliac I74.5
        lower extremities due to stenosis or stricture
            I77.1

Occlusion, occluded—*continued*
    artery—*continued*
        mesenteric (embolic) (thrombotic) K55.0
        perforating — *see* Occlusion, artery, cerebral,
            specified NEC
        peripheral I77.9
            thrombotic or embolic I74.4
        pontine — *see* Occlusion, artery, cerebral,
            specified NEC
        precerebral I65.9
            specified NEC I65.8
            with infarction I63.20
                specified NEC I63.29
                due to
                    embolism I63.10
                        specified NEC I63.19
                    thrombosis I63.00
                        specified NEC I63.09
            basilar — *see* Occlusion, artery, basilar
            carotid — *see* Occlusion, artery, carotid
                with infarction I63.2
                    due to
                        embolism I63.13-
                        thrombosis I63.03-
            puerperal O88.23
            specified NEC I65.8
                with infarction I63.2
                    due to
                        embolism I63.1
                        thrombosis I63.00
            vertebral — *see* Occlusion, artery, vertebral
        renal N28.0
        retinal
            central H34.1-
            partial H34.21-
            branch H34.23-
            transient H34.0-
        spinal — *see* Occlusion, artery, precerebral,
            vertebral
        total (chronic)
            coronary I25.82
            extremities I70.92
        vertebral I65.0-
            with
                infarction I63.21-
                    due to
                        embolism I63.11-
                        thrombosis I63.01-
    basilar artery — *see* Occlusion, artery, basilar
    bile duct (common) (hepatic) (noncalculous) K83.1
    bowel — *see* Obstruction, intestine
    carotid (artery) (common) (internal) — *see*
        Occlusion, artery, carotid
    centric (of teeth) M26.59
        maximum intercuspation discrepancy M26.55
    cerebellar (artery) — *see* Occlusion, artery,
        cerebellar
    cerebral (artery) — *see* Occlusion, artery, cerebral
    cerebrovascular (*see also* Occlusion, artery, cerebral)
        with infarction I63.5
    cervical canal — *see* Stricture, cervix
    cervix (uteri) — *see* Stricture, cervix
    choanal Q30.0
    choroidal (artery) I65.8
    colon — *see* Obstruction, intestine
    communicating posterior artery — *see* Occlusion,
        artery, precerebral, specified NEC
    coronary (artery) (vein) (thrombotic) (*see also*
        Infarct, myocardium)
        chronic total I25.82
        healed or old I25.2
        not resulting in infarction I24.0
        total (chronic) I25.82
    cystic duct — *see* Obstruction, gallbladder
    embolic — *see* Embolism
    fallopian tube N97.1
        congenital Q50.6
    gallbladder (*see also* Obstruction, gallbladder)
        congenital (causing jaundice) Q44.1
    gingiva, traumatic K06.2
    hymen N89.6
        congenital Q52.3

Occlusion, occluded—*continued*
hypophyseal (artery) — *see* Occlusion, artery, precerebral, specified NEC
iliac artery I74.5
intestine — *see* Obstruction, intestine
lacrimal passages — *see* Obstruction, lacrimal
lung J98.4
lymph or lymphatic channel I89.0
mammary duct N64.89
mesenteric artery (embolic) (thrombotic) K55.0
nose J34.89
congenital Q30.0
organ or site, congenital NEC — *see* Atresia, by site
oviduct N97.1
congenital Q50.6
peripheral arteries
due to stricture or stenosis I77.1
upper extremity I74.3
pontine (artery) — *see* Occlusion, artery, precerebral, specified NEC
posterior lingual, of mandibular teeth M26.29
precerebral artery — *see* Occlusion, artery, precerebral
punctum lacrimale — *see* Obstruction, lacrimal
pupil — *see* Membrane, pupillary
pylorus, adult (*see also* Stricture, pylorus) K31.1
renal artery N28.0
retina, retinal
artery — *see* Occlusion, artery, retinal
vein (central) H34.81-
engorgement H34.82-
tributary H34.83-
vessels H34.9
spinal artery — *see* Occlusion, artery, precerebral, vertebral
teeth (mandibular) (posterior lingual) M26.29
thoracic duct I89.0
thrombotic — *see* Thrombosis, artery
traumatic
edentulous (alveolar) ridge K06.2
gingiva K06.2
periodontal K05.5
tubal N97.1
ureter (complete) (partial) N13.5
congenital Q62.10
ureteropelvic junction N13.5
congenital Q62.11
ureterovesical orifice N13.5
congenital Q62.12
urethra — *see* Stricture, urethra
uterus N85.8
vagina N89.5
vascular NEC I99.8
vein — *see* Thrombosis
retinal — *see* Occlusion, retinal, vein
vena cava (inferior) (superior) — *see* Embolism, vena cava
ventricle (brain) NEC G91.1
vertebral (artery) — *see* Occlusion, artery, vertebral
vessel (blood) I99.8
vulva N90.5
Occult
blood in feces (stools) R19.5
Occupational
problems NEC Z56.89
Ochlophobia — *see* Agoraphobia
Ochronosis (endogenous) E70.29
Ocular muscle — *see* condition
Oculogyric crisis or disturbance H51.8
psychogenic F45.8
Oculomotor syndrome H51.9
Oculopathy
syphilitic NEC A52.71
congenital
early A50.01
late A50.30
early (secondary) A51.43
late A52.71
Oddi's sphincter spasm K83.4
Odontalgia K08.8
Odontoameloblastoma — *see* Cyst, calcifying odontogenic
Odontoclasia K03.89

Odontodysplasia, regional K00.4
Odontogenesis imperfecta K00.5
Odontoma (ameloblastic) (complex) (compound) (fibroameloblastic) — *see* Cyst, calcifying odontogenic
Odontomyelitis (closed) (open) K04.0
Odontorrhagia K08.8
Odontosarcoma, ameloblastic C41.1
upper jaw (bone) C41.0
Oedema, oedematous — *see* Edema
Oesophag(o) — *see* Esophag(o)-
Oestriasis — *see* Myiasis
Oguchi's disease H53.63
Ohara's disease — *see* Tularemia
Oidiomycosis — *see* Candidiasis
Oidium albicans infection — *see* Candidiasis
Old age (without mention of debility) R54
dementia F03
Old (previous) myocardial infarction I25.2
Olfactory — *see* condition
Oligemia — *see* Anemia
Oligoastrocytoma
specified site — *see* Neoplasm, malignant, by site
unspecified site C71.9
Oligocythemia D64.9
Oligodendroblastoma
specified site — *see* Neoplasm, malignant, by site
unspecified site C71.9
Oligodendroglioma
anaplastic type
specified site — *see* Neoplasm, malignant, by site
unspecified site C71.9
specified site — *see* Neoplasm, malignant, by site
unspecified site C71.9
Oligodontia — *see* Anodontia
Oligoencephalon Q02
Oligohidrosis L74.4
Oligohydramnios O41.0-
Oligohydrosis L74.4
Oligomenorrhea N91.5
primary N91.3
secondary N91.4
Oligophrenia (*see also* Retardation, mental)
phenylpyruvic E70.0
Oligospermia N46.11
due to
drug therapy N46.121
efferent duct obstruction N46.123
infection N46.122
radiation N46.124
specified cause NEC N46.129
systemic disease N46.125
Oligotrichia — *see* Alopecia
Oliguria R34
with, complicating or following ectopic or molar pregnancy O08.4
postprocedural N99.0
Ollier's disease Q78.4
Omentitis — *see* Peritonitis
Omenotocele — *see* Hernia, abdomen, specified site NEC
Omentum, omental — *see* condition
Omphalitis (congenital) (newborn) P38.9
with mild hemorrhage P38.1
without hemorrhage P38.9
not of newborn L08.82
tetanus A33
Omphalocele Q79.2
Omphalomesenteric duct, persistent Q43.0
Omphalorrhagia, newborn P51.9
Omsk hemorrhagic fever A98.1
Onanism (excessive) F98.8
Onchocerciasis, onchocercosis B73.1
with
eye disease B73.00
endophthalmitis B73.01
eyelid B73.09
glaucoma B73.02
specified NEC B73.09
eye NEC B73.00
eyelid B73.09
Oncocytoma — *see* Neoplasm, benign, by site

Oncovirus, as cause of disease classified elsewhere B97.32
Ondine's curse — *see* Apnea, sleep
Oneirophrenia F23
Onychauxis L60.2
congenital Q84.5
Onychia (*see also* Cellulitis, digit)
with lymphangitis — *see* Lymphangitis, acute, digit
candidal B37.2
dermatophytic B35.1
Onychitis (*see also* Cellulitis, digit)
with lymphangitis — *see* Lymphangitis, acute, digit
Onychocryptosis L60.0
Onychodystrophy L60.3
congenital Q84.6
Onychogryphosis, onychogryposis L60.2
Onycholysis L60.1
Onychomadesis L60.8
Onychomalacia L60.3
Onychomycosis (finger) (toe) B35.1
Onycho-osteodysplasia Q79.8
Onychophagia F98.8
Onychophosis L60.8
Onychoptosis L60.8
Onychorrhexis L60.3
congenital Q84.6
Onychoschizia L60.3
Onyxis (finger) (toe) L60.0
Onyxitis (*see also* Cellulitis, digit)
with lymphangitis — *see* Lymphangitis, acute, digit
Oophoritis (cystic) (infectional) (interstitial) N70.92
with salpingitis N70.93
acute N70.02
with salpingitis N70.03
chronic N70.12
with salpingitis N70.13
complicating abortion — *see* Abortion, by type, complicated by, oophoritis
Oophorocele N83.4
Opacity, opacities
cornea H17.-
central H17.1-
congenital Q13.3
degenerative — *see* Degeneration, cornea
hereditary — *see* Dystrophy, cornea
inflammatory — *see* Keratitis
minor H17.81-
peripheral H17.82-
sequelae of trachoma (healed) B94.0
specified NEC H17.89
enamel (teeth) (fluoride) (nonfluoride) K00.3
lens — *see* Cataract
snowball — *see* Deposit, crystalline
vitreous (humor) NEC H43.39-
congenital Q14.0
membranes and strands H43.31-
Opalescent dentin (hereditary) K00.5
Open, opening
abnormal, organ or site, congenital — *see* Imperfect, closure
angle with
borderline intraocular pressure H40.0
cupping of discs H40.0
glaucoma (primary) — *see* Glaucoma, open angle
bite
anterior M26.220
posterior M26.221
false — *see* Imperfect, closure
margin on tooth restoration K08.51
restoration margins of tooth K08.51
wound — *see* Wound, open
Operational fatigue F48.8
Operative — *see* condition
Operculitis — *see* Periodontitis
Operculum — *see* Break, retina
Ophiasis L63.2
Ophthalmia (*see also* Conjunctivitis) H10.9
actinic rays — *see* Photokeratitis
allergic (acute) — *see* Conjunctivitis, acute, atopic
blennorrhagic (gonococcal) (neonatorum) A54.31
diphtheritic A36.86
Egyptian A71.1

Ophthalmia—*continued*
  electrica — *see* Photokeratitis
  gonococcal (neonatorum) A54.31
  metastatic — *see* Endophthalmitis, purulent
  migraine — *see* Migraine, ophthalmoplegic
  neonatorum, newborn P39.1
    gonococcal A54.31
  nodosa H16.24-
  purulent — *see* Conjunctivitis, acute, mucopurulent
  spring — *see* Conjunctivitis, acute, atopic
  sympathetic — *see* Uveitis, sympathetic
Ophthalmitis — *see* Ophthalmia
Ophthalmocele (congenital) Q15.8
Ophthalmoneuromyelitis G36.0
Ophthalmoplegia (*see also* Strabismus, paralytic)
  anterior internuclear — *see* Ophthalmoplegia, internuclear
  ataxia-areflexia G61.0
  diabetic — *see* E08-E13 with .39
  exophthalmic E05.00
    with thyroid storm E05.01
  external H49.88-
    progressive H49.4-
      with pigmentary retinopathy — *see* Kearns-Sayre syndrome
    total H49.3-
  internal (complete) (total) H52.51-
  internuclear H51.2-
  migraine — *see* Migraine, ophthalmoplegic
  Parinaud's H49.88-
  progressive external — *see* Ophthalmoplegia, external, progressive
  supranuclear, progressive G23.1
  total (external) — *see* Ophthalmoplegia, external, total
Opioid(s)
  abuse — *see* Abuse, drug, opioids
  dependence — *see* Dependence, drug, opioids
Opisthognathism M26.09
Opisthorchiasis (felineus) (viverrini) B66.0
Opitz' disease D73.2
Opiumism — *see* Dependence, drug, opioid
Oppenheim's disease G70.2
Oppenheim-Urbach disease E88.89
Optic nerve — *see* condition
Orbit — *see* condition
Orchioblastoma C62.9-
Orchitis (gangrenous) (nonspecific) (septic) (suppurative) N45.2
  blennorrhagic (gonococcal) (acute) (chronic) A54.23
  chlamydial A56.19
  filarial B74.9
  gonococcal (acute) (chronic) A54.23
  mumps B26.0
  syphilitic A52.76
  tuberculous A18.15
Orf (virus disease) B08.02
Organic (*see also* condition)
  brain syndrome F09
  heart — *see* Disease, heart
  mental disorder F09
  psychosis F09
Orgasm
  anejaculatory N53.13
Oriental
  bilharziasis B65.2
  schistosomiasis B65.2
Orifice — *see* condition
Origin of both great vessels from right ventricle Q20.1
Ormond's disease (with ureteral obstruction) N13.5
  with infection N13.6
Ornithine metabolism disorder E72.4
Ornithinemia (Type I) (Type II) E72.4
Ornithosis A70
Orotaciduria, oroticaciduria (congenital) (hereditary) (pyrimidine deficiency) D53.0
Orotic aciduria (congenital) (hereditary) (pyrimidine deficiency) E79.8
  anemia D53.0
Orthodontics
  adjustment Z46.4
  fitting Z46.4

Orthopnea R06.01
Orthopoxvirus B08.09
  specified NEC B08.09
Os, uterus — *see* condition
Osgood-Schlatter disease or osteochondrosis — *see* Osteochondrosis, juvenile, tibia
Osler(-Weber)-Rendu disease I78.0
Osler's nodes I33.0
Osmidrosis L75.0
Osseous — *see* condition
Ossification
  artery — *see* Arteriosclerosis
  auricle (ear) — *see* Disorder, pinna, specified type NEC
  bronchial J98.09
  cardiac — *see* Degeneration, myocardial
  cartilage (senile) — *see* Disorder, cartilage, specified type NEC
  coronary (artery) — *see* Disease, heart, ischemic, atherosclerotic
  diaphragm J98.6
  ear, middle — *see* Otosclerosis
  falx cerebri G96.19
  fontanel, premature Q75.0
  heart (*see also* Degeneration, myocardial)
    valve — *see* Endocarditis
  larynx J38.7
  ligament — *see* Disorder, tendon, specified type NEC
    posterior longitudinal — *see* Spondylopathy, specified NEC
  meninges (cerebral) (spinal) G96.19
  multiple, eccentric centers — *see* Disorder, bone, development or growth
  muscle (*see also* Calcification, muscle)
    due to burns — *see* Myositis, ossificans, in, burns
    paralytic — *see* Myositis, ossificans, in, quadriplegia
    progressive — *see* Myositis, ossificans, progressiva
    specified NEC M61.50
      ankle M61.57-
      foot M61.57-
      forearm M61.53-
      hand M61.54-
      lower leg M61.56-
      multiple sites M61.59
      pelvic region M61.55-
      shoulder region M61.51-
      specified site NEC M61.58
      thigh M61.55-
      upper arm M61.52-
    traumatic — *see* Myositis, ossificans, traumatica
  myocardium, myocardial — *see* Degeneration, myocardial
  penis N48.89
  periarticular — *see* Disorder, joint, specified type NEC
  pinna — *see* Disorder, pinna, specified type NEC
  rider's bone — *see* Ossification, muscle, specified NEC
  sclera H15.89
  subperiosteal, post-traumatic M89.8x-
  tendon — *see* Disorder, tendon, specified type NEC
  trachea J39.8
  tympanic membrane — *see* Disorder, tympanic membrane, specified NEC
  vitreous (humor) — *see* Deposit, crystalline
Osteitis (*see also* Osteomyelitis)
  alveolar M27.3
  condensans M85.30
    ankle M85.37-
    foot M85.37-
    forearm M85.33-
    hand M85.34-
    lower leg M85.36-
    multiple site M85.39
    neck M85.38
    rib M85.38
    shoulder M85.31-
    skull M85.38
    specified site NEC M85.38
    thigh M85.35-
    toe M85.37-

Osteitis —*continued*
  condensans—*continued*
    upper arm M85.32-
    vertebra M85.38
  deformans M88.9
    in (due to)
      malignant neoplasm of bone C41.9 [M90.60]
      neoplastic disease (*see also* Neoplasm) D49.9 [M90.60]
        carpus D49.9 [M90.64-]
        clavicle D49.9 [M90.61-]
        femur D49.9 [M90.65-]
        fibula D49.9 [M90.66-]
        finger D49.9 [M90.64-]
        humerus D49.9 [M90.62-]
        ilium D49.9 [M90.65-]
        ischium D49.9 [M90.65-]
        metacarpus D49.9 [M90.64-]
        metatarsus D49.9 [M90.67-]
        multiple sites D49.9 [M90.69]
        neck D49.9 [M90.68]
        radius D49.9 [M90.63-]
        rib D49.9 [M90.68]
        scapula D49.9 [M90.61-]
        skull D49.9 [M90.68]
        tarsus D49.9 [M90.67-]
        tibia D49.9 [M90.66-]
        toe D49.9 [M90.67-]
        ulna D49.9 [M90.63-]
        vertebra D49.9 [M90.68]
    skull M88.0
    specified NEC — *see* Paget's disease, bone, by site
    vertebra M88.1
  due to yaws A66.6
  fibrosa NEC — *see* Cyst, bone, by site
    circumscripta — *see* Dysplasia, fibrous, bone NEC
    cystica (generalisata) E21.0
    disseminata Q78.1
    osteoplastica E21.0
  fragilitans Q78.0
  Garr's (sclerosing) — *see* Osteomyelitis, specified type NEC
  jaw (acute) (chronic) (lower) (suppurative) (upper) M27.2
  parathyroid E21.0
  petrous bone (acute) (chronic) — *see* Petrositis
  sclerotic, nonsuppurative — *see* Osteomyelitis, specified type NEC
  tuberculosa A18.09
    cystica D86.89
    multiplex cystoides D86.89
Osteoarthritis M19.90
  ankle M19.07-
  elbow M19.02-
  foot joint M19.07-
  generalized M15.9
    erosive M15.4
    primary M15.0
    specified NEC M15.8
  hand joint M19.04-
    first carpometacarpal joint M18.9-
  hip M16.1-
    bilateral M16.0
    due to hip dysplasia (unilateral) M16.3-
      bilateral M16.2
  interphalangeal
    distal (Heberden) M15.1
    proximal (Bouchard) M15.2
  knee M17.9-
    bilateral M17.0
  shoulder M19.01-
  spine — *see* Spondylosis
  wrist M19.03-
  post-traumatic NEC M19.92
    ankle M19.17-
    elbow M19.12-
    foot joint M19.17-
    hand joint M19.14-
      first carpometacarpal joint M18.3-
        bilateral M18.2

Osteoarthritis—continued
  primary—continued
    hip M16.5-
      bilateral M16.4
    knee M17.3-
      bilateral M17.2
    shoulder M19.11-
    wrist M19.13-
  primary M19.91
    ankle M19.07-
    elbow M19.02-
    foot joint M19.07-
    hand joint M19.04-
      first carpometacarpal joint M18.1-
        bilateral M18.0
    hip M16.1-
      bilateral M16.0
    knee M17.1-
      bilateral M17.0
    shoulder M19.01-
    spine — see Spondylosis
    wrist M19.03-
  secondary M19.93
    ankle M19.27-
    elbow M19.22-
    foot joint M19.27-
    hand joint M19.24-
      first carpometacarpal joint M18.5-
        bilateral M18.4
    hip M16.7
      bilateral M16.6
    knee M17.5
      bilateral M17.4
    multiple M15.3
    shoulder M19.21-
    spine — see Spondylosis
    wrist M19.23-
Osteoarthropathy (hypertrophic) M19.90
  ankle — see Osteoarthritis, primary, ankle
  elbow — see Osteoarthritis, primary, elbow
  foot joint — see Osteoarthritis, primary, foot
  hand joint — see Osteoarthritis, primary, hand joint
  knee joint — see Osteoarthritis, primary, knee
  multiple site — see Osteoarthritis, primary, multiple joint
  pulmonary (see also Osteoarthropathy, specified type NEC)
    hypertrophic — see Osteoarthropathy, hypertrophic, specified type NEC
    secondary hypertrophic — see Osteoarthropathy, specified type NEC
  shoulder — see Osteoarthritis, primary, shoulder
  specified joint NEC — see Osteoarthritis, primary, specified joint NEC
  specified type NEC M89.40
    carpus M89.44-
    clavicle M89.41-
    femur M89.45-
    fibula M89.46-
    finger M89.44-
    humerus M89.42-
    ilium M89.459
    ischium M89.459
    metacarpus M89.44-
    metatarsus M89.47-
    multiple sites M89.49
    neck M89.48
    radius M89.43-
    rib M89.48
    scapula M89.41-
    skull M89.48
    tarsus M89.47-
    tibia M89.46-
    toe M89.47-
    ulna M89.43-
    vertebra M89.48
  secondary — see Osteoarthropathy, specified type NEC
  spine — see Spondylosis
  wrist — see Osteoarthritis, primary, wrist
Osteoarthrosis (degenerative) (hypertrophic) (joint) (see also Osteoarthritis)
  deformans alkaptonurica E70.29 [M36.8]

Osteoarthrosis—continued
  erosive M15.4
  generalized M15.9
    primary M15.0
  polyarticular M15.9
  spine — see Spondylosis
Osteoblastoma — see Neoplasm, bone, benign
  aggressive — see Neoplasm, bone, uncertain behavior
Osteochondroarthrosis deformans endemic — see Disease, Kaschin-Beck
Osteochondritis (see also Osteochondropathy, by site)
  Brailsford's — see Osteochondrosis, juvenile, radius
  dissecans M93.20
    ankle M93.27-
    elbow M93.22-
    foot M93.27-
    hand M93.24-
    hip M93.25-
    knee M93.26-
    multiple sites M93.29
    shoulder joint M93.21-
    specified site NEC M93.28
    wrist M93.23-
  juvenile M92.9
    patellar — see Osteochondrosis, juvenile, patella
  syphilitic (congenital) (early) A50.02 [M90.80]
    ankle A50.02 [M90.87-]
    elbow A50.02 [M90.82-]
    foot A50.02 [M90.87-]
    forearm A50.02 [M90.83-]
    hand A50.02 [M90.84-]
    hip A50.02 [M90.85-]
    knee A50.02 [M90.86-]
    multiple sites A50.02 [M90.89]
    shoulder joint A50.02 [M90.81-]
    specified site NEC A50.02 [M90.88]
Osteochondrodysplasia Q78.9
  with defects of growth of tubular bones and spine Q77.9
    specified NEC Q77.8
  specified NEC Q78.8
Osteochondrodystrophy E78.9
Osteochondrolysis — see Osteochondritis, dissecans
Osteochondroma — see Neoplasm, bone, benign
Osteochondromatosis D48.0
  syndrome Q78.4
Osteochondromyxosarcoma — see Neoplasm, bone, malignant
Osteochondropathy M93.90
  ankle M93.97-
  elbow M93.92-
  foot M93.97-
  hand M93.94-
  hip M93.95-
  Kienböck's disease of adults M93.1
  knee M93.96-
  multiple joints M93.99
  osteochondritis dissecans — see Osteochondritis, dissecans
  osteochondrosis — see Osteochondrosis
  shoulder region M93.91-
  slipped upper femoral epiphysis — see Slipped, epiphysis, upper femoral
  specified joint NEC M93.98
  specified type NEC M93.80
    ankle M93.87-
    elbow M93.82-
    foot M93.87-
    hand M93.84-
    hip M93.85-
    knee M93.86-
    multiple joints M93.89
    shoulder region M93.81-
    specified joint NEC M93.88
    wrist M93.83-
  syphilitic, congenital
    early A50.02 [M90.80]
    late A50.56 [M90.80]
  wrist M93.93-
Osteochondrosarcoma — see Neoplasm, bone, malignant

Osteochondrosis (see also Osteochondropathy, by site)
  acetabulum (juvenile) M91.0
  adult — see Osteochondropathy, specified type NEC, by site
  astragalus (juvenile) — see Osteochondrosis, juvenile, tarsus
  Blount's — see Osteochondrosis, juvenile, tibia
  Buchanan's M91.0
  Burns' — see Osteochondrosis, juvenile, ulna
  calcaneus (juvenile) — see Osteochondrosis, juvenile, tarsus
  capitular epiphysis (femur) (juvenile) — see Legg-Calvé-Perthes disease
  carpal (juvenile) (lunate) (scaphoid) — see Osteochondrosis, juvenile, hand, carpal lunate
    adult M93.1
  coxae juvenilis — see Legg-Calvé-Perthes disease
  deformans juvenilis, coxae — see Legg-Calvé-Perthes disease
  Diaz's — see Osteochondrosis, juvenile, tarsus
  dissecans (knee) (shoulder) — see Osteochondritis, dissecans
  femoral capital epiphysis (juvenile) — see Legg-Calvé-Perthes disease
  femur (head), juvenile — see Legg-Calvé-Perthes disease
  fibula (juvenile) — see Osteochondrosis, juvenile, fibula
  foot NEC (juvenile) M92.8
  Freiberg's — see Osteochondrosis, juvenile, metatarsus
  Haas' (juvenile) — see Osteochondrosis, juvenile, humerus
  Haglund's — see Osteochondrosis, juvenile, tarsus
  hip (juvenile) — see Legg-Calvé-Perthes disease
  humerus (capitulum) (head) (juvenile) — see Osteochondrosis, juvenile, humerus
  ilium, iliac crest (juvenile) M91.0
  ischiopubic synchondrosis M91.0
  Iselin's — see Osteochondrosis, juvenile, metatarsus
  juvenile, juvenilis M92.9
    after congenital dislocation of hip reduction — see Osteochondrosis, juvenile, hip, specified NEC
    arm — see Osteochondrosis, juvenile, upper limb NEC
    capitular epiphysis (femur) — see Legg-Calvé-Perthes disease
    clavicle, sternal epiphysis — see Osteochondrosis, juvenile, upper limb NEC
    coxae — see Legg-Calvé-Perthes disease
    deformans M92.9
    fibula M92.5-
    foot NEC M92.8
    hand M92.20-
      carpal lunate M92.21-
      metacarpal head M92.22-
      specified site NEC M92.29-
    head of femur — see Legg-Calvé-Perthes disease
    hip and pelvis M91.9-
      coxa plana — see Coxa, plana
      femoral head — see Legg-Calvé-Perthes disease
      pelvis M91.0
      pseudocoxalgia — see Pseudocoxalgia
      specified NEC M91.8-
    humerus M92.0-
    limb
      lower NEC M92.8
      upper NEC — see Osteochondrosis, juvenile, upper limb NEC
    medial cuneiform bone — see Osteochondrosis, juvenile, tarsus
    metatarsus M92.7-
    patella M92.4-
    radius M92.1-
    specified site NEC M92.8
    spine M42.00
      cervical region M42.02
      cervicothoracic region M42.03
      lumbar region M42.06
      lumbosacral region M42.07

Osteochondrosis —continued
  juvenile, juvenilis—continued
    spine—continued
      multiple sites M42.09
      occipito-atlanto-axial region M42.01
      sacrococcygeal region M42.08
      thoracic region M42.04
      thoracolumbar region M42.05
    tarsus M92.6-
    tibia M92.5-
    ulna M92.1-
    upper limb NEC M92.3-
    vertebra (body) (epiphyseal plates) (Calvé's)
      (Scheuermann's) — see Osteochondrosis,
      juvenile, spine
  Kienböck's — see Osteochondrosis, juvenile, hand,
    carpal lunate
  adult M93.1
  Köhler's
    patellar — see Osteochondrosis, juvenile, patella
    tarsal navicular — see Osteochondrosis, juvenile,
      tarsus
  Legg-Perthes(-Calvé)(-Waldenström) — see
    Legg-Calvé-Perthes disease
  limb
    lower NEC (juvenile) M92.8
    upper NEC (juvenile) — see Osteochondrosis,
      juvenile, upper limb NEC
  lunate bone (carpal) (juvenile) (see also
    Osteochondrosis, juvenile, hand, carpal
    lunate)
    adult M93.1
  Mauclaire's — see Osteochondrosis, juvenile, hand,
    metacarpal
  metacarpal (head) (juvenile) — see
    Osteochondrosis, juvenile, hand, metacarpal
  metatarsus (fifth) (head) (juvenile) (second) — see
    Osteochondrosis, juvenile, metatarsus
  navicular (juvenile) — see Osteochondrosis,
    juvenile, tarsus
  os
    calcis (juvenile) — see Osteochondrosis, juvenile,
      tarsus
    tibiale externum (juvenile) — see
      Osteochondrosis, juvenile, tarsus
  Osgood-Schlatter — see Osteochondrosis, juvenile,
    tibia
  Panner's — see Osteochondrosis, juvenile, humerus
  patellar center (juvenile) (primary) (secondary) —
    see Osteochondrosis, juvenile, patella
  pelvis (juvenile) M91.0
  Pierson's M91.0
  radius (head) (juvenile) — see Osteochondrosis,
    juvenile, radius
  Scheuermann's — see Osteochondrosis, juvenile,
    spine
  Sever's — see Osteochondrosis, juvenile, tarsus
  Sinding-Larsen — see Osteochondrosis, juvenile,
    patella
  spine M42.9
    adult M42.10
      cervical region M42.12
      cervicothoracic region M42.13
      lumbar region M42.16
      lumbosacral region M42.17
      multiple sites M42.19
      occipito-atlanto-axial region M42.11
      sacrococcygeal region M42.18
      thoracic region M42.14
      thoracolumbar region M42.15
    juvenile — see Osteochondrosis, juvenile, spine
  symphysis pubis (juvenile) M91.0
  syphilitic (congenital) A50.02
  talus (juvenile) — see Osteochondrosis, juvenile,
    tarsus
  tarsus (navicular) (juvenile) — see Osteochondrosis,
    juvenile, tarsus
  tibia (proximal) (tubercle) (juvenile) — see
    Osteochondrosis, juvenile, tibia
  tuberculous — see Tuberculosis, bone
  ulna (lower) (juvenile) — see Osteochondrosis,
    juvenile, ulna
  van Neck's M91.0

Osteochondrosis —continued
  vertebral — see Osteochondrosis, spine
Osteoclastoma D48.0
  malignant — see Neoplasm, bone, malignant
Osteodynia — see Disorder, bone, specified type NEC
Osteodystrophy Q78.9
  azotemic N25.0
  congenital Q78.9
  parathyroid, secondary E21.1
  renal N25.0
Osteofibroma — see Neoplasm, bone, benign
Osteofibrosarcoma — see Neoplasm, bone,
  malignant
Osteogenesis imperfecta Q78.0
Osteogenic — see condition
Osteolysis M89.50
  carpus M89.54-
  clavicle M89.51-
  femur M89.55-
  fibula M89.56-
  finger M89.54-
  humerus M89.52-
  ilium M89.559
  ischium M89.559
  joint prosthesis (periprosthetic) — see
    Complications, joint prosthesis, mechanical,
    periprosthetic, osteolysis, by site
  metacarpus M89.54-
  metatarsus M89.57-
  multiple sites M89.59
  neck M89.58
  periprosthetic — see Complications, joint prosthesis,
    mechanical, periprosthetic, osteolysis, by site
  radius M89.53-
  rib M89.58
  scapula M89.51-
  skull M89.58
  tarsus M89.57-
  tibia M89.56-
  toe M89.57-
  ulna M89.53-
  vertebra M89.58
Osteoma (see also Neoplasm, bone, benign)
  osteoid (see also Neoplasm, bone, benign)
  giant — see Neoplasm, bone, benign
Osteomalacia M83.9
  adult M83.9
    drug-induced NEC M83.5
    due to
      malabsorption (postsurgical) M83.2
      malnutrition M83.3
      specified NEC M83.8
    aluminium-induced M83.4
    infantile — see Rickets
    juvenile — see Rickets
    pelvis M83.8
    puerperal M83.0
    senile M83.1
    vitamin-D-resistant in adults E83.31 [M90.8-]
      carpus E83.31 [M90.84-]
      clavicle E83.31 [M90.81-]
      femur E83.31 [M90.85-]
      fibula E83.31 [M90.86-]
      finger E83.31 [M90.84-]
      humerus E83.31 [M90.82-]
      ilium E83.31 [M90.859]
      ischium E83.31 [M90.859]
      metacarpus E83.31 [M90.84-]
      metatarsus E83.31 [M90.87-]
      multiple sites E83.31 [M90.89]
      neck E83.31 [M90.88]
      radius E83.31 [M90.83-]
      rib E83.31 [M90.88]
      scapula E83.31 [M90.819]
      skull E83.31 [M90.88]
      tarsus E83.31 [M90.879]
      tibia E83.31 [M90.869]
      toe E83.31 [M90.879]
      ulna E83.31 [M90.839]
      vertebra E83.31 [M90.88]

Osteomyelitis (general) (infective) (localized)
  (neonatal) (purulent) (septic) (staphylococcal)
  (streptococcal) (suppurative) (with periostitis)
  M86.9
  acute M86.10
    carpus M86.14-
    clavicle M86.11-
    femur M86.15-
    fibula M86.16-
    finger M86.14-
    hematogenous M86.00
      carpus M86.04-
      clavicle M86.01-
      femur M86.05-
      fibula M86.06-
      finger M86.04-
      humerus M86.02-
      ilium M86.059
      ischium M86.059
      mandible M27.2
      metacarpus M86.04-
      metatarsus M86.07-
      multiple sites M86.09
      neck M86.08
      orbit H05.02-
      petrous bone — see Petrositis
      radius M86.03-
      rib M86.08
      scapula M86.01-
      skull M86.08
      tarsus M86.07-
      tibia M86.06-
      toe M86.07-
      ulna M86.03-
      vertebra — see Osteomyelitis, vertebra
    humerus M86.12-
    ilium M86.159
    ischium M86.159
    mandible M27.2
    metacarpus M86.14-
    metatarsus M86.17-
    multiple sites M86.19
    neck M86.18
    orbit H05.02-
    petrous bone — see Petrositis
    radius M86.13-
    rib M86.18
    scapula M86.11-
    skull M86.18
    tarsus M86.17-
    tibia M86.16-
    toe M86.17-
    ulna M86.13-
    vertebra — see Osteomyelitis, vertebra
  chronic (or old) M86.60
    with draining sinus M86.40
      carpus M86.44-
      clavicle M86.41-
      femur M86.45-
      fibula M86.46-
      finger M86.44-
      humerus M86.42-
      ilium M86.459
      ischium M86.459
      mandible M27.2
      metacarpus M86.44-
      metatarsus M86.47-
      multiple sites M86.49
      neck M86.48
      orbit H05.02-
      petrous bone — see Petrositis
      radius M86.43-
      rib M86.48
      scapula M86.41-
      skull M86.48
      tarsus M86.47-
      tibia M86.46-
      toe M86.47-
      ulna M86.43-
      vertebra — see Osteomyelitis, vertebra
    carpus M86.64-
    clavicle M86.61-
    femur M86.65-

Osteomyelitis —*continued*
  chronic (or old)—*continued*
    fibula M86.66-
    finger M86.64-
    hematogenous NEC M86.50
      carpus M86.54-
      clavicle M86.51-
      femur M86.55-
      fibula M86.56-
      finger M86.54-
      humerus M86.52-
      ilium M86.559
      ischium M86.559
      mandible M27.2
      metacarpus M86.54-
      metatarsus M86.57-
      multifocal M86.30
        carpus M86.34-
        clavicle M86.31-
        femur M86.35-
        fibula M86.36-
        finger M86.34-
        humerus M86.32-
        ilium M86.359
        ischium M86.359
        metacarpus M86.34-
        metatarsus M86.37-
        multiple sites M86.39
        neck M86.38
        radius M86.33-
        rib M86.38
        scapula M86.31-
        skull M86.38
        tarsus M86.37-
        tibia M86.36-
        toe M86.37-
        ulna M86.33-
        vertebra — *see* Osteomyelitis, vertebra
      multiple sites M86.59
      neck M86.58
      orbit H05.02-
      petrous bone — *see* Petrositis
      radius M86.53-
      rib M86.58
      scapula M86.51-
      skull M86.58
      tarsus M86.57-
      tibia M86.56-
      toe M86.57-
      ulna M86.53-
      vertebra — *see* Osteomyelitis, vertebra
    humerus M86.62-
    ilium M86.659
    ischium M86.659
    mandible M27.2
    metacarpus M86.64-
    metatarsus M86.67-
    multifocal — *see* Osteomyelitis, chronic, hematogenous, multifocal
    multiple sites M86.69
    neck M86.68
    orbit H05.02-
    petrous bone — *see* Petrositis
    radius M86.63-
    rib M86.68
    scapula M86.61-
    skull M86.68
    tarsus M86.67-
    tibia M86.66-
    toe M86.67-
    ulna M86.63-
    vertebra — *see* Osteomyelitis, vertebra
  echinococcal B67.2
  Garr's — *see* Osteomyelitis, specified type NEC
  jaw (acute) (chronic) (lower) (neonatal) (suppurative) (upper) M27.2
  nonsuppurating — *see* Osteomyelitis, specified type NEC
  orbit H05.02-
  petrous bone — *see* Petrositis
  Salmonella (arizonae) (cholerae-suis) (enteritidis) (typhimurium) A02.24

Osteomyelitis —*continued*
  sclerosing, nonsuppurative — *see* Osteomyelitis, specified type NEC
  specified type NEC — *see also* subcategory M86.8x-
    mandible M27.2
    orbit H05.02-
    petrous bone — *see* Petrositis
    vertebra — *see* Osteomyelitis, vertebra
  subacute M86.20
    carpus M86.24-
    clavicle M86.21-
    femur M86.25-
    fibula M86.26-
    finger M86.24-
    humerus M86.22-
    mandible M27.2
    metacarpus M86.24-
    metatarsus M86.27-
    multiple sites M86.29
    neck M86.28
    orbit H05.02-
    petrous bone — *see* Petrositis
    radius M86.23-
    rib M86.28
    scapula M86.21-
    skull M86.28
    tarsus M86.27-
    tibia M86.26-
    toe M86.27-
    ulna M86.23-
    vertebra — *see* Osteomyelitis, vertebra
  syphilitic A52.77
    congenital (early) A50.02 [M90.80]
  tuberculous — *see* Tuberculosis, bone
  typhoid A01.05
  vertebra M46.20
    cervical region M46.22
    cervicothoracic region M46.23
    lumbar region M46.26
    lumbosacral region M46.27
    occipito-atlanto-axial region M46.21
    sacrococcygeal region M46.28
    thoracic region M46.24
    thoracolumbar region M46.25

Osteomyelofibrosis D75.89
Osteomyelosclerosis D75.89
Osteonecrosis M87.9
  due to
    drugs — *see* Osteonecrosis, secondary, due to, drugs
    trauma — *see* Osteonecrosis, secondary, due to, trauma
  idiopathic aseptic M87.00
    ankle M87.07-
    carpus M87.03-
    clavicle M87.01-
    femur M87.05-
    fibula M87.06-
    finger M87.04-
    humerus M87.02-
    ilium M87.050
    ischium M87.050
    metacarpus M87.04-
    metatarsus M87.07-
    multiple site M87.09
    neck M87.08
    pelvis M87.050
    radius M87.03-
    rib M87.08
    scapula M87.01-
    skull M87.08
    tarsus M87.07-
    tibia M87.06-
    toe M87.07-
    ulna M87.03-
    vertebra M87.08
  secondary NEC M87.30
    carpus M87.33-
    clavicle M87.31-
    due to
      drugs M87.10
        carpus M87.13-
        clavicle M87.11-

Osteonecrosis—*continued*
  secondary—*continued*
    due to—*continued*
      drugs—*continued*
        femur M87.15-
        fibula M87.16-
        finger M87.14-
        humerus M87.12-
        ilium M87.159
        ischium M87.159
        jaw M87.180
        metacarpus M87.14-
        metatarsus M87.17-
        multiple sites M87.19
        neck M87.18
        radius M87.13-
        rib M87.18
        scapula M87.11-
        skull M87.18
        tarsus M87.17-
        tibia M87.16-
        toe M87.17-
        ulna M87.13-
        vertebra M87.18
      hemoglobinopathy NEC D58.2 [M90.50]
        carpus D58.2 [M90.54-]
        clavicle D58.2 [M90.51-]
        femur D58.2 [M90.55-]
        fibula D58.2 [M90.56-]
        finger D58.2 [M90.54-]
        humerus D58.2 [M90.52-]
        ilium D58.2 [M90.55-]
        ischium D58.2 [M90.55-]
        metacarpus D58.2 [M90.54-]
        metatarsus D58.2 [M90.57-]
        multiple sites D58.2 [M90.58]
        neck D58.2 [M90.58]
        radius D58.2 [M90.53-]
        rib D58.2 [M90.58]
        scapula D58.2 [M90.51-]
        skull D58.2 [M90.58]
        tarsus D58.2 [M90.57-]
        tibia D58.2 [M90.56-]
        toe D58.2 [M90.57-]
        ulna D58.2 [M90.53-]
        vertebra D58.2 [M90.58]
      trauma (previous) M87.20
        carpus M87.23-
        clavicle M87.21-
        femur M87.25-
        fibula M87.26-
        finger M87.24-
        humerus M87.22-
        ilium M87.25-
        ischium M87.25-
        metacarpus M87.24-
        metatarsus M87.27-
        multiple sites M87.29
        neck M87.28
        radius M87.23-
        rib M87.28
        scapula M87.21-
        skull M87.28
        tarsus M87.27-
        tibia M87.26-
        toe M87.27-
        ulna M87.23-
        vertebra M87.28
    femur M87.35-
    fibula M87.36-
    finger M87.34-
    humerus M87.32-
    ilium M87.350
    in
      caisson disease T70.3 [M90.50]
        carpus T70.3 [M90.54-]
        clavicle T70.3 [M90.51-]
        femur T70.3 [M90.55-]
        fibula T70.3 [M90.56-]
        finger T70.3 [M90.54-]
        humerus T70.3 [M90.52-]
        ilium T70.3 [M90.55-]
        ischium T70.3 [M90.55-]

Osteonecrosis—continued
 secondary—continued
  in—continued
   caisson disease—continued
    metacarpus T70.3 [M90.54-]
    metatarsus T70.3 [M90.57-]
    multiple sites T70.3 [M90.59]
    neck T70.3 [M90.58]
    radius T70.3 [M90.53-]
    rib T70.3 [M90.58]
    scapula T70.3 [M90.51-]
    skull T70.3 [M90.58]
    tarsus T70.3 [M90.57-]
    tibia T70.3 [M90.56-]
    toe T70.3 [M90.57-]
    ulna T70.3 [M90.53-]
    vertebra T70.3 [M90.58]
  ischium M87.350
  metacarpus M87.34-
  metatarsus M87.37-
  multiple site M87.39
  neck M87.38
  radius M87.33-
  rib M87.38
  scapula M87.319
  skull M87.38
  tarsus M87.379
  tibia M87.366
  toe M87.379
  ulna M87.33-
  vertebra M87.38
 specified type NEC M87.80
  carpus M87.83-
  clavicle M87.81-
  femur M87.85-
  fibula M87.86-
  finger M87.84-
  humerus M87.82-
  ilium M87.85-
  ischium M87.85-
  metacarpus M87.84-
  metatarsus M87.87-
  multiple sites M87.89
  neck M87.88
  radius M87.83-
  rib M87.88-
  scapula M87.81-
  skull M87.88
  tarsus M87.87-
  tibia M87.86-
  toe M87.87-
  ulna M87.83-
  vertebra M87.88
Osteo-onycho-arthro-dysplasia Q79.8
Osteo-onychodysplasia, hereditary Q79.8
Osteopathia condensans disseminata Q78.8
Osteopathy (see also Osteomyelitis, Osteonecrosis, Osteoporosis)
 after poliomyelitis M89.60
  carpus M89.64-
  clavicle M89.61-
  femur M89.65-
  fibula M89.66-
  finger M89.64-
  humerus M89.62-
  ilium M89.659
  ischium M89.659
  metacarpus M89.64-
  metatarsus M89.67-
  multiple sites M89.69
  neck M89.68
  radius M89.63-
  rib M89.68
  scapula M89.61-
  skull M89.68
  tarsus M89.67-
  tibia M89.66-
  toe M89.67-
  ulna M89.63-
  vertebra M89.68

Osteopathy—continued
 in (due to)
  renal osteodystrophy N25.0
  specified diseases classified elsewhere — see subcategory M90.8
Osteopenia M85.8-
 borderline M85.8-
Osteoperiostitis — see Osteomyelitis, specified type NEC
Osteopetrosis (familial) Q78.2
Osteophyte M25.70
 ankle M25.77-
 elbow M25.72-
 foot joint M25.77-
 hand joint M25.74-
 hip M25.75-
 knee M25.76-
 shoulder M25.71-
 spine M25.78
 vertebrae M25.78
 wrist M25.73-
Osteopoikilosis Q78.8
Osteoporosis (female) (male) M81.0
 with current pathological fracture M80.00
 age-related M81.0
  with current pathologic fracture M80.00
   carpus M80.04-
   clavicle M80.01-
   fibula M80.06-
   finger M80.04-
   humerus M80.02-
   ilium M80.05-
   ischium M80.05-
   metacarpus M80.04-
   metatarsus M80.07-
   pelvis M80.05-
   radius M80.03-
   scapula M80.01-
   tarsus M80.07-
   tibia M80.06-
   toe M80.07-
   ulna M80.03-
   vertebra M80.08
 disuse M81.8
  with current pathological fracture M80.80
   carpus M80.84-
   clavicle M80.81-
   fibula M80.86-
   finger M80.84-
   humerus M80.82-
   ilium M80.85-
   ischium M80.85-
   metacarpus M80.84-
   metatarsus M80.87-
   pelvis M80.85-
   radius M80.83-
   scapula M80.81-
   tarsus M80.87-
   tibia M80.86-
   toe M80.87-
   ulna M80.83-
   vertebra M80.88
 drug-induced — see Osteoporosis, specified type NEC
 idiopathic — see Osteoporosis, specified type NEC
 involutional — see Osteoporosis, age-related
 Lequesne M81.6
 localized M81.6
 postmenopausal M81.0
  with pathological fracture M80.00
   carpus M80.04-
   clavicle M80.01-
   fibula M80.06-
   finger M80.04-
   humerus M80.02-
   ilium M80.05-
   ischium M80.05-
   metacarpus M80.04-
   metatarsus M80.07-
   pelvis M80.05-
   radius M80.03-
   scapula M80.01-
   tarsus M80.07-

Osteoporosis—continued
 postmenopausal—continued
  with pathological fracture—continued
   tibia M80.06-
   toe M80.07-
   ulna M80.03-
   vertebra M80.08
 postoophorectomy — see Osteoporosis, specified type NEC
 postsurgical malabsorption — see Osteoporosis, specified type NEC
 post-traumatic — see Osteoporosis, specified type NEC
 senile — see Osteoporosis, age-related
 specified type NEC M81.8
  with pathological fracture M80.80
   carpus M80.84-
   clavicle M80.81-
   fibula M80.86-
   finger M80.84-
   humerus M80.82-
   ilium M80.85-
   ischium M80.85-
   metacarpus M80.84-
   metatarsus M80.87-
   pelvis M80.85-
   radius M80.83-
   scapula M80.81-
   tarsus M80.87-
   tibia M80.86-
   toe M80.87-
   ulna M80.83-
   vertebra M80.88
Osteopsathyrosis (idiopathica) Q78.0
Osteoradionecrosis, jaw (acute) (chronic) (lower) (suppurative) (upper) M27.2
Osteosarcoma (any form) — see Neoplasm, bone, malignant
Osteosclerosis Q78.2
 acquired M85.8-
 congenita Q77.4
 fragilitas (generalisata) Q78.2
 myelofibrosis D75.81
Osteosclerotic anemia D64.89
Osteosis
 cutis L94.2
 renal fibrocystic N25.0
Österreicher-Turner syndrome Q87.2
Ostium
 atrioventriculare commune Q21.2
 primum (arteriosum) (defect) (persistent) Q21.2
 secundum (arteriosum) (defect) (patent) (persistent) Q21.1
Ostrum-Furst syndrome Q75.8
Otalgia — see subcategory H92.0
Otitis (acute) H66.90
 with effusion (see also Otitis, media, nonsuppurative)
  purulent — see Otitis, media, suppurative
 adhesive — see subcategory H74.1
 chronic (see also Otitis, media, chronic)
  with effusion (see also Otitis, media, nonsuppurative, chronic)
 externa H60.90-
  abscess — see Abscess, ear, external
  acute (noninfective) H60.50-
   actinic H60.51-
   chemical H60.52-
   contact H60.53-
   eczematoid H60.54-
   infective — see Otitis, externa, infective
   reactive H60.55-
   specified NEC H60.59-
  cellulitis — see Cellulitis, ear
  chronic H60.6-
  diffuse — see Otitis, externa, infective, diffuse
  hemorrhagic — see Otitis, externa, infective, hemorrhagic
  in (due to)
   aspergillosis B44.89
   candidiasis B37.84
   erysipelas A46 [H62.40]

Overriding
aorta Q25.4
finger (acquired) — *see* Deformity, finger
congenital Q68.1
toe (acquired) (*see also* Deformity, toe, specified
NEC)
congenital Q66.8
Overstrained R53.83
heart — *see* Hypertrophy, cardiac
Overuse, muscle NEC M70.8-
Overweight E66.3
Overworked R53.83
Oviduct — *see* condition
Ovotestis Q56.0
Ovulation (cycle)
failure or lack of N97.0
pain N94.0
Ovum — *see* condition
Owren's disease or syndrome (parahemophilia)
D68.2
Ox heart — *see* Hypertrophy, cardiac
Oxalosis E72.53
Oxaluria E72.53
Oxycephaly, oxycephalic Q75.0
syphilitic, congenital A50.02
Oxyuriasis B80
Oxyuris vermicularis (infestation) B80
Ozena J31.0

P

Pachyderma, pachydermia L85.9
larynx (verrucosa) J38.7
Pachydermatocele (congenital) Q82.8
Pachydermoperiostosis (*see also* Osteoarthropathy,
hypertrophic, specified type NEC)
clubbed nail M89.40 [L62]
Pachygyria Q04.3
Pachymeningitis (adhesive) (basal) (brain) (cervical)
(chronic)(circumscribed) (external) (fibrous)
(hemorrhagic) (hypertrophic) (internal)
(purulent) (spinal) (suppurative) — *see*
Meningitis
Pachyonychia (congenital) Q84.5
Pacinian tumor — *see* Neoplasm, skin, benign
Pad, knuckle or Garrod's M72.1
Paget-Schroetter syndrome I82.890
Paget's disease
with infiltrating duct carcinoma — *see* Neoplasm,
breast, malignant
bone M88.9
carpus M88.84-
clavicle M88.81-
femur M88.85-
fibula M88.86-
finger M88.84-
humerus M88.82-
ilium M88.85-
in neoplastic disease — *see* Osteitis, deformans,
in neoplastic disease
ischium M88.85-
metacarpus M88.84-
metatarsus M88.87-
multiple sites M88.89
neck M88.88
radius M88.83-
rib M88.88
scapula M88.81-
skull M88.0
tarsus M88.87-
tibia M88.86-
toe M88.87-
ulna M88.83-
vertebra M88.88
breast (female) C50.01-
male C50.02-
extramammary (*see also* Neoplasm, skin, malignant)
anus C21.0
margin C44.51
skin C44.51

Paget's disease—*continued*
intraductal carcinoma — *see* Neoplasm, breast,
malignant
malignant — *see* Neoplasm, skin, malignant
breast (female) C50.01-
male C50.02-
unspecified site (female) C50.01-
male C50.02-
mammary — *see* Paget's disease, breast
nipple — *see* Paget's disease, breast
osteitis deformans — *see* Paget's disease, bone
Pain(s) (*see also* Painful) R52
abdominal R10.9
colic R10.83
generalized R10.84
with acute abdomen R10.0
lower R10.30
left quadrant R10.32
pelvic or perineal R10.2
periumbilical R10.33
right quadrant R10.31
rebound — *see* Tenderness, abdominal, rebound
severe with abdominal rigidity R10.0
tenderness — *see* Tenderness, abdominal
upper R10.10
epigastric R10.13
left quadrant R10.12
right quadrant R10.11
acute R52
due to trauma G89.11
neoplasm related G89.3
postprocedural NEC G89.18
post-thoracotomy G89.12
specified by site code to Pain, by site
adnexa (uteri) R10.2
anginoid — *see* Pain, precordial
anus K62.8
arm — *see* Pain, limb, upper
axillary (axilla) M79.62-
back (postural) M54.9
bladder R39.89
associated with micturition — *see* Micturition,
painful
bone — *see* Disorder, bone, specified type NEC
breast N64.4
broad ligament R10.2
cancer associated (acute) (chronic) G89.3
cecum — *see* Pain, abdominal
cervicobrachial M53.1
chest (central) R07.9
anterior wall R07.89
atypical R07.89
ischemic I20.9
musculoskeletal R07.89
non-cardiac R07.89
on breathing R07.1
pleurodynia R07.81
precordial R07.2
wall (anterior) R07.89
chronic R52
associated with significant psychosocial
dysfunction G89.4
due to trauma G89.21
neoplasm related G89.3
postoperative NEC G89.28
postprocedural NEC G89.28
post-thoracotomy G89.22
specified by site code to Pain, by site
coccyx M53.3
colon — *see* Pain, abdominal
coronary — *see* Angina
costochondral R07.1
diaphragm R07.1
due to cancer G89.3
due to device, implant or graft (*see also*
Complications, by site and type, specified
NEC) T85.84
arterial graft NEC T82.848
breast (implant) T85.84
catheter NEC T85.84
dialysis (renal) T82.848
intraperitoneal T85.84

Pain(s) —*continued*
due to device, implant or graft—*continued*
catheter NEC—*continued*
infusion NEC T82.848
spinal (epidural) (subdural) T85.84
urinary (indwelling) T83.84
electronic (electrode) (pulse generator)
(stimulator)
bone T84.84
cardiac T82.847
nervous system (brain) (peripheral nerve)
(spinal) T85.84
urinary T83.84
fixation, internal (orthopedic) NEC T84.84
gastrointestinal (bile duct) (esophagus) T85.84
genital NEC T83.84
heart NEC T82.847
infusion NEC T85.84
joint prosthesis T84.84
ocular (corneal graft) (orbital implant) NEC
T85.84
orthopedic NEC T84.84
specified NEC T85.84
urinary NEC T83.84
vascular NEC T82.848
ventricular intracranial shunt T85.84
due to malignancy (primary) (secondary) G89.3
ear — *see* subcategory H92.0
epigastric, epigastrium R10.13
eye — *see* Pain, ocular
face, facial R51
atypical G50.1
female genital organs NEC N94.89
finger — *see* Pain, limb, upper
flank — *see* Pain, abdominal
foot — *see* Pain, limb, lower
gallbladder K82.9
gas (intestinal) R14.1
gastric — *see* Pain, abdominal
generalized NOS R52
genital organ
female N94.89
male N50.8
groin — *see* Pain, abdominal, lower
hand — *see* Pain, limb, upper
head — *see* Headache
heart — *see* Pain, precordial
infra-orbital — *see* Neuralgia, trigeminal
intercostal R07.82
intermenstrual N94.0
jaw R68.84
joint M25.50
ankle M25.57-
elbow M25.52-
finger M79.64-
foot M79.67-
hand M79.64-
hip M25.55-
knee M25.56-
shoulder M25.51-
toe M79.67-
wrist M25.53-
kidney N23
laryngeal R07.0
leg — *see* Pain, limb, lower
limb M79.609
lower M79.60-
lower leg M79.66-
thigh M79.65-
toe M79.67-
upper M79.60-
axilla M79.62-
finger M79.64-
forearm M79.63-
hand M79.64-
upper arm M79.62-
loin M54.5
low back M54.5
lumbar region M54.5
mandibular R68.84
mastoid — *see* subcategory H92.0
maxilla R68.84
menstrual (*see also* Dysmenorrhea) N94.6

Pain(s) —continued
  metacarpophalangeal (joint) — see Pain, joint, hand
  metatarsophalangeal (joint) — see Pain, joint, foot
  mouth K13.79
  muscle — see Myalgia
  musculoskeletal (see also Pain, by site) M79.1
  myofascial M79.1
  nasal J34.89
  nasopharynx J39.2
  neck NEC M54.2
  nerve NEC — see Neuralgia
  neuromuscular — see Neuralgia
  nose J34.89
  ocular H57.1-
  ophthalmic — see Pain, ocular
  orbital region — see Pain, ocular
  ovary N94.89
  over heart — see Pain, precordial
  ovulation N94.0
  pelvic (female) R10.2
  penis N48.89
  pericardial — see Pain, precordial
  perineal, perineum R10.2
  pharynx J39.2
  pleura, pleural, pleuritic R07.89
  postoperative NOS G89.18
  postprocedural NOS G89.18
  post-thoracotomy G89.12
  precordial (region) R07.2
  premenstrual N94.3
  psychogenic (persistent) (any site) F45.41
  radicular (spinal) — see Radiculopathy
  rectum K62.8
  respiration R07.1
  retrosternal R07.2
  rheumatoid, muscular — see Myalgia
  rib R07.81
  root (spinal) — see Radiculopathy
  round ligament (stretch) R10.2
  sacroiliac M53.3
  sciatic — see Sciatica
  scrotum N50.8
  seminal vesicle N50.8
  shoulder M25.51-
  spermatic cord N50.8
  spinal root — see Radiculopathy
  spine M54.9
    cervical M54.2
    low back M54.5
      with sciatica M54.4-
    thoracic M54.6
  stomach — see Pain, abdominal
  substernal R07.2
  temporomandibular (joint) M26.62
  testis N50.8
  thoracic spine M54.6
    with radicular and visceral pain M54.14
  throat R07.0
  tibia — see Pain, limb, lower
  toe — see Pain, limb, lower
  tongue K14.6
  tooth K08.8
  trigeminal — see Neuralgia, trigeminal
  tumor associated G89.3
  ureter N23
  urinary (organ) (system) N23
  uterus NEC N94.89
  vagina R10.2
  vertebrogenic (syndrome) M54.89
  vesical R39.89
    associated with micturition — see Micturition, painful
  vulva R10.2
Painful (see also Pain)
  coitus
    female N94.1
    male N53.12
    psychogenic F52.6
  ejaculation (semen) N53.12
    psychogenic F52.6
  erection — see Priapism
  feet syndrome E53.8
  joint replacement (hip) (knee) T84.84

Painful—continued
  menstruation — see Dysmenorrhea
    psychogenic F45.8
  micturition — see Micturition, painful
  respiration R07.1
  scar NEC L90.5
  wire sutures T81.89
Painter's colic — see subcategory T56.0
Palate — see condition
Palatoplegia K13.79
Palatoschisis — see Cleft, palate
Palilalia R48.8
Palliative care Z51.5
Pallor R23.1
  optic disc, temporal — see Atrophy, optic
Palmar (see also condition)
  fascia — see condition
Palpable
  cecum K63.89
  kidney N28.89
  ovary N83.8
  prostate N42.9
  spleen — see Splenomegaly
Palpitations (heart) R00.2
  psychogenic F45.8
Palsy (see also Paralysis) G83.9
  atrophic diffuse (progressive) G12.22
  Bell's (see also Palsy, facial)
    newborn P11.3
  brachial plexus NEC G54.0
    newborn (birth injury) P14.3
  brain — see Palsy, cerebral
  bulbar (progressive) (chronic) G12.22
    of childhood (Fazio-Londe) G12.1
    pseudo NEC G12.29
    supranuclear NEC G12.22
  cerebral (congenital) G80.9
    ataxic G80.4
    athetoid G80.3
    choreathetoid G80.3
    diplegic G80.8
      spastic G80.1
    dyskinetic G80.3
      athetoid G80.3
      choreathetoid G80.3
      distonic G80.3
    dystonic G80.3
    hemiplegic G80.8
      spastic G80.2
    mixed G80.8
    monoplegic G80.8
      spastic G80.1
    paraplegic G80.8
      spastic G80.1
    quadriplegic G80.8
      spastic G80.0
    spastic G80.1
      diplegic G80.1
      hemiplegic G80.2
      monoplegic G80.1
      quadriplegic G80.0
      specified NEC G80.1
      tetrapelgic G80.0
    specified NEC G80.8
    syphilitic A52.12
      congenital A50.49
    tetraplegic G80.8
      spastic G80.0
  cranial nerve (see also Disorder, nerve, cranial)
    multiple G52.7
      in
        infectious disease B99 [G53]
        neoplastic disease (see also Neoplasm)
          D49.9 [G53]
        parasitic disease B89 [G53]
        sarcoidosis D86.82
  creeping G12.22
  diver's T70.3
  Erb's P14.0
  facial G51.0
    newborn (birth injury) P11.3
  glossopharyngeal G52.1
  Klumpke(-Déjérine) P14.1

Palsy—continued
  lead — see subcategory T56.0
  median nerve (tardy) G56.1-
  nerve G58.9
    specified NEC G58.8
  peroneal nerve (acute) (tardy) G57.3-
  pseudobulbar NEC G12.29
  radial nerve (acute) G56.3-
  seventh nerve (see also Palsy, facial)
    newborn P11.3
  shaking — see Parkinsonism
  spastic (cerebral) (spinal) G80.9
  ulnar nerve (tardy) G56.2-
  wasting G12.29
Paludism — see Malaria
Panangiitis M30.0
Panaris, panaritium (see also Cellulitis, digit)
  with lymphangitis — see Lymphangitis, acute, digit
Panarteritis nodosa M30.0
  brain or cerebral I67.7
Pancake heart R93.1
  with cor pulmonale (chronic) I27.81
Pancarditis (acute) (chronic) I51.89
  rheumatic I09.89
    active or acute I01.8
Pancoast's syndrome or tumor C34.1-
Pancolitis, ulcerative (chronic) K51.00
  with
    complication K51.019
      abscess K51.014
      fistula K51.013
      obstruction K51.012
      rectal bleeding K51.011
      specified complication NEC K51.018
Pancreas, pancreatic — see condition
Pancreatitis (annular) (apoplectic) (calcareous)
  (edematous) (hemorrhagic) (malignant)
  (recurrent) (subacute) (suppurative) K85.9
  acute K85.9
    alcohol induced K85.2
    biliary K85.1
    drug induced K85.3
    gallstone K85.1
    idiopathic K85.0
    specified NEC K85.8
  chronic (infectious) K86.1
    alcohol-induced K86.0
    recurrent K86.1
    relapsing K86.1
  cystic (chronic) K86.1
  cytomegaloviral B25.2
  fibrous (chronic) K86.1
  gangrenous K85.8
  gallstone K85.1
  interstitial (chronic) K86.1
    acute K85.8
  mumps B26.3
  recurrent (chronic) K86.1
  relapsing, chronic K86.1
  syphilitic A52.74
Pancreatoblastoma — see Neoplasm, pancreas,
    malignant
Pancreolithiasis K86.8
Pancytolysis D75.89
Pancytopenia (acquired) D61.81
  with malformations D61.09
  congenital D61.09
Panencephalitis, subacute, sclerosing A81.1
Panhematopenia D61.9
  congenital D61.09
  constitutional D61.09
  splenic, primary D73.1
Panhemocytopenia D61.9
  congenital D61.09
  constitutional D61.09
Panhypogonadism E29.1
Panhypopituitarism E23.0
  prepubertal E23.0
Panic (attack) (state) F41.0
  reaction to exceptional stress (transient) F43.0
Panmyelopathy, familial, constitutional D61.09
Panmyelophthisis D61.82
  congenital D61.09

Paralysis, paralytic —*continued*
- deglutition R13.0
  - hysterical F44.4
- dementia A52.17
- descending (spinal) NEC G12.29
- diaphragm (flaccid) J98.6
  - due to accidental dissection of phrenic nerve during procedure — *see* Puncture, accidental complicating surgery
- digestive organs NEC K59.8
- diplegic — *see* Diplegia
- divergence (nuclear) H51.8
- diver's T70.3
- Duchenne's
  - birth injury P14.0
  - due to or associated with
    - motor neuron disease G12.22
    - muscular dystrophy G71.0
  - due to intracranial or spinal birth injury — *see* Palsy, cerebral
- embolic (current episode) I63.4
- Erb(-Duchenne) (birth) (newborn) P14.0
- Erb's syphilitic spastic spinal A52.17
- esophagus K22.8
- eye muscle (extrinsic) H49.9
  - intrinsic (*see also* Paresis, of accommodation)
- facial (nerve) G51.0
  - birth injury P11.3
  - congenital P11.3
  - following operation NEC — *see* Puncture, accidental complicating surgery
  - newborn (birth injury) P11.3
- familial (recurrent) (periodic) G72.3
  - spastic G11.4
- fauces J39.2
- finger G56.9-
- gait R26.1
- gastric nerve (nondiabetic) G52.2
- gaze, conjugate H51.0
- general (progressive) (syphilitic) A52.17
  - juvenile A50.45
- glottis J38.00
  - bilateral J38.02
  - unilateral J38.01
- gluteal G54.1
- Gubler(-Millard) G46.3
- hand — *see* Monoplegia, upper limb
- heart — *see* Arrest, cardiac
- hemiplegic — *see* Hemiplegia
- hyperkalemic periodic (familial) G72.3
- hypoglossal (nerve) G52.3
- hypokalemic periodic G72.3
- hysterical F44.4
- ileus K56.0
- infantile (*see also* Poliomyelitis, paralytic) A80.30
  - bulbar — *see* Poliomyelitis, paralytic
  - cerebral — *see* Palsy, cerebral
  - spastic — *see* Palsy, cerebral, spastic
- infective — *see* Poliomyelitis, paralytic
- inferior nuclear G83.9
- internuclear — *see* Ophthalmoplegia, internuclear
- intestine K56.0
- iris H57.09
  - due to diphtheria (toxin) A36.89
- ischemic, Volkmann's (complicating trauma) T79.6
- Jackson's G83.89
- jake — *see* Poisoning, food, noxious, plant
- Jamaica ginger (jake) G62.2
- juvenile general A50.45
- Klumpke(-Déjérine) (birth) (newborn) P14.1
- labioglossal (laryngeal) (pharyngeal) G12.29
- Landry's G61.0
- laryngeal nerve (recurrent) (superior) (unilateral) J38.00
  - bilateral J38.02
  - unilateral J38.01
- larynx J38.00
  - bilateral J38.02
  - due to diphtheria (toxin) A36.2
  - unilateral J38.01
- lateral G12.21
- lead — *see* subcategory T56.0
- left side — *see* Hemiplegia

Paralysis, paralytic —*continued*
- leg G83.1-
  - both — *see* Paraplegia
  - crossed G83.89
  - hysterical F44.4
  - psychogenic F44.4
  - transient or transitory R29.81
    - traumatic NEC — *see* Injury, nerve, leg
- levator palpebrae superioris — *see* Blepharoptosis, paralytic
- limb — *see* Monoplegia
- lip K13.0
- Lissauer's A52.17
- lower limb — *see* Monoplegia, lower limb
  - both — *see* Paraplegia
- lung J98.4
- median nerve G56.1-
- medullary (tegmental) G83.89
- mesencephalic NEC G83.89
  - tegmental G83.89
- middle alternating G83.89
- Millard-Gubler-Foville G46.3
- monoplegic — *see* Monoplegia
- motor G83.9
- muscle, muscular NEC G72.8
  - due to nerve lesion G58.9
  - eye (extrinsic) H49.9
    - intrinsic — *see* Paresis, of accommodation
    - oblique — *see* Strabismus, paralytic, fourth nerve
  - iris sphincter H21.9
  - ischemic (Volkmann's) (complicating trauma) T79.6
  - progressive G12.21
  - pseudohypertrophic G71.0
- musculocutaneous nerve G56.9-
- musculospiral G56.9-
- nerve (*see also* Disorder, nerve)
  - abducent — *see* Strabismus, paralytic, sixth nerve
  - accessory G52.8
  - auditory (except Deafness) — *see* subcategory H93.3
  - birth injury P14.9
  - cranial or cerebral G52.9
  - facial G51.0
    - birth injury P11.3
    - newborn (birth injury) P11.3
  - fourth or trochlear — *see* Strabismus, paralytic, fourth nerve
  - newborn (birth injury) P14.9
  - oculomotor — *see* Strabismus, paralytic, third nerve
  - phrenic (birth injury) P14.2
  - radial G56.3-
  - seventh or facial G51.0
    - newborn (birth injury) P11.3
  - sixth or abducent — *see* Strabismus, paralytic, sixth nerve
  - syphilitic A52.15
  - third or oculomotor — *see* Strabismus, paralytic, third nerve
  - trigeminal G50.9
  - trochlear — *see* Strabismus, paralytic, fourth nerve
  - ulnar G56.2-
- normokalemic periodic G72.3
- ocular H49.9
  - alternating G83.89
- oculofacial, congenital (Moebius) Q87.0
- oculomotor (external bilateral) (nerve) — *see* Strabismus, paralytic, third nerve
- palate (soft) K13.79
- paratrigeminal G50.9
- periodic (familial) (hyperkalemic) (hypokalemic) (myotonic) (normokalemic) (potassium sensitive) (secondary) G72.3
- peripheral autonomic nervous system — *see* Neuropathy, peripheral, autonomic
- peroneal (nerve) G57.3-
- pharynx J39.2
- phrenic nerve G56.8-
- plantar nerve(s) G57.6-

Paralysis, paralytic —*continued*
- pneumogastric nerve G52.2
- poliomyelitis (current) — *see* Poliomyelitis, paralytic
- popliteal nerve G57.3-
- postepileptic transitory G83.84
- progressive (atrophic) (bulbar) (spinal) G12.22
  - general A52.17
  - infantile acute — *see* Poliomyelitis, paralytic
- pseudobulbar G12.29
- pseudohypertrophic (muscle) G71.0
- psychogenic F44.4
- quadriceps G57.9-
- quadriplegic — *see* Tetraplegia
- radial nerve G56.3-
- rectus muscle (eye) H49.9
- recurrent isolated sleep G47.53
- respiratory (muscle) (system) (tract) R06.81
  - center NEC G93.89
  - congenital P28.89
  - newborn P28.89
- right side — *see* Hemiplegia
- saturnine — *see* subcategory T56.0
- sciatic nerve G57.0-
- senile G83.9
- shaking — *see* Parkinsonism
- shoulder G56.9-
- sleep, recurrent isolated G47.53
- spastic G83.9
  - cerebral — *see* Palsy, cerebral, spastic
  - congenital (cerebral) — *see* Palsy, cerebral, spastic
  - familial G11.4
  - hereditary G11.4
  - quadriplegic G80.0
  - syphilitic (spinal) A52.17
- sphincter, bladder — *see* Paralysis, bladder
- spinal (cord) G83.9
  - accessory nerve G52.8
  - acute — *see* Poliomyelitis, paralytic
  - ascending acute G61.0
  - atrophic (acute) (*see also* Poliomyelitis, paralytic)
    - spastic, syphilitic A52.17
  - congenital NEC — *see* Palsy, cerebral
  - infantile — *see* Poliomyelitis, paralytic
  - hereditary G95.89
  - progressive G12.21
  - sequelae NEC G83.89
- sternomastoid G52.8
- stomach K31.89
  - diabetic — *see* Diabetes, by type, with gastroparesis
  - nerve G52.2
    - diabetic — *see* Diabetes, by type, with gastroparesis
- stroke — *see* Infarct, brain
- subcapsularis G56.8-
- supranuclear G12.29
- sympathetic G90.8
  - cervical G90.09
  - nervous system — *see* Neuropathy, peripheral, autonomic
- syndrome G83.9
  - specified NEC G83.89
- syphilitic spastic spinal (Erb's) A52.17
- thigh G57.9-
- throat J39.2
  - diphtheritic A36.0
  - muscle J39.2
- thrombotic (current episode) I63.3
- thumb G56.9-
- tick — *see* Toxicity, venom, arthropod, specified NEC
- Todd's (postepileptic transitory paralysis) G83.84
- toe G57.6-
- tongue K14.8
- transient R29.5
  - arm or leg NEC R29.81
  - traumatic NEC — *see* Injury, nerve
- trapezius G52.8
- traumatic, transient NEC — *see* Injury, nerve
- trembling — *see* Parkinsonism
- triceps brachii G56.9-
- trigeminal nerve G50.9

Paralysis, paralytic —continued
　trochlear (nerve) — see Strabismus, paralytic, fourth
　　　nerve
　ulnar nerve G56.2-
　upper limb — see Monoplegia, upper limb
　uremic N18.9 [G99.8]
　uveoparotitic D86.89
　uvula K13.79
　　postdiphtheritic A36.0
　vagus nerve G52.2
　vasomotor NEC G90.8
　velum palati K13.79
　vesical — see Paralysis, bladder
　vestibular nerve (except Vertigo) — see subcategory
　　　H93.3
　vocal cords J38.00
　　bilateral J38.02
　　unilateral J38.01
　Volkmann's (complicating trauma) T79.6
　wasting G12.29
　Weber's G46.3
　wrist G56.9-
Paramedial urethrovesical orifice Q64.79
Paramenia N92.6
Parametritis (see also Disease, pelvis, inflammatory)
　　　N73.2
　acute N73.0
　complicating abortion — see Abortion, by type,
　　　complicated by, parametritis
Parametrium, parametric — see condition
Paramnesia — see Amnesia
Paramolar K00.1
Paramyloidosis E85.8
Paramyoclonus multiplex G25.3
Paramyotonia (congenita) G71.19
Parangi — see Yaws
Paranoia (querulans) F22
　senile F03
Paranoid
　dementia (senile) F03
　　praecox — see Schizophrenia
　personality F60.0
　psychosis (climacteric) (involutional) (menopausal)
　　　F22
　　psychogenic (acute) F23
　　senile F03
　reaction (acute) F23
　　chronic F22
　schizophrenia F20.0
　state (climacteric) (involutional) (menopausal)
　　　(simple) F22
　　senile F03
　tendencies F60.0
　traits F60.0
　trends F60.0
　type, psychopathic personality F60.0
Paraparesis — see Paraplegia
Paraphasia R47.02
Paraphilia F65.9
Paraphimosis (congenital) N47.2
　chancroidal A57
Paraphrenia, paraphrenic (late) F22
　schizophrenia F20.0
Paraplegia (lower) G82.20
　ataxic — see Degeneration, combined, spinal cord
　complete G82.21
　congenital (cerebral) G80.8
　　spastic G80.1
　familial spastic G11.4
　functional (hysterical) F44.4
　hereditary, spastic G11.4
　hysterical F44.4
　incomplete G82.22
　Pott's A18.01
　psychogenic F44.4
　spastic
　　Erb's spinal, syphilitic A52.17
　　hereditary G11.4
　　tropical G04.1
　syphilitic (spastic) A52.17
　tropical spastic G04.1
Parapoxvirus B08.60
　specified NEC B08.69

Paraproteinemia D89.2
　benign (familial) D89.2
　monoclonal D47.2
　secondary to malignant disease D47.2
Parapsoriasis L41.9
　en plaques L41.4
　guttata L41.1
　large plaque L41.4
　retiform, retiformis L41.5
　small plaque L41.3
　specified NEC L41.8
　varioliformis (acuta) L41.0
Parasitic (see also condition)
　disease NEC B89
　stomatitis B37.0
　sycosis (beard) (scalp) B35.0
　twin Q89.4
Parasitism B89
　intestinal B82.9
　skin B88.9
　specified — see Infestation
Parasitophobia F40.218
Parasomnia G47.50
　due to
　　alcohol
　　　abuse F10.182
　　　dependence F10.282
　　　use F10.982
　　amphetamines
　　　abuse F15.182
　　　dependence F15.282
　　　use F15.982
　　caffeine
　　　abuse F15.182
　　　dependence F15.282
　　　use F15.982
　　cocaine
　　　abuse F14.182
　　　dependence F14.282
　　　use F14.982
　　drug NEC
　　　abuse F19.182
　　　dependence F19.282
　　　use F19.982
　　opioid
　　　abuse F11.182
　　　dependence F11.282
　　　use F11.982
　　psychoactive substance NEC
　　　abuse F19.182
　　　dependence F19.282
　　　use F19.982
　　sedative, hypnotic, or anxiolytic
　　　abuse F13.182
　　　dependence F13.282
　　　use F13.982
　　stimulant NEC
　　　abuse F15.182
　　　dependence F15.282
　　　use F15.982
　in conditions classified elsewhere G47.54
　nonorganic origin F51.8
　organic G47.50
　specified NEC G47.59
Paraspadias Q54.9
Paraspasmus facialis G51.8
Parasuicide (attempt)
　history of (personal) Z91.5
　　in family Z81.8
Parathyroid gland — see condition
Parathyroid tetany E20.9
Paratrachoma A74.0
Paratyphlitis — see Appendicitis
Paratyphoid (fever) — see Fever, paratyphoid
Paratyphus — see Fever, paratyphoid
Paraurethral duct Q64.79
　nonorganic origin F51.5
Paraurethritis (see also Urethritis)
　gonococcal (acute) (chronic) (with abscess) A54.1
Paravaccinia NEC B08.04
Paravaginitis — see Vaginitis
Parencephalitis (see also Encephalitis)
　sequelae G09

Parent-child conflict — see Conflict, parent-child
　estrangement NEC Z62.890
Paresis (see also Paralysis)
　accommodation — see Paresis, of accommodation
　Bernhardt's G57.1-
　bladder (sphincter) (see also Paralysis, bladder)
　　tabetic A52.17
　bowel, colon or intestine K56.0
　extrinsic muscle, eye H49.9
　general (progressive) (syphilitic) A52.17
　　juvenile A50.45
　heart — see Failure, heart
　insane (syphilitic) A52.17
　juvenile (general) A50.45
　of accommodation H52.52-
　peripheral progressive (idiopathic) G60.3
　pseudohypertrophic G71.0
　senile G83.9
　syphilitic (general) A52.17
　　congenital A50.45
　vesical NEC N31.2
Paresthesia (see also Disturbance, sensation)
　Bernhardt G57.1-
Paretic — see condition
Parinaud's
　conjunctivitis H10.89
　oculoglandular syndrome H10.89
　ophthalmoplegia H49.88-
Parkinsonism (idiopathic) (primary) G20
　with neurogenic orthostatic hypotension
　　　(symptomatic) G90.3
　arteriosclerotic G21.4
　dementia G31.83 [F02.80]
　　with behavioral disturbance G31.83 [F02.81]
　due to
　　drugs NEC G21.19
　　　neuroleptic G21.11
　neuroleptic induced G21.11
　postencephalitic G21.3
　secondary G21.9
　　due to
　　　arteriosclerosis G21.4
　　　drugs NEC G21.19
　　　　neuroleptic G21.11
　　　encephalitis G21.3
　　　external agents NEC G21.2
　　　syphilis A52.19
　　specified NEC G21.8
　syphilitic A52.19
　treatment-induced NEC G21.19
　vascular G21.4
Parkinson's disease, syndrome or tremor — see
　　Parkinsonism
Parodontitis — see Periodontitis
Parodontosis K05.4
Paronychia (see also Cellulitis, digit)
　with lymphangitis — see Lymphangitis, acute, digit
　candidal (chronic) B37.2
　tuberculous (primary) A18.4
Parorexia (psychogenic) F50.8
Parosmia R43.1
　psychogenic F45.8
Parotid gland — see condition
Parotitis, parotiditis (allergic)(nonspecific toxic)
　　　(purulent) (septic) (suppurative) see also
　　　Sialoadenitis
　epidemic — see Mumps
　infectious — see Mumps
　postoperative K91.89
　surgical K91.89
Parrot fever A70
Parrot's disease (early congenital syphilitic
　　　pseudoparalysis) A50.02
Parry-Romberg syndrome G51.8
Parry's disease or syndrome E05.00
　with thyroid storm E05.01
Pars planitis — see Cyclitis
Parsonage(-Aldren)-**Turner syndrome** G54.5
Parson's disease (exophthalmic goiter) E05.00
　with thyroid storm E05.01
Particolored infant Q82.8
Parturition — see Delivery

Perforation, perforated—*continued*
diverticulum (intestine) K57.80
  with bleeding K57.81
  large intestine K57.20
    with
      bleeding K57.21
      small intestine K57.40
        with bleeding K57.41
  small intestine K57.00
    with
      bleeding K57.01
      large intestine K57.40
        with bleeding K57.41
ear drum — *see* Perforation, tympanum
esophagus K22.3
ethmoidal sinus — *see* Sinusitis, ethmoidal
frontal sinus — *see* Sinusitis, frontal
gallbladder K82.2
heart valve — *see* Endocarditis
ileum K63.1
  newborn P78.0
  obstetrical trauma O71.5
  traumatic — *see* Laceration, intestine, small
instrumental, surgical (accidental) (blood vessel)
  (nerve) (organ) — *see* Puncture, accidental
  complicating surgery
intestine NEC K63.1
  with ectopic or molar pregnancy O08.6
  newborn P78.0
  obstetrical trauma O71.5
  traumatic — *see* Laceration, intestine
  ulcerative NEC K63.1
    newborn P78.0
jejunum, jejunal K63.1
  obstetrical trauma O71.5
  traumatic — *see* Laceration, intestine, small
  ulcer — *see* Ulcer, gastrojejunal, with perforation
joint prosthesis — *see* Complications, joint
  prosthesis, mechanical, specified NEC, by site
mastoid (antrum) (cell) — *see* Disorder, mastoid,
  specified NEC
maxillary sinus — *see* Sinusitis, maxillary
membrana tympani — *see* Perforation, tympanum
nasal
  septum J34.89
    congenital Q30.3
    syphilitic A52.73
  sinus J34.89
    congenital Q30.8
    due to sinusitis — *see* Sinusitis
palate (*see also* Cleft, palate) Q35.9
  syphilitic A52.79
palatal vault (*see also* Cleft, palate, hard) Q35.1
  syphilitic A52.79
  congenital A50.59
pars flaccida (ear drum) — *see* Perforation,
  tympanum, attic
pelvic
  floor S31.030
    with
      ectopic or molar pregnancy O08.6
      penetration into retroperitoneal space
        S31.031
      retained foreign body S31.040
        with penetration into retroperitoneal
          space S31.041
    following ectopic or molar pregnancy O08.6
    obstetrical trauma O70.1
  organ S37.99
    adrenal gland S37.818
    bladder — *see* Perforation, bladder
    fallopian tube S37.599
      bilateral S37.592
      unilateral S37.591
    kidney S37.09-
    obstetrical trauma O71.5
    ovary S37.499
      bilateral S37.492
      unilateral S37.491
    prostate S37.828
    specified organ NEC S37.898
    ureter — *see* Perforation, ureter
    urethra — *see* Perforation, urethra

Perforation, perforated—*continued*
pelvic—*continued*
  organ—*continued*
    uterus — *see* Perforation, uterus
perineum — *see* Laceration, perineum
pharynx J39.2
rectum K63.1
  newborn P78.0
  obstetrical trauma O71.5
  traumatic S36.63
root canal space due to endodontic treatment
  M27.51
sigmoid K63.1
  newborn P78.0
  obstetrical trauma O71.5
  traumatic S36.533
sinus (accessory) (chronic) (nasal) J34.89
sphenoidal sinus — *see* Sinusitis, sphenoidal
surgical (accidental) (by instrument) (blood vessel)
  (nerve) (organ) — *see* Puncture, accidental
  complicating surgery
traumatic
  external — *see* Puncture
  eye — *see* Puncture, eyeball
  internal organ — *see* Injury, by site
tympanum, tympanic (membrane) (persistent
  post-traumatic) (postinflammatory) H72.9-
  attic H72.1-
    multiple — *see* Perforation, tympanum,
      multiple
    total — *see* Perforation, tympanum, total
  central H72.0-
    multiple — *see* Perforation, tympanum,
      multiple
    total — *see* Perforation, tympanum, total
  marginal NEC — *see* subcategory H72.2
  multiple H72.81-
  pars flaccida — *see* Perforation, tympanum, attic
  total H72.82-
  traumatic, current episode S09.2-
typhoid, gastrointestinal — *see* Typhoid
ulcer — *see* Ulcer, by site, with perforation
ureter N28.89
  traumatic S37.19
urethra N36.8
  with ectopic or molar pregnancy O08.6
  following ectopic or molar pregnancy O08.6
  obstetrical trauma O71.5
  traumatic S37.39
    at delivery O71.5
uterus
  with ectopic or molar pregnancy O08.6
  by intrauterine contraceptive device T83.39
  following ectopic or molar pregnancy O08.6
  obstetrical trauma O71.1
  traumatic S37.69
    obstetric O71.1
uvula K13.79
  syphilitic A52.79
vagina (*see also* Puncture, vagina) O71.4
Periadenitis mucosa necrotica recurrens K12.0
Periappendicitis (acute) — *see* Appendicitis
Periarteritis nodosa (disseminated) (infectious)
  (necrotizing) M30.0
Periarthritis (joint) (*see also* Enthesopathy)
  Duplay's M75.0-
  gonococcal A54.42
  humeroscapularis — *see* Capsulitis, adhesive
  scapulohumeral — *see* Capsulitis, adhesive
  shoulder — *see* Capsulitis, adhesive
  wrist M77.2-
Periarthrosis (angioneural) — *see* Enthesopathy
Pericapsulitis, adhesive (shoulder) — *see* Capsulitis,
  adhesive
Pericarditis (with decompensation) (with effusion)
  I31.9
  with rheumatic fever (conditions in I00)
    active — *see* Pericarditis, rheumatic
    inactive or quiescent I09.2
  acute (hemorrhagic) (infective) (nonrheumatic)
    (Sicca) I30.9
    with chorea (acute) (rheumatic) (Sydenham's)
      I02.0

Pericarditis—*continued*
acute—*continued*
  benign I30.8
  nonspecific I30.0
  rheumatic I01.0
    with chorea (acute) (Sydenham's) I02.0
adhesive or adherent (chronic) (external) (internal)
  I31.0
  acute — *see* Pericarditis, acute
  rheumatic I09.2
bacterial (acute) (subacute) (with serous or
  seropurulent effusion) I30.1
calcareous I31.1
cholesterol (chronic) I31.8
  acute I30.9
chronic (nonrheumatic) I31.9
  rheumatic I09.2
constrictive (chronic) I31.1
coxsackie B33.23
fibrinocaseous (tuberculous) A18.84
fibrinopurulent I30.1
fibrinous I30.8
fibrous I31.0
gonococcal A54.83
idiopathic I30.0
in systemic lupus erythematosus M32.12
infective I30.1
meningococcal A39.53
neoplastic (chronic) I31.8
  acute I30.9
obliterans, obliterating I31.0
plastic I31.0
pneumococcal I30.1
postinfarction I24.1
purulent I30.1
rheumatic (active) (acute) (with effusion) (with
  pneumonia) I01.0
  with chorea (acute) (rheumatic) (Sydenham's)
    I02.0
  chronic or inactive (with chorea) I09.2
rheumatoid — *see* Rheumatoid, carditis
septic I30.1
serofibrinous I30.8
staphylococcal I30.1
streptococcal I30.1
suppurative I30.1
syphilitic A52.06
tuberculous A18.84
uremic N18.9 [I32]
viral I30.1
Pericardium, pericardial — *see* condition
Pericellulitis — *see* Cellulitis
Pericementitis (chronic) (suppurative) (*see also*
  Periodontitis)
acute K05.20
  generalized K05.22
  localized K05.21
Perichondritis
auricle — *see* Perichondritis, ear
bronchus J98.09
ear (external) H61.00-
  acute H61.01-
  chronic H61.02-
external auditory canal — *see* Perichondritis, ear
larynx J38.7
  syphilitic A52.73
  typhoid A01.09
nose J34.89
pinna — *see* Perichondritis, ear
trachea J39.8
Periclasia K05.4
Pericoronitis — *see* Periodontitis
Pericystitis N30.90
  with hematuria N30.91
Peridiverticulitis (intestine) K57.92
cecum — *see* Diverticulitis, intestine, large
colon — *see* Diverticulitis, intestine, large
duodenum — *see* Diverticulitis, intestine, small
intestine — *see* Diverticulitis, intestine
jejunum — *see* Diverticulitis, intestine, small
rectosigmoid — *see* Diverticulitis, intestine, large
rectum — *see* Diverticulitis, intestine, large
sigmoid — *see* Diverticulitis, intestine, large

Periendocarditis — *see* Endocarditis
Periepididymitis N45.1
Perifolliculitis LØ1.Ø2
  abscedens, caput, scalp L66.3
  capitis, abscedens (et suffodiens) L66.3
  superficial pustular LØ1.Ø2
Perihepatitis K65.8
Perilabyrinthitis (acute) — *see* subcategory H83.Ø
Perimeningitis — *see* Meningitis
Perimetritis — *see* Endometritis
Perimetrosalpingitis — *see* Salpingo-oophoritis
Perineocele N81.81
Perinephric, perinephritic — *see* condition
Perinephritis (*see also* Infection, kidney)
  purulent — *see* Abscess, kidney
Perineum, perineal — *see* condition
Perineuritis NEC — *see* Neuralgia
Periodic — *see* condition
Periodontitis (chronic) (complex) (compound) (local)
  (simplex) KØ5.3Ø
  acute KØ5.2Ø
    generalized KØ5.22
    localized KØ5.21
  apical KØ4.5
    acute (pulpal origin) KØ4.4
  generalized KØ5.32
  localized KØ5.31
Periodontoclasia KØ5.4
Periodontosis (juvenile) KØ5.4
Periods (*see also* Menstruation)
  heavy N92.Ø
  irregular N92.6
  shortened intervals (irregular) N92.1
Perionychia (*see also* Cellulitis, digit)
  with lymphangitis — *see* Lymphangitis, acute, digit
Perioophoritis — *see* Salpingo-oophoritis
Periorchitis N45.2
Periosteum, periosteal — *see* condition
Periostitis (albuminosa) (circumscribed) (diffuse)
  (infective) (monomelic) (*see also* Osteomyelitis)
  alveolar M27.3
  alveolodental M27.3
  dental M27.3
  gonorrheal A54.43
  jaw (lower) (upper) M27.2
  orbit HØ5.Ø3-
  syphilitic A52.77
    congenital (early) A5Ø.Ø2 [M9Ø.8Ø]
    secondary A51.46
  tuberculous — *see* Tuberculosis, bone
  yaws (hypertrophic) (early) (late) A66.6 [M9Ø.8Ø]
Periostosis (hyperplastic) (*see also* Disorder, bone,
  specified type NEC)
  with osteomyelitis — *see* Osteomyelitis, specified
    type NEC
Peripartum
  cardiomyopathy O9Ø.3
Periphlebitis — *see* Phlebitis
Periproctitis K62.8
Periprostatitis — *see* Prostatitis
Perirectal — *see* condition
Perirenal — *see* condition
Perisalpingitis — *see* Salpingo-oophoritis
Perisplenitis (infectional) D73.89
Peristalsis, visible or reversed R19.2
Peritendinitis — *see* Enthesopathy
Peritoneum, peritoneal — *see* condition
Peritonitis (adhesive) (bacterial) (fibrinous)
  (hemorrhagic) (idiopathic) (localized)
  (perforative) (primary) (with adhesions) (with
  effusion) K65.9
  with or following
    abscess K65.1
    appendicitis K35.3
      with perforation or rupture K35.2
      localized K35.3
      generalized K35.2
    diverticular disease (intestine) K57.8Ø
      with bleeding K57.81

Peritonitis—*continued*
  with or following—*continued*
    diverticular disease—*continued*
      large intestine K57.2Ø
        with
          bleeding K57.21
          small intestine K57.4Ø
            with bleeding K57.41
      small intestine K57.ØØ
        with
          bleeding K57.Ø1
          large intestine K57.4Ø
            with bleeding K57.41
    ectopic or molar pregnancy OØ8.Ø
  acute (generalized) K65.Ø
  aseptic T81.61
  bile, biliary K65.3
  chemical T81.61
  chlamydial A74.81
  complicating abortion — *see* Abortion, by type,
    complicated by, pelvic peritonitis
  congenital P78.1
  chronic proliferative K65.8
  diaphragmatic K65.Ø
  diffuse K65.Ø
  diphtheritic A36.89
  disseminated K65.Ø
  due to
    bile K65.3
    foreign
      body or object accidentally left during a
        procedure (instrument) (sponge) (swab)
        T81.599
      substance accidentally left during a procedure
        (chemical) (powder) (talc) T81.61
    talc T81.61
    urine K65.8
  eosinophilic K65.8
    acute K65.Ø
  fibrocaseous (tuberculous) A18.31
  fibropurulent K65.Ø
  following ectopic or molar pregnancy OØ8.Ø
  general(ized) K65.Ø
  gonococcal A54.85
  meconium (newborn) P78.Ø
  neonatal P78.1
    meconium P78.Ø
  pancreatic K65.Ø
  paroxysmal, familial E85.Ø
    benign E85.Ø
  pelvic
    female N73.5
      acute N73.3
      chronic N73.4
        with adhesions N73.6
    male K65.Ø
  periodic, familial E85.Ø
  proliferative, chronic K65.8
  puerperal, postpartum, childbirth O85
  purulent K65.Ø
  septic K65.Ø
  specified NEC K65.8
  spontaneous bacterial K65.2
  subdiaphragmatic K65.Ø
  subphrenic K65.Ø
  suppurative K65.Ø
  syphilitic A52.74
    congenital (early) A5Ø.Ø8 [K67]
  talc T81.61
  tuberculous A18.31
  urine K65.8
Peritonsillar — *see* condition
Peritonsillitis J36
Perityphlitis K37
Periureteritis N28.89
Periurethral — *see* condition
Periurethritis (gangrenous) — *see* Urethritis
Periuterine — *see* condition
Perivaginitis — *see* Vaginitis
Perivasculitis, retinal — *see* Vasculitis, retina
Perivasitis (chronic) N49.1
Perivesiculitis (seminal) — *see* Vesiculitis

Perlèche NEC K13.Ø
  due to
    candidiasis B37.83
    moniliasis B37.83
    riboflavin deficiency E53.Ø
    vitamin B2 (riboflavin) deficiency E53.Ø
Pernicious — *see* condition
Pernio, perniosis T69.1
Perpetrator (of abuse) — *see* Index to External Cause
  of Injury, Perpetrator
Persecution
  delusion F22
  social Z6Ø.5
Perseveration (tonic) R48.8
Persistence, persistent (congenital)
  anal membrane Q42.3
    with fistula Q42.2
  arteria stapedia Q16.3
  atrioventricular canal Q21.2
  branchial cleft Q18.Ø
  bulbus cordis in left ventricle Q21.8
  canal of Cloquet Q14.Ø
  capsule (opaque) Q12.8
  cilioretinal artery or vein Q14.8
  cloaca Q43.7
  communication — *see* Fistula, congenital
  convolutions
    aortic arch Q25.4
    fallopian tube Q5Ø.6
    oviduct Q5Ø.6
    uterine tube Q5Ø.6
  double aortic arch Q25.4
  ductus arteriosus (Botalli) Q25.Ø
  fetal
    circulation P29.3
    form of cervix (uteri) Q51.828
    hemoglobin, hereditary (HPFH) D56.4
  foramen
    Botalli Q21.1
    ovale Q21.1
  Gartner's duct Q52.4
  hemoglobin, fetal (hereditary) (HPFH) D56.4
  hyaloid
    artery (generally incomplete) Q14.Ø
    system Q14.8
  hymen, in pregnancy or childbirth — *see* Pregnancy,
    complicated by, abnormal, vulva
  lanugo Q84.2
  left
    posterior cardinal vein Q26.8
    root with right arch of aorta Q25.4
    superior vena cava Q26.1
  Meckel's diverticulum Q43.Ø
    malignant — *see* Table of Neoplams, small
      intestine, malignant
  mucosal disease (middle ear) — *see* Otitis, media,
    suppurative, chronic, tubotympanic
  nail(s), anomalous Q84.6
  omphalomesenteric duct Q43.Ø
  organ or site not listed — *see* Anomaly, by site
  ostium
    atrioventriculare commune Q21.2
    primum Q21.2
    secundum Q21.1
  ovarian rests in fallopian tube Q5Ø.6
  pancreatic tissue in intestinal tract Q43.8
  primary (deciduous)
    teeth KØØ.6
    vitreous hyperplasia Q14.Ø
  pupillary membrane Q13.89
  right aortic arch Q25.4
  rhesus (Rh) titer — *see* Complication(s), transfusion,
    incompatibility reaction, Rh (factor)
  sinus
    urogenitalis
      female Q52.8
      male Q55.8
    venosus with imperfect incorporation in right
      auricle Q26.8
  thymus (gland) (hyperplasia) E32.Ø
  thyroglossal duct Q89.2
  thyrolingual duct Q89.2
  truncus arteriosus or communis Q2Ø.Ø

Persistence, persistent—*continued*
  tunica vasculosa lentis Q12.2
  umbilical sinus Q64.4
  urachus Q64.4
  vitelline duct Q43.0
Person (with)
  admitted for clinical research, as a control subject
    Z00.6
  awaiting admission to adequate facility elsewhere
    Z75.1
  concern (normal) about sick person in family Z63.6
  consulting on behalf of another Z71.0
  feigning illness Z76.5
  living (in)
    alone Z60.2
    boarding school Z59.3
    residential institution Z59.3
    without
      adequate housing (heating) (space) Z59.1
      housing (permanent) (temporary) Z59.0
      person able to render necessary care Z74.2
      shelter Z59.0
  on waiting list Z75.1
  sick or handicapped in family Z63.6
Personality (disorder) F60.9
  accentuation of traits (type A pattern) Z73.1
  affective F34.0
  aggressive F60.3
  amoral F60.2
  anacastic, anankastic F60.5
  antisocial F60.2
  anxious F60.6
  asocial F60.2
  asthenic F60.7
  avoidant F60.6
  borderline F60.3
  change due to organic condition (enduring) F07.0
  compulsive F60.5
  cycloid F34.0
  cyclothymic F34.0
  dependent F60.7
  depressive F34.1
  dissocial F60.2
  dual F44.81
  eccentric F60.89
  emotionally unstable F60.3
  expansive paranoid F60.0
  explosive F60.3
  fanatic F60.0
  haltose type F60.89
  histrionic F60.4
  hyperthymic F34.0
  hypothymic F34.1
  hysterical F60.4
  immature F60.89
  inadequate F60.7
  labile (emotional) F60.3
  mixed (nonspecific) F60.81
  morally defective F60.2
  multiple F44.81
  narcissistic F60.81
  obsessional F60.5
  obsessive(-compulsive) F60.5
  organic F07.0
  overconscientious F60.5
  paranoid F60.0
  passive(-dependent) F60.7
  passive-aggressive F60.89
  pathologic F60.9
  pattern defect or disturbance F60.9
  pseudopsychopathic (organic) F07.0
  pseudoretarded (organic) F07.0
  psychoinfantile F60.4
  psychoneurotic NEC F60.89
  psychopathic F60.2
  querulant F60.0
  sadistic F60.89
  schizoid F60.1
  self-defeating F60.7
  sensitive paranoid F60.0
  sociopathic (amoral) (antisocial) (asocial) (dissocial)
    F60.2
  specified NEC F60.89

Personality—*continued*
  type A Z73.1
  unstable (emotional) F60.3
Perthes' disease — *see* Legg-Calvé-Perthes disease
Pertussis (*see also* Whooping cough) A37.90
Perversion, perverted
  appetite F50.8
    psychogenic F50.8
  function
    pituitary gland E23.2
      posterior lobe E22.2
  sense of smell and taste R43.8
    psychogenic F45.8
  sexual — *see* Deviation, sexual
Pervious, congenital (*see also* Imperfect, closure)
  ductus arteriosus Q25.0
Pes (congenital) (*see also* Talipes)
  acquired (*see also* Deformity, limb, foot, specified
    NEC)
    planus — *see* Deformity, limb, flat foot
  adductus Q66.8
  cavus Q66.7
  deformity NEC, acquired — *see* Deformity, limb,
    foot, specified NEC
  planus (acquired) (any degree) (*see also* Deformity,
    limb, flat foot)
    rachitic sequelae (late effect) E64.3
  valgus Q66.6
Pest, pestis — *see* Plague
Petechia, petechiae R23.3
  newborn P54.5
Petechial typhus A75.9
Peter's anomaly Q13.4
Petit mal seizure — *see* Epilepsy, generalized,
  idiopathic
Petit's hernia — *see* Hernia, abdomen, specified site
  NEC
Petrellidosis B48.2
Petrositis H70.20-
  acute H70.21-
  chronic H70.22-
Peutz-Jeghers disease or syndrome Q85.8
Peyronie's disease N48.6
Pfeiffer's disease — *see* Mononucleosis, infectious
Phagedena (dry) (moist) (sloughing) (*see also*
  Gangrene)
  geometric L88
  penis N48.29
  tropical — *see* Ulcer, skin
  vulva N76.6
Phagedenic — *see* condition
Phakoma H35.89
Phakomatosis (*see also* specific eponymous
  syndromes) Q85.9
  Bourneville's Q85.1
  specified NEC Q85.8
Phantom limb syndrome (without pain) G54.7
  with pain G54.6
Pharyngeal pouch syndrome D82.1
Pharyngitis (acute) (catarrhal)(gangrenous) (infective)
  (malignant) (membranous) (phlegmonous)
  (pseudomembranous) (simple) (subacute)
  (suppurative) (ulcerative) (viral) J02.9
  with influenza, flu, or grippe — *see* Influenza, with,
    pharyngitis
  aphthous B08.5
  atrophic J31.2
  chlamydial A56.4
  chronic (atrophic) (granular) (hypertrophic) J31.2
  coxsackievirus B08.5
  diphtheritic A36.0
  enteroviral vesicular B08.5
  follicular (chronic) J31.2
  fusospirochetal A69.1
  gonococcal A54.5
  granular (chronic) J31.2
  herpesviral B00.2
  hypertrophic J31.2
  infectional, chronic J31.2
  influenzal — *see* Influenza, with, respiratory
    manifestations NEC
  lymphonodular, acute (enteroviral) B08.8
  pneumococcal J02.8

Pharyngitis—*continued*
  purulent J02.9
  putrid J02.9
  septic J02.0
  sicca J31.2
  specified organism NEC J02.8
  staphylococcal J02.8
  streptococcal J02.0
  syphilitic, congenital (early) A50.03
  tuberculous A15.8
  vesicular, enteroviral B08.5
  viral NEC J02.8
Pharyngoconjunctivitis, viral B30.2
Pharyngolaryngitis (acute) J06.0
  chronic J37.0
Pharyngoplegia J39.2
Pharyngotonsillitis, herpesviral B00.2
Pharyngotracheitis, chronic J42
Pharynx, pharyngeal — *see* condition
Phenomenon
  Arthus' — *see* Arthus' phenomenon
  jaw-winking Q07.8
  lupus erythematosus (LE) cell M32.9
  Raynaud's (secondary) I73.00
    with gangrene I73.01
  vasomotor R55
  vasospastic I73.9
  vasovagal R55
  Wenckebach's I44.1
Phenylketonuria E70.1
  classical E70.0
  maternal E70.1
Pheochromoblastoma
  specified site — *see* Neoplasm, malignant, by site
  unspecified site C74.10
Pheochromocytoma
  malignant
    specified site — *see* Neoplasm, malignant, by site
    unspecified site C74.10
  specified site — *see* Neoplasm, benign, by site
  unspecified site D35.00
Pheohyphomycosis — *see* Chromomycosis
Pheomycosis — *see* Chromomycosis
Phimosis (congenital) (due to infection) N47.1
  chancroidal A57
Phlebectasia (*see also* Varix)
  congenital Q27.4
Phlebitis (infective) (pyemic) (septic) (suppurative)
  I80.9
  antepartum — *see* Thrombophlebitis, antepartum
  blue — *see* Phlebitis, leg, deep
  breast, superficial I80.8
  cavernous (venous) sinus — *see* Phlebitis,
    intracranial (venous) sinus
  cerebral (venous) sinus — *see* Phlebitis, intracranial
    (venous) sinus
  chest wall, superficial I80.8
  cranial (venous) sinus — *see* Phlebitis, intracranial
    (venous) sinus
  deep (vessels) — *see* Phlebitis, leg, deep
  due to implanted device — *see* Complications, by
    site and type, specified NEC
  during or resulting from a procedure T81.72
  femoral vein (superficial) I80.1-
  femoropopliteal vein I80.0-
  gestational — *see* Phlebopathy, gestational
  hepatic veins I80.8
  iliofemoral — *see* Phlebitis, femoral vein
  intracranial (venous) sinus (any) G08
    nonpyogenic I67.6
  intraspinal venous sinuses and veins G08
    nonpyogenic G95.19
  lateral (venous) sinus — *see* Phlebitis, intracranial
    (venous) sinus
  leg I80.3
    antepartum — *see* Thrombophlebitis,
      antepartum
    deep (vessels) NEC I80.20-
      iliac I80.21-
      popliteal vein I80.22-
      specified vessel NEC I80.29-
      tibial vein I80.23-
    femoral vein (superficial) I80.1-

Phlebitis —*continued*
  leg—*continued*
    superficial (vessels) I80.0-
  longitudinal sinus — *see* Phlebitis, intracranial (venous) sinus
  lower limb — *see* Phlebitis, leg
  migrans, migrating (superficial) I82.1
  pelvic
    with ectopic or molar pregnancy O08.0
    following ectopic or molar pregnancy O08.0
    puerperal, postpartum O87.1
  popliteal vein — *see* Phlebitis, leg, deep, popliteal
  portal (vein) K75.1
  postoperative T81.72
  pregnancy — *see* Thrombophlebitis, antepartum
  puerperal, postpartum, childbirth O87.0
    deep O87.1
    pelvic O87.1
    superficial O87.0
  retina — *see* Vasculitis, retina
  saphenous (accessory) (great) (long) (small) — *see* Phlebitis, leg, superficial
  sinus (meninges) — *see* Phlebitis, intracranial (venous) sinus
  specified site NEC I80.8
  syphilitic A52.09
  tibial vein — *see* Phlebitis, leg, deep, tibial
  ulcerative I80.9
    leg — *see* Phlebitis, leg
  umbilicus I80.8
  uterus (septic) — *see* Endometritis
  varicose (leg) (lower limb) — *see* Varix, leg, with, inflammation
Phlebofibrosis I87.8
Phleboliths I87.8
Phlebopathy,
  gestational O22.9-
  puerperal O87.9
Phlebosclerosis I87.8
Phlebothrombosis (*see also* Thrombosis)
  antepartum — *see* Thrombophlebitis, antepartum
  pregnancy — *see* Thrombophlebitis, antepartum
  puerperal — *see* Thrombophlebitis, puerperal
Phlebotomus fever A93.1
Phlegmasia
  alba dolens O87.1
    nonpuerperal — *see* Phlebitis, femoral vein
  cerulea dolens — *see* Phlebitis, leg, deep
Phlegmon — *see* Abscess
Phlegmonous — *see* condition
Phlyctenulosis (allergic) (keratoconjunctivitis) (nontuberculous) (*see also* Keratoconjunctivitis)
  cornea — *see* Keratoconjunctivitis
  tuberculous A18.52
Phobia, phobic F40.9
  animal F40.218
    spiders F40.210
  examination F40.298
  reaction F40.9
  simple F40.298
  social F40.10
    generalized F40.11
  specific (isolated) F40.298
    animal F40.218
      spiders F40.210
    blood F40.230
    injection F40.231
    injury F40.233
    men F40.290
    natural environment F40.228
      thunderstorms F40.220
    situational F40.248
      bridges F40.242
      closed in spaces F40.240
      flying F40.243
      heights F40.241
    specified focus NEC F40.298
    transfusion F40.231
    women F40.291
  specified NEC F40.8
    medical care NEC F40.232
  state F40.9
Phocas' disease — *see* Mastopathy, cystic

Phocomelia Q73.1
  lower limb — *see* Agenesis, leg, with foot present
  upper limb — *see* Agenesis, arm, with hand present
Phoria H50.50
Phosphate-losing tubular disorder N25.0
Phosphatemia E83.39
Phosphaturia E83.39
Photodermatitis (sun) L56.8
  chronic L57.8
  due to drug L56.8
  light other than sun L59.8
Photokeratitis H16.13-
Photophobia H53.19
Photophthalmia — *see* Photokeratitis
Photopsia H53.19
Photoretinitis — *see* Retinopathy, solar
Photosensitivity, photosensitization (sun) skin L56.8
  light other than sun L59.8
Phrenitis — *see* Encephalitis
Phrynoderma (vitamin A deficiency) E50.8
Phthiriasis (pubis) B85.3
  with any infestation classifiable to B85.0-B85.2 B85.4
Phthirus infestation — *see* Phthiriasis
Phthisis (*see also* Tuberculosis)
  bulbi (infectional) — *see* Disorder, globe, degenerated condition, atrophy
  eyeball (due to infection) — *see* Disorder, globe, degenerated condition, atrophy
Phycomycosis — *see* Zygomycosis
Physalopteriasis B81.8
Physical restraint status Z78.1
Phytobezoar T18.9
  intestine T18.3
  stomach T18.2
Pian — *see* Yaws
Pianoma A66.1
Pica F50.8
  in adults F50.8
  infant or child F98.3
Picking, nose F98.8
Pick-Niemann disease — *see* Niemann-Pick disease or syndrome
Pick's
  cerebral atrophy G31.01 [F02.80]
    with behavioral disturbance G31.01 [F02.81]
  disease or syndrome (brain) G31.01 [F02.80]
    with behavioral disturbance G31.01 [F02.81]
Pickwickian syndrome E66.2
Piebaldism E70.39
Piedra (beard) (scalp) B36.8
  black B36.3
  white B36.2
Pierre Robin deformity or syndrome Q87.0
Pierson's disease or osteochondrosis M91.0
Pig-bel A05.2
Pigeon
  breast or chest (acquired) M95.4
    congenital Q67.7
    rachitic sequelae (late effect) E64.3
  breeder's disease or lung J67.2
  fancier's disease or lung J67.2
  toe — *see* Deformity, toe, specified NEC
Pigmentation (abnormal) (anomaly) L81.9
  conjunctiva H11.13-
  cornea (anterior) H18.01-
    posterior H18.05-
    stromal H18.06-
  diminished melanin formation NEC L81.6
  iron L81.8
  lids, congenital Q82.8
  limbus corneae — *see* Pigmentation, cornea
  metals L81.8
  optic papilla, congenital Q14.2
  retina, congenital (grouped) (nevoid) Q14.1
  scrotum, congenital Q82.8
  tattoo L81.8
Piles — *see* Hemorrhoids
Pili
  annulati or torti (congenital) Q84.1
  incarnati L73.1
Pill roller hand (intrinsic) — *see* Parkinsonism

Pilomatrixoma — *see* Neoplasm, skin, benign
  malignant — *see* Neoplasm, skin, malignant
Pilonidal — *see* condition
Pimple R23.8
Pinched nerve — *see* Neuropathy, entrapment
Pindborg tumor — *see* Cyst, calcifying odontogenic
Pineal body or gland — *see* condition
Pinealoblastoma C75.3
Pinealoma D44.5
  malignant C75.3
Pineoblastoma C75.3
Pineocytoma D44.5
Pinguecula H11.15-
Pingueculitis H10.81-
Pinhole meatus (*see also* Stricture, urethra) N35.9
Pink
  disease — *see* subcategory T56.1
  eye — *see* Conjunctivitis, acute, mucopurulent
Pinkus' disease (lichen nitidus) L44.1
Pinpoint
  meatus — *see* Stricture, urethra
  os (uteri) — *see* Stricture, cervix
Pins and needles R20.2
Pinta A67.9
  cardiovascular lesions A67.2
  chancre (primary) A67.0
  erythematous plaques A67.1
  hyperchromic lesions A67.1
  hyperkeratosis A67.1
  lesions A67.9
    cardiovascular A67.2
    hyperchromic A67.1
    intermediate A67.1
    late A67.2
    mixed A67.3
    primary A67.0
    skin (achromic) (cicatricial) (dyschromic) A67.2
      hyperchromic A67.1
      mixed (achromic and hyperchromic) A67.3
  papule (primary) A67.0
  skin lesions (achromic) (cicatricial) (dyschromic) A67.2
    hyperchromic A67.1
    mixed (achromic and hyperchromic) A67.3
  vitiligo A67.2
Pintids A67.1
Pinworm (disease) (infection) (infestation) B80
Piroplasmosis B60.0
Pistol wound — *see* Gunshot wound
Pitchers' elbow — *see* Derangement, joint, specified type NEC, elbow
Pithecoid pelvis Q74.2
  with disproportion (fetopelvic) O33.0
    causing obstructed labor O65.0
Pithiatism F48.8
Pitted — *see* Pitting
Pitting (*see also* Edema) R60.9
  lip R60.0
  nail L60.8
  teeth K00.4
Pituitary gland — *see* condition
Pituitary-snuff-taker's disease J67.8
Pityriasis (capitis) L21.0
  alba L30.5
  circinata (et maculata) L42
  furfuracea L21.0
  Hebra's L26
  lichenoides L41.0
    chronica L41.1
    et varioliformis (acuta) L41.0
  maculata (et circinata) L30.5
  nigra B36.1
  pilaris, Hebra's L44.0
  rosea L42
  rotunda L44.8
  rubra (Hebra) pilaris L44.0
  simplex L30.5
  specified type NEC L30.5
  streptogenes L30.5
  versicolor (scrotal) B36.0
Placenta, placental — *see* Pregnancy, complicated by (care of) (management affected by), specified condition

Placentitis O41.14-
Plagiocephaly Q67.3
Plague A20.9
  abortive A20.8
  ambulatory A20.8
  asymptomatic A20.8
  bubonic A20.0
  cellulocutaneous A20.1
  cutaneobubonic A20.1
  lymphatic gland A20.0
  meningitis A20.3
  pharyngeal A20.8
  pneumonic (primary) (secondary) A20.2
  pulmonary, pulmonic A20.2
  septicemic A20.7
  tonsillar A20.8
    septicemic A20.7
Planning, family
  contraception Z30.9
  procreation Z31.69
Plaque(s)
  artery, arterial — *see* Arteriosclerosis
  calcareous — *see* Calcification
  coronary, lipid rich I25.83
  epicardial I31.8
  erythematous, of pinta A67.1
  Hollenhorst's — *see* Occlusion, artery, retina
  lipid rich, coronary I25.83
  pleural (without asbestos) J92.9
    with asbestos J92.0
  tongue K13.29
Plasmacytoma C90.3-
  extramedullary C90.2-
  medullary C90.0-
  solitary C90.3-
Plasmacytopenia D72.818
Plasmacytosis D72.822
Plaster ulcer — *see* Ulcer, pressure, by site
Plateau iris syndrome (post-iridectomy)
    (postprocedural) H21.82
Platybasia Q75.8
Platyonychia (congenital) Q84.6
  acquired L60.8
Platypelloid pelvis M95.5
  with disproportion (fetopelvic) O33.0
    causing obstructed labor O65.0
  congenital Q74.2
Platyspondylisis Q76.49
Plaut(-Vincent) **disease** (*see also* Vincent's) A69.1
Plethora R23.2
  newborn P61.1
Pleura, pleural — *see* condition
Pleuralgia R07.89
Pleurisy (acute) (adhesive) (chronic) (costal)
    (diaphragmatic) (double) (dry) (fibrinous)
    (fibrous) (interlobar) (latent) (plastic) (primary)
    (residual) (sicca) (sterile) (subacute) (unresolved)
    R09.1
  with
    adherent pleura J86.0
    effusion J90
      chylous, chyliform J94.0
      tuberculous (non primary) A15.6
        primary (progressive) A15.7
    tuberculosis — *see* Pleurisy, tuberculous (non
      primary)
  encysted — *see* Pleurisy, with effusion
  exudative — *see* Pleurisy, with effusion
  fibrinopurulent, fibropurulent — *see* Pyothorax
  hemorrhagic — *see* Hemothorax
  pneumococcal J90
  purulent — *see* Pyothorax
  septic — *see* Pyothorax
  serofibrinous — *see* Pleurisy, with effusion
  seropurulent — *see* Pyothorax
  serous — *see* Pleurisy, with effusion
  staphylococcal J86.9
  streptococcal J90
  suppurative — *see* Pyothorax
  traumatic (post) (current) — *see* Injury, intrathoracic,
    pleura
  tuberculous (with effusion) (non primary) A15.6
    primary (progressive) A15.7

Pleuritis sicca — *see* Pleurisy
Pleurobronchopneumonia — *see* Pneumonia,
  broncho-
Pleurodynia R07.81
  epidemic B33.0
  viral B33.0
Pleuropericarditis (*see also* Pericarditis)
  acute I30.9
Pleuropneumonia (acute) (bilateral) (double) (septic)
    (*see also* Pneumonia) J18.8
  chronic — *see* Fibrosis, lung
Pleuro-pneumonia-like-organism (PPLO), **as cause
    of disease classified elsewhere** B96.0
Pleurorrhea — *see* Pleurisy, with effusion
Plexitis, brachial G54.0
Plica
  polonica B85.0
  syndrome, knee M67.5-
  tonsil J35.8
Plicated tongue K14.5
Plug
  bronchus NEC J98.09
  meconium (newborn) NEC syndrome P76.0
  mucus — *see* Asphyxia, mucus
Plumbism — *see* subcategory T56.0
Plummer's disease E05.20
  with thyroid storm E05.21
Plummer-Vinson syndrome D50.1
Pluricarential syndrome of infancy E40
Plus (and minus) **hand** (intrinsic) — *see* Deformity,
    limb, specified type NEC, forearm
Pneumathemia — *see* Air, embolism
Pneumatic hammer (drill) syndrome T75.21
Pneumatocele (lung) J98.4
  intracranial G93.89
  tension J44.9
Pneumatosis
  cystoides intestinalis K63.89
  intestinalis K63.89
  peritonei K66.8
Pneumaturia R39.89
Pneumoblastoma — *see* Neoplasm, lung, malignant
Pneumocephalus G93.89
Pneumococcemia A40.3
Pneumococcus, pneumococcal — *see* condition
Pneumoconiosis (due to) (inhalation of) J64
  with tuberculosis (any type in A15) J65
  aluminum J63.0
  asbestos J61
  bagasse, bagassosis J67.1
  bauxite J63.1
  beryllium J63.2
  coal miners' (simple) J60
  coalworkers' (simple) J60
  collier's J60
  cotton dust J66.0
  diatomite (diatomaceous earth) J62.8
  dust
    inorganic NEC J63.6
    lime J62.8
    marble J62.8
    organic NEC J66.8
  fumes or vapors (from silo) J68.9
  graphite J63.3
  grinder's J62.8
  kaolin J62.8
  mica J62.8
  millstone maker's J62.8
  mineral fibers NEC J61
  miner's J60
  moldy hay J67.0
  potter's J62.8
  rheumatoid — *see* Rheumatoid, lung
  sandblaster's J62.8
  silica, silicate NEC J62.8
    with carbon J60
  stonemason's J62.8
  talc (dust) J62.0
Pneumocystis carinii pneumonia B59
Pneumocystis jiroveci (pneumonia) B59
Pneumocystosis (with pneumonia) B59
Pneumohemopericardium I31.2

Pneumohemothorax J94.2
  traumatic S27.2
Pneumohydropericardium — *see* Pericarditis
Pneumohydrothorax — *see* Hydrothorax
Pneumomediastinum J98.2
  congenital or perinatal P25.2
Pneumomycosis B49 [J99]
Pneumonia (acute) (Alpenstich) (benign) (bilateral)
    (brain) (cerebral) (circumscribed) (congestive)
    (creeping) (delayed resolution) (double)
    (epidemic) (fever) (flash) (fulminant) (fungoid)
    (granulomatous) (hemorrhagic) (incipient)
    (infantile) (infectious) (infiltration) (insular)
    (intermittent) (latent) (migratory) (organized)
    (overwhelming) (primary (atypical)) (progressive)
    (pseudolobar) (purulent) (resolved) (secondary)
    (senile) (septic) (suppurative) (terminal) (true)
    (unresolved) (vesicular) J18.9
  with
    influenza — *see* Influenza, with, pneumonia
    lung abscess J85.1
      due to specified organism — *see* Pneumonia,
        in (due to)
  adenoviral J12.0
  adynamic J18.2
  alba A50.04
  allergic (eosinophilic) J82
  alveolar — *see* Pneumonia, lobar
  anaerobes J15.8
  anthrax A22.1
  apex, apical — *see* Pneumonia, lobar
  Ascaris B77.81
  aspiration J69.0
    due to
      aspiration of microorganisms
        bacterial J15.9
        viral J12.9
      food (regurgitated) J69.0
      gastric secretions J69.0
      milk (regurgitated) J69.0
      oils, essences J69.1
      solids, liquids NEC J69.8
      vomitus J69.0
    newborn P24.81
      amniotic fluid (clear) P24.11
      blood P24.21
      liquor (amnii) P24.11
      meconium P24.01
      milk P24.31
      mucus P24.11
      food (regurgitated) P24.31
      specified NEC P24.81
      stomach contents P24.31
  atypical NEC J18.9
  bacillus J15.9
    specified NEC J15.8
  bacterial J15.9
    specified NEC J15.8
  Bacteroides (fragilis) (oralis) (melaninogenicus)
    J15.8
  basal, basic, basilar — *see* Pneumonia, by type
  bronchiolitis obliterans organized (BOOP) J84.8
  broncho-, bronchial (confluent) (croupous) (diffuse)
    (disseminated) (hemorrhagic) (involving
    lobes) (lobar) (terminal) J18.0
    allergic (eosinophilic) J82
    aspiration — *see* Pneumonia, aspiration
    bacterial J15.9
      specified NEC J15.8
    chronic — *see* Fibrosis, lung
    diplococcal J13
    Eaton's agent J15.7
    Escherichia coli (E. coli) J15.5
    Friedländer's bacillus J15.0
    Hemophilus influenzae J14
    hypostatic J18.2
    inhalation (*see also* Pneumonia, aspiration
      due to fumes or vapors (chemical) J68.0
      of oils or essences J69.1
    Klebsiella (pneumoniae) J15.0
    lipid, lipoid J69.1
      endogenous J84.8
    Mycoplasma (pneumoniae) J15.7

Pneumonia—*continued*
  broncho-, bronchial—*continued*
    pleuro-pneumonia-like-organisms (PPLO) J15.7
    pneumococcal J13
    Proteus J15.6
    Pseudomonas J15.1
    Serratia marcescens J15.6
    specified organism NEC J16.8
    staphylococcal — *see* Pneumonia, staphylococcal
    streptococcal NEC J15.4
      group B J15.3
      pneumoniae J13
    viral, virus — *see* Pneumonia, viral
  Butyrivibrio (fibriosolvens) J15.8
  Candida B37.1
  caseous — *see* Tuberculosis, pulmonary
  catarrhal — *see* Pneumonia, broncho
  chlamydial J16.0
    congenital P23.1
  cholesterol J84.8
  cirrhotic (chronic) — *see* Fibrosis, lung
  Clostridium (haemolyticum) (novyi) J15.8
  confluent — *see* Pneumonia, broncho
  congenital (infective) P23.9
    due to
      bacterium NEC P23.6
      Chlamydia P23.1
      Escherichia coli P23.4
      Haemophilus influenzae P23.6
      infective organism NEC P23.8
      Klebsiella pneumoniae P23.6
      Mycoplasma P23.6
      Pseudomonas P23.5
      Staphylococcus P23.2
      Streptococcus (except group B) P23.6
        group B P23.3
      viral agent P23.0
    specified NEC P23.8
  croupous — *see* Pneumonia, lobar
  cryptogenic organizing J84.2
  cytomegalic inclusion B25.0
  cytomegaloviral B25.0
  deglutition — *see* Pneumonia, aspiration
  desquamative interstitial J84.8
  diffuse — *see* Pneumonia, broncho
  diplococcal, diplococcus (broncho) (lobar) J13
  disseminated (focal) — *see* Pneumonia, broncho
  Eaton's agent J15.7
  embolic, embolism — *see* Embolism, pulmonary
  Enterobacter J15.6
  eosinophilic J82
  Escherichia coli (E. coli) J15.5
  Eubacterium J15.8
  fibrinous — *see* Pneumonia, lobar
  fibroid, fibrous (chronic) — *see* Fibrosis, lung
  Friedländer's bacillus J15.0
  Fusobacterium (nucleatum) J15.8
  gangrenous J85.0
  giant cell (measles) B05.2
  gonococcal A54.84
  gram-negative bacteria NEC J15.6
    anaerobic J15.8
  Hemophilus influenzae (broncho) (lobar) J14
  human metapneumovirus J12.3
  hypostatic (broncho) (lobar) J18.2
  in (due to)
    actinomycosis A42.0
    adenovirus J12.0
    anthrax A22.1
    ascariasis B77.81
    aspergillosis B44.9
    Bacillus anthracis A22.1
    Bacterium anitratum J15.6
    candidiasis B37.1
    chickenpox B01.2
    Chlamydia J16.0
      neonatal P23.1
    coccidioidomycosis B38.2
      acute B38.0
      chronic B38.1
    cytomegalovirus disease B25.0
    Diplococcus (pneumoniae) J13

Pneumonia—*continued*
  in (due to)—*continued*
    Eaton's agent J15.7
    Enterobacter J15.6
    Escherichia coli (E. coli) J15.5
    Friedländer's bacillus J15.0
    fumes and vapors (chemical) (inhalation) J68.0
    gonorrhea A54.84
    Hemophilus influenzae (H. influenzae) J14
    Herellea J15.6
    histoplasmosis B39.2
      acute B39.0
      chronic B39.1
    human metapneumovirus J12.3
    Klebsiella (pneumoniae) J15.0
    measles B05.2
    Mycoplasma (pneumoniae) J15.7
    nocardiosis, nocardiasis A43.0
    ornithosis A70
    parainfluenza virus J12.2
    pleuro-pneumonia-like-organism (PPLO) J15.7
    pneumococcus J13
    pneumocystosis (Pneumocystis carinii)
        (Pneumocystis jiroveci) B59
    Proteus J15.6
    Pseudomonas NEC J15.1
      pseudomallei A24.1
    psittacosis A70
    Q fever A78
    respiratory syncytial virus J12.1
    rheumatic fever I00 [J17]
    rubella B06.81
    Salmonella (infection) A02.22
      typhi A01.03
    schistosomiasis B65.9 [J17]
    Serratia marcescens J15.6
    specified
      bacterium NEC J15.8
      organism NEC J16.8
    spirochetal NEC A69.8
    Staphylococcus J15.20
      aureus J15.21
      specified NEC J15.29
    Streptococcus J15.4
      group B J15.3
      pneumoniae J13
      specified NEC J15.4
    toxoplasmosis B58.3
    tularemia A21.2
    typhoid (fever) A01.03
    varicella B01.2
    virus — *see* Pneumonia, viral
    whooping cough A37.91
      due to
        Bordetella parapertussis A37.11
        Bordetella pertussis A37.01
        specified NEC A37.81
    Yersinia pestis A20.2
  inhalation of food or vomit — *see* Pneumonia,
      aspiration
  interstitial J84.9
    chronic J84.1
    lymphoid J84.2
    plasma cell B59
    pseudomonas J15.1
    usual J84.1
  Klebsiella (pneumoniae) J15.0
  lipid, lipoid (exogenous) J69.1
    endogenous J84.2
  lobar (disseminated) (double) (interstitial) J18.1
    bacterial J15.9
      specified NEC J15.8
    chronic — *see* Fibrosis, lung
    Escherichia coli (E. coli) J15.5
    Friedländer's bacillus J15.0
    Hemophilus influenzae J14
    hypostatic J18.2
    Klebsiella (pneumoniae) J15.0
    pneumococcal J13
    Proteus J15.6
    Pseudomonas J15.1
    specified organism NEC J16.8

Pneumonia—*continued*
  lobar—*continued*
    staphylococcal — *see* Pneumonia, staphylococcal
    streptococcal NEC J15.4
    Streptococcus pneumoniae J13
    viral, virus — *see* Pneumonia, viral
  lobular — *see* Pneumonia, broncho
  Löffler's J82
  lymphoid interstitial J84.2
  massive — *see* Pneumonia, lobar
  meconium P24.01
  Mycoplasma (pneumoniae) J15.7
  multilobar — *see* Pneumonia, by type
  necrotic J85.0
  neonatal P23.9
    aspiration — *see* Aspiration, by substance, with
        pneumonia
  nitrogen dioxide J68.9
  orthostatic J18.2
  parainfluenza virus J12.2
  parenchymatous — *see* Fibrosis, lung
  passive J18.2
  patchy — *see* Pneumonia, broncho
  Peptococcus J15.8
  Peptostreptococcus J15.8
  plasma cell (of infants) B59
  pleurolobar — *see* Pneumonia, lobar
  pleuro-pneumonia-like organism (PPLO) J15.7
  pneumococcal (broncho) (lobar) J13
  Pneumocystis (carinii) (jiroveci) B59
  postinfectional NEC B99 [J17]
  postmeasles B05.2
  Proteus J15.6
  Pseudomonas J15.1
  psittacosis A70
  radiation J70.0
  respiratory syncytial virus J12.1
  resulting from a procedure J95.89
  rheumatic I00 [J17]
  Salmonella (arizonae) (cholerae-suis) (enteritidis)
      (typhimurium) A02.22
    typhi A01.03
    typhoid fever A01.03
  SARS-associated coronavirus J12.81
  segmented, segmental — *see* Pneumonia, broncho-
  Serratia marcescens J15.6
  specified NEC J18.8
    bacterium NEC J15.8
    organism NEC J16.8
    virus NEC J12.89
  spirochetal NEC A69.8
  staphylococcal (broncho) (lobar) J15.20
    aureus J15.21
    specified NEC J15.29
  static, stasis J18.2
  streptococcal NEC (broncho) (lobar) J15.4
    group
      A J15.4
      B J15.3
      specified NEC J15.4
  Streptococcus pneumoniae J13
  syphilitic, congenital (early) A50.04
  traumatic (complication) (early) (secondary) T79.8
  tuberculous (any) — *see* Tuberculosis, pulmonary
  tularemic A21.2
  varicella B01.2
  Veillonella J15.8
  ventilator associated J95.851
  viral, virus (broncho) (interstitial) (lobar) J12.9
    adenoviral J12.0
    congenital P23.0
    human metapneumovirus J12.3
    parainfluenza J12.2
    respiratory syncytial J12.1
    SARS-associated coronavirus J12.81
    specified NEC J12.89
  white (congenital) A50.04
Pneumonic — *see* condition

Pneumonitis (acute) (primary) (*see also* Pneumonia)
 air-conditioner J67.7
 allergic (due to) J67.9
  organic dust NEC J67.8
  red cedar dust J67.8
  sequoiosis J67.8
  wood dust J67.8
 aspiration J69.0
  due to
   anesthesia J95.4
    during
     labor and delivery O74.0
     pregnancy O29.01-
     puerperium O89.01
   fumes or gases J68.0
   obstetric O74.0
 chemical (due to gases, fumes or vapors)
  (inhalation) J68.0
 cholesterol J84.8
 crack (cocaine) J68.0
 chronic — *see* Fibrosis, lung
 congenital rubella P35.0
 due to
  beryllium J68.0
  cadmium J68.0
  crack (cocaine) J68.0
  detergent J69.8
  fluorocarbon-polymer J68.0
  food, vomit (aspiration) J69.0
  fumes or vapors J68.0
  gases, fumes or vapors (inhalation) J68.0
  inhalation
   blood J69.8
   essences J69.1
   food (regurgitated), milk, vomit J69.0
   oils, essences J69.1
   saliva J69.0
   solids, liquids NEC J69.8
  manganese J68.0
  nitrogen dioxide J68.0
  oils, essences J69.1
  solids, liquids NEC J69.8
  toxoplasmosis (acquired) B58.3
   congenital P37.1
  vanadium J68.0
  ventilator J95.851
 eosinophilic J82
 hypersensitivity J67.9
  air conditioner lung J67.7
  bagassosis J67.1
  bird fancier's lung J67.2
  farmer's lung J67.0
  maltworker's lung J67.4
  maple bark-stripper's lung J67.6
  mushroom worker's lung J67.5
  specified organic dust NEC J67.8
  suberosis J67.3
 interstitial (chronic) J84.1
  lymphoid J84.2
 lymphoid, interstitial J84.2
 meconium P24.01
 postanesthetic J95.4
  correct substance properly administered — *see*
   Table of Drugs and Chemcials, by drug,
   adverse effect
  in labor and delivery O74.0
  in pregnancy O29.01-
  obstetric O74.0
  overdose or wrong substance given or taken (by
   accident) — *see* Table of Drugs and
   Chemicals, by drug, poisoning
  postpartum, puerperal O89.01
 postoperative J95.4
  obstetric O74.0
 radiation J70.0
 rubella, congenital P35.0
 ventilation (air-conditioning) J67.7
 ventilator associated J95.851
 wood-dust J67.8
Pneumonoconiosis — *see* Pneumoconiosis
Pneumoparotid K11.8

Pneumopathy NEC J98.4
 alveolar J84.0
 due to organic dust NEC J66.8
 parietoalveolar J84.0
Pneumopericarditis (*see also* Pericarditis)
 acute I30.9
Pneumopericardium (*see also* Pericarditis)
 congenital P25.3
 newborn P25.3
 traumatic (post) — *see* Injury, heart
Pneumophagia (psychogenic) F45.8
Pneumopleurisy, pneumopleuritis (*see also*
 Pneumonia) J18.8
Pneumopyopericardium I30.1
Pneumopyothorax — *see* Pyopneumothorax
 with fistula J86.0
Pneumorrhagia (*see also* Hemorrhage, lung)
 tuberculous — *see* Tuberculosis, pulmonary
Pneumothorax J93.9
 acute J93.8
 chronic J93.8
 congenital P25.1
 perinatal period P25.1
 postprocedural J95.81
 specified NEC J93.8
 spontaneous NEC J93.1
  newborn P25.1
  tension J93.0
 tense valvular, infectional J93.0
 tension (spontaneous) J93.0
 traumatic S27.0
  with hemothorax S27.2
 tuberculous — *see* Tuberculosis, pulmonary
Podagra (*see also* Gout) M10.9
Podencephalus Q01.9
Poikilocytosis R71.8
Poikiloderma L81.6
 Civatte's L57.3
 congenital Q82.8
 vasculare atrophicans L94.5
Poikilodermatomyositis M33.10
 with
  myopathy M33.12
  respiratory involvement M33.11
  specified organ involvement NEC M33.19
Pointed ear (congenital) Q17.3
Poison ivy, oak, sumac or other plant dermatitis
 (allergic) (contact) L23.7
Poisoning (acute) (*see also* Table of Drugs and
 Chemicals)
 algae and toxins T65.82-
 Bacillus B (aertrycke) (cholerae (suis))
  (paratyphosus) (suipestifer) A02.9
  botulinus A05.1
 bacterial toxins A05.9
 berries, noxious — *see* Poisoning, food, noxious,
  berries
 botulism A05.1
 ciguatera fish T61.0-
 Clostridium botulinum A05.1
 death-cap (Amanita phalloides) (Amanita verna) —
  see Poisoning, food, noxious, mushrooms
 drug — *see* Table of Drugs and Chemicals, by drug,
  poisoning
 epidemic, fish (noxious) — *see* Poisoning, seafood
  bacterial A05.9
 fava bean D55.0
 fish (noxious) T61.9-
  bacterial — *see* Intoxication, foodborne, by agent
  ciguatera fish — *see* Poisoning, ciguatera fish
  scombroid fish — *see* Poisoning, scombroid fish
  specified type NEC T61.77-
 food (acute) (diseased) (infected) (noxious) NEC
  T62.9-
  bacterial — *see* Intoxication, foodborne, by agent
  due to
   Bacillus (aertrycke) (choleraesuis)
    (paratyphosus) (suipestifer) A02.9
    botulinus A05.1
   Clostridium (perfringens) (Welchii) A05.2

Poisoning—*continued*
 food—*continued*
  due to—*continued*
   salmonella (aertrycke) (callinarum)
    (choleraesuis) (enteritidis) (paratyphi)
    (suipestifer) A02.9
   with
    gastroenteritis A02.0
    sepsis A02.1
   staphylococcus A05.0
   Vibrio
    parahaemolyticus A05.3
    vulnificus A05.5
  noxious or naturally toxic T62.9-
   berries — *see* subcategory T62.1-
   fish — *see* Poisoning, seafood
   mushrooms — *see* subcategory T62.0x-
   plants NEC — *see* subcategory T62.2x-
   seafood — *see* Poisoning, seafood
   specified NEC — *see* subcategory T62.8x-
 ichthyotoxism — *see* Poisoning, seafood
 kreotoxism, food A05.9
 latex T65.81-
 lead T56.0-
 mushroom — *see* Poisoning, food, noxious,
  mushroom
 mussels (*see also* Poisoning, shellfish)
  bacterial — *see* Intoxication, foodborne, by agent
 nicotine (tobacco) T65.2-
 noxious foodstuffs — *see* Poisoning, food, noxious
 plants, noxious — *see* Poisoning, food, noxious,
  plants NEC
 ptomaine — *see* Poisoning, food
 radiation J70.0
 Salmonella (arizonae) (cholerae-suis) (enteritidis)
  (typhimurium) A02.9
 scombroid fish T61.1-
 seafood (noxious) T61.9-
  bacterial — *see* Intoxication, foodborne, by agent
  fish — *see* Poisoning, fish
  shellfish — *see* Poisoning, shellfish
  specified NEC — *see* subcategory T61.8x-
 shellfish (amnesic) (azaspiracid) (diarrheic)
  (neurotoxic) (noxious) (paralytic) T61.78-
  bacterial — *see* Intoxication, foodborne, by agent
  ciguatera mollusk — *see* Poisoning, ciguatera fish
 specified substance NEC T65.891
 Staphylococcus, food A05.0
 tobacco (nicotine) T65.2-
 water E87.79
Poker spine — *see* Spondylitis, ankylosing
Poland syndrome Q79.8
Polioencephalitis (acute) (bulbar) A80.9
 inferior G12.22
 influenzal — *see* Influenza, with, encephalopathy
 superior hemorrhagic (acute) (Wernicke's) E51.2
 Wernicke's E51.2
Polioencephalomyelitis (acute) (anterior) A80.9
 with beriberi E51.2
Polioencephalopathy, superior hemorrhagic E51.8
 with
  beriberi E51.11
  pellagra E52
Poliomeningoencephalitis — *see*
 Meningoencephalitis
Poliomyelitis (acute) (anterior) (epidemic) A80.9
 with paralysis (bulbar) — *see* Poliomyelitis, paralytic
 abortive A80.4
 ascending (progressive) — *see* Poliomyelitis,
  paralytic
 bulbar (paralytic) — *see* Poliomyelitis, paralytic
 congenital P35.8
 nonepidemic A80.9
 nonparalytic A80.4
 paralytic A80.30
  specified NEC A80.39
  vaccine-associated A80.0
  wild virus
   imported A80.1
   indigenous A80.2
 spinal, acute A80.9

Poliosis (eyebrow) (eyelashes) L67.1
 circumscripta, acquired L67.1
Pollakiuria R35.Ø
 psychogenic F45.8
Pollinosis J3Ø.1
Pollitzer's disease L73.2
Polyadenitis (*see also* Lymphadenitis)
 malignant A2Ø.Ø
Polyalgia M79.89
Polyangiitis M3Ø.Ø
 microscopic M31.7
 overlap syndrome M3Ø.8
Polyarteritis
 microscopic M31.7
 nodosa M3Ø.Ø
 with lung involvement M3Ø.1
 juvenile M3Ø.2
 related condition NEC M3Ø.8
Polyarthralgia — *see* Pain, joint
Polyarthritis, polyarthropathy (*see also* Arthritis)
 M13.Ø
 due to or associated with other specified conditions
 — *see* Arthritis
 epidemic (Australian) (with exanthema) B33.1
 infective — *see* Arthritis, pyogenic or pyemic
 inflammatory MØ6.4
 juvenile (chronic) (seronegative) MØ8.3
 migratory — *see* Fever, rheumatic
 rheumatic, acute — *see* Fever, rheumatic
Polyarthrosis
 M15.9
 post-traumatic M15.3
 primary M15.Ø
 specified NEC M15.8
Polycarential syndrome of infancy E4Ø
Polychondritis (atrophic) (chronic) (*see also* Disorder,
 cartilage, specified type NEC)
 relapsing M94.1
Polycoria Q13.2
Polycystic (disease)
 degeneration, kidney Q61.3
 autosomal dominant (adult type) Q61.2
 autosomal recessive (infantile type) NEC Q61.19
 kidney Q61.3
 autosomal
 dominant Q61.2
 recessive NEC Q61.19
 autosomal dominant (adult type) Q61.2
 autosomal recessive (childhood type) NEC
 Q61.19
 infantile type NEC Q61.19
 liver Q44.6
 lung J98.4
 congenital Q33.Ø
 ovary, ovaries E28.2
 spleen Q89.Ø9
Polycythemia (secondary) D75.1
 acquired D75.1
 benign (familial) D75.Ø
 due to
 donor twin P61.1
 erythropoietin D75.1
 fall in plasma volume D75.1
 high altitude D75.1
 maternal-fetal transfusion P61.1
 stress D75.1
 emotional D75.1
 erythropoietin D75.1
 familial (benign) D75.Ø
 Gaisböck's (hypertonica) D75.1
 high altitude D75.1
 hypertonica D75.1
 hypoxemic D75.1
 neonatorum P61.1
 nephrogenous D75.1
 relative D75.1
 secondary D75.1
 spurious D75.1
 stress D75.1
 vera D45
Polycytosis cryptogenica D75.1
Polydactylism, polydactyly Q69.9
 toes Q69.2

Polydipsia R63.1
Polydystrophy, pseudo-Hurler E77.Ø
Polyembryoma — *see* Neoplasm, malignant, by site
Polyglandular
 deficiency E31.Ø
 dyscrasia E31.9
 dysfunction E31.9
 syndrome E31.8
Polyhydramnios O4Ø.-
Polymastia Q83.1
Polymenorrhea N92.Ø
Polymyalgia M35.3
 arteritica, giant cell M31.5
 rheumatica M35.3
 with giant cell arteritis M31.5
Polymyositis (acute) (chronic) (hemorrhagic) M33.2Ø
 with
 myopathy M33.22
 respiratory involvement M33.21
 skin involvement — *see* Dermatopolymyositis
 specified organ involvement NEC M33.29
 ossificans (generalisata) (progressiva) —
 see Myositis, ossificans, progressiva
Polyneuritis, polyneuritic (*see also* Polyneuropathy)
 acute (post-)infective G61.Ø
 alcoholic G62.1
 cranialis G52.7
 demyelinating, chronic inflammatory (CIDP) G61.81
 diabetic — *see* Diabetes, polyneuropathy
 diphtheritic A36.83
 due to lack of vitamin NEC E56.9 [G63]
 endemic E51.11
 erythredema — *see* subcategory T56.1
 febrile, acute G61.Ø
 hereditary ataxic G6Ø.1
 idiopathic, acute G61.Ø
 infective (acute) G61.Ø
 inflammatory, chronic demyelinating (CIDP) G61.81
 nutritional E63.9 [G63]
 postinfective (acute) G61.Ø
 specified NEC G62.89
Polyneuropathy (peripheral) G62.9
 alcoholic G62.1
 amyloid (Portuguese) E85.1 [G63]
 arsenical G62.2
 critical illness G62.81
 demyelinating, chronic inflammatory (CIDP) G61.81
 diabetic — *see* Diabetes, polyneuropathy
 drug-induced G62.Ø
 hereditary G6Ø.9
 specified NEC G6Ø.8
 idiopathic G6Ø.9
 progressive G6Ø.3
 in (due to)
 alcohol G62.1
 sequelae G65.2
 amyloidosis, familial (Portuguese) E85.1 [G63]
 antitetanus serum G61.1
 arsenic G62.2
 sequelae G65.2
 avitaminosis NEC E56.9 [G63]
 beriberi E51.11
 collagen vascular disease NEC M35.9 [G63]
 deficiency (of)
 B(-complex) vitamins E53.9 [G63]
 vitamin B6 E53.1 [G63]
 diabetes — *see* Diabetes, polyneuropathy
 diphtheria A36.83
 drug or medicament G62.Ø
 correct substance properly administered —
 see Table of Drugs and Chemicals, by
 drug, adverse effect
 overdose or wrong substance given or taken
 — *see* Table of Drugs and Chemicals, by
 drug, poisoning
 endocrine disease NEC E34.9 [G63]
 herpes zoster BØ2.23
 hypoglycemia E16.2 [G63]
 infectious
 disease NEC B99 [G63]
 mononucleosis B27.91
 lack of vitamin NEC E56.9 [G63]

Polyneuropathy —*continued*
 in (due to)—*continued*
 lead G62.2
 sequelae G65.2
 leprosy A3Ø.9
 Lyme disease A69.22
 metabolic disease NEC E88.9 [G63]
 microscopic polyangiitis M31.7 [G63]
 mumps B26.84
 neoplastic disease (*see also* Neoplasm) D49.9
 [G63]
 nutritional deficiency NEC E63.9 [G63]
 organophosphate compounds G62.2
 sequelae G65.2
 parasitic disease NEC B89 [G63]
 pellagra E52 [G63]
 polyarteritis nodosa M3Ø.Ø
 porphyria E8Ø.2Ø [G63]
 radiation G62.82
 rheumatoid arthritis — *see* Rheumatoid,
 polyneuropathy
 sarcoidosis D86.9
 serum G61.1
 syphilis (late) A52.15
 congenital A5Ø.43
 systemic
 connective tissue disorder M35.9 [G63]
 lupus erythematosus M32.19
 toxic agent NEC G62.2
 triorthocresyl phosphate G62.2
 sequelae G65.2
 tuberculosis A17.89
 uremia N18.9 [G63]
 vitamin B12 deficiency E53.8 [G63]
 with anemia (pernicious) D51.Ø [G63]
 due to dietary deficiency D51.3 [G63]
 zoster BØ2.23
 inflammatory G61.9
 chronic demyelinating (CIDP) G61.81
 sequelae G65.1
 specified NEC G61.89
 lead G62.2
 sequelae G65.2
 nutritional NEC E63.9 [G63]
 postherpetic (zoster) BØ2.23
 progressive G6Ø.3
 radiation-induced G62.82
 sensory (hereditary) (idiopathic) G6Ø.8
 specified NEC G62.89
 syphilitic (late) A52.15
 congenital A5Ø.43
Polyopia H53.8
Polyorchism, polyorchidism Q55.21
Polyosteoarthritis (*see also* Osteoarthritis,
 generalized) M15.9
 post-traumatic M15.3
 specified NEC M15.8
Polyostotic fibrous dysplasia Q78.1
Polyotia Q17.Ø
Polyp, polypus
 accessory sinus J33.8
 adenocarcinoma in — *see* Neoplasm, malignant, by
 site
 adenocarcinoma in situ in — *see* Neoplasm, in situ,
 by site
 adenoid tissue J33.Ø
 adenomatous (*see also* Neoplasm, benign, by site)
 adenocarcinoma in — *see* Neoplasm, malignant,
 by site
 adenocarcinoma in situ in — *see* Neoplasm, in
 situ, by site
 carcinoma in — *see* Neoplasm, malignant, by site
 carcinoma in situ in — *see* Neoplasm, in situ, by
 site
 multiple — *see* Neoplasm, benign, by site
 adenocarcinoma in — *see* Neoplasm,
 malignant, by site
 adenocarcinoma in situ in — *see* Neoplasm, in
 situ, by site
 antrum J33.8
 anus, anal (canal) K62.Ø
 Bartholin's gland N84.3

Polyp, polypus—*continued*
- bladder D41.4
- carcinoma in — *see* Neoplasm, malignant, by site
- carcinoma in situ in — *see* Neoplasm, in situ, by site
- cecum D12.Ø
- cervix (uteri) N84.1
    - in pregnancy or childbirth — *see* Pregnancy, complicated by, abnormal, cervix
    - mucous N84.1
    - nonneoplastic N84.1
- choanal J33.Ø
- cholesterol K82.4
- clitoris N84.3
- colon K63.5
    - adenomatous D12.6
    - ascending D12.2
    - cecum D12.Ø
    - descending D12.4
    - inflammatory K51.4Ø
        - with
            - abscess K51.414
            - complication K51.419
                - specified NEC K51.418
            - fistula K51.413
            - intestinal obstruction K51.412
            - rectal bleeding K51.411
    - sigmoid D12.5
    - transverse D12.3
- corpus uteri N84.Ø
- dental KØ4.Ø
- duodenum K31.7
- ear (middle) H74.4-
- endometrium N84.Ø
- ethmoidal (sinus) J33.8
- fallopian tube N84.8
- female genital tract N84.9
    - specified NEC N84.8
- frontal (sinus) J33.8
- gallbladder K82.4
- gingiva, gum KØ6.8
- labia, labium (majus) (minus) N84.3
- larynx (mucous) J38.1
    - adenomatous D14.1
- malignant — *see* Neoplasm, malignant, by site
- maxillary (sinus) J33.8
- middle ear — *see* Polyp, ear (middle)
- myometrium N84.Ø
- nares
    - anterior J33.9
    - posterior J33.Ø
- nasal (mucous) J33.9
    - cavity J33.Ø
    - septum J33.9
- nasopharyngeal J33.Ø
- nose (mucous) J33.9
- oviduct N84.8
- pharynx J39.2
- placenta O9Ø.89
- prostate — *see* Enlargement, enlarged, prostate
- pudenda, pudendum N84.3
- pulpal (dental) KØ4.Ø
- rectum (nonadenomatous) K62.1
    - adenomatous — *see* Polyp, adenomatous
- septum (nasal) J33.Ø
- sinus (accessory) (ethmoidal) (frontal) (maxillary) (sphenoidal) J33.8
- sphenoidal (sinus) J33.8
- stomach K31.7
    - adenomatous D13.1
- tube, fallopian N84.8
- turbinate, mucous membrane J33.8
- umbilical, newborn P83.6
- ureter N28.89
- urethra N36.2
- uterus (body) (corpus) (mucous) N84.Ø
    - cervix N84.1
    - in pregnancy or childbirth — *see* Pregnancy, complicated by, tumor, uterus
- vagina N84.2
- vocal cord (mucous) J38.1
- vulva N84.3

Polyphagia R63.2
Polyploidy Q92.7

Polypoid — *see* condition
Polyposis (*see also* Polyp)
- coli (adenomatous) D12.6
    - adenocarcinoma in C18.9
    - adenocarcinoma in situ in — *see* Neoplasm, in situ, by site
    - carcinoma in C18.9
- colon (adenomatous) D12.6
- familial D12.6
    - adenocarcinoma in situ in — *see* Neoplasm, in situ, by site
- intestinal (adenomatous) D12.6
- malignant lymphomatous C83.1-
- multiple, adenomatous (*see also* Neoplasm, benign) D36.9
Polyradiculitis — *see* Polyneuropathy
Polyradiculoneuropathy (acute) (postinfective) (segmentally demyelinating) G61.Ø
Polyserositis
- due to pericarditis I31.1
- pericardial I31.1
- periodic, familial E85.Ø
- tuberculous A19.9
    - acute A19.1
    - chronic A19.8
Polysplenia syndrome Q89.Ø9
Polysyndactyly (*see also* Syndactylism, syndactyly) Q7Ø.4
Polytrichia L68.3
Polyunguia Q84.6
Polyuria R35.8
- nocturnal R35.1
- psychogenic F45.8
Pompe's disease (glycogen storage) E74.Ø2
Pompholyx L3Ø.1
Poncet's disease (tuberculous rheumatism) A18.Ø9
Pond fracture — *see* Fracture, skull
Ponos B55.Ø
Pons, pontine — *see* condition
Poor
- aesthetic of existing restoration of tooth KØ8.56
- contractions, labor O62.2
- gingival margin to tooth restoration KØ8.51
- personal hygiene R46.Ø
- prenatal care, affecting management of pregnancy — *see* Pregnancy, complicated by, insufficient, prenatal care
- sucking reflex (newborn) R29.2
- urinary stream R39.12
- vision NEC H54.7
Poradenitis, nostras inguinalis or venerea A55
Porencephaly (congenital) (developmental) (true) QØ4.6
- acquired G93.Ø
- nondevelopmental G93.Ø
- traumatic (post) FØ7.89
Porocephaliasis B88.8
Porokeratosis Q82.8
Poroma, eccrine — *see* Neoplasm, skin, benign
Porphyrisa (South African) E8Ø.2Ø
- acquired E8Ø.2Ø
- acute intermittent (hepatic) (Swedish) E8Ø.21
- cutanea tarda (hereditary) (symptomatic) E8Ø.1
- due to drugs E8Ø.2Ø
    - correct substance properly administered — *see* Table of Drugs and Chemicals, by drug, adverse effect
    - overdose or wrong substance given or taken — *see* Table of Drugs and Chemicals, by drug, poisoning
- erythropoietic (congenital) (hereditary) E8Ø.Ø
- hepatocutaneous type E8Ø.1
- secondary E8Ø.2Ø
- toxic NEC E8Ø.2Ø
- variegata E8Ø.2Ø
Porphyrinuria — *see* Porphyria
Porphyruria — *see* Porphyria
Portal — *see* condition
Port wine nevus, mark, or stain Q82.5
Posada-Wernicke disease B38.7

Positive
- culture (nonspecific)
    - blood R78.81
    - bronchial washings R84.5
    - cerebrospinal fluid R83.5
    - cervix uteri R87.5
    - nasal secretions R84.5
    - nipple discharge R89.5
    - nose R84.5
        - staphylococcus Z22.32
    - peritoneal fluid R85.5
    - pleural fluid R84.5
    - prostatic secretions R86.5
    - saliva R85.5
    - seminal fluid R86.5
    - sputum R84.5
    - synovial fluid R89.5
    - throat scrapings R84.5
    - urine R82.7
    - vagina R87.5
    - vulva R87.5
    - wound secretions R89.5
- PPD (skin test) R76.1
- serology for syphilis A53.Ø
    - false R76.8
    - with signs or symptoms code as Syphilis, by site and stage
- skin test, tuberculin (without active tuberculosis) R76.1
- test, human immunodeficiency virus (HIV) R75
- VDRL A53.Ø
    - with signs or symptoms code by site and stage under Syphilis A53.9
- Wassermann reaction A53.Ø
Postcardiotomy syndrome I97.Ø
Postcaval ureter Q62.62
Postcholecystectomy syndrome K91.5
Postclimacteric bleeding N95.Ø
Postcommissurotomy syndrome I97.Ø
Postconcussional syndrome FØ7.81
Postcontusional syndrome FØ7.81
Postcricoid region — *see* condition
Post-dates (4Ø-42 weeks) (pregnancy) (mother) O48.Ø
- more than 42 weeks gestation O48.1
Postencephalitic syndrome FØ7.89
Posterior — *see* condition
Posterolateral sclerosis (spinal cord) — *see* Degeneration, combined
Postexanthematous — *see* condition
Postfebrile — *see* condition
Postgastrectomy dumping syndrome K91.1
Posthemiplegic chorea — *see* Monoplegia
Posthemorrhagic anemia (chronic) D5Ø.Ø
- acute D62
- newborn P61.3
Postherpetic neuralgia (zoster) BØ2.29
- trigeminal BØ2.22
Posthitis N47.7
Postimmunization complication or reaction — *see* Complications, vaccination
Postinfectious — *see* condition
Postlaminectomy syndrome NEC M96.1
Postleukotomy syndrome FØ7.Ø
Postmastectomy lymphedema (syndrome) I97.2
Postmaturity, postmature (over 42 weeks)
- maternal (over 42 weeks gestation) O48.1
- newborn PØ8.22
Postmeasles complication NEC (*see also* condition) BØ5.89
Postmenopausal
- endometrium (atrophic) N95.8
    - suppurative (*see also* Endometritis) N71.9
- osteoporosis — *see* Osteoporosis, postmenopausal
Postnasal drip RØ9.82
- due to
    - allergic rhinitis — *see* Rhinitis, allergic
    - common cold JØØ
    - gastroesophageal reflux — *see* Reflux, gastroesophageal
    - nasopharyngitis — *see* Nasopharyngitis
    - other know condition code to condition
    - sinusitis — *see* Sinusitis
Postnatal — *see* condition

Postoperative (postprocedural) — *see* Complication, postoperative
  pneumothorax, therapeutic Z98.3
  state NEC Z98.89
Postpancreatectomy hyperglycemia E89.1
Postpartum — *see* Puerperal
Postphlebitic syndrome — *see* Syndrome, postthrombotic
Postpoliomyelitic (*see also* condition)
  osteopathy — *see* Osteopathy, after poliomyelitis
Postpolio (myelitic) **syndrome** G14
Postprocedural (*see also* Postoperative)
  hypoinsulinemia E89.1
Postschizophrenic depression F32.8
Postsurgery status (*see also* Status (post))
  pneumothorax, therapeutic Z98.3
Post-term (40–42 weeks) (pregnancy) (mother) O48.0
  infant P08.21
  more than 42 weeks gestation (mother) O48.1
Post-traumatic brain syndrome, nonpsychotic F07.81
Post-typhoid abscess A01.09
Postures, hysterical F44.2
Postvaccinal reaction or complication — *see* Complications, vaccination
Postvalvulotomy syndrome I97.0
Potain's
  disease (pulmonary edema) — *see* Edema, lung
  syndrome (gastrectasis with dyspepsia) K31.0
Potter's
  asthma J62.8
  facies Q60.6
  lung J62.8
  syndrome (with renal agenesis) Q60.6
Pott's
  curvature (spinal) A18.01
  disease or paraplegia A18.01
  spinal curvature A18.01
  tumor, puffy — *see* Osteomyelitis, specified type NEC
Pouch
  bronchus Q32.4
  Douglas' — *see* condition
  esophagus, esophageal, congenital Q39.6
    acquired K22.5
  gastric K31.4
  Hartmann's K82.8
  pharynx, pharyngeal (congenital) Q38.7
Pouchitis K91.850
Poultrymen's itch B88.0
Poverty NEC Z59.6
  extreme Z59.5
Poxvirus NEC B08.8
Prader-Willi syndrome Q87.1
Preauricular appendage or tag Q17.0
Prebetalipoproteinemia (acquired) (essential) (familial) (hereditary) (primary) (secondary) E78.1
  with chylomicronemia E78.3
Precipitate labor or delivery O62.3
Preclimacteric bleeding (menorrhagia) N92.4
Precocious
  adrenarche E30.1
  menarche E30.1
  menstruation E30.1
  pubarche E30.1
  puberty E30.1
    central E22.8
  sexual development NEC E30.1
  thelarche E30.8
Precocity, sexual (constitutional) (cryptogenic) (female) (idiopathic) (male) E30.1
  with adrenal hyperplasia E25.9
    congenital E25.0
Precordial pain R07.2
Predeciduous teeth K00.2
Prediabetes, prediabetic R73.09
  complicating
    pregnancy — *see* Pregnancy, complicated by, diseases of, specified type or system NEC
    puerperium O99.89
Predislocation status of hip at birth Q65.6

Pre-eclampsia O14.9-
  with pre-existing hypertension — *see* Hypertension, complicating pregnancy, pre-existing, with, pre-eclampsia
  moderate O14.0-
  severe O14.1-
  with HELLP O14.2
Pre-eruptive color change, teeth, tooth K00.8
Pre-excitation atrioventricular conduction I45.6
Pregnancy (childbirth) (labor) (puerperium) (*see also* Delivery and Puerperal)

Note: the tabular must be reviewed for assignment of the final character for trimester

Note: the tabular must be reviewed for assignment of the correct extension for multiple gestations for all chapter 15 codes

---

  abdominal (ectopic) O00.0
    with viable fetus O36.7-
  ampullar O00.1
  broad ligament O00.8
  cervical O00.8
  complicated NOS O26.9-
  complicated by (care of) (management affected by)
    abnormal, abnormality
      cervix O34.4-
        causing obstructed labor O65.5
      cord (umbilical) O69.9
      findings on antenatal screening of mother O28.9
        biochemical O28.1
        cytological O28.2
        chromosomal O28.5
        genetic O28.5
        hematological O28.0
        radiological O28.4
        specified NEC O28.8
        ultrasonic O28.3
      glucose (tolerance) NEC O99.810
      pelvic organs O34.9-
        specified NEC O34.8-
          causing obstructed labor O65.5
      pelvis (bony) (major) NEC O33.0
      perineum O34.7-
      position
        placenta O44.1-
          without hemorrhage O44.0-
        uterus O34.59-
      uterus O34.59-
        causing obstructed labor O65.5
        congenital O34.0-
      vagina O34.6-
        causing obstructed labor O65.5
      vulva O34.7-
        causing obstructed labor O65.5
    abruptio placentae — *see* Abruptio placentae
    abscess or cellulitis
      bladder O23.1-
      breast O91.11-
      genital organ or tract O23.9-
    abuse
      physical O9a.31-
      psychological O9a.51-
      sexual O9a.41-
    adverse effect anesthesia O29.9-
      aspiration pneumonitis O29.01-
      cardiac arrest O29.11-
      cardiac complication NEC O29.19-
      cardiac failure O29.12-
      central nervous system complication NEC O29.29-
      cerebral anoxia O29.21-
      failed or difficult intubation O29.6-
      inhalation of stomach contents or secretions NOS O29.01-
      local, toxic reaction O29.3x
      Mendelson's syndrome O29.01-
      pressure collapse of lung O29.02-
      pulmonary complications NEC O29.09-
      specified NEC O29.8x-

Pregnancy —*continued*
  complicated by—*continued*
    adverse effect anesthesia—*continued*
      spinal and epidural type NEC O29.5x
        induced headache O29.4-
    albuminuria O12.1-
    alcohol use O99.31-
    amnionitis O41.12-
    anaphylactoid syndrome of pregnancy O88.01-
    anemia (conditions in D50–D64) (pre-existing) O99.01-
      postpartum O90.81
    antepartum hemorrhage O46.9-
      with coagulation defect — *see* Hemorrhage, antepartum, with coagulation defect
      specified NEC O46.8x-
    appendicitis O99.61-
    atrophy (yellow) (acute) liver (subacute) O26.61-
    bariatric surgery status O99.84-
    bicornis or bicornuate uterus O34.59-
    biliary problems O99.61-
    breech presentation O32.1
    cardiovascular diseases (conditions in I00–I09, I20–I52, I70–I99) O99.41-
    cerebrovascular disorders (conditions in I60–I69) O99.41-
    cervical shortening O26.87-
    cervicitis O23.51-
    chloasma (gravidarum) O26.89-
    cholestasis (intrahepatic) O26.61-
    cholecystitis O99.61-
    chorioamnionitis O41.12-
    circulatory system disorder (conditions in I00–I09, I20–I99, O99.41-)
    conjoined twins O30.02-
    compound presentation O32.6
    connective system disorders (conditions in M00–M99) O99.89
    contracted pelvis (general) O33.1
      inlet O33.2
      outlet O33.3
    convulsions (eclamptic) (uremic) (*see also* Eclampsia) O15.9
    cracked nipple O92.11-
    cystitis O23.1-
    cystocele O34.8-
    death of fetus (near term) O36.4
      early pregnancy O02.1
      of one fetus or more in multiple gestation O31.2-
    deciduitis O41.14-
    decreased fetal movement O36.81-
    dental problems O99.61-
    diabetes (mellitus) O24.91-
      gestational (pregnancy induced) *see* Diabetes, gestational
      pre-existing O24.31-
        specified NEC O24.81-
        type 1 O24.01-
        type 2 O24.11-
    digestive system disorders (conditions in K00–K93) O99.61-
    diseases of — *see* Pregnancy, complicated by, specified body system disease
      blood NEC (conditions in D65-D77) O99.11-
      liver O26.61-
      specified NEC O99.89
    disorders of — *see* Pregnancy, complicated by, specified body system disorder
      amniotic fluid and membranes O41.9-
        specified NEC O41.8x-
      ear and mastoid process (conditions in H60–H95) O99.89
      eye and adnexa (conditions in H00–H59) O99.89
      liver O26.61-
      skin (conditions in L00–L99) O99.7-
      specified NEC O99.89
    displacement, uterus NEC O34.59-
      causing obstructed labor O65.5
    disproportion (due to) O33.9
      fetal deformities NEC O33.7
      generally contracted pelvis O33.1

Pregnancy —continued
  ectopic—continued
    specified site NEC O00.8
    tubal (ruptured) O00.1
  examination (normal) Z34.9-
    high-risk — see Pregnancy, supervision of,
      high-risk
    first Z34.0-
    specified Z34.8-
  extrauterine — see Pregnancy, ectopic
  fallopian O00.1
  false F45.8
  hidden O09.3-
  high-risk — see Pregnancy, supervision of, high-risk
  incidental finding Z33.1
  interstitial O00.8
  intraligamentous O00.8
  intramural O00.8
  intraperitoneal O00.0
  isthmian O00.1
  mesometric (mural) O00.8
  molar NEC O02.0
    complicated (by) O07.30
      afibrinogenemia O07.1
      cardiac arrest O07.39
      chemical damage of pelvic organ(s) O07.39
      circulatory collapse O07.39
      defibrination syndrome O07.1
      electrolyte imbalance O07.39
      embolism (amniotic fluid) (blood clot)
        (pulmonary) (septic) O07.2
      endometritis O07.0
      genital tract and pelvic infection O07.0
      hemorrhage (delayed) (excessive) O07.1
      infection
        genital tract or pelvic O07.0
        urinary tract O07.39
      intravascular coagulation O07.1
      laceration of pelvic organ(s) O07.39
      metabolic disorder O07.39
      oliguria O07.39
      oophoritis O07.0
      parametritis O07.0
      pelvic peritonitis O07.0
      perforation of pelvic organ(s) O07.39
      renal failure or shutdown O07.39
      salpingitis or salpingo-oophoritis O07.0
      sepsis O07.0
      shock O07.39
        septic O07.0
      specified condition NEC O07.39
      tubular necrosis (renal) O07.39
      uremia O07.39
      urinary infection O07.39
      venous complication NEC O07.39
        embolism O07.2
  hydatidiform (see also Mole, hydatidiform) O01.9
  multiple (gestation) O30.9-
    greater than quadruplets — see Pregnancy,
      multiple (gestation), specified NEC
    specified NEC O30.80-
      with
        two or more monoamniotic fetuses
          O30.82-
        two or more monochorionic fetuses
          O30.81-
      two or more monoamniotic fetuses O30.82-
      two or more monochorionic fetuses O30.81-
      unable to determine number of placenta and
        number of amniotic sacs O30.89-
      unspecified number of placenta and
        unspecified number of amniotic sacs
        O30.80-
  mural O00.8
  normal (supervision of) Z34.9-
    high-risk — see Pregnancy, supervision of,
      high-risk
    first Z34.0-
    specified Z34.8-
  ovarian O00.2
  postmature (40 to 42 weeks) O48.0
    more than 42 weeks gestation O48.1
  post-term (40 to 42 weeks) O48.0

Pregnancy —continued
  prenatal care only Z34.9-
    high-risk — see Pregnancy, supervision of,
      high-risk
    first Z34.0-
    specified Z34.8-
  prolonged (more than 42 weeks gestation) O48.1
  quadruplet O30.20 — see Tabular for required
    trimester
    with
      two or more monoamniotic fetuses O30.22-
      two or more monochorionic fetuses O30.21-
    two or more monoamniotic fetuses O30.22-
    two or more monochorionic fetuses O30.21-
    unable to determine number of placenta and
      number of amniotic sacs O30.29-
    unspecified number of placenta and unspecified
      number of amniotic sacs O30.20-
  quintuplet — see Pregnancy, multiple (gestation),
    specified NEC
  sextuplet — see Pregnancy, multiple (gestation),
    specified NEC
  supervision of
    high-risk O09.9-
      due to (history of)
        ectopic pregnancy O09.1-
        grand multiparity O09.4
        infertility O09.0-
        insufficient prenatal care O09.3-
        in utero procedure during previous
          pregnancy O09.82-
        in vitro fertilization O09.81-
        molar pregnancy O09.1-
        multiple previous pregnancies O09.4-
        older mother
          multigravida O09.52-
          primigravida O09.51-
        poor reproductive or obstetric history NEC
          O09.29-
        pre-term labor O09.21-
        previous
          neonatal death O09.29-
        social problems O09.7-
        specified NEC O09.89-
        very young mother
          multigravida O09.62-
          primigravida O09.61-
      resulting from in vitro fertilization O09.81-
    normal Z34.9-
      first Z34.0-
      specified NEC Z34.8-
      older mother
        multigravida O09.52-
        primigravida O09.51-
      very young mother
        multigravida O09.62-
        primigravida O09.61-
  tubal (with abortion) (with rupture) O00.1
  triplet O30.10 — see Tabular for required trimester
    with
      two or more monoamniotic fetuses O30.12-
      two or more monochrorionic fetuses O30.11-
    two or more monoamniotic fetuses O30.12-
    two or more monochrorionic fetuses O30.11-
    unable to determine number of placenta and
      number of amniotic sacs O30.19-
    unspecified number of placenta and unspecified
      number of amniotic sacs O30.10-
  twin O30.00 — see Tabular for required trimester
    conjoined O30.02-
    dichorionic/diamniotic (two placenta, two
      amniotic sacs) O30.04-
    monochorionic/diamniotic (one placenta, two
      amniotic sacs) O30.03-
    monochorionic/monoamniotic (one placenta,
      one amniotic sac) O30.01-
    unable to determine number of placenta and
      number of amniotic sacs O30.09-
    unspecified number of placenta and unspecified
      number of amniotic sacs O30.00-
Preiser's disease — see Osteonecrosis, secondary, due
  to, trauma, metacarpus
Pre-kwashiorkor — see Malnutrition, severe

Preleukemia (syndrome) D46.9
Preluxation, hip, congenital Q65.6
Premature (see also condition)
  adrenarche E27.0
  aging E34.8
  beats I49.40
    atrial I49.1
    auricular I49.1
    supraventricular I49.1
  birth NEC — see Preterm infant, newborn
  closure, foramen ovale Q21.8
  contraction
    atrial I49.1
    atrioventricular I49.2
    auricular I49.1
    auriculoventricular I49.2
    heart (extrasystole) I49.49
    junctional I49.2
    ventricular I49.3
  delivery (see also Pregnancy, complicated by,
    preterm labor) O60.10
  ejaculation F52.4
  infant NEC — see Preterm infant, newborn
    light-for-dates — see Light for dates
  labor — see Pregnancy, complicated by, preterm
    labor
  lungs P28.0
  menopause E28.319
    asymptomatic E28.319
    symptomatic E28.310
  newborn
    extreme (less than 28 completed weeks) — see
      Immaturity, extreme
    less than 37 completed weeks — see Preterm
      infant, newborn
  puberty E30.1
  rupture membranes or amnion — see Pregnancy,
    complicated by, premature rupture of
    membranes
  senility E34.8
  thelarche E30.8
  ventricular systole I49.3
Prematurity NEC (less than 37 completed weeks) —
  see Preterm infant, newborn
  extreme (less than 28 completed weeks) — see
    Immaturity, extreme
Premenstrual
  dysphoric disorder (PMDD) N94.3
  tension (syndrome) N94.3
Premolarization, cuspids K00.2
Prenatal
  care, normal pregnancy — see Pregnancy, normal
  screening of mother Z36
  teeth K00.6
Preparatory care for subsequent treatment NEC
  for dialysis Z49.01
    peritoneal Z49.02
Prepartum — see condition
Preponderance, left or right ventricular I51.7
Prepuce — see condition
PRES (Posterior Reversible Encephalopathy Syndrome)
  G93.49
Presbycardia R54
Presbycusis, presbyacusia H91.1-
Presbyesophagus K22.8
Presbyophrenia F03
Presbyopia H52.4
Prescription of contraceptives (initial) Z30.019
  emergency (postcoital) Z30.012
  implantable subdermal Z30.019
  injectable Z30.013
  intrauterine contraceptive device Z30.014
  pills Z30.011
  postcoital (emergency) Z30.012
  repeat Z30.40
    implantable subdermal Z30.49
    injectable Z30.42
    pills Z30.41
    specified type NEC Z30.49
  specified type NEC Z30.018
Presence (of)
  ankle-joint implant (functional) (prosthesis) Z96.66-
  aortocoronary (bypass) graft Z95.1

Presence—continued
arterial-venous shunt (dialysis) Z99.2
artificial
    eye (globe) Z97.0
    heart (fully implantable) (mechanical) Z95.812
      valve Z95.2
    larynx Z96.3
    lens (intraocular) Z96.1
    limb (complete) (partial) Z97.1-
      arm Z97.1-
        bilateral Z97.15
      leg Z97.1-
        bilateral Z97.16
audiological implant (functional) Z96.29
bladder implant (functional) Z96.0
bone
    conduction hearing device Z96.29
    implant (functional) NEC Z96.7
    joint (prosthesis) — see Presence, joint implant
cardiac
    defibrillator (functional) (with synchronous
      cardiac pacemaker) Z95.810
    implant or graft Z95.9
      specified type NEC Z95.818
    pacemaker Z95.0
cerebrospinal fluid drainage device Z98.2
cochlear implant (functional) Z96.21
contact lens(es) Z97.3
coronary artery graft or prosthesis Z95.5
CSF shunt Z98.2
dental prosthesis device Z97.2
dentures Z97.2
device (external) NEC Z97.8
    cardiac NEC Z95.818
    heart assist Z95.811
    implanted (functional) Z96.9
      specified NEC Z96.89
    prosthetic Z97.8
ear implant Z96.20
    cochlear implant Z96.21
    myringotomy tube Z96.22
    specified type NEC Z96.29
elbow-joint implant (functional) (prosthesis) Z96.62-
endocrine implant (functional) NEC Z96.49
eustachian tube stent or device (functional) Z96.29
external hearing-aid or device Z97.4
finger-joint implant (functional) (prosthetic) Z96.69-
functional implant Z96.9
    specified NEC Z96.89
graft
    cardiac NEC Z95.818
    vascular NEC Z95.828
hearing-aid or device (external) Z97.4
    implant (bone) (cochlear) (functional) Z96.21
heart assist device Z95.811
heart valve implant (functional) Z95.2
    prosthetic Z95.2
    specified type NEC Z95.4
    xenogenic Z95.3
hip-joint implant (functional) (prosthesis) Z96.64-
implanted device (artificial) (functional) (prosthetic)
    Z96.9
    automatic cardiac defibrillator (with synchronous
      cardiac pacemaker) Z95.810
    cardiac pacemaker Z95.0
    cochlear Z96.21
    dental Z96.5
    heart Z95.812
    heart valve Z95.2
      prosthetic Z95.2
      specified NEC Z95.4
      xenogenic Z95.3
    insulin pump Z96.41
    intraocular lens Z96.1
    joint Z96.60
      ankle Z96.66-
      elbow Z96.62-
      finger Z96.69-
      hip Z96.64-
      knee Z96.65-
      shoulder Z96.61-
      specified NEC Z96.698

Presence—continued
implanted device—continued
    joint—continued
      wrist Z96.63-
    larynx Z96.3
    myringotomy tube Z96.22
    otological Z96.20
      cochlear Z96.21
      eustachian stent Z96.29
      myringotomy Z96.22
      specified NEC Z96.29
      stapes Z96.29
    skin Z96.81
    skull plate Z96.7
    specified NEC Z96.89
    urogenital Z96.0
insulin pump (functional) Z96.41
intestinal bypass or anastomosis Z98.0
intraocular lens (functional) Z96.1
intrauterine contraceptive device (IUD) Z97.5
intravascular implant (functional) (prosthetic) NEC
    Z95.9
    coronary artery Z95.5
    defibrillator (with synchronous cardiac
      pacemaker) Z95.810
    peripheral vessel (with angioplasty) Z95.820
joint implant (prosthetic) (any) Z96.60
    ankle — see Presence, ankle joint implant
    elbow — see Presence, elbow joint implant
    finger — see Presence, finger joint implant
    hip — see Presence, hip joint implant
    knee — see Presence, knee joint implant
    shoulder — see Presence, shoulder joint implant
    specified joint NEC Z96.698
    wrist — see Presence, wrist joint implant
knee-joint implant (functional) (prosthesis) Z96.65-
laryngeal implant (functional) Z96.3
mandibular implant (dental) Z96.5
myringotomy tube(s) Z96.22
orthopedic-joint implant (prosthetic) (any) — see
    Presence, joint implant
otological implant (functional) Z96.29
shoulder-joint implant (functional) (prosthesis)
    Z96.61-
skull-plate implant Z96.7
spectacles Z97.3
stapes implant (functional) Z96.29
systemic lupus erythematosus [SLE] inhibitor
    D68.62
tendon implant (functional) (graft) Z96.7
tooth root(s) implant Z96.5
ureteral stent Z96.0
urethral stent Z96.0
urogenital implant (functional) Z96.0
vascular implant or device Z95.9
    access port device Z95.828
    specified NEC Z95.828
wrist-joint implant (functional) (prosthesis) Z96.63-
Presenile (see also condition)
dementia F03
premature aging E34.8
Presentation, fetal — see Delivery (childbirth) (labor)
    (complicated by), malposition, malpresentation
Prespondylolisthesis (congenital) Q76.2
Pressure
area, skin — see Ulcer, pressure, by site
brachial plexus G54.0
brain G93.5
    injury at birth NEC P11.1
cerebral — see Pressure, brain
chest R07.89
cone, tentorial G93.5
hyposystolic (see also Hypotension)
    incidental reading, without diagnosis of
      hypotension R03.1
increased
    intracranial (benign) G93.2
      injury at birth P11.0
    intraocular H40.0
lumbosacral plexus G54.1
mediastinum J98.5
necrosis (chronic) — see Ulcer, pressure, by site
parental, inappropriate (excessive) Z62.6

Pressure—continued
sore (chronic) — see Ulcer, pressure, by site
spinal cord G95.20
ulcer (chronic) — see Ulcer, pressure, by site
venous, increased I87.8
Pre-syncope R55
Preterm
delivery (see also Pregnancy, complicated by,
    preterm labor) O60.10
infant, newborn P07.30
    with gestation of:
      28-31 weeks P07.31
      32-36 weeks P07.32
labor — see Pregnancy, complicated by, preterm
    labor
Previa
placenta (low) (marginal) (partial) (total) (with
    hemorrhage) O44.1-
    without hemorrhage O44.0-
vasa O69.4
Priapism N48.30
due to
    disease classified elsewhere N48.32
    drug N48.33
    specified cause NEC N48.39
    trauma N48.31
Prickling sensation (skin) R20.2
Prickly heat L74.0
Primary — see condition
Primigravida
elderly, affecting management of pregnancy, labor
    and delivery (supervision only) — see
    Pregnancy, complicated by, elderly,
    primigravida
very young, affecting management of pregnancy,
    labor and delivery (supervision only) — see
    Pregnancy, complicated by, very young,
    primigravida
Primipara
elderly, affecting management of pregnancy, labor
    and delivery (supervision only) — see
    Pregnancy, complicated by, elderly,
    primigravida
very young, affecting management of pregnancy,
    labor and delivery (supervision only) — see
    Pregnancy, complicated by, very young,
    primigravida
Primus varus (bilateral) Q66.3
PRIND (Prolonged reversible ischemic neurologic
    deficit) I63.9
Pringle's disease (tuberous sclerosis) Q85.1
Prinzmetal angina I20.1
Prizefighter ear — see Cauliflower ear
Problem (with) (related to)
academic Z55.8
acculturation Z60.3
adjustment (to)
    change of job Z56.1
    life-cycle transition Z60.0
    pension Z60.0
    retirement Z60.0
adopted child Z62.821
alcoholism in family Z63.72
atypical parenting situation Z62.9
bankruptcy Z59.8
behavioral (adult) F69
    drug seeking Z72.89
birth of sibling affecting child Z62.898
care (of)
    provider dependency Z74.9
      specified NEC Z74.8
    sick or handicapped person in family or
      household Z63.6
child
    abuse (affecting the child) — see Maltreatment,
      child
    custody or support proceedings Z65.3
    in welfare custody Z62.21
    in care of non-parental family member Z62.21
    in foster care Z62.21
    living in orphanage or group home Z62.22
child-rearing Z62.9
    specified NEC Z62.8

Problem—*continued*
communication (developmental) F80.9
conflict or discord (with)
  boss Z56.4
  classmates Z55.4
  counselor Z64.4
  employer Z56.4
  family Z63.9
    specified NEC Z63.8
  probation officer Z64.4
  social worker Z64.4
  teachers Z55.4
  workmates Z56.4
conviction in legal proceedings Z65.0
  with imprisonment Z65.1
counselor Z64.4
creditors Z59.8
digestive K92.9
drug addict in family Z63.72
ear — *see* Disorder, ear
Peconomic Z59.9
  affecting care Z59.9
  specified NEC Z59.8
education Z55.9
  specified NEC Z55.8
employment Z56.9
  change of job Z56.1
  discord Z56.4
  environment Z56.5
  sexual harassment Z56.81
  specified NEC Z56.89
  stress NEC Z56.6
  stressful schedule Z56.3
  threat of job loss Z56.2
  unemployment Z56.0
enuresis, child F98.0
eye H57.9
failed examinations (school) Z55.2
falling Z91.81
family (*see also* Disruption, family) Z63.9 (
  specified NEC Z63.8
feeding (elderly) (infant) R63.3
  newborn P92.9
    breast P92.5
    overfeeding P92.4
    slow P92.2
    specified NEC P92.8
    underfeeding P92.3
  nonorganic F50.8
finance Z59.9
  specified NEC Z59.8
foreclosure on loan Z59.8
foster child Z62.822
frightening experience(s) in childhood Z62.898
genital NEC
  female N94.9
  male N50.9
health care Z75.9
  specified NEC Z75.8
hearing — *see* Deafness
homelessness Z59.0
housing Z59.9
  inadequate Z59.1
  isolated Z59.8
  specified NEC Z59.8
identity (of childhood) F93.8
illegitimate pregnancy (unwanted) Z64.0
illiteracy Z55.0
impaired mobility Z74.09
imprisonment or incarceration Z65.1
inadequate teaching affecting education Z55.8
inappropriate (excessive) parental pressure Z62.6
influencing health status NEC Z78.9
in-law Z63.1
institutionalization, affecting child Z62.22
intrafamilial communication Z63.8
jealousy, child F93.8
landlord Z59.2
language (developmental) F80.9
learning (developmental) F81.9
legal Z65.3
  conviction without imprisonment Z65.0
  imprisonment Z65.1

Problem—*continued*
legal—*continued*
  release from prison Z65.2
life-management Z73.9
  specified NEC Z73.89
life-style Z72.9
  gambling Z72.6
  high-risk sexual behavior (heterosexual) Z72.51
    bisexual Z72.53
    homosexual Z72.52
  inappropriate eating habits Z72.4
  self-damaging behavior NEC Z72.89
  specified NEC Z72.89
  tobacco use Z72.0
literacy Z55.9
  low level Z55.0
  specified NEC Z55.8
living alone Z60.2
lodgers Z59.2
loss of love relationship in childhood Z62.898
marital Z63.0
  involving
    divorce Z63.5
    estrangement Z63.5
    gender identity F66
mastication K08.8
medical
  care, within family Z63.6
  facilities Z75.9
    specified NEC Z75.8
mental F48.9
multiparity Z64.1
negative life events in childhood Z62.9
  altered pattern of family relationships Z62.898
  frightening experience Z62.898
  loss of
    love relationship Z62.898
    self-esteem Z62.898
  physical abuse (alleged) — *see* Maltreatment,
    child
  removal from home Z62.29
  specified event NEC Z62.898
neighbor Z59.2
neurological NEC R29.81
new step-parent affecting child Z62.898
none (feared complaint unfounded) Z71.1
occupational NEC Z56.89
parent-child — *see* Conflict, parent-child
personal hygiene Z91.89
personality F69
phase-of-life transition, adjustment Z60.0
presence of sick or disabled person in family or
  household Z63.79
  needing care Z63.6
primary support group (family) Z63.9
  specified NEC Z63.8
probation officer Z64.4
psychiatric F99
psychosexual (development) F66
psychosocial Z65.9
  specified NEC Z65.8
relationship Z63.9
  childhood F93.8
release from prison Z65.2
removal from home affecting child Z62.29
seeking and accepting known hazardous and
  harmful
  behavioral or psychological interventions Z65.8
  chemical, nutritional or physical interventions
    Z65.8
sexual function (nonorganic) F52.9
sight H54.7
sleep disorder, child F51.9
smell — *see* Disturbance, sensation, smell
social
  environment Z60.9
    specified NEC Z60.8
  exclusion and rejection Z60.4
  worker Z64.4
speech R47.9
  developmental F80.9
  specified NEC R47.89
swallowing — *see* Dysphagia

Problem—*continued*
taste — *see* Disturbance, sensation, taste
tic, child F95.0
underachievement in school Z55.3
unemployment Z56.0
  threatened Z56.2
unwanted pregnancy Z64.0
upbringing Z62.9
  specified NEC Z62.898
urinary N39.9
voice production R47.89
work schedule (stressful) Z56.3
Procedure (surgical)
elective — *see* Surgery, elective
  ear piercing Z41.3
  specified NEC Z41.8
for purpose other than remedying health state
  Z41.9
  specified NEC Z41.8
not done Z53.9
  because of
    administrative reasons Z53.8
    contraindication Z53.09
      smoking Z53.01
    patient's decision Z53.20
      for reasons of belief or group pressure
        Z53.1
      left against medical advice (AMA) Z53.21
        specified reason NEC Z53.29
    specified reason NEC Z53.8
Procidentia (uteri) N81.3
Proctalgia K62.8
fugax K59.4
spasmodic K59.4
Proctitis K62.8
amebic (acute) A06.0
chlamydial A56.3
gonococcal A54.6
granulomatous — *see* Enteritis, regional, large
  intestine
herpetic A60.1
radiation K62.7
tuberculous A18.32
ulcerative (chronic) K51.20
  with
    complication K51.219
      abscess K51.214
      fistula K51.213
      obstruction K51.212
      rectal bleeding K51.211
      specified NEC K51.218
Proctocele
female (without uterine prolapse) N81.6
  with uterine prolapse N81.2
    complete N81.3
male K62.3
Proctocolitis, mucosal — *see* Rectosigmoiditis,
  ulcerative
Proctoptosis K62.3
Proctorrhagia K62.5
Proctosigmoiditis K63.89
ulcerative (chronic) — *see* Rectosigmoiditis,
  ulcerative
Proctospasm K59.4
psychogenic F45.8
Profichet's disease — *see* Disorder, soft tissue,
  specified type NEC
Progeria E34.8
Prognathism (mandibular) (maxillary) M26.19
Progonoma (melanotic) — *see* Neoplasm, benign, by
  site
Progressive — *see* condition
Prolactinoma
specified site — *see* Neoplasm, benign, by site
unspecified site D35.2
Prolapse, prolapsed
anus, anal (canal) (sphincter) K62.2
arm or hand O32.2
  causing obstructed labor O64.4
bladder (mucosa) (sphincter) (acquired)
  congenital Q79.4
  female — *see* Cystocele
  male N32.89

Prolapse, prolapsed—*continued*
breast implant (prosthetic) T85.49
cecostomy K94.19
cecum K63.4
cervix, cervical (hypertrophied) N81.2
anterior lip, obstructing labor O65.5
congenital Q51.828
postpartal, old N81.2
stump N81.85
ciliary body (traumatic) — *see* Laceration, eye(ball),
with prolapse or loss of interocular tissue
colon (pedunculated) K63.4
colostomy K94.09
disc (intervertebral) — *see* Displacement,
intervertebral disc
eye implant (orbital) T85.398
lens (ocular) — *see* Complications, intraocular
lens
fallopian tube N83.4
gastric (mucosa) K31.89
genital, female N81.9
specified NEC N81.89
globe, nontraumatic — *see* Luxation, globe
ileostomy bud K94.19
intervertebral disc — *see* Displacement,
intervertebral disc
intestine (small) K63.4
iris (traumatic) — *see* Laceration, eye(ball), with
prolapse or loss of interocular tissue
nontraumatic H21.89
kidney N28.83
congenital Q63.2
laryngeal muscles or ventricle J38.7
liver K76.8
meatus urinarius N36.8
mitral (valve) I34.1
ocular lens implant — *see* Complications,
intraocular lens
organ or site, congenital NEC — *see* Malposition,
congenital
ovary N83.4
pelvic floor, female N81.89
perineum, female N81.89
rectum (mucosa) (sphincter) K62.3
due to trichuris trichuria B79
spleen D73.89
stomach K31.89
umbilical cord
complicating delivery O69.0
urachus, congenital Q64.4
ureter N28.89
with obstruction N13.5
with infection N13.6
ureterovesical orifice N28.89
urethra (acquired) (infected) (mucosa) N36.8
congenital Q64.71
urinary meatus N36.8
congenital Q64.72
uterovaginal N81.4
complete N81.3
incomplete N81.2
uterus (with prolapse of vagina) N81.4
complete N81.3
congenital Q51.818
first degree N81.2
in pregnancy or childbirth — *see* Pregnancy,
complicated by, abnormal, uterus
incomplete N81.2
postpartal (old) N81.4
second degree N81.2
third degree N81.3
uveal (traumatic) — *see* Laceration, eye(ball), with
prolapse or loss of interocular tissue
vagina (anterior) (wall) — *see* Cystocele
with prolapse of uterus N81.4
complete N81.3
incomplete N81.2
posterior wall N81.6
posthysterectomy N99.3
vitreous (humor) H43.0-
in wound — *see* Laceration, eye(ball), with
prolapse or loss of interocular tissue
womb — *see* Prolapse, uterus

Prolapsus, female N81.9
specified NEC N81.89
Proliferation(s)
primary cutaneous CD30-positive T-cell C86.6
Proliferative — *see* condition
Prolonged, prolongation (of)
bleeding (time) (idiopathic) R79.1
coagulation (time) R79.1
gestation (over 42 completed weeks)
mother O48.1
newborn P08.22
interval I44.0
labor O63.9
first stage O63.0
second stage O63.1
partial thromboplastin time (PTT) R79.1
pregnancy (more than 42 weeks gestation) O48.1
prothrombin time R79.1
QT interval I45.81
uterine contractions in labor O62.4
Prominence, prominent
auricle (congenital) (ear) Q17.5
ischial spine or sacral promontory
with disproportion (fetopelvic) O33.0
causing obstructed labor O65.0
nose (congenital) acquired M95.0
Promiscuity — *see* High, risk, sexual behavior
Pronation
ankle — *see* Deformity, limb, foot, specified NEC
foot (*see also* Deformity, limb, foot, specified NEC)
congenital Q74.2
Prophylactic
administration of
antibiotics, long-term Z79.2
short-term use — *omit code*
drug (*see also* Long-term (current) drug therapy
(use of)) Z79.899
medication Z79.899
organ removal (for neoplasia management) Z40.00
breast Z40.01
ovary Z40.02
specified site NEC Z40.09
surgery Z40.9
for risk factors related to malignant neoplasm —
see Prophylactic, organ removal
specified NEC Z40.8
vaccination Z23
Propionic acidemia E71.121
Proptosis (ocular) (*see also* Exophthalmos)
thyroid — *see* Hyperthyroidism, with goiter
Prosecution, anxiety concerning Z65.3
Prosopagnosia H53.16
Prostadynia N42.81
Prostate, prostatic — *see* condition
Prostatism — *see* Hyperplasia, prostate
Prostatitis (congestive) (suppurative) (with cystitis)
N41.9
acute N41.00
with hematuria N41.01
cavitary N41.8
chronic N41.10
with hematuria N41.11
diverticular N41.8
due to Trichomonas (vaginalis) A59.02
fibrous N41.10
with hematuria N41.11
gonococcal (acute) (chronic) A54.22
granulomatous N41.4
hypertrophic N41.10
with hematuria N41.11
subacute N41.10
with hematuria N41.11
trichomonal A59.02
tuberculous A18.14
Prostatocystitis N41.3
Prostatorrhea N42.89
Prostatosis N42.82
Prostration R53.83
heat (*see also* Heat, exhaustion)
anhydrotic T67.3
due to
salt (and water) depletion T67.4
water depletion T67.3

Prostration—*continued*
nervous F48.8
senile R54
Protanomaly (anomalous trichromat) H53.54
Protanopia (complete) (incomplete) H53.54
Protection (against) (from) — *see* Prophylactic
Protein
deficiency NEC — *see* Malnutrition
malnutrition — *see* Malnutrition
sickness (prophylactic) (therapeutic) T80.6
Proteinemia R77.9
Proteinosis
alveolar (pulmonary) J84.0
lipid or lipoid (of Urbach) E78.89
Proteinuria R80.9
Bence Jones R80.3
complicating pregnancy — *see* Proteinuria,
gestational
gestational O12.1-
with edema O12.2-
idiopathic R80.0
isolated R80.0
with glomerular lesion N06.9
dense deposit disease N06.6
diffuse
crescentic glomerulonephritis N06.7
endocapillary proliferative
glomerulonephritis N06.4
mesangiocapillary glomerulonephritis
N06.5
focal and segmental hyalinosis or sclerosis
N06.1
membranous (diffuse) N06.2
mesangial proliferative (diffuse) N06.3
minimal change N06.0
specified pathology NEC N06.8
orthostatic R80.2
with glomerular lesion — *see* Proteinuria,
isolated, with glomerular lesion
persistent R80.1
with glomerular lesion — *see* Proteinuria,
isolated, with glomerular lesion
postural R80.2
with glomerular lesion — *see* Proteinuria,
isolated, with glomerular lesion
pre-eclamptic — *see* Pre-eclampsia
specified type NEC R80.8
Proteolysis, pathologic D65
Proteus (mirabilis) (morganii), **as cause of disease
classified elsewhere** B96.4
Prothrombin gene mutation D68.52
Protoporphyria, erythropoietic E80.0
Protozoal (*see also* condition)
disease B64
specified NEC B60.8
Protrusion, protrusio
acetabuli M24.7
acetabulum (into pelvis) M24.7
device, implant or graft (*see also* Complications, by
site and type, mechanical) T85.628
arterial graft NEC — *see* Complication,
cardiovascular device, mechanical, vascular
breast (implant) T85.49
catheter NEC T85.628
cystostomy T83.090
dialysis (renal) T82.49
intraperitoneal T85.691
infusion NEC T82.594
spinal (epidural) (subdural) T85.690
urinary, indwelling T83.098
electronic (electrode) (pulse generator)
(stimulator)
bone T84.390
nervous system — *see* Complication,
prosthetic device, mechanical,
electronic nervous system stimulator
fixation, internal (orthopedic) NEC — *see*
Complication, fixation device, mechanical
gastrointestinal — *see* Complications, prosthetic
device, mechanical, gastrointestinal device

Protrusion, protrusio—*continued*
  device, implant or graft—*continued*
    genital NEC T83.498
      intrauterine contraceptive device T83.39
      penile prosthesis T83.490
    heart NEC — *see* Complication, cardiovascular
        device, mechanical
    joint prosthesis — *see* Complications, joint
        prosthesis, mechanical, specified NEC, by
        site
    ocular NEC — *see* Complications, prosthetic
        device, mechanical, ocular device
    orthopedic NEC — *see* Complication, orthopedic,
        device, mechanical
    specified NEC T85.628
    urinary NEC (*see also* Complication,
        genitourinary, device, urinary, mechanical)
        graft T83.29
    vascular NEC — *see* Complication, cardiovascular
        device, mechanical
    ventricular intracranial shunt T85.09
  intervertebral disc — *see* Displacement,
      intervertebral disc
  joint prosthesis — *see* Complications, joint
      prosthesis, mechanical, specified NEC, by site
  nucleus pulposus — *see* Displacement,
      intervertebral disc
Prune belly (syndrome) Q79.4
Prurigo (ferox) (gravis) (Hebrae) (Hebra's) (mitis)
    (simplex) L28.2
  Besnier's L20.0
  estivalis L56.4
  nodularis L28.1
  psychogenic F45.8
Pruritus, pruritic (essential) L29.9
  ani, anus L29.0
    psychogenic F45.8
  anogenital L29.3
    psychogenic F45.8
  due to onchocerca volvulus B73.1
  gravidarum — *see* Pregnancy, complicated by,
        specified pregnancy-related condition NEC
  hiemalis L29.8
  neurogenic (any site) F45.8
  perianal L29.0
  psychogenic (any site) F45.8
  scroti, scrotum L29.1
    psychogenic F45.8
  senile, senilis L29.8
  specified NEC L29.8
    psychogenic F45.8
  Trichomonas A59.9
  vulva, vulvae L29.2
    psychogenic F45.8
Pseudarthrosis, pseudoarthrosis (bone) — *see*
    Nonunion, fracture
  clavicle, congenital Q74.0
  joint, following fusion or arthrodesis M96.0
Pseudoaneurysm — *see* Aneurysm
Pseudoangioma I81
Pseudoangina (pectoris) — *see* Angina
Pseudoarteriosus Q28.8
Pseudoarthrosis — *see* Pseudarthrosis
Pseudobulbar affect (PBA) F48.8
Pseudochromhidrosis L67.8
Pseudocirrhosis, liver, pericardial I31.1
Pseudocowpox B08.03
Pseudocoxalgia M91.3-
Pseudocroup J38.5
Pseudo-Cushing's syndrome, alcohol-induced E24.4
Pseudocyesis F45.8
Pseudocyst
  lung J98.4
  pancreas K86.3
  retina — *see* Cyst, retina
Pseudoelephantiasis neuroarthritica Q82.0
Pseudoexfoliation, capsule (lens) — *see* Cataract,
    specified NEC
Pseudofolliculitis barbae L73.1
Pseudoglioma H44.89

Pseudohemophilia (Bernuth's) (hereditary) (type B)
    D68.0
  Type A D69.8
  vascular D69.8
Pseudohermaphroditism Q56.3
  adrenal E25.8
  female Q56.2
    with adrenocortical disorder E25.8
    without adrenocortical disorder Q56.2
    adrenal, congenital E25.0
  male Q56.1
    with
      adrenocortical disorder E25.8
      androgen resistance E34.51
      cleft scrotum Q56.1
      feminizing testis E34.51
      5-alpha-reductase deficiency E29.1
    without gonadal disorder Q56.1
    adrenal E25.8
Pseudo-Hurler's polydystrophy E77.0
Pseudohydrocephalus G93.2
Pseudohypertrophic muscular dystrophy (Erb's)
    G71.0
Pseudohypertrophy, muscle G71.0
Pseudohypoparathyroidism E20.1
Pseudoinsomnia F51.03
Pseudoleukemia, infantile D64.89
Pseudomembranous — *see* condition
Pseudomenses (newborn) P54.6
Pseudomenstruation (newborn) P54.6
Pseudomeningocele (cerebral) (infective)
    (post-traumatic) G96.19
  postprocedural (spinal) G97.82
Pseudomonas
  aeruginosa, as cause of disease classified elsewhere
      B96.5
  mallei infection A24.0
    as cause of disease classified elsewhere B96.5
  pseudomallei, as cause of disease classified
      elsewhere B96.5
Pseudomyotonia G71.19
Pseudomyxoma peritonei C78.6
Pseudoneuritis, optic (nerve) (disc) (papilla),
    congenital Q14.2
Pseudo-obstruction intestine (acute) (chronic)
    (idiopathic) (intermittent secondary) (primary)
    K59.8
Pseudopapilledema H47.33-
  congenital Q14.2
Pseudoparalysis
  arm or leg R29.81
  atonic, congenital P94.2
Pseudopelade L66.0
Pseudophakia Z96.1
Pseudopolyarthritis, rhizomelic M35.3
Pseudopolycythemia D75.1
Pseudopseudohypoparathyroidism E20.1
Pseudopterygium H11.81-
Pseudoptosis (eyelid) — *see* Blepharochalasis
Pseudopuberty, precocious
  female heterosexual E25.8
  male isosexual E25.8
Pseudorickets (renal) N25.0
Pseudorubella B08.20
Pseudosclerema, newborn P83.8
Pseudosclerosis (brain)
  of Westphal (Strümpell) E83.01
  Jakob's — *see* Creutzfeldt-Jakob disease or
      syndrome
  spastic — *see* Creutzfeldt-Jakob disease or
      syndrome
Pseudotetanus — *see* Convulsions
Pseudotetany R29.0
  hysterical F44.5
Pseudotruncus arteriosus Q25.4
Pseudotuberculosis A28.2
  enterocolitis A04.8
  pasteurella (infection) A28.0
Pseudotumor
  cerebri G93.2
  orbital — *see* Inflammation, orbit
Pseudoxanthoma elasticum Q82.8

Psilosis (sprue) (tropical) K90.1
  nontropical K90.0
Psittacosis A70
Psoitis M60.88
Psoriasis L40.9
  arthropathic L40.50
    arthritis mutilans L40.52
    distal interphalangeal L40.51
    juvenile L40.54
    other specified L40.59
    spondylitis L40.53
  buccal K13.29
  flexural L40.8
  guttate L40.4
  mouth K13.29
  nummular L40.0
  plaque L40.0
  psychogenic F54
  pustular (generalized) L40.1
    palmaris et plantaris L40.3
  specified NEC L40.8
  vulgaris L40.0
Psychasthenia F48.8
Psychiatric disorder or problem F99
Psychogenic (*see also* condition)
  factors associated with physical conditions F54
**Psychological and behavioral factors affecting
    medical condition** F59
Psychoneurosis, psychoneurotic (*see also* Neurosis)
  anxiety (state) F41.1
  depersonalization F48.1
  hypochondriacal F45.21
  hysteria F44.9
  neurasthenic F48.8
  personality NEC F60.89
Psychopathy, psychopathic
  affectionless F94.2
  autistic F84.5
  constitution, post-traumatic F07.81
  personality — *see* Disorder, personality
  sexual — *see* Deviation, sexual
  state F60.2
Psychosexual identity disorder of childhood F64.2
Psychosis, psychotic F29
  acute (transient) F23
    hysterical F44.9
  affective — *see* Disorder, mood
  alcoholic F10.959
    with
      abuse F10.159
      anxiety disorder F10.980
        with
          abuse F10.180
          dependence F10.280
      delirium tremens F10.231
      delusions F10.950
        with
          abuse F10.150
          dependence F10.250
      dementia F10.97
        with dependence F10.27
      dependence F10.259
      hallucinosis F10.951
        with
          abuse F10.151
          dependence F10.251
      mood disorder F10.94
        with
          abuse F10.14
          dependence F10.24
      paranoia F10.950
        with
          abuse F10.150
          dependence F10.250
    persisting amnesia F10.96
      with dependence F10.26
    amnestic confabulatory F10.96
      with dependence F10.26
    delirium tremens F10.231
    Korsakoff's, Korsakov's, Korsakow's F10.26

Psychosis, psychotic—continued
  alcoholic—continued
    paranoid type F10.950
      with
        abuse F10.150
        dependence F10.250
  anergastic — see Psychosis, organic
  arteriosclerotic (simple type) (uncomplicated)
      F01.50
    with behavioral disturbance F01.51
  childhood F84.0
    atypical F84.8
  climacteric — see Psychosis, involutional
  confusional F29
    acute or subacute F05
    reactive F23
  cycloid F23
  depressive — see Disorder, depressive
  disintegrative (childhood) F84.3
  drug-induced — see F11-F19 with .x59
    paranoid and hallucinatory states — see F11-F19
        with .x50 or .x51
  due to or associated with
    addiction, drug — see F11-F19 with .x59
    dependence
        alcohol F10.259
        drug — see F11-F19 with .x59
    epilepsy F06.8
    Huntington's chorea F06.8
    ischemia, cerebrovascular (generalized) F06.8
    multiple sclerosis F06.8
    physical disease F06.8
    presenile dementia F03
    senile dementia F03
    vascular disease (arteriosclerotic) (cerebral)
        F01.50
      with behavioral disturbance F01.51
  epileptic F06.8
  episode F23
    due to or associated with physical condition
        F06.8
  exhaustive F43.0
  hallucinatory, chronic F28
  hypomanic F30.8
  hysterical (acute) F44.9
  induced F24
  infantile F84.0
    atypical F84.8
  infective (acute) (subacute) F05
  involutional F28
    depressive — see Disorder, depressive
    melancholic — see Disorder, depressive
    paranoid (state) F22
  Korsakoff's, Korsakov's, Korsakow's (nonalcoholic)
      F04
    alcoholic F10.96
      in dependence F10.26
    induced by other psychoactive substance — see
        categories F11-F19 with .x5x
  mania, manic (single episode) F30.2
    recurrent type F31.89
  manic-depressive — see Disorder, mood
  menopausal — see Psychosis, involutional
  mixed schizophrenic and affective F25.8
  multi-infarct (cerebrovascular) F01.50
    with behavioral disturbance F01.51
  nonorganic F29
    specified NEC F28
  organic F09
    due to or associated with
        arteriosclerosis (cerebral) — see Psychosis,
            arteriosclerotic
        cerebrovascular disease, arteriosclerotic —
            see Psychosis, arteriosclerotic
        childbirth — see Psychosis, puerperal
        Creutzfeldt-Jakob disease or syndrome — see
            Creutzfeldt-Jakob disease or syndrome
        dependence, alcohol F10.259
        disease
            alcoholic liver F10.259
            brain, arteriosclerotic — see Psychosis,
                arteriosclerotic

Psychosis, psychotic—continued
  organic—continued
    due to or associated with—continued
        disease—continued
            cerebrovascular F01.50
                with behavioral disturbance F01.51
            Creutzfeldt-Jakob — see Creutzfeldt-Jakob
                disease or syndrome
            endocrine or metabolic F06.8
                acute or subacute F05
            liver, alcoholic F10.259
        epilepsy transient (acute) F05
        infection
            brain (intracranial) F06.8
                acute or subacute F05
        intoxication
            alcoholic (acute) F10.259
            drug F11-F19 with .x59
        ischemia, cerebrovascular (generalized) — see
            Psychosis, arteriosclerotic
        puerperium — see Psychosis, puerperal
        trauma, brain (birth) (from electric current)
            (surgical) F06.8
            acute or subacute F05
    infective F06.8
        acute or subacute F05
    post-traumatic F06.8
        acute or subacute F05
  paranoiac F22
  paranoid (climacteric) (involutional) (menopausal)
      F22
    psychogenic (acute) F23
    schizophrenic F20.0
    senile F03
  postpartum F53
  presbyophrenic (type) F03
  presenile F03
  psychogenic (paranoid) F23
    depressive F32.3
  puerperal F53
    specified type — see Psychosis, by type
  reactive (brief) (transient) (emotional stress)
      (psychological trauma) F23
    depressive F32.3
        recurrent F33.3
    excitative type F30.8
  schizoaffective F25.9
    depressive type F25.1
    manic type F25.0
  schizophrenia, schizophrenic — see Schizophrenia
  schizophrenia-like, in epilepsy F06.2
  schizophreniform F20.81
    affective type F25.9
    brief F23
    confusional type F23
    depressive type F25.1
    manic type F25.0
    mixed type F25.8
  senile NEC F03
    depressed or paranoid type F03
    simple deterioration F03
  specified type code to condition
  shared F24
  situational (reactive) F23
  symbiotic (childhood) F84.3
  symptomatic F09
Psychosomatic — see Disorder, psychosomatic
Psychosyndrome, organic F07.9
Psychotic episode due to or associated with
    physical condition F06.8
Pterygium (eye) H11.00-
  amyloid H11.01-
  central H11.02-
  colli Q18.3
  double H11.03-
  peripheral
    progressive H11.05-
    stationary H11.04-
  recurrent H11.06-
Ptilosis (eyelid) — see Madarosis
Ptomaine (poisoning) — see Poisoning, food

Ptosis (see also Blepharoptosis)
  adiposa (false) — see Blepharoptosis
  breast N64.81
  cecum K63.4
  colon K63.4
  congenital (eyelid) Q10.0
    specified site NEC — see Anomaly, by site
  eyelid — see Blepharoptosis
    congenital Q10.0
  gastric K31.89
  intestine K63.4
  kidney N28.83
  liver K76.8
  renal N28.83
  splanchnic K63.4
  spleen D73.89
  stomach K31.89
  viscera K63.4
PTP D69.51
Ptyalism (periodic) K11.7
  hysterical F45.8
  pregnancy — see Pregnancy, complicated by,
      specified pregnancy-related condition NEC
  psychogenic F45.8
Ptyalolithiasis K11.5
Pubarche, precocious E30.1
Pubertas praecox E30.1
Puberty (development state) Z00.3
  bleeding (excessive) N92.2
  delayed E30.0
  precocious (constitutional) (cryptogenic)
      (idiopathic) E30.1
    central E22.8
    due to
        ovarian hyperfunction E28.1
            estrogen E28.0
        testicular hyperfunction E29.0
  premature E30.1
    due to
        adrenal cortical hyperfunction E25.8
        pineal tumor E34.8
        pituitary (anterior) hyperfunction E22.8
Puckering, macula — see Degeneration, macula,
    puckering
Pudenda, pudendum — see condition
Puente's disease (simple glandular cheilitis) K13.0
Puerperal, puerperium (complicated by,
    complications)
  abnormal glucose (tolerance test) O99.815
  abscess
    areola O91.02
        associated with lactation O91.03
    Bartholin's gland O86.19
    breast O91.12
        associated with lactation O91.13
    cervix (uteri) O86.11
    genital organ NEC O86.19
    kidney O86.21
    mammary O91.12
        associated with lactation O91.13
    nipple O91.02
        associated with lactation O91.03
    peritoneum O85
    subareolar O91.12
        associated with lactation O91.13
    urinary tract — see Puerperal, infection, urinary
    uterus O86.12
    vagina (wall) O86.13
    vaginorectal O86.13
    vulvovaginal gland O86.13
  adnexitis O86.19
  afibrinogenemia, or other coagulation defect O72.3
  albuminuria (acute) (subacute) — see Proteinuria,
      gestational
  alcohol use O99.315
  anemia (pre-exisitng) O99.03
  anesthetic death O89.8
  apoplexy O99.43
  bariatric surgery status O99.845
  blood disorder NEC O99.13
  blood dyscrasia O72.3
  cardiomyopathy O90.3

Puerperal, puerperium —continued
  cerebrovascular disorder (conditions in I60-I69)
    O99.43
  cervicitis O86.11
  circulatory system disorder O99.43
  coagulopathy (any) O72.3
  complications O90.9
    specified NEC O90.89
  convulsions — see Eclampsia
  cystitis O86.22
  cystopyelitis O86.29
  delirium NEC F05
  diabetes O24.93
    gestational — see Puerperal, gestational diabetes
    pre-existing O24.33
      specified NEC O24.83
      type 1 O24.03
      type 2 O24.13
  digestive system disorder O99.63
  disease O90.9
    breast NEC O92.29
    cerebrovascular (acute) O99.43
    nonobstetric NEC O99.89
    tubo-ovarian O86.19
    Valsuani's O99.03
  disorder O90.9
    lactation O92.79
    nonobstetric NEC O99.89
  disruption
    cesarean wound O90.0
    episiotomy wound O90.1
    perineal laceration wound O90.1
  drug use O99.325
  eclampsia (with pre-existing hypertension) O15.2
  embolism (pulmonary) (blood clot) — see
    Embolism, obstetric, puerperal
  endocrine, nutritional or metabolic disease NEC
    O99.285
  endophlebitis — see Puerperal, phlebitis
  endotrachelitis O86.19
  failure
    lactation (complete) O92.3
      partial O92.4
    renal, acute O90.4
  fever (of unknown origin) O86.4
    septic O85
  fissure, nipple O92.12
    associated with lactation O92.13
  fistula
    breast (due to mastitis) O91.12
      associated with lactation O91.13
    nipple O91.02
      associated with lactation O91.03
  galactophoritis O91.22
    associated with lactation O91.23
  galactorrhea O92.6
  gastric banding status O99.845
  gastric bypass status O99.845
  gastrointestinal disease NEC O99.63
  gestational diabetes O24.439
    diet controlled O24.430
    insulin (and diet) controlled O24.434
  gonorrhea O98.23
  hematoma, subdural O99.43
  hemiplegia, cerebral O99.35-
    due to cerebrovascular disorder O99.43
  hemorrhage O72.1
    brain O99.43
    bulbar O99.43
    cerebellar O99.43
    cerebral O99.43
    cortical O99.43
    delayed or secondary O72.2
    extradural O99.43
    internal capsule O99.43
    intracranial O99.43
    intrapontine O99.43
    meningeal O99.43
    pontine O99.43
    retained placenta O72.0
    subarachnoid O99.43
    subcortical O99.43

Puerperal, puerperium —continued
  hemorrhage—continued
    subdural O99.43
    third stage O72.0
    uterine, delayed O72.2
    ventricular O99.43
  hemorrhoids O87.2
  hepatorenal syndrome O90.4
  hypertension — see Hypertension, complicating,
    puerperium
  hypertrophy, breast O92.29
  induration breast (fibrous) O92.29
  infection O86.4
    cervix O86.11
    generalized O85
    genital tract NEC O86.19
      obstetric surgical wound O86.0
    kidney (bacillus coli) O86.21
    maternal O98.93
      carrier state NEC O99.835
      gonorrhea O98.23
      human immunodeficiency (HIV) O98.73
      protozoal O98.63
      sexually transmitted NEC O98.33
      specified NEC O98.83
      streptococcus B carrier state O99.825
      syphilis O98.13
      tuberculosis O98.03
      viral hepatitis O98.43
      viral NEC O98.53
    nipple O91.02
      associated with lactation O91.03
    peritoneum O85
    renal O86.21
    specified NEC O86.89
    urinary (asymptomatic) (tract) NEC O86.20
      bladder O86.22
      kidney O86.21
      specified site NEC O86.29
      urethra O86.22
    vagina O86.13
    vein — see Puerperal, phlebitis
  ischemia, cerebral O99.43
  lymphangitis O86.89
    breast O91.22
      associated with lactation O91.23
  malignancy O9A.13
  malnutrition O25.3
  mammillitis O91.02
    associated with lactation O91.03
  mammitis O91.22
    associated with lactation O91.23
  mania F30.8
  mastitis O91.22
    associated with lactation O91.23
    purulent O91.12
      associated with lactation O91.13
  melancholia — see Disorder, depressive
  mental disorder NEC O99.345
  metroperitonitis O85
  metrorrhagia — see Hemorrhage, postpartum
  metrosalpingitis O86.19
  metrovaginitis O86.13
  milk leg O87.1
  monoplegia, cerebral O99.43
  mood disturbance O90.6
  necrosis, liver (acute) (subacute) (conditions in
    subcategory K72.0) O26.63
    with renal failure O90.4
  nervous system disorder O99.355
  obesity (pre-existing prior to pregnancy) O99.215
  obesity surgery status O99.845
  occlusion, precerebral artery O99.43
  paralysis
    bladder (sphincter) O90.89
    cerebral O99.43
  paralytic stroke O99.43
  parametritis O85
  paravaginitis O86.13
  pelviperitonitis O85
  perimetritis O86.19
  perimetrosalpingitis O86.19
  perinephritis O86.21

Puerperal, puerperium —continued
  periphlebitis — see Puerperal phlebitis
  peritoneal infection O85
  peritonitis (pelvic) O85
  perivaginitis O86.13
  phlebitis O87.0
    deep O87.1
    pelvic O87.1
    superficial O87.0
  phlebothrombosis, deep O87.1
  phlegmasia alba dolens O87.1
  placental polyp O90.89
  pneumonia, embolic — see Embolism, obstetric,
    puerperal
  pre-eclampsia — see Pre-eclampsia
  psychosis F53
  pyelitis O86.21
  pyelocystitis O86.29
  pyelonephritis O86.21
  pyelonephrosis O86.21
  pyemia O85
  pyocystitis O86.29
  pyohemia O85
  pyometra O86.19
  pyonephritis O86.21
  pyosalpingitis O86.19
  pyrexia (of unknown origin) O86.4
  renal
    disease NEC O90.89
    failure O90.4
  respiratory disease NEC O99.53
  retention
    decidua — see Retention, decidua
    placenta O72.0
    secundines — see Retention, secundines
  retrated nipple O92.02
  salpingo-ovaritis O86.19
  salpingoperitonitis O85
  secondary perineal tear O90.1
  sepsis (pelvic) O85
  sepsis O85
  septic thrombophlebitis O86.81
  skin disorder NEC O99.73
  specified condition NEC O99.89
  stroke O99.43
  subinvolution (uterus) O90.89
  subluxation of symphysis (pubis) O26.73
  suppuration — see Puerperal, abscess
  tetanus A34
  thelitis O91.02
    associated with lactation O91.03
  thrombocytopenia O72.3
  thrombophlebitis (superficial) O87.0
    deep O87.1
    pelvic O87.1
    septic O86.81
  thrombosis (venous) — see Thrombosis, puerperal
  thyroiditis O90.5
  toxemia (eclamptic) (pre-eclamptic) (with
    convulsions) O15.2
  trauma, non-obstetric O9A.23
    caused by abuse (physical) (suspected) O9A.33
      confirmed O9A.33
      psychological (suspected) O9A.53
        confirmed O9A.53
      sexual (suspected) O9A.43
        confirmed O9A.43
  uremia (due to renal failure) O90.4
  urethritis O86.22
  vaginitis O86.13
  varicose veins (legs) O87.4
    vulva or perineum O87.8
  venous O87.9
  vulvitis O86.19
  vulvovaginitis O86.13
  white leg O87.1
Puerperium — see Puerperal
Pulmolithiasis J98.4
Pulmonary — see condition
Pulpitis (acute) (anachoretic) (chronic) (hyperplastic)
  (putrescent) (suppurative) (ulcerative) K04.0
Pulpless tooth K04.99

Pulse
- alternating R00.8
- bigeminal R00.8
- fast R00.0
- feeble, rapid due to shock following injury T79.4
- rapid R00.0
- weak R09.89

Pulsus alternans or trigeminus R00.8

Punch drunk F07.81

Punctum lacrimale occlusion — *see* Obstruction, lacrimal

Puncture
- abdomen, abdominal
  - wall S31.139
    - with
      - foreign body S31.149
      - penetration into peritoneal cavity S31.639
        - with foreign body S31.649
    - epigastric region S31.132
      - with
        - foreign body S31.142
        - penetration into peritoneal cavity S31.632
          - with foreign body S31.642
    - left
      - lower quadrant S31.134
        - with
          - foreign body S31.144
          - penetration into peritoneal cavity S31.634
            - with foreign body S31.644
      - upper quadrant S31.131
        - with
          - foreign body S31.141
          - penetration into peritoneal cavity S31.631
            - with foreign body S31.641
    - periumbilic region S31.135
      - with
        - foreign body S31.145
        - penetration into peritoneal cavity S31.635
          - with foreign body S31.645
    - right
      - lower quadrant S31.133
        - with
          - foreign body S31.143
          - penetration into peritoneal cavity S31.633
            - with foreign body S31.643
      - upper quadrant S31.130
        - with
          - foreign body S31.140
          - penetration into peritoneal cavity S31.630
            - with foreign body S31.640
- accidental, complicating surgery — *see* Complication, accidental puncture or laceration
- alveolar (process) — *see* Puncture, oral cavity
- ankle S91.039
  - with
    - foreign body S91.049
  - left S91.032
    - with
      - foreign body S91.042
  - right S91.031
    - with
      - foreign body S91.041
- anus S31.833
  - with foreign body S31.834
- arm (upper) S41.139
  - with foreign body S41.149
  - left S41.132
    - with foreign body S41.142
  - lower — *see* Puncture, forearm
  - right S41.131
    - with foreign body S41.141
- auditory canal (external) (meatus) — *see* Puncture, ear
- auricle, ear — *see* Puncture, ear
- axilla — *see* Puncture, arm

Puncture—*continued*
- back (*see also* Puncture, thorax, back)
  - lower S31.030
    - with
      - foreign body S31.040
        - with penetration into retroperitoneal space S31.041
      - penetration into retroperitoneal space S31.031
- bladder (traumatic) S37.29
  - nontraumatic N32.89
- breast S21.039
  - with foreign body S21.049
  - left S21.032
    - with foreign body S21.042
  - right S21.031
    - with foreign body S21.041
- buttock S31.803
  - with foreign body S31.804
  - left S31.823
    - with foreign body S31.824
  - right S31.813
    - with foreign body S31.814
- by
  - device, implant or graft — *see* Complications, by site and type, mechanical
  - foreign body left accidentally in operative wound T81.539
  - instrument (any) during a procedure, accidental — *see* Puncture, accidental complicating surgery
- calf — *see* Puncture, leg
- canaliculus lacrimalis — *see* Puncture, eyelid
- canthus, eye — *see* Puncture, eyelid
- cervical esophagus S11.23
  - with foreign body S11.24
- cheek (external) S01.439
  - with foreign body S01.449
  - left S01.432
    - with foreign body S01.442
  - right S01.431
    - with foreign body S01.441
  - internal — *see* Puncture, oral cavity
- chest wall — *see* Puncture, thorax
- chin — *see* Puncture, head, specified site NEC
- clitoris — *see* Puncture, vulva
- costal region — *see* Puncture, thorax
- digit(s)
  - hand — *see* Puncture, finger
  - foot — *see* Puncture, toe
- ear (canal) (external) S01.339
  - with foreign body S01.349
  - left S01.332
    - with foreign body S01.342
  - right S01.331
    - with foreign body S01.341
  - drum S09.2-
- elbow S51.039
  - with
    - foreign body S51.049
  - left S51.032
    - with
      - foreign body S51.042
  - right S51.031
    - with
      - foreign body S51.041
- epididymis — *see* Puncture, testis
- epigastric region — *see* Puncture, abdomen, wall, epigastric
- epiglottis S11.83
  - with foreign body S11.84
- esophagus
  - cervical S11.23
    - with foreign body S11.24
  - thoracic S27.818
- eyeball S05.6-
  - with foreign body S05.5-
- eyebrow — *see* Puncture, eyelid

Puncture—*continued*
- eyelid S01.13-
  - with foreign body S01.14-
  - left S01.132
    - with foreign body S01.142
  - right S01.131
    - with foreign body S01.141
- face NEC — *see* Puncture, head, specified site NEC
- finger(s) S61.239
  - with
    - damage to nail S61.339
      - with
        - foreign body S61.349
    - foreign body S61.249
  - index S61.238
    - with
      - damage to nail S61.338
        - with
          - foreign body S61.348
      - foreign body S61.248
    - left S61.231
      - with
        - damage to nail S61.331
          - with
            - foreign body S61.341
        - foreign body S61.241
    - right S61.230
      - with
        - damage to nail S61.330
          - with
            - foreign body S61.340
        - foreign body S61.240
  - little S61.238
    - with
      - damage to nail S61.338
        - with
          - foreign body S61.348
      - foreign body S61.248
    - left S61.237
      - with
        - damage to nail S61.337
          - with
            - foreign body S61.347
        - foreign body S61.247
    - right S61.236
      - with
        - damage to nail S61.336
          - with
            - foreign body S61.346
        - foreign body S61.246
  - middle S61.238
    - with
      - damage to nail S61.338
        - with
          - foreign body S61.348
      - foreign body S61.248
    - left S61.233
      - with
        - damage to nail S61.333
          - with
            - foreign body S61.343
        - foreign body S61.243
    - right S61.232
      - with
        - damage to nail S61.332
          - with
            - foreign body S61.342
        - foreign body S61.242
  - ring S61.238
    - with
      - damage to nail S61.338
        - with
          - foreign body S61.348
      - foreign body S61.248
    - left S61.235
      - with
        - damage to nail S61.335
          - with
            - foreign body S61.345
        - foreign body S61.245

Puncture—continued
  finger(s)—continued
    ring—continued
      right S61.234
        with
          damage to nail S61.334
            with
              foreign body S61.344
          foreign body S61.244
  flank S31.139
    with foreign body S31.149
  foot (except toe(s) alone) S91.339
    with foreign body S91.349
    left S91.332
      with foreign body S91.342
    right S91.331
      with foreign body S91.341
    toe — see Puncture, toe
  forearm S51.839
    with
      foreign body S51.849
    elbow only — see Puncture, elbow
    left S51.832
      with
        foreign body S51.842
    right S51.831
      with
        foreign body S51.841
  forehead — see Puncture, head, specified site NEC
  genital organs, external
    female S31.532
      with foreign body S31.542
      vagina — see Puncture, vagina
      vulva — see Puncture, vulva
    male S31.531
      with foreign body S31.541
      penis — see Puncture, penis
      scrotum — see Puncture, scrotum
      testis — see Puncture, testis
  groin — see Puncture, abdomen, wall
  gum — see Puncture, oral cavity
  hand S61.439
    with
      foreign body S61.449
    finger — see Puncture, finger
    left S61.432
      with
        foreign body S61.442
    right S61.431
      with
        foreign body S61.441
    thumb — see Puncture, thumb
  head S01.93
    with foreign body S01.94
    cheek — see Puncture, cheek
    ear — see Puncture, ear
    eyelid — see Puncture, eyelid
    lip — see Puncture, oral cavity
    nose — see Puncture, nose
    oral cavity — see Puncture, oral cavity
    scalp S01.03
      with foreign body S01.04
    specified site NEC S01.83
      with foreign body S01.84
    temporomandibular area — see Puncture, cheek
  heart S26.99
    with hemopericardium S26.09
    without hemopericardium S26.19
  heel — see Puncture, foot
  hip S71.039
    with foreign body S71.049
    left S71.032
      with foreign body S71.042
    right S71.031
      with foreign body S71.041
  hymen — see Puncture, vagina
  hypochondrium — see Puncture, abdomen, wall
  hypogastric region — see Puncture, abdomen, wall
  inguinal region — see Puncture, abdomen, wall
  instep — see Puncture, foot
  internal organs — see Injury, by site
  interscapular region — see Puncture, thorax, back

Puncture—continued
  intestine
    large
      colon S36.599
        ascending S36.590
        descending S36.592
        sigmoid S36.593
        specified site NEC S36.598
        transverse S36.591
      rectum S36.69
    small S36.499
      duodenum S36.490
      specified site NEC S36.498
  intra-abdominal organ S36.99
    gallbladder S36.128
    intestine — see Puncture, intestine
    liver S36.118
    pancreas — see Puncture, pancreas
    peritoneum S36.81
    specified site NEC S36.898
    spleen S36.09
    stomach S36.39
  jaw — see Puncture, head, specified site NEC
  knee S81.039
    with foreign body S81.049
    left S81.032
      with foreign body S81.042
    right S81.031
      with foreign body S81.041
  labium (majus) (minus) — see Puncture, vulva
  lacrimal duct — see Puncture, eyelid
  larynx S11.013
    with foreign body S11.014
  leg (lower) S81.839
    with foreign body S81.849
    foot — see Puncture, foot
    knee — see Puncture, knee
    left S81.832
      with foreign body S81.842
    right S81.831
      with foreign body S81.841
    upper — see Puncture, thigh
  lip S01.531
    with foreign body S01.541
  loin — see Puncture, abdomen, wall
  lower back — see Puncture, back, lower
  lumbar region — see Puncture, back, lower
  malar region — see Puncture, head, specified site NEC
  mammary — see Puncture, breast
  mastoid region — see Puncture, head, specified site NEC
  mouth — see Puncture, oral cavity
  nail
    finger — see Puncture, finger, with damage to nail
    toe — see Puncture, toe, with damage to nail
  nasal (septum) (sinus) — see Puncture, nose
  nasopharynx — see Puncture, head, specified site NEC
  neck S11.93
    with foreign body S11.94
    involving
      cervical esophagus — see Puncture, cervical esophagus
      larynx — see Puncture, larynx
      pharynx — see Puncture, pharynx
      thyroid gland — see Puncture, thyroid gland
      trachea — see Puncture, trachea
    specified site NEC S11.83
      with foreign body S11.84
  nose (septum) (sinus) S01.23
    with foreign body S01.24
  ocular — see Puncture, eyeball
  oral cavity S01.532
    with foreign body S01.542
  orbit S05.4-
  palate — see Puncture, oral cavity
  palm — see Puncture, hand
  pancreas S36.299
    body S36.291
    head S36.290
    tail S36.292

Puncture—continued
  pelvis — see Puncture, back, lower
  penis S31.23
    with foreign body S31.24
  perineum
    female S31.43
      with foreign body S31.44
    male S31.139
      with foreign body S31.149
  periocular area (with or without lacrimal passages) — see Puncture, eyelid
  phalanges
    finger — see Puncture, finger
    toe — see Puncture, toe
  pharynx S11.23
    with foreign body S11.24
  pinna — see Puncture, ear
  popliteal space — see Puncture, knee
  prepuce — see Puncture, penis
  pubic region S31.139
    with foreign body S31.149
  pudendum — see Puncture, genital organs, external
  rectovaginal septum — see Puncture, vagina
  sacral region — see Puncture, back, lower
  sacroiliac region — see Puncture, back, lower
  salivary gland — see Puncture, oral cavity
  scalp S01.03
    with foreign body S01.04
  scapular region — see Puncture, shoulder
  scrotum S31.33
    with foreign body S31.34
  shin — see Puncture, leg
  shoulder S41.039
    with foreign body S41.049
    left S41.032
      with foreign body S41.042
    right S41.031
      with foreign body S41.041
  spermatic cord — see Puncture, testis
  sternal region — see Puncture, thorax, front
  submaxillary region — see Puncture, head, specified site NEC
  submental region — see Puncture, head, specified site NEC
  subungual
    finger(s) — see Puncture, finger, with damage to nail
    toe — see Puncture, toe, with damage to nail
  supraclavicular fossa — see Puncture, neck, specified site NEC
  temple, temporal region — see Puncture, head, specified site NEC
  temporomandibular area — see Puncture, cheek
  testis S31.33
    with foreign body S31.34
  thigh S71.139
    with foreign body S71.149
    left S71.132
      with foreign body S71.142
    right S71.131
      with foreign body S71.141
  thorax, thoracic (wall) S21.93
    with foreign body S21.94
    back S21.23-
      with
        foreign body S21.24-
          with penetration S21.44
        penetration S21.43
    front S21.13-
      with
        foreign body S21.14-
          with penetration S21.34
        penetration S21.33
    breast — see Puncture, breast
  throat — see Puncture, neck
  thumb S61.039
    with
      damage to nail S61.139
        with
          foreign body S61.149
      foreign body S61.049

Puncture—*continued*
  thumb—*continued*
    left S61.Ø32
      with
        damage to nail S61.132
          with
            foreign body S61.142
        foreign body S61.Ø42
    right S61.Ø31
      with
        damage to nail S61.131
          with
            foreign body S61.141
        foreign body S61.Ø41
  thyroid gland S11.13
    with foreign body S11.14
  toe(s) S91.139
    with
      damage to nail S91.239
        with
          foreign body S91.249
      foreign body S91.149
    great S91.133
      with
        damage to nail S91.233
          with
            foreign body S91.243
        foreign body S91.143
      left S91.132
        with
          damage to nail S91.232
            with
              foreign body S91.242
          foreign body S91.142
      right S91.131
        with
          damage to nail S91.231
            with
              foreign body S91.241
          foreign body S91.141
    lesser S91.136
      with
        damage to nail S91.236
          with
            foreign body S91.246
        foreign body S91.146
      left S91.135
        with
          damage to nail S91.235
            with
              foreign body S91.245
          foreign body S91.145
      right S91.134
        with
          damage to nail S91.234
            with
              foreign body S91.244
          foreign body S91.144
  tongue — *see* Puncture, oral cavity
  trachea S11.Ø23
    with foreign body S11.Ø24
  tunica vaginalis — *see* Puncture, testis
  tympanum, tympanic membrane SØ9.2-
  umbilical region S31.135
    with foreign body S31.145
  uvula — *see* Puncture, oral cavity
  vagina S31.43
    with foreign body S31.44
  vocal cords S11.83
    with foreign body S11.84
  vulva S31.43
    with foreign body S31.44
  wrist S61.539
    with
      foreign body S61.549
    left S61.532
      with
        foreign body S61.542
    right S61.531
      with
        foreign body S61.541
PUO (pyrexia of unknown origin) R5Ø.9
Pupillary membrane (persistent) Q13.89

Pupillotonia — *see* Anomaly, pupil, function, tonic pupil
Purpura D69.2
  abdominal D69.Ø
  allergic D69.Ø
  anaphylactoid D69.Ø
  annularis telangiectodes L81.7
  arthritic D69.Ø
  autoerythrocyte sensitization D69.2
  autoimmune D69.Ø
  bacterial D69.Ø
  Bateman's (senile) D69.2
  capillary fragility (hereditary) (idiopathic)D69.8
  cryoglobulinemic D89.1
  Devil's pinches D69.2
  fibrinolytic — *see* Fibrinolysis
  fulminans, fulminous D65
  gangrenous D65
  hemorrhagic, hemorrhagica D69.3
    not due to thrombocytopenia D69.Ø
  Henoch(-Schönlein) (allergic) D69.Ø
  hypergammaglobulinemic (benign) (Waldenström) D89.Ø
  idiopathic (thrombocytopenic) D69.3
    nonthrombocytopenic D69.Ø
  immune thrombocytopenic D69.3
  infectious D69.Ø
  malignant D69.Ø
  neonatorum P54.5
  nervosa D69.Ø
  newborn P54.5
  nonthrombocytopenic D69.2
    hemorrhagic D69.Ø
    idiopathic D69.Ø
  nonthrombopenic D69.2
  peliosis rheumatica D69.Ø
  posttransfusion (post-transfusion) (from (fresh) whole blood or blood products) D69.51
  primary D69.49
  red cell membrane sensitivity D69.2
  rheumatica D69.Ø
  Schönlein(-Henoch) (allergic) D69.Ø
  scorbutic E54 [D77]
  senile D69.2
  simplex D69.2
  symptomatica D69.Ø
  telangiectasia annularis L81.7
  thrombocytopenic D69.49
    congenital D69.42
    hemorrhagic D69.3
    hereditary D69.42
    idiopathic D69.3
    immune D69.3
    neonatal, transitory P61.Ø
    thrombotic M31.1
  thrombohemolytic — *see* Fibrinolysis
  thrombolytic — *see* Fibrinolysis
  thrombopenic D69.49
  thrombotic, thrombocytopenic M31.1
  toxic D69.Ø
  vascular D69.Ø
  visceral symptoms D69.Ø
Purpuric spots R23.3
Purulent — *see* condition
Pus
  in
    stool R19.5
    urine N39.Ø
  tube (rupture) — *see* Salpingo-oophoritis
Pustular rash LØ8.Ø
Pustule (nonmalignant) LØ8.9
  malignant A22.Ø
Pustulosis palmaris et plantaris L4Ø.3
Putnam(-Dana) **disease or syndrome** — *see* Degeneration, combined
Putrescent pulp (dental) KØ4.1
Pyarthritis, pyarthrosis — *see* Arthritis, pyogenic or pyemic
  tuberculous — *see* Tuberculosis, joint
Pyelectasis — *see* Hydronephrosis

Pyelitis (congenital) (uremic) (*see also* Pyelonephritis)
  with
    calculus — *see* category N2Ø
      with hydronephrosis N13.2
    contracted kidney N11.9
  acute N1Ø
  chronic N11.9
    with calculus — *see* category N2Ø
      with hydronephrosis N13.2
  cystica N28.84
  puerperal (postpartum) O86.21
  tuberculous A18.11
Pyelocystitis — *see* Pyelonephritis
Pyelonephritis (*see also* Nephritis, tubulo-interstitial)
  with
    calculus — *see* category N2Ø
      with hydronephrosis N13.2
    contracted kidney N11.9
  acute N1Ø
  calculus — *see* category N2Ø
    with hydronephrosis N13.2
  chronic N11.9
    with calculus — *see* category N2Ø
      with hydronephrosis N13.2
    associated with ureteral obstruction or stricture N11.1
    nonobstructive N11.8
      with reflux (vesicoureteral) N11.Ø
    obstructive N11.1
    specified NEC N11.8
  in (due to)
    brucellosis A23.9 [N16]
    cryoglobulinemia (mixed) D89.1 [N16]
    cystinosis E72.Ø4
    diphtheria A36.84
    glycogen storage disease E74.Ø9 [N16]
    leukemia NEC C95.9- [N16]
    lymphoma NEC C85.9Ø [N16]
    multiple myeloma C9Ø.Ø- [N16]
    obstruction N11.1
    Salmonella infection AØ2.25
    sarcoidosis D86.84
    sepsis A41.9 [N16]
    Sjögren's disease M35.Ø4
    toxoplasmosis B58.83
    transplant rejection T86.91 [N16]
    Wilson's disease E83.Ø1 [N16]
  nonobstructive N12
    with reflux (vesicoureteral) N11.Ø
    chronic N11.8
  syphilitic A52.75
Pyelonephrosis (obstructive) N11.1
  chronic N11.9
Pyelophlebitis I8Ø.8
Pyeloureteritis cystica N28.85
Pyemia, pyemic (fever) (infection) (purulent) (*see also* Sepsis)
  joint — *see* Arthritis, pyogenic or pyemic
  liver K75.1
  pneumococcal A4Ø.3
  portal K75.1
  postvaccinal T88.Ø
  puerperal, postpartum, childbirth O85
  specified organism NEC A41.89
  tuberculous — *see* Tuberculosis, miliary
Pygopagus Q89.4
Pyknoepilepsy, pyknolepsy (idiopathic) — *see* Epilepsy, generalized, idiopathic
Pyknolepsy — *see* Epilepsy, generalized, idiopathic
Pylephlebitis K75.1
Pyle's syndrome Q78.5
Pylethrombophlebitis K75.1
Pylethrombosis K75.1
Pyloritis K29.9Ø
  with bleeding K29.91
Pylorospasm (reflex) NEC K31.3
  congenital or infantile Q4Ø.Ø
  newborn Q4Ø.Ø
  neurotic F45.8
  psychogenic F45.8
Pylorus, pyloric — *see* condition
Pyoarthrosis — *see* Arthritis, pyogenic or pyemic

Pyocele
  mastoid — *see* Mastoiditis, acute
  sinus (accessory) — *see* Sinusitis
  turbinate (bone) J32.9
  urethra (*see also* Urethritis) N34.0
Pyocolpos — *see* Vaginitis
Pyocystitis N30.80
  with hematuria N30.81
Pyoderma, pyodermia L08.0
  gangrenosum L88
  newborn P39.4
  phagedenic L88
  vegetans L08.81
Pyodermatitis L08.0
  vegetans L08.81
Pyogenic — *see* condition
Pyohydronephrosis N13.6
Pyometra, pyometrium, pyometritis — *see*
  Endometritis
Pyomyositis (tropical) — *see* Myositis, infective
Pyonephritis N12
Pyonephrosis N13.6
  tuberculous A18.11
Pyo-oophoritis — *see* Salpingo-oophoritis
Pyo-ovarium — *see* Salpingo-oophoritis
Pyopericarditis, pyopericardium I30.1
Pyophlebitis — *see* Phlebitis
Pyopneumopericardium I30.1
Pyopneumothorax (infective) J86.9
  with fistula J86.0
  tuberculous NEC A15.6
Pyosalpinx, pyosalpingitis (*see also*
  Salpingo-oophoritis)
Pyothorax J86.9
  with fistula J86.0
  tuberculous NEC A15.6
Pyoureter N28.89
  tuberculous A18.11
Pyramidopallidonigral syndrome G20
Pyrexia (of unknown origin) R50.9
  atmospheric T67.0
  during labor NEC O75.2
  heat T67.0
  newborn P81.9
    environmentally-induced P81.0
  persistent R50.9
  puerperal O86.4
Pyroglobulinemia NEC E88.09
Pyromania F63.1
Pyrosis R12
Pyuria (bacterial) N39.0

Q

Q fever A78
  with pneumonia A78
Quadricuspid aortic valve Q23.8
Quadrilateral fever A78
Quadriparesis — *see* Quadriplegia
  meaning muscle weakness M62.81
Quadriplegia G82.50-
  complete
    C1-C4 level G82.51
    C5-C7 level G82.53
  congenital (cerebral) (spinal) G80.8
    spastic G80.0
  embolic (current episode) I63.4
  incomplete
    C1-C4 level G82.52
    C5-C7 level G82.54
  functional R53.2
  thrombotic (current episode) I63.3
  traumatic — code to injury with extension s
    current episode — *see* Injury, spinal (cord),
      cervical
  functional R53.2
Quadruplet, pregnancy — *see* Pregnancy, quadruplet
Quarrelsomeness F60.3
Queensland fever A77.3
Quervain's disease M65.4
  thyroid E06.1

Queyrat's erythroplasia D07.4
  penis D07.4
  specified site — *see* Neoplasm, skin, in situ
  unspecified site D07.4
Quincke's disease or edema T78.3
  hereditary D84.1
Quinsy (gangrenous) J36
Quintan fever A79.0
Quintuplet, pregnancy — *see* Pregnancy, quintuplet

R

Rabbit fever — *see* Tularemia
Rabies A82.9
  contact Z20.3
  exposure to Z20.3
  inoculation reaction — *see* Complications,
    vaccination
  sylvatic A82.0
  urban A82.1
Rachischisis — *see* Spina bifida
Rachitic (*see also* condition)
  deformities of spine (late effect) (sequelae) E64.3
  pelvis (late effect) (sequelae) E64.3
    with disproportion (fetopelvic) O33.0
      causing obstructed labor O65.0
Rachitis, rachitism (acute) (tarda) (*see also* Rickets)
  renalis N25.0
  sequelae E64.3
Radial nerve — *see* condition
Radiation
  burn — *see* Burn
  effects NOS T66
  sickness NOS T66
  therapy, encounter for Z51.0
Radiculitis (pressure) (vertebrogenic) — *see*
  Radiculopathy
Radiculomyelitis (*see also* Encephalitis)
  toxic, due to
    Clostridium tetani A35
    Corynebacterium diphtheriae A36.82
Radiculopathy M54.10
  cervical region M54.12
  cervicothoracic region M54.13
  due to displacement of intervertebral disc — *see*
    Disorder, disc, with, radiculopathy
  leg M54.1-
  lumbar region M54.16
  lumbosacral region M54.17
  occipito-atlanto-axial region M54.11
  postherpetic B02.29
  sacrococcygeal region M54.18
  syphilitic A52.11
  thoracic region (with visceral pain) M54.14
  thoracolumbar region M54.15
Radiodermal burns (acute, chronic, or occupational)
  — *see* Burn
Radiodermatitis L58.9
  acute L58.0
  chronic L58.1
Radiotherapy session Z51.0
Rage, meaning rabies — *see* Rabies
Ragpicker's disease A22.1
Ragsorter's disease A22.1
Raillietiniasis B71.8
Railroad neurosis F48.8
Railway spine F48.8
Raised (*see also* Elevated)
  antibody titer R76.0
Rake teeth, tooth M26.39
Rales R09.89
Ramifying renal pelvis Q63.8
Ramsay-Hunt disease or syndrome (*see also* Hunt's
  disease) B02.21
  meaning dyssynergia cerebellaris myoclonica G11.1
Ranula K11.6
  congenital Q38.4
Rape
  adult
    confirmed T74.21
    suspected T76.21

Rape—*continued*
  alleged, observation or examination, ruled out
    adult Z04.41
    child Z04.42
  child
    confirmed T74.22
    suspected T76.22
Rapid
  feeble pulse, due to shock, following injury T79.4
  heart (beat) R00.0
    psychogenic F45.8
  second stage (delivery) O62.3
  time-zone change syndrome — *see* Disorder, sleep,
    circadian rhythm, psychogenic
Rarefaction, bone— *see* Disorder, bone, density and
  structure, specified NEC
Rash (toxic) R21
  canker A38.9
  diaper L22
  drug (internal use) L27.0
    contact (*see also* Dermatitis, due to, drugs,
      external) L25.1
  following immunization T88.1
  food — *see* Dermatitis, due to, food
  heat L74.0
  napkin (psoriasiform) L22
  nettle — *see* Urticaria
  pustular L08.0
  rose R21
    epidemic B06.9
  scarlet A38.9
  serum (prophylactic) (therapeutic) T80.6
  wandering tongue K14.1
Rasmussen aneurysm — *see* Tuberculosis, pulmonary
Rasmussen encephalitis G04.81
Rat-bite fever A25.9
  due to Streptobacillus moniliformis A25.1
  spirochetal (morsus muris) A25.0
Rathke's pouch tumor D44.3
Raymond (-Cestan) **syndrome** I65.8
Raynaud's disease, phenomenon or syndrome
  (secondary) I73.00
  with gangrene (symmetric) I73.01
RDS (newborn) (type I) P22.0
  type II P22.1
Reaction (*see also* Disorder)
  adaptation — *see* Disorder, adjustment
  adjustment (anxiety) (conduct disorder)
    (depressiveness) (distress) (*see also* Disorder,
    adjustment)
    with
      mutism, elective (child) (adolescent) F94.0
  affective — *see* Disorder, mood
  allergic — *see* Allergy
  anaphylactic — *see* Shock, anaphylactic
  anesthesia — *see* Anesthesia, complication
  antitoxin (prophylactic) (therapeutic) — *see*
    Complications, vaccination
  anxiety F41.1
  Arthus — *see* Arthus' phenomenon
  asthenic F48.8
  combat and operational stress F43.0
  compulsive F42
  conversion F44.9
  crisis, acute F43.0
  deoxyribonuclease (DNA) (DNase) hypersensitivity
    D69.2
  depressive (single episode) F32.9
    affective (single episode) F31.4
      recurrent episode F33.9
    neurotic F34.1
    psychoneurotic F34.1
    psychotic F32.3
    recurrent — *see* Disorder, depressive, recurrent
  dissociative F44.9
  drug NEC T88.7 — This code not for use in the
    inpatient setting
    addictive — *see* Dependence, drug
      transmitted via placenta or breast milk — *see*
        Absorption, drug, addictive, through
        placenta
    allergic — *see* Allergy, drug
    lichenoid L43.2

Reaction—continued
  drug NEC—continued
    newborn P93.8
      gray baby syndrome P93.0
    overdose or poisoning (by accident) — see Table
        of Drugs and Chemicals, by drug,
        poisoning
    photoallergic L56.1
    phototoxic L56.0
    withdrawal — see Dependence, by drug, with,
        withdrawal
      infant of dependent mother P96.1
      newborn P96.1
    wrong substance given or taken (by accident) —
        see Table of Drugs and Chemicals, by drug,
        poisoning
  fear F40.9
    child (abnormal) F93.8
  febrile nonhemolytic transfusion (FNHTR) R50.84
  fluid loss, cerebrospinal G97.1
  foreign
    body NEC — see Granuloma, foreign body
      in operative wound (inadvertently left) — see
          Foreign body, accidentally left during a
          procedure
    substance accidentally left during a procedure
        (chemical) (powder) (talc) T81.60
      aseptic peritonitis T81.61
      body or object (instrument) (sponge) (swab)
          — see Foreign body, accidentally left
          during a procedure
      specified reaction NEC T81.69
  grief — see Disorder, adjustment
  Herxheimer's T88.6
  hyperkinetic — see Hyperkinesia
  hypochondriacal F45.20
  hypoglycemic, due to insulin E16.0
    with coma (diabetic) — see Diabetes, coma
      nondiabetic E15
    therapeutic misadventure — see subcategory
        T38.3
  hypomanic F30.8
  hysterical F44.9
  immunization — see Complications, vaccination
  incompatibility
    ABO blood group (infusion) (transfusion) — see
        Complication(s), transfusion,
        incompatiblity reaction, ABO
      delayed serologic T80.39
    minor blood group (Duffy) (E) (K(ell)) (Kidd)
        (Lewis) (M) (N) (P) (S) T80.89
    Rh (factor) (infusion) (transfusion) T80.4 — see
        Complication(s), transfusion,
        incompatibility reaction, Rh (factor)
  inflammatory — see Infection
  infusion — see Complications, infusion
  inoculation (immune serum) — see Complications,
      vaccination
  insulin T38.3-
  involutional psychotic — see Disorder, depressive
  leukemoid D72.823
    basophilic D72.823
    lymphocytic D72.823
    monocytic D72.823
    myelocytic D72.823
    neutrophilic D72.823
  LSD (acute)
    due to drug abuse — see Abuse, drug,
        hallucinogen
    due to drug dependence — see Dependence,
        drug, hallucinogen
  lumbar puncture G97.1
  manic-depressive — see Disorder, bipolar
  neurasthenic F48.8
  neurogenic — see Neurosis
  neurotic F48.9
  neurotic-depressive F34.1
  nitritoid — see Crisis, nitritoid
  obsessive-compulsive F42
  organic, acute or subacute — see Delirium
  paranoid (acute) F23
    chronic F22
    senile F03

Reaction—continued
  passive dependency F60.7
  phobic F40.9
  post-traumatic stress, uncomplicated Z73.3
  psychogenic F99
  psychoneurotic (see also Neurosis)
    compulsive F42
    depersonalization F48.1
    depressive F34.1
    hypochondriacal F45.20
    neurasthenic F48.8
    obsessive F42
  psychophysiologic — see Disorder, somatoform
  psychosomatic — see Disorder, somatoform
  psychotic — see Psychosis
  scarlet fever toxin — see Complications, vaccination
  schizophrenic F23
    acute (brief) (undifferentiated) F23
    latent F21
    undifferentiated (acute) (brief) F23
  serological for syphilis — see Serology for syphilis
  serum (prophylactic) (therapeutic) T80.6
    anaphylactic (immediate) T80.5
  situational — see Disorder, adjustment
  somatization — see Disorder, somatoform
  spinal puncture G97.1
  stress (severe) F43.9
    acute (agitation) ("daze") (disorientation)
        (disturbance of consciousness) (flight
        reaction) (fugue) F43.0
    specified NEC F43.8
  surgical procedure — see Complications, surgical
      procedure
  tetanus antitoxin — see Complications, vaccination
  toxic, to local anesthesia T81.89
    in labor and delivery O74.4
    in pregnancy O29.3x-
    postpartum, puerperal O89.3
  toxin-antitoxin — see Complications, vaccination
  transfusion (blood) (bone marrow) (lymphocytes)
      (allergic) — see Complications, transfusion
  tuberculin skin test, abnormal R76.1
  vaccination (any) — see Complications, vaccination
  withdrawing, child or adolescent F93.8
Reactive airway disease — see Asthma
Reactive depression — see Reaction, depressive
Rearrangement
  chromosomal
    balanced (in) Q95.9
      abnormal individual (autosomal) Q95.2
        non-sex (autosomal) chromosomes Q95.2
        sex/non-sex chromosomes Q95.3
      specified NEC Q95.8
Recalcitrant patient — see Noncompliance
Recanalization, thrombus — see Thrombosis
Recession, receding
  chamber angle (eye) H21.55-
  chin M26.09
  gingival (generalized) (localized) (postinfective)
      (postoperative) K06.0
Recklinghausen disease Q85.00
  bones E21.0
Reclus' disease (cystic) — see Mastopathy, cystic
Recrudescent typhus (fever) A75.1
Recruitment, auditory H93.21-
Rectalgia K62.8
Rectitis K62.8
Rectocele
  female (without uterine prolapse) N81.6
    with uterine prolapse N81.4
      incomplete N81.2
  in pregnancy — see Pregnancy, complicated by,
      abnormal, pelvic organs or tissues NEC
  male K62.3
Rectosigmoid junction — see condition
Rectosigmoiditis K63.89
  ulcerative (chronic) K51.30
    with
      complication K51.319
        abscess K51.314
        fistula K51.313
        obstruction K51.312

Rectosigmoiditis—continued
  ulcerative—continued
    with—continued
      complication—continued
        rectal bleeding K51.311
        specified NEC K51.318
Rectourethral— see condition
Rectovaginal — see condition
Rectovesical — see condition
Rectum, rectal — see condition
Recurrent — see condition
  pregnancy loss — see Loss (of), pregnancy,
      recurrent
Red bugs B88.0
Red-cedar lung or pneumonitis J67.8
Red tide (see also Table of Drugs and Chemicals) T65.82
Reduced
  mobility Z74.09
  ventilatory or vital capacity R94.2
Redundant, redundancy
  anus (congenital) Q43.8
  clitoris N90.89
  colon (congenital) Q43.8
  foreskin (congenital) N47.8
  intestine (congenital) Q43.8
  labia N90.6
  organ or site, congenital NEC — see Accessory
  panniculus (abdominal) E65
  prepuce (congenital) N47.8
  pylorus K31.89
  rectum (congenital) Q43.8
  scrotum N50.8
  sigmoid (congenital) Q43.8
  skin (of face) L57.4
    eyelids — see Blepharochalasis
  stomach K31.89
Reduplication — see Duplication
Reflex R29.2
  hyperactive gag J39.2
  pupillary, abnormal — see Anomaly, pupil, function
  vasoconstriction I73.9
  vasovagal R55
Reflux K21.9
  acid K21.9
  esophageal K21.9
    with esophagitis K21.0
    newborn P78.83
  gastroesophageal K21.9
    with esophagitis K21.0
  mitral — see Insufficiency, mitral
  ureteral — see Reflux, vesicoureteral
  vesicoureteral (with scarring) N13.70
    with
      nephropathy N13.729
        with hydroureter N13.739
          bilateral N13.732
          unilateral N13.731
        bilateral N13.722
        unilateral N13.721
        without hydroureter N13.729
          bilateral N13.722
          unilateral N13.721
      pyelonephritis (chronic) N11.1
    congenital Q62.7
    without nephropathy N13.71
Reforming, artificial openings — see Attention to,
    artificial, opening
Refractive error — see Disorder, refraction
Refsum's disease or syndrome G60.1
Refusal of
  food, psychogenic F50.8
  treatment (because of) Z53.20
    left against medical advice (AMA) Z53.21
    patient's decision NEC Z53.29
    reasons of belief or group pressure Z53.1
Regional — see condition
Regurgitation R11.10
  aortic (valve) — see Insufficiency, aortic
  food (see also Vomiting)
    with reswallowing — see Rumination
    newborn P92.1
  gastric contents — see Vomiting

Regurgitation—*continued*
  heart — *see* Endocarditis
  mitral (valve) — *see* Insufficiency, mitral
    congenital Q23.3
  myocardial — *see* Endocarditis
  pulmonary (valve) (heart) I37.1
    congenital Q22.2
    syphilitic A52.03
  tricuspid — *see* Insufficiency, tricuspid
  valve, valvular — *see* Endocarditis
    congenital Q24.8
  vesicoureteral — *see* Reflux, vesicoureteral
Reifenstein syndrome E34.52
Reinsertion, contraceptive device Z30.433
Reiter's disease, syndrome, or urethritis M02.30
  ankle M02.37-
  elbow M02.32-
  foot joint M02.37-
  hand joint M02.34-
  hip M02.35-
  knee M02.36-
  multiple site M02.39
  shoulder M02.31-
  vertebra M02.38
  wrist M02.33-
Reichmann's disease or syndrome K31.89
Rejection
  food, psychogenic F50.8
  transplant T86.91
    bone T86.830
      marrow T86.01
    cornea T86.840
    heart T86.21
      with lung(s) T86.31
    intestine T86.890
    kidney T86.11
    liver T86.41
    lung(s) T86.810
      with heart T86.31
    organ (immune or nonimmune cause) T86.91
    pancreas T86.890
    skin (allograft) (autograft) T86.820
    specified NEC T86.890
Relapsing fever A68.9
  Carter's (Asiatic) A68.1
  Dutton's (West African) A68.1
  Koch's A68.9
  louse-borne (epidemic) A68.0
  Novy's (American) A68.1
  Obermeyers's (European) A68.0
  Spirillum A68.9
  tick-borne (endemic) A68.1
Relationship
  occlusal
    open anterior M26.220
    open posterior M26.221
Relaxation
  anus (sphincter) K62.8
    psychogenic F45.8
  arch (foot) (*see also* Deformity, limb, flat foot)
  back ligaments — *see* Instability, joint, spine
  bladder (sphincter) N31.2
  cardioesophageal K21.9
  cervix — *see* Incompetency, cervix
  diaphragm J98.6
  joint (capsule) (ligament) (paralytic) — *see* Flail, joint
    congenital NEC Q74.8
  lumbosacral (joint) — *see* subcategory M53.2
  pelvic floor N81.89
  perineum N81.89
  posture R29.3
  rectum (sphincter) K62.8
  sacroiliac (joint) — *see* subcategory M53.2
  scrotum N50.8
  urethra (sphincter) N36.44
  vesical N31.2
Release from prison, anxiety concerning Z65.2
Remains
  canal of Cloquet Q14.0
  capsule (opaque) Q14.8
Remittent fever (malarial) B54

Remnant
  canal of Cloquet Q14.0
  capsule (opaque) Q14.8
  cervix, cervical stump (acquired) (postoperative)
    N88.8
  cystic duct, postcholecystectomy K91.5
  fingernail L60.8
    congenital Q84.6
  meniscus, knee — *see* Derangement, knee,
    meniscus, specified NEC
  thyroglossal duct Q89.2
  tonsil J35.8
    infected (chronic) J35.01
  urachus Q64.4
Removal (from) (of)
  artificial
    arm Z44.00-
      complete Z44.01-
      partial Z44.02-
    eye Z44.2-
    leg Z44.10-
      complete Z44.11-
      partial Z44.12-
  breast implant Z45.81
  cardiac pulse generator (battery) (end-of-life)
    Z45.010
  catheter (urinary) (indwelling) Z46.6
    from artificial opening — *see* Attention to,
      artificial, opening
    non-vascular Z46.82
    vascular NEC Z45.2
  drains Z48.03
  device Z46.9
    contraceptive Z30.432
    implanted NEC Z45.89
    specified NEC Z46.89
  dressing (nonsurgical) Z48.00
    surgical Z48.01
  external
  fixation device code to fracture with extension d
    prosthesis, prosthetic device Z44.9
      breast Z44.3-
      specified NEC Z44.8
  home in childhood (to foster home or institution)
    Z62.29
  ileostomy Z43.2
  insulin pump Z46.81
  myringotomy device (stent) (tube) Z45.82
  nervous system device NEC Z46.2
    brain neuropacemaker Z46.2
    visual substitution device Z46.2
      implanted Z45.31
  non-vascular catheter Z46.82
  orthodontic device Z46.4
  organ, prophylactic (for neoplasia management) —
    see Prophylactic, organ removal
  staples Z48.02
  stent
    ureteral Z46.6
  suture Z48.02
  urinary device Z46.6
  vascular access device or catheter Z45.2
Ren
  arcuatus Q63.1
  mobile, mobilis N28.89
    congenital Q63.8
  unguliformis Q63.1
Renal — *see* condition
Rendu-Osler-Weber disease or syndrome I78.0
Reninoma D41.0-
Renon-Delille syndrome E23.3
Reovirus, as cause of disease classified elsewhere
  B97.5
Repeated falls NEC R29.6
Replaced chromosome by dicentric ring Q93.2
Replacement by artificial or mechanical device or
    prosthesis of
  bladder Z96.0
  blood vessel NEC Z95.828
  bone NEC Z96.7
  cochlea Z96.21
  coronary artery Z95.5
  eustachian tube Z96.29

Replacement by artificial or mechanical device or
    prosthesis of—*continued*
  eye globe Z97.0
  heart Z95.812
    valve Z95.2
      prosthetic Z95.2
      specified NEC Z95.4
      xenogenic Z95.3
  intestine Z96.89
  joint Z96.60
    hip — *see* Presence, hip joint implant
    knee — *see* Presence, knee joint implant
    specified site NEC Z96.698
  larynx Z96.3
  lens Z96.1
  limb(s) — *see* Presence, artificial, limb
  mandible NEC (for tooth root implant(s)) Z96.5
  organ NEC Z96.89
  peripheral vessel NEC Z95.828
  stapes Z96.29
  teeth Z97.2
  tendon Z96.7
  tissue NEC Z96.89
  tooth root(s) Z96.5
  vessel NEC Z95.828
    coronary (artery) Z95.5
Request for expert evidence Z04.8
Reserve, decreased or low
  cardiac — *see* Disease, heart
  kidney N28.89
Residual (*see also* condition)
  ovary syndrome N99.83
  state, schizophrenic F20.5
  urine R39.19
Resistance, resistant
  activated protein C (to) D68.51
  insulin E88.81
  organism(s), to multiple drugs (MDRO) Z16
  thyroid hormone E07.89
Resorption
  dental (roots) K03.3
    alveoli M26.79
  teeth (external) (internal) (pathological) (roots)
    K03.3
Respiration
  Cheyne-Stokes R06.3
  decreased due to shock, following injury T79.4
  disorder of, psychogenic F45.8
  insufficient, or poor R06.89
    newborn P28.5
  painful R07.1
  sighing, psychogenic F45.8
Respiratory (*see also* condition)
  distress syndrome (newborn) (type I) P22.0
    type II P22.1
  syncytial virus, as cause of disease classified
    elsewhere B97.4
Respite care Z75.5
Response (drug)
  photoallergic L56.1
  phototoxic L56.0
Restless legs (syndrome) G25.81
Restlessness R45.1
Restriction of housing space Z59.1
Restoration (of)
  dental
    aesthetically inadequate or displeasing K08.56
    defective K08.50
      specified NEC K08.59
    failure of marginal integrity K08.51
    failure of periodontal anatomical intergrity
      K08.54
  organ continuity from previous sterilization
    (tuboplasty) (vasoplasty) Z31.0
    aftercare Z31.42
  tooth (existing)
    contours biologically incompatible with oral
      health K08.54
    open margins K08.51
    overhanging K08.52
    poor aesthetic K08.56
    poor gingival margins K08.51

Restoration—*continued*
   unsatisfactory, of tooth K08.50
     specified NEC K08.59
Restorative material (dental)
   allergy to K08.55
   fractured K08.539
     with loss of material K08.531
     without loss of material K08.530
   unrepairable overhanging of K08.52
Rests, ovarian, in fallopian tube Q50.6
Restzustand (schizophrenic) F20.5
Retained (*see also* Retention)
   foreign body fragments (type of) Z18.9
     acrylics Z18.2
     animal quill(s) or spines Z18.31
     cement Z18.83
     concrete Z18.83
     crystalline Z18.83
     depleted isotope Z18.09
     depleted uranium Z18.01
     diethylhexylphthalates Z18.2
     glass Z18.81
     isocyanate Z18.2
     magnetic metal Z18.11
     metal Z18.10
     nonmagnetic metal Z18.12
     nontherapeutic radioactive Z18.09
     organic NEC Z18.39
     plastic Z18.2
     quill(s) (animal) Z18.31
     radioactive (nontherapeutic) NEC Z18.09
     specified NEC Z18.89
     spine(s) (animal) Z18.31
     stone Z18.83
     tooth (teeth) Z18.32
     wood Z18.33
   fragments (type of) Z18.9
     acrylics Z18.2
     animal quill(s) or spines Z18.31
     cement Z18.83
     concrete Z18.83
     crystalline Z18.83
     depleted isotope Z18.09
     depleted uranium Z18.01
     diethylhexylphthalates Z18.2
     glass Z18.81
     isocyanate Z18.2
     magnetic metal Z18.11
     metal Z18.10
     nonmagnetic metal Z18.12
     nontherapeutic radioactive Z18.09
     organic NEC Z18.39
     plastic Z18.2
     quill(s) (animal) Z18.31
     radioactive (nontherapeutic) NEC Z18.09
     specified NEC Z18.89
     spine(s) (animal) Z18.31
     stone Z18.83
     tooth (teeth) Z18.32
     wood Z18.33
Retardation
   development, developmental, specific — *see*
     Disorder, developmental
   endochondral bone growth — *see* Disorder, bone,
     development or growth
   growth R62.50
     due to malnutrition E45
   mental F79
     with
       autistic features F84.9
     mild (I.Q. 50-69) F70
     moderate (I.Q. 35-49) F71
     profound (I.Q. under 20) F73
     severe (I.Q. 20-34) F72
     specified level NEC F78
   motor function, specific F82
   physical (child) R62.50
     due to malnutrition E45
   reading (specific) F81.0
   spelling (specific) (without reading disorder) F81.81
Retching — *see* Vomiting

Retention (*see also* Retained)
   bladder — *see* Retention, urine
   carbon dioxide E87.2
   cholelithiasis K91.89
   cyst — *see* Cyst
   dead
     fetus (at or near term) (mother) O36.4
       early fetal death O02.1
     ovum O02.0
   decidua (fragments) (following delivery) (with
     hemorrhage) O72.2
     without hemorrhage O73.1
   deciduous tooth K00.6
   dental root K08.3
   fecal — *see* Constipation
   fetus
     dead O36.4
       early O02.1
   fluid R60.9
   foreign body (*see also* Foreign body, retained)
     current trauma — code as Foreign body, by site
       or type
   gallstones K91.89
   gastric K31.89
   intrauterine contraceptive device, in pregnancy —
     see Pregnancy, complicated by, retention,
     intrauterine device
   membranes (complicating delivery) (with
     hemorrhage) O72.2
     with abortion — *see* Abortion, by type
     without hemorrhage O73.1
   meniscus — *see* Derangement, meniscus
   menses N94.89
   milk (puerperal, postpartum) O92.79
   nitrogen, extrarenal R39.2
   ovary syndrome N99.83
   placenta (total) (with hemorrhage) O72.0
     without hemorrhage O73.0
     portions or fragments (with hemorrhage) O72.2
       without hemorrhage O73.1
   products of conception
     early pregnancy (dead fetus) O02.1
     following
       delivery (with hemorrhage) O72.2
         without hemorrhage O73.1
   secundines (following delivery) (with hemorrhage)
     O72.0
     without hemorrhage O73.0
     complicating puerperium (delayed hemorrhage)
       O72.2
     partial O72.2
       without hemorrhage O73.1
   smegma, clitoris N90.89
   urine R33.9
     due to hyperplasia (hypertrophy) of prostate —
       see Hyperplasia, prostate
     drug-induced R33.0
     organic R33.8
       drug-induced R33.0
     psychogenic F45.8
     specified NEC R33.8
   water (in tissues) — *see* Edema
Reticulation, dust — *see* Pneumoconiosis
Reticulocytosis R70.1
Reticuloendotheliosis
   acute infantile C96.0
   leukemic C91.4-
   malignant C96.9
   nonlipid C96.0
Reticulohistiocytoma (giant-cell) D76.3
Reticuloid, actinic L57.1
Reticulosis (skin)
   acute of infancy C96.0
   hemophagocytic, familial D76.1
   histiocytic medullary C96.9
   lipomelanotic I89.8
   malignant (midline) C86.0
   nonlipid C96.0
   polymorphic C83.8-
   Sézary — *see* Sézary disease
Retina, retinal (*see also* condition)
   dark area D49.81

Retinitis (*see also* Inflammation, chorioretinal)
   albuminurica N18.9 [H32]
   diabetic — *see* Diabetes, retinitis
   disciformis — *see* Degeneration, macula
   focal — *see* Inflammation, chorioretinal, focal
   gravidarum — *see* Pregnancy, complicated by,
     specified pregnancy-related condition NEC
   juxtapapillaris — *see* Inflammation, chorioretinal,
     focal, juxtapapillary
   luetic — *see* Retinitis, syphilitic
   pigmentosa H35.52
   proliferans — *see* Disorder, globe, degenerative,
     specified type NEC
   proliferating — *see* Disorder, globe, degenerative,
     specified type NEC
   renal N18.9 [H32]
   syphilitic (early) (secondary) A51.43
     central, recurrent A52.71
     congenital (early) A50.01 [H32]
     late A52.71
   tuberculous A18.53
Retinoblastoma C69.2-
   differentiated C69.2-
   undifferentiated C69.2-
Retinochoroiditis (*see also* Inflammation,
   chorioretinal)
   disseminated — *see* Inflammation, chorioretinal,
     disseminated
     syphilitic A52.71
   focal — *see* Inflammation, chorioretinal
   juxtapapillaris — *see* Inflammation, chorioretinal,
     focal, juxtapapillary
Retinopathy (background) (Coats) H35.9
   arteriosclerotic I70.90 [H36]
   atherosclerotic I70.90 [H36]
   central serous — *see* Chorioretinopathy, central
     serous
   diabetic — *see* Diabetes, retinopathy
   exudative H35.02-
   hypertensive H35.03-
   in (due to)
     diabetes — *see* Diabetes, retinopathy
     sickle-cell disorders D57.-[H36]
   of prematurity H35.10-
     stage 0 H35.11-
     stage 1 H35.12-
     stage 2 H35.13-
     stage 3 H35.14-
     stage 4 H35.15-
     stage 5 H35.16-
   pigmentary, congenital — *see* Dystrophy, retina
   proliferative NEC H35.2-
     diabetic — *see* Diabetes, retinopathy,
       proliferative
     sickle-cell D57.- [H36]
   solar H31.02-
Retinoschisis H33.10-
   congenital Q14.1
   specified type NEC H33.19-
Retortamoniasis A07.8
Retractile testis Q55.22
Retraction
   cervix — *see* Retroversion, uterus
   drum (membrane) — *see* Disorder, tympanic
     membrane, specified NEC
   finger — *see* Deformity, finger
   lid H02.539
     left H02.536
       lower H02.535
       upper H02.534
     right H02.533
       lower H02.532
       upper H02.531
   lung J98.4
   mediastinum J98.5
   nipple N64.53
     associated with
       lactation O92.03
       pregnancy O92.01-
       puerperium O92.02
     congenital Q83.8
   palmar fascia M72.0
   pleura — *see* Pleurisy

Retraction—*continued*
ring, uterus (Bandl's) (pathological) O62.4
sternum (congenital) Q76.7
acquired M95.4
uterus — *see* Retroversion, uterus
valve (heart) — *see* Endocarditis
Retrobulbar — *see* condition
Retrocecal — *see* condition
Retrocession — *see* Retroversion
Retrodisplacement — *see* Retroversion
Retroflection, retroflexion — *see* Retroversion
Retrognathia, retrognathism (mandibular)
(maxillary) M26.19
Retrograde menstruation N92.5
Retroperineal — *see* condition
Retroperitoneal — *see* condition
Retroperitonitis K68.9
Retropharyngeal — *see* condition
Retroplacental — *see* condition
Retroposition — *see* Retroversion
Retrosternal thyroid (congenital) Q89.2
Retroversion, retroverted
cervix — *see* Retroversion, uterus
female NEC — *see* Retroversion, uterus
iris H21.89
testis (congenital) Q55.29
uterus (acquired) (acute) (any degree)
(asymptomatic) (cervix) (postinfectional)
(postpartal, old) N85.4
congenital Q51.818
in pregnancy — *see* Pregnancy, complicated by,
abnormal, uterus
Retrovirus, as cause of disease classified elsewhere
B97.30
human
immunodeficiency, type 2 (HIV 2) B97.35
T-cell lymphotropic
type I (HTLV-I) B97.33
type II (HTLV-II) B97.34
lentivirus B97.31
oncovirus B97.32
specified NEC B97.39
Retrusion, premaxilla (developmental) M26.09
Rett's disease or syndrome F84.2
Reverse peristalsis R19.2
Reye's syndrome G93.7
Rh (factor)
hemolytic disease (newborn) P55.0
incompatibility, immunization or sensitization
affecting management of pregnancy NEC
O36.09-
anti-D antibody O36.01-
newborn P55.0
transfusion reaction — *see* Complication(s),
transfusion, incompatibility reaction, Rh
(factor)
negative mother affecting newborn P55.0
titer elevated — *see* Complication(s), transfusion,
incompatibility reaction, Rh (factor)
transfusion reaction — *see* Complication(s),
transfusion, incompatibility reaction, Rh
(factor)
Rhabdomyolysis (idiopathic) NEC M62.82
traumatic T79.6
Rhabdomyoma (*see also* Neoplasm, connective tissue,
benign)
adult — *see* Neoplasm, connective tissue, benign
fetal — *see* Neoplasm, connective tissue, benign
glycogenic — *see* Neoplasm, connective tissue,
benign
Rhabdomyosarcoma (any type) — *see* Neoplasm,
connective tissue, malignant
Rhabdosarcoma — *see* Rhabdomyosarcoma
Rhesus (factor) **incompatibility** — *see* Rh,
incompatibility
Rheumatic (acute) (subacute) (chronic)
adherent pericardium I09.2
coronary arteritis I01.9
degeneration, myocardium I09.0
fever (acute) — *see* Fever, rheumatic
heart — *see* Disease, heart, rheumatic
myocardial degeneration — *see* Degeneration,
myocardium

Rheumatic—*continued*
myocarditis (chronic) (inactive) (with chorea) I09.0
active or acute I01.2
with chorea (acute) (rheumatic) (Sydenham's)
I02.0
pancarditis, acute I01.8
with chorea (acute (rheumatic) Sydenham's) I02.0
pericarditis (active) (acute) (with effusion) (with
pneumonia) I01.0
with chorea (acute) (rheumatic) (Sydenham's)
I02.0
chronic or inactive I09.2
pneumonia I00 [J17]
torticollis M43.6
typhoid fever A01.09
Rheumatism (articular) (neuralgic) (nonarticular)
M79.0
intercostal, meaning Tietze's disease M94.0
gout — *see* Arthritis, rheumatoid
palindromic (any site) M12.30
ankle M12.37-
elbow M12.32-
foot joint M12.37-
hand joint M12.34-
hip M12.35-
knee M12.36-
multiple site M12.39
shoulder M12.31-
specified joint NEC M12.38
wrist M12.33-
sciatic M54.4-
Rheumatoid (*see also* condition)
arthritis (*see also* Arthritis, rheumatoid)
with involvement of organs NEC M05.60
ankle M05.67-
elbow M05.62-
foot joint M05.67-
hand joint M05.64-
hip M05.65-
knee M05.66-
multiple site M05.69
shoulder M05.61-
vertebra — *see* Spondylitis, ankylosing
wrist M05.63-
seronegative — *see* Arthritis, rheumatoid,
seronegative
seropositive — *see* Arthritis, rheumatoid,
seropositive
carditis M05.30
ankle M05.37-
elbow M05.32-
foot joint M05.37-
hand joint M05.34-
hip M05.35-
knee M05.36-
multiple site M05.39
shoulder M05.31-
vertebra — *see* Spondylitis, ankylosing
wrist M05.33-
endocarditis — *see* Rheumatoid, carditis
lung (disease) M05.10
ankle M05.17-
elbow M05.12-
foot joint M05.17-
hand joint M05.14-
hip M05.15-
knee M05.16-
multiple site M05.19
shoulder M05.11-
vertebra — *see* Spondylitis, ankylosing
wrist M05.13-
myocarditis — *see* Rheumatoid, carditis
myopathy M05.40
ankle M05.47-
elbow M05.42-
foot joint M05.47-
hand joint M05.44-
hip M05.45-
knee M05.46-
multiple site M05.49
shoulder M05.41-
vertebra — *see* Spondylitis, ankylosing

Rheumatoid —*continued*
myopathy—*continued*
wrist M05.43-
pericarditis — *see* Rheumatoid, carditis
polyarthritis — *see* Arthritis, rheumatoid
polyneuropathy M05.50
ankle M05.57-
elbow M05.52-
foot joint M05.57-
hand joint M05.54-
hip M05.55-
knee M05.56-
multiple site M05.59
shoulder M05.51-
vertebra— *see* Spondylitis, ankylosing
wrist M05.53-
vasculitis M05.20
ankle M05.27-
elbow M05.22-
foot joint M05.27-
hand joint M05.24-
hip M05.25-
knee M05.26-
multiple site M05.29
shoulder M05.21-
vertebra — *see* Spondylitis, ankylosing
wrist M05.23-
Rhinitis (atrophic) (catarrhal) (chronic) (croupous)
(fibrinous) (granulomatous) (hyperplastic)
(hypertrophic) (membranous) (obstructive)
(purulent) (suppurative) (ulcerative) J31.0
with
sore throat — *see* Nasopharyngitis
acute J00
allergic J30.9
with asthma J45.909
with
exacerbation (acute) J45.901
status asthmaticus J45.902
due to
food J30.5
pollen J30.1
nonseasonal J30.89
perennial J30.89
seasonal NEC J30.2
specified NEC J30.89
infective J00
pneumococcal J00
syphilitic A52.73
congenital A50.05 [J99]
tuberculous A15.8
vasomotor J30.0
Rhinoantritis (chronic) — *see* Sinusitis, maxillary
Rhinodacryolith — *see* Dacryolith
Rhinolith (nasal sinus) J34.89
Rhinomegaly J34.89
Rhinopharyngitis (acute) (subacute) (*see also*
Nasopharyngitis)
chronic J31.1
destructive ulcerating A66.5
mutilans A66.5
Rhinophyma L71.1
Rhinorrhea J34.89
cerebrospinal (fluid) G96.0
paroxysmal — *see* Rhinitis, allergic
spasmodic — *see* Rhinitis, allergic
Rhinosalpingitis — *see* Salpingitis, eustachian
Rhinoscleroma A48.8
Rhinosporidiosis B48.1
Rhinovirus infection NEC B34.8
Rhizomelic chondrodysplasia punctata E71.540
Rhythm
atrioventricular nodal I49.8
disorder I49.9
coronary sinus I49.8
ectopic I49.8
nodal I49.8
escape I49.9
heart, abnormal I49.9
idioventricular I44.2
nodal I49.8

Rhythm—continued
  sleep, inversion G47.2
    nonorganic origin — see Disorder, sleep,
      circadian rhythm, psychogenic
Rhytidosis facialis L98.8
Rib (see also condition)
  cervical Q76.5
Riboflavin deficiency E53.0
Rice bodies (see also Loose, body, joint)
  knee M23.4-
Richter syndrome — see Leukemia, chronic
  lymphocytic, B-cell type
Richter's hernia — see Hernia, abdomen, with
  obstruction
Ricinism — see Poisoning, food, noxious, plant
Rickets (active) (acute) (adolescent) (chest wall)
  (congenital) (current) (infantile) (intestinal) E55.0
  adult — see Osteomalacia
  celiac K90.0
  hypophosphatemic with nephrotic-glycosuric
    dwarfism E72.09
  inactive E64.3
  kidney N25.0
  renal N25.0
  sequelae, any E64.3
  vitamin-D-resistant E83.31 [M90.80]
Rickettsial disease A79.9
  specified type NEC A79.89
Rickettsialpox (Rickettsia akari) A79.1
Rickettsiosis A79.9
  due to
    Ehrlichia sennetsu A79.81
    Rickettsia akari (rickettsialpox) A79.1
  specified type NEC A79.89
  tick-borne A77.9
  vesicular A79.1
Rider's bone — see Ossification, muscle, specified NEC
Ridge, alveolus (see also condition)
  flabby K06.8
Ridged ear, congenital Q17.3
Riedel's
  lobe, liver Q44.7
  struma, thyroiditis or disease E06.5
Rieger's anomaly or syndrome Q13.81
Riehl's melanosis L81.4
Rietti-Greppi-Micheli anemia D56.9
Rieux's hernia — see Hernia, abdomen, specified site
  NEC
Riga (-Fede) **disease** K14.0
Riggs' disease — see Periodontitis
Right middle lobe syndrome J98.11
Rigid, rigidity (see also condition)
  abdominal R19.30
    with severe abdominal pain R10.0
    epigastric R19.36
    generalized R19.37
    left lower quadrant R19.34
    left upper quadrant R19.32
    periumbilic R19.35
    right lower quadrant R19.33
    right upper quadrant R19.31
  articular, multiple, congenital Q68.8
  cervix (uteri) in pregnancy — see Pregnancy,
    complicated by, abnormal, cervix
  hymen (acquired) (congenital) N89.6
  nuchal R29.1
  pelvic floor in pregnancy — see Pregnancy,
    complicated by, abnormal, Pelvic organs or
    tissues NEC
  perineum or vulva in pregnancy — see Pregnancy,
    complicated by, abnormal, vulva
  spine — see Dorsopathy, specified NEC
  vagina in pregnancy — see Pregnancy, complicated
    by, abnormal, vagina
Rigors R68.89
  with fever R50.9
Riley-Day syndrome G90.1
RIND (reversible ischemic neurologic deficit) I63.9
Ring(s)
  aorta (vascular) Q25.4
  Bandl's O62.4
  contraction, complicating delivery O62.4
  esophageal, lower (muscular) K22.2

Ring(s)—continued
  Fleischer's (cornea) H18.04-
  hymenal, tight (acquired) (congenital) N89.6
  Kayser-Fleischer (cornea) H18.04-
  retraction, uterus, pathological O62.4
  Schatzki's (esophagus) (lower) K22.4
    congenital Q39.8
  Soemmerring's — see Cataract, secondary
  vascular (congenital) Q25.8
    aorta Q25.4
Ringed hair (congenital) Q84.1
Ringworm B35.9
  beard B35.0
  black dot B35.0
  body B35.4
  Burmese B35.5
  corporeal B35.4
  foot B35.3
  groin B35.6
  hand B35.2
  honeycomb B35.0
  nails B35.1
  perianal (area) B35.6
  scalp B35.0
  specified NEC B35.8
  Tokelau B35.5
Rise, venous pressure I87.8
Risk, suicidal
  meaning personal history of attempted suicide
    Z91.5
  meaning suicidal ideation — see Ideation, suicidal
Ritter's disease L00
Rivalry, sibling Z62.891
Rivalta's disease A42.2
River blindness B73.01
Robert's pelvis Q74.2
  with disproportion (fetopelvic) O33.0
    causing obstructed labor O65.0
Robin(-Pierre) **syndrome** Q87.0
Robinow-Silvermann-Smith syndrome Q87.1
Robinson's (hidrotic) **ectodermal dysplasia or
  syndrome** Q82.4
Robles' disease — see Onchocerciasis
Rocky Mountain (spotted) **fever** A77.0
Roetheln — see Rubella
Roger's disease Q21.0
Rokitansky-Aschoff sinuses (gallbladder) K82.8
Rolando's fracture (displaced) S62.22-
    nondisplaced S62.22-
Romano-Ward (prolonged QT interval) **syndrome**
  I45.81
Romberg's disease or syndrome G51.8
Roof, mouth — see condition
Rosacea L71.9
  acne L71.9
  keratitis L71.8
  specified NEC L71.8
Rosary, rachitic E55.0
Rose
  cold J30.1
  fever J30.1
  rash R21
    epidemic B06.9
Rosenbach's erysipeloid A26.0
Rosenthal's disease or syndrome D68.1
Roseola B09
  infantum B08.20
    due to human herpesvirus 6 B08.21
    due to human herpesvirus 7 B08.22
Rossbach's disease K31.89
  psychogenic F45.8
Ross River disease or fever B33.1
Rostan's asthma (cardiac) — see Failure, ventricular,
  left
Rotation
  anomalous, incomplete or insufficient, intestine
    Q43.3
  cecum (congenital) Q43.3
  colon (congenital) Q43.3
  spine, incomplete or insufficient — see Dorsopathy,
    deforming, specified NEC
  tooth, teeth, fully erupted M26.35

Rotation—continued
  vertebra, incomplete or insufficient — see
    Dorsopathy, deforming, specified NEC
Rotes Quérol disease or syndrome — see
  Hyperostosis, ankylosing
Roth(-Bernhardt) **disease or syndrome** — see
  Meralgia paraesthetica
Rothmund(-Thomson) **syndrome** Q82.8
Rotor's disease or syndrome E80.6
Round
  back (with wedging of vertebrae) — see Kyphosis
    sequelae (late effect) of rickets E64.3
  worms (large) (infestation) NEC B82.0
    Ascariasis (see also Ascariasis) B77.9
Roussy-Lévy syndrome G60.0
Rubella (German measles) B06.9
  complication NEC B06.09
    neurological B06.00
  congenital P35.0
  contact Z20.4
  exposure to Z20.4
  maternal
    manifest rubella in infant P35.0
    care for (suspected) damage to fetus O35.3
    suspected damage to fetus affecting
      management of pregnancy O35.3
  specified complications NEC B06.89
Rubeola (meaning measles) — see Measles
  meaning rubella — see Rubella
Rubeosis, iris — see Disorder, iris, vascular
Rubinstein-Taybi syndrome Q87.2
Rudimentary (congenital) (see also Agenesis)
  arm — see Defect, reduction, upper limb
  bone Q79.9
  cervix uteri Q51.828
  eye Q11.2
  lobule of ear Q17.3
  patella Q74.1
  respiratory organs in thoracopagus Q89.4
  tracheal bronchus Q32.4
  uterus Q51.818
    in male Q56.1
  vagina Q52.0
Ruled out condition — see Observation, suspected
Rumination R11.10
  with nausea R11.2
  disorder of infancy F98.21
  neurotic F42
  newborn P92.1
  obsessional F42
  psychogenic F42
Runeberg's disease D51.0
Runny nose R09.89
Rupia (syphilitic) A51.39
  congenital A50.06
  tertiary A52.79
Rupture, ruptured
  abscess (spontaneous) — code by site under Abscess
  aneurysm — see Aneurysm
  anus (sphincter) — see Laceration, anus
  aorta, aortic I71.8
    abdominal I71.3
    arch I71.1
    ascending I71.1
    descending I71.8
      abdominal I71.3
      thoracic I71.1
    syphilitic A52.01
    thoracoabdominal I71.5
    thorax, thoracic I71.1
    transverse I71.1
    traumatic — see Injury, aorta, laceration, major
    valve or cusp (see also Endocarditis, aortic) I35.8
  appendix (with peritonitis) K35.2
  arteriovenous fistula, brain I60.8
  artery I77.2
    brain — see Hemorrhage, intracranial,
      intracerebral
    coronary — see Infarct, myocardium
    heart — see Infarct, myocardium
    pulmonary I28.8
    traumatic (complication) — see Injury, blood
      vessel

Rupture, ruptured—*continued*
- bile duct (common) (hepatic) K83.2
  - cystic K82.2
- bladder (sphincter) (nontraumatic) (spontaneous) N32.89
  - following ectopic or molar pregnancy O08.6
  - obstetrical trauma O71.5
  - traumatic S37.29
- blood vessel (*see also* Hemorrhage)
  - brain — *see* Hemorrhage, intracranial, intracerebral
  - heart — *see* Infarct, myocardium
  - traumatic (complication) — *see* Injury, blood vessel, laceration, major, by site
- bone — *see* Fracture
- bowel (nontraumatic) K63.1
- brain
  - aneurysm (congenital) (*see also* Hemorrhage, intracranial, subarachnoid)
    - syphilitic A52.05
  - hemorrhagic — *see* Hemorrhage, intracranial, intracerebral
- capillaries I78.8
- cardiac (auricle) (ventricle) (wall) I23.3
  - with hemopericardium I23.0
  - infectional I40.9
  - traumatic — *see* Injury, heart
- cartilage (articular) (current) (*see also* Sprain)
  - knee S83.3-
  - semilunar — *see* Tear, meniscus
- cecum (with peritonitis) K65.0
  - with peritoneal abscess K35.3
  - traumatic S36.598
- celiac artery, traumatic — *see* Injury, blood vessel, celiac artery, laceration, major
- cerebral aneurysm (congenital) (see Hemorrhage, intracranial, subarachnoid)
- cervix (uteri)
  - with ectopic or molar pregnancy O08.6
  - following ectopic or molar pregnancy O08.6
  - obstetrical trauma O71.3
  - traumatic S37.69
- chordae tendineae NEC I51.1
  - concurrent with acute myocardial infarction — *see* Infarct, myocardium
  - following acute myocardial infarction (current complication) I23.4
- choroid (direct) (indirect) (traumatic) H31.32-
- circle of Willis I60.6
- colon (nontraumatic) K63.1
  - traumatic — *see* Injury, intestine, large
- cornea (traumatic) — *see* Injury, eye, laceration
- coronary (artery) (thrombotic) — *see* Infarct, myocardium
- corpus luteum (infected) (ovary) N83.1
- cyst — *see* Cyst
- cystic duct K82.2
- Descemet's membrane — *see* Change, corneal membrane, Descemet's, rupture
  - traumatic — *see* Injury, eye, laceration
- diaphragm, traumatic — *see* Injury, intrathoracic, diaphragm
- disc — *see* Rupture, intervertebral disc
- diverticulum (intestine) K57.80
  - with bleeding K57.81
  - bladder N32.3
  - large intestine K57.20
    - with
      - bleeding K57.21
      - small intestine K57.40
        - with bleeding K57.41
  - small intestine K57.00
    - with
      - bleeding K57.01
      - large intestine K57.40
        - with bleeding K57.41
- duodenal stump K31.89
- ear drum (nontraumatic) (*see also* Perforation, tympanum)
  - traumatic S09.2-
    - due to blast injury — *see* Injury, blast, ear
- esophagus K22.3

Rupture, ruptured—*continued*
- eye (without prolapse or loss of intraocular tissue) — *see* Injury, eye, laceration
- fallopian tube NEC (nonobstetric) (nontraumatic) N83.8
  - due to pregnancy O00.1
- fontanel P13.1
- gallbladder K82.2
  - traumatic S36.128
- gastric (*see also* Rupture, stomach)
  - vessel K92.2
- globe (eye) (traumatic) — *see* Injury, eye, laceration
- graafian follicle (hematoma) N83.0
- heart — *see* Rupture, cardiac
- hymen (nontraumatic) (nonintentional) N89.8
- internal organ, traumatic — *see* Injury, by site
- intervertebral disc — *see* Displacement, intervertebral disc
  - traumatic — *see* Rupture, traumatic, intervertebral disc
- intestine NEC (nontraumatic) K63.1
  - traumatic — *see* Injury, intestine
- iris (*see also* Abnormality, pupillary)
  - traumatic — *see* Injury, eye, laceration
- joint capsule, traumatic — *see* Sprain
- kidney (traumatic) S37.06-
  - birth injury P15.8
  - nontraumatic N28.89
- lacrimal duct (traumatic) — *see* Injury, eye, specified site NEC
- lens (cataract) (traumatic) — *see* Cataract, traumatic
- ligament, traumatic — *see* Rupture, traumatic, ligament, by site
- liver S36.116
  - birth injury P15.0
- lymphatic vessel I89.8
- marginal sinus (placental) (with hemorrhage) — *see* Hemorrhage, antepartum, specified cause NEC
- membrana tympani (nontraumatic) — *see* Perforation, tympanum
- membranes (spontaneous)
  - artificial
    - delayed delivery following O75.5
  - delayed delivery following — *see* Pregnancy, complicated by, premature rupture of membranes
- meningeal artery I60.8
- meniscus (knee) (*see also* Tear, meniscus)
  - old — *see* Derangement, meniscus
  - site other than knee — code as Sprain
- mesenteric artery, traumatic — *see* Injury, mesenteric, artery, laceration, major
- mesentery (nontraumatic) K66.8
  - traumatic — *see* Injury, intra-abdominal, specified, site NEC
- mitral (valve) I34.8
- muscle (traumatic) (*see also* Strain)
  - diastasis — *see* Diastasis, muscle
  - nontraumatic M62.10
    - ankle M62.17-
    - foot M62.17-
    - forearm M62.13-
    - hand M62.14-
    - lower leg M62.16-
    - pelvic region M62.15-
    - shoulder region M62.11-
    - specified site NEC M62.18
    - thigh M62.15-
    - upper arm M62.12-
  - traumatic — *see* Strain, by site
- musculotendinous junction NEC, nontraumatic — *see* Rupture, tendon, spontaneous
- mycotic aneurysm causing cerebral hemorrhage — *see* Hemorrhage, intracranial, subarachnoid
- myocardium, myocardial — *see* Rupture, cardiac
  - traumatic — *see* Injury, heart
- nontraumatic, meaning hernia — *see* Hernia
- obstructed — *see* Hernia, by site, obstructed
- operation wound — *see* Disruption, wound, operation

Rupture, ruptured—*continued*
- ovary, ovarian N83.8
  - corpus luteum cyst N83.1
  - follicle (graafian) N83.0
- oviduct (nonobstetric) (nontraumatic) N83.8
  - due to pregnancy O00.1
- pancreas (nontraumatic) K86.8
  - traumatic S36.299
- papillary muscle NEC I51.2
  - following acute myocardial infarction (current complication) I23.5
- pelvic
  - floor, complicating delivery O70.1
  - organ NEC, obstetrical trauma O71.5
- perineum (nonobstetric) (nontraumatic) N90.89
  - complicating delivery — *see* Delivery, complicated, by, laceration, anus (sphincter)
- postoperative wound — *see* Disruption, wound, operation
- prostate (traumatic) S37.828
- pulmonary
  - artery I28.8
  - valve (heart) I37.8
  - vein I28.8
  - vessel I28.8
- pus tube — *see* Salpingitis
- pyosalpinx — *see* Salpingitis
- rectum (nontraumatic) K63.1
  - traumatic S36.69
- retina, retinal (traumatic) (without detachment) (*see also* Break, retina)
  - with detachment — *see* Detachment, retina, with retinal, break
- rotator cuff (complete) (incomplete) (nontraumatic) M75.1-
- sclera — *see* Injury, eye, laceration
- sigmoid (nontraumatic) K63.1
  - traumatic S36.593
- spinal cord (*see also* Injury, spinal cord, by region)
  - due to injury at birth P11.5
  - newborn (birth injury) P11.5
- spleen (traumatic) S36.09
  - birth injury P15.1
  - congenital (birth injury) P15.1
  - due to P. vivax malaria B51.0
  - nontraumatic D73.5
  - spontaneous D73.5
- splenic vein R58
  - traumatic — *see* Injury, blood vessel, portal vein
- stomach (nontraumatic) (spontaneous) K31.89
  - traumatic S36.39
- supraspinatus (complete) (incomplete) (nontraumatic) M75.1-
- symphysis pubis
  - obstetric O71.6
  - traumatic S33.4
- synovium (cyst) M66.10
  - ankle M66.17-
  - elbow M66.12-
  - finger M66.14-
  - foot M66.17-
  - forearm M66.13-
  - hand M66.14-
  - pelvic region M66.15-
  - shoulder region M66.11-
  - specified site NEC M66.18
  - thigh M66.15-
  - toe M66.17-
  - upper arm M66.12-
  - wrist M66.13-
- tendon (traumatic) — *see* Strain
  - nontraumatic (spontaneous) M66.9
    - ankle M66.87-
      - extensor M66.20
        - ankle M66.27-
        - foot M66.27-
        - forearm M66.23-
        - hand M66.24-
        - lower leg M66.26-
        - multiple sites M66.29
        - pelvic region M66.25-
        - shoulder region M66.21-

Salpingo-oophoritis—*continued*
  tuberculous (acute) (chronic) A18.17
  venereal (gonococcal) (acute) (chronic) A54.24
Salpingo-ovaritis — *see* Salpingo-oophoritis
Salpingoperitonitis — *see* Salpingo-oophoritis
Salzmann's nodular dystrophy — *see* Degeneration,
    cornea, nodular
Sampson's cyst or tumor N80.1
San Joaquin (Valley) **fever** B38.0
Sandblaster's asthma, lung or pneumoconiosis
    J62.8
Sander's disease (paranoia) F22
Sandfly fever A93.1
Sandhoff's disease E75.01
Sanfilippo (Type B) (Type C) (Type D) **syndrome**
    E76.22
Sanger-Brown ataxia G11.2
Sao Paulo fever or typhus A77.0
Saponification, mesenteric K65.8
Sarcocele (benign)
  syphilitic A52.76
    congenital A50.59
Sarcocystosis A07.8
Sarcoepiplocele — *see* Hernia
Sarcoepiplomphalocele Q79.2
Sarcoid (*see also* Sarcoidosis)
  arthropathy D86.86
  Boeck's D86.9
  Darier-Roussy D86.3
  iridocyclitis D86.83
  meningitis D86.81
  myocarditis D86.85
  myositis D86.87
  pyelonephritis D86.84
  Spiegler-Fendt L08.89
Sarcoidosis D86.9
  with
    cranial nerve palsies D86.82
    hepatic granuloma D86.89
    polyarthritis D86.86
    tubulo-interstitial nephropathy D86.84
  combined sites NEC D86.89
  lung D86.0
    and lymph nodes D86.2
  lymph nodes D86.1
    and lung D86.2
  meninges D86.81
  skin D86.3
  specified type NEC D86.89
Sarcoma (of) (*see also* Neoplasm, connective tissue,
    malignant)
  alveolar soft part — *see* Neoplasm, connective
      tissue, malignant
  ameloblastic C41.1
    upper jaw (bone) C41.0
  botryoid — *see* Neoplasm, connective tissue,
      malignant
  botryoides — *see* Neoplasm, connective tissue,
      malignant
  cerebellar C71.6
    circumscribed (arachnoidal) C71.6
  circumscribed (arachnoidal) cerebellar C71.6
  clear cell (*see also* Neoplasm, connective tissue,
      malignant)
    kidney C64.-
  dendritic cells (accessory cells) C96.4
  embryonal — *see* Neoplasm, connective tissue,
      malignant
  endometrial (stromal) C54.1
    isthmus C54.0
  epithelioid (cell) — *see* Neoplasm, connective tissue,
      malignant
  Ewing's — *see* Neoplasm, bone, malignant
  follicular dendritic cell C96.4
  germinoblastic (diffuse) — *see* Lymphoma, diffuse
      large cell
    follicular — *see* Lymphoma, follicular, specified
        NEC
  giant cell (except of bone) (*see also* Neoplasm,
      connective tissue, malignant)
    bone — *see* Neoplasm, bone, malignant
  glomoid — *see* Neoplasm, connective tissue,
      malignant

Sarcoma —*continued*
  granulocytic C92.3-
  hemangioendothelial — *see* Neoplasm, connective
      tissue, malignant
  hemorrhagic, multiple — *see* Sarcoma, Kaposi's
  histiocytic C96.a
  Hodgkin — *see* Lymphoma, Hodgkin
  immunoblastic (diffuse) — *see* Lymphoma, diffuse
      large cell
  interdigitating dendritic cell C96.4
  Kaposi's
    colon C46.4
    connective tissue C46.1
    gastrointestinal organ C46.4
    lung C46.5-
    lymph node(s) C46.3
    palate (hard) (soft) C46.2
    rectum C46.4
    skin C46.0
    specified site NEC C46.7
    stomach C46.4
    unspecified site C46.9
  Kupffer cell C22.3
  Langerhans cell C96.4
  leptomeningeal — *see* Neoplasm, meninges,
      malignant
  liver NEC C22.4
  lymphangioendothelial — *see* Neoplasm,
      connective tissue, malignant
  lymphoblastic — *see* Lymphoma, lymphoblastic
      (diffuse)
  lymphocytic — *see* Lymphoma, small cell B-cell
  mast cell C96.2
  melanotic — *see* Melanoma
  meningeal — *see* Neoplasm, meninges, malignant
  meningothelial — *see* Neoplasm, meninges,
      malignant
  mesenchymal (*see also* Neoplasm, connective tissue,
      malignant)
    mixed — *see* Neoplasm, connective tissue,
        malignant
  mesothelial — *see* Mesothelioma
  monstrocellular
    specified site — *see* Neoplasm, malignant, by site
    unspecified site C71.9
  myeloid C92.3-
  neurogenic — *see* Neoplasm, nerve, malignant
  odontogenic C41.1
    upper jaw (bone) C41.0
  osteoblastic — *see* Neoplasm, bone, malignant
  osteogenic (*see also* Neoplasm, bone, malignant)
    juxtacortical — *see* Neoplasm, bone, malignant
    periosteal — *see* Neoplasm, bone, malignant
  periosteal (*see also* Neoplasm, bone, malignant)
    osteogenic — *see* Neoplasm, bone, malignant
  pleomorphic cell — *see* Neoplasm, connective
      tissue, malignant
  reticulum cell (diffuse) — *see* Lymphoma, diffuse
      large cell
    nodular — *see* Lymphoma, follicular
    pleomorphic cell type — *see* Lymphoma, diffuse
        large cell
  rhabdoid — *see* Neoplasm, malignant, by site
  round cell — *see* Neoplasm, connective tissue,
      malignant
  small cell — *see* Neoplasm, connective tissue,
      malignant
  soft tissue — *see* Neoplasm, connective tissue,
      malignant
  spindle cell — *see* Neoplasm, connective tissue,
      malignant
  stromal (endometrial) C54.1
    isthmus C54.0
  synovial (*see also* Neoplasm, connective tissue,
      malignant)
    biphasic — *see* Neoplasm, connective tissue,
        malignant
    epithelioid cell — *see* Neoplasm, connective
        tissue, malignant
    spindle cell — *see* Neoplasm, connective tissue,
        malignant

Sarcomatosis
  meningeal — *see* Neoplasm, meninges, malignant
  specified site NEC — *see* Neoplasm, connective
      tissue, malignant
  unspecified site C80.1
Sarcosinemia E72.59
Sarcosporidiosis (intestinal) A07.8
Satiety, early R68.81
Saturnine — *see* condition
Saturnism
  overdose or wrong substance given or taken — *see*
      Table of Drugs and Chemicals, by drug,
      poisoning
Satyriasis F52.8
Sauriasis — *see* Ichthyosis
SBE (subacute bacterial endocarditis) I33.0
Scabs R23.4
Scabies (any site) B86
Scaglietti-Dagnini syndrome E22.0
Scald — *see* Burn
Scalenus anticus (anterior) **syndrome** G54.0
Scales R23.4
Scaling, skin R23.4
Scalp — *see* condition
Scapegoating affecting child Z62.3
Scaphocephaly Q75.0
Scapulalgia M89.8x1
Scapulohumeral myopathy G71.0
Scar, scarring (*see also* Cicatrix) L90.5
  adherent L90.5
  atrophic L90.5
  cervix
    in pregnancy or childbirth — *see* Pregnancy,
        complicated by, abnormal cervix
  cheloid L91.0
  chorioretinal H31.00-
    posterior pole macula H31.01-
    postsurgical H59.81-
    solar retinopathy H31.02-
    specified type NEC H31.09-
  choroid — *see* Scar, chorioretinal
  conjunctiva H11.24-
  cornea H17.9
    xerophthalmic (*see also* Opacity, cornea)
      vitamin A deficiency E50.6
  duodenum, obstructive K31.5
  hypertrophic L91.0
  keloid L91.0
  labia N90.89
  lung (base) J98.4
  macula — *see* Scar, chorioretinal, posterior pole
  muscle M62.89
  myocardium, myocardial I25.2
  painful L90.5
  posterior pole (eye) — *see* Scar, chorioretinal,
      posterior pole
  retina — *see* Scar, chorioretinal
  trachea J39.8
  uterus N85.8
    in pregnancy O34.29
  vagina N89.8
    postoperative N99.2
  vulva N90.89
Scarabiasis B88.2
Scarlatina (anginosa) (maligna) (ulcerosa) A38.9
  myocarditis (acute) A38.1
  old — *see* Myocarditis
  otitis media A38.0
Scarlet fever (albuminuria) (angina) A38.9
Schamberg's disease (progressive pigmentary
    dermatosis) L81.7
Schatzki's ring (acquired) (esophagus) (lower) K22.2
  congenital Q39.8
Schaufenster krankheit I20.8
Schaumann's
  benign lymphogranulomatosis D86.1
  disease or syndrome — *see* Sarcoidosis
Scheie's syndrome E76.03
Schenck's disease B42.1
Scheuermann's disease or osteochondrosis — *see*
    Osteochondrosis, juvenile, spine
Schilder(-Flatau) **disease** G37.0
Schilling-type monocytic leukemia C93.0-

Schimmelbusch's disease, cystic mastitis, or hyperplasia — see Mastopathy, cystic
Schistosoma infestation — see Infestation, Schistosoma
Schistosomiasis B65.9
  with muscle disorder B65.9 [M63.80]
    ankle B65.9 [M63.87-]
    foot B65.9 [M63.87-]
    forearm B65.9 [M63.83-]
    hand B65.9 [M63.84-]
    lower leg B65.9 [M63.86-]
    multiple sites B65.9 [M63.89]
    pelvic region B65.9 [M63.85-]
    shoulder region B65.9 [M63.81-]
    specified site NEC B65.9 [M63.88]
    thigh B65.9 [M63.85-]
    upper arm B65.9 [M63.82-]
  Asiatic B65.2
  bladder B65.0
  chestermani B65.8
  colon B65.1
  cutaneous B65.3
  due to
    S. haematobium B65.0
    S. japonicum B65.2
    S. mansoni B65.1
    S. mattheii B65.8
  Eastern B65.2
  genitourinary tract B65.0
  intestinal B65.1
  lung NEC B65.9 [J99]
    pneumonia B65.9 [J17]
  Manson's (intestinal) B65.1
  oriental B65.2
  pulmonary NEC B65.9 [J99]
    pneumonia B65.9
  Schistosoma
    haematobium B65.0
    japonicum B65.2
    mansoni B65.1
  specified type NEC B65.8
  urinary B65.0
  vesical B65.0
Schizencephaly Q04.6
Schizoaffective psychosis F25.9
Schizodontia K00.2
Schizoid personality F60.1
Schizophrenia, schizophrenic F20.9
  acute (brief) (undifferentiated) F23
  atypical (form) F20.3
  borderline F21
  catalepsy F20.2
  catatonic (type) (excited) (withdrawn) F20.2
  cenesthopathic, cenesthesiopathic F20.89
  childhood type F84.5
  chronic undifferentiated F20.5
  cyclic F25.0
  disorganized (type) F20.1
  flexibilitas cerea F20.2
  hebephrenic (type) F20.1
  incipient F21
  latent F21
  negative type F20.5
  paranoid (type) F20.0
  paraphrenic F20.0
  post-psychotic depression F32.8
  prepsychotic F21
  prodromal F21
  pseudoneurotic F21
  pseudopsychopathic F21
  reaction F23
  residual (state) (type) F20.5
  restzustand F20.5
  schizoaffective (type) — see Psychosis, schizoaffective
  simple (type) F20.89
  simplex F20.89
  specified type NEC F20.89
  stupor F20.2
  syndrome of childhood F84.5
  undifferentiated (type) F20.3
    chronic F20.5
Schizothymia (persistent) F60.1

Schlatter-Osgood disease or osteochondrosis — see Osteochondrosis, juvenile, tibia
Schlatter's tibia — see Osteochondrosis, juvenile, tibia
Schmidt's syndrome (polyglandular, autoimmune) E31.0
Schmincke's carcinoma or tumor — see Neoplasm, nasopharynx, malignant
Schmitz(-Stutzer) **dysentery** A03.0
Schmorl's disease or nodes
  lumbar region M51.46
  lumbosacral region M51.47
  sacrococcygeal region M53.3
  thoracic region M51.44
  thoracolumbar region M51.45
Schneiderian
  carcinoma
    unspecified site C30.0
  papilloma — see Neoplasm, nasopharynx, benign
    specified site — see Neoplasm, benign, by site
    unspecified site D14.0
  specified site — see Neoplasm, malignant, by site
Scholte's syndrome (malignant carcinoid) E34.0
Scholz(-Bielchowsky-Henneberg) **disease or syndrome** E75.25
Schönlein(-Henoch) **disease or purpura** (primary) (rheumatic) D69.0
Schottmuller's disease A01.4
Schroeder's syndrome (endocrine hypertensive) E27.0
Schüller-Christian disease or syndrome C96.5
Schultze's type acroparesthesia, simple I73.89
Schultz's disease or syndrome — see Agranulocytosis
Schwalbe-Ziehen-Oppenheim disease G24.1
Schwannoma (see also Neoplasm, nerve, benign)
  malignant (see also Neoplasm, nerve, malignant)
    with rhabdomyoblastic differentiation — see Neoplasm, nerve, malignant
  melanocytic (9560/0) — see Neoplasm, nerve, benign
  pigmented — see Neoplasm, nerve, benign
Schwannomatosis Q85.03
Schwartz(-Jampel) **syndrome** G71.13
Schwartz-Bartter syndrome E22.2
Schweniger-Buzzi anetoderma L90.1
Sciatic — see condition
Sciatica (infective)
  with lumbago M54.4-
    due to intervertebral disc disorder — see Disorder, disc, with, radiculopathy
  due to displacement of intervertebral disc (with lumbago) — see Disorder, disc, with, radiculopathy
  wallet M54.3-
Scimitar syndrome Q26.8
Sclera — see condition
Sclerectasia H15.84-
Scleredema
  adultorum — see Sclerosis, systemic
  Buschke's — see Sclerosis, systemic
  newborn P83.0
Sclerema (adiposum) (edematosum) (neonatorum) (newborn) P83.0
  adultorum see Sclerosis, systemic
Scleriasis — see Scleroderma
Scleritis H15.00-
  with corneal involvement H15.04-
  anterior H15.01-
  brawny H15.02-
  in (due to) zoster B02.34
  posterior H15.03-
  specified type NEC H15.09-
  syphilitic A52.71
  tuberculous (nodular) A18.51
Sclerochoroiditis H31.8
Scleroconjunctivitis — see Scleritis
Sclerocystic ovary syndrome E28.2
Sclerodactyly, sclerodactylia L94.3
Scleroderma, sclerodermia (acrosclerotic) (diffuse) (generalized) (progressive) (pulmonary) (see also Sclerosis, systemic) M34.9
  circumscribed L94.0

Scleroderma, sclerodermia—continued
  linear L94.1
  localized L94.0
  newborn P83.8
  systemic M34.9
Sclerokeratitis H16.8
  tuberculous A18.52
Scleroma nasi A48.8
Scleromalacia (perforans) H15.05-
Scleromyxedema L98.5
Sclérose en plaques G35
Sclerosis, sclerotic
  adrenal (gland) E27.8
  Alzheimer's — see Disease, Alzheimer's
  amyotrophic (lateral) G12.21
  aorta, aortic I70.0
    valve — see Endocarditis, aortic
  artery, arterial, arteriolar, arteriovascular — see Arteriosclerosis
  ascending multiple G35
  brain (generalized) (lobular) G37.9
    artery, arterial I67.2
    diffuse G37.0
    disseminated G35
    insular G35
    Krabbe's E75.23
    miliary G35
    multiple G35
    presenile (Alzheimer's) — see Disease, Alzheimer's, early onset
    senile (arteriosclerotic) I67.2
    stem, multiple G35
    tuberous Q85.1
  bulbar, multiple G35
  bundle of His I44.39
  cardiac — see Disease, heart, ischemic, atherosclerotic
  cardiorenal — see Hypertension, cardiorenal
  cardiovascular (see also Disease, cardiovascular)
    renal — see Hypertension, cardiorenal
  cerebellar — see Sclerosis, brain
  cerebral — see Sclerosis, brain
  cerebrospinal (disseminated) (multiple) G35
  cerebrovascular I67.2
  choroid — see Degeneration, choroid
  combined (spinal cord) (see also Degeneration, combined)
    multiple G35
  concentric (Balo) G37.5
  cornea — see Opacity, cornea
  coronary (artery) I25.10
    with angina pectoris — see Arteriosclerosis, coronary (artery),
  corpus cavernosum
    female N90.89
    male N48.6
  diffuse (brain) (spinal cord) G37.0
  disseminated G35
  dorsal G35
  dorsolateral (spinal cord) — see Degeneration, combined
  endometrium N85.5
  extrapyramidal G25.9
  eye, nuclear (senile) — see Cataract, senile, nuclear
  focal and segmental (glomerular) (see also N00-N07 with fourth character .1) N05.1
  Friedreich's (spinal cord) G11.1
  funicular (spermatic cord) N50.8
  general (vascular) — see Arteriosclerosis
  gland (lymphatic) I89.8
  hepatic K74.1
    alcoholic K70.2
  hereditary
    cerebellar G11.9
    spinal (Friedreich's ataxia) G11.1
  hippocampal G93.81
  insular G35
  kidney — see Sclerosis, renal
  larynx J38.7
  lateral (amyotrophic) (descending) (primary) (spinal) G12.21
  lens, senile nuclear — see Cataract, senile, nuclear

Sclerosis, sclerotic—*continued*
  liver K74.1
    with fibrosis K74.2
      alcoholic K70.2
    alcoholic K70.2
    cardiac K76.1
  lung — *see* Fibrosis, lung
  mastoid — *see* Mastoiditis, chronic
  mesial temporal G93.81
  mitral I05.8
  Mönckeberg's (medial) — *see* Arteriosclerosis,
      extremities
  multiple (brain stem) (cerebral) (generalized) (spinal
      cord) G35
  myocardium, myocardial — *see* Disease, heart,
      ischemic, atherosclerotic
  nuclear (senile), eye — *see* Cataract, senile, nuclear
  ovary N83.8
  pancreas K86.8
  penis N48.6
  peripheral arteries — *see* Arteriosclerosis,
      extremities
  plaques G35
  pluriglandular E31.8
  polyglandular E31.8
  posterolateral (spinal cord) — *see* Degeneration,
      combined
  presenile (Alzheimer's) — *see* Disease, Alzheimer's,
      early onset
  primary, lateral G12.29
  progressive, systemic M34.0
  pulmonary — *see* Fibrosis, lung
    artery I27.0
    valve (heart) — *see* Endocarditis, pulmonary
  renal N26.9
    with
      cystine storage disease E72.09
      hypertensive heart disease (conditions in I11)
          — *see* Hypertension, cardiorenal
      arteriolar (hyaline) (hyperplastic) — *see*
          Hypertension, kidney
  retina (senile) (vascular) H35.00
  senile (vascular) — *see* Arteriosclerosis
  spinal (cord) (progressive) G95.89
    ascending G61.0
    combined (*see also* Degeneration, combined)
      multiple G35
      syphilitic A52.11
    disseminated G35
    dorsolateral — *see* Degeneration, combined
    hereditary (Friedreich's) (mixed form) G11.1
    lateral (amyotrophic) G12.21
    multiple G35
    posterior (syphilitic) A52.11
  stomach K31.89
  subendocardial, congenital I42.4
  systemic M34.9
    with
      lung involvement M34.81
      myopathy M34.82
      polyneuropathy M34.83
    drug-induced M34.2
    due to chemicals NEC M34.2
    progressive M34.0
    specified NEC M34.89
  temporal (mesial) G93.81
  tricuspid (heart) (valve) I07.8
  tuberous (brain) Q85.1
  tympanic membrane — *see* Disorder, tympanic
      membrane, specified NEC
  valve, valvular (heart) — *see* Endocarditis
  vascular — *see* Arteriosclerosis
  vein I87.8
Scoliosis (acquired) (postural) M41.9
  adolescent (idiopathic) — *see* Scoliosis, idiopathic,
      juvenile
  congenital Q67.5
    due to bony malformation Q76.3
    failure of segmentation (hemivertebra) Q76.3
    hemivertebra fusion Q76.3
    postural Q67.5

Scoliosis—*continued*
  idiopathic M41.20
    adolescent M41.129
      cervical region M41.122
      cervicothoracic region M41.123
      lumbar region M41.126
      lumbosacral region M41.127
      multiple sites M41.129
      thoracic region M41.124
      thoracolumbar region M41.125
    cervical region M41.22
    cervicothoracic region M41.23
    infantile M41.00
      cervical region M41.02
      cervicothoracic region M41.03
      lumbar region M41.06
      lumbosacral region M41.07
      sacrococcygeal region M41.08
      thoracic region M41.04
      thoracolumbar region M41.05
    juvenile M41.119
      cervical region M41.112
      cervicothoracic region M41.113
      lumbar region M41.116
      lumbosacral region M41.117
      multiple sites M41.119
      thoracic region M41.114
      thoracolumbar region M41.115
    lumbar region M41.26
    lumbosacral region M41.27
    thoracic region M41.24
    thoracolumbar region M41.25
  neuromuscular M41.40
    cervical region M41.42
    cervicothoracic region M41.43
    lumbar region M41.46
    lumbosacral region M41.47
    occipito-atlanto-axial region M41.41
    thoracic region M41.44
    thoracolumbar region M41.45
  paralytic — *see* Scoliosis, neuromuscular
  postradiation therapy M96.5
  rachitic (late effect or sequelae) E64.3 [M49.80]
    cervical region E64.3 [M49.82]
    cervicothoracic region E64.3 [M49.83]
    lumbar region E64.3 [M49.86]
    lumbosacral region E64.3 [M49.87]
    multiple sites E64.3 [M49.89]
    occipito-atlanto-axial region E64.3 [M49.81]
    sacrococcygeal region E64.3 [M49.88]
    thoracic region E64.3 [M49.84]
    thoracolumbar region E64.3 [M49.85]
  sciatic M54.4-
  secondary (to) NEC M41.50
    cerebral palsy, Friedreich's ataxia, poliomyelitis,
        neuromuscular disorders — *see* Scoliosis,
        neuromuscular
    cervical region M41.52
    cervicothoracic region M41.53
    lumbar region M41.56
    lumbosacral region M41.57
    thoracic region M41.54
    thoracolumbar region M41.55
  specified form NEC M41.80
    cervical region M41.82
    cervicothoracic region M41.83
    lumbar region M41.86
    lumbosacral region M41.87
    thoracic region M41.84
    thoracolumbar region M41.85
  thoracogenic M41.30
    thoracic region M41.34
    thoracolumbar region M41.35
  tuberculous A18.01
Scoliotic pelvis
  with disproportion (fetopelvic) O33.0
    causing obstructed labor O65.0
Scorbutus, scorbutic (*see also* Scurvy)
  anemia D53.2
Scotoma (arcuate) (Bjerrum) (central) (ring) (*see also*
      Defect, visual field, localized, scotoma)
  scintillating H53.19
Scratch — *see* Abrasion

Scratchy throat R09.89
Screening (for) Z13.9
  alcoholism Z13.89
  anemia Z13.0
  anomaly, congenital Z13.89
  antenatal, of mother Z36
  arterial hypertension Z13.6
  arthropod-borne viral disease NEC Z11.59
  bacteriuria, asymptomatic Z13.89
  behavioral disorder Z13.89
  brain injury, traumatic Z13.850
  bronchitis, chronic Z13.83
  brucellosis Z11.2
  cardiovascular disorder Z13.6
  cataract Z13.5
  chlamydial diseases Z11.8
  cholera Z11.0
  chromosomal abnormalities (nonprocreative) NEC
      Z13.79
  colonoscopy Z12.11
  congenital
    dislocation of hip Z13.89
    eye disorder Z13.5
    malformation or deformation Z13.89
  contamination NEC Z13.88
  cystic fibrosis Z13.228
  dengue fever Z11.59
  dental disorder Z13.84
  depression Z13.89
  developmental handicap Z13.4
    in early childhood Z13.4
  diabetes mellitus Z13.1
  diphtheria Z11.2
  disease or disorder Z13.9
    bacterial NEC Z11.2
      intestinal infectious Z11.0
      respiratory tuberculosis Z11.1
    blood or blood-forming organ Z13.0
    cardiovascular Z13.6
    Chagas' Z11.6
    chlamydial Z11.8
    dental Z13.89
    developmental Z13.4
    digestive tract NEC Z13.818
      lower GI Z13.811
      upper GI Z13.810
    ear Z13.5
    endocrine Z13.29
    eye Z13.5
    genitourinary Z13.89
    heart Z13.6
    human immunodeficiency virus (HIV) infection
        Z11.4
    immunity Z13.0
    infection
      intestinal Z11.0
        specified NEC Z11.6
    infectious Z11.9
    mental Z13.89
    metabolic Z13.228
    neurological Z13.89
    nutritional Z13.21
      metabolic Z13.228
        lipoid disorders Z13.220
    protozoal Z11.6
      intestinal Z11.0
    respiratory Z13.83
    rheumatic Z13.828
    rickettsial Z11.8
    sexually-transmitted NEC Z11.3
      human immunodeficiency virus (HIV) Z11.4
    sickle-cell (trait) Z13.0
    skin Z13.89
    specified NEC Z13.89
    spirochetal Z11.8
    thyroid Z13.29
    vascular Z13.6
    venereal Z11.3
    viral NEC Z11.59
      human immunodeficiency virus (HIV) Z11.4
      intestinal Z11.0
  elevated titer Z13.89
  emphysema Z13.83

Screening —*continued*
  encephalitis, viral (mosquitoor tick-borne) Z11.59
  exposure to contaminants (toxic) Z13.88
  fever
    dengue Z11.59
    hemorrhagic Z11.59
    yellow Z11.59
  filariasis Z11.6
  galactosemia Z13.228
  gastrointestinal condition Z13.818
  genetic (nonprocreative) for procreative
      management *see* Testing, genetic, for
      procreative management
    disease carrier status (nonprocreative) Z13.71
    specified NEC (nonprocreative) Z13.79
  genitourinary condition Z13.89
  glaucoma Z13.5
  gonorrhea Z11.3
  gout Z13.89
  helminthiasis (intestinal) Z11.6
  hematopoietic malignancy Z12.89
  hemoglobinopathies NEC Z13.0
  hemorrhagic fever Z11.59
  Hodgkin disease Z12.89
  human immunodeficiency virus (HIV) Z11.4
  human papillomavirus Z11.51
  hypertension Z13.6
  immunity disorders Z13.0
  infection
    mycotic Z11.8
    parasitic Z11.8
  ingestion of radioactive substance Z13.88
  intestinal
    helminthiasis Z11.6
    infectious disease Z11.0
  leishmaniasis Z11.6
  leprosy Z11.2
  leptospirosis Z11.8
  leukemia Z12.89
  lymphoma Z12.89
  malaria Z11.6
  malnutrition Z13.29
    metabolic Z13.228
    nutritional Z13.21
  measles Z11.59
  mental
    disorder Z13.89
    retardation Z13.4
  metabolic errors, inborn Z13.228
  multiphasic Z13.89
  musculoskeletal disorder Z13.828
    osteoporosis Z13.820
  mycoses Z11.8
  myocardial infarction (acute) Z13.6
  neoplasm (malignant) (of) Z12.9
    bladder Z12.6
    blood Z12.89
    breast Z12.39
      routine mammogram Z12.31
    cervix Z12.4
    colon Z12.11
    genitourinary organs NEC Z12.79
      bladder Z12.6
      cervix Z12.4
      ovary Z12.73
      prostate Z12.5
      testis Z12.71
      vagina Z12.72
    hematopoietic system Z12.89
    intestinal tract Z12.10
      colon Z12.11
      rectum Z12.12
      small intestine Z12.13
    lung Z12.2
    lymph (glands) Z12.89
    nervous system Z12.82
    oral cavity Z12.81
    prostate Z12.5
    rectum Z12.12
    respiratory organs Z12.2
    skin Z12.83
    small intestine Z12.13
    specified site NEC Z12.89

Screening —*continued*
  neoplasm—*continued*
    stomach Z12.0
  nephropathy Z13.89
  nervous system disorders NEC Z13.858
  neurological condition Z13.89
  osteoporosis Z13.820
  parasitic infestation Z11.9
    specified NEC Z11.8
  phenylketonuria Z13.228
  plague Z11.2
  poisoning (chemical) (heavy metal) Z13.88
  poliomyelitis Z11.59
  postnatal, chromosomal abnormalities Z13.89
  prenatal, of mother Z36
  protozoal disease Z11.6
    intestinal Z11.0
  pulmonary tuberculosis Z11.1
  radiation exposure Z13.88
  respiratory condition Z13.83
  respiratory tuberculosis Z11.1
  rheumatoid arthritis Z13.828
  rubella Z11.59
  schistosomiasis Z11.6
  sexually-transmitted disease NEC Z11.3
    human immunodeficiency virus (HIV) Z11.4
  sickle-cell disease or trait Z13.0
  skin condition Z13.89
  sleeping sickness Z11.6
  special Z13.9
    specified NEC Z13.89
  syphilis Z11.3
  tetanus Z11.2
  trachoma Z11.8
  traumatic brain injury Z13.850
  trypanosomiasis Z11.6
  tuberculosis, respiratory Z11.1
  venereal disease Z11.3
  viral encephalitis (mosquitoor tick-borne) Z11.59
  whooping cough Z11.2
  worms, intestinal Z11.6
  yaws Z11.8
  yellow fever Z11.59
Scrofula, scrofulosis (tuberculosis of cervical lymph
    glands) A18.2
Scrofulide (primary) (tuberculous) A18.4
Scrofuloderma, scrofulodermia (any site) (primary)
    A18.4
Scrofulosus lichen (primary) (tuberculous) A18.4
Scrofulous — *see* condition
Scrotal tongue K14.5
Scrotum — *see* condition
Scurvy, scorbutic E54
  anemia D53.2
  gum E54
  infantile E54
  rickets E55.9 [M90.80]
Sealpox B08.62
Seasickness T75.3
Seatworm (infection) (infestation) B80
Sebaceous (*see also* condition)
  cyst — *see* Cyst, sebaceous
Seborrhea, seborrheic L21.9
  capillitii R23.8
  capitis L21.0
  dermatitis L21.9
    infantile L21.1
  eczema L21.9
    infantile L21.1
  sicca L21.0
Seckel's syndrome Q87.1
Seclusion, pupil — *see* Membrane, pupillary
Second hand tobacco smoke exposure (acute)
    (chronic) Z77.22
  in the perinatal period P96.81
Secondary
  dentin (in pulp) K04.3
  neoplasm, secondaries — *see* Table of Neoplasms,
    secondary

Secretion
  antidiuretic hormone, inappropriate E22.2
  catecholamine, by pheochromocytoma E27.5
  hormone
    antidiuretic, inappropriate (syndrome) E22.2
    by
      carcinoid tumor E34.0
      pheochromocytoma E27.5
    ectopic NEC E34.2
  urinary
    excessive R35.8
    suppression R34
Section
  nerve, traumatic — *see* Injury, nerve
Segmentation, incomplete (congenital) (*see also*
    Fusion)
  bone NEC Q78.8
  lumbosacral (joint) (vertebra) Q76.49
Seitelberger's syndrome (infantile neuraxonal
    dystrophy) G31.89
Seizure(s) (*see also* Convulsions) R56.9
  akinetic — *see* Epilepsy, generalized, idiopathic
  atonic — *see* Epilepsy, generalized, idiopathic
  autonomic (hysterical) F44.5
  convulsive — *see* Convulsions
  cortical (focal) (motor) — *see* Epilepsy,
      localization-related, symptomatic, with simple
      partial seizures
  disorder (*see also* Eplepsy) G40.909
  due to stroke — *see* Sequelae (of), disease,
      cerebrovascular, by type, specified NEC
  epileptic — *see* Epilepsy
  febrile (simple) R56.00
    with status epilepticus G40.901
    complex (atypical) (complicated) R56.01
      with status epilepticus G40.901
  grand mal G40.309
    intractable G40.319
      with status epilepticus G40.311
      without status epilepticus G40.319
    not intractable G40.309
      with status epilepticus G40.301
      without status epilepticus G40.309
  heart — *see* Disease, heart
  hysterical F44.5
  intractable G40.919
    with status epilepticus G40.911
  Jacksonian (focal) (motor type) (sensory type) — *see*
      Epilepsy, localization-related, symptomatic,
      with simple partial seizures
  newborn P90
  nonspecific epileptic
    atonic — *see* Epilepsy, generalized, idiopathic
    clonic — *see* Epilepsy, generalized, idiopathic
    myoclonic — *see* Epilepsy, generalized,
        idiopathic
    tonic — *see* Epilepsy, generalized, idiopathic
    tonic-clonic — *see* Epilepsy, generalized,
        idiopathic
  partial, developing into secondarily generalized
      seizures
    complex — *see* Epilepsy, localization-related,
        symptomatic, with complex partial
        seizures
    simple — *see* Epilepsy, localization-related,
        symptomatic, with simple partial seizures
  petit mal G40.309
    intractable G40.319
      with status epilepticus G40.311
      without status epilepticus G40.319
    not intractable G40.309
      with status epilepticus G40.301
      without status epilepticus G40.309
  post traumatic R56.1
  recurrent G40.909
  specified NEC G40.89
  uncinate — *see* Epilepsy, localization-related,
      symptomatic, with complex partial seizures
Selenium deficiency, dietary E59
Self-damaging behavior (life-style) Z72.89
Self-harm (attempted)
  history (personal) Z91.5
    in family Z81.8

Self-mutilation (attempted)
 history (personal) Z91.5
  in family Z81.8
Self-poisoning
 history (personal) Z91.5
  in family Z81.8
 observation following (alleged) attempt Z03.6
Semicoma R40.1
Seminal vesiculitis N49.0
Seminoma C62.9-
 specified site — see Neoplasm, malignant, by site
Senear-Usher disease or syndrome L10.4
Senectus R54
Senescence (without mention of psychosis) R54
Senile, senility (see also condition) R54
 with
  acute confusional state F05
  mental changes NOS F03
  psychosis NEC — see Psychosis, senile
 asthenia R54
 cervix (atrophic) N88.8
 debility R54
 endometrium (atrophic) N85.8
 fallopian tube (atrophic) — see Atrophy, fallopian
  tube
 heart (failure) R54
 ovary (atrophic) — see Atrophy, ovary
 premature E34.8
 vagina, vaginitis (atrophic) N95.2
 wart L82.1
Sensation
 burning (skin) R20.8
  tongue K14.6
 loss of R20.8
 prickling (skin) R20.2
 tingling (skin) R20.2
Sense loss
 smell — see Disturbance, sensation, smell
 taste — see Disturbance, sensation, taste
 touch R20.8
Sensibility disturbance (cortical) (deep) (vibratory)
  R20.9
Sensitive, sensitivity (see also Allergy)
 carotid sinus G90.01
 child (excessive) F93.8
 cold, autoimmune D59.1
 dentin K03.89
 latex Z91.040
 methemoglobin D74.8
 tuberculin, without clinical or radiological
  symptoms R76.1
 visual
  glare H53.71
  impaired contrast H53.72
Sensitiver Beziehungswahn F22
Sensitization, auto-erythrocytic D69.2
Separation
 anxiety, abnormal (of childhood) F93.0
 apophysis, traumatic code as Fracture, by site
 choroid — see Detachment, choroid
 epiphysis, epiphyseal
  nontraumatic (see also Osteochondropathy,
   specified type NEC)
   upper femoral — see Slipped, epiphysis,
    upper femoral
  traumatic code as Fracture, by site
 fracture — see Fracture
 infundibulum cardiac from right ventricle by a
  partition Q24.3
 joint (traumatic) (current) code by site under
  Dislocation
 pubic bone, obstetrical trauma O71.6
 retina, retinal — see Detachment, retina
 symphysis pubis, obstetrical trauma O71.6
 tracheal ring, incomplete, congenital Q32.1
Sepsis (generalized) A41.9
 with
  acute organ dysfunction R65.2
  multiple organ dysfunction R65.2
 actinomycotic A42.7
 adrenal hemorrhage syndrome (meningococcal)
  A39.1
 anaerobic A41.4

Sepsis —continued
 Bacillus anthracis A22.7
 Brucella (see also Brucellosis) A23.9
 candidal B37.7
 cryptogenic A41.9
 due to device, implant or graft T85.79
  arterial graft NEC T82.7
  breast (implant) T85.79
  catheter NEC T85.79
   dialysis (renal) T82.7
    intraperitoneal T85.71
   infusion NEC T82.7
    spinal (epidural) (subdural) T85.79
   urinary (indwelling) T83.51
  ectopic or molar pregnancy O08.82
  electronic (electrode) (pulse generator)
   (stimulator)
   bone T84.7
   cardiac T82.7
   nervous system (brain) (peripheral nerve)
    (spinal) T85.79
   urinary T83.59
  fixation, internal (orthopedic) — see
   Complication, fixation device, infection
  gastrointestinal (bile duct) (esophagus) T85.79
  genital T83.6
  heart NEC T82.7
   valve (prosthesis) T82.6
    graft T82.7
  joint prosthesis — see Complication, joint
   prosthesis, infection
  ocular (corneal graft) (orbital implant) T85.79
  orthopedic NEC T84.7
   fixation device, internal — see Complication,
    fixation device, infection
  specified NEC T85.79
  vascular T82.7
  ventricular intracranial shunt T85.79
 during labor O75.3
 Enterococcus A41.81
 Erysipelothrix (rhusiopathiae) (erysipeloid) A26.7
 Escherichia coli (E. coli) A41.5
 extraintestinal yersiniosis A28.2
 following
  abortion (subsequent episode) O08.0
   current episode — see Abortion
  ectopic or molar pregnancy O08.82
  immunization T88.0
  infusion, therapeutic injection or transfusion NEC
   T80.29
 gangrenous A41.9
 gonococcal A54.8
 Gram-negative (organism) A41.5
  anaerobic A41.4
 Haemophilus influenzae A41.3
 herpesviral B00.7
 intraocular — see Endophthalmitis, purulent
 Listeria monocytogenes A32.7
 localized
  in operation wound T81.4
  skin — see Abscess
 malleus A24.0
 melioidosis A24.1
 meningeal — see Meningitis
 meningococcal A39.4
  acute A39.2
  chronic A39.3
 newborn P36.9
  due to
   anaerobes NEC P36.5
   Escherichia coli P36.4
   Staphylococcus P36.30
    aureus P36.2
    specified NEC P36.39
   Streptococcus P36.10
    group B P36.0
    specified NEC P36.19
  specified NEC P36.8
 Pasteurella multocida A28.0
 pelvic, puerperal, postpartum, childbirth O85
 postprocedural T81.4
 pneumococcal A40.3
 puerperal, postpartum, childbirth (pelvic) O85

Sepsis —continued
 Salmonella (arizonae) (choleraesuis) (enteritidis)
  (typhimurium) A02.1
 severe R65.20
  with septic shock R65.21
 skin, localized — see Abscess
 Shigella (see also Dysentery, bacillary) A03.9
 specified organism NEC A41.89
 Staphylococcus, staphylococcal A41.2
  aureus A41.0
  coagulase-negative A41.1
  specified NEC A41.1
 Streptococcus, streptococcal A40.9
  agalactiae A40.1
  group
   A A40.0
   B A40.1
   D A41.81
  neonatal P36.10
   group B P36.0
   specified NEC P36.19
  pneumoniae A40.3
  pyogenes A40.0
  specified NEC A40.8
 tracheostomy stoma J95.02
 tularemic A21.7
 umbilical, umbilical cord (newborn) — see Sepsis,
  newborn
 Yersinia pestis A20.7
Septate — see Septum
Septic — see condition
 arm — see Cellulitis, upper limb
  with lymphangitis — see Lymphangitis, acute,
   upper limb
 embolus — see Embolism
 finger — see Cellulitis, digit
  with lymphangitis — see Lymphangitis, acute,
   digit
 foot — see Cellulitis, lower limb
  with lymphangitis — see Lymphangitis, acute,
   lower limb
 gallbladder (acute) K81.0
 hand — see Cellulitis, upper limb
  with lymphangitis — see Lymphangitis, acute,
   upper limb
 joint — see Arthritis, pyogenic or pyemic
 leg — see Cellulitis, lower limb
  with lymphangitis — see Lymphangitis, acute,
   lower limb
 nail (see also Cellulitis, digit)
  with lymphangitis — see Lymphangitis, acute,
   digit
 sore (see also Abscess)
  throat J02.0
   streptococcal J02.0
 spleen (acute) D73.89
 teeth, tooth (pulpal origin) K04.4
 throat — see Pharyngitis
 thrombus — see Thrombosis
 toe — see Cellulitis, digit
  with lymphangitis — see Lymphangitis, acute,
   digit
 tonsils, chronic J35.01
  with adenoiditis J35.03
 uterus — see Endometritis
Septicemia A41.9
 meaning sepsis — see Sepsis
Septum, septate (congenital) (see also Anomaly, by
  site)
 anal Q42.3
  with fistula Q42.2
 aqueduct of Sylvius Q03.0
  with spina bifida — see Spina bifida, by site, with
   hydrocephalus
 uterus — see Double, uterus
 vagina Q52.10
  in pregnancy (see also Pregnancy, complicated
   by, abnormal vagina)
   causing obstructed labor O65.5
  longitudinal (with or without obstruction)
   Q52.12
  transverse Q52.11

Sequelae (of) (*see also* condition)
abscess, intracranial or intraspinal (conditions in G06) G09
amputation — code to injury with extension s
burn and corrosion — code to injury with extension s
calcium deficiency E64.8
cerebrovascular disease — *see* Sequelae, disease, cerebrovascular
childbirth O94
contusion — code to injury with extension s
corrosion — *see* Sequelae, burn and corrosion
crushing injury — code to injury with extension s
disease
  cerebrovascular I69.90
    alteration of sensation I69.998
    aphasia I69.920
    apraxia I69.990
    ataxia I69.993
    cognitive defects I69.91
    disturbance of vision I69.998
    dysarthria I69.922
    dysphagia I69.991
    dysphasia I69.921
    facial droop I69.992
    facial weakness I69.992
    fluency disorder I69.923
    hemiplegia I69.95-
    hemorrhage
      intracerebral — *see* Sequelae, hemorrhage, intracerebral
      intracranial, nontraumatic NEC — *see* Sequelae, hemorrhage, intracranial, nontraumatic
      subarachnoid — *see* Sequelae, hemorrhage, subarachnoid
    language deficit I69.928
    monoplegia
      lower limb I69.84-
      upper limb I69.93-
    paralytic syndrome I69.96-
    specified effect NEC I69.998
    specified type NEC I69.80
      alteration of sensation I69.898
      aphasia I69.820
      apraxia I69.890
      ataxia I69.893
      cognitive defects I69.81
      disturbance of vision I69.898
      dysarthria I69.822
      dysphagia I69.891
      dysphasia I69.821
      facial droop I69.892
      facial weakness I69.892
      fluency disorder I69.823
      hemiplegia I69.85-
      language deficit I69.828
      monoplegia
        lower limb I69.84-
        upper limb I69.83-
      paralytic syndrome I69.86-
      specified effect NEC I69.898
    speech deficit I69.928
      speech deficit I69.828
    stroke NOS — *see* Sequelae, stroke NOS
dislocation — code to injury with extension s
encephalitis or encephalomyelitis (conditions in G04) G09
  in infectious disease NEC B94.8
  viral B94.1
external cause — code to injury with extension s
foreign body entering natural orifice — code to injury with extension s
fracture — code to injury with extension s
frostbite — code to injury with extension s
Hansen's disease B92
hemorrhage
  intracerebral I69.10
    alteration of sensation I69.198
    aphasia I69.120
    apraxia I69.190
    ataxia I69.193
    cognitive defects I69.11

Sequelae—*continued*
hemorrhage—*continued*
  intracerebral—*continued*
    disturbance of vision I69.198
    dysarthria I69.122
    dysphagia I69.191
    dysphasia I69.121
    facial droop I69.192
    facial weakness I69.192
    fluency disorder I69.123
    hemiplegia I69.15-
    language deficit NEC I69.128
    monoplegia
      lower limb I69.14-
      upper limb I69.13-
    paralytic syndrome I69.16-
    specified effect NEC I69.198
    speech deficit NEC I69.128
  intracranial, nontraumatic NEC I69.20
    alteration of sensation I69.298
    aphasia I69.220
    apraxia I69.290
    ataxia I69.293
    cognitive defects I69.21
    disturbance of vision I69.298
    dysarthria I69.222
    dysphagia I69.291
    dysphasia I69.221
    facial droop I69.292
    facial weakness I69.292
    fluency disorder I69.223
    hemiplegia I69.25-
    language deficit NEC I69.228
    monoplegia
      lower limb I69.24-
      upper limb I69.23-
    paralytic syndrome I69.26-
    specified effect NEC I69.298
    speech deficit NEC I69.228
  subarachnoid I69.00
    alteration of sensation I69.098
    aphasia I69.020
    apraxia I69.090
    ataxia I69.093
    cognitive defects I69.01
    disturbance of vision I69.098
    dysarthria I69.022
    dysphagia I69.091
    dysphasia I69.021
    facial droop I69.092
    facial weakness I69.092
    fluency disorder I69.023
    hemiplegia I69.05-
    language deficit NEC I69.028
    monoplegia
      lower limb I69.04-
      upper limb I69.03-
    paralytic syndrome I69.06-
    specified effect NEC I69.098
    speech deficit NEC I69.028
hepatitis, viral B94.2
hyperalimentation E68
infarction
  cerebral I69.30
    alteration of sensation I69.398
    aphasia I69.320
    apraxia I69.390
    ataxia I69.393
    cognitive defects I69.31
    disturbance of vision I69.398
    dysarthria I69.322
    dysphagia I69.391
    dysphasia I69.321
    facial droop I69.392
    facial weakness I69.392
    fluency disorder I69.323
    hemiplegia I69.35-
    language deficit NEC I69.328
    monoplegia
      lower limb I69.34-
      upper limb I69.33-
    paralytic syndrome I69.36-
    specified effect NEC I69.398

Sequelae—*continued*
infarction—*continued*
  cerebral—*continued*
    speech deficit NEC I69.328
infection, pyogenic, intracranial or intraspinal G09
infectious disease B94.9
  specified NEC B94.8
injury — code to injury with extension S
leprosy B92
meningitis
  bacterial (conditions in G00) G09
  other or unspecified cause (conditions in G03) G09
muscle (and tendon) injury — code to injury with extension S
myelitis — *see* Sequelae, encephalitis
niacin deficiency E64.8
nutritional deficiency E64.9
  specified NEC E64.8
obstetrical condition O94
parasitic disease B94.9
phlebitis or thrombophlebitis of intracranial or intraspinal venous sinuses and veins (conditions in G08) G09
poisoning — code to poisoning with extension S
  nonmedicinal substance — *see* Sequelae, toxic effect, nonmedicinal substance
poliomyelitis (acute) B91
pregnancy O94
protein-energy malnutrition E64.0
puerperium O94
rickets E64.3
selenium deficiency E64.8
sprain and strain — code to injury with extension s
stroke NOS I69.30
  alteration in sensation I69.398
  aphasia I69.320
  apraxia I69.390
  ataxia I69.393
  cognitive defects I69.31
  disturbance of vision I69.398
  dysarthria I69.322
  dysphagia I69.391
  dysphasia I69.321
  facial droop I69.392
  facial weakness I69.392
  hemiplegia I69.35-
  language deficit NEC I69.328
  monoplegia
    lower limb I69.34-
    upper limb I69.33-
  paralytic syndrome I69.36-
  specified effect NEC I69.398
  speech deficit NEC I69.328
tendon and muscle injury — code to injury with extension S
thiamine deficiency E64.8
trachoma B94.0
tuberculosis B90.9
  bones and joints B90.2
  central nervous system B90.0
  genitourinary B90.1
  pulmonary (respiratory) B90.9
  specified organs NEC B90.8
viral
  encephalitis B94.1
  hepatitis B94.2
vitamin deficiency NEC E64.8
  A E64.1
  B E64.8
  C E64.2
wound, open — code to injury with extension s
Sequestration (*see also* Sequestrum)
lung, congenital Q33.2
Sequestrum
bone — *see* Osteomyelitis, chronic
dental M27.2
jaw bone M27.2
orbit — *see* Osteomyelitis, orbit
sinus (accessory) (nasal) — *see* Sinusitis
Sequoiosis lung or pneumonitis J67.8

Serology for syphilis
  doubtful
    with signs or symptoms code by site and stage
      under Syphilis
    follow-up of latent syphilis — *see* Syphilis, latent
    negative, with signs or symptoms code by site and
      stage under Syphilis
  positive A53.0
    with signs or symptoms code by site and stage
      under Syphilis
  reactivated A53.0
Seroma *(see also* Hematoma)
  traumatic, secondary and recurrent T79.2
Seropurulent — *see* condition
Serositis, multiple K65.8
  pericardial I31.1
  peritoneal K65.8
Serous — *see* condition
Sertoli cell
  benign
    specified site — *see* Neoplasm, benign, by site
    unspecified site
      female D27.9
      male D29.20
  malignant
    specified site — *see* Neoplasm, malignant, by site
    unspecified site (male) C62.9-
      female C56.9
  specified site — *see* Neoplasm, benign, by site
  unspecified site
    female D27.9
    male D29.20
Sertoli-Leydig cell tumor — *see* Neoplasm, benign,
    by site
  specified site — *see* Neoplasm, benign, by site
  unspecified site
    female D27.9
    male D29.20
Serum
  allergy, allergic reaction T80.6
    shock T80.5
  arthritis T80.6
  complication or reaction NEC T80.6
  disease NEC T80.6
  hepatitis *(see also* Hepatitis, viral, type B)
    carrier (suspected) of Z22.51
  intoxication T80.6
  neuritis T80.6
  neuropathy G61.1
  poisoning NEC T80.6
  rash NEC T80.6
  reaction NEC T80.6
  sickness NEC T80.6
  urticaria T80.6
Sesamoiditis — *see* Osteomyelitis, specified type NEC
Sever's disease or osteochondrosis — *see*
    Osteochondrosis, juvenile, tarsus
Severe sepsis R65.20
  with septic shock R65.21
Sex
  chromosome mosaics Q97.8
    lines with various numbers of X chromosomes
      Q97.2
  education Z70.8
  reassignment surgery status Z87.890
Sextuplet pregnancy — *see* Pregnancy, sextuplet
Sexual
  function, disorder of (psychogenic) F52.9
  immaturity (female) (male) E30.0
  impotence (psychogenic) organic origin NEC — *see*
    Dysfunction, sexual, male
  precocity (constitutional) (cryptogenic)(female)
    (idiopathic) (male) E30.1
Sexuality, pathologic — *see* Deviation, sexual
Sézary disease C84.1-
Shadow, lung R91
Shaking palsy or paralysis — *see* Parkinsonism
Shallowness, acetabulum — *see* Derangement, joint,
    specified type NEC, hip
Shaver's disease J63.1
Sheath (tendon) — *see* condition
Sheathing, retinal vessels H35.00

Shedding
  nail L60.8
  premature, primary (deciduous) teeth K00.6
Sheehan's disease or syndrome E23.0
Shelf, rectal K62.8
Shell teeth K00.5
Shellshock (current) F43.0
  lasting state — *see* Disorder, post-traumatic stress
Shield kidney Q63.1
Shift
  auditory threshold (temporary) H93.24-
  mediastinal R93.8
Shifting sleep-work schedule (affecting sleep)
    G47.26
Shiga(-Kruse) **dysentery** A03.0
Shiga's bacillus A03.0
Shigella (dysentery) — *see* Dysentery, bacillary
Shigellosis A03.9
  Group A A03.0
  Group B A03.1
  Group C A03.2
  Group D A03.3
Shin splints T79.6
Shingles — *see* Herpes, zoster
Shipyard disease or eye B30.0
Shirodkar suture, in pregnancy — *see* Pregnancy,
    complicated by, incompetent cervix
Shock R57.9
  with ectopic or molar pregnancy O08.3
  adrenal (cortical) (Addisonian) E27.2
  adverse food reaction (anaphylactic) — *see* Shock,
    anaphylactic, food
  allergic — *see* Shock, anaphylactic
  anaphylactic T78.2
    chemical — *see* Table of Drugs and Chemicals
    due to drug or medicinal substance
      correct substance properly administered
        T88.6
      overdose or wrong substance given or taken
        (by accident) — *see* Table of Drugs and
        Chemicals, by drug, poisoning
    due to food T78.00
      additives T78.06
      dairy products T78.07
      eggs T78.08
      fish T78.03
        shellfish T78.02
      fruit T78.04
      milk T78.07
      nuts T78.05
        peanuts T78.01
      peanuts T78.01
      seeds T78.05
      specified type NEC T78.09
      vegetable T78.04
    following sting(s) — *see* Venom
    immunization T80.5
    serum T80.5
  anaphylactoid — *see* Shock, anaphylactic
  anesthetic
    correct substance properly administered T88.2
    overdose or wrong substance given or taken —
      see Table of Drugs and Chemicals, by drug,
      poisoning
      specified anesthetic — *see* Table of Drugs and
        Chemicals, by drug, poisoning
  cardiogenic R57.0
  chemical substance — *see* Table of Drugs and
    Chemicals
  complicating ectopic or molar pregnancy O08.3
  culture — *see* Disorder, adjustment
  drug
    due to correct substance properly administered
      T88.6
    overdose or wrong substance given or taken (by
      accident) — *see* Table of Drugs and
      Chemicals, by drug, poisoning
  during or after labor and delivery O75.1
  electric T75.4
    (taser) T75.4
  endotoxic R65.21

Shock—*continued*
  following
    ectopic or molar pregnancy O08.3
    injury (immediate) (delayed) T79.4
    labor and delivery O75.1
  food (anaphylactic) — *see* Shock, anaphylactic, food
  from electroshock gun (taser) T75.4
  gram-negative R65.21
  hematologic R57.8
  hemorrhagic
    surgery (intraoperative) (postoperative) T81.1
    trauma T79.4
  hypovolemic R57.1
    surgical T81.1
    traumatic T79.4
  insulin E15
    therapeutic misadventure — *see* subcategory
      T38.3
  kidney N17.0
    traumatic (following crushing) T79.5
  lightning T75.01
  lung J80
  obstetric O75.1
    with ectopic or molar pregnancy O08.3
    following ectopic or molar pregnancy O08.3
  pleural (surgical) T81.1
    due to trauma T79.4
  postoperative T81.1
    with ectopic or molar pregnancy O08.3
    following ectopic or molar pregnancy O08.3
  psychic F43.0
  septic (due to severe sepsis) R65.21
  specified NEC R57.8
  surgical T81.1
  taser gun (taser) T75.4
  therapeutic misadventure NEC T81.1
  thyroxin
    overdose or wrong substance given or taken —
      see Table of Drugs and Chemicals, by drug,
      poisoning
  toxic, syndrome A48.3
  transfusion — *see* Complications, transfusion
  traumatic (immediate) (delayed) T79.4
Shoemaker's chest M95.4
Short, shortening, shortness
  arm (acquired) *(see also* Deformity, limb, unequal
    length)
    congenital Q71.81-
    forearm — *see* Deformity, limb, unequal length
  bowel syndrome K91.2
  breath R06.02
  cervical (complicating pregnancy) O26.87-
    non-gravid uterus N88.3
  common bile duct, congenital Q44.5
  cord (umbilical), complicating delivery O69.3
  cystic duct, congenital Q44.5
  esophagus (congenital) Q39.8
  femur (acquired) — *see* Deformity, limb, unequal
    length, femur
    congenital — *see* Defect, reduction, lower limb,
      longitudinal, femur
  frenum, frenulum, linguae (congenital) Q38.1
  hip (acquired) *(see also* Deformity, limb, unequal
    length)
    congenital Q65.8
  leg (acquired) *(see also* Deformity, limb, unequal
    length)
    congenital Q72.81-
    lower leg *(see also* Deformity, limb, unequal
      length)
  limbed stature, with immunodeficiency D82.2
  lower limb (acquired) *(see also* Deformity, limb,
    unequal length)
    congenital Q72.81-
  organ or site, congenital NEC — *see* Distortion
  palate, congenital Q38.5
  radius (acquired) *(see also* Deformity, limb, unequal
    length)
    congenital — *see* Defect, reduction, upper limb,
      longitudinal, radius
  rib syndrome Q77.2

Short, shortening, shortness—*continued*
  stature (child) (hereditary) (idiopathic) NEC R62.52
    constitutional E34.3
    due to endocrine disorder E34.3
    Laron-type E34.3
  tendon (*see also* Contraction, tendon)
    with contracture of joint — *see* Contraction, joint
    Achilles (acquired) M67.0-
      congenital Q66.8
    congenital Q79.8
  thigh (acquired) (*see also* Deformity, limb, unequal length, femur)
    congenital — *see* Defect, reduction, lower limb, longitudinal, femur
  tibialis anterior (tendon) — *see* Contraction, tendon
  umbilical cord
    complicating delivery O69.3
  upper limb, congenital — *see* Defect, reduction, upper limb, specified type NEC
  urethra N36.8
  uvula, congenital Q38.5
  vagina (congenital) Q52.4
Shortsightedness — *see* Myopia
Shoshin (acute fulminating beriberi) E51.11
Shoulder — *see* condition
Shovel-shaped incisors K00.2
Shower, thromboembolic — *see* Embolism
Shunt
  arterial-venous (dialysis) Z99.2
  arteriovenous, pulmonary (acquired) I28.0
    congenital Q25.7
  cerebral ventricle (communicating) in situ Z98.2
  surgical, prosthetic, with complications — *see* Complications, cardiovascular, device or implant
Shutdown, renal N28.9
Shy-Drager syndrome G90.3
Sialadenitis, sialadenosis (any gland) (chronic) (periodic) (suppurative) — *see* Sialoadenitis
Sialectasia K11.8
Sialidosis E77.1
Sialitis, silitis (any gland) (chronic) (suppurative) — *see* Sialoadenitis
Sialoadenitis (any gland) (periodic) (suppurative) K11.20
  acute K11.21
    recurrent K11.22
  chronic K11.23
Sialoadenopathy K11.9
Sialoangitis — *see* Sialoadenitis
Sialodochitis (fibrinosa) — *see* Sialoadenitis
Sialodocholithiasis K11.5
Sialolithiasis K11.5
Sialometaplasia, necrotizing K11.8
Sialorrhea (*see also* Ptyalism)
  periodic — *see* Sialoadenitis
Sialosis K11.7
Siamese twin Q89.4
Sibling rivalry Z62.891
Sicard's syndrome G52.7
Sicca syndrome M35.00
  with
    keratoconjunctivitis M35.01
    lung involvement M35.02
    myopathy M35.03
    renal tubulo-interstitial disorders M35.04
  specified organ involvement NEC M35.09
Sick R69
  or handicapped person in family Z63.79
    needing care at home Z63.6
  sinus (syndrome) I49.5
Sick-euthyroid syndrome E07.81
Sickle-cell
  anemia — *see* Disease, sickle-cell
  trait D57.3
Sicklemia (*see also* Disease, sickle-cell)
  trait D57.3
Sickness
  air (travel) T75.3
  airplane T75.3
  alpine T70.29
  altitude T70.20
  Andes T70.29

Sickness—*continued*
  aviator's T70.29
  balloon T70.29
  car T75.3
  compressed air T70.3
  decompression T70.3
  green D50.9
  milk — *see* Poisoning, food, noxious
  motion T75.3
  mountain T70.20
    acute D75.1
  protein T80.6
  radiation T66
  roundabout (motion) T75.3
  sea T75.3
  serum NEC T80.6
  sleeping (African) B56.9
    by Trypanosoma B56.9
      brucei
        gambiense B56.0
        rhodesiense B56.1
    East African B56.1
    Gambian B56.0
    Rhodesian B56.1
    West African B56.0
  swing (motion) T75.3
  train (railway) (travel) T75.3
  travel (any vehicle) T75.3
Sideropenia — *see* Anemia, iron deficiency
Siderosilicosis J62.8
Siderosis (lung) J63.4
  eye (globe) — *see* Disorder, globe, degenerative, siderosis
Siemens' syndrome (ectodermal dysplasia) Q82.8
Sighing R06.89
  psychogenic F45.8
Sigmoid (*see also* condition)
  flexure — *see* condition
  kidney Q63.1
Sigmoiditis (*see also* Enteritis) K52.9
  infectious A09
  noninfectious K52.9
Silfverskiöld's syndrome Q78.9
Silicosiderosis J62.8
Silicosis, silicotic (simple) (complicated) J62.8
  with tuberculosis J65
Silicotuberculosis J65
Silo-fillers' disease J68.8
  bronchitis J68.0
  pneumonitis J68.0
  pulmonay edema J68.1
Silver's syndrome Q87.1
Simian malaria B53.1
Simmonds' cachexia or disease E23.0
Simons' disease or syndrome (progressive lipodystrophy) E88.1
Simple, simplex — *see* condition
Simulation, conscious (of illness) Z76.5
Sin Nombre virus disease (Hantavirus (cardio)-pulmonary syndrome) B33.4
Sinding-Larsen disease or osteochondrosis — *see* Osteochondrosis, juvenile, patella
Singapore hemorrhagic fever A91
Singer's node or nodule J38.2
Single
  atrium Q21.2
  coronary artery Q24.5
  umbilical artery Q27.0
  ventricle Q20.4
Singultus R06.6
  epidemicus B33.0
Sinus (*see also* Fistula)
  abdominal K63.89
  arrest I45.5
  arrhythmia I49.8
  bradycardia R00.1
  branchial cleft (internal) (external) Q18.0
  coccygeal — *see* Sinus, pilonidal
  dental K04.6
  dermal (congenital) Q06.8
    with abscess Q06.8
    coccygeal, pilonidal — *see* Sinus, coccygeal
  infected, skin NEC L08.89

Sinus—*continued*
  marginal, ruptured or bleeding — *see* Hemorrhage, antepartum, specified cause NEC
  medial, face and neck Q18.8
  pause I45.5
  pericranii Q01.9
  pilonidal (infected) (rectum) L05.92
    with abscess L05.02
  preauricular Q18.1
  rectovaginal N82.3
  Rokitansky-Aschoff (gallbladder) K82.8
  sacrococcygeal (dermoid) (infected) — *see* Sinus, pilonidal
  tachycardia R00.0
    paroxysmal I47.1
  tarsi syndrome — *see* Syndrome, tarsal tunnel
  testis N50.8
  tract (postinfective) — *see* Fistula
  urachus Q64.4
Sinusitis (accessory) (chronic) (hyperplastic) (nasal) (nonpurulent) (purulent) J32.9
  acute J01.90
    ethmoidal J01.20
      recurrent J01.21
    frontal J01.10
      recurrent J01.11
    involving more than one sinus, other than pansinusitis J01.80
      recurrent J01.81
    maxillary J01.00
      recurrent J01.01
    pansinusitis J01.40
      recurrent J01.41
    recurrent J01.91
    specified NEC J01.80
      recurrent J01.81
    sphenoidal J01.30
      recurrent J01.31
  allergic — *see* Rhinitis, allergic
  due to high altitude T70.1
  ethmoidal J32.2
    acute J01.20
      recurrent J01.21
  frontal J32.1
    acute J01.10
      recurrent J01.11
  influenzal — *see* Influenza, with, respiratory manifestations NEC
  involving more than one sinus but not pansinusitis J32.8
    acute J01.80
      recurrent J01.81
  maxillary J32.0
    acute J01.00
      recurrent J01.01
Sinusitis—*continued*
  sphenoidal J32.3
    acute J01.30
      recurrent J01.31
  tuberculous, any sinus A15.8
Sinusitis-bronchiectasis-situs inversus (syndrome) (triad) Q89.3
Sipple's syndrome E31.22
Sirenomelia (syndrome) Q87.2
Siriasis T67.0
Sirkari's disease B55.0
Siti A65
Situation, psychiatric F99
Situational
  disturbance (transient) — *see* Disorder, adjustment
    acute F43.0
  maladjustment — *see* Disorder, adjustment
  reaction — *see* Disorder, adjustment
    acute F43.0
Situs inversus or transversus (abdominalis) (thoracis) Q89.3
Sixth disease B08.20
  due to human herpesvirus 6 B08.21
  due to human herpesvirus 7 B08.22
Sjögren-Larsson syndrome Q87.1
Sjögren's syndrome or disease — *see* Sicca syndrome
Skeletal — *see* condition

Skene's gland — *see* condition
Skenitis — *see* Urethritis
Skerljevo A65
Skevas-Zerfus disease — *see* Toxicity, venom, marine
　　animal, sea anemone
Skin (*see also* condition)
　clammy R23.1
　donor — *see* Donor, skin
　hidebound M35.9
Slate-dressers' or slate-miners' lung J62.8
Sleep
　apnea — *see* Apnea, sleep
　deprivation Z72.820
　disorder or disturbance G47.9
　　child F51.9
　　nonorganic origin F51.9
　　specified NEC G47.8
　disturbance G47.9
　　nonorganic origin F51.9
　drunkenness F51.5
　rhythm inversion G47.2
　terrors F51.4
　walking F51.3
　　hysterical F44.89
Sleep hygiene
　abuse Z72.821
　inadequate Z72.821
　poor Z72.821
Sleeping sickness — *see* Sickness, sleeping
Sleeplessness — *see* Insomnia
　menopausal N95.1
Sleep-wake schedule disorder G47.2
Slim disease (in HIV infection) B20
Slipped, slipping
　epiphysis (traumatic) (*see also* Osteochondropathy,
　　specified type NEC)
　　capital femoral (traumatic)
　　　acute (on chronic) S79.01-
　　　current traumatic code as Fracture, by site
　　　upper femoral (nontraumatic) M93.00-
　　　　acute M93.01-
　　　　　on chronic M93.03-
　　　　chronic M93.02-
　　intervertebral disc — *see* Displacement,
　　　intervertebral disc
　　ligature, umbilical P51.8
　　patella — *see* Disorder, patella, derangement NEC
　　rib M89.8x8
　　sacroiliac joint — *see* subcategory M53.2
　　tendon — *see* Disorder, tendon
　　ulnar nerve, nontraumatic — *see* Lesion, nerve,
　　　ulnar
　　vertebra NEC — *see* Spondylolisthesis
Slocumb's syndrome E27.0
Sloughing (multiple) (phagedena) (skin) (*see also*
　　Gangrene)
　abscess — *see* Abscess
　appendix K38.8
　fascia — *see* Disorder, soft tissue, specified type NEC
　scrotum N50.8
　tendon — *see* Disorder, tendon
　transplanted organ — *see* Rejection, transplant
　ulcer — *see* Ulcer, skin
Slow
　feeding, newborn P92.2
　flow syndrome, coronary I20.8
　heart(beat) R00.1
Slowing, urinary stream R39.19
Sluder's neuralgia (syndrome) G44.89
Slurred, slurring speech R47.81
Small(ness)
　for gestational age — *see* Small for dates
　introitus, vagina N89.6
　kidney (unknown cause) N27.9
　　bilateral N27.1
　　unilateral N27.0
　ovary (congenital) Q50.39
　pelvis
　　with disproportion (fetopelvic) O33.1
　　　causing obstructed labor O65.1
　uterus N85.8
　white kidney N03.9
Small-and-light-for-dates — *see* Small for dates

Small-for-dates (infant) P05.10
　with weight of
　　499 grams or less P05.11
　　500-749 grams P05.12
　　750-999 grams P05.13
　　1000-1249 grams P05.14
　　1250-1499 grams P05.15
　　1500-1749 grams P05.16
　　1750-1999 grams P05.17
　　2000-2499 grams P05.18
Smallpox B03
Smearing, fecal R15.1
Smith-Lemli-Opitz syndrome Q87.1
Smith's fracture S52.54-
Smoker — *see* Dependence, drug, nicotine
Smoker's
　bronchitis J41.0
　cough J41.0
　palate K13.24
　throat J31.2
　tongue K13.24
Smoking
　passive Z77.22
Smothering spells R06.81
Snaggle teeth, tooth M26.39
Snapping
　finger — *see* Trigger finger
　hip — *see* Derangement, joint, specified type NEC,
　　hip
　　involving the iliotiblial band M76.3-
　knee — *see* Derangement, knee
　　involving the iliotiblial band M76.3-
Sneddon-Wilkinson disease or syndrome L13.1
Sneddon-Wilkinson disease or syndrome
　　(sub-corneal pustular dermatosis) L13.1
Sneezing (intractable) R06.7
Sniffing
　cocaine
　　abuse — *see* Abuse, drug, cocaine
　　dependence — *see* Dependence, drug, cocaine
　gasoline
　　abuse — *see* Abuse, drug, inhalant
　　dependence — *see* Dependence, drug, inhalant
　glue (airplane)
　　abuse — *see* Abuse, drug, inhalant
　　drug dependence — *see* Dependence, drug,
　　　inhalant
Sniffles
　newborn P28.89
Snoring R06.83
Snow blindness — *see* Photokeratitis
Snuffles (non-syphilitic) R06.5
　newborn P28.89
　syphilitic (infant) A50.05 [J99]
Social exclusion Z60.4
　　due to discrimination or persecution (perceived)
　　　Z60.5
　migrant Z59.0
　　acculturation difficulty Z60.3
　rejection Z60.4
　　due to discrimination or persecution Z60.5
　role conflict NEC Z73.5
　skills inadequacy NEC Z73.4
　transplantation Z60.3
Sodoku A25.0
Soemmerring's ring — *see* Cataract, secondary
Soft (*see also* condition)
　nails L60.3
Softening
　bone — *see* Osteomalacia
　brain (necrotic) (progressive) G93.89
　　congenital Q04.8
　　embolic I63.4
　　hemorrhagic — *see* Hemorrhage, intracranial,
　　　intracerebral
　　occlusive I63.5
　　thrombotic I63.3
　cartilage M94.2-
　　patella M22.4-
　cerebellar — *see* Softening, brain
　cerebral — *see* Softening, brain
　cerebrospinal — *see* Softening, brain
　myocardial, heart — *see* Degeneration, myocardial

Softening—*continued*
　spinal cord G95.89
　stomach K31.89
Soldier's
　heart F45.8
　patches I31.0
Solitary
　cyst, kidney N28.1
　kidney, congenital Q60.0
Solvent abuse — *see* Abuse, drug, inhalant
　dependence — *see* Dependence, drug, inhalant
Somatization reaction, somatic reaction — *see*
　　Disorder, somatoform
Somnambulism F51.3
　hysterical F44.89
Somnolence R40.0
　nonorganic origin F51.1
Sonne dysentery A03.3
Soor B37.0
Sore
　bed — *see* Ulcer, pressure, by site
　chiclero B55.1
　Delhi B55.1
　desert — *see* Ulcer, skin
　eye H57.1-
　Lahore B55.1
　mouth K13.79
　　canker K12.0
　muscle M79.1
　Naga — *see* Ulcer, skin
　of skin — *see* Ulcer, skin
　oriental B55.1
　pressure — *see* Ulcer, pressure, by site
　skin L98.9
　soft A57
　throat (acute) (*see also* Pharyngitis)
　　with influenza, flu, or grippe — *see* Influenza,
　　　with, respiratory manifestations NEC
　　chronic J31.2
　　coxsackie (virus) B08.5
　　diphtheritic A36.0
　　herpesviral B00.2
　　influenzal — *see* Influenza, with, respiratory
　　　manifestations NEC
　　septic J02.0
　　streptococcal (ulcerative) J02.0
　　viral NEC J02.8
　　　coxsackie B08.5
　　tropical — *see* Ulcer, skin
　　veldt — *see* Ulcer, skin
Soto's syndrome (cerebral gigantism) Q87.3
South African cardiomyopathy syndrome I42.8
Southeast Asian hemorrhagic fever A91
Spacing abnormal, tooth, teeth, fully erupted M26.30
　excessive, tooth, fully erupted M26.32
Spade-like hand (congenital) Q68.1
Spading nail L60.8
　congenital Q84.6
Spanish collar N47.1
Sparganosis B70.1
Spasm(s), spastic, spasticity (*see also* condition)
　　R25.2
　accommodation — *see* Spasm, of accommodation
　ampulla of Vater K83.4
　anus, ani (sphincter) (reflex) K59.4
　　psychogenic F45.8
　artery I73.9
　　cerebral G45.9
　Bell's G51.3
　bladder (sphincter, external or internal) N32.89
　　psychogenic F45.8
　bronchus, bronchiole J98.01
　cardia K22.0
　cardiac I20.1
　carpopedal — *see* Tetany
　cerebral (arteries) (vascular) G45.9
　cervix, complicating delivery O62.4
　ciliary body (of accommodation) — *see* Spasm, of
　　accommodation
　colon K58.9
　　with diarrhea K58.0
　　psychogenic F45.8
　common duct K83.8

Spasm(s), spastic, spasticity —*continued*
compulsive — *see* Tic
conjugate H51.8
coronary (artery) I20.1
diaphragm (reflex) R06.6
    epidemic B33.0
    psychogenic F45.8
duodenum K59.8
epidemic diaphragmatic (transient) B33.0
esophagus (diffuse) K22.4
    psychogenic F45.8
facial G51.3
fallopian tube N83.8
gastrointestinal (tract) K31.89
    psychogenic F45.8
glottis J38.5
    hysterical F44.4
    psychogenic F45.8
        conversion reaction F44.4
    reflex through recurrent laryngeal nerve J38.5
habit — *see* Tic
heart I20.1
hemifacial (clonic) G51.3
hourglass — *see* Contraction, hourglass
hysterical F44.4
infantile — *see* Epilepsy, generalized, specified NEC
inferior oblique, eye H51.8
intestinal (*see also* Syndrome, irritable bowel) K58.9
    psychogenic F45.8
larynx, laryngeal J38.5
    hysterical F44.4
    psychogenic F45.8
        conversion reaction F44.4
levator palpebrae superioris — *see* Disorder, eyelid
        function
muscle NEC M62.838
    back M62.830
nerve, trigeminal G51.0
nervous F45.8
nodding F98.4
occupational F48.8
oculogyric H51.8
    psychogenic F45.8
of accommodation H52.53-
ophthalmic artery — *see* Occlusion, artery, retina
perineal, female N94.89
peroneo-extensor (*see also* Deformity, limb, flat foot)
pharynx (reflex) J39.2
    hysterical F45.8
    psychogenic F45.8
psychogenic F45.8
pylorus NEC K31.3
    adult hypertrophic K31.89
    congenital or infantile Q40.0
    psychogenic F45.8
rectum (sphincter) K59.4
    psychogenic F45.8
retinal (artery) — *see* Occlusion, artery, retina
sigmoid (*see also* Syndrome, irritable bowel)K58.9
    psychogenic F45.8
sphincter of Oddi K83.4
stomach K31.89
    neurotic F45.8
throat J39.2
    hysterical F45.8
    psychogenic F45.8
tic F95.9
    chronic F95.1
    transient of childhood F95.0
tongue K14.8
torsion (progressive) G24.1
trigeminal nerve — *see* Neuralgia, trigeminal
ureter N13.5
urethra (sphincter) N35.9
uterus N85.8
    complicating labor O62.4
vagina N94.2
    psychogenic F52.5
vascular I73.9
vasomotor I73.9
vein NEC I87.8
viscera — *see* Pain, abdominal
Spasmodic — *see* condition

Spasmophilia — *see* Tetany
Spasmus nutans F98.4
Spastic, spasticity (*see also* Spasm)
    child (cerebral) (congenital) (paralysis) G80.1
Speaker's throat R49.8
Specific, specified — *see* condition
Speech
    defect, disorder, disturbance, impediment R47.9
        psychogenic, in childhood and adolescence
            F98.8
        slurring R47.81
        specified NEC R47.89
Spencer's disease A08.19
Spens' syndrome (syncope with heart block) I45.9
Sperm counts (fertility testing) Z31.41
    postvasectomy Z30.8
    reversal Z31.42
Spermatic cord — *see* condition
Spermatocele N43.40
    congenital Q55.4
    multiple N43.42
    single N43.41
Spermatocystitis N49.0
Spermatocytoma C62.9-
    specified site — *see* Neoplasm, malignant, by site
Spermatorrhea N50.8
Sphacelus — *see* Gangrene
Sphenoidal — *see* condition
Sphenoiditis (chronic) — *see* Sinusitis, sphenoidal
Sphenopalatine ganglion neuralgia G90.09
Sphericity, increased, lens (congenital) Q12.4
Spherocytosis (congenital) (familial) (hereditary)
    D58.0
    hemoglobin disease D58.0
    sickle-cell (disease) D57.8-
Spherophakia Q12.4
Sphincter — *see* condition
Sphincteritis, sphincter of Oddi — *see* Cholangitis
Sphingolipidosis E75.3
    specified NEC E75.29
Sphingomyelinosis E75.3
Spicule tooth K00.2
Spider
    bite — *see* Toxicity, venom, spider
    fingers — *see* Syndrome, Marfan's
    nevus I78.1
    toes — *see* Syndrome, Marfan's
    vascular I78.1
Spiegler-Fendt
    benign lymphocytoma L98.8
    sarcoid L08.0
Spielmeyer-Vogt disease E75.4
Spina bifida (aperta) Q05.9
    with hydrocephalus NEC Q05.4
    cervical Q05.5
        with hydrocephalus Q05.0
    dorsal Q05.6
        with hydrocephalus Q05.1
    lumbar Q05.7
        with hydrocephalus Q05.2
    lumbosacral Q05.7
        with hydrocephalus Q05.2
    occulta Q76.0
    sacral Q05.8
        with hydrocephalus Q05.3
    thoracic Q05.6
        with hydrocephalus Q05.1
    thoracolumbar Q05.6
        with hydrocephalus Q05.1
Spindle, Krukenberg's — *see* Pigmentation, cornea,
        posterior
Spine, spinal — *see* condition
Spiradenoma (eccrine) — *see* Neoplasm, skin, benign
Spirillosis A25.0
Spirillum
    minus A25.0
    obermeieri infection A68.0
Spirochetal — *see* condition
Spirochetosis A69.9
    arthritic, arthritica A69.9
    bronchopulmonary A69.8
    icterohemorrhagic A27.0

Spirochetosis—*continued*
    lung A69.8
Spirometrosis B70.1
Spitting blood — *see* Hemoptysis
Splanchnoptosis K63.4
Spleen, splenic — *see* condition
Splenectasis — *see* Splenomegaly
Splenitis (interstitial) (malignant) (nonspecific) D73.89
    malarial B54
    tuberculous A18.85
Splenocele D73.89
Splenomegaly, splenomegalia (Bengal)
        (cryptogenic) (idiopathic) (tropical) R16.1
    with hepatomegaly R16.2
    cirrhotic D73.2
    congenital Q89.09
    congestive, chronic D73.2
    Egyptian B65.1
    Gaucher's E75.22
    malarial (*see also* Malaria) B54 [D77]
    neutropenic D73.81
    Niemann-Pick — *see* Niemann-Pick disease or
        syndrome
    siderotic D73.2
    syphilitic A52.79
        congenital (early) A50.08 [D77]
Splenopathy D73.9
Splenoptosis D73.89
Splenosis D73.89
Splinter — *see* Foreign body, superficial, by site
Split, splitting
    foot Q72.7-
    heart sounds R01.2
    lip, congenital — *see* Cleft, lip
    nails L60.3
    urinary stream R39.13
Spondylarthrosis — *see* Spondylosis
Spondylitis (chronic) (*see also* Spondylopathy,
        inflammatory)
    ankylopoietica — *see* Spondylitis, ankylosing
    ankylosing (chronic) M45.9
        with lung involvement M45.9 [J99]
            cervical region M45.2
            cervicothoracic region M45.3
            juvenile M08.1
            lumbar region M45.6
            lumbosacral region M45.7
            multiple sites M45.0
            occipito-atlanto-axial region M45.1
            sacrococcygeal region M45.8
            thoracic region M45.4
            thoracolumbar region M45.5
    atrophic (ligamentous) — *see* Spondylitis,
        ankylosing
    deformans (chronic) — *see* Spondylosis
    gonococcal A54.41
    gouty M10.08
    in (due to)
        brucellosis A23.9 [M49.80]
            cervical region A23.9 [M49.82]
            cervicothoracic region A23.9 [M49.83]
            lumbar region A23.9 [M49.86]
            lumbosacral region A23.9 [M49.87]
            multiple sites A23.9 [M49.89]
            occipito-atlanto-axial region A23.9 [M49.81]
            sacrococcygeal region A23.9 [M49.88]
            thoracic region A23.9 [M49.84]
            thoracolumbar region A23.9 [M49.85]
        enterobacteria (*see also* subcategory M49.8)
            A04.9
        tuberculosis A18.01
    infectious NEC — *see* Spondylopathy, infective
    juvenile ankylosing (chronic) M08.1
    Kümmell's — *see* Spondylopathy, traumatic
    Marie-Strümpell — *see* Spondylitis, ankylosing
    muscularis — *see* Spondylopathy, specified NEC
    psoriatic L40.53
    rheumatoid — *see* Spondylitis, ankylosing
    rhizomelica — *see* Spondylitis, ankylosing
    sacroiliac NEC M46.1
    senescent, senile — *see* Spondylosis
    traumatic (chronic) or post-traumatic — *see*
        Spondylopathy, traumatic

Spondylitis—*continued*
  tuberculous A18.01
  typhosa A01.05
Spondylarthrosis — *see* Spondylosis
Spondylolisthesis (acquired) (degenerative) M43.10
  with disproportion (fetopelvic) O33.0
    causing obstructed labor O65.0
  cervical region M43.12
  cervicothoracic region M43.13
  congenital Q76.2
  lumbar region M43.16
  lumbosacral region M43.17
  multiple sites M43.19
  occipito-atlanto-axial region M43.11
  sacrococcygeal region M43.18
  thoracic region M43.14
  thoracolumbar region M43.15
  traumatic (old) M43.10
    acute
      fifth cervical (displaced) S12.430
        nondisplaced S12.431
          specified type NEC (displaced) S12.450
            nondisplaced S12.451
          type III S12.44
      fourth cervical (displaced) S12.330
        nondisplaced S12.331
          specified type NEC (displaced) S12.350
            nondisplaced S12.351
          type III S12.34
      second cervical (displaced) S12.130
        nondisplaced S12.131
          specified type NEC (displaced) S12.150
            nondisplaced S12.151
          type III S12.14
      seventh cervical (displaced) S12.630
        nondisplaced S12.631
          specified type NEC (displaced) S12.650
            nondisplaced S12.651
          type III S12.64
      sixth cervical (displaced) S12.530
        nondisplaced S12.531
          specified type NEC (displaced) S12.550
            nondisplaced S12.551
          type III S12.54
      third cervical (displaced) S12.230
        nondisplaced S12.231
          specified type NEC (displaced) S12.250
            nondisplaced S12.251
          type III S12.24
Spondylolysis (acquired) M43.00
  cervical region M43.02
  cervicothoracic region M43.03
  congenital Q76.2
  lumbar region M43.06
  lumbosacral region M43.07
    with disproportion (fetopelvic) O33.0
      causing obstructed labor O65.8
  multiple sites M43.09
  occipito-atlanto-axial region M43.01
  sacrococcygeal region M43.08
  thoracic region M43.04
  thoracolumbar region M43.05
Spondylopathy M48.9
  infective NEC M46.50
    cervical region M46.52
    cervicothoracic region M46.53
    lumbar region M46.56
    lumbosacral region M46.57
    multiple sites M46.59
    occipito-atlanto-axial region M46.51
    sacrococcygeal region M46.58
    thoracic region M46.54
    thoracolumbar region M46.55
  inflammatory M46.90
    cervical region M46.92
    cervicothoracic region M46.93
    lumbar region M46.96
    lumbosacral region M46.97
    multiple sites M46.99
    occipito-atlanto-axial region M46.91
    sacrococcygeal region M46.98
    specified type NEC M46.80
      cervical region M46.82

Spondylopathy—*continued*
  inflammatory—*continued*
    specified type—*continued*
      cervicothoracic region M46.83
      lumbar region M46.86
      lumbosacral region M46.87
      multiple sites M46.89
      occipito-atlanto-axial region M46.81
      sacrococcygeal region M46.88
      thoracic region M46.84
      thoracolumbar region M46.85
    thoracic region M46.94
    thoracolumbar region M46.95
  neuropathic, in
    syringomyelia and syringobulbia G95.0
    tabes dorsalis A52.11
  specified NEC — *see* subcategory M48.8
  traumatic M48.30
    cervical region M48.32
    cervicothoracic region M48.33
    lumbar region M48.36
    lumbosacral region M48.37
    occipito-atlanto-axial region M48.31
    sacrococcygeal region M48.38
    thoracic region M48.34
    thoracolumbar region M48.35
Spondylosis M47.9
  with
    disproportion (fetopelvic) O33.0
      causing obstructed labor O65.0
    myelopathy NEC M47.10
      cervical region M47.12
      cervicothoracic region M47.13
      lumbar region M47.16
      lumbosacral region M47.17
      occipito-atlanto-axial region M47.11
      sacrococcygeal region M47.18
      thoracic region M47.14
      thoracolumbar region M47.15
    radiculopathy M47.20
      cervical region M47.22
      cervicothoracic region M47.23
      lumbar region M47.26
      lumbosacral region M47.27
      occipito-atlanto-axial region M47.21
      sacrococcygeal region M47.28
      thoracic region M47.24
      thoracolumbar region M47.25
  specified NEC M47.899
    cervical region M47.892
    cervicothoracic region M47.893
    lumbar region M47.896
    lumbosacral region M47.897
    occipito-atlanto-axial region M47.891
    sacrococcygeal region M47.898
    thoracic region M47.894
    thracolumbar region M47.895
  traumatic — *see* Spondylopathy, traumatic
  without myelopathy or radiculopathy M47.819
    cervical region M47.812
    cervicothoracic region M47.813
    lumbar region M47.816
    lumbosacral region M47.817
    occipito-atlanto-axial region M47.811
    sacrococcygeal region M47.818
    thoracic region M47.814
    thoracolumbar region M47.815
Sponge
  inadvertently left in operation wound — *see* Foreign
    body, accidentally left during a procedure
  kidney (medullary) Q61.5
Sponge-diver's disease — *see* Toxicity, venom,
    marine animal, sea anemone
Spongioblastoma (any type) — *see* Neoplasm,
    malignant, by site
  specified site — *see* Neoplasm, malignant, by site
  unspecified site C71.9
Spongioneuroblastoma — *see* Neoplasm, malignant
    by site
Spontaneous (*see also* condition)
  fracture (cause unknown) — *see* Fracture,
    pathological

Spoon nail L60.3
  congenital Q84.6
Sporadic — *see* condition
Sporothrix schenckii infection — *see* Sporotrichosis
Sporotrichosis B42.9
  arthritis B42.82
  disseminated B42.7
  generalized B42.7
  lymphocutaneous (fixed) (progressive) B42.1
  pulmonary B42.0
  specified NEC B42.89
Spots, spotting (in) (of)
  Bitot's (*see also* Pigmentation, conjunctiva)
    in the young child E50.1
      vitamin A deficiency E50.1
  café, au lait L81.3
  Cayenne pepper I78.1
  cotton wool, retina — *see* Occlusion, artery, retina
  de Morgan's (senile angiomas) I78.1
  Fuchs' black (myopic) — *see* Disorder, globe,
    degenerative, myopia
  intermenstrual (regular) N92.0
    irregular N92.1
  Koplik's B05.9
  liver L81.4
  pregnancy O26.85-
  purpuric R23.3
  ruby I78.1
Spotted fever — *see* Fever, spotted N92.3
Sprain (joint) (ligament)
  acromioclavicular joint or ligament S43.5-
  ankle S93.40-
    calcaneofibular ligament S93.41-
    deltoid ligament S93.42-
    internal collateral ligament — *see* Sprain, ankle,
      specified ligament NEC
    specified ligament NEC S93.49-
    talofibular ligament — *see* Sprain, ankle,
      specified ligament NEC
    tibiofibular ligament S93.43-
  anterior longitudinal, cervical S13.4
  atlas, atlanto-axial, atlanto-occipital S13.4
  breast bone — *see* Sprain, sternum
  calcaneofibular — *see* Sprain, ankle
  carpal — *see* Sprain, wrist
  carpometacarpal — *see* Sprain, hand, specified site
    NEC
  cartilage
    costal S23.41
    semilunar (knee) — *see* Sprain, knee, specified
      site NEC
      with current tear — *see* Tear, meniscus
    thyroid region S13.5
    xiphoid — *see* Sprain, sternum
  cervical, cervicodorsal, cervicothoracic S13.4
  chondrosternal S23.421
  coracoclavicular S43.8-
  coracohumeral S43.41-
  coronary, knee — *see* Sprain, knee, specified site
    NEC
  costal cartilage S23.41
  cricoarytenoid articulation or ligament S13.5
  cricothyroid articulation S13.5
  cruciate, knee — *see* Sprain, knee, cruciate
  deltoid, ankle — *see* Sprain, ankle
  dorsal (spine) S23.3
  elbow S53.40-
    radial collateral ligament S53.43-
    radiohumeral S53.41-
    rupture
      radial collateral ligament — *see* Rupture,
        traumatic, ligament, radial collateral
      ulnar collateral ligament — *see* Rupture,
        traumatic, ligament, ulnar collateral
    specified type NEC S53.49-
    ulnar collateral ligament S53.44-
    ulnohumeral S53.42-
  femur, head — *see* Sprain, hip
  fibular collateral, knee — *see* Sprain, knee, collateral
  fibulocalcaneal — *see* Sprain, ankle

Sprain —*continued*
- finger(s) S63.61-
  - index S63.61-
  - interphalangeal (joint) S63.63-
    - index S63.63-
    - little S63.63-
    - middle S63.63-
    - ring S63.63-
  - little S63.61-
  - metacarpophalangeal (joint) S63.65-
  - middle S63.61-
  - ring S63.61-
  - specified site NEC S63.69-
    - index S63.69-
    - little S63.69-
    - middle S63.69-
    - ring S63.69-
- foot S93.60-
  - specified ligament NEC S93.69-
  - tarsal ligament S93.61-
  - tarsometatarsal ligament S93.62-
  - toe — *see* Sprain, toe
- hand S63.9-
  - finger — *see* Sprain, finger
  - specified site NEC — *see* subcategory S63.8
  - thumb — *see* Sprain, thumb
- head S03.9
- hip S73.10-
  - iliofemoral ligament S73.11-
  - ischiocapsular (ligament) S73.12-
  - specified NEC S73.19-
- iliofemoral — *see* Sprain, hip
- innominate
  - acetabulum — *see* Sprain, hip
  - sacral junction S33.6
- internal
  - collateral, ankle — *see* Sprain, ankle
  - semilunar cartilage — *see* Sprain, knee, specified site NEC
- interphalangeal
  - finger — *see* Sprain, finger, interphalangeal (joint)
  - toe — *see* Sprain, toe, interphalangeal joint
- ischiocapsular — *see* Sprain, hip
- ischiofemoral — *see* Sprain, hip
- jaw (articular disc) (cartilage) (meniscus) S03.4
  - old M26.69
- knee S83.9-
  - collateral ligament S83.40-
    - lateral (fibular) S83.42-
    - medial (tibial) S83.41-
  - cruciate ligament S83.50-
    - anterior S83.51-
    - posterior S83.52-
  - lateral (fibular) collateral ligament S83.42-
  - medial (tibial) collateral ligament S83.41-
  - patellar ligament S76.11-
  - specified site NEC S83.8x-
  - superior tibiofibular joint (ligament) S83.6-
- lateral collateral, knee — *see* Sprain, knee, collateral
- lumbar (spine) S33.5
- lumbosacral S33.9
- mandible (articular disc) S03.4
  - old M26.69
- medial collateral, knee — *see* Sprain, knee, collateral
- meniscus
  - jaw S03.4
    - old M26.69
  - knee (*see also* Sprain, knee, specified site NEC)
    - with current tear — *see* Tear, meniscus
      - old — *see* Derangement, knee, meniscus, due to old tear
  - mandible S03.4
    - old M26.69
- metacarpal (distal) (proximal) — *see* Sprain, hand, specified site NEC
- metacarpophalangeal — *see* Sprain, finger, metacarpophalangeal (joint)
- metatarsophalangeal — *see* Sprain, toe, metatarsophalangeal joint
- midcarpal — *see* Sprain, hand, specified site NEC
- midtarsal — *see* Sprain, foot, specified site NEC

Sprain —*continued*
- neck S13.9
  - anterior longitudinal cervical ligament S13.4
  - atlanto-axial joint S13.4
  - atlanto-occipital joint S13.4
  - cervical spine S13.4
  - cricoarytenoid ligament S13.5
  - cricothyroid ligament S13.5
  - specified site NEC S13.8
  - thyroid region (cartilage) S13.5
- nose S03.8
- orbicular, hip — *see* Sprain, hip
- patella — *see* Sprain, knee, specified site NEC
- patellar ligament S76.11-
- pelvis NEC S33.8
- phalanx
  - finger — *see* Sprain, finger
  - toe — *see* Sprain, toe
- pubofemoral — *see* Sprain, hip
- radiocarpal — *see* Sprain, wrist
- radiohumeral — *see* Sprain, elbow
- radius, collateral — *see* Rupture, traumatic, ligament, radial collateral
- rib (cage) S23.41
- rotator cuff (capsule) S43.42-
- sacroiliac (region)
  - chronic or old — *see* subcategory M53.2
  - joint S33.6
- scaphoid (hand) — *see* Sprain, hand, specified site NEC
- scapula(r) — *see* Sprain, shoulder girdle, specified site NEC
- semilunar cartilage (knee) (*see also* Sprain, knee, specified site NEC)
  - with current tear — *see* Tear, meniscus
    - old — *see* Derangement, knee, meniscus, due to old tear
- shoulder joint S43.40-
  - acromioclavicular joint (ligament) — *see* Sprain, acromioclavicular joint
  - blade — *see* Sprain, shoulder, girdle, specified site NEC
  - coracoclavicular joint (ligament) — *see* Sprain, coracoclavicular joint
  - coracohumeral ligament — *see* Sprain, coracohumeral joint
  - girdle S43.9-
    - specified site NEC S43.8-
  - rotator cuff — *see* Sprain, rotator cuff
  - specified site NEC S43.49-
  - sternoclavicular joint (ligament) — *see* Sprain, sternoclavicular joint
- spine
  - cervical S13.4
  - lumbar S33.5
  - thoracic S23.3
- sternoclavicular joint S43.6-
- sternum S23.429
  - chondrosternal joint S23.421
  - specified site NEC S23.428
  - sternoclavicular (joint) (ligament) S23.420
- symphysis
  - jaw S03.4
    - old M26.69
  - mandibular S03.4
    - old M26.69
- talofibular — *see* Sprain, ankle
- tarsal — *see* Sprain, foot, specified site NEC
- tarsometatarsal — *see* Sprain, foot, specified site NEC
- temporomandibular S03.4
  - old M26.69
- thorax S23.9
  - specified site NEC S23.8
  - spine S23.3
- thorax S23.9
  - ribs S23.41
  - specified site NEC S23.8
  - spine S23.3
  - sternum — *see* Sprain, sternum
- thumb S63.60-
  - interphalangeal (joint) S63.62-
  - metacarpophalangeal (joint) S63.64-
  - specified site NEC S63.68-

Sprain —*continued*
- thyroid cartilage or region S13.5
- tibia (proximal end) — *see* Sprain, knee, specified site NEC
- tibial collateral, knee — *see* Sprain, knee, collateral
- tibiofibular
  - distal — *see* Sprain, ankle
  - superior — *see* Sprain, knee, specified site NEC
- toe(s) S93.50-
  - great S93.50-
  - interphalangeal joint S93.51-
    - great S93.51-
    - lesser S93.51-
  - lesser S93.50-
  - metatarsophalangeal joint S93.52-
    - great S93.52-
    - lesser S93.52-
- ulna, collateral — *see* Rupture, traumatic, ligament, ulnar collateral
- ulnohumeral — *see* Sprain, elbow
- wrist S63.50-
  - carpal S63.51-
  - radiocarpal S63.52-
  - specified site NEC S63.59-
- xiphoid cartilage — *see* Sprain, sternum

Sprengel's deformity (congenital) Q74.0
Sprue (tropical) K90.1
- celiac K90.0
- idiopathic K90.0
- meaning thrush B37.0
- nontropical K90.0

Spur, bone (*see also* Enthesopathy)
- calcaneal M77.3-
- iliac crest M76.2-
- nose (septum) J34.89

Spurway's syndrome Q78.0
Sputum
- abnormal (amount) (color) (odor) (purulent) R09.3
- blood-stained R04.2
- excessive (cause unknown) R09.3

Squamous (*see also* condition)
- epithelium in
  - cervical canal (congenital) Q51.828
  - uterine mucosa (congenital) Q51.818

Squashed nose M95.0
- congenital Q67.4

Squeeze, divers' T70.3
Squint (*see also* Strabismus)
- accommodative — *see* Strabismus, convergent concomitant

St. Hubert's disease A82.9
Stab (*see also* Laceration)
- internal organs — *see* Injury, by site

Stafne's cyst or cavity M27.0
Staggering gait R26.0
- hysterical F44.4

Staghorn calculus — *see* Calculus, kidney
Stähli's line (cornea) (pigment) — *see* Pigmentation, cornea, anterior

Stain, staining
- meconium (newborn) P96.83
- port wine Q82.5
- tooth, teeth (hard tissues) (extrinsic) K03.6
  - due to
    - accretions K03.6
    - deposits (betel) (black) (green) (materia alba) (orange) (soft) (tobacco) K03.6
    - metals (copper) (silver) K03.7
    - nicotine K03.6
    - pulpal bleeding K03.7
    - tobacco K03.6
  - intrinsic K00.8

Stammering (*see also* Disorder, fluency) F80.81
Standstill
- auricular I45.5
- cardiac — *see* Arrest, cardiac
- sinoatrial I45.5
- ventricular — *see* Arrest, cardiac

Stannosis J63.5
Stanton's disease — *see* Melioidosis
Staphylitis (acute) (catarrhal) (chronic) (gangrenous) (membranous) (suppurative) (ulcerative) K12.2

Staphylococcal scalded skin syndrome L00
Staphylococcemia A41.2
Staphylococcus, staphylococcal (*see also* condition)
  as cause of disease classified elsewhere B95.8
  aureus, as cause of disease classified elsewhere
    B95.6
  specified NEC, as cause of disease classified
    elsewhere B95.7
Staphyloma (sclera)
  cornea H18.72-
  equatorial H15.81-
  localized (anterior) H15.82-
  posticum H15.83-
  ring H15.85-
Stargardt's disease — *see* Dystrophy, retina
Starvation (inanition) (due to lack of food) T73.0
  edema — *see* Malnutrition, severe
Stasis
  bile (noncalculous) K83.1
  bronchus J98.09
    with infection — *see* Bronchitis
  cardiac — *see* Failure, heart, congestive
  cecum K59.8
  colon K59.8
  dermatitis — *see* Varix, leg, with, inflammation
  duodenal K31.5
  eczema — *see* Varix, leg, with, inflammation
  edema — *see* Hypertension, venous (chronic),
    idiopathic
  foot T69.0-
  ileocecal coil K59.8
  ileum K59.8
  intestinal K59.8
  jejunum K59.8
  kidney N19
  liver (cirrhotic) K76.1
  lymphatic I89.8
  pneumonia J18.2
  pulmonary — *see* Edema, lung
  rectal K59.8
  renal N19
    tubular N17.0
  ulcer — *see* Varix, leg, with, ulcer
    without varicose veins I87.2
  urine — *see* Retention, urine
  venous I87.8
State (of)
  affective and paranoid, mixed, organic psychotic
    F06.8
  agitated R45.1
    acute reaction to stress F43.0
  anxiety (neurotic) F41.1
  apprehension F41.1
  burn-out Z73.0
  climacteric, female Z78.0
    symptomatic N95.1
  compulsive F42
    mixed with obsessional thoughts F42
  confusional (psychogenic) F44.89
    acute (*see also* Delirium)
      with
        arteriosclerotic dementia F01.50
          with behavioral disturbance F01.51
        senility or dementia F05
      alcoholic F10.231
    epileptic F05
    reactive (from emotional stress, psychological
      trauma) F44.89
    subacute — *see* Delirium
  convulsive — *see* Convulsions
  crisis F43.0
  depressive F32.9
    neurotic F34.1
  dissociative F44.9
  emotional shock (stress) R45.7
  hypercoagulation — *see* Hypercoagulable
  locked-in G83.5
  menopausal Z78.0
    symptomatic N95.1
  neurotic F48.9
    with depersonalization F48.1
  obsessional F42
  oneiroid (schizophrenia-like) F23

State—*continued*
  organic
    hallucinatory (nonalcoholic) F06.0
    paranoid(-hallucinatory) F06.2
  panic F41.0
  paranoid F22
    climacteric F22
    involutional F22
    menopausal F22
    organic F06.2
    senile F03
    simple F22
  persistent vegetative R40.3
  phobic F40.9
  postleukotomy F07.0
  pregnant, incidental Z33.1
  psychogenic, twilight F44.89
  psychopathic (constitutional) F60.2
  psychotic, organic (*see also* Psychosis, organic)
    mixed paranoid and affective F06.8
    senile or presenile F03
    transient NEC F06.8
      with
        hallucinations F06.0
        depression F06.31
  residual schizophrenic F20.5
  restlessness R45.1
  stress (emotional) R45.7
  tension (mental) F48.9
    specified NEC F48.8
  transient organic psychotic NEC F06.8
    depressive type F06.31
    hallucinatory type F06.30
  twilight
    epileptic F05
    psychogenic F44.89
  vegetative, persistent R40.3
  vital exhaustion Z73.0
  withdrawal, *see* Withdrawal, state
Status (post) (*see also* Presence (of))
  absence, epileptic — *see* Epilepsy, by type, with
    status epilepticus
  administration of tPA (rtPA) in a different facility
    within the last 24 hours prior to admission to
    current facility Z92.82
  adrenalectomy (unilateral) (bilateral) E89.6
  anastomosis Z98.0
  angioplasty (peripheral) Z98.62
    with implant Z95.820
    coronary artery Z98.61
      with implant Z95.5
  anginosus I20.9
  aortocoronary bypass Z95.1
  arthrodesis Z98.1
  artificial opening (of) Z93.9
    gastrointestinal tract Z93.4
    specified NEC Z93.8
    urinary tract Z93.6
    vagina Z93.8
  asthmaticus — *see* Asthma, by type, with status
    asthmaticus
  awaiting organ transplant Z76.82
  bariatric surgery Z98.84
  bed confinement Z74.01
  bleb, filtering (vitreous), after glaucoma surgery
    Z98.83
  breast implant Z98.82
    removal Z98.86
  cataract extraction Z98.4-
  cholecystectomy Z90.49
  clitorectomy N90.811
    with excision of labia minora N90.812
  colectomy (complete) (partial) Z90.49
  colonization — *see* Carrier (suspected) of
  colostomy Z93.3
  convulsivus idiopathicus — *see* Epilepsy, by type,
    with status epilepticus
  coronary artery angioplasty — *see* Status,
    angioplasty, coronary artery
  cystectomy (urinary bladder) Z90.6

Status —*continued*
  cystostomy Z93.50
    appendico-vesicostomy Z93.52
    cutaneous Z93.51
    specified NEC Z93.59
  delinquent immunization Z28.3
  dental Z98.818
    crown Z98.811
    fillings Z98.811
    restoration Z98.811
    sealant Z98.810
    specified NEC Z98.818
  deployment (current) (military) Z56.82
  dialysis (hemodialysis) (peritoneal) Z99.2
  do not resuscitate (DNR) Z66
  donor — *see* Donor
  embedded fragments — *see* Retained, foreign body
    fragments (type of)
  embedded splinter — *see* Retained, foreign body
    fragments (type of)
  enterostomy Z93.4
  epileptic, epilepticus (*see also* Epilepsy, by type, with
    status epilepticus) G40.901
  estrogen receptor
    negative Z17.0
    positive Z17.1
  female genital cutting — *see* Female genital
    mutilation status
  female genital mutilation — *see* Female genital
    mutilation status
  filtering (vitreous) bleb after glaucoma surgery
    Z98.83
  gastrectomy (complete) (partial) Z90.3
  gastric banding Z98.84
  gastric bypass for obesity Z98.84
  gastrostomy Z93.1
  human immunodeficiency virus (HIV) infection,
    asymptomatic Z21
  hysterectomy (complete) (total) Z90.710
    partial (with remaining cervial stump) Z90.711
  ileostomy Z93.2
  implant
    breast Z98.82
  infibulation N90.813
  intestinal bypass Z98.0
  jejunostomy Z93.4
  laryngectomy Z90.02
  lapsed immunization schedule Z28.3
  lymphaticus E32.8
  marmoratus G80.3
  mastectomy (unilateral) (bilateral) Z90.1-
  military deployment status (current) Z56.82
    in theater or in support of military war,
      peacekeeping and humanitarian
      operations Z56.82
  nephrectomy (unilateral) (bilateral) Z90.5
  nephrostomy Z93.6
  obesity surgery Z98.84
  oophorectomy
    bilateral Z90.722
    unilateral Z90.721
  organ replacement
    by artificial or mechanical device or prosthesis of
      artery Z95.828
      bladder Z96.0
      blood vessel Z95.828
      breast Z97.8
      eye globe Z97.0
      heart Z95.812
        valve Z95.2
      intestine Z97.8
      joint Z96.60
        hip — *see* Presence, hip joint implant
        knee — *see* Presence, knee joint implant
        specified site NEC Z96.698
      kidney Z97.8
      larynx Z96.3
      lens Z96.1
      limbs — *see* Presence, artificial, limb
      liver Z97.8
      lung Z97.8
      pancreas Z97.8

Status—*continued*
  organ replacement—*continued*
    by organ transplant (heterologous)(homologous)
      — *see* Transplant
    pacemaker
      brain Z96.89
      cardiac Z95.0
      specified NEC Z96.89
    pancreatectomy Z90.410
      complete Z90.410
      partial Z90.411
      total Z90.410
    physical restraint Z78.1
    pneumonectomy (complete) (partial) Z90.2
    pneumothorax, therapeutic Z98.3
    postcommotio cerebri F07.81
    postoperative (postprocedural) NEC Z98.89
      breast implant Z98.82
      dental Z98.818
        crown Z98.811
        fillings Z98.811
        restoration Z98.811
        sealant Z98.810
        specified NEC Z98.818
      pneumothorax, therapeutic Z98.3
    postpartum (routine follow-up) Z39.2
      care immediately after delivery Z39.0
    postsurgical (postprocedural) NEC Z98.89
      pneumothorax, therapeutic Z98.3
    pregnancy, incidental Z33.1
    prosthesis coronary angioplasty Z95.5
    pseudophakia Z96.1
    renal dialysis (hemodialysis) (peritoneal) Z99.2
    retained foreign body — *see* Retained, foreign body
      fragments (type of)
    reversed jejunal transposition (for bypass) Z98.0
    salpingo-oophorectomy
      bilateral Z90.722
      unilateral Z90.721
    sex reassignment surgery status Z87.890
    shunt
      arteriovenous (for dialysis) Z99.2
      cerebrospinal fluid Z98.2
      ventricular (communicating) (for drainage) Z98.2
    splenectomy D73.0
    thymicolymphaticus E32.8
    thymicus E32.8
    thymolymphaticus E32.8
    thyroidectomy (hypothyroidism) E89.0
    tooth (teeth) extraction (*see also* Absence, teeth,
      acquired) K08.409
    tPA (rtPA) administration in a different facility within
      the last 24 hours prior to admission to current
      facility Z92.82
    tracheostomy Z93.0
    transplant — *see* Transplant
      organ removed Z98.85
    tubal ligation Z98.51
    underimmunization Z28.3
    ureterostomy Z93.6
    urethrostomy Z93.6
    vagina, artificial Z93.8
    vasectomy Z98.52
    wheelchair confinement Z99.3
Stealing
  child problem F91.8
    in company with others Z72.810
  pathological (compulsive) F63.2
Steam burn — *see* Burn
Steatocystoma multiplex L72.2
Steatohepatitis (nonalcoholic) (NASH) K75.81
Steatoma L72.1
  eyelid (cystic) — *see* Dermatosis, eyelid
  infected — *see* Hordeolum
Steatorrhea (chronic) K90.4
  with lacteal obstruction K90.2
  idiopathic (adult) (infantile) K90.0
  pancreatic K90.3
  primary K90.0
  tropical K90.1

Steatosis E88.89
  heart — *see* Degeneration, myocardial
  kidney N28.89
  liver NEC K76.0
Steele-Richardson-Olszewski disease or syndrome
  G23.1
Steinbrocker's syndrome G90.8
Steinert's disease G71.11
Stein-Leventhal syndrome E28.2
Stein's syndrome E28.2
  STEMI I21.3 (*see also* Infarct, myocardium, ST
    elevation)
Stenocardia I20.8
Stenocephaly Q75.8
Stenosis, stenotic (cicatricial) (*see also* Stricture)
  ampulla of Vater K83.1
  anus, anal (canal) (sphincter) K62.4
    and rectum K62.4
    congenital Q42.3
      with fistula Q42.2
  aorta (ascending) (supraventricular) (congenital)
    Q25.3
    arteriosclerotic I70.0
    calcified I70.0
  aortic (valve) I35.0
    with insufficiency I35.2
    congenital Q23.0
    rheumatic I06.0
      with
        incompetency, insufficiency or
          regurgitation I06.2
          with mitral (valve) disease I08.0
            with tricuspid (valve) disease I08.3
        mitral (valve) disease I08.0
          with tricuspid (valve) disease I08.3
        tricuspid (valve) disease I08.2
          with mitral (valve) disease I08.3
    specified cause NEC I35.0
    syphilitic A52.03
  aqueduct of Sylvius (congenital) Q03.0
    with spina bifida — *see* Spina bifida, by site, with
      hydrocephalus
    acquired G91.1
  artery NEC (*see also* Arteriosclerosis) I77.1
    celiac I77.4
    cerebral — *see* Occlusion, artery, cerebral
    extremities — *see* Arteriosclerosis, extremities
    precerebral — *see* Occlusion, artery, precerebral
    pulmonary (congenital) Q25.6
      acquired I28.8
    renal I70.1
  bile duct (common) (hepatic) K83.1
    congenital Q44.3
  bladder-neck (acquired) N32.0
    congenital Q64.31
  brain G93.89
  bronchus J98.09
    congenital Q32.3
    syphilitic A52.72
  cardia (stomach) K22.2
    congenital Q40.2
  cardiovascular — *see* Disease, cardiovascular
  caudal M48.08
  cervix, cervical (canal) N88.2
    congenital Q51.828
    in pregnancy or childbirth — *see* Pregnancy,
      complicated by, abnormal cervix
  colon (*see also* Obstruction, intestine)
    congenital Q42.9
      specified NEC Q42.8
  colostomy K94.03
  common (bile) duct K83.1
    congenital Q44.3
  coronary (artery) — *see* Disease, heart, ischemic,
    atherosclerotic
  cystic duct — *see* Obstruction, gallbladder
  due to presence of device, implant or graft (*see also*
    Complications, by site and type, specified
    NEC) T85.85
    arterial graft NEC T82.858
    breast (implant) T85.85

Stenosis, stenotis—*continued*
  due to presence of device, implant or
    graft—*continued*
    catheter T83.85
      dialysis (renal) T82.858
        intraperitoneal T85.85
      infusion NEC T82.858
        spinal (epidural) (subdural) T85.85
      urinary (indwelling) T83.85
    fixation, internal (orthopedic) NEC T84.85
    gastrointestinal (bile duct) (esophagus) T85.85
    genital NEC T83.85
    heart NEC T82.857
    joint prosthesis T84.85
    ocular (corneal graft) (orbital implant) NEC
      T85.85
    orthopedic NEC T84.85
    specified NEC T85.85
    urinary NEC T83.85
    vascular NEC T82.858
    ventricular intracranial shunt T85.85
  duodenum K31.5
    congenital Q41.0
  ejaculatory duct NEC N50.8
  endocervical os — *see* Stenosis, cervix
  enterostomy K94.13
  esophagus K22.2
    congenital Q39.3
    syphilitic A52.79
      congenital A50.59 [K23]
  eustachian tube — *see* Obstruction, eustachian tube
  external ear canal (acquired) H61.30-
    congenital Q16.1
    due to
      inflammation H61.32-
      trauma H61.31-
    postprocedural H95.81-
    specified cause NEC H61.39-
  gallbladder — *see* Obstruction, gallbladder
  glottis J38.6
  heart valve (congenital) Q24.8
    aortic Q23.0
    mitral Q23.2
    pulmonary Q22.1
    tricuspid Q22.4
  hepatic duct K83.1
  hymen N89.6
  hypertrophic subaortic (idiopathic) I42.1
  ileum K56.69
    congenital Q41.2
  infundibulum cardia Q24.3
  intervertebral foramina (*see also* Lesion,
    biomechanical, specified NEC)
    connective tissue M99.79
      abdomen M99.79
      cervical region M99.71
      cervicothoracic M99.71
      head region M99.70
      lumbar region M99.73
      lumbosacral M99.73
      occipitocervical M99.70
      sacral region M99.74
      sacrococcygeal M99.74
      sacroiliac M99.74
      specified NEC M99.79
      thoracic region M99.72
      thoracolumbar M99.72
    disc M99.79
      abdomen M99.79
      cervical region M99.71
      cervicothoracic M99.71
      head region M99.70
      lower extremity M99.76
      lumbar region M99.73
      lumbosacral M99.73
      occipitocervical M99.70
      pelvic M99.75
      rib cage M99.78
      sacral region M99.74
      sacrococcygeal M99.74
      sacroiliac M99.74
      specified NEC M99.79
      thoracic region M99.72

Stenosis, stenotic—*continued*
  intervertebral foramina—*continued*
    disc—*continued*
      thoracolumbar M99.72
      upper extremity M99.77
    osseous M99.69
      abdomen M99.69
      cervical region M99.61
      cervicothoracic M99.61
      head region M99.60
      lower extremity M99.66
      lumbar region M99.63
      lumbosacral M99.63
      occipitocervical M99.60
      pelvic M99.65
      rib cage M99.68
      sacral region M99.64
      sacrococcygeal M99.64
      sacroiliac M99.64
      specified NEC M99.69
      thoracic region M99.62
      thoracolumbar M99.62
      upper extremity M99.67
    subluxation — *see* Stenosis, intervertebral foramina, osseous
  intestine (*see also* Obstruction, intestine)
    congenital (small) Q41.9
      large Q42.9
        specified NEC Q42.8
      specified NEC Q41.8
  jejunum K56.69
    congenital Q41.1
  lacrimal (passage)
    canaliculi H04.54-
    congenital Q10.5
    duct H04.55-
    punctum H04.56-
    sac H04.57-
  lacrimonasal duct — *see* Stenosis, lacrimal, duct
    congenital Q10.5
  larynx J38.6
    congenital NEC Q31.8
      subglottic Q31.1
    syphilitic A52.73
      congenital A50.59 [J99]
  mitral (chronic) (inactive) (valve) I05.0
    with
      aortic valve disease I08.0
      incompetency, insufficiency or regurgitation I05.2
    active or acute I01.1
      with rheumatic or Sydenham's chorea I02.0
    congenital Q23.2
    specified cause, except rheumatic I34.2
    syphilitic A52.03
  myocardium, myocardial (*see also* Degeneration, myocardial)
    hypertrophic subaortic (idiopathic) I42.1
  nares (anterior) (posterior) J34.89
    congenital Q30.0
  nasal duct (*see also* Stenosis, lacrimal, duct)
    congenital Q10.5
  nasolacrimal duct (*see also* Stenosis, lacrimal, duct)
    congenital Q10.5
  neural canal (*see also* Lesion, biomechanical, specified NEC)
    connective tissue M99.49
      abdomen M99.49
      cervical region M99.41
      cervicothoracic M99.41
      head region M99.40
      lower extremity M99.46
      lumbar region M99.43
      lumbosacral M99.43
      occipitocervical M99.40
      pelvic M99.45
      rib cage M99.48
      sacral region M99.44
      sacrococcygeal M99.44
      sacroiliac M99.44
      specified NEC M99.49
      thoracic region M99.42
      thoracolumbar M99.42

Stenosis, stenotic—*continued*
  neural canal—*continued*
    connective tissue—*continued*
      upper extremity M99.47
    intervertebral disc M99.59
      abdomen M99.59
      cervical region M99.51
      cervicothoracic M99.51
      head region M99.50
      lower extremity M99.56
      lumbar region M99.53
      lumbosacral M99.53
      occipitocervical M99.50
      pelvic M99.55
      rib cage M99.58
      sacral region M99.54
      sacrococcygeal M99.54
      sacroiliac M99.54
      specified NEC M99.59
      thoracic region M99.52
      thoracolumbar M99.52
      upper extremity M99.57
    osseous M99.39
      abdomen M99.39
      cervical region M99.31
      cervicothoracic M99.31
      head region M99.30
      lower extremity M99.36
      lumbar region M99.33
      lumbosacral M99.33
      pelvic M99.35
      rib cage M99.38
      occipitocervical M99.30
      sacral region M99.34
      sacrococcygeal M99.34
      sacroiliac M99.34
      specified NEC M99.39
      thoracic region M99.32
      thoracolumbar M99.32
      upper extremity M99.37
    subluxation M99.29
      cervical region M99.21
      cervicothoracic M99.21
      head region M99.20
      lower extremity M99.26
      lumbar region M99.23
      lumbosacral M99.23
      occipitocervical M99.20
      pelvic M99.25
      rib cage M99.28
      sacral region M99.24
      sacrococcygeal M99.24
      sacroiliac M99.24
      specified NEC M99.29
      thoracic region M99.22
      thoracolumbar M99.22
      upper extremity M99.27
  oesophagus — *see* Stenosis, esophagus
  organ or site, congenital NEC — *see* Atresia, by site
  papilla of Vater K83.1
  pulmonary (artery) (congenital) Q25.6
    with ventricular septal defect, transposition of aorta, and hypertrophy of right ventricle Q21.3
    acquired I28.8
    in tetralogy of Fallot Q21.3
    infundibular Q24.3
    valve I37.0
      with insufficiency I37.2
      congenital Q22.1
      rheumatic I09.89
        with aortic, mitral or tricuspid (valve) disease I08.8
    subvalvular Q24.3
    supravalvular Q25.6
    vein, acquired I28.8
    vessel NEC I28.8
  pulmonic (congenital) Q22.1
    infundibular Q24.3
    subvalvular Q24.3
  pylorus (hypertrophic) (acquired) K31.1
    adult K31.1
    congenital Q40.0

Stenosis, stenotic—*continued*
  pylorus—*continued*
    infantile Q40.0
  rectum (sphincter) — *see* Stricture, rectum
  renal artery I70.1
    congenital Q27.1
  salivary duct (any) K11.8
  sphincter of Oddi K83.1
  spinal M48.00
    cervical region M48.02
    cervicothoracic region M48.03
    lumbar region M48.06
    lumbosacral region M48.07
    occipito-atlanto-axial region M48.01
    sacrococcygeal region M48.08
    thoracic region M48.04
    thoracolumbar region M48.05
  stomach, hourglass K31.2
  subaortic (congenital) Q24.4
    hypertrophic (idiopathic) I42.1
  subglottic
    congenital Q31.1
    postprocedural J95.5
  trachea J39.8
    congenital Q32.1
    syphilitic A52.73
    tuberculous NEC A15.5
  tracheostomy J95.03
  tricuspid (valve) I07.0
    with
      aortic (valve) disease I08.2
      incompetency, insufficiency or regurgitation I07.2
        with aortic (valve) disease I08.2
          with mitral (valve) disease I08.3
      mitral (valve) disease I08.1
        with aortic (valve) disease I08.3
    congenital Q22.4
    nonrheumatic I36.0
      with insufficiency I36.2
  tubal N97.1
  ureter — *see* Atresia, ureter
  ureteropelvic junction, congenital Q62.11
  ureterovesical orifice, congenital Q62.12
  urethra (valve) (*see also* Stricture, urethra)
    congenital Q64.32
  urinary meatus, congenital Q64.33
  vagina N89.5
    congenital Q52.4
    in pregnancy — *see* Pregnancy, complicated by, abnormal vagina
      causing obstructed labor O65.5
  valve (cardiac) (heart) (*see also* Endocarditis) I38
    congenital Q24.8
      aortic Q23.0
      mitral Q23.2
      pulmonary Q22.1
      tricuspid Q22.4
  vena cava (inferior) (superior) I87.1
    congenital Q26.0
  vesicourethral orifice Q64.31
  vulva N90.5
Stercolith (impaction) K56.41
  appendix K38.1
Stercoraceous, stercoral ulcer K63.3
  anus or rectum K62.6
Stereotypies NEC F98.4
Sterility — *see* Infertility
Sterilization — *see* Encounter (for), sterilization
Sternalgia — *see* Angina
Sternopagus Q89.4
Sternum bifidum Q76.7
Steroid
  effects (adverse) (adrenocortical) (iatrogenic)
    cushingoid E24.2
      correct substance properly administered — *see* Table of Drugs and Chemicals, by drug, adverse effect
      overdose or wrong substance given or taken — *see* Table of Drugs and Chemicals, by drug, poisoning
    diabetes — *see* category E09

Steroid—*continued*
  effects—*continued*
    diabetes—*continued*
      correct substance properly administered
        Table of Drugs and Chemicals, by drug,
        adverse effect
      overdose or wrong substance given or
        taken — *see* Table of Drugs and
        Chemicals, by drug, poisoning
    fever R50.2
    insufficiency E27.3
      correct substance properly administered —
        see Table of Drugs and Chemicals, by
        drug, adverse effect
      overdose or wrong substance given or taken
        — *see* Table of Drugs and Chemicals, by
        drug, poisoning
Stevens-Johnson disease or syndrome L51.1
  toxic epidermal necrolysis overlap L51.3
Stewart-Morel syndrome M85.2
Sticker's disease B08.3
Sticky eye — *see* Conjunctivitis, acute, mucopurulent
Stieda's disease — *see* Bursitis, tibial collateral
Stiff neck — *see* Torticollis
Stiff-man syndrome G25.82
Stiffness, joint NEC M25.60
  ankle M25.67-
  ankylosis — *see* Ankylosis, joint
  contracture — *see* Contraction, joint
  elbow M25.6-
  foot M25.6-
  hand M25.6-
  hip M25.6-
  knee M25.6-
  shoulder M25.1-
  wrist M25.3-
Stigmata congenital syphilis A50.59
Stillbirth P95
Still-Felty syndrome — *see* Felty's syndrome
Still's disease or syndrome (juvenile) M08.20
  adult-onset M06.1
  ankle M08.27-
  elbow M08.22-
  foot joint M08.27-
  hand joint M08.24-
  hip M08.25-
  knee M08.26-
  multiple site M08.29
  shoulder M08.21-
  vertebra M08.28
  wrist M08.23-
Stimulation, ovary E28.1
Sting (venomous) (with allergic or anaphylactic shock)
  — *see* Toxicity, venom
Stippled epiphyses Q78.8
Stitch
  abscess T81.4
  burst (in operation wound) — *see* Disruption,
    wound, operation
Stokes-Adams disease or syndrome I45.9
Stokes' disease E05.00 with thyroid storm E05.01
Stokvis (-Talma) disease D74.8BD>
Stoma malfunction
  colostomy K94.03
  enterostomy K94.13
  gastrostomy K94.23
  ileostomy K94.13
  tracheostomy J95.03
Stomach — *see* condition
Stomatitis (denture) (ulcerative) K12.1
  angular K13.0
    due to dietary or vitamin deficiency E53.0
  aphthous K12.0
  bovine B08.61
  candidal B37.0
  catarrhal K12.1
  diphtheritic A36.89
  due to
    dietary deficiency E53.0
    thrush B37.0
    vitamin deficiency
      B group NEC E53.9
      B2 (riboflavin) E53.0

Stomatitis—*continued*
  epidemic B08.8
  epizootic B08.8
  follicular K12.1
  gangrenous A69.0
  Geotrichum B48.3
  herpesviral, herpetic B00.2
  herpetiformis K12.0
  malignant K12.1
  membranous acute K12.1
  monilial B37.0
  mycotic B37.0
  necrotizing ulcerative A69.0
  parasitic B37.0
  septic K12.1
  spirochetal A69.1
  suppurative (acute) K12.2
  ulceromembranous A69.1
  vesicular K12.1
    with exanthem (enteroviral) B08.4
    virus disease A93.8
  Vincent's A69.1
Stomatocytosis D58.8
Stomatomycosis B37.0
Stomatorrhagia K13.79
Stone(s) (*see also* Calculus)
  bladder (diverticulum) N21.0
  cystine E72.09
  heart syndrome I50.1
  kidney N20.0
  prostate N42.0
  pulpal (dental) K04.2
  renal N20.0
  salivary gland or duct (any) K11.5
  urethra (impacted) N21.1
  urinary (duct) (impacted) (passage) N20.9
    bladder (diverticulum) N21.0
    lower tract N21.9
    specified NEC N21.8
  xanthine E79.8 [N22]
Stonecutter's lung J62.8
Stonemason's asthma, disease, lung or
  pneumoconiosis J62.8
Stoppage
  heart — *see* Arrest, cardiac
  urine — *see* Retention, urine
Storm, thyroid — *see* Thyrotoxicosis
Strabismus (congenital) (nonparalytic) H50.9
  concomitant H50.40
    convergent — *see* Strabismus, convergent
      concomitant
    divergent — *see* Strabismus, divergent
      concomitant
  convergent concomitant H50.00
    accommodative component H50.43
    alternating H50.05
      with
        A pattern H50.06
        specified nonconcomitances NEC H50.08
        V pattern H50.07
    monocular H50.01-
      with
        A pattern H50.02-
        specified nonconcomitances NEC H50.04-
        V pattern H50.03-
      intermittent H50.31-
        alternating H50.32
  cyclotropia H50.1-
  divergent concomitant H50.10
    alternating H50.15
      with
        A pattern H50.16
        specified noncomitances NEC H50.18
        V pattern H50.17
    monocular H50.11-
      with
        A pattern H50.12-
        specified noncomitances NEC H50.14-
        V pattern H50.13-
      intermittent H50.33
        alternating H50.34
  Duane's syndrome H50.81-
  due to adhesions, scars H50.60

Strabismus—*continued*
  heterophoria H50.50
    alternating H50.55
    cyclophoria H50.54
    esophoria H50.51
    exophoria H50.52
    vertical H50.53
  heterotropia H50.40
    intermittent H50.30
  hypertropia H50.2-
  hypotropia — *see* Hypertropia
  latent H50.50
  mechanical H50.60
    Brown's sheath syndrome H50.61-
    specified type NEC H50.69
  monofixation syndrome H50.42
  paralytic H49.9
    abducens nerve H49.2-
    fourth nerve H49.1-
    Kearns-Sayre syndrome H49.81-
    ophthalmoplegia (external)
      progressive H49.4-
        with pigmentary retinopathy H49.81-
      total H49.3-
    sixth nerve H49.2-
    specified type NEC H49.88-
    third nerve H49.0-
    trochlear nerve H49.1-
  specified type NEC H50.89
  vertical H50.2-
Strain
  back S39.012
  cervical S16.1
  eye NEC — *see* Disturbance, vision, subjective
  heart — *see* Disease, heart
  low back S39.012
  mental NOS Z73.3
    work-related Z56.6
  muscle (tendon) — *see* Injury, muscle, by site, strain
  neck S16.1
  postural — *see* Disorder, soft tissue, due to use
  physical NOS Z73.3
    work-related Z56.6
  psychological NEC Z73.3
  tendon — *see* Injury, muscle, by site, strain
Straining, on urination R39.16
Strand, vitreous — *see* Opacity, vitreous, membranes
  and strands
Strangulation, strangulated (*see also* Asphyxia,
  traumatic)
  appendix K38.8
  bladder-neck N32.0
  bowel or colon K56.2
  food or foreign body — *see* Asphyxia, food
  hemorrhoids — *see* Hemorrhoids, with complication
  hernia (*see also* Hernia, by site, with obstruction)
    with gangrene — *see* Hernia, by site, with
      gangrene
  intestine (large) (small) K56.2
    with hernia (*see also* Hernia, by site, with
      obstruction)
      with gangrene — *see* Hernia, by site, with
        gangrene
  mesentery K56.2
  mucus — *see* Asphyxia, mucus
  omentum K56.2
  organ or site, congenital NEC — *see* Atresia, by site
  ovary — *see* Torsion, ovary
  penis N48.89
    foreign body T19.8
  rupture — *see* Hernia, by site, with obstruction
  stomach due to hernia (*see also* Hernia, by site, with
    obstruction)
    with gangrene — *see* Hernia, by site, with
      gangrene
  vesicourethral orifice N32.0
Strangury R30.0
Straw itch B88.0
Strawberry
  gallbladder K82.4
  mark Q82.5
  tongue (red) (white) K14.3

Streak(s)
　macula, angioid H35.33
　ovarian Q50.32
Strephosymbolia F81.0
　secondary to organic lesion R48.8
Streptobacillary fever A25.1
Streptobacillosis A25.1
Streptobacillus moniliformis A25.1
Streptococcus, streptococcal (see also condition)
　as cause of disease classified elsewhere B95.5
　group
　　A, as cause of disease classified elsewhere B95.0
　　B, as cause of disease classified elsewhere B95.1
　　D, as cause of disease classified elsewhere B95.2
　pneumoniae, as cause of disease classified
　　　elsewhere B95.3
　specified NEC, as cause of disease classified
　　　elsewhere B95.4
Streptomycosis B47.1
Streptotrichosis A48.8
Stress F43.9
　family — see Disruption, family
　fetal P84
　　complicating pregnancy O77.9
　　　due to drug administration O77.1
　mental NEC Z73.3
　　work-related Z56.6
　physical NEC Z73.3
　　work-related Z56.6
　polycythemia D75.1
　reaction (see also Reaction, stress) F43.9
　work schedule Z56.3
Stretching, nerve — see Injury, nerve
Striae albicantes, atrophicae or distensae (cutis)
　　L90.6
Stricture (see also Stenosis)
　ampulla of Vater K83.1
　anus (sphincter) K62.4
　　congenital Q42.3
　　　with fistula Q42.2
　　infantile Q42.3
　　　with fistula Q42.2
　aorta (ascending) (congenital) Q25.3
　　arteriosclerotic I70.0
　　calcified I70.0
　　supravalvular, congenital Q25.3
　aortic (valve) — see Stenosis, aortic
　aqueduct of Sylvius (congenital) Q03.0
　　with spina bifida — see Spina bifida, by site, with
　　　　hydrocephalus
　　acquired G91.1
　artery I77.1
　　basilar — see Occlusion, artery, basilar
　　carotid — see Occlusion, artery, carotid
　　celiac I77.4
　　congenital (peripheral) Q27.8
　　　cerebral Q28.3
　　　coronary Q24.5
　　　digestive system Q27.8
　　　lower limb Q27.8
　　　retinal Q14.1
　　　specified site NEC Q27.8
　　　umbilical Q27.0
　　　upper limb Q27.8
　　coronary — see Disease, heart, ischemic,
　　　　atherosclerotic
　　congenital Q24.5
　　precerebral — see Occlusion, artery, precerebral
　　pulmonary (congenital) Q25.6
　　　acquired I28.8
　　renal I70.1
　　vertebral — see Occlusion, artery, vertebral
　auditory canal (external) (congenital)
　　acquired — see Stenosis, external ear canal
　bile duct (common) (hepatic) K83.1
　　congenital Q44.3
　　postoperative K91.89
　bladder N32.89
　　neck N32.0
　bowel — see Obstruction, intestine
　brain G93.89

Stricture —continued
　bronchus J98.09
　　congenital Q32.3
　　syphilitic A52.72
　cardia (stomach) K22.2
　　congenital Q40.2
　cardiac (see also Disease, heart)
　　orifice (stomach) K22.2
　cecum — see Obstruction, intestine
　cervix, cervical (canal) N88.2
　　congenital Q51.828
　　in pregnancy — see Pregnancy, complicated by,
　　　　abnormal cervix
　　　causing obstructed labor O65.5
　colon (see also Obstruction, intestine)
　　congenital Q42.9
　　　specified NEC Q42.8
　colostomy K94.03
　common (bile) duct K83.1
　coronary (artery) — see Disease, heart, ischemic,
　　　atherosclerotic
　cystic duct — see Obstruction, gallbladder
　digestive organs NEC, congenital Q45.8
　duodenum K31.5
　　congenital Q41.0
　ear canal (external) (congenital) Q16.1
　　acquired — see Stricture, auditory canal,
　　　　acquired
　ejaculatory duct N50.8
　enterostomy K94.13
　esophagus K22.2
　　congenital Q39.3
　　syphilitic A52.79
　　　congenital A50.59 [K23]
　eustachian tube (see also Obstruction, eustachian
　　　tube)
　　congenital Q17.8
　fallopian tube N97.1
　　gonococcal A54.24
　　tuberculous A18.17
　gallbladder — see Obstruction, gallbladder
　glottis J38.6
　heart (see also Disease, heart)
　　valve (see also Endocarditis) I38
　　　aortic Q23.0
　　　mitral Q23.4
　　　pulmonary Q22.1
　　　tricuspid Q22.4
　hepatic duct K83.1
　hourglass, of stomach K31.2
　hymen N89.6
　hypopharynx J39.2
　ileum K56.69
　　congenital Q41.2
　intestine (see also Obstruction, intestine)
　　congenital (small) Q41.9
　　　large Q42.9
　　　　specified NEC Q42.8
　　　specified NEC Q41.8
　　ischemic K55.1
　jejunum K56.69
　　congenital Q41.1
　lacrimal passages (see also Stenosis, lacrimal)
　　congenital Q10.5
　larynx J38.6
　　congenital NEC Q31.8
　　　subglottic Q31.1
　　syphilitic A52.73
　　　congenital A50.59 [J99]
　meatus
　　ear (congenital) Q16.1
　　　acquired — see Stricture, auditory canal,
　　　　　acquired
　　osseous (ear) (congenital) Q16.1
　　　acquired — see Stricture, auditory canal,
　　　　　acquired
　　urinarius (see also Stricture, urethra)
　　　congenital Q64.33
　mitral (valve) — see Stenosis, mitral
　myocardium, myocardial I51.5
　　hypertrophic subaortic (idiopathic) I42.1
　nares (anterior) (posterior) J34.89
　　congenital Q30.0

Stricture —continued
　nasal duct (see also Stenosis, lacrimal, duct)
　　congenital Q10.5
　nasolacrimal duct (see also Stenosis, lacrimal, duct)
　　congenital Q10.5
　nasopharynx J39.2
　　syphilitic A52.73
　nose J34.89
　　congenital Q30.0
　nostril (anterior) (posterior) J34.89
　　congenital Q30.0
　　syphilitic A52.73
　　　congenital A50.59 [J99]
　oesophagus — see Stricture, esophagus
　organ or site, congenital NEC — see Atresia, by site
　os uteri — see Stricture, cervix
　osseous meatus (ear) (congenital) Q16.1
　　acquired — see Stricture, auditory canal,
　　　　acquired
　oviduct — see Stricture, fallopian tube
　pelviureteric junction (congenital) Q62.0
　penis, by foreign body T19.8
　pharynx J39.2
　prostate N42.89
　pulmonary, pulmonic
　　artery (congenital) Q25.6
　　　acquired I28.8
　　　noncongenital I28.8
　　infundibulum (congenital) Q24.3
　　valve I37.0
　　　congenital Q22.1
　　vein, acquired I28.8
　　vessel NEC I28.8
　punctum lacrimale (see also Stenosis, lacrimal,
　　　punctum)
　　congenital Q10.5
　pylorus (hypertrophic) K31.1
　　adult K31.1
　　congenital Q40.0
　　infantile Q40.0
　rectosigmoid K56.69
　rectum (sphincter) K62.4
　　congenital Q42.1
　　　with fistula Q42.0
　　due to
　　　chlamydial lymphogranuloma A55
　　　irradiation K91.89
　　　lymphogranuloma venereum A55
　　gonococcal A54.6
　　inflammatory (chlamydial) A55
　　syphilitic A52.74
　　tuberculous A18.32
　renal artery I70.1
　　congenital Q27.1
　salivary duct or gland (any) K11.8
　sigmoid (flexure) — see Obstruction, intestine
　spermatic cord N50.8
　stoma (following) (of)
　　colostomy K94.03
　　enterostomy K94.13
　　gastrostomy K94.23
　　ileostomy K94.13
　　tracheostomy J95.03
　stomach K31.89
　　congenital Q40.2
　　hourglass K31.2
　subaortic Q24.4
　　hypertrophic (acquired) (idiopathic) I42.1
　subglottic J38.6
　syphilitic NEC A52.79
　trachea J39.8
　　congenital Q32.1
　　syphilitic A52.73
　　tuberculous NEC A15.5
　tracheostomy J95.03
　tricuspid (valve) — see Stenosis, tricuspid
　tunica vaginalis N50.8
　ureter (postoperative) N13.5
　　with
　　　hydronephrosis N13.1
　　　　with infection N13.6
　　　pyelonephritis (chronic) N11.1
　　congenital — see Atresia, ureter

Subluxation—continued
  interphalangeal—continued
    thumb S63.12-
      distal joint S63.14-
      proximal joint S63.13-
    toe S93.13-
      great S93.13-
      lesser S93.13-
  joint prosthesis — see Complications, joint
    prosthesis, mechanical, displacement, by site
  knee S83.10-
    cap — see Subluxation, patella
    patella — see Subluxation, patella
    proximal tibia
      anteriorly S83.11-
      laterally S83.14-
      medially S83.13-
      posteriorly S83.12-
    specified type NEC S83.19-
  lens — see Dislocation, lens, partial
  ligament, traumatic — see Sprain, by site
  metacarpal (bone)
    proximal end S63.06-
  metacarpophalangeal (joint)
    finger S63.21-
      index S63.21-
      little S63.21-
      middle S63.21-
      ring S63.21-
    thumb S63.11-
  metatarsophalangeal joint S93.14-
    great toe S93.14-
    lesser toe S93.14-
  midcarpal (joint) S63.03-
  patella S83.00-
    lateral S83.01-
    recurrent (nontraumatic) — see Dislocation,
      patella, recurrent, incomplete
    specified type NEC S83.09-
  pathological — see Dislocation, pathological
  radial head S53.00-
    anterior S53.01-
    nursemaid's elbow S53.03-
    posterior S53.02-
    specified type NEC S53.09-
  radiocarpal (joint) S63.02-
  radioulnar (joint)
    distal S63.01-
    proximal — see Subluxation, elbow
  shoulder
    congenital Q68.8
    girdle S43.30-
      scapula S43.31-
      specified site NEC S43.39-
    traumatic S43.00-
      anterior S43.01-
      inferior S43.03-
      posterior S43.02-
      specified type NEC S43.08-
  sternoclavicular (joint) S43.20-
    anterior S43.21-
    posterior S43.22-
  symphysis (pubis)
  thumb S63.103
    interphalangeal joint — see Subluxation,
      interphalangeal (joint), thumb
    metacarpophalangeal joint — see Subluxation,
      metacarpophalangeal (joint), thumb
  toe(s) S93.10-
    great S93.10-
      interphalangeal joint S93.13-
      metatarsophalangeal joint S93.14-
      interphalangeal joint S93.13-
    lesser S93.10-
      interphalangeal joint S93.13-
      metatarsophalangeal joint S93.14-
    metatarsophalangeal joint S93.149
  ulnohumeral joint — see Subluxation, elbow

Subluxation—continued
  vertebral
    recurrent NEC — see subcategory M43.5
    traumatic
      cervical S13.100
        atlantoaxial joint S13.120
        atlantooccipital joint S13.110
        atloidooccipital joint S13.110
        joint between
          C0 and C1 S13.110
          C1 and C2 S13.120
          C2 and C3 S13.130
          C3 and C4 S13.140
          C4 and C5 S13.150
          C5and C6 S13.160
          C6and C7 S13.170
          C7and T1 S13.180
        occipitoatloid joint S13.110
      lumbar S33.100
        joint between
          L1and L2 S33.110
          L2and L3 S33.120
          L3 and L4 S33.130
          L4and L5 S33.140
      thoracic S23.100
        joint between
          T1and T2 S23.110
          T2and T3 S23.120
          T3 and T4 S23.122
          T4 and T5 S23.130
          T5 and T6 S23.132
          T6 and T7 S23.140
          T7 and T8 S23.142
          T8 and T9 S23.150
          T9 and T10 S23.152
          T10 and T11 S23.160
          T11 and T12 S23.162
          T12 and L1 S23.170
  ulna
    distal end S63.07-
    proximal end — see Subluxation, elbow
  wrist (carpal bone) S63.00-
    carpometacarpal joint — see Subluxation,
      carpometacarpal (joint)
    distal radioulnar joint — see Subluxation,
      radioulnar (joint), distal
    metacarpal bone, proximal — see Subluxation,
      metacarpal (bone), proximal end
    midcarpal — see Subluxation, midcarpal (joint)
    radiocarpal joint — see Subluxation, radiocarpal
      (joint)
    recurrent — see Dislocation, recurrent, wrist
    specified site NEC S63.09-
    ulna — see Subluxation, ulna, distal end
Submaxillary — see condition
Submersion (fatal) (nonfatal) T75.1
Submucous — see condition
Subnormal, subnormality
  accommodation (old age) H52.4
  mental F79
    mild F70
    moderate F71
    profound F73
    severe F72
  temperature (accidental) T68
Subphrenic — see condition
Subscapular nerve — see condition
Subseptus uterus Q51.2
Subsiding appendicitis K36
Substernal thyroid E04.9
  congenital Q89.2
Substitution disorder F44.9
Subtentorial — see condition
Subthyroidism (acquired) (see also Hypothyroidism)
  congenital E03.1
Succenturiate placenta O43.19-
Sucking thumb, child (excessive) F98.8
Sudamen, sudamina L74.1
Sudanese kala-azar B55.0
Sudden
  heart failure — see Failure, heart
  hearing loss — see Deafness, sudden

Sudeck's atrophy, disease, or syndrome — see
  Algoneurodystrophy
Suffocation — see Asphyxia, traumatic
Sugar
  blood
    high (transient) R73.9
    low (transient) E16.2
  in urine R81
Suicide, suicidal (attempted) T14.91
  by poisoning — see Table of Drugs and Chemicals
  history of (personal) Z91.5
    in family Z81.8
  ideation — see Ideation, suicidal
  risk
    meaning personal history of attempted suicide
      Z91.5
    meaning suicidal ideation — see Ideation,
      suicidal
  tendencies
    meaning personal history of attempted suicide
      Z91.5
    meaning suicidal ideation — see Ideation,
      suicidal
  trauma — see nature of injury by site
Suipestifer infection — see Infection, salmonella
Sulfhemoglobinemia, sulphemoglobinemia
  (acquired) (with methemoglobinemia) D74.8
Sumatran mite fever A75.3
Summer — see condition
Sunburn L55.9
  first degree L55.0
  second degree L55.1
  third degree L55.2
SUNCT (short lasting unilateral neuralgiform headache
  with conjunctival injection and tearing) G44.059
  intractable G44.051
  not intractable G44.059
Sunken acetabulum — see Derangement, joint,
  specified type NEC, hip
Sunstroke T67.0
Superfecundation — see Pregnancy, multiple
Superfetation — see Pregnancy, multiple
Superinvolution (uterus) N85.8
Supernumerary (congenital)
  aortic cusps Q23.8
  auditory ossicles Q16.3
  bone Q79.8
  breast Q83.1
  carpal bones Q74.0
  cusps, heart valve NEC Q24.8
    aortic Q23.8
    mitral Q23.2
    pulmonary Q22.3
  digit(s) Q69.9
  ear (lobule) Q17.0
  fallopian tube Q50.6
  finger Q69.0
  hymen Q52.4
  kidney Q63.0
  lacrimonasal duct Q10.6
  lobule (ear) Q17.0
  mitral cusps Q23.2
  muscle Q79.8
  nipple(s) Q83.3
  organ or site not listed — see Accessory
  ossicles, auditory Q16.3
  ovary Q50.31
  oviduct Q50.6
  pulmonary, pulmonic cusps Q22.3
  rib Q76.6
    cervical or first (syndrome) Q76.5
  roots (of teeth) K00.2
  spleen Q89.09
  tarsal bones Q74.2
  teeth K00.1
  testis Q55.29
  thumb Q69.1
  toe Q69.2
  uterus Q51.2
  vagina Q52.1
  vertebra Q76.49

Supervision (of)
  contraceptive — *see* Prescription, contraceptives
  dietary (for) Z71.3
    allergy (food) Z71.3
    colitis Z71.3
    diabetes mellitus Z71.3
    food allergy or intolerance Z71.3
    gastritis Z71.3
    hypercholesterolemia Z71.3
    hypoglycemia Z71.3
    intolerance (food) Z71.3
    obesity Z71.3
    specified NEC Z71.3
  healthy infant or child Z76.2
    foundling Z76.1
  high-risk pregnancy — *see* Pregnancy, complicated
      by, high, risk
  lactation Z39.1
  pregnancy — *see* Pregnancy, supervision of
Supplemental teeth K00.1
Suppression
  binocular vision H53.34
  lactation O92.5
  menstruation N94.89
  ovarian secretion E28.39
  renal N28.9
  urine, urinary secretion R34
Suppuration, suppurative (*see also* condition)
  accessory sinus (chronic) — *see* Sinusitis
  adrenal gland
  antrum (chronic) — *see* Sinusitis, maxillary
  bladder — *see* Cystitis
  brain G06.0
    sequelae G09
  breast N61
    puerperal, postpartum or gestational — *see*
        Mastitis, obstetric, purulent
  dental periosteum M27.3
  ear (middle) (*see also* Otitis, media)
    external NEC — *see* Otitis, externa, infective
    internal — *see* subcategory H83.0
  ethmoidal (chronic) (sinus) — *see* Sinusitis,
      ethmoidal
  fallopian tube — *see* Salpingo-oophoritis
  frontal (chronic) (sinus) — *see* Sinusitis, frontal
  gallbladder (acute) K81.0
  gum K05.20
    generalized K05.22
    localized K05.21
  intracranial G06.0
  joint — *see* Arthritis, pyogenic or pyemic
  labyrinthine — *see* subcategory H83.0
  lung — *see* Abscess, lung
  mammary gland N61
    puerperal, postpartum O91.12
      associated with lactation O91.13
  maxilla, maxillary M27.2
    sinus (chronic) — *see* Sinusitis, maxillary
  muscle — *see* Myositis, infective
  nasal sinus (chronic) — *see* Sinusitis
  pancreas, acute K85.8
  parotid gland — *see* Sialoadenitis
  pelvis, pelvic
    female — *see* Disease, pelvis, inflammatory
    male K65.0
Suppuration, suppurative —*continued*
  pericranial — *see* Osteomyelitis
  salivary duct or gland (any) — *see* Sialoadenitis
  sinus (accessory) (chronic) (nasal) — *see* Sinusitis
  sphenoidal sinus (chronic) — *see* Sinusitis,
      sphenoidal
  thymus (gland) E32.1
  thyroid (gland) E06.0
  tonsil — *see* Tonsillitis
  uterus — *see* Endometritis
Supraeruption of tooth (teeth) M26.34
Supraglottitis J04.30
  with obstruction J04.31
Suprarenal (gland) — *see* condition
Suprascapular nerve — *see* condition
Suprasellar — *see* condition
Surfer's knots or nodules S89.8-

Surgical
  emphysema T81.82
  procedures, complication or misadventure — *see*
      Complications, surgical procedures
  shock T81.1
Surveillance (of) (for) (*see also* Observation)
  alcohol abuse Z71.41
  contraceptive — *see* Prescription, contraceptives
  dietary Z71.3
  drug abuse Z71.51
Susceptibility to disease, genetic Z15.89
  malignant neoplasm Z15.09
    breast Z15.01
    endometrium Z15.04
    ovary Z15.02
    prostate Z15.03
    specified NEC Z15.09
  multiple endocrine neoplasia Z15.81
Suspected condition, ruled out (*see also*
      Observation, suspected)
  amniotic cavity and membrane Z03.71
  cervical shortening Z03.75
  fetal anomaly Z03.73
  fetal growth Z03.74
  maternal and fetal conditions NEC Z03.79
  oligohydramnios Z03.71
  placental problem Z03.72
  polyhydramnios Z03.71
Suspended uterus
  in pregnancy or childbirth — *see* Pregnancy,
      complicated by, abnormal uterus
Sutton's nevus D22.9
Suture
  burst (in operation wound) T81.31
    external operation wound T81.31
    internal operation wound T81.32
  inadvertently left in operation wound — *see* Foreign
      body, accidentally left during a procedure
  removal Z48.02
Swab inadvertently left in operation wound — *see*
    Foreign body, accidentally left during a
    procedure
Swallowed, swallowing
  difficulty — *see* Dysphagia
  foreign body — *see* Foreign body, alimentary tract
Swan-neck deformity (finger) — *see* Deformity,
    finger, swan-neck
Swearing, compulsive F42
  in Gilles de la Tourette's syndrome F95.2
Sweat, sweats
  fetid L75.0
  night R61
Sweating, excessive R61
Sweet's disease or dermatosis L98.2
Swelling (of) R60.9
  abdomen, abdominal (not referable to any
      particular organ) — *see* Mass, abdominal
  ankle — *see* Effusion, joint, ankle
  arm M79.89
    forearm M79.89
  breast N63
  Calabar B74.3
  cervical gland R59.0
  chest, localized R22.2
  ear H93.8-
  extremity (lower) (upper) — *see* Disorder, soft tissue,
      specified type NEC
  finger M79.89
  foot M79.89
  glands R59.9
    generalized R59.1
    localized R59.0
  hand M79.89
  head (localized) R22.0
  inflammatory — *see* Inflammation
  intra-abdominal — *see* Mass, abdominal
  joint — *see* Effusion, joint
  leg M79.89
    lower M79.89
  limb — *see* Disorder, soft tissue, specified type NEC

Swelling—*continued*
  localized (skin) R22.9
    chest R22.2
    head R22.0
    limb
      lower — *see* Mass, localized, limb, lower
      upper — *see* Mass, localized, limb, upper
    neck R22.1
    trunk R22.2
  neck (localized) R22.1
  pelvic — *see* Mass, abdominal
  scrotum N50.8
  splenic — *see* Splenomegaly
  testis N50.8
  toe M79.89
  umbilical R19.09
  wandering, due to Gnathostoma (spinigerum) B83.1
  white — *see* Tuberculosis, arthritis
Swift(-Feer) **disease**
  overdose or wrong substance given or taken — *see*
      Table of Drugs and Chemicals, by drug,
      poisoning
Swimmer's
  cramp T75.1
  ear H60.33-
  itch B65.3
Swimming in the head R42
Swollen — *see* Swelling
Swyer syndrome Q99.1
Sycosis L73.8
  barbae (not parasitic) L73.8
  contagiosa (mycotic) B35.0
  lupoides L73.8
  mycotic B35.0
  parasitic B35.0
  vulgaris L73.8
Sydenham's chorea — *see* Chorea, Sydenham's
Sylvatic yellow fever A95.0
Sylvest's disease B33.0
Symblepharon H11.23-
  congenital Q10.3
Symond's syndrome G93.2
Sympathetic — *see* condition
Sympatheticotonia G90.8
Sympathicoblastoma
  specified site — *see* Neoplasm, malignant, by site
  unspecified site C74.90
Sympathogonioma — *see* Sympathicoblastoma
Symphalangy (fingers) (toes) Q70.9
Symptoms NEC R68.89
  breast NEC N64.59
  development NEC R63.8
  factitious, self-induced — *see* Disorder, factitious
  genital organs, female R10.2
  involving
    abdomen NEC R19.8
    appearance NEC R46.89
    awareness R41.9
      altered mental status R41.82
      amnesia — *see* Amnesia
      borderline intellectual functioning R41.83
      coma — *see* Coma
      disorientation R41.0
      neurologic neglect syndrome R41.4
      senile cognitive decline R41.81
      specified symptom NEC R41.89
    behavior NEC R46.89
    cardiovascular system NEC R09.89
    chest NEC R09.89
    circulatory system NEC R09.89
    cognitive functions R41.9
      altered mental status R41.82
      amnesia — *see* Amnesia
      borderline intellectual functioning R41.83
      coma — *see* Coma
      disorientation R41.0
      neurologic neglect syndrome R41.4
      senile cognitive decline R41.81
      specified symptom NEC R41.89
    development NEC R62.50
    digestive system NEC R19.8

Symptoms NEC—*continued*
  involving—*continued*
    emotional state NEC R45.89
      emotional lability R45.86
    food and fluid intake R63.8
    general perceptions and sensations R44.9
      specified NEC R44.8
    musculoskeletal system R29.91
      specified NEC R29.898
    nervous system R29.90
      specified NEC R29.818
    pelvis NEC R19.8
    respiratory system NEC R09.89
    skin and integument R23.9
    urinary system R39.9
  menopausal N95.1
  metabolism NEC R63.8
  neurotic F48.8
  of infancy R68.19
  pelvis NEC, female R10.2
  skin and integument NEC R23.8
  subcutaneous tissue NEC R23.8
Sympus Q74.2
Syncephalus Q89.4
Synchondrosis
  abnormal (congenital) Q78.8
  ischiopubic M91.0
Synchysis (scintillans) (senile) (vitreous body) H43.89
Syncope (near) (pre-) R55
  anginosa I20.8
  bradycardia R00.1
  cardiac R55
  carotid sinus G90.01
  due to spinal (lumbar) puncture G97.1
  heart R55
  heat T67.1
  laryngeal R05
  psychogenic F48.8
  tussive R05
  vasoconstriction R55
  vasodepressor R55
  vasomotor R55
  vasovagal R55
Syndactylism, syndactyly Q70.9
  complex (with synostosis)
    fingers Q70.0-
    toes Q70.2-
  simple (without synostosis)
    fingers Q70.1-
    toes Q70.3-
Syndrome (*see also* Disease)
  5q minus NOS D46.c
  48,XXXX Q97.1
  49,XXXXX Q97.1
  abdominal
    acute R10.0
    muscle deficiency Q79.4
  abnormal innervation H02.519
    left H02.516
      lower H02.515
      upper H02.514
    right H02.513
      lower H02.512
      upper H02.511
  abstinence, neonatal P96.1
  acid pulmonary aspiration, obstetric O74.0
  acquired immunodeficiency — *see* Human,
    immunodeficiency virus (HIV) disease
  acute abdominal R10.0
  acute respiratory distress (adult) (child) J80
  Adair-Dighton Q78.0
  Adams-Stokes(-Morgagni) I45.9
  adiposogenital E23.6
  adrenal
    hemorrhage (meningococcal) A39.1
    meningococcic A39.1
  adrenocortical — *see* Cushing's syndrome
  adrenogenital E25.9
    congenital, associated with enzyme deficiency
      E25.0
  afferent loop NEC K91.89
  Alagille's Q44.7

Syndrome—*continued*
  alcohol withdrawal (without convulsions) — *see*
    Dependence, alcohol, with, withdrawal
  Alder's D72.0
  Aldrich(-Wiskott) D82.0
  alien hand R41.4
  Alport Q87.81
  alveolar hypoventilation E66.2
  alveolocapillary block J84.1
  amnesic, amnestic (confabulatory) (due to) — *see*
    Disorder, amnesic
  amyostatic (Wilson's disease) E83.01
  androgen insensitivity E34.50
    complete E34.51
    partial E34.52
  androgen resistance (*see also* Syndrome, androgen
    insensitivity) E34.50
  Angelman Q93.5
  anginal — *see* Angina
  ankyloglossia superior Q38.1
  anterior
    chest wall R07.89
    cord G83.82
    spinal artery G95.19
      compression M47.019
        cervical region M47.012
        cervicothoracic region M47.013
        lumbar region M47.016
        occipito-atlanto-axial region M47.011
        thoracic region M47.014
        thoracolumbar region M47.015
    tibial M76.81-
  antibody deficiency D80.9
    agammaglobulinemic D80.1
      hereditary D80.0
    congenital D80.0
    hypogammaglobulinemic D80.1
      hereditary D80.0
  anticardiolipin (-antibody) D68.61
  antiphospholipid (-antibody) D68.61
  aortic
    arch M31.4
    bifurcation I74.0
  aortomesenteric duodenum occlusion K31.5
  apical ballooning (transient left ventricular) I51.81
  arcuate ligament I77.4
  argentaffin, argintaffinoma E34.0
  Arnold-Chiari — *see* Arnold-Chiari disease
  Arrillaga-Ayerza I27.0
  Asherman's N85.6
  aspiration, of newborn — *see* Aspiration, by
    substance, with pneumonia
    meconium P24.01
  ataxia-telangiectasia G11.3
  auriculotemporal G50.8
  autoerythrocyte sensitization (Gardner-Diamond)
    D69.2
  autoimmune polyglandular E31.0
  autoimmune lymphoproliferativee [ALPS] D89.82
  autosomal — *see* Abnormal, autosomes
  Avellis' G83.89
  Ayerza(-Arrillaga) I27.0
  Babinski-Nageotte G83.89
  Bakwin-Krida Q79.8
  bare lymphocyte D81.6
  Barré-Guillain G61.0
  Barré-Liéou M53.0
  Barrett's — *see* Barrett's, esophagus
  Barsony-Polgar K22.4
  Barsony-Teschendorf K22.4
  Barth E78.71
  Bartter's E26.81
  basal cell nevus Q87.89
  Basedow's E05.00
    with thyroid storm E05.01
  basilar artery G45.0
  Batten-Steinert G71.11
  battered
    baby or child — *see* Maltreatment, child, physical
      abuse
    spouse — *see* Maltreatment, adult, physical
      abuse
  Beals Q87.40

Syndrome—*continued*
  Beau's I51.5
  Beck's I65.8
  Benedikt's G83.89
  Béquez César (-Steinbrinck-Chédiak-Higashi) D72.0
  Bernhardt-Roth — *see* Meralgia paresthetica
  Bernheim's I50.9
  big spleen D73.1
  bilateral polycystic ovarian E28.2
  Bing-Horton's G43.809
  Birt-Hogg-Dube syndrome Q87.89
  Björck(-Thorsen) E34.0
  black
    lung J60
    widow spider bite — *see* Toxicity, venom, spider,
      black widow
  Blackfan-Diamond D61.01
  blind loop K90.2
    congenital Q43.8
    postsurgical K91.2
  blue sclera Q78.0
  blue toe I75.02-
  Boder-Sedgewick G11.3
  Boerhaave's K22.3
  Borjeson Forssman Lehmann Q89.8
  Bouillaud's I01.9
  Bourneville(-Pringle) Q85.1
  Bouveret(-Hoffman) I47.9
  brachial plexus G54.0
  bradycardia-tachycardia I49.5
  brain (nonpsychotic) F09
    with psychosis, psychotic reaction F09
    acute or subacute — *see* Delirium
    congenital — *see* Retardation, mental
    organic F09
      post-traumatic (nonpsychotic) F07.81
      psychotic F09
    personality change F07.0
    postcontusional F07.81
    post-traumatic, nonpsychotic F07.81
    psycho-organic F09
    psychotic F06.8
  brain stem stroke G46.3
  Brandt's L08.0
  broad ligament laceration N83.8
  Brock's J98.11
  bronze baby P83.8
  Brown-Sequard G83.81
  bubbly lung P27.0
  Buchem's M85.2
  Budd-Chiari I82.0
  bulbar (progressive) G12.22
  Bürger-Grütz E78.3
  Burke's K86.8
  Burnett's (milk-alkali) E83.52
  burning feet E53.9
  Bywaters' T79.5
  carbohydrate-deficient glycoprotein (CDGS) E77.8
  carcinogenic thrombophlebitis I82.1
  carcinoid E34.0
  cardiac asthma I50.1
  cardiacos negros I27.0
  cardiofaciocutaneous Q87.89
  cardiopulmonary-obesity E66.2
  cardiorenal — *see* Hypertension, cardiorenal
  cardiorespiratory distress (idiopathic), newborn
    P22.0
  cardiovascular renal — *see* Hypertension,
    cardiorenal
  carotid
    artery (hemispheric) (internal) G45.1
      body G90.01
    sinus G90.01
  carpal tunnel G56.0-
  Cassidy(-Scholte) M34.0
  cat- cry Q93.4
  cat eye Q92.8
  cauda equina G83.4
  causalgia — *see* Causalgia
  celiac K90.0
    artery compression I77.4
    axis I77.4
  central pain G89.0

Syndrome—*continued*
cerebellar
hereditary G11.9
stroke G46.4
cerebellomedullary malformation — *see* Spina
bifida
cerebral
artery
anterior G46.1
middle G46.0
posterior G46.2
gigantism E22.0
cervical (root) M53.1
disc — *see* Disorder, disc, cervical, with neuritis
fusion Q76.1
posterior, sympathicus M53.0
rib Q76.5
sympathetic paralysis G90.2
cervicobrachial (diffuse) M53.1
cervicocranial M53.0
cervicodorsal outlet G54.2
cervicothoracic outlet G54.0
Céstan(-Raymond) I65.8
Charcot's (angina cruris) (intermittent claudication)
I73.9
Charcot-Weiss-Baker G90.09
CHARGE Q89.8
Chédiak-Higashi(-Steinbrinck) D72.0
chest wall R07.1
Chiari's (hepatic vein thrombosis) I82.0
Chilaiditi's Q43.3
child maltreatment — *see* Maltreatment, child
chondrocostal junction M94.0
chondroectodermal dysplasia Q77.6
chromosome 4 short arm deletion Q93.3
chromosome 5 short arm deletion Q93.4
chronic
pain G89.4
personality F68.8
Clarke-Hadfield K86.8
Clerambault's automatism G93.89
Clouston's (hidrotic ectodermal dysplasia) Q82.4
clumsiness, clumsy child F82
cluster headache G44.009
intractable G44.001
not intractable G44.009
Coffin-Lowry Q89.8
cold injury (newborn) P80.0
combined immunity deficiency D81.9
compartment (deep) (posterior) (traumatic) T79.A0
abdomen T79.A3
lower extremity (hip, buttock, thigh, leg, foot,
toes) T79.A2
nontraumatic
abdomen M79.A3
lower extremity (hip, buttock, thigh, leg, foot,
toes) M79.A2-
specified site NEC M79.A9
upper extremity (shoulder, arm, forearm,
wrist, hand, fingers) M79.A1-
postprocedural — *see* Syndrome, compartment,
nontraumatic
specified site NEC T79.A9
upper extremity (shoulder, arm, forearm, wrist,
hand, fingers) T79.A1
complex regional pain — *see* Syndrome, pain,
complex regional
compression T79.5
anterior spinal — *see* Syndrome, anterior, spinal
artery, compression
cauda equina G83.4
celiac artery I77.4
vertebral artery M47.029
occipito-atlanto-axial region M47.021
cervical region M47.022
concussion F07.81
congenital
affecting multiple systems NEC Q87.89
central alveolar hypoventilation G47.35
facial diplegia Q87.0
muscular hypertrophy-cerebral Q87.89
oculo-auriculovertebral Q87.0
oculofacial diplegia (Moebius) Q87.0

Syndrome—*continued*
congenital—*continued*
rubella (manifest) P35.0
congestion-fibrosis (pelvic), female N94.89
congestive dysmenorrhea N94.6
Conn's E26.01
connective tissue M35.9
overlap NEC M35.1
conus medullaris G95.81
cord
anterior G83.82
posterior G83.83
coronary
acute NEC I24.9
insufficiency or intermediate I20.0
slow flow I20.8
Costen's (complex) M26.69
costochondral junction M94.0
costoclavicular G54.0
costovertebral E22.0
Cowden Q85.8
craniovertebral M53.0
Creutzfeldt-Jakob — *see* Creutzfeldt-Jakob disease
or syndrome
cri-du-chat Q93.4
crib death R99
cricopharyngeal — *see* Dysphagia
croup J05.0
CRPS I — *see* Syndrome, pain, complex regional I
crush T79.5
cubital tunnel — *see* Lesion, nerve, ulnar
Curschmann (-Batten) (-Steinert) G71.11
Cushing's E24.9
alcohol-induced E24.4
due to
alcohol
drugs E24.2
ectopic ACTH E24.3
overproduction of pituitary ACTH E24.0
drug-induced E24.2
overdose or wrong substance given or taken —
see Table of Drugs and Chemicals, by drug,
poisoning
pituitary-dependent E24.0
specified type NEC E24.8
cryptophthalmos Q87.0
cystic duct stump K91.5
Dana-Putnam D51.0
Danbolt (-Closs) L08.0
Dandy-Walker Q03.0
with spina bifida Q07.01
Danlos' Q79.8
defibrination (Fibrinolysis)
with
antepartum hemorrhage — *see* Hemorrhage,
antepartum
intrapartum hemorrhage — *see* Hemorrhage,
complicating, delivery
newborn P60
postpartum O72.3
Degos' I77.8
Déjérine-Roussy G89.0
delayed sleep phase G47.21
demyelinating G37.9
dependence — *see* F10-F19 with fourth character .2
depersonalization(-derealization) F48.1
De Quervain E34.51
de Toni-Fanconi (-Debré) E72.09
with cystinosis E72.04
diabetes mellitus-hypertension-nephrosis — *see*
Diabetes, nephrosis
diabetes mellitus in newborn infant P70.2
diabetes-nephrosis — *see* Diabetes, nephrosis
diabetic amyotrophy — *see* Diabetes, amyotrophy
Diamond-Blackfan D61.01
Diamond-Gardener D69.2
DIC (diffuse or disseminated intravascular
coagulopathy) D65
di George's D82.1
Dighton's Q78.0
disequilibrium E87.8
Döhle body-panmyelopathic D72.0
dorsolateral medullary G46.4

Syndrome—*continued*
double athetosis G80.3
Down (*see also* Down syndrome) Q90.9
Dresbach's (elliptocytosis) D58.1
Dressler's (postmyocardial infarction) I24.1
postcardiotomy I97.0
drug withdrawal, infant of dependent mother P96.1
dry eye H04.12-
due to abnormality
chromosomal Q99.9
sex
female phenotype Q97.9
male phenotype Q98.9
specified NEC Q99.8
dumping (postgastrectomy) K91.1
nonsurgical K31.89
Dupré's (meningism) R29.1
dysmetabolic X E88.81
dyspraxia, developmental F82
Eagle-Barrett Q79.4
Eaton-Lambert G73.1
not associated with neoplasm G70.8
Ebstein's Q22.5
ectopic ACTH E24.3
eczema-thrombocytopenia D82.0
Eddowes' Q78.0
effort (psychogenic) F45.8
Eisenmenger's I27.89
Ehlers-Danlos Q79.6
Ekman's Q78.0
electric feet E53.8
Ellis-van Creveld Q77.6
empty nest Z60.0
endocrine-hypertensive E27.0
entrapment — *see* Neuropathy, entrapment
eosinophilia-myalgia M35.8
epileptic — *see* Epilepsy
Erdheim-Chester (ECD) E88.89
Erdheim's E22.0
erythrocyte fragmentation D59.4
Evans D69.41
exhaustion F48.8
extrapyramidal G25.9
specified NEC G25.89
eye retraction — *see* Strabismus
eyelid-malar-mandible Q87.0
Faber's D50.9
facial pain, paroxysmal G50.0
Fallot's Q21.3
familial eczema-thrombocytopenia
(Wiskott-Aldrich) D82.0
Fanconi (-de Toni) (-Debré) E72.09
with cystinosis E72.04
Fanconi's (anemia) (congenital pancytopenia)
D61.09
fatigue
chronic R53.82
psychogenic F48.8
faulty bowel habit K59.3
Feil-Klippel (brevicollis) Q76.1
Felty's — *see* Felty's syndrome
fertile eunuch E23.0
fetal
alcohol (dysmorphic) Q86.0
hydantoin Q86.1
Fiedler's I40.1
first arch Q87.0
fish odor E72.8
Fisher's G61.0
Fitzhugh-Curtis
due to
Chlamydia trachomatis A74.81
Neisseria gonorrhorea (gonococcal
peritonitis) A54.85
Fitz's K85.8
Flajani (-Basedow) E05.00
with thyroid storm E05.01
flatback — *see* Flatback syndrome
floppy
baby P94.2
iris (intraoeprative) (IFIS) H21.81
mitral valve I34.1
flush E34.0

Syndrome—*continued*

Foix-Alajouanine G95.19
Fong's Q79.8
foramen magnum G93.5
Foville's (peduncular) G83.89
fragile X Q99.2
Franceschetti Q75.4
Frey's
 auriculotemporal G50.8
 hyperhidrosis L74.52
Friderichsen-Waterhouse A39.1
Froin's G95.89
frontal lobe F07.0
Fukuhara E88.49
functional
 bowel K59.9
 prepubertal castrate E29.1
Gaisböck's D75.1
ganglion (basal ganglia brain) G25.9
 geniculi G51.1
Gardner-Diamond D69.2
gastroesophageal
 junction K22.0
 laceration-hemorrhage K22.6
gastrojejunal loop obstruction K91.89
Gee-Herter-Heubner K90.0
Gelineau's G47.419
 with cataplexy G47.411
genito-anorectal A55
Gerstmann-Sträussler-Scheinker (GSS) A81.82
Gianotti-Crosti L44.4
giant platelet (Bernard-Soulier) D69.1
Gilles de la Tourette's F95.2
goiter-deafness E07.1
Goldberg Q89.8
Goldberg-Maxwell E34.51
Good's D83.8
Gopalan' (burning feet) E53.8
Gorlin's Q87.89
Gougerot-Blum L81.7
Gouley's I31.1
Gower's R55
gray or grey (newborn) P93.0
 platelet D69.1
Gubler-Millard G83.89
Guillain-Barré (-Strohl) G61.0
gustatory sweating G50.8
Hadfield-Clarke K86.8
hair tourniquet — *see* Constriction, external, by site
Hamman's J98.19
hand-foot L27.1
hand-shoulder G90.8
hantavirus (cardio)-pulmonary (HPS) (HCPS) B33.4
happy puppet Q93.5
Harada's H30.81-
Hayem-Faber D50.9
headache NEC G44.89
 complicated NEC G44.59
Heberden's I20.8
Hedinger's E34.0
Hegglin's D72.0
HELLP O14.2
hemolytic-uremic D59.3
hemophagocytic, infection-associated D76.2
Henoch-Schönlein D69.0
hepatic flexure K59.8
hepatorenal K76.7
 following delivery O90.4
 postoperative or postprocedural K91.83
 postpartum, puerperal O90.4
hepatourologic K76.7
Herter (-Gee) (nontropical sprue) K90.0
Heubner-Herter K90.0
Heyd's K76.7
Hilger's G90.09
histamine-like (fish poisoning) — *see* Poisoning, fish
histiocytic D76.3
histiocytosis NEC D76.3
HIV infection, acute B20
Hoffmann-Werdnig G12.0
Hollander-Simons E88.1

Syndrome—*continued*

Hoppe-Goldflam G70.00
 with exacerbation (acute) G70.01
 in crisis G70.01
Horner's G90.2
hungry bone E83.81
hunterian glossitis K14.4
Hutchinson's triad A50.53
hyperabduction G54.0
hyperammonemia-hyperornithinemia-
 homocitrullinemia E72.4
hypereosinophilic (idiopathic) D72.1
hyperimmunoglobulin E (IgE) D82.4
hyperkalemic E87.5
hyperkinetic — *see* Hyperkinesia
hypermobility M35.7
hypernatremia E87.0
hyperosmolarity E87.0
hyperperfusion G97.82
hypersplenic D73.1
hypertransfusion, newborn P61.1
hyperventilation F45.8
hyperviscosity (of serum)
 polycythemic D75.1
 sclerothymic D58.8
hypoglycemic (familial) (neonatal) E16.2
hypokalemic E87.6
hyponatremic E87.1
hypopituitarism E23.0
hypoplastic left-heart Q23.4
hypopotassemia E87.6
hyposmolality E87.1
hypotension, maternal O26.5-
hypothenar hammer I73.89
ICF (intravascular coagulation-fibrinolysis) D65
idiopathic
 cardiorespiratory distress, newborn P22.0
 nephrotic (infantile) N04.9
iliotibial band M76.3-
immobility, immobilization (paraplegic) M62.3
immune reconstitution D89.3
immune reconstitution inflammatory [IRIS] D89.3
immunity deficiency, combined D81.9
immunodeficiency
 acquired — *see* Human, immunodeficiency virus
  (HIV) disease
 combined D81.9
impending coronary I20.0
impingement, shoulder M75.4-
inappropriate secretion of antidiuretic hormone
 E22.2
infant
 of diabetic mother P70.1
 gestational diabetes P70.0
infantilism (pituitary) E23.0
inferior vena cava I87.1
inspissated bile (newborn) P59.1
institutional (childhood) F94.2
insufficient sleep F51.12
intermediate coronary (artery) I20.0
interspinous ligament — *see* Spondylopathy,
 specified NEC
intestinal
 carcinoid E34.0
 knot K56.2
intravascular coagulation-fibrinolysis (ICF) D65
iodine-deficiency, congenital E00.9
 type
  mixed E00.2
  myxedematous E00.1
  neurological E00.0
IRDS (idiopathic respiratory distress, newborn) P22.0
irritable
 bowel K58.9
  with diarrhea K58.0
  psychogenic F45.8
 heart (psychogenic) F45.8
 weakness F48.8
ischemic bowel (transient) K55.9
 chronic K55.1
 due to mesenteric artery insufficiency K55.1
IVC (intravascular coagulopathy) D65
Ivemark's Q89.01

Syndrome—*continued*

Jaccoud's — *see* Arthropathy, postrheumatic,
 chronic
Jackson's G83.89
Jakob-Creutzfeldt — *see* Creutzfeldt-Jakob disease
 or syndrome
jaw-winking Q07.8
Jervell-Lange-Nielsen I45.81
jet lag G47.25
Job's D71
Joseph-Diamond-Blackfan D61.01
jugular foramen G52.7
Kabuki Q89.8
Kanner's (autism) F84.0
Kartagener's Q89.3
Kelly's D50.1
Kimmelstiel-Wilson — *see* Diabetes, specified type,
 with Kimmelsteil-Wilson disease
Klein(e)-Levine G47.13
Klippel-Feil (brevicollis) Q76.1
Köhler-Pellegrini-Steida — *see* Bursitis, tibial
 collateral
König's K59.8
Korsakoff (-Wernicke) (nonalcoholic) F04
 alcoholic F10.26
Kostmann's D70.0
Krabbe's congenital muscle hypoplasia Q79.8
labyrinthine — *see* subcategory H83.2
lacunar NEC G46.7
Lambert-Eaton G73.1
 not associated with neoplasm G70.8
Landau-Kleffner F80.3
Larsen's Q74.8
lateral
 cutaneous nerve of thigh D57.1-
 medullary G46.4
Launois' E22.0
lazy
 leukocyte D70.8
 posture M62.3
Lemiere I80.8
Lennox-Gastaut — *see* Epilepsy, generalized,
 specified NEC
lenticular, progressive E83.01
Leopold-Levi's E05.90
Lev's I44.2
Li-Fraumeni Z15.01
Lichtheim's D51.0
Lightwood's N25.89
Lignac (de Toni) (-Fanconi) (-Debré) E72.09
 with cystinosis E72.04
Likoff's I20.8
limbic epilepsy personality F07.0
liver-kidney K76.7
lobotomy F07.0
Loffler's J82
long arm 18 or 21 deletion Q93.89
long QT I45.81
Louis-Barré G11.3
low
 atmospheric pressure T70.20
 back M54.5
 output (cardiac) I50.9
lower radicular, newborn (birth injury) P14.8
Luetscher's (dehydration) E86.0
Lupus anticoagulant D68.62
Lutembacher's Q21.1
macrophage activation D76.1
 due to infection D76.2
Mal de Debarquement R42
malabsorption K90.9
 postsurgical K91.2
magnesium-deficiency R29.0
malabsorption K90.9
 postsurgical K91.2
malformation, congenital, due to
 alcohol Q86.0
 exogenous cause NEC Q86.8
 hydantoin Q86.1
 warfarin Q86.2
malignant
 carcinoid E34.0
 neuroleptic G21.0

Syndrome—*continued*

Mallory-Weiss K22.6
mandibulofacial dysostosis Q75.4
manic-depressive — *see* Disorder, bipolar, affective
maple-syrup-urine E71.0
Marable's I77.4
Marfan's Q87.40
  with
    cardiovascular manifestations Q87.418
      aortic dilation Q87.410
    ocular manifestations Q87.42
    skeletal manifestations Q87.43
Marie's (acromegaly) E22.0
maternal hypotension — *see* Syndrome,
  hypotension, maternal
May (-Hegglin) D72.0
McArdle (-Schmidt) (-Pearson) E74.04
McQuarrie's E16.2
meconium plug (newborn) P76.0
median arcuate ligament I77.4
Meekeren-Ehlers-Danlos Q79.6
megavitamin-B6 E67.2
Meige G24.4
MELAS E88.41
Mendelson's O74.0
MERFF E88.42
mesenteric
  artery (superior) K55.1
  vascular insufficiency K55.1
metabolic E88.81
metastatic carcinoid E34.0
micrognathia-glossoptosis Q87.0
midbrain NEC G93.89
middle lobe (lung) J98.19
middle radicular G54.0
migraine (*see also* Migraine) G43.909
Mikulicz' K11.8
milk-alkali E83.52
Millard-Gubler G83.89
Miller-Dieker Q93.88
Miller-Fisher G61.0
Minkowski-Chauffard D58.0
Mirizzi's K83.1
MNGIE (Mitochondrial Neurogastrointestinal
  Encephalopathy) E88.49
Möbius, ophthalmoplegic migraine — *see* Migraine,
  ophthalmoplegic
monofixation H50.42
Morel-Moore M85.2
Morel-Morgagni M85.2
Morgagni (-Morel) (-Stewart) M85.2
Morgagni-Adams-Stokes I45.9
mucocutaneous lymph node (acute febrile) (MCLS)
  M30.3
multiple endocrine neoplasia (MEN) — *see*
  Neoplasia, endocrine, multiple (MEN)
multiple operations — *see* Disorder, factitious
Mounier-Kuhn Q32.4
  with bronchiectasis J47.9
    with
      exacerbation (acute) J47.1
      lower respiratory infection J47.0
  acquired J98.09
    with bronchiectasis J47.9
      with
        exacerbation (acute) J47.1
        lower respiratory infection J47.0
myasthenic G70.9
  in
    diabetes mellitus — *see* Diabetes,
      amyotrophy
    endocrine disease NEC E34.9 [G73.3]
    neoplastic disease (*see also* Neoplasm) D49.9
      [G73.3]
    thyrotoxicosis (hyperthyroidism) E05.90
      [G73.3]
      with thyroid storm E05.91 [G73.3]
myelodysplastic D46.9
  with 5q deletion D46.c
  with isolated del(5q) chromosomal abnormality
    D46.c
  specified NEC D46.z
myelopathic pain G89.0

Syndrome—*continued*

myeloproliferative (chronic) D47.1
myofascial pain M79.1
Naffziger's G54.0
nail patella Q87.2
NARP (Neuropathy, Ataxia and Retinitis pigmentosa)
  E88.49
neonatal abstinence P96.1
nephritic (*see also* Nephritis)
  with edema — *see* Nephrosis
  acute N00.9
  chronic N03.9
  rapidly progressive N01.9
nephrotic (congenital) (*see also* Nephrosis) N04.9
  with
    dense deposit disease N04.6
    diffuse
      crescentic glomerulonephritis N04.7
      endocapillary proliferative
        glomerulonephritis N04.4
      membranous glomerulonephritis N04.2
      mesangial proliferative
        glomerulonephritis N04.3
      mesangiocapillary glomerulonephritis
        N04.5
    focal and segmental glomerular lesions N04.1
    minor glomerular abnormality N04.0
    specified morphological changes NEC N04.8
  diabetic — *see* Diabetes, nephrosis
neurologic neglect R41.4
Nezelof's D81.4
Nonne-Milroy-Meige Q82.0
Nothnagel's vasomotor acroparesthesia I73.89
oculomotor H51.9
ophthalmoplegia-cerebellar ataxia — *see*
  Strabismus, paralytic, third nerve
oral-facial-digital Q87.0
organic
  affective F06.30
  amnesic (not alcoholor drug-induced) F04
  brain F09
  depressive F06.31
  hallucinosis F06.0
  personality F07.0
Ormond's N13.5
oro-facial-digital Q87.0
os trigonum Q68.8
Osler-Weber-Rendu I78.0
osteoporosis-osteomalacia M83.8
Osterreicher-Turner Q79.8
otolith — *see* subcategory H81.8
oto-palatal-digital Q87.0
outlet (thoracic) G54.0
ovary
  polycystic E28.2
  resistant E28.39
  sclerocystic E28.2
Owren's D68.2
Paget-Schroetter I82.890
pain (*see also* Pain)
  complex regional I G90.50
    lower limb G90.52-
    specified site NEC G90.59
    upper limb G90.51-
  complex regional II — *see* Causalgia
painful
  bruising D69.2
  feet E53.8
  prostate N42.81
paralysis agitans — *see* Parkinsonism
paralytic G83.9
  specified NEC G83.89
Parinaud's H51.0
parkinsonian — *see* Parkinsonism
Parkinson's — *see* Parkinsonism
paroxysmal facial pain G50.0
Parry's E05.00
  with thyroid storm E05.01
Parsonage(-Aldren)-Turner G54.5
patella clunk M25.86-
Paterson(-Brown) (-Kelly) D50.1
pectoral girdle I77.89
pectoralis minor I77.89

Syndrome—*continued*

Pelger-Huet D72.0
pellagra-cerebellar ataxia-renal aminoaciduria
  E72.02
pellagroid E52
Pellegrini-Stieda — *see* Bursitis, tibial collateral
pelvic congestion-fibrosis, female N94.89
penta X Q97.1
peptic ulcer — *see* Ulcer, peptic
perabduction I77.89
periodic headache, in adults and children G43.c09
  intractable G43.c19
    with status migrainosus G43.c11
    without status migrainosus G43.c19
  not intractable G43.c09
    with status migrainosus G43.c01
    without status migrainosus G43.c09
periurethral fibrosis N13.5
phantom limb (without pain) G54.7
  with pain G54.6
pharyngeal pouch D82.1
Pick's (heart) (liver) I31.1
Pickwickian E66.2
PIE (pulmonary infiltration with eosinophilia) J82
pigmentary pallidal degeneration (progressive)
  G23.0
pineal E34.8
pituitary E22.0
placental transfusion — *see* Pregnancy, complicated
  by, placental transfusion syndromes
plateau iris (post-iridectomy) (postprocedural)
  H21.82
Plummer-Vinson D50.1
pluricarential of infancy E40
plurideficiency E40
pluriglandular (compensatory) E31.20
  autoimmune E31.0
pneumatic hammer T75.21
polyangiitis overlap M30.8
polycarential of infancy E40
polyglandular E31.20
  autoimmune E31.0
polysplenia Q89.09
pontine NEC G93.89
popliteal
  artery entrapment I77.89
  web Q87.89
postcardiac injury
  postcardiotomy I97.0
  postmyocardial infarction I24.1
postcardiotomy I97.0
postcholecystectomy K91.5
postcommissurotomy I97.0
postconcussional F07.81
postcontusional F07.81
postencephalitic F07.89
posterior
  cervical sympathetic M53.0
  cord G83.83
  fossa compression G93.5
  reversible encephalopathy (PRES) G93.49
postgastrectomy (dumping) K91.1
postgastric surgery K91.1
postinfarction I24.1
postlaminectomy NEC M96.1
postleukotomy F07.0
postmastectomy lymphedema I97.2
postmyocardial infarction I24.1
postoperative NEC T81.9
  blind loop K90.2
postpartum panhypopituitary (Sheehan) E23.0
postpolio (myelitic) G14
postthrombotic I87.009
  with
    inflammation I87.02-
      with ulcer I87.03-
    specified complication NEC I87.09-
    ulcer I87.01-
      with inflammation I87.03-
  asymptomatic I87.00-
postvagotomy K91.1
postvalvulotomy I97.0

Syndrome—*continued*
- postviral NEC G93.3
  - fatigue G93.3
- Potain's K31.0
- potassium intoxication E87.5
- precerebral artery (multiple) (bilateral) G45.2
- preinfarction I20.0
- preleukemic D46.9
- premature senility E34:8
- premenstrual dysphoric N94.3
- premenstrual tension N94.3
- Prinzmetal-Massumi R07.1
- prune belly Q79.4
- pseudocarpal tunnel (sublimis) — *see* Syndrome, carpal tunnel
- pseudoparalytica G70.00
  - with exacerbation (acute) G70.01
  - in crisis G70.01
- pseudo -Turner's Q87.1
- psycho-organic (nonpsychotic severity) F07.9
  - acute or subacute F05
  - depressive type F06.31
  - hallucinatory type F06.0
  - nonpsychotic severity F07.0
  - specified NEC F07.89
- pulmonary
  - arteriosclerosis I27.0
  - dysmaturity (Wilson-Mikity) P27.0
  - hypoperfusion (idiopathic) P22.0
  - renal (hemorrhagic) (Goodpasture's) M31.0
- pure
  - motor lacunar G46.5
  - sensory lacunar G46.6
- Putnam-Dana D51.0
- pyramidopallidonigral G20
- pyriformis — *see* Lesion, nerve, sciatic
- QT interval prolongation I45.81
- radicular NEC — *see* Radiculopathy
  - upper limbs, newborn (birth injury) P14.3
- rapid time-zone change G47.25
- Rasmussen G04.81
- Raymond (-Céstan) I65.8
- Raynaud's I73.00
  - with gangrene I73.01
- RDS (respiratory distress syndrome, newborn) P22.0
- reactive airways dysfunction J68.3
- Refsum's G60.1
- Reifenstein E34.52
- renal glomerulohyalinosis-diabetic — *see* Diabetes, nephrosis
- Rendu-Osler-Weber I78.0
- residual ovary N99.83
- resistant ovary E28.39
- respiratory
  - distress
    - acute J80
      - adult J80
      - child J80
    - newborn (idiopathic) (type I) P22.0
      - type II P22.1
- restless legs G25.81
- retinoblastoma (familial) C69.2
- retroperitoneal fibrosis N13.8
- retroviral seroconversion (acute) Z21
- Reye's G93.7
- Richter — *see* Leukemia, chronic lymphocytic, B-cell type
- Ridley's I50.1
- right
  - heart, hypoplastic Q22.6
  - ventricular obstruction — *see* Failure, heart, congestive
- Romano-Ward (prolonged QT interval) I45.81
- rotator cuff, shoulder M75.1-
- Rotes Quérol — *see* Hyperostosis, ankylosing
- Roth — *see* Meralgia paresthetica
- rubella (congenital) P35.0
- Ruvalcaba-Myhre-Smith E71.440
- Rytand-Lipsitch I44.2

Syndrome—*continued*
- salt
  - depletion E87.1
    - due to heat NEC T67.8
      - causing heat exhaustion or prostration T67.4
  - low E87.1
- salt-losing N28.89
- Scaglietti-Dagnini E22.0
- scalenus anticus (anterior) G54.0
- scapulocostal — *see* Mononeuropathy, upper limb, specified site NEC
- scapuloperoneal G71.0
- schizophrenic, of childhood NEC F84.5
- Schnitzler D47.2
- Scholte's E34.0
- Schroeder's E27.0
- Schüller-Christian C96.5
- Schwachman's — *see* Syndrome, Shwachman's
- Schwartz (-Jampel) G71.13
- Schwartz-Bartter E22.2
- scimitar Q26.8
- sclerocystic ovary E28.2
- Seitelberger's G31.89
- septicemic adrenal hemorrhage A39.1
- seroconversion, retroviral (acute) Z21
- serous meningitis G93.2
- severe acute respiratory (SARS) J12.81
- shaken infant T74.4
- shock (traumatic) T79.4
  - kidney N17.0
    - following crush injury T79.5
  - toxic A48.3
- shock-lung J80
- Shone's code to specific anomalies
- short
  - bowel K91.2
  - rib Q77.2
- shoulder-hand — *see* Algoneurodystrophy
- Shwachman's D70.4
- sicca — *see* Sicca syndrome
- sick
  - cell E87.1
  - sinus I49.5
- sick-euthyroid E07.81
- sideropenic D50.1
- Siemens' ectodermal dysplasia Q82.4
- Silfversköld's Q78.9
- Simon's E88.1
- sinus tarsi — *see* Syndrome, tarsal tunnel
- sinusitis-bronchiectasis-situs inversus Q89.3
- Sipple's E31.22
- sirenomelia Q87.2
- Slocumb's E27.0
- slow flow, coronary I20.8
- Sluder's
- Smith-Magenis Q93.88
- Sneddon-Wilkinson L13.1
- Sotos' E22.0
- South African cardiomyopathy I42.8
- spasmodic
  - upward movement, eyes H51.8
  - winking F95.8
- Spen's I45.9
- splenic
  - agenesis Q89.01
  - flexure K59.8
  - neutropenia D73.81
- Spurway's Q78.0
- staphylococcal scalded skin L00
- Stein-Leventhal E28.2
- Stein's E28.2
- Stevens-Johnson syndrome L51.1
  - toxic epidermal necrolysis overlap L51.3
- Stewart-Morel M85.2
- Stickler Q89.8
- stiff baby Q89.8
- stiff man G25.82
- Still-Felty — *see* Felty's syndrome
- Stokes (-Adams) I45.9
- stone heart I50.1
- straight back, congenital Q76.49
- subclavian steal G45.8

Syndrome—*continued*
- subcoracoid-pectoralis minor G54.0
- subcostal nerve compression I77.89
- subphrenic interposition Q43.3
- superior
  - cerebellar artery I63.8
  - mesenteric artery K55.1
  - vena cava I87.1
- supine hypotensive (maternal) — *see* Syndrome, hypotension, maternal
- suprarenal cortical E27.0
- supraspinatus M75.1-
- Susac G93.49
- swallowed blood P78.2
- sweat retention L74.0
- Swyer Q99.1
- Symond's G93.2
- sympathetic
  - cervical paralysis G90.2
  - pelvic, female N94.89
- systemic inflammatory response (SIRS), of non-infectious origin (without organ dysfunction) R65.10
  - with acute organ dysfunction R65.11
- tachycardia-bradycardia I49.5
- takotsubo I51.81
- TAR (thrombocytopenia with absent radius) Q87.2
- tarsal tunnel G57.5-
- teething K00.7
- tegmental G93.89
- telangiectasic-pigmentation-cataract Q82.8
- temporal pyramidal apex — *see* Otitis, media, suppurative, acute
- temporomandibular joint-pain-dysfunction M26.62
- Terry's — *see* Disorder, globe, degenerative, myopia
- testicular feminization (*see also* Syndrome, androgen insensitivity) E34.51
- thalamic pain (hyperesthetic) G89.0
- thoracic outlet (compression) G54.0
- Thorson-Björck E34.0
- thrombocytopenia with absent radius (TAR) Q87.2
- thyroid-adrenocortical insufficiency E31.0
- tibial
  - anterior M76.81-
  - posterior M76.82-
- Tietze's M94.0
- time-zone (rapid) G47.25
- Toni-Fanconi E72.09
  - with cystinosis E72.04
- Touraine's Q79.8
- tourniquet — *see* Constriction, external, by site
- toxic shock A48.3
- transient left ventricular apical ballooning I51.81
- traumatic vasospastic T75.22
- Treacher Collins Q75.4
- triple X, female Q97.0
- trisomy Q92.9
  - 13 Q91.7
    - meiotic nondisjunction Q91.4
    - mitotic nondisjunction Q91.5
    - mosaicism Q91.5
    - translocation Q91.6
  - 18 Q91.3
    - meiotic nondisjunction Q91.0
    - mitotic nondisjunction Q91.1
    - mosaicism Q91.1
    - translocation Q91.2
  - 20(q)(p) Q92.8
  - 21 Q90.9
    - meiotic nondisjunction Q90.0
    - mitotic nondisjunction Q90.1
    - mosaicism Q90.1
    - translocation Q90.2
  - 22 Q92.8
- tropical wet feet T69.0-
- Trousseau's I82.1
- tumor lysis (following antineoplastic chemotherapy) (spontaneous) NEC E88.3
- Twiddler's (due to)
  - automatic implantable defibrillator T82.198
  - cardiac pacemaker T82.198
- Unverricht (-Lundborg) — *see* Epilepsy, generalized, idiopathic

Syndrome—*continued*
  upward gaze H51.8
  uremia, chronic (*see also* Disease, kidney, chronic) N18.9
  urethral N34.3
  urethro-oculo-articular — *see* Reiter's disease
  urohepatic K76.7
  vago-hypoglossal G52.7
  vascular NEC in cerebrovascular disease G46.8
  vasomotor I73.9
  vasospastic (traumatic) T75.22
  vasovagal R55
  van Buchem's M85.2
  van der Hoeve's Q78.0
  VATER Q87.2
  velo-cardio-facial Q93.81
  vena cava (inferior) (superior) (obstruction) I87.1
  vertebral
      artery G45.0
          compression — *see* Syndrome, anterior, spinal artery, compression
      steal G45.0
  vertebro-basilar artery G45.0
  vertebrogenic (pain) M54.89
  vertiginous — *see* Disorder, vestibular function
  Vinson-Plummer D50.1
  virus B34.9
  visceral larva migrans B83.0
  visual disorientation H53.8
  vitamin B6 deficiency E53.1
  vitreal corneal H59.01-
  vitreous (touch) H59.01-
  Vogt-Koyanagi H20.82-
  Volkmann's T79.6
  von Schroetter's I82.890
  von Willebrand (-Jürgen) D68.0
  Waldenström-Kjellberg D50.1
  Wallenberg's I63.9
  water retention E87.79
  Waterhouse (-Friderichsen) A39.1
  Weber-Gubler G83.89
  Weber-Leyden G83.89
  Weber's G83.89
  Wegener's M31.30
      with
          kidney involvement M31.31
          lung involvement M31.30
              with kidney involvement M31.31
  Weingarten's (tropical eosinophilia) J82
  Weiss-Baker G90.09
  Werdnig-Hoffman G12.0
  Wermer's E31.21
  Wernicke-Korsakoff (nonalcoholic) F04
      alcoholic F10.26
  West's — *see* Epilepsy, generalized, specified NEC
  Westphal-Strümpell E83.01
  wet
      feet (maceration) (tropical) T69.0-
      lung, newborn P22.1
  whiplash S13.4
  whistling face Q87.0
  Wilkie's K55.1
  Wilkinson-Sneddon L13.1
  Willebrand (-Jürgens) D68.0
  Wilson's (hepatolenticular degeneration) D83.0
  Wiskott-Aldrich D82.0
  withdrawal — *see* Withdrawal, state
      drug
          infant of dependent mother P96.1
          therapeutic use, newborn P96.2
  Woakes' (ethmoiditis) J33.1
  Wright's (hyperabduction) I77.89
  X I20.9
  XXXX Q97.1
  XXXXX Q97.1
  XXXXY Q98.1
  XXY Q98.0
  yellow nail L60.5
  Zahorsky's B08.5
  Zellweger syndrome E71.510
  Zellweger-like syndrome E71.541

Synechia (anterior) (iris) (posterior) (pupil) (*see also* Adhesions, iris)
  intra-uterine (traumatic) N85.6
Synesthesia R20.8
Syngamiasis, syngamosis B83.3
Synodontia K00.2
Synorchidism, synorchism Q55.1
Synostosis (congenital) Q78.8
  astragalo-scaphoid Q74.2
  radioulnar Q74.0
Synovial sarcoma — *see* Neoplasm, connective tissue, malignant
Synovioma (malignant) (*see also* Neoplasm, connective tissue, malignant)
  benign — *see* Neoplasm, connective tissue, benign
Synoviosarcoma — *see* Neoplasm, connective tissue, malignant
Synovitis (*see also* Tenosynovitis)
  crepitant
      hand M70.0-
      wrist M70.03-
  gonococcal A54.49
  gouty — *see* Gout, idiopathic
  in (due to)
      crystals M65.8-
      gonorrhea A54.49
      syphilis (late) A52.78
      use, overuse, pressure — *see* Disorder, soft tissue, due to use
  infective NEC — *see* Tenosynovitis, infective NEC
  specified NEC — *see* Tenosynovitis, specified type NEC
  syphilitic A52.78
      congenital (early) A50.02
  toxic — *see* Synovitis, transient
  transient M67.3-
      ankle M67.37-
      elbow M67.32-
      foot joint M67.37-
      hand joint M67.34-
      hip M67.35-
      knee M67.36-
      multiple site M67.39
      pelvic region M67.35-
      shoulder M67.31-
      specified joint NEC M67.38
      wrist M67.33-
  traumatic, current — *see* Sprain
  tuberculous — *see* Tuberculosis, synovitis
  villonodular (pigmented) M12.2-
      ankle M12.27-
      elbow M12.22-
      foot joint M12.27-
      hand joint M12.24-
      hip M12.25-
      knee M12.26-
      multiple site M12.29
      pelvic region M12.25-
      shoulder M12.21-
      specified joint NEC M12.28
      wrist M12.23-
Syphilid A51.39
  congenital A50.06
  newborn A50.06
  tubercular (late) A52.79
Syphilis, syphilitic (acquired) A53.9
  abdomen (late) A52.79
  acoustic nerve A52.15
  adenopathy (secondary) A51.49
  adrenal (gland) (with cortical hypofunction) A52.79
  age under 2 years NOS (*see also* Syphilis, congenital, early)
      acquired A51.9
  alopecia (secondary) A51.32
  anemia (late) A52.79 [D63.8]
  aneurysm (aorta) (ruptured) A52.01
      central nervous system A52.05
      congenital A50.54 [I79.0]
  anus (late) A52.74
      primary A51.1
      secondary A51.39

Syphilis, syphilitic—*continued*
  aorta (arch) (abdominal) (thoracic) A52.02
      aneurysm A52.01
  aortic (insufficiency) (regurgitation) (stenosis) A52.03
      aneurysm A52.01
  arachnoid (adhesive) (cerebral) (spinal) A52.13
  asymptomatic — *see* Syphilis, latent
  ataxia (locomotor) A52.11
  atrophoderma maculatum A51.39
  auricular fibrillation A52.06
  bladder (late) A52.76
  bone A52.77
      secondary A51.46
  brain A52.17
  breast (late) A52.79
  bronchus (late) A52.72
  bubo (primary) A51.0
  bulbar palsy A52.19
  bursa (late) A52.78
  cardiac decompensation A52.06
  cardiovascular A52.00
  central nervous system (late) (recurrent) (relapse) (tertiary) A52.3
      with
          ataxia A52.11
          general paralysis A52.17
              juvenile A50.45
          paresis (general) A52.17
              juvenile A50.45
          tabes (dorsalis) A52.11
              juvenile A50.45
          taboparesis A52.11
              juvenile A50.45
      aneurysm A52.05
      congenital A50.40
      juvenile A50.40
      remission in (sustained) A52.3
      serology doubtful, negative, or positive A52.3
      specified nature or site NEC A52.19
      vascular A52.05
  cerebral A52.17
      meningovascular A52.13
      nerves (multiple palsies) A52.15
      sclerosis A52.17
      thrombosis A52.05
  cerebrospinal (tabetic type) A52.12
  cerebrovascular A52.05
  cervix (late) A52.76
  chancre (multiple) A51.0
      extragenital A51.2
      Rollet's A51.0
  Charcot's joint A52.16
  chorioretinitis A51.43
      congenital A50.01
      late A52.71
      prenatal A50.01
  choroiditis — *see* Syphilitic chorioretinitis
  choroidoretinitis — *see* Syphilitic chorioretinitis
  ciliary body (secondary) A51.43
      late A52.71
  colon (late) A52.74
  combined spinal sclerosis A52.11
  condyloma (latum) A51.31
  congenital A50.9
      with
          paresis (general) A50.45
          tabes (dorsalis) A50.45
          taboparesis A50.45
      chorioretinitis, choroiditis A50.01 [H32]
      early, or less than 2 years after birth NEC A50.2
          with manifestations — *see* Syphilis, congenital, early, symptomatic
          latent (without manifestations) A50.1
              negative spinal fluid test A50.1
              serology positive A50.1
          symptomatic A50.09
              cutaneous A50.06
              mucocutaneous A50.07
              oculopathy A50.01
              osteochondropathy A50.02
              pharyngitis A50.03
              pneumonia A50.04

Syphilis, syphilitic —*continued*
  congenital—*continued*
    early, or less than 2 years after birth—*continued*
      symptomatic—*continued*
        rhinitis A50.05
        visceral A50.08
    interstitial keratitis A50.31
    juvenile neurosyphilis A50.45
    late, or 2 years or more after birth NEC A50.7
      chorioretinitis, choroiditis A50.32
      interstitial keratitis A50.31
      juvenile neurosyphilis A50.45
      latent (without manifestations) A50.6
        negative spinal fluid test A50.6
        serology positive A50.6
      symptomatic or with manifestations NEC
        A50.59
        arthropathy A50.55
        cardiovascular A50.54
        Clutton's joints A50.51
        Hutchinson's teeth A50.52
        Hutchinson's triad A50.53
        osteochondropathy A50.56
        saddle nose A50.57
  conjugal A53.9
    tabes A52.11
  conjunctiva (late) A52.71
  contact Z20.2
  cord bladder A52.19
  cornea, late A52.71
  coronary (artery) (sclerosis) A52.06
  coryza, congenital A50.05
  cranial nerve A52.15
    multiple palsies A52.15
  cutaneous — *see* Syphilis, skin
  dacryocystitis (late) A52.71
  degeneration, spinal cord A52.12
  dementia paralytica A52.17
    juvenilis A50.45
  destruction of bone A52.77
  dilatation, aorta A52.01
  due to blood transfusion A53.9
  dura mater A52.13
  ear A52.79
    inner A52.79
      nerve (eighth) A52.15
      neurorecurrence A52.15
  early A51.9
    cardiovascular A52.00
    central nervous system A52.3
    latent (without manifestations) (less than 2 years
      after infection) A51.5
      negative spinal fluid test A51.5
      serological relapse after treatment A51.5
      serology positive A51.5
    relapse (treated, untreated) A51.9
    skin A51.39
    symptomatic A51.9
      extragenital chancre A51.2
      primary, except extragenital chancre A51.0
      secondary (*see also* Syphilis, secondary)
        A51.39
        relapse (treated, untreated) A51.49
    ulcer A51.39
  eighth nerve (neuritis) A52.15
  endemic A65
  endocarditis A52.03
    aortic A52.03
    pulmonary A52.03
  epididymis (late) A52.76
  epiglottis (late) A52.73
  epiphysitis (congenital) (early) A50.02 [M90.80]
  episcleritis (late) A52.71
  esophagus A52.79
  eustachian tube A52.73
  exposure to Z20.2
  eye A52.71
  eyelid (late) (with gumma) A52.71
  fallopian tube (late) A52.76
  fracture A52.77
  gallbladder (late) A52.74
  gastric (polyposis) (late) A52.74

Syphilis, syphilitic—*continued*
  general A53.9
    paralysis A52.17
      juvenile A50.45
  genital (primary) A51.0
  glaucoma A52.71
  gumma NEC A52.79
    cardiovascular system A52.00
    central nervous system A52.3
    congenital A50.59
  heart (block) (decompensation) (disease) (failure)
    A52.06 [I52]
    valve NEC A52.03
  hemianesthesia A52.19
  hemianopsia A52.71
  hemiparesis A52.17
  hemiplegia A52.17
  hepatic artery A52.09
  hepatis A52.74
  hepatomegaly, congenital A50.08
  hereditaria tarda — *see* Syphilis, congenital, late
  hereditary — *see* Syphilis, congenital
  Hutchinson's teeth A50.52
  hyalitis A52.71
  inactive — *see* Syphilis, latent
  infantum — *see* Syphilis, congenital
  inherited — *see* Syphilis, congenital
  internal ear A52.79
  intestine (late) A52.74
  iris, iritis (secondary) A51.43
    late A52.71
  joint (late) A52.77
  keratitis (congenital) (interstitial) (late) A50.31
  kidney (late) A52.75
  lacrimal passages (late) A52.71
  larynx (late) A52.73
  late A52.9
    cardiovascular A52.00
    central nervous system A52.3
    kidney A52.75
    latent or 2 years or more after infection (without
      manifestations) A52.8
      negative spinal fluid test A52.8
      serology positive A52.8
    paresis A52.17
    specified site NEC A52.79
    symptomatic or with manifestations A52.79
    tabes A52.11
  latent A53.0
  with signs or symptoms code by site and stage
    under Syphilis
    central nervous system A52.2
    date of infection unspecified A53.0
    early, or less than 2 years after infection A51.5
    follow-up of latent syphilis A53.0
      date of infection unspecified A53.0
      late, or 2 years or more after infection A52.8
    late, or 2 years or more after infection A52.8
    positive serology (only finding) A53.0
      date of infection unspecified A53.0
      early, or less than 2 years after infection A51.5
      late, or 2 years or more after infection A52.8
  lens (late) A52.71
  leukoderma A51.39
    late A52.79
  lienitis A52.79
  lip A51.39
    chancre (primary) A51.2
    late A52.79
  Lissauer's paralysis A52.17
  liver A52.74
  locomotor ataxia A52.11
  lung A52.72
  lymph gland (early) (secondary) A51.49
    late A52.79
  lymphadenitis (secondary) A51.49
  macular atrophy of skin A51.39
    striated A52.79
  mediastinum (late) A52.73
  meninges (adhesive) (brain) (spinal cord) A52.13
  meningitis A52.13
    acute (secondary) A51.41
    congenital A50.41

Syphilis, syphilitic—*continued*
  meningoencephalitis A52.14
  meningovascular A52.13
    congenital A50.41
  mesarteritis A52.09
    brain A52.04
  middle ear A52.77
  mitral stenosis A52.03
  monoplegia A52.17
  mouth (secondary) A51.39
    late A52.79
  mucocutaneous (secondary) A51.39
    late A52.79
  mucous
    membrane (secondary) A51.39
      late A52.79
    patches A51.39
      congenital A50.07
  mulberry molars A50.52
  muscle A52.78
  myocardium A52.06
  nasal sinus (late) A52.73
  neonatorum — *see* Syphilis, congenital
  nephrotic syndrome (secondary) A51.44
  nerve palsy (any cranial nerve) A52.15
    multiple A52.15
  nervous system, central A52.3
  neuritis A52.15
    acoustic A52.15
  neurorecidive of retina A52.19
  neuroretinitis A52.19
  newborn — *see* Syphilis, congenital
  nodular superficial (late) A52.79
  nonvenereal A65
  nose (late) A52.73
    saddle back deformity A50.57
  occlusive arterial disease A52.09
  oculopathy A52.71
  oesophagus (late) A52.79
  ophthalmic (late) A52.71
  optic nerve (atrophy) (neuritis) (papilla) A52.15
  orbit (late) A52.71
  organic A53.9
  osseous (late) A52.77
  osteochondritis (congenital) (early) A50.02 [M90.80]
  osteoporosis A52.77
  ovary (late) A52.76
  oviduct (late) A52.76
  palate (late) A52.79
  pancreas (late) A52.74
  paralysis A52.17
    general A52.17
      juvenile A50.45
  paresis (general) A52.17
    juvenile A50.45
  paresthesia A52.19
  Parkinson's disease or syndrome A52.19
  paroxysmal tachycardia A52.06
  pemphigus (congenital) A50.06
  penis (chancre) A51.0
    late A52.76
  pericardium A52.06
  perichondritis, larynx (late) A52.73
  periosteum (late) A52.77
    congenital (early) A50.02 [M90.80]
    early (secondary) A51.46
  peripheral nerve A52.79
  petrous bone (late) A52.77
  pharynx (late) A52.73
    secondary A51.39
  pituitary (gland) A52.79
  pleura (late) A52.73
  pneumonia, white A50.04
  pontine lesion A52.17
  portal vein A52.09
  primary A51.0
    anal A51.1
    and secondary — *see* Syphilis, secondary

Syphilis, syphilitic—*continued*
  primary 346
    central nervous system A52.3
    extragenital chancre NEC A51.2
    fingers A51.2
    genital A51.0
    lip A51.2
    specified site NEC A51.2
    tonsils A51.2
  prostate (late) A52.76
  ptosis (eyelid) A52.71
  pulmonary (late) A52.72
    artery A52.09
  pyelonephritis (late) A52.75
  recently acquired, symptomatic A51.9
  rectum (late) A52.74
  respiratory tract (late) A52.73
  retina, late A52.71
  retrobulbar neuritis A52.15
  salpingitis A52.76
  sclera (late) A52.71
  sclerosis
    cerebral A52.17
    coronary A52.06
    multiple A52.11
  scotoma (central) A52.71
  scrotum (late) A52.76
  secondary (and primary) A51.49
    adenopathy A51.49
    anus A51.39
    bone A51.46
    chorioretinitis, choroiditis A51.43
    hepatitis A51.45
    liver A51.45
    lymphadenitis A51.49
    meningitis (acute) A51.41
    mouth A51.39
    mucous membranes A51.39
    periosteum, periostitis A51.46
    pharynx A51.39
    relapse (treated, untreated) A51.49
    skin A51.39
    specified form NEC A51.49
    tonsil A51.39
    ulcer A51.39
    viscera NEC A51.49
    vulva A51.39
  seminal vesicle (late) A52.76
  seronegative with signs or symptoms — code by
    site and stage under Syphilis

Syphilis, syphilitic—*continued*
  seropositive
  with signs or symptoms — code by site and stage
      under Syphilis
    follow-up of latent syphilis — *see* Syphilis, latent
    only finding — *see* Syphilis, latent
  seventh nerve (paralysis) A52.15
  sinus, sinusitis (late) A52.73
  skeletal system A52.77
  skin (with ulceration) (early) (secondary) A51.39
    late or tertiary A52.79
  small intestine A52.74
  spastic spinal paralysis A52.17
  spermatic cord (late) A52.76
  spinal (cord) A52.12
  spleen A52.79
  splenomegaly A52.79
  spondylitis A52.77
  staphyloma A52.71
  stigmata (congenital) A50.59
  stomach A52.74
  synovium A52.78
  tabes dorsalis (late) A52.11
    juvenile A50.45
  tabetic type A52.11
    juvenile A50.45
  taboparesis A52.11
    juvenile A50.45
  tachycardia A52.06
  tendon (late) A52.78
  tertiary A52.9
    with symptoms NEC A52.79
    cardiovascular A52.00
    central nervous system A52.3
    multiple NEC A52.79
    specified site NEC A52.79
  testis A52.76
  thorax A52.73
  throat A52.73
  thymus (gland) (late) A52.79
  thyroid (late) A52.79
  tongue (late) A52.79
  tonsil (lingual) (late) A52.73
    primary A51.2
    secondary A51.39
  trachea (late) A52.73
  tunica vaginalis (late) A52.76
  ulcer (any site) (early) (secondary) A51.39
    late A52.79
    perforating A52.79
      foot A52.11

Syphilis, syphilitic—*continued*
  urethra (late) A52.76
  urogenital (late) A52.76
  uterus (late) A52.76
  uveal tract (secondary) A51.43
    late A52.71
  uveitis (secondary) A51.43
    late A52.71
  uvula (late) (perforated) A52.79
  vagina A51.0
    late A52.76
  valvulitis NEC A52.03
  vascular A52.00
    brain (cerebral) A52.05
  ventriculi A52.74
  vesicae urinariae (late) A52.76
  viscera (abdominal) (late) A52.74
    secondary A51.49
  vitreous (opacities) (late) A52.71
    hemorrhage A52.71
  vulva A51.0
    late A52.76
    secondary A51.39
Syphiloma A52.79
  cardiovascular system A52.00
  central nervous system A52.3
  circulatory system A52.00
  congenital A50.59
Syphilophobia F45.29
Syringadenoma (*see also* Neoplasm, skin, benign)
  papillary — *see* Neoplasm, skin, benign
Syringobulbia G95.0
Syringocystadenoma (*see also* Neoplasm, skin,
  benign)
  papillary — *see* Neoplasm, skin, benign
Syringoma (*see also* Neoplasm, skin, benign)
  chondroid — *see* Neoplasm, skin, benign
Syringomyelia G95.0
Syringomyelitis — *see* Encephalitis
Syringomyelocele — *see* Spina bifida
Syringopontia G95.0
System, systemic (*see also* condition)
  disease, combined — *see* Degeneration, combined
  inflammatory response syndrome (SIRS) of
      non-infectious origin (without organ
      dysfunction) R65.10
    with acute organ dysfunction R65.11
  lupus erythematosus M32.9
    inhibitor present D68.62

T

Tabacism, tabacosis, tabagism (*see also* Poisioning, tobacco)
  meaning dependence (without remission) F17.200
    with
      disorder F17.299
        remission F17.211
        specified disorder NEC F17.298
        withdrawal F17.203
Tabardillo A75.9
  flea-borne A75.2
  louse-borne A75.0
Tabes, tabetic A52.10
  with
    central nervous system syphilis A52.10
    Charcot's joint A52.16
    cord bladder A52.19
    crisis, viscera (any) A52.19
    paralysis, general A52.17
    paresis (general) A52.17
    perforating ulcer (foot) A52.19
  arthropathy (Charcot) A52.16
  bladder A52.19
  bone A52.11
  cerebrospinal A52.12
  congenital A50.45
  conjugal A52.10
  dorsalis A52.11
    juvenile A50.49
  juvenile A50.49
  latent A52.19
  mesenterica A18.39
  paralysis, insane, general A52.17
  spasmodic A52.17
  syphilis (cerebrospinal) A52.12
Taboparalysis A52.17
Taboparesis (remission) A52.17
  juvenile A50.45
TAC (trigeminal autonomic cephalgia) **NEC** G44.099
  intractable G44.091
  not intractable G44.099
Tache noir S60.22-
Tachyalimentation K91.2
Tachyarrhythmia, tachyrhythmia — *see* Tachycardia
Tachycardia R00.0
  atrial I47.1
  auricular I47.1
  AV nodal re-entry (re-entrant) I49.8
  newborn P29.11
  nodal I47.1
  non-paroxysmal AV nodal I45.89
  paroxysmal (sustained) (nonsustained) I47.9
    with sinus bradycardia I49.5
    atrial (PAT) I47.1
    atrioventricular (AV) I47.1
      psychogenic F54
    junctional I47.1
      ectopic I47.1
    nodal I47.1
    psychogenic (atrial) (supraventricular) (ventricular) F54
    supraventricular (sustained) I47.1
      psychogenic F54
    ventricular I47.2
      psychogenic F54
  psychogenic F45.8
  sick sinus I49.5
  sinoauricular NOS R00.0
    paroxysmal I47.1
  sinus [sinusal] NOS R00.0
    paroxysmal I47.1
  supraventricular I47.1
  ventricular (paroxysmal) (sustained) I47.2
    psychogenic F54
Tachygastria K31.89
Tachypnea R06.82
  hysterical F45.8
  newborn (idiopathic) (transitory) P22.1
  psychogenic F45.8
  transitory, of newborn P22.1

TACO (transfusion associated circulatory overload) E87.71
Taenia (infection) (infestation) B68.9
  diminuta B71.0
  echinococcal infestation B67.90
  mediocanellata B68.1
  nana B71.0
  saginata B68.1
  solium (intestinal form) B68.0
    larval form — *see* Cysticercosis
Taeniasis (intestine) — *see* Taenia
Tag (hypertrophied skin) (infected) L91.8
  adenoid J35.8
  anus I84.6
  hemorrhoidal I84.6
  hymen N89.8
  perineal N90.89
  preauricular Q17.0
  rectum I84.6
  sentinel I84.6
  skin L91.8
    accessory (congenital) Q82.8
    anus I84.6
    congenital Q82.8
    preauricular Q17.0
    rectum I84.6
  tonsil J35.8
  urethra, urethral N36.8
  vulva N90.89
Tahyna fever B33.8
Takahara's disease E80.3
Takayasu's disease or syndrome M31.4
Talcosis (pulmonary) J62.0
Talipes (congenital) Q66.8
  acquired, planus — *see* Deformity, limb, flat foot
  asymmetric Q66.8
  calcaneovalgus Q66.4
  calcaneovarus Q66.1
  calcaneus Q66.8
  cavus Q66.7
  equinovalgus Q66.6
  equinovarus Q66.0
  equinus Q66.8
  percavus Q66.7
  planovalgus Q66.6
  planus (acquired) (any degree) (*see also* Deformity, limb, flat foot)
    congenital Q66.5
    due to rickets (sequelae) E64.3
  valgus Q66.6
  varus Q66.3
Tall stature, constitutional E34.4
Talma's disease M62.89
Talon noir S90.3-
  hand S60.22-
  heel S90.3-
  toe S90.1-
Tamponade, heart I31.4
Tanapox (virus disease) B08.71
Tangier disease E78.6
Tantrum, child problem F91.8
Tapeworm (infection) (infestation) — *see* Infestation, tapeworm
Tapia's syndrome G52.7
TAR (thrombocytopenia with absent radius) **syndrome** Q87.2
Tarral-Besnier disease L44.0
Tarsal tunnel syndrome — *see* Syndrome, tarsal tunnel
Tarsalgia — *see* Pain, limb, lower
Tarsitis (eyelid) H01.8
  syphilitic A52.71
  tuberculous A18.4
Tartar (teeth) (dental calculus) K03.6
Tattoo (mark) L81.8
Tauri's disease E74.09
Taurodontism K00.2
Taussig-Bing syndrome Q20.1
Taybi's syndrome Q87.2
Tay-Sachs amaurotic familial idiocy or disease E75.02
TBI (traumatic brain injury) — *see* category S06
Teacher's node or nodule J38.2

Tear, torn (traumatic) (*see also* Laceration)
  with abortion — *see* Abortion
  anus, anal (sphincter) S31.831
    complicating delivery
      with third degree perineal laceration O70.2
        with mucosa O70.3
      without third degree perineal laceration O70.4
    nontraumatic (healed) (old) K62.81
  articular cartilage, old — *see* Derangement, joint, articular cartilage, by site
  bladder
    with ectopic or molar pregnancy O08.6
    following ectopic or molar pregnancy O08.6
    obstetrical O71.5
    traumatic — *see* Injury, bladder
  bowel
    with ectopic or molar pregnancy O08.6
    following ectopic or molar pregnancy O08.6
    obstetrical trauma O71.5
  broad ligament
    with ectopic or molar pregnancy O08.6
    following ectopic or molar pregnancy O08.6
    obstetrical trauma O71.6
  bucket handle (knee) (meniscus) — *see* Tear, meniscus
  capsule, joint — *see* Sprain
  cartilage (*see also* Sprain)
    articular, old — *see* Derangement, joint, articular cartilage, by site
  cervix
    with ectopic or molar pregnancy O08.6
    following ectopic or molar pregnancy O08.6
    obstetrical trauma (current) O71.3
    old N88.1
    traumatic *see* Injury, uterus
  dural G97.41
    nontraumatic G96.11
  internal organ — *see* Injury, by site
  knee cartilage
    articular (current) S83.3-
    old — *see* Derangement, knee, meniscus, due to old tear
  ligament — *see* Sprain
  meniscus (knee) (current injury) S83.209
    bucket-handle S83.20-
    lateral
      bucket-handle S83.25-
      complex S83.27-
      peripheral S83.26-
      specified type NEC S83.28-
    medial
      bucket-handle S83.21-
      complex S83.23-
      peripheral S83.22-
      specified type NEC S83.24-
    old — *see* Derangement, knee, meniscus, due to old tear
    site other than knee code as Sprain
    specified type NEC S83.20-
  muscle — *see* Strain
  pelvic
    floor, complicating delivery O70.1
    organ NEC, obstetrical trauma O71.5
      with ectopic or molar pregnancy O08.6
      following ectopic or molar pregnancy O08.6
  perineal, secondary O90.1
  periurethral tissue, obstetrical trauma O71.82
    with ectopic or molar pregnancy O08.6
    following ectopic or molar pregnancy O08.6
  rectovaginal septum — *see* Laceration, vagina
  retina, retinal (without detachment) (horseshoe) (*see also* Break, retina, horseshoe)
    with detachment — *see* Detachment, retina, with retinal, break
  rotator cuff (complete) (incomplete) (nontraumatic) M75.1-
    traumatic S46.01-
    capsule S43.42-
  semilunar cartilage, knee — *see* Tear, meniscus
  supraspinatus (complete) (incomplete) (nontraumatic) M75.1-
  tendon — *see* Strain

Tear, torn—continued
- tentorial, at birth P10.4
- umbilical cord
  - complicating delivery O69.89
- urethra
  - with ectopic or molar pregnancy O08.6
  - following ectopic or molar pregnancy O08.6
  - obstetrical trauma O71.5
- uterus — see Injury, uterus
- vagina — see Laceration, vagina
- vessel, from catheter — see Puncture, accidental
  - complicating surgery
- vulva, complicating delivery O70.0

Tear-stone — see Dacryolith

Teeth (see also condition)
- grinding
  - psychogenic F45.8
  - sleep related G47.63

Teething (syndrome) K00.7

Telangiectasia, telangiectasis (verrucous) I78.1
- ataxic (cerebellar) (Louis-Bar) G11.3
- familial I78.0
- hemorrhagic, hereditary (congenital) (senile) I78.0
- hereditary, hemorrhagic (congenital) (senile) I78.0
- retina H35.07-
- spider I78.1

Telephone scatologia F65.89

Telescoped bowel or intestine K56.1
- congenital Q43.8

Temperature
- body, high (of unknown origin) R50.9
- cold, trauma from T69.9
  - newborn P80.0
  - specified effect NEC T69.8

Temple — see condition

Temporal — see condition

Temporomandibular joint pain-dysfunction syndrome M26.62

Temporosphenoidal — see condition

Tendency
- bleeding — see Defect, coagulation
- suicide
  - meaning personal history of attempted suicide Z91.5
  - meaning suicidal ideation — see Ideation, suicidal
- to fall R29.6

Tenderness, abdominal R10.819
- epigastric R10.816
- generalized R10.817
- left lower quadrant R10.814
- left upper quadrant R10.812
- periumbilic R10.815
- right lower quadrant R10.813
- right upper quadrant R10.811
- rebound R10.829
  - epigastric R10.826
  - generalized R10.827
  - left lower quadrant R10.824
  - left upper quadrant R10.822
  - periumbilic R10.825
  - right lower quadrant R10.823
  - right upper quadrant R10.821

Tendinitis, tendonitis (see also Enthesopathy)
- Achilles M76.6-
- adhesive — see Tenosynovitis, specified type NEC
  - shoulder — see Capsulitis, adhesive
- bicipital M75.2-
- calcific M65.2-
  - ankle M65.27-
  - foot M65.27-
  - forearm M65.23-
  - hand M65.24-
  - lower leg M65.26-
  - multiple sites M65.29
  - pelvic region M65.25-
  - shoulder M75.3-
  - specified site NEC M65.28
  - thigh M65.25-
  - upper arm M65.22-
- due to use, overuse, pressure (see also Disorder, soft tissue, due to use)

Tendinitis, tendonitis —continued
- due to use, overuse, pressure —continued
  - specified NEC — see Disorder, soft tissue, due to use, specified NEC
- gluteal M76.0-
- patellar M76.5-
- peroneal M76.7-
- psoas M76.1-
- tibal (posterior) M76.82-
  - anterior M76.81-
- trochanteric — see Bursitis, hip, trochanteric

Tendon — see condition

Tendosynovitis — see Tenosynovitis

Tenesmus (rectal) R19.8
- vesical R30.1

Tennis elbow — see Epicondylitis, lateral

Tenonitis (see also Tenosynovitis)
- eye (capsule) H05.04-

Tenontosynovitis — see Tenosynovitis

Tenontothecitis — see Tenosynovitis

Tenophyte — see Disorder, synovium, specified type NEC

Tenosynovitis (see also Synovitis) M65.9
- adhesive — see Tenosynovitis, specified type NEC
  - shoulder — see Capsulitis, adhesive
- bicipital (calcifying) — see Tendinitis, bicipital
- gonococcal A54.49
- in (due to)
  - crystals M65.8-
  - gonorrhea A54.49
  - syphilis (late) A52.78
  - use, overuse, pressure (see also Disorder, soft tissue, due to use)
    - specified NEC — see Disorder, soft tissue, due to use, specified NEC
- infective NEC M65.1-
  - ankle M65.17-
  - foot M65.17-
  - forearm M65.13-
  - hand M65.14-
  - lower leg M65.16-
  - multiple sites M65.19
  - pelvic region M65.15-
  - shoulder region M65.11-
  - specified site NEC M65.18
  - thigh M65.15-
  - upper arm M65.12-
- radial styloid M65.4
- shoulder region M65.81-
  - adhesive — see Capsulitis, adhesive
- specified type NEC M65.88-
  - ankle M65.87-
  - foot M65.87-
  - forearm M65.83-
  - hand M65.84-
  - lower leg M65.86-
  - multiple sites M65.89
  - pelvic region M65.85-
  - shoulder region M65.81-
  - specified site NEC M65.88
  - thigh M65.85-
  - upper arm M65.82-
- tuberculous — see Tuberculosis, tenosynovitis

Tenovaginitis — see Tenosynovitis

Tension
- arterial, high (see also Hypertension)
  - without diagnosis of hypertension R03.0
- headache G44.209
  - intractable G44.201
  - not intractable G44.209
- nervous R45.0
- pneumothorax J93.0
- premenstrual N94.3
- state (mental) F48.9

Tentorium — see condition

Teratencephalus Q89.8

Teratism Q89.7

Teratoblastoma (malignant) — see Neoplasm, malignant, by site

Teratocarcinoma (see also Neoplasm, malignant, by site)
- liver C22.7

Teratoma (solid) (see also Neoplasm, uncertain behavior, by site)
- with embryonal carcinoma, mixed — see Neoplasm, malignant, by site
- with malignant transformation — see Neoplasm, malignant, by site
- adult (cystic) — see Neoplasm, benign, by site
- benign — see Neoplasm, benign, by site
- combined with choriocarcinoma — see Neoplasm, malignant, by site
- cystic (adult) — see Neoplasm, benign, by site
- differentiated — see Neoplasm, benign, by site
- embryonal (see also Neoplasm, malignant, by site)
  - liver C22.7
- immature — see Neoplasm, malignant, by site
- liver C22.7
  - adult, benign, cystic, differentiated type or mature D13.4
- malignant (see also Neoplasm, malignant, by site)
  - anaplastic — see Neoplasm, malignant, by site
  - intermediate — see Neoplasm, malignant, by site
    - specified site — see Neoplasm, malignant, by site
    - unspecified site C62.90
  - undifferentiated — see Neoplasm, malignant, by site
- mature — see Neoplasm, uncertain behavior, by site
  - malignant — see Neoplasm, by site, malignant, by site
- ovary D27.-
  - embryonal, immature or malignant C56.-
- solid — see Neoplasm, uncertain behavior, by site
- testis C62.9-
  - adult, benign, cystic, differentiated type or mature D29.2-
  - scrotal C62.1-
  - undescended C62.0-

Termination
- anomalous (see also Malposition, congenital)
  - right pulmonary vein Q26.3
- pregnancy, elective Z33.2

Ternidens diminutus infestation B81.8

Ternidensiasis B81.8

Terror(s) night (child) F51.4

Terrorism, victim of Z65.4

Terry's syndrome — see Disorder, globe, degenerative, myopia

Tertiary — see condition

Test, tests, testing (for)
- adequacy (for dialysis)
  - hemodialysis Z49.31
  - peritoneal Z49.32
- blood pressure Z01.30
  - abnormal reading — see Blood, pressure
- blood-alcohol Z04.8
  - positive — see Findings, abnormal, in blood
- blood-drug Z04.8
  - positive — see Findings, abnormal, in blood
- blood typing Z01.83
  - Rh typing Z01.83
- cardiac pulse generator (battery) Z45.010
- fertility Z31.41
- genetic
  - disease carrier status for procreative management
    - female Z31.430
    - male Z31.440
  - male partner of patient with recurrent pregnancy loss Z31.441
  - procreative management NEC
    - female Z31.438
    - male Z31.448
- hearing Z01.10
  - with abnormal findings NEC Z01.118
- HIV (human immunodeficiency virus)
  - nonconclusive (in infants) R75
  - positive Z21
  - seropositive Z21
- immunity status Z01.84
- intelligence NEC Z01.89
- laboratory (as part of a general medical examination) Z00.00
  - with abnormal finding Z00.01

Test, tests, testing —continued
- laboratory—continued
  - for medicolegal reason NEC Z04.8
  - male partner of patient with recurrent pregnancy loss Z31.411
  - Mantoux (for tuberculosis) Z11.1
    - abnormal result R76.1
  - pregnancy, positive first pregnancy — see Pregnancy, normal, first
  - procreative Z31.49
    - fertility Z31.41
  - skin, diagnostic
    - allergy Z01.82
      - special screening examination — see Screening, by name of disease
    - Mantoux Z11.1
    - tuberculin Z11.1
  - specified NEC Z01.89
  - tuberculin Z11.1
    - abnormal result R76.1
  - vision Z01.00
    - with abnormal findings Z01.01
  - Wassermann Z11.3
    - positive — see Serology for syphilis, positive
- **Testicle, testicular, testis** (see also condition)
  - feminization syndrome (see also Syndrome, androgen insensitivity) E34.50
  - migrans Q55.29
- **Tetanus, tetanic** (cephalic) (convulsions) A35
  - with
    - abortion A34
    - ectopic or molar pregnancy O08.0
  - following ectopic or molar pregnancy O08.0
  - inoculation reaction (due to serum) — see Complications, vaccination
  - neonatorum A33
  - obstetrical A34
  - puerperal, postpartum, childbirth A34
- **Tetany** (due to) R29.0
  - alkalosis E87.3
  - associated with rickets E55.0
  - convulsions R29.0
    - hysterical F44.5
  - functional (hysterical) F44.5
  - hyperkinetic R29.0
    - hysterical F44.5
  - hyperpnea R06.4
    - hysterical F44.5
    - psychogenic F45.8
  - hyperventilation (see also Hyperventilation) R06.4
    - hysterical F44.5
  - neonatal (without calcium or magnesium deficiency) P71.3
  - parathyroid (gland) E20.9
  - parathyroprival E89.2
  - post-(para)thyroidectomy E89.2
  - postoperative E89.2
  - pseudotetany R29.0
  - psychogenic (conversion reaction) F44.5
- **Tetralogy of Fallot** Q21.3
- **Tetraplegia** (chronic) (see also Quadriplegia) G82.50 -
- **Thailand hemorrhagic fever** A91
- **Thalassanemia** — see Thalassemia
- **Thalassemia** (anemia) (disease) D56.9
  - with other hemoglobinopathy NEC D56.9
  - alpha (major) (severe) (triple gene defect) D56.0
    - minor D56.3
  - beta (severe) D56.1
    - minor D56.3
  - delta-beta (homozygous) D56.2
    - minor D56.3
  - intermedia D56.1
  - major D56.1
  - minor D56.3
  - mixed (with other hemoglobinopathy) D56.9
  - sickle cell — see Disease, sickle cell, thalassemia
  - specified type NEC D56.8
  - trait D56.3
  - variants D56.8
- **Thanatophoric dwarfism or short stature** Q77.1
- **Thaysen-Gee disease** (nontropical sprue) K90.0
- **Thaysen's disease** K90.0

Thecoma D27.-
- luteinized D27.-
- malignant C56.-
Thelarche, premature E30.8
Thelaziasis B83.8
Thelitis N61
- puerperal, postpartum or gestational — see Infection, nipple
Therapeutic — see condition
Therapy
- drug, long-term (current) (prophylactic)
  - agents affecting estrogen receptors and estrogen levels NEC Z79.818
  - anastrozole (Arimidex) Z79.811
  - antibiotics Z79.2
    - short-term use — omit code
  - anticoagulants Z79.01
  - anti-inflammatory Z79.1
  - antiplatelet Z79.02
  - antithrombotics Z79.02
  - aromatase inhibitors Z79.811
  - aspirin Z79.82
  - birth control pill or patch Z79.3
  - contraceptive, oral Z79.3
  - drug, specified NEC Z79.899
  - estrogen receptor downregulators Z79.818
  - Evista Z79.810
  - exemestane (Aromasin) Z79.811
  - Fareston Z79.810
  - fulvestrant (Faslodex) Z79.818
  - gonadotropin-releasing hormone (GnRH) agonist Z79.818
  - goserelin acetate (Zoladex) Z79.818
  - hormone replacement (postmenopausal) Z79.890
  - insulin Z79.4
  - letrozole (Femara) Z79.811
  - leuprolide acetate (leuprorelin) (Lupron) Z79.818
  - megestrol acetate (Megace) Z79.818
  - methadone for pain management Z79.891
  - Nolvadex Z79.810
  - opiate analgesic Z79.891
  - oral contraceptive Z79.3
  - raloxifene (Evista) Z79.810
  - short term — omit code
  - selective estrogen receptor modulators (SERMs) Z79.810
  - steroids
    - inhaled Z79.51
    - systemic Z79.52
  - tamoxifen (Nolvadex) Z79.810
  - toremifene (Fareston) Z79.810
Thermic — see condition
Thermography (abnormal) R93.8
- breast R92.8
Thermoplegia T67.0
Thesaurismosis, glycogen — see Disease, glycogen storage
Thiamin deficiency E51.9
- specified NEC E51.8
Thiaminic deficiency with beriberi E51.11
Thibierge-Weissenbach syndrome — see Sclerosis, systemic
Thickening
- bone — see Hypertrophy, bone
- breast N64.59
- epidermal L85.9
  - specified NEC L85.8
- hymen N89.6
- larynx J38.7
- nail L60.2
  - congenital Q84.5
- periosteal — see Hypertrophy, bone
- pleura J92.9
  - with asbestos J92.0
- skin R23.4
- subepiglottic J38.7
- tongue K14.8
- valve, heart — see Endocarditis
Thigh — see condition
Thinning vertebra — see Spondylopathy, specified NEC

Thirst, excessive R63.1
- due to deprivation of water T73.1
Thomsen disease G71.12
Thoracic (see also condition)
- kidney Q63.2
- outlet syndrome G54.0
Thoracogastroschisis (congenital) Q79.8
Thoracopagus Q89.4
Thorax — see condition
Thorn's syndrome N28.89
Thorson-Björck syndrome E34.0
Threadworm (infection) (infestation) B80
Threatened
- abortion O20.0
  - with subsequent abortion O03.9
- job loss, anxiety concerning Z56.2
- labor (without delivery) O47.9
  - after 37 completed weeks of gestation O47.1
  - before 37 completed weeks of gestation O47.0-
- loss of job, anxiety concerning Z56.2
- miscarriage O20.0
- unemployment, anxiety concerning Z56.2
Three-day fever A93.1
ThresHers' lung J67.0
Thrix annulata (congenital) Q84.1
Throat — see condition
Thrombasthenia (Glanzmann) (hemorrhagic) (hereditary) D69.1
Thromboangiitis I73.1
- obliterans (general) I73.1
  - cerebral I67.8
  - vessels
    - brain I67.8
    - spinal cord I67.8
Thromboarteritis — see Arteritis
Thromboasthenia (Glanzmann) (hemorrhagic) (hereditary) D69.1
Thrombocytasthenia (Glanzmann) D69.1
Thrombocythemia (essential) (hemorrhagic) (idiopathic) (primary) D47.3
Thrombocytopathy (dystrophic) (granulopenic) D69.1
Thrombocytopenia, thrombocytopenic D69.6
- with absent radius (TAR) Q87.2
- congenital D69.42
- dilutional D69.59
- due to
  - drugs D69.59
  - extracorporeal circulation of blood D69.59
  - (massive) blood transfusion D69.59
  - platelet alloimmunization D69.59
- essential D69.3
- heparin induced (HIT) D75.82
- hereditary D69.42
- idiopathic D69.3
- neonatal, transitory P61.0
  - due to
    - exchange transfusion P61.0
    - idiopathic maternal thrombocytopenia P61.0
    - isoimmunization P61.0
- primary NEC D69.49
  - idiopathic D69.3
- puerperal, postpartum O72.3
- secondary D69.59
- transient neonatal P61.0
Thrombocytosis, essential D47.3
- primary D47.3
Thromboembolism — see Embolism
Thrombopathy (Bernard-Soulier) D69.1
- constitutional D68.0
- Willebrand-Jurgens D68.0
Thrombopenia — see Thrombocytopenia
Thrombophilia D68.59
- primary NEC D68.59
- secondary NEC D68.69
- specified NEC D68.69
Thrombophlebitis I80.9
- antepartum O22.2-
  - deep O22.3-
  - superficial O22.2-
- cavernous (venous) sinus G08
  - complicating pregnancy O22.5-
  - nonpyogenic I67.6
- cerebral (sinus) (vein) G08

Thrombophlebitis—continued
cerebral (sinus) (vein) G08
  nonpyogenic I67.6
  sequelae G09
due to implanted device — see Complications, by
  site and type, specified NEC
during or resulting from a procedure NEC T81.72
femoral vein (superficial) I80.1-
femoropopliteal vein I80.0-
hepatic (vein) I80.8
idiopathic, recurrent I82.1
iliofemoral I80.1-
intracranial venous sinus (any) G08
  nonpyogenic I67.6
  sequelae G09
intraspinal venous sinuses and veins G08
  nonpyogenic G95.19
lateral (venous) sinus G08
  nonpyogenic I67.6
leg I80.299
  superficial I80.0-
longitudinal (venous) sinus G08
  nonpyogenic I67.6
lower extremity I80.299
migrans, migrating I82.1
pelvic
  with ectopic or molar pregnancy O08.0
  following ectopic or molar pregnancy O08.0
  puerperal O87.1
popliteal vein — see Phlebitis, leg, deep, popliteal
portal (vein) K75.1
postoperative T81.72
pregnancy — see Thrombophlebitis, antepartum
puerperal, postpartum, childbirth O87.0
  deep O87.1
  pelvic O87.1
  septic O86.81
  superficial O87.0
saphenous (greater) (lesser) I80.0-
sinus (intracranial) G08
  nonpyogenic I67.6
specified site NEC I80.8
tibial vein I80.23-

Thrombosis, thrombotic (bland) (multiple)
  (progressive) (silent) (vessel) I82.90
antepartum — see Thrombophlebitis, antepartum
aorta, aortic I74.10
  abdominal I74.0
  bifurcation I74.0
  saddle I74.0
  specified site NEC I74.19
  terminal I74.0
  thoracic I74.11
  valve — see Endocarditis, aortic
apoplexy I63.3
artery, arteries (postinfectional) I74.9
  auditory, internal — see Occlusion, artery,
    precerebral, specified NEC
  basilar — see Occlusion, artery, basilar
  carotid (common) (internal) — see Occlusion,
    artery, carotid
  cerebellar (anterior inferior) (posterior inferior)
    (superior) — see Occlusion, artery,
    cerebellar
  cerebral — see Occlusion, artery, cerebral
  choroidal (anterior) — see Occlusion, artery,
    cerebral, specified NEC
  communicating, posterior — see Occlusion,
    artery, cerebral, specified NEC
  coronary (see also Infarct, myocardium)
    not resulting in infarction I24.0
  hepatic I74.8
  hypophyseal — see Occlusion, artery, cerebral,
    specified NEC
  iliac I74.5
  limb I74.4
    lower I74.3
    upper I74.2
  meningeal, anterior or posterior — see Occlusion,
    artery, cerebral, specified NEC
  mesenteric (with gangrene) K55.0
  ophthalmic — see Occlusion, artery, retina

Thrombosis, thrombotic —continued
artery, arteries—continued
  pontine — see Occlusion, artery, cerebral,
    specified NEC
  precerebral — see Occlusion, artery, precerebral
  pulmonary (iatrogenic) — see Embolism,
    pulmonary
  renal N28.0
  retinal — see Occlusion, artery, retina
  spinal, anterior or posterior G95.11
  traumatic NEC T14.8
  vertebral — see Occlusion, artery, vertebral
atrium, auricular (see also Infarct, myocardium)
  following acute myocardial infarction (current
    complication) I23.6
  not resulting in infarction I24.0
basilar (artery) — see Occlusion, artery, basilar
brain (artery) (stem) (see also Occlusion, artery,
  cerebral)
  due to syphilis A52.05
  puerperal O99.43
  sinus — see Thrombosis, intracranial venous
    sinus
capillary I78.8
cardiac (see also Infarct, myocardium)
  not resulting in infarction I24.0
  valve — see Endocarditis
carotid (artery) (common) (internal) — see
  Occlusion, artery, carotid
cavernous (venous) sinus — see Thrombosis,
  intracranial venous sinus
cerebellar artery (anterior inferior) (posterior
  inferior) (superior) I65.8
cerebral (artery) — see Occlusion, artery, cerebral
cerebrovenous sinus (see also Thrombosis,
  intracranial venous sinus)
  puerperium O87.3
chronic I82.91
coronary (artery) (vein) (see also Infarct,
  myocardium)
  not resulting in infarction I24.0
corpus cavernosum N48.89
cortical I66.9
deep — see Embolism, vein, lower extremity
due to device, implant or graft (see also
  Complications, by site and type, specified
  NEC) T85.86
  arterial graft NEC T82.868
  breast (implant) T85.86
  catheter NEC T85.86
    dialysis (renal) T82.868
      intraperitoneal T85.86
    infusion NEC T82.868
      spinal (epidural) (subdural) T85.86
    urinary (indwelling) T83.86
  electronic (electrode) (pulse generator)
    (stimulator)
    bone T84.86
    cardiac T82.867
    nervous system (brain) (peripheral nerve)
      (spinal) T85.86
    urinary T83.86
  fixation, internal (orthopedic) NEC T84.86
  gastrointestinal (bile duct) (esophagus) T85.86
  genital NEC T83.86
  heart T82.867
  joint prosthesis T84.86
  ocular (corneal graft) (orbital implant) NEC
    T85.86
  orthopedic NEC T84.86
  specified NEC T85.86
  urinary NEC T83.86
  vascular NEC T82.868
  ventricular intracranial shunt T85.86
during the puerperium — see Thrombosis,
  puerperal
endocardial (see also Infarct, myocardium)
  not resulting in infarction I24.0
eye — see Occlusion, retina
genital organ
  female NEC N94.89
    pregnancy — see Thrombophlebitis,
      antepartum

Thrombosis, thrombotic —continued
genital organ—continued
  male N50.1
gestational — see Phlebopathy, gestational
heart (chamber) (see also Infarct, myocardium)
  not resulting in infarction I24.0
hepatic (vein) I82.0
  artery I74.8
history (of) Z86.71
intestine (with gangrene) K55.0
intracardiac NEC (apical) (atrial) (auricular)
  (ventricular) (old) I51.3
intracranial (arterial) I66.9
  venous sinus (any) G08
    nonpyogenic origin I67.6
    puerperium O87.3
intramural (see also Infarct, myocardium)
  not resulting in infarction I24.0
intraspinal venous sinuses and veins G08
  nonpyogenic G95.19
kidney (artery) N28.0
lateral (venous) sinus — see Thrombosis, intracranial
  venous sinus
leg — see Thrombosis, vein, lower extremity
  arterial I74.3
liver (venous) I82.0
  artery I74.8
  portal vein I81
longitudinal (venous) sinus — see Thrombosis,
  intracranial venous sinus
lower limb — see Thrombosis, vein, lower extremity
lung (iatrogenic) (postoperative) — see Embolism,
  pulmonary
meninges (brain) (arterial) I66.8
mesenteric (artery) (with gangrene) K55.0
  vein (inferior) (superior) I81
mitral I34.8
mural (see also Infarct, myocardium)
  due to syphilis A52.06
  not resulting in infarction I24.0
omentum (with gangrene) K55.0
ophthalmic — see Occlusion, artery, retina
pampiniform plexus (male) N50.1
parietal (see also Infarct, myocardium)
  not resulting in infarction I24.0
penis, superficial vein N48.81
peripheral arteries I74.4
  upper I74.3
personal history (of) Z86.71
portal I81
  due to syphilis A52.09
precerebral artery — see Occlusion, artery,
  precerebral
puerperal, postpartum O87.0
  brain (artery) O99.43
    venous (sinus) O87.3
  cardiac O99.43
  cerebral (artery) O99.43
    venous (sinus) O87.3
  superficial O87.0
pulmonary (artery) (iatrogenic) (postoperative)
  (vein) — see Embolism, pulmonary
renal (artery) N28.0
  vein I82.3
resulting from presence of device, implant or graft
  — see Complications, by site and type,
    specified NEC
retina, retinal — see Occlusion, retina
scrotum N50.1
seminal vesicle N50.1
sigmoid (venous) sinus — see Thrombosis,
  intracranial venous sinus
sinus, intracranial (any) — see Thrombosis,
  intracranial venous sinus
specified site NEC I82.890
  chronic I82.891
spermatic cord N50.1
spinal cord (arterial) G95.11
  due to syphilis A52.09
  pyogenic origin G06.1
spleen, splenic D73.5
  artery I74.8
testis N50.1

Thrombosis, thrombotic —*continued*
  tumor — *see* Neoplasm, unspecified behavior, by
     site
  traumatic NEC T14.8
  tricuspid I07.8
  tunica vaginalis N50.1
  umbilical cord (vessels), complicating delivery O69.5
  vas deferens N50.1
  vein (acute) I82.90
    antecubital I82.61-
      chronic I82.71-
    axillary I82.a1-
      chronic I82.a2-
    basilic I82.61-
      chronic I82.71-
    brachial I82.62-
      chronic I82.72-
    brachiocephalic (innominate) I82.290
      chronic I82.291
    cephalic I82.61-
      chronic I82.71-
    chronic I82.91
    deep (DVT) I82.40-
      calf I82.4z-
        chronic I82.5z-
      lower leg I82.4z-
        chronic I82.5z
      thigh I82.4Y
        chronic I82.5y
      upper extremity I82.70-
      upper leg I82.4y
        chronic I82.5y-
    femoral I82.41-
      chronic I82.51-
    iliac (iliofemoral) I82.42-
      chronic I82.52
    innominate I82.290
      chronic I82.291
    internal jugular I82.c1-
      chronic I82.c2
    lower extremity
      deep I82.40-
        chronic I82.50-
        specified NEC I82.49-
          chronic NEC I82.59-
      distal
        deep I82.4z
      proximal
        deep I82.4y
          chronic I82.5y-
      superficial I82.81-
    popliteal I82.43-
      chronic I82.53-
    radial I82.62-
      chronic I82.72
    renal I82.3
    saphenous (greater) (lesser) I82.81-
    specified NEC I82.890
      chronic NEC I82.891
    subclavian I82.b1-
      chronic I82.b2-
    thoracic NEC I82.290
      chronic I82.291
    tibial I82.44-
      chronic I82.54-
    ulnar I82.62-
      chronic I82.72-
    upper extremity I82.60-
      chronic I82.70-
      deep I82.62-
        chronic I82.72-
      superficial I82.61-
        chronic I82.71-
  vena cava
    inferior I82.220
      chronic I82.221
    superior I82.210
      chronic I82.211
  ventricle (*see also* Infarct, myocardium)
    following acute myocardial infarction (current
      complication) I23.6
    not resulting in infarction I24.0
Thrombus — *see* Thrombosis

Thrush (*see also* Candidiasis)
  oral B37.0
  newborn P37.5
  vaginal B37.3
Thumb (*see also* condition)
  sucking (child problem) F98.8
Thymitis E32.8
Thymoma (benign) D15.0
  malignant C37
Thymus, thymic (gland) — *see* condition
Thyrocele — *see* Goiter
Thyroglossal (*see also* condition)
  cyst Q89.2
  duct, persistent Q89.2
Thyroid (gland) (body) (*see also* condition)
  hormone resistance E07.89
  lingual Q89.2
  nodule (cystic) (nontoxic) (single) E04.1
Thyroiditis E06.9
  acute (nonsuppurative) (pyogenic) (suppurative)
    E06.0
  autoimmune E06.3
  chronic (nonspecific) (sclerosing) E06.5
    with thyrotoxicosis, transient E06.2
    fibrous E06.5
    lymphadenoid E06.3
    lymphocytic E06.3
    lymphoid E06.3
  de Quervain's E06.1
  drug-induced E06.4
  fibrous (chronic) E06.5
  giant-cell (follicular) E06.1
  granulomatous (de Quervain) (subacute) E06.1
  Hashimoto's (struma lymphomatosa) E06.3
  iatrogenic E06.4
  ligneous E06.5
  lymphocytic (chronic) E06.3
  lymphoid E06.3
  lymphomatous E06.3
  nonsuppurative E06.1
  postpartum, puerperal O90.5
  pseudotuberculous E06.1
  pyogenic E06.0
  radiation E06.4
  Riedel's E06.5
  subacute (granulomatous) E06.1
  suppurative E06.0
  tuberculous A18.81
  viral E06.1
  woody E06.5
Thyrolingual duct, persistent Q89.2
Thyromegaly E01.0
Thyrotoxic
  crisis — *see* Thyrotoxicosis
  heart disease or failure (*see also* Thyrotoxicosis)
    E05.90 [I43]
    with thyroid storm E05.91 [I43]
  storm — *see* Thyrotoxicosis
Thyrotoxicosis (recurrent) E05.90
  with
    goiter (diffuse) E05.00
      with thyroid storm E05.01
      adenomatous uninodular E05.10
        with thyroid storm E05.11
      multinodular E05.20
        with thyroid storm E05.21
      nodular E05.20
        with thyroid storm E05.21
      uninodular E05.10
        with thyroid storm E05.11
    thyroid storm E05.91
    infiltrative
      dermopathy E05.00
        with thyroid storm E05.01
      ophthalmopathy E05.00
        with thyroid storm E05.01
    single thyroid nodule E05.10
      with thyroid storm E05.11
    thyroid storm E05.91
  due to
    ectopic thyroid nodule or tissue E05.30
      with thyroid storm E05.31
    ingestion of (excessive) thyroid material E05.40

Thyrotoxicosis —*continued*
  due to—*continued*
    ingestion of thyroid material—*continued*
      with thyroid storm E05.41
    overproduction of thyroid-stimulating hormone
      E05.80
      with thyroid storm E05.81
    specified cause NEC E05.80
      with thyroid storm E05.81
    factitia E05.40
      with thyroid storm E05.41
    heart E05.90 [I43]
      with thyroid storm E05.91 [I43]
      failure E05.90 [I43]
    neonatal (transient) P72.1
    transient with chronic thyroiditis E06.2
Tibia vara — *see* Osteochondrosis, juvenile, tibia
Tic (disorder) F95.9
  breathing F95.8
  child problem F95.0
  compulsive F95.1
  de la Tourette F95.2
  degenerative (generalized) (localized) G25.69
    facial G25.69
  disorder
    chronic
      motor F95.1
      vocal F95.1
    combined vocal and multiple motor F95.2
    transient F95.0
  douloureux G50.0
    atypical G50.1
    postherpetic, postzoster B02.22
  drug-induced G25.61
  eyelid F95.8
  habit F95.9
    chronic F95.1
    transient of childhood F95.0
  lid, transient of childhood F95.0
  motor-verbal F95.2
  occupational F48.8
  orbicularis F95.8
    transient of childhood F95.0
  organic origin G25.69
  postchoreic G25.69
  psychogenic, compulsive F95.1
  salaam R25.8
  spasm (motor or vocal) F95.9
    chronic F95.1
    transient of childhood F95.0
  specified NEC F95.8
Tick-borne — *see* condition
Tietze's disease or syndrome M94.0
Tight, tightness
  anus K62.8
  chest R07.89
  fascia (lata) M62.89
  foreskin (congenital) N47.1
  hymen, hymenal ring N89.6
  introitus (acquired) (congenital) N89.6
  rectal sphincter K62.8
  tendon — *see* Short, tendon
  urethral sphincter N35.9
Tilting vertebra — *see* Dorsopathy, deforming,
  specified NEC
Timidity, child F93.8
Tin-miner's lung J63.5
Tinea (intersecta) (tarsi) B35.9
  amiantacea L44.8
  asbestina B35.0
  barbae B35.0
  beard B35.0
  black dot B35.0
  blanca B36.2
  capitis B35.0
  corporis B35.4
  cruris B35.6
  flava B36.0
  foot B35.3
  furfuracea B36.0
  imbricata (Tokelau) B35.5
  kerion B35.0
  manuum B35.2

Tinea —continued
microsporic — see Dermatophytosis
nigra B36.1
nodosa — see Piedra
pedis B35.3
scalp B35.0
specified site NEC B35.8
sycosis B35.0
tonsurans B35.0
trichophytic — see Dermatophytosis
unguium B35.1
versicolor B36.0
Tingling sensation (skin) R20.2
Tinnitus (audible) (aurium) (subjective) — see
subcategory H93.1
Tipped tooth (teeth) M26.33
Tipping
pelvis M95.5
with disproportion (fetopelvic) O33.0
causing obstructed labor O65.0
tooth (teeth), fully erupted M26.33
Tiredness R53.83
Tissue — see condition
Tobacco (nicotine)
dependence — see Dependence, drug, nicotine
harmful use Z72.0
heart — see Tobacco, toxic effect
maternal use, affecting newborn P04.2
toxic effect — see Table of Drugs and Chemicals, by
substance, poisoning
chewing tobacco — see Table of Drugs and
Chemicals, by substance, poisoning
cigarettes — see Table of Drugs and Chemicals,
by substance, poisoning
use Z72.0
complicating
childbirth O99.334
pregnancy O99.33-
puerperium O99.335
counseling and surveillance Z71.6
withdrawal state — see Dependence, drug, nicotine
Tocopherol deficiency E56.0
Todd's
cirrhosis K74.3
paralysis (postepileptic) (transitory) G83.84
Toe — see condition
Toilet, artificial opening — see Attention to, artificial,
opening
Tokelau (ringworm) B35.5
Tollwut — see Rabies
Tommaselli's disease R31.9
correct substance properly administered — see
Table of Drugs and Chemicals, by drug,
adverse effect
overdose or wrong substance given or taken — see
Table of Drugs and Chemicals, by drug,
poisoning
Tongue (see also condition)
tie Q38.1
Tonic pupil — see Anomaly, pupil, function, tonic pupil
Toni-Fanconi syndrome (cystinosis) E72.09
with cystinosis E72.04
Tonsil — see condition
Tonsillitis (acute) (catarrhal) (croupous) (follicular)
(gangrenous) (infective) (lacunar) (lingual)
(malignant) (membranous) (parenchymatous)
(phlegmonous) (pseudomembranous) (purulent)
(septic) (subacute) (suppurative) (toxic)
(ulcerative) (vesicular) (viral) J03.90
chronic J35.01
with adenoiditis J35.03
diphtheritic A36.0
hypertrophic J35.01
with adenoiditis J35.03
recurrent J03.91
specified organism NEC J03.80
recurrent J03.81
staphylococcal J03.80
recurrent J03.81
streptococcal J03.00
recurrent J03.01
tuberculous A15.8

Tonsillitis —continued
Vincent's A69.1
Tooth, teeth — see condition
Toothache K08.8
Topagnosis R20.8
Tophi — see Gout
TORCH infection — see Infection, congenital
without active infection P00.2
Torn — see Tear
Tornwaldt's cyst or disease J39.2
Torsion
accessory tube — see Torsion, fallopian tube
adnexa (female) — see Torsion, fallopian tube
aorta, acquired I77.1
appendix epididymis N44.04
appendix testis N44.03
bile duct (common) (hepatic) K83.8
congenital Q44.5
bowel, colon or intestine K56.2
cervix — see Malposition, uterus
cystic duct K82.8
dystonia — see Dystonia, torsion
epididymis (appendix) N44.04
fallopian tube N83.52
with ovary N83.53
gallbladder K82.8
congenital Q44.1
hydatid of Morgagni
female N83.52
male N44.03
kidney (pedicle) (leading to infarction) N28.0
Meckel's diverticulum (congenital) Q43.0
malignant — see Table of Neoplasms, small
intestine, malignant
mesentery K56.2
omentum K56.2
organ or site, congenital NEC — see Anomaly, by site
ovary (pedicle) N83.51
with fallopian tube N83.53
congenital Q50.2
oviduct — see Torsion, fallopian tube
penis N48.89
congenital Q55.69
spasm — see Dystonia, torsion
spermatic cord N44.02
extravaginal N44.01
intravaginal N44.02
spleen D73.5
testis, testicle N44.00
appendix N44.03
tibia — see Deformity, limb, specified type NEC,
lower leg
uterus — see Malposition, uterus
Torticollis (intermittent) (spastic) M43.6
congenital (sternomastoid) Q68.0
due to birth injury P15.2
hysterical F44.4
ocular R29.891
psychogenic F45.8
conversion reaction F44.4
rheumatoid M06.88
spasmodic G24.3
traumatic, current S13.4
Tortipelvis G24.1
Tortuous
artery I77.1
organ or site, congenital NEC — see Distortion
retinal vessel, congenital Q14.1
ureter N13.8
urethra N36.8
vein — see Varix
Torture, victim of Z65.4
Torula, torular (histolytica) (infection) — see
Cryptococcosis
Torulosis — see Cryptococcosis
Torus (mandibularis) (palatinus) M27.0
fracture — see Fracture, by site, torus
Touraine's syndrome Q79.8
Tourette's syndrome F95.2
Tourniquet syndrome — see Constriction, external,
by site
Tower skull Q75.0
with exophthalmos Q87.0

Toxemia R68.89
bacterial — see Sepsis
burn — see Burn
eclamptic (with pre-existing hypertension) — see
Eclampsia
erysipelatous — see Erysipelas
fatigue R68.89
food — see Poisoning, food
gastrointestinal K52.1
intestinal K52.1
kidney — see Uremia
malarial — see Malaria
myocardial — see Myocarditis, toxic
of pregnancy — see Pre-eclampsia
pre-eclamptic — see Pre-eclampsia
small intestine K52.1
staphylococcal, due to food A05.0
stasis R68.89
uremic — see Uremia
urinary — see Uremia
Toxemica cerebropathia psychica (nonalcoholic) F04
alcoholic — see Alcohol, amnestic disorder
Toxic (poisoning) (see also condition) T65.91
effect — see Table of Drugs and Chemicals, by
substance, poisoning
shock syndrome A48.3
thyroid (gland) — see Thyrotoxicosis
Toxicemia — see Toxemia
Toxicity — see Table of Drugs and Chemicals, by
substance, poisoning
fava bean D55.0
food, noxious — see Poisoning, food
from drug or nonmedicinal substance — see Table
of Drugs and Chemicals, by drug
Toxicosis (see also Toxemia)
capillary, hemorrhagic D69.0
Toxinfection, gastrointestinal K52.1
Toxocariasis B83.0
Toxoplasma, toxoplasmosis (acquired) B58.9
with
hepatitis B58.1
meningoencephalitis B58.2
ocular involvement B58.00
other organ involvement B58.89
pneumonia, pneumonitis B58.3
congenital (acute) (subacute) (chronic) P37.1
maternal, manifest toxoplasmosis in infant (acute)
(subacute) (chronic) P37.1
**tPA (rtPA) administration in a different facility
within the last 24 hours prior to admission to
current facility** Z92.82
Trabeculation, bladder N32.89
Trachea — see condition
Tracheitis (catarrhal) (infantile) (membranous)
(plastic) (septal) (suppurative) (viral) J04.10
with
bronchitis (15 years of age and above) J40
acute or subacute — see Bronchitis, acute
chronic J42
tuberculous NEC A15.5
under 15 years of age J20.9
laryngitis (acute) J04.2
chronic J37.1
tuberculous NEC A15.5
acute J04.10
with obstruction J04.11
chronic J42
with
bronchitis (chronic) J42
laryngitis (chronic) J37.1
diphtheritic (membranous) A36.89
due to external agent — see Inflammation,
respiratory, upper, due to
syphilitic A52.73
tuberculous A15.5
Trachelitis (nonvenereal) — see Cervicitis
Tracheobronchial — see condition
Tracheobronchitis (15 years of age and above) (see
also Bronchitis)
due to
Bordetella bronchiseptica A37.80
with pneumonia A37.81
Francisella tularensis A21.8

Tracheobronchomegaly Q32.4
  with bronchiectasis J47.9
    with
      exacerbation (acute) J47.1
      lower respiratory infection J47.0
  acquired J98.09
    with bronchiectasis J47.9
      with
        ‛ exacerbation (acute) J47.1
        lower respiratory infection J47.0
Tracheobronchopneumonitis — see Pneumonia, broncho-
Tracheocele (external) (internal) J39.8
  congenital Q32.1
Tracheomalacia J39.8
  congenital Q32.0
Tracheopharyngitis chronic J42
  due to external agent — see Inflammation, respiratory, upper, due to
Tracheostenosis J39.8
Tracheostomy
  complication — see Complication, tracheostomy
  status Z93.0
    attention to Z43.0
    malfunctioning J95.03
Trachoma, trachomatous A71.9
  active (stage) A71.1
  contraction of conjunctiva A71.1
  dubium A71.0
  initial (stage) A71.0
  healed or sequelae B94.0
  pannus A71.1
  Türck's J37.0
Train sickness T75.3
Trait(s)
  Hb-S D57.3
  hemoglobin
    abnormal NEC D58.2
      with thalassemia D56.3
    C — see Disease, hemoglobin C
    S (Hb-S) D57.3
  Lepore D56.3
  personality, accentuated Z73.1
  sickle-cell D57.3
    with elliptocytosis or spherocytosis D57.3
  type A personality Z73.1
Tramp Z59.0
Trance R41.89
  hysterical F44.89
Transection
  abdomen (partial) S38.3
  aorta (incomplete) (see also Injury, aorta)
    complete — see Injury, aorta, laceration, major
  carotid artery (incomplete) (see also Injury, blood vessel, carotid, laceration)
    complete — see Injury, blood vessel, carotid, laceration, major
  celiac artery (incomplete) S35.211
    branch (incomplete) S35.291
      complete S35.292
    complete S35.212
  innominate
    artery (incomplete) (see also Injury, blood vessel, thoracic, innominate, artery, laceration)
      complete — see Injury, blood vessel, thoracic, innominate, artery, laceration, major
    vein (incomplete) (see also Injury, blood vessel, thoracic, innominate, vein, laceration)
      complete — see Injury, blood vessel, thoracic, innominate, vein, laceration, major
  jugular vein (external) (incomplete) (see also Injury, blood vessel, jugular vein, laceration)
    complete — see Injury, blood vessel, jugular vein, laceration, major
    internal (incomplete) (see also Injury, blood vessel, jugular vein, internal, laceration)
      complete — see Injury, blood vessel, jugular vein, internal, laceration, major
  mesenteric artery (incomplete) (see also Injury, mesenteric, artery, laceration)
    complete — see Injury, mesenteric artery, laceration, major

Transection—continued
  pulmonary vessel (incomplete) (see also Injury, blood vessel, thoracic, pulmonary, laceration)
    complete — see Injury, blood vessel, thoracic, pulmonary, laceration, major
  subclavian — see Transection, innominate
  vena cava (incomplete) (see also Injury, vena cava)
    complete — see Injury, vena cava, laceration, major
  vertebral artery (incomplete) (see also Injury, blood vessel, vertebral, laceration)
    complete — see Injury, blood vessel, vertebral, laceration, major
Transaminasemia R74.0
Transfusion
  associated (red blood bell) hemochromatosis E83.111
  blood
    ABO incompatible — see Complication(s), transfusion, incompatibility reaction, ABO
    minor blood group (Duffy) (E) (K(ell)) (Kidd) (Lewis) (M) (N) (P) (S) T80.89
    reaction or complication — see Complications, transfusion
  fetomaternal (mother) — see Pregnancy, complicated by, placenta, transfusion syndrome
  maternofetal (mother) — see Pregnancy, complicated by, placenta, transfusion syndrome
  placental (syndrome) (mother) — see Pregnancy, complicated by, placenta, transfusion syndrome
  reaction (adverse) — see Complications, transfusion
  related acute lung injury (TRALI) J95.84
  twin-to-twin — see Pregnancy, complicated by, placenta, transfusion syndrome, fetus to fetus
Transient (meaning homeless) (see also condition) Z59.0
Translocation
  balanced autosomal Q95.9
    in normal individual Q95.0
  chromosomes NEC Q99.8
    balanced and insertion in normal individual Q95.0
  Down syndrome Q90.2
  trisomy
    13 Q91.6
    18 Q91.2
    21 Q90.2
Translucency, iris — see Degeneration, iris
Transmission of chemical substances through the placenta — see Absorption, chemical, through placenta
Transparency, lung, unilateral J43.0
Transplant(ed) (status) Z94.9
  awaiting organ Z76.82
  bone Z94.6
    marrow Z94.81
  candidate Z76.82
  complication — see Complication, transplant
  cornea Z94.7
  heart Z94.1
    and lung(s) Z94.3
    valve Z95.2
      prosthetic Z95.2
      specified NEC Z95.4
      xenogenic Z95.3
  intestine Z94.82
  kidney Z94.0
  liver Z94.4
  lung(s) Z94.2
    and heart Z94.3
  organ (failure) (infection) (rejection) Z94.9
    removal status Z98.85
  pancreas Z94.83
  skin Z94.5
  social Z60.3
  specified organ or tissue NEC Z94.89
  stem cells Z94.84
  tissue Z94.9
Transplants, ovarian, endometrial N80.1
Transposed — see Transposition

Transposition (congenital) (see also Malposition, congenital)
  abdominal viscera Q89.3
  aorta (dextra) Q20.3
  appendix Q43.8
  colon Q43.8
  corrected Q20.5
  great vessels (complete) (partial) Q20.3
  heart Q24.0
    with complete transposition of viscera Q89.3
  intestine (large) (small) Q43.8
  reversed jejunal (for bypass) (status) Z98.0
  scrotum Q55.23
  stomach Q40.2
    with general transposition of viscera Q89.3
  tooth, teeth, fully erupted M26.30
  vessels, great (complete) (partial) Q20.3
  viscera (abdominal) (thoracic) Q89.3
Transsexualism F64.1
Transverse (see also condition)
  arrest (deep), in labor O64.0
  lie (mother) O32.2
    causing obstructed labor O64.8
Transvestism, transvestitism (dual-role) F64.1
  fetishistic F65.1
Trapped placenta (with hemorrhage) O72.0
  without hemorrhage O73.0
Trauma, traumatism (see also Injury)
  acoustic — see subcategory H83.3
  birth — see Birth, injury
  complicating ectopic or molar pregnancy O08.6
  during delivery O71.9
  following ectopic or molar pregnancy O08.6
  obstetric O71.9
    specified NEC O71.89
Traumatic (see also condition)
  brain injury — see category S06
Treacher Collins syndrome Q75.4
Treitz's hernia — see Hernia, abdomen, specified site NEC
Trematode infestation — see Infestation, fluke
Trematodiasis — see Infestation, fluke
Trembling paralysis — see Parkinsonism
Tremor(s) R25.1
  drug induced G25.1
  essential (benign) G25.0
  familial G25.0
  hereditary G25.0
  hysterical F44.4
  intention G25.2
  medication induced postural G25.1
  mercurial — see subcategory T56.1
  Parkinson's — see Parkinsonism
  psychogenic (conversion reaction) F44.4
  senilis R54
  specified type NEC G25.2
Trench
  fever A79.0
  foot — see Immersion, foot
  mouth A69.1
Treponema pallidum infection — see Syphilis
Treponematosis
  due to
    T. pallidum — see Syphilis
    T. pertenue — see Yaws
Triad
  Hutchinson's (congenital syphilis) A50.53
  Kartagener's Q89.3
  Saint's — see Hernia, diaphragm
Trichiasis (eyelid) H02.059
  with entropion — see Entropion
  left H02.056
    lower H02.055
    upper H02.054
  right H02.053
    lower H02.052
    upper H02.051
Trichinella spiralis (infection) (infestation) B75
Trichinellosis, trichiniasis, trichinelliasis, trichinosis B75
  with muscle disorder B75 [M63.80]
    ankle B75 [M63.87-]
    foot B75 [M63.87-]

Trichinellosis, trichiniasis, trichinelliasis, trichinosis—*continued*
  with muscle disorder—*continued*
      forearm B75 [M63.83-]
      hand B75 [M63.84-]
      lower leg B75 [M63.86-]
      multiple sites B75 [M63.89]
      pelvic region B75 [M63.85-]
      shoulder region B75 [M63.81-]
      specified site NEC B75 [M63.88]
      thigh B75 [M63.85-]
      upper arm B75 [M63.82-]
Trichobezoar T18.9
  intestine T18.3
  stomach T18.2
Trichocephaliasis, trichocephalosis B79
Trichocephalus infestation B79
Trichoclasis L67.8
Trichoepithelioma (*see also* Neoplasm, skin, benign)
  malignant — *see* Neoplasm, skin, malignant
Trichofolliculoma — *see* Neoplasm, skin, benign
Tricholemmoma — *see* Neoplasm, skin, benign
Trichomoniasis A59.9
  bladder A59.03
  cervix A59.09
  intestinal A07.8
  prostate A59.02
  seminal vesicles A59.09
  specified site NEC A59.8
  urethra A59.03
  urogenitalis A59.00
  vagina A59.01
  vulva A59.01
Trichomycosis
  axillaris A48.8
  nodosa, nodularis B36.8
Trichonodosis L67.8
Trichophytid, trichophyton infection — *see* Dermatophytosis
Trichophytobezoar T18.9
  intestine T18.3
  stomach T18.2
Trichophytosis — *see* Dermatophytosis
Trichoptilosis L67.8
Trichorrhexis (nodosa) (invaginata) L67.0
Trichosis axillaris A48.8
Trichosporosis nodosa B36.2
Trichostasis spinulosa (congenital) Q84.1
Trichostrongyliasis, trichostrongylosis (small intestine) B81.2
Trichostrongylus infection B81.2
Trichotillomania F63.3
Trichromat, trichromatopsia, anomalous (congenital) H53.55
Trichuriasis B79
Trichuris trichiura (infection) (infestation) (any site) B79
Tricuspid (valve) — *see* condition
Trifid (*see also* Accessory)
  kidney (pelvis) Q63.8
  tongue Q38.3
Trigeminal neuralgia — *see* Neuralgia, trigeminal
Trigeminy R00.8
Trigger finger (acquired) M65.30
  congenital Q74.0
  index finger M65.32-
  little finger M65.35-
  middle finger M65.33-
  ring finger M65.34-
  thumb M65.31-
Trigonitis (bladder) (chronic) (pseudomembranous) N30.30
  with hematuria N30.31
Trigonocephaly Q75.0
Trilocular heart — *see* Cor triloculare
Trimethylaminuria E72.52
Tripartite placenta O43.19-
Triphalangeal thumb Q74.0
Triple (*see also* Accessory)
  kidneys Q63.0
  uteri Q51.818
  X, female Q97.0

Triplegia G83.89
  congenital G80.8
Triplet (newborn) (*see also* Newborn, triplet)
  complicating pregnancy — *see* Pregnancy, triplet
Triplication — *see* Accessory
Triploidy Q92.7
Trismus R25.2
  neonatorum A33
  newborn A33
Trisomy (syndrome) Q92.9
  autosomes Q92.9
  chromosome specified NEC Q92.8
      partial Q92.2
          due to unbalanced translocation Q92.5
      whole (nonsex chromosome)
          meiotic nondisjunction Q92.0
          mitotic nondisjunction Q92.1
          mosaicism Q92.1
      specified NEC Q92.8
  due to
      dicentrics — *see* Extra, marker chromosomes
      extra rings — *see* Extra, marker chromosomes
      isochromosomes — *see* Extra, marker chromosomes
  specified NEC Q92.8
  whole chromosome Q92.9
      meiotic nondisjunction Q92.0
      mitotic nondisjunction Q92.1
      mosaicism Q92.1
      partial Q92.9
      specified NEC Q92.8
  13 (partial) Q91.7
      meiotic nondisjunction Q91.4
      mitotic nondisjunction Q91.5
      mosaicism Q91.5
      translocation Q91.6
  18 (partial) Q91.3
      meiotic nondisjunction Q91.0
      mitotic nondisjunction Q91.1
      mosaicism Q91.1
      translocation Q91.2
  20 Q92.8
  21 (partial) Q90.9
      meiotic nondisjunction Q90.0
      mitotic nondisjunction Q90.1
      mosaicism Q90.1
      translocation Q90.2
  22 Q92.8
Tritanomaly, tritanopia H53.55
Trombiculosis, trombiculiasis, trombidiosis B88.0
Trophedema (congenital) (hereditary) Q82.0
Trophoblastic disease (*see also* Mole, hydatidiform) O01.9
Tropholymphedema Q82.0
Trophoneurosis NEC G96.8
  disseminated M34.9
Tropical — *see* condition
Trouble (*see also* Disease)
  heart — *see* Disease, heart
  kidney — *see* Disease, renal
  nervous R45.0
  sinus — *see* Sinusitis
Trousseau's syndrome (thrombophlebitis migrans) I82.1
Truancy, childhood
  from school Z72.810
Truncus
  arteriosus (persistent) Q20.0
  communis Q20.0
Trunk — *see* condition
Trypanosomiasis
  African B56.9
      by Trypanosoma brucei
          gambiense B56.0
          rhodesiense B56.1
  American — *see* Chagas' disease
  Brazilian — *see* Chagas' disease
  by Trypanosoma
      brucei gambiense B56.0
      brucei rhodesiense B56.1
      cruzi — *see* Chagas' disease
  gambiensis, Gambian B56.0
  rhodesiensis, Rhodesian B56.1

Trypanosomiasis—*continued*
  South American — *see* Chagas' disease
  where
      African trypanosomiasis is prevalent B56.9
      Chagas' disease is prevalent B57.2
T-shaped incisors K00.2
Tsutsugamushi (disease) (fever) A75.3
Tube, tubal, tubular — *see* condition
Tubercle (*see also* Tuberculosis)
  brain, solitary A17.81
  Darwin's Q17.8
  Ghon, primary infection A15.7
Tuberculid, tuberculide (indurating, subcutaneous) (lichenoid) (miliary) (papulonecrotic) (primary) (skin) A18.4
Tuberculoma (*see also* Tuberculosis)
  brain A17.81
  meninges (cerebral) (spinal) A17.1
  spinal cord A17.81
Tuberculosis, tubercular, tuberculous (calcification) (calcified) (caseous) (chromogenic acid-fast bacilli) (degeneration) (fibrocaseous) (fistula) (interstitial) (isolated circumscribed lesions) (necrosis) (parenchymatous) (ulcerative) A15.9
  with pneumoconiosis (any condition in J60-J64) J65
  abdomen (lymph gland) A18.39
  abscess (respiratory) A15.9
      bone A18.03
          hip A18.02
          knee A18.02
          sacrum A18.01
          specified site NEC A18.03
          spinal A18.01
          vertebra A18.01
      brain A17.81
      breast A18.89
      Cowper's gland A18.15
      dura (mater) (cerebral) (spinal) A17.81
      epidural (cerebral) (spinal) A17.81
      female pelvis A18.17
      frontal sinus A15.8
      genital organs NEC A18.10
      genitourinary A18.10
      gland (lymphatic) — *see* Tuberculosis, lymph gland
      hip A18.02
      intestine A18.32
      ischiorectal A18.32
      joint NEC A18.02
          hip A18.02
          knee A18.02
          specified NEC A18.02
          vertebral A18.01
      kidney A18.11
      knee A18.02
      lumbar (spine) A18.01
      lung — *see* Tuberculosis, pulmonary
      meninges (cerebral) (spinal) A17.0
      muscle A18.09
      perianal (fistula) A18.32
      perinephritic A18.11
      perirectal A18.32
      rectum A18.32
      retropharyngeal A15.8
      sacrum A18.01
      scrofulous A18.2
      scrotum A18.15
      skin (primary) A18.4
      spinal cord A17.81
      spine or vertebra (column) A18.01
      subdiaphragmatic A18.31
      testis A18.15
      urinary A18.13
      uterus A18.17
  accessory sinus — *see* Tuberculosis, sinus
  Addison's disease A18.7
  adenitis — *see* Tuberculosis, lymph gland
  adenoids A15.8
  adenopathy — *see* Tuberculosis, lymph gland
  adherent pericardium A18.84
  adnexa (uteri) A18.17
  adrenal (capsule) (gland) A18.7
  alimentary canal A18.32

Tuberculosis, tubercular, tuberculous —*continued*
anemia A18.89
ankle (joint) (bone) A18.02
anus A18.32
apex, apical — *see* Tuberculosis, pulmonary
appendicitis, appendix A18.32
arachnoid A17.0
artery, arteritis A18.89
   cerebral A18.89
arthritis (chronic) (synovial) A18.02
   spine or vertebra (column) A18.01
articular — *see* Tuberculosis, joint
ascites A18.31
asthma — *see* Tuberculosis, pulmonary
axilla, axillary (gland) A18.2
bladder A18.12
bone A18.03
   hip A18.02
   knee A18.02
   limb NEC A18.03
   sacrum A18.01
   spine or vertebral column A18.01
bowel (miliary) A18.32
brain A17.81
breast A18.89
broad ligament A18.17
bronchi, bronchial, bronchus A15.5
   ectasia, ectasis (bronchiectasis) — *see*
      Tuberculosis, pulmonary
   fistula A15.5
      primary (progressive) A15.7
   gland or node A15.4
      primary (progressive) A15.7
   lymph gland or node A15.4
      primary (progressive) A15.7
bronchiectasis — *see* Tuberculosis, pulmonary
bronchitis A15.5
bronchopleural A15.6
bronchopneumonia, bronchopneumonic — *see*
   Tuberculosis, pulmonary
bronchorrhagia A15.5
bronchotracheal A15.5
bronze disease A18.7
buccal cavity A18.83
bulbourethral gland A18.15
bursa A18.09
cachexia A15.9
cardiomyopathy A18.84
caries — *see* Tuberculosis, bone
cartilage A18.02
   intervertebral A18.01
catarrhal — *see* Tuberculosis, respiratory
cecum A18.32
cellulitis (primary) A18.4
cerebellum A17.81
cerebral, cerebrum A17.81
cerebrospinal A17.81
   meninges A17.0
cervical (lymph gland or node) A18.2
cervicitis, cervix (uteri) A18.16
chest — *see* Tuberculosis, respiratory
chorioretinitis A18.53
choroid, choroiditis A18.53
ciliary body A18.54
colitis A18.32
collier's J65
colliquativa (primary) A18.4
colon A18.32
complex, primary A15.7
congenital P37.0
conjunctiva A18.59
connective tissue (systemic) A18.89
contact Z20.1
cornea (ulcer) A18.52
Cowper's gland A18.15
coxae A18.02
coxalgia A18.02
cul-de-sac of Douglas A18.17
curvature, spine A18.01
cutis (colliquativa) (primary) A18.4
cyst, ovary A18.18
cystitis A18.12
dactylitis A18.03

Tuberculosis, tubercular, tuberculous —*continued*
diarrhea A18.32
diffuse — *see* Tuberculosis, miliary
digestive tract A18.32
disseminated — *see* Tuberculosis, miliary
duodenum A18.32
dura (mater) (cerebral) (spinal) A17.0
   abscess (cerebral) (spinal) A17.81
dysentery A18.32
ear (inner) (middle) A18.6
   bone A18.03
   external (primary) A18.4
   skin (primary) A18.4
elbow A18.02
emphysema — *see* Tuberculosis, pulmonary
empyema A15.6
encephalitis A17.82
endarteritis A18.89
endocarditis A18.84
   aortic A18.84
   mitral A18.84
   pulmonary A18.84
   tricuspid A18.84
endocrine glands NEC A18.82
endometrium A18.17
enteric, enterica, enteritis A18.32
enterocolitis A18.32
epididymis, epididymitis A18.15
epidural abscess (cerebral) (spinal) A17.81
epiglottis A15.5
episcleritis A18.51
erythema (induratum) (nodosum) (primary) A18.4
esophagus A18.83
eustachian tube A18.6
exposure (to) Z20.1
exudative — *see* Tuberculosis, pulmonary
eye A18.50
eyelid (primary) (lupus) A18.4
fallopian tube (acute) (chronic) A18.17
fascia A18.09
fauces A15.8
female pelvic inflammatory disease A18.17
finger A18.03
first infection A15.7
gallbladder A18.83
ganglion A18.09
gastritis A18.83
gastrocolic fistula A18.32
gastroenteritis A18.32
gastrointestinal tract A18.32
general, generalized — *see* Tuberculosis, miliary
genital organs A18.10
genitourinary A18.10
genu A18.02
glandula suprarenalis A18.7
glandular, general A18.2
glottis A15.5
grinder's J65
gum A18.83
hand A18.03
hematogenous — *see* Tuberculosis, miliary
hemoptysis — *see* Tuberculosis, pulmonary
hemorrhage NEC — *see* Tuberculosis, pulmonary
hemothorax A15.6
hepatitis A18.83
hilar lymph nodes A15.4
   primary (progressive) A15.7
hip (joint) (disease) (bone) A18.02
hydropneumothorax A15.6
hydrothorax A15.6
hypoadrenalism A18.7
hypopharynx A15.8
ileocecal (hyperplastic) A18.32
ileocolitis A18.32
ileum A18.32
iliac spine (superior) A18.03
immunological findings only A15.7
indurativa (primary) A18.4
infantile A15.7
infection A15.9
   without clinical manifestations A15.7
infraclavicular gland A18.2

Tuberculosis, tubercular, tuberculous —*continued*
inguinal gland A18.2
inguinalis A18.2
intestine (any part) A18.32
iridocyclitis A18.54
iris, iritis A18.54
ischiorectal A18.32
jaw A18.03
jejunum A18.32
joint A18.02
   vertebral A18.01
keratitis (interstitial) A18.52
keratoconjunctivitis A18.52
kidney A18.11
knee (joint) A18.02
kyphosis, kyphoscoliosis A18.01
laryngitis A15.5
larynx A15.5
leptomeninges, leptomeningitis (cerebral) (spinal)
   A17.0
lichenoides (primary) A18.4
linguae A18.83
lip A18.83
liver A18.83
lordosis A18.01
lung — *see* Tuberculosis, pulmonary
lupus vulgaris A18.4
lymph gland or node (peripheral) A18.2
   abdomen A18.39
   bronchial A15.4
      primary (progressive) A15.7
   cervical A18.2
   hilar A15.4
      primary (progressive) A15.7
   intrathoracic A15.4
      primary (progressive) A15.7
   mediastinal A15.4
      primary (progressive) A15.7
   mesenteric A18.39
   retroperitoneal A18.39
   tracheobronchial A15.4
      primary (progressive) A15.7
lymphadenitis — *see* Tuberculosis, lymph gland
lymphangitis — *see* Tuberculosis, lymph gland
lymphatic (gland) (vessel) — *see* Tuberculosis,
   lymph gland
mammary gland A18.89
marasmus A15.9
mastoiditis A18.03
mediastinal lymph gland or node A15.4
   primary (progressive) A15.7
mediastinitis A15.8
   primary (progressive) A15.7
mediastinum A15.8
   primary (progressive) A15.7
medulla A17.81
melanosis, Addisonian A18.7
meninges, meningitis (basilar) (cerebral)
   (cerebrospinal) (spinal) A17.0
meningoencephalitis A17.82
mesentery, mesenteric (gland or node) A18.39
miliary A19.9
   acute A19.2
      multiple sites A19.1
      single specified site A19.0
   chronic A19.8
   specified NEC A19.8
millstone makers' J65
miner's J65
molder's J65
mouth A18.83
multiple A19.9
   acute A19.1
   chronic A19.8
muscle A18.09
myelitis A17.82
myocardium, myocarditis A18.84
nasal (passage) (sinus) A15.8
nasopharynx A15.8
neck gland A18.2
nephritis A18.11
nerve (mononeuropathy) A17.83
nervous system A17.9

Tuberculosis, tubercular, tuberculous —continued
- nose (septum) A15.8
- ocular A18.50
- omentum A18.31
- oophoritis (acute) (chronic) A18.17
- optic (nerve trunk) (papilla) A18.59
- orbit A18.59
- orchitis A18.15
- organ, specified NEC A18.89
- osseous — see Tuberculosis, bone
- osteitis — see Tuberculosis, bone
- osteomyelitis — see Tuberculosis, bone
- otitis media A18.6
- ovary, ovaritis (acute) (chronic) A18.17
- oviduct (acute) (chronic) A18.17
- pachymeningitis A17.0
- palate (soft) A18.83
- pancreas A18.83
- papulonecrotic(a) (primary) A18.4
- parathyroid glands A18.82
- paronychia (primary) A18.4
- parotid gland or region A18.83
- pelvis (bony) A18.03
- penis A18.15
- peribronchitis A15.5
- pericardium, pericarditis A18.84
- perichondritis, larynx A15.5
- periostitis — see Tuberculosis, bone
- perirectal fistula A18.32
- peritoneum NEC A18.31
- peritonitis A18.31
- pharynx, pharyngitis A15.8
- phlyctenulosis (keratoconjunctivitis) A18.52
- phthisis NEC — see Tuberculosis, pulmonary
- pituitary gland A18.82
- pleura, pleural, pleurisy, pleuritis (fibrinous) (obliterative) (purulent) (simple plastic) (with effusion) A15.6
  - primary (progressive) A15.7
- pneumonia, pneumonic — see Tuberculosis, pulmonary
- pneumothorax (spontaneous) (tense valvular) — see Tuberculosis, pulmonary
- polyneuropathy A17.89
- polyserositis A19.9
  - acute A19.1
  - chronic A19.8
- potter's J65
- prepuce A18.15
- primary (complex) A15.7
- proctitis A18.32
- prostate, prostatitis A18.14
- pulmonalis — see Tuberculosis, pulmonary
- pulmonary (cavitated) (fibrotic) (infiltrative) (nodular) A15.0
  - childhood type or first infection A15.7
  - primary (complex) A15.7
- pyelitis A18.11
- pyelonephritis A18.11
- pyemia — see Tuberculosis, miliary
- pyonephrosis A18.11
- pyopneumothorax A15.6
- pyothorax A15.6
- rectum (fistula) (with abscess) A18.32
- reinfection stage — see Tuberculosis, pulmonary
- renal A18.11
- renis A18.11
- respiratory A15.9
  - primary A15.7
  - specified site NEC A15.8
- retina, retinitis A18.53
- retroperitoneal (lymph gland or node) A18.39
- rheumatism NEC A18.09
- rhinitis A15.8
- sacroiliac (joint) A18.01
- sacrum A18.01
- salivary gland A18.83
- salpingitis (acute) (chronic) A18.17
- sandblaster's J65
- sclera A18.51
- scoliosis A18.01
- scrofulous A18.2
- scrotum A18.15

Tuberculosis, tubercular, tuberculous —continued
- seminal tract or vesicle A18.15
- senile A15.9
- septic — see Tuberculosis, miliary
- shoulder (joint) A18.02
  - blade A18.03
- sigmoid A18.32
- sinus (any nasal) A15.8
  - bone A18.03
  - epididymis A18.15
- skeletal NEC A18.03
- skin (any site) (primary) A18.4
- small intestine A18.32
- soft palate A18.83
- spermatic cord A18.15
- spine, spinal (column) A18.01
  - cord A17.81
  - medulla A17.81
  - membrane A17.0
  - meninges A17.0
- spleen, splenitis A18.85
- spondylitis A18.01
- sternoclavicular joint A18.02
- stomach A18.83
- stonemason's J65
- subcutaneous tissue (cellular) (primary) A18.4
- subcutis (primary) A18.4
- subdeltoid bursa A18.83
- submaxillary (region) A18.83
- supraclavicular gland A18.2
- suprarenal (capsule) (gland) A18.7
- swelling, joint (see also Tuberculosis, joint) A18.02
  - (see also category M01)
- symphysis pubis A18.02
- synovitis A18.09
  - articular A18.02
  - spine or vertebra A18.01
- systemic — see Tuberculosis, miliary
- tarsitis A18.4
- tendon (sheath) — see Tuberculosis, tenosynovitis
- tenosynovitis A18.09
  - spine or vertebra A18.01
- testis A18.15
- throat A15.8
- thymus gland A18.82
- thyroid gland A18.81
- tongue A18.83
- tonsil, tonsillitis A15.8
- trachea, tracheal A15.5
  - lymph gland or node A15.4
    - primary (progressive) A15.7
- tracheobronchial A15.5
  - lymph gland or node A15.4
    - primary (progressive) A15.7
- tubal (acute) (chronic) A18.17
- tunica vaginalis A18.15
- ulcer (skin) (primary) A18.4
  - bowel or intestine A18.32
- specified NEC code under Tuberculosis, by site
- unspecified site A15.9
- ureter A18.11
- urethra, urethral (gland) A18.13
- urinary organ or tract A18.13
- uterus A18.17
- uveal tract A18.54
- uvula A18.83
- vagina A18.18
- vas deferens A18.15
- verruca, verrucosa (cutis) (primary) A18.4
- vertebra (column) A18.01
- vesiculitis A18.15
- vulva A18.18
- wrist (joint) A18.02

Tuberculum
- Carabelli — see Note at K00.2
- occlusal — see Note at K00.2
- paramolare K00.2

Tuberosity, enitre maxillary M26.07

Tuberous sclerosis (brain) Q85.1

Tubo-ovarian — see condition

Tuboplasty, after previous sterilization Z31.0
- aftercare Z31.42

Tubotympanitis, catarrhal (chronic) — see Otitis, media, nonsuppurative, chronic, serous

Tularemia A21.9
- with
  - conjunctivitis A21.1
  - pneumonia A21.2
- abdominal A21.3
- bronchopneumonic A21.2
- conjunctivitis A21.1
- cryptogenic A21.3
- enteric A21.3
- gastrointestinal A21.3
- generalized A21.7
- ingestion A21.3
- intestinal A21.3
- oculoglandular A21.1
- ophthalmic A21.1
- pneumonia (any), pneumonic A21.2
- pulmonary A21.2
- sepsis A21.7
- specified NEC A21.8
- typhoidal A21.7
- ulceroglandular A21.0

Tularensis conjunctivitis A21.1

Tumefaction (see also Swelling)
- liver — see Hypertrophy, liver

Tumor (see also Neoplasm, unspecified behavior, by site)
- acinar cell — see Neoplasm, uncertain behavior, by site
- acinic cell — see Neoplasm, uncertain behavior, by site
- adenocarcinoid — see Neoplasm, malignant, by site
- adenomatoid (see also Neoplasm, benign, by site)
  - odontogenic — see Cyst, calcifying odontogenic
- adnexal (skin) — see Neoplasm, skin, benign, by site
- adrenal
  - cortical (benign) D35.0-
    - malignant C74.0-
  - rest — see Neoplasm, benign, by site
    - pancreas C25.4
    - specified site NEC — see Neoplasm, malignant, by site
    - unspecified site C25.4
- alpha-cell
  - malignant
    - pancreas D13.7
    - specified site NEC — see Neoplasm, benign, by site
  - unspecified site D13.7
- aneurysmal — see Aneurysm
- aortic body D44.7
  - malignant C75.5
- Askin's — see Neoplasm, connective tissue, malignant
- basal cell (see also Neoplasm, skin, uncertain behavior) D48.5
- Bednar — see Neoplasm, skin, malignant
- benign (unclassified) — see Neoplasm, benign, by site
- beta-cell
  - malignant
    - pancreas C25.4
    - specified site NEC — see Neoplasm, malignant, by site
    - unspecified site C25.4
  - pancreas D13.7
  - specified site NEC — see Neoplasm, benign, by site
  - unspecified site D13.7
- Brenner D27.9
  - borderline malignancy D39.1-
  - malignant C56.-
  - proliferating D39.1-
- bronchial alveolar, intravascular D38.1
- Brooke's — see Neoplasm, skin, benign
- brown fat — see Lipoma
- Burkitt — see Lymphoma, Burkitt
- calcifying epithelial odontogenic — see Cyst, calcifying odontogenic
- carcinoid
  - benign D3a.00
    - appendix D3a.020

Tumor—Tumor

Tumor—*continued*
carcinoid—*continued*
benign —*continued*
ascending colon D3a.022
bronchus (lung) D3a.090
cecum D3a.021
colon D3a.029
descending colon D3a.024
duodenum D3a.010
foregut NOS D3a.094
hindgut NOS D3a.096
ileum D3a.012
jejunum D3a.011
kidney D3a.093
large intestine D3a.029
lung (bronchus) D3a.090
midgut NOS D3a.095
rectum D3a.026
sigmoid colon D3a.025
small intestine D3a.019
specified NEC D3a.098
stomach D3a.092
thymus D3a.091
transverse colon D3a.023
malignant C7a.00
appendix C7a.020
ascending colon C7a.022
bronchus (lung) C7a.090
cecum C7a.021
colon C7a.029
descending colon C7a.024
duodenum C7a.010
foregut NOS C7a.094
hindgut NOS C7a.096
ileum C7a.012
jejunum C7a.011
kidney C7a.093
large intestine C7a.029
lung (bronchus) C7a.090
midgut NOS C7a.095
rectum C7a.026
sigmoid colon C7a.025
small intestine C7a.019
specified NEC C7a.098
stomach C7a.092
thymus C7a.091
transverse colon C7a.023
mesentary metastasis C7b.01
secondary C7b.00
bone C7b.03
distant lymph nodes C7b.01
liver C7b.02
peritoneum C7b.04
specified NEC C7b.09
carotid body D44.6
malignant C75.4
cells (*see also* Neoplasm, unspecified behavior, by site)
benign — *see* Neoplasm, benign, by site
malignant — *see* Neoplasm, malignant, by site
uncertain whether benign or malignant — *see* Neoplasm, uncertain behavior, by site
cervix, in pregnancy or childbirth — *see* Pregnancy, complicated by, tumor, cervix
chondromatous giant cell — *see* Neoplasm, bone, benign
chromaffin (*see also* Neoplasm, benign, by site)
malignant — *see* Neoplasm, malignant
Cock's peculiar L72.1
Codman's — *see* Neoplasm, bone, benign
dentigerous, mixed — *see* Cyst, calcifying odontogenic
dermoid (*see also* Neoplasm, benign, by site)
with malignant transformation C56.-
desmoid (extra-abdominal) (*see also* Neoplasm, connective tissue, uncertain behavior)
abdominal — *see* Neoplasm, connective tissue, uncertain behavior
embolus — *see* Neoplasm, secondary, by site
embryonal (mixed) (*see also* Neoplasm, uncertain behavior, by site)
liver C22.7
unspecified site

Tumor—*continued*
embryonal (mixed) —*continued*
unspecified site—*continued*
female C56.-
male C62.90
endodermal sinus
specified site — *see* Neoplasm, malignant, by site
epithelial
benign — *see* Neoplasm, benign by site
malignant — *see* Neoplasm, malignant by site
Ewing's — *see* Neoplasm, bone, malignant by site
fatty — *see* Lipoma
fibroid — *see* Leiomyoma
specified site — *see* Neoplasm, uncertain behavior, by site
unspecified site D37.9
G cell
malignant
pancreas C25.4
specified site NEC — *see* Neoplasm, malignant, by site
unspecified site C25.4
germ cell (*see also* Neoplasm, malignant, by site)
mixed — *see* Neoplasm, malignant, by site
ghost cell, odontogenic — *see* Cyst, calcifying odontogenic
giant cell (*see also* Neoplasm, uncertain behavior, by site)
bone D48.0
malignant — *see* Neoplasm, bone, malignant, by site
chondromatous — *see* Neoplasm, bone, benign
malignant — *see* Neoplasm, malignant, by site
soft parts (*see also* Neoplasm, connective tissue, uncertain behavior)
malignant — *see* Neoplasm, connective tissue, malignant
glomus D18.00
intra-abdominal D18.03
intracranial D18.02
jugulare D44.7
malignant C75.5
skin D18.01
specified site NEC D18.09
gonadal stromal — *see* Neoplasm, uncertain behavior, by site
granular cell (*see also* Neoplasm, connective tissue, benign)
malignant — *see* Neoplasm, connective tissue, malignant
granulosa cell D39.1-
juvenile D39.1-
malignant C56.-
granulosa cell-theca cell D39.1-
malignant C56.-
Grawitz's C64.-
hemorrhoidal — *see* Hemorrhoids
hilar cell D27.-
hilus cell D27.-
Hurthle cell (benign) D34
malignant C73
hydatid — *see* Echinococcus
hypernephroid — *see* Neoplasm, uncertain behavior, by site
interstitial cell (*see also* Neoplasm, uncertain behavior, by site)
benign — *see* Neoplasm, benign, by site
malignant — *see* Neoplasm, malignant, by site
intravascular bronchial alveolar D38.1
islet cell (*see also* Neoplasm, benign, by site)
malignant (*see also* Neoplasm, malignant, by site)
pancreas C25.4
specified site NEC — *see* Neoplasm, malignant, by site
unspecified site C25.4
pancreas D13.7
specified site NEC — *see* Neoplasm, benign, by site
unspecified site D13.7
juxtaglomerular D41.0-
Klatskin's C22.1
Krukenberg's C79.6-

Tumor—*continued*
Leydig cell (*see also* Neoplasm, uncertain behavior, by site)
benign (*see also* Neoplasm, benign, by site)
specified site — *see* Neoplasm, benign, by site
unspecified site
female D27.9
male D29.20
malignant (*see also* Neoplasm, malignant, by site)
specified site — *see* Neoplasm, malignant, by site
unspecified site
female C56.9
male C62.90
specified site — *see* Neoplasm, uncertain behavior , by site
unspecified site
female D39.10
male D40.10
lipid cell, ovary D27.-
lipoid cell, ovary D27.-
malignant (*see also* Neoplasm, malignant, by site) C80.1
fusiform cell (type) C80.1
giant cell (type) C80.1
localized, plasma cell — *see* Plasmacytoma, solitary
mixed NEC C80.1
small cell (type) C80.1
spindle cell (type) C80.1
unclassified C80.1
mast cell D47.0
malignant C96.2
melanotic, neuroectodermal — *see* Neoplasm, benign, by site
Merkel cell — *see* Carcinoma, Merkel cell
mesenchymal
malignant — *see* Neoplasm, connective tissue, malignant
mixed — *see* Neoplasm, connective tissue, uncertain behavior
mesodermal, mixed (*see also* Neoplasm, malignant, by site)
liver C22.4
mesonephric (*see also* Neoplasm, uncertain behavior, by site)
malignant — *see* Neoplasm, malignant, by site
metastatic
from specified site — *see* Neoplasm, malignant, by site
of specified site — *see* Neoplasm, malignant, by site
to specified site — *see* Neoplasm, secondary, by site
mixed NEC (*see also* Neoplasm, benign, by site)
malignant — *see* Neoplasm, malignant, by site
unspecified site C56.9
mucinous of low malignant potential
specified site — *see* Neoplasm, malignant, by site
unspecified site C18.1
mucocarcinoid
specified site — *see* Neoplasm, malignant, by site
mucoepidermoid — *see* Neoplasm, uncertain behavior, by site
Müllerian, mixed
specified site — *see* Neoplasm, malignant, by site
unspecified site C54.9
myoepithelial — *see* Neoplasm, benign, by site
neuroectodermal (peripheral) (primative) (*see also* Neoplasm, malignant, by site)
primitive
specified site — *see* Neoplasm, malignant, by site
unspecified site C71.9
neuroendocrine D3a.8
malignant poorly differentiated C7a.1
secondary NEC C7b.8
specified NEC C7a.8
neurogenic olfactory C30.0
nonencapsulated sclerosing C73

Tumor —*continued*
  odontogenic (adenomatoid) (benign) (calcifying
      epithelial) (keratocystic) (squamous) *(see also*
      Cyst, calcifying odontogenic)
    malignant C41.1
      upper jaw (bone) C41.0
  ovarian stromal D39.1-
  ovary, in pregnancy — *see* Pregnancy, complicated
      by
  pacinian — *see* Neoplasm, skin, benign
  Pancoast's — *see* Pancoast's syndrome
  papillary *(see also* Papilloma)
    cystic D37.9
    mucinous of low malignant potential C56.-
      specified site — *see* Neoplasm, malignant, by
          site
      unspecified site C56.9
    serous of low malignant potential
      specified site — *see* Neoplasm, malignant, by
          site
      unspecified site C56.9
  pelvic, in pregnancy or childbirth — *see* Pregnancy,
      complicated by
  phantom F45.8
  phyllodes D48.6-
    benign D24-
    malignant — *see* Neoplasm, breast, malignant
  Pindborg — *see* Cyst, calcifying odontogenic
  placental site trophoblastic D39.2
  plasma cell (malignant) (localized) — *see*
      Plasmacytoma, solitary
  polyvesicular vitelline
    specifed site — see Neoplasm, malignant, by site
    unspecified site
      female C56.9
      male C62.90
  Pott's puffy — *see* Osteomyelitis, specified NEC
  Rathke's pouch D44.3
  retinal anlage — *see* Neoplasm, benign, by site
  salivary gland type, mixed *(see also* Neoplasm,
      salivary gland, benign)
    malignant — *see* Neoplasm, salivary gland,
        malignant
  Sampson's N80.1
  Schmincke's — *see* Neoplasm, nasopharynx,
      malignant
  sclerosing stromal D27.-
  sebaceous — *see* Cyst, sebaceous
  secondary *(see also* Neoplasm, secondary, by site)
    carcinoid C7b.00
      bone C7b.03
      distant lymph nodes C7b.01
      liver C7b.02
      peritoneum C7b.04
      specified NEC C7b.09
    neuroendocrine NEC C7b.8
  serous of low malignant potential
    specified site — *see* Neoplasm, malignant, by site
    unspecified site C56.9
  Sertoli cell *(see also* Neoplasm, benign, by site)
    with lipid storage
      specified stie — *see* Neoplasm, benign, by site
    specified site — *see* Neoplasm, benign, by site
    unspecified site
      female D27.9
      male D29.20
  Sertoli-Leydig cell *(see also* Neoplasm, benign, by
      site)
    specified site — *see* Neoplasm, benign, by site
    unspecified site
      female D27.9
      male D29.20
  sex cord(-stromal) *(see also* Neoplasm, uncertain
      behavior, by site)
    with annular tubules D39.1-
  skin appendage — *see* Neoplasm, skin, benign
  smooth muscle — *see* Neoplasm, connective tissue,
      uncertain behavior

Tumor —*continued*
  soft tissue
    benign — *see* Neoplasm, connective tissue,
        benign
    malignant — *see* Neoplasm, connective tissue,
        malignant
  sternomastoid (congenital) Q68.0
  stromal
    endometrial D39.0
    gastric D48.1
      benign D21.4
      malignant C16.9
      uncertain behavior D48.1
    gastrointestinal
      benign D21.4
      malignant C49.4
      uncertain behavior D48.1
    intestine
      benign D21.4
      malignant C49.4
      uncertain behavior D48.1
    ovarian D39.1-
    stomach
      benign D21.4
      malignant C16.9
      uncertain behavior D48.1
  testicular D40.10
  sweat gland *(see also* Neoplasm, skin, uncertain
      behavior)
    benign — *see* Neoplasm, skin, benign
    malignant — *see* Neoplasm, skin, malignant
  syphilitic, brain A52.17
  testicular stromal D40.1-
  theca cell D27.-
  theca cell-granulosa cell D39.1-
  Triton, malignant — *see* Neoplasm, nerve,
      malignant
  trophoblastic, placental site D39.2
  turban D23.4
  uterus (body), in pregnancy or childbirth — *see*
      Pregnancy, complicated by, tumor, uterus
  vagina, in pregnancy or childbirth — *see* Pregnancy,
      complicated by
  varicose — *see* Varix
  von Recklinghausen's — *see* Neurofibromatosis
  vulva or perineum, in pregnancy or childbirth — *see*
      Pregnancy, complicated by
    causing obstructed labor O65.5
  Warthin's — *see* Neoplasm, salivary gland, benign
  Wilms' C64.-
  yolk sac *(see also* Neoplasm, malignant, by site)
    specified site — *see* Neoplasm, malignant, by site
    unspecified site
      female C56.9
      male C62.90
Tumor lysis syndrome (following antineoplastic
    chemotherapy) (spontaneous) NEC E88.3
Tumorlet — *see* Neoplasm, uncertain behavior, by site
Tungiasis B88.1
Tunica vasculosa lentis Q12.2
Turban tumor D23.4
Türck's trachoma J37.0
Turner-Kieser syndrome Q79.8
Turner-like syndrome Q87.1
Turner's
  hypoplasia (tooth) K00.4
  syndrome Q96.9
    specified NEC Q96.8
  tooth K00.4
Turner-Ullrich syndrome Q96.9
Tussis convulsiva — *see* Whooping cough
Twiddler's syndrome (due to)
  automatic implantable defibrillatorT82.198
  cardiac pacemaker T82.198
Twilight state
  epileptic F05
  psychogenic F44.89
Twin (newborn) *(see also* Newborn, twin)
  conjoined Q89.4
    pregnancy — *see* Pregnancy, twin, conjoined
Twinning, teeth K00.2
Twist, twisted
  bowel, colon or intestine K56.2

Twist, twisted—*continued*
  hair (congenital) Q84.1
  mesentery K56.2
  omentum K56.2
  organ or site, congenital NEC — *see* Anomaly, by site
  ovarian pedicle — *see* Torsion, ovary
Twitching R25.3
Tylosis (acquired) L84
  buccalis K13.29
  linguae K13.29
  palmaris et plantaris (congenital) (inherited) Q82.8
    acquired L85.1
Tympanism R14.0
Tympanites (abdominal) (intestinal) R14.0
Tympanitis — *see* Myringitis
Tympanosclerosis — *see* subcategory H74.0
Tympanum — *see* condition
Tympany
  abdomen R14.0
  chest R09.89
Type A behavior pattern Z73.1
Typhlitis — *see* Appendicitis
Typhoenteritis — *see* Typhoid
Typhoid (abortive) (ambulant) (any site) (clinical)
    (fever) (hemorrhagic) (infection) (intermittent)
    (malignant) (rheumatic) (Widalnegative) A01.00
  with pneumonia A01.03
  abdominal A01.09
  arthritis A01.04
  carrier (suspected) of Z22.0
  cholecystitis (current) A01.09
  endocarditis A01.02
  heart involvement A01.02
  inoculation reaction — *see* Complications,
      vaccination
  meningitis A01.01
  mesenteric lymph nodes A01.09
  myocarditis A01.02
  osteomyelitis A01.05
  perichondritis, larynx A01.09
  pneumonia A01.03
  spine A01.05
  specified NEC A01.09
  ulcer (perforating) A01.09
Typhomalaria (fever) — *see* Malaria
Typhomania A01.00
Typhoperitonitis A01.09
Typhus (fever) A75.9
  abdominal, abdominalis — *see* Typhoid
  African tick A77.1
  amarillic A95.9
  brain A75.9 [G94]
  cerebral A75.9 [G94]
  classical A75.0
  due to Rickettsia
    prowazekii A75.0
      recrudescent A75.1
    tsutsugamushi A75.3
    typhi A75.2
  endemic (flea-borne) A75.2
  epidemic (louse-borne) A75.0
  exanthematic NEC A75.0
  exanthematicus SAI A75.0
    brillii SAI A75.1
    mexicanus SAI A75.2
    typhus murinus A75.2
  flea-borne A75.2
  India tick A77.1
  Kenya (tick) A77.1
  louse-borne A75.0
  Mexican A75.2
  mite-borne A75.3
  murine A75.2
  North Asian tick-borne A77.2
  petechial A75.9
  Queensland tick A77.3
  rat A75.2
  recrudescent A75.1
  recurrens — *see* Fever, relapsing
  Sao Paulo A77.0
  scrub (China) (India) (Malaysia) (New Guinea) A75.3
  shop (of Malaysia) A75.2
  Siberian tick A77.2

Typhus (fever) A75.9
   tick-borne A77.9
   tropical (mite-borne) A75.3
Tyrosinemia E70.21
   newborn, transitory P74.5
Tyrosinosis E70.21
Tyrosinuria E70.29

U

Uhl's anomaly or disease Q24.8
Ulcer, ulcerated, ulcerating, ulceration, ulcerative
   alveolar process M27.3
   amebic (intestine) A06.1
      skin A06.7
   anastomotic — see Ulcer, gastrojejunal
   anorectal K62.6
   antral — see Ulcer, stomach
   anus (sphincter) (solitary) K62.6
      varicose — see Varicose, ulcer, anus
   aorta — see Aneurysm
   aphthous (oral) (recurrent) K12.0
      genital organ(s)
         female N76.6
         male N50.8
   artery I77.2
   atrophic — see Ulcer, skin
      decubitus — see Ulcer, pressure, by site
   back L98.429
      with
         bone necrosis L98.424
         exposed fat layer L98.422
         muscle necrosis L98.423
         skin breakdown only L98.421
   Barrett's (esophagus) K22.10
      with bleeding K22.11
   bile duct (common) (hepatic) K83.8
   bladder (solitary) (sphincter) NEC N32.89
      bilharzial B65.9 [N33]
      in schistosomiasis (bilharzial) B65.9 [N33]
      submucosal — see Cystitis, interstitial
      tuberculous A18.12
   bleeding K27.4
   bone — see Osteomyelitis, specified type NEC
   bowel — see Ulcer, intestine
   breast N61
   bronchus J98.09
   buccal (cavity) (traumatic) K12.1
   Buruli A31.1
   buttock L98.419
      bone necrosis L98.414
      exposed fat layer L98.412
      muscle necrosis L98.413
      skin breakdown L98.411
   cancerous — see Neoplasm, malignant, by site
   cardia K22.10
      with bleeding K22.11
   cardioesophageal (peptic) K22.10
      with bleeding K22.11
   cecum — see Ulcer, intestine
   cervix (uteri) (decubitus) (trophic) N86
      with cervicitis N72
   chancroidal A57
   chiclero B55.1
   chronic (cause unknown) — see Ulcer, skin
   Cochin-China B55.1
   colon — see Ulcer, intestine
   conjunctiva H10.89
   cornea H16.00-
      with hypopyon H16.03-
      central H16.01-
      dendritic (herpes simplex) B00.52
      marginal H16.04-
      Mooren's H16.05-
      mycotic H16.06-
      perforated H16.07-
      ring H16.02-
      tuberculous (phlyctenular) A18.52
   corpus cavernosum (chronic) N48.5
   crural — see Ulcer, lower limb
   Curling's — see Ulcer, peptic, acute

Ulcer, ulcerated, ulcerating, ulceration, ulcerative—continued
   Cushing's — see Ulcer, peptic, acute
   cystic duct K82.8
   cystitis (interstitial) — see Cystitis, interstitial
   decubitus — see Ulcer, pressure, by site
   dendritic, cornea (herpes simplex) B00.52
   diabetes, diabetic — see Diabetes, ulcer
   Dieulafoy's K25.0
   due to
      infection NEC — see Ulcer, skin
      radiation NEC L59.8
      trophic disturbance (any region) — see Ulcer, skin
      X-ray L58.1
   duodenum, duodenal (eroded) (peptic) K26.9
      with
         hemorrhage K26.4
            and perforation K26.6
         perforation K26.5
      acute K26.3
         with
            hemorrhage K26.0
               and perforation K26.2
            perforation K26.1
      chronic K26.7
         with
            hemorrhage K26.4
               and perforation K26.6
            perforation K26.5
   dysenteric A09
   elusive — see Cystitis, interstitial
   endocarditis (acute) (chronic) (subacute) I28.8
   epiglottis J38.7
   esophagus (peptic) K22.10
      with bleeding K22.11
      due to
         aspirin K22.10
            with bleeding K22.11
         gastrointestinal reflux disease K21.0
         ingestion of chemical or medicament K22.10
            with bleeding K22.11
      fungal K22.10
         with bleeding K22.11
      infective K22.10
         with bleeding K22.11
      varicose — see Varix, esophagus
   eyelid (region) H01.8
   fauces J39.2
   Fenwick (-Hunner) (solitary) — see Cystitis, interstitial
   fistulous — see Ulcer, skin
   foot (indolent) (trophic) — see Ulcer, lower limb
   frambesial, initial A66.0
   frenum (tongue) K14.0
   gallbladder or duct K82.8
   gangrenous — see Gangrene
   gastric — see Ulcer, stomach
   gastrocolic — see Ulcer, gastrojejunal
   gastroduodenal — see Ulcer, peptic
   gastroesophageal — see Ulcer, stomach
   gastrointestinal — see Ulcer, gastrojejunal
   gastrojejunal (peptic) K28.9
      with
         hemorrhage K28.4
            and perforation K28.6
         perforation K28.5
      acute K28.3
         with
            hemorrhage K28.0
               and perforation K28.2
            perforation K28.1
      chronic K28.7
         with
            hemorrhage K28.4
               and perforation K28.6
            perforation K28.5
   gastrojejunocolic — see Ulcer, gastrojejunal
   gingiva K06.8
   gingivitis K05.10
      plaque induced K05.10
      nonplaque induced K05.11
   glottis J38.7

Ulcer, ulcerated, ulcerating, ulceration, ulcerative—continued
   granuloma of pudenda A58
   gum K06.8
   gumma, due to yaws A66.4
   heel — see Ulcer, lower limb
   hemorrhoids — see Hemorrhoids
   Hunner's — see Cystitis, interstitial
   hypopharynx J39.2
   hypopyon (chronic) (subacute) — see Ulcer, cornea, with hypopyon
   hypostaticum — see Ulcer, varicose
   ileum — see Ulcer, intestine
   intestine, intestinal K63.3
      with perforation K63.1
      amebic A06.1
      duodenal — see Ulcer, duodenum
      granulocytopenic (with hemorrhage) — see Neutropenia
      marginal — see Ulcer, gastrojejunal
      perforating K63.1
         newborn P78.0
      primary, small intestine K63.3
      rectum K62.6
      stercoraceous, stercoral K63.3
      tuberculous A18.32
      typhoid (fever) — see Typhoid
      varicose I86.8
   jejunum, jejunal — see Ulcer, gastrojejunal
   keratitis — see Ulcer, cornea
   knee — see Ulcer, lower limb
   labium (majus) (minus) N76.6
   laryngitis — see Laryngitis
   larynx (aphthous) (contact) J38.7
      diphtheritic A36.2
   leg — see Ulcer, lower limb
   lip K13.0
   Lipschütz's N76.6
   lower limb (atrophic) (chronic) (neurogenic) (perforating) (pyogenic) (trophic) (tropical) L97.909
      with
         bone necrosis L97.904
         exposed fat layer L97.902
         muscle necrosis L97.903
         skin breakdown only L97.901
      ankle L97.309
         with
            bone necrosis L97.304
            exposed fat layer L97.302
            muscle necrosis L97.303
            skin breakdown only L97.301
         left L97.329
            with
               bone necrosis L97.324
               exposed fat layer L97.322
               muscle necrosis L97.323
               skin breakdown only L97.321
         right L97.319
            with
               bone necrosis L97.314
               exposed fat layer L97.312
               muscle necrosis L97.313
               skin breakdown only L97.311
      calf L97.209
         with
            bone necrosis L97.204
            exposed fat layer L97.202
            muscle necrosis L97.203
            skin breakdown only L97.201
         left L97.229
            with
               bone necrosis L97.224
               exposed fat layer L97.222
               muscle necrosis L97.223
               skin breakdown only L97.221
         right L97.219
            with
               bone necrosis L97.214
               exposed fat layer L97.212
               muscle necrosis L97.213
               skin breakdown only L97.211

Ulcer, ulcerated, ulcerating, ulceration, ulcerative—continued
lower limb—continued
  decubitus — see Ulcer, pressure, by site
  foot specified NEC L97.509
    with
      bone necrosis L97.504
      exposed fat layer L97.502
      muscle necrosis L97.503
      skin breakdown only L97.501
    left L97.529
      with
        bone necrosis L97.524
        exposed fat layer L97.522
        muscle necrosis L97.523
        skin breakdown only L97.521
    right L97.519
      with
        bone necrosis L97.514
        exposed fat layer L97.512
        muscle necrosis L97.513
        skin breakdown only L97.511
  heel L97.409
    with
      bone necrosis L97.404
      exposed fat layer L97.402
      muscle necrosis L97.403
      skin breakdown only L97.401
    left L97.429
      with
        bone necrosis L97.424
        exposed fat layer L97.422
        muscle necrosis L97.423
        skin breakdown only L97.421
    right L97.419
      with
        bone necrosis L97.414
        exposed fat layer L97.412
        muscle necrosis L97.413
        skin breakdown only L97.411
  left L97.929
    with
      bone necrosis L97.924
      exposed fat layer L97.922
      muscle necrosis L97.923
      skin breakdown only L97.921
  lower leg NOS L97.909
    with
      bone necrosis L97.904
      exposed fat layer L97.902
      muscle necrosis L97.903
      skin breakdown only L97.901
    left L97.929
      with
        bone necrosis L97.924
        exposed fat layer L97.922
        muscle necrosis L97.923
        skin breakdown only L97.921
    right L97.919
      with
        bone necrosis L97.914
        exposed fat layer L97.912
        muscle necrosis L97.913
        skin breakdown only L97.911
  specified site NEC L97.809
    with
      bone necrosis L97.804
      exposed fat layer L97.802
      muscle necrosis L97.803
      skin breakdown only L97.801
    left L97.829
      with
        bone necrosis L97.824
        exposed fat layer L97.822
        muscle necrosis L97.823
        skin breakdown only L97.821
    right L97.819
      with
        bone necrosis L97.814
        exposed fat layer L97.812
        muscle necrosis L97.813
        skin breakdown only L97.811

Ulcer, ulcerated, ulcerating, ulceration, ulcerative—continued
lower limb—continued
  midfoot L97.409
    with
      bone necrosis L97.404
      exposed fat layer L97.402
      muscle necrosis L97.403
      skin breakdown only L97.401
    left L97.429
      with
        bone necrosis L97.424
        exposed fat layer L97.422
        muscle necrosis L97.423
        skin breakdown only L97.421
    right L97.419
      with
        bone necrosis L97.414
        exposed fat layer L97.412
        muscle necrosis L97.413
        skin breakdown only L97.411
  right L97.919
    with
      bone necrosis L97.914
      exposed fat layer L97.912
      muscle necrosis L97.913
      skin breakdown only L97.911
  thigh L97.109
    with
      bone necrosis L97.104
      exposed fat layer L97.102
      muscle necrosis L97.103
      skin breakdown only L97.101
    left L97.129
      with
        bone necrosis L97.124
        exposed fat layer L97.122
        muscle necrosis L97.123
        skin breakdown only L97.121
    right L97.119
      with
        bone necrosis L97.114
        exposed fat layer L97.112
        muscle necrosis L97.113
        skin breakdown only L97.111
  toe L97.509
    with
      bone necrosis L97.504
      exposed fat layer L97.502
      muscle necrosis L97.503
      skin breakdown only L97.501
    left L97.529
      with
        bone necrosis L97.524
        exposed fat layer L97.522
        muscle necrosis L97.523
        skin breakdown only L97.521
    right L97.519
      with
        bone necrosis L97.514
        exposed fat layer L97.512
        muscle necrosis L97.513
        skin breakdown only L97.511
  leprous A30.1
  syphilitic A52.19
  varicose — see Varix, leg, with, ulcer
luetic — see Ulcer, syphilitic
lung J98.4
  tuberculous — see Tuberculosis, pulmonary
malignant — see Neoplasm, malignant, by site
marginal NEC — see Ulcer, gastrojejunal
meatus (urinarius) N34.2
Meckel's diverticulum Q43.0
  malignant — see Table of Neoplasms, small
    intestine, malignant
Meleney's (chronic undermining) — see Ulcer, skin
Mooren's (cornea) — see Ulcer, cornea, Mooren's
mycobacterial (skin) A31.1
nasopharynx J39.2
neck, uterus N86
neurogenic NEC — see Ulcer, skin
nose, nasal (passage) (infective) (septum) J34.0
  skin — see Ulcer, skin

Ulcer, ulcerated, ulcerating, ulceration, ulcerative—continued
nose, nasal —continued
  spirochetal A69.8
  varicose (bleeding) I86.8
oral mucosa (traumatic) K12.1
palate (soft) K12.1
penis (chronic) N48.5
peptic (site unspecified) K27.9
  with
    hemorrhage K27.4
      and perforation K27.6
    perforation K27.5
  acute K27.3
    with
      hemorrhage K27.0
        and perforation K27.2
      perforation K27.1
  chronic K27.7
    with
      hemorrhage K27.4
        and perforation K27.6
      perforation K27.5
  esophagus K22.10
    with bleeding K22.11
  newborn P78.82
perforating K27.5
  skin — see Ulcer, skin
peritonsillar J35.8
phagedenic (tropical) — see Ulcer, skin
pharynx J39.2
phlebitis — see Phlebitis
plaster — see Ulcer, pressure, by site
popliteal space — see Ulcer, lower limb
postpyloric — see Ulcer, duodenum
prepuce N47.7
prepyloric — see Ulcer, stomach
pressure (pressure area) L89.9-
  ankle L89.5-
  back L89.1-
  buttock L89.3-
  coccyx L89.15-
  contiguous site of back, buttock, hip L89.4-
  elbow L89.0-
  face L89.81-
  head L89.81-
  heel L89.6-
  hip L89.2-
  sacral region (tailbone) L89.15-
  specified site NEC L89.89-
  stage 1 (healing) (pre-ulcer skin changes limited
      to persistent focal edema)
    ankle L89.5-
    back L89.1-
    buttock L89.3-
    coccyx L89.15-
    contiguous site of back, buttock, hip L89.4-
    elbow L89.0-
    face L89.81-
    head L89.81-
    heel L89.6-
    hip L89.2-
    sacral region (tailbone) L89.15-
    specified site NEC L89.89-
  stage 2 (healing) (abrasion, blister, partial
      thickness skin loss involving epidermis
      and/or dermis)
    ankle L89.5-
    back L89.1-
    buttock L89.3-
    coccyx L89.15-
    contiguous site of back, buttock, hip L89.4-
    elbow L89.0-
    face L89.81-
    head L89.81-
    heel L89.6-
    hip L89.2-
    sacral region (tailbone) L89.15-
    specified site NEC L89.89-
  stage 3 (healing) (full thickness skin loss
      involving damage or necrosis of
      subcutaneous tissue)
    ankle L89.5-

Ulcer, ulcerated, ulcerating, ulceration, ulcerative—continued
  pressure—continued
    stage 3—continued
      back L89.1-
      buttock L89.3-
      coccyx L89.15-
      contiguous site of back, buttock, hip L89.4-
      elbow L89.0-
      face L89.81-
      head L89.81-
      heel L89.6-
      hip L89.2-
      sacral region (tailbone) L89.15-
      specified site NEC L89.89-
    stage 4 (healing) (necrosis of soft tissues through to underlying muscle, tendon, or bone)
      ankle L89.5-
      back L89.1-
      buttock L89.3-
      coccyx L89.15-
      contiguous site of back, buttock, hip L89.4-
      elbow L89.0-
      face L89.81-
      head L89.81-
      heel L89.6-
      hip L89.2-
      sacral region (tailbone) L89.15-
      specified site NEC L89.89-
    unspecified stage
      ankle L89.5-
      back L89.1-
      buttock L89.3-
      coccyx L89.15-
      contiguous site of back, buttock, hip L89.4-
      elbow L89.0-
      face L89.81-
      head L89.81-
      heel L89.6-
      hip L89.2-
      sacral region (tailbone) L89.15-
      specified site NEC L89.89-
    unstageable
      ankle L89.5-
      back L89.1-
      buttock L89.3-
      coccyx L89.15-
      contiguous site of back, buttock, hip L89.4-
      elbow L89.0-
      face L89.81-
      head L89.81-
      heel L89.6-
      hip L89.2-
      sacral region (tailbone) L89.15-
      specified site NEC L89.89-
  primary of intestine K63.3
    with perforation K63.1
  prostate N41.9
  pyloric — see Ulcer, stomach
  rectosigmoid K63.3
    with perforation K63.1
  rectum (sphincter) (solitary) K62.6
    stercoraceous, stercoral K62.6
    varicose — see Varicose, ulcer, anus
  retina — see Inflammation, chorioretinal
  rodent (see also Neoplasm, skin, malignant)
  sclera — see Scleritis
  scrofulous (tuberculous) A18.2
  scrotum N50.8
    tuberculous A18.15
    varicose I86.1
  seminal vesicle N50.8
  sigmoid — see Ulcer, intestine
  skin (atrophic) (chronic) (neurogenic) (non-healing) (perforating) (pyogenic) (trophic) (tropical) L98.499
    with gangrene — see Gangrene
    amebic A06.7
    back — see Ulcer, back
    buttock — see Ulcer, buttock
    decubitus — see Ulcer, pressure
    lower limb — see Ulcer, lower limb
    mycobacterial A31.1

Ulcer, ulcerated, ulcerating, ulceration, ulcerative—continued
  skin—continued
    specified site NEC L98.499
      with
        bone necrosis L98.494
        exposed fat layer L98.492
        muscle necrosis L98.493
        skin breakdown only L98.491
    tuberculous (primary) A18.4
    varicose — see Ulcer, varicose
  sloughing — see Ulcer, skin
  solitary, anus or rectum (sphincter) K62.6
  sore throat J02.9
    streptococcal J02.0
  spermatic cord N50.8
  spine (tuberculous) A18.01
  stasis (venous) — see Varix, leg, with, ulcer
    without varicose veins I87.2
  stercoraceous, stercoral K63.3
    with perforation K63.1
    anus or rectum K62.6
  stoma, stomal — see Ulcer, gastrojejunal
  stomach (eroded) (peptic) (round) K25.9
    with
      hemorrhage K25.4
        and perforation K25.6
      perforation K25.5
    acute K25.3
      with
        hemorrhage K25.0
          and perforation K25.2
        perforation K25.1
    chronic K25.7
      with
        hemorrhage K25.4
          and perforation K25.6
        perforation K25.5
  stomal — see Ulcer, gastrojejunal
  stomatitis K12.1
  stress — see Ulcer, peptic
  strumous (tuberculous) A18.2
  submucosal, bladder — see Cystitis, interstitial
  syphilitic (any site) (early) (secondary) A51.39
    late A52.79
    perforating A52.79
      foot A52.11
  testis N50.8
  thigh — see Ulcer, lower limb
  throat J39.2
    diphtheritic A36.0
  toe — see Ulcer, lower limb
  tongue (traumatic) K14.0
  tonsil J35.8
    diphtheritic A36.0
  trachea J39.8
  trophic — see Ulcer, skin
  tropical — see Ulcer, skin
  tuberculous — see Tuberculosis, ulcer
  tunica vaginalis N50.8
  turbinate J34.89
  typhoid (perforating) — see Typhoid
  unspecified site — see Ulcer, skin
  urethra (meatus) — see Urethritis
  uterus N85.8
    cervix N86
      with cervicitis N72
    neck N86
      with cervicitis N72
  vagina N76.5
    in Behçet's disease M35.2 [N77.0]
    pessary N89.8
  valve, heart I33.0
  varicose (lower limb, any part) (see also Varix, leg, with, ulcer)
    anus — see Varicose, ulcer, anus
    broad ligament I86.2
    esophagus — see Varix, esophagus
    inflamed or infected — see Varix, leg, with ulcer, with inflammation
    nasal septum I86.8
    perineum I86.3
    rectum — see Varicose, ulcer, anus

Ulcer, ulcerated, ulcerating, ulceration, ulcerative—continued
  varicose—continued
    scrotum I86.1
    specified site NEC I86.8
    sublingual I86.0
    vulva I86.3
  vas deferens N50.8
  vulva (acute) (infectional) N76.6
    in (due to)
      Behçet's disease M35.2 [N77.0]
      herpesviral (herpes simplex) infection A60.04
      tuberculosis A18.18
  vulvobuccal, recurring N76.6
  X-ray L58.1
  yaws A66.4
Ulcerosa scarlatina A38.8
Ulcus (see also Ulcer)
  cutis tuberculosum A18.4
  duodeni — see Ulcer, duodenum
  durum (syphilitic) A51.0
    extragenital A51.2
  gastrojejunale — see Ulcer, gastrojejunal
  hypostaticum — see Ulcer, varicose
  molle (cutis) (skin) A57
  serpens corneae — see Ulcer, cornea, central
  ventriculi — see Ulcer, stomach
Ulegyria Q04.8
Ulerythema
  ophryogenes, congenital Q84.2
  sycosiforme L73.8
Ullrich(-Bonnevie)(-Turner) syndrome Q87.1
Ullrich-Feichtiger syndrome Q87.0
Ulnar — see condition
Ulorrhagia, ulorrhea K06.8
Umbilicus, umbilical — see condition
Unacceptable
  contours of tooth K08.54
  morphology of tooth K08.54
Unavailability (of)
  bed at medical facility Z75.1
  health service-related agencies Z75.4
  medical facilities (at) Z75.3
    due to
      investigation by social service agency Z75.2
      lack of services at home Z75.0
      remoteness from facility Z75.3
      waiting list Z75.1
      home Z75.0
      outpatient clinic Z75.3
    schooling Z55.1
    social service agencies Z75.4
Uncinaria americana infestation B76.9
Uncinariasis B76.9
Uncongenial work Z56.5
Unconscious(ness) — see Coma
Under observation — see Observation
Underachievement in school Z55.3
Underdevelopment (see also Undeveloped)
  nose Q30.1
  sexual E30.0
Underdosing (see also Table of Drugs and Chemicals, categories T36-T50, with final character 6 Z91.14)
  intentional NEC Z91.128
    due to financial hardship of patient Z91.120
  unintentional NEC Z91.138
    due to patient's age related debility Z91.130
Underfeeding, newborn P92.3
Underfill, endodontic M27.53
Underimmunization status Z28.3
Undernourishment — see Malnutrition
Undernutrition — see Malnutrition
Underweight R63.6
  for gestational age — see Light for dates
Underwood's disease P83.0
Undescended (see also Malposition, congenital)
  cecum Q43.3
  colon Q43.3
  testicle — see Cryptorchid
Undeveloped, undevelopment (see also Hypoplasia)
  brain (congenital) Q02

Undeveloped, undevelopment —*continued*
  cerebral (congenital) Q02
  heart Q24.8
  lung Q33.6
  testis E29.1
  uterus E30.0
Undiagnosed (disease) R69
Undulant fever — *see* Brucellosis
Unemployment, anxiety concerning Z56.0
  threatened Z56.2
Unequal length (acquired) (limb) (*see also* Deformity, limb, unequal length)
  leg (*see also* Deformity, limb, unequal length)
    congenital Q72.9-
Unextracted dental root K08.3
Unguis incarnatus L60.0
Unhappiness R45.2
Unicornate uterus Q51.4
Unilateral (*see also* condition)
  development, breast N64.89
  organ or site, congenital NEC — *see* Agenesis, by site
Unilocular heart Q20.8
Union, abnormal (*see also* Fusion)
  larynx and trachea Q34.8
Universal mesentery Q43.3
Unrepairable overhanging of dental restorative materials K08.52
Unsatisfactory
  restoration of tooth K08.50
    specified NEC K08.59
  sample of cytologic smear
    anus R85.615
    cervix R87.615
    vagina R87.625
  surroundings Z59.1
    work Z56.5
Unsoundness of mind — *see* Psychosis
Unstable
  back NEC — *see* Instability, joint, spine
  hip (congenital) Q65.6
    acquired — *see* Derangement, joint, specified type NEC, hip
  joint — *see* Instability, joint
    secondary to removal of joint prosthesis M96.89
  lie (mother) O32.0
  lumbosacral joint (congenital)
    acquired — *see* subcategory M53.2
  sacroiliac — *see* subcategory M53.2
  spine NEC — *see* Instability, joint, spine
Unsteadiness on feet R26.81
Untruthfulness, child problem F91.8
Unverricht (-Lundborg) **disease or epilepsy** — *see* Epilepsy, generalized, idiopathic
Unwanted pregnancy Z64.0
Upbringing, institutional Z62.22
  away from parents NEC Z62.29
  in care of non-parental family member Z62.21
  in foster care Z62.21
  in orphanage or group home Z62.22
  in welfare custody Z62.21
Upper respiratory — *see* condition
Upset
  gastric K30
  gastrointestinal K30
    psychogenic F45.8
  intestinal (large) (small) K59.9
    psychogenic F45.8
  menstruation N93.9
  mental F48.9
  stomach K30
    psychogenic F45.8
Urachus (*see also* condition)
  patent or persistent Q64.4
Urbach-Oppenheim disease E88.89
Urbach's lipoid proteinosis E78.89
Urbach-Wiethe disease E78.89
Urban yellow fever A95.1
Urea
  blood, high — *see* Uremia
  cycle metabolism disorder — *see* Disorder, urea cycle metabolism

Uremia, uremic N19
  with
    ectopic or molar pregnancy O08.4
    polyneuropathy N19 [G63]
  chronic (*see also* Disease, kidney, chronic) N18.9
    due to hypertension — *see* Hypertensive, kidney
  complicating
    ectopic or molar pregnancy O08.4
  congenital P96.0
  extrarenal R39.2
  following ectopic or molar pregnancy O08.4
  newborn P96.0
  prerenal R39.2
Ureter, ureteral — *see* condition
Ureteralgia N23
Ureterectasis — *see* Hydroureter
Ureteritis N28.89
  cystica N28.86
  due to calculus N20.1
    with calculus, kidney N20.2
      with hydronephrosis N13.2
  gonococcal (acute) (chronic) A54.21
  nonspecific N28.89
Ureterocele N28.89
  congenital (orthotopic) Q62.31
    ectopic Q62.32
Ureterolith, ureterolithiasis — *see* Calculus, ureter
Ureterostomy
  attention to Z43.6
  status Z93.6
Urethra, urethral — *see* condition
Urethralgia R39.89
Urethritis (anterior) (posterior) N34.2
  calculous N21.1
  candidal B37.41
  chlamydial A56.01
  diplococcal (gonococcal) A54.01
    with abscess (accessory gland) (periurethral) A54.1
  gonococcal A54.01
    with abscess (accessory gland) (periurethral) A54.1
  nongonococcal N34.1
    Reiter's — *see* Reiter's disease
  nonspecific N34.1
  nonvenereal N34.1
  postmenopausal N34.2
  puerperal O86.29
  Reiter's — *see* Reiter's disease
  specified NEC N34.2
  trichomonal or due to Trichomonas (vaginalis) A59.03
Urethrocele N81.0 with
  cystocele — *see* Cystocele
  prolapse of uterus — *see* Prolapse, uterus
Urethrolithiasis (with colic or infection) N21.1
Urethrorectal — *see* condition
Urethrorrhagia N36.8
Urethrorrhea R36.9
Urethrostomy
  attention to Z43.6
  status Z93.6
Urethrotrigonitis — *see* Trigonitis
Urethrovaginal — *see* condition
Urgency
  fecal R15.2
  hypertensive — *see* Hypertension
  urinary N39.41
Urhidrosis, uridrosis L74.8
Uric acid in blood (increased) E79.0
Uricacidemia (asymptomatic) E79.0
Uricemia (asymptomatic) E79.0
Uricosuria R82.99
Urinary — *see* condition
Urination
  frequent R35.0
  painful R30.9
Urine
  blood in — *see* Hematuria
  discharge, excessive R35.8
  enuresis, nonorganic origin F98.0
  extravasation R39.0
  frequency R35.0

Urine—*continued*
  incontinence R32
    nonorganic origin F98.0
  intermittent stream R39.19
  pus in N39.0
  retention or stasis R33.9
    organic R33.8
      drug-induced R33.0
    psychogenic F45.8
  secretion
    deficient R34
    excessive R35.8
    frequency R35.0
  stream
    intermittent R39.19
    slowing R39.19
    splitting R39.13
    weak R39.12
Urinemia — *see* Uremia
Urinoma, urethra N36.8
Uroarthritis, infectious (Reiter's) — *see* Reiter's disease
Urodialysis R34
Urolithiasis — *see* Calculus, urinary
Uronephrosis — *see* Hydronephrosis
Uropathy N39.9
  obstructive N13.9
    specified NEC N13.8
  reflux N13.9
    specified NEC N13.8
  vesicoureteral reflux-associated — *see* Reflux, vesicoureteral
Urosepsis — code to condition
Urticaria L50.9
  with angioneurotic edema T78.3
    hereditary D84.1
  allergic L50.0
  cholinergic L50.5
  chronic L50.8
  cold, familial L50.2
  contact L50.6
  dermatographic L50.3
  due to
    cold or heat L50.2
    drugs L50.0
    food L50.0
    inhalants L50.0
    plants L50.6
    serum T80.6
  factitial L50.3
  giant T78.3
    hereditary D84.1
  gigantea T78.3
  idiopathic L50.1
  larynx T78.3
    hereditary D84.1
  neonatorum P83.8
  nonallergic L50.1
  papulosa (Hebra) L28.2
  pigmentosa Q82.2
  recurrent periodic L50.8
  serum T80.6
  solar L56.3
  specified type NEC L50.8
  thermal (cold) (heat) L50.2
  vibratory L50.4
  xanthelasmoidea Q82.2
Use (of)
  alcohol F10.99
    with sleep disorder F10.982
    harmful — *see* Abuse, alcohol
  amphetamines — *see* Use, stimulant NEC
  caffeine — *see* Use, stimulant NEC
  cannabis F12.90
    with
      anxiety disorder F12.980
      intoxication F12.929
        with
          delirium F12.921
          perceptual disturbance F12.922
        uncomplicated F12.920
      other specified disorder F12.988
      psychosis F12.959

Use —*continued*
  cannabis—*continued*
    with—*continued*
      psychosis—*continued*
        delusions F12.950
        hallucinations F12.951
      unspecified disorder F12.99
  cocaine F14.90
    with
      anxiety disorder F14.980
      intoxication F14.929
        with
          delirium F14.921
            perceptual disturbance F14.922
        uncomplicated F14.920
      other specified disorder F14.988
      psychosis F14.959
        delusions F14.950
        hallucinations F14.951
      sexual dysfunction F14.981
      sleep disorder F14.982
      unspecifed disorder F14.99
    harmful — *see* Abuse, drug, cocaine
  drug(s) NEC F19.90
    with sleep disorder F19.982
    harmful — *see* Abuse, drug, by type
  hallucinogen NEC F16.90
    with
      anxiety disorder F16.980
      intoxication F16.929
        with
          delirium F16.921
        uncomplicated F16.920
      mood disorder F16.94
      other specified disorder F16.988
      perception disorder (flashbacks) F16.983
      psychosis F16.959
        delusion(s) F16.950
        hallucinations F16.951
      unspecified disorder F16.99
    harmful — *see* Abuse, drug, hallucinogen NEC
  inhalants F18.90
    with
      anxiety disorder F18.980
      intoxication F18.929
        with delirium F18.921
        uncomplicated F18.920
      mood disorder F18.94
      other specified disorder F18.988
      persisting dementia F18.97
      psychosis F18.959
        delusions F18.950
        hallucinations F18.951
      unspecified disorder F18.99
    harmful — *see* Abuse, drug, inhalant
  methadone F11.20
  nonprescribed drugs F19.90
    harmful — *see* Abuse, non-psychoactive
        substance
  opioid F11.90
    with
      disorder F11.99
        mood F11.94
        sleep F11.982
        specified type NEC F11.988
      intoxication F11.929
        with
          delirium F11.921
            perceptual disturbance F11.922
        uncomplicated F11.920
      withdrawal F11.93
    harmful — *see* Abuse, drug, opioid
  patent medicines F19.90
    harmful — *see* Abuse, non-psychoactive
        substance
  psychoactive drug NEC F19.90
    with
      anxiety disorder F19.980
      intoxication F19.929
        with
          delirium F19.921
            perceptual disturbance F19.922
        uncomplicated F19.920

Use —*continued*
  psychoactive drug—*continued*
    with—*continued*
      mood disorder F19.94
      other specifed disorder F19.988
      persisting
        amnestic disorder F19.96
        dementia F19.97
      psychosis F19.959
        delusions F19.950
        hallucinations F19.951
      sexual dysfunction F19.981
      sleep disorder F19.982
      unspecified disorder F19.99
      withdrawal F19.939
        with
          delirium F19.931
            perceptual disturbance F19.932
        uncomplicated F19.930
    with sleep disorder F19.982
    harmful — *see* Abuse, drug NEC, psychoactive
        NEC
  sedative, hypnotic, or anxiolytic F13.90
    with
      anxiety disorder F13.980
      intoxication F13.929
        with
          delirium F13.921
        uncomplicated F13.920
      other specified disorder F13.988
      persisting
        amnestic disorder F13.96
        dementia F13.97
      psychosis F13.959
        delusions F13.950
        hallucinations F13.951
      sexual dysfunction F13.981
      sleep disorder F13.982
      unspecified disorder F13.99
    harmful — *see* Abuse, drug, sedative, hypnotic,
        or anxiolytic
  stimulant NEC F15.90
    with
      anxiety disorder F15.980
      intoxication F15.929
        with
          delirium F15.921
            perceptual disturbance F15.922
        uncomplicated F15.920
      mood disorder F19.94
      other specified disorder F15.988
      psychosis F15.959
        delusions F15.950
        hallucinations F15.951
      sexual dysfunction F15.982
      sleep disorder F15.982
      unspecified disorder F15.99
      withdrawal F15.93
    harmful — *see* Abuse, drug, stimulant NEC
  tobacco Z72.0
  volatile solvents (*see also* Use, inhalant F18.90
    harmful — *see* Abuse, drug, inhalant
  tobacco Z72.0
Usher-Senear disease or syndrome L10.4
Uta B55.1
Uteromegaly N85.2
Uterovaginal — *see* condition
Uterovesical — *see* condition
Uveal — *see* condition
Uveitis (anterior) (*see also* Iridocyclitis)
  acute — *see* Iridocyclitis, acute
  chronic — *see* Iridocyclitis, chronic
  due to toxoplasmosis (acquired) B58.09
    congenital P37.1
  granulomatous — *see* Iridocyclitis, chronic
  heterochromic — *see* Cyclitis, Fuchs' heterochromic
  lens-induced — *see* Iridocyclitis, lens-induced
  posterior — *see* Chorioretinitis
  sympathetic H44.13-
  syphilitic (secondary) A51.43
    congenital (early) A50.01
    late A52.71
  tuberculous A18.54

Uveoencephalitis — *see* Inflammation, chorioretinal
Uveokeratitis — *see* Iridocyclitis
Uveoparotitis D86.89
Uvula — *see* condition
Uvulitis (acute) (catarrhal) (chronic) (membranous) (suppurative) (ulcerative) K12.2

V

Vaccination (prophylactic)
  complication or reaction — *see* Complications, vaccination
  delayed Z28.9
  encounter for Z23
  not done — *see* Immunization, not done, because (of)
Vaccinia (generalized) (localized) T88.1
  congenital P35.8
  without vaccination B08.011
Vacuum, in sinus (accessory) (nasal) J34.89
Vagabond, vagabondage Z59.0
Vagabond's disease B85.1
Vagina, vaginal — *see* condition
Vaginalitis (tunica) (testis) N49.1
Vaginismus (reflex) N94.2
  functional F52.5
  nonorganic F52.5
  psychogenic F52.5
  secondary N94.2
Vaginitis (acute) (circumscribed) (diffuse) (emphysematous) (nonvenereal) (ulcerative) N76.0
  with ectopic or molar pregnancy O08.0
  amebic A06.82
  atrophic, postmenopausal N95.2
  bacterial N76.0
  blennorrhagic (gonococcal) A54.02
  candidal B37.3
  chlamydial A56.02
  chronic N76.1
  due to Trichomonas (vaginalis) A59.01
  following ectopic or molar pregnancy O08.0
  gonococcal A54.02
    with abscess (accessory gland) (periurethral) A54.1
  granuloma A58
  in (due to)
    candidiasis B37.3
    herpesviral (herpes simplex) infection A60.04
    pinworm infection B80 [N77.1]
  monilial B37.3
  mycotic (candidal) B37.3
  postmenopausal atrophic N95.2
  puerperal (postpartum) O86.13
  senile (atrophic) N95.2
  subacute or chronic N76.1
  syphilitic (early) A51.0
    late A52.76
  trichomonal A59.01
  tuberculous A18.18
Vaginosis — *see* Vaginitis
Vagotonia G52.2
Vagrancy Z59.0
VAIN — *see* Neoplasia, intraepithelial, vagina
Vallecula — *see* condition
Valley fever B38.0
Valsuani's disease — *see* Anemia, obstetric
Valve, valvular (formation) (*see also* condition)
  cerebral ventricle (communicating) in situ Z98.2
  cervix, internal os Q51.828
  congenital NEC — *see* Atresia, by site
  ureter (pelvic junction) (vesical orifice) Q62.39
  urethra (congenital) (posterior) Q64.2
Valvulitis (chronic) — *see* Endocarditis
Valvulopathy — *see* Endocarditis
Van Bogaert's leukoencephalopathy (sclerosing) (subacute) A81.1
Van Bogaert-Scherer-Epstein disease or syndrome E75.5
Van Buchem's syndrome M85.2
Van Creveld-von Gierke disease E74.01

Van der Hoeve (-de Kleyn) **syndrome** Q78.0
Van der Woude's syndrome Q38.0
Van Neck's disease or osteochondrosis M91.0
Vanishing lung J44.9
Vapor asphyxia or suffocation T59.9
  specified agent — *see* Table of Drugs and Chemicals
Variance, lethal ball, prosthetic heart valve T82.09
Variants, thalassemic D56.8
Variations in hair color L67.1
Varicella B01.9
  with
    complications NEC B01.89
    encephalitis B01.11
    encephalomyelitis B01.11
    meningitis B01.0
    myelitis B01.12
    pneumonia B01.2
  congenital P35.8
Varices — *see* Varix
Varicocele (scrotum) (thrombosed) I86.1
  ovary I86.2
  perineum I86.3
  spermatic cord (ulcerated) I86.1
Varicose
  aneurysm (ruptured) I77.0
  dermatitis — *see* Varix, leg, with, inflammation
  eczema — *see* Varix, leg, with, inflammation
  phlebitis — *see* Varix, with, inflammation
  tumor — *see* Varix
  ulcer (lower limb, any part) (*see also* Varix, leg, with, ulcer)
    anus — *see* Hemorrhoids, with complication
    esophagus — *see* Varix, esophagus
    inflamed or infected — *see* Varix, leg, with ulcer, with inflammation
    nasal septum I86.8
    perineum I86.3
    rectum — *see* Varicose, ulcer, anus
    scrotum I86.1
    specified site NEC I86.8
  vein — *see* Varix
  vessel — *see* Varix, leg
Varicosis, varicosities, varicosity — *see* Varix
Variola (major) (minor) B03
Varioloid B03
Varix (lower limb) (ruptured) I83.90
  with
    edema I83.899
    inflammation I83.10
      with ulcer (venous) I83.209
    pain I83.819
    specified complication NEC I83.899
    stasis dermatitis I83.10
      with ulcer (venous) I83.209
    swelling I83.899
    ulcer I83.009
      with inflammation I83.209
  aneurysmal I77.0
  anus — *see* Hemorrhoids
  asymptomatic I83.9-
  bladder I86.2
  broad ligament I86.2
  complicating
    childbirth (lower extremity) O87.4
      anus or rectum O87.2
      genital (vagina, vulva or perineum) O87.8
    pregnancy (lower extremity) O22.0-
      anus or rectum O22.4-
      genital (vagina, vulva or perineum) O22.1-
    puerperium (lower extremity) O87.4
      anus or rectum O87.2
      genital (vagina, vulva, perineum) O87.8
  congenital (any site) Q27.8
  esophagus (idiopathic) (primary) (ulcerated) I85.00
    bleeding I85.01
    congenital Q27.8
    in (due to)
      alcoholic liver disease I85.10
        bleeding I85.11
      cirrhosis of liver I85.10
        bleeding I85.11
      portal hypertension I85.10
        bleeding I85.11

Varix —*continued*
  esophagus—*continued*
    in (due to)—*continued*
      schistosomiasis I85.10
        bleeding I85.11
      toxic liver disease I85.10
        bleeding I85.11
    secondary I85.10
      bleeding I85.11
  gastric I86.4
  inflamed or infected I83.10
    ulcerated I83.209
  labia (majora) I86.3
  leg (asymptomatic) I83.90
    with
      edema I83.899
      inflammation I83.10
        with ulcer — *see* Varix, leg, with, ulcer, with inflammation by site
      pain I83.819
      specified complication NEC I83.899
      swelling I83.899
      ulcer I83.009
        with inflammation I83.209
        ankle I83.003
          with inflammation I83.203
        calf I83.002
          with inflammation I83.202
        foot NEC I83.005
          with inflammation I83.205
        heel I83.004
          with inflammation I83.204
        lower leg NEC I83.008
          with inflammation I83.208
        midfoot I83.004
          with inflammation I83.204
        thigh I83.001
          with inflammation I83.201
    bilateral (asymptomatic) I83.93
      with
        edema I83.893
        pain I83.813
        specified complication NEC I83.893
        swelling I83.893
        ulcer I83.009
          with inflammation I83.209
    left (asymptomatic) I83.92
      with
        edema I83.892
        pain I83.812
        specified complication NEC I83.892
        swelling I83.892
        inflammation I83.12
          with ulcer — *see* Varix, leg, with, ulcer, with inflammation by site
        ulcer I83.029
          with inflammation I83.229
          ankle I83.023
            with inflammation I83.223
          calf I83.022
            with inflammation I83.222
          foot NEC I83.025
            with inflammation I83.225
          heel I83.024
            with inflammation I83.224
          lower leg NEC I83.028
            with inflammation I83.228
          midfoot I83.024
            with inflammation I83.224
          thigh I83.021
            with inflammation I83.221
    right (asymptomatic) I83.91
      with
        edema I83.891
        pain I83.811
        specified complication NEC I83.891
        swelling I83.891
        inflammation I83.11
          with ulcer — *see* Varix, leg, with, ulcer, with inflammation by site
        ulcer I83.019
          with inflammation I83.219

Varix —*continued*
  leg—*continued*
    right—*continued*
      with—*continued*
        ulcer—*continued*
          ankle I83.013
            with inflammation I83.213
          calf I83.012
            with inflammation I83.212
          foot NEC I83.015
            with inflammation I83.215
          heel I83.014
            with inflammation I83.214
          lower leg NEC I83.018
            with inflammation I83.218
          midfoot I83.014
            with inflammation I83.214
          thigh I83.011
            with inflammation I83.211
  nasal septum I86.8
  orbit I86.8
    congenital Q27.8
  ovary I86.2
  papillary I78.1
  pelvis I86.2
  perineum I86.3
  pharynx I86.8
  placenta O43.89-
  rectum — *see* Hemorrhoids, internal
  renal papilla I86.8
  retina H35.09
  scrotum (ulcerated) I86.1
  sigmoid colon I86.8
  specified site NEC I86.8
  spinal (cord) (vessels) I86.8
  spleen, splenic (vein) (with phlebolith) I86.8
  stomach I86.4
  sublingual I86.0
  ulcerated I83.009
    inflamed or infected I83.209
  uterine ligament I86.2
  vagina I86.8
  vocal cord I86.8
  vulva I86.3
Vas deferens — *see* condition
Vas deferentitis N49.1
Vasa previa O69.4
  hemorrhage from, affecting newborn P50.0
Vascular (*see also* condition)
  loop on optic papilla Q14.2
  spasm I73.9
  spider I78.1
Vascularization, cornea — *see* Neovascularization, cornea
Vasculitis I77.6
  allergic D69.0
  cryoglobulinemic D89.1
  disseminated I77.6
  hypocomplementemic M31.8
  kidney I77.89
  livedoid L95.0
  nodular L95.8
  retina H35.06-
  rheumatic — *see* Fever, rheumatic
  rheumatoid — *see* Rheumatoid, vasculitis
  skin (limited to) L95.9
    specified NEC L95.8
Vasculopathy, necrotizing M31.9
  cardiac allograft T86.290
  specified NEC M31.8
Vasitis (nodosa) N49.1
  tuberculous A18.15
Vasodilation I73.9
Vasomotor — *see* condition
Vasoplasty, after previous sterilization Z31.0
  aftercare Z31.42
Vasospasm I73.9
  cerebral (artery) G45.9
  coronary I20.9
  nerve
    arm — *see* Mononeuropathy, upper limb
    brachial plexus G54.0
    cervical plexus G54.2

Vasospasm—*continued*
  nerve—*continued*
    leg — *see* Mononeuropathy, lower limb
    peripheral NOS I73.9
    retina (artery) — *see* Occlusion, artery, retina
Vasospastic — *see* condition
Vasovagal attack (paroxysmal) R55
  psychogenic F45.8
VATER syndrome Q87.2
Vater's ampulla — *see* condition
Vegetation, vegetative adenoid (nasal fossa) J35.8
  endocarditis (acute) (any valve) (subacute) I33.0
  heart (mycotic) (valve) I33.0
Veil
  Jackson's Q43.3
Vein, venous — *see* condition
Veldt sore — *see* Ulcer, skin
Velpeau's hernia — *see* Hernia, femoral
Venereal
  bubo A55
  disease A64
  granuloma inguinale A58
  lymphogranuloma (Durand-Nicolas-Favre) A55
Venofibrosis I87.8
Venom, venomous — *see* Table of Drugs and Chemicals, by animal or substance, poisoning
Venous — *see* condition
Ventilator lung, newborn P27.8
Ventral — *see* condition
Ventricle, ventricular (*see also* condition)
  escape I49.3
  inversion Q20.5
Ventriculitis (cerebral) (*see also* Encephalitis) G04.90
Ventriculostomy status Z98.2
Vernet's syndrome G52.7
Verneuil's disease (syphilitic bursitis) A52.78
Verruca (due to HPV) (filiformis) (simplex) (viral) (vulgaris) B07.9
  acuminata A63.0
  necrogenica (primary) (tuberculosa) A18.4
  plana B07.8
  plantaris B07.0
  seborrheica L82.1
    inflamed L82.0
  senile (seborrheic) L82.1
    inflamed L82.0
  tuberculosa (primary) A18.4
  venereal A63.0
Verrucosities — *see* Verruca
Verruga peruana, peruviana A44.1
Version
  with extraction
  cervix — *see* Malposition, uterus
  uterus (postinfectional) (postpartal, old) — *see* Malposition, uterus
Vertebra, vertebral — *see* condition
Vertical talus Q66.8
Vertigo R42
  auditory — *see* Vertigo, aural
  aural H81.31-
  benign paroxysmal (positional) H81.1-
  central (origin) — *see* subcategory H81.4
  cerebral — *see* subcategory H81.4
  Dix and Hallpike (epidemic) — *see* Neuronitis, vestibular
  due to infrasound T75.23
  epidemic A88.1
    Dix and Hallpike — *see* Neuronitis, vestibular
    Pedersen's — *see* Neuronitis, vestibular
    vestibular neuronitis — *see* Neuronitis, vestibular
  hysterical F44.89
  infrasound T75.23
  labyrinthine — *see* subcategory H81.0
  laryngeal R05
  malignant positional — *see* subcategory H81.4
  Ménière's — *see* subcategory H81.0
  menopausal N95.1
  otogenic — *see* Vertigo, aural
  paroxysmal positional, benign — *see* Vertigo, benign paroxysmal
  Pedersen's (epidemic) — *see* Neuronitis, vestibular
  peripheral NEC H81.39-

Vertigo—*continued*
  positional
    benign paroxysmal — *see* Vertigo, benign paroxysmal
    malignant — *see* subcategory H81.4
Very-low-density-lipoprotein-type (VLDL) **hyperlipoproteinemia** E78.1
Vesania — *see* Psychosis
Vesical — *see* condition
Vesicle cutaneous R23.8
  seminal — *see* condition
  skin R23.8
Vesicocolic — *see* condition
Vesicoperineal — *see* condition
Vesicorectal — *see* condition
Vesicourethrorectal — *see* condition
Vesicovaginal — *see* condition
Vesicular — *see* condition
Vesiculitis (seminal) N49.0
  amebic A06.82
  gonorrheal (acute) (chronic) A54.23
  trichomonal A59.09
  tuberculous A18.15
Vestibulitis (ear) (*see also* subcategory) H83.0
  nose (external) J34.89
  vulvar N94.810
Vestibulopathy , acute peripheral (recurrent) — *see* Neuronitis, vestibular
Vestige, vestigial (*see also* Persistence)
  branchial Q18.0
  structures in vitreous Q14.0
Vibration
  adverse effects T75.20
    pneumatic hammer syndrome T75.21
    specified effect NEC T75.29
    vasospastic syndrome T75.22
    vertigo from infrasound T75.23
  exposure (occupational) Z57.7
  vertigo T75.23
Vibriosis A28.9
Victim (of)
  crime Z65.4
  disaster Z65.5
  terrorism Z65.4
  torture Z65.4
  war Z65.5
Vidal's disease L28.0
Villaret's syndrome G52.7
Villous — *see* condition
VIN — *see* Neoplasia, intraepithelial, vulva
Vincent's infection (angina) (gingivitis) A69.1
  stomatitis NEC A69.1
Vinson-Plummer syndrome D50.1
Violence, physical R45.6
Viosterol deficiency — *see* Deficiency, calciferol
Vipoma — *see* Neoplasm, malignant, by site
Viremia B34.9
Virilism (adrenal) E25.9
  congenital E25.0
Virilization (female) (suprarenal) E25.9
  congenital E25.0
  isosexual E28.2
Virulent bubo A57
Virus, viral (*see also* condition)
  as cause of disease classified elsewhere B97.8
  cytomegalovirus B25.9
  human immunodeficiency (HIV) — *see* Human, immunodeficiency virus (HIV) disease
  infection — *see* Infection, virus
  specified NEC B34.8
  West Nile (fever) A92.30
    with
      complications NEC A92.39
      cranial nerve disorders A92.32
      encephalitis A92.31
      encephalomyelitis A92.31
      neurologic manifestation NEC A92.32
      optic neuritis A92.32
      polyradiculitis A92.32
Viscera, visceral — *see* condition
Visceroptosis K63.4
Visible peristalsis R19.2

Vision, visual
  binocular, suppression H53.34
  blurred, blurring H53.8
    hysterical F44.6
  defect, defective NEC H54.7
  disorientation (syndrome) H53.8
  disturbance H53.9
    hysterical F44.6
  double H53.2
  examination Z01.00
    with abnormal findings Z01.01
  field, limitation (defect) — *see* Defect, visual field
  hallucinations R44.1
  halos H53.19
  loss — *see* Loss, vision
    sudden — *see* Disturbance, vision, subjective, loss, sudden
  low (both eyes) — *see* Low, vision
  perception, simultaneous without fusion H53.33
Vitality, lack or want of R53.83
  newborn P96.89
Vitamin deficiency — *see* Deficiency, vitamin
Vitelline duct, persistent Q43.0
Vitiligo L80
  eyelid H02.739
    left H02.736
      lower H02.735
      upper H02.734
    right H02.733
      lower H02.732
      upper H02.731
  pinta A67.2
  vulva N90.89
Vitreal corneal syndrome H59.01-
Vitreoretinopathy, proliferative (*see also* Retinopathy, proliferative)
  with retinal detachment — *see* Detachment, retina, traction
Vitreous (*see also* condition)
  touch syndrome — *see* Complication, postprocedural, following cataract surgery
Vocal cord — *see* condition
Vogt-Koyanagi syndrome H20.82-
Vogt's disease or syndrome G80.3
Vogt-Spielmeyer amaurotic idiocy or disease E75.4
Voice
  change R49.9
    specified NEC R49.8
  loss — *see* Aphonia
Volhynian fever A79.0
Volkmann's ischemic contracture or paralysis (complicating trauma) T79.6
Volvulus (bowel) (colon) (duodenum) (intestine) K56.2
  with perforation K56.2
  congenital Q43.8
  fallopian tube — *see* Torsion, fallopian tube
  oviduct — *see* Torsion, fallopian tube
  stomach (due to absence of gastrocolic ligament) K31.89
Vomiting R11.10
  with nausea R11.2
  asphyxia — *see* Foreign body, by site, causing asphyxia, gastric contents
  bilious (cause unknown) R11.14
    in newborn P92.01
    following gastro-intestinal surgery K91.0
  blood — *see* Hematemesis
  causing asphyxia, choking, or suffocation — *see* Asphyxia, food
  cyclical G43.a09
    intractable G43.a19
      with status migrainosus G43.a11
      without status migrainosus G43.a19
    not intractable G43.a09
      with status migrainosus G43.a01
      without status migrainosus G43.a09
    psychogenic F50.8
  fecal mater R11.13
  following gastrointestinal surgery K91.0
    psychogenic F50.8
  functional K31.89
  hysterical F50.8
  nervous F50.8

Vomiting—continued
  neurotic F50.8
  newborn NEC P92.09
    bilious P92.01
  periodic R11.10
    psychogenic F50.8
  projectile R11.12
  psychogenic F50.8
  uremic — see Uremia
  without nausea R11.11
Vomito negro — see Fever, yellow
Von Bezold's abscess — see Mastoiditis, acute
Von Economo-Cruchet disease A85.8
Von Eulenburg's disease G71.19
Von Gierke's disease E74.01
Von Hippel(-Lindau) **disease or syndrome** Q85.8
Von Jaksch's anemia or disease D64.89
Von Recklinghausen
  disease (neurofibromatosis) Q85.00
    bones E21.0
Von Schroetter's syndrome I82.890
Von Willebrand(-Jurgens)(-Minot) **disease or syndrome** D68.0
Von Zumbusch's disease L40.1
Voyeurism F65.3
Vrolik's disease Q78.0
Vulva — see condition
Vulvismus N94.2
Vulvitis (acute) (allergic) (atrophic) (hypertrophic) (intertriginous) (senile) N76.2 with ectopic or molar pregnancy O08.0
  adhesive, congenital Q52.79
  blennorrhagic (gonococcal) A54.02
  candidal B37.3
Vulvitis (acute) (allergic) (atrophic) (hypertrophic) (intertriginous) (senile) N76.2
  chlamydial A56.02
  due to Haemophilus ducreyi A57
  following ectopic or molar pregnancy O08.0
  gonococcal A54.02
    with abscess (accessory gland) (periurethral) A54.1
  herpesviral A60.04
  leukoplakic N90.4
  monilial B37.3
  puerperal (postpartum) O86.19
  subacute or chronic N76.3
  syphilitic (early) A51.0
    late A52.76
  trichomonal A59.01
  tuberculous A18.18
Vulvodynia N94.819
  specified NEC N94.818
Vulvorectal — see condition
Vulvovaginitis (acute) — see Vaginitis

W

Waiting list, person on Z75.1
  for organ transplant Z76.82
  undergoing social agency investigation Z75.2
Waldenström-Kjellberg syndrome D50.1
Waldenström
  hypergammaglobulinemia D89.0
  syndrome or macroglobulinemia C88.0
Walking
  difficulty R26.2
    psychogenic F44.4
  sleep F51.3
    hysterical F44.89
Wall, abdominal — see condition
Wallenberg's disease or syndrome G46.3
Wallgren's disease I87.8
Wandering
  gallbladder, congenital Q44.1
  kidney, congenital Q63.8
  organ or site, congenital NEC — see Malposition, congenital, by site
  pacemaker (heart) I49.8
  spleen D73.89
War neurosis F48.8

Wart (due to HPV) (filiform) (infectious) (viral) B07.9
  anogenital region (venereal) A63.0
  common B07.8
  external genital organs (venereal) A63.0
  flat B07.8
  Hassal-Henle's (of cornea) H18.49
  Peruvian A44.1
  plantar B07.0
  prosector (tuberculous) A18.4
  seborrheic L82.1
    inflamed L82.0
  senile (seborrheic) L82.1
    inflamed L82.0
  tuberculous A18.4
  venereal A63.0
Warthin's tumor — see Neoplasm, salivary gland, benign
Wassilieff's disease A27.0
Wasting
  disease R64
    due to malnutrition E41
  extreme (due to malnutrition) E41
  muscle NEC — see Atrophy, muscle
Water
  clefts (senile cataract) — see Cataract, senile, incipient
  deprivation of T73.1
  intoxication E87.79
  itch B76.9
  lack of T73.1
  loading E87.70
  on
    brain — see Hydrocephalus
    chest J94.8
  poisoning E87.79
Waterbrash R12
Waterhouse(-Friderichsen) **syndrome or disease** (meningococcal) A39.1
Water-losing nephritis N25.89
Watermelon stomach K31.819
  with hemorrhage K31.811
  without hemorrhage K31.819
Watsoniasis B66.8
Wax in ear — see Impaction, cerumen
Weak, weakening, weakness (generalized) R53.1
  arches (acquired) (see also Deformity, limb, flat foot)
  bladder (sphincter) R32
  facial R29.810
    following
      cerebrovascular disease I69.992
        specified NEC I69.892
      cerebral infarction I69.392
      intracerebral hemorrhage I69.192
      nontraumatic intracranial hemorrhage NEC I69.292
      specified disease NEC I69.892
      stroke I69.392
      subarachnoid hemorrhage I69.092
  foot (double) — see Weak, arches
  heart, cardiac — see Failure, heart
  mind F70
  muscle M62.81
  myocardium — see Failure, heart
  newborn P96.89
  pelvic fundus N81.89
  pubocervical tissue N81.82
  senile R54
  rectovaginal tissue N81.83
  urinary stream R39.12
  valvular — see Endocarditis
Wear, worn (with normal or routine use)
  articular bearing surface of internal joint prosthesis — see Complications, joint prosthesis, mechanical, wear of articular bearing surfaces, by site
  device, implant or graft — see Complications, by site, mechanical complication
  tooth, teeth (approximal) (hard tissues) (interproximal) (occlusal) K03.0

Weather, weathered
  effects of
    cold T69.9
      specified effect NEC T69.8
    hot — see Heat
  skin L57.8
Weaver's syndrome Q87.3
Web, webbed (congenital)
  duodenal Q43.8
  esophagus Q39.4
  fingers Q70.1
  larynx (glottic) (subglottic) Q31.0
  neck (pterygium colli) Q18.3
  Paterson-Kelly D50.1
  popliteal syndrome Q87.89
  toes Q70.3-
Weber-Christian disease M35.6
Weber-Cockayne syndrome (epidermolysis bullosa) Q81.8
Weber-Gubler syndrome G46.3
Weber-Leyden syndrome G46.3
Weber-Osler syndrome I78.0
Weber's paralysis or syndrome G46.3
Wedge-shaped or wedging vertebra — see Collapse, vertebra NEC
Wegener's granulomatosis or syndrome M31.30
  with
    kidney involvement M31.31
    lung involvement M31.30
      with kidney involvement M31.31
Wegner's disease A50.02
Weight
  1000-2499 grams at birth (low) — see Low, birthweight
  999 grams or less at birth (extremely low) — see Low, birthweight, extreme
  gain (abnormal) (excessive) R63.5
    in pregnancy — see Pregnancy, complicated by, excessive weight gain
    low — see Pregnancy, complicated by, insufficient, weight gain
  loss (abnormal) (cause unknown) R63.4
Weightlessness (effect of) T75.82
Weil(l)-Marchesani syndrome Q87.1
Weil's disease A27.0
Weingarten's syndrome J82
Weir Mitchell's disease I73.81
Weiss-Baker syndrome G90.09
Wells' disease L98.3
Wen — see Cyst, sebaceous
Wenckebach's block or phenomenon I44.1
Werdnig-Hoffmann syndrome (muscular atrophy) G12.0
Werlhof's disease D69.3
Wermer's disease or syndrome E31.21
Werner-His disease A79.0
Werner's disease or syndrome E34.8
Wernicke-Korsakoff's syndrome or psychosis (alcoholic) F10.96
  with dependence F10.26 drug-induced
    due to drug abuse — see Abuse, drug, by type, with amnestic disorder
    due to drug dependence — see Dependence, drug, by type, with amnestic disorder
  nonalcoholic F04
Wernicke-Posada disease B38.7
Wernicke's
  developmental aphasia F80.2
  disease or syndrome E51.2
  encephalopathy E51.2
  polioencephalitis, superior E51.2
West African fever B50.8
Westphal-Strümpell syndrome E83.01
West's syndrome — see Epilepsy, generalized, specified NEC
Wet
  feet, tropical (maceration) (syndrome) — see Immersion, foot
  lung (syndrome), newborn P22.1
Wharton's duct — see condition
Wheal — see Urticaria
Wheezing R06.2

Whiplash injury S13.4

Whipple's disease (see also subcategory M14.8-)
K90.81

Whipworm (disease) (infection) (infestation) B79

Whistling face Q87.0

White (see also condition)
  kidney, small N03.9
  leg, puerperal, postpartum, childbirth O87.1
  mouth B37.0
  patches of mouth K13.29
  spot lesions, teeth
    chewing surface K02.51
    pit and fissure surface K02.51
    smooth surface K02.61

Whitehead L70.0

Whitlow (see also Cellulitis, digit)
  with lymphangitis — see Lymphangitis, acute, digit
  herpesviral B00.89

Whitmore's disease or fever — see Melioidosis

Whooping cough A37.90
  with pneumonia A37.91
    due to Bordetella
      bronchiseptica A37.81
      parapertussis A37.11
      pertussis A37.01
      specified organism NEC A37.81
    due to
      Bordetella
        bronchiseptica A37.80
          with pneumonia A37.81
        parapertussis A37.10
          with pneumonia A37.11
        pertussis A37.00
          with pneumonia A37.01
        specified NEC A37.80
          with pneumonia A37.81

Wichman's asthma J38.5

Wide cranial sutures, newborn P96.3

Widening aorta — see Ectasia, aorta
  with aneurysm — see Aneurysm, aorta

Wilkie's disease or syndrome K55.1

Wilkinson-Sneddon disease or syndrome L13.1

Willebrand (-Jürgens) **thrombopathy** D68.0

Willige-Hunt disease or syndrome G23.1

Wilms' tumor C64.-

Wilson-Mikity syndrome P27.0

Wilson's
  disease or syndrome E83.01
  hepatolenticular degeneration E83.01
  lichen ruber L43.9

Window (see also Imperfect, closure)
  aorticopulmonary Q21.4

Winter — see condition

Wiskott-Aldrich syndrome D82.0

Withdrawal state (see also Dependence, drug by type,
  with withdrawal)
  newborn
    correct therapeutic substance properly
      administered P96.2
    infant of dependent mother P96.1
    therapeutic substance, neonatal P96.2

Witts' anemia D50.8

Witzelsucht F07.0

Woakes' ethmoiditis or syndrome J33.1

Wolff-Hirschorn syndrome Q93.3

Wolff-Parkinson-White syndrome I45.6

Wolhynian fever A79.0

Wolman's disease E75.5

Wood lung or pneumonitis J67.8

Woolly, wooly hair (congenital) (nevus) Q84.1

Woolsorter's disease A22.1

Word
  blindness (congenital) (developmental) F81.0
  deafness (congenital) (developmental) H93.25

Worm(s) (infection) (infestation) (see also Infestation,
  helminth)
  guinea B72
  in intestine NEC B82.0

Worm-eaten soles A66.3

Worn out (see also Exhaustion)
  cardiac defibrillator (with synchronous cardiace
    pacemaker) Z45.02

Worn out —continued
  cardiac pacemaker
    battery Z45.010
    lead Z45.018
  device, implant or graft — see Complications, by
    site, mechanical

Worried well Z71.1

Worries R45.82

Wound, open
  abdomen, abdominal
    wall S31.109
      with penetration into peritoneal cavity
        S31.609
      bite — see Bite, abdomen, wall
      epigastric region S31.102
        with penetration into peritoneal cavity
          S31.602
        bite — see Bite, abdomen, wall, epigastric
          region
        laceration — see Laceration, abdomen,
          wall, epigastric region
        puncture — see Puncture, abdomen, wall,
          epigastric region
      laceration — see Laceration, abdomen, wall
      left
        lower quadrant S31.104
          with penetration into peritoneal cavity
            S31.604
          bite — see Bite, abdomen, wall, left,
            lower quadrant
          laceration — see Laceration, abdomen,
            wall, left, lower quadrant
          puncture — see Puncture, abdomen,
            wall, left, lower quadrant
        upper quadrant S31.101
          with penetration into peritoneal cavity
            S31.601
          bite — see Bite, abdomen, wall, left,
            upper quadrant
          laceration — see Laceration, abdomen,
            wall, left, upper quadrant
          puncture — see Puncture, abdomen,
            wall, left, upper quadrant
      periumbilic region S31.105
        with penetration into peritoneal cavity
          S31.605
        bite — see Bite, abdomen, wall,
          periumbilic region
        laceration — see Laceration, abdomen,
          wall, periumbilic region
        puncture — see Puncture, abdomen, wall,
          periumbilic region
      puncture — see Puncture, abdomen, wall
      right
        lower quadrant S31.103
          with penetration into peritoneal cavity
            S31.603
          bite — see Bite, abdomen, wall, right,
            lower quadrant
          laceration — see Laceration, abdomen,
            wall, right, lower quadrant
          puncture — see Puncture, abdomen,
            wall, right, lower quadrant
        upper quadrant S31.100
          with penetration into peritoneal cavity
            S31.600
          bite — see Bite, abdomen, wall, right,
            upper quadrant
          laceration — see Laceration, abdomen,
            wall, right, upper quadrant
          puncture — see Puncture, abdomen,
            wall, right, upper quadrant
    alveolar (process) — see Wound, open, oral cavity
    ankle S91.00-
      bite — see Bite, ankle
      laceration — see Laceration, ankle
      puncture — see Puncture, ankle
    antecubital space — see Wound, open, elbow
    anterior chamber, eye — see Wound, open, ocular

Wound, open—continued
  anus S31.839
    bite S31.835
    laceration — see Laceration, anus
    puncture — see Puncture, anus
  arm (upper) S41.10-
    with amputation — see Amputation, traumatic,
      arm
    bite — see Bite, arm
    forearm — see Wound, open, forearm
    laceration — see Laceration, arm
    puncture — see Puncture, arm
  auditory canal (external) (meatus) — see Wound,
    open, ear
  auricle, ear — see Wound, open, ear
  axilla — see Wound, open, arm
  back (see also Wound, open, thorax, back)
    lower S31.000
      with penetration into retroperitoneal space
        S31.001
      bite — see Bite, back, lower
      laceration — see Laceration, back, lower
      puncture — see Puncture, back, lower
  bite — see Bite
  blood vessel — see Injury, blood vessel
  breast S21.00-
    with amputation — see Amputation, traumatic,
      breast
    bite — see Bite, breast
    laceration — see Laceration, breast
    puncture — see Puncture, breast
  buttock S31.809
    bite — see Bite, buttock
    laceration — see Laceration, buttock
    left S31.829
    puncture — see Puncture, buttock
    right S31.819
  calf — see Wound, open, leg
  canaliculus lacrimalis — see Wound, open, eyelid
  canthus, eye — see Wound, open, eyelid
  cervical esophagus S11.20
    bite S11.25
    laceration — see Laceration, esophagus,
      traumatic, cervical
    puncture — see Puncture, cervical esophagus
  cheek (external) S01.40-
    bite — see Bite, cheek
    laceration — see Laceration, cheek
    puncture — see Puncture, cheek
    internal — see Wound, open, oral cavity
  chest wall — see Wound, open, thorax
  chin — see Wound, open, head, specified site NEC
  choroid — see Wound, open, ocular
  ciliary body (eye) — see Wound, open, ocular
  clitoris S31.40
    with amputation — see Amputation, traumatic,
      clitoris
    bite S31.45
    laceration — see Laceration, vulva
    puncture — see Puncture, vulva
  conjunctiva — see Wound, open, ocular
  cornea — see Wound, open, ocular
  costal region — see Wound, open, thorax
  Descemet's membrane — see Wound, open, ocular
  digit(s)
    foot — see Wound, open, toe
    hand — see Wound, open, finger
  ear (canal) (external) S01.30-
    with amputation — see Amputation, traumatic,
      ear
    bite — see Bite, ear
    laceration — see Laceration, ear
    puncture — see Puncture, ear
    drum S09.2-
  elbow S51.00-
    bite — see Bite, elbow
    laceration — see Laceration, elbow
    puncture — see Puncture, elbow
  epididymis — see Wound, open, testis
  epigastric region S31.102
    with penetration into peritoneal cavity S31.602
    bite — see Bite, abdomen, wall, epigastric region

Wound, open—*continued*
  ocular—*continued*
    orbit (penetrating) (with or without foreign body) S05.4-
    periocular area — *see* Wound, open, eyelid
    specified NEC S05.8x-
  oral cavity S01.502
    bite S01.552
    laceration — *see* Laceration, oral cavity
    puncture — *see* Puncture, oral cavity
  orbit — *see* Wound, open, ocular, orbit
  palate — *see* Wound, open, oral cavity
  palm — *see* Wound, open, hand
  pelvis, pelvic (*see also* Wound, open, back, lower)
    girdle (*see* Wound, open, hip
  penetrating — *see* Puncture, by site
  penis S31.20
    with amputation — *see* Amputation, traumatic, penis
    bite S31.25
    laceration — *see* Laceration, penis
    puncture — *see* Puncture, penis
  perineum
    bite — *see* Bite, perineum
    female S31.502
    laceration — *see* Laceration, perineum
    male S31.501
    puncture — *see* Puncture, perineum
  periocular area (with or without lacrimal passages) — *see* Wound, open, eyelid
  periumbilic region S31.105
    with penetration into peritoneal cavity S31.605
    bite — *see* Bite, abdomen, wall, periumbilic region
    laceration — *see* Laceration, abdomen, wall, periumbilic region
    puncture — *see* Puncture, abdomen, wall, periumbilic region
  phalanges
    finger — *see* Wound, open, finger
    toe — *see* Wound, open, toe
  pharynx S11.20
  pinna — *see* Wound, open, ear
  popliteal space — *see* Wound, open, knee
  prepuce — *see* Wound, open, penis
  pubic region — *see* Wound, open, back, lower
  pudendum — *see* Wound, open, genital organs, external
  puncture wound — *see* Puncture
  rectovaginal septum — *see* Wound, open, vagina
  right
    lower quadrant S31.103
      with penetration into peritoneal cavity S31.603
      bite — *see* Bite, abdomen, wall, right, lower quadrant
      laceration — *see* Laceration, abdomen, wall, right, lower quadrant
      puncture — *see* Puncture, abdomen, wall, right, lower quadrant
    upper quadrant S31.100
      with penetration into peritoneal cavity S31.600
      bite — *see* Bite, abdomen, wall, right, upper quadrant
      laceration — *see* Laceration, abdomen, wall, right, upper quadrant
      puncture — *see* Puncture, abdomen, wall, right, upper quadrant
  sacral region — *see* Wound, open, back, lower
  sacroiliac region — *see* Wound, open, back, lower
  salivary gland — *see* Wound, open, oral cavity
  scalp S01.00
    bite S01.05
    laceration — *see* Laceration, scalp
    puncture — *see* Puncture, scalp
  scalpel, newborn (birth injury) P15.8
  scapular region — *see* Wound, open, shoulder
  sclera — *see* Wound, open, ocular
  scrotum S31.30
    with amputation — *see* Amputation, traumatic, scrotum
    bite S31.35

Wound, open—*continued*
  scrotum—*continued*
    laceration — *see* Laceration, scrotum
    puncture — *see* Puncture, scrotum
  shin — *see* Wound, open, leg
  shoulder S41.00-
    with amputation — *see* Amputation, traumatic, arm
    bite — *see* Bite, shoulder
    laceration — *see* Laceration, shoulder
    puncture — *see* Puncture, shoulder
  skin NOS T14.8
  spermatic cord — *see* Wound, open, testis
  sternal region — *see* Wound, open, thorax, front wall
  submaxillary region — *see* Wound, open, head, specified site NEC
  submental region — *see* Wound, open, head, specified site NEC
  subungual
    finger(s) — *see* Wound, open, finger
    toe(s) — *see* Wound, open, toe
  supraclavicular region — *see* Wound, open, neck, specified site NEC
  temple, temporal region — *see* Wound, open, head, specified site NEC
  temporomandibular area — *see* Wound, open, cheek
  testis S31.30
    with amputation — *see* Amputation, traumatic, testes
    bite S31.35
    laceration — *see* Laceration, testis
    puncture — *see* Puncture, testis
  thigh S71.10-
    with amputation — *see* Amputation, traumatic, hip
    bite — *see* Bite, thigh
    laceration — *see* Laceration, thigh
    puncture — *see* Puncture, thigh
  thorax, thoracic (wall) S21.90
    back S21.20-
      with penetration S21.40
    bite — *see* Bite, thorax
    breast — *see* Wound, open, breast
    front S21.10-
      with pentration S31.30
    laceration — *see* Laceration, thorax
    puncture — *see* Puncture, thorax
  throat — *see* Wound, open, neck
  thumb S61.009
    with
      amputation — *see* Amputation, traumatic, thumb
      damage to nail S61.109
    bite — *see* Bite, thumb
    laceration — *see* Laceration, thumb
    left S61.002
      with
        damage to nail S61.102
      puncture — *see* Puncture, thumb
    right S61.001
      with
        damage to nail S61.101
  thyroid (gland) — *see* Wound, open, neck, thyroid
  toe(s) S91.109
    with
      amputation — *see* Amputation, traumatic, toe
      damage to nail S91.209
    bite — *see* Bite, toe
    great S91.103
      with
        damage to nail S91.203
      left S91.102
        with
          damage to nail S91.202
      right S91.101
        with
          damage to nail S91.201
    laceration — *see* Laceration, toe

Wound, open—*continued*
  toe(s)—*continued*
    lesser S91.106
      with
        damage to nail S91.206
      left S91.105
        with
          damage to nail S91.205
      right S91.104
        with
          damage to nail S91.204
    puncture — *see* Puncture, toe
  tongue — *see* Wound, open, oral cavity
  trachea (cervical region) — *see* Wound, open, neck, trachea
  tunica vaginalis — *see* Wound, open, testis
  tympanum, tympanic membrane S09.2-
    laceration — *see* Laceration, ear, drum
    puncture — *see* Puncture, tympanum
  umbilical region — *see* Wound, open, abdomen, wall, periumbilic region
  uvula — *see* Wound, open, oral cavity
  vagina S31.40
    bite S31.45
    laceration — *see* Laceration, vagina
    puncture — *see* Puncture, vagina
  vocal cord S11.039
    bite — *see* Bite, vocal cord
    laceration S11.031
      with foreign body S11.032
    puncture S11.033
      with foreign body S11.034
  vitreous (humor) — *see* Wound, open, ocular
  vulva S31.40
    with amputation — *see* Amputation, traumatic, vulva
    bite S31.45
    laceration — *see* Laceration, vulva
    puncture — *see* Puncture, vulva
  wrist S61.50-
    bite — *see* Bite, wrist
    laceration — *see* Laceration, wrist
    puncture — *see* Puncture, wrist
Wound, superficial (*see also* specified injury type) — *see* Injury
Wright's syndrome G54.0
Wrist — *see* condition
Wrong drug (by accident) (given in error) — *see* Table of Drugs and Chemicals, by drug, poisoning
Wry neck — *see* Torticollis
Wuchereria (bancrofti) **infestation** B74.0
Wuchereriasis B74.0
Wuchernde Struma Langhans C73

X

Xanthelasma (eyelid) (palpebrarum) H02.60
  left H02.66
    lower H02.65
    upper H02.64
  right H02.63
    lower H02.62
    upper H02.61
Xanthelasmatosis (essential) E78.2
Xanthinuria, hereditary E79.8
Xanthoastrocytoma
  specified site — *see* Neoplasm, malignant, by site
  unspecifed site C71.9
Xanthofibroma — *see* Neoplasm, connective tissue, benign
Xanthogranuloma D76.3
Xanthoma(s), xanthomatosis (primary) (familial) (hereditary) E75.5
  with
    hyperlipoproteinemia
      Type I E78.3
      Type III E78.2
      Type IV E78.1
      Type V E78.3
  cerebrotendinous E75.5
  cutaneotendinous E75.5

Xanthoma(s), xanthomatosis—*continued*
- disseminatum (skin) E78.2
- eruptive E78.2
- hypercholesterinemic E78.0
- hypercholesterolemic E78.0
- hyperlipidemic E78.5
- joint E75.5
- multiple (skin) E78.2
- tendon (sheath) E75.5
- tubo-eruptive E78.2
- tuberosum E78.2
- tuberous E78.2
- verrucous, oral mucosa K13.4

Xanthosis R23.8
Xenophobia F40.10
Xeroderma (*see also* Ichthyosis)
- acquired L85.0
  - eyelid H01.149
    - left H01.146
      - lower H01.145
      - upper H01.144
    - right H01.143
      - lower H01.142
      - upper H01.141
- pigmentosum Q82.1
- vitamin A deficiency E50.8

Xerophthalmia (vitamin A deficiency) E50.7
- unrelated to vitamin A deficiency — *see* Keratoconjunctivitis

Xerosis
- conjunctiva H11.14-
  - with Bitot's spots (*see also* Pigmentation, conjunctiva)
    - vitamin A deficiency E50.1
  - vitamin A deficiency E50.0
- cornea H18.89-
  - with ulceration — *see* Ulcer, cornea
    - vitamin A deficiency E50.3
  - vitamin A deficiency E50.2
- cutis L85.3
- skin L85.3

Xerostomia K11.7
Xiphopagus Q89.4
XO syndrome Q96.9

X-ray (of)
- abnormal findings — *see* Abnormal, diagnostic imaging
- breast (mammogram) (routine) Z12.31
- chest
  - routine (as part of a general medical examination) Z00.00
  - with abnormal findings Z00.01
- routine (as part of a general medical examination) Z00.00
  - with abnormal findings Z00.01

XXXY syndrome Q98.1
XXY syndrome Q98.0

Y

Yaba pox (virus disease) B08.72
Yatapoxvirus B08.70
- specified NEC B08.79

Yawning R06.89
- psychogenic F45.8

Yaws A66.9
- bone lesions A66.6
- butter A66.1
- chancre A66.0
- cutaneous, less than five years after infection A66.2
- early (cutaneous) (macular) (maculopapular) (micropapular) (papular) A66.2
  - frambeside A66.2
  - skin lesions NEC A66.2
- eyelid A66.2
- ganglion A66.6
- gangosis, gangosa A66.5
- gumma, gummata A66.4
  - bone A66.6
- gummatous
  - frambeside A66.4
  - osteitis A66.6
  - periostitis A66.6
- hydrarthrosis (*see also* subcategory M14.8-) A66.6
- hyperkeratosis (early) (late) A66.3
- initial lesions A66.0
- joint lesions (*see also* subcategory M14.8-) A66.6

Yaws—*continued*
- juxta-articular nodules A66.7
- late nodular (ulcerated) A66.4
- latent (without clinical manifestations) (with positive serology) A66.8
- mother A66.0
- mucosal A66.7
- multiple papillomata A66.1
- nodular, late (ulcerated) A66.4
- osteitis A66.6
- papilloma, plantar or palmar A66.1
- periostitis (hypertrophic) A66.6
- specified NEC A66.7
- ulcers A66.4
- wet crab A66.1

Yeast infection (*see also* Candidiasis) B37.9
Yellow
- atrophy (liver) — *see* Failure, hepatic
- fever — *see* Fever, yellow
- jack — *see* Fever, yellow
- jaundice — *see* Jaundice
- nail syndrome L60.5

Yersiniosis (*see also* Infection, Yersinia)
- extraintestinal A28.2
- intestinal A04.6

Z

Zahorsky's syndrome (herpangina) B08.5
Zellweger's syndrome Q87.89
Zenker's diverticulum (esophagus) K22.5
Ziehen-Oppenheim disease G24.1
Zieve's syndrome K70.0
Zinc
- deficiency, dietary E60
- metabolism disorder E83.2

Zollinger-Ellison syndrome E16.4
Zona — *see* Herpes, zoster
Zoophobia F40.218
Zoster (herpes) — *see* Herpes, zoster
Zygomycosis B46.9
- specified NEC B46.8

Zymotic — *see* condition

ICD-1Ø-CM Neoplasm Table

Notes—

The list below gives the code numbers for neoplasms by anatomical site. For each site there are six possible code numbers according to whether the neoplasm in question is malignant, benign, in situ, of uncertain behavior, or of unspecified nature. The description of the neoplasm will often indicate which of the six columns is appropriate; e.g., malignant melanoma of skin, benign fibroadenoma of breast, carcinoma in situ of cervix uteri.

Where such descriptors are not present, the remainder of the Index should be consulted where guidance is given to the appropriate column for each morphological (histological) variety listed; e.g., Mesonephroma—see Neoplasm, malignant; Embryoma (see also Neoplasm, uncertain behavior); Disease, Bowen's—see Neoplasm, skin, in situ. However, the guidance in the Index can be overridden if one of the descriptors mentioned above is present; e.g., malignant adenoma of colon is coded to C18.9 and not to D12.6 as the adjective "malignant" overrides the Index entry "Adenoma (see also Neoplasm, benign)."

Codes listed with a dash -, following the code have a required 5th character for laterality. The tablular list must be reviewed for the complete code.

	Malignant Primary	Malignant Secondary	Ca in situ	Benign	Uncertain	Unspecified Behavior
Neoplasm, neoplastic	C8Ø.1	C79.9	DØ9.9	D36.9	D48.9	D49.9
abdomen, abdominal	C76.2	C79.8-	DØ9.8	D36.7	D48.7	D49.89
cavity	C76.2	C79.8-	DØ9.8	D36.7	D48.7	D49.89
organ	C76.2	C79.8-	DØ9.8	D36.7	D48.7	D49.89
viscera	C76.2	C79.8-	DØ9.8	D36.7	D48.7	D49.89
wall	C44.59	C79.2-	DØ4.5	D23.5	D48.5	D49.2
connective tissue	C49.4	C79.8-	—	D21.4	D48.1	D49.2
abdominopelvic	C76.8	C79.8-	—	D36.7	D48.7	D49.89
accessory sinus—see Neoplasm, sinus						
acoustic nerve	C72.4-	C79.49	—	D33.3	D43.3	D49.7
adenoid (pharynx) (tissue)	C11.1	C79.89	DØØ.Ø8	D1Ø.6	D37.Ø5	D49.Ø
adipose tissue (see also Neoplasm, connective tissue)	C49.4	C79.89	—	D21.9	D48.1	D49.2
adnexa (uterine)	C57.4	C79.89	DØ7.39	D28.7	D39.8	D49.5
adrenal	C74.9-	C79.7-	DØ9.3	D35.Ø-	D44.1-	D49.7
capsule	C74.9-	C79.7-	DØ9.3	D35.Ø-	D44.1-	D49.7
cortex	C74.Ø-	C79.7-	DØ9.3	D35.Ø-	D44.1-	D49.7
gland	C74.9-	C79.7-	DØ9.3	D35.Ø-	D44.1-	D49.7
medulla	C74.1-	C79.7-	DØ9.3	D35.Ø-	D44.1-	D49.7
ala nasi (external)	C44.31	C79.2-	DØ4.39	D23.39	D48.5	D49.2
alimentary canal or tract NEC	C26.9	C78.8Ø	DØ1.9	D13.9	D37.9	D49.Ø
alveolar	CØ3.9	C79.89	DØØ.Ø3	D1Ø.39	D37.Ø9	D49.Ø
mucosa	CØ3.9	C79.89	DØØ.Ø3	D1Ø.39	D37.Ø9	D49.Ø
lower	CØ3.1	C79.89	DØØ.Ø3	D1Ø.39	D37.Ø9	D49.Ø
upper	CØ3.Ø	C79.89	DØØ.Ø3	D1Ø.39	D37.Ø9	D49.Ø
ridge or process	C41.1	C79.51	—	D16.5-	D48.Ø	D49.2
carcinoma	CØ3.9	C79.8-	—	—	—	—
lower	CØ3.1	C79.8-	—	—	—	—
upper	CØ3.Ø	C79.8-	—	—	—	—
lower	C41.1	C79.51	—	D16.5-	D48.Ø	D49.2
mucosa	CØ3.9	C79.89	DØØ.Ø3	D1Ø.39	D37.Ø9	D49.Ø
lower	CØ3.1	C79.89	DØØ.Ø3	D1Ø.39	D37.Ø9	D49.Ø
upper	CØ3.Ø	C79.89	DØØ.Ø3	D1Ø.39	D37.Ø9	D49.Ø
upper	C41.Ø-	C79.51	—	D16.4-	D48.Ø	D49.2
sulcus	CØ6.1	C79.89	DØØ.Ø2	D1Ø.39	D37.Ø9	D49.Ø
alveolus	CØ3.9	C79.89	DØØ.Ø3	D1Ø.39	D37.Ø9	D49.Ø
lower	CØ3.1	C79.89	DØØ.Ø3	D1Ø.39	D37.Ø9	D49.Ø
upper	CØ3.Ø	C79.89	DØØ.Ø3	D1Ø.39	D37.Ø9	D49.Ø
ampulla of Vater	C24.1	C78.89	DØ1.5	D13.5	D37.6	D49.Ø
ankle NEC	C76.5-	C79.89	DØ4.7-	D36.7	D48.7	D49.89
anorectum, anorectal (junction)	C21.8	C78.5	DØ1.3	D12.9	D37.8	D49.Ø
antecubital fossa or space	C76.4-	C79.89	DØ4.6-	D36.7	D48.7	D49.89
antrum (Highmore) (maxillary)	C31.Ø	C78.39	DØ2.3	D14.Ø	D38.5	D49.1
pyloric	C16.3	C78.89	DØØ.2	D13.1	D37.1	D49.Ø
tympanicum	C3Ø.1	C78.39	DØ2.3	D14.Ø	D38.5	D49.1
anus, anal	C21.Ø	C78.5	DØ1.3	D12.9	D37.8	D49.Ø
canal	C21.1	C78.5	DØ1.3	D12.9	D37.8	D49.Ø
cloacogenic zone	C21.2	C78.5	DØ1.3	D12.9	D37.8	D49.Ø
margin	C44.51	C79.2-	DØ4.5	D23.5	D48.5	D49.2
overlapping lesion with rectosigmoid junction or rectum	C21.8	—	—	—	—	—
skin	C44.51	C79.2-	DØ4.5	D23.5	D48.5	D49.2
sphincter	C21.1	C78.5	DØ1.3	D12.9	D37.8	D49.Ø

	Malignant Primary	Malignant Secondary	Ca in situ	Benign	Uncertain	Unspecified Behavior
Neoplasm, neoplastic—*continued*						
aorta (thoracic)	C49.3	C79.89	—	D21.3	D48.1	D49.2
abdominal	C49.4	C79.89	—	D21.4	D48.1	D49.2
aortic body	C75.5	C79.89	—	D35.6	D44.7	D49.7
aponeurosis	C49.9	C79.89	—	D21.9	D48.1	D49.2
palmar	C49.1-	C79.89	—	D21.1-	D48.1	D49.2
plantar	C49.2-	C79.89	—	D21.2-	D48.1	D49.2
appendix	C18.1	C78.5	DØ1.Ø	D12.1	D37.3	D49.Ø
arachnoid	C7Ø.9	C79.49	—	D32.9	D42.9	D49.7
cerebral	C7Ø.Ø	C79.32	—	D32.Ø	D42.Ø	D49.7
spinal	C7Ø.1	C79.49	—	D32.1	D42.1	D49.7
areola	C5Ø.Ø-	C79.81	DØ5.-	D24.-	D48.6-	D49.3
arm NEC	C76.4-	C79.89	DØ4.6-	D36.7	D48.7	D49.89
artery—see Neoplasm, connective tissue						
aryepiglottic fold	C13.1	C79.89	DØØ.Ø8	D1Ø.7	D37.Ø5	D49.Ø
hypopharyngeal aspect	C13.1	C79.89	DØØ.Ø8	D1Ø.7	D37.Ø5	D49.Ø
laryngeal aspect	C32.1	C78.39	DØ2.Ø	D14.1	D38.Ø	D49.1
marginal zone	C13.1	C79.89	DØØ.Ø8	D1Ø.7	D37.Ø5	D49.Ø
arytenoid (cartilage)	C32.3	C78.39	DØ2.Ø	D14.1	D38.Ø	D49.1
fold—see Neoplasm, aryepiglottic						
associated with transplanted organ	C8Ø.2	—	—	—	—	—
atlas	C41.2-	C79.51	—	D16.6-	D48.Ø	D49.2
atrium, cardiac	C38.Ø	C79.89	—	D15.1	D48.7	D49.89
auditory						
canal (external) (skin)	C44.2-	C79.2-	DØ4.2-	D23.2-	D48.5	D49.2
internal	C3Ø.1	C78.39	DØ2.3	D14.Ø	D38.5	D49.1
nerve	C72.4-	C79.49	—	D33.3	D43.3	D49.7
tube	C3Ø.1	C78.39	DØ2.3	D14.Ø	D38.5	D49.1
opening	C11.2	C79.89	DØØ.Ø8	D1Ø.6	D37.Ø5	D49.Ø
auricle, ear	C44.2-					
auricular canal (external)	C44.2-	—	—	—	—	—
internal	C3Ø.1	C78.39	DØ2.3	D14.Ø	D38.5	D49.2
autonomic nerve or nervous system NEC (see Neoplasm, nerve, peripheral)						
axilla, axillary	C76.1	C79.89	DØ9.8	D36.7	D48.7	D49.89
fold	C44.59	C79.2-	DØ4.5	D23.5	D48.5	D49.2
back NEC	C76.8	C79.89	DØ4.5	D36.7	D48.7	D49.89
Bartholin's gland	C51.Ø	C79.82	DØ7.1	D28.Ø	D39.8	D49.5
basal ganglia	C71.Ø	C79.31	—	D33.Ø	D43.Ø	D49.6
basis pedunculi	C71.7	C79.31	—	D33.1	D43.1	D49.6
bile or biliary (tract)	C24.9	C78.89	DØ1.5	D13.5	D37.6	D49.Ø
canaliculi (biliferi) (intrahepatic)	C22.1	C78.7	DØ1.5	D13.4	D37.6	D49.Ø
canals, interlobular	C22.1	C78.89	DØ1.5	D13.4	D37.6	D49.Ø
duct or passage (common) (cystic) (extrahepatic)	C24.Ø	C78.89	DØ1.5	D13.5	D37.6	D49.Ø
interlobular	C22.1	C78.89	DØ1.5	D13.4	D37.6	D49.Ø
intrahepatic	C22.1	C78.7	DØ1.5	D13.4	D37.6	D49.Ø
and extrahepatic	C24.8	C78.89	DØ1.5	D13.5	D37.6	D49.Ø
bladder (urinary)	C67.9	C79.11	DØ9.Ø	D3Ø.3	D41.4	D49.4
dome	C67.1	C79.11	DØ9.Ø	D3Ø.3	D41.4	D49.4
neck	C67.5	C79.11	DØ9.Ø	D3Ø.3	D41.4	D49.4
orifice	C67.9	C79.11	DØ9.Ø	D3Ø.3	D41.4	D49.4
ureteric	C67.6	C79.11	DØ9.Ø	D3Ø.3	D41.4	D49.4
urethral	C67.5	C79.11	DØ9.Ø	D3Ø.3	D41.4	D49.4
overlapping lesion	C67.8	—	—	—	—	—
sphincter	C67.8	C79.11	DØ9.Ø	D3Ø.3	D41.4	D49.4
trigone	C67.Ø	C79.11	DØ9.Ø	D3Ø.3	D41.4	D49.4
urachus	C67.7	C79.11	DØ9.Ø	D3Ø.3	D41.4	D49.4
wall	C67.9	C79.11	DØ9.Ø	D3Ø.3	D41.4	D49.4
anterior	C67.3	C79.11	DØ9.Ø	D3Ø.3	D41.4	D49.4
lateral	C67.2	C79.11	DØ9.Ø	D3Ø.3	D41.4	D49.4
posterior	C67.4	C79.11	DØ9.Ø	D3Ø.3	D41.4	D49.4
blood vessel—see Neoplasm, connective tissue						
bone (periosteum)	C41.9	C79.51	—	D16.9-	D48.Ø	D49.2
acetabulum	C41.4-	C79.51	—	D16.8-	D48.Ø	D49.2

Neoplasm, neoplastic—*continued*

bone—*continued*

	Malignant Primary	Malignant Secondary	Ca in situ	Benign	Uncertain	Unspecified Behavior
ankle	C40.3-	C79.51	—	D16.3-	—	—
arm NEC	C40.0-	C79.51	—	D16.0--	—	—
astragalus	C40.3-	C79.51	—	D16.3-	—	—
atlas	C41.2-	C79.51	—	D16.6-	D48.0	D49.2
axis	C41.2-	C79.51	—	D16.6-	D48.0	D49.2
back NEC	C41.2-	C79.51	—	D16.6-	D48.0	D49.2
calcaneus	C40.3-	C79.51	—	D16.3-	—	—
calvarium	C41.0-	C79.51	—	D16.4-	D48.0	D49.2
carpus (any)	C40.1-	C79.51	—	D16.1-	—	—
cartilage NEC	C41.9	C79.51	—	D16.9-	D48.0	D49.2
clavicle	C41.3	C79.51	—	D16.7-	D48.0	D49.2
clivus	C41.0-	C79.51	—	D16.4-	D48.0	D49.2
coccygeal vertebra	C41.4-	C79.51	—	D16.8-	D48.0	D49.2
coccyx	C41.4-	C79.51	—	D16.8-	D48.0	D49.2
costal cartilage	C41.3	C79.51	—	D16.7-	D48.0	D49.2
costovertebral joint	C41.3	C79.51	—	D16.7-	D48.0	D49.2
cranial	C41.0-	C79.51	—	D16.4-	D48.0	D49.2
cuboid	C40.3-	C79.51	—	D16.3-	—	—
cuneiform	C41.9	C79.51	—	D16.9-	D48.0	D49.2
elbow	C40.0-	C79.51	—	D16.0-	—	—
ethmoid (labyrinth)	C41.0-	C79.51	—	D16.4-	D48.0	D49.2
face	C41.0-	C79.51	—	D16.4-	D48.0	D49.2
femur (any part)	C40.2-	C79.51	—	D16.2-	—	—
fibula (any part)	C40.2-	C79.51	—	D16.2-	—	—
finger (any)	C40.1-	C79.51	—	D16.1-	—	—
foot	C40.3-	C79.51	—	D16.3-	—	—
forearm	C40.0-	C79.51	—	D16.0-	—	—
frontal	C41.0-	C79.51	—	D16.4-	D48.0	D49.2
hand	C40.1-	C79.51	—	D16.1-	—	—
heel	C40.3-	C79.51	—	D16.3-	—	—
hip	C41.4-	C79.51	—	D16.8-	D48.0	D49.2
humerus (any part)	C40.0-	C79.51	—	D16.0-	—	—
hyoid	C41.0-	C79.51	—	D16.4-	D48.0	D49.2
ilium	C41.4-	C79.51	—	D16.8-	D48.0	D49.2
innominate	C41.4-	C79.51	—	D16.8-	D48.0	D49.2
intervertebral cartilage or disc	C41.2-	C79.51	—	D16.6-	D48.0	D49.2
ischium	C41.4-	C79.51	—	D16.8-	D48.0	D49.2
jaw (lower)	C41.1	C79.51	—	D16.5-	D48.0	D49.2
knee	C40.2-	C79.51	—	D16.2-	—	—
leg NEC	C40.2-	C79.51	—	D16.2-	—	—
limb NEC	C40.9-	C79.51	—	D16.9-	—	—
lower (long bones)	C40.2-	C79.51	—	D16.2-	—	—
short bones	C40.3-	C79.51	—	D16.3-	—	—
upper (long bones)	C40.0-	C79.51	—	D16.0-	—	—
short bones	C40.1-	C79.51	—	D16.1-	—	—
malar	C41.0-	C79.51	—	D16.4-	D48.0	D49.2
mandible	C41.1	C79.51	—	D16.5-	D48.0	D49.2
marrow NEC (any bone)	C96.9	C79.52	—	—	—	D47.9
mastoid	C41.0-	C79.51	—	D16.4-	D48.0	D49.2
maxilla, maxillary (superior)	C41.0-	C79.51	—	D16.4-	D48.0	D49.2
inferior	C41.1	C79.51	—	D16.5-	D48.0	D49.2
metacarpus (any)	C40.1-	C79.51	—	D16.1-	—	—
metatarsus (any)	C40.3-	C79.51	—	D16.3-	—	—
overlapping sites	C40.8-	-	—	—	—	—
navicular				—	—	—
ankle	C40.3-	C79.51	—	—	—	—
hand	C40.1-	C79.51	—	—	—	—
nose, nasal	C41.0-	C79.51	—	D16.4-	D48.0	D49.2
occipital	C41.0-	C79.51	—	D16.4-	D48.0	D49.2
orbit	C41.0-	C79.51	—	D16.4-	D48.0	D49.2
parietal	C41.0-	C79.51	—	D16.4-	D48.0	D49.2
patella	C40.2-	C79.51	—	—	—	—
pelvic	C41.4-	C79.51	—	D16.8-	D48.0	D49.2
phalanges				—	—	—
foot	C40.3-	C79.51	—	—	—	—
hand	C40.1-	C79.51	—	—	—	—
pubic	C41.4-	C79.51	—	D16.8-	D48.0	D49.2
radius (any part)	C40.0-	C79.51	—	D16.0-	—	—
rib	C41.3	C79.51	—	D16.7-	D48.0	D49.2
sacral vertebra	C41.4-	C79.51	—	D16.8-	D48.0	D49.2

Neoplasm, neoplastic—*continued*

bone—*continued*

	Malignant Primary	Malignant Secondary	Ca in situ	Benign	Uncertain	Unspecified Behavior
sacrum	C41.4-	C79.51	—	D16.8-	D48.0	D49.2
scaphoid						
of ankle	C40.3-	C79.51	—	—	—	—
of hand	C40.1-	C79.51	—	—	—	—
scapula (any part)	C40.0-	C79.51	—	D16.0-	—	—
sella turcica	C41.0-	C79.51	—	D16.4-	D48.0	D49.2
shoulder	C40.0-	C79.51	—	D16.0-	—	—
skull	C41.0-	C79.51	—	D16.4-	D48.0	D49.2
sphenoid	C41.0-	C79.51	—	D16.4-	D48.0	D49.2
spine, spinal (column)	C41.2-	C79.51	—	D16.6-	D48.0	D49.2
coccyx	C41.4-	C79.51	—	D16.8-	D48.0	D49.2
sacrum	C41.4-	C79.51	—	D16.8-	D48.0	D49.2
sternum	C41.3	C79.51	—	D16.7-	D48.0	D49.2
tarsus (any)	C40.3-	C79.51	—	—	—	—
temporal	C41.0-	C79.51	—	D16.4-	D48.0	D49.2
thumb	C40.1-	C79.51	—	—	—	—
tibia (any part)	C40.2-	C79.51	—	—	—	—
toe (any)	C40.3-	C79.51	—	—	—	—
trapezium	C40.1-	C79.51	—	—	—	—
trapezoid	C40.1-	C79.51	—	—	—	—
turbinate	C41.0-	C79.51	—	D16.4-	D48.0	D49.2
ulna (any part)	C40.0-	C79.51	—	D16.0-	—	—
unciform	C40.1-	C79.51	—	—	—	—
vertebra (column)	C41.2-	C79.51	—	D16.6-	D48.0	D49.2
coccyx	C41.4-	C79.51	—	D16.8-	D48.0	D49.2
sacrum	C41.4-	C79.51	—	D16.8-	D48.0	D49.2
vomer	C41.0-	C79.51	—	D16.4-	D48.0	D49.2
wrist	C40.1-	C79.51	—	—	—	—
xiphoid process	C41.3	C79.51	—	D16.7-	D48.0	D49.2
zygomatic	C41.0-	C79.51	—	D16.4-	D48.0	D49.2
book-leaf (mouth) (ventral surface of tongue and floor of mouth)	C06.89	C79.89	D00.00	D10.39	D37.09	D49.0
bowel —*see* Neoplasm, intestine						
brachial plexus	C47.1-	C79.89	—	D36.12	D48.2	D49.2
brain NEC	C71.9	C79.31	—	D33.2	D43.2	D49.6
basal ganglia	C71.0	C79.31	—	D33.0	D43.0	D49.6
cerebellopontine angle	C71.6	C79.31	—	D33.1	D43.1	D49.6
cerebellum NOS	C71.6	C79.31	—	D33.1	D43.1	D49.6
cerebrum	C71.0	C79.31	—	D33.0	D43.0	D49.6
choroid plexus	C71.7	C79.31	—	D33.1	D43.1	D49.6
corpus callosum	C71.8	C79.31	—	D33.2	D43.2	D49.6
corpus striatum	C71.0	C79.31	—	D33.0	D43.0	D49.6
cortex (cerebral)	C71.0	C79.31	—	D33.0	D43.0	D49.6
frontal lobe	C71.1	C79.31	—	D33.0	D43.0	D49.6
globus pallidus	C71.0	C79.31	—	D33.0	D43.0	D49.6
hippocampus	C71.2	C79.31	—	D33.0	D43.0	D49.6
hypothalamus	C71.0	C79.31	—	D33.0	D43.0	D49.6
internal capsule	C71.0	C79.31	—	D33.0	D43.0	D49.6
medulla oblongata	C71.7	C79.31	—	D33.1	D43.1	D49.6
meninges	C70.0	C79.32	—	D32.0	D42.0	D49.7
midbrain	C71.7	C79.31	—	D33.1	D43.1	D49.6
occipital lobe	C71.4	C79.31	—	D33.0	D43.0	D49.6
overlapping lesion	C71.8	C79.31	—	—	—	—
parietal lobe	C71.3	C79.31	—	D33.0	D43.0	D49.6
peduncle	C71.7	C79.31	—	D33.1	D43.1	D49.6
pons	C71.7	C79.31	—	D33.1	D43.1	D49.6
stem	C71.7	C79.31	—	D33.1	D43.1	D49.6
tapetum	C71.8	C79.31	—	D33.2	D43.2	D49.6
temporal lobe	C71.2	C79.31	—	D33.0	D43.0	D49.6
thalamus	C71.0	C79.31	—	D33.0	D43.0	D49.6
uncus	C71.2	C79.31	—	D33.0	D43.0	D49.6
ventricle (floor)	C71.5	C79.31	—	D33.0	D43.0	D49.6
fourth	C71.7	C79.31	—	D33.1	D43.1	D49.6
branchial (cleft) (cyst) (vestiges)	C10.4	C79.89	D00.08	D10.5	D37.05	D49.0
breast (connective tissue) (glandular tissue) (soft parts)	C50.9-	C79.81	D05.-.	D24.-	D48.6-	D49.3
areola	C50.0-	C79.81	D05.-	D24.-	D48.6-	D49.3
axillary tail	C50.6-	C79.81	D05.-	D24.-	D48.6-	D49.3
central portion	C50.1-	C79.81	D05.-	ICD24.-	D48.6-	D49.3
inner	C50.8-	C79.81	D05.-	D24.-	D48.6-	D49.3

	Malignant Primary	Malignant Secondary	Ca in situ	Benign	Uncertain	Unspecified Behavior
Neoplasm, neoplastic—*continued*						
breast—*continued*						
lower	C50.8-	C79.81	D05.-	D24.-	D48.6-	D49.3
lower-inner quadrant	C50.3	C79.81	D05.-	D24.-	D48.6-	D49.3
lower-outer quadrant	C50.5-	C79.81	D05.-	D24.-	D48.6-	D49.3
mastectomy site (skin)	C44.52	C79.2-	—	—	—	—
specified as breast tissue	C50.8-	C79.81	—	—	—	—
midline	C50.8-	C79.81	D05.-	D24.-	D48.6-	D49.3
nipple	C50.0-	C79.81	D05.-	D24.-	D48.6-	D49.3
outer	C50.8-	C79.81	D05.-	D24.-	D48.6-	D49.3
overlapping lesion	C50.8-	—	—	—	—	—
skin	C44.52	C79.2-	D04.5	D23.5	D48.5	D49.2
tail (axillary)	C50.6-	C79.81	D05.-	D24.-	D48.6-	D49.3
upper	C50.8-	C79.81	D05.-	D24.-	D48.6-	D49.3
upper-inner quadrant	C50.2-	C79.81	D05.-	D24.-	D48.6-	D49.3
upper-outer quadrant	C50.4-	C79.81	D05.-	D24.-	D48.6-	D49.3
broad ligament	C57.1	C79.82	D07.39	D28.2	D39.8	D49.5
bronchiogenic, bronchogenic (lung)	C34.9-	C78.0-	D02.2-	D14.3-	D38.1	D49.1
bronchiole	C34.9-	C78.0-	D02.2-	D14.3-	D38.1	D49.1
bronchus	C34.9-	C78.0-	D02.2-	D14.3-	D38.1	D49.1
carina	C34.0-	C78.0-	D02.2-	D14.3-	D38.1	D49.1
lower lobe of lung	C34.3-	C78.0-	D02.2-	D14.3-	D38.1	D49.1
main	C34.0-	C78.0-	D02.2-	D14.3-	D38.1	D49.1
middle lobe of lung	C34.2	C78.0-	D02.21	D14.31	D38.1	D49.1
overlapping lesion	C34.8-	—	—	—	—	—
upper lobe of lung	C34.1-	C78.0-	D02.2-	D14.3-	D38.1	D49.1
brow	C44.39	C79.2-	D04.39	D23.39	D48.5	D49.2
buccal (cavity)	C06.9	C79.89	D00.00	D10.39	D37.09	D49.0
commissure	C06.0	C79.89	D00.02	D10.39	D37.09	D49.0
groove (lower) (upper)	C06.1	C79.89	D00.02	D10.39	D37.09	D49.0
mucosa	C06.0	C79.89	D00.02	D10.39	D37.09	D49.0
sulcus (lower) (upper)	C06.1	C79.89	D00.02	D10.39	D37.09	D49.0
bulbourethral gland	C68.0	C79.19	D09.19	D30.4	D41.3	D49.5
bursa—*see* Neoplasm, connective tissue						
buttock NEC	C76.3	C79.89	D04.5	D36.7	D48.7	D49.89
calf	C76.5-	C79.89	D04.7-	D36.7	D48.7	D49.89
calvarium	C41.0-	C79.51	—	D16.4-	D48.0	D49.2
calyx, renal	C65.-	C79.0-	D09.19	D30.1-	D41.1-	D49.5
canal						
anal	C21.1	C78.5	D01.3	D12.9	D37.8	D49.0
auditory (external)	C44.2-	C79.2-	D04.2-	D23.2-	D48.5	D49.2
auricular (external)	C44.2-	C79.2-	D04.2-	D23.2-	D48.5	D49.2
canaliculi, biliary (biliferi) (intrahepatic)	C22.1	C78.7	D01.5	D13.4	D37.6	D49.0
canthus (eye) (inner) (outer)	C44.1-	C79.2-	D04.1-	D23.1-	D48.5	D49.2
capillary—*see* Neoplasm, connective tissue						
caput coli	C18.0	C78.5	D01.0	D12.0	D37.4	D49.0
carcinoid see Tumor, carcinoid						
cardia (gastric)	C16.0	C78.89	D00.2	D13.1	D37.1	D49.0
cardiac orifice (stomach)	C16.0	C78.89	D00.2	D13.1	D37.1	D49.0
cardio-esophageal junction	C16.0	C78.89	D00.2	D13.1	D37.1	D49.0
cardio-esophagus	C16.0	C78.89	D00.2	D13.1	D37.1	D49.0
carina (bronchus)	C34.0-	C78.0-	D02.2-	D14.3-	D38.1	D49.1
carotid (artery)	C49.0	C79.89	—	D21.0	D48.1	D49.2
body	C75.4	C79.89	—	D35.5	D44.6-	D49.7
carpus (any bone)	C40.1-	C79.51	—	D16.1-	—	—
cartilage (articular) (joint) NEC (*see also* Neoplasm, bone)	C41.9	C79.51	—	D16.9-	D48.0	D49.2
arytenoid	C32.3	C78.39	D02.0	D14.1	D38.0	D49.1
auricular	C49.0	C79.89	—	D21.0	D48.1	D49.2
bronchi	C34.0-	C78.39	—	D14.3-	D38.1	D49.1
costal	C41.3	C79.51	—	D16.7-	D48.0	D49.2
cricoid	C32.3	C78.39	D02.0	D14.1	D38.0	D49.1
cuneiform	C32.3	C78.39	D02.0	D14.1	D38.0	D49.1
ear (external)	C49.0	C79.89	—	D21.0	D48.1	D49.2
ensiform	C41.3	C79.51	—	D16.7-	D48.0	D49.2
epiglottis	C32.1	C78.39	D02.0	D14.1	D38.0	D49.1
anterior surface	C10.1	C79.89	D00.08	D10.5	D37.05	D49.0
eyelid	C49.0	C79.89	—	D21.0	D48.1	D49.2

	Malignant Primary	Malignant Secondary	Ca in situ	Benign	Uncertain	Unspecified Behavior
Neoplasm, neoplastic—*continued*						
cartilage—*continued*						
intervertebral	C41.2-	C79.51	—	D16.6-	D48.0	D49.2
larynx, laryngeal	C32.3	C78.39	D02.0	D14.1	D38.0	D49.1
nose, nasal	C30.0	C78.39	D02.3	D14.0	D38.5	D49.1
pinna	C49.0	C79.89	—	D21.0	D48.1	D49.2
rib	C41.3	C79.51	—	D16.7-	D48.0	D49.2
semilunar (knee)	C40.2-	C79.51	—	D16.2-	D48.0	D49.2
thyroid	C32.3	C78.39	D02.0	D14.1	D38.0	D49.1
trachea	C33	C78.39	D02.1	D14.2	D38.1	D49.1
cauda equina	C72.1	C79.49	—	D33.4	D43.4	D49.7
cavity						
buccal	C06.9	C79.89	D00.00	D10.30	D37.09	D49.0
nasal	C30.0	C78.39	D02.3	D14.0	D38.5	D49.1
oral	C06.9	C79.89	D00.00	D10.30	D37.09	D49.0
peritoneal	C48.2	C78.6	-	D20.1	D48.4	D49.0
tympanic	C30.1	C78.39	D02.3	D14.0	D38.5	D49.1
cecum	C18.0	C78.5	D01.0	D12.0	D37.4	D49.0
central nervous system	C72.9	C79.40	—	—	—	—
cerebellopontine (angle)	C71.6	C79.31	—	D33.1	D43.1	D49.6
cerebellum, cerebellar	C71.6	C79.31	—	D33.1	D43.1	D49.6
cerebrum, cerebral (cortex) (hemisphere) (white matter)	C71.0	C79.31	—	D33.0	D43.0	D49.6
meninges	C70.0	C79.32	—	D32.0	D42.0	D49.7
peduncle	C71.7	C79.31	—	D33.1	D43.1	D49.6
ventricle	C71.5	C79.31	—	D33.0	D43.0	D49.6
fourth	C71.7	C79.31	—	D33.1	D43.1	D49.6
cervical region	C76.0	C79.89	D09.8	D36.7	D48.7	D49.89
cervix (cervical) (uteri) (uterus)	C53.9	C79.82	D06.9	D26.0	D39.0	D49.5
canal	C53.0	C79.82	D06.0	D26.0	D39.0	D49.5
endocervix (canal) (gland)	C53.0	C79.82	D06.0	D26.0	D39.0	D49.5
exocervix	C53.1	C79.82	D06.1	D26.0	D39.0	D49.5
external os	C53.1	C79.82	D06.1	D26.0	D39.0	D49.5
internal os	C53.0	C79.82	D06.0	D26.0	D39.0	D49.5
nabothian gland	C53.0	C79.82	D06.0	D26.0	D39.0	D49.5
overlapping lesion	C53.8	—	—	—	—	—
squamocolumnar junction	C53.8	C79.82	D06.7	D26.0	D39.0	D49.5
stump	C53.8	C79.82	D06.7	D26.0	D39.0	D49.5
cheek	C76.0	C79.89	D09.8	D36.7	D48.7	D49.89
external	C44.39	C79.2-	D04.39	D23.39	D48.5	D49.2
inner aspect	C06.0	C79.89	D00.02	D10.39	D37.09	D49.0
internal	C06.0	C79.89	D00.02	D10.39	D37.09	D49.0
mucosa	C06.0	C79.89	D00.02	D10.39	D37.09	D49.0
chest (wall) NEC	C76.1	C79.89	D09.8	D36.7	D48.7	D49.89
chiasma opticum	C72.3-	C79.49	—	D33.3	D43.3	D49.7
chin	C44.39	C79.2-	D04.39	D23.39	D48.5	D49.2
choana	C11.3	C79.89	D00.08	D10.6	D37.05	D49.0
cholangiole	C22.1	C78.89	D01.5	D13.4	D37.6	D49.0
choledochal duct	C24.0	C78.89	D01.5	D13.5	D37.6	D49.0
choroid	C69.3-	C79.49	D09.2-	D31.3-	D48.7	D49.81
plexus	C71.5	C79.31	—	D33.0	D43.0	D49.6
ciliary body	C69.4-	C79.49	D09.2-	D31.4-	D48.7	D49.89
clavicle	C41.3	C79.51	—	D16.7-	D48.0	D49.2
clitoris	C51.2	C79.82	D07.1	D28.0	D39.8	D49.5
clivus	C41.0-	C79.51	—	D16.4-	D48.0	D49.2
cloacogenic zone	C21.2	C78.5	D01.3	D12.9	D37.8	D49.0
coccygeal						
body or glomus	C75.5	C79.89	—	D35.6	D44.7	D49.7
vertebra	C41.4-	C79.51	—	D16.8-	D48.0	D49.2
coccyx	C41.4-	C79.51	—	D16.8-	D48.0	D49.2
colon	C18.9	C79.89	—	—	—	—
with rectum	C19	C78.5	D01.1	D12.7	D37.5	D49.0
column, spinal—*see* Neoplasm, spine						
columnella	C44.39	C79.2-	D04.39	D23.39	D48.5	D49.2
commissure						
labial, lip	C00.6	C79.89	D00.01	D10.39	D37.01	D49.0
laryngeal	C32.0	C78.39	D02.0	D14.1	D38.0	D49.1
common (bile) duct	C24.0	C78.89	D01.5	D13.5	D37.6	D49.0
concha	C44.2-	C79.89	—	—	—	—
nose	C30.0	C78.39	D02.3	D14.0	D38.5	D49.1
conjunctiva	C69.0-	C79.49	D09.2-	D31.0	D48.7	D49.89

Neoplasm, neoplastic—*continued*

Note: For neoplasms of connective tissue (blood vessel, bursa, fascia, ligament, muscle, peripheral nerves, sympathetic and parasympathetic nerves and ganglia, synovia, tendon, etc.) or of morphological types that indicate connective tissue, code according to the list under "Neoplasm, connective tissue". For sites that do not appear in this list, code to neoplasm of that site; e.g., liposarcoma, shoulder, leiomyosarcoma, stomach, neurofibroma, chest wall

Note: Morphological types that indicate connective tissue appear in their proper place in the alphabetic index with the instruction "see Neoplasm, connective tissue ...."

	Malignant Primary	Malignant Secondary	Ca in situ	Benign	Uncertain	Unspecified Behavior
connective tissue NEC	C49.9	C79.89	—	D21.9	D48.1	D49.2
abdomen	C49.4	C79.89	—	D21.4	D48.1	D49.2
abdominal wall	C49.4	C79.89	—	D21.4	D48.1	D49.2
ankle	C49.2-	C79.89	—	D21.2-	D48.1	D49.2
antecubital fossa or space	C49.1-	C79.89	—	D21.2-	D48.1	D49.2
arm	C49.1-	C79.89	—	D21.1-	D48.1	D49.2
auricle (ear)	C49.0	C79.89	—	D21.0	D48.1	D49.2
axilla	C49.3	C79.89	—	D21.3	D48.1	D49.2
back	C49.6	C79.89	—	D21.6	D48.1	D49.2
breast—*see* Neoplasm, breast						
buttock	C49.5	C79.89	—	D21.5	D48.1	D49.2
calf	C49.2-	C79.89	—	D21.2-	D48.1	D49.2
cervical region	C49.0	C79.89	—	D21.0	D48.1	D49.2
cheek	C49.0	C79.89	—	D21.0	D48.1	D49.2
chest (wall)	C49.3	C79.89	—	D21.3	D48.1	D49.2
chin	C49.0	C79.89	—	D21.0	D48.1	D49.2
diaphragm	C49.3	C79.89	—	D21.3	D48.1	D49.2
ear (external)	C49.0	C79.89	—	D21.0	D48.1	D49.2
elbow	C49.1-	C79.89	—	D21.1-	D48.1	D49.2
extrarectal	C49.5	C79.89	—	D21.5	D48.1	D49.2
extremity	C49.9	C79.89	—	D21.9	D48.1	D49.2
lower	C49.2-	C79.89	—	D21.2-	D48.1	D49.2
upper	C49.1-	C79.89	—	D21.1-	D48.1	D49.2
eyelid	C49.0	C79.89	—	D21.0	D48.1	D49.2
face.	C49.0	C79.89	—	D21.0	D48.1	D49.2
finger	C49.1-	C79.89	—	D21.1-	D48.1	D49.2
flank	C49.6	C79.89	—	D21.6	D48.1	D49.2
foot	C49.2-	C79.89	—	D21.2-	D48.1	D49.2
forearm	C49.1-	C79.89	—	D21.1-	D48.1	D49.2
forehead	C49.0	C79.89	—	D21.0	D48.1	D49.2
gastric	C49.4	C79.89	—	D21.4	D48.1	D49.2
gastrointestinal	C49.4	C79.89	—	D21.4	D48.1	D49.2
gluteal region	C49.5	C79.89	—	D21.5	D48.1	D49.2
great vessels NEC	C49.3	C79.89	—	D21.3	D48.1	D49.2
groin	C49.5	C79.89	—	D21.5	D48.1	D49.2
hand	C49.1-	C79.89	—	D21.1-	D48.1	D49.2
head	C49.0	C79.89	—	D21.0	D48.1	D49.2
heel	C49.2-	C79.89	—	D21.2-	D48.1	D49.2
hip	C49.2-	C79.89	—	D21.2-	D48.1	D49.2
hypochondrium	C49.4	C79.89	—	D21.4	D48.1	D49.2
iliopsoas muscle	C49.5	C79.89	—	D21.5	D48.1	D49.2
infraclavicular region	C49.3	C79.89	—	D21.3	D48.1	D49.2
inguinal (canal) (region)	C49.5	C79.89	—	D21.5	D48.1	D49.2
intestinal	C49.4	C79.89	—	D21.4	D48.1	D49.2
intrathoracic	C49.3	C79.89	—	D21.3	D48.1	D49.2
ischiorectal fossa	C49.5	C79.89	—	D21.5	D48.1	D49.2
jaw	C03.9	C79.89	D00.03	D10.39	D48.1	D49.0
knee	C49.2-	C79.89	—	D21.2-	D48.1	D49.2
leg	C49.2-	C79.89	—	D21.2-	D48.1	D49.2
limb NEC	C49.9	C79.89	—	D21.9	D48.1	D49.2
lower	C49.2-	C79.89	—	D21.2-	D48.1	D49.2
upper	C49.1-	C79.89	—	D21.1-	D48.1	D49.2
nates	C49.5	C79.89	—	D21.5	D48.1	D49.2
neck	C49.0	C79.89	—	D21.0	D48.1	D49.2
orbit	C69.6-	C79.49	D09.2-	D31.6-	D48.7	D49.89
overlapping lesion	C49.8	—	—	—	—	—
pararectal	C49.5	C79.89	—	D21.5	D48.1	D49.2
para-urethral	C49.5	C79.89	—	D21.5	D48.1	D49.2
paravaginal	C49.5	C79.89	—	D21.5	D48.1	D49.2
pelvis (floor)	C49.5	C79.89	—	D21.5	D48.1	D49.2
pelvo-abdominal	C49.8	C79.89	—	D21.6	D48.1	D49.2
perineum	C49.5	C79.89	—	D21.5	D48.1	D49.2
perirectal (tissue)	C49.5	C79.89	—	D21.5	D48.1	D49.2

Neoplasm, neoplastic—*continued*
connective tissue NEC—*continued*

	Malignant Primary	Malignant Secondary	Ca in situ	Benign	Uncertain	Unspecified Behavior
periurethral (tissue)	C49.5	C79.89	—	D21.5	D48.1	D49.2
popliteal fossa or space	C49.2-	C79.89	—	D21.2-	D48.1	D49.2
presacral	C49.5	C79.89	—	D21.5	D48.1	D49.2
psoas muscle	C49.4	C79.89	—	D21.4	D48.1	D49.2
pterygoid fossa	C49.0	C79.89	—	D21.0	D48.1	D49.2
rectovaginal septum or wall	C49.5	C79.89	—	D21.5	D48.1	D49.2
rectovesical	C49.5	C79.89	—	D21.5	D48.1	D49.2
retroperitoneum	C48.0	C78.6	—	D20.0	D48.3	D49.0
sacrococcygeal region	C49.5	C79.89	—	D21.5	D48.1	D49.2
scalp	C49.0	C79.89	—	D21.0	D48.1	D49.2
scapular region	C49.3	C79.89	—	D21.3	D48.1	D49.2
shoulder	C49.1-	C79.89	—	D21.1-	D48.1	D49.2
skin (dermis) NEC	C44.9	C79.2-	D04.9	D23.9	D48.5	D49.2
stomach	C49.4	C79.89	—	D21.4	D48.1	D49.2
submental	C49.0	C79.89	—	D21.0	D48.1	D49.2
supraclavicular region	C49.0	C79.89	—	D21.0	D48.1	D49.2
temple	C49.0	C79.89	—	D21.0	D48.1	D49.2
temporal region	C49.0	C79.89	—	D21.0	D48.1	D49.2
thigh	C49.2-	C79.89	—	D21.2-	D48.1	D49.2
thoracic (duct) (wall)	C49.3	C79.89	—	D21.3	D48.1	D49.2
thorax	C49.3	C79.89	—	D21.3	D48.1	D49.2
thumb	C49.1-	C79.89	—	D21.1-	D48.1	D49.2
toe	C49.2-	C79.89	—	D21.2-	D48.1	D49.2
trunk	C49.6	C79.89	—	D21.6	D48.1	D49.2
umbilicus	C49.4	C79.89	—	D21.4	D48.1	D49.2
vesicorectal	C49.5	C79.89	—	D21.5	D48.1	D49.2
wrist	C49.1-	C79.89	—	D21.1-	D48.1	D49.2
conus medullaris	C72.0	C79.49	—	D33.4	D43.4	D49.7
cord (true) (vocal)	C32.0	C78.39	D02.0	D14.1	D38.0	D49.1
false	C32.1	C78.39	D02.0	D14.1	D38.0	D49.1
spermatic	C63.1-	C79.82	D07.69	D29.8	D40.8	D49.5
spinal (cervical) (lumbar) (thoracic)	C72.0	C79.49	—	D33.4	D43.4	D49.7
cornea (limbus)	C69.1-	C79.49	D09.2-	D31.1-	D48.7	D49.89
corpus						
albicans	C56.-	C79.6-	D07.39	D27.-	D39.1-	D49.5
callosum, brain	C71.0	C79.31	—	D33.2	D43.2	D49.6
cavernosum	C60.2	C79.82	D07.4	D29.0	D40.8	D49.5
gastric	C16.2	C78.89	D00.-	D13.1	D37.1	D49.0
overlapping sites	C54.8	—	—	—	—	—
penis	C60.2	C79.82	D07.4	D29.0	D40.8	D49.5
striatum, cerebrum	C71.0	C79.31	—	D33.0	D43.0	D49.6
uteri	C54.9	C79.82	D07.0	D26.1	D39.0	D49.5
isthmus	C54.0	C79.82	D07.0	D26.1	D39.0	D49.5
cortex						
adrenal	C74.0-	C79.7-	D09.3	D35.0-	D44.1-	D49.7
cerebral	C71.0	C79.31	—	D33.0	D43.0	D49.6
costal cartilage	C41.3	C79.51	—	D16.7-	D48.0	D49.2
costovertebral joint	C41.3	C79.51	—	D16.7-	D48.0	D49.2
Cowper's gland	C68.0	C79.19	D09.19	D30.4	D41.3	D49.5
cranial (fossa, any)	C71.9	C79.31	—	D33.2	D43.2	D49.6
meninges	C70.0	C79.32	—	D32.0	D42.0	D49.7
nerve	C72.50	C79.49	—	D33.3	D43.3	D49.7
specified NEC	C72.59	C79.49	—	D33.3	D43.3	D49.7
craniobuccal pouch	C75.2	C79.89	D09.3	D35.2	D44.3	D49.7
craniopharyngeal (duct) (pouch)	C75.2	C79.89	D09.3	D35.3	D44.4	D49.7
cricoid	C13.0	C79.89	D00.08	D10.7	D37.05	D49.0
cartilage	C32.3	C79.89	D02.0	D14.1	D38.0	D49.1
cricopharynx	C13.0	C79.89	D00.08	D10.7	D37.05	D49.0
crypt of Morgagni	C21.8	C78.5	D01.3	D12.9	D37.8	D49.0
crystalline lens	C69.4-	C79.49	D09.2-	D31.4-	D48.7	D49.89
cul-de-sac (Douglas')	C48.1	C78.6	—	D20.1	D48.4	D49.0
cuneiform cartilage	C32.3	C78.39	D02.0	D14.1	D38.0	D49.1
cutaneous—*see* Neoplasm, skin						
cutis—*see* Neoplasm, skin						
cystic (bile) duct (common)	C24.0	C78.89	D01.5	D13.5	D37.6	D49.0
dermis—*see* Neoplasm, skin						
diaphragm	C49.3	C79.89	—	D21.3	D48.1	D49.2
digestive organs, system, tube, or tract NEC	C26.9	C78.89	D01.9	D13.9	D37.9	D49.0

Neoplasm, neoplastic—*continued*	Malignant Primary	Malignant Secondary	Ca in situ	Benign	Uncertain	Unspecified Behavior
disc, intervertebral	C41.2-	C79.51	—	D16.6-	D48.0	D49.2
disease, generalized	C80.0	—	—	—	—	—
disseminated	C80.0	—	—	—	—	—
Douglas' cul-de-sac or pouch	C48.1	C78.6	—	D20.1	D48.4	D49.0
duodenojejunal junction	C17.8	C78.4	D01.49	D13.39	D37.2	D49.0
duodenum	C17.0	C78.4	D01.49	D13.2	D37.2	D49.0
dura (cranial) (mater)	C70.9	C79.49	—	D32.9	D42.9	D49.7
cerebral	C70.0	C79.32	—	D32.0	D42.0	D49.7
spinal	C70.1	C79.49	—	D32.1	D42.1	D49.7
ear (external)	C44.2-	C79.89	—	—	—	—
auricle or auris	C44.2-	C79.2-	D04.2-	D23.2-	D48.5	D49.2
canal, external	C44.2-	C79.2-	D04.2-	D23.2-	D48.5	D49.2
cartilage	C49.0	C79.89	-	D21.0	D48.1	D49.2
external meatus	C44.2-	C79.2-	D04.2-	D23.2-	D48.5	D49.2
inner	C30.1	C78.39	D02.3	D14.0	D38.5	D49.1
lobule	C44.2-	C79.2-	D04.2-	D23.2-	D48.5	D49.2
middle	C30.1	C78.39	D02.3	D14.0	D38.5	D49.1
overlapping lesion with accessory sinuses	C31.8	—	—	—	—	—
skin	C44.2-	C79.2-	D04.2-	D23.2-	D48.5	D49.2
earlobe	C44.2-	C79.2-	D04.2-	D23.2-	D48.5	D49.2
ejaculatory duct	C63.7	C79.82	D07.69	D29.8	D40.8	D49.5
elbow NEC	C76.4-	C79.89	D04.6-	D36.7	D48.7	D49.89
endocardium	C38.0	C79.89	—	D15.1	D48.7	D49.89
endocervix (canal) (gland)	C53.0	C79.82	D06.0	D26.0	D39.0	D49.5
endocrine gland NEC	C75.9	C79.89	D09.3	D35.9	D44.9	D49.7
endometrium (gland) (stroma)	C54.1	C79.82	D07.0	D26.1	D39.0	D49.5
ensiform cartilage	C41.3	C79.51	—	D16.7-	D48.0	D49.2
enteric—*see* Neoplasm, intestine						
ependyma (brain)	C71.5	C79.31	—	D33.0	D43.0	D49.6
fourth ventricle	C71.7	C79.31	—	D33.1	D43.1	D49.6
epicardium	C38.0	C79.89	—	D15.1	D48.7	D49.89
epididymis	C63.0-	C79.82	D07.69	D29.3-	D40.8	D49.5
epidural	C72.9	C79.49	—	D33.9	D43.9	D49.7
epiglottis	C32.1	C78.39	D02.0	D14.1	D38.0	D49.1
anterior aspect or surface	C10.1	C79.89	D00.08	D10.5	D37.05	D49.0
cartilage	C32.3	C78.39	D02.0	D14.1	D38.0	D49.1
free border (margin)	C10.1	C79.89	D00.08	D10.5	D37.05	D49.0
junctional region	C10.8	C79.89	D00.08	D10.5	D37.05	D49.0
posterior (laryngeal) surface	C32.1	C78.39	D02.0	D14.1	D38.0	D49.1
suprahyoid portion	C32.1	C78.39	D02.0	D14.1	D38.0	D49.1
esophagogastric junction	C16.0	C78.89	D00.2	D13.1	D37.1	D49.0
esophagus	C15.9	C78.89	D00.1	D13.0	D37.8	D49.0
abdominal	C15.5	C78.89	D00.1	D13.0	D37.8	D49.0
cervical	C15.3	C78.89	D00.1	D13.0	D37.8	D49.0
distal (third)	C15.5	C78.89	D00.1	D13.0	D37.8	D49.0
lower (third)	C15.5	C78.89	D00.1	D13.0	D37.8	D49.0
middle (third)	C15.4	C78.89	D00.1	D13.0	D37.8	D49.0
overlapping lesion	C15.8	—	—	—	—	—
proximal (third)	C15.3	C78.89	D00.1	D13.0	D37.8	D49.0
thoracic	C15.4	C78.89	D00.1	D13.0	D37.8	D49.0
upper (third)	C15.3	C78.89	D00.1	D13.0	D37.8	D49.0
ethmoid (sinus)	C31.1	C78.39	D02.3	D14.0	D38.5	D49.1
bone or labyrinth	C41.0-	C79.51	-	D16.4-	D48.0	D49.2
eustachian tube	C30.1	C78.39	D02.3	D14.0	D38.5	D49.1
exocervix	C53.1	C79.82	D06.1	D26.0	D39.0	D49.5
external						
meatus (ear)	C44.2-	C79.2-	D04.2-	D23.2-	D48.5	D49.2
os, cervix uteri	C53.1	C79.82	D06.1	D26.0	D39.0	D49.5
extradural	C72.9	C79.49	—	D33.9	D43.9	D49.7
extrahepatic (bile) duct	C24.0	C78.89	D01.5	D13.5	D37.6	D49.0
overlapping lesion with gallbladder	C24.8	—	—	—	—	—
extraocular muscle	C69.6-	C79.49	D09.2-	D31.6-	D48.7	D49.89
extrarectal	C76.3	C79.89	D09.8	D36.7	D48.7	D49.89
extremity	C76.8	C79.89	D04.8	D36.7	D48.7	D49.89
lower	C76.5-	C79.89	D04.7-	D36.7	D48.7	D49.89
upper	C76.4-	C79.89	D04.6-	D36.7	D48.7	D49.89
eye NEC	C69.9	C79.49	D09.2-	D31.9	D48.7	D49.89
eyeball	C69.4-	C79.49	D09.2-	D31.4-	D48.7	D49.89
eyebrow	C44.39	C79.2-	D04.39	D23.39	D48.5	D49.2

Neoplasm, neoplastic—*continued*	Malignant Primary	Malignant Secondary	Ca in situ	Benign	Uncertain	Unspecified Behavior
eyelid (lower) (skin) (upper)	C44.1-	—	—	—	—	—
cartilage	C49.0	C79.89	—	D21.0	D48.1	D49.2
face NEC	C76.0	C79.89	D04.39	D36.7	D48.7	D49.89
fallopian tube (accessory)	C57.0-	C79.82	D07.39	D28.2	D39.8	D49.5
falx (cerebella) (cerebri)	C70.0	C79.32	—	D32.0	D42.0	D49.7
fascia (*see also* Neoplasm, connective tissue)						
palmar	C49.1-	C79.89	—	D21.1-	D48.1	D49.2
plantar	C49.2-	C79.89	—	D21.2-	D48.1	D49.2
fatty tissue—*see* Neoplasm, connective tissue						
fauces, faucial NEC	C10.9	C79.89	D00.08	D10.5	D37.05	D49.0
pillars	C09.1	C79.89	D00.08	D10.5	D37.05	D49.0
tonsil	C09.9	C79.89	D00.08	D10.4	D37.05	D49.0
femur (any part)	C40.2-	—	—	D16.2-	—	—
fetal membrane	C58	C79.82	D07.0	D26.7	D39.2	D49.5
fibrous tissue—*see* Neoplasm, connective tissue						
fibula (any part)	C40.2-	C79.51	—	D16.2-	—	—
filum terminale	C72.0	C79.49	—	D33.4	D43.4	D49.7
finger NEC	C76.4-	C79.89	D04.6-	D36.7	D48.7	D49.89
flank NEC	C76.8	C79.89	D04.5	D36.7	D48.7	D49.89
follicle, nabothian	C53.0	C79.82	D06.0	D26.0	D39.0	D49.5
foot NEC	C76.5-	C79.89	D04.7-	D36.7	D48.7	D49.89
forearm NEC	C76.4-	C79.89	D04.6-	D36.7	D48.7	D49.89
forehead (skin)	C44.39	C79.2-	D04.39	D23.39	D48.5	D49.2
foreskin	C60.0	C79.82	D07.4	D29.0	D40.8	D49.5
fornix						
pharyngeal	C11.3	C79.89	D00.08	D10.6	D37.05	D49.0
vagina	C52	C79.82	D07.2	D28.1	D39.8	D49.5
fossa (of)						
anterior (cranial)	C71.9	C79.31	—	D33.2	D43.2	D49.6
cranial	C71.9	C79.31	—	D33.2	D43.2	D49.6
ischiorectal	C76.3	C79.89	D09.8	D36.7	D48.7	D49.89
middle (cranial)	C71.9	C79.31	—	D33.2	D43.2	D49.6
piriform	C12	C79.89	D00.08	D10.7	D37.05	D49.0
pituitary	C75.1	C79.89	D09.3	D35.2	D44.3	D49.7
posterior (cranial)	C71.9	C79.31	—	D33.2	D43.2	D49.6
pterygoid	C49.0	C79.89	—	D21.0	D48.1	D49.2
pyriform	C12	C79.89	D00.08	D10.7	D37.05	D49.0
Rosenmüller	C11.2	C79.89	D00.08	D10.6	D37.05	D49.0
tonsillar	C09.0	C79.89	D00.08	D10.5	D37.05	D49.0
fourchette	C51.9	C79.82	D07.1	D28.0	D39.8	D49.5
frenulum						
labii—*see* Neoplasm, lip, internal						
linguae	C02.2	C79.89	D00.07	D10.1	D37.02	D49.0
frontal						
bone	C41.0-	C79.51	—	D16.4-	D48.0	D49.2
lobe, brain	C71.1	C79.31	—	D33.0	D43.0	D49.6
pole	C71.1	C79.31	—	D33.0	D43.0	D49.6
sinus	C31.2	C78.39	D02.3	D14.0	D38.5	D49.1
fundus						
stomach	C16.1	C78.89	D00.2	D13.1	D37.1	D49.0
uterus	C54.3	C79.82	D07.0	D26.1	D39.0	D49.5
gall duct (extrahepatic)	C24.0	C78.89	D01.5	D13.5	D37.6	D49.0
intrahepatic	C22.1	C78.7	D01.5	D13.4	D37.6	D49.0
gallbladder	C23	C78.89	D01.5	D13.5	D37.6	D49.0
overlapping lesion with extrahepatic bile ducts	C24.8	—	—	—	—	—
ganglia (*see also* Neoplasm, nerve, peripheral)	C47.9	C79.89	—	D36.10	D48.2	D49.2
basal	C71.0	C79.31	—	D33.0	D43.0	D49.6
cranial nerve	C72.50	C79.49	—	D33.3	D43.3	D49.7
Gartner's duct	C52	C79.82	D07.2	D28.1	D39.8	D49.5
gastric—*see* Neoplasm, stomach						
gastrocolic	C26.9	C78.89	D01.9	D13.9	D37.9	D49.0
gastroesophageal junction	C16.0	C78.89	D00.2	D13.1	D37.1	D49.0
gastrointestinal (tract) NEC	C26.9	C78.89	D01.9	D13.9	D37.9	D49.0
generalized	C80.0	—	—	—	—	—

Neoplasm Table

Neoplasm, genital organ or tract—Neoplasm, jejunum

Neoplasm, neoplastic—*continued*	Malignant Primary	Malignant Secondary	Ca in situ	Benign	Uncertain	Unspecified Behavior
genital organ or tract						
female NEC	C57.9	C79.82	D07.30	D28.9	D39.9	D49.5
overlapping lesion	C57.8	—	—	—	—	—
specified site NEC	C57.7	C79.82	D07.39	D28.7	D39.8	D49.5
male NEC	C63.9	C79.82	D07.60	D29.9	D40.9	D49.5
overlapping lesion	C63.8	—	—	—	—	—
specified site NEC	C63.7	C79.82	D07.69	D29.8	D40.8	D49.5
genitourinary tract						
female	C57.9	C79.82	D07.30	D28.9	D39.9	D49.5
male	C63.9	C79.82	D07.60	D29.9	D40.9	D49.5
gingiva (alveolar) (marginal)	C03.9	C79.89	D00.03	D10.39	D37.09	D49.0
lower	C03.1	C79.89	D00.03	D10.39	D37.09	D49.0
mandibular	C03.1	C79.89	D00.03	D10.39	D37.09	D49.0
maxillary	C03.0	C79.89	D00.03	D10.39	D37.09	D49.0
upper	C03.0	C79.89	D00.03	D10.39	D37.09	D49.0
gland, glandular (lymphatic) (system) (*see also* Neoplasm, lymph gland)						
endocrine NEC	C75.9	C79.89	D09.3	D35.9	D44.9	D49.7
salivary—*see* Neoplasm, salivary gland						
glans penis	C60.1	C79.82	D07.4	D29.0	D40.8	D49.5
globus pallidus	C71.0	C79.31	—	D33.0	D43.0	D49.6
glomus						
coccygeal	C75.5	C79.89	—	D35.6	D44.7	D49.7
jugularis	C75.5	C79.89	—	D35.6	D44.7	D49.7
glosso-epiglottic fold (s)	C10.1	C79.89	D00.08	D10.5	D37.05	D49.0
glossopalatine fold	C09.1	C79.89	D00.08	D10.5	D37.05	D49.0
glossopharyngeal sulcus	C09.0	C79.89	D00.08	D10.5	D37.05	D49.0
glottis	C32.0	C78.39	D02.0	D14.1	D38.0	D49.1
gluteal region	C76.3	C79.89	D04.5	D36.7	D48.7	D49.89
great vessels NEC	C49.3	C79.89	-	D21.3	D48.1	D49.2
groin NEC	C76.3	C79.89	D04.5	D36.7	D48.7	D49.89
gum	C03.9	C79.89	D00.03	D10.39	D37.09	D49.0
lower	C03.1	C79.89	D00.03	D10.39	D37.09	D49.0
upper	C03.0	C79.89	D00.03	D10.39	D37.09	D49.0
hand NEC	C76.4-	C79.89	D04.6-	D36.7	D48.7	D49.89
head NEC	C76.0	C79.89	D04.4	D36.7	D48.7	D49.89
heart	C38.0	C79.89	-	D15.1	D48.7	D49.89
heel NEC	C76.5-	C79.89	D04.7-	D36.7	D48.7	D49.89
helix	C44.2-	C79.2-	D04.2-	D23.2-	D48.5	D49.2
hematopoietic, hemopoietic tissue NEC	C96.9	—	—	—	—	—
specified NEC	C96.Z	—	—	—	—	—
hemisphere, cerebral	C71.0	C79.31	—	D33.0	D43.0	D49.6
hemorrhoidal zone	C21.1	C78.5	D01.3	D12.9	D37.8	D49.0
hepatic (*see also* Index to disease, by histology)	C22.9	C78.7	D01.5	D13.4	D37.6	D49.0
duct (bile)	C24.0	C78.89	D01.5	D13.5	D37.6	D49.0
flexure (colon)	C18.3	C78.5	D01.0	D12.3	D37.4	D49.0
primary	C22.8	C78.7	D01.5	D13.4	D37.6	D49.0
hepatoblastoma	C22.2	C78.7	D01.5	D13.4	D37.6	D49.0
hepatoma	C22.0	C78.7	D01.5	D13.4	D37.6	D49.0
hilus of lung	C34.0-	C78.0-	D02.2-	D14.3-	D38.1	D49.1
hip NEC	C76.5-	C79.89	D04.7-	D36.7	D48.7	D49.89
hippocampus, brain	C71.2	C79.31	—	D33.0	D43.0	D49.6
humerus (any part)	C40.0-	C79.51	—	D16.0-	—	—
hymen	C52	C79.82	D07.2	D28.1	D39.8	D49.5
hypopharynx, hypopharyngeal NEC	C13.9	C79.89	D00.08	D10.7	D37.05	D49.0
overlapping lesion	C13.8	—	—	—	—	—
postcricoid region	C13.0	C79.89	D00.08	D10.7	D37.05	D49.0
posterior wall	C13.2	C79.89	D00.08	D10.7	D37.05	D49.0
pyriform fossa (sinus)	C12	C79.89	D00.08	D10.7	D37.05	D49.0
hypophysis	C75.1	C79.89	D09.3	D35.2	D44.3	D49.7
hypothalamus	C71.0	C79.31	—	D33.0	D43.0	D49.6
ileocecum, ileocecal (coil) (junction) (valve)	C18.0	C78.5	D01.0	D12.0	D37.4	D49.0
ileum	C17.2	C78.4	D01.49	D13.39	D37.2	D49.0
ilium	C41.4-	C79.51	—	D16.8-	D48.0	D49.2
immunoproliferative NEC	C88.9	—	—	—	—	—
infraclavicular (region)	C76.1	C79.89	D04.5	D36.7	D48.7	D49.89

Neoplasm, neoplastic—*continued*	Malignant Primary	Malignant Secondary	Ca in situ	Benign	Uncertain	Unspecified Behavior
inguinal (region)	C76.3	C79.89	D04.5	D36.7	D48.7	D49.89
insula	C71.0	C79.31	—	D33.0	D43.0	D49.6
insular tissue (pancreas)	C25.4	C78.89	D01.7	D13.7	D37.8	D49.0
brain	C71.0	C79.31	—	D33.0	D43.0	D49.6
interarytenoid fold	C13.1	C79.89	D00.08	D10.7	D37.05	D49.0
hypopharyngeal aspect	C13.1	C79.89	D00.08	D10.7	D37.05	D49.0
laryngeal aspect	C32.1	C79.89	D02.0	D14.1	D38.0	D49.1
marginal zone	C13.1	C79.89	D00.08	D10.7	D37.05	D49.0
interdental papillae	C03.9	C79.89	D00.03	D10.39	D37.09	D49.0
lower	C03.1	C79.89	D00.03	D10.39	D37.09	D49.0
upper	C03.0	C79.89	D00.03	D10.39	D37.09	D49.0
internal						
capsule	C71.0	C79.31	—	D33.0	D43.0	D49.6
os (cervix)	C53.0	C79.82	D06.0	D26.0	D39.0	D49.5
intervertebral cartilage or disc	C41.2-	C79.51	—	D16.6-	D48.0	D49.2
intestine, intestinal	C26.0	C78.80	D01.40	D13.9	D37.8	D49.0
large	C18.9	C78.5	D01.0	D12.6	D37.4	D49.0
appendix	C18.1	C78.5	D01.0	D12.1	D37.3	D49.0
caput coli	C18.0	C78.5	D01.0	D12.0	D37.4	D49.0
cecum	C18.0	C78.5	D01.0	D12.0	D37.4	D49.0
colon	C18.9	C78.5	D01.0	D12.6	D37.4	D49.0
and rectum	C19	C78.5	D01.1	D12.7	D37.5	D49.0
ascending	C18.2	C78.5	D01.0	D12.2	D37.4	D49.0
caput	C18.0	C78.5	D01.0	D12.0	D37.4	D49.0
descending	C18.6	C78.5	D01.0	D12.4	D37.4	D49.0
distal	C18.6	C78.5	D01.0	D12.4	D37.4	D49.0
left	C18.6	C78.5	D01.0	D12.4	D37.4	D49.0
overlapping lesion	C18.8	—	—	—	—	—
pelvic	C18.7	C78.5	D01.0	D12.5	D37.4	D49.0
right	C18.2	C78.5	D01.0	D12.2	D37.4	D49.0
sigmoid (flexure)	C18.7	C78.5	D01.0	D12.5	D37.4	D49.0
transverse	C18.4	C78.5	D01.0	D12.3	D37.4	D49.0
hepatic flexure	C18.3	C78.5	D01.0	D12.3	D37.4	D49.0
ileocecum, ileocecal (coil) (valve)	C18.0	C78.5	D01.0	D12.0	D37.4	D49.0
overlapping lesion	C18.8	—	—	—	—	—
sigmoid flexure (lower) (upper)	C18.7	C78.5	D01.0	D12.5	D37.4	D49.0
splenic flexure	C18.5	C78.5	D01.0	D12.3	D37.4	D49.0
small	C17.9	C78.4	D01.40	D13.30	D37.2	D49.0
duodenum	C17.0	C78.4	D01.49	D13.2	D37.2	D49.0
ileum	C17.2	C78.4	D01.49	D13.39	D37.2	D49.0
jejunum	C17.1	C78.4	D01.49	D13.39	D37.2	D49.0
overlapping lesion	C17.8	—	—	—	—	—
tract NEC	C26.0	C78.89	D01.40	D13.9	D37.8	D49.0
intra-abdominal	C76.2	C79.89	D09.8	D36.7	D48.7	D49.89
intracranial NEC	C71.9	C79.31	—	D33.2	D43.2	D49.6
intrahepatic (bile) duct	C22.1	C78.7	D01.5	D13.4	D37.6	D49.0
intraocular	C69.4-	C79.49	D09.2-	D31.4-	D48.7	D49.89
intraorbital	C69.6-	C79.49	D09.2-	D31.6-	D48.7	D49.89
intrasellar	C75.1	C79.89	D09.3	D35.2	D44.3	D49.7
intrathoracic (cavity) (organs)	C76.1	C79.89	D09.8	D15.7	D48.7	D49.89
specified NEC	C76.1	C79.89	D09.8	D15.9	—	—
iris	C69.4-	C79.49	D09.2-	D31.4-	D48.7	D49.89
ischiorectal (fossa)	C76.3	C79.89	D09.8	D36.7	D48.7	D49.89
ischium	C41.4-	C79.51	—	D16.8-	D48.0	D49.2
island of Reil	C71.0	C79.31	—	D33.0	D43.0	D49.6
islands or islets of Langerhans	C25.4	C78.89	D01.7	D13.7	D37.8	D49.0
isthmus uteri	C54.0	C79.82	D07.0	D26.1	D39.0	D49.5
jaw	C76.0	C79.89	D09.8	D36.7	D48.7	D49.89
bone	C41.1	C79.51	—	D16.5-	D48.0	D49.2
lower	C41.1	C79.51	—	D16.5-	—	—
upper	C41.0-	C79.51	—	D16.4-	—	—
carcinoma (any type) (lower) (upper)	C76.0	C79.89	—	—	—	—
skin	C44.39	C79.2-	D04.39	D23.39	D48.5	D49.2
soft tissues	C03.9	C79.89	D00.03	D10.39	D37.09	D49.0
lower	C03.1	C79.89	D00.03	D10.39	D37.09	D49.0
upper	C03.0	C79.89	D00.03	D10.39	D37.09	D49.0
jejunum	C17.1	C78.4	D01.49	D13.39	D37.2	D49.0

	Malignant Primary	Malignant Secondary	Ca in situ	Benign	Uncertain	Unspecified Behavior
Neoplasm, neoplastic—*continued*						
joint NEC (*see also* Neoplasm, bone)	C41.9	C79.51	—	D16.9-	D48.0	D49.2
acromioclavicular	C40.0-	C79.51	—	D16.0-	—	—
bursa or synovial membrane—*see* Neoplasm, connective tissue						
costovertebral	C41.3	C79.51	—	D16.7-	D48.0	D49.2
sternocostal	C41.3	C79.51	—	D16.7-	D48.0	D49.2
temporomandibular	C41.1	C79.51	—	D16.5-	D48.0	D49.2
junction						
anorectal	C21.8	C78.5	D01.3	D12.9	D37.8	D49.0
cardioesophageal	C16.0	C78.89	D00.2	D13.1	D37.1	D49.0
esophagogastric	C16.0	C78.89	D00.2	D13.1	D37.1	D49.0
gastroesophageal	C16.0	C78.89	D00.2	D13.1	D37.1	D49.0
hard and soft palate	C05.9	C79.89	D00.00	D10.39	D37.09	D49.0
ileocecal	C18.0	C78.5	D01.0	D12.0	D37.4	D49.0
pelvirectal	C19	C78.5	D01.1	D12.7	D37.5	D49.0
pelviureteric	C65.-	C79.0-	D09.19	D41.1-	D41.1-	D49.5
rectosigmoid	C19	C78.5	D01.1	D12.7	D37.5	D49.0
squamocolumnar, of cervix	C53.8	C79.82	D06.7	D26.0	D39.0	D49.5
Kaposi's sarcoma see Kaposi's, sarcoma						
kidney (parenchymal	C64.-	C79.0-	D09.19	D30.0-	D41.0-	D49.5
calyx	C65.-	C79.0-	D09.19	D30.1-	D41.1-	D49.5
hilus	C65.-	C79.0-	D09.19	D30.1-	D41.1-	D49.5
pelvis	C65.-	C79.0-	D09.19	D30.1-	D41.1-	D49.5
knee NEC	C76.5-	C79.89	D04.7-	D36.7	D48.7	D49.89
labia (skin)	C51.9	C79.82	D07.0	D28.0	D39.8	D49.5
majora	C51.0	C79.82	D07.0	D28.0	D39.8	D49.5
minora	C51.1	C79.82	D07.0	D28.0	D39.8	D49.5
labial (*see also* Neoplasm, lip)	C00.9	C79.89	D00.01	D10.0	D37.01	D49.0
sulcus (lower) (upper)	C06.1	C79.89	D00.02	D10.39	D37.09	D49.0
labium (skin)	C51.9	C79.82	D07.1	D28.0	D39.8	D49.5
majus	C51.0	C79.82	D07.1	D28.0	D39.8	D49.5
minus	C51.1	C79.82	D07.1	D28.0	D39.8	D49.5
lacrimal						
canaliculi	C69.5-	C79.49	D09.2-	D31.5-	D48.7	D49.89
duct (nasal)	C69.5-	C79.49	D09.2-	D31.5-	D48.7	D49.89
gland	C69.5-	C79.49	D09.2-	D31.5-	D48.7	D49.89
punctum	C69.5-	C79.49	D09.2-	D31.5-	D48.7	D49.89
sac	C69.5-	C79.49	D09.2-	D31.5-	D48.7	D49.89
Langerhans, islands or islets	C25.4	C78.89	D01.7	D13.7	D37.8	D49.0
laryngopharynx	C13.9	C79.89	D00.08	D10.7	D37.05	D49.0
larynx, laryngeal NEC	C32.9	C78.39	D02.0	D14.1	D38.0	D49.1
aryepiglottic fold	C32.1	C78.39	D02.0	D14.1	D38.0	D49.1
cartilage (arytenoid) (cricoid) (cuneiform) (thyroid)	C32.3	C78.39	D02.0	D14.1	D38.0	D49.1
commissure (anterior) (posterior)	C32.0	C78.39	D02.0	D14.1	D38.0	D49.1
extrinsic NEC	C32.1	C78.39	D02.0	D14.1	D38.0	D49.1
meaning hypopharynx	C13.9	C79.89	D00.08	D10.7	D37.05	D49.0
interarytenoid fold	C32.1	C78.39	D02.0	D14.1	D38.0	D49.1
intrinsic	C32.0	C78.39	D02.0	D14.1	D38.0	D49.1
overlapping lesion	C32.8	—	—	—	—	—
ventricular band	C32.1	C78.39	D02.0	D14.1	D38.0	D49.1
leg NEC	C76.5-	C79.89	D04.7-	D36.7	D48.7	D49.89
lens, crystalline	C69.4-	C79.49	D09.2-	D31.4-	D48.7	D49.89
lid (lower) (upper)	C44.1-	C79.2-	D04.1-	D23.1-	D48.5	D49.2
ligament (*see also* Neoplasm, connective tissue)						
broad	C57.1	C79.82	D07.39	D28.2	D39.8	D49.5
Mackenrodt's	C57.7	C79.82	D07.39	D28.7	D39.8	D49.5
non-uterine—*see* Neoplasm, connective tissue						
round	C57.2	C79.82	—	D28.2	D39.8	D49.5
sacro-uterine	C57.3	C79.82	—	D28.2	D39.8	D49.5
uterine	C57.3	C79.82	—	D28.2	D39.8	D49.5
utero-ovarian	C57.7	C79.82	D07.39	D28.2	D39.8	D49.5
uterosacral	C57.3	C79.82	—	D28.2	D39.8	D49.5
limb	C76.8	C79.89	D04.8	D36.7	D48.7	D49.89
lower	C76.5-	C79.89	D04.7-	D36.7	D48.7	D49.89
upper	C76.4-	C79.89	D04.6-	D36.7	D48.7	D49.89

	Malignant Primary	Malignant Secondary	Ca in situ	Benign	Uncertain	Unspecified Behavior
Neoplasm, neoplastic—*continued*						
limbus of cornea	C69.1-	C79.49	D09.2-	D31.1-	D48.7	D49.89
lingual NEC (*see also* Neoplasm, tongue)	C02.9	C79.89	D00.07	D10.1	D37.02	D49.0
lingula, lung	C34.1-	C78.0-	D02.2-	D14.3-	D38.1	D49.1
lip	C00.9	C79.89	D00.01	D10.0	D37.01	D49.0
buccal aspect—*see* Neoplasm, lip, internal						
commissure	C00.6	C79.89	D00.01	D10.0	D37.01	D49.0
external	C00.2	C79.89	D00.01	D10.0	D37.01	D49.0
lower	C00.1	C79.89	D00.01	D10.0	D37.01	D49.0
upper	C00.0	C79.89	D00.01	D10.0	D37.01	D49.0
frenulum—*see* Neoplasm, lip, internal						
inner aspect—*see* Neoplasm, lip, internal						
internal	C00.5	C79.89	D00.01	D10.0	D37.01	D49.0
lower	C00.4	C79.89	D00.01	D10.0	D37.01	D49.0
upper	C00.3	C79.89	D00.01	D10.0	D37.01	D49.0
lipstick area	C00.2	C79.89	D00.01	D10.0	D37.01	D49.0
lower	C00.1	C79.89	D00.01	D10.0	D37.01	D49.0
upper	C00.0	C79.89	D00.01	D10.0	D37.01	D49.0
lower	C00.1	C79.89	D00.01	D10.0	D37.01	D49.0
internal	C00.4	C79.89	D00.01	D10.0	D37.01	D49.0
mucosa—*see* Neoplasm, lip, internal						
oral aspect—*see* Neoplasm, lip, internal						
overlapping lesion	C00.8	—	—	—	—	—
with oral cavity or pharynx	C14.8	—	—	—	—	—
skin (commissure) (lower) (upper)	C44.0	C79.2-	D04.0	D23.0	D48.5	D49.2
upper	C00.0	C79.89	D00.01	D10.0	D37.01	D49.0
internal	C00.3	C79.89	D00.01	D10.0	D37.01	D49.0
vermilion border	C00.2	C79.89	D00.01	D10.0	D37.01	D49.0
lower	C00.1	C79.89	D00.01	D10.0	D37.01	D49.0
upper	C00.0	C79.89	D00.01	D10.0	D37.01	D49.0
lipomatous — *see* Lipoma, by site						
liver (*see also* Index to disease, by histology)	C22.9	C78.7	D01.5	D13.4	D37.6	D49.0
primary	C22.8	C78.7	D01.5	D13.4	D37.6	D49.0
lumbosacral plexus	C47.5	C79.49	—	D36.16	D48.2	D49.2
lung	C34.9-	C78.0-	D02.2-	D14.3-	D38.1	D49.1
azygos lobe	C34.1-	C78.0-	D02.2-	D14.3-	D38.1	D49.1
carina	C34.0-	C78.0-	D02.2-	D14.3-	D38.1	D49.1
hilus	C34.0-	C78.0-	D02.2-	D14.3-	D38.1	D49.1
lingula	C34.1-	C78.0-	D02.2-	D14.3-	D38.1	D49.1
lobe NEC	C34.9-	C78.0-	D02.2-	D14.3-	D38.1	D49.1
lower lobe	C34.3-	C78.0-	D02.2-	D14.3-	D38.1	D49.1
main bronchus	C34.0-	C78.0-	D02.2-	D14.3-	D38.1	D49.1
mesothelioma — *see* Mesothelioma						
middle lobe	C34.2	C78.0-	D02.21	D14.31	D38.1	D49.1
overlapping lesion	C34.8-	—	—	—	—	—
upper lobe	C34.1-	C78.0-	D02.2-	D14.3-	D38.1	D49.1
lymph, lymphatic channel NEC	C49.9	C79.89	—	D21.9	D48.1	D49.2
gland (secondary)	—	C77.9	—	D36.0	D48.7	D49.89
abdominal	—	C77.2	—	D36.0	D48.7	D49.89
aortic	—	C77.2	—	D36.0	D48.7	D49.89
arm	—	C77.3	—	D36.0	D48.7	D49.89
auricular (anterior) (posterior)	—	C77.0	—	D36.0	D48.7	D49.89
axilla, axillary	—	C77.3	—	D36.0	D48.7	D49.89
brachial	—	C77.3	—	D36.0	D48.7	D49.89
bronchial	—	C77.1	—	D36.0	D48.7	D49.89
bronchopulmonary	—	C77.1	—	D36.0	D48.7	D49.89
celiac	—	C77.2	—	D36.0	D48.7	D49.89
cervical	—	C77.0	—	D36.0	D48.7	D49.89
cervicofacial	—	C77.0	—	D36.0	D48.7	D49.89
Cloquet	—	C77.4	—	D36.0	D48.7	D49.89
colic	—	C77.2	—	D36.0	D48.7	D49.89
common duct	—	C77.2	—	D36.0	D48.7	D49.89
cubital	—	C77.3	—	D36.0	D48.7	D49.89
diaphragmatic	—	C77.1	—	D36.0	D48.7	D49.89

	Malignant Primary	Malignant Secondary	Ca in situ	Benign	Uncertain	Unspecified Behavior
Neoplasm, neoplastic—*continued*						
lymph, lymphatic channel NEC —*continued*						
gland—*continued*						
epigastric, inferior	—	C77.1	—	D36.0	D48.7	D49.89
epitrochlear	—	C77.3	—	D36.0	D48.7	D49.89
esophageal	—	C77.1	—	D36.0	D48.7	D49.89
face	—	C77.0	—	D36.0	D48.7	D49.89
femoral	—	C77.4	—	D36.0	D48.7	D49.89
gastric	—	C77.2	—	D36.0	D48.7	D49.89
groin	—	C77.4	—	D36.0	D48.7	D49.89
head	—	C77.0	—	D36.0	D48.7	D49.89
hepatic	—	C77.2	—	D36.0	D48.7	D49.89
hilar (pulmonary)	—	C77.1	—	D36.0	D48.7	D49.89
splenic	—	C77.2	—	D36.0	D48.7	D49.89
hypogastric	—	C77.5	—	D36.0	D48.7	D49.89
ileocolic	—	C77.2	—	D36.0	D48.7	D49.89
iliac	—	C77.5	—	D36.0	D48.7	D49.89
infraclavicular	—	C77.3	—	D36.0	D48.7	D49.89
inguina, inguinal	—	C77.4	—	D36.0	D48.7	D49.89
innominate	—	C77.1	—	D36.0	D48.7	D49.89
intercostal	—	C77.1	—	D36.0	D48.7	D49.89
intestinal	—	C77.2	—	D36.0	D48.7	D49.89
intrabdominal	—	C77.2	—	D36.0	D48.7	D49.89
intrapelvic	—	C77.5	—	D36.0	D48.7	D49.89
intrathoracic	—	C77.1	—	D36.0	D48.7	D49.89
jugular	—	C77.0	—	D36.0	D48.7	D49.89
leg	—	C77.4	—	D36.0	D48.7	D49.89
limb						
lower	—	C77.4	—	D36.0	D48.7	D49.89
upper	—	C77.3	—	D36.0	D48.7	D49.89
lower limb	—	C77.4	—	D36.0	D48.7	D49.89
lumbar	—	C77.2	—	D36.0	D48.7	D49.89
mandibular	—	C77.0	—	D36.0	D48.7	D49.89
mediastinal	—	C77.1	—	D36.0	D48.7	D49.89
mesenteric (inferior) (superior)	—	C77.2	—	D36.0	D48.7	D49.89
midcolic	—	C77.2	—	D36.0	D48.7	D49.89
multiple sites in categories C77.0 C77.5	—	C77.8	—	D36.0	D48.7	D49.89
neck	—	C77.0	—	D36.0	D48.7	D49.89
obturator	—	C77.5	—	D36.0	D48.7	D49.89
occipital	—	C77.0	—	D36.0	D48.7	D49.89
pancreatic	—	C77.2	—	D36.0	D48.7	D49.89
para-aortic	—	C77.2	—	D36.0	D48.7	D49.89
paracervical	—	C77.5	—	D36.0	D48.7	D49.89
parametrial	—	C77.5	—	D36.0	D48.7	D49.89
parasternal	—	C77.1	—	D36.0	D48.7	D49.89
parotid	—	C77.0	—	D36.0	D48.7	D49.89
pectoral	—	C77.3	—	D36.0	D48.7	D49.89
pelvic	—	C77.5	—	D36.0	D48.7	D49.89
peri-aortic	—	C77.2	—	D36.0	D48.7	D49.89
peripancreatic	—	C77.2	—	D36.0	D48.7	D49.89
popliteal	—	C77.4	—	D36.0	D48.7	D49.89
porta hepatis	—	C77.2	—	D36.0	D48.7	D49.89
portal	—	C77.2	—	D36.0	D48.7	D49.89
preauricular	—	C77.0	—	D36.0	D48.7	D49.89
prelaryngeal	—	C77.0	—	D36.0	D48.7	D49.89
presymphysial	—	C77.5	—	D36.0	D48.7	D49.89
pretracheal	—	C77.0	—	D36.0	D48.7	D49.89
primary (any site) NEC	—	C96.9	—	—	—	—
pulmonary (hiler)	—	C77.1	—	D36.0	D48.7	D49.89
pyloric	—	C77.2	—	D36.0	D48.7	D49.89
retroperitoneal	—	C77.2	—	D36.0	D48.7	D49.89
retropharyngeal	—	C77.0	—	D36.0	D48.7	D49.89
Rosenmüller's	—	C77.4	—	D36.0	D48.7	D49.89
sacral	—	C77.5	—	D36.0	D48.7	D49.89
scalene	—	C77.0	—	D36.0	D48.7	D49.89
site NEC	—	C77.9	—	D36.0	D48.7	D49.89
splenic (hilar)	—	C77.2	—	D36.0	D48.7	D49.89
subclavicular	—	C77.3	—	D36.0	D48.7	D49.89
subinguinal	—	C77.4	—	D36.0	D48.7	D49.89
sublingual	—	C77.0	—	D36.0	D48.7	D49.89

	Malignant Primary	Malignant Secondary	Ca in situ	Benign	Uncertain	Unspecified Behavior
Neoplasm, neoplastic—*continued*						
lymph, lymphatic channel NEC —*continued*						
gland—*continued*						
submandibular	—	C77.0	—	D36.0	D48.7	D49.89
submaxillary	—	C77.0	—	D36.0	D48.7	D49.89
submental	—	C77.0	—	D36.0	D48.7	D49.89
subscapular	—	C77.3	—	D36.0	D48.7	D49.89
supraclavicular	—	C77.0	—	D36.0	D48.7	D49.89
thoracic	—	C77.1	—	D36.0	D48.7	D49.89
tibial	—	C77.4	—	D36.0	D48.7	D49.89
tracheal	—	C77.1	—	D36.0	D48.7	D49.89
tracheobronchial	—	C77.1	—	D36.0	D48.7	D49.89
upper limb	—	C77.3	—	D36.0	D48.7	D49.89
Virchow's	—	C77.0	—	D36.0	D48.7	D49.89
node (*see also* Neoplasm, lymph gland)						
primary NEC	C96.9	—	—	—	—	—
vessel (*see also* Neoplasm, connective tissue)	C49.9	C79.89	—	D21.9	D48.1	D49.2
Mackenrodt's ligament	C57.7	C79.82	D07.39	D28.7	D39.8	D49.5
malar	C41.0-	C79.51	—	D16.4-	D48.0	D49.2
region—*see* Neoplasm, cheek						
mammary gland—*see* Neoplasm, breast						
mandible	C41.1	C79.51	—	D16.5-	D48.0	D49.2
alveolar						
mucosa (carcinoma)	C03.1	C79.89	D00.03	D10.39	D37.09	D49.0
ridge or process	C41.1	C79.51	—	D16.5-	D48.0	D49.2
marrow (bone) NEC	C96.9	C79.52	—	—	—	D47.9
mastectomy site (skin)	C44.52	C79.2-	—	—	—	—
specified as breast tissue	C50.8-	C79.81	—	—	—	—
mastoid (air cells) (antrum) (cavity)	C30.1	C78.39	D02.3	D14.0	D38.5	D49.1
bone or process	C41.0-	C79.51	—	D16.4-	D48.0	D49.2
maxilla, maxillary (superior)	C41.0-	C79.51	—	D16.4-	D48.0	D49.2
alveolar						
mucosa	C03.0	C79.89	D00.03	D10.39	D37.09	D49.0
ridge or process (carcinoma)	C41.0-	C79.51	—	D16.4-	D48.0	D49.2
antrum	C31.0	C78.39	D02.3	D14.0	D38.5	D49.1
carcinoma	C03.0	C79.51	—	—	—	—
inferior—*see* Neoplasm, mandible						
sinus	C31.0	C78.39	D02.3	D14.0	D38.5	D49.1
meatus external (ear)	C44.2-	C79.2-	D04.2-	D23.2-	D48.5	D49.2
Meckel diverticulum, malignant	C17.3	C78.4	D01.49	D13.39	D37.2	D49.0
mediastinum, mediastinal	C38.3	C78.1	—	D15.2	D38.3	D49.89
anterior	C38.1	C78.1	—	D15.2	D38.3	D49.89
posterior	C38.2	C78.1	—	D15.2	D38.3	D49.89
medulla						
adrenal	C74.1-	C79.7-	D09.3	D35.0-	D44.1-	D49.7
oblongata	C71.7	C79.31	—	D33.1	D43.1	D49.6
meibomian gland	C44.1-	C79.2-	D04.1-	D23.1-	D48.5	D49.2
melanoma—*see* Melanoma						
meninges	C70.9	C79.49	—	D32.9	D42.9	D49.7
brain	C70.0	C79.32	—	D32.0	D42.0	D49.7
cerebral	C70.0	C79.32	—	D32.0	D42.0	D49.7
crainial	C70.0	C79.32	—	D32.0	D42.0	D49.7
intracranial	C70.0	C79.32	—	D32.0	D42.0	D49.7
spinal (cord)	C70.1	C79.49	—	D32.1	D42.1	D49.7
meniscus, knee joint (lateral) (medial)	C40.2-	C79.51	—	D16.2-	D48.0	D49.2
Merkel cell—*see* Carcinoma, Merkel cell						
mesentery, mesenteric	C48.1	C78.6	—	D20.1	D48.4	D49.0
mesoappendix	C48.1	C78.6	—	D20.1	D48.4	D49.0
mesocolon	C48.1	C78.6	—	D20.1	D48.4	D49.0
mesopharynx—*see* Neoplasm, oropharynx						
mesosalpinx	C57.1	C79.82	D07.39	D28.2	D39.8	D49.5
mesothelial tissue—*see* Mesothelioma						
mesothelioma—*see* Mesothelioma						

Neoplasm, neoplastic—*continued*

	Malignant Primary	Malignant Secondary	Ca in situ	Benign	Uncertain	Unspecified Behavior
mesovarium	C57.1	C79.82	D07.39	D28.2	D39.8	D49.5
metacarpus (any bone)	C40.1-	C79.51	—	D16.1-	—	—
metastatic NEC (*see also* Neoplasm, by site, secondary)	—	C79.9	—	—	—	—
metatarsus (any bone)	C40.3-	C79.51	—	D16.3-	—	—
midbrain	C71.7	C79.31	—	D33.1	D43.1	D49.6
milk duct—*see* Neoplasm, breast						
mons						
pubis	C51.9	C79.82	D07.1	D28.0	D39.8	D49.5
veneris	C51.9	C79.82	D07.1	D28.0	D39.8	D49.5
motor tract	C72.9	C79.49	—	D33.9	D43.9	D49.7
brain	C71.9	C79.31	—	D33.2	D43.2	D49.6
cauda equina	C72.1	C79.49	—	D33.4	D43.4	D49.7
spinal	C72.0	C79.49	—	D33.4	D43.4	D49.7
mouth	C06.9	C79.89	D00.00	D10.30	D37.09	D49.0
book-leaf	C06.89	C79.89	—	—	—	—
floor	C04.9	C79.89	D00.06	D10.2	D37.09	D49.0
anterior portion	C04.0	C79.89	D00.06	D10.2	D37.09	D49.0
lateral portion	C04.1	C79.89	D00.06	D10.2	D37.09	D49.0
overlapping lesion	C04.8	—	—	—	—	—
overlapping NEC	C06.80	—	—	—	—	—
roof	C05.9	C79.89	D00.00	D10.39	D37.09	D49.0
specified part NEC	C06.89	C79.89	D00.00	D10.39	D37.09	D49.0
vestibule	C06.1	C79.89	D00.00	D10.39	D37.09	D49.0
mucosa						
alveolar (ridge or process)	C03.9	C79.89	D00.03	D10.39	D37.09	D49.0
lower	C03.1	C79.89	D00.03	D10.39	D37.09	D49.0
upper	C03.0	C79.89	D00.03	D10.39	D37.09	D49.0
buccal	C06.0	C79.89	D00.02	D10.39	D37.09	D49.0
cheek	C06.0	C79.89	D00.02	D10.39	D37.09	D49.0
lip—*see* Neoplasm, lip, internal						
nasal	C30.0	C78.39	D02.3	D14.0	D38.5	D49.1
oral	C06.0	C79.89	D00.02	D10.39	D37.09	D49.0
Müllerian duct						
female	C57.7	C79.82	D07.39	D28.7	D39.8	D49.5
male	C63.7	C79.82	D07.69	D29.8	D40.8	D49.5
muscle (*see also* Neoplasm, connective tissue)						
extraocular	C69.6-	C79.49	D09.2-	D31.6-	D48.7	D49.89
myocardium	C38.0	C79.89	—	D15.1	D48.7	D49.89
myometrium	C54.2	C79.82	D07.0	D26.1	D39.0	D49.5
myopericardium	C38.0	C79.89	—	D15.1	D48.7	D49.89
nabothian gland (follicle)	C53.0	C79.82	D06.0	D26.0	D39.0	D49.5
nail	C44.9	C79.2-	D04.9	D23.9	D48.5	D49.2
finger	C44.6-	C79.2-	D04.6-	D23.6-	D48.5	D49.2
toe	C44.7-	C79.2-	D04.7-	D23.7-	D48.5	D49.2
nares, naris (anterior) (posterior)	C30.0	C78.39	D02.3	D14.0	D38.5	D49.1
nasal—*see* Neoplasm, nose						
nasolabial groove	C44.39	C79.2-	D04.39	D23.39	D48.5	D49.2
nasolacrimal duct	C69.5-	C79.49	D09.2-	D31.5-	D48.7	D49.89
nasopharynx, nasopharyngeal	C11.9	C79.89	D00.08	D10.6	D37.05	D49.0
floor	C11.3	C79.89	D00.08	D10.6	D37.05	D49.0
overlapping lesion	C11.8	—	—	—	—	—
roof	C11.0	C79.89	D00.08	D10.6	D37.05	D49.0
wall	C11.9	C79.89	D00.08	D10.6	D37.05	D49.0
anterior	C11.3	C79.89	D00.08	D10.6	D37.05	D49.0
lateral	C11.2	C79.89	D00.08	D10.6	D37.05	D49.0
posterior	C11.1	C79.89	D00.08	D10.6	D37.05	D49.0
superior	C11.0	C79.89	D00.08	D10.6	D37.05	D49.0
nates	C44.59	C79.2-	D04.5	D23.5	D48.5	D49.2
neck NEC	C76.0	C79.89	D09.8	D36.7	D48.7	D49.89
nerve (ganglion)	C47.9	C79.89	—	D36.10	D48.2	D49.2
abducens	C72.59	C79.49	—	D33.3	D43.3	D49.7
accessory (spinal)	C72.59	C79.49	—	D33.3	D43.3	D49.7
acoustic	C72.4-	C79.49	—	D33.3	D43.3	D49.7
auditory	C72.4-	C79.49	—	D33.3	D43.3	D49.7
autonomic NEC (*see also* Neoplasm, nerve, peripheral)	C47.9	C79.89	—	D36.10	D48.2	D49.2
brachial	C47.1-	C79.89	—	D36.12	D48.2	D49.2
cranial	C72.50	C79.49	—	D33.3	D43.3	D49.7
specified NEC	C72.59	C79.49	—	D33.3	D43.3	D49.7

Neoplasm, neoplastic—*continued*

	Malignant Primary	Malignant Secondary	Ca in situ	Benign	Uncertain	Unspecified Behavior
nerve—*continued*						
facial	C72.59	C79.49	—	D33.3	D43.3	D49.7
femoral	C47.2-	C79.89	—	D36.13	D48.2	D49.2
ganglion NEC (*see also* Neoplasm, nerve, peripheral)	C47.9	C79.89	—	D36.10	D48.2	D49.2
glossopharyngeal	C72.59	C79.49	—	D33.3	D43.3	D49.7
hypoglossal	C72.59	C79.49	—	D33.3	D43.3	D49.7
intercostal	C47.3	C79.89	—	D36.14	D48.2	D49.2
lumbar	C47.6	C79.89	—	D36.17	D48.2	D49.2
median	C47.1-	C79.89	—	D36.12	D48.2	D49.2
obturator	C47.2-	C79.89	—	D36.13	D48.2	D49.2
oculomotor	C72.59	C79.49	—	D33.3	D43.3	D49.7
olfactory	C47.2-	C79.49	—	D33.3	D43.3	D49.7
optic	C72.3-	C79.49	—	D33.3	D43.3	D49.7
parasympathetic NEC	C47.9	C79.89	—	D36.10	D48.2	D49.2
peripheral NEC	C47.9	C79.89	—	D36.10	D48.2	D49.2
abdomen	C47.4	C79.89	—	D36.15	D48.2	D49.2
abdominal wall	C47.4	C79.89	—	D36.15	D48.2	D49.2
ankle	C47.2-	C79.89	—	D36.13	D48.2	D49.2
antecubital fossa or space	C47.1-	C79.89	—	D36.12	D48.2	D49.2
arm	C47.1-	C79.89	—	D36.12	D48.2	D49.2
auricle (ear)	C47.0	C79.89	—	D36.11	D48.2	D49.2
axilla	C47.3	C79.89	—	D36.12	D48.2	D49.2
back	C47.6	C79.89	—	D36.17	D48.2	D49.2
buttock	C47.5	C79.89	—	D36.16	D48.2	D49.2
calf	C47.2-	C79.89	—	D36.13	D48.2	D49.2
cervical region	C47.0	C79.89	—	D36.11	D48.2	D49.2
cheek	C47.0	C79.89	—	D36.11	D48.2	D49.2
chest (wall)	C47.3	C79.89	—	D36.14	D48.2	D49.2
chin	C47.0	C79.89	—	D36.11	D48.2	D49.2
ear (external)	C47.0	C79.89	—	D36.11	D48.2	D49.2
elbow	C47.1-	C79.89	—	D36.12	D48.2	D49.2
extrarectal	C47.5	C79.89	—	D36.16	D48.2	D49.2
extremity	C47.9	C79.89	—	D36.10	D48.2	D49.2
lower	C47.2-	C79.89	—	D36.13	D48.2	D49.2
upper	C47.1-	C79.89	—	D36.12	D48.2	D49.2
eyelid	C47.0	C79.89	—	D36.11	D48.2	D49.2
face	C47.0	C79.89	—	D36.11	D48.2	D49.2
finger	C47.1-	C79.89	—	D36.12	D48.2	D49.2
flank	C47.6	C79.89	—	D36.17	D48.2	D49.2
foot	C47.2-	C79.89	—	D36.13	D48.2	D49.2
forearm	C47.1-	C79.89	—	D36.12	D48.2	D49.2
forehead	C47.0	C79.89	—	D36.11	D48.2	D49.2
gluteal region	C47.5	C79.89	—	D36.16	D48.2	D49.2
groin	C47.5	C79.89	—	D36.16	D48.2	D49.2
hand	C47.1-	C79.89	—	D36.12	D48.2	D49.2
head	C47.0	C79.89	—	D36.11	D48.2	D49.2
heel	C47.2-	C79.89	—	D36.13	D48.2	D49.2
hip	C47.2-	C79.89	—	D36.13	D48.2	D49.2
infraclavicular region	C47.3	C79.89	—	D36.14	D48.2	D49.2
inguinal (canal) (region)	C47.5	C79.89	—	D36.16	D48.2	D49.2
intrathoracic	C47.3	C79.89	—	D36.14	D48.2	D49.2
ischiorectal fossa	C47.5	C79.89	—	D36.16	D48.2	D49.2
knee	C47.2-	C79.89	—	D36.13	D48.2	D49.2
leg	C47.2-	C79.89	—	D36.13	D48.2	D49.2
limb NEC	C47.9	C79.89	—	D36.10	D48.2	D49.2
lower	C47.2-	C79.89	—	D36.13	D48.2	D49.2
upper	C47.1-	C79.89	—	D36.12	D48.2	D49.2
nates	C47.5	C79.89	—	D36.16	D48.2	D49.2
neck	C47.0	C79.89	—	D36.11	D48.2	D49.2
orbit	C69.6-	C79.49	—	D31.6-	D48.7	D49.2
pararectal	C47.5	C79.89	—	D36.16	D48.2	D49.2
paraurethral	C47.5	C79.89	—	D36.16	D48.2	D49.2
paravaginal	C47.5	C79.89	—	D36.16	D48.2	D49.2
pelvis (floor)	C47.5	C79.89	—	D36.16	D48.2	D49.2
pelvoabdominal	C47.8	C79.89	—	D36.17	D48.2	D49.2
perineum	C47.5	C79.89	—	D36.16	D48.2	D49.2
perirectal (tissue)	C47.5	C79.89	—	D36.16	D48.2	D49.2
periurethral (tissue)	C47.5	C79.89	—	D36.16	D48.2	D49.2
popliteal fossa or space	C47.2-	C79.89	—	D36.13	D48.2	D49.2

	Malignant Primary	Malignant Secondary	Ca in situ	Benign	Uncertain	Unspecified Behavior
Neoplasm, neoplastic—*continued*						
nerve—*continued*						
peripheral NEC—*continued*						
presacral	C47.5	C79.89	—	D36.16	D48.2	D49.2
pterygoid fossa	C47.0	C79.89	—	D36.11	D48.2	D49.2
rectovaginal septum or wall	C47.5	C79.89	—	D36.16	D48.2	D49.2
rectovesical	C47.5	C79.89	—	D36.16	D48.2	D49.2
sacrococcygeal region	C47.5	C79.89	—	D36.16	D48.2	D49.2
scalp	C47.0	C79.89	—	D36.11	D48.2	D49.2
scapular region	C47.3	C79.89	—	D36.14	D48.2	D49.2
shoulder	C47.1-	C79.89	—	D36.12	D48.2	D49.2
submental	C47.0	C79.89	—	D36.11	D48.2	D49.2
supraclavicular region	C47.0	C79.89	—	D36.11	D48.2	D49.2
temple	C47.0	C79.89	—	D36.11	D48.2	D49.2
temporal region	C47.0	C79.89	—	D36.11	D48.2	D49.2
thigh	C47.2-	C79.89	—	D36.13	D48.2	D49.2
thoracic (duct) (wall)	C47.3	C79.89	—	D36.14	D48.2	D49.2
thorax	C47.3	C79.89	—	D36.14	D48.2	D49.2
thumb	C47.1-	C79.89	—	D36.12	D48.2	D49.2
toe	C47.2-	C79.89	—	D36.13	D48.2	D49.2
trunk	C47.6	C79.89	—	D36.17	D48.2	D49.2
umbilicus	C47.4	C79.89	—	D36.15	D48.2	D49.2
vesicorectal	C47.5	C79.89	—	D36.16	D48.2	D49.2
wrist	C47.1-	C79.89	—	D36.12	D48.2	D49.2
radial	C47.1-	C79.89	—	D36.12	D48.2	D49.2
sacral	C47.5	C79.89	—	D36.16	D48.2	D49.2
sciatic	C47.2-	C79.89	—	D36.13	D48.2	D49.2
spinal NEC	C47.9	C79.89	—	D36.10	D48.2	D49.2
accessory	C72.59	C79.49	—	D33.3	D43.3	D49.7
sympathetic NEC (*see also* Neoplasm, nerve, peripheral)	C47.9	C79.89	—	D36.10	D48.2	D49.2
trigeminal	C72.59	C79.49	—	D33.3	D43.3	D49.7
trochlear	C72.59	C79.49	—	D33.3	D43.3	D49.7
ulnar	C47.1-	C79.89	—	D36.12	D48.2	D49.2
vagus	C72.59	C79.49	—	D33.3	D43.3	D49.7
nervous system (central)	C72.9	C79.40	—	D33.9	D43.9	D49.7
autonomic—*see* Neoplasm, nerve, peripheral						
parasympathetic—*see* Neoplasm, nerve, peripheral						
specified site NEC	—	C79.49	—	D33.7	D43.8	—
sympathetic—*see* Neoplasm, nerve, peripheral						
nevus see Nevus						
nipple	C50.0-	C79.81	D05.-	D24.-	—	—
nose, nasal	C76.0	C79.89	D09.8	D36.7	D48.7	D49.89
ala (external) (nasi)	C44.31	C79.2-	D04.39	D23.39	D48.5	D49.2
bone	C41.0-	C79.51	—	D16.4-	D48.0	D49.2
cartilage	C30.0	C78.39	D02.3	D14.0	D38.5	D49.1
cavity	C30.0	C78.39	D02.3	D14.0	D38.5	D49.1
choana	C11.3	C79.89	D00.08	D10.6	D37.05	D49.0
external (skin)	C44.31	C79.2-	D04.39	D23.39	D48.5	D49.2
fossa	C30.0	C78.39	D02.3	D14.0	D38.5	D49.1
internal	C30.0	C78.39	D02.3	D14.0	D38.5	D49.1
mucosa	C30.0	C78.39	D02.3	D14.0	D38.5	D49.1
septum	C30.0	C78.39	D02.3	D14.0	D38.5	D49.1
posterior margin	C11.3	C79.89	D00.08	D10.6	D37.05	D49.0
sinus—*see* Neoplasm, sinus						
skin	C44.31	C79.2-	D04.39	D23.39	D48.5	D49.2
turbinate (mucosa)	C30.0	C78.39	D02.3	D14.0	D38.5	D49.1
bone	C41.0-	C79.51	—	D16.4-	D48.0	D49.2
vestibule	C30.0	C78.39	D02.3	D14.0	D38.5	D49.1
nostril	C30.0	C78.39	D02.3	D14.0	D38.5	D49.1
nucleus pulposus	C41.2-	C79.51	—	D16.6-	D48.0	D49.2
occipital			—			
bone	C41.0-	C79.51	—	D16.4-	D48.0	D49.2
lobe or pole, brain	C71.4	C79.31	—	D33.0	D43.0	D49.6
odontogenic—*see* Neoplasm, jaw, bone			—			
olfactory nerve or bulb	C72.2-	C79.49	—	D33.3	D43.3	D49.7
olive (brain)	C71.7	C79.31	—	D33.1	D43.1	D49.6
Neoplasm, neoplastic—*continued*						
omentum	C48.1	C78.6	—	D20.1	D48.4	D49.0
operculum (brain)	C71.0	C79.31	—	D33.0	D43.0	D49.6
optic nerve, chiasm, or tract	C72.3-	C79.49	—	D33.3	D43.3	D49.7
oral (cavity)	C06.9	C79.89	D00.00	D10.30	D37.09	D49.0
ill-defined	C14.8	C79.89	D00.00	D10.30	D37.09	D49.0
mucosa	C06.0	C79.89	D00.02	D10.39	D37.09	D49.0
orbit	C69.6-	C79.49	D09.2-	D31.6-	D48.7	D49.89
autonomic nerve	C69.6-	C79.49	—	D31.6-	D48.7	D49.2
bone	C41.0-	C79.51	—	D16.4-	D48.0	D49.2
eye	C69.6-	C79.49	D09.2-	D31.6-	D48.7	D49.89
peripheral nerves	C69.6-	C79.49	—	D31.6-	D48.7	D49.2
soft parts	C69.6-	C79.49	D09.2-	D31.6-	D48.7	D49.89
organ of Zuckerkandl	C75.5	C79.89	—	D35.6	D44.7	D49.7
oropharynx	C10.9	C79.89	D00.08	D10.5	D37.05	D49.0
branchial cleft (vestige)	C10.4	C79.89	D00.08	D10.5	D37.05	D49.0
junctional region	C10.8	C79.89	D00.08	D10.5	D37.05	D49.0
lateral wall	C10.2	C79.89	D00.08	D10.5	D37.05	D49.0
overlapping lesion	C10.8	—	—	—	—	—
pillars or fauces	C09.1	C79.89	D00.08	D10.5	D37.05	D49.0
posterior wall	C10.3	C79.89	D00.08	D10.5	D37.05	D49.0
vallecula	C10.0	C79.89	D00.08	D10.5	D37.05	D49.0
os						
external	C53.1	C79.82	D06.1	D26.0	D39.0	D49.5
internal	C53.0	C79.82	D06.0	D26.0	D39.0	D49.5
ovary	C56.-	C79.6-	D07.39	D27.-	D39.1-	D49.5
oviduct	C57.0-	C79.82	D07.39	D28.2	D39.8	D49.5
palate	C05.9	C79.89	D00.00	D10.39	D37.09	D49.0
hard	C05.0	C79.89	D00.05	D10.39	D37.09	D49.0
junction of hard and soft palate	C05.9	C79.89	D00.00	D10.39	D37.09	D49.0
overlapping lesions	C05.8	—	—	—	—	—
soft	C05.1	C79.89	D00.04	D10.39	D37.09	D49.0
nasopharyngeal surface	C11.3	C79.89	D00.08	D10.6	D37.05	D49.0
posterior surface	C11.3	C79.89	D00.08	D10.6	D37.05	D49.0
superior surface	C11.3	C79.89	D00.08	D10.6	D37.05	D49.0
palatoglossal arch	C09.1	C79.89	D00.00	D10.5	D37.09	D49.0
palatopharyngeal arch	C09.1	C79.89	D00.00	D10.5	D37.09	D49.0
pallium	C71.0	C79.31	—	D33.0	D43.0	D49.6
palpebra	C44.1-	C79.2-	D04.1-	D23.1-	D48.5	D49.2
pancreas	C25.9	C78.89	D01.7	D13.6	D37.8	D49.0
body	C25.1	C78.89	D01.7	D13.6	D37.8	D49.0
duct (of Santorini) (of Wirsung)	C25.3	C78.89	D01.7	D13.6	D37.8	D49.0
ectopic tissue	C25.7	C78.89	-	D13.6	D37.8	D49.0
head	C25.0	C78.89	D01.7	D13.6	D37.8	D49.0
islet cells	C25.4	C78.89	D01.7	D13.7	D37.8	D49.0
neck	C25.7	C78.89	D01.7	D13.6	D37.8	D49.0
overlapping lesion	C25.8	—	—	—	—	—
tail	C25.2	C78.89	D01.7	D13.6	D37.8	D49.0
para-aortic body	C75.5	C79.89	—	D35.6	D44.7	D49.7
paraganglion NEC	C75.5	C79.89	—	D35.6	D44.7	D49.7
parametrium	C57.3	C79.82	—	D28.2	D39.8	D49.5
paranephric	C48.0	C78.6	—	D20.0	D48.3	D49.0
pararectal	C76.3	C79.89	—	D36.7	D48.7	D49.89
parasagittal (region)	C76.0	C79.89	D09.8	D36.7	D48.7	D49.89
parasellar	C72.9	C79.49	—	D33.9	D43.8	D49.7
parathyroid (gland)	C75.0	C79.89	D09.3	D35.1	D44.2-	D49.7
paraurethral	C76.3	C79.89	—	D36.7	D48.7	D49.89
gland	C68.1	C79.19	D09.19	D30.8	D41.8	D49.5
paravaginal	C76.3	C79.89	—	D36.7	D48.7	D49.89
parenchyma, kidney	C64.-	C79.0-	D09.19	D30.0-	D41.0-	D49.5
parietal						
bone	C41.0-	C79.51	—	D16.4-	D48.0	D49.2
lobe, brain	C71.3	C79.31	—	D33.0	D43.0	D49.6
paroophoron	C57.1	C79.82	D07.39	D28.2	D39.8	D49.5
parotid (duct) (gland)	C07	C79.89	D00.00	D11.0	D37.030	D49.0
parovarium	C57.1	C79.82	D07.39	D28.2	D39.8	D49.5
patella	C40.20	C79.51	—	—	—	—
peduncle, cerebral	C71.7	C79.31	—	D33.1	D43.1	D49.6
pelvirectal junction	C19	C78.5	D01.1	D12.7	D37.5	D49.0
pelvis, pelvic	C76.3	C79.89	D09.8	D36.7	D48.7	D49.89
bone	C41.4-	C79.51	—	D16.8-	D48.0	D49.2
floor	C76.3	C79.89	D09.8	D36.7	D48.7	D49.89

Neoplasm, neoplastic—*continued*

	Malignant Primary	Malignant Secondary	Ca in situ	Benign	Uncertain	Unspecified Behavior
pelvis, pelvic—*continued*						
renal	C65.-	C79.-	D09.19	D30.1-	D41.1-	D49.5
viscera	C76.3	C79.89	D09.8	D36.7	D48.7	D49.89
wall	C76.3	C79.89	D09.8	D36.7	D48.7	D49.89
pelvo-abdominal	C76.8	C79.89	D09.8	D36.7	D48.7	D49.89
penis	C60.9	C79.82	D07.4	D29.0	D40.8	D49.5
body	C60.2	C79.82	D07.4	D29.0	D40.8	D49.5
corpus (cavernosum)	C60.2	C79.82	D07.4	D29.0	D40.8	D49.5
glans	C60.1	C79.82	D07.4	D29.0	D40.8	D49.5
overlapping sites	C60.8	—	—	—	—	—
skin NEC	C60.9	C79.82	D07.4	D29.0	D40.8	D49.5
periadrenal (tissue)	C48.0	C78.6	—	D20.0	D48.3	D49.0
perianal (skin)	C44.51	C79.2-	D04.5	D23.5	D48.5	D49.2
pericardium	C38.0	C79.89	—	D15.1	D48.7	D49.89
perinephric	C48.0	C78.6	—	D20.0	D48.3	D49.0
perineum	C76.3	C79.89	D09.8	D36.7	D48.7	D49.89
periodontal tissue NEC	C03.9	C79.89	D00.03	D10.39	D37.09	D49.0
periosteum—*see* Neoplasm, bone						
peripancreatic	C48.0	C78.6	—	D20.0	D48.3	D49.0
peripheral nerve NEC	C47.9	C79.89	—	D36.10	D48.2	D49.2
perirectal (tissue)	C76.3	C79.89	—	D36.7	D48.7	D49.89
perirenal (tissue)	C48.0	C78.6	—	D20.0	D48.3	D49.0
peritoneum, peritoneal (cavity)	C48.2	C78.6	—	D20.1	D48.4	D49.0
benign mesothelial tissue—*see* Mesothelioma, benign						
overlapping lesion	C48.8	—	—	—	—	—
with digestive organs	C26.9	—	—	—	—	—
parietal	C48.1	C78.6	—	D20.1	D48.4	D49.0
pelvic	C48.1	C78.6	—	D20.1	D48.4	D49.0
specified part NEC	C48.1	C78.6	—	D20.1	D48.4	D49.0
peritonsillar (tissue)	C76.0	C79.89	D09.8	D36.7	D48.7	D49.89
periurethral tissue	C76.3	C79.89	—	D36.7	D48.7	D49.89
phalanges						
foot	C40.3-	C79.51	—	D16.3-	—	—
hand	C40.1-	C79.51	—	D16.1-	—	—
pharynx, pharyngeal	C14.0	C79.89	D00.08	D10.9	D37.05	D49.0
bursa	C11.1	C79.89	D00.08	D10.6	D37.05	D49.0
fornix	C11.3	C79.89	D00.08	D10.6	D37.05	D49.0
recess	C11.2	C79.89	D00.08	D10.6	D37.05	D49.0
region	C14.0	C79.89	D00.08	D10.9	D37.05	D49.0
tonsil	C11.1	C79.89	D00.08	D10.6	D37.05	D49.0
wall (lateral) (posterior)	C14.0	C79.89	D00.08	D10.9	D37.05	D49.0
pia mater	C70.9	C79.40	—	D32.9	D42.9	D49.7
cerebral	C70.0	C79.32	—	D32.0	D42.0	D49.7
cranial	C70.0	C79.32	—	D32.0	D42.0	D49.7
spinal	C70.1	C79.49	—	D32.1	D42.1	D49.7
pillars of fauces	C09.1	C79.89	D00.08	D10.5	D37.05	D49.0
pineal (body) (gland)	C75.3	C79.89	D09.3	D35.4	D44.5	D49.7
pinna (ear) NEC	C44.2-	C79.89	—	—	—	—
piriform fossa or sinus	C12	C79.89	D00.08	D10.7	D37.05	D49.0
pituitary (body) (fossa) (gland) (lobe)	C75.1	C79.89	D09.3	D35.2	D44.3	D49.7
placenta	C58	C79.82	D07.0	D26.7	D39.2	D49.5
pleura, pleural (cavity)	C38.4	C78.2	—	D19.0	D38.2	D49.1
overlapping lesion with heart or mediastinum	C38.8	—	—	—	—	—
parietal	C38.4	C78.2	—	D19.0	D38.2	D49.1
visceral	C38.4	C78.2	—	D19.0	D38.2	D49.1
plexus				—		
brachial	C47.1-	C79.89	—	D36.12	D48.2	D49.2
cervical	C47.0	C79.89	—	D36.11	D48.2	D49.2
choroid	C71.5	C79.31	—	D33.0	D43.0	D49.6
lumbosacral	C47.5	C79.89	—	D36.16	D48.2	D49.2
sacral	C47.5	C79.89	—	D36.16	D48.2	D49.2
pole						
frontal	C71.1	C79.31	—	D33.0	D43.0	D49.6
occipital	C71.4	C79.31	—	D33.0	D43.0	D49.6
pons (varolii)	C71.7	C79.31	—	D33.1	D43.1	D49.6
popliteal fossa or space	C76.5-	C79.89	D04.7-	D36.7	D48.7	D49.89
postcricoid (region)	C13.0	C79.89	D00.08	D10.7	D37.05	D49.0
posterior fossa (cranial)	C71.9	C79.31	—	D33.2	D43.2	D49.6

Neoplasm, neoplastic—*continued*

	Malignant Primary	Malignant Secondary	Ca in situ	Benign	Uncertain	Unspecified Behavior
postnasal space	C11.9	C79.89	D00.08	D10.6	D37.05	D49.0
prepuce	C60.0	C79.82	D07.4	D29.0	D40.8	D49.5
prepylorus	C16.4	C78.89	D00.2	D13.1	D37.1	D49.0
presacral (region)	C76.3	C79.89	—	D36.7	D48.7	D49.89
prostate (gland)	C61	C79.82	D07.5	D29.1	D40.0-	D49.5
utricle	C68.0	C79.19	D09.19	D30.4	D41.3	D49.5
pterygoid fossa	C49.0	C79.89	—	D21.0	D48.1	D49.2
pubic bone	C41.4-	C79.51	—	D16.8-	D48.0	D49.2
pudenda, pudendum (female)	C51.9	C79.82	D07.1	D28.0	D39.8	D49.5
pulmonary (*see also* Neoplasm, lung)	C34.9-	C78.0-	D02.2-	D14.3-	D38.1	D49.1
putamen	C71.0	C79.31	—	D33.0	D43.0	D49.6
pyloric						
antrum	C16.3	C78.89	D00.2	D13.1	D37.1	D49.0
canal	C16.4	C78.89	D00.2	D13.1	D37.1	D49.0
pylorus	C16.4	C78.89	D00.2	D13.1	D37.1	D49.0
pyramid (brain)	C71.7	C79.31	—	D33.1	D43.1	D49.6
pyriform fossa or sinus	C12	C79.89	D00.08	D10.7	D37.05	D49.0
radius (any part)	C40.0-	C79.51	—	D16.0-	—	—
Rathke's pouch	C75.1	C79.89	D09.3	D35.2	D44.3	D49.7
rectosigmoid (junction)	C19	C78.5	D01.1	D12.7	D37.5	D49.0
overlapping lesion with anus or rectum	C21.8	—	—	—	—	—
rectouterine pouch	C48.1	C78.6	—	D20.1	D48.4	D49.0
rectovaginal septum or wall	C76.3	C79.89	D09.8	D36.7	D48.7	D49.89
rectovesical septum	C76.3	C79.89	D09.8	D36.7	D48.7	D49.89
rectum (ampulla)	C20	C78.5	D01.2	D12.8	D37.5	D49.0
and colon	C19	C78.5	D01.1	D12.7	D37.5	D49.0
overlapping lesion with anus or rectosigmoid junction	C21.8					
renal	C64.-	C79.0-	D09.19	D30.0-	D41.0-	D49.5
calyx	C65.-	C79.0-	D09.19	D30.1-	D41.1-	D49.5
hilus	C65.-	C79.0-	D09.19	D30.1-	D41.1-	D49.5
parenchyma	C64.-	C79.0-	D09.19	D30.0--	D41.0-	D49.5
pelvis	C65.-	C79.0-	D09.19	D30.1-	D41.1-	D49.5
respiratory						
organs or system NEC	C39.9	C78.30	D02.4	D14.4	D38.6	D49.1
tract NEC	C39.9	C78.30	D02.4	D14.4	D38.5	D49.1
upper	C39.0	C78.30	D02.4	D14.4	D38.5	D49.1
retina	C69.2-	C79.49	D09.2-	D31.2	D48.7	D49.81
retrobulbar	C69.6-	C79.49	—	D31.6-	D48.7	D49.89
retrocecal	C48.0	C78.6	—	D20.0	D48.3	D49.0
retromolar (area) (triangle) (trigone)	C06.2	C79.89	D00.00	D10.39	D37.09	D49.0
retro-orbital	C76.0	C79.89	D09.8	D36.7	D48.7	D49.89
retroperitoneal (space) (tissue)	C48.0	C78.6	—	D20.0	D48.3	D49.0
retroperitoneum	C48.0	C78.6	—	D20.0	D48.3	D49.0
retropharyngeal	C14.0	C79.89	D00.08	D10.9	D37.05	D49.0
retrovesical (septum)	C76.3	C79.89	D09.8	D36.7	D48.7	D49.89
rhinencephalon	C71.0	C79.31	—	D33.0	D43.0	D49.6
rib	C41.3	C79.51	—	D16.7-	D48.0	D49.2
Rosenmüller's fossa	C11.2	C79.89	D00.08	D10.6	D37.05	D49.0
round ligament	C57.2	C79.82	—	D28.2	D39.8	D49.5
sacrococcyx, sacrococcygeal	C41.4-	C79.51	—	D16.8-	D48.0	D49.2
region	C76.3	C79.89	D09.8	D36.7	D48.7	D49.89
sacrouterine ligament	C57.3	C79.82	—	D28.2	D39.8	D49.5
sacrum, sacral (vertebra)	C41.4-	C79.51	—	D16.8-	D48.0	D49.2
salivary gland or duct (major)	C08.9	C79.89	D00.00	D11.9	D37.039	D49.0
minor NEC	C06.9	C79.89	D00.00	D10.39	D37.04	D49.0
overlapping lesion	C08.9	—	—	—	—	—
parotid	C07	C79.89	D00.00	D11.0	D37.030	D49.0
pluriglandular	C08.9	C79.89	D00.00	D11.9	D37.039	D49.0
sublingual	C08.1	C79.89	D00.00	D11.7	D37.031	D49.0
submandibular	C08.0	C79.89	D00.00	D11.7	D37.032	D49.0
submaxillary	C08.0	C79.89	D00.00	D11.7	D37.032	D49.0
salpinx (uterine)	C57.0-	C79.82	D07.39	D28.2	D39.8	D49.5
Santorini's duct	C25.3	C78.89	D01.7	D13.6	D37.8	D49.0
scalp	C44.4	C79.2-	D04.4	D23.4	D48.5	D49.2
scapula (any part)	C40.0-	C79.51	—	D16.0-	—	—
scapular region	C76.1	C79.89	D09.8	D36.7	D48.7	D49.89
scar NEC (*see also* Neoplasm, skin)	C44.9	C79.2-	D04.9	D23.9	D48.5	D49.2
sciatic nerve	C47.2-	C79.89	—	D36.13	D48.2	D49.2

Neoplasm Table

Neoplasm, sclera—Neoplasm, specified site NEC

	Malignant Primary	Malignant Secondary	Ca in situ	Benign	Uncertain	Unspecified Behavior
Neoplasm, neoplastic—*continued*						
sclera	C69.4-	C79.49	D09.2-	D31.4-	D48.7	D49.89
scrotum (skin)	C63.2	C79.82	D07.61	D29.4	D40.8	D49.5
sebaceous gland—*see* Neoplasm, skin						
sella turcica	C75.1	C79.89	D09.3	D35.2	D44.3	D49.7
bone	C41.0-	C79.51	—	D16.4-	D48.0	D49.2
semilunar cartilage (knee)	C40.2-	C79.51	—	D16.2-	D48.0	D49.2
seminal vesicle	C63.7	C79.82	D07.69	D29.8	D40.8	D49.5
septum						
nasal	C30.0	C78.39	D02.3	D14.0	D38.5	D49.1
posterior margin	C11.3	C79.89	D00.08	D10.6	D37.05	D49.0
rectovaginal	C76.3	C79.89	D09.8	D36.7	D48.7	D49.89
rectovesical	C76.3	C79.89	D09.8	D36.7	D48.7	D49.89
urethrovaginal	C57.9	C79.82	D07.30	D28.9	D39.9	D49.5
vesicovaginal	C57.9	C79.82	D07.30	D28.9	D39.9	D49.5
shoulder NEC	C76.4-	C79.89	D04.6-	D36.7	D48.7	D49.89
sigmoid flexure (lower) (upper)	C18.7	C78.5	D01.0	D12.5	D37.4	D49.0
sinus (accessory)	C31.9	C78.39	D02.3	D14.0	D38.5	D49.1
bone (any)	C41.0-	C79.51	—	D16.4-	D48.0	D49.2
ethmoidal	C31.1	C78.39	D02.3	D14.0	D38.5	D49.1
frontal	C31.2	C78.39	D02.3	D14.0	D38.5	D49.1
maxillary	C31.0	C78.39	D02.3	D14.0	D38.5	D49.1
nasal, paranasal NEC	C31.9	C78.39	D02.3	D14.0	D38.5	D49.1
overlapping lesion	C31.8	—	—	—	—	—
pyriform	C12	C79.89	D00.08	D10.7	D37.05	D49.0
sphenoid	C31.3	C78.39	D02.3	D14.0	D38.5	D49.1
skeleton, skeletal NEC	C41.9	C79.51	—	D16.9-	D48.0	D49.2
Skene's gland	C68.1	C79.19	D09.19	D30.8	D41.8	D49.5
skin NEC	C44.9	C79.2-	D04.9	D23.9	D48.5	D49.2
abdominal wall	C44.59	C79.2-	D04.5	D23.5	D48.5	D49.2
ala nasi	C44.31	C79.2-	D04.39	D23.39	D48.5	D49.2
ankle	C44.7-	C79.2-	D04.7-	D23.7-	D48.5	D49.2
antecubital space	C44.6-	C79.2-	D04.6-	D23.6-	D48.5	D49.2
anus	C44.51	C79.2-	D04.5	D23.5	D48.5	D49.2
arm	C44.6-	C79.2-	D04.6-	D23.6-	D48.5	D49.2
auditory canal (external)	C44.2-	C79.2-	D04.2-	D23.2-	D48.5	D49.2
auricle (ear)	C44.2-	C79.2-	D04.2-	D23.2-	D48.5	D49.2
auricular canal (external)	C44.2-	C79.2-	D04.2-	D23.2-	D48.5	D49.2
axilla, axillary fold	C44.59	C79.2-	D04.5	D23.5	D48.5	D49.2
back	C44.59	C79.2-	D04.5	D23.5	D48.5	D49.2
breast	C44.52	C79.2-	D04.5	D23.5	D48.5	D49.2
brow	C44.39	C79.2-	D04.39	D23.39	D48.5	D49.2
buttock	C44.59	C79.2-	D04.5	D23.5	D48.5	D49.2
calf	C44.7-	C79.2-	D04.7-	D23.7-	D48.5	D49.2
canthus (eye) (inner) (outer)	C44.1-	C79.2-	D04.1-	D23.1-	D48.5	D49.2
cervical region	C44.4	C79.2-	D04.4	D23.4	D48.5	D49.2
cheek (external)	C44.39	C79.2-	D04.39	D23.39	D48.5	D49.2
chest (wall)	C44.59	C79.2-	D04.5	D23.5	D48.5	D49.2
chin	C44.39	C79.2-	D04.39	D23.39	D48.5	D49.2
clavicular area	C44.59	C79.2-	D04.5	D23.5	D48.5	D49.2
clitoris	C51.2	C79.82	D07.1	D28.0	D39.8	D49.5
columnella	C44.39	C79.2-	D04.39	D23.39	D48.5	D49.2
concha	C44.2-	C79.2-	D04.2-	D23.2-	D48.5	D49.2
ear (external)	C44.2-	C79.2-	D04.2-	D23.2-	D48.5	D49.2
elbow	C44.6-	C79.2-	D04.6-	D23.6-	D48.5	D49.2
eyebrow	C44.39	C79.2-	D04.39	D23.39	D48.5	D49.2
eyelid	C44.1-	C79.2-	D04.1-	D23.1-	D48.5	D49.2
face NOS	C44.30	C79.2-	D04.30	D23.30	D48.5	D49.2
female genital organs (external)	C51.9	C79.82	D07.1	D28.0	D39.8	D49.5
clitoris	C51.2	C79.82	D07.1	D28.0	D39.8	D49.5
labium NEC	C51.9	C79.82	D07.1	D28.0	D39.8	D49.5
majus	C51.0	C79.82	D07.1	D28.0	D39.8	D49.5
minus	C51.1	C79.82	D07.1	D28.0	D39.8	D49.5
pudendum	C51.9	C79.82	D07.1	D28.0	D39.8	D49.5
vulva	C51.9	C79.82	D07.1	D28.0	D39.8	D49.5
finger	C44.6-	C79.2-	D04.6-	D23.6-	D48.5	D49.2
flank	C44.59	C79.2-	D04.5	D23.5	D48.5	D49.2
foot	C44.7-	C79.2-	D04.7-	D23.7-	D48.5	D49.2
forearm	C44.6-	C79.2-	D04.6-	D23.6-	D48.5	D49.2
forehead	C44.39	C79.2-	D04.39	D23.39	D48.5	D49.2
glabella	C44.39	C79.2-	D04.39	D23.39	D48.5	D49.2

	Malignant Primary	Malignant Secondary	Ca in situ	Benign	Uncertain	Unspecified Behavior
Neoplasm, neoplastic—*continued*						
vulva—*continued*						
gluteal region	C44.59	C79.2-	D04.5	D23.5	D48.5	D49.2
groin	C44.59	C79.2-	D04.5	D23.5	D48.5	D49.2
hand	C44.6-	C79.2-	D04.6-	D23.6-	D48.5	D49.2
head NEC	C44.4	C79.2-	D04.4	D23.4	D48.5	D49.2
heel	C44.7-	C79.2-	D04.7-	D23.7-	D48.5	D49.2
helix	C44.2-	C79.2-	D04.2-	D23.2-	D48.5	D49.2
hip	C44.7-	C79.2-	D04.7-	D23.7-	D48.5	D49.2
infraclavicular region	C44.59	C79.2-	D04.5	D23.5	D48.5	D49.2
inguinal region	C44.59	C79.2-	D04.5	D23.5	D48.5	D49.2
jaw	C44.39	C79.2-	D04.39	D23.39	D48.5	D49.2
Kaposi's sarcoma—*see* Kaposi's, sarcoma, skin						
knee	C44.7-	C79.2-	D04.7-	D23.7-	D48.5	D49.2
labia						
majora	C51.0	C79.82	D07.1	D28.0	D39.8	D49.5
minora	C51.1	C79.82	D07.1	D28.0	D39.8	D49.5
leg	C44.7-	C79.2-	D04.7-	D23.7-	D48.5	D49.2
lid (lower) (upper)	C44.1-	C79.2-	D04.1-	D23.1-	D48.5	D49.2
limb NEC	C44.9	C79.2-	D04.9	D23.9	D48.5	D49.2
lower	C44.7-	C79.2-	D04.7-	D23.7-	D48.5	D49.2
upper	C44.6-	C79.2-	D04.6-	D23.6-	D48.5	D49.2
lip (lower) (upper)	C44.0	C79.2-	D04.0	D23.0	D48.5	D49.2
male genital organs	C63.9	C79.82	D07.60	D29.9	D40.8	D49.5
penis	C60.9	C79.82	D07.4	D29.0	D40.8	D49.5
prepuce	C60.0	C79.82	D07.4	D29.0	D40.8	D49.5
scrotum	C63.2	C79.82	D07.61	D29.4	D40.8	D49.5
mastectomy site (skin)	C44.52	C79.2-	—	—	—	—
specified as breast tissue	C50.8-	C79.81	—	—	—	—
meatus, acoustic (external)	C44.2-	C79.2-	D04.2-	D23.2-	D48.5	D49.2
melanotic—*see* Melanoma						
Merkel cell—*see* Carcinoma, Merkel cell						
nates	C44.59	C79.2-	D04.5	D23.5	D48.5	D49.2
neck	C44.4	C79.2-	D04.4	D23.4	D48.5	D49.2
nevus—*see* Nevus, skin						
nose (external)	C44.31	C79.2-	D04.39	D23.39	D48.5	D49.2
overlapping lesion	C44.8	—	—	—	—	—
palm	C44.6-	C79.2-	D04.6-	D23.6-	D48.5	D49.2
palpebra	C44.1-	C79.2-	D04.1-	D23.1-	D48.5	D49.2
penis NEC	C60.9	C79.82	D07.4	D29.0	D40.8	D49.5
perianal	C44.51	C79.2-	D04.5	D23.5	D48.5	D49.2
perineum	C44.59	C79.2-	D04.5	D23.5	D48.5	D49.2
pinna	C44.2-	C79.2-	D04.2-	D23.2-	D48.5	D49.2
plantar	C44.7-	C79.2-	D04.7-	D23.7-	D48.5	D49.2
popliteal fossa or space	C44.7-	C79.2-	D04.7-	D23.7-	D48.5	D49.2
prepuce	C60.0	C79.82	D07.4	D29.0	D40.8	D49.5
pubes	C44.59	C79.2-	D04.5	D23.5	D48.5	D49.2
sacrococcygeal region	C44.59	C79.2-	D04.5	D23.5	D48.5	D49.2
scalp	C44.4	C79.2-	D04.4	D23.4	D48.5	D49.2
scapular region	C44.59	C79.2-	D04.5	D23.5	D48.5	D49.2
scrotum	C63.2	C79.82	D07.61	D29.4	D40.8	D49.5
shoulder	C44.6-	C79.2-	D04.6-	D23.6-	D48.5	D49.2
sole (foot)	C44.7-	C79.2-	D04.7-	D23.7-	D48.5	D49.2
specified sites NEC	C44.8	C79.2-	D04.8	D23.9	D48.5	D49.2
submammary fold	C44.59	C79.2-	D04.5	D23.5	D48.5	D49.2
supraclavicular region	C44.4	C79.2-	D04.4	D23.4	D48.5	D49.2
temple	C44.39	C79.2-	D04.39	D23.39	D48.5	D49.2
thigh	C44.7-	C79.2-	D04.7-	D23.7-	D48.5	D49.2
thoracic wall	C44.59	C79.2-	D04.5	D23.5	D48.5	D49.2
thumb	C44.6-	C79.2-	D04.6-	D23.6-	D48.5	D49.2
toe	C44.7-	C79.2-	D04.7-	D23.7-	D48.5	D49.2
tragus	C44.2-	C79.2-	D04.2-	D23.2-	D48.5	D49.2
trunk	C44.59	C79.2-	D04.5	D23.5	D48.5	D49.2
umbilicus	C44.59	C79.2-	D04.5	D23.5	D48.5	D49.2
vulva	C51.9	C79.82	D07.1	D28.0	D39.8	D49.5
wrist	C44.6-	C79.2-	D04.6-	D23.6-	D48.5	D49.2
skull	C41.0-	C79.51	—	D16.4-	D48.0	D49.2
soft parts or tissues—*see* Neoplasm, connective tissue						
specified site NEC	C76.8	C79.89	D09.8	D36.7	D48.7	D49.89

	Malignant Primary	Malignant Secondary	Ca in situ	Benign	Uncertain	Unspecified Behavior
Neoplasm, neoplastic—*continued*						
spermatic cord	C63.1-	C79.82	D07.69	D29.8	D40.8	D49.5
sphenoid	C31.3	C78.39	D02.3	D14.0	D38.5	D49.1
bone	C41.0-	C79.51	—	D16.4-	D48.0	D49.2
sinus	C31.3	C78.39	D02.3	D14.0	D38.5	D49.1
sphincter						
anal	C21.1	C78.5	D01.3	D12.9	D37.8	D49.0
of Oddi	C24.0	C78.89	D01.5	D13.5	D37.6	D49.0
spine, spinal (column)	C41.2-	C79.51	—	D16.6	D48.0	D49.2
bulb	C71.7	C79.31	—	D33.1	D43.1	D49.6
coccyx	C41.4-	C79.51	—	D16.8-	D48.0	D49.2
cord (cervical) (lumbar) (sacral) (thoracic)	C72.0	C79.49	—	D33.4	D43.4	D49.7
dura mater	C70.1	C79.49	—	D32.1	D42.1	D49.7
lumbosacral	C41.2-	C79.51	—	D16.6	D48.0	D49.2
marrow NEC	C96.9	C79.52	—	—	—	D47.9
membrane	C70.1	C79.49	—	D32.1	D42.1	D49.7
meninges	C70.1	C79.49	—	D32.1	D42.1	D49.7
nerve (root)	C47.9	C79.89	—	D36.10	D48.2	D49.2
pia mater	C70.1	C79.49	—	D32.1	D42.1	D49.7
root	C47.9	C79.89	—	D36.10	D48.2	D49.2
sacrum	C41.4-	C79.51	—	D16.8-	D48.0	D49.2
spleen, splenic NEC	C26.1	C78.89	D01.7	D13.9	D37.8	D49.0
flexure (colon)	C18.5	C78.5	D01.0	D12.3	D37.4	D49.0
stem, brain	C71.7	C79.31	—	D33.1	D43.1	D49.6
Stensen's duct	C07	C79.89	D00.00	D11.0	D37.030	D49.0
sternum	C41.3	C79.51	—	D16.7-	D48.0	D49.2
stomach	C16.9	C78.89	D00.2	D13.1	D37.1	D49.0
antrum (pyloric)	C16.3	C78.89	D00.2	D13.1	D37.1	D49.0
body	C16.2	C78.89	D00.2	D13.1	D37.1	D49.0
cardia	C16.0	C78.89	D00.2	D13.1	D37.1	D49.0
cardiac orifice	C16.0	C78.89	D00.2	D13.1	D37.1	D49.0
corpus	C16.2	C78.89	D00.2	D13.1	D37.1	D49.0
fundus	C16.1	C78.89	D00.2	D13.1	D37.1	D49.0
greater curvature NEC	C16.6	C78.89	D00.2	D13.1	D37.1	D49.0
lesser curvature NEC	C16.5	C78.89	D00.2	D13.1	D37.1	D49.0
overlapping lesion	C16.8	—	—	—	—	—
prepylorus	C16.4	C78.89	D00.2	D13.1	D37.1	D49.0
pylorus	C16.4	C78.89	D00.2	D13.1	D37.1	D49.0
wall NEC	C16.9	C78.89	D00.2	D13.1	D37.1	D49.0
anterior NEC	C16.8	C78.89	D00.2	D13.1	D37.1	D49.0
posterior NEC	C16.8	C78.89	D00.2	D13.1	D37.1	D49.0
stroma, endometrial	C54.1	C79.82	D07.0	D26.1	D39.0	D49.5
stump, cervical	C53.8	C79.82	D06.7	D26.0	D39.0	D49.5
subcutaneous (nodule) (tissue) NEC—*see* Neoplasm, connective tissue						
subdural	C70.9	C79.32	-	D32.9	D42.9	D49.7
subglottis, subglottic	C32.2	C78.39	D02.0	D14.1	D38.0	D49.1
sublingual	C04.9	C79.89	D00.06	D10.2	D37.09	D49.0
gland or duct	C08.1	C79.89	D00.00	D11.7	D37.031	D49.0
submandibular gland	C08.0	C79.89	D00.00	D11.7	D37.032	D49.0
submaxillary gland or duct	C08.0	C79.89	D00.00	D11.7	D37.032	D49.0
submental	C76.0	C79.89	D09.8	D36.7	D48.7	D49.89
subpleural	C34.9-	C78.0-	—	D14.3-	D38.1	D49.1
substernal	C38.1	C78.1	—	D15.2	D38.3	D49.89
sudoriferous, sudoriparous gland, site unspecified	C44.9	C79.2-	D04.9	D23.9	D48.5	D49.2
specified site—*see* Neoplasm, skin						
supraclavicular region	C76.0	C79.89	D09.8	D36.7	D48.7	D49.89
supraglottis	C32.1	C78.39	D02.0	D14.1	D38.0	D49.1
suprarenal	C74.9-	C79.7-	D09.3	D35.0-	D44.1-	D49.7
capsule	C74.9-	C79.7-	D09.3	D35.0-	D44.1-	D49.7
cortex	C74.0-	C79.7-	D09.3	D35.0-	D44.1-	D49.7
gland	C74.9-	C79.7-	D09.3	D35.0-	D44.1-	D49.7
medulla	C74.1-	C79.7-	D09.3	D35.0-	D44.1-	D49.7
suprasellar (region)	C71.9	C79.31	—	D33.2	D43.2	D49.6
supratentorial (brain) NEC	C71.0	C79.31	—	D33.0	D43.0	D49.6
sweat gland (apocrine) (eccrine), site unspecified	C44.9	C79.2-	D04.9	D23.9	D48.5	D49.2
specified site—*see* Neoplasm, skin						
sympathetic nerve or nervous system NEC	C47.9	C79.89	—	D36.10	D48.2	D49.2
symphysis pubis	C41.4-	C79.51	—	D16.8-	D48.0	D49.2
synovial membrane—*see* Neoplasm, connective tissue						
tapetum, brain	C71.8	C79.31	—	D33.2	D43.2	D49.6
tarsus (any bone)	C40.3-	C79.51	—	D16.3-		
temple (skin)	C44.39	C79.2-	D04.39	D23.39	D48.5	D49.2
temporal						
bone	C41.0-	C79.51	—	D16.4-	D48.0	D49.2
lobe or pole	C71.2	C79.31	—	D33.0	D43.0	D49.6
region	C76.0	C79.89	D09.8	D36.7	D48.7	D49.89
skin	C44.39	C79.2-	D04.39	D23.39	D48.5	D49.2
tendon (sheath)—*see* Neoplasm, connective tissue						
tentorium (cerebelli)	C70.0	C79.32	—	D32.0	D42.0	D49.7
testis, testes	C62.9	C79.82	D07.69	D29.2	D40.1-	D49.5
descended	C62.1-	C79.82	D07.69	D29.2	D40.1-	D49.5
ectopic	C62.0	C79.82	D07.69	D29.2	D40.1-	D49.5
retained	C62.0	C79.82	D07.69	D29.2	D40.1-	D49.5
scrotal	C62.1-	C79.82	D07.69	D29.2	D40.1-	D49.5
undescended	C62.0	C79.82	D07.69	D29.2	D40.1-	D49.5
unspecified whether descended or undescended	C62.9	C79.82	D07.69	D29.2	D40.1-	D49.5
thalamus	C71.0	C79.31	—	D33.0	D43.0	D49.6
thigh NEC	C76.5-	C79.89	D04.7-	D36.7	D48.7	D49.89
thorax, thoracic (cavity) (organs NEC)	C76.1	C79.89	D09.8	D36.7	D48.7	D49.89
duct	C49.3	C79.89	—	D21.3	D48.1	D49.2
wall NEC	C76.1	C79.89	D09.8	D36.7	D48.7	D49.89
throat	C14.0	C79.89	D00.08	D10.9	D37.05	D49.0
thumb NEC	C76.4-	C79.89	D04.6-	D36.7	D48.7	D49.89
thymus (gland)	C37	C79.89	—	D15.0	D38.4	D49.89
thyroglossal duct	C73	C79.89	D09.3	D34	D44.0	D49.7
thyroid (gland)	C73	C79.89	D09.3	D34	D44.0	D49.7
cartilage	C32.3	C78.39	D02.0	D14.1	D38.0	D49.1
tibia (any part)	C40.2-	C79.51	—	D16.2-	—	—
toe NEC	C76.5-	C79.89	D04.7-	D36.7	D48.7	D49.89
tongue	C02.9	C79.89	D00.07	D10.1	D37.02	D49.0
anterior (two-thirds) NEC	C02.3	C79.89	D00.07	D10.1	D37.02	D49.0
dorsal surface	C02.0	C79.89	D00.07	D10.1	D37.02	D49.0
ventral surface	C02.2	C79.89	D00.07	D10.1	D37.02	D49.0
base (dorsal surface)	C01	C79.89	D00.07	D10.1	D37.02	D49.0
border (lateral)	C02.1	C79.89	D00.07	D10.1	D37.02	D49.0
dorsal surface NEC	C02.0	C79.89	D00.07	D10.1	D37.02	D49.0
fixed part NEC	C01	C79.89	D00.07	D10.1	D37.02	D49.0
foreamen cecum	C02.0	C79.89	D00.07	D10.1	D37.02	D49.0
frenulum linguae	C02.2	C79.89	D00.07	D10.1	D37.02	D49.0
junctional zone	C02.8	C79.89	D00.07	D10.1	D37.02	D49.0
margin (lateral)	C02.1	C79.89	D00.07	D10.1	D37.02	D49.0
midline NEC	C02.0	C79.89	D00.07	D10.1	D37.02	D49.0
mobile part NEC	C02.3	C79.89	D00.07	D10.1	D37.02	D49.0
overlapping lesion	C02.8	—	—	—	—	—
posterior (third)	C01	C79.89	D00.07	D10.1	D37.02	D49.0
root	C01	C79.89	D00.07	D10.1	D37.02	D49.0
surface (dorsal)	C02.0	C79.89	D00.07	D10.1	D37.02	D49.0
base	C01	C79.89	D00.07	D10.1	D37.02	D49.0
ventral	C02.2	C79.89	D00.07	D10.1	D37.02	D49.0
tip	C02.1	C79.89	D00.07	D10.1	D37.02	D49.0
tonsil	C02.4	C79.89	D00.07	D10.1	D37.02	D49.0
tonsil	C09.9	C79.89	D00.08	D10.4	D37.05	D49.0
fauces, faucial	C09.9	C79.89	D00.08	D10.4	D37.05	D49.0
lingual	C02.4	C79.89	D00.07	D10.1	D37.02	D49.0
overlapping sites	C09.8	—	—	—	—	—
palatine	C09.9	C79.89	D00.08	D10.4	D37.05	D49.0
pharyngeal	C11.1	C79.89	D00.08	D10.6	D37.05	D49.0
pillar (anterior) (posterior)	C09.1	C79.89	D00.08	D10.5	D37.05	D49.0
tonsillar fossa	C09.0	C79.89	D00.08	D10.5	D37.05	D49.0
tooth socket NEC	C03.9	C79.89	D00.03	D10.39	D37.09	D49.0
trachea (cartilage) (mucosa)	C33	C78.39	D02.1	D14.2	D38.1	D49.1
overlapping lesion with bronchus or lung	C34.8-					

Neoplasm Table

Neoplasm, tracheobronchial—Neoplasm, Zuckerkandl organ

	Malignant Primary	Malignant Secondary	Ca in situ	Benign	Uncertain	Unspecified Behavior
Neoplasm, neoplastic—*continued*						
tracheobronchial	C34.8-	C78.39	D02.1	D14.2	D38.1	D49.1
overlapping lesion with lung	C34.8-	—	—	—	—	—
tragus	C44.2-	C79.2-	D04.2-	D23.2-	D48.5	D49.2
trunk NEC	C76.8	C79.89	D04.5	D36.7	D48.7	D49.89
tubo-ovarian	C57.8	C79.82	D07.39	D28.7	D39.8	D49.5
tunica vaginalis	C63.7	C79.82	D07.69	D29.8	D40.8	D49.5
turbinate (bone)	C41.0-	C79.51	—	D16.4-	D48.0	D49.2
nasal	C30.0	C78.39	D02.3	D14.0	D38.5	D49.1
tympanic cavity	C30.1	C78.39	D02.3	D14.0	D38.5	D49.1
ulna (any part)	C40.0-	C79.51	—	D16.0-	—	—
umbilicus, umbilical	C44.59	C79.2-	D04.5	D23.5	D48.5	D49.2
uncus, brain	C71.2	C79.31	—	D33.0	D43.0	D49.6
unknown site or unspecified	C80.1	C79.9	D09.9	D36.9	D48.9	D49.9
urachus	C67.7	C79.11	D09.0	D30.3	D41.4	D49.4
ureter, ureteral	C66.-	C79.19	D09.19	D30.2-	D41.2-	D49.5
orifice (bladder)	C67.6	C79.11	D09.0	D30.3	D41.4	D49.4
ureter-bladder (junction)	C67.6	C79.11	D09.0	D30.3	D41.4	D49.4
urethra, urethral (gland)	C68.0	C79.19	D09.19	D30.4	D41.3	D49.5
orifice, internal	C67.5	C79.11	D09.0	D30.3	D41.4	D49.4
urethrovaginal (septum)	C57.9	C79.82	D07.39	D28.9	D39.8	D49.5
urinary organ or system	C68.9	C79.10	D09.10	D30.9	D41.9	D49.5
bladder—*see* Neoplasm, bladder						
overlapping lesion	C68.8	—	—	—	—	—
specified sites NEC	C68.8	C79.19	D09.19	D30.8	D41.8	D49.5
utero-ovarian	C57.8	C79.82	D07.39	D28.7	D39.8	D49.5
ligament	C57.1	C79.82	D07.39	D28.2	D39.8	D49.5
uterosacral ligament	C57.3	C79.82	—	D28.2	D39.8	D49.5
uterus, uteri, uterine	C55	C79.82	D07.0	D26.9	D39.0	D49.5
adnexa NEC	C57.4	C79.82	D07.39	D28.7	D39.8	D49.5
body	C54.9	C79.82	D07.0	D26.1	D39.0	D49.5
cervix	C53.9	C79.82	D06.9	D26.0	D39.0	D49.5
cornu	C54.9	C79.82	D07.0	D26.1	D39.0	D49.5
corpus	C54.9	C79.82	D07.0	D26.1	D39.0	D49.5
endocervix (canal) (gland)	C53.0	C79.82	D06.0	D26.0	D39.0	D49.5
endometrium	C54.1	C79.82	D07.0	D26.1	D39.0	D49.5
exocervix	C53.1	C79.82	D06.1	D26.0	D39.0	D49.5
external os	C53.1	C79.82	D06.1	D26.0	D39.0	D49.5
fundus	C54.3	C79.82	D07.0	D26.1	D39.0	D49.5
internal os	C53.0	C79.82	D06.0	D26.0	D39.0	D49.5
isthmus	C54.0	C79.82	D07.0	D26.1	D39.0	D49.5
ligament	C57.3	C79.82	—	D28.2	D39.8	D49.5
broad	C57.1	C79.82	D07.39	D28.2	D39.8	D49.5
round	C57.2	C79.82	—	D28.2	D39.8	D49.5
lower segment	C54.0	C79.82	D07.0	D26.1	D39.0	D49.5
myometrium	C54.2	C79.82	D07.0	D26.1	D39.0	D49.5
overlapping sites	C54.8	—	—	—	—	—
squamocolumnar junction	C53.8	C79.82	D06.7	D26.0	D39.0	D49.5
tube	C57.0-	C79.82	D07.39	D28.2	D39.8	D49.5
utricle, prostatic	C68.0	C79.19	D09.19	D30.4	D41.3	D49.5
uveal tract	C69.4-	C79.49	D09.2-	D31.4-	D48.7	D49.89
uvula	C05.2	C79.89	D00.04	D10.39	D37.09	D49.0
vagina, vaginal (fornix) (vault) (wall)	C52	C79.82	D07.2	D28.1	D39.8	D49.5
vaginovesical	C57.9	C79.82	D07.30	D28.9	D39.9	D49.5
septum	C57.9	C79.82	D07.30	D28.9	D39.9	D49.5

	Malignant Primary	Malignant Secondary	Ca in situ	Benign	Uncertain	Unspecified Behavior
Neoplasm, neoplastic—*continued*						
vallecula (epiglottis)	C10.0	C79.89	D00.08	D10.5	D37.05	D49.0
vas deferens	C63.1-	C79.82	D07.69	D29.8	D40.8	D49.5
vascular—*see* Neoplasm, connective tissue						
Vater's ampulla	C24.1	C78.89	D01.5	D13.5	D37.6	D49.0
vein, venous—*see* Neoplasm, connective tissue						
vena cava (abdominal) (inferior)	C49.4	C79.89	—	D21.4	D48.1	D49.2
superior	C49.3	C79.89	—	D21.3	D48.1	D49.2
ventricle (cerebral) (floor) (lateral) (third)	C71.5	C79.31	—	D33.0	D43.0	D49.6
cardiac (left) (right)	C38.0	C79.89	—	D15.1	D48.7	D49.89
fourth	C71.7	C79.31	—	D33.1	D43.1	D49.6
ventricular band of larynx	C32.1	C78.39	D02.0	D14.1	D38.0	D49.1
ventriculus—*see* Neoplasm, stomach						
vermillion border—*see* Neoplasm, lip						
vermis, cerebellum	C71.6	C79.31	—	D33.1	D43.1	D49.6
vertebra (column)	C41.2-	C79.51	—	D16.6	D48.0	D49.2
coccyx	C41.4-	C79.51	—	D16.8-	D48.0	D49.2
marrow NEC	C96.9	C79.52	—	—	—	D47.9
sacrum	C41.4-	C79.51	—	D16.8-	D48.0	D49.2
vesical—*see* Neoplasm, bladder						
vesicle, seminal	C63.7	C79.82	D07.69	D29.8	D40.8	D49.5
vesicocervical tissue	C57.9	C79.82	D07.30	D28.9	D39.9	D49.5
vesicorectal	C76.3	C79.82	D09.8	D36.7	D48.7	D49.89
vesicovaginal	C57.9	C79.82	D07.30	D28.9	D39.9	D49.5
septum	C57.9	C79.82	D07.39	D28.9	D39.8	D49.5
vessel (blood)—*see* Neoplasm, connective tissue						
vestibular gland, greater	C51.0	C79.82	D07.1	D28.0	D39.8	D49.5
vestibule						
mouth	C06.1	C79.89	D00.00	D10.39	D37.09	D49.0
nose	C30.0	C78.39	D02.3	D14.0	D38.5	D49.1
Virchow's gland	C77.0	C77.0	—	D36.0	D48.7	D49.89
viscera NEC	C76.8	C79.89	D09.8	D36.7	D48.7	D49.89
vocal cords (true)	C32.0	C78.39	D02.0	D14.1	D38.0	D49.1
false	C32.1	C78.39	D02.0	D14.1	D38.0	D49.1
vomer	C41.0-	C79.51	—	D16.4-	D48.0	D49.2
vulva	C51.9	C79.82	D07.1	D28.0	D39.8	D49.5
vulvovaginal gland	C51.0	C79.82	D07.1	D28.0	D39.8	D49.5
Waldeyer's ring	C14.2	C79.89	D00.08	D10.9	D37.05	D49.0
Wharton's duct	C08.0	C79.89	D00.00	D11.7	D37.032	D49.0
white matter (central) (cerebral)	C71.0	C79.31	—	D33.0	D43.0	D49.6
windpipe	C33	C78.39	D02.1	D14.2	D38.1	D49.1
Wirsung's duct	C25.3	C78.89	D01.7	D13.6	D37.8	D49.0
wolffian (body) (duct)						
female	C57.7	C79.82	D07.39	D28.7	D39.8	D49.5
male	C63.7	C79.82	D07.69	D29.8	D40.8	D49.5
womb—*see* Neoplasm, uterus						
wrist NEC	C76.4-	C79.89	D04.6-	D36.7	D48.7	D49.89
xiphoid process	C41.3	C79.51	—	D16.7-	D48.0	D49.2
Zuckerkandl organ	C75.5	C79.89	—	D35.6	D44.7	D49.7

ICD-10-CM Table of Drugs and Chemicals

Substance	Poisoning, Accidental (unintentional)	Poisoning, Intentional Self-harm	Poisoning, Assault	Poisoning, Undetermined	Adverse Effect	Under-dosing
1-propanol	T51.3x1	T51.3x2	T51.3x3	T51.3x4	—	—
2-Deoxy-5-fluorouridine	T45.1x1	T45.1x2	T45.1x3	T45.1x4	T45.1x5	T45.1x6
2-Methoxyethanol	T52.3x1	T52.3x2	T52.3x3	T52.3x4	—	—
2-propanol	T51.2x1	T51.2x2	T51.2x3	T51.2x4	—	—
2,3,7,8-tetrachlorodi-benzo-p-dioxin	T53.7x1	T53.7x2	T53.7x3	T53.7x4	—	—
2,4-D (dichlorophen-oxyacetic acid)	T60.3x1	T60.3x2	T60.3x3	T60.3x4	—	—
2,4-Dichlorophenoxyacetic acid	T60.3x1	T60.3x2	T60.3x3	T60.3x4	T60.3x5	T60.3x6
2,4-toluene diisocyanate	T65.0x1	T65.0x2	T65.0x3	T65.0x4	—	—
2,4,5-T	T60.3x1	T60.3x2	T60.3x3	T60.3x4	—	—
2,4,5-T (trichloro-phenoxyacetic acid)	T60.1x1	T60.1x2	T60.1x3	T60.1x4	—	—
2,4,5-trichlorophen-oxyacetic acid	T60.3x1	T60.3x2	T60.3x3	T60.3x4	—	—
4-aminobutyric acid	T43.8x1	T43.8x2	T43.8x3	T43.8x4	T43.8x5	T43.8x6
4-aminophenol derivatives	T39.1x1	T39.1x2	T39.1x3	T39.1x4	T39.1x5	T39.1x6
5-Deoxy-5-fluorouridine	T45.1x1	T45.1x2	T45.1x3	T45.1x4	T45.1x5	T45.1x6
5-Methoxypsoralen (5-MOP)	T50.991	T50.992	T50.993	T50.994	T50.995	T50.996
8-aminoquinoline drugs	T37.2x1	T37.2x2	T37.2x3	T37.2x4	T37.2x5	T37.2x6
8-Methoxypsoralen (8-MOP)	T50.991	T50.992	T50.993	T50.994	T50.995	T50.996
14-hydroxydihydro-morphinone	T40.2x1	T40.2x2	T40.2x3	T40.2x4	T40.2x5	T40.2x6
ABOB	T37.5x1	T37.5x2	T37.5x3	T37.5x4	T37.5x5	T37.5x6
Abrine	T62.2x1	T62.2x2	T62.2x3	T62.2x4	—	—
Abrus (seed)	T62.2x1	T62.2x2	T62.2x3	T62.2x4	—	—
Absinthe	T51.0x1	T51.0x2	T51.0x3	T51.0x4	—	—
beverage	T51.0x1	T51.0x2	T51.0x3	T51.0x4	—	—
Acaricide	T60.8x1	T60.8x2	T60.8x3	T60.8x4	—	—
Acebutolol	T44.7x1	T44.7x2	T44.7x3	T44.7x4	T44.7x5	T44.7x6
Acecarbromal	T42.6x1	T42.6x2	T42.6x3	T42.6x4	T42.6x5	T42.6x6
Aceclidine	T44.1x1	T44.1x2	T44.1x3	T44.1x4	T44.1x5	T44.1x6
Acedapsone	T37.0x1	T37.0x2	T37.0x3	T37.0x4	T37.0x5	T37.0x6
Acefylline piperazine	T48.6x1	T48.6x2	T48.6x3	T48.6x4	T48.6x5	T48.6x6
Acemorphan	T40.2x1	T40.2x2	T40.2x3	T40.2x4	T40.2x5	T40.2x6
Acenocoumarin	T45.511	T45.512	T45.513	T45.514	T45.515	T45.516
Acenocoumarol	T45.511	T45.512	T45.513	T45.514	T45.515	T45.516
Acepifylline	T48.6x1	T48.6x2	T48.6x3	T48.6x4	T48.6x5	T48.6x6
Acepromazine	T43.3x1	T43.3x2	T43.3x3	T43.3x4	T43.3x5	T43.3x6
Acesulfamethoxypyridazine	T37.0x1	T37.0x2	T37.0x3	T37.0x4	T37.0x5	T37.0x6
Acetal	T52.8x1	T52.8x2	T52.8x3	T52.8x4	—	—
Acetaldehyde (vapor)	T52.8x1	T52.8x2	T52.8x3	T52.8x4	—	—
liquid	T65.891	T65.892	T65.893	T65.894	—	—
P-Acetamidophenol	T39.1x1	T39.1x2	T39.1x3	T39.1x4	T39.1x5	T39.1x6
Acetaminophen	T39.1x1	T39.1x2	T39.1x3	T39.1x4	T39.1x5	T39.1x6
Acetaminosalol	T39.1x1	T39.1x2	T39.1x3	T39.1x4	T39.1x5	T39.1x6
Acetanilide	T39.1x1	T39.1x2	T39.1x3	T39.1x4	T39.1x5	T39.1x6
Acetarsol	T37.3x1	T37.3x2	T37.3x3	T37.3x4	T37.3x5	T37.3x6
Acetazolamide	T50.2x1	T50.2x2	T50.2x3	T50.2x4	T50.2x5	T50.2x6
Acetiamine	T45.2x1	T45.2x2	T45.2x3	T45.2x4	T45.2x5	T45.2x6
Acetic						
acid	T54.2x1	T54.2x2	T54.2x3	T54.2x4	—	—
with sodium acetate (ointment)	T49.3x1	T49.3x2	T49.3x3	T49.3x4	T49.3x5	T49.3x6
ester (solvent)(vapor)	T52.8x1	T52.8x2	T52.8x3	T52.8x4	—	—
irrigating solution	T50.3x1	T50.3x2	T50.3x3	T50.3x4	T50.3x5	T50.3x6
medicinal (lotion)	T49.2x1	T49.2x2	T49.2x3	T49.2x4	T49.2x5	T49.2x6
anhydride	T65.891	T65.892	T65.893	T65.894	—	—
ether (vapor)	T52.8x1	T52.8x2	T52.8x3	T52.8x4	—	—
Acetohexamide	T38.3x1	T38.3x2	T38.3x3	T38.3x4	T38.3x5	T38.3x6
Acetohydroxamic acid	T50.991	T50.992	T50.993	T50.994	T50.995	T50.996
Acetomenaphthone	T45.7x1	T45.7x2	T45.7x3	T45.7x4	T45.7x5	T45.7x6
Acetomorphine	T40.1x1	T40.1x2	T40.1x3	T40.1x4	T40.1x5	T40.1x6
Acetone (oils)	T52.4x1	T52.4x2	T52.4x3	T52.4x4	—	—
chlorinated	T52.4x1	T52.4x2	T52.4x3	T52.4x4	—	—
vapor	T52.4x1	T52.4x2	T52.4x3	T52.4x4	—	—
Acetonitrile	T52.8x1	T52.8x2	T52.8x3	T52.8x4	—	—
Acetophenazine	T43.3x1	T43.3x2	T43.3x3	T43.3x4	T43.3x5	T43.3x6
Acetophenetedin	T39.1x1	T39.1x2	T39.1x3	T39.1x4	T39.1x5	T39.1x6
Acetophenone	T52.4x1	T52.4x2	T52.4x3	T52.4x4	—	—
Acetorphine	T40.2x1	T40.2x2	T40.2x3	T40.2x4	T40.2x5	T40.2x6
Acetosulfone (sodium)	T37.1x1	T37.1x2	T37.1x3	T37.1x4	T37.1x5	T37.1x6
Acetrizoate (sodium)	T50.8x1	T50.8x2	T50.8x3	T50.8x4	T50.8x5	T50.8x6
Acetylcarbromal	T42.6x1	T42.6x2	T42.6x3	T42.6x4	T42.6x5	T42.6x6
Acetrizoic acid	T50.8x1	T50.8x2	T50.8x3	T50.8x4	T50.8x5	T50.8x6
Acetyl						
bromide	T53.6x1	T53.6x2	T53.6x3	T53.6x4	—	—
chloride	T53.6x1	T53.6x2	T53.6x3	T53.6x4	—	—
Acetylcholine						
chloride	T44.1x1	T44.1x2	T44.1x3	T44.1x4	T44.1x5	T44.1x6
derivative	T44.1x1	T44.1x2	T44.1x3	T44.1x4	T44.1x5	T44.1x6
Acetylcysteine	T48.4x1	T48.4x2	T48.4x3	T48.4x4	T48.4x5	T48.4x6
Acetyldigitoxin	T46.0x1	T46.0x2	T46.0x3	T46.0x4	T46.0x5	T46.0x6
Acetyldigoxin	T46.0x1	T46.0x2	T46.0x3	T46.0x4	T46.0x5	T46.0x6
Acetyldihydrocodeine	T40.2x1	T40.2x2	T40.2x3	T40.2x4	T40.2x5	T40.2x6
Acetyldihydrocodeinone	T40.2x1	T40.2x2	T40.2x3	T40.2x4	T40.2x5	T40.2x6
Acetylene (gas)	T59.891	T59.892	T59.893	T59.894	—	—
dichloride	T53.6x1	T53.6x2	T53.6x3	T53.6x4	—	—
incomplete combustion of— see Carbon, monoxide, industrial fuels or gases						
industrial	T59.891	T59.892	T59.893	T59.894	—	—
tetrachloride	T53.6x1	T53.6x2	T53.6x3	T53.6x4	—	—
vapor	T53.6x1	T53.6x2	T53.6x3	T53.6x4	—	—
Acetylphenylhydrazine	T39.8x1	T39.8x2	T39.8x3	T39.8x4	T39.8x5	T39.8x6
Acetylpheneturide	T42.6x1	T42.6x2	T42.6x3	T42.6x4	T42.6x5	T42.6x6
Acetylsalicylic acid (salts)	T39.011	T39.012	T39.013	T39.014	T39.015	T39.016
enteric coated	T39.011	T39.012	T39.013	T39.014	T39.015	T39.016
Acetylsulfamethoxypyridazine	T37.0x1	T37.0x2	T37.0x3	T37.0x4	T37.0x5	T37.0x6
Achromycin	T36.4x1	T36.4x2	T36.4x3	T36.4x4	T36.4x5	T36.4x6
ophthalmic preparation	T49.5x1	T49.5x2	T49.5x3	T49.5x4	T49.5x5	T49.5x6
topical NEC	T49.0x1	T49.0x2	T49.0x3	T49.0x4	T49.0x5	T49.0x6
Aciclovir	T37.5x1	T37.5x2	T37.5x3	T37.5x4	T37.5x5	T37.5x6
Acid (corrosive) NEC	T54.2x1	T54.2x2	T54.2x3	T54.2x4	—	—
Acidifying agent NEC	T50.901	T50.902	T50.903	T50.904	T50.905	T50.906
Acipimox	T46.6x1	T46.6x2	T46.6x3	T46.6x4	T46.6x5	T46.6x6
Acitretin	T50.991	T50.992	T50.993	T50.994	T50.995	T50.996
Aclarubicin	T45.1x1	T45.1x2	T45.1x3	T45.1x4	T45.1x5	T45.1x6
Aclatonium napadisilate	T48.1x1	T48.1x2	T48.1x3	T48.1x4	T48.1x5	T48.1x6
Aconite (wild)	T46.991	T46.992	T46.993	T46.994	T46.995	T46.996
Aconitine	T46.991	T46.992	T46.993	T46.994	T46.995	T46.996
Aconitum ferox	T46.991	T46.992	T46.993	T46.994	T46.995	T46.996
Acridine	T65.6x1	T65.6x2	T65.6x3	T65.6x4	—	—
vapor	T59.891	T59.892	T59.893	T59.894	—	—
Acriflavine	T37.91	T37.92	T37.93	T37.94	T37.95	T37.96
Acriflavinium chloride	T49.0x1	T49.0x2	T49.0x3	T49.0x4	T49.0x5	T49.0x6
Acrinol	T49.0x1	T49.0x2	T49.0x3	T49.0x4	T49.0x5	T49.0x6
Acrisorcin	T49.0x1	T49.0x2	T49.0x3	T49.0x4	T49.0x5	T49.0x6
Acrivastine	T45.0x1	T45.0x2	T45.0x3	T45.0x4	T45.0x5	T45.0x6
Acrolein (gas)	T59.891	T59.892	T59.893	T59.894	—	—
liquid	T54.1x1	T54.1x2	T54.1x3	T54.1x4	—	—
Acrylamide	T65.891	T65.892	T65.893	T65.894	—	—
Acrylic resin	T49.3x1	T49.3x2	T49.3x3	T49.3x4	T49.3x5	T49.3x6
Acrylonitrile	T65.891	T65.892	T65.893	T65.894	—	—
Actaea spicata	T62.2x1	T62.2x2	T62.2x3	T62.2x4	—	—
berry	T62.1x1	T62.1x2	T62.1x3	T62.1x4	—	—
Acterol	T37.3x1	T37.3x2	T37.3x3	T37.3x4	T37.3x5	T37.3x6
ACTH	T38.811	T38.812	T38.813	T38.814	T38.815	T38.816
Actinomycin C	T45.1x1	T45.1x2	T45.1x3	T45.1x4	T45.1x5	T45.1x6
Actinomycin D	T45.1x1	T45.1x2	T45.1x3	T45.1x4	T45.1x5	T45.1x6
Activated charcoal	T47.6x1	T47.6x2	T47.6x3	T47.6x4	T47.6x5	T47.6x6
Acyclovir	T37.5x1	T37.5x2	T37.5x3	T37.5x4	T37.5x5	T37.5x6
Adenine	T45.2x1	T45.2x2	T45.2x3	T45.2x4	T45.2x5	T45.2x6
arabinoside	T37.5x1	T37.5x2	T37.5x3	T37.5x4	T37.5x5	T37.5x6
Adenosine (phosphate)	T46.2x1	T46.2x2	T46.2x3	T46.2x4	T46.2x5	T46.2x6
ADH	T38.891	T38.892	T38.893	T38.894	T38.895	T38.896
Adhesive NEC	T65.891	T65.892	T65.893	T65.894	—	—
Adicillin	T36.0x1	T36.0x2	T36.0x3	T36.0x4	T36.0x5	T36.0x6
Adiphenine	T44.3x1	T44.3x2	T44.3x3	T44.3x4	T44.3x5	T44.3x6

Substance	Poisoning, Accidental (unintentional)	Poisoning, Intentional Self-harm	Poisoning, Assault	Poisoning, Undetermined	Adverse Effect	Under-dosing
Adipiodone	T50.8x1	T50.8x2	T50.8x3	T50.8x4	T50.8x5	T50.8x6
Adjunct, pharmaceutical	T50.901	T50.902	T50.903	T50.904	T50.905	T50.906
Adrenal (extract, cortex or medulla) (glucocorticoids) (hormones) (mineralocorticoids)	T38.0x1	T38.0x2	T38.0x3	T38.0x4	T38.0x5	T38.0x6
ENT agent	T49.6x1	T49.6x2	T49.6x3	T49.6x4	T49.6x5	T49.6x6
ophthalmic preparation	T49.5x1	T49.5x2	T49.5x3	T49.5x4	T49.5x5	T49.5x6
topical NEC	T49.0x1	T49.0x2	T49.0x3	T49.0x4	T49.0x5	T49.0x6
Adrenaline	T44.5x1	T44.5x2	T44.5x3	T44.5x4	T44.5x5	T44.5x6
Adrenalin—see Adrenaline						
Adrenergic NEC	T44.901	T44.902	T44.903	T44.904	T44.905	T44.906
blocking agent NEC	T44.8x1	T44.8x2	T44.8x3	T44.8x4	T44.8x5	T44.8x6
beta, heart	T44.7x1	T44.7x2	T44.7x3	T44.7x4	T44.7x5	T44.7x6
specified NEC	T44.991	T44.992	T44.993	T44.994	T44.995	T44.996
Adrenochrome						
(mono) semicarbazone	T46.991	T46.992	T46.993	T46.994	T46.995	T46.996
derivative	T46.991	T46.992	T46.993	T46.994	T46.995	T46.996
Adrenocorticotrophic hormone	T38.811	T38.812	T38.813	T38.814	T38.815	T38.816
Adrenocorticotrophin	T38.811	T38.812	T38.813	T38.814	T38.815	T38.816
Adriamycin	T45.1x1	T45.1x2	T45.1x3	T45.1x4	T45.1x5	T45.1x6
Aerosol spray NEC	T65.91	T65.92	T65.93	T65.94	—	—
Aerosporin	T36.8x1	T36.8x2	T36.8x3	T36.8x4	T36.8x5	T36.8x6
ENT agent	T49.6x1	T49.6x2	T49.6x3	T49.6x4	T49.6x5	T49.6x6
ophthalmic preparation	T49.5x1	T49.5x2	T49.5x3	T49.5x4	T49.5x5	T49.5x6
topical NEC	T49.0x1	T49.0x2	T49.0x3	T49.0x4	T49.0x5	T49.0x6
Aethusa cynapium	T62.2x1	T62.2x2	T62.2x3	T62.2x4	—	—
Afghanistan black	T40.7x1	T40.7x2	T40.7x3	T40.7x4	T40.7x5	T40.7x6
Aflatoxin	T64.01	T64.02	T64.03	T64.04	—	—
Afloqualone	T42.8x1	T42.8x2	T42.8x3	T42.8x4	T42.8x5	T42.8x6
African boxwood	T62.2x1	T62.2x2	T62.2x3	T62.2x4	—	—
Agar	T47.4x1	T47.4x2	T47.4x3	T47.4x4	T47.4x5	T47.4x6
Agricultural agent NEC	T65.91	T65.92	T65.93	T65.94	—	—
Agrypnal	T42.3x1	T42.3x2	T42.3x3	T42.3x4	T42.3x5	T42.3x6
AHLG	T50.Z11	T50.Z12	T50.Z13	T50.Z14	T50.Z15	T50.Z16
Air contaminant(s), source/type NOS	T65.91	T65.92	T65.93	T65.94	—	—
Ajmaline	T46.2x1	T46.2x2	T46.2x3	T46.2x4	T46.2x5	T46.2x6
Akritoin	T37.8x1	T37.8x2	T37.8x3	T37.8x4	T37.8x5	T37.8x6
Akee	T62.1x1	T62.1x2	T62.1x3	T62.1x4	—	—
Akrinol	T49.0x1	T49.0x2	T49.0x3	T49.0x4	T49.0x5	T49.0x6
Alacepril	T46.4x1	T46.4x2	T46.4x3	T46.4x4	T46.4x5	T46.4x6
Alantolactone	T37.4x1	T37.4x2	T37.4x3	T37.4x4	T37.4x5	T37.4x6
Albamycin	T36.8x1	T36.8x2	T36.8x3	T36.8x4	T36.8x5	T36.8x6
Albendazole	T37.4x1	T37.4x2	T37.4x3	T37.4x4	T37.4x5	T37.4x6
Albumin						
bovine	T45.8x1	T45.8x2	T45.8x3	T45.8x4	T45.8x5	T45.8x6
human serum	T45.8x1	T45.8x2	T45.8x3	T45.8x4	T45.8x5	T45.8x6
salt-poor	T45.8x1	T45.8x2	T45.8x3	T45.8x4	T45.8x5	T45.8x6
normal human serum	T45.8x1	T45.8x2	T45.8x3	T45.8x4	T45.8x5	T45.8x6
Albuterol	T48.6x1	T48.6x2	T48.6x3	T48.6x4	T48.6x5	T48.6x6
Albutoin	T42.0x1	T42.0x2	T42.0x3	T42.0x4	T42.0x5	T42.0x6
Alclometasone	T49.0x1	T49.0x2	T49.0x3	T49.0x4	T49.0x5	T49.0x6
Alcohol	T51.91	T51.92	T51.93	T51.94	—	—
absolute	T51.0x1	T51.0x2	T51.0x3	T51.0x4	—	—
beverage	T51.0x1	T51.0x2	T51.0x3	T51.0x4	—	—
allyl	T51.8x1	T51.8x2	T51.8x3	T51.8x4	—	—
antifreeze	T51.1x1	T51.1x2	T51.1x3	T51.1x4	—	—
amyl	T51.3x1	T51.3x2	T51.3x3	T51.3x4	—	—
beverage	T51.0x1	T51.0x2	T51.0x3	T51.0x4	—	—
butyl	T51.3x1	T51.3x2	T51.3x3	T51.3x4	—	—
dehydrated	T51.0x1	T51.0x2	T51.0x3	T51.0x4	—	—
beverage	T51.0x1	T51.0x2	T51.0x3	T51.0x4	—	—
denatured	T51.0x1	T51.0x2	T51.0x3	T51.0x4	—	—
deterrent NEC	T50.6x1	T50.6x2	T50.6x3	T50.6x4	T50.6x5	T50.6x6
diagnostic (gastric function)	T50.8x1	T50.8x2	T50.8x3	T50.8x4	T50.8x5	T50.8x6
ethyl	T51.0x1	T51.0x2	T51.0x3	T51.0x4	—	—
beverage	T51.0x1	T51.0x2	T51.0x3	T51.0x4	—	—
grain	T51.0x1	T51.0x2	T51.0x3	T51.0x4	—	—
beverage	T51.0x1	T51.0x2	T51.0x3	T51.0x4	—	—

Substance	Poisoning, Accidental (unintentional)	Poisoning, Intentional Self-harm	Poisoning, Assault	Poisoning, Undetermined	Adverse Effect	Under-dosing
Alcohol—continued						
industrial	T51.0x1	T51.0x2	T51.0x3	T51.0x4	—	—
isopropyl	T51.2x1	T51.2x2	T51.2x3	T51.2x4	—	—
methyl	T51.1x1	T51.1x2	T51.1x3	T51.1x4	—	—
preparation for consumption	T51.0x1	T51.0x2	T51.0x3	T51.0x4	—	—
propyl	T51.3x1	T51.3x2	T51.3x3	T51.3x4	—	—
secondary	T51.2x1	T51.2x2	T51.2x3	T51.2x4	—	—
radiator	T51.1x1	T51.1x2	T51.1x3	T51.1x4	—	—
rubbing	T51.2x1	T51.2x2	T51.2x3	T51.2x4	—	—
specified type NEC	T51.8x1	T51.8x2	T51.8x3	T51.8x4	—	—
surgical	T51.0x1	T51.0x2	T51.0x3	T51.0x4	—	—
vapor (from any type of Alcohol)	T59.891	T59.892	T59.893	T59.894	—	—
wood	T51.1x1	T51.1x2	T51.1x3	T51.1x4	—	—
Alcuronium (chloride)	T48.1x1	T48.1x2	T48.1x3	T48.1x4	T48.1x5	T48.1x6
Aldactone	T50.0x1	T50.0x2	T50.0x3	T50.0x4	T50.0x5	T50.0x6
Aldesulfone sodium	T37.1x1	T37.1x2	T37.1x3	T37.1x4	T37.1x5	T37.1x6
Aldicarb	T60.0x1	T60.0x2	T60.0x3	T60.0x4	—	—
Aldomet	T46.5x1	T46.5x2	T46.5x3	T46.5x4	T46.5x5	T46.5x6
Aldosterone	T50.0x1	T50.0x2	T50.0x3	T50.0x4	T50.0x5	T50.0x6
Aldrin (dust)	T60.1x1	T60.1x2	T60.1x3	T60.1x4	—	—
Aleve—see Naproxen						
Alexitol sodium	T47.1x1	T47.1x2	T47.1x3	T47.1x4	T47.1x5	T47.1x6
Alfacalcidol	T45.2x1	T45.2x2	T45.2x3	T45.2x4	T45.2x5	T45.2x6
Alfadolone	T41.1x1	T41.1x2	T41.1x3	T41.1x4	T41.1x5	T41.1x6
Alfaxalone	T41.1x1	T41.1x2	T41.1x3	T41.1x4	T41.1x5	T41.1x6
Alfentanil	T40.4x1	T40.4x2	T40.4x3	T40.4x4	T40.4x5	T40.4x6
Alfuzosin (hydrochloride)	T44.8x1	T44.8x2	T44.8x3	T44.8x4	T44.8x5	T44.8x6
Algae (harmful) (toxin)	T65.821	T65.822	T65.823	T65.824	—	—
Algeldrate	T47.1x1	T47.1x2	T47.1x3	T47.1x4	T47.1x5	T47.1x6
Algin	T47.8x1	T47.8x2	T47.8x3	T47.8x4	T47.8x5	T47.8x6
Alglucerase	T45.3x1	T45.3x2	T45.3x3	T45.3x4	T45.3x5	T45.3x6
Alidase	T45.3x1	T45.3x2	T45.3x3	T45.3x4	T45.3x5	T45.3x6
Alimemazine	T43.3x1	T43.3x2	T43.3x3	T43.3x4	T43.3x5	T43.3x6
Aliphatic thiocyanates	T65.0x1	T65.0x2	T65.0x3	T65.0x4	—	—
Alizapride	T45.0x1	T45.0x2	T45.0x3	T45.0x4	T45.0x5	T45.0x6
Alkali (caustic)	T54.3x1	T54.3x2	T54.3x3	T54.3x4	—	—
Alkalizing agent NEC	T50.901	T50.902	T50.903	T50.904	T50.905	T50.906
Alkaline antiseptic solution (aromatic)	T49.6x1	T49.6x2	T49.6x3	T49.6x4	T49.6x5	T49.6x6
Alkalinizing agents (medicinal)	T50.901	T50.902	T50.903	T50.904	T50.905	T50.906
Alka-seltzer	T39.011	T39.012	T39.013	T39.014	T39.015	T39.016
Alkavervir	T46.5x1	T46.5x2	T46.5x3	T46.5x4	T46.5x5	T46.5x6
Alkonium (bromide)	T49.0x1	T49.0x2	T49.0x3	T49.0x4	T49.0x5	T49.0x6
Alkylating drug NEC	T45.1x1	T45.1x2	T45.1x3	T45.1x4	T45.1x5	T45.1x6
antimyeloproliferative	T45.1x1	T45.1x2	T45.1x3	T45.1x4	T45.1x5	T45.1x6
lymphatic	T45.1x1	T45.1x2	T45.1x3	T45.1x4	T45.1x5	T45.1x6
Alkylisocyanate	T65.0x1	T65.0x2	T65.0x3	T65.0x4	—	—
Allantoin	T49.4x1	T49.4x2	T49.4x3	T49.4x4	T49.4x5	T49.4x6
Allegron	T43.011	T43.012	T43.013	T43.014	T43.015	T43.016
Allethrin	T49.0x1	T49.0x2	T49.0x3	T49.0x4	T49.0x5	T49.0x6
Allobarbital	T42.3x1	T42.3x2	T42.3x3	T42.3x4	T42.3x5	T42.3x6
Allopurinol	T50.4x1	T50.4x2	T50.4x3	T50.4x4	T50.4x5	T50.4x6
Allyl						
Alcohol	T51.8x1	T51.8x2	T51.8x3	T51.8x4	—	—
disulfide	T46.6x1	T46.6x2	T46.6x3	T46.6x4	T46.6x5	T46.6x6
Allylestrenol	T38.5x1	T38.5x2	T38.5x3	T38.5x4	T38.5x5	T38.5x6
Allylisopropylacetylurea	T42.6x1	T42.6x2	T42.6x3	T42.6x4	T42.6x5	T42.6x6
Allylisopropylmalonylurea	T42.3x1	T42.3x2	T42.3x3	T42.3x4	T42.3x5	T42.3x6
Allylthiourea	T49.3x1	T49.3x2	T49.3x3	T49.3x4	T49.3x5	T49.3x6
Allyltribromide	T42.6x1	T42.6x2	T42.6x3	T42.6x4	T42.6x5	T42.6x6
Allypropymal	T42.3x1	T42.3x2	T42.3x3	T42.3x4	T42.3x5	T42.3x6
Almagate	T47.1x1	T47.1x2	T47.1x3	T47.1x4	T47.1x5	T47.1x6
Almasilate	T47.1x1	T47.1x2	T47.1x3	T47.1x4	T47.1x5	T47.1x6
Almitrine	T50.7x1	T50.7x2	T50.7x3	T50.7x4	T50.7x5	T50.7x6
Aloes	T47.2x1	T47.2x2	T47.2x3	T47.2x4	T47.2x5	T47.2x6
Aloglutamol	T47.1x1	T47.1x2	T47.1x3	T47.1x4	T47.1x5	T47.1x6
Aloin	T47.2x1	T47.2x2	T47.2x3	T47.2x4	T47.2x5	T47.2x6
Aloxidone	T42.2x1	T42.2x2	T42.2x3	T42.2x4	T42.2x5	T42.2x6
Alpha						
Acetyldigoxin	T46.0x1	T46.0x2	T46.0x3	T46.0x4	T46.0x5	T46.0x6
amylase	T45.3x1	T45.3x2	T45.3x3	T45.3x4	T45.3x5	T45.3x6

Substance	Poisoning, Accidental (unintentional)	Poisoning, Intentional Self-harm	Poisoning, Assault	Poisoning, Undetermined	Adverse Effect	Under-dosing
Alpha—*continued*						
tocoferol(acetate)	T45.2x1	T45.2x2	T45.2x3	T45.2x4	T45.2x5	T45.2x6
Alpha-adrenergic blocking drug	T44.6x1	T44.6x2	T44.6x3	T44.6x4	T44.6x5	T44.6x6
Alpha tocopherol	T45.2x1	T45.2x2	T45.2x3	T45.2x4	T45.2x5	T45.2x6
Alphadolone	T41.1x1	T41.1x2	T41.1x3	T41.1x4	T41.1x5	T41.1x6
Alphaprodine	T40.4x1	T40.4x2	T40.4x3	T40.4x4	T40.4x5	T40.4x6
Alphaxalone	T41.1x1	T41.1x2	T41.1x3	T41.1x4	T41.1x5	T41.1x6
Alprazolam	T42.4x1	T42.4x2	T42.4x3	T42.4x4	T42.4x5	T42.4x6
Alprenolol	T44.7x1	T44.7x2	T44.7x3	T44.7x4	T44.7x5	T44.7x6
Alprostadil	T46.7x1	T46.7x2	T46.7x3	T46.7x4	T46.7x5	T46.7x6
Alsactide	T38.811	T38.812	T38.813	T38.814	T38.815	T38.816
Alseroxylon	T46.5x1	T46.5x2	T46.5x3	T46.5x4	T46.5x5	T46.5x6
Alteplase	T45.611	T45.612	T45.613	T45.614	T45.615	T45.616
Altizide	T50.2x1	T50.2x2	T50.2x3	T50.2x4	T50.2x5	T50.2x6
Altretamine	T45.1x1	T45.1x2	T45.1x3	T45.1x4	T45.1x5	T45.1x6
Alum (medicinal)	T49.4x1	T49.4x2	T49.4x3	T49.4x4	T49.4x5	T49.4x6
nonmedicinal (ammonium) (potassium)	T56.891	T56.892	T56.893	T56.894	—	—
Aluminium, aluminum						
acetate	T49.2x1	T49.2x2	T49.2x3	T49.2x4	T49.2x5	T49.2x6
solution	T49.0x1	T49.0x2	T49.0x3	T49.0x4	T49.0x5	T49.0x6
aspirin	T39.011	T39.012	T39.013	T39.014	T39.015	T39.016
bis (acetylsalicylate)	T39.011	T39.012	T39.013	T39.014	T39.015	T39.016
carbonate (gel, basic)	T47.1x1	T47.1x2	T47.1x3	T47.1x4	T47.1x5	T47.1x6
chlorhydroxide-complex	T47.1x1	T47.1x2	T47.1x3	T47.1x4	T47.1x5	T47.1x6
chloride	T49.2x1	T49.2x2	T49.2x3	T49.2x4	T49.2x5	T49.2x6
clofibrate	T46.6x1	T46.6x2	T46.6x3	T46.6x4	T46.6x5	T46.6x6
diacetate	T49.2x1	T49.2x2	T49.2x3	T49.2x4	T49.2x5	T49.2x6
glycinate	T47.1x1	T47.1x2	T47.1x3	T47.1x4	T47.1x5	T47.1x6
hydroxide (gel)	T47.1x1	T47.1x2	T47.1x3	T47.1x4	T47.1x5	T47.1x6
hydroxide-magnesium carb. gel	T47.1x1	T47.1x2	T47.1x3	T47.1x4	T47.1x5	T47.1x6
magnesium silicate	T47.1x1	T47.1x2	T47.1x3	T47.1x4	T47.1x5	T47.1x6
nicotinate	T46.7x1	T46.7x2	T46.7x3	T46.7x4	T46.7x5	T46.7x6
ointment (surgical) (topical)	T49.3x1	T49.3x2	T49.3x3	T49.3x4	T49.3x5	T49.3x6
phosphate	T47.1x1	T47.1x2	T47.1x3	T47.1x4	T47.1x5	T47.1x6
salicylate	T39.091	T39.092	T39.093	T39.094	T39.095	T39.096
silicate	T47.1x1	T47.1x2	T47.1x3	T47.1x4	T47.1x5	T47.1x6
sodium silicate	T47.1x1	T47.1x2	T47.1x3	T47.1x4	T47.1x5	T47.1x6
subacetate	T49.2x1	T49.2x2	T49.2x3	T49.2x4	T49.2x5	T49.2x6
sulfate	T49.0x1	T49.0x2	T49.0x3	T49.0x4	T49.0x5	T49.0x6
tannate	T47.6x1	T47.6x2	T47.6x3	T47.6x4	T47.6x5	T47.6x6
topical NEC	T49.3x1	T49.3x2	T49.3x3	T49.3x4	T49.3x5	T49.3x6
Alurate	T42.3x1	T42.3x2	T42.3x3	T42.3x4	T42.3x5	T42.3x6
Alverine	T44.3x1	T44.3x2	T44.3x3	T44.3x4	T44.3x5	T44.3x6
Alvodine	T40.2x1	T40.2x2	T40.2x3	T40.2x4	T40.2x5	T40.2x6
Amanita phalloides	T62.0x1	T62.0x2	T62.0x3	T62.0x4	—	—
Amanitine	T62.0x1	T62.0x2	T62.0x3	T62.0x4	—	—
Amantadine	T42.8x1	T42.8x2	T42.8x3	T42.8x4	T42.8x5	T42.8x6
Ambazone	T49.6x1	T49.6x2	T49.6x3	T49.6x4	T49.6x5	T49.6x6
Ambenonium (chloride)	T44.0x1	T44.0x2	T44.0x3	T44.0x4	T44.0x5	T44.0x6
Ambroxol	T48.4x1	T48.4x2	T48.4x3	T48.4x4	T48.4x5	T48.4x6
Ambuphylline	T48.6x1	T48.6x2	T48.6x3	T48.6x4	T48.6x5	T48.6x6
Ambutonium bromide	T44.3x1	T44.3x2	T44.3x3	T44.3x4	T44.3x5	T44.3x6
Amcinonide	T49.0x1	T49.0x2	T49.0x3	T49.0x4	T49.0x5	T49.0x6
Amdinocilline	T36.0x1	T36.0x2	T36.0x3	T36.0x4	T36.0x5	T36.0x6
Ametazole	T50.8x1	T50.8x2	T50.8x3	T50.8x4	T50.8x5	T50.8x6
Amethocaine	T41.3x1	T41.3x2	T41.3x3	T41.3x4	T41.3x5	T41.3x6
regional	T41.3x1	T41.3x2	T41.3x3	T41.3x4	T41.3x5	T41.3x6
spinal	T41.3x1	T41.3x2	T41.3x3	T41.3x4	T41.3x5	T41.3x6
Amethopterin	T45.1x1	T45.1x2	T45.1x3	T45.1x4	T45.1x5	T45.1x6
Amezinium metilsulfate	T44.991	T44.992	T44.993	T44.994	T44.995	T44.996
Amfebutamone	T43.291	T43.292	T43.293	T43.294	T43.295	T43.296
Amfepramone	T50.5x1	T50.5x2	T50.5x3	T50.5x4	T50.5x5	T50.5x6
Amfetamine	T43.621	T43.622	T43.623	T43.624	T43.625	T43.626
Amfetaminil	T43.621	T43.622	T43.623	T43.624	T43.625	T43.626
Amfomycin	T36.8x1	T36.8x2	T36.8x3	T36.8x4	T36.8x5	T36.8x6
Amidefrine mesilate	T48.5x1	T48.5x2	T48.5x3	T48.5x4	T48.5x5	T48.5x6
Amidone	T40.3x1	T40.3x2	T40.3x3	T40.3x4	T40.3x5	T40.3x6
Amidopyrine	T39.2x1	T39.2x2	T39.2x3	T39.2x4	T39.2x5	T39.2x6
Amidotrizoate	T50.8x1	T50.8x2	T50.8x3	T50.8x4	T50.8x5	T50.8x6
Amiflamine	T43.1x1	T43.1x2	T43.1x3	T43.1x4	T43.1x5	T43.1x6

Substance	Poisoning, Accidental (unintentional)	Poisoning, Intentional Self-harm	Poisoning, Assault	Poisoning, Undetermined	Adverse Effect	Under-dosing
Amikacin	T36.5x1	T36.5x2	T36.5x3	T36.5x4	T36.5x5	T36.5x6
Amikhelline	T46.3x1	T46.3x2	T46.3x3	T46.3x4	T46.3x5	T46.3x6
Amiloride	T50.2x1	T50.2x2	T50.2x3	T50.2x4	T50.2x5	T50.2x6
Aminacrine	T49.0x1	T49.0x2	T49.0x3	T49.0x4	T49.0x5	T49.0x6
Amineptine	T43.011	T43.012	T43.013	T43.014	T43.015	T43.016
Aminitrozole	T37.3x1	T37.3x2	T37.3x3	T37.3x4	T37.3x5	T37.3x6
Aminoacetic acid (derivatives)	T50.3x1	T50.3x2	T50.3x3	T50.3x4	T50.3x5	T50.3x6
Amino acids	T50.3x1	T50.3x2	T50.3x3	T50.3x4	T50.3x5	T50.3x6
Aminoacridine	T49.0x1	T49.0x2	T49.0x3	T49.0x4	T49.0x5	T49.0x6
Aminobenzoic acid (-p)	T49.3x1	T49.3x2	T49.3x3	T49.3x4	T49.3x5	T49.3x6
Aminocaproic acid	T45.621	T45.622	T45.623	T45.624	T45.625	T45.626
Aminofenazone	T39.2x1	T39.2x2	T39.2x3	T39.2x4	T39.2x5	T39.2x6
Aminoethylisothiourium	T45.8x1	T45.8x2	T45.8x3	T45.8x4	T45.8x5	T45.8x6
Aminoglutethimide	T45.1x1	T45.1x2	T45.1x3	T45.1x4	T45.1x5	T45.1x6
Aminohippuric acid	T50.8x1	T50.8x2	T50.8x3	T50.8x4	T50.8x5	T50.8x6
Aminomethylbenzoic acid	T45.691	T45.692	T45.693	T45.694	T45.695	T45.696
Aminometradine	T50.2x1	T50.2x2	T50.2x3	T50.2x4	T50.2x5	T50.2x6
Aminopentamide	T44.3x1	T44.3x2	T44.3x3	T44.3x4	T44.3x5	T44.3x6
Aminophenazone	T39.2x1	T39.2x2	T39.2x3	T39.2x4	T39.2x5	T39.2x6
Aminophenol	T54.0x1	T54.0x2	T54.0x3	T54.0x4	—	—
Aminophenylpyridone	T43.591	T43.592	T43.593	T43.594	T43.595	T43.596
Aminophylline	T48.6x1	T48.6x2	T48.6x3	T48.6x4	T48.6x5	T48.6x6
Aminopterin sodium	T45.1x1	T45.1x2	T45.1x3	T45.1x4	T45.1x5	T45.1x6
Aminopyrine	T39.2x1	T39.2x2	T39.2x3	T39.2x4	T39.2x5	T39.2x6
Aminorex	T50.5x1	T50.5x2	T50.5x3	T50.5x4	T50.5x5	T50.5x6
Aminosalicylic acid	T37.1x1	T37.1x2	T37.1x3	T37.1x4	T37.1x5	T37.1x6
Aminosalylum	T37.1x1	T37.1x2	T37.1x3	T37.1x4	T37.1x5	T37.1x6
Amiodarone	T46.2x1	T46.2x2	T46.2x3	T46.2x4	T46.2x5	T46.2x6
Amiphenazole	T50.7x1	T50.7x2	T50.7x3	T50.7x4	T50.7x5	T50.7x6
Amiquinsin	T46.5x1	T46.5x2	T46.5x3	T46.5x4	T46.5x5	T46.5x6
Amisometradine	T50.2x1	T50.2x2	T50.2x3	T50.2x4	T50.2x5	T50.2x6
Amisulpride	T43.591	T43.592	T43.593	T43.594	T43.595	T43.596
Amitriptyline	T43.011	T43.012	T43.013	T43.014	T43.015	T43.016
Amitriptylinoxide	T43.011	T43.012	T43.013	T43.014	T43.015	T43.016
Amlexanox	T48.6x1	T48.6x2	T48.6x3	T48.6x4	T48.6x5	T48.6x6
Ammonia (fumes) (gas) (vapor)	T59.891	T59.892	T59.893	T59.894	—	—
aromatic spirit	T48.991	T48.992	T48.993	T48.994	T48.995	T48.996
liquid (household)	T54.3x1	T54.3x2	T54.3x3	T54.3x4	—	—
Ammoniated mercury	T49.0x1	T49.0x2	T49.0x3	T49.0x4	T49.0x5	T49.0x6
Ammonium						
acid tartrate	T49.5x1	T49.5x2	T49.5x3	T49.5x4	T49.5x5	T49.5x6
bromide	T42.6x1	T42.6x2	T42.6x3	T42.6x4	T42.6x5	T42.6x6
carbonate	T54.3x1	T54.3x2	T54.3x3	T54.3x4	—	—
chloride	T50.991	T50.992	T50.993	T50.994	T50.995	T50.996
expectorant	T48.4x1	T48.4x2	T48.4x3	T48.4x4	T48.4x5	T48.4x6
compounds (household) NEC	T54.3x1	T54.3x2	T54.3x3	T54.3x4	—	—
fumes (any usage)	T59.891	T59.892	T59.893	T59.894	—	—
industrial	T54.3x1	T54.3x2	T54.3x3	T54.3x4	—	—
ichthyosulronate	T49.4x1	T49.4x2	T49.4x3	T49.4x4	T49.4x5	T49.4x6
mandelate	T37.91	T37.92	T37.93	T37.94	T37.95	T37.96
sulfamate	T60.3x1	T60.3x2	T60.3x3	T60.3x4	—	—
sulfonate resin	T47.8x1	T47.8x2	T47.8x3	T47.8x4	T47.8x5	T47.8x6
Amobarbital (sodium)	T42.3x1	T42.3x2	T42.3x3	T42.3x4	T42.3x5	T42.3x6
Amodiaquine	T37.2x1	T37.2x2	T37.2x3	T37.2x4	T37.2x5	T37.2x6
Amopyroquin(e)	T37.2x1	T37.2x2	T37.2x3	T37.2x4	T37.2x5	T37.2x6
Amoxapine	T43.011	T43.012	T43.013	T43.014	T43.015	T43.016
Amoxicillin	T36.0x1	T36.0x2	T36.0x3	T36.0x4	T36.0x5	T36.0x6
Amperozide	T43.591	T43.592	T43.593	T43.594	T43.595	T43.596
Amphenidone	T43.591	T43.592	T43.593	T43.594	T43.595	T43.596
Amphetamine NEC	T43.621	T43.622	T43.623	T43.624	T43.625	T43.626
Amphomycin	T36.8x1	T36.8x2	T36.8x3	T36.8x4	T36.8x5	T36.8x6
Amphotalide	T37.4x1	T37.4x2	T37.4x3	T37.4x4	T37.4x5	T37.4x6
Amphotericin B	T36.7x1	T36.7x2	T36.7x3	T36.7x4	T36.7x5	T36.7x6
topical	T49.0x1	T49.0x2	T49.0x3	T49.0x4	T49.0x5	T49.0x6
Ampicillin	T36.0x1	T36.0x2	T36.0x3	T36.0x4	T36.0x5	T36.0x6
Amprotropine	T44.3x1	T44.3x2	T44.3x3	T44.3x4	T44.3x5	T44.3x6
Amsacrine	T45.1x1	T45.1x2	T45.1x3	T45.1x4	T45.1x5	T45.1x6
Amygdaline	T62.2x1	T62.2x2	T62.2x3	T62.2x4	—	—
Amyl						
acetate	T52.8x1	T52.8x2	T52.8x3	T52.8x4	—	—
vapor	T59.891	T59.892	T59.893	T59.894	—	—

Substance	Poisoning, Accidental (unintentional)	Poisoning, Intentional Self-harm	Poisoning, Assault	Poisoning, Undetermined	Adverse Effect	Under-dosing
Amyl—continued						
alcohol	T51.3x1	T51.3x2	T51.3x3	T51.3x4	—	—
chloride	T53.6x1	T53.6x2	T53.6x3	T53.6x4	—	—
formate	T52.8x1	T52.8x2	T52.8x3	T52.8x4	—	—
nitrite	T46.3x1	T46.3x2	T46.3x3	T46.3x4	T46.3x5	T46.3x6
propionate	T65.891	T65.892	T65.893	T65.894	—	—
Amylase	T47.5x1	T47.5x2	T47.5x3	T47.5x4	T47.5x5	T47.5x6
Amyleine, regional	T41.3x1	T41.3x2	T41.3x3	T41.3x4	T41.3x5	T41.3x6
Amylene						
dichloride	T53.6x1	T53.6x2	T53.6x3	T53.6x4	—	—
hydrate	T51.3x1	T51.3x2	T51.3x3	T51.3x4	—	—
Amylmetacresol	T49.6x1	T49.6x2	T49.6x3	T49.6x4	T49.6x5	T49.6x6
Amylobarbitone	T42.3x1	T42.3x2	T42.3x3	T42.3x4	T42.3x5	T42.3x6
Amylocaine, regional	T41.3x1	T41.3x2	T41.3x3	T41.3x4	T41.3x5	T41.3x6
infiltration (subcutaneous)	T41.3x1	T41.3x2	T41.3x3	T41.3x4	T41.3x5	T41.3x6
nerve block (peripheral) (plexus)	T41.3x1	T41.3x2	T41.3x3	T41.3x4	T41.3x5	T41.3x6
spinal	T41.3x1	T41.3x2	T41.3x3	T41.3x4	T41.3x5	T41.3x6
topical (surface)	T41.3x1	T41.3x2	T41.3x3	T41.3x4	T41.3x5	T41.3x6
Amylopectin	T47.6x1	T47.6x2	T47.6x3	T47.6x4	T47.6x5	T47.6x6
Amytal (sodium)	T42.3x1	T42.3x2	T42.3x3	T42.3x4	T42.3x5	T42.3x6
Anabolic steroid	T38.7x1	T38.7x2	T38.7x3	T38.7x4	T38.7x5	T38.7x6
Analeptic NEC	T50.7x1	T50.7x2	T50.7x3	T50.7x4	T50.7x5	T50.7x6
Analgesic NEC	T39.8x1	T39.8x2	T39.8x3	T39.8x4	T39.8x5	T39.8x6
anti-inflammatory NEC	T39.91	T39.92	T39.93	T39.94	T39.95	T39.96
propionic acid derivative	T39.311	T39.312	T39.313	T39.314	T39.315	T39.316
antirheumatic NEC	T39.91	T39.92	T39.93	T39.94	T39.95	T39.96
aromatic NEC	T39.1x1	T39.1x2	T39.1x3	T39.1x4	T39.1x5	T39.1x6
narcotic NEC	T40.601	T40.602	T40.603	T40.604	T40.605	T40.606
combination	T40.601	T40.602	T40.603	T40.604	T40.605	T40.606
obstetric	T40.601	T40.602	T40.603	T40.604	T40.605	T40.606
non-narcotic NEC	T39.91	T39.92	T39.93	T39.94	T39.95	T39.96
combination	T39.91	T39.92	T39.93	T39.94	T39.95	T39.96
pyrazole	T39.2x1	T39.2x2	T39.2x3	T39.2x4	T39.2x5	T39.2x6
specified NEC	T39.8x1	T39.8x2	T39.8x3	T39.8x4	T39.8x5	T39.8x6
Analgin	T39.2x1	T39.2x2	T39.2x3	T39.2x4	T39.2x5	T39.2x6
Anamirta cocculus	T62.1x1	T62.1x2	T62.1x3	T62.1x4	—	—
Ancillin	T36.0x1	T36.0x2	T36.0x3	T36.0x4	T36.0x5	T36.0x6
Ancrod	T45.691	T45.692	T45.693	T45.694	T45.695	T45.696
Androgen	T38.7x1	T38.7x2	T38.7x3	T38.7x4	T38.7x5	T38.7x6
Androgen-estrogen mixture	T38.7x1	T38.7x2	T38.7x3	T38.7x4	T38.7x5	T38.7x6
Androstalone	T38.7x1	T38.7x2	T38.7x3	T38.7x4	T38.7x5	T38.7x6
Androstanolone	T38.7x1	T38.7x2	T38.7x3	T38.7x4	T38.7x5	T38.7x6
Androsterone	T38.7x1	T38.7x2	T38.7x3	T38.7x4	T38.7x5	T38.7x6
Anemone pulsatilla	T62.2x1	T62.2x2	T62.2x3	T62.2x4	—	—
Anesthesia						
caudal	T41.3x1	T41.3x2	T41.3x3	T41.3x4	T41.3x5	T41.3x6
endotracheal	T41.0x1	T41.0x2	T41.0x3	T41.0x4	T41.0x5	T41.0x6
epidural	T41.3x1	T41.3x2	T41.3x3	T41.3x4	T41.3x5	T41.3x6
inhalation	T41.0x1	T41.0x2	T41.0x3	T41.0x4	T41.0x5	T41.0x6
local	T41.3x1	T41.3x2	T41.3x3	T41.3x4	T41.3x5	T41.3x6
mucosal	T41.3x1	T41.3x2	T41.3x3	T41.3x4	T41.3x5	T41.3x6
muscle relaxation	T48.1x1	T48.1x2	T48.1x3	T48.1x4	T48.1x5	T48.1x6
nerve blocking	T41.3x1	T41.3x2	T41.3x3	T41.3x4	T41.3x5	T41.3x6
plexus blocking	T41.3x1	T41.3x2	T41.3x3	T41.3x4	T41.3x5	T41.3x6
potentiated	T41.201	T41.202	T41.203	T41.204	T41.205	T41.206
rectal	T41.201	T41.202	T41.203	T41.204	T41.205	T41.206
general	T41.201	T41.202	T41.203	T41.204	T41.205	T41.206
local	T41.3x1	T41.3x2	T41.3x3	T41.3x4	T41.3x5	T41.3x6
regional	T41.3x1	T41.3x2	T41.3x3	T41.3x4	T41.3x5	T41.3x6
surface	T41.3x1	T41.3x2	T41.3x3	T41.3x4	T41.3x5	T41.3x6
Anesthetic NEC (see also Anesthesia)	T41.41	T41.42	T41.43	T41.44	T41.45	T41.46
with muscle relaxant	T41.201	T41.202	T41.203	T41.204	T41.205	T41.206
general	T41.201	T41.202	T41.203	T41.204	T41.205	T41.206
local	T41.3x1	T41.3x2	T41.3x3	T41.3x4	T41.3x5	T41.3x6
gaseous NEC	T41.0x1	T41.0x2	T41.0x3	T41.0x4	T41.0x5	T41.0x6
general NEC	T41.201	T41.202	T41.203	T41.204	T41.205	T41.206
halogenated hydrocarbon derivatives NEC	T41.0x1	T41.0x2	T41.0x3	T41.0x4	T41.0x5	T41.0x6
infiltration NEC	T41.3x1	T41.3x2	T41.3x3	T41.3x4	T41.3x5	T41.3x6
intravenous NEC	T41.1x1	T41.1x2	T41.1x3	T41.1x4	T41.1x5	T41.1x6

Substance	Poisoning, Accidental (unintentional)	Poisoning, Intentional Self-harm	Poisoning, Assault	Poisoning, Undetermined	Adverse Effect	Under-dosing
Anesthetic NEC —continued						
local NEC	T41.3x1	T41.3x2	T41.3x3	T41.3x4	T41.3x5	T41.3x6
rectal	T41.201	T41.202	T41.203	T41.204	T41.205	T41.206
general	T41.201	T41.202	T41.203	T41.204	T41.205	T41.206
local	T41.3x1	T41.3x2	T41.3x3	T41.3x4	T41.3x5	T41.3x6
regional NEC	T41.3x1	T41.3x2	T41.3x3	T41.3x4	T41.3x5	T41.3x6
spinal NEC	T41.3x1	T41.3x2	T41.3x3	T41.3x4	T41.3x5	T41.3x6
thiobarbiturate	T41.1x1	T41.1x2	T41.1x3	T41.1x4	T41.1x5	T41.1x6
topical	T41.3x1	T41.3x2	T41.3x3	T41.3x4	T41.3x5	T41.3x6
Aneurine	T45.2x1	T45.2x2	T45.2x3	T45.2x4	T45.2x5	T45.2x6
Angio-Conray	T50.8x1	T50.8x2	T50.8x3	T50.8x4	T50.8x5	T50.8x6
Angiotensin	T44.5x1	T44.5x2	T44.5x3	T44.5x4	T44.5x5	T44.5x6
Angiotensinamide	T44.991	T44.992	T44.993	T44.994	T44.995	T44.996
Anhydrohydroxy progesterone	T38.5x1	T38.5x2	T38.5x3	T38.5x4	T38.5x5	T38.5x6
Anhydron	T50.2x1	T50.2x2	T50.2x3	T50.2x4	T50.2x5	T50.2x6
Anileridine	T40.4x1	T40.4x2	T40.4x3	T40.4x4	T40.4x5	T40.4x6
Aniline (dye) (liquid)	T65.3x1	T65.3x2	T65.3x3	T65.3x4	—	—
analgesic	T39.1x1	T39.1x2	T39.1x3	T39.1x4	T39.1x5	T39.1x6
derivatives, therapeutic NEC	T39.1x1	T39.1x2	T39.1x3	T39.1x4	T39.1x5	T39.1x6
vapor	T65.3x1	T65.3x2	T65.3x3	T65.3x4	—	—
Anise oil	T47.5x1	T47.5x2	T47.5x3	T47.5x4	T47.5x5	T47.5x6
Aniscorpine	T44.3x1	T44.3x2	T44.3x3	T44.3x4	T44.3x5	T44.3x6
Anisidine	T65.3x1	T65.3x2	T65.3x3	T65.3x4	—	—
Anisindione	T45.511	T45.512	T45.513	T45.514	T45.515	T45.516
Anisotropine methyl-bromide	T44.3x1	T44.3x2	T44.3x3	T44.3x4	T44.3x5	T44.3x6
Anistreplase	T45.611	T45.612	T45.613	T45.614	T45.615	T45.616
Anorexiant (central)	T50.5x1	T50.5x2	T50.5x3	T50.5x4	T50.5x5	T50.5x6
Anorexic agents	T50.5x1	T50.5x2	T50.5x3	T50.5x4	T50.5x5	T50.5x6
Ansamycin	T36.6x1	T36.6x2	T36.6x3	T36.6x4	T36.6x5	T36.6x6
Ant (bite) (sting)	T63.421	T63.422	T63.423	T63.424	—	—
Antabuse	T50.6x1	T50.6x2	T50.6x3	T50.6x4	T50.6x5	T50.6x6
Ant poison—see Insecticide						
Antacid NEC	T47.1x1	T47.1x2	T47.1x3	T47.1x4	T47.1x5	T47.1x6
Antagonist						
Aldosterone	T50.0x1	T50.0x2	T50.0x3	T50.0x4	T50.0x5	T50.0x6
anticoagulant	T45.7x1	T45.7x2	T45.7x3	T45.7x4	T45.7x5	T45.7x6
extrapyramidal NEC	T44.3x1	T44.3x2	T44.3x3	T44.3x4	T44.3x5	T44.3x6
folic acid	T45.1x1	T45.1x2	T45.1x3	T45.1x4	T45.1x5	T45.1x6
heavy metal	T45.8x1	T45.8x2	T45.8x3	T45.8x4	T45.8x5	T45.8x6
H2 receptor	T47.1x1	T47.1x2	T47.1x3	T47.1x4	T47.1x5	T47.1x6
narcotic analgesic	T50.7x1	T50.7x2	T50.7x3	T50.7x4	T50.7x5	T50.7x6
opiate	T50.7x1	T50.7x2	T50.7x3	T50.7x4	T50.7x5	T50.7x6
pyrimidine	T45.1x1	T45.1x2	T45.1x3	T45.1x4	T45.1x5	T45.1x6
serotonin	T46.5x1	T46.5x2	T46.5x3	T46.5x4	T46.5x5	T46.5x6
Antazolin(e)	T45.0x1	T45.0x2	T45.0x3	T45.0x4	T45.0x5	T45.0x6
Anterior pituitary hormone NEC	T38.811	T38.812	T38.813	T38.814	T38.815	T38.816
Anthelmintic NEC	T37.4x1	T37.4x2	T37.4x3	T37.4x4	T37.4x5	T37.4x6
Anthiolimine	T37.4x1	T37.4x2	T37.4x3	T37.4x4	T37.4x5	T37.4x6
Anthralin	T49.4x1	T49.4x2	T49.4x3	T49.4x4	T49.4x5	T49.4x6
Anthramycin	T45.1x1	T45.1x2	T45.1x3	T45.1x4	T45.1x5	T45.1x6
Antiadrenergic NEC	T44.8x1	T44.8x2	T44.8x3	T44.8x4	T44.8x5	T44.8x6
Antiallergic NEC	T45.0x1	T45.0x2	T45.0x3	T45.0x4	T45.0x5	T45.0x6
Anti-anemic (drug) (preparation)	T45.8x1	T45.8x2	T45.8x3	T45.8x4	T45.8x5	T45.8x6
Antianxiety drug NEC	T43.501	T43.502	T43.503	T43.504	T43.505	T43.506
Antiaris toxicaria	T65.891	T65.892	T65.893	T65.894	—	—
Antiarteriosclerotic drug	T46.6x1	T46.6x2	T46.6x3	T46.6x4	T46.6x5	T46.6x6
Antiasthmatic drug NEC	T48.6x1	T48.6x2	T48.6x3	T48.6x4	T48.6x5	T48.6x6
Antibiotic NEC	T36.91	T36.92	T36.93	T36.94	T36.95	T36.96
aminoglycoside	T36.5x1	T36.5x2	T36.5x3	T36.5x4	T36.5x5	T36.5x6
anticancer	T45.1x1	T45.1x2	T45.1x3	T45.1x4	T45.1x5	T45.1x6
antifungal	T36.7x1	T36.7x2	T36.7x3	T36.7x4	T36.7x5	T36.7x6
antimycobacterial	T36.5x1	T36.5x2	T36.5x3	T36.5x4	T36.5x5	T36.5x6
antineoplastic	T45.1x1	T45.1x2	T45.1x3	T45.1x4	T45.1x5	T45.1x6
cephalosporin (group)	T36.1x1	T36.1x2	T36.1x3	T36.1x4	T36.1x5	T36.1x6
chloramphenicol (group)	T36.2x1	T36.2x2	T36.2x3	T36.2x4	T36.2x5	T36.2x6
ENT	T49.6x1	T49.6x2	T49.6x3	T49.6x4	T49.6x5	T49.6x6
eye	T49.5x1	T49.5x2	T49.5x3	T49.5x4	T49.5x5	T49.5x6
fungicidal (local)	T49.0x1	T49.0x2	T49.0x3	T49.0x4	T49.0x5	T49.0x6
intestinal	T36.8x1	T36.8x2	T36.8x3	T36.8x4	T36.8x5	T36.8x6
b-lactam NEC	T36.1x1	T36.1x2	T36.1x3	T36.1x4	T36.1x5	T36.1x6
local	T49.0x1	T49.0x2	T49.0x3	T49.0x4	T49.0x5	T49.0x6

Substance	Poisoning, Accidental (unintentional)	Poisoning, Intentional Self-harm	Poisoning, Assault	Poisoning, Undetermined	Adverse Effect	Under-dosing
Antibiotic NEC—*continued*						
macrolides	T36.3x1	T36.3x2	T36.3x3	T36.3x4	T36.3x5	T36.3x6
polypeptide	T36.8x1	T36.8x2	T36.8x3	T36.8x4	T36.8x5	T36.8x6
specified NEC	T36.8x1	T36.8x2	T36.8x3	T36.8x4	T36.8x5	T36.8x6
tetracycline (group)	T36.4x1	T36.4x2	T36.4x3	T36.4x4	T36.4x5	T36.4x6
throat	T49.6x1	T49.6x2	T49.6x3	T49.6x4	T49.6x5	T49.6x6
Anticancer agents NEC	T45.1x1	T45.1x2	T45.1x3	T45.1x4	T45.1x5	T45.1x6
Anticholesterolemic drug NEC	T46.6x1	T46.6x2	T46.6x3	T46.6x4	T46.6x5	T46.6x6
Anticholinergic NEC	T44.3x1	T44.3x2	T44.3x3	T44.3x4	T44.3x5	T44.3x6
Anticholinesterase	T44.0x1	T44.0x2	T44.0x3	T44.0x4	T44.0x5	T44.0x6
organophosphorus	T44.0x1	T44.0x2	T44.0x3	T44.0x4	T44.0x5	T44.0x6
insecticide	T60.0x1	T60.0x2	T60.0x3	T60.0x4	—	—
nerve gas	T59.891	T59.892	T59.893	T59.894	—	—
reversible	T44.0x1	T44.0x2	T44.0x3	T44.0x4	T44.0x5	T44.0x6
ophthalmological	T49.5x1	T49.5x2	T49.5x3	T49.5x4	T49.5x5	T49.5x6
Anticoagulant NEC	T45.511	T45.512	T45.513	T45.514	T45.515	T45.516
antagonist	T45.7x1	T45.7x2	T45.7x3	T45.7x4	T45.7x5	T45.7x6
Anti-common-cold drug NEC	T48.5x1	T48.5x2	T48.5x3	T48.5x4	T48.5x5	T48.5x6
Anticonvulsant NEC	T42.6x1	T42.6x2	T42.6x3	T42.6x4	T42.6x5	T42.6x6
barbiturate	T42.3x1	T42.3x2	T42.3x3	T42.3x4	T42.3x5	T42.3x6
combination (with barbiturate)	T42.3x1	T42.3x2	T42.3x3	T42.3x4	T42.3x5	T42.3x6
hydantoin	T42.0x1	T42.0x2	T42.0x3	T42.0x4	T42.0x5	T42.0x6
hypnotic NEC	T42.6x1	T42.6x2	T42.6x3	T42.6x4	T42.6x5	T42.6x6
oxazolidinedione	T42.2x1	T42.2x2	T42.2x3	T42.2x4	T42.2x5	T42.2x6
pyrimidinedione	T42.6x1	T42.6x2	T42.6x3	T42.6x4	T42.6x5	T42.6x6
succinimide	T42.2x1	T42.2x2	T42.2x3	T42.2x4	T42.2x5	T42.2x6
Anti-D immunoglobulin (human)	T50.Z11	T50.Z12	T50.Z13	T50.Z14	T50.Z15	T50.Z16
Antidepressant	T43.201	T43.202	T43.203	T43.204	T43.205	T43.206
selective serotonin norepinephrine reuptake inhibitor	T43.211	T43.212	T43.213	T43.214	T43.215	T43.216
selective serotonin reuptake inhibitor	T43.221	T43.222	T43.223	T43.224	T43.225	T43.226
specified NEC	T43.291	T43.292	T43.293	T43.294	T43.295	T43.296
triazolopyridine	T43.211	T43.212	T43.213	T43.214	T43.215	T43.216
tetracyclic	T43.021	T43.022	T43.023	T43.024	T43.025	T43.026
tricyclic	T43.011	T43.012	T43.013	T43.014	T43.015	T43.016
Antidiabetic NEC	T38.3x1	T38.3x2	T38.3x3	T38.3x4	T38.3x5	T38.3x6
biguanide	T38.3x1	T38.3x2	T38.3x3	T38.3x4	T38.3x5	T38.3x6
and sulfonyl combined	T38.3x1	T38.3x2	T38.3x3	T38.3x4	T38.3x5	T38.3x6
combined	T38.3x1	T38.3x2	T38.3x3	T38.3x4	T38.3x5	T38.3x6
sulfonylurea	T38.3x1	T38.3x2	T38.3x3	T38.3x4	T38.3x5	T38.3x6
Antidiarrheal drug NEC	T47.6x1	T47.6x2	T47.6x3	T47.6x4	T47.6x5	T47.6x6
absorbent	T47.6x1	T47.6x2	T47.6x3	T47.6x4	T47.6x5	T47.6x6
Antidiphtheria serum	T50.Z11	T50.Z12	T50.Z13	T50.Z14	T50.Z15	T50.Z16
Antidiuretic hormone	T38.891	T38.892	T38.893	T38.894	T38.895	T38.896
Antidote NEC	T50.6x1	T50.6x2	T50.6x3	T50.6x4	T50.6x5	T50.6x6
heavy metal	T45.8x1	T45.8x2	T45.8x3	T45.8x4	T45.8x5	T45.8x6
Antiemetic drug	T45.0x1	T45.0x2	T45.0x3	T45.0x4	T45.0x5	T45.0x6
Antiepilepsy agent	T42.71	T42.72	T42.73	T42.74	T42.75	T42.76
combination	T42.5x1	T42.5x2	T42.5x3	T42.5x4	T42.5x5	T42.5x6
mixed	T42.5x1	T42.5x2	T42.5x3	T42.5x4	T42.5x5	T42.5x6
specified, NEC	T42.6x1	T42.6x2	T42.6x3	T42.6x4	T42.6x5	T42.6x6
Antifertility pill	T38.4x1	T38.4x2	T38.4x3	T38.4x4	T38.4x5	T38.4x6
Antifibrinolytic drug	T45.621	T45.622	T45.623	T45.624	T45.625	T45.626
Antifilarial drug	T37.4x1	T37.4x2	T37.4x3	T37.4x4	T37.4x5	T37.4x6
Antiflatulent	T47.5x1	T47.5x2	T47.5x3	T47.5x4	T47.5x5	T47.5x6
Antifreeze	T65.91	T65.92	T65.93	T65.94	—	—
alcohol	T51.1x1	T51.1x2	T51.1x3	T51.1x4	—	—
ethylene glycol	T51.8x1	T51.8x2	T51.8x3	T51.8x4	—	—
Antifungal						
antibiotic (systemic)	T36.7x1	T36.7x2	T36.7x3	T36.7x4	T36.7x5	T36.7x6
anti-infective NEC	T37.91	T37.92	T37.93	T37.94	T37.95	T37.96
disinfectant, local	T49.0x1	T49.0x2	T49.0x3	T49.0x4	T49.0x5	T49.0x6
nonmedicinal (spray)	T60.3x1	T60.3x2	T60.3x3	T60.3x4	—	—
topical	T49.0x1	T49.0x2	T49.0x3	T49.0x4	T49.0x5	T49.0x6
Anti-gastric-secretion drug NEC	T47.1x1	T47.1x2	T47.1x3	T47.1x4	T47.1x5	T47.1x6
Antihallucinogen	T43.501	T43.502	T43.503	T43.504	T43.505	T43.506
Antihelmintics	T37.4x1	T37.4x2	T37.4x3	T37.4x4	T37.4x5	T37.4x6
Antihemophilic						
factor	T45.8x1	T45.8x2	T45.8x3	T45.8x4	T45.8x5	T45.8x6

Substance	Poisoning, Accidental (unintentional)	Poisoning, Intentional Self-harm	Poisoning, Assault	Poisoning, Undetermined	Adverse Effect	Under-dosing
Antihemophilic—*continued*						
fraction	T45.8x1	T45.8x2	T45.8x3	T45.8x4	T45.8x5	T45.8x6
globulin concentrate	T45.7x1	T45.7x2	T45.7x3	T45.7x4	T45.7x5	T45.7x6
human plasma	T45.8x1	T45.8x2	T45.8x3	T45.8x4	T45.8x5	T45.8x6
plasma, dried	T45.7x1	T45.7x2	T45.7x3	T45.7x4	T45.7x5	T45.7x6
Antihemorrhoidal preparation	T49.2x1	T49.2x2	T49.2x3	T49.2x4	T49.2x5	T49.2x6
Antiheparin drug	T45.7x1	T45.7x2	T45.7x3	T45.7x4	T45.7x5	T45.7x6
Antihistamine	T45.0x1	T45.0x2	T45.0x3	T45.0x4	T45.0x5	T45.0x6
Antihookworm drug	T37.4x1	T37.4x2	T37.4x3	T37.4x4	T37.4x5	T37.4x6
Anti-human lymphocytic globulin	T50.Z11	T50.Z12	T50.Z13	T50.Z14	T50.Z15	T50.Z16
Antihypertensive drug NEC	T46.5x1	T46.5x2	T46.5x3	T46.5x4	T46.5x5	T46.5x6
Anti-infective NEC	T37.91	T37.92	T37.93	T37.94	T37.95	T37.96
antibiotics	T36.91	T36.92	T36.93	T36.94	T36.95	T36.96
specified NEC	T36.8x1	T36.8x2	T36.8x3	T36.8x4	T36.8x5	T36.8x6
anthelmintic	T37.4x1	T37.4x2	T37.4x3	T37.4x4	T37.4x5	T37.4x6
antimalarial	T37.2x1	T37.2x2	T37.2x3	T37.2x4	T37.2x5	T37.2x6
antimycobacterial NEC	T37.1x1	T37.1x2	T37.1x3	T37.1x4	T37.1x5	T37.1x6
antibiotics	T36.5x1	T36.5x2	T36.5x3	T36.5x4	T36.5x5	T36.5x6
antiprotozoal NEC	T37.3x1	T37.3x2	T37.3x3	T37.3x4	T37.3x5	T37.3x6
blood	T37.2x1	T37.2x2	T37.2x3	T37.2x4	T37.2x5	T37.2x6
antiviral	T37.5x1	T37.5x2	T37.5x3	T37.5x4	T37.5x5	T37.5x6
arsenical	T37.8x1	T37.8x2	T37.8x3	T37.8x4	T37.8x5	T37.8x6
bismuth, local	T49.0x1	T49.0x2	T49.0x3	T49.0x4	T49.0x5	T49.0x6
ENT	T49.6x1	T49.6x2	T49.6x3	T49.6x4	T49.6x5	T49.6x6
eye NEC	T49.5x1	T49.5x2	T49.5x3	T49.5x4	T49.5x5	T49.5x6
heavy metals NEC	T37.8x1	T37.8x2	T37.8x3	T37.8x4	T37.8x5	T37.8x6
local NEC	T49.0x1	T49.0x2	T49.0x3	T49.0x4	T49.0x5	T49.0x6
specified NEC	T49.0x1	T49.0x2	T49.0x3	T49.0x4	T49.0x5	T49.0x6
mixed	T37.91	T37.92	T37.93	T37.94	T37.95	T37.96
ophthalmic preparation	T49.5x1	T49.5x2	T49.5x3	T49.5x4	T49.5x5	T49.5x6
topical NEC	T49.0x1	T49.0x2	T49.0x3	T49.0x4	T49.0x5	T49.0x6
Anti-inflammatory drug, local, NEC	T49.0x1	T49.0x2	T49.0x3	T49.0x4	T49.0x5	T49.0x6
Antikaluretic	T50.3x1	T50.3x2	T50.3x3	T50.3x4	T50.3x5	T50.3x6
Antiknock (tetraethyl lead)	T56.0x1	T56.0x2	T56.0x3	T56.0x4	—	—
Antilipemic drug NEC	T46.6x1	T46.6x2	T46.6x3	T46.6x4	T46.6x5	T46.6x6
Antimalarial	T37.2x1	T37.2x2	T37.2x3	T37.2x4	T37.2x5	T37.2x6
prophylactic NEC	T37.2x1	T37.2x2	T37.2x3	T37.2x4	T37.2x5	T37.2x6
pyrimidine derivative	T37.2x1	T37.2x2	T37.2x3	T37.2x4	T37.2x5	T37.2x6
Antimetabolite	T45.1x1	T45.1x2	T45.1x3	T45.1x4	T45.1x5	T45.1x6
Antimitotic agent	T45.1x1	T45.1x2	T45.1x3	T45.1x4	T45.1x5	T45.1x6
Antimony (compounds) (vapor) NEC	T56.891	T56.892	T56.893	T56.894	—	—
anti-infectives	T37.8x1	T37.8x2	T37.8x3	T37.8x4	T37.8x5	T37.8x6
dimercaptosuccinate	T37.3x1	T37.3x2	T37.3x3	T37.3x4	T37.3x5	T37.3x6
hydride	T56.891	T56.892	T56.893	T56.894	—	—
pesticide (vapor)	T60.8x1	T60.8x2	T60.8x3	T60.8x4	—	—
potassium (sodium) Tartrate	T37.8x1	T37.8x2	T37.8x3	T37.8x4	T37.8x5	T37.8x6
tartrated	T37.8x1	T37.8x2	T37.8x3	T37.8x4	T37.8x5	T37.8x6
sodium dimercaptosuccinate	T37.3x1	T37.3x2	T37.3x3	T37.3x4	T37.3x5	T37.3x6
Antimuscarinic NEC	T44.3x1	T44.3x2	T44.3x3	T44.3x4	T44.3x5	T44.3x6
Antimycobacterial drug NEC	T37.1x1	T37.1x2	T37.1x3	T37.1x4	T37.1x5	T37.1x6
antibiotics	T36.5x1	T36.5x2	T36.5x3	T36.5x4	T36.5x5	T36.5x6
combination	T37.1x1	T37.1x2	T37.1x3	T37.1x4	T37.1x5	T37.1x6
Antinausea drug	T45.0x1	T45.0x2	T45.0x3	T45.0x4	T45.0x5	T45.0x6
Antinematode drug	T37.4x1	T37.4x2	T37.4x3	T37.4x4	T37.4x5	T37.4x6
Antineoplastic NEC	T45.1x1	T45.1x2	T45.1x3	T45.1x4	T45.1x5	T45.1x6
antibiotics	T45.1x1	T45.1x2	T45.1x3	T45.1x4	T45.1x5	T45.1x6
alkaloidal	T45.1x1	T45.1x2	T45.1x3	T45.1x4	T45.1x5	T45.1x6
combination	T45.1x1	T45.1x2	T45.1x3	T45.1x4	T45.1x5	T45.1x6
estrogen	T38.5x1	T38.5x2	T38.5x3	T38.5x4	T38.5x5	T38.5x6
steroid	T38.7x1	T38.7x2	T38.7x3	T38.7x4	T38.7x5	T38.7x6
Antiparasitic drug, local	T49.0x1	T49.0x2	T49.0x3	T49.0x4	T49.0x5	T49.0x6
Antiparkinsonism drug NEC	T42.8x1	T42.8x2	T42.8x3	T42.8x4	T42.8x5	T42.8x6
Antiperspirant NEC	T49.2x1	T49.2x2	T49.2x3	T49.2x4	T49.2x5	T49.2x6
Antiphlogistic NEC	T39.4x1	T39.4x2	T39.4x3	T39.4x4	T39.4x5	T39.4x6
Antiplatyhelmintic drug	T37.4x1	T37.4x2	T37.4x3	T37.4x4	T37.4x5	T37.4x6
Antiprotozoal drug NEC	T37.3x1	T37.3x2	T37.3x3	T37.3x4	T37.3x5	T37.3x6
blood	T37.2x1	T37.2x2	T37.2x3	T37.2x4	T37.2x5	T37.2x6
local	T49.0x1	T49.0x2	T49.0x3	T49.0x4	T49.0x5	T49.0x6

Substance	Poisoning, Accidental (unintentional)	Poisoning, Intentional Self-harm	Poisoning, Assault	Poisoning, Undetermined	Adverse Effect	Under-dosing
Antipruritic drug NEC	T49.1x1	T49.1x2	T49.1x3	T49.1x4	T49.1x5	T49.1x6
Antipsychotic drug	T43.501	T43.502	T43.503	T43.504	T43.505	T43.506
specified NEC	T43.591	T43.592	T43.593	T43.594	T43.595	T43.596
Antipyretic NEC	T39.8x1	T39.8x2	T39.8x3	T39.8x4	T39.8x5	T39.8x6
Antipyrine	T39.2x1	T39.2x2	T39.2x3	T39.2x4	T39.2x5	T39.2x6
Antirabies hyperimmune serum	T50.Z11	T50.Z12	T50.Z13	T50.Z14	T50.Z15	T50.Z16
Antirheumatic NEC	T39.4x1	T39.4x2	T39.4x3	T39.4x4	T39.4x5	T39.4x6
Antirigidity drug NEC	T42.8x1	T42.8x2	T42.8x3	T42.8x4	T42.8x5	T42.8x6
Antischistosomal drug	T37.4x1	T37.4x2	T37.4x3	T37.4x4	T37.4x5	T37.4x6
Antiscorpion sera	T50.Z11	T50.Z12	T50.Z13	T50.Z14	T50.Z15	T50.Z16
Antiseborrheics	T49.4x1	T49.4x2	T49.4x3	T49.4x4	T49.4x5	T49.4x6
Antiseptics (external) (medicinal)	T49.0x1	T49.0x2	T49.0x3	T49.0x4	T49.0x5	T49.0x6
Antistine	T45.0x1	T45.0x2	T45.0x3	T45.0x4	T45.0x5	T45.0x6
Antitapeworm drug	T37.4x1	T37.4x2	T37.4x3	T37.4x4	T37.4x5	T37.4x6
Antitetanus immunoglobulin	T50.Z11	T50.Z12	T50.Z13	T50.Z14	T50.Z15	T50.Z16
Antithyroid drug NEC	T38.2x1	T38.2x2	T38.2x3	T38.2x4	T38.2x5	T38.2x6
Antitoxin	T50.Z11	T50.Z12	T50.Z13	T50.Z14	T50.Z15	T50.Z16
diphtheria	T50.Z11	T50.Z12	T50.Z13	T50.Z14	T50.Z15	T50.Z16
gas gangrene	T50.Z11	T50.Z12	T50.Z13	T50.Z14	T50.Z15	T50.Z16
tetanus	T50.Z11	T50.Z12	T50.Z13	T50.Z14	T50.Z15	T50.Z16
Antitrichomonal drug	T37.3x1	T37.3x2	T37.3x3	T37.3x4	T37.3x5	T37.3x6
Antituberculars	T37.1x1	T37.1x2	T37.1x3	T37.1x4	T37.1x5	T37.1x6
antibiotics	T36.5x1	T36.5x2	T36.5x3	T36.5x4	T36.5x5	T36.5x6
Antitussive NEC	T48.3x1	T48.3x2	T48.3x3	T48.3x4	T48.3x5	T48.3x6
codeine mixture	T40.2x1	T40.2x2	T40.2x3	T40.2x4	T40.2x5	T40.2x6
opiate	T40.2x1	T40.2x2	T40.2x3	T40.2x4	T40.2x5	T40.2x6
Antivaricose drug	T46.8x1	T46.8x2	T46.8x3	T46.8x4	T46.8x5	T46.8x6
Antivenin, antivenom (sera)	T50.Z11	T50.Z12	T50.Z13	T50.Z14	T50.Z15	T50.Z16
crotaline	T50.Z11	T50.Z12	T50.Z13	T50.Z14	T50.Z15	T50.Z16
spider bite	T50.Z11	T50.Z12	T50.Z13	T50.Z14	T50.Z15	T50.Z16
Antivertigo drug	T45.0x1	T45.0x2	T45.0x3	T45.0x4	T45.0x5	T45.0x6
Antiviral drug NEC	T37.5x1	T37.5x2	T37.5x3	T37.5x4	T37.5x5	T37.5x6
eye	T49.5x1	T49.5x2	T49.5x3	T49.5x4	T49.5x5	T49.5x6
Antiwhipworm drug	T37.4x1	T37.4x2	T37.4x3	T37.4x4	T37.4x5	T37.4x6
Ant poisons—*see* Pesticides						
Antrol (*see also* by specific chemical substance)	T60.91	T60.92	T60.93	T60.94	—	—
fungicide	T60.91	T60.92	T60.93	T60.94	—	—
ANTU (alpha naphthylthiourea)	T60.4x1	T60.4x2	T60.4x3	T60.4x4	—	—
Apalcillin	T36.0x1	T36.0x2	T36.0x3	T36.0x4	T36.0x5	T36.0x6
APC	T48.5x1	T48.5x2	T48.5x3	T48.5x4	T48.5x5	T48.5x6
Aplonidine	T44.4x1	T44.4x2	T44.4x3	T44.4x4	T44.4x5	T44.4x6
Apomorphine	T47.7x1	T47.7x2	T47.7x3	T47.7x4	T47.7x5	T47.7x6
Appetite depressants, central	T50.5x1	T50.5x2	T50.5x3	T50.5x4	T50.5x5	T50.5x6
Apraclonidine (hydrochloride)	T44.4x1	T44.4x2	T44.4x3	T44.4x4	T44.4x5	T44.4x6
Apresoline	T46.5x1	T46.5x2	T46.5x3	T46.5x4	T46.5x5	T46.5x6
Aprindine	T46.2x1	T46.2x2	T46.2x3	T46.2x4	T46.2x5	T46.2x6
Aprobarbital	T42.3x1	T42.3x2	T42.3x3	T42.3x4	T42.3x5	T42.3x6
Apronalide	T42.6x1	T42.6x2	T42.6x3	T42.6x4	T42.6x5	T42.6x6
Aprotinin	T45.621	T45.622	T45.623	T45.624	T45.625	T45.626
Aptocaine	T41.3x1	T41.3x2	T41.3x3	T41.3x4	T41.3x5	T41.3x6
Aqua fortis	T54.2x1	T54.2x2	T54.2x3	T54.2x4	—	—
Ara-A	T37.5x1	T37.5x2	T37.5x3	T37.5x4	T37.5x5	T37.5x6
Ara-C	T45.1x1	T45.1x2	T45.1x3	T45.1x4	T45.1x5	T45.1x6
Arachis oil	T49.3x1	T49.3x2	T49.3x3	T49.3x4	T49.3x5	T49.3x6
cathartic	T47.4x1	T47.4x2	T47.4x3	T47.4x4	T47.4x5	T47.4x6
Aralen	T37.2x1	T37.2x2	T37.2x3	T37.2x4	T37.2x5	T37.2x6
Arecoline	T44.1x1	T44.1x2	T44.1x3	T44.1x4	T44.1x5	T44.1x6
Arginine	T50.991	T50.992	T50.993	T50.994	T50.995	T50.996
glutamate	T50.991	T50.992	T50.993	T50.994	T50.995	T50.996
Argyrol	T49.0x1	T49.0x2	T49.0x3	T49.0x4	T49.0x5	T49.0x6
ENT agent	T49.6x1	T49.6x2	T49.6x3	T49.6x4	T49.6x5	T49.6x6
ophthalmic preparation	T49.5x1	T49.5x2	T49.5x3	T49.5x4	T49.5x5	T49.5x6
Aristocort	T38.0x1	T38.0x2	T38.0x3	T38.0x4	T38.0x5	T38.0x6
ENT agent	T49.6x1	T49.6x2	T49.6x3	T49.6x4	T49.6x5	T49.6x6
ophthalmic preparation	T49.5x1	T49.5x2	T49.5x3	T49.5x4	T49.5x5	T49.5x6
topical NEC	T49.0x1	T49.0x2	T49.0x3	T49.0x4	T49.0x5	T49.0x6
Aromatics, corrosive	T54.1x1	T54.1x2	T54.1x3	T54.1x4	—	—
disinfectants	T54.1x1	T54.1x2	T54.1x3	T54.1x4	—	—
Arsenate of lead	T57.0x1	T57.0x2	T57.0x3	T57.0x4	—	—
herbicide	T57.0x1	T57.0x2	T57.0x3	T57.0x4	—	—
Arsenic, arsenicals (compounds) (dust) (vapor) **NEC**	T57.0x1	T57.0x2	T57.0x3	T57.0x4	—	—
anti-infectives	T37.8x1	T37.8x2	T37.8x3	T37.8x4	T37.8x5	T37.8x6
pesticide (dust) (fumes)	T57.0x1	T57.0x2	T57.0x3	T57.0x4	—	—
Arsine (gas)	T57.0x1	T57.0x2	T57.0x3	T57.0x4	—	—
Arsphenamine (silver)	T37.8x1	T37.8x2	T37.8x3	T37.8x4	T37.8x5	T37.8x6
Arsthinol	T37.3x1	T37.3x2	T37.3x3	T37.3x4	T37.3x5	T37.3x6
Artane	T44.3x1	T44.3x2	T44.3x3	T44.3x4	T44.3x5	T44.3x6
Arthropod (venomous) **NEC**	T63.481	T63.482	T63.483	T63.484	—	—
Articaine	T41.3x1	T41.3x2	T41.3x3	T41.3x4	T41.3x5	T41.3x6
Asbestos	T57.8x1	T57.8x2	T57.8x3	T57.8x4	—	—
Ascaridole	T37.4x1	T37.4x2	T37.4x3	T37.4x4	T37.4x5	T37.4x6
Ascorbic acid	T45.2x1	T45.2x2	T45.2x3	T45.2x4	T45.2x5	T45.2x6
Asiaticoside	T49.0x1	T49.0x2	T49.0x3	T49.0x4	T49.0x5	T49.0x6
Asparaginase	T45.1x1	T45.1x2	T45.1x3	T45.1x4	T45.1x5	T45.1x6
Aspidium (oleoresin)	T37.4x1	T37.4x2	T37.4x3	T37.4x4	T37.4x5	T37.4x6
Aspirin (aluminum) (soluble)	T39.011	T39.012	T39.013	T39.014	T39.015	T39.016
Aspoxicillin	T36.0x1	T36.0x2	T36.0x3	T36.0x4	T36.0x5	T36.0x6
Astemizole	T45.0x1	T45.0x2	T45.0x3	T45.0x4	T45.0x5	T45.0x6
Astringent (local)	T49.2x1	T49.2x2	T49.2x3	T49.2x4	T49.2x5	T49.2x6
specified NEC	T49.2x1	T49.2x2	T49.2x3	T49.2x4	T49.2x5	T49.2x6
Astromicin	T36.5x1	T36.5x2	T36.5x3	T36.5x4	T36.5x5	T36.5x6
Atabrine	T37.8x1	T37.8x2	T37.8x3	T37.8x4	T37.8x5	T37.8x6
Ataractic drug NEC	T43.501	T43.502	T43.503	T43.504	T43.505	T43.506
Atenolol	T44.7x1	T44.7x2	T44.7x3	T44.7x4	T44.7x5	T44.7x6
Atonia drug, intestinal	T47.4x1	T47.4x2	T47.4x3	T47.4x4	T47.4x5	T47.4x6
Atophan	T50.4x1	T50.4x2	T50.4x3	T50.4x4	T50.4x5	T50.4x6
Atracurium besilate	T48.1x1	T48.1x2	T48.1x3	T48.1x4	T48.1x5	T48.1x6
Atropine	T44.3x1	T44.3x2	T44.3x3	T44.3x4	T44.3x5	T44.3x6
derivative	T44.3x1	T44.3x2	T44.3x3	T44.3x4	T44.3x5	T44.3x6
methonitrate	T44.3x1	T44.3x2	T44.3x3	T44.3x4	T44.3x5	T44.3x6
Attapulgite	T47.6x1	T47.6x2	T47.6x3	T47.6x4	T47.6x5	T47.6x6
Auramine	T65.891	T65.892	T65.893	T65.894	—	—
dye	T65.6x1	T65.6x2	T65.6x3	T65.6x4	—	—
fungicide	T60.3x1	T60.3x2	T60.3x3	T60.3x4	—	—
Auranofin	T39.4x1	T39.4x2	T39.4x3	T39.4x4	T39.4x5	T39.4x6
Aurantiin	T46.991	T46.992	T46.993	T46.994	T46.995	T46.996
Aureomycin	T36.4x1	T36.4x2	T36.4x3	T36.4x4	T36.4x5	T36.4x6
ophthalmic preparation	T49.5x1	T49.5x2	T49.5x3	T49.5x4	T49.5x5	T49.5x6
topical NEC	T49.0x1	T49.0x2	T49.0x3	T49.0x4	T49.0x5	T49.0x6
Aurothioglucose	T39.4x1	T39.4x2	T39.4x3	T39.4x4	T39.4x5	T39.4x6
Aurothioglycanide	T39.4x1	T39.4x2	T39.4x3	T39.4x4	T39.4x5	T39.4x6
Aurothiomalate sodium	T39.4x1	T39.4x2	T39.4x3	T39.4x4	T39.4x5	T39.4x6
Aurotioprol	T39.4x1	T39.4x2	T39.4x3	T39.4x4	T39.4x5	T39.4x6
Automobile fuel	T52.0x1	T52.0x2	T52.0x3	T52.0x4	—	—
Autonomic nervous system agent NEC	T44.901	T44.902	T44.903	T44.904	T44.905	T44.906
Avlosulfon	T37.1x1	T37.1x2	T37.1x3	T37.1x4	T37.1x5	T37.1x6
Avomine	T42.6x1	T42.6x2	T42.6x3	T42.6x4	T42.6x5	T42.6x6
Axerophthol	T45.2x1	T45.2x2	T45.2x3	T45.2x4	T45.2x5	T45.2x6
Azacitidine	T45.1x1	T45.1x2	T45.1x3	T45.1x4	T45.1x5	T45.1x6
Azacyclonol	T43.591	T43.592	T43.593	T43.594	T43.595	T43.596
Azadirachta	T60.2x1	T60.2x2	T60.2x3	T60.2x4	—	—
Azanidazole	T37.3x1	T37.3x2	T37.3x3	T37.3x4	T37.3x5	T37.3x6
Azapetine	T46.7x1	T46.7x2	T46.7x3	T46.7x4	T46.7x5	T46.7x6
Azapropazone	T39.2x1	T39.2x2	T39.2x3	T39.2x4	T39.2x5	T39.2x6
Azaribine	T45.1x1	T45.1x2	T45.1x3	T45.1x4	T45.1x5	T45.1x6
Azaserine	T45.1x1	T45.1x2	T45.1x3	T45.1x4	T45.1x5	T45.1x6
Azatadine	T45.0x1	T45.0x2	T45.0x3	T45.0x4	T45.0x5	T45.0x6
Azatepa	T45.1x1	T45.1x2	T45.1x3	T45.1x4	T45.1x5	T45.1x6
Azathioprine	T45.1x1	T45.1x2	T45.1x3	T45.1x4	T45.1x5	T45.1x6
Azelaic acid	T49.0x1	T49.0x2	T49.0x3	T49.0x4	T49.0x5	T49.0x6
Azelastine	T45.0x1	T45.0x2	T45.0x3	T45.0x4	T45.0x5	T45.0x6
Azidocillin	T36.0x1	T36.0x2	T36.0x3	T36.0x4	T36.0x5	T36.0x6
Azidothymidine	T37.5x1	T37.5x2	T37.5x3	T37.5x4	T37.5x5	T37.5x6
Azinphos (ethyl) (methyl)	T60.0x1	T60.0x2	T60.0x3	T60.0x4	—	—
Aziridine (chelating)	T54.1x1	T54.1x2	T54.1x3	T54.1x4	—	—
Azithromycin	T36.3x1	T36.3x2	T36.3x3	T36.3x4	T36.3x5	T36.3x6
Azlocillin	T36.0x1	T36.0x2	T36.0x3	T36.0x4	T36.0x5	T36.0x6
Azobenzene smoke	T65.3x1	T65.3x2	T65.3x3	T65.3x4	—	—
acaricide	T60.8x1	T60.8x2	T60.8x3	T60.8x4	—	—

Substance	Poisoning, Accidental (unintentional)	Poisoning, Intentional Self-harm	Poisoning, Assault	Poisoning, Undetermined	Adverse Effect	Under-dosing
Azosulfamide	T37.0x1	T37.0x2	T37.0x3	T37.0x4	T37.0x5	T37.0x6
AZT	T37.5x1	T37.5x2	T37.5x3	T37.5x4	T37.5x5	T37.5x6
Aztreonam	T36.1x1	T36.1x2	T36.1x3	T36.1x4	T36.1x5	T36.1x6
Azulfidine	T37.0x1	T37.0x2	T37.0x3	T37.0x4	T37.0x5	T37.0x6
Azuresin	T50.8x1	T50.8x2	T50.8x3	T50.8x4	T50.8x5	T50.8x6
Bacampicillin	T36.0x1	T36.0x2	T36.0x3	T36.0x4	T36.0x5	T36.0x6
b-acetyldigoxin	T46.0x1	T46.0x2	T46.0x3	T46.0x4	T46.0x5	T46.0x6
Bacillus						
lactobacillus	T47.8x1	T47.8x2	T47.8x3	T47.8x4	T47.8x5	T47.8x6
subtilis	T47.6x1	T47.6x2	T47.6x3	T47.6x4	T47.6x5	T47.6x6
Bacimycin	T49.0x1	T49.0x2	T49.0x3	T49.0x4	T49.0x5	T49.0x6
ophthalmic preparation	T49.5x1	T49.5x2	T49.5x3	T49.5x4	T49.5x5	T49.5x6
Bacitracin zinc	T49.0x1	T49.0x2	T49.0x3	T49.0x4	T49.0x5	T49.0x6
with neomycin	T49.0x1	T49.0x2	T49.0x3	T49.0x4	T49.0x5	T49.0x6
ENT agent	T49.6x1	T49.6x2	T49.6x3	T49.6x4	T49.6x5	T49.6x6
ophthalmic preparation	T49.5x1	T49.5x2	T49.5x3	T49.5x4	T49.5x5	T49.5x6
topical NEC	T49.0x1	T49.0x2	T49.0x3	T49.0x4	T49.0x5	T49.0x6
Baclofen	T42.8x1	T42.8x2	T42.8x3	T42.8x4	T42.8x5	T42.8x6
b-adrenergic blocking agent, heart	T44.7x1	T44.7x2	T44.7x3	T44.7x4	T44.7x5	T44.7x6
Baking soda	T50.991	T50.992	T50.993	T50.994	T50.995	T50.996
BAL	T45.8x1	T45.8x2	T45.8x3	T45.8x4	T45.8x5	T45.8x6
Bambuterol	T48.6x1	T48.6x2	T48.6x3	T48.6x4	T48.6x5	T48.6x6
Bamethan (sulfate)	T46.7x1	T46.7x2	T46.7x3	T46.7x4	T46.7x5	T46.7x6
Bamifylline	T48.6x1	T48.6x2	T48.6x3	T48.6x4	T48.6x5	T48.6x6
Bamipine	T45.0x1	T45.0x2	T45.0x3	T45.0x4	T45.0x5	T45.0x6
Baneberry—see Actaea spicata						
Banewort—see Belladonna						
Barbenyl	T42.3x1	T42.3x2	T42.3x3	T42.3x4	T42.3x5	T42.3x6
Barbexaclone	T42.6x1	T42.6x2	T42.6x3	T42.6x4	T42.6x5	T42.6x6
Barbital	T42.3x1	T42.3x2	T42.3x3	T42.3x4	T42.3x5	T42.3x6
sodium	T42.3x1	T42.3x2	T42.3x3	T42.3x4	T42.3x5	T42.3x6
Barbitone	T42.3x1	T42.3x2	T42.3x3	T42.3x4	T42.3x5	T42.3x6
Barbiturate NEC	T42.3x1	T42.3x2	T42.3x3	T42.3x4	T42.3x5	T42.3x6
with tranquilizer	T42.3x1	T42.3x2	T42.3x3	T42.3x4	T42.3x5	T42.3x6
anesthetic (intravenous)	T41.1x1	T41.1x2	T41.1x3	T41.1x4	T41.1x5	T41.1x6
Barium (carbonate) (chloride) (sulfite)	T57.8x1	T57.8x2	T57.8x3	T57.8x4	—	—
diagnostic agent	T50.8x1	T50.8x2	T50.8x3	T50.8x4	T50.8x5	T50.8x6
pesticide	T60.4x1	T60.4x2	T60.4x3	T60.4x4		
rodenticide	T60.4x1	T60.4x2	T60.4x3	T60.4x4		
sulfate (medicinal)	T50.8x1	T50.8x2	T50.8x3	T50.8x4	T50.8x5	T50.8x6
Barrier cream	T49.3x1	T49.3x2	T49.3x3	T49.3x4	T49.3x5	T49.3x6
Basic fuchsin	T49.0x1	T49.0x2	T49.0x3	T49.0x4	T49.0x5	T49.0x6
Battery acid or fluid	T54.2x1	T54.2x2	T54.2x3	T54.2x4	—	—
Bay rum	T51.8x1	T51.8x2	T51.8x3	T51.8x4	—	—
b-benzalbutyramide	T46.6x1	T46.6x2	T46.6x3	T46.6x4	T46.6x5	T46.6x6
BCG (vaccine)	T50.A91	T50.A92	T50.A93	T50.A94	T50.A95	T50.A96
BCNU	T45.1x1	T45.1x2	T45.1x3	T45.1x4	T45.1x5	T45.1x6
Bearsfoot	T62.2x1	T62.2x2	T62.2x3	T62.2x4		
Beclamide	T42.6x1	T42.6x2	T42.6x3	T42.6x4	T42.6x5	T42.6x6
Beclomethasone	T44.5x1	T44.5x2	T44.5x3	T44.5x4	T44.5x5	T44.5x6
Bee (sting) (venom)	T63.441	T63.442	T63.443	T63.444	—	—
Befunolol	T49.5x1	T49.5x2	T49.5x3	T49.5x4	T49.5x5	T49.5x6
Bekanamycin	T36.5x1	T36.5x2	T36.5x3	T36.5x4	T36.5x5	T36.5x6
Belladonna (see also Nightshade)						
alkaloids	T44.3x1	T44.3x2	T44.3x3	T44.3x4	T44.3x5	T44.3x6
extract	T44.3x1	T44.3x2	T44.3x3	T44.3x4	T44.3x5	T44.3x6
herb	T44.3x1	T44.3x2	T44.3x3	T44.3x4	T44.3x5	T44.3x6
Bemegride	T50.7x1	T50.7x2	T50.7x3	T50.7x4	T50.7x5	T50.7x6
Benactyzine	T44.3x1	T44.3x2	T44.3x3	T44.3x4	T44.3x5	T44.3x6
Benadryl	T45.0x1	T45.0x2	T45.0x3	T45.0x4	T45.0x5	T45.0x6
Benaprizine	T44.3x1	T44.3x2	T44.3x3	T44.3x4	T44.3x5	T44.3x6
Benazepril	T46.4x1	T46.4x2	T46.4x3	T46.4x4	T46.4x5	T46.4x6
Bencyclane	T46.7x1	T46.7x2	T46.7x3	T46.7x4	T46.7x5	T46.7x6
Bendazol	T46.3x1	T46.3x2	T46.3x3	T46.3x4	T46.3x5	T46.3x6
Bendrofluazide	T50.2x1	T50.2x2	T50.2x3	T50.2x4	T50.2x5	T50.2x6
Bendroflumethiazide	T50.2x1	T50.2x2	T50.2x3	T50.2x4	T50.2x5	T50.2x6
Benemid	T50.4x1	T50.4x2	T50.4x3	T50.4x4	T50.4x5	T50.4x6
Benethamine penicillin	T36.0x1	T36.0x2	T36.0x3	T36.0x4	T36.0x5	T36.0x6
Benisone	T49.0x1	T49.0x2	T49.0x3	T49.0x4	T49.0x5	T49.0x6

Substance	Poisoning, Accidental (unintentional)	Poisoning, Intentional Self-harm	Poisoning, Assault	Poisoning, Undetermined	Adverse Effect	Under-dosing
Benexate	T47.1x1	T47.1x2	T47.1x3	T47.1x4	T47.1x5	T47.1x6
Benfluorex	T46.6x1	T46.6x2	T46.6x3	T46.6x4	T46.6x5	T46.6x6
Benfotiamine	T45.2x1	T45.2x2	T45.2x3	T45.2x4	T45.2x5	T45.2x6
Benomyl	T60.0x1	T60.0x2	T60.0x3	T60.0x4	—	—
Benoquin	T49.8x1	T49.8x2	T49.8x3	T49.8x4	T49.8x5	T49.8x6
Benoxinate	T41.3x1	T41.3x2	T41.3x3	T41.3x4	T41.3x5	T41.3x6
Benperidol	T43.4x1	T43.4x2	T43.4x3	T43.4x4	T43.4x5	T43.4x6
Benproperine	T48.3x1	T48.3x2	T48.3x3	T48.3x4	T48.3x5	T48.3x6
Benserazide	T42.8x1	T42.8x2	T42.8x3	T42.8x4	T42.8x5	T42.8x6
Bentazepam	T42.4x1	T42.4x2	T42.4x3	T42.4x4	T42.4x5	T42.4x6
Bentiromide	T50.8x1	T50.8x2	T50.8x3	T50.8x4	T50.8x5	T50.8x6
Bentonite	T49.3x1	T49.3x2	T49.3x3	T49.3x4	T49.3x5	T49.3x6
Benzalbutyramide	T46.6x1	T46.6x2	T46.6x3	T46.6x4	T46.6x5	T46.6x6
Benzalkonium (chloride)	T49.0x1	T49.0x2	T49.0x3	T49.0x4	T49.0x5	T49.0x6
ophthalmic preparation	T49.5x1	T49.5x2	T49.5x3	T49.5x4	T49.5x5	T49.5x6
Benzamine	T41.3x1	T41.3x2	T41.3x3	T41.3x4	T41.3x5	T41.3x6
lactate	T49.1x1	T49.1x2	T49.1x3	T49.1x4	T49.1x5	T49.1x6
Benzamidosalicylate (calcium)	T37.1x1	T37.1x2	T37.1x3	T37.1x4	T37.1x5	T37.1x6
Benzamphetamine	T50.5x1	T50.5x2	T50.5x3	T50.5x4	T50.5x5	T50.5x6
Benzapril hydrochloride	T46.5x1	T46.5x2	T46.5x3	T46.5x4	T46.5x5	T46.5x6
Benzathine benzylpenicillin	T36.0x1	T36.0x2	T36.0x3	T36.0x4	T36.0x5	T36.0x6
Benzathine penicillin	T36.0x1	T36.0x2	T36.0x3	T36.0x4	T36.0x5	T36.0x6
Benzatropine	T42.8x1	T42.8x2	T42.8x3	T42.8x4	T42.8x5	T42.8x6
Benzbromarone	T50.4x1	T50.4x2	T50.4x3	T50.4x4	T50.4x5	T50.4x6
Benzcarbimine	T45.1x1	T45.1x2	T45.1x3	T45.1x4	T45.1x5	T45.1x6
Benzedrex	T44.991	T44.992	T44.993	T44.994	T44.995	T44.996
Benzedrine (amphetamine)	T43.621	T43.622	T43.623	T43.624	T43.625	T43.626
Benzenamine	T65.3x1	T65.3x2	T65.3x3	T65.3x4	—	—
Benzene	T52.1x1	T52.1x2	T52.1x3	T52.1x4	—	—
homologues (acetyl) (dimethyl)(methyl) (solvent)	T52.2x1	T52.2x2	T52.2x3	T52.2x4	—	—
Benzethonium (chloride)	T49.0x1	T49.0x2	T49.0x3	T49.0x4	T49.0x5	T49.0x6
Benzfetamine	T50.5x1	T50.5x2	T50.5x3	T50.5x4	T50.5x5	T50.5x6
Benzhexol	T44.3x1	T44.3x2	T44.3x3	T44.3x4	T44.3x5	T44.3x6
Benzhydramine (chloride)	T45.0x1	T45.0x2	T45.0x3	T45.0x4	T45.0x5	T45.0x6
Benzidine	T65.891	T65.892	T65.893	T65.894	—	—
Benzilonium bromide	T44.3x1	T44.3x2	T44.3x3	T44.3x4	T44.3x5	T44.3x6
Benzimidazole	T60.3x1	T60.3x2	T60.3x3	T60.3x4	—	—
Benzin(e)—see Ligroin						
Benziodarone	T46.3x1	T46.3x2	T46.3x3	T46.3x4	T46.3x5	T46.3x6
Benznidazole	T37.3x1	T37.3x2	T37.3x3	T37.3x4	T37.3x5	T37.3x6
Benzocaine	T41.3x1	T41.3x2	T41.3x3	T41.3x4	T41.3x5	T41.3x6
Benzodiapin	T42.4x1	T42.4x2	T42.4x3	T42.4x4	T42.4x5	T42.4x6
Benzodiazepine NEC	T42.4x1	T42.4x2	T42.4x3	T42.4x4	T42.4x5	T42.4x6
Benzoic acid	T49.0x1	T49.0x2	T49.0x3	T49.0x4	T49.0x5	T49.0x6
with salicylic acid	T49.0x1	T49.0x2	T49.0x3	T49.0x4	T49.0x5	T49.0x6
Benzoin (tincture)	T48.5x1	T48.5x2	T48.5x3	T48.5x4	T48.5x5	T48.5x6
Benzol (benzene)	T52.1x1	T52.1x2	T52.1x3	T52.1x4	—	—
vapor	T52.0x1	T52.0x2	T52.0x3	T52.0x4	—	—
Benzomorphan	T40.2x1	T40.2x2	T40.2x3	T40.2x4	T40.2x5	T40.2x6
Benzonatate	T48.3x1	T48.3x2	T48.3x3	T48.3x4	T48.3x5	T48.3x6
Benzophenones	T49.3x1	T49.3x2	T49.3x3	T49.3x4	T49.3x5	T49.3x6
Benzopyrone	T46.991	T46.992	T46.993	T46.994	T46.995	T46.996
Benzothiadiazides	T50.2x1	T50.2x2	T50.2x3	T50.2x4	T50.2x5	T50.2x6
Benzoxonium chloride	T49.0x1	T49.0x2	T49.0x3	T49.0x4	T49.0x5	T49.0x6
Benzoyl peroxide	T49.0x1	T49.0x2	T49.0x3	T49.0x4	T49.0x5	T49.0x6
Benzoylpas calcium	T37.1x1	T37.1x2	T37.1x3	T37.1x4	T37.1x5	T37.1x6
Benzperidin	T43.591	T43.592	T43.593	T43.594	T43.595	T43.596
Benzperidol	T43.591	T43.592	T43.593	T43.594	T43.595	T43.596
Benzphetamine	T43.621	T43.622	T43.623	T43.624	T43.625	T43.626
Benzpyrinium bromide	T44.1x1	T44.1x2	T44.1x3	T44.1x4	T44.1x5	T44.1x6
Benzquinamide	T45.0x1	T45.0x2	T45.0x3	T45.0x4	T45.0x5	T45.0x6
Benzthiazide	T50.2x1	T50.2x2	T50.2x3	T50.2x4	T50.2x5	T50.2x6
Benztropine						
anticholinergic	T44.3x1	T44.3x2	T44.3x3	T44.3x4	T44.3x5	T44.3x6
antiparkinson	T42.8x1	T42.8x2	T42.8x3	T42.8x4	T42.8x5	T42.8x6
Benzydamine	T49.0x1	T49.0x2	T49.0x3	T49.0x4	T49.0x5	T49.0x6
Benzyl						
acetate	T52.8x1	T52.8x2	T52.8x3	T52.8x4	—	—
alcohol	T49.0x1	T49.0x2	T49.0x3	T49.0x4	T49.0x5	T49.0x6
benzoate	T49.0x1	T49.0x2	T49.0x3	T49.0x4	T49.0x5	T49.0x6

Substance	Poisoning, Accidental (unintentional)	Poisoning, Intentional Self-harm	Poisoning, Assault	Poisoning, Undetermined	Adverse Effect	Under-dosing
Benzyl—continued						
Benzoic acid	T49.0x1	T49.0x2	T49.0x3	T49.0x4	T49.0x5	T49.0x6
morphine	T40.2x1	T40.2x2	T40.2x3	T40.2x4	T40.2x5	T40.2x6
nicotinate	T46.6x1	T46.6x2	T46.6x3	T46.6x4	T46.6x5	T46.6x6
penicillin	T36.0x1	T36.0x2	T36.0x3	T36.0x4	T36.0x5	T36.0x6
Benzylhydrochlorthiazide	T50.2x1	T50.2x2	T50.2x3	T50.2x4	T50.2x5	T50.2x6
Benzylpenicillin	T36.0x1	T36.0x2	T36.0x3	T36.0x4	T36.0x5	T36.0x6
Benzylthiouracil	T38.2x1	T38.2x2	T38.2x3	T38.2x4	T38.2x5	T38.2x6
Bephenium hydroxy-naphthoate	T37.4x1	T37.4x2	T37.4x3	T37.4x4	T37.4x5	T37.4x6
Bepridil	T46.1x1	T46.1x2	T46.1x3	T46.1x4	T46.1x5	T46.1x6
Bergamot oil	T65.891	T65.892	T65.893	T65.894	—	—
Bergapten	T50.991	T50.992	T50.993	T50.994	T50.995	T50.996
Berries, poisonous	T62.1x1	T62.1x2	T62.1x3	T62.1x4	—	—
Beryllium (compounds)	T56.7x1	T56.7x2	T56.7x3	T56.7x4	—	—
Betacarotene	T45.2x1	T45.2x2	T45.2x3	T45.2x4	T45.2x5	T45.2x6
b-eucaine	T49.1x1	T49.1x2	T49.1x3	T49.1x4	T49.1x5	T49.1x6
Beta-Chlor	T42.6x1	T42.6x2	T42.6x3	T42.6x4	T42.6x5	T42.6x6
Betahistine	T46.7x1	T46.7x2	T46.7x3	T46.7x4	T46.7x5	T46.7x6
Betaine	T47.5x1	T47.5x2	T47.5x3	T47.5x4	T47.5x5	T47.5x6
Betamethasone	T49.0x1	T49.0x2	T49.0x3	T49.0x4	T49.0x5	T49.0x6
topical	T49.0x1	T49.0x2	T49.0x3	T49.0x4	T49.0x5	T49.0x6
Betamicin	T36.8x1	T36.8x2	T36.8x3	T36.8x4	T36.8x5	T36.8x6
Betanidine	T46.5x1	T46.5x2	T46.5x3	T46.5x4	T46.5x5	T46.5x6
Betaxolol	T44.7x1	T44.7x2	T44.7x3	T44.7x4	T44.7x5	T44.7x6
Betazole	T50.8x1	T50.8x2	T50.8x3	T50.8x4	T50.8x5	T50.8x6
Bethanechol	T44.1x1	T44.1x2	T44.1x3	T44.1x4	T44.1x5	T44.1x6
chloride	T44.1x1	T44.1x2	T44.1x3	T44.1x4	T44.1x5	T44.1x6
Bethanidine	T46.5x1	T46.5x2	T46.5x3	T46.5x4	T46.5x5	T46.5x6
Betoxycaine	T41.3x1	T41.3x2	T41.3x3	T41.3x4	T41.3x5	T41.3x6
Betula oil	T49.3x1	T49.3x2	T49.3x3	T49.3x4	T49.3x5	T49.3x6
Bevantolol	T44.7x1	T44.7x2	T44.7x3	T44.7x4	T44.7x5	T44.7x6
Bevonium metilsulfate	T44.3x1	T44.3x2	T44.3x3	T44.3x4	T44.3x5	T44.3x6
Bezafibrate	T46.6x1	T46.6x2	T46.6x3	T46.6x4	T46.6x5	T46.6x6
Bezitramide	T40.4x1	T40.4x2	T40.4x3	T40.4x4	T40.4x5	T40.4x6
b-galactosidase	T47.5x1	T47.5x2	T47.5x3	T47.5x4	T47.5x5	T47.5x6
BHA	T50.991	T50.992	T50.993	T50.994	T50.995	T50.996
Bhang	T40.7x1	T40.7x2	T40.7x3	T40.7x4	T40.7x5	T40.7x6
BHC (medicinal)	T49.0x1	T49.0x2	T49.0x3	T49.0x4	T49.0x5	T49.0x6
nonmedicinal (vapor)	T53.6x1	T53.6x2	T53.6x3	T53.6x4	—	—
Bialamicol	T37.3x1	T37.3x2	T37.3x3	T37.3x4	T37.3x5	T37.3x6
Bibenzonium bromide	T48.3x1	T48.3x2	T48.3x3	T48.3x4	T48.3x5	T48.3x6
Bibrocathol	T49.5x1	T49.5x2	T49.5x3	T49.5x4	T49.5x5	T49.5x6
Bichloride of mercury—see Mercury, chloride						
Bichromates (calcium) (potassium)(sodium) (crystals)	T57.8x1	T57.8x2	T57.8x3	T57.8x4	—	—
fumes	T56.2x1	T56.2x2	T56.2x3	T56.2x4	—	—
Biclotymol	T49.6x1	T49.6x2	T49.6x3	T49.6x4	T49.6x5	T49.6x6
Bicucculine	T50.7x1	T50.7x2	T50.7x3	T50.7x4	T50.7x5	T50.7x6
Bifemelane	T43.291	T43.292	T43.293	T43.294	T43.295	T43.296
Biguanide derivatives, oral	T38.3x1	T38.3x2	T38.3x3	T38.3x4	T38.3x5	T38.3x6
Biligrafin	T50.8x1	T50.8x2	T50.8x3	T50.8x4	T50.8x5	T50.8x6
Bile salts	T47.5x1	T47.5x2	T47.5x3	T47.5x4	T47.5x5	T47.5x6
Bilopaque	T50.8x1	T50.8x2	T50.8x3	T50.8x4	T50.8x5	T50.8x6
Binifibrate	T46.6x1	T46.6x2	T46.6x3	T46.6x4	T46.6x5	T46.6x6
Binitrobenzol	T65.3x1	T65.3x2	T65.3x3	T65.3x4	—	—
Bioflavonoid(s)	T46.991	T46.992	T46.993	T46.994	T46.995	T46.996
Biological substance NEC	T50.901	T50.902	T50.903	T50.904	T50.905	T50.906
Biotin	T45.2x1	T45.2x2	T45.2x3	T45.2x4	T45.2x5	T45.2x6
Biperiden	T44.3x1	T44.3x2	T44.3x3	T44.3x4	T44.3x5	T44.3x6
Bisacodyl	T47.2x1	T47.2x2	T47.2x3	T47.2x4	T47.2x5	T47.2x6
Bisbentiamine	T45.2x1	T45.2x2	T45.2x3	T45.2x4	T45.2x5	T45.2x6
Bisbutiamine	T45.2x1	T45.2x2	T45.2x3	T45.2x4	T45.2x5	T45.2x6
Bisdequalinium (salts) (diacetate)	T49.6x1	T49.6x2	T49.6x3	T49.6x4	T49.6x5	T49.6x6
Bishydroxycoumarin	T45.511	T45.512	T45.513	T45.514	T45.515	T45.516
Bismarsen	T37.8x1	T37.8x2	T37.8x3	T37.8x4	T37.8x5	T37.8x6
Bismuth salts	T47.6x1	T47.6x2	T47.6x3	T47.6x4	T47.6x5	T47.6x6
aluminate	T47.1x1	T47.1x2	T47.1x3	T47.1x4	T47.1x5	T47.1x6
anti-infectives	T37.8x1	T37.8x2	T37.8x3	T37.8x4	T37.8x5	T37.8x6
Bismuth salts—continued	T47.6x1	T47.6x2	T47.6x3	T47.6x4	T47.6x5	T47.6x6
formic iodide	T49.0x1	T49.0x2	T49.0x3	T49.0x4	T49.0x5	T49.0x6
glycolylarsenate	T49.0x1	T49.0x2	T49.0x3	T49.0x4	T49.0x5	T49.0x6
nonmedicinal (compounds) NEC	T65.91	T65.92	T65.93	T65.94	—	—
subcarbonate	T47.6x1	T47.6x2	T47.6x3	T47.6x4	T47.6x5	T47.6x6
subsalicylate	T37.8x1	T37.8x2	T37.8x3	T37.8x4	T37.8x5	T37.8x6
sulfarsphenamine	T37.8x1	T37.8x2	T37.8x3	T37.8x4	T37.8x5	T37.8x6
Bisoprolol	T44.7x1	T44.7x2	T44.7x3	T44.7x4	T44.7x5	T44.7x6
Bisoxatin	T47.2x1	T47.2x2	T47.2x3	T47.2x4	T47.2x5	T47.2x6
Bisulepin (hydrochloride)	T45.0x1	T45.0x2	T45.0x3	T45.0x4	T45.0x5	T45.0x6
Bithionol	T37.8x1	T37.8x2	T37.8x3	T37.8x4	T37.8x5	T37.8x6
Bitolterol	T48.6x1	T48.6x2	T48.6x3	T48.6x4	T48.6x5	T48.6x6
Bitoscanate	T37.4x1	T37.4x2	T37.4x3	T37.4x4	T37.4x5	T37.4x6
Bitter almond oil	T62.8x1	T62.8x2	T62.8x3	T62.8x4	—	—
Bittersweet	T62.2x1	T62.2x2	T62.2x3	T62.2x4	—	—
Black						
flag	T60.91	T60.92	T60.93	T60.94	—	—
henbane	T62.2x1	T62.2x2	T62.2x3	T62.2x4	—	—
leaf (40)	T60.91	T60.92	T60.93	T60.94	—	—
widow spider (bite)	T63.311	T63.312	T63.313	T63.314	—	—
antivenin	T50.Z11	T50.Z12	T50.Z13	T50.Z14	T50.Z15	T50.Z16
Blast furnace gas (carbon monoxide from)	T58.8x1	T58.8x2	T58.8x3	T58.8x4	—	—
Bleach	T54.91	T54.92	T54.93	T54.94	—	—
Bleaching agent (medicinal)	T49.4x1	T49.4x2	T49.4x3	T49.4x4	T49.4x5	T49.4x6
Bleomycin	T45.1x1	T45.1x2	T45.1x3	T45.1x4	T45.1x5	T45.1x6
Blockain	T41.3x1	T41.3x2	T41.3x3	T41.3x4	T41.3x5	T41.3x6
infiltration (subcutaneous)	T41.3x1	T41.3x2	T41.3x3	T41.3x4	T41.3x5	T41.3x6
nerve block (peripheral) (plexus)	T41.3x1	T41.3x2	T41.3x3	T41.3x4	T41.3x5	T41.3x6
topical (surface)	T41.3x1	T41.3x2	T41.3x3	T41.3x4	T41.3x5	T41.3x6
Blood (derivatives) (natural) (plasma) (whole)	T45.8x1	T45.8x2	T45.8x3	T45.8x4	T45.8x5	T45.8x6
dried	T45.8x1	T45.8x2	T45.8x3	T45.8x4	T45.8x5	T45.8x6
drug affecting NEC	T45.91	T45.92	T45.93	T45.94	T45.95	T45.96
expander NEC	T45.8x1	T45.8x2	T45.8x3	T45.8x4	T45.8x5	T45.8x6
fraction NEC	T45.8x1	T45.8x2	T45.8x3	T45.8x4	T45.8x5	T45.8x6
substitute (macromolecular)	T45.8x1	T45.8x2	T45.8x3	T45.8x4	T45.8x5	T45.8x6
Blue velvet	T40.2x1	T40.2x2	T40.2x3	T40.2x4	T40.2x5	T40.2x6
Bone meal	T62.8x1	T62.8x2	T62.8x3	T62.8x4	—	—
Bonine	T45.0x1	T45.0x2	T45.0x3	T45.0x4	T45.0x5	T45.0x6
Bopindolol	T44.7x1	T44.7x2	T44.7x3	T44.7x4	T44.7x5	T44.7x6
Boracic acid	T49.0x1	T49.0x2	T49.0x3	T49.0x4	T49.0x5	T49.0x6
ENT agent	T49.6x1	T49.6x2	T49.6x3	T49.6x4	T49.6x5	T49.6x6
ophthalmic preparation	T49.5x1	T49.5x2	T49.5x3	T49.5x4	T49.5x5	T49.5x6
Borane complex	T57.8x1	T57.8x2	T57.8x3	T57.8x4	—	—
Borate(s)	T57.8x1	T57.8x2	T57.8x3	T57.8x4	—	—
buffer	T50.991	T50.992	T50.993	T50.994	T50.995	T50.996
cleanser	T54.91	T54.92	T54.93	T54.94	—	—
sodium	T57.8x1	T57.8x2	T57.8x3	T57.8x4	—	—
Borax (cleanser)	T54.91	T54.92	T54.93	T54.94	—	—
Bordeaux mixture	T60.3x1	T60.3x2	T60.3x3	T60.3x4	—	—
Boric acid	T49.0x1	T49.0x2	T49.0x3	T49.0x4	T49.0x5	T49.0x6
ENT agent	T49.6x1	T49.6x2	T49.6x3	T49.6x4	T49.6x5	T49.6x6
ophthalmic preparation	T49.5x1	T49.5x2	T49.5x3	T49.5x4	T49.5x5	T49.5x6
Bornaprine	T44.3x1	T44.3x2	T44.3x3	T44.3x4	T44.3x5	T44.3x6
Boron	T57.8x1	T57.8x2	T57.8x3	T57.8x4	—	—
hydride NEC	T57.8x1	T57.8x2	T57.8x3	T57.8x4	—	—
fumes or gas	T57.8x1	T57.8x2	T57.8x3	T57.8x4	—	—
trifluoride	T59.891	T59.892	T59.893	T59.894	—	—
Botox	T48.291	T48.292	T48.293	T48.294	T48.295	T48.296
Botulinus anti-toxin (type A, B)	T50.Z11	T50.Z12	T50.Z13	T50.Z14	T50.Z15	T50.Z16
Brake fluid vapor	T59.891	T59.892	T59.893	T59.894	—	—
Brallobarbital	T42.3x1	T42.3x2	T42.3x3	T42.3x4	T42.3x5	T42.3x6
Bran (wheat)	T47.4x1	T47.4x2	T47.4x3	T47.4x4	T47.4x5	T47.4x6
Brass (fumes)	T56.4x1	T56.4x2	T56.4x3	T56.4x4	—	—
Brasso	T52.0x1	T52.0x2	T52.0x3	T52.0x4	—	—
Bretylium tosilate	T46.2x1	T46.2x2	T46.2x3	T46.2x4	T46.2x5	T46.2x6
Brevital (sodium)	T41.1x1	T41.1x2	T41.1x3	T41.1x4	T41.1x5	T41.1x6
Brinase	T45.3x1	T45.3x2	T45.3x3	T45.3x4	T45.3x5	T45.3x6
British antilewisite	T45.8x1	T45.8x2	T45.8x3	T45.8x4	T45.8x5	T45.8x6
Brodifacoum	T60.4x1	T60.4x2	T60.4x3	T60.4x4		

Substance	Poisoning, Accidental (unintentional)	Poisoning, Intentional Self-harm	Poisoning, Assault	Poisoning, Undetermined	Adverse Effect	Under-dosing
Bromal (hydrate)	T42.6x1	T42.6x2	T42.6x3	T42.6x4	T42.6x5	T42.6x6
Bromazepam	T42.4x1	T42.4x2	T42.4x3	T42.4x4	T42.4x5	T42.4x6
Bromazine	T45.0x1	T45.0x2	T45.0x3	T45.0x4	T45.0x5	T45.0x6
Brombenzylcyanide	T59.3x1	T59.3x2	T59.3x3	T59.3x4	—	—
Bromelains	T45.3x1	T45.3x2	T45.3x3	T45.3x4	T45.3x5	T45.3x6
Bromethalin	T60.4x1	T60.4x2	T60.4x3	T60.4x4	—	—
Bromhexine	T48.4x1	T48.4x2	T48.4x3	T48.4x4	T48.4x5	T48.4x6
Bromide salts	T42.6x1	T42.6x2	T42.6x3	T42.6x4	T42.6x5	T42.6x6
Bromindione	T45.511	T45.512	T45.513	T45.514	T45.515	T45.516
Bromine						
compounds (medicinal)	T42.6x1	T42.6x2	T42.6x3	T42.6x4	T42.6x5	T42.6x6
sedative	T42.6x1	T42.6x2	T42.6x3	T42.6x4	T42.6x5	T42.6x6
vapor	T59.891	T59.892	T59.893	T59.894	—	—
Bromisovalum	T42.6x1	T42.6x2	T42.6x3	T42.6x4	T42.6x5	T42.6x6
Bromisoval	T42.6x1	T42.6x2	T42.6x3	T42.6x4	T42.6x5	T42.6x6
Bromobenzylcyanide	T59.3x1	T59.3x2	T59.3x3	T59.3x4	—	—
Bromochlorosalicylanilide	T49.0x1	T49.0x2	T49.0x3	T49.0x4	T49.0x5	T49.0x6
Bromocriptine	T42.8x1	T42.8x2	T42.8x3	T42.8x4	T42.8x5	T42.8x6
Bromodiphenhydramine	T45.0x1	T45.0x2	T45.0x3	T45.0x4	T45.0x5	T45.0x6
Bromoform	T42.6x1	T42.6x2	T42.6x3	T42.6x4	T42.6x5	T42.6x6
Bromophenol blue reagent	T50.991	T50.992	T50.993	T50.994	T50.995	T50.996
Bromopride	T47.8x1	T47.8x2	T47.8x3	T47.8x4	T47.8x5	T47.8x6
Bromosalicylchloranitide	T49.0x1	T49.0x2	T49.0x3	T49.0x4	T49.0x5	T49.0x6
Bromosalicylhydroxamic acid	T37.1x1	T37.1x2	T37.1x3	T37.1x4	T37.1x5	T37.1x6
Bromo-Seltzer	T39.1x1	T39.1x2	T39.1x3	T39.1x4	T39.1x5	T39.1x6
Bromoxynil	T60.3x1	T60.3x2	T60.3x3	T60.3x4	—	—
Bromperidol	T43.4x1	T43.4x2	T43.4x3	T43.4x4	T43.4x5	T43.4x6
Brompheniramine	T45.0x1	T45.0x2	T45.0x3	T45.0x4	T45.0x5	T45.0x6
Bromsulfophthalein	T50.8x1	T50.8x2	T50.8x3	T50.8x4	T50.8x5	T50.8x6
Bromural	T42.6x1	T42.6x2	T42.6x3	T42.6x4	T42.6x5	T42.6x6
Bromvaletone	T42.6x1	T42.6x2	T42.6x3	T42.6x4	T42.6x5	T42.6x6
Bronchodilator NEC	T48.6x1	T48.6x2	T48.6x3	T48.6x4	T48.6x5	T48.6x6
Brotizolam	T42.4x1	T42.4x2	T42.4x3	T42.4x4	T42.4x5	T42.4x6
Brovincamine	T46.7x1	T46.7x2	T46.7x3	T46.7x4	T46.7x5	T46.7x6
Brown spider (bite) (venom)	T63.391	T63.392	T63.393	T63.394	—	—
Brown recluse spider (bite) (venom)	T63.331	T63.332	T63.333	T63.334	—	—
Broxaterol	T48.6x1	T48.6x2	T48.6x3	T48.6x4	T48.6x5	T48.6x6
Broxuridine	T45.1x1	T45.1x2	T45.1x3	T45.1x4	T45.1x5	T45.1x6
Broxyquinoline	T37.8x1	T37.8x2	T37.8x3	T37.8x4	T37.8x5	T37.8x6
Bruceine	T48.291	T48.292	T48.293	T48.294	T48.295	T48.296
Brucia	T62.2x1	T62.2x2	T62.2x3	T62.2x4	—	—
Brucine	T65.1x1	T65.1x2	T65.1x3	T65.1x4	—	—
Brunswick green—see Copper						
Bruten—see Ibuprofen						
Bryonia	T47.2x1	T47.2x2	T47.2x3	T47.2x4	T47.2x5	T47.2x6
b-sitosterol(s)	T46.6x1	T46.6x2	T46.6x3	T46.6x4	T46.6x5	T46.6x6
Buclizine	T45.0x1	T45.0x2	T45.0x3	T45.0x4	T45.0x5	T45.0x6
Buclosamide	T49.0x1	T49.0x2	T49.0x3	T49.0x4	T49.0x5	T49.0x6
Budesonide	T44.5x1	T44.5x2	T44.5x3	T44.5x4	T44.5x5	T44.5x6
Budralazine	T46.5x1	T46.5x2	T46.5x3	T46.5x4	T46.5x5	T46.5x6
Bufferin	T39.011	T39.012	T39.013	T39.014	T39.015	T39.016
Buflomedil	T46.7x1	T46.7x2	T46.7x3	T46.7x4	T46.7x5	T46.7x6
Buformin	T38.3x1	T38.3x2	T38.3x3	T38.3x4	T38.3x5	T38.3x6
Bufotenine	T40.991	T40.992	T40.993	T40.994	T40.995	T40.996
Bufrolin	T48.6x1	T48.6x2	T48.6x3	T48.6x4	T48.6x5	T48.6x6
Bufylline	T48.6x1	T48.6x2	T48.6x3	T48.6x4	T48.6x5	T48.6x6
Bulk filler	T50.5x1	T50.5x2	T50.5x3	T50.5x4	T50.5x5	T50.5x6
cathartic	T47.4x1	T47.4x2	T47.4x3	T47.4x4	T47.4x5	T47.4x6
Bumetanide	T50.1x1	T50.1x2	T50.1x3	T50.1x4	T50.1x5	T50.1x6
Bunaftine	T46.2x1	T46.2x2	T46.2x3	T46.2x4	T46.2x5	T46.2x6
Bunamiodyl	T50.8x1	T50.8x2	T50.8x3	T50.8x4	T50.8x5	T50.8x6
Bunazosin	T44.6x1	T44.6x2	T44.6x3	T44.6x4	T44.6x5	T44.6x6
Bunitrolol	T44.7x1	T44.7x2	T44.7x3	T44.7x4	T44.7x5	T44.7x6
Buphenine	T46.7x1	T46.7x2	T46.7x3	T46.7x4	T46.7x5	T46.7x6
Bupivacaine	T41.3x1	T41.3x2	T41.3x3	T41.3x4	T41.3x5	T41.3x6
infiltration (subcutaneous)	T41.3x1	T41.3x2	T41.3x3	T41.3x4	T41.3x5	T41.3x6
nerve block (peripheral) (plexus)	T41.3x1	T41.3x2	T41.3x3	T41.3x4	T41.3x5	T41.3x6
spinal	T41.3x1	T41.3x2	T41.3x3	T41.3x4	T41.3x5	T41.3x6
Bupranolol	T44.7x1	T44.7x2	T44.7x3	T44.7x4	T44.7x5	T44.7x6
Buprenorphine	T40.4x1	T40.4x2	T40.4x3	T40.4x4	T40.4x5	T40.4x6

Substance	Poisoning, Accidental (unintentional)	Poisoning, Intentional Self-harm	Poisoning, Assault	Poisoning, Undetermined	Adverse Effect	Under-dosing
Bupropion	T43.291	T43.292	T43.293	T43.294	T43.295	T43.296
Burimamide	T47.1x1	T47.1x2	T47.1x3	T47.1x4	T47.1x5	T47.1x6
Buserelin	T38.891	T38.892	T38.893	T38.894	T38.895	T38.896
Buspirone	T43.591	T43.592	T43.593	T43.594	T43.595	T43.596
Busulfan, busulphan	T45.1x1	T45.1x2	T45.1x3	T45.1x4	T45.1x5	T45.1x6
Butabarbital (sodium)	T42.3x1	T42.3x2	T42.3x3	T42.3x4	T42.3x5	T42.3x6
Butabarbitone	T42.3x1	T42.3x2	T42.3x3	T42.3x4	T42.3x5	T42.3x6
Butabarpal	T42.3x1	T42.3x2	T42.3x3	T42.3x4	T42.3x5	T42.3x6
Butacaine	T41.3x1	T41.3x2	T41.3x3	T41.3x4	T41.3x5	T41.3x6
Butalamine	T46.7x1	T46.7x2	T46.7x3	T46.7x4	T46.7x5	T46.7x6
Butalbital	T42.3x1	T42.3x2	T42.3x3	T42.3x4	T42.3x5	T42.3x6
Butallylonal	T42.3x1	T42.3x2	T42.3x3	T42.3x4	T42.3x5	T42.3x6
Butamben	T41.3x1	T41.3x2	T41.3x3	T41.3x4	T41.3x5	T41.3x6
Butamirate	T48.3x1	T48.3x2	T48.3x3	T48.3x4	T48.3x5	T48.3x6
Butane (distributed in mobile container)	T59.891	T59.892	T59.893	T59.894	—	—
distributed through pipes	T59.891	T59.892	T59.893	T59.894	—	—
incomplete combustion	T58.11	T58.12	T58.13	T58.14	—	—
Butanilicaine	T41.3x1	T41.3x2	T41.3x3	T41.3x4	T41.3x5	T41.3x6
Butanol	T51.3x1	T51.3x2	T51.3x3	T51.3x4	—	—
Butanone, 2-butanone	T52.4x1	T52.4x2	T52.4x3	T52.4x4	—	—
Butantrone	T49.4x1	T49.4x2	T49.4x3	T49.4x4	T49.4x5	T49.4x6
Butaperazine	T43.3x1	T43.3x2	T43.3x3	T43.3x4	T43.3x5	T43.3x6
Butazolidin	T39.2x1	T39.2x2	T39.2x3	T39.2x4	T39.2x5	T39.2x6
Butetamate	T48.6x1	T48.6x2	T48.6x3	T48.6x4	T48.6x5	T48.6x6
Butethal	T42.3x1	T42.3x2	T42.3x3	T42.3x4	T42.3x5	T42.3x6
Butethamate	T44.3x1	T44.3x2	T44.3x3	T44.3x4	T44.3x5	T44.3x6
Buthalitone (sodium)	T41.1x1	T41.1x2	T41.1x3	T41.1x4	T41.1x5	T41.1x6
Butisol (sodium)	T42.3x1	T42.3x2	T42.3x3	T42.3x4	T42.3x5	T42.3x6
Butizide	T50.2x1	T50.2x2	T50.2x3	T50.2x4	T50.2x5	T50.2x6
Butobarbital	T42.3x1	T42.3x2	T42.3x3	T42.3x4	T42.3x5	T42.3x6
sodium	T42.3x1	T42.3x2	T42.3x3	T42.3x4	T42.3x5	T42.3x6
Butobarbitone	T42.3x1	T42.3x2	T42.3x3	T42.3x4	T42.3x5	T42.3x6
Butoconazole (nitrate)	T49.0x1	T49.0x2	T49.0x3	T49.0x4	T49.0x5	T49.0x6
Butorphanol	T40.4x1	T40.4x2	T40.4x3	T40.4x4	T40.4x5	T40.4x6
Butriptyline	T43.011	T43.012	T43.013	T43.014	T43.015	T43.016
Butropium bromide	T44.3x1	T44.3x2	T44.3x3	T44.3x4	T44.3x5	T44.3x6
Buttercups	T62.2x1	T62.2x2	T62.2x3	T62.2x4	—	—
Butter of antimony—see Antimony						
Butyl						
acetate (secondary)	T52.8x1	T52.8x2	T52.8x3	T52.8x4	—	—
alcohol	T51.3x1	T51.3x2	T51.3x3	T51.3x4	—	—
aminobenzoate	T41.3x1	T41.3x2	T41.3x3	T41.3x4	T41.3x5	T41.3x6
butyrate	T52.8x1	T52.8x2	T52.8x3	T52.8x4	—	—
carbinol	T51.3x1	T51.3x2	T51.3x3	T51.3x4	—	—
carbitol	T52.3x1	T52.3x2	T52.3x3	T52.3x4	—	—
cellosolve	T52.3x1	T52.3x2	T52.3x3	T52.3x4	—	—
chloral (hydrate)	T42.6x1	T42.6x2	T42.6x3	T42.6x4	T42.6x5	T42.6x6
formate	T52.8x1	T52.8x2	T52.8x3	T52.8x4	—	—
lactate	T52.8x1	T52.8x2	T52.8x3	T52.8x4	—	—
propionate	T52.8x1	T52.8x2	T52.8x3	T52.8x4	—	—
scopolamine bromide	T44.3x1	T44.3x2	T44.3x3	T44.3x4	T44.3x5	T44.3x6
thiobarbital sodium	T41.1x1	T41.1x2	T41.1x3	T41.1x4	T41.1x5	T41.1x6
Butylated hydroxy-anisole	T50.991	T50.992	T50.993	T50.994	T50.995	T50.996
Butylchloral hydrate	T42.6x1	T42.6x2	T42.6x3	T42.6x4	T42.6x5	T42.6x6
Butyltoluene	T52.2x1	T52.2x2	T52.2x3	T52.2x4	—	—
Butyn	T41.3x1	T41.3x2	T41.3x3	T41.3x4	T41.3x5	T41.3x6
Butyrophenone (-based tranquilizers)	T43.4x1	T43.4x2	T43.4x3	T43.4x4	T43.4x5	T43.4x6
Cabergoline	T42.8x1	T42.8x2	T42.8x3	T42.8x4	T42.8x5	T42.8x6
Cacodyl, cacodylic acid	T57.0x1	T57.0x2	T57.0x3	T57.0x4	—	—
Cactinomycin	T45.1x1	T45.1x2	T45.1x3	T45.1x4	T45.1x5	T45.1x6
Cade oil	T49.4x1	T49.4x2	T49.4x3	T49.4x4	T49.4x5	T49.4x6
Cadexomer iodine	T49.0x1	T49.0x2	T49.0x3	T49.0x4	T49.0x5	T49.0x6
Cadmium (chloride) (fumes) (oxide)	T56.3x1	T56.3x2	T56.3x3	T56.3x4	—	—
sulfide (medicinal) NEC	T49.4x1	T49.4x2	T49.4x3	T49.4x4	T49.4x5	T49.4x6
Cadralazine	T46.5x1	T46.5x2	T46.5x3	T46.5x4	T46.5x5	T46.5x6
Caffeine	T43.611	T43.612	T43.613	T43.614	T43.615	T43.616
Calabar bean	T62.2x1	T62.2x2	T62.2x3	T62.2x4	—	—

Substance	Poisoning, Accidental (unintentional)	Poisoning, Intentional Self-harm	Poisoning, Assault	Poisoning, Undetermined	Adverse Effect	Underdosing
Caladium seguinum	T62.2x1	T62.2x2	T62.2x3	T62.2x4	—	—
Calamine (lotion)	T49.3x1	T49.3x2	T49.3x3	T49.3x4	T49.3x5	T49.3x6
Calcifediol	T45.2x1	T45.2x2	T45.2x3	T45.2x4	T45.2x5	T45.2x6
Calciferol	T45.2x1	T45.2x2	T45.2x3	T45.2x4	T45.2x5	T45.2x6
Calcitonin	T50.991	T50.992	T50.993	T50.994	T50.995	T50.996
Calcitriol	T45.2x1	T45.2x2	T45.2x3	T45.2x4	T45.2x5	T45.2x6
Calcium	T50.3x1	T50.3x2	T50.3x3	T50.3x4	T50.3x5	T50.3x6
actylsalicylate	T39.011	T39.012	T39.013	T39.014	T39.015	T39.016
benzamidosalicylate	T37.1x1	T37.1x2	T37.1x3	T37.1x4	T37.1x5	T37.1x6
bromide	T42.6x1	T42.6x2	T42.6x3	T42.6x4	T42.6x5	T42.6x6
bromolactobionate	T42.6x1	T42.6x2	T42.6x3	T42.6x4	T42.6x5	T42.6x6
carbaspirin	T39.011	T39.012	T39.013	T39.014	T39.015	T39.016
carbimide	T50.6x1	T50.6x2	T50.6x3	T50.6x4	T50.6x5	T50.6x6
carbonate	T47.1x1	T47.1x2	T47.1x3	T47.1x4	T47.1x5	T47.1x6
chloride	T50.991	T50.992	T50.993	T50.994	T50.995	T50.996
anhydrous	T50.991	T50.992	T50.993	T50.994	T50.995	T50.996
cyanide	T57.8x1	T57.8x2	T57.8x3	T57.8x4		
dioctyl sulfosuccinate	T47.4x1	T47.4x2	T47.4x3	T47.4x4	T47.4x5	T47.4x6
disodium edathamil	T45.8x1	T45.8x2	T45.8x3	T45.8x4	T45.8x5	T45.8x6
disodium edetate	T45.8x1	T45.8x2	T45.8x3	T45.8x4	T45.8x5	T45.8x6
dobesilate	T46.991	T46.992	T46.993	T46.994	T46.995	T46.996
EDTA	T45.8x1	T45.8x2	T45.8x3	T45.8x4	T45.8x5	T45.8x6
ferrous citrate	T45.4x1	T45.4x2	T45.4x3	T45.4x4	T45.4x5	T45.4x6
folinate	T45.8x1	T45.8x2	T45.8x3	T45.8x4	T45.8x5	T45.8x6
glubionate	T50.3x1	T50.3x2	T50.3x3	T50.3x4	T50.3x5	T50.3x6
gluconate	T50.3x1	T50.3x2	T50.3x3	T50.3x4	T50.3x5	T50.3x6
gluconogalactogluconate	T50.3x1	T50.3x2	T50.3x3	T50.3x4	T50.3x5	T50.3x6
hydrate, hydroxide	T54.3x1	T54.3x2	T54.3x3	T54.3x4		
hypochlorite	T37.91	T37.92	T37.93	T37.94	T37.95	T37.96
iodide	T48.4x1	T48.4x2	T48.4x3	T48.4x4	T48.4x5	T48.4x6
ipodate	T50.8x1	T50.8x2	T50.8x3	T50.8x4	T50.8x5	T50.8x6
lactate	T50.3x1	T50.3x2	T50.3x3	T50.3x4	T50.3x5	T50.3x6
leucovorin	T45.8x1	T45.8x2	T45.8x3	T45.8x4	T45.8x5	T45.8x6
mandelate	T37.91	T37.92	T37.93	T37.94	T37.95	T37.96
oxide	T54.3x1	T54.3x2	T54.3x3	T54.3x4	—	—
pantothenate	T45.2x1	T45.2x2	T45.2x3	T45.2x4	T45.2x5	T45.2x6
phosphate	T50.3x1	T50.3x2	T50.3x3	T50.3x4	T50.3x5	T50.3x6
salicylate	T39.091	T39.092	T39.093	T39.094	T39.095	T39.096
salts	T50.3x1	T50.3x2	T50.3x3	T50.3x4	T50.3x5	T50.3x6
Calculus-dissolving drug	T50.991	T50.992	T50.993	T50.994	T50.995	T50.996
Calomel	T49.0x1	T49.0x2	T49.0x3	T49.0x4	T49.0x5	T49.0x6
Caloric agent	T50.3x1	T50.3x2	T50.3x3	T50.3x4	T50.3x5	T50.3x6
Calusterone	T38.7x1	T38.7x2	T38.7x3	T38.7x4	T38.7x5	T38.7x6
Camazepam	T42.4x1	T42.4x2	T42.4x3	T42.4x4	T42.4x5	T42.4x6
Camomile	T49.0x1	T49.0x2	T49.0x3	T49.0x4	T49.0x5	T49.0x6
Camoquin	T37.2x1	T37.2x2	T37.2x3	T37.2x4	T37.2x5	T37.2x6
Camphor						
insecticide	T60.2x1	T60.2x2	T60.2x3	T60.2x4	—	—
medicinal	T49.8x1	T49.8x2	T49.8x3	T49.8x4	T49.8x5	T49.8x6
Camylofin	T44.3x1	T44.3x2	T44.3x3	T44.3x4	T44.3x5	T44.3x6
Cancer chemotherapy drug regimen	T45.1x1	T45.1x2	T45.1x3	T45.1x4	T45.1x5	T45.1x6
Candeptin	T49.0x1	T49.0x2	T49.0x3	T49.0x4	T49.0x5	T49.0x6
Candicidin	T49.0x1	T49.0x2	T49.0x3	T49.0x4	T49.0x5	T49.0x6
Cannabinol	T40.7x1	T40.7x2	T40.7x3	T40.7x4	T40.7x5	T40.7x6
Cannabis (derivatives)	T40.7x1	T40.7x2	T40.7x3	T40.7x4	T40.7x5	T40.7x6
Canned heat	T51.1x1	T51.1x2	T51.1x3	T51.1x4	—	—
Canrenoic acid	T50.0x1	T50.0x2	T50.0x3	T50.0x4	T50.0x5	T50.0x6
Canrenone	T50.0x1	T50.0x2	T50.0x3	T50.0x4	T50.0x5	T50.0x6
Cantharides, cantharidin, cantharis	T49.8x1	T49.8x2	T49.8x3	T49.8x4	T49.8x5	T49.8x6
Canthaxanthin	T50.991	T50.992	T50.993	T50.994	T50.995	T50.996
Capillary-active drug NEC	T46.901	T46.902	T46.903	T46.904	T46.905	T46.906
Capreomycin	T36.8x1	T36.8x2	T36.8x3	T36.8x4	T36.8x5	T36.8x6
Capsicum	T49.4x1	T49.4x2	T49.4x3	T49.4x4	T49.4x5	T49.4x6
Captafol	T60.3x1	T60.3x2	T60.3x3	T60.3x4	—	—
Captan	T60.3x1	T60.3x2	T60.3x3	T60.3x4	—	—
Captodiame, captodiamine	T43.591	T43.592	T43.593	T43.594	T43.595	T43.596
Captopril	T46.4x1	T46.4x2	T46.4x3	T46.4x4	T46.4x5	T46.4x6
Caramiphen	T44.3x1	T44.3x2	T44.3x3	T44.3x4	T44.3x5	T44.3x6
Carazolol	T44.7x1	T44.7x2	T44.7x3	T44.7x4	T44.7x5	T44.7x6
Carbachol	T44.1x1	T44.1x2	T44.1x3	T44.1x4	T44.1x5	T44.1x6
Carbacrylamine (resin)	T50.3x1	T50.3x2	T50.3x3	T50.3x4	T50.3x5	T50.3x6
Carbamate (insecticide)	T60.0x1	T60.0x2	T60.0x3	T60.0x4	—	—
Carbamate (sedative)	T42.6x1	T42.6x2	T42.6x3	T42.6x4	T42.6x5	T42.6x6
herbicide	T60.0x1	T60.0x2	T60.0x3	T60.0x4	—	—
insecticide	T60.0x1	T60.0x2	T60.0x3	T60.0x4	—	—
Carbamazepine	T42.1x1	T42.1x2	T42.1x3	T42.1x4	T42.1x5	T42.1x6
Carbamide	T47.3x1	T47.3x2	T47.3x3	T47.3x4	T47.3x5	T47.3x6
peroxide	T49.0x1	T49.0x2	T49.0x3	T49.0x4	T49.0x5	T49.0x6
topical	T49.8x1	T49.8x2	T49.8x3	T49.8x4	T49.8x5	T49.8x6
Carbamylcholine chloride	T44.1x1	T44.1x2	T44.1x3	T44.1x4	T44.1x5	T44.1x6
Carbaril	T49.0x1	T49.0x2	T49.0x3	T49.0x4	T49.0x5	T49.0x6
Carbarsone	T37.3x1	T37.3x2	T37.3x3	T37.3x4	T37.3x5	T37.3x6
Carbaryl	T60.0x1	T60.0x2	T60.0x3	T60.0x4	—	—
Carbaspirin	T39.011	T39.012	T39.013	T39.014	T39.015	T39.016
Carbazochrome (salicylate) (sodium sulfonate)	T49.4x1	T49.4x2	T49.4x3	T49.4x4	T49.4x5	T49.4x6
Carbenicillin	T36.0x1	T36.0x2	T36.0x3	T36.0x4	T36.0x5	T36.0x6
Carbenoxolone	T47.1x1	T47.1x2	T47.1x3	T47.1x4	T47.1x5	T47.1x6
Carbetapentane	T48.3x1	T48.3x2	T48.3x3	T48.3x4	T48.3x5	T48.3x6
Carbethyl salicylate	T39.091	T39.092	T39.093	T39.094	T39.095	T39.096
Carbidopa (with levodopa)	T42.8x1	T42.8x2	T42.8x3	T42.8x4	T42.8x5	T42.8x6
Carbimazole	T38.2x1	T38.2x2	T38.2x3	T38.2x4	T38.2x5	T38.2x6
Carbinol	T51.1x1	T51.1x2	T51.1x3	T51.1x4	—	—
Carbinoxamine	T45.0x1	T45.0x2	T45.0x3	T45.0x4	T45.0x5	T45.0x6
Carbiphene	T39.8x1	T39.8x2	T39.8x3	T39.8x4	T39.8x5	T39.8x6
Carbitol	T52.3x1	T52.3x2	T52.3x3	T52.3x4	—	—
Carbocaine	T41.3x1	T41.3x2	T41.3x3	T41.3x4	T41.3x5	T41.3x6
infiltration (subcutaneous)	T41.3x1	T41.3x2	T41.3x3	T41.3x4	T41.3x5	T41.3x6
nerve block (peripheral) (plexus)	T41.3x1	T41.3x2	T41.3x3	T41.3x4	T41.3x5	T41.3x6
topical (surface)	T41.3x1	T41.3x2	T41.3x3	T41.3x4	T41.3x5	T41.3x6
Carbo medicinalis	T47.6x1	T47.6x2	T47.6x3	T47.6x4	T47.6x5	T47.6x6
Carbomycin	T36.8x1	T36.8x2	T36.8x3	T36.8x4	T36.8x5	T36.8x6
Carbocisteine	T48.4x1	T48.4x2	T48.4x3	T48.4x4	T48.4x5	T48.4x6
Carbocromen	T46.3x1	T46.3x2	T46.3x3	T46.3x4	T46.3x5	T46.3x6
Carbol fuchsin	T49.0x1	T49.0x2	T49.0x3	T49.0x4	T49.0x5	T49.0x6
Carbolic acid (see also Phenol)	T54.0x1	T54.0x2	T54.0x3	T54.0x4	—	—
Carbolonium (bromide)	T48.1x1	T48.1x2	T48.1x3	T48.1x4	T48.1x5	T48.1x6
Carbon						
bisulfide (liquid)	T65.4x1	T65.4x2	T65.4x3	T65.4x4	—	—
vapor	T65.4x1	T65.4x2	T65.4x3	T65.4x4	—	—
dioxide (gas)	T59.7x1	T59.7x2	T59.7x3	T59.7x4	—	—
medicinal	T41.5x1	T41.5x2	T41.5x3	T41.5x4	T41.5x5	T41.5x6
nonmedicinal	T59.7x1	T59.7x2	T59.7x3	T59.7x4	—	—
snow	T49.4x1	T49.4x2	T49.4x3	T49.4x4	T49.4x5	T49.4x6
disulfide (liquid)	T65.4x1	T65.4x2	T65.4x3	T65.4x4	—	—
vapor	T65.4x1	T65.4x2	T65.4x3	T65.4x4	—	—
monoxide (from incomplete combustion)	T58.91	T58.92	T58.93	T58.94		
blast furnace gas	T58.8x1	T58.8x2	T58.8x3	T58.8x4		
butane (distributed in mobile container)	T58.11	T58.12	T58.13	T58.14		
distributed through pipes	T58.11	T58.12	T58.13	T58.14		
charcoal fumes	T58.2x1	T58.2x2	T58.2x3	T58.2x4		
coal	T58.2x1	T58.2x2	T58.2x3	T58.2x4		
gas (piped)	T58.11	T58.12	T58.13	T58.14		
solid (in domestic stoves, fireplaces)	T58.2x1	T58.2x2	T58.2x3	T58.2x4		
coke (in domestic stoves, fireplaces)	T58.2x1	T58.2x2	T58.2x3	T58.2x4		
exhaust gas (motor)	T58.01	T58.02	T58.03	T58.04		
not in transit	T58.01	T58.02	T58.03	T58.04		
combustion engine, any not in watercraft	T58.01	T58.02	T58.03	T58.04		
farm tractor, not in transit	T58.01	T58.02	T58.03	T58.04		
gas engine	T58.01	T58.02	T58.03	T58.04		
motor pump	T58.01	T58.02	T58.03	T58.04		
motor vehicle, not in transit	T58.01	T58.02	T58.03	T58.04		
fuel (in domestic use)	T58.2x1	T58.2x2	T58.2x3	T58.2x4		
gas (piped)	T58.11	T58.12	T58.13	T58.14		
in mobile container	T58.11	T58.12	T58.13	T58.14		
utility	T58.11	T58.12	T58.13	T58.14		

Substance	Poisoning, Accidental (unintentional)	Poisoning, Intentional Self-harm	Poisoning, Assault	Poisoning, Undetermined	Adverse Effect	Under-dosing
Carbon—*continued*						
monoxide—*continued*						
fuel—*continued*						
utility—*continued*						
in mobile container	T58.11	T58.12	T58.13	T58.14	—	—
piped (natural)	T58.11	T58.12	T58.13	T58.14	—	—
illuminating gas	T58.11	T58.12	T58.13	T58.14	—	—
industrial fuels or gases, any	T58.8x1	T58.8x2	T58.8x3	T58.8x4	—	—
kerosene (in domestic stoves, fireplaces)	T58.2x1	T58.2x2	T58.2x3	T58.2x4	—	—
kiln gas or vapor	T58.8x1	T58.8x2	T58.8x3	T58.8x4	—	—
motor exhaust gas, not in transit	T58.Ø1	T58.Ø2	T58.Ø3	T58.Ø4	—	—
piped gas (manufactured) (natural)	T58.11	T58.12	T58.13	T58.14	—	—
producer gas	T58.8x1	T58.8x2	T58.8x3	T58.8x4	—	—
propane (distributed in mobile container)	T58.11	T58.12	T58.13	T58.14	—	—
distributed through pipes	T58.11	T58.12	T58.13	T58.14	—	—
specified source NEC	T58.8x1	T58.8x2	T58.8x3	T58.8x4	—	—
stove gas	T58.11	T58.12	T58.13	T58.14	—	—
piped	T58.11	T58.12	T58.13	T58.14	—	—
utility gas	T58.11	T58.12	T58.13	T58.14	—	—
piped	T58.11	T58.12	T58.13	T58.14	—	—
water gas	T58.8x1	T58.8x2	T58.8x3	T58.8x4	—	—
wood (in domestic stoves, fireplaces)	T58.2x1	T58.2x2	T58.2x3	T58.2x4	—	—
tetrachloride (vapor) NEC	T53.Øx1	T53.Øx2	T53.Øx3	T53.Øx4	—	—
liquid (cleansing agent) NEC	T53.Øx1	T53.Øx2	T53.Øx3	T53.Øx4	—	—
solvent	T53.Øx1	T53.Øx2	T53.Øx3	T53.Øx4	—	—
Carbonic acid gas	T59.7x1	T59.7x2	T59.7x3	T59.7x4	—	—
anhydrase inhibitor NEC	T5Ø.2x1	T5Ø.2x2	T5Ø.2x3	T5Ø.2x4	T5Ø.2x5	T5Ø.2x6
Carbophenothion	T6Ø.Øx1	T6Ø.Øx2	T6Ø.Øx3	T6Ø.Øx4	—	—
Carboplatin	T45.1x1	T45.1x2	T45.1x3	T45.1x4	T45.1x5	T45.1x6
Carboprost	T48.Øx1	T48.Øx2	T48.Øx3	T48.Øx4	T48.Øx5	T48.Øx6
Carboquone	T45.1x1	T45.1x2	T45.1x3	T45.1x4	T45.1x5	T45.1x6
Carbowax	T49.3x1	T49.3x2	T49.3x3	T49.3x4	T49.3x5	T49.3x6
Carboxymethyl-cellulose	T47.4x1	T47.4x2	T47.4x3	T47.4x4	T47.4x5	T47.4x6
Carbrital	T42.3x1	T42.3x2	T42.3x3	T42.3x4	T42.3x5	T42.3x6
Carbromal	T42.6x1	T42.6x2	T42.6x3	T42.6x4	T42.6x5	T42.6x6
Carbutamide	T38.3x1	T38.3x2	T38.3x3	T38.3x4	T38.3x5	T38.3x6
Carbuterol	T48.6x1	T48.6x2	T48.6x3	T48.6x4	T48.6x5	T48.6x6
Cardiac rhythm regulator NEC	T46.2x1	T46.2x2	T46.2x3	T46.2x4	T46.2x5	T46.2x6
specified NEC	T46.2x1	T46.2x2	T46.2x3	T46.2x4	T46.2x5	T46.2x6
Cardiac						
depressants	T46.2x1	T46.2x2	T46.2x3	T46.2x4	T46.2x5	T46.2x6
rhythm regulators	T46.2x1	T46.2x2	T46.2x3	T46.2x4	T46.2x5	T46.2x6
Cardiografin	T5Ø.8x1	T5Ø.8x2	T5Ø.8x3	T5Ø.8x4	T5Ø.8x5	T5Ø.8x6
Cardio-green	T5Ø.8x1	T5Ø.8x2	T5Ø.8x3	T5Ø.8x4	T5Ø.8x5	T5Ø.8x6
Cardiotonic (glycoside) **NEC**	T46.Øx1	T46.Øx2	T46.Øx3	T46.Øx4	T46.Øx5	T46.Øx6
Cardiovascular drug NEC	T46.9Ø1	T46.9Ø2	T46.9Ø3	T46.9Ø4	T46.9Ø5	T46.9Ø6
Cardrase	T5Ø.2x1	T5Ø.2x2	T5Ø.2x3	T5Ø.2x4	T5Ø.2x5	T5Ø.2x6
Carfusin	T49.Øx1	T49.Øx2	T49.Øx3	T49.Øx4	T49.Øx5	T49.Øx6
Carfecillin	T36.Øx1	T36.Øx2	T36.Øx3	T36.Øx4	T36.Øx5	T36.Øx6
Carfenazine	T43.3x1	T43.3x2	T43.3x3	T43.3x4	T43.3x5	T43.3x6
Carindacillin	T36.Øx1	T36.Øx2	T36.Øx3	T36.Øx4	T36.Øx5	T36.Øx6
Carisoprodol	T42.8x1	T42.8x2	T42.8x3	T42.8x4	T42.8x5	T42.8x6
Carmellose	T47.4x1	T47.4x2	T47.4x3	T47.4x4	T47.4x5	T47.4x6
Carminative	T47.5x1	T47.5x2	T47.5x3	T47.5x4	T47.5x5	T47.5x6
Carmofur	T45.1x1	T45.1x2	T45.1x3	T45.1x4	T45.1x5	T45.1x6
Carmustine	T45.1x1	T45.1x2	T45.1x3	T45.1x4	T45.1x5	T45.1x6
Carotene	T45.2x1	T45.2x2	T45.2x3	T45.2x4	T45.2x5	T45.2x6
Carphenazine	T43.3x1	T43.3x2	T43.3x3	T43.3x4	T43.3x5	T43.3x6
Carpipramine	T42.4x1	T42.4x2	T42.4x3	T42.4x4	T42.4x5	T42.4x6
Carprofen	T39.311	T39.312	T39.313	T39.314	T39.315	T39.316
Carpronium chloride	T44.3x1	T44.3x2	T44.3x3	T44.3x4	T44.3x5	T44.3x6
Carrageenan	T47.8x1	T47.8x2	T47.8x3	T47.8x4	T47.8x5	T47.8x6
Carteolol	T44.7x1	T44.7x2	T44.7x3	T44.7x4	T44.7x5	T44.7x6
Carter's Little Pills	T47.2x1	T47.2x2	T47.2x3	T47.2x4	T47.2x5	T47.2x6
Cascara (sagrada)	T47.2x1	T47.2x2	T47.2x3	T47.2x4	T47.2x5	T47.2x6
Cassava	T62.2x1	T62.2x2	T62.2x3	T62.2x4	—	—
Castellani's paint	T49.Øx1	T49.Øx2	T49.Øx3	T49.Øx4	T49.Øx5	T49.Øx6
Castor						
bean	T62.2x1	T62.2x2	T62.2x3	T62.2x4	—	—
oil	T47.2x1	T47.2x2	T47.2x3	T47.2x4	T47.2x5	T47.2x6
Catalase	T45.3x1	T45.3x2	T45.3x3	T45.3x4	T45.3x5	T45.3x6
Caterpillar (sting)	T63.431	T63.432	T63.433	T63.434	—	—
Catha (edulis) (tea)	T43.691	T43.692	T43.693	T43.694	—	—
Cathartic NEC	T47.4x1	T47.4x2	T47.4x3	T47.4x4	T47.4x5	T47.4x6
anthracene derivative	T47.2x1	T47.2x2	T47.2x3	T47.2x4	T47.2x5	T47.2x6
bulk	T47.4x1	T47.4x2	T47.4x3	T47.4x4	T47.4x5	T47.4x6
contact	T47.2x1	T47.2x2	T47.2x3	T47.2x4	T47.2x5	T47.2x6
emollient NEC	T47.4x1	T47.4x2	T47.4x3	T47.4x4	T47.4x5	T47.4x6
irritant NEC	T47.2x1	T47.2x2	T47.2x3	T47.2x4	T47.2x5	T47.2x6
mucilage	T47.4x1	T47.4x2	T47.4x3	T47.4x4	T47.4x5	T47.4x6
saline	T47.3x1	T47.3x2	T47.3x3	T47.3x4	T47.3x5	T47.3x6
vegetable	T47.2x1	T47.2x2	T47.2x3	T47.2x4	T47.2x5	T47.2x6
Cathine	T5Ø.5x1	T5Ø.5x2	T5Ø.5x3	T5Ø.5x4	T5Ø.5x5	T5Ø.5x6
Cathomycin	T36.8x1	T36.8x2	T36.8x3	T36.8x4	T36.8x5	T36.8x6
Cation exchange resin	T5Ø.3x1	T5Ø.3x2	T5Ø.3x3	T5Ø.3x4	T5Ø.3x5	T5Ø.3x6
Caustic(s) NEC	T54.91	T54.92	T54.93	T54.94	—	—
alkali	T54.3x1	T54.3x2	T54.3x3	T54.3x4	—	—
hydroxide	T54.3x1	T54.3x2	T54.3x3	T54.3x4	—	—
potash	T54.3x1	T54.3x2	T54.3x3	T54.3x4	—	—
specified NEC	T54.91	T54.92	T54.93	T54.94	—	—
soda	T54.3x1	T54.3x2	T54.3x3	T54.3x4	—	—
Ceepryn	T49.Øx1	T49.Øx2	T49.Øx3	T49.Øx4	T49.Øx5	T49.Øx6
ENT agent	T49.6x1	T49.6x2	T49.6x3	T49.6x4	T49.6x5	T49.6x6
lozenges	T49.6x1	T49.6x2	T49.6x3	T49.6x4	T49.6x5	T49.6x6
Cefacetrile	T36.1x1	T36.1x2	T36.1x3	T36.1x4	T36.1x5	T36.1x6
Cefaclor	T36.1x1	T36.1x2	T36.1x3	T36.1x4	T36.1x5	T36.1x6
Cefadroxil	T36.1x1	T36.1x2	T36.1x3	T36.1x4	T36.1x5	T36.1x6
Cefalexin	T36.1x1	T36.1x2	T36.1x3	T36.1x4	T36.1x5	T36.1x6
Cefaloglycin	T36.1x1	T36.1x2	T36.1x3	T36.1x4	T36.1x5	T36.1x6
Cefaloridine	T36.1x1	T36.1x2	T36.1x3	T36.1x4	T36.1x5	T36.1x6
Cefalosporins	T36.1x1	T36.1x2	T36.1x3	T36.1x4	T36.1x5	T36.1x6
Cefalotin	T36.1x1	T36.1x2	T36.1x3	T36.1x4	T36.1x5	T36.1x6
Cefamandole	T36.1x1	T36.1x2	T36.1x3	T36.1x4	T36.1x5	T36.1x6
Cefamycin antibiotic	T36.1x1	T36.1x2	T36.1x3	T36.1x4	T36.1x5	T36.1x6
Cefapirin	T36.1x1	T36.1x2	T36.1x3	T36.1x4	T36.1x5	T36.1x6
Cefatrizine	T36.1x1	T36.1x2	T36.1x3	T36.1x4	T36.1x5	T36.1x6
Cefazedone	T36.1x1	T36.1x2	T36.1x3	T36.1x4	T36.1x5	T36.1x6
Cefazolin	T36.1x1	T36.1x2	T36.1x3	T36.1x4	T36.1x5	T36.1x6
Cefbuperazone	T36.1x1	T36.1x2	T36.1x3	T36.1x4	T36.1x5	T36.1x6
Cefetamet	T36.1x1	T36.1x2	T36.1x3	T36.1x4	T36.1x5	T36.1x6
Cefixime	T36.1x1	T36.1x2	T36.1x3	T36.1x4	T36.1x5	T36.1x6
Cefmenoxime	T36.1x1	T36.1x2	T36.1x3	T36.1x4	T36.1x5	T36.1x6
Cefmetazole	T36.1x1	T36.1x2	T36.1x3	T36.1x4	T36.1x5	T36.1x6
Cefminox	T36.1x1	T36.1x2	T36.1x3	T36.1x4	T36.1x5	T36.1x6
Cefonicid	T36.1x1	T36.1x2	T36.1x3	T36.1x4	T36.1x5	T36.1x6
Cefoperazone	T36.1x1	T36.1x2	T36.1x3	T36.1x4	T36.1x5	T36.1x6
Ceforanide	T36.1x1	T36.1x2	T36.1x3	T36.1x4	T36.1x5	T36.1x6
Cefotaxime	T36.1x1	T36.1x2	T36.1x3	T36.1x4	T36.1x5	T36.1x6
Cefotetan	T36.1x1	T36.1x2	T36.1x3	T36.1x4	T36.1x5	T36.1x6
Cefotiam	T36.1x1	T36.1x2	T36.1x3	T36.1x4	T36.1x5	T36.1x6
Cefoxitin	T36.1x1	T36.1x2	T36.1x3	T36.1x4	T36.1x5	T36.1x6
Cefpimizole	T36.1x1	T36.1x2	T36.1x3	T36.1x4	T36.1x5	T36.1x6
Cefpiramide	T36.1x1	T36.1x2	T36.1x3	T36.1x4	T36.1x5	T36.1x6
Cefradine	T36.1x1	T36.1x2	T36.1x3	T36.1x4	T36.1x5	T36.1x6
Cefroxadine	T36.1x1	T36.1x2	T36.1x3	T36.1x4	T36.1x5	T36.1x6
Cefsulodin	T36.1x1	T36.1x2	T36.1x3	T36.1x4	T36.1x5	T36.1x6
Ceftazidime	T36.1x1	T36.1x2	T36.1x3	T36.1x4	T36.1x5	T36.1x6
Cefteram	T36.1x1	T36.1x2	T36.1x3	T36.1x4	T36.1x5	T36.1x6
Ceftezole	T36.1x1	T36.1x2	T36.1x3	T36.1x4	T36.1x5	T36.1x6
Ceftizoxime	T36.1x1	T36.1x2	T36.1x3	T36.1x4	T36.1x5	T36.1x6
Ceftriaxone	T36.1x1	T36.1x2	T36.1x3	T36.1x4	T36.1x5	T36.1x6
Cefuroxime	T36.1x1	T36.1x2	T36.1x3	T36.1x4	T36.1x5	T36.1x6
Cefuzonam	T36.1x1	T36.1x2	T36.1x3	T36.1x4	T36.1x5	T36.1x6
Celestone	T38.Øx1	T38.Øx2	T38.Øx3	T38.Øx4	T38.Øx5	T38.Øx6
topical	T49.Øx1	T49.Øx2	T49.Øx3	T49.Øx4	T49.Øx5	T49.Øx6
Celiprolol	T44.7x1	T44.7x2	T44.7x3	T44.7x4	T44.7x5	T44.7x6
Cellosolve	T52.91	T52.92	T52.93	T52.94	—	—
Cell stimulants and proliferants	T49.8x1	T49.8x2	T49.8x3	T49.8x4	T49.8x5	T49.8x6

Substance	Poisoning, Accidental (unintentional)	Poisoning, Intentional Self-harm	Poisoning, Assault	Poisoning, Undetermined	Adverse Effect	Under-dosing
Cellulose	T47.4x1	T47.4x2	T47.4x3	T47.4x4	T47.4x5	T47.4x6
cathartic	T47.4x1	T47.4x2	T47.4x3	T47.4x4	T47.4x5	T47.4x6
hydroxyethyl	T47.4x1	T47.4x2	T47.4x3	T47.4x4	T47.4x5	T47.4x6
nitrates (topical)	T49.3x1	T49.3x2	T49.3x3	T49.3x4	T49.3x5	T49.3x6
oxidized	T49.4x1	T49.4x2	T49.4x3	T49.4x4	T49.4x5	T49.4x6
Centipede (bite)	T63.411	T63.412	T63.413	T63.414	—	—
Central nervous system						
depressants	T41.201	T41.202	T41.203	T41.204	T41.205	T41.206
anesthetic (general) NEC	T41.201	T41.202	T41.203	T41.204	T41.205	T41.206
gases NEC	T41.0x1	T41.0x2	T41.0x3	T41.0x4	T41.0x5	T41.0x6
intravenous	T41.1x1	T41.1x2	T41.1x3	T41.1x4	T41.1x5	T41.1x6
barbiturates	T42.3x1	T42.3x2	T42.3x3	T42.3x4	T42.3x5	T42.3x6
benzodiazepines	T42.4x1	T42.4x2	T42.4x3	T42.4x4	T42.4x5	T42.4x6
bromides	T42.6x1	T42.6x2	T42.6x3	T42.6x4	T42.6x5	T42.6x6
cannabis sativa	T40.7x1	T40.7x2	T40.7x3	T40.7x4	T40.7x5	T40.7x6
chloral hydrate	T42.6x1	T42.6x2	T42.6x3	T42.6x4	T42.6x5	T42.6x6
ethanol	T51.0x1	T51.0x2	T51.0x3	T51.0x4	—	—
hallucinogenics	T40.901	T40.902	T40.903	T40.904	T40.905	T40.906
hypnotics	T42.71	T42.72	T42.73	T42.74	T42.75	T42.76
specified NEC	T42.6x1	T42.6x2	T42.6x3	T42.6x4	T42.6x5	T42.6x6
muscle relaxants	T42.8x1	T42.8x2	T42.8x3	T42.8x4	T42.8x5	T42.8x6
paraldehyde	T42.6x1	T42.6x2	T42.6x3	T42.6x4	T42.6x5	T42.6x6
sedatives; sedative-hypnotics						
mixed NEC	T42.71	T42.72	T42.73	T42.74	T42.75	T42.76
specified NEC	T42.6x1	T42.6x2	T42.6x3	T42.6x4	T42.6x5	T42.6x6
muscle-tone depressants	T42.8x1	T42.8x2	T42.8x3	T42.8x4	T42.8x5	T42.8x6
stimulants	T43.601	T43.602	T43.603	T43.604	T43.605	T43.606
amphetamines	T43.621	T43.622	T43.623	T43.624	T43.625	T43.626
analeptics	T50.7x1	T50.7x2	T50.7x3	T50.7x4	T50.7x5	T50.7x6
antidepressants	T43.201	T43.202	T43.203	T43.204	T43.205	T43.206
opiate antagonists	T50.7x1	T50.7x2	T50.7x3	T50.7x4	T50.7x5	T50.7x6
specified NEC	T43.691	T43.692	T43.693	T43.694	T43.695	T43.696
Cephalexin	T36.1x1	T36.1x2	T36.1x3	T36.1x4	T36.1x5	T36.1x6
Cephaloglycin	T36.1x1	T36.1x2	T36.1x3	T36.1x4	T36.1x5	T36.1x6
Cephaloridine	T36.1x1	T36.1x2	T36.1x3	T36.1x4	T36.1x5	T36.1x6
Cephalosporins	T36.1x1	T36.1x2	T36.1x3	T36.1x4	T36.1x5	T36.1x6
N (adicillin)	T36.0x1	T36.0x2	T36.0x3	T36.0x4	T36.0x5	T36.0x6
Cephalothin	T36.1x1	T36.1x2	T36.1x3	T36.1x4	T36.1x5	T36.1x6
Cephalotin	T36.1x1	T36.1x2	T36.1x3	T36.1x4	T36.1x5	T36.1x6
Cephradine	T36.1x1	T36.1x2	T36.1x3	T36.1x4	T36.1x5	T36.1x6
Cerbera (odallam)	T62.2x1	T62.2x2	T62.2x3	T62.2x4	—	—
Cerberin	T46.0x1	T46.0x2	T46.0x3	T46.0x4	T46.0x5	T46.0x6
Cerebral stimulants	T43.601	T43.602	T43.603	T43.604	T43.605	T43.606
psychotherapeutic	T43.601	T43.602	T43.603	T43.604	T43.605	T43.606
specified NEC	T43.691	T43.692	T43.693	T43.694	T43.695	T43.696
Cerium oxalate	T45.0x1	T45.0x2	T45.0x3	T45.0x4	T45.0x5	T45.0x6
Cerous oxalate	T45.0x1	T45.0x2	T45.0x3	T45.0x4	T45.0x5	T45.0x6
Ceruletide	T50.8x1	T50.8x2	T50.8x3	T50.8x4	T50.8x5	T50.8x6
Cetalkonium (chloride)	T49.0x1	T49.0x2	T49.0x3	T49.0x4	T49.0x5	T49.0x6
Cethexonium chloride	T49.0x1	T49.0x2	T49.0x3	T49.0x4	T49.0x5	T49.0x6
Cetiedil	T46.7x1	T46.7x2	T46.7x3	T46.7x4	T46.7x5	T46.7x6
Cetirizine	T45.0x1	T45.0x2	T45.0x3	T45.0x4	T45.0x5	T45.0x6
Cetomacrogol	T50.991	T50.992	T50.993	T50.994	T50.995	T50.996
Cetotiamine	T45.2x1	T45.2x2	T45.2x3	T45.2x4	T45.2x5	T45.2x6
Cetoxime	T45.0x1	T45.0x2	T45.0x3	T45.0x4	T45.0x5	T45.0x6
Cetraxate	T47.1x1	T47.1x2	T47.1x3	T47.1x4	T47.1x5	T47.1x6
Cetrimide	T49.0x1	T49.0x2	T49.0x3	T49.0x4	T49.0x5	T49.0x6
Cetrimonium (bromide)	T49.0x1	T49.0x2	T49.0x3	T49.0x4	T49.0x5	T49.0x6
Cetylpyridinium chloride	T49.0x1	T49.0x2	T49.0x3	T49.0x4	T49.0x5	T49.0x6
ENT agent	T49.6x1	T49.6x2	T49.6x3	T49.6x4	T49.6x5	T49.6x6
lozenges	T49.6x1	T49.6x2	T49.6x3	T49.6x4	T49.6x5	T49.6x6
Cevadilla—see Sabadilla						
Cevitamic acid	T45.2x1	T45.2x2	T45.2x3	T45.2x4	T45.2x5	T45.2x6
Chalk, precipitated	T47.1x1	T47.1x2	T47.1x3	T47.1x4	T47.1x5	T47.1x6
Chamomile	T49.0x1	T49.0x2	T49.0x3	T49.0x4	T49.0x5	T49.0x6
Ch'an su	T46.0x1	T46.0x2	T46.0x3	T46.0x4	T46.0x5	T46.0x6
Charcoal	T47.6x1	T47.6x2	T47.6x3	T47.6x4	T47.6x5	T47.6x6
activated	T47.6x1	T47.6x2	T47.6x3	T47.6x4	T47.6x5	T47.6x6
fumes (Carbon monoxide)	T58.2x1	T58.2x2	T58.2x3	T58.2x4	—	—
industrial	T58.8x1	T58.8x2	T58.8x3	T58.8x4	—	—
medicinal (activated)	T47.8x1	T47.8x2	T47.8x3	T47.8x4	T47.8x5	T47.8x6

Substance	Poisoning, Accidental (unintentional)	Poisoning, Intentional Self-harm	Poisoning, Assault	Poisoning, Undetermined	Adverse Effect	Under-dosing
Chaulmosulfone	T37.1x1	T37.1x2	T37.1x3	T37.1x4	T37.1x5	T37.1x6
Chelating agent NEC	T50.6x1	T50.6x2	T50.6x3	T50.6x4	T50.6x5	T50.6x6
Chelidonium majus	T62.2x1	T62.2x2	T62.2x3	T62.2x4	—	—
Chemical substance NEC	T65.91	T65.92	T65.93	T65.94	—	—
Chenodeoxycholic acid	T47.5x1	T47.5x2	T47.5x3	T47.5x4	T47.5x5	T47.5x6
Chenodiol	T47.5x1	T47.5x2	T47.5x3	T47.5x4	T47.5x5	T47.5x6
Chenopodium	T37.4x1	T37.4x2	T37.4x3	T37.4x4	T37.4x5	T37.4x6
Cherry laurel	T62.2x1	T62.2x2	T62.2x3	T62.2x4		
Chinidin(e)	T46.2x1	T46.2x2	T46.2x3	T46.2x4		T46.2x6
Chiniofon	T37.8x1	T37.8x2	T37.8x3	T37.8x4	T37.8x5	T37.8x6
Chlophedianol	T48.3x1	T48.3x2	T48.3x3	T48.3x4	T48.3x5	T48.3x6
Chloral (betaine) (formamide) (hydrate)	T42.6x1	T42.6x2	T42.6x3	T42.6x4	T42.6x5	T42.6x6
Chloral	T42.6x1	T42.6x2	T42.6x3	T42.6x4	T42.6x5	T42.6x6
derivative	T42.6x1	T42.6x2	T42.6x3	T42.6x4	T42.6x5	T42.6x6
hydrate	T42.6x1	T42.6x2	T42.6x3	T42.6x4	T42.6x5	T42.6x6
Chloralamide	T42.6x1	T42.6x2	T42.6x3	T42.6x4	T42.6x5	T42.6x6
Chloralodol	T42.6x1	T42.6x2	T42.6x3	T42.6x4	T42.6x5	T42.6x6
Chloralose	T60.4x1	T60.4x2	T60.4x3	T60.4x4	—	—
Chlorambucil	T45.1x1	T45.1x2	T45.1x3	T45.1x4	T45.1x5	T45.1x6
Chloramine (-T)	T49.0x1	T49.0x2	T49.0x3	T49.0x4	T49.0x5	T49.0x6
Chloramphenicol	T36.2x1	T36.2x2	T36.2x3	T36.2x4	T36.2x5	T36.2x6
ENT agent	T49.6x1	T49.6x2	T49.6x3	T49.6x4	T49.6x5	T49.6x6
ophthalmic preparation	T49.5x1	T49.5x2	T49.5x3	T49.5x4	T49.5x5	T49.5x6
topical NEC	T49.0x1	T49.0x2	T49.0x3	T49.0x4	T49.0x5	T49.0x6
Chloramphencolum	T36.2x1	T36.2x2	T36.2x3	T36.2x4	T36.2x5	T36.2x6
Chlorate (potassium) (sodium) NEC	T60.3x1	T60.3x2	T60.3x3	T60.3x4	—	—
herbicide	T60.3x1	T60.3x2	T60.3x3	T60.3x4	—	—
Chlorazanil	T50.2x1	T50.2x2	T50.2x3	T50.2x4	T50.2x5	T50.2x6
Chlorbenzene, chlorbenzol	T53.7x1	T53.7x2	T53.7x3	T53.7x4	—	—
Chlorbenzoxamine	T44.3x1	T44.3x2	T44.3x3	T44.3x4	T44.3x5	T44.3x6
Chlorbutol	T42.6x1	T42.6x2	T42.6x3	T42.6x4	T42.6x5	T42.6x6
Chlorcyclizine	T45.0x1	T45.0x2	T45.0x3	T45.0x4	T45.0x5	T45.0x6
Chlordan(e) (dust)	T60.1x1	T60.1x2	T60.1x3	T60.1x4	—	—
Chlordantoin	T49.0x1	T49.0x2	T49.0x3	T49.0x4	T49.0x5	T49.0x6
Chlordiazepoxide	T42.4x1	T42.4x2	T42.4x3	T42.4x4	T42.4x5	T42.4x6
Chlordiethyl benzamide	T49.3x1	T49.3x2	T49.3x3	T49.3x4	T49.3x5	T49.3x6
Chloresium	T49.8x1	T49.8x2	T49.8x3	T49.8x4	T49.8x5	T49.8x6
Chlorethiazol	T42.6x1	T42.6x2	T42.6x3	T42.6x4	T42.6x5	T42.6x6
Chlorethyl—see Ethyl chloride						
Chloretone	T42.6x1	T42.6x2	T42.6x3	T42.6x4	T42.6x5	T42.6x6
Chlorex	T53.6x1	T53.6x2	T53.6x3	T53.6x4	—	—
insecticide	T60.1x1	T60.1x2	T60.1x3	T60.1x4	—	—
Chlorfenvinphos	T60.0x1	T60.0x2	T60.0x3	T60.0x4	—	—
Chlorhexadol	T42.6x1	T42.6x2	T42.6x3	T42.6x4	T42.6x5	T42.6x6
Chlorhexamide	T45.1x1	T45.1x2	T45.1x3	T45.1x4	T45.1x5	T45.1x6
Chlorhexidine	T49.0x1	T49.0x2	T49.0x3	T49.0x4	T49.0x5	T49.0x6
Chlorhydroxyquinolin	T49.0x1	T49.0x2	T49.0x3	T49.0x4	T49.0x5	T49.0x6
Chloride of lime (bleach)	T54.3x1	T54.3x2	T54.3x3	T54.3x4	—	—
Chlorimipramine	T43.011	T43.012	T43.013	T43.014	T43.015	T43.016
Chlorinated						
camphene	T53.6x1	T53.6x2	T53.6x3	T53.6x4	—	—
diphenyl	T53.7x1	T53.7x2	T53.7x3	T53.7x4	—	—
hydrocarbons NEC	T53.91	T53.92	T53.93	T53.94	—	—
solvents	T53.91	T53.92	T53.93	T53.94	—	—
lime (bleach)	T54.3x1	T54.3x2	T54.3x3	T54.3x4	—	—
and boric acid solution	T49.0x1	T49.0x2	T49.0x3	T49.0x4	T49.0x5	T49.0x6
naphthalene (insecticide)	T60.1x1	T60.1x2	T60.1x3	T60.1x4	—	—
industrial (non-pesticide)	T53.7x1	T53.7x2	T53.7x3	T53.7x4	—	—
pesticide NEC	T60.8x1	T60.8x2	T60.8x3	T60.8x4	—	—
soda (see also sodium hypochlorite)						
solution	T49.0x1	T49.0x2	T49.0x3	T49.0x4	T49.0x5	T49.0x6
Chlorine (fumes) (gas)	T59.4x1	T59.4x2	T59.4x3	T59.4x4	—	—
bleach	T54.3x1	T54.3x2	T54.3x3	T54.3x4	—	—
compound gas NEC	T59.4x1	T59.4x2	T59.4x3	T59.4x4	—	—
disinfectant	T59.4x1	T59.4x2	T59.4x3	T59.4x4	—	—
releasing agents NEC	T59.4x1	T59.4x2	T59.4x3	T59.4x4	—	—
Chlorisondamine chloride	T46.991	T46.992	T46.993	T46.994	T46.995	T46.996
Chlormadinone	T38.5x1	T38.5x2	T38.5x3	T38.5x4	T38.5x5	T38.5x6

Substance	Poisoning, Accidental (unintentional)	Poisoning, Intentional Self-harm	Poisoning, Assault	Poisoning, Undetermined	Adverse Effect	Under-dosing
Chlormephos	T60.0x1	T60.0x2	T60.0x3	T60.0x4	—	—
Chlormerodrin	T50.2x1	T50.2x2	T50.2x3	T50.2x4	T50.2x5	T50.2x6
Chlormethiazole	T42.6x1	T42.6x2	T42.6x3	T42.6x4	T42.6x5	T42.6x6
Chlormethine	T45.1x1	T45.1x2	T45.1x3	T45.1x4	T45.1x5	T45.1x6
Chlormethylenecycline	T36.4x1	T36.4x2	T36.4x3	T36.4x4	T36.4x5	T36.4x6
Chlormezanone	T42.6x1	T42.6x2	T42.6x3	T42.6x4	T42.6x5	T42.6x6
Chloroacetic acid	T60.3x1	T60.3x2	T60.3x3	T60.3x4	—	—
Chloroacetone	T59.3x1	T59.3x2	T59.3x3	T59.3x4	—	—
Chloroacetophenone	T59.3x1	T59.3x2	T59.3x3	T59.3x4	—	—
Chloroaniline	T53.7x1	T53.7x2	T53.7x3	T53.7x4	—	—
Chlorobenzene, chlorobenzol	T53.7x1	T53.7x2	T53.7x3	T53.7x4	—	—
Chlorobromomethane (fire extinguisher)	T53.6x1	T53.6x2	T53.6x3	T53.6x4	—	—
Chlorobutanol	T49.0x1	T49.0x2	T49.0x3	T49.0x4	T49.0x5	T49.0x6
Chlorocresol	T49.0x1	T49.0x2	T49.0x3	T49.0x4	T49.0x5	T49.0x6
Chlorodehydro-methyltestosterone	T38.7x1	T38.7x2	T38.7x3	T38.7x4	T38.7x5	T38.7x6
Chlorodinitrobenzene	T53.7x1	T53.7x2	T53.7x3	T53.7x4	—	—
dust or vapor	T53.7x1	T53.7x2	T53.7x3	T53.7x4	—	—
Chlorodiphenyl	T53.7x1	T53.7x2	T53.7x3	T53.7x4	—	—
Chloroethane—see Ethyl chloride						
Chloroethylene	T53.6x1	T53.6x2	T53.6x3	T53.6x4	—	—
Chlorofluorocarbons	T53.5x1	T53.5x2	T53.5x3	T53.5x4	—	—
Chloroform (fumes) (vapor)	T53.1x1	T53.1x2	T53.1x3	T53.1x4	—	—
anesthetic	T41.0x1	T41.0x2	T41.0x3	T41.0x4	T41.0x5	T41.0x6
solvent	T53.1x1	T53.1x2	T53.1x3	T53.1x4	—	—
water, concentrated	T41.0x1	T41.0x2	T41.0x3	T41.0x4	T41.0x5	T41.0x6
Chloroguanide	T37.2x1	T37.2x2	T37.2x3	T37.2x4	T37.2x5	T37.2x6
Chloromycetin	T36.2x1	T36.2x2	T36.2x3	T36.2x4	T36.2x5	T36.2x6
ENT agent	T49.6x1	T49.6x2	T49.6x3	T49.6x4	T49.6x5	T49.6x6
ophthalmic preparation	T49.5x1	T49.5x2	T49.5x3	T49.5x4	T49.5x5	T49.5x6
otic solution	T49.6x1	T49.6x2	T49.6x3	T49.6x4	T49.6x5	T49.6x6
topical NEC	T49.0x1	T49.0x2	T49.0x3	T49.0x4	T49.0x5	T49.0x6
Chloronitrobenzene	T53.7x1	T53.7x2	T53.7x3	T53.7x4	—	—
dust or vapor	T53.7x1	T53.7x2	T53.7x3	T53.7x4	—	—
Chlorophacinone	T60.4x1	T60.4x2	T60.4x3	T60.4x4	—	—
Chlorophenol	T53.7x1	T53.7x2	T53.7x3	T53.7x4	—	—
Chlorophenothane	T60.1x1	T60.1x2	T60.1x3	T60.1x4	—	—
Chlorophyll	T50.991	T50.992	T50.993	T50.994	T50.995	T50.996
Chloropicrin (fumes)	T53.6x1	T53.6x2	T53.6x3	T53.6x4	—	—
fumigant	T60.8x1	T60.8x2	T60.8x3	T60.8x4	—	—
fungicide	T60.3x1	T60.3x2	T60.3x3	T60.3x4	—	—
pesticide	T60.8x1	T60.8x2	T60.8x3	T60.8x4	—	—
Chloroprocaine	T41.3x1	T41.3x2	T41.3x3	T41.3x4	T41.3x5	T41.3x6
infiltration (subcutaneous)	T41.3x1	T41.3x2	T41.3x3	T41.3x4	T41.3x5	T41.3x6
nerve block (peripheral) (plexus)	T41.3x1	T41.3x2	T41.3x3	T41.3x4	T41.3x5	T41.3x6
spinal	T41.3x1	T41.3x2	T41.3x3	T41.3x4	T41.3x5	T41.3x6
Chloroptic	T49.5x1	T49.5x2	T49.5x3	T49.5x4	T49.5x5	T49.5x6
Chloropurine	T45.1x1	T45.1x2	T45.1x3	T45.1x4	T45.1x5	T45.1x6
Chloropyramine	T45.0x1	T45.0x2	T45.0x3	T45.0x4	T45.0x5	T45.0x6
Chloropyrifos	T60.0x1	T60.0x2	T60.0x3	T60.0x4	—	—
Chloropyrilene	T45.0x1	T45.0x2	T45.0x3	T45.0x4	T45.0x5	T45.0x6
Chloroquine	T37.2x1	T37.2x2	T37.2x3	T37.2x4	T37.2x5	T37.2x6
Chlorothalonil	T60.3x1	T60.3x2	T60.3x3	T60.3x4	—	—
Chlorothen	T45.0x1	T45.0x2	T45.0x3	T45.0x4	T45.0x5	T45.0x6
Chlorothiazide	T50.2x1	T50.2x2	T50.2x3	T50.2x4	T50.2x5	T50.2x6
Chlorothymol	T49.4x1	T49.4x2	T49.4x3	T49.4x4	T49.4x5	T49.4x6
Chlorotrianisene	T38.5x1	T38.5x2	T38.5x3	T38.5x4	T38.5x5	T38.5x6
Chlorovinyldichloroarsine, not in war	T57.0x1	T57.0x2	T57.0x3	T57.0x4	—	—
Chloroxine	T49.4x1	T49.4x2	T49.4x3	T49.4x4	T49.4x5	T49.4x6
Chloroxylenol	T49.0x1	T49.0x2	T49.0x3	T49.0x4	T49.0x5	T49.0x6
Chlorphenamine	T45.0x1	T45.0x2	T45.0x3	T45.0x4	T45.0x5	T45.0x6
Chlorphenesin	T42.8x1	T42.8x2	T42.8x3	T42.8x4	T42.8x5	T42.8x6
topical (antifungal)	T49.0x1	T49.0x2	T49.0x3	T49.0x4	T49.0x5	T49.0x6
Chlorpheniramine	T45.0x1	T45.0x2	T45.0x3	T45.0x4	T45.0x5	T45.0x6
Chlorphenoxamine	T45.0x1	T45.0x2	T45.0x3	T45.0x4	T45.0x5	T45.0x6
Chlorphentermine	T50.5x1	T50.5x2	T50.5x3	T50.5x4	T50.5x5	T50.5x6
Chlorprocaine—see Chloroprocaine						
Chlorproguanil	T37.2x1	T37.2x2	T37.2x3	T37.2x4	T37.2x5	T37.2x6

Substance	Poisoning, Accidental (unintentional)	Poisoning, Intentional Self-harm	Poisoning, Assault	Poisoning, Undetermined	Adverse Effect	Under-dosing
Chlorpromazine	T43.3x1	T43.3x2	T43.3x3	T43.3x4	T43.3x5	T43.3x6
Chlorpropamide	T38.3x1	T38.3x2	T38.3x3	T38.3x4	T38.3x5	T38.3x6
Chlorprothixene	T43.4x1	T43.4x2	T43.4x3	T43.4x4	T43.4x5	T43.4x6
Chlorquinaldol	T49.0x1	T49.0x2	T49.0x3	T49.0x4	T49.0x5	T49.0x6
Chlorquinol	T49.0x1	T49.0x2	T49.0x3	T49.0x4	T49.0x5	T49.0x6
Chlortalidone	T50.2x1	T50.2x2	T50.2x3	T50.2x4	T50.2x5	T50.2x6
Chlortetracycline	T36.4x1	T36.4x2	T36.4x3	T36.4x4	T36.4x5	T36.4x6
Chlorthalidone	T50.2x1	T50.2x2	T50.2x3	T50.2x4	T50.2x5	T50.2x6
Chlorthiophos	T60.0x1	T60.0x2	T60.0x3	T60.0x4	—	—
Chlorotrianisene	T38.5x1	T38.5x2	T38.5x3	T38.5x4	T38.5x5	T38.5x6
Chlor-Trimeton	T45.0x1	T45.0x2	T45.0x3	T45.0x4	T45.0x5	T45.0x6
Chlorthion	T60.0x1	T60.0x2	T60.0x3	T60.0x4	—	—
Chlorzoxazone	T42.8x1	T42.8x2	T42.8x3	T42.8x4	T42.8x5	T42.8x6
Choke damp	T59.7x1	T59.7x2	T59.7x3	T59.7x4	—	—
Cholagogues	T47.5x1	T47.5x2	T47.5x3	T47.5x4	T47.5x5	T47.5x6
Cholebrine	T50.8x1	T50.8x2	T50.8x3	T50.8x4	T50.8x5	T50.8x6
Cholecalciferol	T45.2x1	T45.2x2	T45.2x3	T45.2x4	T45.2x5	T45.2x6
Cholecystokinin	T50.8x1	T50.8x2	T50.8x3	T50.8x4	T50.8x5	T50.8x6
Cholera vaccine	T50.A91	T50.A92	T50.A93	T50.A94	T50.A95	T50.A96
Choleretic	T47.5x1	T47.5x2	T47.5x3	T47.5x4	T47.5x5	T47.5x6
Cholesterol-lowering agents	T46.6x1	T46.6x2	T46.6x3	T46.6x4	T46.6x5	T46.6x6
Cholestyramine (resin)	T46.6x1	T46.6x2	T46.6x3	T46.6x4	T46.6x5	T46.6x6
Cholic acid	T47.5x1	T47.5x2	T47.5x3	T47.5x4	T47.5x5	T47.5x6
Choline	T48.6x1	T48.6x2	T48.6x3	T48.6x4	T48.6x5	T48.6x6
chloride	T50.991	T50.992	T50.993	T50.994	T50.995	T50.996
dihydrogen citrate	T50.991	T50.992	T50.993	T50.994	T50.995	T50.996
salicylate	T39.091	T39.092	T39.093	T39.094	T39.095	T39.096
theophyllinate	T48.6x1	T48.6x2	T48.6x3	T48.6x4	T48.6x5	T48.6x6
Cholinergic (drug) **NEC**	T44.1x1	T44.1x2	T44.1x3	T44.1x4	T44.1x5	T44.1x6
muscle tone enhancer	T44.1x1	T44.1x2	T44.1x3	T44.1x4	T44.1x5	T44.1x6
organophosphorus	T44.0x1	T44.0x2	T44.0x3	T44.0x4	T44.0x5	T44.0x6
insecticide	T60.0x1	T60.0x2	T60.0x3	T60.0x4	—	—
nerve gas	T59.891	T59.892	T59.893	T59.894	—	—
trimethyl ammonium propanediol	T44.1x1	T44.1x2	T44.1x3	T44.1x4	T44.1x5	T44.1x6
Cholinesterase reactivator	T50.6x1	T50.6x2	T50.6x3	T50.6x4	T50.6x5	T50.6x6
Cholografin	T50.8x1	T50.8x2	T50.8x3	T50.8x4	T50.8x5	T50.8x6
Chorionic gonadotropin	T38.891	T38.892	T38.893	T38.894	T38.895	T38.896
Chromate	T56.2x1	T56.2x2	T56.2x3	T56.2x4	—	—
dust or mist	T56.2x1	T56.2x2	T56.2x3	T56.2x4	—	—
lead (see also lead)	T56.0x1	T56.0x2	T56.0x3	T56.0x4	—	—
paint	T56.0x1	T56.0x2	T56.0x3	T56.0x4	—	—
Chromic						
acid	T56.2x1	T56.2x2	T56.2x3	T56.2x4	—	—
dust or mist	T56.2x1	T56.2x2	T56.2x3	T56.2x4	—	—
phosphate 32P	T45.1x1	T45.1x2	T45.1x3	T45.1x4	T45.1x5	T45.1x6
Chromium	T56.2x1	T56.2x2	T56.2x3	T56.2x4	—	—
compounds—see Chromate						
sesquioxide	T50.8x1	T50.8x2	T50.8x3	T50.8x4	T50.8x5	T50.8x6
Chromomycin A3	T45.1x1	T45.1x2	T45.1x3	T45.1x4	T45.1x5	T45.1x6
Chromonar	T46.3x1	T46.3x2	T46.3x3	T46.3x4	T46.3x5	T46.3x6
Chromyl chloride	T56.2x1	T56.2x2	T56.2x3	T56.2x4	—	—
Chrysarobin	T49.4x1	T49.4x2	T49.4x3	T49.4x4	T49.4x5	T49.4x6
Chrysazin	T47.2x1	T47.2x2	T47.2x3	T47.2x4	T47.2x5	T47.2x6
Chymar	T45.3x1	T45.3x2	T45.3x3	T45.3x4	T45.3x5	T45.3x6
ophthalmic preparation	T49.5x1	T49.5x2	T49.5x3	T49.5x4	T49.5x5	T49.5x6
Chymopapain	T45.3x1	T45.3x2	T45.3x3	T45.3x4	T45.3x5	T45.3x6
Chymotrypsin	T45.3x1	T45.3x2	T45.3x3	T45.3x4	T45.3x5	T45.3x6
ophthalmic preparation	T49.5x1	T49.5x2	T49.5x3	T49.5x4	T49.5x5	T49.5x6
Cianidanol	T50.991	T50.992	T50.993	T50.994	T50.995	T50.996
Cianopramine	T43.011	T43.012	T43.013	T43.014	T43.015	T43.016
Cibenzoline	T46.2x1	T46.2x2	T46.2x3	T46.2x4	T46.2x5	T46.2x6
Ciclacillin	T36.0x1	T36.0x2	T36.0x3	T36.0x4	T36.0x5	T36.0x6
Ciclobarbital—see Hexobarbital						
Ciclonicate	T46.7x1	T46.7x2	T46.7x3	T46.7x4	T46.7x5	T46.7x6
Ciclopirox (olamine)	T49.0x1	T49.0x2	T49.0x3	T49.0x4	T49.0x5	T49.0x6
Ciclosporin	T45.1x1	T45.1x2	T45.1x3	T45.1x4	T45.1x5	T45.1x6
Cicuta maculata or virosa	T62.2x1	T62.2x2	T62.2x3	T62.2x4	—	—
Cicutoxin	T62.2x1	T62.2x2	T62.2x3	T62.2x4	—	—
Cigarette lighter fluid	T52.0x1	T52.0x2	T52.0x3	T52.0x4	—	—
Cigarettes (tobacco)	T65.221	T65.222	T65.223	T65.224	—	—

Substance	Poisoning, Accidental (unintentional)	Poisoning, Intentional Self-harm	Poisoning, Assault	Poisoning, Undetermined	Adverse Effect	Under-dosing
Ciguatoxin	T61.01	T61.02	T61.03	T61.04		
Cilazapril	T46.4x1	T46.4x2	T46.4x3	T46.4x4	T46.4x5	T46.4x6
Cimetidine	T47.0x1	T47.0x2	T47.0x3	T47.0x4	T47.0x5	T47.0x6
Cimetropium bromide	T44.3x1	T44.3x2	T44.3x3	T44.3x4	T44.3x5	T44.3x6
Cinchocaine	T41.3x1	T41.3x2	T41.3x3	T41.3x4	T41.3x5	T41.3x6
topical (surface)	T41.3x1	T41.3x2	T41.3x3	T41.3x4	T41.3x5	T41.3x6
Cinchona	T37.2x1	T37.2x2	T37.2x3	T37.2x4	T37.2x5	T37.2x6
Cinchonine alkaloids	T37.2x1	T37.2x2	T37.2x3	T37.2x4	T37.2x5	T37.2x6
Cinchophen	T50.4x1	T50.4x2	T50.4x3	T50.4x4	T50.4x5	T50.4x6
Cinepazide	T46.7x1	T46.7x2	T46.7x3	T46.7x4	T46.7x5	T46.7x6
Cinnamedrine	T48.5x1	T48.5x2	T48.5x3	T48.5x4	T48.5x5	T48.5x6
Cinnarizine	T45.0x1	T45.0x2	T45.0x3	T45.0x4	T45.0x5	T45.0x6
Cinoxacin	T37.8x1	T37.8x2	T37.8x3	T37.8x4	T37.8x5	T37.8x6
Ciprofibrate	T46.6x1	T46.6x2	T46.6x3	T46.6x4	T46.6x5	T46.6x6
Ciprofloxacin	T36.8x1	T36.8x2	T36.8x3	T36.8x4	T36.8x5	T36.8x6
Cisapride	T47.8x1	T47.8x2	T47.8x3	T47.8x4	T47.8x5	T47.8x6
Cisplatin	T45.1x1	T45.1x2	T45.1x3	T45.1x4	T45.1x5	T45.1x6
Citalopram	T43.221	T43.222	T43.223	T43.224	T43.225	T43.226
Citanest	T41.3x1	T41.3x2	T41.3x3	T41.3x4	T41.3x5	T41.3x6
infiltration (subcutaneous)	T41.3x1	T41.3x2	T41.3x3	T41.3x4	T41.3x5	T41.3x6
nerve block (peripheral) (plexus)	T41.3x1	T41.3x2	T41.3x3	T41.3x4	T41.3x5	T41.3x6
Citric acid	T47.5x1	T47.5x2	T47.5x3	T47.5x4	T47.5x5	T47.5x6
Citrovorum (factor)	T45.8x1	T45.8x2	T45.8x3	T45.8x4	T45.8x5	T45.8x6
Claviceps purpurea	T62.2x1	T62.2x2	T62.2x3	T62.2x4		
Clavulanic acid	T36.1x1	T36.1x2	T36.1x3	T36.1x4	T36.1x5	T36.1x6
Cleaner, cleansing agent NEC	T52.91	T52.92	T52.93	T52.94	—	—
of paint or varnish	T52.91	T52.92	T52.93	T52.94	—	—
Clebopride	T47.8x1	T47.8x2	T47.8x3	T47.8x4	T47.8x5	T47.8x6
Clefamide	T37.3x1	T37.3x2	T37.3x3	T37.3x4	T37.3x5	T37.3x6
Clemastine	T45.0x1	T45.0x2	T45.0x3	T45.0x4	T45.0x5	T45.0x6
Clematis vitalba	T62.2x1	T62.2x2	T62.2x3	T62.2x4		
Clemizole	T45.0x1	T45.0x2	T45.0x3	T45.0x4	T45.0x5	T45.0x6
penicillin	T36.0x1	T36.0x2	T36.0x3	T36.0x4	T36.0x5	T36.0x6
Clenbuterol	T48.6x1	T48.6x2	T48.6x3	T48.6x4	T48.6x5	T48.6x6
Clidinium bromide	T44.3x1	T44.3x2	T44.3x3	T44.3x4	T44.3x5	T44.3x6
Clindamycin	T36.8x1	T36.8x2	T36.8x3	T36.8x4	T36.8x5	T36.8x6
Clinofibrate	T46.6x1	T46.6x2	T46.6x3	T46.6x4	T46.6x5	T46.6x6
Clioquinol	T37.8x1	T37.8x2	T37.8x3	T37.8x4	T37.8x5	T37.8x6
Cliradon	T40.2x1	T40.2x2	T40.2x3	T40.2x4	T40.2x5	T40.2x6
Clobazam	T42.4x1	T42.4x2	T42.4x3	T42.4x4	T42.4x5	T42.4x6
Clobenzorex	T50.5x1	T50.5x2	T50.5x3	T50.5x4	T50.5x5	T50.5x6
Clobetasol	T49.0x1	T49.0x2	T49.0x3	T49.0x4	T49.0x5	T49.0x6
Clobetasone	T49.0x1	T49.0x2	T49.0x3	T49.0x4	T49.0x5	T49.0x6
Clobutinol	T48.3x1	T48.3x2	T48.3x3	T48.3x4	T48.3x5	T48.3x6
Clocortolone	T38.0x1	T38.0x2	T38.0x3	T38.0x4	T38.0x5	T38.0x6
Clodantoin	T49.0x1	T49.0x2	T49.0x3	T49.0x4	T49.0x5	T49.0x6
Clodronic acid	T50.991	T50.992	T50.993	T50.994	T50.995	T50.996
Clofazimine	T37.1x1	T37.1x2	T37.1x3	T37.1x4	T37.1x5	T37.1x6
Clofedanol	T48.3x1	T48.3x2	T48.3x3	T48.3x4	T48.3x5	T48.3x6
Clofenamide	T50.2x1	T50.2x2	T50.2x3	T50.2x4	T50.2x5	T50.2x6
Clofenotane	T49.0x1	T49.0x2	T49.0x3	T49.0x4	T49.0x5	T49.0x6
Clofezone	T39.2x1	T39.2x2	T39.2x3	T39.2x4	T39.2x5	T39.2x6
Clofibrate	T46.6x1	T46.6x2	T46.6x3	T46.6x4	T46.6x5	T46.6x6
Clofibride	T46.6x1	T46.6x2	T46.6x3	T46.6x4	T46.6x5	T46.6x6
Cloforex	T50.5x1	T50.5x2	T50.5x3	T50.5x4	T50.5x5	T50.5x6
Clomethiazole	T42.6x1	T42.6x2	T42.6x3	T42.6x4	T42.6x5	T42.6x6
Clometocillin	T36.0x1	T36.0x2	T36.0x3	T36.0x4	T36.0x5	T36.0x6
Clomifene	T38.5x1	T38.5x2	T38.5x3	T38.5x4	T38.5x5	T38.5x6
Clomiphene	T38.5x1	T38.5x2	T38.5x3	T38.5x4	T38.5x5	T38.5x6
Clomipramine	T43.011	T43.012	T43.013	T43.014	T43.015	T43.016
Clomocycline	T36.4x1	T36.4x2	T36.4x3	T36.4x4	T36.4x5	T36.4x6
Clonazepam	T42.4x1	T42.4x2	T42.4x3	T42.4x4	T42.4x5	T42.4x6
Clonidine	T46.5x1	T46.5x2	T46.5x3	T46.5x4	T46.5x5	T46.5x6
Clonixin	T39.8x1	T39.8x2	T39.8x3	T39.8x4	T39.8x5	T39.8x6
Clopamide	T50.2x1	T50.2x2	T50.2x3	T50.2x4	T50.2x5	T50.2x6
Clopenthixol	T43.4x1	T43.4x2	T43.4x3	T43.4x4	T43.4x5	T43.4x6
Cloperastine	T48.3x1	T48.3x2	T48.3x3	T48.3x4	T48.3x5	T48.3x6
Clophedianol	T48.3x1	T48.3x2	T48.3x3	T48.3x4	T48.3x5	T48.3x6
Cloponone	T36.2x1	T36.2x2	T36.2x3	T36.2x4	T36.2x5	T36.2x6
Cloprednol	T38.0x1	T38.0x2	T38.0x3	T38.0x4	T38.0x5	T38.0x6
Cloral betaine	T42.6x1	T42.6x2	T42.6x3	T42.6x4	T42.6x5	T42.6x6

Substance	Poisoning, Accidental (unintentional)	Poisoning, Intentional Self-harm	Poisoning, Assault	Poisoning, Undetermined	Adverse Effect	Under-dosing
Cloramfenicol	T36.2x1	T36.2x2	T36.2x3	T36.2x4	T36.2x5	T36.2x6
Clorazepate (dipotassium)	T42.4x1	T42.4x2	T42.4x3	T42.4x4	T42.4x5	T42.4x6
Clorexolone	T50.2x1	T50.2x2	T50.2x3	T50.2x4	T50.2x5	T50.2x6
Clorox (bleach)	T54.91	T54.92	T54.93	T54.94	—	—
Clorfenamine	T45.0x1	T45.0x2	T45.0x3	T45.0x4	T45.0x5	T45.0x6
Clorgiline	T43.1x1	T43.1x2	T43.1x3	T43.1x4	T43.1x5	T43.1x6
Clorotepine	T44.3x1	T44.3x2	T44.3x3	T44.3x4	T44.3x5	T44.3x6
Clorprenaline	T48.6x1	T48.6x2	T48.6x3	T48.6x4	T48.6x5	T48.6x6
Clortermine	T50.5x1	T50.5x2	T50.5x3	T50.5x4	T50.5x5	T50.5x6
Clotiapine	T43.591	T43.592	T43.593	T43.594	T43.595	T43.596
Clotiazepam	T42.4x1	T42.4x2	T42.4x3	T42.4x4	T42.4x5	T42.4x6
Clotibric acid	T46.6x1	T46.6x2	T46.6x3	T46.6x4	T46.6x5	T46.6x6
Clotrimazole	T49.0x1	T49.0x2	T49.0x3	T49.0x4	T49.0x5	T49.0x6
Cloxacillin	T36.0x1	T36.0x2	T36.0x3	T36.0x4	T36.0x5	T36.0x6
Cloxazolam	T42.4x1	T42.4x2	T42.4x3	T42.4x4	T42.4x5	T42.4x6
Cloxiquine	T49.0x1	T49.0x2	T49.0x3	T49.0x4	T49.0x5	T49.0x6
Clozapine	T42.4x1	T42.4x2	T42.4x3	T42.4x4	T42.4x5	T42.4x6
Coagulant NEC	T45.7x1	T45.7x2	T45.7x3	T45.7x4	T45.7x5	T45.7x6
Coal (carbon monoxide from) (see also Carbon, monoxide, coal)	T58.2x1	T58.2x2	T58.2x3	T58.2x4		
oil—see Kerosene						
tar	T49.1x1	T49.1x2	T49.1x3	T49.1x4	T49.1x5	T49.1x6
fumes	T59.891	T59.892	T59.893	T59.894		
medicinal (ointment)	T49.4x1	T49.4x2	T49.4x3	T49.4x4	T49.4x5	T49.4x6
analgesics NEC	T39.2x1	T39.2x2	T39.2x3	T39.2x4	T39.2x5	T39.2x6
naphtha (solvent)	T52.0x1	T52.0x2	T52.0x3	T52.0x4		
Cobalamine	T45.2x1	T45.2x2	T45.2x3	T45.2x4	T45.2x5	T45.2x6
Cobalt (nonmedicinal) (fumes) (industrial)	T56.891	T56.892	T56.893	T56.894		
medicinal (trace) (chloride)	T45.8x1	T45.8x2	T45.8x3	T45.8x4	T45.8x5	T45.8x6
Cobra (venom)	T63.041	T63.042	T63.043	T63.044		
Coca (leaf)	T40.5x1	T40.5x2	T40.5x3	T40.5x4		
Cocaine	T40.5x1	T40.5x2	T40.5x3	T40.5x4	T40.5x5	T40.5x6
topical anesthetic	T41.3x1	T41.3x2	T41.3x3	T41.3x4	T41.3x5	T41.3x6
Cocarboxylase	T45.3x1	T45.3x2	T45.3x3	T45.3x4	T45.3x5	T45.3x6
Coccidioidin	T50.8x1	T50.8x2	T50.8x3	T50.8x4	T50.8x5	T50.8x6
Cocculus indicus	T62.1x1	T62.1x2	T62.1x3	T62.1x4		
Cochineal	T65.6x1	T65.6x2	T65.6x3	T65.6x4		
medicinal products	T50.991	T50.992	T50.993	T50.994	T50.995	T50.996
Codeine	T40.2x1	T40.2x2	T40.2x3	T40.2x4	T40.2x5	T40.2x6
Cod-liver oil	T45.2x1	T45.2x2	T45.2x3	T45.2x4	T45.2x5	T45.2x6
Coenzyme A	T50.991	T50.992	T50.993	T50.994	T50.995	T50.996
Coffee	T62.8x1	T62.8x2	T62.8x3	T62.8x4		
Cogalactoisomerase	T50.991	T50.992	T50.993	T50.994	T50.995	T50.996
Cogentin	T44.3x1	T44.3x2	T44.3x3	T44.3x4	T44.3x5	T44.3x6
Coke fumes or gas (carbon monoxide)	T58.2x1	T58.2x2	T58.2x3	T58.2x4		
industrial use	T58.8x1	T58.8x2	T58.8x3	T58.8x4		
Colace	T47.4x1	T47.4x2	T47.4x3	T47.4x4	T47.4x5	T47.4x6
Colaspase	T45.1x1	T45.1x2	T45.1x3	T45.1x4	T45.1x5	T45.1x6
Colchicine	T50.4x1	T50.4x2	T50.4x3	T50.4x4	T50.4x5	T50.4x6
Colchicum	T62.2x1	T62.2x2	T62.2x3	T62.2x4		
Cold cream	T49.3x1	T49.3x2	T49.3x3	T49.3x4	T49.3x5	T49.3x6
Colecalciferol	T45.2x1	T45.2x2	T45.2x3	T45.2x4	T45.2x5	T45.2x6
Colestipol	T46.6x1	T46.6x2	T46.6x3	T46.6x4	T46.6x5	T46.6x6
Colestyramine	T46.6x1	T46.6x2	T46.6x3	T46.6x4	T46.6x5	T46.6x6
Colimycin	T36.8x1	T36.8x2	T36.8x3	T36.8x4	T36.8x5	T36.8x6
Colistimethate	T36.8x1	T36.8x2	T36.8x3	T36.8x4	T36.8x5	T36.8x6
Colistin	T36.8x1	T36.8x2	T36.8x3	T36.8x4	T36.8x5	T36.8x6
sulfate (eye preparation)	T49.5x1	T49.5x2	T49.5x3	T49.5x4	T49.5x5	T49.5x6
Collagen	T50.991	T50.992	T50.993	T50.994	T50.995	T50.996
Collagenase	T49.4x1	T49.4x2	T49.4x3	T49.4x4	T49.4x5	T49.4x6
Collodion	T49.3x1	T49.3x2	T49.3x3	T49.3x4	T49.3x5	T49.3x6
Colocynth	T47.2x1	T47.2x2	T47.2x3	T47.2x4	T47.2x5	T47.2x6
Colophony adhesive	T49.3x1	T49.3x2	T49.3x3	T49.3x4	T49.3x5	T49.3x6
Colorant (see also Dye)	T50.991	T50.992	T50.993	T50.994	T50.995	T50.996
Coloring matter—see Dye(s)						
Combustion gas (after combustion)—see Carbon, monoxide						
prior to combustion	T59.891	T59.892	T59.893	T59.894	—	—

Substance	Poisoning, Accidental (unintentional)	Poisoning, Intentional Self-harm	Poisoning, Assault	Poisoning, Undetermined	Adverse Effect	Under-dosing
Compazine	T43.3x1	T43.3x2	T43.3x3	T43.3x4	T43.3x5	T43.3x6
Compound						
42 (warfarin)	T60.4x1	T60.4x2	T60.4x3	T60.4x4	—	—
269 (endrin)	T60.1x1	T60.1x2	T60.1x3	T60.1x4	—	—
497 (dieldrin)	T60.1x1	T60.1x2	T60.1x3	T60.1x4	—	—
L80 (sodium fluoroacetate)	T60.4x1	T60.4x2	T60.4x3	T60.4x4	—	—
3422 (parathion)	T60.0x1	T60.0x2	T60.0x3	T60.0x4	—	—
3911 (phorate)	T60.0x1	T60.0x2	T60.0x3	T60.0x4	—	—
3956 (toxaphene)	T60.1x1	T60.1x2	T60.1x3	T60.1x4	—	—
4049 (malathion)	T60.0x1	T60.0x2	T60.0x3	T60.0x4	—	—
4069 (malathion)	T60.0x1	T60.0x2	T60.0x3	T60.0x4	—	—
4124 (dicapthon)	T60.0x1	T60.0x2	T60.0x3	T60.0x4	—	—
E (cortisone)	T38.0x1	T38.0x2	T38.0x3	T38.0x4	T38.0x5	T38.0x6
F (hydrocortisone)	T38.0x1	T38.0x2	T38.0x3	T38.0x4	T38.0x5	T38.0x6
Congo red	T50.8x1	T50.8x2	T50.8x3	T50.8x4	T50.8x5	T50.8x6
Coniine, conine	T62.2x1	T62.2x2	T62.2x3	T62.2x4	—	—
Conium (maculatum)	T62.2x1	T62.2x2	T62.2x3	T62.2x4	—	—
Conjugated estrogenic substances	T38.5x1	T38.5x2	T38.5x3	T38.5x4	T38.5x5	T38.5x6
Contac	T48.5x1	T48.5x2	T48.5x3	T48.5x4	T48.5x5	T48.5x6
Contact lens solution	T49.5x1	T49.5x2	T49.5x3	T49.5x4	T49.5x5	T49.5x6
Contraceptive (oral)	T38.4x1	T38.4x2	T38.4x3	T38.4x4	T38.4x5	T38.4x6
vaginal	T49.8x1	T49.8x2	T49.8x3	T49.8x4	T49.8x5	T49.8x6
Contrast medium, radiography	T50.8x1	T50.8x2	T50.8x3	T50.8x4	T50.8x5	T50.8x6
Convallaria glycosides	T46.0x1	T46.0x2	T46.0x3	T46.0x4	T46.0x5	T46.0x6
Convallaria majalis	T62.2x1	T62.2x2	T62.2x3	T62.2x4	—	—
berry	T62.1x1	T62.1x2	T62.1x3	T62.1x4	—	—
Copper (dust) (fumes) (nonmedicinal) **NEC**	T56.4x1	T56.4x2	T56.4x3	T56.4x4	—	—
arsenate, arsenite	T57.0x1	T57.0x2	T57.0x3	T57.0x4	—	—
insecticide	T60.2x1	T60.2x2	T60.2x3	T60.2x4	—	—
emetic	T47.7x1	T47.7x2	T47.7x3	T47.7x4	T47.7x5	T47.7x6
fungicide	T60.3x1	T60.3x2	T60.3x3	T60.3x4	—	—
gluconate	T49.0x1	T49.0x2	T49.0x3	T49.0x4	T49.0x5	T49.0x6
insecticide	T60.2x1	T60.2x2	T60.2x3	T60.2x4	—	—
medicinal (trace)	T45.8x1	T45.8x2	T45.8x3	T45.8x4	T45.8x5	T45.8x6
oleate	T49.0x1	T49.0x2	T49.0x3	T49.0x4	T49.0x5	T49.0x6
sulfate	T56.4x1	T56.4x2	T56.4x3	T56.4x4	—	—
cupric	T56.4x1	T56.4x2	T56.4x3	T56.4x4	—	—
fungicide	T60.3x1	T60.3x2	T60.3x3	T60.3x4	—	—
medicinal						
ear	T49.6x1	T49.6x2	T49.6x3	T49.6x4	T49.6x5	T49.6x6
emetic	T47.7x1	T47.7x2	T47.7x3	T47.7x4	T47.7x5	T47.7x6
eye	T49.5x1	T49.5x2	T49.5x3	T49.5x4	T49.5x5	T49.5x6
cuprous	T56.4x1	T56.4x2	T56.4x3	T56.4x4	—	—
fungicide	T60.3x1	T60.3x2	T60.3x3	T60.3x4	—	—
medicinal						
ear	T49.6x1	T49.6x2	T49.6x3	T49.6x4	T49.6x5	T49.6x6
emetic	T47.7x1	T47.7x2	T47.7x3	T47.7x4	T47.7x5	T47.7x6
eye	T49.5x1	T49.5x2	T49.5x3	T49.5x4	T49.5x5	T49.5x6
Copperhead snake (bite) (venom)	T63.061	T63.062	T63.063	T63.064	—	—
Coral (sting)	T63.691	T63.692	T63.693	T63.694	—	—
snake (bite) (venom)	T63.021	T63.022	T63.023	T63.024	—	—
Corbadrine	T49.6x1	T49.6x2	T49.6x3	T49.6x4	T49.6x5	T49.6x6
Cordran	T49.0x1	T49.0x2	T49.0x3	T49.0x4	T49.0x5	T49.0x6
Cordite	T65.891	T65.892	T65.893	T65.894	—	—
vapor	T59.891	T59.892	T59.893	T59.894	—	—
Corn cures	T49.4x1	T49.4x2	T49.4x3	T49.4x4	T49.4x5	T49.4x6
Cornhusker's lotion	T49.3x1	T49.3x2	T49.3x3	T49.3x4	T49.3x5	T49.3x6
Corn starch	T49.3x1	T49.3x2	T49.3x3	T49.3x4	T49.3x5	T49.3x6
Coronary vasodilator NEC	T46.3x1	T46.3x2	T46.3x3	T46.3x4	T46.3x5	T46.3x6
Corrosive NEC	T54.91	T54.92	T54.93	T54.94	—	—
acid NEC	T54.2x1	T54.2x2	T54.2x3	T54.2x4	—	—
aromatics	T54.1x1	T54.1x2	T54.1x3	T54.1x4	—	—
disinfectant	T54.1x1	T54.1x2	T54.1x3	T54.1x4	—	—
fumes NEC	T54.91	T54.92	T54.93	T54.94	—	—
specified NEC	T54.91	T54.92	T54.93	T54.94	—	—
sublimate	T56.1x1	T56.1x2	T56.1x3	T56.1x4	—	—
Cortate	T38.0x1	T38.0x2	T38.0x3	T38.0x4	T38.0x5	T38.0x6
Cort-Dome	T38.0x1	T38.0x2	T38.0x3	T38.0x4	T38.0x5	T38.0x6
ENT agent	T49.6x1	T49.6x2	T49.6x3	T49.6x4	T49.6x5	T49.6x6

Substance	Poisoning, Accidental (unintentional)	Poisoning, Intentional Self-harm	Poisoning, Assault	Poisoning, Undetermined	Adverse Effect	Under-dosing
Cort-Dome—*continued*						
ophthalmic preparation	T49.5x1	T49.5x2	T49.5x3	T49.5x4	T49.5x5	T49.5x6
topical NEC	T49.0x1	T49.0x2	T49.0x3	T49.0x4	T49.0x5	T49.0x6
Cortef	T38.0x1	T38.0x2	T38.0x3	T38.0x4	T38.0x5	T38.0x6
ENT agent	T49.6x1	T49.6x2	T49.6x3	T49.6x4	T49.6x5	T49.6x6
ophthalmic preparation	T49.5x1	T49.5x2	T49.5x3	T49.5x4	T49.5x5	T49.5x6
topical NEC	T49.0x1	T49.0x2	T49.0x3	T49.0x4	T49.0x5	T49.0x6
Corticosteroid	T38.0x1	T38.0x2	T38.0x3	T38.0x4	T38.0x5	T38.0x6
ENT agent	T49.6x1	T49.6x2	T49.6x3	T49.6x4	T49.6x5	T49.6x6
mineral	T50.0x1	T50.0x2	T50.0x3	T50.0x4	T50.0x5	T50.0x6
ophthalmic	T49.5x1	T49.5x2	T49.5x3	T49.5x4	T49.5x5	T49.5x6
topical NEC	T49.0x1	T49.0x2	T49.0x3	T49.0x4	T49.0x5	T49.0x6
Corticotropin	T38.811	T38.812	T38.813	T38.814	T38.815	T38.816
Cortisol	T49.0x1	T49.0x2	T49.0x3	T49.0x4	T49.0x5	T49.0x6
ENT agent	T49.6x1	T49.6x2	T49.6x3	T49.6x4	T49.6x5	T49.6x6
ophthalmic preparation	T49.5x1	T49.5x2	T49.5x3	T49.5x4	T49.5x5	T49.5x6
topical NEC	T49.0x1	T49.0x2	T49.0x3	T49.0x4	T49.0x5	T49.0x6
Cortisone (acetate)	T38.0x1	T38.0x2	T38.0x3	T38.0x4	T38.0x5	T38.0x6
ENT agent	T49.6x1	T49.6x2	T49.6x3	T49.6x4	T49.6x5	T49.6x6
ophthalmic preparation	T49.5x1	T49.5x2	T49.5x3	T49.5x4	T49.5x5	T49.5x6
topical NEC	T49.0x1	T49.0x2	T49.0x3	T49.0x4	T49.0x5	T49.0x6
Cortivazol	T38.0x1	T38.0x2	T38.0x3	T38.0x4	T38.0x5	T38.0x6
Cortogen	T38.0x1	T38.0x2	T38.0x3	T38.0x4	T38.0x5	T38.0x6
ENT agent	T49.6x1	T49.6x2	T49.6x3	T49.6x4	T49.6x5	T49.6x6
ophthalmic preparation	T49.5x1	T49.5x2	T49.5x3	T49.5x4	T49.5x5	T49.5x6
Cortone	T38.0x1	T38.0x2	T38.0x3	T38.0x4	T38.0x5	T38.0x6
ENT agent	T49.6x1	T49.6x2	T49.6x3	T49.6x4	T49.6x5	T49.6x6
ophthalmic preparation	T49.5x1	T49.5x2	T49.5x3	T49.5x4	T49.5x5	T49.5x6
Cortril	T38.0x1	T38.0x2	T38.0x3	T38.0x4	T38.0x5	T38.0x6
ENT agent	T49.6x1	T49.6x2	T49.6x3	T49.6x4	T49.6x5	T49.6x6
ophthalmic preparation	T49.5x1	T49.5x2	T49.5x3	T49.5x4	T49.5x5	T49.5x6
topical NEC	T49.0x1	T49.0x2	T49.0x3	T49.0x4	T49.0x5	T49.0x6
Corynebacterium parvum	T45.1x1	T45.1x2	T45.1x3	T45.1x4	T45.1x5	T45.1x6
Cosmetic preparation	T49.8x1	T49.8x2	T49.8x3	T49.8x4	T49.8x5	T49.8x6
Cosmetics	T49.8x1	T49.8x2	T49.8x3	T49.8x4	T49.8x5	T49.8x6
Cosyntropin	T38.811	T38.812	T38.813	T38.814	T38.815	T38.816
Cotarnine	T45.7x1	T45.7x2	T45.7x3	T45.7x4	T45.7x5	T45.7x6
Co-trimoxazole	T36.8x1	T36.8x2	T36.8x3	T36.8x4	T36.8x5	T36.8x6
Cottonseed oil	T49.3x1	T49.3x2	T49.3x3	T49.3x4	T49.3x5	T49.3x6
Cough mixture (syrup)	T48.4x1	T48.4x2	T48.4x3	T48.4x4	T48.4x5	T48.4x6
containing opiates	T40.2x1	T40.2x2	T40.2x3	T40.2x4	T40.2x5	T40.2x6
expectorants	T48.4x1	T48.4x2	T48.4x3	T48.4x4	T48.4x5	T48.4x6
Coumadin	T45.511	T45.512	T45.513	T45.514	T45.515	T45.516
rodenticide	T60.4x1	T60.4x2	T60.4x3	T60.4x4	—	—
Coumaphos	T60.0x1	T60.0x2	T60.0x3	T60.0x4	—	—
Coumarin	T45.511	T45.512	T45.513	T45.514	T45.515	T45.516
Coumetarol	T45.511	T45.512	T45.513	T45.514	T45.515	T45.516
Cowbane	T62.2x1	T62.2x2	T62.2x3	T62.2x4	—	—
Cozyme	T45.2x1	T45.2x2	T45.2x3	T45.2x4	T45.2x5	T45.2x6
Crack	T40.5x1	T40.5x2	T40.5x3	T40.5x4	T40.5x5	T40.5x6
Crataegus extract	T46.0x1	T46.0x2	T46.0x3	T46.0x4	T46.0x5	T46.0x6
Creolin	T54.1x1	T54.1x2	T54.1x3	T54.1x4	—	—
disinfectant	T54.1x1	T54.1x2	T54.1x3	T54.1x4	—	—
Creosol (compound)	T49.0x1	T49.0x2	T49.0x3	T49.0x4	T49.0x5	T49.0x6
Creosote (coal tar) (beechwood)	T49.0x1	T49.0x2	T49.0x3	T49.0x4	T49.0x5	T49.0x6
medicinal (expectorant)	T48.4x1	T48.4x2	T48.4x3	T48.4x4	T48.4x5	T48.4x6
syrup	T48.4x1	T48.4x2	T48.4x3	T48.4x4	T48.4x5	T48.4x6
Cresol(s)	T49.0x1	T49.0x2	T49.0x3	T49.0x4	T49.0x5	T49.0x6
and soap solution	T49.0x1	T49.0x2	T49.0x3	T49.0x4	T49.0x5	T49.0x6
Cresyl acetate	T49.0x1	T49.0x2	T49.0x3	T49.0x4	T49.0x5	T49.0x6
Cresylic acid	T49.0x1	T49.0x2	T49.0x3	T49.0x4	T49.0x5	T49.0x6
Crimidine	T60.4x1	T60.4x2	T60.4x3	T60.4x4	—	—
Croconazole	T37.8x1	T37.8x2	T37.8x3	T37.8x4	T37.8x5	T37.8x6
Cromoglicic acid	T48.6x1	T48.6x2	T48.6x3	T48.6x4	T48.6x5	T48.6x6
Cromolyn	T48.6x1	T48.6x2	T48.6x3	T48.6x4	T48.6x5	T48.6x6
Cromonar	T46.3x1	T46.3x2	T46.3x3	T46.3x4	T46.3x5	T46.3x6
Cropropamide	T39.8x1	T39.8x2	T39.8x3	T39.8x4	T39.8x5	T39.8x6
with crotethamide	T50.7x1	T50.7x2	T50.7x3	T50.7x4	T50.7x5	T50.7x6
Crotamiton	T49.0x1	T49.0x2	T49.0x3	T49.0x4	T49.0x5	T49.0x6
Crotethamide	T39.8x1	T39.8x2	T39.8x3	T39.8x4	T39.8x5	T39.8x6
with cropropamide	T50.7x1	T50.7x2	T50.7x3	T50.7x4	T50.7x5	T50.7x6

Substance	Poisoning, Accidental (unintentional)	Poisoning, Intentional Self-harm	Poisoning, Assault	Poisoning, Undetermined	Adverse Effect	Under-dosing
Croton (oil)	T47.2x1	T47.2x2	T47.2x3	T47.2x4	T47.2x5	T47.2x6
chloral	T42.6x1	T42.6x2	T42.6x3	T42.6x4	T42.6x5	T42.6x6
Crude oil	T52.0x1	T52.0x2	T52.0x3	T52.0x4	—	—
Cryogenine	T39.8x1	T39.8x2	T39.8x3	T39.8x4	T39.8x5	T39.8x6
Cryolite (vapor)	T60.1x1	T60.1x2	T60.1x3	T60.1x4	—	—
insecticide	T60.1x1	T60.1x2	T60.1x3	T60.1x4	—	—
Cryptenamine (tannates)	T46.5x1	T46.5x2	T46.5x3	T46.5x4	T46.5x5	T46.5x6
Crystal violet	T49.0x1	T49.0x2	T49.0x3	T49.0x4	T49.0x5	T49.0x6
Cuckoopint	T62.2x1	T62.2x2	T62.2x3	T62.2x4	—	—
Cumetharol	T45.511	T45.512	T45.513	T45.514	T45.515	T45.516
Cupric						
acetate	T60.3x1	T60.3x2	T60.3x3	T60.3x4	—	—
acetoarsenite	T57.0x1	T57.0x2	T57.0x3	T57.0x4	—	—
arsenate	T57.0x1	T57.0x2	T57.0x3	T57.0x4	—	—
gluconate	T49.0x1	T49.0x2	T49.0x3	T49.0x4	T49.0x5	T49.0x6
oleate	T49.0x1	T49.0x2	T49.0x3	T49.0x4	T49.0x5	T49.0x6
sulfate	T56.4x1	T56.4x2	T56.4x3	T56.4x4	—	—
Cuprous sulfate (see also Copper sulfate)	T56.4x1	T56.4x2	T56.4x3	T56.4x4	—	—
Curare, curarine	T48.1x1	T48.1x2	T48.1x3	T48.1x4	T48.1x5	T48.1x6
Cyamemazine	T43.3x1	T43.3x2	T43.3x3	T43.3x4	T43.3x5	T43.3x6
Cyamopsis tetragono-loba	T46.6x1	T46.6x2	T46.6x3	T46.6x4	T46.6x5	T46.6x6
Cyanacetyl hydrazide	T37.1x1	T37.1x2	T37.1x3	T37.1x4	T37.1x5	T37.1x6
Cyanic acid (gas)	T59.891	T59.892	T59.893	T59.894	—	—
Cyanide(s) (compounds) (potassium) (sodium) NEC	T65.0x1	T65.0x2	T65.0x3	T65.0x4	—	—
dust or gas (inhalation) NEC	T57.3x1	T57.3x2	T57.3x3	T57.3x4	—	—
fumigant	T65.0x1	T65.0x2	T65.0x3	T65.0x4	—	—
hydrogen	T57.3x1	T57.3x2	T57.3x3	T57.3x4	—	—
mercuric—see Mercury						
pesticide (dust) (fumes)	T65.0x1	T65.0x2	T65.0x3	T65.0x4	—	—
Cyanoacrylate adhesive	T49.3x1	T49.3x2	T49.3x3	T49.3x4	T49.3x5	T49.3x6
Cyanocobalamin	T45.8x1	T45.8x2	T45.8x3	T45.8x4	T45.8x5	T45.8x6
Cyanogen (chloride) (gas) NEC	T59.891	T59.892	T59.893	T59.894	—	—
Cyclacillin	T36.0x1	T36.0x2	T36.0x3	T36.0x4	T36.0x5	T36.0x6
Cyclaine	T41.3x1	T41.3x2	T41.3x3	T41.3x4	T41.3x5	T41.3x6
Cyclamate	T50.991	T50.992	T50.993	T50.994	T50.995	T50.996
Cyclamen europaeum	T62.2x1	T62.2x2	T62.2x3	T62.2x4	—	—
Cyclandelate	T46.7x1	T46.7x2	T46.7x3	T46.7x4	T46.7x5	T46.7x6
Cyclazocine	T50.7x1	T50.7x2	T50.7x3	T50.7x4	T50.7x5	T50.7x6
Cyclizine	T45.0x1	T45.0x2	T45.0x3	T45.0x4	T45.0x5	T45.0x6
Cyclobarbital	T42.3x1	T42.3x2	T42.3x3	T42.3x4	T42.3x5	T42.3x6
Cyclobarbitone	T42.3x1	T42.3x2	T42.3x3	T42.3x4	T42.3x5	T42.3x6
Cyclobenzaprine	T48.1x1	T48.1x2	T48.1x3	T48.1x4	T48.1x5	T48.1x6
Cyclodrine	T44.3x1	T44.3x2	T44.3x3	T44.3x4	T44.3x5	T44.3x6
Cycloguanil embonate	T37.2x1	T37.2x2	T37.2x3	T37.2x4	T37.2x5	T37.2x6
Cyclohexane	T52.8x1	T52.8x2	T52.8x3	T52.8x4	—	—
Cyclohexanol	T51.8x1	T51.8x2	T51.8x3	T51.8x4	—	—
Cyclohexanone	T52.4x1	T52.4x2	T52.4x3	T52.4x4	—	—
Cycloheximide	T60.3x1	T60.3x2	T60.3x3	T60.3x4	—	—
Cyclohexyl acetate	T52.8x1	T52.8x2	T52.8x3	T52.8x4	—	—
Cycloleucin	T45.1x1	T45.1x2	T45.1x3	T45.1x4	T45.1x5	T45.1x6
Cyclomethycaine	T41.3x1	T41.3x2	T41.3x3	T41.3x4	T41.3x5	T41.3x6
Cyclopentamine	T44.4x1	T44.4x2	T44.4x3	T44.4x4	T44.4x5	T44.4x6
Cyclopenthiazide	T50.2x1	T50.2x2	T50.2x3	T50.2x4	T50.2x5	T50.2x6
Cyclopentolate	T44.3x1	T44.3x2	T44.3x3	T44.3x4	T44.3x5	T44.3x6
Cyclophosphamide	T45.1x1	T45.1x2	T45.1x3	T45.1x4	T45.1x5	T45.1x6
Cycloplegic drug	T49.5x1	T49.5x2	T49.5x3	T49.5x4	T49.5x5	T49.5x6
Cyclopropane	T41.291	T41.292	T41.293	T41.294	T41.295	T41.296
Cyclopyrabital	T39.8x1	T39.8x2	T39.8x3	T39.8x4	T39.8x5	T39.8x6
Cycloserine	T37.1x1	T37.1x2	T37.1x3	T37.1x4	T37.1x5	T37.1x6
Cyclosporin	T45.1x1	T45.1x2	T45.1x3	T45.1x4	T45.1x5	T45.1x6
Cyclothiazide	T50.2x1	T50.2x2	T50.2x3	T50.2x4	T50.2x5	T50.2x6
Cycrimine	T44.3x1	T44.3x2	T44.3x3	T44.3x4	T44.3x5	T44.3x6
Cyhalothrin	T60.1x1	T60.1x2	T60.1x3	T60.1x4	—	—
Cymarin	T46.0x1	T46.0x2	T46.0x3	T46.0x4	T46.0x5	T46.0x6
Cypermethrin	T60.1x1	T60.1x2	T60.1x3	T60.1x4	—	—
Cyphenothrin	T60.2x1	T60.2x2	T60.2x3	T60.2x4	—	—
Cyproheptadine	T45.0x1	T45.0x2	T45.0x3	T45.0x4	T45.0x5	T45.0x6
Cyproterone	T38.6x1	T38.6x2	T38.6x3	T38.6x4	T38.6x5	T38.6x6
Cysteamine	T50.6x1	T50.6x2	T50.6x3	T50.6x4	T50.6x5	T50.6x6

Substance	Poisoning, Accidental (unintentional)	Poisoning, Intentional Self-harm	Poisoning, Assault	Poisoning, Undetermined	Adverse Effect	Under-dosing
Cytarabine	T45.1x1	T45.1x2	T45.1x3	T45.1x4	T45.1x5	T45.1x6
Cytisus						
laburnum	T62.2x1	T62.2x2	T62.2x3	T62.2x4	—	—
scoparius	T62.2x1	T62.2x2	T62.2x3	T62.2x4	—	—
Cytochrome C	T47.5x1	T47.5x2	T47.5x3	T47.5x4	T47.5x5	T47.5x6
Cytomel	T38.1x1	T38.1x2	T38.1x3	T38.1x4	T38.1x5	T38.1x6
Cytosine arabinoside	T45.1x1	T45.1x2	T45.1x3	T45.1x4	T45.1x5	T45.1x6
Cytosine (antineoplastic)	T45.1x1	T45.1x2	T45.1x3	T45.1x4	T45.1x5	T45.1x6
Cytoxan	T45.1x1	T45.1x2	T45.1x3	T45.1x4	T45.1x5	T45.1x6
Cytozyme	T45.7x1	T45.7x2	T45.7x3	T45.7x4	T45.7x5	T45.7x6
Dacarbazine	T45.1x1	T45.1x2	T45.1x3	T45.1x4	T45.1x5	T45.1x6
Dactinomycin	T45.1x1	T45.1x2	T45.1x3	T45.1x4	T45.1x5	T45.1x6
DADPS	T37.1x1	T37.1x2	T37.1x3	T37.1x4	T37.1x5	T37.1x6
Dakin's solution	T49.0x1	T49.0x2	T49.0x3	T49.0x4	T49.0x5	T49.0x6
Dalapon (sodium)	T60.3x1	T60.3x2	T60.3x3	T60.3x4	—	—
Dalmane	T42.4x1	T42.4x2	T42.4x3	T42.4x4	T42.4x5	T42.4x6
Danazol	T38.6x1	T38.6x2	T38.6x3	T38.6x4	T38.6x5	T38.6x6
Danilone	T45.511	T45.512	T45.513	T45.514	T45.515	T45.516
Danthron	T47.2x1	T47.2x2	T47.2x3	T47.2x4	T47.2x5	T47.2x6
Dantrolene	T42.8x1	T42.8x2	T42.8x3	T42.8x4	T42.8x5	T42.8x6
Dantron	T47.2x1	T47.2x2	T47.2x3	T47.2x4	T47.2x5	T47.2x6
Daphne (gnidium) (mezereum)	T62.2x1	T62.2x2	T62.2x3	T62.2x4	—	—
berry	T62.1x1	T62.1x2	T62.1x3	T62.1x4	—	—
Dapsone	T37.1x1	T37.1x2	T37.1x3	T37.1x4	T37.1x5	T37.1x6
Daraprim	T37.2x1	T37.2x2	T37.2x3	T37.2x4	T37.2x5	T37.2x6
Darnel	T62.2x1	T62.2x2	T62.2x3	T62.2x4	—	—
Darvon	T39.8x1	T39.8x2	T39.8x3	T39.8x4	T39.8x5	T39.8x6
Daunomycin	T45.1x1	T45.1x2	T45.1x3	T45.1x4	T45.1x5	T45.1x6
Daunorubicin	T45.1x1	T45.1x2	T45.1x3	T45.1x4	T45.1x5	T45.1x6
DBI	T38.3x1	T38.3x2	T38.3x3	T38.3x4	T38.3x5	T38.3x6
D-Con	T60.91	T60.92	T60.93	T60.94	—	—
insecticide	T60.2x1	T60.2x2	T60.2x3	T60.2x4	—	—
rodenticide	T60.4x1	T60.4x2	T60.4x3	T60.4x4	—	—
DDAVP	T38.891	T38.892	T38.893	T38.894	T38.895	T38.896
DDE (bis(chlorophenyl)-dichloroethylene)	T60.2x1	T60.2x2	T60.2x3	T60.2x4	—	—
DDS	T37.1x1	T37.1x2	T37.1x3	T37.1x4	T37.1x5	T37.1x6
DDT (dust)	T60.1x1	T60.1x2	T60.1x3	T60.1x4	—	—
Deadly nightshade (see also Belladonna)	T62.2x1	T62.2x2	T62.2x3	T62.2x4	—	—
berry	T62.1x1	T62.1x2	T62.1x3	T62.1x4	—	—
Deamino-D-arginine vasopressin	T38.891	T38.892	T38.893	T38.894	T38.895	T38.896
Deanol (aceglumate)	T50.991	T50.992	T50.993	T50.994	T50.995	T50.996
Debrisoquine	T46.5x1	T46.5x2	T46.5x3	T46.5x4	T46.5x5	T46.5x6
Decaborane	T57.8x1	T57.8x2	T57.8x3	T57.8x4	—	—
fumes	T59.891	T59.892	T59.893	T59.894	—	—
Decadron	T38.0x1	T38.0x2	T38.0x3	T38.0x4	T38.0x5	T38.0x6
ENT agent	T49.6x1	T49.6x2	T49.6x3	T49.6x4	T49.6x5	T49.6x6
ophthalmic preparation	T49.5x1	T49.5x2	T49.5x3	T49.5x4	T49.5x5	T49.5x6
topical NEC	T49.0x1	T49.0x2	T49.0x3	T49.0x4	T49.0x5	T49.0x6
Decahydronaphthalene	T52.8x1	T52.8x2	T52.8x3	T52.8x4	—	—
Decalin	T52.8x1	T52.8x2	T52.8x3	T52.8x4	—	—
Decamethonium (bromide)	T48.1x1	T48.1x2	T48.1x3	T48.1x4	T48.1x5	T48.1x6
Decholin	T47.5x1	T47.5x2	T47.5x3	T47.5x4	T47.5x5	T47.5x6
Declomycin	T36.4x1	T36.4x2	T36.4x3	T36.4x4	T36.4x5	T36.4x6
Decongestant, nasal (mucosa)	T48.5x1	T48.5x2	T48.5x3	T48.5x4	T48.5x5	T48.5x6
combination	T48.5x1	T48.5x2	T48.5x3	T48.5x4	T48.5x5	T48.5x6
Deet	T60.8x1	T60.8x2	T60.8x3	T60.8x4	—	—
Deferoxamine	T45.8x1	T45.8x2	T45.8x3	T45.8x4	T45.8x5	T45.8x6
Deflazacort	T38.0x1	T38.0x2	T38.0x3	T38.0x4	T38.0x5	T38.0x6
Deglycyrrhizinized extract of licorice	T48.4x1	T48.4x2	T48.4x3	T48.4x4	T48.4x5	T48.4x6
Dehydrocholic acid	T47.5x1	T47.5x2	T47.5x3	T47.5x4	T47.5x5	T47.5x6
Dehydroemetine	T37.3x1	T37.3x2	T37.3x3	T37.3x4	T37.3x5	T37.3x6
Dekalin	T52.8x1	T52.8x2	T52.8x3	T52.8x4	—	—
Delalutin	T38.5x1	T38.5x2	T38.5x3	T38.5x4	T38.5x5	T38.5x6
Delphinium	T62.2x1	T62.2x2	T62.2x3	T62.2x4	—	—
Deltasone	T38.0x1	T38.0x2	T38.0x3	T38.0x4	T38.0x5	T38.0x6
Deltra	T38.0x1	T38.0x2	T38.0x3	T38.0x4	T38.0x5	T38.0x6
Delvinal	T42.3x1	T42.3x2	T42.3x3	T42.3x4	T42.3x5	T42.3x6

Substance	Poisoning, Accidental (unintentional)	Poisoning, Intentional Self-harm	Poisoning, Assault	Poisoning, Undetermined	Adverse Effect	Under-dosing
Delorazepam	T42.4x1	T42.4x2	T42.4x3	T42.4x4	T42.4x5	T42.4x6
Deltamethrin	T60.1x1	T60.1x2	T60.1x3	T60.1x4	—	—
Demecarium (bromide)	T49.5x1	T49.5x2	T49.5x3	T49.5x4	T49.5x5	T49.5x6
Demeclocycline	T36.4x1	T36.4x2	T36.4x3	T36.4x4	T36.4x5	T36.4x6
Demecolcine	T45.1x1	T45.1x2	T45.1x3	T45.1x4	T45.1x5	T45.1x6
Demegestone	T38.5x1	T38.5x2	T38.5x3	T38.5x4	T38.5x5	T38.5x6
Demelanizing agents	T49.8x1	T49.8x2	T49.8x3	T49.8x4	T49.8x5	T49.8x6
Demephion -O and -S	T60.0x1	T60.0x2	T60.0x3	T60.0x4	—	—
Demerol	T40.2x1	T40.2x2	T40.2x3	T40.2x4	T40.2x5	T40.2x6
Demethylchlortetracycline	T36.4x1	T36.4x2	T36.4x3	T36.4x4	T36.4x5	T36.4x6
Demethyltetracycline	T36.4x1	T36.4x2	T36.4x3	T36.4x4	T36.4x5	T36.4x6
Demeton -O and -S	T60.0x1	T60.0x2	T60.0x3	T60.0x4	—	—
Demulcent (external)	T49.3x1	T49.3x2	T49.3x3	T49.3x4	T49.3x5	T49.3x6
specified NEC	T49.3x1	T49.3x2	T49.3x3	T49.3x4	T49.3x5	T49.3x6
Demulen	T38.4x1	T38.4x2	T38.4x3	T38.4x4	T38.4x5	T38.4x6
Denatured alcohol	T51.0x1	T51.0x2	T51.0x3	T51.0x4	—	—
Dendrid	T49.5x1	T49.5x2	T49.5x3	T49.5x4	T49.5x5	T49.5x6
Dental drug, topical application NEC	T49.7x1	T49.7x2	T49.7x3	T49.7x4	T49.7x5	T49.7x6
Dentifrice	T49.7x1	T49.7x2	T49.7x3	T49.7x4	T49.7x5	T49.7x6
Deodorant spray (feminine hygiene)	T49.8x1	T49.8x2	T49.8x3	T49.8x4	T49.8x5	T49.8x6
Deoxycortone	T50.0x1	T50.0x2	T50.0x3	T50.0x4	T50.0x5	T50.0x6
Deoxyribonuclease (pancreatic)	T45.3x1	T45.3x2	T45.3x3	T45.3x4	T45.3x5	T45.3x6
Depilatory	T49.4x1	T49.4x2	T49.4x3	T49.4x4	T49.4x5	T49.4x6
Deprenalin	T42.8x1	T42.8x2	T42.8x3	T42.8x4	T42.8x5	T42.8x6
Deprenyl	T42.8x1	T42.8x2	T42.8x3	T42.8x4	T42.8x5	T42.8x6
Depressant, appetite	T50.5x1	T50.5x2	T50.5x3	T50.5x4	T50.5x5	T50.5x6
Depressants						
appetite, central	T50.5x1	T50.5x2	T50.5x3	T50.5x4	T50.5x5	T50.5x6
cardiac	T46.2x1	T46.2x2	T46.2x3	T46.2x4	T46.2x5	T46.2x6
Central nervous system (anesthetic) (see also Central nervous system, depressants)	T41.41	T41.42	T41.43	T41.44	T41.45	T41.46
general anesthetic	T41.201	T41.202	T41.203	T41.204	T41.205	T41.206
psychotherapeutic	T43.501	T43.502	T43.503	T43.504	T43.505	T43.506
Deptropine	T45.0x1	T45.0x2	T45.0x3	T45.0x4	T45.0x5	T45.0x6
Dequalinium (chloride)	T49.0x1	T49.0x2	T49.0x3	T49.0x4	T49.0x5	T49.0x6
Derris root	T60.2x1	T60.2x2	T60.2x3	T60.2x4	—	—
Deserpidine	T46.5x1	T46.5x2	T46.5x3	T46.5x4	T46.5x5	T46.5x6
Desferrioxamine	T45.8x1	T45.8x2	T45.8x3	T45.8x4	T45.8x5	T45.8x6
Desipramine	T43.011	T43.012	T43.013	T43.014	T43.015	T43.016
Desianoside	T46.0x1	T46.0x2	T46.0x3	T46.0x4	T46.0x5	T46.0x6
Deslanoside	T46.0x1	T46.0x2	T46.0x3	T46.0x4	T46.0x5	T46.0x6
Desloughing agent	T49.4x1	T49.4x2	T49.4x3	T49.4x4	T49.4x5	T49.4x6
Desmethylimipramine	T43.011	T43.012	T43.013	T43.014	T43.015	T43.016
Desmopressin	T38.891	T38.892	T38.893	T38.894	T38.895	T38.896
Desocodeine	T40.2x1	T40.2x2	T40.2x3	T40.2x4	T40.2x5	T40.2x6
Desogestrel	T38.5x1	T38.5x2	T38.5x3	T38.5x4	T38.5x5	T38.5x6
Desomorphine	T40.2x1	T40.2x2	T40.2x3	T40.2x4	T40.2x5	T40.2x6
Desonide	T49.0x1	T49.0x2	T49.0x3	T49.0x4	T49.0x5	T49.0x6
Desoximetasone	T49.0x1	T49.0x2	T49.0x3	T49.0x4	T49.0x5	T49.0x6
Desoxycorticosteroid	T50.0x1	T50.0x2	T50.0x3	T50.0x4	T50.0x5	T50.0x6
Desoxycortone	T50.0x1	T50.0x2	T50.0x3	T50.0x4	T50.0x5	T50.0x6
Desoxyephedrine	T43.621	T43.622	T43.623	T43.624	T43.625	T43.626
Detaxtran	T46.6x1	T46.6x2	T46.6x3	T46.6x4	T46.6x5	T46.6x6
Detergent (local) (medicinal) NEC	T55.1x1	T55.1x2	T55.1x3	T55.1x4	—	—
external medication	T49.2x1	T49.2x2	T49.2x3	T49.2x4	T49.2x5	T49.2x6
nonmedicinal	T55.1x1	T55.1x2	T55.1x3	T55.1x4	—	—
specified NEC	T55.1x1	T55.1x2	T55.1x3	T55.1x4	—	—
Deterrent, alcohol	T50.6x1	T50.6x2	T50.6x3	T50.6x4	T50.6x5	T50.6x6
Detoxifying agent	T50.6x1	T50.6x2	T50.6x3	T50.6x4	T50.6x5	T50.6x6
Detrothyronine	T38.1x1	T38.1x2	T38.1x3	T38.1x4	T38.1x5	T38.1x6
Dettol (external medication)	T49.0x1	T49.0x2	T49.0x3	T49.0x4	T49.0x5	T49.0x6
Dexamethasone	T38.0x1	T38.0x2	T38.0x3	T38.0x4	T38.0x5	T38.0x6
ENT agent	T49.6x1	T49.6x2	T49.6x3	T49.6x4	T49.6x5	T49.6x6
ophthalmic preparation	T49.5x1	T49.5x2	T49.5x3	T49.5x4	T49.5x5	T49.5x6
topical NEC	T49.0x1	T49.0x2	T49.0x3	T49.0x4	T49.0x5	T49.0x6
Dexamfetamine	T43.621	T43.622	T43.623	T43.624	T43.625	T43.626
Dexamphetamine	T43.621	T43.622	T43.623	T43.624	T43.625	T43.626
Dexbrompheniramine	T45.0x1	T45.0x2	T45.0x3	T45.0x4	T45.0x5	T45.0x6

Substance	Poisoning, Accidental (unintentional)	Poisoning, Intentional Self-harm	Poisoning, Assault	Poisoning, Undetermined	Adverse Effect	Under-dosing
Dexchlorpheniramine	T45.0x1	T45.0x2	T45.0x3	T45.0x4	T45.0x5	T45.0x6
Dexedrine	T43.621	T43.622	T43.623	T43.624	T43.625	T43.626
Dexetimide	T44.3x1	T44.3x2	T44.3x3	T44.3x4	T44.3x5	T44.3x6
Dexfenfluramine	T50.5x1	T50.5x2	T50.5x3	T50.5x4	T50.5x5	T50.5x6
Dexpanthenol	T45.2x1	T45.2x2	T45.2x3	T45.2x4	T45.2x5	T45.2x6
Dextran (40) (70) (150)	T45.8x1	T45.8x2	T45.8x3	T45.8x4	T45.8x5	T45.8x6
Dextriferron	T45.4x1	T45.4x2	T45.4x3	T45.4x4	T45.4x5	T45.4x6
Dextroamphetamine	T43.621	T43.622	T43.623	T43.624	T43.625	T43.626
Dextro calcium pantothenate	T45.2x1	T45.2x2	T45.2x3	T45.2x4	T45.2x5	T45.2x6
Dextromethorphan	T48.3x1	T48.3x2	T48.3x3	T48.3x4	T48.3x5	T48.3x6
Dextromoramide	T40.4x1	T40.4x2	T40.4x3	T40.4x4	T40.4x5	T40.4x6
Dextro pantothenyl alcohol	T45.2x1	T45.2x2	T45.2x3	T45.2x4	T45.2x5	T45.2x6
topical	T49.8x1	T49.8x2	T49.8x3	T49.8x4	T49.8x5	T49.8x6
Dextropropoxyphene	T40.4x1	T40.4x2	T40.4x3	T40.4x4	T40.4x5	T40.4x6
Dextrorphan	T40.2x1	T40.2x2	T40.2x3	T40.2x4	T40.2x5	T40.2x6
Dextrose	T50.3x1	T50.3x2	T50.3x3	T50.3x4	T50.3x5	T50.3x6
concentrated solution, intravenous	T46.8x1	T46.8x2	T46.8x3	T46.8x4	T46.8x5	T46.8x6
Dextrothyroxin	T38.1x1	T38.1x2	T38.1x3	T38.1x4	T38.1x5	T38.1x6
Dextrothyroxine sodium	T38.1x1	T38.1x2	T38.1x3	T38.1x4	T38.1x5	T38.1x6
DFP	T44.0x1	T44.0x2	T44.0x3	T44.0x4	T44.0x5	T44.0x6
DHE	T37.3x1	T37.3x2	T37.3x3	T37.3x4	T37.3x5	T37.3x6
45	T46.5x1	T46.5x2	T46.5x3	T46.5x4	T46.5x5	T46.5x6
Diabinese	T38.3x1	T38.3x2	T38.3x3	T38.3x4	T38.3x5	T38.3x6
Diacetone alcohol	T52.4x1	T52.4x2	T52.4x3	T52.4x4	—	—
Diacetyl monoxime	T50.991	T50.992	T50.993	T50.994	—	—
Diacetylmorphine	T40.1x1	T40.1x2	T40.1x3	T40.1x4	T40.1x5	T40.1x6
Diachylon plaster	T49.4x1	T49.4x2	T49.4x3	T49.4x4	T49.4x5	T49.4x6
Diaethylstilboestrolum	T38.5x1	T38.5x2	T38.5x3	T38.5x4	T38.5x5	T38.5x6
Diagnostic agent NEC	T50.8x1	T50.8x2	T50.8x3	T50.8x4	T50.8x5	T50.8x6
Dial (soap)	T49.2x1	T49.2x2	T49.2x3	T49.2x4	T49.2x5	T49.2x6
sedative	T42.3x1	T42.3x2	T42.3x3	T42.3x4	T42.3x5	T42.3x6
Dialkyl carbonate	T52.91	T52.92	T52.93	T52.94	—	—
Diallylbarbituric acid	T42.3x1	T42.3x2	T42.3x3	T42.3x4	T42.3x5	T42.3x6
Diallymal	T42.3x1	T42.3x2	T42.3x3	T42.3x4	T42.3x5	T42.3x6
Dialysis solution (intraperitoneal)	T50.3x1	T50.3x2	T50.3x3	T50.3x4	T50.3x5	T50.3x6
Diaminodiphenylsulfone	T37.1x1	T37.1x2	T37.1x3	T37.1x4	T37.1x5	T37.1x6
Diamorphine	T40.1x1	T40.1x2	T40.1x3	T40.1x4	T40.1x5	T40.1x6
Diamox	T50.2x1	T50.2x2	T50.2x3	T50.2x4	T50.2x5	T50.2x6
Diamthazole	T49.0x1	T49.0x2	T49.0x3	T49.0x4	T49.0x5	T49.0x6
Dianthone	T47.2x1	T47.2x2	T47.2x3	T47.2x4	T47.2x5	T47.2x6
Diaphenylsulfone	T37.0x1	T37.0x2	T37.0x3	T37.0x4	T37.0x5	T37.0x6
Diasone (sodium)	T37.1x1	T37.1x2	T37.1x3	T37.1x4	T37.1x5	T37.1x6
Diastase	T47.5x1	T47.5x2	T47.5x3	T47.5x4	T47.5x5	T47.5x6
Diatrizoate	T50.8x1	T50.8x2	T50.8x3	T50.8x4	T50.8x5	T50.8x6
Diazepam	T42.4x1	T42.4x2	T42.4x3	T42.4x4	T42.4x5	T42.4x6
Diazinon	T60.0x1	T60.0x2	T60.0x3	T60.0x4	—	—
Diazomethane (gas)	T59.891	T59.892	T59.893	T59.894	—	—
Diazoxide	T46.5x1	T46.5x2	T46.5x3	T46.5x4	T46.5x5	T46.5x6
Dibekacin	T36.5x1	T36.5x2	T36.5x3	T36.5x4	T36.5x5	T36.5x6
Dibenamine	T44.6x1	T44.6x2	T44.6x3	T44.6x4	T44.6x5	T44.6x6
Dibenzepin	T43.011	T43.012	T43.013	T43.014	T43.015	T43.016
Dibenzheptropine	T45.0x1	T45.0x2	T45.0x3	T45.0x4	T45.0x5	T45.0x6
Dibenzyline	T44.6x1	T44.6x2	T44.6x3	T44.6x4	T44.6x5	T44.6x6
Diborane (gas)	T59.891	T59.892	T59.893	T59.894	—	—
Dibromochloropropane	T60.8x1	T60.8x2	T60.8x3	T60.8x4	—	—
Dibromodulcitol	T45.1x1	T45.1x2	T45.1x3	T45.1x4	T45.1x5	T45.1x6
Dibromoethane	T53.6x1	T53.6x2	T53.6x3	T53.6x4	—	—
Dibromomannitol	T45.1x1	T45.1x2	T45.1x3	T45.1x4	T45.1x5	T45.1x6
Dibromopropamidine isethionate	T49.0x1	T49.0x2	T49.0x3	T49.0x4	T49.0x5	T49.0x6
Dibrompropamidine	T49.0x1	T49.0x2	T49.0x3	T49.0x4	T49.0x5	T49.0x6
Dibucaine	T41.3x1	T41.3x2	T41.3x3	T41.3x4	T41.3x5	T41.3x6
topical (surface)	T41.3x1	T41.3x2	T41.3x3	T41.3x4	T41.3x5	T41.3x6
Dibunate sodium	T48.3x1	T48.3x2	T48.3x3	T48.3x4	T48.3x5	T48.3x6
Dibutoline sulfate	T44.3x1	T44.3x2	T44.3x3	T44.3x4	T44.3x5	T44.3x6
Dicamba	T60.3x1	T60.3x2	T60.3x3	T60.3x4	—	—
Dicapthon	T60.0x1	T60.0x2	T60.0x3	T60.0x4	—	—
Dichlobenil	T60.3x1	T60.3x2	T60.3x3	T60.3x4	—	—
Dichlone	T60.3x1	T60.3x2	T60.3x3	T60.3x4	—	—
Dichloralphenozone	T42.6x1	T42.6x2	T42.6x3	T42.6x4	T42.6x5	T42.6x6

Substance	Poisoning, Accidental (unintentional)	Poisoning, Intentional Self-harm	Poisoning, Assault	Poisoning, Undetermined	Adverse Effect	Under-dosing
Dichlorbenzidine	T65.3x1	T65.3x2	T65.3x3	T65.3x4	—	—
Dichlorhydrin	T52.8x1	T52.8x2	T52.8x3	T52.8x4	—	—
Dichlorhydroxyquinoline	T37.8x1	T37.8x2	T37.8x3	T37.8x4	T37.8x5	T37.8x6
Dichlorobenzene	T53.7x1	T53.7x2	T53.7x3	T53.7x4	—	—
Dichlorobenzyl alcohol	T49.6x1	T49.6x2	T49.6x3	T49.6x4	T49.6x5	T49.6x6
Dichlorodifluoromethane	T53.5x1	T53.5x2	T53.5x3	T53.5x4	—	—
Dichloroethane	T52.8x1	T52.8x2	T52.8x3	T52.8x4	—	—
Dichloroethyl sulfide, not in war	T59.891	T59.892	T59.893	T59.894	—	—
Dichloroethylene	T53.6x1	T53.6x2	T53.6x3	T53.6x4	—	—
Dichloroformoxine, not in war	T59.891	T59.892	T59.893	T59.894	—	—
Dichlorohydrin, alpha-dichlorohydrin	T52.8x1	T52.8x2	T52.8x3	T52.8x4	—	—
Dichloromethane (solvent)	T53.4x1	T53.4x2	T53.4x3	T53.4x4	—	—
vapor	T53.4x1	T53.4x2	T53.4x3	T53.4x4	—	—
Dichloronaphthoquinone	T60.3x1	T60.3x2	T60.3x3	T60.3x4	—	—
Dichlorophen	T37.4x1	T37.4x2	T37.4x3	T37.4x4	T37.4x5	T37.4x6
Dichloropropene	T60.3x1	T60.3x2	T60.3x3	T60.3x4	—	—
Dichloropropionic acid	T60.3x1	T60.3x2	T60.3x3	T60.3x4	—	—
Dichlorphenamide	T50.2x1	T50.2x2	T50.2x3	T50.2x4	T50.2x5	T50.2x6
Dichlorvos	T60.0x1	T60.0x2	T60.0x3	T60.0x4	—	—
Diclofenac	T39.391	T39.392	T39.393	T39.394	T39.395	T39.396
Diclofenamide	T50.2x1	T50.2x2	T50.2x3	T50.2x4	T50.2x5	T50.2x6
Diclofensine	T43.291	T43.292	T43.293	T43.294	T43.295	T43.296
Diclonixine	T39.8x1	T39.8x2	T39.8x3	T39.8x4	T39.8x5	T39.8x6
Dicloxacillin	T36.0x1	T36.0x2	T36.0x3	T36.0x4	T36.0x5	T36.0x6
Dicophane	T49.0x1	T49.0x2	T49.0x3	T49.0x4	T49.0x5	T49.0x6
Dicoumarol, dicoumarin, dicumarol	T45.511	T45.512	T45.513	T45.514	T45.515	T45.516
Dicrotophos	T60.0x1	T60.0x2	T60.0x3	T60.0x4	—	—
Dicyanogen (gas)	T65.0x1	T65.0x2	T65.0x3	T65.0x4	—	—
Dicyclomine	T44.3x1	T44.3x2	T44.3x3	T44.3x4	T44.3x5	T44.3x6
Dicycloverine	T44.3x1	T44.3x2	T44.3x3	T44.3x4	T44.3x5	T44.3x6
Dideoxycytidine	T37.5x1	T37.5x2	T37.5x3	T37.5x4	T37.5x5	T37.5x6
Dideoxyinosine	T37.5x1	T37.5x2	T37.5x3	T37.5x4	T37.5x5	T37.5x6
Dieldrin (vapor)	T60.1x1	T60.1x2	T60.1x3	T60.1x4	—	—
Diemal	T42.3x1	T42.3x2	T42.3x3	T42.3x4	T42.3x5	T42.3x6
Dienestrol	T38.5x1	T38.5x2	T38.5x3	T38.5x4	T38.5x5	T38.5x6
Dienoestrol	T38.5x1	T38.5x2	T38.5x3	T38.5x4	T38.5x5	T38.5x6
Dietetic drug NEC	T50.901	T50.902	T50.903	T50.904	T50.905	T50.906
Diethazine	T42.8x1	T42.8x2	T42.8x3	T42.8x4	T42.8x5	T42.8x6
Diethyl						
barbituric acid	T42.3x1	T42.3x2	T42.3x3	T42.3x4	T42.3x5	T42.3x6
carbamazine	T37.4x1	T37.4x2	T37.4x3	T37.4x4	T37.4x5	T37.4x6
carbinol	T51.3x1	T51.3x2	T51.3x3	T51.3x4	—	—
carbonate	T52.8x1	T52.8x2	T52.8x3	T52.8x4	—	—
ether (vapor) (see also ether)	T41.0x1	T41.0x2	T41.0x3	T41.0x4	T41.0x5	T41.0x6
oxide	T52.8x1	T52.8x2	T52.8x3	T52.8x4	—	—
propion	T50.5x1	T50.5x2	T50.5x3	T50.5x4	T50.5x5	T50.5x6
stilbestrol	T38.5x1	T38.5x2	T38.5x3	T38.5x4	T38.5x5	T38.5x6
toluamide (nonmedicinal)	T60.8x1	T60.8x2	T60.8x3	T60.8x4	—	—
medicinal	T49.3x1	T49.3x2	T49.3x3	T49.3x4	T49.3x5	T49.3x6
Diethylcarbamazine	T37.4x1	T37.4x2	T37.4x3	T37.4x4	T37.4x5	T37.4x6
Diethylene						
dioxide	T52.8x1	T52.8x2	T52.8x3	T52.8x4	—	—
glycol (monoacetate) (monobutyl ether) (monoethyl ether)	T52.3x1	T52.3x2	T52.3x3	T52.3x4	—	—
Diethylhexylphthalate	T65.891	T65.892	T65.893	T65.894	—	—
Diethylpropion	T50.5x1	T50.5x2	T50.5x3	T50.5x4	T50.5x5	T50.5x6
Diethylstilbestrol	T38.5x1	T38.5x2	T38.5x3	T38.5x4	T38.5x5	T38.5x6
Diethylstilboestrol	T38.5x1	T38.5x2	T38.5x3	T38.5x4	T38.5x5	T38.5x6
Diethylsulfone-diethylmethane	T42.6x1	T42.6x2	T42.6x3	T42.6x4	T42.6x5	T42.6x6
Diethyltoluamide	T49.0x1	T49.0x2	T49.0x3	T49.0x4	T49.0x5	T49.0x6
Diethyltryptamine (DET)	T40.991	T40.992	T40.993	T40.994	T40.995	T40.996
Difebarbamate	T42.3x1	T42.3x2	T42.3x3	T42.3x4	T42.3x5	T42.3x6
Difencloxazine	T40.2x1	T40.2x2	T40.2x3	T40.2x4	T40.2x5	T40.2x6
Difenidol	T45.0x1	T45.0x2	T45.0x3	T45.0x4	T45.0x5	T45.0x6
Difenoxin	T47.6x1	T47.6x2	T47.6x3	T47.6x4	T47.6x5	T47.6x6
Difetarsone	T37.3x1	T37.3x2	T37.3x3	T37.3x4	T37.3x5	T37.3x6
Diffusin	T45.3x1	T45.3x2	T45.3x3	T45.3x4	T45.3x5	T45.3x6
Diflorasone	T49.0x1	T49.0x2	T49.0x3	T49.0x4	T49.0x5	T49.0x6
Diflubenzuron	T60.1x1	T60.1x2	T60.1x3	T60.1x4	—	—
Diflos	T44.0x1	T44.0x2	T44.0x3	T44.0x4	T44.0x5	T44.0x6
Diflucortolone	T49.0x1	T49.0x2	T49.0x3	T49.0x4	T49.0x5	T49.0x6
Diflunisal	T39.091	T39.092	T39.093	T39.094	T39.095	T39.096
Difluoromethyldopa	T42.8x1	T42.8x2	T42.8x3	T42.8x4	T42.8x5	T42.8x6
Difluorophate	T44.0x1	T44.0x2	T44.0x3	T44.0x4	T44.0x5	T44.0x6
Digestant NEC	T47.5x1	T47.5x2	T47.5x3	T47.5x4	T47.5x5	T47.5x6
Digitalin(e)	T46.0x1	T46.0x2	T46.0x3	T46.0x4	T46.0x5	T46.0x6
Digitalis (leaf)(glycoside)	T46.0x1	T46.0x2	T46.0x3	T46.0x4	T46.0x5	T46.0x6
lanata	T46.0x1	T46.0x2	T46.0x3	T46.0x4	T46.0x5	T46.0x6
purpurea	T46.0x1	T46.0x2	T46.0x3	T46.0x4	T46.0x5	T46.0x6
Digitoxin	T46.0x1	T46.0x2	T46.0x3	T46.0x4	T46.0x5	T46.0x6
Digitoxose	T46.0x1	T46.0x2	T46.0x3	T46.0x4	T46.0x5	T46.0x6
Digoxin	T46.0x1	T46.0x2	T46.0x3	T46.0x4	T46.0x5	T46.0x6
Digoxine	T46.0x1	T46.0x2	T46.0x3	T46.0x4	T46.0x5	T46.0x6
Dihydralazine	T46.5x1	T46.5x2	T46.5x3	T46.5x4	T46.5x5	T46.5x6
Dihydrazine	T46.5x1	T46.5x2	T46.5x3	T46.5x4	T46.5x5	T46.5x6
Dihydrocodein	T40.2x1	T40.2x2	T40.2x3	T40.2x4	T40.2x5	T40.2x6
Dihydrocodeinone	T40.2x1	T40.2x2	T40.2x3	T40.2x4	T40.2x5	T40.2x6
Dihydroergocornine	T46.7x1	T46.7x2	T46.7x3	T46.7x4	T46.7x5	T46.7x6
Dihydroergocristine (mesilate)	T46.7x1	T46.7x2	T46.7x3	T46.7x4	T46.7x5	T46.7x6
Dihydroergokryptine	T46.7x1	T46.7x2	T46.7x3	T46.7x4	T46.7x5	T46.7x6
Dihydroergotamine	T46.5x1	T46.5x2	T46.5x3	T46.5x4	T46.5x5	T46.5x6
Dihydroergotoxine	T46.7x1	T46.7x2	T46.7x3	T46.7x4	T46.7x5	T46.7x6
mesilate	T46.7x1	T46.7x2	T46.7x3	T46.7x4	T46.7x5	T46.7x6
Dihydrohydroxycodeinone	T40.2x1	T40.2x2	T40.2x3	T40.2x4	T40.2x5	T40.2x6
Dihydrohydroxymorphinone	T40.2x1	T40.2x2	T40.2x3	T40.2x4	T40.2x5	T40.2x6
Dihydroisocodeine	T40.2x1	T40.2x2	T40.2x3	T40.2x4	T40.2x5	T40.2x6
Dihydromorphine	T40.2x1	T40.2x2	T40.2x3	T40.2x4	T40.2x5	T40.2x6
Dihydromorphinone	T40.2x1	T40.2x2	T40.2x3	T40.2x4	T40.2x5	T40.2x6
Dihydrostreptomycin	T36.5x1	T36.5x2	T36.5x3	T36.5x4	T36.5x5	T36.5x6
Dihydrotachysterol	T45.2x1	T45.2x2	T45.2x3	T45.2x4	T45.2x5	T45.2x6
Dihydroxyaluminum aminoacetate	T47.1x1	T47.1x2	T47.1x3	T47.1x4	T47.1x5	T47.1x6
Dihydroxyaluminum sodium carbonate	T47.1x1	T47.1x2	T47.1x3	T47.1x4	T47.1x5	T47.1x6
Dihydroxyanthraquinone	T47.2x1	T47.2x2	T47.2x3	T47.2x4	T47.2x5	T47.2x6
Dihydroxycodeinone	T40.2x1	T40.2x2	T40.2x3	T40.2x4	T40.2x5	T40.2x6
Dihydroxypropyl theophylline	T50.2x1	T50.2x2	T50.2x3	T50.2x4	T50.2x5	T50.2x6
Diiodohydroxyquin	T37.8x1	T37.8x2	T37.8x3	T37.8x4	T37.8x5	T37.8x6
topical	T49.0x1	T49.0x2	T49.0x3	T49.0x4	T49.0x5	T49.0x6
Diiodohydroxyquinoline	T37.8x1	T37.8x2	T37.8x3	T37.8x4	T37.8x5	T37.8x6
Diiodotyrosine	T38.2x1	T38.2x2	T38.2x3	T38.2x4	T38.2x5	T38.2x6
Diisopromine	T44.3x1	T44.3x2	T44.3x3	T44.3x4	T44.3x5	T44.3x6
Diisopropylamine	T46.3x1	T46.3x2	T46.3x3	T46.3x4	T46.3x5	T46.3x6
Diisopropylfluorophos-phonate	T44.0x1	T44.0x2	T44.0x3	T44.0x4	T44.0x5	T44.0x6
Dilantin	T42.0x1	T42.0x2	T42.0x3	T42.0x4	T42.0x5	T42.0x6
Dilaudid	T40.2x1	T40.2x2	T40.2x3	T40.2x4	T40.2x5	T40.2x6
Dilazep	T46.3x1	T46.3x2	T46.3x3	T46.3x4	T46.3x5	T46.3x6
Dill	T47.5x1	T47.5x2	T47.5x3	T47.5x4	T47.5x5	T47.5x6
Diloxanide	T37.3x1	T37.3x2	T37.3x3	T37.3x4	T37.3x5	T37.3x6
Diltiazem	T46.1x1	T46.1x2	T46.1x3	T46.1x4	T46.1x5	T46.1x6
Dimazole	T49.0x1	T49.0x2	T49.0x3	T49.0x4	T49.0x5	T49.0x6
Dimefline	T50.7x1	T50.7x2	T50.7x3	T50.7x4	T50.7x5	T50.7x6
Dimefox	T60.0x1	T60.0x2	T60.0x3	T60.0x4	—	—
Dimemorfan	T48.3x1	T48.3x2	T48.3x3	T48.3x4	T48.3x5	T48.3x6
Dimenhydrinate	T45.0x1	T45.0x2	T45.0x3	T45.0x4	T45.0x5	T45.0x6
Dimercaprol (British anti-lewisite)	T45.8x1	T45.8x2	T45.8x3	T45.8x4	T45.8x5	T45.8x6
Dimercaptopropanol	T45.8x1	T45.8x2	T45.8x3	T45.8x4	T45.8x5	T45.8x6
Dimestrol	T38.5x1	T38.5x2	T38.5x3	T38.5x4	T38.5x5	T38.5x6
Dimetane	T45.0x1	T45.0x2	T45.0x3	T45.0x4	T45.0x5	T45.0x6
Dimethicone	T47.1x1	T47.1x2	T47.1x3	T47.1x4	T47.1x5	T47.1x6
Dimethindene	T45.0x1	T45.0x2	T45.0x3	T45.0x4	T45.0x5	T45.0x6
Dimethisoquin	T49.1x1	T49.1x2	T49.1x3	T49.1x4	T49.1x5	T49.1x6
Dimethisterone	T38.5x1	T38.5x2	T38.5x3	T38.5x4	T38.5x5	T38.5x6
Dimethoate	T60.0x1	T60.0x2	T60.0x3	T60.0x4	—	—
Dimethocaine	T41.3x1	T41.3x2	T41.3x3	T41.3x4	T41.3x5	T41.3x6
Dimethoxanate	T48.3x1	T48.3x2	T48.3x3	T48.3x4	T48.3x5	T48.3x6
Dimethyl						
arsine, arsinic acid	T57.0x1	T57.0x2	T57.0x3	T57.0x4	—	—
carbinol	T51.2x1	T51.2x2	T51.2x3	T51.2x4	—	—

Substance	Poisoning, Accidental (unintentional)	Poisoning, Intentional Self-harm	Poisoning, Assault	Poisoning, Undetermined	Adverse Effect	Under-dosing
Dimethyl—*continued*						
carbonate	T52.8x1	T52.8x2	T52.8x3	T52.8x4	—	—
diguanide	T38.3x1	T38.3x2	T38.3x3	T38.3x4	T38.3x5	T38.3x6
ketone	T52.4x1	T52.4x2	T52.4x3	T52.4x4	—	—
vapor	T52.4x1	T52.4x2	T52.4x3	T52.4x4	—	—
meperidine	T40.2x1	T40.2x2	T40.2x3	T40.2x4	T40.2x5	T40.2x6
parathion	T60.0x1	T60.0x2	T60.0x3	T60.0x4	—	—
phthlate	T49.3x1	T49.3x2	T49.3x3	T49.3x4	T49.3x5	T49.3x6
polysiloxane	T47.8x1	T47.8x2	T47.8x3	T47.8x4	T47.8x5	T47.8x6
sulfate (fumes)	T59.891	T59.892	T59.893	T59.894	—	—
liquid	T65.891	T65.892	T65.893	T65.894	—	—
sulfoxide (nonmedicinal)	T52.8x1	T52.8x2	T52.8x3	T52.8x4	—	—
medicinal	T49.4x1	T49.4x2	T49.4x3	T49.4x4	T49.4x5	T49.4x6
tryptamine	T40.991	T40.992	T40.993	T40.994	T40.995	T40.996
tubocurarine	T48.1x1	T48.1x2	T48.1x3	T48.1x4	T48.1x5	T48.1x6
Dimethylamine sulfate	T49.4x1	T49.4x2	T49.4x3	T49.4x4	T49.4x5	T49.4x6
Dimethylformamide	T52.8x1	T52.8x2	T52.8x3	T52.8x4	—	—
Dimethyltubocurarinium chloride	T48.1x1	T48.1x2	T48.1x3	T48.1x4	T48.1x5	T48.1x6
Dimeticone	T47.1x1	T47.1x2	T47.1x3	T47.1x4	T47.1x5	T47.1x6
Dimetilan	T60.0x1	T60.0x2	T60.0x3	T60.0x4	—	—
Dimetindene	T45.0x1	T45.0x2	T45.0x3	T45.0x4	T45.0x5	T45.0x6
Dimetotiazine	T43.3x1	T43.3x2	T43.3x3	T43.3x4	T43.3x5	T43.3x6
Dimorpholamine	T50.7x1	T50.7x2	T50.7x3	T50.7x4	T50.7x5	T50.7x6
Dimoxyline	T46.3x1	T46.3x2	T46.3x3	T46.3x4	T46.3x5	T46.3x6
Dinitrobenzene	T65.3x1	T65.3x2	T65.3x3	T65.3x4	—	—
vapor	T59.891	T59.892	T59.893	T59.894	—	—
Dinitrobenzol	T65.3x1	T65.3x2	T65.3x3	T65.3x4	—	—
vapor	T59.891	T59.892	T59.893	T59.894	—	—
Dinitrobutylphenol	T65.3x1	T65.3x2	T65.3x3	T65.3x4	—	—
Dinitro(-ortho-)cresol (pesticide) (spray)	T65.3x1	T65.3x2	T65.3x3	T65.3x4	—	—
Dinitrocyclohexylphenol	T65.3x1	T65.3x2	T65.3x3	T65.3x4	—	—
Dinitrophenol	T65.3x1	T65.3x2	T65.3x3	T65.3x4	—	—
Dinoprost	T48.0x1	T48.0x2	T48.0x3	T48.0x4	T48.0x5	T48.0x6
Dinoprostone	T48.0x1	T48.0x2	T48.0x3	T48.0x4	T48.0x5	T48.0x6
Dinoseb	T60.3x1	T60.3x2	T60.3x3	T60.3x4	—	—
Dioctyl sulfosuccinate (calcium) (sodium)	T47.4x1	T47.4x2	T47.4x3	T47.4x4	T47.4x5	T47.4x6
Diodone	T50.8x1	T50.8x2	T50.8x3	T50.8x4	T50.8x5	T50.8x6
Diodoquin	T37.8x1	T37.8x2	T37.8x3	T37.8x4	T37.8x5	T37.8x6
Dionin	T40.2x1	T40.2x2	T40.2x3	T40.2x4	T40.2x5	T40.2x6
Diosmin	T46.991	T46.992	T46.993	T46.994	T46.995	T46.996
Dioxane	T52.8x1	T52.8x2	T52.8x3	T52.8x4	—	—
Dioxathion	T60.0x1	T60.0x2	T60.0x3	T60.0x4	—	—
Dioxin	T53.7x1	T53.7x2	T53.7x3	T53.7x4	—	—
Dioxopromethazine	T43.3x1	T43.3x2	T43.3x3	T43.3x4	T43.3x5	T43.3x6
Dioxyline	T46.3x1	T46.3x2	T46.3x3	T46.3x4	T46.3x5	T46.3x6
Dipentene	T52.8x1	T52.8x2	T52.8x3	T52.8x4	—	—
Diperodon	T41.3x1	T41.3x2	T41.3x3	T41.3x4	T41.3x5	T41.3x6
Diphacinone	T60.4x1	T60.4x2	T60.4x3	T60.4x4	—	—
Diphemanil	T44.3x1	T44.3x2	T44.3x3	T44.3x4	T44.3x5	T44.3x6
metilsulfate	T44.3x1	T44.3x2	T44.3x3	T44.3x4	T44.3x5	T44.3x6
Diphenadione	T45.511	T45.512	T45.513	T45.514	T45.515	T45.516
rodenticide	T60.4x1	T60.4x2	T60.4x3	T60.4x4	—	—
Diphenhydramine	T45.0x1	T45.0x2	T45.0x3	T45.0x4	T45.0x5	T45.0x6
Diphenidol	T45.0x1	T45.0x2	T45.0x3	T45.0x4	T45.0x5	T45.0x6
Diphenoxylate	T47.6x1	T47.6x2	T47.6x3	T47.6x4	T47.6x5	T47.6x6
Diphenylamine	T65.3x1	T65.3x2	T65.3x3	T65.3x4	—	—
Diphenylbutazone	T39.2x1	T39.2x2	T39.2x3	T39.2x4	T39.2x5	T39.2x6
Diphenylchloroarsine, not in war	T57.0x1	T57.0x2	T57.0x3	T57.0x4	—	—
Diphenylhydantoin	T42.0x1	T42.0x2	T42.0x3	T42.0x4	T42.0x5	T42.0x6
Diphenylmethane dye	T52.1x1	T52.1x2	T52.1x3	T52.1x4	—	—
Diphenylpyraline	T45.0x1	T45.0x2	T45.0x3	T45.0x4	T45.0x5	T45.0x6
Diphtheria						
antitoxin	T50.Z11	T50.Z12	T50.Z13	T50.Z14	T50.Z15	T50.Z16
toxoid	T50.A91	T50.A92	T50.A93	T50.A94	T50.A95	T50.A96
with tetanus toxoid	T50.A21	T50.A22	T50.A23	T50.A24	T50.A25	T50.A26
with pertussis component	T50.A11	T50.A12	T50.A13	T50.A14	T50.A15	T50.A16
vaccine	T50.A91	T50.A92	T50.A93	T50.A94	T50.A95	T50.A96
combination						

Substance	Poisoning, Accidental (unintentional)	Poisoning, Intentional Self-harm	Poisoning, Assault	Poisoning, Undetermined	Adverse Effect	Under-dosing
Diphtheria—*continued*						
vaccine—*continued*						
combination—*continued*						
including pertussis	T50.A11	T50.A12	T50.A13	T50.A14	T50.A15	T50.A16
without pertussis	T50.A21	T50.A22	T50.A23	T50.A24	T50.A25	T50.A26
Diphylline	T50.2x1	T50.2x2	T50.2x3	T50.2x4	T50.2x5	T50.2x6
Dipipanone	T40.4x1	T40.4x2	T40.4x3	T40.4x4	T40.4x5	T40.4x6
Dipivefrine	T49.5x1	T49.5x2	T49.5x3	T49.5x4	T49.5x5	T49.5x6
Diplovax	T50.B91	T50.B92	T50.B93	T50.B94	T50.B95	T50.B96
Diprophylline	T50.2x1	T50.2x2	T50.2x3	T50.2x4	T50.2x5	T50.2x6
Dipropyline	T48.291	T48.292	T48.293	T48.294	T48.295	T48.296
Dipyridamole	T46.3x1	T46.3x2	T46.3x3	T46.3x4	T46.3x5	T46.3x6
Dipyrone	T39.2x1	T39.2x2	T39.2x3	T39.2x4	T39.2x5	T39.2x6
Diquat (dibromide)	T60.3x1	T60.3x2	T60.3x3	T60.3x4	—	—
Disinfectant	T65.891	T65.892	T65.893	T65.894	—	—
alkaline	T54.3x1	T54.3x2	T54.3x3	T54.3x4	—	—
aromatic	T54.1x1	T54.1x2	T54.1x3	T54.1x4	—	—
intestinal	T37.8x1	T37.8x2	T37.8x3	T37.8x4	T37.8x5	T37.8x6
Disipal	T42.8x1	T42.8x2	T42.8x3	T42.8x4	T42.8x5	T42.8x6
Disodium edetate	T50.6x1	T50.6x2	T50.6x3	T50.6x4	T50.6x5	T50.6x6
Disoprofol	T41.291	T41.292	T41.293	T41.294	T41.295	T41.296
Disopyramide	T46.2x1	T46.2x2	T46.2x3	T46.2x4	T46.2x5	T46.2x6
Distigmine (bromide)	T44.0x1	T44.0x2	T44.0x3	T44.0x4	T44.0x5	T44.0x6
Disulfamide	T50.2x1	T50.2x2	T50.2x3	T50.2x4	T50.2x5	T50.2x6
Disulfanilamide	T37.0x1	T37.0x2	T37.0x3	T37.0x4	T37.0x5	T37.0x6
Disulfiram	T50.6x1	T50.6x2	T50.6x3	T50.6x4	T50.6x5	T50.6x6
Disulfoton	T60.0x1	T60.0x2	T60.0x3	T60.0x4	—	—
Dithiazanine iodide	T37.4x1	T37.4x2	T37.4x3	T37.4x4	T37.4x5	T37.4x6
Dithiocarbamate	T60.0x1	T60.0x2	T60.0x3	T60.0x4	—	—
Dithranol	T49.4x1	T49.4x2	T49.4x3	T49.4x4	T49.4x5	T49.4x6
Diucardin	T50.2x1	T50.2x2	T50.2x3	T50.2x4	T50.2x5	T50.2x6
Diupres	T50.2x1	T50.2x2	T50.2x3	T50.2x4	T50.2x5	T50.2x6
Diuretic NEC	T50.2x1	T50.2x2	T50.2x3	T50.2x4	T50.2x5	T50.2x6
carbonic acid anhydrase inhibitors	T50.2x1	T50.2x2	T50.2x3	T50.2x4	T50.2x5	T50.2x6
benzothiadiazine	T50.2x1	T50.2x2	T50.2x3	T50.2x4	T50.2x5	T50.2x6
furfuryl NEC	T50.2x1	T50.2x2	T50.2x3	T50.2x4	T50.2x5	T50.2x6
mercurial NEC	T50.2x1	T50.2x2	T50.2x3	T50.2x4	T50.2x5	T50.2x6
osmotic	T50.2x1	T50.2x2	T50.2x3	T50.2x4	T50.2x5	T50.2x6
purine NEC	T50.2x1	T50.2x2	T50.2x3	T50.2x4	T50.2x5	T50.2x6
saluretic NEC	T50.2x1	T50.2x2	T50.2x3	T50.2x4	T50.2x5	T50.2x6
sulfonamide	T50.2x1	T50.2x2	T50.2x3	T50.2x4	T50.2x5	T50.2x6
thiazide NEC	T50.2x1	T50.2x2	T50.2x3	T50.2x4	T50.2x5	T50.2x6
xanthine	T50.2x1	T50.2x2	T50.2x3	T50.2x4	T50.2x5	T50.2x6
Diurgin	T50.2x1	T50.2x2	T50.2x3	T50.2x4	T50.2x5	T50.2x6
Diuril	T50.2x1	T50.2x2	T50.2x3	T50.2x4	T50.2x5	T50.2x6
Diuron	T60.3x1	T60.3x2	T60.3x3	T60.3x4	—	—
Divalproex	T42.6x1	T42.6x2	T42.6x3	T42.6x4	T42.6x5	T42.6x6
Divinyl ether	T41.0x1	T41.0x2	T41.0x3	T41.0x4	T41.0x5	T41.0x6
Dixanthogen	T49.0x1	T49.0x2	T49.0x3	T49.0x4	T49.0x5	T49.0x6
Dixyrazine	T43.3x1	T43.3x2	T43.3x3	T43.3x4	T43.3x5	T43.3x6
D-lysergic acid diethylamide	T40.8x1	T40.8x2	T40.8x3	T40.8x4	T40.8x5	T40.8x6
DMCT	T36.4x1	T36.4x2	T36.4x3	T36.4x4	T36.4x5	T36.4x6
DMSO—*see* Dimethyl sulfoxide						
DNBP	T60.3x1	T60.3x2	T60.3x3	T60.3x4	—	—
DNOC	T65.3x1	T65.3x2	T65.3x3	T65.3x4	—	—
DOCA	T38.0x1	T38.0x2	T38.0x3	T38.0x4	T38.0x5	T38.0x6
Dobutamine	T44.5x1	T44.5x2	T44.5x3	T44.5x4	T44.5x5	T44.5x6
Docusate sodium	T47.4x1	T47.4x2	T47.4x3	T47.4x4	T47.4x5	T47.4x6
Dodicin	T49.0x1	T49.0x2	T49.0x3	T49.0x4	T49.0x5	T49.0x6
Dofamium chloride	T49.0x1	T49.0x2	T49.0x3	T49.0x4	T49.0x5	T49.0x6
Dolophine	T40.3x1	T40.3x2	T40.3x3	T40.3x4	T40.3x5	T40.3x6
Doloxene	T39.8x1	T39.8x2	T39.8x3	T39.8x4	T39.8x5	T39.8x6
Domestic gas (after combustion)—*see* Gas, utility						
prior to combustion	T59.891	T59.892	T59.893	T59.894	—	—
Domiodol	T48.4x1	T48.4x2	T48.4x3	T48.4x4	T48.4x5	T48.4x6
Domiphen (bromide)	T49.0x1	T49.0x2	T49.0x3	T49.0x4	T49.0x5	T49.0x6
Domperidone	T45.0x1	T45.0x2	T45.0x3	T45.0x4	T45.0x5	T45.0x6
Dopa	T42.8x1	T42.8x2	T42.8x3	T42.8x4	T42.8x5	T42.8x6

Substance	Poisoning, Accidental (unintentional)	Poisoning, Intentional Self-harm	Poisoning, Assault	Poisoning, Undetermined	Adverse Effect	Under-dosing
Dopamine	T44.991	T44.992	T44.993	T44.994	T44.995	T44.996
Doriden	T42.6x1	T42.6x2	T42.6x3	T42.6x4	T42.6x5	T42.6x6
Dormiral	T42.3x1	T42.3x2	T42.3x3	T42.3x4	T42.3x5	T42.3x6
Dormison	T42.6x1	T42.6x2	T42.6x3	T42.6x4	T42.6x5	T42.6x6
Dornase	T48.4x1	T48.4x2	T48.4x3	T48.4x4	T48.4x5	T48.4x6
Dorsacaine	T41.3x1	T41.3x2	T41.3x3	T41.3x4	T41.3x5	T41.3x6
Dosulepin	T43.011	T43.012	T43.013	T43.014	T43.015	T43.016
Dothiepin	T43.011	T43.012	T43.013	T43.014	T43.015	T43.016
Doxantrazole	T48.6x1	T48.6x2	T48.6x3	T48.6x4	T48.6x5	T48.6x6
Doxapram	T50.7x1	T50.7x2	T50.7x3	T50.7x4	T50.7x5	T50.7x6
Doxazosin	T44.6x1	T44.6x2	T44.6x3	T44.6x4	T44.6x5	T44.6x6
Doxepin	T43.011	T43.012	T43.013	T43.014	T43.015	T43.016
Doxifluridine	T45.1x1	T45.1x2	T45.1x3	T45.1x4	T45.1x5	T45.1x6
Doxorubicin	T45.1x1	T45.1x2	T45.1x3	T45.1x4	T45.1x5	T45.1x6
Doxycycline	T36.4x1	T36.4x2	T36.4x3	T36.4x4	T36.4x5	T36.4x6
Doxylamine	T45.0x1	T45.0x2	T45.0x3	T45.0x4	T45.0x5	T45.0x6
Dramamine	T45.0x1	T45.0x2	T45.0x3	T45.0x4	T45.0x5	T45.0x6
Drano (drain cleaner)	T54.3x1	T54.3x2	T54.3x3	T54.3x4	—	—
Dressing, live pulp	T49.7x1	T49.7x2	T49.7x3	T49.7x4	T49.7x5	T49.7x6
Drocode	T40.2x1	T40.2x2	T40.2x3	T40.2x4	T40.2x5	T40.2x6
Dromoran	T40.2x1	T40.2x2	T40.2x3	T40.2x4	T40.2x5	T40.2x6
Dromostanolone	T38.7x1	T38.7x2	T38.7x3	T38.7x4	T38.7x5	T38.7x6
Dronabinol	T40.7x1	T40.7x2	T40.7x3	T40.7x4	T40.7x5	T40.7x6
Droperidol	T43.591	T43.592	T43.593	T43.594	T43.595	T43.596
Dropropizine	T48.3x1	T48.3x2	T48.3x3	T48.3x4	T48.3x5	T48.3x6
Drostanolone	T38.7x1	T38.7x2	T38.7x3	T38.7x4	T38.7x5	T38.7x6
Drotaverine	T44.3x1	T44.3x2	T44.3x3	T44.3x4	T44.3x5	T44.3x6
Drotrecogin alfa	T45.511	T45.512	T45.513	T45.514	T45.515	T45.516
Drug NEC	T50.901	T50.902	T50.903	T50.904	T50.905	T50.906
specified NEC	T50.991	T50.992	T50.993	T50.994	T50.995	T50.996
DTIC	T45.1x1	T45.1x2	T45.1x3	T45.1x4	T45.1x5	T45.1x6
Duboisine	T44.3x1	T44.3x2	T44.3x3	T44.3x4	T44.3x5	T44.3x6
Dulcolax	T47.2x1	T47.2x2	T47.2x3	T47.2x4	T47.2x5	T47.2x6
Duponol (C) (EP)	T49.2x1	T49.2x2	T49.2x3	T49.2x4	T49.2x5	T49.2x6
Durabolin	T38.7x1	T38.7x2	T38.7x3	T38.7x4	T38.7x5	T38.7x6
Dyclone	T41.3x1	T41.3x2	T41.3x3	T41.3x4	T41.3x5	T41.3x6
Dyclonine	T41.3x1	T41.3x2	T41.3x3	T41.3x4	T41.3x5	T41.3x6
Dydrogesterone	T38.5x1	T38.5x2	T38.5x3	T38.5x4	T38.5x5	T38.5x6
Dye NEC	T65.6x1	T65.6x2	T65.6x3	T65.6x4	—	—
antiseptic	T49.0x1	T49.0x2	T49.0x3	T49.0x4	T49.0x5	T49.0x6
diagnostic agents	T50.8x1	T50.8x2	T50.8x3	T50.8x4	T50.8x5	T50.8x6
pharmaceutical NEC	T50.901	T50.902	T50.903	T50.904	T50.905	T50.906
Dyflos	T44.0x1	T44.0x2	T44.0x3	T44.0x4	T44.0x5	T44.0x6
Dymelor	T38.3x1	T38.3x2	T38.3x3	T38.3x4	T38.3x5	T38.3x6
Dynamite	T65.3x1	T65.3x2	T65.3x3	T65.3x4	—	—
fumes	T59.891	T59.892	T59.893	T59.894		
Dyphylline	T44.3x1	T44.3x2	T44.3x3	T44.3x4	T44.3x5	T44.3x6
Ear drug NEC	T49.6x1	T49.6x2	T49.6x3	T49.6x4	T49.6x5	T49.6x6
Ear preparations	T49.6x1	T49.6x2	T49.6x3	T49.6x4	T49.6x5	T49.6x6
Econazole	T49.0x1	T49.0x2	T49.0x3	T49.0x4	T49.0x5	T49.0x6
Ecothiopate iodide	T49.5x1	T49.5x2	T49.5x3	T49.5x4	T49.5x5	T49.5x6
Echothiophate, echothiopate, ecothiopate	T49.5x1	T49.5x2	T49.5x3	T49.5x4	T49.5x5	T49.5x6
Ecstasy	T43.621	T43.622	T43.623	T43.624	T43.625	T43.626
Ectylurea	T42.6x1	T42.6x2	T42.6x3	T42.6x4	T42.6x5	T42.6x6
Edathamil disodium	T45.8x1	T45.8x2	T45.8x3	T45.8x4	T45.8x5	T45.8x6
Edecrin	T50.1x1	T50.1x2	T50.1x3	T50.1x4	T50.1x5	T50.1x6
Edetate, disodium (calcium)	T45.8x1	T45.8x2	T45.8x3	T45.8x4	T45.8x5	T45.8x6
Edoxudine	T49.5x1	T49.5x2	T49.5x3	T49.5x4	T49.5x5	T49.5x6
Edrophonium	T44.0x1	T44.0x2	T44.0x3	T44.0x4	T44.0x5	T44.0x6
chloride	T44.0x1	T44.0x2	T44.0x3	T44.0x4	T44.0x5	T44.0x6
EDTA	T50.6x1	T50.6x2	T50.6x3	T50.6x4	T50.6x5	T50.6x6
Eflornithine	T37.2x1	T37.2x2	T37.2x3	T37.2x4	T37.2x5	T37.2x6
Efloxate	T46.3x1	T46.3x2	T46.3x3	T46.3x4	T46.3x5	T46.3x6
Elase	T49.8x1	T49.8x2	T49.8x3	T49.8x4	T49.8x5	T49.8x6
Elastase	T47.5x1	T47.5x2	T47.5x3	T47.5x4	T47.5x5	T47.5x6
Elaterium	T47.2x1	T47.2x2	T47.2x3	T47.2x4	T47.2x5	T47.2x6
Elcatonin	T50.991	T50.992	T50.993	T50.994	T50.995	T50.996
Elder	T62.2x1	T62.2x2	T62.2x3	T62.2x4	—	—
berry, (unripe)	T62.1x1	T62.1x2	T62.1x3	T62.1x4	—	—
Electrolyte balance drug	T50.3x1	T50.3x2	T50.3x3	T50.3x4	T50.3x5	T50.3x6
Electrolytes NEC	T50.3x1	T50.3x2	T50.3x3	T50.3x4	T50.3x5	T50.3x6
Electrolytic agent NEC	T50.3x1	T50.3x2	T50.3x3	T50.3x4	T50.3x5	T50.3x6
Elemental diet	T50.901	T50.902	T50.903	T50.904	T50.905	T50.906
Elliptinium acetate	T45.1x1	T45.1x2	T45.1x3	T45.1x4	T45.1x5	T45.1x6
Embramine	T45.0x1	T45.0x2	T45.0x3	T45.0x4	T45.0x5	T45.0x6
Emepronium (salts)	T44.3x1	T44.3x2	T44.3x3	T44.3x4	T44.3x5	T44.3x6
bromide	T44.3x1	T44.3x2	T44.3x3	T44.3x4	T44.3x5	T44.3x6
Emetic NEC	T47.7x1	T47.7x2	T47.7x3	T47.7x4	T47.7x5	T47.7x6
Emetine	T37.3x1	T37.3x2	T37.3x3	T37.3x4	T37.3x5	T37.3x6
Emollient NEC	T49.3x1	T49.3x2	T49.3x3	T49.3x4	T49.3x5	T49.3x6
Emorfazone	T39.8x1	T39.8x2	T39.8x3	T39.8x4	T39.8x5	T39.8x6
Emylcamate	T43.591	T43.592	T43.593	T43.594	T43.595	T43.596
Enalapril	T46.4x1	T46.4x2	T46.4x3	T46.4x4	T46.4x5	T46.4x6
Enalaprilat	T46.4x1	T46.4x2	T46.4x3	T46.4x4	T46.4x5	T46.4x6
Encainide	T46.2x1	T46.2x2	T46.2x3	T46.2x4	T46.2x5	T46.2x6
Endocaine	T41.3x1	T41.3x2	T41.3x3	T41.3x4	T41.3x5	T41.3x6
Endosulfan	T60.2x1	T60.2x2	T60.2x3	T60.2x4	—	—
Endothall	T60.3x1	T60.3x2	T60.3x3	T60.3x4	—	—
Endralazine	T46.5x1	T46.5x2	T46.5x3	T46.5x4	T46.5x5	T46.5x6
Endrin	T60.1x1	T60.1x2	T60.1x3	T60.1x4	—	—
Enflurane	T41.0x1	T41.0x2	T41.0x3	T41.0x4	T41.0x5	T41.0x6
Enhexymal	T42.3x1	T42.3x2	T42.3x3	T42.3x4	T42.3x5	T42.3x6
Enocitabine	T45.1x1	T45.1x2	T45.1x3	T45.1x4	T45.1x5	T45.1x6
Enovid	T38.4x1	T38.4x2	T38.4x3	T38.4x4	T38.4x5	T38.4x6
Enoxacin	T36.8x1	T36.8x2	T36.8x3	T36.8x4	T36.8x5	T36.8x6
Enoxaparin (sodium)	T45.511	T45.512	T45.513	T45.514	T45.515	T45.516
Enpiprazole	T43.591	T43.592	T43.593	T43.594	T43.595	T43.596
Enprofylline	T48.6x1	T48.6x2	T48.6x3	T48.6x4	T48.6x5	T48.6x6
Enprostil	T47.1x1	T47.1x2	T47.1x3	T47.1x4	T47.1x5	T47.1x6
Enterogastrone	T38.891	T38.892	T38.893	T38.894	T38.895	T38.896
ENT preparations (anti-infectives)	T49.6x1	T49.6x2	T49.6x3	T49.6x4	T49.6x5	T49.6x6
Enviomycin	T36.8x1	T36.8x2	T36.8x3	T36.8x4	T36.8x5	T36.8x6
Enzodase	T45.3x1	T45.3x2	T45.3x3	T45.3x4	T45.3x5	T45.3x6
Enzyme NEC	T45.3x1	T45.3x2	T45.3x3	T45.3x4	T45.3x5	T45.3x6
depolymerizing	T49.8x1	T49.8x2	T49.8x3	T49.8x4	T49.8x5	T49.8x6
fibrolytic	T45.3x1	T45.3x2	T45.3x3	T45.3x4	T45.3x5	T45.3x6
gastric	T45.3x1	T45.3x2	T45.3x3	T45.3x4	T45.3x5	T45.3x6
intestinal	T47.5x1	T47.5x2	T47.5x3	T47.5x4	T47.5x5	T47.5x6
local action	T49.4x1	T49.4x2	T49.4x3	T49.4x4	T49.4x5	T49.4x6
proteolytic	T49.4x1	T49.4x2	T49.4x3	T49.4x4	T49.4x5	T49.4x6
thrombolytic	T45.3x1	T45.3x2	T45.3x3	T45.3x4	T45.3x5	T45.3x6
EPAB	T41.3x1	T41.3x2	T41.3x3	T41.3x4	T41.3x5	T41.3x6
Epanutin	T42.0x1	T42.0x2	T42.0x3	T42.0x4	T42.0x5	T42.0x6
Ephedra	T44.991	T44.992	T44.993	T44.994	T44.995	T44.996
Ephedrine	T44.991	T44.992	T44.993	T44.994	T44.995	T44.996
Epichlorhydrin, epichlorohydrin	T52.8x1	T52.8x2	T52.8x3	T52.8x4	—	—
Epicillin	T36.0x1	T36.0x2	T36.0x3	T36.0x4	T36.0x5	T36.0x6
Epiestriol	T38.5x1	T38.5x2	T38.5x3	T38.5x4	T38.5x5	T38.5x6
Epilim—see Sodium valproate						
Epimestrol	T38.5x1	T38.5x2	T38.5x3	T38.5x4	T38.5x5	T38.5x6
Epinephrine	T44.5x1	T44.5x2	T44.5x3	T44.5x4	T44.5x5	T44.5x6
Epirubicin	T45.1x1	T45.1x2	T45.1x3	T45.1x4	T45.1x5	T45.1x6
Epitiostanol	T38.7x1	T38.7x2	T38.7x3	T38.7x4	T38.7x5	T38.7x6
Epitizide	T50.2x1	T50.2x2	T50.2x3	T50.2x4	T50.2x5	T50.2x6
EPN	T60.0x1	T60.0x2	T60.0x3	T60.0x4	—	—
EPO	T45.8x1	T45.8x2	T45.8x3	T45.8x4	T45.8x5	T45.8x6
Epoetin alpha	T45.8x1	T45.8x2	T45.8x3	T45.8x4	T45.8x5	T45.8x6
Epomediol	T50.991	T50.992	T50.993	T50.994	T50.995	T50.996
Epoprostenol	T45.521	T45.522	T45.523	T45.524	T45.525	T45.526
Epoxy resin	T65.891	T65.892	T65.893	T65.894	—	—
Eprazinone	T48.4x1	T48.4x2	T48.4x3	T48.4x4	T48.4x5	T48.4x6
Epsilon amino-caproic acid	T45.621	T45.622	T45.623	T45.624	T45.625	T45.626
Epsom salt	T47.3x1	T47.3x2	T47.3x3	T47.3x4	T47.3x5	T47.3x6
Eptazocine	T40.4x1	T40.4x2	T40.4x3	T40.4x4	T40.4x5	T40.4x6
Equanil	T43.591	T43.592	T43.593	T43.594	T43.595	T43.596
Equisetum	T62.2x1	T62.2x2	T62.2x3	T62.2x4	—	—
diuretic	T50.2x1	T50.2x2	T50.2x3	T50.2x4	T50.2x5	T50.2x6
Ergobasine	T48.0x1	T48.0x2	T48.0x3	T48.0x4	T48.0x5	T48.0x6
Ergocalciferol	T45.2x1	T45.2x2	T45.2x3	T45.2x4	T45.2x5	T45.2x6
Ergoloid mesylates	T46.7x1	T46.7x2	T46.7x3	T46.7x4	T46.7x5	T46.7x6
Ergometrine	T48.0x1	T48.0x2	T48.0x3	T48.0x4	T48.0x5	T48.0x6

Substance	Poisoning, Accidental (unintentional)	Poisoning, Intentional Self-harm	Poisoning, Assault	Poisoning, Undetermined	Adverse Effect	Under-dosing
Ergonovine	T48.0x1	T48.0x2	T48.0x3	T48.0x4	T48.0x5	T48.0x6
Ergot NEC	T64.81	T64.82	T64.83	T64.84	—	—
derivative	T48.0x1	T48.0x2	T48.0x3	T48.0x4	T48.0x5	T48.0x6
medicinal (alkaloids)	T48.0x1	T48.0x2	T48.0x3	T48.0x4	T48.0x5	T48.0x6
prepared	T48.0x1	T48.0x2	T48.0x3	T48.0x4	T48.0x5	T48.0x6
Ergotamine	T46.5x1	T46.5x2	T46.5x3	T46.5x4	T46.5x5	T46.5x6
Ergotocine	T48.0x1	T48.0x2	T48.0x3	T48.0x4	T48.0x5	T48.0x6
Ergotrate	T48.0x1	T48.0x2	T48.0x3	T48.0x4	T48.0x5	T48.0x6
Eritrityl tetranitrate	T46.3x1	T46.3x2	T46.3x3	T46.3x4	T46.3x5	T46.3x6
Erythrityl tetranitrate	T46.3x1	T46.3x2	T46.3x3	T46.3x4	T46.3x5	T46.3x6
Erythrol tetranitrate	T46.3x1	T46.3x2	T46.3x3	T46.3x4	T46.3x5	T46.3x6
Erythromycin (salts)	T36.3x1	T36.3x2	T36.3x3	T36.3x4	T36.3x5	T36.3x6
ophthalmic preparation	T49.5x1	T49.5x2	T49.5x3	T49.5x4	T49.5x5	T49.5x6
topical NEC	T49.0x1	T49.0x2	T49.0x3	T49.0x4	T49.0x5	T49.0x6
Erythropoietin	T45.8x1	T45.8x2	T45.8x3	T45.8x4	T45.8x5	T45.8x6
human	T45.8x1	T45.8x2	T45.8x3	T45.8x4	T45.8x5	T45.8x6
Escin	T46.991	T46.992	T46.993	T46.994	T46.995	T46.996
Esculin	T45.2x1	T45.2x2	T45.2x3	T45.2x4	T45.2x5	T45.2x6
Esculoside	T45.2x1	T45.2x2	T45.2x3	T45.2x4	T45.2x5	T45.2x6
ESDT (ether-soluble tar distillate)	T49.1x1	T49.1x2	T49.1x3	T49.1x4	T49.1x5	T49.1x6
Eserine	T49.5x1	T49.5x2	T49.5x3	T49.5x4	T49.5x5	T49.5x6
Esflurbiprofen	T39.311	T39.312	T39.313	T39.314	T39.315	T39.316
Eskabarb	T42.3x1	T42.3x2	T42.3x3	T42.3x4	T42.3x5	T42.3x6
Eskalith	T43.8x1	T43.8x2	T43.8x3	T43.8x4	T43.8x5	T43.8x6
Esmolol	T44.7x1	T44.7x2	T44.7x3	T44.7x4	T44.7x5	T44.7x6
Estanozolol	T38.7x1	T38.7x2	T38.7x3	T38.7x4	T38.7x5	T38.7x6
Estazolam	T42.4x1	T42.4x2	T42.4x3	T42.4x4	T42.4x5	T42.4x6
Estradiol	T38.5x1	T38.5x2	T38.5x3	T38.5x4	T38.5x5	T38.5x6
with testosterone	T38.7x1	T38.7x2	T38.7x3	T38.7x4	T38.7x5	T38.7x6
benzoate	T38.5x1	T38.5x2	T38.5x3	T38.5x4	T38.5x5	T38.5x6
Estramustine	T45.1x1	T45.1x2	T45.1x3	T45.1x4	T45.1x5	T45.1x6
Estriol	T38.5x1	T38.5x2	T38.5x3	T38.5x4	T38.5x5	T38.5x6
Estrogen	T38.5x1	T38.5x2	T38.5x3	T38.5x4	T38.5x5	T38.5x6
with progesterone	T38.5x1	T38.5x2	T38.5x3	T38.5x4	T38.5x5	T38.5x6
conjugated	T38.5x1	T38.5x2	T38.5x3	T38.5x4	T38.5x5	T38.5x6
Estrone	T38.5x1	T38.5x2	T38.5x3	T38.5x4	T38.5x5	T38.5x6
Estropipate	T38.5x1	T38.5x2	T38.5x3	T38.5x4	T38.5x5	T38.5x6
Etacrynate sodium	T50.1x1	T50.1x2	T50.1x3	T50.1x4	T50.1x5	T50.1x6
Etacrynic acid	T50.1x1	T50.1x2	T50.1x3	T50.1x4	T50.1x5	T50.1x6
Etafedrine	T48.6x1	T48.6x2	T48.6x3	T48.6x4	T48.6x5	T48.6x6
Etafenone	T46.3x1	T46.3x2	T46.3x3	T46.3x4	T46.3x5	T46.3x6
Etambutol	T37.1x1	T37.1x2	T37.1x3	T37.1x4	T37.1x5	T37.1x6
Etamiphyllin	T48.6x1	T48.6x2	T48.6x3	T48.6x4	T48.6x5	T48.6x6
Etamivan	T50.7x1	T50.7x2	T50.7x3	T50.7x4	T50.7x5	T50.7x6
Etamsylate	T45.7x1	T45.7x2	T45.7x3	T45.7x4	T45.7x5	T45.7x6
Etebenecid	T50.4x1	T50.4x2	T50.4x3	T50.4x4	T50.4x5	T50.4x6
Ethacridine	T49.0x1	T49.0x2	T49.0x3	T49.0x4	T49.0x5	T49.0x6
Ethacrynic acid	T50.1x1	T50.1x2	T50.1x3	T50.1x4	T50.1x5	T50.1x6
Ethadione	T42.2x1	T42.2x2	T42.2x3	T42.2x4	T42.2x5	T42.2x6
Ethambutol	T37.1x1	T37.1x2	T37.1x3	T37.1x4	T37.1x5	T37.1x6
Ethamide	T50.2x1	T50.2x2	T50.2x3	T50.2x4	T50.2x5	T50.2x6
Ethamivan	T50.7x1	T50.7x2	T50.7x3	T50.7x4	T50.7x5	T50.7x6
Ethamsylate	T45.7x1	T45.7x2	T45.7x3	T45.7x4	T45.7x5	T45.7x6
Ethanol	T51.0x1	T51.0x2	T51.0x3	T51.0x4	—	—
beverage	T51.0x1	T51.0x2	T51.0x3	T51.0x4	—	—
Ethanolamine oleate	T46.8x1	T46.8x2	T46.8x3	T46.8x4	T46.8x5	T46.8x6
Ethaverine	T44.3x1	T44.3x2	T44.3x3	T44.3x4	T44.3x5	T44.3x6
Ethchlorvynol	T42.6x1	T42.6x2	T42.6x3	T42.6x4	T42.6x5	T42.6x6
Ethebenecid	T50.4x1	T50.4x2	T50.4x3	T50.4x4	T50.4x5	T50.4x6
Ether (vapor)	T41.0x1	T41.0x2	T41.0x3	T41.0x4	T41.0x5	T41.0x6
anesthetic	T41.0x1	T41.0x2	T41.0x3	T41.0x4	T41.0x5	T41.0x6
divinyl	T41.0x1	T41.0x2	T41.0x3	T41.0x4	T41.0x5	T41.0x6
ethyl (medicinal)	T41.0x1	T41.0x2	T41.0x3	T41.0x4	T41.0x5	T41.0x6
nonmedicinal	T52.8x1	T52.8x2	T52.8x3	T52.8x4	—	—
petroleum—*see* Ligroin						
solvent	T52.8x1	T52.8x2	T52.8x3	T52.8x4	—	—
Ethiazide	T50.2x1	T50.2x2	T50.2x3	T50.2x4	T50.2x5	T50.2x6
Ethidium chloride (vapor)	T59.891	T59.892	T59.893	T59.894	—	—
Ethinamate	T42.6x1	T42.6x2	T42.6x3	T42.6x4	T42.6x5	T42.6x6

Substance	Poisoning, Accidental (unintentional)	Poisoning, Intentional Self-harm	Poisoning, Assault	Poisoning, Undetermined	Adverse Effect	Under-dosing
Ethinylestradiol, ethinyloestradiol	T38.5x1	T38.5x2	T38.5x3	T38.5x4	T38.5x5	T38.5x6
with						
levonorgestrel	T38.4x1	T38.4x2	T38.4x3	T38.4x4	T38.4x5	T38.4x6
norethisterone	T38.4x1	T38.4x2	T38.4x3	T38.4x4	T38.4x5	T38.4x6
Ethiodized oil (131 I)	T50.8x1	T50.8x2	T50.8x3	T50.8x4	T50.8x5	T50.8x6
Ethion	T60.0x1	T60.0x2	T60.0x3	T60.0x4	—	—
Ethionamide	T37.1x1	T37.1x2	T37.1x3	T37.1x4	T37.1x5	T37.1x6
Ethioniamide	T37.1x1	T37.1x2	T37.1x3	T37.1x4	T37.1x5	T37.1x6
Ethisterone	T38.5x1	T38.5x2	T38.5x3	T38.5x4	T38.5x5	T38.5x6
Ethobral	T42.3x1	T42.3x2	T42.3x3	T42.3x4	T42.3x5	T42.3x6
Ethocaine (infiltration) (topical)	T41.3x1	T41.3x2	T41.3x3	T41.3x4	T41.3x5	T41.3x6
nerve block (peripheral) (plexus)	T41.3x1	T41.3x2	T41.3x3	T41.3x4	T41.3x5	T41.3x6
spinal	T41.3x1	T41.3x2	T41.3x3	T41.3x4	T41.3x5	T41.3x6
Ethoheptazine	T40.4x1	T40.4x2	T40.4x3	T40.4x4	T40.4x5	T40.4x6
Ethopropazine	T44.3x1	T44.3x2	T44.3x3	T44.3x4	T44.3x5	T44.3x6
Ethosuximide	T42.2x1	T42.2x2	T42.2x3	T42.2x4	T42.2x5	T42.2x6
Ethotoin	T42.0x1	T42.0x2	T42.0x3	T42.0x4	T42.0x5	T42.0x6
Ethoxazene	T37.91	T37.92	T37.93	T37.94	T37.95	T37.96
Ethoxazorutoside	T46.991	T46.992	T46.993	T46.994	T46.995	T46.996
2-Ethoxyethanol	T52.3x1	T52.3x2	T52.3x3	T52.3x4	—	—
Ethoxzolamide	T50.2x1	T50.2x2	T50.2x3	T50.2x4	T50.2x5	T50.2x6
Ethyl						
acetate	T52.8x1	T52.8x2	T52.8x3	T52.8x4	—	—
alcohol	T51.0x1	T51.0x2	T51.0x3	T51.0x4	—	—
beverage	T51.0x1	T51.0x2	T51.0x3	T51.0x4	—	—
aldehyde (vapor)	T59.891	T59.892	T59.893	T59.894	—	—
liquid	T52.8x1	T52.8x2	T52.8x3	T52.8x4	—	—
aminobenzoate	T41.3x1	T41.3x2	T41.3x3	T41.3x4	T41.3x5	T41.3x6
aminophenothiazine	T43.3x1	T43.3x2	T43.3x3	T43.3x4	T43.3x5	T43.3x6
benzoate	T52.8x1	T52.8x2	T52.8x3	T52.8x4	—	—
biscoumacetate	T45.511	T45.512	T45.513	T45.514	T45.515	T45.516
bromide (anesthetic)	T41.0x1	T41.0x2	T41.0x3	T41.0x4	T41.0x5	T41.0x6
carbamate	T45.1x1	T45.1x2	T45.1x3	T45.1x4	T45.1x5	T45.1x6
carbinol	T51.2x1	T51.2x2	T51.2x3	T51.2x4	—	—
carbonate	T52.8x1	T52.8x2	T52.8x3	T52.8x4	—	—
chaulmoograte	T37.1x1	T37.1x2	T37.1x3	T37.1x4	T37.1x5	T37.1x6
chloride (anesthetic)	T41.0x1	T41.0x2	T41.0x3	T41.0x4	T41.0x5	T41.0x6
anesthetic (local)	T41.3x1	T41.3x2	T41.3x3	T41.3x4	T41.3x5	T41.3x6
inhaled	T41.0x1	T41.0x2	T41.0x3	T41.0x4	T41.0x5	T41.0x6
local	T49.4x1	T49.4x2	T49.4x3	T49.4x4	T49.4x5	T49.4x6
solvent	T53.6x1	T53.6x2	T53.6x3	T53.6x4	—	—
dibunate	T48.3x1	T48.3x2	T48.3x3	T48.3x4	T48.3x5	T48.3x6
dichloroarsine (vapor)	T57.0x1	T57.0x2	T57.0x3	T57.0x4	—	—
estranol	T38.7x1	T38.7x2	T38.7x3	T38.7x4	T38.7x5	T38.7x6
ether (*see also* ether)	T52.8x1	T52.8x2	T52.8x3	T52.8x4	—	—
formate NEC (solvent)	T52.0x1	T52.0x2	T52.0x3	T52.0x4	—	—
fumarate	T49.4x1	T49.4x2	T49.4x3	T49.4x4	T49.4x5	T49.4x6
hydroxyisobutyrate NEC (solvent)	T52.8x1	T52.8x2	T52.8x3	T52.8x4	—	—
iodoacetate	T59.3x1	T59.3x2	T59.3x3	T59.3x4	—	—
lactate NEC (solvent)	T52.8x1	T52.8x2	T52.8x3	T52.8x4	—	—
loflazepate	T42.4x1	T42.4x2	T42.4x3	T42.4x4	T42.4x5	T42.4x6
mercuric chloride	T56.1x1	T56.1x2	T56.1x3	T56.1x4	—	—
methylcarbinol	T51.8x1	T51.8x2	T51.8x3	T51.8x4	—	—
morphine	T40.2x1	T40.2x2	T40.2x3	T40.2x4	T40.2x5	T40.2x6
noradrenaline	T48.6x1	T48.6x2	T48.6x3	T48.6x4	T48.6x5	T48.6x6
oxybutyrate NEC (solvent)	T52.8x1	T52.8x2	T52.8x3	T52.8x4	—	—
Ethylene (gas)	T59.891	T59.892	T59.893	T59.894	—	—
anesthetic (general)	T41.0x1	T41.0x2	T41.0x3	T41.0x4	T41.0x5	T41.0x6
chlorohydrin	T52.8x1	T52.8x2	T52.8x3	T52.8x4	—	—
vapor	T53.6x1	T53.6x2	T53.6x3	T53.6x4	—	—
dichloride	T52.8x1	T52.8x2	T52.8x3	T52.8x4	—	—
vapor	T53.6x1	T53.6x2	T53.6x3	T53.6x4	—	—
dinitrate	T52.3x1	T52.3x2	T52.3x3	T52.3x4	—	—
glycol(s)	T52.8x1	T52.8x2	T52.8x3	T52.8x4	—	—
dinitrate	T52.3x1	T52.3x2	T52.3x3	T52.3x4	—	—
monobutyl ether	T52.3x1	T52.3x2	T52.3x3	T52.3x4	—	—
imine	T54.1x1	T54.1x2	T54.1x3	T54.1x4	—	—
oxide (fumigant) (nonmedicinal)	T59.891	T59.892	T59.893	T59.894	—	—
medicinal	T49.0x1	T49.0x2	T49.0x3	T49.0x4	T49.0x5	T49.0x6
Ethylenediamine theophylline	T48.6x1	T48.6x2	T48.6x3	T48.6x4	T48.6x5	T48.6x6

Substance	Poisoning, Accidental (unintentional)	Poisoning, Intentional Self-harm	Poisoning, Assault	Poisoning, Undetermined	Adverse Effect	Underdosing
Ethylenediaminetetraacetic acid	T50.6x1	T50.6x2	T50.6x3	T50.6x4	T50.6x5	T50.6x6
Ethylenedinitrilotetra-acetate	T50.6x1	T50.6x2	T50.6x3	T50.6x4	T50.6x5	T50.6x6
Ethylestrenol	T38.7x1	T38.7x2	T38.7x3	T38.7x4	T38.7x5	T38.7x6
Ethylhydroxycellulose	T47.4x1	T47.4x2	T47.4x3	T47.4x4	T47.4x5	T47.4x6
Ethylidene						
chloride NEC	T53.6x1	T53.6x2	T53.6x3	T53.6x4	—	—
diacetate	T60.3x1	T60.3x2	T60.3x3	T60.3x4	—	—
dicoumarin	T45.511	T45.512	T45.513	T45.514	T45.515	T45.516
dicoumarol	T45.511	T45.512	T45.513	T45.514	T45.515	T45.516
diethyl ether	T52.0x1	T52.0x2	T52.0x3	T52.0x4	—	—
Ethylmorphine	T40.2x1	T40.2x2	T40.2x3	T40.2x4	T40.2x5	T40.2x6
Ethylnorepinephrine	T48.6x1	T48.6x2	T48.6x3	T48.6x4	T48.6x5	T48.6x6
Ethylparachlorophen-oxyisobutyrate	T46.6x1	T46.6x2	T46.6x3	T46.6x4	T46.6x5	T46.6x6
Ethynodiol	T38.4x1	T38.4x2	T38.4x3	T38.4x4	T38.4x5	T38.4x6
with mestranol diacetate	T38.4x1	T38.4x2	T38.4x3	T38.4x4	T38.4x5	T38.4x6
Etidocaine	T41.3x1	T41.3x2	T41.3x3	T41.3x4	T41.3x5	T41.3x6
infiltration (subcutaneous)	T41.3x1	T41.3x2	T41.3x3	T41.3x4	T41.3x5	T41.3x6
nerve (peripheral) (plexus)	T41.3x1	T41.3x2	T41.3x3	T41.3x4	T41.3x5	T41.3x6
Etidronate	T50.991	T50.992	T50.993	T50.994	T50.995	T50.996
Etidronic acid (disodium salt)	T50.991	T50.992	T50.993	T50.994	T50.995	T50.996
Etifoxine	T42.6x1	T42.6x2	T42.6x3	T42.6x4	T42.6x5	T42.6x6
Etilefrine	T44.4x1	T44.4x2	T44.4x3	T44.4x4	T44.4x5	T44.4x6
Etilfen	T42.3x1	T42.3x2	T42.3x3	T42.3x4	T42.3x5	T42.3x6
Etinodiol	T38.4x1	T38.4x2	T38.4x3	T38.4x4	T38.4x5	T38.4x6
Etiroxate	T46.6x1	T46.6x2	T46.6x3	T46.6x4	T46.6x5	T46.6x6
Etizolam	T42.4x1	T42.4x2	T42.4x3	T42.4x4	T42.4x5	T42.4x6
Etodolac	T39.391	T39.392	T39.393	T39.394	T39.395	T39.396
Etofamide	T37.3x1	T37.3x2	T37.3x3	T37.3x4	T37.3x5	T37.3x6
Etofibrate	T46.6x1	T46.6x2	T46.6x3	T46.6x4	T46.6x5	T46.6x6
Etofylline	T46.7x1	T46.7x2	T46.7x3	T46.7x4	T46.7x5	T46.7x6
clofibrate	T46.6x1	T46.6x2	T46.6x3	T46.6x4	T46.6x5	T46.6x6
Etoglucid	T45.1x1	T45.1x2	T45.1x3	T45.1x4	T45.1x5	T45.1x6
Etomidate	T41.1x1	T41.1x2	T41.1x3	T41.1x4	T41.1x5	T41.1x6
Etomide	T39.8x1	T39.8x2	T39.8x3	T39.8x4	T39.8x5	T39.8x6
Etomidoline	T44.3x1	T44.3x2	T44.3x3	T44.3x4	T44.3x5	T44.3x6
Etoposide	T45.1x1	T45.1x2	T45.1x3	T45.1x4	T45.1x5	T45.1x6
Etorphine	T40.2x1	T40.2x2	T40.2x3	T40.2x4	T40.2x5	T40.2x6
Etoval	T42.3x1	T42.3x2	T42.3x3	T42.3x4	T42.3x5	T42.3x6
Etozolin	T50.1x1	T50.1x2	T50.1x3	T50.1x4	T50.1x5	T50.1x6
Etretinate	T50.991	T50.992	T50.993	T50.994	T50.995	T50.996
Etryptamine	T43.691	T43.692	T43.693	T43.694	T43.695	T43.696
Etybenzatropine	T44.3x1	T44.3x2	T44.3x3	T44.3x4	T44.3x5	T44.3x6
Etynodiol	T38.4x1	T38.4x2	T38.4x3	T38.4x4	T38.4x5	T38.4x6
Eucaine	T41.3x1	T41.3x2	T41.3x3	T41.3x4	T41.3x5	T41.3x6
Eucalyptus oil	T49.7x1	T49.7x2	T49.7x3	T49.7x4	T49.7x5	T49.7x6
Eucatropine	T49.5x1	T49.5x2	T49.5x3	T49.5x4	T49.5x5	T49.5x6
Eucodal	T40.2x1	T40.2x2	T40.2x3	T40.2x4	T40.2x5	T40.2x6
Euneryl	T42.3x1	T42.3x2	T42.3x3	T42.3x4	T42.3x5	T42.3x6
Euphthalmine	T44.3x1	T44.3x2	T44.3x3	T44.3x4	T44.3x5	T44.3x6
Eurax	T49.0x1	T49.0x2	T49.0x3	T49.0x4	T49.0x5	T49.0x6
Euresol	T49.4x1	T49.4x2	T49.4x3	T49.4x4	T49.4x5	T49.4x6
Euthroid	T38.1x1	T38.1x2	T38.1x3	T38.1x4	T38.1x5	T38.1x6
Evans blue	T50.8x1	T50.8x2	T50.8x3	T50.8x4	T50.8x5	T50.8x6
Evipal	T42.3x1	T42.3x2	T42.3x3	T42.3x4	T42.3x5	T42.3x6
sodium	T41.1x1	T41.1x2	T41.1x3	T41.1x4	T41.1x5	T41.1x6
Evipan	T42.3x1	T42.3x2	T42.3x3	T42.3x4	T42.3x5	T42.3x6
sodium	T41.1x1	T41.1x2	T41.1x3	T41.1x4	T41.1x5	T41.1x6
Exalamide	T49.0x1	T49.0x2	T49.0x3	T49.0x4	T49.0x5	T49.0x6
Exalgin	T39.1x1	T39.1x2	T39.1x3	T39.1x4	T39.1x5	T39.1x6
Excipients, pharmaceutical	T50.901	T50.902	T50.903	T50.904	T50.905	T50.906
Exhaust gas (engine) (motor vehicle)	T58.01	T58.02	T58.03	T58.04	—	—
Ex-Lax (phenolphthalein)	T47.2x1	T47.2x2	T47.2x3	T47.2x4	T47.2x5	T47.2x6
Expectorant NEC	T48.4x1	T48.4x2	T48.4x3	T48.4x4	T48.4x5	T48.4x6
Extended insulin zinc suspension	T38.3x1	T38.3x2	T38.3x3	T38.3x4	T38.3x5	T38.3x6
External medications (skin) (mucous membrane)	T49.91	T49.92	T49.93	T49.94	T49.95	T49.96
dental agent	T49.7x1	T49.7x2	T49.7x3	T49.7x4	T49.7x5	T49.7x6

Substance	Poisoning, Accidental (unintentional)	Poisoning, Intentional Self-harm	Poisoning, Assault	Poisoning, Undetermined	Adverse Effect	Underdosing
External medications —continued						
ENT agent	T49.6x1	T49.6x2	T49.6x3	T49.6x4	T49.6x5	T49.6x6
ophthalmic preparation	T49.5x1	T49.5x2	T49.5x3	T49.5x4	T49.5x5	T49.5x6
specified NEC	T49.8x1	T49.8x2	T49.8x3	T49.8x4	T49.8x5	T49.8x6
Extrapyramidal antagonist NEC	T44.3x1	T44.3x2	T44.3x3	T44.3x4	T44.3x5	T44.3x6
Eye agents (anti-infective)	T49.5x1	T49.5x2	T49.5x3	T49.5x4	T49.5x5	T49.5x6
Eye drug NEC	T49.5x1	T49.5x2	T49.5x3	T49.5x4	T49.5x5	T49.5x6
FAC (fluorouracil + doxorubicin + cyclophosphamide)	T45.1x1	T45.1x2	T45.1x3	T45.1x4	T45.1x5	T45.1x6
Factor						
I (fibrinogen)	T45.8x1	T45.8x2	T45.8x3	T45.8x4	T45.8x5	T45.8x6
III (thromboplastin)	T45.8x1	T45.8x2	T45.8x3	T45.8x4	T45.8x5	T45.8x6
VIII (antihemophilic factor) (concentrate)	T45.8x1	T45.8x2	T45.8x3	T45.8x4	T45.8x5	T45.8x6
IX complex	T45.7x1	T45.7x2	T45.7x3	T45.7x4	T45.7x5	T45.7x6
human	T45.8x1	T45.8x2	T45.8x3	T45.8x4	T45.8x5	T45.8x6
Famotidine	T47.0x1	T47.0x2	T47.0x3	T47.0x4	T47.0x5	T47.0x6
Fat suspension, intravenous	T50.991	T50.992	T50.993	T50.994	T50.995	T50.996
Fazadinium bromide	T48.1x1	T48.1x2	T48.1x3	T48.1x4	T48.1x5	T48.1x6
Febarbamate	T42.3x1	T42.3x2	T42.3x3	T42.3x4	T42.3x5	T42.3x6
Fecal softener	T47.4x1	T47.4x2	T47.4x3	T47.4x4	T47.4x5	T47.4x6
Fedrilate	T48.3x1	T48.3x2	T48.3x3	T48.3x4	T48.3x5	T48.3x6
Felodipine	T46.1x1	T46.1x2	T46.1x3	T46.1x4	T46.1x5	T46.1x6
Felypressin	T38.891	T38.892	T38.893	T38.894	T38.895	T38.896
Femoxetine	T43.221	T43.222	T43.223	T43.224	T43.225	T43.226
Fenalcomine	T46.3x1	T46.3x2	T46.3x3	T46.3x4	T46.3x5	T46.3x6
Fenamisal	T37.1x1	T37.1x2	T37.1x3	T37.1x4	T37.1x5	T37.1x6
Fenazone	T39.2x1	T39.2x2	T39.2x3	T39.2x4	T39.2x5	T39.2x6
Fenbendazole	T37.4x1	T37.4x2	T37.4x3	T37.4x4	T37.4x5	T37.4x6
Fenbutrazate	T50.5x1	T50.5x2	T50.5x3	T50.5x4	T50.5x5	T50.5x6
Fencamfamine	T43.691	T43.692	T43.693	T43.694	T43.695	T43.696
Fendiline	T46.1x1	T46.1x2	T46.1x3	T46.1x4	T46.1x5	T46.1x6
Fenetylline	T43.691	T43.692	T43.693	T43.694	T43.695	T43.696
Fenflumizole	T39.391	T39.392	T39.393	T39.394	T39.395	T39.396
Fenfluramine	T50.5x1	T50.5x2	T50.5x3	T50.5x4	T50.5x5	T50.5x6
Fenobarbital	T42.3x1	T42.3x2	T42.3x3	T42.3x4	T42.3x5	T42.3x6
Fenofibrate	T46.6x1	T46.6x2	T46.6x3	T46.6x4	T46.6x5	T46.6x6
Fenoprofen	T39.311	T39.312	T39.313	T39.314	T39.315	T39.316
Fenoterol	T48.6x1	T48.6x2	T48.6x3	T48.6x4	T48.6x5	T48.6x6
Fenoverine	T44.3x1	T44.3x2	T44.3x3	T44.3x4	T44.3x5	T44.3x6
Fenoxazoline	T48.5x1	T48.5x2	T48.5x3	T48.5x4	T48.5x5	T48.5x6
Fenproporex	T50.5x1	T50.5x2	T50.5x3	T50.5x4	T50.5x5	T50.5x6
Fenquizone	T50.2x1	T50.2x2	T50.2x3	T50.2x4	T50.2x5	T50.2x6
Fentanyl	T40.4x1	T40.4x2	T40.4x3	T40.4x4	T40.4x5	T40.4x6
Fentazin	T43.3x1	T43.3x2	T43.3x3	T43.3x4	T43.3x5	T43.3x6
Fenthion	T60.0x1	T60.0x2	T60.0x3	T60.0x4	—	—
Fenticlor	T49.0x1	T49.0x2	T49.0x3	T49.0x4	T49.0x5	T49.0x6
Fenylbutazone	T39.2x1	T39.2x2	T39.2x3	T39.2x4	T39.2x5	T39.2x6
Feprazone	T39.2x1	T39.2x2	T39.2x3	T39.2x4	T39.2x5	T39.2x6
Fer de lance (bite) (venom)	T63.061	T63.062	T63.063	T63.064	—	—
Ferric (see also Iron)						
chloride	T45.4x1	T45.4x2	T45.4x3	T45.4x4	T45.4x5	T45.4x6
citrate	T45.4x1	T45.4x2	T45.4x3	T45.4x4	T45.4x5	T45.4x6
hydroxide						
colloidal	T45.4x1	T45.4x2	T45.4x3	T45.4x4	T45.4x5	T45.4x6
polymaltose	T45.4x1	T45.4x2	T45.4x3	T45.4x4	T45.4x5	T45.4x6
pyrophosphate	T45.4x1	T45.4x2	T45.4x3	T45.4x4	T45.4x5	T45.4x6
Ferritin	T45.4x1	T45.4x2	T45.4x3	T45.4x4	T45.4x5	T45.4x6
Ferrocholinate	T45.4x1	T45.4x2	T45.4x3	T45.4x4	T45.4x5	T45.4x6
Ferrodextrane	T45.4x1	T45.4x2	T45.4x3	T45.4x4	T45.4x5	T45.4x6
Ferropolimaler	T45.4x1	T45.4x2	T45.4x3	T45.4x4	T45.4x5	T45.4x6
Ferrous (see also Iron)						
phosphate	T45.4x1	T45.4x2	T45.4x3	T45.4x4	T45.4x5	T45.4x6
salt	T45.4x1	T45.4x2	T45.4x3	T45.4x4	T45.4x5	T45.4x6
with folic acid	T45.4x1	T45.4x2	T45.4x3	T45.4x4	T45.4x5	T45.4x6
Ferrous fumerate, gluconate, lactate, salt NEC, sulfate (medicinal)	T45.4x1	T45.4x2	T45.4x3	T45.4x4	T45.4x5	T45.4x6
Ferrovanadium (fumes)	T59.891	T59.892	T59.893	T59.894	—	—
Ferrum—see Iron						

Substance	Poisoning, Accidental (unintentional)	Poisoning, Intentional Self-harm	Poisoning, Assault	Poisoning, Undetermined	Adverse Effect	Under-dosing
Fertilizers NEC	T65.891	T65.892	T65.893	T65.894	—	—
with herbicide mixture	T60.3x1	T60.3x2	T60.3x3	T60.3x4	—	—
Fetoxilate	T47.6x1	T47.6x2	T47.6x3	T47.6x4	T47.6x5	T47.6x6
Fiber, dietary	T47.4x1	T47.4x2	T47.4x3	T47.4x4	T47.4x5	T47.4x6
Fiberglass	T65.831	T65.832	T65.833	T65.834	—	—
Fibrinogen (human)	T45.8x1	T45.8x2	T45.8x3	T45.8x4	T45.8x5	T45.8x6
Fibrinolysin (human)	T45.691	T45.692	T45.693	T45.694	T45.695	T45.696
Fibrinolysis-affecting drug	T45.601	T45.602	T45.603	T45.604	T45.605	T45.606
Fibrinolysis inhibitor NEC	T45.621	T45.622	T45.623	T45.624	T45.625	T45.626
Fibrinolytic drug	T45.611	T45.612	T45.613	T45.614	T45.615	T45.616
Filix mas	T37.4x1	T37.4x2	T37.4x3	T37.4x4	T37.4x5	T37.4x6
Filtering cream	T49.3x1	T49.3x2	T49.3x3	T49.3x4	T49.3x5	T49.3x6
Fiorinal	T39.011	T39.012	T39.013	T39.014	T39.015	T39.016
Firedamp	T59.891	T59.892	T59.893	T59.894	—	—
Fish, noxious, nonbacterial	T61.771	T61.772	T61.773	T61.774	—	—
ciguatera	T61.01	T61.02	T61.03	T61.04	—	—
scombroid	T61.11	T61.12	T61.13	T61.14	—	—
shell	T61.781	T61.782	T61.783	T61.784	—	—
Flagyl	T37.3x1	T37.3x2	T37.3x3	T37.3x4	T37.3x5	T37.3x6
Flavine adenine dinucleotide	T45.2x1	T45.2x2	T45.2x3	T45.2x4	T45.2x5	T45.2x6
Flavodic acid	T46.991	T46.992	T46.993	T46.994	T46.995	T46.996
Flavoxate	T44.3x1	T44.3x2	T44.3x3	T44.3x4	T44.3x5	T44.3x6
Flaxedil	T48.1x1	T48.1x2	T48.1x3	T48.1x4	T48.1x5	T48.1x6
Flaxseed (medicinal)	T49.3x1	T49.3x2	T49.3x3	T49.3x4	T49.3x5	T49.3x6
Flecainide	T46.2x1	T46.2x2	T46.2x3	T46.2x4	T46.2x5	T46.2x6
Fleroxacin	T36.8x1	T36.8x2	T36.8x3	T36.8x4	T36.8x5	T36.8x6
Floctafenine	T39.8x1	T39.8x2	T39.8x3	T39.8x4	T39.8x5	T39.8x6
Flomax	T44.6x1	T44.6x2	T44.6x3	T44.6x4	T44.6x5	T44.6x6
Flomoxef	T36.1x1	T36.1x2	T36.1x3	T36.1x4	T36.1x5	T36.1x6
Flopropione	T44.3x1	T44.3x2	T44.3x3	T44.3x4	T44.3x5	T44.3x6
Florantyrone	T47.5x1	T47.5x2	T47.5x3	T47.5x4	T47.5x5	T47.5x6
Floraquin	T37.8x1	T37.8x2	T37.8x3	T37.8x4	T37.8x5	T37.8x6
Florinef	T38.0x1	T38.0x2	T38.0x3	T38.0x4	T38.0x5	T38.0x6
ENT agent	T49.6x1	T49.6x2	T49.6x3	T49.6x4	T49.6x5	T49.6x6
ophthalmic preparation	T49.5x1	T49.5x2	T49.5x3	T49.5x4	T49.5x5	T49.5x6
topical NEC	T49.0x1	T49.0x2	T49.0x3	T49.0x4	T49.0x5	T49.0x6
Flowers of sulfur	T49.4x1	T49.4x2	T49.4x3	T49.4x4	T49.4x5	T49.4x6
Floxuridine	T45.1x1	T45.1x2	T45.1x3	T45.1x4	T45.1x5	T45.1x6
Fluanisone	T43.4x1	T43.4x2	T43.4x3	T43.4x4	T43.4x5	T43.4x6
Flubendazole	T37.4x1	T37.4x2	T37.4x3	T37.4x4	T37.4x5	T37.4x6
Fluclorolone acetonide	T49.0x1	T49.0x2	T49.0x3	T49.0x4	T49.0x5	T49.0x6
Flucloxacillin	T36.0x1	T36.0x2	T36.0x3	T36.0x4	T36.0x5	T36.0x6
Fluconazole	T37.8x1	T37.8x2	T37.8x3	T37.8x4	T37.8x5	T37.8x6
Flucytosine	T37.8x1	T37.8x2	T37.8x3	T37.8x4	T37.8x5	T37.8x6
Fludeoxyglucose (18F)	T50.8x1	T50.8x2	T50.8x3	T50.8x4	T50.8x5	T50.8x6
Fludiazepam	T42.4x1	T42.4x2	T42.4x3	T42.4x4	T42.4x5	T42.4x6
Fludrocortisone	T50.0x1	T50.0x2	T50.0x3	T50.0x4	T50.0x5	T50.0x6
ENT agent	T49.6x1	T49.6x2	T49.6x3	T49.6x4	T49.6x5	T49.6x6
ophthalmic preparation	T49.5x1	T49.5x2	T49.5x3	T49.5x4	T49.5x5	T49.5x6
topical NEC	T49.0x1	T49.0x2	T49.0x3	T49.0x4	T49.0x5	T49.0x6
Fludroxycortide	T49.0x1	T49.0x2	T49.0x3	T49.0x4	T49.0x5	T49.0x6
Flufenamic acid	T39.391	T39.392	T39.393	T39.394	T39.395	T39.396
Fluindione	T45.511	T45.512	T45.513	T45.514	T45.515	T45.516
Flumequine	T37.8x1	T37.8x2	T37.8x3	T37.8x4	T37.8x5	T37.8x6
Flumethasone	T49.0x1	T49.0x2	T49.0x3	T49.0x4	T49.0x5	T49.0x6
Flumethiazide	T50.2x1	T50.2x2	T50.2x3	T50.2x4	T50.2x5	T50.2x6
Flumidin	T37.5x1	T37.5x2	T37.5x3	T37.5x4	T37.5x5	T37.5x6
Flunarizine	T46.7x1	T46.7x2	T46.7x3	T46.7x4	T46.7x5	T46.7x6
Flunidazole	T37.8x1	T37.8x2	T37.8x3	T37.8x4	T37.8x5	T37.8x6
Flunisolide	T48.6x1	T48.6x2	T48.6x3	T48.6x4	T48.6x5	T48.6x6
Flunitrazepam	T42.4x1	T42.4x2	T42.4x3	T42.4x4	T42.4x5	T42.4x6
Fluocinolone (acetonide)	T49.0x1	T49.0x2	T49.0x3	T49.0x4	T49.0x5	T49.0x6
Fluocinolone	T49.0x1	T49.0x2	T49.0x3	T49.0x4	T49.0x5	T49.0x6
Fluocinonide	T49.0x1	T49.0x2	T49.0x3	T49.0x4	T49.0x5	T49.0x6
Fluocortin (butyl)	T49.0x1	T49.0x2	T49.0x3	T49.0x4	T49.0x5	T49.0x6
Fluocortolone	T49.0x1	T49.0x2	T49.0x3	T49.0x4	T49.0x5	T49.0x6
Fluohydrocortisone	T38.0x1	T38.0x2	T38.0x3	T38.0x4	T38.0x5	T38.0x6
ENT agent	T49.6x1	T49.6x2	T49.6x3	T49.6x4	T49.6x5	T49.6x6
ophthalmic preparation	T49.5x1	T49.5x2	T49.5x3	T49.5x4	T49.5x5	T49.5x6
topical NEC	T49.0x1	T49.0x2	T49.0x3	T49.0x4	T49.0x5	T49.0x6
Fluonid	T49.0x1	T49.0x2	T49.0x3	T49.0x4	T49.0x5	T49.0x6

Substance	Poisoning, Accidental (unintentional)	Poisoning, Intentional Self-harm	Poisoning, Assault	Poisoning, Undetermined	Adverse Effect	Under-dosing
Fluopromazine	T43.3x1	T43.3x2	T43.3x3	T43.3x4	T43.3x5	T43.3x6
Fluoroacetate, fluoracetate	T60.8x1	T60.8x2	T60.8x3	T60.8x4	—	—
Fluorescein	T50.8x1	T50.8x2	T50.8x3	T50.8x4	T50.8x5	T50.8x6
Fluorhydrocortisone	T50.0x1	T50.0x2	T50.0x3	T50.0x4	T50.0x5	T50.0x6
Fluoride (nonmedicinal) (pesticide) (sodium) **NEC**	T60.8x1	T60.8x2	T60.8x3	T60.8x4	—	—
hydrogen—*see* Hydrofluoric acid						
medicinal NEC	T50.991	T50.992	T50.993	T50.994	T50.995	T50.996
dental use	T49.7x1	T49.7x2	T49.7x3	T49.7x4	T49.7x5	T49.7x6
not pesticide NEC	T54.91	T54.92	T54.93	T54.94	—	—
stannous	T49.7x1	T49.7x2	T49.7x3	T49.7x4	T49.7x5	T49.7x6
Fluorinated corticosteroids	T38.0x1	T38.0x2	T38.0x3	T38.0x4	T38.0x5	T38.0x6
Fluorine (gas)	T59.5x1	T59.5x2	T59.5x3	T59.5x4	—	—
salt—*see* Fluoride(s)						
Fluoristan	T49.7x1	T49.7x2	T49.7x3	T49.7x4	T49.7x5	T49.7x6
Fluormetholone	T49.0x1	T49.0x2	T49.0x3	T49.0x4	T49.0x5	T49.0x6
Fluoroacetate	T60.4x1	T60.4x2	T60.4x3	T60.4x4	—	—
Fluorocarbon monomer	T53.6x1	T53.6x2	T53.6x3	T53.6x4	—	—
Fluorocytosine	T37.8x1	T37.8x2	T37.8x3	T37.8x4	T37.8x5	T37.8x6
Fluorodeoxyuridine	T45.1x1	T45.1x2	T45.1x3	T45.1x4	T45.1x5	T45.1x6
Fluorometholone	T49.0x1	T49.0x2	T49.0x3	T49.0x4	T49.0x5	T49.0x6
ophthalmic preparation	T49.5x1	T49.5x2	T49.5x3	T49.5x4	T49.5x5	T49.5x6
Fluorophosphate insecticide	T60.0x1	T60.0x2	T60.0x3	T60.0x4	—	—
Fluorosol	T46.3x1	T46.3x2	T46.3x3	T46.3x4	T46.3x5	T46.3x6
Fluorouracil	T45.1x1	T45.1x2	T45.1x3	T45.1x4	T45.1x5	T45.1x6
Fluorphenylalanine	T49.5x1	T49.5x2	T49.5x3	T49.5x4	T49.5x5	T49.5x6
Fluothane	T41.0x1	T41.0x2	T41.0x3	T41.0x4	T41.0x5	T41.0x6
Fluoxetine	T43.221	T43.222	T43.223	T43.224	T43.225	T43.226
Fluoxymesterone	T38.7x1	T38.7x2	T38.7x3	T38.7x4	T38.7x5	T38.7x6
Flupenthixol	T43.4x1	T43.4x2	T43.4x3	T43.4x4	T43.4x5	T43.4x6
Flupentixol	T43.4x1	T43.4x2	T43.4x3	T43.4x4	T43.4x5	T43.4x6
Fluphenazine	T43.3x1	T43.3x2	T43.3x3	T43.3x4	T43.3x5	T43.3x6
Fluprednidene	T49.0x1	T49.0x2	T49.0x3	T49.0x4	T49.0x5	T49.0x6
Fluprednisolone	T38.0x1	T38.0x2	T38.0x3	T38.0x4	T38.0x5	T38.0x6
Fluradoline	T39.8x1	T39.8x2	T39.8x3	T39.8x4	T39.8x5	T39.8x6
Flurandrenolide	T49.0x1	T49.0x2	T49.0x3	T49.0x4	T49.0x5	T49.0x6
Flurandrenolone	T49.0x1	T49.0x2	T49.0x3	T49.0x4	T49.0x5	T49.0x6
Flurazepam	T42.4x1	T42.4x2	T42.4x3	T42.4x4	T42.4x5	T42.4x6
Flurbiprofen	T39.311	T39.312	T39.313	T39.314	T39.315	T39.316
Flurobate	T49.0x1	T49.0x2	T49.0x3	T49.0x4	T49.0x5	T49.0x6
Fluroxene	T41.0x1	T41.0x2	T41.0x3	T41.0x4	T41.0x5	T41.0x6
Fluspirilene	T43.591	T43.592	T43.593	T43.594	T43.595	T43.596
Flutamide	T38.6x1	T38.6x2	T38.6x3	T38.6x4	T38.6x5	T38.6x6
Flutazolam	T42.4x1	T42.4x2	T42.4x3	T42.4x4	T42.4x5	T42.4x6
Fluticasone propionate	T49.1x1	T49.1x2	T49.1x3	T49.1x4	T49.1x5	T49.1x6
Flutoprazepam	T42.4x1	T42.4x2	T42.4x3	T42.4x4	T42.4x5	T42.4x6
Flutropium bromide	T48.6x1	T48.6x2	T48.6x3	T48.6x4	T48.6x5	T48.6x6
Fluvoxamine	T43.221	T43.222	T43.223	T43.224	T43.225	T43.226
Folacin	T45.8x1	T45.8x2	T45.8x3	T45.8x4	T45.8x5	T45.8x6
Folic acid	T45.8x1	T45.8x2	T45.8x3	T45.8x4	T45.8x5	T45.8x6
with ferrous salt	T45.2x1	T45.2x2	T45.2x3	T45.2x4	T45.2x5	T45.2x6
antagonist	T45.1x1	T45.1x2	T45.1x3	T45.1x4	T45.1x5	T45.1x6
Folinic acid	T45.8x1	T45.8x2	T45.8x3	T45.8x4	T45.8x5	T45.8x6
Folium stramoniae	T48.6x1	T48.6x2	T48.6x3	T48.6x4	T48.6x5	T48.6x6
Follicle-stimulating hormone, human	T38.811	T38.812	T38.813	T38.814	T38.815	T38.816
Folpet	T60.3x1	T60.3x2	T60.3x3	T60.3x4	—	—
Fominoben	T48.3x1	T48.3x2	T48.3x3	T48.3x4	T48.3x5	T48.3x6
Food, foodstuffs, noxious, nonbacterial, NEC	T62.91	T62.92	T62.93	T62.94		
berries	T62.1x1	T62.1x2	T62.1x3	T62.1x4	—	—
fish	T61.771	T61.772	T61.773	T61.774	—	—
mushrooms	T62.0x1	T62.0x2	T62.0x3	T62.0x4	—	—
plants	T62.2x1	T62.2x2	T62.2x3	T62.2x4	—	—
seafood	T61.91	T61.92	T61.93	T61.94	—	—
specified NEC	T61.8x1	T61.8x2	T61.8x3	T61.8x4	—	—
seeds	T62.2x1	T62.2x2	T62.2x3	T62.2x4	—	—
specified type NEC	I62.8x1	T62.8x2	T62.8x3	T62.8x4	—	—
shellfish	T61.781	T61.782	T61.783	T61.784	—	—
specified NEC	T62.8x1	T62.8x2	T62.8x3	T62.8x4	—	—
Fool's parsley	T62.2x1	T62.2x2	T62.2x3	T62.2x4	—	—

Substance	Poisoning, Accidental (unintentional)	Poisoning, Intentional Self-harm	Poisoning, Assault	Poisoning, Undetermined	Adverse Effect	Under-dosing
Formaldehyde (solution), **gas or vapor**	T59.2x1	T59.2x2	T59.2x3	T59.2x4	—	—
fungicide	T60.3x1	T60.3x2	T60.3x3	T60.3x4	—	—
Formalin	T59.2x1	T59.2x2	T59.2x3	T59.2x4	—	—
fungicide	T60.3x1	T60.3x2	T60.3x3	T60.3x4	—	—
vapor	T59.2x1	T59.2x2	T59.2x3	T59.2x4	—	—
Formic acid	T54.2x1	T54.2x2	T54.2x3	T54.2x4	—	—
vapor	T59.891	T59.892	T59.893	T59.894	—	—
Foscarnet sodium	T37.5x1	T37.5x2	T37.5x3	T37.5x4	T37.5x5	T37.5x6
Fosfestrol	T38.5x1	T38.5x2	T38.5x3	T38.5x4	T38.5x5	T38.5x6
Fosfomycin	T36.8x1	T36.8x2	T36.8x3	T36.8x4	T36.8x5	T36.8x6
Fosfonet sodium	T37.5x1	T37.5x2	T37.5x3	T37.5x4	T37.5x5	T37.5x6
Fosinopril	T46.4x1	T46.4x2	T46.4x3	T46.4x4	T46.4x5	T46.4x6
sodium	T46.4x1	T46.4x2	T46.4x3	T46.4x4	T46.4x5	T46.4x6
Fowler's solution	T57.0x1	T57.0x2	T57.0x3	T57.0x4	—	—
Foxglove	T62.2x1	T62.2x2	T62.2x3	T62.2x4	—	—
Framycetin	T36.5x1	T36.5x2	T36.5x3	T36.5x4	T36.5x5	T36.5x6
Frangula	T47.2x1	T47.2x2	T47.2x3	T47.2x4	T47.2x5	T47.2x6
extract	T47.2x1	T47.2x2	T47.2x3	T47.2x4	T47.2x5	T47.2x6
Frei antigen	T50.8x1	T50.8x2	T50.8x3	T50.8x4	T50.8x5	T50.8x6
Freon	T53.5x1	T53.5x2	T53.5x3	T53.5x4	—	—
Fructose	T50.3x1	T50.3x2	T50.3x3	T50.3x4	T50.3x5	T50.3x6
Frusemide	T50.1x1	T50.1x2	T50.1x3	T50.1x4	T50.1x5	T50.1x6
FSH	T38.811	T38.812	T38.813	T38.814	T38.815	T38.816
Ftorafur	T45.1x1	T45.1x2	T45.1x3	T45.1x4	T45.1x5	T45.1x6
Fuel						
automobile	T52.0x1	T52.0x2	T52.0x3	T52.0x4	—	—
exhaust gas, not in transit	T58.01	T58.02	T58.03	T58.04	—	—
vapor NEC	T52.0x1	T52.0x2	T52.0x3	T52.0x4	—	—
gas (domestic use) (*see also* Carbon, monoxide, fuel, utility)	T59.891	T59.892	T59.893	T59.894	—	—
utility	T59.891	T59.892	T59.893	T59.894	—	—
incomplete combustion of—*see* Carbon, monoxide, fuel, utility						
in mobile container	T59.891	T59.892	T59.893	T59.894	—	—
piped (natural)	T59.891	T59.892	T59.893	T59.894	—	—
industrial, incomplete combustion	T58.8x1	T58.8x2	T58.8x3	T58.8x4	—	—
Fugillin	T36.8x1	T36.8x2	T36.8x3	T36.8x4	T36.8x5	T36.8x6
Fulminate of mercury	T56.1x1	T56.1x2	T56.1x3	T56.1x4	—	—
Fulvicin	T36.7x1	T36.7x2	T36.7x3	T36.7x4	T36.7x5	T36.7x6
Fumadil	T36.8x1	T36.8x2	T36.8x3	T36.8x4	T36.8x5	T36.8x6
Fumagillin	T36.8x1	T36.8x2	T36.8x3	T36.8x4	T36.8x5	T36.8x6
Fumaric acid	T49.4x1	T49.4x2	T49.4x3	T49.4x4	T49.4x5	T49.4x6
Fumes (from)	T59.91	T59.92	T59.93	T59.94	—	—
carbon monoxide—*see* Carbon, monoxide						
charcoal (domestic use)—*see* Charcoal, fumes						
chloroform—*see* Chloroform						
coke (in domestic stoves, fireplaces)—*see* Coke fumes						
corrosive NEC	T59.891	T59.892	T59.893	T59.894	—	—
ether—*see* Ether						
freons	T53.5x1	T53.5x2	T53.5x3	T53.5x4	—	—
hydrocarbons	T59.891	T59.892	T59.893	T59.894	—	—
petroleum (liquefied)	T59.891	T59.892	T59.893	T59.894	—	—
distributed through pipes (pure or mixed with air)	T59.891	T59.892	T59.893	T59.894	—	—
lead—*see* Lead						
metal—*see* Metals, or the specified metal						
nitrogen dioxide	T59.0x1	T59.0x2	T59.0x3	T59.0x4	—	—
pesticides—*see* Pesticides						
petroleum (liquefied)	T59.891	T59.892	T59.893	T59.894	—	—
distributed through pipes (pure or mixed with air)	T59.891	T59.892	T59.893	T59.894	—	—
polyester	T59.891	T59.892	T59.893	T59.894	—	—
specified source NEC	T59.91	T59.92	T59.93	T59.94	—	—
sulfur dioxide	T59.1x1	T59.1x2	T59.1x3	T59.1x4	—	—
Fumigant NEC	T60.91	T60.92	T60.93	T60.94	—	—
Fungi, noxious, used as food	T62.0x1	T62.0x2	T62.0x3	T62.0x4	—	—
Fungicide NEC (nonmedicinal)	T60.3x1	T60.3x2	T60.3x3	T60.3x4	—	—
Fungizone	T36.7x1	T36.7x2	T36.7x3	T36.7x4	T36.7x5	T36.7x6
topical	T49.0x1	T49.0x2	T49.0x3	T49.0x4	T49.0x5	T49.0x6
Furacin	T49.0x1	T49.0x2	T49.0x3	T49.0x4	T49.0x5	T49.0x6
Furadantin	T37.91	T37.92	T37.93	T37.94	T37.95	T37.96
Furazolidone	T37.8x1	T37.8x2	T37.8x3	T37.8x4	T37.8x5	T37.8x6
Furazolium chloride	T49.0x1	T49.0x2	T49.0x3	T49.0x4	T49.0x5	T49.0x6
Furfural	T52.8x1	T52.8x2	T52.8x3	T52.8x4	—	—
Furnace (coal burning) (domestic), **gas from**	T58.2x1	T58.2x2	T58.2x3	T58.2x4	—	—
industrial	T58.8x1	T58.8x2	T58.8x3	T58.8x4	—	—
Furniture polish	T65.891	T65.892	T65.893	T65.894	—	—
Furosemide	T50.1x1	T50.1x2	T50.1x3	T50.1x4	T50.1x5	T50.1x6
Furoxone	T37.91	T37.92	T37.93	T37.94	T37.95	T37.96
Fursultiamine	T45.2x1	T45.2x2	T45.2x3	T45.2x4	T45.2x5	T45.2x6
Fusafungine	T36.8x1	T36.8x2	T36.8x3	T36.8x4	T36.8x5	T36.8x6
Fusel oil (any) (amyl) (butyl) (propyl), **vapor**	T51.3x1	T51.3x2	T51.3x3	T51.3x4	—	—
Fusidate (ethanolamine) (sodium)	T36.8x1	T36.8x2	T36.8x3	T36.8x4	T36.8x5	T36.8x6
Fusidic acid	T36.8x1	T36.8x2	T36.8x3	T36.8x4	T36.8x5	T36.8x6
Fytic acid, nonasodium	T50.6x1	T50.6x2	T50.6x3	T50.6x4	T50.6x5	T50.6x6
GABA	T43.8x1	T43.8x2	T43.8x3	T43.8x4	T43.8x5	T43.8x6
Gadopentetic acid	T50.8x1	T50.8x2	T50.8x3	T50.8x4	T50.8x5	T50.8x6
Galactose	T50.3x1	T50.3x2	T50.3x3	T50.3x4	T50.3x5	T50.3x6
b-**Galactosidase**	T47.5x1	T47.5x2	T47.5x3	T47.5x4	T47.5x5	T47.5x6
Galantamine	T44.0x1	T44.0x2	T44.0x3	T44.0x4	T44.0x5	T44.0x6
Gallamine (triethiodide)	T48.1x1	T48.1x2	T48.1x3	T48.1x4	T48.1x5	T48.1x6
Gallium citrate	T50.991	T50.992	T50.993	T50.994	T50.995	T50.996
Gallopamil	T46.1x1	T46.1x2	T46.1x3	T46.1x4	T46.1x5	T46.1x6
Gamboge	T47.2x1	T47.2x2	T47.2x3	T47.2x4	T47.2x5	T47.2x6
Gamimune	T50.Z11	T50.Z12	T50.Z13	T50.Z14	T50.Z15	T50.Z16
Gamma-aminobutyric acid	T43.8x1	T43.8x2	T43.8x3	T43.8x4	T43.8x5	T43.8x6
Gamma-benzene hexachloride (medicinal)	T49.0x1	T49.0x2	T49.0x3	T49.0x4	T49.0x5	T49.0x6
nonmedicinal, vapor	T53.6x1	T53.6x2	T53.6x3	T53.6x4	—	—
Gamma-BHC (medicinal)	T49.0x1	T49.0x2	T49.0x3	T49.0x4	T49.0x5	T49.0x6
Gamma globulin	T50.Z11	T50.Z12	T50.Z13	T50.Z14	T50.Z15	T50.Z16
Gamulin	T50.Z11	T50.Z12	T50.Z13	T50.Z14	T50.Z15	T50.Z16
Ganciclovir (sodium)	T37.5x1	T37.5x2	T37.5x3	T37.5x4	T37.5x5	T37.5x6
Ganglionic blocking drug NEC	T44.2x1	T44.2x2	T44.2x3	T44.2x4	T44.2x5	T44.2x6
specified NEC	T44.2x1	T44.2x2	T44.2x3	T44.2x4	T44.2x5	T44.2x6
Ganja	T40.7x1	T40.7x2	T40.7x3	T40.7x4	T40.7x5	T40.7x6
Garamycin	T36.8x1	T36.8x2	T36.8x3	T36.8x4	T36.8x5	T36.8x6
ophthalmic preparation	T49.5x1	T49.5x2	T49.5x3	T49.5x4	T49.5x5	T49.5x6
topical NEC	T49.0x1	T49.0x2	T49.0x3	T49.0x4	T49.0x5	T49.0x6
Gardenal	T42.3x1	T42.3x2	T42.3x3	T42.3x4	T42.3x5	T42.3x6
Gardepanyl	T42.3x1	T42.3x2	T42.3x3	T42.3x4	T42.3x5	T42.3x6
Gas	T59.91	T59.92	T59.93	T59.94	—	—
acetylene	T59.891	T59.892	T59.893	T59.894	—	—
incomplete combustion of—*see* Carbon, monoxide, industrial fuels or gases						
air contaminants, source or type not specified	T59.91	T59.92	T59.93	T59.94	—	—
anesthetic	T41.0x1	T41.0x2	T41.0x3	T41.0x4	T41.0x5	T41.0x6
blast furnace	T58.8x1	T58.8x2	T58.8x3	T58.8x4	—	—
butane—*see* butane						
carbon monoxide—*see* Carbon, monoxide						
chlorine	T59.4x1	T59.4x2	T59.4x3	T59.4x4	—	—
coal	T58.2x1	T58.2x2	T58.2x3	T58.2x4	—	—
cyanide	T57.3x1	T57.3x2	T57.3x3	T57.3x4	—	—
dicyanogen	T65.0x1	T65.0x2	T65.0x3	T65.0x4	—	—
domestic—*see* Domestic gas						
exhaust	T58.01	T58.02	T58.03	T58.04	—	—
from utility (for cooking, heating, or lighting) (after combustion)—*see* Carbon, monoxide, fuel, utility						
prior to combustion	T59.891	T59.892	T59.893	T59.894	—	—

Substance	Poisoning, Accidental (unintentional)	Poisoning, Intentional Self-harm	Poisoning, Assault	Poisoning, Undetermined	Adverse Effect	Under-dosing
Gas—*continued*						
from wood or coal-burning stove or fireplace	T58.2x1	T58.2x2	T58.2x3	T58.2x4	—	—
fuel (domestic use) (after combustion) (*see also* Carbon, monoxide, fuel)						
industrial use	T58.8x1	T58.8x2	T58.8x3	T58.8x4	—	—
prior to combustion	T59.891	T59.892	T59.893	T59.894	—	—
utility	T59.891	T59.892	T59.893	T59.894	—	—
incomplete combustion of—*see* Carbon, monoxide, fuel, utility						
in mobile container	T59.891	T59.892	T59.893	T59.894	—	—
piped (natural)	T59.891	T59.892	T59.893	T59.894	—	—
garage	T58.01	T58.02	T58.03	T58.04	—	—
hydrocarbon NEC	T59.891	T59.892	T59.893	T59.894	—	—
incomplete combustion of—*see* Carbon, monoxide, fuel, utility						
liquefied—*see* butane						
piped	T59.891	T59.892	T59.893	T59.894	—	—
hydrocyanic acid	T57.3x1	T57.3x2	T57.3x3	T57.3x4	—	—
illuminating (after combustion)	T58.11	T58.12	T58.13	T58.14	—	—
prior to combustion	T59.891	T59.892	T59.893	T59.894	—	—
incomplete combustion, any—*see* Carbon, monoxide						
kiln	T58.8x1	T58.8x2	T58.8x3	T58.8x4	—	—
lacrimogenic	T59.3x1	T59.3x2	T59.3x3	T59.3x4	—	—
liquefied petroleum—*see* Butane						
marsh	T59.891	T59.892	T59.893	T59.894	—	—
motor exhaust, not in transit	T58.01	T58.02	T58.03	T58.04	—	—
mustard, not in war	T59.891	T59.892	T59.893	T59.894	—	—
natural	T59.891	T59.892	T59.893	T59.894	—	—
nerve, not in war	T59.91	T59.92	T59.93	T59.94	—	—
oil	T52.0x1	T52.0x2	T52.0x3	T52.0x4	—	—
petroleum (liquefied) (distributed in mobile containers)	T59.891	T59.892	T59.893	T59.894	—	—
piped (pure or mixed with air)	T59.891	T59.892	T59.893	T59.894	—	—
piped (manufactured) (natural) NEC	T59.891	T59.892	T59.893	T59.894	—	—
producer	T58.8x1	T58.8x2	T58.8x3	T58.8x4	—	—
propane—*see* propane						
refrigerant (chlorofluorocarbon)	T53.5x1	T53.5x2	T53.5x3	T53.5x4	—	—
not chlorofluorocarbon	T59.891	T59.892	T59.893	T59.894	—	—
sewer	T59.91	T59.92	T59.93	T59.94	—	—
specified source NEC	T59.91	T59.92	T59.93	T59.94	—	—
stove (after combustion)	T58.11	T58.12	T58.13	T58.14	—	—
prior to combustion	T59.891	T59.892	T59.893	T59.894	—	—
tear	T59.3x1	T59.3x2	T59.3x3	T59.3x4	—	—
utility (for cooking, heating, or lighting) (piped) NEC	T59.891	T59.892	T59.893	T59.894	—	—
incomplete combustion of—*see* Carbon, monoxide, fuel, utilty						
in mobile container	T59.891	T59.892	T59.893	T59.894	—	—
piped (natural)	T59.891	T59.892	T59.893	T59.894	—	—
water	T58.8x1	T58.8x2	T58.8x3	T58.8x4	—	—
incomplete combustion of—*see* Carbon, monoxide, fuel, utility						
Gaseous substance—*see* Gas						
Gasoline, gasoline	T52.0x1	T52.0x2	T52.0x3	T52.0x4	—	—
vapor	T52.0x1	T52.0x2	T52.0x3	T52.0x4	—	—
Gastric enzymes	T47.5x1	T47.5x2	T47.5x3	T47.5x4	T47.5x5	T47.5x6
Gastrografin	T50.8x1	T50.8x2	T50.8x3	T50.8x4	T50.8x5	T50.8x6
Gastrointestinal drug	T47.91	T47.92	T47.93	T47.94	T47.95	T47.96
biological	T47.8x1	T47.8x2	T47.8x3	T47.8x4	T47.8x5	T47.8x6
specified NEC	T47.8x1	T47.8x2	T47.8x3	T47.8x4	T47.8x5	T47.8x6
Gaultheria procumbens	T62.2x1	T62.2x2	T62.2x3	T62.2x4	—	—
Gelatin (intravenous)	T45.8x1	T45.8x2	T45.8x3	T45.8x4	T45.8x5	T45.8x6
absorbable (sponge)	T45.7x1	T45.7x2	T45.7x3	T45.7x4	T45.7x5	T45.7x6
Gefarnate	T44.3x1	T44.3x2	T44.3x3	T44.3x4	T44.3x5	T44.3x6

Substance	Poisoning, Accidental (unintentional)	Poisoning, Intentional Self-harm	Poisoning, Assault	Poisoning, Undetermined	Adverse Effect	Under-dosing
Gelfilm	T49.8x1	T49.8x2	T49.8x3	T49.8x4	T49.8x5	T49.8x6
Gelfoam	T45.7x1	T45.7x2	T45.7x3	T45.7x4	T45.7x5	T45.7x6
Gelsemine	T50.991	T50.992	T50.993	T50.994	T50.995	T50.996
Gelsemium (sempervirens)	T62.2x1	T62.2x2	T62.2x3	T62.2x4	—	—
Gemeprost	T48.0x1	T48.0x2	T48.0x3	T48.0x4	T48.0x5	T48.0x6
Gemfibrozil	T46.6x1	T46.6x2	T46.6x3	T46.6x4	T46.6x5	T46.6x6
Gemonil	T42.3x1	T42.3x2	T42.3x3	T42.3x4	T42.3x5	T42.3x6
Gentamicin	T36.5x1	T36.5x2	T36.5x3	T36.5x4	T36.5x5	T36.5x6
ophthalmic preparation	T49.5x1	T49.5x2	T49.5x3	T49.5x4	T49.5x5	T49.5x6
topical NEC	T49.0x1	T49.0x2	T49.0x3	T49.0x4	T49.0x5	T49.0x6
Gentian	T47.5x1	T47.5x2	T47.5x3	T47.5x4	T47.5x5	T47.5x6
violet	T49.0x1	T49.0x2	T49.0x3	T49.0x4	T49.0x5	T49.0x6
Gepefrine	T44.4x1	T44.4x2	T44.4x3	T44.4x4	T44.4x5	T44.4x6
Gestonorone caproate	T38.5x1	T38.5x2	T38.5x3	T38.5x4	T38.5x5	T38.5x6
Gexane	T49.0x1	T49.0x2	T49.0x3	T49.0x4	T49.0x5	T49.0x6
Gila monster (venom)	T63.111	T63.112	T63.113	T63.114	—	—
Ginger	T47.5x1	T47.5x2	T47.5x3	T47.5x4	T47.5x5	T47.5x6
jamaica	T62.2x1	T62.2x2	T62.2x3	T62.2x4	—	—
Gitalin	T46.0x1	T46.0x2	T46.0x3	T46.0x4	T46.0x5	T46.0x6
amorphous	T46.0x1	T46.0x2	T46.0x3	T46.0x4	T46.0x5	T46.0x6
Gitaloxin	T46.0x1	T46.0x2	T46.0x3	T46.0x4	T46.0x5	T46.0x6
Gitoxin	T46.0x1	T46.0x2	T46.0x3	T46.0x4	T46.0x5	T46.0x6
Glafenine	T39.8x1	T39.8x2	T39.8x3	T39.8x4	T39.8x5	T39.8x6
Glandular extract (medicinal) NEC	T50.Z91	T50.Z92	T50.Z93	T50.Z94	T50.Z95	T50.Z96
Glaucarubin	T37.3x1	T37.3x2	T37.3x3	T37.3x4	T37.3x5	T37.3x6
Glibenclamide	T38.3x1	T38.3x2	T38.3x3	T38.3x4	T38.3x5	T38.3x6
Glibornuride	T38.3x1	T38.3x2	T38.3x3	T38.3x4	T38.3x5	T38.3x6
Gliclazide	T38.3x1	T38.3x2	T38.3x3	T38.3x4	T38.3x5	T38.3x6
Glimidine	T38.3x1	T38.3x2	T38.3x3	T38.3x4	T38.3x5	T38.3x6
Glipizide	T38.3x1	T38.3x2	T38.3x3	T38.3x4	T38.3x5	T38.3x6
Gliquidone	T38.3x1	T38.3x2	T38.3x3	T38.3x4	T38.3x5	T38.3x6
Glisolamide	T38.3x1	T38.3x2	T38.3x3	T38.3x4	T38.3x5	T38.3x6
Glisoxepide	T38.3x1	T38.3x2	T38.3x3	T38.3x4	T38.3x5	T38.3x6
Globin zinc insulin	T38.3x1	T38.3x2	T38.3x3	T38.3x4	T38.3x5	T38.3x6
Globulin						
antilymphocytic	T50.Z11	T50.Z12	T50.Z13	T50.Z14	T50.Z15	T50.Z16
antirhesus	T50.Z11	T50.Z12	T50.Z13	T50.Z14	T50.Z15	T50.Z16
antivenin	T50.Z11	T50.Z12	T50.Z13	T50.Z14	T50.Z15	T50.Z16
antiviral	T50.Z11	T50.Z12	T50.Z13	T50.Z14	T50.Z15	T50.Z16
Glucagon	T38.3x1	T38.3x2	T38.3x3	T38.3x4	T38.3x5	T38.3x6
Glucocorticoids	T38.0x1	T38.0x2	T38.0x3	T38.0x4	T38.0x5	T38.0x6
Glucocorticosteroid	T38.0x1	T38.0x2	T38.0x3	T38.0x4	T38.0x5	T38.0x6
Gluconic acid	T50.991	T50.992	T50.993	T50.994	T50.995	T50.996
Glucosamine sulfate	T39.4x1	T39.4x2	T39.4x3	T39.4x4	T39.4x5	T39.4x6
Glucose	T50.3x1	T50.3x2	T50.3x3	T50.3x4	T50.3x5	T50.3x6
with sodium chloride	T50.3x1	T50.3x2	T50.3x3	T50.3x4	T50.3x5	T50.3x6
Glucosulfone sodium	T37.1x1	T37.1x2	T37.1x3	T37.1x4	T37.1x5	T37.1x6
Glucurolactone	T47.8x1	T47.8x2	T47.8x3	T47.8x4	T47.8x5	T47.8x6
Glue NEC	T52.8x1	T52.8x2	T52.8x3	T52.8x4	—	—
Glutamic acid	T47.5x1	T47.5x2	T47.5x3	T47.5x4	T47.5x5	T47.5x6
Glutaral (medicinal)	T49.0x1	T49.0x2	T49.0x3	T49.0x4	T49.0x5	T49.0x6
nonmedicinal	T65.891	T65.892	T65.893	T65.894	—	—
Glutaraldehyde (nonmedicinal)	T65.891	T65.892	T65.893	T65.894	—	—
medicinal	T49.0x1	T49.0x2	T49.0x3	T49.0x4	T49.0x5	T49.0x6
Glutathione	T50.6x1	T50.6x2	T50.6x3	T50.6x4	T50.6x5	T50.6x6
Glutethimide	T42.6x1	T42.6x2	T42.6x3	T42.6x4	T42.6x5	T42.6x6
Glyburide	T38.3x1	T38.3x2	T38.3x3	T38.3x4	T38.3x5	T38.3x6
Glycerin	T47.4x1	T47.4x2	T47.4x3	T47.4x4	T47.4x5	T47.4x6
Glycerol	T47.4x1	T47.4x2	T47.4x3	T47.4x4	T47.4x5	T47.4x6
borax	T49.6x1	T49.6x2	T49.6x3	T49.6x4	T49.6x5	T49.6x6
intravenous	T50.3x1	T50.3x2	T50.3x3	T50.3x4	T50.3x5	T50.3x6
iodinated	T48.4x1	T48.4x2	T48.4x3	T48.4x4	T48.4x5	T48.4x6
Glycerophosphate	T50.991	T50.992	T50.993	T50.994	T50.995	T50.996
Glyceryl						
gualacolate	T48.4x1	T48.4x2	T48.4x3	T48.4x4	T48.4x5	T48.4x6
nitrate	T46.3x1	T46.3x2	T46.3x3	T46.3x4	T46.3x5	T46.3x6
triacetate (topical)	T49.0x1	T49.0x2	T49.0x3	T49.0x4	T49.0x5	T49.0x6
trinitrate	T46.3x1	T46.3x2	T46.3x3	T46.3x4	T46.3x5	T46.3x6
Glycine	T50.3x1	T50.3x2	T50.3x3	T50.3x4	T50.3x5	T50.3x6
Glyclopyramide	T38.3x1	T38.3x2	T38.3x3	T38.3x4	T38.3x5	T38.3x6

Substance	Poisoning, Accidental (unintentional)	Poisoning, Intentional Self-harm	Poisoning, Assault	Poisoning, Undetermined	Adverse Effect	Under-dosing
Glycobiarsol	T37.3x1	T37.3x2	T37.3x3	T37.3x4	T37.3x5	T37.3x6
Glycols (ether)	T52.3x1	T52.3x2	T52.3x3	T52.3x4	—	—
Glyconiazide	T37.1x1	T37.1x2	T37.1x3	T37.1x4	T37.1x5	T37.1x6
Glycopyrrolate	T44.3x1	T44.3x2	T44.3x3	T44.3x4	T44.3x5	T44.3x6
Glycopyrronium	T44.3x1	T44.3x2	T44.3x3	T44.3x4	T44.3x5	T44.3x6
bromide	T44.3x1	T44.3x2	T44.3x3	T44.3x4	T44.3x5	T44.3x6
Glycyclamide	T38.3x1	T38.3x2	T38.3x3	T38.3x4	T38.3x5	T38.3x6
Glycyrrhiza extract	T48.4x1	T48.4x2	T48.4x3	T48.4x4	T48.4x5	T48.4x6
Glycyrrhizic acid	T48.4x1	T48.4x2	T48.4x3	T48.4x4	T48.4x5	T48.4x6
Glycyrrhizinate potassium	T48.4x1	T48.4x2	T48.4x3	T48.4x4	T48.4x5	T48.4x6
Glymidine sodium	T38.3x1	T38.3x2	T38.3x3	T38.3x4	T38.3x5	T38.3x6
Glyphosate	T60.3x1	T60.3x2	T60.3x3	T60.3x4	—	—
Glyphylline	T48.6x1	T48.6x2	T48.6x3	T48.6x4	T48.6x5	T48.6x6
Gold						
colloidal (I98Au)	T45.1x1	T45.1x2	T45.1x3	T45.1x4	T45.1x5	T45.1x6
salts	T39.4x1	T39.4x2	T39.4x3	T39.4x4	T39.4x5	T39.4x6
Golden sulfide of antimony	T56.891	T56.892	T56.893	T56.894	—	—
Goldylocks	T62.2x1	T62.2x2	T62.2x3	T62.2x4	—	—
Gonadal tissue extract	T38.901	T38.902	T38.903	T38.904	T38.905	T38.906
female	T38.5x1	T38.5x2	T38.5x3	T38.5x4	T38.5x5	T38.5x6
male	T38.7x1	T38.7x2	T38.7x3	T38.7x4	T38.7x5	T38.7x6
Gonadorelin	T38.891	T38.892	T38.893	T38.894	T38.895	T38.896
Gonadotropin	T38.891	T38.892	T38.893	T38.894	T38.895	T38.896
chorionic	T38.891	T38.892	T38.893	T38.894	T38.895	T38.896
pituitary	T38.811	T38.812	T38.813	T38.814	T38.815	T38.816
Goserelin	T45.1x1	T45.1x2	T45.1x3	T45.1x4	T45.1x5	T45.1x6
Grain alcohol	T51.0x1	T51.0x2	T51.0x3	T51.0x4	—	—
Gramicidin	T49.0x1	T49.0x2	T49.0x3	T49.0x4	T49.0x5	T49.0x6
Granisetron	T45.0x1	T45.0x2	T45.0x3	T45.0x4	T45.0x5	T45.0x6
Gratiola officinalis	T62.2x1	T62.2x2	T62.2x3	T62.2x4	—	—
Grease	T65.891	T65.892	T65.893	T65.894	—	—
Green hellebore	T62.2x1	T62.2x2	T62.2x3	T62.2x4	—	—
Green soap	T49.2x1	T49.2x2	T49.2x3	T49.2x4	T49.2x5	T49.2x6
Grifulvin	T36.7x1	T36.7x2	T36.7x3	T36.7x4	T36.7x5	T36.7x6
Griseofulvin	T36.7x1	T36.7x2	T36.7x3	T36.7x4	T36.7x5	T36.7x6
Growth hormone	T38.811	T38.812	T38.813	T38.814	T38.815	T38.816
Guaiacol derivatives	T48.4x1	T48.4x2	T48.4x3	T48.4x4	T48.4x5	T48.4x6
Guaiac reagent	T50.991	T50.992	T50.993	T50.994	T50.995	T50.996
Guaifenesin	T48.4x1	T48.4x2	T48.4x3	T48.4x4	T48.4x5	T48.4x6
Guaimesal	T48.4x1	T48.4x2	T48.4x3	T48.4x4	T48.4x5	T48.4x6
Guaiphenesin	T48.4x1	T48.4x2	T48.4x3	T48.4x4	T48.4x5	T48.4x6
Guamecycline	T36.4x1	T36.4x2	T36.4x3	T36.4x4	T36.4x5	T36.4x6
Guanabenz	T46.5x1	T46.5x2	T46.5x3	T46.5x4	T46.5x5	T46.5x6
Guanacline	T46.5x1	T46.5x2	T46.5x3	T46.5x4	T46.5x5	T46.5x6
Guanadrel	T46.5x1	T46.5x2	T46.5x3	T46.5x4	T46.5x5	T46.5x6
Guanatol	T37.2x1	T37.2x2	T37.2x3	T37.2x4	T37.2x5	T37.2x6
Guanethidine	T46.5x1	T46.5x2	T46.5x3	T46.5x4	T46.5x5	T46.5x6
Guanfacine	T46.5x1	T46.5x2	T46.5x3	T46.5x4	T46.5x5	T46.5x6
Guano	T65.891	T65.892	T65.893	T65.894	—	—
Guanochlor	T46.5x1	T46.5x2	T46.5x3	T46.5x4	T46.5x5	T46.5x6
Guanoclor	T46.5x1	T46.5x2	T46.5x3	T46.5x4	T46.5x5	T46.5x6
Guanoctine	T46.5x1	T46.5x2	T46.5x3	T46.5x4	T46.5x5	T46.5x6
Guanoxabenz	T46.5x1	T46.5x2	T46.5x3	T46.5x4	T46.5x5	T46.5x6
Guanoxan	T46.5x1	T46.5x2	T46.5x3	T46.5x4	T46.5x5	T46.5x6
Guar gum (medicinal)	T46.6x1	T46.6x2	T46.6x3	T46.6x4	T46.6x5	T46.6x6
Hachimycin	T36.7x1	T36.7x2	T36.7x3	T36.7x4	T36.7x5	T36.7x6
Hair						
dye	T49.4x1	T49.4x2	T49.4x3	T49.4x4	T49.4x5	T49.4x6
preparation NEC	T49.4x1	T49.4x2	T49.4x3	T49.4x4	T49.4x5	T49.4x6
Halazepam	T42.4x1	T42.4x2	T42.4x3	T42.4x4	T42.4x5	T42.4x6
Halcinolone	T49.0x1	T49.0x2	T49.0x3	T49.0x4	T49.0x5	T49.0x6
Halcinonide	T49.0x1	T49.0x2	T49.0x3	T49.0x4	T49.0x5	T49.0x6
Halethazole	T49.0x1	T49.0x2	T49.0x3	T49.0x4	T49.0x5	T49.0x6
Hallucinogen NEC	T40.901	T40.902	T40.903	T40.904	T40.905	T40.906
Halofantrine	T37.2x1	T37.2x2	T37.2x3	T37.2x4	T37.2x5	T37.2x6
Halofenate	T46.6x1	T46.6x2	T46.6x3	T46.6x4	T46.6x5	T46.6x6
Halometasone	T49.0x1	T49.0x2	T49.0x3	T49.0x4	T49.0x5	T49.0x6
Haloperidol	T43.4x1	T43.4x2	T43.4x3	T43.4x4	T43.4x5	T43.4x6
Haloprogin	T49.0x1	T49.0x2	T49.0x3	T49.0x4	T49.0x5	T49.0x6
Halotex	T49.0x1	T49.0x2	T49.0x3	T49.0x4	T49.0x5	T49.0x6
Halothane	T41.0x1	T41.0x2	T41.0x3	T41.0x4	T41.0x5	T41.0x6

Substance	Poisoning, Accidental (unintentional)	Poisoning, Intentional Self-harm	Poisoning, Assault	Poisoning, Undetermined	Adverse Effect	Under-dosing
Haloxazolam	T42.4x1	T42.4x2	T42.4x3	T42.4x4	T42.4x5	T42.4x6
Halquinols	T49.0x1	T49.0x2	T49.0x3	T49.0x4	T49.0x5	T49.0x6
Hamamelis	T49.2x1	T49.2x2	T49.2x3	T49.2x4	T49.2x5	T49.2x6
Haptendextran	T45.8x1	T45.8x2	T45.8x3	T45.8x4	T45.8x5	T45.8x6
Harmonyl	T46.5x1	T46.5x2	T46.5x3	T46.5x4	T46.5x5	T46.5x6
Hartmann's solution	T50.3x1	T50.3x2	T50.3x3	T50.3x4	T50.3x5	T50.3x6
Hashish	T40.7x1	T40.7x2	T40.7x3	T40.7x4	T40.7x5	T40.7x6
Hawaiian wood rose seeds	T40.991	T40.992	T40.993	T40.994	T40.995	T40.996
HCB	T60.3x1	T60.3x2	T60.3x3	T60.3x4	—	—
HCH	T53.6x1	T53.6x2	T53.6x3	T53.6x4	—	—
medicinal	T49.0x1	T49.0x2	T49.0x3	T49.0x4	T49.0x5	T49.0x6
HCN	T57.3x1	T57.3x2	T57.3x3	T57.3x4	—	—
Headache cures, drugs, powders NEC	T50.901	T50.902	T50.903	T50.904	T50.905	T50.906
Heavenly Blue (morning glory)	T40.991	T40.992	T40.993	T40.994	T40.995	T40.996
Heavy metal antidote	T45.8x1	T45.8x2	T45.8x3	T45.8x4	T45.8x5	T45.8x6
Hedaquinium	T49.0x1	T49.0x2	T49.0x3	T49.0x4	T49.0x5	T49.0x6
Hedge hyssop	T62.2x1	T62.2x2	T62.2x3	T62.2x4	—	—
Heet	T49.8x1	T49.8x2	T49.8x3	T49.8x4	T49.8x5	T49.8x6
Helium	T48.991	T48.992	T48.993	T48.994	T48.995	T48.996
Helenin	T37.4x1	T37.4x2	T37.4x3	T37.4x4	T37.4x5	T37.4x6
Hellebore (black) (green) (white)	T62.2x1	T62.2x2	T62.2x3	T62.2x4	—	—
Hematin	T45.8x1	T45.8x2	T45.8x3	T45.8x4	T45.8x5	T45.8x6
Hematinic preparation	T45.8x1	T45.8x2	T45.8x3	T45.8x4	T45.8x5	T45.8x6
Hemlock	T62.2x1	T62.2x2	T62.2x3	T62.2x4	—	—
Hemostatic	T49.4x1	T49.4x2	T49.4x3	T49.4x4	T49.4x5	T49.4x6
drug, systemic	T45.7x1	T45.7x2	T45.7x3	T45.7x4	T45.7x5	T45.7x6
Hemostyptic	T49.4x1	T49.4x2	T49.4x3	T49.4x4	T49.4x5	T49.4x6
Henbane	T62.2x1	T62.2x2	T62.2x3	T62.2x4	—	—
Heparin (sodium)	T45.511	T45.512	T45.513	T45.514	T45.515	T45.516
action reverser	T45.7x1	T45.7x2	T45.7x3	T45.7x4	T45.7x5	T45.7x6
Heparin-fraction	T45.511	T45.512	T45.513	T45.514	T45.515	T45.516
Heparinoid (systemic)	T45.511	T45.512	T45.513	T45.514	T45.515	T45.516
Hepatic secretion stimulant	T47.8x1	T47.8x2	T47.8x3	T47.8x4	T47.8x5	T47.8x6
Hepatitis B						
immune globulin	T50.Z11	T50.Z12	T50.Z13	T50.Z14	T50.Z15	T50.Z16
vaccine	T50.B91	T50.B92	T50.B93	T50.B94	T50.B95	T50.B96
Hepronicate	T46.7x1	T46.7x2	T46.7x3	T46.7x4	T46.7x5	T46.7x6
Heptabarb	T42.3x1	T42.3x2	T42.3x3	T42.3x4	T42.3x5	T42.3x6
Heptabarbitone	T42.3x1	T42.3x2	T42.3x3	T42.3x4	T42.3x5	T42.3x6
Heptabarbital, heptabarbitone	T42.3x1	T42.3x2	T42.3x3	T42.3x4	T42.3x5	T42.3x6
Heptachlor	T60.1x1	T60.1x2	T60.1x3	T60.1x4	—	—
Heptalgin	T40.2x1	T40.2x2	T40.2x3	T40.2x4	T40.2x5	T40.2x6
Heptaminol	T46.3x1	T46.3x2	T46.3x3	T46.3x4	T46.3x5	T46.3x6
Herbicide NEC	T60.3x1	T60.3x2	T60.3x3	T60.3x4	—	—
Heroin	T40.1x1	T40.1x2	T40.1x3	T40.1x4	T40.1x5	T40.1x6
Herplex	T49.5x1	T49.5x2	T49.5x3	T49.5x4	T49.5x5	T49.5x6
HES	T45.8x1	T45.8x2	T45.8x3	T45.8x4	T45.8x5	T45.8x6
Hesperidin	T46.991	T46.992	T46.993	T46.994	T46.995	T46.996
Hetacillin	T36.0x1	T36.0x2	T36.0x3	T36.0x4	T36.0x5	T36.0x6
Hetastarch	T45.8x1	T45.8x2	T45.8x3	T45.8x4	T45.8x5	T45.8x6
HETP	T60.0x1	T60.0x2	T60.0x3	T60.0x4	—	—
Hexachlorobenzene (vapor)	T60.3x1	T60.3x2	T60.3x3	T60.3x4	—	—
Hexachlorocyclohexane	T53.6x1	T53.6x2	T53.6x3	T53.6x4	—	—
Hexachlorophene	T49.0x1	T49.0x2	T49.0x3	T49.0x4	T49.0x5	T49.0x6
Hexadiline	T46.3x1	T46.3x2	T46.3x3	T46.3x4	T46.3x5	T46.3x6
Hexadimethrine (bromide)	T45.7x1	T45.7x2	T45.7x3	T45.7x4	T45.7x5	T45.7x6
Hexadylamine	T46.3x1	T46.3x2	T46.3x3	T46.3x4	T46.3x5	T46.3x6
Hexaethyl tetraphosphate	T60.0x1	T60.0x2	T60.0x3	T60.0x4	—	—
Hexafluorenium bromide	T48.1x1	T48.1x2	T48.1x3	T48.1x4	T48.1x5	T48.1x6
Hexafluronium (bromide)	T48.1x1	T48.1x2	T48.1x3	T48.1x4	T48.1x5	T48.1x6
Hexahydrobenzol	T52.8x1	T52.8x2	T52.8x3	T52.8x4	—	—
Hexahydrocresol (s)	T51.8x1	T51.8x2	T51.8x3	T51.8x4	—	—
arsenide	T57.0x1	T57.0x2	T57.0x3	T57.0x4	—	—
arseniurated	T57.0x1	T57.0x2	T57.0x3	T57.0x4	—	—
cyanide	T57.3x1	T57.3x2	T57.3x3	T57.3x4	—	—
gas	T59.891	T59.892	T59.893	T59.894	—	—
Fluoride (liquid)	T57.8x1	T57.8x2	T57.8x3	T57.8x4	—	—
vapor	T59.891	T59.892	T59.893	T59.894	—	—
phophorated	T60.0x1	T60.0x2	T60.0x3	T60.0x4	—	—
sulfate	T57.8x1	T57.8x2	T57.8x3	T57.8x4	—	—

Substance	Poisoning, Accidental (unintentional)	Poisoning, Intentional Self-harm	Poisoning, Assault	Poisoning, Undetermined	Adverse Effect	Under-dosing
Hexahydrocresol (s)—*continued*						
sulfide (gas)	T59.6x1	T59.6x2	T59.6x3	T59.6x4	—	—
arseniurated	T57.0x1	T57.0x2	T57.0x3	T57.0x4	—	—
sulfurated	T57.8x1	T57.8x2	T57.8x3	T57.8x4	—	—
Hexahydrophenol	T51.8x1	T51.8x2	T51.8x3	T51.8x4	—	—
Hexa-germ	T49.2x1	T49.2x2	T49.2x3	T49.2x4	T49.2x5	T49.2x6
Hexalen	T51.8x1	T51.8x2	T51.8x3	T51.8x4	—	—
Hexamethonium bromide	T44.2x1	T44.2x2	T44.2x3	T44.2x4	T44.2x5	T44.2x6
Hexamethylene	T52.8x1	T52.8x2	T52.8x3	T52.8x4	—	—
Hexamethylmelamine	T45.1x1	T45.1x2	T45.1x3	T45.1x4	T45.1x5	T45.1x6
Hexamidine	T49.0x1	T49.0x2	T49.0x3	T49.0x4	T49.0x5	T49.0x6
Hexamine (mandelate)	T37.8x1	T37.8x2	T37.8x3	T37.8x4	T37.8x5	T37.8x6
Hexanone, 2-hexanone	T52.4x1	T52.4x2	T52.4x3	T52.4x4	—	—
Hexanuorenium	T48.1x1	T48.1x2	T48.1x3	T48.1x4	T48.1x5	T48.1x6
Hexapropymate	T42.6x1	T42.6x2	T42.6x3	T42.6x4	T42.6x5	T42.6x6
Hexasonium iodide	T44.3x1	T44.3x2	T44.3x3	T44.3x4	T44.3x5	T44.3x6
Hexcarbacholine bromide	T48.1x1	T48.1x2	T48.1x3	T48.1x4	T48.1x5	T48.1x6
Hexemal	T42.3x1	T42.3x2	T42.3x3	T42.3x4	T42.3x5	T42.3x6
Hexestrol	T38.5x1	T38.5x2	T38.5x3	T38.5x4	T38.5x5	T38.5x6
Hexethal (sodium)	T42.3x1	T42.3x2	T42.3x3	T42.3x4	T42.3x5	T42.3x6
Hexetidine	T37.8x1	T37.8x2	T37.8x3	T37.8x4	T37.8x5	T37.8x6
Hexobarbital	T42.3x1	T42.3x2	T42.3x3	T42.3x4	T42.3x5	T42.3x6
rectal	T41.291	T41.292	T41.293	T41.294	T41.295	T41.296
sodium	T41.1x1	T41.1x2	T41.1x3	T41.1x4	T41.1x5	T41.1x6
Hexobendine	T46.3x1	T46.3x2	T46.3x3	T46.3x4	T46.3x5	T46.3x6
Hexocyclium	T44.3x1	T44.3x2	T44.3x3	T44.3x4	T44.3x5	T44.3x6
metilsulfate	T44.3x1	T44.3x2	T44.3x3	T44.3x4	T44.3x5	T44.3x6
Hexoestrol	T38.5x1	T38.5x2	T38.5x3	T38.5x4	T38.5x5	T38.5x6
Hexone	T52.4x1	T52.4x2	T52.4x3	T52.4x4	—	—
Hexoprenaline	T48.6x1	T48.6x2	T48.6x3	T48.6x4	T48.6x5	T48.6x6
Hexylcaine	T41.3x1	T41.3x2	T41.3x3	T41.3x4	T41.3x5	T41.3x6
Hexylresorcinol	T52.2x1	T52.2x2	T52.2x3	T52.2x4	—	—
HGH (human growth hormone)	T38.811	T38.812	T38.813	T38.814	T38.815	T38.816
Hinkle's pills	T47.2x1	T47.2x2	T47.2x3	T47.2x4	T47.2x5	T47.2x6
Histalog	T50.8x1	T50.8x2	T50.8x3	T50.8x4	T50.8x5	T50.8x6
Histamine (phosphate)	T50.8x1	T50.8x2	T50.8x3	T50.8x4	T50.8x5	T50.8x6
Histoplasmin	T50.8x1	T50.8x2	T50.8x3	T50.8x4	T50.8x5	T50.8x6
Holly berries	T62.2x1	T62.2x2	T62.2x3	T62.2x4	—	—
Homatropine	T44.3x1	T44.3x2	T44.3x3	T44.3x4	T44.3x5	T44.3x6
methylbromide	T44.3x1	T44.3x2	T44.3x3	T44.3x4	T44.3x5	T44.3x6
Homochlorcyclizine	T45.0x1	T45.0x2	T45.0x3	T45.0x4	T45.0x5	T45.0x6
Homosalate	T49.3x1	T49.3x2	T49.3x3	T49.3x4	T49.3x5	T49.3x6
Homo-tet	T50.Z11	T50.Z12	T50.Z13	T50.Z14	T50.Z15	T50.Z16
Hormone	T38.801	T38.802	T38.803	T38.804	T38.805	T38.806
adrenal cortical steroids	T38.0x1	T38.0x2	T38.0x3	T38.0x4	T38.0x5	T38.0x6
androgenic	T38.7x1	T38.7x2	T38.7x3	T38.7x4	T38.7x5	T38.7x6
anterior pituitary NEC	T38.811	T38.812	T38.813	T38.814	T38.815	T38.816
antidiabetic agents	T38.3x1	T38.3x2	T38.3x3	T38.3x4	T38.3x5	T38.3x6
antidiuretic	T38.891	T38.892	T38.893	T38.894	T38.895	T38.896
cancer therapy	T45.1x1	T45.1x2	T45.1x3	T45.1x4	T45.1x5	T45.1x6
follicle stimulating	T38.811	T38.812	T38.813	T38.814	T38.815	T38.816
gonadotropic	T38.891	T38.892	T38.893	T38.894	T38.895	T38.896
pituitary	T38.811	T38.812	T38.813	T38.814	T38.815	T38.816
growth	T38.811	T38.812	T38.813	T38.814	T38.815	T38.816
luteinizing	T38.811	T38.812	T38.813	T38.814	T38.815	T38.816
ovarian	T38.5x1	T38.5x2	T38.5x3	T38.5x4	T38.5x5	T38.5x6
oxytocic	T48.0x1	T48.0x2	T48.0x3	T48.0x4	T48.0x5	T48.0x6
parathyroid (derivatives)	T50.991	T50.992	T50.993	T50.994	T50.995	T50.996
pituitary (posterior) NEC	T38.891	T38.892	T38.893	T38.894	T38.895	T38.896
anterior	T38.811	T38.812	T38.813	T38.814	T38.815	T38.816
specified, NEC	T38.891	T38.892	T38.893	T38.894	T38.895	T38.896
thyroid	T38.1x1	T38.1x2	T38.1x3	T38.1x4	T38.1x5	T38.1x6
Hornet (sting)	T63.451	T63.452	T63.453	T63.454	—	—
Horse anti-human lymphocytic serum	T50.Z11	T50.Z12	T50.Z13	T50.Z14	T50.Z15	T50.Z16
Horticulture agent NEC	T65.91	T65.92	T65.93	T65.94	—	—
with pesticide	T60.91	T60.92	T60.93	T60.94	—	—
Human						
albumin	T45.8x1	T45.8x2	T45.8x3	T45.8x4	T45.8x5	T45.8x6
growth hormone (HGH)	T38.811	T38.812	T38.813	T38.814	T38.815	T38.816
immune serum	T50.Z11	T50.Z12	T50.Z13	T50.Z14	T50.Z15	T50.Z16

Substance	Poisoning, Accidental (unintentional)	Poisoning, Intentional Self-harm	Poisoning, Assault	Poisoning, Undetermined	Adverse Effect	Under-dosing
Hyaluronidase	T45.3x1	T45.3x2	T45.3x3	T45.3x4	T45.3x5	T45.3x6
Hyazyme	T45.3x1	T45.3x2	T45.3x3	T45.3x4	T45.3x5	T45.3x6
Hycodan	T40.2x1	T40.2x2	T40.2x3	T40.2x4	T40.2x5	T40.2x6
Hydantoin derivative NEC	T42.0x1	T42.0x2	T42.0x3	T42.0x4	T42.0x5	T42.0x6
Hydeltra	T38.0x1	T38.0x2	T38.0x3	T38.0x4	T38.0x5	T38.0x6
Hydergine	T44.6x1	T44.6x2	T44.6x3	T44.6x4	T44.6x5	T44.6x6
Hydrabamine penicillin	T36.0x1	T36.0x2	T36.0x3	T36.0x4	T36.0x5	T36.0x6
Hydralazine	T46.5x1	T46.5x2	T46.5x3	T46.5x4	T46.5x5	T46.5x6
Hydrargaphen	T49.0x1	T49.0x2	T49.0x3	T49.0x4	T49.0x5	T49.0x6
Hydrargyri aminochloridum	T49.0x1	T49.0x2	T49.0x3	T49.0x4	T49.0x5	T49.0x6
Hydrastine	T48.291	T48.292	T48.293	T48.294	T48.295	T48.296
Hydrazine	T54.1x1	T54.1x2	T54.1x3	T54.1x4	—	—
monoamine oxidase inhibitors	T43.1x1	T43.1x2	T43.1x3	T43.1x4	T43.1x5	T43.1x6
Hydrazoic acid, azides	T54.2x1	T54.2x2	T54.2x3	T54.2x4		
Hydriodic acid	T48.4x1	T48.4x2	T48.4x3	T48.4x4	T48.4x5	T48.4x6
Hydrocarbon gas	T59.891	T59.892	T59.893	T59.894		
incomplete combustion of— *see* Carbon, monoxide, fuel, utility						
liquefied (mobile container)	T59.891	T59.892	T59.893	T59.894	—	—
piped (natural)	T59.891	T59.892	T59.893	T59.894	—	—
Hydrochloric acid (liquid)	T54.2x1	T54.2x2	T54.2x3	T54.2x4	—	—
medicinal (digestant)	T47.5x1	T47.5x2	T47.5x3	T47.5x4	T47.5x5	T47.5x6
vapor	T59.891	T59.892	T59.893	T59.894	—	—
Hydrochlorothiazide	T50.2x1	T50.2x2	T50.2x3	T50.2x4	T50.2x5	T50.2x6
Hydrocodone	T40.2x1	T40.2x2	T40.2x3	T40.2x4	T40.2x5	T40.2x6
Hydrocortisone (derivatives)	T49.0x1	T49.0x2	T49.0x3	T49.0x4	T49.0x5	T49.0x6
aceponate	T49.0x1	T49.0x2	T49.0x3	T49.0x4	T49.0x5	T49.0x6
ENT agent	T49.6x1	T49.6x2	T49.6x3	T49.6x4	T49.6x5	T49.6x6
ophthalmic preparation	T49.5x1	T49.5x2	T49.5x3	T49.5x4	T49.5x5	T49.5x6
topical NEC	T49.0x1	T49.0x2	T49.0x3	T49.0x4	T49.0x5	T49.0x6
Hydrocortone	T38.0x1	T38.0x2	T38.0x3	T38.0x4	T38.0x5	T38.0x6
ENT agent	T49.6x1	T49.6x2	T49.6x3	T49.6x4	T49.6x5	T49.6x6
ophthalmic preparation	T49.5x1	T49.5x2	T49.5x3	T49.5x4	T49.5x5	T49.5x6
topical NEC	T49.0x1	T49.0x2	T49.0x3	T49.0x4	T49.0x5	T49.0x6
Hydrocyanic acid (liquid)	T57.3x1	T57.3x2	T57.3x3	T57.3x4	—	—
gas	T65.0x1	T65.0x2	T65.0x3	T65.0x4	—	—
Hydroflumethiazide	T50.2x1	T50.2x2	T50.2x3	T50.2x4	T50.2x5	T50.2x6
Hydrofluoric acid (liquid)	T54.2x1	T54.2x2	T54.2x3	T54.2x4	—	—
vapor	T59.891	T59.892	T59.893	T59.894	—	—
Hydrogen	T59.891	T59.892	T59.893	T59.894	—	—
arsenide	T57.0x1	T57.0x2	T57.0x3	T57.0x4	—	—
arseniureted	T57.0x1	T57.0x2	T57.0x3	T57.0x4	—	—
cyanide (salts)	T57.3x1	T57.3x2	T57.3x3	T57.3x4	—	—
gas	T57.3x1	T57.3x2	T57.3x3	T57.3x4	—	—
chloride	T57.8x1	T57.8x2	T57.8x3	T57.8x4	—	—
cyanide (gas)	T57.3x1	T57.3x2	T57.3x3	T57.3x4	—	—
Fluoride	T59.5x1	T59.5x2	T59.5x3	T59.5x4	—	—
vapor	T59.5x1	T59.5x2	T59.5x3	T59.5x4	—	—
peroxide	T49.0x1	T49.0x2	T49.0x3	T49.0x4	T49.0x5	T49.0x6
phosphureted	T57.1x1	T57.1x2	T57.1x3	T57.1x4	—	—
sulfide	T59.6x1	T59.6x2	T59.6x3	T59.6x4	—	—
arseniureted	T57.0x1	T57.0x2	T57.0x3	T57.0x4	—	—
sulfureted	T59.6x1	T59.6x2	T59.6x3	T59.6x4	—	—
Hydromethylpyridine	T46.7x1	T46.7x2	T46.7x3	T46.7x4	T46.7x5	T46.7x6
Hydromorphinol	T40.2x1	T40.2x2	T40.2x3	T40.2x4	T40.2x5	T40.2x6
Hydromorphinone	T40.2x1	T40.2x2	T40.2x3	T40.2x4	T40.2x5	T40.2x6
Hydromorphone	T40.2x1	T40.2x2	T40.2x3	T40.2x4	T40.2x5	T40.2x6
Hydromox	T50.2x1	T50.2x2	T50.2x3	T50.2x4	T50.2x5	T50.2x6
Hydrophilic lotion	T49.3x1	T49.3x2	T49.3x3	T49.3x4	T49.3x5	T49.3x6
Hydroquinidine	T46.2x1	T46.2x2	T46.2x3	T46.2x4	T46.2x5	T46.2x6
Hydroquinone	T52.2x1	T52.2x2	T52.2x3	T52.2x4	—	—
vapor	T59.891	T59.892	T59.893	T59.894	—	—
Hydrosulfuric acid (gas)	T59.6x1	T59.6x2	T59.6x3	T59.6x4	—	—
Hydrotalcite	T47.1x1	T47.1x2	T47.1x3	T47.1x4	T47.1x5	T47.1x6
Hydrous wool fat	T49.3x1	T49.3x2	T49.3x3	T49.3x4	T49.3x5	T49.3x6
Hydroxide, caustic	T54.3x1	T54.3x2	T54.3x3	T54.3x4	—	—
Hydroxocobalamin	T45.8x1	T45.8x2	T45.8x3	T45.8x4	T45.8x5	T45.8x6
Hydroxyamphetamine	T49.5x1	T49.5x2	T49.5x3	T49.5x4	T49.5x5	T49.5x6
Hydroxycarbamide	T45.1x1	T45.1x2	T45.1x3	T45.1x4	T45.1x5	T45.1x6
Hydroxychloroquine	T37.8x1	T37.8x2	T37.8x3	T37.8x4	T37.8x5	T37.8x6

Substance	Poisoning, Accidental (unintentional)	Poisoning, Intentional Self-harm	Poisoning, Assault	Poisoning, Undetermined	Adverse Effect	Under-dosing
Hydroxydihydrocodeinone	T40.2x1	T40.2x2	T40.2x3	T40.2x4	T40.2x5	T40.2x6
Hydroxyestrone	T38.5x1	T38.5x2	T38.5x3	T38.5x4	T38.5x5	T38.5x6
Hydroxyethyl starch	T45.8x1	T45.8x2	T45.8x3	T45.8x4	T45.8x5	T45.8x6
Hydroxymethylpentanone	T52.4x1	T52.4x2	T52.4x3	T52.4x4	—	—
Hydroxyphenamate	T43.591	T43.592	T43.593	T43.594	T43.595	T43.596
Hydroxyphenylbutazone	T39.2x1	T39.2x2	T39.2x3	T39.2x4	T39.2x5	T39.2x6
Hydroxyprogesterone	T38.5x1	T38.5x2	T38.5x3	T38.5x4	T38.5x5	T38.5x6
caproate	T38.5x1	T38.5x2	T38.5x3	T38.5x4	T38.5x5	T38.5x6
Hydroxyquinoline (derivatives) NEC	T37.8x1	T37.8x2	T37.8x3	T37.8x4	T37.8x5	T37.8x6
Hydroxystilbamidine	T37.3x1	T37.3x2	T37.3x3	T37.3x4	T37.3x5	T37.3x6
Hydroxytoluene (nonmedicinal)	T54.0x1	T54.0x2	T54.0x3	T54.0x4	—	—
medicinal	T49.0x1	T49.0x2	T49.0x3	T49.0x4	T49.0x5	T49.0x6
Hydroxyurea	T45.1x1	T45.1x2	T45.1x3	T45.1x4	T45.1x5	T45.1x6
Hydroxyzine	T43.591	T43.592	T43.593	T43.594	T43.595	T43.596
Hyoscine	T44.3x1	T44.3x2	T44.3x3	T44.3x4	T44.3x5	T44.3x6
Hyoscyamine	T44.3x1	T44.3x2	T44.3x3	T44.3x4	T44.3x5	T44.3x6
Hyoscyamus	T44.3x1	T44.3x2	T44.3x3	T44.3x4	T44.3x5	T44.3x6
dry extract	T44.3x1	T44.3x2	T44.3x3	T44.3x4	T44.3x5	T44.3x6
Hypaque	T50.8x1	T50.8x2	T50.8x3	T50.8x4	T50.8x5	T50.8x6
Hypertussis	T50.Z11	T50.Z12	T50.Z13	T50.Z14	T50.Z15	T50.Z16
Hypnotic	T42.71	T42.72	T42.73	T42.74	T42.75	T42.76
anticonvulsant	T42.71	T42.72	T42.73	T42.74	T42.75	T42.76
specified NEC	T42.6x1	T42.6x2	T42.6x3	T42.6x4	T42.6x5	T42.6x6
Hypochlorite	T49.0x1	T49.0x2	T49.0x3	T49.0x4	T49.0x5	T49.0x6
Hypophysis, posterior	T38.891	T38.892	T38.893	T38.894	T38.895	T38.896
Hypotensive NEC	T46.5x1	T46.5x2	T46.5x3	T46.5x4	T46.5x5	T46.5x6
Hypromellose	T49.5x1	T49.5x2	T49.5x3	T49.5x4	T49.5x5	T49.5x6
Ibacitabine	T37.5x1	T37.5x2	T37.5x3	T37.5x4	T37.5x5	T37.5x6
Ibopamine	T44.991	T44.992	T44.993	T44.994	T44.995	T44.996
Ibufenac	T39.311	T39.312	T39.313	T39.314	T39.315	T39.316
Ibuprofen	T39.311	T39.312	T39.313	T39.314	T39.315	T39.316
Ibuproxam	T39.311	T39.312	T39.313	T39.314	T39.315	T39.316
Ibuterol	T48.6x1	T48.6x2	T48.6x3	T48.6x4	T48.6x5	T48.6x6
Ichthammol	T49.0x1	T49.0x2	T49.0x3	T49.0x4	T49.0x5	T49.0x6
Ichthyol	T49.4x1	T49.4x2	T49.4x3	T49.4x4	T49.4x5	T49.4x6
Idarubicin	T45.1x1	T45.1x2	T45.1x3	T45.1x4	T45.1x5	T45.1x6
Idoxuridine	T37.5x1	T37.5x2	T37.5x3	T37.5x4	T37.5x5	T37.5x6
IDU	T49.5x1	T49.5x2	T49.5x3	T49.5x4	T49.5x5	T49.5x6
Idrocilamide	T42.8x1	T42.8x2	T42.8x3	T42.8x4	T42.8x5	T42.8x6
Ifenprodil	T46.7x1	T46.7x2	T46.7x3	T46.7x4	T46.7x5	T46.7x6
Ifosfamide	T45.1x1	T45.1x2	T45.1x3	T45.1x4	T45.1x5	T45.1x6
Iletin	T38.3x1	T38.3x2	T38.3x3	T38.3x4	T38.3x5	T38.3x6
Ilex	T62.2x1	T62.2x2	T62.2x3	T62.2x4	—	—
Illuminating gas (after combustion)	T58.11	T58.12	T58.13	T58.14		
prior to combustion	T59.891	T59.892	T59.893	T59.894	—	—
Ilopan	T45.2x1	T45.2x2	T45.2x3	T45.2x4	T45.2x5	T45.2x6
Iloprost	T46.7x1	T46.7x2	T46.7x3	T46.7x4	T46.7x5	T46.7x6
Ilotycin	T36.3x1	T36.3x2	T36.3x3	T36.3x4	T36.3x5	T36.3x6
ophthalmic preparation	T49.5x1	T49.5x2	T49.5x3	T49.5x4	T49.5x5	T49.5x6
topical NEC	T49.0x1	T49.0x2	T49.0x3	T49.0x4	T49.0x5	T49.0x6
Imidazole-4-carboxamide	T45.1x1	T45.1x2	T45.1x3	T45.1x4	T45.1x5	T45.1x6
Imipenem	T36.0x1	T36.0x2	T36.0x3	T36.0x4	T36.0x5	T36.0x6
Imipramine	T43.011	T43.012	T43.013	T43.014	T43.015	T43.016
Immu-G	T50.Z11	T50.Z12	T50.Z13	T50.Z14	T50.Z15	T50.Z16
Immuglobin	T50.Z11	T50.Z12	T50.Z13	T50.Z14	T50.Z15	T50.Z16
Immune						
globulin	T50.Z11	T50.Z12	T50.Z13	T50.Z14	T50.Z15	T50.Z16
serum globulin	T50.Z11	T50.Z12	T50.Z13	T50.Z14	T50.Z15	T50.Z16
Immunoglobin human (intravenous) (normal)	T50.Z11	T50.Z12	T50.Z13	T50.Z14	T50.Z15	T50.Z16
unmodified	T50.Z11	T50.Z12	T50.Z13	T50.Z14	T50.Z15	T50.Z16
Immunosuppressive drug	T45.1x1	T45.1x2	T45.1x3	T45.1x4	T45.1x5	T45.1x6
Immu-tetanus	T50.Z11	T50.Z12	T50.Z13	T50.Z14	T50.Z15	T50.Z16
Indalpine	T43.221	T43.222	T43.223	T43.224	T43.225	T43.226
Indanazoline	T48.5x1	T48.5x2	T48.5x3	T48.5x4	T48.5x5	T48.5x6
Indandione (derivatives)	T45.511	T45.512	T45.513	T45.514	T45.515	T45.516
Indapamide	T46.5x1	T46.5x2	T46.5x3	T46.5x4	T46.5x5	T46.5x6
Indendione (derivatives)	T45.511	T45.512	T45.513	T45.514	T45.515	T45.516
Indenolol	T44.7x1	T44.7x2	T44.7x3	T44.7x4	T44.7x5	T44.7x6

Substance	Poisoning, Accidental (unintentional)	Poisoning, Intentional Self-harm	Poisoning, Assault	Poisoning, Undetermined	Adverse Effect	Under-dosing
Inderal	T44.7x1	T44.7x2	T44.7x3	T44.7x4	T44.7x5	T44.7x6
Indian hemp	T40.7x1	T40.7x2	T40.7x3	T40.7x4	T40.7x5	T40.7x6
Indian						
hemp	T40.991	T40.992	T40.993	T40.994	T40.995	T40.996
tobacco	T62.2x1	T62.2x2	T62.2x3	T62.2x4	—	—
Indigo carmine	T50.8x1	T50.8x2	T50.8x3	T50.8x4	T50.8x5	T50.8x6
Indobufen	T45.521	T45.522	T45.523	T45.524	T45.525	T45.526
Indocin	T39.2x1	T39.2x2	T39.2x3	T39.2x4	T39.2x5	T39.2x6
Indocyanine green	T50.8x1	T50.8x2	T50.8x3	T50.8x4	T50.8x5	T50.8x6
Indometacin	T39.391	T39.392	T39.393	T39.394	T39.395	T39.396
Indomethacin	T39.391	T39.392	T39.393	T39.394	T39.395	T39.396
farnesil	T39.4x1	T39.4x2	T39.4x3	T39.4x4	T39.4x5	T39.4x6
Indoramin	T44.6x1	T44.6x2	T44.6x3	T44.6x4	T44.6x5	T44.6x6
Industrial						
alcohol	T51.91	T51.92	T51.93	T51.94	—	—
fumes	T59.891	T59.892	T59.893	T59.894	—	—
solvents (fumes) (vapors)	T52.91	T52.92	T52.93	T52.94	—	—
Influenza vaccine	T50.B91	T50.B92	T50.B93	T50.B94	T50.B95	T50.B96
Ingested substance NEC	T65.91	T65.92	T65.93	T65.94		
INH	T37.1x1	T37.1x2	T37.1x3	T37.1x4	T37.1x5	T37.1x6
Inhalation, gas (noxious)—*see* Gas						
Inhibitor						
fibrinolysis	T45.621	T45.622	T45.623	T45.624	T45.625	T45.626
monoamine oxidase NEC	T43.1x1	T43.1x2	T43.1x3	T43.1x4	T43.1x5	T43.1x6
hydrazine	T43.1x1	T43.1x2	T43.1x3	T43.1x4	T43.1x5	T43.1x6
postsynaptic	T43.8x1	T43.8x2	T43.8x3	T43.8x4	T43.8x5	T43.8x6
prothrombin synthesis	T45.511	T45.512	T45.513	T45.514	T45.515	T45.516
Ink	T65.891	T65.892	T65.893	T65.894		
Inosine pranobex	T37.5x1	T37.5x2	T37.5x3	T37.5x4	T37.5x5	T37.5x6
Inositol	T50.991	T50.992	T50.993	T50.994	T50.995	T50.996
nicotinate	T46.7x1	T46.7x2	T46.7x3	T46.7x4	T46.7x5	T46.7x6
Inproquone	T45.1x1	T45.1x2	T45.1x3	T45.1x4	T45.1x5	T45.1x6
Insect (sting), venomous	T63.481	T63.482	T63.483	T63.484	—	—
ant	T63.421	T63.422	T63.423	T63.424	—	—
bee	T63.441	T63.442	T63.443	T63.444	—	—
caterpillar	T63.431	T63.432	T63.433	T63.434	—	—
hornet	T63.451	T63.452	T63.453	T63.454	—	—
wasp	T63.461	T63.462	T63.463	T63.464	—	—
Insecticide NEC	T60.91	T60.92	T60.93	T60.94		
carbamate	T60.0x1	T60.0x2	T60.0x3	T60.0x4	—	—
chlorinated	T60.1x1	T60.1x2	T60.1x3	T60.1x4	—	—
mixed	T60.91	T60.92	T60.93	T60.94		
organochlorine	T60.1x1	T60.1x2	T60.1x3	T60.1x4	—	—
organophosphorus	T60.0x1	T60.0x2	T60.0x3	T60.0x4	—	—
Insular tissue extract	T38.3x1	T38.3x2	T38.3x3	T38.3x4	T38.3x5	T38.3x6
Insulin NEC	T38.3x1	T38.3x2	T38.3x3	T38.3x4	T38.3x5	T38.3x6
defalan	T38.3x1	T38.3x2	T38.3x3	T38.3x4	T38.3x5	T38.3x6
human	T38.3x1	T38.3x2	T38.3x3	T38.3x4	T38.3x5	T38.3x6
injection, soluble	T38.3x1	T38.3x2	T38.3x3	T38.3x4	T38.3x5	T38.3x6
biphasic	T38.3x1	T38.3x2	T38.3x3	T38.3x4	T38.3x5	T38.3x6
intermediate acting	T38.3x1	T38.3x2	T38.3x3	T38.3x4	T38.3x5	T38.3x6
protamine zinc	T38.3x1	T38.3x2	T38.3x3	T38.3x4	T38.3x5	T38.3x6
slow acting	T38.3x1	T38.3x2	T38.3x3	T38.3x4	T38.3x5	T38.3x6
zinc						
protamine injection	T38.3x1	T38.3x2	T38.3x3	T38.3x4	T38.3x5	T38.3x6
suspension (amorphous) (crystalline)	T38.3x1	T38.3x2	T38.3x3	T38.3x4	T38.3x5	T38.3x6
Insulin (amorphous) (globin) (isophane) (Lente) (NPH) (prolamine) (Semilente) (Ultralente) (zinc)	T38.3x1	T38.3x2	T38.3x3	T38.3x4	T38.3x5	T38.3x6
Interferon (alpha) (beta) (gamma)	T37.5x1	T37.5x2	T37.5x3	T37.5x4	T37.5x5	T37.5x6
Intestinal motility control drug	T47.6x1	T47.6x2	T47.6x3	T47.6x4	T47.6x5	T47.6x6
biological	T47.8x1	T47.8x2	T47.8x3	T47.8x4	T47.8x5	T47.8x6
Intranarcon	T41.1x1	T41.1x2	T41.1x3	T41.1x4	T41.1x5	T41.1x6
Intravenous						
amino acids	T50.991	T50.992	T50.993	T50.994	T50.995	T50.996
fat suspension	T50.991	T50.992	T50.993	T50.994	T50.995	T50.996
Inulin	T50.8x1	T50.8x2	T50.8x3	T50.8x4	T50.8x5	T50.8x6
Invert sugar	T50.3x1	T50.3x2	T50.3x3	T50.3x4	T50.3x5	T50.3x6

Substance	Poisoning, Accidental (unintentional)	Poisoning, Intentional Self-harm	Poisoning, Assault	Poisoning, Undetermined	Adverse Effect	Under-dosing
Inza—see Naproxen						
Iobenzamic acid	T50.8x1	T50.8x2	T50.8x3	T50.8x4	T50.8x5	T50.8x6
Iocarmic acid	T50.8x1	T50.8x2	T50.8x3	T50.8x4	T50.8x5	T50.8x6
Iocetamic acid	T50.8x1	T50.8x2	T50.8x3	T50.8x4	T50.8x5	T50.8x6
Iodamide	T50.8x1	T50.8x2	T50.8x3	T50.8x4	T50.8x5	T50.8x6
Iodide NEC (see also Iodine)	T49.0x1	T49.0x2	T49.0x3	T49.0x4	T49.0x5	T49.0x6
mercury (ointment)	T49.0x1	T49.0x2	T49.0x3	T49.0x4	T49.0x5	T49.0x6
methylate	T49.0x1	T49.0x2	T49.0x3	T49.0x4	T49.0x5	T49.0x6
potassium (expectorant) NEC	T48.4x1	T48.4x2	T48.4x3	T48.4x4	T48.4x5	T48.4x6
Iodinated						
contrast medium	T50.8x1	T50.8x2	T50.8x3	T50.8x4	T50.8x5	T50.8x6
glycerol	T48.4x1	T48.4x2	T48.4x3	T48.4x4	T48.4x5	T48.4x6
human serum albumin (131I)	T50.8x1	T50.8x2	T50.8x3	T50.8x4	T50.8x5	T50.8x6
Iodine (antiseptic, external) (tincture) NEC	T49.0x1	T49.0x2	T49.0x3	T49.0x4	T49.0x5	T49.0x6
solution	T49.0x1	T49.0x2	T49.0x3	T49.0x4	T49.0x5	T49.0x6
125 (see also Radiation sickness, and Exposure to radioactivce isotopes)	T50.8x1	T50.8x2	T50.8x3	T50.8x4	T50.8x5	T50.8x6
therapeutic	T50.991	T50.992	T50.993	T50.994	T50.995	T50.996
131 (see also Radiation sickness, and Exposure to radioactivce isotopes)	T50.8x1	T50.8x2	T50.8x3	T50.8x4	T50.8x5	T50.8x6
therapeutic	T38.2x1	T38.2x2	T38.2x3	T38.2x4	T38.2x5	T38.2x6
diagnostic	T50.8x1	T50.8x2	T50.8x3	T50.8x4	T50.8x5	T50.8x6
for thyroid conditions (antithyroid)	T38.2x1	T38.2x2	T38.2x3	T38.2x4	T38.2x5	T38.2x6
vapor	T59.891	T59.892	T59.893	T59.894	—	—
Iodinated glycerol	T48.4x1	T48.4x2	T48.4x3	T48.4x4	T48.4x5	T48.4x6
Iodipamide	T50.8x1	T50.8x2	T50.8x3	T50.8x4	T50.8x5	T50.8x6
Iodized (poppy seed) oil	T50.8x1	T50.8x2	T50.8x3	T50.8x4	T50.8x5	T50.8x6
Iodobismitol	T37.8x1	T37.8x2	T37.8x3	T37.8x4	T37.8x5	T37.8x6
Iodochlorhydroxyquin	T37.8x1	T37.8x2	T37.8x3	T37.8x4	T37.8x5	T37.8x6
topical	T49.0x1	T49.0x2	T49.0x3	T49.0x4	T49.0x5	T49.0x6
Iodochlorhydroxyquinoline	T37.8x1	T37.8x2	T37.8x3	T37.8x4	T37.8x5	T37.8x6
Iodocholesterol (131I)	T50.8x1	T50.8x2	T50.8x3	T50.8x4	T50.8x5	T50.8x6
Iodoform	T49.0x1	T49.0x2	T49.0x3	T49.0x4	T49.0x5	T49.0x6
Iodohippuric acid	T50.8x1	T50.8x2	T50.8x3	T50.8x4	T50.8x5	T50.8x6
Iodopanoic acid	T50.8x1	T50.8x2	T50.8x3	T50.8x4	T50.8x5	T50.8x6
Iodophthalein (sodium)	T50.8x1	T50.8x2	T50.8x3	T50.8x4	T50.8x5	T50.8x6
Iodopyracet	T50.8x1	T50.8x2	T50.8x3	T50.8x4	T50.8x5	T50.8x6
Iodoquinol	T37.8x1	T37.8x2	T37.8x3	T37.8x4	T37.8x5	T37.8x6
Iodoxamic acid	T50.8x1	T50.8x2	T50.8x3	T50.8x4	T50.8x5	T50.8x6
Iofendylate	T50.8x1	T50.8x2	T50.8x3	T50.8x4	T50.8x5	T50.8x6
Ioglycamic acid	T50.8x1	T50.8x2	T50.8x3	T50.8x4	T50.8x5	T50.8x6
Iohexol	T50.8x1	T50.8x2	T50.8x3	T50.8x4	T50.8x5	T50.8x6
Ion exchange resin						
anion	T47.8x1	T47.8x2	T47.8x3	T47.8x4	T47.8x5	T47.8x6
cation	T50.3x1	T50.3x2	T50.3x3	T50.3x4	T50.3x5	T50.3x6
cholestyramine	T46.6x1	T46.6x2	T46.6x3	T46.6x4	T46.6x5	T46.6x6
intestinal	T47.8x1	T47.8x2	T47.8x3	T47.8x4	T47.8x5	T47.8x6
Iopamidol	T50.8x1	T50.8x2	T50.8x3	T50.8x4	T50.8x5	T50.8x6
Iopanoic acid	T50.8x1	T50.8x2	T50.8x3	T50.8x4	T50.8x5	T50.8x6
Iophenoic acid	T50.8x1	T50.8x2	T50.8x3	T50.8x4	T50.8x5	T50.8x6
Iopodate, sodium	T50.8x1	T50.8x2	T50.8x3	T50.8x4	T50.8x5	T50.8x6
Iopodic acid	T50.8x1	T50.8x2	T50.8x3	T50.8x4	T50.8x5	T50.8x6
Iopromide	T50.8x1	T50.8x2	T50.8x3	T50.8x4	T50.8x5	T50.8x6
Iopydol	T50.8x1	T50.8x2	T50.8x3	T50.8x4	T50.8x5	T50.8x6
Iotalamic acid	T50.8x1	T50.8x2	T50.8x3	T50.8x4	T50.8x5	T50.8x6
Iothalamate	T50.8x1	T50.8x2	T50.8x3	T50.8x4	T50.8x5	T50.8x6
Iothiouracil	T38.2x1	T38.2x2	T38.2x3	T38.2x4	T38.2x5	T38.2x6
Iotrol	T50.8x1	T50.8x2	T50.8x3	T50.8x4	T50.8x5	T50.8x6
Iotrolan	T50.8x1	T50.8x2	T50.8x3	T50.8x4	T50.8x5	T50.8x6
Iotroxate	T50.8x1	T50.8x2	T50.8x3	T50.8x4	T50.8x5	T50.8x6
Iotroxic acid	T50.8x1	T50.8x2	T50.8x3	T50.8x4	T50.8x5	T50.8x6
Ioversol	T50.8x1	T50.8x2	T50.8x3	T50.8x4	T50.8x5	T50.8x6
Ioxaglate	T50.8x1	T50.8x2	T50.8x3	T50.8x4	T50.8x5	T50.8x6
Ioxaglic acid	T50.8x1	T50.8x2	T50.8x3	T50.8x4	T50.8x5	T50.8x6
Ioxitalamic acid	T50.8x1	T50.8x2	T50.8x3	T50.8x4	T50.8x5	T50.8x6
Ipecac	T47.7x1	T47.7x2	T47.7x3	T47.7x4	T47.7x5	T47.7x6
Ipecacuanha	T48.4x1	T48.4x2	T48.4x3	T48.4x4	T48.4x5	T48.4x6
Ipodate, calcium	T50.8x1	T50.8x2	T50.8x3	T50.8x4	T50.8x5	T50.8x6

Substance	Poisoning, Accidental (unintentional)	Poisoning, Intentional Self-harm	Poisoning, Assault	Poisoning, Undetermined	Adverse Effect	Under-dosing
Ipral	T42.3x1	T42.3x2	T42.3x3	T42.3x4	T42.3x5	T42.3x6
Ipratropium (bromide)	T48.6x1	T48.6x2	T48.6x3	T48.6x4	T48.6x5	T48.6x6
Ipriflavone	T46.3x1	T46.3x2	T46.3x3	T46.3x4	T46.3x5	T46.3x6
Iprindole	T43.011	T43.012	T43.013	T43.014	T43.015	T43.016
Iproclozide	T43.1x1	T43.1x2	T43.1x3	T43.1x4	T43.1x5	T43.1x6
Iprofenin	T50.8x1	T50.8x2	T50.8x3	T50.8x4	T50.8x5	T50.8x6
Iproheptine	T49.2x1	T49.2x2	T49.2x3	T49.2x4	T49.2x5	T49.2x6
Iproniazid	T43.1x1	T43.1x2	T43.1x3	T43.1x4	T43.1x5	T43.1x6
Iproplatin	T45.1x1	T45.1x2	T45.1x3	T45.1x4	T45.1x5	T45.1x6
Iproveratril	T46.1x1	T46.1x2	T46.1x3	T46.1x4	T46.1x5	T46.1x6
Iron (compounds) (medicinal) NEC	T45.4x1	T45.4x2	T45.4x3	T45.4x4	T45.4x5	T45.4x6
ammonium	T45.4x1	T45.4x2	T45.4x3	T45.4x4	T45.4x5	T45.4x6
dextran injection	T45.4x1	T45.4x2	T45.4x3	T45.4x4	T45.4x5	T45.4x6
nonmedicinal	T56.891	T56.892	T56.893	T56.894	—	—
salts	T45.4x1	T45.4x2	T45.4x3	T45.4x4	T45.4x5	T45.4x6
sorbitex	T45.4x1	T45.4x2	T45.4x3	T45.4x4	T45.4x5	T45.4x6
sorbitol citric acid complex	T45.4x1	T45.4x2	T45.4x3	T45.4x4	T45.4x5	T45.4x6
Irrigating fluid (vaginal)	T49.8x1	T49.8x2	T49.8x3	T49.8x4	T49.8x5	T49.8x6
eye	T49.5x1	T49.5x2	T49.5x3	T49.5x4	T49.5x5	T49.5x6
Isepamicin	T36.5x1	T36.5x2	T36.5x3	T36.5x4	T36.5x5	T36.5x6
Isoaminile (citrate)	T48.3x1	T48.3x2	T48.3x3	T48.3x4	T48.3x5	T48.3x6
Isoamyl nitrite	T46.3x1	T46.3x2	T46.3x3	T46.3x4	T46.3x5	T46.3x6
Isobenzan	T60.1x1	T60.1x2	T60.1x3	T60.1x4	—	—
Isobutyl acetate	T52.8x1	T52.8x2	T52.8x3	T52.8x4	—	—
Isocarboxazid	T43.1x1	T43.1x2	T43.1x3	T43.1x4	T43.1x5	T43.1x6
Isoconazole	T49.0x1	T49.0x2	T49.0x3	T49.0x4	T49.0x5	T49.0x6
Isocyanate	T65.0x1	T65.0x2	T65.0x3	T65.0x4	—	—
Isoephedrine	T44.991	T44.992	T44.993	T44.994	T44.995	T44.996
Isoetarine	T48.6x1	T48.6x2	T48.6x3	T48.6x4	T48.6x5	T48.6x6
Isoethadione	T42.2x1	T42.2x2	T42.2x3	T42.2x4	T42.2x5	T42.2x6
Isoetharine	T44.5x1	T44.5x2	T44.5x3	T44.5x4	T44.5x5	T44.5x6
Isoflurane	T41.0x1	T41.0x2	T41.0x3	T41.0x4	T41.0x5	T41.0x6
Isoflurophate	T44.0x1	T44.0x2	T44.0x3	T44.0x4	T44.0x5	T44.0x6
Isomaltose, ferric complex	T45.4x1	T45.4x2	T45.4x3	T45.4x4	T45.4x5	T45.4x6
Isometheptene	T44.3x1	T44.3x2	T44.3x3	T44.3x4	T44.3x5	T44.3x6
Isoniazid	T37.1x1	T37.1x2	T37.1x3	T37.1x4	T37.1x5	T37.1x6
with						
rifampicin	T36.6x1	T36.6x2	T36.6x3	T36.6x4	T36.6x5	T36.6x6
thioacetazone	T37.1x1	T37.1x2	T37.1x3	T37.1x4	T37.1x5	T37.1x6
Isonicotinic acid hydrazide	T37.1x1	T37.1x2	T37.1x3	T37.1x4	T37.1x5	T37.1x6
Isonipecaine	T40.4x1	T40.4x2	T40.4x3	T40.4x4	T40.4x5	T40.4x6
Isopentaquine	T37.2x1	T37.2x2	T37.2x3	T37.2x4	T37.2x5	T37.2x6
Isophane insulin	T38.3x1	T38.3x2	T38.3x3	T38.3x4	T38.3x5	T38.3x6
Isophorone	T65.891	T65.892	T65.893	T65.894	—	—
Isophosphamide	T45.1x1	T45.1x2	T45.1x3	T45.1x4	T45.1x5	T45.1x6
Isopregnenone	T38.5x1	T38.5x2	T38.5x3	T38.5x4	T38.5x5	T38.5x6
Isoprenaline	T48.6x1	T48.6x2	T48.6x3	T48.6x4	T48.6x5	T48.6x6
Isopromethazine	T43.3x1	T43.3x2	T43.3x3	T43.3x4	T43.3x5	T43.3x6
Isopropamide	T44.3x1	T44.3x2	T44.3x3	T44.3x4	T44.3x5	T44.3x6
iodide	T44.3x1	T44.3x2	T44.3x3	T44.3x4	T44.3x5	T44.3x6
Isopropanol	T51.2x1	T51.2x2	T51.2x3	T51.2x4	—	—
Isopropyl						
acetate	T52.8x1	T52.8x2	T52.8x3	T52.8x4	—	—
alcohol	T51.2x1	T51.2x2	T51.2x3	T51.2x4	—	—
medicinal	T49.4x1	T49.4x2	T49.4x3	T49.4x4	T49.4x5	T49.4x6
ether	T52.8x1	T52.8x2	T52.8x3	T52.8x4	—	—
Isopropylaminophenazone	T39.2x1	T39.2x2	T39.2x3	T39.2x4	T39.2x5	T39.2x6
Isoproterenol	T48.6x1	T48.6x2	T48.6x3	T48.6x4	T48.6x5	T48.6x6
Isosorbide dinitrate	T46.3x1	T46.3x2	T46.3x3	T46.3x4	T46.3x5	T46.3x6
Isothipendyl	T45.0x1	T45.0x2	T45.0x3	T45.0x4	T45.0x5	T45.0x6
Isotretinoin	T50.991	T50.992	T50.993	T50.994	T50.995	T50.996
Isoxazolyl penicillin	T36.0x1	T36.0x2	T36.0x3	T36.0x4	T36.0x5	T36.0x6
Isoxicam	T39.391	T39.392	T39.393	T39.394	T39.395	T39.396
Isoxsuprine	T46.7x1	T46.7x2	T46.7x3	T46.7x4	T46.7x5	T46.7x6
Ispagula	T47.4x1	T47.4x2	T47.4x3	T47.4x4	T47.4x5	T47.4x6
husk	T47.4x1	T47.4x2	T47.4x3	T47.4x4	T47.4x5	T47.4x6
Isradipine	T46.1x1	T46.1x2	T46.1x3	T46.1x4	T46.1x5	T46.1x6
I-thyroxine sodium	T38.1x1	T38.1x2	T38.1x3	T38.1x4	T38.1x5	T38.1x6
Itraconazole	T37.8x1	T37.8x2	T37.8x3	T37.8x4	T37.8x5	T37.8x6
Itramin tosilate	T46.3x1	T46.3x2	T46.3x3	T46.3x4	T46.3x5	T46.3x6
Ivermectin	T37.4x1	T37.4x2	T37.4x3	T37.4x4	T37.4x5	T37.4x6

Drug and Chemical Table

Izoniazid–Levocabastine (hydrochloride)

Substance	Poisoning, Accidental (unintentional)	Poisoning, Intentional Self-harm	Poisoning, Assault	Poisoning, Undetermined	Adverse Effect	Under-dosing
Izoniazid	T37.1x1	T37.1x2	T37.1x3	T37.1x4	T37.1x5	T37.1x6
with thioacetazone	T37.1x1	T37.1x2	T37.1x3	T37.1x4		T37.1x6
Jalap	T47.2x1	T47.2x2	T47.2x3	T47.2x4	T47.2x5	T47.2x6
Jamaica ginger	T62.2x1	T62.2x2	T62.2x3	T62.2x4	—	—
Jamaica						
dogwood (bark)	T39.8x1	T39.8x2	T39.8x3	T39.8x4	T39.8x5	T39.8x6
ginger	T65.891	T65.892	T65.893	T65.894	—	—
Jatropha	T62.2x1	T62.2x2	T62.2x3	T62.2x4	—	—
curcas	T62.2x1	T62.2x2	T62.2x3	T62.2x4	—	—
Jectofer	T45.4x1	T45.4x2	T45.4x3	T45.4x4	T45.4x5	T45.4x6
Jellyfish (sting)	T63.621	T63.622	T63.623	T63.624	—	—
Jequirity (bean)	T62.2x1	T62.2x2	T62.2x3	T62.2x4	—	—
Jimson weed (stramonium)	T62.2x1	T62.2x2	T62.2x3	T62.2x4	—	—
seeds	T62.2x1	T62.2x2	T62.2x3	T62.2x4	—	—
Josamycin	T36.3x1	T36.3x2	T36.3x3	T36.3x4	T36.3x5	T36.3x6
Juniper tar	T49.1x1	T49.1x2	T49.1x3	T49.1x4	T49.1x5	T49.1x6
Kallidinogenase	T46.7x1	T46.7x2	T46.7x3	T46.7x4	T46.7x5	T46.7x6
Kallikrein	T46.7x1	T46.7x2	T46.7x3	T46.7x4	T46.7x5	T46.7x6
Kanamycin	T36.5x1	T36.5x2	T36.5x3	T36.5x4	T36.5x5	T36.5x6
Kantrex	T36.5x1	T36.5x2	T36.5x3	T36.5x4	T36.5x5	T36.5x6
Kaolin	T47.6x1	T47.6x2	T47.6x3	T47.6x4	T47.6x5	T47.6x6
light	T47.6x1	T47.6x2	T47.6x3	T47.6x4	T47.6x5	T47.6x6
Karaya (gum)	T47.4x1	T47.4x2	T47.4x3	T47.4x4	T47.4x5	T47.4x6
Kebuzone	T39.2x1	T39.2x2	T39.2x3	T39.2x4	T39.2x5	T39.2x6
Kelevan	T60.1x1	T60.1x2	T60.1x3	T60.1x4	—	—
Kemithal	T41.1x1	T41.1x2	T41.1x3	T41.1x4	T41.1x5	T41.1x6
Kenacort	T38.0x1	T38.0x2	T38.0x3	T38.0x4	T38.0x5	T38.0x6
Keratolytic drug NEC	T49.4x1	T49.4x2	T49.4x3	T49.4x4	T49.4x5	T49.4x6
anthracene	T49.4x1	T49.4x2	T49.4x3	T49.4x4	T49.4x5	T49.4x6
Keratoplastic NEC	T49.4x1	T49.4x2	T49.4x3	T49.4x4	T49.4x5	T49.4x6
Kerosene, kerosine (fuel) (solvent) **NEC**	T52.0x1	T52.0x2	T52.0x3	T52.0x4	—	—
insecticide	T52.0x1	T52.0x2	T52.0x3	T52.0x4	—	—
vapor	T52.0x1	T52.0x2	T52.0x3	T52.0x4	—	—
Ketamine	T41.291	T41.292	T41.293	T41.294	T41.295	T41.296
Ketazolam	T42.4x1	T42.4x2	T42.4x3	T42.4x4	T42.4x5	T42.4x6
Ketazon	T39.2x1	T39.2x2	T39.2x3	T39.2x4	T39.2x5	T39.2x6
Ketobemidone	T40.4x1	T40.4x2	T40.4x3	T40.4x4	T40.4x5	T40.4x6
Ketoconazole	T49.0x1	T49.0x2	T49.0x3	T49.0x4	T49.0x5	T49.0x6
Ketols	T52.4x1	T52.4x2	T52.4x3	T52.4x4	—	—
Ketone oils	T52.4x1	T52.4x2	T52.4x3	T52.4x4	—	—
Ketoprofen	T39.311	T39.312	T39.313	T39.314	T39.315	T39.316
Ketorolac	T39.8x1	T39.8x2	T39.8x3	T39.8x4	T39.8x5	T39.8x6
Ketotifen	T45.0x1	T45.0x2	T45.0x3	T45.0x4	T45.0x5	T45.0x6
Khat	T43.691	T43.692	T43.693	T43.694	—	—
Khellin	T46.3x1	T46.3x2	T46.3x3	T46.3x4	T46.3x5	T46.3x6
Khelloside	T46.3x1	T46.3x2	T46.3x3	T46.3x4	T46.3x5	T46.3x6
Kiln gas or vapor (carbon monoxide)	T58.8x1	T58.8x2	T58.8x3	T58.8x4	—	—
Kitasamycin	T36.3x1	T36.3x2	T36.3x3	T36.3x4	T36.3x5	T36.3x6
Konsyl	T47.4x1	T47.4x2	T47.4x3	T47.4x4	T47.4x5	T47.4x6
Kosam seed	T62.2x1	T62.2x2	T62.2x3	T62.2x4	—	—
Krait (venom)	T63.091	T63.092	T63.093	T63.094	—	—
Kwell (insecticide)	T60.1x1	T60.1x2	T60.1x3	T60.1x4	—	—
anti-infective (topical)	T49.0x1	T49.0x2	T49.0x3	T49.0x4	T49.0x5	T49.0x6
Labetalol	T44.8x1	T44.8x2	T44.8x3	T44.8x4	T44.8x5	T44.8x6
Laburnum (seeds)	T62.2x1	T62.2x2	T62.2x3	T62.2x4	—	—
leaves	T62.2x1	T62.2x2	T62.2x3	T62.2x4	—	—
Lachesine	T49.5x1	T49.5x2	T49.5x3	T49.5x4	T49.5x5	T49.5x6
Lacidipine	T46.5x1	T46.5x2	T46.5x3	T46.5x4	T46.5x5	T46.5x6
Lacquer	T65.6x1	T65.6x2	T65.6x3	T65.6x4	—	—
Lacrimogenic gas	T59.3x1	T59.3x2	T59.3x3	T59.3x4	—	—
Lactated potassic saline	T50.3x1	T50.3x2	T50.3x3	T50.3x4	T50.3x5	T50.3x6
Lactic acid	T49.8x1	T49.8x2	T49.8x3	T49.8x4	T49.8x5	T49.8x6
Lactobacillus						
acidophilus	T47.6x1	T47.6x2	T47.6x3	T47.6x4	T47.6x5	T47.6x6
compound	T47.6x1	T47.6x2	T47.6x3	T47.6x4	T47.6x5	T47.6x6
bifidus, lyophilized	T47.6x1	T47.6x2	T47.6x3	T47.6x4	T47.6x5	T47.6x6
bulgaricus	T47.6x1	T47.6x2	T47.6x3	T47.6x4	T47.6x5	T47.6x6
sporogenes	T47.6x1	T47.6x2	T47.6x3	T47.6x4	T47.6x5	T47.6x6
Lactoflavin	T45.2x1	T45.2x2	T45.2x3	T45.2x4	T45.2x5	T45.2x6

Substance	Poisoning, Accidental (unintentional)	Poisoning, Intentional Self-harm	Poisoning, Assault	Poisoning, Undetermined	Adverse Effect	Under-dosing
Lactose (as excipient)	T50.901	T50.902	T50.903	T50.904	T50.905	T50.906
Lactuca (virosa) (extract)	T42.6x1	T42.6x2	T42.6x3	T42.6x4	T42.6x5	T42.6x6
Lactucarium	T42.6x1	T42.6x2	T42.6x3	T42.6x4	T42.6x5	T42.6x6
Lactulose	T47.3x1	T47.3x2	T47.3x3	T47.3x4	T47.3x5	T47.3x6
Laevo—*see* Levo						
Lanatosides	T46.0x1	T46.0x2	T46.0x3	T46.0x4	T46.0x5	T46.0x6
Lanolin	T49.3x1	T49.3x2	T49.3x3	T49.3x4	T49.3x5	T49.3x6
Largactil	T43.3x1	T43.3x2	T43.3x3	T43.3x4	T43.3x5	T43.3x6
Larkspur	T62.2x1	T62.2x2	T62.2x3	T62.2x4	—	—
Laroxyl	T43.011	T43.012	T43.013	T43.014	T43.015	T43.016
Lassar's paste	T49.4x1	T49.4x2	T49.4x3	T49.4x4	T49.4x5	T49.4x6
Lasix	T50.1x1	T50.1x2	T50.1x3	T50.1x4	T50.1x5	T50.1x6
Latamoxef	T36.1x1	T36.1x2	T36.1x3	T36.1x4	T36.1x5	T36.1x6
Latex	T65.811	T65.812	T65.813	T65.814	—	—
Lathyrus (seed)	T62.2x1	T62.2x2	T62.2x3	T62.2x4	—	—
Laudanum	T40.0x1	T40.0x2	T40.0x3	T40.0x4	T40.0x5	T40.0x6
Laudexium	T48.1x1	T48.1x2	T48.1x3	T48.1x4	T48.1x5	T48.1x6
Laughing gas	T41.0x1	T41.0x2	T41.0x3	T41.0x4	T41.0x5	T41.0x6
Laurel, black or cherry	T62.2x1	T62.2x2	T62.2x3	T62.2x4	—	—
Laurolinium	T49.0x1	T49.0x2	T49.0x3	T49.0x4	T49.0x5	T49.0x6
Lauryl sulfoacetate	T49.2x1	T49.2x2	T49.2x3	T49.2x4	T49.2x5	T49.2x6
Laxative NEC	T47.4x1	T47.4x2	T47.4x3	T47.4x4	T47.4x5	T47.4x6
L-dopa	T42.8x1	T42.8x2	T42.8x3	T42.8x4	T42.8x5	T42.8x6
Lead (dust) (fumes) (vapor) **NEC**	T56.0x1	T56.0x2	T56.0x3	T56.0x4		
acetate	T49.2x1	T49.2x2	T49.2x3	T49.2x4	T49.2x5	T49.2x6
alkyl (fuel additive)	T56.0x1	T56.0x2	T56.0x3	T56.0x4		
anti-infectives	T37.8x1	T37.8x2	T37.8x3	T37.8x4	T37.8x5	T37.8x6
antiknock compound (tetraethyl)	T56.0x1	T56.0x2	T56.0x3	T56.0x4		
arsenate, arsenite (dust)(herbicide) (insecticide) (vapor)	T57.0x1	T57.0x2	T57.0x3	T57.0x4		
carbonate	T56.0x1	T56.0x2	T56.0x3	T56.0x4	—	—
paint	T56.0x1	T56.0x2	T56.0x3	T56.0x4	—	—
chromate	T56.0x1	T56.0x2	T56.0x3	T56.0x4		
paint	T56.0x1	T56.0x2	T56.0x3	T56.0x4		
dioxide	T56.0x1	T56.0x2	T56.0x3	T56.0x4		
inorganic	T56.0x1	T56.0x2	T56.0x3	T56.0x4		
iodide	T56.0x1	T56.0x2	T56.0x3	T56.0x4		
pigment (paint)	T56.0x1	T56.0x2	T56.0x3	T56.0x4		
monoxide (dust)	T56.0x1	T56.0x2	T56.0x3	T56.0x4		
paint	T56.0x1	T56.0x2	T56.0x3	T56.0x4		
organic	T56.0x1	T56.0x2	T56.0x3	T56.0x4		
oxide	T56.0x1	T56.0x2	T56.0x3	T56.0x4		
paint	T56.0x1	T56.0x2	T56.0x3	T56.0x4		
paint	T56.0x1	T56.0x2	T56.0x3	T56.0x4		
salts	T56.0x1	T56.0x2	T56.0x3	T56.0x4		
specified compound NEC	T56.0x1	T56.0x2	T56.0x3	T56.0x4		
tetra-ethyl	T56.0x1	T56.0x2	T56.0x3	T56.0x4		
Lebanese red	T40.991	T40.992	T40.993	T40.994	T40.995	T40.996
Lefetamine	T39.8x1	T39.8x2	T39.8x3	T39.8x4	T39.8x5	T39.8x6
Lenperone	T43.4x1	T43.4x2	T43.4x3	T43.4x4	T43.4x5	T43.4x6
Lente lietin (insulin)	T38.3x1	T38.3x2	T38.3x3	T38.3x4	T38.3x5	T38.3x6
Leptazol	T50.7x1	T50.7x2	T50.7x3	T50.7x4	T50.7x5	T50.7x6
Leptophos	T60.0x1	T60.0x2	T60.0x3	T60.0x4	—	—
Leritine	T40.2x1	T40.2x2	T40.2x3	T40.2x4	T40.2x5	T40.2x6
Letosteine	T48.4x1	T48.4x2	T48.4x3	T48.4x4	T48.4x5	T48.4x6
Letter	T38.1x1	T38.1x2	T38.1x3	T38.1x4	T38.1x5	T38.1x6
Lettuce opium	T42.6x1	T42.6x2	T42.6x3	T42.6x4	T42.6x5	T42.6x6
Leucinocaine	T41.3x1	T41.3x2	T41.3x3	T41.3x4	T41.3x5	T41.3x6
Leucocianidol	T46.991	T46.992	T46.993	T46.994	T46.995	T46.996
Leucovorin (factor)	T45.8x1	T45.8x2	T45.8x3	T45.8x4	T45.8x5	T45.8x6
Leukeran	T45.1x1	T45.1x2	T45.1x3	T45.1x4	T45.1x5	T45.1x6
Leuprolide	T38.891	T38.892	T38.893	T38.894	T38.895	T38.896
Levalbuterol	T48.6x1	T48.6x2	T48.6x3	T48.6x4	T48.6x5	T48.6x6
Levallorphan	T50.7x1	T50.7x2	T50.7x3	T50.7x4	T50.7x5	T50.7x6
Levamisole	T37.4x1	T37.4x2	T37.4x3	T37.4x4	T37.4x5	T37.4x6
Levanil	T42.6x1	T42.6x2	T42.6x3	T42.6x4	T42.6x5	T42.6x6
Levarterenol	T44.4x1	T44.4x2	T44.4x3	T44.4x4	T44.4x5	T44.4x6
Levdropropizine	T48.3x1	T48.3x2	T48.3x3	T48.3x4	T48.3x5	T48.3x6
Levobunolol	T49.5x1	T49.5x2	T49.5x3	T49.5x4	T49.5x5	T49.5x6
Levocabastine (hydrochloride)	T45.0x1	T45.0x2	T45.0x3	T45.0x4	T45.0x5	T45.0x6

Substance	Poisoning, Accidental (unintentional)	Poisoning, Intentional Self-harm	Poisoning, Assault	Poisoning, Undetermined	Adverse Effect	Under-dosing
Levocarnitine	T50.991	T50.992	T50.993	T50.994	T50.995	T50.996
Levodopa	T42.8x1	T42.8x2	T42.8x3	T42.8x4	T42.8x5	T42.8x6
with carbidopa	T42.8x1	T42.8x2	T42.8x3	T42.8x4	T42.8x5	T42.8x6
Levo-dromoran	T40.2x1	T40.2x2	T40.2x3	T40.2x4	T40.2x5	T40.2x6
Levoglutamide	T50.991	T50.992	T50.993	T50.994	T50.995	T50.996
Levoid	T38.1x1	T38.1x2	T38.1x3	T38.1x4	T38.1x5	T38.1x6
Levo-iso-methadone	T40.3x1	T40.3x2	T40.3x3	T40.3x4	T40.3x5	T40.3x6
Levomepromazine	T43.3x1	T43.3x2	T43.3x3	T43.3x4	T43.3x5	T43.3x6
Levonordefrin	T49.6x1	T49.6x2	T49.6x3	T49.6x4	T49.6x5	T49.6x6
Levonorgestrel	T38.4x1	T38.4x2	T38.4x3	T38.4x4	T38.4x5	T38.4x6
with ethinylestradiol	T38.5x1	T38.5x2	T38.5x3	T38.5x4	T38.5x5	T38.5x6
Levopromazine	T43.3x1	T43.3x2	T43.3x3	T43.3x4	T43.3x5	T43.3x6
Levoprome	T42.6x1	T42.6x2	T42.6x3	T42.6x4	T42.6x5	T42.6x6
Levopropoxyphene	T40.4x1	T40.4x2	T40.4x3	T40.4x4	T40.4x5	T40.4x6
Levopropylhexedrine	T50.5x1	T50.5x2	T50.5x3	T50.5x4	T50.5x5	T50.5x6
Levoproxyphylline	T48.6x1	T48.6x2	T48.6x3	T48.6x4	T48.6x5	T48.6x6
Levorphanol	T40.4x1	T40.4x2	T40.4x3	T40.4x4	T40.4x5	T40.4x6
Levothyroxine	T38.1x1	T38.1x2	T38.1x3	T38.1x4	T38.1x5	T38.1x6
sodium	T38.1x1	T38.1x2	T38.1x3	T38.1x4	T38.1x5	T38.1x6
Levsin	T44.3x1	T44.3x2	T44.3x3	T44.3x4	T44.3x5	T44.3x6
Levulose	T50.3x1	T50.3x2	T50.3x3	T50.3x4	T50.3x5	T50.3x6
Lewisite (gas), not in war	T57.0x1	T57.0x2	T57.0x3	T57.0x4	—	—
Librium	T42.4x1	T42.4x2	T42.4x3	T42.4x4	T42.4x5	T42.4x6
Lidex	T49.0x1	T49.0x2	T49.0x3	T49.0x4	T49.0x5	T49.0x6
Lidocaine	T41.3x1	T41.3x2	T41.3x3	T41.3x4	T41.3x5	T41.3x6
regional	T41.3x1	T41.3x2	T41.3x3	T41.3x4	T41.3x5	T41.3x6
spinal	T41.3x1	T41.3x2	T41.3x3	T41.3x4	T41.3x5	T41.3x6
Lidofenin	T50.8x1	T50.8x2	T50.8x3	T50.8x4	T50.8x5	T50.8x6
Lidoflazine	T46.1x1	T46.1x2	T46.1x3	T46.1x4	T46.1x5	T46.1x6
Lighter fluid	T52.0x1	T52.0x2	T52.0x3	T52.0x4	—	—
Lignin hemicellulose	T47.6x1	T47.6x2	T47.6x3	T47.6x4	T47.6x5	T47.6x6
Lignocaine	T41.3x1	T41.3x2	T41.3x3	T41.3x4	T41.3x5	T41.3x6
regional	T41.3x1	T41.3x2	T41.3x3	T41.3x4	T41.3x5	T41.3x6
spinal	T41.3x1	T41.3x2	T41.3x3	T41.3x4	T41.3x5	T41.3x6
Ligroin(e) (solvent)	T52.0x1	T52.0x2	T52.0x3	T52.0x4	—	—
vapor	T59.891	T59.892	T59.893	T59.894	—	—
Ligustrum vulgare	T62.2x1	T62.2x2	T62.2x3	T62.2x4	—	—
Lily of the valley	T62.2x1	T62.2x2	T62.2x3	T62.2x4	—	—
Lime (chloride)	T54.3x1	T54.3x2	T54.3x3	T54.3x4	—	—
Limonene	T52.8x1	T52.8x2	T52.8x3	T52.8x4	—	—
Lincomycin	T36.8x1	T36.8x2	T36.8x3	T36.8x4	T36.8x5	T36.8x6
Lindane (insecticide) (nonmedicinal) (vapor)	T53.6x1	T53.6x2	T53.6x3	T53.6x4	—	—
medicinal	T49.0x1	T49.0x2	T49.0x3	T49.0x4	T49.0x5	T49.0x6
Liniments NEC	T49.91	T49.92	T49.93	T49.94	T49.95	T49.96
Linoleic acid	T46.6x1	T46.6x2	T46.6x3	T46.6x4	T46.6x5	T46.6x6
Linolenic acid	T46.6x1	T46.6x2	T46.6x3	T46.6x4	T46.6x5	T46.6x6
Linseed	T47.4x1	T47.4x2	T47.4x3	T47.4x4	T47.4x5	T47.4x6
Liothyronine	T38.1x1	T38.1x2	T38.1x3	T38.1x4	T38.1x5	T38.1x6
Liotrix	T38.1x1	T38.1x2	T38.1x3	T38.1x4	T38.1x5	T38.1x6
Lipancreatin	T47.5x1	T47.5x2	T47.5x3	T47.5x4	T47.5x5	T47.5x6
Lipo-alprostadil	T46.7x1	T46.7x2	T46.7x3	T46.7x4	T46.7x5	T46.7x6
Lipo-Lutin	T38.5x1	T38.5x2	T38.5x3	T38.5x4	T38.5x5	T38.5x6
Lipotropic drug NEC	T50.901	T50.902	T50.903	T50.904	T50.905	T50.906
Liquefied petroleum gases	T59.891	T59.892	T59.893	T59.894	—	—
piped (pure or mixed with air)	T59.891	T59.892	T59.893	T59.894	—	—
Liquid						
paraffin	T47.4x1	T47.4x2	T47.4x3	T47.4x4	T47.4x5	T47.4x6
substance NEC	T65.91	T65.92	T65.93	T65.94	—	—
Liquid petrolatum	T47.4x1	T47.4x2	T47.4x3	T47.4x4	T47.4x5	T47.4x6
substance	T65.91	T65.92	T65.93	T65.94	—	—
specified NEC	T65.891	T65.892	T65.893	T65.894	—	—
Liquor creosolis compositus	T65.891	T65.892	T65.893	T65.894	—	—
Liquorice	T48.4x1	T48.4x2	T48.4x3	T48.4x4	T48.4x5	T48.4x6
extract	T47.8x1	T47.8x2	T47.8x3	T47.8x4	T47.8x5	T47.8x6
Lisinopril	T46.4x1	T46.4x2	T46.4x3	T46.4x4	T46.4x5	T46.4x6
Lisuride	T42.8x1	T42.8x2	T42.8x3	T42.8x4	T42.8x5	T42.8x6
Lithane	T43.8x1	T43.8x2	T43.8x3	T43.8x4	T43.8x5	T43.8x6
Lithium	T56.891	T56.892	T56.893	T56.894	—	—
gluconate	T43.591	T43.592	T43.593	T43.594	T43.595	T43.596
salts (carbonate)	T43.591	T43.592	T43.593	T43.594	T43.595	T43.596
Lithonate	T43.8x1	T43.8x2	T43.8x3	T43.8x4	T43.8x5	T43.8x6
Liver						
extract	T45.8x1	T45.8x2	T45.8x3	T45.8x4	T45.8x5	T45.8x6
for parenteral use	T45.8x1	T45.8x2	T45.8x3	T45.8x4	T45.8x5	T45.8x6
fraction 1	T45.8x1	T45.8x2	T45.8x3	T45.8x4	T45.8x5	T45.8x6
hydrolysate	T45.8x1	T45.8x2	T45.8x3	T45.8x4	T45.8x5	T45.8x6
Lizard (bite) (venom)	T63.121	T63.122	T63.123	T63.124	—	—
LMD	T45.8x1	T45.8x2	T45.8x3	T45.8x4	T45.8x5	T45.8x6
Lobelia	T62.2x1	T62.2x2	T62.2x3	T62.2x4	—	—
Lobeline	T50.7x1	T50.7x2	T50.7x3	T50.7x4	T50.7x5	T50.7x6
Local action drug NEC	T49.8x1	T49.8x2	T49.8x3	T49.8x4	T49.8x5	T49.8x6
Locorten	T49.0x1	T49.0x2	T49.0x3	T49.0x4	T49.0x5	T49.0x6
Lofepramine	T43.011	T43.012	T43.013	T43.014	T43.015	T43.016
Lolium temulentum	T62.2x1	T62.2x2	T62.2x3	T62.2x4	—	—
Lomotil	T47.6x1	T47.6x2	T47.6x3	T47.6x4	T47.6x5	T47.6x6
Lomustine	T45.1x1	T45.1x2	T45.1x3	T45.1x4	T45.1x5	T45.1x6
Lonidamine	T45.1x1	T45.1x2	T45.1x3	T45.1x4	T45.1x5	T45.1x6
Loperamide	T47.6x1	T47.6x2	T47.6x3	T47.6x4	T47.6x5	T47.6x6
Loprazolam	T42.4x1	T42.4x2	T42.4x3	T42.4x4	T42.4x5	T42.4x6
Lorajmine	T46.2x1	T46.2x2	T46.2x3	T46.2x4	T46.2x5	T46.2x6
Loratidine	T45.0x1	T45.0x2	T45.0x3	T45.0x4	T45.0x5	T45.0x6
Lorazepam	T42.4x1	T42.4x2	T42.4x3	T42.4x4	T42.4x5	T42.4x6
Lorcainide	T46.2x1	T46.2x2	T46.2x3	T46.2x4	T46.2x5	T46.2x6
Lormetazepam	T42.4x1	T42.4x2	T42.4x3	T42.4x4	T42.4x5	T42.4x6
Lotions NEC	T49.91	T49.92	T49.93	T49.94	T49.95	T49.96
Lotusate	T42.3x1	T42.3x2	T42.3x3	T42.3x4	T42.3x5	T42.3x6
Lovastatin	T46.6x1	T46.6x2	T46.6x3	T46.6x4	T46.6x5	T46.6x6
Loxapine	T43.591	T43.592	T43.593	T43.594	T43.595	T43.596
Lowila	T49.2x1	T49.2x2	T49.2x3	T49.2x4	T49.2x5	T49.2x6
Lozenges (throat)	T49.6x1	T49.6x2	T49.6x3	T49.6x4	T49.6x5	T49.6x6
LSD	T40.8x1	T40.8x2	T40.8x3	T40.8x4	T40.8x5	T40.8x6
L-tryptophan—see amino acid						
Lubricant, eye	T49.5x1	T49.5x2	T49.5x3	T49.5x4	T49.5x5	T49.5x6
Lubricating oil NEC	T52.0x1	T52.0x2	T52.0x3	T52.0x4	—	—
Lucanthone	T37.4x1	T37.4x2	T37.4x3	T37.4x4	T37.4x5	T37.4x6
Luminal	T42.3x1	T42.3x2	T42.3x3	T42.3x4	T42.3x5	T42.3x6
Lung irritant (gas) NEC	T59.91	T59.92	T59.93	T59.94	—	—
Luteinizing hormone	T38.811	T38.812	T38.813	T38.814	T38.815	T38.816
Lutocylol	T38.5x1	T38.5x2	T38.5x3	T38.5x4	T38.5x5	T38.5x6
Lutromone	T38.5x1	T38.5x2	T38.5x3	T38.5x4	T38.5x5	T38.5x6
Lututrin	T48.291	T48.292	T48.293	T48.294	T48.295	T48.296
Lye (concentrated)	T54.3x1	T54.3x2	T54.3x3	T54.3x4	—	—
Lygranum (skin test)	T50.8x1	T50.8x2	T50.8x3	T50.8x4	T50.8x5	T50.8x6
Lymecycline	T36.4x1	T36.4x2	T36.4x3	T36.4x4	T36.4x5	T36.4x6
Lymphogranuloma venereum antigen	T50.8x1	T50.8x2	T50.8x3	T50.8x4	T50.8x5	T50.8x6
Lynestrenol	T38.4x1	T38.4x2	T38.4x3	T38.4x4	T38.4x5	T38.4x6
Lypressin	T38.891	T38.892	T38.893	T38.894	T38.895	T38.896
Lyovac sodium edecrin	T50.1x1	T50.1x2	T50.1x3	T50.1x4	T50.1x5	T50.1x6
Lysergic acid diethylamide	T40.8x1	T40.8x2	T40.8x3	T40.8x4	T40.8x5	T40.8x6
Lysergide	T40.8x1	T40.8x2	T40.8x3	T40.8x4	T40.8x5	T40.8x6
Lysine vasopressin	T38.891	T38.892	T38.893	T38.894	T38.895	T38.896
Lysol	T54.1x1	T54.1x2	T54.1x3	T54.1x4	—	—
Lysozyme	T49.0x1	T49.0x2	T49.0x3	T49.0x4	T49.0x5	T49.0x6
Lytta (vitatta)	T49.8x1	T49.8x2	T49.8x3	T49.8x4	T49.8x5	T49.8x6
Mace	T59.3x1	T59.3x2	T59.3x3	T59.3x4	—	—
Macrogol	T50.991	T50.992	T50.993	T50.994	T50.995	T50.996
Macrolide						
anabolic drug	T38.7x1	T38.7x2	T38.7x3	T38.7x4	T38.7x5	T38.7x6
antibiotic	T36.3x1	T36.3x2	T36.3x3	T36.3x4	T36.3x5	T36.3x6
Mafenide	T49.0x1	T49.0x2	T49.0x3	T49.0x4	T49.0x5	T49.0x6
Magaldrate	T47.1x1	T47.1x2	T47.1x3	T47.1x4	T47.1x5	T47.1x6
Magic mushroom	T40.991	T40.992	T40.993	T40.994	T40.995	T40.996
Magnamycin	T36.8x1	T36.8x2	T36.8x3	T36.8x4	T36.8x5	T36.8x6
Magnesia magma	T47.1x1	T47.1x2	T47.1x3	T47.1x4	T47.1x5	T47.1x6
Magnesium NEC	T56.891	T56.892	T56.893	T56.894	—	—
carbonate	T47.1x1	T47.1x2	T47.1x3	T47.1x4	T47.1x5	T47.1x6
citrate	T47.4x1	T47.4x2	T47.4x3	T47.4x4	T47.4x5	T47.4x6
hydroxide	T47.1x1	T47.1x2	T47.1x3	T47.1x4	T47.1x5	T47.1x6
oxide	T47.1x1	T47.1x2	T47.1x3	T47.1x4	T47.1x5	T47.1x6
peroxide	T49.0x1	T49.0x2	T49.0x3	T49.0x4	T49.0x5	T49.0x6

Substance	Poisoning, Accidental (unintentional)	Poisoning, Intentional Self-harm	Poisoning, Assault	Poisoning, Undetermined	Adverse Effect	Under-dosing
Magnesium NEC—*continued*						
salicylate	T39.091	T39.092	T39.093	T39.094	T39.095	T39.096
silicofluoride	T50.3x1	T50.3x2	T50.3x3	T50.3x4	T50.3x5	T50.3x6
sulfate	T47.4x1	T47.4x2	T47.4x3	T47.4x4	T47.4x5	T47.4x6
thiosulfate	T45.0x1	T45.0x2	T45.0x3	T45.0x4	T45.0x5	T45.0x6
trisilicate	T47.1x1	T47.1x2	T47.1x3	T47.1x4	T47.1x5	T47.1x6
Malathion (medicinal)	T49.0x1	T49.0x2	T49.0x3	T49.0x4	T49.0x5	T49.0x6
insecticide	T60.0x1	T60.0x2	T60.0x3	T60.0x4	—	—
Male fern extract	T37.4x1	T37.4x2	T37.4x3	T37.4x4	T37.4x5	T37.4x6
M-AMSA	T45.1x1	T45.1x2	T45.1x3	T45.1x4	T45.1x5	T45.1x6
Mandelic acid	T37.8x1	T37.8x2	T37.8x3	T37.8x4	T37.8x5	T37.8x6
Manganese (dioxide) (salts)	T57.2x1	T57.2x2	T57.2x3	T57.2x4	—	—
medicinal	T50.991	T50.992	T50.993	T50.994	T50.995	T50.996
Mannitol	T47.3x1	T47.3x2	T47.3x3	T47.3x4	T47.3x5	T47.3x6
hexanitrate	T46.3x1	T46.3x2	T46.3x3	T46.3x4	T46.3x5	T46.3x6
Mannomustine	T45.1x1	T45.1x2	T45.1x3	T45.1x4	T45.1x5	T45.1x6
MAO inhibitors	T43.1x1	T43.1x2	T43.1x3	T43.1x4	T43.1x5	T43.1x6
Mapharsen	T37.8x1	T37.8x2	T37.8x3	T37.8x4	T37.8x5	T37.8x6
Maphenide	T49.0x1	T49.0x2	T49.0x3	T49.0x4	T49.0x5	T49.0x6
Maprotiline	T43.021	T43.022	T43.023	T43.024	T43.025	T43.026
Marcaine	T41.3x1	T41.3x2	T41.3x3	T41.3x4	T41.3x5	T41.3x6
infiltration (subcutaneous)	T41.3x1	T41.3x2	T41.3x3	T41.3x4	T41.3x5	T41.3x6
nerve block (peripheral) (plexus)	T41.3x1	T41.3x2	T41.3x3	T41.3x4	T41.3x5	T41.3x6
Marezine	T45.0x1	T45.0x2	T45.0x3	T45.0x4	T45.0x5	T45.0x6
Marihuana	T40.7x1	T40.7x2	T40.7x3	T40.7x4	T40.7x5	T40.7x6
Marijuana	T40.7x1	T40.7x2	T40.7x3	T40.7x4	T40.7x5	T40.7x6
Marine (sting)	T63.691	T63.692	T63.693	T63.694	—	—
animals (sting)	T63.691	T63.692	T63.693	T63.694	—	—
plants (sting)	T63.711	T63.712	T63.713	T63.714	—	—
Marplan	T43.1x1	T43.1x2	T43.1x3	T43.1x4	T43.1x5	T43.1x6
Marsh gas	T59.891	T59.892	T59.893	T59.894	—	—
Marsilid	T43.1x1	T43.1x2	T43.1x3	T43.1x4	T43.1x5	T43.1x6
Matulane	T45.1x1	T45.1x2	T45.1x3	T45.1x4	T45.1x5	T45.1x6
Mazindol	T50.5x1	T50.5x2	T50.5x3	T50.5x4	T50.5x5	T50.5x6
MCPA	T60.3x1	T60.3x2	T60.3x3	T60.3x4	—	—
MDMA	T43.621	T43.622	T43.623	T43.624	T43.625	T43.626
Meadow saffron	T62.2x1	T62.2x2	T62.2x3	T62.2x4	—	—
Measles virus vaccine (attenuated)	T50.B91	T50.B92	T50.B93	T50.B94	T50.B95	T50.B96
Meat, noxious	T62.8x1	T62.8x2	T62.8x3	T62.8x4	—	—
Meballymal	T42.3x1	T42.3x2	T42.3x3	T42.3x4	T42.3x5	T42.3x6
Mebanazine	T43.1x1	T43.1x2	T43.1x3	T43.1x4	T43.1x5	T43.1x6
Mebaral	T42.3x1	T42.3x2	T42.3x3	T42.3x4	T42.3x5	T42.3x6
Mebendazole	T37.4x1	T37.4x2	T37.4x3	T37.4x4	T37.4x5	T37.4x6
Mebeverine	T44.3x1	T44.3x2	T44.3x3	T44.3x4	T44.3x5	T44.3x6
Mebhydrolin	T45.0x1	T45.0x2	T45.0x3	T45.0x4	T45.0x5	T45.0x6
Mebumal	T42.3x1	T42.3x2	T42.3x3	T42.3x4	T42.3x5	T42.3x6
Mebutamate	T43.591	T43.592	T43.593	T43.594	T43.595	T43.596
Mecamylamine	T44.2x1	T44.2x2	T44.2x3	T44.2x4	T44.2x5	T44.2x6
Mechlorethamine	T45.1x1	T45.1x2	T45.1x3	T45.1x4	T45.1x5	T45.1x6
Mecillinam	T36.0x1	T36.0x2	T36.0x3	T36.0x4	T36.0x5	T36.0x6
Meclizine (hydrochloride)	T45.0x1	T45.0x2	T45.0x3	T45.0x4	T45.0x5	T45.0x6
Meclocycline	T36.4x1	T36.4x2	T36.4x3	T36.4x4	T36.4x5	T36.4x6
Meclofenamate	T39.391	T39.392	T39.393	T39.394	T39.395	T39.396
Meclofenamic acid	T39.391	T39.392	T39.393	T39.394	T39.395	T39.396
Meclofenoxate	T43.691	T43.692	T43.693	T43.694	T43.695	T43.696
Meclozine	T45.0x1	T45.0x2	T45.0x3	T45.0x4	T45.0x5	T45.0x6
Mecobalamin	T45.8x1	T45.8x2	T45.8x3	T45.8x4	T45.8x5	T45.8x6
Mecoprop	T60.3x1	T60.3x2	T60.3x3	T60.3x4	—	—
Mecrilate	T49.3x1	T49.3x2	T49.3x3	T49.3x4	T49.3x5	T49.3x6
Mecysteine	T48.4x1	T48.4x2	T48.4x3	T48.4x4	T48.4x5	T48.4x6
Medazepam	T42.4x1	T42.4x2	T42.4x3	T42.4x4	T42.4x5	T42.4x6
Medicament NEC	T50.901	T50.902	T50.903	T50.904	T50.905	T50.906
Medinal	T42.3x1	T42.3x2	T42.3x3	T42.3x4	T42.3x5	T42.3x6
Medomin	T42.3x1	T42.3x2	T42.3x3	T42.3x4	T42.3x5	T42.3x6
Medrogestone	T38.5x1	T38.5x2	T38.5x3	T38.5x4	T38.5x5	T38.5x6
Medroxalol	T44.8x1	T44.8x2	T44.8x3	T44.8x4	T44.8x5	T44.8x6
Medroxyprogesterone acetate (depot)	T38.5x1	T38.5x2	T38.5x3	T38.5x4	T38.5x5	T38.5x6
Medrysone	T49.0x1	T49.0x2	T49.0x3	T49.0x4	T49.0x5	T49.0x6
Mefenamic acid	T39.391	T39.392	T39.393	T39.394	T39.395	T39.396

Substance	Poisoning, Accidental (unintentional)	Poisoning, Intentional Self-harm	Poisoning, Assault	Poisoning, Undetermined	Adverse Effect	Under-dosing
Mefenorex	T50.5x1	T50.5x2	T50.5x3	T50.5x4	T50.5x5	T50.5x6
Mefloquine	T37.2x1	T37.2x2	T37.2x3	T37.2x4	T37.2x5	T37.2x6
Mefruside	T50.2x1	T50.2x2	T50.2x3	T50.2x4	T50.2x5	T50.2x6
Megahallucinogen	T40.901	T40.902	T40.903	T40.904	T40.905	T40.906
Megestrol	T38.5x1	T38.5x2	T38.5x3	T38.5x4	T38.5x5	T38.5x6
Meglumine						
antimoniate	T37.8x1	T37.8x2	T37.8x3	T37.8x4	T37.8x5	T37.8x6
diatrizoate	T50.8x1	T50.8x2	T50.8x3	T50.8x4	T50.8x5	T50.8x6
iodipamide	T50.8x1	T50.8x2	T50.8x3	T50.8x4	T50.8x5	T50.8x6
iotroxate	T50.8x1	T50.8x2	T50.8x3	T50.8x4	T50.8x5	T50.8x6
MEK (methyl ethyl ketone)	T52.4x1	T52.4x2	T52.4x3	T52.4x4	—	—
Meladrazine	T44.3x1	T44.3x2	T44.3x3	T44.3x4	T44.3x5	T44.3x6
Meladinin	T49.3x1	T49.3x2	T49.3x3	T49.3x4	T49.3x5	T49.3x6
Melaleuca alternifolia oil	T49.0x1	T49.0x2	T49.0x3	T49.0x4	T49.0x5	T49.0x6
Melanizing agents	T49.3x1	T49.3x2	T49.3x3	T49.3x4	T49.3x5	T49.3x6
Melanocyte-stimulating hormone	T38.891	T38.892	T38.893	T38.894	T38.895	T38.896
Melarsonyl potassium	T37.3x1	T37.3x2	T37.3x3	T37.3x4	T37.3x5	T37.3x6
Melarsoprol	T37.3x1	T37.3x2	T37.3x3	T37.3x4	T37.3x5	T37.3x6
Melia azedarach	T62.2x1	T62.2x2	T62.2x3	T62.2x4	—	—
Melitracen	T43.011	T43.012	T43.013	T43.014	T43.015	T43.016
Mellaril	T43.3x1	T43.3x2	T43.3x3	T43.3x4	T43.3x5	T43.3x6
Meloxine	T49.3x1	T49.3x2	T49.3x3	T49.3x4	T49.3x5	T49.3x6
Melperone	T43.4x1	T43.4x2	T43.4x3	T43.4x4	T43.4x5	T43.4x6
Melphalan	T45.1x1	T45.1x2	T45.1x3	T45.1x4	T45.1x5	T45.1x6
Memantine	T43.8x1	T43.8x2	T43.8x3	T43.8x4	T43.8x5	T43.8x6
Menadiol	T45.7x1	T45.7x2	T45.7x3	T45.7x4	T45.7x5	T45.7x6
sodium sulfate	T45.7x1	T45.7x2	T45.7x3	T45.7x4	T45.7x5	T45.7x6
Menadione	T45.7x1	T45.7x2	T45.7x3	T45.7x4	T45.7x5	T45.7x6
sodium bisulfite	T45.7x1	T45.7x2	T45.7x3	T45.7x4	T45.7x5	T45.7x6
Menaphthone	T45.7x1	T45.7x2	T45.7x3	T45.7x4	T45.7x5	T45.7x6
Menaquinone	T45.7x1	T45.7x2	T45.7x3	T45.7x4	T45.7x5	T45.7x6
Menatetrenone	T45.7x1	T45.7x2	T45.7x3	T45.7x4	T45.7x5	T45.7x6
Meningococcal vaccine	T50.A91	T50.A92	T50.A93	T50.A94	T50.A95	T50.A96
Menningovax (-AC) (-C)	T50.A91	T50.A92	T50.A93	T50.A94	T50.A95	T50.A96
Menotropins	T38.811	T38.812	T38.813	T38.814	T38.815	T38.816
Menthol	T48.5x1	T48.5x2	T48.5x3	T48.5x4	T48.5x5	T48.5x6
Mepacrine	T37.2x1	T37.2x2	T37.2x3	T37.2x4	T37.2x5	T37.2x6
Meparfynol	T42.6x1	T42.6x2	T42.6x3	T42.6x4	T42.6x5	T42.6x6
Mepartricin	T36.7x1	T36.7x2	T36.7x3	T36.7x4	T36.7x5	T36.7x6
Mepazine	T43.3x1	T43.3x2	T43.3x3	T43.3x4	T43.3x5	T43.3x6
Mepenzolate	T44.3x1	T44.3x2	T44.3x3	T44.3x4	T44.3x5	T44.3x6
bromide	T44.3x1	T44.3x2	T44.3x3	T44.3x4	T44.3x5	T44.3x6
Meperidine	T40.4x1	T40.4x2	T40.4x3	T40.4x4	T40.4x5	T40.4x6
Mephebarbital	T42.3x1	T42.3x2	T42.3x3	T42.3x4	T42.3x5	T42.3x6
Mephenamin(e)	T42.8x1	T42.8x2	T42.8x3	T42.8x4	T42.8x5	T42.8x6
Mephenesin	T42.8x1	T42.8x2	T42.8x3	T42.8x4	T42.8x5	T42.8x6
Mephenhydramine	T45.0x1	T45.0x2	T45.0x3	T45.0x4	T45.0x5	T45.0x6
Mephenoxalone	T42.8x1	T42.8x2	T42.8x3	T42.8x4	T42.8x5	T42.8x6
Mephentermine	T44.991	T44.992	T44.993	T44.994	T44.995	T44.996
Mephenytoin	T42.0x1	T42.0x2	T42.0x3	T42.0x4	T42.0x5	T42.0x6
with phenobarbital	T42.3x1	T42.3x2	T42.3x3	T42.3x4	T42.3x5	T42.3x6
Mephobarbital	T42.3x1	T42.3x2	T42.3x3	T42.3x4	T42.3x5	T42.3x6
Mephosfolan	T60.0x1	T60.0x2	T60.0x3	T60.0x4	—	—
Mepindolol	T44.7x1	T44.7x2	T44.7x3	T44.7x4	T44.7x5	T44.7x6
Mepiperphenidol	T44.3x1	T44.3x2	T44.3x3	T44.3x4	T44.3x5	T44.3x6
Mepitiostane	T38.7x1	T38.7x2	T38.7x3	T38.7x4	T38.7x5	T38.7x6
Mepivacaine	T41.3x1	T41.3x2	T41.3x3	T41.3x4	T41.3x5	T41.3x6
epidural	T41.3x1	T41.3x2	T41.3x3	T41.3x4	T41.3x5	T41.3x6
Meprednisone	T38.0x1	T38.0x2	T38.0x3	T38.0x4	T38.0x5	T38.0x6
Meprobam	T43.591	T43.592	T43.593	T43.594	T43.595	T43.596
Meprobamate	T43.591	T43.592	T43.593	T43.594	T43.595	T43.596
Meproscillarin	T46.0x1	T46.0x2	T46.0x3	T46.0x4	T46.0x5	T46.0x6
Meprylcaine	T41.3x1	T41.3x2	T41.3x3	T41.3x4	T41.3x5	T41.3x6
Meptazinol	T39.8x1	T39.8x2	T39.8x3	T39.8x4	T39.8x5	T39.8x6
Mepyramine	T45.0x1	T45.0x2	T45.0x3	T45.0x4	T45.0x5	T45.0x6
Mequitazine	T43.3x1	T43.3x2	T43.3x3	T43.3x4	T43.3x5	T43.3x6
Meralluride	T50.2x1	T50.2x2	T50.2x3	T50.2x4	T50.2x5	T50.2x6
Merbaphen	T50.2x1	T50.2x2	T50.2x3	T50.2x4	T50.2x5	T50.2x6
Merbromin	T49.0x1	T49.0x2	T49.0x3	T49.0x4	T49.0x5	T49.0x6
Mercaptobenzothiazole salts	T49.0x1	T49.0x2	T49.0x3	T49.0x4	T49.0x5	T49.0x6

Substance	Poisoning, Accidental (unintentional)	Poisoning, Intentional Self-harm	Poisoning, Assault	Poisoning, Undetermined	Adverse Effect	Under-dosing
Mercaptomerin	T50.2x1	T50.2x2	T50.2x3	T50.2x4	T50.2x5	T50.2x6
Mercaptopurine	T45.1x1	T45.1x2	T45.1x3	T45.1x4	T45.1x5	T45.1x6
Mercumatilin	T50.2x1	T50.2x2	T50.2x3	T50.2x4	T50.2x5	T50.2x6
Mercuramide	T50.2x1	T50.2x2	T50.2x3	T50.2x4	T50.2x5	T50.2x6
Mercurochrome	T49.0x1	T49.0x2	T49.0x3	T49.0x4	T49.0x5	T49.0x6
Mercurophylline	T50.2x1	T50.2x2	T50.2x3	T50.2x4	T50.2x5	T50.2x6
Mercury, mercurial, mercuric, mercurous (compounds) (cyanide) (fumes) (nonmedicinal) (vapor) NEC	T56.1x1	T56.1x2	T56.1x3	T56.1x4	—	—
ammoniated	T49.0x1	T49.0x2	T49.0x3	T49.0x4	T49.0x5	T49.0x6
anti-infective						
local	T49.0x1	T49.0x2	T49.0x3	T49.0x4	T49.0x5	T49.0x6
systemic	T37.8x1	T37.8x2	T37.8x3	T37.8x4	T37.8x5	T37.8x6
topical	T49.0x1	T49.0x2	T49.0x3	T49.0x4	T49.0x5	T49.0x6
chloride (ammoniated)	T49.0x1	T49.0x2	T49.0x3	T49.0x4	T49.0x5	T49.0x6
fungicide	T56.1x1	T56.1x2	T56.1x3	T56.1x4	—	—
diuretic NEC	T50.2x1	T50.2x2	T50.2x3	T50.2x4	T50.2x5	T50.2x6
fungicide	T56.1x1	T56.1x2	T56.1x3	T56.1x4	—	—
organic (fungicide)	T56.1x1	T56.1x2	T56.1x3	T56.1x4	—	—
oxide, yellow	T49.0x1	T49.0x2	T49.0x3	T49.0x4	T49.0x5	T49.0x6
Mersalyl	T50.2x1	T50.2x2	T50.2x3	T50.2x4	T50.2x5	T50.2x6
Merthiolate	T49.0x1	T49.0x2	T49.0x3	T49.0x4	T49.0x5	T49.0x6
ophthalmic preparation	T49.5x1	T49.5x2	T49.5x3	T49.5x4	T49.5x5	T49.5x6
Meruvax	T50.B91	T50.B92	T50.B93	T50.B94	T50.B95	T50.B96
Mesalazine	T47.8x1	T47.8x2	T47.8x3	T47.8x4	T47.8x5	T47.8x6
Mescal buttons	T40.991	T40.992	T40.993	T40.994	T40.995	T40.996
Mescaline	T40.991	T40.992	T40.993	T40.994	T40.995	T40.996
Mesna	T48.4x1	T48.4x2	T48.4x3	T48.4x4	T48.4x5	T48.4x6
Mesoglycan	T46.6x1	T46.6x2	T46.6x3	T46.6x4	T46.6x5	T46.6x6
Mesoridazine	T43.3x1	T43.3x2	T43.3x3	T43.3x4	T43.3x5	T43.3x6
Mestanolone	T38.7x1	T38.7x2	T38.7x3	T38.7x4	T38.7x5	T38.7x6
Mesterolone	T38.7x1	T38.7x2	T38.7x3	T38.7x4	T38.7x5	T38.7x6
Mestranol	T38.5x1	T38.5x2	T38.5x3	T38.5x4	T38.5x5	T38.5x6
Mesulergine	T42.8x1	T42.8x2	T42.8x3	T42.8x4	T42.8x5	T42.8x6
Mesulfen	T49.0x1	T49.0x2	T49.0x3	T49.0x4	T49.0x5	T49.0x6
Mesuximide	T42.2x1	T42.2x2	T42.2x3	T42.2x4	T42.2x5	T42.2x6
Metabutethamine	T41.3x1	T41.3x2	T41.3x3	T41.3x4	T41.3x5	T41.3x6
Metactesylacetate	T49.0x1	T49.0x2	T49.0x3	T49.0x4	T49.0x5	T49.0x6
Metacycline	T36.4x1	T36.4x2	T36.4x3	T36.4x4	T36.4x5	T36.4x6
Metaldehyde (snail killer) NEC	T60.8x1	T60.8x2	T60.8x3	T60.8x4	—	—
Metals (heavy) (nonmedicinal)	T56.91	T56.92	T56.93	T56.94	—	—
dust, fumes, or vapor NEC	T56.91	T56.92	T56.93	T56.94	—	—
light NEC	T56.91	T56.92	T56.93	T56.94	—	—
dust, fumes, or vapor NEC	T56.91	T56.92	T56.93	T56.94	—	—
specified NEC	T56.891	T56.892	T56.893	T56.894	—	—
thallium	T56.811	T56.812	T56.813	T56.814	—	—
Metamfetamine	T43.621	T43.622	T43.623	T43.624	T43.625	T43.626
Metamizole sodium	T39.2x1	T39.2x2	T39.2x3	T39.2x4	T39.2x5	T39.2x6
Metampicillin	T36.0x1	T36.0x2	T36.0x3	T36.0x4	T36.0x5	T36.0x6
Metamucil	T47.4x1	T47.4x2	T47.4x3	T47.4x4	T47.4x5	T47.4x6
Metaphen	T49.0x1	T49.0x2	T49.0x3	T49.0x4	T49.0x5	T49.0x6
Metandienone	T38.7x1	T38.7x2	T38.7x3	T38.7x4	T38.7x5	T38.7x6
Metandrostenolone	T38.7x1	T38.7x2	T38.7x3	T38.7x4	T38.7x5	T38.7x6
Metaphos	T60.0x1	T60.0x2	T60.0x3	T60.0x4	—	—
Metapramine	T43.011	T43.012	T43.013	T43.014	T43.015	T43.016
Metaproterenol	T48.291	T48.292	T48.293	T48.294	T48.295	T48.296
Metaraminol	T44.4x1	T44.4x2	T44.4x3	T44.4x4	T44.4x5	T44.4x6
Metaxalone	T42.8x1	T42.8x2	T42.8x3	T42.8x4	T42.8x5	T42.8x6
Metenolone	T38.7x1	T38.7x2	T38.7x3	T38.7x4	T38.7x5	T38.7x6
Metergoline	T42.8x1	T42.8x2	T42.8x3	T42.8x4	T42.8x5	T42.8x6
Metescufylline	T46.991	T46.992	T46.993	T46.994	T46.995	T46.996
Metetoin	T42.0x1	T42.0x2	T42.0x3	T42.0x4	T42.0x5	T42.0x6
Metformin	T38.3x1	T38.3x2	T38.3x3	T38.3x4	T38.3x5	T38.3x6
Methacholine	T44.1x1	T44.1x2	T44.1x3	T44.1x4	T44.1x5	T44.1x6
Methacycline	T36.4x1	T36.4x2	T36.4x3	T36.4x4	T36.4x5	T36.4x6
Methadone	T40.3x1	T40.3x2	T40.3x3	T40.3x4	T40.3x5	T40.3x6
Methallenestril	T38.5x1	T38.5x2	T38.5x3	T38.5x4	T38.5x5	T38.5x6
Methallenoestril	T38.5x1	T38.5x2	T38.5x3	T38.5x4	T38.5x5	T38.5x6
Methamphetamine	T43.621	T43.622	T43.623	T43.624	T43.625	T43.626
Methampyrone	T39.2x1	T39.2x2	T39.2x3	T39.2x4	T39.2x5	T39.2x6

Substance	Poisoning, Accidental (unintentional)	Poisoning, Intentional Self-harm	Poisoning, Assault	Poisoning, Undetermined	Adverse Effect	Under-dosing
Methandienone	T38.7x1	T38.7x2	T38.7x3	T38.7x4	T38.7x5	T38.7x6
Methandriol	T38.7x1	T38.7x2	T38.7x3	T38.7x4	T38.7x5	T38.7x6
Methandrostenolone	T38.7x1	T38.7x2	T38.7x3	T38.7x4	T38.7x5	T38.7x6
Methane	T59.891	T59.892	T59.893	T59.894	—	—
Methanethiol	T59.891	T59.892	T59.893	T59.894	—	—
Methaniazide	T37.1x1	T37.1x2	T37.1x3	T37.1x4	T37.1x5	T37.1x6
Methanol (vapor)	T51.1x1	T51.1x2	T51.1x3	T51.1x4	—	—
Methantheline	T44.3x1	T44.3x2	T44.3x3	T44.3x4	T44.3x5	T44.3x6
Methanthelinium bromide	T44.3x1	T44.3x2	T44.3x3	T44.3x4	T44.3x5	T44.3x6
Methaphenilene	T45.0x1	T45.0x2	T45.0x3	T45.0x4	T45.0x5	T45.0x6
Methapyrilene	T45.0x1	T45.0x2	T45.0x3	T45.0x4	T45.0x5	T45.0x6
Methaqualone (compound)	T42.6x1	T42.6x2	T42.6x3	T42.6x4	T42.6x5	T42.6x6
Metharbital	T42.3x1	T42.3x2	T42.3x3	T42.3x4	T42.3x5	T42.3x6
Methazolamide	T50.2x1	T50.2x2	T50.2x3	T50.2x4	T50.2x5	T50.2x6
Methdilazine	T43.3x1	T43.3x2	T43.3x3	T43.3x4	T43.3x5	T43.3x6
Methedrine	T43.621	T43.622	T43.623	T43.624	T43.625	T43.626
Methenamine (mandelate)	T37.8x1	T37.8x2	T37.8x3	T37.8x4	T37.8x5	T37.8x6
Methenolone	T38.7x1	T38.7x2	T38.7x3	T38.7x4	T38.7x5	T38.7x6
Methergine	T48.0x1	T48.0x2	T48.0x3	T48.0x4	T48.0x5	T48.0x6
Methetoin	T42.0x1	T42.0x2	T42.0x3	T42.0x4	T42.0x5	T42.0x6
Methiacil	T38.2x1	T38.2x2	T38.2x3	T38.2x4	T38.2x5	T38.2x6
Methicillin	T36.0x1	T36.0x2	T36.0x3	T36.0x4	T36.0x5	T36.0x6
Methimazole	T38.2x1	T38.2x2	T38.2x3	T38.2x4	T38.2x5	T38.2x6
Methiodal sodium	T50.8x1	T50.8x2	T50.8x3	T50.8x4	T50.8x5	T50.8x6
Methionine	T50.991	T50.992	T50.993	T50.994	T50.995	T50.996
Methisazone	T37.5x1	T37.5x2	T37.5x3	T37.5x4	T37.5x5	T37.5x6
Methisoprinol	T37.5x1	T37.5x2	T37.5x3	T37.5x4	T37.5x5	T37.5x6
Methitural	T42.3x1	T42.3x2	T42.3x3	T42.3x4	T42.3x5	T42.3x6
Methixene	T44.3x1	T44.3x2	T44.3x3	T44.3x4	T44.3x5	T44.3x6
Methobarbital, methobarbitone	T42.3x1	T42.3x2	T42.3x3	T42.3x4	T42.3x5	T42.3x6
Methocarbamol	T42.8x1	T42.8x2	T42.8x3	T42.8x4	T42.8x5	T42.8x6
skeletal muscle relaxant	T48.1x1	T48.1x2	T48.1x3	T48.1x4	T48.1x5	T48.1x6
Methohexital	T41.1x1	T41.1x2	T41.1x3	T41.1x4	T41.1x5	T41.1x6
Methohexitone	T41.1x1	T41.1x2	T41.1x3	T41.1x4	T41.1x5	T41.1x6
Methoin	T42.0x1	T42.0x2	T42.0x3	T42.0x4	T42.0x5	T42.0x6
Methopholine	T39.8x1	T39.8x2	T39.8x3	T39.8x4	T39.8x5	T39.8x6
Methopromazine	T43.3x1	T43.3x2	T43.3x3	T43.3x4	T43.3x5	T43.3x6
Methorate	T48.3x1	T48.3x2	T48.3x3	T48.3x4	T48.3x5	T48.3x6
Methoserpidine	T46.5x1	T46.5x2	T46.5x3	T46.5x4	T46.5x5	T46.5x6
Methotrexate	T45.1x1	T45.1x2	T45.1x3	T45.1x4	T45.1x5	T45.1x6
Methotrimeprazine	T43.3x1	T43.3x2	T43.3x3	T43.3x4	T43.3x5	T43.3x6
Methoxa-Dome	T49.3x1	T49.3x2	T49.3x3	T49.3x4	T49.3x5	T49.3x6
Methoxamine	T44.4x1	T44.4x2	T44.4x3	T44.4x4	T44.4x5	T44.4x6
Methoxsalen	T50.991	T50.992	T50.993	T50.994	T50.995	T50.996
Methoxyaniline	T65.3x1	T65.3x2	T65.3x3	T65.3x4	—	—
Methoxybenzyl penicillin	T36.0x1	T36.0x2	T36.0x3	T36.0x4	T36.0x5	T36.0x6
Methoxychlor	T53.7x1	T53.7x2	T53.7x3	T53.7x4	—	—
Methoxy-DDT	T53.7x1	T53.7x2	T53.7x3	T53.7x4	—	—
Methoxyflurane	T41.0x1	T41.0x2	T41.0x3	T41.0x4	T41.0x5	T41.0x6
Methoxyphenamine	T48.6x1	T48.6x2	T48.6x3	T48.6x4	T48.6x5	T48.6x6
Methoxypromazine	T43.3x1	T43.3x2	T43.3x3	T43.3x4	T43.3x5	T43.3x6
Methscopolamine bromide	T44.3x1	T44.3x2	T44.3x3	T44.3x4	T44.3x5	T44.3x6
Methsuximide	T42.2x1	T42.2x2	T42.2x3	T42.2x4	T42.2x5	T42.2x6
Methyclothiazide	T50.2x1	T50.2x2	T50.2x3	T50.2x4	T50.2x5	T50.2x6
Methyl						
acetate	T52.4x1	T52.4x2	T52.4x3	T52.4x4	—	—
acetone	T52.4x1	T52.4x2	T52.4x3	T52.4x4	—	—
acrylate	T65.891	T65.892	T65.893	T65.894	—	—
alcohol	T51.1x1	T51.1x2	T51.1x3	T51.1x4	—	—
aminophenol	T65.3x1	T65.3x2	T65.3x3	T65.3x4	—	—
amphetamine	T43.621	T43.622	T43.623	T43.624	T43.625	T43.626
androstanolone	T38.7x1	T38.7x2	T38.7x3	T38.7x4	T38.7x5	T38.7x6
atropine	T44.3x1	T44.3x2	T44.3x3	T44.3x4	T44.3x5	T44.3x6
benzene	T52.2x1	T52.2x2	T52.2x3	T52.2x4	—	—
benzoate	T52.8x1	T52.8x2	T52.8x3	T52.8x4	—	—
benzol	T52.2x1	T52.2x2	T52.2x3	T52.2x4	—	—
bromide (gas)	T59.891	T59.892	T59.893	T59.894	—	—
fumigant	T60.8x1	T60.8x2	T60.8x3	T60.8x4	—	—
butanol	T51.3x1	T51.3x2	T51.3x3	T51.3x4	—	—
carbonate	T52.8x1	T52.8x2	T52.8x3	T52.8x4	—	—
carbinol	T51.1x1	T51.1x2	T51.1x3	T51.1x4	—	—

Substance	Poisoning, Accidental (unintentional)	Poisoning, Intentional Self-harm	Poisoning, Assault	Poisoning, Undetermined	Adverse Effect	Under-dosing
Methyl—*continued*						
CCNU	T45.1x1	T45.1x2	T45.1x3	T45.1x4	T45.1x5	T45.1x6
cellosolve	T52.91	T52.92	T52.93	T52.94	—	—
cellulose	T47.4x1	T47.4x2	T47.4x3	T47.4x4	T47.4x5	T47.4x6
chloride (gas)	T59.891	T59.892	T59.893	T59.894	—	—
chloroformate	T59.3x1	T59.3x2	T59.3x3	T59.3x4	—	—
cyclohexane	T52.8x1	T52.8x2	T52.8x3	T52.8x4	—	—
cyclohexanol	T51.8x1	T51.8x2	T51.8x3	T51.8x4	—	—
cyclohexanone	T52.8x1	T52.8x2	T52.8x3	T52.8x4	—	—
cyclohexyl acetate	T52.8x1	T52.8x2	T52.8x3	T52.8x4	—	—
demeton	T60.0x1	T60.0x2	T60.0x3	T60.0x4	—	—
dihydromorphinone	T40.2x1	T40.2x2	T40.2x3	T40.2x4	T40.2x5	T40.2x6
ergometrine	T48.0x1	T48.0x2	T48.0x3	T48.0x4	T48.0x5	T48.0x6
ergonovine	T48.0x1	T48.0x2	T48.0x3	T48.0x4	T48.0x5	T48.0x6
ethyl ketone	T52.4x1	T52.4x2	T52.4x3	T52.4x4	—	—
glucamine antimonate	T37.8x1	T37.8x2	T37.8x3	T37.8x4	T37.8x5	T37.8x6
hydrazine	T65.891	T65.892	T65.893	T65.894	—	—
iodide	T65.891	T65.892	T65.893	T65.894	—	—
isobutyl ketone	T52.4x1	T52.4x2	T52.4x3	T52.4x4	—	—
isothiocyanate	T60.3x1	T60.3x2	T60.3x3	T60.3x4	—	—
mercaptan	T59.891	T59.892	T59.893	T59.894	—	—
morphine NEC	T40.2x1	T40.2x2	T40.2x3	T40.2x4	T40.2x5	T40.2x6
nicotinate	T49.4x1	T49.4x2	T49.4x3	T49.4x4	T49.4x5	T49.4x6
paraben	T49.0x1	T49.0x2	T49.0x3	T49.0x4	T49.0x5	T49.0x6
parafynol	T42.6x1	T42.6x2	T42.6x3	T42.6x4	T42.6x5	T42.6x6
parathion	T60.0x1	T60.0x2	T60.0x3	T60.0x4	—	—
propylcarbinol	T51.3x1	T51.3x2	T51.3x3	T51.3x4	—	—
peridol	T43.4x1	T43.4x2	T43.4x3	T43.4x4	T43.4x5	T43.4x6
phenidate	T43.631	T43.632	T43.633	T43.634	T43.635	T43.636
prednisolone	T38.0x1	T38.0x2	T38.0x3	T38.0x4	T38.0x5	T38.0x6
ENT agent	T49.6x1	T49.6x2	T49.6x3	T49.6x4	T49.6x5	T49.6x6
ophthalmic preparation	T49.5x1	T49.5x2	T49.5x3	T49.5x4	T49.5x5	T49.5x6
topical NEC	T49.0x1	T49.0x2	T49.0x3	T49.0x4	T49.0x5	T49.0x6
propylcarbinol	T51.8x1	T51.8x2	T51.8x3	T51.8x4	—	—
rosaniline NEC	T49.0x1	T49.0x2	T49.0x3	T49.0x4	T49.0x5	T49.0x6
salicylate	T49.2x1	T49.2x2	T49.2x3	T49.2x4	T49.2x5	T49.2x6
sulfate (fumes)	T59.891	T59.892	T59.893	T59.894	—	—
liquid	T52.8x1	T52.8x2	T52.8x3	T52.8x4	—	—
sulfonal	T42.6x1	T42.6x2	T42.6x3	T42.6x4	T42.6x5	T42.6x6
testosterone	T38.7x1	T38.7x2	T38.7x3	T38.7x4	T38.7x5	T38.7x6
thiouracil	T38.2x1	T38.2x2	T38.2x3	T38.2x4	T38.2x5	T38.2x6
Methylamphetamine	T43.621	T43.622	T43.623	T43.624	T43.625	T43.626
Methylated spirit	T51.1x1	T51.1x2	T51.1x3	T51.1x4	—	—
Methylatropine nitrate	T44.3x1	T44.3x2	T44.3x3	T44.3x4	T44.3x5	T44.3x6
Methylbenactyzium bromide	T44.3x1	T44.3x2	T44.3x3	T44.3x4	T44.3x5	T44.3x6
Methylbenzethonium chloride	T49.0x1	T49.0x2	T49.0x3	T49.0x4	T49.0x5	T49.0x6
Methylcellulose	T47.4x1	T47.4x2	T47.4x3	T47.4x4	T47.4x5	T47.4x6
laxative	T47.4x1	T47.4x2	T47.4x3	T47.4x4	T47.4x5	T47.4x6
Methylchlorophenoxyacetic acid	T60.3x1	T60.3x2	T60.3x3	T60.3x4	—	—
Methyldopa	T46.5x1	T46.5x2	T46.5x3	T46.5x4	T46.5x5	T46.5x6
Methyldopate	T46.5x1	T46.5x2	T46.5x3	T46.5x4	T46.5x5	T46.5x6
Methylene						
blue	T50.6x1	T50.6x2	T50.6x3	T50.6x4	T50.6x5	T50.6x6
chloride or dichloride (solvent) NEC	T53.4x1	T53.4x2	T53.4x3	T53.4x4	—	—
Methylenedioxyamphetamine	T43.621	T43.622	T43.623	T43.624	T43.625	T43.626
Methylenedioxymethamphetamine	T43.621	T43.622	T43.623	T43.624	T43.625	T43.626
Methylergometrine	T48.0x1	T48.0x2	T48.0x3	T48.0x4	T48.0x5	T48.0x6
Methylergonovine	T48.0x1	T48.0x2	T48.0x3	T48.0x4	T48.0x5	T48.0x6
Methylestrenolone	T38.5x1	T38.5x2	T38.5x3	T38.5x4	T38.5x5	T38.5x6
Methylethyl cellulose	T50.991	T50.992	T50.993	T50.994	T50.995	T50.996
Methylhexabital	T42.3x1	T42.3x2	T42.3x3	T42.3x4	T42.3x5	T42.3x6
Methylmorphine	T40.2x1	T40.2x2	T40.2x3	T40.2x4	T40.2x5	T40.2x6
Methylparaben (ophthalmic)	T49.5x1	T49.5x2	T49.5x3	T49.5x4	T49.5x5	T49.5x6
Methylparafynol	T42.6x1	T42.6x2	T42.6x3	T42.6x4	T42.6x5	T42.6x6
Methylpentynol, methylpenthynol	T42.6x1	T42.6x2	T42.6x3	T42.6x4	T42.6x5	T42.6x6
Methylphenidate	T43.631	T43.632	T43.633	T43.634	T43.635	T43.636
Methylphenobarbital	T42.3x1	T42.3x2	T42.3x3	T42.3x4	T42.3x5	T42.3x6
Methylpolysiloxane	T47.1x1	T47.1x2	T47.1x3	T47.1x4	T47.1x5	T47.1x6
Methylprednisolone	T49.0x1	T49.0x2	T49.0x3	T49.0x4	T49.0x5	T49.0x6
Methylrosaniline	T49.0x1	T49.0x2	T49.0x3	T49.0x4	T49.0x5	T49.0x6
Methylrosanilinium chloride	T49.0x1	T49.0x2	T49.0x3	T49.0x4	T49.0x5	T49.0x6
Methyltestosterone	T38.7x1	T38.7x2	T38.7x3	T38.7x4	T38.7x5	T38.7x6
Methylthionine chloride	T50.6x1	T50.6x2	T50.6x3	T50.6x4	T50.6x5	T50.6x6
Methylthioninium chloride	T50.6x1	T50.6x2	T50.6x3	T50.6x4	T50.6x5	T50.6x6
Methylthiouracil	T38.2x1	T38.2x2	T38.2x3	T38.2x4	T38.2x5	T38.2x6
Methyprylon	T42.6x1	T42.6x2	T42.6x3	T42.6x4	T42.6x5	T42.6x6
Methysergide	T46.5x1	T46.5x2	T46.5x3	T46.5x4	T46.5x5	T46.5x6
Metiamide	T47.1x1	T47.1x2	T47.1x3	T47.1x4	T47.1x5	T47.1x6
Meticillin	T36.0x1	T36.0x2	T36.0x3	T36.0x4	T36.0x5	T36.0x6
Meticrane	T50.2x1	T50.2x2	T50.2x3	T50.2x4	T50.2x5	T50.2x6
Metildigoxin	T46.0x1	T46.0x2	T46.0x3	T46.0x4	T46.0x5	T46.0x6
Metipranolol	T49.5x1	T49.5x2	T49.5x3	T49.5x4	T49.5x5	T49.5x6
Metirosine	T46.5x1	T46.5x2	T46.5x3	T46.5x4	T46.5x5	T46.5x6
Metisazone	T37.5x1	T37.5x2	T37.5x3	T37.5x4	T37.5x5	T37.5x6
Metixene	T44.3x1	T44.3x2	T44.3x3	T44.3x4	T44.3x5	T44.3x6
Metizoline	T48.5x1	T48.5x2	T48.5x3	T48.5x4	T48.5x5	T48.5x6
Metoclopramide	T45.0x1	T45.0x2	T45.0x3	T45.0x4	T45.0x5	T45.0x6
Metofenazate	T43.3x1	T43.3x2	T43.3x3	T43.3x4	T43.3x5	T43.3x6
Metofoline	T39.8x1	T39.8x2	T39.8x3	T39.8x4	T39.8x5	T39.8x6
Metolazone	T50.2x1	T50.2x2	T50.2x3	T50.2x4	T50.2x5	T50.2x6
Metopon	T40.2x1	T40.2x2	T40.2x3	T40.2x4	T40.2x5	T40.2x6
Metoprine	T45.1x1	T45.1x2	T45.1x3	T45.1x4	T45.1x5	T45.1x6
Metoprolol	T44.7x1	T44.7x2	T44.7x3	T44.7x4	T44.7x5	T44.7x6
Metrifonate	T60.0x1	T60.0x2	T60.0x3	T60.0x4	—	—
Metrizamide	T50.8x1	T50.8x2	T50.8x3	T50.8x4	T50.8x5	T50.8x6
Metrizoic acid	T50.8x1	T50.8x2	T50.8x3	T50.8x4	T50.8x5	T50.8x6
Metronidazole	T37.8x1	T37.8x2	T37.8x3	T37.8x4	T37.8x5	T37.8x6
Metycaine	T41.3x1	T41.3x2	T41.3x3	T41.3x4	T41.3x5	T41.3x6
infiltration (subcutaneous)	T41.3x1	T41.3x2	T41.3x3	T41.3x4	T41.3x5	T41.3x6
nerve block (peripheral) (plexus)	T41.3x1	T41.3x2	T41.3x3	T41.3x4	T41.3x5	T41.3x6
topical (surface)	T41.3x1	T41.3x2	T41.3x3	T41.3x4	T41.3x5	T41.3x6
Metyrapone	T50.8x1	T50.8x2	T50.8x3	T50.8x4	T50.8x5	T50.8x6
Mevinphos	T60.0x1	T60.0x2	T60.0x3	T60.0x4	—	—
Mexazolam	T42.4x1	T42.4x2	T42.4x3	T42.4x4	T42.4x5	T42.4x6
Mexenone	T49.3x1	T49.3x2	T49.3x3	T49.3x4	T49.3x5	T49.3x6
Mexiletine	T46.2x1	T46.2x2	T46.2x3	T46.2x4	T46.2x5	T46.2x6
Mezereon	T62.2x1	T62.2x2	T62.2x3	T62.2x4	—	—
berries	T62.1x1	T62.1x2	T62.1x3	T62.1x4	—	—
Mezlocillin	T36.0x1	T36.0x2	T36.0x3	T36.0x4	T36.0x5	T36.0x6
Mianserin	T43.021	T43.022	T43.023	T43.024	T43.025	T43.026
Micatin	T49.0x1	T49.0x2	T49.0x3	T49.0x4	T49.0x5	T49.0x6
Miconazole	T49.0x1	T49.0x2	T49.0x3	T49.0x4	T49.0x5	T49.0x6
Micronomicin	T36.5x1	T36.5x2	T36.5x3	T36.5x4	T36.5x5	T36.5x6
Midazolam	T42.4x1	T42.4x2	T42.4x3	T42.4x4	T42.4x5	T42.4x6
Midecamycin	T36.3x1	T36.3x2	T36.3x3	T36.3x4	T36.3x5	T36.3x6
Mifepristone	T38.6x1	T38.6x2	T38.6x3	T38.6x4	T38.6x5	T38.6x6
Milk of magnesia	T47.1x1	T47.1x2	T47.1x3	T47.1x4	T47.1x5	T47.1x6
Millipede (tropical) (venomous)	T63.411	T63.412	T63.413	T63.414	—	—
Miltown	T43.591	T43.592	T43.593	T43.594	T43.595	T43.596
Milverine	T44.3x1	T44.3x2	T44.3x3	T44.3x4	T44.3x5	T44.3x6
Minaprine	T43.291	T43.292	T43.293	T43.294	T43.295	T43.296
Minaxolone	T41.291	T41.292	T41.293	T41.294	T41.295	T41.296
Mineral						
acids	T54.2x1	T54.2x2	T54.2x3	T54.2x4	—	—
oil (laxative)(medicinal)	T47.4x1	T47.4x2	T47.4x3	T47.4x4	T47.4x5	T47.4x6
emulsion	T47.2x1	T47.2x2	T47.2x3	T47.2x4	T47.2x5	T47.2x6
nonmedicinal	T52.0x1	T52.0x2	T52.0x3	T52.0x4	—	—
topical	T49.3x1	T49.3x2	T49.3x3	T49.3x4	T49.3x5	T49.3x6
salt NEC	T50.3x1	T50.3x2	T50.3x3	T50.3x4	T50.3x5	T50.3x6
spirits	T52.0x1	T52.0x2	T52.0x3	T52.0x4	—	—
Mineralocorticosteroid	T50.0x1	T50.0x2	T50.0x3	T50.0x4	T50.0x5	T50.0x6
Minocycline	T36.4x1	T36.4x2	T36.4x3	T36.4x4	T36.4x5	T36.4x6
Minoxidil	T46.7x1	T46.7x2	T46.7x3	T46.7x4	T46.7x5	T46.7x6
Miokamycin	T36.3x1	T36.3x2	T36.3x3	T36.3x4	T36.3x5	T36.3x6
Miotic drug	T49.5x1	T49.5x2	T49.5x3	T49.5x4	T49.5x5	T49.5x6
Mipafox	T60.0x1	T60.0x2	T60.0x3	T60.0x4	—	—
Mirex	T60.1x1	T60.1x2	T60.1x3	T60.1x4	—	—
Mirtazapine	T43.021	T43.022	T43.023	T43.024	T43.025	T43.026

Substance	Poisoning, Accidental (unintentional)	Poisoning, Intentional Self-harm	Poisoning, Assault	Poisoning, Undetermined	Adverse Effect	Under-dosing
Misonidazole	T37.3x1	T37.3x2	T37.3x3	T37.3x4	T37.3x5	T37.3x6
Misoprostol	T47.1x1	T47.1x2	T47.1x3	T47.1x4	T47.1x5	T47.1x6
Mithramycin	T45.1x1	T45.1x2	T45.1x3	T45.1x4	T45.1x5	T45.1x6
Mitobronitol	T45.1x1	T45.1x2	T45.1x3	T45.1x4	T45.1x5	T45.1x6
Mitoguazone	T45.1x1	T45.1x2	T45.1x3	T45.1x4	T45.1x5	T45.1x6
Mitolactol	T45.1x1	T45.1x2	T45.1x3	T45.1x4	T45.1x5	T45.1x6
Mitomycin	T45.1x1	T45.1x2	T45.1x3	T45.1x4	T45.1x5	T45.1x6
Mitopodozide	T45.1x1	T45.1x2	T45.1x3	T45.1x4	T45.1x5	T45.1x6
Mitotane	T45.1x1	T45.1x2	T45.1x3	T45.1x4	T45.1x5	T45.1x6
Mitoxantrone	T45.1x1	T45.1x2	T45.1x3	T45.1x4	T45.1x5	T45.1x6
Mivacurium chloride	T48.1x1	T48.1x2	T48.1x3	T48.1x4	T48.1x5	T48.1x6
Miyari bacteria	T47.6x1	T47.6x2	T47.6x3	T47.6x4	T47.6x5	T47.6x6
Moclobemide	T43.1x1	T43.1x2	T43.1x3	T43.1x4	T43.1x5	T43.1x6
Moderil	T46.5x1	T46.5x2	T46.5x3	T46.5x4	T46.5x5	T46.5x6
Mofebutazone	T39.2x1	T39.2x2	T39.2x3	T39.2x4	T39.2x5	T39.2x6
Mogadon—*see* Nitrazepam						
Molindone	T43.591	T43.592	T43.593	T43.594	T43.595	T43.596
Molsidomine	T46.3x1	T46.3x2	T46.3x3	T46.3x4	T46.3x5	T46.3x6
Mometasone	T49.0x1	T49.0x2	T49.0x3	T49.0x4	T49.0x5	T49.0x6
Monistat	T49.0x1	T49.0x2	T49.0x3	T49.0x4	T49.0x5	T49.0x6
Monkshood	T62.2x1	T62.2x2	T62.2x3	T62.2x4	—	—
Monoamine oxidase inhibitor NEC	T43.1x1	T43.1x2	T43.1x3	T43.1x4	T43.1x5	T43.1x6
hydrazine	T43.1x1	T43.1x2	T43.1x3	T43.1x4	T43.1x5	T43.1x6
Monobenzone	T49.4x1	T49.4x2	T49.4x3	T49.4x4	T49.4x5	T49.4x6
Monochloroacetic acid	T60.3x1	T60.3x2	T60.3x3	I60.3x4	—	—
Monochlorobenzene	T53.7x1	T53.7x2	T53.7x3	T53.7x4	—	—
Monoethanolamine	T46.8x1	T46.8x2	T46.8x3	T46.8x4	T46.8x5	T46.8x6
oleate	T46.8x1	T46.8x2	T46.8x3	T46.8x4	T46.8x5	T46.8x6
Monooctanoin	T50.991	T50.992	T50.993	T50.994	T50.995	T50.996
Monophenylbutazone	T39.2x1	T39.2x2	T39.2x3	T39.2x4	T39.2x5	T39.2x6
Monosodium glutamate	T65.891	T65.892	T65.893	T65.894	—	—
Monosulfiram	T49.0x1	T49.0x2	T49.0x3	T49.0x4	T49.0x5	T49.0x6
Monoxide, carbon—*see* Carbon, monoxide						
Monoxidine hydrochloride	T46.1x1	T46.1x2	T46.1x3	T46.1x4	T46.1x5	T46.1x6
Monuron	T60.3x1	T60.3x2	T60.3x3	T60.3x4	—	—
Moperone	T43.4x1	T43.4x2	T43.4x3	T43.4x4	T43.4x5	T43.4x6
Mopidamol	T45.1x1	T45.1x2	T45.1x3	T45.1x4	T45.1x5	T45.1x6
MOPP (mechloreth-amine + vincristine + prednisone + procarbazine)	T45.1x1	T45.1x2	T45.1x3	T45.1x4	T45.1x5	T45.1x6
Morfin	T40.2x1	T40.2x2	T40.2x3	T40.2x4	T40.2x5	T40.2x6
Morinamide	T37.1x1	T37.1x2	T37.1x3	T37.1x4	T37.1x5	T37.1x6
Morning glory seeds	T40.991	T40.992	T40.993	T40.994	T40.995	T40.996
Moroxydine	T37.5x1	T37.5x2	T37.5x3	T37.5x4	T37.5x5	T37.5x6
Morphazinamide	T37.1x1	T37.1x2	T37.1x3	T37.1x4	T37.1x5	T37.1x6
Morphine	T40.2x1	T40.2x2	T40.2x3	T40.2x4	T40.2x5	T40.2x6
antagonist	T50.7x1	T50.7x2	T50.7x3	T50.7x4	T50.7x5	T50.7x6
Morpholinylethylmorphine	T40.2x1	T40.2x2	T40.2x3	T40.2x4	T40.2x5	T40.2x6
Morsuximide	T42.2x1	T42.2x2	T42.2x3	T42.2x4	T42.2x5	T42.2x6
Mosapramine	T43.591	T43.592	T43.593	T43.594	T43.595	T43.596
Moth balls (*see also* Pesticides)	T60.2x1	T60.2x2	T60.2x3	T60.2x4	—	—
naphthalene	T60.2x1	T60.2x2	T60.2x3	T60.2x4	—	—
paradichlorobenzene	T60.1x1	T60.1x2	T60.1x3	T60.1x4	—	—
Motor exhaust gas	T58.01	T58.02	T58.03	T58.04	—	—
Mouthwash (antiseptic) (zinc chloride)	T49.6x1	T49.6x2	T49.6x3	T49.6x4	T49.6x5	T49.6x6
Moxastine	T45.0x1	T45.0x2	T45.0x3	T45.0x4	T45.0x5	T45.0x6
Moxaverine	T44.3x1	T44.3x2	T44.3x3	T44.3x4	T44.3x5	T44.3x6
Moxisylyte	T46.7x1	T46.7x2	T46.7x3	T46.7x4	T46.7x5	T46.7x6
Mucilage, plant	T47.4x1	T47.4x2	T47.4x3	T47.4x4	T47.4x5	T47.4x6
Mucolytic drug	T48.4x1	T48.4x2	T48.4x3	T48.4x4	T48.4x5	T48.4x6
Mucomyst	T48.4x1	T48.4x2	T48.4x3	T48.4x4	T48.4x5	T48.4x6
Mucous membrane agents (external)	T49.91	T49.92	T49.93	T49.94	T49.95	T49.96
specified NEC	T49.8x1	T49.8x2	T49.8x3	T49.8x4	T49.8x5	T49.8x6
Mumps						
immune globulin (human)	T50.Z11	T50.Z12	T50.Z13	T50.Z14	T50.Z15	T50.Z16
skin test antigen	T50.8x1	T50.8x2	T50.8x3	T50.8x4	T50.8x5	T50.8x6
vaccine	T50.B91	T50.B92	T50.B93	T50.B94	T50.B95	T50.B96
Mumpsvax	T50.B91	T50.B92	T50.B93	T50.B94	T50.B95	T50.B96

Substance	Poisoning, Accidental (unintentional)	Poisoning, Intentional Self-harm	Poisoning, Assault	Poisoning, Undetermined	Adverse Effect	Under-dosing
Mupirocin	T49.0x1	T49.0x2	T49.0x3	T49.0x4	T49.0x5	T49.0x6
Muriatic acid—*see* Hydrochloric acid						
Muromonab-CD3	T45.1x1	T45.1x2	T45.1x3	T45.1x4	T45.1x5	T45.1x6
Muscle relaxant—*see* Relaxant, muscle						
Muscle-action drug NEC	T48.201	T48.202	T48.203	T48.204	T48.205	T48.206
Muscle affecting agents NEC	T48.201	T48.202	T48.203	T48.204	T48.205	T48.206
oxytocic	T48.0x1	T48.0x2	T48.0x3	T48.0x4	T48.0x5	T48.0x6
relaxants	T48.201	T48.202	T48.203	T48.204	T48.205	T48.206
central nervous system	T42.8x1	T42.8x2	T42.8x3	T42.8x4	T42.8x5	T42.8x6
skeletal	T48.1x1	T48.1x2	T48.1x3	T48.1x4	T48.1x5	T48.1x6
smooth	T44.3x1	T44.3x2	T44.3x3	T44.3x4	T44.3x5	T44.3x6
Muscle-tone depressant, central NEC	T42.8x1	T42.8x2	T42.8x3	T42.8x4	T42.8x5	T42.8x6
specified NEC	T42.8x1	T42.8x2	T42.8x3	T42.8x4	T42.8x5	T42.8x6
Mushroom, noxious	T62.0x1	T62.0x2	T62.0x3	T62.0x4	—	—
Mussel, noxious	T61.781	T61.782	T61.783	T61.784	—	—
Mustard (emetic)	T47.7x1	T47.7x2	T47.7x3	T47.7x4	T47.7x5	T47.7x6
black	T47.7x1	T47.7x2	T47.7x3	T47.7x4	T47.7x5	T47.7x6
gas, not in war	T59.91	T59.92	T59.93	T59.94	—	—
nitrogen	T45.1x1	T45.1x2	T45.1x3	T45.1x4	T45.1x5	T45.1x6
Mustine	T45.1x1	T45.1x2	T45.1x3	T45.1x4	T45.1x5	T45.1x6
M-vac	T45.1x1	T45.1x2	T45.1x3	T45.1x4	T45.1x5	T45.1x6
Mycifradin	T36.8x1	T36.8x2	T36.8x3	T36.8x4	T36.8x5	T36.8x6
topical	T49.0x1	T49.0x2	T49.0x3	T49.0x4	T49.0x5	T49.0x6
Mycitracin	T36.8x1	T36.8x2	T36.8x3	T36.8x4	T36.8x5	T36.8x6
ophthalmic preparation	T49.5x1	T49.5x2	T49.5x3	T49.5x4	T49.5x5	T49.5x6
Mycostatin	T36.7x1	T36.7x2	T36.7x3	T36.7x4	T36.7x5	T36.7x6
topical	T49.0x1	T49.0x2	T49.0x3	T49.0x4	T49.0x5	T49.0x6
Mycotoxins	T64.81	T64.82	T64.83	T64.84	—	—
aflatoxin	T64.01	T64.02	T64.03	T64.04	—	—
specified NEC	T64.81	T64.82	T64.83	T64.84	—	—
Mydriacyl	T44.3x1	T44.3x2	T44.3x3	T44.3x4	T44.3x5	T44.3x6
Mydriatic drug	T49.5x1	T49.5x2	T49.5x3	T49.5x4	T49.5x5	T49.5x6
Myelobromal	T45.1x1	T45.1x2	T45.1x3	T45.1x4	T45.1x5	T45.1x6
Myleran	T45.1x1	T45.1x2	T45.1x3	T45.1x4	T45.1x5	T45.1x6
Myochrysin(e)	T39.2x1	T39.2x2	T39.2x3	T39.2x4	T39.2x5	T39.2x6
Myoneural blocking agents	T48.1x1	T48.1x2	T48.1x3	T48.1x4	T48.1x5	T48.1x6
Myralact	T49.0x1	T49.0x2	T49.0x3	T49.0x4	T49.0x5	T49.0x6
Myristica fragrans	T62.2x1	T62.2x2	T62.2x3	T62.2x4	—	—
Myristicin	T65.891	T65.892	T65.893	T65.894	—	—
Mysoline	T42.3x1	T42.3x2	T42.3x3	T42.3x4	T42.3x5	T42.3x6
Nabilone	T40.7x1	T40.7x2	T40.7x3	T40.7x4	T40.7x5	T40.7x6
Nabumetone	T39.391	T39.392	T39.393	T39.394	T39.395	T39.396
Nadolol	T44.7x1	T44.7x2	T44.7x3	T44.7x4	T44.7x5	T44.7x6
Nafcillin	T36.0x1	T36.0x2	T36.0x3	T36.0x4	T36.0x5	T36.0x6
Nafoxidine	T38.6x1	T38.6x2	T38.6x3	T38.6x4	T38.6x5	T38.6x6
Naftazone	T46.991	T46.992	T46.993	T46.994	T46.995	T46.996
Naftidrofuryl (oxalate)	T46.7x1	T46.7x2	T46.7x3	T46.7x4	T46.7x5	T46.7x6
Naftifine	T49.0x1	T49.0x2	T49.0x3	T49.0x4	T49.0x5	T49.0x6
Nail polish remover	T52.91	T52.92	T52.93	T52.94	—	—
Nalbuphine	T40.4x1	T40.4x2	T40.4x3	T40.4x4	T40.4x5	T40.4x6
Naled	T60.0x1	T60.0x2	T60.0x3	T60.0x4	—	—
Nalidixic acid	T37.8x1	T37.8x2	T37.8x3	T37.8x4	T37.8x5	T37.8x6
Nalorphine	T50.7x1	T50.7x2	T50.7x3	T50.7x4	T50.7x5	T50.7x6
Naloxone	T50.7x1	T50.7x2	T50.7x3	T50.7x4	T50.7x5	T50.7x6
Naltrexone	T50.7x1	T50.7x2	T50.7x3	T50.7x4	T50.7x5	T50.7x6
Namenda	T43.8x1	T43.8x2	T43.8x3	T43.8x4	T43.8x5	T43.8x6
Nandrolone	T38.7x1	T38.7x2	T38.7x3	T38.7x4	T38.7x5	T38.7x6
Naphazoline	T48.5x1	T48.5x2	T48.5x3	T48.5x4	T48.5x5	T48.5x6
Naphtha (painters') (petroleum)	T52.0x1	T52.0x2	T52.0x3	T52.0x4	—	—
solvent	T52.0x1	T52.0x2	T52.0x3	T52.0x4	—	—
vapor	T52.0x1	T52.0x2	T52.0x3	T52.0x4	—	—
Naphthalene (non-chlorinated)	T60.2x1	T60.2x2	T60.2x3	T60.2x4	—	—
chlorinated	T60.1x1	T60.1x2	T60.1x3	T60.1x4	—	—
vapor	T60.1x1	T60.1x2	T60.1x3	T60.1x4	—	—
insecticide or moth repellent	T60.2x1	T60.2x2	T60.2x3	T60.2x4	—	—
chlorinated	T60.1x1	T60.1x2	T60.1x3	T60.1x4	—	—
vapor	T60.2x1	T60.2x2	T60.2x3	T60.2x4	—	—
chlorinated	T60.1x1	T60.1x2	T60.1x3	T60.1x4	—	—

Substance	Poisoning, Accidental (unintentional)	Poisoning, Intentional Self-harm	Poisoning, Assault	Poisoning, Undetermined	Adverse Effect	Under-dosing
Naphthol	T65.891	T65.892	T65.893	T65.894	—	—
Naphthylamine	T65.891	T65.892	T65.893	T65.894	—	—
Naphthylthiourea (ANTU)	T60.4x1	T60.4x2	T60.4x3	T60.4x4	—	—
Naprosyn—see Naproxen						
Naproxen	T39.311	T39.312	T39.313	T39.314	T39.315	T39.316
Narcotic (drug)	T40.601	T40.602	T40.603	T40.604	T40.605	T40.606
analgesic NEC	T39.8x1	T39.8x2	T39.8x3	T39.8x4	T39.8x5	T39.8x6
antagonist	T50.7x1	T50.7x2	T50.7x3	T50.7x4	T50.7x5	T50.7x6
specified NEC	T40.691	T40.692	T40.693	T40.694	T40.695	T40.696
Narcotine	T48.3x1	T48.3x2	T48.3x3	T48.3x4	T48.3x5	T48.3x6
Nardil	T43.1x1	T43.1x2	T43.1x3	T43.1x4	T43.1x5	T43.1x6
Nasal drug NEC	T49.6x1	T49.6x2	T49.6x3	T49.6x4	T49.6x5	T49.6x6
Natamycin	T49.0x1	T49.0x2	T49.0x3	T49.0x4	T49.0x5	T49.0x6
Natrium cyanide—see Cyanide(s)						
Natural						
blood (product)	T45.8x1	T45.8x2	T45.8x3	T45.8x4	T45.8x5	T45.8x6
gas (piped)	T59.891	T59.892	T59.893	T59.894	—	—
incomplete combustion	T58.11	T58.12	T58.13	T58.14	—	—
Nealbarbital	T42.3x1	T42.3x2	T42.3x3	T42.3x4	T42.3x5	T42.3x6
Nectadon	T48.3x1	T48.3x2	T48.3x3	T48.3x4	T48.3x5	T48.3x6
Nedocromil	T48.6x1	T48.6x2	T48.6x3	T48.6x4	T48.6x5	T48.6x6
Nefopam	T39.8x1	T39.8x2	T39.8x3	T39.8x4	T39.8x5	T39.8x6
Nematocyst (sting)	T63.691	T63.692	T63.693	T63.694	—	—
Nembutal	T42.3x1	T42.3x2	T42.3x3	T42.3x4	T42.3x5	T42.3x6
Nemonapride	T43.591	T43.592	T43.593	T43.594	T43.595	T43.596
Neoarsphenamine	T37.8x1	T37.8x2	T37.8x3	T37.8x4	T37.8x5	T37.8x6
Neocinchophen	T50.4x1	T50.4x2	T50.4x3	T50.4x4	T50.4x5	T50.4x6
Neomycin (derivatives)	T36.5x1	T36.5x2	T36.5x3	T36.5x4	T36.5x5	T36.5x6
with						
bacitracin	T49.0x1	T49.0x2		T49.0x4	T49.0x5	T49.0x6
neostigmine	T44.0x1	T44.0x2	T44.0x3	T44.0x4	T44.0x5	T44.0x6
ENT agent	T49.6x1	T49.6x2	T49.6x3	T49.6x4	T49.6x5	T49.6x6
ophthalmic preparation	T49.5x1	T49.5x2	T49.5x3	T49.5x4	T49.5x5	T49.5x6
topical NEC	T49.0x1	T49.0x2	T49.0x3	T49.0x4	T49.0x5	T49.0x6
Neonal	T42.3x1	T42.3x2	T42.3x3	T42.3x4	T42.3x5	T42.3x6
Neoprontosil	T37.0x1	T37.0x2	T37.0x3	T37.0x4	T37.0x5	T37.0x6
Neosalvarsan	T37.8x1	T37.8x2	T37.8x3	T37.8x4	T37.8x5	T37.8x6
Neosilversalvarsan	T37.8x1	T37.8x2	T37.8x3	T37.8x4	T37.8x5	T37.8x6
Neosporin	T36.8x1	T36.8x2	T36.8x3	T36.8x4	T36.8x5	T36.8x6
ENT agent	T49.6x1	T49.6x2	T49.6x3	T49.6x4	T49.6x5	T49.6x6
opthalmic preparation	T49.5x1	T49.5x2	T49.5x3	T49.5x4	T49.5x5	T49.5x6
topical NEC	T49.0x1	T49.0x2	T49.0x3	T49.0x4	T49.0x5	T49.0x6
Neostigmine bromide	T44.0x1	T44.0x2	T44.0x3	T44.0x4	T44.0x5	T44.0x6
Neraval	T42.3x1	T42.3x2	T42.3x3	T42.3x4	T42.3x5	T42.3x6
Neravan	T42.3x1	T42.3x2	T42.3x3	T42.3x4	T42.3x5	T42.3x6
Nerium oleander	T62.2x1	T62.2x2	T62.2x3	T62.2x4	—	—
Nerve gas, not in war	T59.891	T59.892	T59.893	T59.894	—	—
Nesacaine	T41.3x1	T41.3x2	T41.3x3	T41.3x4	T41.3x5	T41.3x6
infiltration (subcutaneous)	T41.3x1	T41.3x2	T41.3x3	T41.3x4	T41.3x5	T41.3x6
nerve block (peripheral) (plexus)	T41.3x1	T41.3x2	T41.3x3	T41.3x4	T41.3x5	T41.3x6
Netilmicin	T36.5x1	T36.5x2	T36.5x3	T36.5x4	T36.5x5	T36.5x6
Neurobarb	T42.3x1	T42.3x2	T42.3x3	T42.3x4	T42.3x5	T42.3x6
Neuroleptic drug NEC	T43.501	T43.502	T43.503	T43.504	T43.505	T43.506
Neuromuscular blocking drug	T48.1x1	T48.1x2	T48.1x3	T48.1x4	T48.1x5	T48.1x6
Neutral insulin injection	T38.3x1	T38.3x2	T38.3x3	T38.3x4	T38.3x5	T38.3x6
Neutral spirits	T51.0x1	T51.0x2	T51.0x3	T51.0x4	—	—
beverage	T51.0x1	T51.0x2	T51.0x3	T51.0x4	—	—
Niacin	T46.7x1	T46.7x2	T46.7x3	T46.7x4	T46.7x5	T46.7x6
Niacinamide	T45.2x1	T45.2x2	T45.2x3	T45.2x4	T45.2x5	T45.2x6
Nialamide	T43.1x1	T43.1x2	T43.1x3	T43.1x4	T43.1x5	T43.1x6
Niaprazine	T42.6x1	T42.6x2	T42.6x3	T42.6x4	T42.6x5	T42.6x6
Nicametate	T46.7x1	T46.7x2	T46.7x3	T46.7x4	T46.7x5	T46.7x6
Nicardipine	T46.1x1	T46.1x2	T46.1x3	T46.1x4	T46.1x5	T46.1x6
Nicergoline	T46.7x1	T46.7x2	T46.7x3	T46.7x4	T46.7x5	T46.7x6
Nickel (carbonyl) (tetra-carbonyl)(fumes) (vapor)	T56.891	T56.892	T56.893	T56.894	—	—
Nickelocene	T56.891	T56.892	T56.893	T56.894	—	—
Niclosamide	T37.4x1	T37.4x2	T37.4x3	T37.4x4	T37.4x5	T37.4x6
Nicofuranose	T46.7x1	T46.7x2	T46.7x3	T46.7x4	T46.7x5	T46.7x6
Nicomorphine	T40.2x1	T40.2x2	T40.2x3	T40.2x4	T40.2x5	T40.2x6
Nicorandil	T46.3x1	T46.3x2	T46.3x3	T46.3x4	T46.3x5	T46.3x6
Nicotiana (plant)	T62.2x1	T62.2x2	T62.2x3	T62.2x4	—	—
Nicotinamide	T45.2x1	T45.2x2	T45.2x3	T45.2x4	T45.2x5	T45.2x6
Nicotine (insecticide) (spray) (sulfate) NEC	T60.2x1	T60.2x2	T60.2x3	T60.2x4	—	—
from tobacco	T65.291	T65.292	T65.293	T65.294	—	—
cigarettes	T65.221	T65.222	T65.223	T65.224	—	—
not insecticide	T65.291	T65.292	T65.293	T65.294	—	—
Nicotinic acid	T46.7x1	T46.7x2	T46.7x3	T46.7x4	T46.7x5	T46.7x6
Nicotinyl alcohol	T46.7x1	T46.7x2	T46.7x3	T46.7x4	T46.7x5	T46.7x6
Nicoumalone	T45.511	T45.512	T45.513	T45.514	T45.515	T45.516
Nifedipine	T46.1x1	T46.1x2	T46.1x3	T46.1x4	T46.1x5	T46.1x6
Nifenazone	T39.2x1	T39.2x2	T39.2x3	T39.2x4	T39.2x5	T39.2x6
Nifuraldezone	T37.91	T37.92	T37.93	T37.94	T37.95	T37.96
Nifuratel	T37.8x1	T37.8x2	T37.8x3	T37.8x4	T37.8x5	T37.8x6
Nifurtimox	T37.3x1	T37.3x2	T37.3x3	T37.3x4	T37.3x5	T37.3x6
Nifurtoinol	T37.8x1	T37.8x2	T37.8x3	T37.8x4	T37.8x5	T37.8x6
Nightshade, deadly (solanum) (see also Belladonna)	T62.2x1	T62.2x2	T62.2x3	T62.2x4	—	—
berry	T62.1x1	T62.1x2	T62.1x3	T62.1x4	—	—
Nikethamide	T50.7x1	T50.7x2	T50.7x3	T50.7x4	T50.7x5	T50.7x6
Nilstat	T36.7x1	T36.7x2	T36.7x3	T36.7x4	T36.7x5	T36.7x6
topical	T49.0x1	T49.0x2	T49.0x3	T49.0x4	T49.0x5	T49.0x6
Nilutamide	T38.6x1	T38.6x2	T38.6x3	T38.6x4	T38.6x5	T38.6x6
Nimesulide	T39.391	T39.392	T39.393	T39.394	T39.395	T39.396
Nimetazepam	T42.4x1	T42.4x2	T42.4x3	T42.4x4	T42.4x5	T42.4x6
Nimodipine	T46.1x1	T46.1x2	T46.1x3	T46.1x4	T46.1x5	T46.1x6
Nimorazole	T37.3x1	T37.3x2	T37.3x3	T37.3x4	T37.3x5	T37.3x6
Nimustine	T45.1x1	T45.1x2	T45.1x3	T45.1x4	T45.1x5	T45.1x6
Niridazole	T37.4x1	T37.4x2	T37.4x3	T37.4x4	T37.4x5	T37.4x6
Nisentil	T40.2x1	T40.2x2	T40.2x3	T40.2x4	T40.2x5	T40.2x6
Nisoldipine	T46.1x1	T46.1x2	T46.1x3	T46.1x4	T46.1x5	T46.1x6
Nitramine	T65.3x1	T65.3x2	T65.3x3	T65.3x4	—	—
Nitrate, organic	T46.3x1	T46.3x2	T46.3x3	T46.3x4	T46.3x5	T46.3x6
Nitrazepam	T42.4x1	T42.4x2	T42.4x3	T42.4x4	T42.4x5	T42.4x6
Nitrefazole	T50.6x1	T50.6x2	T50.6x3	T50.6x4	T50.6x5	T50.6x6
Nitrendipine	T46.1x1	T46.1x2	T46.1x3	T46.1x4	T46.1x5	T46.1x6
Nitric						
acid (liquid)	T54.2x1	T54.2x2	T54.2x3	T54.2x4	—	—
vapor	T59.891	T59.892	T59.893	T59.894	—	—
oxide (gas)	T59.0x1	T59.0x2	T59.0x3	T59.0x4	—	—
Nitrimidazine	T37.3x1	T37.3x2	T37.3x3	T37.3x4	T37.3x5	T37.3x6
Nitrite, amyl (medicinal) (vapor)	T46.3x1	T46.3x2	T46.3x3	T46.3x4	T46.3x5	T46.3x6
Nitroaniline	T65.3x1	T65.3x2	T65.3x3	T65.3x4	—	—
vapor	T59.891	T59.892	T59.893	T59.894	—	—
Nitrobenzene, nitrobenzol	T65.3x1	T65.3x2	T65.3x3	T65.3x4	—	—
vapor	T65.3x1	T65.3x2	T65.3x3	T65.3x4	—	—
Nitrocellulose	T65.891	T65.892	T65.893	T65.894	—	—
lacquer	T65.891	T65.892	T65.893	T65.894	—	—
Nitrodiphenyl	T65.3x1	T65.3x2	T65.3x3	T65.3x4	—	—
Nitrofural	T49.0x1	T49.0x2	T49.0x3	T49.0x4	T49.0x5	T49.0x6
Nitrofurantoin	T37.8x1	T37.8x2	T37.8x3	T37.8x4	T37.8x5	T37.8x6
Nitrofurazone	T49.0x1	T49.0x2	T49.0x3	T49.0x4	T49.0x5	T49.0x6
Nitrogen	T59.0x1	T59.0x2	T59.0x3	T59.0x4	—	—
mustard	T45.1x1	T45.1x2	T45.1x3	T45.1x4	T45.1x5	T45.1x6
Nitroglycerin, nitro-glycerol (medicinal)	T46.3x1	T46.3x2	T46.3x3	T46.3x4	T46.3x5	T46.3x6
nonmedicinal	T65.5x1	T65.5x2	T65.5x3	T65.5x4	—	—
fumes	T65.5x1	T65.5x2	T65.5x3	T65.5x4	—	—
Nitroglycol	T52.3x1	T52.3x2	T52.3x3	T52.3x4	—	—
Nitrohydrochloric acid	T54.2x1	T54.2x2	T54.2x3	T54.2x4	—	—
Nitromersol	T49.0x1	T49.0x2	T49.0x3	T49.0x4	T49.0x5	T49.0x6
Nitronaphthalene	T65.891	T65.892	T65.893	T65.894	—	—
Nitrophenol	T54.0x1	T54.0x2	T54.0x3	T54.0x4	—	—
Nitropropane	T52.8x1	T52.8x2	T52.8x3	T52.8x4	—	—
Nitroprusside	T46.5x1	T46.5x2	T46.5x3	T46.5x4	T46.5x5	T46.5x6
Nitrosodimethylamine	T65.3x1	T65.3x2	T65.3x3	T65.3x4	—	—
Nitrothiazol	T37.4x1	T37.4x2	T37.4x3	T37.4x4	T37.4x5	T37.4x6
Nitrotoluene, nitrotoluol	T65.3x1	T65.3x2	T65.3x3	T65.3x4	—	—
vapor	T65.3x1	T65.3x2	T65.3x3	T65.3x4	—	—

Substance	Poisoning, Accidental (unintentional)	Poisoning, Intentional Self-harm	Poisoning, Assault	Poisoning, Undetermined	Adverse Effect	Under-dosing
Nitrous						
acid (liquid)	T54.2x1	T54.2x2	T54.2x3	T54.2x4	—	—
fumes	T59.891	T59.892	T59.893	T59.894	—	—
ether spirit	T46.3x1	T46.3x2	T46.3x3	T46.3x4	T46.3x5	T46.3x6
oxide	T41.0x1	T41.0x2	T41.0x3	T41.0x4	T41.0x5	T41.0x6
Nitroxoline	T37.8x1	T37.8x2	T37.8x3	T37.8x4	T37.8x5	T37.8x6
Nitrozone	T49.0x1	T49.0x2	T49.0x3	T49.0x4	T49.0x5	T49.0x6
Nizatidine	T47.0x1	T47.0x2	T47.0x3	T47.0x4	T47.0x5	T47.0x6
Nizofenone	T43.8x1	T43.8x2	T43.8x3	T43.8x4	T43.8x5	T43.8x6
Noctec	T42.6x1	T42.6x2	T42.6x3	T42.6x4	T42.6x5	T42.6x6
Noludar	T42.6x1	T42.6x2	T42.6x3	T42.6x4	T42.6x5	T42.6x6
Noptil	T42.3x1	T42.3x2	T42.3x3	T42.3x4	T42.3x5	T42.3x6
Nomegestrol	T38.5x1	T38.5x2	T38.5x3	T38.5x4	T38.5x5	T38.5x6
Nomifensine	T43.291	T43.292	T43.293	T43.294	T43.295	T43.296
Nonoxinol	T49.8x1	T49.8x2	T49.8x3	T49.8x4	T49.8x5	T49.8x6
Nonylphenoxy (polyethoxy-ethanol)	T49.8x1	T49.8x2	T49.8x3	T49.8x4	T49.8x5	T49.8x6
Noptil	T42.3x1	T42.3x2	T42.3x3	T42.3x4	T42.3x5	T42.3x6
Noradrenaline	T44.4x1	T44.4x2	T44.4x3	T44.4x4	T44.4x5	T44.4x6
Noramidopyrine	T39.2x1	T39.2x2	T39.2x3	T39.2x4	T39.2x5	T39.2x6
methanesulfonate sodium	T39.2x1	T39.2x2	T39.2x3	T39.2x4	T39.2x5	T39.2x6
Norbormide	T60.4x1	T60.4x2	T60.4x3	T60.4x4	—	—
Nordazepam	T42.4x1	T42.4x2	T42.4x3	T42.4x4	T42.4x5	T42.4x6
Norepinephrine	T44.4x1	T44.4x2	T44.4x3	T44.4x4	T44.4x5	T44.4x6
Norethandrolone	T38.7x1	T38.7x2	T38.7x3	T38.7x4	T38.7x5	T38.7x6
Norethindrone	T38.4x1	T38.4x2	T38.4x3	T38.4x4	T38.4x5	T38.4x6
Norethisterone (acetate)(enantate)	T38.4x1	T38.4x2	T38.4x3	T38.4x4	T38.4x5	T38.4x6
with ethinylestradiol	T38.5x1	T38.5x2	T38.5x3	T38.5x4	T38.5x5	T38.5x6
Noretynodrel	T38.5x1	T38.5x2	T38.5x3	T38.5x4	T38.5x5	T38.5x6
Norfenefrine	T44.4x1	T44.4x2	T44.4x3	T44.4x4	T44.4x5	T44.4x6
Norfloxacin	T36.8x1	T36.8x2	T36.8x3	T36.8x4	T36.8x5	T36.8x6
Norgestrel	T38.4x1	T38.4x2	T38.4x3	T38.4x4	T38.4x5	T38.4x6
Norgestrienone	T38.4x1	T38.4x2	T38.4x3	T38.4x4	T38.4x5	T38.4x6
Norlestrin	T38.4x1	T38.4x2	T38.4x3	T38.4x4	T38.4x5	T38.4x6
Norlutin	T38.4x1	T38.4x2	T38.4x3	T38.4x4	T38.4x5	T38.4x6
Normal serum albumin (human), salt-poor	T45.8x1	T45.8x2	T45.8x3	T45.8x4	T45.8x5	T45.8x6
Normethandrone	T38.5x1	T38.5x2	T38.5x3	T38.5x4	T38.5x5	T38.5x6
Normison—see Benzodiazepines						
Normorphine	T40.2x1	T40.2x2	T40.2x3	T40.2x4	T40.2x5	T40.2x6
Norpseudoephedrine	T50.5x1	T50.5x2	T50.5x3	T50.5x4	T50.5x5	T50.5x6
Nortestosterone (furanpropionate)	T38.7x1	T38.7x2	T38.7x3	T38.7x4	T38.7x5	T38.7x6
Nortriptyline	T43.011	T43.012	T43.013	T43.014	T43.015	T43.016
Noscapine	T48.3x1	T48.3x2	T48.3x3	T48.3x4	T48.3x5	T48.3x6
Nose preparations	T49.6x1	T49.6x2	T49.6x3	T49.6x4	T49.6x5	T49.6x6
Novobiocin	T36.5x1	T36.5x2	T36.5x3	T36.5x4	T36.5x5	T36.5x6
Novocain (infiltration) (topical)	T41.3x1	T41.3x2	T41.3x3	T41.3x4	T41.3x5	T41.3x6
nerve block (peripheral) (plexus)	T41.3x1	T41.3x2	T41.3x3	T41.3x4	T41.3x5	T41.3x6
spinal	T41.3x1	T41.3x2	T41.3x3	T41.3x4	T41.3x5	T41.3x6
Noxious foodstuff	T62.91	T62.92	T62.93	T62.94		
specified NEC	T62.8x1	T62.8x2	T62.8x3	T62.8x4	—	—
Noxiptiline	T43.011	T43.012	T43.013	T43.014	T43.015	T43.016
Noxytiolin	T49.0x1	T49.0x2	T49.0x3	T49.0x4	T49.0x5	T49.0x6
NPH Iletin (insulin)	T38.3x1	T38.3x2	T38.3x3	T38.3x4	T38.3x5	T38.3x6
Numorphan	T40.2x1	T40.2x2	T40.2x3	T40.2x4	T40.2x5	T40.2x6
Nunol	T42.3x1	T42.3x2	T42.3x3	T42.3x4	T42.3x5	T42.3x6
Nupercaine (spinal anesthetic)	T41.3x1	T41.3x2	T41.3x3	T41.3x4	T41.3x5	T41.3x6
topical (surface)	T41.3x1	T41.3x2	T41.3x3	T41.3x4	T41.3x5	T41.3x6
Nutmeg oil (liniment)	T49.3x1	T49.3x2	T49.3x3	T49.3x4	T49.3x5	T49.3x6
Nutritional supplement	T50.901	T50.902	T50.903	T50.904	T50.905	T50.906
Nux vomica	T65.1x1	T65.1x2	T65.1x3	T65.1x4	—	—
Nydrazid	T37.1x1	T37.1x2	T37.1x3	T37.1x4	T37.1x5	T37.1x6
Nylidrin	T46.7x1	T46.7x2	T46.7x3	T46.7x4	T46.7x5	T46.7x6
Nystatin	T36.7x1	T36.7x2	T36.7x3	T36.7x4	T36.7x5	T36.7x6
topical	T49.0x1	T49.0x2	T49.0x3	T49.0x4	T49.0x5	T49.0x6
Nytol	T45.0x1	T45.0x2	T45.0x3	T45.0x4	T45.0x5	T45.0x6
Oblivion	T42.6x1	T42.6x2	T42.6x3	T42.6x4	T42.6x5	T42.6x6
Obidoxime chloride	T50.6x1	T50.6x2	T50.6x3	T50.6x4	T50.6x5	T50.6x6
Octafonium (chloride)	T49.3x1	T49.3x2	T49.3x3	T49.3x4	T49.3x5	T49.3x6

Substance	Poisoning, Accidental (unintentional)	Poisoning, Intentional Self-harm	Poisoning, Assault	Poisoning, Undetermined	Adverse Effect	Under-dosing
Octamethyl pyrophos-phoramide	T60.0x1	T60.0x2	T60.0x3	T60.0x4	—	—
Octanoin	T50.991	T50.992	T50.993	T50.994	T50.995	T50.996
Octatropine methylbromide	T44.3x1	T44.3x2	T44.3x3	T44.3x4	T44.3x5	T44.3x6
Octotiamine	T45.2x1	T45.2x2	T45.2x3	T45.2x4	T45.2x5	T45.2x6
Octoxinol (9)	T49.8x1	T49.8x2	T49.8x3	T49.8x4	T49.8x5	T49.8x6
Octreotide	T38.991	T38.992	T38.993	T38.994	T38.995	T38.996
Octyl nitrite	T46.3x1	T46.3x2	T46.3x3	T46.3x4	T46.3x5	T46.3x6
Oestradiol	T38.5x1	T38.5x2	T38.5x3	T38.5x4	T38.5x5	T38.5x6
Oestriol	T38.5x1	T38.5x2	T38.5x3	T38.5x4	T38.5x5	T38.5x6
Oestrogen	T38.5x1	T38.5x2	T38.5x3	T38.5x4	T38.5x5	T38.5x6
Oestrone	T38.5x1	T38.5x2	T38.5x3	T38.5x4	T38.5x5	T38.5x6
Ofloxacin	T36.8x1	T36.8x2	T36.8x3	T36.8x4	T36.8x5	T36.8x6
Oil (of)	T65.891	T65.892	T65.893	T65.894	—	—
bitter almond	T62.8x1	T62.8x2	T62.8x3	T62.8x4	—	—
cloves	T49.7x1	T49.7x2	T49.7x3	T49.7x4	T49.7x5	T49.7x6
colors	T65.6x1	T65.6x2	T65.6x3	T65.6x4	—	—
fumes	T59.891	T59.892	T59.893	T59.894	—	—
lubricating	T52.0x1	T52.0x2	T52.0x3	T52.0x4	—	—
Niobe	T52.8x1	T52.8x2	T52.8x3	T52.8x4	—	—
vitriol (liquid)	T54.2x1	T54.2x2	T54.2x3	T54.2x4	—	—
fumes	T54.2x1	T54.2x2	T54.2x3	T54.2x4	—	—
wintergreen (bitter) NEC	T49.3x1	T49.3x2	T49.3x3	T49.3x4	T49.3x5	T49.3x6
Oily preparation (for skin)	T49.3x1	T49.3x2	T49.3x3	T49.3x4	T49.3x5	T49.3x6
Ointment NEC	T49.3x1	T49.3x2	T49.3x3	T49.3x4	T49.3x5	T49.3x6
Olanzapine	T43.591	T43.592	T43.593	T43.594	T43.595	T43.596
Oleander	T62.2x1	T62.2x2	T62.2x3	T62.2x4	—	—
Oleandomycin	T36.3x1	T36.3x2	T36.3x3	T36.3x4	T36.3x5	T36.3x6
Oleandrin	T46.0x1	T46.0x2	T46.0x3	T46.0x4	T46.0x5	T46.0x6
Oleic acid	T46.6x1	T46.6x2	T46.6x3	T46.6x4	T46.6x5	T46.6x6
Oleovitamin A	T45.2x1	T45.2x2	T45.2x3	T45.2x4	T45.2x5	T45.2x6
Oleum ricini	T47.2x1	T47.2x2	T47.2x3	T47.2x4	T47.2x5	T47.2x6
Olive oil (medicinal) **NEC**	T47.4x1	T47.4x2	T47.4x3	T47.4x4	T47.4x5	T47.4x6
Olivomycin	T45.1x1	T45.1x2	T45.1x3	T45.1x4	T45.1x5	T45.1x6
Olsalazine	T47.8x1	T47.8x2	T47.8x3	T47.8x4	T47.8x5	T47.8x6
Omeprazole	T47.1x1	T47.1x2	T47.1x3	T47.1x4	T47.1x5	T47.1x6
OMPA	T60.0x1	T60.0x2	T60.0x3	T60.0x4	—	—
Ondansetron	T45.0x1	T45.0x2	T45.0x3	T45.0x4	T45.0x5	T45.0x6
Oncovin	T45.1x1	T45.1x2	T45.1x3	T45.1x4	T45.1x5	T45.1x6
Ophthaine	T41.3x1	T41.3x2	T41.3x3	T41.3x4	T41.3x5	T41.3x6
Ophthetic	T41.3x1	T41.3x2	T41.3x3	T41.3x4	T41.3x5	T41.3x6
Opiate NEC	T40.601	T40.602	T40.603	T40.604	T40.605	T40.606
antagonists	T50.7x1	T50.7x2	T50.7x3	T50.7x4	T50.7x5	T50.7x6
Opipramol	T43.011	T43.012	T43.013	T43.014	T43.015	T43.016
Opium alkaloids (total)	T40.0x1	T40.0x2	T40.0x3	T40.0x4	T40.0x5	T40.0x6
standardized powdered	T40.0x1	T40.0x2	T40.0x3	T40.0x4	T40.0x5	T40.0x6
tincture (camphorated)	T40.0x1	T40.0x2	T40.0x3	T40.0x4	T40.0x5	T40.0x6
Oracon	T38.4x1	T38.4x2	T38.4x3	T38.4x4	T38.4x5	T38.4x6
Oragrafin	T50.8x1	T50.8x2	T50.8x3	T50.8x4	T50.8x5	T50.8x6
Oral contraceptives	T38.4x1	T38.4x2	T38.4x3	T38.4x4	T38.4x5	T38.4x6
Oral rehydration salts	T50.3x1	T50.3x2	T50.3x3	T50.3x4	T50.3x5	T50.3x6
Orazamide	T50.991	T50.992	T50.993	T50.994	T50.995	T50.996
Orciprenaline	T48.291	T48.292	T48.293	T48.294	T48.295	T48.296
Organidin	T48.4x1	T48.4x2	T48.4x3	T48.4x4	T48.4x5	T48.4x6
Organonitrate NEC	T46.3x1	T46.3x2	T46.3x3	T46.3x4	T46.3x5	T46.3x6
Organophosphates	T60.0x1	T60.0x2	T60.0x3	T60.0x4	—	—
Orimune	T50.B91	T50.B92	T50.B93	T50.B94	T50.B95	T50.B96
Orinase	T38.3x1	T38.3x2	T38.3x3	T38.3x4	T38.3x5	T38.3x6
Ormeloxifene	T38.6x1	T38.6x2	T38.6x3	T38.6x4	T38.6x5	T38.6x6
Ornidazole	T37.3x1	T37.3x2	T37.3x3	T37.3x4	T37.3x5	T37.3x6
Ornithine aspartate	T50.991	T50.992	T50.993	T50.994	T50.995	T50.996
Ornoprostil	T47.1x1	T47.1x2	T47.1x3	T47.1x4	T47.1x5	T47.1x6
Orphenadrine (hydrochloride)	T42.8x1	T42.8x2	T42.8x3	T42.8x4	T42.8x5	T42.8x6
Ortal (sodium)	T42.3x1	T42.3x2	T42.3x3	T42.3x4	T42.3x5	T42.3x6
Orthoboric acid	T49.0x1	T49.0x2	T49.0x3	T49.0x4	T49.0x5	T49.0x6
ENT agent	T49.6x1	T49.6x2	T49.6x3	T49.6x4	T49.6x5	T49.6x6
ophthalmic preparation	T49.5x1	T49.5x2	T49.5x3	T49.5x4	T49.5x5	T49.5x6
Orthocaine	T41.3x1	T41.3x2	T41.3x3	T41.3x4	T41.3x5	T41.3x6
Orthodichlorobenzene	T53.7x1	T53.7x2	T53.7x3	T53.7x4	—	—
Ortho-Novum	T38.4x1	T38.4x2	T38.4x3	T38.4x4	T38.4x5	T38.4x6
Orthotolidine (reagent)	T54.2x1	T54.2x2	T54.2x3	T54.2x4	—	—

Substance	Poisoning, Accidental (unintentional)	Poisoning, Intentional Self-harm	Poisoning, Assault	Poisoning, Undetermined	Adverse Effect	Underdosing
Osmic acid (liquid)	T54.2x1	T54.2x2	T54.2x3	T54.2x4	—	—
fumes	T54.2x1	T54.2x2	T54.2x3	T54.2x4		
Osmotic diuretics	T50.2x1	T50.2x2	T50.2x3	T50.2x4	T50.2x5	T50.2x6
Otilonium bromide	T44.3x1	T44.3x2	T44.3x3	T44.3x4	T44.3x5	T44.3x6
Ouabain(e)	T46.0x1	T46.0x2	T46.0x3	T46.0x4	T46.0x5	T46.0x6
Ovarian						
hormone	T38.5x1	T38.5x2	T38.5x3	T38.5x4	T38.5x5	T38.5x6
stimulant	T38.5x1	T38.5x2	T38.5x3	T38.5x4	T38.5x5	T38.5x6
Ovral	T38.4x1	T38.4x2	T38.4x3	T38.4x4	T38.4x5	T38.4x6
Ovulen	T38.4x1	T38.4x2	T38.4x3	T38.4x4	T38.4x5	T38.4x6
Oxacillin	T36.0x1	T36.0x2	T36.0x3	T36.0x4	T36.0x5	T36.0x6
Oxalic acid	T54.2x1	T54.2x2	T54.2x3	T54.2x4	—	—
ammonium salt	T50.991	T50.992	T50.993	T50.994	T50.995	T50.996
Oxamniquine	T37.4x1	T37.4x2	T37.4x3	T37.4x4	T37.4x5	T37.4x6
Oxanamide	T43.591	T43.592	T43.593	T43.594	T43.595	T43.596
Oxandrolone	T38.7x1	T38.7x2	T38.7x3	T38.7x4	T38.7x5	T38.7x6
Oxantel	T37.4x1	T37.4x2	T37.4x3	T37.4x4	T37.4x5	T37.4x6
Oxapium iodide	T44.3x1	T44.3x2	T44.3x3	T44.3x4	T44.3x5	T44.3x6
Oxaprotiline	T43.021	T43.022	T43.023	T43.024	T43.025	T43.026
Oxaprozin	T39.311	T39.312	T39.313	T39.314	T39.315	T39.316
Oxatomide	T45.0x1	T45.0x2	T45.0x3	T45.0x4	T45.0x5	T45.0x6
Oxazepam	T42.4x1	T42.4x2	T42.4x3	T42.4x4	T42.4x5	T42.4x6
Oxazimedrine	T50.5x1	T50.5x2	T50.5x3	T50.5x4	T50.5x5	T50.5x6
Oxazolam	T42.4x1	T42.4x2	T42.4x3	T42.4x4	T42.4x5	T42.4x6
Oxazolidine derivatives	T42.2x1	T42.2x2	T42.2x3	T42.2x4	T42.2x5	T42.2x6
Ox bile extract	T47.5x1	T47.5x2	T47.5x3	T47.5x4	T47.5x5	T47.5x6
Oxcarbazepine	T42.1x1	T42.1x2	T42.1x3	T42.1x4	T42.1x5	T42.1x6
Oxedrine	T44.4x1	T44.4x2	T44.4x3	T44.4x4	T44.4x5	T44.4x6
Oxeladin (citrate)	T48.3x1	T48.3x2	T48.3x3	T48.3x4	T48.3x5	T48.3x6
Oxendolone	T38.5x1	T38.5x2	T38.5x3	T38.5x4	T38.5x5	T38.5x6
Oxetacaine	T41.3x1	T41.3x2	T41.3x3	T41.3x4	T41.3x5	T41.3x6
Oxethazine	T41.3x1	T41.3x2	T41.3x3	T41.3x4	T41.3x5	T41.3x6
Oxetorone	T39.8x1	T39.8x2	T39.8x3	T39.8x4	T39.8x5	T39.8x6
Oxiconazole	T49.0x1	T49.0x2	T49.0x3	T49.0x4	T49.0x5	T49.0x6
Oxidizing agent NEC	T54.91	T54.92	T54.93	T54.94	—	—
Oxipurinol	T50.4x1	T50.4x2	T50.4x3	T50.4x4	T50.4x5	T50.4x6
Oxitriptan	T43.291	T43.292	T43.293	T43.294	T43.295	T43.296
Oxitropium bromide	T48.6x1	T48.6x2	T48.6x3	T48.6x4	T48.6x5	T48.6x6
Oxodipine	T46.1x1	T46.1x2	T46.1x3	T46.1x4	T46.1x5	T46.1x6
Oxolamine	T48.3x1	T48.3x2	T48.3x3	T48.3x4	T48.3x5	T48.3x6
Oxolinic acid	T37.8x1	T37.8x2	T37.8x3	T37.8x4	T37.8x5	T37.8x6
Oxomemazine	T43.3x1	T43.3x2	T43.3x3	T43.3x4	T43.3x5	T43.3x6
Oxophenarsine	T37.3x1	T37.3x2	T37.3x3	T37.3x4	T37.3x5	T37.3x6
Oxprenolol	T44.7x1	T44.7x2	T44.7x3	T44.7x4	T44.7x5	T44.7x6
Oxsoralen	T49.3x1	T49.3x2	T49.3x3	T49.3x4	T49.3x5	T49.3x6
Oxtriphylline	T48.6x1	T48.6x2	T48.6x3	T48.6x4	T48.6x5	T48.6x6
Oxybate sodium	T41.291	T41.292	T41.293	T41.294	T41.295	T41.296
Oxybuprocaine	T41.3x1	T41.3x2	T41.3x3	T41.3x4	T41.3x5	T41.3x6
Oxybutynin	T44.3x1	T44.3x2	T44.3x3	T44.3x4	T44.3x5	T44.3x6
Oxychlorosene	T49.0x1	T49.0x2	T49.0x3	T49.0x4	T49.0x5	T49.0x6
Oxycodone	T40.2x1	T40.2x2	T40.2x3	T40.2x4	T40.2x5	T40.2x6
Oxyfedrine	T46.3x1	T46.3x2	T46.3x3	T46.3x4	T46.3x5	T46.3x6
Oxygen	T41.5x1	T41.5x2	T41.5x3	T41.5x4	T41.5x5	T41.5x6
Oxylone	T49.0x1	T49.0x2	T49.0x3	T49.0x4	T49.0x5	T49.0x6
ophthalmic preparation	T49.5x1	T49.5x2	T49.5x3	T49.5x4	T49.5x5	T49.5x6
Oxymesterone	T38.7x1	T38.7x2	T38.7x3	T38.7x4	T38.7x5	T38.7x6
Oxymetazoline	T48.5x1	T48.5x2	T48.5x3	T48.5x4	T48.5x5	T48.5x6
Oxymetholone	T38.7x1	T38.7x2	T38.7x3	T38.7x4	T38.7x5	T38.7x6
Oxymorphone	T40.2x1	T40.2x2	T40.2x3	T40.2x4	T40.2x5	T40.2x6
Oxypertine	T43.591	T43.592	T43.593	T43.594	T43.595	T43.596
Oxyphenbutazone	T39.2x1	T39.2x2	T39.2x3	T39.2x4	T39.2x5	T39.2x6
Oxyphencyclimine	T44.3x1	T44.3x2	T44.3x3	T44.3x4	T44.3x5	T44.3x6
Oxyphenisatine	T47.2x1	T47.2x2	T47.2x3	T47.2x4	T47.2x5	T47.2x6
Oxyphenonium bromide	T44.3x1	T44.3x2	T44.3x3	T44.3x4	T44.3x5	T44.3x6
Oxypolygelatin	T45.8x1	T45.8x2	T45.8x3	T45.8x4	T45.8x5	T45.8x6
Oxyquinoline (derivatives)	T37.8x1	T37.8x2	T37.8x3	T37.8x4	T37.8x5	T37.8x6
Oxytetracycline	T36.4x1	T36.4x2	T36.4x3	T36.4x4	T36.4x5	T36.4x6
Oxytocic drug NEC	T48.0x1	T48.0x2	T48.0x3	T48.0x4	T48.0x5	T48.0x6
Oxytocin (synthetic)	T48.0x1	T48.0x2	T48.0x3	T48.0x4	T48.0x5	T48.0x6
Ozone	T59.891	T59.892	T59.893	T59.894	—	—
PABA	T49.3x1	T49.3x2	T49.3x3	T49.3x4	T49.3x5	T49.3x6

Substance	Poisoning, Accidental (unintentional)	Poisoning, Intentional Self-harm	Poisoning, Assault	Poisoning, Undetermined	Adverse Effect	Underdosing
Packed red cells	T45.8x1	T45.8x2	T45.8x3	T45.8x4	T45.8x5	T45.8x6
Padimate	T49.3x1	T49.3x2	T49.3x3	T49.3x4	T49.3x5	T49.3x6
Paint NEC	T65.6x1	T65.6x2	T65.6x3	T65.6x4	—	—
cleaner	T52.91	T52.92	T52.93	T52.94	—	—
fumes NEC	T59.891	T59.892	T59.893	T59.894	—	—
lead (fumes)	T56.0x1	T56.0x2	T56.0x3	T56.0x4	—	—
solvent NEC	T52.8x1	T52.8x2	T52.8x3	T52.8x4	—	—
stripper	T52.8x1	T52.8x2	T52.8x3	T52.8x4	—	—
Palfium	T40.2x1	T40.2x2	T40.2x3	T40.2x4	T40.2x5	T40.2x6
Palm kernel oil	T50.991	T50.992	T50.993	T50.994	T50.995	T50.996
Paludrine	T37.2x1	T37.2x2	T37.2x3	T37.2x4	T37.2x5	T37.2x6
PAM (pralidoxime)	T50.6x1	T50.6x2	T50.6x3	T50.6x4	T50.6x5	T50.6x6
Pamaquine (naphthoute)	T37.2x1	T37.2x2	T37.2x3	T37.2x4	T37.2x5	T37.2x6
Panadol	T39.1x1	T39.1x2	T39.1x3	T39.1x4	T39.1x5	T39.1x6
Pancreatic						
digestive secretion stimulant	T47.8x1	T47.8x2	T47.8x3	T47.8x4	T47.8x5	T47.8x6
dornase	T45.3x1	T45.3x2	T45.3x3	T45.3x4	T45.3x5	T45.3x6
Pancreatin	T47.5x1	T47.5x2	T47.5x3	T47.5x4	T47.5x5	T47.5x6
Pancrelipase	T47.5x1	T47.5x2	T47.5x3	T47.5x4	T47.5x5	T47.5x6
Pancuronium (bromide)	T48.1x1	T48.1x2	T48.1x3	T48.1x4	T48.1x5	T48.1x6
Pangamic acid	T45.2x1	T45.2x2	T45.2x3	T45.2x4	T45.2x5	T45.2x6
Panthenol	T45.2x1	T45.2x2	T45.2x3	T45.2x4	T45.2x5	T45.2x6
topical	T49.8x1	T49.8x2	T49.8x3	T49.8x4	T49.8x5	T49.8x6
Pantopon	T40.0x1	T40.0x2	T40.0x3	T40.0x4	T40.0x5	T40.0x6
Pantothenic acid	T45.2x1	T45.2x2	T45.2x3	T45.2x4	T45.2x5	T45.2x6
Panwarfin	T45.511	T45.512	T45.513	T45.514	T45.515	T45.516
Papain	T47.5x1	T47.5x2	T47.5x3	T47.5x4	T47.5x5	T47.5x6
digestant	T47.5x1	T47.5x2	T47.5x3	T47.5x4	T47.5x5	T47.5x6
Papaveretum	T40.0x1	T40.0x2	T40.0x3	T40.0x4	T40.0x5	T40.0x6
Papaverine	T44.3x1	T44.3x2	T44.3x3	T44.3x4	T44.3x5	T44.3x6
Para-acetamidophenol	T39.1x1	T39.1x2	T39.1x3	T39.1x4	T39.1x5	T39.1x6
Para-aminobenzoic acid	T49.3x1	T49.3x2	T49.3x3	T49.3x4	T49.3x5	T49.3x6
Para-aminophenol derivatives	T39.1x1	T39.1x2	T39.1x3	T39.1x4	T39.1x5	T39.1x6
Para-aminosalicylic acid	T37.1x1	T37.1x2	T37.1x3	T37.1x4	T37.1x5	T37.1x6
Paracetaldehyde	T42.6x1	T42.6x2	T42.6x3	T42.6x4	T42.6x5	T42.6x6
Paracetamol	T39.1x1	T39.1x2	T39.1x3	T39.1x4	T39.1x5	T39.1x6
Parachlorophenol (camphorated)	T49.0x1	T49.0x2	T49.0x3	T49.0x4	T49.0x5	T49.0x6
Paracodin	T40.2x1	T40.2x2	T40.2x3	T40.2x4	T40.2x5	T40.2x6
Paradione	T42.2x1	T42.2x2	T42.2x3	T42.2x4	T42.2x5	T42.2x6
Paraffin(s) (wax)	T52.0x1	T52.0x2	T52.0x3	T52.0x4	—	—
liquid (medicinal)	T47.4x1	T47.4x2	T47.4x3	T47.4x4	T47.4x5	T47.4x6
nonmedicinal	T52.0x1	T52.0x2	T52.0x3	T52.0x4	—	—
Paraformaldehyde	T60.3x1	T60.3x2	T60.3x3	T60.3x4	—	—
Paraldehyde	T42.6x1	T42.6x2	T42.6x3	T42.6x4	T42.6x5	T42.6x6
Paramethadione	T42.2x1	T42.2x2	T42.2x3	T42.2x4	T42.2x5	T42.2x6
Paramethasone	T38.0x1	T38.0x2	T38.0x3	T38.0x4	T38.0x5	T38.0x6
acetate	T49.0x1	T49.0x2	T49.0x3	T49.0x4	T49.0x5	T49.0x6
Paraoxon	T60.0x1	T60.0x2	T60.0x3	T60.0x4	—	—
Paraquat	T60.3x1	T60.3x2	T60.3x3	T60.3x4	—	—
Parasympatholytic NEC	T44.3x1	T44.3x2	T44.3x3	T44.3x4	T44.3x5	T44.3x6
Parasympathomimetic drug NEC	T44.1x1	T44.1x2	T44.1x3	T44.1x4	T44.1x5	T44.1x6
Parathion	T60.0x1	T60.0x2	T60.0x3	T60.0x4	—	—
Parathormone	T50.991	T50.992	T50.993	T50.994	T50.995	T50.996
Parathyroid extract	T50.991	T50.992	T50.993	T50.994	T50.995	T50.996
Paratyphoid vaccine	T50.A91	T50.A92	T50.A93	T50.A94	T50.A95	T50.A96
Paredrine	T44.4x1	T44.4x2	T44.4x3	T44.4x4	T44.4x5	T44.4x6
Paregoric	T40.0x1	T40.0x2	T40.0x3	T40.0x4	T40.0x5	T40.0x6
Pargyline	T46.5x1	T46.5x2	T46.5x3	T46.5x4	T46.5x5	T46.5x6
Paris green	T57.0x1	T57.0x2	T57.0x3	T57.0x4	—	—
insecticide	T57.0x1	T57.0x2	T57.0x3	T57.0x4	—	—
Parnate	T43.1x1	T43.1x2	T43.1x3	T43.1x4	T43.1x5	T43.1x6
Paromomycin	T36.5x1	T36.5x2	T36.5x3	T36.5x4	T36.5x5	T36.5x6
Paroxypropione	T45.1x1	T45.1x2	T45.1x3	T45.1x4	T45.1x5	T45.1x6
Parzone	T40.2x1	T40.2x2	T40.2x3	T40.2x4	T40.2x5	T40.2x6
PAS	T37.1x1	T37.1x2	T37.1x3	T37.1x4	T37.1x5	T37.1x6
Pasiniazid	T37.1x1	T37.1x2	T37.1x3	T37.1x4	T37.1x5	T37.1x6
PBB (polybrominated biphenyls)	T65.891	T65.892	T65.893	T65.894	—	—
PCB	T65.891	T65.892	T65.893	T65.894	—	—

Substance	Poisoning, Accidental (unintentional)	Poisoning, Intentional Self-harm	Poisoning, Assault	Poisoning, Undetermined	Adverse Effect	Under-dosing
PCP (pentachlorophenol)	T60.1x1	T60.1x2	T60.1x3	T60.1x4	—	—
fungicide	T60.3x1	T60.3x2	T60.3x3	T60.3x4	—	—
herbicide	T60.3x1	T60.3x2	T60.3x3	T60.3x4	—	—
insecticide	T60.1x1	T60.1x2	T60.1x3	T60.1x4	—	—
phencyclidine	T40.991	T40.992	T40.993	T40.994	T40.995	T40.996
Peach kernel oil (emulsion)	T47.4x1	T47.4x2	T47.4x3	T47.4x4	T47.4x5	T47.4x6
Peanut oil (emulsion) **NEC**	T47.4x1	T47.4x2	T47.4x3	T47.4x4	T47.4x5	T47.4x6
topical	T49.3x1	T49.3x2	T49.3x3	T49.3x4	T49.3x5	T49.3x6
Pearly Gates (morning glory seeds)	T40.991	T40.992	T40.993	T40.994	T40.995	T40.996
Pecazine	T43.3x1	T43.3x2	T43.3x3	T43.3x4	T43.3x5	T43.3x6
Pectin	T47.6x1	T47.6x2	T47.6x3	T47.6x4	T47.6x5	T47.6x6
Pefloxacin	T37.8x1	T37.8x2	T37.8x3	T37.8x4	T37.8x5	T37.8x6
Pegademase, bovine	T50.Z91	T50.Z92	T50.Z93	T50.Z94	T50.Z95	T50.Z96
Pelletierine tannate	T37.4x1	T37.4x2	T37.4x3	T37.4x4	T37.4x5	T37.4x6
Pemirolast (potassium)	T48.6x1	T48.6x2	T48.6x3	T48.6x4	T48.6x5	T48.6x6
Pemoline	T50.7x1	T50.7x2	T50.7x3	T50.7x4	T50.7x5	T50.7x6
Pempidine	T44.2x1	T44.2x2	T44.2x3	T44.2x4	T44.2x5	T44.2x6
Penamecillin	T36.0x1	T36.0x2	T36.0x3	T36.0x4	T36.0x5	T36.0x6
Penbutolol	T44.7x1	T44.7x2	T44.7x3	T44.7x4	T44.7x5	T44.7x6
Penethamate	T36.0x1	T36.0x2	T36.0x3	T36.0x4	T36.0x5	T36.0x6
Penfluridol	T43.591	T43.592	T43.593	T43.594	T43.595	T43.596
Penflutizide	T50.2x1	T50.2x2	T50.2x3	T50.2x4	T50.2x5	T50.2x6
Pengitoxin	T46.0x1	T46.0x2	T46.0x3	T46.0x4	T46.0x5	T46.0x6
Penicillamine	T50.6x1	T50.6x2	T50.6x3	T50.6x4	T50.6x5	T50.6x6
Penicillin (any)	T36.0x1	T36.0x2	T36.0x3	T36.0x4	T36.0x5	I36.0x6
Penicillinase	T45.3x1	T45.3x2	T45.3x3	T45.3x4	T45.3x5	T45.3x6
Penicilloyl polylysine	T50.8x1	T50.8x2	T50.8x3	T50.8x4	T50.8x5	T50.8x6
Penimepicycline	T36.4x1	T36.4x2	T36.4x3	T36.4x4	T36.4x5	T36.4x6
Pentachloroethane	T53.6x1	T53.6x2	T53.6x3	T53.6x4	—	—
Pentachloronaphthalene	T53.7x1	T53.7x2	T53.7x3	T53.7x4	—	—
Pentachlorophenol (pesticide)	T60.3x1	T60.3x2	T60.3x3	T60.3x4	—	—
herbicide	T60.3x1	T60.3x2	T60.3x3	T60.3x4	—	—
insecticide	T60.1x1	T60.1x2	T60.1x3	T60.1x4	—	—
Pentaerythritol tetranitrate	T46.3x1	T46.3x2	T46.3x3	T46.3x4	T46.3x5	T46.3x6
Pentaerythritol	T46.3x1	T46.3x2	T46.3x3	T46.3x4	T46.3x5	T46.3x6
chloral	T42.6x1	T42.6x2	T42.6x3	T42.6x4	T42.6x5	T42.6x6
tetranitrate NEC	T46.3x1	T46.3x2	T46.3x3	T46.3x4	T46.3x5	T46.3x6
Pentaerythrityl tetranitrate	T46.3x1	T46.3x2	T46.3x3	T46.3x4	T46.3x5	T46.3x6
Pentagastrin	T50.8x1	T50.8x2	T50.8x3	T50.8x4	T50.8x5	T50.8x6
Pentalin	T53.6x1	T53.6x2	T53.6x3	T53.6x4	—	—
Pentamethonium bromide	T44.2x1	T44.2x2	T44.2x3	T44.2x4	T44.2x5	T44.2x6
Pentamidine	T37.3x1	T37.3x2	T37.3x3	T37.3x4	T37.3x5	T37.3x6
Pentanol	T51.3x1	T51.3x2	T51.3x3	T51.3x4	—	—
Pentapyrrolinium (bitartrate)	T44.2x1	T44.2x2	T44.2x3	T44.2x4	T44.2x5	T44.2x6
Pentaquine	T37.2x1	T37.2x2	T37.2x3	T37.2x4	T37.2x5	T37.2x6
Pentazocine	T40.4x1	T40.4x2	T40.4x3	T40.4x4	T40.4x5	T40.4x6
Pentetrazole	T50.7x1	T50.7x2	T50.7x3	T50.7x4	T50.7x5	T50.7x6
Penthienate bromide	T44.3x1	T44.3x2	T44.3x3	T44.3x4	T44.3x5	T44.3x6
Pentifylline	T46.7x1	T46.7x2	T46.7x3	T46.7x4	T46.7x5	T46.7x6
Pentobarbital	T42.3x1	T42.3x2	T42.3x3	T42.3x4	T42.3x5	T42.3x6
sodium	T42.3x1	T42.3x2	T42.3x3	T42.3x4	T42.3x5	T42.3x6
Pentobarbitone	T42.3x1	T42.3x2	T42.3x3	T42.3x4	T42.3x5	T42.3x6
Pentolonium tartrate	T44.2x1	T44.2x2	T44.2x3	T44.2x4	T44.2x5	T44.2x6
Pentosan polysulfate (sodium)	T45.511	T45.512	T45.513	T45.514	T45.515	T45.516
Pentostatin	T45.1x1	T45.1x2	T45.1x3	T45.1x4	T45.1x5	T45.1x6
Pentothal	T41.1x1	T41.1x2	T41.1x3	T41.1x4	T41.1x5	T41.1x6
Pentoxifylline	T46.7x1	T46.7x2	T46.7x3	T46.7x4	T46.7x5	T46.7x6
Pentoxyverine	T48.3x1	T48.3x2	T48.3x3	T48.3x4	T48.3x5	T48.3x6
Pentrinat	T46.3x1	T46.3x2	T46.3x3	T46.3x4	T46.3x5	T46.3x6
Pentylenetetrazole	T50.7x1	T50.7x2	T50.7x3	T50.7x4	T50.7x5	T50.7x6
Pentylsalicylamide	T37.1x1	T37.1x2	T37.1x3	T37.1x4	T37.1x5	T37.1x6
Pentymal	T42.3x1	T42.3x2	T42.3x3	T42.3x4	T42.3x5	T42.3x6
Peplomycin	T45.1x1	T45.1x2	T45.1x3	T45.1x4	T45.1x5	T45.1x6
Peppermint (oil)	T47.5x1	T47.5x2	T47.5x3	T47.5x4	T47.5x5	T47.5x6
Pepsin	T47.5x1	T47.5x2	T47.5x3	T47.5x4	T47.5x5	T47.5x6
digestant	T47.5x1	T47.5x2	T47.5x3	T47.5x4	T47.5x5	T47.5x6
Pepstatin	T47.1x1	T47.1x2	T47.1x3	T47.1x4	T47.1x5	T47.1x6
Peptavlon	T50.8x1	T50.8x2	T50.8x3	T50.8x4	T50.8x5	T50.8x6
Perazine	T43.3x1	T43.3x2	T43.3x3	T43.3x4	T43.3x5	T43.3x6

Substance	Poisoning, Accidental (unintentional)	Poisoning, Intentional Self-harm	Poisoning, Assault	Poisoning, Undetermined	Adverse Effect	Under-dosing
Percaine (spinal)	T41.3x1	T41.3x2	T41.3x3	T41.3x4	T41.3x5	T41.3x6
topical (surface)	T41.3x1	T41.3x2	T41.3x3	T41.3x4	T41.3x5	T41.3x6
Perchloroethylene	T53.3x1	T53.3x2	T53.3x3	T53.3x4	—	—
vapor	T53.3x1	T53.3x2	T53.3x3	T53.3x4	—	—
medicinal	T37.4x1	T37.4x2	T37.4x3	T37.4x4	T37.4x5	T37.4x6
Percodan	T40.2x1	T40.2x2	T40.2x3	T40.2x4	T40.2x5	T40.2x6
Percogesic	T40.2x1	T40.2x2	T40.2x3	T40.2x4	T40.2x5	T40.2x6
Percorten	T38.0x1	T38.0x2	T38.0x3	T38.0x4	T38.0x5	T38.0x6
Pergolide	T42.8x1	T42.8x2	T42.8x3	T42.8x4	T42.8x5	T42.8x6
Pergonal	T38.811	T38.812	T38.813	T38.814	T38.815	T38.816
Perhexilene	T46.3x1	T46.3x2	T46.3x3	T46.3x4	T46.3x5	T46.3x6
Perhexiline (maleate)	T46.3x1	T46.3x2	T46.3x3	T46.3x4	T46.3x5	T46.3x6
Periactin	T45.0x1	T45.0x2	T45.0x3	T45.0x4	T45.0x5	T45.0x6
Periciazine	T43.3x1	T43.3x2	T43.3x3	T43.3x4	T43.3x5	T43.3x6
Periclor	T42.6x1	T42.6x2	T42.6x3	T42.6x4	T42.6x5	T42.6x6
Perindopril	T46.4x1	T46.4x2	T46.4x3	T46.4x4	T46.4x5	T46.4x6
Perisoxal	T39.8x1	T39.8x2	T39.8x3	T39.8x4	T39.8x5	T39.8x6
Peritrate	T46.3x1	T46.3x2	T46.3x3	T46.3x4	T46.3x5	T46.3x6
Peritoneal dialysis solution	T50.3x1	T50.3x2	T50.3x3	T50.3x4	T50.3x5	T50.3x6
Perlapine	T42.4x1	T42.4x2	T42.4x3	T42.4x4	T42.4x5	T42.4x6
Permanganate	T65.891	T65.892	T65.893	T65.894	—	—
Permethrin	T60.1x1	T60.1x2	T60.1x3	T60.1x4	—	—
Pernocton	T42.3x1	T42.3x2	T42.3x3	T42.3x4	T42.3x5	T42.3x6
Pernoston	T42.3x1	T42.3x2	T42.3x3	T42.3x4	T42.3x5	T42.3x6
Peronin(e)	T40.2x1	T40.2x2	T40.2x3	T40.2x4	T40.2x5	T40.2x6
Perphenazine	T43.3x1	T43.3x2	T43.3x3	T43.3x4	T43.3x5	T43.3x6
Pertofrane	T43.011	T43.012	T43.013	T43.014	T43.015	T43.016
Pertussis vaccine	T50.A11	T50.A12	T50.A13	T50.A14	T50.A15	T50.A16
Pertussis						
immune serum (human)	T50.Z11	T50.Z12	T50.Z13	T50.Z14	T50.Z15	T50.Z16
vaccine (with diphtheria toxoid) (with tetanus toxoid)	T50.A11	T50.A12	T50.A13	T50.A14	T50.A15	T50.A16
Peruvian balsam	T49.0x1	T49.0x2	T49.0x3	T49.0x4	T49.0x5	T49.0x6
Peruvoside	T46.0x1	T46.0x2	T46.0x3	T46.0x4	T46.0x5	T46.0x6
Pesticide (dust) (fumes) (vapor) **NEC**	T60.91	T60.92	T60.93	T60.94		
arsenic	T57.0x1	T57.0x2	T57.0x3	T57.0x4	—	—
chlorinated	T60.1x1	T60.1x2	T60.1x3	T60.1x4	—	—
cyanide	T65.0x1	T65.0x2	T65.0x3	T65.0x4	—	—
kerosene	T52.0x1	T52.0x2	T52.0x3	T52.0x4	—	—
mixture (of compounds)	T60.91	T60.92	T60.93	T60.94		
naphthalene	T60.2x1	T60.2x2	T60.2x3	T60.2x4	—	—
organochlorine (compounds)	T60.1x1	T60.1x2	T60.1x3	T60.1x4	—	—
petroleum (distillate) (products) NEC	T52.0x1	T52.0x2	T52.0x3	T52.0x4	—	—
specified ingredient NEC	T60.8x1	T60.8x2	T60.8x3	T60.8x4	—	—
strychnine	T65.1x1	T65.1x2	T65.1x3	T65.1x4	—	—
thallium	T60.4x1	T60.4x2	T60.4x3	T60.4x4	—	—
Pethidine	T40.4x1	T40.4x2	T40.4x3	T40.4x4	T40.4x5	T40.4x6
Petrichloral	T42.6x1	T42.6x2	T42.6x3	T42.6x4	T42.6x5	T42.6x6
Petrol	T52.0x1	T52.0x2	T52.0x3	T52.0x4	—	—
vapor	T52.0x1	T52.0x2	T52.0x3	T52.0x4	—	—
Petrolatum	T49.3x1	T49.3x2	T49.3x3	T49.3x4	T49.3x5	T49.3x6
hydrophilic	T49.3x1	T49.3x2	T49.3x3	T49.3x4	T49.3x5	T49.3x6
liquid	T47.4x1	T47.4x2	T47.4x3	T47.4x4	T47.4x5	T47.4x6
topical	T49.3x1	T49.3x2	T49.3x3	T49.3x4	T49.3x5	T49.3x6
nonmedicinal	T52.0x1	T52.0x2	T52.0x3	T52.0x4	—	—
red veterinary	T49.3x1	T49.3x2	T49.3x3	T49.3x4	T49.3x5	T49.3x6
white	T49.3x1	T49.3x2	T49.3x3	T49.3x4	T49.3x5	T49.3x6
Petroleum (products) **NEC**	T52.0x1	T52.0x2	T52.0x3	T52.0x4	—	—
benzine(s)—*see* Ligroin						
ether—*see* Ligroin						
jelly—*see* Petrolatum						
naphtha—*see* Ligroin						
pesticide	T60.8x1	T60.8x2	T60.8x3	T60.8x4	—	—
solids	T52.0x1	T52.0x2	T52.0x3	T52.0x4	—	—
solvents	T52.0x1	T52.0x2	T52.0x3	T52.0x4	—	—
vapor	T52.0x1	T52.0x2	T52.0x3	T52.0x4	—	—
Peyote	T40.991	T40.992	T40.993	T40.994	T40.995	T40.996
Phanodorm, phanodorn	T42.3x1	T42.3x2	T42.3x3	T42.3x4	T42.3x5	T42.3x6
Phanquinone	T37.3x1	T37.3x2	T37.3x3	T37.3x4	T37.3x5	T37.3x6

Substance	Poisoning, Accidental (unintentional)	Poisoning, Intentional Self-harm	Poisoning, Assault	Poisoning, Undetermined	Adverse Effect	Under-dosing
Phanquone	T37.3x1	T37.3x2	T37.3x3	T37.3x4	T37.3x5	T37.3x6
Pharmaceutical						
adjunct NEC	T50.901	T50.902	T50.903	T50.904	T50.905	T50.906
excipient NEC	T50.901	T50.902	T50.903	T50.904	T50.905	T50.906
sweetener	T50.901	T50.902	T50.903	T50.904	T50.905	T50.906
viscous agent	T50.901	T50.902	T50.903	T50.904	T50.905	T50.906
Phemitone	T42.3x1	T42.3x2	T42.3x3	T42.3x4	T42.3x5	T42.3x6
Phenacaine	T41.3x1	T41.3x2	T41.3x3	T41.3x4	T41.3x5	T41.3x6
Phenacemide	T42.6x1	T42.6x2	T42.6x3	T42.6x4	T42.6x5	T42.6x6
Phenacetin	T39.1x1	T39.1x2	T39.1x3	T39.1x4	T39.1x5	T39.1x6
Phenadoxone	T40.2x1	T40.2x2	T40.2x3	T40.2x4	T40.2x5	T40.2x6
Phenaglycodol	T43.591	T43.592	T43.593	T43.594	T43.595	T43.596
Phenantoin	T42.0x1	T42.0x2	T42.0x3	T42.0x4	T42.0x5	T42.0x6
Phenaphthazine reagent	T50.991	T50.992	T50.993	T50.994	T50.995	T50.996
Phenazocine	T40.4x1	T40.4x2	T40.4x3	T40.4x4	T40.4x5	T40.4x6
Phenazone	T39.2x1	T39.2x2	T39.2x3	T39.2x4	T39.2x5	T39.2x6
Phenazopyridine	T37.8x1	T37.8x2	T37.8x3	T37.8x4	T37.8x5	T37.8x6
Phenbenicillin	T36.0x1	T36.0x2	T36.0x3	T36.0x4	T36.0x5	T36.0x6
Phenbutrazate	T50.5x1	T50.5x2	T50.5x3	T50.5x4	T50.5x5	T50.5x6
Phencyclidine	T41.1x1	T41.1x2	T41.1x3	T41.1x4	T41.1x5	T41.1x6
Phendimetrazine	T50.5x1	T50.5x2	T50.5x3	T50.5x4	T50.5x5	T50.5x6
Phenelzine	T43.1x1	T43.1x2	T43.1x3	T43.1x4	T43.1x5	T43.1x6
Phenemal	T42.3x1	T42.3x2	T42.3x3	T42.3x4	T42.3x5	T42.3x6
Phenergan	T42.6x1	T42.6x2	T42.6x3	T42.6x4	T42.6x5	T42.6x6
Pheneticillin	T36.0x1	T36.0x2	T36.0x3	T36.0x4	T36.0x5	T36.0x6
Pheneturide	T42.6x1	T42.6x2	T42.6x3	T42.6x4	T42.6x5	T42.6x6
Phenformin	T38.3x1	T38.3x2	T38.3x3	T38.3x4	T38.3x5	T38.3x6
Phenglutarimide	T44.3x1	T44.3x2	T44.3x3	T44.3x4	T44.3x5	T44.3x6
Phenicarbazide	T39.8x1	T39.8x2	T39.8x3	T39.8x4	T39.8x5	T39.8x6
Phenindamine	T45.0x1	T45.0x2	T45.0x3	T45.0x4	T45.0x5	T45.0x6
Phenindione	T45.511	T45.512	T45.513	T45.514	T45.515	T45.516
Pheniprazine	T43.1x1	T43.1x2	T43.1x3	T43.1x4	T43.1x5	T43.1x6
Pheniramine	T45.0x1	T45.0x2	T45.0x3	T45.0x4	T45.0x5	T45.0x6
Phenisatin	T47.2x1	T47.2x2	T47.2x3	T47.2x4	T47.2x5	T47.2x6
Phenmetrazine	T50.5x1	T50.5x2	T50.5x3	T50.5x4	T50.5x5	T50.5x6
Phenobal	T42.3x1	T42.3x2	T42.3x3	T42.3x4	T42.3x5	T42.3x6
Phenobarbital	T42.3x1	T42.3x2	T42.3x3	T42.3x4	T42.3x5	T42.3x6
with						
mephenytoin	T42.3x1	T42.3x2	T42.3x3	T42.3x4	T42.3x5	T42.3x6
phenytoin	T42.3x1	T42.3x2	T42.3x3	T42.3x4	T42.3x5	T42.3x6
sodium	T42.3x1	T42.3x2	T42.3x3	T42.3x4	T42.3x5	T42.3x6
Phenobarbitone	T42.3x1	T42.3x2	T42.3x3	T42.3x4	T42.3x5	T42.3x6
Phenobutiodil	T50.8x1	T50.8x2	T50.8x3	T50.8x4	T50.8x5	T50.8x6
Phenoctide	T49.0x1	T49.0x2	T49.0x3	T49.0x4	T49.0x5	T49.0x6
Phenol	T49.0x1	T49.0x2	T49.0x3	T49.0x4	T49.0x5	T49.0x6
disinfectant	T54.0x1	T54.0x2	T54.0x3	T54.0x4	—	—
in oil injection	T46.8x1	T46.8x2	T46.8x3	T46.8x4	T46.8x5	T46.8x6
medicinal	T49.1x1	T49.1x2	T49.1x3	T49.1x4	T49.1x5	T49.1x6
nonmedicinal NEC	T54.0x1	T54.0x2	T54.0x3	T54.0x4	—	—
pesticide	T60.8x1	T60.8x2	T60.8x3	T60.8x4	—	—
red	T50.8x1	T50.8x2	T50.8x3	T50.8x4	T50.8x5	T50.8x6
Phenolic preparation	T49.1x1	T49.1x2	T49.1x3	T49.1x4	T49.1x5	T49.1x6
Phenolphthalein	T47.2x1	T47.2x2	T47.2x3	T47.2x4	T47.2x5	T47.2x6
Phenolsulfonphthalein	T50.8x1	T50.8x2	T50.8x3	T50.8x4	T50.8x5	T50.8x6
Phenomorphan	T40.2x1	T40.2x2	T40.2x3	T40.2x4	T40.2x5	T40.2x6
Phenonyl	T42.3x1	T42.3x2	T42.3x3	T42.3x4	T42.3x5	T42.3x6
Phenoperidine	T40.4x1	T40.4x2	T40.4x3	T40.4x4	T40.4x5	T40.4x6
Phenopyrazone	T46.991	T46.992	T46.993	T46.994	T46.995	T46.996
Phenoquin	T50.4x1	T50.4x2	T50.4x3	T50.4x4	T50.4x5	T50.4x6
Phenothiazine (psychotropic) NEC	T43.3x1	T43.3x2	T43.3x3	T43.3x4	T43.3x5	T43.3x6
insecticide	T60.2x1	T60.2x2	T60.2x3	T60.2x4	—	—
Phenothrin	T49.0x1	T49.0x2	T49.0x3	T49.0x4	T49.0x5	T49.0x6
Phenoxybenzamine	T46.7x1	T46.7x2	T46.7x3	T46.7x4	T46.7x5	T46.7x6
Phenoxyethanol	T49.0x1	T49.0x2	T49.0x3	T49.0x4	T49.0x5	T49.0x6
Phenoxymethyl penicillin	T36.0x1	T36.0x2	T36.0x3	T36.0x4	T36.0x5	T36.0x6
Phenprobamate	T42.8x1	T42.8x2	T42.8x3	T42.8x4	T42.8x5	T42.8x6
Phenprocoumon	T45.511	T45.512	T45.513	T45.514	T45.515	T45.516
Phensuximide	T42.2x1	T42.2x2	T42.2x3	T42.2x4	T42.2x5	T42.2x6
Phentermine	T50.5x1	T50.5x2	T50.5x3	T50.5x4	T50.5x5	T50.5x6
Phenthicillin	T36.0x1	T36.0x2	T36.0x3	T36.0x4	T36.0x5	T36.0x6

Substance	Poisoning, Accidental (unintentional)	Poisoning, Intentional Self-harm	Poisoning, Assault	Poisoning, Undetermined	Adverse Effect	Under-dosing
Phentolamine	T46.7x1	T46.7x2	T46.7x3	T46.7x4	T46.7x5	T46.7x6
Phenyl						
butazone	T39.2x1	T39.2x2	T39.2x3	T39.2x4	T39.2x5	T39.2x6
enediamine	T65.3x1	T65.3x2	T65.3x3	T65.3x4	—	—
hydrazine	T65.3x1	T65.3x2	T65.3x3	T65.3x4	—	—
antineoplastic	T45.1x1	T45.1x2	T45.1x3	T45.1x4	T45.1x5	T45.1x6
mercuric compounds—*see* Mercury						
salicylate	T49.3x1	T49.3x2	T49.3x3	T49.3x4	T49.3x5	T49.3x6
Phenylalanine mustard	T45.1x1	T45.1x2	T45.1x3	T45.1x4	T45.1x5	T45.1x6
Phenylbutazone	T39.2x1	T39.2x2	T39.2x3	T39.2x4	T39.2x5	T39.2x6
Phenylenediamine	T65.3x1	T65.3x2	T65.3x3	T65.3x4	—	—
Phenylephrine	T44.4x1	T44.4x2	T44.4x3	T44.4x4	T44.4x5	T44.4x6
Phenylethylbiguanide	T38.3x1	T38.3x2	T38.3x3	T38.3x4	T38.3x5	T38.3x6
Phenylmercuric						
acetate	T49.0x1	T49.0x2	T49.0x3	T49.0x4	T49.0x5	T49.0x6
borate	T49.0x1	T49.0x2	T49.0x3	T49.0x4	T49.0x5	T49.0x6
nitrate	T49.0x1	T49.0x2	T49.0x3	T49.0x4	T49.0x5	T49.0x6
Phenylmethylbarbitone	T42.3x1	T42.3x2	T42.3x3	T42.3x4	T42.3x5	T42.3x6
Phenylpropanol	T47.5x1	T47.5x2	T47.5x3	T47.5x4	T47.5x5	T47.5x6
Phenylpropanolamine	T44.991	T44.992	T44.993	T44.994	T44.995	T44.996
Phenylsulfthion	T60.0x1	T60.0x2	T60.0x3	T60.0x4	—	—
Phenyltoloxamine	T45.0x1	T45.0x2	T45.0x3	T45.0x4	T45.0x5	T45.0x6
Phenyramidol, phenyramidon	T39.8x1	T39.8x2	T39.8x3	T39.8x4	T39.8x5	T39.8x6
Phenytoin	T42.0x1	T42.0x2	T42.0x3	T42.0x4	T42.0x5	T42.0x6
with Phenobarbital	T42.3x1	T42.3x2	T42.3x3	T42.3x4	T42.3x5	T42.3x6
pHisoHex	T49.2x1	T49.2x2	T49.2x3	T49.2x4	T49.2x5	T49.2x6
Pholcodine	T48.3x1	T48.3x2	T48.3x3	T48.3x4	T48.3x5	T48.3x6
Pholedrine	T46.991	T46.992	T46.993	T46.994	T46.995	T46.996
Phorate	T60.0x1	T60.0x2	T60.0x3	T60.0x4	—	—
Phosdrin	T60.0x1	T60.0x2	T60.0x3	T60.0x4	—	—
Phosfolan	T60.0x1	T60.0x2	T60.0x3	T60.0x4	—	—
Phosgene (gas)	T59.891	T59.892	T59.893	T59.894	—	—
Phosphamidon	T60.0x1	T60.0x2	T60.0x3	T60.0x4	—	—
Phosphate	T65.891	T65.892	T65.893	T65.894	—	—
laxative	T47.4x1	T47.4x2	T47.4x3	T47.4x4	T47.4x5	T47.4x6
organic	T60.0x1	T60.0x2	T60.0x3	T60.0x4	—	—
solvent	T52.91	T52.92	T52.93	T52.94	—	—
tricresyl	T65.891	T65.892	T65.893	T65.894	—	—
Phosphine	T57.1x1	T57.1x2	T57.1x3	T57.1x4	—	—
fumigant	T57.1x1	T57.1x2	T57.1x3	T57.1x4	—	—
Phospholine	T49.5x1	T49.5x2	T49.5x3	T49.5x4	T49.5x5	T49.5x6
Phosphoric acid	T54.2x1	T54.2x2	T54.2x3	T54.2x4	—	—
Phosphorus (compound) NEC	T57.1x1	T57.1x2	T57.1x3	T57.1x4	—	—
pesticide	T60.0x1	T60.0x2	T60.0x3	T60.0x4	—	—
Phthalates	T65.891	T65.892	T65.893	T65.894	—	—
Phthalic anhydride	T65.891	T65.892	T65.893	T65.894	—	—
Phthalimidoglutarimide	T42.6x1	T42.6x2	T42.6x3	T42.6x4	T42.6x5	T42.6x6
Phthalylsulfathiazole	T37.0x1	T37.0x2	T37.0x3	T37.0x4	T37.0x5	T37.0x6
Phylloquinone	T45.7x1	T45.7x2	T45.7x3	T45.7x4	T45.7x5	T45.7x6
Physeptone	T40.3x1	T40.3x2	T40.3x3	T40.3x4	T40.3x5	T40.3x6
Physostigma venenosum	T62.2x1	T62.2x2	T62.2x3	T62.2x4	—	—
Physostigmine	T49.5x1	T49.5x2	T49.5x3	T49.5x4	T49.5x5	T49.5x6
Phytolacca decandra	T62.2x1	T62.2x2	T62.2x3	T62.2x4	—	—
berries	T62.1x1	T62.1x2	T62.1x3	T62.1x4	—	—
Phytomenadione	T45.7x1	T45.7x2	T45.7x3	T45.7x4	T45.7x5	T45.7x6
Phytonadione	T45.7x1	T45.7x2	T45.7x3	T45.7x4	T45.7x5	T45.7x6
Picoperine	T48.3x1	T48.3x2	T48.3x3	T48.3x4	T48.3x5	T48.3x6
Picosulfate (sodium)	T47.2x1	T47.2x2	T47.2x3	T47.2x4	T47.2x5	T47.2x6
Picric (acid)	T54.2x1	T54.2x2	T54.2x3	T54.2x4	—	—
Picrotoxin	T50.7x1	T50.7x2	T50.7x3	T50.7x4	T50.7x5	T50.7x6
Piketoprofen	T49.0x1	T49.0x2	T49.0x3	T49.0x4	T49.0x5	T49.0x6
Pilocarpine	T44.1x1	T44.1x2	T44.1x3	T44.1x4	T44.1x5	T44.1x6
Pilocarpus (jaborandi) extract	T44.1x1	T44.1x2	T44.1x3	T44.1x4	T44.1x5	T44.1x6
Pilsicainide (hydrochloride)	T46.2x1	T46.2x2	T46.2x3	T46.2x4	T46.2x5	T46.2x6
Pimaricin	T36.7x1	T36.7x2	T36.7x3	T36.7x4	T36.7x5	T36.7x6
Pimeclone	T50.7x1	T50.7x2	T50.7x3	T50.7x4	T50.7x5	T50.7x6
Pimelic ketone	T52.8x1	T52.8x2	T52.8x3	T52.8x4	—	—
Pimethixene	T45.0x1	T45.0x2	T45.0x3	T45.0x4	T45.0x5	T45.0x6
Piminodine	T40.2x1	T40.2x2	T40.2x3	T40.2x4	T40.2x5	T40.2x6
Pimozide	T43.591	T43.592	T43.593	T43.594	T43.595	T43.596

Substance	Poisoning, Accidental (unintentional)	Poisoning, Intentional Self-harm	Poisoning, Assault	Poisoning, Undetermined	Adverse Effect	Under-dosing
Pinacidil	T46.5x1	T46.5x2	T46.5x3	T46.5x4	T46.5x5	T46.5x6
Pinaverium bromide	T44.3x1	T44.3x2	T44.3x3	T44.3x4	T44.3x5	T44.3x6
Pinazepam	T42.4x1	T42.4x2	T42.4x3	T42.4x4	T42.4x5	T42.4x6
Pindolol	T44.7x1	T44.7x2	T44.7x3	T44.7x4	T44.7x5	T44.7x6
Pindone	T60.4x1	T60.4x2	T60.4x3	T60.4x4	—	—
Pine oil (disinfectant)	T65.891	T65.892	T65.893	T65.894	—	—
Pinkroot	T37.4x1	T37.4x2	T37.4x3	T37.4x4	T37.4x5	T37.4x6
Pipadone	T40.2x1	T40.2x2	T40.2x3	T40.2x4	T40.2x5	T40.2x6
Pipamazine	T45.0x1	T45.0x2	T45.0x3	T45.0x4	T45.0x5	T45.0x6
Pipamperone	T43.4x1	T43.4x2	T43.4x3	T43.4x4	T43.4x5	T43.4x6
Pipazetate	T48.3x1	T48.3x2	T48.3x3	T48.3x4	T48.3x5	T48.3x6
Pipemidic acid	T37.8x1	T37.8x2	T37.8x3	T37.8x4	T37.8x5	T37.8x6
Pipenzolate bromide	T44.3x1	T44.3x2	T44.3x3	T44.3x4	T44.3x5	T44.3x6
Piperacetazine	T43.3x1	T43.3x2	T43.3x3	T43.3x4	T43.3x5	T43.3x6
Piperacillin	T36.0x1	T36.0x2	T36.0x3	T36.0x4	T36.0x5	T36.0x6
Piperazine	T37.4x1	T37.4x2	T37.4x3	T37.4x4	T37.4x5	T37.4x6
estrone sulfate	T38.5x1	T38.5x2	T38.5x3	T38.5x4	T38.5x5	T38.5x6
Piper cubeba	T62.2x1	T62.2x2	T62.2x3	T62.2x4	—	—
Piperidione	T48.3x1	T48.3x2	T48.3x3	T48.3x4	T48.3x5	T48.3x6
Piperidolate	T44.3x1	T44.3x2	T44.3x3	T44.3x4	T44.3x5	T44.3x6
Piperocaine	T41.3x1	T41.3x2	T41.3x3	T41.3x4	T41.3x5	T41.3x6
infiltration (subcutaneous)	T41.3x1	T41.3x2	T41.3x3	T41.3x4	T41.3x5	T41.3x6
nerve block (peripheral) (plexus)	T41.3x1	T41.3x2	T41.3x3	T41.3x4	T41.3x5	T41.3x6
topical (surface)	T41.3x1	T41.3x2	T41.3x3	T41.3x4	T41.3x5	T41.3x6
Piperonyl butoxide	T60.8x1	T60.8x2	T60.8x3	T60.8x4	—	—
Pipethanate	T44.3x1	T44.3x2	T44.3x3	T44.3x4	T44.3x5	T44.3x6
Pipobroman	T45.1x1	T45.1x2	T45.1x3	T45.1x4	T45.1x5	T45.1x6
Pipotiazine	T43.3x1	T43.3x2	T43.3x3	T43.3x4	T43.3x5	T43.3x6
Pipoxizine	T45.0x1	T45.0x2	T45.0x3	T45.0x4	T45.0x5	T45.0x6
Pipradrol	T43.691	T43.692	T43.693	T43.694	T43.695	T43.696
Piprinhydrinate	T45.0x1	T45.0x2	T45.0x3	T45.0x4	T45.0x5	T45.0x6
Pirarubicin	T45.1x1	T45.1x2	T45.1x3	T45.1x4	T45.1x5	T45.1x6
Pirazinamide	T37.1x1	T37.1x2	T37.1x3	T37.1x4	T37.1x5	T37.1x6
Pirbuterol	T48.6x1	T48.6x2	T48.6x3	T48.6x4	T48.6x5	T48.6x6
Pirenzepine	T47.1x1	T47.1x2	T47.1x3	T47.1x4	T47.1x5	T47.1x6
Piretanide	T50.1x1	T50.1x2	T50.1x3	T50.1x4	T50.1x5	T50.1x6
Piribedil	T42.8x1	T42.8x2	T42.8x3	T42.8x4	T42.8x5	T42.8x6
Piridoxilate	T46.3x1	T46.3x2	T46.3x3	T46.3x4	T46.3x5	T46.3x6
Piritramide	T40.4x1	T40.4x2	T40.4x3	T40.4x4	T40.4x5	T47.8x6
Piromidic acid	T37.8x1	T37.8x2	T37.8x3	T37.8x4	T37.8x5	T37.8x6
Piroxicam	T39.391	T39.392	T39.393	T39.394	T39.395	T39.396
beta-cyclodextrin complex	T39.8x1	T39.8x2	T39.8x3	T39.8x4	T39.8x5	T39.8x6
Pirozadil	T46.6x1	T46.6x2	T46.6x3	T46.6x4	T46.6x5	T46.6x6
Piscidia (bark) (erythrina)	T39.8x1	T39.8x2	T39.8x3	T39.8x4	T39.8x5	T39.8x6
Pitch	T65.891	T65.892	T65.893	T65.894	—	—
Pitkin's solution	T41.3x1	T41.3x2	T41.3x3	T41.3x4	T41.3x5	T41.3x6
Pitocin	T48.0x1	T48.0x2	T48.0x3	T48.0x4	T48.0x5	T48.0x6
Pitressin (tannate)	T38.891	T38.892	T38.893	T38.894	T38.895	T38.896
Pituitary extracts (posterior)	T38.891	T38.892	T38.893	T38.894	T38.895	T38.896
anterior	T38.811	T38.812	T38.813	T38.814	T38.815	T38.816
Pituitrin	T38.891	T38.892	T38.893	T38.894	T38.895	T38.896
Pivampicillin	T36.0x1	T36.0x2	T36.0x3	T36.0x4	T36.0x5	T36.0x6
Pivmecillinam	T36.0x1	T36.0x2	T36.0x3	T36.0x4	T36.0x5	T36.0x6
Placental hormone	T38.891	T38.892	T38.893	T38.894	T38.895	T38.896
Placidyl	T42.6x1	T42.6x2	T42.6x3	T42.6x4	T42.6x5	T42.6x6
Plague vaccine	T50.A91	T50.A92	T50.A93	T50.A94	T50.A95	T50.A96
Plant						
food or fertilizer NEC	T65.891	T65.892	T65.893	T65.894	—	—
containing herbicide	T60.3x1	T60.3x2	T60.3x3	T60.3x4	—	—
noxious, used as food	T62.2x1	T62.2x2	T62.2x3	T62.2x4	—	—
berries	T62.1x1	T62.1x2	T62.1x3	T62.1x4	—	—
seeds	T62.2x1	T62.2x2	T62.2x3	T62.2x4	—	—
specified type NEC	T62.2x1	T62.2x2	T62.2x3	T62.2x4	—	—
Plasma	T45.8x1	T45.8x2	T45.8x3	T45.8x4	T45.8x5	T45.8x6
expander NEC	T45.8x1	T45.8x2	T45.8x3	T45.8x4	T45.8x5	T45.8x6
protein fraction (human)	T45.8x1	T45.8x2	T45.8x3	T45.8x4	T45.8x5	T45.8x6
Plasmanate	T45.8x1	T45.8x2	T45.8x3	T45.8x4	T45.8x5	T45.8x6
Plasminogen (tissue) activator	T45.611	T45.612	T45.613	T45.614	T45.615	T45.616
Plaster dressing	T49.3x1	T49.3x2	T49.3x3	T49.3x4	T49.3x5	T49.3x6
Plastic dressing	T49.3x1	T49.3x2	T49.3x3	T49.3x4	T49.3x5	T49.3x6
Plegicil	T43.3x1	T43.3x2	T43.3x3	T43.3x4	T43.3x5	T43.3x6
Plicamycin	T45.1x1	T45.1x2	T45.1x3	T45.1x4	T45.1x5	T45.1x6
Podophyllotoxin	T49.8x1	T49.8x2	T49.8x3	T49.8x4	T49.8x5	T49.8x6
Podophyllum (resin)	T49.4x1	T49.4x2	T49.4x3	T49.4x4	T49.4x5	T49.4x6
Poison NEC	T65.91	T65.92	T65.93	T65.94	—	—
Poisonous berries	T62.1x1	T62.1x2	T62.1x3	T62.1x4	—	—
Pokeweed (any part)	T62.2x1	T62.2x2	T62.2x3	T62.2x4	—	—
Poldine metilsulfate	T44.3x1	T44.3x2	T44.3x3	T44.3x4	T44.3x5	T44.3x6
Polidexide (sulfate)	T46.6x1	T46.6x2	T46.6x3	T46.6x4	T46.6x5	T46.6x6
Polidocanol	T46.8x1	T46.8x2	T46.8x3	T46.8x4	T46.8x5	T46.8x6
Poliomyelitis vaccine	T50.B91	T50.B92	T50.B93	T50.B94	T50.B95	T50.B96
Polish (car) (floor) (furni-ture) (metal) (porcelain) (silver)	T65.891	T65.892	T65.893	T65.894		
abrasive	T65.891	T65.892	T65.893	T65.894		
porcelain	T65.891	T65.892	T65.893	T65.894		
Poloxalkol	T47.4x1	T47.4x2	T47.4x3	T47.4x4	T47.4x5	T47.4x6
Poloxamer	T47.4x1	T47.4x2	T47.4x3	T47.4x4	T47.4x5	T47.4x6
Polyaminostyrene resins	T50.3x1	T50.3x2	T50.3x3	T50.3x4	T50.3x5	T50.3x6
Polycarbophil	T47.4x1	T47.4x2	T47.4x3	T47.4x4	T47.4x5	T47.4x6
Polychlorinated biphenyl	T65.891	T65.892	T65.893	T65.894		
Polycycline	T36.4x1	T36.4x2	T36.4x3	T36.4x4	T36.4x5	T36.4x6
Polyester fumes	T59.891	T59.892	T59.893	T59.894		
Polyester resin hardener	T52.91	T52.92	T52.93	T52.94		
fumes	T59.891	T59.892	T59.893	T59.894		
Polyestradiol phosphate	T38.5x1	T38.5x2	T38.5x3	T38.5x4	T38.5x5	T38.5x6
Polyethanolamine alkyl sulfate	T49.2x1	T49.2x2	T49.2x3	T49.2x4	T49.2x5	T49.2x6
Polyethylene adhesive	T49.3x1	T49.3x2	T49.3x3	T49.3x4	T49.3x5	T49.3x6
Polyferose	T45.4x1	T45.4x2	T45.4x3	T45.4x4	T45.4x5	T45.4x6
Polygeline	T45.8x1	T45.8x2	T45.8x3	T45.8x4	T45.8x5	T45.8x6
Polymyxin	T36.8x1	T36.8x2	T36.8x3	T36.8x4	T36.8x5	T36.8x6
B	T36.8x1	T36.8x2	T36.8x3	T36.8x4	T36.8x5	T36.8x6
ENT agent	T49.6x1	T49.6x2	T49.6x3	T49.6x4	T49.6x5	T49.6x6
ophthalmic preparation	T49.5x1	T49.5x2	T49.5x3	T49.5x4	T49.5x5	T49.5x6
topical NEC	T49.0x1	T49.0x2	T49.0x3	T49.0x4	T49.0x5	T49.0x6
E sulfate (eye preparation)	T49.5x1	T49.5x2	T49.5x3	T49.5x4	T49.5x5	T49.5x6
Polynoxylin	T49.0x1	T49.0x2	T49.0x3	T49.0x4	T49.0x5	T49.0x6
Polyoestradiol phosphate	T38.5x1	T38.5x2	T38.5x3	T38.5x4	T38.5x5	T38.5x6
Polyoxymethyleneurea	T49.0x1	T49.0x2	T49.0x3	T49.0x4	T49.0x5	T49.0x6
Polysilane	T47.8x1	T47.8x2	T47.8x3	T47.8x4	T47.8x5	T47.8x6
Polytetrafluoroethylene (inhaled)	T59.891	T59.892	T59.893	T59.894		
Polythiazide	T50.2x1	T50.2x2	T50.2x3	T50.2x4	T50.2x5	T50.2x6
Polyvidone	T45.8x1	T45.8x2	T45.8x3	T45.8x4	T45.8x5	T45.8x6
Polyvinylpyrrolidone	T45.8x1	T45.8x2	T45.8x3	T45.8x4	T45.8x5	T45.8x6
Pontocaine (hydrochloride) (infiltration) (topical)	T41.3x1	T41.3x2	T41.3x3	T41.3x4	T41.3x5	T41.3x6
nerve block (peripheral) (plexus)	T41.3x1	T41.3x2	T41.3x3	T41.3x4	T41.3x5	T41.3x6
spinal	T41.3x1	T41.3x2	T41.3x3	T41.3x4	T41.3x5	T41.3x6
Porfiromycin	T45.1x1	T45.1x2	T45.1x3	T45.1x4	T45.1x5	T45.1x6
Posterior pituitary hormone NEC	T38.891	T38.892	T38.893	T38.894	T38.895	T38.896
Pot	T40.7x1	T40.7x2	T40.7x3	T40.7x4	T40.7x5	T40.7x6
Potash (caustic)	T54.3x1	T54.3x2	T54.3x3	T54.3x4	—	—
Potassic saline injection (lactated)	T50.3x1	T50.3x2	T50.3x3	T50.3x4	T50.3x5	T50.3x6
Potassium (salts) NEC	T50.3x1	T50.3x2	T50.3x3	T50.3x4	T50.3x5	T50.3x6
aminobenzoate	T45.8x1	T45.8x2	T45.8x3	T45.8x4	T45.8x5	T45.8x6
aminosalicylate	T37.1x1	T37.1x2	T37.1x3	T37.1x4	T37.1x5	T37.1x6
antimony ' tartrate'	T37.8x1	T37.8x2	T37.8x3	T37.8x4	T37.8x5	T37.8x6
arsenite (solution)	T57.0x1	T57.0x2	T57.0x3	T57.0x4	—	—
bichromate	T56.2x1	T56.2x2	T56.2x3	T56.2x4	—	—
bisulfate	T47.3x1	T47.3x2	T47.3x3	T47.3x4	T47.3x5	T47.3x6
bromide	T42.6x1	T42.6x2	T42.6x3	T42.6x4	T42.6x5	T42.6x6
canrenoate	T50.0x1	T50.0x2	T50.0x3	T50.0x4	T50.0x5	T50.0x6
carbonate	T54.3x1	T54.3x2	T54.3x3	T54.3x4	—	—
chlorate NEC	T65.891	T65.892	T65.893	T65.894	—	—
chloride	T50.3x1	T50.3x2	T50.3x3	T50.3x4	T50.3x5	T50.3x6
citrate	T50.991	T50.992	T50.993	T50.994	T50.995	T50.996
cyanide	T65.0x1	T65.0x2	T65.0x3	T65.0x4	—	—
ferric hexacyanoferrate (medicinal)	T50.6x1	T50.6x2	T50.6x3	T50.6x4	T50.6x5	T50.6x6
nonmedicinal	T65.891	T65.892	T65.893	T65.894	—	—
Fluoride	T57.8x1	T57.8x2	T57.8x3	T57.8x4	—	—

Substance	Poisoning, Accidental (unintentional)	Poisoning, Intentional Self-harm	Poisoning, Assault	Poisoning, Undetermined	Adverse Effect	Under-dosing
Potassium (salts) NEC—continued						
glucaldrate	T47.1x1	T47.1x2	T47.1x3	T47.1x4	T47.1x5	T47.1x6
hydroxide	T54.3x1	T54.3x2	T54.3x3	T54.3x4	—	—
iodate	T49.0x1	T49.0x2	T49.0x3	T49.0x4	T49.0x5	T49.0x6
iodide	T48.4x1	T48.4x2	T48.4x3	T48.4x4	T48.4x5	T48.4x6
nitrate	T57.8x1	T57.8x2	T57.8x3	T57.8x4	—	—
oxalate	T65.891	T65.892	T65.893	T65.894	—	—
perchlorate (nonmedicinal) NEC	T65.891	T65.892	T65.893	T65.894	—	—
antithyroid	T38.2x1	T38.2x2	T38.2x3	T38.2x4	T38.2x5	T38.2x6
medicinal	T38.2x1	T38.2x2	T38.2x3	T38.2x4	T38.2x5	T38.2x6
Permanganate (nonmedicinal)	T65.891	T65.892	T65.893	T65.894	—	—
medicinal	T49.0x1	T49.0x2	T49.0x3	T49.0x4	T49.0x5	T49.0x6
sulfate	T47.2x1	T47.2x2	T47.2x3	T47.2x4	T47.2x5	T47.2x6
Potassium-removing resin	T50.3x1	T50.3x2	T50.3x3	T50.3x4	T50.3x5	T50.3x6
Potassium-retaining drug	T50.3x1	T50.3x2	T50.3x3	T50.3x4	T50.3x5	T50.3x6
Povidone	T45.8x1	T45.8x2	T45.8x3	T45.8x4	T45.8x5	T45.8x6
iodine	T49.0x1	T49.0x2	T49.0x3	T49.0x4	T49.0x5	T49.0x6
Practolol	T44.7x1	T44.7x2	T44.7x3	T44.7x4	T44.7x5	T44.7x6
Prajmalium bitartrate	T46.2x1	T46.2x2	T46.2x3	T46.2x4	T46.2x5	T46.2x6
Pralidoxime (iodide)	T50.6x1	T50.6x2	T50.6x3	T50.6x4	T50.6x5	T50.6x6
chloride	T50.6x1	T50.6x2	T50.6x3	T50.6x4	T50.6x5	T50.6x6
Pramiverine	T44.3x1	T44.3x2	T44.3x3	T44.3x4	T44.3x5	T44.3x6
Pramocaine	T49.1x1	T49.1x2	T49.1x3	T49.1x4	T49.1x5	T49.1x6
Pramoxine	T49.1x1	T49.1x2	T49.1x3	T49.1x4	T49.1x5	T49.1x6
Prasterone	T38.7x1	T38.7x2	T38.7x3	T38.7x4	T38.7x5	T38.7x6
Pravastatin	T46.6x1	T46.6x2	T46.6x3	T46.6x4	T46.6x5	T46.6x6
Prazepam	T42.4x1	T42.4x2	T42.4x3	T42.4x4	T42.4x5	T42.4x6
Praziquantel	T37.4x1	T37.4x2	T37.4x3	T37.4x4	T37.4x5	T37.4x6
Prazitone	T43.291	T43.292	T43.293	T43.294	T43.295	T43.296
Prazosin	T44.6x1	T44.6x2	T44.6x3	T44.6x4	T44.6x5	T44.6x6
Prednicarbate	T49.0x1	T49.0x2	T49.0x3	T49.0x4	T49.0x5	T49.0x6
Prednimustine	T45.1x1	T45.1x2	T45.1x3	T45.1x4	T45.1x5	T45.1x6
Prednisolone	T49.0x1	T49.0x2	T49.0x3	T49.0x4	T49.0x5	T49.0x6
ENT agent	T49.6x1	T49.6x2	T49.6x3	T49.6x4	T49.6x5	T49.6x6
ophthalmic preparation	T49.5x1	T49.5x2	T49.5x3	T49.5x4	T49.5x5	T49.5x6
steaglate	T49.0x1	T49.0x2	T49.0x3	T49.0x4	T49.0x5	T49.0x6
topical NEC	T49.0x1	T49.0x2	T49.0x3	T49.0x4	T49.0x5	T49.0x6
Prednisone	T38.0x1	T38.0x2	T38.0x3	T38.0x4	T38.0x5	T38.0x6
Prednylidene	T38.0x1	T38.0x2	T38.0x3	T38.0x4	T38.0x5	T38.0x6
Pregnandiol	T38.5x1	T38.5x2	T38.5x3	T38.5x4	T38.5x5	T38.5x6
Pregneninolone	T38.5x1	T38.5x2	T38.5x3	T38.5x4	T38.5x5	T38.5x6
Preludin	T43.691	T43.692	T43.693	T43.694	T43.695	T43.696
Premarin	T38.5x1	T38.5x2	T38.5x3	T38.5x4	T38.5x5	T38.5x6
Premedication anesthetic	T41.201	T41.202	T41.203	T41.204	T41.205	T41.206
Prenalterol	T44.5x1	T44.5x2	T44.5x3	T44.5x4	T44.5x5	T44.5x6
Prenoxdiazine	T48.3x1	T48.3x2	T48.3x3	T48.3x4	T48.3x5	T48.3x6
Prenylamine	T46.3x1	T46.3x2	T46.3x3	T46.3x4	T46.3x5	T46.3x6
Preparation, local	T49.4x1	T49.4x2	T49.4x3	T49.4x4	T49.4x5	T49.4x6
Preparation H	T49.8x1	T49.8x2	T49.8x3	T49.8x4	T49.8x5	T49.8x6
Preservative (nonmedicinal)	T65.891	T65.892	T65.893	T65.894	—	—
medicinal	T50.901	T50.902	T50.903	T50.904	T50.905	T50.906
Prethcamide	T50.7x1	T50.7x2	T50.7x3	T50.7x4	T50.7x5	T50.7x6
Pride of China	T62.2x1	T62.2x2	T62.2x3	T62.2x4	—	—
Pridinol	T44.3x1	T44.3x2	T44.3x3	T44.3x4	T44.3x5	T44.3x6
Prifinium bromide	T44.3x1	T44.3x2	T44.3x3	T44.3x4	T44.3x5	T44.3x6
Prilocaine	T41.3x1	T41.3x2	T41.3x3	T41.3x4	T41.3x5	T41.3x6
infiltration (subcutaneous)	T41.3x1	T41.3x2	T41.3x3	T41.3x4	T41.3x5	T41.3x6
nerve block (peripheral) (plexus)	T41.3x1	T41.3x2	T41.3x3	T41.3x4	T41.3x5	T41.3x6
regional	T41.3x1	T41.3x2	T41.3x3	T41.3x4	T41.3x5	T41.3x6
Primaquine	T37.2x1	T37.2x2	T37.2x3	T37.2x4	T37.2x5	T37.2x6
Primidone	T42.6x1	T42.6x2	T42.6x3	T42.6x4	T42.6x5	T42.6x6
Primula (veris)	T62.2x1	T62.2x2	T62.2x3	T62.2x4	—	—
Prinadol	T40.2x1	T40.2x2	T40.2x3	T40.2x4	T40.2x5	T40.2x6
Priscol, Priscoline	T44.6x1	T44.6x2	T44.6x3	T44.6x4	T44.6x5	T44.6x6
Pristinamycin	T36.3x1	T36.3x2	T36.3x3	T36.3x4	T36.3x5	T36.3x6
Privet	T62.2x1	T62.2x2	T62.2x3	T62.2x4	—	—
berries	T62.1x1	T62.1x2	T62.1x3	T62.1x4	—	—
Privine	T44.4x1	T44.4x2	T44.4x3	T44.4x4	T44.4x5	T44.4x6
Pro-Banthine	T44.3x1	T44.3x2	T44.3x3	T44.3x4	T44.3x5	T44.3x6
Probarbital	T42.3x1	T42.3x2	T42.3x3	T42.3x4	T42.3x5	T42.3x6
Probenecid	T50.4x1	T50.4x2	T50.4x3	T50.4x4	T50.4x5	T50.4x6

Substance	Poisoning, Accidental (unintentional)	Poisoning, Intentional Self-harm	Poisoning, Assault	Poisoning, Undetermined	Adverse Effect	Under-dosing
Probucol	T46.6x1	T46.6x2	T46.6x3	T46.6x4	T46.6x5	T46.6x6
Procainamide	T46.2x1	T46.2x2	T46.2x3	T46.2x4	T46.2x5	T46.2x6
Procaine	T41.3x1	T41.3x2	T41.3x3	T41.3x4	T41.3x5	T41.3x6
benzylpenicillin	T36.0x1	T36.0x2	T36.0x3	T36.0x4	T36.0x5	T36.0x6
nerve block (peripheral) (plexus)	T41.3x1	T41.3x2	T41.3x3	T41.3x4	T41.3x5	T41.3x6
penicillin G	T36.0x1	T36.0x2	T36.0x3	T36.0x4	T36.0x5	T36.0x6
regional	T41.3x1	T41.3x2	T41.3x3	T41.3x4	T41.3x5	T41.3x6
spinal	T41.3x1	T41.3x2	T41.3x3	T41.3x4	T41.3x5	T41.3x6
Procalmidol	T43.591	T43.592	T43.593	T43.594	T43.595	T43.596
Procarbazine	T45.1x1	T45.1x2	T45.1x3	T45.1x4	T45.1x5	T45.1x6
Procaterol	T44.5x1	T44.5x2	T44.5x3	T44.5x4	T44.5x5	T44.5x6
Prochlorperazine	T43.3x1	T43.3x2	T43.3x3	T43.3x4	T43.3x5	T43.3x6
Procyclidine	T44.3x1	T44.3x2	T44.3x3	T44.3x4	T44.3x5	T44.3x6
Producer gas	T58.8x1	T58.8x2	T58.8x3	T58.8x4	—	—
Profadol	T40.4x1	T40.4x2	T40.4x3	T40.4x4	T40.4x5	T40.4x6
Profenamine	T44.3x1	T44.3x2	T44.3x3	T44.3x4	T44.3x5	T44.3x6
Profenil	T44.3x1	T44.3x2	T44.3x3	T44.3x4	T44.3x5	T44.3x6
Proflavine	T49.0x1	T49.0x2	T49.0x3	T49.0x4	T49.0x5	T49.0x6
Progabide	T42.6x1	T42.6x2	T42.6x3	T42.6x4	T42.6x5	T42.6x6
Progestin	T38.5x1	T38.5x2	T38.5x3	T38.5x4	T38.5x5	T38.5x6
oral contraceptive	T38.4x1	T38.4x2	T38.4x3	T38.4x4	T38.4x5	T38.4x6
Progesterone	T38.5x1	T38.5x2	T38.5x3	T38.5x4	T38.5x5	T38.5x6
Progestogen NEC	T38.5x1	T38.5x2	T38.5x3	T38.5x4	T38.5x5	T38.5x6
Progestone	T38.5x1	T38.5x2	T38.5x3	T38.5x4	T38.5x5	T38.5x6
Proglumide	T47.1x1	T47.1x2	T47.1x3	T47.1x4	T47.1x5	T47.1x6
Proguanil	T37.2x1	T37.2x2	T37.2x3	T37.2x4	T37.2x5	T37.2x6
Prolactin	T38.811	T38.812	T38.813	T38.814	T38.815	T38.816
Prolintane	T43.691	T43.692	T43.693	T43.694	T43.695	T43.696
Proloid	T38.1x1	T38.1x2	T38.1x3	T38.1x4	T38.1x5	T38.1x6
Proluton	T38.5x1	T38.5x2	T38.5x3	T38.5x4	T38.5x5	T38.5x6
Promacetin	T37.1x1	T37.1x2	T37.1x3	T37.1x4	T37.1x5	T37.1x6
Promazine	T43.3x1	T43.3x2	T43.3x3	T43.3x4	T43.3x5	T43.3x6
Promedol	T40.2x1	T40.2x2	T40.2x3	T40.2x4	T40.2x5	T40.2x6
Promegestone	T38.5x1	T38.5x2	T38.5x3	T38.5x4	T38.5x5	T38.5x6
Promethazine (teoclate)	T43.3x1	T43.3x2	T43.3x3	T43.3x4	T43.3x5	T43.3x6
Promin	T37.1x1	T37.1x2	T37.1x3	T37.1x4	T37.1x5	T37.1x6
Pronase	T45.3x1	T45.3x2	T45.3x3	T45.3x4	T45.3x5	T45.3x6
Pronestyl (hydrochloride)	T46.2x1	T46.2x2	T46.2x3	T46.2x4	T46.2x5	T46.2x6
Pronetalol	T44.7x1	T44.7x2	T44.7x3	T44.7x4	T44.7x5	T44.7x6
Prontosil	T37.0x1	T37.0x2	T37.0x3	T37.0x4	T37.0x5	T37.0x6
Propachlor	T60.3x1	T60.3x2	T60.3x3	T60.3x4	—	—
Propafenone	T46.2x1	T46.2x2	T46.2x3	T46.2x4	T46.2x5	T46.2x6
Propallylonal	T42.3x1	T42.3x2	T42.3x3	T42.3x4	T42.3x5	T42.3x6
Propamidine	T49.0x1	T49.0x2	T49.0x3	T49.0x4	T49.0x5	T49.0x6
Propane (distributed in mobile container)	T59.891	T59.892	T59.893	T59.894	—	—
distributed through pipes	T59.891	T59.892	T59.893	T59.894	—	—
incomplete combustion	T58.11	T58.12	T58.13	T58.14	—	—
Propanidid	T41.291	T41.292	T41.293	T41.294	T41.295	T41.296
Propanil	T60.3x1	T60.3x2	T60.3x3	T60.3x4	—	—
1-Propanol	T51.3x1	T51.3x2	T51.3x3	T51.3x4	—	—
2-Propanol	T51.2x1	T51.2x2	T51.2x3	T51.2x4	—	—
Propantheline	T44.3x1	T44.3x2	T44.3x3	T44.3x4	T44.3x5	T44.3x6
bromide	T44.3x1	T44.3x2	T44.3x3	T44.3x4	T44.3x5	T44.3x6
Proparacaine	T41.3x1	T41.3x2	T41.3x3	T41.3x4	T41.3x5	T41.3x6
Propatylnitrate	T46.3x1	T46.3x2	T46.3x3	T46.3x4	T46.3x5	T46.3x6
Propicillin	T36.0x1	T36.0x2	T36.0x3	T36.0x4	T36.0x5	T36.0x6
Propiolactone	T49.0x1	T49.0x2	T49.0x3	T49.0x4	T49.0x5	T49.0x6
Propiomazine	T45.0x1	T45.0x2	T45.0x3	T45.0x4	T45.0x5	T45.0x6
Propionaldehyde (medicinal)	T42.6x1	T42.6x2	T42.6x3	T42.6x4	T42.6x5	T42.6x6
Propionate (calcium) (sodium)	T49.0x1	T49.0x2	T49.0x3	T49.0x4	T49.0x5	T49.0x6
Propion gel	T49.0x1	T49.0x2	T49.0x3	T49.0x4	T49.0x5	T49.0x6
Propitocaine	T41.3x1	T41.3x2	T41.3x3	T41.3x4	T41.3x5	T41.3x6
infiltration (subcutaneous)	T41.3x1	T41.3x2	T41.3x3	T41.3x4	T41.3x5	T41.3x6
nerve block (peripheral) (plexus)	T41.3x1	T41.3x2	T41.3x3	T41.3x4	T41.3x5	T41.3x6
Propofol	T41.291	T41.292	T41.293	T41.294	T41.295	T41.296
Propoxur	T60.0x1	T60.0x2	T60.0x3	T60.0x4	—	—
Propoxycaine	T41.3x1	T41.3x2	T41.3x3	T41.3x4	T41.3x5	T41.3x6
infiltration (subcutaneous)	T41.3x1	T41.3x2	T41.3x3	T41.3x4	T41.3x5	T41.3x6
nerve block (peripheral) (plexus)	T41.3x1	T41.3x2	T41.3x3	T41.3x4	T41.3x5	T41.3x6
topical (surface)	T41.3x1	T41.3x2	T41.3x3	T41.3x4	T41.3x5	T41.3x6

Substance	Poisoning, Accidental (unintentional)	Poisoning, Intentional Self-harm	Poisoning, Assault	Poisoning, Undetermined	Adverse Effect	Under-dosing
Propoxyphene	T40.4x1	T40.4x2	T40.4x3	T40.4x4	T40.4x5	T40.4x6
Propranolol	T44.7x1	T44.7x2	T44.7x3	T44.7x4	T44.7x5	T44.7x6
Propyl						
alcohol	T51.3x1	T51.3x2	T51.3x3	T51.3x4	—	—
carbinol	T51.3x1	T51.3x2	T51.3x3	T51.3x4	—	—
hexadrine	T44.4x1	T44.4x2	T44.4x3	T44.4x4	T44.4x5	T44.4x6
iodone	T50.8x1	T50.8x2	T50.8x3	T50.8x4	T50.8x5	T50.8x6
thiouracil	T38.2x1	T38.2x2	T38.2x3	T38.2x4	T38.2x5	T38.2x6
Propylaminopheno-thiazine	T43.3x1	T43.3x2	T43.3x3	T43.3x4	T43.3x5	T43.3x6
Propylene	T59.891	T59.892	T59.893	T59.894	—	—
Propylhexedrine	T48.5x1	T48.5x2	T48.5x3	T48.5x4	T48.5x5	T48.5x6
Propyliodone	T50.8x1	T50.8x2	T50.8x3	T50.8x4	T50.8x5	T50.8x6
Propylthiouracil	T38.2x1	T38.2x2	T38.2x3	T38.2x4	T38.2x5	T38.2x6
Propylparaben (ophthalmic)	T49.5x1	T49.5x2	T49.5x3	T49.5x4	T49.5x5	T49.5x6
Propyphenazone	T39.2x1	T39.2x2	T39.2x3	T39.2x4	T39.2x5	T39.2x6
Proquazone	T39.391	T39.392	T39.393	T39.394	T39.395	T39.396
Proscillaridin	T46.0x1	T46.0x2	T46.0x3	T46.0x4	T46.0x5	T46.0x6
Prostacyclin	T45.521	T45.522	T45.523	T45.524	T45.525	T45.526
Prostaglandin (I2)	T45.521	T45.522	T45.523	T45.524	T45.525	T45.526
E1	T46.7x1	T46.7x2	T46.7x3	T46.7x4	T46.7x5	T46.7x6
E2	T48.0x1	T48.0x2	T48.0x3	T48.0x4	T48.0x5	T48.0x6
F2 alpha	T48.0x1	T48.0x2	T48.0x3	T48.0x4	T48.0x5	T48.0x6
Prostigmin	T44.0x1	T44.0x2	T44.0x3	T44.0x4	T44.0x5	T44.0x6
Prosultiamine	T45.2x1	T45.2x2	T45.2x3	T45.2x4	T45.2x5	T45.2x6
Protamine sulfate	T45.7x1	T45.7x2	T45.7x3	T45.7x4	T45.7x5	T45.7x6
zinc insulin	T38.3x1	T38.3x2	T38.3x3	T38.3x4	T38.3x5	T38.3x6
Protease	T47.5x1	T47.5x2	T47.5x3	T47.5x4	T47.5x5	T47.5x6
Protectant, skin NEC	T49.3x1	T49.3x2	T49.3x3	T49.3x4	T49.3x5	T49.3x6
Protein hydrolysate	T50.991	T50.992	T50.993	T50.994	T50.995	T50.996
Prothiaden—see Dothiepin hydrochloride						
Prothionamide	T37.1x1	T37.1x2	T37.1x3	T37.1x4	T37.1x5	T37.1x6
Prothipendyl	T43.591	T43.592	T43.593	T43.594	T43.595	T43.596
Prothoate	T60.0x1	T60.0x2	T60.0x3	T60.0x4	—	—
Prothrombin						
activator	T45.7x1	T45.7x2	T45.7x3	T45.7x4	T45.7x5	T45.7x6
synthesis inhibitor	T45.511	T45.512	T45.513	T45.514	T45.515	T45.516
Protionamide	T37.1x1	T37.1x2	T37.1x3	T37.1x4	T37.1x5	T37.1x6
Protirelin	T38.891	T38.892	T38.893	T38.894	T38.895	T38.896
Protokylol	T48.6x1	T48.6x2	T48.6x3	T48.6x4	T48.6x5	T48.6x6
Protopam	T50.6x1	T50.6x2	T50.6x3	T50.6x4	T50.6x5	T50.6x6
Protoveratrine(s) (A) (B)	T46.5x1	T46.5x2	T46.5x3	T46.5x4	T46.5x5	T46.5x6
Protriptyline	T43.011	T43.012	T43.013	T43.014	T43.015	T43.016
Provera	T38.5x1	T38.5x2	T38.5x3	T38.5x4	T38.5x5	T38.5x6
Provitamin A	T45.2x1	T45.2x2	T45.2x3	T45.2x4	T45.2x5	T45.2x6
Proxibarbal	T42.3x1	T42.3x2	T42.3x3	T42.3x4	T42.3x5	T42.3x6
Proxymetacaine	T41.3x1	T41.3x2	T41.3x3	T41.3x4	T41.3x5	T41.3x6
Proxyphylline	T48.6x1	T48.6x2	T48.6x3	T48.6x4	T48.6x5	T48.6x6
Prozac—see Fluoxetine hydrochloride						
Prunus						
laurocerasus	T62.2x1	T62.2x2	T62.2x3	T62.2x4	—	—
virginiana	T62.2x1	T62.2x2	T62.2x3	T62.2x4	—	—
Prussian blue						
commercial	T65.891	T65.892	T65.893	T65.894	—	—
therapeutic	T50.6x1	T50.6x2	T50.6x3	T50.6x4	T50.6x5	T50.6x6
Prussic acid	T65.0x1	T65.0x2	T65.0x3	T65.0x4	—	—
vapor	T57.3x1	T57.3x2	T57.3x3	T57.3x4	—	—
Pseudoephedrine	T44.991	T44.992	T44.993	T44.994	T44.995	T44.996
Psilocin	T40.991	T40.992	T40.993	T40.994	T40.995	T40.996
Psilocybin	T40.991	T40.992	T40.993	T40.994	T40.995	T40.996
Psilocybine	T40.991	T40.992	T40.993	T40.994	T40.995	T40.996
Psoralene (nonmedicinal)	T65.891	T65.892	T65.893	T65.894	—	—
Psoralens (medicinal)	T50.991	T50.992	T50.993	T50.994	T50.995	T50.996
PSP (phenolsulfonphthalein)	T50.8x1	T50.8x2	T50.8x3	T50.8x4	T50.8x5	T50.8x6
Psychodysleptic drug NEC	T40.901	T40.902	T40.903	T40.904	T40.905	T40.906
Psychostimulant	T43.601	T43.602	T43.603	T43.604	T43.605	T43.606
amphetamine	T43.621	T43.622	T43.623	T43.624	T43.625	T43.626
caffeine	T43.611	T43.612	T43.613	T43.614	T43.615	T43.616
methylphenidate	T43.631	T43.632	T43.633	T43.634	T43.635	T43.636
specified NEC	T43.691	T43.692	T43.693	T43.694	T43.695	T43.696
Psychotherapeutic drug NEC	T43.91	T43.92	T43.93	T43.94	T43.95	T43.96
antidepressants (see also Antidepressant)	T43.201	T43.202	T43.203	T43.204	T43.205	T43.206
specified NEC	T43.8x1	T43.8x2	T43.8x3	T43.8x4	T43.8x5	T43.8x6
tranquilizers NEC	T43.501	T43.502	T43.503	T43.504	T43.505	T43.506
Psychotomimetic agents	T40.901	T40.902	T40.903	T40.904	T40.905	T40.906
Psychotropic drug NEC	T43.91	T43.92	T43.93	T43.94	T43.95	T43.96
specified NEC	T43.8x1	T43.8x2	T43.8x3	T43.8x4	T43.8x5	T43.8x6
Psyllium hydrophilic mucilloid	T47.4x1	T47.4x2	T47.4x3	T47.4x4	T47.4x5	T47.4x6
Pteroylglutamic acid	T45.8x1	T45.8x2	T45.8x3	T45.8x4	T45.8x5	T45.8x6
Pteroyltriglutamate	T45.1x1	T45.1x2	T45.1x3	T45.1x4	T45.1x5	T45.1x6
PTFE—see Polytetrafluoroethylene						
Pulp						
devitalizing paste	T49.7x1	T49.7x2	T49.7x3	T49.7x4	T49.7x5	T49.7x6
dressing	T49.7x1	T49.7x2	T49.7x3	T49.7x4	T49.7x5	T49.7x6
Pulsatilla	T62.2x1	T62.2x2	T62.2x3	T62.2x4	—	—
Pumpkin seed extract	T37.4x1	T37.4x2	T37.4x3	T37.4x4	T37.4x5	T37.4x6
Purex (bleach)	T54.91	T54.92	T54.93	T54.94	—	—
Purgative NEC (see also Cathartic)	T47.4x1	T47.4x2	T47.4x3	T47.4x4	T47.4x5	T47.4x6
Purine analogue (antineoplastic)	T45.1x1	T45.1x2	T45.1x3	T45.1x4	T45.1x5	T45.1x6
Purine diuretics	T50.2x1	T50.2x2	T50.2x3	T50.2x4	T50.2x5	T50.2x6
Purinethol	T45.1x1	T45.1x2	T45.1x3	T45.1x4	T45.1x5	T45.1x6
PVP	T45.8x1	T45.8x2	T45.8x3	T45.8x4	T45.8x5	T45.8x6
Pyrabital	T39.8x1	T39.8x2	T39.8x3	T39.8x4	T39.8x5	T39.8x6
Pyramidon	T39.2x1	T39.2x2	T39.2x3	T39.2x4	T39.2x5	T39.2x6
Pyrantel	T37.4x1	T37.4x2	T37.4x3	T37.4x4	T37.4x5	T37.4x6
Pyrathiazine	T45.0x1	T45.0x2	T45.0x3	T45.0x4	T45.0x5	T45.0x6
Pyrazinamide	T37.1x1	T37.1x2	T37.1x3	T37.1x4	T37.1x5	T37.1x6
Pyrazinoic acid (amide)	T37.1x1	T37.1x2	T37.1x3	T37.1x4	T37.1x5	T37.1x6
Pyrazole (derivatives)	T39.2x1	T39.2x2	T39.2x3	T39.2x4	T39.2x5	T39.2x6
Pyrazolone analgesic NEC	T39.2x1	T39.2x2	T39.2x3	T39.2x4	T39.2x5	T39.2x6
Pyrethrin, pyrethrum (nonmedicinal)	T60.2x1	T60.2x2	T60.2x3	T60.2x4	—	—
Pyrethrum extract	T49.0x1	T49.0x2	T49.0x3	T49.0x4	T49.0x5	T49.0x6
Pyribenzamine	T45.0x1	T45.0x2	T45.0x3	T45.0x4	T45.0x5	T45.0x6
Pyridine	T52.8x1	T52.8x2	T52.8x3	T52.8x4	—	—
aldoxime methiodide	T50.6x1	T50.6x2	T50.6x3	T50.6x4	T50.6x5	T50.6x6
aldoxime methyl chloride	T50.6x1	T50.6x2	T50.6x3	T50.6x4	T50.6x5	T50.6x6
vapor	T59.891	T59.892	T59.893	T59.894	—	—
Pyridium	T49.1x1	T49.1x2	T49.1x3	T49.1x4	T49.1x5	T49.1x6
Pyridostigmine bromide	T44.0x1	T44.0x2	T44.0x3	T44.0x4	T44.0x5	T44.0x6
Pyridoxal phosphate	T45.2x1	T45.2x2	T45.2x3	T45.2x4	T45.2x5	T45.2x6
Pyridoxine	T45.2x1	T45.2x2	T45.2x3	T45.2x4	T45.2x5	T45.2x6
Pyrilamine	T45.0x1	T45.0x2	T45.0x3	T45.0x4	T45.0x5	T45.0x6
Pyrimethamine	T37.2x1	T37.2x2	T37.2x3	T37.2x4	T37.2x5	T37.2x6
with sulfadoxine	T37.2x1	T37.2x2	T37.2x3	T37.2x4	T37.2x5	T37.2x6
Pyrimidine antagonist	T45.1x1	T45.1x2	T45.1x3	T45.1x4	T45.1x5	T45.1x6
Pyriminil	T60.4x1	T60.4x2	T60.4x3	T60.4x4	—	—
Pyrithione zinc	T49.4x1	T49.4x2	T49.4x3	T49.4x4	T49.4x5	T49.4x6
Pyrithyldione	T42.6x1	T42.6x2	T42.6x3	T42.6x4	T42.6x5	T42.6x6
Pyrogallic acid	T49.0x1	T49.0x2	T49.0x3	T49.0x4	T49.0x5	T49.0x6
Pyrogallol	T49.0x1	T49.0x2	T49.0x3	T49.0x4	T49.0x5	T49.0x6
Pyroxylin	T49.3x1	T49.3x2	T49.3x3	T49.3x4	T49.3x5	T49.3x6
Pyrrobutamine	T45.0x1	T45.0x2	T45.0x3	T45.0x4	T45.0x5	T45.0x6
Pyrrolizidine alkaloids	T62.8x1	T62.8x2	T62.8x3	T62.8x4	—	—
Pyrvinium chloride	T37.4x1	T37.4x2	T37.4x3	T37.4x4	T37.4x5	T37.4x6
PZI	T38.3x1	T38.3x2	T38.3x3	T38.3x4	T38.3x5	T38.3x6
Quaalude	T42.6x1	T42.6x2	T42.6x3	T42.6x4	T42.6x5	T42.6x6
Quarternary ammonium						
anti-infective	T49.0x1	T49.0x2	T49.0x3	T49.0x4	T49.0x5	T49.0x6
ganglion blocking	T44.2x1	T44.2x2	T44.2x3	T44.2x4	T44.2x5	T44.2x6
parasympatholytic	T44.3x1	T44.3x2	T44.3x3	T44.3x4	T44.3x5	T44.3x6
Quazepam	T42.4x1	T42.4x2	T42.4x3	T42.4x4	T42.4x5	T42.4x6
Quicklime	T54.3x1	T54.3x2	T54.3x3	T54.3x4	—	—
Quillaja extract	T48.4x1	T48.4x2	T48.4x3	T48.4x4	T48.4x5	T48.4x6
Quinacrine	T37.2x1	T37.2x2	T37.2x3	T37.2x4	T37.2x5	T37.2x6
Quinaglute	T46.2x1	T46.2x2	T46.2x3	T46.2x4	T46.2x5	T46.2x6
Quinalbarbital	T42.3x1	T42.3x2	T42.3x3	T42.3x4	T42.3x5	T42.3x6
Quinalbarbitone sodium	T42.3x1	T42.3x2	T42.3x3	T42.3x4	T42.3x5	T42.3x6
Quinalphos	T60.0x1	T60.0x2	T60.0x3	T60.0x4	—	—

Drug and Chemical Table

Quinapril–Safflower oil

Substance	Poisoning, Accidental (unintentional)	Poisoning, Intentional Self-harm	Poisoning, Assault	Poisoning, Undetermined	Adverse Effect	Under-dosing
Quinapril	T46.4x1	T46.4x2	T46.4x3	T46.4x4	T46.4x5	T46.4x6
Quinestradiol	T38.5x1	T38.5x2	T38.5x3	T38.5x4	T38.5x5	T38.5x6
Quinestradol	T38.5x1	T38.5x2	T38.5x3	T38.5x4	T38.5x5	T38.5x6
Quinestrol	T38.5x1	T38.5x2	T38.5x3	T38.5x4	T38.5x5	T38.5x6
Quinethazone	T50.2x1	T50.2x2	T50.2x3	T50.2x4	T50.2x5	T50.2x6
Quingestanol	T38.4x1	T38.4x2	T38.4x3	T38.4x4	T38.4x5	T38.4x6
Quinidine	T46.2x1	T46.2x2	T46.2x3	T46.2x4	T46.2x5	T46.2x6
Quinine	T37.2x1	T37.2x2	T37.2x3	T37.2x4	T37.2x5	T37.2x6
Quiniobine	T37.8x1	T37.8x2	T37.8x3	T37.8x4	T37.8x5	T37.8x6
Quinisocaine	T49.1x1	T49.1x2	T49.1x3	T49.1x4	T49.1x5	T49.1x6
Quinocide	T37.2x1	T37.2x2	T37.2x3	T37.2x4	T37.2x5	T37.2x6
Quinoline (derivatives) NEC	T37.8x1	T37.8x2	T37.8x3	T37.8x4	T37.8x5	T37.8x6
Quinupramine	T43.011	T43.012	T43.013	T43.014	T43.015	T43.016
Quotane	T41.3x1	T41.3x2	T41.3x3	T41.3x4	T41.3x5	T41.3x6
Rabies						
immune globulin (human)	T50.Z11	T50.Z12	T50.Z13	T50.Z14	T50.Z15	T50.Z16
vaccine	T50.B91	T50.B92	T50.B93	T50.B94	T50.B95	T50.B96
Racemoramide	T40.2x1	T40.2x2	T40.2x3	T40.2x4	T40.2x5	T40.2x6
Racemorphan	T40.2x1	T40.2x2	T40.2x3	T40.2x4	T40.2x5	T40.2x6
Racepinefrin	T44.5x1	T44.5x2	T44.5x3	T44.5x4	T44.5x5	T44.5x6
Raclopride	T43.591	T43.592	T43.593	T43.594	T43.595	T43.596
Radiator alcohol	T51.1x1	T51.1x2	T51.1x3	T51.1x4	—	—
Radioactive drug NEC	T50.8x1	T50.8x2	T50.8x3	T50.8x4	T50.8x5	T50.8x6
Radio-opaque (drugs) (materials)	T50.8x1	T50.8x2	T50.8x3	T50.8x4	T50.8x5	T50.8x6
Ramifenazone	T39.2x1	T39.2x2	T39.2x3	T39.2x4	T39.2x5	T39.2x6
Ramipril	T46.4x1	T46.4x2	T46.4x3	T46.4x4	T46.4x5	T46.4x6
Ranitidine	T47.0x1	T47.0x2	T47.0x3	T47.0x4	T47.0x5	T47.0x6
Ranunculus	T62.2x1	T62.2x2	T62.2x3	T62.2x4	—	—
Rat poison NEC	T60.4x1	T60.4x2	T60.4x3	T60.4x4	—	—
Rattlesnake (venom)	T63.011	T63.012	T63.013	T63.014	—	—
Raubasine	T46.7x1	T46.7x2	T46.7x3	T46.7x4	T46.7x5	T46.7x6
Raudixin	T46.5x1	T46.5x2	T46.5x3	T46.5x4	T46.5x5	T46.5x6
Rautensin	T46.5x1	T46.5x2	T46.5x3	T46.5x4	T46.5x5	T46.5x6
Rautina	T46.5x1	T46.5x2	T46.5x3	T46.5x4	T46.5x5	T46.5x6
Rautotal	T46.5x1	T46.5x2	T46.5x3	T46.5x4	T46.5x5	T46.5x6
Rauwiloid	T46.5x1	T46.5x2	T46.5x3	T46.5x4	T46.5x5	T46.5x6
Rauwoldin	T46.5x1	T46.5x2	T46.5x3	T46.5x4	T46.5x5	T46.5x6
Rauwolfia (alkaloids)	T46.5x1	T46.5x2	T46.5x3	T46.5x4	T46.5x5	T46.5x6
Razoxane	T45.1x1	T45.1x2	T45.1x3	T45.1x4	T45.1x5	T45.1x6
Realgar	T57.0x1	T57.0x2	T57.0x3	T57.0x4	—	—
Recombinant (R)—see specific protein						
Red blood cells, packed	T45.8x1	T45.8x2	T45.8x3	T45.8x4	T45.8x5	T45.8x6
Red squill (scilliroside)	T60.4x1	T60.4x2	T60.4x3	T60.4x4	—	—
Reducing agent, industrial NEC	T65.891	T65.892	T65.893	T65.894	—	—
Refrigerant gas (chlorofluoro-carbon)	T53.5x1	T53.5x2	T53.5x3	T53.5x4	—	—
not chlorofluorocarbon	T59.891	T59.892	T59.893	T59.894	—	—
Regroton	T50.2x1	T50.2x2	T50.2x3	T50.2x4	T50.2x5	T50.2x6
Rehydration salts (oral)	T50.3x1	T50.3x2	T50.3x3	T50.3x4	T50.3x5	T50.3x6
Rela	T42.8x1	T42.8x2	T42.8x3	T42.8x4	T42.8x5	T42.8x6
Relaxant, muscle						
anesthetic	T48.1x1	T48.1x2	T48.1x3	T48.1x4	T48.1x5	T48.1x6
central nervous system	T42.8x1	T42.8x2	T42.8x3	T42.8x4	T42.8x5	T42.8x6
skeletal NEC	T48.1x1	T48.1x2	T48.1x3	T48.1x4	T48.1x5	T48.1x6
smooth NEC	T44.3x1	T44.3x2	T44.3x3	T44.3x4	T44.3x5	T44.3x6
Remoxipride	T43.591	T43.592	T43.593	T43.594	T43.595	T43.596
Renese	T50.2x1	T50.2x2	T50.2x3	T50.2x4	T50.2x5	T50.2x6
Renografin	T50.8x1	T50.8x2	T50.8x3	T50.8x4	T50.8x5	T50.8x6
Replacement solution	T50.3x1	T50.3x2	T50.3x3	T50.3x4	T50.3x5	T50.3x6
Reproterol	T48.6x1	T48.6x2	T48.6x3	T48.6x4	T48.6x5	T48.6x6
Rescinnamine	T46.5x1	T46.5x2	T46.5x3	T46.5x4	T46.5x5	T46.5x6
Reserpin(e)	T46.5x1	T46.5x2	T46.5x3	T46.5x4	T46.5x5	T46.5x6
Resorcin, resorcinol (nonmedicinal)	T65.891	T65.892	T65.893	T65.894	—	—
medicinal	T49.4x1	T49.4x2	T49.4x3	T49.4x4	T49.4x5	T49.4x6
Respaire	T48.4x1	T48.4x2	T48.4x3	T48.4x4	T48.4x5	T48.4x6
Respiratory drug NEC	T48.901	T48.902	T48.903	T48.904	T48.905	T48.906
antiasthmatic NEC	T48.6x1	T48.6x2	T48.6x3	T48.6x4	T48.6x5	T48.6x6
anti-common-cold NEC	T48.5x1	T48.5x2	T48.5x3	T48.5x4	T48.5x5	T48.5x6
expectorant NEC	T48.4x1	T48.4x2	T48.4x3	T48.4x4	T48.4x5	T48.4x6

Substance	Poisoning, Accidental (unintentional)	Poisoning, Intentional Self-harm	Poisoning, Assault	Poisoning, Undetermined	Adverse Effect	Under-dosing
Respiratory drug NEC —continued						
stimulant	T48.901	T48.902	T48.903	T48.904	T48.905	T48.906
Retinoic acid	T49.0x1	T49.0x2	T49.0x3	T49.0x4	T49.0x5	T49.0x6
Retinol	T45.2x1	T45.2x2	T45.2x3	T45.2x4	T45.2x5	T45.2x6
Rh (D) immune globulin (human)	T50.Z11	T50.Z12	T50.Z13	T50.Z14	T50.Z15	T50.Z16
Rhodine	T39.011	T39.012	T39.013	T39.014	T39.015	T39.016
RhoGAM	T50.Z11	T50.Z12	T50.Z13	T50.Z14	T50.Z15	T50.Z16
Rhubarb						
dry extract	T47.2x1	T47.2x2	T47.2x3	T47.2x4	T47.2x5	T47.2x6
tincture, compound	T47.2x1	T47.2x2	T47.2x3	T47.2x4	T47.2x5	T47.2x6
Ribavirin	T37.5x1	T37.5x2	T37.5x3	T37.5x4	T37.5x5	T37.5x6
Riboflavin	T45.2x1	T45.2x2	T45.2x3	T45.2x4	T45.2x5	T45.2x6
Ribostamycin	T36.5x1	T36.5x2	T36.5x3	T36.5x4	T36.5x5	T36.5x6
Ricin	T62.2x1	T62.2x2	T62.2x3	T62.2x4	—	—
Ricinus communis	T62.2x1	T62.2x2	T62.2x3	T62.2x4	—	—
Rickettsial vaccine NEC	T50.A91	T50.A92	T50.A93	T50.A94	T50.A95	T50.A96
Rifabutin	T36.6x1	T36.6x2	T36.6x3	T36.6x4	T36.6x5	T36.6x6
Rifamide	T36.6x1	T36.6x2	T36.6x3	T36.6x4	T36.6x5	T36.6x6
Rifampicin	T36.6x1	T36.6x2	T36.6x3	T36.6x4	T36.6x5	T36.6x6
with isoniazid	T37.1x1	T37.1x2	T37.1x3	T37.1x4	T37.1x5	T37.1x6
Rifampin	T36.6x1	T36.6x2	T36.6x3	T36.6x4	T36.6x5	T36.6x6
Rifamycin	T36.6x1	T36.6x2	T36.6x3	T36.6x4	T36.6x5	T36.6x6
Rifaximin	T36.6x1	T36.6x2	T36.6x3	T36.6x4	T36.6x5	T36.6x6
Rimantadine	T37.5x1	T37.5x2	T37.5x3	T37.5x4	T37.5x5	T37.5x6
Rimazolium metilsulfate	T39.8x1	T39.8x2	T39.8x3	T39.8x4	T39.8x5	T39.8x6
Rimifon	T37.1x1	T37.1x2	T37.1x3	T37.1x4	T37.1x5	T37.1x6
Rimiterol	T48.6x1	T48.6x2	T48.6x3	T48.6x4	T48.6x5	T48.6x6
Ringer (lactate) solution	T50.3x1	T50.3x2	T50.3x3	T50.3x4	T50.3x5	T50.3x6
Ristocetin	T36.8x1	T36.8x2	T36.8x3	T36.8x4	T36.8x5	T36.8x6
Ritalin	T43.631	T43.632	T43.633	T43.634	T43.635	T43.636
Ritodrine	T44.5x1	T44.5x2	T44.5x3	T44.5x4	T44.5x5	T44.5x6
Roach killer—see Insecticide						
Rociverine	T44.3x1	T44.3x2	T44.3x3	T44.3x4	T44.3x5	T44.3x6
Rocky Mountain spotted fever vaccine	T50.A91	T50.A92	T50.A93	T50.A94	T50.A95	T50.A96
Rodenticide NEC	T60.4x1	T60.4x2	T60.4x3	T60.4x4	—	—
Rohypnol	T42.4x1	T42.4x2	T42.4x3	T42.4x4	T42.4x5	T42.4x6
Rokitamycin	T36.3x1	T36.3x2	T36.3x3	T36.3x4	T36.3x5	T36.3x6
Rolaids	T47.1x1	T47.1x2	T47.1x3	T47.1x4	T47.1x5	T47.1x6
Rolitetracycline	T36.4x1	T36.4x2	T36.4x3	T36.4x4	T36.4x5	T36.4x6
Romilar	T48.3x1	T48.3x2	T48.3x3	T48.3x4	T48.3x5	T48.3x6
Ronifibrate	T46.6x1	T46.6x2	T46.6x3	T46.6x4	T46.6x5	T46.6x6
Rosaprostol	T47.1x1	T47.1x2	T47.1x3	T47.1x4	T47.1x5	T47.1x6
Rose bengal sodium (131I)	T50.8x1	T50.8x2	T50.8x3	T50.8x4	T50.8x5	T50.8x6
Rose water ointment	T49.3x1	T49.3x2	T49.3x3	T49.3x4	T49.3x5	T49.3x6
Rosoxacin	T37.8x1	T37.8x2	T37.8x3	T37.8x4	T37.8x5	T37.8x6
Rotenone	T60.2x1	T60.2x2	T60.2x3	T60.2x4	—	—
Rotoxamine	T45.0x1	T45.0x2	T45.0x3	T45.0x4	T45.0x5	T45.0x6
Rough-on-rats	T60.4x1	T60.4x2	T60.4x3	T60.4x4	—	—
Roxatidine	T47.0x1	T47.0x2	T47.0x3	T47.0x4	T47.0x5	T47.0x6
Roxithromycin	T36.3x1	T36.3x2	T36.3x3	T36.3x4	T36.3x5	T36.3x6
Rt-PA	T45.611	T45.612	T45.613	T45.614	T45.615	T45.616
Rubbing alcohol	T51.2x1	T51.2x2	T51.2x3	T51.2x4	—	—
Rubefacient	T49.4x1	T49.4x2	T49.4x3	T49.4x4	T49.4x5	T49.4x6
Rubella vaccine	T50.B91	T50.B92	T50.B93	T50.B94	T50.B95	T50.B96
Rubeola vaccine	T50.B91	T50.B92	T50.B93	T50.B94	T50.B95	T50.B96
Rubidium chloride Rb82	T50.8x1	T50.8x2	T50.8x3	T50.8x4	T50.8x5	T50.8x6
Rubidomycin	T45.1x1	T45.1x2	T45.1x3	T45.1x4	T45.1x5	T45.1x6
Rue	T62.2x1	T62.2x2	T62.2x3	T62.2x4	—	—
Rufocromomycin	T45.1x1	T45.1x2	T45.1x3	T45.1x4	T45.1x5	T45.1x6
Russel's viper venin	T45.7x1	T45.7x2	T45.7x3	T45.7x4	T45.7x5	T45.7x6
Ruta (graveolens)	T62.2x1	T62.2x2	T62.2x3	T62.2x4	—	—
Rutinum	T46.991	T46.992	T46.993	T46.994	T46.995	T46.996
Rutoside	T46.991	T46.992	T46.993	T46.994	T46.995	T46.996
Sabadilla (plant)	T62.2x1	T62.2x2	T62.2x3	T62.2x4	—	—
pesticide	T60.2x1	T60.2x2	T60.2x3	T60.2x4	—	—
Saccharated iron oxide	T45.8x1	T45.8x2	T45.8x3	T45.8x4	T45.8x5	T45.8x6
Saccharin	T50.901	T50.902	T50.903	T50.904	T50.905	T50.906
Saccharomyces boulardii	T47.6x1	T47.6x2	T47.6x3	T47.6x4	T47.6x5	T47.6x6
Safflower oil	T46.6x1	T46.6x2	T46.6x3	T46.6x4	T46.6x5	T46.6x6

Substance	Poisoning, Accidental (unintentional)	Poisoning, Intentional Self-harm	Poisoning, Assault	Poisoning, Undetermined	Adverse Effect	Under-dosing
Safrazine	T43.1x1	T43.1x2	T43.1x3	T43.1x4	T43.1x5	T43.1x6
Salazosulfapyridine	T37.0x1	T37.0x2	T37.0x3	T37.0x4	T37.0x5	T37.0x6
Salbutamol	T48.6x1	T48.6x2	T48.6x3	T48.6x4	T48.6x5	T48.6x6
Salicylamide	T39.091	T39.092	T39.093	T39.094	T39.095	T39.096
Salicylate NEC	T39.091	T39.092	T39.093	T39.094	T39.095	T39.096
methyl	T49.3x1	T49.3x2	T49.3x3	T49.3x4	T49.3x5	T49.3x6
theobromine calcium	T50.2x1	T50.2x2	T50.2x3	T50.2x4	T50.2x5	T50.2x6
Salicylazosulfapyridine	T37.0x1	T37.0x2	T37.0x3	T37.0x4	T37.0x5	T37.0x6
Salicylhydroxamic acid	T49.0x1	T49.0x2	T49.0x3	T49.0x4	T49.0x5	T49.0x6
Salicylic acid	T49.4x1	T49.4x2	T49.4x3	T49.4x4	T49.4x5	T49.4x6
with benzoic acid	T49.4x1	T49.4x2	T49.4x3	T49.4x4	T49.4x5	T49.4x6
congeners	T39.091	T39.092	T39.093	T39.094	T39.095	T39.096
derivative	T39.091	T39.092	T39.093	T39.094	T39.095	T39.096
salts	T39.091	T39.092	T39.093	T39.094	T39.095	T39.096
Salinazid	T37.1x1	T37.1x2	T37.1x3	T37.1x4	T37.1x5	T37.1x6
Salmeterol	T48.6x1	T48.6x2	T48.6x3	T48.6x4	T48.6x5	T48.6x6
Salol	T49.3x1	T49.3x2	T49.3x3	T49.3x4	T49.3x5	T49.3x6
Salsalate	T39.091	T39.092	T39.093	T39.094	T39.095	T39.096
Salt substitute	T50.901	T50.902	T50.903	T50.904	T50.905	T50.906
Salt-replacing drug	T50.901	T50.902	T50.903	T50.904	T50.905	T50.906
Salt-retaining mineralo-corticoid	T50.0x1	T50.0x2	T50.0x3	T50.0x4	T50.0x5	T50.0x6
Saluretic NEC	T50.2x1	T50.2x2	T50.2x3	T50.2x4	T50.2x5	T50.2x6
Saluron	T50.2x1	T50.2x2	T50.2x3	T50.2x4	T50.2x5	T50.2x6
Salvarsan 606 (neosilver) (silver)	T37.8x1	T37.8x2	T37.8x3	T37.8x4	T37.8x5	T37.8x6
Sambucus canadensis	T62.2x1	T62.2x2	T62.2x3	T62.2x4	—	—
berry	T62.1x1	T62.1x2	T62.1x3	T62.1x4	—	—
Sandril	T46.5x1	T46.5x2	T46.5x3	T46.5x4	T46.5x5	T46.5x6
Sanguinaria canadensis	T62.2x1	T62.2x2	T62.2x3	T62.2x4	—	—
Saniflush (cleaner)	T54.2x1	T54.2x2	T54.2x3	T54.2x4	—	—
Santonin	T37.4x1	T37.4x2	T37.4x3	T37.4x4	T37.4x5	T37.4x6
Santyl	T49.8x1	T49.8x2	T49.8x3	T49.8x4	T49.8x5	T49.8x6
Saralasin	T46.5x1	T46.5x2	T46.5x3	T46.5x4	T46.5x5	T46.5x6
Sarcolysin	T45.1x1	T45.1x2	T45.1x3	T45.1x4	T45.1x5	T45.1x6
Sarkomycin	T45.1x1	T45.1x2	T45.1x3	T45.1x4	T45.1x5	T45.1x6
Saroten	T43.011	T43.012	T43.013	T43.014	T43.015	T43.016
Saturnine—see Lead						
Savin (oil)	T49.4x1	T49.4x2	T49.4x3	T49.4x4	T49.4x5	T49.4x6
Scammony	T47.2x1	T47.2x2	T47.2x3	T47.2x4	T47.2x5	T47.2x6
S-Carboxymethyl-cysteine	T48.4x1	T48.4x2	T48.4x3	T48.4x4	T48.4x5	T48.4x6
Scarlet red	T49.8x1	T49.8x2	T49.8x3	T49.8x4	T49.8x5	T49.8x6
Scheele's green	T57.0x1	T57.0x2	T57.0x3	T57.0x4	—	—
insecticide	T57.0x1	T57.0x2	T57.0x3	T57.0x4	—	—
Schizontozide (blood) (tissue)	T37.2x1	T37.2x2	T37.2x3	T37.2x4	T37.2x5	T37.2x6
Schradan	T60.0x1	T60.0x2	T60.0x3	T60.0x4	—	—
Schweinfurth green	T57.0x1	T57.0x2	T57.0x3	T57.0x4	—	—
insecticide	T57.0x1	T57.0x2	T57.0x3	T57.0x4	—	—
Scilla, rat poison	T60.4x1	T60.4x2	T60.4x3	T60.4x4	—	—
Scillaren	T60.4x1	T60.4x2	T60.4x3	T60.4x4	—	—
Sclerosing agent	T46.8x1	T46.8x2	T46.8x3	T46.8x4	T46.8x5	T46.8x6
Scombrotoxin	T61.11	T61.12	T61.13	T61.14	—	—
Scopolamine	T44.3x1	T44.3x2	T44.3x3	T44.3x4	T44.3x5	T44.3x6
Scopolia extract	T44.3x1	T44.3x2	T44.3x3	T44.3x4	T44.3x5	T44.3x6
Scouring powder	T65.891	T65.892	T65.893	T65.894	—	—
Sea						
anemone (sting)	T63.631	T63.632	T63.633	T63.634	—	—
cucumber (sting)	T63.691	T63.692	T63.693	T63.694	—	—
snake (bite) (venom)	T63.091	T63.092	T63.093	T63.094	—	—
urchin spine (puncture)	T63.691	T63.692	T63.693	T63.694	—	—
Seafood	T61.91	T61.92	T61.93	T61.94	—	—
specified NEC	T61.8x1	T61.8x2	T61.8x3	T61.8x4	—	—
Secbutabarbital	T42.3x1	T42.3x2	T42.3x3	T42.3x4	T42.3x5	T42.3x6
Secbutabarbitone	T42.3x1	T42.3x2	T42.3x3	T42.3x4	T42.3x5	T42.3x6
Secnidazole	T37.3x1	T37.3x2	T37.3x3	T37.3x4	T37.3x5	T37.3x6
Secobarbital	T42.3x1	T42.3x2	T42.3x3	T42.3x4	T42.3x5	T42.3x6
Seconal	T42.3x1	T42.3x2	T42.3x3	T42.3x4	T42.3x5	T42.3x6
Secretin	T50.8x1	T50.8x2	T50.8x3	T50.8x4	T50.8x5	T50.8x6
Sedative NEC	T42.71	T42.72	T42.73	T42.74	142.75	T42.76
mixed NEC	T42.6x1	T42.6x2	T42.6x3	T42.6x4	T42.6x5	T42.6x6
Sedormid	T42.6x1	T42.6x2	T42.6x3	T42.6x4	T42.6x5	T42.6x6
Seed disinfectant or dressing	T60.8x1	T60.8x2	T60.8x3	T60.8x4	—	—
Seeds (poisonous)	T62.2x1	T62.2x2	T62.2x3	T62.2x4	—	—
disinfectant or dressing	T65.891	T65.892	T65.893	T65.894		
Selegiline	T42.8x1	T42.8x2	T42.8x3	T42.8x4	T42.8x5	T42.8x6
Selenium NEC	T56.891	T56.892	T56.893	T56.894		
disulfide or sulfide	T49.4x1	T49.4x2	T49.4x3	T49.4x4	T49.4x5	T49.4x6
fumes	T59.891	T59.892	T59.893	T59.894		
sulfide	T49.4x1	T49.4x2	T49.4x3	T49.4x4	T49.4x5	T49.4x6
Selenomethionine (75Se)	T50.8x1	T50.8x2	T50.8x3	T50.8x4	T50.8x5	T50.8x6
Selsun	T49.4x1	T49.4x2	T49.4x3	T49.4x4	T49.4x5	T49.4x6
Semustine	T45.1x1	T45.1x2	T45.1x3	T45.1x4	T45.1x5	T45.1x6
Senega syrup	T48.4x1	T48.4x2	T48.4x3	T48.4x4	T48.4x5	T48.4x6
Senna	T47.2x1	T47.2x2	T47.2x3	T47.2x4	T47.2x5	T47.2x6
Sennoside A+B	T47.2x1	T47.2x2	T47.2x3	T47.2x4	T47.2x5	T47.2x6
Septisol	T49.2x1	T49.2x2	T49.2x3	T49.2x4	T49.2x5	T49.2x6
Seractide	T38.811	T38.812	T38.813	T38.814	T38.815	T38.816
Serax	T42.4x1	T42.4x2	T42.4x3	T42.4x4	T42.4x5	T42.4x6
Serenesil	T42.6x1	T42.6x2	T42.6x3	T42.6x4	T42.6x5	T42.6x6
Serenium (hydrochloride)	T37.91	T37.92	T37.93	T37.94	T37.95	T37.96
Serepax—see Oxazepam						
Sermorelin	T38.891	T38.892	T38.893	T38.894	T38.895	T38.896
Sernyl	T41.1x1	T41.1x2	T41.1x3	T41.1x4	T41.1x5	T41.1x6
Serotonin	T50.991	T50.992	T50.993	T50.994	T50.995	T50.996
Serpasil	T46.5x1	T46.5x2	T46.5x3	T46.5x4	T46.5x5	T46.5x6
Serrapeptase	T45.3x1	T45.3x2	T45.3x3	T45.3x4	T45.3x5	T45.3x6
Serum						
antibotulinus	T50.Z11	T50.Z12	T50.Z13	T50.Z14	T50.Z15	T50.Z16
anticytotoxic	T50.Z11	T50.Z12	T50.Z13	T50.Z14	T50.Z15	T50.Z16
antidiphtheria	T50.Z11	T50.Z12	T50.Z13	T50.Z14	T50.Z15	T50.Z16
antimeningococcus	T50.Z11	T50.Z12	T50.Z13	T50.Z14	T50.Z15	T50.Z16
anti-Rh	T50.Z11	T50.Z12	T50.Z13	T50.Z14	T50.Z15	T50.Z16
anti-snake-bite	T50.Z11	T50.Z12	T50.Z13	T50.Z14	T50.Z15	T50.Z16
antitetanic	T50.Z11	T50.Z12	T50.Z13	T50.Z14	T50.Z15	T50.Z16
antitoxic	T50.Z11	T50.Z12	T50.Z13	T50.Z14	T50.Z15	T50.Z16
complement (inhibitor)	T45.8x1	T45.8x2	T45.8x3	T45.8x4	T45.8x5	T45.8x6
convalescent	T50.Z11	T50.Z12	T50.Z13	T50.Z14	T50.Z15	T50.Z16
hemolytic complement	T45.8x1	T45.8x2	T45.8x3	T45.8x4	T45.8x5	T45.8x6
immune (human)	T50.Z11	T50.Z12	T50.Z13	T50.Z14	T50.Z15	T50.Z16
protective NEC	T50.Z11	T50.Z12	T50.Z13	T50.Z14	T50.Z15	T50.Z16
Setastine	T45.0x1	T45.0x2	T45.0x3	T45.0x4	T45.0x5	T45.0x6
Setoperone	T43.591	T43.592	T43.593	T43.594	T43.595	T43.596
Sewer gas	T59.891	T59.892	T59.893	T59.894	—	—
Shampoo	T54.91	T54.92	T54.93	T54.94	—	—
Shellfish, noxious, nonbacterial	T61.781	T61.782	T61.783	T61.784	—	—
Silibinin	T50.991	T50.992	T50.993	T50.994	T50.995	T50.996
Silicone NEC	T65.891	T65.892	T65.893	T65.894	—	—
medicinal	T49.3x1	T49.3x2	T49.3x3	T49.3x4	T49.3x5	T49.3x6
Silvadene	T49.0x1	T49.0x2	T49.0x3	T49.0x4	T49.0x5	T49.0x6
Silver	T49.0x1	T49.0x2	T49.0x3	T49.0x4	T49.0x5	T49.0x6
anti-infectives	T49.0x1	T49.0x2	T49.0x3	T49.0x4	T49.0x5	T49.0x6
arsphenamine	T37.8x1	T37.8x2	T37.8x3	T37.8x4	T37.8x5	T37.8x6
colloidal	T49.0x1	T49.0x2	T49.0x3	T49.0x4	T49.0x5	T49.0x6
nitrate	T49.0x1	T49.0x2	T49.0x3	T49.0x4	T49.0x5	T49.0x6
ophthalmic preparation	T49.5x1	T49.5x2	T49.5x3	T49.5x4	T49.5x5	T49.5x6
toughened (keratolytic)	T49.4x1	T49.4x2	T49.4x3	T49.4x4	T49.4x5	T49.4x6
nonmedicinal (dust)	T56.891	T56.892	T56.893	T56.894	—	—
protein	T49.5x1	T49.5x2	T49.5x3	T49.5x4	T49.5x5	T49.5x6
salvarsan	T37.8x1	T37.8x2	T37.8x3	T37.8x4	T37.8x5	T37.8x6
sulfadiazine	T49.4x1	T49.4x2	T49.4x3	T49.4x4	T49.4x5	T49.4x6
Silymarin	T50.991	T50.992	T50.993	T50.994	T50.995	T50.996
Simaldrate	T47.1x1	T47.1x2	T47.1x3	T47.1x4	T47.1x5	T47.1x6
Simazine	T60.3x1	T60.3x2	T60.3x3	T60.3x4	—	—
Simethicone	T47.1x1	T47.1x2	T47.1x3	T47.1x4	T47.1x5	T47.1x6
Simfibrate	T46.6x1	T46.6x2	T46.6x3	T46.6x4	T46.6x5	T46.6x6
Simvastatin	T46.6x1	T46.6x2	T46.6x3	T46.6x4	T46.6x5	T46.6x6
Sincalide	T50.8x1	T50.8x2	T50.8x3	T50.8x4	T50.8x5	T50.8x6
Sinequan	T43.011	T43.012	T43.013	T43.014	T43.015	T43.016
Singoserp	T46.5x1	T46.5x2	T46.5x3	T46.5x4	T46.5x5	T46.5x6
Sintrom	T45.511	T45.512	T45.513	T45.514	T45.515	T45.516
Sisomicin	T36.5x1	T36.5x2	T36.5x3	T36.5x4	T36.5x5	T36.5x6
Sitosterols	T46.6x1	T46.6x2	T46.6x3	T46.6x4	T46.6x5	T46.6x6
Skeletal muscle relaxants	T48.1x1	T48.1x2	T48.1x3	T48.1x4	T48.1x5	T48.1x6

Drug and Chemical Table

Skin—Sodium

Substance	Poisoning, Accidental (unintentional)	Poisoning, Intentional Self-harm	Poisoning, Assault	Poisoning, Undetermined	Adverse Effect	Under-dosing
Skin						
agents (external)	T49.91	T49.92	T49.93	T49.94	T49.95	T49.96
specified NEC	T49.8x1	T49.8x2	T49.8x3	T49.8x4	T49.8x5	T49.8x6
test antigen	T50.8x1	T50.8x2	T50.8x3	T50.8x4	T50.8x5	T50.8x6
Sleep-eze	T45.0x1	T45.0x2	T45.0x3	T45.0x4	T45.0x5	T45.0x6
Sleeping draught, pill	T42.71	T42.72	T42.73	T42.74	T42.75	T42.76
Smallpox vaccine	T50.B11	T50.B12	T50.B13	T50.B14	T50.B15	T50.B16
Smelter fumes NEC	T56.91	T56.92	T56.93	T56.94	—	—
Smog	T59.1x1	T59.1x2	T59.1x3	T59.1x4	—	—
Smoke NEC	T59.811	T59.812	T59.813	T59.814	—	—
Smooth muscle relaxant	T44.3x1	T44.3x2	T44.3x3	T44.3x4	T44.3x5	T44.3x6
Snail killer NEC	T60.8x1	T60.8x2	T60.8x3	T60.8x4	—	—
Snake venom or bite	T63.001	T63.002	T63.003	T63.004	—	—
hemocoagulase	T45.7x1	T45.7x2	T45.7x3	T45.7x4	T45.7x5	T45.7x6
Snuff	T65.211	T65.212	T65.213	T65.214	—	—
Soap (powder) (product)	T54.91	T54.92	T54.93	T54.94	—	—
enema	T47.4x1	T47.4x2	T47.4x3	T47.4x4	T47.4x5	T47.4x6
medicinal, soft	T49.2x1	T49.2x2	T49.2x3	T49.2x4	T49.2x5	T49.2x6
superfatted	T49.2x1	T49.2x2	T49.2x3	T49.2x4	T49.2x5	T49.2x6
Sobrerol	T48.4x1	T48.4x2	T48.4x3	T48.4x4	T48.4x5	T48.4x6
Soda (caustic)	T54.3x1	T54.3x2	T54.3x3	T54.3x4	—	—
bicarb	T47.1x1	T47.1x2	T47.1x3	T47.1x4	T47.1x5	T47.1x6
chlorinated—see Sodium, hypochlorite						
Sodium						
acetosulfone	T37.1x1	T37.1x2	T37.1x3	T37.1x4	T37.1x5	T37.1x6
acetrizoate	T50.8x1	T50.8x2	T50.8x3	T50.8x4	T50.8x5	T50.8x6
acid phosphate	T50.3x1	T50.3x2	T50.3x3	T50.3x4	T50.3x5	T50.3x6
alginate	T47.8x1	T47.8x2	T47.8x3	T47.8x4	T47.8x5	T47.8x6
amidotrizoate	T50.8x1	T50.8x2	T50.8x3	T50.8x4	T50.8x5	T50.8x6
aminopterin	T45.1x1	T45.1x2	T45.1x3	T45.1x4	T45.1x5	T45.1x6
amylosulfate	T47.8x1	T47.8x2	T47.8x3	T47.8x4	T47.8x5	T47.8x6
amytal	T42.3x1	T42.3x2	T42.3x3	T42.3x4	T42.3x5	T42.3x6
antimony gluconate	T37.3x1	T37.3x2	T37.3x3	T37.3x4	T37.3x5	T37.3x6
arsenate	T57.0x1	T57.0x2	T57.0x3	T57.0x4	—	—
aurothiomalate	T39.4x1	T39.4x2	T39.4x3	T39.4x4	T39.4x5	T39.4x6
aurothiosulfate	T39.4x1	T39.4x2	T39.4x3	T39.4x4	T39.4x5	T39.4x6
barbiturate	T42.3x1	T42.3x2	T42.3x3	T42.3x4	T42.3x5	T42.3x6
basic phosphate	T47.4x1	T47.4x2	T47.4x3	T47.4x4	T47.4x5	T47.4x6
bicarbonate	T47.1x1	T47.1x2	T47.1x3	T47.1x4	T47.1x5	T47.1x6
bichromate	T57.8x1	T57.8x2	T57.8x3	T57.8x4	—	—
biphosphate	T50.3x1	T50.3x2	T50.3x3	T50.3x4	T50.3x5	T50.3x6
bisulfate	T65.891	T65.892	T65.893	T65.894	—	—
borate						
cleanser	T57.8x1	T57.8x2	T57.8x3	T57.8x4	—	—
eye	T49.5x1	T49.5x2	T49.5x3	T49.5x4	T49.5x5	T49.5x6
therapeutic	T49.8x1	T49.8x2	T49.8x3	T49.8x4	T49.8x5	T49.8x6
bromide	T42.6x1	T42.6x2	T42.6x3	T42.6x4	T42.6x5	T42.6x6
cacodylate (nonmedicinal) NEC	T50.8x1	T50.8x2	T50.8x3	T50.8x4	T50.8x5	T50.8x6
anti-infective	T37.8x1	T37.8x2	T37.8x3	T37.8x4	T37.8x5	T37.8x6
herbicide	T60.3x1	T60.3x2	T60.3x3	T60.3x4	—	—
calcium edetate	T45.8x1	T45.8x2	T45.8x3	T45.8x4	T45.8x5	T45.8x6
carbonate NEC	T54.3x1	T54.3x2	T54.3x3	T54.3x4	—	—
chlorate NEC	T65.891	T65.892	T65.893	T65.894	—	—
herbicide	T54.91	T54.92	T54.93	T54.94	—	—
chloride	T50.3x1	T50.3x2	T50.3x3	T50.3x4	T50.3x5	T50.3x6
with glucose	T50.3x1	T50.3x2	T50.3x3	T50.3x4	T50.3x5	T50.3x6
chromate	T65.891	T65.892	T65.893	T65.894	—	—
citrate	T50.991	T50.992	T50.993	T50.994	T50.995	T50.996
cromoglicate	T48.6x1	T48.6x2	T48.6x3	T48.6x4	T48.6x5	T48.6x6
cyanide	T57.8x1	T57.8x2	T57.8x3	T57.8x4	—	—
cyclamate	T50.3x1	T50.3x2	T50.3x3	T50.3x4	T50.3x5	T50.3x6
dehydrocholate	T45.8x1	T45.8x2	T45.8x3	T45.8x4	T45.8x5	T45.8x6
diatrizoate	T50.8x1	T50.8x2	T50.8x3	T50.8x4	T50.8x5	T50.8x6
dibunate	T48.4x1	T48.4x2	T48.4x3	T48.4x4	T48.4x5	T48.4x6
dioctyl sulfosuccinate	T47.4x1	T47.4x2	T47.4x3	T47.4x4	T47.4x5	T47.4x6
dipantoyl ferrate	T45.8x1	T45.8x2	T45.8x3	T45.8x4	T45.8x5	T45.8x6
edetate	T45.8x1	T45.8x2	T45.8x3	T45.8x4	T45.8x5	T45.8x6
ethacrynate	T50.1x1	T50.1x2	T50.1x3	T50.1x4	T50.1x5	T50.1x6
feredetate	T45.8x1	T45.8x2	T45.8x3	T45.8x4	T45.8x5	T45.8x6
fluoride—see Fluoride						

Substance	Poisoning, Accidental (unintentional)	Poisoning, Intentional Self-harm	Poisoning, Assault	Poisoning, Undetermined	Adverse Effect	Under-dosing
Sodium—continued						
fluoroacetate (dust) (pesticide)	T60.4x1	T60.4x2	T60.4x3	T60.4x4	—	—
free salt	T50.3x1	T50.3x2	T50.3x3	T50.3x4	T50.3x5	T50.3x6
fusidate	T36.8x1	T36.8x2	T36.8x3	T36.8x4	T36.8x5	T36.8x6
glucaldrate	T47.1x1	T47.1x2	T47.1x3	T47.1x4	T47.1x5	T47.1x6
glucosulfone	T37.1x1	T37.1x2	T37.1x3	T37.1x4	T37.1x5	T37.1x6
glutamate	T45.8x1	T45.8x2	T45.8x3	T45.8x4	T45.8x5	T45.8x6
hydrogen carbonate	T50.3x1	T50.3x2	T50.3x3	T50.3x4	T50.3x5	T50.3x6
hydroxide	T54.3x1	T54.3x2	T54.3x3	T54.3x4	—	—
hypochlorite (bleach) NEC	T54.3x1	T54.3x2	T54.3x3	T54.3x4	—	—
disinfectant	T54.3x1	T54.3x2	T54.3x3	T54.3x4	—	—
medicinal (anti-infective) (external)	T49.0x1	T49.0x2	T49.0x3	T49.0x4	T49.0x5	T49.0x6
vapor	T54.3x1	T54.3x2	T54.3x3	T54.3x4	—	—
hyposulfite	T49.0x1	T49.0x2	T49.0x3	T49.0x4	T49.0x5	T49.0x6
indigotin disulfonate	T50.8x1	T50.8x2	T50.8x3	T50.8x4	T50.8x5	T50.8x6
iodide	T50.991	T50.992	T50.993	T50.994	T50.995	T50.996
I-131	T50.8x1	T50.8x2	T50.8x3	T50.8x4	T50.8x5	T50.8x6
therapeutic	T38.2x1	T38.2x2	T38.2x3	T38.2x4	T38.2x5	T38.2x6
iodohippurate (131I)	T50.8x1	T50.8x2	T50.8x3	T50.8x4	T50.8x5	T50.8x6
iopodate	T50.8x1	T50.8x2	T50.8x3	T50.8x4	T50.8x5	T50.8x6
iothalamate	T50.8x1	T50.8x2	T50.8x3	T50.8x4	T50.8x5	T50.8x6
iron edetate	T45.4x1	T45.4x2	T45.4x3	T45.4x4	T45.4x5	T45.4x6
lactate (compound solution)	T45.8x1	T45.8x2	T45.8x3	T45.8x4	T45.8x5	T45.8x6
lauryl (sulfate)	T49.2x1	T49.2x2	T49.2x3	T49.2x4	T49.2x5	T49.2x6
L-triiodothyronine	T38.1x1	T38.1x2	T38.1x3	T38.1x4	T38.1x5	T38.1x6
magnesium citrate	T50.991	T50.992	T50.993	T50.994	T50.995	T50.996
mersalate	T50.2x1	T50.2x2	T50.2x3	T50.2x4	T50.2x5	T50.2x6
metasilicate	T65.891	T65.892	T65.893	T65.894	—	—
metrizoate	T50.8x1	T50.8x2	T50.8x3	T50.8x4	T50.8x5	T50.8x6
monofluoroacetate (pesticide)	T60.1x1	T60.1x2	T60.1x3	T60.1x4	—	—
morrhuate	T46.8x1	T46.8x2	T46.8x3	T46.8x4	T46.8x5	T46.8x6
nafcillin	T36.0x1	T36.0x2	T36.0x3	T36.0x4	T36.0x5	T36.0x6
nitrate(oxidizing agent)	T65.891	T65.892	T65.893	T65.894	—	—
nitrite	T50.6x1	T50.6x2	T50.6x3	T50.6x4	T50.6x5	T50.6x6
nitroferricyanide	T46.5x1	T46.5x2	T46.5x3	T46.5x4	T46.5x5	T46.5x6
nitroprusside	T46.5x1	T46.5x2	T46.5x3	T46.5x4	T46.5x5	T46.5x6
oxalate	T65.891	T65.892	T65.893	T65.894	—	—
oxide/peroxide	T65.891	T65.892	T65.893	T65.894	—	—
oxybate	T41.291	T41.292	T41.293	T41.294	T41.295	T41.296
para-aminohippurate	T50.8x1	T50.8x2	T50.8x3	T50.8x4	T50.8x5	T50.8x6
perborate (nonmedicinal) NEC	T65.891	T65.892	T65.893	T65.894	—	—
medicinal	T49.0x1	T49.0x2	T49.0x3	T49.0x4	T49.0x5	T49.0x6
soap	T55.0x1	T55.0x2	T55.0x3	T55.0x4	—	—
percarbonate—see Sodium, perborate						
pertechnetate Tc99m	T50.8x1	T50.8x2	T50.8x3	T50.8x4	T50.8x5	T50.8x6
phosphate						
cellulose	T45.8x1	T45.8x2	T45.8x3	T45.8x4	T45.8x5	T45.8x6
dibasic	T47.2x1	T47.2x2	T47.2x3	T47.2x4	T47.2x5	T47.2x6
monobasic	T47.2x1	T47.2x2	T47.2x3	T47.2x4	T47.2x5	T47.2x6
phytate	T50.6x1	T50.6x2	T50.6x3	T50.6x4	T50.6x5	T50.6x6
picosulfate	T47.2x1	T47.2x2	T47.2x3	T47.2x4	T47.2x5	T47.2x6
polyhydroxyaluminium monocarbonate	T47.1x1	T47.1x2	T47.1x3	T47.1x4	T47.1x5	T47.1x6
polystyrene sulfonate	T50.3x1	T50.3x2	T50.3x3	T50.3x4	T50.3x5	T50.3x6
propionate	T49.0x1	T49.0x2	T49.0x3	T49.0x4	T49.0x5	T49.0x6
propyl hydroxybenzoate	T50.991	T50.992	T50.993	T50.994	T50.995	T50.996
psylliate	T46.8x1	T46.8x2	T46.8x3	T46.8x4	T46.8x5	T46.8x6
removing resins	T50.3x1	T50.3x2	T50.3x3	T50.3x4	T50.3x5	T50.3x6
salicylate	T39.091	T39.092	T39.093	T39.094	T39.095	T39.096
salt NEC	T50.3x1	T50.3x2	T50.3x3	T50.3x4	T50.3x5	T50.3x6
selenate	T60.2x1	T60.2x2	T60.2x3	T60.2x4	—	—
stibogluconate	T37.3x1	T37.3x2	T37.3x3	T37.3x4	T37.3x5	T37.3x6
sulfate	T47.4x1	T47.4x2	T47.4x3	T47.4x4	T47.4x5	T47.4x6
sulfoxone	T37.1x1	T37.1x2	T37.1x3	T37.1x4	T37.1x5	T37.1x6
tetradecyl sulfate	T46.8x1	T46.8x2	T46.8x3	T46.8x4	T46.8x5	T46.8x6
thiopental	T41.1x1	T41.1x2	T41.1x3	T41.1x4	T41.1x5	T41.1x6
thiosalicylate	T39.091	T39.092	T39.093	T39.094	T39.095	T39.096
thiosulfate	T50.6x1	T50.6x2	T50.6x3	T50.6x4	T50.6x5	T50.6x6
tolbutamide	T38.3x1	T38.3x2	T38.3x3	T38.3x4	T38.3x5	T38.3x6

Substance	Poisoning, Accidental (unintentional)	Poisoning, Intentional Self-harm	Poisoning, Assault	Poisoning, Undetermined	Adverse Effect	Under-dosing
Sodium—*continued*						
tyropanoate	T50.8x1	T50.8x2	T50.8x3	T50.8x4	T50.8x5	T50.8x6
valproate	T42.6x1	T42.6x2	T42.6x3	T42.6x4	T42.6x5	T42.6x6
versenate	T50.6x1	T50.6x2	T50.6x3	T50.6x4	T50.6x5	T50.6x6
Sodium-free salt	T50.901	T50.902	T50.903	T50.904	T50.905	T50.906
Sodium-removing resin	T50.3x1	T50.3x2	T50.3x3	T50.3x4	T50.3x5	T50.3x6
Soft soap	T54.91	T54.92	T54.93	T54.94	—	—
Solanine	T62.2x1	T62.2x2	T62.2x3	T62.2x4	—	—
berries	T62.1x1	T62.1x2	T62.1x3	T62.1x4	—	—
Solanum dulcamara	T62.2x1	T62.2x2	T62.2x3	T62.2x4	—	—
berries	T62.1x1	T62.1x2	T62.1x3	T62.1x4	—	—
Solapsone	T37.1x1	T37.1x2	T37.1x3	T37.1x4	T37.1x5	T37.1x6
Solar lotion	T49.3x1	T49.3x2	T49.3x3	T49.3x4	T49.3x5	T49.3x6
Solasulfone	T37.1x1	T37.1x2	T37.1x3	T37.1x4	T37.1x5	T37.1x6
Soldering fluid	T65.891	T65.892	T65.893	T65.894	—	—
Solid substance	T65.91	T65.92	T65.93	T65.94	—	—
specified NEC	T65.891	T65.892	T65.893	T65.894	—	—
Solvent, industrial NEC	T52.91	T52.92	T52.93	T52.94	—	—
naphtha	T52.0x1	T52.0x2	T52.0x3	T52.0x4	—	—
petroleum	T52.0x1	T52.0x2	T52.0x3	T52.0x4	—	—
specified NEC	T52.91	T52.92	T52.93	T52.94	—	—
Soma	T42.8x1	T42.8x2	T42.8x3	T42.8x4	T42.8x5	T42.8x6
Somatorelin	T38.891	T38.892	T38.893	T38.894	T38.895	T38.896
Somatostatin	T38.991	T38.992	T38.993	T38.994	T38.995	T38.996
Somatotropin	T38.811	T38.812	T38.813	T38.814	T38.815	T38.816
Somatrem	T38.811	T38.812	T38.813	T38.814	T38.815	T38.816
Somatropin	T38.811	T38.812	T38.813	T38.814	T38.815	T38.816
Sominex	T45.0x1	T45.0x2	T45.0x3	T45.0x4	T45.0x5	T45.0x6
Somnos	T42.6x1	T42.6x2	T42.6x3	T42.6x4	T42.6x5	T42.6x6
Somonal	T42.3x1	T42.3x2	T42.3x3	T42.3x4	T42.3x5	T42.3x6
Soneryl	T42.3x1	T42.3x2	T42.3x3	T42.3x4	T42.3x5	T42.3x6
Soothing syrup	T50.901	T50.902	T50.903	T50.904	T50.905	T50.906
Sopor	T42.6x1	T42.6x2	T42.6x3	T42.6x4	T42.6x5	T42.6x6
Soporific	T42.71	T42.72	T42.73	T42.74	T42.75	T42.76
Soporific drug	T42.71	T42.72	T42.73	T42.74	T42.75	T42.76
specified type NEC	T42.6x1	T42.6x2	T42.6x3	T42.6x4	T42.6x5	T42.6x6
Sorbide nitrate	T46.3x1	T46.3x2	T46.3x3	T46.3x4	T46.3x5	T46.3x6
Sorbitol	T47.4x1	T47.4x2	T47.4x3	T47.4x4	T47.4x5	T47.4x6
Sotalol	T44.7x1	T44.7x2	T44.7x3	T44.7x4	T44.7x5	T44.7x6
Sotradecol	T46.8x1	T46.8x2	T46.8x3	T46.8x4	T46.8x5	T46.8x6
Soysterol	T46.6x1	T46.6x2	T46.6x3	T46.6x4	T46.6x5	T46.6x6
Spacoline	T44.3x1	T44.3x2	T44.3x3	T44.3x4	T44.3x5	T44.3x6
Spanish fly	T49.8x1	T49.8x2	T49.8x3	T49.8x4	T49.8x5	T49.8x6
Sparine	T43.3x1	T43.3x2	T43.3x3	T43.3x4	T43.3x5	T43.3x6
Sparteine	T48.0x1	T48.0x2	T48.0x3	T48.0x4	T48.0x5	T48.0x6
Spasmolytic						
anticholinergics	T44.3x1	T44.3x2	T44.3x3	T44.3x4	T44.3x5	T44.3x6
autonomic	T44.3x1	T44.3x2	T44.3x3	T44.3x4	T44.3x5	T44.3x6
bronchial NEC	T48.6x1	T48.6x2	T48.6x3	T48.6x4	T48.6x5	T48.6x6
quaternary ammonium	T44.3x1	T44.3x2	T44.3x3	T44.3x4	T44.3x5	T44.3x6
skeletal muscle NEC	T48.1x1	T48.1x2	T48.1x3	T48.1x4	T48.1x5	T48.1x6
Spectinomycin	T36.5x1	T36.5x2	T36.5x3	T36.5x4	T36.5x5	T36.5x6
Speed	T43.621	T43.622	T43.623	T43.624	T43.625	T43.626
Spermicide	T49.8x1	T49.8x2	T49.8x3	T49.8x4	T49.8x5	T49.8x6
Spider (bite) (venom)	T63.391	T63.392	T63.393	T63.394	—	—
antivenin	T50.Z11	T50.Z12	T50.Z13	T50.Z14	T50.Z15	T50.Z16
Spigelia (root)	T37.4x1	T37.4x2	T37.4x3	T37.4x4	T37.4x5	T37.4x6
Spindle inactivator	T50.4x1	T50.4x2	T50.4x3	T50.4x4	T50.4x5	T50.4x6
Spiperone	T43.4x1	T43.4x2	T43.4x3	T43.4x4	T43.4x5	T43.4x6
Spiramycin	T36.3x1	T36.3x2	T36.3x3	T36.3x4	T36.3x5	T36.3x6
Spirapril	T46.4x1	T46.4x2	T46.4x3	T46.4x4	T46.4x5	T46.4x6
Spirilene	T43.591	T43.592	T43.593	T43.594	T43.595	T43.596
Spirit(s) (neutral) **NEC**	T51.0x1	T51.0x2	T51.0x3	T51.0x4	—	—
beverage	T51.0x1	T51.0x2	T51.0x3	T51.0x4	—	—
industrial	T51.0x1	T51.0x2	T51.0x3	T51.0x4	—	—
mineral	T52.0x1	T52.0x2	T52.0x3	T52.0x4	—	—
of salt—*see* Hydrochloric acid						
surgical	T51.0x1	T51.0x2	T51.0x3	T51.0x4	—	—
Spironolactone	T50.0x1	T50.0x2	T50.0x3	T50.0x4	T50.0x5	T50.0x6
Spiroperidol	T43.4x1	T43.4x2	T43.4x3	T43.4x4	T43.4x5	T43.4x6
Sponge, absorbable (gelatin)	T45.7x1	T45.7x2	T45.7x3	T45.7x4	T45.7x5	T45.7x6

Substance	Poisoning, Accidental (unintentional)	Poisoning, Intentional Self-harm	Poisoning, Assault	Poisoning, Undetermined	Adverse Effect	Under-dosing
Sporostacin	T49.0x1	T49.0x2	T49.0x3	T49.0x4	T49.0x5	T49.0x6
Spray (aerosol)	T65.91	T65.92	T65.93	T65.94	—	—
cosmetic	T65.891	T65.892	T65.893	T65.894	—	—
medicinal NEC	T50.901	T50.902	T50.903	T50.904	T50.905	T50.906
pesticides—*see* Pesticides						
specified content—*see* specific substance						
Spurge flax	T62.2x1	T62.2x2	T62.2x3	T62.2x4	—	—
Spurges	T62.2x1	T62.2x2	T62.2x3	T62.2x4	—	—
Sputum viscosity-lowering drug	T48.4x1	T48.4x2	T48.4x3	T48.4x4	T48.4x5	T48.4x6
Squill	T46.0x1	T46.0x2	T46.0x3	T46.0x4	T46.0x5	T46.0x6
rat poison	T60.4x1	T60.4x2	T60.4x3	T60.4x4	—	—
Squirting cucumber (cathartic)	T47.2x1	T47.2x2	T47.2x3	T47.2x4	T47.2x5	T47.2x6
Stains	T65.6x1	T65.6x2	T65.6x3	T65.6x4	—	—
Stannous fluoride	T49.7x1	T49.7x2	T49.7x3	T49.7x4	T49.7x5	T49.7x6
Stanolone	T38.7x1	T38.7x2	T38.7x3	T38.7x4	T38.7x5	T38.7x6
Stanozolol	T38.7x1	T38.7x2	T38.7x3	T38.7x4	T38.7x5	T38.7x6
Staphisagria or stavesacre (pediculicide)	T49.0x1	T49.0x2	T49.0x3	T49.0x4	T49.0x5	T49.0x6
Starch	T50.901	T50.902	T50.903	T50.904	T50.905	T50.906
Stelazine	T43.3x1	T43.3x2	T43.3x3	T43.3x4	T43.3x5	T43.3x6
Stemetil	T43.3x1	T43.3x2	T43.3x3	T43.3x4	T43.3x5	T43.3x6
Stepronin	T48.4x1	T48.4x2	T48.4x3	T48.4x4	T48.4x5	T48.4x6
Sterculia	T47.4x1	T47.4x2	T47.4x3	T47.4x4	T47.4x5	T47.4x6
Sternutator gas	T59.891	T59.892	T59.893	T59.894	—	—
Steroid	T38.0x1	T38.0x2	T38.0x3	T38.0x4	T38.0x5	T38.0x6
anabolic	T38.7x1	T38.7x2	T38.7x3	T38.7x4	T38.7x5	T38.7x6
androgenic	T38.7x1	T38.7x2	T38.7x3	T38.7x4	T38.7x5	T38.7x6
antineoplastic, hormone	T38.7x1	T38.7x2	T38.7x3	T38.7x4	T38.7x5	T38.7x6
estrogen	T38.5x1	T38.5x2	T38.5x3	T38.5x4	T38.5x5	T38.5x6
ENT agent	T49.6x1	T49.6x2	T49.6x3	T49.6x4	T49.6x5	T49.6x6
ophthalmic preparation	T49.5x1	T49.5x2	T49.5x3	T49.5x4	T49.5x5	T49.5x6
topical NEC	T49.0x1	T49.0x2	T49.0x3	T49.0x4	T49.0x5	T49.0x6
Stibine	T56.891	T56.892	T56.893	T56.894	—	—
Stibogluconate	T37.3x1	T37.3x2	T37.3x3	T37.3x4	T37.3x5	T37.3x6
Stibophen	T37.4x1	T37.4x2	T37.4x3	T37.4x4	T37.4x5	T37.4x6
Stilbamidine (isetionate)	T37.3x1	T37.3x2	T37.3x3	T37.3x4	T37.3x5	T37.3x6
Stilbestrol	T38.5x1	T38.5x2	T38.5x3	T38.5x4	T38.5x5	T38.5x6
Stilboestrol	T38.5x1	T38.5x2	T38.5x3	T38.5x4	T38.5x5	T38.5x6
Stimulant						
central nervous system (*see also* Psychostimulant)	T43.601	T43.602	T43.603	T43.604	T43.605	T43.606
analeptics	T50.7x1	T50.7x2	T50.7x3	T50.7x4	T50.7x5	T50.7x6
opiate antagonist	T50.7x1	T50.7x2	T50.7x3	T50.7x4	T50.7x5	T50.7x6
psychotherapeutic NEC (*see also* Psychotherapeutic drug)	T43.601	T43.602	T43.603	T43.604	T43.605	T43.606
specified NEC	T43.691	T43.692	T43.693	T43.694	T43.695	T43.696
respiratory	T48.901	T48.902	T48.903	T48.904	T48.905	T48.906
Stone-dissolving drug	T50.901	T50.902	T50.903	T50.904	T50.905	T50.906
Storage battery (cells) (acid)	T54.2x1	T54.2x2	T54.2x3	T54.2x4	—	—
Stovaine	T41.3x1	T41.3x2	T41.3x3	T41.3x4	T41.3x5	T41.3x6
infiltration (subcutaneous)	T41.3x1	T41.3x2	T41.3x3	T41.3x4	T41.3x5	T41.3x6
nerve block (peripheral) (plexus)	T41.3x1	T41.3x2	T41.3x3	T41.3x4	T41.3x5	T41.3x6
spinal	T41.3x1	T41.3x2	T41.3x3	T41.3x4	T41.3x5	T41.3x6
topical (surface)	T41.3x1	T41.3x2	T41.3x3	T41.3x4	T41.3x5	T41.3x6
Stovarsal	T37.8x1	T37.8x2	T37.8x3	T37.8x4	T37.8x5	T37.8x6
Stove gas—*see* Gas, stove						
Stoxil	T49.5x1	T49.5x2	T49.5x3	T49.5x4	T49.5x5	T49.5x6
Stramonium	T48.6x1	T48.6x2	T48.6x3	T48.6x4	T48.6x5	T48.6x6
natural state	T62.2x1	T62.2x2	T62.2x3	T62.2x4	—	—
Streptodornase	T45.3x1	T45.3x2	T45.3x3	T45.3x4	T45.3x5	T45.3x6
Streptoduocin	T36.5x1	T36.5x2	T36.5x3	T36.5x4	T36.5x5	T36.5x6
Streptokinase	T45.611	T45.612	T45.613	T45.614	T45.615	T45.616
Streptomycin (derivative)	T36.5x1	T36.5x2	T36.5x3	T36.5x4	T36.5x5	T36.5x6
Streptonivicin	T36.5x1	T36.5x2	T36.5x3	T36.5x4	T36.5x5	T36.5x6
Streptovarycin	T36.5x1	T36.5x2	T36.5x3	T36.5x4	T36.5x5	T36.5x6
Streptozocin	T45.1x1	T45.1x2	T45.1x3	l45.1x4	T45.1x5	T45.1x6
Streptozotocin	T45.1x1	T45.1x2	T45.1x3	T45.1x4	T45.1x5	T45.1x6
Stripper (paint) (solvent)	T52.8x1	T52.8x2	T52.8x3	T52.8x4	—	—
Strobane	T60.1x1	T60.1x2	T60.1x3	T60.1x4	—	—
Strofantina	T46.0x1	T46.0x2	T46.0x3	T46.0x4	T46.0x5	T46.0x6

Drug and Chemical Table

Strophanthin (g) (k)–Suxibuzone

Substance	Poisoning, Accidental (unintentional)	Poisoning, Intentional Self-harm	Poisoning, Assault	Poisoning, Undetermined	Adverse Effect	Under-dosing
Strophanthin (g) (k)	T46.0x1	T46.0x2	T46.0x3	T46.0x4	T46.0x5	T46.0x6
Strophanthus	T46.0x1	T46.0x2	T46.0x3	T46.0x4	T46.0x5	T46.0x6
Strophantin	T46.0x1	T46.0x2	T46.0x3	T46.0x4	T46.0x5	T46.0x6
Strophantin-g	T46.0x1	T46.0x2	T46.0x3	T46.0x4	T46.0x5	T46.0x6
Strychnine (nonmedicinal) (pesticide) (salts)	T65.1x1	T65.1x2	T65.1x3	T65.1x4	—	—
medicinal	T48.291	T48.292	T48.293	T48.294	T48.295	T48.296
Strychnos (ignatii)—see Strychnine						
Styramate	T42.8x1	T42.8x2	T42.8x3	T42.8x4	T42.8x5	T42.8x6
Styrene	T65.891	T65.892	T65.893	T65.894	—	—
Succinimide, antiepileptic or anticonvulsant	T42.2x1	T42.2x2	T42.2x3	T42.2x4	T42.2x5	T42.2x6
mercuric—see Mercury						
Succinylcholine	T48.1x1	T48.1x2	T48.1x3	T48.1x4	T48.1x5	T48.1x6
Succinylsulfathiazole	T37.0x1	T37.0x2	T37.0x3	T37.0x4	T37.0x5	T37.0x6
Sucralfate	T47.1x1	T47.1x2	T47.1x3	T47.1x4	T47.1x5	T47.1x6
Sucrose	T50.3x1	T50.3x2	T50.3x3	T50.3x4	T50.3x5	T50.3x6
Sufentanil	T40.4x1	T40.4x2	T40.4x3	T40.4x4	T40.4x5	T40.4x6
Sulbactam	T36.0x1	T36.0x2	T36.0x3	T36.0x4	T36.0x5	T36.0x6
Sulbenicillin	T36.0x1	T36.0x2	T36.0x3	T36.0x4	T36.0x5	T36.0x6
Sulbentine	T49.0x1	T49.0x2	T49.0x3	T49.0x4	T49.0x5	T49.0x6
Sulfacetamide	T49.5x1	T49.5x2	T49.5x3	T49.5x4	T49.5x5	T49.5x6
ophthalmic preparation	T49.5x1	T49.5x2	T49.5x3	T49.5x4	T49.5x5	T49.5x6
Sulfachlorpyridazine	T37.0x1	T37.0x2	T37.0x3	T37.0x4	T37.0x5	T37.0x6
Sulfacitine	T37.0x1	T37.0x2	T37.0x3	T37.0x4	T37.0x5	T37.0x6
Sulfadiasulfone sodium	T37.0x1	T37.0x2	T37.0x3	T37.0x4	T37.0x5	T37.0x6
Sulfadiazine	T37.0x1	T37.0x2	T37.0x3	T37.0x4	T37.0x5	T37.0x6
silver (topical)	T49.0x1	T49.0x2	T49.0x3	T49.0x4	T49.0x5	T49.0x6
Sulfadimethoxine	T37.0x1	T37.0x2	T37.0x3	T37.0x4	T37.0x5	T37.0x6
Sulfadimidine	T37.0x1	T37.0x2	T37.0x3	T37.0x4	T37.0x5	T37.0x6
Sulfadoxine	T37.0x1	T37.0x2	T37.0x3	T37.0x4	T37.0x5	T37.0x6
with pyrimethamine	T37.2x1	T37.2x2	T37.2x3	T37.2x4	T37.2x5	T37.2x6
Sulfaethidole	T37.0x1	T37.0x2	T37.0x3	T37.0x4	T37.0x5	T37.0x6
Sulfafurazole	T37.0x1	T37.0x2	T37.0x3	T37.0x4	T37.0x5	T37.0x6
Sulfaguanidine	T37.0x1	T37.0x2	T37.0x3	T37.0x4	T37.0x5	T37.0x6
Sulfalene	T37.0x1	T37.0x2	T37.0x3	T37.0x4	T37.0x5	T37.0x6
Sulfaloxate	T37.0x1	T37.0x2	T37.0x3	T37.0x4	T37.0x5	T37.0x6
Sulfaloxic acid	T37.0x1	T37.0x2	T37.0x3	T37.0x4	T37.0x5	T37.0x6
Sulfamazone	T39.2x1	T39.2x2	T39.2x3	T39.2x4	T39.2x5	T39.2x6
Sulfamerazine	T37.0x1	T37.0x2	T37.0x3	T37.0x4	T37.0x5	T37.0x6
Sulfameter	T37.0x1	T37.0x2	T37.0x3	T37.0x4	T37.0x5	T37.0x6
Sulfamethazine	T37.0x1	T37.0x2	T37.0x3	T37.0x4	T37.0x5	T37.0x6
Sulfamethizole	T37.0x1	T37.0x2	T37.0x3	T37.0x4	T37.0x5	T37.0x6
Sulfamethoxazole	T37.0x1	T37.0x2	T37.0x3	T37.0x4	T37.0x5	T37.0x6
with trimethoprim	T36.8x1	T36.8x2	T36.8x3	T36.8x4	T36.8x5	T36.8x6
Sulfamethoxydiazine	T37.0x1	T37.0x2	T37.0x3	T37.0x4	T37.0x5	T37.0x6
Sulfamethoxypyridazine	T37.0x1	T37.0x2	T37.0x3	T37.0x4	T37.0x5	T37.0x6
Sulfamethylthiazole	T37.0x1	T37.0x2	T37.0x3	T37.0x4	T37.0x5	T37.0x6
Sulfametoxydiazine	T37.0x1	T37.0x2	T37.0x3	T37.0x4	T37.0x5	T37.0x6
Sulfamidopyrine	T39.2x1	T39.2x2	T39.2x3	T39.2x4	T39.2x5	T39.2x6
Sulfamonomethoxine	T37.0x1	T37.0x2	T37.0x3	T37.0x4	T37.0x5	T37.0x6
Sulfamoxole	T37.0x1	T37.0x2	T37.0x3	T37.0x4	T37.0x5	T37.0x6
Sulfamylon	T49.0x1	T49.0x2	T49.0x3	T49.0x4	T49.0x5	T49.0x6
Sulfan blue (diagnostic dye)	T50.8x1	T50.8x2	T50.8x3	T50.8x4	T50.8x5	T50.8x6
Sulfanilamide	T37.0x1	T37.0x2	T37.0x3	T37.0x4	T37.0x5	T37.0x6
Sulfanilylguanidine	T37.0x1	T37.0x2	T37.0x3	T37.0x4	T37.0x5	T37.0x6
Sulfaperin	T37.0x1	T37.0x2	T37.0x3	T37.0x4	T37.0x5	T37.0x6
Sulfaphenazole	T37.0x1	T37.0x2	T37.0x3	T37.0x4	T37.0x5	T37.0x6
Sulfaphenylthiazole	T37.0x1	T37.0x2	T37.0x3	T37.0x4	T37.0x5	T37.0x6
Sulfaproxyline	T37.0x1	T37.0x2	T37.0x3	T37.0x4	T37.0x5	T37.0x6
Sulfapyridine	T37.0x1	T37.0x2	T37.0x3	T37.0x4	T37.0x5	T37.0x6
Sulfapyrimidine	T37.0x1	T37.0x2	T37.0x3	T37.0x4	T37.0x5	T37.0x6
Sulfarsphenamine	T37.8x1	T37.8x2	T37.8x3	T37.8x4	T37.8x5	T37.8x6
Sulfasalazine	T37.0x1	T37.0x2	T37.0x3	T37.0x4	T37.0x5	T37.0x6
Sulfasuxidine	T37.0x1	T37.0x2	T37.0x3	T37.0x4	T37.0x5	T37.0x6
Sulfasymazine	T37.0x1	T37.0x2	T37.0x3	T37.0x4	T37.0x5	T37.0x6
Sulfated amylopectin	T47.8x1	T47.8x2	T47.8x3	T47.8x4	T47.8x5	T47.8x6
Sulfathiazole	T37.0x1	T37.0x2	T37.0x3	T37.0x4	T37.0x5	T37.0x6
Sulfatostearate	T49.2x1	T49.2x2	T49.2x3	T49.2x4	T49.2x5	T49.2x6
Sulfinpyrazone	T50.4x1	T50.4x2	T50.4x3	T50.4x4	T50.4x5	T50.4x6
Sulfiram	T49.0x1	T49.0x2	T49.0x3	T49.0x4	T49.0x5	T49.0x6
Sulfisomidine	T37.0x1	T37.0x2	T37.0x3	T37.0x4	T37.0x5	T37.0x6
Sulfisoxazole	T37.0x1	T37.0x2	T37.0x3	T37.0x4	T37.0x5	T37.0x6
ophthalmic preparation	T49.5x1	T49.5x2	T49.5x3	T49.5x4	T49.5x5	T49.5x6
Sulfobromophthalein (sodium)	T50.8x1	T50.8x2	T50.8x3	T50.8x4	T50.8x5	T50.8x6
Sulfobromphthalein	T50.8x1	T50.8x2	T50.8x3	T50.8x4	T50.8x5	T50.8x6
Sulfogaiacol	T48.4x1	T48.4x2	T48.4x3	T48.4x4	T48.4x5	T48.4x6
Sulfomyxin	T36.8x1	T36.8x2	T36.8x3	T36.8x4	T36.8x5	T36.8x6
Sulfonal	T42.6x1	T42.6x2	T42.6x3	T42.6x4	T42.6x5	T42.6x6
Sulfonamide NEC	T37.0x1	T37.0x2	T37.0x3	T37.0x4	T37.0x5	T37.0x6
eye	T49.5x1	T49.5x2	T49.5x3	T49.5x4	T49.5x5	T49.5x6
Sulfonazide	T37.1x1	T37.1x2	T37.1x3	T37.1x4	T37.1x5	T37.1x6
Sulfones	T37.1x1	T37.1x2	T37.1x3	T37.1x4	T37.1x5	T37.1x6
Sulfonethylmethane	T42.6x1	T42.6x2	T42.6x3	T42.6x4	T42.6x5	T42.6x6
Sulfonmethane	T42.6x1	T42.6x2	T42.6x3	T42.6x4	T42.6x5	T42.6x6
Sulfonphthal, sulfonphthol	T50.8x1	T50.8x2	T50.8x3	T50.8x4	T50.8x5	T50.8x6
Sulfonylurea derivatives, oral	T38.3x1	T38.3x2	T38.3x3	T38.3x4	T38.3x5	T38.3x6
Sulforidazine	T43.3x1	T43.3x2	T43.3x3	T43.3x4	T43.3x5	T43.3x6
Sulfoxone	T37.1x1	T37.1x2	T37.1x3	T37.1x4	T37.1x5	T37.1x6
Sulfur, sulfurated, sulfuric, sulfurous, sulfuryl (compounds NEC) (medicinal)	T49.4x1	T49.4x2	T49.4x3	T49.4x4	T49.4x5	T49.4x6
acid	T54.2x1	T54.2x2	T54.2x3	T54.2x4	—	—
dioxide (gas)	T59.1x1	T59.1x2	T59.1x3	T59.1x4	—	—
ether—see Ether(s)						
hydrogen	T59.6x1	T59.6x2	T59.6x3	T59.6x4	—	—
medicinal (keratolytic) (ointment) NEC	T49.4x1	T49.4x2	T49.4x3	T49.4x4	T49.4x5	T49.4x6
ointment	T49.0x1	T49.0x2	T49.0x3	T49.0x4	T49.0x5	T49.0x6
pesticide (vapor)	T60.91	T60.92	T60.93	T60.94	—	—
vapor NEC	T59.891	T59.892	T59.893	T59.894	—	—
Sulfuric acid	T54.2x1	T54.2x2	T54.2x3	T54.2x4	—	—
Sulglicotide	T47.1x1	T47.1x2	T47.1x3	T47.1x4	T47.1x5	T47.1x6
Sulindac	T39.391	T39.392	T39.393	T39.394	T39.395	T39.396
Sulisatin	T47.2x1	T47.2x2	T47.2x3	T47.2x4	T47.2x5	T47.2x6
Sulisobenzone	T49.3x1	T49.3x2	T49.3x3	T49.3x4	T49.3x5	T49.3x6
Sulkowitch's reagent	T50.8x1	T50.8x2	T50.8x3	T50.8x4	T50.8x5	T50.8x6
Sulmetozine	T44.3x1	T44.3x2	T44.3x3	T44.3x4	T44.3x5	T44.3x6
Suloctidil	T46.7x1	T46.7x2	T46.7x3	T46.7x4	T46.7x5	T46.7x6
Sulph (see also Sulf)						
Sulphadiazine	T37.0x1	T37.0x2	T37.0x3	T37.0x4	T37.0x5	T37.0x6
Sulphadimethoxine	T37.0x1	T37.0x2	T37.0x3	T37.0x4	T37.0x5	T37.0x6
Sulphadimidine	T37.0x1	T37.0x2	T37.0x3	T37.0x4	T37.0x5	T37.0x6
Sulphadione	T37.1x1	T37.1x2	T37.1x3	T37.1x4	T37.1x5	T37.1x6
Sulphafurazole	T37.0x1	T37.0x2	T37.0x3	T37.0x4	T37.0x5	T37.0x6
Sulphamethizole	T37.0x1	T37.0x2	T37.0x3	T37.0x4	T37.0x5	T37.0x6
Sulphamethoxazole	T37.0x1	T37.0x2	T37.0x3	T37.0x4	T37.0x5	T37.0x6
Sulphan blue	T50.8x1	T50.8x2	T50.8x3	T50.8x4	T50.8x5	T50.8x6
Sulphaphenazole	T37.0x1	T37.0x2	T37.0x3	T37.0x4	T37.0x5	T37.0x6
Sulphapyridine	T37.0x1	T37.0x2	T37.0x3	T37.0x4	T37.0x5	T37.0x6
Sulphasalazine	T37.0x1	T37.0x2	T37.0x3	T37.0x4	T37.0x5	T37.0x6
Sulphinpyrazone	T50.4x1	T50.4x2	T50.4x3	T50.4x4	T50.4x5	T50.4x6
Sulpiride	T43.591	T43.592	T43.593	T43.594	T43.595	T43.596
Sulprostone	T48.0x1	T48.0x2	T48.0x3	T48.0x4	T48.0x5	T48.0x6
Sulpyrine	T39.2x1	T39.2x2	T39.2x3	T39.2x4	T39.2x5	T39.2x6
Sultamicillin	T36.0x1	T36.0x2	T36.0x3	T36.0x4	T36.0x5	T36.0x6
Sulthiame	T42.6x1	T42.6x2	T42.6x3	T42.6x4	T42.6x5	T42.6x6
Sultiame	T42.6x1	T42.6x2	T42.6x3	T42.6x4	T42.6x5	T42.6x6
Sultopride	T43.591	T43.592	T43.593	T43.594	T43.595	T43.596
Sumatriptan	T39.8x1	T39.8x2	T39.8x3	T39.8x4	T39.8x5	T39.8x6
Sunflower seed oil	T46.6x1	T46.6x2	T46.6x3	T46.6x4	T46.6x5	T46.6x6
Superinone	T48.4x1	T48.4x2	T48.4x3	T48.4x4	T48.4x5	T48.4x6
Suprofen	T39.311	T39.312	T39.313	T39.314	T39.315	T39.316
Suramin (sodium)	T37.4x1	T37.4x2	T37.4x3	T37.4x4	T37.4x5	T37.4x6
Surfacaine	T41.3x1	T41.3x2	T41.3x3	T41.3x4	T41.3x5	T41.3x6
Surital	T41.1x1	T41.1x2	T41.1x3	T41.1x4	T41.1x5	T41.1x6
Sutilains	T45.3x1	T45.3x2	T45.3x3	T45.3x4	T45.3x5	T45.3x6
Suxamethonium (chloride)	T48.1x1	T48.1x2	T48.1x3	T48.1x4	T48.1x5	T48.1x6
Suxethonium (chloride)	T48.1x1	T48.1x2	T48.1x3	T48.1x4	T48.1x5	T48.1x6
Suxibuzone	T39.2x1	T39.2x2	T39.2x3	T39.2x4	T39.2x5	T39.2x6

Substance	Poisoning, Accidental (unintentional)	Poisoning, Intentional Self-harm	Poisoning, Assault	Poisoning, Undetermined	Adverse Effect	Under-dosing
Sweet oil (birch)	T49.3x1	T49.3x2	T49.3x3	T49.3x4	T49.3x5	T49.3x6
Sweet niter spirit	T46.3x1	T46.3x2	T46.3x3	T46.3x4	T46.3x5	T46.3x6
Sweetener	T50.901	T50.902	T50.903	T50.904	T50.905	T50.906
Sym-dichloroethyl ether	T53.6x1	T53.6x2	T53.6x3	T53.6x4	—	—
Sympatholytic NEC	T44.8x1	T44.8x2	T44.8x3	T44.8x4	T44.8x5	T44.8x6
haloalkylamine	T44.8x1	T44.8x2	T44.8x3	T44.8x4	T44.8x5	T44.8x6
Sympathomimetic NEC	T44.901	T44.902	T44.903	T44.904	T44.905	T44.906
anti-common-cold	T48.5x1	T48.5x2	T48.5x3	T48.5x4	T48.5x5	T48.5x6
bronchodilator	T48.6x1	T48.6x2	T48.6x3	T48.6x4	T48.6x5	T48.6x6
specified NEC	T44.991	T44.992	T44.993	T44.994	T44.995	T44.996
Synagis	T50.B91	T50.B92	T50.B93	T50.B94	T50.B95	T50.B96
Synalar	T49.0x1	T49.0x2	T49.0x3	T49.0x4	T49.0x5	T49.0x6
Synthroid	T38.1x1	T38.1x2	T38.1x3	T38.1x4	T38.1x5	T38.1x6
Syntocinon	T48.0x1	T48.0x2	T48.0x3	T48.0x4	T48.0x5	T48.0x6
Syrosingopine	T46.5x1	T46.5x2	T46.5x3	T46.5x4	T46.5x5	T46.5x6
Systemic drug	T45.91	T45.92	T45.93	T45.94	T45.95	T45.96
specified NEC	T45.8x1	T45.8x2	T45.8x3	T45.8x4	T45.8x5	T45.8x6
Tablets (*see also* specified substance)	T50.901	T50.902	T50.903	T50.904	T50.905	T50.906
Tace	T38.5x1	T38.5x2	T38.5x3	T38.5x4	T38.5x5	T38.5x6
Tacrine	T44.0x1	T44.0x2	T44.0x3	T44.0x4	T44.0x5	T44.0x6
Talampicillin	T36.0x1	T36.0x2	T36.0x3	T36.0x4	T36.0x5	T36.0x6
Talbutal	T42.3x1	T42.3x2	T42.3x3	T42.3x4	T42.3x5	T42.3x6
Talc powder	T49.3x1	T49.3x2	T49.3x3	T49.3x4	T49.3x5	T49.3x6
Talcum	T49.3x1	T49.3x2	T49.3x3	T49.3x4	T49.3x5	T49.3x6
Taleranol	T38.6x1	T38.6x2	T38.6x3	T38.6x4	T38.6x5	T38.6x6
Tamoxifen	T38.6x1	T38.6x2	T38.6x3	T38.6x4	T38.6x5	T38.6x6
Tamsulosin	T44.6x1	T44.6x2	T44.6x3	T44.6x4	T44.6x5	T44.6x6
Tandearil, tanderil	T39.2x1	T39.2x2	T39.2x3	T39.2x4	T39.2x5	T39.2x6
Tannic acid	T49.2x1	T49.2x2	T49.2x3	T49.2x4	T49.2x5	T49.2x6
medicinal (astringent)	T49.2x1	T49.2x2	T49.2x3	T49.2x4	T49.2x5	T49.2x6
Tannin—*see* Tannic acid						
Tansy	T62.2x1	T62.2x2	T62.2x3	T62.2x4	—	—
TAO	T36.3x1	T36.3x2	T36.3x3	T36.3x4	T36.3x5	T36.3x6
Tapazole	T38.2x1	T38.2x2	T38.2x3	T38.2x4	T38.2x5	T38.2x6
Tar NEC	T52.0x1	T52.0x2	T52.0x3	T52.0x4	—	—
camphor	T60.1x1	T60.1x2	T60.1x3	T60.1x4	—	—
distillate	T49.1x1	T49.1x2	T49.1x3	T49.1x4	T49.1x5	T49.1x6
fumes	T59.891	T59.892	T59.893	T59.894	—	—
medicinal	T49.1x1	T49.1x2	T49.1x3	T49.1x4	T49.1x5	T49.1x6
ointment	T49.1x1	T49.1x2	T49.1x3	T49.1x4	T49.1x5	T49.1x6
Taractan	T43.591	T43.592	T43.593	T43.594	T43.595	T43.596
Tarantula (venomous)	T63.321	T63.322	T63.323	T63.324	—	—
Tartar emetic	T37.8x1	T37.8x2	T37.8x3	T37.8x4	T37.8x5	T37.8x6
Tartaric acid	T65.891	T65.892	T65.893	T65.894	—	—
Tartrated antimony (anti-infective)	T37.8x1	T37.8x2	T37.8x3	T37.8x4	T37.8x5	T37.8x6
Tartrate, laxative	T47.4x1	T47.4x2	T47.4x3	T47.4x4	T47.4x5	T47.4x6
Tauromustine	T45.1x1	T45.1x2	T45.1x3	T45.1x4	T45.1x5	T45.1x6
TCA—*see* Trichloroacetic acid						
TCDD	T65.891	T65.892	T65.893	T65.894		
TDI (vapor)	T65.0x1		T65.0x3	T65.0x4		
Tear						
gas	T59.3x1	T59.3x2	T59.3x3	T59.3x4	—	—
solution	T49.5x1	T49.5x2	T49.5x3	T49.5x4	T49.5x5	T49.5x6
Teclothiazide	T50.2x1	T50.2x2	T50.2x3	T50.2x4	T50.2x5	T50.2x6
Teclozan	T37.3x1	T37.3x2	T37.3x3	T37.3x4	T37.3x5	T37.3x6
Tegafur	T45.1x1	T45.1x2	T45.1x3	T45.1x4	T45.1x5	T45.1x6
Tegretol	T42.1x1	T42.1x2	T42.1x3	T42.1x4	T42.1x5	T42.1x6
Teicoplanin	T36.8x1	T36.8x2	T36.8x3	T36.8x4	T36.8x5	T36.8x6
Telepaque	T50.8x1	T50.8x2	T50.8x3	T50.8x4	T50.8x5	T50.8x6
Tellurium	T56.891	T56.892	T56.893	T56.894	—	—
fumes	T56.891	T56.892	T56.893	T56.894	—	—
TEM	T45.1x1	T45.1x2	T45.1x3	T45.1x4	T45.1x5	T45.1x6
Temazepam	T42.4x1	T42.4x2	T42.4x3	T42.4x4	T42.4x5	T42.4x6
Temocillin	T36.0x1	T36.0x2	T36.0x3	T36.0x4	T36.0x5	T36.0x6
Tenamfetamine	T43.621	T43.622	T43.623	T43.624	T43.625	T43.626
Teniposide	T45.1x1	T45.1x2	T45.1x3	T45.1x4	T45.1x5	T45.1x6
Tenitramine	T46.3x1	T46.3x2	T46.3x3	T46.3x4	T46.3x5	T46.3x6
Tenoglicin	T48.4x1	T48.4x2	T48.4x3	T48.4x4	T48.4x5	T48.4x6
Tenonitrozole	T37.3x1	T37.3x2	T37.3x3	T37.3x4	T37.3x5	T37.3x6

Substance	Poisoning, Accidental (unintentional)	Poisoning, Intentional Self-harm	Poisoning, Assault	Poisoning, Undetermined	Adverse Effect	Under-dosing
Tenoxicam	T39.391	T39.392	T39.393	T39.394	T39.395	T39.396
TEPA	T45.1x1	T45.1x2	T45.1x3	T45.1x4	T45.1x5	T45.1x6
TEPP	T60.0x1	T60.0x2	T60.0x3	T60.0x4	—	—
Teprotide	T46.5x1	T46.5x2	T46.5x3	T46.5x4	T46.5x5	T46.5x6
Terazosin	T44.6x1	T44.6x2	T44.6x3	T44.6x4	T44.6x5	T44.6x6
Terbufos	T60.0x1	T60.0x2	T60.0x3	T60.0x4	—	—
Terbutaline	T48.6x1	T48.6x2	T48.6x3	T48.6x4	T48.6x5	T48.6x6
Terconazole	T49.0x1	T49.0x2	T49.0x3	T49.0x4	T49.0x5	T49.0x6
Terfenadine	T45.0x1	T45.0x2	T45.0x3	T45.0x4	T45.0x5	T45.0x6
Teriparatide (acetate)	T50.991	T50.992	T50.993	T50.994	T50.995	T50.996
Terizidone	T37.1x1	T37.1x2	T37.1x3	T37.1x4	T37.1x5	T37.1x6
Terlipressin	T38.891	T38.892	T38.893	T38.894	T38.895	T38.896
Terodiline	T46.3x1	T46.3x2	T46.3x3	T46.3x4	T46.3x5	T46.3x6
Teroxalene	T37.4x1	T37.4x2	T37.4x3	T37.4x4	T37.4x5	T37.4x6
Terpin(cis) hydrate	T48.4x1	T48.4x2	T48.4x3	T48.4x4	T48.4x5	T48.4x6
Terramycin	T36.4x1	T36.4x2	T36.4x3	T36.4x4	T36.4x5	T36.4x6
Tertatolol	T44.7x1	T44.7x2	T44.7x3	T44.7x4	T44.7x5	T44.7x6
Tessalon	T48.3x1	T48.3x2	T48.3x3	T48.3x4	T48.3x5	T48.3x6
Testolactone	T38.7x1	T38.7x2	T38.7x3	T38.7x4	T38.7x5	T38.7x6
Testosterone	T38.7x1	T38.7x2	T38.7x3	T38.7x4	T38.7x5	T38.7x6
Tetanus toxoid or vaccine	T50.A91	T50.A92	T50.A93	T50.A94	T50.A95	T50.A96
antitoxin	T50.Z11	T50.Z12	T50.Z13	T50.Z14	T50.Z15	T50.Z16
immune globulin (human)	T50.Z11	T50.Z12	T50.Z13	T50.Z14	T50.Z15	T50.Z16
toxoid	T50.A91	T50.A92	T50.A93	T50.A94	T50.A95	T50.A96
with diphtheria toxoid	T50.A21	T50.A22	T50.A23	T50.A24	T50.A25	T50.A26
with pertussis	T50.A11	T50.A12	T50.A13	T50.A14	T50.A15	T50.A16
Tetrabenazine	T43.591	T43.592	T43.593	T43.594	T43.595	T43.596
Tetracaine	T41.3x1	T41.3x2	T41.3x3	T41.3x4	T41.3x5	T41.3x6
nerve block (peripheral) (plexus)	T41.3x1	T41.3x2	T41.3x3	T41.3x4	T41.3x5	T41.3x6
regional	T41.3x1	T41.3x2	T41.3x3	T41.3x4	T41.3x5	T41.3x6
spinal	T41.3x1	T41.3x2	T41.3x3	T41.3x4	T41.3x5	T41.3x6
Tetrachlorethylene—*see* Tetrachloroethylene						
Tetrachlormethiazide	T50.2x1	T50.2x2	T50.2x3	T50.2x4	T50.2x5	T50.2x6
Tetrachloroethane	T53.6x1	T53.6x2	T53.6x3	T53.6x4	—	—
vapor	T53.6x1	T53.6x2	T53.6x3	T53.6x4	—	—
paint or varnish	T53.6x1	T53.6x2	T53.6x3	T53.6x4	—	—
Tetrachloroethylene (liquid)	T53.3x1	T53.3x2	T53.3x3	T53.3x4	—	—
medicinal	T37.4x1	T37.4x2	T37.4x3	T37.4x4	T37.4x5	T37.4x6
vapor	T53.3x1	T53.3x2	T53.3x3	T53.3x4	—	—
Tetrachloromethane—*see* Carbon tetrachloride						
Tetracosactide	T38.811	T38.812	T38.813	T38.814	T38.815	T38.816
Tetracosactrin	T38.811	T38.812	T38.813	T38.814	T38.815	T38.816
Tetracycline	T36.4x1	T36.4x2	T36.4x3	T36.4x4	T36.4x5	T36.4x6
ophthalmic preparation	T49.5x1	T49.5x2	T49.5x3	T49.5x4	T49.5x5	T49.5x6
topical NEC	T49.0x1	T49.0x2	T49.0x3	T49.0x4	T49.0x5	T49.0x6
Tetradifon	T60.8x1	T60.8x2	T60.8x3	T60.8x4	—	—
Tetradotoxin	T61.771	T61.772	T61.773	T61.774	—	—
Tetraethyl						
lead	T56.0x1	T56.0x2	T56.0x3	T56.0x4	—	—
pyrophosphate	T60.0x1	T60.0x2	T60.0x3	T60.0x4	—	—
Tetraethylammonium chloride	T44.2x1	T44.2x2	T44.2x3	T44.2x4	T44.2x5	T44.2x6
Tetraethylthiuram disulfide	T50.6x1	T50.6x2	T50.6x3	T50.6x4	T50.6x5	T50.6x6
Tetrahydroaminoacridine	T44.0x1	T44.0x2	T44.0x3	T44.0x4	T44.0x5	T44.0x6
Tetrahydrocannabinol	T40.7x1	T40.7x2	T40.7x3	T40.7x4	T40.7x5	T40.7x6
Tetrahydrofuran	T52.8x1	T52.8x2	T52.8x3	T52.8x4	—	—
Tetrahydronaphthalene	T52.8x1	T52.8x2	T52.8x3	T52.8x4	—	—
Tetrahydrozoline	T49.5x1	T49.5x2	T49.5x3	T49.5x4	T49.5x5	T49.5x6
Tetralin	T52.8x1	T52.8x2	T52.8x3	T52.8x4	—	—
Tetramethrin	T60.2x1	T60.2x2	T60.2x3	T60.2x4	—	—
Tetramethylthiuram (disulfide) NEC	T60.3x1	T60.3x2	T60.3x3	T60.3x4	—	—
medicinal	T49.0x1	T49.0x2	T49.0x3	T49.0x4	T49.0x5	T49.0x6
Tetramisole	T37.4x1	T37.4x2	T37.4x3	T37.4x4	T37.4x5	T37.4x6
Tetranicotinoyl fructose	T46.7x1	T46.7x2	T46.7x3	T46.7x4	T46.7x5	T46.7x6
Tetronal	T42.6x1	T42.6x2	T42.6x3	T42.6x4	T42.6x5	T42.6x6
Tetrazepam	T42.4x1	T42.4x2	T42.4x3	T42.4x4	T42.4x5	T42.4x6
Tetryl	T65.3x1	T65.3x2	T65.3x3	T65.3x4	—	—
Tetrylammonium chloride	T44.2x1	T44.2x2	T44.2x3	T44.2x4	T44.2x5	T44.2x6
Tetryzoline	T49.5x1	T49.5x2	T49.5x3	T49.5x4	T49.5x5	T49.5x6

Substance	Poisoning, Accidental (unintentional)	Poisoning, Intentional Self-harm	Poisoning, Assault	Poisoning, Undetermined	Adverse Effect	Under-dosing
Thalidomide	T45.1x1	T45.1x2	T45.1x3	T45.1x4	T45.1x5	T45.1x6
Thallium (compounds) (dust) NEC	T56.811	T56.812	T56.813	T56.814	—	—
pesticide	T60.4x1	T60.4x2	T60.4x3	T60.4x4	—	—
THC	T40.7x1	T40.7x2	T40.7x3	T40.7x4	T40.7x5	T40.7x6
Thebacon	T48.3x1	T48.3x2	T48.3x3	T48.3x4	T48.3x5	T48.3x6
Thebaine	T40.2x1	T40.2x2	T40.2x3	T40.2x4	T40.2x5	T40.2x6
Thenoic acid	T49.6x1	T49.6x2	T49.6x3	T49.6x4	T49.6x5	T49.6x6
Thenyldiamine	T45.0x1	T45.0x2	T45.0x3	T45.0x4	T45.0x5	T45.0x6
Theobromine (calcium salicylate)	T48.6x1	T48.6x2	T48.6x3	T48.6x4	T48.6x5	T48.6x6
sodium salicylate	T48.6x1	T48.6x2	T48.6x3	T48.6x4	T48.6x5	T48.6x6
Theophyllamine	T48.6x1	T48.6x2	T48.6x3	T48.6x4	T48.6x5	T48.6x6
Theophylline	T48.6x1	T48.6x2	T48.6x3	T48.6x4	T48.6x5	T48.6x6
aminobenzoic acid	T48.6x1	T48.6x2	T48.6x3	T48.6x4	T48.6x5	T48.6x6
ethylenediamine	T48.6x1	T48.6x2	T48.6x3	T48.6x4	T48.6x5	T48.6x6
piperazine p-aminobenzoate	T48.6x1	T48.6x2	T48.6x3	T48.6x4	T48.6x5	T48.6x6
Thiabendazole	T37.4x1	T37.4x2	T37.4x3	T37.4x4	T37.4x5	T37.4x6
Thialbarbital	T41.1x1	T41.1x2	T41.1x3	T41.1x4	T41.1x5	T41.1x6
Thiamazole	T38.2x1	T38.2x2	T38.2x3	T38.2x4	T38.2x5	T38.2x6
Thiambutosine	T37.1x1	T37.1x2	T37.1x3	T37.1x4	T37.1x5	T37.1x6
Thiamine	T45.2x1	T45.2x2	T45.2x3	T45.2x4	T45.2x5	T45.2x6
Thiamphenicol	T36.2x1	T36.2x2	T36.2x3	T36.2x4	T36.2x5	T36.2x6
Thiamylal	T41.1x1	T41.1x2	T41.1x3	T41.1x4	T41.1x5	T41.1x6
sodium	T41.1x1	T41.1x2	T41.1x3	T41.1x4	T41.1x5	T41.1x6
Thiazesim	T43.291	T43.292	T43.293	T43.294	T43.295	T43.296
Thiazides (diuretics)	T50.2x1	T50.2x2	T50.2x3	T50.2x4	T50.2x5	T50.2x6
Thiazinamium metilsulfate	T43.3x1	T43.3x2	T43.3x3	T43.3x4	T43.3x5	T43.3x6
Thiethylperazine	T43.3x1	T43.3x2	T43.3x3	T43.3x4	T43.3x5	T43.3x6
Thimerosal	T49.0x1	T49.0x2	T49.0x3	T49.0x4	T49.0x5	T49.0x6
ophthalmic preparation	T49.5x1	T49.5x2	T49.5x3	T49.5x4	T49.5x5	T49.5x6
Thioacetazone	T37.1x1	T37.1x2	T37.1x3	T37.1x4	T37.1x5	T37.1x6
with isoniazid	T37.1x1	T37.1x2	T37.1x3	T37.1x4	T37.1x5	T37.1x6
Thiobarbital sodium	T41.1x1	T41.1x2	T41.1x3	T41.1x4	T41.1x5	T41.1x6
Thiobarbiturate anesthetic	T41.1x1	T41.1x2	T41.1x3	T41.1x4	T41.1x5	T41.1x6
Thiobismol	T37.8x1	T37.8x2	T37.8x3	T37.8x4	T37.8x5	T37.8x6
Thiobutabarbital sodium	T41.1x1	T41.1x2	T41.1x3	T41.1x4	T41.1x5	T41.1x6
Thiocarbamate (insecticide)	T60.0x1	T60.0x2	T60.0x3	T60.0x4	—	—
Thiocarbamide	T38.2x1	T38.2x2	T38.2x3	T38.2x4	T38.2x5	T38.2x6
Thiocarbarsone	T37.8x1	T37.8x2	T37.8x3	T37.8x4	T37.8x5	T37.8x6
Thiocarlide	T37.1x1	T37.1x2	T37.1x3	T37.1x4	T37.1x5	T37.1x6
Thioctamide	T50.991	T50.992	T50.993	T50.994	T50.995	T50.996
Thioctic acid	T50.991	T50.992	T50.993	T50.994	T50.995	T50.996
Thiofos	T60.0x1	T60.0x2	T60.0x3	T60.0x4	—	—
Thioglycolate	T49.4x1	T49.4x2	T49.4x3	T49.4x4	T49.4x5	T49.4x6
Thioglycolic acid	T65.891	T65.892	T65.893	T65.894	—	—
Thioguanine	T45.1x1	T45.1x2	T45.1x3	T45.1x4	T45.1x5	T45.1x6
Thiomercaptomerin	T50.2x1	T50.2x2	T50.2x3	T50.2x4	T50.2x5	T50.2x6
Thiomerin	T50.2x1	T50.2x2	T50.2x3	T50.2x4	T50.2x5	T50.2x6
Thiomersal	T49.0x1	T49.0x2	T49.0x3	T49.0x4	T49.0x5	T49.0x6
Thionazin	T60.0x1	T60.0x2	T60.0x3	T60.0x4	—	—
Thiopental (sodium)	T41.1x1	T41.1x2	T41.1x3	T41.1x4	T41.1x5	T41.1x6
Thiopentone (sodium)	T41.1x1	T41.1x2	T41.1x3	T41.1x4	T41.1x5	T41.1x6
Thiopropazate	T43.3x1	T43.3x2	T43.3x3	T43.3x4	T43.3x5	T43.3x6
Thioproperazine	T43.3x1	T43.3x2	T43.3x3	T43.3x4	T43.3x5	T43.3x6
Thioridazine	T43.3x1	T43.3x2	T43.3x3	T43.3x4	T43.3x5	T43.3x6
Thiosinamine	T49.3x1	T49.3x2	T49.3x3	T49.3x4	T49.3x5	T49.3x6
Thiotepa	T45.1x1	T45.1x2	T45.1x3	T45.1x4	T45.1x5	T45.1x6
Thiothixene	T43.4x1	T43.4x2	T43.4x3	T43.4x4	T43.4x5	T43.4x6
Thiouracil (benzyl) (methyl) (propyl)	T38.2x1	T38.2x2	T38.2x3	T38.2x4	T38.2x5	T38.2x6
Thiourea	T38.2x1	T38.2x2	T38.2x3	T38.2x4	T38.2x5	T38.2x6
Thiphenamil	T44.3x1	T44.3x2	T44.3x3	T44.3x4	T44.3x5	T44.3x6
Thiram	T60.3x1	T60.3x2	T60.3x3	T60.3x4	—	—
medicinal	T49.2x1	T49.2x2	T49.2x3	T49.2x4	T49.2x5	T49.2x6
Thonzylamine (systemic)	T45.0x1	T45.0x2	T45.0x3	T45.0x4	T45.0x5	T45.0x6
mucosal decongestant	T48.5x1	T48.5x2	T48.5x3	T48.5x4	T48.5x5	T48.5x6
Thorazine	T43.3x1	T43.3x2	T43.3x3	T43.3x4	T43.3x5	T43.3x6
Thorium dioxide suspension	T50.8x1	T50.8x2	T50.8x3	T50.8x4	T50.8x5	T50.8x6
Thornapple	T62.2x1	T62.2x2	T62.2x3	T62.2x4	—	—
Throat drug NEC	T49.6x1	T49.6x2	T49.6x3	T49.6x4	T49.6x5	T49.6x6
Thrombin	T45.7x1	T45.7x2	T45.7x3	T45.7x4	T45.7x5	T45.7x6
Thrombolysin	T45.611	T45.612	T45.613	T45.614	T45.615	T45.616

Substance	Poisoning, Accidental (unintentional)	Poisoning, Intentional Self-harm	Poisoning, Assault	Poisoning, Undetermined	Adverse Effect	Under-dosing
Thromboplastin	T45.7x1	T45.7x2	T45.7x3	T45.7x4	T45.7x5	T45.7x6
Thurfyl nicotinate	T46.7x1	T46.7x2	T46.7x3	T46.7x4	T46.7x5	T46.7x6
Thymol	T49.0x1	T49.0x2	T49.0x3	T49.0x4	T49.0x5	T49.0x6
Thymopentin	T37.5x1	T37.5x2	T37.5x3	T37.5x4	T37.5x5	T37.5x6
Thymoxamine	T46.7x1	T46.7x2	T46.7x3	T46.7x4	T46.7x5	T46.7x6
Thymus extract	T38.891	T38.892	T38.893	T38.894	T38.895	T38.896
Thyreotrophic hormone	T38.811	T38.812	T38.813	T38.814	T38.815	T38.816
Thyroglobulin	T38.1x1	T38.1x2	T38.1x3	T38.1x4	T38.1x5	T38.1x6
Thyroid (hormone)	T38.1x1	T38.1x2	T38.1x3	T38.1x4	T38.1x5	T38.1x6
Thyrolar	T38.1x1	T38.1x2	T38.1x3	T38.1x4	T38.1x5	T38.1x6
Thyrotrophin	T38.811	T38.812	T38.813	T38.814	T38.815	T38.816
Thyrotropic hormone	T38.811	T38.812	T38.813	T38.814	T38.815	T38.816
Thyroxine	T38.1x1	T38.1x2	T38.1x3	T38.1x4	T38.1x5	T38.1x6
Tiabendazole	T37.4x1	T37.4x2	T37.4x3	T37.4x4	T37.4x5	T37.4x6
Tiamizide	T50.2x1	T50.2x2	T50.2x3	T50.2x4	T50.2x5	T50.2x6
Tianeptine	T43.291	T43.292	T43.293	T43.294	T43.295	T43.296
Tiapamil	T46.1x1	T46.1x2	T46.1x3	T46.1x4	T46.1x5	T46.1x6
Tiapride	T43.591	T43.592	T43.593	T43.594	T43.595	T43.596
Tiaprofenic acid	T39.311	T39.312	T39.313	T39.314	T39.315	T39.316
Tiaramide	T39.8x1	T39.8x2	T39.8x3	T39.8x4	T39.8x5	T39.8x6
Ticarcillin	T36.0x1	T36.0x2	T36.0x3	T36.0x4	T36.0x5	T36.0x6
Ticlatone	T49.0x1	T49.0x2	T49.0x3	T49.0x4	T49.0x5	T49.0x6
Ticlopidine	T45.521	T45.522	T45.523	T45.524	T45.525	T45.526
Ticrynafen	T50.1x1	T50.1x2	T50.1x3	T50.1x4	T50.1x5	T50.1x6
Tidiacic	T50.991	T50.992	T50.993	T50.994	T50.995	T50.996
Tiemonium	T44.3x1	T44.3x2	T44.3x3	T44.3x4	T44.3x5	T44.3x6
iodide	T44.3x1	T44.3x2	T44.3x3	T44.3x4	T44.3x5	T44.3x6
Tienilic acid	T50.1x1	T50.1x2	T50.1x3	T50.1x4	T50.1x5	T50.1x6
Tifenamil	T44.3x1	T44.3x2	T44.3x3	T44.3x4	T44.3x5	T44.3x6
Tigan	T45.0x1	T45.0x2	T45.0x3	T45.0x4	T45.0x5	T45.0x6
Tigloidine	T44.3x1	T44.3x2	T44.3x3	T44.3x4	T44.3x5	T44.3x6
Tilactase	T47.5x1	T47.5x2	T47.5x3	T47.5x4	T47.5x5	T47.5x6
Tiletamine	T41.291	T41.292	T41.293	T41.294	T41.295	T41.296
Tilidine	T40.4x1	T40.4x2	T40.4x3	T40.4x4	T40.4x5	T40.4x6
Timepidium bromide	T44.3x1	T44.3x2	T44.3x3	T44.3x4	T44.3x5	T44.3x6
Timiperone	T43.4x1	T43.4x2	T43.4x3	T43.4x4	T43.4x5	T43.4x6
Timolol	T44.7x1	T44.7x2	T44.7x3	T44.7x4	T44.7x5	T44.7x6
Tin (chloride) (dust) (oxide) NEC	T56.6x1	T56.6x2	T56.6x3	T56.6x4	—	—
anti-infectives	T37.8x1	T37.8x2	T37.8x3	T37.8x4	T37.8x5	T37.8x6
Tincture, iodine—see Iodine						
Tindal	T43.3x1	T43.3x2	T43.3x3	T43.3x4	T43.3x5	T43.3x6
Tinidazole	T37.3x1	T37.3x2	T37.3x3	T37.3x4	T37.3x5	T37.3x6
Tinoridine	T39.8x1	T39.8x2	T39.8x3	T39.8x4	T39.8x5	T39.8x6
Tiocarlide	T37.1x1	T37.1x2	T37.1x3	T37.1x4	T37.1x5	T37.1x6
Tioclomarol	T45.511	T45.512	T45.513	T45.514	T45.515	T45.516
Tioconazole	T49.0x1	T49.0x2	T49.0x3	T49.0x4	T49.0x5	T49.0x6
Tioguanine	T45.1x1	T45.1x2	T45.1x3	T45.1x4	T45.1x5	T45.1x6
Tiopronin	T50.991	T50.992	T50.993	T50.994	T50.995	T50.996
Tiotixene	T43.4x1	T43.4x2	T43.4x3	T43.4x4	T43.4x5	T43.4x6
Tioxolone	T49.4x1	T49.4x2	T49.4x3	T49.4x4	T49.4x5	T49.4x6
Tipepidine	T48.3x1	T48.3x2	T48.3x3	T48.3x4	T48.3x5	T48.3x6
Tiquizium bromide	T44.3x1	T44.3x2	T44.3x3	T44.3x4	T44.3x5	T44.3x6
Tiratricol	T38.1x1	T38.1x2	T38.1x3	T38.1x4	T38.1x5	T38.1x6
Tisopurine	T50.4x1	T50.4x2	T50.4x3	T50.4x4	T50.4x5	T50.4x6
Titanium (compounds) (vapor)	T56.891	T56.892	T56.893	T56.894	—	—
dioxide	T49.3x1	T49.3x2	T49.3x3	T49.3x4	T49.3x5	T49.3x6
ointment	T49.3x1	T49.3x2	T49.3x3	T49.3x4	T49.3x5	T49.3x6
oxide	T49.3x1	T49.3x2	T49.3x3	T49.3x4	T49.3x5	T49.3x6
tetrachloride	T56.891	T56.892	T56.893	T56.894	—	—
Titanocene	T56.891	T56.892	T56.893	T56.894	—	—
Titroid	T38.1x1	T38.1x2	T38.1x3	T38.1x4	T38.1x5	T38.1x6
Tizanidine	T42.8x1	T42.8x2	T42.8x3	T42.8x4	T42.8x5	T42.8x6
TMTD	T60.3x1	T60.3x2	T60.3x3	T60.3x4	—	—
TNT (fumes)	T65.3x1	T65.3x2	T65.3x3	T65.3x4	—	—
TNT	T65.891	T65.892	T65.893	T65.894	—	—
fumes	T59.891	T59.892	T59.893	T59.894	—	—
Toadstool	T62.0x1	T62.0x2	T62.0x3	T62.0x4	—	—
Tobacco NEC	T65.291	T65.292	T65.293	T65.294	—	—
cigarettes	T65.221	T65.222	T65.223	T65.224	—	—
Indian	T62.2x1	T62.2x2	T62.2x3	T62.2x4	—	—
smoke, second-hand	T59.811	T59.812	T59.813	T59.814	—	—

Substance	Poisoning, Accidental (unintentional)	Poisoning, Intentional Self-harm	Poisoning, Assault	Poisoning, Undetermined	Adverse Effect	Under-dosing
Tobramycin	T36.5x1	T36.5x2	T36.5x3	T36.5x4	T36.5x5	T36.5x6
Tocainide	T46.2x1	T46.2x2	T46.2x3	T46.2x4	T46.2x5	T46.2x6
Tocoferol	T45.2x1	T45.2x2	T45.2x3	T45.2x4	T45.2x5	T45.2x6
Tocopherol	T45.2x1	T45.2x2	T45.2x3	T45.2x4	T45.2x5	T45.2x6
acetate	T45.2x1	T45.2x2	T45.2x3	T45.2x4	T45.2x5	T45.2x6
Tocosamine	T48.0x1	T48.0x2	T48.0x3	T48.0x4	T48.0x5	T48.0x6
Todralazine	T46.5x1	T46.5x2	T46.5x3	T46.5x4	T46.5x5	T46.5x6
Tofisopam	T42.4x1	T42.4x2	T42.4x3	T42.4x4	T42.4x5	T42.4x6
Tofranil	T43.011	T43.012	T43.013	T43.014	T43.015	T43.016
Toilet deodorizer	T65.891	T65.892	T65.893	T65.894	—	—
Tolamolol	T44.7x1	T44.7x2	T44.7x3	T44.7x4	T44.7x5	T44.7x6
Tolazamide	T38.3x1	T38.3x2	T38.3x3	T38.3x4	T38.3x5	T38.3x6
Tolazoline	T46.7x1	T46.7x2	T46.7x3	T46.7x4	T46.7x5	T46.7x6
Tolbutamide (sodium)	T38.3x1	T38.3x2	T38.3x3	T38.3x4	T38.3x5	T38.3x6
Tolciclate	T49.0x1	T49.0x2	T49.0x3	T49.0x4	T49.0x5	T49.0x6
Tolmetin	T39.391	T39.392	T39.393	T39.394	T39.395	T39.396
Tolnaftate	T49.0x1	T49.0x2	T49.0x3	T49.0x4	T49.0x5	T49.0x6
Tolonidine	T46.5x1	T46.5x2	T46.5x3	T46.5x4	T46.5x5	T46.5x6
Toloxatone	T42.6x1	T42.6x2	T42.6x3	T42.6x4	T42.6x5	T42.6x6
Tolperisone	T44.3x1	T44.3x2	T44.3x3	T44.3x4	T44.3x5	T44.3x6
Tolserol	T42.8x1	T42.8x2	T42.8x3	T42.8x4	T42.8x5	T42.8x6
Toluene (liquid)	T52.2x1	T52.2x2	T52.2x3	T52.2x4	—	—
diisocyanate	T65.0x1	T65.0x2	T65.0x3	T65.0x4	—	—
Toluidine	T65.891	T65.892	T65.893	T65.894	—	—
vapor	T59.891	T59.892	T59.893	T59.894	—	—
Toluol (liquid)	T52.2x1	T52.2x2	T52.2x3	T52.2x4	—	—
vapor	T52.2x1	T52.2x2	T52.2x3	T52.2x4	—	—
Toluylenediamine	T65.3x1	T65.3x2	T65.3x3	T65.3x4	—	—
Tolylene-2,4-diisocyanate	T65.0x1	T65.0x2	T65.0x3	T65.0x4	—	—
Tonic NEC	T50.901	T50.902	T50.903	T50.904	T50.905	T50.906
Topical action drug NEC	T49.91	T49.92	T49.93	T49.94	T49.95	T49.96
ear, nose or throat	T49.6x1	T49.6x2	T49.6x3	T49.6x4	T49.6x5	T49.6x6
eye	T49.5x1	T49.5x2	T49.5x3	T49.5x4	T49.5x5	T49.5x6
skin	T49.4x1	T49.4x2	T49.4x3	T49.4x4	T49.4x5	T49.4x6
specified NEC	T49.8x1	T49.8x2	T49.8x3	T49.8x4	T49.8x5	T49.8x6
Toquizine	T44.3x1	T44.3x2	T44.3x3	T44.3x4	T44.3x5	T44.3x6
Toremifene	T38.6x1	T38.6x2	T38.6x3	T38.6x4	T38.6x5	T38.6x6
Tosylchloramide sodium	T49.8x1	T49.8x2	T49.8x3	T49.8x4	T49.8x5	T49.8x6
Toxaphene (dust) (spray)	T60.1x1	T60.1x2	T60.1x3	T60.1x4	—	—
Toxin, diphtheria (Schick Test)	T50.8x1	T50.8x2	T50.8x3	T50.8x4	T50.8x5	T50.8x6
Toxoid						
combined	T50.A21	T50.A22	T50.A23	T50.A24	T50.A25	T50.A26
diphtheria	T50.A91	T50.A92	T50.A93	T50.A94	T50.A95	T50.A96
tetanus	T50.A91	T50.A92	T50.A93	T50.A94	T50.A95	T50.A96
Trace element NEC	T45.8x1	T45.8x2	T45.8x3	T45.8x4	T45.8x5	T45.8x6
Tractor fuel NEC	T52.0x1	T52.0x2	T52.0x3	T52.0x4	—	—
Tragacanth	T50.991	T50.992	T50.993	T50.994	T50.995	T50.996
Tramadol	T40.4x1	T40.4x2	T40.4x3	T40.4x4	T40.4x5	T40.4x6
Tramazoline	T48.5x1	T48.5x2	T48.5x3	T48.5x4	T48.5x5	T48.5x6
Tranexamic acid	T45.621	T45.622	T45.623	T45.624	T45.625	T45.626
Tranilast	T45.0x1	T45.0x2	T45.0x3	T45.0x4	T45.0x5	T45.0x6
Tranquilizer NEC	T43.501	T43.502	T43.503	T43.504	T43.505	T43.506
with hypnotic or sedative	T42.6x1	T42.6x2	T42.6x3	T42.6x4	T42.6x5	T42.6x6
benzodiazepine NEC	T42.4x1	T42.4x2	T42.4x3	T42.4x4	T42.4x5	T42.4x6
butyrophenone NEC	T43.4x1	T43.4x2	T43.4x3	T43.4x4	T43.4x5	T43.4x6
carbamate	T43.591	T43.592	T43.593	T43.594	T43.595	T43.596
dimethylamine	T43.3x1	T43.3x2	T43.3x3	T43.3x4	T43.3x5	T43.3x6
ethylamine	T43.3x1	T43.3x2	T43.3x3	T43.3x4	T43.3x5	T43.3x6
hydroxyzine	T43.591	T43.592	T43.593	T43.594	T43.595	T43.596
major NEC	T43.501	T43.502	T43.503	T43.504	T43.505	T43.506
penothiazine NEC	T43.3x1	T43.3x2	T43.3x3	T43.3x4	T43.3x5	T43.3x6
phenothiazine-based	T43.3x1	T43.3x2	T43.3x3	T43.3x4	T43.3x5	T43.3x6
piperazine NEC	T43.3x1	T43.3x2	T43.3x3	T43.3x4	T43.3x5	T43.3x6
piperidine	T43.3x1	T43.3x2	T43.3x3	T43.3x4	T43.3x5	T43.3x6
propylamine	T43.3x1	T43.3x2	T43.3x3	T43.3x4	T43.3x5	T43.3x6
specified NEC	T43.591	T43.592	T43.593	T43.594	T43.595	T43.596
thioxanthene NEC	T43.591	T43.592	T43.593	T43.594	T43.595	T43.596
Trantoin	T37.91	T37.92	T37.93	T37.94	T37.95	T37.96
Tranxene	T42.4x1	T42.4x2	T42.4x3	T42.4x4	T42.4x5	T42.4x6
Tranylcypromine	T43.1x1	T43.1x2	T43.1x3	T43.1x4	T43.1x5	T43.1x6
Trapidil	T46.3x1	T46.3x2	T46.3x3	T46.3x4	T46.3x5	T46.3x6
Trasentine	T44.3x1	T44.3x2	T44.3x3	T44.3x4	T44.3x5	T44.3x6
Travert	T50.3x1	T50.3x2	T50.3x3	T50.3x4	T50.3x5	T50.3x6
Trazodone	T43.211	T43.212	T43.213	T43.214	T43.215	T43.216
Trecator	T37.1x1	T37.1x2	T37.1x3	T37.1x4	T37.1x5	T37.1x6
Treosulfan	T45.1x1	T45.1x2	T45.1x3	T45.1x4	T45.1x5	T45.1x6
Tretamine	T45.1x1	T45.1x2	T45.1x3	T45.1x4	T45.1x5	T45.1x6
Tretinoin	T49.0x1	T49.0x2	T49.0x3	T49.0x4	T49.0x5	T49.0x6
Tretoquinol	T48.6x1	T48.6x2	T48.6x3	T48.6x4	T48.6x5	T48.6x6
Triacetin	T49.0x1	T49.0x2	T49.0x3	T49.0x4	T49.0x5	T49.0x6
Triacetoxyanthracene	T49.4x1	T49.4x2	T49.4x3	T49.4x4	T49.4x5	T49.4x6
Triacetyloleandomycin	T36.3x1	T36.3x2	T36.3x3	T36.3x4	T36.3x5	T36.3x6
Triamcinolone	T49.0x1	T49.0x2	T49.0x3	T49.0x4	T49.0x5	T49.0x6
ENT agent	T49.6x1	T49.6x2	T49.6x3	T49.6x4	T49.6x5	T49.6x6
hexacetonide	T49.0x1	T49.0x2	T49.0x3	T49.0x4	T49.0x5	T49.0x6
ophthalmic preparation	T49.5x1	T49.5x2	T49.5x3	T49.5x4	T49.5x5	T49.5x6
topical NEC	T49.0x1	T49.0x2	T49.0x3	T49.0x4	T49.0x5	T49.0x6
Triampyzine	T44.3x1	T44.3x2	T44.3x3	T44.3x4	T44.3x5	T44.3x6
Triamterene	T50.2x1	T50.2x2	T50.2x3	T50.2x4	T50.2x5	T50.2x6
Triazine (herbicide)	T60.3x1	T60.3x2	T60.3x3	T60.3x4	—	—
Triaziquone	T45.1x1	T45.1x2	T45.1x3	T45.1x4	T45.1x5	T45.1x6
Triazolam	T42.4x1	T42.4x2	T42.4x3	T42.4x4	T42.4x5	T42.4x6
Triazole (herbicide)	T60.3x1	T60.3x2	T60.3x3	T60.3x4	—	—
Tribenoside	T46.991	T46.992	T46.993	T46.994	T46.995	T46.996
Tribromacetaldehyde	T42.6x1	T42.6x2	T42.6x3	T42.6x4	T42.6x5	T42.6x6
Tribromoethanol, rectal	T41.291	T41.292	T41.293	T41.294	T41.295	T41.296
Tribromomethane	T42.6x1	T42.6x2	T42.6x3	T42.6x4	T42.6x5	T42.6x6
Trichlorethane	T53.2x1	T53.2x2	T53.2x3	T53.2x4	—	—
Trichlorethylene	T53.2x1	T53.2x2	T53.2x3	T53.2x4	—	—
Trichlorfon	T60.0x1	T60.0x2	T60.0x3	T60.0x4	—	—
Trichlormethiazide	T50.2x1	T50.2x2	T50.2x3	T50.2x4	T50.2x5	T50.2x6
Trichlormethine	T45.1x1	T45.1x2	T45.1x3	T45.1x4	T45.1x5	T45.1x6
Trichloroacetic acid, Trichloracetic acid	T54.2x1	T54.2x2	T54.2x3	T54.2x4	—	—
medicinal	T49.4x1	T49.4x2	T49.4x3	T49.4x4	T49.4x5	T49.4x6
Trichloroethane	T53.2x1	T53.2x2	T53.2x3	T53.2x4	—	—
Trichloroethanol	T42.6x1	T42.6x2	T42.6x3	T42.6x4	T42.6x5	T42.6x6
Trichloroethylene (liquid) (vapor)	T53.2x1	T53.2x2	T53.2x3	T53.2x4	—	—
anesthetic (gas)	T41.0x1	T41.0x2	T41.0x3	T41.0x4	T41.0x5	T41.0x6
vapor NEC	T53.2x1	T53.2x2	T53.2x3	T53.2x4	—	—
Trichloroethyl phosphate	T42.6x1	T42.6x2	T42.6x3	T42.6x4	T42.6x5	T42.6x6
Trichlorofluoromethane NEC	T53.5x1	T53.5x2	T53.5x3	T53.5x4	—	—
Trichloronat(e)	T60.0x1	T60.0x2	T60.0x3	T60.0x4	—	—
Trichloropropane	T53.6x1	T53.6x2	T53.6x3	T53.6x4	—	—
Trichlorotriethylamine	T45.1x1	T45.1x2	T45.1x3	T45.1x4	T45.1x5	T45.1x6
Trichomonacides NEC	T37.3x1	T37.3x2	T37.3x3	T37.3x4	T37.3x5	T37.3x6
Trichomycin	T36.7x1	T36.7x2	T36.7x3	T36.7x4	T36.7x5	T36.7x6
Triclobisonium chloride	T49.0x1	T49.0x2	T49.0x3	T49.0x4	T49.0x5	T49.0x6
Triclocarban	T49.0x1	T49.0x2	T49.0x3	T49.0x4	T49.0x5	T49.0x6
Triclofos	T42.6x1	T42.6x2	T42.6x3	T42.6x4	T42.6x5	T42.6x6
Triclosan	T49.0x1	T49.0x2	T49.0x3	T49.0x4	T49.0x5	T49.0x6
Tricresyl phosphate	T65.891	T65.892	T65.893	T65.894	—	—
solvent	T52.91	T52.92	T52.93	T52.94	—	—
Tricyclamol chloride	T44.3x1	T44.3x2	T44.3x3	T44.3x4	T44.3x5	T44.3x6
Tridesilon	T49.0x1	T49.0x2	T49.0x3	T49.0x4	T49.0x5	T49.0x6
Tridihexethyl iodide	T44.3x1	T44.3x2	T44.3x3	T44.3x4	T44.3x5	T44.3x6
Tridione	T42.2x1	T42.2x2	T42.2x3	T42.2x4	T42.2x5	T42.2x6
Trientine	T45.8x1	T45.8x2	T45.8x3	T45.8x4	T45.8x5	T45.8x6
Triethanolamine NEC	T54.3x1	T54.3x2	T54.3x3	T54.3x4	—	—
detergent	T54.3x1	T54.3x2	T54.3x3	T54.3x4	—	—
trinitrate (biphosphate)	T46.3x1	T46.3x2	T46.3x3	T46.3x4	T46.3x5	T46.3x6
Triethanomelamine	T45.1x1	T45.1x2	T45.1x3	T45.1x4	T45.1x5	T45.1x6
Triethylenemelamine	T45.1x1	T45.1x2	T45.1x3	T45.1x4	T45.1x5	T45.1x6
Triethylenephosphoramide	T45.1x1	T45.1x2	T45.1x3	T45.1x4	T45.1x5	T45.1x6
Triethylenethiophosphoramide	T45.1x1	T45.1x2	T45.1x3	T45.1x4	T45.1x5	T45.1x6
Trifluoperazine	T43.3x1	T43.3x2	T43.3x3	T43.3x4	T43.3x5	T43.3x6
Trifluoroethyl vinyl ether	T41.0x1	T41.0x2	T41.0x3	T41.0x4	T41.0x5	T41.0x6
Trifluperidol	T43.4x1	T43.4x2	T43.4x3	T43.4x4	T43.4x5	T43.4x6
Triflupromazine	T43.3x1	T43.3x2	T43.3x3	T43.3x4	T43.3x5	T43.3x6
Trifluridine	T37.5x1	T37.5x2	T37.5x3	T37.5x4	T37.5x5	T37.5x6
Triflusal	T45.521	T45.522	T45.523	T45.524	T45.525	T45.526
Trihexyphenidyl	T44.3x1	T44.3x2	T44.3x3	T44.3x4	T44.3x5	T44.3x6

Drug and Chemical Table

Triiodothyronine–Vaccine NEC

Substance	Poisoning, Accidental (unintentional)	Poisoning, Intentional Self-harm	Poisoning, Assault	Poisoning, Undetermined	Adverse Effect	Underdosing
Triiodothyronine	T38.1x1	T38.1x2	T38.1x3	T38.1x4	T38.1x5	T38.1x6
Trilene	T41.0x1	T41.0x2	T41.0x3	T41.0x4	T41.0x5	T41.0x6
Trilostane	T38.991	T38.992	T38.993	T38.994	T38.995	T38.996
Trimebutine	T44.3x1	T44.3x2	T44.3x3	T44.3x4	T44.3x5	T44.3x6
Trimecaine	T41.3x1	T41.3x2	T41.3x3	T41.3x4	T41.3x5	T41.3x6
Trimeprazine (tartrate)	T44.3x1	T44.3x2	T44.3x3	T44.3x4	T44.3x5	T44.3x6
Trimetaphan camsilate	T44.2x1	T44.2x2	T44.2x3	T44.2x4	T44.2x5	T44.2x6
Trimetazidine	T46.7x1	T46.7x2	T46.7x3	T46.7x4	T46.7x5	T46.7x6
Trimethadione	T42.2x1	T42.2x2	T42.2x3	T42.2x4	T42.2x5	T42.2x6
Trimethaphan	T44.2x1	T44.2x2	T44.2x3	T44.2x4	T44.2x5	T44.2x6
Trimethidinium	T44.2x1	T44.2x2	T44.2x3	T44.2x4	T44.2x5	T44.2x6
Trimethobenzamide	T45.0x1	T45.0x2	T45.0x3	T45.0x4	T45.0x5	T45.0x6
Trimethoprim	T37.8x1	T37.8x2	T37.8x3	T37.8x4	T37.8x5	T37.8x6
with sulfamethoxazole	T36.8x1	T36.8x2	T36.8x3	T36.8x4	T36.8x5	T36.8x6
Trimethylcarbinol	T51.3x1	T51.3x2	T51.3x3	T51.3x4	—	—
Trimethylpsoralen	T49.3x1	T49.3x2	T49.3x3	T49.3x4	T49.3x5	T49.3x6
Trimeton	T45.0x1	T45.0x2	T45.0x3	T45.0x4	T45.0x5	T45.0x6
Trimetrexate	T45.1x1	T45.1x2	T45.1x3	T45.1x4	T45.1x5	T45.1x6
Trimipramine	T43.011	T43.012	T43.013	T43.014	T43.015	T43.016
Trimustine	T45.1x1	T45.1x2	T45.1x3	T45.1x4	T45.1x5	T45.1x6
Trinitrine	T46.3x1	T46.3x2	T46.3x3	T46.3x4	T46.3x5	T46.3x6
Trinitrobenzol	T65.3x1	T65.3x2	T65.3x3	T65.3x4	—	—
Trinitrophenol	T65.3x1	T65.3x2	T65.3x3	T65.3x4	—	—
Trinitrotoluene (fumes)	T65.3x1	T65.3x2	T65.3x3	T65.3x4	—	—
Trinitrotoluene	T65.891	T65.892	T65.893	T65.894	—	—
fumes	T59.891	T59.892	T59.893	T59.894	—	—
Trional	T42.6x1	T42.6x2	T42.6x3	T42.6x4	T42.6x5	T42.6x6
Triorthocresyl phosphate	T65.891	T65.892	T65.893	T65.894	—	—
Trioxide of arsenic	T57.0x1	T57.0x2	T57.0x3	T57.0x4	—	—
Trioxysalen	T49.4x1	T49.4x2	T49.4x3	T49.4x4	T49.4x5	T49.4x6
Tripamide	T50.2x1	T50.2x2	T50.2x3	T50.2x4	T50.2x5	T50.2x6
Triparanol	T46.6x1	T46.6x2	T46.6x3	T46.6x4	T46.6x5	T46.6x6
Tripelennamine	T45.0x1	T45.0x2	T45.0x3	T45.0x4	T45.0x5	T45.0x6
Triperiden	T44.3x1	T44.3x2	T44.3x3	T44.3x4	T44.3x5	T44.3x6
Triperidol	T43.4x1	T43.4x2	T43.4x3	T43.4x4	T43.4x5	T43.4x6
Triphenylphosphate	T65.891	T65.892	T65.893	T65.894	—	—
Triple						
bromides	T42.6x1	T42.6x2	T42.6x3	T42.6x4	T42.6x5	T42.6x6
carbonate	T47.1x1	T47.1x2	T47.1x3	T47.1x4	T47.1x5	T47.1x6
vaccine						
DPT	T50.A11	T50.A12	T50.A13	T50.A14	T50.A15	T50.A16
including pertussis	T50.A11	T50.A12	T50.A13	T50.A14	T50.A15	T50.A16
MMR	T50.B91	T50.B92	T50.B93	T50.B94	T50.B95	T50.B96
Triprolidine	T45.0x1	T45.0x2	T45.0x3	T45.0x4	T45.0x5	T45.0x6
Trisodium hydrogen edetate	T50.6x1	T50.6x2	T50.6x3	T50.6x4	T50.6x5	T50.6x6
Trisoralen	T49.3x1	T49.3x2	T49.3x3	T49.3x4	T49.3x5	T49.3x6
Trisulfapyrimidines	T37.0x1	T37.0x2	T37.0x3	T37.0x4	T37.0x5	T37.0x6
Trithiozine	T44.3x1	T44.3x2	T44.3x3	T44.3x4	T44.3x5	T44.3x6
Tritiozine	T44.3x1	T44.3x2	T44.3x3	T44.3x4	T44.3x5	T44.3x6
Tritoqualine	T45.0x1	T45.0x2	T45.0x3	T45.0x4	T45.0x5	T45.0x6
Trofosfamide	T45.1x1	T45.1x2	T45.1x3	T45.1x4	T45.1x5	T45.1x6
Troleandomycin	T36.3x1	T36.3x2	T36.3x3	T36.3x4	T36.3x5	T36.3x6
Trolnitrate (phosphate)	T46.3x1	T46.3x2	T46.3x3	T46.3x4	T46.3x5	T46.3x6
Tromantadine	T37.5x1	T37.5x2	T37.5x3	T37.5x4	T37.5x5	T37.5x6
Trometamol	T50.2x1	T50.2x2	T50.2x3	T50.2x4	T50.2x5	T50.2x6
Tromethamine	T50.2x1	T50.2x2	T50.2x3	T50.2x4	T50.2x5	T50.2x6
Tronothane	T41.3x1	T41.3x2	T41.3x3	T41.3x4	T41.3x5	T41.3x6
Tropacine	T44.3x1	T44.3x2	T44.3x3	T44.3x4	T44.3x5	T44.3x6
Tropatepine	T44.3x1	T44.3x2	T44.3x3	T44.3x4	T44.3x5	T44.3x6
Tropicamide	T44.3x1	T44.3x2	T44.3x3	T44.3x4	T44.3x5	T44.3x6
Trospium chloride	T44.3x1	T44.3x2	T44.3x3	T44.3x4	T44.3x5	T44.3x6
Troxerutin	T46.991	T46.992	T46.993	T46.994	T46.995	T46.996
Troxidone	T42.2x1	T42.2x2	T42.2x3	T42.2x4	T42.2x5	T42.2x6
Tryparsamide	T37.3x1	T37.3x2	T37.3x3	T37.3x4	T37.3x5	T37.3x6
Trypsin	T45.3x1	T45.3x2	T45.3x3	T45.3x4	T45.3x5	T45.3x6
Tryptizol	T43.011	T43.012	T43.013	T43.014	T43.015	T43.016
TSH	T38.811	T38.812	T38.813	T38.814	T38.815	T38.816
Tuaminoheptane	T48.5x1	T48.5x2	T48.5x3	T48.5x4	T48.5x5	T48.5x6
Tuberculin, purified protein derivative (PPD)	T50.8x1	T50.8x2	T50.8x3	T50.8x4	T50.8x5	T50.8x6
Tubocurare	T48.1x1	T48.1x2	T48.1x3	T48.1x4	T48.1x5	T48.1x6

Substance	Poisoning, Accidental (unintentional)	Poisoning, Intentional Self-harm	Poisoning, Assault	Poisoning, Undetermined	Adverse Effect	Underdosing
Tubocurarine (chloride)	T48.1x1	T48.1x2	T48.1x3	T48.1x4	T48.1x5	T48.1x6
Tulobuterol	T48.6x1	T48.6x2	T48.6x3	T48.6x4	T48.6x5	T48.6x6
Turpentine (spirits of)	T52.8x1	T52.8x2	T52.8x3	T52.8x4	—	—
vapor	T52.8x1	T52.8x2	T52.8x3	T52.8x4	—	—
Tybamate	T43.591	T43.592	T43.593	T43.594	T43.595	T43.596
Tyloxapol	T48.4x1	T48.4x2	T48.4x3	T48.4x4	T48.4x5	T48.4x6
Tymazoline	T48.5x1	T48.5x2	T48.5x3	T48.5x4	T48.5x5	T48.5x6
Typhoid-paratyphoid vaccine	T50.A91	T50.A92	T50.A93	T50.A94	T50.A95	T50.A96
Typhus vaccine	T50.A91	T50.A92	T50.A93	T50.A94	T50.A95	T50.A96
Tyropanoate	T50.8x1	T50.8x2	T50.8x3	T50.8x4	T50.8x5	T50.8x6
Tyrothricin	T49.6x1	T49.6x2	T49.6x3	T49.6x4	T49.6x5	T49.6x6
ENT agent	T49.6x1	T49.6x2	T49.6x3	T49.6x4	T49.6x5	T49.6x6
ophthalmic preparation	T49.5x1	T49.5x2	T49.5x3	T49.5x4	T49.5x5	T49.5x6
Ufenamate	T39.391	T39.392	T39.393	T39.394	T39.395	T39.396
Ultraviolet light protectant	T49.3x1	T49.3x2	T49.3x3	T49.3x4	T49.3x5	T49.3x6
Undecenoic acid	T49.0x1	T49.0x2	T49.0x3	T49.0x4	T49.0x5	T49.0x6
Undecoylium	T49.0x1	T49.0x2	T49.0x3	T49.0x4	T49.0x5	T49.0x6
Undecylenic acid (derivatives)	T49.0x1	T49.0x2	T49.0x3	T49.0x4	T49.0x5	T49.0x6
Unna's boot	T49.3x1	T49.3x2	T49.3x3	T49.3x4	T49.3x5	T49.3x6
Unsaturated fatty acid	T46.6x1	T46.6x2	T46.6x3	T46.6x4	T46.6x5	T46.6x6
Uracil mustard	T45.1x1	T45.1x2	T45.1x3	T45.1x4	T45.1x5	T45.1x6
Uramustine	T45.1x1	T45.1x2	T45.1x3	T45.1x4	T45.1x5	T45.1x6
Urapidil	T46.5x1	T46.5x2	T46.5x3	T46.5x4	T46.5x5	T46.5x6
Urari	T48.1x1	T48.1x2	T48.1x3	T48.1x4	T48.1x5	T48.1x6
Urate oxidase	T50.4x1	T50.4x2	T50.4x3	T50.4x4	T50.4x5	T50.4x6
Urea	T47.3x1	T47.3x2	T47.3x3	T47.3x4	T47.3x5	T47.3x6
peroxide	T49.0x1	T49.0x2	T49.0x3	T49.0x4	T49.0x5	T49.0x6
stibamine	T37.4x1	T37.4x2	T37.4x3	T37.4x4	T37.4x5	T37.4x6
topical	T49.8x1	T49.8x2	T49.8x3	T49.8x4	T49.8x5	T49.8x6
Urethane	T45.1x1	T45.1x2	T45.1x3	T45.1x4	T45.1x5	T45.1x6
Urginea (maritima) (scilla)—see Squill						
Uric acid metabolism drug NEC	T50.4x1	T50.4x2	T50.4x3	T50.4x4	T50.4x5	T50.4x6
Uricosuric agent	T50.4x1	T50.4x2	T50.4x3	T50.4x4	T50.4x5	T50.4x6
Urinary anti-infective	T37.8x1	T37.8x2	T37.8x3	T37.8x4	T37.8x5	T37.8x6
Urofollitropin	T38.811	T38.812	T38.813	T38.814	T38.815	T38.816
Urokinase	T45.611	T45.612	T45.613	T45.614	T45.615	T45.616
Urokon	T50.8x1	T50.8x2	T50.8x3	T50.8x4	T50.8x5	T50.8x6
Urotropin	T37.91	T37.92	T37.93	T37.94	T37.95	T37.96
Ursodeoxycholic acid	T50.991	T50.992	T50.993	T50.994	T50.995	T50.996
Ursodiol	T50.991	T50.992	T50.993	T50.994	T50.995	T50.996
Uterine relaxing factor	T44.5x1	T44.5x2	T44.5x3	T44.5x4	T44.5x5	T44.5x6
Urtica	T62.2x1	T62.2x2	T62.2x3	T62.2x4	—	—
Utility gas—see Gas, utility						
Vaccine NEC	T50.Z91	T50.Z92	T50.Z93	T50.Z94	T50.Z95	T50.Z96
antineoplastic	T50.Z91	T50.Z92	T50.Z93	T50.Z94	T50.Z95	T50.Z96
bacterial NEC	T50.A91	T50.A92	T50.A93	T50.A94	T50.A95	T50.A96
with						
other bacterial component	T50.A21	T50.A22	T50.A23	T50.A24	T50.A25	T50.A26
pertussis component	T50.A11	T50.A12	T50.A13	T50.A14	T50.A15	T50.A16
viral-rickettsial component	T50.A21	T50.A22	T50.A23	T50.A24	T50.A25	T50.A26
mixed NEC	T50.A21	T50.A22	T50.A23	T50.A24	T50.A25	T50.A26
BCG	T50.A91	T50.A92	T50.A93	T50.A94	T50.A95	T50.A96
cholera	T50.A91	T50.A92	T50.A93	T50.A94	T50.A95	T50.A96
diphtheria	T50.A91	T50.A92	T50.A93	T50.A94	T50.A95	T50.A96
with tetanus	T50.A21	T50.A22	T50.A23	T50.A24	T50.A25	T50.A26
and pertussis	T50.A11	T50.A12	T50.A13	T50.A14	T50.A15	T50.A16
influenza	T50.B91	T50.B92	T50.B93	T50.B94	T50.B95	T50.B96
measles	T50.B91	T50.B92	T50.B93	T50.B94	T50.B95	T50.B96
with mumps and rubella	T50.B91	T50.B92	T50.B93	T50.B94	T50.B95	T50.B96
meningococcal	T50.A91	T50.A92	T50.A93	T50.A94	T50.A95	T50.A96
mumps	T50.B91	T50.B92	T50.B93	T50.B94	T50.B95	T50.B96
paratyphoid	T50.A91	T50.A92	T50.A93	T50.A94	T50.A95	T50.A96
pertussis	T50.A11	T50.A12	T50.A13	T50.A14	T50.A15	T50.A16
with diphtheria	T50.A11	T50.A12	T50.A13	T50.A14	T50.A15	T50.A16
and tetanus	T50.A11	T50.A12	T50.A13	T50.A14	T50.A15	T50.A16
with other component	T50.A11	T50.A12	T50.A13	T50.A14	T50.A15	T50.A16
plague	T50.A91	T50.A92	T50.A93	T50.A94	T50.A95	T50.A96
poliomyelitis	T50.B91	T50.B92	T50.B93	T50.B94	T50.B95	T50.B96
poliovirus	T50.B91	T50.B92	T50.B93	T50.B94	T50.B95	T50.B96
rabies	T50.B91	T50.B92	T50.B93	T50.B94	T50.B95	T50.B96

Substance	Poisoning, Accidental (unintentional)	Poisoning, Intentional Self-harm	Poisoning, Assault	Poisoning, Undetermined	Adverse Effect	Under-dosing
Vaccine NEC—*continued*						
respiratory syncytial virus	T50.B91	T50.B92	T50.B93	T50.B94	T50.B95	T50.B96
rickettsial NEC	T50.A91	T50.A92	T50.A93	T50.A94	T50.A95	T50.A96
with						
bacterial component	T50.A21	T50.A22	T50.A23	T50.A24	T50.A25	T50.A26
Rocky Mountain spotted fever	T50.A91	T50.A92	T50.A93	T50.A94	T50.A95	T50.A96
rubella	T50.B91	T50.B92	T50.B93	T50.B94	T50.B95	T50.B96
sabin oral	T50.B91	T50.B92	T50.B93	T50.B94	T50.B95	T50.B96
smallpox	T50.B11	T50.B12	T50.B13	T50.B14	T50.B15	T50.B16
TAB	T50.A91	T50.A92	T50.A93	T50.A94	T50.A95	T50.A96
tetanus	T50.A91	T50.A92	T50.A93	T50.A94	T50.A95	T50.A96
typhoid	T50.A91	T50.A92	T50.A93	T50.A94	T50.A95	T50.A96
typhus	T50.A91	T50.A92	T50.A93	T50.A94	T50.A95	T50.A96
viral NEC	T50.B91	T50.B92	T50.B93	T50.B94	T50.B95	T50.B96
yellow fever	T50.B91	T50.B92	T50.B93	T50.B94	T50.B95	T50.B96
Vaccinia immune globulin	T50.Z11	T50.Z12	T50.Z13	T50.Z14	T50.Z15	T50.Z16
Vaginal contraceptives	T49.8x1	T49.8x2	T49.8x3	T49.8x4	T49.8x5	T49.8x6
Valerian						
root	T42.6x1	T42.6x2	T42.6x3	T42.6x4	T42.6x5	T42.6x6
tincture	T42.6x1	T42.6x2	T42.6x3	T42.6x4	T42.6x5	T42.6x6
Valethamate bromide	T44.3x1	T44.3x2	T44.3x3	T44.3x4	T44.3x5	T44.3x6
Valisone	T49.0x1	T49.0x2	T49.0x3	T49.0x4	T49.0x5	T49.0x6
Valium	T42.4x1	T42.4x2	T42.4x3	T42.4x4	T42.4x5	T42.4x6
Valmid	T42.6x1	T42.6x2	T42.6x3	T42.6x4	T42.6x5	T42.6x6
Valnoctamide	T42.6x1	T42.6x2	T42.6x3	T42.6x4	T42.6x5	T42.6x6
Valproate (sodium)	T42.6x1	T42.6x2	T42.6x3	T42.6x4	T42.6x5	T42.6x6
Valproic acid	T42.6x1	T42.6x2	T42.6x3	T42.6x4	T42.6x5	T42.6x6
Valpromide	T42.6x1	T42.6x2	T42.6x3	T42.6x4	T42.6x5	T42.6x6
Vanadium	T56.891	T56.892	T56.893	T56.894	—	—
Vancomycin	T36.8x1	T36.8x2	T36.8x3	T36.8x4	T36.8x5	T36.8x6
Vapor (*see also* Gas)	T59.91	T59.92	T59.93	T59.94	—	—
kiln (carbon monoxide)	T58.8x1	T58.8x2	T58.8x3	T58.8x4	—	—
lead—*see* lead						
specified source NEC	T59.91	T59.92	T59.93	T59.94	—	—
Varicose reduction drug	T46.8x1	T46.8x2	T46.8x3	T46.8x4	T46.8x5	T46.8x6
Varnish	T65.4x1	T65.4x2	T65.4x3	T65.4x4	—	—
cleaner	T52.91	T52.92	T52.93	T52.94	—	—
Vaseline	T49.3x1	T49.3x2	T49.3x3	T49.3x4	T49.3x5	T49.3x6
Vasodilan	T46.7x1	T46.7x2	T46.7x3	T46.7x4	T46.7x5	T46.7x6
Vasodilator						
coronary NEC	T46.3x1	T46.3x2	T46.3x3	T46.3x4	T46.3x5	T46.3x6
peripheral NEC	T46.7x1	T46.7x2	T46.7x3	T46.7x4	T46.7x5	T46.7x6
Vasopressin	T38.891	T38.892	T38.893	T38.894	T38.895	T38.896
Vasopressor drugs	T38.891	T38.892	T38.893	T38.894	T38.895	T38.896
Vecuronium bromide	T48.1x1	T48.1x2	T48.1x3	T48.1x4	T48.1x5	T48.1x6
Vegetable extract, astringent	T49.2x1	T49.2x2	T49.2x3	T49.2x4	T49.2x5	T49.2x6
Venlafaxine	T43.211	T43.212	T43.213	T43.214	T43.215	T43.216
Venom, venomous (bite) (sting)	T63.91	T63.92	T63.93	T63.94	—	—
ant	T63.421	T63.422	T63.423	T63.424	—	—
amphibian NEC	T63.831	T63.832	T63.833	T63.834	—	—
animal NEC	T63.891	T63.892	T63.893	T63.894	—	—
arthropod NEC	T63.481	T63.482	T63.483	T63.484	—	—
bee	T63.441	T63.442	T63.443	T63.444	—	—
centipede	T63.411	T63.412	T63.413	T63.414	—	—
fish	T63.591	T63.592	T63.593	T63.594	—	—
frog	T63.811	T63.812	T63.813	T63.814	—	—
hornet	T63.451	T63.452	T63.453	T63.454	—	—
insect NEC	T63.481	T63.482	T63.483	T63.484	—	—
lizard	T63.121	T63.122	T63.123	T63.124	—	—
marine						
animals	T63.691	T63.692	T63.693	T63.694	—	—
bluebottle	T63.611	T63.612	T63.613	T63.614	—	—
jellyfish NEC	T63.621	T63.622	T63.623	T63.624	—	—
Portuguese Man-o-war	T63.611	T63.612	T63.613	T63.614	—	—
sea anemone	T63.631	T63.632	T63.633	T63.634	—	—
specified NEC	T63.691	T63.692	T63.693	T63.694	—	—
fish	T63.591	T63.592	T63.593	T63.594	—	—
sting ray	T63.511	T63.512	T63.513	T63.514	—	—
plants	T63.711	T63.712	T63.713	T63.714	—	—
millipede (tropical)	T63.411	T63.412	T63.413	T63.414	—	—
plant NEC	T63.791	T63.792	T63.793	T63.794	—	—

Substance	Poisoning, Accidental (unintentional)	Poisoning, Intentional Self-harm	Poisoning, Assault	Poisoning, Undetermined	Adverse Effect	Under-dosing
Venom, venomous—*continued*						
plant NEC—*continued*						
marine	T63.711	T63.712	T63.713	T63.714	—	—
reptile	T63.191	T63.192	T63.193	T63.194	—	—
gila monster	T63.111	T63.112	T63.113	T63.114	—	—
lizard NEC	T63.121	T63.122	T63.123	T63.124	—	—
scorpion	T63.2x1	T63.2x2	T63.2x3	T63.2x4	—	—
snake	T63.001	T63.002	T63.003	T63.004	—	—
African NEC	T63.081	T63.082	T63.083	T63.084	—	—
American (North) (South) NEC	T63.061	T63.062	T63.063	T63.064	—	—
Asian	T63.081	T63.082	T63.083	T63.084	—	—
Australian	T63.071	T63.072	T63.073	T63.074	—	—
cobra	T63.041	T63.042	T63.043	T63.044	—	—
coral snake	T63.021	T63.022	T63.023	T63.024	—	—
rattlesnake	T63.011	T63.012	T63.013	T63.014	—	—
specified NEC	T63.091	T63.092	T63.093	T63.094	—	—
taipan	T63.031	T63.032	T63.033	T63.034	—	—
specified NEC	T63.891	T63.892	T63.893	T63.894	—	—
spider	T63.301	T63.302	T63.303	T63.304	—	—
black widow	T63.311	T63.312	T63.313	T63.314	—	—
brown recluse	T63.331	T63.332	T63.333	T63.334	—	—
specified NEC	T63.391	T63.392	T63.393	T63.394	—	—
tarantula	T63.321	T63.322	T63.323	T63.324	—	—
sting ray	T63.511	T63.512	T63.513	T63.514	—	—
toad	T63.821	T63.822	T63.823	T63.824	—	—
wasp	T63.461	T63.462	T63.463	T63.464	—	—
Venous sclerosing drug NEC	T46.8x1	T46.8x2	T46.8x3	T46.8x4	T46.8x5	T46.8x6
Ventolin—*see* Albuterol						
Verapamil	T46.1x1	T46.1x2	T46.1x3	T46.1x4	T46.1x5	T46.1x6
Veramon	T42.3x1	T42.3x2	T42.3x3	T42.3x4	T42.3x5	T42.3x6
Veratrine	T46.5x1	T46.5x2	T46.5x3	T46.5x4	T46.5x5	T46.5x6
Veratrum						
album	T62.2x1	T62.2x2	T62.2x3	T62.2x4	—	—
alkaloids	T46.5x1	T46.5x2	T46.5x3	T46.5x4	T46.5x5	T46.5x6
viride	T62.2x1	T62.2x2	T62.2x3	T62.2x4	—	—
Verdigris	T60.3x1	T60.3x2	T60.3x3	T60.3x4	—	—
Veronal	T42.3x1	T42.3x2	T42.3x3	T42.3x4	T42.3x5	T42.3x6
Veroxil	T37.4x1	T37.4x2	T37.4x3	T37.4x4	T37.4x5	T37.4x6
Versenate	T50.6x1	T50.6x2	T50.6x3	T50.6x4	T50.6x5	T50.6x6
Versidyne	T39.8x1	T39.8x2	T39.8x3	T39.8x4	T39.8x5	T39.8x6
Vetrabutine	T48.0x1	T48.0x2	T48.0x3	T48.0x4	T48.0x5	T48.0x6
Vidarabine	T37.5x1	T37.5x2	T37.5x3	T37.5x4	T37.5x5	T37.5x6
Vienna						
green	T57.0x1	T57.0x2	T57.0x3	T57.0x4	—	—
insecticide	T60.2x1	T60.2x2	T60.2x3	T60.2x4	—	—
red	T57.0x1	T57.0x2	T57.0x3	T57.0x4	—	—
pharmaceutical dye	T50.991	T50.992	T50.993	T50.994	T50.995	T50.996
Vigabatrin	T42.6x1	T42.6x2	T42.6x3	T42.6x4	T42.6x5	T42.6x6
Viloxazine	T43.291	T43.292	T43.293	T43.294	T43.295	T43.296
Viminol	T39.8x1	T39.8x2	T39.8x3	T39.8x4	T39.8x5	T39.8x6
Vinbarbital, vinbarbitone	T42.3x1	T42.3x2	T42.3x3	T42.3x4	T42.3x5	T42.3x6
Vinblastine	T45.1x1	T45.1x2	T45.1x3	T45.1x4	T45.1x5	T45.1x6
Vinburnine	T46.7x1	T46.7x2	T46.7x3	T46.7x4	T46.7x5	T46.7x6
Vincamine	T45.1x1	T45.1x2	T45.1x3	T45.1x4	T45.1x5	T45.1x6
Vincristine	T45.1x1	T45.1x2	T45.1x3	T45.1x4	T45.1x5	T45.1x6
Vindesine	T45.1x1	T45.1x2	T45.1x3	T45.1x4	T45.1x5	T45.1x6
Vinesthene, vinethene	T41.0x1	T41.0x2	T41.0x3	T41.0x4	T41.0x5	T41.0x6
Vinorelbine tartrate	T45.1x1	T45.1x2	T45.1x3	T45.1x4	T45.1x5	T45.1x6
Vinpocetine	T46.7x1	T46.7x2	T46.7x3	T46.7x4	T46.7x5	T46.7x6
Vinyl						
acetate	T65.891	T65.892	T65.893	T65.894	—	—
bital	T42.3x1	T42.3x2	T42.3x3	T42.3x4	T42.3x5	T42.3x6
Vinyl—*continued*						
bromide	T65.891	T65.892	T65.893	T65.894	—	—
chloride	T59.891	T59.892	T59.893	T59.894	—	—
ether	T41.0x1	T41.0x2	T41.0x3	T41.0x4	T41.0x5	T41.0x6
Vinylbital	T42.3x1	T42.3x2	T42.3x3	T42.3x4	T42.3x5	T42.3x6
Vinylidene chloride	T65.891	T65.892	T65.893	T65.894	—	—
Vioform	T37.8x1	T37.8x2	T37.8x3	T37.8x4	T37.8x5	T37.8x6
topical	T49.0x1	T49.0x2	T49.0x3	T49.0x4	T49.0x5	T49.0x6
Viomycin	T36.8x1	T36.8x2	T36.8x3	T36.8x4	T36.8x5	T36.8x6

Substance	Poisoning, Accidental (unintentional)	Poisoning, Intentional Self-harm	Poisoning, Assault	Poisoning, Undetermined	Adverse Effect	Under-dosing
Viosterol	T45.2x1	T45.2x2	T45.2x3	T45.2x4	T45.2x5	T45.2x6
Viper (venom)	T63.091	T63.092	T63.093	T63.094	—	—
Viprynium	T37.4x1	T37.4x2	T37.4x3	T37.4x4	T37.4x5	T37.4x6
Viquidil	T46.7x1	T46.7x2	T46.7x3	T46.7x4	T46.7x5	T46.7x6
Viral vaccine NEC	T50.B91	T50.B92	T50.B93	T50.B94	T50.B95	T50.B96
Virginiamycin	T36.8x1	T36.8x2	T36.8x3	T36.8x4	T36.8x5	T36.8x6
Virugon	T37.5x1	T37.5x2	T37.5x3	T37.5x4	T37.5x5	T37.5x6
Viscous agent	T50.901	T50.902	T50.903	T50.904	T50.905	T50.906
Visine	T49.5x1	T49.5x2	T49.5x3	T49.5x4	T49.5x5	T49.5x6
Visnadine	T46.3x1	T46.3x2	T46.3x3	T46.3x4	T46.3x5	T46.3x6
Vitamin NEC	T45.2x1	T45.2x2	T45.2x3	T45.2x4	T45.2x5	T45.2x6
A	T45.2x1	T45.2x2	T45.2x3	T45.2x4	T45.2x5	T45.2x6
B NEC	T45.2x1	T45.2x2	T45.2x3	T45.2x4	T45.2x5	T45.2x6
nicotinic acid	T46.7x1	T46.7x2	T46.7x3	T46.7x4	T46.7x5	T46.7x6
B1	T45.2x1	T45.2x2	T45.2x3	T45.2x4	T45.2x5	T45.2x6
B2	T45.2x1	T45.2x2	T45.2x3	T45.2x4	T45.2x5	T45.2x6
B6	T45.2x1	T45.2x2	T45.2x3	T45.2x4	T45.2x5	T45.2x6
B12	T45.2x1	T45.2x2	T45.2x3	T45.2x4	T45.2x5	T45.2x6
B15	T45.2x1	T45.2x2	T45.2x3	T45.2x4	T45.2x5	T45.2x6
C	T45.2x1	T45.2x2	T45.2x3	T45.2x4	T45.2x5	T45.2x6
D	T45.2x1	T45.2x2	T45.2x3	T45.2x4	T45.2x5	T45.2x6
D2	T45.2x1	T45.2x2	T45.2x3	T45.2x4	T45.2x5	T45.2x6
D3	T45.2x1	T45.2x2	T45.2x3	T45.2x4	T45.2x5	T45.2x6
E	T45.2x1	T45.2x2	T45.2x3	T45.2x4	T45.2x5	T45.2x6
E acetate	T45.2x1	T45.2x2	T45.2x3	T45.2x4	T45.2x5	T45.2x6
hematopoietic	T45.8x1	T45.8x2	T45.8x3	T45.8x4	T45.8x5	T45.8x6
K NEC	T45.7x1	T45.7x2	T45.7x3	T45.7x4	T45.7x5	T45.7x6
K1	T45.7x1	T45.7x2	T45.7x3	T45.7x4	T45.7x5	T45.7x6
K2	T45.7x1	T45.7x2	T45.7x3	T45.7x4	T45.7x5	T45.7x6
PP	T45.2x1	T45.2x2	T45.2x3	T45.2x4	T45.2x5	T45.2x6
ulceroprotectant	T47.1x1	T47.1x2	T47.1x3	T47.1x4	T47.1x5	T47.1x6
Vleminckx's solution	T49.4x1	T49.4x2	T49.4x3	T49.4x4	T49.4x5	T49.4x6
Voltaren—see Diclofenac sodium						
Warfarin	T45.511	T45.512	T45.513	T45.514	T45.515	T45.516
rodenticide	T60.4x1	T60.4x2	T60.4x3	T60.4x4	—	—
sodium	T60.4x1	T60.4x2	T60.4x3	T60.4x4	—	—
Wasp (sting)	T63.461	T63.462	T63.463	T63.464		
Water						
balance drug	T50.3x1	T50.3x2	T50.3x3	T50.3x4	T50.3x5	T50.3x6
distilled	T50.3x1	T50.3x2	T50.3x3	T50.3x4	T50.3x5	T50.3x6
gas—see Gas, water						
incomplete combustion of— see Carbon, monoxide, fuel, utility						
hemlock	T62.2x1	T62.2x2	T62.2x3	T62.2x4	—	—
moccasin (venom)	T63.061	T63.062	T63.063	T63.064	—	—
purified	T50.3x1	T50.3x2	T50.3x3	T50.3x4	T50.3x5	T50.3x6
Wax (paraffin) (petroleum)	T52.0x1	T52.0x2	T52.0x3	T52.0x4	—	—
automobile	T65.891	T65.892	T65.893	T65.894	—	—
floor	T52.0x1	T52.0x2	T52.0x3	T52.0x4	—	—
Weed killers NEC	T60.3x1	T60.3x2	T60.3x3	T60.3x4	—	—
Welldorm	T42.6x1	T42.6x2	T42.6x3	T42.6x4	T42.6x5	T42.6x6
White						
arsenic	T57.0x1	T57.0x2	T57.0x3	T57.0x4	—	—
hellebore	T62.2x1	T62.2x2	T62.2x3	T62.2x4	—	—
lotion (keratolytic)	T49.4x1	T49.4x2	T49.4x3	T49.4x4	T49.4x5	T49.4x6
spirit	T52.0x1	T52.0x2	T52.0x3	T52.0x4	—	—
Whitewash	T65.891	T65.892	T65.893	T65.894	—	—
Whole Blood (human)	T45.8x1	T45.8x2	T45.8x3	T45.8x4	—	T45.8x6
Wild						
black cherry	T62.2x1	T62.2x2	T62.2x3	T62.2x4	—	—
poisonous plants NEC	T62.2x1	T62.2x2	T62.2x3	T62.2x4	—	—
Window cleaning fluid	T65.891	T65.892	T65.893	T65.894	—	—
Wintergreen (oil)	T49.3x1	T49.3x2	T49.3x3	T49.3x4	T49.3x5	T49.3x6
Witch hazel	T49.2x1	T49.2x2	T49.2x3	T49.2x4	T49.2x5	T49.2x6
Wisterine	T62.2x1	T62.2x2	T62.2x3	T62.2x4	—	—
Witch hazel	T49.2x1	T49.2x2	T49.2x3	T49.2x4	T49.2x5	T49.2x6
Wood alcohol or spirit	T51.1x1	T51.1x2	T51.1x3	T51.1x4	—	—
Wool fat (hydrous)	T49.3x1	T49.3x2	T49.3x3	T49.3x4	T49.3x5	T49.3x6
Woorali	T48.1x1	T48.1x2	T48.1x3	T48.1x4	T48.1x5	T48.1x6
Wormseed, American	T37.4x1	T37.4x2	T37.4x3	T37.4x4	T37.4x5	T37.4x6

Substance	Poisoning, Accidental (unintentional)	Poisoning, Intentional Self-harm	Poisoning, Assault	Poisoning, Undetermined	Adverse Effect	Under-dosing
Xamoterol	T44.5x1	T44.5x2	T44.5x3	T44.5x4	T44.5x5	T44.5x6
Xanthine diuretics	T50.2x1	T50.2x2	T50.2x3	T50.2x4	T50.2x5	T50.2x6
Xanthinol nicotinate	T46.7x1	T46.7x2	T46.7x3	T46.7x4	T46.7x5	T46.7x6
Xanthotoxin	T49.3x1	T49.3x2	T49.3x3	T49.3x4	T49.3x5	T49.3x6
Xantinol nicotinate	T46.7x1	T46.7x2	T46.7x3	T46.7x4	T46.7x5	T46.7x6
Xantocillin	T36.0x1	T36.0x2	T36.0x3	T36.0x4	T36.0x5	T36.0x6
Xenon (127Xe) (133Xe)	T50.8x1	T50.8x2	T50.8x3	T50.8x4	T50.8x5	T50.8x6
Xenysalate	T49.4x1	T49.4x2	T49.4x3	T49.4x4	T49.4x5	T49.4x6
Xibornol	T37.8x1	T37.8x2	T37.8x3	T37.8x4	T37.8x5	T37.8x6
Xigris	T45.511	T45.512	T45.513	T45.514	T45.515	T45.516
Xipamide	T50.2x1	T50.2x2	T50.2x3	T50.2x4	T50.2x5	T50.2x6
Xylene (vapor)	T52.2x1	T52.2x2	T52.2x3	T52.2x4	—	—
Xylocaine (infiltration) (topical)	T41.3x1	T41.3x2	T41.3x3	T41.3x4	T41.3x5	T41.3x6
nerve block (peripheral) (plexus)	T41.3x1	T41.3x2	T41.3x3	T41.3x4	T41.3x5	T41.3x6
spinal	T41.3x1	T41.3x2	T41.3x3	T41.3x4	T41.3x5	T41.3x6
Xylol (vapor)	T52.2x1	T52.2x2	T52.2x3	T52.2x4	—	—
Xylometazoline	T48.5x1	T48.5x2	T48.5x3	T48.5x4	T48.5x5	T48.5x6
Yeast	T45.2x1	T45.2x2	T45.2x3	T45.2x4	T45.2x5	T45.2x6
dried	T45.2x1	T45.2x2	T45.2x3	T45.2x4	T45.2x5	T45.2x6
Yellow						
fever vaccine	T50.B91	T50.B92	T50.B93	T50.B94	T50.B95	T50.B96
jasmine	T62.2x1	T62.2x2	T62.2x3	T62.2x4	—	—
phenolphthalein	T47.2x1	T47.2x2	T47.2x3	T47.2x4	T47.2x5	T47.2x6
Yew	T62.2x1	T62.2x2	T62.2x3	T62.2x4	—	—
Yohimbic acid	T40.991	T40.992	T40.993	T40.994	T40.995	T40.996
Zactane	T39.8x1	T39.8x2	T39.8x3	T39.8x4	T39.8x5	T39.8x6
Zalcitabine	T37.5x1	T37.5x2	T37.5x3	T37.5x4	T37.5x5	T37.5x6
Zaroxolyn	T50.2x1	T50.2x2	T50.2x3	T50.2x4	T50.2x5	T50.2x6
Zephiran (topical)	T49.0x1	T49.0x2	T49.0x3	T49.0x4	T49.0x5	T49.0x6
ophthalmic preparation	T49.5x1	T49.5x2	T49.5x3	T49.5x4	T49.5x5	T49.5x6
Zeranol	T38.7x1	T38.7x2	T38.7x3	T38.7x4	T38.7x5	T38.7x6
Zerone	T51.1x1	T51.1x2	T51.1x3	T51.1x4	—	—
Zidovudine	T37.5x1	T37.5x2	T37.5x3	T37.5x4	T37.5x5	T37.5x6
Zimeldine	T43.221	T43.222	T43.223	T43.224	T43.225	T43.226
Zinc (compounds) (fumes) (vapor) NEC	T56.5x1	T56.5x2	T56.5x3	T56.5x4	—	—
anti-infectives	T49.0x1	T49.0x2	T49.0x3	T49.0x4	T49.0x5	T49.0x6
antivaricose	T46.8x1	T46.8x2	T46.8x3	T46.8x4	T46.8x5	T46.8x6
bacitracin	T49.0x1	T49.0x2	T49.0x3	T49.0x4	T49.0x5	T49.0x6
chloride (mouthwash)	T49.6x1	T49.6x2	T49.6x3	T49.6x4	T49.6x5	T49.6x6
chromate	T56.5x1	T56.5x2	T56.5x3	T56.5x4	—	—
gelatin	T49.3x1	T49.3x2	T49.3x3	T49.3x4	T49.3x5	T49.3x6
oxide	T49.3x1	T49.3x2	T49.3x3	T49.3x4	T49.3x5	T49.3x6
plaster	T49.3x1	T49.3x2	T49.3x3	T49.3x4	T49.3x5	T49.3x6
peroxide	T49.0x1	T49.0x2	T49.0x3	T49.0x4	T49.0x5	T49.0x6
pesticides	T56.5x1	T56.5x2	T56.5x3	T56.5x4	—	—
phosphide	T60.4x1	T60.4x2	T60.4x3	T60.4x4	—	—
pyrithionate	T49.4x1	T49.4x2	T49.4x3	T49.4x4	T49.4x5	T49.4x6
stearate	T49.3x1	T49.3x2	T49.3x3	T49.3x4	T49.3x5	T49.3x6
sulfate	T49.5x1	T49.5x2	T49.5x3	T49.5x4	T49.5x5	T49.5x6
ENT agent	T49.6x1	T49.6x2	T49.6x3	T49.6x4	T49.6x5	T49.6x6
ophthalmic solution	T49.5x1	T49.5x2	T49.5x3	T49.5x4	T49.5x5	T49.5x6
topical NEC	T49.0x1	T49.0x2	T49.0x3	T49.0x4	T49.0x5	T49.0x6
undecylenate	T49.0x1	T49.0x2	T49.0x3	T49.0x4	T49.0x5	T49.0x6
Zineb	T60.0x1	T60.0x2	T60.0x3	T60.0x4	—	—
Zinostatin	T45.1x1	T45.1x2	T45.1x3	T45.1x4	T45.1x5	T45.1x6
Zipeprol	T48.3x1	T48.3x2	T48.3x3	T48.3x4	T48.3x5	T48.3x6
Zofenopril	T46.4x1	T46.4x2	T46.4x3	T46.4x4	T46.4x5	T46.4x6
Zolpidem	T42.6x1	T42.6x2	T42.6x3	T42.6x4	T42.6x5	T42.6x6
Zomepirac	T39.391	T39.392	T39.393	T39.394	T39.395	T39.396
Zopiclone	T42.6x1	T42.6x2	T42.6x3	T42.6x4	T42.6x5	T42.6x6
Zorubicin	T45.1x1	T45.1x2	T45.1x3	T45.1x4	T45.1x5	T45.1x6
Zotepine	T43.591	T43.592	T43.593	T43.594	T43.595	T43.596
Zovant	T45.511	T45.512	T45.513	T45.514	T45.515	T45.516
Zoxazolamine	T42.8x1	T42.8x2	T42.8x3	T42.8x4	T42.8x5	T42.8x6
Zuclopenthixol	T43.4x1	T43.4x2	T43.4x3	T43.4x4	T43.4x5	T43.4x6
Zygadenus (venenosus)	T62.2x1	T62.2x2	T62.2x3	T62.2x4	—	—
Zyprexa	T43.591	T43.592	T43.593	T43.594	T43.595	T43.596

ICD-1Ø-CM Index to External Causes

A

Abandonment (causing exposure to weather conditions) (with intent to injure or kill) NEC X58
Abuse (adult) (child) (mental) (physical) (sexual) X58
Accident (to) X58
  aircraft (in transit) (powered) (see also Accident, transport, aircraft)
    due to, caused by cataclysm — see Forces of nature, by type
  animal-rider — see Accident, transport, animal-rider
  animal-drawn vehicle — see Accident, transport, animal-drawn vehicle occupant
  automobile — see Accident, transport, car occupant
  bare foot water skiier V94.4
  boat, boating (see also Accident, watercraft)
    striking swimmer
      powered V94.11
      unpowered V94.12
  bus — see Accident, transport, bus occupant
  cable car, not on rails V98.Ø
    on rails — see Accident, transport, streetcar occupant
  car — see Accident, transport, car occupant
  caused by, due to
    animal NEC W64
    chain hoist W24.Ø
    cold (excessive) — see Exposure, cold
    corrosive liquid, substance — see Table of Drugs and Chemicals
    cutting or piercing instrument — see Contact, with, by type of instrument
    drive belt W24.Ø
    electric
      current — see Exposure, electric current
      motor (see also Contact, with, by type of machine) W31.3
        current (of) W86.8
    environmental factor NEC X58
    explosive material — see Explosion
    fire, flames — see Exposure, fire
    firearm missile — see Discharge, firearm by type
    heat (excessive) — see Heat
    hot — see Contact, with, hot
    ignition — see Ignition
    lifting device W24.Ø
    lightning — see subcategory T75.Ø
      causing fire — see Exposure, fire
    machine, machinery — see Contact, with, by type of machine
    natural factor NEC X58
    pulley (block) W24.Ø
    radiation — see Radiation
    steam X13.1
      inhalation X13.Ø
      pipe X16
    thunderbolt — see subcategory T75.Ø
      causing fire — see Exposure, fire
    transmission device W24.1
  coach — see Accident, transport, bus occupant
  coal car — see Accident, transport, industrial vehicle occupant
  diving (see also Fall, into, water)
    with
      drowning or submersion — see Drowning
  forklift — see Accident, transport, industrial vehicle occupant
  heavy transport vehicle NOS — see Accident, transport, truck occupant
  ice yacht V98.2
  in
    medical, surgical procedure
      as, or due to misadventure — see Misadventure

Accident— continued
  in— continued
    medical, surgical procedure— continued
      causing an abnormal reaction or later complication without mention of misadventure (see also Complication of or following, by type of procedure) Y84.9
  land yacht V98.1
  late effect of — see WØØ-X58 with 7th character S
  logging car — see Accident, transport, industrial vehicle occupant
  machine, machinery (see also Contact, with, by type of machine)
    on board watercraft V93.69
      explosion — see Explosion, in, watercraft
      fire — see Burn, on board watercraft
      powered craft V93.63
        ferry boat V93.61
        fishing boat V93.62
        jetskis V93.63
        liner V93.61
        merchant ship V93.6Ø
        passenger ship V93.61
        sailboat V93.64
  mine tram — see Accident, transport, industrial vehicle occupant
  mobility scooter (motorized) — see Accident, transport, pedestrian, conveyance, specified type NEC
  motor scooter — see Accident, transport, motorcyclist
  motor vehicle NOS (traffic) (see also Accident, transport) V89.2
    nontraffic V89.Ø
    three-wheeled NOS — see Accident, transport, three-wheeled motor vehicle occupant
  motorcycle NOS — see Accident, transport, motorcyclist
  nonmotor vehicle NOS (nontraffic) (see also Accident, transport) V89.1
    traffic NOS V89.3
  nontraffic (victim's mode of transport NOS) V88.9
    collision (between) V88.7
      bus and truck V88.5
      car and:
        bus V88.3
        pickup V88.2
        three-wheeled motor vehicle V88.Ø
        train V88.6
        truck V88.4
        two-wheeled motor vehicle V88.Ø
        van V88.2
      specified vehicle NEC and:
        three-wheeled motor vehicle V88.1
        two-wheeled motor vehicle V88.1
    known mode of transport — see Accident, transport, by type of vehicle
    noncollision V88.8
  on board watercraft V93.89
    powered craft V93.83
      ferry boat V93.81
      fishing boat V93.82
      jetskis V93.83
      liner V93.81
      merchant ship V93.8Ø
      passenger ship V93.81
    unpowered craft V93.88
      canoe V93.85
      inflatable V93.86
        in tow
          recreational V94.31
          specified NEC V94.32
      kayak V93.85
      sailboat V93.84
      surf-board V93.88
      water skis V93.87

Accident— continued
  on board watercraft— continued
    unpowered craft— continued
      windsurfer V93.88
  parachutist V97.29
    entangled in object V97.21
    injured on landing V97.22
  pedal cycle — see Accident, transport, pedal cyclist
  pedestrian (on foot)
    with
      another pedestrian W51
        with fall WØ3
          due to ice or snow WØØ.Ø
      on pedestrian conveyance NEC VØØ.Ø9
      roller skater (in-line) VØØ.Ø1
      skate boarder VØØ.Ø2
      transport vehicle — see Accident, transport
    on pedestrian conveyance — see Accident, transport, pedestrian, conveyance
  pick-up truck or van — see Accident, transport, pickup truck occupant
  quarry truck — see Accident, transport, industrial vehicle occupant
  railway vehicle (any) (in motion) — see Accident, transport, railway vehicle occupant
    due to cataclysm — see Forces of nature, by type
  scooter (non-motorized) — see Accident, transport, pedestrian, conveyance, scooter
  sequelae of — see WØØ-X58 with 7th character S
  skateboard — see Accident, transport, pedestrian, conveyance, skateboard
  ski(ing) — see Accident, transport, pedestrian, conveyance
    lift V98.3
  specified cause NEC X58
  streetcar — see Accident, transport, streetcar occupant
  traffic (victim's mode of transport NOS) V87.9
    collision (between) V87.7
      bus and truck V87.5
      car and:
        bus V87.3
        pickup V87.2
        three-wheeled motor vehicle V87.Ø
        train V87.6
        truck V87.4
        two-wheeled motor vehicle V87.Ø
        van V87.2
      specified vehicle NEC and:
        three-wheeled motor vehicle V87.1
        two-wheeled motor vehicle V87.1
    known mode of transport — see Accident, transport, by type of vehicle
    noncollision V87.8
  transport (involving injury to) V99
    18 wheeler — see Accident, transport, truck occupant
    agricultural vehicle occupant (nontraffic) V84.9
      driver V84.5
      hanger-on V84.7
      passenger V84.6
      traffic V84.3
        driver V84.Ø
        hanger-on V84.2
        passenger V84.1
      while boarding or alighting V84.4
    aircraft NEC V97.89
      military NEC V97.818
        with civlian aircraft V97.81Ø
        civilian injured by V97.811
      occupant injured (in)
        nonpowered craft accident V96.9
          balloon V96.ØØ
            collision V96.Ø3
            crash V96.Ø1
            explosion V96.Ø5
            fire V96.Ø4

Accident— *continued*
  transport— *continued*
    bus occupant— *continued*
      driver— *continued*
        collision— *continued*
          two wheeled motor vehicle (traffic) V72.5
            nontraffic V72.0
          van (traffic) V73.5
            nontraffic V73.0
        noncollision accident (traffic) V78.5
          nontraffic V78.0
      noncollision accident (traffic) V78.9
        nontraffic V78.3
        while boarding or alighting V78.4
      nontraffic V79.3
      hanger-on
        collision (with)
          animal (traffic) V70.7
            being ridden (traffic) V76.7
              nontraffic V76.2
            nontraffic V70.2
          animal-drawn vehicle (traffic) V76.7
            nontraffic V76.2
          bus (traffic) V74.7
            nontraffic V74.2
          car (traffic) V73.7
            nontraffic V73.2
          pedal cycle (traffic) V71.7
            nontraffic V71.2
          pickup truck (traffic) V73.7
            nontraffic V73.2
          railway vehicle (traffic) V75.7
            nontraffic V75.2
          specified vehicle NEC (traffic) V76.7
            nontraffic V76.2
          stationary object (traffic) V77.7
            nontraffic V77.2
          streetcar (traffic) V76.7
            nontraffic V76.2
          three wheeled motor vehicle (traffic) V72.7
            nontraffic V72.2
          truck (traffic) V74.7
            nontraffic V74.2
          two wheeled motor vehicle (traffic) V72.7
            nontraffic V72.2
          van (traffic) V73.7
            nontraffic V73.2
        noncollision accident (traffic) V78.7
          nontraffic V78.2
      passenger
        collision (with)
          animal (traffic) V70.6
            being ridden (traffic) V76.6
              nontraffic V76.1
            nontraffic V70.1
          animal-drawn vehicle (traffic) V76.6
            nontraffic V76.1
          bus (traffic) V74.6
            nontraffic V74.1
          car (traffic) V73.6
            nontraffic V73.1
          motor vehicle NOS (traffic) V79.50
            nontraffic V79.10
            specified type NEC (traffic) V79.59
              nontraffic V79.19
          pedal cycle (traffic) V71.6
            nontraffic V71.1
          pickup truck (traffic) V73.6
            nontraffic V73.1
          railway vehicle (traffic) V75.6
            nontraffic V75.1
          specified vehicle NEC (traffic) V76.6
            nontraffic V76.1
          stationary object (traffic) V77.6
            nontraffic V77.1
          streetcar (traffic) V76.6
            nontraffic V76.1
          three wheeled motor vehicle (traffic) V72.6
            nontraffic V72.1

Accident— *continued*
  transport— *continued*
    bus occupant— *continued*
      passenger— *continued*
        collision— *continued*
          truck (traffic) V74.6
            nontraffic V74.1
          two wheeled motor vehicle (traffic) V72.6
            nontraffic V72.1
          van (traffic) V73.6
            nontraffic V73.1
        noncollision accident (traffic) V78.6
          nontraffic V78.1
      specified type NEC V79.88
      military vehicle V79.81
    cable car, not on rails V98.0
      on rails — *see* Accident, transport, streetcar occupant
    car occupant V49.9
      ambulance occupant — *see* Accident, transport, ambulance occupant
      collision (with)
        animal (traffic) V40.9
          being ridden (traffic) V46.9
            nontraffic V46.3
              while boarding or alighting V46.4
          nontraffic V40.3
          while boarding or alighting V40.4
        animal-drawn vehicle (traffic) V46.9
          nontraffic V46.3
          while boarding or alighting V46.4
        bus (traffic) V44.9
          nontraffic V44.3
          while boarding or alighting V44.4
        car (traffic) V43.92
          nontraffic V43.32
          while boarding or alighting V43.42
        motor vehicle NOS (traffic) V49.60
          nontraffic V49.20
          specified type NEC (traffic) V49.69
            nontraffic V49.29
        pedal cycle (traffic) V41.9
          nontraffic V41.3
          while boarding or alighting V41.4
        pickup truck (traffic) V43.93
          nontraffic V43.33
          while boarding or alighting V43.43
        railway vehicle (traffic) V45.9
          nontraffic V45.3
          while boarding or alighting V45.4
        specified vehicle NEC (traffic) V46.9
          nontraffic V46.3
          while boarding or alighting V46.4
        sport utility vehicle (traffic) V43.91
          nontraffic V43.31
          while boarding or alighting V43.41
        stationary object (traffic) V47.92
          nontraffic V47.32
          while boarding or alighting V47.4
        streetcar (traffic) V46.9
          nontraffic V46.3
          while boarding or alighting V46.4
        three wheeled motor vehicle (traffic) V42.9
          nontraffic V42.3
          while boarding or alighting V42.4
        truck (traffic) V44.9
          nontraffic V44.3
          while boarding or alighting V44.4
        two wheeled motor vehicle (traffic) V42.9
          nontraffic V42.3
          while boarding or alighting V42.4
        van (traffic) V43.94
          nontraffic V43.34
          while boarding or alighting V43.44
      driver
        collision (with)
          animal (traffic) V40.5
            being ridden (traffic) V46.5
              nontraffic V46.0
            nontraffic V40.0
          animal-drawn vehicle (traffic) V46.5

Accident— *continued*
  transport— *continued*
    car occupant— *continued*
      driver— *continued*
        collision— *continued*
          animal-drawn vehicle— *continued*
            nontraffic V46.0
          bus (traffic) V44.5
            nontraffic V44.0
          car (traffic) V43.52
            nontraffic V43.02
          motor vehicle NOS (traffic) V49.40
            nontraffic V49.00
            specified type NEC (traffic) V49.49
              nontraffic V49.09
          pedal cycle (traffic) V41.5
            nontraffic V41.0
          pickup truck (traffic) V43.53
            nontraffic V43.03
          railway vehicle (traffic) V45.5
            nontraffic V45.0
          specified vehicle NEC (traffic) V46.5
            nontraffic V46.0
          sport utility vehicle (traffic) V43.51
            nontraffic V43.01
          stationary object (traffic) V47.52
            nontraffic V47.02
          streetcar (traffic) V46.5
            nontraffic V46.0
          three wheeled motor vehicle (traffic) V42.5
            nontraffic V42.0
          truck (traffic) V44.5
            nontraffic V44.0
          two wheeled motor vehicle (traffic) V42.5
            nontraffic V42.0
          van (traffic) V43.54
            nontraffic V43.04
        noncollision accident (traffic) V48.5
          nontraffic V48.0
      noncollision accident (traffic) V48.9
        nontraffic V48.3
        while boarding or alighting V48.4
      nontraffic V49.3
      hanger-on
        collision (with)
          animal (traffic) V40.7
            being ridden (traffic) V46.7
              nontraffic V46.2
            nontraffic V40.2
          animal-drawn vehicle (traffic) V46.7
            nontraffic V46.2
          bus (traffic) V44.7
            nontraffic V44.2
          car (traffic) V43.72
            nontraffic V43.22
          pedal cycle (traffic) V41.7
            nontraffic V41.2
          pickup truck (traffic) V43.73
            nontraffic V43.23
          railway vehicle (traffic) V45.7
            nontraffic V45.2
          specified vehicle NEC (traffic) V46.7
            nontraffic V46.2
          sport utility vehicle (traffic) V43.71
            nontraffic V43.21
          stationary object (traffic) V47.7
            nontraffic V47.2
          streetcar (traffic) V46.7
            nontraffic V46.2
          three wheeled motor vehicle (traffic) V42.7
            nontraffic V42.2
          truck (traffic) V44.7
            nontraffic V44.2
          two wheeled motor vehicle (traffic) V42.7
            nontraffic V42.2
          van (traffic) V43.74
            nontraffic V43.24
        noncollision accident (traffic) V48.7
          nontraffic V48.2

Accident— *continued*
 transport— *continued*
  motorcyclist— *continued*
   passenger— *continued*
    noncollision accident (traffic) V28.5
     nontraffic V28.1
   specified type NEC V29.88
    military vehicle V29.81
  motor vehicle NEC occupant (traffic) V86.39
   driver V86.09
   hanger-on V86.29
   nontraffic V86.99
    driver V86.59
    hanger-on V86.79
    passenger V86.69
   passenger V86.19
   while boarding or alighting V86.49
  occupant (of)
   aircraft (powered) V95.9
    fixed wing
     commercial — *see* Accident, transport,
      aircraft, occupant, powered,
      fixed wing, commercial
     private — *see* Accident, transport,
      aircraft, occupant, powered,
      fixed wing, private
    nonpowered V96.9
    specified NEC V95.8
   airport battery-powered vehicle — *see*
    Accident, transport, industrial vehicle
    occupant
   all-terrain vehicle (ATV) — *see* Accident,
    transport, all-terrain vehicle occupant
   animal-drawn vehicle — *see* Accident,
    transport, animal-drawn vehicle
    occupant
   automobile — *see* Accident, transport, car
    occupant
   balloon V96.00
   battery-powered vehicle — *see* Accident,
    transport, industrial vehicle occupant
   bicycle — *see* Accident, transport, pedal
    cyclist
    motorized — *see* Accident, transport,
     motorcycle rider
   boat NEC — *see* Accident, watercraft
   bulldozer — *see* Accident, transport,
    construction vehicle occupant
   bus — *see* Accident, transport, bus occupant
   cable car (on rails) (*see also* Accident,
    transport, streetcar occupant)
    not on rails V98.0
   car (*see also* Accident, transport, car occupant)
    cable (on rails) (*see also* Accident,
     transport, streetcar occupant)
     not on rails V98.0
    coach — *see* Accident, transport, bus
     occupant
   coal-car — *see* Accident, transport, industrial
    vehicle occupant
   digger — *see* Accident, transport,
    construction vehicle occupant
   dump truck — *see* Accident, transport,
    construction vehicle occupant
   earth-leveler — *see* Accident, transport,
    construction vehicle occupant
   farm machinery (self-propelled) — *see*
    Accident, transport, agricultural vehicle
    occupant
   forklift — *see* Accident, transport, industrial
    vehicle occupant
   glider (unpowered) V96.20
    hang V96.10
    powered (microlight) (ultralight) — *see*
     Accident, transport, aircraft,
     occupant, powered, glider
   glider (unpowered) NEC V96.20
   hang-glider V96.10
   harvester — *see* Accident, transport,
    agricultural vehicle occupant
   heavy (transport) vehicle — *see* Accident,
    transport, truck occupant

Accident— *continued*
 transport— *continued*
  occupant— *continued*
   helicopter — *see* Accident, transport, aircraft,
    occupant, helicopter
   ice-yacht V98.2
   kite (carrying person) V96.8
   land-yacht V98.1
   logging car — *see* Accident, transport,
    industrial vehicle occupant
   mechanical shovel — *see* Accident, transport,
    construction vehicle occupant
   microlight — *see* Accident, transport, aircraft,
    occupant, powered, glider
   minibus — *see* Accident, transport, car
    occupant
   minivan — *see* Accident, transport, car
    occupant
   moped — *see* Accident, transport, motorcycle
   motor scooter — *see* Accident, transport,
    motorcycle
   motorcycle (with sidecar) — *see* Accident,
    transport, motorcycle
   pedal cycle (*see also* Accident, transport, pedal
    cyclist)
   pick-up (truck) — *see* Accident, transport,
    pickup truck occupant
   railway (train) (vehicle) (subterranean)
    (elevated) — *see* Accident, transport,
    railway vehicle occupant
   rickshaw — *see* Accident, transport, pedal
    cycle
    pedal driven — *see* Accident, transport,
     pedal cyclist
   road-roller — *see* Accident, transport,
    construction vehicle occupant
   ship NOS V94.9
   ski-lift (chair) (gondola) V98.3
   snowmobile — *see* Accident, transport,
    snowmobile occupant
   spacecraft, spaceship — *see* Accident,
    transport, aircraft, occupant, spacecraft
   sport utility vehicle — *see* Accident, transport,
    car occupant
   streetcar (interurban) (operating on public
    street or highway) — *see* Accident,
    transport, streetcar occupant
   SUV — *see* Accident, transport, car occupant
   téléférique V98.0
   three-wheeled vehicle (motorized) (*see also*
    Accident, transport, three-wheeled
    motor vehicle occupant)
    nonmotorized — *see* Accident, transport,
     pedal cycle
   tractor (farm) (and trailer) — *see* Accident,
    transport, agricultural vehicle occupant
   train — *see* Accident, transport, railway
    vehicle occupant
   tram — *see* Accident, transport, streetcar
    occupant
    in mine or quarry — *see* Accident,
     transport, industrial vehicle
     occupant
   tricycle — *see* Accident, transport, pedal cycle
    motorized — *see* Accident, transport,
     three-wheeled motor vehicle
   trolley — *see* Accident, transport, streetcar
    occupant
    in mine or quarry — *see* Accident,
     transport, industrial vehicle
     occupant
   tub, in mine or quarry — *see* Accident,
    transport, industrial vehicle occupant
   ultralight — *see* Accident, transport, aircraft,
    occupant, powered, glider
   van — *see* Accident, transport, van occupant
   vehicle NEC V89.9
    heavy transport — *see* Accident,
     transport, truck occupant
    motor (traffic) NEC V89.2
     nontraffic NEC V89.0

Accident— *continued*
 transport— *continued*
  occupant— *continued*
   watercraft NOS V94.9
    causing drowning B — *see* Drowning,
     resulting from accident to boat
  parachutist V97.29
   after accident to aircraft — *see* Accident,
    transport, aircraft
  entangled in object V97.21
  injured on landing V97.22
  pedal cyclist V19.9
   collision (with)
    animal (traffic) V10.9
     being ridden (traffic) V16.9
      nontraffic V16.2
       while boarding or alighting V16.3
     nontraffic V10.2
      while boarding or alighting V10.3
    animal-drawn vehicle (traffic) V16.9
     nontraffic V16.2
      while boarding or alighting V16.3
    bus (traffic) V14.9
     nontraffic V14.2
      while boarding or alighting V14.3
    car (traffic) V13.9
     nontraffic V13.2
      while boarding or alighting V13.3
    motor vehicle NOS (traffic) V19.60
     nontraffic V19.20
      specified type NEC (traffic) V19.69
       nontraffic V19.29
    pedal cycle (traffic) V11.9
     nontraffic V11.2
      while boarding or alighting V11.3
    pickup truck (traffic) V13.9
     nontraffic V13.2
      while boarding or alighting V13.3
    railway vehicle (traffic) V15.9
     nontraffic V15.2
      while boarding or alighting V15.3
    specified vehicle NEC (traffic) V16.9
     nontraffic V16.2
      while boarding or alighting V16.3
    stationary object (traffic) V17.9
     nontraffic V17.2
      while boarding or alighting V17.3
    streetcar (traffic) V16.9
     nontraffic V16.2
      while boarding or alighting V16.3
    three wheeled motor vehicle (traffic)
     V12.9
     nontraffic V12.2
      while boarding or alighting V12.3
    truck (traffic) V14.9
     nontraffic V14.2
      while boarding or alighting V14.3
    two wheeled motor vehicle (traffic) V12.9
     nontraffic V12.2
      while boarding or alighting V12.3
    van (traffic) V13.9
     nontraffic V13.2
      while boarding or alighting V13.3
   driver
    collision (with)
     animal (traffic) V10.4
      being ridden (traffic) V16.4
       nontraffic V16.0
      nontraffic V10.0
     animal-drawn vehicle (traffic) V16.4
      nontraffic V16.0
     bus (traffic) V14.4
      nontraffic V14.0
     car (traffic) V13.4
      nontraffic V13.0
     motor vehicle NOS (traffic) V19.40
      nontraffic V19.00
       specified type NEC (traffic) V19.49
        nontraffic V19.09
     pedal cycle (traffic) V11.4
      nontraffic V11.0
     pickup truck (traffic) V13.4
      nontraffic V13.0

Accident— *continued*
　transport— *continued*
　　pedal cyclist— *continued*
　　　driver— *continued*
　　　　collision— *continued*
　　　　　railway vehicle (traffic) V15.4
　　　　　　nontraffic V15.0
　　　　　specified vehicle NEC (traffic) V16.4
　　　　　　nontraffic V16.0
　　　　　stationary object (traffic) V17.4
　　　　　　nontraffic V17.0
　　　　　streetcar (traffic) V16.4
　　　　　　nontraffic V16.0
　　　　　three wheeled motor vehicle (traffic)
　　　　　　V12.4
　　　　　　nontraffic V12.0
　　　　　truck (traffic) V14.4
　　　　　　nontraffic V14.0
　　　　　two wheeled motor vehicle (traffic)
　　　　　　V12.4
　　　　　　nontraffic V12.0
　　　　　van (traffic) V13.4
　　　　　　nontraffic V13.0
　　　　noncollision accident (traffic) V18.4
　　　　　nontraffic V18.0
　　　noncollision accident (traffic) V18.9
　　　　nontraffic V18.2
　　　while boarding or alighting V18.3
　　nontraffic V19.3
　　passenger
　　　collision (with)
　　　　animal (traffic) V10.5
　　　　　being ridden (traffic) V16.5
　　　　　　nontraffic V16.1
　　　　　nontraffic V10.1
　　　　animal-drawn vehicle (traffic) V16.5
　　　　　nontraffic V16.1
　　　　bus (traffic) V14.5
　　　　　nontraffic V14.1
　　　　car (traffic) V13.5
　　　　　nontraffic V13.1
　　　　motor vehicle NOS (traffic) V19.50
　　　　　nontraffic V19.10
　　　　　specified type NEC (traffic) V19.59
　　　　　　nontraffic V19.19
　　　　pedal cycle (traffic) V11.5
　　　　　nontraffic V11.1
　　　　pickup truck (traffic) V13.5
　　　　　nontraffic V13.1
　　　　railway vehicle (traffic) V15.5
　　　　　nontraffic V15.1
　　　　specified vehicle NEC (traffic) V16.5
　　　　　nontraffic V16.1
　　　　stationary object (traffic) V17.5
　　　　　nontraffic V17.1
　　　　streetcar (traffic) V16.5
　　　　　nontraffic V16.1
　　　　three wheeled motor vehicle (traffic)
　　　　　V12.5
　　　　　nontraffic V12.1
　　　　truck (traffic) V14.5
　　　　　nontraffic V14.1
　　　　two wheeled motor vehicle (traffic)
　　　　　V12.5
　　　　　nontraffic V12.1
　　　　van (traffic) V13.5
　　　　　nontraffic V13.1
　　　noncollision accident (traffic) V18.5
　　　　nontraffic V18.1
　　specified type NEC V19.88
　　military vehicle V19.81
　pedestrian
　　conveyance (occupant) V09.9
　　　babystroller V00.828
　　　　collision (with) V09.9
　　　　　animal being ridden or animal
　　　　　　drawn vehicle V06.99
　　　　　　nontraffic V06.09
　　　　　　traffic V06.19
　　　　　bus or heavy transport V04.99
　　　　　　nontraffic V04.09
　　　　　　traffic V04.19

Accident— *continued*
　transport— *continued*
　　pedestrian— *continued*
　　　conveyance— *continued*
　　　　babystroller— *continued*
　　　　　collision— *continued*
　　　　　　car V03.99
　　　　　　　nontraffic V03.09
　　　　　　　traffic V03.19
　　　　　　pedal cycle V01.99
　　　　　　　nontraffic V01.09
　　　　　　　traffic V01.19
　　　　　　pick-up truck or van V03.99
　　　　　　　nontraffic V03.09
　　　　　　　traffic V03.19
　　　　　　railway (train) (vehicle) V05.99
　　　　　　　nontraffic V05.09
　　　　　　　traffic V05.19
　　　　　　streetcar V06.99
　　　　　　　nontraffic V06.09
　　　　　　　traffic V06.19
　　　　　　stationary object V00.822
　　　　　　two or three-wheeled motor
　　　　　　　vehicle V02.99
　　　　　　　nontraffic V02.09
　　　　　　　traffic V02.19
　　　　　　vehicle V09.9
　　　　　　　animal-drawn V06.99
　　　　　　　　nontraffic V06.09
　　　　　　　　traffic V06.19
　　　　　　　motor
　　　　　　　　nontraffic V09.00
　　　　　　　　traffic V09.20
　　　　　fall V00.821
　　　　　nontraffic V09.1
　　　　　　involving motor vehicle NEC
　　　　　　　V09.00
　　　　　traffic V09.3
　　　　　　involving motor vehicle NEC
　　　　　　　V09.20
　　　　flat-bottomed NEC V00.388
　　　　　collision (with) V09.9
　　　　　　animal being ridden or animal
　　　　　　　drawn vehicle V06.99
　　　　　　　nontraffic V06.09
　　　　　　　traffic V06.19
　　　　　　bus or heavy transport V04.99
　　　　　　　nontraffic V04.09
　　　　　　　traffic V04.19
　　　　　　car V03.99
　　　　　　　nontraffic V03.09
　　　　　　　traffic V03.19
　　　　　　pedal cycle V01.99
　　　　　　　nontraffic V01.09
　　　　　　　traffic V01.19
　　　　　　pick-up truck or van V03.99
　　　　　　　nontraffic V03.09
　　　　　　　traffic V03.19
　　　　　　railway (train) (vehicle) V05.99
　　　　　　　nontraffic V05.09
　　　　　　　traffic V05.19
　　　　　　stationary object V00.382
　　　　　　streetcar V06.99
　　　　　　　nontraffic V06.09
　　　　　　　traffic V06.19
　　　　　　two or three-wheeled motor
　　　　　　　vehicle V02.99
　　　　　　　nontraffic V02.09
　　　　　　　traffic V02.19
　　　　　　vehicle V09.9
　　　　　　　animal-drawn V06.99
　　　　　　　　nontraffic V06.09
　　　　　　　　traffic V06.19
　　　　　　　motor
　　　　　　　　nontraffic V09.00
　　　　　　　　traffic V09.20
　　　　　fall V00.381
　　　　　nontraffic V09.1
　　　　　　involving motor vehicle NEC
　　　　　　　V09.00

Accident— *continued*
　transport— *continued*
　　pedestrian— *continued*
　　　conveyance— *continued*
　　　　flat-bottomed— *continued*
　　　　　snow
　　　　　　board — *see* Accident, transport,
　　　　　　　pedestrian, conveyance, snow
　　　　　　　board
　　　　　　ski — *see* Accident, transport,
　　　　　　　pedestrian, conveyance, skis
　　　　　　　(snow)
　　　　　traffic V09.3
　　　　　　involving motor vehicle NEC
　　　　　　　V09.20
　　　　gliding type NEC V00.288
　　　　　collision (with) V09.9
　　　　　　animal being ridden or animal
　　　　　　　drawn vehicle V06.99
　　　　　　　nontraffic V06.09
　　　　　　　traffic V06.19
　　　　　　bus or heavy transport V04.99
　　　　　　　nontraffic V04.09
　　　　　　　traffic V04.19
　　　　　　car V03.99
　　　　　　　nontraffic V03.09
　　　　　　　traffic V03.19
　　　　　　pedal cycle V01.99
　　　　　　　nontraffic V01.09
　　　　　　　traffic V01.19
　　　　　　pick-up truck or van V03.99
　　　　　　　nontraffic V03.09
　　　　　　　traffic V03.19
　　　　　　railway (train) (vehicle) V05.99
　　　　　　　nontraffic V05.09
　　　　　　　traffic V05.19
　　　　　　stationary object V00.282
　　　　　　streetcar V06.99
　　　　　　　nontraffic V06.09
　　　　　　　traffic V06.19
　　　　　　two or three-wheeled motor
　　　　　　　vehicle V02.99
　　　　　　　nontraffic V02.09
　　　　　　　traffic V02.19
　　　　　　vehicle V09.9
　　　　　　　animal-drawn V06.99
　　　　　　　　nontraffic V06.09
　　　　　　　　traffic V06.19
　　　　　　　motor
　　　　　　　　nontraffic V09.00
　　　　　　　　traffic V09.20
　　　　　fall V00.281
　　　　　heelies — *see* Accident, transport,
　　　　　　pedestrian, conveyance, heelies
　　　　　ice skate — *see* Accident, transport,
　　　　　　pedestrian, conveyance, ice
　　　　　　skate
　　　　　nontraffic V09.1
　　　　　　involving motor vehicle NEC
　　　　　　　V09.00
　　　　　sled — *see* Accident, transport,
　　　　　　pedestrian, conveyance, sled
　　　　　traffic V09.3
　　　　　　involving motor vehicle NEC
　　　　　　　V09.20
　　　　　wheelies — *see* Accident,
　　　　　　transport, pedestrian,
　　　　　　conveyance, heelies
　　　　heelies V00.158
　　　　　colliding with stationary object
　　　　　　V00.152
　　　　　fall V00.151
　　　　ice skates V00.218
　　　　　collision (with) V09.9
　　　　　　animal being ridden or animal
　　　　　　　drawn vehicle V06.99
　　　　　　　nontraffic V06.09
　　　　　　　traffic V06.19
　　　　　　bus or heavy transport V04.99
　　　　　　　nontraffic V04.09
　　　　　　　traffic V04.19
　　　　　　car V03.99
　　　　　　　nontraffic V03.09

Accident— *continued*
  transport— *continued*
    pedestrian— *continued*
      conveyance— *continued*
        ice skates — *continued*
          collision— *continued*
            car— *continued*
              traffic V03.19
            pedal cycle V01.99
              nontraffic V01.09
              traffic V01.19
            pick-up truck or van V03.99
              nontraffic V03.09
              traffic V03.19
            railway (train) (vehicle) V05.99
              nontraffic V05.09
              traffic V05.19
            streetcar V06.99
              nontraffic V06.09
              traffic V06.19
            stationary object V00.212
            two or three-wheeled motor
              vehicle V02.99
              nontraffic V02.09
              traffic V02.19
            vehicle V09.9
              animal-drawn V06.99
                nontraffic V06.09
                traffic V06.19
              motor
                nontraffic V09.00
                traffic V09.20
          fall V00.211
          nontraffic V09.1
            involving motor vehicle NEC
              V09.00
          traffic V09.3
            involving motor vehicle NEC
              V09.20
        motorized mobility scooter V00.838
          collision with stationary object
            V00.832
          fall from V00.831
        nontraffic V09.1
          involving motor vehicle V09.00
            military V09.01
            specified type NEC V09.09
        rolling shoes V00.158
        roller skates (non in-line) V00.128
          collision (with) V09.9
            animal being ridden or animal
              drawn vehicle V06.91
              nontraffic V06.01
              traffic V06.11
            bus or heavy transport V04.91
              nontraffic V04.01
              traffic V04.11
            car V03.91
              nontraffic V03.01
              traffic V03.11
            pedal cycle V01.91
              nontraffic V01.01
              traffic V01.11
            pick-up truck or van V03.91
              nontraffic V03.01
              traffic V03.11
            railway (train) (vehicle) V05.91
              nontraffic V05.01
              traffic V05.11
            streetcar V06.91
              nontraffic V06.01
              traffic V06.11
            stationary object V00.122
            two or three-wheeled motor
              vehicle V02.91
              nontraffic V02.01
              traffic V02.11
            vehicle V09.9
              animal-drawn V06.91
                nontraffic V06.01
                traffic V06.11
              motor
                nontraffic V09.00

Accident— *continued*
  transport— *continued*
    pedestrian— *continued*
      conveyance— *continued*
        roller skates— *continued*
          collision— *continued*
            vehicle— *continued*
              motor— *continued*
                traffic V09.20
            fall V00.121
            in-line V00.118
              collision)(*see also* Accident,
                transport, pedestrian,
                conveyance occupant, roller
                skates, collision)
                with stationary object V00.112
              fall V00.111
            nontraffic V09.1
              involving motor vehicle NEC
                V09.00
            traffic V09.3
              involving motor vehicle NEC
                V09.20
        rolling type NEC V00.188
          collision (with) V09.9
            animal being ridden or animal
              drawn vehicle V06.99
              nontraffic V06.09
              traffic V06.19
            bus or heavy transport V04.99
              nontraffic V04.09
              traffic V04.19
            car V03.99
              nontraffic V03.09
              traffic V03.19
            pedal cycle V01.99
              nontraffic V01.09
              traffic V01.19
            pick-up truck or van V03.99
              nontraffic V03.09
              traffic V03.19
            railway (train) (vehicle) V05.99
              nontraffic V05.09
              traffic V05.19
            stationary object V00.182
            streetcar V06.99
              nontraffic V06.09
              traffic V06.19
            two or three-wheeled motor
              vehicle V02.99
              nontraffic V02.09
              traffic V02.19
            vehicle V09.9
              animal-drawn V06.99
                nontraffic V06.09
                traffic V06.19
              motor
                nontraffic V09.00
                traffic V09.20
          fall V00.181
        in-line roller skate — *see* Accident,
          transport, pedestrian,
          conveyance, roller skate, in-line
        nontraffic V09.1
          involving motor vehicle NEC
            V09.00
        roller skate — *see* Accident, transport,
          pedestrian, conveyance, roller
          skate
        scooter (non-motorized) — *see*
          Accident, transport, pedestrian,
          conveyance, scooter
        skateboard — *see* Accident, transport,
          pedestrian, conveyance,
          skateboard
        traffic V09.3
          involving motor vehicle NEC
            V09.20
        scooter (non-motorized) V00.148
          collision (with) V09.9
            animal being ridden or animal
              drawn vehicle V06.99
              nontraffic V06.09

Accident— *continued*
  transport— *continued*
    pedestrian— *continued*
      conveyance— *continued*
        scooter— *continued*
          collision— *continued*
            animal being ridden or animal
              drawn vehicle— *continued*
              traffic V06.19
            bus or heavy transport V04.99
              nontraffic V04.09
              traffic V04.19
            car V03.99
              nontraffic V03.09
              traffic V03.19
            pedal cycle V01.99
              nontraffic V01.09
              traffic V01.19
            pick-up truck or van V03.99
              nontraffic V03.09
              traffic V03.19
            railway (train) (vehicle) V05.99
              nontraffic V05.09
              traffic V05.19
            streetcar V06.99
              nontraffic V06.09
              traffic V06.19
            stationary object V00.142
            two or three-wheeled motor
              vehicle V02.99
              nontraffic V02.09
              traffic V02.19
            vehicle V09.9
              animal-drawn V06.99
                nontraffic V06.09
                traffic V06.19
              motor
                nontraffic V09.00
                traffic V09.20
          fall V00.141
          nontraffic V09.1
            involving motor vehicle NEC
              V09.00
          traffic V09.3
            involving motor vehicle NEC
              V09.20
        skate board V00.138
          collision (with) V09.9
            animal being ridden or animal
              drawn vehicle V06.92
              nontraffic V06.02
              traffic V06.12
            bus or heavy transport V04.92
              nontraffic V04.02
              traffic V04.12
            car V03.92
              nontraffic V03.02
              traffic V03.12
            pedal cycle V01.92
              nontraffic V01.02
              traffic V01.12
            pick-up truck or van V03.92
              nontraffic V03.02
              traffic V03.12
            railway (train) (vehicle) V05.92
              nontraffic V05.02
              traffic V05.12
            streetcar V06.92
              nontraffic V06.02
              traffic V06.12
            stationary object V00.132
            two or three-wheeled motor
              vehicle V02.92
              nontraffic V02.02
              traffic V02.12
            vehicle V09.9
              animal-drawn V06.92
                nontraffic V06.02
                traffic V06.12
              motor
                nontraffic V09.00
                traffic V09.20
          fall V00.131

Accident— *continued*
  transport— *continued*
    pedestrian— *continued*
      on foot— *continued*
        collision— *continued*
          animal being ridden or animal drawn vehicle— *continued*
            traffic V06.10
          bus or heavy transport V04.90
            nontraffic V04.00
            traffic V04.10
          car V03.90
            nontraffic V03.00
            traffic V03.10
          pedal cycle V01.90
            nontraffic V01.00
            traffic V01.10
          pick-up truck or van V03.90
            nontraffic V03.00
            traffic V03.10
          railway (train) (vehicle) V05.90
            nontraffic V05.00
            traffic V05.10
          streetcar V06.90
            nontraffic V06.00
            traffic V06.10
          two or three-wheeled motor vehicle V02.90
            nontraffic V02.00
            traffic V02.10
          vehicle V09.9
           animal-drawn V06.90
            nontraffic V06.00
            traffic V06.10
           motor
            nontraffic V09.00
            traffic V09.20
        nontraffic V09.1
         involving motor vehicle V09.00
          military V09.01
          specified type NEC V09.09
        traffic V09.3
         involving motor vehicle V09.20
          military V09.21
          specified type NEC V09.29
      person NEC (unknown way or transportation) V99
        collision (between)
          bus (with)
           heavy transport vehicle (traffic) V87.5
            nontraffic V88.5
          car (with)
           nontraffic V88.5
           bus (traffic) V87.3
            nontraffic V88.3
           heavy transport vehicle (traffic) V87.4
            nontraffic V88.4
           pick-up truck or van (traffic) V87.2
            nontraffic V88.2
           train or railway vehicle (traffic) V87.6
            nontraffic V88.6
           two-or three-wheeled motor vehicle (traffic) V87.0
            nontraffic V88.0
          motor vehicle (traffic) NEC V87.7
           nontraffic V88.7
          two-or three-wheeled vehicle (with) (traffic)
           motor vehicle NEC V87.1
            nontraffic V88.1
          nonmotor vehicle (collision) (noncollision) (traffic) V87.9
           nontraffic V88.9
      pickup truck occupant V59.9
        collision (with)
          animal (traffic) V50.9
           being ridden (traffic) V56.9
            nontraffic V56.3
             while boarding or alighting V56.4
           nontraffic V50.3
           while boarding or alighting V50.4
          animal-drawn vehicle (traffic) V56.9
           nontraffic V56.3
           while boarding or alighting V56.4

Accident— *continued*
  transport— *continued*
    pickup truck occupant— *continued*
      collision— *continued*
        bus (traffic) V54.9
          nontraffic V54.3
          while boarding or alighting V54.4
        car (traffic) V53.9
          nontraffic V53.3
          while boarding or alighting V53.4
        motor vehicle NOS (traffic) V59.60
          nontraffic V59.20
          specified type NEC (traffic) V59.69
           nontraffic V59.29
        pedal cycle (traffic) V51.9
          nontraffic V51.3
          while boarding or alighting V51.4
        pickup truck (traffic) V53.9
          nontraffic V53.3
          while boarding or alighting V53.4
        railway vehicle (traffic) V55.9
          nontraffic V55.3
          while boarding or alighting V55.4
        specified vehicle NEC (traffic) V56.9
          nontraffic V56.3
          while boarding or alighting V56.4
        stationary object (traffic) V57.9
          nontraffic V57.3
          while boarding or alighting V57.4
        streetcar (traffic) V56.9
          nontraffic V56.3
          while boarding or alighting V56.4
        three wheeled motor vehicle (traffic) V52.9
          nontraffic V52.3
          while boarding or alighting V52.4
        truck (traffic) V54.9
          nontraffic V54.3
          while boarding or alighting V54.4
        two wheeled motor vehicle (traffic) V52.9
          nontraffic V52.3
          while boarding or alighting V52.4
        van (traffic) V53.9
          nontraffic V53.3
          while boarding or alighting V53.4
      driver
        collision (with)
          animal (traffic) V50.5
           being ridden (traffic) V56.5
            nontraffic V56.0
           nontraffic V50.0
          animal-drawn vehicle (traffic) V56.5
           nontraffic V56.0
          bus (traffic) V54.5
           nontraffic V54.0
          car (traffic) V53.5
           nontraffic V53.0
          motor vehicle NOS (traffic) V59.40
           nontraffic V59.00
           specified type NEC (traffic) V59.49
            nontraffic V59.09
          pedal cycle (traffic) V51.5
           nontraffic V51.0
          pickup truck (traffic) V53.5
           nontraffic V53.0
          railway vehicle (traffic) V55.5
           nontraffic V55.0
          specified vehicle NEC (traffic) V56.5
           nontraffic V56.0
          stationary object (traffic) V57.5
           nontraffic V57.0
          streetcar (traffic) V56.5
           nontraffic V56.0
          three wheeled motor vehicle (traffic) V52.5
           nontraffic V52.0
          truck (traffic) V54.5
           nontraffic V54.0
          two wheeled motor vehicle (traffic) V52.5
           nontraffic V52.0
          van (traffic) V53.5
           nontraffic V53.0

Accident— *continued*
  transport— *continued*
    pickup truck occupant— *continued*
      driver— *continued*
        noncollision accident (traffic) V58.5
          nontraffic V58.0
        noncollision accident (traffic) V58.9
          nontraffic V58.3
          while boarding or alighting V58.4
      nontraffic V59.3
      hanger-on
        collision (with)
          animal (traffic) V50.7
           being ridden (traffic) V56.7
            nontraffic V56.2
           nontraffic V50.2
          animal-drawn vehicle (traffic) V56.7
           nontraffic V56.2
          bus (traffic) V54.7
           nontraffic V54.2
          car (traffic) V53.7
           nontraffic V53.2
          pedal cycle (traffic) V51.7
           nontraffic V51.2
          pickup truck (traffic) V53.7
           nontraffic V53.2
          railway vehicle (traffic) V55.7
           nontraffic V55.2
          specified vehicle NEC (traffic) V56.7
           nontraffic V56.2
          stationary object (traffic) V57.7
           nontraffic V57.2
          streetcar (traffic) V56.7
           nontraffic V56.2
          three wheeled motor vehicle (traffic) V52.7
           nontraffic V52.2
          truck (traffic) V54.7
           nontraffic V54.2
          two wheeled motor vehicle (traffic) V52.7
           nontraffic V52.2
          van (traffic) V53.7
           nontraffic V53.2
        noncollision accident (traffic) V58.7
          nontraffic V58.2
      passenger
        collision (with)
          animal (traffic) V50.6
           being ridden (traffic) V56.6
            nontraffic V56.1
           nontraffic V50.1
          animal-drawn vehicle (traffic) V56.6
           nontraffic V56.1
          bus (traffic) V54.6
           nontraffic V54.1
          car (traffic) V53.6
           nontraffic V53.1
          motor vehicle NOS (traffic) V59.50
           nontraffic V59.10
           specified type NEC (traffic) V59.59
            nontraffic V59.19
          pedal cycle (traffic) V51.6
           nontraffic V51.1
          pickup truck (traffic) V53.6
           nontraffic V53.1
          railway vehicle (traffic) V55.6
           nontraffic V55.1
          specified vehicle NEC (traffic) V56.6
           nontraffic V56.1
          stationary object (traffic) V57.6
           nontraffic V57.1
          streetcar (traffic) V56.6
           nontraffic V56.1
          three wheeled motor vehicle (traffic) V52.6
           nontraffic V52.1
          truck (traffic) V54.6
           nontraffic V54.1
          two wheeled motor vehicle (traffic) V52.6
           nontraffic V52.1
          van (traffic) V53.6

Accident— *continued*
  transport— *continued*
    three-wheeled motor vehicle
      occupant— *continued*
        passenger— *continued*
          collision— *continued*
            motor vehicle— *continued*
              specified type— *continued*
                nontraffic V39.19
             pedal cycle (traffic) V31.6
              nontraffic V31.1
             pickup truck (traffic) V33.6
              nontraffic V33.1
             railway vehicle (traffic) V35.6
              nontraffic V35.1
             specified vehicle NEC (traffic) V36.6
              nontraffic V36.1
             stationary object (traffic) V37.6
              nontraffic V37.1
             streetcar (traffic) V36.6
              nontraffic V36.1
             three wheeled motor vehicle (traffic)
              V32.6
              nontraffic V32.1
             truck (traffic) V34.6
              nontraffic V34.1
             two wheeled motor vehicle (traffic)
              V32.6
              nontraffic V32.1
             van (traffic) V33.6
              nontraffic V33.1
           noncollision accident (traffic) V38.6
            nontraffic V38.1
         specified type NEC V39.89
        military vehicle V39.81
    tractor (farm) (and trailer) — *see* Accident,
      transport, agricultural vehicle occupant
    tram — *see* Accident, transport, streetcar
    in mine or quarry — *see* Accident, transport,
      industrial vehicle occupant
    trolley — *see* Accident, transport, streetcar
    in mine or quarry — *see* Accident, transport,
      industrial vehicle occupant
    truck (heavy) occupant V69.9
      collision (with)
        animal (traffic) V60.9
          being ridden (traffic) V66.9
            nontraffic V66.3
              while boarding or alighting V66.4
          nontraffic V60.3
            while boarding or alighting V60.4
        animal-drawn vehicle (traffic) V66.9
          nontraffic V66.3
          while boarding or alighting V66.4
        bus (traffic) V64.9
          nontraffic V64.3
          while boarding or alighting V64.4
        car (traffic) V63.9
          nontraffic V63.3
          while boarding or alighting V63.4
        motor vehicle NOS (traffic) V69.60
          nontraffic V69.20
          specified type NEC (traffic) V69.69
            nontraffic V69.29
        pedal cycle (traffic) V61.9
          nontraffic V61.3
          while boarding or alighting V61.4
        pickup truck (traffic) V63.9
          nontraffic V63.3
          while boarding or alighting V63.4
        railway vehicle (traffic) V65.9
          nontraffic V65.3
          while boarding or alighting V65.4
        specified vehicle NEC (traffic) V66.9
          nontraffic V66.3
          while boarding or alighting V66.4
        stationary object (traffic) V67.9
          nontraffic V67.3
          while boarding or alighting V67.4
        streetcar (traffic) V66.9
          nontraffic V66.3
          while boarding or alighting V66.4

Accident— *continued*
  transport— *continued*
    truck (heavy) occupant— *continued*
      collision— *continued*
        three wheeled motor vehicle (traffic)
          V62.9
          nontraffic V62.3
          while boarding or alighting V62.4
        truck (traffic) V64.9
          nontraffic V64.3
          while boarding or alighting V64.4
        two wheeled motor vehicle (traffic) V62.9
          nontraffic V62.3
          while boarding or alighting V62.4
        van (traffic) V63.9
          nontraffic V63.3
          while boarding or alighting V63.4
      driver
        collision (with)
          animal (traffic) V60.5
            being ridden (traffic) V66.5
              nontraffic V66.0
            nontraffic V60.0
          animal-drawn vehicle (traffic) V66.5
            nontraffic V66.0
          bus (traffic) V64.5
            nontraffic V64.0
          car (traffic) V63.5
            nontraffic V63.0
          motor vehicle NOS (traffic) V69.40
            nontraffic V69.00
            specified type NEC (traffic) V69.49
              nontraffic V69.09
          pedal cycle (traffic) V61.5
            nontraffic V61.0
          pickup truck (traffic) V63.5
            nontraffic V63.0
          railway vehicle (traffic) V65.5
            nontraffic V65.0
          specified vehicle NEC (traffic) V66.5
            nontraffic V66.0
          stationary object (traffic) V67.5
            nontraffic V67.0
          streetcar (traffic) V66.5
            nontraffic V66.0
          three wheeled motor vehicle (traffic)
            V62.5
            nontraffic V62.0
          truck (traffic) V64.5
            nontraffic V64.0
          two wheeled motor vehicle (traffic)
            V62.5
            nontraffic V62.0
          van (traffic) V63.5
            nontraffic V63.0
        noncollision accident (traffic) V68.5
          nontraffic V68.0
      dump — *see* Accident, transport, construction
        vehicle occupant
      hanger-on
        collision (with)
          animal (traffic) V60.7
            being ridden (traffic) V66.7
              nontraffic V66.2
            nontraffic V60.2
          animal-drawn vehicle (traffic) V66.7
            nontraffic V66.2
          bus (traffic) V64.7
            nontraffic V64.2
          car (traffic) V63.7
            nontraffic V63.2
          pedal cycle (traffic) V61.7
            nontraffic V61.2
          pickup truck (traffic) V63.7
            nontraffic V63.2
          railway vehicle (traffic) V65.7
            nontraffic V65.2
          specified vehicle NEC (traffic) V66.7
            nontraffic V66.2
          stationary object (traffic) V67.7
            nontraffic V67.2
          streetcar (traffic) V66.7
            nontraffic V66.2

Accident— *continued*
  transport— *continued*
    truck (heavy) occupant— *continued*
      hanger-on— *continued*
        collision— *continued*
          three wheeled motor vehicle (traffic)
            V62.7
            nontraffic V62.2
          truck (traffic) V64.7
            nontraffic V64.2
          two wheeled motor vehicle (traffic)
            V62.7
            nontraffic V62.2
          van (traffic) V63.7
            nontraffic V63.2
        noncollision accident (traffic) V68.7
          nontraffic V68.2
      noncollision accident (traffic) V68.9
        nontraffic V68.3
        while boarding or alighting V68.4
      nontraffic V69.3
      passenger
        collision (with)
          animal (traffic) V60.6
            being ridden (traffic) V66.6
              nontraffic V66.1
            nontraffic V60.1
          animal-drawn vehicle (traffic) V66.6
            nontraffic V66.1
          bus (traffic) V64.6
            nontraffic V64.1
          car (traffic) V63.6
            nontraffic V63.1
          motor vehicle NOS (traffic) V69.50
            nontraffic V69.10
            specified type NEC (traffic) V69.59
              nontraffic V69.19
          pedal cycle (traffic) V61.6
            nontraffic V61.1
          pickup truck (traffic) V63.6
            nontraffic V63.1
          railway vehicle (traffic) V65.6
            nontraffic V65.1
          specified vehicle NEC (traffic) V66.6
            nontraffic V66.1
          stationary object (traffic) V67.6
            nontraffic V67.1
          streetcar (traffic) V66.6
            nontraffic V66.1
          three wheeled motor vehicle (traffic)
            V62.6
            nontraffic V62.1
          truck (traffic) V64.6
            nontraffic V64.1
          two wheeled motor vehicle (traffic)
            V62.6
            nontraffic V62.1
          van (traffic) V63.6
            nontraffic V63.1
        noncollision accident (traffic) V68.6
          nontraffic V68.1
      pickup — *see* Accident, transport, pickup
        truck occupant
      specified type NEC V69.88
      military vehicle V69.81
    van occupant V59.9
      collision (with)
        animal (traffic) V50.9
          being ridden (traffic) V56.9
            nontraffic V56.3
              while boarding or alighting V56.4
            nontraffic V50.3
            while boarding or alighting V50.4
          animal-drawn vehicle (traffic) V56.9
            nontraffic V56.3
            while boarding or alighting V56.4
          bus (traffic) V54.9
            nontraffic V54.3
            while boarding or alighting V54.4
          car (traffic) V53.9
            nontraffic V53.3
            while boarding or alighting V53.4
          motor vehicle NOS (traffic) V59.60

Accident— *continued*
  transport— *continued*
    van occupant— *continued*
      collision— *continued*
        motor vehicle— *continued*
          nontraffic V59.20
          specified type NEC (traffic) V59.69
            nontraffic V59.29
        pedal cycle (traffic) V51.9
          nontraffic V51.3
          while boarding or alighting V51.4
        pickup truck (traffic) V53.9
          nontraffic V53.3
          while boarding or alighting V53.4
        railway vehicle (traffic) V55.9
          nontraffic V55.3
          while boarding or alighting V55.4
        specified vehicle NEC (traffic) V56.9
          nontraffic V56.3
          while boarding or alighting V56.4
        stationary object (traffic) V57.9
          nontraffic V57.3
          while boarding or alighting V57.4
        streetcar (traffic) V56.9
          nontraffic V56.3
          while boarding or alighting V56.4
        three wheeled motor vehicle (traffic) V52.9
          nontraffic V52.3
          while boarding or alighting V52.4
        truck (traffic) V54.9
          nontraffic V54.3
          while boarding or alighting V54.4
        two wheeled motor vehicle (traffic) V52.9
          nontraffic V52.3
          while boarding or alighting V52.4
        van (traffic) V53.9
          nontraffic V53.3
          while boarding or alighting V53.4
    driver
      collision (with)
        animal (traffic) V50.5
          being ridden (traffic) V56.5
            nontraffic V56.0
          nontraffic V50.0
        animal-drawn vehicle (traffic) V56.5
          nontraffic V56.0
        bus (traffic) V54.5
          nontraffic V54.0
        car (traffic) V53.5
          nontraffic V53.0
        motor vehicle NOS (traffic) V59.40
          nontraffic V59.00
          specified type NEC (traffic) V59.49
            nontraffic V59.09
        pedal cycle (traffic) V51.5
          nontraffic V51.0
        pickup truck (traffic) V53.5
          nontraffic V53.0
        railway vehicle (traffic) V55.5
          nontraffic V55.0
        specified vehicle NEC (traffic) V56.5
          nontraffic V56.0
        stationary object (traffic) V57.5
          nontraffic V57.0
        streetcar (traffic) V56.5
          nontraffic V56.0
        three wheeled motor vehicle (traffic) V52.5
          nontraffic V52.0
        truck (traffic) V54.5
          nontraffic V54.0
        two wheeled motor vehicle (traffic) V52.5
          nontraffic V52.0
        van (traffic) V53.5
          nontraffic V53.0
      noncollision accident (traffic) V58.5
        nontraffic V58.0
    noncollision accident (traffic) V58.9
      nontraffic V58.3
      while boarding or alighting V58.4
    nontraffic V59.3

Accident— *continued*
  transport— *continued*
    van occupant— *continued*
      hanger-on
        collision (with)
          animal (traffic) V50.7
            being ridden (traffic) V56.7
              nontraffic V56.2
            nontraffic V50.2
          animal-drawn vehicle (traffic) V56.7
            nontraffic V56.2
          bus (traffic) V54.7
            nontraffic V54.2
          car (traffic) V53.7
            nontraffic V53.2
          pedal cycle (traffic) V51.7
            nontraffic V51.2
          pickup truck (traffic) V53.7
            nontraffic V53.2
          railway vehicle (traffic) V55.7
            nontraffic V55.2
          specified vehicle NEC (traffic) V56.7
            nontraffic V56.2
          stationary object (traffic) V57.7
            nontraffic V57.2
          streetcar (traffic) V56.7
            nontraffic V56.2
          three wheeled motor vehicle (traffic) V52.7
            nontraffic V52.2
          truck (traffic) V54.7
            nontraffic V54.2
          two wheeled motor vehicle (traffic) V52.7
            nontraffic V52.2
          van (traffic) V53.7
            nontraffic V53.2
        noncollision accident (traffic) V58.7
          nontraffic V58.2
      passenger
        collision (with)
          animal (traffic) V50.6
            being ridden (traffic) V56.6
              nontraffic V56.1
            nontraffic V50.1
          animal-drawn vehicle (traffic) V56.6
            nontraffic V56.1
          bus (traffic) V54.6
            nontraffic V54.1
          car (traffic) V53.6
            nontraffic V53.1
          motor vehicle NOS (traffic) V59.50
            nontraffic V59.10
            specified type NEC (traffic) V59.59
              nontraffic V59.19
          pedal cycle (traffic) V51.6
            nontraffic V51.1
          pickup truck (traffic) V53.6
            nontraffic V53.1
          railway vehicle (traffic) V55.6
            nontraffic V55.1
          specified vehicle NEC (traffic) V56.6
            nontraffic V56.1
          stationary object (traffic) V57.6
            nontraffic V57.1
          streetcar (traffic) V56.6
            nontraffic V56.1
          three wheeled motor vehicle (traffic) V52.6
            nontraffic V52.1
          truck (traffic) V54.6
            nontraffic V54.1
          two wheeled motor vehicle (traffic) V52.6
            nontraffic V52.1
          van (traffic) V53.6
            nontraffic V53.1
        noncollision accident (traffic) V58.6
          nontraffic V58.1
    specified type NEC V59.88
    military vehicle V59.81
    watercraft occupant — *see* Accident, watercraft

Accident— *continued*
  vehicle NEC V89.9
    animal-drawn NEC — *see* Accident, transport, animal-drawn vehicle occupant
  special
    agricultural — *see* Accident, transport, agricultural vehicle occupant
    construction — *see* Accident, transport, construction vehicle occupant
    industrial — *see* Accident, transport, industrial vehicle occupant
    three-wheeled NEC (motorized) — *see* Accident, transport, three-wheeled motor vehicle occupant
  watercraft V94.9
    causing
      drowning B — *see* Drowning, due to, accident to, watercraft
      injury NEC V91.89
        crushed between craft and object V91.19
          powered craft V91.13
            ferry boat V91.11
            fishing boat V91.12
            jetskis V91.13
            liner V91.11
            merchant ship V91.10
            passenger ship V91.11
          unpowered craft V91.18
            canoe V91.15
            inflatable V91.16
            kayak V91.15
            sailboat V91.14
            surf-board V91.18
            windsurfer V91.18
        fall on board V91.29
          powered craft V91.23
            ferry boat V91.21
            fishing boat V91.22
            jetskis V91.23
            liner V91.21
            merchant ship V91.20
            passenger ship V91.21
          unpowered craft
            canoe V91.25
            inflatable V91.26
            kayak V91.25
            sailboat V91.24
        fire on board causing burn V91.09
          powered craft V91.03
            ferry boat V91.01
            fishing boat V91.02
            jetskis V91.03
            liner V91.01
            merchant ship V91.00
            passenger ship V91.01
          unpowered craft V91.08
            canoe V91.05
            inflatable V91.06
            kayak V91.05
            sailboat V91.04
            surf-board V91.08
            water skis V91.07
            windsurfer V91.08
        hit by falling object V91.39
          powered craft V91.33
            ferry boat V91.31
            fishing boat V91.32
            jetskis V91.33
            liner V91.31
            merchant ship V91.30
            passenger ship V91.31
          unpowered craft V91.38
            canoe V91.35
            inflatable V91.36
            kayak V91.35
            sailboat V91.34
            surf-board V91.38
            water skis V91.37
            windsurfer V91.38
        specified type NEC V91.89
          powered craft V91.83
            ferry boat V91.81
            fishing boat V91.82

Assault— *continued*
wound Y09
cutting — *see* Assault, cutting or piercing instrument
gunshot — *see* Assault, firearm
knife X99.1
piercing — *see* Assault, cutting or piercing instrument
puncture — *see* Assault, cutting or piercing instrument
stab — *see* Assault, cutting or piercing instrument
Attack by mammals NEC W55.89
Avalanche B — *see* Landslide
Aviator's disease — *see* Air, pressure

B

Barotitis, barodontalgia, barosinusitis, barotrauma (otitic) (sinus) — *see* Air, pressure
Battered (baby) (child) (person) (syndrome) X58
Bayonet wound W26.1
in
legal intervention — *see* Legal, intervention, sharp object, bayonet
war operations — *see* War operations, combat
stated as undetermined whether accidental or intentional Y28.8
suicide (attempt) X78.2
Bean in nose - *see* categories T17 and T18
Bed set on fire NEC — *see* Exposure, fire, uncontrolled, building, bed
Beheading (by guillotine)
homicide X99.9
legal execution Y35.91
Bending, injury in — *see* Overexertion
Bends — *see* Air, pressure, change
Bite, bitten by
alligator W58.01
arthropod (nonvenomous) NEC W57
bull W55.21
cat W55.01
cow W55.21
crocodile W58.11
dog W54.0
goat W55.31
hoof stock NEC W55.31
horse W55.11
human being (accidentally) W50.3
with intent to injure or kill Y04.1
as, or caused by, a crowd or human stampede (with fall) W52
assault Y04.1
homicide (attempt) Y04.1
in
fight Y04.1
insect (nonvenomous) W57
lizard (nonvenomous) W59.01
millipede W57
mammal NEC W55.81
marine W56.81
marine animal (nonvenomous) W56.81
moray eel W56.51
mouse W53.01
person(s) (accidentally) W50.3
with intent to injure or kill Y04.1
as, or caused by, a crowd or human stampede (with fall) W52
assault Y04.1
homicide (attempt) Y04.1
in
fight Y04.1
pig W55.41
raccoon W55.51
rat W53.11
reptile W59.81
lizard W59.01
snake W59.11
turtle W59.21
terrestrial W59.81
rodent W53.81
mouse W53.01

Bite, bitten by— *continued*
rodent— *continued*
rat W53.11
specified NEC W53.81
squirrel W53.21
shark W56.41
sheep W55.31
snake (nonvenomous) W59.11
spider (nonvenomous) W57
squirrel W53.21
Blast (air) **in war operations** - *see* War operations, blast
Blizzard X37.2
Blood alcohol level Y90.9
less than 20mg/100ml Y90.0
presence in blood, level not specified Y90.9
20-39mg/100ml Y90.1
40-59mg/100ml Y90.2
60-79mg/100ml Y90.3
80-99mg/100ml Y90.4
100-119mg/100ml Y90.5
120-199mg/100ml Y90.6
200-239mg/100ml Y90.7
Blow X58
by law-enforcing agent, police (on duty) — *see* Legal, intervention, manhandling
blunt object — *see* Legal, intervention, blunt object
Blowing up — *see* Explosion
Brawl (hand) (fists) (foot) Y04.0
Breakage (accidental) (part of)
ladder (causing fall) W11
scaffolding (causing fall) W12
Broken
glass, contact with — *see* Contact, with, glass
power line (causing electric shock) W85
Bumping against, into (accidentally)
object W22.8
with fall — *see* Fall, due to, bumping against, object
caused by crowd or human stampede (with fall) W52
sports equipment W21.9
person(s) W51
with fall W03
due to ice or snow W00.0
assault Y04.2
caused by, a crowd or human stampede (with fall) W52
homicide (attempt) Y04.2
sports equipment W21.9
Burn, burned, burning (accidental) (by) (from) (on)
acid NEC — *see* Table of Drugs and Chemicals
bed linen — *see* Exposure, fire, uncontrolled, in building, bed
blowtorch X08.8
with ignition of clothing NEC X06.2
nightwear X05
bonfire, campfire (controlled) (*see also* Exposure, fire, controlled, not in building)
uncontrolled — *see* Exposure, fire, uncontrolled, not in building
candle X08.8
with ignition of clothing NEC X06.2
nightwear X05
caustic liquid, substance (external) (internal) NEC — *see* Table of Drugs and Chemicals
chemical (external) (internal) (*see also* Table of Drugs and Chemicals)
in war operations — *see* War operations. fire
cigar(s) or cigarette(s) X08.8
with ignition of clothing NEC X06.2
nightwear X05
clothes, clothing NEC (from controlled fire) X06.2
with conflagration — *see* Exposure, fire, uncontrolled, building
not in building or structure — *see* Exposure, fire, uncontrolled, not in building
cooker (hot) X15.8
stated as undetermined whether accidental or intentional Y27.3
suicide (attempt) X77.3

Burn, burned, burning— *continued*
electric blanket X16
engine (hot) X17
fire, flames — *see* Exposure, fire
flare, Very pistol — *see* Discharge, firearm NEC
heat
from appliance (electrical) (household) X15.8
cooker X15.8
hotplate X15.2
kettle X15.8
light bulb X15.8
saucepan X15.3
skillet X15.3
stove X15.0
stated as undetermined whether accidental or intentional Y27.3
suicide (attempt) X77.3
toaster X15.1
in local application or packing during medical or surgical procedure Y63.5
heating
appliance, radiator or pipe X16
homicide (attempt) — *see* Assault, burning
hot
air X14.1
cooker X15.8
drink X10.0
engine X17
fat X10.2
fluid NEC X12
food X10.1
gases X14.1
heating appliance X16
household appliance NEC X15.8
kettle X15.8
liquid NEC X12
machinery X17
metal (molten) (liquid) NEC X18
object (not producing fire or flames) NEC X19
oil (cooking) X10.2
pipe(s) X16
radiator X16
saucepan (glass) (metal) X15.3
stove (kitchen) X15.0
substance NEC X19
caustic or corrosive NEC — *see* Table of Drugs and Chemicals
toaster X15.1
tool X17
vapor X13.1
water (tap) — *see* Contact, with, hot, tap water
hotplate X15.2
suicide (attempt) X77.3
ignition — *see* Ignition
in war operations — *see* War operations, fire
inflicted by other person X97
by hot objects, hot vapor, and steam — *see* Assault, burning, hot object
internal, from swallowed caustic, corrosive liquid, substance — *see* Table of Drugs and Chemicals
iron (hot) X15.8
stated as undetermined whether accidental or intentional Y27.3
suicide (attempt) X77.3
kettle (hot) X15.8
stated as undetermined whether accidental or intentional Y27.3
suicide (attempt) X77.3
lamp (flame) X08.8
with ignition of clothing NEC X06.2
nightwear X05
lighter (cigar) (cigarette) X08.8
with ignition of clothing NEC X06.2
nightwear X05
lightning — *see* subcategory T75.0
causing fire — *see* Exposure, fire
liquid (boiling) (hot) NEC X12
stated as undetermined whether accidental or intentional Y27.2
suicide (attempt) X77.2
local application of externally applied substance in medical or surgical care Y63.5

Burn, burned, burning— *continued*
on board watercraft
due to
accident to watercraft V91.09
powered craft V91.03
ferry boat V91.01
fishing boat V91.02
jetskis V91.03
liner V91.01
merchant ship V91.00
passenger ship V91.01
unpowered craft V91.08
canoe V91.05
inflatable V91.06
kayak V91.05
sailboat V91.04
surf-board V91.08
water skis V91.07
windsurfer V91.08
fire on board V93.09
ferry boat V93.01
fishing boat V93.02
jetskis V93.03
liner V93.01
merchant ship V93.00
passenger ship V93.01
powered craft NEC V93.03
sailboat V93.04
specified heat source NEC on board V93.19
ferry boat V93.11
fishing boat V93.12
jetskis V93.13
liner V93.11
merchant ship V93.10
passenger ship V93.11
powered craft NEC V93.13
sailboat V93.14
machinery (hot) X17
matches X08.8
with ignition of clothing NEC X06.2
nightwear X05
mattress — *see* Exposure, fire, uncontrolled,
building, bed
medicament, externally applied Y63.5
metal (hot) (liquid) (molten) NEC X18
nightwear (nightclothes, nightdress, gown,
pajamas, robe) X05
object (hot) NEC X19
pipe (hot) X16
smoking X08.8
with ignition of clothing NEC X06.2
nightwear X05
powder — *see* Powder burn
radiator (hot) X16
saucepan (hot) (glass) (metal) X15.3
stated as undetermined whether accidental or
intentional Y27.3
suicide (attempt) X77.3
self-inflicted X76
stated as undetermined whether accidental or
intentional Y26
steam X13.1
pipe X16
stated as undetermined whether accidental or
intentional Y27.8
stated as undetermined whether accidental or
intentional Y27.0
suicide (attempt) X77.0
stove (hot) (kitchen) X15.0
stated as undetermined whether accidental or
intentional Y27.3
suicide (attempt) X77.3
substance (hot) NEC X19
boiling X12
stated as undetermined whether accidental or
intentional Y27.2
suicide (attempt) X77.2
molten (metal) X18
suicide (attempt) NEC X76
hot
household appliance X77.3
object X77.9

Burn, burned, burning— *continued*
therapeutic misadventure
heat in local application or packing during
medical or surgical procedure Y63.5
overdose of radiation Y63.2
toaster (hot) X15.1
stated as undetermined whether accidental or
intentional Y27.3
suicide (attempt) X77.3
tool (hot) X17
torch, welding X08.8
with ignition of clothing NEC X06.2
nightwear X05
trash fire (controlled) — *see* Exposure, fire,
controlled, not in building
uncontrolled — *see* Exposure, fire, uncontrolled,
not in building
vapor (hot) X13.1
stated as undetermined whether accidental or
intentional Y27.0
suicide (attempt) X77.0
Very pistol — *see* Discharge, firearm NEC
Butted by animal W55.82
bull W55.22
cow W55.22
goat W55.32
horse W55.12
pig W55.42
sheep W55.32

C

Caisson disease — *see* Air, pressure, change
Campfire (exposure to) (controlled) (*see also* Exposure,
fire, controlled, not in building)
uncontrolled — *see* Exposure, fire, uncontrolled, not
in building
Capital punishment (any means) Y35.91
Car sickness T75.3
Casualty (not due to war) NEC X58
war — *see* War operations
Cat
bite W55.01
scratch W55.03
Cataclysm, cataclysmic (any injury) NEC — *see* Forces
of nature
Catching fire — *see* Exposure, fire
Caught
between
folding object W23.0
objects (moving) (stationary and moving) W23.0
and machinery — *see* Contact, with, by type
of machine
stationary W23.1
sliding door and door frame W23.0
by, in
machinery (moving parts of) — *see* Contact,
with, by type of machine
washing-machine wringer W23.0
under packing crate (due to losing grip) W23.1
Cave-in caused by cataclysmic earth surface
movement or eruption — *see* Landslide
Change(s) in air pressure — *see* Air, pressure, change
Choked, choking (on) (any object except food or
vomitus)
food (bone) (seed) — *see* categories T17 and T18
vomitus — *see* subcategories T17.81, T18.81.
Civil insurrection — *see* War operations
Cloudburst (any injury) X37.8
Cold, exposure to (accidental) (excessive) (extreme)
(natural) (place) **NEC** — *see* Exposure, cold
Collapse
building W20.1
burning (uncontrolled fire) X00.2
dam or man-made structure (causing earth
movement) X36.0
machinery — *see* Contact, with, by type of machine
structure W20.1
burning (uncontrolled fire) X00.2

Collision (accidental) NEC (*see also* Accident, transport)
V89.9
pedestrian W51
with fall W03
due to ice or snow W00.0
involving pedestrian conveyance — *see*
Accident, transport, pedestrian,
conveyance
and
crowd or human stampede (with fall) W52
object W22.8
with fall — *see* Fall, due to, bumping
against, object
person(s) — *see* Collision, pedestrian
Collision— *continued*
transport vehicle NEC V89.9
and
avalanche, fallen or not moving — *see*
Accident, transport
falling or moving B — *see* Landslide
landslide, fallen or not moving — *see*
Accident, transport
falling or moving B — *see* Landslide
due to cataclysm — *see* Forces of nature, by type
intentional, purposeful suicide (attempt) — *see*
Suicide, collision
Combustion, spontaneous — *see* Ignition
Complication (delayed) **of or following** (medical or
surgical procedure) Y84.9
with misadventure — *see* Misadventure
amputation of limb(s) Y83.5
anastomosis (arteriovenous) (blood vessel)
(gastrojejunal) (tendon) (natural or artificial
material) Y83.2
aspiration (of fluid) Y84.4
tissue Y84.8
biopsy Y84.8
blood
sampling Y84.7
transfusion
procedure Y84.8
bypass Y83.2
catheterization (urinary) Y84.6
cardiac Y84.0
colostomy Y83.3
cystostomy Y83.3
dialysis (kidney) Y84.1
drug — *see* Table of Drugs and Chemicals
due to misadventure — *see* Misadventure
duodenostomy Y83.3
electroshock therapy Y84.3
external stoma, creation of Y83.3
formation of external stoma Y83.3
gastrostomy Y83.3
graft Y83.2
hypothermia (medically-induced) Y84.8
implant, implantation (of)
artificial
internal device (cardiac pacemaker)
(electrodes in brain) (heart valve
prosthesis) (orthopedic) Y83.1
material or tissue (for anastomosis or bypass)
Y83.2
with creation of external stoma Y83.3
natural tissues (for anastomosis or bypass) Y83.2
with creation of external stoma Y83.3
infusion
procedure Y84.8
injection — *see* Table of Drugs and Chemicals
procedure Y84.8
insertion of gastric or duodenal sound Y84.5
insulin-shock therapy Y84.3
paracentesis (abdominal) (thoracic) (aspirative)
Y84.4
procedures other than surgical operation — *see*
Complication of or following, by type of
procedure
radiological procedure or therapy Y84.2
removal of organ (partial) (total) NEC Y83.6
sampling
blood Y84.7
fluid NEC Y84.4
tissue Y84.8

Complication (delayed) **of or following**— *continued*
  shock therapy Y84.3
  surgical operation NEC (*see also* Complication of or
      following, by type of operation) Y83.9
    reconstructive NEC Y83.4
      with
        anastomosis, bypass or graft Y83.2
        formation of external stoma Y83.3
    specified NEC Y83.8
  transfusion (*see also* Table of Drugs and Chemicals)
    procedure Y84.8
  transplant, transplantation (heart) (kidney) (liver)
      (whole organ, any) Y83.0
    partial organ Y83.4
  ureterostomy Y83.3
  vaccination (*see also* Table of Drugs and Chemicals)
    procedure Y84.8
Compression
  divers' squeeze — *see* Air, pressure, change
  trachea by
    food (lodged in esophagus) — *see* categories T17
        and T18
    vomitus (lodged in esophagus) — *see*
        subcategories T17.81, T18.81.
Conflagration — *see* Exposure, fire, uncontrolled
Constriction (external)
  hair W49.01
  jewelry W49.04
  ring W49.04
  rubber band W49.03
  specified item NEC W49.09
  string W49.02
  thread W49.02
Contact (accidental)
  with
    abrasive wheel (metalworking) W31.1
    alligator W58.09
      bite W58.01
      crushing W58.03
      strike W58.02
    amphibian W62.9
      frog W62.0
      toad W62.1
    animal (nonvenomous) NEC W64
      marine W56.89
        bite W56.81
        dolphin — *see* Contact, with, dolphin
        fish NEC — *see* Contact, with, fish
        mammal — *see* Contact, with, mammal,
            marine
        orca — *see* Contact, with, orca
        sea lion — *see* Contact, with, sea lion
        shark — *see* Contact, with, shark
        strike W56.82
    animate mechanical force NEC W64
    arrow W21.89
      not thrown, projected or falling W45.8
    arthropods (nonvenomous) W57
    axe W27.0
    band-saw (industrial) W31.2
    bayonet — *see* Bayonet wound
    bee(s) X58
    bench-saw (industrial) W31.2
    bird W61.99
      bite W61.91
      chicken — *see* Contact, with, chicken
      duck — *see* Contact, with, duck
      goose — *see* Contact, with, goose
      macaw — *see* Contact, with, macaw
      parrot — *see* Contact, with, parrot
      psittacine — *see* Contact, with, psittacine
      strike W61.92
      turkey — *see* Contact, with, turkey
    blender W29.0
    boiling water X12
      stated as undetermined whether accidental or
          intentional Y27.2
      suicide (attempt) X77.2
    bore, earth-drilling or mining (land) (seabed)
        W31.0
    buffalo — *see* Contact, with, hoof stock NEC
    bull W55.29

Contact— *continued*
  with— *continued*
    bull— *continued*
      bite W55.21
      gored W55.22
      strike W55.22
    bumper cars W31.81
    camel — *see* Contact, with, hoof stock NEC
    can
      lid W45.2
      opener W27.4
        powered W29.0
    cat W55.09
      bite W55.01
      scratch W55.03
    caterpillar (venomous) X58
    centipede (venomous) X58
    chain
      hoist W24.0
        agricultural operations W30.89
      saw W29.3
    chicken W61.39
      peck W61.33
      strike W61.32
    chisel W27.0
    circular saw W31.2
    cobra X58
    combine (harvester) W30.0
    conveyer belt W24.1
    cooker (hot) X15.8
      stated as undetermined whether accidental or
          intentional Y27.3
      suicide (attempt) X77.3
    coral X58
    cotton gin W31.82
    cow W55.29
      bite W55.21
      strike W55.22
    crane W24.0
      agricultural operations W30.89
    crocodile W58.19
      bite W58.11
      crushing W58.13
      strike W58.12
    dagger W26.1
      stated as undetermined whether accidental or
          intentional Y28.2
      suicide (attempt) X78.2
    dairy equipment W31.82
    dart W21.89
      not thrown, projected or falling W45.8
    deer — *see* Contact, with, hoof stock NEC
    derrick W24.0
      agricultural operations W30.89
        hay W30.2
    dog W54.8
      bite W54.0
      strike W54.1
    dolphin W56.09
      bite W56.01
      strike W56.02
    donkey — *see* Contact, with, hoof stock NEC
    drill (powered) W29.8
      earth (land) (seabed) W31.0
      nonpowered W27.8
    drive belt W24.0
      agricultural operations W30.89
    dry ice — *see* Exposure, cold, man-made
    dryer (spin) (clothes) (powered) W29.2
    duck W61.69
      bite W61.61
      strike W61.62
    earth(-)
      drilling machine (industrial) W31.0
      scraping machine in stationary use W31.83
    edge of stiff paper W45.1
    electric
      beater W29.0
      blanket X16
      fan W29.2
        commercial W31.82
      knife W29.1
      mixer W29.0

Contact— *continued*
  with— *continued*
    elevator (building) W24.0
      agricultural operations W30.89
        grain W30.3
    engine(s), hot NEC X17
    excavating machine W31.0
    farm machine W30.9
    feces — *see* Contact, with, by type of animal
    fer de lance X58
    fish W56.59
      bite W56.51
      shark — *see* Contact, with, shark
      strike W56.52
    flying horses W31.81
    forging (metalworking) machine W31.1
    fork W27.4
    forklift (truck) W24.0
      agricultural operations W30.89
    frog W62.0
    garden
      cultivator (powered) W29.3
        riding W30.89
      fork W27.1
    gas turbine W31.3
    Gila monster X58
    giraffe — *see* Contact, with, hoof stock NEC
    glass (sharp) (broken) W25
      with subsequent fall W18.02
      assault X99.0
      due to fall — *see* Fall, by type
      stated as undetermined whether accidental or
          intentional Y28.0
      suicide (attempt) X78.0
    goat W55.39
      bite W55.31
      strike W55.32
    goose W61.59
      bite W61.51
      strike W61.52
    hand
      saw W27.0
      tool (not powered) NEC W27.8
        powered W29.8
    harvester W30.0
    hay-derrick W30.2
    heat NEC X19
      from appliance (electrical) (household) — *see*
          Contact, with, hot, household appliance
      heating appliance X16
    heating
      appliance (hot) X16
      pad (electric) X16
    hedge-trimmer (powered) W29.3
    hoe W27.1
    hoist (chain) (shaft) NEC W24.0
      agricultural W30.89
    hoof stock NEC W55.39
      bite W55.31
      strike W55.32
    hornet(s) X58
    horse W55.19
      bite W55.11
      strike W55.12
    hot
      air X14.1
        inhalation X14.0
      cooker X15.8
      drinks X10.0
      engine X17
      fats X10.2
      fluids NEC X12
        assault X98.2
        suicide (attempt) X77.2
        undetermined whether accidental or
            intentional Y27.2
      food X10.1
      gases X14.1
        inhalation X14.0
      heating appliance X16
      household appliance X15.8
        assault X98.3
        cooker X15.8

Contact— *continued*
  with— *continued*
    hot— *continued*
      household appliance— *continued*
        hotplate X15.2
        kettle X15.8
        light bulb X15.8
        object NEC X19
          assault X98.8
          stated as undetermined whether
            accidental or intentional Y27.9
          suicide (attempt) X77.8
        saucepan X15.3
        skillet X15.3
        stove X15.0
        stated as undetermined whether
          accidental or intentional Y27.3
        suicide (attempt) X77.3
        toaster X15.1
      kettle X15.8
      light bulb X15.8
      liquid NEC (*see also* Burning) X12
        drinks X10.0
        stated as undetermined whether
          accidental or intentional Y27.2
        suicide (attempt) X77.2
        tap water X11.8
          stated as undetermined whether
            accidental or intentional Y27.1
          suicide (attempt) X77.1
      machinery X17
      metal (molten) (liquid) NEC X18
      object (not producing fire or flames) NEC X19
      oil (cooking) X10.2
      pipe X16
      plate X15.2
      radiator X16
      saucepan (glass) (metal) X15.3
      skillet X15.3
      stove (kitchen) X15.0
      substance NEC X19
      tap-water X11.8
        assault X98.1
        heated on stove X12
          stated as undetermined whether
            accidental or intentional Y27.2
          suicide (attempt) X77.2
        in bathtub X11.0
        running X11.1
        stated as undetermined whether
          accidental or intentional Y27.1
        suicide (attempt) X77.1
      toaster X15.1
      tool X17
      vapors X13.1
        inhalation X13.0
      water (tap) X11.8
        boiling X12
          stated as undetermined whether
            accidental or intentional Y27.2
          suicide (attempt) X77.2
        heated on stove X12
          stated as undetermined whether
            accidental or intentional Y27.2
          suicide (attempt) X77.2
        in bathtub X11.0
        running X11.1
        stated as undetermined whether
          accidental or intentional Y27.1
        suicide (attempt) X77.1
    hotplate X15.2
    ice-pick W27.4
    insect (nonvenomous) NEC W57
    kettle (hot) X15.8
    knife W26.0
      assault X99.1
      electric W29.1
      stated as undetermined whether accidental or
        intentional Y28.1
      suicide (attempt) X78.1
    lathe (metalworking) W31.1
      turnings W45.8
      woodworking W31.2

Contact— *continued*
  with— *continued*
    lawnmower (powered) (ridden) W28
      causing electrocution W86.8
        suicide (attempt) X83.1
      unpowered W27.1
    lift, lifting (devices) W24.0
      agricultural operations W30.89
      shaft W24.0
    liquefied gas — *see* Exposure, cold, man-made
    liquid air, hydrogen, nitrogen — *see* Exposure,
      cold, man-made
    lizard (nonvenomous) W59.09
      bite W59.01
      strike W59.02
    llama — *see* Contact, with, hoof stock NEC
    macaw W61.19
      bite W61.11
      strike W61.12
    machine, machinery W31.9
      abrasive wheel W31.1
      agricultural including animal-powered W30.9
        combine harvester W30.0
        grain storage elevator W30.3
        hay derrick W30.2
        power take-off device W30.1
        reaper W30.0
        specified NEC W30.89
        thresher W30.0
        transport vehicle, stationary W30.81
      band saw W31.2
      bench saw W31.2
      circular saw W31.2
      commercial NEC W31.82
      drilling, metal (industrial) W31.1
      earth-drilling W31.0
      earthmoving or scraping W31.89
      excavating W31.89
      forging machine W31.1
      gas turbine W31.3
      hot X17
      internal combustion engine W31.3
      land drill W31.0
      lathe W31.1
      lifting (devices) W24.0
      metal drill W31.1
      metalworking (industrial) W31.1
      milling, metal W31.1
      mining W31.0
      molding W31.2
      overhead plane W31.2
      power press, metal W31.1
      prime mover W31.3
      printing W31.89
      radial saw W31.2
      recreational W31.81
      roller-coaster W31.81
      rolling mill, metal W31.1
      sander W31.2
      seabed drill W31.0
      shaft
        hoist W31.0
        lift W31.0
      specified NEC W31.89
      spinning W31.89
      steam engine W31.3
      transmission W24.1
      undercutter W31.0
      water driven turbine W31.3
      weaving W31.89
      woodworking or forming (industrial) W31.2
    mammal (feces) (urine) W55.89
      bull — *see* Contact, with, bull
      cat — *see* Contact, with, cat
      cow — *see* Contact, with, cow
      goat — *see* Contact, with, goat
      hoof stock — *see* Contact, with, hoof stock
      horse — *see* Contact, with, horse
      marine W56.39
        dolphin — *see* Contact, with, dolphin
        orca — *see* Contact, with, orca
        sea lion — *see* Contact, with, sea lion
        specified NEC W56.39

Contact— *continued*
  with— *continued*
    mammal— *continued*
      marine— *continued*
        specified— *continued*
          bite W56.31
          strike W56.32
      pig — *see* Contact, with, pig
      raccoon — *see* Contact, with, raccoon
      rodent — *see* Contact, with, rodent
      sheep — *see* Contact, with, sheep
      specified NEC W55.89
        bite W55.81
        strike W55.82
    marine
      animal W56.89
        bite W56.81
        dolphin — *see* Contact, with, dolphin
        fish NEC — *see* Contact, with, fish
        mammal — *see* Contact, with, mammal,
          marine
        orca — *see* Contact, with, orca
        sea lion — *see* Contact, with, sea lion
        shark — *see* Contact, with, shark
        strike W56.82
    meat
      grinder (domestic) W29.0
        industrial W31.82
        nonpowered W27.4
      slicer (domestic) W29.0
        industrial W31.82
    merry go round W31.81
    metal, hot (liquid) (molten) NEC X18
    millipede W57
    nail W45.0
      gun W29.4
    needle (sewing) W27.3
      hypodermic W46.0
        contaminated W46.1
    object (blunt) NEC
      hot NEC X19
      legal intervention — *see* Legal, intervention,
        blunt object
      sharp NEC W45.8
        inflicted by other person NEC W45.8
          stated as
            intentional homicide (attempt) —
              see Assault, cutting or piercing
              instrument
            legal intervention — *see* Legal,
              intervention, sharp object
            self-inflicted X78.9
    orca W56.29
      bite W56.21
      strike W56.22
    overhead plane W31.2
    paper (as sharp object) W45.1
    paper-cutter W27.5
    parrot W61.09
      bite W61.01
      strike W61.02
    pig W55.49
      bite W55.41
      strike W55.42
    pipe, hot X16
    pitchfork W27.1
    plane (metal) (wood) W27.0
      overhead W31.2
    plant thorns, spines, sharp leaves or other
      mechanisms W60
    powered
      garden cultivator W29.3
      household appliance, implement, or machine
        W29.8
      saw (industrial) W31.2
        hand W29.8
    printing machine W31.89
    psittacine bird W61.29
      bite W61.21
      macaw — *see* Contace, with, macaw
      parrot — *see* Contact, with, parrot
      strike W61.22

Contact— *continued*
  with— *continued*
    pulley (block) (transmission) W24.0
      agricultural operations W30.89
    raccoon W55.59
      bite W55.51
      strike W55.52
    radial-saw (industrial) W31.2
    radiator (hot) X16
    rake W27.1
    rattlesnake X58
    reaper W30.0
    reptile W59.89
      lizard — *see* Contact, with, lizard
      snake — *see* Contact, with, snake
      specified NEC W59.89
        bite W59.81
        crushing W59.83
        strike W59.82
      turtle — *see* Contact, with, turtle
    rivet gun (powered) W29.4
    road scraper — *see* Accident, transport, construction vehicle
    rodent (feces) (urine) W53.89
      bite W53.81
      mouse W53.09
        bite W53.01
      rat W53.19
        bite W53.11
      specified NEC W53.89
        bite W53.81
      squirrel W53.29
        bite W53.21
    roller coaster W31.81
    rope NEC W24.0
      agricultural operations W30.89
    saliva — *see* Contact, with, by type of animal
    sander W29.8
      industrial W31.2
    saucepan (hot) (glass) (metal) X15.3
    saw W27.0
      band (industrial) W31.2
      bench (industrial) W31.2
      chain W29.3
      hand W27.0
    sawing machine, metal W31.1
    scissors W27.2
    scorpion X58
    screwdriver W27.0
      powered W29.8
    sea
      anemone, cucumber or urchin (spine) X58
      lion W56.19
        bite W56.11
        strike W56.12
    serpent — *see* Contact, with, snake, by type
    sewing-machine (electric) (powered) W29.2
      not powered W27.8
    shaft (hoist) (lift) (transmission) NEC W24.0
      agricultural W30.89
    shark W56.49
      bite W56.41
      strike W56.42
    shears (hand) W27.2
      powered (industrial) W31.1
        domestic W29.2
    sheep W55.39
      bite W55.31
      strike W55.32
    shovel W27.8
      steam — *see* Accident, transport, construction vehicle
    snake (nonvenomous) W59.19
      bite W59.11
      crushing W59.13
      strike W59.12
    spade W27.1
    spider (venomous) X58
    spin-drier W29.2
    spinning machine W31.89
    splinter W45.8
    sports equipment W21.9
    staple gun (powered) W29.8

Contact— *continued*
  with— *continued*
    steam X13.1
      engine W31.3
      inhalation X13.0
      pipe X16
      shovel W31.89
    stove (hot) (kitchen) X15.0
    substance, hot NEC X19
      molten (metal) X18
    sword W26.1
      assault X99.2
      stated as undetermined whether accidental or intentional Y28.2
      suicide (attempt) X78.2
    tarantula X58
    thresher W30.0
    tin can lid W45.2
    toad W62.1
    toaster (hot) X15.1
    tool W27.8
      hand (not powered) W27.8
        auger W27.0
        axe W27.0
        can opener W27.4
        chisel W27.0
        fork W27.4
        garden W27.1
        handsaw W27.0
        hoe W27.1
        ice-pick W27.4
        kitchen utensil W27.4
        manual
          lawn mower W27.1
          sewing machine W27.1
        meat grinder W27.4
        needle (sewing) W27.3
          hypodermic W46.0
            contaminated W46.1
        paper cutter W27.5
        pitchfork W27.1
        rake W27.1
        scissors W27.2
        screwdriver W27.0
        specified NEC W27.8
        workbench W27.0
      hot X17
      powered W29.8
        blender W29.0
          commercial W31.82
        can opener W29.0
          commercial W31.82
        chainsaw W29.3
        clothes dryer W29.2
          commercial W31.82
        dishwasher W29.2
          commercial W31.82
        edger W29.3
        electric fan W29.2
          commercial W31.82
        electric knife W29.1
        food processor W29.0
          commercial W31.82
        garbage disposal W29.0
          commercial W31.82
        garden tool W29.3
        hedge trimmer W29.3
        ice maker W29.0
          commercial W31.82
        kitchen appliance W29.0
          commercial W31.82
        lawn mower W28
        meat grinder W29.0
          commercial W31.82
        mixer W29.0
          commercial W31.82
        rototiller W29.3
        sewing machine W29.2
          commercial W31.82
        washing machine W29.2
          commercial W31.82
    transmission device (belt, cable, chain, gear, pinion, shaft) W24.1

Contact— *continued*
  with— *continued*
    transmission device— *continued*
      agricultural operations W30.89
    turbine (gas) (water-driven) W31.3
    turkey W61.49
      peck W61.43
      strike W61.42
    turtle (nonvenomous) W59.29
      bite W59.21
      strike W59.22
      terrestrial W59.89
        bite W59.81
        crushing W59.83
        strike W59.82
    under-cutter W31.0
    urine — *see* Contact, with, by type of animal
    vehicle
      agricultural use (transport) — *see* Accident, transport, agricultural vehicle
        not on public highway W30.81
      industrial use (transport) — *see* Accident, transport, industrial vehicle
        not on public highway W31.83
      off-road use (transport) — *see* Accident, transport, all-terrain or off-road vehicle
        not on public highway W31.83
      special construction use (transport) — *see* Accident, transport, construction vehicle
        not on public highway W31.83
    venomous
      animal X58
      arthropods X58
      lizard X58
      marine animal NEC X58
      marine plant NEC X58
      millipedes (tropical) X58
      plant(s) X58
      snake X58
      spider X58
      viper X58
    washing-machine (powered) W29.2
    wasp X58
    weaving-machine W31.89
    winch W24.0
      agricultural operations W30.89
    wire NEC W24.0
      agricultural operations W30.89
    wood slivers W45.8
    yellow jacket X58
    zebra — *see* Contact, with, hoof stock NEC
Coup de soleil X32
Crash
  aircraft (in transit) (powered) V95.9
    balloon V96.01
    fixed wing NEC (private) V95.21
      commercial V95.31
    glider V96.21
      hang V96.11
      powered V95.11
    helicopter V95.01
    in war operations — *see* War operations, destruction of aircraft
    microlight V95.11
    nonpowered V96.9
      specified NEC V96.8
    powered NEC V95.8
    stated as
      homicide (attempt) Y08.81
      suicide (attempt) X83.0
    ultralight V95.11
  spacecraft V95.41
  transport vehicle NEC (*see also* Accident, transport) V89.9
    homicide (attempt) Y03.8
    motor NEC (traffic) V89.2
      homicide (attempt) Y03.8
      suicide (attempt) — *see* Suicide, collision
Cruelty (mental) (physical) (sexual) X58
Crushed (accidentally) X58
  between objects (moving) (stationary and moving) W23.0

Crushed— *continued*
  between objects— *continued*
    stationary W23.1
  by
    alligator W58.03
    avalanche NEC B — *see* Landslide
    cave-in W20.0
      caused by cataclysmic earth surface
        movement B — *see* Landslide
    crocodile W58.13
    crowd or human stampede W52
    falling
      aircraft V97.39
        in war operations — *see* War operations,
          destruction of aircraft
      earth, material W20.0
        caused by cataclysmic earth surface
          movement — *see* Landslide
      object NEC W20.8
    landslide NEC B — *see* Landslide
    lizard (nonvenomous) W59.09
    machinery — *see* Contact, with, by type of
      machine
    reptile NEC W59.89
    snake (nonvenomous) W59.13
  in
    machinery — *see* Contact, with, by type of
      machine
Cut, cutting (any part of body) (accidental) (*see also*
  Contact, with, by object or machine)
  during medical or surgical treatment as
    misadventure — *see* Misadventure, cut, by
    type of procedure
  homicide (attempt) — *see* Assault, cutting or
    piercing instrument
  inflicted by other person — *see* Assault, cutting or
    piercing instrument
  legal
    execution Y35.91
    intervention — *see* Legal, intervention, sharp
      object
  machine NEC (*see also* Contact, with, by type of
    machine) W31.9
  self-inflicted — *see* Suicide, cutting or piercing
    instrument
  suicide (attempt) — *see* Suicide, cutting or piercing
    instrument
Cyclone (any injury) X37.1

D

Decapitation (accidental circumstances) NEC X58
  homicide X99.9
  legal execution (by guillotine) Y35.91
Dehydration from lack of water X58
Deprivation X58
Derailment (accidental)
  railway (rolling stock) (train) (vehicle) (without
    antecedent collision) V81.7
    with antecedent collision — *see* Accident,
      transport, railway vehicle occupant
  streetcar (without antecedent collision) V82.7
    with antecedent collision — *see* Accident,
      transport, streetcar occupant
Descent
  parachute (voluntary) (without accident to aircraft)
    V97.29
    due to accident to aircraft — *see* Accident,
      transport, aircraft
Desertion X58
Destitution X58
Disability, late effect or sequela of injury — *see*
  Sequelae
Discharge (accidental)
  airgun W34.010
    assault X95.01
    homicide (attempt) X95.01
    stated as undetermined whether accidental or
      intentional Y24.0
    suicide (attempt) X74.01
  BB gun — *see* Discharge, airgun

Discharge— *continued*
  firearm (accidental) W34.00
    assault X95.9
    handgun (pistol) (revolver) W32.0
      assault X93
      homicide (attempt) X93
      legal intervention — *see* Legal, intervention,
        firearm, handgun
      stated as undetermined whether accidental or
        intentional Y22
      suicide (attempt) X72
    homicide (attempt) X95.9
    hunting rifle W33.02
      assault X94.1
      homicide (attempt) X94.1
      legal intervention
        injuring
          bystander Y35.032
          law enforcement personnel Y35.031
          suspect Y35.033
      stated as undetermined whether accidental or
        intentional Y23.1
      suicide (attempt) X73.1
    larger W33.00
      assault X94.9
      homicide (attempt) X94.9
      hunting rifle — *see* Discharge, firearm,
        hunting rifle
      legal intervention — *see* Legal, intervention,
        firearm by type of firearm
      machine gun — *see* Discharge, firearm,
        machine gun
      shotgun — *see* Discharge, firearm, shotgun
    specified NEC W33.09
      assault X94.8
      homicide (attempt) X94.8
      legal intervention
        injuring
          bystander Y35.092
          law enforcement personnel
            Y35.091
          suspect Y35.093
      stated as undetermined whether
        accidental or intentional Y23.8
      suicide (attempt) X73.8
    stated as undetermined whether accidental or
      intentional Y23.9
    suicide (attempt) X73.9
    legal intervention
      injuring
        bystander Y35.002
        law enforcement personnel Y35.001
        suspect Y35.003
    using rubber bullet
      injuring
        bystander Y35.042
        law enforcement personnel Y35.041
        suspect Y35.043
    machine gun W33.03
      assault X94.2
      homicide (attempt) X94.2
      legal intervention — *see* Legal, intervention,
        firearm, machine gun
      stated as undetermined whether accidental or
        intentional Y23.3
      suicide (attempt) X73.2
    pellet gun — *see* Discharge, airgun
    shotgun W33.01
      assault X94.0
      homicide (attempt) X94.0
      legal intervention — *see* Legal, intervention,
        firearm, specified NEC
      stated as undetermined whether accidental or
        intentional Y23.0
      suicide (attempt) X73.0
    specified NEC W34.09
      assault X95.8
      homicide (attempt) X95.8
      legal intervention — *see* Legal, intervention,
        firearm, specified NEC
      stated as undetermined whether accidental or
        intentional Y24.8
      suicide (attempt) X74.8

Discharge— *continued*
  firearm— *continued*
    stated as undetermined whether accidental or
      intentional Y24.9
    suicide (attempt) X74.9
    Very pistol W34.09
      assault X95.8
      homicide (attempt) X95.8
      stated as undetermined whether accidental or
        intentional Y24.8
      suicide (attempt) X74.8
  firework(s) W39
    stated as undetermined whether accidental or
      intentional Y25
  gas-operated gun NEC W34.018
    airgun — *see* Discharge, airgun
    assault X95.09
    homicide (attempt) X95.09
    paintball gun — *see* Discharge, paintball gun
    stated as undetermined whether accidental or
      intentional Y24.8
    suicide (attempt) X74.09
  gun NEC (*see also* Discharge, firearm NEC)
    air — *see* Discharge, airgun
    BB — *see* Discharge, airgun
    for single hand use — *see* Discharge, firearm,
      handgun
    hand — *see* Discharge, firearm, handgun
    machine — *see* Discharge, firearm, machine gun
    other specified — *see* Discharge, firearm NEC
    paintball — *see* Discharge, paintball gun
    pellet — *see* Discharge, airgun
  handgun — *see* Discharge, firearm, handgun
  machine gun — *see* Discharge, firearm, machine
    gun
  paintball gun W34.011
    assault X95.02
    homicide (attempt) X95.02
    stated as undetermined whether accidental or
      intentional Y24.8
    suicide (attempt) X74.02
  pistol — *see* Discharge, firearm, handgun
    flare — *see* Discharge, firearm, Very pistol
    pellet — *see* Discharge, airgun
    Very — *see* Discharge, firearm, Very pistol
  revolver — *see* Discharge, firearm, handgun
  rifle (hunting) — *see* Discharge, firearm, hunting
    rifle
  shotgun — *see* Discharge, firearm, shotgun
  spring-operated gun NEC W34.018
    assault X95.09
    homicide (attempt) X95.09
    stated as undetermined whether accidental or
      intentional Y24.8
    suicide (attempt) X74.09
Disease
  Andes W94.11
  aviator's — *see* Air, pressure
  range W94.11
Diver's disease, palsy, paralysis, squeeze — *see* Air,
  pressure
Diving (into water) — *see* Accident, diving
Dog bite W54.0
Dragged by transport vehicle NEC (*see also* Accident,
  transport) V09.9
Drinking poison (accidental) — *see* Table of Drugs
  and Chemicals
Dropped (accidentally) **while being carried or**
  supported by other person W04
Drowning (accidental) W74
  assault X92.9
  due to
    accident (to)
      machinery — *see* Contact, with, by type of
        machine
      watercraft V90.89
        burning V90.29
          powered V90.23
            merchant ship V90.20
            passenger ship V90.21
            fishing boat V90.22
            jetskis V90.23
          unpowered V90.28

Drowning — continued
  due to — continued
    accident — continued
      watercraft — continued
        burning — continued
          unpowered — continued
            canoe V90.25
            inflatable V90.26
            kayak V90.25
            sailboat V90.24
            water skis V90.27
        crushed V90.39
          powered V90.33
            merchant ship V90.30
            passenger ship V90.31
            fishing boat V90.32
            jetskis V90.33
          unpowered V90.38
            canoe V90.35
            inflatable V90.36
            kayak V90.35
            sailboat V90.34
            water skis V90.37
        overturning V90.09
          powered V90.03
            merchant ship V90.00
            passenger ship V90.01
            fishing boat V90.02
            jetskis V90.03
          unpowered V90.08
            canoe V90.05
            inflatable V90.06
            kayak V90.05
            sailboat V90.04
        sinking V90.19
          powered V90.13
            merchant ship V90.10
            passenger ship V90.11
            fishing boat V90.12
            jetskis V90.13
          unpowered V90.18
            canoe V90.15
            inflatable V90.16
            kayak V90.15
            sailboat V90.14
        specified type NEC V90.89
          powered V90.83
            merchant ship V90.80
            passenger ship V90.81
            fishing boat V90.82
            jetskis V90.83
          unpowered V90.88
            canoe V90.85
            inflatable V90.86
            kayak V90.85
            sailboat V90.84
            water skis V90.87
    avalanche B — see Landslide
    cataclysmic
      earth surface movement NEC B — see Forces
        of nature, earth movement
      storm B — see Forces of nature, cataclysmic
        storm
    cloudburst X37.8
    cyclone X37.1
    fall overboard (from) V92.09
      powered craft V92.03
        ferry boat V92.01
        liner V92.01
        merchant ship V92.00
        passenger ship V92.01
        fishing boat V92.02
        jetskis V92.03
      unpowered craft V92.08
        canoe V92.05
        inflatable V92.06
        kayak V92.05
        sailboat V92.04
        surf-board V92.08
        water skis V92.07
        windsurfer V92.08

Drowning — continued
  due to — continued
    fall overboard — continued
      resulting from
        accident to watercraft — see Drowning,
          due to, accident to, watercraft
        being washed overboard (from) V92.29
          powered craft V92.23
            ferry boat V92.21
            liner V92.21
            merchant ship V92.20
            passenger ship V92.21
            fishing boat V92.22
            jetskis V92.23
          unpowered craft V92.28
            canoe V92.25
            inflatable V92.26
            kayak V92.25
            sailboat V92.24
            surf-board V92.28
            water skis V92.27
            windsurfer V92.28
        motion of watercraft V92.19
          powered craft V92.13
            ferry boat V92.11
            liner V92.11
            merchant ship V92.10
            passenger ship V92.11
            fishing boat V92.12
            jetskis V92.13
          unpowered craft
            canoe V92.15
            inflatable V92.16
            kayak V92.15
            sailboat V92.14
    hurricane X37.0
    jumping into water from watercraft (involved in
      accident) (see also Drowning, due to,
      accident to, watercraft)
      without accident to or on watercraft W16.711
    tidal wave NEC B — see Forces of nature, tidal
      wave
    torrential rain X37.8
  following
    fall
      into
        bathtub W16.211
        bucket W16.221
        fountain — see Drowning, following, fall,
          into, water, specified NEC
        quarry — see Drowning, following, fall,
          into, water, specified NEC
        reservoir — see Drowning, following, fall,
          into, water, specified NEC
        swimming-pool W16.011
          striking
            bottom W16.021
            wall W16.031
          stated as undetermined whether
            accidental or intentional Y21.3
          suicide (attempt) X71.2
        water NOS W16.41
          natural (lake) (open sea) (river)
            (stream) (pond) W16.111
            striking
              bottom W16.121
              side W16.131
          specified NEC W16.311
            striking
              bottom W16.321
              wall W16.331
        overboard NEC — see Drowning, due to, fall
          overboard
    jump or dive
      from boat W16.711
        striking bottom W16.721
      into
        fountain — see Drowning, following, jump
          or dive, into, water, specified NEC
        quarry — see Drowning, following, jump
          or dive, into, water, specified NEC

Drowning — continued
  following — continued
    jump or dive — continued
      into — continued
        reservoir — see Drowning, following,
          jump or dive, into, water, specified
          NEC
        swimming-pool W16.511
          striking
            bottom W16.521
            wall W16.531
          suicide (attempt) X71.2
        water NOS W16.91
          natural (lake) (open sea) (river)
            (stream) (pond) W16.611
          specified NEC W16.811
            striking
              bottom W16.821
              wall W16.831
            striking bottom W16.621
  homicide (attempt) X92.9
  in
    bathtub (accidental) W65
      assault X92.0
      following fall W16.211
        stated as undetermined whether
          accidental or intentional Y21.1
      stated as undetermined whether accidental or
        intentional Y21.0
      suicide (attempt) X71.0
    lake — see Drowning, in, natural water
    natural water (lake) (open sea) (river) (stream)
      (pond) W69
      assault X92.3
      following
        dive or jump W16.611
          striking bottom W16.621
        fall W16.111
          striking
            bottom W16.121
            side W16.131
      stated as undetermined whether accidental or
        intentional Y21.4
      suicide (attempt) X71.3
    quarry — see Drowning, in, specified place NEC
    quenching tank — see Drowning, in, specified
      place NEC
    reservoir — see Drowning, in, specified place
      NEC
    river — see Drowning, in, natural water
    sea — see Drowning, in, natural water
    specified place NEC W73
      assault X92.8
      following
        dive or jump W16.811
          striking
            bottom W16.821
            wall W16.831
        fall W16.311
          striking
            bottom W16.321
            wall W16.331
      stated as undetermined whether accidental or
        intentional Y21.8
      suicide (attempt) X71.8
    stream — see Drowning, in, natural water
    swimming-pool W67
      assault X92.1
        following fall X92.2
      following
        dive or jump W16.511
          striking
            bottom W16.521
            wall W16.531
        fall W16.011
          striking
            bottom W16.021
            wall W16.031
      stated as undetermined whether accidental or
        intentional Y21.2
        following fall Y21.3
      suicide (attempt) X71.1
        following fall X71.2

Drowning — *continued*
  in— *continued*
    war operations — *see* War operations, restriction of airway
    resulting from accident to watercraftCsee Drowning, due to, accident, watercraft
    self-inflicted X71.9
    stated as undetermined whether accidental or intentional Y21.9
    suicide (attempt) X71.9

E

Earth (surface) **movement NEC B** — *see* Forces of nature, earth movement
Earth falling (on) W20.0
  caused by cataclysmic earth surface movement or eruption B — *see* Landslide
Earthquake (any injury) X34
Effect(s) (adverse) **of**
  air pressure (any) — *see* Air, pressure
  cold, excessive (exposure to) — *see* Exposure, cold
  heat (excessive) — *see* Heat
  hot place (weather) B — *see* Heat
  insolation X30
  late — *see* Sequelae
  motion — *see* Motion
  nuclear explosion or weapon in war operations — *see* War operations, nuclear weapon
  radiation — *see* Radiation
  travel — *see* Travel
Electric shock (accidental) (by) (in) — *see* Exposure, electric current
Electrocution (accidental) — *see* Exposure, electric current
Endotracheal tube wrongly placed during anesthetic procedure
Entanglement
  in
    bed linen, causing suffocation — *see* category T71
    wheel of pedal cycle V19.88
Entry of foreign body or material - *see* Foreign body
Environmental pollution related condition- *see* Z57
Execution, legal (any method) Y35.91
Exhaustion
  cold — *see* Exposure, cold
  due to excessive exertion — *see* Overexertion
  heat — *see* Heat
Explosion (accidental) (of) (with secondary fire) W40.9
  acetylene W40.1
  aerosol can W36.1
  air tank (compressed) (in machinery) W36.2
  aircraft (in transit) (powered) NEC V95.9
    balloon V96.05
    fixed wing NEC (private) V95.25
      commercial V95.35
    glider V96.25
      hang V96.15
      powered V95.15
    helicopter V95.05
    in war operations — *see* War operations, destruction of aircraft
    microlight V95.15
    nonpowered V96.9
      specified NEC V96.8
    powered NEC V95.8
    stated as
      homicide (attempt) Y03.8
      suicide (attempt) X83.0
    ultralight V95.15
  anesthetic gas in operating room W40.1
  antipersonnel bomb W40.8
    assault X96.0
    homicide (attempt) X96.0
    suicide (attempt) X75
  assault X96.9
  bicycle tire W37.0
  blasting (cap) (materials) W40.0
  boiler (machinery), not on transport vehicle W35
    on watercraft — *see* Explosion, in, watercraft

Explosion — *continued*
  butane W40.1
  caused by other person X96.9
  coal gas W40.1
  detonator W40.0
  dump (munitions) W40.8
  dynamite W40.0
    in
      assault X96.8
      homicide (attempt) X96.8
      legal intervention
        injuring
          bystander Y35.112
          law enforcement personnel Y35.111
          suspect Y35.113
      suicide (attempt) X75
  explosive (material) W40.9
    gas W40.1
    in blasting operation W40.0
    specified NEC W40.8
      in
        assault X96.8
        homicide (attempt) X96.8
        legal intervention
          injuring
            bystander Y35.192
            law enforcement personnel Y35.191
            suspect Y35.193
        suicide (attempt) X75
  factory (munitions) W40.8
  fertilizer bomb W40.8
    assault X96.3
    homicide (attempt) X96.3
    suicide (attempt) X75
  firearm (parts) NEC W34.19
    airgun W34.110
    BB gun W34.110
    gas, air or spring-operated gun NEC W34.118
    hangun W32.1
    hunting rifle W33.12
    larger firearm W33.10
      specified NEC W33.19
    machine gun W33.13
    paintball gun W34.111
    pellet gun W34.110
    shotgun W33.11
    Very pistol [flare] W34.19
  fire-damp W40.1
  fireworks W39
  gas (coal) (explosive) W40.1
    cylinder W36.9
      aerosol can W36.1
      air tank W36.2
      pressurized W36.3
      specified NEC W36.8
  gasoline (fumes) (tank) not in moving motor vehicle W40.1
    bomb W40.8
      assault X96.1
      homicide (attempt) X96.1
      suicide (attempt) X75
    in motor vehicle — *see* Accident, transport, by type of vehicle
  grain store W40.8
  grenade W40.8
    in
      assault X96.8
      homicide (attempt) X96.8
      legal intervention
        injuring
          bystander Y35.192
          law enforcement personnel Y35.191
          suspect Y35.193
      suicide (attempt) X75
  handgun (parts) — *see* Explosion, firearm, hangun (parts)
  homicide (attempt) X96.9
    antipersonnel bomb — *see* Explosion, antipersonnel bomb
    fertilizer bomb — *see* Explosion, fertilizer bomb
    gasoline bomb — *see* Explosion, gasoline bomb
    letter bomb — *see* Explosion, letter bomb

Explosion — *continued*
  homicide— *continued*
    pipe bomb — *see* Explosion, pipe bomb
    specified NEC X96.8
  hose, pressurized W37.8
  hot water heater, tank (in machinery) W35
    on watercraft — *see* Explosion, in, watercraft
  in, on
    dump W40.8
    factory W40.8
    mine (of explosive gases) NEC W40.1
    watercraft V93.59
      powered craft V93.53
        ferry boat V93.51
        fishing boat V93.52
        jetskis V93.53
        liner V93.51
        merchant ship V93.50
        passenger ship V93.51
        sailboat V93.54
  letter bomb W40.8
    assault X96.2
    homicide (attempt) X96.2
    suicide (attempt) X75
  machinery (*see also* Contact, with, by type of machine)
    on board watercraft — *see* Explosion, in, watercraft
    pressure vessel — *see* Explosion, by type of vessel
  methane W40.1
  mine W40.1
  missile NEC W40.8
  mortar bomb W40.8
    in
      assault X96.8
      homicide (attempt) X96.8
      legal intervention
        injuring
          bystander Y35.192
          law enforcement personnel Y35.191
          suspect Y35.193
      suicide (attempt) X75
  munitions (dump) (factory) W40.8
  pipe, pressurized W37.8
    bomb W40.8
      assault X96.4
      homicide (attempt) X96.4
      suicide (attempt) X75
  pressure, pressurized
    cooker W38
    gas tank (in machinery) W36.3
    hose W37.8
    pipe W37.8
    specified device NEC W38
    tire W37.8
      bicycle W37.0
    vessel (in machinery) W38
  propane W40.1
  self-inflicted X75
  shell (artillery) NEC W40.8
    during war operations — *see* War operations, explosion
    in
      legal intervention
        injuring
          bystander Y35.122
          law enforcement personnel Y35.121
          suspect Y35.123
    war — *see* War operations, explosion
  spacecraft V95.45
  steam or water lines (in machinery) W37.8
  stove W40.9
  stated as undetermined whether accidental or intentional Y25
  suicide (attempt) X75
  tire, pressurized W37.8
    bicycle W37.0
  undetermined whether accidental or intentional Y25
  vehicle tire NEC W37.8
    bicycle W37.0
  war operations — *see* War operations, explosion

F

Factors, supplemental
alcohol
blood level
less than 20mg/100ml Y90.0
presence in blood, level not specified Y90.9
20-39mg/100ml Y90.1
40-59mg/100ml Y90.2
60-79mg/100ml Y90.3
80-99mg/100ml Y90.4
100-119mg/100ml Y90.5
120-199mg/100ml Y90.6
200-239mg/100ml Y90.7
240 mg/100ml or more Y90.8
presence in blood, but level not specified Y90.9
environmental-pollution-related condition — see Z57
nosocomial condition Y95
work-related condition Y99.0
Failure
in suture or ligature during surgical procedure Y65.2
mechanical, of instrument or apparatus (any) (during any medical or surgical procedure) Y65.8
sterile precautions (during medical and surgical care) — see Misadventure, failure, sterile precautions, by type of procedure
to
introduce tube or instrument Y65.4
endotracheal tube during anesthesia Y65.3
make curve (transport vehicle) NEC — see Accident, transport
remove tube or instrument Y65.4
Fall, falling (accidental) W19
building W20.1
burning (uncontrolled fire) X00.3
down
embankment W17.81
escalator W10.0
hill W17.81
ladder W11
ramp W10.2
stairs, steps W10.9
due to
bumping against
object W18.00
sharp glass W18.02
specified NEC W18.09
sports equipment W18.01
person W03
due to ice or snow W00.0
on pedestrian conveyance — see Accident, transport, pedestrian, conveyance
collision with another person W03
due to ice or snow W00.0
involving pedestrian conveyance — see Accident, transport, pedestrian, conveyance
grocery cart tipping over W17.82
ice or snow W00.9
from one level to another W00.2
on stairs or steps W00.1
involving pedestrian conveyance — see Accident, transport, pedestrian, conveyance
on same level W00.0
slipping (on moving sidewalk) W01.0
with subsequent striking against object W01.10
furniture W01.190
sharp object W01.119
glass W01.110
power tool or machine W01.111
specified NEC W01.118
specified NEC W01.198
striking against
object W18.00
sharp glass W18.02
specified NEC W18.09
sports equipment W18.01
person W03

Fall, falling— continued
due to— continued
striking against— continued
person— continued
due to ice or snow W00.0
on pedestrian conveyance — see Accident, transport, pedestrian, conveyance
earth (with asphyxia or suffocation (by pressure)) — see Earth, falling
from, off, out of
aircraft NEC (with accident to aircraft NEC) V97.0
while boarding or alighting V97.1
balcony W13.0
bed W06
boat, ship, watercraft NEC (with drowning or submersion) — see Drowning, due to, fall overboard
with hitting bottom or object V94.0
bridge W13.1
building W13.9
burning (uncontrolled fire) X00.3
cavity W17.2
chair W07
cliff W15
dock W17.4
embankment W17.81
escalator W10.0
flagpole W13.8
furniture NEC W08
grocery cart W17.82
haystack W17.89
high place NEC W17.89
stated as undetermined whether accidental or intentional Y30
hole W17.2
incline W10.2
ladder W11
machine, machinery (see also Contact, with, by type of machine)
not in operation W17.89
manhole W17.1
motorized mobility scooter W05.2
one level to another NEC W17.89
intentional, purposeful, suicide (attempt) X80
stated as undetermined whether accidental or intentional Y30
pit W17.2
playground equipment W09.8
jungle gym W09.2
slide W09.0
swing W09.1
quarry W17.89
railing W13.9
ramp W10.2
roof W13.2
scaffolding W12
scooter (nonmotorized) W05.1
motorized mobility W05.2
stairs, steps W10.9
curb W10.1
due to ice or snow W00.1
escalator W10.0
incline W10.2
ramp W10.2
sidewalk curb W10.1
specified NEC W10.8
stepladder W11
storm drain W17.1
streetcar NEC V82.6
with antecedent collision — see Accident, transport, streetcar occupant
while boarding or alighting V82.4
structure NEC W13.8
burning (uncontrolled fire) X00.3
table W08
toilet W18.11
with subsequent striking against object W18.12
train NEC V81.6
during derailment (without antecedent collision) V81.7

Fall, falling— continued
from, off, out of — continued
train— continued
during derailment — continued
with antecedent collision — see Accident, transport, railway vehicle occupant
while boarding or alighting V81.4
transport vehicle after collision — see Accident, transport, by type of vehicle, collision
tree W14
vehicle (in motion) NEC (see also Accident, transport) V89.9
motor NEC (see also Accident, transport, occupant, by type of vehicle) V87.8
stationary W17.89
while boarding or alighting B — see Accident, transport, by type of vehicle, while boarding or alighting
viaduct W13.8
wall W13.8
watercraft (see also Drowning, due to, fall overboard)
with hitting bottom or object V94.0
well W17.0
wheelchair, non-moving W05.0
powered — see Accident, transport, pedestrian, conveyance occupant, specified type NEC
window W13.4
in, on
aircraft NEC V97.0
with accident to aircraft V97.0
while boarding or alighting V97.1
bathtub (empty) W18.2
filled W16.212
causing drowning W16.211
escalator W10.0
incline W10.2
ladder W11
machine, machinery — see Contact, with, by type of machine
object, edged, pointed or sharp (with cut) — see Fall, by type
playground equipment W09.8
jungle gym W09.2
slide W09.0
swing W09.1
ramp W10.2
scaffolding W12
shower W18.2
causing drowning W16.211
staircase, stairs, steps W10.9
curb W10.1
due to ice or snow W00.1
escalator W10.0
incline W10.2
specified NEC W10.8
streetcar (without antecedent collision) V82.5
with antecedent collision — see Accident, transport, streetcar occupant
while boarding or alighting V82.4
train (without antecedent collision) V81.5
with antecedent collision — see Accident, transport, railway vehicle occupant
during derailment (without antecedent collision) V81.7
with antecedent collision — see Accident, transport, railway vehicle occupant
while boarding or alighting V81.4
transport vehicle after collision — see Accident, transport, by type of vehicle, collision
watercraft V93.39
due to
accident to craft V91.29
powered craft V91.23
ferry boat V91.21
fishing boat V91.22
jetskis V91.23
liner V91.21
merchant ship V91.20
passenger ship V91.21
unpowered craft
canoe V91.25

Fall, falling— *continued*
  in on— *continued*
    watercraft— *continued*
      due to— *continued*
        accident to craft— *continued*
          unpowered craft— *continued*
            inflatable V91.26
            kayak V91.25
            sailboat V91.24
        powered craft V93.33
          ferry boat V93.31
          fishing boat V93.32
          jetskis V93.33
          liner V93.31
          merchant ship V93.30
          passenger ship V93.31
        unpowered craft V93.38
          canoe V93.35
          inflatable V93.36
          kayak V93.35
          sailboat V93.34
          surf-board V93.38
          windsurfer V93.38
  into
    cavity W17.2
    dock W17.4
    fire — *see* Exposure, fire, by type
    haystack W17.89
    hole W17.2
    lake — *see* Fall, into, water
    manhole W17.1
    moving part of machinery — *see* Contact, with,
      by type of machine
    ocean — *see* Fall, into, water
    opening in surface NEC W17.89
    pit W17.2
    pond — *see* Fall, into, water
    quarry W17.89
    lake — *see* Fall, into, water
    river — *see* Fall, into, water
    shaft W17.89
    storm drain W17.1
    stream — *see* Fall, into, water
    swimming pool (*see also* Fall, into, water, in,
      swimming pool)
      empty W17.3
    tank W17.89
    water W16.42
      causing drowning W16.41
      from watercraft — *see* Drowning, due to, fall
        overboard
      hitting diving board W21.4
      in
        bathtub W16.212
          causing drowning W16.211
        bucket W16.222
          causing drowning W16.221
        natural body of water W16.112
          causing drowning W16.111
          striking
            bottom W16.122
              causing drowning W16.121
            side W16.132
              causing drowning W16.131
        specified water NEC W16.312
          causing drowning W16.311
          striking
            bottom W16.322
              causing drowning W16.321
            wall W16.332
              causing drowning W16.331
        swimming pool W16.012
          causing drowning W16.011
          striking
            bottom W16.022
              causing drowning W16.021
            wall W16.032
              causing drowning W16.031
        utility bucket W16.222
          causing drowning W16.221
    well W17.0
  involving
    bed W06

Fall, falling— *continued*
  involving— *continued*
    chair W07
    furniture NEC W08
    glass — *see* Fall, by type
    playground equipment W09.8
      jungle gym W09.2
      slide W09.0
      swing W09.1
    roller blades — *see* Accident, transport,
      pedestrian, conveyance
    skateboard(s) — *see* Accident, transport,
      pedestrian, conveyance
    skates (ice) (in line) (roller) — *see* Accident,
      transport, pedestrian, conveyance
    skis — *see* Accident, transport, pedestrian,
      conveyance
    table W08
    wheelchair, non-moving W05.0
      powered — *see* Accident, transport,
        pedestrian, conveyance, specified type
        NEC
  object — *see* Struck by, object, falling
  off
    toilet W18.11
      with subsequent striking against object
        W18.12
  on same level W18.30
    due to
      specified NEC W18.39
      stepping on an object W18.31
  out of
    bed W06
    building NEC W13.8
    chair W07
    furniture NEC W08
    wheelchair, non-moving W05.0
      powered — *see* Accident, transport,
        pedestrian, conveyance, specified type
        NEC
    window W13.4
  over
    animal W01.0
    cliff W15
    embankment W17.81
    small object W01.0
  rock W20.8
  same level W18.30
    from
      being crushed, pushed, or stepped on by a
        crowd or human stampede W52
      collision, pushing, shoving, by or with other
        person W03
      slipping, stumbling, tripping W01.0
    involving ice or snow W00.0
      involving skates (ice) (roller), skateboard, skis
        — *see* Accident, transport, pedestrian,
        conveyance
  snowslide (avalanche) B — *see* Landslide
  stone W20.8
  structure W20.1
    burning (uncontrolled fire) X00.3
  through
    bridge W13.1
    floor W13.3
    roof W13.2
    wall W13.8
    window W13.4
  timber W20.8
  tree (caused by lightning) W20.8
  while being carried or supported by other person(s)
    W04
Fallen on by
  animal (not being ridden) NEC W55.89
Felo-de-se — *see* Suicide
Fight (hand) (fists) (foot) — *see* Assault, fight
Fire (accidental) — *see* Exposure, fire
Firearm discharge — *see* Discharge, firearm
Fireball effects from nuclear explosion in war
  operations — *see* War operations, nuclear
  weapons
Fireworks (explosion) W39
Flash burns from explosion — *see* Explosion

Flood (any injury) (caused by) X38
  collapse of man-made structure causing earth
    movement X36.0
  tidal wave — *see* Forces of nature, tidal wave
Food (any type) **in**
  air passages (with asphyxia, obstruction, or
    suffocation) — *see* categories T17 and T18
  alimentary tract causing asphyxia (due to
    compression of trachea) — *see* categories T17
    and T18
Forces of nature X39.8
  avalanche X36.1
    causing transport accident — *see* Accident,
      transport, by type of vehicle
  blizzard X37.2
  cataclysmic storm X37.9
    with flood X38
    blizzard X37.2
    cloudburst X37.8
    cyclone X37.1
    dust storm X37.3
    hurricane X37.0
    specified storm NEC X37.8
    storm surge X37.0
    tornado X37.1
    twister X37.1
    typhoon X37.0
  cloudburst X37.8
  cold (natural) X31
  cyclone X37.1
  dam collapse causing earth movement X36.0
  dust storm X37.3
  earth movement X36.1
    earthquake X34
    caused by dam or structure collapse X36.0
  earthquake X34
  flood (caused by) X38
    dam collapse X36.0
    tidal wave B — *see* Forces of nature, tidal wave
  heat (natural) X30
  hurricane X37.0
  landslide X36.1
    causing transport accident — *see* Accident,
      transport, by type of vehicle
  lightning — *see* subcategory T75.0
    causing fire — *see* Exposure, fire
  mudslide X36.1
    causing transport accident — *see* Accident,
      transport, by type of vehicle
  radiation (natural) X39.08
    radon X39.01
  radon X39.01
  specified force NEC X39.8
  storm surge X37.0
  structure collapse causing earth movement X36.0
  sunlight X32
  tidal wave X37.41
    due to
      earthquake X37.41
      landslide X37.43
      storm X37.42
      volcanic eruption X37.41
  tornado X37.1
  tsunami X37.41
  twister X37.1
  typhoon X37.0
  volcanic eruption X35
Foreign body entering through skin W45.8
  can lid W45.2
  nail W45.0
  paper W45.1
  specified NEC W45.8
  splinter W45.8
Forest fire (exposure to) — *see* Exposure, fire,
  uncontrolled, not in building
Found injured X58
  from exposure (to) — *see* Exposure
  on
    highway, road(way), street V89.9
    railway right of way V81.9
Fracture (circumstances unknown or unspecified) X58
  due to specified cause NEC X58
Freezing — *see* Exposure, cold

Incident, adverse— *continued*
  device— *continued*
    urology Y73.8
      accessory Y73.2
      diagnostic Y73.0
      miscellaneous Y73.8
      monitoring Y73.0
      prosthetic Y73.2
      rehabilitative Y73.1
      surgical Y73.3
      therapeutic Y73.1
Incineration (accidental) — *see* Exposure, fire
Infanticide — *see* Assault
Infrasound waves (causing injury) W49.9
Ingestion
  foreign body (causing injury) (with obstruction) — *see* Foreign body, alimentary canal
  poisonous
    plant(s) X58
    substance NEC — *see* Table of Drugs and Chemicals
Inhalation
  excessively cold substance, man-made — *see* Exposure, cold, man-made
  food (any type) (into respiratory tract) (with asphyxia, obstruction respiratory tract, suffocation) — *see* categories T17 and T18
  foreign body — *see* Foreign body, aspiration
  gastric contents (with asphyxia, obstruction respiratory passage, suffocation) — *see* subcategories T17.81, T18.81.
  hot air or gases X14.0
  liquid air, hydrogen, nitrogen W93.12
    suicide (attempt) X83.2
  steam X13.0
    assault X98.0
    stated as undetermined whether accidental or intentional Y27.0
    suicide (attempt) X77.0
  toxic gas — *see* Table of Drugs and Chemicals
  vomitus (with asphyxia, obstruction respiratory passage, suffocation) — *see* subcategories T17.81, T18.81.
Injury, injured (accidental(ly)) NOS X58
  by, caused by, from
    assault — *see* Assault
    law-enforcing agent, police, in course of legal intervention — *see* Legal intervention
    suicide (attempt) X83.8
  due to, in
    civil insurrection — *see* War operations
    fight (*see also* Assault, fight) Y04.0
    war operations — *see* War operations
  homicide (*see also* Assault) Y09
  inflicted (by)
    in course of arrest (attempted), suppression of disturbance, maintenance of order, by law-enforcing agents — *see* Legal intervention
    other person
      stated as
        accidental X58
        intentional, homicide (attempt) — *see* Assault
        undetermined whether accidental or intentional Y33
  purposely (inflicted) by other person(s) — *see* Assault
  self-inflicted X83.8
    stated as accidental X58
  specified cause NEC X58
  undetermined whether accidental or intentional Y33
Insolation, effects X30
Insufficient nourishment X58
Interruption of respiration (by)
  food (lodged in esophagus) — *see* categories T17 and T18
  vomitus (lodged in esophagus) — *see* subcategories T17.81, T18.81.
Intervention, legal — *see* Legal intervention

Intoxication
  drug — *see* Table of Drugs and Chemicals
  poison — *see* Table of Drugs and Chemicals

J

Jammed (accidentally)
  between objects (moving) (stationary and moving) W23.0
    stationary W23.1
Jumped, jumping
  before moving object NEC X81.8
    motor vehicle X81.0
    subway train X81.1
    train X81.1
    undetermined whether accidental or intentional Y31
  from
    boat (into water) voluntarily, without accident (to or on boat) W16.712
      with
        accident to or on boat — *see* Accident, watercraft
        drowning or submersion W16.711
          suicide (attempt) X71.3
        striking bottom W16.722
          causing drowning W16.721
    building (*see also* Jumped, from, high place) W13.9
      burning (uncontrolled fire) X00.5
    high place NEC W17.89
      suicide (attempt) X80
      undetermined whether accidental or intentional Y30
    structure (*see also* Jumped, from, high place) W13.9
      burning (uncontrolled fire) X00.5
  into water W16.92
    causing drowning W16.91
    from, off watercraft — *see* Jumped, from, boat
    in
      natural body W16.612
        causing drowning W16.611
        striking bottom W16.622
          causing drowning W16.621
      specified place NEC W16.812
        causing drowning W16.811
        striking
          bottom W16.822
            causing drowning W16.821
          wall W16.832
            causing drowning W16.831
      swimming pool W16.512
        causing drowning W16.511
        striking
          bottom W16.522
            causing drowning W16.521
          wall W16.532
            causing drowning W16.531
    suicide (attempt) X71.3

K

Kicked by
  animal NEC W55.82
  person(s) (accidentally) W50.1
    with intent to injure or kill Y04.0
    as, or caused by, a crowd or human stampede (with fall) W52
    assault Y04.0
    homicide (attempt) Y04.0
    in
      fight Y04.0
      legal intervention
        injuring
          bystander Y35.812
          law enforcement personnel Y35.811
          suspect Y35.813

Kicking against
  object W22.8
    sports equipment W21.9
    stationary wW22.09
      sports equipment W21.89
  person — *see* Striking against, person
  sports equipment W21.9
Killed, killing (accidentally) **NOS** (*see also* Injury) X58
  in
    action — *see* War operations
    brawl, fight (hand) (fists) (foot) Y04.0
      by weapon (*see also* Assault)
        cutting, piercing — *see* Assault, cutting or piercing instrument
        firearm — *see* Discharge, firearm, by type, homicide
  self
    stated as
      accident NOS X58
      suicide — *see* Suicide
      undetermined whether accidental or intentional Y33
Knocked down (accidentally) (by) NOS X58
  animal (not being ridden) NEC (*see also* Struck by, by type of animal)
  crowd or human stampede W52
  person W51
    in brawl, fight Y04.0
  transport vehicle NEC (*see also* Accident, transport) V09.9

L

Laceration NEC — *see* Injury
Lack of
  care (helpless person) (infant) (newborn) X58
  food except as result of abandonment or neglect X58
    due to abandonment or neglect X58
  water except as result of transport accident X58
    due to transport accident B — *see* Accident, transport, by type
  helpless person, infant, newborn X58
Landslide (falling on transport vehicle) X36.1
  caused by collapse of man-made structure X36.0
Late effect — *see* Sequelae
Legal
  execution Y35.91
  intervention (by)
    baton — *see* Legal, intervention, blunt object, baton
    bayonet — *see* Legal, intervention, sharp object, bayonet
    blow — *see* Legal, intervention, manhandling
    blunt object
      baton
        injuring
          bystander Y35.312
          law enforcement personnel Y35.311
          suspect Y35.313
      injuring
        bystander Y35.302
        law enforcement personnel Y35.301
        suspect Y35.303
      specified NEC
        injuring
          bystander Y35.392
          law enforcement personnel Y35.391
          suspect Y35.393
      stave
        injuring
          bystander Y35.392
          law enforcement personnel Y35.391
          suspect Y35.393
    bomb — *see* Legal, intervention, explosive
    cutting or piercing instrument — *see* Legal, intervention, sharp object
    dynamite — *see* Legal, intervention, explosive, dynamite
    execution, any method Y35.91

Legal— *continued*
  intervention— *continued*
    explosive(s)
      dynamite
        injuring
          bystander Y35.112
          law enforcement personnel Y35.111
          suspect Y35.113
      grenade
        injuring
          bystander Y35.192
          law enforcement personnel Y35.191
          suspect Y35.193
      injuring
        bystander Y35.102
        law enforcement personnel Y35.101
        suspect Y35.103
      mortar bomb
        injuring
          bystander Y35.192
          law enforcement personnel Y35.191
          suspect Y35.193
      shell
        injuring
          bystander Y35.122
          law enforcement personnel Y35.121
          suspect Y35.123
      specified NEC
        injuring
          bystander Y35.192
          law enforcement personnel Y35.191
          suspect Y35.193
    firearm(s) (discharge)
      handgun
        injuring
          bystander Y35.022
          law enforcement personnel Y35.021
          suspect Y35.023
      injuring
        bystander Y35.002
        law enforcement personnel Y35.001
        suspect Y35.003
      machine gun
        injuring
          bystander Y35.012
          law enforcement personnel Y35.011
          suspect Y35.013
      rifle pellet
        injuring
          bystander Y35.032
          law enforcement personnel Y35.031
          suspect Y35.033
      rubber bullet
        injuring
          bystander Y35.042
          law enforcement personnel Y35.041
          suspect Y35.043
      shotgun — *see* Legal, intervention, firearm, specified NEC
      specified NEC
        injuring
          bystander Y35.092
          law enforcement personnel Y35.091
          suspect Y35.093
    gas (asphyxiation) (poisoning)
      injuring
        bystander Y35.202
        law enforcement personnel Y35.201
        suspect Y35.203
      specified NEC
        injuring
          bystander Y35.292
          law enforcement personnel Y35.291
          suspect Y35.293
      tear gas
        injuring
          bystander Y35.212
          law enforcement personnel Y35.211
          suspect Y35.213
    grenade — *see* Legal, intervention, explosive, grenade
    injuring
      bystander Y35.92

Legal— *continued*
  intervention— *continued*
    injuring— *continued*
      law enforcement personnel Y35.91
      suspect Y35.93
    late effect (of) — *see* Y35 with 7th character S
    manhandling
      injuring
        bystander Y35.812
        law enforcement personnel Y35.811
        suspect Y35.813
    sequelae (of) — *see* Y35 with 7th character S
    sharp objects
      bayonet
        injuring
          bystander Y35.412
          law enforcement personnel Y35.411
          suspect Y35.413
      injuring
        bystander Y35.402
        law enforcement personnel Y35.401
        suspect Y35.403
      specified NEC
        injuring
          bystander Y35.492
          law enforcement personnel Y35.491
          suspect Y35.493
    specified means NEC
      injuring
        bystander Y35.892
        law enforcement personnel Y35.891
        suspect Y35.893
    stabbing — *see* Legal, intervention, sharp object
    stave — *see* Legal, intervention, blunt object, stave
    tear gas — *see* Legal, intervention, gas, tear gas
    truncheon — *see* Legal, intervention, blunt object, stave
Lightning (shock) (stroke) (struck by) — *see* subcategory T75.0
  causing fire — *see* Exposure, fire
Loss of control (transport vehicle) **NEC** — *see* Accident, transport
Lost at sea NOS — *see* Drowning, due to, fall overboard
Low
  pressure (effects) — *see* Air, pressure, low
  temperature (effects) — *see* Exposure, cold
Lying before train, vehicle or other moving object X81.8
  subway train X81.1
  train X81.1
  undetermined whether accidental or intentional Y31
Lynching — *see* Assault

M

Malfunction (mechanism or component) (of)
  firearm W34.10
    airgun W34.110
    BB gun W34.110
    gas, air or spring-operated gun NEC W34.118
    handgun W32.1
    hunting rifle W33.12
    larger firearm W33.10
      specified NEC W33.19
    machine gun W33.13
    paintball gun W34.111
    pellet gun W34.110
    shotgun W33.11
    specified NEC W34.19
    Very pistol [flare] W34.19
  handgun — *see* Malfunction, firearm, handgun
Maltreatment — *see* Perpetrator
Mangled (accidentally) NOS X58
Manhandling (in brawl, fight) Y04.0
  legal intervention — *see* Legal, intervention, manhandling
Manslaughter (nonaccidental) — *see* Assault
Mauled by animal NEC W55.89

Medical procedure, complication of (delayed or as an abnormal reaction without mention of misadventure) — *see* Complication of or following, by specified type of procedure
  due to or as a result of misadventure — *see* Misadventure
Melting (due to fire) (*see also* Exposure, fire)
  apparel NEC X06.3
  clothes, clothing NEC X06.3
  nightwear X05
  fittings or furniture (burning building) (uncontrolled fire) X00.8
  nightwear X05
  plastic jewelry X06.1
Mental cruelty X58
Military operations (injuries to military and civilians occuring during peacetime on military property and during routine military exercises and operations) (by) (from) (involving) Y37.90-
  air blast Y37.20-
  aircraft
    destruction — *see* Military operations, destruction of aircraft
    airway restriction — *see* Military operations, restriction of airways
    asphyxiation — *see* Military operations, restriction of airways
  biological weapons Y37.6x-
  blast Y37.20-
  blast fragments Y37.20-
  blast wave Y37.20-
  blast wind Y37.20-
  bomb Y37.20-
    dirty Y37.50-
    gasoline Y37.31-
    incendiary Y37.31-
    petrol Y37.31-
  bullet Y37.43-
    incendiary Y37.32-
    rubber Y37.41-
  chemical weapons Y37.7x-
  combat
    hand to hand (unarmed) combat Y37.44-
    using blunt or piercing object Y37.45-
  conflagration — *see* Military operations, fire
  conventional warfare NEC Y37.49-
  depth-charge Y37.01-
  destruction of aircraft Y37.10-
    due to
      air to air missile Y37.11-
      collision with other aircraft Y37.12-
      detonation (accidental) of onboard munitions and explosives Y37.14-
      enemy fire or explosives Y37.11-
      explosive placed on aircraft Y37.11-
      onboard fire Y37.13-
      rocket propelled grenade [RPG] Y37.11-
      small arms fire Y37.11-
      surface to air missile Y37.11-
    specified NEC Y37.19-
  detonation (accidental) of
    onboard marine weapons Y37.05-
    own munitions or munitions launch device Y37.24-
  dirty bomb Y37.50-
  explosion (of) Y37.20-
    aerial bomb Y37.21-
    bomb NOS Y37.20-*see also* Military operations, bomb(s)
    own munitions or munitions launch device (accidental) Y37.24-
    fragments Y37.20-
    grenade Y37.29-
    guided missile Y37.22-
    improvised explosive device [IED] (person-borne) (roadside) (vehicle-borne) Y37.23-
    land mine Y37.29-
    marine mine (at sea) (in harbor) Y37.02-
    marine weapon Y37.00-
      specified NEC Y37.09-
    sea-based artillery shell Y37.03-
    specified NEC Y37.29-
    torpedo Y37.04-

Military operations— *continued*
  fire Y37.30-
    specified NEC Y37.39-
  firearms
    discharge Y37.43-
    pellets Y37.42-
  flamethrower Y37.33-
  fragments (from) (of)
    improvised explosive device [IED] (person-borne)
      (roadside) (vehicle-borne) Y37.26-
    munitions Y37.25-
    specified NEC Y37.29-
    weapons Y37.27-
  friendly fire Y37.92-
  hand to hand (unarmed) combat Y37.44-
  hot substances — *see* Military operations, fire
  incendiary bullet Y37.32-
  nuclear weapon (effects of) Y37.50-
    acute radiation exposure Y37.54-
    blast pressure Y37.51-
    direct blast Y37.51-
    direct heat Y37.53-
    fallout exposure Y37.54-
    fireball Y37.53-
    indirect blast (struck or crushed by blast debris)
      (being thrown by blast) Y37.52-
    ionizing radiation (immediate exposure) Y37.54-
    nuclear radiation Y37.54-
    radiation
      ionizing (immediate exposure) Y37.54-
      nuclear Y37.54-
      thermal Y37.53-
    specified NEC Y37.59-
    secondary effects Y37.54-
    thermal radiation Y37.53-
  restriction of air (airway)
    intentional Y37.46-
    unintentional Y37.47-
  rubber bullets Y37.41-
  shrapnel NOS Y37.29-
  suffocation — *see* Military operations, restriction of
    airways
  unconventional warfare NEC Y37.7x-
  underwater blast NOS Y37.00-
  warfare
    conventional NEC Y37.49-
    unconventional NEC Y37.7x-
  weapons
    biological weapons Y37.6x-
    chemical Y37.7x-
    nuclear (effects of) Y37.50-
      acute radiation exposure Y37.54-
      blast pressure Y37.51-
      direct blast Y37.51-
      direct heat Y37.53-
      fallout exposure Y37.54-
      fireball Y37.53-
      indirect blast (struck or crushed by blast
        debris) (being thrown by blast) Y37.52-
      radiation
        ionizing (immediate exposure) Y37.54-
        nuclear Y37.54-
        thermal Y37.53-
      secondary effects Y37.54-
      specified NEC Y37.59-
      indirect blast (struck or crushed by blast
        debris) (being thrown by blast) Y37.52-
    of mass destruction [WMD] Y37.91-
  weapon of mass destruction [WMD] Y37.91-
Misadventure(s) **to patient**(s) **during surgical or**
  medical care Y69
  contaminated medical or biological substance
    (blood, drug, fluid) Y64.9
    administered (by) NEC Y64.9
      immunization Y64.1
      infusion Y64.0
      injection Y64.1
      specified means NEC Y64.8
      transfusion Y64.0
      vaccination Y64.1
  excessive amount of blood or other fluid during
    transfusion or infusion Y63.0

Misadventure(s) **to patient**(s) **during surgical or**
  medical care — *continued*
  failure
    in dosage Y63.9
      electroshock therapy Y63.4
      inappropriate temperature (too hot or too
        cold) in local application and packing
        Y63.5
      infusion
        excessive amount of fluid Y63.0
        incorrect dilution of fluid Y63.1
      insulin-shock therapy Y63.4
      nonadministration of necessary drug or
        biological substance Y63.62
      overdose — *see* Table of Drugs and Chemicals
        radiation, in therapy Y63.2
      radiation
        overdose Y63.2
      specified procedure NEC Y63.8
      transfusion
        excessive amount of blood Y63.0
    mechanical, of instrument or apparatus (any)
      (during any procedure) Y65.8
    sterile precautions (during procedure) Y62.9
      aspiration of fluid or tissue (by puncture or
        catheterization, except heart) Y62.6
      biopsy (except needle aspiration) Y62.8
        needle (aspirating) Y62.6
      blood sampling Y62.6
      catheterization Y62.6
        heart Y62.5
      dialysis (kidney) Y62.2
      endoscopic examination Y62.4
      enema Y62.8
      immunization Y62.3
      infusion Y62.1
      injection Y62.3
      needle biopsy Y62.6
      paracentesis (abdominal) (thoracic) Y62.6
      perfusion Y62.2
      puncture (lumbar) Y62.6
      removal of catheter or packing Y62.8
      specified procedure NEC Y62.8
      surgical operation Y62.0
      transfusion Y62.1
      vaccination Y62.3
    suture or ligature during surgical procedure
      Y65.2
    to introduce or to remove tube or instrument B
      — *see* Failure, to
  hemorrhage — *see* Misadventure, cut, by type of
    procedure
  inadvertent exposure of patient to radiation Y63.3
  inappropriate
    operation performed — *see* Inappropriate
      operation performed
    temperature (too hot or too cold) in local
      application or packing Y63.5
  infusion (*see also* Misadventure, by type, infusion)
    Y69
    excessive amount of fluid Y63.0
    incorrect dilution of fluid Y63.1
    wrong fluid Y65.1
  mismatched blood in transfusion Y65.0
  nonadministration of necessary drug or biological
    substance Y63.62
  overdose — *see* Table of Drugs and Chemicals
    radiation (in therapy) Y63.2
  perforation — *see* Misadventure, cut, by type of
    procedure
  performance of inappropriate operation — *see*
    Inappropriate operation performed
  puncture — *see* Misadventure, cut, by type of
    procedure
  specified type NEC Y65.8
    failure
      suture or ligature during surgical operation
        Y65.2
      to introduce or to remove tube or instrument
        B — *see* Failure, to
    infusion of wrong fluid Y65.1
    performance of inappropriate operation — *see*
      Inappropriate operation performed

Misadventure(s) **to patient**(s) **during surgical or**
  medical care — *continued*
  specified type— *continued*
    transfusion of mismatched blood Y65.0
    wrong
      fluid in infusion Y65.1
      placement of endotracheal tube during
        anesthetic procedure Y65.3
  transfusion — *see* Misadventure, by type,
    transfusion
    excessive amount of blood Y63.0
    mismatched blood Y65.0
  wrong
    drug given in error — *see* Table of Drugs and
      Chemicals
    fluid in infusion Y65.1
    placement of endotracheal tube during
      anesthetic procedure Y65.3
Mismatched blood in transfusion Y65.0
Motion sickness T75.3
Mountain sickness W94.11
Mudslide (of cataclysmic nature) — *see* Landslide
Murder (attempt) — *see* Assault

N

Nail, contact with W45.0
  gun W29.4
Neglect (criminal) (homicidal intent) X58
Noise (causing injury) (pollution) W42.9
  supersonic W42.0
Nonadministration (of)
  drug or biological substance (necessary) Y63.62
  surgical and medical care Y66
Nosocomial condition Y95

O

Object
  falling
    from, in, on, hitting
      machinery — *see* Contact, with, by type of
        machine
    set in motion by
      accidental explosion or rupture of pressure vessel
        W38
      firearm — *see* Discharge, firearm, by type
      machine(ry) — *see* Contact, with, by type of
        machine
Overdose (drug) — *see* Table of Drugs and Chemicals
  radiation Y63.2
Overexertion — *see* category Y93
Overexposure (accidental) (to)
  cold (*see also* Exposure, cold) X31
    due to man-made conditions — *see* Exposure,
      cold, man-made
  heat (*see also* Heat) X30
  radiation — *see* Radiation
  radioactivity W88.0
  sun (sunburn) X32
  weather NEC B — *see* Forces of nature
  wind NEC B — *see* Forces of nature
Overheated — *see* Heat
Overturning (accidental)
  machinery — *see* Contact, with, by type of machine
  transport vehicle NEC (*see also* Accident, transport)
    V89.9
  watercraft (causing drowning, submersion) (*see also*
    Drowning, due to, accident to, watercraft,
    overturning)
    causing injury except drowning or submersion B
      — *see* Accident, watercraft, causing, injury
      NEC

P

Parachute descent (voluntary) (without accident to aircraft) V97.29
  due to accident to aircraft — *see* Accident, transport, aircraft
Pecked by bird W61.99
Perforation during medical or surgical treatment as misadventure — *see* Misadventure, cut, by type of procedure
Perpetrator, perpetration, of assault, maltreatment and neglect (by) Y07.9
  boyfriend Y07.03
  brother Y07.410
    stepbrother Y07.435
  coach Y07.53
  cousin
    female Y07.491
    male Y07.490
  daycare provider Y07.519
    at-home
      adult care Y07.512
      childcare Y07.510
    care center
      adult care Y07.513
      childcare Y07.511
  family member NEC Y07.499
  father Y07.11
    adoptive Y07.13
    foster Y07.420
    stepfather Y07.430
  foster father Y07.420
  foster mother Y07.421
  girl friend Y07.04
  healthcare provider Y07.529
    mental health Y07.521
    specified NEC Y07.528
  husband Y07.01
  instructor Y07.53
  mother Y07.12
    adoptive Y07.14
    foster Y07.421
    stepmother Y07.433
  nonfamily member Y07.50
    specifed NEC Y07.59
  nurse Y07.528
  occupational therapist Y07.528
  partner of parent
    female Y07.434
    male Y07.432
  physical therapist Y07.528
  sister Y07.411
  speech therapist Y07.528
  stepbrother Y07.435
  stepfather Y07.430
  stepmother Y07.433
  stepsister Y07.436
  teacher Y07.53
  wife Y07.02
Piercing — *see* Contact, with, by type of object or machine
Pinched
  between objects (moving) (stationary and moving) W23.0
    stationary W23.1
Pinned under machine(ry) — *see* Contact, with, by type of machine
Place of occurrence Y92.9
  abandoned house Y92.89
  airplane Y92.813
  airport Y92.520
  ambulatory health services establishment NEC Y92.538
  ambulatory surgery center Y92.530
  amusement park Y92.831
  apartment (co-op) — *see* Place of occurrence, residence, apartment
  assembly hall Y92.29
  bank Y92.510
  barn Y92.71
  baseball field Y92.320
  basketball court Y92.310

Place of occurrence — *continued*
  beach Y92.832
  boarding house — *see* Place of occurrence, residence, boarding house
  boat Y92.814
  bowling alley Y92.39
  bridge Y92.89
  building under construction Y92.61
  bus Y92.811
    station Y92.521
  cafe Y92.511
  campsite Y92.833
  campus — *see* Place of occurrence, school
  canal Y92.89
  car Y92.810
  casino Y92.59
  children's home — *see* Place of occurrence, residence, institutional, orphanage
  church Y92.22
  cinema Y92.26
  clubhouse Y92.29
  coal pit Y92.64
  college (community) Y92.214
  condominium — *see* Place of occurrence, residence, apartment
  construction area — *see* Place of occurrence, industrial and construction area
  convalescent home — *see* Place of occurrence, residence, institutional, nursing home
  court-house Y92.240
  cricket ground Y92.328
  cultural building Y92.258
    art gallery Y92.250
    museum Y92.251
    music hall Y92.252
    opera house Y92.253
    specified NEC Y92.258
    theater Y92.254
  dancehall Y92.252
  day nursery Y92.210
  dentist office Y92.531
  derelict house Y92.89
  desert Y92.820
  dock NOS Y92.89
  dockyard Y92.62
  doctor's office Y92.531
  dormitory — *see* Place of occurrence, residence, institutional, school dormitory
  dry dock Y92.62
  factory (building) (premises) Y92.63
  farm (land under cultivation) (outbuildings) Y92.79
    barn Y92.71
    chicken coop Y92.72
    field Y92.73
    hen house Y92.72
    house — *see* Place of occurrence, residence, house
    orchard Y92.74
    specified NEC Y92.79
  football field Y92.321
  forest Y92.821
  freeway Y92.411
  gallery Y92.250
  garage (commercial) Y92.59
    boarding house Y92.044
    military base Y92.135
    mobile home Y92.025
    nursing home Y92.124
    orphanage Y92.114
    private house Y92.015
    reform school Y92.155
  gas station Y92.524
  gasworks Y92.69
  golf course Y92.39
  gravel pit Y92.64
  grocery Y92.512
  gymnasium Y92.39
  handball court Y92.318
  harbor Y92.89
  harness racing course Y92.39
  healthcare provider office Y92.531
  highway (interstate) Y92.411
  hill Y92.828

Place of occurrence — *continued*
  hockey rink Y92.330
  home — *see* Place of occurrence, residence
  hospice — *see* Place of occurrence, residence, institutional, nursing home
  hospital Y92.239
    cafeteria Y92.233
    corridor Y92.232
    operating room Y92.234
    patient
      bathroom Y92.231
      room Y92.230
    specified NEC Y92.238
  hotel Y92.59
  house (*see also* Place of occurrence, residence)
    abandoned Y92.89
    under construction Y92.61
  industrial and construction area (yard) Y92.69
    building under construction Y92.61
    dock Y92.62
    dry dock Y92.62
    factory Y92.63
    gasworks Y92.69
    mine Y92.64
    oil rig Y92.65
    pit Y92.64
    power station Y92.69
    shipyard Y92.62
    specified NEC Y92.69
    tunnel under construction Y92.69
    workshop Y92.69
  kindergarten Y92.211
  lacrosse field Y92.328
  lake Y92.828
  library Y92.241
  mall Y92.59
  market Y92.512
  marsh Y92.828
  military
    base — *see* Place of occurrence, residence, institutional, military base
    training ground Y92.84
  mine Y92.64
  mosque Y92.22
  motel Y92.59
  motorway (interstate) Y92.411
  mountain Y92.828
  movie-house Y92.26
  museum Y92.251
  music-hall Y92.252
  not applicable Y92.9
  nuclear power station Y92.69
  nursing home — *see* Place of occurrence, residence, institutional, nursing home
  office building Y92.59
  offshore installation Y92.65
  oil rig Y92.65
  old people's home — *see* Place of occurrence, residence, institutional, specified NEC
  opera-house Y92.253
  orphanage — *see* Place of occurrence, residence, institutional, orphanage
  outpatient surgery center Y92.530
  park (public) Y92.830
    amusement Y92.831
  parking garage Y92.89
    lot Y92.481
  pavement Y92.480
  physician office Y92.531
  polo field Y92.328
  pond Y92.828
  post office Y92.242
  power station Y92.69
  prairie Y92.828
  prison — *see* Place of occurrence, residence, institutional, prison
  public
    administration building Y92.248
      city hall Y92.243
      courthouse Y92.240
      library Y92.241
      post office Y92.242
      specified NEC Y92.248

Place of occurrence — *continued*
trade area— *continued*
television station Y92.59
warehouse Y92.59
trailer park, residential — *see* Place of occurrence, residence, mobile home
trailer site NOS Y92.89
train Y92.815
station Y92.522
truck Y92.812
tunnel under construction Y92.69
university Y92.214
urgent (health) care center Y92.532
vehicle (transport) Y92.818
airplane Y92.813
boat Y92.814
bus Y92.811
car Y92.810
specified NEC Y92.818
subway car Y92.816
train Y92.815
truck Y92.812
warehouse Y92.59
water reservoir Y92.89
wilderness area Y92.828
desert Y92.820
forest Y92.821
marsh Y92.828
mountain Y92.828
prairie Y92.828
specified NEC Y92.828
swamp Y92.828
workshop Y92.69
yard, private Y92.096
boarding house Y92.046
single family house Y92.017
mobile home Y92.027
youth center Y92.29
zoo (zoological garden) Y92.834
Plumbism — *see* Table of Drugs and Chemicals, lead
Poisoning (accidental) (by) (*see also* Table of Drugs and Chemicals)
by plant, thorns, spines, sharp leaves or other mechanisms NEC X58
carbon monoxide
generated by
motor vehicle — *see* Accident, transport
watercraft (in transit) (not in transit) V93.89
ferry boat V93.81
fishing boat V93.82
jet skis V93.83
liner V93.81
merchant ship V93.80
passenger ship V93.81
powered craft NEC V93.83
caused by injection of poisons into skin by plant thorns, spines, sharp leaves X58
marine or sea plants (venomous) X58
exhaust gas
generated by
motor vehicle — *see* Accident, transport
watercraft (in transit) (not in transit) V93.89
ferry boat V93.81
fishing boat V93.82
jet skis V93.83
liner V93.81
merchant ship V93.80
passenger ship V93.81
powered craft NEC V93.83
fumes or smoke due to
explosion (*see also* Explosion) W40.9
fire — *see* Exposure, fire
ignition — *see* Ignition
gas
in legal intervention — *see* Legal, intervention, gas
legal execution Y35.91
in war operations — *see* War operations
legal
execution Y35.91
intervention by gas — *see* Legal, intervention, gas

Powder burn (by) (from)
airgun W34.110
BB gun W34.110
firearm NEC W34.19
gas, air or spring-operated gun NEC W34.118
handgun W32.1
hunting rifle W33.12
larger firearm W33.10
specified NEC W33.19
machine gun W33.13
paintball gun W34.111
pellet gun W34.110
shotgun W33.11
Very pistol [flare] W34.19
Premature cessation (of) **surgical and medical care** Y66
Privation (food) (water) X58
Procedure (operation)
correct, on wrong side or body part (wrong side) (wrong site) Y65.53
intended for another patient done on wrong patient Y65.52
performed on patient not scheduled for surgery Y65.52
performed on wrong patient Y65.52
wrong, performed on correct patient Y65.51
Prolonged
sitting in transport vehicle — *see* Travel, by type of vehicle
stay in
high altitude as cause of anoxia, barodontalgia, barotitis or hypoxia W94.11
weightless environment X52
Pulling, excessive — *see* Overexertion
Puncture, puncturing (*see also* Contact, with, by type of object or machine)
by
plant thorns, spines, sharp leaves or other mechanisms NEC W60
during medical or surgical treatment as misadventure — *see* Misadventure, cut, by type of procedure
Pushed, pushing (accidental) (injury in) (overexertion) (*see also* Overexertion)
by other person(s) (accidental) W51
with fall W03
due to ice or snow W00.0
as, or caused by, a crowd or human stampede (with fall) W52
before moving object NEC Y02.8
motor vehicle Y02.0
subway train Y02.1
train Y02.1
from
high place NEC
in accidental circumstances W17.89
stated as
intentional, homicide (attempt) Y01
undetermined whether accidental or intentional Y30
transport vehicle NEC (*see also* Accident, transport) V89.9
stated as
intentional, homicide (attempt) Y08.89

R

Radiation (exposure to)
arc lamps W89.0
atomic power plant (malfunction) NEC W88.1
complication of or abnormal reaction to medical radiotherapy Y84.2
electromagnetic, ionizing W88.0
gamma rays W88.1
in
war operations (from or following nuclear explosion) — *see* War operations
inadvertent exposure of patient (receiving test or therapy) Y63.3
infrared (heaters and lamps) W90.1
excessive heat from W92

Radiation— *continued*
ionized, ionizing (particles, artificially accelerated)
radioisotopes W88.1
specified NEC W88.8
x-rays W88.0
isotopes, radioactive — *see* Radiation, radioactive isotopes
laser(s) W90.2
in war operations — *see* War operations
misadventure in medical care Y63.2
light sources (man-made visible and ultraviolet) W89.9
natural X32
specified NEC W89.8
tanning bed W89.1
welding light W89.0
man-made visible light W89.9
specified NEC W89.8
tanning bed W89.1
welding light W89.0
microwave W90.8
misadventure in medical or surgical procedure Y63.2
natural NEC X39.08
radon X39.01
overdose (in medical or surgical procedure) Y63.2
radar W90.0
radioactive isotopes (any) W88.1
atomic power plant malfunction W88.1
misadventure in medical or surgical treatment Y63.2
radiofrequency W90.0
radium NEC W88.1
sun X32
ultraviolet (light) (man-made) W89.9
natural X32
specified NEC W89.8
tanning bed W89.1
welding light W89.0
welding arc, torch, or light W89.0
excessive heat from W92
x-rays (hard) (soft) W88.0
Range disease W94.11
Rape (attempted) T74.2-
Rat bite W53.11
Reaction, abnormal to medical procedure (*see also* Complication of or following, by type of procedure) Y84.9
with misadventure — *see* Misadventure
biologicals — *see* Table of Drugs and Chemicals
drugs — *see* Table of Drugs and Chemicals
vaccine — *see* Table of Drugs and Chemicals
Recoil
airgun W34.110
BB gun W34.110
firearm NEC W34.19
gas, air or spring-operated gun NEC W34.118
handgun W32.1
hunting rifle W33.12
larger firearm W33.10
specified NEC W33.19
machine gun W33.13
paintball gun W34.111
pellet W34.110
shotgun W33.11
Very pistol [flare] W34.19
Reduction in
atmospheric pressure — *see* Air, pressure, change
Rock falling on or hitting (accidentally) (person) W20.8
in cave-in W20.0
Run over (accidentally) (by)
animal (not being ridden) NEC W55.89
machinery — *see* Contact, with, by specified type of machine
transport vehicle NEC (*see also* Accident, transport) V09.9
intentional homicide (attempt) Y03.0
motor NEC V09.20
intentional homicide (attempt) Y03.0
Running
before moving object X81.8
motor vehicle X81.0

Running off, away
animal (being ridden) (*see also* Accident, transport) V80.918
not being ridden W55.89
animal-drawn vehicle NEC (*see also* Accident, transport) V80.928
highway, road(way), street
transport vehicle NEC (*see also* Accident, transport) V89.9
Rupture pressurized devices — *see* Explosion, by type of device

S

Saturnism — *see* Table of Drugs and Chemicals, lead
Scald, scalding (accidental) (by) (from) (in) X19
air (hot) X14.1
gases (hot) X14.1
homicide (attempt) — *see* Assault, burning, hot object
inflicted by other person
stated as intentional, homicide (attempt) — *see* Assault, burning, hot object
liquid (boiling) (hot) NEC X12
stated as undetermined whether accidental or intentional Y27.2
suicide (attempt) X77.2
local application of externally applied substance in medical or surgical care Y63.5
metal (molten) (liquid) (hot) NEC X18
self-inflicted X77.9
stated as undetermined whether accidental or intentional Y27.8
steam X13.1
assault X98.0
stated as undetermined whether accidental or intentional Y27.0
suicide (attempt) X77.0
suicide (attempt) X77.9
vapor (hot) X13.1
assault X98.0
stated as undetermined whether accidental or intentional Y27.0
suicide (attempt) X77.0
Scratched by
cat W55.03
person(s) (accidentally) W50.4
with intent to injure or kill Y04.0
as, or caused by, a crowd or human stampede (with fall) W52
assault Y04.0
homicide (attempt) Y04.0
in
fight Y04.0
legal intervention
injuring
bystander Y35.892
law enforcement personnel Y35.891
suspect Y35.893
Seasickness T75.3
Self-harm NEC (*see also* External cause by type, undetermined whether accidental or intentional)
intentional — *see* Suicide
poisoning NEC — *see* Table of drugs and biologicals, accident
Self-inflicted (injury) NEC (*see also* External cause by type, undetermined whether accidental or intentional)
intentional — *see* Suicide
poisoning NEC — *see* Table of drugs and biologicals, accident
Sequelae (of)
accident NEC — *see* W00-X58 with 7th character S
assault (homicidal) (any means) — *see* X92-Y08 with 7th character S
homicide, attempt (any means) — *see* X92-Y08 with 7th character S
injury undetermined whether accidentally or purposely inflicted — *see* Y21-Y33 with 7th character S

Sequelae — *continued*
intentional self-harm (classifiable to X71-X83) — *see* X71-X83 with 7th character S
legal intervention — *see* Y35 with 7th character S
motor vehicle accident — *see* V00-V99 with 7th character S
suicide, attempt (any means) — *see* X71-X83 with 7th character S
transport accident — *see* V00-V99 with 7th character S
war operations — *see* War operations
Shock
electric — *see* Exposure, electric current
from electric appliance (any) (faulty) W86.8
domestic W86.0
suicide (attempt) X83.1
Shooting, shot (accidental(ly)) (*see also* Discharge, firearm, by type)
herself or himself — *see* Discharge, firearm by type, self-inflicted
homicide (attempt) — *see* Discharge, firearm by type, homicide
in war operations — *see* War operations
inflicted by other person — *see* Discharge, firearm by type, homicide
accidental — *see* Discharge, firearm, by type of firearm
legal
execution Y35.91
intervention — *see* Legal, intervention, firearm
self-inflicted — *see* Discharge, firearm by type, suicide
accidental — *see* Discharge, firearm, by type of firearm
suicide (attempt) — *see* Discharge, firearm by type, suicide
Shoving (accidentally) **by other person** — *see* Pushing, by other person
Sickness
alpine W94.11
motion — *see* Motion
mountain W94.11
Sinking (accidental)
watercraft (causing drowning, submersion) (*see also* Drowning, due to, accident to, watercraft, sinking)
causing injury except drowning or submersion B — *see* Accident, watercraft, causing, injury NEC
Siriasis X32
Slashed wrists — *see* Cut, self-inflicted
Slipping (accidental) (on same level) (with fall) W01.0
on
ice W00.0
with skates — *see* Accident, transport, pedestrian, conveyance
mud W01.0
oil W01.0
snow W00.0
with skis — *see* Accident, transport, pedestrian, conveyance
surface (slippery) (wet) NEC W01.0
without fall W18.40
due to
specified NEC W18.49
stepping from one level to another W18.43
stepping into hole or opening W18.42
stepping on object W18.41
Sliver, wood, contact with W45.8
Smoldering (due to fire) — *see* Exposure, fire
Sodomy (attempted) **by force** T74.2-
Sound waves (causing injury) W42.9
supersonic W42.0
Splinter, contact with W45.8
Stab, stabbing B *see* Cut
Starvation X58
Status of external cause Y99.9
child assisting in compenstated work for family Y99.8
civilian activity done for financial or other compensation Y99.0
civilian activity done for income or pay Y99.0

Status of external cause — *continued*
family member assisting in compensated work for other family member Y99.8
hobby not done for income Y99.8
leisure activity Y99.8
military activity Y99.1
off-duty activity of military personnel Y99.8
recreation or sport not for income or while a student Y99.8
specified NEC Y99.8
student activity Y99.8
volunteer activity Y99.2
Stepped on
by
animal (not being ridden) NEC W55.89
crowd or human stampede W52
person W50.0
Stepping on
object W22.8
with fall W18.31
sports equipment W21.9
stationary W22.09
sports equipment W21.89
person W51
by crowd or human stampede W52
sports equipment W21.9
Sting
arthropod, nonvenomous W57
insect, nonvenomous W57
Storm (cataclysmic) B — *see* Forces of nature, cataclysmic storm
Straining, excessive — *see* Overexertion
Strangling — *see* Strangulation
Strangulation (accidental) — *see* category T71
Strenuous movements — *see* Repetitive movements
Striking against
airbag (automobile) W22.10
driver side W22.11
front passenger side W22.12
specified NEC W22.19
bottom when
diving or jumping into water (in) W16.822
causing drowning W16.821
from boat W16.722
causing drowning W16.721
natural body W16.622
causing drowning W16.821
swimming pool W16.522
causing drowning W16.521
falling into water (in) W16.322
causing drowning W16.321
fountain — *see* Striking against, bottom when, falling into water, specified NEC
natural body W16.122
causing drowning W16.121
reservoir — *see* Striking against, bottom when, falling into water, specified NEC
specified NEC W16.322
causing drowning W16.321
swimming pool W16.022
causing drowning W16.021
diving board (swimming-pool) W21.4
object W22.8
with
drowning or submersion — *see* Drowning
fall — *see* Fall, due to, bumping against, object
caused by crowd or human stampede (with fall) W52
furniture W22.03
lamppost W22.02
sports equipment W21.9
stationary W22.09
sports equipment W21.89
wall W22.01
person(s) W51
with fall W03
due to ice or snow W00.0
as, or caused by, a crowd or human stampede (with fall) W52
assault Y04.2
homicide (attempt) Y04.2
sports equipment W21.9

Striking against— *continued*
  wall (when) W22.01
    diving or jumping into water (in) W16.832
      causing drowning W16.831
      swimming pool W16.532
        causing drowning W16.531
    falling into water (in) W16.332
      causing drowning W16.331
      fountain — *see* Striking against, wall when,
        falling into water, specified NEC
      natural body W16.132
        causing drowning W16.131
      reservoir — *see* Striking against, wall when,
        falling into water, specified NEC
      specified NEC W16.332
        causing drowning W16.331
      swimming pool W16.032
        causing drowning W16.031
  swimming pool (when) W22.042
    causing drowning W22.041
    diving or jumping into water W16.532
      causing drowning W16.531
    falling into water W16.032
      causing drowning W16.031
Struck (accidentally) **by**
  airbag (automobile) W22.10
    driver side W22.11
    front passenger side W22.12
    specified NEC W22.19
  alligator W58.02
  animal (not being ridden) NEC W55.89
  avalanche B — *see* Landslide
  ball (hit) (thrown) W21.00
    assault Y08.09
    baseball W21.03
    basketball W21.05
    golf ball W21.04
    football W21.01
    soccer W21.02
    softball W21.07
    specified NEC W21.09
    volleyball W21.06
  bat or racquet
    baseball bat W21.11
      assault Y08.02
    golf club W21.13
      assault Y08.09
    specified NEC W21.19
      assault Y08.09
    tennis racquet W21.12
      assault Y08.09
  bullet (*see also* Discharge, firearm by type)
    in war operations — *see* War operations
  crocodile W58.12
  dog W54.1
  flare, Very pistol — *see* Discharge, firearm NEC
  hailstones X39.8
  hockey (ice)
    field
      puck W21.221
      stick W21.211
    puck W21.220
    stick W21.210
      assault Y08.01
  landslide B — *see* Landslide
  law-enforcement agent (on duty) — *see* Legal,
    intervention, manhandling
    with blunt object — *see* Legal, intervention,
      blunt object
  lightning — *see* subcategory T75.0
    causing fire — *see* Exposure, fire
  machine — *see* Contact, with, by type of machine
  mammal NEC W55.89
    marine W56.82
  marine animal W56.82
  missile
    firearm — *see* Discharge, firearm by type
    in war operations — *see* War operations, missile
  object W22.8
    blunt W22.8
      assault Y00
      suicide (attempt) X79

Struck (accidentally) **by**— *continued*
  object— *continued*
    blunt— *continued*
      undetermined whether accidental or
        intentional Y29
    falling W20.8
      from, in, on
        building W20.1
          burning (uncontrolled fire) X00.4
        cataclysmic
          earth surface movement NEC B — *see*
            Landslide
          storm B — *see* Forces of nature,
            cataclysmic storm
        cave-in W20.0
        earthquake X34
        machine (in operation) — *see* Contact,
          with, by type of machine
        structure W20.1
          burning X00.4
        transport vehicle (in motion) — *see*
          Accident, transport, by type of
          vehicle
        watercraft V93.49
          due to
            accident to craft V91.39
              powered craft V91.33
                ferry boat V91.31
                fishing boat V91.32
                jetskis V91.33
                liner V91.31
                merchant ship V91.30
                passenger ship V91.31
             unpowered craft V91.38
                canoe V91.35
                inflatable V91.36
                kayak V91.35
                sailboat V91.34
                surf-board V91.38
                windsurfer V91.38
            powered craft V93.43
              ferry boat V93.41
              fishing boat V93.42
              jetskis V93.43
              liner V93.41
              merchant ship V93.40
              passenger ship V93.41
            unpowered craft V93.48
              sailboat V93.44
              surf-board V93.48
              windsurfer V93.48
    moving NEC W20.8
    projected W20.8
      assault Y00
      in sports W21.9
        assault Y08.09
        ball W21.00
          baseball W21.03
          basketball W21.05
          football W21.01
          golf ball W21.04
          soccer W21.02
          softball W21.07
          specified NEC W21.09
          volleyball W21.06
        bat or racquet
          baseball bat W21.11
            assault Y08.02
          golf club W21.13
            assault Y08.09
          specified NEC W21.19
            assault Y08.09
          tennis racquet W21.12
            assault Y08.09
        hockey (ice)
          field
            puck W21.221
            stick W21.211
          puck W21.220
          stick W21.210
            assault Y08.01
      specified NEC W21.89
    set in motion by explosion — *see* Explosion

Struck (accidentally) **by**— *continued*
  object— *continued*
    thrown W20.8
      assault Y00
      in sports W21.9
        assault Y08.09
        ball W21.00
          baseball W21.03
          basketball W21.05
          football W21.01
          golf ball W21.04
          soccer W21.02
          soft ball W21.07
          specified NEC W21.09
          volleyball W21.06
        bat or racquet
          baseball bat W21.11
            assault Y08.02
          golf club W21.13
            assault Y08.09
          specified NEC W21.19
            assault Y08.09
          tennis racquet W21.12
            assault Y08.09
        hockey (ice)
          field
            puck W21.221
            stick W21.211
          puck W21.220
          stick W21.210
            assault Y08.01
        specified NEC W21.89
  other person(s) W50.0
    with
      blunt object W22.8
        intentional, homicide (attempt) Y00
        sports equipment W21.9
        undetermined whether accidental or
          intentional Y29
      fall W03
        due to ice or snow W00.0
    as, or caused by, a crowd or human stampede
      (with fall) W52
    assault Y04.2
    homicide (attempt) Y04.2
    in legal intervention
      injuring
        bystander Y35.812
        law enforcement personnel Y35.811
        suspect Y35.813
    sports equipment W21.9
  police (on duty) — *see* Legal, intervention,
    manhandling
    with blunt object — *see* Legal, intervention,
      blunt object
  sports equipment W21.9
    assault Y08.09
    ball W21.00
      baseball W21.03
      basketball W21.05
      football W21.01
      golf ball W21.04
      soccer W21.02
      soft ball W21.07
      specified NEC W21.09
      volleyball W21.06
    bat or racquet
      baseball bat W21.11
        assault Y08.02
      golf club W21.13
        assault Y08.09
      specified NEC W21.19
      tennis racquet W21.12
        assault Y08.09
    cleats (shoe) W21.31
    foot wear NEC W21.39
    football helmet W21.81
    hockey (ice)
      field
        puck W21.221
        stick W21.211
      puck W21.220
      stick W21.210

ICD-10-CM Tabular List of Diseases and Injuries

Chapter 1. Certain Infectious and Parasitic Diseases (A00-B99)

INCLUDES diseases generally recognized as communicable or transmissible
Use additional code for any associated drug resistance (Z16)

EXCLUDES 1 carrier or suspected carrier of infectious disease (Z22-)
certain localized infections—see body system-related chapters
infectious and parasitic diseases complicating pregnancy, childbirth and the puerperium (O98-)
influenza and other acute respiratory infections (J00-J22)

EXCLUDES 2 infectious and parasitic diseases specific to the perinatal period (P35-P39)

This chapter contains the following blocks:
A00-A09 Intestinal infectious diseases
A15-A19 Tuberculosis
A20-A28 Certain zoonotic bacterial diseases
A30-A49 Other bacterial diseases
A50-A64 Infections with a predominantly sexual mode of transmission
A65-A69 Other spirochetal diseases
A70-A74 Other diseases caused by chlamydiae
A75-A79 Rickettsioses
A80-A89 Viral infections of the central nervous system
A90-A99 Arthropod-borne viral fevers and viral hemorrhagic fevers
B00-B09 Viral infections characterized by skin and mucous membrane lesions
B10 Other human herpesviruses
B15-B19 Viral hepatitis
B20 Human immunodeficiency virus [HIV] disease
B25-B34 Other viral diseases
B35-B49 Mycoses
B50-B64 Protozoal diseases
B65-B83 Helminthiases
B85-B89 Pediculosis, acariasis and other infestations
B90-B94 Sequelae of infectious and parasitic diseases
B95-B97 Bacterial, viral and other infectious agents
B99 Other infectious diseases

Intestinal Infectious Diseases (A00-A09)

✓4ᵗʰ A00 Cholera
    A00.0 Cholera due to Vibrio cholerae 01, biovar cholerae
        Classical cholera
    A00.1 Cholera due to Vibrio cholerae 01, biovar eltor
        Cholera eltor
    A00.9 Cholera, unspecified

✓4ᵗʰ A01 Typhoid and paratyphoid fevers
  ✓5ᵗʰ A01.0 Typhoid fever
      Infection due to Salmonella typhi
      A01.00 Typhoid fever, unspecified
      A01.01 Typhoid meningitis
      A01.02 Typhoid fever with heart involvement
        Typhoid endocarditis
        Typhoid myocarditis
      A01.03 Typhoid pneumonia
      A01.04 Typhoid arthritis
      A01.05 Typhoid osteomyelitis
      A01.09 Typhoid fever with other complications
    A01.1 Paratyphoid fever A
    A01.2 Paratyphoid fever B
    A01.3 Paratyphoid fever C
    A01.4 Paratyphoid fever, unspecified
      Infection due to Salmonella paratyphi NOS

✓4ᵗʰ A02 Other salmonella infections
    INCLUDES infection or foodborne intoxication due to any Salmonella species other than S. typhi and S. paratyphi
    A02.0 Salmonella enteritis
      Salmonellosis
    A02.1 Salmonella sepsis
  ✓5ᵗʰ A02.2 Localized salmonella infections
      A02.20 Localized salmonella infection, unspecified
      A02.21 Salmonella meningitis
      A02.22 Salmonella pneumonia
      A02.23 Salmonella arthritis
      A02.24 Salmonella osteomyelitis
      A02.25 Salmonella pyelonephritis
        Salmonella tubulo-interstitial nephropathy

      A02.29 Salmonella with other localized infection
    A02.8 Other specified salmonella infections
    A02.9 Salmonella infection, unspecified

✓4ᵗʰ A03 Shigellosis
    A03.0 Shigellosis due to Shigella dysenteriae
      Group A shigellosis [Shiga-Kruse dysentery]
    A03.1 Shigellosis due to Shigella flexneri
      Group B shigellosis
    A03.2 Shigellosis due to Shigella boydii
      Group C shigellosis
    A03.3 Shigellosis due to Shigella sonnei
      Group D shigellosis
    A03.8 Other shigellosis
    A03.9 Shigellosis, unspecified
      Bacillary dysentery NOS

✓4ᵗʰ A04 Other bacterial intestinal infections
    EXCLUDES 1 bacterial foodborne intoxications, NEC (A05-)
        tuberculous enteritis (A18.32)
    A04.0 Enteropathogenic Escherichia coli infection
    A04.1 Enterotoxigenic Escherichia coli infection
    A04.2 Enteroinvasive Escherichia coli infection
    A04.3 Enterohemorrhagic Escherichia coli infection
    A04.4 Other intestinal Escherichia coli infections
      Escherichia coli enteritis NOS
    A04.5 Campylobacter enteritis
    A04.6 Enteritis due to Yersinia enterocolitica
      EXCLUDES 1 extraintestinal yersiniosis (A28.2)
    A04.7 Enterocolitis due to Clostridium difficile
      Foodborne intoxication by Clostridium difficile
      Pseudomembraneous colitis
    A04.8 Other specified bacterial intestinal infections
    A04.9 Bacterial intestinal infection, unspecified
      Bacterial enteritis NOS

✓4ᵗʰ A05 Other bacterial foodborne intoxications, not elsewhere classified
    EXCLUDES 1 Escherichia coli infection (A04.0-A04.4)
        foodborne intoxication by Clostridium difficile (A04.7)
        listeriosis (A32-)
        salmonella foodborne intoxication and infection (A02-)
        toxic effect of noxious foodstuffs (T61-T62)
    A05.0 Foodborne staphylococcal intoxication
    A05.1 Botulism food poisoning
      Botulism NOS
      Classical foodborne intoxication due to Clostridium botulinum
      EXCLUDES 1 infant botulism (A48.51)
        wound botulism (A48.52)
    A05.2 Foodborne Clostridium perfringens [Clostridium welchii] intoxication
      Enteritis necroticans
      Pig-bel
    A05.3 Foodborne Vibrio parahaemolyticus intoxication
    A05.4 Foodborne Bacillus cereus intoxication
    A05.5 Foodborne Vibrio vulnificus intoxication
    A05.8 Other specified bacterial foodborne intoxications
    A05.9 Bacterial foodborne intoxication, unspecified

✓4ᵗʰ A06 Amebiasis
    INCLUDES infection due to Entamoeba histolytica
    EXCLUDES 1 other protozoal intestinal diseases (A07-)
    EXCLUDES 2 acanthamebiasis (B60.1-)
        Naegleriasis (B60.2)
    A06.0 Acute amebic dysentery
      Acute amebiasis
      Intestinal amebiasis NOS
    A06.1 Chronic intestinal amebiasis
    A06.2 Amebic nondysenteric colitis
    A06.3 Ameboma of intestine
      Ameboma NOS
    A06.4 Amebic liver abscess
      Hepatic amebiasis
    A06.5 Amebic lung abscess
      Amebic abscess of lung (and liver)
    A06.6 Amebic brain abscess
      Amebic abscess of brain (and liver) (and lung)
    A06.7 Cutaneous amebiasis

✓ Appropriate additional character required   ✓x7ᵗʰ Requires 7th character, placeholder x must fill empty characters

Certain Infectious and Parasitic Diseases

A06.8–A18.16

☑5ᵗʰ **A06.8 Amebic infection of other sites**

     A06.81 Amebic cystitis

     A06.82 Other amebic genitourinary infections
         Amebic balanitis
         Amebic vesiculitis
         Amebic vulvovaginitis

     A06.89 Other amebic infections
         Amebic appendicitis
         Amebic splenic abscess

A06.9 Amebiasis, unspecified

☑4ᵗʰ **A07 Other protozoal intestinal diseases**

     A07.0 Balantidiasis
         Balantidial dysentery

     A07.1 Giardiasis [lambliasis]

     A07.2 Cryptosporidiosis

     A07.3 Isosporiasis
         Infection due to Isospora belli and Isospora hominis
         Intestinal coccidiosis
         Isosporosis

     A07.4 Cyclosporiasis

     A07.8 Other specified protozoal intestinal diseases
         Intestinal microsporidiosis
         Intestinal trichomoniasis
         Sarcocystosis
         Sarcosporidiosis

     A07.9 Protozoal intestinal disease, unspecified
         Flagellate diarrhea   Protozoal diarrhea
         Protozoal colitis   Protozoal dysentery

☑4ᵗʰ **A08 Viral and other specified intestinal infections**

     EXCLUDES 1   *influenza with involvement of gastrointestinal tract (J09.03, J09.13, J10.2, J11.2)*

     A08.0 Rotaviral enteritis

☑5ᵗʰ **A08.1 Acute gastroenteropathy due to Norwalk agent and other small round viruses**

     A08.11 Acute gastroenteropathy due to Norwalk agent
         Acute gastroenteropathy due to Norovirus
         Acute gastroenteropathy due to Norwalk-like agent

     A08.19 Acute gastroenteropathy due to other small round viruses
         Acute gastroenteropathy due to small round virus [SRV] NOS

     A08.2 Adenoviral enteritis

☑5ᵗʰ **A08.3 Other viral enteritis**

     A08.31 Calicivirus enteritis

     A08.32 Astrovirus enteritis

     A08.39 Other viral enteritis
         Coxsackie virus enteritis
         Echovirus enteritis
         Enterovirus enteritis NEC
         Torovirus enteritis

     A08.4 Viral intestinal infection, unspecified
         Viral enteritis NOS
         Viral gastroenteritis NOS
         Viral gastroenteropathy NOS

     A08.8 Other specified intestinal infections

A09 Infectious gastroenteritis and colitis, unspecified
     Infectious colitis NOS
     Infectious enteritis NOS
     Infectious gastroenteritis NOS

     EXCLUDES 1   *colitis NOS (K52.9)*
         diarrhea NOS (R19.7)
         enteritis NOS (K52.9)
         gastroenteritis NOS (K52.9)
         noninfective gastroenteritis and colitis, unspecified (K52.9)

Tuberculosis (A15-A19)

INCLUDES   infections due to Mycobacterium tuberculosis and Mycobacterium bovis

EXCLUDES 1   *congenital tuberculosis (P37.0)*
     pneumoconiosis associated with tuberculosis, any type in A15 (J65)
     sequelae of tuberculosis (B90-)
     silicotuberculosis (J65)

☑4ᵗʰ **A15 Respiratory tuberculosis**

     A15.0 Tuberculosis of lung
         Tuberculous bronchiectasis
         Tuberculous fibrosis of lung
         Tuberculous pneumonia
         Tuberculous pneumothorax

     A15.4 Tuberculosis of intrathoracic lymph nodes
         Tuberculosis of hilar lymph nodes
         Tuberculosis of mediastinal lymph nodes
         Tuberculosis of tracheobronchial lymph nodes
         EXCLUDES 1   *tuberculosis specified as primary (A15.7)*

     A15.5 Tuberculosis of larynx, trachea and bronchus
         Tuberculosis of bronchus
         Tuberculosis of glottis
         Tuberculosis of larynx
         Tuberculosis of trachea

     A15.6 Tuberculous pleurisy
         Tuberculosis of pleura Tuberculous empyema
         EXCLUDES 1   *primary respiratory tuberculosis (A15.7)*

     A15.7 Primary respiratory tuberculosis

     A15.8 Other respiratory tuberculosis
         Mediastinal tuberculosis
         Nasopharyngeal tuberculosis
         Tuberculosis of nose
         Tuberculosis of sinus [any nasal]

     A15.9 Respiratory tuberculosis unspecified

☑4ᵗʰ **A17 Tuberculosis of nervous system**

     A17.0 Tuberculous meningitis
         Tuberculosis of meninges (cerebral)(spinal)
         Tuberculous leptomeningitis
         EXCLUDES 1   *tuberculous meningoencephalitis (A17.82)*

     A17.1 Meningeal tuberculoma
         Tuberculoma of meninges (cerebral) (spinal)
         EXCLUDES 2   *tuberculoma of brain and spinal cord (A17.81)*

☑5ᵗʰ **A17.8 Other tuberculosis of nervous system**

     A17.81 Tuberculoma of brain and spinal cord
         Tuberculous abscess of brain and spinal cord

     A17.82 Tuberculous meningoencephalitis
         Tuberculous myelitis

     A17.83 Tuberculous neuritis
         Tuberculous mononeuropathy

     A17.89 Other tuberculosis of nervous system
         Tuberculous polyneuropathy

     A17.9 Tuberculosis of nervous system, unspecified

☑4ᵗʰ **A18 Tuberculosis of other organs**

☑5ᵗʰ **A18.0 Tuberculosis of bones and joints**

     A18.01 Tuberculosis of spine
         Pott's disease or curvature of spine
         Tuberculous arthritis
         Tuberculous osteomyelitis of spine
         Tuberculous spondylitis

     A18.02 Tuberculous arthritis of other joints
         Tuberculosis of hip (joint)
         Tuberculosis of knee (joint)

     A18.03 Tuberculosis of other bones
         Tuberculous mastoiditis
         Tuberculous osteomyelitis

     A18.09 Other musculoskeletal tuberculosis
         Tuberculous myositis
         Tuberculous synovitis
         Tuberculous tenosynovitis

☑5ᵗʰ **A18.1 Tuberculosis of genitourinary system**

     A18.10 Tuberculosis of genitourinary system, unspecified

     A18.11 Tuberculosis of kidney and ureter

     A18.12 Tuberculosis of bladder

     A18.13 Tuberculosis of other urinary organs
         Tuberculous urethritis

     A18.14 Tuberculosis of prostate

     A18.15 Tuberculosis of other male genital organs

     A18.16 Tuberculosis of cervix

EXCLUDES 1   Not coded here   *EXCLUDES 2*   Not included here   *Manifestation Code*

A18.17   **Tuberculous female pelvic inflammatory disease**
Tuberculous endometritis
Tuberculous oophoritis and salpingitis

A18.18   **Tuberculosis of other female genital organs**
Tuberculous ulceration of vulva

A18.2   **Tuberculous peripheral lymphadenopathy**
Tuberculous adenitis

> EXCLUDES 2   *tuberculosis of bronchial and mediastinal lymph*
>   *nodes (A15.4)*
> *tuberculosis of mesenteric and retroperitoneal lymph*
>   *nodes (A18.39)*
> *tuberculous tracheobronchial adenopathy (A15.4)*

✓5th **A18.3**   **Tuberculosis of intestines, peritoneum and mesenteric glands**

A18.31   **Tuberculous peritonitis**
Tuberculous ascites

A18.32   **Tuberculous enteritis**
Tuberculosis of anus and rectum
Tuberculosis of intestine (large) (small)

A18.39   **Retroperitoneal tuberculosis**
Tuberculosis of mesenteric glands
Tuberculosis of retroperitoneal (lymph glands)

A18.4   **Tuberculosis of skin and subcutaneous tissue**
Erythema induratum, tuberculous
Lupus excedens
Lupus vulgaris NOS
Lupus vulgaris of eyelid
Scrofuloderma
Tuberculosis of external ear

> EXCLUDES 2   *lupus erythematosus (L93-)*
> *lupus NOS (M32.9)*
> *systemic (M32-)*

✓5th **A18.5**   **Tuberculosis of eye**

> EXCLUDES 2   *lupus vulgaris of eyelid (A18.4)*

A18.50   **Tuberculosis of eye, unspecified**

A18.51   **Tuberculous episcleritis**

A18.52   **Tuberculous keratitis**
Tuberculous interstitial keratitis
Tuberculous keratoconjunctivitis (interstitial)
     (phlyctenular)

A18.53   **Tuberculous chorioretinitis**

A18.54   **Tuberculous iridocyclitis**

A18.59   **Other tuberculosis of eye**
Tuberculous conjunctivitis

A18.6   **Tuberculosis of (inner) (middle) ear**
Tuberculous otitis media

> EXCLUDES 2   *tuberculosis of external ear (A18.4)*
> *tuberculous mastoiditis (A18.03)*

A18.7   **Tuberculosis of adrenal glands**
Tuberculous Addison's disease

✓5th **A18.8**   **Tuberculosis of other specified organs**

A18.81   **Tuberculosis of thyroid gland**

A18.82   **Tuberculosis of other endocrine glands**
Tuberculosis of pituitary gland
Tuberculosis of thymus gland

A18.83   **Tuberculosis of digestive tract organs, not elsewhere classified**

> EXCLUDES 1   *tuberculosis of intestine (A18.32)*

A18.84   **Tuberculosis of heart**
Tuberculous cardiomyopathy
Tuberculous endocarditis
Tuberculous myocarditis
Tuberculous pericarditis

A18.85   **Tuberculosis of spleen**

A18.89   **Tuberculosis of other sites**
Tuberculosis of muscle
Tuberculous cerebral arteritis

✓4th **A19**   **Miliary tuberculosis**

> INCLUDES   disseminated tuberculosis
> generalized tuberculosis
> tuberculous polyserositis

A19.0   **Acute miliary tuberculosis of a single specified site**

A19.1   **Acute miliary tuberculosis of multiple sites**

A19.2   **Acute miliary tuberculosis, unspecified**

A19.8   **Other miliary tuberculosis**

A19.9   **Miliary tuberculosis, unspecified**

Certain zoonotic bacterial diseases (A20-A28)

✓4th **A20**   **Plague**

> INCLUDES   infection due to Yersinia pestis

A20.0   **Bubonic plague**

A20.1   **Cellulocutaneous plague**

A20.2   **Pneumonic plague**

A20.3   **Plague meningitis**

A20.7   **Septicemic plague**

A20.8   **Other forms of plague**
Abortive plague
Asymptomatic plague
Pestis minor

A20.9   **Plague, unspecified**

✓4th **A21**   **Tularemia**

> INCLUDES   deer-fly fever
> infection due to Francisella tularensis
> rabbit fever

A21.0   **Ulceroglandular tularemia**

A21.1   **Oculoglandular tularemia**
Ophthalmic tularemia

A21.2   **Pulmonary tularemia**

A21.3   **Gastrointestinal tularemia**
Abdominal tularemia

A21.7   **Generalized tularemia**

A21.8   **Other forms of tularemia**

A21.9   **Tularemia, unspecified**

✓4th **A22**   **Anthrax**

> INCLUDES   infection due to Bacillus anthracis

A22.0   **Cutaneous anthrax**
Malignant carbuncle
Malignant pustule

A22.1   **Pulmonary anthrax**
Inhalation anthrax
Ragpicker's disease
Woolsorter's disease

A22.2   **Gastrointestinal anthrax**

A22.7   **Anthrax sepsis**

A22.8   **Other forms of anthrax**
Anthrax meningitis

A22.9   **Anthrax, unspecified**

✓4th **A23**   **Brucellosis**
Malta fever
Mediterranean fever
Undulant fever

A23.0   **Brucellosis due to Brucella melitensis**

A23.1   **Brucellosis due to Brucella abortus**

A23.2   **Brucellosis due to Brucella suis**

A23.3   **Brucellosis due to Brucella canis**

A23.8   **Other brucellosis**

A23.9   **Brucellosis, unspecified**

✓4th **A24**   **Glanders and melioidosis**

A24.0   **Glanders**
Infection due to Pseudomonas mallei
Malleus

A24.1   **Acute and fulminating melioidosis**
Melioidosis pneumonia
Melioidosis sepsis

A24.2   **Subacute and chronic melioidosis**

A24.3   **Other melioidosis**

A24.9   **Melioidosis, unspecified**
Infection due to Pseudomonas pseudomallei NOS
Whitmore's disease

✓4th **A25**   **Rat-bite fevers**

A25.0   **Spirillosis**
Sodoku

A25.1   **Streptobacillosis**
Epidemic arthritic erythema
Haverhill fever
Streptobacillary rat-bite fever

A25.9   **Rat-bite fever, unspecified**

✓4th **A26**   **Erysipeloid**

A26.0   **Cutaneous erysipeloid**
Erythema migrans

A26.7   **Erysipelothrix sepsis**

A26.8   **Other forms of erysipeloid**

☑ Appropriate additional character required   ☑x7th Requires 7th character, placeholder x must fill empty characters

A26.9   **Erysipeloid, unspecified**

☑4ᵗʰ **A27**   **Leptospirosis**

A27.0   **Leptospirosis icterohemorrhagica**
Leptospiral or spirochetal jaundice (hemorrhagic)
Weil's disease

☑5ᵗʰ   A27.8   **Other forms of leptospirosis**

A27.81   **Aseptic meningitis in leptospirosis**
A27.89   **Other forms of leptospirosis**

A27.9   **Leptospirosis, unspecified**

☑4ᵗʰ **A28**   **Other zoonotic bacterial diseases, not elsewhere classified**

A28.0   **Pasteurellosis**

A28.1   **Cat-scratch disease**
Cat-scratch fever

A28.2   **Extraintestinal yersiniosis**
EXCLUDES 1   *enteritis due to Yersinia enterocolitica (A04.6)*
plague (A20-)

A28.8   **Other specified zoonotic bacterial diseases, not elsewhere classified**

A28.9   **Zoonotic bacterial disease, unspecified**

Other bacterial diseases (A30-A49)

☑4ᵗʰ **A30**   **Leprosy [Hansen's disease]**
INCLUDES   infection due to Mycobacterium leprae
EXCLUDES 1   *sequelae of leprosy (B92)*

A30.0   **Indeterminate leprosy**
I leprosy

A30.1   **Tuberculoid leprosy**
TT leprosy

A30.2   **Borderline tuberculoid leprosy**
BT leprosy

A30.3   **Borderline leprosy**
BB leprosy

A30.4   **Borderline lepromatous leprosy**
BL leprosy

A30.5   **Lepromatous leprosy**
LL leprosy

A30.8   **Other forms of leprosy**

A30.9   **Leprosy, unspecified**

☑4ᵗʰ **A31**   **Infection due to other mycobacteria**
EXCLUDES 2   *leprosy (A30-)*
tuberculosis (A15-A19)

A31.0   **Pulmonary mycobacterial infection**
Infection due to Mycobacterium avium
Infection due to Mycobacterium intracellulare [Battey bacillus]
Infection due to Mycobacterium kansasii

A31.1   **Cutaneous mycobacterial infection**
Buruli ulcer
Infection due to Mycobacterium marinum
Infection due to Mycobacterium ulcerans

A31.2   **Disseminated mycobacterium avium-intracellulare complex (DMAC)**
MAC sepsis

A31.8   **Other mycobacterial infections**

A31.9   **Mycobacterial infection, unspecified**
Atypical mycobacterial infection NOS
Mycobacteriosis NOS

☑4ᵗʰ **A32**   **Listeriosis**
INCLUDES   listerial foodborne infection
EXCLUDES 1   *neonatal (disseminated) listeriosis (P37.2)*

A32.0   **Cutaneous listeriosis**

☑5ᵗʰ   A32.1   **Listerial meningitis and meningoencephalitis**

A32.11   **Listerial meningitis**
A32.12   **Listerial meningoencephalitis**

A32.7   **Listerial sepsis**

☑5ᵗʰ   A32.8   **Other forms of listeriosis**

A32.81   **Oculoglandular listeriosis**
A32.82   **Listerial endocarditis**
A32.89   **Other forms of listeriosis**
Listerial cerebral arteritis

A32.9   **Listeriosis, unspecified**

A33   **Tetanus neonatorum**

A34   **Obstetrical tetanus**

A35   **Other tetanus**
Tetanus NOS
EXCLUDES 1   *obstetrical tetanus (A34)*
tetanus neonatorum (A33)

☑4ᵗʰ **A36**   **Diphtheria**

A36.0   **Pharyngeal diphtheria**
Diphtheritic membranous angina
Tonsillar diphtheria

A36.1   **Nasopharyngeal diphtheria**

A36.2   **Laryngeal diphtheria**
Diphtheritic laryngotracheitis

A36.3   **Cutaneous diphtheria**
EXCLUDES 2   *erythrasma (L08.1)*

☑5ᵗʰ   A36.8   **Other diphtheria**

A36.81   **Diphtheritic cardiomyopathy**
Diphtheritic myocarditis
A36.82   **Diphtheritic radiculomyelitis**
A36.83   **Diphtheritic polyneuritis**
A36.84   **Diphtheritic tubulo-interstitial nephropathy**
A36.85   **Diphtheritic cystitis**
A36.86   **Diphtheritic conjunctivitis**
A36.89   **Other diphtheritic complications**
Diphtheritic peritonitis

A36.9   **Diphtheria, unspecified**

☑4ᵗʰ **A37**   **Whooping cough**

☑5ᵗʰ   A37.0   **Whooping cough due to Bordetella pertussis**

A37.00   **Whooping cough due to Bordetella pertussis without pneumonia**
A37.01   **Whooping cough due to Bordetella pertussis with pneumonia**

☑5ᵗʰ   A37.1   **Whooping cough due to Bordetella parapertussis**

A37.10   **Whooping cough due to Bordetella parapertussis without pneumonia**
A37.11   **Whooping cough due to Bordetella parapertussis with pneumonia**

☑5ᵗʰ   A37.8   **Whooping cough due to other Bordetella species**

A37.80   **Whooping cough due to other Bordetella species without pneumonia**
A37.81   **Whooping cough due to other Bordetella species with pneumonia**

☑5ᵗʰ   A37.9   **Whooping cough, unspecified species**

A37.90   **Whooping cough, unspecified species without pneumonia**
A37.91   **Whooping cough, unspecified species with pneumonia**

☑4ᵗʰ **A38**   **Scarlet fever**
INCLUDES   scarlatina
EXCLUDES 2   *streptococcal sore throat (J02.0)*

A38.0   **Scarlet fever with otitis media**
A38.1   **Scarlet fever with myocarditis**
A38.8   **Scarlet fever with other complications**
A38.9   **Scarlet fever, uncomplicated**
Scarlet fever, NOS

☑4ᵗʰ **A39**   **Meningococcal infection**

A39.0   **Meningococcal meningitis**

A39.1   **Waterhouse-Friderichsen syndrome**
Meningococcal hemorrhagic adrenalitis
Meningococcic adrenal syndrome

A39.2   **Acute meningococcemia**
A39.3   **Chronic meningococcemia**
A39.4   **Meningococcemia, unspecified**

☑5ᵗʰ   A39.5   **Meningococcal heart disease**

A39.50   **Meningococcal carditis, unspecified**
A39.51   **Meningococcal endocarditis**
A39.52   **Meningococcal myocarditis**
A39.53   **Meningococcal pericarditis**

☑5ᵗʰ   A39.8   **Other meningococcal infections**

A39.81   **Meningococcal encephalitis**
A39.82   **Meningococcal retrobulbar neuritis**
A39.83   **Meningococcal arthritis**
A39.84   **Postmeningococcal arthritis**

EXCLUDES 1   Not coded here   EXCLUDES 2   Not included here   *Manifestation Code*

A39.89 Other meningococcal infections
Meningococcal conjunctivitis

A39.9 Meningococcal infection, unspecified
Meningococcal disease NOS

☑4ᵗʰ **A40 Streptococcal sepsis**
Code first: postprocedural streptococcal sepsis (T81.4)
streptococcal sepsis during labor (O75.3)
streptococcal sepsis following abortion or ectopic or molar
pregnancy (O03-O07, O08.0)
streptococcal sepsis following immunization (T88.0)
streptococcal sepsis following infusion, transfusion or
therapeutic injection (T80.2-)

    EXCLUDES 1 *neonatal (P36.0-P36.1)*
puerperal sepsis (O85)
sepsis due to Streptococcus, group D (A41.81)

A40.0 Sepsis due to streptococcus, group A

A40.1 Sepsis due to streptococcus, group B

A40.3 Sepsis due to Streptococcus pneumoniae
Pneumococcal sepsis

A40.8 Other streptococcal sepsis

A40.9 Streptococcal sepsis, unspecified

☑4ᵗʰ **A41 Other sepsis**
Code first: postprocedural sepsis (T81.4)
sepsis during labor (O75.3)
sepsis following abortion, ectopic or molar pregnancy
(O03-O07, O08.0)
sepsis following immunization (T88.0)
sepsis following infusion, transfusion or therapeutic
injection (T80.2-)

    EXCLUDES 1 *bacteremia NOS (R78.81)*
neonatal (P36-)
puerperal sepsis (O85)
sepsis NOS (A41.9)
streptococcal sepsis (A40-)

    EXCLUDES 2 *sepsis (due to) (in) actinomycotic (A42.7)*
sepsis (due to) (in) anthrax (A22.7)
sepsis (due to) (in) candidal (B37.7)
sepsis (due to) (in) Erysipelothrix (A26.7)
sepsis (due to) (in) extraintestinal yersiniosis (A28.2)
sepsis (due to) (in) gonococcal (A54.86)
sepsis (due to) (in) herpesviral (B00.7)
sepsis (due to) (in) listerial (A32.7)
sepsis (due to) (in) melioidosis (A24.1)
sepsis (due to) (in) meningococcal (A39.2-A39.4)
sepsis (due to) (in) plague (A20.7)
sepsis (due to) (in) tularemia (A21.7)
toxic shock syndrome (A48.3)

A41.0 Sepsis due to Staphylococcus aureus

A41.1 Sepsis due to other specified staphylococcus
Coagulase negative staphylococcus sepsis
Sepsis due to other specified staphylococcus

A41.2 Sepsis due to unspecified staphylococcus

A41.3 Sepsis due to Hemophilus influenzae

A41.4 Sepsis due to anaerobes
    EXCLUDES 1 *gas gangrene (A48.0)*

☑5ᵗʰ **A41.5 Sepsis due to other Gram-negative organisms**
A41.50 Gram-negative sepsis, unspecified
Gram-negative sepsis NOS

A41.51 Sepsis due to Escherichia coli [E. coli]

A41.52 Sepsis due to Pseudomonas
Pseudomonas aeroginosa

A41.53 Sepsis due to Serratia

A41.59 Other Gram-negative sepsis

☑5ᵗʰ **A41.8 Other specified sepsis**
A41.81 Sepsis due to Enterococcus

A41.89 Other specified sepsis

A41.9 Sepsis, unspecified
Septicemia NOS

☑4ᵗʰ **A42 Actinomycosis**
    EXCLUDES 1 *actinomycetoma (B47.1)*

A42.0 Pulmonary actinomycosis

A42.1 Abdominal actinomycosis

A42.2 Cervicofacial actinomycosis

A42.7 Actinomycotic sepsis

☑5ᵗʰ **A42.8 Other forms of actinomycosis**
A42.81 Actinomycotic meningitis

A42.82 Actinomycotic encephalitis

A42.89 Other forms of actinomycosis

A42.9 Actinomycosis, unspecified

☑4ᵗʰ **A43 Nocardiosis**
A43.0 Pulmonary nocardiosis

A43.1 Cutaneous nocardiosis

A43.8 Other forms of nocardiosis

A43.9 Nocardiosis, unspecified

☑4ᵗʰ **A44 Bartonellosis**
A44.0 Systemic bartonellosis
Oroya fever

A44.1 Cutaneous and mucocutaneous bartonellosis
Verruga peruana

A44.8 Other forms of bartonellosis

A44.9 Bartonellosis, unspecified

A46 Erysipelas
    EXCLUDES 1 *postpartum or puerperal erysipelas (O86.89)*

☑4ᵗʰ **A48 Other bacterial diseases, not elsewhere classified**
    EXCLUDES 1 *actinomycetoma (B47.1)*

A48.0 Gas gangrene
Clostridial cellulitis
Clostridial myonecrosis

A48.1 Legionnaires' disease

A48.2 Nonpneumonic Legionnaires' disease [Pontiac fever]

A48.3 Toxic shock syndrome
Use additional code to identify the organism (B95, B96)
    EXCLUDES 1 *endotoxic shock NOS (R57.8)*
sepsis NOS (A41.9)

A48.4 Brazilian purpuric fever
Systemic Hemophilus aegyptius infection

☑5ᵗʰ **A48.5 Other specified botulism**
Non-foodborne intoxication due to toxins of Clostridium
botulinum [C. botulinum]
    EXCLUDES 1 *food poisoning due to toxins of Clostridium*
botulinum (A05.1)

A48.51 Infant botulism

A48.52 Wound botulism
Non-foodborne botulism NOS
Use additional code for associated wound

A48.8 Other specified bacterial diseases

☑4ᵗʰ **A49 Bacterial infection of unspecified site**
    EXCLUDES 1 *bacterial agents as the cause of diseases classified elsewhere*
(B95-B96)
chlamydial infection NOS (A74.9)
meningococcal infection NOS (A39.9)
rickettsial infection NOS (A79.9)
spirochetal infection NOS (A69.9)

A49.0 Staphylococcal infection, unspecified site

A49.1 Streptococcal infection, unspecified site

A49.2 Hemophilus influenzae infection, unspecified site

A49.3 Mycoplasma infection, unspecified site

A49.8 Other bacterial infections of unspecified site

A49.9 Bacterial infection, unspecified
    EXCLUDES 1 *bacteremia NOS (R78.81)*

Infections with a predominantly sexual mode of transmission (A50-A64)

    EXCLUDES 1 *human immunodeficiency virus [HIV] disease (B20)*
nonspecific and nongonococcal urethritis (N34.1)
Reiter's disease (M02.3-)

☑4ᵗʰ **A50 Congenital syphilis**
☑5ᵗʰ **A50.0 Early congenital syphilis, symptomatic**
Any congenital syphilitic condition specified as early or
manifest less than two years after birth.

A50.01 Early congenital syphilitic oculopathy

A50.02 Early congenital syphilitic osteochondropathy

A50.03 Early congenital syphilitic pharyngitis
Early congenital syphilitic laryngitis

A50.04 Early congenital syphilitic pneumonia

A50.05 Early congenital syphilitic rhinitis

A50.06 Early cutaneous congenital syphilis

A50.07 Early mucocutaneous congenital syphilis

A50.08 Early visceral congenital syphilis

A50.09 Other early congenital syphilis, symptomatic

☑ Appropriate additional character required   ✓x7ᵗʰ Requires 7th character, placeholder x must fill empty characters

Certain Infectious and Parasitic Diseases

A50.1–A53.0

A50.1   **Early congenital syphilis, latent**
Congenital syphilis without clinical manifestations, with positive serological reaction and negative spinal fluid test, less than two years after birth.

A50.2   **Early congenital syphilis, unspecified**
Congenital syphilis NOS less than two years after birth.

√5ᵗʰ   **A50.3**   **Late congenital syphilitic oculopathy**
EXCLUDES 1   *Hutchinson's triad (A50.53)*

     A50.30   **Late congenital syphilitic oculopathy, unspecified**

     A50.31   **Late congenital syphilitic interstitial keratitis**

     A50.32   **Late congenital syphilitic chorioretinitis**

     A50.39   **Other late congenital syphilitic oculopathy**

√5ᵗʰ   **A50.4**   **Late congenital neurosyphilis [juvenile neurosyphilis]**
Use additional code to identify any associated mental disorder
EXCLUDES 1   *Hutchinson's triad (A50.53)*

     A50.40   **Late congenital neurosyphilis, unspecified**
Juvenile neurosyphilis NOS

     A50.41   **Late congenital syphilitic meningitis**

     A50.42   **Late congenital syphilitic encephalitis**

     A50.43   **Late congenital syphilitic polyneuropathy**

     A50.44   **Late congenital syphilitic optic nerve atrophy**

     A50.45   **Juvenile general paresis**
Dementia paralytica juvenilis
Juvenile tabetoparetic neurosyphilis

     A50.49   **Other late congenital neurosyphilis**
Juvenile tabes dorsalis

√5ᵗʰ   **A50.5**   **Other late congenital syphilis, symptomatic**
Any congenital syphilitic condition specified as late or manifest two years or more after birth.

     A50.51   **Clutton's joints**

     A50.52   **Hutchinson's teeth**

     A50.53   **Hutchinson's triad**

     A50.54   **Late congenital cardiovascular syphilis**

     A50.55   **Late congenital syphilitic arthropathy**

     A50.56   **Late congenital syphilitic osteochondropathy**

     A50.57   **Syphilitic saddle nose**

     A50.59   **Other late congenital syphilis, symptomatic**

A50.6   **Late congenital syphilis, latent**
Congenital syphilis without clinical manifestations, with positive serological reaction and negative spinal fluid test, two years or more after birth.

A50.7   **Late congenital syphilis, unspecified**
Congenital syphilis NOS two years or more after birth.

A50.9   **Congenital syphilis, unspecified**

√4ᵗʰ   **A51**   **Early syphilis**

A51.0   **Primary genital syphilis**
Syphilitic chancre NOS

A51.1   **Primary anal syphilis**

A51.2   **Primary syphilis of other sites**

√5ᵗʰ   **A51.3**   **Secondary syphilis of skin and mucous membranes**

     A51.31   **Condyloma latum**

     A51.32   **Syphilitic alopecia**

     A51.39   **Other secondary syphilis of skin**
Syphilitic leukoderma
Syphilitic mucous patch
EXCLUDES 1   *late syphilitic leukoderma (A52.79)*

√5ᵗʰ   **A51.4**   **Other secondary syphilis**

     A51.41   **Secondary syphilitic meningitis**

     A51.42   **Secondary syphilitic female pelvic disease**

     A51.43   **Secondary syphilitic oculopathy**
Secondary syphilitic chorioretinitis
Secondary syphilitic iridocyclitis, iritis
Secondary syphilitic uveitis

     A51.44   **Secondary syphilitic nephritis**

     A51.45   **Secondary syphilitic hepatitis**

     A51.46   **Secondary syphilitic osteopathy**

     A51.49   **Other secondary syphilitic conditions**
Secondary syphilitic lymphadenopathy
Secondary syphilitic myositis

A51.5   **Early syphilis, latent**
Syphilis (acquired) without clinical manifestations, with positive serological reaction and negative spinal fluid test, less than two years after infection.

A51.9   **Early syphilis, unspecified**

√4ᵗʰ   **A52**   **Late syphilis**

√5ᵗʰ   **A52.0**   **Cardiovascular and cerebrovascular syphilis**

     A52.00   **Cardiovascular syphilis, unspecified**

     A52.01   **Syphilitic aneurysm of aorta**

     A52.02   **Syphilitic aortitis**

     A52.03   **Syphilitic endocarditis**
Syphilitic aortic valve incompetence or stenosis
Syphilitic mitral valve stenosis
Syphilitic pulmonary valve regurgitation

     A52.04   **Syphilitic cerebral arteritis**

     A52.05   **Other cerebrovascular syphilis**
Syphilitic cerebral aneurysm (ruptured) (non-ruptured)
Syphilitic cerebral thrombosis

     A52.06   **Other syphilitic heart involvement**
Syphilitic coronary artery disease
Syphilitic myocarditis
Syphilitic pericarditis

     A52.09   **Other cardiovascular syphilis**

√5ᵗʰ   **A52.1**   **Symptomatic neurosyphilis**

     A52.10   **Symptomatic neurosyphilis, unspecified**

     A52.11   **Tabes dorsalis**
Locomotor ataxia (progressive)
Tabetic neurosyphilis

     A52.12   **Other cerebrospinal syphilis**

     A52.13   **Late syphilitic meningitis**

     A52.14   **Late syphilitic encephalitis**

     A52.15   **Late syphilitic neuropathy**
Late syphilitic acoustic neuritis
Late syphilitic optic (nerve) atrophy
Late syphilitic polyneuropathy
Late syphilitic retrobulbar neuritis

     A52.16   **Charcôt's arthropathy (tabetic)**

     A52.17   **General paresis**
Dementia paralytica

     A52.19   **Other symptomatic neurosyphilis**
Syphilitic parkinsonism

A52.2   **Asymptomatic neurosyphilis**

A52.3   **Neurosyphilis, unspecified**
Gumma (syphilitic)
Syphilis (late)
Syphiloma

√5ᵗʰ   **A52.7**   **Other symptomatic late syphilis**

     A52.71   **Late syphilitic oculopathy**
Late syphilitic chorioretinitis
Late syphilitic episcleritis

     A52.72   **Syphilis of lung and bronchus**

     A52.73   **Symptomatic late syphilis of other respiratory organs**

     A52.74   **Syphilis of liver and other viscera**
Late syphilitic peritonitis

     A52.75   **Syphilis of kidney and ureter**
Syphilitic glomerular disease

     A52.76   **Other genitourinary symptomatic late syphilis**
Late syphilitic female pelvic inflammatory disease

     A52.77   **Syphilis of bone and joint**

     A52.78   **Syphilis of other musculoskeletal tissue**
Late syphilitic bursitis
Syphilis [stage unspecified] of bursa
Syphilis [stage unspecified] of muscle
Syphilis [stage unspecified] of synovium
Syphilis [stage unspecified] of tendon

     A52.79   **Other symptomatic late syphilis**
Late syphilitic leukoderma
Syphilis of adrenal gland
Syphilis of pituitary gland
Syphilis of thyroid gland
Syphilitic splenomegaly
EXCLUDES 1   *syphilitic leukoderma (secondary) (A51.39)*

A52.8   **Late syphilis, latent**
Syphilis (acquired) without clinical manifestations, with positive serological reaction and negative spinal fluid test, two years or more after infection

A52.9   **Late syphilis, unspecified**

√4ᵗʰ   **A53**   **Other and unspecified syphilis**

     A53.0   **Latent syphilis, unspecified as early or late**
Latent syphilis NOS
Positive serological reaction for syphilis

EXCLUDES 1   Not coded here   EXCLUDES 2   Not included here   *Manifestation Code*

A53.9 Syphilis, unspecified
Infection due to Treponema pallidum NOS
Syphilis (acquired) NOS
EXCLUDES 1 *syphilis NOS under two years of age (A50.2)*

✓4th **A54 Gonococcal infection**

✓5th **A54.0 Gonococcal infection of lower genitourinary tract without periurethral or accessory gland abscess**
EXCLUDES 1 *gonococcal infection with genitourinary gland abscess (A54.1)*
gonococcal infection with periurethral abscess (A54.1)

A54.00 Gonococcal infection of lower genitourinary tract, unspecified

A54.01 Gonococcal cystitis and urethritis, unspecified

A54.02 Gonococcal vulvovaginitis, unspecified

A54.03 Gonococcal cervicitis, unspecified

A54.09 Other gonococcal infection of lower genitourinary tract

A54.1 Gonococcal infection of lower genitourinary tract with periurethral and accessory gland abscess
Gonococcal Bartholin's gland abscess

✓5th **A54.2 Gonococcal pelviperitonitis and other gonococcal genitourinary infection**

A54.21 Gonococcal infection of kidney and ureter

A54.22 Gonococcal prostatitis

A54.23 Gonococcal infection of other male genital organs
Gonococcal epididymitis
Gonococcal orchitis

A54.24 Gonococcal female pelvic inflammatory disease
Gonococcal pelviperitonitis
EXCLUDES 1 *gonococcal peritonitis (A54.85)*

A54.29 Other gonococcal genitourinary infections

✓5th **A54.3 Gonococcal infection of eye**

A54.30 Gonococcal infection of eye, unspecified

A54.31 Gonococcal conjunctivitis
Ophthalmia neonatorum due to gonococcus

A54.32 Gonococcal iridocyclitis

A54.33 Gonococcal keratitis

A54.39 Other gonococcal eye infection
Gonococcal endophthalmia

✓5th **A54.4 Gonococcal infection of musculoskeletal system**

A54.40 Gonococcal infection of musculoskeletal system, unspecified

A54.41 Gonococcal spondylopathy

A54.42 Gonococcal arthritis
EXCLUDES 2 *gonococcal infection of spine (A54.41)*

A54.43 Gonococcal osteomyelitis
EXCLUDES 2 *gonococcal infection of spine (A54.41)*

A54.49 Gonococcal infection of other musculoskeletal tissue
Gonococcal bursitis
Gonococcal myositis
Gonococcal synovitis
Gonococcal tenosynovitis

A54.5 Gonococcal pharyngitis

A54.6 Gonococcal infection of anus and rectum

✓5th **A54.8 Other gonococcal infections**

A54.81 Gonococcal meningitis

A54.82 Gonococcal brain abscess

A54.83 Gonococcal heart infection
Gonococcal endocarditis
Gonococcal myocarditis
Gonococcal pericarditis

A54.84 Gonococcal pneumonia

A54.85 Gonococcal peritonitis
EXCLUDES 1 *gonococcal pelviperitonitis (A54.24)*

A54.86 Gonococcal sepsis

A54.89 Other gonococcal infections
Gonococcal keratoderma
Gonococcal lymphadenitis

A54.9 Gonococcal infection, unspecified

A55 Chlamydial lymphogranuloma (venereum)
Climatic or tropical bubo
Durand-Nicolas-Favre disease
Esthiomene
Lymphogranuloma inguinale

✓4th **A56 Other sexually transmitted chlamydial diseases**
INCLUDES sexually transmitted diseases due to Chlamydia trachomatis
EXCLUDES 1 *neonatal chlamydial conjunctivitis (P39.1)*
neonatal chlamydial pneumonia (P23.1)
EXCLUDES 2 *chlamydial lymphogranuloma (A55)*
conditions classified to A74-

✓5th **A56.0 Chlamydial infection of lower genitourinary tract**

A56.00 Chlamydial infection of lower genitourinary tract, unspecified

A56.01 Chlamydial cystitis and urethritis

A56.02 Chlamydial vulvovaginitis

A56.09 Other chlamydial infection of lower genitourinary tract
Chlamydial cervicitis

✓5th **A56.1 Chlamydial infection of pelviperitoneum and other genitourinary organs**

A56.11 Chlamydial female pelvic inflammatory disease

A56.19 Other chlamydial genitourinary infection
Chlamydial epididymitis
Chlamydial orchitis

A56.2 Chlamydial infection of genitourinary tract, unspecified

A56.3 Chlamydial infection of anus and rectum

A56.4 Chlamydial infection of pharynx

A56.8 Sexually transmitted chlamydial infection of other sites

A57 Chancroid
Ulcus molle

A58 Granuloma inguinale
Donovanosis

✓4th **A59 Trichomoniasis**
EXCLUDES 2 *intestinal trichomoniasis (A07.8)*

✓5th **A59.0 Urogenital trichomoniasis**

A59.00 Urogenital trichomoniasis, unspecified
Fluor (vaginalis) due to Trichomonas
Leukorrhea (vaginalis) due to Trichomonas

A59.01 Trichomonal vulvovaginitis

A59.02 Trichomonal prostatitis

A59.03 Trichomonal cystitis and urethritis

A59.09 Other urogenital trichomoniasis
Trichomonas cervicitis

A59.8 Trichomoniasis of other sites

A59.9 Trichomoniasis, unspecified

✓4th **A60 Anogenital herpesviral [herpes simplex] infections**

✓5th **A60.0 Herpesviral infection of genitalia and urogenital tract**

A60.00 Herpesviral infection of urogenital system, unspecified

A60.01 Herpesviral infection of penis

A60.02 Herpesviral infection of other male genital organs

A60.03 Herpesviral cervicitis

A60.04 Herpesviral vulvovaginitis
Herpesviral [herpes simplex] ulceration
Herpesviral [herpes simplex] vaginitis
Herpesviral [herpes simplex] vulvitis

A60.09 Herpesviral infection of other urogenital tract

A60.1 Herpesviral infection of perianal skin and rectum

A60.9 Anogenital herpesviral infection, unspecified

✓4th **A63 Other predominantly sexually transmitted diseases, not elsewhere classified**
EXCLUDES 2 *molluscum contagiosum (B08.1)*
papilloma of cervix (D26.0)

A63.0 Anogenital (venereal) warts
Anogenital warts due to (human) papillomavirus [HPV]
Condyloma acuminatum

A63.8 Other specified predominantly sexually transmitted diseases

A64 Unspecified sexually transmitted disease

Other spirochetal diseases (A65-A69)

EXCLUDES 2 *leptospirosis (A27-)*
syphilis (A50-A53)

A65 Nonvenereal syphilis
Bejel
Endemic syphilis
Njovera

Certain Infectious and Parasitic Diseases

A66–A77.0

☑4th **A66 Yaws**

INCLUDES   bouba
      frambesia (tropica)
      pian

A66.0 Initial lesions of yaws
  Chancre of yaws
  Frambesia, initial or primary
  Initial frambesial ulcer
  Mother yaw

A66.1 Multiple papillomata and wet crab yaws
  Frambesioma
  Pianoma
  Plantar or palmar papilloma of yaws

A66.2 Other early skin lesions of yaws
  Cutaneous yaws, less than five years after infection
  Early yaws (cutaneous) (macular) (maculopapular)
    (micropapular) (papular)
  Frambeside of early yaws

A66.3 Hyperkeratosis of yaws
  Ghoul hand
  Hyperkeratosis, palmar or plantar (early) (late) due to yaws
  Worm-eaten soles

A66.4 Gummata and ulcers of yaws
  Gummatous frambeside
  Nodular late yaws (ulcerated)

A66.5 Gangosa
  Rhinopharyngitis mutilans

A66.6 Bone and joint lesions of yaws
  Yaws ganglion
  Yaws goundou
  Yaws gumma, bone
  Yaws gummatous osteitis or periostitis
  Yaws hydrarthrosis
  Yaws osteitis
  Yaws periostitis (hypertrophic)

A66.7 Other manifestations of yaws
  Juxta-articular nodules of yaws
  Mucosal yaws

A66.8 Latent yaws
  Yaws without clinical manifestations, with positive serology

A66.9 Yaws, unspecified

☑4th **A67 Pinta [carate]**

A67.0 Primary lesions of pinta
  Chancre (primary) of pinta
  Papule (primary) of pinta

A67.1 Intermediate lesions of pinta
  Erythematous plaques of pinta
  Hyperchromic lesions of pinta
  Hyperkeratosis of pinta
  Pintids

A67.2 Late lesions of pinta
  Achromic skin lesions of pinta
  Cicatricial skin lesions of pinta
  Dyschromic skin lesions of pinta

A67.3 Mixed lesions of pinta
  Achromic with hyperchromic skin lesions of pinta [carate]

A67.9 Pinta, unspecified

☑4th **A68 Relapsing fevers**

INCLUDES   recurrent fever

EXCLUDES 2   *Lyme disease (A69.2-)*

A68.0 Louse-borne relapsing fever
  Relapsing fever due to Borrelia recurrentis

A68.1 Tick-borne relapsing fever
  Relapsing fever due to any Borrelia species other than Borrelia recurrentis

A68.9 Relapsing fever, unspecified

☑4th **A69 Other spirochetal infections**

A69.0 Necrotizing ulcerative stomatitis
  Cancrum oris
  Fusospirochetal gangrene
  Noma
  Stomatitis gangrenosa

A69.1 Other Vincent's infections
  Fusospirochetal pharyngitis
  Necrotizing ulcerative (acute) gingivitis
  Necrotizing ulcerative (acute) gingivostomatitis
  Spirochetal stomatitis
  Trench mouth
  Vincent's angina
  Vincent's gingivitis

☑5th **A69.2 Lyme disease**
  Erythema chronicum migrans due to Borrelia burgdorferi

  A69.20 Lyme disease, unspecified

  A69.21 Meningitis due to Lyme disease

  A69.22 Other neurologic disorders in Lyme disease
    Cranial neuritis
    Meningoencephalitis
    Polyneuropathy

  A69.23 Arthritis due to Lyme disease

  A69.29 Other conditions associated with Lyme disease
    Myopericarditis due to Lyme disease

A69.8 Other specified spirochetal infections

A69.9 Spirochetal infection, unspecified

Other diseases caused by chlamydiae (A70-A74)

EXCLUDES 1   *sexually transmitted chlamydial diseases (A55-A56)*

A70 Chlamydia psittaci infections
  Ornithosis
  Parrot fever
  Psittacosis

☑4th **A71 Trachoma**

EXCLUDES 1   *sequelae of trachoma (B94.0)*

A71.0 Initial stage of trachoma
  Trachoma dubium

A71.1 Active stage of trachoma
  Granular conjunctivitis (trachomatous)
  Trachomatous follicular conjunctivitis
  Trachomatous pannus

A71.9 Trachoma, unspecified

☑4th **A74 Other diseases caused by chlamydiae**

EXCLUDES 1   *neonatal chlamydial conjunctivitis (P39.1)*
    neonatal chlamydial pneumonia (P23.1)
    Reiter's disease (M02.3-)
    sexually transmitted chlamydial diseases (A55-A56)

EXCLUDES 2   *chlamydial pneumonia (J16.0)*

A74.0 Chlamydial conjunctivitis
  Paratrachoma

☑5th **A74.8 Other chlamydial diseases**

  A74.81 Chlamydial peritonitis

  A74.89 Other chlamydial diseases

A74.9 Chlamydial infection, unspecified
  Chlamydiosis NOS

Rickettsioses (A75-A79)

☑4th **A75 Typhus fever**

EXCLUDES 1   *rickettsiosis due to Ehrlichia sennetsu (A79.81)*

A75.0 Epidemic louse-borne typhus fever due to Rickettsia prowazekii
  Classical typhus (fever)
  Epidemic (louse-borne) typhus

A75.1 Recrudescent typhus [Brill's disease]
  Brill-Zinsser disease

A75.2 Typhus fever due to Rickettsia typhi
  Murine (flea-borne) typhus

A75.3 Typhus fever due to Rickettsia tsutsugamushi
  Scrub (mite-borne) typhus
  Tsutsugamushi fever

A75.9 Typhus fever, unspecified
  Typhus (fever) NOS

☑4th **A77 Spotted fever [tick-borne rickettsioses]**

A77.0 Spotted fever due to Rickettsia rickettsii
  Rocky Mountain spotted fever
  Sao Paulo fever

EXCLUDES 1 Not coded here   EXCLUDES 2 Not included here   *Manifestation Code*

                                            © 2011 Ingenix

A77.1 Spotted fever due to Rickettsia conorii
  African tick typhus
  Boutonneuse fever
  India tick typhus
  Kenya tick typhus
  Marseilles fever
  Mediterranean tick fever

A77.2 Spotted fever due to Rickettsia siberica
  North Asian tick fever
  Siberian tick typhus

A77.3 Spotted fever due to Rickettsia australis
  Queensland tick typhus

✓5th **A77.4 Ehrlichiosis**
  EXCLUDES 1   *Rickettsiosis due to Ehrlichia sennetsu (A79.81)*
  A77.40 Ehrlichiosis, unspecified
  A77.41 Ehrlichiosis chafeensis [E. chafeensis]
  A77.49 Other ehrlichiosis

A77.8 Other spotted fevers

A77.9 Spotted fever, unspecified
  Tick-borne typhus NOS

A78 Q fever
  Infection due to Coxiella burnetii
  Nine Mile fever
  Quadrilateral fever

✓4th **A79 Other rickettsioses**
  A79.0 Trench fever
    Quintan fever
    Wolhynian fever
  A79.1 Rickettsialpox due to Rickettsia akari
    Kew Garden fever
    Vesicular rickettsiosis
✓5th **A79.8 Other specified rickettsioses**
    A79.81 Rickettsiosis due to Ehrlichia sennetsu
    A79.89 Other specified rickettsioses
  A79.9 Rickettsiosis, unspecified
    Rickettsial infection NOS

Viral and prion infections of the central nervous system (A80-A89)

  EXCLUDES 1   *postpolio syndrome (G14)*
    sequelae of poliomyelitis (B91)
    sequelae of viral encephalitis (B94.1)

✓4th **A80 Acute poliomyelitis**
  A80.0 Acute paralytic poliomyelitis, vaccine-associated
  A80.1 Acute paralytic poliomyelitis, wild virus, imported
  A80.2 Acute paralytic poliomyelitis, wild virus, indigenous
✓5th **A80.3 Acute paralytic poliomyelitis, other and unspecified**
    A80.30 Acute paralytic poliomyelitis, unspecified
    A80.39 Other acute paralytic poliomyelitis
  A80.4 Acute nonparalytic poliomyelitis
  A80.9 Acute poliomyelitis, unspecified

✓4th **A81 Atypical virus infections of central nervous system**
  INCLUDES   diseases of the central nervous system caused by prions
  Use additional code to identify:
    dementia with behavioral disturbance (F02.81)
    dementia without behavioral disturbance (F02.80)
✓5th **A81.0 Creutzfeldt-Jakob disease**
    A81.00 Creutzfeldt-Jakob disease, unspecified
      Jakob-Creutzfeldt disease, unspecified
    A81.01 Variant Creutzfeldt-Jakob disease
      vCJD
    A81.09 Other Creutzfeldt-Jakob disease
      CJD
      Familial Creutzfeldt-Jakob disease
      Iatrogenic Creutzfeldt-Jakob disease
      Sporadic Creutzfeldt-Jakob disease
      Subacute spongiform encephalopathy (with dementia)
  A81.1 Subacute sclerosing panencephalitis
    Dawson's inclusion body encephalitis
    Van Bogaert's sclerosing leukoencephalopathy
  A81.2 Progressive multifocal leukoencephalopathy
    Multifocal leukoencephalopathy NOS
✓5th **A81.8 Other atypical virus infections of central nervous system**
    A81.81 Kuru

A81.82 Gerstmann-Sträussler-Scheinker syndrome
  GSS syndrome
A81.83 Fatal familial insomnia
  FFI
A81.89 Other atypical virus infections of central nervous system

A81.9 Atypical virus infection of central nervous system, unspecified
  Prion diseases of the central nervous system NOS

✓4th **A82 Rabies**
  A82.0 Sylvatic rabies
  A82.1 Urban rabies
  A82.9 Rabies, unspecified

✓4th **A83 Mosquito-borne viral encephalitis**
  INCLUDES   mosquito-borne viral meningoencephalitis
  EXCLUDES 2   *Venezuelan equine encephalitis (A92.2)*
    West Nile fever (A92.3-)
    West Nile virus (A92.3-)
  A83.0 Japanese encephalitis
  A83.1 Western equine encephalitis
  A83.2 Eastern equine encephalitis
  A83.3 St Louis encephalitis
  A83.4 Australian encephalitis
    Kunjin virus disease
  A83.5 California encephalitis
    California meningoencephalitis
    La Crosse encephalitis
  A83.6 Rocio virus disease
  A83.8 Other mosquito-borne viral encephalitis
  A83.9 Mosquito-borne viral encephalitis, unspecified

✓4th **A84 Tick-borne viral encephalitis**
  INCLUDES   tick-borne viral meningoencephalitis
  A84.0 Far Eastern tick-borne encephalitis [Russian spring-summer encephalitis]
  A84.1 Central European tick-borne encephalitis
  A84.8 Other tick-borne viral encephalitis
    Louping ill
    Powassan virus disease
  A84.9 Tick-borne viral encephalitis, unspecified

✓4th **A85 Other viral encephalitis, not elsewhere classified**
  INCLUDES   specified viral encephalomyelitis NEC
    specified viral meningoencephalitis NEC
  EXCLUDES 1   *benign myalgic encephalomyelitis (G93.3)*
    encephalitis due to:
      cytomegalovirus (B25.8)
      herpesvirus NEC (B10.0-)
      herpesvirus [herpes simplex] (B00.4)
      measles virus (B05.0)
      mumps virus (B26.2)
      poliomyelitis virus (A80-)
      zoster (B02.0)
    lymphocytic choriomeningitis (A87.2)
  A85.0 Enteroviral encephalitis
    Enteroviral encephalomyelitis
  A85.1 Adenoviral encephalitis
    Adenoviral meningoencephalitis
  A85.2 Arthropod-borne viral encephalitis, unspecified
    EXCLUDES 1   *West nile virus with encephalitis (A92.31)*
  A85.8 Other specified viral encephalitis
    Encephalitis lethargica
    Von Economo-Cruchet disease

A86 Unspecified viral encephalitis
  Viral encephalomyelitis NOS
  Viral meningoencephalitis NOS

A87 Viral meningitis
  EXCLUDES 1   *meningitis due to:*
    herpesvirus [herpes simplex] (B00.3)
    measles virus (B05.1)
    mumps virus (B26.1)
    poliomyelitis virus (A80-)
    zoster (B02.1)
  A87.0 Enteroviral meningitis
    Coxsackievirus meningitis
    Echovirus meningitis
  A87.1 Adenoviral meningitis

✓ Appropriate additional character required   ✓x7th Requires 7th character, placeholder x must fill empty characters

Certain Infectious and Parasitic Diseases

A87.2–B01.12

A87.2   **Lymphocytic choriomeningitis**
Lymphocytic meningoencephalitis

A87.8   **Other viral meningitis**

A87.9   **Viral meningitis, unspecified**

✓4ᵗʰ **A88**   **Other viral infections of central nervous system, not elsewhere classified**
> EXCLUDES 1   *viral encephalitis NOS (A86)*
> *viral meningitis NOS (A87.9)*

A88.0   **Enteroviral exanthematous fever [Boston exanthem]**

A88.1   **Epidemic vertigo**

A88.8   **Other specified viral infections of central nervous system**

A89   **Unspecified viral infection of central nervous system**

Arthropod-borne viral fevers and viral hemorrhagic fevers (A90-A99)

A90   **Dengue fever [classical dengue]**
> EXCLUDES 1   *dengue hemorrhagic fever (A91)*

A91   **Dengue hemorrhagic fever**

✓4ᵗʰ **A92**   **Other mosquito-borne viral fevers**
> EXCLUDES 1   *Ross River disease (B33.1)*

A92.0   **Chikungunya virus disease**
Chikungunya (hemorrhagic) fever

A92.1   **O'nyong-nyong fever**

A92.2   **Venezuelan equine fever**
Venezuelan equine encephalitis
Venezuelan equine encephalomyelitis virus disease

✓5ᵗʰ **A92.3**   **West Nile virus infection**
West Nile fever

     A92.30   **West Nile virus infection, unspecified**
West Nile fever NOS
West Nile fever without complications
West Nile virus NOS

     A92.31   **West Nile virus infection with encephalitis**
West Nile encephalitis
West Nile encephalomyelitis

     A92.32   **West Nile virus infection with other neurologic manifestation**
Use additional code to specify the neurologic manifestation

     A92.39   **West Nile virus infection with other complications**
Use additional code to specify the other conditions

A92.4   **Rift Valley fever**

A92.8   **Other specified mosquito-borne viral fevers**

A92.9   **Mosquito-borne viral fever, unspecified**

✓4ᵗʰ **A93**   **Other arthropod-borne viral fevers, not elsewhere classified**

A93.0   **Oropouche virus disease**
Oropouche fever

A93.1   **Sandfly fever**
Pappataci fever
Phlebotomus fever

A93.2   **Colorado tick fever**

A93.8   **Other specified arthropod-borne viral fevers**
Piry virus disease
Vesicular stomatitis virus disease [Indiana fever]

A94   **Unspecified arthropod-borne viral fever**
Arboviral fever NOS
Arbovirus infection NOS

✓4ᵗʰ **A95**   **Yellow fever**

A95.0   **Sylvatic yellow fever**
Jungle yellow fever

A95.1   **Urban yellow fever**

A95.9   **Yellow fever, unspecified**

✓4ᵗʰ **A96**   **Arenaviral hemorrhagic fever**

A96.0   **Junin hemorrhagic fever**
Argentinian hemorrhagic fever

A96.1   **Machupo hemorrhagic fever**
Bolivian hemorrhagic fever

A96.2   **Lassa fever**

A96.8   **Other arenaviral hemorrhagic fevers**

A96.9   **Arenaviral hemorrhagic fever, unspecified**

✓4ᵗʰ **A98**   **Other viral hemorrhagic fevers, not elsewhere classified**
> EXCLUDES 1   *chikungunya hemorrhagic fever (A92.0)*
> *dengue hemorrhagic fever (A91)*

A98.0   **Crimean-Congo hemorrhagic fever**
Central Asian hemorrhagic fever

A98.1   **Omsk hemorrhagic fever**

A98.2   **Kyasanur Forest disease**

A98.3   **Marburg virus disease**

A98.4   **Ebola virus disease**

A98.5   **Hemorrhagic fever with renal syndrome**
Epidemic hemorrhagic fever
Korean hemorrhagic fever
Russian hemorrhagic fever
Hantaan virus disease
Hantavirus disease with renal manifestations
Nephropathia epidemica
Songo fever
> EXCLUDES 1   *hantavirus (cardio)-pulmonary syndrome (B33.4)*

A98.8   **Other specified viral hemorrhagic fevers**

A99   **Unspecified viral hemorrhagic fever**

Viral infections characterized by skin and mucous membrane lesions (B00-B09)

✓4ᵗʰ **B00**   **Herpesviral [herpes simplex] infections**
> EXCLUDES 1   *congenital herpesviral infections (P35.2)*
> EXCLUDES 2   *anogenital herpesviral infection (A60-)*
> *gammaherpesviral mononucleosis (B27.0-)*
> *herpangina (B08.5)*

B00.0   **Eczema herpeticum**
Kaposi's varicelliform eruption

B00.1   **Herpesviral vesicular dermatitis**
Herpes simplex facialis
Herpes simplex labialis
Herpes simplex otitis externa
Vesicular dermatitis of ear
Vesicular dermatitis of lip

B00.2   **Herpesviral gingivostomatitis and pharyngotonsillitis**
Herpesviral pharyngitis

B00.3   **Herpesviral meningitis**

B00.4   **Herpesviral encephalitis**
Herpesviral meningoencephalitis
Simian B disease
> EXCLUDES 1   *herpesviral encephalitis due to herpesvirus 6 and 7 (B10.01, B10.09)*
> *non-simplex herpesviral encephalitis (B10.0-)*

✓5ᵗʰ **B00.5**   **Herpesviral ocular disease**

     B00.50   **Herpesviral ocular disease, unspecified**

     B00.51   **Herpesviral iridocyclitis**
Herpesviral iritis
Herpesviral uveitis, anterior

     B00.52   **Herpesviral keratitis**
Herpesviral keratoconjunctivitis

     B00.53   **Herpesviral conjunctivitis**

     B00.59   **Other herpesviral disease of eye**
Herpesviral dermatitis of eyelid

B00.7   **Disseminated herpesviral disease**
Herpesviral sepsis

✓5ᵗʰ **B00.8**   **Other forms of herpesviral infections**

     B00.81   **Herpesviral hepatitis**

     B00.82   **Herpes simplex myelitis**

     B00.89   **Other herpesviral infection**
Herpesviral whitlow

B00.9   **Herpesviral infection, unspecified**
Herpes simplex infection NOS

✓4ᵗʰ **B01**   **Varicella [chickenpox]**

B01.0   **Varicella meningitis**

✓5ᵗʰ **B01.1**   **Varicella encephalitis, myelitis and encephalomyelitis**
Postchickenpox encephalitis, myelitis and encephalomyelitis

     B01.11   **Varicella encephalitis and encephalomyelitis**
Postchickenpox encephalitis and encephalomyelitis

     B01.12   **Varicella myelitis**
Postchickenpox myelitis

EXCLUDES 1   Not coded here   EXCLUDES 2   Not included here   *Manifestation Code*

B01.2   **Varicella pneumonia**

☑5th   B01.8   **Varicella with other complications**

   B01.81   **Varicella keratitis**

   B01.89   **Other varicella complications**

B01.9   **Varicella without complication**
   Varicella NOS

☑4th   **B02   Zoster [herpes zoster]**
   INCLUDES   shingles
             zona

B02.0   **Zoster encephalitis**
   Zoster meningoencephalitis

B02.1   **Zoster meningitis**

☑5th   B02.2   **Zoster with other nervous system involvement**

   B02.21   **Postherpetic geniculate ganglionitis**

   B02.22   **Postherpetic trigeminal neuralgia**

   B02.23   **Postherpetic polyneuropathy**

   B02.24   **Postherpetic myelitis**
      Herpes zoster myelitis

   B02.29   **Other postherpetic nervous system involvement**
      Postherpetic radiculopathy

☑5th   B02.3   **Zoster ocular disease**

   B02.30   **Zoster ocular disease, unspecified**

   B02.31   **Zoster conjunctivitis**

   B02.32   **Zoster iridocyclitis**

   B02.33   **Zoster keratitis**
      Herpes zoster keratoconjunctivitis

   B02.34   **Zoster scleritis**

   B02.39   **Other herpes zoster eye disease**
      Zoster blepharitis

B02.7   **Disseminated zoster**

B02.8   **Zoster with other complications**
   Herpes zoster otitis externa

B02.9   **Zoster without complications**
   Zoster NOS

B03   **Smallpox**
   NOTE   In 1980 the 33rd World Health Assembly declared that
          smallpox had been eradicated.
          The classification is maintained for surveillance purposes.

B04   **Monkeypox**

☑4th   **B05   Measles**
   INCLUDES   morbilli
   EXCLUDES 1   subacute sclerosing panencephalitis (A81.1)

B05.0   **Measles complicated by encephalitis**
   Postmeasles encephalitis

B05.1   **Measles complicated by meningitis**
   Postmeasles meningitis

B05.2   **Measles complicated by pneumonia**
   Postmeasles pneumonia

B05.3   **Measles complicated by otitis media**
   Postmeasles otitis media

B05.4   **Measles with intestinal complications**

☑5th   B05.8   **Measles with other complications**

   B05.81   **Measles keratitis and keratoconjunctivitis**

   B05.89   **Other measles complications**

B05.9   **Measles without complication**
   Measles NOS

☑4th   **B06   Rubella [German measles]**
   EXCLUDES 1   congenital rubella (P35.0)

☑5th   B06.0   **Rubella with neurological complications**

   B06.00   **Rubella with neurological complication, unspecified**

   B06.01   **Rubella encephalitis**
      Rubella meningoencephalitis

   B06.02   **Rubella meningitis**

   B06.09   **Other neurological complications of rubella**

☑5th   B06.8   **Rubella with other complications**

   B06.81   **Rubella pneumonia**

   B06.82   **Rubella arthritis**

   B06.89   **Other rubella complications**

☑5th   B06.9   **Rubella without complication**
   Rubella NOS

☑4th   **B07   Viral warts**
   INCLUDES   verruca simplex
             verruca vulgaris
             viral warts due to human papillomavirus
   EXCLUDES 2   anogenital (venereal) warts (A63.0)
               papilloma of bladder (D41.4)
               papilloma of cervix (D26.0)
               papilloma larynx (D14.1)

B07.0   **Plantar wart**
   Verruca plantaris

B07.8   **Other viral warts**
   Common wart
   Flat wart
   Verruca plana

B07.9   **Viral wart, unspecified**

☑4th   **B08   Other viral infections characterized by skin and mucous membrane lesions, not elsewhere classified**
   EXCLUDES 1   vesicular stomatitis virus disease (A93.8)

☑5th   B08.0   **Other orthopoxvirus infections**
   EXCLUDES 2   monkeypox (B04)

☑6th   B08.01   **Cowpox and vaccinia not from vaccine**

   B08.010   **Cowpox**

   B08.011   **Vaccinia not from vaccine**
      EXCLUDES 1   vaccinia (from vaccination)
                  (generalized) (T88.1)

   B08.02   **Orf virus disease**
      Contagious pustular dermatitis
      Ecthyma contagiosum

   B08.03   **Pseudocowpox [milker's node]**

   B08.04   **Paravaccinia, unspecified**

   B08.09   **Other orthopoxvirus infections**
      Orthopoxvirus infection NOS

B08.1   **Molluscum contagiosum**

☑5th   B08.2   **Exanthema subitum [sixth disease]**
   Roseola infantum

   B08.20   **Exanthema subitum [sixth disease], unspecified**
      Roseola infantum, unspecified

   B08.21   **Exanthema subitum [sixth disease] due to human herpesvirus 6**
      Roseola infantum due to human herpesvirus 6

   B08.22   **Exanthema subitum [sixth disease] due to human herpesvirus 7**
      Roseola infantum due to human herpesvirus 7

B08.3   **Erythema infectiosum [fifth disease]**

B08.4   **Enteroviral vesicular stomatitis with exanthem**
   Hand, foot and mouth disease

B08.5   **Enteroviral vesicular pharyngitis**
   Herpangina

☑5th   B08.6   **Parapoxvirus infections**

   B08.60   **Parapoxvirus infection, unspecified**

   B08.61   **Bovine stomatitis**

   B08.62   **Sealpox**

   B08.69   **Other parapoxvirus infections**

☑5th   B08.7   **Yatapoxvirus infections**

   B08.70   **Yatapoxvirus infection, unspecified**

   B08.71   **Tanapox virus disease**

   B08.72   **Yaba pox virus disease**
      Yaba monkey tumor disease

   B08.79   **Other yatapoxvirus infections**

B08.8   **Other specified viral infections characterized by skin and mucous membrane lesions**
   Enteroviral lymphonodular pharyngitis
   Foot-and-mouth disease
   Poxvirus NEC

B09   **Unspecified viral infection characterized by skin and mucous membrane lesions**
   Viral enanthema NOS
   Viral exanthema NOS

Certain Infectious and Parasitic Diseases

B10–B27.90

Other human herpesviruses (B10)

☑4ᵗʰ B10 Other human herpesviruses

EXCLUDES 2   cytomegalovirus (B25.9)
      Epstein-Barr virus (B27.0-)
      herpes NOS (B00.9)
      herpes simplex (B00-)
      herpes zoster (B02-)
      human herpesvirus NOS (B00-)
      human herpesvirus 1 and 2 (B00-)
      human herpesvirus 3 (B01-, B02-)
      human herpesvirus 4 (B27.0-)
      human herpesvirus 5 (B25-)
      varicella (B01-)
      zoster (B02-)

☑5ᵗʰ B10.0 Other human herpesvirus encephalitis

EXCLUDES 2   herpes encephalitis NOS (B00.4)
      herpes simplex encephalitis (B00.4)
      human herpesvirus encephalitis (B00.4)
      simian B herpes virus encephalitis (B00.4)

B10.01 Human herpesvirus 6 encephalitis
B10.09 Other human herpesvirus encephalitis
      Human herpesvirus 7 encephalitis

☑5ᵗʰ B10.8 Other human herpesvirus infection
B10.81 Human herpesvirus 6 infection
B10.82 Human herpesvirus 7 infection
B10.89 Other human herpesvirus infection
      Human herpesvirus 8 infection
      Kaposi's sarcoma-associated herpesvirus infection

Viral hepatitis (B15-B19)

EXCLUDES 1   sequelae of viral hepatitis (B94.2)
EXCLUDES 2   cytomegaloviral hepatitis (B25.1)
      herpesviral [herpes simplex] hepatitis (B00.81)

☑4ᵗʰ B15 Acute hepatitis A
B15.0 Hepatitis A with hepatic coma
B15.9 Hepatitis A without hepatic coma
      Hepatitis A (acute)(viral) NOS

☑4ᵗʰ B16 Acute hepatitis B
B16.0 Acute hepatitis B with delta-agent with hepatic coma
B16.1 Acute hepatitis B with delta-agent without hepatic coma
B16.2 Acute hepatitis B without delta-agent with hepatic coma
B16.9 Acute hepatitis B without delta-agent and without hepatic coma
      Hepatitis B (acute) (viral) NOS

☑4ᵗʰ B17 Other acute viral hepatitis
B17.0 Acute delta-(super) infection of hepatitis B carrier
☑5ᵗʰ B17.1 Acute hepatitis C
      B17.10 Acute hepatitis C without hepatic coma
          Acute hepatitis C NOS
      B17.11 Acute hepatitis C with hepatic coma
B17.2 Acute hepatitis E
B17.8 Other specified acute viral hepatitis
      Hepatitis non-A non-B (acute) (viral) NEC
B17.9 Acute viral hepatitis, unspecified
      Acute hepatitis NOS

☑4ᵗʰ B18 Chronic viral hepatitis
B18.0 Chronic viral hepatitis B with delta-agent
B18.1 Chronic viral hepatitis B without delta-agent
      Chronic (viral) hepatitis B
B18.2 Chronic viral hepatitis C
B18.8 Other chronic viral hepatitis
B18.9 Chronic viral hepatitis, unspecified

☑4ᵗʰ B19 Unspecified viral hepatitis
B19.0 Unspecified viral hepatitis with hepatic coma
☑5ᵗʰ B19.1 Unspecified viral hepatitis B
      B19.10 Unspecified viral hepatitis B without hepatic coma
          Unspecified viral hepatitis B NOS
      B19.11 Unspecified viral hepatitis B with hepatic coma
☑5ᵗʰ B19.2 Unspecified viral hepatitis C
      B19.20 Unspecified viral hepatitis C without hepatic coma
          Viral hepatitis C NOS
      B19.21 Unspecified viral hepatitis C with hepatic coma
B19.9 Unspecified viral hepatitis without hepatic coma
      Viral hepatitis NOS

Human immunodeficiency virus [HIV] disease (B20)

B20 Human immunodeficiency virus [HIV] disease

INCLUDES   acquired immune deficiency syndrome [AIDS]
      AIDS-related complex [ARC]
      HIV infection, symptomatic

Code first human immunodeficiency [HIV] disease complicating pregnancy, childbirth and the puerperium, if applicable (O98.7-)

Use additional code(s) to identify all manifestations of HIV infection

EXCLUDES 1   asymptomatic human immunodeficiency virus [HIV] infection status (Z21)
      exposure to HIV virus (Z20.6)
      inconclusive serologic evidence of HIV (R75)

Other viral diseases (B25-B34)

☑4ᵗʰ B25 Cytomegaloviral disease
EXCLUDES 1   congenital cytomegalovirus infection (P35.1)
      cytomegaloviral mononucleosis (B27.1-)
B25.0 Cytomegaloviral pneumonitis
B25.1 Cytomegaloviral hepatitis
B25.2 Cytomegaloviral pancreatitis
B25.8 Other cytomegaloviral diseases
      Cytomegaloviral encephalitis
B25.9 Cytomegaloviral disease, unspecified

☑4ᵗʰ B26 Mumps
INCLUDES   epidemic parotitis
      infectious parotitis
B26.0 Mumps orchitis
B26.1 Mumps meningitis
B26.2 Mumps encephalitis
B26.3 Mumps pancreatitis
☑5ᵗʰ B26.8 Mumps with other complications
      B26.81 Mumps hepatitis
      B26.82 Mumps myocarditis
      B26.83 Mumps nephritis
      B26.84 Mumps polyneuropathy
      B26.85 Mumps arthritis
      B26.89 Other mumps complications
B26.9 Mumps without complication
      Mumps NOS
      Mumps parotitis NOS

☑4ᵗʰ B27 Infectious mononucleosis
INCLUDES   glandular fever
      monocytic angina
      Pfeiffer's disease
☑5ᵗʰ B27.0 Gammaherpesviral mononucleosis
      Mononucleosis due to Epstein-Barr virus
      B27.00 Gammaherpesviral mononucleosis without complication
      B27.01 Gammaherpesviral mononucleosis with polyneuropathy
      B27.02 Gammaherpesviral mononucleosis with meningitis
      B27.09 Gammaherpesviral mononucleosis with other complications
          Hepatomegaly in gammaherpesviral mononucleosis
☑5ᵗʰ B27.1 Cytomegaloviral mononucleosis
      B27.10 Cytomegaloviral mononucleosis without complications
      B27.11 Cytomegaloviral mononucleosis with polyneuropathy
      B27.12 Cytomegaloviral mononucleosis with meningitis
      B27.19 Cytomegaloviral mononucleosis with other complication
          Hepatomegaly in cytomegaloviral mononucleosis
☑5ᵗʰ B27.8 Other infectious mononucleosis
      B27.80 Other infectious mononucleosis without complication
      B27.81 Other infectious mononucleosis with polyneuropathy
      B27.82 Other infectious mononucleosis with meningitis
      B27.89 Other infectious mononucleosis with other complication
          Hepatomegaly in other infectious mononucleosis
☑5ᵗʰ B27.9 Infectious mononucleosis, unspecified
      B27.90 Infectious mononucleosis, unspecified without complication

---

EXCLUDES 1 Not coded here   **EXCLUDES 2** Not included here   *Manifestation Code*

B27.91 Infectious mononucleosis, unspecified with polyneuropathy

B27.92 Infectious mononucleosis, unspecified with meningitis

B27.99 Infectious mononucleosis, unspecified with other complication
Hepatomegaly in unspecified infectious mononucleosis

✓4ᵗʰ **B30 Viral conjunctivitis**
> EXCLUDES 1 herpesviral [herpes simplex] ocular disease (B00.5)
> ocular zoster (B02.3)

B30.0 Keratoconjunctivitis due to adenovirus
Epidemic keratoconjunctivitis
Shipyard eye

B30.1 Conjunctivitis due to adenovirus
Acute adenoviral follicular conjunctivitis
Swimming-pool conjunctivitis

B30.2 Viral pharyngoconjunctivitis

B30.3 Acute epidemic hemorrhagic conjunctivitis (enteroviral)
Conjunctivitis due to coxsackievirus 24
Conjunctivitis due to enterovirus 70
Hemorrhagic conjunctivitis (acute)(epidemic)

B30.8 Other viral conjunctivitis
Newcastle conjunctivitis

B30.9 Viral conjunctivitis, unspecified

✓4ᵗʰ **B33 Other viral diseases, not elsewhere classified**

B33.0 Epidemic myalgia
Bornholm disease

B33.1 Ross River disease
Epidemic polyarthritis and exanthema
Ross River fever

✓5ᵗʰ **B33.2 Viral carditis**
Coxsackie (virus) carditis

B33.20 Viral carditis, unspecified
B33.21 Viral endocarditis
B33.22 Viral myocarditis
B33.23 Viral pericarditis
B33.24 Viral cardiomyopathy

B33.3 Retrovirus infections, not elsewhere classified
Retrovirus infection NOS

B33.4 Hantavirus (cardio)-pulmonary syndrome [HPS] [HCPS]
Hantavirus disease with pulmonary manifestations
Sin nombre virus disease
Use additional code to identify any associated acute kidney failure (N17.9)
> EXCLUDES 1 hantavirus disease with renal manifestations (A98.5)
> hemorrhagic fever with renal manifestations (A98.5)

B33.8 Other specified viral diseases
> EXCLUDES 1 anogenital human papillomavirus infection (A63.0)
> viral warts due to human papillomavirus infection (B07)

✓4ᵗʰ **B34 Viral infection of unspecified site**
> EXCLUDES 1 anogenital human papillomavirus infection (A63.0)
> cytomegaloviral disease NOS (B25.9)
> herpesvirus [herpes simplex] infection NOS (B00.9)
> retrovirus infection NOS (B33.3)
> viral agents as the cause of diseases classified elsewhere (B97-)
> viral warts due to human papillomavirus infection (B07)

B34.0 Adenovirus infection, unspecified

B34.1 Enterovirus infection, unspecified
Coxsackievirus infection NOS
Echovirus infection NOS

B34.2 Coronavirus infection, unspecified
> EXCLUDES 1 pneumonia due to SARS-associated coronavirus (J12.3)

B34.3 Parvovirus infection, unspecified

B34.4 Papovavirus infection, unspecified

B34.8 Other viral infections of unspecified site

B34.9 Viral infection, unspecified
Viremia NOS

Mycoses (B35-B49)
> EXCLUDES 2 hypersensitivity pneumonitis due to organic dust (J67-)
> mycosis fungoides (C84.0-)

✓4ᵗʰ **B35 Dermatophytosis**
> INCLUDES favus
> infections due to species of Epidermophyton, Micro-sporum and Trichophyton
> tinea, any type except those in B36-

B35.0 Tinea barbae and tinea capitis
Beard ringworm
Kerion
Scalp ringworm
Sycosis, mycotic

B35.1 Tinea unguium
Dermatophytic onychia
Dermatophytosis of nail
Onychomycosis
Ringworm of nails

B35.2 Tinea manuum
Dermatophytosis of hand
Hand ringworm

B35.3 Tinea pedis
Athlete's foot
Dermatophytosis of foot
Foot ringworm

B35.4 Tinea corporis
Ringworm of the body

B35.5 Tinea imbricata
Tokelau

B35.6 Tinea cruris
Dhobi itch
Groin ringworm
Jock itch

B35.8 Other dermatophytoses
Disseminated dermatophytosis
Granulomatous dermatophytosis

B35.9 Dermatophytosis, unspecified
Ringworm NOS

✓4ᵗʰ **B36 Other superficial mycoses**

B36.0 Pityriasis versicolor
Tinea flava
Tinea versicolor

B36.1 Tinea nigra
Keratomycosis nigricans palmaris
Microsporosis nigra
Pityriasis nigra

B36.2 White piedra
Tinea blanca

B36.3 Black piedra

B36.8 Other specified superficial mycoses

B36.9 Superficial mycosis, unspecified

✓4ᵗʰ **B37 Candidiasis**
> INCLUDES candidosis
> moniliasis
> EXCLUDES 1 neonatal candidiasis (P37.5)

B37.0 Candidal stomatitis
Oral thrush

B37.1 Pulmonary candidiasis
Candidal bronchitis
Candidal pneumonia

B37.2 Candidiasis of skin and nail
Candidal onychia
Candidal paronychia
> EXCLUDES 2 diaper dermatitis (L22)

B37.3 Candidiasis of vulva and vagina
Candidal vulvovaginitis
Monilial vulvovaginitis
Vaginal thrush

✓5ᵗʰ **B37.4 Candidiasis of other urogenital sites**
B37.41 Candidal cystitis and urethritis
B37.42 Candidal balanitis
B37.49 Other urogenital candidiasis
Candidal pyelonephritis

B37.5 Candidal meningitis

B37.6 Candidal endocarditis

B37.7 Candidal sepsis
Disseminated candidiasis
Systemic candidiasis

☑ Appropriate additional character required   ✓x7ᵗʰ Requires 7th character, placeholder x must fill empty characters

Certain Infectious and Parasitic Diseases

B37.8–B49

✓5ᵗʰ **B37.8** **Candidiasis of other sites**
    B37.81 **Candidal esophagitis**
    B37.82 **Candidal enteritis**
        Candidal proctitis
    B37.83 **Candidal cheilitis**
    B37.84 **Candidal otitis externa**
    B37.89 **Other sites of candidiasis**
        Candidal osteomyelitis
B37.9 **Candidiasis, unspecified**
    Thrush NOS

✓4ᵗʰ **B38** **Coccidioidomycosis**
B38.0 **Acute pulmonary coccidioidomycosis**
B38.1 **Chronic pulmonary coccidioidomycosis**
B38.2 **Pulmonary coccidioidomycosis, unspecified**
B38.3 **Cutaneous coccidioidomycosis**
B38.4 **Coccidioidomycosis meningitis**
B38.7 **Disseminated coccidioidomycosis**
    Generalized coccidioidomycosis
✓5ᵗʰ **B38.8** **Other forms of coccidioidomycosis**
    B38.81 **Prostatic coccidioidomycosis**
    B38.89 **Other forms of coccidioidomycosis**
B38.9 **Coccidioidomycosis, unspecified**

✓4ᵗʰ **B39** **Histoplasmosis**
    Code first associated AIDS (B20)
    Use additional code for any associated manifestations, such as:
        endocarditis (I39)
        meningitis (G02)
        pericarditis (I32)
        retinitits (H32)
B39.0 **Acute pulmonary histoplasmosis capsulati**
B39.1 **Chronic pulmonary histoplasmosis capsulati**
B39.2 **Pulmonary histoplasmosis capsulati, unspecified**
B39.3 **Disseminated histoplasmosis capsulati**
    Generalized histoplasmosis capsulati
B39.4 **Histoplasmosis capsulati, unspecified**
    American histoplasmosis
B39.5 **Histoplasmosis duboisii**
    African histoplasmosis
B39.9 **Histoplasmosis, unspecified**

✓4ᵗʰ **B40** **Blastomycosis**
    EXCLUDES 1 *Brazilian blastomycosis (B41-)*
                 keloidal blastomycosis (B48.0)
B40.0 **Acute pulmonary blastomycosis**
B40.1 **Chronic pulmonary blastomycosis**
B40.2 **Pulmonary blastomycosis, unspecified**
B40.3 **Cutaneous blastomycosis**
B40.7 **Disseminated blastomycosis**
    Generalized blastomycosis
✓5ᵗʰ **B40.8** **Other forms of blastomycosis**
    B40.81 **Blastomycotic meningoencephalitis**
        Meningomyelitis due to blastomycosis
    B40.89 **Other forms of blastomycosis**
B40.9 **Blastomycosis, unspecified**

✓4ᵗʰ **B41** **Paracoccidioidomycosis**
    INCLUDES Brazilian blastomycosis
               Lutz' disease
B41.0 **Pulmonary paracoccidioidomycosis**
B41.7 **Disseminated paracoccidioidomycosis**
    Generalized paracoccidioidomycosis
B41.8 **Other forms of paracoccidioidomycosis**
B41.9 **Paracoccidioidomycosis, unspecified**

✓4ᵗʰ **B42** **Sporotrichosis**
B42.0 **Pulmonary sporotrichosis**
B42.1 **Lymphocutaneous sporotrichosis**
B42.7 **Disseminated sporotrichosis**
    Generalized sporotrichosis
✓5ᵗʰ **B42.8** **Other forms of sporotrichosis**
    B42.81 **Cerebral sporotrichosis**
        Meningitis due to sporotrichosis
    B42.82 **Sporotrichosis arthritis**
    B42.89 **Other forms of sporotrichosis**
B42.9 **Sporotrichosis, unspecified**

✓4ᵗʰ **B43** **Chromomycosis and pheomycotic abscess**
B43.0 **Cutaneous chromomycosis**
    Dermatitis verrucosa
B43.1 **Pheomycotic brain abscess**
    Cerebral chromomycosis
B43.2 **Subcutaneous pheomycotic abscess and cyst**
B43.8 **Other forms of chromomycosis**
B43.9 **Chromomycosis, unspecified**

✓4ᵗʰ **B44** **Aspergillosis**
    INCLUDES aspergilloma
B44.0 **Invasive pulmonary aspergillosis**
B44.1 **Other pulmonary aspergillosis**
B44.2 **Tonsillar aspergillosis**
B44.7 **Disseminated aspergillosis**
    Generalized aspergillosis
✓5ᵗʰ **B44.8** **Other forms of aspergillosis**
    B44.81 **Allergic bronchopulmonary aspergillosis**
    B44.89 **Other forms of aspergillosis**
B44.9 **Aspergillosis, unspecified**

✓4ᵗʰ **B45** **Cryptococcosis**
B45.0 **Pulmonary cryptococcosis**
B45.1 **Cerebral cryptococcosis**
    Cryptococcal meningitis
    Cryptococcosis meningocerebralis
B45.2 **Cutaneous cryptococcosis**
B45.3 **Osseous cryptococcosis**
B45.7 **Disseminated cryptococcosis**
    Generalized cryptococcosis
B45.8 **Other forms of cryptococcosis**
B45.9 **Cryptococcosis, unspecified**

✓4ᵗʰ **B46** **Zygomycosis**
B46.0 **Pulmonary mucormycosis**
B46.1 **Rhinocerebral mucormycosis**
B46.2 **Gastrointestinal mucormycosis**
B46.3 **Cutaneous mucormycosis**
    Subcutaneous mucormycosis
B46.4 **Disseminated mucormycosis**
    Generalized mucormycosis
B46.5 **Mucormycosis, unspecified**
B46.8 **Other zygomycoses**
    Entomophthoromycosis
B46.9 **Zygomycosis, unspecified**
    Phycomycosis NOS

✓4ᵗʰ **B47** **Mycetoma**
B47.0 **Eumycetoma**
    Madura foot, mycotic
    Maduromycosis
B47.1 **Actinomycetoma**
B47.9 **Mycetoma, unspecified**
    Madura foot NOS

✓4ᵗʰ **B48** **Other mycoses, not elsewhere classified**
B48.0 **Lobomycosis**
    Keloidal blastomycosis
    Lobo's disease
B48.1 **Rhinosporidiosis**
B48.2 **Allescheriasis**
    Infection due to Pseudallescheria boydii
    EXCLUDES 1 *eumycetoma (B47.0)*
B48.3 **Geotrichosis**
    Geotrichum stomatitis
B48.4 **Penicillosis**
B48.8 **Other specified mycoses**
    Adiaspiromycosis
    Infection of tissue and organs by Alternaria
    Infection of tissue and organs by Drechslera
    Infection of tissue and organs by Fusarium
    Infection of tissue and organs by saprophytic fungi NEC

B49 **Unspecified mycosis**
    Fungemia NOS

EXCLUDES 1 Not coded here   EXCLUDES 2 Not included here   *Manifestation Code*

Protozoal diseases (B50-B64)

EXCLUDES1   amebiasis (A06-)
other protozoal intestinal diseases (A07-)

✓4th **B50   Plasmodium falciparum malaria**
    INCLUDES   mixed infections of Plasmodium falciparum with any other Plasmodium species

    B50.0   Plasmodium falciparum malaria with cerebral complications
       Cerebral malaria NOS

    B50.8   Other severe and complicated Plasmodium falciparum malaria
       Severe or complicated Plasmodium falciparum malaria NOS

    B50.9   Plasmodium falciparum malaria, unspecified

✓4th **B51   Plasmodium vivax malaria**
    INCLUDES   mixed infections of Plasmodium vivax with other Plasmodium species, except Plasmodium falciparum
    EXCLUDES1   plasmodium vivax with Plasmodium falciparum (B50-)

    B51.0   Plasmodium vivax malaria with rupture of spleen

    B51.8   Plasmodium vivax malaria with other complications

    B51.9   Plasmodium vivax malaria without complication
       Plasmodium vivax malaria NOS

✓4th **B52   Plasmodium malariae malaria**
    INCLUDES   mixed infections of Plasmodium malariae with other Plasmodium species, except Plasmodium falciparum and Plasmodium vivax
    EXCLUDES1   Plasmodium falciparum (B50-)
               Plasmodium vivax (B51-)

    B52.0   Plasmodium malariae malaria with nephropathy

    B52.8   Plasmodium malariae malaria with other complications

    B52.9   Plasmodium malariae malaria without complication
       Plasmodium malariae malaria NOS

✓4th **B53   Other specified malaria**

    B53.0   Plasmodium ovale malaria
       EXCLUDES1   Plasmodium ovale with Plasmodium falciparum (B50-)
                 Plasmodium ovale with Plasmodium malariae (B52-)
                 Plasmodium ovale with Plasmodium vivax (B51-)

    B53.1   Malaria due to simian plasmodia
       EXCLUDES1   Malaria due to simian plasmodia with Plasmodium falciparum (B50-)
                 Malaria due to simian plasmodia with Plasmodium malariae (B52-)
                 Malaria due to simian plasmodia with Plasmodium ovale (B53.0)
                 Malaria due to simian plasmodia with Plasmodium vivax (B51-)

    B53.8   Other malaria, not elsewhere classified

    B54   Unspecified malaria

✓4th **B55   Leishmaniasis**

    B55.0   Visceral leishmaniasis
       Kala-azar
       Post-kala-azar dermal leishmaniasis

    B55.1   Cutaneous leishmaniasis

    B55.2   Mucocutaneous leishmaniasis

    B55.9   Leishmaniasis, unspecified

✓4th **B56   African trypanosomiasis**

    B56.0   Gambiense trypanosomiasis
       Infection due to Trypanosoma brucei gambiense
       West African sleeping sickness

    B56.1   Rhodesiense trypanosomiasis
       East African sleeping sickness
       Infection due to Trypanosoma brucei rhodesiense

    B56.9   African trypanosomiasis, unspecified
       Sleeping sickness NOS

✓4th **B57   Chagas' disease**
    INCLUDES   American trypanosomiasis
            infection due to Trypanosoma cruzi

    B57.0   Acute Chagas' disease with heart involvement
       Acute Chagas' disease with myocarditis

    B57.1   Acute Chagas' disease without heart involvement
       Acute Chagas' disease NOS

    B57.2   Chagas' disease (chronic) with heart involvement
       American trypanosomiasis NOS
       Chagas' disease (chronic) NOS
       Chagas' disease (chronic) with myocarditis
       Trypanosomiasis NOS

✓5th **B57.3   Chagas' disease (chronic) with digestive system involvement**

       B57.30   Chagas' disease with digestive system involvement, unspecified

       B57.31   Megaesophagus in Chagas' disease

       B57.32   Megacolon in Chagas' disease

       B57.39   Other digestive system involvement in Chagas' disease

✓5th **B57.4   Chagas' disease (chronic) with nervous system involvement**

       B57.40   Chagas' disease with nervous system involvement, unspecified

       B57.41   Meningitis in Chagas' disease

       B57.42   Meningoencephalitis in Chagas' disease

       B57.49   Other nervous system involvement in Chagas' disease

    B57.5   Chagas' disease (chronic) with other organ involvement

✓4th **B58   Toxoplasmosis**
    INCLUDES   infection due to Toxoplasma gondii
    EXCLUDES1   congenital toxoplasmosis (P37.1)

✓5th **B58.0   Toxoplasma oculopathy**

       B58.00   Toxoplasma oculopathy, unspecified

       B58.01   Toxoplasma chorioretinitis

       B58.09   Other toxoplasma oculopathy
            Toxoplasma uveitis

    B58.1   Toxoplasma hepatitis

    B58.2   Toxoplasma meningoencephalitis

    B58.3   Pulmonary toxoplasmosis

✓5th **B58.8   Toxoplasmosis with other organ involvement**

       B58.81   Toxoplasma myocarditis

       B58.82   Toxoplasma myositis

       B58.83   Toxoplasma tubulo-interstitial nephropathy
            Toxoplasma pyelonephritis

       B58.89   Toxoplasmosis with other organ involvement

    B58.9   Toxoplasmosis, unspecified

    B59   Pneumocystosis
       Pneumonia due to Pneumocystis carinii
       Pneumonia due to Pneumocystis jiroveci

✓4th **B60   Other protozoal diseases, not elsewhere classified**
    EXCLUDES1   cryptosporidiosis (A07.2)
             intestinal microsporidiosis (A07.8)
             isosporiasis (A07.3)

    B60.0   Babesiosis
       Piroplasmosis

✓5th **B60.1   Acanthamebiasis**

       B60.10   Acanthamebiasis, unspecified

       B60.11   Meningoencephalitis due to Acanthamoeba (culbertsoni)

       B60.12   Conjunctivitis due to Acanthamoeba

       B60.13   Keratoconjunctivitis due to Acanthamoeba

       B60.19   Other acanthamebic disease

    B60.2   Naegleriasis
       Primary amebic meningoencephalitis

    B60.8   Other specified protozoal diseases
       Microsporidiosis

    B64   Unspecified protozoal disease

Helminthiases (B65-B83)

✓4th **B65   Schistosomiasis [bilharziasis]**
    INCLUDES   snail fever

    B65.0   Schistosomiasis due to Schistosoma haematobium [urinary schistosomiasis]

    B65.1   Schistosomiasis due to Schistosoma mansoni [intestinal schistosomiasis]

    B65.2   Schistosomiasis due to Schistosoma japonicum
       Asiatic schistosomiasis

    B65.3   Cercarial dermatitis
       Swimmer's itch

☑ Appropriate additional character required   ✓x7th Requires 7th character, placeholder x must fill empty characters

B65.8 **Other schistosomiasis**
     Infection due to Schistosoma intercalatum
     Infection due to Schistosoma mattheei
     Infection due to Schistosoma mekongi

B65.9 **Schistosomiasis, unspecified**

✓4ᵗʰ **B66 Other fluke infections**

B66.0 **Opisthorchiasis**
     Infection due to cat liver fluke
     Infection due to Opisthorchis (felineus)(viverrini)

B66.1 **Clonorchiasis**
     Chinese liver fluke disease
     Infection due to Clonorchis sinensis
     Oriental liver fluke disease

B66.2 **Dicroceliasis**
     Infection due to Dicrocoelium dendriticum
     Lancet fluke infection

B66.3 **Fascioliasis**
     Infection due to Fasciola gigantica
     Infection due to Fasciola hepatica
     Infection due to Fasciola indica
     Sheep liver fluke disease

B66.4 **Paragonimiasis**
     Infection due to Paragonimus species
     Lung fluke disease
     Pulmonary distomiasis

B66.5 **Fasciolopsiasis**
     Infection due to Fasciolopsis buski
     Intestinal distomiasis

B66.8 **Other specified fluke infections**
     Echinostomiasis
     Heterophyiasis
     Metagonimiasis
     Nanophyetiasis
     Watsoniasis

B66.9 **Fluke infection, unspecified**

✓4ᵗʰ **B67 Echinococcosis**
     INCLUDES   hydatidosis

B67.0 **Echinococcus granulosus infection of liver**

B67.1 **Echinococcus granulosus infection of lung**

B67.2 **Echinococcus granulosus infection of bone**

✓5ᵗʰ B67.3 **Echinococcus granulosus infection, other and multiple sites**

     B67.31 **Echinococcus granulosus infection, thyroid gland**

     B67.32 **Echinococcus granulosus infection, multiple sites**

     B67.39 **Echinococcus granulosus infection, other sites**

B67.4 **Echinococcus granulosus infection, unspecified**
     Dog tapeworm (infection)

B67.5 **Echinococcus multilocularis infection of liver**

✓5ᵗʰ B67.6 **Echinococcus multilocularis infection, other and multiple sites**

     B67.61 **Echinococcus multilocularis infection, multiple sites**

     B67.69 **Echinococcus multilocularis infection, other sites**

B67.7 **Echinococcus multilocularis infection, unspecified**

B67.8 **Echinococcosis, unspecified, of liver**

✓5ᵗʰ B67.9 **Echinococcosis, other and unspecified**

     B67.90 **Echinococcosis, unspecified**
         Echinococcosis NOS

     B67.99 **Other echinococcosis**

✓4ᵗʰ **B68 Taeniasis**
     EXCLUDES 1   cysticercosis (B69-)

B68.0 **Taenia solium taeniasis**
     Pork tapeworm (infection)

B68.1 **Taenia saginata taeniasis**
     Beef tapeworm (infection)
     Infection due to adult tapeworm Taenia saginata

B68.9 **Taeniasis, unspecified**

✓4ᵗʰ **B69 Cysticercosis**
     INCLUDES   cysticerciasis infection due to larval form of Taenia solium

B69.0 **Cysticercosis of central nervous system**

B69.1 **Cysticercosis of eye**

✓5ᵗʰ B69.8 **Cysticercosis of other sites**

     B69.81 **Myositis in cysticercosis**

     B69.89 **Cysticercosis of other sites**

B69.9 **Cysticercosis, unspecified**

✓4ᵗʰ **B70 Diphyllobothriasis and sparganosis**

B70.0 **Diphyllobothriasis**
     Diphyllobothrium (adult) (latum) (pacificum) infection
     Fish tapeworm (infection)
     EXCLUDES 2   larval diphyllobothriasis (B70.1)

B70.1 **Sparganosis**
     Infection due to Sparganum (mansoni) (proliferum)
     Infection due to Spirometra larva
     Larval diphyllobothriasis
     Spirometrosis

✓4ᵗʰ **B71 Other cestode infections**

B71.0 **Hymenolepiasis**
     Dwarf tapeworm infection
     Rat tapeworm (infection)

B71.1 **Dipylidiasis**

B71.8 **Other specified cestode infections**
     Coenurosis

B71.9 **Cestode infection, unspecified**
     Tapeworm (infection) NOS

B72 Dracunculiasis
     INCLUDES   guinea worm infection
         infection due to Dracunculus medinensis

B73 Onchocerciasis
     INCLUDES   onchocerca volvulus infection
         onchocercosis
         river blindness

✓5ᵗʰ B73.0 **Onchocerciasis with eye disease**

     B73.00 **Onchocerciasis with eye involvement, unspecified**

     B73.01 **Onchocerciasis with endophthalmitis**

     B73.02 **Onchocerciasis with glaucoma**

     B73.09 **Onchocerciasis with other eye involvement**
         Infestation of eyelid due to onchocerciasis

B73.1 **Onchocerciasis without eye disease**

✓4ᵗʰ **B74 Filariasis**
     EXCLUDES 2   onchocerciasis (B73)
         tropical (pulmonary) eosinophilia NOS (J82)

B74.0 **Filariasis due to Wuchereria bancrofti**
     Bancroftian elephantiasis
     Bancroftian filariasis

B74.1 **Filariasis due to Brugia malayi**

B74.2 **Filariasis due to Brugia timori**

B74.3 **Loiasis**
     Calabar swelling
     Eyeworm disease of Africa
     Loa loa infection

B74.4 **Mansonelliasis**
     Infection due to Mansonella ozzardi
     Infection due to Mansonella perstans
     Infection due to Mansonella streptocerca

B74.8 **Other filariases**
     Dirofilariasis

B74.9 **Filariasis, unspecified**

B75 Trichinellosis
     INCLUDES   infection due to Trichinella species
         trichiniasis

✓4ᵗʰ **B76 Hookworm diseases**
     INCLUDES   uncinariasis

B76.0 **Ancylostomiasis**
     Infection due to Ancylostoma species

B76.1 **Necatoriasis**
     Infection due to Necator americanus

B76.8 **Other hookworm diseases**

B76.9 **Hookworm disease, unspecified**
     Cutaneous larva migrans NOS

✓4ᵗʰ **B77 Ascariasis**
     INCLUDES   ascaridiasis
         roundworm infection

B77.0 **Ascariasis with intestinal complications**

✓5ᵗʰ B77.8 **Ascariasis with other complications**

     B77.81 **Ascariasis pneumonia**

     B77.89 **Ascariasis with other complications**

B77.9 **Ascariasis, unspecified**

✓4ᵗʰ **B78 Strongyloidiasis**
     EXCLUDES 1   trichostrongyliasis (B81.2)

B78.0 **Intestinal strongyloidiasis**

EXCLUDES 1   Not coded here   EXCLUDES 2   Not included here   *Manifestation Code*

B78.1   **Cutaneous strongyloidiasis**

B78.7   **Disseminated strongyloidiasis**

B78.9   **Strongyloidiasis, unspecified**

B79   **Trichuriasis**

INCLUDES   trichocephaliasis
whipworm (disease)(infection)

B80   **Enterobiasis**

INCLUDES   oxyuriasis
pinworm infection
threadworm infection

✓4th **B81**   **Other intestinal helminthiases, not elsewhere classified**

EXCLUDES 1   angiostrongyliasis due to Parastrongylus cantonensis (B83.2)

B81.0   **Anisakiasis**
Infection due to Anisakis larva

B81.1   **Intestinal capillariasis**
Capillariasis NOS
Infection due to Capillaria philippinensis
EXCLUDES 2   hepatic capillariasis (B83.8)

B81.2   **Trichostrongyliasis**

B81.3   **Intestinal angiostrongyliasis**
Angiostrongyliasis due to Parastrongylus costaricensis

B81.4   **Mixed intestinal helminthiases**
Infection due to intestinal helminths classified to more than
one of the categories B65.0-B81.3 and B81.8
Mixed helminthiasis NOS

B81.8   **Other specified intestinal helminthiases**
Infection due to Oesophagostomum species
[esophagostomiasis]
Infection due to Ternidens diminutus [ternidensiasis]

✓4th **B82**   **Unspecified intestinal parasitism**

B82.0   **Intestinal helminthiasis, unspecified**

B82.9   **Intestinal parasitism, unspecified**

✓4th **B83**   **Other helminthiases**

EXCLUDES 1   capillariasis NOS (B81.1)
EXCLUDES 2   intestinal capillariasis (B81.1)

B83.0   **Visceral larva migrans**
Toxocariasis

B83.1   **Gnathostomiasis**
Wandering swelling

B83.2   **Angiostrongyliasis due to Parastrongylus cantonensis**
Eosinophilic meningoencephalitis due to Parastrongylus
cantonensis
EXCLUDES 2   intestinal angiostrongyliasis (B81.3)

B83.3   **Syngamiasis**
Syngamosis

B83.4   **Internal hirudiniasis**
EXCLUDES 2   external hirudiniasis (B88.3)

B83.8   **Other specified helminthiases**
Acanthocephaliasis
Gongylonemiasis
Hepatic capillariasis
Metastrongyliasis
Thelaziasis

B83.9   **Helminthiasis, unspecified**
Worms NOS
EXCLUDES 1   intestinal helminthiasis NOS (B82.0)

Pediculosis, acariasis and other infestations (B85-B89)

✓4th **B85**   **Pediculosis and phthiriasis**

B85.0   **Pediculosis due to Pediculus humanus capitis**
Head-louse infestation

B85.1   **Pediculosis due to Pediculus humanus corporis**
Body-louse infestation

B85.2   **Pediculosis, unspecified**

B85.3   **Phthiriasis**
Infestation by crab-louse
Infestation by Phthirus pubis

B85.4   **Mixed pediculosis and phthiriasis**
Infestation classifiable to more than one of the categories
B85.0- B85.3

B86   **Scabies**
Sarcoptic itch

✓4th **B87**   **Myiasis**
INCLUDES   infestation by larva of flies

B87.0   **Cutaneous myiasis**
Creeping myiasis

B87.1   **Wound myiasis**
Traumatic myiasis

B87.2   **Ocular myiasis**

B87.3   **Nasopharyngeal myiasis**
Laryngeal myiasis

B87.4   **Aural myiasis**

✓5th B87.8   **Myiasis of other sites**

B87.81   **Genitourinary myiasis**

B87.82   **Intestinal myiasis**

B87.89   **Myiasis of other sites**

B87.9   **Myiasis, unspecified**

✓4th **B88**   **Other infestations**

B88.0   **Other acariasis**
Acarine dermatitis
Dermatitis due to Demodex species
Dermatitis due to Dermanyssus gallinae
Dermatitis due to Liponyssoides sanguineus
Trombiculosis
EXCLUDES 2   scabies (B86)

B88.1   **Tungiasis [sandflea infestation]**

B88.2   **Other arthropod infestations**
Scarabiasis

B88.3   **External hirudiniasis**
Leech infestation NOS
EXCLUDES 2   internal hirudiniasis (B83.4)

B88.8   **Other specified infestations**
Ichthyoparasitism due to Vandellia cirrhosa
Linguatulosis
Porocephaliasis

B88.9   **Infestation, unspecified**
Infestation (skin) NOS
Infestation by mites NOS
Skin parasites NOS

B89   **Unspecified parasitic disease**

Sequelae of infectious and parasitic diseases (B90-B94)

NOTE   Categories B90-B94 are to be used to indicate conditions in
categories A00-B89 as the cause of sequelae, which are themselves
classified elsewhere. The "sequelae" include conditions specified as
such; they also include residuals of diseases classifiable to the
above categories if there is evidence that the disease itself is no
longer present. Codes from these categories are not to be used for
chronic infections. Code chronic current infections to active
infectious disease as appropriate.

Code first condition resulting from (sequela) the infectious or parasitic disease

✓4th **B90**   **Sequelae of tuberculosis**

B90.0   **Sequelae of central nervous system tuberculosis**

B90.1   **Sequelae of genitourinary tuberculosis**

B90.2   **Sequelae of tuberculosis of bones and joints**

B90.8   **Sequelae of tuberculosis of other organs**
EXCLUDES 2   sequelae of respiratory tuberculosis (B90.9)

B90.9   **Sequelae of respiratory and unspecified tuberculosis**
Sequelae of tuberculosis NOS

B91   **Sequelae of poliomyelitis**
EXCLUDES 1   postpolio syndrome (G14)

B92   **Sequelae of leprosy**

✓4th **B94**   **Sequelae of other and unspecified infectious and parasitic
diseases**

B94.0   **Sequelae of trachoma**

B94.1   **Sequelae of viral encephalitis**

B94.2   **Sequelae of viral hepatitis**

B94.8   **Sequelae of other specified infectious and parasitic
diseases**

B94.9   **Sequelae of unspecified infectious and parasitic disease**

Bacterial and viral infectious agents (B95-B97)

> **NOTE**   These categories are provided for use as supplementary or additional codes to identify the infectious agent(s) in diseases classified elsewhere.

☑4ᵗʰ B95 Streptococcus, Staphylococcus, and Enterococcus as the cause of diseases classified elsewhere

- **B95.0** Streptococcus, group A, as the cause of diseases classified elsewhere
- **B95.1** Streptococcus, group B, as the cause of diseases classified elsewhere
- **B95.2** Enterococcus as the cause of diseases classified elsewhere
- **B95.3** Streptococcus pneumoniae as the cause of diseases classified elsewhere
- **B95.4** Other streptococcus as the cause of diseases classified elsewhere
- **B95.5** Unspecified streptococcus as the cause of diseases classified elsewhere
- **B95.6** Staphylococcus aureus as the cause of diseases classified elsewhere
- **B95.7** Other staphylococcus as the cause of diseases classified elsewhere
- **B95.8** Unspecified staphylococcus as the cause of diseases classified elsewhere

☑4ᵗʰ B96 Other bacterial agents as the cause of diseases classified elsewhere

- **B96.0** Mycoplasma pneumoniae [M. pneumoniae] as the cause of diseases classified elsewhere
  - Pleuro-pneumonia-like-organism [PPLO]
- **B96.1** Klebsiella pneumoniae [K. pneumoniae] as the cause of diseases classified elsewhere
- **B96.2** Escherichia coli [E. coli] as the cause of diseases classified elsewhere
- **B96.3** Hemophilus influenzae [H. influenzae] as the cause of diseases classified elsewhere
- **B96.4** Proteus (mirabilis) (morganii) as the cause of diseases classified elsewhere
- **B96.5** Pseudomonas (aeruginosa) (mallei) (pseudomallei) as the cause of diseases classified elsewhere
- **B96.6** Bacteroides fragilis [B. fragilis] as the cause of diseases classified elsewhere
- **B96.7** Clostridium perfringens [C. perfringens] as the cause of diseases classified elsewhere
- **☑5ᵗʰ B96.8** Other specified bacterial agents as the cause of diseases classified elsewhere
  - **B96.81** Helicobacter pylori [H. pylori] as the cause of diseases classified elsewhere
  - **B96.82** Vibrio vulnificus as the cause of diseases classified elsewhere
  - **B96.89** Other specified bacterial agents as the cause of diseases classified elsewhere

☑4ᵗʰ B97 Viral agents as the cause of diseases classified elsewhere

- **B97.0** Adenovirus as the cause of diseases classified elsewhere
- **☑5ᵗʰ B97.1** Enterovirus as the cause of diseases classified elsewhere
  - **B97.10** Unspecified enterovirus as the cause of diseases classified elsewhere
  - **B97.11** Coxsackievirus as the cause of diseases classified elsewhere
  - **B97.12** Echovirus as the cause of diseases classified elsewhere
  - **B97.19** Other enterovirus as the cause of diseases classified elsewhere
- **☑5ᵗʰ B97.2** Coronavirus as the cause of diseases classified elsewhere
  - **B97.21** SARS-associated coronavirus as the cause of diseases classified elsewhere
    - *EXCLUDES 1*   pneumonia due to SARS-associated coronavirus (J12.81)
  - **B97.29** Other coronavirus as the cause of diseases classified elsewhere
- **☑5ᵗʰ B97.3** Retrovirus as the cause of diseases classified elsewhere
  - *EXCLUDES 1*   human immunodeficiency virus [HIV} disease (B20)
  - **B97.30** Unspecified retrovirus as the cause of diseases classified elsewhere
  - **B97.31** Lentivirus as the cause of diseases classified elsewhere
  - **B97.32** Oncovirus as the cause of diseases classified elsewhere
  - **B97.33** Human T-cell lymphotrophic virus, type I [HTLV-I] as the cause of diseases classified elsewhere
  - **B97.34** Human T-cell lymphotrophic virus, type II [HTLV-II] as the cause of diseases classified elsewhere
  - **B97.35** Human immunodeficiency virus, type 2 [HIV 2] as the cause of diseases classified elsewhere
  - **B97.39** Other retrovirus as the cause of diseases classified elsewhere
- **B97.4** Respiratory syncytial virus as the cause of diseases classified elsewhere
- **B97.5** Reovirus as the cause of diseases classified elsewhere
- **B97.6** Parvovirus as the cause of diseases classified elsewhere
- **B97.7** Papillomavirus as the cause of diseases classified elsewhere
- **☑5ᵗʰ B97.8** Other viral agents as the cause of diseases classified elsewhere
  - **B97.81** Human metapneumovirus as the cause of diseases classified elsewhere
  - **B97.89** Other viral agents as the cause of diseases classified elsewhere

Other infectious diseases (B99)

☑4ᵗʰ B99 Other and unspecified infectious diseases

- **B99.8** Other infectious disease
- **B99.9** Unspecified infectious disease

EXCLUDES 1 Not coded here   *EXCLUDES 2* Not included here   **Manifestation Code**

Chapter 2. Neoplasms (C00-D49)

This chapter contains the following broad groups of neoplasms:

C00-C14	Malignant neoplasms of lip, oral cavity and pharynx
C15-C26	Malignant neoplasms of digestive organs
C30-C39	Malignant neoplasms of respiratory and intrathoracic organs
C40-C41	Malignant neoplasms of bone and articular cartilage
C43-C44	Malignant neoplasms of skin
C45-C49	Malignant neoplasms of mesothelial and soft tissue
C50	Malignant neoplasms of breast
C51-C58	Malignant neoplasms of female genital organs
C60-C63	Malignant neoplasms of male genital organs
C64-C68	Malignant neoplasms of urinary tract
C69-C72	Malignant neoplasms of eye, brain and other parts of central nervous system
C73-C75	Malignant neoplasms of thyroid and other endocrine glands
C7a	Malignant neuroendocrine tumors
C7b	Secondary neuroendocrine tumors
C76-C80	Malignant neoplasms of ill-defined, other secondary and unspecified sites
C81-C96	Malignant neoplasms of lymphoid, hematopoietic and related tissue
D00-D09	In situ neoplasms
D10-D36	Benign neoplasms, except benign neuroendocrine tumors
D3a	Benign neuroendocrine tumors
D37-D48	Neoplasms of uncertain behavior, polycythemia vera and myelodysplastic syndromes
D49	Neoplasms of unspecified behavior

NOTE

Functional activity
All neoplasms are classified in this chapter, whether they are functionally active or not. An additional code from Chapter 4 may be used, to identify functional activity associated with any neoplasm.

Morphology [Histology]
Chapter 2 classifies neoplasms primarily by site (topography), with broad groupings for behavior, malignant, in situ, benign, etc. The Table of Neoplasms should be used to identify the correct topography code. In a few cases, such as for malignant melanoma and certain neuroendocrine tumors, the morphology (histologic type) is included in the category and codes. To identify the morphology for the majority of Chapter 2 codes that do not include the histologic type, comprehensive separate morphology codes are provided. These morphology codes are derived from the International Classification of Diseases for Oncology (ICD-O).

Primary malignant neoplasms overlapping site boundaries
A primary malignant neoplasm that overlaps two or more contiguous (next to each other) sites should be classified to the subcategory/code .8 ("overlapping lesion"), unless the combination is specifically indexed elsewhere. For multiple neoplasms of the same site that are not contiguous, such as tumors in different quadrants of the same breast, codes for each site should be assigned.

Malignant neoplasm of ectopic tissue
Malignant neoplasms of ectopic tissue are to be coded to the site mentioned, e.g., ectopic pancreatic malignant neoplasms are coded to pancreas, unspecified (C25.9).

MALIGNANT NEOPLASMS (C00-C96)

Use additional morphology codes with behavior code /3

NOTE Malignant neoplasms, stated or presumed to be primary (of specified sites), and certain specified histologies, except neuroendocrine, and of lymphoid, hematopoietic and related tissue (C00-C75)

Malignant neoplasm of lip, oral cavity and pharynx (C00-C14)

✓4ᵗʰ **C00 Malignant neoplasm of lip**

> EXCLUDES 1 *malignant neoplasm of skin of lip (C43.0, C44.0)*
> *Merkel cell carcinoma of lip (C4a.0)*

Use additional code to identify:
alcohol abuse and dependence (F10-)
history of tobacco use (Z87.891)
tobacco dependence (F17-)
tobacco use (Z72.0)

C00.0 Malignant neoplasm of external upper lip
Malignant neoplasm of lipstick area of upper lip
Malignant neoplasm of upper lip NOS
Malignant neoplasm of vermilion border of upper lip

C00.1 Malignant neoplasm of external lower lip
Malignant neoplasm of lower lip NOS
Malignant neoplasm of lipstick area of lower lip
Malignant neoplasm of vermilion border of lower lip

C00.2 Malignant neoplasm of external lip, unspecified
Malignant neoplasm of vermilion border of lip NOS

C00.3 Malignant neoplasm of upper lip, inner aspect
Malignant neoplasm of buccal aspect of upper lip
Malignant neoplasm of frenulum of upper lip
Malignant neoplasm of mucosa of upper lip
Malignant neoplasm of oral aspect of upper lip

C00.4 Malignant neoplasm of lower lip, inner aspect
Malignant neoplasm of buccal aspect of lower lip
Malignant neoplasm of frenulum of lower lip
Malignant neoplasm of mucosa of lower lip
Malignant neoplasm of oral aspect of lower lip

C00.5 Malignant neoplasm of lip, unspecified, inner aspect
Malignant neoplasm of buccal aspect of lip, unspecified
Malignant neoplasm of frenulum of lip, unspecified
Malignant neoplasm of mucosa of lip, unspecified
Malignant neoplasm of oral aspect of lip, unspecified

C00.6 Malignant neoplasm of commissure of lip, unspecified

C00.8 Malignant neoplasm of overlapping sites of lip

C00.9 Malignant neoplasm of lip, unspecified

C01 Malignant neoplasm of base of tongue
Malignant neoplasm of dorsal surface of base of tongue NOS
Malignant neoplasm of fixed part of tongue NOS
Malignant neoplasm of posterior third of tongue
Use additional code to identify:
alcohol abuse and dependence (F10-)
history of tobacco use (Z87.891)
tobacco dependence (F17-)
tobacco use (Z72.0)

✓4ᵗʰ **C02 Malignant neoplasm of other and unspecified parts of tongue**
Use additional code to identify:
alcohol abuse and dependence (F10-)
history of tobacco use (Z87.891)
tobacco dependence (F17-)
tobacco use (Z72.0)

C02.0 Malignant neoplasm of dorsal surface of tongue
Malignant neoplasm of anterior two-thirds of tongue, dorsal surface
> EXCLUDES 2 *malignant neoplasm of dorsal surface of base of tongue (C01)*

C02.1 Malignant neoplasm of border of tongue
Malignant neoplasm of tip of tongue

C02.2 Malignant neoplasm of ventral surface of tongue
Malignant neoplasm of anterior two-thirds of tongue, ventral surface
Malignant neoplasm of frenulum linguae

C02.3 Malignant neoplasm of anterior two-thirds of tongue, part unspecified
Malignant neoplasm of middle third of tongue NOS
Malignant neoplasm of mobile part of tongue NOS

C02.4 Malignant neoplasm of lingual tonsil
> EXCLUDES 2 *malignant neoplasm of tonsil NOS (C09.9)*

C02.8 Malignant neoplasm of overlapping sites of tongue
Malignant neoplasm of two or more contiguous sites of tongue

C02.9 Malignant neoplasm of tongue, unspecified

✓4ᵗʰ **C03 Malignant neoplasm of gum**
> INCLUDES malignant neoplasm of alveolar (ridge) mucosa
> malignant neoplasm of gingiva
> EXCLUDES 2 *malignant odontogenic neoplasms (C41.0-C41.1)*

Use additional code to identify:
alcohol abuse and dependence (F10-)
history of tobacco use (Z87.891)
tobacco dependence (F17-)
tobacco use (Z72.0)

C03.0 Malignant neoplasm of upper gum

C03.1 Malignant neoplasm of lower gum

C03.9 Malignant neoplasm of gum, unspecified

Neoplasms

C04–C12

✓4th **C04 Malignant neoplasm of floor of mouth**
Use additional code to identify:
    alcohol abuse and dependence (F10-)
    history of tobacco use (Z87.891)
    tobacco dependence (F17-)
    tobacco use (Z72.0)

  C04.0 Malignant neoplasm of anterior floor of mouth
    Malignant neoplasm of anterior to the premolar-canine junction

  C04.1 Malignant neoplasm of lateral floor of mouth

  C04.8 Malignant neoplasm of overlapping sites of floor of mouth

  C04.9 Malignant neoplasm of floor of mouth, unspecified

✓4th **C05 Malignant neoplasm of palate**
  EXCLUDES 1   *Kaposi's sarcoma of palate (C46.2)*
Use additional code to identify:
    alcohol abuse and dependence (F10-)
    history of tobacco use (Z87.891)
    tobacco dependence (F17-)
    tobacco use (Z72.0)

  C05.0 Malignant neoplasm of hard palate

  C05.1 Malignant neoplasm of soft palate
    EXCLUDES 2   *malignant neoplasm of nasopharyngeal surface of soft palate (C11.3)*

  C05.2 Malignant neoplasm of uvula

  C05.8 Malignant neoplasm of overlapping sites of palate

  C05.9 Malignant neoplasm of palate, unspecified
    Malignant neoplasm of roof of mouth

✓4th **C06 Malignant neoplasm of other and unspecified parts of mouth**
Use additional code to identify:
    alcohol abuse and dependence (F10-)
    history of tobacco use (Z87.891)
    tobacco dependence (F17-)
    tobacco use (Z72.0)

  C06.0 Malignant neoplasm of cheek mucosa
    Malignant neoplasm of buccal mucosa NOS
    Malignant neoplasm of internal cheek

  C06.1 Malignant neoplasm of vestibule of mouth
    Malignant neoplasm of buccal sulcus (upper) (lower)
    Malignant neoplasm of labial sulcus (upper) (lower)

  C06.2 Malignant neoplasm of retromolar area

✓5th **C06.8 Malignant neoplasm of overlapping sites of other and unspecified parts of mouth**

    C06.80 Malignant neoplasm of overlapping sites of unspecified parts of mouth

    C06.89 Malignant neoplasm of overlapping sites of other parts of mouth
      "book leaf" neoplasm [ventral surface of tongue and floor of mouth]

  C06.9 Malignant neoplasm of mouth, unspecified
    Malignant neoplasm of minor salivary gland, unspecified site
    Malignant neoplasm of oral cavity NOS

C07 Malignant neoplasm of parotid gland
Use additional code to identify:
    alcohol abuse and dependence (F10-)
    exposure to environmental tobacco smoke (Z77.22)
    exposure to tobacco smoke in the perinatal period (P96.81)
    history of tobacco use (Z87.891)
    occupational exposure to environmental tobacco smoke (Z57.31)
    tobacco dependence (F17-)
    tobacco use (Z72.0)

✓4th **C08 Malignant neoplasm of other and unspecified major salivary glands**
  INCLUDES   malignant neoplasm of salivary ducts
  EXCLUDES 1   *malignant neoplasms of specified minor salivary glands which are classified according to their anatomical location*
  EXCLUDES 2   *malignant neoplasms of minor salivary glands NOS (C06.9)*
      malignant neoplasm of parotid gland (C07)
Use additional code to identify:
    alcohol abuse and dependence (F10-)
    exposure to environmental tobacco smoke (Z77.22)
    exposure to tobacco smoke in the perinatal period (P96.81)
    history of tobacco use (Z87.891)
    occupational exposure to environmental tobacco smoke (Z57.31)
    tobacco dependence (F17-)
    tobacco use (Z72.0)

  C08.0 Malignant neoplasm of submandibular gland
    Malignant neoplasm of submaxillary gland

  C08.1 Malignant neoplasm of sublingual gland

  C08.9 Malignant neoplasm of major salivary gland, unspecified
    Malignant neoplasm of salivary gland (major) NOS

✓4th **C09 Malignant neoplasm of tonsil**
  EXCLUDES 2   *malignant neoplasm of lingual tonsil (C02.4)*
      malignant neoplasm of pharyngeal tonsil (C11.1)
Use additional code to identify:
    alcohol abuse and dependence (F10-)
    exposure to environmental tobacco smoke (Z77.22)
    exposure to tobacco smoke in the perinatal period (P96.81)
    history of tobacco use (Z87.891)
    occupational exposure to environmental tobacco smoke (Z57.31)
    tobacco dependence (F17-)
    tobacco use (Z72.0)

  C09.0 Malignant neoplasm of tonsillar fossa

  C09.1 Malignant neoplasm of tonsillar pillar (anterior) (posterior)

  C09.8 Malignant neoplasm of overlapping sites of tonsil

  C09.9 Malignant neoplasm of tonsil, unspecified
    Malignant neoplasm of tonsil NOS
    Malignant neoplasm of faucial tonsils
    Malignant neoplasm of palatine tonsils

✓4th **C10 Malignant neoplasm of oropharynx**
  EXCLUDES 2   *malignant neoplasm of tonsil (C09-)*
Use additional code to identify:
    alcohol abuse and dependence (F10-)
    exposure to environmental tobacco smoke (Z77.22)
    exposure to tobacco smoke in the perinatal period (P96.81)
    history of tobacco use (Z87.891)
    occupational exposure to environmental tobacco smoke (Z57.31)
    tobacco dependence (F17-)
    tobacco use (Z72.0)

  C10.0 Malignant neoplasm of vallecula

  C10.1 Malignant neoplasm of anterior surface of epiglottis
    Malignant neoplasm of epiglottis, free border [margin]
    Malignant neoplasm of glossoepiglottic fold(s)
    EXCLUDES 2   *malignant neoplasm of epiglottis (suprahyoid portion) NOS (C32.1)*

  C10.2 Malignant neoplasm of lateral wall of oropharynx

  C10.3 Malignant neoplasm of posterior wall of oropharynx

  C10.4 Malignant neoplasm of branchial cleft
    Malignant neoplasm of branchial cyst [site of neoplasm]

  C10.8 Malignant neoplasm of overlapping sites of oropharynx
    Malignant neoplasm of junctional region of oropharynx

  C10.9 Malignant neoplasm of oropharynx, unspecified

✓4th **C11 Malignant neoplasm of nasopharynx**
Use additional code to identify:
    exposure to environmental tobacco smoke (Z77.22)
    exposure to tobacco smoke in the perinatal period (P96.81)
    history of tobacco use (Z87.891)
    occupational exposure to environmental tobacco smoke (Z57.31)
    tobacco dependence (F17-)
    tobacco use (Z72.0)

  C11.0 Malignant neoplasm of superior wall of nasopharynx
    Malignant neoplasm of roof of nasopharynx

  C11.1 Malignant neoplasm of posterior wall of nasopharynx
    Malignant neoplasm of adenoid
    Malignant neoplasm of pharyngeal tonsil

  C11.2 Malignant neoplasm of lateral wall of nasopharynx
    Malignant neoplasm of fossa of Rosenmüller
    Malignant neoplasm of opening of auditory tube
    Malignant neoplasm of pharyngeal recess

  C11.3 Malignant neoplasm of anterior wall of nasopharynx
    Malignant neoplasm of floor of nasopharynx
    Malignant neoplasm of nasopharyngeal (anterior) (posterior) surface of soft palate
    Malignant neoplasm of posterior margin of nasal choana
    Malignant neoplasm of posterior margin of nasal septum

  C11.8 Malignant neoplasm of overlapping sites of nasopharynx

  C11.9 Malignant neoplasm of nasopharynx, unspecified
    Malignant neoplasm of nasopharyngeal wall NOS

C12 Malignant neoplasm of pyriform sinus
  Malignant neoplasm of pyriform fossa
Use additional code to identify:
    exposure to environmental tobacco smoke (Z77.22)
    exposure to tobacco smoke in the perinatal period (P96.81)
    history of tobacco use (Z87.891)
    occupational exposure to environmental tobacco smoke (Z57.31)
    tobacco dependence (F17-)
    tobacco use (Z72.0)

EXCLUDES 1   Not coded here   EXCLUDES 2   Not included here   *Manifestation Code*

☑4ᵗʰ **C13 Malignant neoplasm of hypopharynx**
> *EXCLUDES 2* *malignant neoplasm of pyriform sinus (C12)*
> Use additional code to identify:
> exposure to environmental tobacco smoke (Z77.22)
> exposure to tobacco smoke in the perinatal period (P96.81)
> history of tobacco use (Z87.891)
> occupational exposure to environmental tobacco smoke (Z57.31)
> tobacco dependence (F17-)
> tobacco use (Z72.Ø)

C13.Ø Malignant neoplasm of postcricoid region

C13.1 Malignant neoplasm of aryepiglottic fold, hypopharyngeal aspect
> Malignant neoplasm of aryepiglottic fold NOS
> Malignant neoplasm of interarytenoid fold NOS
> Malignant neoplasm of aryepiglottic fold marginal zone
> Malignant neoplasm of interarytenoid fold marginal zone
> *EXCLUDES 2* *malignant neoplasm of aryepiglottic fold or interarytenoid fold, laryngeal aspect (C32.1)*

C13.2 Malignant neoplasm of posterior wall of hypopharynx

C13.8 Malignant neoplasm of overlapping sites of hypopharynx

C13.9 Malignant neoplasm of hypopharynx, unspecified
> Malignant neoplasm of hypopharyngeal wall NOS

☑4ᵗʰ **C14 Malignant neoplasm of other and ill-defined sites in the lip, oral cavity and pharynx**
> *EXCLUDES 1* *malignant neoplasm of oral cavity NOS (CØ6.9)*
> Use additional code to identify:
> alcohol abuse and dependence (F1Ø-)
> exposure to environmental tobacco smoke (Z77.22)
> exposure to tobacco smoke in the perinatal period (P96.81)
> history of tobacco use (Z87.891)
> occupational exposure to environmental tobacco smoke (Z57.31)
> tobacco dependence (F17-)
> tobacco use (Z72.Ø)

C14.Ø Malignant neoplasm of pharynx, unspecified

C14.2 Malignant neoplasm of Waldeyer's ring

C14.8 Malignant neoplasm of overlapping sites of lip, oral cavity and pharynx
> Primary malignant neoplasm of two or more contiguous sites of lip, oral cavity and pharynx
> *EXCLUDES 1* *"book leaf" neoplasm [ventral surface of tongue and floor of mouth] (CØ6.89)*

Malignant neoplasm of digestive organs (C15-C26)
> *EXCLUDES 1* *Kaposi's sarcoma of gastrointestinal sites (C46.4)*

☑4ᵗʰ **C15 Malignant neoplasm of esophagus**
> Use additional code to identify:
> alcohol abuse and dependence (F1Ø-)

C15.3 Malignant neoplasm of upper third of esophagus

C15.4 Malignant neoplasm of middle third of esophagus

C15.5 Malignant neoplasm of lower third of esophagus
> *EXCLUDES 1* *malignant neoplasm of cardio-esophageal junction (C16.Ø)*

C15.8 Malignant neoplasm of overlapping sites of esophagus

C15.9 Malignant neoplasm of esophagus, unspecified

☑4ᵗʰ **C16 Malignant neoplasm of stomach**
> Use additional code to identify:
> alcohol abuse and dependence (F1Ø-)
> *EXCLUDES 2* *malignant carcinoid tumor of the stomach (C7a.Ø92)*

C16.Ø Malignant neoplasm of cardia
> Malignant neoplasm of cardiac orifice
> Malignant neoplasm of cardio-esophageal junction
> Malignant neoplasm of esophagus and stomach
> Malignant neoplasm of gastro-esophageal junction

C16.1 Malignant neoplasm of fundus of stomach

C16.2 Malignant neoplasm of body of stomach

C16.3 Malignant neoplasm of pyloric antrum
> Malignant neoplasm of gastric antrum

C16.4 Malignant neoplasm of pylorus
> Malignant neoplasm of prepylorus
> Malignant neoplasm of pyloric canal

C16.5 Malignant neoplasm of lesser curvature of stomach, unspecified
> Malignant neoplasm of lesser curvature of stomach, not classifiable to C16.1-C16.4

C16.6 Malignant neoplasm of greater curvature of stomach, unspecified
> Malignant neoplasm of greater curvature of stomach, not classifiable to C16.Ø-C16.4

C16.8 Malignant neoplasm of overlapping sites of stomach

C16.9 Malignant neoplasm of stomach, unspecified
> Gastric cancer NOS

☑4ᵗʰ **C17 Malignant neoplasm of small intestine**
> *EXCLUDES 1* *malignant carcinoid tumors of the small intestine (C7a.Ø1)*

C17.Ø Malignant neoplasm of duodenum

C17.1 Malignant neoplasm of jejunum

C17.2 Malignant neoplasm of ileum
> *EXCLUDES 1* *malignant neoplasm of ileocecal valve (C18.Ø)*

C17.3 Meckel's diverticulum, malignant
> *EXCLUDES 1* *Meckel's diverticulum, congenital (Q43.Ø)*

C17.8 Malignant neoplasm of overlapping sites of small intestine

C17.9 Malignant neoplasm of small intestine, unspecified

☑4ᵗʰ **C18 Malignant neoplasm of colon**
> *EXCLUDES 1* *malignant carcinoid tumors of the colon (C7a.Ø2-)*

C18.Ø Malignant neoplasm of cecum
> Malignant neoplasm of ileocecal valve

C18.1 Malignant neoplasm of appendix

C18.2 Malignant neoplasm of ascending colon

C18.3 Malignant neoplasm of hepatic flexure

C18.4 Malignant neoplasm of transverse colon

C18.5 Malignant neoplasm of splenic flexure

C18.6 Malignant neoplasm of descending colon

C18.7 Malignant neoplasm of sigmoid colon
> Malignant neoplasm of sigmoid (flexure)
> *EXCLUDES 1* *malignant neoplasm of rectosigmoid junction (C19)*

C18.8 Malignant neoplasm of overlapping sites of colon

C18.9 Malignant neoplasm of colon, unspecified
> Malignant neoplasm of large intestine NOS

C19 Malignant neoplasm of rectosigmoid junction
> Malignant neoplasm of colon with rectum
> Malignant neoplasm of rectosigmoid (colon)
> *EXCLUDES 1* *malignant carcinoid tumors of the colon (C7a.Ø2-)*

C2Ø Malignant neoplasm of rectum
> Malignant neoplasm of rectal ampulla
> *EXCLUDES 1* *malignant carcinoid tumor of the rectum (C7a.Ø26)*

☑4ᵗʰ **C21 Malignant neoplasm of anus and anal canal**
> *EXCLUDES 2* *malignant carcinoid tumors of the colon (C7a.Ø2-)*
> *malignant melanoma of anal margin (C43.51)*
> *malignant melanoma of anal skin (C43.51)*
> *malignant melanoma of perianal skin (C43.51)*
> *malignant neoplasm of anal margin (C44.51)*
> *malignant neoplasm of anal skin (C44.51)*
> *malignant neoplasm of perianal skin (C44.51)*

C21.Ø Malignant neoplasm of anus, unspecified

C21.1 Malignant neoplasm of anal canal
> Malignant neoplasm of anal sphincter

C21.2 Malignant neoplasm of cloacogenic zone

C21.8 Malignant neoplasm of overlapping sites of rectum, anus and anal canal
> Malignant neoplasm of anorectal junction
> Malignant neoplasm of anorectum
> Primary malignant neoplasm of two or more contiguous sites of rectum, anus and anal canal

☑4ᵗʰ **C22 Malignant neoplasm of liver and intrahepatic bile ducts**
> *EXCLUDES 1* *malignant neoplasm of biliary tract NOS (C24.9)*
> *secondary malignant neoplasm of liver and intrahepatic bile duct (C78.7)*
> Use additional code to identify:
> alcohol abuse and dependence (F1Ø-)
> hepatitis B (B16-, B18.Ø-B18.1)
> hepatitis C (B17.1-, B18.2)

C22.Ø Liver cell carcinoma
> Hepatocellular carcinoma
> Hepatoma

C22.1 Intrahepatic bile duct carcinoma
> Cholangiocarcinoma
> *EXCLUDES 1* *malignant neoplasm of hepatic duct (C24.Ø)*

C22.2 Hepatoblastoma

C22.3 Angiosarcoma of liver
> Kupffer cell sarcoma

C22.4   **Other sarcomas of liver**

C22.7   **Other specified carcinomas of liver**

C22.8   **Malignant neoplasm of liver, primary, unspecified as to type**

C22.9   **Malignant neoplasm of liver, not specified as primary or secondary**

C23   Malignant neoplasm of gallbladder

✓4ᵗʰ **C24   Malignant neoplasm of other and unspecified parts of biliary tract**

> EXCLUDES 1   *malignant neoplasm of intrahepatic bile duct (C22.1)*

C24.0   **Malignant neoplasm of extrahepatic bile duct**
Malignant neoplasm of biliary duct or passage NOS
Malignant neoplasm of common bile duct
Malignant neoplasm of cystic duct
Malignant neoplasm of hepatic duct

C24.1   **Malignant neoplasm of ampulla of Vater**

C24.8   **Malignant neoplasm of overlapping sites of biliary tract**
Malignant neoplasm involving both intrahepatic and extrahepatic bile ducts
Primary malignant neoplasm of two or more contiguous sites of biliary tract

C24.9   **Malignant neoplasm of biliary tract, unspecified**

✓4ᵗʰ **C25   Malignant neoplasm of pancreas**
Use additional code to identify:
alcohol abuse and dependence (F10-)

C25.0   **Malignant neoplasm of head of pancreas**

C25.1   **Malignant neoplasm of body of pancreas**

C25.2   **Malignant neoplasm of tail of pancreas**

C25.3   **Malignant neoplasm of pancreatic duct**

C25.4   **Malignant neoplasm of endocrine pancreas**
Malignant neoplasm of islets of Langerhans
Use additional code to identify any functional activity

C25.7   **Malignant neoplasm of other parts of pancreas**
Malignant neoplasm of neck of pancreas

C25.8   **Malignant neoplasm of overlapping sites of pancreas**

C25.9   **Malignant neoplasm of pancreas, unspecified**

✓4ᵗʰ **C26   Malignant neoplasm of other and ill-defined digestive organs**

> EXCLUDES 1   *malignant neoplasm of peritoneum and retroperitoneum (C48-)*

C26.0   **Malignant neoplasm of intestinal tract, part unspecified**
Malignant neoplasm of intestine NOS

C26.1   **Malignant neoplasm of spleen**
> EXCLUDES 1   *Hodgkin lymphoma (C81-)*
> *non-Hodgkin lymphoma (C82-C85)*

C26.9   **Malignant neoplasm of ill-defined sites within the digestive system**
Malignant neoplasm of alimentary canal or tract NOS
Malignant neoplasm of gastrointestinal tract NOS
> EXCLUDES 1   *malignant neoplasm of abdominal NOS (C76.2)*
> *malignant neoplasm of intra-abdominal NOS (C76.2)*

Malignant neoplasm of respiratory and intrathoracic organs (C30-C39)

> INCLUDES   malignant neoplasm of middle ear
> EXCLUDES 1   *mesothelioma (C45-)*

✓4ᵗʰ **C30   Malignant neoplasm of nasal cavity and middle ear**

C30.0   **Malignant neoplasm of nasal cavity**
Malignant neoplasm of cartilage of nose
Malignant neoplasm of nasal concha
Malignant neoplasm of internal nose
Malignant neoplasm of septum of nose
Malignant neoplasm of vestibule of nose
> EXCLUDES 1   *malignant neoplasm of nasal bone (C41.0)*
> *malignant neoplasm of nose NOS (C76.0)*
> *malignant neoplasm of olfactory bulb (C72.2-)*
> *malignant neoplasm of posterior margin of nasal septum and choana (C11.3)*
> *malignant neoplasm of skin of nose (C43.31, C44.31)*
> *malignant neoplasm of turbinates (C41.0)*

C30.1   **Malignant neoplasm of middle ear**
Malignant neoplasm of antrum tympanicum
Malignant neoplasm of auditory tube
Malignant neoplasm of eustachian tube
Malignant neoplasm of inner ear
Malignant neoplasm of mastoid air cells
Malignant neoplasm of tympanic cavity
> EXCLUDES 1   *malignant neoplasm of auricular canal (external) (C43.2-,C44.2-)*
> *malignant neoplasm of bone of ear (meatus) (C41.0)*
> *malignant neoplasm of cartilage of ear (C49.0)*
> *malignant neoplasm of skin of (external) ear (C43.2-, C44.2-)*

✓4ᵗʰ **C31   Malignant neoplasm of accessory sinuses**

C31.0   **Malignant neoplasm of maxillary sinus**
Malignant neoplasm of antrum (Highmore) (maxillary)

C31.1   **Malignant neoplasm of ethmoidal sinus**

C31.2   **Malignant neoplasm of frontal sinus**

C31.3   **Malignant neoplasm of sphenoid sinus**

C31.8   **Malignant neoplasm of overlapping sites of accessory sinuses**

C31.9   **Malignant neoplasm of accessory sinus, unspecified**

✓4ᵗʰ **C32   Malignant neoplasm of larynx**
Use additional code to identify:
alcohol abuse and dependence (F10-)
exposure to environmental tobacco smoke (Z77.22)
exposure to tobacco smoke in the perinatal period (P96.81)
history of tobacco use (Z87.891)
occupational exposure to environmental tobacco smoke (Z57.31)
tobacco dependence (F17-)
tobacco use (Z72.0)

C32.0   **Malignant neoplasm of glottis**
Malignant neoplasm of intrinsic larynx
Malignant neoplasm of laryngeal commissure (anterior)(posterior)
Malignant neoplasm of vocal cord (true) NOS

C32.1   **Malignant neoplasm of supraglottis**
Malignant neoplasm of aryepiglottic fold or interarytenoid fold, laryngeal aspect
Malignant neoplasm of epiglottis (suprahyoid portion) NOS
Malignant neoplasm of extrinsic larynx
Malignant neoplasm of false vocal cord
Malignant neoplasm of posterior (laryngeal) surface of epiglottis
Malignant neoplasm of ventricular bands
> EXCLUDES 2   *malignant neoplasm of anterior surface of epiglottis (C10.1)*
> *malignant neoplasm of aryepiglottic fold or interarytenoid fold:*
> *NOS (C13.1)*
> *hypopharyngeal aspect (C13.1)*
> *marginal zone (C13.1)*

C32.2   **Malignant neoplasm of subglottis**

C32.3   **Malignant neoplasm of laryngeal cartilage**

C32.8   **Malignant neoplasm of overlapping sites of larynx**

C32.9   **Malignant neoplasm of larynx, unspecified**

EXCLUDES 1   Not coded here   EXCLUDES 2   Not included here   *Manifestation Code*

C33   Malignant neoplasm of trachea
   Use additional code to identify:
      exposure to environmental tobacco smoke (Z77.22)
      exposure to tobacco smoke in the perinatal period (P96.81)
      history of tobacco use (Z87.891)
      occupational exposure to environmental tobacco smoke (Z57.31)
      tobacco dependence (F17-)
      tobacco use (Z72.0)

☑4ᵗʰ **C34   Malignant neoplasm of bronchus and lung**
   EXCLUDES 1   *Kaposi's sarcoma of lung (C46.5-)*
               malignant carcinoid tumor of the bronchus and lung (C7a.090)
   Use additional code to identify:
      exposure to environmental tobacco smoke (Z77.22)
      exposure to tobacco smoke in the perinatal period (P96.81)
      history of tobacco use (Z87.891)
      occupational exposure to environmental tobacco smoke (Z57.31)
      tobacco dependence (F17-)
      tobacco use (Z72.0)

☑5ᵗʰ **C34.0   Malignant neoplasm of main bronchus**
      Malignant neoplasm of carina
      Malignant neoplasm of hilus (of lung)
      C34.00   Malignant neoplasm of unspecified main bronchus
      C34.01   Malignant neoplasm of right main bronchus
      C34.02   Malignant neoplasm of left main bronchus

☑5ᵗʰ **C34.1   Malignant neoplasm of upper lobe, bronchus or lung**
      C34.10   Malignant neoplasm of upper lobe, unspecified bronchus or lung
      C34.11   Malignant neoplasm of upper lobe, right bronchus or lung
      C34.12   Malignant neoplasm of upper lobe, left bronchus or lung

   C34.2   Malignant neoplasm of middle lobe, bronchus or lung

☑5ᵗʰ **C34.3   Malignant neoplasm of lower lobe, bronchus or lung**
      C34.30   Malignant neoplasm of lower lobe, unspecified bronchus or lung
      C34.31   Malignant neoplasm of lower lobe, right bronchus or lung
      C34.32   Malignant neoplasm of lower lobe, left bronchus or lung

☑5ᵗʰ **C34.8   Malignant neoplasm of overlapping sites of bronchus and lung**
      C34.80   Malignant neoplasm of overlapping sites of unspecified bronchus and lung
      C34.81   Malignant neoplasm of overlapping sites of right bronchus and lung
      C34.82   Malignant neoplasm of overlapping sites of left bronchus and lung

☑5ᵗʰ **C34.9   Malignant neoplasm of unspecified part of bronchus or lung**
      C34.90   Malignant neoplasm of unspecified part of unspecified bronchus or lung
         Lung cancer NOS
      C34.91   Malignant neoplasm of unspecified part of right bronchus or lung
      C34.92   Malignant neoplasm of unspecified part of left bronchus or lung

C37   Malignant neoplasm of thymus
   EXCLUDES 1   *malignant carcinoid tumor of the thymus (C7a.091)*

☑4ᵗʰ **C38   Malignant neoplasm of heart, mediastinum and pleura**
   EXCLUDES 1   *mesothelioma (C45-)*

   C38.0   Malignant neoplasm of heart
      Malignant neoplasm of pericardium
      EXCLUDES 1   *malignant neoplasm of great vessels (C49.3)*

   C38.1   Malignant neoplasm of anterior mediastinum
   C38.2   Malignant neoplasm of posterior mediastinum
   C38.3   Malignant neoplasm of mediastinum, part unspecified
   C38.4   Malignant neoplasm of pleura
   C38.8   Malignant neoplasm of overlapping sites of heart, mediastinum and pleura

☑4ᵗʰ **C39   Malignant neoplasm of other and ill-defined sites in the respiratory system and intrathoracic organs**
   EXCLUDES 1   *intrathoracic malignant neoplasm NOS (C76.1)*
               thoracic malignant neoplasm NOS (C76.1)
   Use additional code to identify:
      exposure to environmental tobacco smoke (Z77.22)
      exposure to tobacco smoke in the perinatal period (P96.81)
      history of tobacco use (Z87.891)
      occupational exposure to environmental tobacco smoke (Z57.31)
      tobacco dependence (F17-)
      tobacco use (Z72.0)

   C39.0   Malignant neoplasm of upper respiratory tract, part unspecified
   C39.9   Malignant neoplasm of lower respiratory tract, part unspecified
      Malignant neoplasm of respiratory tract NOS

Malignant neoplasm of bone and articular cartilage (C40-C41)

   INCLUDES   malignant neoplasm of cartilage (articular) (joint)
            malignant neoplasm of periosteum
   EXCLUDES 1   *malignant neoplasm of bone marrow NOS (C96.9)*
               malignant neoplasm of synovia (C49-)

☑4ᵗʰ **C40   Malignant neoplasm of bone and articular cartilage of limbs**
   Use additional code to identify major osseous defect, if applicable (M89.7-)

☑5ᵗʰ **C40.0   Malignant neoplasm of scapula and long bones of upper limb**
      C40.00   Malignant neoplasm of scapula and long bones of unspecified upper limb
      C40.01   Malignant neoplasm of scapula and long bones of right upper limb
      C40.02   Malignant neoplasm of scapula and long bones of left upper limb

☑5ᵗʰ **C40.1   Malignant neoplasm of short bones of upper limb**
      C40.10   Malignant neoplasm of short bones of unspecified upper limb
      C40.11   Malignant neoplasm of short bones of right upper limb
      C40.12   Malignant neoplasm of short bones of left upper limb

☑5ᵗʰ **C40.2   Malignant neoplasm of long bones of lower limb**
      C40.20   Malignant neoplasm of long bones of unspecified lower limb
      C40.21   Malignant neoplasm of long bones of right lower limb
      C40.22   Malignant neoplasm of long bones of left lower limb

☑5ᵗʰ **C40.3   Malignant neoplasm of short bones of lower limb**
      C40.30   Malignant neoplasm of short bones of unspecified lower limb
      C40.31   Malignant neoplasm of short bones of right lower limb
      C40.32   Malignant neoplasm of short bones of left lower limb

☑5ᵗʰ **C40.8   Malignant neoplasm of overlapping sites of bone and articular cartilage of limb**
      C40.80   Malignant neoplasm of overlapping sites of bone and articular cartilage of unspecified limb
      C40.81   Malignant neoplasm of overlapping sites of bone and articular cartilage of right limb
      C40.82   Malignant neoplasm of overlapping sites of bone and articular cartilage of left limb

☑5ᵗʰ **C40.9   Malignant neoplasm of unspecified bones and articular cartilage of limb**
      C40.90   Malignant neoplasm of unspecified bones and articular cartilage of unspecified limb
      C40.91   Malignant neoplasm of unspecified bones and articular cartilage of right limb
      C40.92   Malignant neoplasm of unspecified bones and articular cartilage of left limb

☑4th C41 Malignant neoplasm of bone and articular cartilage of other and unspecified sites

EXCLUDES 1   *malignant neoplasm of bones of limbs (C40-)*
malignant neoplasm of cartilage of:
    ear (C49.0)
    eyelid (C49.0)
    larynx (C32.3)
    limbs (C40-)
    nose (C30.0)

C41.0 Malignant neoplasm of bones of skull and face
Malignant neoplasm of maxilla (superior)
Malignant neoplasm of orbital bone
EXCLUDES 2   *carcinoma, any type except intraosseous or odontogenic of:*
    maxillary sinus (C31.0)
    upper jaw (C03.0)
    malignant neoplasm of jaw bone (lower) (C41.1)

C41.1 Malignant neoplasm of mandible
Malignant neoplasm of inferior maxilla
Malignant neoplasm of lower jaw bone
EXCLUDES 2   *carcinoma, any type except intraosseous or odontogenic of:*
    jaw NOS (C03.9)
    lower (C03.1)
    malignant neoplasm of upper jaw bone (C41.0)

C41.2 Malignant neoplasm of vertebral column
EXCLUDES 1   *malignant neoplasm of sacrum and coccyx (C41.4)*

C41.3 Malignant neoplasm of ribs, sternum and clavicle

C41.4 Malignant neoplasm of pelvic bones, sacrum and coccyx

C41.9 Malignant neoplasm of bone and articular cartilage, unspecified

Melanoma and other malignant neoplasms of skin (C43-C44)

☑4th C43 Malignant melanoma of skin

EXCLUDES 1   *melanoma in situ (D03-)*
EXCLUDES 2   *malignant melanoma of skin of genital organs (C51-C52, C60-, C63-)*
    Merkel cell carcinoma (C4a-)
    sites other than skin—code to malignant neoplasm of the site

C43.0 Malignant melanoma of lip
EXCLUDES 1   *malignant neoplasm of vermilion border of lip (C00.0-C00.2)*

☑5th C43.1 Malignant melanoma of eyelid, including canthus
  C43.10 Malignant melanoma of unspecified eyelid, including canthus
  C43.11 Malignant melanoma of right eyelid, including canthus
  C43.12 Malignant melanoma of left eyelid, including canthus

☑5th C43.2 Malignant melanoma of ear and external auricular canal
  C43.20 Malignant melanoma of unspecified ear and external auricular canal
  C43.21 Malignant melanoma of right ear and external auricular canal
  C43.22 Malignant melanoma of left ear and external auricular canal

☑5th C43.3 Malignant melanoma of other and unspecified parts of face
  C43.30 Malignant melanoma of unspecified part of face
  C43.31 Malignant melanoma of nose
  C43.39 Malignant melanoma of other parts of face

C43.4 Malignant melanoma of scalp and neck

☑5th C43.5 Malignant melanoma of trunk
EXCLUDES 2   *malignant neoplasm of anus NOS (C21.0)*
    malignant neoplasm of scrotum (C63.2)
  C43.51 Malignant melanoma of anal skin
  Malignant melanoma of anal margin
  Malignant melanoma of perianal skin
  C43.52 Malignant melanoma of skin of breast
  C43.59 Malignant melanoma of other part of trunk

☑5th C43.6 Malignant melanoma of upper limb, including shoulder
  C43.60 Malignant melanoma of unspecified upper limb, including shoulder
  C43.61 Malignant melanoma of right upper limb, including shoulder
  C43.62 Malignant melanoma of left upper limb, including shoulder

☑5th C43.7 Malignant melanoma of lower limb, including hip
  C43.70 Malignant melanoma of unspecified lower limb, including hip
  C43.71 Malignant melanoma of right lower limb, including hip
  C43.72 Malignant melanoma of left lower limb, including hip

C43.8 Malignant melanoma of overlapping sites of skin

C43.9 Malignant melanoma of skin, unspecified
Malignant melanoma of unspecified site of skin

☑4th C4a Merkel cell carcinoma

C4a.0 Merkel cell carcinoma of lip
EXCLUDES 1   *malignant neoplasm of vermilion border of lip (C00.0-C00.2)*

☑5th C4a.1 Merkel cell carcinoma of eyelid, including canthus
  C4a.10 Merkel cell carcinoma of unspecified eyelid, including canthus
  C4a.11 Merkel cell carcinoma of right eyelid, including canthus
  C4a.12 Merkel cell carcinoma of left eyelid, including canthus

☑5th C4a.2 Merkel cell carcinoma of ear and external auricular canal
  C4a.20 Merkel cell carcinoma of unspecified ear and external auricular canal
  C4a.21 Merkel cell carcinoma of right ear and external auricular canal
  C4a.22 Merkel cell carcinoma of left ear and external auricular canal

☑5th C4a.3 Merkel cell carcinoma of other and unspecified parts of face
  C4a.30 Merkel cell carcinoma of unspecified part of face
  C4a.31 Merkel cell carcinoma of nose
  C4a.39 Merkel cell carcinoma of other parts of face

C4a.4 Merkel cell carcinoma of scalp and neck

☑5th C4a.5 Merkel cell carcinoma of trunk
EXCLUDES 2   *malignant neoplasm of anus NOS (C21.0)*
    malignant neoplasm of scrotum (C63.2)
  C4a.51 Merkel cell carcinoma of anal skin
  Merkel cell carcinoma of anal margin
  Merkel cell carcinoma of perianal skin
  C4a.52 Merkel cell carcinoma of skin of breast
  C4a.59 Merkel cell carcinoma of other part of trunk

☑5th C4a.6 Merkel cell carcinoma of upper limb, including shoulder
  C4a.60 Merkel cell carcinoma of unspecified upper limb, including shoulder
  C4a.61 Merkel cell carcinoma of right upper limb, including shoulder
  C4a.62 Merkel cell carcinoma of left upper limb, including shoulder

☑5th C4a.7 Merkel cell carcinoma of lower limb, including hip
  C4a.70 Merkel cell carcinoma of unspecified lower limb, including hip
  C4a.71 Merkel cell carcinoma of right lower limb, including hip
  C4a.72 Merkel cell carcinoma of left lower limb, including hip

C4a.8 Merkel cell carcinoma of overlapping sites

C4a.9 Merkel cell carcinoma, unspecified
Merkel cell carcinoma of unspecified site

☑4th C44 Other malignant neoplasm of skin
INCLUDES   malignant neoplasm of sebaceous glands
    malignant neoplasm of sweat glands
EXCLUDES 1   *Kaposi's sarcoma of skin (C46.0)*
    malignant melanoma of skin (C43-)
    malignant neoplasm of skin of genital organs (C51-C52, C60-, C63.2)
    Merkel cell carcinoma (C4a-)

C44.0 Malignant neoplasm of skin of lip
EXCLUDES 1   *malignant neoplasm of lip (C00-)*

☑5th C44.1 Malignant neoplasm of skin of eyelid, including canthus
EXCLUDES 1   *connective tissue of eyelid (C49.0)*
  C44.10 Malignant neoplasm of skin of unspecified eyelid, including canthus
  C44.11 Malignant neoplasm of skin of right eyelid, including canthus
  C44.12 Malignant neoplasm of skin of left eyelid, including canthus

---

EXCLUDES 1   Not coded here   EXCLUDES 2   Not included here   *Manifestation Code*

☑5ᵗʰ **C44.2** **Malignant neoplasm of skin of ear and external auricular canal**
EXCLUDES 1 *connective tissue of ear (C49.0)*

C44.20 **Malignant neoplasm of skin of unspecified ear and external auricular canal**

C44.21 **Malignant neoplasm of skin of right ear and external auricular canal**

C44.22 **Malignant neoplasm of skin of left ear and external auricular canal**

☑5ᵗʰ **C44.3** **Malignant neoplasm of skin of other and unspecified parts of face**

C44.30 **Malignant neoplasm of skin of unspecified part of face**

C44.31 **Malignant neoplasm of skin of nose**

C44.39 **Malignant neoplasm of skin of other parts of face**

C44.4 **Malignant neoplasm of skin of scalp and neck**

☑5ᵗʰ **C44.5** **Malignant neoplasm of skin of trunk**
EXCLUDES 1 *anus NOS (C21.0)*
scrotum (C63.2)

C44.51 **Malignant neoplasm of anal skin**
Malignant neoplasm of anal margin
Malignant neoplasm of perianal skin

C44.52 **Malignant neoplasm of skin of breast**

C44.59 **Malignant neoplasm of other part of trunk**

☑5ᵗʰ **C44.6** **Malignant neoplasm of skin of upper limb, including shoulder**

C44.60 **Malignant neoplasm of skin of unspecified upper limb, including shoulder**

C44.61 **Malignant neoplasm of skin of right upper limb, including shoulder**

C44.62 **Malignant neoplasm of skin of left upper limb, including shoulder**

☑5ᵗʰ **C44.7** **Malignant neoplasm of skin of lower limb, including hip**

C44.70 **Malignant neoplasm of skin of unspecified lower limb, including hip**

C44.71 **Malignant neoplasm of skin of right lower limb, including hip**

C44.72 **Malignant neoplasm of skin of left lower limb, including hip**

C44.8 **Malignant neoplasm of overlapping sites of skin**

C44.9 **Malignant neoplasm of skin, unspecified**
Malignant neoplasm of unspecified site of skin

Malignant neoplasms of mesothelial and soft tissue (C45-C49)

☑4ᵗʰ **C45** **Mesothelioma**

C45.0 **Mesothelioma of pleura**
EXCLUDES 1 *other malignant neoplasm of pleura (C38.4)*

C45.1 **Mesothelioma of peritoneum**
Mesothelioma of cul-de-sac
Mesothelioma of mesentery
Mesothelioma of mesocolon
Mesothelioma of omentum
Mesothelioma of peritoneum (parietal) (pelvic)
EXCLUDES 1 *other malignant neoplasm of soft tissue of peritoneum (C48-)*

C45.2 **Mesothelioma of pericardium**
EXCLUDES 1 *other malignant neoplasm of pericardium (C38.0)*

C45.7 **Mesothelioma of other sites**

C45.9 **Mesothelioma, unspecified**

☑4ᵗʰ **C46** **Kaposi's sarcoma**
Code first any human immunodeficiency virus [HIV] disease (B20)

C46.0 **Kaposi's sarcoma of skin**

C46.1 **Kaposi's sarcoma of soft tissue**
Kaposi's sarcoma of blood vessel
Kaposi's sarcoma of connective tissue
Kaposi's sarcoma of fascia
Kaposi's sarcoma of ligament
Kaposi's sarcoma of lymphatic(s) NEC
Kaposi's sarcoma of muscle
EXCLUDES 2 *Kaposi's sarcoma of lymph glands and nodes (C46.3)*

C46.2 **Kaposi's sarcoma of palate**

C46.3 **Kaposi's sarcoma of lymph nodes**

C46.4 **Kaposi's sarcoma of gastrointestinal sites**

☑5ᵗʰ **C46.5** **Kaposi's sarcoma of lung**

C46.50 **Kaposi's sarcoma of unspecified lung**

C46.51 **Kaposi's sarcoma of right lung**

C46.52 **Kaposi's sarcoma of left lung**

C46.7 **Kaposi's sarcoma of other sites**

C46.9 **Kaposi's sarcoma, unspecified**
Kaposi's sarcoma of unspecified site

☑4ᵗʰ **C47** **Malignant neoplasm of peripheral nerves and autonomic nervous system**
INCLUDES malignant neoplasm of sympathetic and parasympathetic nerves and ganglia
EXCLUDES 1 *Kaposi's sarcoma of soft tissue (C46.1)*

C47.0 **Malignant neoplasm of peripheral nerves of head, face and neck**
EXCLUDES 1 *malignant neoplasm of peripheral nerves of orbit (C69.6-)*

☑5ᵗʰ **C47.1** **Malignant neoplasm of peripheral nerves of upper limb, including shoulder**

C47.10 **Malignant neoplasm of peripheral nerves of unspecified upper limb, including shoulder**

C47.11 **Malignant neoplasm of peripheral nerves of right upper limb, including shoulder**

C47.12 **Malignant neoplasm of peripheral nerves of left upper limb, including shoulder**

☑5ᵗʰ **C47.2** **Malignant neoplasm of peripheral nerves of lower limb, including hip**

C47.20 **Malignant neoplasm of peripheral nerves of unspecified lower limb, including hip**

C47.21 **Malignant neoplasm of peripheral nerves of right lower limb, including hip**

C47.22 **Malignant neoplasm of peripheral nerves of left lower limb, including hip**

C47.3 **Malignant neoplasm of peripheral nerves of thorax**

C47.4 **Malignant neoplasm of peripheral nerves of abdomen**

C47.5 **Malignant neoplasm of peripheral nerves of pelvis**

C47.6 **Malignant neoplasm of peripheral nerves of trunk, unspecified**
Malignant neoplasm of peripheral nerves of unspecified part of trunk

C47.8 **Malignant neoplasm of overlapping sites of peripheral nerves and autonomic nervous system**

C47.9 **Malignant neoplasm of peripheral nerves and autonomic nervous system, unspecified**
Malignant neoplasm of unspecified site of peripheral nerves and autonomic nervous system

☑4ᵗʰ **C48** **Malignant neoplasm of retroperitoneum and peritoneum**
EXCLUDES 1 *Kaposi's sarcoma of connective tissue (C46.1)*
mesothelioma (C45-)

C48.0 **Malignant neoplasm of retroperitoneum**

C48.1 **Malignant neoplasm of specified parts of peritoneum**
Malignant neoplasm of cul-de-sac
Malignant neoplasm of mesentery
Malignant neoplasm of mesocolon
Malignant neoplasm of omentum
Malignant neoplasm of parietal peritoneum
Malignant neoplasm of pelvic peritoneum

C48.2 **Malignant neoplasm of peritoneum, unspecified**

C48.8 **Malignant neoplasm of overlapping sites of retroperitoneum and peritoneum**

✓4th **C49   Malignant neoplasm of other connective and soft tissue**
> INCLUDES   malignant neoplasm of blood vessel
> malignant neoplasm of bursa
> malignant neoplasm of cartilage
> malignant neoplasm of fascia
> malignant neoplasm of fat
> malignant neoplasm of ligament, except uterine
> malignant neoplasm of lymphatic vessel
> malignant neoplasm of muscle
> malignant neoplasm of synovia
> malignant neoplasm of tendon (sheath)
>
> EXCLUDES 1   *malignant neoplasm of cartilage (of):*
> > *articular (C40-C41)*
> > *larynx (C32.3)*
> > *nose (C30.0)*
> > *malignant neoplasm of connective tissue of internal organs—code to malignant neoplasm of the site*
> > *malignant stromal tumors—code to malignant neoplasm of the site*
>
> EXCLUDES 2   *Kaposi's sarcoma of soft tissue (C46.1)*
> > *malignant neoplasm of heart (C38.0)*
> > *malignant neoplasm of peripheral nerves and autonomic nervous system (C47-)*
> > *malignant neoplasm of peritoneum (C48.2)*
> > *malignant neoplasm of retroperitoneum (C48.0)*
> > *malignant neoplasm of uterine ligament (C57.3)*
> > *mesothelioma (C45-)*

C49.0   Malignant neoplasm of connective and soft tissue of head, face and neck
> Malignant neoplasm of connective tissue of ear
> Malignant neoplasm of connective tissue of eyelid
> EXCLUDES 1   *connective tissue of orbit (C69.6-)*

✓5th **C49.1   Malignant neoplasm of connective and soft tissue of upper limb, including shoulder**
> **C49.10   Malignant neoplasm of connective and soft tissue of unspecified upper limb, including shoulder**
> **C49.11   Malignant neoplasm of connective and soft tissue of right upper limb, including shoulder**
> **C49.12   Malignant neoplasm of connective and soft tissue of left upper limb, including shoulder**

✓5th **C49.2   Malignant neoplasm of connective and soft tissue of lower limb, including hip**
> **C49.20   Malignant neoplasm of connective and soft tissue of unspecified lower limb, including hip**
> **C49.21   Malignant neoplasm of connective and soft tissue of right lower limb, including hip**
> **C49.22   Malignant neoplasm of connective and soft tissue of left lower limb, including hip**

C49.3   Malignant neoplasm of connective and soft tissue of thorax
> Malignant neoplasm of axilla
> Malignant neoplasm of diaphragm
> Malignant neoplasm of great vessels
> EXCLUDES 1   *malignant neoplasm of breast (C50-)*
> > *malignant neoplasm of heart (C38.0)*
> > *malignant neoplasm of mediastinum (C38.1-C38.3)*
> > *malignant neoplasm of thymus (C37)*

C49.4   Malignant neoplasm of connective and soft tissue of abdomen
> Malignant neoplasm of abdominal wall
> Malignant neoplasm of hypochondrium

C49.5   Malignant neoplasm of connective and soft tissue of pelvis
> Malignant neoplasm of buttock
> Malignant neoplasm of groin
> Malignant neoplasm of perineum

C49.6   Malignant neoplasm of connective and soft tissue of trunk, unspecified
> Malignant neoplasm of back NOS

C49.8   Malignant neoplasm of overlapping sites of connective and soft tissue
> Primary malignant neoplasm of two or more contiguous sites of connective and soft tissue

C49.9   Malignant neoplasm of connective and soft tissue, unspecified

Malignant neoplasm of breast (C50)

✓4th **C50   Malignant neoplasm of breast**
> INCLUDES   connective tissue of breast
> Paget's disease of breast
> Paget's disease of nipple
> Use additional code to identify estrogen receptor status (Z17.0, Z17.1)
> EXCLUDES 1   *skin of breast (C44.52)*

✓5th **C50.0   Malignant neoplasm of nipple and areola**
> ✓6th **C50.01   Malignant neoplasm of nipple and areola, female**
> > **C50.011   Malignant neoplasm of nipple and areola, right female breast**
> > **C50.012   Malignant neoplasm of nipple and areola, left female breast**
> > **C50.019   Malignant neoplasm of nipple and areola, unspecified female breast**
> ✓6th **C50.02   Malignant neoplasm of nipple and areola, male**
> > **C50.021   Malignant neoplasm of nipple and areola, right male breast**
> > **C50.022   Malignant neoplasm of nipple and areola, left male breast**
> > **C50.029   Malignant neoplasm of nipple and areola, unspecified male breast**

✓5th **C50.1   Malignant neoplasm of central portion of breast**
> ✓6th **C50.11   Malignant neoplasm of central portion of breast, female**
> > **C50.111   Malignant neoplasm of central portion of right female breast**
> > **C50.112   Malignant neoplasm of central portion of left female breast**
> > **C50.119   Malignant neoplasm of central portion of unspecified female breast**
> ✓6th **C50.12   Malignant neoplasm of central portion of breast, male**
> > **C50.121   Malignant neoplasm of central portion of right male breast**
> > **C50.122   Malignant neoplasm of central portion of left male breast**
> > **C50.129   Malignant neoplasm of central portion of unspecified male breast**

✓5th **C50.2   Malignant neoplasm of upper-inner quadrant of breast**
> ✓6th **C50.21   Malignant neoplasm of upper-inner quadrant of breast, female**
> > **C50.211   Malignant neoplasm of upper-inner quadrant of right female breast**
> > **C50.212   Malignant neoplasm of upper-inner quadrant of left female breast**
> > **C50.219   Malignant neoplasm of upper-inner quadrant of unspecified female breast**
> ✓6th **C50.22   Malignant neoplasm of upper-inner quadrant of breast, male**
> > **C50.221   Malignant neoplasm of upper-inner quadrant of right male breast**
> > **C50.222   Malignant neoplasm of upper-inner quadrant of left male breast**
> > **C50.229   Malignant neoplasm of upper-inner quadrant of unspecified male breast**

✓5th **C50.3   Malignant neoplasm of lower-inner quadrant of breast**
> ✓6th **C50.31   Malignant neoplasm of lower-inner quadrant of breast, female**
> > **C50.311   Malignant neoplasm of lower-inner quadrant of right female breast**
> > **C50.312   Malignant neoplasm of lower-inner quadrant of left female breast**
> > **C50.319   Malignant neoplasm of lower-inner quadrant of unspecified female breast**
> ✓6th **C50.32   Malignant neoplasm of lower-inner quadrant of breast, male**
> > **C50.321   Malignant neoplasm of lower-inner quadrant of right male breast**
> > **C50.322   Malignant neoplasm of lower-inner quadrant of left male breast**
> > **C50.329   Malignant neoplasm of lower-inner quadrant of unspecified male breast**

✓5th **C50.4 Malignant neoplasm of upper-outer quadrant of breast**
  ✓6th **C50.41 Malignant neoplasm of upper-outer quadrant of breast, female**
    C50.411 Malignant neoplasm of upper-outer quadrant of right female breast
    C50.412 Malignant neoplasm of upper-outer quadrant of left female breast
    C50.419 Malignant neoplasm of upper-outer quadrant of unspecified female breast
  ✓6th **C50.42 Malignant neoplasm of upper-outer quadrant of breast, male**
    C50.421 Malignant neoplasm of upper-outer quadrant of right male breast
    C50.422 Malignant neoplasm of upper-outer quadrant of left male breast
    C50.429 Malignant neoplasm of upper-outer quadrant of unspecified male breast

✓5th **C50.5 Malignant neoplasm of lower-outer quadrant of breast**
  ✓6th **C50.51 Malignant neoplasm of lower-outer quadrant of breast, female**
    C50.511 Malignant neoplasm of lower-outer quadrant of right female breast
    C50.512 Malignant neoplasm of lower-outer quadrant of left female breast
    C50.519 Malignant neoplasm of lower-outer quadrant of unspecified female breast
  ✓6th **C50.52 Malignant neoplasm of lower-outer quadrant of breast, male**
    C50.521 Malignant neoplasm of lower-outer quadrant of right male breast
    C50.522 Malignant neoplasm of lower-outer quadrant of left male breast
    C50.529 Malignant neoplasm of lower-outer quadrant of unspecified male breast

✓5th **C50.6 Malignant neoplasm of axillary tail of breast**
  ✓6th **C50.61 Malignant neoplasm of axillary tail of breast, female**
    C50.611 Malignant neoplasm of axillary tail of right female breast
    C50.612 Malignant neoplasm of axillary tail of left female breast
    C50.619 Malignant neoplasm of axillary tail of unspecified female breast
  ✓6th **C50.62 Malignant neoplasm of axillary tail of breast, male**
    C50.621 Malignant neoplasm of axillary tail of right male breast
    C50.622 Malignant neoplasm of axillary tail of left male breast
    C50.629 Malignant neoplasm of axillary tail of unspecified male breast

✓5th **C50.8 Malignant neoplasm of overlapping sites of breast**
  ✓6th **C50.81 Malignant neoplasm of overlapping sites of breast, female**
    C50.811 Malignant neoplasm of overlapping sites of right female breast
    C50.812 Malignant neoplasm of overlapping sites of left female breast
    C50.819 Malignant neoplasm of overlapping sites of unspecified female breast
  ✓6th **C50.82 Malignant neoplasm of overlapping sites of breast, male**
    C50.821 Malignant neoplasm of overlapping sites of right male breast
    C50.822 Malignant neoplasm of overlapping sites of left male breast
    C50.829 Malignant neoplasm of overlapping sites of unspecified male breast

✓5th **C50.9 Malignant neoplasm of breast of unspecified site**
  ✓6th **C50.91 Malignant neoplasm of breast of unspecified site, female**
    C50.911 Malignant neoplasm of unspecified site of right female breast
    C50.912 Malignant neoplasm of unspecified site of left female breast
    C50.919 Malignant neoplasm of unspecified site of unspecified female breast

  ✓6th **C50.92 Malignant neoplasm of breast of unspecified site, male**
    C50.921 Malignant neoplasm of unspecified site of right male breast
    C50.922 Malignant neoplasm of unspecified site of left male breast
    C50.929 Malignant neoplasm of unspecified site of unspecified male breast

Malignant neoplasm of female genital organs (C51-C58)

INCLUDES   malignant neoplasm of skin of female genital organs

✓4th **C51 Malignant neoplasm of vulva**
  EXCLUDES 1   *carcinoma in situ of vulva (D07.1)*
  C51.0 Malignant neoplasm of labium majus
    Malignant neoplasm of Bartholin's [greater vestibular] gland
  C51.1 Malignant neoplasm of labium minus
  C51.2 Malignant neoplasm of clitoris
  C51.8 Malignant neoplasm of overlapping sites of vulva
  C51.9 Malignant neoplasm of vulva, unspecified
    Malignant neoplasm of external female genitalia NOS
    Malignant neoplasm of pudendum

C52 Malignant neoplasm of vagina
  EXCLUDES 1   *carcinoma in situ of vagina (D07.2)*

✓4th **C53 Malignant neoplasm of cervix uteri**
  EXCLUDES 1   *carcinoma in situ of cervix uteri (D06-)*
  C53.0 Malignant neoplasm of endocervix
  C53.1 Malignant neoplasm of exocervix
  C53.8 Malignant neoplasm of overlapping sites of cervix uteri
  C53.9 Malignant neoplasm of cervix uteri, unspecified

✓4th **C54 Malignant neoplasm of corpus uteri**
  C54.0 Malignant neoplasm of isthmus uteri
    Malignant neoplasm of lower uterine segment
  C54.1 Malignant neoplasm of endometrium
  C54.2 Malignant neoplasm of myometrium
  C54.3 Malignant neoplasm of fundus uteri
  C54.8 Malignant neoplasm of overlapping sites of corpus uteri
  C54.9 Malignant neoplasm of corpus uteri, unspecified

C55 Malignant neoplasm of uterus, part unspecified

✓4th **C56 Malignant neoplasm of ovary**
  Use additional code to identify any functional activity
  C56.1 Malignant neoplasm of right ovary
  C56.2 Malignant neoplasm of left ovary
  C56.9 Malignant neoplasm of unspecified ovary

✓4th **C57 Malignant neoplasm of other and unspecified female genital organs**
  ✓5th **C57.0 Malignant neoplasm of fallopian tube**
    Malignant neoplasm of oviduct
    Malignant neoplasm of uterine tube
    C57.00 Malignant neoplasm of unspecified fallopian tube
    C57.01 Malignant neoplasm of right fallopian tube
    C57.02 Malignant neoplasm of left fallopian tube
  ✓5th **C57.1 Malignant neoplasm of broad ligament**
    C57.10 Malignant neoplasm of unspecified broad ligament
    C57.11 Malignant neoplasm of right broad ligament
    C57.12 Malignant neoplasm of left broad ligament
  ✓5th **C57.2 Malignant neoplasm of round ligament**
    C57.20 Malignant neoplasm of unspecified round ligament
    C57.21 Malignant neoplasm of right round ligament
    C57.22 Malignant neoplasm of left round ligament
  C57.3 Malignant neoplasm of parametrium
    Malignant neoplasm of uterine ligament NOS
  C57.4 Malignant neoplasm of uterine adnexa, unspecified
  C57.7 Malignant neoplasm of other specified female genital organs
    Malignant neoplasm of wolffian body or duct

C57.8 Malignant neoplasm of overlapping sites of female genital organs
Primary malignant neoplasm of two or more contiguous sites of the female genital organs whose point of origin cannot be determined
Primary tubo-ovarian malignant neoplasm whose point of origin cannot be determined
Primary utero-ovarian malignant neoplasm whose point of origin cannot be determined

C57.9 Malignant neoplasm of female genital organ, unspecified
Malignant neoplasm of female genitourinary tract NOS

C58 Malignant neoplasm of placenta
INCLUDES choriocarcinoma NOS
chorionepithelioma NOS
EXCLUDES 1 chorioadenoma (destruens) (D39.2)
hydatidiform mole NOS (O01.9)
invasive hydatidiform mole (D39.2)
male choriocarcinoma NOS (C62.9-)
malignant hydatidiform mole (D39.2)

Malignant neoplasms of male genital organs (C60-C63)
INCLUDES malignant neoplasm of skin of male genital organs

✓4ᵗʰ **C60 Malignant neoplasm of penis**
C60.0 Malignant neoplasm of prepuce
Malignant neoplasm of foreskin
C60.1 Malignant neoplasm of glans penis
C60.2 Malignant neoplasm of body of penis
Malignant neoplasm of corpus cavernosum
C60.8 Malignant neoplasm of overlapping sites of penis
C60.9 Malignant neoplasm of penis, unspecified
Malignant neoplasm of skin of penis NOS

C61 Malignant neoplasm of prostate
EXCLUDES 1 malignant neoplasm of seminal vesicle (C63.7)

✓4ᵗʰ **C62 Malignant neoplasm of testis**
Use additional code to identify any functional activity

✓5ᵗʰ **C62.0 Malignant neoplasm of undescended testis**
Malignant neoplasm of ectopic testis
Malignant neoplasm of retained testis
C62.00 Malignant neoplasm of unspecified undescended testis
C62.01 Malignant neoplasm of undescended right testis
C62.02 Malignant neoplasm of undescended left testis

✓5ᵗʰ **C62.1 Malignant neoplasm of descended testis**
Malignant neoplasm of scrotal testis
C62.10 Malignant neoplasm of unspecified descended testis
C62.11 Malignant neoplasm of descended right testis
C62.12 Malignant neoplasm of descended left testis

✓5ᵗʰ **C62.9 Malignant neoplasm of testis, unspecified whether descended or undescended**
C62.90 Malignant neoplasm of unspecified testis, unspecified whether descended or undescended
Malignant neoplasm of testis NOS
C62.91 Malignant neoplasm of right testis, unspecified whether descended or undescended
C62.92 Malignant neoplasm of left testis, unspecified whether descended or undescended

✓4ᵗʰ **C63 Malignant neoplasm of other and unspecified male genital organs**
✓5ᵗʰ **C63.0 Malignant neoplasm of epididymis**
C63.00 Malignant neoplasm of unspecified epididymis
C63.01 Malignant neoplasm of right epididymis
C63.02 Malignant neoplasm of left epididymis
✓5ᵗʰ **C63.1 Malignant neoplasm of spermatic cord**
C63.10 Malignant neoplasm of unspecified spermatic cord
C63.11 Malignant neoplasm of right spermatic cord
C63.12 Malignant neoplasm of left spermatic cord
C63.2 Malignant neoplasm of scrotum
Malignant neoplasm of skin of scrotum
C63.7 Malignant neoplasm of other specified male genital organs
Malignant neoplasm of seminal vesicle
Malignant neoplasm of tunica vaginalis

C63.8 Malignant neoplasm of overlapping sites of male genital organs
Primary malignant neoplasm of two or more contiguous sites of male genital organs whose point of origin cannot be determined

C63.9 Malignant neoplasm of male genital organ, unspecified
Malignant neoplasm of male genitourinary tract NOS

Malignant neoplasm of urinary tract (C64-C68)

✓4ᵗʰ **C64 Malignant neoplasm of kidney, except renal pelvis**
EXCLUDES 1 *malignant carcinoid tumor of the kidney (C7a.093)*
malignant neoplasm of renal calyces (C65-)
malignant neoplasm of renal pelvis (C65-)
C64.1 Malignant neoplasm of right kidney, except renal pelvis
C64.2 Malignant neoplasm of left kidney, except renal pelvis
C64.9 Malignant neoplasm of unspecified kidney, except renal pelvis

✓4ᵗʰ **C65 Malignant neoplasm of renal pelvis**
INCLUDES malignant neoplasm of pelviureteric junction
malignant neoplasm of renal calyces
C65.1 Malignant neoplasm of right renal pelvis
C65.2 Malignant neoplasm of left renal pelvis
C65.9 Malignant neoplasm of unspecified renal pelvis

✓4ᵗʰ **C66 Malignant neoplasm of ureter**
EXCLUDES 1 *malignant neoplasm of ureteric orifice of bladder (C67.6)*
C66.1 Malignant neoplasm of right ureter
C66.2 Malignant neoplasm of left ureter
C66.9 Malignant neoplasm of unspecified ureter

✓4ᵗʰ **C67 Malignant neoplasm of bladder**
C67.0 Malignant neoplasm of trigone of bladder
C67.1 Malignant neoplasm of dome of bladder
C67.2 Malignant neoplasm of lateral wall of bladder
C67.3 Malignant neoplasm of anterior wall of bladder
C67.4 Malignant neoplasm of posterior wall of bladder
C67.5 Malignant neoplasm of bladder neck
Malignant neoplasm of internal urethral orifice
C67.6 Malignant neoplasm of ureteric orifice
C67.7 Malignant neoplasm of urachus
C67.8 Malignant neoplasm of overlapping sites of bladder
C67.9 Malignant neoplasm of bladder, unspecified

✓4ᵗʰ **C68 Malignant neoplasm of other and unspecified urinary organs**
EXCLUDES 1 *malignant neoplasm of female genitourinary tract NOS (C57.9)*
malignant neoplasm of male genitourinary tract NOS (C63.9)
C68.0 Malignant neoplasm of urethra
EXCLUDES 1 *malignant neoplasm of urethral orifice of bladder (C67.5)*
C68.1 Malignant neoplasm of paraurethral glands
C68.8 Malignant neoplasm of overlapping sites of urinary organs
Primary malignant neoplasm of two or more contiguous sites of urinary organs whose point of origin cannot be determined
C68.9 Malignant neoplasm of urinary organ, unspecified
Malignant neoplasm of urinary system NOS

Malignant neoplasms of eye, brain and other parts of central nervous system (C69-C72)

✓4ᵗʰ **C69 Malignant neoplasm of eye and adnexa**
EXCLUDES 1 *malignant neoplasm of connective tissue of eyelid (C49.0)*
malignant neoplasm of eyelid (skin) (C43.1-, C44.1-)
malignant neoplasm of optic nerve (C72.3-)
✓5ᵗʰ **C69.0 Malignant neoplasm of conjunctiva**
C69.00 Malignant neoplasm of unspecified conjunctiva
C69.01 Malignant neoplasm of right conjunctiva
C69.02 Malignant neoplasm of left conjunctiva
✓5ᵗʰ **C69.1 Malignant neoplasm of cornea**
C69.10 Malignant neoplasm of unspecified cornea
C69.11 Malignant neoplasm of right cornea
C69.12 Malignant neoplasm of left cornea

EXCLUDES 1 Not coded here   EXCLUDES 2 Not included here   *Manifestation Code*

☑5ᵗʰ **C69.2 Malignant neoplasm of retina**
EXCLUDES 1 *dark area on retina (D49.81)*
neoplasm of unspecified behavior of retina and choroid (D49.81)
retinal freckle (D49.81)
C69.20 Malignant neoplasm of unspecified retina
C69.21 Malignant neoplasm of right retina
C69.22 Malignant neoplasm of left retina

☑5ᵗʰ **C69.3 Malignant neoplasm of choroid**
C69.30 Malignant neoplasm of unspecified choroid
C69.31 Malignant neoplasm of right choroid
C69.32 Malignant neoplasm of left choroid

☑5ᵗʰ **C69.4 Malignant neoplasm of ciliary body**
Malignant neoplasm of eyeball
C69.40 Malignant neoplasm of unspecified ciliary body
C69.41 Malignant neoplasm of right ciliary body
C69.42 Malignant neoplasm of left ciliary body

☑5ᵗʰ **C69.5 Malignant neoplasm of lacrimal gland and duct**
Malignant neoplasm of lacrimal sac
Malignant neoplasm of nasolacrimal duct
C69.50 Malignant neoplasm of unspecified lacrimal gland and duct
C69.51 Malignant neoplasm of right lacrimal gland and duct
C69.52 Malignant neoplasm of left lacrimal gland and duct

☑5ᵗʰ **C69.6 Malignant neoplasm of orbit**
Malignant neoplasm of connective tissue of orbit
Malignant neoplasm of extraocular muscle
Malignant neoplasm of peripheral nerves of orbit
Malignant neoplasm of retrobulbar tissue
Malignant neoplasm of retro-ocular tissue
EXCLUDES 1 *malignant neoplasm of orbital bone (C41.0)*
C69.60 Malignant neoplasm of unspecified orbit
C69.61 Malignant neoplasm of right orbit
C69.62 Malignant neoplasm of left orbit

☑5ᵗʰ **C69.8 Malignant neoplasm of overlapping sites of eye and adnexa**
C69.80 Malignant neoplasm of overlapping sites of unspecified eye and adnexa
C69.81 Malignant neoplasm of overlapping sites of right eye and adnexa
C69.82 Malignant neoplasm of overlapping sites of left eye and adnexa

☑5ᵗʰ **C69.9 Malignant neoplasm of unspecified site of eye**
C69.90 Malignant neoplasm of unspecified site of unspecified eye
C69.91 Malignant neoplasm of unspecified site of right eye
C69.92 Malignant neoplasm of unspecified site of left eye

☑4ᵗʰ **C70 Malignant neoplasm of meninges**
C70.0 Malignant neoplasm of cerebral meninges
C70.1 Malignant neoplasm of spinal meninges
C70.9 Malignant neoplasm of meninges, unspecified

☑4ᵗʰ **C71 Malignant neoplasm of brain**
EXCLUDES 1 *malignant neoplasm of cranial nerves (C72.2-C72.5)*
retrobulbar malignant neoplasm (C69.6-)
C71.0 Malignant neoplasm of cerebrum, except lobes and ventricles
Malignant neoplasm of supratentorial NOS
C71.1 Malignant neoplasm of frontal lobe
C71.2 Malignant neoplasm of temporal lobe
C71.3 Malignant neoplasm of parietal lobe
C71.4 Malignant neoplasm of occipital lobe
C71.5 Malignant neoplasm of cerebral ventricle
EXCLUDES 1 *malignant neoplasm of fourth cerebral ventricle (C71.7)*
C71.6 Malignant neoplasm of cerebellum
C71.7 Malignant neoplasm of brain stem
Malignant neoplasm of fourth cerebral ventricle
Infratentorial malignant neoplasm NOS
C71.8 Malignant neoplasm of overlapping sites of brain
C71.9 Malignant neoplasm of brain, unspecified

☑4ᵗʰ **C72 Malignant neoplasm of spinal cord, cranial nerves and other parts of central nervous system**
EXCLUDES 1 *malignant neoplasm of meninges (C70-)*
malignant neoplasm of peripheral nerves and autonomic nervous system (C47-)
C72.0 Malignant neoplasm of spinal cord
C72.1 Malignant neoplasm of cauda equina
☑5ᵗʰ **C72.2 Malignant neoplasm of olfactory nerve**
Malignant neoplasm of olfactory bulb
C72.20 Malignant neoplasm of unspecified olfactory nerve
C72.21 Malignant neoplasm of right olfactory nerve
C72.22 Malignant neoplasm of left olfactory nerve
☑5ᵗʰ **C72.3 Malignant neoplasm of optic nerve**
C72.30 Malignant neoplasm of unspecified optic nerve
C72.31 Malignant neoplasm of right optic nerve
C72.32 Malignant neoplasm of left optic nerve
☑5ᵗʰ **C72.4 Malignant neoplasm of acoustic nerve**
C72.40 Malignant neoplasm of unspecified acoustic nerve
C72.41 Malignant neoplasm of right acoustic nerve
C72.42 Malignant neoplasm of left acoustic nerve
☑5ᵗʰ **C72.5 Malignant neoplasm of other and unspecified cranial nerves**
C72.50 Malignant neoplasm of unspecified cranial nerve
Malignant neoplasm of cranial nerve NOS
C72.59 Malignant neoplasm of other cranial nerves
C72.9 Malignant neoplasm of central nervous system, unspecified
Malignant neoplasm of unspecified site of central nervous system
Malignant neoplasm of nervous system NOS

Malignant neoplasm of thyroid and other endocrine glands (C73-C75)

C73 Malignant neoplasm of thyroid gland
Use additional code to identify any functional activity

☑4ᵗʰ **C74 Malignant neoplasm of adrenal gland**
☑5ᵗʰ **C74.0 Malignant neoplasm of cortex of adrenal gland**
C74.00 Malignant neoplasm of cortex of unspecified adrenal gland
C74.01 Malignant neoplasm of cortex of right adrenal gland
C74.02 Malignant neoplasm of cortex of left adrenal gland
☑5ᵗʰ **C74.1 Malignant neoplasm of medulla of adrenal gland**
C74.10 Malignant neoplasm of medulla of unspecified adrenal gland
C74.11 Malignant neoplasm of medulla of right adrenal gland
C74.12 Malignant neoplasm of medulla of left adrenal gland
☑5ᵗʰ **C74.9 Malignant neoplasm of unspecified part of adrenal gland**
C74.90 Malignant neoplasm of unspecified part of unspecified adrenal gland
C74.91 Malignant neoplasm of unspecified part of right adrenal gland
C74.92 Malignant neoplasm of unspecified part of left adrenal gland

☑4ᵗʰ **C75 Malignant neoplasm of other endocrine glands and related structures**
EXCLUDES 1 *malignant carcinoid tumors (C7a.0-)*
malignant neoplasm of adrenal gland (C74-)
malignant neoplasm of endocrine pancreas (C25.4)
malignant neoplasm of islets of Langerhans (C25.4)
malignant neoplasm of ovary (C56-)
malignant neoplasm of testis (C62-)
malignant neoplasm of thymus (C37)
malignant neoplasm of thyroid gland (C73)
malignant neuroendocrine tumors (C7a-)
C75.0 Malignant neoplasm of parathyroid gland
C75.1 Malignant neoplasm of pituitary gland
C75.2 Malignant neoplasm of craniopharyngeal duct
C75.3 Malignant neoplasm of pineal gland
C75.4 Malignant neoplasm of carotid body
C75.5 Malignant neoplasm of aortic body and other paraganglia
C75.8 Malignant neoplasm with pluriglandular involvement, unspecified

C75.9 **Malignant neoplasm of endocrine gland, unspecified**

Malignant neuroendocrine tumors (C7a)

✓4th **C7a Malignant neuroendocrine tumors**
Code also any associated multiple endocrine neoplasia [MEN] syndromes (E31.2-)
Use additional code to identify any associated endocrine syndrome, such as:
carcinoid syndrome (E34.0)
EXCLUDES 2 *malignant pancreatic islet cell tumors (C25.4)*
Merkel cell carcinoma (C4a-)

✓5th **C7a.0 Malignant carcinoid tumors**
C7a.00 **Malignant carcinoid tumor of unspecified site**
✓6th C7a.01 **Malignant carcinoid tumors of the small intestine**
C7a.010 **Malignant carcinoid tumor of the duodenum**
C7a.011 **Malignant carcinoid tumor of the jejunum**
C7a.012 **Malignant carcinoid tumor of the ileum**
C7a.019 **Malignant carcinoid tumor of the small intestine, unspecified portion**
✓6th C7a.02 **Malignant carcinoid tumors of the appendix, large intestine, and rectum**
C7a.020 **Malignant carcinoid tumor of the appendix**
C7a.021 **Malignant carcinoid tumor of the cecum**
C7a.022 **Malignant carcinoid tumor of the ascending colon**
C7a.023 **Malignant carcinoid tumor of the transverse colon**
C7a.024 **Malignant carcinoid tumor of the descending colon**
C7a.025 **Malignant carcinoid tumor of the sigmoid colon**
C7a.026 **Malignant carcinoid tumor of the rectum**
C7a.029 **Malignant carcinoid tumor of the large intestine, unspecified portion**
Malignant carcinoid tumor of the colon NOS
✓6th C7a.09 **Malignant carcinoid tumors of other sites**
C7a.090 **Malignant carcinoid tumor of the bronchus and lung**
C7a.091 **Malignant carcinoid tumor of the thymus**
C7a.092 **Malignant carcinoid tumor of the stomach**
C7a.093 **Malignant carcinoid tumor of the kidney**
C7a.094 **Malignant carcinoid tumor of the foregut NOS**
C7a.095 **Malignant carcinoid tumor of the midgut NOS**
C7a.096 **Malignant carcinoid tumor of the hindgut NOS**
C7a.098 **Malignant carcinoid tumors of other sites**
C7a.1 **Malignant poorly differentiated neuroendocrine tumors**
High grade neuroendocrine carcinoma, any site
Malignant poorly differentiated neuroendocrine tumor NOS
Malignant poorly differentiated neuroendocrine carcinoma, any site
C7a.8 **Other malignant neuroendocrine tumors**

Secondary neuroendocrine tumors (C7b)

✓4th **C7b Secondary neuroendocrine tumors**
Use additional code to identify any functional activity
✓5th **C7b.0 Secondary carcinoid tumors**
C7b.00 **Secondary carcinoid tumors, unspecified site**
C7b.01 **Secondary carcinoid tumors of distant lymph nodes**
Mesentery metastasis of carcinoid tumor
C7b.02 **Secondary carcinoid tumors of liver**
C7b.03 **Secondary carcinoid tumors of bone**
C7b.04 **Secondary carcinoid tumors of peritoneum**
C7b.09 **Secondary carcinoid tumors of other sites**

C7b.1 **Secondary Merkel cell carcinoma**
Merkel cell carcinoma nodal presentation
Merkel cell carcinoma visceral metastatic presentation
C7b.8 **Other secondary neuroendocrine tumors**

Malignant neoplasms of ill-defined, other secondary and unspecified sites (C76-C80)

✓4th **C76 Malignant neoplasm of other and ill-defined sites**
EXCLUDES 1 *malignant neoplasm of female genitourinary tract NOS (C57.9)*
malignant neoplasm of male genitourinary tract NOS (C63.9)
malignant neoplasm of lymphoid, hematopoietic and related tissue (C81-C96)
malignant neoplasm of skin (C44-)
malignant neoplasm of unspecified site NOS (C80.1)
C76.0 **Malignant neoplasm of head, face and neck**
Malignant neoplasm of cheek NOS
Malignant neoplasm of nose NOS
C76.1 **Malignant neoplasm of thorax**
Intrathoracic malignant neoplasm NOS
Malignant neoplasm of axilla NOS
Thoracic malignant neoplasm NOS
C76.2 **Malignant neoplasm of abdomen**
C76.3 **Malignant neoplasm of pelvis**
Malignant neoplasm of groin NOS
Malignant neoplasm of sites overlapping systems within the pelvis
Rectovaginal (septum) malignant neoplasm
Rectovesical (septum) malignant neoplasm
✓5th C76.4 **Malignant neoplasm of upper limb**
C76.40 **Malignant neoplasm of unspecified upper limb**
C76.41 **Malignant neoplasm of right upper limb**
C76.42 **Malignant neoplasm of left upper limb**
✓5th C76.5 **Malignant neoplasm of lower limb**
C76.50 **Malignant neoplasm of unspecified lower limb**
C76.51 **Malignant neoplasm of right lower limb**
C76.52 **Malignant neoplasm of left lower limb**
C76.8 **Malignant neoplasm of other specified ill-defined sites**
Malignant neoplasm of overlapping ill-defined sites

✓4th **C77 Secondary and unspecified malignant neoplasm of lymph nodes**
EXCLUDES 1 *malignant neoplasm of lymph nodes, specified as primary (C81-C88, C96-)*
mesentery metastasis of carcinoid tumor (C7b.01)
secondary carcinoid tumors of distant lymph nodes (C7b.01)
C77.0 **Secondary and unspecified malignant neoplasm of lymph nodes of head, face and neck**
Secondary and unspecified malignant neoplasm of supraclavicular lymph nodes
C77.1 **Secondary and unspecified malignant neoplasm of intrathoracic lymph nodes**
C77.2 **Secondary and unspecified malignant neoplasm of intra-abdominal lymph nodes**
C77.3 **Secondary and unspecified malignant neoplasm of axilla and upper limb lymph nodes**
Secondary and unspecified malignant neoplasm of pectoral lymph nodes
C77.4 **Secondary and unspecified malignant neoplasm of inguinal and lower limb lymph nodes**
C77.5 **Secondary and unspecified malignant neoplasm of intrapelvic lymph nodes**
C77.8 **Secondary and unspecified malignant neoplasm of lymph nodes of multiple regions**
C77.9 **Secondary and unspecified malignant neoplasm of lymph node, unspecified**

✓4th **C78 Secondary malignant neoplasm of respiratory and digestive organs**
EXCLUDES 1 *lymph node metastases (C77.0)*
secondary carcinoid tumors of liver (C7b.02)
secondary carcinoid tumors of peritoneum (C7b.04)
✓5th C78.0 **Secondary malignant neoplasm of lung**
C78.00 **Secondary malignant neoplasm of unspecified lung**
C78.01 **Secondary malignant neoplasm of right lung**
C78.02 **Secondary malignant neoplasm of left lung**
C78.1 **Secondary malignant neoplasm of mediastinum**
C78.2 **Secondary malignant neoplasm of pleura**

EXCLUDES 1 Not coded here   EXCLUDES 2 Not included here   *Manifestation Code*

✓5th **C78.3** **Secondary malignant neoplasm of other and unspecified respiratory organs**

　　C78.30 Secondary malignant neoplasm of unspecified respiratory organ

　　C78.39 Secondary malignant neoplasm of other respiratory organs

C78.4 Secondary malignant neoplasm of small intestine

C78.5 Secondary malignant neoplasm of large intestine and rectum

C78.6 Secondary malignant neoplasm of retroperitoneum and peritoneum

C78.7 Secondary malignant neoplasm of liver and intrahepatic bile duct

✓5th **C78.8** **Secondary malignant neoplasm of other and unspecified digestive organs**

　　C78.80 Secondary malignant neoplasm of unspecified digestive organ

　　C78.89 Secondary malignant neoplasm of other digestive organs

✓4th **C79** **Secondary malignant neoplasm of other and unspecified sites**

　　EXCLUDES 1　*lymph node metastases (C77.0)*
　　　　secondary carcinoid tumors (C7b-)
　　　　secondary neuroendocrine tumors (C7b-)

✓5th **C79.0** **Secondary malignant neoplasm of kidney and renal pelvis**

　　C79.00 Secondary malignant neoplasm of unspecified kidney and renal pelvis

　　C79.01 Secondary malignant neoplasm of right kidney and renal pelvis

　　C79.02 Secondary malignant neoplasm of left kidney and renal pelvis

✓5th **C79.1** **Secondary malignant neoplasm of bladder and other and unspecified urinary organs**

　　C79.10 Secondary malignant neoplasm of unspecified urinary organs

　　C79.11 Secondary malignant neoplasm of bladder

　　C79.19 Secondary malignant neoplasm of other urinary organs

C79.2 Secondary malignant neoplasm of skin

　　EXCLUDES 1　*secondary Merkel cell carcinoma (C7b.1)*

✓5th **C79.3** **Secondary malignant neoplasm of brain and cerebral meninges**

　　C79.31 Secondary malignant neoplasm of brain

　　C79.32 Secondary malignant neoplasm of cerebral meninges

✓5th **C79.4** **Secondary malignant neoplasm of other and unspecified parts of nervous system**

　　C79.40 Secondary malignant neoplasm of unspecified part of nervous system

　　C79.49 Secondary malignant neoplasm of other parts of nervous system

✓5th **C79.5** **Secondary malignant neoplasm of bone and bone marrow**

　　EXCLUDES 1　*secondary carcinoid tumors of bone (C7b.03)*

　　C79.51 Secondary malignant neoplasm of bone

　　C79.52 Secondary malignant neoplasm of bone marrow

✓5th **C79.6** **Secondary malignant neoplasm of ovary**

　　C79.60 Secondary malignant neoplasm of unspecified ovary

　　C79.61 Secondary malignant neoplasm of right ovary

　　C79.62 Secondary malignant neoplasm of left ovary

✓5th **C79.7** **Secondary malignant neoplasm of adrenal gland**

　　C79.70 Secondary malignant neoplasm of unspecified adrenal gland

　　C79.71 Secondary malignant neoplasm of right adrenal gland

　　C79.72 Secondary malignant neoplasm of left adrenal gland

✓5th **C79.8** **Secondary malignant neoplasm of other specified sites**

　　C79.81 Secondary malignant neoplasm of breast

　　C79.82 Secondary malignant neoplasm of genital organs

　　C79.89 Secondary malignant neoplasm of other specified sites

C79.9 **Secondary malignant neoplasm of unspecified site**

　　Metastatic cancer NOS
　　Metastatic disease NOS
　　EXCLUDES 1　*carcinomatosis NOS (C80.0)*
　　　　generalized cancer NOS (C80.0)
　　　　malignant (primary) neoplasm of unspecified site (C80.1)

✓4th **C80** **Malignant neoplasm without specification of site**

　　EXCLUDES 1　*malignant carcinoid tumor of unspecified site (C7a.00)*
　　　　malignant neoplasm of specified multiple sites—code to each site

C80.0 **Disseminated malignant neoplasm, unspecified**

　　Carcinomatosis NOS
　　Generalized cancer, unspecified site (primary) (secondary)
　　Generalized malignancy, unspecified site (primary) (secondary)

C80.1 **Malignant (primary) neoplasm, unspecified**

　　Cancer NOS
　　Cancer unspecified site (primary)
　　Carcinoma unspecified site (primary)
　　Malignancy unspecified site (primary)
　　EXCLUDES 1　*secondary malignant neoplasm of unspecified site (C79.9)*

C80.2 **Malignant neoplasm associated with transplanted organ**

　　Code first complication of transplanted organ (T86-)
　　Use additional code to identify the specific malignancy

Malignant neoplasms of lymphoid, hematopoietic and related tissue (C81-C96)

　　EXCLUDES 2　*Kaposi's sarcoma of lymph nodes (C46.3)*
　　　　secondary and unspecified neoplasm of lymph nodes (C77-)
　　　　secondary neoplasm of bone marrow (C79.52)
　　　　secondary neoplasm of spleen (C78.89)

✓4th **C81** **Hodgkin lymphoma**

　　EXCLUDES 1　*personal history of Hodgkin lymphoma (Z85.71)*

✓5th **C81.0** **Nodular lymphocyte predominant Hodgkin lymphoma**

　　C81.00 Nodular lymphocyte predominant Hodgkin lymphoma, unspecified site

　　C81.01 Nodular lymphocyte predominant Hodgkin lymphoma, lymph nodes of head, face, and neck

　　C81.02 Nodular lymphocyte predominant Hodgkin lymphoma, intrathoracic lymph nodes

　　C81.03 Nodular lymphocyte predominant Hodgkin lymphoma, intra-abdominal lymph nodes

　　C81.04 Nodular lymphocyte predominant Hodgkin lymphoma, lymph nodes of axilla and upper limb

　　C81.05 Nodular lymphocyte predominant Hodgkin lymphoma, lymph nodes of inguinal region and lower limb

　　C81.06 Nodular lymphocyte predominant Hodgkin lymphoma, intrapelvic lymph nodes

　　C81.07 Nodular lymphocyte predominant Hodgkin lymphoma, spleen

　　C81.08 Nodular lymphocyte predominant Hodgkin lymphoma, lymph nodes of multiple sites

　　C81.09 Nodular lymphocyte predominant Hodgkin lymphoma, extranodal and solid organ sites

✓5th **C81.1** **Nodular sclerosis classical Hodgkin lymphoma**

　　C81.10 Nodular sclerosis classical Hodgkin lymphoma, unspecified site

　　C81.11 Nodular sclerosis classical Hodgkin lymphoma, lymph nodes of head, face, and neck

　　C81.12 Nodular sclerosis classical Hodgkin lymphoma, intrathoracic lymph nodes

　　C81.13 Nodular sclerosis classical Hodgkin lymphoma, intra-abdominal lymph nodes

　　C81.14 Nodular sclerosis classical Hodgkin lymphoma, lymph nodes of axilla and upper limb

　　C81.15 Nodular sclerosis classical Hodgkin lymphoma, lymph nodes of inguinal region and lower limb

　　C81.16 Nodular sclerosis classical Hodgkin lymphoma, intrapelvic lymph nodes

　　C81.17 Nodular sclerosis classical Hodgkin lymphoma, spleen

　　C81.18 Nodular sclerosis classical Hodgkin lymphoma, lymph nodes of multiple sites

---

✓ Appropriate additional character required　　　　✓x7th Requires 7th character, placeholder x must fill empty characters

C81.19   Nodular sclerosis classical Hodgkin lymphoma, extranodal and solid organ sites

✓5ᵗʰ   **C81.2**   **Mixed cellularity classical Hodgkin lymphoma**

C81.20   Mixed cellularity classical Hodgkin lymphoma, unspecified site

C81.21   Mixed cellularity classical Hodgkin lymphoma, lymph nodes of head, face, and neck

C81.22   Mixed cellularity classical Hodgkin lymphoma, intrathoracic lymph nodes

C81.23   Mixed cellularity classical Hodgkin lymphoma, intra-abdominal lymph nodes

C81.24   Mixed cellularity classical Hodgkin lymphoma, lymph nodes of axilla and upper limb

C81.25   Mixed cellularity classical Hodgkin lymphoma, lymph nodes of inguinal region and lower limb

C81.26   Mixed cellularity classical Hodgkin lymphoma, intrapelvic lymph nodes

C81.27   Mixed cellularity classical Hodgkin lymphoma, spleen

C81.28   Mixed cellularity classical Hodgkin lymphoma, lymph nodes of multiple sites

C81.29   Mixed cellularity classical Hodgkin lymphoma, extranodal and solid organ sites

✓5ᵗʰ   **C81.3**   **Lymphocyte-depleted classical Hodgkin lymphoma**

C81.30   Lymphocyte-depleted classical Hodgkin lymphoma, unspecified site

C81.31   Lymphocyte-depleted classical Hodgkin lymphoma, lymph nodes of head, face, and neck

C81.32   Lymphocyte-depleted classical Hodgkin lymphoma, intrathoracic lymph nodes

C81.33   Lymphocyte-depleted classical Hodgkin lymphoma, intra-abdominal lymph nodes

C81.34   Lymphocyte-depleted classical Hodgkin lymphoma, lymph nodes of axilla and upper limb

C81.35   Lymphocyte-depleted classical Hodgkin lymphoma, lymph nodes of inguinal region and lower limb

C81.36   Lymphocyte-depleted classical Hodgkin lymphoma, intrapelvic lymph nodes

C81.37   Lymphocyte-depleted classical Hodgkin lymphoma, spleen

C81.38   Lymphocyte-depleted classical Hodgkin lymphoma, lymph nodes of multiple sites

C81.39   Lymphocyte-depleted classical Hodgkin lymphoma, extranodal and solid organ sites

✓5ᵗʰ   **C81.4**   **Lymphocyte-rich classical Hodgkin lymphoma**

> EXCLUDES 1   *nodular lymphocyte predominant Hodgkin lymphoma (C81.0-)*

C81.40   Lymphocyte-rich classical Hodgkin lymphoma, unspecified site

C81.41   Lymphocyte-rich classical Hodgkin lymphoma, lymph nodes of head, face, and neck

C81.42   Lymphocyte-rich classical Hodgkin lymphoma, intrathoracic lymph nodes

C81.43   Lymphocyte-rich classical Hodgkin lymphoma, intra-abdominal lymph nodes

C81.44   Lymphocyte-rich classical Hodgkin lymphoma, lymph nodes of axilla and upper limb

C81.45   Lymphocyte-rich classical Hodgkin lymphoma, lymph nodes of inguinal region and lower limb

C81.46   Lymphocyte-rich classical Hodgkin lymphoma, intrapelvic lymph nodes

C81.47   Lymphocyte-rich classical Hodgkin lymphoma, spleen

C81.48   Lymphocyte-rich classical Hodgkin lymphoma, lymph nodes of multiple sites

C81.49   Lymphocyte-rich classical Hodgkin lymphoma, extranodal and solid organ sites

✓5ᵗʰ   **C81.7**   **Other classical Hodgkin lymphoma**

Classical Hodgkin lymphoma NOS

C81.70   Other classical Hodgkin lymphoma, unspecified site

C81.71   Other classical Hodgkin lymphoma, lymph nodes of head, face, and neck

C81.72   Other classical Hodgkin lymphoma, intrathoracic lymph nodes

C81.73   Other classical Hodgkin lymphoma, intra-abdominal lymph nodes

C81.74   Other classical Hodgkin lymphoma, lymph nodes of axilla and upper limb

C81.75   Other classical Hodgkin lymphoma, lymph nodes of inguinal region and lower limb

C81.76   Other classical Hodgkin lymphoma, intrapelvic lymph nodes

C81.77   Other classical Hodgkin lymphoma, spleen

C81.78   Other classical Hodgkin lymphoma, lymph nodes of multiple sites

C81.79   Other classical Hodgkin lymphoma, extranodal and solid organ sites

✓5ᵗʰ   **C81.9**   **Hodgkin lymphoma, unspecified**

C81.90   Hodgkin lymphoma, unspecified, unspecified site

C81.91   Hodgkin lymphoma, unspecified, lymph nodes of head, face, and neck

C81.92   Hodgkin lymphoma, unspecified, intrathoracic lymph nodes

C81.93   Hodgkin lymphoma, unspecified, intra-abdominal lymph nodes

C81.94   Hodgkin lymphoma, unspecified, lymph nodes of axilla and upper limb

C81.95   Hodgkin lymphoma, unspecified, lymph nodes of inguinal region and lower limb

C81.96   Hodgkin lymphoma, unspecified, intrapelvic lymph nodes

C81.97   Hodgkin lymphoma, unspecified, spleen

C81.98   Hodgkin lymphoma, unspecified, lymph nodes of multiple sites

C81.99   Hodgkin lymphoma, unspecified, extranodal and solid organ sites

✓4ᵗʰ   **C82**   **Follicular lymphoma**

> INCLUDES   follicular lymphoma with or without diffuse areas
>
> EXCLUDES 1   *mature T/NK-cell lymphomas (C84.-)*
> *personal history of non-Hodgkin lymphoma (Z85.72)*

✓5ᵗʰ   **C82.0**   **Follicular lymphoma grade I**

C82.00   Follicular lymphoma grade I, unspecified site

C82.01   Follicular lymphoma grade I, lymph nodes of head, face, and neck

C82.02   Follicular lymphoma grade I, intrathoracic lymph nodes

C82.03   Follicular lymphoma grade I, intra-abdominal lymph nodes

C82.04   Follicular lymphoma grade I, lymph nodes of axilla and upper limb

C82.05   Follicular lymphoma grade I, lymph nodes of inguinal region and lower limb

C82.06   Follicular lymphoma grade I, intrapelvic lymph nodes

C82.07   Follicular lymphoma grade I, spleen

C82.08   Follicular lymphoma grade I, lymph nodes of multiple sites

C82.09   Follicular lymphoma grade I, extranodal and solid organ sites

✓5ᵗʰ   **C82.1**   **Follicular lymphoma grade II**

C82.10   Follicular lymphoma grade II, unspecified site

C82.11   Follicular lymphoma grade II, lymph nodes of head, face, and neck

C82.12   Follicular lymphoma grade II, intrathoracic lymph nodes

C82.13   Follicular lymphoma grade II, intra-abdominal lymph nodes

C82.14   Follicular lymphoma grade II, lymph nodes of axilla and upper limb

C82.15   Follicular lymphoma grade II, lymph nodes of inguinal region and lower limb

C82.16   Follicular lymphoma grade II, intrapelvic lymph nodes

C82.17   Follicular lymphoma grade II, spleen

C82.18   Follicular lymphoma grade II, lymph nodes of multiple sites

C82.19   Follicular lymphoma grade II, extranodal and solid organ sites

✓5ᵗʰ   **C82.2**   **Follicular lymphoma grade III, unspecified**

C82.20   Follicular lymphoma grade III, unspecified, unspecified site

C82.21   Follicular lymphoma grade III, unspecified, lymph nodes of head, face, and neck

---

EXCLUDES 1   Not coded here   EXCLUDES 2   Not included here   *Manifestation Code*

C82.22 Follicular lymphoma grade III, unspecified, intrathoracic lymph nodes

C82.23 Follicular lymphoma grade III, unspecified, intra-abdominal lymph nodes

C82.24 Follicular lymphoma grade III, unspecified, lymph nodes of axilla and upper limb

C82.25 Follicular lymphoma grade III, unspecified, lymph nodes of inguinal region and lower limb

C82.26 Follicular lymphoma grade III, unspecified, intrapelvic lymph nodes

C82.27 Follicular lymphoma grade III, unspecified, spleen

C82.28 Follicular lymphoma grade III, unspecified, lymph nodes of multiple sites

C82.29 Follicular lymphoma grade III, unspecified, extranodal and solid organ sites

√5th **C82.3** **Follicular lymphoma grade IIIa**

C82.30 Follicular lymphoma grade IIIa, unspecified site

C82.31 Follicular lymphoma grade IIIa, lymph nodes of head, face, and neck

C82.32 Follicular lymphoma grade IIIa, intrathoracic lymph nodes

C82.33 Follicular lymphoma grade IIIa, intra-abdominal lymph nodes

C82.34 Follicular lymphoma grade IIIa, lymph nodes of axilla and upper limb

C82.35 Follicular lymphoma grade IIIa, lymph nodes of inguinal region and lower limb

C82.36 Follicular lymphoma grade IIIa, intrapelvic lymph nodes

C82.37 Follicular lymphoma grade IIIa, spleen

C82.38 Follicular lymphoma grade IIIa, lymph nodes of multiple sites

C82.39 Follicular lymphoma grade IIIa, extranodal and solid organ sites

√5th **C82.4** **Follicular lymphoma grade IIIb**

C82.40 Follicular lymphoma grade IIIb, unspecified site

C82.41 Follicular lymphoma grade IIIb, lymph nodes of head, face, and neck

C82.42 Follicular lymphoma grade IIIb, intrathoracic lymph nodes

C82.43 Follicular lymphoma grade IIIb, intra-abdominal lymph nodes

C82.44 Follicular lymphoma grade IIIb, lymph nodes of axilla and upper limb

C82.45 Follicular lymphoma grade IIIb, lymph nodes of inguinal region and lower limb

C82.46 Follicular lymphoma grade IIIb, intrapelvic lymph nodes

C82.47 Follicular lymphoma grade IIIb, spleen

C82.48 Follicular lymphoma grade IIIb, lymph nodes of multiple sites

C82.49 Follicular lymphoma grade IIIb, extranodal and solid organ sites

√5th **C82.5** **Diffuse follicle center lymphoma**

C82.50 Diffuse follicle center lymphoma, unspecified site

C82.51 Diffuse follicle center lymphoma, lymph nodes of head, face, and neck

C82.52 Diffuse follicle center lymphoma, intrathoracic lymph nodes

C82.53 Diffuse follicle center lymphoma, intra-abdominal lymph nodes

C82.54 Diffuse follicle center lymphoma, lymph nodes of axilla and upper limb

C82.55 Diffuse follicle center lymphoma, lymph nodes of inguinal region and lower limb

C82.56 Diffuse follicle center lymphoma, intrapelvic lymph nodes

C82.57 Diffuse follicle center lymphoma, spleen

C82.58 Diffuse follicle center lymphoma, lymph nodes of multiple sites

C82.59 Diffuse follicle center lymphoma, extranodal and solid organ sites

√5th **C82.6** **Cutaneous follicle center lymphoma**

C82.60 Cutaneous follicle center lymphoma, unspecified site

C82.61 Cutaneous follicle center lymphoma, lymph nodes of head, face, and neck

C82.62 Cutaneous follicle center lymphoma, intrathoracic lymph nodes

C82.63 Cutaneous follicle center lymphoma, intra-abdominal lymph nodes

C82.64 Cutaneous follicle center lymphoma, lymph nodes of axilla and upper limb

C82.65 Cutaneous follicle center lymphoma, lymph nodes of inguinal region and lower limb

C82.66 Cutaneous follicle center lymphoma, intrapelvic lymph nodes

C82.67 Cutaneous follicle center lymphoma, spleen

C82.68 Cutaneous follicle center lymphoma, lymph nodes of multiple sites

C82.69 Cutaneous follicle center lymphoma, extranodal and solid organ sites

√5th **C82.8** **Other types of follicular lymphoma**

C82.80 Other types of follicular lymphoma, unspecified site

C82.81 Other types of follicular lymphoma, lymph nodes of head, face, and neck

C82.82 Other types of follicular lymphoma, intrathoracic lymph nodes

C82.83 Other types of follicular lymphoma, intra-abdominal lymph nodes

C82.84 Other types of follicular lymphoma, lymph nodes of axilla and upper limb

C82.85 Other types of follicular lymphoma, lymph nodes of inguinal region and lower limb

C82.86 Other types of follicular lymphoma, intrapelvic lymph nodes

C82.87 Other types of follicular lymphoma, spleen

C82.88 Other types of follicular lymphoma, lymph nodes of multiple sites

C82.89 Other types of follicular lymphoma, extranodal and solid organ sites

√5th **C82.9** **Follicular lymphoma, unspecified**

C82.90 Follicular lymphoma, unspecified, unspecified site

C82.91 Follicular lymphoma, unspecified, lymph nodes of head, face, and neck

C82.92 Follicular lymphoma, unspecified, intrathoracic lymph nodes

C82.93 Follicular lymphoma, unspecified, intra-abdominal lymph nodes

C82.94 Follicular lymphoma, unspecified, lymph nodes of axilla and upper limb

C82.95 Follicular lymphoma, unspecified, lymph nodes of inguinal region and lower limb

C82.96 Follicular lymphoma, unspecified, intrapelvic lymph nodes

C82.97 Follicular lymphoma, unspecified, spleen

C82.98 Follicular lymphoma, unspecified, lymph nodes of multiple sites

C82.99 Follicular lymphoma, unspecified, extranodal and solid organ sites

√4th **C83** **Non-follicular lymphoma**

EXCLUDES 1 *personal history of non-Hodgkin lymphoma (Z85.72)*

√5th **C83.0** **Small cell B-cell lymphoma**

Lymphoplasmacytic lymphoma
Nodal marginal zone lymphoma
Non-leukemic variant of B-CLL
Splenic marginal zone lymphoma

EXCLUDES 1 *chronic lymphocytic leukemia (C91.1)*
mature T/NK-cell lymphomas (C84.-)
Waldenström macroglobulinemia (C88.0)

C83.00 Small cell B-cell lymphoma, unspecified site

C83.01 Small cell B-cell lymphoma, lymph nodes of head, face, and neck

C83.02 Small cell B-cell lymphoma, intrathoracic lymph nodes

C83.03 Small cell B-cell lymphoma, intra-abdominal lymph nodes

C83.04 Small cell B-cell lymphoma, lymph nodes of axilla and upper limb

C83.05 Small cell B-cell lymphoma, lymph nodes of inguinal region and lower limb

C83.06 Small cell B-cell lymphoma, intrapelvic lymph nodes

C83.07   **Small cell B-cell lymphoma, spleen**
C83.08   **Small cell B-cell lymphoma, lymph nodes of multiple sites**
C83.09   **Small cell B-cell lymphoma, extranodal and solid organ sites**

☑5ᵗʰ **C83.1   Mantle cell lymphoma**
Centrocytic lymphoma
Malignant lymphomatous polyposis
C83.10   **Mantle cell lymphoma, unspecified site**
C83.11   **Mantle cell lymphoma, lymph nodes of head, face, and neck**
C83.12   **Mantle cell lymphoma, intrathoracic lymph nodes**
C83.13   **Mantle cell lymphoma, intra-abdominal lymph nodes**
C83.14   **Mantle cell lymphoma, lymph nodes of axilla and upper limb**
C83.15   **Mantle cell lymphoma, lymph nodes of inguinal region and lower limb**
C83.16   **Mantle cell lymphoma, intrapelvic lymph nodes**
C83.17   **Mantle cell lymphoma, spleen**
C83.18   **Mantle cell lymphoma, lymph nodes of multiple sites**
C83.19   **Mantle cell lymphoma, extranodal and solid organ sites**

☑5ᵗʰ **C83.3   Diffuse large B-cell lymphoma**
Anaplastic diffuse large B-cell lymphoma
CD30-positive diffuse large B-cell lymphoma
Centroblastic diffuse large B-cell lymphoma
Diffuse large B-cell lymphoma, subtype not specified
Immunoblastic diffuse large B-cell lymphoma
Plasmablastic diffuse large B-cell lymphoma
T-cell rich diffuse large B-cell lymphoma
EXCLUDES 1   mediastinal (thymic) large B-cell lymphoma (C85.2-)
mature T/NK-cell lymphomas (C84.-)
C83.30   **Diffuse large B-cell lymphoma, unspecified site**
C83.31   **Diffuse large B-cell lymphoma, lymph nodes of head, face, and neck**
C83.32   **Diffuse large B-cell lymphoma, intrathoracic lymph nodes**
C83.33   **Diffuse large B-cell lymphoma, intra-abdominal lymph nodes**
C83.34   **Diffuse large B-cell lymphoma, lymph nodes of axilla and upper limb**
C83.35   **Diffuse large B-cell lymphoma, lymph nodes of inguinal region and lower limb**
C83.36   **Diffuse large B-cell lymphoma, intrapelvic lymph nodes**
C83.37   **Diffuse large B-cell lymphoma, spleen**
C83.38   **Diffuse large B-cell lymphoma, lymph nodes of multiple sites**
C83.39   **Diffuse large B-cell lymphoma, extranodal and solid organ sites**

☑5ᵗʰ **C83.5   Lymphoblastic (diffuse) lymphoma**
B-precursor lymphoma
Lymphoblastic B-cell lymphoma
Lymphoblastic lymphoma NOS
Lymphoblastic T-cell lymphoma
T-precursor lymphoma
C83.50   **Lymphoblastic (diffuse) lymphoma, unspecified site**
C83.51   **Lymphoblastic (diffuse) lymphoma, lymph nodes of head, face, and neck**
C83.52   **Lymphoblastic (diffuse) lymphoma, intrathoracic lymph nodes**
C83.53   **Lymphoblastic (diffuse) lymphoma, intra-abdominal lymph nodes**
C83.54   **Lymphoblastic (diffuse) lymphoma, lymph nodes of axilla and upper limb**
C83.55   **Lymphoblastic (diffuse) lymphoma, lymph nodes of inguinal region and lower limb**
C83.56   **Lymphoblastic (diffuse) lymphoma, intrapelvic lymph nodes**
C83.57   **Lymphoblastic (diffuse) lymphoma, spleen**
C83.58   **Lymphoblastic (diffuse) lymphoma, lymph nodes of multiple sites**
C83.59   **Lymphoblastic (diffuse) lymphoma, extranodal and solid organ sites**

☑5ᵗʰ **C83.7   Burkitt lymphoma**
Atypical Burkitt lymphoma
Burkitt-like lymphoma
EXCLUDES 1   mature B-cell leukemia Burkitt type (C91.a-)
C83.70   **Burkitt lymphoma, unspecified site**
C83.71   **Burkitt lymphoma, lymph nodes of head, face, and neck**
C83.72   **Burkitt lymphoma, intrathoracic lymph nodes**
C83.73   **Burkitt lymphoma, intra-abdominal lymph nodes**
C83.74   **Burkitt lymphoma, lymph nodes of axilla and upper limb**
C83.75   **Burkitt lymphoma, lymph nodes of inguinal region and lower limb**
C83.76   **Burkitt lymphoma, intrapelvic lymph nodes**
C83.77   **Burkitt lymphoma, spleen**
C83.78   **Burkitt lymphoma, lymph nodes of multiple sites**
C83.79   **Burkitt lymphoma, extranodal and solid organ sites**

☑5ᵗʰ **C83.8   Other non-follicular lymphoma**
Intravascular large B-cell lymphoma
Lymphoid granulomatosis
Primary effusion B-cell lymphoma
EXCLUDES 1   mediastinal (thymic) large B-cell lymphoma (C85.2-)
T-cell rich B-cell lymphoma (C83.3-)
C83.80   **Other non-follicular lymphoma, unspecified site**
C83.81   **Other non-follicular lymphoma, lymph nodes of head, face, and neck**
C83.82   **Other non-follicular lymphoma, intrathoracic lymph nodes**
C83.83   **Other non-follicular lymphoma, intra-abdominal lymph nodes**
C83.84   **Other non-follicular lymphoma, lymph nodes of axilla and upper limb**
C83.85   **Other non-follicular lymphoma, lymph nodes of inguinal region and lower limb**
C83.86   **Other non-follicular lymphoma, intrapelvic lymph nodes**
C83.87   **Other non-follicular lymphoma, spleen**
C83.88   **Other non-follicular lymphoma, lymph nodes of multiple sites**
C83.89   **Other non-follicular lymphoma, extranodal and solid organ sites**

☑5ᵗʰ **C83.9   Non-follicular lymphoma, unspecified**
C83.90   **Non-follicular lymphoma, unspecified, unspecified site**
C83.91   **Non-follicular lymphoma, unspecified, lymph nodes of head, face, and neck**
C83.92   **Non-follicular lymphoma, unspecified, intrathoracic lymph nodes**
C83.93   **Non-follicular lymphoma, unspecified, intra-abdominal lymph nodes**
C83.94   **Non-follicular lymphoma, unspecified, lymph nodes of axilla and upper limb**
C83.95   **Non-follicular lymphoma, unspecified, lymph nodes of inguinal region and lower limb**
C83.96   **Non-follicular lymphoma, unspecified, intrapelvic lymph nodes**
C83.97   **Non-follicular lymphoma, unspecified, spleen**
C83.98   **Non-follicular lymphoma, unspecified, lymph nodes of multiple sites**
C83.99   **Non-follicular lymphoma, unspecified, extranodal and solid organ sites**

☑4ᵗʰ **C84   Mature T/NK-cell lymphomas**
EXCLUDES 1   personal history of non-Hodgkin lymphoma (Z85.72)
☑5ᵗʰ **C84.0   Mycosis fungoides**
EXCLUDES 1   peripheral T-cell lymphoma, not classified (C84.4-)
C84.00   **Mycosis fungoides, unspecified site**
C84.01   **Mycosis fungoides, lymph nodes of head, face, and neck**
C84.02   **Mycosis fungoides, intrathoracic lymph nodes**
C84.03   **Mycosis fungoides, intra-abdominal lymph nodes**
C84.04   **Mycosis fungoides, lymph nodes of axilla and upper limb**
C84.05   **Mycosis fungoides, lymph nodes of inguinal region and lower limb**
C84.06   **Mycosis fungoides, intrapelvic lymph nodes**
C84.07   **Mycosis fungoides, spleen**

C84.08 Mycosis fungoides, lymph nodes of multiple sites

C84.09 Mycosis fungoides, extranodal and solid organ sites

√5th **C84.1** **Sézary disease**

C84.10 Sézary disease, unspecified site

C84.11 Sézary disease, lymph nodes of head, face, and neck

C84.12 Sézary disease, intrathoracic lymph nodes

C84.13 Sézary disease, intra-abdominal lymph nodes

C84.14 Sézary disease, lymph nodes of axilla and upper limb

C84.15 Sézary disease, lymph nodes of inguinal region and lower limb

C84.16 Sézary disease, intrapelvic lymph nodes

C84.17 Sézary disease, spleen

C84.18 Sézary disease, lymph nodes of multiple sites

C84.19 Sézary disease, extranodal and solid organ sites

√5th **C84.4** **Peripheral T-cell lymphoma, not classified**
Lennert's lymphoma
Lymphoepithelioid lymphoma
Mature T-cell lymphoma, not elsewhere classified

C84.40 Peripheral T-cell lymphoma, not classified, unspecified site

C84.41 Peripheral T-cell lymphoma, not classified, lymph nodes of head, face, and neck

C84.42 Peripheral T-cell lymphoma, not classified, intrathoracic lymph nodes

C84.43 Peripheral T-cell lymphoma, not classified, intra-abdominal lymph nodes

C84.44 Peripheral T-cell lymphoma, not classified, lymph nodes of axilla and upper limb

C84.45 Peripheral T-cell lymphoma, not classified, lymph nodes of inguinal region and lower limb

C84.46 Peripheral T-cell lymphoma, not classified, intrapelvic lymph nodes

C84.47 Peripheral T-cell lymphoma, not classified, spleen

C84.48 Peripheral T-cell lymphoma, not classified, lymph nodes of multiple sites

C84.49 Peripheral T-cell lymphoma, not classified, extranodal and solid organ sites

√5th **C84.6** **Anaplastic large cell lymphoma, ALK-positive**
Anaplastic large cell lymphoma, CD30-positive

C84.60 Anaplastic large cell lymphoma, ALK-positive, unspecified site

C84.61 Anaplastic large cell lymphoma, ALK-positive, lymph nodes of head, face, and neck

C84.62 Anaplastic large cell lymphoma, ALK-positive, intrathoracic lymph nodes

C84.63 Anaplastic large cell lymphoma, ALK-positive, intra-abdominal lymph nodes

C84.64 Anaplastic large cell lymphoma, ALK-positive, lymph nodes of axilla and upper limb

C84.65 Anaplastic large cell lymphoma, ALK-positive, lymph nodes of inguinal region and lower limb

C84.66 Anaplastic large cell lymphoma, ALK-positive, intrapelvic lymph nodes

C84.67 Anaplastic large cell lymphoma, ALK-positive, spleen

C84.68 Anaplastic large cell lymphoma, ALK-positive, lymph nodes of multiple sites

C84.69 Anaplastic large cell lymphoma, ALK-positive, extranodal and solid organ sites

√5th **C84.7** **Anaplastic large cell lymphoma, ALK-negative**

EXCLUDES 1   *primary cutaneous CD30-positive T-cell proliferations (C86.6-)*

C84.70 Anaplastic large cell lymphoma, ALK-negative, unspecified site

C84.71 Anaplastic large cell lymphoma, ALK-negative, lymph nodes of head, face, and neck

C84.72 Anaplastic large cell lymphoma, ALK-negative, intrathoracic lymph nodes

C84.73 Anaplastic large cell lymphoma, ALK-negative, intra-abdominal lymph nodes

C84.74 Anaplastic large cell lymphoma, ALK-negative, lymph nodes of axilla and upper limb

C84.75 Anaplastic large cell lymphoma, ALK-negative, lymph nodes of inguinal region and lower limb

C84.76 Anaplastic large cell lymphoma, ALK-negative, intrapelvic lymph nodes

C84.77 Anaplastic large cell lymphoma, ALK-negative, spleen

C84.78 Anaplastic large cell lymphoma, ALK-negative, lymph nodes of multiple sites

C84.79 Anaplastic large cell lymphoma, ALK-negative, extranodal and solid organ sites

√5th **C84.a** **Cutaneous T-cell lymphoma, unspecified**

C84.a0 Cutaneous T-cell lymphoma, unspecified, unspecified site

C84.a1 Cutaneous T-cell lymphoma, unspecified lymph nodes of head, face, and neck

C84.a2 Cutaneous T-cell lymphoma, unspecified, intrathoracic lymph nodes

C84.a3 Cutaneous T-cell lymphoma, unspecified, intra-abdominal lymph nodes

C84.a4 Cutaneous T-cell lymphoma, unspecified, lymph nodes of axilla and upper limb

C84.a5 Cutaneous T-cell lymphoma, unspecified, lymph nodes of inguinal region and lower limb

C84.a6 Cutaneous T-cell lymphoma, unspecified, intrapelvic lymph nodes

C84.a7 Cutaneous T-cell lymphoma, unspecified, spleen

C84.a8 Cutaneous T-cell lymphoma, unspecified, lymph nodes of multiple sites

C84.a9 Cutaneous T-cell lymphoma, unspecified, extranodal and solid organ sites

√5th **C84.z** **Other mature T/NK-cell lymphomas**

NOTE   If T-cell lineage or involvement is mentioned in conjunction with a specific lymphoma, code to the more specific description.

EXCLUDES 1   *angioimmunoblastic T-cell lymphoma (C86.5)*
blastic NK-cell lymphoma (C86.4)
enteropathy-type T-cell lymphoma (C86.2)
extranodal NK-cell lymphoma, nasal type (C86.0)
hepatosplenic T-cell lymphoma (C86.1)
primary cutaneous CD30-positive T-cell proliferations (C86.6)
subcutaneous panniculitis-like T-cell lymphoma (C86.3)
T-cell leukemia (C91.1-)

C84.z0 Other mature T/NK-cell lymphomas, unspecified site

C84.z1 Other mature T/NK-cell lymphomas, lymph nodes of head, face, and neck

C84.z2 Other mature T/NK-cell lymphomas, intrathoracic lymph nodes

C84.z3 Other mature T/NK-cell lymphomas, intra-abdominal lymph nodes

C84.z4 Other mature T/NK-cell lymphomas, lymph nodes of axilla and upper limb

C84.z5 Other mature T/NK-cell lymphomas, lymph nodes of inguinal region and lower limb

C84.z6 Other mature T/NK-cell lymphomas, intrapelvic lymph nodes

C84.z7 Other mature T/NK-cell lymphomas, spleen

C84.z8 Other mature T/NK-cell lymphomas, lymph nodes of multiple sites

C84.z9 Other mature T/NK-cell lymphomas, extranodal and solid organ sites

√5th **C84.9** **Mature T/NK-cell lymphomas, unspecified**
NK/T cell lymphoma NOS

EXCLUDES 1   *mature T-cell lymphoma, not elsewhere classified (C84.4-)*

C84.90 Mature T/NK-cell lymphomas, unspecified, unspecified site

C84.91 Mature T/NK-cell lymphomas, unspecified, lymph nodes of head, face, and neck

C84.92 Mature T/NK-cell lymphomas, unspecified, intrathoracic lymph nodes

C84.93 Mature T/NK-cell lymphomas, unspecified, intra-abdominal lymph nodes

C84.94 Mature T/NK-cell lymphomas, unspecified, lymph nodes of axilla and upper limb

C84.95 Mature T/NK-cell lymphomas, unspecified, lymph nodes of inguinal region and lower limb

C84.96 Mature T/NK-cell lymphomas, unspecified, intrapelvic lymph nodes

---

☑ Appropriate additional character required   √x7th Requires 7th character, placeholder x must fill empty characters

Neoplasms

C84.97–C90.00

C84.97   Mature T/NK-cell lymphomas, unspecified, spleen
C84.98   Mature T/NK-cell lymphomas, unspecified, lymph nodes of multiple sites
C84.99   Mature T/NK-cell lymphomas, unspecified, extranodal and solid organ sites

√4th **C85   Other specified and unspecified types of non-Hodgkin lymphoma**
        EXCLUDES 1   *other specified types of T/NK-cell lymphoma (C86-)*
                      personal history of non-Hodgkin lymphoma (Z85.72)

√5th **C85.1   Unspecified B-cell lymphoma**
        NOTE   If B-cell lineage or involvement is mentioned in conjunction with a specific lymphoma, code to the more specific description.
        C85.10   Unspecified B-cell lymphoma, unspecified site
        C85.11   Unspecified B-cell lymphoma, lymph nodes of head, face, and neck
        C85.12   Unspecified B-cell lymphoma, intrathoracic lymph nodes
        C85.13   Unspecified B-cell lymphoma, intra-abdominal lymph nodes
        C85.14   Unspecified B-cell lymphoma, lymph nodes of axilla and upper limb
        C85.15   Unspecified B-cell lymphoma, lymph nodes of inguinal region and lower limb
        C85.16   Unspecified B-cell lymphoma, intrapelvic lymph nodes
        C85.17   Unspecified B-cell lymphoma, spleen
        C85.18   Unspecified B-cell lymphoma, lymph nodes of multiple sites
        C85.19   Unspecified B-cell lymphoma, extranodal and solid organ sites

√5th **C85.2   Mediastinal (thymic) large B-cell lymphoma**
        C85.20   Mediastinal (thymic) large B-cell lymphoma, unspecified site
        C85.21   Mediastinal (thymic) large B-cell lymphoma, lymph nodes of head, face, and neck
        C85.22   Mediastinal (thymic) large B-cell lymphoma, intrathoracic lymph nodes
        C85.23   Mediastinal (thymic) large B-cell lymphoma, intra-abdominal lymph nodes
        C85.24   Mediastinal (thymic) large B-cell lymphoma, lymph nodes of axilla and upper limb
        C85.25   Mediastinal (thymic) large B-cell lymphoma, lymph nodes of inguinal region and lower limb
        C85.26   Mediastinal (thymic) large B-cell lymphoma, intrapelvic lymph nodes
        C85.27   Mediastinal (thymic) large B-cell lymphoma, spleen
        C85.28   Mediastinal (thymic) large B-cell lymphoma, lymph nodes of multiple sites
        C85.29   Mediastinal (thymic) large B-cell lymphoma, extranodal and solid organ sites

√5th **C85.8   Other specified types of non-Hodgkin lymphoma**
        C85.80   Other specified types of non-Hodgkin lymphoma, unspecified site
        C85.81   Other specified types of non-Hodgkin lymphoma, lymph nodes of head, face, and neck
        C85.82   Other specified types of non-Hodgkin lymphoma, intrathoracic lymph nodes
        C85.83   Other specified types of non-Hodgkin lymphoma, intra-abdominal lymph nodes
        C85.84   Other specified types of non-Hodgkin lymphoma, lymph nodes of axilla and upper limb
        C85.85   Other specified types of non-Hodgkin lymphoma, lymph nodes of inguinal region and lower limb
        C85.86   Other specified types of non-Hodgkin lymphoma, intrapelvic lymph nodes
        C85.87   Other specified types of non-Hodgkin lymphoma, spleen
        C85.88   Other specified types of non-Hodgkin lymphoma, lymph nodes of multiple sites
        C85.89   Other specified types of non-Hodgkin lymphoma, extranodal and solid organ sites

√5th **C85.9   Non-Hodgkin lymphoma, unspecified**
        Lymphoma NOS
        Malignant lymphoma NOS
        Non-Hodgkin lymphoma NOS

C85.90   Non-Hodgkin lymphoma, unspecified, unspecified site
C85.91   Non-Hodgkin lymphoma, unspecified, lymph nodes of head, face, and neck
C85.92   Non-Hodgkin lymphoma, unspecified, intrathoracic lymph nodes
C85.93   Non-Hodgkin lymphoma, unspecified, intra-abdominal lymph nodes
C85.94   Non-Hodgkin lymphoma, unspecified, lymph nodes of axilla and upper limb
C85.95   Non-Hodgkin lymphoma, unspecified, lymph nodes of inguinal region and lower limb
C85.96   Non-Hodgkin lymphoma, unspecified, intrapelvic lymph nodes
C85.97   Non-Hodgkin lymphoma, unspecified, spleen
C85.98   Non-Hodgkin lymphoma, unspecified, lymph nodes of multiple sites
C85.99   Non-Hodgkin lymphoma, unspecified, extranodal and solid organ sites

√4th **C86   Other specified types of T/NK-cell lymphoma**
        EXCLUDES 1   *anaplastic large cell lymphoma, ALK negative (C84.7-)*
                      anaplastic large cell lymphoma, ALK positive (C84.6-)
                      mature T/NK-cell lymphomas (C84-)
                      other specified types of non-Hodgkin lymphoma (C85.8-)
        C86.0   Extranodal NK/T-cell lymphoma, nasal type
        C86.1   Hepatosplenic T-cell lymphoma
                 Alpha-beta and gamma delta types
        C86.2   Enteropathy-type (intestinal) T-cell lymphoma
                 Enteropathy associated T-cell lymphoma
        C86.3   Subcutaneous panniculitis-like T-cell lymphoma
        C86.4   Blastic NK-cell lymphoma
        C86.5   Angioimmunoblastic T-cell lymphoma
                 Angioimmunoblastic lymphadenopathy with dysproteinemia [AILD]
        C86.6   Primary cutaneous CD30-positive T-cell proliferations
                 Lymphomatoid papulosis
                 Primary cutaneous anaplastic large cell lymphoma
                 Primary cutaneous CD30-positive T-cell lymphoma

√4th **C88   Malignant immunoproliferative diseases and certain other B-cell lymphomas**
        EXCLUDES 1   *B-cell lymphoma, unspecified C85.1-*
                      personal history of other malignant neoplasms of lymphoid, hematopoietic and related tissues (Z85.79)
        C88.0   Waldenström macroglobulinemia
                 Lymphoplasmacytic lymphoma with IgM-production
                 Macroglobulinemia (idiopathic) (primary)
                 EXCLUDES 1   *small cell B-cell lymphoma (C83.0)*
        C88.2   Heavy chain disease
                 Franklin disease
                 Gamma heavy chain disease
                 Mu heavy chain disease
        C88.3   Immunoproliferative small intestinal disease
                 Alpha heavy chain disease
                 Mediterranean lymphoma
        C88.4   Extranodal marginal zone B-cell lymphoma of mucosa-associated lymphoid tissue [MALT-lymphoma]
                 Lymphoma of skin-associated lymphoid tissue [SALT-lymphoma]
                 Lymphoma of bronchial-associated lymphoid tissue [BALT-lymphoma]
                 EXCLUDES 1   *high malignant (diffuse large B-cell) lymphoma (C83.3-)*
        C88.8   Other malignant immunoproliferative diseases
        C88.9   Malignant immunoproliferative disease, unspecified
                 Immunoproliferative disease NOS

√4th **C90   Multiple myeloma and malignant plasma cell neoplasms**
        EXCLUDES 1   *personal history of other malignant neoplasms of lymphoid, hematopoietic and related tissues (Z85.79)*
√5th **C90.0   Multiple myeloma**
                 Kahler's disease
                 Medullary plasmacytoma
                 Myelomatosis
                 Plasma cell myeloma
                 EXCLUDES 1   *solitary myeloma (C90.3-)*
                               solitary plasmactyoma (C90.3-)
        C90.00   Multiple myeloma not having achieved remission
                  Multiple myeloma with failed remission
                  Multiple myeloma NOS

EXCLUDES 1   Not coded here   EXCLUDES 2   Not included here   *Manifestation Code*

    C90.01   **Multiple myeloma in remission**
    C90.02   **Multiple myeloma in relapse**

√5th   **C90.1**   **Plasma cell leukemia**
    Plasmacytic leukemia

    C90.10   **Plasma cell leukemia not having achieved remission**
        Plasma cell leukemia with failed remission
        Plasma cell leukemia NOS

    C90.11   **Plasma cell leukemia in remission**
    C90.12   **Plasma cell leukemia in relapse**

√5th   **C90.2**   **Extramedullary plasmacytoma**
    C90.20   **Extramedullary plasmacytoma not having achieved remission**
        Extramedullary plasmacytoma with failed remission
        Extramedullary plasmacytoma NOS

    C90.21   **Extramedullary plasmacytoma in remission**
    C90.22   **Extramedullary plasmacytoma in relapse**

√5th   **C90.3**   **Solitary plasmacytoma**
    Localized malignant plasma cell tumor NOS
    Plasmacytoma NOS
    Solitary myeloma

    C90.30   **Solitary plasmacytoma not having achieved remission**
        Solitary plasmacytoma with failed remission
        Solitary plasmacytoma NOS

    C90.31   **Solitary plasmacytoma in remission**
    C90.32   **Solitary plasmacytoma in relapse**

√4th   **C91**   **Lymphoid leukemia**
    EXCLUDES 1   *personal history of leukemia (Z85.6)*

√5th   **C91.0**   **Acute lymphoblastic leukemia [ALL]**
    NOTE   Code C91.0 should only be used for T-cell and B-cell precursor leukemia

    C91.00   **Acute lymphoblastic leukemia not having achieved remission**
        Acute lymphoblastic leukemia with failed remission
        Acute lymphoblastic leukemia NOS

    C91.01   **Acute lymphoblastic leukemia, in remission**
    C91.02   **Acute lymphoblastic leukemia, in relapse**

√5th   **C91.1**   **Chronic lymphocytic leukemia of B-cell type**
    Lymphoplasmacytic leukemia
    Richter syndrome
    EXCLUDES 1   *lymphoplasmacytic lymphoma (C83.0-)*

    C91.10   **Chronic lymphocytic leukemia of B-cell type not having achieved remission**
        Chronic lymphocytic leukemia of B-cell type with failed remission
        Chronic lymphocytic leukemia of B-cell type NOS

    C91.11   **Chronic lymphocytic leukemia of B-cell type in remission**
    C91.12   **Chronic lymphocytic leukemia of B-cell type in relapse**

√5th   **C91.3**   **Prolymphocytic leukemia of B-cell type**
    C91.30   **Prolymphocytic leukemia of B-cell type not having achieved remission**
        Prolymphocytic leukemia of B-cell type with failed remission
        Prolymphocytic leukemia of B-cell type NOS

    C91.31   **Prolymphocytic leukemia of B-cell type, in remission**
    C91.32   **Prolymphocytic leukemia of B-cell type, in relapse**

√5th   **C91.4**   **Hairy cell leukemia**
    Leukemic reticuloendotheliosis

    C91.40   **Hairy cell leukemia not having achieved remission**
        Hairy cell leukemia with failed remission
        Hairy cell leukemia NOS

    C91.41   **Hairy cell leukemia, in remission**
    C91.42   **Hairy cell leukemia, in relapse**

√5th   **C91.5**   **Adult T-cell lymphoma/leukemia (HTLV-1-associated)**
    Acute variant of adult T-cell lymphoma/leukemia (HTLV-1-associated)
    Chronic variant of adult T-cell lymphoma/leukemia (HTLV-1-associated)
    Lymphomatoid variant of adult T-cell lymphoma/leukemia (HTLV-1-associated)
    Smouldering variant of adult T-cell lymphoma/leukemia (HTLV-1-associated)

    C91.50   **Adult T-cell lymphoma/leukemia (HTLV-1-associated) not having achieved remission**
        Adult T-cell lymphoma/leukemia (HTLV-1-associated) with failed remission
        Adult T-cell lymphoma/leukemia (HTLV-1-associated) NOS

    C91.51   **Adult T-cell lymphoma/leukemia (HTLV-1-associated), in remission**
    C91.52   **Adult T-cell lymphoma/leukemia (HTLV-1-associated), in relapse**

√5th   **C91.6**   **Prolymphocytic leukemia of T-cell type**
    C91.60   **Prolymphocytic leukemia of T-cell type not having achieved remission**
        Prolymphocytic leukemia of T-cell type with failed remission
        Prolymphocytic leukemia of T-cell type NOS

    C91.61   **Prolymphocytic leukemia of T-cell type, in remission**
    C91.62   **Prolymphocytic leukemia of T-cell type, in relapse**

√5th   **C91.a**   **Mature B-cell leukemia Burkitt-type**
    EXCLUDES 1   *Burkitt lymphoma (C83.7-)*

    C91.a0   **Mature B-cell leukemia Burkitt-type not having achieved remission**
        Mature B-cell leukemia Burkitt-type with failed remission
        Mature B-cell leukemia Burkitt-type NOS

    C91.a1   **Mature B-cell leukemia Burkitt-type, in remission**
    C91.a2   **Mature B-cell leukemia Burkitt-type, in relapse**

√5th   **C91.z**   **Other lymphoid leukemia**
    T-cell large granular lymphocytic leukemia (associated with rheumatoid arthritis)

    C91.z0   **Other lymphoid leukemia not having achieved remission**
        Other lymphoid leukemia with failed remission
        Other lymphoid leukemia NOS

    C91.z1   **Other lymphoid leukemia, in remission**
    C91.z2   **Other lymphoid leukemia, in relapse**

√5th   **C91.9**   **Lymphoid leukemia, unspecified**
    C91.90   **Lymphoid leukemia, unspecified not having achieved remission**
        Lymphoid leukemia with failed remission
        Lymphoid leukemia NOS

    C91.91   **Lymphoid leukemia, unspecified, in remission**
    C91.92   **Lymphoid leukemia, unspecified, in relapse**

√4th   **C92**   **Myeloid leukemia**
    INCLUDES   granulocytic leukemia
        myelogenous leukemia
    EXCLUDES 1   *personal history of leukemia (Z85.6)*

√5th   **C92.0**   **Acute myeloblastic leukemia**
    Acute myeloblastic leukemia, minimal differentiation
    Acute myeloblastic leukemia (with maturation)
    Acute myeloblastic leukemia 1/ETO
    Acute myeloblastic leukemia M0
    Acute myeloblastic leukemia M1
    Acute myeloblastic leukemia M2
    Acute myeloblastic leukemia with t(8;21)
    Acute myeloblastic leukemia (without a FAB classification) NOS
    Refractory anemia with excess blasts in transformation [RAEB T]
    EXCLUDES 1   *acute exacerbation of chronic myeloid leukemia (C92.10)*
        refractory anemia with excess of blasts not in transformation (D46.2-)

    C92.00   **Acute myeloblastic leukemia, not having achieved remission**
        Acute myeloblastic leukemia with failed remission
        Acute myeloblastic leukemia NOS

    C92.01   **Acute myeloblastic leukemia, in remission**
    C92.02   **Acute myeloblastic leukemia, in relapse**

☑ Appropriate additional character required   √x7th Requires 7th character, placeholder x must fill empty characters

✓5th **C92.1 Chronic myeloid leukemia, BCR/ABL-positive**
Chronic myelogenous leukemia, Philadelphia chromosome (Ph1) positive
Chronic myelogenous leukemia, t(9;22) (q34;q11)
Chronic myelogenous leukemia with crisis of blast cells
> EXCLUDES 1   atypical chronic myeloid leukemia BCR/ABL-negative (C92.2-)
> chronic myelomonocytic leukemia (C93.1-)
> chronic myeloproliferative disease (D47.1)

C92.10 Chronic myeloid leukemia, BCR/ABL-positive, not having achieved remission
Chronic myeloid leukemia, BCR/ABL-positive with failed remission
Chronic myeloid leukemia, BCR/ABL-positive NOS

C92.11 Chronic myeloid leukemia, BCR/ABL-positive, in remission

C92.12 Chronic myeloid leukemia, BCR/ABL-positive, in relapse

✓5th **C92.2 Atypical chronic myeloid leukemia, BCR/ABL-negative**
C92.20 Atypical chronic myeloid leukemia, BCR/ABL-negative, not having achieved remission
Atypical chronic myeloid leukemia, BCR/ABL-negative with failed remission
Atypical chronic myeloid leukemia, BCR/ABL-negative NOS

C92.21 Atypical chronic myeloid leukemia, BCR/ABL-negative, in remission

C92.22 Atypical chronic myeloid leukemia, BCR/ABL-negative, in relapse

✓5th **C92.3 Myeloid sarcoma**
A malignant tumor of immature myeloid cells
Chloroma
Granulocytic sarcoma
C92.30 Myeloid sarcoma, not having achieved remission
Myeloid sarcoma with failed remission
Myeloid sarcoma NOS

C92.31 Myeloid sarcoma, in remission

C92.32 Myeloid sarcoma, in relapse

✓5th **C92.4 Acute promyelocytic leukemia**
AML M3
AML Me with t(15;17) and variants
C92.40 Acute promyelocytic leukemia, not having achieved remission
Acute promyelocytic leukemia with failed remission
Acute promyelocytic leukemia NOS

C92.41 Acute promyelocytic leukemia, in remission

C92.42 Acute promyelocytic leukemia, in relapse

✓5th **C92.5 Acute myelomonocytic leukemia**
AML M4
AML M4 Eo with inv(16) or t(16;16)
C92.50 Acute myelomonocytic leukemia, not having achieved remission
Acute myelomonocytic leukemia with failed remission
Acute myelomonocytic leukemia NOS

C92.51 Acute myelomonocytic leukemia, in remission

C92.52 Acute myelomonocytic leukemia, in relapse

✓5th **C92.6 Acute myeloid leukemia with 11q23-abnormality**
Acute myeloid leukemia with variation of MLL-gene
C92.60 Acute myeloid leukemia with 11q23-abnormality not having achieved remission
Acute myeloid leukemia with 11q23-abnormality with failed remission
Acute myeloid leukemia with 11q23-abnormality NOS

C92.61 Acute myeloid leukemia with 11q23-abnormality in remission

C92.62 Acute myeloid leukemia with 11q23-abnormality in relapse

✓5th **C92.a Acute myeloid leukemia with multilineage dysplasia**
Acute myeloid leukemia with dysplasia of remaining hematopoesis and/or myelodysplastic disease in its history
C92.a0 Acute myeloid leukemia with multilineage dysplasia, not having achieved remission
Acute myeloid leukemia with multilineage dysplasia with failed remission
Acute myeloid leukemia with multilineage dysplasia NOS

C92.a1 Acute myeloid leukemia with multilineage dysplasia, in remission

C92.a2 Acute myeloid leukemia with multilineage dysplasia, in relapse

✓5th **C92.z Other myeloid leukemia**
C92.z0 Other myeloid leukemia not having achieved remission
Myeloid leukemia NEC with failed remission
Myeloid leukemia NEC

C92.z1 Other myeloid leukemia, in remission

C92.z2 Other myeloid leukemia, in relapse

✓5th **C92.9 Myeloid leukemia, unspecified**
C92.90 Myeloid leukemia, unspecified, not having achieved remission
Myeloid leukemia, unspecified with failed remission
Myeloid leukemia, unspecified NOS

C92.91 Myeloid leukemia, unspecified in remission

C92.92 Myeloid leukemia, unspecified in relapse

✓4th **C93 Monocytic leukemia**
> INCLUDES   monocytoid leukemia
> EXCLUDES 1   personal history of leukemia (Z85.6)

✓5th **C93.0 Acute monoblastic/monocytic leukemia**
AML M5
AML M5a
AML M5b
C93.00 Acute monoblastic/monocytic leukemia, not having achieved remission
Acute monoblastic/monocytic leukemia with failed remission
Acute monoblastic/monocytic leukemia NOS

C93.01 Acute monoblastic/monocytic leukemia, in remission

C93.02 Acute monoblastic/monocytic leukemia, in relapse

✓5th **C93.1 Chronic myelomonocytic leukemia**
Chronic monocytic leukemia
CMML-1
CMML-2
CMML with eosinophilia
C93.10 Chronic myelomonocytic leukemia not having achieved remission
Chronic myelomonocytic leukemia with failed remission
Chronic myelomonocytic leukemia NOS

C93.11 Chronic myelomonocytic leukemia, in remission

C93.12 Chronic myelomonocytic leukemia, in relapse

✓5th **C93.3 Juvenile myelomonocytic leukemia**
C93.30 Juvenile myelomonocytic leukemia, not having achieved remission
Juvenile myelomonocytic leukemia with failed remission
Juvenile myelomonocytic leukemia NOS

C93.31 Juvenile myelomonocytic leukemia, in remission

C93.32 Juvenile myelomonocytic leukemia, in relapse

✓5th **C93.z Other monocytic leukemia**
C93.z0 Other monocytic leukemia, not in remission
Other monocytic leukemia NOS

C93.z1 Other monocytic leukemia, in remission

✓5th **C93.9 Monocytic leukemia, unspecified**
C93.90 Monocytic leukemia, unspecified, not having achieved remission
Monocytic leukemia, unspecified with failed remission
Monocytic leukemia, unspecified NOS

C93.91 Monocytic leukemia, unspecified in remission

C93.92 Monocytic leukemia, unspecified in relapse

✓4th **C94 Other leukemias of specified cell type**
> EXCLUDES 1   leukemic reticuloendotheliosis (C91.4-)
> myelodysplastic syndromes (D46-)
> personal history of leukemia (Z85.6)
> plasma cell leukemia (C90.1-)

✓5th **C94.0 Acute erythroid leukemia**
Acute myeloid leukemia M6(a)(b)
Erythroleukemia
C94.00 Acute erythroid leukemia, not having achieved remission
Acute erythroid leukemia with failed remission
Acute erythroid leukemia NOS

C94.01 Acute erythroid leukemia, in remission

EXCLUDES 1   Not coded here   EXCLUDES 2   Not included here   *Manifestation Code*

C94.02 **Acute erythroid leukemia, in relapse**

✓5ᵗʰ C94.2 **Acute megakaryoblastic leukemia**
Acute myeloid leukemia M7
Acute megakaryocytic leukemia

C94.20 **Acute megakaryoblastic leukemia not having achieved remission**
Acute megakaryoblastic leukemia with failed remission
Acute megakaryoblastic leukemia NOS

C94.21 **Acute megakaryoblastic leukemia, in remission**
C94.22 **Acute megakaryoblastic leukemia, in relapse**

✓5ᵗʰ C94.3 **Mast cell leukemia**
C94.30 **Mast cell leukemia not having achieved remission**
Mast cell leukemia with failed remission
Mast cell leukemia NOS
C94.31 **Mast cell leukemia, in remission**
C94.32 **Mast cell leukemia, in relapse**

✓5ᵗʰ C94.4 **Acute panmyelosis with myelofibrosis**
Acute myelofibrosis
EXCLUDES 1 *myelofibrosis NOS (D75.81)*
secondary myelofibrosis NOS (D75.81)
C94.40 **Acute panmyelosis with myelofibrosis not having achieved remission**
Acute myelofibrosis NOS
Acute panmyelosis with myelofibrosis with failed remission
Acute panmyelosis NOS
C94.41 **Acute panmyelosis with myelofibrosis, in remission**
C94.42 **Acute panmyelosis with myelofibrosis, in relapse**

C94.6 **Myelodysplastic disease, not classified**
Myeloproliferative diease, not classified

✓5ᵗʰ C94.8 **Other specified leukemias**
Aggressive NK-cell leukemia
Acute basophilic leukemia
C94.80 **Other specified leukemias not having achieved remission**
Other specified leukemia with failed remission
Other specified leukemias NOS
C94.81 **Other specified leukemias, in remission**
C94.82 **Other specified leukemias, in relapse**

✓4ᵗʰ C95 **Leukemia of unspecified cell type**
EXCLUDES 1 *personal history of leukemia (Z85.6)*

✓5ᵗʰ C95.0 **Acute leukemia of unspecified cell type**
Acute bilineal leukemia
Acute mixed lineage leukemia
Biphenotypic acute leukemia
Stem cell leukemia of unclear lineage
EXCLUDES 1 *acute exacerbation of unspecified chronic leukemia (C95.10)*
C95.00 **Acute leukemia of unspecified cell type not having achieved remission**
Acute leukemia of unspecified cell type with failed remission
Acute leukemia NOS
C95.01 **Acute leukemia of unspecified cell type, in remission**
C95.02 **Acute leukemia of unspecified cell type, in relapse**

✓5ᵗʰ C95.1 **Chronic leukemia of unspecified cell type**
C95.10 **Chronic leukemia of unspecified cell type not having achieved remission**
Chronic leukemia of unspecified cell type with failed remission
Chronic leukemia NOS
C95.11 **Chronic leukemia of unspecified cell type, in remission**
C95.12 **Chronic leukemia of unspecified cell type, in relapse**

✓5ᵗʰ C95.9 **Leukemia, unspecified**
C95.90 **Leukemia, unspecified not having achieved remission**
Leukemia, unspecified with failed remission
Leukemia NOS
C95.91 **Leukemia, unspecified, in remission**
C95.92 **Leukemia, unspecified, in relapse**

✓4ᵗʰ C96 **Other and unspecified malignant neoplasms of lymphoid, hematopoietic and related tissue**
EXCLUDES 1 *personal history of other malignant neoplasms of lymphoid, hematopoietic and related tissues (Z85.79)*

C96.0 **Multifocal and multisystemic (disseminated) Langerhans-cell histiocytosis**
Histiocytosis X, multisystemic
Letterer-Siwe disease
EXCLUDES 1 *multifocal and unisystemic Langerhans-cell histiocytosis (C96.5)*
unifocal Langerhans-cell histiocytosis (C96.6)

C96.2 **Malignant mast cell tumor**
Aggressive systemic mastocytosis
Mast cell sarcoma
EXCLUDES 1 *indolent mastocytosis (D47.0)*
mast cell leukemia (C94.30)
mastocytosis (congenital) (cutaneous) (Q82.2)

C96.4 **Sarcoma of dendritic cells (accessory cells)**
Follicular dendritic cell sarcoma
Interdigitating dendritic cell sarcoma
Langerhans cell sarcoma

C96.5 **Multifocal and unisystemic Langerhans-cell histiocytosis**
Hand-Schüller-Christian disease
Histiocytosis X, multifocal
EXCLUDES 1 *multifocal and multisystemic (disseminated) Langerhans-cell histiocytosis (C96.0)*
unifocal Langerhans-cell histiocytosis (C96.6)

C96.6 **Unifocal Langerhans-cell histiocytosis**
Eosinophilic granuloma
Histiocytosis X, unifocal
Histiocytosis X NOS
Langerhans-cell histiocytosis NOS
EXCLUDES 1 *multifocal and multisysemic (disseminated) Langerhans-cell histiocytosis (C96.0)*
multifocal and unisystemic Langerhans-cell histiocytosis (C96.5)

C96.a **Histiocytic sarcoma**
Malignant histiocytosis

C96.z **Other specified malignant neoplasms of lymphoid, hematopoietic and related tissue**

C96.9 **Malignant neoplasm of lymphoid, hematopoietic and related tissue, unspecified**

In situ neoplasms (D00-D09)

INCLUDES Bowen's disease
erythroplasia
grade III intraepithelial neoplasia
Queyrat's erythroplasia
Use additional morphology codes with behavior code /2

✓4ᵗʰ D00 **Carcinoma in situ of oral cavity, esophagus and stomach**
EXCLUDES 1 *melanoma in situ (D03-)*

✓5ᵗʰ D00.0 **Carcinoma in situ of lip, oral cavity and pharynx**
EXCLUDES 1 *carcinoma in situ of aryepiglottic fold or interarytenoid fold, laryngeal aspect (D02.0)*
carcinoma in situ of epiglottis NOS (D02.0)
carcinoma in situ of epiglottis suprahyoid portion (D02.0)
carcinoma in situ of skin of lip (D03.0, D04.0)
Use additional code to identify:
exposure to environmental tobacco smoke (Z77.22)
exposure to tobacco smoke in the perinatal period (P96.81)
history of tobacco use (Z87.891)
occupational exposure to environmental tobacco smoke (Z57.31)
tobacco dependence (F17-)
tobacco use (Z72.0)
D00.00 **Carcinoma in situ of oral cavity, unspecified site**
D00.01 **Carcinoma in situ of labial mucosa and vermilion border**
D00.02 **Carcinoma in situ of buccal mucosa**
D00.03 **Carcinoma in situ of gingiva and edentulous alveolar ridge**
D00.04 **Carcinoma in situ of soft palate**
D00.05 **Carcinoma in situ of hard palate**
D00.06 **Carcinoma in situ of floor of mouth**
D00.07 **Carcinoma in situ of tongue**

D00.08 **Carcinoma in situ of pharynx**
Carcinoma in situ of aryepiglottic fold NOS
Carcinoma in situ of hypopharyngeal aspect of aryepiglottic fold
Carcinoma in situ of marginal zone of aryepiglottic fold

D00.1 **Carcinoma in situ of esophagus**

D00.2 **Carcinoma in situ of stomach**

√4ᵗʰ **D01** **Carcinoma in situ of other and unspecified digestive organs**
EXCLUDES 1   *melanoma in situ (D03-)*

D01.0 **Carcinoma in situ of colon**
EXCLUDES 1   *carcinoma in situ of rectosigmoid junction (D01.1)*

D01.1 **Carcinoma in situ of rectosigmoid junction**

D01.2 **Carcinoma in situ of rectum**

D01.3 **Carcinoma in situ of anus and anal canal**
EXCLUDES 1   *carcinoma in situ of anal margin (D04.5)*
carcinoma in situ of anal skin (D04.5)
carcinoma in situ of perianal skin (D04.5)

√5ᵗʰ **D01.4** **Carcinoma in situ of other and unspecified parts of intestine**
EXCLUDES 1   *carcinoma in situ of ampulla of Vater (D01.5)*

D01.40 **Carcinoma in situ of unspecified part of intestine**

D01.49 **Carcinoma in situ of other parts of intestine**

D01.5 **Carcinoma in situ of liver, gallbladder and bile ducts**
Carcinoma in situ of ampulla of Vater

D01.7 **Carcinoma in situ of other specified digestive organs**
Carcinoma in situ of pancreas

D01.9 **Carcinoma in situ of digestive organ, unspecified**

√4ᵗʰ **D02** **Carcinoma in situ of middle ear and respiratory system**
EXCLUDES 1   *melanoma in situ (D03-)*
Use additional code to identify:
exposure to environmental tobacco smoke (Z77.22)
exposure to tobacco smoke in the perinatal period (P96.81)
history of tobacco use (Z87.891)
occupational exposure to environmental tobacco smoke (Z57.31)
tobacco dependence (F17-)
tobacco use (Z72.0)

D02.0 **Carcinoma in situ of larynx**
Carcinoma in situ of aryepiglottic fold or interarytenoid fold, laryngeal aspect
Carcinoma in situ of epiglottis (suprahyoid portion)
EXCLUDES 1   *carcinoma in situ of aryepiglottic fold or interarytenoid fold NOS (D00.08)*
carcinoma in situ of hypopharyngeal aspect (D00.08)
carcinoma in situ of marginal zone (D00.08)

D02.1 **Carcinoma in situ of trachea**

√5ᵗʰ **D02.2** **Carcinoma in situ of bronchus and lung**

D02.20 **Carcinoma in situ of unspecified bronchus and lung**

D02.21 **Carcinoma in situ of right bronchus and lung**

D02.22 **Carcinoma in situ of left bronchus and lung**

D02.3 **Carcinoma in situ of other parts of respiratory system**
Carcinoma in situ of accessory sinuses
Carcinoma in situ of middle ear
Carcinoma in situ of nasal cavities
EXCLUDES 1   *carcinoma in situ of ear (external) (skin) (D04.2-)*
carcinoma in situ of nose NOS (D09.8)
carcinoma in situ of skin of nose (D04.3)

D02.4 **Carcinoma in situ of respiratory system, unspecified**

√4ᵗʰ **D03** **Melanoma in situ**

D03.0 **Melanoma in situ of lip**

√5ᵗʰ **D03.1** **Melanoma in situ of eyelid, including canthus**

D03.10 **Melanoma in situ of unspecified eyelid, including canthus**

D03.11 **Melanoma in situ of right eyelid, including canthus**

D03.12 **Melanoma in situ of left eyelid, including canthus**

√5ᵗʰ **D03.2** **Melanoma in situ of ear and external auricular canal**

D03.20 **Melanoma in situ of unspecified ear and external auricular canal**

D03.21 **Melanoma in situ of right ear and external auricular canal**

D03.22 **Melanoma in situ of left ear and external auricular canal**

√5ᵗʰ **D03.3** **Melanoma in situ of other and unspecified parts of face**

D03.30 **Melanoma in situ of unspecified part of face**

D03.39 **Melanoma in situ of other parts of face**

D03.4 **Melanoma in situ of scalp and neck**

√5ᵗʰ **D03.5** **Melanoma in situ of trunk**

D03.51 **Melanoma in situ of anal skin**
Melanoma in situ of anal margin
Melanoma in situ of perianal skin

D03.52 **Melanoma in situ of breast (skin) (soft tissue)**

D03.59 **Melanoma in situ of other part of trunk**

√5ᵗʰ **D03.6** **Melanoma in situ of upper limb, including shoulder**

D03.60 **Melanoma in situ of unspecified upper limb, including shoulder**

D03.61 **Melanoma in situ of right upper limb, including shoulder**

D03.62 **Melanoma in situ of left upper limb, including shoulder**

√5ᵗʰ **D03.7** **Melanoma in situ of lower limb, including hip**

D03.70 **Melanoma in situ of unspecified lower limb, including hip**

D03.71 **Melanoma in situ of right lower limb, including hip**

D03.72 **Melanoma in situ of left lower limb, including hip**

D03.8 **Melanoma in situ of other sites**
Melanoma in situ of scrotum
EXCLUDES 1   *carcinoma in situ of scrotum (D07.61)*

D03.9 **Melanoma in situ, unspecified**

√4ᵗʰ **D04** **Carcinoma in situ of skin**
EXCLUDES 1   *erythroplasia of Queyrat (penis) NOS (D07.4)*
melanoma in situ (D03-)

D04.0 **Carcinoma in situ of skin of lip**
EXCLUDES 1   *carcinoma in situ of vermilion border of lip (D00.01)*

√5ᵗʰ **D04.1** **Carcinoma in situ of skin of eyelid, including canthus**

D04.10 **Carcinoma in situ of skin of unspecified eyelid, including canthus**

D04.11 **Carcinoma in situ of skin of right eyelid, including canthus**

D04.12 **Carcinoma in situ of skin of left eyelid, including canthus**

√5ᵗʰ **D04.2** **Carcinoma in situ of skin of ear and external auricular canal**

D04.20 **Carcinoma in situ of skin of unspecified ear and external auricular canal**

D04.21 **Carcinoma in situ of skin of right ear and external auricular canal**

D04.22 **Carcinoma in situ of skin of left ear and external auricular canal**

√5ᵗʰ **D04.3** **Carcinoma in situ of skin of other and unspecified parts of face**

D04.30 **Carcinoma in situ of skin of unspecified part of face**

D04.39 **Carcinoma in situ of skin of other parts of face**

D04.4 **Carcinoma in situ of skin of scalp and neck**

D04.5 **Carcinoma in situ of skin of trunk**
Carcinoma in situ of anal margin
Carcinoma in situ of anal skin
Carcinoma in situ of perianal skin
Carcinoma in situ of skin of breast
EXCLUDES 1   *carcinoma in situ of anus NOS (D01.3)*
carcinoma in situ of scrotum (D07.61)
carcinoma in situ of skin of genital organs (D07-)

√5ᵗʰ **D04.6** **Carcinoma in situ of skin of upper limb, including shoulder**

D04.60 **Carcinoma in situ of skin of unspecified upper limb, including shoulder**

D04.61 **Carcinoma in situ of skin of right upper limb, including shoulder**

D04.62 **Carcinoma in situ of skin of left upper limb, including shoulder**

√5ᵗʰ **D04.7** **Carcinoma in situ of skin of lower limb, including hip**

D04.70 **Carcinoma in situ of skin of unspecified lower limb, including hip**

D04.71 **Carcinoma in situ of skin of right lower limb, including hip**

D04.72 **Carcinoma in situ of skin of left lower limb, including hip**

D04.8 **Carcinoma in situ of skin of other sites**

D04.9 **Carcinoma in situ of skin, unspecified**

√4ᵗʰ **D05** **Carcinoma in situ of breast**
EXCLUDES 1   *carcinoma in situ of skin of breast (D04.5)*
melanoma in situ of breast (skin) (D03.5)
Paget's disease of breast or nipple (C50-)

√5ᵗʰ **D05.0** **Lobular carcinoma in situ of breast**

D05.00 **Lobular carcinoma in situ of unspecified breast**

EXCLUDES 1 Not coded here   EXCLUDES 2 Not included here   ***Manifestation Code***

D05.01   Lobular carcinoma in situ of right breast
D05.02   Lobular carcinoma in situ of left breast
✓5th D05.1   **Intraductal carcinoma in situ of breast**
D05.10   Intraductal carcinoma in situ of unspecified breast
D05.11   Intraductal carcinoma in situ of right breast
D05.12   Intraductal carcinoma in situ of left breast
✓5th D05.8   **Other specified type of carcinoma in situ of breast**
D05.80   Other specified type of carcinoma in situ of unspecified breast
D05.81   Other specified type of carcinoma in situ of right breast
D05.82   Other specified type of carcinoma in situ of left breast
✓5th D05.9   **Unspecified type of carcinoma in situ of breast**
D05.90   Unspecified type of carcinoma in situ of unspecified breast
D05.91   Unspecified type of carcinoma in situ of right breast
D05.92   Unspecified type of carcinoma in situ of left breast

✓4th **D06   Carcinoma in situ of cervix uteri**
INCLUDES   cervical adenocarcinoma in situ
cervical intraepithelial glandular neoplasia
cervical intraepithelial neoplasia III [CIN III]
severe dysplasia of cervix uteri
EXCLUDES 1   *cervical intraepithelial neoplasia II [CIN II] (N87.1)*
cytologic evidence of malignancy of cervix without histologic confirmation (R87.614)
high grade squamous intraepithelial lesion (HGSIL) of cervix (R87.613)
melanoma in situ of cervix (D03.5)
moderate cervical dysplasia (N87.1)
D06.0   Carcinoma in situ of endocervix
D06.1   Carcinoma in situ of exocervix
D06.7   Carcinoma in situ of other parts of cervix
D06.9   Carcinoma in situ of cervix, unspecified

✓4th **D07   Carcinoma in situ of other and unspecified genital organs**
EXCLUDES 1   *melanoma in situ of trunk (D03.5)*
D07.0   Carcinoma in situ of endometrium
D07.1   Carcinoma in situ of vulva
Severe dysplasia of vulva
Vulvar intraepithelial neoplasia III [VIN III]
EXCLUDES 1   *moderate dysplasia of vulva (N90.1)*
vulvar intraepithelial neoplasia II [VIN II] (N90.1)
D07.2   Carcinoma in situ of vagina
Severe dysplasia of vagina
Vaginal intraepithelial neoplasia III [VAIN III]
EXCLUDES 1   *moderate dysplasia of vagina (N89.1)*
vaginal intraepithelial neoplasia II [VIN II] (N89.1)
✓5th D07.3   **Carcinoma in situ of other and unspecified female genital organs**
D07.30   Carcinoma in situ of unspecified female genital organs
D07.39   Carcinoma in situ of other female genital organs
D07.4   Carcinoma in situ of penis
Erythroplasia of Queyrat NOS
D07.5   Carcinoma in situ of prostate
Prostatic intraepithelial neoplasia III [PIN III]
Severe dysplasia of prostate
EXCLUDES 1   *dysplasia (mild) (moderate) of prostate (N42.3)*
✓5th D07.6   **Carcinoma in situ of other and unspecified male genital organs**
D07.60   Carcinoma in situ of unspecified male genital organs
D07.61   Carcinoma in situ of scrotum
D07.69   Carcinoma in situ of other male genital organs

✓4th **D09   Carcinoma in situ of other and unspecified sites**
EXCLUDES 1   *melanoma in situ (D03-)*
D09.0   Carcinoma in situ of bladder
✓5th D09.1   **Carcinoma in situ of other and unspecified urinary organs**
D09.10   Carcinoma in situ of unspecified urinary organ
D09.19   Carcinoma in situ of other urinary organs
✓5th D09.2   **Carcinoma in situ of eye**
EXCLUDES 1   *carcinoma in situ of skin of eyelid (D04.1-)*
D09.20   Carcinoma in situ of unspecified eye
D09.21   Carcinoma in situ of right eye
D09.22   Carcinoma in situ of left eye

D09.3   Carcinoma in situ of thyroid and other endocrine glands
EXCLUDES 1   *carcinoma in situ of endocrine pancreas (D01.7)*
carcinoma in situ of ovary (D07.39)
carcinoma in situ of testis (D07.69)
D09.8   Carcinoma in situ of other specified sites
D09.9   Carcinoma in situ, unspecified

Benign neoplasms, except benign neuroendocrine tumors (D10-D36)

Use additional morphology codes with behavior code /0

✓4th **D10   Benign neoplasm of mouth and pharynx**
D10.0   **Benign neoplasm of lip**
Benign neoplasm of lip (frenulum) (inner aspect) (mucosa) (vermilion border)
EXCLUDES 1   *benign neoplasm of skin of lip (D22.0, D23.0)*
D10.1   **Benign neoplasm of tongue**
Benign neoplasm of lingual tonsil
D10.2   **Benign neoplasm of floor of mouth**
✓5th D10.3   **Other and unspecified parts of mouth**
D10.30   Benign neoplasm of unspecified part of mouth
D10.39   Benign neoplasm of other parts of mouth
Benign neoplasm of minor salivary gland NOS
EXCLUDES 1   *benign odontogenic neoplasms (D16.4-D16.5)*
benign neoplasm of mucosa of lip (D10.0)
benign neoplasm of nasopharyngeal surface of soft palate (D10.6)
D10.4   **Benign neoplasm of tonsil**
Benign neoplasm of tonsil (faucial) (palatine)
EXCLUDES 1   *benign neoplasm of lingual tonsil (D10.1)*
benign neoplasm of pharyngeal tonsil (D10.6)
benign neoplasm of tonsillar fossa (D10.5)
benign neoplasm of tonsillar pillars (D10.5)
D10.5   **Benign neoplasm of other parts of oropharynx**
Benign neoplasm of epiglottis, anterior aspect
Benign neoplasm of tonsillar fossa
Benign neoplasm of tonsillar pillars
Benign neoplasm of vallecula
EXCLUDES 1   *benign neoplasm of epiglottis NOS (D14.1)*
benign neoplasm of epiglottis, suprahyoid portion (D14.1)
D10.6   **Benign neoplasm of nasopharynx**
Benign neoplasm of pharyngeal tonsil
Benign neoplasm of posterior margin of septum and choanae
D10.7   **Benign neoplasm of hypopharynx**
D10.9   **Benign neoplasm of pharynx, unspecified**

✓4th **D11   Benign neoplasm of major salivary glands**
EXCLUDES 1   *benign neoplasms of specified minor salivary glands which are classified according to their anatomical location*
benign neoplasms of minor salivary glands NOS (D10.39)
D11.0   **Benign neoplasm of parotid gland**
D11.7   **Benign neoplasm of other major salivary glands**
Benign neoplasm of sublingual salivary gland
Benign neoplasm of submandibular salivary gland
D11.9   **Benign neoplasm of major salivary gland, unspecified**

✓4th **D12   Benign neoplasm of colon, rectum, anus and anal canal**
EXCLUDES 1   *benign carcinoid tumors of the large intestine, and rectum (D3a.02-)*
D12.0   **Benign neoplasm of cecum**
Benign neoplasm of ileocecal valve
D12.1   **Benign neoplasm of appendix**
EXCLUDES 1   *benign carcinoid tumor of the appendix (D3a.020)*
D12.2   **Benign neoplasm of ascending colon**
D12.3   **Benign neoplasm of transverse colon**
Benign neoplasm of hepatic flexure
Benign neoplasm of splenic flexure
D12.4   **Benign neoplasm of descending colon**
D12.5   **Benign neoplasm of sigmoid colon**
D12.6   **Benign neoplasm of colon, unspecified**
Adenomatosis of colon
Benign neoplasm of large intestine NOS
Polyposis (hereditary) of colon
EXCLUDES 1   *inflammatory polyp of colon (K51.4-)*
polyp of colon NOS (K63.5)
D12.7   **Benign neoplasm of rectosigmoid junction**

✔ Appropriate additional character required
✓x7th Requires 7th character, placeholder x must fill empty characters

D12.8   **Benign neoplasm of rectum**
> *EXCLUDES 1*   *benign carcinoid tumor of the rectum (D3a.026)*

D12.9   **Benign neoplasm of anus and anal canal**
Benign neoplasm of anus NOS
> *EXCLUDES 1*   *benign neoplasm of anal margin (D22.5, D23.5)*
> *benign neoplasm of anal skin (D22.5, D23.5)*
> *benign neoplasm of perianal skin (D22.5, D23.5)*

✓4th **D13**   **Benign neoplasm of other and ill-defined parts of digestive system**
> *EXCLUDES 1*   *benign stromal tumors of digestive system (D21.4)*

D13.0   **Benign neoplasm of esophagus**

D13.1   **Benign neoplasm of stomach**
> *EXCLUDES 1*   *benign carcinoid tumor of the stomach (D3a.092)*

D13.2   **Benign neoplasm of duodenum**
> *EXCLUDES 1*   *benign carcinoid tumor of the duodenum (D3a.010)*

✓5th **D13.3**   **Benign neoplasm of other and unspecified parts of small intestine**
> *EXCLUDES 1*   *benign carcinoid tumors of the small intestine (D3a.01-)*
> *benign neoplasm of ileocecal valve (D12.0)*

     D13.30   **Benign neoplasm of unspecified part of small intestine**

     D13.39   **Benign neoplasm of other parts of small intestine**

D13.4   **Benign neoplasm of liver**
Benign neoplasm of intrahepatic bile ducts

D13.5   **Benign neoplasm of extrahepatic bile ducts**

D13.6   **Benign neoplasm of pancreas**
> *EXCLUDES 1*   *benign neoplasm of endocrine pancreas (D13.7)*

D13.7   **Benign neoplasm of endocrine pancreas**
Islet cell tumor
Benign neoplasm of islets of Langerhans
Use additional code to identify any functional activity

D13.9   **Benign neoplasm of ill-defined sites within the digestive system**
Benign neoplasm of digestive system NOS
Benign neoplasm of intestine NOS
Benign neoplasm of spleen

✓4th **D14**   **Benign neoplasm of middle ear and respiratory system**

D14.0   **Benign neoplasm of middle ear, nasal cavity and accessory sinuses**
Benign neoplasm of cartilage of nose
> *EXCLUDES 1*   *benign neoplasm of auricular canal (external) (D22.2-, D23.2-)*
> *benign neoplasm of bone of ear (D16.4)*
> *benign neoplasm of bone of nose (D16.4)*
> *benign neoplasm of cartilage of ear (D21.0)*
> *benign neoplasm of ear (external)(skin) (D22.2-, D23.2-)*
> *benign neoplasm of nose NOS (D36.7)*
> *benign neoplasm of skin of nose (D22.39, D23.39)*
> *benign neoplasm of olfactory bulb (D33.3)*
> *benign neoplasm of posterior margin of septum and choanae (D10.6)*
> *polyp of accessory sinus (J33.8)*
> *polyp of ear (middle) (H74.4)*
> *polyp of nasal (cavity) (J33-)*

D14.1   **Benign neoplasm of larynx**
Adenomatous polyp of larynx
Benign neoplasm of epiglottis (suprahyoid portion)
> *EXCLUDES 1*   *benign neoplasm of epiglottis, anterior aspect (D10.5)*
> *polyp (nonadenomatous) of vocal cord or larynx (J38.1)*

D14.2   **Benign neoplasm of trachea**

✓5th **D14.3**   **Benign neoplasm of bronchus and lung**
> *EXCLUDES 1*   *benign carcinoid tumor of the bronchus and lung (D3a.090)*

     D14.30   **Benign neoplasm of unspecified bronchus and lung**

     D14.31   **Benign neoplasm of right bronchus and lung**

     D14.32   **Benign neoplasm of left bronchus and lung**

D14.4   **Benign neoplasm of respiratory system, unspecified**

✓4th **D15**   **Benign neoplasm of other and unspecified intrathoracic organs**
> *EXCLUDES 1*   *benign neoplasm of mesothelial tissue (D19-)*

D15.0   **Benign neoplasm of thymus**
> *EXCLUDES 1*   *benign carcinoid tumor of the thymus (D3a.091)*

D15.1   **Benign neoplasm of heart**
> *EXCLUDES 1*   *benign neoplasm of great vessels (D21.3)*

D15.2   **Benign neoplasm of mediastinum**

D15.7   **Benign neoplasm of other specified intrathoracic organs**

D15.9   **Benign neoplasm of intrathoracic organ, unspecified**

✓4th **D16**   **Benign neoplasm of bone and articular cartilage**
> *EXCLUDES 1*   *benign neoplasm of connective tissue of ear (D21.0)*
> *benign neoplasm of connective tissue of eyelid (D21.0)*
> *benign neoplasm of connective tissue of larynx (D14.1)*
> *benign neoplasm of connective tissue of nose (D14.0)*
> *benign neoplasm of synovia (D21-)*

✓5th **D16.0**   **Benign neoplasm of scapula and long bones of upper limb**

     D16.00   **Benign neoplasm of scapula and long bones of unspecified upper limb**

     D16.01   **Benign neoplasm of scapula and long bones of right upper limb**

     D16.02   **Benign neoplasm of scapula and long bones of left upper limb**

✓5th **D16.1**   **Benign neoplasm of short bones of upper limb**

     D16.10   **Benign neoplasm of short bones of unspecified upper limb**

     D16.11   **Benign neoplasm of short bones of right upper limb**

     D16.12   **Benign neoplasm of short bones of left upper limb**

✓5th **D16.2**   **Benign neoplasm of long bones of lower limb**

     D16.20   **Benign neoplasm of long bones of unspecified lower limb**

     D16.21   **Benign neoplasm of long bones of right lower limb**

     D16.22   **Benign neoplasm of long bones of left lower limb**

✓5th **D16.3**   **Benign neoplasm of short bones of lower limb**

     D16.30   **Benign neoplasm of short bones of unspecified lower limb**

     D16.31   **Benign neoplasm of short bones of right lower limb**

     D16.32   **Benign neoplasm of short bones of left lower limb**

D16.4   **Benign neoplasm of bones of skull and face**
Benign neoplasm of maxilla (superior)
Benign neoplasm of orbital bone
Keratocyst of maxilla
Keratocystic odontogenic tumor of maxilla
> *EXCLUDES 1*   *benign neoplasm of lower jaw bone (D16.5)*

D16.5   **Benign neoplasm of lower jaw bone**
Keratocyst of mandible
Keratocystic odontogenic tumor of mandible

D16.6   **Benign neoplasm of vertebral column**
> *EXCLUDES 1*   *benign neoplasm of sacrum and coccyx (D16.8)*

D16.7   **Benign neoplasm of ribs, sternum and clavicle**

D16.8   **Benign neoplasm of pelvic bones, sacrum and coccyx**

D16.9   **Benign neoplasm of bone and articular cartilage, unspecified**

✓4th **D17**   **Benign lipomatous neoplasm**

D17.0   **Benign lipomatous neoplasm of skin and subcutaneous tissue of head, face and neck**

D17.1   **Benign lipomatous neoplasm of skin and subcutaneous tissue of trunk**

✓5th **D17.2**   **Benign lipomatous neoplasm of skin and subcutaneous tissue of limb**

     D17.20   **Benign lipomatous neoplasm of skin and subcutaneous tissue of unspecified limb**

     D17.21   **Benign lipomatous neoplasm of skin and subcutaneous tissue of right arm**

     D17.22   **Benign lipomatous neoplasm of skin and subcutaneous tissue of left arm**

     D17.23   **Benign lipomatous neoplasm of skin and subcutaneous tissue of right leg**

     D17.24   **Benign lipomatous neoplasm of skin and subcutaneous tissue of left leg**

✓5th **D17.3**   **Benign lipomatous neoplasm of skin and subcutaneous tissue of other and unspecified sites**

     D17.30   **Benign lipomatous neoplasm of skin and subcutaneous tissue of unspecified sites**

     D17.39   **Benign lipomatous neoplasm of skin and subcutaneous tissue of other sites**

D17.4   **Benign lipomatous neoplasm of intrathoracic organs**

D17.5   **Benign lipomatous neoplasm of intra-abdominal organs**
> *EXCLUDES 1*   *benign lipomatous neoplasm of peritoneum and retroperitoneum (D17.7)*

EXCLUDES 1   Not coded here   *EXCLUDES 2*   Not included here   *Manifestation Code*

D17.6 Benign lipomatous neoplasm of spermatic cord
D17.7 Benign lipomatous neoplasm of other sites
Benign lipomatous neoplasm of peritoneum
Benign lipomatous neoplasm of retroperitoneum
D17.9 Benign lipomatous neoplasm, unspecified
Lipoma NOS

✓4th **D18 Hemangioma and lymphangioma, any site**
EXCLUDES 1 *benign neoplasm of glomus jugulare (D35.6)*
blue or pigmented nevus (D22-)
nevus NOS (D22-)
vascular nevus (Q82.5)
✓5th **D18.0 Hemangioma**
Angioma NOS
Cavernous nevus
D18.00 Hemangioma unspecified site
D18.01 Hemangioma of skin and subcutaneous tissue
D18.02 Hemangioma of intracranial structures
D18.03 Hemangioma of intra-abdominal structures
D18.09 Hemangioma of other sites
D18.1 Lymphangioma, any site

✓4th **D19 Benign neoplasm of mesothelial tissue**
D19.0 Benign neoplasm of mesothelial tissue of pleura
D19.1 Benign neoplasm of mesothelial tissue of peritoneum
D19.7 Benign neoplasm of mesothelial tissue of other sites
D19.9 Benign neoplasm of mesothelial tissue, unspecified
Benign mesothelioma NOS

✓4th **D20 Benign neoplasm of soft tissue of retroperitoneum and peritoneum**
EXCLUDES 1 *benign lipomatous neoplasm of peritoneum and retroperitoneum (D17.7)*
benign neoplasm of mesothelial tissue (D19-)
D20.0 Benign neoplasm of soft tissue of retroperitoneum
D20.1 Benign neoplasm of soft tissue of peritoneum

✓4th **D21 Other benign neoplasms of connective and other soft tissue**
INCLUDES benign neoplasm of blood vessel
benign neoplasm of bursa
benign neoplasm of cartilage
benign neoplasm of fascia
benign neoplasm of fat
benign neoplasm of ligament, except uterine
benign neoplasm of lymphatic channel
benign neoplasm of muscle
benign neoplasm of synovia
benign neoplasm of tendon (sheath)
benign stromal tumors
EXCLUDES 1 *benign neoplasm of articular cartilage (D16-)*
benign neoplasm of cartilage of larynx (D14.1)
benign neoplasm of cartilage of nose (D14.0)
benign neoplasm of connective tissue of breast (D24-)
benign neoplasm of peripheral nerves and autonomic nervous system (D36.1-)
benign neoplasm of peritoneum (D20.1)
benign neoplasm of retroperitoneum (D20.0)
benign neoplasm of uterine ligament, any (D28.2)
benign neoplasm of vascular tissue (D18-)
hemangioma (D18.0-)
lipomatous neoplasm (D17-)
lymphangioma (D18.1)
uterine leiomyoma (D25-)
D21.0 Benign neoplasm of connective and other soft tissue of head, face and neck
Benign neoplasm of connective tissue of ear
Benign neoplasm of connective tissue of eyelid
EXCLUDES 1 *benign neoplasm of connective tissue of orbit (D31.6-)*
✓5th **D21.1 Benign neoplasm of connective and other soft tissue of upper limb, including shoulder**
D21.10 Benign neoplasm of connective and other soft tissue of unspecified upper limb, including shoulder
D21.11 Benign neoplasm of connective and other soft tissue of right upper limb, including shoulder
D21.12 Benign neoplasm of connective and other soft tissue of left upper limb, including shoulder
✓5th **D21.2 Benign neoplasm of connective and other soft tissue of lower limb, including hip**
D21.20 Benign neoplasm of connective and other soft tissue of unspecified lower limb, including hip

D21.21 Benign neoplasm of connective and other soft tissue of right lower limb, including hip
D21.22 Benign neoplasm of connective and other soft tissue of left lower limb, including hip
D21.3 Benign neoplasm of connective and other soft tissue of thorax
Benign neoplasm of axilla
Benign neoplasm of diaphragm
Benign neoplasm of great vessels
EXCLUDES 1 *benign neoplasm of heart (D15.1)*
benign neoplasm of mediastinum (D15.2)
benign neoplasm of thymus (D15.0)
D21.4 Benign neoplasm of connective and other soft tissue of abdomen
Benign stromal tumors of abdomen
D21.5 Benign neoplasm of connective and other soft tissue of pelvis
EXCLUDES 1 *benign neoplasm of any uterine ligament (D28.2)*
uterine leiomyoma (D25-)
D21.6 Benign neoplasm of connective and other soft tissue of trunk, unspecified
Benign neoplasm of back NOS
D21.9 Benign neoplasm of connective and other soft tissue, unspecified

✓4th **D22 Melanocytic nevi**
INCLUDES atypical nevus
blue hairy pigmented nevus
nevus NOS
D22.0 Melanocytic nevi of lip
✓5th **D22.1 Melanocytic nevi of eyelid, including canthus**
D22.10 Melanocytic nevi of unspecified eyelid, including canthus
D22.11 Melanocytic nevi of right eyelid, including canthus
D22.12 Melanocytic nevi of left eyelid, including canthus
✓5th **D22.2 Melanocytic nevi of ear and external auricular canal**
D22.20 Melanocytic nevi of unspecified ear and external auricular canal
D22.21 Melanocytic nevi of right ear and external auricular canal
D22.22 Melanocytic nevi of left ear and external auricular canal
✓5th **D22.3 Melanocytic nevi of other and unspecified parts of face**
D22.30 Melanocytic nevi of unspecified part of face
D22.39 Melanocytic nevi of other parts of face
D22.4 Melanocytic nevi of scalp and neck
D22.5 Melanocytic nevi of trunk
Melanocytic nevi of anal margin
Melanocytic nevi of anal skin
Melanocytic nevi of perianal skin
Melanocytic nevi of skin of breast
✓5th **D22.6 Melanocytic nevi of upper limb, including shoulder**
D22.60 Melanocytic nevi of unspecified upper limb, including shoulder
D22.61 Melanocytic nevi of right upper limb, including shoulder
D22.62 Melanocytic nevi of left upper limb, including shoulder
✓5th **D22.7 Melanocytic nevi of lower limb, including hip**
D22.70 Melanocytic nevi of unspecified lower limb, including hip
D22.71 Melanocytic nevi of right lower limb, including hip
D22.72 Melanocytic nevi of left lower limb, including hip
D22.9 Melanocytic nevi, unspecified

✓4th **D23 Other benign neoplasms of skin**
INCLUDES benign neoplasm of hair follicles
benign neoplasm of sebaceous glands
benign neoplasm of sweat glands
EXCLUDES 1 *benign lipomatous neoplasms of skin (D17.0-D17.3)*
melanocytic nevi (D22-)
D23.0 Other benign neoplasm of skin of lip
EXCLUDES 1 *benign neoplasm of vermilion border of lip (D10.0)*
✓5th **D23.1 Other benign neoplasm of skin of eyelid, including canthus**
D23.10 Other benign neoplasm of skin of unspecified eyelid, including canthus
D23.11 Other benign neoplasm of skin of right eyelid, including canthus

D23.12 **Other benign neoplasm of skin of left eyelid, including canthus**

√5th D23.2 **Other benign neoplasm of skin of ear and external auricular canal**

D23.20 **Other benign neoplasm of skin of unspecified ear and external auricular canal**

D23.21 **Other benign neoplasm of skin of right ear and external auricular canal**

D23.22 **Other benign neoplasm of skin of left ear and external auricular canal**

√5th D23.3 **Other benign neoplasm of skin of other and unspecified parts of face**

D23.30 **Other benign neoplasm of skin of unspecified part of face**

D23.39 **Other benign neoplasm of skin of other parts of face**

D23.4 **Other benign neoplasm of skin of scalp and neck**

D23.5 **Other benign neoplasm of skin of trunk**
Other benign neoplasm of anal margin
Other benign neoplasm of anal skin
Other benign neoplasm of perianal skin
Other benign neoplasm of skin of breast
EXCLUDES 1 *benign neoplasm of anus NOS (D12.9)*

√5th D23.6 **Other benign neoplasm of skin of upper limb, including shoulder**

D23.60 **Other benign neoplasm of skin of unspecified upper limb, including shoulder**

D23.61 **Other benign neoplasm of skin of right upper limb, including shoulder**

D23.62 **Other benign neoplasm of skin of left upper limb, including shoulder**

√5th D23.7 **Other benign neoplasm of skin of lower limb, including hip**

D23.70 **Other benign neoplasm of skin of unspecified lower limb, including hip**

D23.71 **Other benign neoplasm of skin of right lower limb, including hip**

D23.72 **Other benign neoplasm of skin of left lower limb, including hip**

D23.9 **Other benign neoplasm of skin, unspecified**

√4th D24 **Benign neoplasm of breast**
INCLUDES benign neoplasm of connective tissue of breast
benign neoplasm of soft parts of breast
fibroadenoma of breast
EXCLUDES 2 *adenofibrosis of breast (N60.2)*
benign cyst of breast (N60-)
benign mammary dysplasia (N60-)
benign neoplasm of skin of breast (D22.5, D23.5)
fibrocystic disease of breast (N60-)

D24.1 **Benign neoplasm of right breast**

D24.2 **Benign neoplasm of left breast**

D24.9 **Benign neoplasm of unspecified breast**

√4th D25 **Leiomyoma of uterus**
INCLUDES uterine fibroid
uterine fibromyoma
uterine myoma

D25.0 **Submucous leiomyoma of uterus**

D25.1 **Intramural leiomyoma of uterus**
Interstitial leiomyoma of uterus

D25.2 **Subserosal leiomyoma of uterus**
Subperitoneal leiomyoma of uterus

D25.9 **Leiomyoma of uterus, unspecified**

√4th D26 **Other benign neoplasms of uterus**

D26.0 **Other benign neoplasm of cervix uteri**

D26.1 **Other benign neoplasm of corpus uteri**

D26.7 **Other benign neoplasm of other parts of uterus**

D26.9 **Other benign neoplasm of uterus, unspecified**

√4th D27 **Benign neoplasm of ovary**
Use additional code to identify any functional activity
EXCLUDES 2 *corpus albicans cyst (N83.2)*
corpus luteum cyst (N83.1)
endometrial cyst (N80.1)
follicular (atretic) cyst (N83.0)
graafian follicle cyst (N83.0)
ovarian cyst NEC (N83.2)
ovarian retention cyst (N83.2)

D27.0 **Benign neoplasm of right ovary**

D27.1 **Benign neoplasm of left ovary**

D27.9 **Benign neoplasm of unspecified ovary**

√4th D28 **Benign neoplasm of other and unspecified female genital organs**
INCLUDES adenomatous polyp
benign neoplasm of skin of female genital organs
benign teratoma
EXCLUDES 1 *epoophoron cyst (Q50.5)*
fimbrial cyst (Q50.4)
Gartner's duct cyst (Q52.4)
parovarian cyst (Q50.5)

D28.0 **Benign neoplasm of vulva**

D28.1 **Benign neoplasm of vagina**

D28.2 **Benign neoplasm of uterine tubes and ligaments**
Benign neoplasm of fallopian tube
Benign neoplasm of uterine ligament (broad) (round)

D28.7 **Benign neoplasm of other specified female genital organs**

D28.9 **Benign neoplasm of female genital organ, unspecified**

√4th D29 **Benign neoplasm of male genital organs**
INCLUDES benign neoplasm of skin of male genital organs

D29.0 **Benign neoplasm of penis**

D29.1 **Benign neoplasm of prostate**
EXCLUDES 1 *enlarged prostate (N40-)*

√5th D29.2 **Benign neoplasm of testis**
Use additional code to identify any functional activity

D29.20 **Benign neoplasm of unspecified testis**

D29.21 **Benign neoplasm of right testis**

D29.22 **Benign neoplasm of left testis**

√5th D29.3 **Benign neoplasm of epididymis**

D29.30 **Benign neoplasm of unspecified epididymis**

D29.31 **Benign neoplasm of right epididymis**

D29.32 **Benign neoplasm of left epididymis**

D29.4 **Benign neoplasm of scrotum**
Benign neoplasm of skin of scrotum

D29.8 **Benign neoplasm of other specified male genital organs**
Benign neoplasm of seminal vesicle
Benign neoplasm of spermatic cord
Benign neoplasm of tunica vaginalis

D29.9 **Benign neoplasm of male genital organ, unspecified**

√4th D30 **Benign neoplasm of urinary organs**

√5th D30.0 **Benign neoplasm of kidney**
EXCLUDES 1 *benign carcinoid tumor of the kidney (D3a.093)*
benign neoplasm of renal calyces (D30.1-)
benign neoplasm of renal pelvis (D30.1-)

D30.00 **Benign neoplasm of unspecified kidney**

D30.01 **Benign neoplasm of right kidney**

D30.02 **Benign neoplasm of left kidney**

√5th D30.1 **Benign neoplasm of renal pelvis**

D30.10 **Benign neoplasm of unspecified renal pelvis**

D30.11 **Benign neoplasm of right renal pelvis**

D30.12 **Benign neoplasm of left renal pelvis**

√5th D30.2 **Benign neoplasm of ureter**
EXCLUDES 1 *benign neoplasm of ureteric orifice of bladder (D30.3)*

D30.20 **Benign neoplasm of unspecified ureter**

D30.21 **Benign neoplasm of right ureter**

D30.22 **Benign neoplasm of left ureter**

D30.3 **Benign neoplasm of bladder**
Benign neoplasm of ureteric orifice of bladder
Benign neoplasm of urethral orifice of bladder

D30.4 **Benign neoplasm of urethra**
EXCLUDES 1 *benign neoplasm of urethral orifice of bladder (D30.3)*

D30.8 **Benign neoplasm of other specified urinary organs**
Benign neoplasm of paraurethral glands

D30.9 **Benign neoplasm of urinary organ, unspecified**
Benign neoplasm of urinary system NOS

√4th D31 **Benign neoplasm of eye and adnexa**
EXCLUDES 1 *benign neoplasm of connective tissue of eyelid (D21.0)*
benign neoplasm of optic nerve (D33.3)
benign neoplasm of skin of eyelid (D22.1-, D23.1-)

√5th D31.0 **Benign neoplasm of conjunctiva**

D31.00 **Benign neoplasm of unspecified conjunctiva**

D31.01 **Benign neoplasm of right conjunctiva**

D31.02 **Benign neoplasm of left conjunctiva**

√5th D31.1 **Benign neoplasm of cornea**

D31.10 **Benign neoplasm of unspecified cornea**

EXCLUDES 1 Not coded here   EXCLUDES 2 Not included here   *Manifestation Code*

D31.11   Benign neoplasm of right cornea
D31.12   Benign neoplasm of left cornea
✓5th D31.2   Benign neoplasm of retina
EXCLUDES 1   *dark area on retina (D49.81)*
              hemangioma of retina (D49.81)
              neoplasm of unspecified behavior of retina and choroid (D49.81)
              retinal freckle (D49.81)

D31.20   Benign neoplasm of unspecified retina
D31.21   Benign neoplasm of right retina
D31.22   Benign neoplasm of left retina
✓5th D31.3   Benign neoplasm of choroid
D31.30   Benign neoplasm of unspecified choroid
D31.31   Benign neoplasm of right choroid
D31.32   Benign neoplasm of left choroid
✓5th D31.4   Benign neoplasm of ciliary body
D31.40   Benign neoplasm of unspecified ciliary body
D31.41   Benign neoplasm of right ciliary body
D31.42   Benign neoplasm of left ciliary body
✓5th D31.5   Benign neoplasm of lacrimal gland and duct
              Benign neoplasm of lacrimal sac
              Benign neoplasm of nasolacrimal duct
D31.50   Benign neoplasm of unspecified lacrimal gland and duct
D31.51   Benign neoplasm of right lacrimal gland and duct
D31.52   Benign neoplasm of left lacrimal gland and duct
✓5th D31.6   Benign neoplasm of unspecified site of orbit
              Benign neoplasm of connective tissue of orbit
              Benign neoplasm of extraocular muscle
              Benign neoplasm of peripheral nerves of orbit
              Benign neoplasm of retrobulbar tissue
              Benign neoplasm of retro-ocular tissue
EXCLUDES 1   *benign neoplasm of orbital bone (D16.4)*
D31.60   Benign neoplasm of unspecified site of unspecified orbit
D31.61   Benign neoplasm of unspecified site of right orbit
D31.62   Benign neoplasm of unspecified site of left orbit
✓5th D31.9   Benign neoplasm of unspecified part of eye
D31.90   Benign neoplasm of unspecified part of unspecified eye
D31.91   Benign neoplasm of unspecified part of right eye
D31.92   Benign neoplasm of unspecified part of left eye

✓4th D32   Benign neoplasm of meninges
D32.0   Benign neoplasm of cerebral meninges
D32.1   Benign neoplasm of spinal meninges
D32.9   Benign neoplasm of meninges, unspecified
         Meningioma NOS

✓4th D33   Benign neoplasm of brain and other parts of central nervous system
EXCLUDES 1   *angioma (D18.0-)*
              benign neoplasm of meninges (D32-)
              benign neoplasm of peripheral nerves and autonomic nervous system (D36.1-)
              hemangioma (D18.0-)
              neurofibromatosis (Q85.0-)
              retro-ocular benign neoplasm (D31.6-)
D33.0   Benign neoplasm of brain, supratentorial
         Benign neoplasm of cerebral ventricle
         Benign neoplasm of cerebrum
         Benign neoplasm of frontal lobe
         Benign neoplasm of occipital lobe
         Benign neoplasm of parietal lobe
         Benign neoplasm of temporal lobe
EXCLUDES 1   *benign neoplasm of fourth ventricle (D33.1)*
D33.1   Benign neoplasm of brain, infratentorial
         Benign neoplasm of brain stem
         Benign neoplasm of cerebellum
         Benign neoplasm of fourth ventricle
D33.2   Benign neoplasm of brain, unspecified
D33.3   Benign neoplasm of cranial nerves
         Benign neoplasm of olfactory bulb
D33.4   Benign neoplasm of spinal cord
D33.7   Benign neoplasm of other specified parts of central nervous system
D33.9   Benign neoplasm of central nervous system, unspecified
         Benign neoplasm of nervous system (central) NOS

D34   Benign neoplasm of thyroid gland
       Use additional code to identify any functional activity

✓4th D35   Benign neoplasm of other and unspecified endocrine glands
       Use additional code to identify any functional activity
EXCLUDES 1   *benign neoplasm of endocrine pancreas (D13.7)*
              benign neoplasm of ovary (D27-)
              benign neoplasm of testis (D29.2-)
              benign neoplasm of thymus (D15.0)
✓5th D35.0   Benign neoplasm of adrenal gland
D35.00   Benign neoplasm of unspecified adrenal gland
D35.01   Benign neoplasm of right adrenal gland
D35.02   Benign neoplasm of left adrenal gland
D35.1   Benign neoplasm of parathyroid gland
D35.2   Benign neoplasm of pituitary gland
D35.3   Benign neoplasm of craniopharyngeal duct
D35.4   Benign neoplasm of pineal gland
D35.5   Benign neoplasm of carotid body
D35.6   Benign neoplasm of aortic body and other paraganglia
         Benign tumor of glomus jugulare
D35.7   Benign neoplasm of other specified endocrine glands
D35.9   Benign neoplasm of endocrine gland, unspecified
         Benign neoplasm of unspecified endocrine gland

✓4th D36   Benign neoplasm of other and unspecified sites
D36.0   Benign neoplasm of lymph nodes
EXCLUDES 1   *lymphangioma (D18.1)*
✓5th D36.1   Benign neoplasm of peripheral nerves and autonomic nervous system
EXCLUDES 1   *benign neoplasm of peripheral nerves of orbit (D31.6-)*
              neurofibromatosis (Q85.0-)
D36.10   Benign neoplasm of peripheral nerves and autonomic nervous system, unspecified
D36.11   Benign neoplasm of peripheral nerves and autonomic nervous system of face, head, and neck
D36.12   Benign neoplasm of peripheral nerves and autonomic nervous system, upper limb, including shoulder
D36.13   Benign neoplasm of peripheral nerves and autonomic nervous system of lower limb, including hip
D36.14   Benign neoplasm of peripheral nerves and autonomic nervous system of thorax
D36.15   Benign neoplasm of peripheral nerves and autonomic nervous system of abdomen
D36.16   Benign neoplasm of peripheral nerves and autonomic nervous system of pelvis
D36.17   Benign neoplasm of peripheral nerves and autonomic nervous system of trunk, unspecified
D36.7   Benign neoplasm of other specified sites
         Benign neoplasm of nose NOS
D36.9   Benign neoplasm, unspecified site

Benign neuroendocrine tumors (D3a)

✓4th D3a   Benign neuroendocrine tumors
       Code also any associated multiple endocrine neoplasia [MEN] syndromes (E31.2-)
       Use additional code to identify any associated endocrine syndrome, such as:
       carcinoid syndrome (E34.0)
EXCLUDES 2   *benign pancreatic islet cell tumors (D13.7)*
✓5th D3a.0   Benign carcinoid tumors
D3a.00   Benign carcinoid tumor of unspecified site
          Carcinoid tumor NOS
✓6th D3a.01   Benign carcinoid tumors of the small intestine
D3a.010   Benign carcinoid tumor of the duodenum
D3a.011   Benign carcinoid tumor of the jejunum
D3a.012   Benign carcinoid tumor of the ileum
D3a.019   Benign carcinoid tumor of the small intestine, unspecified portion
✓6th D3a.02   Benign carcinoid tumors of the appendix, large intestine, and rectum
D3a.020   Benign carcinoid tumor of the appendix
D3a.021   Benign carcinoid tumor of the cecum

✓ Appropriate additional character required   ✓x7th Requires 7th character, placeholder x must fill empty characters

D3a.022   **Benign carcinoid tumor of the ascending colon**

D3a.023   **Benign carcinoid tumor of the transverse colon**

D3a.024   **Benign carcinoid tumor of the descending colon**

D3a.025   **Benign carcinoid tumor of the sigmoid colon**

D3a.026   **Benign carcinoid tumor of the rectum**

D3a.029   **Benign carcinoid tumor of the large intestine, unspecified portion**
Benign carcinoid tumor of the colon NOS

√6th **D3a.09**   **Benign carcinoid tumors of other sites**

D3a.090   **Benign carcinoid tumor of the bronchus and lung**

D3a.091   **Benign carcinoid tumor of the thymus**

D3a.092   **Benign carcinoid tumor of the stomach**

D3a.093   **Benign carcinoid tumor of the kidney**

D3a.094   **Benign carcinoid tumor of the foregut NOS**

D3a.095   **Benign carcinoid tumor of the midgut NOS**

D3a.096   **Benign carcinoid tumor of the hindgut NOS**

D3a.098   **Benign carcinoid tumors of other sites**

D3a.8   **Other benign neuroendocrine tumors**
Neuroendocrine tumor NOS

Neoplasms of uncertain behavior, polycythemia vera and myelodysplastic syndromes (D37-D48)

NOTE   Categories D37-D44, and D48 classify by site neoplasms of uncertain behavior, i.e., histologic confirmation whether the neoplasm is malignant or benign cannot be made. Use additional morphology codes with behavior code /1.

EXCLUDES 1   *neoplasms of unspecified behavior (D49-)*

√4th **D37**   **Neoplasm of uncertain behavior of oral cavity and digestive organs**

EXCLUDES 1   *stromal tumors of uncertain behavior of digestive system (D48.1)*

√5th **D37.0**   **Neoplasm of uncertain behavior of lip, oral cavity and pharynx**

EXCLUDES 1   *neoplasm of uncertain behavior of aryepiglottic fold or interarytenoid fold, laryngeal aspect (D38.0)*
neoplasm of uncertain behavior of epiglottis NOS (D38.0)
neoplasm of uncertain behavior of skin of lip (D48.5)
neoplasm of uncertain behavior of suprahyoid portion of epiglottis (D38.0)

D37.01   **Neoplasm of uncertain behavior of lip**
Neoplasm of uncertain behavior of vermilion border of lip

D37.02   **Neoplasm of uncertain behavior of tongue**

√6th **D37.03**   **Neoplasm of uncertain behavior of the major salivary glands**

D37.030   **Neoplasm of uncertain behavior of the parotid salivary glands**

D37.031   **Neoplasm of uncertain behavior of the sublingual salivary glands**

D37.032   **Neoplasm of uncertain behavior of the submandibular salivary glands**

D37.039   **Neoplasm of uncertain behavior of the major salivary glands, unspecified**

D37.04   **Neoplasm of uncertain behavior of the minor salivary glands**
Neoplasm of uncertain behavior of submucosal salivary glands of lip
Neoplasm of uncertain behavior of submucosal salivary glands of cheek
Neoplasm of uncertain behavior of submucosal salivary glands of hard palate
Neoplasm of uncertain behavior of submucosal salivary glands of soft palate

D37.05   **Neoplasm of uncertain behavior of pharynx**
Neoplasm of uncertain behavior of aryepiglottic fold of pharynx NOS
Neoplasm of uncertain behavior of hypopharyngeal aspect of aryepiglottic fold of pharynx
Neoplasm of uncertain behavior of marginal zone of aryepiglottic fold of pharynx

D37.09   **Neoplasm of uncertain behavior of other specified sites of the oral cavity**

D37.1   **Neoplasm of uncertain behavior of stomach**

D37.2   **Neoplasm of uncertain behavior of small intestine**

D37.3   **Neoplasm of uncertain behavior of appendix**

D37.4   **Neoplasm of uncertain behavior of colon**

D37.5   **Neoplasm of uncertain behavior of rectum**
Neoplasm of uncertain behavior of rectosigmoid junction

D37.6   **Neoplasm of uncertain behavior of liver, gallbladder and bile ducts**
Neoplasm of uncertain behavior of ampulla of Vater

D37.8   **Neoplasm of uncertain behavior of other specified digestive organs**
Neoplasm of uncertain behavior of anal canal
Neoplasm of uncertain behavior of anal sphincter
Neoplasm of uncertain behavior of anus NOS
Neoplasm of uncertain behavior of esophagus
Neoplasm of uncertain behavior of intestine NOS
Neoplasm of uncertain behavior of pancreas

EXCLUDES 1   *neoplasm of uncertain behavior of anal margin (D48.5)*
neoplasm of uncertain behavior of anal skin (D48.5)
neoplasm of uncertain behavior of perianal skin (D48.5)

D37.9   **Neoplasm of uncertain behavior of digestive organ, unspecified**

√4th **D38**   **Neoplasm of uncertain behavior of middle ear and respiratory and intrathoracic organs**

EXCLUDES 1   *neoplasm of uncertain behavior of heart (D48.7)*

D38.0   **Neoplasm of uncertain behavior of larynx**
Neoplasm of uncertain behavior of aryepiglottic fold or interarytenoid fold, laryngeal aspect
Neoplasm of uncertain behavior of epiglottis (suprahyoid portion)

EXCLUDES 1   *neoplasm of uncertain behavior of aryepiglottic fold or interarytenoid fold NOS (D37.05)*
neoplasm of uncertain behavior of hypopharyngeal aspect of aryepiglottic fold (D37.05)
neoplasm of uncertain behavior of marginal zone of aryepiglottic fold (D37.05)

D38.1   **Neoplasm of uncertain behavior of trachea, bronchus and lung**

D38.2   **Neoplasm of uncertain behavior of pleura**

D38.3   **Neoplasm of uncertain behavior of mediastinum**

D38.4   **Neoplasm of uncertain behavior of thymus**

D38.5   **Neoplasm of uncertain behavior of other respiratory organs**
Neoplasm of uncertain behavior of accessory sinuses
Neoplasm of uncertain behavior of cartilage of nose
Neoplasm of uncertain behavior of middle ear
Neoplasm of uncertain behavior of nasal cavities

EXCLUDES 1   *neoplasm of uncertain behavior of ear (external) (skin) (D48.5)*
neoplasm of uncertain behavior of nose NOS (D48.7)
neoplasm of uncertain behavior of skin of nose (D48.5)

D38.6   **Neoplasm of uncertain behavior of respiratory organ, unspecified**

√4th **D39**   **Neoplasm of uncertain behavior of female genital organs**

D39.0   **Neoplasm of uncertain behavior of uterus**

√5th **D39.1**   **Neoplasm of uncertain behavior of ovary**
Use additional code to identify any functional activity

D39.10   **Neoplasm of uncertain behavior of unspecified ovary**

D39.11   **Neoplasm of uncertain behavior of right ovary**

D39.12   **Neoplasm of uncertain behavior of left ovary**

D39.2   **Neoplasm of uncertain behavior of placenta**
Chorioadenoma destruens
Invasive hydatidiform mole
Malignant hydatidiform mole

EXCLUDES 1   *hydatidiform mole NOS (O01.9)*

EXCLUDES 1   Not coded here   EXCLUDES 2   Not included here   *Manifestation Code*

D39.8 Neoplasm of uncertain behavior of other specified female genital organs
  Neoplasm of uncertain behavior of skin of female genital organs

D39.9 Neoplasm of uncertain behavior of female genital organ, unspecified

☑4th **D40 Neoplasm of uncertain behavior of male genital organs**
  D40.0 Neoplasm of uncertain behavior of prostate
  ☑5th **D40.1 Neoplasm of uncertain behavior of testis**
    D40.10 Neoplasm of uncertain behavior of unspecified testis
    D40.11 Neoplasm of uncertain behavior of right testis
    D40.12 Neoplasm of uncertain behavior of left testis
  D40.8 Neoplasm of uncertain behavior of other specified male genital organs
    Neoplasm of uncertain behavior of skin of male genital organs
  D40.9 Neoplasm of uncertain behavior of male genital organ, unspecified

☑4th **D41 Neoplasm of uncertain behavior of urinary organs**
  ☑5th **D41.0 Neoplasm of uncertain behavior of kidney**
    EXCLUDES 1 *neoplasm of uncertain behavior of renal pelvis (D41.1-)*
    D41.00 Neoplasm of uncertain behavior of unspecified kidney
    D41.01 Neoplasm of uncertain behavior of right kidney
    D41.02 Neoplasm of uncertain behavior of left kidney
  ☑5th **D41.1 Neoplasm of uncertain behavior of renal pelvis**
    D41.10 Neoplasm of uncertain behavior of unspecified renal pelvis
    D41.11 Neoplasm of uncertain behavior of right renal pelvis
    D41.12 Neoplasm of uncertain behavior of left renal pelvis
  ☑5th **D41.2 Neoplasm of uncertain behavior of ureter**
    D41.20 Neoplasm of uncertain behavior of unspecified ureter
    D41.21 Neoplasm of uncertain behavior of right ureter
    D41.22 Neoplasm of uncertain behavior of left ureter
  D41.3 Neoplasm of uncertain behavior of urethra
  D41.4 Neoplasm of uncertain behavior of bladder
  D41.8 Neoplasm of uncertain behavior of other specified urinary organs
  D41.9 Neoplasm of uncertain behavior of unspecified urinary organ

☑4th **D42 Neoplasm of uncertain behavior of meninges**
  D42.0 Neoplasm of uncertain behavior of cerebral meninges
  D42.1 Neoplasm of uncertain behavior of spinal meninges
  D42.9 Neoplasm of uncertain behavior of meninges, unspecified

☑4th **D43 Neoplasm of uncertain behavior of brain and central nervous system**
  EXCLUDES 1 *neoplasm of uncertain behavior of peripheral nerves and autonomic nervous system (D48.2)*
  D43.0 Neoplasm of uncertain behavior of brain, supratentorial
    Neoplasm of uncertain behavior of cerebral ventricle
    Neoplasm of uncertain behavior of cerebrum
    Neoplasm of uncertain behavior of frontal lobe
    Neoplasm of uncertain behavior of occipital lobe
    Neoplasm of uncertain behavior of parietal lobe
    Neoplasm of uncertain behavior of temporal lobe
    EXCLUDES 1 *neoplasm of uncertain behavior of fourth ventricle (D43.1)*
  D43.1 Neoplasm of uncertain behavior of brain, infratentorial
    Neoplasm of uncertain behavior of brain stem
    Neoplasm of uncertain behavior of cerebellum
    Neoplasm of uncertain behavior of fourth ventricle
  D43.2 Neoplasm of uncertain behavior of brain, unspecified
  D43.3 Neoplasm of uncertain behavior of cranial nerves
  D43.4 Neoplasm of uncertain behavior of spinal cord
  D43.8 Neoplasm of uncertain behavior of other specified parts of central nervous system
  D43.9 Neoplasm of uncertain behavior of central nervous system, unspecified
    Neoplasm of uncertain behavior of nervous system (central) NOS

☑4th **D44 Neoplasm of uncertain behavior of endocrine glands**
  EXCLUDES 1 *multiple endocrine adenomatosis (E31.2-)*
    multiple endocrine neoplasia (E31.2-)
    neoplasm of uncertain behavior of endocrine pancreas (D37.8)
    neoplasm of uncertain behavior of ovary (D39.1-)
    neoplasm of uncertain behavior of testis (D40.1-)
    neoplasm of uncertain behavior of thymus (D38.4)
  D44.0 Neoplasm of uncertain behavior of thyroid gland
  ☑5th **D44.1 Neoplasm of uncertain behavior of adrenal gland**
    Use additional code to identify any functional activity
    D44.10 Neoplasm of uncertain behavior of unspecified adrenal gland
    D44.11 Neoplasm of uncertain behavior of right adrenal gland
    D44.12 Neoplasm of uncertain behavior of left adrenal gland
  D44.2 Neoplasm of uncertain behavior of parathyroid gland
  D44.3 Neoplasm of uncertain behavior of pituitary gland
    Use additional code to identify any functional activity
  D44.4 Neoplasm of uncertain behavior of craniopharyngeal duct
  D44.5 Neoplasm of uncertain behavior of pineal gland
  D44.6 Neoplasm of uncertain behavior of carotid body
  D44.7 Neoplasm of uncertain behavior of aortic body and other paraganglia
  D44.9 Neoplasm of uncertain behavior of unspecified endocrine gland

D45 Polycythemia vera
  EXCLUDES 1 *familial polycythemia (D75.0)*
    secondary polycythemia (D75.1)

☑4th **D46 Myelodysplastic syndromes**
  Code first (T36-T50) to identify drug, if drug induced
  EXCLUDES 2 *drug-induced aplastic anemia (D61.1)*
  D46.0 Refractory anemia without ring sideroblasts, so stated
    Refractory anemia without sideroblasts, without excess of blasts
  D46.1 Refractory anemia with ring sideroblasts
    RARS
  ☑5th **D46.2 Refractory anemia with excess of blasts**
    D46.20 Refractory anemia with excess of blasts, unspecified
      RAEB NOS
    D46.21 Refractory anemia with excess of blasts 1
      RAEB 1
    D46.22 Refractory anemia with excess of blasts 2
      RAEB 2
  D46.a Refractory cytopenia with multilineage dysplasia
  D46.b Refractory cytopenia with multilineage dysplasia and ring sideroblasts
    RCMD RS
  D46.c Myelodysplastic syndrome with isolated del(5q) chromosomal abnormality
    Myelodysplastic syndrome with 5q deletion
    5q minus syndrome NOS
  D46.4 Refractory anemia, unspecified
  D46.z Other myelodysplastic syndromes
    EXCLUDES 1 *chronic myelomonocytic leukemia (C93.1-)*
  D46.9 Myelodysplastic syndrome, unspecified
    Myelodysplasia NOS

☑4th **D47 Other neoplasms of uncertain behavior of lymphoid, hematopoietic and related tissue**
  D47.0 Histiocytic and mast cell tumors of uncertain behavior
    Indolent systemic mastocytosis
    Mast cell tumor NOS
    Mastocytoma NOS
    EXCLUDES 1 *malignant mast cell tumor (C96.2)*
      mastocytosis (congenital) (cutaneous) (Q82.2)
  D47.1 Chronic myeloproliferative disease
    Chronic neutrophilic leukemia
    Myeloproliferative disease, unspecified
    EXCLUDES 1 *atypical chronic myeloid leukemia BCR/ABL-negative (C92.2-)*
      chronic myeloid leukemia BCR/ABL-positive (C92.1-)
      myelofibrosis NOS (D75.81)
      myelophthisic anemia (D61.82)
      myelophthisis (D61.82)
      secondary myelofibrosis NOS (D75.81)

☑ Appropriate additional character required   ☑x7th Requires 7th character, placeholder x must fill empty characters

D47.2 Monoclonal gammopathy
Monoclonal gammopathy of undetermined significance [MGUS]

D47.3 Essential (hemorrhagic) thrombocythemia
Essential thrombocytosis
Idiopathic hemorrhagic thrombocythemia

D47.4 Osteomyelofibrosis
Chronic idiopathic myelofibrosis
Myelofibrosis (idiopathic) (with myeloid metaplasia)
Myelosclerosis (megakaryocytic) with myeloid metaplasia
Secondary myelofibrosis in myeloproliferative disease
EXCLUDES 1 *acute myelofibrosis (C94.4-)*

√5ᵗʰ **D47.z Other specified neoplasms of uncertain behavior of lymphoid, hematopoietic and related tissue**

D47.z1 Post-transplant lymphoproliferative disorder (PTLD)
Code first complications of transplanted organs and tissue (T86-)

D47.z9 Other specified neoplasms of uncertain behavior of lymphoid, hematopoietic and related tissue
Histiocytic tumors of uncertain behavior

D47.9 Neoplasm of uncertain behavior of lymphoid, hematopoietic and related tissue, unspecified
Lymphoproliferative disease NOS

√4ᵗʰ **D48 Neoplasm of uncertain behavior of other and unspecified sites**
EXCLUDES 1 *neurofibromatosis (nonmalignant) (Q85.0-)*

D48.0 Neoplasm of uncertain behavior of bone and articular cartilage
EXCLUDES 1 *neoplasm of uncertain behavior of cartilage of ear (D48.1)*
neoplasm of uncertain behavior of cartilage of larynx (D38.0)
neoplasm of uncertain behavior of cartilage of nose (D38.5)
neoplasm of uncertain behavior of connective tissue of eyelid (D48.1)
neoplasm of uncertain behavior of synovia (D48.1)

D48.1 Neoplasm of uncertain behavior of connective and other soft tissue
Neoplasm of uncertain behavior of connective tissue of ear
Neoplasm of uncertain behavior of connective tissue of eyelid
Stromal tumors of uncertain behavior of digestive system
EXCLUDES 1 *neoplasm of uncertain behavior of articular cartilage (D48.0)*
neoplasm of uncertain behavior of cartilage of larynx (D38.0)
neoplasm of uncertain behavior of cartilage of nose (D38.5)
neoplasm of uncertain behavior of connective tissue of breast (D48.6-)

D48.2 Neoplasm of uncertain behavior of peripheral nerves and autonomic nervous system
EXCLUDES 1 *neoplasm of uncertain behavior of peripheral nerves of orbit (D48.7)*

D48.3 Neoplasm of uncertain behavior of retroperitoneum

D48.4 Neoplasm of uncertain behavior of peritoneum

D48.5 Neoplasm of uncertain behavior of skin
Neoplasm of uncertain behavior of anal margin
Neoplasm of uncertain behavior of anal skin
Neoplasm of uncertain behavior of perianal skin
Neoplasm of uncertain behavior of skin of breast
EXCLUDES 1 *neoplasm of uncertain behavior of anus NOS (D37.8)*
neoplasm of uncertain behavior of skin of genital organs (D39.8, D40.7)
neoplasm of uncertain behavior of vermilion border of lip (D37.0)

√5ᵗʰ **D48.6 Neoplasm of uncertain behavior of breast**
Neoplasm of uncertain behavior of connective tissue of breast
Cystosarcoma phyllodes
EXCLUDES 1 *neoplasm of uncertain behavior of skin of breast (D48.5)*

D48.60 Neoplasm of uncertain behavior of unspecified breast

D48.61 Neoplasm of uncertain behavior of right breast

D48.62 Neoplasm of uncertain behavior of left breast

D48.7 Neoplasm of uncertain behavior of other specified sites
Neoplasm of uncertain behavior of eye
Neoplasm of uncertain behavior of heart
Neoplasm of uncertain behavior of peripheral nerves of orbit
EXCLUDES 1 *neoplasm of uncertain behavior of connective tissue (D48.1)*
neoplasm of uncertain behavior of skin of eyelid (D48.5)

D48.9 Neoplasm of uncertain behavior, unspecified

Neoplasm of uncertain behavior (D49)

√4ᵗʰ **D49 Neoplasms of unspecified behavior**
NOTE Category D49 classifies by site neoplasms of unspecified morphology and behavior. The term "mass", unless otherwise stated, is not to be regarded as a neoplastic growth.
INCLUDES "growth" NOS
neoplasm NOS
new growth NOS
tumor NOS
EXCLUDES 1 *neoplasms of uncertain behavior (D37-D44, D48)*

D49.0 Neoplasm of unspecified behavior of digestive system
EXCLUDES 1 *neoplasm of unspecified behavior of margin of anus (D49.2)*
neoplasm of unspecified behavior of perianal skin (D49.2)
neoplasm of unspecified behavior of skin of anus (D49.2)

D49.1 Neoplasm of unspecified behavior of respiratory system

D49.2 Neoplasm of unspecified behavior of bone, soft tissue, and skin
EXCLUDES 1 *neoplasm of unspecified behavior of anal canal (D49.0)*
neoplasm of unspecified behavior of anus NOS (D49.0)
neoplasm of unspecified behavior of bone marrow (D49.9)
neoplasm of unspecified behavior of cartilage of larynx (D49.1)
neoplasm of unspecified behavior of cartilage of nose (D49.1)
neoplasm of unspecified behavior of connective tissue of breast (D49.3)
neoplasm of unspecified behavior of skin of genital organs (D49.5)
neoplasm of unspecified behavior of vermilion border of lip (D49.0)

D49.3 Neoplasm of unspecified behavior of breast
EXCLUDES 1 *neoplasm of unspecified behavior of skin of breast (D49.2)*

D49.4 Neoplasm of unspecified behavior of bladder

D49.5 Neoplasm of unspecified behavior of other genitourinary organs

D49.6 Neoplasm of unspecified behavior of brain
EXCLUDES 1 *neoplasm of unspecified behavior of cerebral meninges (D49.7)*
neoplasm of unspecified behavior of cranial nerves (D49.7)

D49.7 Neoplasm of unspecified behavior of endocrine glands and other parts of nervous system
EXCLUDES 1 *neoplasm of unspecified behavior of peripheral, sympathetic, and parasympathetic nerves and ganglia (D49.2)*

√5ᵗʰ **D49.8 Neoplasm of unspecified behavior of other specified sites**
EXCLUDES 1 *neoplasm of unspecified behavior of eyelid (skin) (D49.2)*
neoplasm of unspecified behavior of eyelid cartilage (D49.2)
neoplasm of unspecified behavior of great vessels (D49.2)
neoplasm of unspecified behavior of optic nerve (D49.7)

D49.81 Neoplasm of unspecified behavior of retina and choroid
Dark area on retina
Retinal freckle

D49.89 Neoplasm of unspecified behavior of other specified sites

D49.9 Neoplasm of unspecified behavior of unspecified site

EXCLUDES 1 Not coded here *EXCLUDES 2* Not included here **Manifestation Code**

Chapter 3. Diseases of the Blood and Blood-forming Organs and Certain Disorders Involving the Immune Mechanism (D50-D89)

EXCLUDES 2　autoimmune disease (systemic) NOS (M35.9)
　　　　certain conditions originating in the perinatal period (P00-P96)
　　　　complications of pregnancy, childbirth and the puerperium (O00-O99)
　　　　congenital malformations, deformations and chromosomal abnormalities (Q00-Q99)
　　　　endocrine, nutritional and metabolic diseases (E00-E88)
　　　　human immunodeficiency virus [HIV] disease (B20)
　　　　injury, poisoning and certain other consequences of external causes (S00-T88)
　　　　neoplasms (C00-D49)
　　　　symptoms, signs and abnormal clinical and laboratory findings, not elsewhere classified (R00-R94)

This chapter contains the following blocks:
D50-D53　Nutritional anemias
D55-D59　Hemolytic anemias
D60-D64　Aplastic and other anemias and other bone marrow failure syndromes
D65-D69　Coagulation defects, purpura and other hemorrhagic conditions
D70-D77　Other disorders of blood and blood-forming organs
D78　　　Intraoperative and postprocedural complications of spleen
D80-D89　Certain disorders involving the immune mechanism

Nutritional anemias (D50-D53)

☑4th **D50　Iron deficiency anemia**
　　INCLUDES　asiderotic anemia
　　　　hypochromic anemia
　　D50.0　Iron deficiency anemia secondary to blood loss (chronic)
　　　　Posthemorrhagic anemia (chronic)
　　　　EXCLUDES 1　acute posthemorrhagic anemia (D62)
　　　　　　congenital anemia from fetal blood loss (P61.3)
　　D50.1　Sideropenic dysphagia
　　　　Kelly-Paterson syndrome
　　　　Plummer-Vinson syndrome
　　D50.8　Other iron deficiency anemias
　　　　Iron deficiency anemia due to inadequate dietary iron intake
　　D50.9　Iron deficiency anemia, unspecified

☑4th **D51　Vitamin B12 deficiency anemia**
　　EXCLUDES 1　vitamin B12 deficiency (E53.8)
　　D51.0　Vitamin B12 deficiency anemia due to intrinsic factor deficiency
　　　　Addison anemia
　　　　Biermer anemia
　　　　Pernicious (congenital) anemia
　　　　Congenital intrinsic factor deficiency
　　D51.1　Vitamin B12 deficiency anemia due to selective vitamin B12 malabsorption with proteinuria
　　　　Imerslund (Gräsbeck) syndrome
　　　　Megaloblastic hereditary anemia
　　D51.2　Transcobalamin II deficiency
　　D51.3　Other dietary vitamin B12 deficiency anemia
　　　　Vegan anemia
　　D51.8　Other vitamin B12 deficiency anemias
　　D51.9　Vitamin B12 deficiency anemia, unspecified

☑4th **D52　Folate deficiency anemia**
　　EXCLUDES 1　folate deficiency without anemia (E53.8)
　　D52.0　Dietary folate deficiency anemia
　　　　Nutritional megaloblastic anemia
　　D52.1　Drug-induced folate deficiency anemia
　　　　Code first (T36-T50) to identify drug
　　D52.8　Other folate deficiency anemias
　　D52.9　Folate deficiency anemia, unspecified
　　　　Folic acid deficiency anemia NOS

☑4th **D53　Other nutritional anemias**
　　INCLUDES　megaloblastic anemia unresponsive to vitamin B12 or folate therapy
　　D53.0　Protein deficiency anemia
　　　　Amino-acid deficiency anemia
　　　　Orotaciduric anemia
　　　　EXCLUDES 1　Lesch-Nyhan syndrome (E79.1)
　　D53.1　Other megaloblastic anemias, not elsewhere classified
　　　　Megaloblastic anemia NOS
　　　　EXCLUDES 1　Di Guglielmo's disease (C94.0)

　　D53.2　Scorbutic anemia
　　　　EXCLUDES 1　scurvy (E54)
　　D53.8　Other specified nutritional anemias
　　　　Anemia associated with deficiency of copper
　　　　Anemia associated with deficiency of molybdenum
　　　　Anemia associated with deficiency of zinc
　　　　EXCLUDES 1　nutritional deficiencies without anemia, such as:
　　　　　　copper deficiency NOS (E61.0)
　　　　　　molybdenum deficiency NOS (E61.5)
　　　　　　zinc deficiency NOS (E60)
　　D53.9　Nutritional anemia, unspecified
　　　　Simple chronic anemia
　　　　EXCLUDES 1　anemia NOS (D64.9)

Hemolytic anemias (D55-D59)

☑4th **D55　Anemia due to enzyme disorders**
　　EXCLUDES 1　drug-induced enzyme deficiency anemia (D59.2)
　　D55.0　Anemia due to glucose-6-phosphate dehydrogenase [G6PD] deficiency
　　　　Favism
　　　　G6PD deficiency anemia
　　D55.1　Anemia due to other disorders of glutathione metabolism
　　　　Anemia (due to) enzyme deficiencies, except G6PD, related to the hexose monophosphate [HMP] shunt pathway
　　　　Anemia (due to) hemolytic nonspherocytic (hereditary), type I
　　D55.2　Anemia due to disorders of glycolytic enzymes
　　　　Hemolytic nonspherocytic (hereditary) anemia, type II
　　　　Hexokinase deficiency anemia
　　　　Pyruvate kinase [PK] deficiency anemia
　　　　Triose-phosphate isomerase deficiency anemia
　　　　EXCLUDES 1　disorders of glycolysis not associated with anemia (E74.8)
　　D55.3　Anemia due to disorders of nucleotide metabolism
　　D55.8　Other anemias due to enzyme disorders
　　D55.9　Anemia due to enzyme disorder, unspecified

☑4th **D56　Thalassemia**
　　EXCLUDES 1　sickle-cell thalassemia (D57.4-)
　　D56.0　Alpha thalassemia
　　　　Alpha thalassemia major
　　　　Hemoglobin H disease
　　　　Severe alpha thalassemia
　　　　Triple gene defect alpha thalassemia
　　　　EXCLUDES 1　alpha thalassemia minor (D56.3)
　　　　　　asymptomatic alpha thalassemia (D56.3)
　　　　　　hydrops fetalis due to hemolytic disease (P56-)
　　D56.1　Beta thalassemia
　　　　Beta thalassemia major
　　　　Cooley's anemia
　　　　Homozygous beta thalassemia
　　　　Severe beta thalassemia
　　　　Thalassemia intermedia
　　　　EXCLUDES 1　beta thalassemia minor (D56.3)
　　　　　　delta-beta thalassemia (D56.2)
　　　　　　sickle-cell beta thalassemia (D57.4-)
　　D56.2　Delta-beta thalassemia
　　　　Homozygous delta-beta thalassemia
　　　　EXCLUDES 1　delta-beta thalassemia minor (D56.3)
　　D56.3　Thalassemia minor
　　　　Alpha thalassemia minor
　　　　Alpha thalassemia trait
　　　　Beta thalassemia minor
　　　　Delta-beta thalassemia minor
　　　　EXCLUDES 1　alpha thalassemia (D56.0)
　　　　　　beta thalassemia (D56.1)
　　　　　　delta-beta thalassemia (D56.2)
　　D56.4　Hereditary persistence of fetal hemoglobin [HPFH]
　　D56.8　Other thalassemias
　　　　Hb-Bart's disease
　　　　EXCLUDES 1　sickle cell anemia (D57-)
　　　　　　sickle-cell thalassemia (D57.4)
　　D56.9　Thalassemia, unspecified
　　　　Mediterranean anemia (with other hemoglobinopathy)
　　　　Thalassemia (minor) (mixed) (with other hemoglobinopathy)

☑ Appropriate additional character required　　　　☑x7th Requires 7th character, placeholder x must fill empty characters

Diseases of the Blood and Blood-forming Organs

D57–D61.3

✓4ᵗʰ **D57 Sickle-cell disorders**
Use additional code for any associated fever (R50.81)
EXCLUDES 1   *other hemoglobinopathies (D58-)*

✓5ᵗʰ **D57.0 Hb-SS disease with crisis**
Sickle-cell disease NOS with crisis
Hb-SS disease with vasoocclusive pain

     D57.00 Hb-SS disease with crisis, unspecified
     D57.01 Hb-SS disease with acute chest syndrome
     D57.02 Hb-SS disease with splenic sequestration

D57.1 Sickle-cell disease without crisis
Hb-SS disease without crisis
Sickle-cell anemia NOS
Sickle-cell disease NOS
Sickle-cell disorder NOS

✓5ᵗʰ **D57.2 Sickle-cell/Hb-C disease**
Hb-SC disease
Hb-S/Hb-C disease

     D57.20 Sickle-cell/Hb-C disease without crisis
     ✓6ᵗʰ **D57.21 Sickle-cell/Hb-C disease with crisis**
         D57.211 Sickle-cell/Hb-C disease with acute chest syndrome
         D57.212 Sickle-cell/Hb-C disease with splenic sequestration
         D57.219 Sickle-cell/Hb-C disease with crisis, unspecified
             Sickle-cell/Hb-C disease with crisis NOS

D57.3 Sickle-cell trait
Hb-S trait
Heterozygous hemoglobin S

✓5ᵗʰ **D57.4 Sickle-cell thalassemia**
Sickle-cell beta thalassemia
Thalassemia Hb-S disease

     D57.40 Sickle-cell thalassemia without crisis
         Sickle-cell thalassemia NOS
     ✓6ᵗʰ **D57.41 Sickle-cell thalassemia with crisis**
         Sickle-cell thalassemia with vasoocclusive pain
         D57.411 Sickle-cell thalassemia with acute chest syndrome
         D57.412 Sickle-cell thalassemia with splenic sequestration
         D57.419 Sickle-cell thalassemia with crisis, unspecified
             Sickle-cell thalassemia with crisis NOS

✓5ᵗʰ **D57.8 Other sickle-cell disorders**
Hb-SD disease
Hb-SE disease

     D57.80 Other sickle-cell disorders without crisis
     ✓6ᵗʰ **D57.81 Other sickle-cell disorders with crisis**
         D57.811 Other sickle-cell disorders with acute chest syndrome
         D57.812 Other sickle-cell disorders with splenic sequestration
         D57.819 Other sickle-cell disorders with crisis, unspecified
             Other sickle-cell disorders with crisis NOS

✓4ᵗʰ **D58 Other hereditary hemolytic anemias**
EXCLUDES 1   *hemolytic anemia of the newborn (P55-)*

D58.0 Hereditary spherocytosis
Acholuric (familial) jaundice
Congenital (spherocytic) hemolytic icterus
Minkowski-Chauffard syndrome

D58.1 Hereditary elliptocytosis
Elliptocytosis (congenital)
Ovalocytosis (congenital) (hereditary)

D58.2 Other hemoglobinopathies
Abnormal hemoglobin NOS
Congenital Heinz body anemia
Hb-C disease
Hb-D disease
Hb-E disease
Hemoglobinopathy NOS
Unstable hemoglobin hemolytic disease
EXCLUDES 1   *familial polycythemia (D75.0)*
         Hb-M disease (D74.0)
         hereditary persistence of fetal hemoglobin [HPFH] (D56.4)
         high-altitude polycythemia (D75.1)
         methemoglobinemia (D74-)

D58.8 Other specified hereditary hemolytic anemias
Stomatocytosis

D58.9 Hereditary hemolytic anemia, unspecified

✓4ᵗʰ **D59 Acquired hemolytic anemia**

D59.0 Drug-induced autoimmune hemolytic anemia
Code first (T36-T50) to identify drug

D59.1 Other autoimmune hemolytic anemias
Autoimmune hemolytic disease (cold type) (warm type)
Chronic cold hemagglutinin disease
Cold agglutinin disease
Cold agglutinin hemoglobinuria
Cold type (secondary) (symptomatic) hemolytic anemia
Warm type (secondary) (symptomatic) hemolytic anemia
EXCLUDES 1   *Evans syndrome (D69.41)*
         hemolytic disease of newborn (P55-)
         paroxysmal cold hemoglobinuria (D59.6)

D59.2 Drug-induced nonautoimmune hemolytic anemia
Drug-induced enzyme deficiency anemia
Code first (T36-T50) to identify drug

D59.3 Hemolytic-uremic syndrome

D59.4 Other nonautoimmune hemolytic anemias
Mechanical hemolytic anemia
Microangiopathic hemolytic anemia
Toxic hemolytic anemia

D59.5 Paroxysmal nocturnal hemoglobinuria [Marchiafava-Micheli]
EXCLUDES 1   *hemoglobinuria NOS (R82.3)*

D59.6 Hemoglobinuria due to hemolysis from other external causes
Hemoglobinuria from exertion
March hemoglobinuria
Paroxysmal cold hemoglobinuria
Use additional code (Chapter 20) to identify external cause
EXCLUDES 1   *hemoglobinuria NOS (R82.3)*

D59.8 Other acquired hemolytic anemias

D59.9 Acquired hemolytic anemia, unspecified
Idiopathic hemolytic anemia, chronic

Aplastic and other anemias and other bone marrow failure syndromes (D60-D64)

✓4ᵗʰ **D60 Acquired pure red cell aplasia [erythroblastopenia]**
INCLUDES   red cell aplasia (acquired) (adult) (with thymoma)
EXCLUDES 1   *congenital red cell aplasia (D61.01)*

D60.0 Chronic acquired pure red cell aplasia

D60.1 Transient acquired pure red cell aplasia

D60.8 Other acquired pure red cell aplasias

D60.9 Acquired pure red cell aplasia, unspecified

✓4ᵗʰ **D61 Other aplastic anemias and other bone marrow failure syndromes**
EXCLUDES 1   *neutropenia (D70-)*

✓5ᵗʰ **D61.0 Constitutional aplastic anemia**
     D61.01 Constitutional (pure) red blood cell aplasia
         Blackfan-Diamond syndrome
         Congenital (pure) red cell aplasia
         Familial hypoplastic anemia
         Primary (pure) red cell aplasia
         Red cell (pure) aplasia of infants
         EXCLUDES 1   *acquired red cell aplasia (D60.9)*
     D61.09 Other constitutional aplastic anemia
         Fanconi's anemia
         Pancytopenia with malformations

D61.1 Drug-induced aplastic anemia
Code first (T36-T50) to identify drug

D61.2 Aplastic anemia due to other external agents
Code first (T51-T65) to identify cause

D61.3 Idiopathic aplastic anemia

☑5ᵗʰ **D61.8 Other specified aplastic anemias and other bone marrow failure syndromes**

  D61.81 Pancytopenia
    EXCLUDES 1 *pancytopenia (due to) (with):*
      aplastic anemia (D61-)
      bone marrow infiltration (D61.82)
      congenital (pure) red cell aplasia (D61.01)
      drug induced (D61.1)
      hairy cell leukemia (C91.4-)
      human immunodeficiency virus disease (B20-)
      leukoerythroblastic anemia (M61.82)
      myelodysplastic syndromes (D46-)
      myeloproliferative disease (D47.1)

  D61.82 Myelophthisis
    Leukoerythroblastic anemia
    Myelophthisic anemia
    Panmyelophthisis
    Code also the underlying disorder, such as:
      malignant neoplasm of breast (C50-)
      tuberculosis (A15-)
    EXCLUDES 1 *idiopathic myelofibrosis (D47.1)*
      myelofibrosis NOS (D75.81)
      myelofibrosis with myeloid metaplasia (D47.4)
      primary myelofibrosis (D47.1)
      secondary myelofibrosis (D75.81)

  D61.89 Other specified aplastic anemias and other bone marrow failure syndromes

D61.9 Aplastic anemia, unspecified
  Hypoplastic anemia NOS
  Medullary hypoplasia

D62 Acute posthemorrhagic anemia
  EXCLUDES 1 *anemia due to chronic blood loss (D50.0)*
    blood loss anemia NOS (D50.0)
    congenital anemia from fetal blood loss (P61.3)

☑4ᵗʰ **D63 Anemia in chronic diseases classified elsewhere**

  D63.0 Anemia in neoplastic disease
    Code first neoplasm (C00-D49)
    EXCLUDES 1 *anemia due to antineoplastic chemotherapy (D64.81)*
      aplastic anemia due to antineoplastic chemotherapy (D61.1)

  D63.1 Anemia in chronic kidney disease
    Erythropoietin resistant anemia (EPO resistant anemia)
    Code first underlying chronic kidney disease (CKD) (N18-)

  D63.8 Anemia in other chronic diseases classified elsewhere
    Code first underlying disease, such as:
      diphyllobothriasis (B70.0)
      hookworm disease (B76.0-B76.9)
      hypothyroidism (E00.0-E03.9)
      malaria (B50.0-B54)
      symptomatic late syphilis (A52.79)
      tuberculosis (A18.89)

☑4ᵗʰ **D64 Other anemias**
  EXCLUDES 1 *refractory anemia (D46-)*
    refractory anemia with excess blasts in transformation [RAEB T] (C92.0-)

  D64.0 Hereditary sideroblastic anemia
    Sex-linked hypochromic sideroblastic anemia

  D64.1 Secondary sideroblastic anemia due to disease
    Code first underlying disease

  D64.2 Secondary sideroblastic anemia due to drugs and toxins
    Code first (T36-T65) to identify drug or toxin

  D64.3 Other sideroblastic anemias
    Sideroblastic anemia NOS
    Pyridoxine-responsive sideroblastic anemia NEC

  D64.4 Congenital dyserythropoietic anemia
    Dyshematopoietic anemia (congenital)
    EXCLUDES 1 *Blackfan-Diamond syndrome (D61.01)*
      Di Guglielmo's disease (C94.0)

☑5ᵗʰ **D64.8 Other specified anemias**

  D64.81 Anemia due to antineoplastic chemotherapy
    Antineoplastic chemotherapy induced anemia
    EXCLUDES 1 *anemia in neoplastic disease (D63.0)*
      aplastic anemia due to antineoplastic chemotherapy (D61.1)

  D64.89 Other specified anemias
    Infantile pseudoleukemia

D64.9 Anemia, unspecified

Coagulation defects, purpura and other hemorrhagic conditions (D65-D69)

D65 Disseminated intravascular coagulation [defibrination syndrome]
  Afibrinogenemia, acquired
  Consumption coagulopathy
  Diffuse or disseminated intravascular coagulation [DIC]
  Fibrinolytic hemorrhage, acquired
  Fibrinolytic purpura
  Purpura fulminans
  EXCLUDES 1 *disseminated intravascular coagulation (complicating):*
    abortion or ectopic or molar pregnancy (O00-O07, O08.1)
    in newborn (P60)
    pregnancy, childbirth and the puerperium (O45.0, O46.0, O67.0, O72.3)

D66 Hereditary factor VIII deficiency
  Classical hemophilia
  Deficiency factor VIII (with functional defect)
  Hemophilia NOS
  Hemophilia A
  EXCLUDES 1 *factor VIII deficiency with vascular defect (D68.0)*

D67 Hereditary factor IX deficiency
  Christmas disease
  Factor IX deficiency (with functional defect)
  Hemophilia B
  Plasma thromboplastin component [PTC] deficiency

☑4ᵗʰ **D68 Other coagulation defects**
  EXCLUDES 1 *abnormal coagulation profile (R79.1)*
    coagulation defects complicating:
    abortion or ectopic or molar pregnancy (O00-O07, O08.1)
    pregnancy, childbirth and the puerperium (O45.0, O46.0, O67.0, O72.3)

  D68.0 Von Willebrand's disease
    Angiohemophilia
    Factor VIII deficiency with vascular defect
    Vascular hemophilia
    EXCLUDES 1 *capillary fragility (hereditary) (D69.8)*
      factor VIII deficiency NOS (D66)
      factor VIII deficiency with functional defect (D66)

  D68.1 Hereditary factor XI deficiency
    Hemophilia C
    Plasma thromboplastin antecedent [PTA] deficiency
    Rosenthal's disease

  D68.2 Hereditary deficiency of other clotting factors
    AC globulin deficiency
    Congenital afibrinogenemia
    Deficiency of factor I [fibrinogen]
    Deficiency of factor II [prothrombin]
    Deficiency of factor V [labile]
    Deficiency of factor VII [stable]
    Deficiency of factor X [Stuart-Prower]
    Deficiency of factor XII [Hageman]
    Deficiency of factor XIII [fibrin stabilizing]
    Dysfibrinogenemia (congenital)
    Hypoproconvertinemia
    Owren's disease
    Proaccelerin deficiency

☑5ᵗʰ **D68.3 Hemorrhagic disorder due to circulating anticoagulants**

  D68.31 Hemorrhagic disorder due to intrinsic circulating anticoagulants
    Hemorrhagic disorder due to intrinsic increase in antithrombin
    Hemorrhagic disorder due to intrinsic increase in anti-VIIIa
    Hemorrhagic disorder due to intrinsic increase in anti-IXa
    Hemorrhagic disorder due to intrinsic increase in anti-Xa
    Hemorrhagic disorder due to intrinsic increase in anti-XIa
    Hyperheparinemia

☑ Appropriate additional character required   ☑x7ᵗʰ Requires 7th character, placeholder x must fill empty characters

D68.32 Hemorrhagic disorder due to extrinsic circulating anticoagulants
Drug-induced hemorrhagic disorder
Code first (T45.5-) to identify any administered anticoagulant

D68.4 Acquired coagulation factor deficiency
Deficiency of coagulation factor due to liver disease
Deficiency of coagulation factor due to vitamin K deficiency
EXCLUDES 1 vitamin K deficiency of newborn (P53)

✓5th **D68.5 Primary thrombophilia**
Primary hypercoagulable states
EXCLUDES 1 lupus anticoagulant (D68.62)
thrombotic thrombocytopenic purpura (M31.1)

D68.51 Activated protein C resistance
Factor V Leiden mutation
D68.52 Prothrombin gene mutation
D68.59 Other primary thrombophilia
Antithrombin III deficiency
Hypercoagulable state NOS
Primary hypercoagulable state NEC
Primary thrombophilia NEC
Protein C deficiency
Protein S deficiency
Thrombophilia NOS

✓5th **D68.6 Other thrombophilia**
Other hypercoagulable states
EXCLUDES 1 diffuse or disseminated intravascular coagulation [DIC] (D65)
heparin induced thrombocytopenia (HIT) (D75.82)
hyperhomocysteinemia (E72.11)

D68.61 Anticardiolipin syndrome
Antiphospholipid syndrome
EXCLUDES 1 lupus anticoagulant syndrome (D68.62)
D68.62 Lupus anticoagulant syndrome
Lupus anticoagulant
Presence of systemic lupus erythematosus [SLE] inhibitor
EXCLUDES 1 anticardiolipin syndrome (D68.61)
antiphospholipid syndrome (D68.61)
D68.69 Other thrombophilia
Hypercoagulable states NEC
Secondary hypercoagulable state NOS

D68.8 Other specified coagulation defects
EXCLUDES 1 hemorrhagic disease of newborn (P53)

D68.9 Coagulation defect, unspecified

✓4th **D69 Purpura and other hemorrhagic conditions**
EXCLUDES 1 benign hypergammaglobulinemic purpura (D89.Ø)
cryoglobulinemic purpura (D89.1)
essential (hemorrhagic) thrombocythemia (D47.3)
hemorrhagic thrombocythemia (D47.3)
purpura fulminans (D65)
thrombotic thrombocytopenic purpura (M31.1)
Waldenström hypergammaglobulinemic purpura (D89.Ø)

D69.Ø Allergic purpura
Allergic vasculitis
Nonthrombocytopenic hemorrhagic purpura
Nonthrombocytopenic idiopathic purpura
Purpura anaphylactoid
Purpura Henoch(-Schönlein)
Purpura rheumatica
Vascular purpura
EXCLUDES 1 thrombocytopenic hemorrhagic purpura (D69.3)

D69.1 Qualitative platelet defects
Bernard-Soulier [giant platelet] syndrome
Glanzmann's disease
Grey platelet syndrome
Thromboasthenia (hemorrhagic) (hereditary)
Thrombocytopathy
EXCLUDES 1 von Willebrand's disease (D68.Ø)

D69.2 Other nonthrombocytopenic purpura
Purpura NOS
Purpura simplex
Senile purpura

D69.3 Immune thrombocytopenic purpura
Hemorrhagic (thrombocytopenic) purpura
Idiopathic thrombocytopenic purpura
Tidal platelet dysgenesis

✓5th **D69.4 Other primary thrombocytopenia**
EXCLUDES 1 transient neonatal thrombocytopenia (P61.Ø)
Wiskott-Aldrich syndrome (D82.Ø)
D69.41 Evans syndrome
D69.42 Congenital and hereditary thrombocytopenia purpura
Congenital thrombocytopenia
Hereditary thrombocytopenia
Code first congenital or hereditary disorder, such as:
thrombocytopenia with absent radius (TAR syndrome) (Q87.2)
D69.49 Other primary thrombocytopenia
Megakaryocytic hypoplasia
Primary thrombocytopenia NOS

✓5th **D69.5 Secondary thrombocytopenia**
EXCLUDES 1 heparin induced thrombocytopenia (HIT) (D75.82)
transient thrombocytopenia of newborn (P61.Ø)
D69.51 Posttransfusion purpura
Posttransfusion purpura from whole blood (fresh) or blood products
PTP
D69.59 Other secondary thrombocytopenia

D69.6 Thrombocytopenia, unspecified
D69.8 Other specified hemorrhagic conditions
Capillary fragility (hereditary)
Vascular pseudohemophilia
D69.9 Hemorrhagic condition, unspecified

Other disorders of blood and blood-forming organs (D7Ø-D77)

✓4th **D7Ø Neutropenia**
INCLUDES agranulocytosis
decreased absolute neurophile count (ANC)
Use additional code for any associated:
fever (R5Ø.81)
mucositis (J34.81, K12.3-, K92.81, N76.81)
EXCLUDES 1 neutropenic splenomegaly (D73.81)
transient neonatal neutropenia (P61.5)
D7Ø.Ø Congenital agranulocytosis
Congenital neutropenia
Infantile genetic agranulocytosis
Kostmann's disease
D7Ø.1 Agranulocytosis secondary to cancer chemotherapy
Code first (T45.1-) to identify drug
Code also underlying neoplasm
D7Ø.2 Other drug-induced agranulocytosis
Code first (T36-T5Ø) to identify drug
D7Ø.3 Neutropenia due to infection
D7Ø.4 Cyclic neutropenia
Cyclic hematopoiesis
Periodic neutropenia
D7Ø.8 Other neutropenia
D7Ø.9 Neutropenia, unspecified

D71 Functional disorders of polymorphonuclear neutrophils
Cell membrane receptor complex [CR3] defect
Chronic (childhood) granulomatous disease
Congenital dysphagocytosis
Progressive septic granulomatosis

✓4th **D72 Other disorders of white blood cells**
EXCLUDES 1 basophilia (D72.824)
immunity disorders (D8Ø-D89)
neutropenia (D7Ø)
preleukemia (syndrome) (D46.9)
D72.Ø Genetic anomalies of leukocytes
Alder (granulation) (granulocyte) anomaly
Alder syndrome
Hereditary leukocytic hypersegmentation
Hereditary leukocytic hyposegmentation
Hereditary leukomelanopathy
May-Hegglin (granulation) (granulocyte) anomaly
May-Hegglin syndrome
Pelger-Huët (granulation) (granulocyte) anomaly
Pelger-Huët syndrome
EXCLUDES 1 Chédiak (-Steinbrinck)-Higashi syndrome (E7Ø.33Ø)

EXCLUDES 1 Not coded here   *EXCLUDES 2* Not included here   *Manifestation Code*

D72.1 Eosinophilia
Allergic eosinophilia
Hereditary eosinophilia
EXCLUDES 1   *Löffler's syndrome (J82)*
pulmonary eosinophilia (J82)

✓5th **D72.8 Other specified disorders of white blood cells**
EXCLUDES 1   *leukemia (C91-C95)*

✓6th **D72.81 Decreased white blood cell count**
EXCLUDES 1   *neutropenia (D70-)*

D72.810 Lymphocytopenia
Decreased lymphocytes

D72.818 Other decreased white blood cell count
Basophilic leukopenia
Eosinophilic leukopenia
Monocytopenia
Other decreased leukocytes
Plasmacytopenia

D72.819 Decreased white blood cell count, unspecified
Decreased leukocytes, unspecified
Leukocytopenia, unspecified
Leukopenia
EXCLUDES 1   *malignant leukopenia (D70.9)*

✓6th **D72.82 Elevated white blood cell count**
EXCLUDES 1   *eosinophilia (D72.1)*

D72.820 Lymphocytosis (symptomatic)
Elevated lymphocytes

D72.821 Monocytosis (symptomatic)
EXCLUDES 1   *infectious mononucleosis (B27-)*

D72.822 Plasmacytosis

D72.823 Leukemoid reaction
Basophilic leukemoid reaction
Leukemoid reaction NOS
Lymphocytic leukemoid reaction
Monocytic leukemoid reaction
Myelocytic leukemoid reaction
Neutrophilic leukemoid reaction

D72.824 Basophilia

D72.825 Bandemia
Bandemia without diagnosis of specific infection
EXCLUDES 1   *confirmed infection—code to infection*
leukemia (C91-, C92-, C93-, C94-, C95-)

D72.828 Other elevated white blood cell count

D72.829 Elevated white blood cell count, unspecified
Elevated leukocytes, unspecified
Leukocytosis, unspecified

D72.89 Other specified disorders of white blood cells
Abnormality of white blood cells NEC

D72.9 Disorder of white blood cells, unspecified
Abnormal leukocyte differential NOS

✓4th **D73 Diseases of spleen**

D73.0 Hyposplenism
Atrophy of spleen
EXCLUDES 1   *asplenia (congenital) (Q89.01)*
postsurgical absence of spleen (Z90.81)

D73.1 Hypersplenism
EXCLUDES 1   *neutropenic splenomegaly (D73.81)*
primary splenic neutropenia (D73.81)
splenitis, splenomegaly in late syphilis (A52.79)
splenitis, splenomegaly in tuberculosis (A18.85)
splenomegaly NOS (R16.1)
splenomegaly congenital (Q89.0)

D73.2 Chronic congestive splenomegaly

D73.3 Abscess of spleen

D73.4 Cyst of spleen

D73.5 Infarction of spleen
Splenic rupture, nontraumatic
Torsion of spleen
EXCLUDES 1   *rupture of spleen due to Plasmodium vivax malaria (B51.0)*
traumatic rupture of spleen (S36.03-)

✓5th **D73.8 Other diseases of spleen**

D73.81 Neutropenic splenomegaly
Werner-Schultz disease

D73.89 Other diseases of spleen
Fibrosis of spleen NOS
Perisplenitis
Splenitis NOS

D73.9 Disease of spleen, unspecified

✓4th **D74 Methemoglobinemia**

D74.0 Congenital methemoglobinemia
Congenital NADH-methemoglobin reductase deficiency
Hemoglobin-M [Hb-M] disease
Methemoglobinemia, hereditary

D74.8 Other methemoglobinemias
Acquired methemoglobinemia (with sulfhemoglobinemia)
Toxic methemoglobinemia

D74.9 Methemoglobinemia, unspecified

✓4th **D75 Other and unspecified diseases of blood and blood-forming organs**
EXCLUDES 2   *acute lymphadenitis (L04-)*
chronic lymphadenitis (I88.1)
enlarged lymph nodes (R59-)
hypergammaglobulinemia NOS (D89.2)
lymphadenitis NOS (I88.9)
mesenteric lymphadenitis (acute) (chronic) (I88.0)

D75.0 Familial erythrocytosis
Benign polycythemia
Familial polycythemia
EXCLUDES 1   *hereditary ovalocytosis (D58.1)*

D75.1 Secondary polycythemia
Acquired polycythemia
Emotional polycythemia
Erythrocytosis NOS
Hypoxemic polycythemia
Nephrogenous polycythemia
Polycythemia due to erythropoietin
Polycythemia due to fall in plasma volume
Polycythemia due to high altitude
Polycythemia due to stress
Polycythemia NOS
Relative polycythemia
EXCLUDES 1   *polycythemia neonatorum (P61.1)*
polycythemia vera (D45)

✓5th **D75.8 Other specified diseases of blood and blood-forming organs**

D75.81 Myelofibrosis
Myelofibrosis NOS
Secondary myelofibrosis NOS
Code first the underlying disorder, such as:
malignant neoplasm of breast (C50-)
Use additional code, if applicable, for associated therapy-related myelodysplastic syndrome (D46-)
Use additional external cause code, if due to antineoplastic chemotherapy (T45.1-)
EXCLUDES 1   *acute myelofibrosis (C94.4-)*
idiopathic myelofibrosis (D47.1)
leukoerythroblastic anemia (D61.82)
myelofibrosis with myeloid metaplasia (D47.4)
myelophthisic anemia (D61.82)
myelophthisis (D61.82)
primary myelofibrosis (D47.1)

D75.82 Heparin induced thrombocytopenia (HIT)

D75.89 Other specified diseases of blood and blood-forming organs

D75.9 Disease of blood and blood-forming organs, unspecified

✓ Appropriate additional character required   ✓x7th Requires 7th character, placeholder x must fill empty characters

✓4th **D76 Other specified diseases with participation of lymphoreticular and reticulohistiocytic tissue**

EXCLUDES 1 *(Abt-) Letterer-Siwe disease (C96.0)*
eosinophilic granuloma (C96.6)
Hand-Schüller-Christian disease (C96.5)
histiocytic sarcoma (C96.a)
histiocytosis X, multifocal (C96.5)
histiocytosis X, unifocal (C96.6)
malignant histiocytosis (C96.a)
Langerhans-cell histiocytosis, multifocal (C96.5)
Langerhans-cell histiocytosis NOS (C96.6)
Langerhans-cell histiocytosis, unifocal (C96.6)
leukemic reticuloendotheliosis or reticulosis (C91.4-)
lipomelanotic reticuloendotheliosis or reticulosis (I89.8)

D76.1 Hemophagocytic lymphohistiocytosis
Familial hemophagocytic reticulosis
Histiocytoses of mononuclear phagocytes

D76.2 Hemophagocytic syndrome, infection-associated
Use additional code to identify infectious agent or disease

D76.3 Other histiocytosis syndromes
Reticulohistiocytoma (giant-cell)
Sinus histiocytosis with massive lymphadenopathy
Xanthogranuloma

D77 Other disorders of blood and blood-forming organs in diseases classified elsewhere

Code first underlying disease, such as:
amyloidosis (E85-)
congenital early syphilis (A50.0)
echinococcosis (B67.0-B67.9)
malaria (B50.0-B54)
schistosomiasis [bilharziasis] (B65.0-B65.9)
vitamin C deficiency (E54)

EXCLUDES 1 *rupture of spleen due to Plasmodium vivax malaria (B51.0)*
splenitis, splenomegaly in:
late syphilis (A52.79)
tuberculosis (A18.85)

Intraoperative and postprocedural complications of the spleen (D78)

✓4th **D78 Intraoperative and postprocedural complications of the spleen**

✓5th **D78.0 Intraoperative hemorrhage and hematoma of spleen complicating a procedure**

EXCLUDES 1 *intraoperative hemorrhage and hematoma of spleen due to accidental puncture or laceration during a procedure (D78.1-)*

D78.01 Intraoperative hemorrhage and hematoma of spleen complicating a procedure on the spleen

D78.02 Intraoperative hemorrhage and hematoma of spleen complicating other procedure

✓5th **D78.1 Accidental puncture and laceration of spleen during a procedure**

D78.11 Accidental puncture and laceration of spleen during a procedure on the spleen

D78.12 Accidental puncture and laceration of spleen during other procedure

✓5th **D78.2 Postprocedural hemorrhage and hematoma of spleen following a procedure**

D78.21 Postprocedural hemorrhage and hematoma of spleen following a procedure on the spleen

D78.22 Postprocedural hemorrhage and hematoma of spleen following other procedure

✓5th **D78.8 Other intraoperative and postprocedural complications of spleen**
Use additional code, if applicable, to further specify disorder

D78.81 Other intraoperative complications of spleen

D78.89 Other postprocedural complications of spleen

Certain disorders involving the immune mechanism (D80-D89)

INCLUDES defects in the complement system
immunodeficiency disorders, except human immunodeficiency virus [HIV] disease
sarcoidosis

EXCLUDES 1 *autoimmune disease (systemic) NOS (M35.9)*
functional disorders of polymorphonuclear neutrophils (D71)
human immunodeficiency virus [HIV] disease (B20)

✓4th **D80 Immunodeficiency with predominantly antibody defects**

D80.0 Hereditary hypogammaglobulinemia
Autosomal recessive agammaglobulinemia (Swiss type)
X-linked agammaglobulinemia [Bruton] (with growth hormone deficiency)

D80.1 Nonfamilial hypogammaglobulinemia
Agammaglobulinemia with immunoglobulin-bearing B-lymphocytes
Common variable agammaglobulinemia [CVAgamma]
Hypogammaglobulinemia NOS

D80.2 Selective deficiency of immunoglobulin A [IgA]

D80.3 Selective deficiency of immunoglobulin G [IgG] subclasses

D80.4 Selective deficiency of immunoglobulin M [IgM]

D80.5 Immunodeficiency with increased immunoglobulin M [IgM]

D80.6 Antibody deficiency with near-normal immunoglobulins or with hyperimmunoglobulinemia

D80.7 Transient hypogammaglobulinemia of infancy

D80.8 Other immunodeficiencies with predominantly antibody defects
Kappa light chain deficiency

D80.9 Immunodeficiency with predominantly antibody defects, unspecified

✓4th **D81 Combined immunodeficiencies**

EXCLUDES 1 *autosomal recessive agammaglobulinemia (Swiss type) (D80.0)*

D81.0 Severe combined immunodeficiency [SCID] with reticular dysgenesis

D81.1 Severe combined immunodeficiency [SCID] with low T- and B-cell numbers

D81.2 Severe combined immunodeficiency [SCID] with low or normal B-cell numbers

D81.3 Adenosine deaminase [ADA] deficiency

D81.4 Nezelof's syndrome

D81.5 Purine nucleoside phosphorylase [PNP] deficiency

D81.6 Major histocompatibility complex class I deficiency
Bare lymphocyte syndrome

D81.7 Major histocompatibility complex class II deficiency

✓5th **D81.8 Other combined immunodeficiencies**

✓6th **D81.81 Biotin-dependent carboxylase deficiency**
Multiple carboxylase deficiency

EXCLUDES 1 *biotin-dependent carboxylase deficiency due to dietary deficiency of biotin (E53.8)*

D81.810 Biotinidase deficiency

D81.818 Other biotin-dependent carboxylase deficiency
Holocarboxylase synthetase deficiency
Other multiple carboxylase deficiency

D81.819 Biotin-dependent carboxylase deficiency, unspecified
Multiple carboxylase deficiency, unspecified

D81.89 Other combined immunodeficiencies

D81.9 Combined immunodeficiency, unspecified
Severe combined immunodeficiency disorder [SCID] NOS

✓4th **D82 Immunodeficiency associated with other major defects**

EXCLUDES 1 *ataxia telangiectasia [Louis-Bar] (G11.3)*

D82.0 Wiskott-Aldrich syndrome
Immunodeficiency with thrombocytopenia and eczema

D82.1 Di George's syndrome
Pharyngeal pouch syndrome
Thymic alymphoplasia
Thymic aplasia or hypoplasia with immunodeficiency

D82.2 Immunodeficiency with short-limbed stature

D82.3 Immunodeficiency following hereditary defective response to Epstein-Barr virus
X-linked lymphoproliferative disease

D82.4 Hyperimmunoglobulin E [IgE] syndrome

EXCLUDES 1 Not coded here   EXCLUDES 2 Not included here   *Manifestation Code*

D82.8   Immunodeficiency associated with other specified major defects

D82.9   Immunodeficiency associated with major defect, unspecified

☑4ᵗʰ **D83   Common variable immunodeficiency**

D83.0   Common variable immunodeficiency with predominant abnormalities of B-cell numbers and function

D83.1   Common variable immunodeficiency with predominant immunoregulatory T-cell disorders

D83.2   Common variable immunodeficiency with autoantibodies to B- or T-cells

D83.8   Other common variable immunodeficiencies

D83.9   Common variable immunodeficiency, unspecified

☑4ᵗʰ **D84   Other immunodeficiencies**

D84.0   Lymphocyte function antigen-1 [LFA-1] defect

D84.1   Defects in the complement system
C1 esterase inhibitor [C1-INH] deficiency

D84.8   Other specified immunodeficiencies

D84.9   Immunodeficiency, unspecified

☑4ᵗʰ **D86   Sarcoidosis**

D86.0   Sarcoidosis of lung

D86.1   Sarcoidosis of lymph nodes

D86.2   Sarcoidosis of lung with sarcoidosis of lymph nodes

D86.3   Sarcoidosis of skin

☑5ᵗʰ **D86.8   Sarcoidosis of other sites**

D86.81   Sarcoid meningitis

D86.82   Multiple cranial nerve palsies in sarcoidosis

D86.83   Sarcoid iridocyclitis

D86.84   Sarcoid pyelonephritis
Tubulo-interstitial nephropathy in sarcoidosis

D86.85   Sarcoid myocarditis

D86.86   Sarcoid arthropathy
Polyarthritis in sarcoidosis

D86.87   Sarcoid myositis

D86.89   Sarcoidosis of other sites
Hepatic granuloma
Uveoparotid fever [Heerfordt]

D86.9   Sarcoidosis, unspecified

☑4ᵗʰ **D89   Other disorders involving the immune mechanism, not elsewhere classified**
EXCLUDES 1   *hyperglobulinemia NOS (R77.1)*
monoclonal gammopathy (of undetermined significance) (D47.2)
EXCLUDES 2   *transplant failure and rejection (T86-)*

D89.0   Polyclonal hypergammaglobulinemia
Benign hypergammaglobulinemic purpura
Polyclonal gammopathy NOS

D89.1   Cryoglobulinemia
Cryoglobulinemic purpura
Cryoglobulinemic vasculitis
Essential cryoglobulinemia
Idiopathic cryoglobulinemia
Mixed cryoglobulinemia
Primary cryoglobulinemia
Secondary cryoglobulinemia

D89.2   Hypergammaglobulinemia, unspecified

D89.3   Immune reconstitution syndrome
Immune reconstitution inflammatory syndrome [IRIS]
Code first (T36-T50) to identify drug, if drug induced

☑5ᵗʰ **D89.8   Other specified disorders involving the immune mechanism, not elsewhere classified**

☑6ᵗʰ **D89.81   Graft-versus-host disease**
Code first underlying cause, such as:
complications of transplanted organs and tissue (T86-)
complications of blood transfusion (T80.89)
Use additional code to identify associated manifestations, such as:
desquamative dermatitis (L30.8)
diarrhea (R19.7)
elevated bilirubin (R17)
hair loss (L65.9)

D89.810   Acute graft-versus-host disease

D89.811   Chronic graft-versus-host disease

D89.812   Acute on chronic graft-versus-host disease

D89.813   Graft-versus-host disease, unspecified

D89.82   Autoimmune lymphoproliferative syndrome [ALPS]

D89.89   Other specified disorders involving the immune mechanism, not elsewhere classified
EXCLUDES 1   *human immunodeficiency virus disease (B20)*

D89.9   Disorder involving the immune mechanism, unspecified
Immune disease NOS

☑ Appropriate additional character required   ☑x7ᵗʰ Requires 7th character, placeholder x must fill empty characters

Chapter 4. Endocrine, Nutritional and Metabolic Diseases (E00-E89)

NOTE   All neoplasms, whether functionally active or not, are classified in Chapter 2. Appropriate codes in this chapter (i.e. E05.8, E07.0, E16-E31, E34-) may be used as additional codes to indicate either functional activity by neoplasms and ectopic endocrine tissue or hyperfunction and hypofunction of endocrine glands associated with neoplasms and other conditions classified elsewhere.

EXCLUDES 1   *transitory endocrine and metabolic disorders specific to newborn (P70-P74)*

This chapter contains the following blocks:

E00-E07	Disorders of thyroid gland
E08-E13	Diabetes mellitus
E15-E16	Other disorders of glucose regulation and pancreatic internal secretion
E20-E35	Disorders of other endocrine glands
E36	Intraoperative complications of endocrine system
E40-E46	Malnutrition
E50-E64	Other nutritional deficiencies
E65-E68	Overweight, obesity and other hyperalimentation
E70-E88	Metabolic disorders
E89	Postprocedural endocrine and metabolic complications and disorders, not elsewhere classified

Disorders of thyroid gland (E00-E07)

✓4ᵗʰ E00   Congenital iodine-deficiency syndrome

Use additional code (F70-F79) to identify associated mental retardation

EXCLUDES 1   *subclinical iodine-deficiency hypothyroidism (E02)*

E00.0   Congenital iodine-deficiency syndrome, neurological type
Endemic cretinism, neurological type

E00.1   Congenital iodine-deficiency syndrome, myxedematous type
Endemic hypothyroid cretinism
Endemic cretinism, myxedematous type

E00.2   Congenital iodine-deficiency syndrome, mixed type
Endemic cretinism, mixed type

E00.9   Congenital iodine-deficiency syndrome, unspecified
Congenital iodine-deficiency hypothyroidism NOS
Endemic cretinism NOS

✓4ᵗʰ E01   Iodine-deficiency related thyroid disorders and allied conditions

EXCLUDES 1   *congenital iodine-deficiency syndrome (E00-)*
subclinical iodine-deficiency hypothyroidism (E02)

E01.0   Iodine-deficiency related diffuse (endemic) goiter

E01.1   Iodine-deficiency related multinodular (endemic) goiter
Iodine-deficiency related nodular goiter

E01.2   Iodine-deficiency related (endemic) goiter, unspecified
Endemic goiter NOS

E01.8   Other iodine-deficiency related thyroid disorders and allied conditions
Acquired iodine-deficiency hypothyroidism NOS

E02   Subclinical iodine-deficiency hypothyroidism

✓4ᵗʰ E03   Other hypothyroidism

EXCLUDES 1   *iodine-deficiency related hypothyroidism (E00-E02)*
postprocedural hypothyroidism (E89.0)

E03.0   Congenital hypothyroidism with diffuse goiter
Congenital parenchymatous goiter (nontoxic)
Congenital goiter (nontoxic) NOS
EXCLUDES 1   *transitory congenital goiter with normal function (P72.0)*

E03.1   Congenital hypothyroidism without goiter
Aplasia of thyroid (with myxedema)
Congenital atrophy of thyroid
Congenital hypothyroidism NOS

E03.2   Hypothyroidism due to medicaments and other exogenous substances
Code first (T36-T65) to identify drug or substance

E03.3   Postinfectious hypothyroidism

E03.4   Atrophy of thyroid (acquired)
EXCLUDES 1   *congenital atrophy of thyroid (E03.1)*

E03.5   Myxedema coma

E03.8   Other specified hypothyroidism

E03.9   Hypothyroidism, unspecified
Myxedema NOS

✓4ᵗʰ E04   Other nontoxic goiter

EXCLUDES 1   *congenital goiter (NOS) (diffuse) (parenchymatous) (E03.0)*
iodine-deficiency related goiter (E00-E02)

E04.0   Nontoxic diffuse goiter
Diffuse (colloid) nontoxic goiter
Simple nontoxic goiter

E04.1   Nontoxic single thyroid nodule
Colloid nodule (cystic) (thyroid)
Nontoxic uninodular goiter
Thyroid (cystic) nodule NOS

E04.2   Nontoxic multinodular goiter
Cystic goiter NOS
Multinodular (cystic) goiter NOS

E04.8   Other specified nontoxic goiter

E04.9   Nontoxic goiter, unspecified
Goiter NOS
Nodular goiter (nontoxic) NOS

✓4ᵗʰ E05   Thyrotoxicosis [hyperthyroidism]

EXCLUDES 1   *chronic thyroiditis with transient thyrotoxicosis (E06.2)*
neonatal thyrotoxicosis (P72.1)

✓5ᵗʰ E05.0   Thyrotoxicosis with diffuse goiter
Exophthalmic or toxic goiter NOS
Graves' disease
Toxic diffuse goiter

E05.00   Thyrotoxicosis with diffuse goiter without thyrotoxic crisis or storm

E05.01   Thyrotoxicosis with diffuse goiter with thyrotoxic crisis or storm

✓5ᵗʰ E05.1   Thyrotoxicosis with toxic single thyroid nodule
Thyrotoxicosis with toxic uninodular goiter

E05.10   Thyrotoxicosis with toxic single thyroid nodule without thyrotoxic crisis or storm

E05.11   Thyrotoxicosis with toxic single thyroid nodule with thyrotoxic crisis or storm

✓5ᵗʰ E05.2   Thyrotoxicosis with toxic multinodular goiter
Toxic nodular goiter NOS

E05.20   Thyrotoxicosis with toxic multinodular goiter without thyrotoxic crisis or storm

E05.21   Thyrotoxicosis with toxic multinodular goiter with thyrotoxic crisis or storm

✓5ᵗʰ E05.3   Thyrotoxicosis from ectopic thyroid tissue

E05.30   Thyrotoxicosis from ectopic thyroid tissue without thyrotoxic crisis or storm

E05.31   Thyrotoxicosis from ectopic thyroid tissue with thyrotoxic crisis or storm

✓5ᵗʰ E05.4   Thyrotoxicosis factitia

E05.40   Thyrotoxicosis factitia without thyrotoxic crisis or storm

E05.41   Thyrotoxicosis factitia with thyrotoxic crisis or storm

✓5ᵗʰ E05.8   Other thyrotoxicosis
Overproduction of thyroid-stimulating hormone

E05.80   Other thyrotoxicosis without thyrotoxic crisis or storm

E05.81   Other thyrotoxicosis with thyrotoxic crisis or storm

✓5ᵗʰ E05.9   Thyrotoxicosis, unspecified
Hyperthyroidism NOS

E05.90   Thyrotoxicosis, unspecified without thyrotoxic crisis or storm

E05.91   Thyrotoxicosis, unspecified with thyrotoxic crisis or storm

✓4ᵗʰ E06   Thyroiditis

EXCLUDES 1   *postpartum thyroiditis (O90.5)*

E06.0   Acute thyroiditis
Abscess of thyroid
Pyogenic thyroiditis
Suppurative thyroiditis
Use additional code (B95-B97) to identify infectious agent

E06.1   Subacute thyroiditis
de Quervain thyroiditis
Giant-cell thyroiditis
Granulomatous thyroiditis
Nonsuppurative thyroiditis
Viral thyroiditis
EXCLUDES 1   *autoimmune thyroiditis (E06.3)*

E06.2   Chronic thyroiditis with transient thyrotoxicosis
EXCLUDES 1   *autoimmune thyroiditis (E06.3)*

EXCLUDES 1   Not coded here   *EXCLUDES 2*   Not included here   ***Manifestation Code***

E06.3 **Autoimmune thyroiditis**
Hashimoto's thyroiditis
Hashitoxicosis (transient)
Lymphadenoid goiter
Lymphocytic thyroiditis
Struma lymphomatosa

E06.4 **Drug-induced thyroiditis**
Code first (T36-T50) to identify drug

E06.5 **Other chronic thyroiditis**
Chronic fibrous thyroiditis
Chronic thyroiditis NOS
Ligneous thyroiditis
Riedel thyroiditis

E06.9 **Thyroiditis, unspecified**

✓4th **E07 Other disorders of thyroid**

E07.0 **Hypersecretion of calcitonin**
C-cell hyperplasia of thyroid
Hypersecretion of thyrocalcitonin

E07.1 **Dyshormogenetic goiter**
Familial dyshormogenetic goiter
Pendred's syndrome
EXCLUDES 1   *transitory congenital goiter with normal function (P72.0)*

✓5th E07.8 **Other specified disorders of thyroid**
E07.81 **Sick-euthyroid syndrome**
Euthyroid sick-syndrome
E07.89 **Other specified disorders of thyroid**
Abnormality of thyroid-binding globulin
Hemorrhage of thyroid
Infarction of thyroid

E07.9 **Disorder of thyroid, unspecified**

Diabetes mellitus (E08-E13)

✓4th **E08 Diabetes mellitus due to underlying condition**
Code first the underlying condition, such as:
Congenital rubella (P35.0)
Cushing's syndrome (E24-)
Cystic fibrosis (E84-)
Malignant neoplasm (C00-C96)
Malnutrition (E40-E46)
Pancreatitis and other diseases of the pancreas (K85-, K86-)
Use additional code to identify any insulin use (Z79.4)
EXCLUDES 1   *drug or chemical induced diabetes mellitus (E09.-)*
gestational diabetes (O24.4-)
neonatal diabetes mellitus (P70.2)
postpancreatectomy diabetes mellitus (E13.-)
postprocedural diabetes mellitus (E13.-)
secondary diabetes mellitus NEC (E13.-)
type 1 diabetes mellitus (E10.-)
type 2 diabetes mellitus (E11.-)

✓5th E08.0 **Diabetes mellitus due to underlying condition with hyperosmolarity**
E08.00 **Diabetes mellitus due to underlying condition with hyperosmolarity without nonketotic hyperglycemic-hyperosmolar coma (NKHHC)**
E08.01 **Diabetes mellitus due to underlying condition with hyperosmolarity with coma**

✓5th E08.1 **Diabetes mellitus due to underlying condition with ketoacidosis**
E08.10 **Diabetes mellitus due to underlying condition with ketoacidosis without coma**
E08.11 **Diabetes mellitus due to underlying condition with ketoacidosis with coma**

✓5th E08.2 **Diabetes mellitus due to underlying condition with kidney complications**
E08.21 **Diabetes mellitus due to underlying condition with diabetic nephropathy**
Diabetes mellitus due to underlying condition with intercapillary glomerulosclerosis
Diabetes mellitus due to underlying condition with intracapillary glomerulonephrosis
Diabetes mellitus due to underlying condition with Kimmelstiel-Wilson disease

E08.22 **Diabetes mellitus due to underlying condition with diabetic chronic kidney disease**
Diabetes mellitus due to underlying condition with chronic kidney disease due to conditions classified to .21 and .22
Use additional code to identify stage of chronic kidney disease (N18.1-N18.6)

E08.29 **Diabetes mellitus due to underlying condition with other diabetic kidney complication**
Renal tubular degeneration in diabetes mellitus due to underlying condition

✓5th E08.3 **Diabetes mellitus due to underlying condition with ophthalmic complications**
✓6th E08.31 **Diabetes mellitus due to underlying condition with unspecified diabetic retinopathy**
E08.311 **Diabetes mellitus due to underlying condition with unspecified diabetic retinopathy with macular edema**
E08.319 **Diabetes mellitus due to underlying condition with unspecified diabetic retinopathy without macular edema**
✓6th E08.32 **Diabetes mellitus due to underlying condition with mild nonproliferative diabetic retinopathy**
Diabetes mellitus due to underlying condition with nonproliferative diabetic retinopathy NOS
E08.321 **Diabetes mellitus due to underlying condition with mild nonproliferative diabetic retinopathy with macular edema**
E08.329 **Diabetes mellitus due to underlying condition with mild nonproliferative diabetic retinopathy without macular edema**
✓6th E08.33 **Diabetes mellitus due to underlying condition with moderate nonproliferative diabetic retinopathy**
E08.331 **Diabetes mellitus due to underlying condition with moderate nonproliferative diabetic retinopathy with macular edema**
E08.339 **Diabetes mellitus due to underlying condition with moderate nonproliferative diabetic retinopathy without macular edema**
✓6th E08.34 **Diabetes mellitus due to underlying condition with severe nonproliferative diabetic retinopathy**
E08.341 **Diabetes mellitus due to underlying condition with severe nonproliferative diabetic retinopathy with macular edema**
E08.349 **Diabetes mellitus due to underlying condition with severe nonproliferative diabetic retinopathy without macular edema**
✓6th E08.35 **Diabetes mellitus due to underlying condition with proliferative diabetic retinopathy**
E08.351 **Diabetes mellitus due to underlying condition with proliferative diabetic retinopathy with macular edema**
E08.359 **Diabetes mellitus due to underlying condition with proliferative diabetic retinopathy without macular edema**
E08.36 **Diabetes mellitus due to underlying condition with diabetic cataract**
E08.39 **Diabetes mellitus due to underlying condition with other diabetic ophthalmic complication**

✓5th E08.4 **Diabetes mellitus due to underlying condition with neurological complications**
E08.40 **Diabetes mellitus due to underlying condition with diabetic neuropathy, unspecified**
E08.41 **Diabetes mellitus due to underlying condition with diabetic mononeuropathy**
E08.42 **Diabetes mellitus due to underlying condition with diabetic polyneuropathy**
Diabetes mellitus due to underlying condition with diabetic neuralgia
E08.43 **Diabetes mellitus due to underlying condition with diabetic autonomic (poly)neuropathy**
Diabetes mellitus due to underlying condition with diabetic gastroparesis

---

☑ Appropriate additional character required   ✓x7th Requires 7th character, placeholder x must fill empty characters

Endocrine, Nutritional and Metabolic Diseases

E08.44–E09.349

E08.44   **Diabetes mellitus due to underlying condition with diabetic amyotrophy**

E08.49   **Diabetes mellitus due to underlying condition with other diabetic neurological complication**

✓5ᵗʰ   E08.5   **Diabetes mellitus due to underlying condition with circulatory complications**

E08.51   **Diabetes mellitus due to underlying condition with diabetic peripheral angiopathy without gangrene**

E08.52   **Diabetes mellitus due to underlying condition with diabetic peripheral angiopathy with gangrene**
Diabetes mellitus due to underlying condition with diabetic gangrene

E08.59   **Diabetes mellitus due to underlying condition with other circulatory complications**

✓5ᵗʰ   E08.6   **Diabetes mellitus due to underlying condition with other specified complications**

✓6ᵗʰ   E08.61   **Diabetes mellitus due to underlying condition with diabetic arthropathy**

E08.610   **Diabetes mellitus due to underlying condition with diabetic neuropathic arthropathy**
Diabetes mellitus due to underlying condition with Charcôt's joints

E08.618   **Diabetes mellitus due to underlying condition with other diabetic arthropathy**

✓6ᵗʰ   E08.62   **Diabetes mellitus due to underlying condition with skin complications**

E08.620   **Diabetes mellitus due to underlying condition with diabetic dermatitis**
Diabetes mellitus due to underlying condition with diabetic necrobiosis lipoidica

E08.621   **Diabetes mellitus due to underlying condition with foot ulcer**
Use additional code to identify site of ulcer (L97.4-, L97.5-)

E08.622   **Diabetes mellitus due to underlying condition with other skin ulcer**
Use additional code to identify site of ulcer (L97.1-L97.9, L98.41-L98.49)

E08.628   **Diabetes mellitus due to underlying condition with other skin complications**

✓6ᵗʰ   E08.63   **Diabetes mellitus due to underlying condition with oral complications**

E08.630   **Diabetes mellitus due to underlying condition with periodontal disease**

E08.638   **Diabetes mellitus due to underlying condition with other oral complications**

✓6ᵗʰ   E08.64   **Diabetes mellitus due to underlying condition with hypoglycemia**

E08.641   **Diabetes mellitus due to underlying condition with hypoglycemia with coma**

E08.649   **Diabetes mellitus due to underlying condition with hypoglycemia without coma**

E08.65   **Diabetes mellitus due to underlying condition with hyperglycemia**

E08.69   **Diabetes mellitus due to underlying condition with other specified complication**
Use additional code to identify complication

E08.8   **Diabetes mellitus due to underlying condition with unspecified complications**

E08.9   **Diabetes mellitus due to underlying condition without complications**

✓4ᵗʰ   **E09   Drug or chemical induced diabetes mellitus**
Code first (T36-T65) to identify drug or chemical
Use additional code to identify any insulin use (Z79.4)
EXCLUDES 1   *diabetes mellitus due to underlying condition (E08.-)*
gestational diabetes (O24.4-)
neonatal diabetes mellitus (P70.2)
postpancreatectomy diabetes mellitus (E13.-)
postprocedural diabetes mellitus (E13.-)
secondary diabetes mellitus NEC (E13.-)
type 1 diabetes mellitus (E10.-)
type 2 diabetes mellitus (E11.-)

✓5ᵗʰ   E09.0   **Drug or chemical induced diabetes mellitus with hyperosmolarity**

E09.00   **Drug or chemical induced diabetes mellitus with hyperosmolarity without nonketotic hyperglycemic-hyperosmolar coma (NKHHC)**

E09.01   **Drug or chemical induced diabetes mellitus with hyperosmolarity with coma**

✓5ᵗʰ   E09.1   **Drug or chemical induced diabetes mellitus with ketoacidosis**

E09.10   **Drug or chemical induced diabetes mellitus with ketoacidosis without coma**

E09.11   **Drug or chemical induced diabetes mellitus with ketoacidosis with coma**

✓5ᵗʰ   E09.2   **Drug or chemical induced diabetes mellitus with kidney complications**

E09.21   **Drug or chemical induced diabetes mellitus with diabetic nephropathy**
Drug or chemical induced diabetes mellitus with intercapillary glomerulosclerosis
Drug or chemical induced diabetes mellitus with intracapillary glomerulonephrosis
Drug or chemical induced diabetes mellitus with Kimmelstiel-Wilson disease

E09.22   **Drug or chemical induced diabetes mellitus with diabetic chronic kidney disease**
Drug or chemical induced diabetes mellitus with chronic kidney disease due to conditions classified to .21 and .22
Use additional code to identify stage of chronic kidney disease (N18.1-N18.6)

E09.29   **Drug or chemical induced diabetes mellitus with other diabetic kidney complication**
Drug or chemical induced diabetes mellitus with renal tubular degeneration

✓5ᵗʰ   E09.3   **Drug or chemical induced diabetes mellitus with ophthalmic complications**

✓6ᵗʰ   E09.31   **Drug or chemical induced diabetes mellitus with unspecified diabetic retinopathy**

E09.311   **Drug or chemical induced diabetes mellitus with unspecified diabetic retinopathy with macular edema**

E09.319   **Drug or chemical induced diabetes mellitus with unspecified diabetic retinopathy without macular edema**

✓6ᵗʰ   E09.32   **Drug or chemical induced diabetes mellitus with mild nonproliferative diabetic retinopathy**
Drug or chemical induced diabetes mellitus with nonproliferative diabetic retinopathy NOS

E09.321   **Drug or chemical induced diabetes mellitus with mild nonproliferative diabetic retinopathy with macular edema**

E09.329   **Drug or chemical induced diabetes mellitus with mild nonproliferative diabetic retinopathy without macular edema**

✓6ᵗʰ   E09.33   **Drug or chemical induced diabetes mellitus with moderate nonproliferative diabetic retinopathy**

E09.331   **Drug or chemical induced diabetes mellitus with moderate nonproliferative diabetic retinopathy with macular edema**

E09.339   **Drug or chemical induced diabetes mellitus with moderate nonproliferative diabetic retinopathy without macular edema**

✓6ᵗʰ   E09.34   **Drug or chemical induced diabetes mellitus with severe nonproliferative diabetic retinopathy**

E09.341   **Drug or chemical induced diabetes mellitus with severe nonproliferative diabetic retinopathy with macular edema**

E09.349   **Drug or chemical induced diabetes mellitus with severe nonproliferative diabetic retinopathy without macular edema**

✓6th E09.35 Drug or chemical induced diabetes mellitus with proliferative diabetic retinopathy
    E09.351 Drug or chemical induced diabetes mellitus with proliferative diabetic retinopathy with macular edema
    E09.359 Drug or chemical induced diabetes mellitus with proliferative diabetic retinopathy without macular edema
    E09.36 Drug or chemical induced diabetes mellitus with diabetic cataract
    E09.39 Drug or chemical induced diabetes mellitus with other diabetic ophthalmic complication

✓5th E09.4 Drug or chemical induced diabetes mellitus with neurological complications
    E09.40 Drug or chemical induced diabetes mellitus with neurological complications with diabetic neuropathy, unspecified
    E09.41 Drug or chemical induced diabetes mellitus with neurological complications with diabetic mononeuropathy
    E09.42 Drug or chemical induced diabetes mellitus with neurological complications with diabetic polyneuropathy
      Drug or chemical induced diabetes mellitus with diabetic neuralgia
    E09.43 Drug or chemical induced diabetes mellitus with neurological complications with diabetic autonomic (poly)neuropathy
      Drug or chemical induced diabetes mellitus with diabetic gastroparesis
    E09.44 Drug or chemical induced diabetes mellitus with neurological complications with diabetic amyotrophy
    E09.49 Drug or chemical induced diabetes mellitus with neurological complications with other diabetic neurological complication

✓5th E09.5 Drug or chemical induced diabetes mellitus with circulatory complications
    E09.51 Drug or chemical induced diabetes mellitus with diabetic peripheral angiopathy without gangrene
    E09.52 Drug or chemical induced diabetes mellitus with diabetic peripheral angiopathy with gangrene
      Drug or chemical induced diabetes mellitus with diabetic gangrene
    E09.59 Drug or chemical induced diabetes mellitus with other circulatory complications

✓5th E09.6 Drug or chemical induced diabetes mellitus with other specified complications
    ✓6th E09.61 Drug or chemical induced diabetes mellitus with diabetic arthropathy
      E09.610 Drug or chemical induced diabetes mellitus with diabetic neuropathic arthropathy
        Drug or chemical induced diabetes mellitus with Charcôt's joints
      E09.618 Drug or chemical induced diabetes mellitus with other diabetic arthropathy
    ✓6th E09.62 Drug or chemical induced diabetes mellitus with skin complications
      E09.620 Drug or chemical induced diabetes mellitus with diabetic dermatitis
        Drug or chemical induced diabetes mellitus with diabetic necrobiosis lipoidica
      E09.621 Drug or chemical induced diabetes mellitus with foot ulcer
        Use additional code to identify site of ulcer (L97.4-, L97.5-)
      E09.622 Drug or chemical induced diabetes mellitus with other skin ulcer
        Use additional code to identify site of ulcer (L97.1-L97.9, L98.41-L98.49)
      E09.628 Drug or chemical induced diabetes mellitus with other skin complications
    ✓6th E09.63 Drug or chemical induced diabetes mellitus with oral complications
      E09.630 Drug or chemical induced diabetes mellitus with periodontal disease

      E09.638 Drug or chemical induced diabetes mellitus with other oral complications
    ✓6th E09.64 Drug or chemical induced diabetes mellitus with hypoglycemia
      E09.641 Drug or chemical induced diabetes mellitus with hypoglycemia with coma
      E09.649 Drug or chemical induced diabetes mellitus with hypoglycemia without coma
    E09.65 Drug or chemical induced diabetes mellitus with hyperglycemia
    E09.69 Drug or chemical induced diabetes mellitus with other specified complication
      Use additional code to identify complication

E09.8 Drug or chemical induced diabetes mellitus with unspecified complications

E09.9 Drug or chemical induced diabetes mellitus without complications

✓4th E10 Type 1 diabetes mellitus
    INCLUDES   brittle diabetes (mellitus)
        diabetes (mellitus) due to autoimmune process
        diabetes (mellitus) due to immune mediated pancreatic islet beta-cell destruction
        idiopathic diabetes (mellitus)
        juvenile onset diabetes (mellitus)
        ketosis-prone diabetes (mellitus)
    EXCLUDES 1   *diabetes mellitus due to underlying condition (E08.-)*
        drug or chemical induced diabetes mellitus (E09.-)
        gestational diabetes (O24.4-)
        hyperglycemia NOS (R73.9)
        neonatal diabetes mellitus (P70.2)
        postpancreatectomy diabetes mellitus (E13.-)
        postprocedural diabetes mellitus (E13.-)
        secondary diabetes mellitus NEC (E13.-)
        type 2 diabetes mellitus (E11.-)

✓5th E10.1 Type 1 diabetes mellitus with ketoacidosis
    E10.10 Type 1 diabetes mellitus with ketoacidosis without coma
    E10.11 Type 1 diabetes mellitus with ketoacidosis with coma

✓5th E10.2 Type 1 diabetes mellitus with kidney complications
    E10.21 Type 1 diabetes mellitus with diabetic nephropathy
      Type 1 diabetes mellitus with intercapillary glomerulosclerosis
      Type 1 diabetes mellitus with intracapillary glomerulonephrosis
      Type 1 diabetes mellitus with Kimmelstiel-Wilson disease
    E10.22 Type 1 diabetes mellitus with diabetic chronic kidney disease
      Type 1 diabetes mellitus with chronic kidney disease due to conditions classified to .21 and .22
      Use additional code to identify stage of chronic kidney disease (N18.1-N18.6)
    E10.29 Type 1 diabetes mellitus with other diabetic kidney complication
      Type 1 diabetes mellitus with renal tubular degeneration

✓5th E10.3 Type 1 diabetes mellitus with ophthalmic complications
    ✓6th E10.31 Type 1 diabetes mellitus with unspecified diabetic retinopathy
      E10.311 Type 1 diabetes mellitus with unspecified diabetic retinopathy with macular edema
      E10.319 Type 1 diabetes mellitus with unspecified diabetic retinopathy without macular edema
    ✓6th E10.32 Type 1 diabetes mellitus with mild nonproliferative diabetic retinopathy
      Type 1 diabetes mellitus with nonproliferative diabetic retinopathy NOS
      E10.321 Type 1 diabetes mellitus with mild nonproliferative diabetic retinopathy with macular edema
      E10.329 Type 1 diabetes mellitus with mild nonproliferative diabetic retinopathy without macular edema

---

✔ Appropriate additional character required   ✓x7th Requires 7th character, placeholder x must fill empty characters

✓6th **E10.33** **Type 1 diabetes mellitus with moderate nonproliferative diabetic retinopathy**

     E10.331 Type 1 diabetes mellitus with moderate nonproliferative diabetic retinopathy with macular edema

     E10.339 Type 1 diabetes mellitus with moderate nonproliferative diabetic retinopathy without macular edema

✓6th **E10.34** **Type 1 diabetes mellitus with severe nonproliferative diabetic retinopathy**

     E10.341 Type 1 diabetes mellitus with severe nonproliferative diabetic retinopathy with macular edema

     E10.349 Type 1 diabetes mellitus with severe nonproliferative diabetic retinopathy without macular edema

✓6th **E10.35** **Type 1 diabetes mellitus with proliferative diabetic retinopathy**

     E10.351 Type 1 diabetes mellitus with proliferative diabetic retinopathy with macular edema

     E10.359 Type 1 diabetes mellitus with proliferative diabetic retinopathy without macular edema

     E10.36 **Type 1 diabetes mellitus with diabetic cataract**

     E10.39 **Type 1 diabetes mellitus with other diabetic ophthalmic complication**

✓5th **E10.4** **Type 1 diabetes mellitus with neurological complications**

     E10.40 **Type 1 diabetes mellitus with diabetic neuropathy, unspecified**

     E10.41 **Type 1 diabetes mellitus with diabetic mononeuropathy**

     E10.42 **Type 1 diabetes mellitus with diabetic polyneuropathy**

         Type 1 diabetes mellitus with diabetic neuralgia

     E10.43 **Type 1 diabetes mellitus with diabetic autonomic (poly)neuropathy**

         Type 1 diabetes mellitus with diabetic gastroparesis

     E10.44 **Type 1 diabetes mellitus with diabetic amyotrophy**

     E10.49 **Type 1 diabetes mellitus with other diabetic neurological complication**

✓5th **E10.5** **Type 1 diabetes mellitus with circulatory complications**

     E10.51 **Type 1 diabetes mellitus with diabetic peripheral angiopathy without gangrene**

     E10.52 **Type 1 diabetes mellitus with diabetic peripheral angiopathy with gangrene**

         Type 1 diabetes mellitus with diabetic gangrene

     E10.59 **Type 1 diabetes mellitus with other circulatory complications**

✓5th **E10.6** **Type 1 diabetes mellitus with other specified complications**

     ✓6th **E10.61** **Type 1 diabetes mellitus with diabetic arthropathy**

         E10.610 **Type 1 diabetes mellitus with diabetic neuropathic arthropathy**

             Type 1 diabetes mellitus with Charcôt's joints

         E10.618 **Type 1 diabetes mellitus with other diabetic arthropathy**

     ✓6th **E10.62** **Type 1 diabetes mellitus with skin complications**

         E10.620 **Type 1 diabetes mellitus with diabetic dermatitis**

             Type 1 diabetes mellitus with diabetic necrobiosis lipoidica

         E10.621 **Type 1 diabetes mellitus with foot ulcer**

             Use additional code to identify site of ulcer (L97.4-, L97.5-)

         E10.622 **Type 1 diabetes mellitus with other skin ulcer**

             Use additional code to identify site of ulcer (L97.1-L97.9, L98.41-L98.49)

         E10.628 **Type 1 diabetes mellitus with other skin complications**

     ✓6th **E10.63** **Type 1 diabetes mellitus with oral complications**

         E10.630 **Type 1 diabetes mellitus with periodontal disease**

         E10.638 **Type 1 diabetes mellitus with other oral complications**

✓6th **E10.64** **Type 1 diabetes mellitus with hypoglycemia**

     E10.641 **Type 1 diabetes mellitus with hypoglycemia with coma**

     E10.649 **Type 1 diabetes mellitus with hypoglycemia without coma**

     E10.65 **Type 1 diabetes mellitus with hyperglycemia**

     E10.69 **Type 1 diabetes mellitus with other specified complication**

         Use additional code to identify complication

     E10.8 **Type 1 diabetes mellitus with unspecified complications**

     E10.9 **Type 1 diabetes mellitus without complications**

✓4th **E11** **Type 2 diabetes mellitus**

     INCLUDES   diabetes (mellitus) due to insulin secretory defect
                diabetes NOS
                insulin resistant diabetes (mellitus)

     Use additional code to identify any insulin use (Z79.4)

     EXCLUDES 1   *diabetes mellitus due to underlying condition (E08.-)*
                drug or chemical induced diabetes mellitus (E09.-)
                gestational diabetes (O24.4-)
                neonatal diabetes mellitus (P70.2)
                postpancreatectomy diabetes mellitus (E13.-)
                postprocedural diabetes mellitus (E13.-)
                secondary diabetes mellitus NEC (E13.-)
                type 1 diabetes mellitus (E10.-)

✓5th **E11.0** **Type 2 diabetes mellitus with hyperosmolarity**

     E11.00 **Type 2 diabetes mellitus with hyperosmolarity without nonketotic hyperglycemic-hyperosmolar coma (NKHHC)**

     E11.01 **Type 2 diabetes mellitus with hyperosmolarity with coma**

✓5th **E11.2** **Type 2 diabetes mellitus with kidney complications**

     E11.21 **Type 2 diabetes mellitus with diabetic nephropathy**

         Type 2 diabetes mellitus with intercapillary glomerulosclerosis
         Type 2 diabetes mellitus with intracapillary glomerulonephrosis
         Type 2 diabetes mellitus with Kimmelstiel-Wilson disease

     E11.22 **Type 2 diabetes mellitus with diabetic chronic kidney disease**

         Type 2 diabetes mellitus with chronic kidney disease due to conditions classified to .21 and .22
         Use additional code to identify stage of chronic kidney disease (N18.1-N18.6)

     E11.29 **Type 2 diabetes mellitus with other diabetic kidney complication**

         Type 2 diabetes mellitus with renal tubular degeneration

✓5th **E11.3** **Type 2 diabetes mellitus with ophthalmic complications**

     ✓6th **E11.31** **Type 2 diabetes mellitus with unspecified diabetic retinopathy**

         E11.311 **Type 2 diabetes mellitus with unspecified diabetic retinopathy with macular edema**

         E11.319 **Type 2 diabetes mellitus with unspecified diabetic retinopathy without macular edema**

     ✓6th **E11.32** **Type 2 diabetes mellitus with mild nonproliferative diabetic retinopathy**

         Type 2 diabetes mellitus with nonproliferative diabetic retinopathy NOS

         E11.321 **Type 2 diabetes mellitus with mild nonproliferative diabetic retinopathy with macular edema**

         E11.329 **Type 2 diabetes mellitus with mild nonproliferative diabetic retinopathy without macular edema**

     ✓6th **E11.33** **Type 2 diabetes mellitus with moderate nonproliferative diabetic retinopathy**

         E11.331 **Type 2 diabetes mellitus with moderate nonproliferative diabetic retinopathy with macular edema**

         E11.339 **Type 2 diabetes mellitus with moderate nonproliferative diabetic retinopathy without macular edema**

EXCLUDES 1   Not coded here   EXCLUDES 2   Not included here   *Manifestation Code*

✓6th **E11.34 Type 2 diabetes mellitus with severe nonproliferative diabetic retinopathy**

    E11.341 Type 2 diabetes mellitus with severe nonproliferative diabetic retinopathy with macular edema

    E11.349 Type 2 diabetes mellitus with severe nonproliferative diabetic retinopathy without macular edema

✓6th **E11.35 Type 2 diabetes mellitus with proliferative diabetic retinopathy**

    E11.351 Type 2 diabetes mellitus with proliferative diabetic retinopathy with macular edema

    E11.359 Type 2 diabetes mellitus with proliferative diabetic retinopathy without macular edema

E11.36 Type 2 diabetes mellitus with diabetic cataract

E11.39 Type 2 diabetes mellitus with other diabetic ophthalmic complication

✓5th **E11.4 Type 2 diabetes mellitus with neurological complications**

E11.40 Type 2 diabetes mellitus with diabetic neuropathy, unspecified

E11.41 Type 2 diabetes mellitus with diabetic mononeuropathy

E11.42 Type 2 diabetes mellitus with diabetic polyneuropathy
    Type 2 diabetes mellitus with diabetic neuralgia

E11.43 Type 2 diabetes mellitus with diabetic autonomic (poly)neuropathy
    Type 2 diabetes mellitus with diabetic gastroparesis

E11.44 Type 2 diabetes mellitus with diabetic amyotrophy

E11.49 Type 2 diabetes mellitus with other diabetic neurological complication

✓5th **E11.5 Type 2 diabetes mellitus with circulatory complications**

E11.51 Type 2 diabetes mellitus with diabetic peripheral angiopathy without gangrene

E11.52 Type 2 diabetes mellitus with diabetic peripheral angiopathy with gangrene
    Type 2 diabetes mellitus with diabetic gangrene

E11.59 Type 2 diabetes mellitus with other circulatory complications

✓5th **E11.6 Type 2 diabetes mellitus with other specified complications**

✓6th **E11.61 Type 2 diabetes mellitus with diabetic arthropathy**

    E11.610 Type 2 diabetes mellitus with diabetic neuropathic arthropathy
      Type 2 diabetes mellitus with Charcôt's joints

    E11.618 Type 2 diabetes mellitus with other diabetic arthropathy

✓6th **E11.62 Type 2 diabetes mellitus with skin complications**

    E11.620 Type 2 diabetes mellitus with diabetic dermatitis
      Type 2 diabetes mellitus with diabetic necrobiosis lipoidica

    E11.621 Type 2 diabetes mellitus with foot ulcer
      Use additional code to identify site of ulcer (L97.4-, L97.5-)

    E11.622 Type 2 diabetes mellitus with other skin ulcer
      Use additional code to identify site of ulcer (L97.1-L97.9, L98.41-L98.49)

    E11.628 Type 2 diabetes mellitus with other skin complications

✓6th **E11.63 Type 2 diabetes mellitus with oral complications**

    E11.630 Type 2 diabetes mellitus with periodontal disease

    E11.638 Type 2 diabetes mellitus with other oral complications

✓6th **E11.64 Type 2 diabetes mellitus with hypoglycemia**

    E11.641 Type 2 diabetes mellitus with hypoglycemia with coma

    E11.649 Type 2 diabetes mellitus with hypoglycemia without coma

E11.65 Type 2 diabetes mellitus with hyperglycemia

E11.69 Type 2 diabetes mellitus with other specified complication
    Use additional code to identify complication

E11.8 Type 2 diabetes mellitus with unspecified complications

E11.9 Type 2 diabetes mellitus without complications

✓4th **E13 Other specified diabetes mellitus**
    Diabetes mellitus due to genetic defects of beta-cell function
    Diabetes mellitus due to genetic defects in insulin action
    Postpancreatectomy diabetes mellitus
    Postprocedural diabetes mellitus
    Secondary diabetes mellitus NEC
    Use additional code to identify any insulin use (Z79.4)

    EXCLUDES 1 *diabetes (mellitus) due to autoimmune process (E10-)*
      diabetes (mellitus) due to immune mediated pancreatic islet beta-cell destruction (E10-)
      diabetes mellitus due to underlying condition (E08-)
      drug or chemical induced diabetes mellitus (E09-)
      gestational diabetes (O24.4-)
      neonatal diabetes mellitus (P70.2)
      type 2 diabetes mellitus (E11-)

✓5th **E13.0 Other specified diabetes mellitus with hyperosmolarity**

    E13.00 Other specified diabetes mellitus with hyperosmolarity without nonketotic hyperglycemic-hyperosmolar coma (NKHHC)

    E13.01 Other specified diabetes mellitus with hyperosmolarity with coma

✓5th **E13.1 Other specified diabetes mellitus with ketoacidosis**

    E13.10 Other specified diabetes mellitus with ketoacidosis without coma

    E13.11 Other specified diabetes mellitus with ketoacidosis with coma

✓5th **E13.2 Other specified diabetes mellitus with kidney complications**

    E13.21 Other specified diabetes mellitus with diabetic nephropathy
      Other specified diabetes mellitus with intercapillary glomerulosclerosis
      Other specified diabetes mellitus with intracapillary glomerulonephrosis
      Other specified diabetes mellitus with Kimmelstiel-Wilson disease

    E13.22 Other specified diabetes mellitus with diabetic chronic kidney disease
      Other specified diabetes mellitus with chronic kidney disease due to conditions classified to .21 and .22
      Use additional code to identify stage of chronic kidney disease (N18.1-N18.6)

    E13.29 Other specified diabetes mellitus with other diabetic kidney complication
      Other specified diabetes mellitus with renal tubular degeneration

✓5th **E13.3 Other specified diabetes mellitus with ophthalmic complications**

    ✓6th **E13.31 Other specified diabetes mellitus with unspecified diabetic retinopathy**

      E13.311 Other specified diabetes mellitus with unspecified diabetic retinopathy with macular edema

      E13.319 Other specified diabetes mellitus with unspecified diabetic retinopathy without macular edema

    ✓6th **E13.32 Other specified diabetes mellitus with mild nonproliferative diabetic retinopathy**
      Other specified diabetes mellitus with nonproliferative diabetic retinopathy NOS

      E13.321 Other specified diabetes mellitus with mild nonproliferative diabetic retinopathy with macular edema

      E13.329 Other specified diabetes mellitus with mild nonproliferative diabetic retinopathy without macular edema

    ✓6th **E13.33 Other specified diabetes mellitus with moderate nonproliferative diabetic retinopathy**

      E13.331 Other specified diabetes mellitus with moderate nonproliferative diabetic retinopathy with macular edema

      E13.339 Other specified diabetes mellitus with moderate nonproliferative diabetic retinopathy without macular edema

Endocrine, Nutritional and Metabolic Diseases

E13.34–E21.0

√6ᵗʰ **E13.34** **Other specified diabetes mellitus with severe nonproliferative diabetic retinopathy**

E13.341 Other specified diabetes mellitus with severe nonproliferative diabetic retinopathy with macular edema

E13.349 Other specified diabetes mellitus with severe nonproliferative diabetic retinopathy without macular edema

√6ᵗʰ **E13.35** **Other specified diabetes mellitus with proliferative diabetic retinopathy**

E13.351 Other specified diabetes mellitus with proliferative diabetic retinopathy with macular edema

E13.359 Other specified diabetes mellitus with proliferative diabetic retinopathy without macular edema

E13.36 **Other specified diabetes mellitus with diabetic cataract**

E13.39 **Other specified diabetes mellitus with other diabetic ophthalmic complication**

√5ᵗʰ **E13.4** **Other specified diabetes mellitus with neurological complications**

E13.40 **Other specified diabetes mellitus with diabetic neuropathy, unspecified**

E13.41 **Other specified diabetes mellitus with diabetic mononeuropathy**

E13.42 **Other specified diabetes mellitus with diabetic polyneuropathy**
Other specified diabetes mellitus with diabetic neuralgia

E13.43 **Other specified diabetes mellitus with diabetic autonomic (poly)neuropathy**
Other specified diabetes mellitus with diabetic gastroparesis

E13.44 **Other specified diabetes mellitus with diabetic amyotrophy**

E13.49 **Other specified diabetes mellitus with other diabetic neurological complication**

√5ᵗʰ **E13.5** **Other specified diabetes mellitus with circulatory complications**

E13.51 **Other specified diabetes mellitus with diabetic peripheral angiopathy without gangrene**

E13.52 **Other specified diabetes mellitus with diabetic peripheral angiopathy with gangrene**
Other specified diabetes mellitus with diabetic gangrene

E13.59 **Other specified diabetes mellitus with other circulatory complications**

√5ᵗʰ **E13.6** **Other specified diabetes mellitus with other specified complications**

√6ᵗʰ **E13.61** **Other specified diabetes mellitus with diabetic arthropathy**

E13.610 **Other specified diabetes mellitus with diabetic neuropathic arthropathy**
Other specified diabetes mellitus with Charcôt's joints

E13.618 **Other specified diabetes mellitus with other diabetic arthropathy**

√6ᵗʰ **E13.62** **Other specified diabetes mellitus with skin complications**

E13.620 **Other specified diabetes mellitus with diabetic dermatitis**
Other specified diabetes mellitus with diabetic necrobiosis lipoidica

E13.621 **Other specified diabetes mellitus with foot ulcer**
Use additional code to identify site of ulcer (L97.4-, L97.5-)

E13.622 **Other specified diabetes mellitus with other skin ulcer**
Use additional code to identify site of ulcer (L97.1-L97.9, L98.41-L98.49)

E13.628 **Other specified diabetes mellitus with other skin complications**

√6ᵗʰ **E13.63** **Other specified diabetes mellitus with oral complications**

E13.630 **Other specified diabetes mellitus with periodontal disease**

E13.638 **Other specified diabetes mellitus with other oral complications**

√6ᵗʰ **E13.64** **Other specified diabetes mellitus with hypoglycemia**

E13.641 **Other specified diabetes mellitus with hypoglycemia with coma**

E13.649 **Other specified diabetes mellitus with hypoglycemia without coma**

E13.65 **Other specified diabetes mellitus with hyperglycemia**

E13.69 **Other specified diabetes mellitus with other specified complication**
Use additional code to identify complication

E13.8 **Other specified diabetes mellitus with unspecified complications**

E13.9 **Other specified diabetes mellitus without complications**

Other disorders of glucose regulation and pancreatic internal secretion (E15-E16)

E15 **Nondiabetic hypoglycemic coma**
INCLUDES drug-induced insulin coma in nondiabetic
hyperinsulinism with hypoglycemic coma
hypoglycemic coma NOS

√4ᵗʰ **E16** **Other disorders of pancreatic internal secretion**

E16.0 **Drug-induced hypoglycemia without coma**
Code first (T36-T50) to identify drug

E16.1 **Other hypoglycemia**
Functional hyperinsulinism
Functional nonhyperinsulinemic hypoglycemia
Hyperinsulinism NOS
Hyperplasia of pancreatic islet beta cells NOS
EXCLUDES 1 *hypoglycemia in infant of diabetic mother (P70.1)*
neonatal hypoglycemia (P70.4)

E16.2 **Hypoglycemia, unspecified**

E16.3 **Increased secretion of glucagon**
Hyperplasia of pancreatic endocrine cells with glucagon excess

E16.4 **Increased secretion of gastrin**
Hypergastrinemia
Hyperplasia of pancreatic endocrine cells with gastrin excess
Zollinger-Ellison syndrome

E16.8 **Other specified disorders of pancreatic internal secretion**
Increased secretion from endocrine pancreas of growth hormone-releasing hormone
Increased secretion from endocrine pancreas of pancreatic polypeptide
Increased secretion from endocrine pancreas of somatostatin
Increased secretion from endocrine pancreas of vasoactive-intestinal polypeptide

E16.9 **Disorder of pancreatic internal secretion, unspecified**
Islet-cell hyperplasia NOS
Pancreatic endocrine cell hyperplasia NOS

Disorders of other endocrine glands (E20-E35)

EXCLUDES 1 *galactorrhea (N64.3)*
gynecomastia (N62)

√4ᵗʰ **E20** **Hypoparathyroidism**
EXCLUDES 1 *Di George's syndrome (D82.1)*
postprocedural hypoparathyroidism (E89.2)
tetany NOS (R29.0)
transitory neonatal hypoparathyroidism (P71.4)

E20.0 **Idiopathic hypoparathyroidism**

E20.1 **Pseudohypoparathyroidism**

E20.8 **Other hypoparathyroidism**

E20.9 **Hypoparathyroidism, unspecified**
Parathyroid tetany

√4ᵗʰ **E21** **Hyperparathyroidism and other disorders of parathyroid gland**
EXCLUDES 1 *adult osteomalacia (M83-)*
ectopic hyperparathyroidism (E34.2)
familial hypocalciuric hypercalcemia (E83.52)
hungry bone syndrome (E83.81)
infantile and juvenile osteomalacia (E55.0)

E21.0 **Primary hyperparathyroidism**
Hyperplasia of parathyroid
Osteitis fibrosa cystica generalisata [von Recklinghausen's disease of bone]

EXCLUDES 1 Not coded here   EXCLUDES 2 Not included here   *Manifestation Code*

E21.1 Secondary hyperparathyroidism, not elsewhere classified
EXCLUDES 1 secondary hyperparathyroidism of renal origin (N25.81)

E21.2 Other hyperparathyroidism
Tertiary hyperparathyroidism
EXCLUDES 1 familial hypocalciuric hypercalcemia (E83.52)

E21.3 Hyperparathyroidism, unspecified

E21.4 Other specified disorders of parathyroid gland

E21.5 Disorder of parathyroid gland, unspecified

☑4th **E22** Hyperfunction of pituitary gland
EXCLUDES 1 Cushing's syndrome (E24-)
Nelson's syndrome (E24.1)
overproduction of ACTH not associated with Cushing's disease (E27.0)
overproduction of pituitary ACTH (E24.0)
overproduction of thyroid-stimulating hormone (E05.8-)

E22.0 Acromegaly and pituitary gigantism
Overproduction of growth hormone
EXCLUDES 1 constitutional gigantism (E34.4)
constitutional tall stature (E34.4)
increased secretion from endocrine pancreas of growth hormone-releasing hormone (E16.8)

E22.1 Hyperprolactinemia

E22.2 Syndrome of inappropriate secretion of antidiuretic hormone

E22.8 Other hyperfunction of pituitary gland
Central precocious puberty

E22.9 Hyperfunction of pituitary gland, unspecified

☑4th **E23** Hypofunction and other disorders of the pituitary gland
INCLUDES the listed conditions whether the disorder is in the pituitary or the hypothalamus
EXCLUDES 1 postprocedural hypopituitarism (E89.3)

E23.0 Hypopituitarism
Fertile eunuch syndrome
Hypogonadotropic hypogonadism
Idiopathic growth hormone deficiency
Isolated deficiency of gonadotropin
Isolated deficiency of growth hormone
Isolated deficiency of pituitary hormone
Kallmann's syndrome
Lorain-Levi short stature
Necrosis of pituitary gland (postpartum)
Panhypopituitarism
Pituitary cachexia
Pituitary insufficiency NOS
Pituitary short stature
Sheehan's syndrome
Simmonds' disease

E23.1 Drug-induced hypopituitarism
Code first (T36-T50) to identify drug

E23.2 Diabetes insipidus
EXCLUDES 1 nephrogenic diabetes insipidus (N25.1)

E23.3 Hypothalamic dysfunction, not elsewhere classified
EXCLUDES 1 Prader-Willi syndrome (Q87.1)
Russell-Silver syndrome (Q87.1)

E23.6 Other disorders of pituitary gland
Abscess of pituitary
Adiposogenital dystrophy

E23.7 Disorder of pituitary gland, unspecified

☑4th **E24** Cushing's syndrome
EXCLUDES 1 congenital adrenal hyperplasia (E25.0)

E24.0 Pituitary-dependent Cushing's disease
Overproduction of pituitary ACTH
Pituitary-dependent hypercorticalism

E24.1 Nelson's syndrome

E24.2 Drug-induced Cushing's syndrome
Code first (T36-T50) to identify drug

E24.3 Ectopic ACTH syndrome

E24.4 Alcohol-induced pseudo-Cushing's syndrome

E24.8 Other Cushing's syndrome

E24.9 Cushing's syndrome, unspecified

☑4th **E25** Adrenogenital disorders
Adrenogenital syndromes, virilizing or feminizing, whether acquired or due to adrenal hyperplasia
Consequent on inborn enzyme defects in hormone synthesis
Female adrenal pseudohermaphroditism
Female heterosexual precocious pseudopuberty
Male isosexual precocious pseudopuberty
Male macrogenitosomia praecox
Male sexual precocity with adrenal hyperplasia
Male virilization (female)
EXCLUDES 1 indeterminate sex and pseudohermaphroditism (Q56)
chromosomal abnormalities (Q90-Q99)

E25.0 Congenital adrenogenital disorders associated with enzyme deficiency
Congenital adrenal hyperplasia
21-Hydroxylase deficiency
Salt-losing congenital adrenal hyperplasia

E25.8 Other adrenogenital disorders
Idiopathic adrenogenital disorder

E25.9 Adrenogenital disorder, unspecified
Adrenogenital syndrome NOS

☑4th **E26** Hyperaldosteronism
☑5th **E26.0** Primary hyperaldosteronism
E26.01 Conn's syndrome
Code also adrenal adenoma (D35.0)
E26.02 Glucocorticoid-remediable aldosteronism
Familial aldosteronism type I
E26.09 Other primary hyperaldosteronism
Primary aldosteronism due to adrenal hyperplasia (bilateral)

E26.1 Secondary hyperaldosteronism
☑5th **E26.8** Other hyperaldosteronism
E26.81 Bartter's syndrome
E26.89 Other hyperaldosteronism

E26.9 Hyperaldosteronism, unspecified
Aldosteronism NOS
Hyperaldosteronism NOS

☑4th **E27** Other disorders of adrenal gland
E27.0 Other adrenocortical overactivity
Overproduction of ACTH, not associated with Cushing's disease
Premature adrenarche
EXCLUDES 1 Cushing's syndrome (E24-)

E27.1 Primary adrenocortical insufficiency
Addison's disease
Autoimmune adrenalitis
EXCLUDES 1 Addison only phenotype adrenoleukodystrophy (E71.428)
amyloidosis (E85-)
tuberculous Addison's disease (A18.7)
Waterhouse-Friderichsen syndrome (A39.1)

E27.2 Addisonian crisis
Adrenal crisis
Adrenocortical crisis

E27.3 Drug-induced adrenocortical insufficiency
Code first (T36-T50) to identify drug

☑5th **E27.4** Other and unspecified adrenocortical insufficiency
EXCLUDES 1 adrenoleukodystrophy [Addison-Schilder] (E71.528)
Waterhouse-Friderichsen syndrome (A39.1)
E27.40 Unspecified adrenocortical insufficiency
Adrenocortical insufficiency NOS
Hypoaldosteronism
E27.49 Other adrenocortical insufficiency
Adrenal hemorrhage
Adrenal infarction

E27.5 Adrenomedullary hyperfunction
Adrenomedullary hyperplasia
Catecholamine hypersecretion

E27.8 Other specified disorders of adrenal gland
Abnormality of cortisol-binding globulin

E27.9 Disorder of adrenal gland, unspecified

☑4th **E28** Ovarian dysfunction
EXCLUDES 1 isolated gonadotropin deficiency (E23.0)
postprocedural ovarian failure (E89.4-)

E28.0 Estrogen excess

E28.1 Androgen excess
Hypersecretion of ovarian androgens

E28.2   Polycystic ovarian syndrome
Sclerocystic ovary syndrome
Stein-Leventhal syndrome

✓5ᵗʰ **E28.3   Primary ovarian failure**
EXCLUDES 1   *pure gonadal dysgenesis (Q99.1)*
Turner's syndrome (Q96-)

✓6ᵗʰ   **E28.31   Premature menopause**
E28.310   Symptomatic premature menopause
Symptoms such as flushing,
sleeplessness, headache, lack of
concentration, associated with
premature menopause
E28.319   Asymptomatic premature menopause
Premature menopause NOS

E28.39   Other primary ovarian failure
Decreased estrogen
Resistant ovary syndrome

E28.8   Other ovarian dysfunction
Ovarian hyperfunction NOS
EXCLUDES 1   *postprocedural ovarian failure (E89.4-)*

E28.9   Ovarian dysfunction, unspecified

✓4ᵗʰ **E29   Testicular dysfunction**
EXCLUDES 1   *androgen insensitivity syndrome (E34.5-)*
azoospermia or oligospermia NOS (N46.0-N46.1)
isolated gonadotropin deficiency (E23.0)
Klinefelter's syndrome (Q98.0-Q98.2, Q98.4)

E29.0   Testicular hyperfunction
Hypersecretion of testicular hormones

E29.1   Testicular hypofunction
Defective biosynthesis of testicular androgen NOS
5-delta-Reductase deficiency (with male
pseudohermaphroditism)
Testicular hypogonadism NOS
EXCLUDES 1   *postprocedural testicular hypofunction (E89.5)*

E29.8   Other testicular dysfunction

E29.9   Testicular dysfunction, unspecified

✓4ᵗʰ **E30   Disorders of puberty, not elsewhere classified**
E30.0   Delayed puberty
Constitutional delay of puberty
Delayed sexual development

E30.1   Precocious puberty
Precocious menstruation
EXCLUDES 1   *Albright (-McCune) (-Sternberg) syndrome (Q78.1)*
central precocious puberty (E22.8)
congenital adrenal hyperplasia (E25.0)
female heterosexual precocious pseudopuberty
(E25-)
male isosexual precocious pseudopuberty (E25-)

E30.8   Other disorders of puberty
Premature thelarche

E30.9   Disorder of puberty, unspecified

✓4ᵗʰ **E31   Polyglandular dysfunction**
EXCLUDES 1   *ataxia telangiectasia [Louis-Bar] (G11.3)*
dystrophia myotonica [Steinert] (G71.11)
pseudohypoparathyroidism (E20.1)

E31.0   Autoimmune polyglandular failure
Schmidt's syndrome

E31.1   Polyglandular hyperfunction
EXCLUDES 1   *multiple endocrine adenomatosis (E31.2-)*
multiple endocrine neoplasia (E31.2-)

✓5ᵗʰ **E31.2   Multiple endocrine neoplasia [MEN] syndromes**
Multiple endocrine adenomatosis
Code also any associated malignancies and other conditions
associated with the syndromes

**E31.20   Multiple endocrine neoplasia [MEN] syndrome,
unspecified**
Multiple endocrine adenomatosis NOS
Multiple endocrine neoplasia [MEN] syndrome NOS

E31.21   Multiple endocrine neoplasia [MEN] type I
Wermer's syndrome

E31.22   Multiple endocrine neoplasia [MEN] type IIA
Sipple's syndrome

E31.23   Multiple endocrine neoplasia [MEN] type IIB

E31.8   Other polyglandular dysfunction

E31.9   Polyglandular dysfunction, unspecified

✓4ᵗʰ **E32   Diseases of thymus**
EXCLUDES 1   *aplasia or hypoplasia of thymus with immunodeficiency*
(D82.1)
myasthenia gravis (G70.0)

E32.0   Persistent hyperplasia of thymus
Hypertrophy of thymus

E32.1   Abscess of thymus

E32.8   Other diseases of thymus
EXCLUDES 1   *aplasia or hypoplasia with immunodeficiency (D82.1)*
thymoma (D15.0)

E32.9   Disease of thymus, unspecified

✓4ᵗʰ **E34   Other endocrine disorders**
EXCLUDES 1   *pseudohypoparathyroidism (E20.1)*

E34.0   Carcinoid syndrome
NOTE   May be used as an additional code to identify
functional activity associated with a carcinoid
tumor.

E34.1   Other hypersecretion of intestinal hormones

E34.2   Ectopic hormone secretion, not elsewhere classified
EXCLUDES 1   *ectopic ACTH syndrome (E24.3)*

E34.3   Short stature due to endocrine disorder
Constitutional short stature
Laron-type short stature
EXCLUDES 1   *achondroplastic short stature (Q77.4)*
hypochondroplastic short stature (Q77.4)
nutritional short stature (E45)
pituitary short stature (E23.0)
progeria (E34.8)
renal short stature (N25.0)
Russell-Silver syndrome (Q87.1)
short-limbed stature with immunodeficiency (D82.2)
short stature in specific dysmorphic syndromes—
code to syndrome—see Alphabetical Index
short stature NOS (R62.52)

E34.4   Constitutional tall stature
Constitutional gigantism

✓5ᵗʰ **E34.5   Androgen insensitivity syndrome**
E34.50   Androgen insensitivity syndrome, unspecified
Androgen insensitivity NOS

E34.51   Complete androgen insensitivity syndrome
Complete androgen insensitivity
de Quervain syndrome
Goldberg-Maxwell syndrome

E34.52   Partial androgen insensitivity syndrome
Partial androgen insensitivity
Reifenstein syndrome

E34.8   Other specified endocrine disorders
Pineal gland dysfunction
Progeria
EXCLUDES 2   *pseudohypoparathyroidism (E20.1)*

E34.9   Endocrine disorder, unspecified
Endocrine disturbance NOS
Hormone disturbance NOS

**E35   Disorders of endocrine glands in diseases classified
elsewhere**
Code first underlying disease, such as:
late congenital syphilis of thymus gland [Dubois disease] (A50.5)
tuberculous calcification of adrenal gland (B90.8)
EXCLUDES 1   *Echinococcus granulosus infection of thyroid gland (B67.3)*
meningococcal hemorrhagic adrenalitis (A39.1)
syphilis of endocrine gland (A52.79)
tuberculosis of:
adrenal gland, except calcification (A18.7)
endocrine gland NEC (A18.82)
thyroid gland (A18.81)
Waterhouse-Friderichsen syndrome (A39.1)

✓4ᵗʰ **E36   Intraoperative complications of endocrine system**
EXCLUDES 2   *postprocedural endocrine and metabolic complications and*
disorders, not elsewhere classified (E89-)

✓5ᵗʰ **E36.0   Intraoperative hemorrhage and hematoma of an endocrine
system organ or structure complicating a procedure**
EXCLUDES 1   *intraoperative hemorrhage and hematoma of an*
endocrine system organ or structure due to
accidental puncture or laceration during a
procedure (E36.1-)

**E36.01   Intraoperative hemorrhage and hematoma of an
endocrine system organ or structure complicating
an endocrine system procedure**

EXCLUDES 1 Not coded here   EXCLUDES 2 Not included here   *Manifestation Code*

E36.02 **Intraoperative hemorrhage and hematoma of an endocrine system organ or structure complicating other procedure**

✓5ᵗʰ E36.1 **Accidental puncture and laceration of an endocrine system organ or structure during a procedure**

E36.11 **Accidental puncture and laceration of an endocrine system organ or structure during an endocrine system procedure**

E36.12 **Accidental puncture and laceration of an endocrine system organ or structure during other procedure**

E36.8 **Other intraoperative complications of endocrine system**
Use additional code, if applicable, to further specify disorder

Malnutrition (E40-E46)

EXCLUDES 1 *intestinal malabsorption (K90-)*
sequelae of protein-calorie malnutrition (E64.0)
EXCLUDES 2 *nutritional anemias (D50-D53)*
starvation (T73.0)

E40 **Kwashiorkor**
Severe malnutrition with nutritional edema with dyspigmentation of skin and hair
EXCLUDES 1 *marasmic kwashiorkor (E42)*

E41 **Nutritional marasmus**
Severe malnutrition with marasmus
EXCLUDES 1 *marasmic kwashiorkor (E42)*

E42 **Marasmic kwashiorkor**
Intermediate form severe protein-calorie malnutrition
Severe protein-calorie malnutrition with signs of both kwashiorkor and marasmus

E43 **Unspecified severe protein-calorie malnutrition**
Starvation edema

✓4ᵗʰ E44 **Protein-calorie malnutrition of moderate and mild degree**
E44.0 **Moderate protein-calorie malnutrition**
E44.1 **Mild protein-calorie malnutrition**

E45 **Retarded development following protein-calorie malnutrition**
Nutritional short stature
Nutritional stunting
Physical retardation due to malnutrition

E46 **Unspecified protein-calorie malnutrition**
Malnutrition NOS
Protein-calorie imbalance NOS
EXCLUDES 1 *nutritional deficiency NOS (E63.9)*

Other nutritional deficiencies (E50-E64)

EXCLUDES 2 *nutritional anemias (D50-D53)*

✓4ᵗʰ E50 **Vitamin A deficiency**
EXCLUDES 1 *sequelae of vitamin A deficiency (E64.1)*
E50.0 **Vitamin A deficiency with conjunctival xerosis**
E50.1 **Vitamin A deficiency with Bitot's spot and conjunctival xerosis**
Bitot's spot in the young child
E50.2 **Vitamin A deficiency with corneal xerosis**
E50.3 **Vitamin A deficiency with corneal ulceration and xerosis**
E50.4 **Vitamin A deficiency with keratomalacia**
E50.5 **Vitamin A deficiency with night blindness**
E50.6 **Vitamin A deficiency with xerophthalmic scars of cornea**
E50.7 **Other ocular manifestations of vitamin A deficiency**
Xerophthalmia NOS
E50.8 **Other manifestations of vitamin A deficiency**
Follicular keratosis
Xeroderma
E50.9 **Vitamin A deficiency, unspecified**
Hypovitaminosis A NOS

✓4ᵗʰ E51 **Thiamine deficiency**
EXCLUDES 1 *sequelae of thiamine deficiency (E64.8)*
✓5ᵗʰ E51.1 **Beriberi**
E51.11 **Dry beriberi**
Beriberi NOS
Beriberi with polyneuropathy
E51.12 **Wet beriberi**
Beriberi with cardiovascular manifestations
Cardiovascular beriberi
Shoshin disease

E51.2 **Wernicke's encephalopathy**
E51.8 **Other manifestations of thiamine deficiency**
E51.9 **Thiamine deficiency, unspecified**

E52 **Niacin deficiency [pellagra]**
Niacin (-tryptophan) deficiency
Nicotinamide deficiency
Pellagra (alcoholic)
EXCLUDES 1 *sequelae of niacin deficiency (E64.8)*

✓4ᵗʰ E53 **Deficiency of other B group vitamins**
EXCLUDES 1 *sequelae of vitamin B deficiency (E64.8)*
E53.0 **Riboflavin deficiency**
Ariboflavinosis
Vitamin B2 deficiency
E53.1 **Pyridoxine deficiency**
Vitamin B6 deficiency
EXCLUDES 1 *pyridoxine-responsive sideroblastic anemia (D64.3)*
E53.8 **Deficiency of other specified B group vitamins**
Biotin deficiency
Cyanocobalamin deficiency
Folate deficiency
Folic acid deficiency
Pantothenic acid deficiency
Vitamin B12 deficiency
EXCLUDES 1 *folate deficiency anemia (D52-)*
vitamin B12 deficiency anemia (D51-)
E53.9 **Vitamin B deficiency, unspecified**

E54 **Ascorbic acid deficiency**
Deficiency of vitamin C
Scurvy
EXCLUDES 1 *scorbutic anemia (D53.2)*
sequelae of vitamin C deficiency (E64.2)

✓4ᵗʰ E55 **Vitamin D deficiency**
EXCLUDES 1 *adult osteomalacia (M83-)*
osteoporosis (M80-)
sequelae of rickets (E64.3)
E55.0 **Rickets, active**
Infantile Osteomalacia
Juvenile Osteomalacia
EXCLUDES 1 *celiac rickets (K90.0)*
Crohn's rickets (K50-)
hereditary vitamin D-dependent rickets (E83.32)
inactive rickets (E64.3)
renal rickets (N25.0)
sequelae of rickets (E64.3)
vitamin D-resistant rickets (E83.31)
E55.9 **Vitamin D deficiency, unspecified**
Avitaminosis D

✓4ᵗʰ E56 **Other vitamin deficiencies**
EXCLUDES 1 *sequelae of other vitamin deficiencies (E64.8)*
E56.0 **Deficiency of vitamin E**
E56.1 **Deficiency of vitamin K**
EXCLUDES 1 *deficiency of coagulation factor due to vitamin K deficiency (D68.4)*
vitamin K deficiency of newborn (P53)
E56.8 **Deficiency of other vitamins**
E56.9 **Vitamin deficiency, unspecified**

E58 **Dietary calcium deficiency**
EXCLUDES 1 *disorders of calcium metabolism (E83.5)*
sequelae of calcium deficiency (E64.8)

E59 **Dietary selenium deficiency**
Keshan disease
EXCLUDES 1 *sequelae of selenium deficiency (E64.8)*

E60 **Dietary zinc deficiency**

✓4ᵗʰ E61 **Deficiency of other nutrient elements**
EXCLUDES 1 *disorders of mineral metabolism (E83-)*
iodine deficiency related thyroid disorders (E00-E02)
sequelae of malnutrition and other nutritional deficiencies (E64-)
E61.0 **Copper deficiency**
E61.1 **Iron deficiency**
EXCLUDES 1 *iron deficiency anemia (D50-)*
E61.2 **Magnesium deficiency**
E61.3 **Manganese deficiency**
E61.4 **Chromium deficiency**
E61.5 **Molybdenum deficiency**

☑ Appropriate additional character required   ✓x7ᵗʰ Requires 7th character, placeholder x must fill empty characters

Endocrine, Nutritional and Metabolic Diseases

E61.6–E71.2

E61.6   **Vanadium deficiency**

E61.7   **Deficiency of multiple nutrient elements**

E61.8   **Deficiency of other specified nutrient elements**

E61.9   **Deficiency of nutrient element, unspecified**

√4th **E63   Other nutritional deficiencies**

> EXCLUDES 1   dehydration (E86.0)
> failure to thrive, adult (R62.7)
> failure to thrive, child (R62.51)
> feeding problems in newborn (P92-)
> sequelae of malnutrition and other nutritional deficiencies
> (E64-)

E63.0   **Essential fatty acid [EFA] deficiency**

E63.1   **Imbalance of constituents of food intake**

E63.8   **Other specified nutritional deficiencies**

E63.9   **Nutritional deficiency, unspecified**

√4th **E64   Sequelae of malnutrition and other nutritional deficiencies**

> NOTE   This category is to be used to indicate conditions in categories E43, E44, E46, E50-E63 as the cause of sequelae, which are themselves classified elsewhere. The 'sequelae' include conditions specified as such; they also include the late effects of diseases classifiable to the above categories if the disease itself is no longer present

> Code first condition resulting from (sequela) of malnutrition and other nutritional deficiencies

E64.0   **Sequelae of protein-calorie malnutrition**

> EXCLUDES 2   retarded development following protein-calorie malnutrition (E45)

E64.1   **Sequelae of vitamin A deficiency**

E64.2   **Sequelae of vitamin C deficiency**

E64.3   **Sequelae of rickets**

E64.8   **Sequelae of other nutritional deficiencies**

E64.9   **Sequelae of unspecified nutritional deficiency**

Overweight, obesity and other hyperalimentation (E65-E68)

E65   Localized adiposity

> Fat pad

√4th **E66   Overweight and obesity**

> Code first obesity complicating pregnancy, childbirth and the puerperium, if applicable (O99.21-)
> Use additional code to identify body mass index (BMI), if known (Z68-)

> EXCLUDES 1   adiposogenital dystrophy (E23.6)
> lipomatosis NOS (E88.2)
> lipomatosis dolorosa [Dercum] (E88.2)
> Prader-Willi syndrome (Q87.1)

√5th   E66.0   **Obesity due to excess calories**

E66.01   **Morbid (severe) obesity due to excess calories**

> EXCLUDES 1   morbid (severe) obesity with alveolar hypoventilation (E66.2)

E66.09   **Other obesity due to excess calories**

E66.1   **Drug-induced obesity**

> Code first (T36-T50) to identify drug

E66.2   **Morbid (severe) obesity with alveolar hypoventilation**

> Pickwickian syndrome

E66.3   **Overweight**

E66.8   **Other obesity**

E66.9   **Obesity, unspecified**

> Obesity NOS

√4th **E67   Other hyperalimentation**

> EXCLUDES 1   hyperalimentation NOS (R63.2)
> sequelae of hyperalimentation (E68)

E67.0   **Hypervitaminosis A**

E67.1   **Hypercarotinemia**

E67.2   **Megavitamin-B6 syndrome**

E67.3   **Hypervitaminosis D**

E67.8   **Other specified hyperalimentation**

E68   Sequelae of hyperalimentation

> Code first condition resulting from (sequela) of hyperalimentation

Metabolic disorders (E70-E88)

> EXCLUDES 1   androgen insensitivity syndrome (E34.5-)
> congenital adrenal hyperplasia (E25.0)
> Ehlers-Danlos syndrome (Q79.6)
> hemolytic anemias attributable to enzyme disorders (D55-)
> Marfan's syndrome (Q87.4)
> 5-alpha-reductase deficiency (E29.1)

√4th **E70   Disorders of aromatic amino-acid metabolism**

E70.0   **Classical phenylketonuria**

E70.1   **Other hyperphenylalaninemias**

√5th   E70.2   **Disorders of tyrosine metabolism**

> EXCLUDES 1   transitory tyrosinemia of newborn (P74.5)

E70.20   **Disorder of tyrosine metabolism, unspecified**

E70.21   **Tyrosinemia**

> Hypertyrosinemia

E70.29   **Other disorders of tyrosine metabolism**

> Alkaptonuria
> Ochronosis

√5th   E70.3   **Albinism**

E70.30   **Albinism, unspecified**

√6th   E70.31   **Ocular albinism**

E70.310   **X-linked ocular albinism**

E70.311   **Autosomal recessive ocular albinism**

E70.318   **Other ocular albinism**

E70.319   **Ocular albinism, unspecified**

√6th   E70.32   **Oculocutaneous albinism**

> EXCLUDES 1   Chediak-Higashi syndrome (E70.330)
> Hermansky-Pudlak syndrome (E70.331)

E70.320   **Tyrosinase negative oculocutaneous albinism**

> Albinism I
> Oculocutaneous albinism ty-neg

E70.321   **Tyrosinase positive oculocutaneous albinism**

> Albinism II
> Oculocutaneous albinism ty-pos

E70.328   **Other oculocutaneous albinism**

> Cross syndrome

E70.329   **Oculocutaneous albinism, unspecified**

√6th   E70.33   **Albinism with hematologic abnormality**

E70.330   **Chediak-Higashi syndrome**

E70.331   **Hermansky-Pudlak syndrome**

E70.338   **Other albinism with hematologic abnormality**

E70.339   **Albinism with hematologic abnormality, unspecified**

E70.39   **Other specified albinism**

> Piebaldism

√5th   E70.4   **Disorders of histidine metabolism**

E70.40   **Disorders of histidine metabolism, unspecified**

E70.41   **Histidinemia**

E70.49   **Other disorders of histidine metabolism**

E70.5   **Disorders of tryptophan metabolism**

E70.8   **Other disorders of aromatic amino-acid metabolism**

E70.9   **Disorder of aromatic amino-acid metabolism, unspecified**

√4th **E71   Disorders of branched-chain amino-acid metabolism and fatty-acid metabolism**

E71.0   **Maple-syrup-urine disease**

√5th   E71.1   **Other disorders of branched-chain amino-acid metabolism**

√6th   E71.11   **Branched-chain organic acidurias**

E71.110   **Isovaleric acidemia**

E71.111   **3-methylglutaconic aciduria**

E71.118   **Other branched-chain organic acidurias**

√6th   E71.12   **Disorders of propionate metabolism**

E71.120   **Methylmalonic acidemia**

E71.121   **Propionic acidemia**

E71.128   **Other disorders of propionate metabolism**

E71.19   **Other disorders of branched-chain amino-acid metabolism**

> Hyperleucine-isoleucinemia
> Hypervalinemia

E71.2   **Disorder of branched-chain amino-acid metabolism, unspecified**

✓5th **E71.3　Disorders of fatty-acid metabolism**
　　　EXCLUDES 1　*peroxisomal disorders (E71.5)*
　　　　　　　Refsum's disease (G60.1)
　　　　　　　Schilder's disease (G37.0)
　　　EXCLUDES 2　*carnitine deficiency due to inborn error of*
　　　　　　　metabolism (E71.42)
　　E71.30　**Disorder of fatty-acid metabolism, unspecified**
✓6th　E71.31　**Disorders of fatty-acid oxidation**
　　　　E71.310　**Long chain/very long chain acyl CoA dehydrogenase deficiency**
　　　　　　　LCAD
　　　　　　　VLCAD
　　　　E71.311　**Medium chain acyl CoA dehydrogenase deficiency**
　　　　　　　MCAD
　　　　E71.312　**Short chain acyl CoA dehydrogenase deficiency**
　　　　　　　SCAD
　　　　E71.313　**Glutaric aciduria type II**
　　　　　　　Glutaric aciduria type II A
　　　　　　　Glutaric aciduria type II B
　　　　　　　Glutaric aciduria type II C
　　　　　　　EXCLUDES 1　*glutaric aciduria (type 1) NOS (E72.3)*
　　　　E71.314　**Muscle carnitine palmitoyltransferase deficiency**
　　　　E71.318　**Other disorders of fatty-acid oxidation**
　　E71.32　**Disorders of ketone metabolism**
　　E71.39　**Other disorders of fatty-acid metabolism**
✓5th **E71.4　Disorders of carnitine metabolism**
　　　EXCLUDES 1　*muscle carnitine palmitoyltransferase deficiency (E71.314)*
　　E71.40　**Disorder of carnitine metabolism, unspecified**
　　E71.41　**Primary carnitine deficiency**
　　E71.42　**Carnitine deficiency due to inborn errors of metabolism**
　　　　　Code also associated inborn error or metabolism
　　E71.43　**Iatrogenic carnitine deficiency**
　　　　　Carnitine deficiency due to:
　　　　　　hemodialysis
　　　　　　valproic acid therapy
✓6th　E71.44　**Other secondary carnitine deficiency**
　　　　E71.440　**Ruvalcaba-Myhre-Smith syndrome**
　　　　E71.448　**Other secondary carnitine deficiency**
✓5th **E71.5　Peroxisomal disorders**
　　　EXCLUDES 1　*Schilder's disease (G37.0)*
　　E71.50　**Peroxisomal disorder, unspecified**
✓6th　E71.51　**Disorders of peroxisome biogenesis**
　　　　　Group 1 peroxisomal disorders
　　　　　EXCLUDES 1　*Refsum's disease (G60.1)*
　　　　E71.510　**Zellweger syndrome**
　　　　E71.511　**Neonatal adrenoleukodystrophy**
　　　　　　　EXCLUDES 1　*X-linked adrenoleukodystrophy (E71.52-)*
　　　　E71.518　**Other disorders of peroxisome biogenesis**
✓6th　E71.52　**X-linked adrenoleukodystrophy**
　　　　E71.520　**Childhood cerebral X-linked adrenoleukodystrophy**
　　　　E71.521　**Adolescent X-linked adrenoleukodystrophy**
　　　　E71.522　**Adrenomyeloneuropathy**
　　　　E71.528　**Other X-linked adrenoleukodystrophy**
　　　　　　　Addison only phenotype adrenoleukodystrophy
　　　　　　　Addison-Schilder adrenoleukodystrophy
　　　　E71.529　**X-linked adrenoleukodystrophy, unspecified type**
　　E71.53　**Other group 2 peroxisomal disorders**
✓6th　E71.54　**Other peroxisomal disorders**
　　　　E71.540　**Rhizomelic chondrodysplasia punctata**
　　　　　　　EXCLUDES 1　*chondrodysplasia punctata NOS (Q77.3)*
　　　　E71.541　**Zellweger-like syndrome**
　　　　E71.542　**Other group 3 peroxisomal disorders**
　　　　E71.548　**Other peroxisomal disorders**

✓4th **E72　Other disorders of amino-acid metabolism**
　　　EXCLUDES 1　*disorders of:*
　　　　　　aromatic amino-acid metabolism (E70-)
　　　　　　branched-chain amino-acid metabolism (E71.0-E71.2)
　　　　　　fatty-acid metabolism (E71.3)
　　　　　　purine and pyrimidine metabolism (E79-)
　　　　　　gout (M1a-, M10-)
✓5th　E72.0　**Disorders of amino-acid transport**
　　　　EXCLUDES 1　*disorders of tryptophan metabolism (E70.5)*
　　　E72.00　**Disorders of amino-acid transport, unspecified**
　　　E72.01　**Cystinuria**
　　　E72.02　**Hartnup's disease**
　　　E72.03　**Lowe's syndrome**
　　　　　Use additional code for associated glaucoma (H42)
　　　E72.04　**Cystinosis**
　　　　　Fanconi (-de Toni) (-Debré) syndrome with cystinosis
　　　　　EXCLUDES 1　*Fanconi (-de Toni) (-Debré) syndrome without cystinosis (E72.09)*
　　　E72.09　**Other disorders of amino-acid transport**
　　　　　Fanconi (-de Toni) (-Debré) syndrome, unspecified
✓5th　E72.1　**Disorders of sulfur-bearing amino-acid metabolism**
　　　　EXCLUDES 1　*cystinosis (E72.04)*
　　　　　　cystinuria (E72.01)
　　　　　　transcobalamin II deficiency (D51.2)
　　　E72.10　**Disorders of sulfur-bearing amino-acid metabolism, unspecified**
　　　E72.11　**Homocystinuria**
　　　　　Cystathionine synthase deficiency
　　　E72.12　**Methylenetetrahydrofolate reductase deficiency**
　　　E72.19　**Other disorders of sulfur-bearing amino-acid metabolism**
　　　　　Cystathioninuria
　　　　　Methioninemia
　　　　　Sulfite oxidase deficiency
✓5th　E72.2　**Disorders of urea cycle metabolism**
　　　　EXCLUDES 1　*disorders of ornithine metabolism (E72.4)*
　　　E72.20　**Disorder of urea cycle metabolism, unspecified**
　　　　　Hyperammonemia
　　　　　EXCLUDES 1　*hyperammonemia- hyperornithinemia-homocitrullinemia syndrome (E72.4)*
　　　　　　transient hyperammonemia of newborn (P74.6)
　　　E72.21　**Argininemia**
　　　E72.22　**Arginosuccinic aciduria**
　　　E72.23　**Citrullinemia**
　　　E72.29　**Other disorders of urea cycle metabolism**
　　E72.3　**Disorders of lysine and hydroxylysine metabolism**
　　　　Glutaric aciduria NOS
　　　　Glutaric aciduria (type I)
　　　　Hydroxylysinemia
　　　　Hyperlysinemia
　　　　EXCLUDES 1　*glutaric aciduria type II (E71.313)*
　　　　　　Refsum's disease (G60.1)
　　　　　　Zellweger syndrome (E71.510)
　　E72.4　**Disorders of ornithine metabolism**
　　　　Hyperammonemia-hyperornithinemia-homocitrullinemia syndrome
　　　　Ornithinemia (types I, II)
　　　　Ornithine transcarbamylase deficiency
　　　　EXCLUDES 1　*hereditary choroidal dystrophy (H31.2-)*
✓5th　E72.5　**Disorders of glycine metabolism**
　　　E72.50　**Disorder of glycine metabolism, unspecified**
　　　E72.51　**Non-ketotic hyperglycinemia**
　　　E72.52　**Trimethylaminuria**
　　　E72.53　**Hyperoxaluria**
　　　　　Oxalosis
　　　　　Oxaluria
　　　E72.59　**Other disorders of glycine metabolism**
　　　　　D-glycericacidemia
　　　　　Hyperhydroxyprolinemia
　　　　　Hyperprolinemia (types I, II)
　　　　　Sarcosinemia
　　E72.8　**Other specified disorders of amino-acid metabolism**
　　　　Disorders of beta-amino-acid metabolism
　　　　Disorders of gamma-glutamyl cycle
　　E72.9　**Disorder of amino-acid metabolism, unspecified**

☑ Appropriate additional character required　　　　✓x7th Requires 7th character, placeholder x must fill empty characters

Endocrine, Nutritional and Metabolic Diseases

E73–E77.8

✓4th **E73**   **Lactose intolerance**
     E73.0   **Congenital lactase deficiency**
     E73.1   **Secondary lactase deficiency**
     E73.8   **Other lactose intolerance**
     E73.9   **Lactose intolerance, unspecified**

✓4th **E74**   **Other disorders of carbohydrate metabolism**
     EXCLUDES 1   *diabetes mellitus (E08-E13)*
                 hypoglycemia NOS (E16.2)
                 increased secretion of glucagon (E16.3)
                 mucopolysaccharidosis (E76.0-E76.3)

   ✓5th **E74.0**   **Glycogen storage disease**
       E74.00   **Glycogen storage disease, unspecified**
       E74.01   **von Gierke disease**
            Type I glycogen storage disease
       E74.02   **Pompe disease**
            Cardiac glycogenosis
            Type II glycogen storage disease
       E74.03   **Cori disease**
            Forbes disease
            Type III glycogen storage disease
       E74.04   **McArdle disease**
            Type V glycogen storage disease
       E74.09   **Other glycogen storage disease**
            Andersen disease
            Hers disease
            Tauri disease
            Glycogen storage disease, types 0, IV, VI-XI
            Liver phosphorylase deficiency
            Muscle phosphofructokinase deficiency

   ✓5th **E74.1**   **Disorders of fructose metabolism**
       EXCLUDES 1   *muscle phosphofructokinase deficiency (E74.09)*
       E74.10   **Disorder of fructose metabolism, unspecified**
       E74.11   **Essential fructosuria**
            Fructokinase deficiency
       E74.12   **Hereditary fructose intolerance**
            Fructosemia
       E74.19   **Other disorders of fructose metabolism**
            Fructose-1, 6-diphosphatase deficiency

   ✓5th **E74.2**   **Disorders of galactose metabolism**
       E74.20   **Disorders of galactose metabolism, unspecified**
       E74.21   **Galactosemia**
       E74.29   **Other disorders of galactose metabolism**
            Galactokinase deficiency

   ✓5th **E74.3**   **Other disorders of intestinal carbohydrate absorption**
       EXCLUDES 2   *lactose intolerance (E73-)*
       E74.31   **Sucrase-isomaltase deficiency**
       E74.39   **Other disorders of intestinal carbohydrate absorption**
            Disorder of intestinal carbohydrate absorption NOS
            Glucose-galactose malabsorption
            Sucrase deficiency

     E74.4   **Disorders of pyruvate metabolism and gluconeogenesis**
         Deficiency of phosphoenolpyruvate carboxykinase
         Deficiency of pyruvate carboxylase
         Deficiency of pyruvate dehydrogenase
       EXCLUDES 1   *disorders of pyruvate metabolism and*
                 gluconeogenesis with anemia (D55-)
                 Leigh's syndrome (G31.82)

     E74.8   **Other specified disorders of carbohydrate metabolism**
         Essential pentosuria
         Renal glycosuria

     E74.9   **Disorder of carbohydrate metabolism, unspecified**

✓4th **E75**   **Disorders of sphingolipid metabolism and other lipid storage disorders**
     EXCLUDES 1   *mucolipidosis, types I-III (E77.0-E77.1)*
                 Refsum's disease (G60.1)

   ✓5th **E75.0**   **GM2 gangliosidosis**
       E75.00   **GM2 gangliosidosis, unspecified**
       E75.01   **Sandhoff disease**
       E75.02   **Tay-Sachs disease**
       E75.09   **Other GM2 gangliosidosis**
            Adult GM2 gangliosidosis
            Juvenile GM2 gangliosidosis

   ✓5th **E75.1**   **Other and unspecified gangliosidosis**
       E75.10   **Unspecified gangliosidosis**
            Gangliosidosis NOS
       E75.11   **Mucolipidosis IV**

     E75.19   **Other gangliosidosis**
         GM1 gangliosidosis
         GM3 gangliosidosis

   ✓5th **E75.2**   **Other sphingolipidosis**
       EXCLUDES 1   *adrenoleukodystrophy [Addison-Schilder] (E71.528)*
       E75.21   **Fabry (-Anderson) disease**
       E75.22   **Gaucher disease**
       E75.23   **Krabbe disease**
       ✓6th **E75.24**   **Niemann-Pick disease**
          E75.240   **Niemann-Pick disease type A**
          E75.241   **Niemann-Pick disease type B**
          E75.242   **Niemann-Pick disease type C**
          E75.243   **Niemann-Pick disease type D**
          E75.248   **Other Niemann-Pick disease**
          E75.249   **Niemann-Pick disease, unspecified**
       E75.25   **Metachromatic leukodystrophy**
       E75.29   **Other sphingolipidosis**
            Farber's syndrome
            Sulfatase deficiency
            Sulfatide lipidosis

     E75.3   **Sphingolipidosis, unspecified**
     E75.4   **Neuronal ceroid lipofuscinosis**
         Batten disease
         Bielschowsky-Jansky disease
         Kufs disease
         Spielmeyer-Vogt disease
     E75.5   **Other lipid storage disorders**
         Cerebrotendinous cholesterosis [van
            Bogaert-Scherer-Epstein]
         Wolman's disease
     E75.6   **Lipid storage disorder, unspecified**

✓4th **E76**   **Disorders of glycosaminoglycan metabolism**
   ✓5th **E76.0**   **Mucopolysaccharidosis, type I**
       E76.01   **Hurler's syndrome**
       E76.02   **Hurler-Scheie syndrome**
       E76.03   **Scheie's syndrome**
     E76.1   **Mucopolysaccharidosis, type II**
         Hunter's syndrome
   ✓5th **E76.2**   **Other mucopolysaccharidoses**
       ✓6th **E76.21**   **Morquio mucopolysaccharidoses**
          E76.210   **Morquio A mucopolysaccharidoses**
             Classic Morquio syndrome
             Morquio syndrome A
             Mucopolysaccharidosis, type IVA
          E76.211   **Morquio B mucopolysaccharidoses**
             Morquio-like mucopolysaccharidoses
             Morquio-like syndrome
             Morquio syndrome B
             Mucopolysaccharidosis, type IVB
          E76.219   **Morquio mucopolysaccharidoses, unspecified**
             Morquio syndrome
             Mucopolysaccharidosis, type IV
       E76.22   **Sanfilippo mucopolysaccharidoses**
            Mucopolysaccharidosis, type III (A) (B) (C) (D)
            Sanfilippo A syndrome
            Sanfilippo B syndrome
            Sanfilippo C syndrome
            Sanfilippo D syndrome
       E76.29   **Other mucopolysaccharidoses**
            beta-Glucuronidase deficiency
            Maroteaux-Lamy (mild) (severe) syndrome
            Mucopolysaccharidosis, types VI, VII
     E76.3   **Mucopolysaccharidosis, unspecified**
     E76.8   **Other disorders of glucosaminoglycan metabolism**
     E76.9   **Glucosaminoglycan metabolism disorder, unspecified**

✓4th **E77**   **Disorders of glycoprotein metabolism**
     E77.0   **Defects in post-translational modification of lysosomal enzymes**
         Mucolipidosis II [I-cell disease]
         Mucolipidosis III [pseudo-Hurler polydystrophy]
     E77.1   **Defects in glycoprotein degradation**
         Aspartylglucosaminuria
         Fucosidosis
         Mannosidosis
         Sialidosis [mucolipidosis I]
     E77.8   **Other disorders of glycoprotein metabolism**

EXCLUDES 1   Not coded here   EXCLUDES 2   Not included here   *Manifestation Code*

E77.9   Disorder of glycoprotein metabolism, unspecified

☑4ᵗʰ **E78   Disorders of lipoprotein metabolism and other lipidemias**
EXCLUDES 1   *sphingolipidosis (E75.0-E75.3)*

E78.0   **Pure hypercholesterolemia**
Familial hypercholesterolemia
Fredrickson's hyperlipoproteinemia, type IIa
Hyperbetalipoproteinemia
Hyperlipidemia, Group A
Low-density-lipoprotein-type [LDL] hyperlipoproteinemia

E78.1   **Pure hyperglyceridemia**
Elevated fasting triglycerides
Endogenous hyperglyceridemia
Fredrickson's hyperlipoproteinemia, type IV
Hyperlipidemia, group B
Hyperprebetalipoproteinemia
Very-low-density-lipoprotein-type [VLDL]
hyperlipoproteinemia

E78.2   **Mixed hyperlipidemia**
Broad- or floating-betalipoproteinemia
Combined hyperlipidemia NOS
Elevated cholesterol with elevated triglycerides NEC
Fredrickson's hyperlipoproteinemia, type IIb or III
Hyperbetalipoproteinemia with prebetalipoproteinemia
Hypercholesteremia with endogenous hyperglyceridemia
Hyperlipidemia, group C
Tubo-eruptive xanthoma
Xanthoma tuberosum
EXCLUDES 1   *cerebrotendinous cholesterosis [van*
Bogaert-Scherer- Epstein] (E75.5)
familial combined hyperlipidemia (E78.4)

E78.3   **Hyperchylomicronemia**
Chylomicron retention disease
Fredrickson's hyperlipoproteinemia, type I or V
Hyperlipidemia, group D
Mixed hyperglyceridemia

E78.4   **Other hyperlipidemia**
Familial combined hyperlipidemia

E78.5   **Hyperlipidemia, unspecified**

E78.6   **Lipoprotein deficiency**
Abetalipoproteinemia
Depressed HDL cholesterol
High-density lipoprotein deficiency
Hypoalphalipoproteinemia
Hypobetalipoproteinemia (familial)
Lecithin cholesterol acyltransferase deficiency
Tangier disease

☑5ᵗʰ E78.7   **Disorders of bile acid and cholesterol metabolism**
EXCLUDES 1   *Niemann-Pick disease type C (E75.242)*

E78.70   **Disorder of bile acid and cholesterol metabolism, unspecified**

E78.71   **Barth syndrome**

E78.72   **Smith-Lemli-Opitz syndrome**

E78.79   **Other disorders of bile acid and cholesterol metabolism**

☑5ᵗʰ E78.8   **Other disorders of lipoprotein metabolism**

E78.81   **Lipoid dermatoarthritis**

E78.89   **Other lipoprotein metabolism disorders**

E78.9   **Disorder of lipoprotein metabolism, unspecified**

☑4ᵗʰ **E79   Disorders of purine and pyrimidine metabolism**
EXCLUDES 1   *Ataxia-telangiectasia (G11.3)*
Bloom's syndrome (Q82.8)
Cockayne's syndrome (Q87.1)
calculus of kidney (N20.0)
combined immunodeficiency disorders (D81-)
Fanconi's anemia (D61.09)
gout (M1a-, M10-)
orotaciduric anemia (D53.0)
progeria (E34.8)
Werner's syndrome (E34.8)
xeroderma pigmentosum (Q82.1)

E79.0   **Hyperuricemia without signs of inflammatory arthritis and tophaceous disease**
Asymptomatic hyperuricemia

E79.1   **Lesch-Nyhan syndrome**
HGPRT deficiency

E79.2   **Myoadenylate deaminase deficiency**

E79.8   **Other disorders of purine and pyrimidine metabolism**
Hereditary xanthinuria

E79.9   **Disorder of purine and pyrimidine metabolism, unspecified**

☑4ᵗʰ **E80   Disorders of porphyrin and bilirubin metabolism**
INCLUDES   defects of catalase and peroxidase

E80.0   **Hereditary erythropoietic porphyria**
Congenital erythropoietic porphyria
Erythropoietic protoporphyria

E80.1   **Porphyria cutanea tarda**

☑5ᵗʰ E80.2   **Other and unspecified porphyria**

E80.20   **Unspecified porphyria**
Porphyria NOS

E80.21   **Acute intermittent (hepatic) porphyria**

E80.29   **Other porphyria**
Hereditary coproporphyria

E80.3   **Defects of catalase and peroxidase**
Acatalasia [Takahara]

E80.4   **Gilbert syndrome**

E80.5   **Crigler-Najjar syndrome**

E80.6   **Other disorders of bilirubin metabolism**
Dubin-Johnson syndrome
Rotor's syndrome

E80.7   **Disorder of bilirubin metabolism, unspecified**

☑4ᵗʰ **E83   Disorders of mineral metabolism**
EXCLUDES 1   *dietary mineral deficiency (E58-E61)*
parathyroid disorders (E20-E21)
vitamin D deficiency (E55-)

☑5ᵗʰ E83.0   **Disorders of copper metabolism**

E83.00   **Disorder of copper metabolism, unspecified**

E83.01   **Wilson's disease**
Code also associated Kayser Fleischer ring (H18.04-)

E83.09   **Other disorders of copper metabolism**
Menkes' (kinky hair) (steely hair) disease

☑5ᵗʰ E83.1   **Disorders of iron metabolism**
EXCLUDES 1   *iron deficiency anemia (D50-)*
sideroblastic anemia (D64.0-D64.3)

E83.10   **Disorder of iron metabolism, unspecified**

☑6ᵗʰ E83.11   **Hemochromatosis**

E83.110   **Hereditary hemochromatosis**
Bronzed diabetes
Pigmentary cirrhosis (of liver)
Primary (hereditary) hemochromatosis

E83.111   **Hemochromatosis due to repeated red blood cell transfusions**
Iron overload due to repeated red blood cell transfusions
Transfusion (red blood cell) associated hemochromatosis

E83.118   **Other hemochromatosis**

E83.119   **Hemochromatosis, unspecified**

E83.19   **Other disorders of iron metabolism**

E83.2   **Disorders of zinc metabolism**
Acrodermatitis enteropathica

☑5ᵗʰ E83.3   **Disorders of phosphorus metabolism and phosphatases**
EXCLUDES 1   *adult osteomalacia (M83-)*
osteoporosis (M80-)

E83.30   **Disorder of phosphorus metabolism, unspecified**

E83.31   **Familial hypophosphatemia**
Vitamin D-resistant osteomalacia
Vitamin D-resistant rickets
EXCLUDES 1   *vitamin D-deficiency rickets (E55.0)*

E83.32   **Hereditary vitamin D-dependent rickets (type 1) (type 2)**
25-hydroxyvitamin D 1-alpha-hydroxylase deficiency
Pseudovitamin D deficiency
Vitamin D receptor defect

E83.39   **Other disorders of phosphorus metabolism**
Acid phosphatase deficiency
Hypophosphatasia

☑5ᵗʰ E83.4   **Disorders of magnesium metabolism**

E83.40   **Disorders of magnesium metabolism, unspecified**

E83.41   **Hypermagnesemia**

E83.42   **Hypomagnesemia**

E83.49   **Other disorders of magnesium metabolism**

☑5ᵗʰ E83.5   **Disorders of calcium metabolism**
EXCLUDES 1   *chondrocalcinosis (M11.1-M11.2)*
hungry bone syndrome (E83.81)
hyperparathyroidism (E21.0-E21.3)

E83.50   **Unspecified disorder of calcium metabolism**

☑ Appropriate additional character required   ☑x7ᵗʰ Requires 7th character, placeholder x must fill empty characters

    E83.51 Hypocalcemia
    E83.52 Hypercalcemia
        Familial hypocalciuric hypercalcemia
    E83.59 Other disorders of calcium metabolism
        Idiopathic hypercalciuria
✓5ᵗʰ **E83.8 Other disorders of mineral metabolism**
    E83.81 Hungry bone syndrome
    E83.89 Other disorders of mineral metabolism
E83.9 Disorder of mineral metabolism, unspecified

✓4ᵗʰ **E84 Cystic fibrosis**
    INCLUDES mucoviscidosis
E84.0 Cystic fibrosis with pulmonary manifestations
    Use additional code to identify any infectious organism
        present, such as:
        Pseudomonas (B96.5)
✓5ᵗʰ **E84.1 Cystic fibrosis with intestinal manifestations**
    E84.11 Meconium ileus in cystic fibrosis
        EXCLUDES 1 *meconium ileus not due to cystic fibrosis*
            (P76.0)
    E84.19 Cystic fibrosis with other intestinal manifestations
        Distal intestinal obstruction syndrome
E84.8 Cystic fibrosis with other manifestations
E84.9 Cystic fibrosis, unspecified

✓4ᵗʰ **E85 Amyloidosis**
    EXCLUDES 1 *Alzheimer's disease (G30.0-)*
E85.0 Non-neuropathic heredofamilial amyloidosis
    Familial Mediterranean fever
    Hereditary amyloid nephropathy
E85.1 Neuropathic heredofamilial amyloidosis
    Amyloid polyneuropathy (Portuguese)
E85.2 Heredofamilial amyloidosis, unspecified
E85.3 Secondary systemic amyloidosis
    Hemodialysis-associated amyloidosis
E85.4 Organ-limited amyloidosis
    Localized amyloidosis
E85.8 Other amyloidosis
E85.9 Amyloidosis, unspecified

✓4ᵗʰ **E86 Volume depletion**
    EXCLUDES 1 *dehydration of newborn (P74.1)*
        hypovolemic shock NOS (R57.1)
        postprocedural hypovolemic shock (T81.1)
        traumatic hypovolemic shock (T79.4)
E86.0 Dehydration
E86.1 Hypovolemia
    Depletion of volume of plasma
E86.9 Volume depletion, unspecified

✓4ᵗʰ **E87 Other disorders of fluid, electrolyte and acid-base balance**
    EXCLUDES 1 *diabetes insipidus (E23.2)*
        electrolyte imbalance associated with hyperemesis
          gravidarum (O21.1)
        electrolyte imbalance following ectopic or molar pregnancy
          (O08.5)
        familial periodic paralysis (G72.3)
E87.0 Hyperosmolality and hypernatremia
    Sodium [Na] excess
    Sodium [Na] overload
E87.1 Hypo-osmolality and hyponatremia
    Sodium [Na] deficiency
    EXCLUDES 1 *syndrome of inappropriate secretion of antidiuretic*
        hormone (E22.2)
E87.2 Acidosis
    Acidosis NOS
    Lactic acidosis
    Metabolic acidosis
    Respiratory acidosis
    EXCLUDES 1 *diabetic acidosis—see categories E08-E13 with*
        ketoacidosis
E87.3 Alkalosis
    Alkalosis NOS
    Metabolic alkalosis
    Respiratory alkalosis
E87.4 Mixed disorder of acid-base balance
E87.5 Hyperkalemia
    Potassium [K] excess
    Potassium [K] overload

E87.6 Hypokalemia
    Potassium [K] deficiency
✓5ᵗʰ **E87.7 Fluid overload**
    EXCLUDES 1 *edema NOS (R60.9)*
        fluid retention (R60.9)
    E87.70 Fluid overload, unspecified
    E87.71 Transfusion associated circulatory overload
        Fluid overload due to transfusion (blood) (blood
          components)
        TACO
    E87.79 Other fluid overload
E87.8 Other disorders of electrolyte and fluid balance, not elsewhere classified
    Electrolyte imbalance NOS
    Hyperchloremia
    Hypochloremia

✓4ᵗʰ **E88 Other and unspecified metabolic disorders**
    Use additional codes for associated conditions
    EXCLUDES 1 *histiocytosis X (chronic) (C96.6)*
✓5ᵗʰ **E88.0 Disorders of plasma-protein metabolism, not elsewhere classified**
    EXCLUDES 1 *disorder of lipoprotein metabolism (E78-)*
        monoclonal gammopathy (of undetermined
          significance) (D47.2)
        polyclonal hypergammaglobulinemia (D89.0)
        Waldenström's macroglobulinemia (C88.0)
    E88.01 Alpha-1-antitrypsin deficiency
        AAT deficiency
    E88.09 Other disorders of plasma-protein metabolism, not elsewhere classified
        Bisalbuminemia
E88.1 Lipodystrophy, not elsewhere classified
    Lipodystrophy NOS
    EXCLUDES 1 *Whipple's disease (K90.81)*
E88.2 Lipomatosis, not elsewhere classified
    Lipomatosis NOS
    Lipomatosis (Check) dolorosa [Dercum]
E88.3 Tumor lysis syndrome
    Tumor lysis syndrome (spontaneous)
    Tumor lysis syndrome following antineoplastic drug
        chemotherapy
    Code first (T45.1-) to identify drug, if drug induced
✓5ᵗʰ **E88.4 Mitochondrial metabolism disorders**
    EXCLUDES 1 *disorders of pyruvate metabolism (E74.4)*
        Kearns-Sayre syndrome (H49.81)
        Leber's disease (H47.22)
        Leigh's encephalopathy (G31.82)
        Mitochondrial myopathy, NEC (G71.3)
        Reye's syndrome (G93.7)
    E88.40 Mitochondrial metabolism disorder, unspecified
    E88.41 MELAS syndrome
        Mitochondrial myopathy, encephalopathy, lactic
          acidosis and stroke-like episodes
    E88.42 MERRF syndrome
        Myoclonic epilepsy associated with ragged-red
          fibers
        Code also myoclonic epilepsy (G40.3-)
    E88.49 Other mitochondrial metabolism disorders
✓5ᵗʰ **E88.8 Other specified metabolic disorders**
    E88.81 Metabolic syndrome
        Dysmetabolic syndrome X
        Use additional codes for associated manifestations,
          such as:
          obesity (E66.-)
    E88.89 Other specified metabolic disorders
        Launois-Bensaude adenolipomatosis
E88.9 Metabolic disorder, unspecified

✓4ᵗʰ **E89 Postprocedural endocrine and metabolic complications and disorders, not elsewhere classified**
    EXCLUDES 2 *intraoperative complications of endocrine system organ or structure (E36.0-, E36.1-, E36.8)*
E89.0 Postprocedural hypothyroidism
    Postirradiation hypothyroidism
    Postsurgical hypothyroidism

EXCLUDES 1 Not coded here   EXCLUDES 2 Not included here   *Manifestation Code*

E89.1 **Postprocedural hypoinsulinemia**
Postpancreatectomy hyperglycemia
Postsurgical hypoinsulinemia
Use additional code, if applicable, to identify:
  acquired absence of pancreas (Z90.41-)
    diabetes mellitus (postpancreatectomy) (postprocedural)
    (E13.-)
    insulin use (Z79.4)
  EXCLUDES 1 *transient postprocedural hyperglycemia (R73.9)*
               transient postprocedural hypoglycemia (E16.2)

E89.2 **Postprocedural hypoparathyroidism**
Parathyroprival tetany

E89.3 **Postprocedural hypopituitarism**
Postirradiation hypopituitarism

√5th E89.4 **Postprocedural ovarian failure**

   E89.40 **Asymptomatic postprocedural ovarian failure**
Postprocedural ovarian failure NOS

   E89.41 **Symptomatic postprocedural ovarian failure**
Symptoms such as flushing, sleeplessness,
headache, lack of concentration, associated
with postprocedural menopause

E89.5 **Postprocedural testicular hypofunction**

E89.6 **Postprocedural adrenocortical (-medullary) hypofunction**

√5th E89.8 **Other postprocedural endocrine and metabolic
complications and disorders**

   √6th E89.81 **Postprocedural hemorrhage and hematoma of an
endocrine system organ or structure following a
procedure**

      E89.810 **Postprocedural hemorrhage and
hematoma of an endocrine system
organ or structure following an
endocrine system procedure**

      E89.811 **Postprocedural hemorrhage and
hematoma of an endocrine system
organ or structure following other
procedure**

   E89.89 **Other postprocedural endocrine and metabolic
complications and disorders**
Use additional code, if applicable, to further specify
disorder

Chapter 5. Mental and Behavioral Disorders (F01-F99)

INCLUDES   disorders of psychological development
EXCLUDES 2   *symptoms, signs and abnormal clinical laboratory findings, not elsewhere classified (R00-R99)*

This chapter contains the following blocks:

F01-F09	Mental disorders due to known physiological conditions
F10-F19	Mental and behavioral disorders due to psychoactive substance use
F20-F29	Schizophrenia, schizotypal and delusional, and other non-mood psychotic disorders
F30-F39	Mood [affective] disorders
F40-F48	Anxiety, dissociative, stress-related, somatoform and other nonpsychotic mental disorders
F50-F59	Behavioral syndromes associated with physiological disturbances and physical factors
F60-F69	Disorders of adult personality and behavior
F70-F79	Mental retardation
F80-F89	Pervasive and specific developmental disorders
F90-F98	Behavioral and emotional disorders with onset usually occurring in childhood and adolescence
F99	Unspecified mental disorder

Mental disorders due to known physiological conditions (F01-F09)

NOTE   This block comprises a range of mental disorders grouped together on the basis of their having in common a demonstrable etiology in cerebral disease, brain injury, or other insult leading to cerebral dysfunction. The dysfunction may be primary, as in diseases, injuries, and insults that affect the brain directly and selectively; or secondary, as in systemic diseases and disorders that attack the brain only as one of the multiple organs or systems of the body that are involved.

✓4ᵗʰ **F01**   **Vascular dementia**

Vascular dementia as a result of infarction of the brain due to vascular disease, including hypertensive cerebrovascular disease.

INCLUDES   arteriosclerotic dementia

Code first the underlying physiological condition or sequelae of cerebrovascular disease.

    ✓5ᵗʰ **F01.5**   **Vascular dementia**

       F01.50   **Vascular dementia without behavioral disturbance**

       F01.51   **Vascular dementia with behavioral disturbance**
          Vascular dementia with aggressive behavior
          Vascular dementia with combative behavior
          Vascular dementia with violent behavior
          Vascular dementia with wandering off

✓4ᵗʰ **F02**   **Dementia in other diseases classified elsewhere**

Code first the underlying physiological condition, such as:
    Alzheimer's (G30-)
    cerebral lipidosis (E75.4)
    Creutzfeldt-Jakob disease (A81.0-)
    dementia with Lewy bodies (G31.83)
    epilepsy and recurrent seizures (G40-)
    frontotemporal dementia (G31.09)
    hepatolenticular degeneration (E83.0)
    human immunodeficiency virus [HIV] disease (B20)
    hypercalcemia (E83.52)
    hypothyroidism, acquired (E00-E03-)
    intoxications (T36-T65)
    Jakob-Creutzfeldt disease (A81.0-)
    multiple sclerosis (G35)
    neurosyphilis (A52.17)
    niacin deficiency [pellagra] (E52)
    Parkinson's disease (G20)
    Pick's disease (G31.01)
    polyarteritis nodosa (M30.0)
    systemic lupus erythematosus (M32-)
    trypanosomiasis (B56-, B57-)
    vitamin B deficiency (E53.8)
EXCLUDES 1   *dementia with Parkinsonism (G31.83)*
EXCLUDES 2   *dementia in alcohol and psychoactive substance disorders (F10-F19, with .17, .27, .97)*
          vascular dementia (F01.5-)

✓5ᵗʰ **F02.8**   **Dementia in other diseases classified elsewhere**

    F02.80   *Dementia in other diseases classified elsewhere, without behavioral disturbance*
       Dementia in other diseases classified elsewhere NOS

    F02.81   *Dementia in other diseases classified elsewhere, with behavioral disturbance*
       Dementia in other diseases classified elsewhere with aggressive behavior
       Dementia in other diseases classified elsewhere with combative behavior
       Dementia in other diseases classified elsewhere with violent behavior
       Dementia in other diseases classified elsewhere with wandering off

F03   **Unspecified dementia**

Presenile dementia NOS
Presenile psychosis NOS
Primary degenerative dementia NOS
Senile dementia NOS
Senile dementia depressed or paranoid type
Senile psychosis NOS
EXCLUDES 1   *senility NOS (R41.81)*
EXCLUDES 2   *senile dementia with delirium or acute confusional state (F05)*

F04   **Amnestic disorder due to known physiological condition**

Korsakov's psychosis or syndrome, nonalcoholic
Code first the underlying physiological condition
EXCLUDES 1   *amnesia NOS (R41.3)*
          anterograde amnesia (R41.1)
          dissociative amnesia (F44.0)
          retrograde amnesia (R41.2)
EXCLUDES 2   *alcohol-induced or unspecified Korsakov's syndrome (F10.26, F10.96)*
          Korsakov's syndrome induced by other psychoactive substances (F13.26, F13.96, F19.16, F19.26, F19.96)

F05   **Delirium due to known physiological condition**

Acute or subacute brain syndrome
Acute or subacute confusional state (nonalcoholic)
Acute or subacute infective psychosis
Acute or subacute organic reaction
Acute or subacute psycho-organic syndrome
Delirium of mixed etiology
Delirium superimposed on dementia
Sundowning
Code first the underlying physiological condition
EXCLUDES 1   *delirium NOS (R41.0)*
EXCLUDES 2   *delirium tremens alcohol-induced or unspecified (F10.231, F10.921)*

✓4ᵗʰ **F06**   **Other mental disorders due to known physiological condition**

INCLUDES   mental disorders due to endocrine disorder
          mental disorders due to exogenous hormone
          mental disorders due to exogenous toxic substance
          mental disorders due to primary cerebral disease
          mental disorders due to somatic illness
          mental disorders due to systemic disease affecting the brain
Code first the underlying physiological condition
EXCLUDES 1   *unspecified dementia (F03)*
EXCLUDES 2   *delirium due to known physiological condition (F05)*
          dementia as classified in F01-F02
          other mental disorders associated with alcohol and other psychoactive substances (F10-F19)

    F06.0   **Psychotic disorder with hallucinations due to known physiological condition**

       Organic hallucinatory state (nonalcoholic)
EXCLUDES 2   *hallucinations and perceptual disturbance induced by alcohol and other psychoactive substances (F10-F19 with .151, .251, .951)*
          schizophrenia (F20-)

    F06.1   **Catatonic disorder due to known physiological condition**

EXCLUDES 1   *catatonic stupor (R40.1)*
          stupor NOS (R40.1)
EXCLUDES 2   *catatonic schizophrenia (F20.2)*
          dissociative stupor (F44.2)

F06.2 Psychotic disorder with delusions due to known physiological condition
Paranoid and paranoid-hallucinatory organic states
Schizophrenia-like psychosis in epilepsy
EXCLUDES 2 *alcohol and drug-induced psychotic disorder (F10-F19 with .150, .250, .950)*
brief psychotic disorder (F23)
delusional disorder (F22)
schizophrenia (F20-)

✓5th F06.3 Mood disorder due to known physiological condition
EXCLUDES 2 *mood disorders due to alcohol and other psychoactive substances (F10-F19 with .14, .24, .94)*
mood disorders, not due to known physiological condition or unspecified (F30-F39)
F06.30 Mood disorder due to known physiological condition, unspecified
F06.31 Mood disorder due to known physiological condition with depressive features
F06.32 Mood disorder due to known physiological condition with major depressive-like episode
F06.33 Mood disorder due to known physiological condition with manic features
F06.34 Mood disorder due to known physiological condition with mixed features

F06.4 Anxiety disorder due to known physiological condition
EXCLUDES 2 *anxiety disorders due to alcohol and other psychoactive substances (F10-F19 with .180, .280, .980)*
anxiety disorders, not due to known physiological condition or unspecified (F40-, F41-)

F06.8 Other specified mental disorders due to known physiological condition
Epileptic psychosis NOS
Organic dissociative disorder
Organic emotionally labile [asthenic] disorder

✓4th F07 Personality and behavioral disorders due to known physiological condition
Code first the underlying physiological condition
F07.0 Personality change due to known physiological condition
Frontal lobe syndrome
Limbic epilepsy personality syndrome
Lobotomy syndrome
Organic personality disorder
Organic pseudopsychopathic personality
Organic pseudoretarded personality
Postleucotomy syndrome
Code first underlying physiological condition
EXCLUDES 1 *mild cognitive impairment (G31.84)*
postconcussional syndrome (F07.81)
postencephalitic syndrome (F07.89)
signs and symptoms involving emotional state (R45-)
EXCLUDES 2 *specific personality disorder (F60-)*

✓5th F07.8 Other personality and behavioral disorders due to known physiological condition
F07.81 Postconcussional syndrome
Postcontusional syndrome (encephalopathy)
Post-traumatic brain syndrome, nonpsychotic
Use additional code to identify associated post-traumatic headache (G44.3-)
EXCLUDES 1 *current concussion (brain) (S06.0-)*
F07.89 Other personality and behavioral disorders due to known physiological condition
Postencephalitic syndrome
Right hemispheric organic affective disorder
F07.9 Unspecified personality and behavioral disorder due to known physiological condition
Organic psychosyndrome

F09 Unspecified mental disorder due to known physiological condition
Mental disorder NOS due to known physiological condition
Organic brain syndrome NOS
Organic mental disorder NOS
Organic psychosis NOS
Symptomatic psychosis NOS
Code first the underlying physiological condition
EXCLUDES 1 *psychosis NOS (F29)*

Mental and behavioral disorders due to psychoactive substance use (F10-F19)

✓4th F10 Alcohol related disorders
Use additional code for blood alcohol level, if applicable (Y90-)
✓5th F10.1 Alcohol abuse
EXCLUDES 1 *alcohol dependence (F10.2-)*
alcohol use, unspecified (F10.9-)
F10.10 Alcohol abuse, uncomplicated
✓6th F10.12 Alcohol abuse with intoxication
F10.120 Alcohol abuse with intoxication, uncomplicated
F10.121 Alcohol abuse with intoxication delirium
F10.129 Alcohol abuse with intoxication, unspecified
F10.14 Alcohol abuse with alcohol-induced mood disorder
✓6th F10.15 Alcohol abuse with alcohol-induced psychotic disorder
F10.150 Alcohol abuse with alcohol-induced psychotic disorder with delusions
F10.151 Alcohol abuse with alcohol-induced psychotic disorder with hallucinations
F10.159 Alcohol abuse with alcohol-induced psychotic disorder, unspecified
✓6th F10.18 Alcohol abuse with other alcohol-induced disorders
F10.180 Alcohol abuse with alcohol-induced anxiety disorder
F10.181 Alcohol abuse with alcohol-induced sexual dysfunction
F10.182 Alcohol abuse with alcohol-induced sleep disorder
F10.188 Alcohol abuse with other alcohol-induced disorder
F10.19 Alcohol abuse with unspecified alcohol-induced disorder
✓5th F10.2 Alcohol dependence
EXCLUDES 1 *alcohol abuse (F10.1-)*
alcohol use, unspecified (F10.9-)
EXCLUDES 2 *toxic effect of alcohol (T51.0-)*
F10.20 Alcohol dependence, uncomplicated
F10.21 Alcohol dependence, in remission
✓6th F10.22 Alcohol dependence with intoxication
Acute drunkenness (in alcoholism)
EXCLUDES 1 *alcohol dependence with withdrawal (F10.23-)*
F10.220 Alcohol dependence with intoxication, uncomplicated
F10.221 Alcohol dependence with intoxication delirium
F10.229 Alcohol dependence with intoxication, unspecified
✓6th F10.23 Alcohol dependence with withdrawal
EXCLUDES 1 *Alcohol dependence with intoxication (F10.22-)*
F10.230 Alcohol dependence with withdrawal, uncomplicated
F10.231 Alcohol dependence with withdrawal delirium
F10.232 Alcohol dependence with withdrawal with perceptual disturbance
F10.239 Alcohol dependence with withdrawal, unspecified
F10.24 Alcohol dependence with alcohol-induced mood disorder
✓6th F10.25 Alcohol dependence with alcohol-induced psychotic disorder
F10.250 Alcohol dependence with alcohol-induced psychotic disorder with delusions
F10.251 Alcohol dependence with alcohol-induced psychotic disorder with hallucinations
F10.259 Alcohol dependence with alcohol-induced psychotic disorder, unspecified

✓ Appropriate additional character required   ✓x7th Requires 7th character, placeholder x must fill empty characters

F10.26   Alcohol dependence with alcohol-induced persisting amnestic disorder

F10.27   Alcohol dependence with alcohol-induced persisting dementia

√6th F10.28   Alcohol dependence with other alcohol-induced disorders

    F10.280   Alcohol dependence with alcohol-induced anxiety disorder

    F10.281   Alcohol dependence with alcohol-induced sexual dysfunction

    F10.282   Alcohol dependence with alcohol-induced sleep disorder

    F10.288   Alcohol dependence with other alcohol-induced disorder

F10.29   Alcohol dependence with unspecified alcohol-induced disorder

√5th F10.9   Alcohol use, unspecified

    EXCLUDES 1   alcohol abuse (F10.1-)
           alcohol dependence (F10.2-)

√6th F10.92   Alcohol use, unspecified with intoxication

    F10.920   Alcohol use, unspecified with intoxication, uncomplicated

    F10.921   Alcohol use, unspecified with intoxication delirium

    F10.929   Alcohol use, unspecified with intoxication, unspecified

F10.94   Alcohol use, unspecified with alcohol-induced mood disorder

√6th F10.95   Alcohol use, unspecified with alcohol-induced psychotic disorder

    F10.950   Alcohol use, unspecified with alcohol-induced psychotic disorder with delusions

    F10.951   Alcohol use, unspecified with alcohol-induced psychotic disorder with hallucinations

    F10.959   Alcohol use, unspecified with alcohol-induced psychotic disorder, unspecified

F10.96   Alcohol use, unspecified with alcohol-induced persisting amnestic disorder

F10.97   Alcohol use, unspecified with alcohol-induced persisting dementia

√6th F10.98   Alcohol use, unspecified with other alcohol-induced disorders

    F10.980   Alcohol use, unspecified with alcohol-induced anxiety disorder

    F10.981   Alcohol use, unspecified with alcohol-induced sexual dysfunction

    F10.982   Alcohol use, unspecified with alcohol-induced sleep disorder

    F10.988   Alcohol use, unspecified with other alcohol-induced disorder

F10.99   Alcohol use, unspecified with unspecified alcohol-induced disorder

√4th **F11**   **Opioid related disorders**

√5th F11.1   Opioid abuse

    EXCLUDES 1   opioid dependence (F11.2-)
           opioid use, unspecified (F11.9-)

F11.10   Opioid abuse, uncomplicated

√6th F11.12   Opioid abuse with intoxication

    F11.120   Opioid abuse with intoxication, uncomplicated

    F11.121   Opioid abuse with intoxication delirium

    F11.122   Opioid abuse with intoxication with perceptual disturbance

    F11.129   Opioid abuse with intoxication, unspecified

F11.14   Opioid abuse with opioid-induced mood disorder

√6th F11.15   Opioid abuse with opioid-induced psychotic disorder

    F11.150   Opioid abuse with opioid-induced psychotic disorder with delusions

    F11.151   Opioid abuse with opioid-induced psychotic disorder with hallucinations

    F11.159   Opioid abuse with opioid-induced psychotic disorder, unspecified

√6th F11.18   Opioid abuse with other opioid-induced disorder

    F11.181   Opioid abuse with opioid-induced sexual dysfunction

    F11.182   Opioid abuse with opioid-induced sleep disorder

    F11.188   Opioid abuse with other opioid-induced disorder

F11.19   Opioid abuse with unspecified opioid-induced disorder

√5th F11.2   Opioid dependence

    EXCLUDES 1   opioid abuse (F11.1-)
           opioid use, unspecified (F11.9-)

    EXCLUDES 2   opioid poisoning (T40.0-T40.2-)

F11.20   Opioid dependence, uncomplicated

F11.21   Opioid dependence, in remission

√6th F11.22   Opioid dependence with intoxication

    EXCLUDES 1   opioid dependence with withdrawal (F11.23)

    F11.220   Opioid dependence with intoxication, uncomplicated

    F11.221   Opioid dependence with intoxication delirium

    F11.222   Opioid dependence with intoxication with perceptual disturbance

    F11.229   Opioid dependence with intoxication, unspecified

F11.23   Opioid dependence with withdrawal

    EXCLUDES 1   opioid dependence with intoxication (F11.22-)

F11.24   Opioid dependence with opioid-induced mood disorder

√6th F11.25   Opioid dependence with opioid-induced psychotic disorder

    F11.250   Opioid dependence with opioid-induced psychotic disorder with delusions

    F11.251   Opioid dependence with opioid-induced psychotic disorder with hallucinations

    F11.259   Opioid dependence with opioid-induced psychotic disorder, unspecified

√6th F11.28   Opioid dependence with other opioid-induced disorder

    F11.281   Opioid dependence with opioid-induced sexual dysfunction

    F11.282   Opioid dependence with opioid-induced sleep disorder

    F11.288   Opioid dependence with other opioid-induced disorder

F11.29   Opioid dependence with unspecified opioid-induced disorder

√5th F11.9   Opioid use, unspecified

    EXCLUDES 1   opioid abuse (F11.1-)
           opioid dependence (F11.2-)

F11.90   Opioid use, unspecified, uncomplicated

√6th F11.92   Opioid use, unspecified with intoxication

    EXCLUDES 1   opioid use, unspecified with withdrawal (F11.93)

    F11.920   Opioid use, unspecified with intoxication, uncomplicated

    F11.921   Opioid use, unspecified with intoxication delirium

    F11.922   Opioid use, unspecified with intoxication with perceptual disturbance

    F11.929   Opioid use, unspecified with intoxication, unspecified

F11.93   Opioid use, unspecified with withdrawal

    EXCLUDES 1   opioid use, unspecified with intoxication (F11.92-)

F11.94   Opioid use, unspecified with opioid-induced mood disorder

√6th F11.95   Opioid use, unspecified with opioid-induced psychotic disorder

    F11.950   Opioid use, unspecified with opioid-induced psychotic disorder with delusions

    F11.951   Opioid use, unspecified with opioid-induced psychotic disorder with hallucinations

---

EXCLUDES 1   Not coded here   EXCLUDES 2   Not included here   *Manifestation Code*

F11.959   **Opioid use, unspecified with opioid-induced psychotic disorder, unspecified**

√6th   F11.98   **Opioid use, unspecified with other specified opioid-induced disorder**

F11.981   **Opioid use, unspecified with opioid-induced sexual dysfunction**

F11.982   **Opioid use, unspecified with opioid-induced sleep disorder**

F11.988   **Opioid use, unspecified with other opioid-induced disorder**

F11.99   **Opioid use, unspecified with unspecified opioid-induced disorder**

√4th   **F12   Cannabis related disorders**

INCLUDES   marijuana

√5th   F12.1   **Cannabis abuse**

EXCLUDES 1   *cannabis dependence (F12.2-)*
cannabis use, unspecified (F12.9-)

F12.10   **Cannabis abuse, uncomplicated**

√6th   F12.12   **Cannabis abuse with intoxication**

F12.120   **Cannabis abuse with intoxication, uncomplicated**

F12.121   **Cannabis abuse with intoxication delirium**

F12.122   **Cannabis abuse with intoxication with perceptual disturbance**

F12.129   **Cannabis abuse with intoxication, unspecified**

√6th   F12.15   **Cannabis abuse with psychotic disorder**

F12.150   **Cannabis abuse with psychotic disorder with delusions**

F12.151   **Cannabis abuse with psychotic disorder with hallucinations**

F12.159   **Cannabis abuse with psychotic disorder, unspecified**

√6th   F12.18   **Cannabis abuse with other cannabis-induced disorder**

F12.180   **Cannabis abuse with cannabis-induced anxiety disorder**

F12.188   **Cannabis abuse with other cannabis-induced disorder**

F12.19   **Cannabis abuse with unspecified cannabis-induced disorder**

√5th   F12.2   **Cannabis dependence**

EXCLUDES 1   *cannabis abuse (F12.1-)*
cannabis use, unspecified (F12.9-)

EXCLUDES 2   *cannabis poisoning (T40.7-)*

F12.20   **Cannabis dependence, uncomplicated**

F12.21   **Cannabis dependence, in remission**

√6th   F12.22   **Cannabis dependence with intoxication**

F12.220   **Cannabis dependence with intoxication, uncomplicated**

F12.221   **Cannabis dependence with intoxication delirium**

F12.222   **Cannabis dependence with intoxication with perceptual disturbance**

F12.229   **Cannabis dependence with intoxication, unspecified**

√6th   F12.25   **Cannabis dependence with psychotic disorder**

F12.250   **Cannabis dependence with psychotic disorder with delusions**

F12.251   **Cannabis dependence with psychotic disorder with hallucinations**

F12.259   **Cannabis dependence with psychotic disorder, unspecified**

√6th   F12.28   **Cannabis dependence with other cannabis-induced disorder**

F12.280   **Cannabis dependence with cannabis-induced anxiety disorder**

F12.288   **Cannabis dependence with other cannabis-induced disorder**

F12.29   **Cannabis dependence with unspecified cannabis-induced disorder**

√5th   F12.9   **Cannabis use, unspecified**

EXCLUDES 1   *cannabis abuse (F12.1-)*
cannabis dependence (F12.2-)

F12.90   **Cannabis use, unspecified, uncomplicated**

√6th   F12.92   **Cannabis use, unspecified with intoxication**

F12.920   **Cannabis use, unspecified with intoxication, uncomplicated**

F12.921   **Cannabis use, unspecified with intoxication delirium**

F12.922   **Cannabis use, unspecified with intoxication with perceptual disturbance**

F12.929   **Cannabis use, unspecified with intoxication, unspecified**

√6th   F12.95   **Cannabis use, unspecified with psychotic disorder**

F12.950   **Cannabis use, unspecified with psychotic disorder with delusions**

F12.951   **Cannabis use, unspecified with psychotic disorder with hallucinations**

F12.959   **Cannabis use, unspecified with psychotic disorder, unspecified**

√6th   F12.98   **Cannabis use, unspecified with other cannabis-induced disorder**

F12.980   **Cannabis use, unspecified with anxiety disorder**

F12.988   **Cannabis use, unspecified with other cannabis-induced disorder**

F12.99   **Cannabis use, unspecified with unspecified cannabis-induced disorder**

√4th   **F13   Sedative, hypnotic, or anxiolytic related disorders**

√5th   F13.1   **Sedative, hypnotic or anxiolytic-related abuse**

EXCLUDES 1   *sedative, hypnotic or anxiolytic-related dependence (F13.2-)*
sedative, hypnotic, or anxiolytic use, unspecified (F13.9-)

F13.10   **Sedative, hypnotic or anxiolytic abuse, uncomplicated**

√6th   F13.12   **Sedative, hypnotic or anxiolytic abuse with intoxication**

F13.120   **Sedative, hypnotic or anxiolytic abuse with intoxication, uncomplicated**

F13.121   **Sedative, hypnotic or anxiolytic abuse with intoxication delirium**

F13.129   **Sedative, hypnotic or anxiolytic abuse with intoxication, unspecified**

F13.14   **Sedative, hypnotic or anxiolytic abuse with sedative, hypnotic or anxiolytic-induced mood disorder**

√6th   F13.15   **Sedative, hypnotic or anxiolytic abuse with sedative, hypnotic or anxiolytic-induced psychotic disorder**

F13.150   **Sedative, hypnotic or anxiolytic abuse with sedative, hypnotic or anxiolytic-induced psychotic disorder with delusions**

F13.151   **Sedative, hypnotic or anxiolytic abuse with sedative, hypnotic or anxiolytic-induced psychotic disorder with hallucinations**

F13.159   **Sedative, hypnotic or anxiolytic abuse with sedative, hypnotic or anxiolytic-induced psychotic disorder, unspecified**

√6th   F13.18   **Sedative, hypnotic or anxiolytic abuse with other sedative, hypnotic or anxiolytic-induced disorders**

F13.180   **Sedative, hypnotic or anxiolytic abuse with sedative, hypnotic or anxiolytic-induced anxiety disorder**

F13.181   **Sedative, hypnotic or anxiolytic abuse with sedative, hypnotic or anxiolytic-induced sexual dysfunction**

F13.182   **Sedative, hypnotic or anxiolytic abuse with sedative, hypnotic or anxiolytic-induced sleep disorder**

F13.188   **Sedative, hypnotic or anxiolytic abuse with other sedative, hypnotic or anxiolytic-induced disorder**

F13.19   **Sedative, hypnotic or anxiolytic abuse with unspecified sedative, hypnotic or anxiolytic-induced disorder**

☑ Appropriate additional character required   √x7th Requires 7th character, placeholder x must fill empty characters

☑5ᵗʰ F13.2 Sedative, hypnotic or anxiolytic-related dependence

EXCLUDES 1   *sedative, hypnotic or anxiolytic-related abuse (F13.1-)*
     sedative, hypnotic, or anxiolytic use, unspecified (F13.9-)

EXCLUDES 2   *sedative, hypnotic, or anxiolytic poisoning (T42-)*

F13.20 Sedative, hypnotic or anxiolytic dependence, uncomplicated

F13.21 Sedative, hypnotic or anxiolytic dependence, in remission

☑6ᵗʰ F13.22 Sedative, hypnotic or anxiolytic dependence with intoxication

     EXCLUDES 1   *sedative, hypnotic or anxiolytic dependence with withdrawal (F13.23-)*

     F13.220 Sedative, hypnotic or anxiolytic dependence with intoxication, uncomplicated

     F13.221 Sedative, hypnotic or anxiolytic dependence with intoxication delirium

     F13.229 Sedative, hypnotic or anxiolytic dependence with intoxication, unspecified

☑6ᵗʰ F13.23 Sedative, hypnotic or anxiolytic dependence with withdrawal

     EXCLUDES 1   *sedative, hypnotic or anxiolytic dependence with intoxication (F13.22-)*

     F13.230 Sedative, hypnotic or anxiolytic dependence with withdrawal, uncomplicated

     F13.231 Sedative, hypnotic or anxiolytic dependence with withdrawal delirium

     F13.232 Sedative, hypnotic or anxiolytic dependence with withdrawal with perceptual disturbance

     F13.239 Sedative, hypnotic or anxiolytic dependence with withdrawal, unspecified

F13.24 Sedative, hypnotic or anxiolytic dependence with sedative, hypnotic or anxiolytic-induced mood disorder

☑6ᵗʰ F13.25 Sedative, hypnotic or anxiolytic dependence with sedative, hypnotic or anxiolytic-induced psychotic disorder

     F13.250 Sedative, hypnotic or anxiolytic dependence with sedative, hypnotic or anxiolytic-induced psychotic disorder with delusions

     F13.251 Sedative, hypnotic or anxiolytic dependence with sedative, hypnotic or anxiolytic-induced psychotic disorder with hallucinations

     F13.259 Sedative, hypnotic or anxiolytic dependence with sedative, hypnotic or anxiolytic-induced psychotic disorder, unspecified

F13.26 Sedative, hypnotic or anxiolytic dependence with sedative, hypnotic or anxiolytic-induced persisting amnestic disorder

F13.27 Sedative, hypnotic or anxiolytic dependence with sedative, hypnotic or anxiolytic-induced persisting dementia

☑6ᵗʰ F13.28 Sedative, hypnotic or anxiolytic dependence with other sedative, hypnotic or anxiolytic-induced disorders

     F13.280 Sedative, hypnotic or anxiolytic dependence with sedative, hypnotic or anxiolytic-induced anxiety disorder

     F13.281 Sedative, hypnotic or anxiolytic dependence with sedative, hypnotic or anxiolytic-induced sexual dysfunction

     F13.282 Sedative, hypnotic or anxiolytic dependence with sedative, hypnotic or anxiolytic-induced sleep disorder

     F13.288 Sedative, hypnotic or anxiolytic dependence with other sedative, hypnotic or anxiolytic-induced disorder

F13.29 Sedative, hypnotic or anxiolytic dependence with unspecified sedative, hypnotic or anxiolytic-induced disorder

☑5ᵗʰ F13.9 Sedative, hypnotic or anxiolytic-related use, unspecified

EXCLUDES 1   *sedative, hypnotic or anxiolytic-related abuse (F13.1-)*
     sedative, hypnotic or anxiolytic-related dependence (F13.2-)

F13.90 Sedative, hypnotic, or anxiolytic use, unspecified, uncomplicated

☑6ᵗʰ F13.92 Sedative, hypnotic or anxiolytic use, unspecified with intoxication

     EXCLUDES 1   *sedative, hypnotic or anxiolytic use, unspecified with withdrawal (F13.93-)*

     F13.920 Sedative, hypnotic or anxiolytic use, unspecified with intoxication, uncomplicated

     F13.921 Sedative, hypnotic or anxiolytic use, unspecified with intoxication delirium

     F13.929 Sedative, hypnotic or anxiolytic use, unspecified with intoxication, unspecified

☑6ᵗʰ F13.93 Sedative, hypnotic or anxiolytic use, unspecified with withdrawal

     EXCLUDES 1   *sedative, hypnotic or anxiolytic use, unspecified with intoxication (F13.92-)*

     F13.930 Sedative, hypnotic or anxiolytic use, unspecified with withdrawal, uncomplicated

     F13.931 Sedative, hypnotic or anxiolytic use, unspecified with withdrawal delirium

     F13.932 Sedative, hypnotic or anxiolytic use, unspecified with withdrawal with perceptual disturbances

     F13.939 Sedative, hypnotic or anxiolytic use, unspecified with withdrawal, unspecified

F13.94 Sedative, hypnotic or anxiolytic use, unspecified with sedative, hypnotic or anxiolytic-induced mood disorder

☑6ᵗʰ F13.95 Sedative, hypnotic or anxiolytic use, unspecified with sedative, hypnotic or anxiolytic-induced psychotic disorder

     F13.950 Sedative, hypnotic or anxiolytic use, unspecified with sedative, hypnotic or anxiolytic-induced psychotic disorder with delusions

     F13.951 Sedative, hypnotic or anxiolytic use, unspecified with sedative, hypnotic or anxiolytic-induced psychotic disorder with hallucinations

     F13.959 Sedative, hypnotic or anxiolytic use, unspecified with sedative, hypnotic or anxiolytic-induced psychotic disorder, unspecified

F13.96 Sedative, hypnotic or anxiolytic use, unspecified with sedative, hypnotic or anxiolytic-induced persisting amnestic disorder

F13.97 Sedative, hypnotic or anxiolytic use, unspecified with sedative, hypnotic or anxiolytic-induced persisting dementia

☑6ᵗʰ F13.98 Sedative, hypnotic or anxiolytic use, unspecified with other sedative, hypnotic or anxiolytic-induced disorders

     F13.980 Sedative, hypnotic or anxiolytic use, unspecified with sedative, hypnotic or anxiolytic-induced anxiety disorder

     F13.981 Sedative, hypnotic or anxiolytic use, unspecified with sedative, hypnotic or anxiolytic-induced sexual dysfunction

     F13.982 Sedative, hypnotic or anxiolytic use, unspecified with sedative, hypnotic or anxiolytic-induced sleep disorder

     F13.988 Sedative, hypnotic or anxiolytic use, unspecified with other sedative, hypnotic or anxiolytic-induced disorder

F13.99 Sedative, hypnotic or anxiolytic use, unspecified with unspecified sedative, hypnotic or anxiolytic-induced disorder

---

EXCLUDES 1 Not coded here   EXCLUDES 2 Not included here   *Manifestation Code*

✓4th **F14 Cocaine related disorders**
  EXCLUDES 2 *other stimulant-related disorders (F15-)*
✓5th **F14.1 Cocaine abuse**
    EXCLUDES 1 *cocaine dependence (F14.2-)*
                cocaine use, unspecified (F14.9-)
    F14.10 Cocaine abuse, uncomplicated
✓6th **F14.12 Cocaine abuse with intoxication**
      F14.120 Cocaine abuse with intoxication, uncomplicated
      F14.121 Cocaine abuse with intoxication with delirium
      F14.122 Cocaine abuse with intoxication with perceptual disturbance
      F14.129 Cocaine abuse with intoxication, unspecified
    F14.14 Cocaine abuse with cocaine-induced mood disorder
✓6th **F14.15 Cocaine abuse with cocaine-induced psychotic disorder**
      F14.150 Cocaine abuse with cocaine-induced psychotic disorder with delusions
      F14.151 Cocaine abuse with cocaine-induced psychotic disorder with hallucinations
      F14.159 Cocaine abuse with cocaine-induced psychotic disorder, unspecified
✓6th **F14.18 Cocaine abuse with other cocaine-induced disorder**
      F14.180 Cocaine abuse with cocaine-induced anxiety disorder
      F14.181 Cocaine abuse with cocaine-induced sexual dysfunction
      F14.182 Cocaine abuse with cocaine-induced sleep disorder
      F14.188 Cocaine abuse with other cocaine-induced disorder
    F14.19 Cocaine abuse with unspecified cocaine-induced disorder
✓5th **F14.2 Cocaine dependence**
    EXCLUDES 1 *cocaine abuse (F14.1-)*
                cocaine use, unspecified (F14.9-)
    EXCLUDES 2 *cocaine poisoning (T40.5-)*
    F14.20 Cocaine dependence, uncomplicated
    F14.21 Cocaine dependence, in remission
✓6th **F14.22 Cocaine dependence with intoxication**
      EXCLUDES 1 *cocaine dependence with withdrawal (F14.23)*
      F14.220 Cocaine dependence with intoxication, uncomplicated
      F14.221 Cocaine dependence with intoxication delirium
      F14.222 Cocaine dependence with intoxication with perceptual disturbance
      F14.229 Cocaine dependence with intoxication, unspecified
    F14.23 Cocaine dependence with withdrawal
      EXCLUDES 1 *cocaine dependence with intoxication (F14.22-)*
    F14.24 Cocaine dependence with cocaine-induced mood disorder
✓6th **F14.25 Cocaine dependence with cocaine-induced psychotic disorder**
      F14.250 Cocaine dependence with cocaine-induced psychotic disorder with delusions
      F14.251 Cocaine dependence with cocaine-induced psychotic disorder with hallucinations
      F14.259 Cocaine dependence with cocaine-induced psychotic disorder, unspecified
✓6th **F14.28 Cocaine dependence with other cocaine-induced disorder**
      F14.280 Cocaine dependence with cocaine-induced anxiety disorder
      F14.281 Cocaine dependence with cocaine-induced sexual dysfunction
      F14.282 Cocaine dependence with cocaine-induced sleep disorder

      F14.288 Cocaine dependence with other cocaine-induced disorder
    F14.29 Cocaine dependence with unspecified cocaine-induced disorder
✓5th **F14.9 Cocaine use, unspecified**
    EXCLUDES 1 *cocaine abuse (F14.1-)*
                cocaine dependence (F14.2-)
    F14.90 Cocaine use, unspecified, uncomplicated
✓6th **F14.92 Cocaine use, unspecified with intoxication**
      F14.920 Cocaine use, unspecified with intoxication, uncomplicated
      F14.921 Cocaine use, unspecified with intoxication delirium
      F14.922 Cocaine use, unspecified with intoxication with perceptual disturbance
      F14.929 Cocaine use, unspecified with intoxication, unspecified
    F14.94 Cocaine use, unspecified with cocaine-induced mood disorder
✓6th **F14.95 Cocaine use, unspecified with cocaine-induced psychotic disorder**
      F14.950 Cocaine use, unspecified with cocaine-induced psychotic disorder with delusions
      F14.951 Cocaine use, unspecified with cocaine-induced psychotic disorder with hallucinations
      F14.959 Cocaine use, unspecified with cocaine-induced psychotic disorder, unspecified
✓6th **F14.98 Cocaine use, unspecified with other specified cocaine-induced disorder**
      F14.980 Cocaine use, unspecified with cocaine-induced anxiety disorder
      F14.981 Cocaine use, unspecified with cocaine-induced sexual dysfunction
      F14.982 Cocaine use, unspecified with cocaine-induced sleep disorder
      F14.988 Cocaine use, unspecified with other cocaine-induced disorder
    F14.99 Cocaine use, unspecified with unspecified cocaine-induced disorder

✓4th **F15 Other stimulant related disorders**
  Amphetamine-related disorders
  Caffeine
  EXCLUDES 2 *cocaine-related disorders (F14-)*
✓5th **F15.1 Other stimulant abuse**
    EXCLUDES 1 *other stimulant dependence (F15.2-)*
                other stimulant use, unspecified (F15.9-)
    F15.10 Other stimulant abuse, uncomplicated
✓6th **F15.12 Other stimulant abuse with intoxication**
      F15.120 Other stimulant abuse with intoxication, uncomplicated
      F15.121 Other stimulant abuse with intoxication delirium
      F15.122 Other stimulant abuse with intoxication with perceptual disturbance
      F15.129 Other stimulant abuse with intoxication, unspecified
    F15.14 Other stimulant abuse with stimulant-induced mood disorder
✓6th **F15.15 Other stimulant abuse with stimulant-induced psychotic disorder**
      F15.150 Other stimulant abuse with stimulant-induced psychotic disorder with delusions
      F15.151 Other stimulant abuse with stimulant-induced psychotic disorder with hallucinations
      F15.159 Other stimulant abuse with stimulant-induced psychotic disorder, unspecified
✓6th **F15.18 Other stimulant abuse with other stimulant-induced disorder**
      F15.180 Other stimulant abuse with stimulant-induced anxiety disorder

    F15.181 **Other stimulant abuse with stimulant-induced sexual dysfunction**

    F15.182 **Other stimulant abuse with stimulant-induced sleep disorder**

    F15.188 **Other stimulant abuse with other stimulant-induced disorder**

  F15.19 **Other stimulant abuse with unspecified stimulant-induced disorder**

☑5th F15.2 **Other stimulant dependence**

    EXCLUDES 1 *other stimulant abuse (F15.1-)*
    other stimulant use, unspecified (F15.9-)

  F15.20 **Other stimulant dependence, uncomplicated**

  F15.21 **Other stimulant dependence, in remission**

☑6th F15.22 **Other stimulant dependence with intoxication**

    EXCLUDES 1 *other stimulant dependence with withdrawal (F15.23)*

    F15.220 **Other stimulant dependence with intoxication, uncomplicated**

    F15.221 **Other stimulant dependence with intoxication delirium**

    F15.222 **Other stimulant dependence with intoxication with perceptual disturbance**

    F15.229 **Other stimulant dependence with intoxication, unspecified**

  F15.23 **Other stimulant dependence with withdrawal**

    EXCLUDES 1 *other stimulant dependence with intoxication (F15.22-)*

  F15.24 **Other stimulant dependence with stimulant-induced mood disorder**

☑6th F15.25 **Other stimulant dependence with stimulant-induced psychotic disorder**

    F15.250 **Other stimulant dependence with stimulant-induced psychotic disorder with delusions**

    F15.251 **Other stimulant dependence with stimulant-induced psychotic disorder with hallucinations**

    F15.259 **Other stimulant dependence with stimulant-induced psychotic disorder, unspecified**

☑6th F15.28 **Other stimulant dependence with other stimulant-induced disorder**

    F15.280 **Other stimulant dependence with stimulant-induced anxiety disorder**

    F15.281 **Other stimulant dependence with stimulant-induced sexual dysfunction**

    F15.282 **Other stimulant dependence with stimulant-induced sleep disorder**

    F15.288 **Other stimulant dependence with other stimulant-induced disorder**

  F15.29 **Other stimulant dependence with unspecified stimulant-induced disorder**

☑5th F15.9 **Other stimulant use, unspecified**

    EXCLUDES 1 *other stimulant abuse (F15.1-)*
    other stimulant dependence (F15.2-)

  F15.90 **Other stimulant use, unspecified, uncomplicated**

☑6th F15.92 **Other stimulant use, unspecified with intoxication**

    EXCLUDES 1 *other stimulant use, unspecified with withdrawal (F15.93)*

    F15.920 **Other stimulant use, unspecified with intoxication, uncomplicated**

    F15.921 **Other stimulant use, unspecified with intoxication delirium**

    F15.922 **Other stimulant use, unspecified with intoxication with perceptual disturbance**

    F15.929 **Other stimulant use, unspecified with intoxication, unspecified**

  F15.93 **Other stimulant use, unspecified with withdrawal**

    EXCLUDES 1 *other stimulant use, unspecified with intoxication (F15.92-)*

  F15.94 **Other stimulant use, unspecified with stimulant-induced mood disorder**

☑6th F15.95 **Other stimulant use, unspecified with stimulant-induced psychotic disorder**

    F15.950 **Other stimulant use, unspecified with stimulant-induced psychotic disorder with delusions**

    F15.951 **Other stimulant use, unspecified with stimulant-induced psychotic disorder with hallucinations**

    F15.959 **Other stimulant use, unspecified with stimulant-induced psychotic disorder, unspecified**

☑6th F15.98 **Other stimulant use, unspecified with other stimulant-induced disorder**

    F15.980 **Other stimulant use, unspecified with stimulant-induced anxiety disorder**

    F15.981 **Other stimulant use, unspecified with stimulant-induced sexual dysfunction**

    F15.982 **Other stimulant use, unspecified with stimulant-induced sleep disorder**

    F15.988 **Other stimulant use, unspecified with other stimulant-induced disorder**

  F15.99 **Other stimulant use, unspecified with unspecified stimulant-induced disorder**

☑4th **F16 Hallucinogen related disorders**

    INCLUDES ecstasy
    PCP
    phencyclidine

☑5th F16.1 **Hallucinogen abuse**

    EXCLUDES 1 *hallucinogen dependence (F16.2-)*
    hallucinogen use, unspecified (F16.9-)

  F16.10 **Hallucinogen abuse, uncomplicated**

☑6th F16.12 **Hallucinogen abuse with intoxication**

    F16.120 **Hallucinogen abuse with intoxication, uncomplicated**

    F16.121 **Hallucinogen abuse with intoxication with delirium**

    F16.122 **Hallucinogen abuse with intoxication with perceptual disturbance**

    F16.129 **Hallucinogen abuse with intoxication, unspecified**

  F16.14 **Hallucinogen abuse with hallucinogen-induced mood disorder**

☑6th F16.15 **Hallucinogen abuse with hallucinogen-induced psychotic disorder**

    F16.150 **Hallucinogen abuse with hallucinogen-induced psychotic disorder with delusions**

    F16.151 **Hallucinogen abuse with hallucinogen-induced psychotic disorder with hallucinations**

    F16.159 **Hallucinogen abuse with hallucinogen-induced psychotic disorder, unspecified**

☑6th F16.18 **Hallucinogen abuse with other hallucinogen-induced disorder**

    F16.180 **Hallucinogen abuse with hallucinogen-induced anxiety disorder**

    F16.183 **Hallucinogen abuse with hallucinogen persisting perception disorder (flashbacks)**

    F16.188 **Hallucinogen abuse with other hallucinogen-induced disorder**

  F16.19 **Hallucinogen abuse with unspecified hallucinogen-induced disorder**

☑5th F16.2 **Hallucinogen dependence**

    EXCLUDES 1 *hallucinogen abuse (F16.1-)*
    hallucinogen use, unspecified (F16.9-)

  F16.20 **Hallucinogen dependence, uncomplicated**

  F16.21 **Hallucinogen dependence, in remission**

☑6th F16.22 **Hallucinogen dependence with intoxication**

    F16.220 **Hallucinogen dependence with intoxication, uncomplicated**

    F16.221 **Hallucinogen dependence with intoxication with delirium**

    F16.229 **Hallucinogen dependence with intoxication, unspecified**

  F16.24 **Hallucinogen dependence with hallucinogen-induced mood disorder**

EXCLUDES 1 Not coded here   EXCLUDES 2 Not included here   *Manifestation Code*

✓6ᵗʰ **F16.25 Hallucinogen dependence with hallucinogen-induced psychotic disorder**
    F16.250 Hallucinogen dependence with hallucinogen-induced psychotic disorder with delusions
    F16.251 Hallucinogen dependence with hallucinogen-induced psychotic disorder with hallucinations
    F16.259 Hallucinogen dependence with hallucinogen-induced psychotic disorder, unspecified

✓6ᵗʰ **F16.28 Hallucinogen dependence with other hallucinogen-induced disorder**
    F16.280 Hallucinogen dependence with hallucinogen-induced anxiety disorder
    F16.283 Hallucinogen dependence with hallucinogen persisting perception disorder (flashbacks)
    F16.288 Hallucinogen dependence with other hallucinogen-induced disorder

    F16.29 Hallucinogen dependence with unspecified hallucinogen-induced disorder

✓5ᵗʰ **F16.9 Hallucinogen use, unspecified**
    EXCLUDES 1 *hallucinogen abuse (F16.1-)*
        hallucinogen dependence (F16.2-)

    F16.90 Hallucinogen use, unspecified, uncomplicated

✓6ᵗʰ **F16.92 Hallucinogen use, unspecified with intoxication**
    F16.920 Hallucinogen use, unspecified with intoxication, uncomplicated
    F16.921 Hallucinogen use, unspecified with intoxication with delirium
    F16.929 Hallucinogen use, unspecified with intoxication, unspecified

    F16.94 Hallucinogen use, unspecified with hallucinogen-induced mood disorder

✓6ᵗʰ **F16.95 Hallucinogen use, unspecified with hallucinogen-induced psychotic disorder**
    F16.950 Hallucinogen use, unspecified with hallucinogen-induced psychotic disorder with delusions
    F16.951 Hallucinogen use, unspecified with hallucinogen-induced psychotic disorder with hallucinations
    F16.959 Hallucinogen use, unspecified with hallucinogen-induced psychotic disorder, unspecified

✓6ᵗʰ **F16.98 Hallucinogen use, unspecified with other specified hallucinogen-induced disorder**
    F16.980 Hallucinogen use, unspecified with hallucinogen-induced anxiety disorder
    F16.983 Hallucinogen use, unspecified with hallucinogen persisting perception disorder (flashbacks)
    F16.988 Hallucinogen use, unspecified with other hallucinogen-induced disorder

    F16.99 Hallucinogen use, unspecified with unspecified hallucinogen-induced disorder

✓4ᵗʰ **F17 Nicotine dependence**
    EXCLUDES 1 *history of tobacco dependence (Z87.891)*
        tobacco use NOS (Z72.0)
    EXCLUDES 2 *tobacco use (smoking) during pregnancy, childbirth and the puerperium (O99.33-)*
        toxic effect of nicotine (T65.2-)

✓5ᵗʰ **F17.2 Nicotine dependence**

✓6ᵗʰ **F17.20 Nicotine dependence, unspecified**
    F17.200 Nicotine dependence, unspecified, uncomplicated
    F17.201 Nicotine dependence, unspecified, in remission
    F17.203 Nicotine dependence unspecified, with withdrawal
    F17.208 Nicotine dependence, unspecified, with other nicotine-induced disorders
    F17.209 Nicotine dependence, unspecified, with unspecified nicotine-induced disorders

✓6ᵗʰ **F17.21 Nicotine dependence, cigarettes**
    F17.210 Nicotine dependence, cigarettes, uncomplicated

    F17.211 Nicotine dependence, cigarettes, in remission
    F17.213 Nicotine dependence, cigarettes, with withdrawal
    F17.218 Nicotine dependence, cigarettes, with other nicotine-induced disorders
    F17.219 Nicotine dependence, cigarettes, with unspecified nicotine-induced disorders

✓6ᵗʰ **F17.22 Nicotine dependence, chewing tobacco**
    F17.220 Nicotine dependence, chewing tobacco, uncomplicated
    F17.221 Nicotine dependence, chewing tobacco, in remission
    F17.223 Nicotine dependence, chewing tobacco, with withdrawal
    F17.228 Nicotine dependence, chewing tobacco, with other nicotine-induced disorders
    F17.229 Nicotine dependence, chewing tobacco, with unspecified nicotine-induced disorders

✓6ᵗʰ **F17.29 Nicotine dependence, other tobacco product**
    F17.290 Nicotine dependence, other tobacco product, uncomplicated
    F17.291 Nicotine dependence, other tobacco product, in remission
    F17.293 Nicotine dependence, other tobacco product, with withdrawal
    F17.298 Nicotine dependence, other tobacco product, with other nicotine-induced disorders
    F17.299 Nicotine dependence, other tobacco product, with unspecified nicotine-induced disorders

✓4ᵗʰ **F18 Inhalant related disorders**
    INCLUDES volatile solvents

✓5ᵗʰ **F18.1 Inhalant abuse**
    EXCLUDES 1 *inhalant dependence (F18.2-)*
        inhalant use, unspecified (F18.9-)

    F18.10 Inhalant abuse, uncomplicated

✓6ᵗʰ **F18.12 Inhalant abuse with intoxication**
    F18.120 Inhalant abuse with intoxication, uncomplicated
    F18.121 Inhalant abuse with intoxication delirium
    F18.129 Inhalant abuse with intoxication, unspecified

    F18.14 Inhalant abuse with inhalant-induced mood disorder

✓6ᵗʰ **F18.15 Inhalant abuse with inhalant-induced psychotic disorder**
    F18.150 Inhalant abuse with inhalant-induced psychotic disorder with delusions
    F18.151 Inhalant abuse with inhalant-induced psychotic disorder with hallucinations
    F18.159 Inhalant abuse with inhalant-induced psychotic disorder, unspecified

    F18.17 Inhalant abuse with inhalant-induced dementia

✓6ᵗʰ **F18.18 Inhalant abuse with other inhalant-induced disorders**
    F18.180 Inhalant abuse with inhalant-induced anxiety disorder
    F18.188 Inhalant abuse with other inhalant-induced disorder

    F18.19 Inhalant abuse with unspecified inhalant-induced disorder

✓5ᵗʰ **F18.2 Inhalant dependence**
    EXCLUDES 1 *inhalant abuse (F18.1-)*
        inhalant use, unspecified (F18.9-)

    F18.20 Inhalant dependence, uncomplicated
    F18.21 Inhalant dependence, in remission

✓6ᵗʰ **F18.22 Inhalant dependence with intoxication**
    F18.220 Inhalant dependence with intoxication, uncomplicated
    F18.221 Inhalant dependence with intoxication delirium
    F18.229 Inhalant dependence with intoxication, unspecified

---

✓ Appropriate additional character required   ✓ₓ7ᵗʰ Requires 7th character, placeholder x must fill empty characters

F18.24   Inhalant dependence with inhalant-induced mood disorder

☑6ᵗʰ F18.25   Inhalant dependence with inhalant-induced psychotic disorder

    F18.250   Inhalant dependence with inhalant-induced psychotic disorder with delusions

    F18.251   Inhalant dependence with inhalant-induced psychotic disorder with hallucinations

    F18.259   Inhalant dependence with inhalant-induced psychotic disorder, unspecified

F18.27   Inhalant dependence with inhalant-induced dementia

☑6ᵗʰ F18.28   Inhalant dependence with other inhalant-induced disorders

    F18.280   Inhalant dependence with inhalant-induced anxiety disorder

    F18.288   Inhalant dependence with other inhalant-induced disorder

F18.29   Inhalant dependence with unspecified inhalant-induced disorder

☑5ᵗʰ F18.9   **Inhalant use, unspecified**

    EXCLUDES 1   inhalant abuse (F18.1-)
                  inhalant dependence (F18.2-)

F18.90   Inhalant use, unspecified, uncomplicated

☑6ᵗʰ F18.92   Inhalant use, unspecified with intoxication

    F18.920   Inhalant use, unspecified with intoxication, uncomplicated

    F18.921   Inhalant use, unspecified with intoxication with delirium

    F18.929   Inhalant use, unspecified with intoxication, unspecified

F18.94   Inhalant use, unspecified with inhalant-induced mood disorder

☑6ᵗʰ F18.95   Inhalant use, unspecified with inhalant-induced psychotic disorder

    F18.950   Inhalant use, unspecified with inhalant-induced psychotic disorder with delusions

    F18.951   Inhalant use, unspecified with inhalant-induced psychotic disorder with hallucinations

    F18.959   Inhalant use, unspecified with inhalant-induced psychotic disorder, unspecified

F18.97   Inhalant use, unspecified with inhalant-induced persisting dementia

☑6ᵗʰ F18.98   Inhalant use, unspecified with other inhalant-induced disorders

    F18.980   Inhalant use, unspecified with inhalant-induced anxiety disorder

    F18.988   Inhalant use, unspecified with other inhalant-induced disorder

F18.99   Inhalant use, unspecified with unspecified inhalant-induced disorder

☑4ᵗʰ **F19   Other psychoactive substance related disorders**

    INCLUDES   polysubstance drug use (indiscriminate drug use)

☑5ᵗʰ F19.1   **Other psychoactive substance abuse**

    EXCLUDES 1   other psychoactive substance dependence (F19.2-)
                  other psychoactive substance use, unspecified (F19.9-)

F19.10   Other psychoactive substance abuse, uncomplicated

☑6ᵗʰ F19.12   Other psychoactive substance abuse with intoxication

    F19.120   Other psychoactive substance abuse with intoxication, uncomplicated

    F19.121   Other psychoactive substance abuse with intoxication delirium

    F19.122   Other psychoactive substance abuse with intoxication with perceptual disturbances

    F19.129   Other psychoactive substance abuse with intoxication, unspecified

F19.14   Other psychoactive substance abuse with psychoactive substance-induced mood disorder

☑6ᵗʰ F19.15   Other psychoactive substance abuse with psychoactive substance-induced psychotic disorder

    F19.150   Other psychoactive substance abuse with psychoactive substance-induced psychotic disorder with delusions

    F19.151   Other psychoactive substance abuse with psychoactive substance-induced psychotic disorder with hallucinations

    F19.159   Other psychoactive substance abuse with psychoactive substance-induced psychotic disorder, unspecified

F19.16   Other psychoactive substance abuse with psychoactive substance-induced persisting amnestic disorder

F19.17   Other psychoactive substance abuse with psychoactive substance-induced persisting dementia

☑6ᵗʰ F19.18   Other psychoactive substance abuse with other psychoactive substance-induced disorders

    F19.180   Other psychoactive substance abuse with psychoactive substance-induced anxiety disorder

    F19.181   Other psychoactive substance abuse with psychoactive substance-induced sexual dysfunction

    F19.182   Other psychoactive substance abuse with psychoactive substance-induced sleep disorder

    F19.188   Other psychoactive substance abuse with other psychoactive substance-induced disorder

F19.19   Other psychoactive substance abuse with unspecified psychoactive substance-induced disorder

☑5ᵗʰ F19.2   **Other psychoactive substance dependence**

    EXCLUDES 1   other psychoactive substance abuse (F19.1-)
                  other psychoactive substance use, unspecified (F19.9-)

F19.20   Other psychoactive substance dependence, uncomplicated

F19.21   Other psychoactive substance dependence, in remission

☑6ᵗʰ F19.22   Other psychoactive substance dependence with intoxication

    EXCLUDES 1   other psychoactive substance dependence with withdrawal (F19.23-)

    F19.220   Other psychoactive substance dependence with intoxication, uncomplicated

    F19.221   Other psychoactive substance dependence with intoxication delirium

    F19.222   Other psychoactive substance dependence with intoxication with perceptual disturbance

    F19.229   Other psychoactive substance dependence with intoxication, unspecified

☑6ᵗʰ F19.23   Other psychoactive substance dependence with withdrawal

    EXCLUDES 1   other psychoactive substance dependence with intoxication (F19.22-)

    F19.230   Other psychoactive substance dependence with withdrawal, uncomplicated

    F19.231   Other psychoactive substance dependence with withdrawal delirium

    F19.232   Other psychoactive substance dependence with withdrawal with perceptual disturbance

    F19.239   Other psychoactive substance dependence with withdrawal, unspecified

F19.24   Other psychoactive substance dependence with psychoactive substance-induced mood disorder

---

EXCLUDES 1   Not coded here   EXCLUDES 2   Not included here   *Manifestation Code*

✓6th **F19.25 Other psychoactive substance dependence with psychoactive substance-induced psychotic disorder**

    F19.250 Other psychoactive substance dependence with psychoactive substance-induced psychotic disorder with delusions

    F19.251 Other psychoactive substance dependence with psychoactive substance-induced psychotic disorder with hallucinations

    F19.259 Other psychoactive substance dependence with psychoactive substance-induced psychotic disorder, unspecified

F19.26 Other psychoactive substance dependence with psychoactive substance-induced persisting amnestic disorder

F19.27 Other psychoactive substance dependence with psychoactive substance-induced persisting dementia

✓6th **F19.28 Other psychoactive substance dependence with other psychoactive substance-induced disorders**

    F19.280 Other psychoactive substance dependence with psychoactive substance-induced anxiety disorder

    F19.281 Other psychoactive substance dependence with psychoactive substance-induced sexual dysfunction

    F19.282 Other psychoactive substance dependence with psychoactive substance-induced sleep disorder

    F19.288 Other psychoactive substance dependence with other psychoactive substance-induced disorder

F19.29 Other psychoactive substance dependence with unspecified psychoactive substance-induced disorder

✓5th **F19.9 Other psychoactive substance use, unspecified**

    EXCLUDES 1 *other psychoactive substance abuse (F19.1-)*
           other psychoactive substance dependence (F19.2-)

F19.90 Other psychoactive substance use, unspecified, uncomplicated

✓6th **F19.92 Other psychoactive substance use, unspecified with intoxication**

    EXCLUDES 1 *other psychoactive substance use, unspecified with withdrawal (F19.93)*

    F19.920 Other psychoactive substance use, unspecified with intoxication, uncomplicated

    F19.921 Other psychoactive substance use, unspecified with intoxication with delirium

    F19.922 Other psychoactive substance use, unspecified with intoxication with perceptual disturbance

    F19.929 Other psychoactive substance use, unspecified with intoxication, unspecified

✓6th **F19.93 Other psychoactive substance use, unspecified with withdrawal**

    EXCLUDES 1 *other psychoactive substance use, unspecified with intoxication (F19.92-)*

    F19.930 Other psychoactive substance use, unspecified with withdrawal, uncomplicated

    F19.931 Other psychoactive substance use, unspecified with withdrawal delirium

    F19.932 Other psychoactive substance use, unspecified with withdrawal with perceptual disturbance

    F19.939 Other psychoactive substance use, unspecified with withdrawal, unspecified

F19.94 Other psychoactive substance use, unspecified with psychoactive substance-induced mood disorder

✓6th **F19.95 Other psychoactive substance use, unspecified with psychoactive substance-induced psychotic disorder**

    F19.950 Other psychoactive substance use, unspecified with psychoactive substance-induced psychotic disorder with delusions

    F19.951 Other psychoactive substance use, unspecified with psychoactive substance-induced psychotic disorder with hallucinations

    F19.959 Other psychoactive substance use, unspecified with psychoactive substance-induced psychotic disorder, unspecified

F19.96 Other psychoactive substance use, unspecified with psychoactive substance-induced persisting amnestic disorder

F19.97 Other psychoactive substance use, unspecified with psychoactive substance-induced persisting dementia

✓6th **F19.98 Other psychoactive substance use, unspecified with other psychoactive substance-induced disorders**

    F19.980 Other psychoactive substance use, unspecified with psychoactive substance-induced anxiety disorder

    F19.981 Other psychoactive substance use, unspecified with psychoactive substance-induced sexual dysfunction

    F19.982 Other psychoactive substance use, unspecified with psychoactive substance-induced sleep disorder

    F19.988 Other psychoactive substance use, unspecified with other psychoactive substance-induced disorder

F19.99 Other psychoactive substance use, unspecified with unspecified psychoactive substance-induced disorder

Schizophrenia, schizotypal, delusional, and other non-mood psychotic disorders (F20-F29)

✓4th **F20 Schizophrenia**

    EXCLUDES 1 *brief psychotic disorder (F23)*
           cyclic schizophrenia (F25.0)
           mood [affective] disorders with psychotic symptoms (F30.2, F31.2, F31.5, F31.64, F32.3, F33.3)
           schizoaffective disorder (F25-)
           schizophrenic reaction NOS (F23)

    EXCLUDES 2 *schizophrenic reaction in:*
           alcoholism (F10.15-, F10.25-, F10.95-)
           brain disease (F06.2)
           epilepsy (F06.2)
           psychoactive drug use (F11-F19 with .15. .25, .95)
           schizotypal disorder (F21)

F20.0 Paranoid schizophrenia
    Paraphrenic schizophrenia
    EXCLUDES 1 *involutional paranoid state (F22)*
           paranoia (F22)

F20.1 Disorganized schizophrenia
    Hebephrenic schizophrenia
    Hebephrenia

F20.2 Catatonic schizophrenia
    Schizophrenic catalepsy
    Schizophrenic catatonia
    Schizophrenic flexibilitas cerea
    EXCLUDES 1 *catatonic stupor (R40.1)*

F20.3 Undifferentiated schizophrenia
    Atypical schizophrenia
    EXCLUDES 1 *acute schizophrenia-like psychotic disorder (F23)*
    EXCLUDES 2 *post-schizophrenic depression (F32.8)*

F20.5 Residual schizophrenia
    Restzustand (schizophrenic)
    Schizophrenic residual state

✓5th **F20.8 Other schizophrenia**

    F20.81 Schizophreniform disorder
        Schizophreniform psychosis NOS

Mental and Behavioral Disorders

F20.89–F31.74

F20.89   Other schizophrenia
     Cenesthopathic schizophrenia
     Simple schizophrenia

F20.9   Schizophrenia, unspecified

F21   Schizotypal disorder
     Borderline schizophrenia
     Latent schizophrenia
     Latent schizophrenic reaction
     Prepsychotic schizophrenia
     Prodromal schizophrenia
     Pseudoneurotic schizophrenia
     Pseudopsychopathic schizophrenia
     Schizotypal personality disorder
     EXCLUDES 2   *Asperger's syndrome (F84.5)*
                schizoid personality disorder (F60.1)

F22   Delusional disorders
     Delusional dysmorphophobia
     Involutional paranoid state
     Paranoia
     Paranoia querulans
     Paranoid psychosis
     Paranoid state
     Paraphrenia (late)
     Sensitiver Beziehungswahn
     EXCLUDES 1   *mood [affective] disorders with psychotic symptoms (F30.2,*
                F31.2, F31.5, F31.64, F32.3, F33.3)
                paranoid schizophrenia (F20.0)
     EXCLUDES 2   *paranoid personality disorder (F60.0)*
                paranoid psychosis, psychogenic (F23)
                paranoid reaction (F23)

F23   Brief psychotic disorder
     Paranoid reaction
     Psychogenic paranoid psychosis
     EXCLUDES 2   *mood [affective] disorders with psychotic symptoms (F30.2,*
                F31.2, F31.5, F31.64, F32.3, F33.3)

F24   Shared psychotic disorder
     Folie à deux
     Induced paranoid disorder
     Induced psychotic disorder

✓4ᵗʰ F25   Schizoaffective disorders
     EXCLUDES 1   *mood [affective] disorders with psychotic symptoms (F30.2,*
                F31.2, F31.5, F31.64, F32.3, F33.3)
                schizophrenia (F20-)

F25.0   Schizoaffective disorder, bipolar type
     Cyclic schizophrenia
     Schizoaffective disorder, manic type
     Schizoaffective disorder, mixed type
     Schizoaffective psychosis, bipolar type
     Schizophreniform psychosis, manic type

F25.1   Schizoaffective disorder, depressive type
     Schizoaffective psychosis, depressive type
     Schizophreniform psychosis, depressive type

F25.8   Other schizoaffective disorders

F25.9   Schizoaffective disorder, unspecified
     Schizoaffective psychosis NOS

F28   Other psychotic disorder not due to a substance or known physiological condition
     Chronic hallucinatory psychosis

F29   Unspecified psychosis not due to a substance or known physiological condition
     Psychosis NOS
     EXCLUDES 1   *mental disorder NOS (F99)*
                unspecified mental disorder due to known physiological
                condition (F09)

Mood [affective] disorders (F30-F39)

✓4ᵗʰ F30   Manic episode
     INCLUDES   bipolar disorder, single manic episode
                mixed affective episode
     EXCLUDES 1   *bipolar disorder (F31-)*
                major depressive disorder, single episode (F32-)
                major depressive disorder, recurrent (F33-)

✓5ᵗʰ F30.1   Manic episode without psychotic symptoms

F30.10   Manic episode without psychotic symptoms, unspecified

F30.11   Manic episode without psychotic symptoms, mild

F30.12   Manic episode without psychotic symptoms, moderate

F30.13   Manic episode, severe, without psychotic symptoms

F30.2   Manic episode, severe with psychotic symptoms
     Manic stupor
     Mania with mood-congruent psychotic symptoms
     Mania with mood-incongruent psychotic symptoms

F30.3   Manic episode in partial remission

F30.4   Manic episode in full remission

F30.8   Other manic episodes
     Hypomania

F30.9   Manic episode, unspecified
     Mania NOS

✓4ᵗʰ F31   Bipolar disorder
     INCLUDES   manic-depressive illness
                manic-depressive psychosis
                manic-depressive reaction
     EXCLUDES 1   *bipolar disorder, single manic episode (F30-)*
                major depressive disorder, single episode (F32-)
                major depressive disorder, recurrent (F33-)
     EXCLUDES 2   *cyclothymia (F34.0)*

F31.0   Bipolar disorder, current episode hypomanic

✓5ᵗʰ F31.1   Bipolar disorder, current episode manic without psychotic features

F31.10   Bipolar disorder, current episode manic without psychotic features, unspecified

F31.11   Bipolar disorder, current episode manic without psychotic features, mild

F31.12   Bipolar disorder, current episode manic without psychotic features, moderate

F31.13   Bipolar disorder, current episode manic without psychotic features, severe

F31.2   Bipolar disorder, current episode manic severe with psychotic features
     Bipolar disorder, current episode manic with mood-congruent psychotic symptoms
     Bipolar disorder, current episode manic with mood-incongruent psychotic symptoms

✓5ᵗʰ F31.3   Bipolar disorder, current episode depressed, mild or moderate severity

F31.30   Bipolar disorder, current episode depressed, mild or moderate severity, unspecified

F31.31   Bipolar disorder, current episode depressed, mild

F31.32   Bipolar disorder, current episode depressed, moderate

F31.4   Bipolar disorder, current episode depressed, severe, without psychotic features

F31.5   Bipolar disorder, current episode depressed, severe, with psychotic features
     Bipolar disorder, current episode depressed with mood-incongruent psychotic symptoms
     Bipolar disorder, current episode depressed with mood-congruent psychotic symptoms

✓5ᵗʰ F31.6   Bipolar disorder, current episode mixed

F31.60   Bipolar disorder, current episode mixed, unspecified

F31.61   Bipolar disorder, current episode mixed, mild

F31.62   Bipolar disorder, current episode mixed, moderate

F31.63   Bipolar disorder, current episode mixed, severe, without psychotic features

F31.64   Bipolar disorder, current episode mixed, severe, with psychotic features
     Bipolar disorder, current episode mixed with mood-congruent psychotic symptoms
     Bipolar disorder, current episode mixed with mood-incongruent psychotic symptoms

✓5ᵗʰ F31.7   Bipolar disorder, currently in remission

F31.70   Bipolar disorder, currently in remission, most recent episode unspecified

F31.71   Bipolar disorder, in partial remission, most recent episode hypomanic

F31.72   Bipolar disorder, in full remission, most recent episode hypomanic

F31.73   Bipolar disorder, in partial remission, most recent episode manic

F31.74   Bipolar disorder, in full remission, most recent episode manic

---

EXCLUDES 1   Not coded here   EXCLUDES 2   Not included here   *Manifestation Code*

F31.75   **Bipolar disorder, in partial remission, most recent episode depressed**

F31.76   **Bipolar disorder, in full remission, most recent episode depressed**

F31.77   **Bipolar disorder, in partial remission, most recent episode mixed**

F31.78   **Bipolar disorder, in full remission, most recent episode mixed**

✓5th   **F31.8**   **Other bipolar disorders**

     F31.81   **Bipolar II disorder**

     F31.89   **Other bipolar disorder**
         Recurrent manic episodes NOS

  F31.9   **Bipolar disorder, unspecified**

✓4th   **F32**   **Major depressive disorder, single episode**

     INCLUDES   single episode of agitated depression
         single episode of depressive reaction
         single episode of major depression
         single episode of psychogenic depression
         single episode of reactive depression
         single episode of vital depression

     EXCLUDES 1   *bipolar disorder (F31-)*
         manic episode (F30-)
         recurrent depressive disorder (F33-)

     EXCLUDES 2   *adjustment disorder (F43.2)*

  F32.0   **Major depressive disorder, single episode, mild**

  F32.1   **Major depressive disorder, single episode, moderate**

  F32.2   **Major depressive disorder, single episode, severe without psychotic features**

  F32.3   **Major depressive disorder, single episode, severe with psychotic features**
     Single episode of major depression with mood-congruent psychotic symptoms
     Single episode of major depression with mood-incongruent psychotic symptoms
     Single episode of major depression with psychotic symptoms
     Single episode of psychogenic depressive psychosis
     Single episode of psychotic depression
     Single episode of reactive depressive psychosis

  F32.4   **Major depressive disorder, single episode, in partial remission**

  F32.5   **Major depressive disorder, single episode, in full remission**

  F32.8   **Other depressive episodes**
     Atypical depression
     Post-schizophrenic depression
     Single episode of 'masked' depression NOS

  F32.9   **Major depressive disorder, single episode, unspecified**
     Depression NOS
     Depressive disorder NOS
     Major depression NOS

✓4th   **F33**   **Major depressive disorder, recurrent**
     Recurrent episodes of depressive reaction
     Recurrent episodes of endogenous depression
     Recurrent episodes of major depression
     Recurrent episodes of psychogenic depression
     Recurrent episodes of reactive depression
     Recurrent episodes of seasonal depressive disorder
     Recurrent episodes of vital depression

     EXCLUDES 1   *bipolar disorder (F31-)*
         manic episode (F30-)

  F33.0   **Major depressive disorder, recurrent, mild**

  F33.1   **Major depressive disorder, recurrent, moderate**

  F33.2   **Major depressive disorder, recurrent severe without psychotic features**

  F33.3   **Major depressive disorder, recurrent, severe with psychotic symptoms**
     Endogenous depression with psychotic symptoms
     Recurrent severe episodes of major depression with mood-congruent psychotic symptoms
     Recurrent severe episodes of major depression with mood-incongruent psychotic symptoms
     Recurrent severe episodes of major depression with psychotic symptoms
     Recurrent severe episodes of psychogenic depressive psychosis
     Recurrent severe episodes of psychotic depression
     Recurrent severe episodes of reactive depressive psychosis

✓5th   **F33.4**   **Major depressive disorder, recurrent, in remission**

     F33.40   **Major depressive disorder, recurrent, in remission, unspecified**

     F33.41   **Major depressive disorder, recurrent, in partial remission**

     F33.42   **Major depressive disorder, recurrent, in full remission**

  F33.8   **Other recurrent depressive disorders**
     Recurrent brief depressive episodes

  F33.9   **Major depressive disorder, recurrent, unspecified**
     Monopolar depression NOS

✓4th   **F34**   **Persistent mood [affective] disorders**

  F34.0   **Cyclothymic disorder**
     Affective personality disorder
     Cycloid personality
     Cyclothymia
     Cyclothymic personality

  F34.1   **Dysthymic disorder**
     Depressive neurosis
     Depressive personality disorder
     Dysthymia
     Neurotic depression
     Persistent anxiety depression

     EXCLUDES 2   *anxiety depression (mild or not persistent) (F41.8)*

  F34.8   **Other persistent mood [affective] disorders**

  F34.9   **Persistent mood [affective] disorder, unspecified**

  F39   **Unspecified mood [affective] disorder**
     Affective psychosis NOS

Anxiety, dissociative, stress-related, somatoform and other nonpsychotic mental disorders (F40-F48)

✓4th   **F40**   **Phobic anxiety disorders**

✓5th   **F40.0**   **Agoraphobia**

     F40.00   **Agoraphobia, unspecified**

     F40.01   **Agoraphobia with panic disorder**
         Panic disorder with agoraphobia
         EXCLUDES 1   *panic disorder without agoraphobia (F41.0)*

     F40.02   **Agoraphobia without panic disorder**

✓5th   **F40.1**   **Social phobias**
     Anthropophobia
     Social anxiety disorder of childhood
     Social neurosis

     F40.10   **Social phobia, unspecified**

     F40.11   **Social phobia, generalized**

✓5th   **F40.2**   **Specific (isolated) phobias**
     EXCLUDES 2   *dysmorphophobia (nondelusional) (F45.22)*
         nosophobia (F45.22)

     ✓6th   **F40.21**   **Animal type phobia**

         F40.210   **Arachnophobia**
             Fear of spiders

         F40.218   **Other animal type phobia**

     ✓6th   **F40.22**   **Natural environment type phobia**

         F40.220   **Fear of thunderstorms**

         F40.228   **Other natural environment type phobia**

     ✓6th   **F40.23**   **Blood, injection, injury type phobia**

         F40.230   **Fear of blood**

         F40.231   **Fear of injections and transfusions**

         F40.232   **Fear of other medical care**

         F40.233   **Fear of injury**

     ✓6th   **F40.24**   **Situational type phobia**

         F40.240   **Claustrophobia**

         F40.241   **Acrophobia**

         F40.242   **Fear of bridges**

         F40.243   **Fear of flying**

         F40.248   **Other situational type phobia**

     ✓6th   **F40.29**   **Other specified phobia**

         F40.290   **Androphobia**
             Fear of men

         F40.291   **Gynephobia**
             Fear of women

         F40.298   **Other specified phobia**

  F40.8   **Other phobic anxiety disorders**
     Phobic anxiety disorder of childhood

  F40.9   **Phobic anxiety disorder, unspecified**
     Phobia NOS
     Phobic state NOS

Mental and Behavioral Disorders

F41–F48.1

✓4ᵗʰ F41   Other anxiety disorders

> EXCLUDES 2   *anxiety in:*
> *acute stress reaction (F43.0)*
> *transient adjustment reaction (F43.2)*
> *neurasthenia (F48.8)*
> *psychophysiologic disorders (F45-)*
> *separation anxiety (F93.0)*

F41.0   Panic disorder [episodic paroxysmal anxiety] without agoraphobia
Panic attack
Panic state
> EXCLUDES 1   *panic disorder with agoraphobia (F40.01)*

F41.1   Generalized anxiety disorder
Anxiety neurosis
Anxiety reaction
Anxiety state
Overanxious disorder
> EXCLUDES 2   *neurasthenia (F48.8)*

F41.3   Other mixed anxiety disorders

F41.8   Other specified anxiety disorders
Anxiety depression (mild or not persistent)
Anxiety hysteria
Mixed anxiety and depressive disorder

F41.9   Anxiety disorder, unspecified
Anxiety NOS

F42   Obsessive-compulsive disorder
Anancastic neurosis
Obsessive-compulsive neurosis
> EXCLUDES 2   *obsessive-compulsive personality (disorder) (F60.5)*
> *obsessive-compulsive symptoms occurring in:*
> *depression (F32-F33)*
> *schizophrenia (F20-)*

✓4ᵗʰ F43   Reaction to severe stress, and adjustment disorders

F43.0   Acute stress reaction
Acute crisis reaction
Acute reaction to stress
Combat and operational stress reaction
Combat fatigue
Crisis state
Psychic shock

✓5ᵗʰ F43.1   Post-traumatic stress disorder (PTSD)
Traumatic neurosis
     F43.10   Post-traumatic stress disorder, unspecified
     F43.11   Post-traumatic stress disorder, acute
     F43.12   Post-traumatic stress disorder, chronic

✓5ᵗʰ F43.2   Adjustment disorders
Culture shock
Grief reaction
Hospitalism in children
> EXCLUDES 2   *separation anxiety disorder of childhood (F93.0)*

     F43.20   Adjustment disorder, unspecified
     F43.21   Adjustment disorder with depressed mood
     F43.22   Adjustment disorder with anxiety
     F43.23   Adjustment disorder with mixed anxiety and depressed mood
     F43.24   Adjustment disorder with disturbance of conduct
     F43.25   Adjustment disorder with mixed disturbance of emotions and conduct
     F43.29   Adjustment disorder with other symptoms

F43.8   Other reactions to severe stress

F43.9   Reaction to severe stress, unspecified

✓4ᵗʰ F44   Dissociative and conversion disorders
> INCLUDES   conversion hysteria
> conversion reaction
> hysteria
> hysterical psychosis
> EXCLUDES 2   *malingering [conscious simulation] (Z76.5)*

F44.0   Dissociative amnesia
> EXCLUDES 1   *amnesia NOS (R41.3)*
> *anterograde amnesia (R41.1)*
> *retrograde amnesia (R41.2)*
> EXCLUDES 2   *alcohol-or other psychoactive substance-induced*
> *amnestic disorder (F10, F13, F19 with .26, .96)*
> *amnestic disorder due to known physiological*
> *condition (F04)*
> *postictal amnesia in epilepsy (G40-)*

F44.1   Dissociative fugue
> EXCLUDES 2   *postictal fugue in epilepsy (G40-)*

F44.2   Dissociative stupor
> EXCLUDES 1   *catatonic stupor (R40.1)*
> *stupor NOS (R40.1)*
> EXCLUDES 2   *catatonic disorder due to known physiological*
> *condition (F06.1)*
> *depressive stupor (F32, F33)*
> *manic stupor (F30, F31)*

F44.4   Conversion disorder with motor symptom or deficit
Dissociative motor disorders
Psychogenic aphonia
Psychogenic dysphonia

F44.5   Conversion disorder with seizures or convulsions
Dissociative convulsions

F44.6   Conversion disorder with sensory symptom or deficit
Dissociative anesthesia and sensory loss
Psychogenic deafness

F44.7   Conversion disorder with mixed symptom presentation

✓5ᵗʰ F44.8   Other dissociative and conversion disorders
     F44.81   Dissociative identity disorder
         Multiple personality disorder
     F44.89   Other dissociative and conversion disorders
         Ganser's syndrome
         Psychogenic confusion
         Psychogenic twilight state
         Trance and possession disorders

F44.9   Dissociative and conversion disorder, unspecified
Dissociative disorder NOS

✓4ᵗʰ F45   Somatoform disorders
> EXCLUDES 2   *dissociative and conversion disorders (F44-)*
> *factitious disorders (F68.1-)*
> *hair-plucking (F63.3)*
> *lalling (F80.0)*
> *lisping (F80.0)*
> *malingering [conscious simulation] (Z76.5)*
> *nail-biting (F98.8)*
> *psychological or behavioral factors associated with disorders*
> *or diseases classified elsewhere (F54)*
> *sexual dysfunction, not due to a substance or known*
> *physiological condition (F52-)*
> *thumb-sucking (F98.8)*
> *tic disorders (in childhood and adolescence) (F95-)*
> *Tourette's syndrome (F95.2)*
> *trichotillomania (F63.3)*

F45.0   Somatization disorder
Briquet's disorder
Multiple psychosomatic disorder

F45.1   Undifferentiated somatoform disorder
Undifferentiated psychosomatic disorder

✓5ᵗʰ F45.2   Hypochondriacal disorders
> EXCLUDES 2   *delusional dysmorphophobia (F22)*
> *fixed delusions about bodily functions or shape (F22)*

     F45.20   Hypochondriacal disorder, unspecified
     F45.21   Hypochondriasis
         Hypochondriacal neurosis
     F45.22   Body dysmorphic disorder
         Dysmorphophobia (nondelusional)
         Nosophobia
     F45.29   Other hypochondriacal disorders

✓5ᵗʰ F45.4   Pain disorders related to psychological factors
> EXCLUDES 1   *pain NOS (R52)*

     F45.41   Pain disorder exclusively related to psychological factors
         Somatoform pain disorder (persistent)
     F45.42   Pain disorder with related psychological factors
         Code also associated acute or chronic pain (G89-)

F45.8   Other somatoform disorders
Psychogenic dysmenorrhea
Psychogenic dysphagia, including "globus hystericus"
Psychogenic pruritus
Psychogenic torticollis
Somatoform autonomic dysfunction
Teeth grinding
> EXCLUDES 1   *sleep related teeth grinding (G47.63)*

F45.9   Somatoform disorder, unspecified
Psychosomatic disorder NOS

✓4ᵗʰ F48   Other nonpsychotic mental disorders
F48.1   Depersonalization-derealization syndrome

EXCLUDES 1   Not coded here   EXCLUDES 2   Not included here   *Manifestation Code*

F48.8 **Other specified nonpsychotic mental disorders**
Dhat syndrome
Neurasthenia
Occupational neurosis, including writer's cramp
Psychasthenia
Psychasthenic neurosis
Psychogenic syncope

F48.9 **Nonpsychotic mental disorder, unspecified**
Neurosis NOS

Behavioral syndromes associated with physiological disturbances and physical factors (F50-F59)

✓4ᵗʰ **F50** **Eating disorders**
EXCLUDES 1 *anorexia NOS (R63.0)*
feeding difficulties (R63.3)
polyphagia (R63.2)
EXCLUDES 2 *feeding disorder in infancy or childhood (F98.2-)*

✓5ᵗʰ **F50.0** **Anorexia nervosa**
EXCLUDES 1 *loss of appetite (R63.0)*
psychogenic loss of appetite (F50.8)

F50.00 **Anorexia nervosa, unspecified**
F50.01 **Anorexia nervosa, restricting type**
F50.02 **Anorexia nervosa, binge eating/purging type**
EXCLUDES 1 *bulimia nervosa (F50.2)*

F50.2 **Bulimia nervosa**
Bulimia NOS
Hyperorexia nervosa
EXCLUDES 1 *anorexia nervosa, binge eating/purging type (F50.02)*

F50.8 **Other eating disorders**
Pica in adults
Psychogenic loss of appetite
EXCLUDES 2 *pica of infancy and childhood (F98.3)*

F50.9 **Eating disorder, unspecified**
Atypical anorexia nervosa
Atypical bulimia nervosa

✓4ᵗʰ **F51** **Sleep disorders not due to a substance or known physiological condition**
EXCLUDES 2 *organic sleep disorders (G47-)*

✓5ᵗʰ **F51.0** **Insomnia not due to a substance or known physiological condition**
EXCLUDES 2 *alcohol related insomnia (F10.182, F10.282, F10.982)*
drug related insomnia (F11.182, F11.282, F11.982, F13.182, F13.282, F13.982, F14.182, F14.282, F14.982, F15.182, F15.282, F15.982, F19.182, F19.282, F19.982)
insomnia NOS (G47.0-)
insomnia due to known physiological condition (G47.0-)
organic insomnia (G47.0-)
sleep deprivation (Z72.820)

F51.01 **Primary insomnia**
Idiopathic insomnia
F51.02 **Adjustment insomnia**
F51.03 **Paradoxical insomnia**
F51.04 **Psychophysiologic insomnia**
F51.05 **Insomnia due to other mental disorder**
Code also associated mental disorder
F51.09 **Other insomnia not due to a substance or known physiological condition**

✓5ᵗʰ **F51.1** **Hypersomnia not due to a substance or known physiological condition**
EXCLUDES 2 *alcohol related hypersomnia (F10.182, F10.282, F10.982)*
drug related hypersomnia (F11.182, F11.282, F11.982, F13.182, F13.282, F13.982, F14.182, F14.282, F14.982, F15.182, F15.282, F15.982, F19.182, F19.282, F19.982)
hypersomnia NOS (G47.10)
hypersomnia due to known physiological condition (G47.10)
idiopathic hypersomnia (G47.11, G47.12)
narcolepsy (G47.4-)

F51.11 **Primary hypersomnia**
F51.12 **Insufficient sleep syndrome**
EXCLUDES 1 *sleep deprivation (Z72.820)*
F51.13 **Hypersomnia due to other mental disorder**

F51.19 **Other hypersomnia not due to a substance or known physiological condition**
F51.3 **Sleepwalking [somnambulism]**
F51.4 **Sleep terrors [night terrors]**
F51.5 **Nightmare disorder**
Dream anxiety disorder
F51.8 **Other sleep disorders not due to a substance or known physiological condition**
F51.9 **Sleep disorder not due to a substance or known physiological condition, unspecified**
Emotional sleep disorder NOS

✓4ᵗʰ **F52** **Sexual dysfunction not due to a substance or known physiological condition**
EXCLUDES 2 *Dhat syndrome (F48.8)*

F52.0 **Hypoactive sexual desire disorder**
Anhedonia (sexual)
Lack or loss of sexual desire
EXCLUDES 1 *decreased libido (R68.82)*

F52.1 **Sexual aversion disorder**
Sexual aversion and lack of sexual enjoyment

✓5ᵗʰ **F52.2** **Sexual arousal disorders**
Failure of genital response
F52.21 **Male erectile disorder**
Psychogenic impotence
EXCLUDES 1 *impotence of organic origin (N52-)*
impotence NOS (N52-)
F52.22 **Female sexual arousal disorder**
Frigidity

✓5ᵗʰ **F52.3** **Orgasmic disorder**
Inhibited orgasm
Psychogenic anorgasmy
F52.31 **Female orgasmic disorder**
F52.32 **Male orgasmic disorder**

F52.4 **Premature ejaculation**
F52.5 **Vaginismus not due to a substance or known physiological condition**
Psychogenic vaginismus
EXCLUDES 2 *vaginismus (due to a known physiological condition) (N94.2)*

F52.6 **Dyspareunia not due to a substance or known physiological condition**
Psychogenic dyspareunia
EXCLUDES 2 *dyspareunia (due to a known physiological condition) (N94.1)*

F52.8 **Other sexual dysfunction not due to a substance or known physiological condition**
Excessive sexual drive
Nymphomania
Satyriasis

F52.9 **Unspecified sexual dysfunction not due to a substance or known physiological condition**
Sexual dysfunction NOS

F53 **Puerperal psychosis**
Postpartum depression
EXCLUDES 1 *mood disorders with psychotic features (F30.2, F31.2, F31.5, F31.64, F32.3, F33.3)*
postpartum dysphoria (O90.6)
psychosis in schizophrenia, schizotypal, delusional, and other psychotic disorders (F20-F29)

F54 **Psychological and behavioral factors associated with disorders or diseases classified elsewhere**
Psychological factors affecting physical conditions
Code first the associated physical disorder, such as:
asthma (J45-)
dermatitis (L23-L25)
gastric ulcer (K25-)
mucous colitis (K58-)
ulcerative colitis (K51-)
urticaria (L50-)
EXCLUDES 2 *tension-type headache (G44.2)*

✓4ᵗʰ **F55** **Abuse of non-psychoactive substances**
EXCLUDES 2 *abuse of psychoactive substances (F10-F19)*
F55.0 **Abuse of antacids**
F55.1 **Abuse of herbal or folk remedies**
F55.2 **Abuse of laxatives**
F55.3 **Abuse of steroids or hormones**
F55.4 **Abuse of vitamins**

✓ Appropriate additional character required   √x7ᵗʰ Requires 7th character, placeholder x must fill empty characters

Mental and Behavioral Disorders

F55.8–F68.12

F55.8   Abuse of other non-psychoactive substances

F59   **Unspecified behavioral syndromes associated with physiological disturbances and physical factors**
     Psychogenic physiological dysfunction NOS

Disorders of adult personality and behavior (F60-F69)

☑4ᵗʰ **F60**   **Specific personality disorders**

   F60.0   **Paranoid personality disorder**
     Expansive paranoid personality (disorder)
     Fanatic personality (disorder)
     Querulant personality (disorder)
     Paranoid personality (disorder)
     Sensitive paranoid personality (disorder)
     EXCLUDES 2   *paranoia (F22)*
           paranoia querulans (F22)
           paranoid psychosis (F22)
           paranoid schizophrenia (F20.0)
           paranoid state (F22)

   F60.1   **Schizoid personality disorder**
     EXCLUDES 2   *Asperger's syndrome (F84.5)*
           delusional disorder (F22)
           schizoid disorder of childhood (F84.5)
           schizophrenia (F20-)
           schizotypal disorder (F21)

   F60.2   **Antisocial personality disorder**
     Amoral personality (disorder)
     Asocial personality (disorder)
     Dissocial personality disorder
     Psychopathic personality (disorder)
     Sociopathic personality (disorder)
     EXCLUDES 1   *conduct disorders (F91-)*
     EXCLUDES 2   *borderline personality disorder (F60.3)*

   F60.3   **Borderline personality disorder**
     Aggressive personality (disorder)
     Emotionally unstable personality disorder
     Explosive personality (disorder)
     EXCLUDES 2   *antisocial personality disorder (F60.2)*

   F60.4   **Histrionic personality disorder**
     Hysterical personality (disorder)
     Psychoinfantile personality (disorder)

   F60.5   **Obsessive-compulsive personality disorder**
     Anankastic personality (disorder)
     Compulsive personality (disorder)
     Obsessional personality (disorder)
     EXCLUDES 2   *obsessive-compulsive disorder (F42)*

   F60.6   **Avoidant personality disorder**
     Anxious personality disorder

   F60.7   **Dependent personality disorder**
     Asthenic personality (disorder)
     Inadequate personality (disorder)
     Passive personality (disorder)

  ☑5ᵗʰ **F60.8**   **Other specific personality disorders**
     F60.81   **Narcissistic personality disorder**
     F60.89   **Other specific personality disorders**
         Eccentric personality disorder
         "Haltlose" type personality disorder
         Immature personality disorder
         Passive-aggressive personality disorder
         Psychoneurotic personality disorder
         Self-defeating personality disorder

   F60.9   **Personality disorder, unspecified**
     Character disorder NOS
     Character neurosis NOS
     Pathological personality NOS

☑4ᵗʰ **F63**   **Impulse disorders**
   EXCLUDES 2   *habitual excessive use of alcohol or psychoactive substances (F10-F19)*
           impulse disorders involving sexual behavior (F65-)

   F63.0   **Pathological gambling**
     Compulsive gambling
     EXCLUDES 1   *gambling and betting NOS (Z72.6)*
     EXCLUDES 2   *excessive gambling by manic patients (F30, F31)*
           gambling in antisocial personality disorder (F60.2)

   F63.1   **Pyromania**
     Pathological fire-setting
     EXCLUDES 2   *fire-setting (by) (in):*
           adult with antisocial personality disorder (F60.2)
           alcohol or psychoactive substance intoxication (F10-F19)
           conduct disorders (F91-)
           mental disorders due to known physiological condition (F01-F09)
           schizophrenia (F20-)

   F63.2   **Kleptomania**
     Pathological stealing
     EXCLUDES 1   *shoplifting as the reason for observation for suspected mental disorder (Z03.8)*
     EXCLUDES 2   *depressive disorder with stealing (F31-F33)*
           stealing due to underlying mental condition—code to mental condition
           stealing in mental disorders due to known physiological condition (F01-F09)

   F63.3   **Trichotillomania**
     Hair plucking
     EXCLUDES 2   *other stereotyped movement disorder (F98.4)*

  ☑5ᵗʰ **F63.8**   **Other impulse disorders**
     F63.81   **Intermittent explosive disorder**
     F63.89   **Other impulse disorders**

   F63.9   **Impulse disorder, unspecified**
     Impulse control disorder NOS

☑4ᵗʰ **F64**   **Gender identity disorders**

   F64.1   **Gender identity disorder in adolescence and adulthood**
     Dual role transvestism
     Transsexualism
     Use additional code to identify sex reassignment status (Z87.890)
     EXCLUDES 1   *gender identity disorder in childhood (F64.2)*
     EXCLUDES 2   *fetishistic transvestism (F65.1)*

   F64.2   **Gender identity disorder of childhood**
     EXCLUDES 1   *gender identity disorder in adolescence and adulthood (F64.1)*
     EXCLUDES 2   *sexual maturation disorder (F66)*

   F64.8   **Other gender identity disorders**

   F64.9   **Gender identity disorder, unspecified**
     Gender-role disorder NOS

☑4ᵗʰ **F65**   **Paraphilias**

   F65.0   **Fetishism**

   F65.1   **Transvestic fetishism**
     Fetishistic transvestism

   F65.2   **Exhibitionism**

   F65.3   **Voyeurism**

   F65.4   **Pedophilia**

  ☑5ᵗʰ **F65.5**   **Sadomasochism**
     F65.50   **Sadomasochism, unspecified**
     F65.51   **Sexual masochism**
     F65.52   **Sexual sadism**

  ☑5ᵗʰ **F65.8**   **Other paraphilias**
     F65.81   **Frotteurism**
     F65.89   **Other paraphilias**
         Necrophilia

   F65.9   **Paraphilia, unspecified**
     Sexual deviation NOS

  F66   **Other sexual disorders**
     Sexual maturation disorder
     Sexual relationship disorder

☑4ᵗʰ **F68**   **Other disorders of adult personality and behavior**
  ☑5ᵗʰ **F68.1**   **Factitious disorder**
     Compensation neurosis
     Elaboration of physical symptoms for psychological reasons
     Hospital hopper syndrome
     Münchhausen's syndrome
     Peregrinating patient
     EXCLUDES 2   *factitial dermatitis (L98.1)*
           person feigning illness (with obvious motivation) (Z76.5)

     F68.10   **Factitious disorder, unspecified**
     F68.11   **Factitious disorder with predominantly psychological signs and symptoms**
     F68.12   **Factitious disorder with predominantly physical signs and symptoms**

EXCLUDES 1 Not coded here   *EXCLUDES 2* Not included here   *Manifestation Code*

F68.13 **Factitious disorder with combined psychological and physical signs and symptoms**

F68.8 **Other specified disorders of adult personality and behavior**

F69 Unspecified disorder of adult personality and behavior

Mental retardation (F70-F79)

Code first any associated physical or developmental disorders

EXCLUDES 1 *borderline intellectual functioning, IQ above 70 to 84 (R41.83)*

F70 Mild mental retardation
IQ level 50-55 to approximately 70
Mild mental subnormality

F71 Moderate mental retardation
IQ level 35-40 to 50-55
Moderate mental subnormality

F72 Severe mental retardation
IQ 20-25 to 35-40
Severe mental subnormality

F73 Profound mental retardation
IQ level below 20-25
Profound mental subnormality

F78 Other mental retardation

F79 Unspecified mental retardation
Mental deficiency NOS
Mental subnormality NOS

Pervasive and specific developmental disorders (F80-F89)

☑4ᵗʰ **F80 Specific developmental disorders of speech and language**

F80.0 **Phonological disorder**
Dyslalia
Functional speech articulation disorder
Lalling
Lisping
Phonological developmental disorder
Speech articulation developmental disorder

EXCLUDES 1 *speech articulation impairment due to aphasia NOS (R47.01)*
speech articulation impairment due to apraxia (R48.2)

EXCLUDES 2 *speech articulation impairment due to hearing loss (F80.4)*
speech articulation impairment due to mental retardation (F70-F79)
speech articulation impairment with expressive language developmental disorder (F80.1)
speech articulation impairment with mixed receptive expressive language developmental disorder (F80.2)

F80.1 **Expressive language disorder**
Developmental dysphasia or aphasia, expressive type

EXCLUDES 1 *mixed receptive-expressive language disorder (F80.2)*
dysphasia and aphasia NOS (R47-)

EXCLUDES 2 *acquired aphasia with epilepsy [Landau-Kleffner] (F80.3)*
selective mutism (F94.0)
mental retardation (F70-F79)
pervasive developmental disorders (F84-)

F80.2 **Mixed receptive-expressive language disorder**
Developmental dysphasia or aphasia, receptive type
Developmental Wernicke's aphasia

EXCLUDES 1 *central auditory processing disorder (H93.25)*
dysphasia or aphasia NOS (R47-)
expressive language disorder (F80.1)
expressive type dysphasia or aphasia (F80.1)
word deafness (H93.25)

EXCLUDES 2 *acquired aphasia with epilepsy [Landau-Kleffner] (F80.3)*
pervasive developmental disorders (F84-)
selective mutism (F94.0)
mental retardation (F70-F79)

F80.3 **Acquired aphasia with epilepsy [Landau-Kleffner]**

EXCLUDES 1 *aphasia NOS (R47.01)*

EXCLUDES 2 *pervasive developmental disorders (F84-)*

F80.4 **Speech and language development delay due to hearing loss**
Code also type of hearing loss (H90-, H91-)

☑5ᵗʰ F80.8 **Other developmental disorders of speech and language**

F80.81 **Childhood onset fluency disorder**
Cluttering NOS
Stuttering NOS

EXCLUDES 1 *adult onset fluency disorder (F98.5)*
fluency disorder in conditions classified elsewhere (R47.82)
fluency disorder (stuttering) following cerebrovascular disease (I69. with final characters-23)

F80.89 **Other developmental disorders of speech and language**

F80.9 **Developmental disorder of speech and language, unspecified**
Communication disorder NOS
Language disorder NOS

☑4ᵗʰ **F81 Specific developmental disorders of scholastic skills**

F81.0 **Specific reading disorder**
"Backward reading"
Developmental dyslexia
Specific reading retardation

EXCLUDES 1 *alexia NOS (R48.0)*
dyslexia NOS (R48.0)

F81.2 **Mathematics disorder**
Developmental acalculia
Developmental arithmetical disorder
Developmental Gerstmann's syndrome

EXCLUDES 1 *acalculia NOS (R48.8)*

EXCLUDES 2 *arithmetical difficulties associated with a reading disorder (F81.0)*
arithmetical difficulties associated with a spelling disorder (F81.81)
arithmetical difficulties due to inadequate teaching (Z55.8)

☑5ᵗʰ F81.8 **Other developmental disorders of scholastic skills**

F81.81 **Disorder of written expression**
Specific spelling disorder

F81.89 **Other developmental disorders of scholastic skills**

F81.9 **Developmental disorder of scholastic skills, unspecified**
Knowledge acquisition disability NOS
Learning disability NOS
Learning disorder NOS

F82 Specific developmental disorder of motor function
Clumsy child syndrome
Developmental coordination disorder
Developmental dyspraxia

EXCLUDES 1 *abnormalities of gait and mobility (R26-)*
lack of coordination (R27-)

EXCLUDES 2 *lack of coordination secondary to mental retardation (F70-F79)*

☑4ᵗʰ **F84 Pervasive developmental disorders**
Use additional code to identify any associated medical condition and mental retardation

F84.0 **Autistic disorder**
Infantile autism
Infantile psychosis
Kanner's syndrome

EXCLUDES 1 *Asperger's syndrome (F84.5)*

F84.2 **Rett's syndrome**

EXCLUDES 1 *Asperger's syndrome (F84.5)*
Autistic disorder (F84.0)
Other childhood disintegrative disorder (F84.3)

F84.3 **Other childhood disintegrative disorder**
Dementia infantilis
Disintegrative psychosis
Heller's syndrome
Symbiotic psychosis
Use additional code to identify any associated neurological condition

EXCLUDES 1 *Asperger's syndrome (F84.5)*
Autistic disorder (F84.0)
Rett's syndrome (F84.2)

F84.5 **Asperger's syndrome**
Asperger's disorder
Autistic psychopathy
Schizoid disorder of childhood

☑ Appropriate additional character required   ☑x7ᵗʰ Requires 7th character, placeholder x must fill empty characters

F84.8 Other pervasive developmental disorders
Overactive disorder associated with mental retardation and stereotyped movements

F84.9 Pervasive developmental disorder, unspecified
Atypical autism

F88 Other disorders of psychological development
Developmental agnosia

F89 Unspecified disorder of psychological development
Developmental disorder NOS

Behavioral and emotional disorders with onset usually occurring in childhood and adolescence (F90-F98)

NOTE   Codes within categories F90-F98 may be used regardless of the age of a patient. These disorders generally have onset within the childhood or adolescent years, but may continue throughout life or not be diagnosed until adulthood

✓4th F90 Attention-deficit hyperactivity disorders
INCLUDES attention deficit disorder with hyperactivity
attention deficit syndrome with hyperactivity
EXCLUDES 2 anxiety disorders (F40-, F41-)
mood [affective] disorders (F30-F39)
pervasive developmental disorders (F84-)
schizophrenia (F20-)

F90.0 Attention-deficit hyperactivity disorder, predominantly inattentive type

F90.1 Attention-deficit hyperactivity disorder, predominantly hyperactive type

F90.2 Attention-deficit hyperactivity disorder, combined type

F90.8 Attention-deficit hyperactivity disorder, other type

F90.9 Attention-deficit hyperactivity disorder, unspecified type
Attention-deficit hyperactivity disorder of childhood or adolescence NOS
Attention-deficit hyperactivity disorder NOS

✓4th F91 Conduct disorders
EXCLUDES 1 antisocial behavior (Z72.81-)
antisocial personality disorder (F60.2)
EXCLUDES 2 conduct problems associated with attention-deficit hyperactivity disorder (F90-)
mood [affective] disorders (F30-F39)
pervasive developmental disorders (F84-)
schizophrenia (F20-)

F91.0 Conduct disorder confined to family context

F91.1 Conduct disorder, childhood-onset type
Unsocialized conduct disorder
Conduct disorder, solitary aggressive type
Unsocialized aggressive disorder

F91.2 Conduct disorder, adolescent-onset type
Socialized conduct disorder
Conduct disorder, group type

F91.3 Oppositional defiant disorder

F91.8 Other conduct disorders

F91.9 Conduct disorder, unspecified
Behavioral disorder NOS
Conduct disorder NOS
Disruptive behavior disorder NOS

✓4th F93 Emotional disorders with onset specific to childhood

F93.0 Separation anxiety disorder of childhood
EXCLUDES 2 mood [affective] disorders (F30-F39)
nonpsychotic mental disorders (F40-F48)
phobic anxiety disorder of childhood (F40.8)
social phobia (F40.1)

F93.8 Other childhood emotional disorders
Identity disorder
EXCLUDES 2 gender identity disorder of childhood (F64.2)

F93.9 Childhood emotional disorder, unspecified

✓4th F94 Disorders of social functioning with onset specific to childhood and adolescence

F94.0 Selective mutism
Elective mutism
EXCLUDES 2 pervasive developmental disorders (F84-)
schizophrenia (F20-)
specific developmental disorders of speech and language (F80-)
transient mutism as part of separation anxiety in young children (F93.0)

F94.1 Reactive attachment disorder of childhood
Use additional code to identify any associated failure to thrive or growth retardation
EXCLUDES 1 disinhibited attachment disorder of childhood (F94.2)
normal variation in pattern of selective attachment
EXCLUDES 2 Asperger's syndrome (F84.5)
maltreatment syndromes (T74-)
sexual or physical abuse in childhood, resulting in psychosocial problems (Z62.81-)

F94.2 Disinhibited attachment disorder of childhood
Affectionless psychopathy
Institutional syndrome
EXCLUDES 1 reactive attachment disorder of childhood (F94.1)
EXCLUDES 2 Asperger's syndrome (F84.5)
attention-deficit hyperactivity disorders (F90-)
hospitalism in children (F43.2-)

F94.8 Other childhood disorders of social functioning

F94.9 Childhood disorder of social functioning, unspecified

✓4th F95 Tic disorder

F95.0 Transient tic disorder

F95.1 Chronic motor or vocal tic disorder

F95.2 Tourette's disorder
Combined vocal and multiple motor tic disorder [de la Tourette]
Tourette's syndrome

F95.8 Other tic disorders

F95.9 Tic disorder, unspecified
Tic NOS

✓4th F98 Other behavioral and emotional disorders with onset usually occurring in childhood and adolescence
EXCLUDES 2 breath-holding spells (R06.89)
gender identity disorder of childhood (F64.2)
Kleine-Levin syndrome (G47.13)
obsessive-compulsive disorder (F42)
sleep disorders not due to a substance or known physiological condition (F51-)

F98.0 Enuresis not due to a substance or known physiological condition
Enuresis (primary) (secondary) of nonorganic origin
Functional enuresis
Psychogenic enuresis
Urinary incontinence of nonorganic origin
EXCLUDES 1 enuresis NOS (R32)

F98.1 Encopresis not due to a substance or known physiological condition
Functional encopresis
Incontinence of feces of nonorganic origin
Psychogenic encopresis
Use additional code to identify the cause of any coexisting constipation
EXCLUDES 1 encopresis NOS (R15-)

✓5th F98.2 Other feeding disorders of infancy and childhood
EXCLUDES 1 feeding difficulties (R63.3)
EXCLUDES 2 anorexia nervosa and other eating disorders (F50-)
feeding problems of newborn (P92-)
pica of infancy or childhood (F98.3)

F98.21 Rumination disorder of infancy

F98.29 Other feeding disorders of infancy and early childhood

F98.3 Pica of infancy and childhood

F98.4 Stereotyped movement disorders
Stereotype/habit disorder
EXCLUDES 1 abnormal involuntary movements (R25-)
EXCLUDES 2 compulsions in obsessive-compulsive disorder (F42)
hair plucking (F63.3)
movement disorders of organic origin (G20-G25)
nail-biting (F98.8)
nose-picking (F98.8)
stereotypies that are part of a broader psychiatric condition (F01-F95)
thumb-sucking (F98.8)
tic disorders (F95-)
trichotillomania (F63.3)

F98.5　Adult onset fluency disorder
　　EXCLUDES 1　*childhood onset fluency disorder (F80.81)*
　　　　　　　dysphasia (R47.02)
　　　　　　　fluency disorder in conditions classified elsewhere
　　　　　　　　(R47.82)
　　　　　　　fluency disorder (stuttering) following
　　　　　　　　cerebrovascular disease (I69. with final
　　　　　　　　characters -23)
　　　　　　　tic disorders (F95.-)

F98.8　Other specified behavioral and emotional disorders with onset usually occurring in childhood and adolescence
　　Excessive masturbation
　　Nail-biting
　　Nose-picking
　　Thumb-sucking

F98.9　Unspecified behavioral and emotional disorders with onset usually occurring in childhood and adolescence

Unspecified mental disorder (F99)

F99　Mental disorder, not otherwise specified
　　Mental illness NOS
　　EXCLUDES 1　*unspecified mental disorder due to known physiological*
　　　　　　　condition (F09)

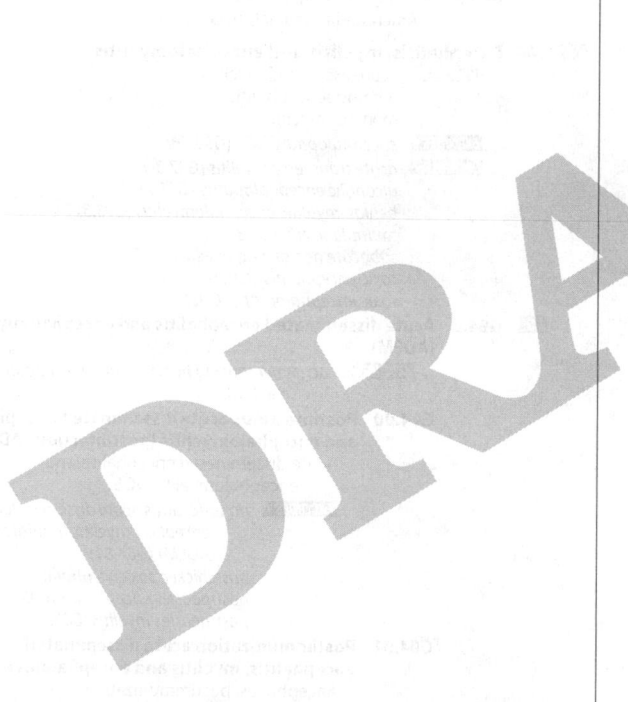

☑ Appropriate additional character required　　　　√x7th Requires 7th character, placeholder x must fill empty characters

Diseases of the Nervous System

G00–G04.31

Chapter 6. Diseases of the Nervous System (G00-G99)

> EXCLUDES 2   certain conditions originating in the perinatal period (P04-P96)
> certain infectious and parasitic diseases (A00-B99)
> complications of pregnancy, childbirth and the puerperium (O00-O99)
> congenital malformations, deformations, and chromosomal abnormalities (Q00-Q99)
> endocrine, nutritional and metabolic diseases (E00-E88)
> injury, poisoning and certain other consequences of external causes (S00-T88)
> neoplasms (C00-D49)
> symptoms, signs and abnormal clinical and laboratory findings, not elsewhere classified (R00-R94)

This chapter contains the following blocks:

G00-G09	Inflammatory diseases of the central nervous system
G10-G14	Systemic atrophies primarily affecting the central nervous system
G20-G26	Extrapyramidal and movement disorders
G30-G32	Other degenerative diseases of the nervous system
G35-G37	Demyelinating diseases of the central nervous system
G40-G47	Episodic and paroxysmal disorders
G50-G59	Nerve, nerve root and plexus disorders
G60-G65	Polyneuropathies and other disorders of the peripheral nervous system
G70-G73	Diseases of myoneural junction and muscle
G80-G83	Cerebral palsy and other paralytic syndromes
G89-G99	Other disorders of the nervous system

Inflammatory diseases of the central nervous system (G00-G09)

✓4th G00   Bacterial meningitis, not elsewhere classified

> INCLUDES   bacterial arachnoiditis
> bacterial leptomeningitis
> bacterial meningitis
> bacterial pachymeningitis

> EXCLUDES 1   bacterial:
>   meningoencephalitis (G04.2)
>   meningomyelitis (G04.2)

G00.0   Hemophilus meningitis
Meningitis due to Hemophilus influenzae

G00.1   Pneumococcal meningitis

G00.2   Streptococcal meningitis
Use additional code to further identify organism (B95.0-B95.5)

G00.3   Staphylococcal meningitis
Use additional code to further identify organism (B95.6-B95.8)

G00.8   Other bacterial meningitis
Meningitis due to Escherichia coli
Meningitis due to Friedländer's bacillus
Meningitis due to Klebsiella
Use additional code to further identify organism (B96-)

G00.9   Bacterial meningitis, unspecified
Meningitis due to gram-negative bacteria, unspecified
Purulent meningitis NOS
Pyogenic meningitis NOS
Suppurative meningitis NOS

G01   Meningitis in bacterial diseases classified elsewhere

> Code first underlying disease
> EXCLUDES 1   meningitis (in):
>   gonococcal (A54.81)
>   leptospirosis (A27.81)
>   listeriosis (A32.11)
>   Lyme disease (A69.21)
>   meningococcal (A39.0)
>   neurosyphilis (A52.13)
>   tuberculosis (A17.0)
> meningoencephalitis and meningomyelitis in bacterial diseases classified elsewhere (G05)

G02   Meningitis in other infectious and parasitic diseases classified elsewhere

> Code first underlying disease, such as:
> poliovirus infection (A80-)
> EXCLUDES 1   meningitis (due to):
>   candidal (B37.5)
>   coccidioidomycosis (B38.4)
>   cryptococcal meningitis (B45.1)
>   herpesviral [herpes simplex] (B00.3)
>   infectious mononucleosis (B27)
>   measles (B05.1)
>   mumps (B26.1)
>   rubella (B06.02)
>   varicella [chickenpox] (B01.0)
>   zoster (B02.1)
> meningoencephalitis and meningomyelitis in other infectious and parasitic diseases classified elsewhere (G05)

✓4th G03   Meningitis due to other and unspecified causes

> INCLUDES   arachnoiditis NOS
> leptomeningitis NOS
> meningitis NOS
> pachymeningitis NOS

> EXCLUDES 1   meningoencephalitis (G04-)
> meningomyelitis (G04-)

G03.0   Nonpyogenic meningitis
Aseptic meningitis
Nonbacterial meningitis

G03.1   Chronic meningitis

G03.2   Benign recurrent meningitis [Mollaret]

G03.8   Meningitis due to other specified causes

G03.9   Meningitis, unspecified
Arachnoiditis (spinal) NOS

✓4th G04   Encephalitis, myelitis and encephalomyelitis

> INCLUDES   acute ascending myelitis
> meningoencephalitis
> meningomyelitis

> EXCLUDES 1   encephalopathy NOS (G93.40)
> EXCLUDES 2   acute transverse myelitis (G37.3-)
> alcoholic encephalopathy (G31.2)
> benign myalgic encephalomyelitis (G93.3)
> multiple sclerosis (G35)
> subacute necrotizing myelitis (G37.4)
> toxic encephalitis (G92)
> toxic encephalopathy (G92)

✓5th G04.0   Acute disseminated encephalitis and encephalomyelitis (ADEM)

> EXCLUDES 1   acute necrotizing hemorrhagic encephalopathy (G04.3-)

G04.00   Postinfectious acute disseminated encephalitis and encephalomyelitis (postinfectious ADEM)
Acute disseminated encephalitis and encephalomyelitis NOS

> EXCLUDES 1   noninfectious acute disseminated encephalomyelitis (noninfectious ADEM) (G04.81)
> postchickenpox encephalitis (B01.1)
> postmeasles encephalitis (B05.0)
> postmeasles myelitis (B05.1)

G04.01   Postimmunization acute disseminated encephalitis, myelitis and encephalomyelitis
Encephalitis, postimmunization
Encephalomyelitis, postimmunization
Use additional code to identify the vaccine (T50.A-, T50.B-, T50.Z-)

G04.1   Tropical spastic paraplegia

G04.2   Bacterial meningoencephalitis and meningomyelitis, not elsewhere classified

✓5th G04.3   Acute necrotizing hemorrhagic encephalopathy

> EXCLUDES 1   acute disseminated encephalitis and encephalomyelitis (G04.0-)

G04.30   Postinfectious acute necrotizing hemorrhagic encephalopathy
Acute necrotizing hemorrhagic encephalopathy NOS

G04.31   Postimmunization acute necrotizing hemorrhagic encephalopathy
Use additional code to identify the vaccine (T50.A-, T50.B-, T50.Z-)

EXCLUDES 1   Not coded here   EXCLUDES 2   Not included here   *Manifestation Code*

✓5th **G04.8 Other encephalitis, myelitis and encephalomyelitis**
Code also any associated seizure (G40.-, R56.9)

G04.81 Other encephalitis and encephalomyelitis
Noninfectious acute disseminated
encephalomyelitis (noninfectious ADEM)

G04.89 Other myelitis

✓5th **G04.9 Encephalitis, myelitis and encephalomyelitis, unspecified**

G04.90 Encephalitis and encephalomyelitis, unspecified
Ventriculitis (cerebral) NOS

G04.91 Myelitis, unspecified

✓4th **G05 Encephalitis, myelitis and encephalomyelitis in diseases classified elsewhere**
Code first underlying disease, such as:
poliovirus (A80-)
suppurative otitis media (H66.01-H66.4)
trichinellosis (B75)

EXCLUDES 1 *encephalitis, myelitis and encephalomyelitis (in):*
adenoviral (A85.1)
congenital (P37.1)
cytomegaloviral (B25.8)
enteroviral (A85.0)
herpesviral [herpes simplex] (B00.4)
listerial (A32.12)
measles (B05.0)
meningococcal (A39.81)
mumps (B26.2)
postchickenpox (B01.1)
rubella (B06.01)
systemic lupus erythematosus (M32.19)
toxoplasmosis (B58.2)
zoster (B02.0)
eosinophilic meningoencephalitis (B83.2)

G05.3 Encephalitis and encephalomyelitis in diseases classified elsewhere
Meningoencephalitis in diseases classified elsewhere

G05.4 Myelitis in diseases classified elsewhere
Meningomyelitis in diseases classified elsewhere

✓4th **G06 Intracranial and intraspinal abscess and granuloma**
Use additional code (B95-B97) to identify infectious agent

G06.0 Intracranial abscess and granuloma
Brain [any part] abscess (embolic)
Cerebellar abscess (embolic)
Cerebral abscess (embolic)
Intracranial epidural abscess or granuloma
Intracranial extradural abscess or granuloma
Intracranial subdural abscess or granuloma
Otogenic abscess (embolic)

EXCLUDES 1 *tuberculous intracranial abscess and granuloma (A17.81)*

G06.1 Intraspinal abscess and granuloma
Abscess (embolic) of spinal cord [any part]
Intraspinal epidural abscess or granuloma
Intraspinal extradural abscess or granuloma
Intraspinal subdural abscess or granuloma

EXCLUDES 1 *tuberculous intraspinal abscess and granuloma (A17.81)*

G06.2 Extradural and subdural abscess, unspecified

G07 Intracranial and intraspinal abscess and granuloma in diseases classified elsewhere
Code first, underlying disease, such as:
schistosomiasis granuloma of brain (B65-)

EXCLUDES 1 *abscess of brain:*
amebic (A06.6)
chromomycotic (B43.1)
gonococcal (A54.82)
tuberculous (A17.81)
tuberculoma of meninges (A17.1)

G08 Intracranial and intraspinal phlebitis and thrombophlebitis
Septic embolism of intracranial or intraspinal venous sinuses and veins
Septic endophlebitis of intracranial or intraspinal venous sinuses and veins
Septic phlebitis of intracranial or intraspinal venous sinuses and veins
Septic thrombophlebitis of intracranial or intraspinal venous sinuses and veins
Septic thrombosis of intracranial or intraspinal venous sinuses and veins

EXCLUDES 1 *intracranial phlebitis and thrombophlebitis complicating:*
abortion, ectopic or molar pregnancy (O00-O07, O08.7)
pregnancy, childbirth and the puerperium (O22.5, O87.3)
nonpyogenic intracranial phlebitis and thrombophlebitis (I67.6)
nonpyogenic intraspinal phlebitis and thrombophlebitis (G95.1)

G09 Sequelae of inflammatory diseases of central nervous system
NOTE Category G09 is to be used to indicate conditions whose primary classification is to G00-G08 as the cause of sequelae, themselves classifiable elsewhere. The "sequelae" include conditions specified as residuals.
Code first condition resulting from (sequela) of inflammatory diseases of central nervous system

Systemic atrophies primarily affecting the central nervous system (G10-G14)

G10 Huntington's disease
Huntington's chorea
Huntington's dementia

✓4th **G11 Hereditary ataxia**
EXCLUDES 2 *cerebral palsy (G80-)*
hereditary and idiopathic neuropathy (G60-)
metabolic disorders (E70-E88)

G11.0 Congenital nonprogressive ataxia

G11.1 Early-onset cerebellar ataxia
Early-onset cerebellar ataxia with essential tremor
Early-onset cerebellar ataxia with myoclonus [Hunt's ataxia]
Early-onset cerebellar ataxia with retained tendon reflexes
Friedreich's ataxia (autosomal recessive)
X-linked recessive spinocerebellar ataxia

G11.2 Late-onset cerebellar ataxia

G11.3 Cerebellar ataxia with defective DNA repair
Ataxia telangiectasia [Louis-Bar]

EXCLUDES 2 *Cockayne's syndrome (Q87.1)*
other disorders of purine and pyrimidine metabolism (E79-)
xeroderma pigmentosum (Q82.1)

G11.4 Hereditary spastic paraplegia

G11.8 Other hereditary ataxias

G11.9 Hereditary ataxia, unspecified
Hereditary cerebellar ataxia NOS
Hereditary cerebellar degeneration
Hereditary cerebellar disease
Hereditary cerebellar syndrome

✓4th **G12 Spinal muscular atrophy and related syndromes**

G12.0 Infantile spinal muscular atrophy, type I [Werdnig-Hoffman]

G12.1 Other inherited spinal muscular atrophy
Adult form spinal muscular atrophy
Childhood form, type II spinal muscular atrophy
Distal spinal muscular atrophy
Juvenile form, type III spinal muscular atrophy [Kugelberg-Welander]
Progressive bulbar palsy of childhood [Fazio-Londe]
Scapuloperoneal form spinal muscular atrophy

✓5th **G12.2 Motor neuron disease**

G12.20 Motor neuron disease, unspecified

G12.21 Amyotrophic lateral sclerosis
Progressive spinal muscle atrophy

G12.22 Progressive bulbar palsy

G12.29 Other motor neuron disease
Familial motor neuron disease
Primary lateral sclerosis

G12.8 Other spinal muscular atrophies and related syndromes

G12.9 Spinal muscular atrophy, unspecified

☑4ᵗʰ **G13** **Systemic atrophies primarily affecting central nervous system in diseases classified elsewhere**

    G13.0 *Paraneoplastic neuromyopathy and neuropathy*
        Carcinomatous neuromyopathy
        Sensorial paraneoplastic neuropathy [Denny Brown]
        Code first underlying neoplasm (C00-D49)

    G13.1 *Other systemic atrophy primarily affecting central nervous system in neoplastic disease*
        Paraneoplastic limbic encephalopathy
        Code first underlying neoplasm (C00-D49)

    G13.8 *Systemic atrophy primarily affecting central nervous system in other diseases classified elsewhere*
        Code first underlying disease, such as:
        cerebellar ataxia (in):
        hypothyroidism (E03-)
        myxedematous congenital iodine deficiency (E00.1)

G14 **Postpolio syndrome**
    Postpolio myelitic syndrome
    EXCLUDES 1 *sequelae of poliomyelitis (B91)*

Extrapyramidal and movement disorders (G20-G26)

G20 **Parkinson's disease**
    Hemiparkinsonism
    Idiopathic Parkinsonism or Parkinson's disease
    Paralysis agitans
    Parkinsonism or Parkinson's disease NOS
    Primary Parkinsonism or Parkinson's disease
    EXCLUDES 1 *dementia with Parkinsonism (G31.83)*

☑4ᵗʰ **G21** **Secondary parkinsonism**
    EXCLUDES 1 *dementia with Parkinsonism (G31.83)*
               Huntington's disease (G10)
               Shy-Drager syndrome (G90.3)
               syphilitic Parkinsonism (A52.19)

    G21.0 **Malignant neuroleptic syndrome**
        Code first (T43.3-T43.5) to identify drug
        EXCLUDES 1 *neuroleptic induced parkinsonism (G21.11)*

    ☑5ᵗʰ **G21.1** **Other drug-induced secondary parkinsonism**
        G21.11 **Neuroleptic induced parkinsonism**
            Code first (T43.3-T43.5) to identify drug
            EXCLUDES 1 *malignant neuroleptic syndrome (G21.0)*
        G21.19 **Other drug induced secondary parkinsonism**
            Code first (T36-T50) to identify drug

    G21.2 **Secondary parkinsonism due to other external agents**
        Code first (T51-T65) to identify external agent

    G21.3 **Postencephalitic parkinsonism**
    G21.4 **Vascular parkinsonism**
    G21.8 **Other secondary parkinsonism**
    G21.9 **Secondary parkinsonism, unspecified**

☑4ᵗʰ **G23** **Other degenerative diseases of basal ganglia**
    EXCLUDES 2 *multi-system degeneration of the autonomic nervous system (G90.3)*

    G23.0 **Hallervorden-Spatz disease**
        Pigmentary pallidal degeneration

    G23.1 **Progressive supranuclear ophthalmoplegia [Steele-Richardson-Olszewski]**
    G23.2 **Striatonigral degeneration**
    G23.8 **Other specified degenerative diseases of basal ganglia**
        Calcification of basal ganglia
    G23.9 **Degenerative disease of basal ganglia, unspecified**

☑4ᵗʰ **G24** **Dystonia**
    INCLUDES dyskinesia
    EXCLUDES 2 *athetoid cerebral palsy (G80.3)*

    ☑5ᵗʰ **G24.0** **Drug induced dystonia**
        Code first (T36-T50) to identify drug
        G24.01 **Drug induced subacute dyskinesia**
            Drug induced blepharospasm
            Drug induced orofacial dyskinesia
            Neuroleptic induced tardive dyskinesia
            Tardive dyskinesia
        G24.02 **Drug induced acute dystonia**
            Acute dystonic reaction to drugs
            Neuroleptic induced acute dystonia
        G24.09 **Other drug induced dystonia**

    G24.1 **Genetic torsion dystonia**
        Dystonia deformans progressiva
        Dystonia musculorum deformans
        Familial torsion dystonia
        Idiopathic familial dystonia
        Idiopathic (torsion) dystonia NOS
        (Schwalbe-) Ziehen-Oppenheim disease

    G24.2 **Idiopathic nonfamilial dystonia**

    G24.3 **Spasmodic torticollis**
        EXCLUDES 1 *congenital torticollis (Q68.0)*
               hysterical torticollis (F44.4)
               ocular torticollis (R29.891)
               psychogenic torticollis (F45.8)
               torticollis NOS (M43.6)
               traumatic recurrent torticollis (S13.4)

    G24.4 **Idiopathic orofacial dystonia**
        Orofacial dyskinesia
        EXCLUDES 1 *drug induced orofacial dyskinesia (G24.01)*

    G24.5 **Blepharospasm**
        EXCLUDES 1 *drug induced blepharospasm (G24.01)*

    G24.8 **Other dystonia**
        Acquired torsion dystonia NOS

    G24.9 **Dystonia, unspecified**
        Dyskinesia NOS

☑4ᵗʰ **G25** **Other extrapyramidal and movement disorders**
    EXCLUDES 2 *sleep related movement disorders (G47.6-)*

    G25.0 **Essential tremor**
        Familial tremor
        EXCLUDES 1 *tremor NOS (R25.1)*

    G25.1 **Drug-induced tremor**
        Code first (T36-T50) to identify drug

    G25.2 **Other specified forms of tremor**
        Intention tremor

    G25.3 **Myoclonus**
        Drug-induced myoclonus
        Palatal myoclonus
        Code first (T36-T50) to identify drug, if drug-induced
        EXCLUDES 1 *facial myokymia (G51.4)*
               myoclonic epilepsy (G40-)

    G25.4 **Drug-induced chorea**
        Code first (T36-T50) to identify drug

    G25.5 **Other chorea**
        Chorea NOS
        EXCLUDES 1 *chorea NOS with heart involvement (I02.0)*
               Huntington's chorea (G10)
               rheumatic chorea (I02-)
               Sydenham's chorea (I02-)

    ☑5ᵗʰ **G25.6** **Drug induced tics and other tics of organic origin**
        G25.61 **Drug induced tics**
            Code first (T36-T50) to identify drug
        G25.69 **Other tics of organic origin**
            EXCLUDES 1 *habit spasm (F95.9)*
                  tic NOS (F95.9)
                  Tourette's syndrome (F95.2)

    ☑5ᵗʰ **G25.7** **Other and unspecified drug induced movement disorders**
        Code first (T36-T50) to identify drug
        G25.70 **Drug induced movement disorder, unspecified**
        G25.71 **Drug induced akathisia**
            Drug induced acathisia
            Neuroleptic induced acute akathisia
        G25.79 **Other drug induced movement disorders**

    ☑5ᵗʰ **G25.8** **Other specified extrapyramidal and movement disorders**
        G25.81 **Restless legs syndrome**
        G25.82 **Stiff-man syndrome**
        G25.89 **Other specified extrapyramidal and movement disorders**

    G25.9 **Extrapyramidal and movement disorder, unspecified**

G26 **Extrapyramidal and movement disorders in diseases classified elsewhere**
    Code first underlying disease

EXCLUDES 1 Not coded here   EXCLUDES 2 Not included here   *Manifestation Code*

Other degenerative diseases of the nervous system (G30-G32)

☑4th G30   Alzheimer's disease

INCLUDES   Alzheimer's dementia senile and presenile forms
Use additional code to identify:
   delirium, if applicable (F05)
   dementia with behavioral disturbance (F02.81)
   dementia without behavioral disturbance (F02.80)

EXCLUDES 1   senile degeneration of brain NEC (G31.1)
   senile dementia NOS (F03)
   senility NOS (R41.81)

G30.0   Alzheimer's disease with early onset
G30.1   Alzheimer's disease with late onset
G30.8   Other Alzheimer's disease
G30.9   Alzheimer's disease, unspecified

☑4th G31   Other degenerative diseases of nervous system, not elsewhere classified

Use additional code to identify:
   dementia with behavioral disturbance (F02.81)
   dementia without behavioral disturbance (F02.80)

EXCLUDES 2   Reye's syndrome (G93.7)

☑5th G31.0   Frontotemporal dementia

G31.01   Pick's disease
   Circumscribed brain atrophy
   Progressive isolated aphasia

G31.09   Other frontotemporal dementia
   Frontal dementia

G31.1   Senile degeneration of brain, not elsewhere classified

EXCLUDES 1   Alzheimer's disease (G30-)
   senility NOS (R41.81)

G31.2   Degeneration of nervous system due to alcohol
   Alcoholic cerebellar ataxia
   Alcoholic cerebellar degeneration
   Alcoholic cerebral degeneration
   Alcoholic encephalopathy
   Dysfunction of the autonomic nervous system due to alcohol
   Code also associated alcoholism (F10-)

☑5th G31.8   Other specified degenerative diseases of nervous system

G31.81   Alpers disease
   Grey-matter degeneration

G31.82   Leigh's disease
   Subacute necrotizing encephalopathy

G31.83   Dementia with Lewy bodies
   Dementia with Parkinsonism
   Lewy body dementia
   Lewy body disease

G31.84   Mild cognitive impairment, so stated

EXCLUDES 1   age related cognitive decline (R41.81)
   altered mental status (R41.82)
   cerebral degeneration (G31.9)
   change in mental status (R41.82)
   cognitive deficits following (sequelae of)
      cerebral hemorrhage or infarction
      (I69.01, I69.11, I69.21, I69.31, I69.81,
      I69.91)
   cognitive impairment due to intracranial or
      head injury (S06-)
   dementia (F01-, F02-, F03)
   mild memory disturbance (F06.8)
   neurologic neglect syndrome (R41.4)
   personality change, nonpsychotic (F68.8)

G31.89   Other specified degenerative diseases of nervous system

G31.9   Degenerative disease of nervous system, unspecified

☑4th G32   Other degenerative disorders of nervous system in diseases classified elsewhere

G32.0   **Subacute combined degeneration of spinal cord in diseases classified elsewhere**
   Dana-Putnam syndrome
   Sclerosis of spinal cord (combined) (dorsolateral)
      (posterolateral)
   Code first underlying disease, such as:
   vitamin B12 deficiency (E53.8)
   vitamin B12 deficiency:
      anemia (D51.9)
      dietary (D51.3)
      pernicious (D51.0)

EXCLUDES 1   syphilitic combined degeneration of spinal cord
   (A52.11)

G32.8   **Other specified degenerative disorders of nervous system in diseases classified elsewhere**
   Degenerative encephalopathy in diseases classified elsewhere
   Code first underlying disease, such as:
   cerebral degeneration (due to):
      amyloid (E85-)
      hypothyroidism (E00-, E03-)
      neoplasm (C00-D49)
      vitamin B deficiency, except thiamine (E52-E53-)

EXCLUDES 1   superior hemorrhagic polioencephalitis [Wernicke's
   encephalopathy] (E51.2)

Demyelinating diseases of the central nervous system (G35-G37)

G35   Multiple sclerosis
   Disseminated multiple sclerosis
   Generalized multiple sclerosis
   Multiple sclerosis NOS
   Multiple sclerosis of brain stem
   Multiple sclerosis of cord

☑4th G36   Other acute disseminated demyelination

EXCLUDES 1   postinfectious encephalitis and encephalomyelitis NOS
   (G04.020)

G36.0   Neuromyelitis optica [Devic]
   Demyelination in optic neuritis

EXCLUDES 1   optic neuritis NOS (H46)

G36.1   Acute and subacute hemorrhagic leukoencephalitis [Hurst]
G36.8   Other specified acute disseminated demyelination
G36.9   Acute disseminated demyelination, unspecified

☑4th G37   Other demyelinating diseases of central nervous system

G37.0   Diffuse sclerosis of central nervous system
   Periaxial encephalitis
   Schilder's disease

EXCLUDES 1   X linked adrenoleukodystrophy (E71.52-)

G37.1   Central demyelination of corpus callosum
G37.2   Central pontine myelinolysis
G37.3   Acute transverse myelitis in demyelinating disease of central nervous system
   Acute transverse myelitis NOS
   Acute transverse myelopathy

EXCLUDES 1   multiple sclerosis (G35)
   neuromyelitis optica [Devic] (G36.0)

G37.4   Subacute necrotizing myelitis of central nervous system
G37.5   Concentric sclerosis [Balo] of central nervous system
G37.8   Other specified demyelinating diseases of central nervous system
G37.9   Demyelinating disease of central nervous system, unspecified

Episodic and paroxysmal disorders (G40-G47)

☑4th G40   Epilepsy and recurrent seizures

NOTE   The following terms are to be considered equivalent to intractable: pharmacoresistant (pharmacologically resistant), treatment resistant, refractory (medically) and poorly controlled

EXCLUDES 1   conversion disorder with seizures (F44.5)
   convulsions NOS (R56.9)
   hippocampal sclerosis (G93.81)
   Landau-Kleffner syndrome (F80.3)
   mesial temporal sclerosis (G93.81)
   post traumatic seizures (R56.1)
   seizure (convulsive) NOS (R56.9)
   seizure of newborn (P90)
   temporal sclerosis (G93.81)
   Todd's paralysis (G83.8)

☑5th G40.0   Localization-related (focal) (partial) idiopathic epilepsy and epileptic syndromes with seizures of localized onset
   Benign childhood epilepsy with centrotemporal EEG spikes
   Childhood epilepsy with occipital EEG paroxysms

EXCLUDES 1   adult onset localization-related epilepsy (G40.1-,
   G40.2-)

☑6th G40.00   Localization-related (focal) (partial) idiopathic epilepsy and epileptic syndromes with seizures of localized onset, not intractable
   Localization-related (focal) (partial) idiopathic epilepsy and epileptic syndromes with seizures of localized onset without intractability

---

☑ Appropriate additional character required   ☑x7th Requires 7th character, placeholder x must fill empty characters

G40.001 Localization-related (focal) (partial) idiopathic epilepsy and epileptic syndromes with seizures of localized onset, not intractable, with status epilepticus

G40.009 Localization-related (focal) (partial) idiopathic epilepsy and epileptic syndromes with seizures of localized onset, not intractable, without status epilepticus

Localization-related (focal) (partial) idiopathic epilepsy and epileptic syndromes with seizures of localized onset NOS

√6ᵗʰ **G40.01** Localization-related (focal) (partial) idiopathic epilepsy and epileptic syndromes with seizures of localized onset, intractable

G40.011 Localization-related (focal) (partial) idiopathic epilepsy and epileptic syndromes with seizures of localized onset, intractable, with status epilepticus

G40.019 Localization-related (focal) (partial) idiopathic epilepsy and epileptic syndromes with seizures of localized onset, intractable, without status epilepticus

√5ᵗʰ **G40.1** Localization-related (focal) (partial) symptomatic epilepsy and epileptic syndromes with simple partial seizures

Attacks without alteration of consciousness
Simple partial seizures developing into secondarily generalized seizures

√6ᵗʰ **G40.10** Localization-related (focal) (partial) symptomatic epilepsy and epileptic syndromes with simple partial seizures, not intractable

Localization-related (focal) (partial) symptomatic epilepsy and epileptic syndromes with simple partial seizures without intractability

G40.101 Localization-related (focal) (partial) symptomatic epilepsy and epileptic syndromes with simple partial seizures, not intractable, with status epilepticus

G40.109 Localization-related (focal) (partial) symptomatic epilepsy and epileptic syndromes with simple partial seizures, not intractable, without status epilepticus

Localization-related (focal) (partial) symptomatic epilepsy and epileptic syndromes with simple partial seizures NOS

√6ᵗʰ **G40.11** Localization-related (focal) (partial) symptomatic epilepsy and epileptic syndromes with simple partial seizures, intractable

G40.111 Localization-related (focal) (partial) symptomatic epilepsy and epileptic syndromes with simple partial seizures, intractable, with status epilepticus

G40.119 Localization-related (focal) (partial) symptomatic epilepsy and epileptic syndromes with simple partial seizures, intractable, without status epilepticus

√5ᵗʰ **G40.2** Localization-related (focal) (partial) symptomatic epilepsy and epileptic syndromes with complex partial seizures

Attacks with alteration of consciousness, often with automatisms
Complex partial seizures developing into secondarily generalized seizures

√6ᵗʰ **G40.20** Localization-related (focal) (partial) symptomatic epilepsy and epileptic syndromes with complex partial seizures, not intractable

Localization-related (focal) (partial) symptomatic epilepsy and epileptic syndromes with complex partial seizures without intractability

G40.201 Localization-related (focal) (partial) symptomatic epilepsy and epileptic syndromes with complex partial seizures, not intractable, with status epilepticus

G40.209 Localization-related (focal) (partial) symptomatic epilepsy and epileptic syndromes with complex partial seizures, not intractable, without status epilepticus

Localization-related (focal) (partial) symptomatic epilepsy and epileptic syndromes with complex partial seizures NOS

√6ᵗʰ **G40.21** Localization-related (focal) (partial) symptomatic epilepsy and epileptic syndromes with complex partial seizures, intractable

G40.211 Localization-related (focal) (partial) symptomatic epilepsy and epileptic syndromes with complex partial seizures, intractable, with status epilepticus

G40.219 Localization-related (focal) (partial) symptomatic epilepsy and epileptic syndromes with complex partial seizures, intractable, without status epilepticus

√5ᵗʰ **G40.3** Generalized idiopathic epilepsy and epileptic syndromes

Benign myoclonic epilepsy in infancy
Benign neonatal convulsions (familial)
Childhood absence epilepsy [pyknolepsy]
Epilepsy with grand mal seizures on awakening
Grand mal seizure NOS
Juvenile absence epilepsy
Juvenile myoclonic epilepsy [impulsive petit mal]
Nonspecific atonic epileptic seizures
Nonspecific clonic epileptic seizures
Nonspecific myoclonic epileptic seizures
Nonspecific tonic epileptic seizures
Nonspecific tonic-clonic epileptic seizures
Petit mal seizure NOS
Code also MERRF syndrome, if applicable, (E88.42)

√6ᵗʰ **G40.30** Generalized idiopathic epilepsy and epileptic syndromes, not intractable

Generalized idiopathic epilepsy and epileptic syndromes without intractability

G40.301 Generalized idiopathic epilepsy and epileptic syndromes, not intractable, with status epilepticus

G40.309 Generalized idiopathic epilepsy and epileptic syndromes, not intractable, without status epilepticus

Generalized idiopathic epilepsy and epileptic syndromes NOS

√6ᵗʰ **G40.31** Generalized idiopathic epilepsy and epileptic syndromes, intractable

G40.311 Generalized idiopathic epilepsy and epileptic syndromes, intractable, with status epilepticus

G40.319 Generalized idiopathic epilepsy and epileptic syndromes, intractable, without status epilepticus

√5ᵗʰ **G40.4** Other generalized epilepsy and epileptic syndromes

Epilepsy with myoclonic absences
Epilepsy with myoclonic-astatic seizures
Infantile spasms
Lennox-Gastaut syndrome
Salaam attacks
Symptomatic early myoclonic encephalopathy
West's syndrome

√6ᵗʰ **G40.40** Other generalized epilepsy and epileptic syndromes, not intractable

Other generalized epilepsy and epileptic syndromes without intractability
Other generalized epilepsy and epileptic syndromes NOS

G40.401 Other generalized epilepsy and epileptic syndromes, not intractable, with status epilepticus

G40.409 Other generalized epilepsy and epileptic syndromes, not intractable, without status epilepticus

✓6th **G40.41　Other generalized epilepsy and epileptic syndromes, intractable**
　　　　　　G40.411　Other generalized epilepsy and epileptic syndromes, intractable, with status epilepticus
　　　　　　G40.419　Other generalized epilepsy and epileptic syndromes, intractable, without status epilepticus

✓5th **G40.5　Special epileptic syndromes**
　　　　Epilepsia partialis continua [Kozhevnikof]
　　　　Epileptic seizures related to alcohol
　　　　Epileptic seizures related to drugs
　　　　Epileptic seizures related to hormonal changes
　　　　Epileptic seizures related to sleep deprivation
　　　　Epileptic seizures related to stress

✓6th **G40.50　Special epileptic syndromes, not intractable**
　　　　　Special epileptic syndromes without intractability
　　　　　　G40.501　Special epileptic syndromes, not intractable, with status epilepticus
　　　　　　G40.509　Special epileptic syndromes, not intractable, without status epilepticus
　　　　　　　Special epileptic syndromes NOS

✓6th **G40.51　Special epileptic syndromes, intractable**
　　　　　　G40.511　Special epileptic syndromes, intractable, with status epilepticus
　　　　　　G40.519　Special epileptic syndromes, intractable, without status epilepticus

✓5th **G40.8　Other epilepsy and seizures**
　　　　Epilepsies and epileptic syndromes undetermined as to whether they are focal or generalized

✓6th **G40.80　Other epilepsy, not intractable**
　　　　　Other epilepsy without intractability
　　　　　　G40.801　Other epilepsy, not intractable, with status epilepticus
　　　　　　G40.809　Other epilepsy, not intractable, without status epilepticus
　　　　　　　Other epilepsy NOS

✓6th **G40.81　Other epilepsy, intractable**
　　　　　　G40.811　Other epilepsy, intractable, with status epilepticus
　　　　　　G40.819　Other epilepsy, intractable, without status epilepticus

G40.89　Other seizures
　　　　EXCLUDES 1　*post traumatic seizures (R56.1)*
　　　　　　　　　recurrent seizures NOS (G40.909)
　　　　　　　　　seizure NOS (R56.9)

✓5th **G40.9　Epilepsy, unspecified**
✓6th **G40.90　Epilepsy, unspecified, not intractable**
　　　　　Epilepsy, unspecified, without intractability
　　　　　　G40.901　Epilepsy, unspecified, not intractable, with status epilepticus
　　　　　　G40.909　Epilepsy, unspecified, not intractable, without status epilepticus
　　　　　　　Epilepsy NOS
　　　　　　　Epileptic convulsions NOS
　　　　　　　Epileptic fits NOS
　　　　　　　Epileptic seizures NOS
　　　　　　　Recurrent seizures NOS

✓6th **G40.91　Epilepsy, unspecified, intractable**
　　　　　Intractable seizure disorder NOS
　　　　　　G40.911　Epilepsy, unspecified, intractable, with status epilepticus
　　　　　　G40.919　Epilepsy, unspecified, intractable, without status epilepticus

✓4th **G43　Migraine**
　　NOTE　The following terms are to be considered equivalent to intractable: pharmacoresistant (pharmacologically resistant), treatment resistant, refractory (medically) and poorly controlled
　　EXCLUDES 1　*headache NOS (R51)*
　　　　　　　headache syndromes (G44-)
　　　　　　　lower half migraine (G44.00)

✓5th **G43.0　Migraine without aura**
　　　　Common migraine
　　　　EXCLUDES 1　*chronic migraine without aura (G43.7)*

✓6th **G43.00　Migraine without aura, not intractable**
　　　　　　G43.001　Migraine without aura, not intractable, with status migrainosus

　　　　　　G43.009　Migraine without aura, not intractable, without status migrainosus
　　　　　　　Migraine without aura NOS

✓6th **G43.01　Migraine without aura, intractable**
　　　　　　G43.011　Migraine without aura, intractable, with status migrainosus
　　　　　　G43.019　Migraine without aura, intractable, without status migrainosus

✓5th **G43.1　Migraine with aura**
　　　　Basilar migraine
　　　　Classical migraine
　　　　Migraine equivalents
　　　　Migraine preceded or accompanied by transient focal neurological phenomena
　　　　Migraine triggered seizures
　　　　Migraine with acute-onset aura
　　　　Migraine with aura without headache (migraine equivalents)
　　　　Migraine with prolonged aura
　　　　Migraine with typical aura
　　　　Retinal migraine
　　　　Code also any associated seizure (G40-, R56.9)
　　　　EXCLUDES 1　*persistent migraine aura (G43.5-, G43.6-)*

✓6th **G43.10　Migraine with aura, not intractable**
　　　　　　G43.101　Migraine with aura, not intractable, with status migrainosus
　　　　　　G43.109　Migraine with aura, not intractable, without status migrainosus
　　　　　　　Migraine with aura NOS

✓6th **G43.11　Migraine with aura, intractable**
　　　　　　G43.111　Migraine with aura, intractable, with status migrainosus
　　　　　　G43.119　Migraine with aura, intractable, without status migrainosus

✓5th **G43.4　Hemiplegic migraine**
　　　　Familial migraine
　　　　Sporadic migraine

✓6th **G43.40　Hemiplegic migraine, not intractable**
　　　　　　G43.401　Hemiplegic migraine, not intractable, with status migrainosus
　　　　　　G43.409　Hemiplegic migraine, not intractable, without status migrainosus
　　　　　　　Hemiplegic migraine NOS

✓6th **G43.41　Hemiplegic migraine, intractable**
　　　　　　G43.411　Hemiplegic migraine, intractable, with status migrainosus
　　　　　　G43.419　Hemiplegic migraine, intractable, without status migrainosus

✓5th **G43.5　Persistent migraine aura without cerebral infarction**
✓6th **G43.50　Persistent migraine aura without cerebral infarction, not intractable**
　　　　　　G43.501　Persistent migraine aura without cerebral infarction, not intractable, with status migrainosus
　　　　　　G43.509　Persistent migraine aura without cerebral infarction, not intractable, without status migrainosus
　　　　　　　Persistent migraine aura NOS

✓6th **G43.51　Persistent migraine aura without cerebral infarction, intractable**
　　　　　　G43.511　Persistent migraine aura without cerebral infarction, intractable, with status migrainosus
　　　　　　G43.519　Persistent migraine aura without cerebral infarction, intractable, without status migrainosus

✓5th **G43.6　Persistent migraine aura with cerebral infarction**
　　　　Code also the type of cerebral infarction (I63-)
✓6th **G43.60　Persistent migraine aura with cerebral infarction, not intractable**
　　　　　　G43.601　Persistent migraine aura with cerebral infarction, not intractable, with status migrainosus
　　　　　　G43.609　Persistent migraine aura with cerebral infarction, not intractable, without status migrainosus

---

✓ Appropriate additional character required　　　　✓x7th Requires 7th character, placeholder x must fill empty characters

✓6th **G43.61 Persistent migraine aura with cerebral infarction, intractable**
     G43.611 Persistent migraine aura with cerebral infarction, intractable, with status migrainosus
     G43.619 Persistent migraine aura with cerebral infarction, intractable, without status migrainosus

✓5th **G43.7 Chronic migraine without aura**
     Transformed migraine
     EXCLUDES 1   *migraine without aura (G43.0-)*

     ✓6th **G43.70 Chronic migraine without aura, not intractable**
        G43.701 Chronic migraine without aura, not intractable, with status migrainosus
        G43.709 Chronic migraine without aura, not intractable, without status migrainosus
          Chronic migraine without aura NOS

     ✓6th **G43.71 Chronic migraine without aura, intractable**
        G43.711 Chronic migraine without aura, intractable, with status migrainosus
        G43.719 Chronic migraine without aura, intractable, without status migrainosus

✓5th **G43.a Cyclical vomiting**
     ✓6th **G43.a0 Cyclical vomiting, not intractable**
        G43.a01 Cyclical vomiting, not intractable, with status migrainosus
        G43.a09 Cyclical vomiting, not intractable, without status migrainosus
          Cyclical vomiting NOS

     ✓6th **G43.a1 Cyclical vomiting, intractable**
        G43.a11 Cyclical vomiting, intractable, with status migrainosus
        G43.a19 Cyclical vomiting, intractable, without status migrainosus

✓5th **G43.b Ophthalmoplegic migraine**
     ✓6th **G43.b0 Ophthalmoplegic migraine, not intractable**
        G43.b01 Ophthalmoplegic migraine, not intractable, with status migrainosus
        G43.b09 Ophthalmoplegic migraine, not intractable, without status migrainosus
          Ophthalmoplegic migraine NOS

     ✓6th **G43.b1 Ophthalmoplegic migraine, intractable**
        G43.b11 Ophthalmoplegic migraine, intractable, with status migrainosus
        G43.b19 Ophthalmoplegic migraine, intractable, without status migrainosus

✓5th **G43.c Periodic headache syndromes in child or adult**
     ✓6th **G43.c0 Periodic headache syndromes in child or adult, not intractable**
        G43.c01 Periodic headache syndromes in child or adult, not intractable, with status migrainosus
        G43.c09 Periodic headache syndromes in child or adult, not intractable, without status migrainosus
          Periodic headache syndromes in child or adult NOS

     ✓6th **G43.c1 Periodic headache syndromes in child or adult, intractable**
        G43.c11 Periodic headache syndromes in child or adult, intractable, with status migrainosus
        G43.c19 Periodic headache syndromes in child or adult, intractable, without status migrainosus

✓5th **G43.d Menstrual migraine**
     Menstrual headache
     Menstrually related migraine
     Pre-menstrual headache
     Pre-menstrual migraine
     Pure menstrual migraine
     Code also associated premenstrual tension syndrome (N94.3)

     ✓6th **G43.d0 Menstrual migraine, not intractable**
        G43.d01 Menstrual migraine, not intractable, with status migrainosus
        G43.d09 Menstrual migraine, not intractable, without status migrainosus
          Menstrual migraine NOS

     ✓6th **G43.d1 Menstrual migraine, intractable**
        G43.d11 Menstrual migraine, intractable, with status migrainosus
        G43.d19 Menstrual migraine, intractable, without status migrainosus

✓5th **G43.8 Other migraine**
     ✓6th **G43.80 Other migraine, not intractable**
        G43.801 Other migraine, not intractable, with status migrainosus
        G43.809 Other migraine, not intractable, without status migrainosus

     ✓6th **G43.81 Other migraine, intractable**
        G43.811 Other migraine, intractable, with status migrainosus
        G43.819 Other migraine, intractable, without status migrainosus

✓5th **G43.9 Migraine, unspecified**
     ✓6th **G43.90 Migraine, unspecified, not intractable**
        G43.901 Migraine, unspecified, not intractable, with status migrainosus
          Status migrainosus NOS
        G43.909 Migraine, unspecified, not intractable, without status migrainosus
          Migraine NOS

     ✓6th **G43.91 Migraine, unspecified, intractable**
        G43.911 Migraine, unspecified, intractable, with status migrainosus
        G43.919 Migraine, unspecified, intractable, without status migrainosus

✓4th **G44 Other headache syndromes**
     EXCLUDES 1   *headache NOS (R51)*
     EXCLUDES 2   *atypical facial pain (G50.1)*
          headache due to lumbar puncture (G97.1)
          migraines (G43-)
          trigeminal neuralgia (G50.0)

✓5th **G44.0 Cluster headaches and other trigeminal autonomic cephalgias (TAC)**
     ✓6th **G44.00 Cluster headache syndrome, unspecified**
        Ciliary neuralgia
        Cluster headache NOS
        Histamine cephalgia
        Lower half migraine
        Migrainous neuralgia
        G44.001 Cluster headache syndrome, unspecified, intractable
        G44.009 Cluster headache syndrome, unspecified, not intractable
          Cluster headache syndrome NOS

     ✓6th **G44.01 Episodic cluster headache**
        G44.011 Episodic cluster headache, intractable
        G44.019 Episodic cluster headache, not intractable
          Episodic cluster headache NOS

     ✓6th **G44.02 Chronic cluster headache**
        G44.021 Chronic cluster headache, intractable
        G44.029 Chronic cluster headache, not intractable
          Chronic cluster headache NOS

     ✓6th **G44.03 Episodic paroxysmal hemicrania**
        Paroxysmal hemicrania NOS
        G44.031 Episodic paroxysmal hemicrania, intractable
        G44.039 Episodic paroxysmal hemicrania, not intractable
          Episodic paroxysmal hemicrania NOS

     ✓6th **G44.04 Chronic paroxysmal hemicrania**
        G44.041 Chronic paroxysmal hemicrania, intractable
        G44.049 Chronic paroxysmal hemicrania, not intractable
          Chronic paroxysmal hemicrania NOS

     ✓6th **G44.05 Short lasting unilateral neuralgiform headache with conjunctival injection and tearing (SUNCT)**
        G44.051 Short lasting unilateral neuralgiform headache with conjunctival injection and tearing (SUNCT), intractable

---

EXCLUDES 1   Not coded here   EXCLUDES 2   Not included here   *Manifestation Code*

G44.059　Short lasting unilateral neuralgiform headache with conjunctival injection and tearing (SUNCT), not intractable
Short lasting unilateral neuralgiform headache with conjunctival injection and tearing (SUNCT) NOS

✓6th **G44.09　Other trigeminal autonomic cephalgias (TAC)**

G44.091　Other trigeminal autonomic cephalgias (TAC), intractable

G44.099　Other trigeminal autonomic cephalgias (TAC), not intractable

✓5th **G44.1　Vascular headache, not elsewhere classified**

G44.10　Vascular headache, not elsewhere classified, not intractable
Vascular headache NOS

G44.11　Vascular headache, not elsewhere classified, intractable

✓5th **G44.2　Tension-type headache**

✓6th **G44.20　Tension-type headache, unspecified**

G44.201　Tension-type headache, unspecified, intractable

G44.209　Tension-type headache, unspecified, not intractable
Tension headache NOS

✓6th **G44.21　Episodic tension-type headache**

G44.211　Episodic tension-type headache, intractable

G44.219　Episodic tension-type headache, not intractable
Episodic tension-type headache NOS

✓6th **G44.22　Chronic tension-type headache**

G44.221　Chronic tension-type headache, intractable

G44.229　Chronic tension-type headache, not intractable
Chronic tension-type headache NOS

✓5th **G44.3　Post-traumatic headache**
Code first: postconcussional syndrome (F07.81)

✓6th **G44.30　Post-traumatic headache, unspecified**

G44.301　Post-traumatic headache, unspecified, intractable

G44.309　Post-traumatic headache, unspecified, not intractable
Post-traumatic headache NOS

✓6th **G44.31　Acute post-traumatic headache**

G44.311　Acute post-traumatic headache, intractable

G44.319　Acute post-traumatic headache, not intractable
Acute post-traumatic headache NOS

✓6th **G44.32　Chronic post-traumatic headache**

G44.321　Chronic post-traumatic headache, intractable

G44.329　Chronic post-traumatic headache, not intractable
Chronic post-traumatic headache NOS

✓5th **G44.4　Drug-induced headache, not elsewhere classified**
Medication overuse headache
Code first (T36-T50) to identify drug

G44.40　Drug-induced headache, not elsewhere classified, not intractable

G44.41　Drug-induced headache, not elsewhere classified, intractable

✓5th **G44.5　Complicated headache syndromes**

G44.51　Hemicrania continua

G44.52　New daily persistent headache (NDPH)

G44.53　Primary thunderclap headache

G44.59　Other complicated headache syndrome

✓5th **G44.8　Other specified headache syndromes**

G44.81　Hypnic headache

G44.82　Headache associated with sexual activity
Orgasmic headache
Preorgasmic headache

G44.83　Primary cough headache

G44.84　Primary exertional headache

G44.85　Primary stabbing headache

G44.89　Other headache syndrome

✓4th **G45　Transient cerebral ischemic attacks and related syndromes**
EXCLUDES 1　neonatal cerebral ischemia (P91.0)
transient retinal artery occlusion (H34.0-)

G45.0　Vertebro-basilar artery syndrome

G45.1　Carotid artery syndrome (hemispheric)

G45.2　Multiple and bilateral precerebral artery syndromes

G45.3　Amaurosis fugax

G45.4　Transient global amnesia
EXCLUDES 1　amnesia NOS (R41.3)

G45.8　Other transient cerebral ischemic attacks and related syndromes

G45.9　Transient cerebral ischemic attack, unspecified
Spasm of cerebral artery
TIA
Transient cerebral ischemia NOS

✓4th **G46　Vascular syndromes of brain in cerebrovascular diseases**
Code first underlying cerebrovascular disease (I60-I69)

G46.0　Middle cerebral artery syndrome

G46.1　Anterior cerebral artery syndrome

G46.2　Posterior cerebral artery syndrome

G46.3　Brain stem stroke syndrome
Benedikt syndrome
Claude syndrome
Foville syndrome
Millard-Gubler syndrome
Wallenberg syndrome
Weber syndrome

G46.4　Cerebellar stroke syndrome

G46.5　Pure motor lacunar syndrome

G46.6　Pure sensory lacunar syndrome

G46.7　Other lacunar syndromes

G46.8　Other vascular syndromes of brain in cerebrovascular diseases

✓4th **G47　Sleep disorders**
EXCLUDES 2　nightmares (F51.5)
nonorganic sleep disorders (F51-)
sleep terrors (F51.4)
sleepwalking (F51.3)

✓5th **G47.0　Insomnia**
EXCLUDES 2　alcohol related insomnia (F10.182, F10.282, F10.982)
drug related insomnia (F11.182, F11.282, F13.182, F13.282, F13.982, F14.182, F14.282, F14.982, F15.182, F15.282, F15.982, F19.182, F19.282, F19.982)
idiopathic insomnia (F51.01)
insomnia due to a mental disorder (F51.05)
insomnia not due to a substance or known physiological condition (F51.0-)
nonorganic insomnia (F51.0-)
primary insomnia (F51.01)
sleep apnea (G47.3-)

G47.00　Insomnia, unspecified
Insomnia NOS

G47.01　Insomnia due to medical condition
Code also associated medical condition

G47.09　Other insomnia

✓5th **G47.1　Hypersomnia**
EXCLUDES 2　alcohol-related hypersomnia (F10.182, F10.282, F10.982)
drug-related hypersomnia (F11.182, F11.282, F11.982, F13.182, F13.282, F13.982, F14.182, F14.282, F14.982, F15.182, F15.282, F15.982, F19.182, F19.282, F19.982)
hypersomnia due to a mental disorder (F51.13)
hypersomnia not due to a substance or known physiological condition (F51.11)
primary hypersomnia (F51.11)
sleep apnea (G47.3-)

G47.10　Hypersomnia, unspecified
Hypersomnia NOS

G47.11　Idiopathic hypersomnia with long sleep time
Idiopathic hypersomnia NOS

G47.12　Idiopathic hypersomnia without long sleep time

G47.13　Recurrent hypersomnia
Kleine-Levin syndrome
Menstrual related hypersomnia

G47.14　Hypersomnia due to medical condition
Code also associated medical condition

☑ Appropriate additional character required　　　✓x7th Requires 7th character, placeholder x must fill empty characters

G47.19   **Other hypersomnia**

✓5ᵗʰ   **G47.2**   **Circadian rhythm sleep disorders**
Disorders of the sleep wake schedule
Inversion of nyctohemeral rhythm
Inversion of sleep rhythm

G47.20   **Circadian rhythm sleep disorder, unspecified type**
Sleep wake schedule disorder NOS

G47.21   **Circadian rhythm sleep disorder, delayed sleep phase type**
Delayed sleep phase syndrome

G47.22   **Circadian rhythm sleep disorder, advanced sleep phase type**

G47.23   **Circadian rhythm sleep disorder, irregular sleep wake type**
Irregular sleep-wake pattern

G47.24   **Circadian rhythm sleep disorder, free running type**

G47.25   **Circadian rhythm sleep disorder, jet lag type**

G47.26   **Circadian rhythm sleep disorder, shift work type**

G47.27   **Circadian rhythm sleep disorder in conditions classified elsewhere**
Code first underlying condition

G47.29   **Other circadian rhythm sleep disorder**

✓5ᵗʰ   **G47.3**   **Sleep apnea**
Code also any associated underlying condition
EXCLUDES 1   *apnea NOS R06.81*
Cheyne-Stokes breathing (R06.3)
pickwickian syndrome (E66.2)
sleep apnea of newborn (P28.3)

G47.30   **Sleep apnea, unspecified**
Sleep apnea NOS

G47.31   **Primary central sleep apnea**

G47.32   **High altitude periodic breathing**

G47.33   **Obstructive sleep apnea (adult) (pediatric)**
EXCLUDES 1   *obstructive sleep apnea of newborn (P28.3)*

G47.34   **Idiopathic sleep related nonobstructive alveolar hypoventilation**
Sleep related hypoxia

G47.35   **Congenital central alveolar hypoventilation syndrome**

G47.36   **Sleep related hypoventilation in conditions classified elsewhere**
Sleep related hypoxemia in conditions classified elsewhere
Code first underlying condition

G47.37   **Central sleep apnea in conditions classified elsewhere**
Code first underlying condition

G47.39   **Other sleep apnea**

✓5ᵗʰ   **G47.4**   **Narcolepsy and cataplexy**

✓6ᵗʰ   G47.41   **Narcolepsy**

G47.411   **Narcolepsy with cataplexy**

G47.419   **Narcolepsy without cataplexy**
Narcolepsy NOS

✓6ᵗʰ   G47.42   **Narcolepsy in conditions classified elsewhere**

G47.421   **Narcolepsy in conditions classified elsewhere with cataplexy**

G47.429   **Narcolepsy in conditions classified elsewhere without cataplexy**

✓5ᵗʰ   **G47.5**   **Parasomnia**
EXCLUDES 1   *alcohol induced parasomnia (F10.182, F10.282, F10.982)*
drug induced parasomnia (F11.182, F11.282, F11.982, F13.182, F13.282, F13.982, F14.182, F14.282, F14.982, F15.182, F15.282, F15.982, F19.182, F19.282, F19.982)
parasomnia not due to a substance or known physiological condition (F51.8)

G47.50   **Parasomnia, unspecified**
Parasomnia NOS

G47.51   **Confusional arousals**

G47.52   **REM sleep behavior disorder**

G47.53   **Recurrent isolated sleep paralysis**

G47.54   **Parasomnia in conditions classified elsewhere**
Code first underlying condition

G47.59   **Other parasomnia**

✓5ᵗʰ   **G47.6**   **Sleep related movement disorders**
EXCLUDES 2   *restless legs syndrome (G25.81)*

G47.61   **Periodic limb movement disorder**

G47.62   **Sleep related leg cramps**

G47.63   **Sleep related bruxism**
EXCLUDES 1   *psychogenic bruxism (F45.8)*

G47.69   **Other sleep related movement disorders**

G47.8   **Other sleep disorders**

G47.9   **Sleep disorder, unspecified**
Sleep disorder NOS

Nerve, nerve root and plexus disorders (G50-G59)

EXCLUDES 1   *current traumatic nerve, nerve root and plexus disorders—see Injury, nerve by body region*
neuralgia NOS (M79.2)
neuritis NOS (M79.2)
peripheral neuritis in pregnancy (O26.82-)
radiculitis NOS (M54.1-)

✓4ᵗʰ   **G50**   **Disorders of trigeminal nerve**
INCLUDES   disorders of 5th cranial nerve

G50.0   **Trigeminal neuralgia**
Syndrome of paroxysmal facial pain
Tic douloureux

G50.1   **Atypical facial pain**

G50.8   **Other disorders of trigeminal nerve**

G50.9   **Disorder of trigeminal nerve, unspecified**

✓4ᵗʰ   **G51**   **Facial nerve disorders**
INCLUDES   disorders of 7th cranial nerve

G51.0   **Bell's palsy**
Facial palsy

G51.1   **Geniculate ganglionitis**
EXCLUDES 1   *postherpetic geniculate ganglionitis (B02.21)*

G51.2   **Melkersson's syndrome**
Melkersson-Rosenthal syndrome

G51.3   **Clonic hemifacial spasm**

G51.4   **Facial myokymia**

G51.8   **Other disorders of facial nerve**

G51.9   **Disorder of facial nerve, unspecified**

✓4ᵗʰ   **G52**   **Disorders of other cranial nerves**
EXCLUDES 2   *disorders of acoustic [8th] nerve (H93.3)*
disorders of optic [2nd] nerve (H46, H47.0)
paralytic strabismus due to nerve palsy (H49.0-H49.2)

G52.0   **Disorders of olfactory nerve**
Disorders of 1st cranial nerve

G52.1   **Disorders of glossopharyngeal nerve**
Disorder of 9th cranial nerve
Glossopharyngeal neuralgia

G52.2   **Disorders of vagus nerve**
Disorders of pneumogastric [10th] nerve

G52.3   **Disorders of hypoglossal nerve**
Disorders of 12th cranial nerve

G52.7   **Disorders of multiple cranial nerves**
Polyneuritis cranialis

G52.8   **Disorders of other specified cranial nerves**

G52.9   **Cranial nerve disorder, unspecified**

G53   ***Cranial nerve disorders in diseases classified elsewhere***
Code first underlying disease, such as:
neoplasm (C00-D49)
EXCLUDES 1   *multiple cranial nerve palsy in sarcoidosis (D86.82)*
multiple cranial nerve palsy in syphilis (A52.15)
postherpetic geniculate ganglionitis (B02.21)
postherpetic trigeminal neuralgia (B02.22)

✓4ᵗʰ   **G54**   **Nerve root and plexus disorders**
EXCLUDES 1   *current traumatic nerve root and plexus disorders—see nerve injury by body region*
intervertebral disc disorders (M50-M51)
neuralgia or neuritis NOS (M79.2)
neuritis or radiculitis:
brachial NOS (M54.13)
lumbar NOS (M54.16)
lumbosacral NOS (M54.17)
thoracic NOS (M54.14)
radiculitis NOS (M54.10)
radiculopathy NOS (M54.10)
spondylosis (M47-)

G54.0   **Brachial plexus disorders**
Thoracic outlet syndrome

G54.1   **Lumbosacral plexus disorders**

G54.2   **Cervical root disorders, not elsewhere classified**

EXCLUDES 1   Not coded here   EXCLUDES 2   Not included here   ***Manifestation Code***

G54.3 **Thoracic root disorders, not elsewhere classified**

G54.4 **Lumbosacral root disorders, not elsewhere classified**

G54.5 **Neuralgic amyotrophy**
Parsonage-Aldren-Turner syndrome
Shoulder-girdle neuritis
EXCLUDES 1 *neuralgic amyotrophy in diabetes mellitus (E08-E13 with .44)*

G54.6 **Phantom limb syndrome with pain**

G54.7 **Phantom limb syndrome without pain**
Phantom limb syndrome NOS

G54.8 **Other nerve root and plexus disorders**

G54.9 **Nerve root and plexus disorder, unspecified**

G55 ***Nerve root and plexus compressions in diseases classified elsewhere***
Code first underlying disease, such as:
neoplasm (C00-D49)
EXCLUDES 1 *nerve root compression (due to) (in) ankylosing spondylitis (M45-)*
nerve root compression (due to) (in) dorsopathies (M53-, M54-)
nerve root compression (due to) (in) intervertebral disc disorders (M50.1-, M51.1-)
nerve root compression (due to) (in) spondylopathies (M46-, M48-)
nerve root compression (due to) (in) spondylosis (M47.0-M47.2-)

✓4th G56 **Mononeuropathies of upper limb**
EXCLUDES 1 *current traumatic nerve disorder—see nerve injury by body region*

✓5th G56.0 **Carpal tunnel syndrome**
G56.00 **Carpal tunnel syndrome, unspecified upper limb**
G56.01 **Carpal tunnel syndrome, right upper limb**
G56.02 **Carpal tunnel syndrome, left upper limb**

✓5th G56.1 **Other lesions of median nerve**
G56.10 **Other lesions of median nerve, unspecified upper limb**
G56.11 **Other lesions of median nerve, right upper limb**
G56.12 **Other lesions of median nerve, left upper limb**

✓5th G56.2 **Lesion of ulnar nerve**
Tardy ulnar nerve palsy
G56.20 **Lesion of ulnar nerve, unspecified upper limb**
G56.21 **Lesion of ulnar nerve, right upper limb**
G56.22 **Lesion of ulnar nerve, left upper limb**

✓5th G56.3 **Lesion of radial nerve**
G56.30 **Lesion of radial nerve, unspecified upper limb**
G56.31 **Lesion of radial nerve, right upper limb**
G56.32 **Lesion of radial nerve, left upper limb**

✓5th G56.4 **Causalgia of upper limb**
Complex regional pain syndrome II of upper limb
EXCLUDES 1 *complex regional pain syndrome I of lower limb (G90.52-)*
complex regional pain syndrome I of upper limb (G90.51-)
complex regional pain syndrome II of lower limb (G57.7-)
reflex sympathetic dystrophy of lower limb (G90.52-)
reflex sympathetic dystrophy of upper limb (G90.51-)
G56.40 **Causalgia of unspecified upper limb**
G56.41 **Causalgia of right upper limb**
G56.42 **Causalgia of left upper limb**

✓5th G56.8 **Other specified mononeuropathies of upper limb**
Interdigital neuroma of upper limb
G56.80 **Other specified mononeuropathies of unspecified upper limb**
G56.81 **Other specified mononeuropathies of right upper limb**
G56.82 **Other specified mononeuropathies of left upper limb**

✓5th G56.9 **Unspecified mononeuropathy of upper limb**
G56.90 **Unspecified mononeuropathy of unspecified upper limb**
G56.91 **Unspecified mononeuropathy of right upper limb**
G56.92 **Unspecified mononeuropathy of left upper limb**

✓4th G57 **Mononeuropathies of lower limb**
EXCLUDES 1 *current traumatic nerve disorder—see nerve injury by body region*

✓5th G57.0 **Lesion of sciatic nerve**
EXCLUDES 1 *sciatica NOS (M54.3-)*
EXCLUDES 2 *sciatica attributed to intervertebral disc disorder (M51.1-)*
G57.00 **Lesion of sciatic nerve, unspecified lower limb**
G57.01 **Lesion of sciatic nerve, right lower limb**
G57.02 **Lesion of sciatic nerve, left lower limb**

✓5th G57.1 **Meralgia paresthetica**
Lateral cutaneous nerve of thigh syndrome
G57.10 **Meralgia paresthetica, unspecified lower limb**
G57.11 **Meralgia paresthetica, right lower limb**
G57.12 **Meralgia paresthetica, left lower limb**

✓5th G57.2 **Lesion of femoral nerve**
G57.20 **Lesion of femoral nerve, unspecified lower limb**
G57.21 **Lesion of femoral nerve, right lower limb**
G57.22 **Lesion of femoral nerve, left lower limb**

✓5th G57.3 **Lesion of lateral popliteal nerve**
Peroneal nerve palsy
G57.30 **Lesion of lateral popliteal nerve, unspecified lower limb**
G57.31 **Lesion of lateral popliteal nerve, right lower limb**
G57.32 **Lesion of lateral popliteal nerve, left lower limb**

✓5th G57.4 **Lesion of medial popliteal nerve**
G57.40 **Lesion of medial popliteal nerve, unspecified lower limb**
G57.41 **Lesion of medial popliteal nerve, right lower limb**
G57.42 **Lesion of medial popliteal nerve, left lower limb**

✓5th G57.5 **Tarsal tunnel syndrome**
G57.50 **Tarsal tunnel syndrome, unspecified lower limb**
G57.51 **Tarsal tunnel syndrome, right lower limb**
G57.52 **Tarsal tunnel syndrome, left lower limb**

✓5th G57.6 **Lesion of plantar nerve**
Morton's metatarsalgia
G57.60 **Lesion of plantar nerve, unspecified lower limb**
G57.61 **Lesion of plantar nerve, right lower limb**
G57.62 **Lesion of plantar nerve, left lower limb**

✓5th G57.7 **Causalgia of lower limb**
Complex regional pain syndrome II of lower limb
EXCLUDES 1 *complex regional pain syndrome I of lower limb (G90.52-)*
complex regional pain syndrome I of upper limb (G90.51-)
complex regional pain syndrome II of upper limb (G56.4-)
reflex sympathetic dystrophy of lower limb (G90.52-)
reflex sympathetic dystrophy of upper limb (G90.51-)
G57.70 **Causalgia of unspecified lower limb**
G57.71 **Causalgia of right lower limb**
G57.72 **Causalgia of left lower limb**

✓5th G57.8 **Other specified mononeuropathies of lower limb**
Interdigital neuroma of lower limb
G57.80 **Other specified mononeuropathies of unspecified lower limb**
G57.81 **Other specified mononeuropathies of right lower limb**
G57.82 **Other specified mononeuropathies of left lower limb**

✓5th G57.9 **Unspecified mononeuropathy of lower limb**
G57.90 **Unspecified mononeuropathy of unspecified lower limb**
G57.91 **Unspecified mononeuropathy of right lower limb**
G57.92 **Unspecified mononeuropathy of left lower limb**

✓4th G58 **Other mononeuropathies**
G58.0 **Intercostal neuropathy**
G58.7 **Mononeuritis multiplex**
G58.8 **Other specified mononeuropathies**
G58.9 **Mononeuropathy, unspecified**

G59 ***Mononeuropathy in diseases classified elsewhere***
Code first underlying disease
EXCLUDES 1 *diabetic mononeuropathy (E09-E14 with .41)*
syphilitic nerve paralysis (A52.19)
syphilitic neuritis (A52.15)
tuberculous mononeuropathy (A17.83)

☑ Appropriate additional character required   ✓x7th Requires 7th character, placeholder x must fill empty characters

Diseases of the Nervous System

G60–G71.8

Polyneuropathies and other disorders of the peripheral nervous system (G60-G65)

> EXCLUDES 1   neuralgia NOS (M79.2)
> neuritis NOS (M79.2)
> peripheral neuritis in pregnancy (O26.82-)
> radiculitis NOS (M54.10)

✓4ᵗʰ **G60   Hereditary and idiopathic neuropathy**

    G60.0   Hereditary motor and sensory neuropathy
        Charcôt-Marie-Tooth disease
        Déjérine-Sottas disease
        Hereditary motor and sensory neuropathy, types I-IV
        Hypertrophic neuropathy of infancy
        Peroneal muscular atrophy (axonal type) (hypertrophic type)
        Roussy-Levy syndrome

    G60.1   Refsum's disease
        Infantile Refsum disease

    G60.2   Neuropathy in association with hereditary ataxia

    G60.3   Idiopathic progressive neuropathy

    G60.8   Other hereditary and idiopathic neuropathies
        Dominantly inherited sensory neuropathy
        Morvan's disease
        Nelaton's syndrome
        Recessively inherited sensory neuropathy

    G60.9   Hereditary and idiopathic neuropathy, unspecified

✓4ᵗʰ **G61   Inflammatory polyneuropathy**

    G61.0   Guillain-Barre syndrome
        Acute (post-)infective polyneuritis
        Miller Fisher syndrome

    G61.1   Serum neuropathy
        Code first (T50.9-) to identify serum

    ✓5ᵗʰ **G61.8   Other inflammatory polyneuropathies**
        G61.81   Chronic inflammatory demyelinating polyneuritis
        G61.89   Other inflammatory polyneuropathies

    G61.9   Inflammatory polyneuropathy, unspecified

✓4ᵗʰ **G62   Other and unspecified polyneuropathies**

    G62.0   Drug-induced polyneuropathy
        Code first (T36-T50) to identify drug

    G62.1   Alcoholic polyneuropathy

    G62.2   Polyneuropathy due to other toxic agents
        Code first (T51-T65) to identify toxic agent.

    ✓5ᵗʰ **G62.8   Other specified polyneuropathies**
        G62.81   Critical illness polyneuropathy
            Acute motor neuropathy
        G62.82   Radiation-induced polyneuropathy
            Use additional external cause code (W88-W90, X39.0-) to identify cause
        G62.89   Other specified polyneuropathies

    G62.9   Polyneuropathy, unspecified
        Neuropathy NOS

G63   Polyneuropathy in diseases classified elsewhere
    Code first underlying disease, such as:
        amyloidosis (E85-)
        endocrine disease, except diabetes (E00-E07, E15-E16, E20-E34)
        metabolic diseases (E70-E88)
        neoplasm (C00-D49)
        nutritional deficiency (E40-E64)

> EXCLUDES 1   *polyneuropathy (in):*
> *diabetes mellitus (E08-E13 with .42)*
> *diphtheria (A36.83)*
> *infectious mononucleosis (B27.0-B27.9 with 1)*
> *Lyme disease (A69.22)*
> *mumps (B26.84)*
> *postherpetic (B02.23)*
> *rheumatoid arthritis (M05.33)*
> *scleroderma (M34.83)*
> *systemic lupus erythematosus (M32.19)*

G64   Other disorders of peripheral nervous system
    Disorder of peripheral nervous system NOS

✓4ᵗʰ **G65   Sequelae of inflammatory and toxic polyneuropathies**
    Code first condition resulting from (sequela) of inflammatory and toxic polyneuropathies

    G65.0   Sequelae of Guillain-Barré syndrome
    G65.1   Sequelae of other inflammatory polyneuropathy
    G65.2   Sequelae of toxic polyneuropathy

Diseases of myoneural junction and muscle (G70-G73)

✓4ᵗʰ **G70   Myasthenia gravis and other myoneural disorders**

> EXCLUDES 1   botulism (A05.1, A48.51-A48.52)
> transient neonatal myasthenia gravis (P94.0)

    ✓5ᵗʰ **G70.0   Myasthenia gravis**
        G70.00   Myasthenia gravis without (acute) exacerbation
            Myasthenia gravis NOS
        G70.01   Myasthenia gravis with (acute) exacerbation
            Myasthenia gravis in crisis

    G70.1   Toxic myoneural disorders
        Code first (T51-T65) to identify toxic agent.

    G70.2   Congenital and developmental myasthenia

    G70.8   Other specified myoneural disorders

    G70.9   Myoneural disorder, unspecified

✓4ᵗʰ **G71   Primary disorders of muscles**

> EXCLUDES 2   *arthrogryposis multiplex congenita (Q74.3)*
> *metabolic disorders (E70-E88)*
> *myositis (M60-)*

    G71.0   Muscular dystrophy
        Autosomal recessive, childhood type, muscular dystrophy resembling Duchenne or Becker muscular dystrophy
        Benign [Becker] muscular dystrophy
        Benign scapuloperoneal muscular dystrophy with early contractures [Emery-Dreifuss]
        Distal muscular dystrophy
        Facioscapulohumeral muscular dystrophy
        Limb-girdle muscular dystrophy
        Ocular muscular dystrophy
        Oculopharyngeal muscular dystrophy
        Scapuloperoneal muscular dystrophy
        Severe [Duchenne] muscular dystrophy

> EXCLUDES 1   *congenital muscular dystrophy NOS (G71.2)*
> *congenital muscular dystrophy with specific morphological abnormalities of the muscle fiber (G71.2)*

    ✓5ᵗʰ **G71.1   Myotonic disorders**
        G71.11   Myotonic muscular dystrophy
            Dystrophia myotonica [Steinert]
            Myotonia atrophica
            Myotonic dystrophy
            Proximal myotonic myopathy (PROMM)
            Steinert disease
        G71.12   Myotonia congenita
            Acetazolamide responsive myotonia congenita
            Dominant myotonia congenita [Thomsen disease]
            Myotonia levior
            Recessive myotonia congenita [Becker disease]
        G71.13   Myotonic chondrodystrophy
            Chondrodystrophic myotonia
            Congenital myotonic chondrodystrophy
            Schwartz-Jampel disease
        G71.14   Drug induced myotonia
            Code first (T36-T50) to identify drug
        G71.19   Other specified myotonic disorders
            Myotonia fluctuans
            Myotonia permanens
            Neuromyotonia [Isaacs]
            Paramyotonia congenita (of von Eulenburg)
            Pseudomyotonia
            Symptomatic myotonia

    G71.2   Congenital myopathies
        Central core disease
        Congenital muscular dystrophy NOS
        Congenital muscular dystrophy with specific morphological abnormalities of the muscle fiber
        Fiber-type disproportion
        Minicore disease
        Multicore disease
        Myotubular (centronuclear) myopathy
        Nemaline myopathy

> EXCLUDES 1   *arthrogryposis multiplex congenita (Q74.3)*

    G71.3   Mitochondrial myopathy, not elsewhere classified

> EXCLUDES 1   *Kearns-Sayre syndrome (H49.81)*
> *Leber's disease (H47.21)*
> *Leigh's encephalopathy (G31.82)*
> *mitochondrial metabolism disorders (E88.4-)*
> *Reye's syndrome (G93.7)*

    G71.8   Other primary disorders of muscles

EXCLUDES 1   Not coded here   EXCLUDES 2   Not included here   *Manifestation Code*

G71.9 Primary disorder of muscle, unspecified
Hereditary myopathy NOS

✓4th **G72 Other and unspecified myopathies**
EXCLUDES 1 *arthrogryposis multiplex congenita (Q74.3)*
dermatopolymyositis (M33-)
ischemic infarction of muscle (M62.2-)
myositis (M60-)
polymyositis (M33.2-)

G72.0 Drug-induced myopathy
Code first (T36-T50) to identify drug

G72.1 Alcoholic myopathy
Use additional code to identify alcoholism (F10-)

G72.2 Myopathy due to other toxic agents
Code first (T51-T65) to identify toxic agent.

G72.3 Periodic paralysis
Familial periodic paralysis
Hyperkalemic periodic paralysis (familial)
Hypokalemic periodic paralysis (familial)
Myotonic periodic paralysis (familial)
Normokalemic paralysis (familial)
Potassium sensitive periodic paralysis
EXCLUDES 1 *paramyotonia congenita (of von Eulenburg) (G71.19)*

✓5th **G72.4 Inflammatory and immune myopathies, not elsewhere classified**
G72.41 Inclusion body myositis [IBM]
G72.49 Other inflammatory and immune myopathies, not elsewhere classified
Inflammatory myopathy NOS

✓5th **G72.8 Other specified myopathies**
G72.81 Critical illness myopathy
Acute necrotizing myopathy
Acute quadriplegic myopathy
Intensive care (ICU) myopathy
Myopathy of critical illness
G72.89 Other specified myopathies

G72.9 Myopathy, unspecified

✓4th **G73 Disorders of myoneural junction and muscle in diseases classified elsewhere**
G73.1 Lambert-Eaton syndrome
Code first underlying disease, such as:
malignant neoplasm of lung (C34-)
other neoplastic disease (C00-D49)
EXCLUDES 1 *Lambert-Eaton syndrome not associated with neoplasm (G70.8)*

G73.3 Myasthenic syndromes in other diseases classified elsewhere
Code first underlying disease, such as:
neoplasm (C00-D49)
thyrotoxicosis (E05-)

G73.7 Myopathy in diseases classified elsewhere
Code first underlying disease, such as:
hyperparathyroidism (E21.0, E21.3)
hypoparathyroidism (E20-)
glycogen storage disease (E74.0)
lipid storage disorders (E75-)
EXCLUDES 1 *myopathy in:*
rheumatoid arthritis (M05.4-)
sarcoidosis (D86.87)
scleroderma (M34.82)
sicca syndrome [Sjögren] (M35.03)
systemic lupus erythematosus (M32.19)

Cerebral palsy and other paralytic syndromes (G80-G83)

✓4th **G80 Cerebral palsy**
EXCLUDES 1 *hereditary spastic paraplegia (G11.4)*
G80.0 Spastic quadriplegic cerebral palsy
Congenital spastic paralysis (cerebral)
G80.1 Spastic diplegic cerebral palsy
Spastic cerebral palsy NOS
G80.2 Spastic hemiplegic cerebral palsy
G80.3 Athetoid cerebral palsy
Double athetosis (syndrome)
Dyskinetic cerebral palsy
Dystonic cerebral palsy
Vogt disease
G80.4 Ataxic cerebral palsy

G80.8 Other cerebral palsy
Mixed cerebral palsy syndromes
G80.9 Cerebral palsy, unspecified
Cerebral palsy NOS

✓4th **G81 Hemiplegia and hemiparesis**
NOTE This category is to be used only when hemiplegia (complete)(incomplete) is reported without further specification, or is stated to be old or longstanding but of unspecified cause. The category is also for use in multiple coding to identify these types of hemiplegia resulting from any cause.
EXCLUDES 1 *congenital cerebral palsy (G80-)*
hemiplegia and hemiparesis due to sequela of cerebrovascular disease (I69.05-, I69.15-, I69.25-, I69.35-, I69.45-, I69.85-, I69.95-)

✓5th **G81.0 Flaccid hemiplegia**
G81.00 Flaccid hemiplegia affecting unspecified side
G81.01 Flaccid hemiplegia affecting right dominant side
G81.02 Flaccid hemiplegia affecting left dominant side
G81.03 Flaccid hemiplegia affecting right nondominant side
G81.04 Flaccid hemiplegia affecting left nondominant side

✓5th **G81.1 Spastic hemiplegia**
G81.10 Spastic hemiplegia affecting unspecified side
G81.11 Spastic hemiplegia affecting right dominant side
G81.12 Spastic hemiplegia affecting left dominant side
G81.13 Spastic hemiplegia affecting right nondominant side
G81.14 Spastic hemiplegia affecting left nondominant side

✓5th **G81.9 Hemiplegia, unspecified**
G81.90 Hemiplegia, unspecified affecting unspecified side
G81.91 Hemiplegia, unspecified affecting right dominant side
G81.92 Hemiplegia, unspecified affecting left dominant side
G81.93 Hemiplegia, unspecified affecting right nondominant side
G81.94 Hemiplegia, unspecified affecting left nondominant side

✓4th **G82 Paraplegia (paraparesis) and quadriplegia (quadriparesis)**
NOTE This category is to be used only when the listed conditions are reported without further specification, or are stated to be old or longstanding but of unspecified cause. The category is also for use in multiple coding to identify these conditions resulting from any cause
EXCLUDES 1 *congenital cerebral palsy (G80-)*
functional quadriplegia (R53.2)
hysterical paralysis (F44.4)

✓5th **G82.2 Paraplegia**
Paralysis of both lower limbs NOS
Paraparesis (lower) NOS
Paraplegia (lower) NOS
G82.20 Paraplegia, unspecified
G82.21 Paraplegia, complete
G82.22 Paraplegia, incomplete

✓5th **G82.5 Quadriplegia**
G82.50 Quadriplegia, unspecified
G82.51 Quadriplegia, C1-C4 complete
G82.52 Quadriplegia, C1-C4 incomplete
G82.53 Quadriplegia, C5-C7 complete
G82.54 Quadriplegia, C5-C7 incomplete

✓4th **G83 Other paralytic syndromes**
NOTE This category is to be used only when the listed conditions are reported without further specification, or are stated to be old or longstanding but of unspecified cause. The category is also for use in multiple coding to identify these conditions resulting from any cause.
INCLUDES paralysis (complete) (incomplete), except as in G80-G82
G83.0 Diplegia of upper limbs
Diplegia (upper)
Paralysis of both upper limbs

✓ Appropriate additional character required   ✓x7th Requires 7th character, placeholder x must fill empty characters

✓5th **G83.1 Monoplegia of lower limb**
Paralysis of lower limb
EXCLUDES 1 *monoplegia of lower limbs due to sequela of cerebrovascular disease (I69.04-, I69.14-, I69.24-, I69.34-, I69.44-, I69.84-, I69.94-)*

G83.10 **Monoplegia of lower limb affecting unspecified side**

G83.11 **Monoplegia of lower limb affecting right dominant side**

G83.12 **Monoplegia of lower limb affecting left dominant side**

G83.13 **Monoplegia of lower limb affecting right nondominant side**

G83.14 **Monoplegia of lower limb affecting left nondominant side**

✓5th **G83.2 Monoplegia of upper limb**
Paralysis of upper limb
EXCLUDES 1 *monoplegia of upper limbs due to sequela of cerebrovascular disease (I69.03-, I69.13-, I69.23-, I69.33-, I69.43-, I69.83-, I69.93-)*

G83.20 **Monoplegia of upper limb affecting unspecified side**

G83.21 **Monoplegia of upper limb affecting right dominant side**

G83.22 **Monoplegia of upper limb affecting left dominant side**

G83.23 **Monoplegia of upper limb affecting right nondominant side**

G83.24 **Monoplegia of upper limb affecting left nondominant side**

✓5th **G83.3 Monoplegia, unspecified**

G83.30 **Monoplegia, unspecified affecting unspecified side**

G83.31 **Monoplegia, unspecified affecting right dominant side**

G83.32 **Monoplegia, unspecified affecting left dominant side**

G83.33 **Monoplegia, unspecified affecting right nondominant side**

G83.34 **Monoplegia, unspecified affecting left nondominant side**

G83.4 Cauda equina syndrome
Neurogenic bladder due to cauda equina syndrome
EXCLUDES 1 *cord bladder NOS (G95.8)*
neurogenic bladder NOS (N31.9)

G83.5 Locked-in state

✓5th **G83.8 Other specified paralytic syndromes**
EXCLUDES 1 *paralytic syndromes due to current spinal cord injury—code to spinal cord injury (S14, S24, S34)*

G83.81 **Brown-Séquard syndrome**

G83.82 **Anterior cord syndrome**

G83.83 **Posterior cord syndrome**

G83.84 **Todd's paralysis (postepileptic)**

G83.89 **Other specified paralytic syndromes**

G83.9 Paralytic syndrome, unspecified

Other disorders of the nervous system (G89-G99)

✓4th **G89 Pain, not elsewhere classified**
Code also related psychological factors associated with pain (F45.42)
EXCLUDES 1 *generalized pain NOS (R52)*
pain disorders exclusively related to psychological factors (F45.41)
pain NOS (R52)
EXCLUDES 2 *atypical face pain (G50.1)*
headache syndromes (G44-)
localized pain, unspecified type—code to pain by site, such as:
abdomen pain (R10-)
back pain (M54.9)
breast pain (N64.4)
chest pain (R07.1-R07.9)
ear pain (H92.0-)
eye pain (H57.1)
headache (R51)
joint pain (M25.5-)
limb pain (M79.6-)
lumbar region pain (M54.5)
painful urination (R30.9)
pelvic and perineal pain (R10.2)
renal colic (N23)
shoulder pain (M25.51-)
spine pain (M54-)
throat pain (R07.0)
tongue pain (K14.6)
tooth pain (K08.8)
migraines (G43-)
myalgia (M79.1)
pain from prosthetic devices, implants, and grafts (T82.84, T83.84, T84.84, T85.84)
phantom limb syndrome with pain (G54.6)
vulvar vestibulitis (N94.810)
vulvodynia (N94.81-)

G89.0 Central pain syndrome
Déjérine-Roussy syndrome
Myelopathic pain syndrome
Thalamic pain syndrome (hyperesthetic)

✓5th **G89.1 Acute pain, not elsewhere classified**

G89.11 **Acute pain due to trauma**

G89.12 **Acute post-thoracotomy pain**
Post-thoracotomy pain NOS

G89.18 **Other acute postprocedural pain**
Postoperative pain NOS
Postprocedural pain NOS

✓5th **G89.2 Chronic pain, not elsewhere classified**
EXCLUDES 1 *causalgia, lower limb (G57.7-)*
causalgia, upper limb (G56.4-)
central pain syndrome (G89.0)
chronic pain syndrome (G89.4)
complex regional pain syndrome II, lower limb (G57.7-)
complex regional pain syndrome II, upper limb (G56.4-)
neoplasm related chronic pain (G89.3)
reflex sympathetic dystrophy (G90.5-)

G89.21 **Chronic pain due to trauma**

G89.22 **Chronic post-thoracotomy pain**

G89.28 **Other chronic postprocedural pain**
Other chronic postoperative pain

G89.3 Neoplasm related pain (acute) (chronic)
Cancer associated pain
Pain due to malignancy (primary) (secondary)
Tumor associated pain

G89.4 Chronic pain syndrome
Chronic pain associated with significant psychosocial dysfunction

✓4th **G90 Disorders of autonomic nervous system**
EXCLUDES 1 *dysfunction of the autonomic nervous system due to alcohol (G31.2)*

✓5th **G90.0 Idiopathic peripheral autonomic neuropathy**

G90.01 **Carotid sinus syncope**
Carotid sinus syndrome

G90.09 **Other idiopathic peripheral autonomic neuropathy**
Idiopathic peripheral autonomic neuropathy NOS

G90.1 Familial dysautonomia [Riley-Day]

EXCLUDES 1 Not coded here   EXCLUDES 2 Not included here   *Manifestation Code*

G90.2 Horner's syndrome
Bernard(-Horner) syndrome
Cervical sympathetic dystrophy or paralysis

G90.3 Multi-system degeneration of the autonomic nervous system
Neurogenic orthostatic hypotension [Shy-Drager]
EXCLUDES 1 *orthostatic hypotension NOS (I95.1)*

G90.4 Autonomic dysreflexia
Use additional code to identify the cause, such as:
fecal impaction (K56.41)
pressure ulcer (pressure area) (L89-)
urinary tract infection (N39.0)

√5th **G90.5 Complex regional pain syndrome I (CRPS I)**
Reflex sympathetic dystrophy
EXCLUDES 1 *causalgia of lower limb (G57.7-)*
causalgia of upper limb (G56.4-)
complex regional pain syndrome II of lower limb (G57.7-)
complex regional pain syndrome II of upper limb (G56.4-)

G90.50 Complex regional pain syndrome I, unspecified
√6th **G90.51 Complex regional pain syndrome I of upper limb**
G90.511 Complex regional pain syndrome I of right upper limb
G90.512 Complex regional pain syndrome I of left upper limb
G90.513 Complex regional pain syndrome I of upper limb, bilateral
G90.519 Complex regional pain syndrome I of unspecified upper limb
√6th **G90.52 Complex regional pain syndrome I of lower limb**
G90.521 Complex regional pain syndrome I of right lower limb
G90.522 Complex regional pain syndrome I of left lower limb
G90.523 Complex regional pain syndrome I of lower limb, bilateral
G90.529 Complex regional pain syndrome I of unspecified lower limb
G90.59 Complex regional pain syndrome I of other specified site

G90.8 Other disorders of autonomic nervous system
G90.9 Disorder of the autonomic nervous system, unspecified

√4th **G91 Hydrocephalus**
INCLUDES acquired hydrocephalus
EXCLUDES 1 *Arnold-Chiari syndrome with hydrocephalus (Q07-)*
congenital hydrocephalus (Q03-)
spina bifida with hydrocephalus (Q05-)

G91.0 Communicating hydrocephalus
Secondary normal pressure hydrocephalus
G91.1 Obstructive hydrocephalus
G91.2 (Idiopathic) normal pressure hydrocephalus
Normal pressure hydrocephalus NOS
G91.3 Post-traumatic hydrocephalus, unspecified
G91.4 Hydrocephalus in diseases classified elsewhere
Code first underlying condition, such as:
congenital syphilis (A50.4-)
neoplasm (C00-D49)
EXCLUDES 1 *hydrocephalus due to congenital toxoplasmosis (P37.1)*
G91.8 Other hydrocephalus
G91.9 Hydrocephalus, unspecified

G92 Toxic encephalopathy
Toxic encephalitis
Toxic metabolic encephalopathy
Code first (T51-T65) to identify toxic agent

√4th **G93 Other disorders of brain**
G93.0 Cerebral cysts
Arachnoid cyst
Porencephalic cyst, acquired
EXCLUDES 1 *acquired periventricular cysts of newborn (P91.1)*
congenital cerebral cysts (Q04.6)

G93.1 Anoxic brain damage, not elsewhere classified
EXCLUDES 1 *cerebral anoxia due to anesthesia during labor and delivery (O74.3)*
cerebral anoxia due to anesthesia during the puerperium (O89.2)
neonatal anoxia (P28.9)

G93.2 Benign intracranial hypertension
EXCLUDES 1 *hypertensive encephalopathy (I67.4)*

G93.3 Postviral fatigue syndrome
Benign myalgic encephalomyelitis
EXCLUDES 1 *chronic fatigue syndrome NOS (R53.82)*

√5th **G93.4 Other and unspecified encephalopathy**
EXCLUDES 1 *alcoholic encephalopathy (G31.2)*
encephalopathy in diseases classified elsewhere (G94)
hypertensive encephalopathy (I67.4)
toxic (metabolic) encephalopathy (G92)
G93.40 Encephalopathy, unspecified
G93.41 Metabolic encephalopathy
Septic encephalopathy
G93.49 Other encephalopathy
Encephalopathy NEC

G93.5 Compression of brain
Arnold-Chiari type 1 compression of brain
Compression of brain (stem)
Herniation of brain (stem)
EXCLUDES 1 *diffuse traumatic compression of brain (S06.2-)*
focal traumatic compression of brain (S06.3-)

G93.6 Cerebral edema
EXCLUDES 1 *cerebral edema due to birth injury (P11.0)*
traumatic cerebral edema (S06.1-)

G93.7 Reye's syndrome
Code first (T39.0-), if salicylates-induced

√5th **G93.8 Other specified disorders of brain**
G93.81 Temporal sclerosis
Hippocampal sclerosis
Mesial temporal sclerosis
G93.89 Other specified disorders of brain
Postradiation encephalopathy

G93.9 Disorder of brain, unspecified

G94 Other disorders of brain in diseases classified elsewhere
Code first underlying disease
EXCLUDES 1 *encephalopathy in congenital syphilis (A50.49)*
encephalopathy in influenza (J09.090, J09.190, J10.81, J11.81)
encephalopathy in syphilis (A52.19)
hydrocephalus in diseases classified elsewhere (G91.4)

√4th **G95 Other and unspecified diseases of spinal cord**
EXCLUDES 2 *myelitis (G04-)*
G95.0 Syringomyelia and syringobulbia
√5th **G95.1 Vascular myelopathies**
EXCLUDES 2 *intraspinal phlebitis and thrombophlebitis, except non-pyogenic (G08)*
G95.11 Acute infarction of spinal cord (embolic) (nonembolic)
Anoxia of spinal cord
Arterial thrombosis of spinal cord
G95.19 Other vascular myelopathies
Edema of spinal cord
Hematomyelia
Nonpyogenic intraspinal phlebitis and thrombophlebitis
Subacute necrotic myelopathy
√5th **G95.2 Other and unspecified cord compression**
G95.20 Unspecified cord compression
G95.29 Other cord compression
√5th **G95.8 Other specified diseases of spinal cord**
EXCLUDES 1 *neurogenic bladder NOS (N31.9)*
neurogenic bladder due to cauda equina syndrome (G83.4)
neuromuscular dysfunction of bladder without spinal cord lesion (N31-)
G95.81 Conus medullaris syndrome
G95.89 Other specified diseases of spinal cord
Cord bladder NOS
Drug-induced myelopathy
Radiation-induced myelopathy
EXCLUDES 1 *myelopathy NOS (G95.9)*

☑ Appropriate additional character required

√x7th Requires 7th character, placeholder x must fill empty characters

G95.9 Disease of spinal cord, unspecified
Myelopathy NOS

☑️4ᵗʰ **G96 Other disorders of central nervous system**

G96.0 Cerebrospinal fluid leak
> **EXCLUDES 1**   cerebrospinal fluid leak from spinal puncture (G97.0)

☑️5ᵗʰ **G96.1 Disorders of meninges, not elsewhere classified**

G96.11 Dural tear
> **EXCLUDES 1**   accidental puncture or laceration of dura during a procedure (G97.41)

G96.12 Meningeal adhesions (cerebral) (spinal)

G96.19 Other disorders of meninges, not elsewhere classified

G96.8 Other specified disorders of central nervous system

G96.9 Disorder of central nervous system, unspecified

☑️4ᵗʰ **G97 Intraoperative and postprocedural complications and disorders of nervous system, not elsewhere classified**
> **EXCLUDES 2**   intraoperative and postprocedural cerebrovascular infarction (I97.81-, I97.82-)

G97.0 Cerebrospinal fluid leak from spinal puncture

G97.1 Other reaction to spinal and lumbar puncture
Headache due to lumbar puncture

G97.2 Intracranial hypotension following ventricular shunting

☑️5ᵗʰ **G97.3 Intraoperative hemorrhage and hematoma of a nervous system organ or structure complicating a procedure**
> **EXCLUDES 1**   intraoperative hemorrhage and hematoma of a nervous system organ or structure due to accidental puncture and laceration during a procedure (G97.4-)

G97.31 Intraoperative hemorrhage and hematoma of a nervous system organ or structure complicating a nervous system procedure

G97.32 Intraoperative hemorrhage and hematoma of a nervous system organ or structure complicating other procedure

☑️5ᵗʰ **G97.4 Accidental puncture and laceration of a nervous system organ or structure during a procedure**

G97.41 Accidental puncture or laceration of dura during a procedure
Incidental (inadvertent) durotomy

G97.48 Accidental puncture and laceration of other nervous system organ or structure during a nervous system procedure

G97.49 Accidental puncture and laceration of other nervous system organ or structure during other procedure

☑️5ᵗʰ **G97.5 Postprocedural hemorrhage and hematoma of a nervous system organ or structure following a procedure**

G97.51 Postprocedural hemorrhage and hematoma of a nervous system organ or structure following a nervous system procedure

G97.52 Postprocedural hemorrhage and hematoma of a nervous system organ or structure following other procedure

☑️5ᵗʰ **G97.8 Other intraoperative and postprocedural complications and disorders of nervous system**
Use additional code to further specify disorder

G97.81 Other intraoperative complications of nervous system

G97.82 Other postprocedural complications and disorders of nervous system

☑️4ᵗʰ **G98 Other disorders of nervous system not elsewhere classified**
> **INCLUDES**   nervous system disorder NOS

G98.0 Neurogenic arthritis, not elsewhere classified
Nonsyphilitic neurogenic arthropathy NEC
Nonsyphilitic neurogenic spondylopathy NEC
> **EXCLUDES 1**   spondylopathy (in):
>   syringomyelia and syringobulbia (G95.0)
>   tabes dorsalis (A52.11)

G98.8 Other disorders of nervous system
Nervous system disorder NOS

☑️4ᵗʰ **G99 Other disorders of nervous system in diseases classified elsewhere**

G99.0 Autonomic neuropathy in diseases classified elsewhere
Code first underlying disease, such as:
amyloidosis (E85-)
gout (M1a-, M10-)
hyperthyroidism (E05-)
> **EXCLUDES 1**   diabetic autonomic neuropathy (E09-14 with .43)

G99.2 Myelopathy in diseases classified elsewhere
Code first underlying disease, such as:
neoplasm (C00-D49)
> **EXCLUDES 1**   myelopathy in:
>   intervertebral disease (M50.0-, M51.0-)
>   spondylosis (M47.0-, M47.1-)

G99.8 Other specified disorders of nervous system in diseases classified elsewhere
Code first underlying disorder, such as:
amyloidosis (E85-)
avitaminosis (E56.9)
> **EXCLUDES 1**   nervous system involvement in:
>   cysticercosis (B69.0)
>   rubella (B06.0-)
>   syphilis (A52.1-)

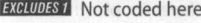

EXCLUDES 1 Not coded here   **EXCLUDES 2** Not included here   *Manifestation Code*

Chapter 7. Diseases of the Eye and Adnexa (H00-H59)

NOTE   Use an external cause code following the code for the eye condition, if applicable, to identify the cause of the eye condition

EXCLUDES 2   certain conditions originating in the perinatal period (P04-P96)
certain infectious and parasitic diseases (A00-B99)
complications of pregnancy, childbirth and the puerperium (O00-O99)
congenital malformations, deformations, and chromosomal abnormalities (Q00-Q99)
diabetes mellitus related eye conditions (E09.3-, E10.3-, E11.3-, E13.3-)
endocrine, nutritional and metabolic diseases (E00-E88)
injury (trauma) of eye and orbit (S05-)
injury, poisoning and certain other consequences of external causes (S00-T88)
neoplasms (C00-D49)
symptoms, signs and abnormal clinical and laboratory findings, not elsewhere classified (R00-R94)
syphilis related eye disorders (A50.01, A50.3-, A51.43, A52.71)

This chapter contains the following blocks:

H00-H05   Disorders of eyelid, lacrimal system and orbit
H10-H11   Disorders of conjunctiva
H15-H22   Disorders of sclera, cornea, iris and ciliary body
H25-H28   Disorders of lens
H30-H36   Disorders of choroid and retina
H40-H42   Glaucoma
H43-H44   Disorders of vitreous body and globe
H46-H47   Disorders of optic nerve and visual pathways
H49-H52   Disorders of ocular muscles, binocular movement, accommodation and refraction
H53-H54   Visual disturbances and blindness
H55-H57   Other disorders of eye and adnexa
H59   Intraoperative and postprocedural complications and disorders of eye and adnexa, not elsewhere classified

Disorders of eyelid, lacrimal system and orbit (H00-H05)

EXCLUDES 2   open wound of eyelid (S01.1-)
superficial injury of eyelid (S00.1-, S00.2-)

✓4th H00 Hordeolum and chalazion

   ✓5th H00.0 Hordeolum (externum) (internum) of eyelid

     ✓6th H00.01 Hordeolum externum
       Hordeolum NOS
       Stye
       H00.011 Hordeolum externum right upper eyelid
       H00.012 Hordeolum externum right lower eyelid
       H00.013 Hordeolum externum right eye, unspecified eyelid
       H00.014 Hordeolum externum left upper eyelid
       H00.015 Hordeolum externum left lower eyelid
       H00.016 Hordeolum externum left eye, unspecified eyelid
       H00.019 Hordeolum externum unspecified eye, unspecified eyelid

     ✓6th H00.02 Hordeolum internum
       Infection of meibomian gland
       H00.021 Hordeolum internum right upper eyelid
       H00.022 Hordeolum internum right lower eyelid
       H00.023 Hordeolum internum right eye, unspecified eyelid
       H00.024 Hordeolum internum left upper eyelid
       H00.025 Hordeolum internum left lower eyelid
       H00.026 Hordeolum internum left eye, unspecified eyelid
       H00.029 Hordeolum internum unspecified eye, unspecified eyelid

     ✓6th H00.03 Abscess of eyelid
       Furuncle of eyelid
       H00.031 Abscess of right upper eyelid
       H00.032 Abscess of right lower eyelid
       H00.033 Abscess of eyelid right eye, unspecified eyelid
       H00.034 Abscess of left upper eyelid
       H00.035 Abscess of left lower eyelid
       H00.036 Abscess of eyelid left eye, unspecified eyelid
       H00.039 Abscess of eyelid unspecified eye, unspecified eyelid

   ✓5th H00.1 Chalazion
     Meibomian (gland) cyst
     EXCLUDES 2   infected meibomian gland (H00.02-)
     H00.11 Chalazion right upper eyelid
     H00.12 Chalazion right lower eyelid
     H00.13 Chalazion right eye, unspecified eyelid
     H00.14 Chalazion left upper eyelid
     H00.15 Chalazion left lower eyelid
     H00.16 Chalazion left eye, unspecified eyelid
     H00.19 Chalazion unspecified eye, unspecified eyelid

✓4th H01 Other inflammation of eyelid

   ✓5th H01.0 Blepharitis
     EXCLUDES 1   blepharoconjunctivitis (H10.5-)

     ✓6th H01.00 Unspecified blepharitis
       H01.001 Unspecified blepharitis right upper eyelid
       H01.002 Unspecified blepharitis right lower eyelid
       H01.003 Unspecified blepharitis right eye, unspecified eyelid
       H01.004 Unspecified blepharitis left upper eyelid
       H01.005 Unspecified blepharitis left lower eyelid
       H01.006 Unspecified blepharitis left eye, unspecified eyelid
       H01.009 Unspecified blepharitis unspecified eye, unspecified eyelid

     ✓6th H01.01 Ulcerative blepharitis
       H01.011 Ulcerative blepharitis right upper eyelid
       H01.012 Ulcerative blepharitis right lower eyelid
       H01.013 Ulcerative blepharitis right eye, unspecified eyelid
       H01.014 Ulcerative blepharitis left upper eyelid
       H01.015 Ulcerative blepharitis left lower eyelid
       H01.016 Ulcerative blepharitis left eye, unspecified eyelid
       H01.019 Ulcerative blepharitis unspecified eye, unspecified eyelid

     ✓6th H01.02 Squamous blepharitis
       H01.021 Squamous blepharitis right upper eyelid
       H01.022 Squamous blepharitis right lower eyelid
       H01.023 Squamous blepharitis right eye, unspecified eyelid
       H01.024 Squamous blepharitis left upper eyelid
       H01.025 Squamous blepharitis left lower eyelid
       H01.026 Squamous blepharitis left eye, unspecified eyelid
       H01.029 Squamous blepharitis unspecified eye, unspecified eyelid

   ✓5th H01.1 Noninfectious dermatoses of eyelid

     ✓6th H01.11 Allergic dermatitis of eyelid
       Contact dermatitis of eyelid
       H01.111 Allergic dermatitis of right upper eyelid
       H01.112 Allergic dermatitis of right lower eyelid
       H01.113 Allergic dermatitis of right eye, unspecified eyelid
       H01.114 Allergic dermatitis of left upper eyelid
       H01.115 Allergic dermatitis of left lower eyelid
       H01.116 Allergic dermatitis of left eye, unspecified eyelid
       H01.119 Allergic dermatitis of unspecified eye, unspecified eyelid

     ✓6th H01.12 Discoid lupus erythematosus of eyelid
       H01.121 Discoid lupus erythematosus of right upper eyelid
       H01.122 Discoid lupus erythematosus of right lower eyelid
       H01.123 Discoid lupus erythematosus of right eye, unspecified eyelid
       H01.124 Discoid lupus erythematosus of left upper eyelid
       H01.125 Discoid lupus erythematosus of left lower eyelid
       H01.126 Discoid lupus erythematosus of left eye, unspecified eyelid
       H01.129 Discoid lupus erythematosus of unspecified eye, unspecified eyelid

---

✓ Appropriate additional character required   ✓x7th Requires 7th character, placeholder x must fill empty characters

✓6ᵗʰ **H01.13 Eczematous dermatitis of eyelid**

     H01.131   **Eczematous dermatitis of right upper eyelid**

     H01.132   **Eczematous dermatitis of right lower eyelid**

     H01.133   **Eczematous dermatitis of right eye, unspecified eyelid**

     H01.134   **Eczematous dermatitis of left upper eyelid**

     H01.135   **Eczematous dermatitis of left lower eyelid**

     H01.136   **Eczematous dermatitis of left eye, unspecified eyelid**

     H01.139   **Eczematous dermatitis of unspecified eye, unspecified eyelid**

✓6ᵗʰ **H01.14 Xeroderma of eyelid**

     H01.141   **Xeroderma of right upper eyelid**

     H01.142   **Xeroderma of right lower eyelid**

     H01.143   **Xeroderma of right eye, unspecified eyelid**

     H01.144   **Xeroderma of left upper eyelid**

     H01.145   **Xeroderma of left lower eyelid**

     H01.146   **Xeroderma of left eye, unspecified eyelid**

     H01.149   **Xeroderma of unspecified eye, unspecified eyelid**

H01.8 Other specified inflammations of eyelid

H01.9 Unspecified inflammation of eyelid
     Inflammation of eyelid NOS

✓4ᵗʰ **H02 Other disorders of eyelid**

     EXCLUDES 1   *congenital malformations of eyelid (Q10.0–Q10.3)*

✓5ᵗʰ **H02.0 Entropion and trichiasis of eyelid**

✓6ᵗʰ **H02.00 Unspecified entropion of eyelid**

     H02.001   **Unspecified entropion of right upper eyelid**

     H02.002   **Unspecified entropion of right lower eyelid**

     H02.003   **Unspecified entropion of right eye, unspecified eyelid**

     H02.004   **Unspecified entropion of left upper eyelid**

     H02.005   **Unspecified entropion of left lower eyelid**

     H02.006   **Unspecified entropion of left eye, unspecified eyelid**

     H02.009   **Unspecified entropion of unspecified eye, unspecified eyelid**

✓6ᵗʰ **H02.01 Cicatricial entropion of eyelid**

     H02.011   **Cicatricial entropion of right upper eyelid**

     H02.012   **Cicatricial entropion of right lower eyelid**

     H02.013   **Cicatricial entropion of right eye, unspecified eyelid**

     H02.014   **Cicatricial entropion of left upper eyelid**

     H02.015   **Cicatricial entropion of left lower eyelid**

     H02.016   **Cicatricial entropion of left eye, unspecified eyelid**

     H02.019   **Cicatricial entropion of unspecified eye, unspecified eyelid**

✓6ᵗʰ **H02.02 Mechanical entropion of eyelid**

     H02.021   **Mechanical entropion of right upper eyelid**

     H02.022   **Mechanical entropion of right lower eyelid**

     H02.023   **Mechanical entropion of right eye, unspecified eyelid**

     H02.024   **Mechanical entropion of left upper eyelid**

     H02.025   **Mechanical entropion of left lower eyelid**

     H02.026   **Mechanical entropion of left eye, unspecified eyelid**

     H02.029   **Mechanical entropion of unspecified eye, unspecified eyelid**

✓6ᵗʰ **H02.03 Senile entropion of eyelid**

     H02.031   **Senile entropion of right upper eyelid**

     H02.032   **Senile entropion of right lower eyelid**

     H02.033   **Senile entropion of right eye, unspecified eyelid**

     H02.034   **Senile entropion of left upper eyelid**

     H02.035   **Senile entropion of left lower eyelid**

     H02.036   **Senile entropion of left eye, unspecified eyelid**

     H02.039   **Senile entropion of unspecified eye, unspecified eyelid**

✓6ᵗʰ **H02.04 Spastic entropion of eyelid**

     H02.041   **Spastic entropion of right upper eyelid**

     H02.042   **Spastic entropion of right lower eyelid**

     H02.043   **Spastic entropion of right eye, unspecified eyelid**

     H02.044   **Spastic entropion of left upper eyelid**

     H02.045   **Spastic entropion of left lower eyelid**

     H02.046   **Spastic entropion of left eye, unspecified eyelid**

     H02.049   **Spastic entropion of unspecified eye, unspecified eyelid**

✓6ᵗʰ **H02.05 Trichiasis without entropian**

     H02.051   **Trichiasis without entropian right upper eyelid**

     H02.052   **Trichiasis without entropian right lower eyelid**

     H02.053   **Trichiasis without entropian right eye, unspecified eyelid**

     H02.054   **Trichiasis without entropian left upper eyelid**

     H02.055   **Trichiasis without entropian left lower eyelid**

     H02.056   **Trichiasis without entropian left eye, unspecified eyelid**

     H02.059   **Trichiasis without entropian unspecified eye, unspecified eyelid**

✓5ᵗʰ **H02.1 Ectropion of eyelid**

✓6ᵗʰ **H02.10 Unspecified ectropion of eyelid**

     H02.101   **Unspecified ectropion of right upper eyelid**

     H02.102   **Unspecified ectropion of right lower eyelid**

     H02.103   **Unspecified ectropion of right eye, unspecified eyelid**

     H02.104   **Unspecified ectropion of left upper eyelid**

     H02.105   **Unspecified ectropion of left lower eyelid**

     H02.106   **Unspecified ectropion of left eye, unspecified eyelid**

     H02.109   **Unspecified ectropion of unspecified eye, unspecified eyelid**

✓6ᵗʰ **H02.11 Cicatricial ectropion of eyelid**

     H02.111   **Cicatricial ectropion of right upper eyelid**

     H02.112   **Cicatricial ectropion of right lower eyelid**

     H02.113   **Cicatricial ectropion of right eye, unspecified eyelid**

     H02.114   **Cicatricial ectropion of left upper eyelid**

     H02.115   **Cicatricial ectropion of left lower eyelid**

     H02.116   **Cicatricial ectropion of left eye, unspecified eyelid**

     H02.119   **Cicatricial ectropion of unspecified eye, unspecified eyelid**

✓6ᵗʰ **H02.12 Mechanical ectropion of eyelid**

     H02.121   **Mechanical ectropion of right upper eyelid**

     H02.122   **Mechanical ectropion of right lower eyelid**

     H02.123   **Mechanical ectropion of right eye, unspecified eyelid**

     H02.124   **Mechanical ectropion of left upper eyelid**

     H02.125   **Mechanical ectropion of left lower eyelid**

     H02.126   **Mechanical ectropion of left eye, unspecified eyelid**

EXCLUDES 1 Not coded here   EXCLUDES 2 Not included here   *Manifestation Code*

H02.129   Mechanical ectropion of unspecified eye, unspecified eyelid

☑6th H02.13 Senile ectropion of eyelid
- H02.131   Senile ectropion of right upper eyelid
- H02.132   Senile ectropion of right lower eyelid
- H02.133   Senile ectropion of right eye, unspecified eyelid
- H02.134   Senile ectropion of left upper eyelid
- H02.135   Senile ectropion of left lower eyelid
- H02.136   Senile ectropion of left eye, unspecified eyelid
- H02.139   Senile ectropion of unspecified eye, unspecified eyelid

☑6th H02.14 Spastic ectropion of eyelid
- H02.141   Spastic ectropion of right upper eyelid
- H02.142   Spastic ectropion of right lower eyelid
- H02.143   Spastic ectropion of right eye, unspecified eyelid
- H02.144   Spastic ectropion of left upper eyelid
- H02.145   Spastic ectropion of left lower eyelid
- H02.146   Spastic ectropion of left eye, unspecified eyelid
- H02.149   Spastic ectropion of unspecified eye, unspecified eyelid

☑5th H02.2 Lagophthalmos

☑6th H02.20 Unspecified lagophthalmos
- H02.201   Unspecified lagophthalmos right upper eyelid
- H02.202   Unspecified lagophthalmos right lower eyelid
- H02.203   Unspecified lagophthalmos right eye, unspecified eyelid
- H02.204   Unspecified lagophthalmos left upper eyelid
- H02.205   Unspecified lagophthalmos left lower eyelid
- H02.206   Unspecified lagophthalmos left eye, unspecified eyelid
- H02.209   Unspecified lagophthalmos unspecified eye, unspecified eyelid

☑6th H02.21 Cicatricial lagophthalmos
- H02.211   Cicatricial lagophthalmos right upper eyelid
- H02.212   Cicatricial lagophthalmos right lower eyelid
- H02.213   Cicatricial lagophthalmos right eye, unspecified eyelid
- H02.214   Cicatricial lagophthalmos left upper eyelid
- H02.215   Cicatricial lagophthalmos left lower eyelid
- H02.216   Cicatricial lagophthalmos left eye, unspecified eyelid
- H02.219   Cicatricial lagophthalmos unspecified eye, unspecified eyelid

☑6th H02.22 Mechanical lagophthalmos
- H02.221   Mechanical lagophthalmos right upper eyelid
- H02.222   Mechanical lagophthalmos right lower eyelid
- H02.223   Mechanical lagophthalmos right eye, unspecified eyelid
- H02.224   Mechanical lagophthalmos left upper eyelid
- H02.225   Mechanical lagophthalmos left lower eyelid
- H02.226   Mechanical lagophthalmos left eye, unspecified eyelid
- H02.229   Mechanical lagophthalmos unspecified eye, unspecified eyelid

☑6th H02.23 Paralytic lagophthalmos
- H02.231   Paralytic lagophthalmos right upper eyelid
- H02.232   Paralytic lagophthalmos right lower eyelid
- H02.233   Paralytic lagophthalmos right eye, unspecified eyelid
- H02.234   Paralytic lagophthalmos left upper eyelid
- H02.235   Paralytic lagophthalmos left lower eyelid
- H02.236   Paralytic lagophthalmos left eye, unspecified eyelid
- H02.239   Paralytic lagophthalmos unspecified eye, unspecified eyelid

☑5th H02.3 Blepharochalasis
        Pseudoptosis
- H02.30   Blepharochalasis unspecified eye, unspecified eyelid
- H02.31   Blepharochalasis right upper eyelid
- H02.32   Blepharochalasis right lower eyelid
- H02.33   Blepharochalasis right eye, unspecified eyelid
- H02.34   Blepharochalasis left upper eyelid
- H02.35   Blepharochalasis left lower eyelid
- H02.36   Blepharochalasis left eye, unspecified eyelid

☑5th H02.4 Ptosis of eyelid

☑6th H02.40 Unspecified ptosis of eyelid
- H02.401   Unspecified ptosis of right eyelid
- H02.402   Unspecified ptosis of left eyelid
- H02.403   Unspecified ptosis of bilateral eyelids
- H02.409   Unspecified ptosis of unspecified eyelid

☑6th H02.41 Mechanical ptosis of eyelid
- H02.411   Mechanical ptosis of right eyelid
- H02.412   Mechanical ptosis of left eyelid
- H02.413   Mechanical ptosis of bilateral eyelids
- H02.419   Mechanical ptosis of unspecified eyelid

☑6th H02.42 Myogenic ptosis of eyelid
- H02.421   Myogenic ptosis of right eyelid
- H02.422   Myogenic ptosis of left eyelid
- H02.423   Myogenic ptosis of bilateral eyelids
- H02.429   Myogenic ptosis of unspecified eyelid

☑6th H02.43 Paralytic ptosis of eyelid
        Neurogenic ptosis of eyelid
- H02.431   Paralytic ptosis of right eyelid
- H02.432   Paralytic ptosis of left eyelid
- H02.433   Paralytic ptosis of bilateral eyelids
- H02.439   Paralytic ptosis unspecified eyelid

☑5th H02.5 Other disorders affecting eyelid function
    EXCLUDES 2 *blepharospasm (G24.5)*
                  organic tic (G25.69)
                  psychogenic tic (F95-)

☑6th H02.51 Abnormal innervation syndrome
- H02.511   Abnormal innervation syndrome right upper eyelid
- H02.512   Abnormal innervation syndrome right lower eyelid
- H02.513   Abnormal innervation syndrome right eye, unspecified eyelid
- H02.514   Abnormal innervation syndrome left upper eyelid
- H02.515   Abnormal innervation syndrome left lower eyelid
- H02.516   Abnormal innervation syndrome left eye, unspecified eyelid
- H02.519   Abnormal innervation syndrome unspecified eye, unspecified eyelid

☑6th H02.52 Blepharophimosis
        Ankyloblepharon
- H02.521   Blepharophimosis right upper eyelid
- H02.522   Blepharophimosis right lower eyelid
- H02.523   Blepharophimosis right eye, unspecified eyelid
- H02.524   Blepharophimosis left upper eyelid
- H02.525   Blepharophimosis left lower eyelid
- H02.526   Blepharophimosis left eye, unspecified eyelid
- H02.529   Blepharophimosis unspecified eye, unspecified lid

☑6th H02.53 Eyelid retraction
        Eyelid lag
- H02.531   Eyelid retraction right upper eyelid
- H02.532   Eyelid retraction right lower eyelid

☑ Appropriate additional character required   ☑x7th Requires 7th character, placeholder x must fill empty characters

Diseases of the Eye and Adnexa

H02.533–H02.869

H02.533   Eyelid retraction right eye, unspecified eyelid
H02.534   Eyelid retraction left upper eyelid
H02.535   Eyelid retraction left lower eyelid
H02.536   Eyelid retraction left eye, unspecified eyelid
H02.539   Eyelid retraction unspecified eye, unspecified lid

H02.59   Other disorders affecting eyelid function
Deficient blink reflex
Sensory disorders

✓5th   **H02.6   Xanthelasma of eyelid**
H02.60   Xanthelasma of unspecified eye, unspecified eyelid
H02.61   Xanthelasma of right upper eyelid
H02.62   Xanthelasma of right lower eyelid
H02.63   Xanthelasma of right eye, unspecified eyelid
H02.64   Xanthelasma of left upper eyelid
H02.65   Xanthelasma of left lower eyelid
H02.66   Xanthelasma of left eye, unspecified eyelid

✓5th   **H02.7   Other and unspecified degenerative disorders of eyelid and periocular area**
H02.70   Unspecified degenerative disorders of eyelid and periocular area

✓6th   H02.71   Chloasma of eyelid and periocular area
Dyspigmentation of eyelid
Hyperpigmentation of eyelid
H02.711   Chloasma of right upper eyelid and periocular area
H02.712   Chloasma of right lower eyelid and periocular area
H02.713   Chloasma of right eye, unspecified eyelid and periocular area
H02.714   Chloasma of left upper eyelid and periocular area
H02.715   Chloasma of left lower eyelid and periocular area
H02.716   Chloasma of left eye, unspecified eyelid and periocular area
H02.719   Chloasma of unspecified eye, unspecified eyelid and periocular area

✓6th   H02.72   Madarosis of eyelid and periocular area
Hypotrichosis of eyelid
H02.721   Madarosis of right upper eyelid and periocular area
H02.722   Madarosis of right lower eyelid and periocular area
H02.723   Madarosis of right eye, unspecified eyelid and periocular area
H02.724   Madarosis of left upper eyelid and periocular area
H02.725   Madarosis of left lower eyelid and periocular area
H02.726   Madarosis of left eye, unspecified eyelid and periocular area
H02.729   Madarosis of unspecified eye, unspecified eyelid and periocular area

✓6th   H02.73   Vitiligo of eyelid and periocular area
Hypopigmentation of eyelid
H02.731   Vitiligo of right upper eyelid and periocular area
H02.732   Vitiligo of right lower eyelid and periocular area
H02.733   Vitiligo of right eye, unspecified eyelid and periocular area
H02.734   Vitiligo of left upper eyelid and periocular area
H02.735   Vitiligo of left lower eyelid and periocular area
H02.736   Vitiligo of left eye, unspecified eyelid and periocular area
H02.739   Vitiligo of unspecified eye, unspecified eyelid and periocular area

H02.79   Other degenerative disorders of eyelid and periocular area

✓5th   **H02.8   Other specified disorders of eyelid**
✓6th   H02.81   Retained foreign body in eyelid
Use additional code to identify the type of retained foreign body (Z18.-)
EXCLUDES 1   laceration of eyelid with foreign body (S01.12-)
retained intraocular foreign body (H44.6-, H44.7-)
superficial foreign body of eyelid and periocular area (S00.25-)
H02.811   Retained foreign body in right upper eyelid
H02.812   Retained foreign body in right lower eyelid
H02.813   Retained foreign body in right eye, unspecified eyelid
H02.814   Retained foreign body in left upper eyelid
H02.815   Retained foreign body in left lower eyelid
H02.816   Retained foreign body in left eye, unspecified eyelid
H02.819   Retained foreign body in unspecified eye, unspecified eyelid

✓6th   H02.82   Cysts of eyelid
Sebaceous cyst of eyelid
H02.821   Cysts of right upper eyelid
H02.822   Cysts of right lower eyelid
H02.823   Cysts of right eye, unspecified eyelid
H02.824   Cysts of left upper eyelid
H02.825   Cysts of left lower eyelid
H02.826   Cysts of left eye, unspecified eyelid
H02.829   Cysts of unspecified eye, unspecified eyelid

✓6th   H02.83   Dermatochalasis of eyelid
H02.831   Dermatochalasis of right upper eyelid
H02.832   Dermatochalasis of right lower eyelid
H02.833   Dermatochalasis of right eye, unspecified eyelid
H02.834   Dermatochalasis of left upper eyelid
H02.835   Dermatochalasis of left lower eyelid
H02.836   Dermatochalasis of left eye, unspecified eyelid
H02.839   Dermatochalasis of unspecified eye, unspecified eyelid

✓6th   H02.84   Edema of eyelid
Hyperemia of eyelid
H02.841   Edema of right upper eyelid
H02.842   Edema of right lower eyelid
H02.843   Edema of right eye, unspecified eyelid
H02.844   Edema of left upper eyelid
H02.845   Edema of left lower eyelid
H02.846   Edema of left eye, unspecified eyelid
H02.849   Edema of unspecified eye, unspecified eyelid

✓6th   H02.85   Elephantiasis of eyelid
H02.851   Elephantiasis of right upper eyelid
H02.852   Elephantiasis of right lower eyelid
H02.853   Elephantiasis of right eye, unspecified eyelid
H02.854   Elephantiasis of left upper eyelid
H02.855   Elephantiasis of left lower eyelid
H02.856   Elephantiasis of left eye, unspecified eyelid
H02.859   Elephantiasis of unspecified eye, unspecified eyelid

✓6th   H02.86   Hypertrichosis of eyelid
H02.861   Hypertrichosis of right upper eyelid
H02.862   Hypertrichosis of right lower eyelid
H02.863   Hypertrichosis of right eye, unspecified eyelid
H02.864   Hypertrichosis of left upper eyelid
H02.865   Hypertrichosis of left lower eyelid
H02.866   Hypertrichosis of left eye, unspecified eyelid
H02.869   Hypertrichosis of unspecified eye, unspecified eyelid

---

EXCLUDES 1   Not coded here   EXCLUDES 2   Not included here   *Manifestation Code*

✓6ᵗʰ **H02.87 Vascular anomalies of eyelid**
    H02.871 Vascular anomalies of right upper eyelid
    H02.872 Vascular anomalies of right lower eyelid
    H02.873 Vascular anomalies of right eye, unspecified eyelid
    H02.874 Vascular anomalies of left upper eyelid
    H02.875 Vascular anomalies of left lower eyelid
    H02.876 Vascular anomalies of left eye, unspecified eyelid
    H02.879 Vascular anomalies of unspecified eye, unspecified eyelid

H02.89 Other specified disorders of eyelid
    Hemorrhage of eyelid

H02.9 Unspecified disorder of eyelid
    Disorder of eyelid NOS

✓4ᵗʰ **H04 Disorders of lacrimal system**
    EXCLUDES 1   *congenital malformations of lacrimal system (Q10.4-Q10.6)*

✓5ᵗʰ **H04.0 Dacryoadenitis**
    ✓6ᵗʰ **H04.00 Unspecified dacryoadenitis**
        H04.001 Unspecified dacryoadenitis, right lacrimal gland
        H04.002 Unspecified dacryoadenitis, left lacrimal gland
        H04.003 Unspecified dacryoadenitis, bilateral lacrimal glands
        H04.009 Unspecified dacryoadenitis, unspecified lacrimal gland

    ✓6ᵗʰ **H04.01 Acute dacryoadenitis**
        H04.011 Acute dacryoadenitis, right lacrimal gland
        H04.012 Acute dacryoadenitis, left lacrimal gland
        H04.013 Acute dacryoadenitis, bilateral lacrimal glands
        H04.019 Acute dacryoadenitis, unspecified lacrimal gland

    ✓6ᵗʰ **H04.02 Chronic dacryoadenitis**
        H04.021 Chronic dacryoadenitis, right lacrimal gland
        H04.022 Chronic dacryoadenitis, left lacrimal gland
        H04.023 Chronic dacryoadenitis, bilateral lacrimal glands
        H04.029 Chronic dacryoadenitis, unspecified lacrimal gland

    ✓6ᵗʰ **H04.03 Chronic enlargement of lacrimal gland**
        H04.031 Chronic enlargement of right lacrimal gland
        H04.032 Chronic enlargement of left lacrimal gland
        H04.033 Chronic enlargement of bilateral lacrimal glands
        H04.039 Chronic enlargement of unspecified lacrimal gland

✓5ᵗʰ **H04.1 Other disorders of lacrimal gland**
    ✓6ᵗʰ **H04.11 Dacryops**
        H04.111 Dacryops of right lacrimal gland
        H04.112 Dacryops of left lacrimal gland
        H04.113 Dacryops of bilateral lacrimal glands
        H04.119 Dacryops of unspecified lacrimal gland

    ✓6ᵗʰ **H04.12 Dry eye syndrome**
        Tear film insufficiency, NOS
        H04.121 Dry eye syndrome of right lacrimal gland
        H04.122 Dry eye syndrome of left lacrimal gland
        H04.123 Dry eye syndrome of bilateral lacrimal glands
        H04.129 Dry eye syndrome of unspecified lacrimal gland

    ✓6ᵗʰ **H04.13 Lacrimal cyst**
        Lacrimal cystic degeneration
        H04.131 Lacrimal cyst, right lacrimal gland
        H04.132 Lacrimal cyst, left lacrimal gland
        H04.133 Lacrimal cyst, bilateral lacrimal glands
        H04.139 Lacrimal cyst, unspecified lacrimal gland

✓6ᵗʰ **H04.14 Primary lacrimal gland atrophy**
    H04.141 Primary lacrimal gland atrophy, right lacrimal gland
    H04.142 Primary lacrimal gland atrophy, left lacrimal gland
    H04.143 Primary lacrimal gland atrophy, bilateral lacrimal glands
    H04.149 Primary lacrimal gland atrophy, unspecified lacrimal gland

✓6ᵗʰ **H04.15 Secondary lacrimal gland atrophy**
    H04.151 Secondary lacrimal gland atrophy, right lacrimal gland
    H04.152 Secondary lacrimal gland atrophy, left lacrimal gland
    H04.153 Secondary lacrimal gland atrophy, bilateral lacrimal glands
    H04.159 Secondary lacrimal gland atrophy, unspecified lacrimal gland

✓6ᵗʰ **H04.16 Lacrimal gland dislocation**
    H04.161 Lacrimal gland dislocation, right lacrimal gland
    H04.162 Lacrimal gland dislocation, left lacrimal gland
    H04.163 Lacrimal gland dislocation, bilateral lacrimal glands
    H04.169 Lacrimal gland dislocation, unspecified lacrimal gland

H04.19 Other specified disorders of lacrimal gland

✓5ᵗʰ **H04.2 Epiphora**
    ✓6ᵗʰ **H04.20 Unspecified epiphora**
        H04.201 Unspecified epiphora, right lacrimal gland
        H04.202 Unspecified epiphora, left lacrimal gland
        H04.203 Unspecified epiphora, bilateral lacrimal glands
        H04.209 Unspecified epiphora, unspecified lacrimal gland

    ✓6ᵗʰ **H04.21 Epiphora due to excess lacrimation**
        H04.211 Epiphora due to excess lacrimation, right lacrimal gland
        H04.212 Epiphora due to excess lacrimation, left lacrimal gland
        H04.213 Epiphora due to excess lacrimation, bilateral lacrimal glands
        H04.219 Epiphora due to excess lacrimation, unspecified lacrimal gland

    ✓6ᵗʰ **H04.22 Epiphora due to insufficient drainage**
        H04.221 Epiphora due to insufficient drainage, right lacrimal gland
        H04.222 Epiphora due to insufficient drainage, left lacrimal gland
        H04.223 Epiphora due to insufficient drainage, bilateral lacrimal glands
        H04.229 Epiphora due to insufficient drainage, unspecified lacrimal gland

✓5ᵗʰ **H04.3 Acute and unspecified inflammation of lacrimal passages**
    EXCLUDES 1   *neonatal dacryocystitis (P39.1)*
    ✓6ᵗʰ **H04.30 Unspecified dacryocystitis**
        H04.301 Unspecified dacryocystitis of right lacrimal passage
        H04.302 Unspecified dacryocystitis of left lacrimal passage
        H04.303 Unspecified dacryocystitis of bilateral lacrimal passages
        H04.309 Unspecified dacryocystitis of unspecified lacrimal passage

    ✓6ᵗʰ **H04.31 Phlegmonous dacryocystitis**
        H04.311 Phlegmonous dacryocystitis of right lacrimal passage
        H04.312 Phlegmonous dacryocystitis of left lacrimal passage
        H04.313 Phlegmonous dacryocystitis of bilateral lacrimal passages
        H04.319 Phlegmonous dacryocystitis of unspecified lacrimal passage

---

✓ Appropriate additional character required   ✓x7ᵗʰ Requires 7th character, placeholder x must fill empty characters

✓6th **H04.32 Acute dacryocystitis**
Acute dacryopericystitis

H04.321 Acute dacryocystitis of right lacrimal passage

H04.322 Acute dacryocystitis of left lacrimal passage

H04.323 Acute dacryocystitis of bilateral lacrimal passages

H04.329 Acute dacryocystitis of unspecified lacrimal passage

✓6th **H04.33 Acute lacrimal canaliculitis**

H04.331 Acute lacrimal canaliculitis of right lacrimal passage

H04.332 Acute lacrimal canaliculitis of left lacrimal passage

H04.333 Acute lacrimal canaliculitis of bilateral lacrimal passages

H04.339 Acute lacrimal canaliculitis of unspecified lacrimal passage

✓5th **H04.4 Chronic inflammation of lacrimal passages**

✓6th **H04.41 Chronic dacryocystitis**

H04.411 Chronic dacryocystitis of right lacrimal passage

H04.412 Chronic dacryocystitis of left lacrimal passage

H04.413 Chronic dacryocystitis of bilateral lacrimal passages

H04.419 Chronic dacryocystitis of unspecified lacrimal passage

✓6th **H04.42 Chronic lacrimal canaliculitis**

H04.421 Chronic lacrimal canaliculitis of right lacrimal passage

H04.422 Chronic lacrimal canaliculitis of left lacrimal passage

H04.423 Chronic lacrimal canaliculitis of bilateral lacrimal passages

H04.429 Chronic lacrimal canaliculitis of unspecified lacrimal passage

✓6th **H04.43 Chronic lacrimal mucocele**

H04.431 Chronic lacrimal mucocele of right lacrimal passage

H04.432 Chronic lacrimal mucocele of left lacrimal passage

H04.433 Chronic lacrimal mucocele of bilateral lacrimal passages

H04.439 Chronic lacrimal mucocele of unspecified lacrimal passage

✓5th **H04.5 Stenosis and insufficiency of lacrimal passages**

✓6th **H04.51 Dacryolith**

H04.511 Dacryolith of right lacrimal passage

H04.512 Dacryolith of left lacrimal passage

H04.513 Dacryolith of bilateral lacrimal passages

H04.519 Dacryolith of unspecified lacrimal passage

✓6th **H04.52 Eversion of lacrimal punctum**

H04.521 Eversion of right lacrimal punctum

H04.522 Eversion of left lacrimal punctum

H04.523 Eversion of bilateral lacrimal punctum

H04.529 Eversion of unspecified lacrimal punctum

✓6th **H04.53 Neonatal obstruction of nasolacrimal duct**

EXCLUDES 1   *congenital stenosis and stricture of lacrimal duct (Q10.5)*

H04.531 Neonatal obstruction of right nasolacrimal duct

H04.532 Neonatal obstruction of left nasolacrimal duct

H04.533 Neonatal obstruction of bilateral nasolacrimal duct

H04.539 Neonatal obstruction of unspecified nasolacrimal duct

✓6th **H04.54 Stenosis of lacrimal canaliculi**

H04.541 Stenosis of right lacrimal canaliculi

H04.542 Stenosis of left lacrimal canaliculi

H04.543 Stenosis of bilateral lacrimal canaliculi

H04.549 Stenosis of unspecified lacrimal canaliculi

✓6th **H04.55 Acquired stenosis of nasolacrimal duct**

H04.551 Acquired stenosis of right nasolacrimal duct

H04.552 Acquired stenosis of left nasolacrimal duct

H04.553 Acquired stenosis of bilateral nasolacrimal duct

H04.559 Acquired stenosis of unspecified nasolacrimal duct

✓6th **H04.56 Stenosis of lacrimal punctum**

H04.561 Stenosis of right lacrimal punctum

H04.562 Stenosis of left lacrimal punctum

H04.563 Stenosis of bilateral lacrimal punctum

H04.569 Stenosis of unspecified lacrimal punctum

✓6th **H04.57 Stenosis of lacrimal sac**

H04.571 Stenosis of right lacrimal sac

H04.572 Stenosis of left lacrimal sac

H04.573 Stenosis of bilateral lacrimal sac

H04.579 Stenosis of unspecified lacrimal sac

✓5th **H04.6 Other changes of lacrimal passages**

✓6th **H04.61 Lacrimal fistula**

H04.611 Lacrimal fistula right lacrimal passage

H04.612 Lacrimal fistula left lacrimal passage

H04.613 Lacrimal fistula bilateral lacrimal passages

H04.619 Lacrimal fistula unspecified lacrimal passage

H04.69 Other changes of lacrimal passages

✓5th **H04.8 Other disorders of lacrimal system**

✓6th **H04.81 Granuloma of lacrimal passages**

H04.811 Granuloma of right lacrimal passage

H04.812 Granuloma of left lacrimal passage

H04.813 Granuloma of bilateral lacrimal passages

H04.819 Granuloma of unspecified lacrimal passage

H04.89 Other disorders of lacrimal system

H04.9 Disorder of lacrimal system, unspecified

✓4th **H05 Disorders of orbit**

EXCLUDES 1   *congenital malformation of orbit (Q10.7)*

✓5th **H05.0 Acute inflammation of orbit**

H05.00 Unspecified acute inflammation of orbit

✓6th **H05.01 Cellulitis of orbit**
Abscess of orbit

H05.011 Cellulitis of right orbit

H05.012 Cellulitis of left orbit

H05.013 Cellulitis of bilateral orbits

H05.019 Cellulitis of unspecified orbit

✓6th **H05.02 Osteomyelitis of orbit**

H05.021 Osteomyelitis of right orbit

H05.022 Osteomyelitis of left orbit

H05.023 Osteomyelitis of bilateral orbits

H05.029 Osteomyelitis of unspecified orbit

✓6th **H05.03 Periostitis of orbit**

H05.031 Periostitis of right orbit

H05.032 Periostitis of left orbit

H05.033 Periostitis of bilateral orbits

H05.039 Periostitis of unspecified orbit

✓6th **H05.04 Tenonitis of orbit**

H05.041 Tenonitis of right orbit

H05.042 Tenonitis of left orbit

H05.043 Tenonitis of bilateral orbits

H05.049 Tenonitis of unspecified orbit

✓5th **H05.1 Chronic inflammatory disorders of orbit**

H05.10 Unspecified chronic inflammatory disorders of orbit

✓6th **H05.11 Granuloma of orbit**
Pseudotumor (inflammatory) of orbit

H05.111 Granuloma of right orbit

H05.112 Granuloma of left orbit

H05.113 Granuloma of bilateral orbits

H05.119 Granuloma of unspecified orbit

✓6th **H05.12 Orbital myositis**

H05.121 Orbital myositis, right orbit

H05.122 Orbital myositis, left orbit
H05.123 Orbital myositis, bilateral
H05.129 Orbital myositis, unspecified orbit

✓5th **H05.2 Exophthalmic conditions**
H05.20 Unspecified exophthalmos
✓6th H05.21 Displacement (lateral) of globe
H05.211 Displacement (lateral) of globe, right eye
H05.212 Displacement (lateral) of globe, left eye
H05.213 Displacement (lateral) of globe, bilateral
H05.219 Displacement (lateral) of globe, unspecified eye
✓6th H05.22 Edema of orbit
Orbital congestion
H05.221 Edema of right orbit
H05.222 Edema of left orbit
H05.223 Edema of bilateral orbit
H05.229 Edema of unspecified orbit
✓6th H05.23 Hemorrhage of orbit
H05.231 Hemorrhage of right orbit
H05.232 Hemorrhage of left orbit
H05.233 Hemorrhage of bilateral orbit
H05.239 Hemorrhage of unspecified orbit
✓6th H05.24 Constant exophthalmos
H05.241 Constant exophthalmos, right eye
H05.242 Constant exophthalmos, left eye
H05.243 Constant exophthalmos, bilateral
H05.249 Constant exophthalmos, unspecified eye
✓6th H05.25 Intermittent exophthalmos
H05.251 Intermittent exophthalmos, right eye
H05.252 Intermittent exophthalmos, left eye
H05.253 Intermittent exophthalmos, bilateral
H05.259 Intermittent exophthalmos, unspecified eye
✓6th H05.26 Pulsating exophthalmos
H05.261 Pulsating exophthalmos, right eye
H05.262 Pulsating exophthalmos, left eye
H05.263 Pulsating exophthalmos, bilateral
H05.269 Pulsating exophthalmos, unspecified eye

✓5th **H05.3 Deformity of orbit**
EXCLUDES 1 *congenital deformity of orbit (Q10.7)*
hypertelorism (Q75.2)
H05.30 Unspecified deformity of orbit
✓6th H05.31 Atrophy of orbit
H05.311 Atrophy of right orbit
H05.312 Atrophy of left orbit
H05.313 Atrophy of bilateral orbit
H05.319 Atrophy of unspecified orbit
✓6th H05.32 Deformity of orbit due to bone disease
Code also associated bone disease
H05.321 Deformity of right orbit due to bone disease
H05.322 Deformity of left orbit due to bone disease
H05.323 Deformity of bilateral orbits due to bone disease
H05.329 Deformity of unspecified orbit due to bone disease
✓6th H05.33 Deformity of orbit due to trauma or surgery
H05.331 Deformity of right orbit due to trauma or surgery
H05.332 Deformity of left orbit due to trauma or surgery
H05.333 Deformity of bilateral orbits due to trauma or surgery
H05.339 Deformity of unspecified orbit due to trauma or surgery
✓6th H05.34 Enlargement of orbit
H05.341 Enlargement of right orbit
H05.342 Enlargement of left orbit
H05.343 Enlargement of bilateral orbits
H05.349 Enlargement of unspecified orbit
✓6th H05.35 Exostosis of orbit
H05.351 Exostosis of right orbit

H05.352 Exostosis of left orbit
H05.353 Exostosis of bilateral orbits
H05.359 Exostosis of unspecified orbit

✓5th **H05.4 Enophthalmos**
✓6th H05.40 Unspecified enophthalmos
H05.401 Unspecified enophthalmos, right eye
H05.402 Unspecified enophthalmos, left eye
H05.403 Unspecified enophthalmos, bilateral
H05.409 Unspecified enophthalmos, unspecified eye
✓6th H05.41 Enophthalmos due to atrophy of orbital tissue
H05.411 Enophthalmos due to atrophy of orbital tissue, right eye
H05.412 Enophthalmos due to atrophy of orbital tissue, left eye
H05.413 Enophthalmos due to atrophy of orbital tissue, bilateral
H05.419 Enophthalmos due to atrophy of orbital tissue, unspecified eye
✓6th H05.42 Enophthalmos due to trauma or surgery
H05.421 Enophthalmos due to trauma or surgery, right eye
H05.422 Enophthalmos due to trauma or surgery, left eye
H05.423 Enophthalmos due to trauma or surgery, bilateral
H05.429 Enophthalmos due to trauma or surgery, unspecified eye

✓5th **H05.5 Retained (old) foreign body following penetrating wound of orbit**
Use additional code to identify the type of retained foreign body (Z18.-)
Retrobulbar foreign body
EXCLUDES 1 *current penetrating wound of orbit (S05.4-)*
EXCLUDES 2 *retained foreign body of eyelid (H02.81-)*
retained intraocular foreign body (H44.6-, H44.7-)
H05.50 Retained (old) foreign body following penetrating wound of unspecified orbit
H05.51 Retained (old) foreign body following penetrating wound of right orbit
H05.52 Retained (old) foreign body following penetrating wound of left orbit
H05.53 Retained (old) foreign body following penetrating wound of bilateral orbits

✓5th **H05.8 Other disorders of orbit**
✓6th H05.81 Cyst of orbit
Encephalocele of orbit
H05.811 Cyst of right orbit
H05.812 Cyst of left orbit
H05.813 Cyst of bilateral orbits
H05.819 Cyst of unspecified orbit
✓6th H05.82 Myopathy of extraocular muscles
H05.821 Myopathy of extraocular muscles, right orbit
H05.822 Myopathy of extraocular muscles, left orbit
H05.823 Myopathy of extraocular muscles, bilateral
H05.829 Myopathy of extraocular muscles, unspecified orbit
H05.89 Other disorders of orbit
H05.9 Unspecified disorder of orbit

Disorders of conjunctiva (H10-H11)

✓4th **H10 Conjunctivitis**
EXCLUDES 1 *keratoconjunctivitis (H16.2-)*
✓5th **H10.0 Mucopurulent conjunctivitis**
✓6th H10.01 Acute follicular conjunctivitis
H10.011 Acute follicular conjunctivitis, right eye
H10.012 Acute follicular conjunctivitis, left eye
H10.013 Acute follicular conjunctivitis, bilateral
H10.019 Acute follicular conjunctivitis, unspecified eye
✓6th H10.02 Other mucopurulent conjunctivitis
H10.021 Other mucopurulent conjunctivitis, right eye

	H10.022	**Other mucopurulent conjunctivitis, left eye**
	H10.023	**Other mucopurulent conjunctivitis, bilateral**
	H10.029	**Other mucopurulent conjunctivitis, unspecified eye**

✓5th **H10.1** **Acute atopic conjunctivitis**
Acute papillary conjunctivitis

H10.10	**Acute atopic conjunctivitis, unspecified eye**
H10.11	**Acute atopic conjunctivitis, right eye**
H10.12	**Acute atopic conjunctivitis, left eye**
H10.13	**Acute atopic conjunctivitis, bilateral**

✓5th **H10.2** **Other acute conjunctivitis**

✓6th **H10.21** **Acute toxic conjunctivitis**
Acute chemical conjunctivitis
Code first (T51-T65) to identify chemical and intent
EXCLUDES 1   burn and corrosion of eye and adnexa (T26-)

H10.211	**Acute toxic conjunctivitis, right eye**
H10.212	**Acute toxic conjunctivitis, left eye**
H10.213	**Acute toxic conjunctivitis, bilateral**
H10.219	**Acute toxic conjunctivitis, unspecified eye**

✓6th **H10.22** **Pseudomembranous conjunctivitis**

H10.221	**Pseudomembranous conjunctivitis, right eye**
H10.222	**Pseudomembranous conjunctivitis, left eye**
H10.223	**Pseudomembranous conjunctivitis, bilateral**
H10.229	**Pseudomembranous conjunctivitis, unspecified eye**

✓6th **H10.23** **Serous conjunctivitis, except viral**
EXCLUDES 1   viral conjunctivitis (B30-)

H10.231	**Serous conjunctivitis, except viral, right eye**
H10.232	**Serous conjunctivitis, except viral, left eye**
H10.233	**Serous conjunctivitis, except viral, bilateral**
H10.239	**Serous conjunctivitis, except viral, unspecified eye**

✓5th **H10.3** **Unspecified acute conjunctivitis**
EXCLUDES 1   ophthalmia neonatorum NOS (P39.1)

H10.30	**Unspecified acute conjunctivitis, unspecified eye**
H10.31	**Unspecified acute conjunctivitis, right eye**
H10.32	**Unspecified acute conjunctivitis, left eye**
H10.33	**Unspecified acute conjunctivitis, bilateral**

✓5th **H10.4** **Chronic conjunctivitis**

✓6th **H10.40** **Unspecified chronic conjunctivitis**

H10.401	**Unspecified chronic conjunctivitis, right eye**
H10.402	**Unspecified chronic conjunctivitis, left eye**
H10.403	**Unspecified chronic conjunctivitis, bilateral**
H10.409	**Unspecified chronic conjunctivitis, unspecified eye**

✓6th **H10.41** **Chronic giant papillary conjunctivitis**

H10.411	**Chronic giant papillary conjunctivitis, right eye**
H10.412	**Chronic giant papillary conjunctivitis, left eye**
H10.413	**Chronic giant papillary conjunctivitis, bilateral**
H10.419	**Chronic giant papillary conjunctivitis, unspecified eye**

✓6th **H10.42** **Simple chronic conjunctivitis**

H10.421	**Simple chronic conjunctivitis, right eye**
H10.422	**Simple chronic conjunctivitis, left eye**
H10.423	**Simple chronic conjunctivitis, bilateral**
H10.429	**Simple chronic conjunctivitis, unspecified eye**

✓6th **H10.43** **Chronic follicular conjunctivitis**

H10.431	**Chronic follicular conjunctivitis, right eye**
H10.432	**Chronic follicular conjunctivitis, left eye**

	H10.433	**Chronic follicular conjunctivitis, bilateral**
	H10.439	**Chronic follicular conjunctivitis, unspecified eye**

   H10.44 **Vernal conjunctivitis**
EXCLUDES 1   vernal keratoconjunctivitis with limbar and corneal involvement (H16.26-)

   H10.45 **Other chronic allergic conjunctivitis**

✓5th **H10.5** **Blepharoconjunctivitis**

✓6th **H10.50** **Unspecified blepharoconjunctivitis**

H10.501	**Unspecified blepharoconjunctivitis, right eye**
H10.502	**Unspecified blepharoconjunctivitis, left eye**
H10.503	**Unspecified blepharoconjunctivitis, bilateral**
H10.509	**Unspecified blepharoconjunctivitis, unspecified eye**

✓6th **H10.51** **Ligneous conjunctivitis**

H10.511	**Ligneous conjunctivitis, right eye**
H10.512	**Ligneous conjunctivitis, left eye**
H10.513	**Ligneous conjunctivitis, bilateral**
H10.519	**Ligneous conjunctivitis, unspecified eye**

✓6th **H10.52** **Angular blepharoconjunctivitis**

H10.521	**Angular blepharoconjunctivitis, right eye**
H10.522	**Angular blepharoconjunctivitis, left eye**
H10.523	**Angular blepharoconjunctivitis, bilateral**
H10.529	**Angular blepharoconjunctivitis, unspecified eye**

✓6th **H10.53** **Contact blepharoconjunctivitis**

H10.531	**Contact blepharoconjunctivitis, right eye**
H10.532	**Contact blepharoconjunctivitis, left eye**
H10.533	**Contact blepharoconjunctivitis, bilateral**
H10.539	**Contact blepharoconjunctivitis, unspecified eye**

✓5th **H10.8** **Other conjunctivitis**

✓6th **H10.81** **Pingueculitis**
EXCLUDES 1   pinguecula (H11.15-)

H10.811	**Pingueculitis, right eye**
H10.812	**Pingueculitis, left eye**
H10.813	**Pingueculitis, bilateral**
H10.819	**Pingueculitis, unspecified eye**

   H10.89 **Other conjunctivitis**

   H10.9 **Unspecified conjunctivitis**

✓4th **H11** **Other disorders of conjunctiva**
EXCLUDES 1   keratoconjunctivitis (H16.2-)

✓5th **H11.0** **Pterygium of eye**
EXCLUDES 1   pseudopterygium (H11.81-)

✓6th **H11.00** **Unspecified pterygium of eye**

H11.001	**Unspecified pterygium of right eye**
H11.002	**Unspecified pterygium of left eye**
H11.003	**Unspecified pterygium of eye, bilateral**
H11.009	**Unspecified pterygium of unspecified eye**

✓6th **H11.01** **Amyloid pterygium**

H11.011	**Amyloid pterygium of right eye**
H11.012	**Amyloid pterygium of left eye**
H11.013	**Amyloid pterygium of eye, bilateral**
H11.019	**Amyloid pterygium of unspecified eye**

✓6th **H11.02** **Central pterygium of eye**

H11.021	**Central pterygium of right eye**
H11.022	**Central pterygium of left eye**
H11.023	**Central pterygium of eye, bilateral**
H11.029	**Central pterygium of unspecified eye**

✓6th **H11.03** **Double pterygium of eye**

H11.031	**Double pterygium of right eye**
H11.032	**Double pterygium of left eye**
H11.033	**Double pterygium of eye, bilateral**
H11.039	**Double pterygium of unspecified eye**

EXCLUDES 1 Not coded here   *EXCLUDES 2* Not included here   ***Manifestation Code***

✓6th **H11.04 Peripheral pterygium of eye, stationary**
- **H11.041** Peripheral pterygium, stationary, right eye
- **H11.042** Peripheral pterygium, stationary, left eye
- **H11.043** Peripheral pterygium, stationary, bilateral
- **H11.049** Peripheral pterygium, stationary, unspecified eye

✓6th **H11.05 Peripheral pterygium of eye, progressive**
- **H11.051** Peripheral pterygium, progressive, right eye
- **H11.052** Peripheral pterygium, progressive, left eye
- **H11.053** Peripheral pterygium, progressive, bilateral
- **H11.059** Peripheral pterygium, progressive, unspecified eye

✓6th **H11.06 Recurrent pterygium of eye**
- **H11.061** Recurrent pterygium of right eye
- **H11.062** Recurrent pterygium of left eye
- **H11.063** Recurrent pterygium of eye, bilateral
- **H11.069** Recurrent pterygium of unspecified eye

✓5th **H11.1 Conjunctival degenerations and deposits**
> EXCLUDES 2 *pseudopterygium (H11.81)*
- **H11.10** Unspecified conjunctival degenerations

✓6th **H11.11 Conjunctival deposits**
- **H11.111** Conjunctival deposits, right eye
- **H11.112** Conjunctival deposits, left eye
- **H11.113** Conjunctival deposits, bilateral
- **H11.119** Conjunctival deposits, unspecified eye

✓6th **H11.12 Conjunctival concretions**
- **H11.121** Conjunctival concretions, right eye
- **H11.122** Conjunctival concretions, left eye
- **H11.123** Conjunctival concretions, bilateral
- **H11.129** Conjunctival concretions, unspecified eye

✓6th **H11.13 Conjunctival pigmentations**
> Conjunctival argyrosis [argyria]
- **H11.131** Conjunctival pigmentations, right eye
- **H11.132** Conjunctival pigmentations, left eye
- **H11.133** Conjunctival pigmentations, bilateral
- **H11.139** Conjunctival pigmentations, unspecified eye

✓6th **H11.14 Conjunctival xerosis, unspecified**
> EXCLUDES 1 *xerosis of conjunctiva due to vitamin A deficiency (E50.0, E50.1)*
- **H11.141** Conjunctival xerosis, unspecified, right eye
- **H11.142** Conjunctival xerosis , unspecified, left eye
- **H11.143** Conjunctival xerosis, unspecified, bilateral
- **H11.149** Conjunctival xerosis, unspecified, unspecified eye

✓6th **H11.15 Pinguecula**
> EXCLUDES 1 *pingueculitis (H10.81-)*
- **H11.151** Pinguecula, right eye
- **H11.152** Pinguecula, left eye
- **H11.153** Pinguecula, bilateral
- **H11.159** Pinguecula, unspecified eye

✓5th **H11.2 Conjunctival scars**
✓6th **H11.21 Conjunctival adhesions and strands (localized)**
- **H11.211** Conjunctival adhesions and strands (localized), right eye
- **H11.212** Conjunctival adhesions and strands (localized), left eye
- **H11.213** Conjunctival adhesions and strands (localized), bilateral
- **H11.219** Conjunctival adhesions and strands (localized), unspecified eye

✓6th **H11.22 Conjunctival granuloma**
- **H11.221** Conjunctival granuloma, right eye
- **H11.222** Conjunctival granuloma, left eye
- **H11.223** Conjunctival granuloma, bilateral
- **H11.229** Conjunctival granuloma, unspecified

✓6th **H11.23 Symblepharon**
- **H11.231** Symblepharon, right eye
- **H11.232** Symblepharon, left eye
- **H11.233** Symblepharon, bilateral
- **H11.239** Symblepharon, unspecified eye

✓6th **H11.24 Scarring of conjunctiva**
- **H11.241** Scarring of conjunctiva, right eye
- **H11.242** Scarring of conjunctiva, left eye
- **H11.243** Scarring of conjunctiva, bilateral
- **H11.249** Scarring of conjunctiva, unspecified eye

✓5th **H11.3 Conjunctival hemorrhage**
> Subconjunctival hemorrhage
- **H11.30** Conjunctival hemorrhage, unspecified eye
- **H11.31** Conjunctival hemorrhage, right eye
- **H11.32** Conjunctival hemorrhage, left eye
- **H11.33** Conjunctival hemorrhage, bilateral

✓5th **H11.4 Other conjunctival vascular disorders and cysts**
✓6th **H11.41 Vascular abnormalities of conjunctiva**
> Conjunctival aneurysm
- **H11.411** Vascular abnormalities of conjunctiva, right eye
- **H11.412** Vascular abnormalities of conjunctiva, left eye
- **H11.413** Vascular abnormalities of conjunctiva, bilateral
- **H11.419** Vascular abnormalities of conjunctiva, unspecified eye

✓6th **H11.42 Conjunctival edema**
- **H11.421** Conjunctival edema, right eye
- **H11.422** Conjunctival edema, left eye
- **H11.423** Conjunctival edema, bilateral
- **H11.429** Conjunctival edema, unspecified eye

✓6th **H11.43 Conjunctival hyperemia**
- **H11.431** Conjunctival hyperemia, right eye
- **H11.432** Conjunctival hyperemia, left eye
- **H11.433** Conjunctival hyperemia, bilateral
- **H11.439** Conjunctival hyperemia, unspecified eye

✓6th **H11.44 Conjunctival cysts**
- **H11.441** Conjunctival cysts, right eye
- **H11.442** Conjunctival cysts, left eye
- **H11.443** Conjunctival cysts, bilateral
- **H11.449** Conjunctival cysts, unspecified eye

✓5th **H11.8 Other specified disorders of conjunctiva**
✓6th **H11.81 Pseudopterygium of conjunctiva**
- **H11.811** Pseudopterygium of conjunctiva, right eye
- **H11.812** Pseudopterygium of conjunctiva, left eye
- **H11.813** Pseudopterygium of conjunctiva, bilateral
- **H11.819** Pseudopterygium of conjunctiva, unspecified eye

✓6th **H11.82 Conjunctivochalasis**
- **H11.821** Conjunctivochalasis, right eye
- **H11.822** Conjunctivochalasis, left eye
- **H11.823** Conjunctivochalasis, bilateral
- **H11.829** Conjunctivochalasis, unspecified eye
- **H11.89** Other specified disorders of conjunctiva

H11.9 Unspecified disorder of conjunctiva

Disorders of sclera, cornea, iris and ciliary body (H15-H22)

✓4th **H15 Disorders of sclera**
✓5th **H15.0 Scleritis**
✓6th **H15.00 Unspecified scleritis**
- **H15.001** Unspecified scleritis, right eye
- **H15.002** Unspecified scleritis, left eye
- **H15.003** Unspecified scleritis, bilateral
- **H15.009** Unspecified scleritis, unspecified eye

✓6th **H15.01 Anterior scleritis**
- **H15.011** Anterior scleritis, right eye
- **H15.012** Anterior scleritis, left eye
- **H15.013** Anterior scleritis, bilateral

☑ Appropriate additional character required   ✓x7th Requires 7th character, placeholder x must fill empty characters

H15.019   Anterior scleritis, unspecified eye
✓6ᵗʰ   H15.02   Brawny scleritis
    H15.021   Brawny scleritis, right eye
    H15.022   Brawny scleritis, left eye
    H15.023   Brawny scleritis, bilateral
    H15.029   Brawny scleritis, unspecified eye
✓6ᵗʰ   H15.03   Posterior scleritis
    Sclerotenonitis
    H15.031   Posterior scleritis, right eye
    H15.032   Posterior scleritis, left eye
    H15.033   Posterior scleritis, bilateral
    H15.039   Posterior scleritis, unspecified eye
✓6ᵗʰ   H15.04   Scleritis with corneal involvement
    H15.041   Scleritis with corneal involvement, right eye
    H15.042   Scleritis with corneal involvement, left eye
    H15.043   Scleritis with corneal involvement, bilateral
    H15.049   Scleritis with corneal involvement, unspecified eye
✓6ᵗʰ   H15.05   Scleromalacia perforans
    H15.051   Scleromalacia perforans, right eye
    H15.052   Scleromalacia perforans, left eye
    H15.053   Scleromalacia perforans, bilateral
    H15.059   Scleromalacia perforans, unspecified eye
✓6ᵗʰ   H15.09   Other scleritis
    Scleral abscess
    H15.091   Other scleritis, right eye
    H15.092   Other scleritis, left eye
    H15.093   Other scleritis, bilateral
    H15.099   Other scleritis, unspecified eye
✓5ᵗʰ   H15.1   Episcleritis
✓6ᵗʰ   H15.10   Unspecified episcleritis
    H15.101   Unspecified episcleritis, right eye
    H15.102   Unspecified episcleritis, left eye
    H15.103   Unspecified episcleritis, bilateral
    H15.109   Unspecified episcleritis, unspecified eye
✓6ᵗʰ   H15.11   Episcleritis periodica fugax
    H15.111   Episcleritis periodica fugax, right eye
    H15.112   Episcleritis periodica fugax, left eye
    H15.113   Episcleritis periodica fugax, bilateral
    H15.119   Episcleritis periodica fugax, unspecified eye
✓6ᵗʰ   H15.12   Nodular episcleritis
    H15.121   Nodular episcleritis, right eye
    H15.122   Nodular episcleritis, left eye
    H15.123   Nodular episcleritis, bilateral
    H15.129   Nodular episcleritis, unspecified eye
✓5ᵗʰ   H15.8   Other disorders of sclera
    EXCLUDES 2   blue sclera (Q13.5)
              degenerative myopia (H44.2-)
✓6ᵗʰ   H15.81   Equatorial staphyloma
    H15.811   Equatorial staphyloma, right eye
    H15.812   Equatorial staphyloma, left eye
    H15.813   Equatorial staphyloma, bilateral
    H15.819   Equatorial staphyloma, unspecified eye
✓6ᵗʰ   H15.82   Localized anterior staphyloma
    H15.821   Localized anterior staphyloma, right eye
    H15.822   Localized anterior staphyloma, left eye
    H15.823   Localized anterior staphyloma, bilateral
    H15.829   Localized anterior staphyloma, unspecified eye
✓6ᵗʰ   H15.83   Staphyloma posticum
    H15.831   Staphyloma posticum, right eye
    H15.832   Staphyloma posticum, left eye
    H15.833   Staphyloma posticum, bilateral
    H15.839   Staphyloma posticum, unspecified eye
✓6ᵗʰ   H15.84   Scleral ectasia
    H15.841   Scleral ectasia, right eye
    H15.842   Scleral ectasia, left eye
    H15.843   Scleral ectasia, bilateral
    H15.849   Scleral ectasia, unspecified eye
✓6ᵗʰ   H15.85   Ring staphyloma

H15.851   Ring staphyloma, right eye
H15.852   Ring staphyloma, left eye
H15.853   Ring staphyloma, bilateral
H15.859   Ring staphyloma, unspecified eye
    H15.89   Other disorders of sclera
  H15.9   Unspecified disorder of sclera
✓4ᵗʰ   **H16**   **Keratitis**
✓5ᵗʰ   H16.0   Corneal ulcer
✓6ᵗʰ   H16.00   Unspecified corneal ulcer
    H16.001   Unspecified corneal ulcer, right eye
    H16.002   Unspecified corneal ulcer, left eye
    H16.003   Unspecified corneal ulcer, bilateral
    H16.009   Unspecified corneal ulcer, unspecified eye
✓6ᵗʰ   H16.01   Central corneal ulcer
    H16.011   Central corneal ulcer, right eye
    H16.012   Central corneal ulcer, left eye
    H16.013   Central corneal ulcer, bilateral
    H16.019   Central corneal ulcer, unspecified eye
✓6ᵗʰ   H16.02   Ring corneal ulcer
    H16.021   Ring corneal ulcer, right eye
    H16.022   Ring corneal ulcer, left eye
    H16.023   Ring corneal ulcer, bilateral
    H16.029   Ring corneal ulcer, unspecified eye
✓6ᵗʰ   H16.03   Corneal ulcer with hypopyon
    H16.031   Corneal ulcer with hypopyon, right eye
    H16.032   Corneal ulcer with hypopyon, left eye
    H16.033   Corneal ulcer with hypopyon, bilateral
    H16.039   Corneal ulcer with hypopyon, unspecified eye
✓6ᵗʰ   H16.04   Marginal corneal ulcer
    H16.041   Marginal corneal ulcer, right eye
    H16.042   Marginal corneal ulcer, left eye
    H16.043   Marginal corneal ulcer, bilateral
    H16.049   Marginal corneal ulcer, unspecified eye
✓6ᵗʰ   H16.05   Mooren's corneal ulcer
    H16.051   Mooren's corneal ulcer, right eye
    H16.052   Mooren's corneal ulcer, left eye
    H16.053   Mooren's corneal ulcer, bilateral
    H16.059   Mooren's corneal ulcer, unspecified eye
✓6ᵗʰ   H16.06   Mycotic corneal ulcer
    H16.061   Mycotic corneal ulcer, right eye
    H16.062   Mycotic corneal ulcer, left eye
    H16.063   Mycotic corneal ulcer, bilateral
    H16.069   Mycotic corneal ulcer, unspecified eye
✓6ᵗʰ   H16.07   Perforated corneal ulcer
    H16.071   Perforated corneal ulcer, right eye
    H16.072   Perforated corneal ulcer, left eye
    H16.073   Perforated corneal ulcer, bilateral
    H16.079   Perforated corneal ulcer, unspecified eye
✓5ᵗʰ   H16.1   Other and unspecified superficial keratitis without conjunctivitis
✓6ᵗʰ   H16.10   Unspecified superficial keratitis
    H16.101   Unspecified superficial keratitis, right eye
    H16.102   Unspecified superficial keratitis, left eye
    H16.103   Unspecified superficial keratitis, bilateral
    H16.109   Unspecified superficial keratitis, unspecified eye
✓6ᵗʰ   H16.11   Macular keratitis
    Areolar keratitis
    Nummular keratitis
    Stellate keratitis
    Striate keratitis
    H16.111   Macular keratitis, right eye
    H16.112   Macular keratitis, left eye
    H16.113   Macular keratitis, bilateral
    H16.119   Macular keratitis, unspecified eye
✓6ᵗʰ   H16.12   Filamentary keratitis
    H16.121   Filamentary keratitis, right eye
    H16.122   Filamentary keratitis, left eye
    H16.123   Filamentary keratitis, bilateral
    H16.129   Filamentary keratitis, unspecified eye

EXCLUDES 1   Not coded here   EXCLUDES 2   Not included here   *Manifestation Code*

✓6th **H16.13** **Photokeratitis**
   Snow blindness
   Welders keratitis
   H16.131 **Photokeratitis, right eye**
   H16.132 **Photokeratitis, left eye**
   H16.133 **Photokeratitis, bilateral**
   H16.139 **Photokeratitis, unspecified eye**
✓6th **H16.14** **Punctate keratitis**
   H16.141 **Punctate keratitis, right eye**
   H16.142 **Punctate keratitis, left eye**
   H16.143 **Punctate keratitis, bilateral**
   H16.149 **Punctate keratitis, unspecified eye**
✓5th **H16.2** **Keratoconjunctivitis**
✓6th **H16.20** **Unspecified keratoconjunctivitis**
   Superficial keratitis with conjunctivitis NOS
   H16.201 **Unspecified keratoconjunctivitis, right eye**
   H16.202 **Unspecified keratoconjunctivitis, left eye**
   H16.203 **Unspecified keratoconjunctivitis, bilateral**
   H16.209 **Unspecified keratoconjunctivitis, unspecified eye**
✓6th **H16.21** **Exposure keratoconjunctivitis**
   H16.211 **Exposure keratoconjunctivitis, right eye**
   H16.212 **Exposure keratoconjunctivitis, left eye**
   H16.213 **Exposure keratoconjunctivitis, bilateral**
   H16.219 **Exposure keratoconjunctivitis, unspecified eye**
✓6th **H16.22** **Keratoconjunctivitis sicca, not specified as Sjögren's**
   EXCLUDES 1 *Sjögren's syndrome (M35.01)*
   H16.221 **Keratoconjunctivitis sicca, not specified as Sjögren's, right eye**
   H16.222 **Keratoconjunctivitis sicca, not specified as Sjögren's, left eye**
   H16.223 **Keratoconjunctivitis sicca, not specified as Sjögren's, bilateral**
   H16.229 **Keratoconjunctivitis sicca, not specified as Sjögren's, unspecified eye**
✓6th **H16.23** **Neurotrophic keratoconjunctivitis**
   H16.231 **Neurotrophic keratoconjunctivitis, right eye**
   H16.232 **Neurotrophic keratoconjunctivitis, left eye**
   H16.233 **Neurotrophic keratoconjunctivitis, bilateral**
   H16.239 **Neurotrophic keratoconjunctivitis, unspecified eye**
✓6th **H16.24** **Ophthalmia nodosa**
   H16.241 **Ophthalmia nodosa, right eye**
   H16.242 **Ophthalmia nodosa, left eye**
   H16.243 **Ophthalmia nodosa, bilateral**
   H16.249 **Ophthalmia nodosa, unspecified eye**
✓6th **H16.25** **Phlyctenular keratoconjunctivitis**
   H16.251 **Phlyctenular keratoconjunctivitis, right eye**
   H16.252 **Phlyctenular keratoconjunctivitis, left eye**
   H16.253 **Phlyctenular keratoconjunctivitis, bilateral**
   H16.259 **Phlyctenular keratoconjunctivitis, unspecified eye**
✓6th **H16.26** **Vernal keratoconjunctivitis, with limbar and corneal involvement**
   EXCLUDES 1 *vernal conjunctivitis without limbar and corneal involvement (H10.44)*
   H16.261 **Vernal keratoconjunctivitis, with limbar and corneal involvement, right eye**
   H16.262 **Vernal keratoconjunctivitis, with limbar and corneal involvement, left eye**
   H16.263 **Vernal keratoconjunctivitis, with limbar and corneal involvement, bilateral**
   H16.269 **Vernal keratoconjunctivitis, with limbar and corneal involvement, unspecified eye**

✓6th **H16.29** **Other keratoconjunctivitis**
   H16.291 **Other keratoconjunctivitis, right eye**
   H16.292 **Other keratoconjunctivitis, left eye**
   H16.293 **Other keratoconjunctivitis, bilateral**
   H16.299 **Other keratoconjunctivitis, unspecified eye**
✓5th **H16.3** **Interstitial and deep keratitis**
✓6th **H16.30** **Unspecified interstitial keratitis**
   H16.301 **Unspecified interstitial keratitis, right eye**
   H16.302 **Unspecified interstitial keratitis, left eye**
   H16.303 **Unspecified interstitial keratitis, bilateral**
   H16.309 **Unspecified interstitial keratitis, unspecified eye**
✓6th **H16.31** **Corneal abscess**
   H16.311 **Corneal abscess, right eye**
   H16.312 **Corneal abscess, left eye**
   H16.313 **Corneal abscess, bilateral**
   H16.319 **Corneal abscess, unspecified eye**
✓6th **H16.32** **Diffuse interstitial keratitis**
   Cogan's syndrome
   H16.321 **Diffuse interstitial keratitis, right eye**
   H16.322 **Diffuse interstitial keratitis, left eye**
   H16.323 **Diffuse interstitial keratitis, bilateral**
   H16.329 **Diffuse interstitial keratitis, unspecified eye**
✓6th **H16.33** **Sclerosing keratitis**
   H16.331 **Sclerosing keratitis, right eye**
   H16.332 **Sclerosing keratitis, left eye**
   H16.333 **Sclerosing keratitis, bilateral**
   H16.339 **Sclerosing keratitis, unspecified eye**
✓6th **H16.39** **Other interstitial and deep keratitis**
   H16.391 **Other interstitial and deep keratitis, right eye**
   H16.392 **Other interstitial and deep keratitis, left eye**
   H16.393 **Other interstitial and deep keratitis, bilateral**
   H16.399 **Other interstitial and deep keratitis, unspecified eye**
✓5th **H16.4** **Corneal neovascularization**
✓6th **H16.40** **Unspecified corneal neovascularization**
   H16.401 **Unspecified corneal neovascularization, right eye**
   H16.402 **Unspecified corneal neovascularization, left eye**
   H16.403 **Unspecified corneal neovascularization, bilateral**
   H16.409 **Unspecified corneal neovascularization, unspecified eye**
✓6th **H16.41** **Ghost vessels (corneal)**
   H16.411 **Ghost vessels (corneal), right eye**
   H16.412 **Ghost vessels (corneal), left eye**
   H16.413 **Ghost vessels (corneal), bilateral**
   H16.419 **Ghost vessels (corneal), unspecified eye**
✓6th **H16.42** **Pannus (corneal)**
   H16.421 **Pannus (corneal), right eye**
   H16.422 **Pannus (corneal), left eye**
   H16.423 **Pannus (corneal), bilateral**
   H16.429 **Pannus (corneal), unspecified eye**
✓6th **H16.43** **Localized vascularization of cornea**
   H16.431 **Localized vascularization of cornea, right eye**
   H16.432 **Localized vascularization of cornea, left eye**
   H16.433 **Localized vascularization of cornea, bilateral**
   H16.439 **Localized vascularization of cornea, unspecified eye**
✓6th **H16.44** **Deep vascularization of cornea**
   H16.441 **Deep vascularization of cornea, right eye**
   H16.442 **Deep vascularization of cornea, left eye**
   H16.443 **Deep vascularization of cornea, bilateral**

☑ Appropriate additional character required   √x7th Requires 7th character, placeholder x must fill empty characters

H16.449   Deep vascularization of cornea, unspecified eye

H16.8   **Other keratitis**

H16.9   **Unspecified keratitis**

✓4th **H17**   **Corneal scars and opacities**

✓5th   H17.0   **Adherent leukoma**

H17.00   Adherent leukoma, unspecified eye

H17.01   Adherent leukoma, right eye

H17.02   Adherent leukoma, left eye

H17.03   Adherent leukoma, bilateral

✓5th   H17.1   **Central corneal opacity**

H17.10   Central corneal opacity, unspecified eye

H17.11   Central corneal opacity, right eye

H17.12   Central corneal opacity, left eye

H17.13   Central corneal opacity, bilateral

✓5th   H17.8   **Other corneal scars and opacities**

✓6th   H17.81   Minor opacity of cornea

Corneal nebula

H17.811   Minor opacity of cornea, right eye

H17.812   Minor opacity of cornea, left eye

H17.813   Minor opacity of cornea, bilateral

H17.819   Minor opacity of cornea, unspecified eye

✓6th   H17.82   Peripheral opacity of cornea

H17.821   Peripheral opacity of cornea, right eye

H17.822   Peripheral opacity of cornea, left eye

H17.823   Peripheral opacity of cornea, bilateral

H17.829   Peripheral opacity of cornea, unspecified eye

H17.89   Other corneal scars and opacities

H17.9   **Unspecified corneal scar and opacity**

✓4th **H18**   **Other disorders of cornea**

✓5th   H18.0   **Corneal pigmentations and deposits**

✓6th   H18.00   Unspecified corneal deposit

H18.001   Unspecified corneal deposit, right eye

H18.002   Unspecified corneal deposit, left eye

H18.003   Unspecified corneal deposit, bilateral

H18.009   Unspecified corneal deposit, unspecified eye

✓6th   H18.01   Anterior corneal pigmentations

Staehli's line

H18.011   Anterior corneal pigmentations, right eye

H18.012   Anterior corneal pigmentations, left eye

H18.013   Anterior corneal pigmentations, bilateral

H18.019   Anterior corneal pigmentations, unspecified eye

✓6th   H18.02   Argentous corneal deposits

H18.021   Argentous corneal deposits, right eye

H18.022   Argentous corneal deposits, left eye

H18.023   Argentous corneal deposits, bilateral

H18.029   Argentous corneal deposits, unspecified eye

✓6th   H18.03   Corneal deposits in metabolic disorders

Code also associated metabolic disorder

H18.031   Corneal deposits in metabolic disorders, right eye

H18.032   Corneal deposits in metabolic disorders, left eye

H18.033   Corneal deposits in metabolic disorders, bilateral

H18.039   Corneal deposits in metabolic disorders, unspecified eye

✓6th   H18.04   Kayser-Fleischer ring

Code also associated Wilson's disease (E83.01)

H18.041   Kayser-Fleischer ring, right eye

H18.042   Kayser-Fleischer ring, left eye

H18.043   Kayser-Fleischer ring, bilateral

H18.049   Kayser-Fleischer ring, unspecified eye

✓6th   H18.05   Posterior corneal pigmentations

Krukenberg's spindle

H18.051   Posterior corneal pigmentations, right eye

H18.052   Posterior corneal pigmentations, left eye

H18.053   Posterior corneal pigmentations, bilateral

H18.059   Posterior corneal pigmentations, unspecified eye

✓6th   H18.06   Stromal corneal pigmentations

Hematocornea

H18.061   Stromal corneal pigmentations, right eye

H18.062   Stromal corneal pigmentations, left eye

H18.063   Stromal corneal pigmentations, bilateral

H18.069   Stromal corneal pigmentations, unspecified eye

✓5th   H18.1   **Bullous keratopathy**

H18.10   Bullous keratopathy, unspecified eye

H18.11   Bullous keratopathy, right eye

H18.12   Bullous keratopathy, left eye

H18.13   Bullous keratopathy, bilateral

✓5th   H18.2   **Other and unspecified corneal edema**

H18.20   Unspecified corneal edema

✓6th   H18.21   Corneal edema secondary to contact lens

EXCLUDES 2   *other corneal disorders due to contact lens (H18.82-)*

H18.211   Corneal edema secondary to contact lens, right eye

H18.212   Corneal edema secondary to contact lens, left eye

H18.213   Corneal edema secondary to contact lens, bilateral

H18.219   Corneal edema secondary to contact lens, unspecified eye

✓6th   H18.22   Idiopathic corneal edema

H18.221   Idiopathic corneal edema, right eye

H18.222   Idiopathic corneal edema, left eye

H18.223   Idiopathic corneal edema, bilateral

H18.229   Idiopathic corneal edema, unspecified eye

✓6th   H18.23   Secondary corneal edema

H18.231   Secondary corneal edema, right eye

H18.232   Secondary corneal edema, left eye

H18.233   Secondary corneal edema, bilateral

H18.239   Secondary corneal edema, unspecified eye

✓5th   H18.3   **Changes of corneal membranes**

H18.30   Unspecified corneal membrane change

✓6th   H18.31   Folds and rupture in Bowman's membrane

H18.311   Folds and rupture in Bowman's membrane, right eye

H18.312   Folds and rupture in Bowman's membrane, left eye

H18.313   Folds and rupture in Bowman's membrane, bilateral

H18.319   Folds and rupture in Bowman's membrane, unspecified eye

✓6th   H18.32   Folds in Descemet's membrane

H18.321   Folds in Descemet's membrane, right eye

H18.322   Folds in Descemet's membrane, left eye

H18.323   Folds in Descemet's membrane, bilateral

H18.329   Folds in Descemet's membrane, unspecified eye

✓6th   H18.33   Rupture in Descemet's membrane

H18.331   Rupture in Descemet's membrane, right eye

H18.332   Rupture in Descemet's membrane, left eye

H18.333   Rupture in Descemet's membrane, bilateral

H18.339   Rupture in Descemet's membrane, unspecified eye

✓5th   H18.4   **Corneal degeneration**

EXCLUDES 1   *Mooren's ulcer (H16.0-)*

recurrent erosion of cornea (H18.83-)

H18.40   Unspecified corneal degeneration

EXCLUDES 1   Not coded here   EXCLUDES 2   Not included here   *Manifestation Code*

✓6th **H18.41** **Arcus senilis**
　　　　Senile corneal changes
　　　H18.411　**Arcus senilis, right eye**
　　　H18.412　**Arcus senilis, left eye**
　　　H18.413　**Arcus senilis, bilateral**
　　　H18.419　**Arcus senilis, unspecified eye**
✓6th **H18.42** **Band keratopathy**
　　　H18.421　**Band keratopathy, right eye**
　　　H18.422　**Band keratopathy, left eye**
　　　H18.423　**Band keratopathy, bilateral**
　　　H18.429　**Band keratopathy, unspecified eye**
　H18.43 **Other calcerous corneal degeneration**
✓6th **H18.44** **Keratomalacia**
　　　EXCLUDES 1　*keratomalacia due to vitamin A deficiency (E50.4)*
　　　H18.441　**Keratomalacia, right eye**
　　　H18.442　**Keratomalacia, left eye**
　　　H18.443　**Keratomalacia, bilateral**
　　　H18.449　**Keratomalacia, unspecified eye**
✓6th **H18.45** **Nodular corneal degeneration**
　　　H18.451　**Nodular corneal degeneration, right eye**
　　　H18.452　**Nodular corneal degeneration, left eye**
　　　H18.453　**Nodular corneal degeneration, bilateral**
　　　H18.459　**Nodular corneal degeneration, unspecified eye**
✓6th **H18.46** **Peripheral corneal degeneration**
　　　H18.461　**Peripheral corneal degeneration, right eye**
　　　H18.462　**Peripheral corneal degeneration, left eye**
　　　H18.463　**Peripheral corneal degeneration, bilateral**
　　　H18.469　**Peripheral corneal degeneration, unspecified eye**
　H18.49 **Other corneal degeneration**
✓5th **H18.5** **Hereditary corneal dystrophies**
　H18.50 **Unspecified hereditary corneal dystrophies**
　H18.51 **Endothelial corneal dystrophy**
　　　　Fuchs' dystrophy
　H18.52 **Epithelial (juvenile) corneal dystrophy**
　H18.53 **Granular corneal dystrophy**
　H18.54 **Lattice corneal dystrophy**
　H18.55 **Macular corneal dystrophy**
　H18.59 **Other hereditary corneal dystrophies**
✓5th **H18.6** **Keratoconus**
✓6th **H18.60** **Keratoconus, unspecified**
　　　H18.601　**Keratoconus, unspecified, right eye**
　　　H18.602　**Keratoconus, unspecified, left eye**
　　　H18.603　**Keratoconus, unspecified, bilateral**
　　　H18.609　**Keratoconus, unspecified, unspecified eye**
✓6th **H18.61** **Keratoconus, stable**
　　　H18.611　**Keratoconus, stable, right eye**
　　　H18.612　**Keratoconus, stable, left eye**
　　　H18.613　**Keratoconus, stable, bilateral**
　　　H18.619　**Keratoconus, stable, unspecified eye**
✓6th **H18.62** **Keratoconus, unstable**
　　　　Acute hydrops
　　　H18.621　**Keratoconus, unstable, right eye**
　　　H18.622　**Keratoconus, unstable, left eye**
　　　H18.623　**Keratoconus, unstable, bilateral**
　　　H18.629　**Keratoconus, unstable, unspecified eye**
✓5th **H18.7** **Other and unspecified corneal deformities**
　　　EXCLUDES 1　*congenital malformations of cornea (Q13.3-Q13.4)*
　H18.70 **Unspecified corneal deformity**
✓6th **H18.71** **Corneal ectasia**
　　　H18.711　**Corneal ectasia, right eye**
　　　H18.712　**Corneal ectasia, left eye**
　　　H18.713　**Corneal ectasia, bilateral**
　　　H18.719　**Corneal ectasia, unspecified eye**
✓6th **H18.72** **Corneal staphyloma**
　　　H18.721　**Corneal staphyloma, right eye**
　　　H18.722　**Corneal staphyloma, left eye**
　　　H18.723　**Corneal staphyloma, bilateral**
　　　H18.729　**Corneal staphyloma, unspecified eye**

✓6th **H18.73** **Descemetocele**
　　　H18.731　**Descemetocele, right eye**
　　　H18.732　**Descemetocele, left eye**
　　　H18.733　**Descemetocele, bilateral**
　　　H18.739　**Descemetocele, unspecified eye**
✓6th **H18.79** **Other corneal deformities**
　　　H18.791　**Other corneal deformities, right eye**
　　　H18.792　**Other corneal deformities, left eye**
　　　H18.793　**Other corneal deformities, bilateral**
　　　H18.799　**Other corneal deformities, unspecified eye**
✓5th **H18.8** **Other specified disorders of cornea**
✓6th **H18.81** **Anesthesia and hypoesthesia of cornea**
　　　H18.811　**Anesthesia and hypoesthesia of cornea, right eye**
　　　H18.812　**Anesthesia and hypoesthesia of cornea, left eye**
　　　H18.813　**Anesthesia and hypoesthesia of cornea, bilateral**
　　　H18.819　**Anesthesia and hypoesthesia of cornea, unspecified eye**
✓6th **H18.82** **Corneal disorder due to contact lens**
　　　EXCLUDES 2　*corneal edema due to contact lens (H18.21-)*
　　　H18.821　**Corneal disorder due to contact lens, right eye**
　　　H18.822　**Corneal disorder due to contact lens, left eye**
　　　H18.823　**Corneal disorder due to contact lens, bilateral**
　　　H18.829　**Corneal disorder due to contact lens, unspecified eye**
✓6th **H18.83** **Recurrent erosion of cornea**
　　　H18.831　**Recurrent erosion of cornea, right eye**
　　　H18.832　**Recurrent erosion of cornea, left eye**
　　　H18.833　**Recurrent erosion of cornea, bilateral**
　　　H18.839　**Recurrent erosion of cornea, unspecified eye**
✓6th **H18.89** **Other specified disorders of cornea**
　　　H18.891　**Other specified disorders of cornea, right eye**
　　　H18.892　**Other specified disorders of cornea, left eye**
　　　H18.893　**Other specified disorders of cornea, bilateral**
　　　H18.899　**Other specified disorders of cornea, unspecified eye**
　H18.9 **Unspecified disorder of cornea**
✓4th **H20** **Iridocyclitis**
✓5th **H20.0** **Acute and subacute iridocyclitis**
　　　　Acute anterior uveitis
　　　　Acute cyclitis
　　　　Acute iritis
　　　　Subacute anterior uveitis
　　　　Subacute cyclitis
　　　　Subacute iritis
　　　EXCLUDES 1　*iridocyclitis, iritis, uveitis (due to) (in) diabetes mellitus (E08-E13 with .39)*
　　　　　iridocyclitis, iritis, uveitis (due to) (in) diphtheria (A36.89)
　　　　　iridocyclitis, iritis, uveitis (due to) (in) gonococcal (A54.32)
　　　　　iridocyclitis, iritis, uveitis (due to) (in) herpes (simplex) (B00.51)
　　　　　iridocyclitis, iritis, uveitis (due to) (in) herpes zoster (B02.32)
　　　　　iridocyclitis, iritis, uveitis (due to) (in) late congenital syphilis (A50.39)
　　　　　iridocyclitis, iritis, uveitis (due to) (in) late syphilis (A52.71)
　　　　　iridocyclitis, iritis, uveitis (due to) (in) sarcoidosis (D86.83)
　　　　　iridocyclitis, iritis, uveitis (due to) (in) syphilis (A51.43)
　　　　　iridocyclitis, iritis, uveitis (due to) (in) toxoplasmosis (B58.09)
　　　　　iridocyclitis, iritis, uveitis (due to) (in) tuberculosis (A18.54)
　　　H20.00　**Unspecified acute and subacute iridocyclitis**

✓ Appropriate additional character required　　　✓x7th Requires 7th character, placeholder x must fill empty characters

Diseases of the Eye and Adnexa

H20.01–H21.302

✓6th **H20.01 Primary iridocyclitis**
- H20.011 Primary iridocyclitis, right eye
- H20.012 Primary iridocyclitis, left eye
- H20.013 Primary iridocyclitis, bilateral
- H20.019 Primary iridocyclitis, unspecified eye

✓6th **H20.02 Recurrent acute iridocyclitis**
- H20.021 Recurrent acute iridocyclitis, right eye
- H20.022 Recurrent acute iridocyclitis, left eye
- H20.023 Recurrent acute iridocyclitis, bilateral
- H20.029 Recurrent acute iridocyclitis, unspecified eye

✓6th **H20.03 Secondary infectious iridocyclitis**
- H20.031 Secondary infectious iridocyclitis, right eye
- H20.032 Secondary infectious iridocyclitis, left eye
- H20.033 Secondary infectious iridocyclitis, bilateral
- H20.039 Secondary infectious iridocyclitis, unspecified eye

✓6th **H20.04 Secondary noninfectious iridocyclitis**
- H20.041 Secondary noninfectious iridocyclitis, right eye
- H20.042 Secondary noninfectious iridocyclitis, left eye
- H20.043 Secondary noninfectious iridocyclitis, bilateral
- H20.049 Secondary noninfectious iridocyclitis, unspecified eye

✓6th **H20.05 Hypopyon**
- H20.051 Hypopyon, right eye
- H20.052 Hypopyon, left eye
- H20.053 Hypopyon, bilateral
- H20.059 Hypopyon, unspecified eye

✓5th **H20.1 Chronic iridocyclitis**
Use additional code for any associated cataract (H26.21-)
EXCLUDES 2   posterior cyclitis (H30.2-)
- H20.10 Chronic iridocyclitis, unspecified eye
- H20.11 Chronic iridocyclitis, right eye
- H20.12 Chronic iridocyclitis, left eye
- H20.13 Chronic iridocyclitis, bilateral

✓5th **H20.2 Lens-induced iridocyclitis**
- H20.20 Lens-induced iridocyclitis, unspecified eye
- H20.21 Lens-induced iridocyclitis, right eye
- H20.22 Lens-induced iridocyclitis, left eye
- H20.23 Lens-induced iridocyclitis, bilateral

✓5th **H20.8 Other iridocyclitis**
EXCLUDES 2   glaucomatocyclitis crises (H40.4-)
     posterior cyclitis (H30.2-)
     sympathetic uveitis (H44.13-)

✓6th **H20.81 Fuchs' heterochromic cyclitis**
- H20.811 Fuchs' heterochromic cyclitis, right eye
- H20.812 Fuchs' heterochromic cyclitis, left eye
- H20.813 Fuchs' heterochromic cyclitis, bilateral
- H20.819 Fuchs' heterochromic cyclitis, unspecified eye

✓6th **H20.82 Vogt-Koyanagi syndrome**
- H20.821 Vogt-Koyanagi syndrome, right eye
- H20.822 Vogt-Koyanagi syndrome, left eye
- H20.823 Vogt-Koyanagi syndrome, bilateral
- H20.829 Vogt-Koyanagi syndrome, unspecified eye

H20.9 Unspecified iridocyclitis
Uveitis NOS

✓4th **H21 Other disorders of iris and ciliary body**
EXCLUDES 2   sympathetic uveitis (H44.1-)

✓5th **H21.0 Hyphema**
EXCLUDES 1   traumatic hyphema (S05.1-)
- H21.00 Hyphema, unspecified eye
- H21.01 Hyphema, right eye
- H21.02 Hyphema, left eye
- H21.03 Hyphema, bilateral

✓5th **H21.1 Other vascular disorders of iris and ciliary body**
Neovascularization of iris or ciliary body
Rubeosis iridis
Rubeosis of iris

✓6th **H21.1x Other vascular disorders of iris and ciliary body**
- H21.1x1 Other vascular disorders of iris and ciliary body, right eye
- H21.1x2 Other vascular disorders of iris and ciliary body, left eye
- H21.1x3 Other vascular disorders of iris and ciliary body, bilateral
- H21.1x9 Other vascular disorders of iris and ciliary body, unspecified eye

✓5th **H21.2 Degeneration of iris and ciliary body**

✓6th **H21.21 Degeneration of chamber angle**
- H21.211 Degeneration of chamber angle, right eye
- H21.212 Degeneration of chamber angle, left eye
- H21.213 Degeneration of chamber angle, bilateral
- H21.219 Degeneration of chamber angle, unspecified eye

✓6th **H21.22 Degeneration of ciliary body**
- H21.221 Degeneration of ciliary body, right eye
- H21.222 Degeneration of ciliary body, left eye
- H21.223 Degeneration of ciliary body, bilateral
- H21.229 Degeneration of ciliary body, unspecified eye

✓6th **H21.23 Degeneration of iris (pigmentary)**
Translucency of iris
- H21.231 Degeneration of iris (pigmentary), right eye
- H21.232 Degeneration of iris (pigmentary), left eye
- H21.233 Degeneration of iris (pigmentary), bilateral
- H21.239 Degeneration of iris (pigmentary), unspecified eye

✓6th **H21.24 Degeneration of pupillary margin**
- H21.241 Degeneration of pupillary margin, right eye
- H21.242 Degeneration of pupillary margin, left eye
- H21.243 Degeneration of pupillary margin, bilateral
- H21.249 Degeneration of pupillary margin, unspecified eye

✓6th **H21.25 Iridoschisis**
- H21.251 Iridoschisis, right eye
- H21.252 Iridoschisis, left eye
- H21.253 Iridoschisis, bilateral
- H21.259 Iridoschisis, unspecified eye

✓6th **H21.26 Iris atrophy (essential) (progressive)**
- H21.261 Iris atrophy (essential) (progressive), right eye
- H21.262 Iris atrophy (essential) (progressive), left eye
- H21.263 Iris atrophy (essential) (progressive), bilateral
- H21.269 Iris atrophy (essential) (progressive), unspecified eye

✓6th **H21.27 Miotic pupillary cyst**
- H21.271 Miotic pupillary cyst, right eye
- H21.272 Miotic pupillary cyst, left eye
- H21.273 Miotic pupillary cyst, bilateral
- H21.279 Miotic pupillary cyst, unspecified eye

H21.29 Other iris atrophy

✓5th **H21.3 Cyst of iris, ciliary body and anterior chamber**
EXCLUDES 2   miotic pupillary cyst (H21.27-)

✓6th **H21.30 Idiopathic cysts of iris, ciliary body or anterior chamber**
Cyst of iris, ciliary body or anterior chamber NOS
- H21.301 Idiopathic cysts of iris, ciliary body or anterior chamber, right eye
- H21.302 Idiopathic cysts of iris, ciliary body or anterior chamber, left eye

---

EXCLUDES 1   Not coded here   EXCLUDES 2   Not included here   *Manifestation Code*

H21.303 Idiopathic cysts of iris, ciliary body or anterior chamber, bilateral
H21.309 Idiopathic cysts of iris, ciliary body or anterior chamber, unspecified eye

✓6th H21.31 **Exudative cysts of iris or anterior chamber**
H21.311 Exudative cysts of iris or anterior chamber, right eye
H21.312 Exudative cysts of iris or anterior chamber, left eye
H21.313 Exudative cysts of iris or anterior chamber, bilateral
H21.319 Exudative cysts of iris or anterior chamber, unspecified eye

✓6th H21.32 **Implantation cysts of iris, ciliary body or anterior chamber**
H21.321 Implantation cysts of iris, ciliary body or anterior chamber, right eye
H21.322 Implantation cysts of iris, ciliary body or anterior chamber, left eye
H21.323 Implantation cysts of iris, ciliary body or anterior chamber, bilateral
H21.329 Implantation cysts of iris, ciliary body or anterior chamber, unspecified eye

✓6th H21.33 **Parasitic cyst of iris, ciliary body or anterior chamber**
H21.331 Parasitic cyst of iris, ciliary body or anterior chamber, right eye
H21.332 Parasitic cyst of iris, ciliary body or anterior chamber, left eye
H21.333 Parasitic cyst of iris, ciliary body or anterior chamber, bilateral
H21.339 Parasitic cyst of iris, ciliary body or anterior chamber, unspecified eye

✓6th H21.34 **Primary cyst of pars plana**
H21.341 Primary cyst of pars plana, right eye
H21.342 Primary cyst of pars plana, left eye
H21.343 Primary cyst of pars plana, bilateral
H21.349 Primary cyst of pars plana, unspecified eye

✓6th H21.35 **Exudative cyst of pars plana**
H21.351 Exudative cyst of pars plana, right eye
H21.352 Exudative cyst of pars plana, left eye
H21.353 Exudative cyst of pars plana, bilateral
H21.359 Exudative cyst of pars plana, unspecified eye

✓5th H21.4 **Pupillary membranes**
Iris bombé
Pupillary occlusion
Pupillary seclusion
EXCLUDES 1 *congenital pupillary membranes (Q13.8)*
H21.40 Pupillary membranes, unspecified eye
H21.41 Pupillary membranes, right eye
H21.42 Pupillary membranes, left eye
H21.43 Pupillary membranes, bilateral

✓5th H21.5 **Other and unspecified adhesions and disruptions of iris and ciliary body**
EXCLUDES 1 *corectopia (Q13.2)*

✓6th H21.50 **Unspecified adhesions of iris**
Synechia (iris) NOS
H21.501 Unspecified adhesions of iris, right eye
H21.502 Unspecified adhesions of iris, left eye
H21.503 Unspecified adhesions of iris, bilateral
H21.509 Unspecified adhesions of iris and ciliary body, unspecified eye

✓6th H21.51 **Anterior synechiae (iris)**
H21.511 Anterior synechiae (iris), right eye
H21.512 Anterior synechiae (iris), left eye
H21.513 Anterior synechiae (iris), bilateral
H21.519 Anterior synechiae (iris), unspecified eye

✓6th H21.52 **Goniosynechiae**
H21.521 Goniosynechiae, right eye
H21.522 Goniosynechiae, left eye
H21.523 Goniosynechiae, bilateral
H21.529 Goniosynechiae, unspecified eye

✓6th H21.53 **Iridodialysis**
H21.531 Iridodialysis, right eye
H21.532 Iridodialysis, left eye

H21.533 Iridodialysis, bilateral
H21.539 Iridodialysis, unspecified eye

✓6th H21.54 **Posterior synechiae (iris)**
H21.541 Posterior synechiae (iris), right eye
H21.542 Posterior synechiae (iris), left eye
H21.543 Posterior synechiae (iris), bilateral
H21.549 Posterior synechiae (iris), unspecified eye

✓6th H21.55 **Recession of chamber angle**
H21.551 Recession of chamber angle, right eye
H21.552 Recession of chamber angle, left eye
H21.553 Recession of chamber angle, bilateral
H21.559 Recession of chamber angle, unspecified eye

✓6th H21.56 **Pupillary abnormalities**
Deformed pupil
Ectopic pupil
Rupture of sphincter, pupil
EXCLUDES 1 *congenital deformity of pupil (Q13.2-)*
H21.561 Pupillary abnormality, right eye
H21.562 Pupillary abnormality, left eye
H21.563 Pupillary abnormality, bilateral
H21.569 Pupillary abnormality, unspecified eye

✓5th H21.8 **Other specified disorders of iris and ciliary body**
H21.81 **Floppy iris syndrome**
Intraoperative floppy iris syndrome (IFIS)
Code first (T36-T50) to identify drug
H21.82 **Plateau iris syndrome (post-iridectomy) (postprocedural)**
H21.89 **Other specified disorders of iris and ciliary body**
H21.9 **Unspecified disorder of iris and ciliary body**

H22 **Disorders of iris and ciliary body in diseases classified elsewhere**
Code first underlying disease, such as:
gout (M1a-, M10-)

Disorders of lens (H25-H28)

✓4th H25 **Age-related cataract**
Senile cataract
EXCLUDES 2 *capsular glaucoma with pseudoexfoliation of lens (H40.1-)*

✓5th H25.0 **Age-related incipient cataract**
✓6th H25.01 **Cortical age-related cataract**
H25.011 Cortical age-related cataract, right eye
H25.012 Cortical age-related cataract, left eye
H25.013 Cortical age-related cataract, bilateral
H25.019 Cortical age-related cataract, unspecified eye

✓6th H25.03 **Anterior subcapsular polar age-related cataract**
H25.031 Anterior subcapsular polar age-related cataract, right eye
H25.032 Anterior subcapsular polar age-related cataract, left eye
H25.033 Anterior subcapsular polar age-related cataract, bilateral
H25.039 Anterior subcapsular polar age-related cataract, unspecified eye

✓6th H25.04 **Posterior subcapsular polar age-related cataract**
H25.041 Posterior subcapsular polar age-related cataract, right eye
H25.042 Posterior subcapsular polar age-related cataract, left eye
H25.043 Posterior subcapsular polar age-related cataract, bilateral
H25.049 Posterior subcapsular polar age-related cataract, unspecified eye

✓6th H25.09 **Other age-related incipient cataract**
Coronary age-related cataract
Punctate age-related cataract
Water clefts
H25.091 Other age-related incipient cataract, right eye
H25.092 Other age-related incipient cataract, left eye
H25.093 Other age-related incipient cataract, bilateral

    H25.099   Other age-related incipient cataract, unspecified eye

✓5th **H25.1**   **Age-related nuclear cataract**
    Cataracta brunescens
    Nuclear sclerosis cataract

    H25.10   **Age-related nuclear cataract, unspecified eye**
    H25.11   **Age-related nuclear cataract, right eye**
    H25.12   **Age-related nuclear cataract, left eye**
    H25.13   **Age-related nuclear cataract, bilateral**

✓5th **H25.2**   **Age-related cataract, morgagnian type**
    Age-related hypermature cataract

    H25.20   **Age-related cataract, morgagnian type, unspecified eye**
    H25.21   **Age-related cataract, morgagnian type, right eye**
    H25.22   **Age-related cataract, morgagnian type, left eye**
    H25.23   **Age-related cataract, morgagnian type, bilateral**

✓5th **H25.8**   **Other age-related cataract**

    ✓6th **H25.81**   **Combined forms of age-related cataract**
        H25.811   **Combined forms of age-related cataract, right eye**
        H25.812   **Combined forms of age-related cataract, left eye**
        H25.813   **Combined forms of age-related cataract, bilateral**
        H25.819   **Combined forms of age-related cataract, unspecified eye**

    H25.89   **Other age-related cataract**

    H25.9   **Unspecified age-related cataract**

✓4th **H26**   **Other cataract**
    EXCLUDES 1   congenital cataract (Q12.0)

✓5th **H26.0**   **Infantile and juvenile cataract**

    ✓6th **H26.00**   **Unspecified infantile and juvenile cataract**
        H26.001   **Unspecified infantile and juvenile cataract, right eye**
        H26.002   **Unspecified infantile and juvenile cataract, left eye**
        H26.003   **Unspecified infantile and juvenile cataract, bilateral**
        H26.009   **Unspecified infantile and juvenile cataract, unspecified eye**

    ✓6th **H26.01**   **Infantile and juvenile cortical, lamellar, or zonular cataract**
        H26.011   **Infantile and juvenile cortical, lamellar, or zonular cataract, right eye**
        H26.012   **Infantile and juvenile cortical, lamellar, or zonular cataract, left eye**
        H26.013   **Infantile and juvenile cortical, lamellar, or zonular cataract, bilateral**
        H26.019   **Infantile and juvenile cortical, lamellar, or zonular cataract, unspecified eye**

    ✓6th **H26.03**   **Infantile and juvenile nuclear cataract**
        H26.031   **Infantile and juvenile nuclear cataract, right eye**
        H26.032   **Infantile and juvenile nuclear cataract, left eye**
        H26.033   **Infantile and juvenile nuclear cataract, bilateral**
        H26.039   **Infantile and juvenile nuclear cataract, unspecified eye**

    ✓6th **H26.04**   **Anterior subcapsular polar infantile and juvenile cataract**
        H26.041   **Anterior subcapsular polar infantile and juvenile cataract, right eye**
        H26.042   **Anterior subcapsular polar infantile and juvenile cataract, left eye**
        H26.043   **Anterior subcapsular polar infantile and juvenile cataract, bilateral**
        H26.049   **Anterior subcapsular polar infantile and juvenile cataract, unspecified eye**

    ✓6th **H26.05**   **Posterior subcapsular polar infantile and juvenile cataract**
        H26.051   **Posterior subcapsular polar infantile and juvenile cataract, right eye**
        H26.052   **Posterior subcapsular polar infantile and juvenile cataract, left eye**
        H26.053   **Posterior subcapsular polar infantile and juvenile cataract, bilateral**

        H26.059   **Posterior subcapsular polar infantile and juvenile cataract, unspecified eye**

    ✓6th **H26.06**   **Combined forms of infantile and juvenile cataract**
        H26.061   **Combined forms of infantile and juvenile cataract, right eye**
        H26.062   **Combined forms of infantile and juvenile cataract, left eye**
        H26.063   **Combined forms of infantile and juvenile cataract, bilateral**
        H26.069   **Combined forms of infantile and juvenile cataract, unspecified eye**

    H26.09   **Other infantile and juvenile cataract**

✓5th **H26.1**   **Traumatic cataract**
    Use additional code (Chapter 20) to identify external cause

    ✓6th **H26.10**   **Unspecified traumatic cataract**
        H26.101   **Unspecified traumatic cataract, right eye**
        H26.102   **Unspecified traumatic cataract, left eye**
        H26.103   **Unspecified traumatic cataract, bilateral**
        H26.109   **Unspecified traumatic cataract, unspecified eye**

    ✓6th **H26.11**   **Localized traumatic opacities**
        H26.111   **Localized traumatic opacities, right eye**
        H26.112   **Localized traumatic opacities, left eye**
        H26.113   **Localized traumatic opacities, bilateral**
        H26.119   **Localized traumatic opacities, unspecified eye**

    ✓6th **H26.12**   **Partially resolved traumatic cataract**
        H26.121   **Partially resolved traumatic cataract, right eye**
        H26.122   **Partially resolved traumatic cataract, left eye**
        H26.123   **Partially resolved traumatic cataract, bilateral**
        H26.129   **Partially resolved traumatic cataract, unspecified eye**

    ✓6th **H26.13**   **Total traumatic cataract**
        H26.131   **Total traumatic cataract, right eye**
        H26.132   **Total traumatic cataract, left eye**
        H26.133   **Total traumatic cataract, bilateral**
        H26.139   **Total traumatic cataract, unspecified eye**

✓5th **H26.2**   **Complicated cataract**

    H26.20   **Unspecified complicated cataract**
    Cataracta complicata NOS

    ✓6th **H26.21**   **Cataract with neovascularization**
    Code also associated condition, such as:
        chronic iridocyclitis (H20.1-)
        H26.211   **Cataract with neovascularization, right eye**
        H26.212   **Cataract with neovascularization, left eye**
        H26.213   **Cataract with neovascularization, bilateral**
        H26.219   **Cataract with neovascularization, unspecified eye**

    ✓6th **H26.22**   **Cataract secondary to ocular disorders (degenerative) (inflammatory)**
    Code also associated ocular disorder
        H26.221   **Cataract secondary to ocular disorders (degenerative) (inflammatory), right eye**
        H26.222   **Cataract secondary to ocular disorders (degenerative) (inflammatory), left eye**
        H26.223   **Cataract secondary to ocular disorders (degenerative) (inflammatory), bilateral**
        H26.229   **Cataract secondary to ocular disorders (degenerative) (inflammatory), unspecified eye**

    ✓6th **H26.23**   **Glaucomatous flecks (subcapsular)**
    Code first underlying glaucoma (H40-H42)
        H26.231   **Glaucomatous flecks (subcapsular), right eye**
        H26.232   **Glaucomatous flecks (subcapsular), left eye**
        H26.233   **Glaucomatous flecks (subcapsular), bilateral**

    EXCLUDES 1   Not coded here   *EXCLUDES 2*   Not included here   *Manifestation Code*

         H26.239 **Glaucomatous flecks (subcapsular), unspecified eye**

✓5th **H26.3 Drug-induced cataract**
     Toxic cataract
     Code first (T36-T50) to identify drug
     H26.30 **Drug-induced cataract, unspecified eye**
     H26.31 **Drug-induced cataract, right eye**
     H26.32 **Drug-induced cataract, left eye**
     H26.33 **Drug-induced cataract, bilateral**

✓5th **H26.4 Secondary cataract**
     H26.40 **Unspecified secondary cataract**
     ✓6th H26.41 **Soemmering's ring**
         H26.411 **Soemmering's ring, right eye**
         H26.412 **Soemmering's ring, left eye**
         H26.413 **Soemmering's ring, bilateral**
         H26.419 **Soemmering's ring, unspecified eye**
     ✓6th H26.49 **Other secondary cataract**
         H26.491 **Other secondary cataract, right eye**
         H26.492 **Other secondary cataract, left eye**
         H26.493 **Other secondary cataract, bilateral**
         H26.499 **Other secondary cataract, unspecified eye**

     H26.8 **Other specified cataract**
     H26.9 **Unspecified cataract**

✓4th **H27 Other disorders of lens**
     EXCLUDES 1   congenital lens malformations (Q12-)
         mechanical complications of intraocular lens implant (T85.2)
         pseudophakia (Z96.1)

✓5th **H27.0 Aphakia**
     Acquired absence of lens
     Acquired aphakia
     Aphakia due to trauma
     EXCLUDES 1   cataract extraction status (Z98.4-)
         congenital absence of lens (Q12.3)
         congenital aphakia (Q12.3)
     H27.00 **Aphakia, unspecified eye**
     H27.01 **Aphakia, right eye**
     H27.02 **Aphakia, left eye**
     H27.03 **Aphakia, bilateral**

✓5th **H27.1 Dislocation of lens**
     H27.10 **Unspecified dislocation of lens**
     ✓6th H27.11 **Subluxation of lens**
         H27.111 **Subluxation of lens, right eye**
         H27.112 **Subluxation of lens, left eye**
         H27.113 **Subluxation of lens, bilateral**
         H27.119 **Subluxation of lens, unspecified eye**
     ✓6th H27.12 **Anterior dislocation of lens**
         H27.121 **Anterior dislocation of lens, right eye**
         H27.122 **Anterior dislocation of lens, left eye**
         H27.123 **Anterior dislocation of lens, bilateral**
         H27.129 **Anterior dislocation of lens, unspecified eye**
     ✓6th H27.13 **Posterior dislocation of lens**
         H27.131 **Posterior dislocation of lens, right eye**
         H27.132 **Posterior dislocation of lens, left eye**
         H27.133 **Posterior dislocation of lens, bilateral**
         H27.139 **Posterior dislocation of lens, unspecified eye**
     H27.8 **Other specified disorders of lens**
     H27.9 **Unspecified disorder of lens**

H28 Cataract in diseases classified elsewhere
     Code first underlying disease, such as:
         hypoparathyroidism (E20-)
         myotonia (G71.1-)
         myxedema (E03-)
         protein-calorie malnutrition (E40-E46)
     EXCLUDES 1   cataract in diabetes mellitus (E08.33, E09.33, E10.33, E11.33, E13.33)

Disorders of choroid and retina (H30-H36)

✓4th **H30 Chorioretinal inflammation**
     ✓5th **H30.0 Focal chorioretinal inflammation**
         Focal chorioretinitis
         Focal choroiditis
         Focal retinitis
         Focal retinochoroiditis
         ✓6th H30.00 **Unspecified focal chorioretinal inflammation**
             Focal chorioretinitis NOS
             Focal choroiditis NOS
             Focal retinitis NOS
             Focal retinochoroiditis NOS
             H30.001 **Unspecified focal chorioretinal inflammation, right eye**
             H30.002 **Unspecified focal chorioretinal inflammation, left eye**
             H30.003 **Unspecified focal chorioretinal inflammation, bilateral**
             H30.009 **Unspecified focal chorioretinal inflammation, unspecified eye**
         ✓6th H30.01 **Focal chorioretinal inflammation, juxtapapillary**
             H30.011 **Focal chorioretinal inflammation, juxtapapillary, right eye**
             H30.012 **Focal chorioretinal inflammation, juxtapapillary, left eye**
             H30.013 **Focal chorioretinal inflammation, juxtapapillary, bilateral**
             H30.019 **Focal chorioretinal inflammation, juxtapapillary, unspecified eye**
         ✓6th H30.02 **Focal chorioretinal inflammation of posterior pole**
             H30.021 **Focal chorioretinal inflammation of posterior pole, right eye**
             H30.022 **Focal chorioretinal inflammation of posterior pole, left eye**
             H30.023 **Focal chorioretinal inflammation of posterior pole, bilateral**
             H30.029 **Focal chorioretinal inflammation of posterior pole, unspecified eye**
         ✓6th H30.03 **Focal chorioretinal inflammation, peripheral**
             H30.031 **Focal chorioretinal inflammation, peripheral, right eye**
             H30.032 **Focal chorioretinal inflammation, peripheral, left eye**
             H30.033 **Focal chorioretinal inflammation, peripheral, bilateral**
             H30.039 **Focal chorioretinal inflammation, peripheral, unspecified eye**
         ✓6th H30.04 **Focal chorioretinal inflammation, macular or paramacular**
             H30.041 **Focal chorioretinal inflammation, macular or paramacular, right eye**
             H30.042 **Focal chorioretinal inflammation, macular or paramacular, left eye**
             H30.043 **Focal chorioretinal inflammation, macular or paramacular, bilateral**
             H30.049 **Focal chorioretinal inflammation, macular or paramacular, unspecified eye**
     ✓5th **H30.1 Disseminated chorioretinal inflammation**
         Disseminated chorioretinitis
         Disseminated choroiditis
         Disseminated retinitis
         Disseminated retinochoroiditis
         EXCLUDES 2   exudative retinopathy (H35.02-)
         ✓6th H30.10 **Unspecified disseminated chorioretinal inflammation**
             Disseminated chorioretinitis NOS
             Disseminated choroiditis NOS
             Disseminated retinitis NOS
             Disseminated retinochoroiditis NOS
             H30.101 **Unspecified disseminated chorioretinal inflammation, right eye**
             H30.102 **Unspecified disseminated chorioretinal inflammation, left eye**
             H30.103 **Unspecified disseminated chorioretinal inflammation, bilateral**
             H30.109 **Unspecified disseminated chorioretinal inflammation, unspecified eye**

✔ Appropriate additional character required   ✓x7th Requires 7th character, placeholder x must fill empty characters

Diseases of the Eye and Adnexa

H30.11–H31.301

√6th **H30.11** **Disseminated chorioretinal inflammation of posterior pole**
- H30.111 **Disseminated chorioretinal inflammation of posterior pole, right eye**
- H30.112 **Disseminated chorioretinal inflammation of posterior pole, left eye**
- H30.113 **Disseminated chorioretinal inflammation of posterior pole, bilateral**
- H30.119 **Disseminated chorioretinal inflammation of posterior pole, unspecified eye**

√6th **H30.12** **Disseminated chorioretinal inflammation, peripheral**
- H30.121 **Disseminated chorioretinal inflammation, peripheral right eye**
- H30.122 **Disseminated chorioretinal inflammation, peripheral, left eye**
- H30.123 **Disseminated chorioretinal inflammation, peripheral, bilateral**
- H30.129 **Disseminated chorioretinal inflammation, peripheral, unspecified eye**

√6th **H30.13** **Disseminated chorioretinal inflammation, generalized**
- H30.131 **Disseminated chorioretinal inflammation, generalized, right eye**
- H30.132 **Disseminated chorioretinal inflammation, generalized, left eye**
- H30.133 **Disseminated chorioretinal inflammation, generalized, bilateral**
- H30.139 **Disseminated chorioretinal inflammation, generalized, unspecified eye**

√6th **H30.14** **Acute posterior multifocal placoid pigment epitheliopathy**
- H30.141 **Acute posterior multifocal placoid pigment epitheliopathy, right eye**
- H30.142 **Acute posterior multifocal placoid pigment epitheliopathy, left eye**
- H30.143 **Acute posterior multifocal placoid pigment epitheliopathy, bilateral**
- H30.149 **Acute posterior multifocal placoid pigment epitheliopathy, unspecified eye**

√5th **H30.2** **Posterior cyclitis**
Pars planitis
- H30.20 **Posterior cyclitis, unspecified eye**
- H30.21 **Posterior cyclitis, right eye**
- H30.22 **Posterior cyclitis, left eye**
- H30.23 **Posterior cyclitis, bilateral**

√5th **H30.8** **Other chorioretinal inflammations**

√6th **H30.81** **Harada's disease**
- H30.811 **Harada's disease, right eye**
- H30.812 **Harada's disease, left eye**
- H30.813 **Harada's disease, bilateral**
- H30.819 **Harada's disease, unspecified eye**

√6th **H30.89** **Other chorioretinal inflammations**
- H30.891 **Other chorioretinal inflammations, right eye**
- H30.892 **Other chorioretinal inflammations, left eye**
- H30.893 **Other chorioretinal inflammations, bilateral**
- H30.899 **Other chorioretinal inflammations, unspecified eye**

√5th **H30.9** **Unspecified chorioretinal inflammation**
Chorioretinitis NOS
Choroiditis NOS
Neuroretinitis NOS
Retinitis NOS
Retinochoroiditis NOS
- H30.90 **Unspecified chorioretinal inflammation, unspecified eye**
- H30.91 **Unspecified chorioretinal inflammation, right eye**
- H30.92 **Unspecified chorioretinal inflammation, left eye**
- H30.93 **Unspecified chorioretinal inflammation, bilateral**

√4th **H31** **Other disorders of choroid**

√5th **H31.0** **Chorioretinal scars**
EXCLUDES 2 *postsurgical chorioretinal scars (H59.81-)*

√6th **H31.00** **Unspecified chorioretinal scars**
- H31.001 **Unspecified chorioretinal scars, right eye**
- H31.002 **Unspecified chorioretinal scars, left eye**
- H31.003 **Unspecified chorioretinal scars, bilateral**
- H31.009 **Unspecified chorioretinal scars, unspecified eye**

√6th **H31.01** **Macula scars of posterior pole (postinflammatory) (post-traumatic)**
EXCLUDES 1 *postprocedural choriorentinal scar (H59.81-)*
- H31.011 **Macula scars of posterior pole (postinflammatory) (post-traumatic), right eye**
- H31.012 **Macula scars of posterior pole (postinflammatory) (post-traumatic), left eye**
- H31.013 **Macula scars of posterior pole (postinflammatory) (post-traumatic), bilateral**
- H31.019 **Macula scars of posterior pole (postinflammatory) (post-traumatic), unspecified eye**

√6th **H31.02** **Solar retinopathy**
- H31.021 **Solar retinopathy, right eye**
- H31.022 **Solar retinopathy, left eye**
- H31.023 **Solar retinopathy, bilateral**
- H31.029 **Solar retinopathy, unspecified eye**

√6th **H31.09** **Other chorioretinal scars**
- H31.091 **Other chorioretinal scars, right eye**
- H31.092 **Other chorioretinal scars, left eye**
- H31.093 **Other chorioretinal scars, bilateral**
- H31.099 **Other chorioretinal scars, unspecified eye**

√5th **H31.1** **Choroidal degeneration**
EXCLUDES 2 *angioid streaks of macula (H35.33)*

√6th **H31.10** **Unspecified choroidal degeneration**
Choroidal sclerosis NOS
- H31.101 **Choroidal degeneration, unspecified, right eye**
- H31.102 **Choroidal degeneration, unspecified, left eye**
- H31.103 **Choroidal degeneration, unspecified, bilateral**
- H31.109 **Choroidal degeneration, unspecified, unspecified eye**

√6th **H31.11** **Age-related choroidal atrophy**
- H31.111 **Age-related choroidal atrophy, right eye**
- H31.112 **Age-related choroidal atrophy, left eye**
- H31.113 **Age-related choroidal atrophy, bilateral**
- H31.119 **Age-related choroidal atrophy, unspecified eye**

√6th **H31.12** **Diffuse secondary atrophy of choroid**
- H31.121 **Diffuse secondary atrophy of choroid, right eye**
- H31.122 **Diffuse secondary atrophy of choroid, left eye**
- H31.123 **Diffuse secondary atrophy of choroid, bilateral**
- H31.129 **Diffuse secondary atrophy of choroid, unspecified eye**

√5th **H31.2** **Hereditary choroidal dystrophy**
EXCLUDES 2 *hyperornithinemia (E72.4)*
ornithinemia (E72.4)
- H31.20 **Hereditary choroidal dystrophy, unspecified**
- H31.21 **Choroideremia**
- H31.22 **Choroidal dystrophy (central areolar) (generalized) (peripapillary)**
- H31.23 **Gyrate atrophy, choroid**
- H31.29 **Other hereditary choroidal dystrophy**

√5th **H31.3** **Choroidal hemorrhage and rupture**

√6th **H31.30** **Unspecified choroidal hemorrhage**
- H31.301 **Unspecified choroidal hemorrhage, right eye**

EXCLUDES 1   Not coded here   EXCLUDES 2   Not included here   *Manifestation Code*

           H31.302   **Unspecified choroidal hemorrhage, left eye**

           H31.303   **Unspecified choroidal hemorrhage, bilateral**

           H31.309   **Unspecified choroidal hemorrhage, unspecified eye**

     ✓6ᵗʰ   **H31.31   Expulsive choroidal hemorrhage**

           H31.311   **Expulsive choroidal hemorrhage, right eye**

           H31.312   **Expulsive choroidal hemorrhage, left eye**

           H31.313   **Expulsive choroidal hemorrhage, bilateral**

           H31.319   **Expulsive choroidal hemorrhage, unspecified eye**

     ✓6ᵗʰ   **H31.32   Choroidal rupture**

           H31.321   **Choroidal rupture, right eye**

           H31.322   **Choroidal rupture, left eye**

           H31.323   **Choroidal rupture, bilateral**

           H31.329   **Choroidal rupture, unspecified eye**

✓5ᵗʰ   **H31.4   Choroidal detachment**

     ✓6ᵗʰ   **H31.40   Unspecified choroidal detachment**

           H31.401   **Unspecified choroidal detachment, right eye**

           H31.402   **Unspecified choroidal detachment, left eye**

           H31.403   **Unspecified choroidal detachment, bilateral**

           H31.409   **Unspecified choroidal detachment, unspecified eye**

     ✓6ᵗʰ   **H31.41   Hemorrhagic choroidal detachment**

           H31.411   **Hemorrhagic choroidal detachment, right eye**

           H31.412   **Hemorrhagic choroidal detachment, left eye**

           H31.413   **Hemorrhagic choroidal detachment, bilateral**

           H31.419   **Hemorrhagic choroidal detachment, unspecified eye**

     ✓6ᵗʰ   **H31.42   Serous choroidal detachment**

           H31.421   **Serous choroidal detachment, right eye**

           H31.422   **Serous choroidal detachment, left eye**

           H31.423   **Serous choroidal detachment, bilateral**

           H31.429   **Serous choroidal detachment, unspecified eye**

    H31.8   **Other specified disorders of choroid**

    H31.9   **Unspecified disorder of choroid**

H32   Chorioretinal disorders in diseases classified elsewhere

Code first underlying disease, such as:
congenital toxoplasmosis (P37.1)
histoplasmosis (B39-)
leprosy (A30-)

EXCLUDES 1   *chorioretinitis (in):*
toxoplasmosis (acquired) (B58.01)
tuberculosis (A18.53)

✓4ᵗʰ   H33   Retinal detachments and breaks

EXCLUDES 1   *detachment of retinal pigment epithelium (H35.72-, H35.73-)*

✓5ᵗʰ   **H33.0   Retinal detachment with retinal break**

    Rhegmatogenous retinal detachment

    EXCLUDES 1   *serous retinal detachment (without retinal break) (H33.2-)*

     ✓6ᵗʰ   **H33.00   Unspecified retinal detachment with retinal break**

           H33.001   **Unspecified retinal detachment with retinal break, right eye**

           H33.002   **Unspecified retinal detachment with retinal break, left eye**

           H33.003   **Unspecified retinal detachment with retinal break, bilateral**

           H33.009   **Unspecified retinal detachment with retinal break, unspecified eye**

     ✓6ᵗʰ   **H33.01   Retinal detachment with single break**

           H33.011   **Retinal detachment with single break, right eye**

           H33.012   **Retinal detachment with single break, left eye**

           H33.013   **Retinal detachment with single break, bilateral**

           H33.019   **Retinal detachment with single break, unspecified eye**

     ✓6ᵗʰ   **H33.02   Retinal detachment with multiple breaks**

           H33.021   **Retinal detachment with multiple breaks, right eye**

           H33.022   **Retinal detachment with multiple breaks, left eye**

           H33.023   **Retinal detachment with multiple breaks, bilateral**

           H33.029   **Retinal detachment with multiple breaks, unspecified eye**

     ✓6ᵗʰ   **H33.03   Retinal detachment with giant retinal tear**

           H33.031   **Retinal detachment with giant retinal tear, right eye**

           H33.032   **Retinal detachment with giant retinal tear, left eye**

           H33.033   **Retinal detachment with giant retinal tear, bilateral**

           H33.039   **Retinal detachment with giant retinal tear, unspecified eye**

     ✓6ᵗʰ   **H33.04   Retinal detachment with retinal dialysis**

           H33.041   **Retinal detachment with retinal dialysis, right eye**

           H33.042   **Retinal detachment with retinal dialysis, left eye**

           H33.043   **Retinal detachment with retinal dialysis, bilateral**

           H33.049   **Retinal detachment with retinal dialysis, unspecified eye**

     ✓6ᵗʰ   **H33.05   Total retinal detachment**

           H33.051   **Total retinal detachment, right eye**

           H33.052   **Total retinal detachment, left eye**

           H33.053   **Total retinal detachment, bilateral**

           H33.059   **Total retinal detachment, unspecified eye**

✓5ᵗʰ   **H33.1   Retinoschisis and retinal cysts**

    EXCLUDES 1   *congenital retinoschisis (Q14.1)*
                 microcystoid degeneration of retina (H35.42-)

     ✓6ᵗʰ   **H33.10   Unspecified retinoschisis**

           H33.101   **Unspecified retinoschisis, right eye**

           H33.102   **Unspecified retinoschisis, left eye**

           H33.103   **Unspecified retinoschisis, bilateral**

           H33.109   **Unspecified retinoschisis, unspecified eye**

     ✓6ᵗʰ   **H33.11   Cyst of ora serrata**

           H33.111   **Cyst of ora serrata, right eye**

           H33.112   **Cyst of ora serrata, left eye**

           H33.113   **Cyst of ora serrata, bilateral**

           H33.119   **Cyst of ora serrata, unspecified eye**

     ✓6ᵗʰ   **H33.12   Parasitic cyst of retina**

           H33.121   **Parasitic cyst of retina, right eye**

           H33.122   **Parasitic cyst of retina, left eye**

           H33.123   **Parasitic cyst of retina, bilateral**

           H33.129   **Parasitic cyst of retina, unspecified eye**

     ✓6ᵗʰ   **H33.19   Other retinoschisis and retinal cysts**

        Pseudocyst of retina

           H33.191   **Other retinoschisis and retinal cysts, right eye**

           H33.192   **Other retinoschisis and retinal cysts, left eye**

           H33.193   **Other retinoschisis and retinal cysts, bilateral**

           H33.199   **Other retinoschisis and retinal cysts, unspecified eye**

✓5ᵗʰ   **H33.2   Serous retinal detachment**

    Retinal detachment NOS

    Retinal detachment without retinal break

    EXCLUDES 1   *central serous chorioretinopathy (H35.71-)*

    H33.20   **Serous retinal detachment, unspecified eye**

    H33.21   **Serous retinal detachment, right eye**

    H33.22   **Serous retinal detachment, left eye**

    H33.23   **Serous retinal detachment, bilateral**

☑ Appropriate additional character required   ✓x7ᵗʰ Requires 7th character, placeholder x must fill empty characters

☑5th H33.3 Retinal breaks without detachment
> EXCLUDES 1   chorioretinal scars after surgery for detachment
> (H59.81-)
> peripheral retinal degeneration without break
> (H35.4-)

☑6th H33.30 Unspecified retinal break
- H33.301   Unspecified retinal break, right eye
- H33.302   Unspecified retinal break, left eye
- H33.303   Unspecified retinal break, bilateral
- H33.309   Unspecified retinal break, unspecified eye

☑6th H33.31 Horseshoe tear of retina without detachment
> Operculum of retina without detachment
- H33.311   Horseshoe tear of retina without detachment, right eye
- H33.312   Horseshoe tear of retina without detachment, left eye
- H33.313   Horseshoe tear of retina without detachment, bilateral
- H33.319   Horseshoe tear of retina without detachment, unspecified eye

☑6th H33.32 Round hole of retina without detachment
- H33.321   Round hole, right eye
- H33.322   Round hole, left eye
- H33.323   Round hole, bilateral
- H33.329   Round hole, unspecified eye

☑6th H33.33 Multiple defects of retina without detachment
- H33.331   Multiple defects of retina without detachment, right eye
- H33.332   Multiple defects of retina without detachment, left eye
- H33.333   Multiple defects of retina without detachment, bilateral
- H33.339   Multiple defects of retina without detachment, unspecified eye

☑5th H33.4 Traction detachment of retina
> Proliferative vitreo-retinopathy with retinal detachment
- H33.40   Traction detachment of retina, unspecified eye
- H33.41   Traction detachment of retina, right eye
- H33.42   Traction detachment of retina, left eye
- H33.43   Traction detachment of retina, bilateral

H33.8 Other retinal detachments

☑4th H34 Retinal vascular occlusions
> EXCLUDES 1   amaurosis fugax (G45.3)

☑5th H34.0 Transient retinal artery occlusion
- H34.00   Transient retinal artery occlusion, unspecified eye
- H34.01   Transient retinal artery occlusion, right eye
- H34.02   Transient retinal artery occlusion, left eye
- H34.03   Transient retinal artery occlusion, bilateral

☑5th H34.1 Central retinal artery occlusion
- H34.10   Central retinal artery occlusion, unspecified eye
- H34.11   Central retinal artery occlusion, right eye
- H34.12   Central retinal artery occlusion, left eye
- H34.13   Central retinal artery occlusion, bilateral

☑5th H34.2 Other retinal artery occlusions

☑6th H34.21 Partial retinal artery occlusion
> Hollenhorst's plaque
> Retinal microembolism
- H34.211   Partial retinal artery occlusion, right eye
- H34.212   Partial retinal artery occlusion, left eye
- H34.213   Partial retinal artery occlusion, bilateral
- H34.219   Partial retinal artery occlusion, unspecified eye

☑6th H34.23 Retinal artery branch occlusion
- H34.231   Retinal artery branch occlusion, right eye
- H34.232   Retinal artery branch occlusion, left eye
- H34.233   Retinal artery branch occlusion, bilateral
- H34.239   Retinal artery branch occlusion, unspecified eye

☑5th H34.8 Other retinal vascular occlusions

☑6th H34.81 Central retinal vein occlusion
- H34.811   Central retinal vein occlusion, right eye
- H34.812   Central retinal vein occlusion, left eye
- H34.813   Central retinal vein occlusion, bilateral
- H34.819   Central retinal vein occlusion, unspecified eye

☑6th H34.82 Venous engorgement
> Incipient retinal vein occlusion
> Partial retinal vein occlusion
- H34.821   Venous engorgement, right eye
- H34.822   Venous engorgement, left eye
- H34.823   Venous engorgement, bilateral
- H34.829   Venous engorgement, unspecified eye

☑6th H34.83 Tributary (branch) retinal vein occlusion
- H34.831   Tributary (branch) retinal vein occlusion, right eye
- H34.832   Tributary (branch) retinal vein occlusion, left eye
- H34.833   Tributary (branch) retinal vein occlusion, bilateral
- H34.839   Tributary (branch) retinal vein occlusion, unspecified eye

H34.9 Unspecified retinal vascular occlusion

☑4th H35 Other retinal disorders
> EXCLUDES 2   diabetic retinal disorders (E08.311- E08.359, E09.311- E09.359,
> E10.311- E10.359, E11.311- E11.359, E13.311- E13.359)

☑5th H35.0 Background retinopathy and retinal vascular changes
> Code also any associated hypertension (I10-)
- H35.00   Unspecified background retinopathy

☑6th H35.01 Changes in retinal vascular appearance
> Retinal vascular sheathing
- H35.011   Changes in retinal vascular appearance, right eye
- H35.012   Changes in retinal vascular appearance, left eye
- H35.013   Changes in retinal vascular appearance, bilateral
- H35.019   Changes in retinal vascular appearance, unspecified eye

☑6th H35.02 Exudative retinopathy
> Coats retinopathy
- H35.021   Exudative retinopathy, right eye
- H35.022   Exudative retinopathy, left eye
- H35.023   Exudative retinopathy, bilateral
- H35.029   Exudative retinopathy, unspecified eye

☑6th H35.03 Hypertensive retinopathy
- H35.031   Hypertensive retinopathy, right eye
- H35.032   Hypertensive retinopathy, left eye
- H35.033   Hypertensive retinopathy, bilateral
- H35.039   Hypertensive retinopathy, unspecified eye

☑6th H35.04 Retinal micro-aneurysms, unspecified
- H35.041   Retinal micro-aneurysms, unspecified, right eye
- H35.042   Retinal micro-aneurysms, unspecified, left eye
- H35.043   Retinal micro-aneurysms, unspecified, bilateral
- H35.049   Retinal micro-aneurysms, unspecified, unspecified eye

☑6th H35.05 Retinal neovascularization, unspecified
- H35.051   Retinal neovascularization, unspecified, right eye
- H35.052   Retinal neovascularization, unspecified, left eye
- H35.053   Retinal neovascularization, unspecified, bilateral
- H35.059   Retinal neovascularization, unspecified, unspecified eye

☑6th H35.06 Retinal vasculitis
> Eales disease
> Retinal perivasculitis
- H35.061   Retinal vasculitis, right eye
- H35.062   Retinal vasculitis, left eye
- H35.063   Retinal vasculitis, bilateral
- H35.069   Retinal vasculitis, unspecified eye

☑6th H35.07 Retinal telangiectasis
- H35.071   Retinal telangiectasis, right eye
- H35.072   Retinal telangiectasis, left eye
- H35.073   Retinal telangiectasis, bilateral

EXCLUDES 1   Not coded here   EXCLUDES 2   Not included here   *Manifestation Code*

H35.079   Retinal telangiectasis, unspecified eye
H35.09   **Other intraretinal microvascular abnormalities**
Retinal varices
✓5th   H35.1   **Retinopathy of prematurity**
✓6th   H35.10   **Retinopathy of prematurity, unspecified**
Retinopathy of prematurity NOS
H35.101   **Retinopathy of prematurity, unspecified, right eye**
H35.102   **Retinopathy of prematurity, unspecified, left eye**
H35.103   **Retinopathy of prematurity, unspecified, bilateral**
H35.109   **Retinopathy of prematurity, unspecified, unspecified eye**
✓6th   H35.11   **Retinopathy of prematurity, stage 0**
H35.111   **Retinopathy of prematurity, stage 0, right eye**
H35.112   **Retinopathy of prematurity, stage 0, left eye**
H35.113   **Retinopathy of prematurity, stage 0, bilateral**
H35.119   **Retinopathy of prematurity, stage 0, unspecified eye**
✓6th   H35.12   **Retinopathy of prematurity, stage 1**
H35.121   **Retinopathy of prematurity, stage 1, right eye**
H35.122   **Retinopathy of prematurity, stage 1, left eye**
H35.123   **Retinopathy of prematurity, stage 1, bilateral**
H35.129   **Retinopathy of prematurity, stage 1, unspecified eye**
✓6th   H35.13   **Retinopathy of prematurity, stage 2**
H35.131   **Retinopathy of prematurity, stage 2, right eye**
H35.132   **Retinopathy of prematurity, stage 2, left eye**
H35.133   **Retinopathy of prematurity, stage 2, bilateral**
H35.139   **Retinopathy of prematurity, stage 2, unspecified eye**
✓6th   H35.14   **Retinopathy of prematurity, stage 3**
H35.141   **Retinopathy of prematurity, stage 3, right eye**
H35.142   **Retinopathy of prematurity, stage 3, left eye**
H35.143   **Retinopathy of prematurity, stage 3, bilateral**
H35.149   **Retinopathy of prematurity, stage 3, unspecified eye**
✓6th   H35.15   **Retinopathy of prematurity, stage 4**
H35.151   **Retinopathy of prematurity, stage 4, right eye**
H35.152   **Retinopathy of prematurity, stage 4, left eye**
H35.153   **Retinopathy of prematurity, stage 4, bilateral**
H35.159   **Retinopathy of prematurity, stage 4, unspecified eye**
✓6th   H35.16   **Retinopathy of prematurity, stage 5**
H35.161   **Retinopathy of prematurity, stage 5, right eye**
H35.162   **Retinopathy of prematurity, stage 5, left eye**
H35.163   **Retinopathy of prematurity, stage 5, bilateral**
H35.169   **Retinopathy of prematurity, stage 5, unspecified eye**
✓6th   H35.17   **Retrolental fibroplasia**
H35.171   **Retrolental fibroplasia, right eye**
H35.172   **Retrolental fibroplasia, left eye**
H35.173   **Retrolental fibroplasia, bilateral**
H35.179   **Retrolental fibroplasia, unspecified eye**
✓5th   H35.2   **Other non-diabetic proliferative retinopathy**
Proliferative vitreo-retinopathy
EXCLUDES 1   *proliferative vitreo-retinopathy with retinal detachment (H33.4-)*

H35.20   **Other non-diabetic proliferative retinopathy, unspecified eye**
H35.21   **Other non-diabetic proliferative retinopathy, right eye**
H35.22   **Other non-diabetic proliferative retinopathy, left eye**
H35.23   **Other non-diabetic proliferative retinopathy, bilateral**
✓5th   H35.3   **Degeneration of macula and posterior pole**
H35.30   **Unspecified macular degeneration (age-related)**
H35.31   **Nonexudative age-related macular degeneration**
Atrophic age-related macular degeneration
H35.32   **Exudative age-related macular degeneration**
H35.33   **Angioid streaks of macula**
✓6th   H35.34   **Macular cyst, hole, or pseudohole**
H35.341   **Macular cyst, hole, or pseudohole, right eye**
H35.342   **Macular cyst, hole, or pseudohole, left eye**
H35.343   **Macular cyst, hole, or pseudohole, bilateral**
H35.349   **Macular cyst, hole, or pseudohole, unspecified eye**
✓6th   H35.35   **Cystoid macular degeneration**
EXCLUDES 1   *cystoid macular edema following cataract surgery (H59.03-)*
H35.351   **Cystoid macular degeneration, right eye**
H35.352   **Cystoid macular degeneration, left eye**
H35.353   **Cystoid macular degeneration, bilateral**
H35.359   **Cystoid macular degeneration, unspecified eye**
✓6th   H35.36   **Drusen (degenerative) of macula**
H35.361   **Drusen (degenerative) of macula, right eye**
H35.362   **Drusen (degenerative) of macula, left eye**
H35.363   **Drusen (degenerative) of macula, bilateral**
H35.369   **Drusen (degenerative) of macula, unspecified eye**
✓6th   H35.37   **Puckering of macula**
H35.371   **Puckering of macula, right eye**
H35.372   **Puckering of macula, left eye**
H35.373   **Puckering of macula, bilateral**
H35.379   **Puckering of macula, unspecified eye**
✓6th   H35.38   **Toxic maculopathy**
H35.381   **Toxic maculopathy, right eye**
H35.382   **Toxic maculopathy, left eye**
H35.383   **Toxic maculopathy, bilateral**
H35.389   **Toxic maculopathy, unspecified eye**
✓5th   H35.4   **Peripheral retinal degeneration**
EXCLUDES 1   *hereditary retinal degeneration (dystrophy) (H35.5-)*
peripheral retinal degeneration with retinal break (H33.3-)
H35.40   **Unspecified peripheral retinal degeneration**
✓6th   H35.41   **Lattice degeneration of retina**
Palisade degeneration of retina
H35.411   **Lattice degeneration of retina, right eye**
H35.412   **Lattice degeneration of retina, left eye**
H35.413   **Lattice degeneration of retina, bilateral**
H35.419   **Lattice degeneration of retina, unspecified eye**
✓6th   H35.42   **Microcystoid degeneration of retina**
H35.421   **Microcystoid degeneration of retina, right eye**
H35.422   **Microcystoid degeneration of retina, left eye**
H35.423   **Microcystoid degeneration of retina, bilateral**
H35.429   **Microcystoid degeneration of retina, unspecified eye**
✓6th   H35.43   **Paving stone degeneration of retina**
H35.431   **Paving stone degeneration of retina, right eye**
H35.432   **Paving stone degeneration of retina, left eye**

☑ Appropriate additional character required   ✓x7th Requires 7th character, placeholder x must fill empty characters

H35.433 Paving stone degeneration of retina, bilateral

H35.439 Paving stone degeneration of retina, unspecified eye

✓6th **H35.44** Age-related reticular degeneration of retina

    H35.441 Age-related reticular degeneration of retina, right eye

    H35.442 Age-related reticular degeneration of retina, left eye

    H35.443 Age-related reticular degeneration of retina, bilateral

    H35.449 Age-related reticular degeneration of retina, unspecified eye

✓6th **H35.45** Secondary pigmentary degeneration

    H35.451 Secondary pigmentary degeneration, right eye

    H35.452 Secondary pigmentary degeneration, left eye

    H35.453 Secondary pigmentary degeneration, bilateral

    H35.459 Secondary pigmentary degeneration, unspecified eye

✓6th **H35.46** Secondary vitreoretinal degeneration

    H35.461 Secondary vitreoretinal degeneration, right eye

    H35.462 Secondary vitreoretinal degeneration, left eye

    H35.463 Secondary vitreoretinal degeneration, bilateral

    H35.469 Secondary vitreoretinal degeneration, unspecified eye

✓5th **H35.5** Hereditary retinal dystrophy

    EXCLUDES 1   dystrophies primarily involving Bruch's membrane (H31.1-)

    H35.50 Unspecified hereditary retinal dystrophy

    H35.51 Vitreoretinal dystrophy

    H35.52 Pigmentary retinal dystrophy

        Albipunctate retinal dystrophy

        Retinitis pigmentosa

        Tapetoretinal dystrophy

    H35.53 Other dystrophies primarily involving the sensory retina

        Stargardt's disease

    H35.54 Dystrophies primarily involving the retinal pigment epithelium

        Vitelliform retinal dystrophy

✓5th **H35.6** Retinal hemorrhage

    H35.60 Retinal hemorrhage, unspecified eye

    H35.61 Retinal hemorrhage, right eye

    H35.62 Retinal hemorrhage, left eye

    H35.63 Retinal hemorrhage, bilateral

✓5th **H35.7** Separation of retinal layers

    EXCLUDES 1   retinal detachment (serous) (H33.2-)

                rhegmatogenous retinal detachment (H33.0-)

    H35.70 Unspecified separation of retinal layers

✓6th **H35.71** Central serous chorioretinopathy

    H35.711 Central serous chorioretinopathy, right eye

    H35.712 Central serous chorioretinopathy, left eye

    H35.713 Central serous chorioretinopathy, bilateral

    H35.719 Central serous chorioretinopathy, unspecified eye

✓6th **H35.72** Serous detachment of retinal pigment epithelium

    H35.721 Serous detachment of retinal pigment epithelium, right eye

    H35.722 Serous detachment of retinal pigment epithelium, left eye

    H35.723 Serous detachment of retinal pigment epithelium, bilateral

    H35.729 Serous detachment of retinal pigment epithelium, unspecified eye

✓6th **H35.73** Hemorrhagic detachment of retinal pigment epithelium

    H35.731 Hemorrhagic detachment of retinal pigment epithelium, right eye

H35.732 Hemorrhagic detachment of retinal pigment epithelium, left eye

H35.733 Hemorrhagic detachment of retinal pigment epithelium, bilateral

H35.739 Hemorrhagic detachment of retinal pigment epithelium, unspecified eye

✓5th **H35.8** Other specified retinal disorders

    EXCLUDES 2   retinal hemorrhage (H35.6-)

    H35.81 Retinal edema

        Retinal cotton wool spots

    H35.82 Retinal ischemia

    H35.89 Other specified retinal disorders

    H35.9 Unspecified retinal disorder

H36 **Retinal disorders in diseases classified elsewhere**

    Code first underlying disease, such as:

        lipid storage disorders (E75-)

        sickle-cell disorders (D57-)

    EXCLUDES 1   arteriosclerotic retinopathy (H35.0-)

                diabetic retinopathy (E08.3-, E09.3-, E10.3-, E11.3-, E13.3-)

Glaucoma (H40-H42)

✓4th **H40** Glaucoma

    EXCLUDES 1   absolute glaucoma (H44.51-)

                congenital glaucoma (Q15.0)

                traumatic glaucoma due to birth injury (P15.3)

    H40.0 Glaucoma suspect

        Ocular hypertension

✓5th **H40.1** Open-angle glaucoma

    H40.10 Unspecified open-angle glaucoma

    H40.11 Primary open-angle glaucoma

        Chronic simple glaucoma

    ✓6th **H40.12** Low-tension glaucoma

        H40.121 Low-tension glaucoma, right eye

        H40.122 Low-tension glaucoma, left eye

        H40.123 Low-tension glaucoma, bilateral

        H40.129 Low-tension glaucoma, unspecified eye

    ✓6th **H40.13** Pigmentary glaucoma

        H40.131 Pigmentary glaucoma, right eye

        H40.132 Pigmentary glaucoma, left eye

        H40.133 Pigmentary glaucoma, bilateral

        H40.139 Pigmentary glaucoma, unspecified eye

    ✓6th **H40.14** Capsular glaucoma with pseudoexfoliation of lens

        H40.141 Capsular glaucoma with pseudoexfoliation of lens, right eye

        H40.142 Capsular glaucoma with pseudoexfoliation of lens, left eye

        H40.143 Capsular glaucoma with pseudoexfoliation of lens, bilateral

        H40.149 Capsular glaucoma with pseudoexfoliation of lens, unspecified eye

    ✓6th **H40.15** Residual stage of open-angle glaucoma

        H40.151 Residual stage of open-angle glaucoma, right eye

        H40.152 Residual stage of open-angle glaucoma, left eye

        H40.153 Residual stage of open-angle glaucoma, bilateral

        H40.159 Residual stage of open-angle glaucoma, unspecified eye

✓5th **H40.2** Primary angle-closure glaucoma

    EXCLUDES 1   aqueous misdirection (H40.83-)

                malignant glaucoma (H40.83-)

    H40.20 Unspecified primary angle-closure glaucoma

    ✓6th **H40.21** Acute angle-closure glaucoma

        H40.211 Acute angle-closure glaucoma, right eye

        H40.212 Acute angle-closure glaucoma, left eye

        H40.213 Acute angle-closure glaucoma, bilateral

        H40.219 Acute angle-closure glaucoma, unspecified eye

    ✓6th **H40.22** Chronic angle-closure glaucoma

        H40.221 Chronic angle-closure glaucoma, right eye

        H40.222 Chronic angle-closure glaucoma, left eye

EXCLUDES 1   Not coded here   *EXCLUDES 2*   Not included here   *Manifestation Code*

        H40.223 **Chronic angle-closure glaucoma, bilateral**
        H40.229 **Chronic angle-closure glaucoma, unspecified eye**
    ✓6ᵗʰ H40.23 **Intermittent angle-closure glaucoma**
        H40.231 **Intermittent angle-closure glaucoma, right eye**
        H40.232 **Intermittent angle-closure glaucoma, left eye**
        H40.233 **Intermittent angle-closure glaucoma, bilateral**
        H40.239 **Intermittent angle-closure glaucoma, unspecified eye**
    ✓6ᵗʰ H40.24 **Residual stage of angle-closure glaucoma**
        H40.241 **Residual stage of angle-closure glaucoma, right eye**
        H40.242 **Residual stage of angle-closure glaucoma, left eye**
        H40.243 **Residual stage of angle-closure glaucoma, bilateral**
        H40.249 **Residual stage of angle-closure glaucoma, unspecified eye**
  ✓5ᵗʰ H40.3 **Glaucoma secondary to eye trauma**
      Code also underlying condition
      H40.30 **Glaucoma secondary to eye trauma, unspecified eye**
      H40.31 **Glaucoma secondary to eye trauma, right eye**
      H40.32 **Glaucoma secondary to eye trauma, left eye**
      H40.33 **Glaucoma secondary to eye trauma, bilateral**
  ✓5ᵗʰ H40.4 **Glaucoma secondary to eye inflammation**
      Code also underlying condition
      H40.40 **Glaucoma secondary to eye inflammation, unspecified eye**
      H40.41 **Glaucoma secondary to eye inflammation, right eye**
      H40.42 **Glaucoma secondary to eye inflammation, left eye**
      H40.43 **Glaucoma secondary to eye inflammation, bilateral**
  ✓5ᵗʰ H40.5 **Glaucoma secondary to other eye disorders**
      Code also underlying eye disorder
      H40.50 **Glaucoma secondary to other eye disorders, unspecified eye**
      H40.51 **Glaucoma secondary to other eye disorders, right eye**
      H40.52 **Glaucoma secondary to other eye disorders, left eye**
      H40.53 **Glaucoma secondary to other eye disorders, bilateral**
  ✓5ᵗʰ H40.6 **Glaucoma secondary to drugs**
      Code first (T36-T50) to identify drug
      H40.60 **Glaucoma secondary to drugs, unspecified eye**
      H40.61 **Glaucoma secondary to drugs, right eye**
      H40.62 **Glaucoma secondary to drugs, left eye**
      H40.63 **Glaucoma secondary to drugs, bilateral**
  ✓5ᵗʰ H40.8 **Other glaucoma**
    ✓6ᵗʰ H40.81 **Glaucoma with increased episcleral venous pressure**
        H40.811 **Glaucoma with increased episcleral venous pressure, right eye**
        H40.812 **Glaucoma with increased episcleral venous pressure, left eye**
        H40.813 **Glaucoma with increased episcleral venous pressure, bilateral**
        H40.819 **Glaucoma with increased episcleral venous pressure, unspecified eye**
    ✓6ᵗʰ H40.82 **Hypersecretion glaucoma**
        H40.821 **Hypersecretion glaucoma, right eye**
        H40.822 **Hypersecretion glaucoma, left eye**
        H40.823 **Hypersecretion glaucoma, bilateral**
        H40.829 **Hypersecretion glaucoma, unspecified eye**
    ✓6ᵗʰ H40.83 **Aqueous misdirection**
      Malignant glaucoma
        H40.831 **Aqueous misdirection, right eye**
        H40.832 **Aqueous misdirection, left eye**
        H40.833 **Aqueous misdirection, bilateral**
        H40.839 **Aqueous misdirection, unspecified eye**

      H40.89 **Other specified glaucoma**
  H40.9 **Unspecified glaucoma**
H42 *Glaucoma in diseases classified elsewhere*
    Code first underlying condition, such as:
      amyloidosis (E85-)
      aniridia (Q13.1)
      Lowe's syndrome (E72.03)
      Reiger's anomaly (Q13.81)
      specified metabolic disorder (E70-E88)
    EXCLUDES 1 *glaucoma (in):*
      diabetes mellitus (E08.39, E09.39, E10.39, E11.39, E13.39)
      onchocerciasis (B73.02)
      syphilis (A52.71)
      tuberculous (A18.59)

Disorders of vitreous body and globe (H43-H44)

✓4ᵗʰ **H43** **Disorders of vitreous body**
  ✓5ᵗʰ **H43.0** **Vitreous prolapse**
      EXCLUDES 1 *vitreous syndrome following cataract surgery (H59.0-)*
        traumatic vitreous prolapse (S05.2-)
      H43.00 **Vitreous prolapse, unspecified eye**
      H43.01 **Vitreous prolapse, right eye**
      H43.02 **Vitreous prolapse, left eye**
      H43.03 **Vitreous prolapse, bilateral**
  ✓5ᵗʰ **H43.1** **Vitreous hemorrhage**
      H43.10 **Vitreous hemorrhage, unspecified eye**
      H43.11 **Vitreous hemorrhage, right eye**
      H43.12 **Vitreous hemorrhage, left eye**
      H43.13 **Vitreous hemorrhage, bilateral**
  ✓5ᵗʰ **H43.2** **Crystalline deposits in vitreous body**
      H43.20 **Crystalline deposits in vitreous body, unspecified eye**
      H43.21 **Crystalline deposits in vitreous body, right eye**
      H43.22 **Crystalline deposits in vitreous body, left eye**
      H43.23 **Crystalline deposits in vitreous body, bilateral**
  ✓5ᵗʰ **H43.3** **Other vitreous opacities**
    ✓6ᵗʰ H43.31 **Vitreous membranes and strands**
        H43.311 **Vitreous membranes and strands, right eye**
        H43.312 **Vitreous membranes and strands, left eye**
        H43.313 **Vitreous membranes and strands, bilateral**
        H43.319 **Vitreous membranes and strands, unspecified eye**
    ✓6ᵗʰ H43.39 **Other vitreous opacities**
      Vitreous floaters
        H43.391 **Other vitreous opacities, right eye**
        H43.392 **Other vitreous opacities, left eye**
        H43.393 **Other vitreous opacities, bilateral**
        H43.399 **Other vitreous opacities, unspecified eye**
  ✓5ᵗʰ **H43.8** **Other disorders of vitreous body**
      EXCLUDES 1 *proliferative vitreo-retinopathy with retinal detachment (H33.4-)*
      EXCLUDES 2 *vitreous abscess (H44.02-)*
    ✓6ᵗʰ H43.81 **Vitreous degeneration**
      Vitreous detachment
        H43.811 **Vitreous degeneration, right eye**
        H43.812 **Vitreous degeneration, left eye**
        H43.813 **Vitreous degeneration, bilateral**
        H43.819 **Vitreous degeneration, unspecified eye**
      H43.89 **Other disorders of vitreous body**
    H43.9 **Unspecified disorder of vitreous body**
✓4ᵗʰ **H44** **Disorders of globe**
    INCLUDES disorders affecting multiple structures of eye
  ✓5ᵗʰ **H44.0** **Purulent endophthalmitis**
      Use additional code to identify organism
      EXCLUDES 1 *bleb associated endophthalmitis (H59.4-)*
    ✓6ᵗʰ H44.00 **Unspecified purulent endophthalmitis**
        H44.001 **Unspecified purulent endophthalmitis, right eye**
        H44.002 **Unspecified purulent endophthalmitis, left eye**

☑ Appropriate additional character required   ✓x7ᵗʰ Requires 7th character, placeholder x must fill empty characters

H44.003 Unspecified purulent endophthalmitis, bilateral

H44.009 Unspecified purulent endophthalmitis, unspecified eye

√6th **H44.01 Panophthalmitis (acute)**

    H44.011 Panophthalmitis (acute), right eye

    H44.012 Panophthalmitis (acute), left eye

    H44.013 Panophthalmitis (acute), bilateral

    H44.019 Panophthalmitis (acute), unspecified eye

√6th **H44.02 Vitreous abscess (chronic)**

    H44.021 Vitreous abscess (chronic), right eye

    H44.022 Vitreous abscess (chronic), left eye

    H44.023 Vitreous abscess (chronic), bilateral

    H44.029 Vitreous abscess (chronic), unspecified eye

√5th **H44.1 Other endophthalmitis**

    EXCLUDES 1 *bleb associated endophthalmitis (H59.4-)*

    EXCLUDES 2 *ophthalmia nodosa (H16.2-)*

√6th **H44.11 Panuveitis**

    H44.111 Panuveitis, right eye

    H44.112 Panuveitis, left eye

    H44.113 Panuveitis, bilateral

    H44.119 Panuveitis, unspecified eye

√6th **H44.12 Parasitic endophthalmitis, unspecified**

    H44.121 Parasitic endophthalmitis, unspecified, right eye

    H44.122 Parasitic endophthalmitis, unspecified, left eye

    H44.123 Parasitic endophthalmitis, unspecified, bilateral

    H44.129 Parasitic endophthalmitis, unspecified, unspecified eye

√6th **H44.13 Sympathetic uveitis**

    H44.131 Sympathetic uveitis, right eye

    H44.132 Sympathetic uveitis, left eye

    H44.133 Sympathetic uveitis, bilateral

    H44.139 Sympathetic uveitis, unspecified eye

    H44.19 Other endophthalmitis

√5th **H44.2 Degenerative myopia**

    Malignant myopia

    H44.20 Degenerative myopia, unspecified eye

    H44.21 Degenerative myopia, right eye

    H44.22 Degenerative myopia, left eye

    H44.23 Degenerative myopia, bilateral

√5th **H44.3 Other and unspecified degenerative disorders of globe**

    H44.30 Unspecified degenerative disorder of globe

√6th **H44.31 Chalcosis**

    H44.311 Chalcosis, right eye

    H44.312 Chalcosis, left eye

    H44.313 Chalcosis, bilateral

    H44.319 Chalcosis, unspecified eye

√6th **H44.32 Siderosis of eye**

    H44.321 Siderosis of eye, right eye

    H44.322 Siderosis of eye, left eye

    H44.323 Siderosis of eye, bilateral

    H44.329 Siderosis of eye, unspecified eye

√6th **H44.39 Other degenerative disorders of globe**

    H44.391 Other degenerative disorders of globe, right eye

    H44.392 Other degenerative disorders of globe, left eye

    H44.393 Other degenerative disorders of globe, bilateral

    H44.399 Other degenerative disorders of globe, unspecified eye

√5th **H44.4 Hypotony of eye**

    H44.40 Unspecified hypotony of eye

√6th **H44.41 Flat anterior chamber hypotony of eye**

    H44.411 Flat anterior chamber hypotony of right eye

    H44.412 Flat anterior chamber hypotony of left eye

    H44.413 Flat anterior chamber hypotony of eye, bilateral

H44.419 Flat anterior chamber hypotony of unspecified eye

√6th **H44.42 Hypotony of eye due to ocular fistula**

    H44.421 Hypotony of right eye due to ocular fistula

    H44.422 Hypotony of left eye due to ocular fistula

    H44.423 Hypotony of eye due to ocular fistula, bilateral

    H44.429 Hypotony of unspecified eye due to ocular fistula

√6th **H44.43 Hypotony of eye due to other ocular disorders**

    H44.431 Hypotony of eye due to other ocular disorders, right eye

    H44.432 Hypotony of eye due to other ocular disorders, left eye

    H44.433 Hypotony of eye due to other ocular disorders, bilateral

    H44.439 Hypotony of eye due to other ocular disorders, unspecified eye

√6th **H44.44 Primary hypotony of eye**

    H44.441 Primary hypotony of right eye

    H44.442 Primary hypotony of left eye

    H44.443 Primary hypotony of eye, bilateral

    H44.449 Primary hypotony of unspecified eye

√5th **H44.5 Degenerated conditions of globe**

    H44.50 Unspecified degenerated conditions of globe

√6th **H44.51 Absolute glaucoma**

    H44.511 Absolute glaucoma, right eye

    H44.512 Absolute glaucoma, left eye

    H44.513 Absolute glaucoma, bilateral

    H44.519 Absolute glaucoma, unspecified eye

√6th **H44.52 Atrophy of globe**

    Phthisis bulbi

    H44.521 Atrophy of globe, right eye

    H44.522 Atrophy of globe, left eye

    H44.523 Atrophy of globe, bilateral

    H44.529 Atrophy of globe, unspecified eye

√6th **H44.53 Leucocoria**

    H44.531 Leucocoria, right eye

    H44.532 Leucocoria, left eye

    H44.533 Leucocoria, bilateral

    H44.539 Leucocoria, unspecified eye

√5th **H44.6 Retained (old) intraocular foreign body, magnetic**

    Use additional code to identify magnetic foreign body (Z18.11)

    EXCLUDES 1 *current intraocular foreign body (S05-)*

    EXCLUDES 2 *retained foreign body in eyelid (H02.81-)*

        retained (old) foreign body following penetrating wound of orbit (H05.5-)

        retained (old) intraocular foreign body, nonmagnetic (H44.7-)

√6th **H44.60 Unspecified retained (old) intraocular foreign body, magnetic**

    H44.601 Unspecified retained (old) intraocular foreign body, magnetic, right eye

    H44.602 Unspecified retained (old) intraocular foreign body, magnetic, left eye

    H44.603 Unspecified retained (old) intraocular foreign body, magnetic, bilateral

    H44.609 Unspecified retained (old) intraocular foreign body, magnetic, unspecified eye

√6th **H44.61 Retained (old) magnetic foreign body in anterior chamber**

    H44.611 Retained (old) magnetic foreign body in anterior chamber, right eye

    H44.612 Retained (old) magnetic foreign body in anterior chamber, left eye

    H44.613 Retained (old) magnetic foreign body in anterior chamber, bilateral

    H44.619 Retained (old) magnetic foreign body in anterior chamber, unspecified eye

√6th **H44.62 Retained (old) magnetic foreign body in iris or ciliary body**

    H44.621 Retained (old) magnetic foreign body in iris or ciliary body, right eye

---

H44.622 Retained (old) magnetic foreign body in iris or ciliary body, left eye

H44.623 Retained (old) magnetic foreign body in iris or ciliary body, bilateral

H44.629 Retained (old) magnetic foreign body in iris or ciliary body, unspecified eye

✓6th **H44.63** Retained (old) magnetic foreign body in lens

H44.631 Retained (old) magnetic foreign body in lens, right eye

H44.632 Retained (old) magnetic foreign body in lens, left eye

H44.633 Retained (old) magnetic foreign body in lens, bilateral

H44.639 Retained (old) magnetic foreign body in lens, unspecified eye

✓6th **H44.64** Retained (old) magnetic foreign body in posterior wall of globe

H44.641 Retained (old) magnetic foreign body in posterior wall of globe, right eye

H44.642 Retained (old) magnetic foreign body in posterior wall of globe, left eye

H44.643 Retained (old) magnetic foreign body in posterior wall of globe, bilateral

H44.649 Retained (old) magnetic foreign body in posterior wall of globe, unspecified eye

✓6th **H44.65** Retained (old) magnetic foreign body in vitreous body

H44.651 Retained (old) magnetic foreign body in vitreous body, right eye

H44.652 Retained (old) magnetic foreign body in vitreous body, left eye

H44.653 Retained (old) magnetic foreign body in vitreous body, bilateral

H44.659 Retained (old) magnetic foreign body in vitreous body, unspecified eye

✓6th **H44.69** Retained (old) intraocular foreign body, magnetic, in other or multiple sites

H44.691 Retained (old) intraocular foreign body, magnetic, in other or multiple sites, right eye

H44.692 Retained (old) intraocular foreign body, magnetic, in other or multiple sites, left eye

H44.693 Retained (old) intraocular foreign body, magnetic, in other or multiple sites, bilateral

H44.699 Retained (old) intraocular foreign body, magnetic, in other or multiple sites, unspecified eye

✓5th **H44.7** Retained (old) intraocular foreign body, nonmagnetic

Use additional code to identify nonmagnetic foreign body (Z18.01-Z18.10, Z18.12, Z18.2-Z18.9)

EXCLUDES 1 *current intraocular foreign body (S05-)*

EXCLUDES 2 *retained foreign body in eyelid (H02.81-)*

retained (old) foreign body following penetrating wound of orbit (H05.5-)

retained (old) intraocular foreign body, magnetic (H44.6-)

✓6th **H44.70** Unspecified retained (old) intraocular foreign body, nonmagnetic

H44.701 Unspecified retained (old) intraocular foreign body, nonmagnetic, right eye

H44.702 Unspecified retained (old) intraocular foreign body, nonmagnetic, left eye

H44.703 Unspecified retained (old) intraocular foreign body, nonmagnetic, bilateral

H44.709 Unspecified retained (old) intraocular foreign body, nonmagnetic, unspecified eye

Retained (old) intraocular foreign body NOS

✓6th **H44.71** Retained (nonmagnetic) (old) foreign body in anterior chamber

H44.711 Retained (nonmagnetic) (old) foreign body in anterior chamber, right eye

H44.712 Retained (nonmagnetic) (old) foreign body in anterior chamber, left eye

H44.713 Retained (nonmagnetic) (old) foreign body in anterior chamber, bilateral

H44.719 Retained (nonmagnetic) (old) foreign body in anterior chamber, unspecified eye

✓6th **H44.72** Retained (nonmagnetic) (old) foreign body in iris or ciliary body

H44.721 Retained (nonmagnetic) (old) foreign body in iris or ciliary body, right eye

H44.722 Retained (nonmagnetic) (old) foreign body in iris or ciliary body, left eye

H44.723 Retained (nonmagnetic) (old) foreign body in iris or ciliary body, bilateral

H44.729 Retained (nonmagnetic) (old) foreign body in iris or ciliary body, unspecified eye

✓6th **H44.73** Retained (nonmagnetic) (old) foreign body in lens

H44.731 Retained (nonmagnetic) (old) foreign body in lens, right eye

H44.732 Retained (nonmagnetic) (old) foreign body in lens, left eye

H44.733 Retained (nonmagnetic) (old) foreign body in lens, bilateral

H44.739 Retained (nonmagnetic) (old) foreign body in lens, unspecified eye

✓6th **H44.74** Retained (nonmagnetic) (old) foreign body in posterior wall of globe

H44.741 Retained (nonmagnetic) (old) foreign body in posterior wall of globe, right eye

H44.742 Retained (nonmagnetic) (old) foreign body in posterior wall of globe, left eye

H44.743 Retained (nonmagnetic) (old) foreign body in posterior wall of globe, bilateral

H44.749 Retained (nonmagnetic) (old) foreign body in posterior wall of globe, unspecified eye

✓6th **H44.75** Retained (nonmagnetic) (old) foreign body in vitreous body

H44.751 Retained (nonmagnetic) (old) foreign body in vitreous body, right eye

H44.752 Retained (nonmagnetic) (old) foreign body in vitreous body, left eye

H44.753 Retained (nonmagnetic) (old) foreign body in vitreous body, bilateral

H44.759 Retained (nonmagnetic) (old) foreign body in vitreous body, unspecified eye

✓6th **H44.79** Retained (old) intraocular foreign body, nonmagnetic, in other or multiple sites

H44.791 Retained (old) intraocular foreign body, nonmagnetic, in other or multiple sites, right eye

H44.792 Retained (old) intraocular foreign body, nonmagnetic, in other or multiple sites, left eye

H44.793 Retained (old) intraocular foreign body, nonmagnetic, in other or multiple sites, bilateral

H44.799 Retained (old) intraocular foreign body, nonmagnetic, in other or multiple sites, unspecified eye

✓5th **H44.8** Other disorders of globe

✓6th **H44.81** Hemophthalmos

H44.811 Hemophthalmos, right eye

H44.812 Hemophthalmos, left eye

H44.813 Hemophthalmos, bilateral

H44.819 Hemophthalmos, unspecified eye

✓6th **H44.82** Luxation of globe

H44.821 Luxation of globe, right eye

H44.822 Luxation of globe, left eye

H44.823 Luxation of globe, bilateral

H44.829 Luxation of globe, unspecified eye

H44.89 Other disorders of globe

H44.9 Unspecified disorder of globe

✔ Appropriate additional character required   ✓x7th Requires 7th character, placeholder x must fill empty characters

Disorders of optic nerve and visual pathways (H46-H47)

☑4ᵗʰ **H46 Optic neuritis**
> EXCLUDES 2   ischemic optic neuropathy (H47.01-)
> neuromyelitis optica [Devic] (G36.0)

☑5ᵗʰ **H46.0 Optic papillitis**
- **H46.00 Optic papillitis, unspecified eye**
- **H46.01 Optic papillitis, right eye**
- **H46.02 Optic papillitis, left eye**
- **H46.03 Optic papillitis, bilateral**

☑5ᵗʰ **H46.1 Retrobulbar neuritis**
> Retrobulbar neuritis NOS
> EXCLUDES 1   syphilitic retrobulbar neuritis (A52.15)
- **H46.10 Retrobulbar neuritis, unspecified eye**
- **H46.11 Retrobulbar neuritis, right eye**
- **H46.12 Retrobulbar neuritis, left eye**
- **H46.13 Retrobulbar neuritis, bilateral**

H46.2 Nutritional optic neuropathy

H46.3 Toxic optic neuropathy
> Code first (T51-T65) to identify cause

H46.8 Other optic neuritis

H46.9 Unspecified optic neuritis

☑4ᵗʰ **H47 Other disorders of optic [2nd] nerve and visual pathways**

☑5ᵗʰ **H47.0 Disorders of optic nerve, not elsewhere classified**

☑6ᵗʰ **H47.01 Ischemic optic neuropathy**
- **H47.011 Ischemic optic neuropathy, right eye**
- **H47.012 Ischemic optic neuropathy, left eye**
- **H47.013 Ischemic optic neuropathy, bilateral**
- **H47.019 Ischemic optic neuropathy, unspecified eye**

☑6ᵗʰ **H47.02 Hemorrhage in optic nerve sheath**
- **H47.021 Hemorrhage in optic nerve sheath, right eye**
- **H47.022 Hemorrhage in optic nerve sheath, left eye**
- **H47.023 Hemorrhage in optic nerve sheath, bilateral**
- **H47.029 Hemorrhage in optic nerve sheath, unspecified eye**

☑6ᵗʰ **H47.03 Optic nerve hypoplasia**
- **H47.031 Optic nerve hypoplasia, right eye**
- **H47.032 Optic nerve hypoplasia, left eye**
- **H47.033 Optic nerve hypoplasia, bilateral**
- **H47.039 Optic nerve hypoplasia, unspecified eye**

☑6ᵗʰ **H47.09 Other disorders of optic nerve, not elsewhere classified**
> Compression of optic nerve
- **H47.091 Other disorders of optic nerve, not elsewhere classified, right eye**
- **H47.092 Other disorders of optic nerve, not elsewhere classified, left eye**
- **H47.093 Other disorders of optic nerve, not elsewhere classified, bilateral**
- **H47.099 Other disorders of optic nerve, not elsewhere classified, unspecified eye**

☑5ᵗʰ **H47.1 Papilledema**
- **H47.10 Unspecified papilledema**
- **H47.11 Papilledema associated with increased intracranial pressure**
- **H47.12 Papilledema associated with decreased ocular pressure**
- **H47.13 Papilledema associated with retinal disorder**

☑6ᵗʰ **H47.14 Foster-Kennedy syndrome**
- **H47.141 Foster-Kennedy syndrome, right eye**
- **H47.142 Foster-Kennedy syndrome, left eye**
- **H47.143 Foster-Kennedy syndrome, bilateral**
- **H47.149 Foster-Kennedy syndrome, unspecified eye**

☑5ᵗʰ **H47.2 Optic atrophy**
- **H47.20 Unspecified optic atrophy**

☑6ᵗʰ **H47.21 Primary optic atrophy**
- **H47.211 Primary optic atrophy, right eye**
- **H47.212 Primary optic atrophy, left eye**
- **H47.213 Primary optic atrophy, bilateral**
- **H47.219 Primary optic atrophy, unspecified eye**

H47.22 Hereditary optic atrophy
> Leber's optic atrophy

☑6ᵗʰ **H47.23 Glaucomatous optic atrophy**
- **H47.231 Glaucomatous optic atrophy, right eye**
- **H47.232 Glaucomatous optic atrophy, left eye**
- **H47.233 Glaucomatous optic atrophy, bilateral**
- **H47.239 Glaucomatous optic atrophy, unspecified eye**

☑6ᵗʰ **H47.29 Other optic atrophy**
> Temporal pallor of optic disc
- **H47.291 Other optic atrophy, right eye**
- **H47.292 Other optic atrophy, left eye**
- **H47.293 Other optic atrophy, bilateral**
- **H47.299 Other optic atrophy, unspecified eye**

☑5ᵗʰ **H47.3 Other disorders of optic disc**

☑6ᵗʰ **H47.31 Coloboma of optic disc**
- **H47.311 Coloboma of optic disc, right eye**
- **H47.312 Coloboma of optic disc, left eye**
- **H47.313 Coloboma of optic disc, bilateral**
- **H47.319 Coloboma of optic disc, unspecified eye**

☑6ᵗʰ **H47.32 Drusen of optic disc**
- **H47.321 Drusen of optic disc, right eye**
- **H47.322 Drusen of optic disc, left eye**
- **H47.323 Drusen of optic disc, bilateral**
- **H47.329 Drusen of optic disc, unspecified eye**

☑6ᵗʰ **H47.33 Pseudopapilledema of optic disc**
- **H47.331 Pseudopapilledema of optic disc, right eye**
- **H47.332 Pseudopapilledema of optic disc, left eye**
- **H47.333 Pseudopapilledema of optic disc, bilateral**
- **H47.339 Pseudopapilledema of optic disc, unspecified eye**

☑6ᵗʰ **H47.39 Other disorders of optic disc**
- **H47.391 Other disorders of optic disc, right eye**
- **H47.392 Other disorders of optic disc, left eye**
- **H47.393 Other disorders of optic disc, bilateral**
- **H47.399 Other disorders of optic disc, unspecified eye**

☑5ᵗʰ **H47.4 Disorders of optic chiasm**
> Code also underlying condition
- **H47.41 Disorders of optic chiasm in (due to) inflammatory disorders**
- **H47.42 Disorders of optic chiasm in (due to) neoplasm**
- **H47.43 Disorders of optic chiasm in (due to) vascular disorders**
- **H47.49 Disorders of optic chiasm in (due to) other disorders**

☑5ᵗʰ **H47.5 Disorders of other visual pathways**
> Disorders of optic tracts, geniculate nuclei and optic radiations
> Code also underlying condition

☑6ᵗʰ **H47.51 Disorders of visual pathways in (due to) inflammatory disorders**
- **H47.511 Disorders of visual pathways in (due to) inflammatory disorders, right side**
- **H47.512 Disorders of visual pathways in (due to) inflammatory disorders, left side**
- **H47.519 Disorders of visual pathways in (due to) inflammatory disorders, unspecified side**

☑6ᵗʰ **H47.52 Disorders of visual pathways in (due to) neoplasm**
- **H47.521 Disorders of visual pathways in (due to) neoplasm, right side**
- **H47.522 Disorders of visual pathways in (due to) neoplasm, left side**
- **H47.529 Disorders of visual pathways in (due to) neoplasm, unspecified side**

☑6ᵗʰ **H47.53 Disorders of visual pathways in (due to) vascular disorders**
- **H47.531 Disorders of visual pathways in (due to) vascular disorders, right side**
- **H47.532 Disorders of visual pathways in (due to) vascular disorders, left side**
- **H47.539 Disorders of visual pathways in (due to) vascular disorders, unspecified side**

EXCLUDES 1   Not coded here   EXCLUDES 2   Not included here   *Manifestation Code*

☑5ᵗʰ H47.6   Disorders of visual cortex
Code also underlying condition
EXCLUDES 1   injury to visual cortex S04.04

☑6ᵗʰ H47.61   Cortical blindness
H47.611   Cortical blindness, right side of brain
H47.612   Cortical blindness, left side of brain
H47.619   Cortical blindness, unspecified side of brain

☑6ᵗʰ H47.62   Disorders of visual cortex in (due to) inflammatory disorders
H47.621   Disorders of visual cortex in (due to) inflammatory disorders, right side of brain
H47.622   Disorders of visual cortex in (due to) inflammatory disorders, left side of brain
H47.629   Disorders of visual cortex in (due to) inflammatory disorders, unspecified side of brain

☑6ᵗʰ H47.63   Disorders of visual cortex in (due to) neoplasm
H47.631   Disorders of visual cortex in (due to) neoplasm, right side of brain
H47.632   Disorders of visual cortex in (due to) neoplasm, left side of brain
H47.639   Disorders of visual cortex in (due to) neoplasm, unspecified side of brain

☑6ᵗʰ H47.64   Disorders of visual cortex in (due to) vascular disorders
H47.641   Disorders of visual cortex in (due to) vascular disorders, right side of brain
H47.642   Disorders of visual cortex in (due to) vascular disorders, left side of brain
H47.649   Disorders of visual cortex in (due to) vascular disorders, unspecified side of brain

H47.9   Unspecified disorder of visual pathways

Disorders of ocular muscles, binocular movement, accommodation and refraction (H49-H52)
EXCLUDES 2   nystagmus and other irregular eye movements (H55)

☑4ᵗʰ H49   Paralytic strabismus
EXCLUDES 2   internal ophthalmoplegia (H52.51-)
internuclear ophthalmoplegia (H51.2-)
progressive supranuclear ophthalmoplegia (G23.1)

☑5ᵗʰ H49.0   Third [oculomotor] nerve palsy
H49.00   Third [oculomotor] nerve palsy, unspecified eye
H49.01   Third [oculomotor] nerve palsy, right eye
H49.02   Third [oculomotor] nerve palsy, left eye
H49.03   Third [oculomotor] nerve palsy, bilateral

☑5ᵗʰ H49.1   Fourth [trochlear] nerve palsy
H49.10   Fourth [trochlear] nerve palsy, unspecified eye
H49.11   Fourth [trochlear] nerve palsy, right eye
H49.12   Fourth [trochlear] nerve palsy, left eye
H49.13   Fourth [trochlear] nerve palsy, bilateral

☑5ᵗʰ H49.2   Sixth [abducent] nerve palsy
H49.20   Sixth [abducent] nerve palsy, unspecified eye
H49.21   Sixth [abducent] nerve palsy, right eye
H49.22   Sixth [abducent] nerve palsy, left eye
H49.23   Sixth [abducent] nerve palsy, bilateral

☑5ᵗʰ H49.3   Total (external) ophthalmoplegia
H49.30   Total (external) ophthalmoplegia, unspecified eye
H49.31   Total (external) ophthalmoplegia, right eye
H49.32   Total (external) ophthalmoplegia, left eye
H49.33   Total (external) ophthalmoplegia, bilateral

☑5ᵗʰ H49.4   Progressive external ophthalmoplegia
EXCLUDES 1   Kearns-Sayre syndrome (H49.81-)
H49.40   Progressive external ophthalmoplegia, unspecified eye
H49.41   Progressive external ophthalmoplegia, right eye
H49.42   Progressive external ophthalmoplegia, left eye
H49.43   Progressive external ophthalmoplegia, bilateral

☑5ᵗʰ H49.8   Other paralytic strabismus
☑6ᵗʰ H49.81   Kearns-Sayre syndrome
Progressive external ophthalmoplegia with pigmentary retinopathy
Use additional code for other manifestation, such as: heart block (I45.9)
H49.811   Kearns-Sayre syndrome, right eye
H49.812   Kearns-Sayre syndrome, left eye
H49.813   Kearns-Sayre syndrome, bilateral
H49.819   Kearns-Sayre syndrome, unspecified eye

☑6ᵗʰ H49.88   Other paralytic strabismus
External ophthalmoplegia NOS
H49.881   Other paralytic strabismus, right eye
H49.882   Other paralytic strabismus, left eye
H49.883   Other paralytic strabismus, bilateral
H49.889   Other paralytic strabismus, unspecified eye

H49.9   Unspecified paralytic strabismus

☑4ᵗʰ H50   Other strabismus
☑5ᵗʰ H50.0   Esotropia
Convergent concomitant strabismus
EXCLUDES 1   intermittent esotropia (H50.31-, H50.32)
H50.00   Unspecified esotropia
☑6ᵗʰ H50.01   Monocular esotropia
H50.011   Monocular esotropia, right eye
H50.012   Monocular esotropia, left eye
☑6ᵗʰ H50.02   Monocular esotropia with A pattern
H50.021   Monocular esotropia with A pattern, right eye
H50.022   Monocular esotropia with A pattern, left eye
☑6ᵗʰ H50.03   Monocular esotropia with V pattern
H50.031   Monocular esotropia with V pattern, right eye
H50.032   Monocular esotropia with V pattern, left eye
☑6ᵗʰ H50.04   Monocular esotropia with other noncomitancies
H50.041   Monocular esotropia with other noncomitancies, right eye
H50.042   Monocular esotropia with other noncomitancies, left eye
H50.05   Alternating esotropia
H50.06   Alternating esotropia with A pattern
H50.07   Alternating esotropia with V pattern
H50.08   Alternating esotropia with other noncomitancies

☑5ᵗʰ H50.1   Exotropia
Divergent concomitant strabismus
EXCLUDES 1   intermittent exotropia (H50.33-, H50.34)
H50.10   Unspecified exotropia
☑6ᵗʰ H50.11   Monocular exotropia
H50.111   Monocular exotropia, right eye
H50.112   Monocular exotropia, left eye
☑6ᵗʰ H50.12   Monocular exotropia with A pattern
H50.121   Monocular exotropia with A pattern, right eye
H50.122   Monocular exotropia with A pattern, left eye
☑6ᵗʰ H50.13   Monocular exotropia with V pattern
H50.131   Monocular exotropia with V pattern, right eye
H50.132   Monocular exotropia with V pattern, left eye
☑6ᵗʰ H50.14   Monocular exotropia with other noncomitancies
H50.141   Monocular exotropia with other noncomitancies, right eye
H50.142   Monocular exotropia with other noncomitancies, left eye
H50.15   Alternating exotropia
H50.16   Alternating exotropia with A pattern
H50.17   Alternating exotropia with V pattern
H50.18   Alternating exotropia with other noncomitancies

☑5ᵗʰ H50.2   Vertical strabismus
Hypertropia
H50.21   Vertical strabismus, right eye
H50.22   Vertical strabismus, left eye

☑ Appropriate additional character required   ☑7ᵗʰ Requires 7th character, placeholder x must fill empty characters

√5th **H50.3** **Intermittent heterotropia**
    H50.30 **Unspecified intermittent heterotropia**
    √6th **H50.31** **Intermittent monocular esotropia**
        H50.311 **Intermittent monocular esotropia, right eye**
        H50.312 **Intermittent monocular esotropia, left eye**
    H50.32 **Intermittent alternating esotropia**
    √6th **H50.33** **Intermittent monocular exotropia**
        H50.331 **Intermittent monocular exotropia, right eye**
        H50.332 **Intermittent monocular exotropia, left eye**
    H50.34 **Intermittent alternating exotropia**
√5th **H50.4** **Other and unspecified heterotropia**
    H50.40 **Unspecified heterotropia**
    √6th **H50.41** **Cyclotropia**
        H50.411 **Cyclotropia, right eye**
        H50.412 **Cyclotropia, left eye**
    H50.42 **Monofixation syndrome**
    H50.43 **Accommodative component in esotropia**
√5th **H50.5** **Heterophoria**
    H50.50 **Unspecified heterophoria**
    H50.51 **Esophoria**
    H50.52 **Exophoria**
    H50.53 **Vertical heterophoria**
    H50.54 **Cyclophoria**
    H50.55 **Alternating heterophoria**
√5th **H50.6** **Mechanical strabismus**
    H50.60 **Mechanical strabismus, unspecified**
    √6th **H50.61** **Brown's sheath syndrome**
        H50.611 **Brown's sheath syndrome, right eye**
        H50.612 **Brown's sheath syndrome, left eye**
    H50.69 **Other mechanical strabismus**
        Strabismus due to adhesions
        Traumatic limitation of duction of eye muscle
√5th **H50.8** **Other specified strabismus**
    √6th **H50.81** **Duane's syndrome**
        H50.811 **Duane's syndrome, right eye**
        H50.812 **Duane's syndrome, left eye**
    H50.89 **Other specified strabismus**
    H50.9 **Unspecified strabismus**
√4th **H51** **Other disorders of binocular movement**
    H51.0 **Palsy (spasm) of conjugate gaze**
    √5th **H51.1** **Convergence insufficiency and excess**
        H51.11 **Convergence insufficiency**
        H51.12 **Convergence excess**
    √5th **H51.2** **Internuclear ophthalmoplegia**
        H51.20 **Internuclear ophthalmoplegia, unspecified eye**
        H51.21 **Internuclear ophthalmoplegia, right eye**
        H51.22 **Internuclear ophthalmoplegia, left eye**
        H51.23 **Internuclear ophthalmoplegia, bilateral**
    H51.8 **Other specified disorders of binocular movement**
    H51.9 **Unspecified disorder of binocular movement**
√4th **H52** **Disorders of refraction and accommodation**
    √5th **H52.0** **Hypermetropia**
        H52.00 **Hypermetropia, unspecified eye**
        H52.01 **Hypermetropia, right eye**
        H52.02 **Hypermetropia, left eye**
        H52.03 **Hypermetropia, bilateral**
    √5th **H52.1** **Myopia**
        EXCLUDES 1   *degenerative myopia (H44.2-)*
        H52.10 **Myopia, unspecified eye**
        H52.11 **Myopia, right eye**
        H52.12 **Myopia, left eye**
        H52.13 **Myopia, bilateral**
    √5th **H52.2** **Astigmatism**
        √6th **H52.20** **Unspecified astigmatism**
            H52.201 **Unspecified astigmatism, right eye**
            H52.202 **Unspecified astigmatism, left eye**
            H52.203 **Unspecified astigmatism, bilateral**
            H52.209 **Unspecified astigmatism, unspecified eye**

√6th **H52.21** **Irregular astigmatism**
    H52.211 **Irregular astigmatism, right eye**
    H52.212 **Irregular astigmatism, left eye**
    H52.213 **Irregular astigmatism, bilateral**
    H52.219 **Irregular astigmatism, unspecified eye**
√6th **H52.22** **Regular astigmatism**
    H52.221 **Regular astigmatism, right eye**
    H52.222 **Regular astigmatism, left eye**
    H52.223 **Regular astigmatism, bilateral**
    H52.229 **Regular astigmatism, unspecified eye**
√5th **H52.3** **Anisometropia and aniseikonia**
    H52.31 **Anisometropia**
    H52.32 **Aniseikonia**
    H52.4 **Presbyopia**
√5th **H52.5** **Disorders of accommodation**
    √6th **H52.51** **Internal ophthalmoplegia (complete) (total)**
        H52.511 **Internal ophthalmoplegia (complete) (total), right eye**
        H52.512 **Internal ophthalmoplegia (complete) (total), left eye**
        H52.513 **Internal ophthalmoplegia (complete) (total), bilateral**
        H52.519 **Internal ophthalmoplegia (complete) (total), unspecified eye**
    √6th **H52.52** **Paresis of accommodation**
        H52.521 **Paresis of accommodation, right eye**
        H52.522 **Paresis of accommodation, left eye**
        H52.523 **Paresis of accommodation, bilateral**
        H52.529 **Paresis of accommodation, unspecified eye**
    √6th **H52.53** **Spasm of accommodation**
        H52.531 **Spasm of accommodation, right eye**
        H52.532 **Spasm of accommodation, left eye**
        H52.533 **Spasm of accommodation, bilateral**
        H52.539 **Spasm of accommodation, unspecified eye**
    H52.6 **Other disorders of refraction**
    H52.7 **Unspecified disorder of refraction**

Visual disturbances and blindness (H53-H54)

√4th **H53** **Visual disturbances**
    √5th **H53.0** **Amblyopia ex anopsia**
        EXCLUDES 1   *amblyopia due to vitamin A deficiency (E50.5)*
        √6th **H53.00** **Unspecified amblyopia**
            H53.001 **Unspecified amblyopia, right eye**
            H53.002 **Unspecified amblyopia, left eye**
            H53.003 **Unspecified amblyopia, bilateral**
            H53.009 **Unspecified amblyopia, unspecified eye**
        √6th **H53.01** **Deprivation amblyopia**
            H53.011 **Deprivation amblyopia, right eye**
            H53.012 **Deprivation amblyopia, left eye**
            H53.013 **Deprivation amblyopia, bilateral**
            H53.019 **Deprivation amblyopia, unspecified eye**
        √6th **H53.02** **Refractive amblyopia**
            H53.021 **Refractive amblyopia, right eye**
            H53.022 **Refractive amblyopia, left eye**
            H53.023 **Refractive amblyopia, bilateral**
            H53.029 **Refractive amblyopia, unspecified eye**
        √6th **H53.03** **Strabismic amblyopia**
            EXCLUDES 1   *strabismus (H50-)*
            H53.031 **Strabismic amblyopia, right eye**
            H53.032 **Strabismic amblyopia, left eye**
            H53.033 **Strabismic amblyopia, bilateral**
            H53.039 **Strabismic amblyopia, unspecified eye**
    √5th **H53.1** **Subjective visual disturbances**
        EXCLUDES 1   *subjective visual disturbances due to vitamin A deficiency (E50.5)*
            visual hallucinations (R44.1)
        H53.10 **Unspecified subjective visual disturbances**
        H53.11 **Day blindness**
            Hemeralopia

√6th **H53.12** **Transient visual loss**
  Scintillating scotoma
  EXCLUDES 1 *amaurosis fugax (G45.3-)*
     transient retinal artery occlusion (H34.0-)
  H53.121 **Transient visual loss, right eye**
  H53.122 **Transient visual loss, left eye**
  H53.123 **Transient visual loss, bilateral**
  H53.129 **Transient visual loss, unspecified eye**

√6th **H53.13** **Sudden visual loss**
  H53.131 **Sudden visual loss, right eye**
  H53.132 **Sudden visual loss, left eye**
  H53.133 **Sudden visual loss, bilateral**
  H53.139 **Sudden visual loss, unspecified eye**

√6th **H53.14** **Visual discomfort**
  Asthenopia
  Photophobia
  H53.141 **Visual discomfort, right eye**
  H53.142 **Visual discomfort, left eye**
  H53.143 **Visual discomfort, bilateral**
  H53.149 **Visual discomfort, unspecified**

H53.15 **Visual distortions of shape and size**
  Metamorphopsia

H53.16 **Psychophysical visual disturbances**
  Prosopagnosia
  Visual object agnosia

H53.19 **Other subjective visual disturbances**
  Visual halos

H53.2 **Diplopia**
 Double vision

√5th **H53.3** **Other and unspecified disorders of binocular vision**
 H53.30 **Unspecified disorder of binocular vision**
 H53.31 **Abnormal retinal correspondence**
 H53.32 **Fusion with defective stereopsis**
 H53.33 **Simultaneous visual perception without fusion**
 H53.34 **Suppression of binocular vision**

√5th **H53.4** **Visual field defects**
 H53.40 **Unspecified visual field defects**
 √6th **H53.41** **Scotoma involving central area**
  Central scotoma
  H53.411 **Scotoma involving central area, right eye**
  H53.412 **Scotoma involving central area, left eye**
  H53.413 **Scotoma involving central area, bilateral**
  H53.419 **Scotoma involving central area, unspecified eye**

 √6th **H53.42** **Scotoma of blind spot area**
  Enlarged blind spot
  H53.421 **Scotoma of blind spot area, right eye**
  H53.422 **Scotoma of blind spot area, left eye**
  H53.423 **Scotoma of blind spot area, bilateral**
  H53.429 **Scotoma of blind spot area, unspecified eye**

 √6th **H53.43** **Sector or arcuate defects**
  Arcuate scotoma
  Bjerrum scotoma
  H53.431 **Sector or arcuate defects, right eye**
  H53.432 **Sector or arcuate defects, left eye**
  H53.433 **Sector or arcuate defects, bilateral**
  H53.439 **Sector or arcuate defects, unspecified eye**

 √6th **H53.45** **Other localized visual field defect**
  Peripheral visual field defect
  Ring scotoma NOS
  Scotoma NOS
  H53.451 **Other localized visual field defect, right eye**
  H53.452 **Other localized visual field defect, left eye**
  H53.453 **Other localized visual field defect, bilateral**
  H53.459 **Other localized visual field defect, unspecified eye**

 √6th **H53.46** **Homonymous bilateral field defects**
  Homonymous hemianop(s)ia
  Quadrant anop(s)ia

  H53.461 **Homonymous bilateral field defects, right side**
  H53.462 **Homonymous bilateral field defects, left side**
  H53.469 **Homonymous bilateral field defects, unspecified side**
    Homonymous bilateral field defects NOS

 H53.47 **Heteronymous bilateral field defects**
  Heteronymous hemianop(s)ia

 √6th **H53.48** **Generalized contraction of visual field**
  H53.481 **Generalized contraction of visual field, right eye**
  H53.482 **Generalized contraction of visual field, left eye**
  H53.483 **Generalized contraction of visual field, bilateral**
  H53.489 **Generalized contraction of visual field, unspecified eye**

√5th **H53.5** **Color vision deficiencies**
 Color blindness
 EXCLUDES 2 *day blindness (H53.11)*
 H53.50 **Unspecified color vision deficiencies**
  Color blindness NOS
 H53.51 **Achromatopsia**
 H53.52 **Acquired color vision deficiency**
 H53.53 **Deuteranomaly**
  Deuteranopia
 H53.54 **Protanomaly**
  Protanopia
 H53.55 **Tritanomaly**
  Tritanopia
 H53.59 **Other color vision deficiencies**

√5th **H53.6** **Night blindness**
 EXCLUDES 1 *night blindness due to vitamin A deficiency (E50.5)*
 H53.60 **Unspecified night blindness**
 H53.61 **Abnormal dark adaptation curve**
 H53.62 **Acquired night blindness**
 H53.63 **Congenital night blindness**
 H53.69 **Other night blindness**

√5th **H53.7** **Vision sensitivity deficiencies**
 H53.71 **Glare sensitivity**
 H53.72 **Impaired contrast sensitivity**

H53.8 **Other visual disturbances**

H53.9 **Unspecified visual disturbance**

√4th **H54** **Blindness and low vision**
 NOTE For definition of visual impairment categories see table below
 Code first any associated underlying cause of the blindness
 EXCLUDES 1 *amaurosis fugax (G45.3)*

 H54.0 **Blindness, both eyes**
  Visual impairment categories 3, 4, 5 in both eyes.

 √5th **H54.1** **Blindness, one eye, low vision other eye**
  Visual impairment categories 3, 4, 5 in one eye, with categories 1 or 2 in the other eye.
  H54.10 **Blindness, one eye, low vision other eye, unspecified eyes**
  H54.11 **Blindness, right eye, low vision left eye**
  H54.12 **Blindness, left eye, low vision right eye**

 H54.2 **Low vision, both eyes**
  Visual impairment categories 1 or 2 in both eyes.

 H54.3 **Unqualified visual loss, both eyes**
  Visual impairment category 9 in both eyes.

 √5th **H54.4** **Blindness, one eye**
  Visual impairment categories 3, 4, 5 in one eye [normal vision in other eye]
  H54.40 **Blindness, one eye, unspecified eye**
  H54.41 **Blindness, right eye, normal vision left eye**
  H54.42 **Blindness, left eye, normal vision right eye**

 √5th **H54.5** **Low vision, one eye**
  Visual impairment categories 1 or 2 in one eye [normal vision in other eye].
  H54.50 **Low vision, one eye, unspecified eye**
  H54.51 **Low vision, right eye, normal vision left eye**
  H54.52 **Low vision, left eye, normal vision right eye**

✔ Appropriate additional character required √x7th Requires 7th character, placeholder x must fill empty characters

✓5th **H54.6 Unqualified visual loss, one eye**
Visual impairment category 9 in one eye [normal vision in other eye].

    H54.60 Unqualified visual loss, one eye, unspecified

    H54.61 Unqualified visual loss, right eye, normal vision left eye

    H54.62 Unqualified visual loss, left eye, normal vision right eye

H54.7 Unspecified visual loss
Visual impairment category 9 NOS

H54.8 Legal blindness, as defined in USA
Blindness NOS according to USA definition

    EXCLUDES 1 *legal blindness with specification of impairment level (H54.0-H54.7)*

NOTE   The following table gives a classification of severity of visual impairment recommended by a WHO Study Group on the Prevention of Blindness, Geneva, 6-10 November 1972.[1]

The term "low vision" in category H54 comprises categories 1 and 2 of the table, the term "blindness" categories 3, 4 and 5, and the term "unqualified visual loss" category 9.

If the extent of the visual field is taken into account, patients with a field no greater than 10 but greater than 5 around central fixation should be placed in category 3 and patients with a field no greater than 5 around central fixation should be placed in category 4, even if the central acuity is not impaired.

Category of visual impairment	Visual acuity with best possible correction	
	Maximum less than:	Minimum equal to or better than:
1	6/18 3/10 (0.3) 20/70	6/60 1/10 (0.1) 20/200
2	6/60 1/10 (0.1) 20/200	3/60 1/20 (0.5) 20/400
3	3/60 1/20 (0.05) 20/400	1/60 (finger counting at one meter) 1/50 (0.02) 5/300 (20/1200)
4	1/60 (finger counting at one meter) 1/50 (0.02) 5/300	Light perception
5	No light perception	
9	Undetermined or unspecified	

Other disorders of eye and adnexa (H55-H59)

✓4th **H55 Nystagmus and other irregular eye movements**

✓5th **H55.0 Nystagmus**

    H55.00 Unspecified nystagmus

    H55.01 Congenital nystagmus

    H55.02 Latent nystagmus

    H55.03 Visual deprivation nystagmus

    H55.04 Dissociated nystagmus

    H55.09 Other forms of nystagmus

✓5th **H55.8 Other irregular eye movements**

    H55.81 Saccadic eye movements

    H55.89 Other irregular eye movements

✓4th **H57 Other disorders of eye and adnexa**

✓5th **H57.0 Anomalies of pupillary function**

    H57.00 Unspecified anomaly of pupillary function

    H57.01 Argyll Robertson pupil, atypical

      EXCLUDES 1 *syphilitic Argyll Robertson pupil (A52.19)*

    H57.02 Anisocoria

    H57.03 Miosis

    H57.04 Mydriasis

✓6th **H57.05 Tonic pupil**

    H57.051 Tonic pupil, right eye

    H57.052 Tonic pupil, left eye

    H57.053 Tonic pupil, bilateral

    H57.059 Tonic pupil, unspecified eye

    H57.09 Other anomalies of pupillary function

✓5th **H57.1 Ocular pain**

    H57.10 Ocular pain, unspecified eye

    H57.11 Ocular pain, right eye

    H57.12 Ocular pain, left eye

    H57.13 Ocular pain, bilateral

H57.8 Other specified disorders of eye and adnexa

H57.9 Unspecified disorder of eye and adnexa

✓4th **H59 Intraoperative and postprocedural complications and disorders of eye and adnexa, not elsewhere classified**

    EXCLUDES 1 *mechanical complication of intraocular lens (T85.2)*
mechanical complication of other ocular prosthetic devices, implants and grafts (T85.3)
pseudophakia (Z96.1)
secondary cataracts (H26.4-)

✓5th **H59.0 Disorders of the eye following cataract surgery**

✓6th **H59.01 Keratopathy (bullous aphakic) following cataract surgery**
Vitreal corneal syndrome
Vitreous (touch) syndrome

    H59.011 Keratopathy (bullous aphakic) following cataract surgery, right eye

    H59.012 Keratopathy (bullous aphakic) following cataract surgery, left eye

    H59.013 Keratopathy (bullous aphakic) following cataract surgery, bilateral

    H59.019 Keratopathy (bullous aphakic) following cataract surgery, unspecified eye

✓6th **H59.02 Cataract (lens) fragments in eye following cataract surgery**

    H59.021 Cataract (lens) fragments in eye following cataract surgery, right eye

    H59.022 Cataract (lens) fragments in eye following cataract surgery, left eye

    H59.023 Cataract (lens) fragments in eye following cataract surgery, bilateral

    H59.029 Cataract (lens) fragments in eye following cataract surgery, unspecified eye

✓6th **H59.03 Cystoid macular edema following cataract surgery**

    H59.031 Cystoid macular edema following cataract surgery, right eye

    H59.032 Cystoid macular edema following cataract surgery, left eye

    H59.033 Cystoid macular edema following cataract surgery, bilateral

    H59.039 Cystoid macular edema following cataract surgery, unspecified eye

✓6th **H59.09 Other disorders of the eye following cataract surgery**

    H59.091 Other disorders of the right eye following cataract surgery

    H59.092 Other disorders of the left eye following cataract surgery

    H59.093 Other disorders of the eye following cataract surgery, bilateral

    H59.099 Other disorders of unspecified eye following cataract surgery

✓5th **H59.1 Intraoperative hemorrhage and hematoma of eye and adnexa complicating a procedure**

    EXCLUDES 1 *intraoperative hemorrhage and hematoma of eye and adnexa due to accidental puncture or laceration during a procedure (H59.2-)*

✓6th **H59.11 Intraoperative hemorrhage and hematoma of eye and adnexa complicating an ophthalmic procedure**

    H59.111 Intraoperative hemorrhage and hematoma of right eye and adnexa complicating an ophthalmic procedure

    H59.112 Intraoperative hemorrhage and hematoma of left eye and adnexa complicating an ophthalmic procedure

    H59.113 Intraoperative hemorrhage and hematoma of eye and adnexa complicating an ophthalmic procedure, bilateral

---

EXCLUDES 1 Not coded here   EXCLUDES 2 Not included here   *Manifestation Code*

H59.119   Intraoperative hemorrhage and hematoma of unspecified eye and adnexa complicating an ophthalmic procedure

✓6ᵗʰ   H59.12   Intraoperative hemorrhage and hematoma of eye and adnexa complicating other procedure

H59.121   Intraoperative hemorrhage and hematoma of right eye and adnexa complicating other procedure

H59.122   Intraoperative hemorrhage and hematoma of left eye and adnexa complicating other procedure

H59.123   Intraoperative hemorrhage and hematoma of eye and adnexa complicating other procedure, bilateral

H59.129   Intraoperative hemorrhage and hematoma of unspecified eye and adnexa complicating other procedure

✓5ᵗʰ   H59.2   Accidental puncture and laceration of eye and adnexa during a procedure

✓6ᵗʰ   H59.21   Accidental puncture and laceration of eye and adnexa during an ophthalmic procedure

H59.211   Accidental puncture and laceration of right eye and adnexa during an ophthalmic procedure

H59.212   Accidental puncture and laceration of left eye and adnexa during an ophthalmic procedure

H59.213   Accidental puncture and laceration of eye and adnexa during an ophthalmic procedure, bilateral

H59.219   Accidental puncture and laceration of unspecified eye and adnexa during an ophthalmic procedure

✓6ᵗʰ   H59.22   Accidental puncture and laceration of eye and adnexa during other procedure

H59.221   Accidental puncture and laceration of right eye and adnexa during other procedure

H59.222   Accidental puncture and laceration of left eye and adnexa during other procedure

H59.223   Accidental puncture and laceration of eye and adnexa during other procedure, bilateral

H59.229   Accidental puncture and laceration of unspecified eye and adnexa during other procedure

✓5ᵗʰ   H59.3   Postprocedural hemorrhage and hematoma of eye and adnexa following a procedure

✓6ᵗʰ   H59.31   Postprocedural hemorrhage and hematoma of eye and adnexa following an ophthalmic procedure

H59.311   Postprocedural hemorrhage and hematoma of right eye and adnexa following an ophthalmic procedure

H59.312   Postprocedural hemorrhage and hematoma of left eye and adnexa following an ophthalmic procedure

H59.313   Postprocedural hemorrhage and hematoma of eye and adnexa following an ophthalmic procedure, bilateral

H59.319   Postprocedural hemorrhage and hematoma of unspecified eye and adnexa following an ophthalmic procedure

✓6ᵗʰ   H59.32   Postprocedural hemorrhage and hematoma of eye and adnexa following other procedure

H59.321   Postprocedural hemorrhage and hematoma of right eye and adnexa following other procedure

H59.322   Postprocedural hemorrhage and hematoma of left eye and adnexa following other procedure

H59.323   Postprocedural hemorrhage and hematoma of eye and adnexa following other procedure, bilateral

H59.329   Postprocedural hemorrhage and hematoma of unspecified eye and adnexa following other procedure

✓6ᵗʰ   H59.4   Inflammation (infection) of postprocedural bleb
Postprocedural blebitis

EXCLUDES 1   filtering (vitreous) bleb after glaucoma surgery status (Z98.83)

H59.40   Inflammation (infection) of postprocedural bleb, unspecified

H59.41   Inflammation (infection) of postprocedural bleb, stage 1

H59.42   Inflammation (infection) of postprocedural bleb, stage 2

H59.43   Inflammation (infection) of postprocedural bleb, stage 3
Bleb endophthalmitis

✓6ᵗʰ   H59.8   Other intraoperative and postprocedural complications and disorders of eye and adnexa, not elsewhere classified

✓6ᵗʰ   H59.81   Chorioretinal scars after surgery for detachment

H59.811   Chorioretinal scars after surgery for detachment, right eye

H59.812   Chorioretinal scars after surgery for detachment, left eye

H59.813   Chorioretinal scars after surgery for detachment, bilateral

H59.819   Chorioretinal scars after surgery for detachment, unspecified eye

H59.88   Other intraoperative complications of eye and adnexa, not elsewhere classified

H59.89   Other postprocedural complications and disorders of eye and adnexa, not elsewhere classified

---

✔ Appropriate additional character required   ✓x7ᵗʰ Requires 7th character, placeholder x must fill empty characters

Chapter 8. Diseases of the Ear and Mastoid Process (H60–H95)

NOTE   Use an external cause code following the code for the ear condition, if applicable, to identify the cause of the ear condition

EXCLUDES 2   certain conditions originating in the perinatal period (P04–P96)
certain infectious and parasitic diseases (A00–B99)
complications of pregnancy, childbirth and the puerperium (O00–O99)
congenital malformations, deformations and chromosomal abnormalities (Q00–Q99)
endocrine, nutritional and metabolic diseases (E00–E88)
injury, poisoning and certain other consequences of external causes (S00–T88)
neoplasms (C00–D49)
symptoms, signs and abnormal clinical and laboratory findings, not elsewhere classified (R00–R94)

This chapter contains the following blocks:
H60–H62   Diseases of external ear
H65–H75   Diseases of middle ear and mastoid
H80–H83   Diseases of inner ear
H90–H94   Other disorders of ear
H95   Intraoperative and postprocedural complications and disorders of ear and mastoid process, not elsewhere classified

Diseases of external ear (H60–H62)

☑4th H60 Otitis externa

☑5th H60.0 Abscess of external ear
Boil of external ear
Carbuncle of auricle or external auditory canal
Furuncle of external ear
H60.00   Abscess of external ear, unspecified ear
H60.01   Abscess of right external ear
H60.02   Abscess of left external ear
H60.03   Abscess of external ear, bilateral

☑5th H60.1 Cellulitis of external ear
Cellulitis of auricle
Cellulitis of external auditory canal
H60.10   Cellulitis of external ear, unspecified ear
H60.11   Cellulitis of right external ear
H60.12   Cellulitis of left external ear
H60.13   Cellulitis of external ear, bilateral

☑5th H60.2 Malignant otitis externa
H60.20   Malignant otitis externa, unspecified ear
H60.21   Malignant otitis externa, right ear
H60.22   Malignant otitis externa, left ear
H60.23   Malignant otitis externa, bilateral

☑5th H60.3 Other infective otitis externa
   ☑6th H60.31 Diffuse otitis externa
     H60.311   Diffuse otitis externa, right ear
     H60.312   Diffuse otitis externa, left ear
     H60.313   Diffuse otitis externa, bilateral
     H60.319   Diffuse otitis externa, unspecified ear
   ☑6th H60.32 Hemorrhagic otitis externa
     H60.321   Hemorrhagic otitis externa, right ear
     H60.322   Hemorrhagic otitis externa, left ear
     H60.323   Hemorrhagic otitis externa, bilateral
     H60.329   Hemorrhagic otitis externa, unspecified ear
   ☑6th H60.33 Swimmer's ear
     H60.331   Swimmer's ear, right ear
     H60.332   Swimmer's ear, left ear
     H60.333   Swimmer's ear, bilateral
     H60.339   Swimmer's ear, unspecified ear
   ☑6th H60.39 Other infective otitis externa
     H60.391   Other infective otitis externa, right ear
     H60.392   Other infective otitis externa, left ear
     H60.393   Other infective otitis externa, bilateral
     H60.399   Other infective otitis externa, unspecified ear

☑5th H60.4 Cholesteatoma of external ear
Keratosis obturans of external ear (canal)
EXCLUDES 2   cholesteatoma of middle ear (H71-)
recurrent cholesteatoma of postmastoidectomy cavity (H95.0-)
H60.40   Cholesteatoma of external ear, unspecified ear
H60.41   Cholesteatoma of right external ear

H60.42   Cholesteatoma of left external ear
H60.43   Cholesteatoma of external ear, bilateral

☑5th H60.5 Acute noninfective otitis externa
   ☑6th H60.50 Unspecified acute noninfective otitis externa
Acute otitis externa NOS
     H60.501   Unspecified acute noninfective otitis externa, right ear
     H60.502   Unspecified acute noninfective otitis externa, left ear
     H60.503   Unspecified acute noninfective otitis externa, bilateral
     H60.509   Unspecified acute noninfective otitis externa, unspecified ear
   ☑6th H60.51 Acute actinic otitis externa
     H60.511   Acute actinic otitis externa, right ear
     H60.512   Acute actinic otitis externa, left ear
     H60.513   Acute actinic otitis externa, bilateral
     H60.519   Acute actinic otitis externa, unspecified ear
   ☑6th H60.52 Acute chemical otitis externa
     H60.521   Acute chemical otitis externa, right ear
     H60.522   Acute chemical otitis externa, left ear
     H60.523   Acute chemical otitis externa, bilateral
     H60.529   Acute chemical otitis externa, unspecified ear
   ☑6th H60.53 Acute contact otitis externa
     H60.531   Acute contact otitis externa, right ear
     H60.532   Acute contact otitis externa, left ear
     H60.533   Acute contact otitis externa, bilateral
     H60.539   Acute contact otitis externa, unspecified ear
   ☑6th H60.54 Acute eczematoid otitis externa
     H60.541   Acute eczematoid otitis externa, right ear
     H60.542   Acute eczematoid otitis externa, left ear
     H60.543   Acute eczematoid otitis externa, bilateral
     H60.549   Acute eczematoid otitis externa, unspecified ear
   ☑6th H60.55 Acute reactive otitis externa
     H60.551   Acute reactive otitis externa, right ear
     H60.552   Acute reactive otitis externa, left ear
     H60.553   Acute reactive otitis externa, bilateral
     H60.559   Acute reactive otitis externa, unspecified ear
   ☑6th H60.59 Other noninfective acute otitis externa
     H60.591   Other noninfective acute otitis externa, right ear
     H60.592   Other noninfective acute otitis externa, left ear
     H60.593   Other noninfective acute otitis externa, bilateral
     H60.599   Other noninfective acute otitis externa, unspecified ear

☑5th H60.6 Unspecified chronic otitis externa
H60.60   Unspecified chronic otitis externa, unspecified ear
H60.61   Unspecified chronic otitis externa, right ear
H60.62   Unspecified chronic otitis externa, left ear
H60.63   Unspecified chronic otitis externa, bilateral

☑5th H60.8 Other otitis externa
   ☑6th H60.8x Other otitis externa
     H60.8x1   Other otitis externa, right ear
     H60.8x2   Other otitis externa, left ear
     H60.8x3   Other otitis externa, bilateral
     H60.8x9   Other otitis externa, unspecified ear

☑5th H60.9 Unspecified otitis externa
H60.90   Unspecified otitis externa, unspecified ear
H60.91   Unspecified otitis externa, right ear
H60.92   Unspecified otitis externa, left ear
H60.93   Unspecified otitis externa, bilateral

EXCLUDES 1 Not coded here   **EXCLUDES 2** Not included here   *Manifestation Code*

✓4th **H61　Other disorders of external ear**

✓5th **H61.0　Chondritis and perichondritis of external ear**
Chondrodermatitis nodularis chronica helicis
Perichondritis of auricle
Perichondritis of pinna

✓6th **H61.00　Unspecified perichondritis of external ear**
H61.001　Unspecified perichondritis of right external ear
H61.002　Unspecified perichondritis of left external ear
H61.003　Unspecified perichondritis of external ear, bilateral
H61.009　Unspecified perichondritis of external ear, unspecified ear

✓6th **H61.01　Acute perichondritis of external ear**
H61.011　Acute perichondritis of right external ear
H61.012　Acute perichondritis of left external ear
H61.013　Acute perichondritis of external ear, bilateral
H61.019　Acute perichondritis of external ear, unspecified ear

✓6th **H61.02　Chronic perichondritis of external ear**
H61.021　Chronic perichondritis of right external ear
H61.022　Chronic perichondritis of left external ear
H61.023　Chronic perichondritis of external ear, bilateral
H61.029　Chronic perichondritis of external ear, unspecified ear

✓6th **H61.03　Chondritis of external ear**
Chondritis of auricle
Chondritis of pinna
H61.031　Chondritis of right external ear
H61.032　Chondritis of left external ear
H61.033　Chondritis of external ear, bilateral
H61.039　Chondritis of external ear, unspecified ear

✓5th **H61.1　Noninfective disorders of pinna**
EXCLUDES 2　*cauliflower ear (M95.1-)*
gouty tophi of ear (M1a-, M10-)

✓6th **H61.10　Unspecified noninfective disorders of pinna**
Disorder of pinna NOS
H61.101　Unspecified noninfective disorders of pinna, right ear
H61.102　Unspecified noninfective disorders of pinna, left ear
H61.103　Unspecified noninfective disorders of pinna, bilateral
H61.109　Unspecified noninfective disorders of pinna, unspecified ear

✓6th **H61.11　Acquired deformity of pinna**
Acquired deformity of auricle
EXCLUDES 2　*cauliflower ear (M95.1-)*
H61.111　Acquired deformity of pinna, right ear
H61.112　Acquired deformity of pinna, left ear
H61.113　Acquired deformity of pinna, bilateral
H61.119　Acquired deformity of pinna, unspecified ear

✓6th **H61.12　Hematoma of pinna**
Hematoma of auricle
H61.121　Hematoma of pinna, right ear
H61.122　Hematoma of pinna, left ear
H61.123　Hematoma of pinna, bilateral
H61.129　Hematoma of pinna, unspecified ear

✓6th **H61.19　Other noninfective disorders of pinna**
H61.191　Noninfective disorders of pinna, right ear
H61.192　Noninfective disorders of pinna, left ear
H61.193　Noninfective disorders of pinna, bilateral
H61.199　Noninfective disorders of pinna, unspecified ear

✓5th **H61.2　Impacted cerumen**
Wax in ear
H61.20　Impacted cerumen, unspecified ear

H61.21　Impacted cerumen, right ear
H61.22　Impacted cerumen, left ear
H61.23　Impacted cerumen, bilateral

✓5th **H61.3　Acquired stenosis of external ear canal**
Collapse of external ear canal
EXCLUDES 1　*postprocedural stenosis of external ear canal (H95.81-)*

✓6th **H61.30　Acquired stenosis of external ear canal, unspecified**
H61.301　Acquired stenosis of right external ear canal, unspecified
H61.302　Acquired stenosis of left external ear canal, unspecified
H61.303　Acquired stenosis of external ear canal, unspecified, bilateral
H61.309　Acquired stenosis of external ear canal, unspecified, unspecified ear

✓6th **H61.31　Acquired stenosis of external ear canal secondary to trauma**
H61.311　Acquired stenosis of right external ear canal secondary to trauma
H61.312　Acquired stenosis of left external ear canal secondary to trauma
H61.313　Acquired stenosis of external ear canal secondary to trauma, bilateral
H61.319　Acquired stenosis of external ear canal secondary to trauma, unspecified ear

✓6th **H61.32　Acquired stenosis of external ear canal secondary to inflammation and infection**
H61.321　Acquired stenosis of right external ear canal secondary to inflammation and infection
H61.322　Acquired stenosis of left external ear canal secondary to inflammation and infection
H61.323　Acquired stenosis of external ear canal secondary to inflammation and infection, bilateral
H61.329　Acquired stenosis of external ear canal secondary to inflammation and infection, unspecified ear

✓6th **H61.39　Other acquired stenosis of external ear canal**
H61.391　Other acquired stenosis of right external ear canal
H61.392　Other acquired stenosis of left external ear canal
H61.393　Other acquired stenosis of external ear canal, bilateral
H61.399　Other acquired stenosis of external ear canal, unspecified ear

✓5th **H61.8　Other specified disorders of external ear**
✓6th **H61.81　Exostosis of external canal**
H61.811　Exostosis of right external canal
H61.812　Exostosis of left external canal
H61.813　Exostosis of external canal, bilateral
H61.819　Exostosis of external canal, unspecified ear

✓6th **H61.89　Other specified disorders of external ear**
H61.891　Other specified disorders of right external ear
H61.892　Other specified disorders of left external ear
H61.893　Other specified disorders of external ear, bilateral
H61.899　Other specified disorders of external ear, unspecified ear

✓5th **H61.9　Disorder of external ear, unspecified**
H61.90　Disorder of external ear, unspecified, unspecified ear
H61.91　Disorder of right external ear, unspecified
H61.92　Disorder of left external ear, unspecified
H61.93　Disorder of external ear, unspecified, bilateral

✓ Appropriate additional character required　　　　✓x7th Requires 7th character, placeholder x must fill empty characters

☑4ᵗʰ H62   Disorders of external ear in diseases classified elsewhere

☑5ᵗʰ H62.4   Otitis externa in other diseases classified elsewhere

Code first underlying disease, such as:
erysipelas (A46)
impetigo (L01.0)

EXCLUDES 1   otitis externa (in):
candidiasis (B37.84)
herpes viral [herpes simplex] (B00.1)
herpes zoster (B02.8)

H62.40   Otitis externa in other diseases classified elsewhere, unspecified ear

H62.41   Otitis externa in other diseases classified elsewhere, right ear

H62.42   Otitis externa in other diseases classified elsewhere, left ear

H62.43   Otitis externa in other diseases classified elsewhere, bilateral

☑5ᵗʰ H62.8   Other disorders of external ear in diseases classified elsewhere

Code first underlying disease, such as:
gout (M1a-, M10-)

☑6ᵗʰ H62.8x   Other disorders of external ear in diseases classified elsewhere

H62.8x1   Other disorders of right external ear in diseases classified elsewhere

H62.8x2   Other disorders of left external ear in diseases classified elsewhere

H62.8x3   Other disorders of external ear in diseases classified elsewhere, bilateral

H62.8x9   Other disorders of external ear in diseases classified elsewhere, unspecified ear

Diseases of middle ear and mastoid (H65-H75)

☑4ᵗʰ H65   Nonsuppurative otitis media

INCLUDES   nonsuppurative otitis media with myringitis

Use additional code for any associated perforated tympanic membrane (H72-)
Use additional code to identify:
exposure to environmental tobacco smoke (Z77.22)
exposure to tobacco smoke in the perinatal period (P96.81)
history of tobacco use (Z87.891)
occupational exposure to environmental tobacco smoke (Z57.31)
tobacco dependence (F17-)
tobacco use (Z72.0)

☑5ᵗʰ H65.0   Acute serous otitis media

Acute and subacute secretory otitis

H65.00   Acute serous otitis media, unspecified ear

H65.01   Acute serous otitis media, right ear

H65.02   Acute serous otitis media, left ear

H65.03   Acute serous otitis media, bilateral

H65.04   Acute serous otitis media, recurrent, right ear

H65.05   Acute serous otitis media, recurrent, left ear

H65.06   Acute serous otitis media, recurrent, bilateral

H65.07   Acute serous otitis media, recurrent, unspecified ear

☑5ᵗʰ H65.1   Other acute nonsuppurative otitis media

EXCLUDES 1   otitic barotrauma (T70.0)
otitis media (acute) NOS (H66.9)

☑6ᵗʰ H65.11   Acute and subacute allergic otitis media (mucoid) (sanguinous) (serous)

H65.111   Acute and subacute allergic otitis media (mucoid) (sanguinous) (serous), right ear

H65.112   Acute and subacute allergic otitis media (mucoid) (sanguinous) (serous), left ear

H65.113   Acute and subacute allergic otitis media (mucoid) (sanguinous) (serous), bilateral

H65.114   Acute and subacute allergic otitis media (mucoid) (sanguinous) (serous), recurrent, right ear

H65.115   Acute and subacute allergic otitis media (mucoid) (sanguinous) (serous), recurrent, left ear

H65.116   Acute and subacute allergic otitis media (mucoid) (sanguinous) (serous), recurrent, bilateral

H65.117   Acute and subacute allergic otitis media (mucoid) (sanguinous) (serous), recurrent, unspecified ear

H65.119   Acute and subacute allergic otitis media (mucoid) (sanguinous) (serous), unspecified ear

☑6ᵗʰ H65.19   Other acute nonsuppurative otitis media

Acute and subacute mucoid otitis media
Acute and subacute nonsuppurative otitis media NOS
Acute and subacute sanguinous otitis media
Acute and subacute seromucinous otitis media

H65.191   Other acute nonsuppurative otitis media, right ear

H65.192   Other acute nonsuppurative otitis media, left ear

H65.193   Other acute nonsuppurative otitis media, bilateral

H65.194   Other acute nonsuppurative otitis media, recurrent, right ear

H65.195   Other acute nonsuppurative otitis media, recurrent, left ear

H65.196   Other acute nonsuppurative otitis media, recurrent, bilateral

H65.197   Other acute nonsuppurative otitis media recurrent, unspecified ear

H65.199   Other acute nonsuppurative otitis media, unspecified ear

☑5ᵗʰ H65.2   Chronic serous otitis media

Chronic tubotympanal catarrh

H65.20   Chronic serous otitis media, unspecified ear

H65.21   Chronic serous otitis media, right ear

H65.22   Chronic serous otitis media, left ear

H65.23   Chronic serous otitis media, bilateral

☑5ᵗʰ H65.3   Chronic mucoid otitis media

Chronic mucinous otitis media
Chronic secretory otitis media
Chronic transudative otitis media
Glue ear

EXCLUDES 1   adhesive middle ear disease (H74.1)

H65.30   Chronic mucoid otitis media, unspecified ear

H65.31   Chronic mucoid otitis media, right ear

H65.32   Chronic mucoid otitis media, left ear

H65.33   Chronic mucoid otitis media, bilateral

☑5ᵗʰ H65.4   Other chronic nonsuppurative otitis media

☑6ᵗʰ H65.41   Chronic allergic otitis media

H65.411   Chronic allergic otitis media, right ear

H65.412   Chronic allergic otitis media, left ear

H65.413   Chronic allergic otitis media, bilateral

H65.419   Chronic allergic otitis media, unspecified ear

☑6ᵗʰ H65.49   Other chronic nonsuppurative otitis media

Chronic exudative otitis media
Chronic nonsuppurative otitis media NOS
Chronic otitis media with effusion (nonpurulent)
Chronic seromucinous otitis media

H65.491   Other chronic nonsuppurative otitis media, right ear

H65.492   Other chronic nonsuppurative otitis media, left ear

H65.493   Other chronic nonsuppurative otitis media, bilateral

H65.499   Other chronic nonsuppurative otitis media, unspecified ear

☑5ᵗʰ H65.9   Unspecified nonsuppurative otitis media

Allergic otitis media NOS
Catarrhal otitis media NOS
Exudative otitis media NOS
Mucoid otitis media NOS
Otitis media with effusion (nonpurulent) NOS
Secretory otitis media NOS
Seromucinous otitis media NOS
Serous otitis media NOS
Transudative otitis media NOS

H65.90   Unspecified nonsuppurative otitis media, unspecified ear

H65.91   Unspecified nonsuppurative otitis media, right ear

H65.92   Unspecified nonsuppurative otitis media, left ear

EXCLUDES 1   Not coded here   EXCLUDES 2   Not included here   **Manifestation Code**

H65.93   Unspecified nonsuppurative otitis media, bilateral

☑4ᵗʰ **H66 Suppurative and unspecified otitis media**
    INCLUDES suppurative and unspecified otitis media with myringitis
    Use additional code for any associated perforated tympanic
        membrane (H72-)
    Use additional code to identify:
        exposure to environmental tobacco smoke (Z77.22)
        exposure to tobacco smoke in the perinatal period (P96.81)
        history of tobacco use (Z87.891)
        occupational exposure to environmental tobacco smoke (Z57.31)
        tobacco dependence (F17-)
        tobacco use (Z72.0)

☑5ᵗʰ **H66.0 Acute suppurative otitis media**
    ☑6ᵗʰ **H66.00 Acute suppurative otitis media without
        spontaneous rupture of ear drum**
        **H66.001 Acute suppurative otitis media without
            spontaneous rupture of ear drum, right
            ear**
        **H66.002 Acute suppurative otitis media without
            spontaneous rupture of ear drum, left
            ear**
        **H66.003 Acute suppurative otitis media without
            spontaneous rupture of ear drum,
            bilateral**
        **H66.004 Acute suppurative otitis media without
            spontaneous rupture of ear drum,
            recurrent, right ear**
        **H66.005 Acute suppurative otitis media without
            spontaneous rupture of ear drum,
            recurrent, left ear**
        **H66.006 Acute suppurative otitis media without
            spontaneous rupture of ear drum,
            recurrent, bilateral**
        **H66.007 Acute suppurative otitis media without
            spontaneous rupture of ear drum,
            recurrent, unspecified ear**
        **H66.009 Acute suppurative otitis media without
            spontaneous rupture of ear drum,
            unspecified ear**
    ☑6ᵗʰ **H66.01 Acute suppurative otitis media with spontaneous
        rupture of ear drum**
        **H66.011 Acute suppurative otitis media with
            spontaneous rupture of ear drum, right
            ear**
        **H66.012 Acute suppurative otitis media with
            spontaneous rupture of ear drum, left
            ear**
        **H66.013 Acute suppurative otitis media with
            spontaneous rupture of ear drum,
            bilateral**
        **H66.014 Acute suppurative otitis media with
            spontaneous rupture of ear drum,
            recurrent, right ear**
        **H66.015 Acute suppurative otitis media with
            spontaneous rupture of ear drum,
            recurrent, left ear**
        **H66.016 Acute suppurative otitis media with
            spontaneous rupture of ear drum,
            recurrent, bilateral**
        **H66.017 Acute suppurative otitis media with
            spontaneous rupture of ear drum,
            recurrent, unspecified ear**
        **H66.019 Acute suppurative otitis media with
            spontaneous rupture of ear drum,
            unspecified ear**

☑5ᵗʰ **H66.1 Chronic tubotympanic suppurative otitis media**
    Benign chronic suppurative otitis media
    Chronic tubotympanic disease
    **H66.10 Chronic tubotympanic suppurative otitis media,
        unspecified**
    **H66.11 Chronic tubotympanic suppurative otitis media,
        right ear**
    **H66.12 Chronic tubotympanic suppurative otitis media,
        left ear**
    **H66.13 Chronic tubotympanic suppurative otitis media,
        bilateral**

☑5ᵗʰ **H66.2 Chronic atticoantral suppurative otitis media**
    Chronic atticoantral disease
    **H66.20 Chronic atticoantral suppurative otitis media,
        unspecified ear**
    **H66.21 Chronic atticoantral suppurative otitis media,
        right ear**
    **H66.22 Chronic atticoantral suppurative otitis media, left
        ear**
    **H66.23 Chronic atticoantral suppurative otitis media,
        bilateral**

☑5ᵗʰ **H66.3 Other chronic suppurative otitis media**
    Chronic suppurative otitis media NOS
    EXCLUDES 1 *tuberculous otitis media (A18.6)*
    ☑6ᵗʰ **H66.3x Other chronic suppurative otitis media**
        **H66.3x1 Other chronic suppurative otitis media,
            right ear**
        **H66.3x2 Other chronic suppurative otitis media,
            left ear**
        **H66.3x3 Other chronic suppurative otitis media,
            bilateral**
        **H66.3x9 Other chronic suppurative otitis media,
            unspecified ear**

☑5ᵗʰ **H66.4 Suppurative otitis media, unspecified**
    Purulent otitis media NOS
    **H66.40 Suppurative otitis media, unspecified, unspecified
        ear**
    H66.41 Suppurative otitis media, unspecified, right ear
    H66.42 Suppurative otitis media, unspecified, left ear
    H66.43 Suppurative otitis media, unspecified, bilateral

☑5ᵗʰ **H66.9 Otitis media, unspecified**
    Otitis media NOS
    Acute otitis media NOS
    Chronic otitis media NOS
    H66.90 Otitis media, unspecified, unspecified ear
    H66.91 Otitis media, unspecified. right ear
    H66.92 Otitis media, unspecified, left ear
    H66.93 Otitis media, unspecified, bilateral

☑4ᵗʰ **H67 Otitis media in diseases classified elsewhere**
    Code first underlying disease, such as:
        viral disease NEC (B00-B34)
    Use additional code for any associated perforated tympanic
        membrane (H72-)
    EXCLUDES 1 otitis media in:
        influenza (J09.092, J09.192, J10.83, J11.83)
        measles (B05.3)
        scarlet fever (A38.0)
        tuberculosis (A18.6)
    H67.1 *Otitis media in diseases classified elsewhere, right ear*
    H67.2 *Otitis media in diseases classified elsewhere, left ear*
    H67.3 *Otitis media in diseases classified elsewhere, bilateral*
    H67.9 *Otitis media in diseases classified elsewhere, unspecified
        ear*

☑4ᵗʰ **H68 Eustachian salpingitis and obstruction**
    ☑5ᵗʰ **H68.0 Eustachian salpingitis**
        ☑6ᵗʰ **H68.00 Unspecified Eustachian salpingitis**
            **H68.001 Unspecified Eustachian salpingitis, right
                ear**
            **H68.002 Unspecified Eustachian salpingitis, left
                ear**
            **H68.003 Unspecified Eustachian salpingitis,
                bilateral**
            **H68.009 Unspecified Eustachian salpingitis,
                unspecified ear**
        ☑6ᵗʰ **H68.01 Acute Eustachian salpingitis**
            H68.011 Acute Eustachian salpingitis, right ear
            H68.012 Acute Eustachian salpingitis, left ear
            H68.013 Acute Eustachian salpingitis, bilateral
            **H68.019 Acute Eustachian salpingitis,
                unspecified ear**
        ☑6ᵗʰ **H68.02 Chronic Eustachian salpingitis**
            H68.021 Chronic Eustachian salpingitis, right ear
            H68.022 Chronic Eustachian salpingitis, left ear
            H68.023 Chronic Eustachian salpingitis, bilateral
            **H68.029 Chronic Eustachian salpingitis,
                unspecified ear**

☑ Appropriate additional character required   ☑7ᵗʰ Requires 7th character, placeholder x must fill empty characters

√5th **H68.1 Obstruction of Eustachian tube**
Stenosis of Eustachian tube
Stricture of Eustachian tube

    √6th **H68.10 Unspecified obstruction of Eustachian tube**
       H68.101 Unspecified obstruction of Eustachian tube, right ear
       H68.102 Unspecified obstruction of Eustachian tube, left ear
       H68.103 Unspecified obstruction of Eustachian tube, bilateral
       H68.109 Unspecified obstruction of Eustachian tube, unspecified ear

    √6th **H68.11 Osseous obstruction of Eustachian tube**
       H68.111 Osseous obstruction of Eustachian tube, right ear
       H68.112 Osseous obstruction of Eustachian tube, left ear
       H68.113 Osseous obstruction of Eustachian tube, bilateral
       H68.119 Osseous obstruction of Eustachian tube, unspecified ear

    √6th **H68.12 Intrinsic cartilagenous obstruction of Eustachian tube**
       H68.121 Intrinsic cartilagenous obstruction of Eustachian tube, right ear
       H68.122 Intrinsic cartilagenous obstruction of Eustachian tube, left ear
       H68.123 Intrinsic cartilagenous obstruction of Eustachian tube, bilateral
       H68.129 Intrinsic cartilagenous obstruction of Eustachian tube, unspecified ear

    √6th **H68.13 Extrinsic cartilagenous obstruction of Eustachian tube**
Compression of Eustachian tube
       H68.131 Extrinsic cartilagenous obstruction of Eustachian tube, right ear
       H68.132 Extrinsic cartilagenous obstruction of Eustachian tube, left ear
       H68.133 Extrinsic cartilagenous obstruction of Eustachian tube, bilateral
       H68.139 Extrinsic cartilagenous obstruction of Eustachian tube, unspecified ear

√4th **H69 Other and unspecified disorders of Eustachian tube**
    √5th **H69.0 Patulous Eustachian tube**
       H69.00 Patulous Eustachian tube, unspecified ear
       H69.01 Patulous Eustachian tube, right ear
       H69.02 Patulous Eustachian tube, left ear
       H69.03 Patulous Eustachian tube, bilateral

    √5th **H69.8 Other specified disorders of Eustachian tube**
       H69.80 Other specified disorders of Eustachian tube, unspecified ear
       H69.81 Other specified disorders of Eustachian tube, right ear
       H69.82 Other specified disorders of Eustachian tube, left ear
       H69.83 Other specified disorders of Eustachian tube, bilateral

    √5th **H69.9 Unspecified Eustachian tube disorder**
       H69.90 Unspecified Eustachian tube disorder, unspecified ear
       H69.91 Unspecified Eustachian tube disorder, right ear
       H69.92 Unspecified Eustachian tube disorder, left ear
       H69.93 Unspecified Eustachian tube disorder, bilateral

√4th **H70 Mastoiditis and related conditions**
    √5th **H70.0 Acute mastoiditis**
Abscess of mastoid
Empyema of mastoid
    √6th **H70.00 Acute mastoiditis without complications**
       H70.001 Acute mastoiditis without complications, right ear
       H70.002 Acute mastoiditis without complications, left ear
       H70.003 Acute mastoiditis without complications, bilateral
       H70.009 Acute mastoiditis without complications, unspecified ear

    √6th **H70.01 Subperiosteal abscess of mastoid**
       H70.011 Subperiosteal abscess of mastoid, right ear
       H70.012 Subperiosteal abscess of mastoid, left ear
       H70.013 Subperiosteal abscess of mastoid, bilateral
       H70.019 Subperiosteal abscess of mastoid, unspecified ear

    √6th **H70.09 Acute mastoiditis with other complications**
       H70.091 Acute mastoiditis with other complications, right ear
       H70.092 Acute mastoiditis with other complications, left ear
       H70.093 Acute mastoiditis with other complications, bilateral
       H70.099 Acute mastoiditis with other complications, unspecified ear

    √5th **H70.1 Chronic mastoiditis**
Caries of mastoid
Fistula of mastoid
EXCLUDES 1   tuberculous mastoiditis (A18.03)
       H70.10 Chronic mastoiditis, unspecified ear
       H70.11 Chronic mastoiditis, right ear
       H70.12 Chronic mastoiditis, left ear
       H70.13 Chronic mastoiditis, bilateral

    √5th **H70.2 Petrositis**
Inflammation of petrous bone
    √6th **H70.20 Unspecified petrositis**
       H70.201 Unspecified petrositis, right ear
       H70.202 Unspecified petrositis, left ear
       H70.203 Unspecified petrositis, bilateral
       H70.209 Unspecified petrositis, unspecified ear

    √6th **H70.21 Acute petrositis**
       H70.211 Acute petrositis, right ear
       H70.212 Acute petrositis, left ear
       H70.213 Acute petrositis, bilateral
       H70.219 Acute petrositis, unspecified ear

    √6th **H70.22 Chronic petrositis**
       H70.221 Chronic petrositis, right ear
       H70.222 Chronic petrositis, left ear
       H70.223 Chronic petrositis, bilateral
       H70.229 Chronic petrositis, unspecified ear

    √5th **H70.8 Other mastoiditis and related conditions**
EXCLUDES 1   preauricular sinus and cyst (Q18.1)
               sinus, fistula, and cyst of branchial cleft (Q18.0)
    √6th **H70.81 Postauricular fistula**
       H70.811 Postauricular fistula, right ear
       H70.812 Postauricular fistula, left ear
       H70.813 Postauricular fistula, bilateral
       H70.819 Postauricular fistula, unspecified ear

    √6th **H70.89 Other mastoiditis and related conditions**
       H70.891 Other mastoiditis and related conditions, right ear
       H70.892 Other mastoiditis and related conditions, left ear
       H70.893 Other mastoiditis and related conditions, bilateral
       H70.899 Other mastoiditis and related conditions, unspecified ear

    √5th **H70.9 Unspecified mastoiditis**
       H70.90 Unspecified mastoiditis, unspecified ear
       H70.91 Unspecified mastoiditis, right ear
       H70.92 Unspecified mastoiditis, left ear
       H70.93 Unspecified mastoiditis, bilateral

√4th **H71 Cholesteatoma of middle ear**
EXCLUDES 2   cholesteatoma of external ear (H60.4-)
               recurrent cholesteatoma of postmastoidectomy cavity (H95.0-)
    √5th **H71.0 Cholesteatoma of attic**
       H71.00 Cholesteatoma of attic, unspecified ear
       H71.01 Cholesteatoma of attic, right ear
       H71.02 Cholesteatoma of attic, left ear
       H71.03 Cholesteatoma of attic, bilateral

EXCLUDES 1 Not coded here   *EXCLUDES 2* Not included here   *Manifestation Code*

✓5ᵗʰ **H71.1** **Cholesteatoma of tympanum**
    H71.10 **Cholesteatoma of tympanum, unspecified ear**
    H71.11 **Cholesteatoma of tympanum, right ear**
    H71.12 **Cholesteatoma of tympanum, left ear**
    H71.13 **Cholesteatoma of tympanum, bilateral**

✓5ᵗʰ **H71.2** **Cholesteatoma of mastoid**
    H71.20 **Cholesteatoma of mastoid, unspecified ear**
    H71.21 **Cholesteatoma of mastoid, right ear**
    H71.22 **Cholesteatoma of mastoid, left ear**
    H71.23 **Cholesteatoma of mastoid, bilateral**

✓5ᵗʰ **H71.3** **Diffuse cholesteatosis**
    H71.30 **Diffuse cholesteatosis, unspecified ear**
    H71.31 **Diffuse cholesteatosis, right ear**
    H71.32 **Diffuse cholesteatosis, left ear**
    H71.33 **Diffuse cholesteatosis, bilateral**

✓5ᵗʰ **H71.9** **Unspecified cholesteatoma**
    H71.90 **Unspecified cholesteatoma, unspecified ear**
    H71.91 **Unspecified cholesteatoma, right ear**
    H71.92 **Unspecified cholesteatoma, left ear**
    H71.93 **Unspecified cholesteatoma, bilateral**

✓4ᵗʰ **H72** **Perforation of tympanic membrane**
    INCLUDES persistent post-traumatic perforation of ear drum
                postinflammatory perforation of ear drum
    Code first any associated otitis media (H65-, H66.1-, H66.2-, H66.3-,
        H66.4-, H66.9-, H67-)
    EXCLUDES 1 *acute suppurative otitis media with rupture of the tympanic*
        membrane (H66.01-)
        traumatic rupture of ear drum (S09.2-)

✓5ᵗʰ **H72.0** **Central perforation of tympanic membrane**
    H72.00 **Central perforation of tympanic membrane, unspecified ear**
    H72.01 **Central perforation of tympanic membrane, right ear**
    H72.02 **Central perforation of tympanic membrane, left ear**
    H72.03 **Central perforation of tympanic membrane, bilateral**

✓5ᵗʰ **H72.1** **Attic perforation of tympanic membrane**
    Perforation of pars flaccida
    H72.10 **Attic perforation of tympanic membrane, unspecified ear**
    H72.11 **Attic perforation of tympanic membrane, right ear**
    H72.12 **Attic perforation of tympanic membrane, left ear**
    H72.13 **Attic perforation of tympanic membrane, bilateral**

✓5ᵗʰ **H72.2** **Other marginal perforations of tympanic membrane**
  ✓6ᵗʰ **H72.2x** **Other marginal perforations of tympanic membrane**
    H72.2x1 **Other marginal perforations of tympanic membrane, right ear**
    H72.2x2 **Other marginal perforations of tympanic membrane, left ear**
    H72.2x3 **Other marginal perforations of tympanic membrane, bilateral**
    H72.2x9 **Other marginal perforations of tympanic membrane, unspecified ear**

✓5ᵗʰ **H72.8** **Other perforations of tympanic membrane**
  ✓6ᵗʰ **H72.81** **Multiple perforations of tympanic membrane**
    H72.811 **Multiple perforations of tympanic membrane, right ear**
    H72.812 **Multiple perforations of tympanic membrane, left ear**
    H72.813 **Multiple perforations of tympanic membrane, bilateral**
    H72.819 **Multiple perforations of tympanic membrane, unspecified ear**
  ✓6ᵗʰ **H72.82** **Total perforations of tympanic membrane**
    H72.821 **Total perforations of tympanic membrane, right ear**
    H72.822 **Total perforations of tympanic membrane, left ear**
    H72.823 **Total perforations of tympanic membrane, bilateral**
    H72.829 **Total perforations of tympanic membrane, unspecified ear**

✓5ᵗʰ **H72.9** **Unspecified perforation of tympanic membrane**
    H72.90 **Unspecified perforation of tympanic membrane, unspecified ear**
    H72.91 **Unspecified perforation of tympanic membrane, right ear**
    H72.92 **Unspecified perforation of tympanic membrane, left ear**
    H72.93 **Unspecified perforation of tympanic membrane, bilateral**

✓4ᵗʰ **H73** **Other disorders of tympanic membrane**
  ✓5ᵗʰ **H73.0** **Acute myringitis**
    EXCLUDES 1 *acute myringitis with otitis media (H65, H66)*
  ✓6ᵗʰ **H73.00** **Unspecified acute myringitis**
    Acute tympanitis NOS
    H73.001 **Acute myringitis, right ear**
    H73.002 **Acute myringitis, left ear**
    H73.003 **Acute myringitis, bilateral**
    H73.009 **Acute myringitis, unspecified ear**
  ✓6ᵗʰ **H73.01** **Bullous myringitis**
    H73.011 **Bullous myringitis, right ear**
    H73.012 **Bullous myringitis, left ear**
    H73.013 **Bullous myringitis, bilateral**
    H73.019 **Bullous myringitis, unspecified ear**
  ✓6ᵗʰ **H73.09** **Other acute myringitis**
    H73.091 **Other acute myringitis, right ear**
    H73.092 **Other acute myringitis, left ear**
    H73.093 **Other acute myringitis, bilateral**
    H73.099 **Other acute myringitis, unspecified ear**

  ✓5ᵗʰ **H73.1** **Chronic myringitis**
    Chronic tympanitis
    EXCLUDES 1 *chronic myringitis with otitis media (H65, H66)*
    H73.10 **Chronic myringitis, unspecified ear**
    H73.11 **Chronic myringitis, right ear**
    H73.12 **Chronic myringitis, left ear**
    H73.13 **Chronic myringitis, bilateral**

  ✓5ᵗʰ **H73.2** **Unspecified myringitis**
    H73.20 **Unspecified myringitis, unspecified ear**
    H73.21 **Unspecified myringitis, right ear**
    H73.22 **Unspecified myringitis, left ear**
    H73.23 **Unspecified myringitis, bilateral**

  ✓5ᵗʰ **H73.8** **Other specified disorders of tympanic membrane**
  ✓6ᵗʰ **H73.81** **Atrophic flaccid tympanic membrane**
    H73.811 **Atrophic flaccid tympanic membrane, right ear**
    H73.812 **Atrophic flaccid tympanic membrane, left ear**
    H73.813 **Atrophic flaccid tympanic membrane, bilateral**
    H73.819 **Atrophic flaccid tympanic membrane, unspecified ear**
  ✓6ᵗʰ **H73.82** **Atrophic nonflaccid tympanic membrane**
    H73.821 **Atrophic nonflaccid tympanic membrane, right ear**
    H73.822 **Atrophic nonflaccid tympanic membrane, left ear**
    H73.823 **Atrophic nonflaccid tympanic membrane, bilateral**
    H73.829 **Atrophic nonflaccid tympanic membrane, unspecified ear**
  ✓6ᵗʰ **H73.89** **Other specified disorders of tympanic membrane**
    H73.891 **Other specified disorders of tympanic membrane, right ear**
    H73.892 **Other specified disorders of tympanic membrane, left ear**
    H73.893 **Other specified disorders of tympanic membrane, bilateral**
    H73.899 **Other specified disorders of tympanic membrane, unspecified ear**

  ✓5ᵗʰ **H73.9** **Unspecified disorder of tympanic membrane**
    H73.90 **Unspecified disorder of tympanic membrane, unspecified ear**
    H73.91 **Unspecified disorder of tympanic membrane, right ear**
    H73.92 **Unspecified disorder of tympanic membrane, left ear**

☑ Appropriate additional character required   ✓x7ᵗʰ Requires 7th character, placeholder x must fill empty characters

Diseases of the Ear and Mastoid Process

H73.93–H81.09

H73.93   **Unspecified disorder of tympanic membrane, bilateral**

√4th **H74   Other disorders of middle ear mastoid**
    EXCLUDES 2   *mastoiditis (H70-)*

√5th **H74.0   Tympanosclerosis**
    H74.01   **Tympanosclerosis, right ear**
    H74.02   **Tympanosclerosis, left ear**
    H74.03   **Tympanosclerosis, bilateral**
    H74.09   **Tympanosclerosis, unspecified ear**

√5th **H74.1   Adhesive middle ear disease**
    Adhesive otitis
    EXCLUDES 1   *glue ear (H65.3-)*
    H74.11   **Adhesive right middle ear disease**
    H74.12   **Adhesive left middle ear disease**
    H74.13   **Adhesive middle ear disease, bilateral**
    H74.19   **Adhesive middle ear disease, unspecified ear**

√5th **H74.2   Discontinuity and dislocation of ear ossicles**
    H74.20   **Discontinuity and dislocation of ear ossicles, unspecified ear**
    H74.21   **Discontinuity and dislocation of right ear ossicles**
    H74.22   **Discontinuity and dislocation of left ear ossicles**
    H74.23   **Discontinuity and dislocation of ear ossicles, bilateral**

√5th **H74.3   Other acquired abnormalities of ear ossicles**
   √6th **H74.31   Ankylosis of ear ossicles**
    H74.311   **Ankylosis of ear ossicles, right ear**
    H74.312   **Ankylosis of ear ossicles, left ear**
    H74.313   **Ankylosis of ear ossicles, bilateral**
    H74.319   **Ankylosis of ear ossicles, unspecified ear**
   √6th **H74.32   Partial loss of ear ossicles**
    H74.321   **Partial loss of ear ossicles, right ear**
    H74.322   **Partial loss of ear ossicles, left ear**
    H74.323   **Partial loss of ear ossicles, bilateral**
    H74.329   **Partial loss of ear ossicles, unspecified ear**
   √6th **H74.39   Other acquired abnormalities of ear ossicles**
    H74.391   **Other acquired abnormalities of right ear ossicles**
    H74.392   **Other acquired abnormalities of left ear ossicles**
    H74.393   **Other acquired abnormalities of ear ossicles, bilateral**
    H74.399   **Other acquired abnormalities of ear ossicles, unspecified ear**

√5th **H74.4   Polyp of middle ear**
    H74.40   **Polyp of middle ear, unspecified ear**
    H74.41   **Polyp of right middle ear**
    H74.42   **Polyp of left middle ear**
    H74.43   **Polyp of middle ear, bilateral**

√5th **H74.8   Other specified disorders of middle ear and mastoid**
   √6th **H74.8x   Other specified disorders of middle ear and mastoid**
    H74.8x1   **Other specified disorders of right middle ear and mastoid**
    H74.8x2   **Other specified disorders of left middle ear and mastoid**
    H74.8x3   **Other specified disorders of middle ear and mastoid, bilateral**
    H74.8x9   **Other specified disorders of middle ear and mastoid, unspecified ear**

√5th **H74.9   Unspecified disorder of middle ear and mastoid**
    H74.90   **Unspecified disorder of middle ear and mastoid, unspecified ear**
    H74.91   **Unspecified disorder of right middle ear and mastoid**
    H74.92   **Unspecified disorder of left middle ear and mastoid**
    H74.93   **Unspecified disorder of middle ear and mastoid, bilateral**

√4th **H75   Other disorders of middle ear and mastoid in diseases classified elsewhere**
    Code first underlying disease

√5th **H75.0   Mastoiditis in infectious and parasitic diseases classified elsewhere**
    EXCLUDES 1   *mastoiditis (in):*
      syphilis (A52.77)
      tuberculosis (A18.03)
    H75.00   *Mastoiditis in infectious and parasitic diseases classified elsewhere, unspecified ear*
    H75.01   *Mastoiditis in infectious and parasitic diseases classified elsewhere, right ear*
    H75.02   *Mastoiditis in infectious and parasitic diseases classified elsewhere, left ear*
    H75.03   *Mastoiditis in infectious and parasitic diseases classified elsewhere, bilateral*

√5th **H75.8   Other specified disorders of middle ear and mastoid in diseases classified elsewhere**
    H75.80   *Other specified disorders of middle ear and mastoid in diseases classified elsewhere, unspecified ear*
    H75.81   *Other specified disorders of right middle ear and mastoid in diseases classified elsewhere*
    H75.82   *Other specified disorders of left middle ear and mastoid in diseases classified elsewhere*
    H75.83   *Other specified disorders of middle ear and mastoid in diseases classified elsewhere, bilateral*

Diseases of inner ear (H80-H83)

√4th **H80   Otosclerosis**
    INCLUDES   Otospongiosis

√5th **H80.0   Otosclerosis involving oval window, nonobliterative**
    H80.00   **Otosclerosis involving oval window, nonobliterative, unspecified ear**
    H80.01   **Otosclerosis involving oval window, nonobliterative, right ear**
    H80.02   **Otosclerosis involving oval window, nonobliterative, left ear**
    H80.03   **Otosclerosis involving oval window, nonobliterative, bilateral**

√5th **H80.1   Otosclerosis involving oval window, obliterative**
    H80.10   **Otosclerosis involving oval window, obliterative, unspecified ear**
    H80.11   **Otosclerosis involving oval window, obliterative, right ear**
    H80.12   **Otosclerosis involving oval window, obliterative, left ear**
    H80.13   **Otosclerosis involving oval window, obliterative, bilateral**

√5th **H80.2   Cochlear otosclerosis**
    Otosclerosis involving otic capsule
    Otosclerosis involving round window
    H80.20   **Cochlear otosclerosis, unspecified ear**
    H80.21   **Cochlear otosclerosis, right ear**
    H80.22   **Cochlear otosclerosis, left ear**
    H80.23   **Cochlear otosclerosis, bilateral**

√5th **H80.8   Other otosclerosis**
    H80.80   **Other otosclerosis, unspecified ear**
    H80.81   **Other otosclerosis, right ear**
    H80.82   **Other otosclerosis, left ear**
    H80.83   **Other otosclerosis, bilateral**

√5th **H80.9   Unspecified otosclerosis**
    H80.90   **Unspecified otosclerosis, unspecified ear**
    H80.91   **Unspecified otosclerosis, right ear**
    H80.92   **Unspecified otosclerosis, left ear**
    H80.93   **Unspecified otosclerosis, bilateral**

√4th **H81   Disorders of vestibular function**
    EXCLUDES 1   *epidemic vertigo (A88.1)*
      vertigo NOS (R42)

√5th **H81.0   Ménière's disease**
    Labyrinthine hydrops
    Ménière's syndrome or vertigo
    H81.01   **Ménière's disease, right ear**
    H81.02   **Ménière's disease, left ear**
    H81.03   **Ménière's disease, bilateral**
    H81.09   **Ménière's disease, unspecified ear**

EXCLUDES 1   Not coded here   EXCLUDES 2   Not included here   *Manifestation Code*

√5th **H81.1 Benign paroxysmal vertigo**
    H81.10 Benign paroxysmal vertigo, unspecified ear
    H81.11 Benign paroxysmal vertigo, right ear
    H81.12 Benign paroxysmal vertigo, left ear
    H81.13 Benign paroxysmal vertigo, bilateral

√5th **H81.2 Vestibular neuronitis**
    H81.20 Vestibular neuronitis, unspecified ear
    H81.21 Vestibular neuronitis, right ear
    H81.22 Vestibular neuronitis, left ear
    H81.23 Vestibular neuronitis, bilateral

√5th **H81.3 Other peripheral vertigo**
  √6th **H81.31 Aural vertigo**
    H81.311 Aural vertigo, right ear
    H81.312 Aural vertigo, left ear
    H81.313 Aural vertigo, bilateral
    H81.319 Aural vertigo, unspecified ear
  √6th **H81.39 Other peripheral vertigo**
    Lermoyez' syndrome
    Otogenic vertigo
    Peripheral vertigo NOS
    H81.391 Other peripheral vertigo, right ear
    H81.392 Other peripheral vertigo, left ear
    H81.393 Other peripheral vertigo, bilateral
    H81.399 Other peripheral vertigo, unspecified ear

√5th **H81.4 Vertigo of central origin**
    Central positional nystagmus
    H81.41 Vertigo of central origin, right ear
    H81.42 Vertigo of central origin, left ear
    H81.43 Vertigo of central origin, bilateral
    H81.49 Vertigo of central origin, unspecified ear

√5th **H81.8 Other disorders of vestibular function**
  √6th **H81.8x Other disorders of vestibular function**
    H81.8x1 Other disorders of vestibular function, right ear
    H81.8x2 Other disorders of vestibular function, left ear
    H81.8x3 Other disorders of vestibular function, bilateral
    H81.8x9 Other disorders of vestibular function, unspecified ear

√5th **H81.9 Unspecified disorder of vestibular function**
    Vertiginous syndrome NOS
    H81.90 Unspecified disorder of vestibular function, unspecified ear
    H81.91 Unspecified disorder of vestibular function, right ear
    H81.92 Unspecified disorder of vestibular function, left ear
    H81.93 Unspecified disorder of vestibular function, bilateral

√4th **H82 Vertiginous syndromes in diseases classified elsewhere**
    Code first underlying disease
    EXCLUDES 1 *epidemic vertigo (A88.1)*
    H82.1 *Vertiginous syndromes in diseases classified elsewhere, right ear*
    H82.2 *Vertiginous syndromes in diseases classified elsewhere, left ear*
    H82.3 *Vertiginous syndromes in diseases classified elsewhere, bilateral*
    H82.9 *Vertiginous syndromes in diseases classified elsewhere, unspecified ear*

√4th **H83 Other diseases of inner ear**
  √5th **H83.0 Labyrinthitis**
    H83.01 Labyrinthitis, right ear
    H83.02 Labyrinthitis, left ear
    H83.03 Labyrinthitis, bilateral
    H83.09 Labyrinthitis, unspecified ear
  √5th **H83.1 Labyrinthine fistula**
    H83.11 Labyrinthine fistula, right ear
    H83.12 Labyrinthine fistula, left ear
    H83.13 Labyrinthine fistula, bilateral
    H83.19 Labyrinthine fistula, unspecified ear

√5th **H83.2 Labyrinthine dysfunction**
    Labyrinthine hypersensitivity
    Labyrinthine hypofunction
    Labyrinthine loss of function
  √6th **H83.2x Labyrinthine dysfunction**
    H83.2x1 Labyrinthine dysfunction, right ear
    H83.2x2 Labyrinthine dysfunction, left ear
    H83.2x3 Labyrinthine dysfunction, bilateral
    H83.2x9 Labyrinthine dysfunction, unspecified ear

√5th **H83.3 Noise effects on inner ear**
    Acoustic trauma of inner ear
    Noise-induced hearing loss of inner ear
  √6th **H83.3x Noise effects on inner ear**
    H83.3x1 Noise effects on right inner ear
    H83.3x2 Noise effects on left inner ear
    H83.3x3 Noise effects on inner ear, bilateral
    H83.3x9 Noise effects on inner ear, unspecified ear

√5th **H83.8 Other specified diseases of inner ear**
  √6th **H83.8x Other specified diseases of inner ear**
    H83.8x1 Other specified diseases of right inner ear
    H83.8x2 Other specified diseases of left inner ear
    H83.8x3 Other specified diseases of inner ear, bilateral
    H83.8x9 Other specified diseases of inner ear, unspecified ear

√5th **H83.9 Unspecified disease of inner ear**
    H83.90 Unspecified disease of inner ear, unspecified ear
    H83.91 Unspecified disease of right inner ear
    H83.92 Unspecified disease of left inner ear
    H83.93 Unspecified disease of inner ear, bilateral

Other disorders of ear (H90-H94)

√4th **H90 Conductive and sensorineural hearing loss**
    EXCLUDES 1 *deaf nonspeaking NEC (H91.3)*
    deafness NOS (H91.9-)
    hearing loss NOS (H91.9-)
    noise-induced hearing loss (H83.3-)
    ototoxic hearing loss (H91.0-)
    sudden (idiopathic) hearing loss (H91.2-)
    H90.0 Conductive hearing loss, bilateral
  √5th H90.1 Conductive hearing loss, unilateral with unrestricted hearing on the contralateral side
    H90.11 Conductive hearing loss, unilateral, right ear, with unrestricted hearing on the contralateral side
    H90.12 Conductive hearing loss, unilateral, left ear, with unrestricted hearing on the contralateral side
    H90.2 Conductive hearing loss, unspecified
    Conductive deafness NOS
    H90.3 Sensorineural hearing loss, bilateral
  √5th H90.4 Sensorineural hearing loss, unilateral with unrestricted hearing on the contralateral side
    H90.41 Sensorineural hearing loss, unilateral, right ear, with unrestricted hearing on the contralateral side
    H90.42 Sensorineural hearing loss, unilateral, left ear, with unrestricted hearing on the contralateral side
    H90.5 Unspecified sensorineural hearing loss
    Central hearing loss NOS
    Congenital deafness NOS
    Neural hearing loss NOS
    Perceptive hearing loss NOS
    Sensorineural deafness NOS
    Sensory hearing loss NOS
    EXCLUDES 1 *abnormal auditory perception (H93.2-)*
    psychogenic deafness (F44.6)
    H90.6 Mixed conductive and sensorineural hearing loss, bilateral
  √5th H90.7 Mixed conductive and sensorineural hearing loss, unilateral with unrestricted hearing on the contralateral side
    H90.71 Mixed conductive and sensorineural hearing loss, unilateral, right ear, with unrestricted hearing on the contralateral side
    H90.72 Mixed conductive and sensorineural hearing loss, unilateral, left ear, with unrestricted hearing on the contralateral side

☑ Appropriate additional character required   √x7th Requires 7th character, placeholder x must fill empty characters

H90.8   Mixed conductive and sensorineural hearing loss, unspecified

✓4th **H91**   **Other and unspecified hearing loss**
     EXCLUDES 1   *abnormal auditory perception (H93.2-)*
                 hearing loss as classified in H90-
                  impacted cerumen (H61.2-)
                  noise-induced hearing loss (H83.3-)
                  psychogenic deafness (F44.6)
                  transient ischemic deafness (H93.01-)

     ✓5th **H91.0**   **Ototoxic hearing loss**
            Code first (T36-T65) to identify toxic agent
            H91.01   Ototoxic hearing loss, right ear
            H91.02   Ototoxic hearing loss, left ear
            H91.03   Ototoxic hearing loss, bilateral
            H91.09   Ototoxic hearing loss, unspecified ear

     ✓5th **H91.1**   **Presbycusis**
            Presbyacusia
            H91.10   Presbycusis, unspecified ear
            H91.11   Presbycusis, right ear
            H91.12   Presbycusis, left ear
            H91.13   Presbycusis, bilateral

     ✓5th **H91.2**   **Sudden idiopathic hearing loss**
            Sudden hearing loss NOS
            H91.20   Sudden idiopathic hearing loss, unspecified ear
            H91.21   Sudden idiopathic hearing loss, right ear
            H91.22   Sudden idiopathic hearing loss, left ear
            H91.23   Sudden idiopathic hearing loss, bilateral

     H91.3   **Deaf nonspeaking, not elsewhere classified**

     ✓5th **H91.8**   **Other specified hearing loss**
       ✓6th **H91.8x**   **Other specified hearing loss**
            H91.8x1   Other specified hearing loss, right ear
            H91.8x2   Other specified hearing loss, left ear
            H91.8x3   Other specified hearing loss, bilateral
            H91.8x9   Other specified hearing loss, unspecified ear

     ✓5th **H91.9**   **Unspecified hearing loss**
            Congenital deafness NOS
            Deafness NOS
            High frequency deafness
            Low frequency deafness
            H91.90   Unspecified hearing loss, unspecified ear
            H91.91   Unspecified hearing loss, right ear
            H91.92   Unspecified hearing loss, left ear
            H91.93   Unspecified hearing loss, bilateral

✓4th **H92**   **Otalgia and effusion of ear**
     ✓5th **H92.0**   **Otalgia**
            H92.01   Otalgia, right ear
            H92.02   Otalgia, left ear
            H92.03   Otalgia, bilateral
            H92.09   Otalgia, unspecified ear

     ✓5th **H92.1**   **Otorrhea**
         EXCLUDES 1   *leakage of cerebrospinal fluid through ear (G96.0)*
            H92.10   Otorrhea, unspecified ear
            H92.11   Otorrhea, right ear
            H92.12   Otorrhea, left ear
            H92.13   Otorrhea, bilateral

     ✓5th **H92.2**   **Otorrhagia**
         EXCLUDES 1   *traumatic otorrhagia—code to injury*
            H92.20   Otorrhagia, unspecified ear
            H92.21   Otorrhagia, right ear
            H92.22   Otorrhagia, left ear
            H92.23   Otorrhagia, bilateral

✓4th **H93**   **Other disorders of ear, not elsewhere classified**
     ✓5th **H93.0**   **Degenerative and vascular disorders of ear**
         EXCLUDES 1   *presbycusis (H91.1)*
       ✓6th **H93.01**   **Transient ischemic deafness**
            H93.011   Transient ischemic deafness, right ear
            H93.012   Transient ischemic deafness, left ear
            H93.013   Transient ischemic deafness, bilateral
            H93.019   Transient ischemic deafness, unspecified ear
       ✓6th **H93.09**   **Unspecified degenerative and vascular disorders of ear**
            H93.091   Unspecified degenerative and vascular disorders of right ear

---

            H93.092   Unspecified degenerative and vascular disorders of left ear
            H93.093   Unspecified degenerative and vascular disorders of ear, bilateral
            H93.099   Unspecified degenerative and vascular disorders of unspecified ear

     ✓5th **H93.1**   **Tinnitus**
            H93.11   Tinnitus, right ear
            H93.12   Tinnitus, left ear
            H93.13   Tinnitus, bilateral
            H93.19   Tinnitus, unspecified ear

     ✓5th **H93.2**   **Other abnormal auditory perceptions**
         EXCLUDES 2   *auditory hallucinations (R44.0)*
       ✓6th **H93.21**   **Auditory recruitment**
            H93.211   Auditory recruitment, right ear
            H93.212   Auditory recruitment, left ear
            H93.213   Auditory recruitment, bilateral
            H93.219   Auditory recruitment, unspecified ear
       ✓6th **H93.22**   **Diplacusis**
            H93.221   Diplacusis, right ear
            H93.222   Diplacusis, left ear
            H93.223   Diplacusis, bilateral
            H93.229   Diplacusis, unspecified ear
       ✓6th **H93.23**   **Hyperacusis**
            H93.231   Hyperacusis, right ear
            H93.232   Hyperacusis, left ear
            H93.233   Hyperacusis, bilateral
            H93.239   Hyperacusis, unspecified ear
       ✓6th **H93.24**   **Temporary auditory threshold shift**
            H93.241   Temporary auditory threshold shift, right ear
            H93.242   Temporary auditory threshold shift, left ear
            H93.243   Temporary auditory threshold shift, bilateral
            H93.249   Temporary auditory threshold shift, unspecified ear
       H93.25   **Central auditory processing disorder**
            Congenital auditory imperception
            Word deafness
            EXCLUDES 1   *mixed receptive-expressive language disorder (F80.2)*
       ✓6th **H93.29**   **Other abnormal auditory perceptions**
            H93.291   Other abnormal auditory perceptions, right ear
            H93.292   Other abnormal auditory perceptions, left ear
            H93.293   Other abnormal auditory perceptions, bilateral
            H93.299   Other abnormal auditory perceptions, unspecified ear

     ✓5th **H93.3**   **Disorders of acoustic nerve**
            Disorder of 8th cranial nerve
         EXCLUDES 1   *acoustic neuroma (D33.3)*
                     syphilitic acoustic neuritis (A52.15)
       ✓6th **H93.3x**   **Disorders of acoustic nerve**
            H93.3x1   Disorders of right acoustic nerve
            H93.3x2   Disorders of left acoustic nerve
            H93.3x3   Disorders of bilateral acoustic nerves
            H93.3x9   Disorders of unspecified acoustic nerve

     ✓5th **H93.8**   **Other specified disorders of ear**
       ✓6th **H93.8x**   **Other specified disorders of ear**
            H93.8x1   Other specified disorders of right ear
            H93.8x2   Other specified disorders of left ear
            H93.8x3   Other specified disorders of ear, bilateral
            H93.8x9   Other specified disorders of ear, unspecified ear

     ✓5th **H93.9**   **Unspecified disorder of ear**
            H93.90   Unspecified disorder of ear, unspecified ear
            H93.91   Unspecified disorder of right ear
            H93.92   Unspecified disorder of left ear
            H93.93   Unspecified disorder of ear, bilateral

EXCLUDES 1   Not coded here   EXCLUDES 2   Not included here   *Manifestation Code*

✓4th **H94 Other disorders of ear in diseases classified elsewhere**

✓5th **H94.0 Acoustic neuritis in infectious and parasitic diseases classified elsewhere**

Code first underlying disease, such as:
parasitic disease (B65-B89)

EXCLUDES 1 *acoustic neuritis (in):*
herpes zoster (B02.29)
syphilis (A52.15)

H94.00 *Acoustic neuritis in infectious and parasitic diseases classified elsewhere, unspecified ear*

H94.01 *Acoustic neuritis in infectious and parasitic diseases classified elsewhere, right ear*

H94.02 *Acoustic neuritis in infectious and parasitic diseases classified elsewhere, left ear*

H94.03 *Acoustic neuritis in infectious and parasitic diseases classified elsewhere, bilateral*

✓5th **H94.8 Other specified disorders of ear in diseases classified elsewhere**

Code first underlying disease, such as:
congenital syphilis (A50.0)

EXCLUDES 1 *aural myiasis (B87.4)*
syphilitic labyrinthitis (A52.79)

H94.80 *Other specified disorders of ear in diseases classified elsewhere, unspecified ear*

H94.81 *Other specified disorders of right ear in diseases classified elsewhere*

H94.82 *Other specified disorders of left ear in diseases classified elsewhere*

H94.83 *Other specified disorders of ear in diseases classified elsewhere, bilateral*

Intraoperative and postprocedural complications and disorders of ear and mastoid process, not elsewhere classified (H95)

✓4th **H95 Intraoperative and postprocedural complications and disorders of ear and mastoid process, not elsewhere classified**

✓5th **H95.0 Recurrent cholesteatoma of postmastoidectomy cavity**

H95.00 **Recurrent cholesteatoma of postmastoidectomy cavity, unspecified ear**

H95.01 **Recurrent cholesteatoma of postmastoidectomy cavity, right ear**

H95.02 **Recurrent cholesteatoma of postmastoidectomy cavity, left ear**

H95.03 **Recurrent cholesteatoma of postmastoidectomy cavity, bilateral ears**

✓5th **H95.1 Other disorders of ear and mastoid process following mastoidectomy**

✓6th H95.11 **Chronic inflammation of postmastoidectomy cavity**

H95.111 **Chronic inflammation of postmastoidectomy cavity, right ear**

H95.112 **Chronic inflammation of postmastoidectomy cavity, left ear**

H95.113 **Chronic inflammation of postmastoidectomy cavity, bilateral ears**

H95.119 **Chronic inflammation of postmastoidectomy cavity, unspecified ear**

✓6th H95.12 **Granulation of postmastoidectomy cavity**

H95.121 **Granulation of postmastoidectomy cavity, right ear**

H95.122 **Granulation of postmastoidectomy cavity, left ear**

H95.123 **Granulation of postmastoidectomy cavity, bilateral ears**

H95.129 **Granulation of postmastoidectomy cavity, unspecified ear**

✓6th H95.13 **Mucosal cyst of postmastoidectomy cavity**

H95.131 **Mucosal cyst of postmastoidectomy cavity, right ear**

H95.132 **Mucosal cyst of postmastoidectomy cavity, left ear**

H95.133 **Mucosal cyst of postmastoidectomy cavity, bilateral ears**

H95.139 **Mucosal cyst of postmastoidectomy cavity, unspecified ear**

✓6th H95.19 **Other disorders following mastoidectomy**

H95.191 **Other disorders following mastoidectomy, right ear**

H95.192 **Other disorders following mastoidectomy, left ear**

H95.193 **Other disorders following mastoidectomy, bilateral ears**

H95.199 **Other disorders following mastoidectomy, unspecified ear**

✓5th **H95.2 Intraoperative hemorrhage and hematoma of ear and mastoid process complicating a procedure**

EXCLUDES 1 *intraoperative hemorrhage and hematoma of ear and mastoid process due to accidental puncture or laceration during a procedure (H95.3-)*

H95.21 **Intraoperative hemorrhage and hematoma of ear and mastoid process complicating a procedure on the ear and mastoid process**

H95.22 **Intraoperative hemorrhage and hematoma of ear and mastoid process complicating other procedure**

✓5th **H95.3 Accidental puncture and laceration of ear and mastoid process during a procedure**

H95.31 **Accidental puncture and laceration of the ear and mastoid process during a procedure on the ear and mastoid process**

H95.32 **Accidental puncture and laceration of the ear and mastoid process during other procedure**

✓5th **H95.4 Postprocedural hemorrhage and hematoma of ear and mastoid process following a procedure**

H95.41 **Postprocedural hemorrhage and hematoma of ear and mastoid process following a procedure on the ear and mastoid process**

H95.42 **Postprocedural hemorrhage and hematoma of ear and mastoid process following other procedure**

✓5th **H95.8 Other intraoperative and postprocedural complications and disorders of the ear and mastoid process, not elsewhere classified**

EXCLUDES 2 *postprocedural complications and disorders following mastoidectomy (H95.0-, H95.1-)*

✓6th H95.81 **Postprocedural stenosis of external ear canal**

H95.811 **Postprocedural stenosis of right external ear canal**

H95.812 **Postprocedural stenosis of left external ear canal**

H95.813 **Postprocedural stenosis of external ear canal, bilateral**

H95.819 **Postprocedural stenosis of unspecified external ear canal**

H95.88 **Other intraoperative complications and disorders of the ear and mastoid process, not elsewhere classified**

Use additional code, if applicable, to further specify disorder

H95.89 **Other postprocedural complications and disorders of the ear and mastoid process, not elsewhere classified**

Use additional code, if applicable, to further specify disorder

---

✔ Appropriate additional character required   ✓x7th Requires 7th character, placeholder x must fill empty characters

Chapter 9. Diseases of the Circulatory System (I00-I99)

EXCLUDES 2   certain conditions originating in the perinatal period (P04-P96)
certain infectious and parasitic diseases (A00-B99)
complications of pregnancy, childbirth and the puerperium (O00-O99)
congenital malformations, deformations, and chromosomal abnormalities (Q00-Q99)
endocrine, nutritional and metabolic diseases (E00-E88)
injury, poisoning and certain other consequences of external causes (S00-T88)
neoplasms (C00-D49)
symptoms, signs and abnormal clinical and laboratory findings, not elsewhere classified (R00-R94)
systemic connective tissue disorders (M30-M36)
transient cerebral ischemic attacks and related syndromes (G45-)

This chapter contains the following blocks:
I00-I02   Acute rheumatic fever
I05-I09   Chronic rheumatic heart diseases
I10-I15   Hypertensive diseases
I20-I25   Ischemic heart diseases
I26-I28   Pulmonary heart disease and diseases of pulmonary circulation
I30-I52   Other forms of heart disease
I60-I69   Cerebrovascular diseases
I70-I79   Diseases of arteries, arterioles and capillaries
I80-I89   Diseases of veins, lymphatic vessels and lymph nodes, not elsewhere classified
I95-I99   Other and unspecified disorders of the circulatory system

Acute rheumatic fever (I00-I02)

I00   Rheumatic fever without heart involvement
     INCLUDES   arthritis, rheumatic, acute or subacute
     EXCLUDES 1   rheumatic fever with heart involvement (I01.0–I01.9)

✓4ᵗʰ **I01   Rheumatic fever with heart involvement**
     EXCLUDES 1   chronic diseases of rheumatic origin (I05-I09) unless rheumatic fever is also present or there is evidence of reactivation or activity of the rheumatic process.

     I01.0   Acute rheumatic pericarditis
         Any condition in I00 with pericarditis
         Rheumatic pericarditis (acute)
         EXCLUDES 1   acute pericarditis not specified as rheumatic (I30-)

     I01.1   Acute rheumatic endocarditis
         Any condition in I00 with endocarditis or valvulitis
         Acute rheumatic valvulitis

     I01.2   Acute rheumatic myocarditis
         Any condition in I00 with myocarditis

     I01.8   Other acute rheumatic heart disease
         Any condition in I00 with other or multiple types of heart involvement
         Acute rheumatic pancarditis

     I01.9   Acute rheumatic heart disease, unspecified
         Any condition in I00 with unspecified type of heart involvement
         Rheumatic carditis, acute
         Rheumatic heart disease, active or acute

✓4ᵗʰ **I02   Rheumatic chorea**
     INCLUDES   Sydenham's chorea
     EXCLUDES 1   chorea NOS (G25.5)
               Huntington's chorea (G10)

     I02.0   Rheumatic chorea with heart involvement
         Chorea NOS with heart involvement
         Rheumatic chorea with heart involvement of any type classifiable under I01-

     I02.9   Rheumatic chorea without heart involvement
         Rheumatic chorea NOS

Chronic rheumatic heart diseases (I05-I09)

✓4ᵗʰ **I05   Rheumatic mitral valve diseases**
     INCLUDES   conditions classifiable to both I05.0 and I05.2-I05.9, whether specified as rheumatic or not
     EXCLUDES 1   mitral valve disease specified as nonrheumatic (I34-)
               mitral valve disease with aortic and/or tricuspid valve involvement (I08-)

     I05.0   Rheumatic mitral stenosis
         Mitral (valve) obstruction (rheumatic)

     I05.1   Rheumatic mitral insufficiency
         Rheumatic mitral incompetence
         Rheumatic mitral regurgitation
         EXCLUDES 1   mitral insufficiency not specified as rheumatic (I34.0)

     I05.2   Rheumatic mitral stenosis with insufficiency
         Rheumatic mitral stenosis with incompetence or regurgitation

     I05.8   Other rheumatic mitral valve diseases
         Rheumatic mitral (valve) failure

     I05.9   Rheumatic mitral valve disease, unspecified
         Rheumatic mitral (valve) disorder (chronic) NOS

✓4ᵗʰ **I06   Rheumatic aortic valve diseases**
     EXCLUDES 1   aortic valve disease not specified as rheumatic (I35-)
               aortic valve disease with mitral and/or tricuspid valve involvement (I08-)

     I06.0   Rheumatic aortic stenosis
         Rheumatic aortic (valve) obstruction

     I06.1   Rheumatic aortic insufficiency
         Rheumatic aortic incompetence
         Rheumatic aortic regurgitation

     I06.2   Rheumatic aortic stenosis with insufficiency
         Rheumatic aortic stenosis with incompetence or regurgitation

     I06.8   Other rheumatic aortic valve diseases

     I06.9   Rheumatic aortic valve disease, unspecified
         Rheumatic aortic (valve) disease NOS

✓4ᵗʰ **I07   Rheumatic tricuspid valve diseases**
     INCLUDES   rheumatic tricuspid valve diseases specified as rheumatic or unspecified
     EXCLUDES 1   tricuspid valve disease specified as nonrheumatic (I36-)
               tricuspid valve disease with aortic and/or mitral valve involvement (I08-)

     I07.0   Rheumatic tricuspid stenosis
         Tricuspid (valve) stenosis (rheumatic)

     I07.1   Rheumatic tricuspid insufficiency
         Tricuspid (valve) insufficiency (rheumatic)

     I07.2   Rheumatic tricuspid stenosis and insufficiency

     I07.8   Other rheumatic tricuspid valve diseases

     I07.9   Rheumatic tricuspid valve disease, unspecified
         Rheumatic tricuspid valve disorder NOS

✓4ᵗʰ **I08   Multiple valve diseases**
     INCLUDES   multiple valve diseases specified as rheumatic or unspecified
     EXCLUDES 1   endocarditis, valve unspecified (I38)
               multiple valve disease specified a nonrheumatic (I34-, I35-, I36-, I37-, I38-, Q22-, Q23-, Q24.8-)
               rheumatic valve disease NOS (I09.1)

     I08.0   Rheumatic disorders of both mitral and aortic valves
         Involvement of both mitral and aortic valves specified as rheumatic or unspecified

     I08.1   Rheumatic disorders of both mitral and tricuspid valves

     I08.2   Rheumatic disorders of both aortic and tricuspid valves

     I08.3   Combined rheumatic disorders of mitral, aortic and tricuspid valves

     I08.8   Other rheumatic multiple valve diseases

     I08.9   Rheumatic multiple valve disease, unspecified

✓4ᵗʰ **I09   Other rheumatic heart diseases**
     I09.0   Rheumatic myocarditis
         EXCLUDES 1   myocarditis not specified as rheumatic (I51.4)

     I09.1   Rheumatic diseases of endocardium, valve unspecified
         Rheumatic endocarditis (chronic)
         Rheumatic valvulitis (chronic)
         EXCLUDES 1   endocarditis, valve unspecified (I38)

     I09.2   Chronic rheumatic pericarditis
         Adherent pericardium, rheumatic
         Chronic rheumatic mediastinopericarditis
         Chronic rheumatic myopericarditis
         EXCLUDES 1   chronic pericarditis not specified as rheumatic (I31-)

✓5ᵗʰ **I09.8   Other specified rheumatic heart diseases**
         I09.81   Rheumatic heart failure
               Use additional code to identify type of heart failure (I50-)

         I09.89   Other specified rheumatic heart diseases
               Rheumatic disease of pulmonary valve

     I09.9   Rheumatic heart disease, unspecified
         Rheumatic carditis
         EXCLUDES 1   rheumatoid carditis (M05.31)

EXCLUDES 1   Not coded here   EXCLUDES 2   Not included here   ***Manifestation Code***

Hypertensive diseases (I10-I15)

Use additional code to identify:
  exposure to environmental tobacco smoke (Z77.22)
  history of tobacco use (Z87.891)
  occupational exposure to environmental tobacco smoke (Z57.31)
  tobacco dependence (F17-)
  tobacco use (Z72.0)

  EXCLUDES 1 *hypertensive disease complicating pregnancy, childbirth and the puerperium (O10-O11, O13-O16)*
  neonatal hypertension (P29.2)
  primary pulmonary hypertension (I27.0)

I10 Essential (primary) hypertension

  INCLUDES high blood pressure
  hypertension (arterial) (benign) (essential) (malignant) (primary) (systemic)

  EXCLUDES 1 *hypertensive disease complicating pregnancy, childbirth and the puerperium (O10-O11, O13-O16)*

  EXCLUDES 2 *essential (primary) hypertension involving vessels of brain (I60-I69)*
  essential (primary) hypertension involving vessels of eye (H35.0)

✓4th I11 Hypertensive heart disease

  INCLUDES any condition in I51.4-I51.9 due to hypertension

  I11.0 Hypertensive heart disease with heart failure
  Hypertensive heart failure
  Use additional code to identify type of heart failure (I50-)

  I11.9 Hypertensive heart disease without heart failure
  Hypertensive heart disease NOS

✓4th I12 Hypertensive chronic kidney disease

  INCLUDES any condition in N18- and N26- due to hypertension
  arteriosclerosis of kidney
  arteriosclerotic nephritis (chronic) (interstitial)
  hypertensive nephropathy
  nephrosclerosis

  EXCLUDES 1 *hypertension due to kidney disease (I15.0, I15.1)*
  renovascular hypertension (I15.0)
  secondary hypertension (I15-)

  EXCLUDES 2 *acute kidney failure (N17-)*

  I12.0 Hypertensive chronic kidney disease with stage 5 chronic kidney disease or end stage renal disease
  Use additional code to identify the stage of chronic kidney disease (N18.5, N18.6)

  I12.9 Hypertensive chronic kidney disease with stage 1 through stage 4 chronic kidney disease, or unspecified chronic kidney disease
  Hypertensive chronic kidney disease NOS
  Hypertensive renal disease NOS
  Use additional code to identify the stage of chronic kidney disease (N18.1-N18.4, N18.9)

✓4th I13 Hypertensive heart and chronic kidney disease

  INCLUDES any condition in I11- with any condition in I12-
  cardiorenal disease
  cardiovascular renal disease

  I13.0 Hypertensive heart and chronic kidney disease with heart failure and stage 1 through stage 4 chronic kidney disease, or unspecified chronic kidney disease
  Use additional code to identify type of heart failure (I50-)
  Use additional code to identify stage of chronic kidney disease (N18.1-N18.4, N18.9)

✓5th I13.1 Hypertensive heart and chronic kidney disease without heart failure

  I13.10 Hypertensive heart and chronic kidney disease without heart failure, with stage 1 through stage 4 chronic kidney disease, or unspecified chronic kidney disease
  Hypertensive heart disease and hypertensive chronic kidney disease NOS
  Use additional code to identify the stage of chronic kidney disease (N18.1-N18.4, N18.9)

  I13.11 Hypertensive heart and chronic kidney disease without heart failure, with stage 5 chronic kidney disease, or end stage renal disease
  Use additional code to identify the stage of chronic kidney disease (N18.5, N18.6)

  I13.2 Hypertensive heart and chronic kidney disease with heart failure and with stage 5 chronic kidney disease, or end stage renal disease
  Use additional code to identify type of heart failure (I50-)
  Use additional code to identify the stage of chronic kidney disease (N18.5, N18.6)

✓4th I15 Secondary hypertension

  Code also underlying condition

  EXCLUDES 1 *postprocedural hypertension (I97.3)*

  EXCLUDES 2 *secondary hypertension involving vessels of brain (I60-I69)*
  secondary hypertension involving vessels of eye (H35.0)

  I15.0 Renovascular hypertension
  I15.1 Hypertension secondary to other renal disorders
  I15.2 Hypertension secondary to endocrine disorders
  I15.8 Other secondary hypertension
  I15.9 Secondary hypertension, unspecified

Ischemic heart diseases (I20-I25)

Use additional code to identify presence of hypertension (I10-I15)

✓4th I20 Angina pectoris

Use additional code to identify:
  exposure to environmental tobacco smoke (Z77.22)
  history of tobacco use (Z87.891)
  occupational exposure to environmental tobacco smoke (Z57.31)
  tobacco dependence (F17-)
  tobacco use (Z72.0)

  EXCLUDES 1 *angina pectoris with atherosclerotic heart disease of native coronary arteries (I25.1-)*
  atherosclerosis of coronary artery bypass graft(s) and coronary artery of transplanted heart with angina pectoris (I25.7-)
  postinfarction angina (I23.7)

  I20.0 Unstable angina
  Accelerated angina
  Crescendo angina
  De novo effort angina
  Intermediate coronary syndrome
  Preinfarction syndrome
  Worsening effort angina

  I20.1 Angina pectoris with documented spasm
  Angiospastic angina
  Prinzmetal angina
  Spasm-induced angina
  Variant angina

  I20.8 Other forms of angina pectoris
  Angina equivalent
  Angina of effort
  Coronary slow flow syndrome
  Stenocardia
  Use additional code(s) for symptoms associated with angina equivalent

  I20.9 Angina pectoris, unspecified
  Angina NOS
  Anginal syndrome
  Cardiac angina
  Ischemic chest pain

☑ Appropriate additional character required √x7th Requires 7th character, placeholder x must fill empty characters

✓4th **I21**   **ST elevation (STEMI) and non-ST elevation (NSTEMI) myocardial infarction**

INCLUDES cardiac infarction
coronary (artery) embolism
coronary (artery) occlusion
coronary (artery) rupture
coronary (artery) thrombosis
infarction of heart, myocardium, or ventricle
myocardial infarction specified as acute or with a stated duration of 4 weeks (28 days) or less from onset

Use additional code, if applicable, to identify:
exposure to environmental tobacco smoke (Z77.22)
history of tobacco use (Z87.891)
occupational exposure to environmental tobacco smoke (Z57.31)
status post administration of tPA (rtPA) in a different facility within the last 24 hours prior to admission to current facility (Z92.82)
tobacco dependence (F17-)
tobacco use (Z72.0)

Use additional code, if known, to identify:
body mass index (BMI) (Z68-)

EXCLUDES 2 *old myocardial infarction (I25.2)*
postmyocardial infarction syndrome (I24.1)
subsequent myocardial infarction (I22-)

✓5th **I21.0**   **ST elevation (STEMI) myocardial infarction of anterior wall**

I21.01   **ST elevation (STEMI) myocardial infarction involving left main coronary artery**

I21.02   **ST elevation (STEMI) myocardial infarction involving left anterior descending coronary artery**
ST elevation (STEMI) myocardial infarction involving diagonal coronary artery

I21.09   **ST elevation (STEMI) myocardial infarction involving other coronary artery of anterior wall**
Acute transmural myocardial infarction of anterior wall
Anteroapical transmural (Q wave) infarction (acute)
Anterolateral transmural (Q wave) infarction (acute)
Anteroseptal transmural (Q wave) infarction (acute)
Transmural (Q wave) infarction (acute) (of) anterior (wall) NOS

✓5th **I21.1**   **ST elevation (STEMI) myocardial infarction of inferior wall**

I21.11   **ST elevation (STEMI) myocardial infarction involving right coronary artery**
Inferoposterior transmural (Q wave) infarction (acute)

I21.19   **ST elevation (STEMI) myocardial infarction involving other coronary artery of inferior wall**
Acute transmural myocardial infarction of inferior wall
Inferolateral transmural (Q wave) infarction (acute)
Transmural (Q wave) infarction (acute) (of) diaphragmatic wall
Transmural (Q wave) infarction (acute) (of) inferior (wall) NOS

EXCLUDES 2 *ST elevation (STEMI) myocardial infarction involving left circumflex coronary artery (I21.21)*

✓5th **I21.2**   **ST elevation (STEMI) myocardial infarction of other sites**

I21.21   **ST elevation (STEMI) myocardial infarction involving left circumflex coronary artery**
ST elevation (STEMI) myocardial infarction involving oblique marginal coronary artery

I21.29   **ST elevation (STEMI) myocardial infarction involving other sites**
Acute transmural myocardial infarction of other sites
Apical-lateral transmural (Q wave) infarction (acute)
Basal-lateral transmural (Q wave) infarction (acute)
High lateral transmural (Q wave) infarction (acute)
Lateral (wall) NOS transmural (Q wave) infarction (acute)
Posterior (true) transmural (Q wave) infarction (acute)
Posterobasal transmural (Q wave) infarction (acute)
Posterolateral transmural (Q wave) infarction (acute)
Posteroseptal transmural (Q wave) infarction (acute)
Septal transmural (Q wave) infarction (acute) NOS

I21.3   **ST elevation (STEMI) myocardial infarction of unspecified site**
Acute transmural myocardial infarction of unspecified site
Myocardial infarction (acute) NOS
Transmural (Q wave) myocardial infarction NOS

I21.4   **Non-ST elevation (NSTEMI) myocardial infarction**
Acute subendocardial myocardial infarction
Non-Q wave myocardial infarction NOS
Nontransmural myocardial infarction NOS

✓4th **I22**   **Subsequent ST elevation (STEMI) and non-ST elevation (NSTEMI) myocardial infarction**

NOTE A code from category I22 must be used in conjunction with a code from category I21. The I22 code should be sequenced first, if it the reason for encounter, or, it should be sequenced after the I21 code if the subsequent MI occurs during the encounter for the initial MI.

INCLUDES acute myocardial infarction occurring within four weeks (28 days) of a previous acute myocardial infarction, regardless of site
cardiac infarction
coronary (artery) embolism
coronary (artery) occlusion
coronary (artery) rupture
coronary (artery) thrombosis
infarction of heart, myocardium, or ventricle
recurrent myocardial infarction
reinfarction of myocardium
rupture of heart, myocardium, or ventricle

Use additional code, if applicable, to identify:
exposure to environmental tobacco smoke (Z77.22)
history of tobacco use (Z87.891)
occupational exposure to environmental tobacco smoke (Z57.31)
status post administration of tPA (rtPA) in a different facility within the last 24 hours prior to admission to current facility (Z92.82)
tobacco dependence (F17-)
tobacco use (Z72.0)

Use additional code, if known, to identify:
body mass index (BMI) (Z68-)

I22.0   **Subsequent ST elevation (STEMI) myocardial infarction of anterior wall**
Subsequent acute transmural myocardial infarction of anterior wall
Subsequent transmural (Q wave) infarction (acute)(of) anterior (wall) NOS
Subsequent anteroapical transmural (Q wave) infarction (acute)
Subsequent anterolateral transmural (Q wave) infarction (acute)
Subsequent anteroseptal transmural (Q wave) infarction (acute)

I22.1   **Subsequent ST elevation (STEMI) myocardial infarction of inferior wall**
Subsequent acute transmural myocardial infarction of inferior wall
Subsequent transmural (Q wave) infarction (acute)(of) diaphragmatic wall
Subsequent transmural (Q wave) infarction (acute)(of) inferior (wall) NOS
Subsequent inferolateral transmural (Q wave) infarction (acute)
Subsequent inferoposterior transmural (Q wave) infarction (acute)

I22.2   **Subsequent non-ST elevation (NSTEMI) myocardial infarction**
Subsequent acute subendocardial myocardial infarction
Subsequent non-Q wave myocardial infarction NOS
Subsequent nontransmural myocardial infarction NOS

EXCLUDES 1 Not coded here   EXCLUDES 2 Not included here   *Manifestation Code*

I22.8 **Subsequent ST elevation (STEMI) myocardial infarction of other sites**
Subsequent acute transmural myocardial infarction of other sites
Subsequent apical-lateral transmural (Q wave) myocardial infarction (acute)
Subsequent basal-lateral transmural (Q wave) myocardial infarction (acute)
Subsequent high lateral transmural (Q wave) myocardial infarction (acute)
Subsequent transmural (Q wave) myocardial infarction (acute)(of) lateral (wall) NOS
Subsequent posterior (true)transmural (Q wave) myocardial infarction (acute)
Subsequent posterobasal transmural (Q wave) myocardial infarction (acute)
Subsequent posterolateral transmural (Q wave) myocardial infarction (acute)
Subsequent posteroseptal transmural (Q wave) myocardial infarction (acute)
Subsequent septal NOS transmural (Q wave) myocardial infarction (acute)

I22.9 **Subsequent ST elevation (STEMI) myocardial infarction of unspecified site**
Subsequent acute myocardial infarction of unspecified site
Subsequent myocardial infarction (acute) NOS

✓4ᵗʰ **I23** **Certain current complications following ST elevation (STEMI) and non-ST elevation (NSTEMI) myocardial infarction (within the 28 day period)**

> **NOTE** A code from category I23 must be used in conjunction with a code from category I21 or category I22. The I23 code should be sequenced first, if it is the reason for encounter, or, it should be sequenced after the I21 or I22 code if the complication of the MI occurs during the encounter for the MI.

I23.0 **Hemopericardium as current complication following acute myocardial infarction**
> **EXCLUDES 1** hemopericardium not specified as current complication following acute myocardial infarction (I31.2)

I23.1 **Atrial septal defect as current complication following acute myocardial infarction**
> **EXCLUDES 1** acquired atrial septal defect not specified as current complication following acute myocardial infarction (I51.0)

I23.2 **Ventricular septal defect as current complication following acute myocardial infarction**
> **EXCLUDES 1** acquired ventricular septal defect not specified as current complication following acute myocardial infarction (I51.0)

I23.3 **Rupture of cardiac wall without hemopericardium as current complication following acute myocardial infarction**

I23.4 **Rupture of chordae tendineae as current complication following acute myocardial infarction**
> **EXCLUDES 1** rupture of chordae tendineae not specified as current complication following acute myocardial infarction (I51.1)

I23.5 **Rupture of papillary muscle as current complication following acute myocardial infarction**
> **EXCLUDES 1** rupture of papillary muscle not specified as current complication following acute myocardial infarction (I51.2)

I23.6 **Thrombosis of atrium, auricular appendage, and ventricle as current complications following acute myocardial infarction**
> **EXCLUDES 1** thrombosis of atrium, auricular appendage, and ventricle not specified as current complication following acute myocardial infarction (I51.3)

I23.7 **Postinfarction angina**

I23.8 **Other current complications following acute myocardial infarction**

✓4ᵗʰ **I24** **Other acute ischemic heart diseases**
> **EXCLUDES 1** angina pectoris (I20-)
> transient myocardial ischemia in newborn (P29.4)

I24.0 **Acute coronary thrombosis not resulting in myocardial infarction**
Acute coronary (artery) (vein) embolism not resulting in myocardial infarction
Acute coronary (artery) (vein) occlusion not resulting in myocardial infarction
Acute coronary (artery) (vein) thromboembolism not resulting in myocardial infarction
> **EXCLUDES 1** atherosclerotic heart disease (I25.1-)

I24.1 **Dressler's syndrome**
Postmyocardial infarction syndrome
> **EXCLUDES 1** postinfarction angina (I23.7)

I24.8 **Other forms of acute ischemic heart disease**

I24.9 **Acute ischemic heart disease, unspecified**
> **EXCLUDES 1** ischemic heart disease (chronic) NOS (I25.9)

✓4ᵗʰ **I25** **Chronic ischemic heart disease**
Use additional code to identify:
chronic total occlusion of coronary artery (I25.82)
exposure to environmental tobacco smoke (Z77.22)
history of tobacco use (Z87.891)
occupational exposure to environmental tobacco smoke (Z57.31)
tobacco dependence (F17-)
tobacco use (Z72.0)

I25.1 **Atherosclerotic heart disease of native coronary artery**
Atherosclerotic cardiovascular disease
Coronary (artery) atheroma
Coronary (artery) atherosclerosis
Coronary (artery) disease
Coronary (artery) sclerosis
Use additional code, if applicable, to identify coronary atherosclerosis due to lipid rich plaque (I25.83)
> **EXCLUDES 2** atheroembolism (I75-)
> atherosclerosis of coronary artery bypass graft(s) and transplanted heart (I25.7-)

I25.10 **Atherosclerotic heart disease of native coronary artery without angina pectoris**
Atherosclerotic heart disease NOS

✓6ᵗʰ **I25.11** **Atherosclerotic heart disease of native coronary artery with angina pectoris**

I25.110 **Atherosclerotic heart disease of native coronary artery with unstable angina pectoris**
> **EXCLUDES 1** unstable angina without atherosclerotic heart disease (I20.0)

I25.111 **Atherosclerotic heart disease of native coronary artery with angina pectoris with documented spasm**
> **EXCLUDES 1** angina pectoris with documented spasm without atherosclerotic heart disease (I20.1)

I25.118 **Atherosclerotic heart disease of native coronary artery with other forms of angina pectoris**
> **EXCLUDES 1** other forms of angina pectoris without atherosclerotic heart disease (I20.8)

I25.119 **Atherosclerotic heart disease of native coronary artery with unspecified angina pectoris**
Atherosclerotic heart disease with angina NOS
Atherosclerotic heart disease with ischemic chest pain
> **EXCLUDES 1** unspecified angina pectoris without atherosclerotic heart disease (I20.9)

I25.2 **Old myocardial infarction**
Healed myocardial infarction
Past myocardial infarction diagnosed by ECG or other investigation, but currently presenting no symptoms

I25.3 **Aneurysm of heart**
Mural aneurysm
Ventricular aneurysm

☑ Appropriate additional character required   ✓x7ᵗʰ Requires 7th character, placeholder x must fill empty characters

✓5ᵗʰ **I25.4**   **Coronary artery aneurysm and dissection**

     I25.41   **Coronary artery aneurysm**

       Coronary arteriovenous fistula, acquired

       EXCLUDES 1   *congenital coronary (artery) aneurysm (Q24.5)*

     I25.42   **Coronary artery dissection**

I25.5   **Ischemic cardiomyopathy**

     EXCLUDES 2   *coronary atherosclerosis (I25.1-, I25.7-)*

I25.6   **Silent myocardial ischemia**

✓5ᵗʰ **I25.7**   **Atherosclerosis of coronary artery bypass graft(s) and coronary artery of transplanted heart with angina pectoris**

     Use additional code, if applicable, to identify coronary atherosclerosis due to lipid rich plaque (I25.83)

     EXCLUDES 1   *atherosclerosis of bypass graft(s) of transplanted heart without angina pectoris (I25.812)*

         atherosclerosis of coronary artery bypass graft(s) without angina pectoris (I25.810)

         atherosclerosis of native coronary artery of transplanted heart without angina pectoris (I25.811)

         embolism or thrombus of coronary artery bypass graft(s) (T82.8-)

    ✓6ᵗʰ **I25.70**   **Atherosclerosis of coronary artery bypass graft(s), unspecified, with angina pectoris**

     I25.700   **Atherosclerosis of coronary artery bypass graft(s), unspecified, with unstable angina pectoris**

       EXCLUDES 1   *unstable angina pectoris without atherosclerosis of coronary artery bypass graft (I20.0)*

     I25.701   **Atherosclerosis of coronary artery bypass graft(s), unspecified, with angina pectoris with documented spasm**

       EXCLUDES 1   *angina pectoris with documented spasm without atherosclerosis of coronary artery bypass graft (I20.1)*

     I25.708   **Atherosclerosis of coronary artery bypass graft(s), unspecified, with other forms of angina pectoris**

       EXCLUDES 1   *other forms of angina pectoris without atherosclerosis of coronary artery bypass graft (I20.8)*

     I25.709   **Atherosclerosis of coronary artery bypass graft(s), unspecified, with unspecified angina pectoris**

       EXCLUDES 1   *unspecified angina pectoris without atherosclerosis of coronary artery bypass graft (I20.9)*

    ✓6ᵗʰ **I25.71**   **Atherosclerosis of autologous vein coronary artery bypass graft(s) with angina pectoris**

     I25.710   **Atherosclerosis of autologous vein coronary artery bypass graft(s) with unstable angina pectoris**

       EXCLUDES 1   *unstable angina without atherosclerosis of autologous vein coronary artery bypass graft(s) (I20.0)*

     I25.711   **Atherosclerosis of autologous vein coronary artery bypass graft(s) with angina pectoris with documented spasm**

       EXCLUDES 1   *angina pectoris with documented spasm without atherosclerosis of autologous vein coronary artery bypass graft(s) (I20.1)*

     I25.718   **Atherosclerosis of autologous vein coronary artery bypass graft(s) with other forms of angina pectoris**

       EXCLUDES 1   *other forms of angina pectoris without atherosclerosis of autologous vein coronary artery bypass graft(s) (I20.8)*

     I25.719   **Atherosclerosis of autologous vein coronary artery bypass graft(s) with unspecified angina pectoris**

       EXCLUDES 1   *unspecified angina pectoris without atherosclerosis of autologous vein coronary artery bypass graft(s) (I20.9)*

    ✓6ᵗʰ **I25.72**   **Atherosclerosis of autologous artery coronary artery bypass graft(s) with angina pectoris**

     Atherosclerosis of internal mammary artery graft with angina pectoris

     I25.720   **Atherosclerosis of autologous artery coronary artery bypass graft(s) with unstable angina pectoris**

       EXCLUDES 1   *unstable angina without atherosclerosis of autologous artery coronary artery bypass graft(s) (I20.0)*

     I25.721   **Atherosclerosis of autologous artery coronary artery bypass graft(s) with angina pectoris with documented spasm**

       EXCLUDES 1   *angina pectoris with documented spasm without atherosclerosis of autologous artery coronary artery bypass graft(s) (I20.1)*

     I25.728   **Atherosclerosis of autologous artery coronary artery bypass graft(s) with other forms of angina pectoris**

       EXCLUDES 1   *other forms of angina pectoris without atherosclerosis of autologous artery coronary artery bypass graft(s) (I20.8)*

     I25.729   **Atherosclerosis of autologous artery coronary artery bypass graft(s) with unspecified angina pectoris**

       EXCLUDES 1   *unspecified angina pectoris without atherosclerosis of autologous artery coronary artery bypass graft(s) (I20.9)*

    ✓6ᵗʰ **I25.73**   **Atherosclerosis of nonautologous biological coronary artery bypass graft(s) with angina pectoris**

     I25.730   **Atherosclerosis of nonautologous biological coronary artery bypass graft(s) with unstable angina pectoris**

       EXCLUDES 1   *unstable angina without atherosclerosis of nonautologous biological coronary artery bypass graft(s) (I20.0)*

     I25.731   **Atherosclerosis of nonautologous biological coronary artery bypass graft(s) with angina pectoris with documented spasm**

       EXCLUDES 1   *angina pectoris with documented spasm without atherosclerosis of nonautologous biological coronary artery bypass graft(s) (I20.1)*

     I25.738   **Atherosclerosis of nonautologous biological coronary artery bypass graft(s) with other forms of angina pectoris**

       EXCLUDES 1   *other forms of angina pectoris without atherosclerosis of nonautologous biological coronary artery bypass graft(s) (I20.8)*

     I25.739   **Atherosclerosis of nonautologous biological coronary artery bypass graft(s) with unspecified angina pectoris**

       EXCLUDES 1   *unspecified angina pectoris without atherosclerosis of nonautologous biological coronary artery bypass graft(s) (I20.9)*

EXCLUDES 1 Not coded here   **EXCLUDES 2** Not included here   *Manifestation Code*

✓6th **I25.75** **Atherosclerosis of native coronary artery of transplanted heart with angina pectoris**

> **EXCLUDES 1** *atherosclerosis of native coronary artery of transplanted heart without angina pectoris (I25.811)*

I25.750 **Atherosclerosis of native coronary artery of transplanted heart with unstable angina**

I25.751 **Atherosclerosis of native coronary artery of transplanted heart with angina pectoris with documented spasm**

I25.758 **Atherosclerosis of native coronary artery of transplanted heart with other forms of angina pectoris**

I25.759 **Atherosclerosis of native coronary artery of transplanted heart with unspecified angina pectoris**

✓6th **I25.76** **Atherosclerosis of bypass graft of coronary artery of transplanted heart with angina pectoris**

> **EXCLUDES 1** *atherosclerosis of bypass graft of coronary artery of transplanted heart without angina pectoris (I25.812)*

I25.760 **Atherosclerosis of bypass graft of coronary artery of transplanted heart with unstable angina**

I25.761 **Atherosclerosis of bypass graft of coronary artery of transplanted heart with angina pectoris with documented spasm**

I25.768 **Atherosclerosis of bypass graft of coronary artery of transplanted heart with other forms of angina pectoris**

I25.769 **Atherosclerosis of bypass graft of coronary artery of transplanted heart with unspecified angina pectoris**

✓6th **I25.79** **Atherosclerosis of other coronary artery bypass graft(s) with angina pectoris**

I25.790 **Atherosclerosis of other coronary artery bypass graft(s) with unstable angina pectoris**

> **EXCLUDES 1** *unstable angina without atherosclerosis of other coronary artery bypass graft(s) (I20.0)*

I25.791 **Atherosclerosis of other coronary artery bypass graft(s) with angina pectoris with documented spasm**

> **EXCLUDES 1** *angina pectoris with documented spasm without atherosclerosis of other coronary artery bypass graft(s) (I20.1)*

I25.798 **Atherosclerosis of other coronary artery bypass graft(s) with other forms of angina pectoris**

> **EXCLUDES 1** *other forms of angina pectoris without atherosclerosis of other coronary artery bypass graft(s)(I20.8)*

I25.799 **Atherosclerosis of other coronary artery bypass graft(s) with unspecified angina pectoris**

> **EXCLUDES 1** *unspecified angina pectoris without atherosclerosis of other coronary artery bypass graft(s) (I20.9)*

✓5th **I25.8** **Other forms of chronic ischemic heart disease**

✓6th **I25.81** **Atherosclerosis of other coronary vessels without angina pectoris**

> Use additional code, if applicable, to identify coronary atherosclerosis due to lipid rich plaque (I25.83)

> **EXCLUDES 1** *atherosclerotic heart disease of native coronary artery without angina pectoris (I25.10)*

I25.810 **Atherosclerosis of coronary artery bypass graft(s) without angina pectoris**

> Atherosclerosis of coronary artery bypass graft NOS

> **EXCLUDES 1** *atherosclerosis of coronary bypass graft(s) with angina pectoris (I25.70--I25.73-, I25.79-)*

I25.811 **Atherosclerosis of native coronary artery of transplanted heart without angina pectoris**

> Atherosclerosis of native coronary artery of transplanted heart NOS

> **EXCLUDES 1** *atherosclerosis of native coronary artery of transplanted heart with angina pectoris (I25.75-)*

I25.812 **Atherosclerosis of bypass graft of coronary artery of transplanted heart without angina pectoris**

> Atherosclerosis of bypass graft of transplanted heart NOS

> **EXCLUDES 1** *atherosclerosis of bypass graft of transplanted heart with angina pectoris (I25.76)*

I25.82 **Chronic total occlusion of coronary artery**

> Complete occlusion of coronary artery
> Total occlusion of coronary artery
> Code first coronary atherosclerosis (I25.1-, I25.7-, I25.81-)

> **EXCLUDES 1** *acute coronary occlusion with myocardial infarction (I21-, I22-)*
> *acute coronary occlusion without myocardial infarction (I24.0)*

I25.83 **Coronary atherosclerosis due to lipid rich plaque**

> Code first coronary atherosclerosis (I25.1-, I25.7-, I25.81-)

I25.89 **Other forms of chronic ischemic heart disease**

I25.9 **Chronic ischemic heart disease, unspecified**

> Ischemic heart disease (chronic) NOS

Pulmonary heart disease and diseases of pulmonary circulation (I26-I28)

✓4th **I26** **Pulmonary embolism**

> Pulmonary (acute) (artery)(vein) infarction
> Pulmonary (acute) (artery)(vein) thromboembolism
> Pulmonary (acute) (artery)(vein) thrombosis

> **EXCLUDES 2** *chronic pulmonary embolism (I27.82)*
> *personal history of pulmonary embolism (Z86.71)*
> *pulmonary embolism due to trauma (T79.0, T79.1)*
> *pulmonary embolism due to complications of surgical and medical care (T80.0, T81.7-, T82.8-)*
> *pulmonary embolism complicating:*
>   *abortion, ectopic or molar pregnancy (O00-O07, O08.2)*
>   *pregnancy, childbirth and the puerperium (O88-)*
>   *septic (non-pulmonary) arterial embolism (I76)*

✓5th **I26.0** **Pulmonary embolism with acute cor pulmonale**

I26.01 **Septic pulmonary embolism with acute cor pulmonale**

> Code first underlying infection

I26.09 **Other pulmonary embolism with acute cor pulmonale**

> Acute cor pulmonale NOS

✓5th **I26.9** **Pulmonary embolism without acute cor pulmonale**

I26.90 **Septic pulmonary embolism without acute cor pulmonale**

> Code first underlying infection

I26.99   **Other pulmonary embolism without acute cor pulmonale**
Acute pulmonary embolism NOS
Pulmonary embolism NOS

✓4th **I27**   **Other pulmonary heart diseases**

I27.0   **Primary pulmonary hypertension**
EXCLUDES 1   *pulmonary hypertension NOS (I27.2)*
secondary pulmonary hypertension (I27.2)

I27.1   **Kyphoscoliotic heart disease**

I27.2   **Other secondary pulmonary hypertension**
Pulmonary hypertension NOS
Code also associated underlying condition

✓5th **I27.8**   **Other specified pulmonary heart diseases**

I27.81   **Cor pulmonale (chronic)**
Cor pulmonale NOS
EXCLUDES 1   *acute cor pulmonale (I26.0-)*

I27.82   **Chronic pulmonary embolism**
Use additional code, if applicable, for associated long-term (current) use of anticoagulants (Z79.01)
EXCLUDES 1   *personal history of pulmonary embolism (Z86.71)*

I27.89   **Other specified pulmonary heart diseases**
Eisenmenger's complex
Eisenmenger's syndrome
EXCLUDES 1   *Eisenmenger's defect (Q21.8)*

I27.9   **Pulmonary heart disease, unspecified**
Chronic cardiopulmonary disease

✓4th **I28**   **Other diseases of pulmonary vessels**

I28.0   **Arteriovenous fistula of pulmonary vessels**
EXCLUDES 1   *congenital arteriovenous fistula (Q25.7)*

I28.1   **Aneurysm of pulmonary artery**
EXCLUDES 1   *congenital aneurysm (Q25.7)*

I28.8   **Other diseases of pulmonary vessels**
Pulmonary arteritis
Pulmonary endarteritis
Rupture of pulmonary vessels
Stenosis of pulmonary vessels
Stricture of pulmonary vessels

I28.9   **Disease of pulmonary vessels, unspecified**

Other forms of heart disease (I30-I52)

✓4th **I30**   **Acute pericarditis**
INCLUDES   acute mediastinopericarditis
acute myopericarditis
acute pericardial effusion
acute pleuropericarditis
acute pneumopericarditis
EXCLUDES 1   *Dressler's syndrome (I24.1)*
rheumatic pericarditis (acute) (I01.0)

I30.0   **Acute nonspecific idiopathic pericarditis**

I30.1   **Infective pericarditis**
Pneumococcal pericarditis
Pneumopyopericardium
Purulent pericarditis
Pyopericarditis
Pyopericardium
Pyopneumopericardium
Staphylococcal pericarditis
Streptococcal pericarditis
Suppurative pericarditis
Viral pericarditis
Use additional code (B95-B97) to identify infectious agent

I30.8   **Other forms of acute pericarditis**

I30.9   **Acute pericarditis, unspecified**

✓4th **I31**   **Other diseases of pericardium**
EXCLUDES 1   *diseases of pericardium specified as rheumatic (I09.2)*
postcardiotomy syndrome (I97.0)
traumatic injury to pericardium (S26-)

I31.0   **Chronic adhesive pericarditis**
Accretio cordis
Adherent pericardium
Adhesive mediastinopericarditis

I31.1   **Chronic constrictive pericarditis**
Concretio cordis
Pericardial calcification

I31.2   **Hemopericardium, not elsewhere classified**
EXCLUDES 1   *hemopericardium as current complication following acute myocardial infarction (I23.0)*

I31.3   **Pericardial effusion (noninflammatory)**
Chylopericardium
EXCLUDES 1   *acute pericardial effusion (I30.9)*

I31.4   **Cardiac tamponade**
Code first underlying cause

I31.8   **Other specified diseases of pericardium**
Epicardial plaques
Focal pericardial adhesions

I31.9   **Disease of pericardium, unspecified**
Pericarditis (chronic) NOS

I32   *Pericarditis in diseases classified elsewhere*
Code first underlying disease
EXCLUDES 1   *pericarditis (in):*
coxsackie (virus) (B33.23)
gonococcal (A54.83)
meningococcal (A39.53)
rheumatoid (arthritis) (M05.31)
syphilitic (A52.06)
systemic lupus erythematosus (M32.12)
tuberculosis (A18.84)

✓4th **I33**   **Acute and subacute endocarditis**
EXCLUDES 1   *acute rheumatic endocarditis (I01.1)*
endocarditis NOS (I38)

I33.0   **Acute and subacute infective endocarditis**
Bacterial endocarditis (acute) (subacute)
Infective endocarditis (acute) (subacute) NOS
Endocarditis lenta (acute) (subacute)
Malignant endocarditis (acute) (subacute)
Purulent endocarditis (acute) (subacute)
Septic endocarditis (acute) (subacute)
Ulcerative endocarditis (acute) (subacute)
Vegetative endocarditis (acute) (subacute)
Use additional code (B95-B97) to identify infectious agent

I33.9   **Acute and subacute endocarditis, unspecified**
Acute endocarditis NOS
Acute myoendocarditis NOS
Acute periendocarditis NOS
Subacute endocarditis NOS
Subacute myoendocarditis NOS
Subacute periendocarditis NOS

✓4th **I34**   **Nonrheumatic mitral valve disorders**
EXCLUDES 1   *mitral valve disease (I05.9)*
mitral valve failure (I05.8)
mitral valve stenosis (I05.0)
mitral valve disorder of unspecified cause with diseases of aortic and/or tricuspid valve(s) (I08-)
mitral valve disorder of unspecified cause with mitral stenosis or obstruction (I05.0)
mitral valve disorder specified as congenital (Q23.2, Q23.3)
mitral valve disorder specified as rheumatic (I05-)

I34.0   **Nonrheumatic mitral (valve) insufficiency**
Nonrheumatic mitral (valve) incompetence NOS
Nonrheumatic mitral (valve) regurgitation NOS

I34.1   **Nonrheumatic mitral (valve) prolapse**
Floppy nonrheumatic mitral valve syndrome
EXCLUDES 1   *Marfan's syndrome (Q87.4-)*

I34.2   **Nonrheumatic mitral (valve) stenosis**

I34.8   **Other nonrheumatic mitral valve disorders**

I34.9   **Nonrheumatic mitral valve disorder, unspecified**

✓4th **I35**   **Nonrheumatic aortic valve disorders**
EXCLUDES 1   *aortic valve disorder of unspecified cause but with diseases of mitral and/or tricuspid valve(s) (I08-)*
aortic valve disorder specified as congenital (Q23.0, Q23.1)
aortic valve disorder specified as rheumatic (I06-)
hypertrophic subaortic stenosis (I42.1)

I35.0   **Nonrheumatic aortic (valve) stenosis**

I35.1   **Nonrheumatic aortic (valve) insufficiency**
Nonrheumatic aortic (valve) incompetence NOS
Nonrheumatic aortic (valve) regurgitation NOS

I35.2   **Nonrheumatic aortic (valve) stenosis with insufficiency**

I35.8   **Other nonrheumatic aortic valve disorders**

I35.9   **Nonrheumatic aortic valve disorder, unspecified**

EXCLUDES 1   Not coded here   EXCLUDES 2   Not included here   *Manifestation Code*

☑4ᵗʰ **I36 Nonrheumatic tricuspid valve disorders**

> EXCLUDES 1 *tricuspid valve disorders of unspecified cause (I07-)*
> *tricuspid valve disorders specified as congenital (Q22.4, Q22.8, Q22.9)*
> *tricuspid valve disorders specified as rheumatic (I07-)*
> *tricuspid valve disorders with aortic and/or mitral valve involvement (I08-)*

I36.0 Nonrheumatic tricuspid (valve) stenosis

I36.1 Nonrheumatic tricuspid (valve) insufficiency
Nonrheumatic tricuspid (valve) incompetence
Nonrheumatic tricuspid (valve) regurgitation

I36.2 Nonrheumatic tricuspid (valve) stenosis with insufficiency

I36.8 Other nonrheumatic tricuspid valve disorders

I36.9 Nonrheumatic tricuspid valve disorder, unspecified

☑4ᵗʰ **I37 Nonrheumatic pulmonary valve disorders**

> EXCLUDES 1 *pulmonary valve disorder specified as congenital (Q22.1, Q22.2, Q22.3)*
> *pulmonary valve disorder specified as rheumatic (I09.89)*

I37.0 Nonrheumatic pulmonary valve stenosis

I37.1 Nonrheumatic pulmonary valve insufficiency
Nonrheumatic pulmonary valve incompetence
Nonrheumatic pulmonary valve regurgitation

I37.2 Nonrheumatic pulmonary valve stenosis with insufficiency

I37.8 Other nonrheumatic pulmonary valve disorders

I37.9 Nonrheumatic pulmonary valve disorder, unspecified

I38 Endocarditis, valve unspecified

> INCLUDES endocarditis (chronic) NOS
> valvular incompetence NOS
> valvular insufficiency NOS
> valvular regurgitation NOS
> valvular stenosis NOS
> valvulitis (chronic) NOS

> EXCLUDES 1 *congenital insufficiency of cardiac valve NOS (Q24.8)*
> *congenital stenosis of cardiac valve NOS (Q24.8)*
> *endocardial fibroelastosis (I42.4)*
> *endocarditis specified as rheumatic (I09.1)*

I39 Endocarditis and heart valve disorders in diseases classified elsewhere

> Code first underlying disease, such as:
> Q fever (A78)

> EXCLUDES 1 *endocardial involvement in:*
> *candidiasis (B37.6)*
> *gonococcal infection (A54.83)*
> *Libman-Sacks disease (M32.11)*
> *listerosis (A32.82)*
> *meningococcal infection (A39.51)*
> *rheumatoid arthritis (M05.31)*
> *syphilis (A52.03)*
> *tuberculosis (A18.84)*
> *typhoid fever (A01.02)*

☑4ᵗʰ **I40 Acute myocarditis**

> INCLUDES subacute myocarditis
> EXCLUDES 1 *acute rheumatic myocarditis (I01.2)*

I40.0 Infective myocarditis
Septic myocarditis
Use additional code (B95-B97) to identify infectious agent

I40.1 Isolated myocarditis
Fiedler's myocarditis
Giant cell myocarditis
Idiopathic myocarditis

I40.8 Other acute myocarditis

I40.9 Acute myocarditis, unspecified

I41 Myocarditis in diseases classified elsewhere

> Code first underlying disease, such as:
> typhus (A75.0-A75.9)

> EXCLUDES 1 *myocarditis (in):*
> *Chagas' disease (chronic) (B57.2)*
> *acute (B57.0)*
> *coxsackie (virus) infection (B33.22)*
> *diphtheritic (A36.81)*
> *gonococcal (A54.83)*
> *influenzal (J09.091, J09.191, J10.82, J11.82)*
> *meningococcal (A39.52)*
> *mumps (B26.82)*
> *rheumatoid arthritis (M05.31)*
> *sarcoid (D86.85)*
> *syphilis (A52.06)*
> *toxoplasmosis (B58.81)*
> *tuberculous (A18.84)*

☑4ᵗʰ **I42 Cardiomyopathy**

> INCLUDES myocardiopathy
> Code first cardiomyopathy complicating pregnancy and puerperium (O99.4)

> EXCLUDES 1 *ischemic cardiomyopathy (I25.5)*
> *peripartum cardiomyopathy (O90.3)*

I42.0 Dilated cardiomyopathy
Congestive cardiomyopathy

I42.1 Obstructive hypertrophic cardiomyopathy
Hypertrophic subaortic stenosis

I42.2 Other hypertrophic cardiomyopathy
Nonobstructive hypertrophic cardiomyopathy

I42.3 Endomyocardial (eosinophilic) disease
Endomyocardial (tropical) fibrosis
Löffler's endocarditis

I42.4 Endocardial fibroelastosis
Congenital cardiomyopathy
Elastomyofibrosis

I42.5 Other restrictive cardiomyopathy
Constrictive cardiomyopathy NOS

I42.6 Alcoholic cardiomyopathy
Code also presence of alcoholism (F10-)

I42.7 Cardiomyopathy due to drug and external agent
Code first (T36-T65) to identify cause

I42.8 Other cardiomyopathies

I42.9 Cardiomyopathy, unspecified
Cardiomyopathy (primary) (secondary) NOS

I43 Cardiomyopathy in diseases classified elsewhere

> Code first underlying disease, such as:
> amyloidosis (E85-)
> glycogen storage disease (E74.0)
> gout (M10.0-)
> thyrotoxicosis (E05.0-E05.9-)

> EXCLUDES 1 *cardiomyopathy (in):*
> *coxsackie (virus) (B33.24)*
> *diphtheria (A36.81)*
> *sarcoidosis (D86.85)*
> *tuberculosis (A18.84)*

☑4ᵗʰ **I44 Atrioventricular and left bundle-branch block**

I44.0 Atrioventricular block, first degree

I44.1 Atrioventricular block, second degree
Atrioventricular block, type I and II
Möbitz block, type I and II
Second degree block, type I and II
Wenckebach's block

I44.2 Atrioventricular block, complete
Complete heart block NOS
Third degree block

☑5ᵗʰ **I44.3 Other and unspecified atrioventricular block**
Atrioventricular block NOS

    I44.30 Unspecified atrioventricular block

    I44.39 Other atrioventricular block

I44.4 Left anterior fascicular block

I44.5 Left posterior fascicular block

☑5ᵗʰ **I44.6 Other and unspecified fascicular block**

    I44.60 Unspecified fascicular block
       Left bundle-branch hemiblock NOS

    I44.69 Other fascicular block

I44.7 Left bundle-branch block, unspecified

☑ Appropriate additional character required   ☑x7ᵗʰ Requires 7th character, placeholder x must fill empty characters

√4th **I45**   **Other conduction disorders**

     I45.0   **Right fascicular block**

√5th   **I45.1**   **Other and unspecified right bundle-branch block**

         I45.10   **Unspecified right bundle-branch block**
            Right bundle-branch block NOS

         I45.19   **Other right bundle-branch block**

     I45.2   **Bifascicular block**

     I45.3   **Trifascicular block**

     I45.4   **Nonspecific intraventricular block**
         Bundle-branch block NOS

     I45.5   **Other specified heart block**
         Sinoatrial block
         Sinoauricular block
         EXCLUDES 1   *heart block NOS (I45.9)*

     I45.6   **Pre-excitation syndrome**
         Accelerated atrioventricular conduction
         Accessory atrioventricular conduction
         Anomalous atrioventricular excitation
         Lown-Ganong-Levine syndrome
         Pre-excitation atrioventricular conduction
         Wolff-Parkinson-White syndrome

√5th   **I45.8**   **Other specified conduction disorders**

         I45.81   **Long QT syndrome**

         I45.89   **Other specified conduction disorders**
            Atrioventricular [AV] dissociation
            Interference dissociation
            Isorhythmic dissociation
            Nonparoxysmal AV nodal tachycardia

     I45.9   **Conduction disorder, unspecified**
         Heart block NOS
         Stokes-Adams syndrome

√4th **I46**   **Cardiac arrest**
     EXCLUDES 1   *cardiogenic shock (R57.0)*

     I46.2   **Cardiac arrest due to underlying cardiac condition**
         Code first underlying cardiac condition

     I46.8   **Cardiac arrest due to other underlying condition**
         Code first underlying condition

     I46.9   **Cardiac arrest, cause unspecified**

√4th **I47**   **Paroxysmal tachycardia**
     Code first tachycardia complicating:
         abortion or ectopic or molar pregnancy (O00-O07, O08.8)
         obstetric surgery and procedures (O75.4)
     EXCLUDES 1   *tachycardia:*
         NOS (R00.0)
         sinoauricular NOS (R00.0)
         sinus [sinusal] NOS (R00.0)

     I47.0   **Re-entry ventricular arrhythmia**

     I47.1   **Supraventricular tachycardia**
         Atrial paroxysmal tachycardia
         Atrioventricular [AV] paroxysmal tachycardia
         Junctional paroxysmal tachycardia
         Nodal paroxysmal tachycardia

     I47.2   **Ventricular tachycardia**

     I47.9   **Paroxysmal tachycardia, unspecified**
         Bouveret (-Hoffman) syndrome

√4th **I48**   **Atrial fibrillation and flutter**

     I48.0   **Atrial fibrillation**

     I48.1   **Atrial flutter**

√4th **I49**   **Other cardiac arrhythmias**
     Code first cardiac arrhythmia complicating:
         abortion or ectopic or molar pregnancy (O00-O07, O08.8)
         obstetric surgery and procedures (O75.4)
     EXCLUDES 1   *bradycardia:*
         NOS (R00.1)
         sinoatrial (R00.1)
         sinus (R00.1)
         vagal (R00.1)
         neonatal dysrhythmia (P29.1)

√5th   **I49.0**   **Ventricular fibrillation and flutter**

         I49.01   **Ventricular fibrillation**

         I49.02   **Ventricular flutter**

     I49.1   **Atrial premature depolarization**
         Atrial premature beats

     I49.2   **Junctional premature depolarization**

     I49.3   **Ventricular premature depolarization**

√5th   **I49.4**   **Other and unspecified premature depolarization**

         I49.40   **Unspecified premature depolarization**
            Premature beats NOS

         I49.49   **Other premature depolarization**
            Ectopic beats
            Extrasystoles
            Extrasystolic arrhythmias
            Premature contractions

     I49.5   **Sick sinus syndrome**
         Tachycardia-bradycardia syndrome

     I49.8   **Other specified cardiac arrhythmias**
         Coronary sinus rhythm disorder
         Ectopic rhythm disorder
         Nodal rhythm disorder

     I49.9   **Cardiac arrhythmia, unspecified**
         Arrhythmia (cardiac) NOS

√4th **I50**   **Heart failure**
     Code first:
         heart failure complicating abortion or ectopic or molar pregnancy
            (O00-O07, O08.8)
         heart failure following surgery (I97.13-)
         heart failure due to hypertension (I11.0)
         heart failure due to hypertension with chronic kidney disease (I13-)
         obstetric surgery and procedures (O75.4)
         rheumatic heart failure (I09.81)
     EXCLUDES 1   *cardiac arrest (I46-)*
            neonatal cardiac failure (P29.0)

     I50.1   **Left ventricular failure**
         Cardiac asthma
         Edema of lung with heart disease NOS
         Edema of lung with heart failure
         Left heart failure
         Pulmonary edema with heart disease NOS
         Pulmonary edema with heart failure
         EXCLUDES 1   *edema of lung without heart disease or heart failure*
            (J81-)
            pulmonary edema without heart disease or failure
            (J81-)

√5th   **I50.2**   **Systolic (congestive) heart failure**
         EXCLUDES 1   *combined systolic (congestive) and diastolic*
            (congestive) heart failure (I50.4-)

         I50.20   **Unspecified systolic (congestive) heart failure**

         I50.21   **Acute systolic (congestive) heart failure**

         I50.22   **Chronic systolic (congestive) heart failure**

         I50.23   **Acute on chronic systolic (congestive) heart failure**

√5th   **I50.3**   **Diastolic (congestive) heart failure**
         EXCLUDES 1   *combined systolic (congestive) and diastolic*
            (congestive) heart failure (I50.4-)

         I50.30   **Unspecified diastolic (congestive) heart failure**

         I50.31   **Acute diastolic (congestive) heart failure**

         I50.32   **Chronic diastolic (congestive) heart failure**

         I50.33   **Acute on chronic diastolic (congestive) heart failure**

√5th   **I50.4**   **Combined systolic (congestive) and diastolic (congestive) heart failure**

         I50.40   **Unspecified combined systolic (congestive) and diastolic (congestive) heart failure**

         I50.41   **Acute combined systolic (congestive) and diastolic (congestive) heart failure**

         I50.42   **Chronic combined systolic (congestive) and diastolic (congestive) heart failure**

         I50.43   **Acute on chronic combined systolic (congestive) and diastolic (congestive) heart failure**

     I50.9   **Heart failure, unspecified**
         Biventricular (heart) failure NOS
         Cardiac, heart or myocardial failure NOS
         Congestive heart disease
         Congestive heart failure NOS
         Right ventricular failure (secondary to left heart failure)
         EXCLUDES 1   *fluid overload (E87.70)*

EXCLUDES 1   Not coded here   EXCLUDES 2   Not included here   ***Manifestation Code***

✓4th I51　Complications and ill-defined descriptions of heart disease
EXCLUDES 1　*any condition in I51.4-I51.9 due to hypertension (I11-)*
　　　　　any condition in I51.4-I51.9 due to hypertension and chronic kidney disease (I13-)
　　　　　heart disease specified as rheumatic (I00-I09)

I51.0　Cardiac septal defect, acquired
　　Acquired septal atrial defect (old)
　　Acquired septal auricular defect (old)
　　Acquired septal ventricular defect (old)
　　EXCLUDES 1　*cardiac septal defect as current complication following acute myocardial infarction (I23.1, I23.2)*

I51.1　Rupture of chordae tendineae, not elsewhere classified
　　EXCLUDES 1　*rupture of chordae tendineae as current complication following acute myocardial infarction (I23.4)*

I51.2　Rupture of papillary muscle, not elsewhere classified
　　EXCLUDES 1　*rupture of papillary muscle as current complication following acute myocardial infarction (I23.5)*

I51.3　Intracardiac thrombosis, not elsewhere classified
　　Apical thrombosis (old)
　　Atrial thrombosis (old)
　　Auricular thrombosis (old)
　　Mural thrombosis (old)
　　Ventricular thrombosis (old)
　　EXCLUDES 1　*intracardiac thrombosis as current complication following acute myocardial infarction (I23.6)*

I51.4　Myocarditis, unspecified
　　Chronic (interstitial) myocarditis
　　Myocardial fibrosis
　　Myocarditis NOS
　　EXCLUDES 1　*acute or subacute myocarditis (I40-)*

I51.5　Myocardial degeneration
　　Fatty degeneration of heart or myocardium
　　Myocardial disease
　　Senile degeneration of heart or myocardium

I51.7　Cardiomegaly
　　Cardiac dilatation
　　Cardiac hypertrophy
　　Ventricular dilatation

✓5th **I51.8　Other ill-defined heart diseases**
　　I51.81　Takotsubo syndrome
　　　　Reversible left ventricular dysfunction following sudden emotional stress
　　　　Stress induced cardiomyopathy
　　　　Takotsubo cardiomyopathy
　　　　Transient left ventricular apical ballooning syndrome
　　I51.89　Other ill-defined heart diseases
　　　　Carditis (acute)(chronic)
　　　　Pancarditis (acute)(chronic)

I51.9　Heart disease, unspecified

I52　*Other heart disorders in diseases classified elsewhere*
Code first underlying disease, such as:
　　congenital syphilis (A50.5)
　　mucopolysaccharidosis (E76.3)
　　schistosomiasis (B65.0-B65.9)
　　EXCLUDES 1　*heart disease (in):*
　　　　gonococcal infection (A54.83)
　　　　meningococcal infection (A39.50)
　　　　rheumatoid arthritis (M05.31)
　　　　syphilis (A52.06)

Cerebrovascular diseases (I60-I69)
Use additional code to identify presence of:
　　alcohol abuse and dependence (F10-)
　　exposure to environmental tobacco smoke (Z77.22)
　　history of tobacco use (Z87.891)
　　hypertension (I10-I15)
　　occupational exposure to environmental tobacco smoke (Z57.31)
　　tobacco dependence (F17-)
　　tobacco use (Z72.0)
　　EXCLUDES 1　*transient cerebral ischemic attacks and related syndromes (G45-)*
　　　　traumatic intracranial hemorrhage (S06-)

✓4th I60　Nontraumatic subarachnoid hemorrhage
INCLUDES　ruptured cerebral aneurysm
EXCLUDES 1　*sequelae of subarachnoid hemorrhage (I69.0-)*
　　　　syphilitic ruptured cerebral aneurysm (A52.05)

✓5th **I60.0　Nontraumatic subarachnoid hemorrhage from carotid siphon and bifurcation**
　　I60.00　Nontraumatic subarachnoid hemorrhage from unspecified carotid siphon and bifurcation
　　I60.01　Nontraumatic subarachnoid hemorrhage from right carotid siphon and bifurcation
　　I60.02　Nontraumatic subarachnoid hemorrhage from left carotid siphon and bifurcation

✓5th **I60.1　Nontraumatic subarachnoid hemorrhage from middle cerebral artery**
　　I60.10　Nontraumatic subarachnoid hemorrhage from unspecified middle cerebral artery
　　I60.11　Nontraumatic subarachnoid hemorrhage from right middle cerebral artery
　　I60.12　Nontraumatic subarachnoid hemorrhage from left middle cerebral artery

✓5th **I60.2　Nontraumatic subarachnoid hemorrhage from anterior communicating artery**
　　I60.20　Nontraumatic subarachnoid hemorrhage from unspecified anterior communicating artery
　　I60.21　Nontraumatic subarachnoid hemorrhage from right anterior communicating artery
　　I60.22　Nontraumatic subarachnoid hemorrhage from left anterior communicating artery

✓5th **I60.3　Nontraumatic subarachnoid hemorrhage from posterior communicating artery**
　　I60.30　Nontraumatic subarachnoid hemorrhage from unspecified posterior communicating artery
　　I60.31　Nontraumatic subarachnoid hemorrhage from right posterior communicating artery
　　I60.32　Nontraumatic subarachnoid hemorrhage from left posterior communicating artery

I60.4　Nontraumatic subarachnoid hemorrhage from basilar artery

✓5th **I60.5　Nontraumatic subarachnoid hemorrhage from vertebral artery**
　　I60.50　Nontraumatic subarachnoid hemorrhage from unspecified vertebral artery
　　I60.51　Nontraumatic subarachnoid hemorrhage from right vertebral artery
　　I60.52　Nontraumatic subarachnoid hemorrhage from left vertebral artery

I60.6　Nontraumatic subarachnoid hemorrhage from other intracranial arteries

I60.7　Nontraumatic subarachnoid hemorrhage from unspecified intracranial artery
　　Ruptured (congenital) berry aneurysm
　　Ruptured (congenital) cerebral aneurysm
　　Subarachnoid hemorrhage (nontraumatic) from cerebral artery NOS
　　Subarachnoid hemorrhage (nontraumatic) from communicating artery NOS

I60.8　Other nontraumatic subarachnoid hemorrhage
　　Meningeal hemorrhage
　　Rupture of cerebral arteriovenous malformation

I60.9　Nontraumatic subarachnoid hemorrhage, unspecified

✓4th I61　Nontraumatic intracerebral hemorrhage
EXCLUDES 1　*sequelae of intracerebral hemorrhage (I69.1-)*

I61.0　Nontraumatic intracerebral hemorrhage in hemisphere, subcortical
　　Deep intracerebral hemorrhage (nontraumatic)

I61.1　Nontraumatic intracerebral hemorrhage in hemisphere, cortical
　　Cerebral lobe hemorrhage (nontraumatic)
　　Superficial intracerebral hemorrhage (nontraumatic)

I61.2　Nontraumatic intracerebral hemorrhage in hemisphere, unspecified

I61.3　Nontraumatic intracerebral hemorrhage in brain stem

I61.4　Nontraumatic intracerebral hemorrhage in cerebellum

I61.5　Nontraumatic intracerebral hemorrhage, intraventricular

I61.6　Nontraumatic intracerebral hemorrhage, multiple localized

I61.8　Other nontraumatic intracerebral hemorrhage

I61.9　Nontraumatic intracerebral hemorrhage, unspecified

✓4th I62　Other and unspecified nontraumatic intracranial hemorrhage
EXCLUDES 1　*sequelae of intracranial hemorrhage (I69.2)*

✓5th **I62.0　Nontraumatic subdural hemorrhage**
　　I62.00　Nontraumatic subdural hemorrhage, unspecified

☑ Appropriate additional character required

✓x7th Requires 7th character, placeholder x must fill empty characters

I62.01	**Nontraumatic acute subdural hemorrhage**
I62.02	**Nontraumatic subacute subdural hemorrhage**
I62.03	**Nontraumatic chronic subdural hemorrhage**
I62.1	**Nontraumatic extradural hemorrhage**
	Nontraumatic epidural hemorrhage
I62.9	**Nontraumatic intracranial hemorrhage, unspecified**

√4th **I63**   **Cerebral infarction**

INCLUDES   occlusion and stenosis of cerebral and precerebral arteries, resulting in cerebral infarction

Use additional code, if applicable, to identify status post administration of tPA (rtPA) in a different facility within the last 24 hours prior to admission to current facility (Z92.82)

EXCLUDES 1   *sequelae of cerebral infarction (I69.3-)*

√5th **I63.0**   **Cerebral infarction due to thrombosis of precerebral arteries**

     I63.00   **Cerebral infarction due to thrombosis of unspecified precerebral artery**

     √6th   I63.01   **Cerebral infarction due to thrombosis of vertebral artery**

         I63.011   **Cerebral infarction due to thrombosis of right vertebral artery**

         I63.012   **Cerebral infarction due to thrombosis of left vertebral artery**

         I63.019   **Cerebral infarction due to thrombosis of unspecified vertebral artery**

     I63.02   **Cerebral infarction due to thrombosis of basilar artery**

     √6th   I63.03   **Cerebral infarction due to thrombosis of carotid artery**

         I63.031   **Cerebral infarction due to thrombosis of right carotid artery**

         I63.032   **Cerebral infarction due to thrombosis of left carotid artery**

         I63.039   **Cerebral infarction due to thrombosis of unspecified carotid artery**

     I63.09   **Cerebral infarction due to thrombosis of other precerebral artery**

√5th **I63.1**   **Cerebral infarction due to embolism of precerebral arteries**

     I63.10   **Cerebral infarction due to embolism of unspecified precerebral artery**

     √6th   I63.11   **Cerebral infarction due to embolism of vertebral artery**

         I63.111   **Cerebral infarction due to embolism of right vertebral artery**

         I63.112   **Cerebral infarction due to embolism of left vertebral artery**

         I63.119   **Cerebral infarction due to embolism of unspecified vertebral artery**

     I63.12   **Cerebral infarction due to embolism of basilar artery**

     √6th   I63.13   **Cerebral infarction due to embolism of carotid artery**

         I63.131   **Cerebral infarction due to embolism of right carotid artery**

         I63.132   **Cerebral infarction due to embolism of left carotid artery**

         I63.139   **Cerebral infarction due to embolism of unspecified carotid artery**

     I63.19   **Cerebral infarction due to embolism of other precerebral artery**

√5th **I63.2**   **Cerebral infarction due to unspecified occlusion or stenosis of precerebral arteries**

     I63.20   **Cerebral infarction due to unspecified occlusion or stenosis of unspecified precerebral arteries**

     √6th   I63.21   **Cerebral infarction due to unspecified occlusion or stenosis of vertebral arteries**

         I63.211   **Cerebral infarction due to unspecified occlusion or stenosis of right vertebral arteries**

         I63.212   **Cerebral infarction due to unspecified occlusion or stenosis of left vertebral arteries**

         I63.219   **Cerebral infarction due to unspecified occlusion or stenosis of unspecified vertebral arteries**

     I63.22   **Cerebral infarction due to unspecified occlusion or stenosis of basilar arteries**

√6th **I63.23**   **Cerebral infarction due to unspecified occlusion or stenosis of carotid arteries**

     I63.231   **Cerebral infarction due to unspecified occlusion or stenosis of right carotid arteries**

     I63.232   **Cerebral infarction due to unspecified occlusion or stenosis of left carotid arteries**

     I63.239   **Cerebral infarction due to unspecified occlusion or stenosis of unspecified carotid arteries**

   I63.29   **Cerebral infarction due to unspecified occlusion or stenosis of other precerebral arteries**

√5th **I63.3**   **Cerebral infarction due to thrombosis of cerebral arteries**

     I63.30   **Cerebral infarction due to thrombosis of unspecified cerebral artery**

     √6th   I63.31   **Cerebral infarction due to thrombosis of middle cerebral artery**

         I63.311   **Cerebral infarction due to thrombosis of right middle cerebral artery**

         I63.312   **Cerebral infarction due to thrombosis of left middle cerebral artery**

         I63.319   **Cerebral infarction due to thrombosis of unspecified middle cerebral artery**

     √6th   I63.32   **Cerebral infarction due to thrombosis of anterior cerebral artery**

         I63.321   **Cerebral infarction due to thrombosis of right anterior cerebral artery**

         I63.322   **Cerebral infarction due to thrombosis of left anterior cerebral artery**

         I63.329   **Cerebral infarction due to thrombosis of unspecified anterior cerebral artery**

     √6th   I63.33   **Cerebral infarction due to thrombosis of posterior cerebral artery**

         I63.331   **Cerebral infarction due to thrombosis of right posterior cerebral artery**

         I63.332   **Cerebral infarction due to thrombosis of left posterior cerebral artery**

         I63.339   **Cerebral infarction due to thrombosis of unspecified posterior cerebral artery**

     √6th   I63.34   **Cerebral infarction due to thrombosis of cerebellar artery**

         I63.341   **Cerebral infarction due to thrombosis of right cerebellar artery**

         I63.342   **Cerebral infarction due to thrombosis of left cerebellar artery**

         I63.349   **Cerebral infarction due to thrombosis of unspecified cerebellar artery**

   I63.39   **Cerebral infarction due to thrombosis of other cerebral artery**

√5th **I63.4**   **Cerebral infarction due to embolism of cerebral arteries**

     I63.40   **Cerebral infarction due to embolism of unspecified cerebral artery**

     √6th   I63.41   **Cerebral infarction due to embolism of middle cerebral artery**

         I63.411   **Cerebral infarction due to embolism of right middle cerebral artery**

         I63.412   **Cerebral infarction due to embolism of left middle cerebral artery**

         I63.419   **Cerebral infarction due to embolism of unspecified middle cerebral artery**

     √6th   I63.42   **Cerebral infarction due to embolism of anterior cerebral artery**

         I63.421   **Cerebral infarction due to embolism of right anterior cerebral artery**

         I63.422   **Cerebral infarction due to embolism of left anterior cerebral artery**

         I63.429   **Cerebral infarction due to embolism of unspecified anterior cerebral artery**

     √6th   I63.43   **Cerebral infarction due to embolism of posterior cerebral artery**

         I63.431   **Cerebral infarction due to embolism of right posterior cerebral artery**

         I63.432   **Cerebral infarction due to embolism of left posterior cerebral artery**

         I63.439   **Cerebral infarction due to embolism of unspecified posterior cerebral artery**

EXCLUDES 1   Not coded here   EXCLUDES 2   Not included here   *Manifestation Code*

✓6th **I63.44** **Cerebral infarction due to embolism of cerebellar artery**

I63.441 **Cerebral infarction due to embolism of right cerebellar artery**

I63.442 **Cerebral infarction due to embolism of left cerebellar artery**

I63.449 **Cerebral infarction due to embolism of unspecified cerebellar artery**

I63.49 **Cerebral infarction due to embolism of other cerebral artery**

✓5th **I63.5** **Cerebral infarction due to unspecified occlusion or stenosis of cerebral arteries**

I63.50 **Cerebral infarction due to unspecified occlusion or stenosis of unspecified cerebral artery**

✓6th **I63.51** **Cerebral infarction due to unspecified occlusion or stenosis of middle cerebral artery**

I63.511 **Cerebral infarction due to unspecified occlusion or stenosis of right middle cerebral artery**

I63.512 **Cerebral infarction due to unspecified occlusion or stenosis of left middle cerebral artery**

I63.519 **Cerebral infarction due to unspecified occlusion or stenosis of unspecified middle cerebral artery**

✓6th **I63.52** **Cerebral infarction due to unspecified occlusion or stenosis of anterior cerebral artery**

I63.521 **Cerebral infarction due to unspecified occlusion or stenosis of right anterior cerebral artery**

I63.522 **Cerebral infarction due to unspecified occlusion or stenosis of left anterior cerebral artery**

I63.529 **Cerebral infarction due to unspecified occlusion or stenosis of unspecified anterior cerebral artery**

✓6th **I63.53** **Cerebral infarction due to unspecified occlusion or stenosis of posterior cerebral artery**

I63.531 **Cerebral infarction due to unspecified occlusion or stenosis of right posterior cerebral artery**

I63.532 **Cerebral infarction due to unspecified occlusion or stenosis of left posterior cerebral artery**

I63.539 **Cerebral infarction due to unspecified occlusion or stenosis of unspecified posterior cerebral artery**

✓6th **I63.54** **Cerebral infarction due to unspecified occlusion or stenosis of cerebellar artery**

I63.541 **Cerebral infarction due to unspecified occlusion or stenosis of right cerebellar artery**

I63.542 **Cerebral infarction due to unspecified occlusion or stenosis of left cerebellar artery**

I63.549 **Cerebral infarction due to unspecified occlusion or stenosis of unspecified cerebellar artery**

I63.59 **Cerebral infarction due to unspecified occlusion or stenosis of other cerebral artery**

I63.6 **Cerebral infarction due to cerebral venous thrombosis, nonpyogenic**

I63.8 **Other cerebral infarction**

I63.9 **Cerebral infarction, unspecified**
Stroke NOS

✓4th **I65** **Occlusion and stenosis of precerebral arteries, not resulting in cerebral infarction**

INCLUDES embolism of precerebral artery
narrowing of precerebral artery
obstruction (complete) (partial) of precerebral artery
thrombosis of precerebral artery

EXCLUDES 1 *insufficiency, NOS, of precerebral artery (G45-)*
insufficiency of precerebral arteries causing cerebral infarction (I63.0-I63.2)

✓5th **I65.0** **Occlusion and stenosis of vertebral artery**

I65.01 **Occlusion and stenosis of right vertebral artery**

I65.02 **Occlusion and stenosis of left vertebral artery**

I65.03 **Occlusion and stenosis of bilateral vertebral arteries**

I65.09 **Occlusion and stenosis of unspecified vertebral artery**

I65.1 **Occlusion and stenosis of basilar artery**

✓5th **I65.2** **Occlusion and stenosis of carotid artery**

I65.21 **Occlusion and stenosis of right carotid artery**

I65.22 **Occlusion and stenosis of left carotid artery**

I65.23 **Occlusion and stenosis of bilateral carotid arteries**

I65.29 **Occlusion and stenosis of unspecified carotid artery**

I65.8 **Occlusion and stenosis of other precerebral arteries**

I65.9 **Occlusion and stenosis of unspecified precerebral artery**
Occlusion and stenosis of precerebral artery NOS

✓4th **I66** **Occlusion and stenosis of cerebral arteries, not resulting in cerebral infarction**

INCLUDES embolism of cerebral artery
narrowing of cerebral artery
obstruction (complete) (partial) of cerebral artery
thrombosis of cerebral artery

EXCLUDES 1 *occlusion and stenosis of cerebral artery causing cerebral infarction (I63.3-I63.5)*

✓5th **I66.0** **Occlusion and stenosis of middle cerebral artery**

I66.01 **Occlusion and stenosis of right middle cerebral artery**

I66.02 **Occlusion and stenosis of left middle cerebral artery**

I66.03 **Occlusion and stenosis of bilateral middle cerebral arteries**

I66.09 **Occlusion and stenosis of unspecified middle cerebral artery**

✓5th **I66.1** **Occlusion and stenosis of anterior cerebral artery**

I66.11 **Occlusion and stenosis of right anterior cerebral artery**

I66.12 **Occlusion and stenosis of left anterior cerebral artery**

I66.13 **Occlusion and stenosis of bilateral anterior cerebral arteries**

I66.19 **Occlusion and stenosis of unspecified anterior cerebral artery**

✓5th **I66.2** **Occlusion and stenosis of posterior cerebral artery**

I66.21 **Occlusion and stenosis of right posterior cerebral artery**

I66.22 **Occlusion and stenosis of left posterior cerebral artery**

I66.23 **Occlusion and stenosis of bilateral posterior cerebral arteries**

I66.29 **Occlusion and stenosis of unspecified posterior cerebral artery**

I66.3 **Occlusion and stenosis of cerebellar arteries**

I66.8 **Occlusion and stenosis of other cerebral arteries**
Occlusion and stenosis of perforating arteries

I66.9 **Occlusion and stenosis of unspecified cerebral artery**

✓4th **I67** **Other cerebrovascular diseases**

EXCLUDES 1 *sequelae of the listed conditions (I69.8)*

I67.0 **Dissection of cerebral arteries, nonruptured**

EXCLUDES 1 *ruptured cerebral arteries (I60.7)*

I67.1 **Cerebral aneurysm, nonruptured**
Cerebral aneurysm NOS
Cerebral arteriovenous fistula, acquired
Internal carotid artery aneurysm, intracranial portion
Internal carotid artery aneurysm, NOS

EXCLUDES 1 *congenital cerebral aneurysm, nonruptured (Q28-)*
ruptured cerebral aneurysm (I60.7)

I67.2 **Cerebral atherosclerosis**
Atheroma of cerebral and precerebral arteries

I67.3 **Progressive vascular leukoencephalopathy**
Binswanger's disease

I67.4 **Hypertensive encephalopathy**

I67.5 **Moyamoya disease**

I67.6 **Nonpyogenic thrombosis of intracranial venous system**
Nonpyogenic thrombosis of cerebral vein
Nonpyogenic thrombosis of intracranial venous sinus

EXCLUDES 1 *nonpyogenic thrombosis of intracranial venous system causing infarction (I63.6)*

☑ Appropriate additional character required   ✓x7th Requires 7th character, placeholder x must fill empty characters

Diseases of the Circulatory System

I67.7–I69.069

I67.7 **Cerebral arteritis, not elsewhere classified**
Granulomatous angiitis of the nervous system
EXCLUDES 1 *allergic granulomatous angiitis (M30.1)*

I67.8 **Other specified cerebrovascular diseases**
Acute cerebrovascular insufficiency NOS
Cerebral ischemia (chronic)

I67.9 **Cerebrovascular disease, unspecified**

✓4th **I68** **Cerebrovascular disorders in diseases classified elsewhere**

I68.0 *Cerebral amyloid angiopathy*
Code first underlying amyloidosis (E85-)

I68.2 *Cerebral arteritis in other diseases classified elsewhere*
Code first underlying disease
EXCLUDES 1 *cerebral arteritis (in):*
listerosis (A32.89)
systemic lupus erythematosus (M32.19)
syphilis (A52.04)
tuberculosis (A18.89)

I68.8 *Other cerebrovascular disorders in diseases classified elsewhere*
Code first underlying disease
EXCLUDES 1 *syphilitic cerebral aneurysm (A52.05)*

✓4th **I69** **Sequelae of cerebrovascular disease**
NOTE   Category I69 is to be used to indicate conditions in I60-I67 as the cause of sequelae. The "sequelae" include conditions specified as such or as residuals which may occur at any time after the onset of the causal condition
EXCLUDES 1 *personal history of cerebral infarction without residual deficit (Z86.73)*
personal history of prolonged reversible ischemic neurologic deficit (PRIND) (Z86.73)
personal history of reversible ischemic neurologcial deficit (RIND) (Z86.73)
sequelae of traumatic intracranial injury (S06-)
transient ischemic attack (TIA) (G45.9)

✓5th **I69.0** **Sequelae of nontraumatic subarachnoid hemorrhage**

I69.00 **Unspecified sequelae of nontraumatic subarachnoid hemorrhage**

I69.01 **Cognitive deficits following nontraumatic subarachnoid hemorrhage**

✓6th **I69.02** **Speech and language deficits following nontraumatic subarachnoid hemorrhage**

I69.020 **Aphasia following nontraumatic subarachnoid hemorrhage**

I69.021 **Dysphasia following nontraumatic subarachnoid hemorrhage**

I69.022 **Dysarthria following nontraumatic subarachnoid hemorrhage**

I69.023 **Fluency disorder following nontraumatic subarachnoid hemorrhage**
Stuttering following nontraumatic subarachnoid hemorrhage

I69.028 **Other speech and language deficits following nontraumatic subarachnoid hemorrhage**

✓6th **I69.03** **Monoplegia of upper limb following nontraumatic subarachnoid hemorrhage**

I69.031 **Monoplegia of upper limb following nontraumatic subarachnoid hemorrhage affecting right dominant side**

I69.032 **Monoplegia of upper limb following nontraumatic subarachnoid hemorrhage affecting left dominant side**

I69.033 **Monoplegia of upper limb following nontraumatic subarachnoid hemorrhage affecting right non-dominant side**

I69.034 **Monoplegia of upper limb following nontraumatic subarachnoid hemorrhage affecting left non-dominant side**

I69.039 **Monoplegia of upper limb following nontraumatic subarachnoid hemorrhage affecting unspecified side**

✓6th **I69.04** **Monoplegia of lower limb following nontraumatic subarachnoid hemorrhage**

I69.041 **Monoplegia of lower limb following nontraumatic subarachnoid hemorrhage affecting right dominant side**

I69.042 **Monoplegia of lower limb following nontraumatic subarachnoid hemorrhage affecting left dominant side**

I69.043 **Monoplegia of lower limb following nontraumatic subarachnoid hemorrhage affecting right non-dominant side**

I69.044 **Monoplegia of lower limb following nontraumatic subarachnoid hemorrhage affecting left non-dominant side**

I69.049 **Monoplegia of lower limb following nontraumatic subarachnoid hemorrhage affecting unspecified side**

✓6th **I69.05** **Hemiplegia and hemiparesis following nontraumatic subarachnoid hemorrhage**

I69.051 **Hemiplegia and hemiparesis following nontraumatic subarachnoid hemorrhage affecting right dominant side**

I69.052 **Hemiplegia and hemiparesis following nontraumatic subarachnoid hemorrhage affecting left dominant side**

I69.053 **Hemiplegia and hemiparesis following nontraumatic subarachnoid hemorrhage affecting right non-dominant side**

I69.054 **Hemiplegia and hemiparesis following nontraumatic subarachnoid hemorrhage affecting left non-dominant side**

I69.059 **Hemiplegia and hemiparesis following nontraumatic subarachnoid hemorrhage affecting unspecified side**

✓6th **I69.06** **Other paralytic syndrome following nontraumatic subarachnoid hemorrhage**
Use additional code to identify type of paralytic syndrome, such as:
locked-in state (G83.5)
quadriplegia (G82.5-)
EXCLUDES 1 *hemiplegia/hemiparesis following nontraumatic subarachnoid hemorrhage (I69.05-)*
monoplegia of lower limb following nontraumatic subarachnoid hemorrhage (I69.04-)
monoplegia of upper limb following nontraumatic subarachnoid hemorrhage (I69.03-)

I69.061 **Other paralytic syndrome following nontraumatic subarachnoid hemorrhage affecting right dominant side**

I69.062 **Other paralytic syndrome following nontraumatic subarachnoid hemorrhage affecting left dominant side**

I69.063 **Other paralytic syndrome following nontraumatic subarachnoid hemorrhage affecting right non-dominant side**

I69.064 **Other paralytic syndrome following nontraumatic subarachnoid hemorrhage affecting left non-dominant side**

I69.065 **Other paralytic syndrome following nontraumatic subarachnoid hemorrhage, bilateral**

I69.069 **Other paralytic syndrome following nontraumatic subarachnoid hemorrhage affecting unspecified side**

EXCLUDES 1 Not coded here   EXCLUDES 2 Not included here   *Manifestation Code*

✓6th **I69.09 Other sequelae of nontraumatic subarachnoid hemorrhage**

I69.090 Apraxia following nontraumatic subarachnoid hemorrhage

I69.091 Dysphagia following nontraumatic subarachnoid hemorrhage
Use additional code to identify the type of dysphagia, if known (R13.1-)

I69.092 Facial weakness following nontraumatic subarachnoid hemorrhage
Facial droop following nontraumatic subarachnoid hemorrhage

I69.093 Ataxia following nontraumatic subarachnoid hemorrhage

I69.098 Other sequelae following nontraumatic subarachnoid hemorrhage
Alterations of sensation following nontraumatic subarachnoid hemorrhage
Disturbance of vision following nontraumatic subarachnoid hemorrhage
Use additional code to identify the sequelae

✓5th **I69.1 Sequelae of nontraumatic intracerebral hemorrhage**

I69.10 Unspecified sequelae of nontraumatic intracerebral hemorrhage

I69.11 Cognitive deficits following nontraumatic intracerebral hemorrhage

✓6th **I69.12 Speech and language deficits following nontraumatic intracerebral hemorrhage**

I69.120 Aphasia following nontraumatic intracerebral hemorrhage

I69.121 Dysphasia following nontraumatic intracerebral hemorrhage

I69.122 Dysarthria following nontraumatic intracerebral hemorrhage

I69.123 Fluency disorder following nontraumatic intracerebral hemorrhage
Stuttering following nontraumatic subarachnoid hemorrhage

I69.128 Other speech and language deficits following nontraumatic intracerebral hemorrhage

✓6th **I69.13 Monoplegia of upper limb following nontraumatic intracerebral hemorrhage**

I69.131 Monoplegia of upper limb following nontraumatic intracerebral hemorrhage affecting right dominant side

I69.132 Monoplegia of upper limb following nontraumatic intracerebral hemorrhage affecting left dominant side

I69.133 Monoplegia of upper limb following nontraumatic intracerebral hemorrhage affecting right non-dominant side

I69.134 Monoplegia of upper limb following nontraumatic intracerebral hemorrhage affecting left non-dominant side

I69.139 Monoplegia of upper limb following nontraumatic intracerebral hemorrhage affecting unspecified side

✓6th **I69.14 Monoplegia of lower limb following nontraumatic intracerebral hemorrhage**

I69.141 Monoplegia of lower limb following nontraumatic intracerebral hemorrhage affecting right dominant side

I69.142 Monoplegia of lower limb following nontraumatic intracerebral hemorrhage affecting left dominant side

I69.143 Monoplegia of lower limb following nontraumatic intracerebral hemorrhage affecting right non-dominant side

I69.144 Monoplegia of lower limb following nontraumatic intracerebral hemorrhage affecting left non-dominant side

I69.149 Monoplegia of lower limb following nontraumatic intracerebral hemorrhage affecting unspecified side

✓6th **I69.15 Hemiplegia and hemiparesis following nontraumatic intracerebral hemorrhage**

I69.151 Hemiplegia and hemiparesis following nontraumatic intracerebral hemorrhage affecting right dominant side

I69.152 Hemiplegia and hemiparesis following nontraumatic intracerebral hemorrhage affecting left dominant side

I69.153 Hemiplegia and hemiparesis following nontraumatic intracerebral hemorrhage affecting right non-dominant side

I69.154 Hemiplegia and hemiparesis following nontraumatic intracerebral hemorrhage affecting left non-dominant side

I69.159 Hemiplegia and hemiparesis following nontraumatic intracerebral hemorrhage affecting unspecified side

✓6th **I69.16 Other paralytic syndrome following nontraumatic intracerebral hemorrhage**
Use additional code to identify type of paralytic syndrome, such as:
locked-in state (G83.5)
quadriplegia (G82.5-)

EXCLUDES 1 *hemiplegia/hemiparesis following nontraumatic intracerebral hemorrhage (I69.15-)*
monoplegia of lower limb following nontraumatic intracerebral hemorrhage (I69.14-)
monoplegia of upper limb following nontraumatic intracerebral hemorrhage (I69.13-)

I69.161 Other paralytic syndrome following nontraumatic intracerebral hemorrhage affecting right dominant side

I69.162 Other paralytic syndrome following nontraumatic intracerebral hemorrhage affecting left dominant side

I69.163 Other paralytic syndrome following nontraumatic intracerebral hemorrhage affecting right non-dominant side

I69.164 Other paralytic syndrome following nontraumatic intracerebral hemorrhage affecting left non-dominant side

I69.165 Other paralytic syndrome following nontraumatic intracerebral hemorrhage, bilateral

I69.169 Other paralytic syndrome following nontraumatic intracerebral hemorrhage affecting unspecified side

✓6th **I69.19 Other sequelae of nontraumatic intracerebral hemorrhage**

I69.190 Apraxia following nontraumatic intracerebral hemorrhage

I69.191 Dysphagia following nontraumatic intracerebral hemorrhage
Use additional code to identify the type of dysphagia, if known (R13.1-)

I69.192 Facial weakness following nontraumatic intracerebral hemorrhage
Facial droop following nontraumatic intracerebral hemorrhage

I69.193 Ataxia following nontraumatic intracerebral hemorrhage

I69.198 Other sequelae of nontraumatic intracerebral hemorrhage
Alteration of sensations following nontraumatic intracerebral hemorrhage
Disturbance of vision following nontraumatic intracerebral hemorrhage
Use additional code to identify the sequelae

✓5th **I69.2 Sequelae of other nontraumatic intracranial hemorrhage**

I69.20 Unspecified sequelae of other nontraumatic intracranial hemorrhage

I69.21 Cognitive deficits following other nontraumatic intracranial hemorrhage

---

✔ Appropriate additional character required

✓x7th Requires 7th character, placeholder x must fill empty characters

✓6ᵗʰ I69.22 Speech and language deficits following other nontraumatic intracranial hemorrhage

    I69.220 Aphasia following other nontraumatic intracranial hemorrhage

    I69.221 Dysphasia following other nontraumatic intracranial hemorrhage

    I69.222 Dysarthria following other nontraumatic intracranial hemorrhage

    I69.223 Fluency disorder following other nontraumatic intracranial hemorrhage
        Stuttering following nontraumatic subarachnoid hemorrhage

    I69.228 Other speech and language deficits following other nontraumatic intracranial hemorrhage

✓6ᵗʰ I69.23 Monoplegia of upper limb following other nontraumatic intracranial hemorrhage

    I69.231 Monoplegia of upper limb following other nontraumatic intracranial hemorrhage affecting right dominant side

    I69.232 Monoplegia of upper limb following other nontraumatic intracranial hemorrhage affecting left dominant side

    I69.233 Monoplegia of upper limb following other nontraumatic intracranial hemorrhage affecting right non-dominant side

    I69.234 Monoplegia of upper limb following other nontraumatic intracranial hemorrhage affecting left non-dominant side

    I69.239 Monoplegia of upper limb following other nontraumatic intracranial hemorrhage affecting unspecified side

✓6ᵗʰ I69.24 Monoplegia of lower limb following other nontraumatic intracranial hemorrhage

    I69.241 Monoplegia of lower limb following other nontraumatic intracranial hemorrhage affecting right dominant side

    I69.242 Monoplegia of lower limb following other nontraumatic intracranial hemorrhage affecting left dominant side

    I69.243 Monoplegia of lower limb following other nontraumatic intracranial hemorrhage affecting right non-dominant side

    I69.244 Monoplegia of lower limb following other nontraumatic intracranial hemorrhage affecting left non-dominant side

    I69.249 Monoplegia of lower limb following other nontraumatic intracranial hemorrhage affecting unspecified side

✓6ᵗʰ I69.25 Hemiplegia and hemiparesis following other nontraumatic intracranial hemorrhage

    I69.251 Hemiplegia and hemiparesis following other nontraumatic intracranial hemorrhage affecting right dominant side

    I69.252 Hemiplegia and hemiparesis following other nontraumatic intracranial hemorrhage affecting left dominant side

    I69.253 Hemiplegia and hemiparesis following other nontraumatic intracranial hemorrhage affecting right non-dominant side

    I69.254 Hemiplegia and hemiparesis following other nontraumatic intracranial hemorrhage affecting left non-dominant side

    I69.259 Hemiplegia and hemiparesis following other nontraumatic intracranial hemorrhage affecting unspecified side

✓6ᵗʰ I69.26 Other paralytic syndrome following other nontraumatic intracranial hemorrhage
    Use additional code to identify type of paralytic syndrome, such as:
    locked-in state (G83.5)
    quadriplegia (G82.5-)

    EXCLUDES 1   *hemiplegia/hemiparesis following other nontraumatic intracranial hemorrhage (I69.25-)*
        monoplegia of lower limb following other nontraumatic intracranial hemorrhage (I69.24-)
        monoplegia of upper limb following other nontraumatic intracranial hemorrhage (I69.23-)

    I69.261 Other paralytic syndrome following other nontraumatic intracranial hemorrhage affecting right dominant side

    I69.262 Other paralytic syndrome following other nontraumatic intracranial hemorrhage affecting left dominant side

    I69.263 Other paralytic syndrome following other nontraumatic intracranial hemorrhage affecting right non-dominant side

    I69.264 Other paralytic syndrome following other nontraumatic intracranial hemorrhage affecting left non-dominant side

    I69.265 Other paralytic syndrome following other nontraumatic intracranial hemorrhage, bilateral

    I69.269 Other paralytic syndrome following other nontraumatic intracranial hemorrhage affecting unspecified side

✓6ᵗʰ I69.29 Other sequelae of other nontraumatic intracranial hemorrhage

    I69.290 Apraxia following other nontraumatic intracranial hemorrhage

    I69.291 Dysphagia following other nontraumatic intracranial hemorrhage
        Use additional code to identify the type of dysphagia, if known (R13.1-)

    I69.292 Facial weakness following other nontraumatic intracranial hemorrhage
        Facial droop following other nontraumatic intracranial hemorrhage

    I69.293 Ataxia following other nontraumatic intracranial hemorrhage

    I69.298 Other sequelae of other nontraumatic intracranial hemorrhage
        Alteration of sensation following other nontraumatic intracranial hemorrhage
        Disturbance of vision following other nontraumatic intracranial hemorrhage
        Use additional code to identify the sequelae

✓5ᵗʰ I69.3 Sequelae of cerebral infarction
    Sequelae of stroke NOS

    I69.30 Unspecified sequelae of cerebral infarction

    I69.31 Cognitive deficits following cerebral infarction

    ✓6ᵗʰ I69.32 Speech and language deficits following cerebral infarction

        I69.320 Aphasia following cerebral infarction

        I69.321 Dysphasia following cerebral infarction

        I69.322 Dysarthria following cerebral infarction

        I69.323 Fluency disorder following cerebral infarction
            Stuttering following nontraumatic subarachnoid hemorrhage

        I69.328 Other speech and language deficits following cerebral infarction

---

EXCLUDES 1   Not coded here   EXCLUDES 2   Not included here   ***Manifestation Code***

✓6th **I69.33 Monoplegia of upper limb following cerebral infarction**

    I69.331 Monoplegia of upper limb following cerebral infarction affecting right dominant side

    I69.332 Monoplegia of upper limb following cerebral infarction affecting left dominant side

    I69.333 Monoplegia of upper limb following cerebral infarction affecting right non-dominant side

    I69.334 Monoplegia of upper limb following cerebral infarction affecting left non-dominant side

    I69.339 Monoplegia of upper limb following cerebral infarction affecting unspecified side

✓6th **I69.34 Monoplegia of lower limb following cerebral infarction**

    I69.341 Monoplegia of lower limb following cerebral infarction affecting right dominant side

    I69.342 Monoplegia of lower limb following cerebral infarction affecting left dominant side

    I69.343 Monoplegia of lower limb following cerebral infarction affecting right non-dominant side

    I69.344 Monoplegia of lower limb following cerebral infarction affecting left non-dominant side

    I69.349 Monoplegia of lower limb following cerebral infarction affecting unspecified side

✓6th **I69.35 Hemiplegia and hemiparesis following cerebral infarction**

    I69.351 Hemiplegia and hemiparesis following cerebral infarction affecting right dominant side

    I69.352 Hemiplegia and hemiparesis following cerebral infarction affecting left dominant side

    I69.353 Hemiplegia and hemiparesis following cerebral infarction affecting right non-dominant side

    I69.354 Hemiplegia and hemiparesis following cerebral infarction affecting left non-dominant side

    I69.359 Hemiplegia and hemiparesis following cerebral infarction affecting unspecified side

✓6th **I69.36 Other paralytic syndrome following cerebral infarction**

    Use additional code to identify type of paralytic syndrome, such as:

    locked-in state (G83.5)

    quadriplegia (G82.5-)

    EXCLUDES 1   *hemiplegia/hemiparesis following cerebral infarction (I69.35-)*

    monoplegia of lower limb following cerebral infarction (I69.34-)

    monoplegia of upper limb following cerebral infarction (I69.33-)

    I69.361 Other paralytic syndrome following cerebral infarction affecting right dominant side

    I69.362 Other paralytic syndrome following cerebral infarction affecting left dominant side

    I69.363 Other paralytic syndrome following cerebral infarction affecting right non-dominant side

    I69.364 Other paralytic syndrome following cerebral infarction affecting left non-dominant side

    I69.365 Other paralytic syndrome following cerebral infarction, bilateral

    I69.369 Other paralytic syndrome following cerebral infarction affecting unspecified side

✓6th **I69.39 Other sequelae of cerebral infarction**

    I69.390 Apraxia following cerebral infarction

    I69.391 Dysphagia following cerebral infarction

    Use additional code to identify the type of dysphagia, if known (R13.1-)

    I69.392 Facial weakness following cerebral infarction

    Facial droop following cerebral infarction

    I69.393 Ataxia following cerebral infarction

    I69.398 Other sequelae of cerebral infarction

    Alteration of sensation following cerebral infarction

    Disturbance of vision following cerebral infarction

    Use additional code to identify the sequelae

✓5th **I69.8 Sequelae of other cerebrovascular diseases**

    EXCLUDES 1   *sequelae of traumatic intracranial injury (S06-)*

    I69.80 Unspecified sequelae of other cerebrovascular disease

    I69.81 Cognitive deficits following other cerebrovascular disease

✓6th **I69.82 Speech and language deficits following other cerebrovascular disease**

    I69.820 Aphasia following other cerebrovascular disease

    I69.821 Dysphasia following other cerebrovascular disease

    I69.822 Dysarthria following other cerebrovascular disease

    I69.823 Fluency disorder following other cerebrovascular disease

    Stuttering following nontraumatic subarachnoid hemorrhage

    I69.828 Other speech and language deficits following other cerebrovascular disease

✓6th **I69.83 Monoplegia of upper limb following other cerebrovascular disease**

    I69.831 Monoplegia of upper limb following other cerebrovascular disease affecting right dominant side

    I69.832 Monoplegia of upper limb following other cerebrovascular disease affecting left dominant side

    I69.833 Monoplegia of upper limb following other cerebrovascular disease affecting right non-dominant side

    I69.834 Monoplegia of upper limb following other cerebrovascular disease affecting left non-dominant side

    I69.839 Monoplegia of upper limb following other cerebrovascular disease affecting unspecified side

✓6th **I69.84 Monoplegia of lower limb following other cerebrovascular disease**

    I69.841 Monoplegia of lower limb following other cerebrovascular disease affecting right dominant side

    I69.842 Monoplegia of lower limb following other cerebrovascular disease affecting left dominant side

    I69.843 Monoplegia of lower limb following other cerebrovascular disease affecting right non-dominant side

    I69.844 Monoplegia of lower limb following other cerebrovascular disease affecting left non-dominant side

    I69.849 Monoplegia of lower limb following other cerebrovascular disease affecting unspecified side

✓6th **I69.85 Hemiplegia and hemiparesis following other cerebrovascular disease**

    I69.851 Hemiplegia and hemiparesis following other cerebrovascular disease affecting right dominant side

    I69.852 Hemiplegia and hemiparesis following other cerebrovascular disease affecting left dominant side

---

✓ Appropriate additional character required   ✓x7th Requires 7th character, placeholder x must fill empty characters

Diseases of the Circulatory System

I69.853–I69.963

I69.853   **Hemiplegia and hemiparesis following other cerebrovascular disease affecting right non-dominant side**

I69.854   **Hemiplegia and hemiparesis following other cerebrovascular disease affecting left non-dominant side**

I69.859   **Hemiplegia and hemiparesis following other cerebrovascular disease affecting unspecified side**

√6th   **I69.86   Other paralytic syndrome following other cerebrovascular disease**

Use additional code to identify type of paralytic syndrome, such as:
locked-in state (G83.5)
quadriplegia (G82.5-)

> EXCLUDES 1   *hemiplegia/hemiparesis following other cerebrovascular disease (I69.85-)*
> *monoplegia of lower limb following other cerebrovascular disease (I69.84-)*
> *monoplegia of upper limb following other cerebrovascular disease (I69.83-)*

I69.861   **Other paralytic syndrome following other cerebrovascular disease affecting right dominant side**

I69.862   **Other paralytic syndrome following other cerebrovascular disease affecting left dominant side**

I69.863   **Other paralytic syndrome following other cerebrovascular disease affecting right non-dominant side**

I69.864   **Other paralytic syndrome following other cerebrovascular disease affecting left non-dominant side**

I69.865   **Other paralytic syndrome following other cerebrovascular disease, bilateral**

I69.869   **Other paralytic syndrome following other cerebrovascular disease affecting unspecified side**

√6th   **I69.89   Other sequelae of other cerebrovascular disease**

I69.890   **Apraxia following other cerebrovascular disease**

I69.891   **Dysphagia following other cerebrovascular disease**

Use additional code to identify the type of dysphagia, if known (R13.1-)

I69.892   **Facial weakness following other cerebrovascular disease**

Facial droop following other cerebrovascular disease

I69.893   **Ataxia following other cerebrovascular disease**

I69.898   **Other sequelae of other cerebrovascular disease**

Alteration of sensation following other cerebrovascular disease
Disturbance of vision following other cerebrovascular disease
Use additional code to identify the sequelae

√5th   **I69.9   Sequelae of unspecified cerebrovascular diseases**

> EXCLUDES 1   *sequelae of stroke (I63.3)*
> *sequelae of traumatic intracranial injury (S06-)*

I69.90   **Unspecified sequelae of unspecified cerebrovascular disease**

I69.91   **Cognitive deficits following unspecified cerebrovascular disease**

√6th   **I69.92   Speech and language deficits following unspecified cerebrovascular disease**

I69.920   **Aphasia following unspecified cerebrovascular disease**

I69.921   **Dysphasia following unspecified cerebrovascular disease**

I69.922   **Dysarthria following unspecified cerebrovascular disease**

I69.923   **Fluency disorder following unspecified cerebrovascular disease**

Stuttering following nontraumatic subarachnoid hemorrhage

I69.928   **Other speech and language deficits following unspecified cerebrovascular disease**

√6th   **I69.93   Monoplegia of upper limb following unspecified cerebrovascular disease**

I69.931   **Monoplegia of upper limb following unspecified cerebrovascular disease affecting right dominant side**

I69.932   **Monoplegia of upper limb following unspecified cerebrovascular disease affecting left dominant side**

I69.933   **Monoplegia of upper limb following unspecified cerebrovascular disease affecting right non-dominant side**

I69.934   **Monoplegia of upper limb following unspecified cerebrovascular disease affecting left non-dominant side**

I69.939   **Monoplegia of upper limb following unspecified cerebrovascular disease affecting unspecified side**

√6th   **I69.94   Monoplegia of lower limb following unspecified cerebrovascular disease**

I69.941   **Monoplegia of lower limb following unspecified cerebrovascular disease affecting right dominant side**

I69.942   **Monoplegia of lower limb following unspecified cerebrovascular disease affecting left dominant side**

I69.943   **Monoplegia of lower limb following unspecified cerebrovascular disease affecting right non-dominant side**

I69.944   **Monoplegia of lower limb following unspecified cerebrovascular disease affecting left non-dominant side**

I69.949   **Monoplegia of lower limb following unspecified cerebrovascular disease affecting unspecified side**

√6th   **I69.95   Hemiplegia and hemiparesis following unspecified cerebrovascular disease**

I69.951   **Hemiplegia and hemiparesis following unspecified cerebrovascular disease affecting right dominant side**

I69.952   **Hemiplegia and hemiparesis following unspecified cerebrovascular disease affecting left dominant side**

I69.953   **Hemiplegia and hemiparesis following unspecified cerebrovascular disease affecting right non-dominant side**

I69.954   **Hemiplegia and hemiparesis following unspecified cerebrovascular disease affecting left non-dominant side**

I69.959   **Hemiplegia and hemiparesis following unspecified cerebrovascular disease affecting unspecified side**

√6th   **I69.96   Other paralytic syndrome following unspecified cerebrovascular disease**

Use additional code to identify type of paralytic syndrome, such as:
locked-in state (G83.5)
quadriplegia (G82.5-)

> EXCLUDES 1   *hemiplegia/hemiparesis following unspecified cerebrovascular disease (I69.95-)*
> *monoplegia of lower limb following unspecified cerebrovascular disease (I69.94-)*
> *monoplegia of upper limb following unspecified cerebrovascular disease (I69.93-)*

I69.961   **Other paralytic syndrome following unspecified cerebrovascular disease affecting right dominant side**

I69.962   **Other paralytic syndrome following unspecified cerebrovascular disease affecting left dominant side**

I69.963   **Other paralytic syndrome following unspecified cerebrovascular disease affecting right non-dominant side**

EXCLUDES 1   Not coded here   EXCLUDES 2   Not included here   *Manifestation Code*

I69.964 Other paralytic syndrome following unspecified cerebrovascular disease affecting left non-dominant side

I69.965 Other paralytic syndrome following unspecified cerebrovascular disease, bilateral

I69.969 Other paralytic syndrome following unspecified cerebrovascular disease affecting unspecified side

✓6th **I69.99** Other sequelae of unspecified cerebrovascular disease

I69.990 Apraxia following unspecified cerebrovascular disease

I69.991 Dysphagia following unspecified cerebrovascular disease
　　Use additional code to identify the type of dysphagia, if known (R13.1-)

I69.992 Facial weakness following unspecified cerebrovascular disease
　　Facial droop following unspecified cerebrovascular disease

I69.993 Ataxia following unspecified cerebrovascular disease

I69.998 Other sequelae following unspecified cerebrovascular disease
　　Alteration in sensation following unspecified cerebrovascular disease
　　Disturbance of vision following unspecified cerebrovascular disease
　　Use additional code to identify the sequelae

Diseases of arteries, arterioles and capillaries (I70-I79)

✓4th **I70** **Atherosclerosis**

INCLUDES　andarteritis deformans or obliterans
　　　　arteriolosclerosis
　　　　arterial degeneration
　　　　arteriosclerosis
　　　　arteriosclerotic vascular disease
　　　　arteriovascular degeneration
　　　　atheroma
　　　　senile arteritis
　　　　senile endarteritis
　　　　vascular degeneration
Use additional code to identify:
　exposure to environmental tobacco smoke (Z77.22)
　history of tobacco use (Z87.891)
　occupational exposure to environmental tobacco smoke (Z57.31)
　tobacco dependence (F17-)
　tobacco use (Z72.0)

EXCLUDES 2　*arteriosclerotic cardiovascular disease (I25.1-)*
　　　　arteriosclerotic heart disease (I25.1-)
　　　　atheroembolism (I75-)
　　　　cerebral atherosclerosis (I67.2)
　　　　coronary atherosclerosis (I25.1-)
　　　　mesenteric atherosclerosis (K55.1)
　　　　precerebral atherosclerosis (I67.2)
　　　　primary pulmonary atherosclerosis (I27.0)

I70.0 **Atherosclerosis of aorta**

I70.1 **Atherosclerosis of renal artery**
　Goldblatt's kidney
　EXCLUDES 2　*atherosclerosis of renal arterioles (I12-)*

I70.2 **Atherosclerosis of native arteries of the extremities**
　Mönckeberg's (medial) sclerosis
　Use additional code, if applicable, to identify chronic total occlusion of artery of extremity (I70.92)
　EXCLUDES 2　*atherosclerosis of bypass graft of extremities (I70.30-I70.79)*

✓6th **I70.20** **Unspecified atherosclerosis of native arteries of extremities**

I70.201 Unspecified atherosclerosis of native arteries of extremities, right leg

I70.202 Unspecified atherosclerosis of native arteries of extremities, left leg

I70.203 Unspecified atherosclerosis of native arteries of extremities, bilateral legs

I70.208 Unspecified atherosclerosis of native arteries of extremities, other extremity

I70.209 Unspecified atherosclerosis of native arteries of extremities, unspecified extremity

✓6th **I70.21** **Atherosclerosis of native arteries of extremities with intermittent claudication**

I70.211 Atherosclerosis of native arteries of extremities with intermittent claudication, right leg

I70.212 Atherosclerosis of native arteries of extremities with intermittent claudication, left leg

I70.213 Atherosclerosis of native arteries of extremities with intermittent claudication, bilateral legs

I70.218 Atherosclerosis of native arteries of extremities with intermittent claudication, other extremity

I70.219 Atherosclerosis of native arteries of extremities with intermittent claudication, unspecified extremity

✓6th **I70.22** **Atherosclerosis of native arteries of extremities with rest pain**
　Includes any condition classifiable to I70.21-

I70.221 Atherosclerosis of native arteries of extremities with rest pain, right leg

I70.222 Atherosclerosis of native arteries of extremities with rest pain, left leg

I70.223 Atherosclerosis of native arteries of extremities with rest pain, bilateral legs

I70.228 Atherosclerosis of native arteries of extremities with rest pain, other extremity

I70.229 Atherosclerosis of native arteries of extremities with rest pain, unspecified extremity

✓6th **I70.23** **Atherosclerosis of native arteries of right leg with ulceration**
　Includes any condition classifiable to I70.211 and I70.221
　Use additional code to identify severity of ulcer (L97- with fifth character 1)

I70.231 Atherosclerosis of native arteries of right leg with ulceration of thigh

I70.232 Atherosclerosis of native arteries of right leg with ulceration of calf

I70.233 Atherosclerosis of native arteries of right leg with ulceration of ankle

I70.234 Atherosclerosis of native arteries of right leg with ulceration of heel and midfoot
　　Atherosclerosis of native arteries of right leg with ulceration of plantar surface of midfoot

I70.235 Atherosclerosis of native arteries of right leg with ulceration of other part of foot
　　Atherosclerosis of native arteries of right leg extremities with ulceration of toe

I70.238 Atherosclerosis of native arteries of right leg with ulceration of other part of lower right leg

I70.239 Atherosclerosis of native arteries of right leg with ulceration of unspecified site

✓6th **I70.24** **Atherosclerosis of native arteries of left leg with ulceration**
　Includes any condition classifiable to I70.212 and I70.222
　Use additional code to identify severity of ulcer (L97- with fifth character 2)

I70.241 Atherosclerosis of native arteries of left leg with ulceration of thigh

I70.242 Atherosclerosis of native arteries of left leg with ulceration of calf

I70.243 Atherosclerosis of native arteries of left leg with ulceration of ankle

---

✓ Appropriate additional character required　　　　✓x7th Requires 7th character, placeholder x must fill empty characters

I70.244   **Atherosclerosis of native arteries of left leg with ulceration of heel and midfoot**
Atherosclerosis of native arteries of left leg with ulceration of plantar surface of midfoot

I70.245   **Atherosclerosis of native arteries of left leg with ulceration of other part of foot**
Atherosclerosis of native arteries of left leg extremities with ulceration of toe

I70.248   **Atherosclerosis of native arteries of left leg with ulceration of other part of lower left leg**

I70.249   **Atherosclerosis of native arteries of left leg with ulceration of unspecified site**

I70.25   **Atherosclerosis of native arteries of other extremities with ulceration**
Includes any condition classifiable to I70.218 and I70.228
Use additional code to identify the severity of the ulcer (L98.49-)

✓6th **I70.26**   **Atherosclerosis of native arteries of extremities with gangrene**
Includes any condition classifiable to I70.21-, I70.22-, I70.23-, I70.24-, and I70.25-
Use additional code to identify the severity of any ulcer (L98.49-), if applicable

I70.261   **Atherosclerosis of native arteries of extremities with gangrene, right leg**

I70.262   **Atherosclerosis of native arteries of extremities with gangrene, left leg**

I70.263   **Atherosclerosis of native arteries of extremities with gangrene, bilateral legs**

I70.268   **Atherosclerosis of native arteries of extremities with gangrene, other extremity**

I70.269   **Atherosclerosis of native arteries of extremities with gangrene, unspecified extremity**

✓6th **I70.29**   **Other atherosclerosis of native arteries of extremities**

I70.291   **Other atherosclerosis of native arteries of extremities, right leg**

I70.292   **Other atherosclerosis of native arteries of extremities, left leg**

I70.293   **Other atherosclerosis of native arteries of extremities, bilateral legs**

I70.298   **Other atherosclerosis of native arteries of extremities, other extremity**

I70.299   **Other atherosclerosis of native arteries of extremities, unspecified extremity**

✓5th **I70.3**   **Atherosclerosis of unspecified type of bypass graft(s) of the extremities**
Use additional code, if applicable, to identify chronic total occlusion of artery of extremity (I70.92)
EXCLUDES 1   *embolism or thrombus of bypass graft(s) of extremities (T82.8-)*

✓6th **I70.30**   **Unspecified atherosclerosis of unspecified type of bypass graft(s) of the extremities**

I70.301   **Unspecified atherosclerosis of unspecified type of bypass graft(s) of the extremities, right leg**

I70.302   **Unspecified atherosclerosis of unspecified type of bypass graft(s) of the extremities, left leg**

I70.303   **Unspecified atherosclerosis of unspecified type of bypass graft(s) of the extremities, bilateral legs**

I70.308   **Unspecified atherosclerosis of unspecified type of bypass graft(s) of the extremities, other extremity**

I70.309   **Unspecified atherosclerosis of unspecified type of bypass graft(s) of the extremities, unspecified extremity**

✓6th **I70.31**   **Atherosclerosis of unspecified type of bypass graft(s) of the extremities with intermittent claudication**

I70.311   **Atherosclerosis of unspecified type of bypass graft(s) of the extremities with intermittent claudication, right leg**

I70.312   **Atherosclerosis of unspecified type of bypass graft(s) of the extremities with intermittent claudication, left leg**

I70.313   **Atherosclerosis of unspecified type of bypass graft(s) of the extremities with intermittent claudication, bilateral legs**

I70.318   **Atherosclerosis of unspecified type of bypass graft(s) of the extremities with intermittent claudication, other extremity**

I70.319   **Atherosclerosis of unspecified type of bypass graft(s) of the extremities with intermittent claudication, unspecified extremity**

✓6th **I70.32**   **Atherosclerosis of unspecified type of bypass graft(s) of the extremities with rest pain**
Includes any condition classifiable to I70.31-

I70.321   **Atherosclerosis of unspecified type of bypass graft(s) of the extremities with rest pain, right leg**

I70.322   **Atherosclerosis of unspecified type of bypass graft(s) of the extremities with rest pain, left leg**

I70.323   **Atherosclerosis of unspecified type of bypass graft(s) of the extremities with rest pain, bilateral legs**

I70.328   **Atherosclerosis of unspecified type of bypass graft(s) of the extremities with rest pain, other extremity**

I70.329   **Atherosclerosis of unspecified type of bypass graft(s) of the extremities with rest pain, unspecified extremity**

✓6th **I70.33**   **Atherosclerosis of unspecified type of bypass graft(s) of the right leg with ulceration**
Includes any condition classifiable to I70.311 and I70.321
Use additional code to identify severity of ulcer (L97- with fifth character 1)

I70.331   **Atherosclerosis of unspecified type of bypass graft(s) of the right leg with ulceration of thigh**

I70.332   **Atherosclerosis of unspecified type of bypass graft(s) of the right leg with ulceration of calf**

I70.333   **Atherosclerosis of unspecified type of bypass graft(s) of the right leg with ulceration of ankle**

I70.334   **Atherosclerosis of unspecified type of bypass graft(s) of the right leg with ulceration of heel and midfoot**
Atherosclerosis of unspecified type of bypass graft(s) of right leg with ulceration of plantar surface of midfoot

I70.335   **Atherosclerosis of unspecified type of bypass graft(s) of the right leg with ulceration of other part of foot**
Atherosclerosis of unspecified type of bypass graft(s) of the right leg with ulceration of toe

I70.338   **Atherosclerosis of unspecified type of bypass graft(s) of the right leg with ulceration of other part of lower leg**

I70.339   **Atherosclerosis of unspecified type of bypass graft(s) of the right leg with ulceration of unspecified site**

EXCLUDES 1   Not coded here   EXCLUDES 2   Not included here   *Manifestation Code*

✓6ᵗʰ **I70.34 Atherosclerosis of unspecified type of bypass graft(s) of the left leg with ulceration**
  Includes any condition classifiable to I70.312 and I70.322
  Use additional code to identify severity of ulcer (L97- with fifth character 2)

  I70.341 Atherosclerosis of unspecified type of bypass graft(s) of the left leg with ulceration of thigh

  I70.342 Atherosclerosis of unspecified type of bypass graft(s) of the left leg with ulceration of calf

  I70.343 Atherosclerosis of unspecified type of bypass graft(s) of the left leg with ulceration of ankle

  I70.344 Atherosclerosis of unspecified type of bypass graft(s) of the left leg with ulceration of heel and midfoot
    Atherosclerosis of unspecified type of bypass graft(s) of left leg with ulceration of plantar surface of midfoot

  I70.345 Atherosclerosis of unspecified type of bypass graft(s) of the left leg with ulceration of other part of foot
    Atherosclerosis of unspecified type of bypass graft(s) of the left leg with ulceration of toe

  I70.348 Atherosclerosis of unspecified type of bypass graft(s) of the left leg with ulceration of other part of lower leg

  I70.349 Atherosclerosis of unspecified type of bypass graft(s) of the left leg with ulceration of unspecified site

I70.35 Atherosclerosis of unspecified type of bypass graft(s) of other extremity with ulceration
  Includes any condition classifiable to I70.318 and I70.328
  Use additional code to identify severity of ulcer (L98.49-)

✓6ᵗʰ **I70.36 Atherosclerosis of unspecified type of bypass graft(s) of the extremities with gangrene**
  Includes any condition classifiable to I70.31-, I70.32-, I70.33-, I70.34-, I70.35
  Use additional code to identify the severity of any ulcer (L98.49-), if applicable

  I70.361 Atherosclerosis of unspecified type of bypass graft(s) of the extremities with gangrene, right leg

  I70.362 Atherosclerosis of unspecified type of bypass graft(s) of the extremities with gangrene, left leg

  I70.363 Atherosclerosis of unspecified type of bypass graft(s) of the extremities with gangrene, bilateral legs

  I70.368 Atherosclerosis of unspecified type of bypass graft(s) of the extremities with gangrene, other extremity

  I70.369 Atherosclerosis of unspecified type of bypass graft(s) of the extremities with gangrene, unspecified extremity

✓6ᵗʰ **I70.39 Other atherosclerosis of unspecified type of bypass graft(s) of the extremities**

  I70.391 Other atherosclerosis of unspecified type of bypass graft(s) of the extremities, right leg

  I70.392 Other atherosclerosis of unspecified type of bypass graft(s) of the extremities, left leg

  I70.393 Other atherosclerosis of unspecified type of bypass graft(s) of the extremities, bilateral legs

  I70.398 Other atherosclerosis of unspecified type of bypass graft(s) of the extremities, other extremity

  I70.399 Other atherosclerosis of unspecified type of bypass graft(s) of the extremities, unspecified extremity

✓5ᵗʰ **I70.4 Atherosclerosis of autologous vein bypass graft(s) of the extremities**
  Use additional code, if applicable, to identify chronic total occlusion of artery of extremity (I70.92)

✓6ᵗʰ **I70.40 Unspecified atherosclerosis of autologous vein bypass graft(s) of the extremities**

  I70.401 Unspecified atherosclerosis of autologous vein bypass graft(s) of the extremities, right leg

  I70.402 Unspecified atherosclerosis of autologous vein bypass graft(s) of the extremities, left leg

  I70.403 Unspecified atherosclerosis of autologous vein bypass graft(s) of the extremities, bilateral legs

  I70.408 Unspecified atherosclerosis of autologous vein bypass graft(s) of the extremities, other extremity

  I70.409 Unspecified atherosclerosis of autologous vein bypass graft(s) of the extremities, unspecified extremity

✓6ᵗʰ **I70.41 Atherosclerosis of autologous vein bypass graft(s) of the extremities with intermittent claudication**

  I70.411 Atherosclerosis of autologous vein bypass graft(s) of the extremities with intermittent claudication, right leg

  I70.412 Atherosclerosis of autologous vein bypass graft(s) of the extremities with intermittent claudication, left leg

  I70.413 Atherosclerosis of autologous vein bypass graft(s) of the extremities with intermittent claudication, bilateral legs

  I70.418 Atherosclerosis of autologous vein bypass graft(s) of the extremities with intermittent claudication, other extremity

  I70.419 Atherosclerosis of autologous vein bypass graft(s) of the extremities with intermittent claudication, unspecified extremity

✓6ᵗʰ **I70.42 Atherosclerosis of autologous vein bypass graft(s) of the extremities with rest pain**
  Includes any condition classifiable to I70.41-

  I70.421 Atherosclerosis of autologous vein bypass graft(s) of the extremities with rest pain, right leg

  I70.422 Atherosclerosis of autologous vein bypass graft(s) of the extremities with rest pain, left leg

  I70.423 Atherosclerosis of autologous vein bypass graft(s) of the extremities with rest pain, bilateral legs

  I70.428 Atherosclerosis of autologous vein bypass graft(s) of the extremities with rest pain, other extremity

  I70.429 Atherosclerosis of autologous vein bypass graft(s) of the extremities with rest pain, unspecified extremity

✓6ᵗʰ **I70.43 Atherosclerosis of autologous vein bypass graft(s) of the right leg with ulceration**
  Includes any condition classifiable to I70.411 and I70.421
  Use additional code to identify severity of ulcer (L97- with fifth character 1)

  I70.431 Atherosclerosis of autologous vein bypass graft(s) of the right leg with ulceration of thigh

  I70.432 Atherosclerosis of autologous vein bypass graft(s) of the right leg with ulceration of calf

  I70.433 Atherosclerosis of autologous vein bypass graft(s) of the right leg with ulceration of ankle

  I70.434 Atherosclerosis of autologous vein bypass graft(s) of the right leg with ulceration of heel and midfoot
    Atherosclerosis of autologous vein bypass graft(s) of right leg with ulceration of plantar surface of midfoot

---

☑ Appropriate additional character required   ✓x7ᵗʰ Requires 7th character, placeholder x must fill empty characters

Diseases of the Circulatory System

I70.435–I70.529

I70.435   **Atherosclerosis of autologous vein bypass graft(s) of the right leg with ulceration of other part of foot**
    Atherosclerosis of autologous vein bypass graft(s) of right leg with ulceration of toe

I70.438   **Atherosclerosis of autologous vein bypass graft(s) of the right leg with ulceration of other part of lower leg**

I70.439   **Atherosclerosis of autologous vein bypass graft(s) of the right leg with ulceration of unspecified site**

✓6ᵗʰ   **I70.44**   **Atherosclerosis of autologous vein bypass graft(s) of the left leg with ulceration**
    Includes any condition classifiable to I70.412 and I70.422
    Use additional code to identify severity of ulcer (L97- with fifth character 2)

I70.441   **Atherosclerosis of autologous vein bypass graft(s) of the left leg with ulceration of thigh**

I70.442   **Atherosclerosis of autologous vein bypass graft(s) of the left leg with ulceration of calf**

I70.443   **Atherosclerosis of autologous vein bypass graft(s) of the left leg with ulceration of ankle**

I70.444   **Atherosclerosis of autologous vein bypass graft(s) of the left leg with ulceration of heel and midfoot**
    Atherosclerosis of autologous vein bypass graft(s) of left leg with ulceration of plantar surface of midfoot

I70.445   **Atherosclerosis of autologous vein bypass graft(s) of the left leg with ulceration of other part of foot**
    Atherosclerosis of autologous vein bypass graft(s) of left leg with ulceration of toe

I70.448   **Atherosclerosis of autologous vein bypass graft(s) of the left leg with ulceration of other part of lower leg**

I70.449   **Atherosclerosis of autologous vein bypass graft(s) of the left leg with ulceration of unspecified site**

I70.45   **Atherosclerosis of autologous vein bypass graft(s) of other extremity with ulceration**
    Includes any condition classifiable to I70.418, I70.428, and I70.438
    Use additional code to identify severity of ulcer (L98.49)

✓6ᵗʰ   **I70.46**   **Atherosclerosis of autologous vein bypass graft(s) of the extremities with gangrene**
    Includes any condition classifiable to I70.41-, I70.42-, and I70.43-, I70.44-, I70.45
    Use additional code to identify the severity of any ulcer (L98.49-), if applicable

I70.461   **Atherosclerosis of autologous vein bypass graft(s) of the extremities with gangrene, right leg**

I70.462   **Atherosclerosis of autologous vein bypass graft(s) of the extremities with gangrene, left leg**

I70.463   **Atherosclerosis of autologous vein bypass graft(s) of the extremities with gangrene, bilateral legs**

I70.468   **Atherosclerosis of autologous vein bypass graft(s) of the extremities with gangrene, other extremity**

I70.469   **Atherosclerosis of autologous vein bypass graft(s) of the extremities with gangrene, unspecified extremity**

✓6ᵗʰ   **I70.49**   **Other atherosclerosis of autologous vein bypass graft(s) of the extremities**

I70.491   **Other atherosclerosis of autologous vein bypass graft(s) of the extremities, right leg**

I70.492   **Other atherosclerosis of autologous vein bypass graft(s) of the extremities, left leg**

I70.493   **Other atherosclerosis of autologous vein bypass graft(s) of the extremities, bilateral legs**

I70.498   **Other atherosclerosis of autologous vein bypass graft(s) of the extremities, other extremity**

I70.499   **Other atherosclerosis of autologous vein bypass graft(s) of the extremities, unspecified extremity**

✓5ᵗʰ   **I70.5**   **Atherosclerosis of nonautologous biological bypass graft(s) of the extremities**
    Use additional code, if applicable, to identify chronic total occlusion of artery of extremity (I70.92)

✓6ᵗʰ   **I70.50**   **Unspecified atherosclerosis of nonautologous biological bypass graft(s) of the extremities**

I70.501   **Unspecified atherosclerosis of nonautologous biological bypass graft(s) of the extremities, right leg**

I70.502   **Unspecified atherosclerosis of nonautologous biological bypass graft(s) of the extremities, left leg**

I70.503   **Unspecified atherosclerosis of nonautologous biological bypass graft(s) of the extremities, bilateral legs**

I70.508   **Unspecified atherosclerosis of nonautologous biological bypass graft(s) of the extremities, other extremity**

I70.509   **Unspecified atherosclerosis of nonautologous biological bypass graft(s) of the extremities, unspecified extremity**

✓6ᵗʰ   **I70.51**   **Atherosclerosis of nonautologous biological bypass graft(s) of the extremities with intermittent claudication**

I70.511   **Atherosclerosis of nonautologous biological bypass graft(s) of the extremities with intermittent claudication, right leg**

I70.512   **Atherosclerosis of nonautologous biological bypass graft(s) of the extremities with intermittent claudication, left leg**

I70.513   **Atherosclerosis of nonautologous biological bypass graft(s) of the extremities with intermittent claudication, bilateral legs**

I70.518   **Atherosclerosis of nonautologous biological bypass graft(s) of the extremities with intermittent claudication, other extremity**

I70.519   **Atherosclerosis of nonautologous biological bypass graft(s) of the extremities with intermittent claudication, unspecified extremity**

✓6ᵗʰ   **I70.52**   **Atherosclerosis of nonautologous biological bypass graft(s) of the extremities with rest pain**
    Includes any condition classifiable to I70.51-

I70.521   **Atherosclerosis of nonautologous biological bypass graft(s) of the extremities with rest pain, right leg**

I70.522   **Atherosclerosis of nonautologous biological bypass graft(s) of the extremities with rest pain, left leg**

I70.523   **Atherosclerosis of nonautologous biological bypass graft(s) of the extremities with rest pain, bilateral legs**

I70.528   **Atherosclerosis of nonautologous biological bypass graft(s) of the extremities with rest pain, other extremity**

I70.529   **Atherosclerosis of nonautologous biological bypass graft(s) of the extremities with rest pain, unspecified extremity**

☑6ᵗʰ **I70.53 Atherosclerosis of nonautologous biological bypass graft(s) of the right leg with ulceration**
Includes any condition classifiable to I70.511 and I70.521
Use additional code to identify severity of ulcer (L97- with fifth character 1)

I70.531 Atherosclerosis of nonautologous biological bypass graft(s) of the right leg with ulceration of thigh

I70.532 Atherosclerosis of nonautologous biological bypass graft(s) of the right leg with ulceration of calf

I70.533 Atherosclerosis of nonautologous biological bypass graft(s) of the right leg with ulceration of ankle

I70.534 Atherosclerosis of nonautologous biological bypass graft(s) of the right leg with ulceration of heel and midfoot
Atherosclerosis of nonautologous biological bypass graft(s) of right leg with ulceration of plantar surface of midfoot

I70.535 Atherosclerosis of nonautologous biological bypass graft(s) of the right leg with ulceration of other part of foot
Atherosclerosis of nonautologous biological bypass graft(s) of the right leg with ulceration of toe

I70.538 Atherosclerosis of nonautologous biological bypass graft(s) of the right leg with ulceration of other part of lower leg

I70.539 Atherosclerosis of nonautologous biological bypass graft(s) of the right leg with ulceration of unspecified site

☑6ᵗʰ **I70.54 Atherosclerosis of nonautologous biological bypass graft(s) of the left leg with ulceration**
Includes any condition classifiable to I70.512 and I70.522
Use additional code to identify severity of ulcer (L97- with fifth character 2)

I70.541 Atherosclerosis of nonautologous biological bypass graft(s) of the left leg with ulceration of thigh

I70.542 Atherosclerosis of nonautologous biological bypass graft(s) of the left leg with ulceration of calf

I70.543 Atherosclerosis of nonautologous biological bypass graft(s) of the left leg with ulceration of ankle

I70.544 Atherosclerosis of nonautologous biological bypass graft(s) of the left leg with ulceration of heel and midfoot
Atherosclerosis of nonautologous biological bypass graft(s) of left leg with ulceration of plantar surface of midfoot

I70.545 Atherosclerosis of nonautologous biological bypass graft(s) of the left leg with ulceration of other part of foot
Atherosclerosis of nonautologous biological bypass graft(s) of the left leg with ulceration of toe

I70.548 Atherosclerosis of nonautologous biological bypass graft(s) of the left leg with ulceration of other part of lower leg

I70.549 Atherosclerosis of nonautologous biological bypass graft(s) of the left leg with ulceration of unspecified site

I70.55 Atherosclerosis of nonautologous biological bypass graft(s) of other extremity with ulceration
Includes any condition classifiable to I70.518, I70.528, and I70.538
Use additional code to identify severity of ulcer (L98.49)

☑6ᵗʰ **I70.56 Atherosclerosis of nonautologous biological bypass graft(s) of the extremities with gangrene**
Includes any condition classifiable to I70.51-, I70.52-, and I70.53-, I70.54-, I70.55
Use additional code to identify the severity of any ulcer (L98.49-), if applicable

I70.561 Atherosclerosis of nonautologous biological bypass graft(s) of the extremities with gangrene, right leg

I70.562 Atherosclerosis of nonautologous biological bypass graft(s) of the extremities with gangrene, left leg

I70.563 Atherosclerosis of nonautologous biological bypass graft(s) of the extremities with gangrene, bilateral legs

I70.568 Atherosclerosis of nonautologous biological bypass graft(s) of the extremities with gangrene, other extremity

I70.569 Atherosclerosis of nonautologous biological bypass graft(s) of the extremities with gangrene, unspecified extremity

☑6ᵗʰ **I70.59 Other atherosclerosis of nonautologous biological bypass graft(s) of the extremities**

I70.591 Other atherosclerosis of nonautologous biological bypass graft(s) of the extremities, right leg

I70.592 Other atherosclerosis of nonautologous biological bypass graft(s) of the extremities, left leg

I70.593 Other atherosclerosis of nonautologous biological bypass graft(s) of the extremities, bilateral legs

I70.598 Other atherosclerosis of nonautologous biological bypass graft(s) of the extremities, other extremity

I70.599 Other atherosclerosis of nonautologous biological bypass graft(s) of the extremities, unspecified extremity

☑5ᵗʰ **I70.6 Atherosclerosis of nonbiological bypass graft(s) of the extremities**
Use additional code, if applicable, to identify chronic total occlusion of artery of extremity (I70.92)

☑6ᵗʰ **I70.60 Unspecified atherosclerosis of nonbiological bypass graft(s) of the extremities**

I70.601 Unspecified atherosclerosis of nonbiological bypass graft(s) of the extremities, right leg

I70.602 Unspecified atherosclerosis of nonbiological bypass graft(s) of the extremities, left leg

I70.603 Unspecified atherosclerosis of nonbiological bypass graft(s) of the extremities, bilateral legs

I70.608 Unspecified atherosclerosis of nonbiological bypass graft(s) of the extremities, other extremity

I70.609 Unspecified atherosclerosis of nonbiological bypass graft(s) of the extremities, unspecified extremity

☑6ᵗʰ **I70.61 Atherosclerosis of nonbiological bypass graft(s) of the extremities with intermittent claudication**

I70.611 Atherosclerosis of nonbiological bypass graft(s) of the extremities with intermittent claudication, right leg

I70.612 Atherosclerosis of nonbiological bypass graft(s) of the extremities with intermittent claudication, left leg

I70.613 Atherosclerosis of nonbiological bypass graft(s) of the extremities with intermittent claudication, bilateral legs

I70.618 Atherosclerosis of nonbiological bypass graft(s) of the extremities with intermittent claudication, other extremity

---

☑ Appropriate additional character required   ☑x7ᵗʰ Requires 7th character, placeholder x must fill empty characters

I70.619   **Atherosclerosis of nonbiological bypass graft(s) of the extremities with intermittent claudication, unspecified extremity**

☑6ᵗʰ **I70.62**   **Atherosclerosis of nonbiological bypass graft(s) of the extremities with rest pain**
> Includes any condition classifiable to I70.61-

I70.621   **Atherosclerosis of nonbiological bypass graft(s) of the extremities with rest pain, right leg**

I70.622   **Atherosclerosis of nonbiological bypass graft(s) of the extremities with rest pain, left leg**

I70.623   **Atherosclerosis of nonbiological bypass graft(s) of the extremities with rest pain, bilateral legs**

I70.628   **Atherosclerosis of nonbiological bypass graft(s) of the extremities with rest pain, other extremity**

I70.629   **Atherosclerosis of nonbiological bypass graft(s) of the extremities with rest pain, unspecified extremity**

☑6ᵗʰ **I70.63**   **Atherosclerosis of nonbiological bypass graft(s) of the right leg with ulceration**
> Includes any condition classifiable to I70.611 and I70.621
> Use additional code to identify severity of ulcer (L97- with fifth character 1)

I70.631   **Atherosclerosis of nonbiological bypass graft(s) of the right leg with ulceration of thigh**

I70.632   **Atherosclerosis of nonbiological bypass graft(s) of the right leg with ulceration of calf**

I70.633   **Atherosclerosis of nonbiological bypass graft(s) of the right leg with ulceration of ankle**

I70.634   **Atherosclerosis of nonbiological bypass graft(s) of the right leg with ulceration of heel and midfoot**
> Atherosclerosis of nonbiological bypass graft(s) of right leg with ulceration of plantar surface of midfoot

I70.635   **Atherosclerosis of nonbiological bypass graft(s) of the right leg with ulceration of other part of foot**
> Atherosclerosis of nonbiological bypass graft(s) of the right leg with ulceration of toe

I70.638   **Atherosclerosis of nonbiological bypass graft(s) of the right leg with ulceration of other part of lower leg**

I70.639   **Atherosclerosis of nonbiological bypass graft(s) of the right leg with ulceration of unspecified site**

☑6ᵗʰ **I70.64**   **Atherosclerosis of nonbiological bypass graft(s) of the left leg with ulceration**
> Includes any condition classifiable to I70.612 and I70.622
> Use additional code to identify severity of ulcer (L97- with fifth character 2)

I70.641   **Atherosclerosis of nonbiological bypass graft(s) of the left leg with ulceration of thigh**

I70.642   **Atherosclerosis of nonbiological bypass graft(s) of the left leg with ulceration of calf**

I70.643   **Atherosclerosis of nonbiological bypass graft(s) of the left leg with ulceration of ankle**

I70.644   **Atherosclerosis of nonbiological bypass graft(s) of the left leg with ulceration of heel and midfoot**
> Atherosclerosis of nonbiological bypass graft(s) of left leg with ulceration of plantar surface of midfoot

I70.645   **Atherosclerosis of nonbiological bypass graft(s) of the left leg with ulceration of other part of foot**
> Atherosclerosis of nonbiological bypass graft(s) of the left leg with ulceration of toe

I70.648   **Atherosclerosis of nonbiological bypass graft(s) of the left leg with ulceration of other part of lower leg**

I70.649   **Atherosclerosis of nonbiological bypass graft(s) of the left leg with ulceration of unspecified site**

I70.65   **Atherosclerosis of nonbiological bypass graft(s) of other extremity with ulceration**
> Includes any condition classifiable to I70.618 and I70.628
> Use additional code to identify severity of ulcer (L98.49)

☑6ᵗʰ **I70.66**   **Atherosclerosis of nonbiological bypass graft(s) of the extremities with gangrene**
> Includes any condition classifiable to I70.61-, I70.62-, I70.63-, I70.64-, I70.65
> Use additional code to identify the severity of any ulcer (L98.49-), if applicable

I70.661   **Atherosclerosis of nonbiological bypass graft(s) of the extremities with gangrene, right leg**

I70.662   **Atherosclerosis of nonbiological bypass graft(s) of the extremities with gangrene, left leg**

I70.663   **Atherosclerosis of nonbiological bypass graft(s) of the extremities with gangrene, bilateral legs**

I70.668   **Atherosclerosis of nonbiological bypass graft(s) of the extremities with gangrene, other extremity**

I70.669   **Atherosclerosis of nonbiological bypass graft(s) of the extremities with gangrene, unspecified extremity**

☑6ᵗʰ **I70.69**   **Other atherosclerosis of nonbiological bypass graft(s) of the extremities**

I70.691   **Other atherosclerosis of nonbiological bypass graft(s) of the extremities, right leg**

I70.692   **Other atherosclerosis of nonbiological bypass graft(s) of the extremities, left leg**

I70.693   **Other atherosclerosis of nonbiological bypass graft(s) of the extremities, bilateral legs**

I70.698   **Other atherosclerosis of nonbiological bypass graft(s) of the extremities, other extremity**

I70.699   **Other atherosclerosis of nonbiological bypass graft(s) of the extremities, unspecified extremity**

☑5ᵗʰ **I70.7**   **Atherosclerosis of other type of bypass graft(s) of the extremities**
> Use additional code, if applicable, to identify chronic total occlusion of artery of extremity (I70.92)

☑6ᵗʰ **I70.70**   **Unspecified atherosclerosis of other type of bypass graft(s) of the extremities**

I70.701   **Unspecified atherosclerosis of other type of bypass graft(s) of the extremities, right leg**

I70.702   **Unspecified atherosclerosis of other type of bypass graft(s) of the extremities, left leg**

I70.703   **Unspecified atherosclerosis of other type of bypass graft(s) of the extremities, bilateral legs**

I70.708   **Unspecified atherosclerosis of other type of bypass graft(s) of the extremities, other extremity**

I70.709   **Unspecified atherosclerosis of other type of bypass graft(s) of the extremities, unspecified extremity**

EXCLUDES 1 Not coded here   **EXCLUDES 2** Not included here   *Manifestation Code*

✓6th **I70.71** **Atherosclerosis of other type of bypass graft(s) of the extremities with intermittent claudication**

I70.711 **Atherosclerosis of other type of bypass graft(s) of the extremities with intermittent claudication, right leg**

I70.712 **Atherosclerosis of other type of bypass graft(s) of the extremities with intermittent claudication, left leg**

I70.713 **Atherosclerosis of other type of bypass graft(s) of the extremities with intermittent claudication, bilateral legs**

I70.718 **Atherosclerosis of other type of bypass graft(s) of the extremities with intermittent claudication, other extremity**

I70.719 **Atherosclerosis of other type of bypass graft(s) of the extremities with intermittent claudication, unspecified extremity**

✓6th **I70.72** **Atherosclerosis of other type of bypass graft(s) of the extremities with rest pain**

Includes any condition classifiable to I70.71-

I70.721 **Atherosclerosis of other type of bypass graft(s) of the extremities with rest pain, right leg**

I70.722 **Atherosclerosis of other type of bypass graft(s) of the extremities with rest pain, left leg**

I70.723 **Atherosclerosis of other type of bypass graft(s) of the extremities with rest pain, bilateral legs**

I70.728 **Atherosclerosis of other type of bypass graft(s) of the extremities with rest pain, other extremity**

I70.729 **Atherosclerosis of other type of bypass graft(s) of the extremities with rest pain, unspecified extremity**

✓6th **I70.73** **Atherosclerosis of other type of bypass graft(s) of the right leg with ulceration**

Includes any condition classifiable to I70.711 and I70.721

Use additional code to identify severity of ulcer (L97- with fifth character 1)

I70.731 **Atherosclerosis of other type of bypass graft(s) of the right leg with ulceration of thigh**

I70.732 **Atherosclerosis of other type of bypass graft(s) of the right leg with ulceration of calf**

I70.733 **Atherosclerosis of other type of bypass graft(s) of the right leg with ulceration of ankle**

I70.734 **Atherosclerosis of other type of bypass graft(s) of the right leg with ulceration of heel and midfoot**

Atherosclerosis of other type of bypass graft(s) of right leg with ulceration of plantar surface of midfoot

I70.735 **Atherosclerosis of other type of bypass graft(s) of the right leg with ulceration of other part of foot**

Atherosclerosis of other type of bypass graft(s) of right leg with ulceration of toe

I70.738 **Atherosclerosis of other type of bypass graft(s) of the right leg with ulceration of other part of lower leg**

I70.739 **Atherosclerosis of other type of bypass graft(s) of the right leg with ulceration of unspecified site**

✓6th **I70.74** **Atherosclerosis of other type of bypass graft(s) of the left leg with ulceration**

Includes any condition classifiable to I70.712 and I70.722

Use additional code to identify severity of ulcer (L97- with fifth character 2)

I70.741 **Atherosclerosis of other type of bypass graft(s) of the left leg with ulceration of thigh**

I70.742 **Atherosclerosis of other type of bypass graft(s) of the left leg with ulceration of calf**

I70.743 **Atherosclerosis of other type of bypass graft(s) of the left leg with ulceration of ankle**

I70.744 **Atherosclerosis of other type of bypass graft(s) of the left leg with ulceration of heel and midfoot**

Atherosclerosis of other type of bypass graft(s) of left leg with ulceration of plantar surface of midfoot

I70.745 **Atherosclerosis of other type of bypass graft(s) of the left leg with ulceration of other part of foot**

Atherosclerosis of other type of bypass graft(s) of left leg with ulceration of toe

I70.748 **Atherosclerosis of other type of bypass graft(s) of the left leg with ulceration of other part of lower leg**

I70.749 **Atherosclerosis of other type of bypass graft(s) of the left leg with ulceration of unspecified site**

I70.75 **Atherosclerosis of other type of bypass graft(s) of other extremity with ulceration**

Includes any condition classifiable to I70.718 and I70.728

Use additional code to identify severity of ulcer (L98.49)

✓6th **I70.76** **Atherosclerosis of other type of bypass graft(s) of the extremities with gangrene**

Includes any condition classifiable to I70.71-, I70.72-, I70.73-, I70.74-, I70.75

Use additional code to identify the severity of any ulcer (L98.49-), if applicable

I70.761 **Atherosclerosis of other type of bypass graft(s) of the extremities with gangrene, right leg**

I70.762 **Atherosclerosis of other type of bypass graft(s) of the extremities with gangrene, left leg**

I70.763 **Atherosclerosis of other type of bypass graft(s) of the extremities with gangrene, bilateral legs**

I70.768 **Atherosclerosis of other type of bypass graft(s) of the extremities with gangrene, other extremity**

I70.769 **Atherosclerosis of other type of bypass graft(s) of the extremities with gangrene, unspecified extremity**

✓6th **I70.79** **Other atherosclerosis of other type of bypass graft(s) of the extremities**

I70.791 **Other atherosclerosis of other type of bypass graft(s) of the extremities, right leg**

I70.792 **Other atherosclerosis of other type of bypass graft(s) of the extremities, left leg**

I70.793 **Other atherosclerosis of other type of bypass graft(s) of the extremities, bilateral legs**

I70.798 **Other atherosclerosis of other type of bypass graft(s) of the extremities, other extremity**

I70.799 **Other atherosclerosis of other type of bypass graft(s) of the extremities, unspecified extremity**

I70.8 **Atherosclerosis of other arteries**

✓5th **I70.9** **Other and unspecified atherosclerosis**

I70.90 **Unspecified atherosclerosis**

I70.91 **Generalized atherosclerosis**

I70.92 **Chronic total occlusion of artery of the extremities**

Complete occlusion of artery of the extremities

Total occlusion of artery of the extremities

Code first atherosclerosis of arteries of the extremities (I70.2-, I70.3-, I70.4-, I70.5-, I70.6-, I70.7-)

EXCLUDES 1 *acute occlusion of artery of the extremity (I70.2-, I70.3-, I70.4-)*

✓4th **I71 Aortic aneurysm and dissection**

    EXCLUDES 1   *aortic ectasia (I77.81-)*
          syphilitic aortic aneurysm (A52.Ø1)
          traumatic aortic aneurysm (S25.Ø9, S35.Ø9)

  ✓5th **I71.Ø Dissection of aorta**

      I71.ØØ   Dissection of unspecified site of aorta

      I71.Ø1   Dissection of thoracic aorta

      I71.Ø2   Dissection of abdominal aorta

      I71.Ø3   Dissection of thoracoabdominal aorta

  I71.1 Thoracic aortic aneurysm, ruptured

  I71.2 Thoracic aortic aneurysm, without rupture

  I71.3 Abdominal aortic aneurysm, ruptured

  I71.4 Abdominal aortic aneurysm, without rupture

  I71.5 Thoracoabdominal aortic aneurysm, ruptured

  I71.6 Thoracoabdominal aortic aneurysm, without rupture

  I71.8 Aortic aneurysm of unspecified site, ruptured

      Rupture of aorta NOS

  I71.9 Aortic aneurysm of unspecified site, without rupture

      Aneurysm of aorta
      Dilatation of aorta
      Hyaline necrosis of aorta

✓4th **I72 Other aneurysm**

    INCLUDES   aneurysm (cirsoid) (false) (ruptured)

    EXCLUDES 2   *acquired aneurysm (I77.Ø)*
          aneurysm (of) aorta (I71-)
          aneurysm (of) arteriovenous NOS (Q27.3-)
          carotid artery dissection (I77.71)
          cerebral (nonruptured) aneurysm (I67.1)
          coronary aneurysm (I25.4)
          coronary artery dissection (I25.42)
          dissection of artery NEC (I77.79)
          heart aneurysm (I25.3)
          iliac artery dissection (I77.72)
          pulmonary artery aneurysm (I28.1)
          renal artery dissection (I77.73)
          retinal aneurysm (H35.Ø)
          ruptured cerebral aneurysm (I6Ø.7)
          varicose aneurysm (I77.Ø)
          vertebral artery dissection (I77.74)

  I72.Ø Aneurysm of carotid artery (common) (external) (internal, extracranial portion)

      EXCLUDES 1   *aneurysm of internal carotid artery, intracranial portion (I67.1)*
             aneurysm of internal carotid artery NOS (I67.1)

  I72.1 Aneurysm of artery of upper extremity

  I72.2 Aneurysm of renal artery

  I72.3 Aneurysm of iliac artery

  I72.4 Aneurysm of artery of lower extremity

  I72.8 Aneurysm of other specified arteries

  I72.9 Aneurysm of unspecified site

✓4th **I73 Other peripheral vascular diseases**

    EXCLUDES 2   *chilblains (T69.1)*
          frostbite (T33- T34)
          immersion hand or foot (T69.Ø-)
          spasm of cerebral artery (G45.9)

  ✓5th **I73.Ø Raynaud's syndrome**

      Raynaud's disease
      Raynaud's phenomenon (secondary)

      I73.ØØ   Raynaud's syndrome without gangrene

      I73.Ø1   Raynaud's syndrome with gangrene

  I73.1 Thromboangiitis obliterans [Buerger's disease]

  ✓5th **I73.8 Other specified peripheral vascular diseases**

      EXCLUDES 1   *diabetic (peripheral) angiopathy (E08-E13 with .51-.52)*

      I73.81   Erythromelalgia

      I73.89   Other specified peripheral vascular diseases

         Acrocyanosis
         Erythrocyanosis
         Simple acroparesthesia [Schultze's type]
         Vasomotor acroparesthesia [Nothnagel's type]

  I73.9 Peripheral vascular disease, unspecified

      Intermittent claudication
      Peripheral angiopathy NOS
      Spasm of artery

      EXCLUDES 1   *atherosclerosis of the extremities (I7Ø.2--I7Ø.7-)*

✓4th **I74 Arterial embolism and thrombosis**

    Embolic infarction
    Embolic occlusion
    Thrombotic infarction
    Thrombotic occlusion

    Code first embolism and thrombosis complicating:
      abortion or ectopic or molar pregnancy (OØØ-OØ7, OØ8.2)
      pregnancy, childbirth and the puerperium (O88-)

    EXCLUDES 2   *atheroembolism (I75-)*
          embolism and thrombosis:
            basilar (I63.Ø-I63.2, I65.1)
            carotid (I63.Ø-I63.2, I65.2)
            cerebral (I63.3-I63.5, I66-)
            coronary (I21-I25)
            mesenteric (K55.Ø)
            ophthalmic (H34-)
            precerebral NOS (I63.Ø-I63.2, I65.9)
            pulmonary (I26-)
            renal (N28.Ø)
            retinal (H34-)
            septic (I76)
            vertebral (I63.Ø-I63.2, I65.Ø)

  I74.Ø Embolism and thrombosis of abdominal aorta

      Aortic bifurcation syndrome
      Aortoiliac obstruction
      Leriche's syndrome
      Saddle embolus

  ✓5th **I74.1 Embolism and thrombosis of other and unspecified parts of aorta**

      I74.1Ø   Embolism and thrombosis of unspecified parts of aorta

      I74.11   Embolism and thrombosis of thoracic aorta

      I74.19   Embolism and thrombosis of other parts of aorta

  I74.2 Embolism and thrombosis of arteries of the upper extremities

  I74.3 Embolism and thrombosis of arteries of the lower extremities

  I74.4 Embolism and thrombosis of arteries of extremities, unspecified

      Peripheral arterial embolism NOS

  I74.5 Embolism and thrombosis of iliac artery

  I74.8 Embolism and thrombosis of other arteries

  I74.9 Embolism and thrombosis of unspecified artery

✓4th **I75 Atheroembolism**

    Atherothrombotic microembolism
    Cholesterol embolism

  ✓5th **I75.Ø Atheroembolism of extremities**

    ✓6th **I75.Ø1   Atheroembolism of upper extremity**

      I75.Ø11   Atheroembolism of right upper extremity

      I75.Ø12   Atheroembolism of left upper extremity

      I75.Ø13   Atheroembolism of bilateral upper extremities

      I75.Ø19   Atheroembolism of unspecified upper extremity

    ✓6th **I75.Ø2   Atheroembolism of lower extremity**

      I75.Ø21   Atheroembolism of right lower extremity

      I75.Ø22   Atheroembolism of left lower extremity

      I75.Ø23   Atheroembolism of bilateral lower extremities

      I75.Ø29   Atheroembolism of unspecified lower extremity

  ✓5th **I75.8 Atheroembolism of other sites**

      I75.81   Atheroembolism of kidney

         Use additional code for any associated acute kidney failure and chronic kidney disease (N17-, N18-)

      I75.89   Atheroembolism of other site

I76 Septic arterial embolism

    Code first underlying infection, such as:
      infective endocarditis (I33.Ø)
      lung abscess (J85-)

    Use additional code to identify the site of the embolism (I74-)

    EXCLUDES 2   *septic pulmonary embolism (I26.Ø1, I26.9Ø)*

    EXCLUDES 1 Not coded here   EXCLUDES 2 Not included here   *Manifestation Code*

✓4th I77 Other disorders of arteries and arterioles
> EXCLUDES 2 *collagen (vascular) diseases (M30-M36)*
> *hypersensitivity angiitis (M31.0)*
> *pulmonary artery (I28-)*

I77.0 Arteriovenous fistula, acquired
Aneurysmal varix
Arteriovenous aneurysm, acquired
> EXCLUDES 1 *arteriovenous aneurysm NOS (Q27.3-)*
> *presence of arteriovenous shunt (fistula) for dialysis (Z99.2)*
> *traumatic—see injury of blood vessel by body region*
> EXCLUDES 2 *cerebral (I67.1)*
> *coronary (I25.4)*

I77.1 Stricture of artery
Narrowing of artery

I77.2 Rupture of artery
Erosion of artery
Fistula of artery
Ulcer of artery
> EXCLUDES 1 *traumatic rupture of artery—see injury of blood vessel by body region*

I77.3 Arterial fibromuscular dysplasia
Fibromuscular hyperplasia (of) carotid artery
Fibromuscular hyperplasia (of) renal artery

I77.4 Celiac artery compression syndrome

I77.5 Necrosis of artery

I77.6 Arteritis, unspecified
Aortitis NOS
Endarteritis NOS
> EXCLUDES 1 *arteritis or endarteritis:*
> *aortic arch (M31.4)*
> *cerebral NEC (I67.7)*
> *coronary (I25.89)*
> *deformans (I70-)*
> *giant cell (M31.5., M31.6)*
> *obliterans (I70-)*
> *senile (I70-)*

✓5th I77.7 Other arterial dissection
> EXCLUDES 2 *dissection of aorta (I71.0-)*
> *dissection of coronary artery (I25.42)*

I77.71 Dissection of carotid artery
I77.72 Dissection of iliac artery
I77.73 Dissection of renal artery
I77.74 Dissection of vertebral artery
I77.79 Dissection of other artery

✓5th I77.8 Other specified disorders of arteries and arterioles
✓6th I77.81 Aortic ectasia
Ectasis aorta
> EXCLUDES 1 *aortic aneurysm and dissection (I71.0-)*

I77.810 Thoracic aortic ectasia
I77.811 Abdominal aortic ectasia
I77.812 Thoracoabdominal aortic ectasia
I77.819 Aortic ectasia, unspecified site
I77.89 Other specified disorders of arteries and arterioles

I77.9 Disorder of arteries and arterioles, unspecified

✓4th I78 Diseases of capillaries
I78.0 Hereditary hemorrhagic telangiectasia
Rendu-Osler-Weber disease

I78.1 Nevus, non-neoplastic
Araneus nevus
Senile nevus
Spider nevus
Stellar nevus
> EXCLUDES 1 *nevus NOS (D22-)*
> *vascular NOS (Q82.5)*
> EXCLUDES 2 *blue nevus (D22-)*
> *flammeus nevus (Q82.5)*
> *hairy nevus (D22-)*
> *melanocytic nevus (D22-)*
> *pigmented nevus (D22-)*
> *portwine nevus (Q82.5)*
> *sanguineous nevus (Q82.5)*
> *strawberry nevus (Q82.5)*
> *verrucous nevus (Q82.5)*

I78.8 Other diseases of capillaries
I78.9 Disease of capillaries, unspecified

✓4th I79 Disorders of arteries, arterioles and capillaries in diseases classified elsewhere

I79.0 Aneurysm of aorta in diseases classified elsewhere
Code first underlying disease
> EXCLUDES 1 *syphilitic aneurysm (A52.01)*

I79.1 Aortitis in diseases classified elsewhere
Code first underlying disease
> EXCLUDES 1 *syphilitic aortitis (A52.02)*

I79.8 Other disorders of arteries, arterioles and capillaries in diseases classified elsewhere
Code first underlying disease, such as:
amyloidosis (E85-)
> EXCLUDES 1 *diabetic (peripheral) angiopathy (E08-E13 with .51-.52)*
> *endarteritis:*
> *syphilitic (A52.09)*
> *tuberculous (A18.89)*

Diseases of veins, lymphatic vessels and lymph nodes, not elsewhere classified. (I80-I89)

✓4th I80 Phlebitis and thrombophlebitis
> INCLUDES endophlebitis
> inflammation, vein
> periphlebitis
> suppurative phlebitis

Code first phlebitis and thrombophlebitis complicating:
abortion, ectopic or molar pregnancy (O00-O07, O08.7)
pregnancy, childbirth and the puerperium (O22-, O87-)
> EXCLUDES 1 *venous embolism and thrombosis of lower extremities ((I82.4-, I82.5-, I82.81-)*

✓5th I80.0 Phlebitis and thrombophlebitis of superficial vessels of lower extremities
Phlebitis and thrombophlebitis of femoropopliteal vein

I80.00 Phlebitis and thrombophlebitis of superficial vessels of unspecified lower extremity
I80.01 Phlebitis and thrombophlebitis of superficial vessels of right lower extremity
I80.02 Phlebitis and thrombophlebitis of superficial vessels of left lower extremity
I80.03 Phlebitis and thrombophlebitis of superficial vessels of lower extremities, bilateral

✓5th I80.1 Phlebitis and thrombophlebitis of femoral vein
I80.10 Phlebitis and thrombophlebitis of unspecified femoral vein
I80.11 Phlebitis and thrombophlebitis of right femoral vein
I80.12 Phlebitis and thrombophlebitis of left femoral vein
I80.13 Phlebitis and thrombophlebitis of femoral vein, bilateral

✓5th I80.2 Phlebitis and thrombophlebitis of other and unspecified deep vessels of lower extremities
✓6th I80.20 Phlebitis and thrombophlebitis of unspecified deep vessels of lower extremities
I80.201 Phlebitis and thrombophlebitis of unspecified deep vessels of right lower extremity
I80.202 Phlebitis and thrombophlebitis of unspecified deep vessels of left lower extremity
I80.203 Phlebitis and thrombophlebitis of unspecified deep vessels of lower extremities, bilateral
I80.209 Phlebitis and thrombophlebitis of unspecified deep vessels of unspecified lower extremity

✓6th I80.21 Phlebitis and thrombophlebitis of iliac vein
I80.211 Phlebitis and thrombophlebitis of right iliac vein
I80.212 Phlebitis and thrombophlebitis of left iliac vein
I80.213 Phlebitis and thrombophlebitis of iliac vein, bilateral
I80.219 Phlebitis and thrombophlebitis of unspecified iliac vein

Diseases of the Circulatory System

I80.22–I82.499

✓6ᵗʰ **I80.22 Phlebitis and thrombophlebitis of popliteal vein**

     I80.221 Phlebitis and thrombophlebitis of right popliteal vein

     I80.222 Phlebitis and thrombophlebitis of left popliteal vein

     I80.223 Phlebitis and thrombophlebitis of popliteal vein, bilateral

     I80.229 Phlebitis and thrombophlebitis of unspecified popliteal vein

✓6ᵗʰ **I80.23 Phlebitis and thrombophlebitis of tibial vein**

     I80.231 Phlebitis and thrombophlebitis of right tibial vein

     I80.232 Phlebitis and thrombophlebitis of left tibial vein

     I80.233 Phlebitis and thrombophlebitis of tibial vein, bilateral

     I80.239 Phlebitis and thrombophlebitis of unspecified tibial vein

✓6ᵗʰ **I80.29 Phlebitis and thrombophlebitis of other deep vessels of lower extremities**

     I80.291 Phlebitis and thrombophlebitis of other deep vessels of right lower extremity

     I80.292 Phlebitis and thrombophlebitis of other deep vessels of left lower extremity

     I80.293 Phlebitis and thrombophlebitis of other deep vessels of lower extremity, bilateral

     I80.299 Phlebitis and thrombophlebitis of other deep vessels of unspecified lower extremity

I80.3 Phlebitis and thrombophlebitis of lower extremities, unspecified

I80.8 Phlebitis and thrombophlebitis of other sites

I80.9 Phlebitis and thrombophlebitis of unspecified site

I81 Portal vein thrombosis

Portal (vein) obstruction

EXCLUDES 2   *hepatic vein thrombosis (I82.0)*
phlebitis of portal vein (K75.1)

✓4ᵗʰ **I82 Other venous embolism and thrombosis**

Code first venous embolism and thrombosis complicating:
abortion, ectopic or molar pregnancy (O00-O07, O08.7)
pregnancy, childbirth and the puerperium (O22-, O87-)

EXCLUDES 2   *venous embolism and thrombosis (of):*
cerebral (I63.6, I67.6)
coronary (I21-I25)
intracranial and intraspinal, septic or NOS (G08)
intracranial, nonpyogenic (I67.6)
intraspinal, nonpyogenic (G95.1)
mesenteric (K55.0)
portal (I81)
pulmonary (I26-)

I82.0 Budd-Chiari syndrome

Hepatic vein thrombosis

I82.1 Thrombophlebitis migrans

✓5ᵗʰ **I82.2 Embolism and thrombosis of vena cava and other thoracic veins**

✓6ᵗʰ **I82.21 Embolism and thrombosis of superior vena cava**

     I82.210 Acute embolism and thrombosis of superior vena cava

Embolism and thrombosis of superior vena cava NOS

     I82.211 Chronic embolism and thrombosis of superior vena cava

✓6ᵗʰ **I82.22 Embolism and thrombosis of inferior vena cava**

     I82.220 Acute embolism and thrombosis of inferior vena cava

Embolism and thrombosis of inferior vena cava NOS

     I82.221 Chronic embolism and thrombosis of inferior vena cava

✓6ᵗʰ **I82.29 Embolism and thrombosis of other thoracic veins**

Embolism and thrombosis of brachiocephalic (innominate) vein

     I82.290 Acute embolism and thrombosis of other thoracic veins

     I82.291 Chronic embolism and thrombosis of other thoracic veins

I82.3 Embolism and thrombosis of renal vein

✓5ᵗʰ **I82.4 Acute embolism and thrombosis of deep veins of lower extremity**

✓6ᵗʰ **I82.40 Acute embolism and thrombosis of unspecified deep veins of lower extremity**

Deep vein thrombosis NOS
DVT NOS

EXCLUDES 1   *acute embolism and thrombosis of unspecified deep veins of distal lower extremity (I82.4b-)*
acute embolism and thrombosis of unspecified deep veins of proximal lower extremity (I82.4a-)

     I82.401 Acute embolism and thrombosis of unspecified deep veins of right lower extremity

     I82.402 Acute embolism and thrombosis of unspecified deep veins of left lower extremity

     I82.403 Acute embolism and thrombosis of unspecified deep veins of lower extremity, bilateral

     I82.409 Acute embolism and thrombosis of unspecified deep veins of unspecified lower extremity

✓6ᵗʰ **I82.41 Acute embolism and thrombosis of femoral vein**

     I82.411 Acute embolism and thrombosis of right femoral vein

     I82.412 Acute embolism and thrombosis of left femoral vein

     I82.413 Acute embolism and thrombosis of femoral vein, bilateral

     I82.419 Acute embolism and thrombosis of unspecified femoral vein

✓6ᵗʰ **I82.42 Acute embolism and thrombosis of iliac vein**

     I82.421 Acute embolism and thrombosis of right iliac vein

     I82.422 Acute embolism and thrombosis of left iliac vein

     I82.423 Acute embolism and thrombosis of iliac vein, bilateral

     I82.429 Acute embolism and thrombosis of unspecified iliac vein

✓6ᵗʰ **I82.43 Acute embolism and thrombosis of popliteal vein**

     I82.431 Acute embolism and thrombosis of right popliteal vein

     I82.432 Acute embolism and thrombosis of left popliteal vein

     I82.433 Acute embolism and thrombosis of popliteal vein, bilateral

     I82.439 Acute embolism and thrombosis of unspecified popliteal vein

✓6ᵗʰ **I82.44 Acute embolism and thrombosis of tibial vein**

     I82.441 Acute embolism and thrombosis of right tibial vein

     I82.442 Acute embolism and thrombosis of left tibial vein

     I82.443 Acute embolism and thrombosis of tibial vein, bilateral

     I82.449 Acute embolism and thrombosis of unspecified tibial vein

✓6ᵗʰ **I82.49 Acute embolism and thrombosis of other specified deep vein of lower extremity**

     I82.491 Acute embolism and thrombosis of other specified deep vein of right lower extremity

     I82.492 Acute embolism and thrombosis of other specified deep vein of left lower extremity

     I82.493 Acute embolism and thrombosis of other specified deep vein of lower extremity, bilateral

     I82.499 Acute embolism and thrombosis of other specified deep vein of unspecified lower extremity

---

EXCLUDES 1   Not coded here   EXCLUDES 2   Not included here   *Manifestation Code*

✓6ᵗʰ **I82.4y** **Acute embolism and thrombosis of unspecified deep veins of proximal lower extremity**
Acute embolism and thrombosis of deep vein of thigh NOS
Acute embolism and thrombosis of deep vein of upper leg NOS

I82.4y1 **Acute embolism and thrombosis of unspecified deep veins of right proximal lower extremity**

I82.4y2 **Acute embolism and thrombosis of unspecified deep veins of left proximal lower extremity**

I82.4y3 **Acute embolism and thrombosis of unspecified deep veins of proximal lower extremity, bilateral**

I82.4y9 **Acute embolism and thrombosis of unspecified deep veins of unspecified proximal lower extremity**

✓6ᵗʰ **I82.4z** **Acute embolism and thrombosis of unspecified deep veins of distal lower extremity**
Acute embolism and thrombosis of deep vein of calf NOS
Acute embolism and thrombosis of deep vein of lower leg NOS

I82.4z1 **Acute embolism and thrombosis of unspecified deep veins of right distal lower extremity**

I82.4z2 **Acute embolism and thrombosis of unspecified deep veins of left distal lower extremity**

I82.4z3 **Acute embolism and thrombosis of unspecified deep veins of distal lower extremity, bilateral**

I82.4z9 **Acute embolism and thrombosis of unspecified deep veins of unspecified distal lower extremity**

✓5ᵗʰ **I82.5** **Chronic embolism and thrombosis of deep veins of lower extremity**
Use additional code, if applicable, for associated long-term (current) use of anticoagulants (Z79.01)
EXCLUDES 1 *personal history of venous embolism and thrombosis (Z86.71)*

✓6ᵗʰ **I82.50** **Chronic embolism and thrombosis of unspecified deep veins of lower extremity**
EXCLUDES 1 *chronic embolism and thrombosis of unspecified deep veins of distal lower extremity (I82.5b-)*
chronic embolism and thrombosis of unspecified deep veins of proximal lower extremity (I82.5a-)

I82.501 **Chronic embolism and thrombosis of unspecified deep veins of right lower extremity**

I82.502 **Chronic embolism and thrombosis of unspecified deep veins of left lower extremity**

I82.503 **Chronic embolism and thrombosis of unspecified deep veins of lower extremity, bilateral**

I82.509 **Chronic embolism and thrombosis of unspecified deep veins of unspecified lower extremity**

✓6ᵗʰ **I82.51** **Chronic embolism and thrombosis of femoral vein**

I82.511 **Chronic embolism and thrombosis of right femoral vein**

I82.512 **Chronic embolism and thrombosis of left femoral vein**

I82.513 **Chronic embolism and thrombosis of femoral vein, bilateral**

I82.519 **Chronic embolism and thrombosis of unspecified femoral vein**

✓6ᵗʰ **I82.52** **Chronic embolism and thrombosis of iliac vein**

I82.521 **Chronic embolism and thrombosis of right iliac vein**

I82.522 **Chronic embolism and thrombosis of left iliac vein**

I82.523 **Chronic embolism and thrombosis of iliac vein, bilateral**

I82.529 **Chronic embolism and thrombosis of unspecified iliac vein**

✓6ᵗʰ **I82.53** **Chronic embolism and thrombosis of popliteal vein**

I82.531 **Chronic embolism and thrombosis of right popliteal vein**

I82.532 **Chronic embolism and thrombosis of left popliteal vein**

I82.533 **Chronic embolism and thrombosis of popliteal vein, bilateral**

I82.539 **Chronic embolism and thrombosis of unspecified popliteal vein**

✓6ᵗʰ **I82.54** **Chronic embolism and thrombosis of tibial vein**

I82.541 **Chronic embolism and thrombosis of right tibial vein**

I82.542 **Chronic embolism and thrombosis of left tibial vein**

I82.543 **Chronic embolism and thrombosis of tibial vein, bilateral**

I82.549 **Chronic embolism and thrombosis of unspecified tibial vein**

✓6ᵗʰ **I82.59** **Chronic embolism and thrombosis of other specified deep vein of lower extremity**

I82.591 **Chronic embolism and thrombosis of other specified deep vein of right lower extremity**

I82.592 **Chronic embolism and thrombosis of other specified deep vein of left lower extremity**

I82.593 **Chronic embolism and thrombosis of other specified deep vein of lower extremity, bilateral**

I82.599 **Chronic embolism and thrombosis of other specified deep vein of unspecified lower extremity**

✓6ᵗʰ **I82.5y** **Chronic embolism and thrombosis of unspecified deep veins of proximal lower extremity**
Chronic embolism and thrombosis of deep veins of thigh NOS
Chronic embolism and thrombosis of deep veins of upper leg NOS

I82.5y1 **Chronic embolism and thrombosis of unspecified deep veins of right proximal lower extremity**

I82.5y2 **Chronic embolism and thrombosis of unspecified deep veins of left proximal lower extremity**

I82.5y3 **Chronic embolism and thrombosis of unspecified deep veins of proximal lower extremity, bilateral**

I82.5y9 **Chronic embolism and thrombosis of unspecified deep veins of unspecified proximal lower extremity**

✓6ᵗʰ **I82.5z** **Chronic embolism and thrombosis of unspecified deep veins of distal lower extremity**
Chronic embolism and thrombosis of deep veins of calf NOS
Chronic embolism and thrombosis of deep veins of lower leg NOS

I82.5z1 **Chronic embolism and thrombosis of unspecified deep veins of right distal lower extremity**

I82.5z2 **Chronic embolism and thrombosis of unspecified deep veins of left distal lower extremity**

I82.5Z3 **Chronic embolism and thrombosis of unspecified deep veins of distal lower extremity, bilateral**

I82.5z9 **Chronic embolism and thrombosis of unspecified deep veins of unspecified distal lower extremity**

✓5ᵗʰ **I82.6** **Acute embolism and thrombosis of veins of upper extremity**

✓6ᵗʰ **I82.60** **Acute embolism and thrombosis of unspecified veins of upper extremity**

I82.601 **Acute embolism and thrombosis of unspecified veins of right upper extremity**

✓ Appropriate additional character required   ✓x7ᵗʰ Requires 7th character, placeholder x must fill empty characters

Diseases of the Circulatory System

I82.602–I82.811

I82.602   Acute embolism and thrombosis of unspecified veins of left upper extremity

I82.603   Acute embolism and thrombosis of unspecified veins of upper extremity, bilateral

I82.609   Acute embolism and thrombosis of unspecified veins of unspecified upper extremity

✓6th **I82.61**   **Acute embolism and thrombosis of superficial veins of upper extremity**
Acute embolism and thrombosis of antecubital vein
Acute embolism and thrombosis of basilic vein
Acute embolism and thrombosis of cephalic vein

I82.611   Acute embolism and thrombosis of superficial veins of right upper extremity

I82.612   Acute embolism and thrombosis of superficial veins of left upper extremity

I82.613   Acute embolism and thrombosis of superficial veins of upper extremity, bilateral

I82.619   Acute embolism and thrombosis of superficial veins of unspecified upper extremity

✓6th **I82.62**   **Acute embolism and thrombosis of deep veins of upper extremity**
Acute embolism and thrombosis of brachial vein
Acute embolism and thrombosis of radial vein
Acute embolism and thrombosis of ulnar vein

I82.621   Acute embolism and thrombosis of deep veins of right upper extremity

I82.622   Acute embolism and thrombosis of deep veins of left upper extremity

I82.623   Acute embolism and thrombosis of deep veins of upper extremity, bilateral

I82.629   Acute embolism and thrombosis of deep veins of unspecified upper extremity

✓5th **I82.7**   **Chronic embolism and thrombosis of veins of upper extremity**
Use additional code, if applicable, for associated long-term (current) use of anticoagulants (Z79.01)
EXCLUDES 1   *personal history of venous embolism and thrombosis (Z86.71)*

✓6th **I82.70**   **Chronic embolism and thrombosis of unspecified veins of upper extremity**

I82.701   Chronic embolism and thrombosis of unspecified veins of right upper extremity

I82.702   Chronic embolism and thrombosis of unspecified veins of left upper extremity

I82.703   Chronic embolism and thrombosis of unspecified veins of upper extremity, bilateral

I82.709   Chronic embolism and thrombosis of unspecified veins of unspecified upper extremity

✓6th **I82.71**   **Chronic embolism and thrombosis of superficial veins of upper extremity**
Chronic embolism and thrombosis of antecubital vein
Chronic embolism and thrombosis of basilic vein
Chronic embolism and thrombosis of cephalic vein

I82.711   Chronic embolism and thrombosis of superficial veins of right upper extremity

I82.712   Chronic embolism and thrombosis of superficial veins of left upper extremity

I82.713   Chronic embolism and thrombosis of superficial veins of upper extremity, bilateral

I82.719   Chronic embolism and thrombosis of superficial veins of unspecified upper extremity

✓6th **I82.72**   **Chronic embolism and thrombosis of deep veins of upper extremity**
Chronic embolism and thrombosis of brachial vein
Chronic embolism and thrombosis of radial vein
Chronic embolism and thrombosis of ulnar vein

I82.721   Chronic embolism and thrombosis of deep veins of right upper extremity

I82.722   Chronic embolism and thrombosis of deep veins of left upper extremity

I82.723   Chronic embolism and thrombosis of deep veins of upper extremity, bilateral

I82.729   Chronic embolism and thrombosis of deep veins of unspecified upper extremity

✓5th **I82.a**   **Embolism and thrombosis of axillary vein**

✓6th **I82.a1**   **Acute embolism and thrombosis of axillary vein**

I82.a11   Acute embolism and thrombosis of right axillary vein

I82.a12   Acute embolism and thrombosis of left axillary vein

I82.a13   Acute embolism and thrombosis of axillary vein, bilateral

I82.a19   Acute embolism and thrombosis of unspecified axillary vein

✓6th **I82.a2**   **Chronic embolism and thrombosis of axillary vein**

I82.a21   Chronic embolism and thrombosis of right axillary vein

I82.a22   Chronic embolism and thrombosis of left axillary vein

I82.a23   Chronic embolism and thrombosis of axillary vein, bilateral

I82.a29   Chronic embolism and thrombosis of unspecified axillary vein

✓5th **I82.b**   **Embolism and thrombosis of subclavian vein**

✓6th **I82.b1**   **Acute embolism and thrombosis of subclavian vein**

I82.b11   Acute embolism and thrombosis of right subclavian vein

I82.b12   Acute embolism and thrombosis of left subclavian vein

I82.b13   Acute embolism and thrombosis of subclavian vein, bilateral

I82.b19   Acute embolism and thrombosis of unspecified subclavian vein

✓6th **I82.b2**   **Chronic embolism and thrombosis of subclavian vein**

I82.b21   Chronic embolism and thrombosis of right subclavian vein

I82.b22   Chronic embolism and thrombosis of left subclavian vein

I82.b23   Chronic embolism and thrombosis of subclavian vein, bilateral

I82.b29   Chronic embolism and thrombosis of unspecified subclavian vein

✓5th **I82.c**   **Embolism and thrombosis of internal jugular vein**

✓6th **I82.c1**   **Acute embolism and thrombosis of internal jugular vein**

I82.c11   Acute embolism and thrombosis of right internal jugular vein

I82.c12   Acute embolism and thrombosis of left internal jugular vein

I82.c13   Acute embolism and thrombosis of internal jugular vein, bilateral

I82.c19   Acute embolism and thrombosis of unspecified internal jugular vein

✓6th **I82.c2**   **Chronic embolism and thrombosis of internal jugular vein**

I82.c21   Chronic embolism and thrombosis of right internal jugular vein

I82.c22   Chronic embolism and thrombosis of left internal jugular vein

I82.c23   Chronic embolism and thrombosis of internal jugular vein, bilateral

I82.c29   Chronic embolism and thrombosis of unspecified internal jugular vein

✓5th **I82.8**   **Embolism and thrombosis of other specified veins**
Use additional code, if applicable, for associated long-term (current) use of anticoagulants (Z79.01)

✓6th **I82.81**   **Embolism and thrombosis of superficial veins of lower extremities**
Embolism and thrombosis of saphenous vein (greater) (lesser)

I82.811   Embolism and thrombosis of superficial veins of right lower extremities

---

EXCLUDES 1   Not coded here   **EXCLUDES 2**   Not included here   *Manifestation Code*

I82.812 **Embolism and thrombosis of superficial veins of left lower extremities**

I82.813 **Embolism and thrombosis of superficial veins of lower extremities, bilateral**

I82.819 **Embolism and thrombosis of superficial veins of unspecified lower extremities**

√6ᵗʰ I82.89 **Embolism and thrombosis of other specified veins**

I82.890 **Acute embolism and thrombosis of other specified veins**

I82.891 **Chronic embolism and thrombosis of other specified veins**

√5ᵗʰ I82.9 **Embolism and thrombosis of unspecified vein**

I82.90 **Acute embolism and thrombosis of unspecified vein**
Embolism of vein NOS
Thrombosis (vein) NOS

I82.91 **Chronic embolism and thrombosis of unspecified vein**

√4ᵗʰ **I83** **Varicose veins of lower extremities**

EXCLUDES 1 *varicose veins complicating pregnancy (O22.0-)*
varicose veins complicating the puerperium (O87.4)

√5ᵗʰ I83.0 **Varicose veins of lower extremities with ulcer**
Use additional code to identify severity of ulcer (L97-)

√6ᵗʰ I83.00 **Varicose veins of unspecified lower extremity with ulcer**

I83.001 **Varicose veins of unspecified lower extremity with ulcer of thigh**

I83.002 **Varicose veins of unspecified lower extremity with ulcer of calf**

I83.003 **Varicose veins of unspecified lower extremity with ulcer of ankle**

I83.004 **Varicose veins of unspecified lower extremity with ulcer of heel and midfoot**
Varicose veins of unspecified lower extremity with ulcer of plantar surface of midfoot

I83.005 **Varicose veins of unspecified lower extremity with ulcer other part of foot**
Varicose veins of unspecified lower extremity with ulcer of toe

I83.008 **Varicose veins of unspecified lower extremity with ulcer other part of lower leg**

I83.009 **Varicose veins of unspecified lower extremity with ulcer of unspecified site**

√6ᵗʰ I83.01 **Varicose veins of right lower extremity with ulcer**

I83.011 **Varicose veins of right lower extremity with ulcer of thigh**

I83.012 **Varicose veins of right lower extremity with ulcer of calf**

I83.013 **Varicose veins of right lower extremity with ulcer of ankle**

I83.014 **Varicose veins of right lower extremity with ulcer of heel and midfoot**
Varicose veins of right lower extremity with ulcer of plantar surface of midfoot

I83.015 **Varicose veins of right lower extremity with ulcer other part of foot**
Varicose veins of right lower extremity with ulcer of toe

I83.018 **Varicose veins of right lower extremity with ulcer other part of lower leg**

I83.019 **Varicose veins of right lower extremity with ulcer of unspecified site**

√6ᵗʰ I83.02 **Varicose veins of left lower extremity with ulcer**

I83.021 **Varicose veins of left lower extremity with ulcer of thigh**

I83.022 **Varicose veins of left lower extremity with ulcer of calf**

I83.023 **Varicose veins of left lower extremity with ulcer of ankle**

I83.024 **Varicose veins of left lower extremity with ulcer of heel and midfoot**
Varicose veins of left lower extremity with ulcer of plantar surface of midfoot

I83.025 **Varicose veins of left lower extremity with ulcer other part of foot**
Varicose veins of left lower extremity with ulcer of toe

I83.028 **Varicose veins of left lower extremity with ulcer other part of lower leg**

I83.029 **Varicose veins of left lower extremity with ulcer of unspecified site**

√5ᵗʰ I83.1 **Varicose veins of lower extremities with inflammation**
Stasis dermatitis

I83.10 **Varicose veins of unspecified lower extremity with inflammation**

I83.11 **Varicose veins of right lower extremity with inflammation**

I83.12 **Varicose veins of left lower extremity with inflammation**

√5ᵗʰ I83.2 **Varicose veins of lower extremities with both ulcer and inflammation**
Use additional code to identify severity of ulcer (L97-)

√6ᵗʰ I83.20 **Varicose veins of unspecified lower extremity with both ulcer and inflammation**

I83.201 **Varicose veins of unspecified lower extremity with both ulcer of thigh and inflammation**

I83.202 **Varicose veins of unspecified lower extremity with both ulcer of calf and inflammation**

I83.203 **Varicose veins of unspecified lower extremity with both ulcer of ankle and inflammation**

I83.204 **Varicose veins of unspecified lower extremity with both ulcer of heel and midfoot and inflammation**
Varicose veins of unspecified lower extremity with both ulcer of plantar surface of midfoot and inflammation

I83.205 **Varicose veins of unspecified lower extremity with both ulcer other part of foot and inflammation**
Varicose veins of unspecified lower extremity with both ulcer of toe and inflammation

I83.208 **Varicose veins of unspecified lower extremity with both ulcer of other part of lower extremity and inflammation**

I83.209 **Varicose veins of unspecified lower extremity with both ulcer of unspecified site and inflammation**

√6ᵗʰ I83.21 **Varicose veins of right lower extremity with both ulcer and inflammation**

I83.211 **Varicose veins of right lower extremity with both ulcer of thigh and inflammation**

I83.212 **Varicose veins of right lower extremity with both ulcer of calf and inflammation**

I83.213 **Varicose veins of right lower extremity with both ulcer of ankle and inflammation**

I83.214 **Varicose veins of right lower extremity with both ulcer of heel and midfoot and inflammation**
Varicose veins of right lower extremity with both ulcer of plantar surface of midfoot and inflammation

I83.215 **Varicose veins of right lower extremity with both ulcer other part of foot and inflammation**
Varicose veins of right lower extremity with both ulcer of toe and inflammation

I83.218 **Varicose veins of right lower extremity with both ulcer of other part of lower extremity and inflammation**

I83.219 **Varicose veins of right lower extremity with both ulcer of unspecified site and inflammation**

☑ Appropriate additional character required

√x7ᵗʰ Requires 7th character, placeholder x must fill empty characters

Diseases of the Circulatory System *(left margin)*

I83.22–I86.8 *(left margin)*

√6th **I83.22** **Varicose veins of left lower extremity with both ulcer and inflammation**

I83.221 **Varicose veins of left lower extremity with both ulcer of thigh and inflammation**

I83.222 **Varicose veins of left lower extremity with both ulcer of calf and inflammation**

I83.223 **Varicose veins of left lower extremity with both ulcer of ankle and inflammation**

I83.224 **Varicose veins of left lower extremity with both ulcer of heel and midfoot and inflammation**
Varicose veins of left lower extremity with both ulcer of plantar surface of midfoot and inflammation

I83.225 **Varicose veins of left lower extremity with both ulcer other part of foot and inflammation**
Varicose veins of left lower extremity with both ulcer of toe and inflammation

I83.228 **Varicose veins of left lower extremity with both ulcer of other part of lower extremity and inflammation**

I83.229 **Varicose veins of left lower extremity with both ulcer of unspecified site and inflammation**

√5th **I83.8** **Varicose veins of lower extremities with other complications**

√6th **I83.81** **Varicose veins of lower extremities with pain**

I83.811 **Varicose veins of right lower extremities with pain**

I83.812 **Varicose veins of left lower extremities with pain**

I83.813 **Varicose veins of bilateral lower extremities with pain**

I83.819 **Varicose veins of unspecified lower extremities with pain**

√6th **I83.89** **Varicose veins of lower extremities with other complications**
Varicose veins of lower extremities with edema
Varicose veins of lower extremities with swelling

I83.891 **Varicose veins of right lower extremities with other complications**

I83.892 **Varicose veins of left lower extremities with other complications**

I83.893 **Varicose veins of bilateral lower extremities with other complications**

I83.899 **Varicose veins of unspecified lower extremities with other complications**

√5th **I83.9** **Asymptomatic varicose veins of lower extremities**
Phlebectasia of lower extremities
Varicose veins of lower extremities
Varix of lower extremities

I83.90 **Asymptomatic varicose veins of unspecified lower extremity**
Varicose veins NOS

I83.91 **Asymptomatic varicose veins of right lower extremity**

I83.92 **Asymptomatic varicose veins of left lower extremity**

I83.93 **Asymptomatic varicose veins of bilateral lower extremities**

√4th **I84** **Hemorrhoids**
INCLUDES   piles
varicose veins of anus and rectum
EXCLUDES 1   *hemorrhoids complicating childbirth and the puerperium (O87.2)*
hemorrhoids complicating pregnancy (O22.4)

√5th **I84.0** **Thrombosed hemorrhoids**

I84.00 **Unspecified thrombosed hemorrhoids**
Thrombosed hemorrhoids, unspecified whether internal or external

I84.01 **Internal thrombosed hemorrhoids**

I84.02 **External thrombosed hemorrhoids**

I84.03 **Internal and external thrombosed hemorrhoids**

√5th **I84.1** **Hemorrhoids with other complications**

√6th **I84.10** **Unspecified hemorrhoids with other complications**

I84.101 **Unspecified bleeding hemorrhoids**

I84.102 **Unspecified prolapsed hemorrhoids**

I84.103 **Unspecified strangulated hemorrhoids**

I84.104 **Unspecified ulcerated hemorrhoids**

√6th **I84.11** **Internal hemorrhoids with other complications**

I84.111 **Internal bleeding hemorrhoids**

I84.112 **Internal prolapsed hemorrhoids**

I84.113 **Internal strangulated hemorrhoids**

I84.114 **Internal ulcerated hemorrhoids**

√6th **I84.12** **External hemorrhoids with other complications**

I84.121 **External bleeding hemorrhoids**

I84.122 **External prolapsed hemorrhoids**

I84.123 **External strangulated hemorrhoids**

I84.124 **External ulcerated hemorrhoids**

√6th **I84.13** **Internal and external hemorrhoids with other complications**

I84.131 **Internal and external bleeding hemorrhoids**

I84.132 **Internal and external prolapsed hemorrhoids**

I84.133 **Internal and external strangulated hemorrhoids**

I84.134 **Internal and external ulcerated hemorrhoids**

√5th **I84.2** **Hemorrhoids without complication**

I84.20 **Unspecified hemorrhoids without complication**
Hemorrhoids NOS

I84.21 **Internal hemorrhoids without complication**
Internal hemorrhoids NOS

I84.22 **External hemorrhoids without complication**
External hemorrhoids NOS

I84.23 **Internal and external hemorrhoids without complication**
Internal and external hemorrhoids NOS

I84.6 **Residual hemorrhoidal skin tags**
Skin tags of anus or rectum

√4th **I85** **Esophageal varices**
Use additional code to identify:
alcohol abuse and dependence (F10-)

√5th **I85.0** **Esophageal varices**
Idiopathic esophageal varices
Primary esophageal varices

I85.00 **Esophageal varices without bleeding**
Esophageal varices NOS

I85.01 **Esophageal varices with bleeding**

√5th **I85.1** **Secondary esophageal varices**
Esophageal varices secondary to alcoholic liver disease
Esophageal varices secondary to cirrhosis of liver
Esophageal varices secondary to schistosomiasis
Esophageal varices secondary to toxic liver disease
Code first underlying disease

I85.10 **Secondary esophageal varices without bleeding**

I85.11 **Secondary esophageal varices with bleeding**

√4th **I86** **Varicose veins of other sites**
EXCLUDES 1   *varicose veins of unspecified site (I83.9-)*
EXCLUDES 2   *retinal varices (H35.0-)*

I86.0 **Sublingual varices**

I86.1 **Scrotal varices**
Varicocele

I86.2 **Pelvic varices**

I86.3 **Vulval varices**
EXCLUDES 1   *vulval varices complicating childbirth and the puerperium (O87.8)*
vulval varices complicating pregnancy (O22.1-)

I86.4 **Gastric varices**

I86.8 **Varicose veins of other specified sites**
Varicose ulcer of nasal septum

EXCLUDES 1   Not coded here   EXCLUDES 2   Not included here   *Manifestation Code*

✓4th **I87** **Other disorders of veins**

✓5th **I87.0** **Postthrombotic syndrome**
Chronic venous hypertension due to deep vein thrombosis
Postphlebitic syndrome
EXCLUDES 1 *chronic venous hypertension without deep vein thrombosis (I87.3-)*

✓6th **I87.00** **Postthrombotic syndrome without complications**
Asymptomatic postthrombotic syndrome

I87.001 **Postthrombotic syndrome without complications of right lower extremity**

I87.002 **Postthrombotic syndrome without complications of left lower extremity**

I87.003 **Postthrombotic syndrome without complications of bilateral lower extremity**

I87.009 **Postthrombotic syndrome without complications of unspecified extremity**
Postthrombotic syndrome NOS

✓6th **I87.01** **Postthrombotic syndrome with ulcer**
Use additional code to specify site and severity of ulcer (L97-)

I87.011 **Postthrombotic syndrome with ulcer of right lower extremity**

I87.012 **Postthrombotic syndrome with ulcer of left lower extremity**

I87.013 **Postthrombotic syndrome with ulcer of bilateral lower extremity**

I87.019 **Postthrombotic syndrome with ulcer of unspecified lower extremity**

✓6th **I87.02** **Postthrombotic syndrome with inflammation**

I87.021 **Postthrombotic syndrome with inflammation of right lower extremity**

I87.022 **Postthrombotic syndrome with inflammation of left lower extremity**

I87.023 **Postthrombotic syndrome with inflammation of bilateral lower extremity**

I87.029 **Postthrombotic syndrome with inflammation of unspecified lower extremity**

✓6th **I87.03** **Postthrombotic syndrome with ulcer and inflammation**
Use additional code to specify site and severity of ulcer (L97-)

I87.031 **Postthrombotic syndrome with ulcer and inflammation of right lower extremity**

I87.032 **Postthrombotic syndrome with ulcer and inflammation of left lower extremity**

I87.033 **Postthrombotic syndrome with ulcer and inflammation of bilateral lower extremity**

I87.039 **Postthrombotic syndrome with ulcer and inflammation of unspecified lower extremity**

✓6th **I87.09** **Postthrombotic syndrome with other complications**

I87.091 **Postthrombotic syndrome with other complications of right lower extremity**

I87.092 **Postthrombotic syndrome with other complications of left lower extremity**

I87.093 **Postthrombotic syndrome with other complications of bilateral lower extremity**

I87.099 **Postthrombotic syndrome with other complications of unspecified lower extremity**

I87.1 **Compression of vein**
Stricture of vein
Vena cava syndrome (inferior) (superior)
EXCLUDES 2 *compression of pulmonary vein (I28.8)*

I87.2 **Venous insufficiency (chronic) (peripheral)**

✓5th **I87.3** **Chronic venous hypertension (idiopathic)**
Stasis edema
EXCLUDES 1 *chronic venous hypertension due to deep vein thrombosis (I87.0-)*
varicose veins of lower extremities (I83-)

✓6th **I87.30** **Chronic venous hypertension (idiopathic) without complications**
Asymptomatic chronic venous hypertension (idiopathic)

I87.301 **Chronic venous hypertension (idiopathic) without complications of right lower extremity**

I87.302 **Chronic venous hypertension (idiopathic) without complications of left lower extremity**

I87.303 **Chronic venous hypertension (idiopathic) without complications of bilateral lower extremity**

I87.309 **Chronic venous hypertension (idiopathic) without complications of unspecified lower extremity**
Chronic venous hypertension NOS

✓6th **I87.31** **Chronic venous hypertension (idiopathic) with ulcer**
Use additional code to specify site and severity of ulcer (L97-)

I87.311 **Chronic venous hypertension (idiopathic) with ulcer of right lower extremity**

I87.312 **Chronic venous hypertension (idiopathic) with ulcer of left lower extremity**

I87.313 **Chronic venous hypertension (idiopathic) with ulcer of bilateral lower extremity**

I87.319 **Chronic venous hypertension (idiopathic) with ulcer of unspecified lower extremity**

✓6th **I87.32** **Chronic venous hypertension (idiopathic) with inflammation**

I87.321 **Chronic venous hypertension (idiopathic) with inflammation of right lower extremity**

I87.322 **Chronic venous hypertension (idiopathic) with inflammation of left lower extremity**

I87.323 **Chronic venous hypertension (idiopathic) with inflammation of bilateral lower extremity**

I87.329 **Chronic venous hypertension (idiopathic) with inflammation of unspecified lower extremity**

✓6th **I87.33** **Chronic venous hypertension (idiopathic) with ulcer and inflammation**
Use additional code to specify site and severity of ulcer (L97-)

I87.331 **Chronic venous hypertension (idiopathic) with ulcer and inflammation of right lower extremity**

I87.332 **Chronic venous hypertension (idiopathic) with ulcer and inflammation of left lower extremity**

I87.333 **Chronic venous hypertension (idiopathic) with ulcer and inflammation of bilateral lower extremity**

I87.339 **Chronic venous hypertension (idiopathic) with ulcer and inflammation of unspecified lower extremity**

✓6th **I87.39** **Chronic venous hypertension (idiopathic) with other complications**

I87.391 **Chronic venous hypertension (idiopathic) with other complications of right lower extremity**

I87.392 **Chronic venous hypertension (idiopathic) with other complications of left lower extremity**

I87.393 **Chronic venous hypertension (idiopathic) with other complications of bilateral lower extremity**

☑ Appropriate additional character required   ✓x7th Requires 7th character, placeholder x must fill empty characters

    I87.399   **Chronic venous hypertension (idiopathic) with other complications of unspecified lower extremity**

   I87.8   **Other specified disorders of veins**
     Phlebosclerosis
     Venofibrosis

   I87.9   **Disorder of vein, unspecified**

✓4ᵗʰ **I88**   **Nonspecific lymphadenitis**
     EXCLUDES 1   *acute lymphadenitis, except mesenteric (L04-)*
       enlarged lymph nodes NOS (R59-)
       human immunodeficiency virus [HIV] disease resulting in generalized lymphadenopathy (B20)

   I88.0   **Nonspecific mesenteric lymphadenitis**
     Mesenteric lymphadenitis (acute)(chronic)

   I88.1   **Chronic lymphadenitis, except mesenteric**
     Adenitis
     Lymphadenitis

   I88.8   **Other nonspecific lymphadenitis**

   I88.9   **Nonspecific lymphadenitis, unspecified**
     Lymphadenitis NOS

✓4ᵗʰ **I89**   **Other noninfective disorders of lymphatic vessels and lymph nodes**
     EXCLUDES 1   *chylocele, tunica vaginalis (nonfilarial) NOS (N50.8)*
       enlarged lymph nodes NOS (R59-)
       filarial chylocele (B74-)
       hereditary lymphedema (Q82.0)

   I89.0   **Lymphedema, not elsewhere classified**
     Elephantiasis (nonfilarial) NOS
     Lymphangiectasis
     Obliteration, lymphatic vessel
     Praecox lymphedema
     Secondary lymphedema
     EXCLUDES 1   *postmastectomy lymphedema (I97.2)*

   I89.1   **Lymphangitis**
     Chronic lymphangitis
     Lymphangitis NOS
     Subacute lymphangitis
     EXCLUDES 1   *acute lymphangitis (L03-)*

   I89.8   **Other specified noninfective disorders of lymphatic vessels and lymph nodes**
     Chylocele (nonfilarial)
     Chylous ascites
     Chylous cyst
     Lipomelanotic reticulosis
     Lymph node or vessel fistula
     Lymph node or vessel infarction
     Lymph node or vessel rupture

   I89.9   **Noninfective disorder of lymphatic vessels and lymph nodes, unspecified**
     Disease of lymphatic vessels NOS

Other and unspecified disorders of the circulatory system (I95-I99)

✓4ᵗʰ **I95**   **Hypotension**
     EXCLUDES 1   *cardiovascular collapse (R57.9)*
       maternal hypotension syndrome (O26.5-)
       nonspecific low blood pressure reading NOS (R03.1)

   I95.0   **Idiopathic hypotension**

   I95.1   **Orthostatic hypotension**
     Hypotension, postural
     EXCLUDES 1   *neurogenic orthostatic hypotension [Shy-Drager] (G90.3)*
       orthostatic hypotension due to drugs (I95.2)

   I95.2   **Hypotension due to drugs**
     Orthostatic hypotension due to drugs
     Code first (T36-T50) to identify drug

   I95.3   **Hypotension of hemodialysis**
     Intra-dialytic hypotension

✓5ᵗʰ **I95.8**   **Other hypotension**
   I95.81   **Postprocedural hypotension**
   I95.89   **Other hypotension**
     Chronic hypotension

   I95.9   **Hypotension, unspecified**

I96   **Gangrene, not elsewhere classified**
     Gangrenous cellulitis
     EXCLUDES 1   *gangrene in:*
       atherosclerosis of native arteries of the extremities (I70.24)
       diabetes mellitus (E08-E13)
       hernia (K40.1, K40.4, K41.1, K41.4, K42.1, K43.1-, K44.1, K45.1, K46.1)
       other peripheral vascular diseases (I73-)
       gangrene of certain specified sites—see Alphabetical Index
       gas gangrene (A48.0)
       pyoderma gangrenosum (L88)

✓4ᵗʰ **I97**   **Intraoperative and postprocedural complications and disorders of circulatory system, not elsewhere classified**
     EXCLUDES 2   *postprocedural shock (T81.1)*

   I97.0   **Postcardiotomy syndrome**

✓5ᵗʰ **I97.1**   **Other postprocedural cardiac functional disturbances**
     EXCLUDES 2   *acute pulmonary insufficiency following thoracic surgery (J95.1)*
       intraoperative cardiac functional disturbances (I97.7-)

   ✓6ᵗʰ **I97.11**   **Postprocedural cardiac insufficiency**
     I97.110   **Postprocedural cardiac insufficiency following cardiac surgery**
     I97.111   **Postprocedural cardiac insufficiency following other surgery**

   ✓6ᵗʰ **I97.12**   **Postprocedural cardiac arrest**
     I97.120   **Postprocedural cardiac arrest following cardiac surgery**
     I97.121   **Postprocedural cardiac arrest following other surgery**

   ✓6ᵗʰ **I97.13**   **Postprocedural heart failure**
     Use additional code to identify the heart failure (I50-)
     I97.130   **Postprocedural heart failure following cardiac surgery**
     I97.131   **Postprocedural heart failure following other surgery**

   ✓6ᵗʰ **I97.19**   **Other postprocedural cardiac functional disturbances**
     Use additional code, if applicable, to further specify disorder
     I97.190   **Other postprocedural cardiac functional disturbances following cardiac surgery**
     I97.191   **Other postprocedural cardiac functional disturbances following other surgery**

   I97.2   **Postmastectomy lymphedema syndrome**
     Elephantiasis due to mastectomy
     Obliteration of lymphatic vessels

   I97.3   **Postprocedural hypertension**

✓5ᵗʰ **I97.4**   **Intraoperative hemorrhage and hematoma of a circulatory system organ or structure complicating a procedure**
     EXCLUDES 1   *intraoperative hemorrhage and hematoma of a circulatory system organ or structure due to accidental puncture and laceration during a procedure (I97.5-)*
     EXCLUDES 2   *intraoperative cerebrovascular hemorrhage complicating a procedure (G97.3-)*

   ✓6ᵗʰ **I97.41**   **Intraoperative hemorrhage and hematoma of a circulatory system organ or structure complicating a circulatory system procedure**
     I97.410   **Intraoperative hemorrhage and hematoma of a circulatory system organ or structure complicating a cardiac catheterization**
     I97.411   **Intraoperative hemorrhage and hematoma of a circulatory system organ or structure complicating a cardiac bypass**
     I97.418   **Intraoperative hemorrhage and hematoma of a circulatory system organ or structure complicating other circulatory system procedure**

   I97.42   **Intraoperative hemorrhage and hematoma of a circulatory system organ or structure complicating other procedure**

EXCLUDES 1   Not coded here   EXCLUDES 2   Not included here   *Manifestation Code*

✓5th **I97.5** **Accidental puncture and laceration of a circulatory system organ or structure during a procedure**

EXCLUDES 2 *accidental puncture and laceration of brain during a procedure (G97.4-)*

I97.51 **Accidental puncture and laceration of a circulatory system organ or structure during a circulatory system procedure**

I97.52 **Accidental puncture and laceration of a circulatory system organ or structure during other procedure**

✓5th **I97.6** **Postprocedural hemorrhage and hematoma of a circulatory system organ or structure following a procedure**

EXCLUDES 2 *postprocedural cerebrovascular hemorrhage complicating a procedure (G97.5-)*

✓6th **I97.61** **Postprocedural hemorrhage and hematoma of a circulatory system organ or structure following a circulatory system procedure**

I97.610 **Postprocedural hemorrhage and hematoma of a circulatory system organ or structure following a cardiac catheterization**

I97.611 **Postprocedural hemorrhage and hematoma of a circulatory system organ or structure following cardiac bypass**

I97.618 **Postprocedural hemorrhage and hematoma of a circulatory system organ or structure following other circulatory system procedure**

I97.62 **Postprocedural hemorrhage and hematoma of a circulatory system organ or structure following other procedure**

✓5th **I97.7** **Intraoperative cardiac functional disturbances**

EXCLUDES 2 *acute pulmonary insufficiency following thoracic surgery (J95.1)*
postprocedural cardiac functional disturbances (I97.1-)

✓6th **I97.71** **Intraoperative cardiac arrest**

I97.710 **Intraoperative cardiac arrest during cardiac surgery**

I97.711 **Intraoperative cardiac arrest during other surgery**

✓6th **I97.79** **Other intraoperative cardiac functional disturbances**

Use additional code, if applicable, to further specify disorder

I97.790 **Other intraoperative cardiac functional disturbances during cardiac surgery**

I97.791 **Other intraoperative cardiac functional disturbances during other surgery**

✓5th **I97.8** **Other intraoperative and postprocedural complications and disorders of the circulatory system, not elsewhere classified**

Use additional code, if applicable, to further specify disorder

✓6th **I97.81** **Intraoperative cerebrovascular infarction**

I97.810 **Intraoperative cerebrovascular infarction during cardiac surgery**

I97.811 **Intraoperative cerebrovascular infarction during other surgery**

✓6th **I97.82** **Postprocedural cerebrovascular infarction**

I97.820 **Postprocedural cerebrovascular infarction during cardiac surgery**

I97.821 **Postprocedural cerebrovascular infarction during other surgery**

I97.88 **Other intraoperative complications of the circulatory system, not elsewhere classified**

I97.89 **Other postprocedural complications and disorders of the circulatory system, not elsewhere classified**

✓4th **I99** **Other and unspecified disorders of circulatory system**

I99.8 **Other disorder of circulatory system**

I99.9 **Unspecified disorder of circulatory system**

Diseases of the Respiratory System *(left margin)*

J00–J03.91 *(left margin)*

Chapter 10. Diseases of the Respiratory System (J00-J99)

NOTE   When a respiratory condition is described as occurring in more than one site and is not specifically indexed, it should be classified to the lower anatomic site (e.g. tracheobronchitis to bronchitis in J40).

Use additional code, where applicable, to identify:
    exposure to environmental tobacco smoke (Z77.22)
    exposure to tobacco smoke in the perinatal period (P96.81)
    history of tobacco use (Z87.891)
    occupational exposure to environmental tobacco smoke (Z57.31)
    tobacco dependence (F17-)
    tobacco use (Z72.0)

EXCLUDES 2   *certain conditions originating in the perinatal period (P04-P96)*
certain infectious and parasitic diseases (A00-B99)
complications of pregnancy, childbirth and the puerperium (O00-O99)
congenital malformations, deformations and chromosomal abnormalities (Q00-Q99)
endocrine, nutritional and metabolic diseases (E00-E88)
injury, poisoning and certain other consequences of external causes (S00-T88)
neoplasms (C00-D49)
smoke inhalation (T59.81-)
symptoms, signs and abnormal clinical and laboratory findings, not elsewhere classified (R00-R94)

This chapter contains the following blocks:
J00-J06   Acute upper respiratory infections
J09-J18   Influenza and pneumonia
J20-J22   Other acute lower respiratory infections
J30-J39   Other diseases of upper respiratory tract
J40-J47   Chronic lower respiratory diseases
J60-J70   Lung diseases due to external agents
J80-J84   Other respiratory diseases principally affecting the interstitium
J85-J86   Suppurative and necrotic conditions of the lower respiratory tract
J90-J94   Other diseases of the pleura
J95   Intraoperative and postprocedural complications and disorders of respiratory system, not elsewhere classified
J96-J99   Other diseases of the respiratory system

Acute upper respiratory infections (J00-J06)

EXCLUDES 1   *chronic obstructive pulmonary disease with acute lower respiratory infection (J44.0)*
influenza (J09-J11)

J00   **Acute nasopharyngitis (common cold)**
Acute rhinitis
Coryza (acute)
Infective nasopharyngitis NOS
Infective rhinitis
Nasal catarrh, acute
Nasopharyngitis NOS

EXCLUDES 1   *acute pharyngitis (J02-)*
acute sore throat NOS (J02.9)
pharyngitis NOS (J02.9)
rhinitis NOS (J31.0)
sore throat NOS (J02.9)

EXCLUDES 2   *allergic rhinitis (J30.1-J30.9)*
chronic pharyngitis (J31.2)
chronic rhinitis (J31.0)
chronic sore throat (J31.2)
nasopharyngitis, chronic (J31.1)
vasomotor rhinitis (J30.0)

✓4ᵗʰ J01   **Acute sinusitis**
   INCLUDES   acute abscess of sinus
            acute empyema of sinus
            acute infection of sinus
            acute inflammation of sinus
            acute suppuration of sinus
Use additional code (B95-B97) to identify infectious agent
   EXCLUDES 1   *sinusitis NOS (J32.9)*
   EXCLUDES 2   *chronic sinusitis (J32.0-J32.8)*

   ✓5ᵗʰ J01.0   **Acute maxillary sinusitis**
        Acute antritis
        J01.00   **Acute maxillary sinusitis, unspecified**
        J01.01   **Acute recurrent maxillary sinusitis**
   ✓5ᵗʰ J01.1   **Acute frontal sinusitis**
        J01.10   **Acute frontal sinusitis, unspecified**
        J01.11   **Acute recurrent frontal sinusitis**

✓5ᵗʰ J01.2   **Acute ethmoidal sinusitis**
    J01.20   **Acute ethmoidal sinusitis, unspecified**
    J01.21   **Acute recurrent ethmoidal sinusitis**
✓5ᵗʰ J01.3   **Acute sphenoidal sinusitis**
    J01.30   **Acute sphenoidal sinusitis, unspecified**
    J01.31   **Acute recurrent sphenoidal sinusitis**
✓5ᵗʰ J01.4   **Acute pansinusitis**
    J01.40   **Acute pansinusitis, unspecified**
    J01.41   **Acute recurrent pansinusitis**
✓5ᵗʰ J01.8   **Other acute sinusitis**
    J01.80   **Other acute sinusitis**
         Acute sinusitis involving more than one sinus but not pansinusitis
    J01.81   **Other acute recurrent sinusitis**
         Acute recurrent sinusitis involving more than one sinus but not pansinusitis
✓5ᵗʰ J01.9   **Acute sinusitis, unspecified**
    J01.90   **Acute sinusitis, unspecified**
    J01.91   **Acute recurrent sinusitis, unspecified**

✓4ᵗʰ J02   **Acute pharyngitis**
   INCLUDES   acute sore throat
   EXCLUDES 1   *acute laryngopharyngitis (J06.0)*
peritonsillar abscess (J36)
pharyngeal abscess (J39.1)
retropharyngeal abscess (J39.0)
   EXCLUDES 2   *chronic pharyngitis (J31.2)*

   J02.0   **Streptococcal pharyngitis**
       Septic pharyngitis
       Streptococcal sore throat
      EXCLUDES 1   *scarlet fever (A38-)*

   J02.8   **Acute pharyngitis due to other specified organisms**
       Use additional code (B95-B97) to identify infectious agent
      EXCLUDES 1   *acute pharyngitis due to coxsackie virus (B08.5)*
acute pharyngitis due to gonococcus (A54.5)
acute pharyngitis due to herpes [simplex] virus (B00.2)
acute pharyngitis due to infectious mononucleosis (B27.-)
acute pharyngitis due to influenza virus (J09.02, J09.12, J10.1, J11.1)
enteroviral vesicular pharyngitis (B08.5)

   J02.9   **Acute pharyngitis, unspecified**
       Gangrenous pharyngitis (acute)
       Infective pharyngitis (acute) NOS
       Pharyngitis (acute) NOS
       Sore throat (acute) NOS
       Suppurative pharyngitis (acute)
       Ulcerative pharyngitis (acute)

✓4ᵗʰ J03   **Acute tonsillitis**
   EXCLUDES 1   *acute sore throat (J02-)*
hypertrophy of tonsils (J35.1)
peritonsillar abscess (J36)
sore throat NOS (J02.9)
streptococcal sore throat (J02.0)
   EXCLUDES 2   *chronic tonsillitis (J35.0)*

   ✓5ᵗʰ J03.0   **Streptococcal tonsillitis**
      J03.00   **Acute streptococcal tonsillitis, unspecified**
      J03.01   **Acute recurrent streptococcal tonsillitis**
   ✓5ᵗʰ J03.8   **Acute tonsillitis due to other specified organisms**
       Use additional code (B95-B97) to identify infectious agent
      EXCLUDES 1   *diphtheritic tonsillitis (A36.0)*
herpesviral pharyngotonsillitis (B00.2)
streptococcal tonsillitis (J03.0)
tuberculous tonsillitis (A15.8)
Vincent's tonsillitis (A69.1)
      J03.80   **Acute tonsillitis due to other specified organisms**
      J03.81   **Acute recurrent tonsillitis due to other specified organisms**
   ✓5ᵗʰ J03.9   **Acute tonsillitis, unspecified**
       Follicular tonsillitis (acute)
       Gangrenous tonsillitis (acute)
       Infective tonsillitis (acute)
       Tonsillitis (acute) NOS
       Ulcerative tonsillitis (acute)
      J03.90   **Acute tonsillitis, unspecified**
      J03.91   **Acute recurrent tonsillitis, unspecified**

EXCLUDES 1 Not coded here   **EXCLUDES 2** Not included here   ***Manifestation Code***

✓4ᵗʰ **J04 Acute laryngitis and tracheitis**

Use additional code (B95-B97) to identify infectious agent

EXCLUDES 1 *acute laryngitis due to influenza virus (J09.02, J09.12, J10.1, J11.1)*

acute obstructive laryngitis [croup] and epiglottitis (J05-)

EXCLUDES 2 *laryngismus (stridulus) (J38.5)*

J04.0 Acute laryngitis

Edematous laryngitis (acute)

Laryngitis (acute) NOS

Subglottic laryngitis (acute)

Suppurative laryngitis (acute)

Ulcerative laryngitis (acute)

EXCLUDES 1 *acute obstructive laryngitis (J05.0)*

EXCLUDES 2 *chronic laryngitis (J37.0)*

✓5ᵗʰ **J04.1 Acute tracheitis**

Acute viral tracheitis

Catarrhal tracheitis (acute)

Tracheitis (acute) NOS

EXCLUDES 2 *chronic tracheitis (J42)*

J04.10   Acute tracheitis without obstruction

J04.11   Acute tracheitis with obstruction

✓5ᵗʰ **J04.2 Acute laryngotracheitis**

Laryngotracheitis NOS

Tracheitis (acute) with laryngitis (acute)

EXCLUDES 1 *acute obstructive laryngotracheitis (J05.0)*

EXCLUDES 2 *chronic laryngotracheitis (J37.1)*

✓5ᵗʰ **J04.3 Supraglottitis, unspecified**

J04.30   Supraglottitis, unspecified, without obstruction

J04.31   Supraglottitis, unspecified, with obstruction

✓4ᵗʰ **J05 Acute obstructive laryngitis [croup] and epiglottitis**

Use additional code (B95-B97) to identify infectious agent

J05.0 Acute obstructive laryngitis [croup]

Obstructive laryngitis (acute) NOS

Obstructive laryngotracheitis NOS

✓5ᵗʰ **J05.1 Acute epiglottitis**

EXCLUDES 2 *epiglottitis, chronic (J37.0)*

J05.10   Acute epiglottitis without obstruction

Epiglottitis NOS

J05.11   Acute epiglottitis with obstruction

✓4ᵗʰ **J06 Acute upper respiratory infections of multiple and unspecified sites**

EXCLUDES 1 *acute respiratory infection NOS (J22)*

influenza virus (J09-J11)

streptococcal pharyngitis (J02.0)

J06.0 Acute laryngopharyngitis

J06.9 Acute upper respiratory infection, unspecified

Upper respiratory disease, acute

Upper respiratory infection NOS

Influenza and pneumonia (J09-J18)

EXCLUDES 1 *allergic or eosinophilic pneumonia (J82)*

aspiration pneumonia NOS (J69.0)

congenital pneumonia (P23.9)

lipid pneumonia (J69.1)

meconium pneumonia (P24.01)

neonatal aspiration pneumonia (P24-)

pneumonia due to solids and liquids (J69-)

rheumatic pneumonia (I00)

ventilator associated pneumonia (J95.851)

✓4ᵗʰ **J09 Influenza due to certain identified influenza viruses**

EXCLUDES 1 *influenza due to other identified influenza virus (J10.-)*

influenza due to unidentified influenza virus (J11.-)

✓5ᵗʰ **J09.0 Influenza due to identified avian influenza virus**

Avian influenza

Bird flu

Influenza A/H5N1

✓6ᵗʰ **J09.01   Influenza due to identified avian influenza virus with pneumonia**

Code also associated lung abscess, if applicable (J85.1)

J09.010   Influenza due to identified avian influenza virus with identified avian influenza pneumonia

J09.018   Influenza due to identified avian influenza virus with other specified type of pneumonia

Code also the specified type of pneumonia

J09.019   Influenza due to identified avian influenza virus with unspecified type of pneumonia

J09.02   Influenza due to identified avian influenza virus with other respiratory manifestations

Influenza due to identified avian influenza virus NOS

Influenza due to identified avian influenza virus with laryngitis

Influenza due to identified avian influenza virus with pharyngitis

Influenza due to identified avian influenza virus with upper respiratory symptoms

Use additional code for associated pleural effusion, if applicable (J91.8)

Use additional code for associated sinusitis, if applicable (J01.-)

J09.03   Influenza due to identified avian influenza virus with gastrointestinal manifestations

Influenza due to identified avian influenza virus gastroenteritis

EXCLUDES 1 *'intestinal flu' [viral gastroenteritis] (A08.-)*

✓6ᵗʰ **J09.09   Influenza due to identified avian influenza virus with other manifestations**

J09.090   Influenza due to identified avian influenza virus with encephalopathy

J09.091   Influenza due to identified avian influenza virus with myocarditis

J09.092   Influenza due to identified avian influenza virus with otitis media

Use additional code for any associated perforated tympanic membrane (H72.-)

J09.098   Influenza due to identified avian influenza virus with other manifestations

Use additional codes to identfy the manifestations

✓5ᵗʰ **J09.1 Influenza due to identified novel H1N1 influenza virus**

2009 H1N1 [swine] influenza virus

Novel 2009 influenza H1N1

Novel H1N1 influenza

Novel influenza A/H1N1

Swine flu

✓6ᵗʰ **J09.11   Influenza due to identified novel H1N1 influenza virus with pneumonia**

Code also associated lung abscess, if applicable (J85.1)

J09.110   Influenza due to identified novel H1N1 influenza virus with identified novel H1N1 influenza pneumonia

J09.118   Influenza due to identified novel H1N1 influenza virus with other specified type of pneumonia

J09.119   Influenza due to identified novel H1N1 influenza virus with unspecified type of pneumonia

J09.12   Influenza due to identified novel H1N1 influenza virus with other respiratory manifestations

Influenza due to identified novel H1N1 influenza virus NOS

Influenza due to identified novel H1N1 influenza virus with laryngitis

Influenza due to identified novel H1N1 influenza virus with pharyngitis

Influenza due to identified novel H1N1 influenza virus with upper respiratory symptoms

Use additional code for associated pleural effusion, if applicable (J91.8)

Use additional code for associated sinusitis, if applicable (J01.-)

J09.13   Influenza due to identified novel H1N1 influenza virus with gastrointestinal manifestations

Influenza due to identified novel H1N1 influenza virus gastroenteritis

EXCLUDES 1 *'intestinal flu' [viral gastroenteritis] (A08.-)*

✓6th **J09.19 Influenza due to identified novel H1N1 influenza virus with other manifestations**

J09.190 Influenza due to identified novel H1N1 influenza virus with encephalopathy

J09.191 Influenza due to identified novel H1N1 influenza virus with myocarditis

J09.192 Influenza due to identified novel H1N1 influenza virus with otitis media
  Use additional code for any associated perforated tympanic membrane (H72.-)

J09.198 Influenza due to identified novel H1N1 influenza virus with other manifestations
  Use additional codes to identify the manifestations

✓4th **J10 Influenza due to other identified nfluenza virus**
  Use additional code to identify the virus (B97-)
  EXCLUDES 2 influenza due to avian influenza virus (J09.0-)
    influenza due to novel (2009) H1N1 influenza virus (J09.1-)
    influenza due to swine flu (J09.1-)
    influenza due to unidentifed influenza virus (J11.-)

✓5th **J10.0 Influenza due to other identified influenza virus with pneumonia**
  Code also associated lung abscess, if applicable (J85.1)

J10.00 Influenza due to other identified influenza virus with unspecified type of pneumonia

J10.01 Influenza due to other identified influenza virus with the same other identified influenza virus pneumonia

J10.08 Influenza due to other identified influenza virus with other specified pneumonia
  Code also the specified type of pneumonia

J10.1 Influenza due to other identified influenza virus with other respiratory manifestations
  Influenza due to other identified influenza virus NOS
  Influenza due to other identified influenza virus with laryngitis
  Influenza due to other identified influenza virus with pharyngitis
  Influenza due to other identified influenza virus with upper respiratory symptoms
  Use additional code for associated pleural effusion, if applicable (J91.8)
  Use additional code for associated sinusitis, if applicable (J01.-)

J10.2 Influenza due to other identified influenza virus with gastrointestinal manifestations
  Influenza due to other identified influenza virus gastroenteritis
  EXCLUDES 1 'intestinal flu' [viral gastroenteritis] (A08.-)

✓5th **J10.8 Influenza due to other identified influenza virus with other manifestations**

J10.81 Influenza due to other identified influenza virus with encephalopathy

J10.82 Influenza due to other identified influenza virus with myocarditis

J10.83 Influenza due to other identified influenza virus with otitis media
  Use additional code for any associated perforated tympanic membrane (H72.-)

J10.89 Influenza due to other identified influenza virus with other manifestations
  Use additional codes to identify the manifestations

✓4th **J11 Influenza due to unidentified influenza virus**

✓5th **J11.0 Influenza due to unidentified influenza virus with pneumonia**
  Code also associated lung abscess, if applicable (J85.1)

J11.00 Influenza due to unidentified influenza virus with unspecified type of pneumonia
  Influenza with pneumonia NOS

J11.08 Influenza due to unidentified influenza virus with specified pneumonia
  Code also specified pneumonia

J11.1 Influenza due to unidentified influenza virus with other respiratory manifestations
  Influenza NOS
  Influenzal laryngitis NOS
  Influenzal pharyngitis NOS
  Influenza with upper respiratory symptoms NOS
  Use additional code for associated pleural effusion, if applicable (J91.8)
  Use additional code for associated sinusitis, if applicable (J01.-)

J11.2 Influenza due to unidentified influenza virus with gastrointestinal manifestations
  Influenza gastroenteritis NOS
  EXCLUDES 1 'intestinal flu' [viral gastroenteritis] (A08.-)

✓5th **J11.8 Influenza due to unidentified influenza virus with other manifestations**

J11.81 Influenza due to unidentified influenza virus with encephalopathy
  Influenzal encephalopathy NOS

J11.82 Influenza due to unidentified influenza virus with myocarditis
  Influenzal myocarditis NOS

J11.83 Influenza due to unidentified influenza virus with otitis media
  Influenzal otitis media NOS
  Use additional code for any associated perforated tympanic membrane (H72.-)

J11.89 Influenza due to unidentified influenza virus with other manifestations
  Use additional codes to identify the manifestations

✓4th **J12 Viral pneumonia, not elsewhere classified**
  INCLUDES bronchopneumonia due to viruses other than influenza viruses
  Code first associated influenza, if applicable (J09.01-, J09.11-, J10.0-, J11.0-)
  Code also associated abscess, if applicable (J85.1)
  EXCLUDES 1 aspiration pneumonia due to anesthesia during labor and delivery (O74.0)
    aspiration pneumonia due to anesthesia during pregnancy (O29)
    aspiration pneumonia due to anesthesia during puerperium (O89.0)
    aspiration pneumonia due to solids and liquids (J69-)
    aspiration pneumonia NOS (J69.0)
    congenital pneumonia (P23.0)
    congenital rubella pneumonitis (P35.0)
    interstitial pneumonia NOS (J84.9)
    lipid pneumonia (J69.1)
    neonatal aspiration pneumonia (P24-)

J12.0 Adenoviral pneumonia

J12.1 Respiratory syncytial virus pneumonia

J12.2 Parainfluenza virus pneumonia

J12.3 Human metapneumovirus pneumonia

✓5th **J12.8 Other viral pneumonia**

J12.81 Pneumonia due to SARS-associated coronavirus
  Severe acute respiratory syndrome NOS

J12.89 Other viral pneumonia

J12.9 Viral pneumonia, unspecified

J13 Pneumonia due to Streptococcus pneumoniae
  Bronchopneumonia due to S. pneumoniae
  Code first associated influenza, if applicable (J09.01-, J09.11-, J10.0-, J11.0-)
  Code also associated lung abscess, if applicable (J85.1)
  EXCLUDES 1 congenital pneumonia due to S. pneumoniae (P23.6)
    lobar pneumonia, unspecified organism (J18.1)
    pneumonia due to other streptococci (J15.3-J15.4)

J14 Pneumonia due to Hemophilus influenzae
  Bronchopneumonia due to H. influenzae
  Code first associated influenza, if applicable (J09.01-, J09.11-, J10.0-, J11.0-)
  Code also associated lung abscess, if applicable (J85.1)
  EXCLUDES 1 congenital pneumonia due to H. influenzae (P23.6)

EXCLUDES 1 Not coded here EXCLUDES 2 Not included here *Manifestation Code*

☑4ᵗʰ J15   Bacterial pneumonia, not elsewhere classified
Bronchopneumonia due to bacteria other than S. pneumoniae and H. influenzae
Code first associated influenza, if applicable (J09.01-, J09.11-, J10.0-, -J11.0-)
Code also associated lung abscess, if applicable (J85.1)
EXCLUDES 1   *chlamydial pneumonia (J16.0)*
congenital pneumonia (P23-)
Legionnaires' disease (A48.1)
spirochetal pneumonia (A69.8)

J15.0   **Pneumonia due to Klebsiella pneumoniae**
J15.1   **Pneumonia due to Pseudomonas**
☑5ᵗʰ J15.2   **Pneumonia due to staphylococcus**
J15.20   **Pneumonia due to staphylococcus, unspecified**
J15.21   **Pneumonia due to staphylococcus aureus**
J15.29   **Pneumonia due to other staphylococcus**
J15.3   **Pneumonia due to streptococcus, group B**
J15.4   **Pneumonia due to other streptococci**
EXCLUDES 1   *pneumonia due to streptococcus, group B (J15.3)*
pneumonia due to Streptococcus pneumoniae (J13)
J15.5   **Pneumonia due to Escherichia coli**
J15.6   **Pneumonia due to other aerobic Gram-negative bacteria**
Pneumonia due to Serratia marcescens
J15.7   **Pneumonia due to Mycoplasma pneumoniae**
J15.8   **Pneumonia due to other specified bacteria**
J15.9   **Unspecified bacterial pneumonia**
Pneumonia due to gram-positive bacteria

☑4ᵗʰ J16   Pneumonia due to other infectious organisms, not elsewhere classified
Code first associated influenza, if applicable (J09.01-, J09.11-, J10.0-, -J11.0-)
Code also associated lung abscess, if applicable (J85.1)
EXCLUDES 1   *congenital pneumonia (P23-)*
ornithosis (A70)
pneumocystosis (B59)
pneumonia NOS (J18.9)

J16.0   **Chlamydial pneumonia**
J16.8   **Pneumonia due to other specified infectious organisms**

J17   Pneumonia in diseases classified elsewhere
Code first underlying disease, such as:
Q fever (A78)
rheumatic fever (I00)
schistosomiasis (B65.0-B65.9)
EXCLUDES 1   *candidial pneumonia (B37.1)*
chlamydial pneumonia (J16.0)
gonorrheal pneumonia (A54.84)
histoplasmosis pneumonia (B39.0-B39.2)
measles pneumonia (B05.2)
nocardiosis pneumonia (A43.0)
pneumocystosis (B59)
pneumonia due to Pneumocystis carinii (B59)
pneumonia due to Pneumocystis jiroveci (B59)
pneumonia in actinomycosis (A42.0)
pneumonia in anthrax (A22.1)
pneumonia in ascariasis (B77.81)
pneumonia in aspergillosis (B44.0-B44.1)
pneumonia in coccidioidomycosis (B38.0-B38.2)
pneumonia in cytomegalovirus disease (B25.0)
pneumonia in toxoplasmosis (B58.3)
rubella pneumonia (B06.81)
salmonella pneumonia (A02.22)
spirochetal infection NEC with pneumonia (A69.8)
tularemia pneumonia (A21.2)
typhoid fever with pneumonia (A01.03)
varicella pneumonia (B01.2)
whooping cough with pneumonia (A37 with fifth-character 1)

☑4ᵗʰ J18   Pneumonia, unspecified organism
Code first associated influenza, if applicable (J09.01-, J09.11-, J10.0-, -J11.0-)
EXCLUDES 1   *abscess of lung with pneumonia (J85.1)*
aspiration pneumonia due to anesthesia during labor and delivery (O74.0)
aspiration pneumonia due to anesthesia during pregnancy (O29)
aspiration pneumonia due to anesthesia during puerperium (O89.0)
aspiration pneumonia due to solids and liquids (J69-)
aspiration pneumonia NOS (J69.0)
congenital pneumonia (P23.0)
drug-induced interstitial lung disorder (J70.2-J70.4)
interstitial pneumonia NOS (J84.9)
lipid pneumonia (J69.1)
neonatal aspiration pneumonia (P24-)
pneumonitis due to external agents (J67-J70)
pneumonitis due to fumes and vapors (J68.0)
usual interstitial pneumonia (J84.1)

J18.0   **Bronchopneumonia, unspecified organism**
EXCLUDES 1   *hypostatic bronchopneumonia (J18.2)*
lipid pneumonia (J69.1)
EXCLUDES 2   *acute bronchiolitis (J21-)*
chronic bronchiolitis (J44.9)
J18.1   **Lobar pneumonia, unspecified organism**
J18.2   **Hypostatic pneumonia, unspecified organism**
Hypostatic bronchopneumonia
Passive pneumonia
J18.8   **Other pneumonia, unspecified organism**
J18.9   **Pneumonia, unspecified organism**

Other acute lower respiratory infections (J20-J22)
EXCLUDES 1   *chronic obstructive pulmonary disease with acute lower respiratory infection (J44.0)*

☑4ᵗʰ J20   Acute bronchitis
INCLUDES   acute and subacute bronchitis (with) bronchospasm
acute and subacute bronchitis (with) tracheitis
acute and subacute bronchitis (with) tracheobronchitis, acute
acute and subacute fibrinous bronchitis
acute and subacute membranous bronchitis
acute and subacute purulent bronchitis
acute and subacute septic bronchitis
EXCLUDES 2   *acute bronchitis with bronchiectasis (J47.0)*
acute bronchitis with chronic obstructive asthma (J44.0)
acute bronchitis with chronic obstructive pulmonary disease (J44.0)
allergic bronchitis NOS (J45.909-)
bronchitis due to chemicals, fumes and vapors (J68.0)
bronchitis NOS (J40)
chronic bronchitis NOS (J42)
chronic mucopurulent bronchitis (J41.1)
chronic obstructive bronchitis (J44-)
chronic obstructive tracheobronchitis (J44-)
chronic simple bronchitis (J41.0)
chronic tracheobronchitis (J42)
tracheobronchitis NOS (J40)

J20.0   **Acute bronchitis due to Mycoplasma pneumoniae**
J20.1   **Acute bronchitis due to Hemophilus influenzae**
J20.2   **Acute bronchitis due to streptococcus**
J20.3   **Acute bronchitis due to coxsackievirus**
J20.4   **Acute bronchitis due to parainfluenza virus**
J20.5   **Acute bronchitis due to respiratory syncytial virus**
J20.6   **Acute bronchitis due to rhinovirus**
J20.7   **Acute bronchitis due to echovirus**
J20.8   **Acute bronchitis due to other specified organisms**
J20.9   **Acute bronchitis, unspecified**

☑4ᵗʰ J21   Acute bronchiolitis
Acute bronchiolitis with bronchospasm
J21.0   **Acute bronchiolitis due to respiratory syncytial virus**
J21.1   **Acute bronchiolitis due to human metapneumovirus**
J21.8   **Acute bronchiolitis due to other specified organisms**
J21.9   **Acute bronchiolitis, unspecified**
Bronchiolitis (acute)
EXCLUDES 1   *chronic bronchiolitis (J44-)*

J22   **Unspecified acute lower respiratory infection**
Acute (lower) respiratory (tract) infection NOS
   EXCLUDES 1   *upper respiratory infection (acute) (J06.9)*

Other diseases of upper respiratory tract (J30-J39)

✓4th **J30**   **Vasomotor and allergic rhinitis**
   INCLUDES   spasmodic rhinorrhea
   EXCLUDES 1   *allergic rhinitis with asthma (bronchial) (J45.909)*
               rhinitis NOS (J31.0)

   J30.0   **Vasomotor rhinitis**
   J30.1   **Allergic rhinitis due to pollen**
       Allergy NOS due to pollen
       Hay fever
       Pollinosis
   J30.2   **Other seasonal allergic rhinitis**
   J30.5   **Allergic rhinitis due to food**
✓5th   **J30.8**   **Other allergic rhinitis**
     J30.81   **Allergic rhinitis due to animal (cat) (dog) hair and dander**
     J30.89   **Other allergic rhinitis**
            Perennial allergic rhinitis
   J30.9   **Allergic rhinitis, unspecified**

✓4th **J31**   **Chronic rhinitis, nasopharyngitis and pharyngitis**
   Use additional code to identify:
     exposure to environmental tobacco smoke (Z77.22)
     exposure to tobacco smoke in the perinatal period (P96.81)
     history of tobacco use (Z87.891)
     occupational exposure to environmental tobacco smoke (Z57.31)
     tobacco dependence (F17-)
     tobacco use (Z72.0)

   J31.0   **Chronic rhinitis**
       Atrophic rhinitis (chronic)
       Granulomatous rhinitis (chronic)
       Hypertrophic rhinitis (chronic)
       Obstructive rhinitis (chronic)
       Ozena
       Purulent rhinitis (chronic)
       Rhinitis (chronic) NOS
       Ulcerative rhinitis (chronic)
     EXCLUDES 1   *allergic rhinitis (J30.1-J30.9)*
               vasomotor rhinitis (J30.0)
   J31.1   **Chronic nasopharyngitis**
     EXCLUDES 2   *acute nasopharyngitis (J00)*
   J31.2   **Chronic pharyngitis**
       Atrophic pharyngitis (chronic)
       Chronic sore throat
       Granular pharyngitis (chronic)
       Hypertrophic pharyngitis (chronic)
     EXCLUDES 2   *acute pharyngitis (J02.9)*

✓4th **J32**   **Chronic sinusitis**
   INCLUDES   sinus abscess
           sinus empyema
           sinus infection
           sinus suppuration
   Use additional code to identify:
     exposure to environmental tobacco smoke (Z77.22)
     exposure to tobacco smoke in the perinatal period (P96.81)
     history of tobacco use (Z87.891)
     infectious agent (B95-B97)
     occupational exposure to environmental tobacco smoke (Z57.31)
     tobacco dependence (F17-)
     tobacco use (Z72.0)
   EXCLUDES 2   *acute sinusitis (J01-)*

   J32.0   **Chronic maxillary sinusitis**
       Antritis (chronic)
       Maxillary sinusitis NOS
   J32.1   **Chronic frontal sinusitis**
       Frontal sinusitis NOS
   J32.2   **Chronic ethmoidal sinusitis**
       Ethmoidal sinusitis NOS
     EXCLUDES 1   *Woakes' ethmoiditis (J33.1)*
   J32.3   **Chronic sphenoidal sinusitis**
       Sphenoidal sinusitis NOS
   J32.4   **Chronic pansinusitis**
       Pansinusitis NOS
   J32.8   **Other chronic sinusitis**
       Sinusitis (chronic) involving more than one sinus but not pansinusitis

   J32.9   **Chronic sinusitis, unspecified**
       Sinusitis (chronic) NOS

✓4th **J33**   **Nasal polyp**
   Use additional code to identify:
     exposure to environmental tobacco smoke (Z77.22)
     exposure to tobacco smoke in the perinatal period (P96.81)
     history of tobacco use (Z87.891)
     occupational exposure to environmental tobacco smoke (Z57.31)
     tobacco dependence (F17-)
     tobacco use (Z72.0)
   EXCLUDES 1   *adenomatous polyps (D14.0)*

   J33.0   **Polyp of nasal cavity**
       Choanal polyp
       Nasopharyngeal polyp
   J33.1   **Polypoid sinus degeneration**
       Woakes' syndrome or ethmoiditis
   J33.8   **Other polyp of sinus**
       Accessory polyp of sinus
       Ethmoidal polyp of sinus
       Maxillary polyp of sinus
       Sphenoidal polyp of sinus
   J33.9   **Nasal polyp, unspecified**

✓4th **J34**   **Other and unspecified disorders of nose and nasal sinuses**
   EXCLUDES 2   *varicose ulcer of nasal septum (I86.8)*
   J34.0   **Abscess, furuncle and carbuncle of nose**
       Cellulitis of nose
       Necrosis of nose
       Ulceration of nose
   J34.1   **Cyst and mucocele of nose and nasal sinus**
   J34.2   **Deviated nasal septum**
       Deflection or deviation of septum (nasal) (acquired)
     EXCLUDES 1   *congenital deviated nasal septum (Q67.4)*
   J34.3   **Hypertrophy of nasal turbinates**
✓5th   **J34.8**   **Other specified disorders of nose and nasal sinuses**
     J34.81   **Nasal mucositis (ulcerative)**
           Code also type of associated therapy, such as:
             antineoplastic and immunosuppressive drugs (T45.1x-)
             radiological procedure and radiotherapy (Y84.2)
       EXCLUDES 2   *gastrointestinal mucositis (ulcerative) (K92.81)*
                mucositis (ulcerative) of vagina and vulva (N76.81)
                oral mucositis (ulcerative) (K12.3-)
     J34.89   **Other specified disorders of nose and nasal sinuses**
           Perforation of nasal septum NOS
           Rhinolith
   J34.9   **Unspecified disorder of nose and nasal sinuses**

✓4th **J35**   **Chronic diseases of tonsils and adenoids**
   Use additional code to identify:
     exposure to environmental tobacco smoke (Z77.22)
     exposure to tobacco smoke in the perinatal period (P96.81)
     history of tobacco use (Z87.891)
     occupational exposure to environmental tobacco smoke (Z57.31)
     tobacco dependence (F17-)
     tobacco use (Z72.0)
✓5th   **J35.0**   **Chronic tonsillitis and adenoiditis**
     EXCLUDES 2   *acute tonsillitis (J03-)*
     J35.01   **Chronic tonsillitis**
     J35.02   **Chronic adenoiditis**
     J35.03   **Chronic tonsillitis and adenoiditis**
   J35.1   **Hypertrophy of tonsils**
       Enlargement of tonsils
     EXCLUDES 1   *hypertrophy of tonsils with tonsillitis (J35.0-)*
   J35.2   **Hypertrophy of adenoids**
       Enlargement of adenoids
     EXCLUDES 1   *hypertrophy of adenoids with adenoiditis (J35.0-)*
   J35.3   **Hypertrophy of tonsils with hypertrophy of adenoids**
     EXCLUDES 1   *hypertrophy of tonsils and adenoids with tonsillitis and adenoiditis (J35.03)*
   J35.8   **Other chronic diseases of tonsils and adenoids**
       Adenoid vegetations
       Amygdalolith
       Calculus, tonsil
       Cicatrix of tonsil (and adenoid)
       Tonsillar tag
       Ulcer of tonsil

EXCLUDES 1   Not coded here   EXCLUDES 2   Not included here   *Manifestation Code*

J35.9　**Chronic disease of tonsils and adenoids, unspecified**
　　　Disease (chronic) of tonsils and adenoids NOS

J36　**Peritonsillar abscess**
　　INCLUDES　abscess of tonsil
　　　　peritonsillar cellulitis
　　　　quinsy
　　Use additional code (B95-B97) to identify infectious agent
　　EXCLUDES 1　*acute tonsillitis (J03-)*
　　　　chronic tonsillitis (J35.0)
　　　　retropharyngeal abscess (J39.0)
　　　　tonsillitis NOS (J03.9-)

✓4th J37　**Chronic laryngitis and laryngotracheitis**
　　Use additional code to identify:
　　　exposure to environmental tobacco smoke (Z77.22)
　　　exposure to tobacco smoke in the perinatal period (P96.81)
　　　history of tobacco use (Z87.891)
　　　infectious agent (B95-B97)
　　　occupational exposure to environmental tobacco smoke (Z57.31)
　　　tobacco dependence (F17-)
　　　tobacco use (Z72.0)
　　J37.0　**Chronic laryngitis**
　　　　Catarrhal laryngitis
　　　　Hypertrophic laryngitis
　　　　Sicca laryngitis
　　　　EXCLUDES 2　*acute laryngitis (J04.0)*
　　　　　obstructive (acute) laryngitis (J05.0)
　　J37.1　**Chronic laryngotracheitis**
　　　　Laryngitis, chronic, with tracheitis (chronic)
　　　　Tracheitis, chronic, with laryngitis
　　　　EXCLUDES 1　*chronic tracheitis (J42)*
　　　　EXCLUDES 2　*acute laryngotracheitis (J04.2)*
　　　　　acute tracheitis (J04.1)

✓4th J38　**Diseases of vocal cords and larynx, not elsewhere classified**
　　Use additional code to identify:
　　　exposure to environmental tobacco smoke (Z77.22)
　　　exposure to tobacco smoke in the perinatal period (P96.81)
　　　history of tobacco use (Z87.891)
　　　occupational exposure to environmental tobacco smoke (Z57.31)
　　　tobacco dependence (F17-)
　　　tobacco use (Z72.0)
　　EXCLUDES 1　*congenital laryngeal stridor (P28.89)*
　　　　obstructive laryngitis (acute) (J05.0)
　　　　postprocedural subglottic stenosis (J95.5)
　　　　stridor (R06.1)
　　　　ulcerative laryngitis (J04.0)
　　✓5th J38.0　**Paralysis of vocal cords and larynx**
　　　　Laryngoplegia
　　　　Paralysis of glottis
　　　　J38.00　**Paralysis of vocal cords and larynx, unspecified**
　　　　J38.01　**Paralysis of vocal cords and larynx, unilateral**
　　　　J38.02　**Paralysis of vocal cords and larynx, bilateral**
　　J38.1　**Polyp of vocal cord and larynx**
　　　　EXCLUDES 1　*adenomatous polyps (D14.1)*
　　J38.2　**Nodules of vocal cords**
　　　　Chorditis (fibrinous)(nodosa)(tuberosa)
　　　　Singer's nodes
　　　　Teacher's nodes
　　J38.3　**Other diseases of vocal cords**
　　　　Abscess of vocal cords
　　　　Cellulitis of vocal cords
　　　　Granuloma of vocal cords
　　　　Leukokeratosis of vocal cords
　　　　Leukoplakia of vocal cords
　　J38.4　**Edema of larynx**
　　　　Edema (of) glottis
　　　　Subglottic edema
　　　　Supraglottic edema
　　　　EXCLUDES 1　*acute obstructive laryngitis [croup] (J05.0)*
　　　　　edematous laryngitis (J04.0)
　　J38.5　**Laryngeal spasm**
　　　　Laryngismus (stridulus)
　　J38.6　**Stenosis of larynx**

J38.7　**Other diseases of larynx**
　　　　Abscess of larynx
　　　　Cellulitis of larynx
　　　　Disease of larynx NOS
　　　　Necrosis of larynx
　　　　Pachyderma of larynx
　　　　Perichondritis of larynx
　　　　Ulcer of larynx

✓4th J39　**Other diseases of upper respiratory tract**
　　EXCLUDES 1　*acute respiratory infection NOS (J22)*
　　　　acute upper respiratory infection (J06.9)
　　　　upper respiratory inflammation due to chemicals, gases, fumes or vapors (J68.2)
　　J39.0　**Retropharyngeal and parapharyngeal abscess**
　　　　Peripharyngeal abscess
　　　　EXCLUDES 1　*peritonsillar abscess (J36)*
　　J39.1　**Other abscess of pharynx**
　　　　Cellulitis of pharynx
　　　　Nasopharyngeal abscess
　　J39.2　**Other diseases of pharynx**
　　　　Cyst of pharynx
　　　　Edema of pharynx
　　　　EXCLUDES 2　*chronic pharyngitis (J31.2)*
　　　　　ulcerative pharyngitis (J02.9)
　　J39.3　**Upper respiratory tract hypersensitivity reaction, site unspecified**
　　　　EXCLUDES 1　*hypersensitivity reaction of upper respiratory tract, such as:*
　　　　　extrinsic allergic alveolitis (J67.9)
　　　　　pneumoconiosis (J60-J67.9)
　　J39.8　**Other specified diseases of upper respiratory tract**
　　J39.9　**Disease of upper respiratory tract, unspecified**

Chronic lower respiratory diseases (J40-J47)

　　EXCLUDES 1　*bronchitis due to chemicals, gases, fumes and vapors (J68.0)*
　　EXCLUDES 2　*cystic fibrosis (E84-)*

J40　**Bronchitis, not specified as acute or chronic**
　　　Bronchitis NOS
　　　Bronchitis with tracheitis NOS
　　　Catarrhal bronchitis
　　　Tracheobronchitis NOS
　　Use additional code to identify:
　　　exposure to environmental tobacco smoke (Z77.22)
　　　exposure to tobacco smoke in the perinatal period (P96.81)
　　　history of tobacco use (Z87.891)
　　　occupational exposure to environmental tobacco smoke (Z57.31)
　　　tobacco dependence (F17-)
　　　tobacco use (Z72.0)
　　EXCLUDES 1　*allergic bronchitis NOS (J45.909-)*
　　　　asthmatic bronchitis NOS (J45.9-)
　　　　bronchitis due to chemicals, gases, fumes and vapors (J68.0)

✓4th J41　**Simple and mucopurulent chronic bronchitis**
　　Use additional code to identify:
　　　exposure to environmental tobacco smoke (Z77.22)
　　　exposure to tobacco smoke in the perinatal period (P96.81)
　　　history of tobacco use (Z87.891)
　　　occupational exposure to environmental tobacco smoke (Z57.31)
　　　tobacco dependence (F17-)
　　　tobacco use (Z72.0)
　　EXCLUDES 1　*chronic bronchitis NOS (J42)*
　　　　chronic obstructive bronchitis (J44-)
　　J41.0　**Simple chronic bronchitis**
　　J41.1　**Mucopurulent chronic bronchitis**
　　J41.8　**Mixed simple and mucopurulent chronic bronchitis**

J42   Unspecified chronic bronchitis
Chronic bronchitis NOS
Chronic tracheitis
Chronic tracheobronchitis
Use additional code to identify:
   exposure to environmental tobacco smoke (Z77.22)
   exposure to tobacco smoke in the perinatal period (P96.81)
   history of tobacco use (Z87.891)
   occupational exposure to environmental tobacco smoke (Z57.31)
   tobacco dependence (F17-)
   tobacco use (Z72.0)
   EXCLUDES 1   *chronic asthmatic bronchitis (J44-)*
      chronic bronchitis with airways obstruction (J44-)
      chronic emphysematous bronchitis (J44-)
      chronic obstructive pulmonary disease NOS (J44.9)
      simple and mucopurulent chronic bronchitis (J41-)

✓4th   J43   Emphysema
Use additional code to identify:
   exposure to environmental tobacco smoke (Z77.22)
   history of tobacco use (Z87.891)
   occupational exposure to environmental tobacco smoke (Z57.31)
   tobacco dependence (F17-)
   tobacco use (Z72.0)
   EXCLUDES 1   *compensatory emphysema (J98.3)*
      emphysema due to inhalation of chemicals, gases, fumes or
        vapors (J68.4)
      emphysema with chronic (obstructive) bronchitis (J44-)
      emphysematous (obstructive) bronchitis (J44-)
      interstitial emphysema (J98.2)
      mediastinal emphysema (J98.2)
      neonatal interstitial emphysema (P25.0)
      surgical (subcutaneous) emphysema (T81.82)
      traumatic subcutaneous emphysema (T79.7)

J43.0   Unilateral pulmonary emphysema [MacLeod's syndrome]
Swyer-James syndrome
Unilateral emphysema
Unilateral hyperlucent lung
Unilateral pulmonary artery functional hypoplasia
Unilateral transparency of lung

J43.1   Panlobular emphysema
Panacinar emphysema

J43.2   Centrilobular emphysema

J43.8   Other emphysema

J43.9   Emphysema, unspecified
Bullous emphysema (lung)(pulmonary)
Emphysema (lung)(pulmonary) NOS
Emphysematous bleb
Vesicular emphysema (lung)(pulmonary)

✓4th   J44   Other chronic obstructive pulmonary disease
   INCLUDES   asthma with chronic obstructive pulmonary disease
      chronic asthmatic (obstructive) bronchitis
      chronic bronchitis with airways obstruction
      chronic bronchitis with emphysema
      chronic emphysematous bronchitis
      chronic obstructive asthma
      chronic obstructive bronchitis
      chronic obstructive tracheobronchitis
Code also type of asthma, if applicable (J45-)
Use additional code to identify:
   exposure to environmental tobacco smoke (Z77.22)
   history of tobacco use (Z87.891)
   occupational exposure to environmental tobacco smoke (Z57.31)
   tobacco dependence (F17-)
   tobacco use (Z72.0)
   EXCLUDES 1   *bronchiectasis (J47-)*
      chronic bronchitis NOS (J42)
      chronic simple and mucopurulent bronchitis (J41-)
      chronic tracheitis (J42)
      chronic tracheobronchitis (J42)
      emphysema without chronic bronchitis (J43-)
      lung diseases due to external agents (J60-J70)

J44.0   Chronic obstructive pulmonary disease with acute lower respiratory infection
Use additional code to identify the infection

J44.1   Chronic obstructive pulmonary disease with (acute) exacerbation
Decompensated COPD
Decompensated COPD with (acute) exacerbation
   EXCLUDES 2   *chronic obstructive pulmonary disease [COPD] with*
      acute bronchitis (J44.0)

J44.9   Chronic obstructive pulmonary disease, unspecified
Chronic obstructive airway disease NOS
Chronic obstructive lung disease NOS

✓4th   J45   Asthma
Allergic (predominantly) asthma
Allergic bronchitis NOS
Allergic rhinitis with asthma
Atopic asthma
Extrinsic allergic asthma
Hay fever with asthma
Idiosyncratic asthma
Intrinsic nonallergic asthma
Nonallergic asthma
Use additional code to identify:
   exposure to environmental tobacco smoke (Z77.22)
   exposure to tobacco smoke in the perinatal period (P96.81)
   history of tobacco use (Z87.891)
   occupational exposure to environmental tobacco smoke (Z57.31)
   tobacco dependence (F17-)
   tobacco use (Z72.0)
   EXCLUDES 1   *detergent asthma (J69.8)*
      eosinophilic asthma (J82)
      lung diseases due to external agents (J60-J70)
      miner's asthma (J60)
      wheezing NOS (R06.2)
      wood asthma (J67.8)
   EXCLUDES 2   *asthma with chronic obstructive pulmonary disease*
      chronic asthmatic (obstructive) bronchitis
      chronic obstructive asthma

✓5th   J45.2   Mild intermittent asthma
   J45.20   Mild intermittent asthma, uncomplicated
      Mild intermittent asthma NOS
   J45.21   Mild intermittent asthma with (acute) exacerbation
   J45.22   Mild intermittent asthma with status asthmaticus

✓5th   J45.3   Mild persistent asthma
   J45.30   Mild persistent asthma, uncomplicated
      Mild persistent asthma NOS
   J45.31   Mild persistent asthma with (acute) exacerbation
   J45.32   Mild persistent asthma with status asthmaticus

✓5th   J45.4   Moderate persistent asthma
   J45.40   Moderate persistent asthma, uncomplicated
      Moderate persistent asthma NOS
   J45.41   Moderate persistent asthma with (acute) exacerbation
   J45.42   Moderate persistent asthma with status asthmaticus

✓5th   J45.5   Severe persistent asthma
   J45.50   Severe persistent asthma, uncomplicated
      Severe persistent asthma NOS
   J45.51   Severe persistent asthma with (acute) exacerbation
   J45.52   Severe persistent asthma with status asthmaticus

✓5th   J45.9   Other and unspecified asthma
   ✓6th   J45.90   Unspecified asthma
      Asthmatic bronchitis NOS
      Childhood asthma NOS
      Late onset asthma
      J45.901   Unspecified asthma with (acute) exacerbation
      J45.902   Unspecified asthma with status asthmaticus
      J45.909   Unspecified asthma, uncomplicated
        Asthma NOS
   ✓6th   J45.99   Other asthma
      J45.990   Exercise induced bronchospasm
      J45.991   Cough variant asthma
      J45.998   Other asthma

EXCLUDES 1   Not coded here   *EXCLUDES 2*   Not included here   ***Manifestation Code***

✓4th **J47** **Bronchiectasis**
    INCLUDES bronchiolectasis
    Use additional code to identify:
      exposure to environmental tobacco smoke (Z77.22)
      exposure to tobacco smoke in the perinatal period (P96.81)
      history of tobacco use (Z87.891)
      occupational exposure to environmental tobacco smoke (Z57.31)
      tobacco dependence (F17-)
      tobacco use (Z72.0)
      EXCLUDES 1 *congenital bronchiectasis (Q33.4)*
              tuberculous bronchiectasis (current disease) (A15.0)

    J47.0 **Bronchiectasis with acute lower respiratory infection**
          Bronchiectasis with acute bronchitis
    J47.1 **Bronchiectasis with (acute) exacerbation**
    J47.9 **Bronchiectasis, uncomplicated**
          Bronchiectasis NOS

Lung diseases due to external agents (J60-J70)

  EXCLUDES 2 *asthma (J45-)*
            malignant neoplasm of bronchus and lung (C34-)

J60 **Coalworker's pneumoconiosis**
    Anthracosilicosis
    Anthracosis
    Black lung disease
    Coalworker's lung
    EXCLUDES 1 *coalworker pneumoconiosis with tuberculosis, any type in A15 (J65)*

J61 **Pneumoconiosis due to asbestos and other mineral fibers**
    Asbestosis
    EXCLUDES 1 *pleural plaque with asbestosis (J92.0)*
            pneumoconiosis with tuberculosis, any type in A15 (J65)

✓4th **J62** **Pneumoconiosis due to dust containing silica**
    INCLUDES silicotic fibrosis (massive) of lung
    EXCLUDES 1 *pneumoconiosis with tuberculosis, any type in A15 (J65)*

    J62.0 **Pneumoconiosis due to talc dust**
    J62.8 **Pneumoconiosis due to other dust containing silica**
          Silicosis NOS

✓4th **J63** **Pneumoconiosis due to other inorganic dusts**
    EXCLUDES 1 *pneumoconiosis with tuberculosis, any type in A15 (J65)*

    J63.0 **Aluminosis (of lung)**
    J63.1 **Bauxite fibrosis (of lung)**
    J63.2 **Berylliosis**
    J63.3 **Graphite fibrosis (of lung)**
    J63.4 **Siderosis**
    J63.5 **Stannosis**
    J63.6 **Pneumoconiosis due to other specified inorganic dusts**

J64 **Unspecified pneumoconiosis**
    EXCLUDES 1 *pneumonoconiosis with tuberculosis, any type in A15 (J65)*

J65 **Pneumoconiosis associated with tuberculosis**
    Any condition in J60-J64 with tuberculosis, any type in A15
    silicotuberculosis

✓4th **J66** **Airway disease due to specific organic dust**
    EXCLUDES 2 *allergic alveolitis (J67-)*
            asbestosis (J61)
            bagassosis (J67.1)
            farmer's lung (J67.0)
            hypersensitivity pneumonitis due to organic dust (J67-)
            reactive airways dysfunction syndrome (J68.3)

    J66.0 **Byssinosis**
          Airway disease due to cotton dust
    J66.1 **Flax-dressers' disease**
    J66.2 **Cannabinosis**
    J66.8 **Airway disease due to other specific organic dusts**

✓4th **J67** **Hypersensitivity pneumonitis due to organic dust**
    INCLUDES allergic alveolitis and pneumonitis due to inhaled organic
              dust and particles of fungal, actinomycetic or other
              origin
    EXCLUDES 1 *pneumonitis due to inhalation of chemicals, gases, fumes or*
              vapors (J68.0)

    J67.0 **Farmer's lung**
          Harvester's lung
          Haymaker's lung
          Moldy hay disease

    J67.1 **Bagassosis**
          Bagasse disease
          Bagasse pneumonitis
    J67.2 **Bird fancier's lung**
          Budgerigar fancier's disease or lung
          Pigeon fancier's disease or lung
    J67.3 **Suberosis**
          Corkhandler's disease or lung
          Corkworker's disease or lung
    J67.4 **Maltworker's lung**
          Alveolitis due to Aspergillus clavatus
    J67.5 **Mushroom-worker's lung**
    J67.6 **Maple-bark-stripper's lung**
          Alveolitis due to Cryptostroma corticale
          Cryptostromosis
    J67.7 **Air conditioner and humidifier lung**
          Allergic alveolitis due to fungal, thermophilic actinomycetes
            and other organisms growing in ventilation [air
            conditioning] systems
    J67.8 **Hypersensitivity pneumonitis due to other organic dusts**
          Cheese-washer's lung
          Coffee-worker's lung
          Fish-meal worker's lung
          Furrier's lung
          Sequoiosis
    J67.9 **Hypersensitivity pneumonitis due to unspecified organic dust**
          Allergic alveolitis (extrinsic) NOS
          Hypersensitivity pneumonitis NOS

✓4th **J68** **Respiratory conditions due to inhalation of chemicals, gases, fumes and vapors**
    Code first (T51-T65) to identify cause

    J68.0 **Bronchitis and pneumonitis due to chemicals, gases, fumes and vapors**
          Chemical bronchitis (acute)
    J68.1 **Pulmonary edema due to chemicals, gases, fumes and vapors**
          Chemical pulmonary edema (acute) (chronic)
          EXCLUDES 1 *pulmonary edema (acute) (chronic) NOS (J81-)*
    J68.2 **Upper respiratory inflammation due to chemicals, gases, fumes and vapors, not elsewhere classified**
    J68.3 **Other acute and subacute respiratory conditions due to chemicals, gases, fumes and vapors**
          Reactive airways dysfunction syndrome
    J68.4 **Chronic respiratory conditions due to chemicals, gases, fumes and vapors**
          Emphysema (diffuse) (chronic) due to inhalation of chemicals,
            gases, fumes and vapors
          Obliterative bronchiolitis (chronic) (subacute) due to
            inhalation of chemicals, gases, fumes and vapors
          Pulmonary fibrosis (chronic) due to inhalation of chemicals,
            gases, fumes and vapors
          EXCLUDES 1 *chronic pulmonary edema due to chemicals, gases,*
               fumes and vapors (J68.1)
    J68.8 **Other respiratory conditions due to chemicals, gases, fumes and vapors**
    J68.9 **Unspecified respiratory condition due to chemicals, gases, fumes and vapors**

✓4th **J69** **Pneumonitis due to solids and liquids**
    EXCLUDES 1 *neonatal aspiration syndromes (P24-)*

    J69.0 **Pneumonitis due to inhalation of food and vomit**
          Aspiration pneumonia NOS
          Aspiration pneumonia (due to) food (regurgitated)
          Aspiration pneumonia (due to) gastric secretions
          Aspiration pneumonia (due to) milk
          Aspiration pneumonia (due to) vomit
          Code also any associated foreign body in respiratory tract
            (T17-)
          EXCLUDES 1 *chemical pneumonitis due to anesthesia*
               [Mendelson's syndrome] (J95.4)
               obstetric aspiration pneumonitis (O74.0)
    J69.1 **Pneumonitis due to inhalation of oils and essences**
          Exogenous lipoid pneumonia
          Lipid pneumonia NOS
          Code first (T51-T65) to identify substance
          EXCLUDES 1 *endogenous lipoid pneumonia (J84.2)*

✓ Appropriate additional character required   ✓x7th Requires 7th character, placeholder x must fill empty characters

J69.8   **Pneumonitis due to inhalation of other solids and liquids**
     Pneumonitis due to aspiration of blood
     Pneumonitis due to aspiration of detergent
     Code first (T51-T65) to identify substance

✓4th **J70**   **Respiratory conditions due to other external agents**

   J70.0   **Acute pulmonary manifestations due to radiation**
     Radiation pneumonitis
     Use additional code (W88-W90, X39.0-) to identify the external cause

   J70.1   **Chronic and other pulmonary manifestations due to radiation**
     Fibrosis of lung following radiation
     Use additional code (W88-W90, X39.0-) to identify the external cause

   J70.2   **Acute drug-induced interstitial lung disorders**
     Code first (T36-T50) to identify drug
     EXCLUDES 1   *interstitial pneumonia NOS (J84.9)*
           lymphoid interstitial pneumonia (J84.2)

   J70.3   **Chronic drug-induced interstitial lung disorders**
     Code first (T36-T50 with 7th character S) to identify drug
     EXCLUDES 1   *interstitial pneumonia NOS (J84.9)*
           lymphoid interstitial pneumonia (J84.2)

   J70.4   **Drug-induced interstitial lung disorders, unspecified**
     Code first (T36-T50) to identify drug
     EXCLUDES 1   *interstitial pneumonia NOS (J84.9)*
           lymphoid interstitial pneumonia (J84.2)

   J70.8   **Respiratory conditions due to other specified external agents**
     Code first (T51-T65) to identify the external agent

   J70.9   **Respiratory conditions due to unspecified external agent**
     Code first (T51-T65) to identify the external agent

Other respiratory diseases principally affecting the interstitium (J80-J84)

J80   **Acute respiratory distress syndrome**
     Acute respiratory distress syndrome in adult or child
     Adult hyaline membrane disease
     EXCLUDES 1   *respiratory distress syndrome in newborn (perinatal) (P22.0)*

✓4th **J81**   **Pulmonary edema**
     Use additional code to identify:
     exposure to environmental tobacco smoke (Z77.22)
     history of tobacco use (Z87.891)
     occupational exposure to environmental tobacco smoke (Z57.31)
     tobacco dependence (F17-)
     tobacco use (Z72.0)
     EXCLUDES 1   *chemical (acute) pulmonary edema (J68.1)*
           hypostatic pneumonia (J18.2)
           passive pneumonia (J18.2)
           pulmonary edema due to external agents (J60-J70)
           pulmonary edema with heart disease NOS (I50.1)
           pulmonary edema with heart failure (I50.1)

   J81.0   **Acute pulmonary edema**
     Acute edema of lung

   J81.1   **Chronic pulmonary edema**
     Pulmonary congestion (chronic) (passive)
     Pulmonary edema NOS

J82   **Pulmonary eosinophilia, not elsewhere classified**
     Allergic pneumonia
     Eosinophilic asthma
     Eosinophilic pneumonia
     Löffler's pneumonia
     Tropical (pulmonary) eosinophilia NOS
     EXCLUDES 1   *pulmonary eosinophilia due to aspergillosis (B44-)*
           pulmonary eosinophilia due to drugs (J70.2-J70.4)
           pulmonary eosinophilia due to specified parasitic infection (B50-B83)
           pulmonary eosinophilia due to systemic connective tissue disorders (M30-M36)

✓4th **J84**   **Other interstitial pulmonary diseases**
     EXCLUDES 1   *drug-induced interstitial lung disorders (J70.2-J70.4)*
           interstitial emphysema (J98.2)
           lung diseases due to external agents (J60-J70)

   J84.0   **Alveolar and parieto-alveolar conditions**
     Alveolar proteinosis
     Pulmonary alveolar microlithiasis

   J84.1   **Other interstitial pulmonary diseases with fibrosis**
     Cirrhosis of lung
     Diffuse pulmonary fibrosis
     Fibrosing alveolitis (cryptogenic)
     Hamman-Rich syndrome
     Idiopathic pulmonary fibrosis
     Induration of lung
     Usual interstitial pneumonia
     EXCLUDES 1   *pulmonary fibrosis (chronic) due to inhalation of chemicals, gases, fumes or vapors (J68.4)*
           pulmonary fibrosis (chronic) following radiation (J70.1)

   J84.2   **Lymphoid interstitial pneumonia**
     Endogenous lipoid pneumonia
     Lymphoid interstitial pneumonitis
     EXCLUDES 1   *exogenous lipoid pneumonia (J69.1)*
           unspecified lipoid pneumonia (J69.1)

   J84.8   **Other specified interstitial pulmonary diseases**

   J84.9   **Interstitial pulmonary disease, unspecified**
     Interstitial pneumonia NOS

Suppurative and necrotic conditions of the lower respiratory tract (J85-J86)

✓4th **J85**   **Abscess of lung and mediastinum**
     Use additional code (B95-B97) to identify infectious agent.

   J85.0   **Gangrene and necrosis of lung**

   J85.1   **Abscess of lung with pneumonia**
     Code also the type of pneumonia

   J85.2   **Abscess of lung without pneumonia**
     Abscess of lung NOS

   J85.3   **Abscess of mediastinum**

✓4th **J86**   **Pyothorax**
     Use additional code (B95-B97) to identify infectious agent.
     EXCLUDES 1   *abscess of lung (J85-)*
           pyothorax due to tuberculosis (A15.6)

   J86.0   **Pyothorax with fistula**
     Bronchocutaneous fistula
     Bronchopleural fistula
     Hepatopleural fistula
     Mediastinal fistula
     Pleural fistula
     Thoracic fistula
     Any condition classifiable to J86.9 with fistula

   J86.9   **Pyothorax without fistula**
     Abscess of pleura
     Abscess of thorax
     Empyema (chest) (lung) (pleura)
     Fibrinopurulent pleurisy
     Purulent pleurisy
     Pyopneumothorax
     Septic pleurisy
     Seropurulent pleurisy
     Suppurative pleurisy

Other diseases of the pleura (J90-J94)

J90   **Pleural effusion, not elsewhere classified**
     Encysted pleurisy
     Pleural effusion NOS
     Pleurisy with effusion (exudative) (serous)
     EXCLUDES 1   *chylous (pleural) effusion (J94.0)*
           malignant pleural effusion (J91.0))
           pleurisy NOS (R09.1)
           tuberculous pleural effusion (A15.6)

✓4th **J91**   **Pleural effusion in conditions classified elsewhere**
     EXCLUDES 2   *pleural effusion in heart failure (I50-)*
           pleural effusion in systemic lupus erythematosus (M32.13)

   J91.0   **Malignant pleural effusion**
     Code first underlying neoplasm

   J91.8   **Pleural effusion in other conditions classified elsewhere**
     Code first underlying disease, such as:
     filariasis (B74.0-B74.9)
     influenza (J09.02, J09.12, J10.1, J11.1)

EXCLUDES 1   Not coded here   EXCLUDES 2   Not included here   *Manifestation Code*

✓4th **J92 Pleural plaque**
INCLUDES pleural thickening
J92.0 Pleural plaque with presence of asbestos
J92.9 Pleural plaque without asbestos
Pleural plaque NOS

✓4th **J93 Pneumothorax**
EXCLUDES 1 congenital or perinatal pneumothorax (P25.1)
postprocedural pneumothorax (J95.81)
traumatic pneumothorax (S27.0)
tuberculous (current disease) pneumothorax (A15-)
pyopneumothorax (J86-)
J93.0 Spontaneous tension pneumothorax
J93.1 Other spontaneous pneumothorax
J93.8 Other pneumothorax
EXCLUDES 1 postprocedural pneumothorax (J95.81)
J93.9 Pneumothorax, unspecified

✓4th **J94 Other pleural conditions**
EXCLUDES 1 pleurisy NOS (R09.1)
traumatic hemopneumothorax (S27.2)
traumatic hemothorax (S27.1)
tuberculous pleural conditions (current disease) (A15-)
J94.0 Chylous effusion
Chyliform effusion
J94.1 Fibrothorax
J94.2 Hemothorax
Hemopneumothorax
J94.8 Other specified pleural conditions
Hydropneumothorax
Hydrothorax
J94.9 Pleural condition, unspecified

Intraoperative and postprocedural complications and disorders of respiratory system, not elsewhere classified (J95)

✓4th **J95 Intraoperative and postprocedural complications and disorders of respiratory system, not elsewhere classified**
EXCLUDES 2 aspiration pneumonia (J69-)
emphysema (subcutaneous) resulting from a procedure (T81.82)
hypostatic pneumonia (J18.2)
pulmonary manifestations due to radiation (J70.0- J70.1)
✓5th **J95.0 Tracheostomy complications**
J95.00 Unspecified tracheostomy complication
J95.01 Hemorrhage from tracheostomy stoma
J95.02 Infection of tracheostomy stoma
Use additional code to identify type of infection, such as:
cellulitis of neck (L03.8)
sepsis (A40, A41-)
J95.03 Malfunction of tracheostomy stoma
Mechanical complication of tracheostomy stoma
Obstruction of tracheostomy airway
Tracheal stenosis due to tracheostomy
J95.04 Tracheo-esophageal fistula following tracheostomy
J95.09 Other tracheostomy complication
J95.1 Acute pulmonary insufficiency following thoracic surgery
EXCLUDES 2 functional disturbances following cardiac surgery (I97.0, I97.1-)
J95.2 Acute pulmonary insufficiency following nonthoracic surgery
EXCLUDES 2 functional disturbances following cardiac surgery (I97.0, I97.1-)
J95.3 Chronic pulmonary insufficiency following surgery
EXCLUDES 2 functional disturbances following cardiac surgery (I97.0, I97.1-)
J95.4 Chemical pneumonitis due to anesthesia [Mendelson's syndrome]
Code first appropriate code from category T41
EXCLUDES 1 aspiration pneumonitis due to anesthesia complicating labor and delivery (O74.0)
aspiration pneumonitis due to anesthesia complicating pregnancy (O29)
aspiration pneumonitis due to anesthesia complicating the puerperium (O89.01)
J95.5 Postprocedural subglottic stenosis

✓5th **J95.6 Intraoperative hemorrhage and hematoma of a respiratory system organ or structure complicating a procedure**
EXCLUDES 1 intraoperative hemorrhage and hematoma of a respiratory system organ or structure due to accidental puncture and laceration during procedure (J95.7-)
J95.61 Intraoperative hemorrhage and hematoma of a respiratory system organ or structure complicating a respiratory system procedure
J95.62 Intraoperative hemorrhage and hematoma of a respiratory system organ or structure complicating other procedure
✓5th **J95.7 Accidental puncture and laceration of a respiratory system organ or structure during a procedure**
EXCLUDES 2 postprocedural pneumothorax (J95.8)
J95.71 Accidental puncture and laceration of a respiratory system organ or structure during a respiratory system procedure
J95.72 Accidental puncture and laceration of a respiratory system organ or structure during other procedure
✓5th **J95.8 Other intraoperative and postprocedural complications and disorders of respiratory system, not elsewhere classified**
J95.81 Postprocedural pneumothorax
J95.82 Postprocedural respiratory failure
✓6th **J95.83 Postprocedural hemorrhage and hematoma of a respiratory system organ or structure following a procedure**
J95.830 Postprocedural hemorrhage and hematoma of a respiratory system organ or structure following a respiratory system procedure
J95.831 Postprocedural hemorrhage and hematoma of a respiratory system organ or structure following other procedure
J95.84 Transfusion-related acute lung injury (TRALI)
✓6th **J95.85 Complication of respirator [ventilator]**
J95.850 Mechanical complication of respirator
EXCLUDES 1 encounter for respirator [ventilator] dependence during power failure (Z99.12)
J95.851 Ventilator associated pneumonia
Ventilator associated pneumonitis
Use additional code to identify the organism, if known (B95.-, B96.-, B97.-)
EXCLUDES 1 ventilator lung in newborn (P27.8)
J95.859 Other complication of respirator [ventilator]
J95.88 Other intraoperative complications of respiratory system, not elsewhere classified
J95.89 Other postprocedural complications and disorders of respiratory system, not elsewhere classified
Use additional code to identify disorder, such as:
aspiration pneumonia (J69-)
bacterial or viral pneumonia (J12-J18)
EXCLUDES 2 acute pulmonary insufficiency following thoracic surgery (J95.1)
postprocedural subglottic stenosis (J95.5)

Other diseases of the respiratory system (J96-J99)

✓4th **J96 Respiratory failure, not elsewhere classified**
EXCLUDES 1 acute respiratory distress syndrome (J80)
cardiorespiratory failure (R09.2)
newborn respiratory distress syndrome (P22.0)
postprocedural respiratory failure (J95.82)
respiratory arrest (R09.2)
respiratory arrest of newborn (P28.81)
respiratory failure of newborn (P28.5)
✓5th **J96.0 Acute respiratory failure**
J96.00 Acute respiratory failure, unspecified whether with hypoxia or hypercapnia
J96.01 Acute respiratory failure with hypoxia
J96.02 Acute respiratory failure with hypercapnia
✓5th **J96.1 Chronic respiratory failure**

✓ Appropriate additional character required

✓x7th Requires 7th character, placeholder x must fill empty characters

Diseases of the Respiratory System

J96.10   **Chronic respiratory failure, unspecified whether with hypoxia or hypercapnia**

J96.11   **Chronic respiratory failure with hypoxia**

J96.12   **Chronic respiratory failure with hypercapnia**

√5ᵗʰ **J96.2**   **Acute and chronic respiratory failure**
Acute on chronic respiratory failure

J96.20   **Acute and chronic respiratory failure, unspecified whether with hypoxia or hypercapnia**

J96.21   **Acute and chronic respiratory failure with hypoxia**

J96.22   **Acute and chronic respiratory failure with hypercapnia**

√5ᵗʰ **J96.9**   **Respiratory failure, unspecified**

J96.90   **Respiratory failure, unspecified, unspecified whether with hypoxia or hypercapnia**

J96.91   **Respiratory failure, unspecified with hypoxia**

J96.92   **Respiratory failure, unspecified with hypercapnia**

J98   **Other respiratory disorders**
Use additional code to identify:
exposure to environmental tobacco smoke (Z77.22)
exposure to tobacco smoke in the perinatal period (P96.81)
history of tobacco use (Z87.891)
occupational exposure to environmental tobacco smoke (Z57.31)
tobacco dependence (F17-)
tobacco use (Z72.0)
EXCLUDES 1   *newborn apnea (P28.4)*
newborn sleep apnea (P28.3)
EXCLUDES 2   *apnea NOS (R06.81)*
sleep apnea (G47.3-)

√5ᵗʰ **J98.0**   **Diseases of bronchus, not elsewhere classified**

J98.01   **Acute bronchospasm**
EXCLUDES 1   *acute bronchiolitis with bronchospasm (J21-)*
acute bronchitis with bronchospasm (J20-)
asthma (J45-)
exercise induced bronchospasm (J45.990)

J98.09   **Other diseases of bronchus, not elsewhere classified**
Broncholithiasis
Calcification of bronchus
Stenosis of bronchus
Tracheobronchial collapse
Tracheobronchial dyskinesia
Ulcer of bronchus

√5ᵗʰ **J98.1**   **Pulmonary collapse**
EXCLUDES 1   *therapeutic collapse of lung status (Z98.3)*

J98.11   **Atelectasis**
EXCLUDES 1   *newborn atelectasis*
tuberculous atelectasis (current disease) (A15)

J98.19   **Other pulmonary collapse**

J98.2   **Interstitial emphysema**
Mediastinal emphysema
EXCLUDES 1   *emphysema NOS (J43.9)*
emphysema in newborn (P25.0)
surgical emphysema (subcutaneous) (T81.82)
traumatic subcutaneous emphysema (T79.7)

J98.3   **Compensatory emphysema**

J98.4   **Other disorders of lung**
Calcification of lung
Cystic lung disease (acquired)
Lung disease NOS
Pulmolithiasis

J98.5   **Diseases of mediastinum, not elsewhere classified**
Fibrosis of mediastinum
Hernia of mediastinum
Retraction of mediastinum
Mediastinitis
EXCLUDES 2   *abscess of mediastinum (J85.3)*

J98.6   **Disorders of diaphragm**
Diaphragmatitis
Paralysis of diaphragm
Relaxation of diaphragm
EXCLUDES 1   *congenital malformation of diaphragm NEC (Q79.1)*
congenital diaphragmatic hernia (Q79.0)
EXCLUDES 2   *diaphragmatic hernia (K44-)*

J98.8   **Other specified respiratory disorders**

J98.9   **Respiratory disorder, unspecified**
Respiratory disease (chronic) NOS

J99   *Respiratory disorders in diseases classified elsewhere*
Code first underlying disease, such as:
amyloidosis (E85-)
ankylosing spondylitis (M45)
congenital syphilis (A50.5)
cryoglobulinemia (D89.1)
early congenital syphilis (A50.0)
hemosiderosis (E83.19)
schistosomiasis (B65.0-B65.9)
EXCLUDES 1   *respiratory disorders in:*
amebiasis (A06.5)
blastomycosis (B40.0-B40.2)
candidiasis (B37.1)
coccidioidomycosis (B38.0-B38.2)
cystic fibrosis with pulmonary manifestations (E84.0)
dermatomyositis (M33.01, M33.11)
histoplasmosis (B39.0-B39.2)
late syphilis (A52.72, A52.73)
polymyositis (M33.21)
sicca syndrome (M35.02)
systemic lupus erythematosus (M32.13)
systemic sclerosis (M34.81)
Wegener's granulomatosis (M31.30-M31.31)

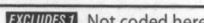

EXCLUDES 1   Not coded here   EXCLUDES 2   Not included here   *Manifestation Code*

Chapter 11. Diseases of the Digestive System (K00-K94)

EXCLUDES 2 *certain conditions originating in the perinatal period (P04-P96)*
certain infectious and parasitic diseases (A00-B99)
complications of pregnancy, childbirth and the puerperium (O00-O99)
congenital malformations, deformations and chromosomal abnormalities (Q00-Q99)
endocrine, nutritional and metabolic diseases (E00-E88)
injury, poisoning and certain other consequences of external causes (S00-T88)
neoplasms (C00-D49)
symptoms, signs and abnormal clinical and laboratory findings, not elsewhere classified (R00-R94)

This chapter contains the following blocks:

K00-K14	Diseases of oral cavity and salivary glands
K20-K31	Diseases of esophagus, stomach and duodenum
K35-K38	Diseases of appendix
K40-K46	Hernia
K50-K52	Noninfective enteritis and colitis
K55-K63	Other diseases of intestines
K65-K68	Diseases of peritoneum and retroperitoneum
K70-K77	Diseases of liver
K80-K87	Disorders of gallbladder, biliary tract and pancreas
K90-K94	Other diseases of the digestive system

Diseases of oral cavity and salivary glands (K00-K14)

☑4ᵗʰ **K00 Disorders of tooth development and eruption**

EXCLUDES 2 *embedded and impacted teeth (K01-)*

K00.0 Anodontia
Hypodontia
Oligodontia
EXCLUDES 1 *acquired absence of teeth (K08.1-)*

K00.1 Supernumerary teeth
Distomolar
Fourth molar
Mesiodens
Paramolar
Supplementary teeth
EXCLUDES 2 *supernumerary roots (K00.2)*

K00.2 Abnormalities of size and form of teeth
Concrescence of teeth
Dens evaginatus
Dens in dente
Dens invaginatus
Enamel pearls
Fusion of teeth
Gemination of teeth
Macrodontia
Microdontia
Peg-shaped [conical] teeth
Supernumerary roots
Taurodontism
Tuberculum paramolare
EXCLUDES 1 *abnormalities of teeth due to congenital syphilis (A50.5)*
tuberculum Carabelli, which is regarded as a normal variation and should not be coded

K00.3 Mottled teeth
Dental fluorosis
Mottling of enamel
Nonfluoride enamel opacities
EXCLUDES 2 *deposits [accretions] on teeth (K03.6)*

K00.4 Disturbances in tooth formation
Aplasia and hypoplasia of cementum
Dilaceration of tooth
Enamel hypoplasia (neonatal) (postnatal) (prenatal)
Regional odontodysplasia
Turner's tooth
EXCLUDES 1 *Hutchinson's teeth and mulberry molars in congenital syphilis (A50.5)*
EXCLUDES 2 *mottled teeth (K00.3)*

K00.5 Hereditary disturbances in tooth structure, not elsewhere classified
Amelogenesis imperfecta
Dentinogenesis imperfecta
Odontogenesis imperfecta
Dentinal dysplasia
Shell teeth

K00.6 Disturbances in tooth eruption
Dentia praecox
Natal tooth
Neonatal tooth
Premature eruption of tooth
Premature shedding of primary [deciduous] tooth
Prenatal teeth
Retained [persistent] primary tooth
EXCLUDES 2 *embedded and impacted teeth (K01-)*

K00.7 Teething syndrome

K00.8 Other disorders of tooth development
Color changes during tooth formation
Intrinsic staining of teeth NOS
EXCLUDES 2 *posteruptive color changes (K03.7)*

K00.9 Disorder of tooth development, unspecified
Disorder of odontogenesis NOS

☑4ᵗʰ **K01 Embedded and impacted teeth**
EXCLUDES 1 *abnormal position of fully erupted teeth (M26.3-)*

K01.0 Embedded teeth

K01.1 Impacted teeth

☑4ᵗʰ **K02 Dental caries**
Dental cavities
Tooth decay

K02.3 Arrested dental caries
Arrested coronal and root caries

☑5ᵗʰ **K02.5 Dental caries on pit and fissure surface**
Dental caries on chewing surface of tooth

K02.51 Dental caries on pit and fissure surface limited to enamel
White spot lesions [initial caries] on pit and fissure surface of tooth

K02.52 Dental caries on pit and fissure surface penetrating into dentin

K02.53 Dental caries on pit and fissure surface penetrating into pulp

☑5ᵗʰ **K02.6 Dental caries on smooth surface**

K02.61 Dental caries on smooth surface limited to enamel
White spot lesions [initial caries] on smooth surface of tooth

K02.62 Dental caries on smooth surface penetrating into dentin

K02.63 Dental caries on smooth surface penetrating into pulp

K02.7 Dental root caries

K02.9 Dental caries, unspecified

☑4ᵗʰ **K03 Other diseases of hard tissues of teeth**
EXCLUDES 2 *bruxism (F45.8)*
dental caries (K02-)
teeth-grinding NOS (F45.8)

K03.0 Excessive attrition of teeth
Approximal wear of teeth
Occlusal wear of teeth

K03.1 Abrasion of teeth
Dentifrice abrasion of teeth
Habitual abrasion of teeth
Occupational abrasion of teeth
Ritual abrasion of teeth
Traditional abrasion of teeth
Wedge defect NOS

K03.2 Erosion of teeth
Erosion of teeth due to diet
Erosion of teeth due to drugs and medicaments
Erosion of teeth due to persistent vomiting
Erosion of teeth NOS
Idiopathic erosion of teeth
Occupational erosion of teeth

K03.3 Pathological resorption of teeth
Internal granuloma of pulp
Resorption of teeth (external)

K03.4 Hypercementosis
Cementation hyperplasia

K03.5 Ankylosis of teeth

☑ Appropriate additional character required ☑x7ᵗʰ Requires 7th character, placeholder x must fill empty characters

K03.6 **Deposits [accretions] on teeth**
Betel deposits [accretions] on teeth
Black deposits [accretions] on teeth
Extrinsic staining of teeth NOS
Green deposits [accretions] on teeth
Materia alba deposits [accretions] on teeth
Orange deposits [accretions] on teeth
Staining of teeth NOS
Subgingival dental calculus
Supragingival dental calculus
Tobacco deposits [accretions] on teeth

K03.7 **Posteruptive color changes of dental hard tissues**
EXCLUDES 2 *deposits [accretions] on teeth (K03.6)*

✓5ᵗʰ **K03.8** **Other specified diseases of hard tissues of teeth**
K03.81 **Cracked tooth**
EXCLUDES 1 *asymptomatic craze lines in enamel—omit code*
broken or fractured tooth due to trauma (S02.5)
K03.89 **Other specified diseases of hard tissues of teeth**

K03.9 **Disease of hard tissues of teeth, unspecified**

✓4ᵗʰ **K04** **Diseases of pulp and periapical tissues**
K04.0 **Pulpitis**
Acute pulpitis
Chronic (hyperplastic) (ulcerative) pulpitis
Irreversible pulpitis
Reversible pulpitis

K04.1 **Necrosis of pulp**
Pulpal gangrene

K04.2 **Pulp degeneration**
Denticles
Pulpal calcifications
Pulpal stones

K04.3 **Abnormal hard tissue formation in pulp**
Secondary or irregular dentine

K04.4 **Acute apical periodontitis of pulpal origin**
Acute apical periodontitis NOS
EXCLUDES 1 *acute periodontitis (K05.2-)*

K04.5 **Chronic apical periodontitis**
Apical or periapical granuloma
Apical periodontitis NOS
EXCLUDES 1 *chronic periodontitis (K05.3-)*

K04.6 **Periapical abscess with sinus**
Dental abscess with sinus
Dentoalveolar abscess with sinus

K04.7 **Periapical abscess without sinus**
Dental abscess without sinus
Dentoalveolar abscess without sinus
Periapical abscess without sinus

K04.8 **Radicular cyst**
Apical (periodontal) cyst
Periapical cyst
Residual radicular cyst
EXCLUDES 2 *lateral periodontal cyst (K09.0)*

✓5ᵗʰ **K04.9** **Other and unspecified diseases of pulp and periapical tissues**
K04.90 **Unspecified diseases of pulp and periapical tissues**
K04.99 **Other diseases of pulp and periapical tissues**

✓4ᵗʰ **K05** **Gingivitis and periodontal diseases**
Use additional code to identify:
alcohol abuse and dependence (F10-)
exposure to environmental tobacco smoke (Z77.22)
exposure to tobacco smoke in the perinatal period (P96.81)
history of tobacco use (Z87.891)
occupational exposure to environmental tobacco smoke (Z57.31)
tobacco dependence (F17-)
tobacco use (Z72.0)
✓5ᵗʰ **K05.0** **Acute gingivitis**
EXCLUDES 1 *acute necrotizing ulcerative gingivitis (A69.1)*
herpesviral [herpes simplex] gingivostomatitis (B00.2)
K05.00 **Acute gingivitis, plaque induced**
Acute gingivitis NOS
K05.01 **Acute gingivitis, non-plaque induced**

✓5ᵗʰ **K05.1** **Chronic gingivitis**
Desquamative gingivitis (chronic)
Gingivitis (chronic) NOS
Hyperplastic gingivitis (chronic)
Simple marginal gingivitis (chronic)
Ulcerative gingivitis (chronic)
K05.10 **Chronic gingivitis, plaque induced**
Chronic gingivitis NOS
Gingivitis NOS
K05.11 **Chronic gingivitis, non-plaque induced**

✓5ᵗʰ **K05.2** **Aggressive periodontitis**
Acute pericoronitis
EXCLUDES 1 *acute apical periodontitis (K04.4)*
periapical abscess (K04.7)
periapical abscess with sinus (K04.6)
K05.20 **Aggressive periodontitis, unspecified**
K05.21 **Aggressive periodontitis, localized**
Periodontal abscess
K05.22 **Aggressive periodontitis, generalized**

✓5ᵗʰ **K05.3** **Chronic periodontitis**
Chronic pericoronitis
Complex periodontitis
Periodontitis NOS
Simplex periodontitis
EXCLUDES 1 *chronic apical periodontitis (K04.5)*
K05.30 **Chronic periodontitis, unspecified**
K05.31 **Chronic periodontitis, localized**
K05.32 **Chronic periodontitis, generalized**

K05.4 **Periodontosis**
Juvenile periodontosis

K05.5 **Other periodontal diseases**
EXCLUDES 2 *leukoplakia of gingiva (K13.21)*

K05.6 **Periodontal disease, unspecified**

✓4ᵗʰ **K06** **Other disorders of gingiva and edentulous alveolar ridge**
EXCLUDES 2 *acute gingivitis (K05.0)*
atrophy of edentulous alveolar ridge (K08.2)
chronic gingivitis (K05.1)
gingivitis NOS (K05.1)

K06.0 **Gingival recession**
Gingival recession (generalized) (localized) (postinfective) (postprocedural)

K06.1 **Gingival enlargement**
Gingival fibromatosis

K06.2 **Gingival and edentulous alveolar ridge lesions associated with trauma**
Irritative hyperplasia of edentulous ridge [denture hyperplasia]
Use additional code (Chapter 20) to identify external cause or denture status (Z97.2)

K06.8 **Other specified disorders of gingiva and edentulous alveolar ridge**
Fibrous epulis
Flabby alveolar ridge
Giant cell epulis
Peripheral giant cell granuloma of gingiva
Pyogenic granuloma of gingiva
EXCLUDES 2 *gingival cyst (K09.0)*

K06.9 **Disorder of gingiva and edentulous alveolar ridge, unspecified**

✓4ᵗʰ **K08** **Other disorders of teeth and supporting structures**
EXCLUDES 2 *dentofacial anomalies [including malocclusion] (M26-)*
disorders of jaw (M27-)

K08.0 **Exfoliation of teeth due to systemic causes**
Code also underlying systemic condition

✓5ᵗʰ **K08.1** **Complete loss of teeth**
Acquired loss of teeth, complete
EXCLUDES 1 *congenital absence of teeth (K00.0)*
exfoliation of teeth due to systemic causes (K08.0)
partial loss of teeth (K08.4-)

✓6ᵗʰ **K08.10** **Complete loss of teeth, unspecified cause**
K08.101 **Complete loss of teeth, unspecified cause, class I**
K08.102 **Complete loss of teeth, unspecified cause, class II**
K08.103 **Complete loss of teeth, unspecified cause, class III**
K08.104 **Complete loss of teeth, unspecified cause, class IV**

EXCLUDES 1 Not coded here   EXCLUDES 2 Not included here   *Manifestation Code*

K08.109 Complete loss of teeth, unspecified cause, unspecified class
Edentulism NOS

✓6ᵗʰ **K08.11** **Complete loss of teeth due to trauma**

K08.111 Complete loss of teeth due to trauma, class I

K08.112 Complete loss of teeth due to trauma, class II

K08.113 Complete loss of teeth due to trauma, class III

K08.114 Complete loss of teeth due to trauma, class IV

K08.119 Complete loss of teeth due to trauma, unspecified class

✓6ᵗʰ **K08.12** **Complete loss of teeth due to periodontal diseases**

K08.121 Complete loss of teeth due to periodontal diseases, class I

K08.122 Complete loss of teeth due to periodontal diseases, class II

K08.123 Complete loss of teeth due to periodontal diseases, class III

K08.124 Complete loss of teeth due to periodontal diseases, class IV

K08.129 Complete loss of teeth due to periodontal diseases, unspecified class

✓6ᵗʰ **K08.13** **Complete loss of teeth due to caries**

K08.131 Complete loss of teeth due to caries, class I

K08.132 Complete loss of teeth due to caries, class II

K08.133 Complete loss of teeth due to caries, class III

K08.134 Complete loss of teeth due to caries, class IV

K08.139 Complete loss of teeth due to caries, unspecified class

✓6ᵗʰ **K08.19** **Complete loss of teeth due to other specified cause**

K08.191 Complete loss of teeth due to other specified cause, class I

K08.192 Complete loss of teeth due to other specified cause, class II

K08.193 Complete loss of teeth due to other specified cause, class III

K08.194 Complete loss of teeth due to other specified cause, class IV

K08.199 Complete loss of teeth due to other specified cause, unspecified class

✓5ᵗʰ **K08.2** **Atrophy of edentulous alveolar ridge**

K08.20 **Unspecified atrophy of edentulous alveolar ridge**
Atrophy of the mandible NOS
Atrophy of the maxilla NOS

K08.21 **Minimal atrophy of the mandible**
Minimal atrophy of the edentulous mandible

K08.22 **Moderate atrophy of the mandible**
Moderate atrophy of the edentulous mandible

K08.23 **Severe atrophy of the mandible**
Severe atrophy of the edentulous mandible

K08.24 **Minimal atrophy of maxilla**
Minimal atrophy of the edentulous maxilla

K08.25 **Moderate atrophy of the maxilla**
Moderate atrophy of the edentulous maxilla

K08.26 **Severe atrophy of the maxilla**
Severe atrophy of the edentulous maxilla

K08.3 **Retained dental root**

✓5ᵗʰ **K08.4** **Partial loss of teeth**
Acquired loss of teeth, partial
EXCLUDES 1 *complete loss of teeth (K08.1-)*
congenital absence of teeth (K00.0)
EXCLUDES 2 *exfoliation of teeth due to systemic causes (K08.0)*

✓6ᵗʰ **K08.40** **Partial loss of teeth, unspecified cause**

K08.401 Partial loss of teeth, unspecified cause, class I

K08.402 Partial loss of teeth, unspecified cause, class II

K08.403 Partial loss of teeth, unspecified cause, class III

K08.404 Partial loss of teeth, unspecified cause, class IV

K08.409 Partial loss of teeth, unspecified cause, unspecified class
Tooth extraction status NOS

✓6ᵗʰ **K08.41** **Partial loss of teeth due to trauma**

K08.411 Partial loss of teeth due to trauma, class I

K08.412 Partial loss of teeth due to trauma, class II

K08.413 Partial loss of teeth due to trauma, class III

K08.414 Partial loss of teeth due to trauma, class IV

K08.419 Partial loss of teeth due to trauma, unspecified class

✓6ᵗʰ **K08.42** **Partial loss of teeth due to periodontal diseases**

K08.421 Partial loss of teeth due to periodontal diseases, class I

K08.422 Partial loss of teeth due to periodontal diseases, class II

K08.423 Partial loss of teeth due to periodontal diseases, class III

K08.424 Partial loss of teeth due to periodontal diseases, class IV

K08.429 Partial loss of teeth due to periodontal diseases, unspecified class

✓6ᵗʰ **K08.43** **Partial loss of teeth due to caries**

K08.431 Partial loss of teeth due to caries, class I

K08.432 Partial loss of teeth due to caries, class II

K08.433 Partial loss of teeth due to caries, class III

K08.434 Partial loss of teeth due to caries, class IV

K08.439 Partial loss of teeth due to caries, unspecified class

✓6ᵗʰ **K08.49** **Partial loss of teeth due to other specified cause**

K08.491 Partial loss of teeth due to other specified cause, class I

K08.492 Partial loss of teeth due to other specified cause, class II

K08.493 Partial loss of teeth due to other specified cause, class III

K08.494 Partial loss of teeth due to other specified cause, class IV

K08.499 Partial loss of teeth due to other specified cause, unspecified class

✓5ᵗʰ **K08.5** **Unsatisfactory restoration of tooth**
Defective bridge, crown, filling
Defective dental restoration
EXCLUDES 1 *dental restoration status (Z98.811)*
EXCLUDES 2 *endosseous dental implant failure (M27.6-)*
unsatisfactory endodontic treatment (M27.5-)

K08.50 **Unsatisfactory restoration of tooth, unspecified**
Defective dental restoration NOS

K08.51 **Open restoration margins of tooth**
Dental restoration failure of marginal integrity
Open margin on tooth restoration
Poor gingival margin to tooth restoration

K08.52 **Unrepairable overhanging of dental restorative materials**
Overhanging of tooth restoration

✓6ᵗʰ **K08.53** **Fractured dental restorative material**
EXCLUDES 1 *cracked tooth (K03.81)*
traumatic fracture of tooth (S02.5)

K08.530 **Fractured dental restorative material without loss of material**

K08.531 **Fractured dental restorative material with loss of material**

K08.539 **Fractured dental restorative material, unspecified**

K08.54 **Contour of existing restoration of tooth biologically incompatible with oral health**
Dental restoration failure of periodontal anatomical integrity
Unacceptable contours of existing restoration of tooth
Unacceptable morphology of existing restoration of tooth

☑ Appropriate additional character required   ✓x7ᵗʰ Requires 7th character, placeholder x must fill empty characters

Diseases of the Digestive System

K08.55–K12.39

K08.55   Allergy to existing dental restorative material
Use additional code to identify the specific type of allergy

K08.56   Poor aesthetic of existing restoration of tooth
Dental restoration aesthetically inadequate or displeasing

K08.59   Other unsatisfactory restoration of tooth
Other defective dental restoration

K08.8   Other specified disorders of teeth and supporting structures
Enlargement of alveolar ridge NOS
Irregular alveolar process
Toothache NOS

K08.9   Disorder of teeth and supporting structures, unspecified

☑4ᵗʰ **K09   Cysts of oral region, not elsewhere classified**
INCLUDES   lesions showing histological features both of aneurysmal cyst and of another fibro-osseous lesion
EXCLUDES 2   cysts of jaw (M27.0-, M27.4-)
radicular cyst (K04.8)

K09.0   Developmental odontogenic cysts
Dentigerous cyst
Eruption cyst
Follicular cyst
Gingival cyst
Lateral periodontal cyst
Primordial cyst
EXCLUDES 2   keratocysts (D16.4, D16.5)
odontogenic keratocystic tumors (D16.4, D16.5)

K09.1   Developmental (nonodontogenic) cysts of oral region
Cyst (of) incisive canal
Cyst (of) palatine of papilla
Globulomaxillary cyst
Median palatal cyst
Nasoalveolar cyst
Nasolabial cyst
Nasopalatine duct cyst

K09.8   Other cysts of oral region, not elsewhere classified
Dermoid cyst
Epidermoid cyst
Lymphoepithelial cyst
Epstein's pearl

K09.9   Cyst of oral region, unspecified

☑4ᵗʰ **K11   Diseases of salivary glands**
Use additional code to identify:
alcohol abuse and dependence (F10-)
exposure to environmental tobacco smoke (Z77.22)
exposure to tobacco smoke in the perinatal period (P96.81)
history of tobacco use (Z87.891)
occupational exposure to environmental tobacco smoke (Z57.31)
tobacco dependence (F17-)
tobacco use (Z72.0)

K11.0   Atrophy of salivary gland

K11.1   Hypertrophy of salivary gland

☑5ᵗʰ **K11.2   Sialoadenitis**
Parotitis
EXCLUDES 1   epidemic parotitis (B26-)
mumps (B26-)
uveoparotid fever [Heerfordt] (D86.89)

K11.20   Sialoadenitis, unspecified

K11.21   Acute sialoadenitis
EXCLUDES 1   acute recurrent sialoadenitis (K11.22)

K11.22   Acute recurrent sialoadenitis

K11.23   Chronic sialoadenitis

K11.3   Abscess of salivary gland

K11.4   Fistula of salivary gland
EXCLUDES 1   congenital fistula of salivary gland (Q38.4)

K11.5   Sialolithiasis
Calculus of salivary gland or duct
Stone of salivary gland or duct

K11.6   Mucocele of salivary gland
Mucous extravasation cyst of salivary gland
Mucous retention cyst of salivary gland
Ranula

K11.7   Disturbances of salivary secretion
Hypoptyalism
Ptyalism
Xerostomia
EXCLUDES 2   dry mouth NOS (R68.2)

K11.8   Other diseases of salivary glands
Benign lymphoepithelial lesion of salivary gland
Mikulicz' disease
Necrotizing sialometaplasia
Sialectasia
Stenosis of salivary duct
Stricture of salivary duct
EXCLUDES 1   sicca syndrome [Sjögren] (M35.0-)

K11.9   Disease of salivary gland, unspecified
Sialoadenopathy NOS

☑4ᵗʰ **K12   Stomatitis and related lesions**
Use additional code to identify:
alcohol abuse and dependence (F10-)
exposure to environmental tobacco smoke (Z77.22)
exposure to tobacco smoke in the perinatal period (P96.81)
history of tobacco use (Z87.891)
occupational exposure to environmental tobacco smoke (Z57.31)
tobacco dependence (F17-)
tobacco use (Z72.0)
EXCLUDES 1   cancrum oris (A69.0)
cheilitis (K13.0)
gangrenous stomatitis (A69.0)
herpesviral [herpes simplex] gingivostomatitis (B00.2)
noma (A69.0)

K12.0   Recurrent oral aphthae
Aphthous stomatitis (major) (minor)
Bednar's aphthae
Periadenitis mucosa necrotica recurrens
Recurrent aphthous ulcer
Stomatitis herpetiformis

K12.1   Other forms of stomatitis
Stomatitis NOS
Denture stomatitis
Ulcerative stomatitis
Vesicular stomatitis
EXCLUDES 1   acute necrotizing ulcerative stomatitis (A69.1)
Vincent's stomatitis (A69.1)

K12.2   Cellulitis and abscess of mouth
Cellulitis of mouth (floor)
Submandibular abscess
EXCLUDES 2   abscess of salivary gland (K11.3)
abscess of tongue (K14.0)
periapical abscess (K04.6-K04.7)
periodontal abscess (K05.21)
peritonsillar abscess (J36)

☑5ᵗʰ **K12.3   Oral mucositis (ulcerative)**
Mucositis (oral) (oropharyneal)
EXCLUDES 2   gastrointestinal mucositis (ulcerative) (K92.81)
mucositis (ulcerative) of vagina and vulva (N76.81)
nasal mucositis (ulcerative) (J34.81)

K12.30   Oral mucositis (ulcerative), unspecified

K12.31   Oral mucositis (ulcerative) due to antineoplastic therapy
Code also type of associated therapy, such as:
antineoplastic and immunosuppressive drugs (T45.1x-)
radiological procedure and radiotherapy (Y84.2)

K12.32   Oral mucositis (ulcerative) due to other drugs
Code also drug (T36-T50)

K12.33   Oral mucositis (ulcerative) due to radiation
Use additional external cause code (W88-W90, X39.0-) to identify cause

K12.39   Other oral mucositis (ulcerative)
Viral oral mucositis (ulcerative)

EXCLUDES 1   Not coded here   EXCLUDES 2   Not included here   *Manifestation Code*

☑4th **K13   Other diseases of lip and oral mucosa**
    INCLUDES   epithelial disturbances of tongue
    Use additional code to identify:
        alcohol abuse and dependence (F10-)
        exposure to environmental tobacco smoke (Z77.22)
        exposure to tobacco smoke in the perinatal period (P96.81)
        history of tobacco use (Z87.891)
        occupational exposure to environmental tobacco smoke (Z57.31)
        tobacco dependence (F17-)
        tobacco use (Z72.0)
    EXCLUDES 2   certain disorders of gingiva and edentulous alveolar ridge
                (K05-K06)
            cysts of oral region (K09-)
            diseases of tongue (K14-)
            stomatitis and related lesions (K12-)

    K13.0   Diseases of lips
            Abscess of lips
            Angular cheilitis
            Cellulitis of lips
            Cheilitis NOS
            Cheilodynia
            Cheilosis
            Exfoliative cheilitis
            Fistula of lips
            Glandular cheilitis
            Hypertrophy of lips
            Perlèche NEC
            EXCLUDES 1   ariboflavinosis (E53.0)
                    cheilitis due to radiation-related disorders (L55-L59)
                    congenital fistula of lips (Q38.0)
                    congenital hypertrophy of lips (Q18.6)
                    Perlèche due to candidiasis (B37.83)
                    Perlèche due to riboflavin deficiency (E53.0)

    K13.1   Cheek and lip biting
☑5th **K13.2   Leukoplakia and other disturbances of oral epithelium,
            including tongue**
            EXCLUDES 1   carcinoma in situ of oral epithelium (D00.0-)
                    hairy leukoplakia (K13.3)
            K13.21   Leukoplakia of oral mucosa, including tongue
                    Leukokeratosis of oral mucosa
                    Leukoplakia of gingiva, lips, tongue
                    EXCLUDES 1   hairy leukoplakia (K13.3)
                            leukokeratosis nicotina palati (K13.24)
            K13.22   Minimal keratinized residual ridge mucosa
                    Minimal keratinization of alveolar ridge mucosa
            K13.23   Excessive keratinized residual ridge mucosa
                    Excessive keratinization of alveolar ridge mucosa
            K13.24   Leukokeratosis nicotina palati
                    Smoker's palate
            **K13.29   Other disturbances of oral epithelium, including
                    tongue**
                    Erythroplakia of mouth or tongue
                    Focal epithelial hyperplasia of mouth or tongue
                    Leukoedema of mouth or tongue
                    Other oral epithelium disturbances

    K13.3   Hairy leukoplakia
    K13.4   Granuloma and granuloma-like lesions of oral mucosa
            Eosinophilic granuloma
            Granuloma pyogenicum
            Verrucous xanthoma
    K13.5   Oral submucous fibrosis
            Submucous fibrosis of tongue
    K13.6   Irritative hyperplasia of oral mucosa
            EXCLUDES 2   irritative hyperplasia of edentulous ridge [denture
                    hyperplasia] (K06.2)
☑5th **K13.7   Other and unspecified lesions of oral mucosa**
            K13.70   Unspecified lesions of oral mucosa
            K13.79   Other lesions of oral mucosa
                    Focal oral mucinosis

☑4th **K14   Diseases of tongue**
    Use additional code to identify:
        alcohol abuse and dependence (F10-)
        exposure to environmental tobacco smoke (Z77.22)
        history of tobacco use (Z87.891)
        occupational exposure to environmental tobacco smoke (Z57.31)
        tobacco dependence (F17-)
        tobacco use (Z72.0)
        EXCLUDES 2   erythroplakia (K13.29)
                focal epithelial hyperplasia (K13.29)
                leukedema of tongue (K13.29)
                leukoplakia of tongue (K13.21)
                hairy leukoplakia (K13.3)
                macroglossia (congenital) (Q38.2)
                submucous fibrosis of tongue (K13.5)

    K14.0   Glossitis
            Abscess of tongue
            Ulceration (traumatic) of tongue
            EXCLUDES 1   atrophic glossitis (K14.4)
    K14.1   Geographic tongue
            Benign migratory glossitis
            Glossitis areata exfoliativa
    K14.2   Median rhomboid glossitis
    K14.3   Hypertrophy of tongue papillae
            Black hairy tongue
            Coated tongue
            Hypertrophy of foliate papillae
            Lingua villosa nigra
    K14.4   Atrophy of tongue papillae
            Atrophic glossitis
    K14.5   Plicated tongue
            Fissured tongue
            Furrowed tongue
            Scrotal tongue
            EXCLUDES 1   fissured tongue, congenital (Q38.3)
    K14.6   Glossodynia
            Glossopyrosis
            Painful tongue
    K14.8   Other diseases of tongue
            Atrophy of tongue
            Crenated tongue
            Enlargement of tongue
            Glossocele
            Glossoptosis
            Hypertrophy of tongue
    K14.9   Disease of tongue, unspecified
            Glossopathy NOS

Diseases of esophagus, stomach and duodenum (K20-K31)
    EXCLUDES 2   hiatus hernia (K44-)

☑4th **K20   Esophagitis**
    Use additional code to identify:
        alcohol abuse and dependence (F10-)
        EXCLUDES 1   erosion of esophagus (K22.1-)
                esophagitis with gastro-esophageal reflux disease (K21.0)
                reflux esophagitis (K21.0)
                ulcerative esophagitis (K22.1-)
        EXCLUDES 2   eosinophilic gastritis or gastroenteritis (K52.81)
    K20.0   Eosinophilic esophagitis
    K20.8   Other esophagitis
            Abscess of esophagus
    K20.9   Esophagitis, unspecified
            Esophagitis NOS

☑4th **K21   Gastro-esophageal reflux disease**
    EXCLUDES 1   newborn esophageal reflux (P78.83)
    K21.0   Gastro-esophageal reflux disease with esophagitis
            Reflux esophagitis
    K21.9   Gastro-esophageal reflux disease without esophagitis
            Esophageal reflux NOS

☑4th **K22   Other diseases of esophagus**
    EXCLUDES 2   esophageal varices (I85-)
    K22.0   Achalasia of cardia
            Achalasia NOS
            Cardiospasm
            EXCLUDES 1   congenital cardiospasm (Q39.5)

☑ Appropriate additional character required   ☑x7th Requires 7th character, placeholder x must fill empty characters

Diseases of the Digestive System

K22.1–K29.00

✓5th **K22.1 Ulcer of esophagus**
Barrett's ulcer
Erosion of esophagus
Fungal ulcer of esophagus
Peptic ulcer of esophagus
Ulcer of esophagus due to ingestion of chemicals
Ulcer of esophagus due to ingestion of drugs and medicaments
Ulcerative esophagitis
Code first (T36-T65) to identify drug or chemical
EXCLUDES 1 *Barrett's esophagus (K22.7)*

K22.10 Ulcer of esophagus without bleeding
Ulcer of esophagus NOS

K22.11 Ulcer of esophagus with bleeding
EXCLUDES 2 *bleeding esophageal varices (I85.01, I85.11)*

K22.2 Esophageal obstruction
Compression of esophagus
Constriction of esophagus
Stenosis of esophagus
Stricture of esophagus
EXCLUDES 1 *congenital stenosis or stricture of esophagus (Q39.3)*

K22.3 Perforation of esophagus
Rupture of esophagus
EXCLUDES 1 *traumatic perforation of (thoracic) esophagus (S27.8-)*

K22.4 Dyskinesia of esophagus
Corkscrew esophagus
Diffuse esophageal spasm
Spasm of esophagus
EXCLUDES 1 *cardiospasm (K22.0)*

K22.5 Diverticulum of esophagus, acquired
Esophageal pouch, acquired
EXCLUDES 1 *diverticulum of esophagus (congenital) (Q39.6)*

K22.6 Gastro-esophageal laceration-hemorrhage syndrome
Mallory-Weiss syndrome

✓5th **K22.7 Barrett's esophagus**
Barrett's disease
Barrett's syndrome
EXCLUDES 1 *Barrett's ulcer (K22.1)*
malignant neoplasm of esophagus (C15-)

K22.70 Barrett's esophagus without dysplasia
Barrett's esophagus NOS

✓6th **K22.71 Barrett's esophagus with dysplasia**
K22.710 Barrett's esophagus with low grade dysplasia
K22.711 Barrett's esophagus with high grade dysplasia
K22.719 Barrett's esophagus with dysplasia, unspecified

K22.8 Other specified diseases of esophagus
Hemorrhage of esophagus NOS
EXCLUDES 2 *esophageal varices (I85-)*
Paterson-Kelly syndrome (D50.1)

K22.9 Disease of esophagus, unspecified

K23 Disorders of esophagus in diseases classified elsewhere
Code first underlying disease, such as:
congenital syphilis (A50.5)
EXCLUDES 1 *late syphilis (A52.79)*
megaesophagus due to Chagas' disease (B57.31)
tuberculosis (A18.83)

✓4th **K25 Gastric ulcer**
INCLUDES erosion (acute) of stomach
pylorus ulcer (peptic)
stomach ulcer (peptic)
Use additional code to identify:
alcohol abuse and dependence (F10-)
EXCLUDES 1 *acute gastritis (K29.0-)*
peptic ulcer NOS (K27-)

K25.0 Acute gastric ulcer with hemorrhage
K25.1 Acute gastric ulcer with perforation
K25.2 Acute gastric ulcer with both hemorrhage and perforation
K25.3 Acute gastric ulcer without hemorrhage or perforation
K25.4 Chronic or unspecified gastric ulcer with hemorrhage
K25.5 Chronic or unspecified gastric ulcer with perforation
K25.6 Chronic or unspecified gastric ulcer with both hemorrhage and perforation
K25.7 Chronic gastric ulcer without hemorrhage or perforation

K25.9 Gastric ulcer, unspecified as acute or chronic, without hemorrhage or perforation

✓4th **K26 Duodenal ulcer**
INCLUDES erosion (acute) of duodenum
duodenum ulcer (peptic)
postpyloric ulcer (peptic)
Use additional code to identify:
alcohol abuse and dependence (F10-)
EXCLUDES 1 *peptic ulcer NOS (K27-)*

K26.0 Acute duodenal ulcer with hemorrhage
K26.1 Acute duodenal ulcer with perforation
K26.2 Acute duodenal ulcer with both hemorrhage and perforation
K26.3 Acute duodenal ulcer without hemorrhage or perforation
K26.4 Chronic or unspecified duodenal ulcer with hemorrhage
K26.5 Chronic or unspecified duodenal ulcer with perforation
K26.6 Chronic or unspecified duodenal ulcer with both hemorrhage and perforation
K26.7 Chronic duodenal ulcer without hemorrhage or perforation
K26.9 Duodenal ulcer, unspecified as acute or chronic, without hemorrhage or perforation

✓4th **K27 Peptic ulcer, site unspecified**
INCLUDES gastroduodenal ulcer NOS
peptic ulcer NOS
Use additional code to identify:
alcohol abuse and dependence (F10-)
EXCLUDES 1 *peptic ulcer of newborn (P78.82)*

K27.0 Acute peptic ulcer, site unspecified, with hemorrhage
K27.1 Acute peptic ulcer, site unspecified, with perforation
K27.2 Acute peptic ulcer, site unspecified, with both hemorrhage and perforation
K27.3 Acute peptic ulcer, site unspecified, without hemorrhage or perforation
K27.4 Chronic or unspecified peptic ulcer, site unspecified, with hemorrhage
K27.5 Chronic or unspecified peptic ulcer, site unspecified, with perforation
K27.6 Chronic or unspecified peptic ulcer, site unspecified, with both hemorrhage and perforation
K27.7 Chronic peptic ulcer, site unspecified, without hemorrhage or perforation
K27.9 Peptic ulcer, site unspecified, unspecified as acute or chronic, without hemorrhage or perforation

✓4th **K28 Gastrojejunal ulcer**
INCLUDES anastomotic ulcer (peptic) or erosion
gastrocolic ulcer (peptic) or erosion
gastrointestinal ulcer (peptic) or erosion
gastrojejunal ulcer (peptic) or erosion
jejunal ulcer (peptic) or erosion
marginal ulcer (peptic) or erosion
stomal ulcer (peptic) or erosion
Use additional code to identify:
alcohol abuse and dependence (F10-)
EXCLUDES 1 *primary ulcer of small intestine (K63.3)*

K28.0 Acute gastrojejunal ulcer with hemorrhage
K28.1 Acute gastrojejunal ulcer with perforation
K28.2 Acute gastrojejunal ulcer with both hemorrhage and perforation
K28.3 Acute gastrojejunal ulcer without hemorrhage or perforation
K28.4 Chronic or unspecified gastrojejunal ulcer with hemorrhage
K28.5 Chronic or unspecified gastrojejunal ulcer with perforation
K28.6 Chronic or unspecified gastrojejunal ulcer with both hemorrhage and perforation
K28.7 Chronic gastrojejunal ulcer without hemorrhage or perforation
K28.9 Gastrojejunal ulcer, unspecified as acute or chronic, without hemorrhage or perforation

✓4th **K29 Gastritis and duodenitis**
EXCLUDES 1 *eosinophilic gastritis or gastroenteritis (K52.81)*
Zollinger-Ellison syndrome (E16.4)

✓5th **K29.0 Acute gastritis**
Use additional code to identify:
alcohol abuse and dependence (F10-)
EXCLUDES 1 *erosion (acute) of stomach (K25-)*

K29.00 Acute gastritis without bleeding

EXCLUDES 1 Not coded here   **EXCLUDES 2** Not included here   *Manifestation Code*

    K29.01   **Acute gastritis with bleeding**

√5ᵗʰ   **K29.2**   **Alcoholic gastritis**
    Use additional code to identify:
      alcohol abuse and dependence (F10-)
    K29.20   **Alcoholic gastritis without bleeding**
    K29.21   **Alcoholic gastritis with bleeding**

√5ᵗʰ   **K29.3**   **Chronic superficial gastritis**
    K29.30   **Chronic superficial gastritis without bleeding**
    K29.31   **Chronic superficial gastritis with bleeding**

√5ᵗʰ   **K29.4**   **Chronic atrophic gastritis**
    Gastric atrophy
    K29.40   **Chronic atrophic gastritis without bleeding**
    K29.41   **Chronic atrophic gastritis with bleeding**

√5ᵗʰ   **K29.5**   **Unspecified chronic gastritis**
    Chronic antral gastritis
    Chronic fundal gastritis
    K29.50   **Unspecified chronic gastritis without bleeding**
    K29.51   **Unspecified chronic gastritis with bleeding**

√5ᵗʰ   **K29.6**   **Other gastritis**
    Giant hypertrophic gastritis
    Granulomatous gastritis
    Ménétrier's disease
    K29.60   **Other gastritis without bleeding**
    K29.61   **Other gastritis with bleeding**

√5ᵗʰ   **K29.7**   **Gastritis, unspecified**
    K29.70   **Gastritis, unspecified, without bleeding**
    K29.71   **Gastritis, unspecified, with bleeding**

√5ᵗʰ   **K29.8**   **Duodenitis**
    K29.80   **Duodenitis without bleeding**
    K29.81   **Duodenitis with bleeding**

√5ᵗʰ   **K29.9**   **Gastroduodenitis, unspecified**
    K29.90   **Gastroduodenitis, unspecified, without bleeding**
    K29.91   **Gastroduodenitis, unspecified, with bleeding**

K30   **Functional dyspepsia**
    Indigestion
    EXCLUDES 1   dyspepsia NOS (R10.13)
         heartburn (R12)
         nervous dyspepsia (F45.8)
         neurotic dyspepsia (F45.8)
         psychogenic dyspepsia (F45.8)

√4ᵗʰ   **K31**   **Other diseases of stomach and duodenum**
    INCLUDES   functional disorders of stomach
    EXCLUDES 2   diabetic gastroparesis (E08.43, E09.43, E10.43, E11.43, E13.43)
         diverticulum of duodenum (K57.00-K57.11)

    K31.0   **Acute dilatation of stomach**
      Acute distention of stomach

    K31.1   **Adult hypertrophic pyloric stenosis**
      Pyloric stenosis NOS
      EXCLUDES 1   congenital or infantile pyloric stenosis (Q40.0)

    K31.2   **Hourglass stricture and stenosis of stomach**
      EXCLUDES 1   congenital hourglass stomach (Q40.2)
         hourglass contraction of stomach (K31.89)

    K31.3   **Pylorospasm, not elsewhere classified**
      EXCLUDES 1   congenital or infantile pylorospasm (Q40.0)
         neurotic pylorospasm (F45.8)
         psychogenic pylorospasm (F45.8)

    K31.4   **Gastric diverticulum**
      EXCLUDES 1   congenital diverticulum of stomach (Q40.2)

    K31.5   **Obstruction of duodenum**
      Constriction of duodenum
      Duodenal ileus (chronic)
      Stenosis of duodenum
      Stricture of duodenum
      Volvulus of duodenum
      EXCLUDES 1   congenital stenosis of duodenum (Q41.0)

    K31.6   **Fistula of stomach and duodenum**
      Gastrocolic fistula
      Gastrojejunocolic fistula

    K31.7   **Polyp of stomach and duodenum**
      EXCLUDES 1   adenomatous polyp of stomach (D13.1)

√5ᵗʰ   **K31.8**   **Other specified diseases of stomach and duodenum**
      √6ᵗʰ   **K31.81**   **Angiodysplasia of stomach and duodenum**
          K31.811   **Angiodysplasia of stomach and duodenum with bleeding**

          K31.819   **Angiodysplasia of stomach and duodenum without bleeding**
            Angiodysplasia of stomach and duodenum NOS

      K31.82   **Dieulafoy lesion (hemorrhagic) of stomach and duodenum**
        EXCLUDES 2   Dieulafoy lesion of intestine (K63.81)

      K31.83   **Achlorhydria**
      K31.89   **Other diseases of stomach and duodenum**

    K31.9   **Disease of stomach and duodenum, unspecified**

Diseases of appendix (K35-K38)

√4ᵗʰ   **K35**   **Acute appendicitis**
    K35.2   **Acute appendicitis with generalized peritonitis**
      Appendicitis (acute) with generalized (diffuse) peritonitis
        following rupture or perforation of appendix
      Appendicitis with peritonitis NOS
      Perforated appendix NOS
      Ruptured appendix NOS

    K35.3   **Acute appendicitis with localized peritonitis**
      Acute appendicitis with localized peritonitis with or without
        rupture or perforation of appendix
      Acute appendicitis with peritoneal abscess

√5ᵗʰ   **K35.8**   **Other and unspecified acute appendicitis**
      K35.80   **Unspecified acute appendicitis**
        Acute appendicitis NOS
        Acute appendicitis without (localized) (generalized)
          peritonitis
      K35.89   **Other acute appendicitis**

    K36   **Other appendicitis**
      Chronic appendicitis
      Recurrent appendicitis

    K37   **Unspecified appendicitis**
      EXCLUDES 1   unspecified appendicitis with peritonitis (K35.2-K35.3)

√4ᵗʰ   **K38**   **Other diseases of appendix**
    K38.0   **Hyperplasia of appendix**
    K38.1   **Appendicular concretions**
      Fecalith of appendix
      Stercolith of appendix
    K38.2   **Diverticulum of appendix**
    K38.3   **Fistula of appendix**
    K38.8   **Other specified diseases of appendix**
      Intussusception of appendix
    K38.9   **Disease of appendix, unspecified**

Hernia (K40-K46)

    NOTE   Hernia with both gangrene and obstruction is classified to hernia with gangrene.
    INCLUDES   acquired hernia
      congenital [except diaphragmatic or hiatus] hernia
      recurrent hernia

√4ᵗʰ   **K40**   **Inguinal hernia**
    INCLUDES   bubonocele
      direct inguinal hernia
      double inguinal hernia
      indirect inguinal hernia
      inguinal hernia NOS
      oblique inguinal hernia
      scrotal hernia

√5ᵗʰ   **K40.0**   **Bilateral inguinal hernia, with obstruction, without gangrene**
      Inguinal hernia (bilateral) causing obstruction without gangrene
      Incarcerated inguinal hernia (bilateral) without gangrene
      Irreducible inguinal hernia (bilateral) without gangrene
      Strangulated inguinal hernia (bilateral) without gangrene
      K40.00   **Bilateral inguinal hernia, with obstruction, without gangrene, not specified as recurrent**
        Bilateral inguinal hernia, with obstruction, without gangrene NOS
      K40.01   **Bilateral inguinal hernia, with obstruction, without gangrene, recurrent**

√5ᵗʰ   **K40.1**   **Bilateral inguinal hernia, with gangrene**
      K40.10   **Bilateral inguinal hernia, with gangrene, not specified as recurrent**
        Bilateral inguinal hernia, with gangrene NOS

K40.11 Bilateral inguinal hernia, with gangrene, recurrent

✓5th **K40.2** Bilateral inguinal hernia, without obstruction or gangrene

K40.20 Bilateral inguinal hernia, without obstruction or gangrene, not specified as recurrent
Bilateral inguinal hernia NOS

K40.21 Bilateral inguinal hernia, without obstruction or gangrene, recurrent

✓5th **K40.3** Unilateral inguinal hernia, with obstruction, without gangrene
Inguinal hernia (unilateral) causing obstruction without gangrene
Incarcerated inguinal hernia (unilateral) without gangrene
Irreducible inguinal hernia (unilateral) without gangrene
Strangulated inguinal hernia (unilateral) without gangrene

K40.30 Unilateral inguinal hernia, with obstruction, without gangrene, not specified as recurrent
Inguinal hernia, with obstruction NOS
Unilateral inguinal hernia, with obstruction, without gangrene NOS

K40.31 Unilateral inguinal hernia, with obstruction, without gangrene, recurrent

✓5th **K40.4** Unilateral inguinal hernia, with gangrene

K40.40 Unilateral inguinal hernia, with gangrene, not specified as recurrent
Inguinal hernia with gangrene NOS
Unilateral inguinal hernia with gangrene NOS

K40.41 Unilateral inguinal hernia, with gangrene, recurrent

✓5th **K40.9** Unilateral inguinal hernia, without obstruction or gangrene

K40.90 Unilateral inguinal hernia, without obstruction or gangrene, not specified as recurrent
Inguinal hernia NOS
Unilateral inguinal hernia NOS

K40.91 Unilateral inguinal hernia, without obstruction or gangrene, recurrent

✓4th **K41 Femoral hernia**

✓5th **K41.0** Bilateral femoral hernia, with obstruction, without gangrene
Femoral hernia (bilateral) causing obstruction, without gangrene
Incarcerated femoral hernia (bilateral), without gangrene
Irreducible femoral hernia (bilateral), without gangrene
Strangulated femoral hernia (bilateral), without gangrene

K41.00 Bilateral femoral hernia, with obstruction, without gangrene, not specified as recurrent
Bilateral femoral hernia, with obstruction, without gangrene NOS

K41.01 Bilateral femoral hernia, with obstruction, without gangrene, recurrent

✓5th **K41.1** Bilateral femoral hernia, with gangrene

K41.10 Bilateral femoral hernia, with gangrene, not specified as recurrent
Bilateral femoral hernia, with gangrene NOS

K41.11 Bilateral femoral hernia, with gangrene, recurrent

✓5th **K41.2** Bilateral femoral hernia, without obstruction or gangrene

K41.20 Bilateral femoral hernia, without obstruction or gangrene, not specified as recurrent
Bilateral femoral hernia NOS

K41.21 Bilateral femoral hernia, without obstruction or gangrene, recurrent

✓5th **K41.3** Unilateral femoral hernia, with obstruction, without gangrene
Femoral hernia (unilateral) causing obstruction, without gangrene
Incarcerated femoral hernia (unilateral), without gangrene
Irreducible femoral hernia (unilateral), without gangrene
Strangulated femoral hernia (unilateral), without gangrene

K41.30 Unilateral femoral hernia, with obstruction, without gangrene, not specified as recurrent
Femoral hernia, with obstruction NOS
Unilateral femoral hernia, with obstruction NOS

K41.31 Unilateral femoral hernia, with obstruction, without gangrene, recurrent

✓5th **K41.4** Unilateral femoral hernia, with gangrene

K41.40 Unilateral femoral hernia, with gangrene, not specified as recurrent
Femoral hernia, with gangrene NOS
Unilateral femoral hernia, with gangrene NOS

K41.41 Unilateral femoral hernia, with gangrene, recurrent

✓5th **K41.9** Unilateral femoral hernia, without obstruction or gangrene

K41.90 Unilateral femoral hernia, without obstruction or gangrene, not specified as recurrent
Femoral hernia NOS
Unilateral femoral hernia NOS

K41.91 Unilateral femoral hernia, without obstruction or gangrene, recurrent

✓4th **K42 Umbilical hernia**
INCLUDES paraumbilical hernia
EXCLUDES 1 omphalocele (Q79.2)

K42.0 Umbilical hernia with obstruction, without gangrene
Umbilical hernia causing obstruction, without gangrene
Incarcerated umbilical hernia, without gangrene
Irreducible umbilical hernia, without gangrene
Strangulated umbilical hernia, without gangrene

K42.1 Umbilical hernia with gangrene
Gangrenous umbilical hernia

K42.9 Umbilical hernia without obstruction or gangrene
Umbilical hernia NOS

✓4th **K43 Ventral hernia**

✓5th **K43.0** Ventral hernia with obstruction, without gangrene
Ventral hernia causing obstruction, without gangrene
Incarcerated ventral hernia, without gangrene
Irreducible ventral hernia, without gangrene
Strangulated ventral hernia, without gangrene

K43.00 Ventral hernia, unspecified, with obstruction, without gangrene

K43.01 Incisional hernia, with obstruction, without gangrene

K43.09 Other ventral hernia, with obstruction, without gangrene
Epigastric hernia

✓5th **K43.1** Ventral hernia with gangrene
Gangrenous ventral hernia

K43.10 Ventral hernia, unspecified, with gangrene

K43.11 Incisional hernia, with gangrene

K43.19 Other ventral hernia, with gangrene
Epigastric hernia

✓5th **K43.9** Ventral hernia without obstruction or gangrene

K43.90 Ventral hernia, unspecified, without obstruction or gangrene
Ventral hernia NOS

K43.91 Incisional hernia, without obstruction or gangrene

K43.99 Other ventral hernia, without obstruction or gangrene
Epigastric hernia

✓4th **K44 Diaphragmatic hernia**
INCLUDES hiatus hernia (esophageal) (sliding)
paraesophageal hernia
EXCLUDES 1 congenital diaphragmatic hernia (Q79.0)
congenital hiatus hernia (Q40.1)

K44.0 Diaphragmatic hernia with obstruction, without gangrene
Diaphragmatic hernia causing obstruction
Incarcerated diaphragmatic hernia
Irreducible diaphragmatic hernia
Strangulated diaphragmatic hernia

K44.1 Diaphragmatic hernia with gangrene
Gangrenous diaphragmatic hernia

K44.9 Diaphragmatic hernia without obstruction or gangrene
Diaphragmatic hernia NOS

✓4th **K45 Other abdominal hernia**
INCLUDES abdominal hernia, specified site NEC
lumbar hernia
obturator hernia
pudendal hernia
retroperitoneal hernia
sciatic hernia

K45.0 Other specified abdominal hernia with obstruction, without gangrene
Other specified abdominal hernia causing obstruction
Other specified incarcerated abdominal hernia
Other specified irreducible abdominal hernia
Other specified strangulated abdominal hernia

K45.1 Other specified abdominal hernia with gangrene
Any condition listed under K4 specified as gangrenous

EXCLUDES 1 Not coded here   EXCLUDES 2 Not included here   *Manifestation Code*

K45.8 **Other specified abdominal hernia without obstruction or gangrene**

☑4ᵗʰ **K46 Unspecified abdominal hernia**
INCLUDES enterocele
epiplocele
hernia NOS
interstitial hernia
intestinal hernia
intra-abdominal hernia
EXCLUDES 1 *vaginal enterocele (N81.5)*

K46.0 **Unspecified abdominal hernia with obstruction, without gangrene**
Unspecified abdominal hernia causing obstruction
Unspecified incarcerated abdominal hernia
Unspecified irreducible abdominal hernia
Unspecified strangulated abdominal hernia

K46.1 **Unspecified abdominal hernia with gangrene**
Any condition listed under K46 specified as gangrenous

K46.9 **Unspecified abdominal hernia without obstruction or gangrene**
Abdominal hernia NOS

Noninfective enteritis and colitis (K50-K52)

INCLUDES noninfective inflammatory bowel disease
EXCLUDES 1 *irritable bowel syndrome (K58-)*
megacolon (K59.3)

☑4ᵗʰ **K50 Crohn's disease [regional enteritis]**
INCLUDES granulomatous enteritis
EXCLUDES 1 *ulcerative colitis (K51-)*
Use additional code to identify manifestations, such as:
pyoderma gangrenosum (L88)

☑5ᵗʰ **K50.0 Crohn's disease of small intestine**
Crohn's disease [regional enteritis] of duodenum
Crohn's disease [regional enteritis] of ileum
Crohn's disease [regional enteritis] of jejunum
Regional ileitis
Terminal ileitis
EXCLUDES 1 *Crohn's disease of both small and large intestine (K50.8-)*

K50.00 **Crohn's disease of small intestine without complications**

☑6ᵗʰ K50.01 **Crohn's disease of small intestine with complications**

K50.011 **Crohn's disease of small intestine with rectal bleeding**

K50.012 **Crohn's disease of small intestine with intestinal obstruction**

K50.013 **Crohn's disease of small intestine with fistula**

K50.014 **Crohn's disease of small intestine with abscess**

K50.018 **Crohn's disease of small intestine with other complication**

K50.019 **Crohn's disease of small intestine with unspecified complications**

☑5ᵗʰ **K50.1 Crohn's disease of large intestine**
Crohn's disease [regional enteritis] of colon
Crohn's disease [regional enteritis] of large bowel
Crohn's disease [regional enteritis] of rectum
Granulomatous colitis
Regional colitis
EXCLUDES 1 *Crohn's disease of both small and large intestine (K50.8)*

K50.10 **Crohn's disease of large intestine without complications**

☑6ᵗʰ K50.11 **Crohn's disease of large intestine with complications**

K50.111 **Crohn's disease of large intestine with rectal bleeding**

K50.112 **Crohn's disease of large intestine with intestinal obstruction**

K50.113 **Crohn's disease of large intestine with fistula**

K50.114 **Crohn's disease of large intestine with abscess**

K50.118 **Crohn's disease of large intestine with other complication**

K50.119 **Crohn's disease of large intestine with unspecified complications**

☑5ᵗʰ **K50.8 Crohn's disease of both small and large intestine**

K50.80 **Crohn's disease of both small and large intestine without complications**

☑6ᵗʰ K50.81 **Crohn's disease of both small and large intestine with complications**

K50.811 **Crohn's disease of both small and large intestine with rectal bleeding**

K50.812 **Crohn's disease of both small and large intestine with intestinal obstruction**

K50.813 **Crohn's disease of both small and large intestine with fistula**

K50.814 **Crohn's disease of both small and large intestine with abscess**

K50.818 **Crohn's disease of both small and large intestine with other complication**

K50.819 **Crohn's disease of both small and large intestine with unspecified complications**

☑5ᵗʰ **K50.9 Crohn's disease, unspecified**

K50.90 **Crohn's disease, unspecified, without complications**
Crohn's disease NOS
Regional enteritis NOS

☑6ᵗʰ K50.91 **Crohn's disease, unspecified, with complications**

K50.911 **Crohn's disease, unspecified, with rectal bleeding**

K50.912 **Crohn's disease, unspecified, with intestinal obstruction**

K50.913 **Crohn's disease, unspecified, with fistula**

K50.914 **Crohn's disease, unspecified, with abscess**

K50.918 **Crohn's disease, unspecified, with other complication**

K50.919 **Crohn's disease, unspecified, with unspecified complications**

☑4ᵗʰ **K51 Ulcerative colitis**
Use additional code to identify manifestations, such as:
pyoderma gangrenosum (L88)
EXCLUDES 1 *Crohn's disease [regional enteritis] (K50-)*

☑5ᵗʰ **K51.0 Ulcerative (chronic) pancolitis**
Backwash ileitis

K51.00 **Ulcerative (chronic) pancolitis without complications**
Ulcerative (chronic) pancolitis NOS

☑6ᵗʰ K51.01 **Ulcerative (chronic) pancolitis with complications**

K51.011 **Ulcerative (chronic) pancolitis with rectal bleeding**

K51.012 **Ulcerative (chronic) pancolitis with intestinal obstruction**

K51.013 **Ulcerative (chronic) pancolitis with fistula**

K51.014 **Ulcerative (chronic) pancolitis with abscess**

K51.018 **Ulcerative (chronic) pancolitis with other complication**

K51.019 **Ulcerative (chronic) pancolitis with unspecified complications**

☑5ᵗʰ **K51.2 Ulcerative (chronic) proctitis**

K51.20 **Ulcerative (chronic) proctitis without complications**
Ulcerative (chronic) proctitis NOS

☑6ᵗʰ K51.21 **Ulcerative (chronic) proctitis with complications**

K51.211 **Ulcerative (chronic) proctitis with rectal bleeding**

K51.212 **Ulcerative (chronic) proctitis with intestinal obstruction**

K51.213 **Ulcerative (chronic) proctitis with fistula**

K51.214 **Ulcerative (chronic) proctitis with abscess**

K51.218 **Ulcerative (chronic) proctitis with other complication**

K51.219 **Ulcerative (chronic) proctitis with unspecified complications**

☑5ᵗʰ **K51.3 Ulcerative (chronic) rectosigmoiditis**

K51.30 **Ulcerative (chronic) rectosigmoiditis without complications**
Ulcerative (chronic) rectosigmoiditis NOS

☑ Appropriate additional character required ☑x7ᵗʰ Requires 7th character, placeholder x must fill empty characters

√6ᵗʰ K51.31 Ulcerative (chronic) rectosigmoiditis with complications
    K51.311 Ulcerative (chronic) rectosigmoiditis with rectal bleeding
    K51.312 Ulcerative (chronic) rectosigmoiditis with intestinal obstruction
    K51.313 Ulcerative (chronic) rectosigmoiditis with fistula
    K51.314 Ulcerative (chronic) rectosigmoiditis with abscess
    K51.318 Ulcerative (chronic) rectosigmoiditis with other complication
    K51.319 Ulcerative (chronic) rectosigmoiditis with unspecified complications

√5ᵗʰ K51.4 Inflammatory polyps of colon
    EXCLUDES 1   adenomatous polyp of colon (D12.6)
         polyposis of colon (D12.6)
         polyps of colon NOS (K63.5)
    K51.40 Inflammatory polyps of colon without complications
         Inflammatory polyps of colon NOS
    √6ᵗʰ K51.41 Inflammatory polyps of colon with complications
        K51.411 Inflammatory polyps of colon with rectal bleeding
        K51.412 Inflammatory polyps of colon with intestinal obstruction
        K51.413 Inflammatory polyps of colon with fistula
        K51.414 Inflammatory polyps of colon with abscess
        K51.418 Inflammatory polyps of colon with other complication
        K51.419 Inflammatory polyps of colon with unspecified complications

√5ᵗʰ K51.5 Left sided colitis
     Left hemicolitis
    K51.50 Left sided colitis without complications
         Left sided colitis NOS
    √6ᵗʰ K51.51 Left sided colitis with complications
        K51.511 Left sided colitis with rectal bleeding
        K51.512 Left sided colitis with intestinal obstruction
        K51.513 Left sided colitis with fistula
        K51.514 Left sided colitis with abscess
        K51.518 Left sided colitis with other complication
        K51.519 Left sided colitis with unspecified complications

√5ᵗʰ K51.8 Other ulcerative colitis
    K51.80 Other ulcerative colitis without complications
    √6ᵗʰ K51.81 Other ulcerative colitis with complications
        K51.811 Other ulcerative colitis with rectal bleeding
        K51.812 Other ulcerative colitis with intestinal obstruction
        K51.813 Other ulcerative colitis with fistula
        K51.814 Other ulcerative colitis with abscess
        K51.818 Other ulcerative colitis with other complication
        K51.819 Other ulcerative colitis with unspecified complications

√5ᵗʰ K51.9 Ulcerative colitis, unspecified
    K51.90 Ulcerative colitis, unspecified, without complications
    √6ᵗʰ K51.91 Ulcerative colitis, unspecified, with complications
        K51.911 Ulcerative colitis, unspecified with rectal bleeding
        K51.912 Ulcerative colitis, unspecified with intestinal obstruction
        K51.913 Ulcerative colitis, unspecified with fistula
        K51.914 Ulcerative colitis, unspecified with abscess
        K51.918 Ulcerative colitis, unspecified with other complication
        K51.919 Ulcerative colitis, unspecified with unspecified complications

√4ᵗʰ K52 Other and unspecified noninfective gastroenteritis and colitis
    K52.0 Gastroenteritis and colitis due to radiation
    K52.1 Toxic gastroenteritis and colitis
         Code first (T51-T65) to identify toxic agent
    K52.2 Allergic and dietetic gastroenteritis and colitis
         Food hypersensitivity gastroenteritis or colitis
         Use additional code to identify type of food allergy (Z91.01-, Z91.02-)
    √5ᵗʰ K52.8 Other specified noninfective gastroenteritis and colitis
        K52.81 Eosinophilic gastritis or gastroenteritis
             Eosinophilic enteritis
            EXCLUDES 1   eosinophilic esophagitis (K20.0)
        K52.82 Eosinophilic colitis
        K52.89 Other specified noninfective gastroenteritis and colitis
             Collagenous colitis
             Lymphocytic colitis
             Microscopic colitis (collagenous or lymphocytic)
    K52.9 Noninfective gastroenteritis and colitis, unspecified
         Colitis NOS
         Enteritis NOS
         Gastroenteritis NOS
         Ileitis NOS
         Jejunitis NOS
         Sigmoiditis NOS
        EXCLUDES 1   diarrhea NOS (R19.7)
             functional diarrhea (K59.1)
             infectious gastroenteritis and colitis NOS (A09)
             neonatal diarrhea (noninfective) (P78.3)
             psychogenic diarrhea (F45.8)

Other diseases of intestines (K55-K63)

√4ᵗʰ K55 Vascular disorders of intestine
    EXCLUDES 1   necrotizing enterocolitis of newborn (P77-)
    K55.0 Acute vascular disorders of intestine
         Acute fulminant ischemic colitis
         Acute intestinal infarction
         Acute small intestine ischemia
         Infarction of appendices epiploicae
         Mesenteric (artery) (vein) embolism
         Mesenteric (artery) (vein) infarction
         Mesenteric (artery) (vein) thrombosis
         Necrosis of intestine
         Subacute ischemic colitis
    K55.1 Chronic vascular disorders of intestine
         Chronic ischemic colitis
         Chronic ischemic enteritis
         Chronic ischemic enterocolitis
         Ischemic stricture of intestine
         Mesenteric atherosclerosis
         Mesenteric vascular insufficiency
    √5ᵗʰ K55.2 Angiodysplasia of colon
        K55.20 Angiodysplasia of colon without hemorrhage
        K55.21 Angiodysplasia of colon with hemorrhage
    K55.8 Other vascular disorders of intestine
    K55.9 Vascular disorder of intestine, unspecified
         Ischemic colitis
         Ischemic enteritis
         Ischemic enterocolitis

√4ᵗʰ K56 Paralytic ileus and intestinal obstruction without hernia
    EXCLUDES 1   congenital stricture or stenosis of intestine (Q41-Q42)
         cystic fibrosis with meconium ileus (E84.11)
         intestinal obstruction with hernia (K40-K46)
         ischemic stricture of intestine (K55.1)
         meconium ileus NOS (P76.0)
         neonatal intestinal obstructions classifiable to P76-
         obstruction of duodenum (K31.5)
         postprocedural intestinal obstruction (K91.3)
         stenosis of anus or rectum (K62.4)
    K56.0 Paralytic ileus
         Paralysis of bowel
         Paralysis of colon
         Paralysis of intestine
        EXCLUDES 1   gallstone ileus (K56.3)
             ileus NOS (K56.7)
             obstructive ileus NOS (K56.69)

EXCLUDES 1 Not coded here   **EXCLUDES 2** Not included here   *Manifestation Code*

K56.1 Intussusception
Intussusception or invagination of bowel
Intussusception or invagination of colon
Intussusception or invagination of intestine
Intussusception or invagination of rectum
EXCLUDES 2 *intussusception of appendix (K38.8)*

K56.2 Volvulus
Strangulation of colon or intestine
Torsion of colon or intestine
Twist of colon or intestine
EXCLUDES 2 *volvulus of duodenum (K31.5)*

K56.3 Gallstone ileus
Obstruction of intestine by gallstone

✓5th **K56.4 Other impaction of intestine**
  K56.41 Fecal impaction
    EXCLUDES 1 *constipation (K59.0-)*
    incomplete defecation (R15.0)
  K56.49 Other impaction of intestine

K56.5 Intestinal adhesions [bands] with obstruction (postprocedural) (postinfection)
Abdominal hernia due to adhesions with obstruction
Peritoneal adhesions [bands] with intestinal obstruction (postprocedural) (postinfection)

✓5th **K56.6 Other and unspecified intestinal obstruction**
  K56.60 Unspecified intestinal obstruction
    Intestinal obstruction NOS
    EXCLUDES 1 *intestinal obstruction due to specified condition—code to condition*
  K56.69 Other intestinal obstruction
    Enterostenosis NOS
    Obstructive ileus NOS
    Occlusion of colon or intestine NOS
    Stenosis of colon or intestine NOS
    Stricture of colon or intestine NOS
    EXCLUDES 1 *intestinal obstruction due to specified condition—code to condition*

K56.7 Ileus, unspecified
EXCLUDES 1 *obstructive ileus (K56.69)*

✓4th **K57 Diverticular disease of intestine**
EXCLUDES 1 *congenital diverticulum of intestine (Q43.8)*
Meckel's diverticulum (Q43.0)
EXCLUDES 2 *diverticulum of appendix (K38.2)*

✓5th **K57.0 Diverticulitis of small intestine with perforation and abscess**
Diverticulitis of small intestine with peritonitis
EXCLUDES 1 *diverticulitis of both small and large intestine with perforation and abscess (K57.4-)*
  K57.00 Diverticulitis of small intestine with perforation and abscess without bleeding
  K57.01 Diverticulitis of small intestine with perforation and abscess with bleeding

✓5th **K57.1 Diverticular disease of small intestine without perforation or abscess**
EXCLUDES 1 *diverticular disease of both small and large intestine without perforation or abscess (K57.5-)*
  K57.10 Diverticulosis of small intestine without perforation or abscess without bleeding
    Diverticular disease of small intestine NOS
  K57.11 Diverticulosis of small intestine without perforation or abscess with bleeding
  K57.12 Diverticulitis of small intestine without perforation or abscess without bleeding
  K57.13 Diverticulitis of small intestine without perforation or abscess with bleeding

✓5th **K57.2 Diverticulitis of large intestine with perforation and abscess**
Diverticulitis of colon with peritonitis
EXCLUDES 1 *diverticulitis of both small and large intestine with perforation and abscess (K57.4-)*
  K57.20 Diverticulitis of large intestine with perforation and abscess without bleeding
  K57.21 Diverticulitis of large intestine with perforation and abscess with bleeding

✓5th **K57.3 Diverticular disease of large intestine without perforation or abscess**
EXCLUDES 1 *diverticular disease of both small and large intestine without perforation or abscess (K57.5-)*
  K57.30 Diverticulosis of large intestine without perforation or abscess without bleeding
    Diverticular disease of colon NOS
  K57.31 Diverticulosis of large intestine without perforation or abscess with bleeding
  K57.32 Diverticulitis of large intestine without perforation or abscess without bleeding
  K57.33 Diverticulitis of large intestine without perforation or abscess with bleeding

✓5th **K57.4 Diverticulitis of both small and large intestine with perforation and abscess**
Diverticulitis of both small and large intestine with peritonitis
  K57.40 Diverticulitis of both small and large intestine with perforation and abscess without bleeding
  K57.41 Diverticulitis of both small and large intestine with perforation and abscess with bleeding

✓5th **K57.5 Diverticular disease of both small and large intestine without perforation or abscess**
  K57.50 Diverticulosis of both small and large intestine without perforation or abscess without bleeding
    Diverticular disease of both small and large intestine NOS
  K57.51 Diverticulosis of both small and large intestine without perforation or abscess with bleeding
  K57.52 Diverticulitis of both small and large intestine without perforation or abscess without bleeding
  K57.53 Diverticulitis of both small and large intestine without perforation or abscess with bleeding

✓5th **K57.8 Diverticulitis of intestine, part unspecified, with perforation and abscess**
Diverticulitis of intestine NOS with peritonitis
  K57.80 Diverticulitis of intestine, part unspecified, with perforation and abscess without bleeding
  K57.81 Diverticulitis of intestine, part unspecified, with perforation and abscess with bleeding

✓5th **K57.9 Diverticular disease of intestine, part unspecified, without perforation or abscess**
  K57.90 Diverticulosis of intestine, part unspecified, without perforation or abscess without bleeding
    Diverticular disease of intestine NOS
  K57.91 Diverticulosis of intestine, part unspecified, without perforation or abscess with bleeding
  K57.92 Diverticulitis of intestine, part unspecified, without perforation or abscess without bleeding
  K57.93 Diverticulitis of intestine, part unspecified, without perforation or abscess with bleeding

✓4th **K58 Irritable bowel syndrome**
INCLUDES *irritable colon*
spastic colon
K58.0 Irritable bowel syndrome with diarrhea
K58.9 Irritable bowel syndrome without diarrhea
Irritable bowel syndrome NOS

✓4th **K59 Other functional intestinal disorders**
EXCLUDES 1 *change in bowel habit NOS (R19.4)*
intestinal malabsorption (K90-)
psychogenic intestinal disorders (F45.8)
EXCLUDES 2 *functional disorders of stomach (K31-)*

✓5th **K59.0 Constipation**
EXCLUDES 1 *fecal impaction (K56.41)*
incomplete defecation (R15.0)
  K59.00 Constipation, unspecified
  K59.01 Slow transit constipation
  K59.02 Outlet dysfunction constipation
  K59.09 Other constipation

K59.1 Functional diarrhea
EXCLUDES 1 *diarrhea NOS (R19.7)*
irritable bowel syndrome with diarrhea (K58.0)

K59.2 Neurogenic bowel, not elsewhere classified

✓ Appropriate additional character required   ✓x7th Requires 7th character, placeholder x must fill empty characters

K59.3 **Megacolon, not elsewhere classified**
Dilatation of colon
Toxic megacolon
Code first (T51-T65) to identify toxic agent
> EXCLUDES 1   *congenital megacolon (aganglionic) (Q43.1)*
> *Hirschsprung's disease (Q43.1)*
> *megacolon in Chagas' disease (B57.32)*

K59.4 **Anal spasm**
Proctalgia fugax

K59.8 **Other specified functional intestinal disorders**
Atony of colon
Pseudo-obstruction (acute) (chronic) of intestine

K59.9 **Functional intestinal disorder, unspecified**

✓4ᵗʰ **K60** **Fissure and fistula of anal and rectal regions**
> EXCLUDES 1   *fissure and fistula of anal and rectal regions with abscess or cellulitis (K61-)*
> EXCLUDES 2   *anal sphincter tear (healed) (nontraumatic) (old) (K62.81)*

K60.0 **Acute anal fissure**

K60.1 **Chronic anal fissure**

K60.2 **Anal fissure, unspecified**

K60.3 **Anal fistula**

K60.4 **Rectal fistula**
Fistula of rectum to skin
> EXCLUDES 1   *rectovaginal fistula (N82.3)*
> *vesicorectal fistual (N32.1)*

K60.5 **Anorectal fistula**

✓4ᵗʰ **K61** **Abscess of anal and rectal regions**
> INCLUDES   abscess of anal and rectal regions
> cellulitis of anal and rectal regions

K61.0 **Anal abscess**
Perianal abscess
> EXCLUDES 1   *intrasphincteric abscess (K61.4)*

K61.1 **Rectal abscess**
Perirectal abscess
> EXCLUDES 1   *ischiorectal abscess (K61.3)*

K61.2 **Anorectal abscess**

K61.3 **Ischiorectal abscess**
Abscess of ischiorectal fossa

K61.4 **Intrasphincteric abscess**

✓4ᵗʰ **K62** **Other diseases of anus and rectum**
> INCLUDES   anal canal
> EXCLUDES 2   *colostomy and enterostomy malfunction (K94.0-, K94.1-)*
> *fecal incontinence (R15)*
> *hemorrhoids (I84-)*

K62.0 **Anal polyp**

K62.1 **Rectal polyp**
> EXCLUDES 1   *adenomatous polyp (D12.8)*

K62.2 **Anal prolapse**
Prolapse of anal canal

K62.3 **Rectal prolapse**
Prolapse of rectal mucosa

K62.4 **Stenosis of anus and rectum**
Stricture of anus (sphincter)

K62.5 **Hemorrhage of anus and rectum**
> EXCLUDES 1   *gastrointestinal bleeding NOS (K92.2)*
> *melena (K92.1)*
> *neonatal rectal hemorrhage (P54.2)*

K62.6 **Ulcer of anus and rectum**
Solitary ulcer of anus and rectum
Stercoral ulcer of anus and rectum
> EXCLUDES 1   *fissure and fistula of anus and rectum (K60-)*
> *ulcerative colitis (K51-)*

K62.7 **Radiation proctitis**
Use additional code to identify the type of radiation (W90-)

✓5ᵗʰ **K62.8** **Other specified diseases of anus and rectum**
> EXCLUDES 2   *ulcerative proctitis (K51.2)*

K62.81 **Anal sphincter tear (healed) (nontraumatic) (old)**
Tear of anus, nontraumatic
Use additional code for any associated fecal incontinence (R15-)
> EXCLUDES 2   *anal fissure (K60-)*
> *anal sphincter tear (healed) (old) complicating delivery (O34.7-)*
> *traumatic tear of anal sphincter (S31.831)*

K62.82 **Dysplasia of anus**
Anal intraepithelial neoplasia I and II (AIN I and II) (histologically confirmed)
Dysplasia of anus NOS
Mild and moderate dysplasia of anus (histologically confirmed)
> EXCLUDES 1   *abnormal results from anal cytologic examination without histologic confirmation (R85.61-)*
> *anal intraepithelial neoplasia III (D01.3)*
> *carcinoma in situ of anus (D01.3)*
> *HGSIL of anus (R85.613)*
> *severe dysplasia of anus (D01.3)*

K62.89 **Other specified diseases of anus and rectum**
Proctitis NOS
Use additional code for any associated fecal incontinence (R15-)

K62.9 **Disease of anus and rectum, unspecified**

✓4ᵗʰ **K63** **Other diseases of intestine**

K63.0 **Abscess of intestine**
> EXCLUDES 1   *abscess of intestine with Crohn's disease (K50.04, K50.14, K50.84, K50.94,)*
> *abscess of intestine with diverticular disease (K57.0, K57.2, K57.4, K57.8)*
> *abscess of intestine with ulcerative colitis (K51.04, K51.14, K51.24, K51.34, K51.44, K51.54, K51.84, K51.94)*
> EXCLUDES 2   *abscess of anal and rectal regions (K61-)*
> *abscess of appendix (K35.2)*

K63.1 **Perforation of intestine (nontraumatic)**
Perforation (nontraumatic) of rectum
> EXCLUDES 1   *perforation (nontraumatic) of duodenum (K26-)*
> *perforation (nontraumatic) of intestine with diverticular disease (K57.0, K57.2, K57.4, K57.8)*
> EXCLUDES 2   *perforation (nontraumatic) of appendix (K35.2, K35.3)*

K63.2 **Fistula of intestine**
> EXCLUDES 1   *fistula of duodenum (K31.6)*
> *fistula of intestine with Crohn's disease (K50.03, K50.13, K50.83, K50.93,)*
> *fistula of intestine with ulcerative colitis (K51.03, K51.13, K51.23, K51.33, K51.43, K51.53, K51.83, K51.93)*
> EXCLUDES 2   *fistula of anal and rectal regions (K60-)*
> *fistula of appendix (K38.3)*
> *intestinal-genital fistula, female (N82.2-N82.4)*
> *vesicointestinal fistula (N32.1)*

K63.3 **Ulcer of intestine**
Primary ulcer of small intestine
> EXCLUDES 1   *duodenal ulcer (K26-)*
> *gastrointestinal ulcer (K28-)*
> *gastrojejunal ulcer (K28-)*
> *jejunal ulcer (K28-)*
> *peptic ulcer, site unspecified (K27-)*
> *ulcer of intestine with perforation (K63.1)*
> *ulcer of anus or rectum (K62.6)*
> *ulcerative colitis (K51-)*

K63.4 **Enteroptosis**

K63.5 **Polyp of colon**
> EXCLUDES 1   *adenomatous polyp of colon (D12.6)*
> *inflammatory polyp of colon (K51.4-)*
> *polyposis of colon (D12.6)*

✓5ᵗʰ **K63.8** **Other specified diseases of intestine**

K63.81 **Dieulafoy lesion of intestine**
> EXCLUDES 2   *Dieulafoy lesion of stomach and duodenum (K31.82)*

K63.89 **Other specified diseases of intestine**

K63.9 **Disease of intestine, unspecified**

Diseases of peritoneum and retroperitoneum (K65-K68)

☑4ᵗʰ **K65 Peritonitis**
　　Use additional code (B95-B97), to identify infectious agent
　　EXCLUDES 1　*acute appendicitis with generalized peritonitis (K35.2)*
　　　　aseptic peritonitis (T81.6)
　　　　benign paroxysmal peritonitis (E85.0)
　　　　chemical peritonitis (T81.6)
　　　　diverticulitis of both small and large intestine with peritonitis (K57.4-)
　　　　diverticulitis of colon with peritonitis (K57.2-)
　　　　diverticulitis of intestine, NOS, with peritonitis (K57.8-)
　　　　diverticulitis of small intestine with peritonitis (K57.0-)
　　　　gonococcal peritonitis (A54.85)
　　　　neonatal peritonitis (P78.0-P78.1)
　　　　pelvic peritonitis, female (N73.3-N73.5)
　　　　periodic familial peritonitis (E85.0)
　　　　peritonitis due to talc or other foreign substance (T81.6)
　　　　peritonitis in chlamydia (A74.81)
　　　　peritonitis in diphtheria (A36.89)
　　　　peritonitis in syphilis (late) (A52.74)
　　　　peritonitis in tuberculosis (A18.31)
　　　　peritonitis with or following abortion or ectopic or molar pregnancy (O00-O07, O08.0)
　　　　peritonitis with or following appendicitis (K35-)
　　　　peritonitis with or following diverticular disease of intestine (K57-)
　　　　puerperal peritonitis (O85)
　　　　retroperitoneal infections (K68-)

　　K65.0 Generalized (acute) peritonitis
　　　　Pelvic peritonitis (acute), male
　　　　Subphrenic peritonitis (acute)
　　　　Suppurative peritonitis (acute)

　　K65.1 Peritoneal abscess
　　　　Abdominopelvic abscess
　　　　Abscess (of) omentum
　　　　Abscess (of) peritoneum
　　　　Mesenteric abscess
　　　　Retrocecal abscess
　　　　Subdiaphragmatic abscess
　　　　Subhepatic abscess
　　　　Subphrenic abscess

　　K65.2 Spontaneous bacterial peritonitis
　　　　EXCLUDES 1　*bacterial peritonitis NOS K65.9*

　　K65.3 Choleperitonitis
　　　　Peritonitis due to bile

　　K65.4 Sclerosing mesenteritis
　　　　Fat necrosis of peritoneum
　　　　(Idiopathic) sclerosing mesenteric fibrosis
　　　　Mesenteric lipodystrophy
　　　　Mesenteric panniculitis
　　　　Retractile mesenteritis

　　K65.8 Other peritonitis
　　　　Chronic proliferative peritonitis
　　　　Peritonitis due to urine

　　K65.9 Peritonitis, unspecified
　　　　Bacterial peritonitis NOS

☑4ᵗʰ **K66 Other disorders of peritoneum**
　　EXCLUDES 2　*ascites (R18-)*
　　　　peritoneal effusion (chronic) (R18.8)

　　K66.0 Peritoneal adhesions (postprocedural) (postinfection)
　　　　Adhesions (of) abdominal (wall)
　　　　Adhesions (of) diaphragm
　　　　Adhesions (of) intestine
　　　　Adhesions (of) male pelvis
　　　　Adhesions (of) omentum
　　　　Adhesions (of) stomach
　　　　Adhesive bands
　　　　Mesenteric adhesions
　　　　EXCLUDES 1　*female pelvic adhesions [bands] (N73.6)*
　　　　　　peritoneal adhesions with intestinal obstruction (K56.5)

　　K66.1 Hemoperitoneum
　　　　EXCLUDES 1　*traumatic hemoperitoneum (S36.8-)*

　　K66.8 Other specified disorders of peritoneum

　　K66.9 Disorder of peritoneum, unspecified

K67 **Disorders of peritoneum in infectious diseases classified elsewhere**
　　Code first underlying disease, such as :
　　　congenital syphilis (A50.0)
　　　helminthiasis (B65.0–B83.9)
　　　EXCLUDES 1　*peritonitis in chlamydia (A74.81)*
　　　　peritonitis in diphtheria (A36.89)
　　　　peritonitis in gonococcal (A54.85)
　　　　peritonitis in syphilis (late) (A52.74)
　　　　peritonitis in tuberculosis (A18.31)

☑4ᵗʰ **K68 Disorders of retroperitoneum**
　☑5ᵗʰ **K68.1 Retroperitoneal abscess**
　　　　K68.11 Postprocedural retroperitoneal abscess
　　　　K68.12 Psoas muscle abscess
　　　　K68.19 Other retroperitoneal abscess
　　K68.9 Other disorders of retroperitoneum

Diseases of liver (K70-K77)

EXCLUDES 1　*jaundice NOS (R17)*
EXCLUDES 2　*hemochromatosis (E83.11-)*
　　Reye's syndrome (G93.7)
　　vira lhepatitis (B15-B19)
　　Wilson's disease (E83.0)

☑4ᵗʰ **K70 Alcoholic liver disease**
　　Use additional code to identify:
　　　alcohol abuse and dependence (F10-)
　　K70.0 Alcoholic fatty liver
　☑5ᵗʰ **K70.1 Alcoholic hepatitis**
　　　　K70.10 Alcoholic hepatitis without ascites
　　　　K70.11 Alcoholic hepatitis with ascites
　　K70.2 Alcoholic fibrosis and sclerosis of liver
　☑5ᵗʰ **K70.3 Alcoholic cirrhosis of liver**
　　　　Alcoholic cirrhosis NOS
　　　　K70.30 Alcoholic cirrhosis of liver without ascites
　　　　K70.31 Alcoholic cirrhosis of liver with ascites
　☑5ᵗʰ **K70.4 Alcoholic hepatic failure**
　　　　Acute alcoholic hepatic failure
　　　　Alcoholic hepatic failure NOS
　　　　Chronic alcoholic hepatic failure
　　　　Subacute alcoholic hepatic failure
　　　　K70.40 Alcoholic hepatic failure without coma
　　　　K70.41 Alcoholic hepatic failure with coma
　　K70.9 Alcoholic liver disease, unspecified

☑4ᵗʰ **K71 Toxic liver disease**
　　INCLUDES　drug-induced idiosyncratic (unpredictable) liver disease
　　　　drug-induced toxic (predictable) liver disease
　　Code first (T36-T65) to identify drug or toxic agent
　　EXCLUDES 2　*alcoholic liver disease (K70-)*
　　　　Budd-Chiari syndrome (I82.0)

　　K71.0 Toxic liver disease with cholestasis
　　　　Cholestasis with hepatocyte injury
　　　　"Pure" cholestasis

　☑5ᵗʰ **K71.1 Toxic liver disease with hepatic necrosis**
　　　　Hepatic failure (acute) (chronic) due to drugs
　　　　K71.10 Toxic liver disease with hepatic necrosis, without coma
　　　　K71.11 Toxic liver disease with hepatic necrosis, with coma

　　K71.2 Toxic liver disease with acute hepatitis

　　K71.3 Toxic liver disease with chronic persistent hepatitis

　　K71.4 Toxic liver disease with chronic lobular hepatitis

　☑5ᵗʰ **K71.5 Toxic liver disease with chronic active hepatitis**
　　　　Toxic liver disease with lupoid hepatitis
　　　　K71.50 Toxic liver disease with chronic active hepatitis without ascites
　　　　K71.51 Toxic liver disease with chronic active hepatitis with ascites

　　K71.6 Toxic liver disease with hepatitis, not elsewhere classified

　　K71.7 Toxic liver disease with fibrosis and cirrhosis of liver

　　K71.8 Toxic liver disease with other disorders of liver
　　　　Toxic liver disease with focal nodular hyperplasia
　　　　Toxic liver disease with hepatic granulomas
　　　　Toxic liver disease with peliosis hepatis
　　　　Toxic liver disease with veno-occlusive disease of liver

　　K71.9 Toxic liver disease, unspecified

☑ Appropriate additional character required　　　　√x7ᵗʰ Requires 7th character, placeholder x must fill empty characters

Diseases of the Digestive System

K72–K80.00

✓4ᵗʰ **K72   Hepatic failure, not elsewhere classified**
> INCLUDES   acute hepatitis NEC, with hepatic failure
>   fulminant hepatitis NEC, with hepatic failure
>   hepatic encephalopathy NOS
>   liver (cell) necrosis with hepatic failure
>   malignant hepatitis NEC, with hepatic failure
>   yellow liver atrophy or dystrophy
> EXCLUDES 1   *alcoholic hepatic failure (K70.4)*
>   *hepatic failure complicating abortion or ectopic or molar*
>   *pregnancy (O00-O07, O08.8)*
>   *hepatic failure complicating pregnancy, childbirth and the*
>   *puerperium (O26.6)*
>   *hepatic failure with toxic liver disease (K71.1-)*
>   *icterus of newborn (P55-P59)*
>   *postprocedural hepatic failure (K91.81)*
>   *viral hepatitis with hepatic coma (B15-B19)*

   ✓5ᵗʰ **K72.0   Acute and subacute hepatic failure**
       K72.00   Acute and subacute hepatic failure without coma
       K72.01   Acute and subacute hepatic failure with coma
   ✓5ᵗʰ **K72.1   Chronic hepatic failure**
       K72.10   Chronic hepatic failure without coma
       K72.11   Chronic hepatic failure with coma
   ✓5ᵗʰ **K72.9   Hepatic failure, unspecified**
       K72.90   Hepatic failure, unspecified without coma
       K72.91   Hepatic failure, unspecified with coma
          Hepatic coma NOS

✓4ᵗʰ **K73   Chronic hepatitis, not elsewhere classified**
> EXCLUDES 1   *alcoholic hepatitis (chronic) (K70.1-)*
>   *drug-induced hepatitis (chronic) (K71-)*
>   *granulomatous hepatitis (chronic) NEC (K75.3)*
>   *reactive, nonspecific hepatitis (chronic) (K75.2)*
>   *viral hepatitis (chronic) (B15-B19)*

   K73.0   Chronic persistent hepatitis, not elsewhere classified
   K73.1   Chronic lobular hepatitis, not elsewhere classified
   K73.2   Chronic active hepatitis, not elsewhere classified
       Lupoid hepatitis NEC
   K73.8   Other chronic hepatitis, not elsewhere classified
   K73.9   Chronic hepatitis, unspecified

✓4ᵗʰ **K74   Fibrosis and cirrhosis of liver**
> Code also, if applicable, viral hepatitis (acute) (chronic) (B15-B19)
> EXCLUDES 1   *alcoholic cirrhosis (of liver) (K70.3)*
>   *alcoholic fibrosis of liver (K70.2)*
>   *cardiac sclerosis of liver (K76.1)*
>   *cirrhosis (of liver) with toxic liver disease (K71.7)*
>   *congenital cirrhosis (of liver) (P78.81)*
>   *pigmentary cirrhosis (of liver) (E83.110)*

   K74.0   Hepatic fibrosis
   K74.1   Hepatic sclerosis
   K74.2   Hepatic fibrosis with hepatic sclerosis
   K74.3   Primary biliary cirrhosis
       Chronic nonsuppurative destructive cholangitis
   K74.4   Secondary biliary cirrhosis
   K74.5   Biliary cirrhosis, unspecified
   ✓5ᵗʰ **K74.6   Other and unspecified cirrhosis of liver**
       K74.60   Unspecified cirrhosis of liver
          Cirrhosis (of liver) NOS
       K74.69   Other cirrhosis of liver
          Cryptogenic cirrhosis (of liver)
          Macronodular cirrhosis (of liver)
          Micronodular cirrhosis (of liver)
          Mixed type cirrhosis (of liver)
          Portal cirrhosis (of liver)
          Postnecrotic cirrhosis (of liver)

✓4ᵗʰ **K75   Other inflammatory liver diseases**
> EXCLUDES 2   *toxic liver disease (K71-)*

   K75.0   Abscess of liver
       Cholangitic hepatic abscess
       Hematogenic hepatic abscess
       Hepatic abscess NOS
       Lymphogenic hepatic abscess
       Pylephlebitic hepatic abscess
>   EXCLUDES 1   *amebic liver abscess (A06.4)*
>   *cholangitis without liver abscess (K83.0)*
>   *pylephlebitis without liver abscess (K75.1)*
   K75.1   Phlebitis of portal vein
       Pylephlebitis
>   EXCLUDES 1   *pylephlebitic liver abscess (K75.0)*

   K75.2   Nonspecific reactive hepatitis
>   EXCLUDES 1   *acute or subacute hepatitis (K72.0-)*
>   *chronic hepatitis NEC (K73-)*
>   *viral hepatitis (B15-B19)*
   K75.3   Granulomatous hepatitis, not elsewhere classified
>   EXCLUDES 1   *acute or subacute hepatitis (K72.0-)*
>   *chronic hepatitis NEC (K73-)*
>   *viral hepatitis (B15-B19)*
   K75.4   Autoimmune hepatitis
   ✓5ᵗʰ **K75.8   Other specified inflammatory liver diseases**
       K75.81   Nonalcoholic steatohepatitis (NASH)
       K75.89   Other specified inflammatory liver diseases
   K75.9   Inflammatory liver disease, unspecified
       Hepatitis NOS
>   EXCLUDES 1   *acute or subacute hepatitis (K72.0-)*
>   *chronic hepatitis NEC (K73-)*
>   *viral hepatitis (B15-B19)*

✓4ᵗʰ **K76   Other diseases of liver**
> EXCLUDES 2   *alcoholic liver disease (K70-)*
>   *amyloid degeneration of liver (E85-)*
>   *cystic disease of liver (congenital) (Q44.6)*
>   *hepatic vein thrombosis (I82.0)*
>   *hepatomegaly NOS (R16.0)*
>   *pigmentary cirrhosis (of liver) (E83.110)*
>   *portal vein thrombosis (I81)*
>   *toxic liver disease (K71-)*

   K76.0   Fatty (change of) liver, not elsewhere classified
       Nonalcoholic fatty liver disease (NAFLD)
>   EXCLUDES 1   *nonalcoholic steatohepatitis (NASH) (K75.81)*
   K76.1   Chronic passive congestion of liver
       Cardiac cirrhosis
       Cardiac sclerosis
   K76.2   Central hemorrhagic necrosis of liver
>   EXCLUDES 1   *liver necrosis with hepatic failure (K72-)*
   K76.3   Infarction of liver
   K76.4   Peliosis hepatis
       Hepatic angiomatosis
   K76.5   Hepatic veno-occlusive disease
>   EXCLUDES 1   *Budd-Chiari syndrome (I82.0)*
   K76.6   Portal hypertension
       Use additional code for any associated complications, such as:
          portal hypertensive gastropathy (K31.89)
   K76.7   Hepatorenal syndrome
>   EXCLUDES 1   *hepatorenal syndrome following labor and delivery*
>   *(O90.4)*
>   *postprocedural hepatorenal syndrome (K91.82)*
   K76.8   Other specified diseases of liver
       Cyst (simple) of liver
       Focal nodular hyperplasia of liver
       Hepatoptosis
   K76.9   Liver disease, unspecified

K77   *Liver disorders in diseases classified elsewhere*
> Code first underlying disease, such as:
>   *amyloidosis (E85-)*
>   *congenital syphilis (A50.0, A50.5)*
>   *congenital toxoplasmosis (P37.1)*
>   *schistosomiasis (B65.0-B65.9)*
>   EXCLUDES 1   *alcoholic hepatitis (K70.1-)*
>   *alcoholic liver disease (K70-)*
>   *cytomegaloviral hepatitis (B25.1)*
>   *herpesviral [herpes simplex] hepatitis (B00.81)*
>   *infectious mononucleosis with liver disease*
>   *(B27.0-B27.9 with .9)*
>   *mumps hepatitis (B26.81)*
>   *sarcoidosis with liver disease (D86.89)*
>   *secondary syphilis with liver disease (A51.45)*
>   *syphilis (late) with liver disease (A52.74)*
>   *toxoplasmosis (acquired) hepatitis (B58.1)*
>   *tuberculosis with liver disease (A18.83)*

Disorders of gallbladder, biliary tract and pancreas (K80-K87)

✓4ᵗʰ **K80   Cholelithiasis**
   ✓5ᵗʰ **K80.0   Calculus of gallbladder with acute cholecystitis**
       Any condition listed in K80.2 with acute cholecystitis
       K80.00   Calculus of gallbladder with acute cholecystitis
            without obstruction

EXCLUDES 1   Not coded here   EXCLUDES 2   Not included here   *Manifestation Code*

K80.01　Calculus of gallbladder with acute cholecystitis with obstruction

☑5ᵗʰ　K80.1　**Calculus of gallbladder with other cholecystitis**

　　K80.10　**Calculus of gallbladder with chronic cholecystitis without obstruction**
　　　　　　Cholelithiasis with cholecystitis NOS

　　K80.11　**Calculus of gallbladder with chronic cholecystitis with obstruction**

　　K80.12　**Calculus of gallbladder with acute and chronic cholecystitis without obstruction**

　　K80.13　**Calculus of gallbladder with acute and chronic cholecystitis with obstruction**

　　K80.18　**Calculus of gallbladder with other cholecystitis without obstruction**

　　K80.19　**Calculus of gallbladder with other cholecystitis with obstruction**

☑5ᵗʰ　K80.2　**Calculus of gallbladder without cholecystitis**
　　　　Cholecystolithiasis without cholecystitis
　　　　Cholelithiasis (without cholecystitis)
　　　　Colic (recurrent) of gallbladder (without cholecystitis)
　　　　Gallstone (impacted) of cystic duct (without cholecystitis)
　　　　Gallstone (impacted) of gallbladder (without cholecystitis)

　　K80.20　**Calculus of gallbladder without cholecystitis without obstruction**

　　K80.21　**Calculus of gallbladder without cholecystitis with obstruction**

☑5ᵗʰ　K80.3　**Calculus of bile duct with cholangitis**
　　　　Any condition listed in K80.5 with cholangitis

　　K80.30　**Calculus of bile duct with cholangitis, unspecified, without obstruction**

　　K80.31　**Calculus of bile duct with cholangitis, unspecified, with obstruction**

　　K80.32　**Calculus of bile duct with acute cholangitis without obstruction**

　　K80.33　**Calculus of bile duct with acute cholangitis with obstruction**

　　K80.34　**Calculus of bile duct with chronic cholangitis without obstruction**

　　K80.35　**Calculus of bile duct with chronic cholangitis with obstruction**

　　K80.36　**Calculus of bile duct with acute and chronic cholangitis without obstruction**

　　K80.37　**Calculus of bile duct with acute and chronic cholangitis with obstruction**

☑5ᵗʰ　K80.4　**Calculus of bile duct with cholecystitis**
　　　　Any condition listed in K80.5 with cholecystitis (with cholangitis)

　　K80.40　**Calculus of bile duct with cholecystitis, unspecified, without obstruction**

　　K80.41　**Calculus of bile duct with cholecystitis, unspecified, with obstruction**

　　K80.42　**Calculus of bile duct with acute cholecystitis without obstruction**

　　K80.43　**Calculus of bile duct with acute cholecystitis with obstruction**

　　K80.44　**Calculus of bile duct with chronic cholecystitis without obstruction**

　　K80.45　**Calculus of bile duct with chronic cholecystitis with obstruction**

　　K80.46　**Calculus of bile duct with acute and chronic cholecystitis without obstruction**

　　K80.47　**Calculus of bile duct with acute and chronic cholecystitis with obstruction**

☑5ᵗʰ　K80.5　**Calculus of bile duct without cholangitis or cholecystitis**
　　　　Choledocholithiasis (without cholangitis or cholecystitis)
　　　　Gallstone (impacted) of bile duct NOS (without cholangitis or cholecystitis)
　　　　Gallstone (impacted) of common duct (without cholangitis or cholecystitis)
　　　　Gallstone (impacted) of hepatic duct (without cholangitis or cholecystitis)
　　　　Hepatic cholelithiasis (without cholangitis or cholecystitis)
　　　　Hepatic colic (recurrent) (without cholangitis or cholecystitis)

　　K80.50　**Calculus of bile duct without cholangitis or cholecystitis without obstruction**

　　K80.51　**Calculus of bile duct without cholangitis or cholecystitis with obstruction**

☑5ᵗʰ　K80.6　**Calculus of gallbladder and bile duct with cholecystitis**

　　K80.60　**Calculus of gallbladder and bile duct with cholecystitis, unspecified, without obstruction**

　　K80.61　**Calculus of gallbladder and bile duct with cholecystitis, unspecified, with obstruction**

　　K80.62　**Calculus of gallbladder and bile duct with acute cholecystitis without obstruction**

　　K80.63　**Calculus of gallbladder and bile duct with acute cholecystitis with obstruction**

　　K80.64　**Calculus of gallbladder and bile duct with chronic cholecystitis without obstruction**

　　K80.65　**Calculus of gallbladder and bile duct with chronic cholecystitis with obstruction**

　　K80.66　**Calculus of gallbladder and bile duct with acute and chronic cholecystitis without obstruction**

　　K80.67　**Calculus of gallbladder and bile duct with acute and chronic cholecystitis with obstruction**

•　☑5ᵗʰ　K80.7　**Calculus of gallbladder and bile duct without cholecystitis**

　　K80.70　**Calculus of gallbladder and bile duct without cholecystitis without obstruction**

　　K80.71　**Calculus of gallbladder and bile duct without cholecystitis with obstruction**

☑5ᵗʰ　K80.8　**Other cholelithiasis**

　　K80.80　**Other cholelithiasis without obstruction**

　　K80.81　**Other cholelithiasis with obstruction**

☑4ᵗʰ　**K81**　**Cholecystitis**
　　EXCLUDES 1 *cholecystitis with cholelithiasis (K80-)*

　　K81.0　**Acute cholecystitis**
　　　　Abscess of gallbladder
　　　　Angiocholecystitis
　　　　Emphysematous (acute) cholecystitis
　　　　Empyema of gallbladder
　　　　Gangrene of gallbladder
　　　　Gangrenous cholecystitis
　　　　Suppurative cholecystitis

　　K81.1　**Chronic cholecystitis**

　　K81.2　**Acute cholecystitis with chronic cholecystitis**

　　K81.9　**Cholecystitis, unspecified**

☑4ᵗʰ　**K82**　**Other diseases of gallbladder**
　　EXCLUDES 1 *nonvisualization of gallbladder (R93.2)*
　　　　　　　　postcholecystectomy syndrome (K91.5)

　　K82.0　**Obstruction of gallbladder**
　　　　Occlusion of cystic duct or gallbladder without cholelithiasis
　　　　Stenosis of cystic duct or gallbladder without cholelithiasis
　　　　Stricture of cystic duct or gallbladder without cholelithiasis
　　　　EXCLUDES 1 *obstruction of gallbladder with cholelithiasis (K80-)*

　　K82.1　**Hydrops of gallbladder**
　　　　Mucocele of gallbladder

　　K82.2　**Perforation of gallbladder**
　　　　Rupture of cystic duct or gallbladder

　　K82.3　**Fistula of gallbladder**
　　　　Cholecystocolic fistula
　　　　Cholecystoduodenal fistula

　　K82.4　**Cholesterolosis of gallbladder**
　　　　Strawberry gallbladder
　　　　EXCLUDES 1 *cholesterolosis of gallbladder with cholecystitis (K81-)*
　　　　　　　　cholesterolosis of gallbladder with cholelithiasis (K80-)

　　K82.8　**Other specified diseases of gallbladder**
　　　　Adhesions of cystic duct or gallbladder
　　　　Atrophy of cystic duct or gallbladder
　　　　Cyst of cystic duct or gallbladder
　　　　Dyskinesia of cystic duct or gallbladder
　　　　Hypertrophy of cystic duct or gallbladder
　　　　Nonfunctioning of cystic duct or gallbladder
　　　　Ulcer of cystic duct or gallbladder

　　K82.9　**Disease of gallbladder, unspecified**

☑ Appropriate additional character required　　　　☑x7ᵗʰ Requires 7th character, placeholder x must fill empty characters

Diseases of the Digestive System

K83–K91.61

☑4ᵗʰ **K83 Other diseases of biliary tract**

EXCLUDES 1   *postcholecystectomy syndrome (K91.5)*

EXCLUDES 2   *conditions involving the gallbladder (K81-K82)*
                conditions involving the cystic duct (K81-K82)

K83.0 Cholangitis
Ascending cholangitis
Cholangitis NOS
Primary cholangitis
Recurrent cholangitis
Sclerosing cholangitis
Secondary cholangitis
Stenosing cholangitis
Suppurative cholangitis

EXCLUDES 1   *cholangitic liver abscess (K75.0)*
                cholangitis with choledocholithiasis (K80.3-, K80.4-)
                chronic nonsuppurative destructive cholangitis (K74.3)

K83.1 Obstruction of bile duct
Occlusion of bile duct without cholelithiasis
Stenosis of bile duct without cholelithiasis
Stricture of bile duct without cholelithiasis

EXCLUDES 1   *congenital obstruction of bile duct (Q44.3)*
                obstruction of bile duct with cholelithiasis (K80-)

K83.2 Perforation of bile duct
Rupture of bile duct

K83.3 Fistula of bile duct
Choledochoduodenal fistula

K83.4 Spasm of sphincter of Oddi

K83.5 Biliary cyst

K83.8 Other specified diseases of biliary tract
Adhesions of biliary tract
Atrophy of biliary tract
Hypertrophy of biliary tract
Ulcer of biliary tract

K83.9 Disease of biliary tract, unspecified

☑4ᵗʰ **K85 Acute pancreatitis**
Abscess of pancreas
Acute necrosis of pancreas
Acute (recurrent) pancreatitis
Gangrene of (gangrenous) pancreas
Hemorrhagic pancreatitis
Infective necrosis of pancreas
Subacute pancreatitis
Suppurative pancreatitis

K85.0 Idiopathic acute pancreatitis

K85.1 Biliary acute pancreatitis
Gallstone pancreatitis

K85.2 Alcohol induced acute pancreatitis

EXCLUDES 2   *alcohol induced chronic pancreatitis (K86.0)*

K85.3 Drug induced acute pancreatitis
Use additional code to identify:
drug abuse and dependence (F11- F17)

K85.8 Other acute pancreatitis

K85.9 Acute pancreatitis, unspecified
Pancreatitis NOS

☑4ᵗʰ **K86 Other diseases of pancreas**

EXCLUDES 2   *fibrocystic disease of pancreas (E84-)*
                islet cell tumor (of pancreas) (D13.7)
                pancreatic steatorrhea (K90.3)

K86.0 Alcohol-induced chronic pancreatitis
Use additional code to identify:
alcohol abuse and dependence (F10-)

EXCLUDES 2   *alcohol induced acute pancreatitis (K85.2)*

K86.1 Other chronic pancreatitis
Chronic pancreatitis NOS
Infectious chronic pancreatitis
Recurrent chronic pancreatitis
Relapsing chronic pancreatitis

K86.2 Cyst of pancreas

K86.3 Pseudocyst of pancreas

K86.8 Other specified diseases of pancreas
Aseptic pancreatic necrosis
Atrophy of pancreas
Calculus of pancreas
Cirrhosis of pancreas
Fibrosis of pancreas
Pancreatic fat necrosis
Pancreatic infantilism
Pancreatic necrosis NOS

K86.9 Disease of pancreas, unspecified

K87   *Disorders of gallbladder, biliary tract and pancreas in diseases classified elsewhere*
Code first underlying disease

EXCLUDES 1   *cytomegaloviral pancreatitis (B25.2)*
                mumps pancreatitis (B26.3)
                syphilitic gallbladder (A52.74)
                syphilitic pancreas (A52.74)
                tuberculosis of gallbladder (A18.83)
                tuberculosis of pancreas (A18.83)

Other diseases of the digestive system (K90-K94)

☑4ᵗʰ **K90 Intestinal malabsorption**

EXCLUDES 1   *intestinal malabsorption following gastrointestinal surgery (K91.2)*

K90.0 Celiac disease
Gluten-sensitive enteropathy
Idiopathic steatorrhea
Nontropical sprue

K90.1 Tropical sprue
Sprue NOS
Tropical steatorrhea

K90.2 Blind loop syndrome, not elsewhere classified
Blind loop syndrome NOS

EXCLUDES 1   *congenital blind loop syndrome (Q43.8)*
                postsurgical blind loop syndrome (K91.2)

K90.3 Pancreatic steatorrhea

K90.4 Malabsorption due to intolerance, not elsewhere classified
Malabsorption due to intolerance to carbohydrate
Malabsorption due to intolerance to fat
Malabsorption due to intolerance to protein
Malabsorption due to intolerance to starch

EXCLUDES 2   *gluten-sensitive enteropathy (K90.0)*
                lactose intolerance (E73-)

☑5ᵗʰ **K90.8 Other intestinal malabsorption**

K90.81 Whipple's disease

K90.89 Other intestinal malabsorption

K90.9 Intestinal malabsorption, unspecified

☑4ᵗʰ **K91 Intraoperative and postprocedural complications and disorders of digestive system, not elsewhere classified**

EXCLUDES 2   *complications of artificial opening of digestive system (K94-)*
                gastrojejunal ulcer (K28-)
                postprocedural (radiation) retroperitoneal abscess (K68.11)
                radiation colitis (K52.0)
                radiation gastroenteritis (K52.0)
                radiation proctitis (K62.7)

K91.0 Vomiting following gastrointestinal surgery

K91.1 Postgastric surgery syndromes
Dumping syndrome
Postgastrectomy syndrome
Postvagotomy syndrome

K91.2 Postsurgical malabsorption, not elsewhere classified
Postsurgical blind loop syndrome

EXCLUDES 1   *malabsorption osteomalacia in adults (M83.2)*
                malabsorption osteoporosis, postsurgical (M80.8-, M81.8)

K91.3 Postprocedural intestinal obstruction

K91.5 Postcholecystectomy syndrome

☑5ᵗʰ **K91.6 Intraoperative hemorrhage and hematoma of a digestive system organ or structure complicating a procedure**

EXCLUDES 1   *intraoperative hemorrhage and hematoma of a digestive system organ or structure due to accidental puncture and laceration during a procedure (K91.7-)*

K91.61 Intraoperative hemorrhage and hematoma of a digestive system organ or structure complicating a digestive sytem procedure

---

EXCLUDES 1   Not coded here   EXCLUDES 2   Not included here   *Manifestation Code*

K91.62 **Intraoperative hemorrhage and hematoma of a digestive system organ or structure complicating other procedure**

✓5ᵗʰ **K91.7** **Accidental puncture and laceration of a digestive system organ or structure during a procedure**

K91.71 **Accidental puncture and laceration of a digestive system organ or structure during a digestive system procedure**

K91.72 **Accidental puncture and laceration of a digestive system organ or structure during other procedure**

✓5ᵗʰ **K91.8** **Other intraoperative and postprocedural complications and disorders of digestive system**

K91.81 **Other intraoperative complications of digestive system**

K91.82 **Postprocedural hepatic failure**

K91.83 **Postprocedural hepatorenal syndrome**

✓6ᵗʰ **K91.84** **Postprocedural hemorrhage and hematoma of a digestive system organ or structure following a procedure**

K91.840 **Postprocedural hemorrhage and hematoma of a digestive system organ or structure following a digestive system procedure**

K91.841 **Postprocedural hemorrhage and hematoma of a digestive system organ or structure following other procedure**

✓6ᵗʰ **K91.85** **Complications of intestinal pouch**

K91.850 **Pouchitis**
Inflammation of internal ileoanal pouch

K91.858 **Other complications of intestinal pouch**

K91.89 **Other postprocedural complications and disorders of digestive system**
Use additional code, if applicable, to further specify disorder
EXCLUDES 2 *postprocedural retroperitoneal abscess (K68.11)*

✓4ᵗʰ **K92** **Other diseases of digestive system**
EXCLUDES 1 *neonatal gastrointestinal hemorrhage (P54.0-P54.3)*

K92.0 **Hematemesis**

K92.1 **Melena**
EXCLUDES 1 *occult blood in feces (R19.5)*

K92.2 **Gastrointestinal hemorrhage, unspecified**
Gastric hemorrhage NOS
Intestinal hemorrhage NOS
EXCLUDES 1 *acute hemorrhagic gastritis (K29.01)*
hemorrhage of anus and rectum (K62.5)
angiodysplasia of stomach with hemorrhage (K31.811)
diverticular disease with hemorrhage (K57-)
gastritis and duodenitis with hemorrhage (K29-)
peptic ulcer with hemorrhage (K25-K28)

✓5ᵗʰ **K92.8** **Other specified diseases of the digestive system**

K92.81 **Gastrointestinal mucositis (ulcerative)**
Code also type of associated therapy, such as:
antineoplastic and immunosuppressive drugs (T45.1x-)
radiological procedure and radiotherapy (Y84.2)
EXCLUDES 2 *mucositis (ulcerative) of vagina and vulva (N76.81)*
nasal mucositis (ulcerative) (J34.81)
oral mucositis (ulcerative) (K12.3-)

K92.89 **Other specified diseases of the digestive system**

K92.9 **Disease of digestive system, unspecified**

✓4ᵗʰ **K94** **Complications of artificial openings of the digestive system**

✓5ᵗʰ **K94.0** **Colostomy complications**

K94.00 **Colostomy complication, unspecified**

K94.01 **Colostomy hemorrhage**

K94.02 **Colostomy infection**
Use additional code to specify type of infection, such as:
cellulitis of abdominal wall (L03.311)
sepsis (A40-, A41-)

K94.03 **Colostomy malfunction**
Mechanical complication of colostomy

K94.09 **Other complications of colostomy**

✓5ᵗʰ **K94.1** **Enterostomy complications**

K94.10 **Enterostomy complication, unspecified**

K94.11 **Enterostomy hemorrhage**

K94.12 **Enterostomy infection**
Use additional code to specify type of infection, such as:
cellulitis of abdominal wall (L03.311)
sepsis (A40-, A41-)

K94.13 **Enterostomy malfunction**
Mechanical complication of enterostomy

K94.19 **Other complications of enterostomy**

✓5ᵗʰ **K94.2** **Gastrostomy complications**

K94.20 **Gastrostomy complication, unspecified**

K94.21 **Gastrostomy hemorrhage**

K94.22 **Gastrostomy infection**
Use additional code to specify type of infection, such as:
cellulitis of abdominal wall (L03.311)
sepsis (A40-, A41-)

K94.23 **Gastrostomy malfunction**
Mechanical complication of gastrostomy

K94.29 **Other complications of gastrostomy**

✓5ᵗʰ **K94.3** **Esophagostomy complications**

K94.30 **Esophagostomy complications, unspecified**

K94.31 **Esophagostomy hemorrhage**

K94.32 **Esophagostomy infection**
Use additional code to identify the infection

K94.33 **Esophagostomy malfunction**
Mechanical complication of esophagostomy

K94.39 **Other complications of esophagostomy**

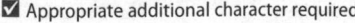

Chapter 12. Diseases of the Skin and Subcutaneous Tissue (L00-L99)

EXCLUDES 2   certain conditions originating in the perinatal period (P04-P96)
certain infectious and parasitic diseases (A00-B99)
complications of pregnancy, childbirth and the puerperium (O00-O99)
congenital malformations, deformations, and chromosomal abnormalities (Q00-Q99)
endocrine, nutritional and metabolic diseases (E00-E88)
lipomelanotic reticulosis (I89.8)
neoplasms (C00-D49)
symptoms, signs and abnormal clinical and laboratory findings, not elsewhere classified (R00-R94)
systemic connective tissue disorders (M30-M36)
viral warts (B07-)

This chapter contains the following blocks:

L00-L08   Infections of the skin and subcutaneous tissue
L10-L14   Bullous disorders
L20-L30   Dermatitis and eczema
L40-L45   Papulosquamous disorders
L49-L54   Urticaria and erythema
L55-L59   Radiation-related disorders of the skin and subcutaneous tissue
L60-L75   Disorders of skin appendages
L76   Intraoperative and postprocedural complications of skin and subcutaneous tissue
L80-L99   Other disorders of the skin and subcutaneous tissue

Infections of the skin and subcutaneous tissue (L00-L08)

Use additional code (B95-B97) to identify infectious agent

EXCLUDES 2   hordeolum (H00.0)
infective dermatitis (L30.3)
local infections of skin classified in Chapter 1
lupus panniculitis (L93.2)
panniculitis NOS (M79.3)
panniculitis of neck and back (M54.0-)
Perlèche NOS (K13.0)
Perlèche due to candidiasis (B37.0)
Perlèche due to riboflavin deficiency (E53.0)
pyogenic granuloma (L98.0)
relapsing panniculitis [Weber-Christian] (M35.6)
viral warts (B07-)
zoster (B02-)

L00   Staphylococcal scalded skin syndrome
Ritter's disease
Use additional code to identify percentage of skin exfoliation (L49-)
EXCLUDES 1   bullous impetigo (L01.03)
pemphigus neonatorum (L01.03)
toxic epidermal necrolysis [Lyell] (L51.2)

✓4th **L01   Impetigo**
EXCLUDES 1   impetigo herpetiformis (L40.1)
    ✓5th **L01.0   Impetigo**
       Impetigo contagiosa
       Impetigo vulgaris
       L01.00   Impetigo, unspecified
          Impetigo NOS
       L01.01   Non-bullous impetigo
       L01.02   Bockhart's impetigo
          Impetigo follicularis
          Perifolliculitis NOS
          Superficial pustular perifolliculitis
       L01.03   Bullous impetigo
          Impetigo neonatorum
          Pemphigus neonatorum
       L01.09   Other impetigo
          Ulcerative impetigo
    L01.1   Impetiginization of other dermatoses

✓4th **L02   Cutaneous abscess, furuncle and carbuncle**
Use additional code to identify organism (B95-B96)
EXCLUDES 2   abscess of anus and rectal regions (K61-)
abscess of female genital organs (external) (N76.4)
abscess of male genital organs (external) (N48.2, N49-)
    ✓5th **L02.0   Cutaneous abscess, furuncle and carbuncle of face**
       EXCLUDES 1   abscess of ear, external (H60.0)
          abscess of eyelid (H00.03-)
          abscess of head [any part, except face] (L02.8)
          abscess of lacrimal gland (H04.0)
          abscess of lacrimal passages (H04.3)
          abscess of mouth (K12.2)
          abscess of nose (J34.0)
          abscess of orbit (H05.0)
          submandibular abscess (K12.2)
       L02.01   Cutaneous abscess of face
       L02.02   Furuncle of face
          Boil of face
          Folliculitis of face
       L02.03   Carbuncle of face
    ✓5th **L02.1   Cutaneous abscess, furuncle and carbuncle of neck**
       L02.11   Cutaneous abscess of neck
       L02.12   Furuncle of neck
          Boil of neck
          Folliculitis of neck
       L02.13   Carbuncle of neck
    ✓5th **L02.2   Cutaneous abscess, furuncle and carbuncle of trunk**
       EXCLUDES 1   non-newborn omphalitis (L08.82)
          omphalitis of newborn (P38-)
       EXCLUDES 2   abscess of breast (N61)
          abscess of buttocks (L02.3)
          abscess of female external genital organs (N76.4)
          abscess of hip (L02.4)
          abscess of male external genital organs (N48.2, N49-)
       ✓6th **L02.21   Cutaneous abscess of trunk**
          L02.211   Cutaneous abscess of abdominal wall
          L02.212   Cutaneous abscess of back [any part, except buttock]
          L02.213   Cutaneous abscess of chest wall
          L02.214   Cutaneous abscess of groin
          L02.215   Cutaneous abscess of perineum
          L02.216   Cutaneous abscess of umbilicus
          L02.219   Cutaneous abscess of trunk, unspecified
       ✓6th **L02.22   Furuncle of trunk**
          Boil of trunk
          Folliculitis of trunk
          L02.221   Furuncle of abdominal wall
          L02.222   Furuncle of back [any part, except buttock]
          L02.223   Furuncle of chest wall
          L02.224   Furuncle of groin
          L02.225   Furuncle of perineum
          L02.226   Furuncle of umbilicus
          L02.229   Furuncle of trunk, unspecified
       ✓6th **L02.23   Carbuncle of trunk**
          L02.231   Carbuncle of abdominal wall
          L02.232   Carbuncle of back [any part, except buttock]
          L02.233   Carbuncle of chest wall
          L02.234   Carbuncle of groin
          L02.235   Carbuncle of perineum
          L02.236   Carbuncle of umbilicus
          L02.239   Carbuncle of trunk, unspecified
    ✓5th **L02.3   Cutaneous abscess, furuncle and carbuncle of buttock**
       EXCLUDES 1   pilonidal cyst with abscess (L05.01)
       L02.31   Cutaneous abscess of buttock
          Cutaneous abscess of gluteal region
       L02.32   Furuncle of buttock
          Boil of buttock
          Folliculitis of buttock
          Furuncle of gluteal region
       L02.33   Carbuncle of buttock
          Carbuncle of gluteal region

EXCLUDES 1   Not coded here   EXCLUDES 2   Not included here   *Manifestation Code*

✓5ᵗʰ **L02.4 Cutaneous abscess, furuncle and carbuncle of limb**
    EXCLUDES 2   *cutaneous abscess, furuncle and carbuncle of groin (L02.214, L02.224, L02.234)*
            cutaneous abscess, furuncle and carbuncle of hand (L02.5-)
            cutaneous abscess, furuncle and carbuncle of foot (L02.6-)

✓6ᵗʰ **L02.41 Cutaneous abscess of limb**
     L02.411 Cutaneous abscess of right axilla
     L02.412 Cutaneous abscess of left axilla
     L02.413 Cutaneous abscess of right upper limb
     L02.414 Cutaneous abscess of left upper limb
     L02.415 Cutaneous abscess of right lower limb
     L02.416 Cutaneous abscess of left lower limb
     L02.419 Cutaneous abscess of limb, unspecified

✓6ᵗʰ **L02.42 Furuncle of limb**
     Boil of limb
     Folliculitis of limb
     L02.421 Furuncle of right axilla
     L02.422 Furuncle of left axilla
     L02.423 Furuncle of right upper limb
     L02.424 Furuncle of left upper limb
     L02.425 Furuncle of right lower limb
     L02.426 Furuncle of left lower limb
     L02.429 Furuncle of limb, unspecified

✓6ᵗʰ **L02.43 Carbuncle of limb**
     L02.431 Carbuncle of right axilla
     L02.432 Carbuncle of left axilla
     L02.433 Carbuncle of right upper limb
     L02.434 Carbuncle of left upper limb
     L02.435 Carbuncle of right lower limb
     L02.436 Carbuncle of left lower limb
     L02.439 Carbuncle of limb, unspecified

✓5ᵗʰ **L02.5 Cutaneous abscess, furuncle and carbuncle of hand**
✓6ᵗʰ **L02.51 Cutaneous abscess of hand**
     L02.511 Cutaneous abscess of right hand
     L02.512 Cutaneous abscess of left hand
     L02.519 Cutaneous abscess of unspecified hand
✓6ᵗʰ **L02.52 Furuncle hand**
     Boil of hand
     Folliculitis of hand
     L02.521 Furuncle right hand
     L02.522 Furuncle left hand
     L02.529 Furuncle unspecified hand
✓6ᵗʰ **L02.53 Carbuncle of hand**
     L02.531 Carbuncle of right hand
     L02.532 Carbuncle of left hand
     L02.539 Carbuncle of unspecified hand

✓5ᵗʰ **L02.6 Cutaneous abscess, furuncle and carbuncle of foot**
✓6ᵗʰ **L02.61 Cutaneous abscess of foot**
     L02.611 Cutaneous abscess of right foot
     L02.612 Cutaneous abscess of left foot
     L02.619 Cutaneous abscess of unspecified foot
✓6ᵗʰ **L02.62 Furuncle of foot**
     Boil of foot
     Folliculitis of foot
     L02.621 Furuncle of right foot
     L02.622 Furuncle of left foot
     L02.629 Furuncle of unspecified foot
✓6ᵗʰ **L02.63 Carbuncle of foot**
     L02.631 Carbuncle of right foot
     L02.632 Carbuncle of left foot
     L02.639 Carbuncle of unspecified foot

✓5ᵗʰ **L02.8 Cutaneous abscess, furuncle and carbuncle of other sites**
✓6ᵗʰ **L02.81 Cutaneous abscess of other sites**
     L02.811 Cutaneous abscess of head [any part, except face]
     L02.818 Cutaneous abscess of other sites
✓6ᵗʰ **L02.82 Furuncle of other sites**
     Boil of other sites
     Folliculitis of other sites
     L02.821 Furuncle of head [any part, except face]
     L02.828 Furuncle of other sites
✓6ᵗʰ **L02.83 Carbuncle of other sites**
     L02.831 Carbuncle of head [any part, except face]

     L02.838 Carbuncle of other sites
✓5ᵗʰ **L02.9 Cutaneous abscess, furuncle and carbuncle, unspecified**
     L02.91 Cutaneous abscess, unspecified
     L02.92 Furuncle, unspecified
         Boil NOS
         Furunculosis NOS
     L02.93 Carbuncle, unspecified

✓4ᵗʰ **L03 Cellulitis and acute lymphangitis**
    EXCLUDES 2   *cellulitis of anal and rectal region (K61-)*
            cellulitis of external auditory canal (H60.1)
            cellulitis of eyelid (H00.03-)
            cellulitis of female external genital organs (N76.4)
            cellulitis of lacrimal apparatus (H04.3)
            cellulitis of male external genital organs (N48.2, N49-)
            cellulitis of mouth (K12.2)
            cellulitis of nose (J34.0)
            eosinophilic cellulitis [Wells] (L98.3)
            febrile neutrophilic dermatosis [Sweet] (L98.2)
            lymphangitis (chronic) (subacute) (I89.1)

✓5ᵗʰ **L03.0 Cellulitis and acute lymphangitis of finger and toe**
     Infection of nail
     Onychia
     Paronychia
     Perionychia
    ✓6ᵗʰ **L03.01 Cellulitis of finger**
         Felon
         Whitlow
        EXCLUDES 1   *herpetic whitlow (B00.89)*
         L03.011 Cellulitis of right finger
         L03.012 Cellulitis of left finger
         L03.019 Cellulitis of unspecified finger
    ✓6ᵗʰ **L03.02 Acute lymphangitis of finger**
         Hangnail with lymphangitis of finger
         L03.021 Acute lymphangitis of right finger
         L03.022 Acute lymphangitis of left finger
         L03.029 Acute lymphangitis of unspecified finger
    ✓6ᵗʰ **L03.03 Cellulitis of toe**
         L03.031 Cellulitis of right toe
         L03.032 Cellulitis of left toe
         L03.039 Cellulitis of unspecified toe
    ✓6ᵗʰ **L03.04 Acute lymphangitis of toe**
         Hangnail with lymphangitis of toe
         L03.041 Acute lymphangitis of right toe
         L03.042 Acute lymphangitis of left toe
         L03.049 Acute lymphangitis of unspecified toe

✓5ᵗʰ **L03.1 Cellulitis and acute lymphangitis of other parts of limb**
    ✓6ᵗʰ **L03.11 Cellulitis of other parts of limb**
        EXCLUDES 2   *cellulitis of fingers (L03.01-)*
                  cellulitis of toes (L03.03-)
                  groin (L03.314)
         L03.111 Cellulitis of right axilla
         L03.112 Cellulitis of left axilla
         L03.113 Cellulitis of right upper limb
         L03.114 Cellulitis of left upper limb
         L03.115 Cellulitis of right lower limb
         L03.116 Cellulitis of left lower limb
         L03.119 Cellulitis of unspecified part of limb
    ✓6ᵗʰ **L03.12 Acute lymphangitis of other parts of limb**
        EXCLUDES 2   *acute lymphangitis of fingers (L03.02-)*
                  acute lymphangitis of groin (L03.324)
                  acute lymphangitis of toes (L03.04-)
         L03.121 Acute lymphangitis of right axilla
         L03.122 Acute lymphangitis of left axilla
         L03.123 Acute lymphangitis of right upper limb
         L03.124 Acute lymphangitis of left upper limb
         L03.125 Acute lymphangitis of right lower limb
         L03.126 Acute lymphangitis of left lower limb
         L03.129 Acute lymphangitis of unspecified part of limb

---

✓ Appropriate additional character required   ✓×7ᵗʰ Requires 7th character, placeholder x must fill empty characters

Diseases of the Skin and Subcutaneous Tissue

L03.2–L11.9

✓5th **L03.2**   **Cellulitis and acute lymphangitis of face and neck**
   ✓6th   **L03.21**   **Cellulitis and acute lymphangitis of face**
         L03.211   **Cellulitis of face**
             EXCLUDES 2   *cellulitis of ear (H60.1-)*
                      cellulitis of eyelid (H00.03-)
                      cellulitis of head (L03.811)
                      cellulitis of lacrimal apparatus (H04.3)
                      cellulitis of lip (K13.0)
                      cellulitis of mouth (K12.2)
                      cellulitis of nose (internal) (J34.0)
                      cellulitis of orbit (H05.0)
                      cellulitis of scalp (L03.811)
         L03.212   **Acute lymphangitis of face**
   ✓6th   **L03.22**   **Cellulitis and acute lymphangitis of neck**
         L03.221   **Cellulitis of neck**
         L03.222   **Acute lymphangitis of neck**

✓5th **L03.3**   **Cellulitis and acute lymphangitis of trunk**
   ✓6th   **L03.31**   **Cellulitis of trunk**
         EXCLUDES 2   *cellulitis of anal and rectal regions (K61-)*
                cellulitis of breast NOS (N61)
                cellulitis of female external genital organs (N76.4)
                cellulitis of male external genital organs (N48.2, N49-)
                omphalitis of newborn (P38-)
                puerperal cellulitis of breast (O91.2)
         L03.311   **Cellulitis of abdominal wall**
             EXCLUDES 2   *cellulitis of umbilicus (L03.316)*
                      cellulitis of groin (L03.314)
         L03.312   **Cellulitis of back [any part except buttock]**
         L03.313   **Cellulitis of chest wall**
         L03.314   **Cellulitis of groin**
         L03.315   **Cellulitis of perineum**
         L03.316   **Cellulitis of umbilicus**
         L03.317   **Cellulitis of buttock**
         L03.319   **Cellulitis of trunk, unspecified**
   ✓6th   **L03.32**   **Acute lymphangitis of trunk**
         L03.321   **Acute lymphangitis of abdominal wall**
         L03.322   **Acute lymphangitis of back [any part except buttock]**
         L03.323   **Acute lymphangitis of chest wall**
         L03.324   **Acute lymphangitis of groin**
         L03.325   **Acute lymphangitis of perineum**
         L03.326   **Acute lymphangitis of umbilicus**
         L03.327   **Acute lymphangitis of buttock**
         L03.329   **Acute lymphangitis of trunk, unspecified**

✓5th **L03.8**   **Cellulitis and acute lymphangitis of other sites**
   ✓6th   **L03.81**   **Cellulitis of other sites**
         L03.811   **Cellulitis of head [any part, except face]**
             Cellulitis of scalp
             EXCLUDES 2   *cellulitis of face (L03.211)*
         L03.818   **Cellulitis of other sites**
   ✓6th   **L03.89**   **Acute lymphangitis of other sites**
         L03.891   **Acute lymphangitis of head [any part, except face]**
         L03.898   **Acute lymphangitis of other sites**
✓5th **L03.9**   **Cellulitis and acute lymphangitis, unspecified**
         L03.90   **Cellulitis, unspecified**
         L03.91   **Acute lymphangitis, unspecified**
             EXCLUDES 1   *lymphangitis NOS (I89.1)*

✓4th **L04**   **Acute lymphadenitis**
     INCLUDES   abscess (acute) of lymph nodes, except mesenteric
                acute lymphadenitis, except mesenteric
     EXCLUDES 1   *chronic or subacute lymphadenitis, except mesenteric (I88.1)*
                enlarged lymph nodes (R59-)
                human immunodeficiency virus [HIV] disease resulting in generalized lymphadenopathy (B20)
                lymphadenitis NOS (I88.9)
                nonspecific mesenteric lymphadenitis (I88.0)
         L04.0   **Acute lymphadenitis of face, head and neck**
         L04.1   **Acute lymphadenitis of trunk**

         L04.2   **Acute lymphadenitis of upper limb**
             Acute lymphadenitis of axilla
             Acute lymphadenitis of shoulder
         L04.3   **Acute lymphadenitis of lower limb**
             Acute lymphadenitis of hip
             EXCLUDES 2   *acute lymphadenitis of groin (L04.1)*
         L04.8   **Acute lymphadenitis of other sites**
         L04.9   **Acute lymphadenitis, unspecified**

✓4th **L05**   **Pilonidal cyst and sinus**
   ✓5th   **L05.0**   **Pilonidal cyst and sinus with abscess**
         L05.01   **Pilonidal cyst with abscess**
             Parasacral dimple with abscess
             Pilonidal abscess
             Pilonidal dimple with abscess
             Postanal dimple with abscess
         L05.02   **Pilonidal sinus with abscess**
             Coccygeal fistula with abscess
             Coccygeal sinus with abscess
             Pilonidal fistula with abscess
   ✓5th   **L05.9**   **Pilonidal cyst and sinus without abscess**
         L05.91   **Pilonidal cyst without abscess**
             Parasacral dimple
             Pilonidal dimple
             Postanal dimple .
             Pilonidal cyst NOS
         L05.92   **Pilonidal sinus without abscess**
             Coccygeal fistula
             Coccygeal sinus without abscess
             Pilonidal fistula

✓4th **L08**   **Other local infections of skin and subcutaneous tissue**
         L08.0   **Pyoderma**
             Purulent dermatitis
             Septic dermatitis
             Suppurative dermatitis
             EXCLUDES 1   *pyoderma gangrenosum (L88)*
                      pyoderma vegetans (L08.81)
         L08.1   **Erythrasma**
   ✓5th   **L08.8**   **Other specified local infections of the skin and subcutaneous tissue**
         L08.81   **Pyoderma vegetans**
             EXCLUDES 1   *pyoderma gangrenosum (L88)*
                      pyoderma NOS (L08.0)
         L08.82   **Omphalitis not of newborn**
             EXCLUDES 1   *omphalitis of newborn (P38-)*
         L08.89   **Other specified local infections of the skin and subcutaneous tissue**
         L08.9   **Local infection of the skin and subcutaneous tissue, unspecified**

Bullous disorders (L10-L14)

   EXCLUDES 1   *benign familial pemphigus [Hailey-Hailey] (Q82.8)*
                staphylococcal scalded skin syndrome (L00)
                toxic epidermal necrolysis [Lyell] (L51.2)

✓4th **L10**   **Pemphigus**
     EXCLUDES 1   *pemphigus neonatorum (L01.03)*
         L10.0   **Pemphigus vulgaris**
         L10.1   **Pemphigus vegetans**
         L10.2   **Pemphigus foliaceous**
         L10.3   **Brazilian pemphigus [fogo selvagem]**
         L10.4   **Pemphigus erythematosus**
             Senear-Usher syndrome
         L10.5   **Drug-induced pemphigus**
             Code first (T36-T50) to identify drug
   ✓5th   **L10.8**   **Other pemphigus**
         L10.81   **Paraneoplastic pemphigus**
         L10.89   **Other pemphigus**
         L10.9   **Pemphigus, unspecified**

✓4th **L11**   **Other acantholytic disorders**
         L11.0   **Acquired keratosis follicularis**
             EXCLUDES 1   *keratosis follicularis (congenital) [Darier-White] (Q82.8)*
         L11.1   **Transient acantholytic dermatosis [Grover]**
         L11.8   **Other specified acantholytic disorders**
         L11.9   **Acantholytic disorder, unspecified**

EXCLUDES 1   Not coded here   EXCLUDES 2   Not included here   *Manifestation Code*

✓4th **L12 Pemphigoid**

> EXCLUDES 1 *herpes gestationis (O26.4-)*
> *impetigo herpetiformis (L40.1)*

L12.0 Bullous pemphigoid

L12.1 Cicatricial pemphigoid
  Benign mucous membrane pemphigoid

L12.2 Chronic bullous disease of childhood
  Juvenile dermatitis herpetiformis

✓5th **L12.3 Acquired epidermolysis bullosa**
> EXCLUDES 1 *epidermolysis bullosa (congenital) (Q81-)*

  L12.30 Acquired epidermolysis bullosa, unspecified

  L12.31 Epidermolysis bullosa due to drug
    Code first (T36-T50) to identify drug

  L12.35 Other acquired epidermolysis bullosa

L12.8 Other pemphigoid

L12.9 Pemphigoid, unspecified

✓4th **L13 Other bullous disorders**

L13.0 Dermatitis herpetiformis
  Duhring's disease
  Hydroa herpetiformis
> EXCLUDES 1 *juvenile dermatitis herpetiformis (L12.2)*
> *senile dermatitis herpetiformis (L12.0)*

L13.1 Subcorneal pustular dermatitis
  Sneddon-Wilkinson disease

L13.8 Other specified bullous disorders

L13.9 Bullous disorder, unspecified

L14 Bullous disorders in diseases classified elsewhere
  Code first underlying disease

Dermatitis and eczema (L20-L30)

> NOTE In this block the terms dermatitis and eczema are used synonymously and interchangeably.

> EXCLUDES 2 *chronic (childhood) granulomatous disease (D71)*
> *dermatitis gangrenosa (L88)*
> *dermatitis herpetiformis (L13.0)*
> *dry skin dermatitis (L85.3)*
> *factitial dermatitis (L98.1)*
> *perioral dermatitis (L71.0)*
> *radiation-related disorders of the skin and subcutaneous tissue (L55-L59)*
> *stasis dermatitis (I83.1-I83.2)*

✓4th **L20 Atopic dermatitis**

L20.0 Besnier's prurigo

✓5th **L20.8 Other atopic dermatitis**
> EXCLUDES 2 *circumscribed neurodermatitis (L28.0)*

  L20.81 Atopic neurodermatitis
    Diffuse neurodermatitis

  L20.82 Flexural eczema

  L20.83 Infantile (acute) (chronic) eczema

  L20.84 Intrinsic (allergic) eczema

  L20.89 Other atopic dermatitis

L20.9 Atopic dermatitis, unspecified

✓4th **L21 Seborrheic dermatitis**

> EXCLUDES 2 *infective dermatitis (L30.3)*
> *seborrheic keratosis (L82-)*

L21.0 Seborrhea capitis
  Cradle cap

L21.1 Seborrheic infantile dermatitis

L21.8 Other seborrheic dermatitis

L21.9 Seborrheic dermatitis, unspecified
  Seborrhea NOS

L22 Diaper dermatitis
  Diaper erythema
  Diaper rash
  Psoriasiform diaper rash

✓4th **L23 Allergic contact dermatitis**
  Code first (T36-T65), to identify drug or substance
> EXCLUDES 1 *allergy NOS (T78.40)*
> *contact dermatitis NOS (L25.9)*
> *dermatitis NOS (L30.9)*

> EXCLUDES 2 *dermatitis due to substances taken internally (L27-)*
> *dermatitis of eyelid (H01.1-)*
> *diaper dermatitis (L22)*
> *eczema of external ear (H60.5-)*
> *irritant contact dermatitis (L24-)*
> *perioral dermatitis (L71.0)*
> *radiation-related disorders of the skin and subcutaneous tissue (L55-L59)*

L23.0 Allergic contact dermatitis due to metals
  Allergic contact dermatitis due to chromium
  Allergic contact dermatitis due to nickel

L23.1 Allergic contact dermatitis due to adhesives

L23.2 Allergic contact dermatitis due to cosmetics

L23.3 Allergic contact dermatitis due to drugs in contact with skin
> EXCLUDES 2 *dermatitis due to ingested drugs and medicaments (L27.0-L27.1)*

L23.4 Allergic contact dermatitis due to dyes

L23.5 Allergic contact dermatitis due to other chemical products
  Allergic contact dermatitis due to cement
  Allergic contact dermatitis due to insecticide
  Allergic contact dermatitis due to plastic
  Allergic contact dermatitis due to rubber

L23.6 Allergic contact dermatitis due to food in contact with the skin
> EXCLUDES 2 *dermatitis due to ingested food (L27.2)*

L23.7 Allergic contact dermatitis due to plants, except food
> EXCLUDES 2 *allergy NOS due to pollen (J30.1)*

✓5th **L23.8 Allergic contact dermatitis due to other agents**

  L23.81 Allergic contact dermatitis due to animal (cat) (dog) dander
    Allergic contact dermatitis due to animal (cat) (dog) hair

  L23.89 Allergic contact dermatitis due to other agents

L23.9 Allergic contact dermatitis, unspecified cause
  Allergic contact eczema NOS

✓4th **L24 Irritant contact dermatitis**
  Code first (T36-T65) to identify drug or substance
> EXCLUDES 1 *allergy NOS (T78.40)*
> *contact dermatitis NOS (L25.9)*
> *dermatitis NOS (L30.9)*

> EXCLUDES 2 *allergic contact dermatitis (L23-)*
> *dermatitis due to substances taken internally (L27-)*
> *dermatitis of eyelid (H01.1-)*
> *diaper dermatitis (L22)*
> *eczema of external ear (H60.5-)*
> *perioral dermatitis (L71.0)*
> *radiation-related disorders of the skin and subcutaneous tissue (L55-L59)*

L24.0 Irritant contact dermatitis due to detergents

L24.1 Irritant contact dermatitis due to oils and greases

L24.2 Irritant contact dermatitis due to solvents
  Irritant contact dermatitis due to chlorocompound
  Irritant contact dermatitis due to cyclohexane
  Irritant contact dermatitis due to ester
  Irritant contact dermatitis due to glycol
  Irritant contact dermatitis due to hydrocarbon
  Irritant contact dermatitis due to ketone

L24.3 Irritant contact dermatitis due to cosmetics

L24.4 Irritant contact dermatitis due to drugs in contact with skin

L24.5 Irritant contact dermatitis due to other chemical products
  Irritant contact dermatitis due to cement
  Irritant contact dermatitis due to insecticide
  Irritant contact dermatitis due to plastic
  Irritant contact dermatitis due to rubber

L24.6 Irritant contact dermatitis due to food in contact with skin
> EXCLUDES 2 *dermatitis due to ingested food (L27.2)*

L24.7 Irritant contact dermatitis due to plants, except food
> EXCLUDES 2 *allergy NOS to pollen (J30.1)*

✓5th **L24.8 Irritant contact dermatitis due to other agents**

  L24.81 Irritant contact dermatitis due to metals
    Irritant contact dermatitis due to chromium
    Irritant contact dermatitis due to nickel

✓ Appropriate additional character required   ✓x7th Requires 7th character, placeholder x must fill empty characters

L24.89   **Irritant contact dermatitis due to other agents**
     Irritant contact dermatitis due to dyes

L24.9   **Irritant contact dermatitis, unspecified cause**
     Irritant contact eczema NOS

✓4ᵗʰ **L25**   **Unspecified contact dermatitis**
     Code first (T36-T65), to identify drug or substance
     EXCLUDES 1   *allergic contact dermatitis (L23-)*
         allergy NOS (T78.40)
         dermatitis NOS (L30.9)
         irritant contact dermatitis (L24-)
     EXCLUDES 2   *dermatitis due to ingested substances (L27-)*
         dermatitis of eyelid (H01.1-)
         eczema of external ear (H60.5-)
         perioral dermatitis (L71.0)
         radiation-related disorders of the skin and subcutaneous
           tissue (L55-L59)

L25.0   **Unspecified contact dermatitis due to cosmetics**

L25.1   **Unspecified contact dermatitis due to drugs in contact with skin**
     EXCLUDES 2   *dermatitis due to ingested drugs and medicaments*
           (L27.0-L27.1)

L25.2   **Unspecified contact dermatitis due to dyes**

L25.3   **Unspecified contact dermatitis due to other chemical products**
     Unspecified contact dermatitis due to cement
     Unspecified contact dermatitis due to insecticide

L25.4   **Unspecified contact dermatitis due to food in contact with skin**
     EXCLUDES 2   *dermatitis due to ingested food (L27.2)*

L25.5   **Unspecified contact dermatitis due to plants, except food**
     EXCLUDES 1   *nettle rash (L50.9)*
     EXCLUDES 2   *allergy NOS due to pollen (J30.1)*

L25.8   **Unspecified contact dermatitis due to other agents**

L25.9   **Unspecified contact dermatitis, unspecified cause**
     Contact dermatitis (occupational) NOS
     Contact eczema (occupational) NOS

L26   **Exfoliative dermatitis**
     Hebra's pityriasis
     EXCLUDES 1   *Ritter's disease (L00)*

✓4ᵗʰ **L27**   **Dermatitis due to substances taken internally**
     Code first (T36-T65), to identify drug or substance
     EXCLUDES 1   *allergy NOS (T78.40)*
     EXCLUDES 2   *adverse food reaction, except dermatitis (T78.0-T78.1)*
         contact dermatitis (L23-L25)
         drug photoallergic response (L56.1)
         drug phototoxic response (L56.0)
         urticaria (L50-)

L27.0   **Generalized skin eruption due to drugs and medicaments taken internally**

L27.1   **Localized skin eruption due to drugs and medicaments taken internally**

L27.2   **Dermatitis due to ingested food**
     EXCLUDES 2   *dermatitis due to food in contact with skin (L23.6, L24.6, L25.4)*

L27.8   **Dermatitis due to other substances taken internally**

L27.9   **Dermatitis due to unspecified substance taken internally**

✓4ᵗʰ **L28**   **Lichen simplex chronicus and prurigo**

L28.0   **Lichen simplex chronicus**
     Circumscribed neurodermatitis
     Lichen NOS

L28.1   **Prurigo nodularis**

L28.2   **Other prurigo**
     Prurigo NOS
     Prurigo Hebra
     Prurigo mitis
     Urticaria papulosa

✓4ᵗʰ **L29**   **Pruritus**
     EXCLUDES 1   *neurotic excoriation (L98.1)*
         psychogenic pruritus (F45.8)

L29.0   **Pruritus ani**

L29.1   **Pruritus scroti**

L29.2   **Pruritus vulvae**

L29.3   **Anogenital pruritus, unspecified**

L29.8   **Other pruritus**

L29.9   **Pruritus, unspecified**
     Itch NOS

✓4ᵗʰ **L30**   **Other and unspecified dermatitis**
     EXCLUDES 2   *contact dermatitis (L23-L25)*
         dry skin dermatitis (L85.3)
         small plaque parapsoriasis (L41.3)
         stasis dermatitis (I83.1-.2)

L30.0   **Nummular dermatitis**

L30.1   **Dyshidrosis [pompholyx]**

L30.2   **Cutaneous autosensitization**
     Candidid [levurid]
     Dermatophytid
     Eczematid

L30.3   **Infective dermatitis**
     Infectious eczematoid dermatitis

L30.4   **Erythema intertrigo**

L30.5   **Pityriasis alba**

L30.8   **Other specified dermatitis**

L30.9   **Dermatitis, unspecified**
     Eczema NOS

Papulosquamous disorders (L40-L45)

✓4ᵗʰ **L40**   **Psoriasis**

L40.0   **Psoriasis vulgaris**
     Nummular psoriasis
     Plaque psoriasis

L40.1   **Generalized pustular psoriasis**
     Impetigo herpetiformis
     Von Zumbusch's disease

L40.2   **Acrodermatitis continua**

L40.3   **Pustulosis palmaris et plantaris**

L40.4   **Guttate psoriasis**

✓5ᵗʰ **L40.5**   **Arthropathic psoriasis**

     L40.50   **Arthropathic psoriasis, unspecified**

     L40.51   **Distal interphalangeal psoriatic arthropathy**

     L40.52   **Psoriatic arthritis mutilans**

     L40.53   **Psoriatic spondylitis**

     L40.54   **Psoriatic juvenile arthropathy**

     L40.59   **Other psoriatic arthropathy**

L40.8   **Other psoriasis**
     Flexural psoriasis

L40.9   **Psoriasis, unspecified**

✓4ᵗʰ **L41**   **Parapsoriasis**
     EXCLUDES 1   *poikiloderma vasculare atrophicans (L94.5)*

L41.0   **Pityriasis lichenoides et varioliformis acuta**
     Mucha-Habermann disease

L41.1   **Pityriasis lichenoides chronica**

L41.2   **Lymphomatoid papulosis**

L41.3   **Small plaque parapsoriasis**

L41.4   **Large plaque parapsoriasis**

L41.5   **Retiform parapsoriasis**

L41.8   **Other parapsoriasis**

L41.9   **Parapsoriasis, unspecified**

L42   **Pityriasis rosea**

✓4ᵗʰ **L43**   **Lichen planus**
     EXCLUDES 1   *lichen planopilaris (L66.1)*

L43.0   **Hypertrophic lichen planus**

L43.1   **Bullous lichen planus**

L43.2   **Lichenoid drug reaction**
     Code first (T36-T50) to identify drug

L43.3   **Subacute (active) lichen planus**
     Lichen planus tropicus

L43.8   **Other lichen planus**

L43.9   **Lichen planus, unspecified**

✓4ᵗʰ **L44**   **Other papulosquamous disorders**

L44.0   **Pityriasis rubra pilaris**

L44.1   **Lichen nitidus**

L44.2   **Lichen striatus**

L44.3   **Lichen ruber moniliformis**

L44.4   **Infantile papular acrodermatitis [Gianotti-Crosti]**

L44.8   **Other specified papulosquamous disorders**

L44.9   **Papulosquamous disorder, unspecified**

L45   *Papulosquamous disorders in diseases classified elsewhere*
     Code first underlying disease

EXCLUDES 1 Not coded here   **EXCLUDES 2** Not included here   *Manifestation Code*

Urticaria and erythema (L49-L54)

EXCLUDES 1   *Lyme disease (A69.2-)*
               rosacea (L71-)

✓4th **L49**   **Exfoliation due to erythematous conditions according to extent of body surface involved**

Code first erythematous condition causing exfoliation, such as:
   Ritter's disease (L00)
   (Staphylococcal) scalded skin syndrom (L00)
   Stevens-Johnson syndrome (L51.1)
   Stevens-Johnson syndrome-toxic epidermal necrolysis overlap
     syndrome (L51.3)
   toxic epidermal necrolysis (L51.2)

L49.0   **Exfoliation due to erythematous condition involving less than 10**
         percent of body surface
         Exfoliation due to erythematous condition NOS

L49.1   **Exfoliation due to erythematous condition involving 10-19 percent of body surface**

L49.2   **Exfoliation due to erythematous condition involving 20-29 percent of body surface**

L49.3   **Exfoliation due to erythematous condition involving 30-39 percent of body surface**

L49.4   **Exfoliation due to erythematous condition involving 40-49 percent of body surface**

L49.5   **Exfoliation due to erythematous condition involving 50-59 percent of body surface**

L49.6   **Exfoliation due to erythematous condition involving 60-69 percent of body surface**

L49.7   **Exfoliation due to erythematous condition involving 70-79 percent of body surface**

L49.8   **Exfoliation due to erythematous condition involving 80-89 percent of body surface**

L49.9   **Exfoliation due to erythematous condition involving 90 or more percent of body surface**

✓4th **L50**   **Urticaria**

EXCLUDES 1   *allergic contact dermatitis (L23-)*
               angioneurotic edema (T78.3)
               giant urticaria (T78.3)
               hereditary angio-edema (D84.1)
               Quincke's edema (T78.3)
               serum urticaria (T80.6)
               solar urticaria (L56.3)
               urticaria neonatorum (P83.8)
               urticaria papulosa (L28.2)
               urticaria pigmentosa (Q82.2)

L50.0   **Allergic urticaria**
L50.1   **Idiopathic urticaria**
L50.2   **Urticaria due to cold and heat**
L50.3   **Dermatographic urticaria**
L50.4   **Vibratory urticaria**
L50.5   **Cholinergic urticaria**
L50.6   **Contact urticaria**
L50.8   **Other urticaria**
         Chronic urticaria
         Recurrent periodic urticaria
L50.9   **Urticaria, unspecified**

✓4th **L51**   **Erythema multiforme**

Code first (T36-T50) to identify drug, if drug-induced
Use additional code to identify associated manifestations, such as:
   arthropathy associated with dermatological disorders (M14.8-)
   conjunctival edema (H11.42)
   conjunctivitis (H10.22-)
   corneal scars and opacities (H17-)
   corneal ulcer (H16.0-)
   edema of eyelid (H02.84)
   inflammation of eyelid (H01.8)
   keratoconjunctivitis sicca (H16.22-)
   mechanical lagophthalmos (H02.22-)
   stomatitis (K12-)
   symblepharon (H11.23-)
Use additional code to identify percentage of skin exfoliation (L49-)

EXCLUDES 1   *staphylococcal scalded skin syndrome (L00)*
               Ritter's disease (L00)

L51.0   **Nonbullous erythema multiforme**
L51.1   **Stevens-Johnson syndrome**
L51.2   **Toxic epidermal necrolysis [Lyell]**

L51.3   **Stevens-Johnson syndrome-toxic epidermal necrolysis overlap syndrome**
         SJS-TEN overlap syndrome
L51.8   **Other erythema multiforme**
L51.9   **Erythema multiforme, unspecified**
         Erythema iris
         Erythema multiforme major NOS
         Erythema multiforme minor NOS
         Herpes iris

L52   **Erythema nodosum**

EXCLUDES 1   *tuberculous erythema nodosum (A18.4)*

✓4th **L53**   **Other erythematous conditions**

EXCLUDES 1   *erythema ab igne (L59.0)*
               erythema due to external agents in contact with skin (L23-L25)
               erythema intertrigo (L30.4)

L53.0   **Toxic erythema**
         Code first (T36-T65) to identify external agent
         EXCLUDES 1   *neonatal erythema toxicum (P83.1)*

L53.1   **Erythema annulare centrifugum**
L53.2   **Erythema marginatum**
L53.3   **Other chronic figurate erythema**
L53.8   **Other specified erythematous conditions**
L53.9   **Erythematous condition, unspecified**
         Erythema NOS
         Erythroderma NOS

L54   *Erythema in diseases classified elsewhere*
         Code first underlying disease

Radiation-related disorders of the skin and subcutaneous tissue (L55-L59)

✓4th **L55**   **Sunburn**
L55.0   **Sunburn of first degree**
L55.1   **Sunburn of second degree**
L55.2   **Sunburn of third degree**
L55.9   **Sunburn, unspecified**

✓4th **L56**   **Other acute skin changes due to ultraviolet radiation**
         Use additional code to identify the source of the ultraviolet radiation
         (W89, X32)
L56.0   **Drug phototoxic response**
         Code first (T36-T50) to identify drug
L56.1   **Drug photoallergic response**
         Code first (T36-T50) to identify drug
L56.2   **Photocontact dermatitis [berloque dermatitis]**
L56.3   **Solar urticaria**
L56.4   **Polymorphous light eruption**
L56.5   **Disseminated superficial actinic porokeratosis (DSAP)**
L56.8   **Other specified acute skin changes due to ultraviolet radiation**
L56.9   **Acute skin change due to ultraviolet radiation, unspecified**

✓4th **L57**   **Skin changes due to chronic exposure to nonionizing radiation**
         Use additional code to identify the source of the ultraviolet radiation
         (W89, X32)
L57.0   **Actinic keratosis**
         Keratosis NOS
         Senile keratosis
         Solar keratosis
L57.1   **Actinic reticuloid**
L57.2   **Cutis rhomboidalis nuchae**
L57.3   **Poikiloderma of Civatte**
L57.4   **Cutis laxa senilis**
         Elastosis senilis
L57.5   **Actinic granuloma**
L57.8   **Other skin changes due to chronic exposure to nonionizing radiation**
         Farmer's skin
         Sailor's skin
         Solar dermatitis
L57.9   **Skin changes due to chronic exposure to nonionizing radiation, unspecified**

✓4th **L58**   **Radiodermatitis**
         Use additional code to identify the source of the radiation (W88, W90)
L58.0   **Acute radiodermatitis**
L58.1   **Chronic radiodermatitis**
L58.9   **Radiodermatitis, unspecified**

✓ Appropriate additional character required   ✓x7th Requires 7th character, placeholder x must fill empty characters

Diseases of the Skin and Subcutaneous Tissue

L59–L75.9

✓4ᵗʰ **L59** **Other disorders of skin and subcutaneous tissue related to radiation**
     L59.0   **Erythema ab igne [dermatitis ab igne]**
     L59.8   **Other specified disorders of the skin and subcutaneous tissue related to radiation**
     L59.9   **Disorder of the skin and subcutaneous tissue related to radiation, unspecified**

Disorders of skin appendages (L60-L75)

     EXCLUDES 1   congenital malformations of integument (Q84-)

✓4ᵗʰ **L60** **Nail disorders**
     EXCLUDES 2   clubbing of nails (R68.3)
                 onychia and paronychia (L03.0-)
     L60.0   **Ingrowing nail**
     L60.1   **Onycholysis**
     L60.2   **Onychogryphosis**
     L60.3   **Nail dystrophy**
     L60.4   **Beau's lines**
     L60.5   **Yellow nail syndrome**
     L60.8   **Other nail disorders**
     L60.9   **Nail disorder, unspecified**

   L62   *Nail disorders in diseases classified elsewhere*
       Code first underlying disease, such as:
       pachydermoperiostosis (M89.4-)

✓4ᵗʰ **L63** **Alopecia areata**
     L63.0   **Alopecia (capitis) totalis**
     L63.1   **Alopecia universalis**
     L63.2   **Ophiasis**
     L63.8   **Other alopecia areata**
     L63.9   **Alopecia areata, unspecified**

✓4ᵗʰ **L64** **Androgenic alopecia**
     INCLUDES   male-pattern baldness
     L64.0   **Drug-induced androgenic alopecia**
             Code first (T36-T50) to identify drug
     L64.8   **Other androgenic alopecia**
     L64.9   **Androgenic alopecia, unspecified**

✓4ᵗʰ **L65** **Other nonscarring hair loss**
     EXCLUDES 1   trichotillomania (F63.3)
     L65.0   **Telogen effluvium**
     L65.1   **Anagen effluvium**
     L65.2   **Alopecia mucinosa**
     L65.8   **Other specified nonscarring hair loss**
     L65.9   **Nonscarring hair loss, unspecified**
             Alopecia NOS

✓4ᵗʰ **L66** **Cicatricial alopecia [scarring hair loss]**
     L66.0   **Pseudopelade**
     L66.1   **Lichen planopilaris**
             Follicular lichen planus
     L66.2   **Folliculitis decalvans**
     L66.3   **Perifolliculitis capitis abscedens**
     L66.4   **Folliculitis ulerythematosa reticulata**
     L66.8   **Other cicatricial alopecia**
     L66.9   **Cicatricial alopecia, unspecified**

✓4ᵗʰ **L67** **Hair color and hair shaft abnormalities**
     EXCLUDES 1   monilethrix (Q84.1)
                 pili annulati (Q84.1)
                 telogen effluvium (L65.0)
     L67.0   **Trichorrhexis nodosa**
     L67.1   **Variations in hair color**
             Canities
             Greyness, hair (premature)
             Heterochromia of hair
             Poliosis circumscripta, acquired
             Poliosis NOS
     L67.8   **Other hair color and hair shaft abnormalities**
             Fragilitas crinium
     L67.9   **Hair color and hair shaft abnormality, unspecified**

✓4ᵗʰ **L68** **Hypertrichosis**
     INCLUDES   excess hair
     EXCLUDES 1   congenital hypertrichosis (Q84.2)
                 persistent lanugo (Q84.2)
     L68.0   **Hirsutism**
     L68.1   **Acquired hypertrichosis lanuginosa**

     L68.2   **Localized hypertrichosis**
     L68.3   **Polytrichia**
     L68.8   **Other hypertrichosis**
     L68.9   **Hypertrichosis, unspecified**

✓4ᵗʰ **L70** **Acne**
     EXCLUDES 2   acne keloid (L73.0)
     L70.0   **Acne vulgaris**
     L70.1   **Acne conglobata**
     L70.2   **Acne varioliformis**
             Acne necrotica miliaris
     L70.3   **Acne tropica**
     L70.4   **Infantile acne**
     L70.5   **Acné excoriée des jeunes filles**
             Picker's acne
     L70.8   **Other acne**
     L70.9   **Acne, unspecified**

✓4ᵗʰ **L71** **Rosacea**
     L71.0   **Perioral dermatitis**
     L71.1   **Rhinophyma**
     L71.8   **Other rosacea**
     L71.9   **Rosacea, unspecified**

✓4ᵗʰ **L72** **Follicular cysts of skin and subcutaneous tissue**
     L72.0   **Epidermal cyst**
     L72.1   **Trichodermal cyst**
             Pilar cyst
             Sebaceous cyst
     L72.2   **Steatocystoma multiplex**
     L72.8   **Other follicular cysts of the skin and subcutaneous tissue**
     L72.9   **Follicular cyst of the skin and subcutaneous tissue, unspecified**

✓4ᵗʰ **L73** **Other follicular disorders**
     L73.0   **Acne keloid**
     L73.1   **Pseudofolliculitis barbae**
     L73.2   **Hidradenitis suppurativa**
     L73.8   **Other specified follicular disorders**
             Sycosis barbae
     L73.9   **Follicular disorder, unspecified**

✓4ᵗʰ **L74** **Eccrine sweat disorders**
     EXCLUDES 2   generalized hyperhidrosis (R61)
     L74.0   **Miliaria rubra**
     L74.1   **Miliaria crystallina**
     L74.2   **Miliaria profunda**
             Miliaria tropicalis
     L74.3   **Miliaria, unspecified**
     L74.4   **Anhidrosis**
             Hypohidrosis
     ✓5ᵗʰ   L74.5   **Focal hyperhidrosis**
         ✓6ᵗʰ   L74.51   **Primary focal hyperhidrosis**
                 L74.510   **Primary focal hyperhidrosis, axilla**
                 L74.511   **Primary focal hyperhidrosis, face**
                 L74.512   **Primary focal hyperhidrosis, palms**
                 L74.513   **Primary focal hyperhidrosis, soles**
                 L74.519   **Primary focal hyperhidrosis, unspecified**
         L74.52   **Secondary focal hyperhidrosis**
             Frey's syndrome
     L74.8   **Other eccrine sweat disorders**
     L74.9   **Eccrine sweat disorder, unspecified**
             Sweat gland disorder NOS

✓4ᵗʰ **L75** **Apocrine sweat disorders**
     EXCLUDES 1   dyshidrosis (L30.1)
                 hidradenitis suppurativa (L73.2)
     L75.0   **Bromhidrosis**
     L75.1   **Chromhidrosis**
     L75.2   **Apocrine miliaria**
             Fox-Fordyce disease
     L75.8   **Other apocrine sweat disorders**
     L75.9   **Apocrine sweat disorder, unspecified**

EXCLUDES 1   Not coded here   EXCLUDES 2   Not included here   *Manifestation Code*

Intraoperative and postprocedural complications of skin and subcutaneous tissue (L76)

✓4th **L76 Intraoperative and postprocedural complications of skin and subcutaneous tissue**

✓5th **L76.0 Intraoperative hemorrhage and hematoma of skin and subcutaneous tissue complicating a procedure**

> EXCLUDES 1 *intraoperative hemorrhage and hematoma of skin and subcutaneous tissue due to accidental puncture and laceration during a procedure (L76.1-)*

     L76.01 Intraoperative hemorrhage and hematoma of skin and subcutaneous tissue complicating a dermatologic procedure

     L76.02 Intraoperative hemorrhage and hematoma of skin and subcutaneous tissue complicating other procedure

✓5th **L76.1 Accidental puncture and laceration of skin and subcutaneous tissue during a procedure**

     L76.11 Accidental puncture and laceration of skin and subcutaneous tissue during a dermatologic procedure

     L76.12 Accidental puncture and laceration of skin and subcutaneous tissue during other procedure

✓5th **L76.2 Postprocedural hemorrhage and hematoma of skin and subcutaneous tissue following a procedure**

     L76.21 Postprocedural hemorrhage and hematoma of skin and subcutaneous tissue following a dermatologic procedure

     L76.22 Postprocedural hemorrhage and hematoma of skin and subcutaneous tissue following other procedure

✓5th **L76.8 Other intraoperative and postprocedural complications of skin and subcutaneous tissue**

> Use additional code, if applicable, to further specify disorder

     L76.81 Other intraoperative complications of skin and subcutaneous tissue

     L76.82 Other postprocedural complications of skin and subcutaneous tissue

Other disorders of the skin and subcutaneous tissue (L80-L99)

L80 Vitiligo

> EXCLUDES 2 *vitiligo of eyelids (H02.73-)*
> *vitiligo of vulva (N90.89)*

✓4th **L81 Other disorders of pigmentation**

> EXCLUDES 1 *birthmark NOS (Q82.5)*
> *Peutz-Jeghers syndrome (Q85.8)*
> EXCLUDES 2 *nevus—see Alphabetical Index*

     L81.0 Postinflammatory hyperpigmentation
     L81.1 Chloasma
     L81.2 Freckles
     L81.3 Café au lait spots
     L81.4 Other melanin hyperpigmentation
        Lentigo
     L81.5 Leukoderma, not elsewhere classified
     L81.6 Other disorders of diminished melanin formation
     L81.7 Pigmented purpuric dermatosis
        Angioma serpiginosum
     L81.8 Other specified disorders of pigmentation
        Iron pigmentation
        Tattoo pigmentation
     L81.9 Disorder of pigmentation, unspecified

✓4th **L82 Seborrheic keratosis**

> INCLUDES dermatosis papulosa nigra
> Leser-Trélat disease
> EXCLUDES 2 *seborrheic dermatitis (L21-)*

     L82.0 Inflamed seborrheic keratosis
     L82.1 Other seborrheic keratosis
        Seborrheic keratosis NOS

L83 Acanthosis nigricans
     Confluent and reticulated papillomatosis

L84 Corns and callosities
     Callus
     Clavus

✓4th **L85 Other epidermal thickening**

> EXCLUDES 2 *hypertrophic disorders of the skin (L91-)*

     L85.0 Acquired ichthyosis
> EXCLUDES 1 *congenital ichthyosis (Q80-)*

     L85.1 Acquired keratosis [keratoderma] palmaris et plantaris
> EXCLUDES 1 *inherited keratosis palmaris et plantaris (Q82.8)*

     L85.2 Keratosis punctata (palmaris et plantaris)

     L85.3 Xerosis cutis
        Dry skin dermatitis

     L85.8 Other specified epidermal thickening
        Cutaneous horn

     L85.9 Epidermal thickening, unspecified

L86 *Keratoderma in diseases classified elsewhere*

> Code first underlying disease, such as:
> Reiter's disease (M02.3-)
> EXCLUDES 1 *gonococcal keratoderma (A54.89)*
> *gonococcal keratosis (A54.89)*
> *keratoderma due to vitamin A deficiency (E50.8)*
> *keratosis due to vitamin A deficiency (E50.8)*
> *xeroderma due to vitamin A deficiency (E50.8)*

✓4th **L87 Transepidermal elimination disorders**

> EXCLUDES 1 *granuloma annulare (perforating) (L92.0)*

     L87.0 Keratosis follicularis et parafollicularis in cutem penetrans
        Kyrle disease
        Hyperkeratosis follicularis penetrans

     L87.1 Reactive perforating collagenosis
     L87.2 Elastosis perforans serpiginosa
     L87.8 Other transepidermal elimination disorders
     L87.9 Transepidermal elimination disorder, unspecified

L88 Pyoderma gangrenosum
     Dermatitis gangrenosa
     Phagedenic pyoderma

L89 Pressure ulcer
     Bed sore
     Decubitus ulcer
     Plaster ulcer
     Pressure area
     Pressure sore

> Code first any associated gangrene (I96)
> EXCLUDES 2 *decubitus (trophic) ulcer of cervix (uteri) (N86)*
> *diabetic ulcers (E08.621, E08.622, E09.621, E09.622, E10.621, E10.622, E11.621, E11.622, E13.621, E13.622)*
> *non-pressure chronic ulcer of skin (L97-)*
> *skin infections (L00-L08)*
> *varicose ulcer (I83.0, I83.2)*

✓5th **L89.0 Pressure ulcer of elbow**

✓6th **L89.00 Pressure ulcer of unspecified elbow**

     L89.000 Pressure ulcer of unspecified elbow, unstageable

     L89.001 Pressure ulcer of unspecified elbow, stage 1
        Healing pressure ulcer of unspecified elbow, stage 1
        Pressure pre-ulcer skin changes limited to persistent focal edema, unspecified elbow

     L89.002 Pressure ulcer of unspecified elbow, stage 2
        Healing pressure ulcer of unspecified elbow, stage 2
        Pressure ulcer with abrasion, blister, partial thickness skin loss involving epidermis and/or dermis, unspecified elbow

     L89.003 Pressure ulcer of unspecified elbow, stage 3
        Healing pressure ulcer of unspecified elbow, stage 3
        Pressure ulcer with full thickness skin loss involving damage or necrosis of subcutaneous tissue, unspecified elbow

---

☑ Appropriate additional character required   ✓x7th Requires 7th character, placeholder x must fill empty characters

L89.004   Pressure ulcer of unspecified elbow, stage 4

Healing pressure ulcer of unspecified elbow, stage 4

Pressure ulcer with necrosis of soft tissues through to underlying muscle, tendon, or bone, unspecified elbow

L89.009   Pressure ulcer of unspecified elbow, unspecified stage

Healing pressure ulcer of elbow NOS

Healing pressure ulcer of unspecified elbow, unspecified stage

✓6ᵗʰ **L89.01   Pressure ulcer of right elbow**

L89.010   Pressure ulcer of right elbow, unstageable

L89.011   Pressure ulcer of right elbow, stage 1

Healing pressure ulcer of right elbow, stage 1

Pressure pre-ulcer skin changes limited to persistent focal edema, right elbow

L89.012   Pressure ulcer of right elbow, stage 2

Healing pressure ulcer of right elbow, stage 2

Pressure ulcer with abrasion, blister, partial thickness skin loss involving epidermis and/or dermis, right elbow

L89.013   Pressure ulcer of right elbow, stage 3

Healing pressure ulcer of right elbow, stage 3

Pressure ulcer with full thickness skin loss involving damage or necrosis of subcutaneous tissue, right elbow

L89.014   Pressure ulcer of right elbow, stage 4

Healing pressure ulcer of right elbow, stage 4

Pressure ulcer with necrosis of soft tissues through to underlying muscle, tendon, or bone, right elbow

L89.019   Pressure ulcer of right elbow, unspecified stage

Healing pressure right of elbow NOS

Healing pressure ulcer of unspecified elbow, unspecified stage

✓6ᵗʰ **L89.02   Pressure ulcer of left elbow**

L89.020   Pressure ulcer of left elbow, unstageable

L89.021   Pressure ulcer of left elbow, stage 1

Healing pressure ulcer of left elbow, stage 1

Pressure pre-ulcer skin changes limited to persistent focal edema, left elbow

L89.022   Pressure ulcer of left elbow, stage 2

Healing pressure ulcer of left elbow, stage 2

Pressure ulcer with abrasion, blister, partial thickness skin loss involving epidermis and/or dermis, left elbow

L89.023   Pressure ulcer of left elbow, stage 3

Healing pressure ulcer of left elbow, stage 3

Pressure ulcer with full thickness skin loss involving damage or necrosis of subcutaneous tissue, left elbow

L89.024   Pressure ulcer of left elbow, stage 4

Healing pressure ulcer of left elbow, stage 4

Pressure ulcer with necrosis of soft tissues through to underlying muscle, tendon, or bone, left elbow

L89.029   Pressure ulcer of left elbow, unspecified stage

Healing pressure ulcer of left of elbow NOS

Healing pressure ulcer of unspecified elbow, unspecified stage

✓5ᵗʰ **L89.1   Pressure ulcer of back**

✓6ᵗʰ **L89.10   Pressure ulcer of unspecified part of back**

L89.100   Pressure ulcer of unspecified part of back, unstageable

L89.101   Pressure ulcer of unspecified part of back, stage 1

Healing pressure ulcer of unspecified part of back, stage 1

Pressure pre-ulcer skin changes limited to persistent focal edema, unspecified part of back

L89.102   Pressure ulcer of unspecified part of back, stage 2

Healing pressure ulcer of unspecified part of back, stage 2

Pressure ulcer with abrasion, blister, partial thickness skin loss involving epidermis and/or dermis, unspecified part of back

L89.103   Pressure ulcer of unspecified part of back, stage 3

Healing pressure ulcer of unspecified part of back, stage 3

Pressure ulcer with full thickness skin loss involving damage or necrosis of subcutaneous tissue, unspecified part of back

L89.104   Pressure ulcer of unspecified part of back, stage 4

Healing pressure ulcer of unspecified part of back, stage 4

Pressure ulcer with necrosis of soft tissues through to underlying muscle, tendon, or bone, unspecified part of back

L89.109   Pressure ulcer of unspecified part of back, unspecified stage

Healing pressure ulcer of unspecified part of back NOS

Healing pressure ulcer of unspecified part of back, unspecified stage

✓6ᵗʰ **L89.11   Pressure ulcer of right upper back**

Pressure ulcer of right shoulder blade

L89.110   Pressure ulcer of right upper back, unstageable

L89.111   Pressure ulcer of right upper back, stage 1

Healing pressure ulcer of right upper back, stage 1

Pressure pre-ulcer skin changes limited to persistent focal edema, right upper back

L89.112   Pressure ulcer of right upper back, stage 2

Healing pressure ulcer of right upper back, stage 2

Pressure ulcer with abrasion, blister, partial thickness skin loss involving epidermis and/or dermis, right upper back

L89.113   Pressure ulcer of right upper back, stage 3

Healing pressure ulcer of right upper back, stage 3

Pressure ulcer with full thickness skin loss involving damage or necrosis of subcutaneous tissue, right upper back

L89.114   Pressure ulcer of right upper back, stage 4

Healing pressure ulcer of right upper back, stage 4

Pressure ulcer with necrosis of soft tissues through to underlying muscle, tendon, or bone, right upper back

---

EXCLUDES 1   Not coded here   EXCLUDES 2   Not included here   *Manifestation Code*

L89.119 Pressure ulcer of right upper back, unspecified stage
Healing pressure ulcer of right upper back NOS
Healing pressure ulcer of right upper back, unspecified stage

☑6th **L89.12 Pressure ulcer of left upper back**
Pressure ulcer of left shoulder blade

L89.120 Pressure ulcer of left upper back, unstageable

L89.121 Pressure ulcer of left upper back, stage 1
Healing pressure ulcer of left upper back, stage 1
Pressure pre-ulcer skin changes limited to persistent focal edema, left upper back

L89.122 Pressure ulcer of left upper back, stage 2
Healing pressure ulcer of left upper back, stage 2
Pressure ulcer with abrasion, blister, partial thickness skin loss involving epidermis and/or dermis, left upper back

L89.123 Pressure ulcer of left upper back, stage 3
Healing pressure ulcer of left upper back, stage 3
Pressure ulcer with full thickness skin loss involving damage or necrosis of subcutaneous tissue, left upper back

L89.124 Pressure ulcer of left upper back, stage 4
Healing pressure ulcer of left upper back, stage 4
Pressure ulcer with necrosis of soft tissues through to underlying muscle, tendon, or bone, left upper back

L89.129 Pressure ulcer of left upper back, unspecified stage
Healing pressure ulcer of left upper back NOS
Healing pressure ulcer of left upper back, unspecified stage

☑6th **L89.13 Pressure ulcer of right lower back**

L89.130 Pressure ulcer of right lower back, unstageable

L89.131 Pressure ulcer of right lower back, stage 1
Healing pressure ulcer of right lower back, stage 1
Pressure pre-ulcer skin changes limited to persistent focal edema, right lower back

L89.132 Pressure ulcer of right lower back, stage 2
Healing pressure ulcer of right lower back, stage 2
Pressure ulcer with abrasion, blister, partial thickness skin loss involving epidermis and/or dermis, right lower back

L89.133 Pressure ulcer of right lower back, stage 3
Healing pressure ulcer of right lower back, stage 3
Pressure ulcer with full thickness skin loss involving damage or necrosis of subcutaneous tissue, right lower back

L89.134 Pressure ulcer of right lower back, stage 4
Healing pressure ulcer of right lower back, stage 4
Pressure ulcer with necrosis of soft tissues through to underlying muscle, tendon, or bone, right lower back

L89.139 Pressure ulcer of right lower back, unspecified stage
Healing pressure ulcer of right lower back NOS
Healing pressure ulcer of right lower back, unspecified stage

☑6th **L89.14 Pressure ulcer of left lower back**

L89.140 Pressure ulcer of left lower back, unstageable

L89.141 Pressure ulcer of left lower back, stage 1
Healing pressure ulcer of left lower back, stage 1
Pressure pre-ulcer skin changes limited to persistent focal edema, left lower back

L89.142 Pressure ulcer of left lower back, stage 2
Healing pressure ulcer of left lower back, stage 2
Pressure ulcer with abrasion, blister, partial thickness skin loss involving epidermis and/or dermis, left lower back

L89.143 Pressure ulcer of left lower back, stage 3
Healing pressure ulcer of left lower back, stage 3
Pressure ulcer with full thickness skin loss involving damage or necrosis of subcutaneous tissue, left lower back

L89.144 Pressure ulcer of left lower back, stage 4
Healing pressure ulcer of left lower back, stage 4
Pressure ulcer with necrosis of soft tissues through to underlying muscle, tendon, or bone, left lower back

L89.149 Pressure ulcer of left lower back, unspecified stage
Healing pressure ulcer of left lower back NOS
Healing pressure ulcer of left lower back, unspecified stage

☑6th **L89.15 Pressure ulcer of sacral region**
Pressure ulcer of coccyx
Pressure ulcer of tailbone

L89.150 Pressure ulcer of sacral region, unstageable

L89.151 Pressure ulcer of sacral region, stage 1
Healing pressure ulcer of sacral region, stage 1
Pressure pre-ulcer skin changes limited to persistent focal edema, sacral region

L89.152 Pressure ulcer of sacral region, stage 2
Healing pressure ulcer of sacral region, stage 2
Pressure ulcer with abrasion, blister, partial thickness skin loss involving epidermis and/or dermis, sacral region

L89.153 Pressure ulcer of sacral region, stage 3
Healing pressure ulcer of sacral region, stage 3
Pressure ulcer with full thickness skin loss involving damage or necrosis of subcutaneous tissue, sacral region

L89.154 Pressure ulcer of sacral region, stage 4
Healing pressure ulcer of sacral region, stage 4
Pressure ulcer with necrosis of soft tissues through to underlying muscle, tendon, or bone, sacral region

L89.159 Pressure ulcer of sacral region, unspecified stage
Healing pressure ulcer of sacral region NOS
Healing pressure ulcer of sacral region, unspecified stage

☑ Appropriate additional character required   ☑x7th Requires 7th character, placeholder x must fill empty characters

✓5th **L89.2   Pressure ulcer of hip**
  ✓6th **L89.20   Pressure ulcer of unspecified hip**
    L89.200   Pressure ulcer of unspecified hip, unstageable
    L89.201   Pressure ulcer of unspecified hip, stage 1
      Healing pressure ulcer of unspecified hip back, stage 1
      Pressure pre-ulcer skin changes limited to persistent focal edema, unspecified hip
    L89.202   Pressure ulcer of unspecified hip, stage 2
      Healing pressure ulcer of unspecified hip, stage 2
      Pressure ulcer with abrasion, blister, partial thickness skin loss involving epidermis and/or dermis, unspecified hip
    L89.203   Pressure ulcer of unspecified hip, stage 3
      Healing pressure ulcer of unspecified hip, stage 3
      Pressure ulcer with full thickness skin loss involving damage or necrosis of subcutaneous tissue, unspecified hip
    L89.204   Pressure ulcer of unspecified hip, stage 4
      Healing pressure ulcer of unspecified hip, stage 4
      Pressure ulcer with necrosis of soft tissues through to underlying muscle, tendon, or bone, unspecified hip
    L89.209   Pressure ulcer of unspecified hip, unspecified stage
      Healing pressure ulcer of unspecified hip NOS
      Healing pressure ulcer of unspecified hip, unspecified stage
  ✓6th **L89.21   Pressure ulcer of right hip**
    L89.210   Pressure ulcer of right hip, unstageable
    L89.211   Pressure ulcer of right hip, stage 1
      Healing pressure ulcer of right hip back, stage 1
      Pressure pre-ulcer skin changes limited to persistent focal edema, right hip
    L89.212   Pressure ulcer of right hip, stage 2
      Healing pressure ulcer of right hip, stage 2
      Pressure ulcer with abrasion, blister, partial thickness skin loss involving epidermis and/or dermis, right hip
    L89.213   Pressure ulcer of right hip, stage 3
      Healing pressure ulcer of right hip, stage 3
      Pressure ulcer with full thickness skin loss involving damage or necrosis of subcutaneous tissue, right hip
    L89.214   Pressure ulcer of right hip, stage 4
      Healing pressure ulcer of right hip, stage 4
      Pressure ulcer with necrosis of soft tissues through to underlying muscle, tendon, or bone, right hip
    L89.219   Pressure ulcer of right hip, unspecified stage
      Healing pressure ulcer of right hip NOS
      Healing pressure ulcer of right hip, unspecified stage
  ✓6th **L89.22   Pressure ulcer of left hip**
    L89.220   Pressure ulcer of left hip, unstageable
    L89.221   Pressure ulcer of left hip, stage 1
      Healing pressure ulcer of left hip back, stage 1
      Pressure pre-ulcer skin changes limited to persistent focal edema, left hip

    L89.222   Pressure ulcer of left hip, stage 2
      Healing pressure ulcer of left hip, stage 2
      Pressure ulcer with abrasion, blister, partial thickness skin loss involving epidermis and/or dermis, left hip
    L89.223   Pressure ulcer of left hip, stage 3
      Healing pressure ulcer of left hip, stage 3
      Pressure ulcer with full thickness skin loss involving damage or necrosis of subcutaneous tissue, left hip
    L89.224   Pressure ulcer of left hip, stage 4
      Healing pressure ulcer of left hip, stage 4
      Pressure ulcer with necrosis of soft tissues through to underlying muscle, tendon, or bone, left hip
    L89.229   Pressure ulcer of left hip, unspecified stage
      Healing pressure ulcer of left hip NOS
      Healing pressure ulcer of left hip, unspecified stage
✓5th **L89.3   Pressure ulcer of buttock**
  ✓6th **L89.30   Pressure ulcer of unspecified buttock**
    L89.300   Pressure ulcer of unspecified buttock, unstageable
    L89.301   Pressure ulcer of unspecified buttock, stage 1
      Healing pressure ulcer of unspecified buttock, stage 1
      Pressure pre-ulcer skin changes limited to persistent focal edema, unspecified buttock
    L89.302   Pressure ulcer of unspecified buttock, stage 2
      Healing pressure ulcer of unspecified buttock, stage 2
      Pressure ulcer with abrasion, blister, partial thickness skin loss involving epidermis and/or dermis, unspecified buttock
    L89.303   Pressure ulcer of unspecified buttock, stage 3
      Healing pressure ulcer of unspecified buttock, stage 3
      Pressure ulcer with full thickness skin loss involving damage or necrosis of subcutaneous tissue, unspecified buttock
    L89.304   Pressure ulcer of unspecified buttock, stage 4
      Healing pressure ulcer of unspecified buttock, stage 4
      Pressure ulcer with necrosis of soft tissues through to underlying muscle, tendon, or bone, unspecified buttock
    L89.309   Pressure ulcer of unspecified buttock, unspecified stage
      Healing pressure ulcer of unspecified buttock NOS
      Healing pressure ulcer of unspecified buttock, unspecified stage
  ✓6th **L89.31   Pressure ulcer of right buttock**
    L89.310   Pressure ulcer of right buttock, unstageable
    L89.311   Pressure ulcer of right buttock, stage 1
      Healing pressure ulcer of right buttock, stage 1
      Pressure pre-ulcer skin changes limited to persistent focal edema, right buttock
    L89.312   Pressure ulcer of right buttock, stage 2
      Healing pressure ulcer of right buttock, stage 2
      Pressure ulcer with abrasion, blister, partial thickness skin loss involving epidermis and/or dermis, right buttock

---

EXCLUDES 1 Not coded here   EXCLUDES 2 Not included here   *Manifestation Code*

L89.313 **Pressure ulcer of right buttock, stage 3**
Healing pressure ulcer of right buttock, stage 3
Pressure ulcer with full thickness skin loss involving damage or necrosis of subcutaneous tissue, right buttock

L89.314 **Pressure ulcer of right buttock, stage 4**
Healing pressure ulcer of right buttock, stage 4
Pressure ulcer with necrosis of soft tissues through to underlying muscle, tendon, or bone, right buttock

L89.319 **Pressure ulcer of right buttock, unspecified stage**
Healing pressure ulcer of right buttock NOS
Healing pressure ulcer of right buttock, unspecified stage

✓6ᵗʰ **L89.32** **Pressure ulcer of left buttock**

L89.320 **Pressure ulcer of left buttock, unstageable**

L89.321 **Pressure ulcer of left buttock, stage 1**
Healing pressure ulcer of left buttock, stage 1
Pressure pre-ulcer skin changes limited to persistent focal edema, left buttock

L89.322 **Pressure ulcer of left buttock, stage 2**
Healing pressure ulcer of left buttock, stage 2
Pressure ulcer with abrasion, blister, partial thickness skin loss involving epidermis and/or dermis, left buttock

L89.323 **Pressure ulcer of left buttock, stage 3**
Healing pressure ulcer of left buttock, stage 3
Pressure ulcer with full thickness skin loss involving damage or necrosis of subcutaneous tissue, left buttock

L89.324 **Pressure ulcer of left buttock, stage 4**
Healing pressure ulcer of left buttock, stage 4
Pressure ulcer with necrosis of soft tissues through to underlying muscle, tendon, or bone, left buttock

L89.329 **Pressure ulcer of left buttock, unspecified stage**
Healing pressure ulcer of left buttock NOS
Healing pressure ulcer of left buttock, unspecified stage

✓5ᵗʰ **L89.4** **Pressure ulcer of contiguous site of back, buttock and hip**

L89.40 **Pressure ulcer of contiguous site of back, buttock and hip, unspecified stage**
Healing pressure ulcer of contiguous site of back, buttock and hip NOS
Healing pressure ulcer of contiguous site of back, buttock and hip, unspecified stage

L89.41 **Pressure ulcer of contiguous site of back, buttock and hip, stage 1**
Healing pressure ulcer of contiguous site of back, buttock and hip, stage 1
Pressure pre-ulcer skin changes limited to persistent focal edema, contiguous site of back, buttock and hip

L89.42 **Pressure ulcer of contiguous site of back, buttock and hip, stage 2**
Healing pressure ulcer of contiguous site of back, buttock and hip, stage 2
Pressure ulcer with abrasion, blister, partial thickness skin loss involving epidermis and/or dermis, contiguous site of back, buttock and hip

L89.43 **Pressure ulcer of contiguous site of back, buttock and hip, stage 3**
Healing pressure ulcer of contiguous site of back, buttock and hip, stage 3
Pressure ulcer with full thickness skin loss involving damage or necrosis of subcutaneous tissue, contiguous site of back, buttock and hip

L89.44 **Pressure ulcer of contiguous site of back, buttock and hip, stage 4**
Healing pressure ulcer of contiguous site of back, buttock and hip, stage 4
Pressure ulcer with necrosis of soft tissues through to underlying muscle, tendon, or bone, contiguous site of back, buttock and hip

L89.45 **Pressure ulcer of contiguous site of back, buttock and hip, unstageable**

✓5ᵗʰ **L89.5** **Pressure ulcer of ankle**

✓6ᵗʰ **L89.50** **Pressure ulcer of unspecified ankle**

L89.500 **Pressure ulcer of unspecified ankle, unstageable**

L89.501 **Pressure ulcer of unspecified ankle, stage 1**
Healing pressure ulcer of unspecified ankle, stage 1
Pressure pre-ulcer skin changes limited to persistent focal edema, unspecified ankle

L89.502 **Pressure ulcer of unspecified ankle, stage 2**
Healing pressure ulcer of unspecified ankle, stage 2
Pressure ulcer with abrasion, blister, partial thickness skin loss involving epidermis and/or dermis, unspecified ankle

L89.503 **Pressure ulcer of unspecified ankle, stage 3**
Healing pressure ulcer of unspecified ankle, stage 3
Pressure ulcer with full thickness skin loss involving damage or necrosis of subcutaneous tissue, unspecified ankle

L89.504 **Pressure ulcer of unspecified ankle, stage 4**
Healing pressure ulcer of unspecified ankle, stage 4
Pressure ulcer with necrosis of soft tissues through to underlying muscle, tendon, or bone, unspecified ankle

L89.509 **Pressure ulcer of unspecified ankle, unspecified stage**
Healing pressure ulcer of unspecified ankle NOS
Healing pressure ulcer of unspecified ankle, unspecified stage

✓6ᵗʰ **L89.51** **Pressure ulcer of right ankle**

L89.510 **Pressure ulcer of right ankle, unstageable**

L89.511 **Pressure ulcer of right ankle, stage 1**
Healing pressure ulcer of right ankle, stage 1
Pressure pre-ulcer skin changes limited to persistent focal edema, right ankle

L89.512 **Pressure ulcer of right ankle, stage 2**
Healing pressure ulcer of right ankle, stage 2
Pressure ulcer with abrasion, blister, partial thickness skin loss involving epidermis and/or dermis, right ankle

L89.513 **Pressure ulcer of right ankle, stage 3**
Healing pressure ulcer of right ankle, stage 3
Pressure ulcer with full thickness skin loss involving damage or necrosis of subcutaneous tissue, right ankle

L89.514 Pressure ulcer of right ankle, stage 4
Healing pressure ulcer of right ankle, stage 4
Pressure ulcer with necrosis of soft tissues through to underlying muscle, tendon, or bone, right ankle

L89.519 Pressure ulcer of right ankle, unspecified stage
Healing pressure ulcer of right ankle NOS
Healing pressure ulcer of right ankle, unspecified stage

√6ᵗʰ **L89.52 Pressure ulcer of left ankle**

L89.520 Pressure ulcer of left ankle, unstageable

L89.521 Pressure ulcer of left ankle, stage 1
Healing pressure ulcer of left ankle, stage 1
Pressure pre-ulcer skin changes limited to persistnt focal edema, left ankle

L89.522 Pressure ulcer of left ankle, stage 2
Healing pressure ulcer of left ankle, stage 2
Pressure ulcer with abrasion, blister, partial thickness skin loss involving epidermis and/or dermis, left ankle

L89.523 Pressure ulcer of left ankle, stage 3
Healing pressure ulcer of left ankle, stage 3
Pressure ulcer with full thickness skin loss involving damage or necrosis of subcutaneous tissue, left ankle

L89.524 Pressure ulcer of left ankle, stage 4
Healing pressure ulcer of left ankle, stage 4
Pressure ulcer with necrosis of soft tissues through to underlying muscle, tendon, or bone, left ankle

L89.529 Pressure ulcer of left ankle, unspecified stage
Healing pressure ulcer of left ankle NOS
Healing pressure ulcer of left ankle, unspecified stage

√5ᵗʰ **L89.6 Pressure ulcer of heel**

√6ᵗʰ **L89.60 Pressure ulcer of unspecified heel**

L89.600 Pressure ulcer of unspecified heel, unstageable

L89.601 Pressure ulcer of unspecified heel, stage 1
Healing pressure ulcer of unspecified heel, stage 1
Pressure pre-ulcer skin changes limited to persistent focal edema, unspecified heel

L89.602 Pressure ulcer of unspecified heel, stage 2
Healing pressure ulcer of unspecified heel, stage 2
Pressure ulcer with abrasion, blister, partial thickness skin loss involving epidermis and/or dermis, unspecified heel

L89.603 Pressure ulcer of unspecified heel, stage 3
Healing pressure ulcer of unspecified heel, stage 3
Pressure ulcer with full thickness skin loss involving damage or necrosis of subcutaneous tissue, unspecified heel

L89.604 Pressure ulcer of unspecified heel, stage 4
Healing pressure ulcer of unspecified heel, stage 4
Pressure ulcer with necrosis of soft tissues through to underlying muscle, tendon, or bone, unspecified heel

L89.609 Pressure ulcer of unspecified heel, unspecified stage
Healing pressure ulcer of unspecified heel NOS
Healing pressure ulcer of unspecified heel, unspecified stage

√6ᵗʰ **L89.61 Pressure ulcer of right heel**

L89.610 Pressure ulcer of right heel, unstageable

L89.611 Pressure ulcer of right heel, stage 1
Healing pressure ulcer of right heel, stage 1
Pressure pre-ulcer skin changes limited to persistent focal edema, right heel

L89.612 Pressure ulcer of right heel, stage 2
Healing pressure ulcer of right heel, stage 2
Pressure ulcer with abrasion, blister, partial thickness skin loss involving epidermis and/or dermis, right heel

L89.613 Pressure ulcer of right heel, stage 3
Healing pressure ulcer of right heel, stage 3
Pressure ulcer with full thickness skin loss involving damage or necrosis of subcutaneous tissue, right heel

L89.614 Pressure ulcer of right heel, stage 4
Healing pressure ulcer of right heel, stage 4
Pressure ulcer with necrosis of soft tissues through to underlying muscle, tendon, or bone, right heel

L89.619 Pressure ulcer of right heel, unspecified stage
Healing pressure ulcer of right heel NOS
Healing pressure ulcer of unspecified heel, right stage

√6ᵗʰ **L89.62 Pressure ulcer of left heel**

L89.620 Pressure ulcer of left heel, unstageable

L89.621 Pressure ulcer of left heel, stage 1
Healing pressure ulcer of left heel, stage 1
Pressure pre-ulcer skin changes limited to persistent focal edema, left heel

L89.622 Pressure ulcer of left heel, stage 2
Healing pressure ulcer of left heel, stage 2
Pressure ulcer with abrasion, blister, partial thickness skin loss involving epidermis and/or dermis, left heel

L89.623 Pressure ulcer of left heel, stage 3
Healing pressure ulcer of left heel, stage 3
Pressure ulcer with full thickness skin loss involving damage or necrosis of subcutaneous tissue, left heel

L89.624 Pressure ulcer of left heel, stage 4
Healing pressure ulcer of left heel, stage 4
Pressure ulcer with necrosis of soft tissues through to underlying muscle, tendon, or bone, left heel

L89.629 Pressure ulcer of left heel, unspecified stage
Healing pressure ulcer of left heel NOS
Healing pressure ulcer of left heel, unspecified stage

√5ᵗʰ **L89.8 Pressure ulcer of other site**

√6ᵗʰ **L89.81 Pressure ulcer of head**
Pressure ulcer of face

L89.810 Pressure ulcer of head, unstageable

L89.811 Pressure ulcer of head, stage 1
Healing pressure ulcer of head, stage 1
Pressure pre-ulcer skin changes limited to persistent focal edema, head

L89.812 Pressure ulcer of head, stage 2
Healing pressure ulcer of head, stage 2
Pressure ulcer with abrasion, blister, partial thickness skin loss involving epidermis and/or dermis, head

---

EXCLUDES 1 Not coded here   EXCLUDES 2 Not included here   *Manifestation Code*

L89.813 **Pressure ulcer of head, stage 3**
Healing pressure ulcer of head, stage 3
Pressure ulcer with full thickness skin loss involving damage or necrosis of subcutaneous tissue, head

L89.814 **Pressure ulcer of head, stage 4**
Healing pressure ulcer of head, stage 4
Pressure ulcer with necrosis of soft tissues through to underlying muscle, tendon, or bone, head

L89.819 **Pressure ulcer of head, unspecified stage**
Healing pressure ulcer of head NOS
Healing pressure ulcer of head, unspecified stage

✓6th **L89.89 Pressure ulcer of other site**

L89.890 **Pressure ulcer of other site, unstageable**

L89.891 **Pressure ulcer of other site, stage 1**
Healing pressure ulcer of other site, stage 1
Pressure pre-ulcer skin changes limited to persistent focal edema, other site

L89.892 **Pressure ulcer of other site, stage 2**
Healing pressure ulcer of other site, stage 2
Pressure ulcer with abrasion, blister, partial thickness skin loss involving epidermis and/or dermis, other site

L89.893 **Pressure ulcer of other site, stage 3**
Healing pressure ulcer of other site, stage 3
Pressure ulcer with full thickness skin loss involving damage or necrosis of subcutaneous tissue, other site

L89.894 **Pressure ulcer of other site, stage 4**
Healing pressure ulcer of other site, stage 4
Pressure ulcer with necrosis of soft tissues through to underlying muscle, tendon, or bone, other site

L89.899 **Pressure ulcer of other site, unspecified stage**
Healing pressure ulcer of other site NOS
Healing pressure ulcer of other site, unspecified stage

✓5th **L89.9 Pressure ulcer of unspecified site**

L89.90 **Pressure ulcer of unspecified site, unspecified stage**
Healing pressure ulcer of unspecified site NOS
Healing pressure ulcer of unspecified site, unspecified stage

L89.91 **Pressure ulcer of unspecified site, stage 1**
Healing pressure ulcer of unspecified site, stage 1
Pressure pre-ulcer skin changes limited to persistent focal edema, unspecified site

L89.92 **Pressure ulcer of unspecified site, stage 2**
Healing pressure ulcer of unspecified site, stage 2
Pressure ulcer with abrasion, blister, partial thickness skin loss involving epidermis and/or dermis, unspecified site

L89.93 **Pressure ulcer of unspecified site, stage 3**
Healing pressure ulcer of unspecified site, stage 3
Pressure ulcer with full thickness skin loss involving damage or necrosis of subcutaneous tissue, unspecified site

L89.94 **Pressure ulcer of unspecified site, stage 4**
Healing pressure ulcer of unspecified site, stage 4
Pressure ulcer with necrosis of soft tissues through to underlying muscle, tendon, or bone, unspecified site

L89.95 **Pressure ulcer of unspecified site, unstageable**

✓4th **L90 Atrophic disorders of skin**

L90.0 **Lichen sclerosus et atrophicus**
EXCLUDES 2 *lichen sclerosus of external female genital organs (N90.4)*
lichen sclerosus of external male genital organs (N48.0)

L90.1 **Anetoderma of Schweninger-Buzzi**

L90.2 **Anetoderma of Jadassohn-Pellizzari**

L90.3 **Atrophoderma of Pasini and Pierini**

L90.4 **Acrodermatitis chronica atrophicans**

L90.5 **Scar conditions and fibrosis of skin**
Adherent scar (skin)
Cicatrix
Disfigurement of skin due to scar
Fibrosis of skin NOS
Scar NOS
EXCLUDES 2 *hypertrophic scar (L91.0)*
keloid scar (L91.0)

L90.6 **Striae atrophicae**

L90.8 **Other atrophic disorders of skin**

L90.9 **Atrophic disorder of skin, unspecified**

✓4th **L91 Hypertrophic disorders of skin**

L91.0 **Hypertrophic scar**
Keloid
Keloid scar
EXCLUDES 2 *acne keloid (L73.0)*
scar NOS (L90.5)

L91.8 **Other hypertrophic disorders of the skin**

L91.9 **Hypertrophic disorder of the skin, unspecified**

✓4th **L92 Granulomatous disorders of skin and subcutaneous tissue**
EXCLUDES 2 *actinic granuloma (L57.5)*

L92.0 **Granuloma annulare**
Perforating granuloma annulare

L92.1 **Necrobiosis lipoidica, not elsewhere classified**
EXCLUDES 1 *necrobiosis lipoidica associated with diabetes mellitus (E08-E13 with .620)*

L92.2 **Granuloma faciale [eosinophilic granuloma of skin]**

L92.3 **Foreign body granuloma of the skin and subcutaneous tissue**
Use additional code to identify the type of retained foreign body (Z18.-)

L92.8 **Other granulomatous disorders of the skin and subcutaneous tissue**

L92.9 **Granulomatous disorder of the skin and subcutaneous tissue, unspecified**

✓4th **L93 Lupus erythematosus**
EXCLUDES 1 *lupus exedens (A18.4)*
lupus vulgaris (A18.4)
scleroderma (M34-)
systemic lupus erythematosus (M32-)

L93.0 **Discoid lupus erythematosus**
Lupus erythematosus NOS

L93.1 **Subacute cutaneous lupus erythematosus**

L93.2 **Other local lupus erythematosus**
Lupus erythematosus profundus
Lupus panniculitis

✓4th **L94 Other localized connective tissue disorders**
EXCLUDES 1 *systemic connective tissue disorders (M30-M36)*

L94.0 **Localized scleroderma [morphea]**
Circumscribed scleroderma

L94.1 **Linear scleroderma**
En coup de sabre lesion

L94.2 **Calcinosis cutis**

L94.3 **Sclerodactyly**

L94.4 **Gottron's papules**

L94.5 **Poikiloderma vasculare atrophicans**

L94.6 **Ainhum**

L94.8 **Other specified localized connective tissue disorders**

L94.9 **Localized connective tissue disorder, unspecified**

✓4th **L95 Vasculitis limited to skin, not elsewhere classified**
EXCLUDES 1 *angioma serpiginosum (L81.7)*
Henoch(-Schönlein) purpura (D69.0)
hypersensitivity angiitis (M31.0)
lupus panniculitis (L93.2)
panniculitis NOS (M79.3)
panniculitis of neck and back (M54.0-)
polyarteritis nodosa (M30.0)
relapsing panniculitis (M35.6)
rheumatoid vasculitis (M05.2)
serum sickness (T80.6)
urticaria (L50-)
Wegener's granulomatosis (M31.3-)

L95.0 **Livedoid vasculitis**
Atrophie blanche (en plaque)

L95.1 **Erythema elevatum diutinum**

Diseases of the Skin and Subcutaneous Tissue

L95.8–L97.404

L95.8   **Other vasculitis limited to the skin**

L95.9   **Vasculitis limited to the skin, unspecified**

✓4th **L97   Non-pressure chronic ulcer of lower limb, not elsewhere classified**

Chronic ulcer of skin NOS
Non-healing ulcer of skin
Non-infected sinus of skin
Trophic ulcer NOS
Tropical ulcer NOS
Ulcer of skin NOS

NOTE   A code from L97 may be used as a principal or first listed code if no underlying condition is documented as the cause of the ulcer. If one of the underlying conditions listed below is documented with a lower extremity ulcer a causal condition should be assumed.

Code first any associated underlying condition:
atherosclerosis of the lower extremities (I70.23-, I70.24-, I70.33-, I70.34-, I70.43-, I70.44-, I70.53-, I70.54-, I70.63-, I70.64-, I70.73-, I70.74-)
chronic venous hypertension (I87.31-, I87.33-)
diabetic ulcers (E08.621, E08.622, E09.621, E09.622, E10.621, E10.622, E11.621, E11.622, E13.621, E13.622)
postphlebitic syndrome (I87.01-, I87.03-)
postthrombotic syndrome (I87.01-, I87.03-)
varicose ulcer (I83.0-, I83.2-)

Code first any associated gangrene (I96)

EXCLUDES 2   *pressure ulcer (pressure area) (L89-)*
skin infections (L00-L08)
specific infections classified to A00-B99

✓5th **L97.1   Non-pressure chronic ulcer of thigh**

    ✓6th **L97.10   Non-pressure chronic ulcer of unspecified thigh**

      L97.101   **Non-pressure chronic ulcer of unspecified thigh limited to breakdown of skin**

      L97.102   **Non-pressure chronic ulcer of unspecified thigh with fat layer exposed**

      L97.103   **Non-pressure chronic ulcer of unspecified thigh with necrosis of muscle**

      L97.104   **Non-pressure chronic ulcer of unspecified thigh with necrosis of bone**

      L97.109   **Non-pressure chronic ulcer of unspecified thigh with unspecified severity**

    ✓6th **L97.11   Non-pressure chronic ulcer of right thigh**

      L97.111   **Non-pressure chronic ulcer of right thigh limited to breakdown of skin**

      L97.112   **Non-pressure chronic ulcer of right thigh with fat layer exposed**

      L97.113   **Non-pressure chronic ulcer of right thigh with necrosis of muscle**

      L97.114   **Non-pressure chronic ulcer of right thigh with necrosis of bone**

      L97.119   **Non-pressure chronic ulcer of right thigh with unspecified severity**

    ✓6th **L97.12   Non-pressure chronic ulcer of left thigh**

      L97.121   **Non-pressure chronic ulcer of left thigh limited to breakdown of skin**

      L97.122   **Non-pressure chronic ulcer of left thigh with fat layer exposed**

      L97.123   **Non-pressure chronic ulcer of left thigh with necrosis of muscle**

      L97.124   **Non-pressure chronic ulcer of left thigh with necrosis of bone**

      L97.129   **Non-pressure chronic ulcer of left thigh with unspecified severity**

✓5th **L97.2   Non-pressure chronic ulcer of calf**

    ✓6th **L97.20   Non-pressure chronic ulcer of unspecified calf**

      L97.201   **Non-pressure chronic ulcer of unspecified calf limited to breakdown of skin**

      L97.202   **Non-pressure chronic ulcer of unspecified calf with fat layer exposed**

      L97.203   **Non-pressure chronic ulcer of unspecified calf with necrosis of muscle**

      L97.204   **Non-pressure chronic ulcer of unspecified calf with necrosis of bone**

      L97.209   **Non-pressure chronic ulcer of unspecified calf with unspecified severity**

    ✓6th **L97.21   Non-pressure chronic ulcer of right calf**

      L97.211   **Non-pressure chronic ulcer of right calf limited to breakdown of skin**

      L97.212   **Non-pressure chronic ulcer of right calf with fat layer exposed**

      L97.213   **Non-pressure chronic ulcer of right calf with necrosis of muscle**

      L97.214   **Non-pressure chronic ulcer of right calf with necrosis of bone**

      L97.219   **Non-pressure chronic ulcer of right calf with unspecified severity**

    ✓6th **L97.22   Non-pressure chronic ulcer of left calf**

      L97.221   **Non-pressure chronic ulcer of left calf limited to breakdown of skin**

      L97.222   **Non-pressure chronic ulcer of left calf with fat layer exposed**

      L97.223   **Non-pressure chronic ulcer of left calf with necrosis of muscle**

      L97.224   **Non-pressure chronic ulcer of left calf with necrosis of bone**

      L97.229   **Non-pressure chronic ulcer of left calf with unspecified severity**

✓5th **L97.3   Non-pressure chronic ulcer of ankle**

    ✓6th **L97.30   Non-pressure chronic ulcer of unspecified ankle**

      L97.301   **Non-pressure chronic ulcer of unspecified ankle limited to breakdown of skin**

      L97.302   **Non-pressure chronic ulcer of unspecified ankle with fat layer exposed**

      L97.303   **Non-pressure chronic ulcer of unspecified ankle with necrosis of muscle**

      L97.304   **Non-pressure chronic ulcer of unspecified ankle with necrosis of bone**

      L97.309   **Non-pressure chronic ulcer of unspecified ankle with unspecified severity**

    ✓6th **L97.31   Non-pressure chronic ulcer of right ankle**

      L97.311   **Non-pressure chronic ulcer of right ankle limited to breakdown of skin**

      L97.312   **Non-pressure chronic ulcer of right ankle with fat layer exposed**

      L97.313   **Non-pressure chronic ulcer of right ankle with necrosis of muscle**

      L97.314   **Non-pressure chronic ulcer of right ankle with necrosis of bone**

      L97.319   **Non-pressure chronic ulcer of right ankle with unspecified severity**

    ✓6th **L97.32   Non-pressure chronic ulcer of left ankle**

      L97.321   **Non-pressure chronic ulcer of left ankle limited to breakdown of skin**

      L97.322   **Non-pressure chronic ulcer of left ankle with fat layer exposed**

      L97.323   **Non-pressure chronic ulcer of left ankle with necrosis of muscle**

      L97.324   **Non-pressure chronic ulcer of left ankle with necrosis of bone**

      L97.329   **Non-pressure chronic ulcer of left ankle with unspecified severity**

✓5th **L97.4   Non-pressure chronic ulcer of heel and midfoot**

Non-pressure chronic ulcer of plantar surface of midfoot

    ✓6th **L97.40   Non-pressure chronic ulcer of unspecified heel and midfoot**

      L97.401   **Non-pressure chronic ulcer of unspecified heel and midfoot limited to breakdown of skin**

      L97.402   **Non-pressure chronic ulcer of unspecified heel and midfoot with fat layer exposed**

      L97.403   **Non-pressure chronic ulcer of unspecified heel and midfoot with necrosis of muscle**

      L97.404   **Non-pressure chronic ulcer of unspecified heel and midfoot with necrosis of bone**

EXCLUDES 1 Not coded here   **EXCLUDES 2** Not included here   *Manifestation Code*

L97.409 Non-pressure chronic ulcer of unspecified heel and midfoot with unspecified severity

√6ᵗʰ L97.41 Non-pressure chronic ulcer of right heel and midfoot

L97.411 Non-pressure chronic ulcer of right heel and midfoot limited to breakdown of skin

L97.412 Non-pressure chronic ulcer of right heel and midfoot with fat layer exposed

L97.413 Non-pressure chronic ulcer of right heel and midfoot with necrosis of muscle

L97.414 Non-pressure chronic ulcer of right heel and midfoot with necrosis of bone

L97.419 Non-pressure chronic ulcer of right heel and midfoot with unspecified severity

√6ᵗʰ L97.42 Non-pressure chronic ulcer of left heel and midfoot

L97.421 Non-pressure chronic ulcer of left heel and midfoot limited to breakdown of skin

L97.422 Non-pressure chronic ulcer of left heel and midfoot with fat layer exposed

L97.423 Non-pressure chronic ulcer of left heel and midfoot with necrosis of muscle

L97.424 Non-pressure chronic ulcer of left heel and midfoot with necrosis of bone

L97.429 Non-pressure chronic ulcer of left heel and midfoot with unspecified severity

√5ᵗʰ L97.5 Non-pressure chronic ulcer of other part of foot
Non-pressure chronic ulcer of toe

√6ᵗʰ L97.50 Non-pressure chronic ulcer of other part of unspecified foot

L97.501 Non-pressure chronic ulcer of other part of unspecified foot limited to breakdown of skin

L97.502 Non-pressure chronic ulcer of other part of unspecified foot with fat layer exposed

L97.503 Non-pressure chronic ulcer of other part of unspecified foot with necrosis of muscle

L97.504 Non-pressure chronic ulcer of other part of unspecified foot with necrosis of bone

L97.509 Non-pressure chronic ulcer of other part of unspecified foot with unspecified severity

√6ᵗʰ L97.51 Non-pressure chronic ulcer of other part of right foot

L97.511 Non-pressure chronic ulcer of other part of right foot limited to breakdown of skin

L97.512 Non-pressure chronic ulcer of other part of right foot with fat layer exposed

L97.513 Non-pressure chronic ulcer of other part of right foot with necrosis of muscle

L97.514 Non-pressure chronic ulcer of other part of right foot with necrosis of bone

L97.519 Non-pressure chronic ulcer of other part of right foot with unspecified severity

√6ᵗʰ L97.52 Non-pressure chronic ulcer of other part of left foot

L97.521 Non-pressure chronic ulcer of other part of left foot limited to breakdown of skin

L97.522 Non-pressure chronic ulcer of other part of left foot with fat layer exposed

L97.523 Non-pressure chronic ulcer of other part of left foot with necrosis of muscle

L97.524 Non-pressure chronic ulcer of other part of left foot with necrosis of bone

L97.529 Non-pressure chronic ulcer of other part of left foot with unspecified severity

√5ᵗʰ L97.8 Non-pressure chronic ulcer of other part of lower leg

√6ᵗʰ L97.80 Non-pressure chronic ulcer of other part of unspecified lower leg

L97.801 Non-pressure chronic ulcer of other part of unspecified lower leg limited to breakdown of skin

L97.802 Non-pressure chronic ulcer of other part of unspecified lower leg with fat layer exposed

L97.803 Non-pressure chronic ulcer of other part of unspecified lower leg with necrosis of muscle

L97.804 Non-pressure chronic ulcer of other part of unspecified lower leg with necrosis of bone

L97.809 Non-pressure chronic ulcer of other part of unspecified lower leg with unspecified severity

√6ᵗʰ L97.81 Non-pressure chronic ulcer of other part of right lower leg

L97.811 Non-pressure chronic ulcer of other part of right lower leg limited to breakdown of skin

L97.812 Non-pressure chronic ulcer of other part of right lower leg with fat layer exposed

L97.813 Non-pressure chronic ulcer of other part of right lower leg with necrosis of muscle

L97.814 Non-pressure chronic ulcer of other part of right lower leg with necrosis of bone

L97.819 Non-pressure chronic ulcer of other part of right lower leg with unspecified severity

√6ᵗʰ L97.82 Non-pressure chronic ulcer of other part of left lower leg

L97.821 Non-pressure chronic ulcer of other part of left lower leg limited to breakdown of skin

L97.822 Non-pressure chronic ulcer of other part of left lower leg with fat layer exposed

L97.823 Non-pressure chronic ulcer of other part of left lower leg with necrosis of muscle

L97.824 Non-pressure chronic ulcer of other part of left lower leg with necrosis of bone

L97.829 Non-pressure chronic ulcer of other part of left lower leg with unspecified severity

√5ᵗʰ L97.9 Non-pressure chronic ulcer of unspecified part of lower leg

√6ᵗʰ L97.90 Non-pressure chronic ulcer of unspecified part of unspecified lower leg

L97.901 Non-pressure chronic ulcer of unspecified part of unspecified lower leg limited to breakdown of skin

L97.902 Non-pressure chronic ulcer of unspecified part of unspecified lower leg with fat layer exposed

L97.903 Non-pressure chronic ulcer of unspecified part of unspecified lower leg with necrosis of muscle

L97.904 Non-pressure chronic ulcer of unspecified part of unspecified lower leg with necrosis of bone

L97.909 Non-pressure chronic ulcer of unspecified part of unspecified lower leg with unspecified severity

√6ᵗʰ L97.91 Non-pressure chronic ulcer of unspecified part of right lower leg

L97.911 Non-pressure chronic ulcer of unspecified part of right lower leg limited to breakdown of skin

L97.912 Non-pressure chronic ulcer of unspecified part of right lower leg with fat layer exposed

L97.913 Non-pressure chronic ulcer of unspecified part of right lower leg with necrosis of muscle

L97.914 Non-pressure chronic ulcer of unspecified part of right lower leg with necrosis of bone

L97.919 Non-pressure chronic ulcer of unspecified part of right lower leg with unspecified severity

✔ Appropriate additional character required

√x7ᵗʰ Requires 7th character, placeholder x must fill empty characters

✓6th **L97.92** **Non-pressure chronic ulcer of unspecified part of left lower leg**

     L97.921 **Non-pressure chronic ulcer of unspecified part of left lower leg limited to breakdown of skin**

     L97.922 **Non-pressure chronic ulcer of unspecified part of left lower leg with fat layer exposed**

     L97.923 **Non-pressure chronic ulcer of unspecified part of left lower leg with necrosis of muscle**

     L97.924 **Non-pressure chronic ulcer of unspecified part of left lower leg with necrosis of bone**

     L97.929 **Non-pressure chronic ulcer of unspecified part of left lower leg with unspecified severity**

✓4th **L98** **Other disorders of skin and subcutaneous tissue, not elsewhere classified**

     L98.0 **Pyogenic granuloma**

         EXCLUDES 2   *pyogenic granuloma of gingiva (K06.8)*
                 pyogenic granuloma of maxillary alveolar ridge (K04.5)
                 pyogenic granuloma of oral mucosa (K13.4)

     L98.1 **Factitial dermatitis**
         Neurotic excoriation

     L98.2 **Febrile neutrophilic dermatosis [Sweet]**

     L98.3 **Eosinophilic cellulitis [Wells]**

✓5th **L98.4** **Non-pressure chronic ulcer of skin, not elsewhere classified**
         Chronic ulcer of skin NOS
         Tropical ulcer NOS
         Ulcer of skin NOS

         EXCLUDES 2   *pressure ulcer (pressure area) (L89-)*
                 gangrene (I96)
                 skin infections (L00-L08)
                 specific infections classified to A00-B99
                 ulcer of lower limb NEC (L97-)
                 varicose ulcer (I83.0-I82.2)

✓6th **L98.41** **Non-pressure chronic ulcer of buttock**

     L98.411 **Non-pressure chronic ulcer of buttock limited to breakdown of skin**

     L98.412 **Non-pressure chronic ulcer of buttock with fat layer exposed**

     L98.413 **Non-pressure chronic ulcer of buttock with necrosis of muscle**

     L98.414 **Non-pressure chronic ulcer of buttock with necrosis of bone**

     L98.419 **Non-pressure chronic ulcer of buttock with unspecified severity**

✓6th **L98.42** **Non-pressure chronic ulcer of back**

     L98.421 **Non-pressure chronic ulcer of back limited to breakdown of skin**

     L98.422 **Non-pressure chronic ulcer of back with fat layer exposed**

     L98.423 **Non-pressure chronic ulcer of back with necrosis of muscle**

     L98.424 **Non-pressure chronic ulcer of back with necrosis of bone**

     L98.429 **Non-pressure chronic ulcer of back with unspecified severity**

✓6th **L98.49** **Non-pressure chronic ulcer of skin of other sites**
         Non-pressure chronic ulcer of skin NOS

     L98.491 **Non-pressure chronic ulcer of skin of other sites limited to breakdown of skin**

     L98.492 **Non-pressure chronic ulcer of skin of other sites with fat layer exposed**

     L98.493 **Non-pressure chronic ulcer of skin of other sites with necrosis of muscle**

     L98.494 **Non-pressure chronic ulcer of skin of other sites with necrosis of bone**

     L98.499 **Non-pressure chronic ulcer of skin of other sites with unspecified severity**

     L98.5 **Mucinosis of the skin**
         Focal mucinosis
         Lichen myxedematosus

         EXCLUDES 1   *focal oral mucinosis (K13.79)*
                 myxedema (E03.9)

     L98.6 **Other infiltrative disorders of the skin and subcutaneous tissue**

         EXCLUDES 1   *hyalinosis cutis et mucosae (E78.89)*

     L98.8 **Other specified disorders of the skin and subcutaneous tissue**

     L98.9 **Disorder of the skin and subcutaneous tissue, unspecified**

L99 ***Other disorders of skin and subcutaneous tissue in diseases classified elsewhere***

     Code first underlying disease, such as:
         amyloidosis (E85-)

     EXCLUDES 1   *skin disorders in diabetes (E08-E13 with .62)*
                 skin disorders in gonorrhea (A54.89)
                 skin disorders in syphilis (A51.31, A52.79)

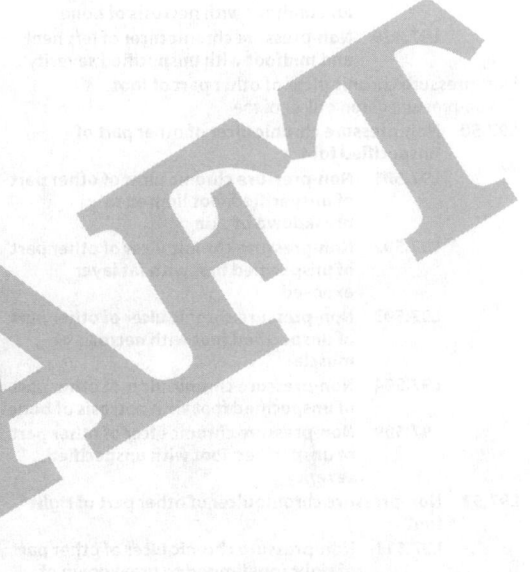

Chapter 13. Diseases of the Musculoskeletal System and Connective Tissue (M00-M99)

NOTE Use an external cause code following the code for the musculoskeletal condition, if applicable, to identify the cause of the musculoskeletal condition

EXCLUDES 2 *arthropathic psoriasis (L40.5-)*
certain conditions originating in the perinatal period (P04-P96)
certain infectious and parasitic diseases (A00-B99)
compartment syndrome (traumatic) (T79.a-)
complications of pregnancy, childbirth and the puerperium (O00-O99)
congenital malformations, deformations, and chromosomal abnormalities (Q00-Q99)
endocrine, nutritional and metabolic diseases (E00-E88)
injury, poisoning and certain other consequences of external causes (S00-T88)
neoplasms (C00-D49)
symptoms, signs and abnormal clinical and laboratory findings, not elsewhere classified (R00-R94)

This chapter contains the following blocks:

M00-M02 Infectious arthropathies
M05-M14 Inflammatory polyarthropathies
M15-M19 Osteoarthritis
M20-M25 Other joint disorders
M26-M27 Dentofacial anomalies [including malocclusion] and other disorders of jaw
M30-M36 Systemic connective tissue disorders
M40-M43 Deforming dorsopathies
M45-M49 Spondylopathies
M50-M54 Other dorsopathies
M60-M63 Disorders of muscles
M65-M67 Disorders of synovium and tendon
M70-M79 Other soft tissue disorders
M80-M85 Disorders of bone density and structure
M86-M90 Other osteopathies
M91-M94 Chondropathies
M95 Other disorders of the musculoskeletal system and connective tissue
M96 Intraoperative and postprocedural complications and disorders of musculoskeletal system, not elsewhere classified
M99 Biomechanical lesions, not elsewhere classified

ARTHROPATHIES (M00-M25)

Disorders affecting predominantly peripheral (limb) joints

Infectious arthropathies (M00-M02)

This block comprises arthropathies due to microbiological agents. Distinction is made between the following types of etiological relationship:

a) direct infection of joint, where organisms invade synovial tissue and microbial antigen is present in the joint;
b) indirect infection, which may be of two types: a reactive arthropathy, where microbial infection of the body is established but neither organisms nor antigens can be identified in the joint, and a postinfective arthropathy, where microbial antigen is present but recovery of an organism is inconstant and evidence of local multiplication is lacking.

√4th **M00 Pyogenic arthritis**
√5th **M00.0 Staphylococcal arthritis and polyarthritis**
Use additional code (B95.6-B95.7) to identify bacterial agent
M00.00 Staphylococcal arthritis, unspecified joint
√6th **M00.01 Staphylococcal arthritis, shoulder**
M00.011 Staphylococcal arthritis, right shoulder
M00.012 Staphylococcal arthritis, left shoulder
M00.019 Staphylococcal arthritis, unspecified shoulder
√6th **M00.02 Staphylococcal arthritis, elbow**
M00.021 Staphylococcal arthritis, right elbow
M00.022 Staphylococcal arthritis, left elbow
M00.029 Staphylococcal arthritis, unspecified elbow
√6th **M00.03 Staphylococcal arthritis, wrist**
Staphylococcal arthritis of carpal bones
M00.031 Staphylococcal arthritis, right wrist
M00.032 Staphylococcal arthritis, left wrist
M00.039 Staphylococcal arthritis, unspecified wrist

√6th **M00.04 Staphylococcal arthritis, hand**
Staphylococcal arthritis of metacarpus and phalanges
M00.041 Staphylococcal arthritis, right hand
M00.042 Staphylococcal arthritis, left hand
M00.049 Staphylococcal arthritis, unspecified hand
√6th **M00.05 Staphylococcal arthritis, hip**
M00.051 Staphylococcal arthritis, right hip
M00.052 Staphylococcal arthritis, left hip
M00.059 Staphylococcal arthritis, unspecified hip
√6th **M00.06 Staphylococcal arthritis, knee**
M00.061 Staphylococcal arthritis, right knee
M00.062 Staphylococcal arthritis, left knee
M00.069 Staphylococcal arthritis, unspecified knee
√6th **M00.07 Staphylococcal arthritis, ankle and foot**
Staphylococcal arthritis, tarsus, metatarsus and phalanges
M00.071 Staphylococcal arthritis, right ankle and foot
M00.072 Staphylococcal arthritis, left ankle and foot
M00.079 Staphylococcal arthritis, unspecified ankle and foot
M00.08 Staphylococcal arthritis, vertebrae
M00.09 Staphylococcal polyarthritis
√5th **M00.1 Pneumococcal arthritis and polyarthritis**
M00.10 Pneumococcal arthritis, unspecified joint
√6th **M00.11 Pneumococcal arthritis, shoulder**
M00.111 Pneumococcal arthritis, right shoulder
M00.112 Pneumococcal arthritis, left shoulder
M00.119 Pneumococcal arthritis, unspecified shoulder
√6th **M00.12 Pneumococcal arthritis, elbow**
M00.121 Pneumococcal arthritis, right elbow
M00.122 Pneumococcal arthritis, left elbow
M00.129 Pneumococcal arthritis, unspecified elbow
√6th **M00.13 Pneumococcal arthritis, wrist**
Pneumococcal arthritis of carpal bones
M00.131 Pneumococcal arthritis, right wrist
M00.132 Pneumococcal arthritis, left wrist
M00.139 Pneumococcal arthritis, unspecified wrist
√6th **M00.14 Pneumococcal arthritis, hand**
Pneumococcal arthritis of metacarpus and phalanges
M00.141 Pneumococcal arthritis, right hand
M00.142 Pneumococcal arthritis, left hand
M00.149 Pneumococcal arthritis, unspecified hand
√6th **M00.15 Pneumococcal arthritis, hip**
M00.151 Pneumococcal arthritis, right hip
M00.152 Pneumococcal arthritis, left hip
M00.159 Pneumococcal arthritis, unspecified hip
√6th **M00.16 Pneumococcal arthritis, knee**
M00.161 Pneumococcal arthritis, right knee
M00.162 Pneumococcal arthritis, left knee
M00.169 Pneumococcal arthritis, unspecified knee
√6th **M00.17 Pneumococcal arthritis, ankle and foot**
Pneumococcal arthritis, tarsus, metatarsus and phalanges
M00.171 Pneumococcal arthritis, right ankle and foot
M00.172 Pneumococcal arthritis, left ankle and foot
M00.179 Pneumococcal arthritis, unspecified ankle and foot
M00.18 Pneumococcal arthritis, vertebrae
M00.19 Pneumococcal polyarthritis
√5th **M00.2 Other streptococcal arthritis and polyarthritis**
Use additional code (B95.0-B95.2, B95.4-B95.5) to identify bacterial agent
M00.20 Other streptococcal arthritis, unspecified joint

☑ Appropriate additional character required   √x7th Requires 7th character, placeholder x must fill empty characters

✓6ᵗʰ **M00.21** Other streptococcal arthritis, shoulder
    M00.211 Other streptococcal arthritis, right shoulder
    M00.212 Other streptococcal arthritis, left shoulder
    M00.219 Other streptococcal arthritis, unspecified shoulder
✓6ᵗʰ **M00.22** Other streptococcal arthritis, elbow
    M00.221 Other streptococcal arthritis, right elbow
    M00.222 Other streptococcal arthritis, left elbow
    M00.229 Other streptococcal arthritis, unspecified elbow
✓6ᵗʰ **M00.23** Other streptococcal arthritis, wrist
    Other streptococcal arthritis of carpal bones
    M00.231 Other streptococcal arthritis, right wrist
    M00.232 Other streptococcal arthritis, left wrist
    M00.239 Other streptococcal arthritis, unspecified wrist
✓6ᵗʰ **M00.24** Other streptococcal arthritis, hand
    Other streptococcal arthritis metacarpus and phalanges
    M00.241 Other streptococcal arthritis, right hand
    M00.242 Other streptococcal arthritis, left hand
    M00.249 Other streptococcal arthritis, unspecified hand
✓6ᵗʰ **M00.25** Other streptococcal arthritis, hip
    M00.251 Other streptococcal arthritis, right hip
    M00.252 Other streptococcal arthritis, left hip
    M00.259 Other streptococcal arthritis, unspecified hip
✓6ᵗʰ **M00.26** Other streptococcal arthritis, knee
    M00.261 Other streptococcal arthritis, right knee
    M00.262 Other streptococcal arthritis, left knee
    M00.269 Other streptococcal arthritis, unspecified knee
✓6ᵗʰ **M00.27** Other streptococcal arthritis, ankle and foot
    Other streptococcal arthritis, tarsus, metatarsus and phalanges
    M00.271 Other streptococcal arthritis, right ankle and foot
    M00.272 Other streptococcal arthritis, left ankle and foot
    M00.279 Other streptococcal arthritis, unspecified ankle and foot
    M00.28 Other streptococcal arthritis, vertebrae
    M00.29 Other streptococcal polyarthritis
✓5ᵗʰ **M00.8** Arthritis and polyarthritis due to other bacteria
    Use additional code (B96) to identify bacteria
    M00.80 Arthritis due to other bacteria, unspecified joint
✓6ᵗʰ **M00.81** Arthritis due to other bacteria, shoulder
    M00.811 Arthritis due to other bacteria, right shoulder
    M00.812 Arthritis due to other bacteria, left shoulder
    M00.819 Arthritis due to other bacteria, unspecified shoulder
✓6ᵗʰ **M00.82** Arthritis due to other bacteria, elbow
    M00.821 Arthritis due to other bacteria, right elbow
    M00.822 Arthritis due to other bacteria, left elbow
    M00.829 Arthritis due to other bacteria, unspecified elbow
✓6ᵗʰ **M00.83** Arthritis due to other bacteria, wrist
    Arthritis due to other bacteria, carpal bones
    M00.831 Arthritis due to other bacteria, right wrist
    M00.832 Arthritis due to other bacteria, left wrist
    M00.839 Arthritis due to other bacteria, unspecified wrist
✓6ᵗʰ **M00.84** Arthritis due to other bacteria, hand
    Arthritis due to other bacteria, metacarpus and phalanges
    M00.841 Arthritis due to other bacteria, right hand
    M00.842 Arthritis due to other bacteria, left hand

M00.849 Arthritis due to other bacteria, unspecified hand
✓6ᵗʰ **M00.85** Arthritis due to other bacteria, hip
    M00.851 Arthritis due to other bacteria, right hip
    M00.852 Arthritis due to other bacteria, left hip
    M00.859 Arthritis due to other bacteria, unspecified hip
✓6ᵗʰ **M00.86** Arthritis due to other bacteria, knee
    M00.861 Arthritis due to other bacteria, right knee
    M00.862 Arthritis due to other bacteria, left knee
    M00.869 Arthritis due to other bacteria, unspecified knee
✓6ᵗʰ **M00.87** Arthritis due to other bacteria, ankle and foot
    Arthritis due to other bacteria, tarsus, metatarsus, and phalanges
    M00.871 Arthritis due to other bacteria, right ankle and foot
    M00.872 Arthritis due to other bacteria, left ankle and foot
    M00.879 Arthritis due to other bacteria, unspecified ankle and foot
    M00.88 Arthritis due to other bacteria, vertebrae
    M00.89 Polyarthritis due to other bacteria
M00.9 Pyogenic arthritis, unspecified
    Infective arthritis NOS

✓4ᵗʰ **M01** **Direct infections of joint in infectious and parasitic diseases classified elsewhere**
    Code first underlying disease, such as:
    leprosy [Hansen's disease] (A30-)
    mycoses (B35-B49)
    O'nyong-nyong fever (A92.1)
    paratyphoid fever (A01.1-A01.4)
    EXCLUDES 1   *arthritis, arthropathy (in):*
      gonococcal (A54.42)
      Lyme disease (A69.23)
      meningococcal (A39.83)
      mumps (B26.85)
      postinfective (M02-)
      postmeningococcal (A39.84)
      reactive (M04.0-)
      rubella (B06.82)
      sarcoidosis (D86.86)
      spine (A18.01)
      typhoid fever (A01.04)
      tuberculosis (A18.02)
    M01.x0 *Direct infection of unspecified joint in infectious and parasitic diseases classified elsewhere*
✓6ᵗʰ **M01.x1** **Direct infection of shoulder joint in infectious and parasitic diseases classified elsewhere**
    M01.x11 *Direct infection of right shoulder in infectious and parasitic diseases classified elsewhere*
    M01.x12 *Direct infection of left shoulder in infectious and parasitic diseases classified elsewhere*
    M01.x19 *Direct infection of unspecified shoulder in infectious and parasitic diseases classified elsewhere*
✓6ᵗʰ **M01.x2** **Direct infection of elbow in infectious and parasitic diseases classified elsewhere**
    M01.x21 *Direct infection of right elbow in infectious and parasitic diseases classified elsewhere*
    M01.x22 *Direct infection of left elbow in infectious and parasitic diseases classified elsewhere*
    M01.x29 *Direct infection of unspecified elbow in infectious and parasitic diseases classified elsewhere*
✓6ᵗʰ **M01.x3** **Direct infection of wrist in infectious and parasitic diseases classified elsewhere**
    Direct infection of carpal bones in infectious and parasitic diseases classified elsewhere
    M01.x31 *Direct infection of right wrist in infectious and parasitic diseases classified elsewhere*

EXCLUDES 1   Not coded here   EXCLUDES 2   Not included here   *Manifestation Code*

M01.x32   *Direct infection of left wrist in infectious and parasitic diseases classified elsewhere*

M01.x39   *Direct infection of unspecified wrist in infectious and parasitic diseases classified elsewhere*

✓6ᵗʰ   **M01.x4**   **Direct infection of hand in infectious and parasitic diseases classified elsewhere**
Direct infection of metacarpus and phalanges in infectious and parasitic diseases classified elsewhere

M01.x41   *Direct infection of right hand in infectious and parasitic diseases classified elsewhere*

M01.x42   *Direct infection of left hand in infectious and parasitic diseases classified elsewhere*

M01.x49   *Direct infection of unspecified hand in infectious and parasitic diseases classified elsewhere*

✓6ᵗʰ   **M01.x5**   **Direct infection of hip in infectious and parasitic diseases classified elsewhere**

M01.x51   *Direct infection of right hip in infectious and parasitic diseases classified elsewhere*

M01.x52   *Direct infection of left hip in infectious and parasitic diseases classified elsewhere*

M01.x59   *Direct infection of unspecified hip in infectious and parasitic diseases classified elsewhere*

✓6ᵗʰ   **M01.x6**   **Direct infection of knee in infectious and parasitic diseases classified elsewhere**

M01.x61   *Direct infection of right knee in infectious and parasitic diseases classified elsewhere*

M01.x62   *Direct infection of left knee in infectious and parasitic diseases classified elsewhere*

M01.x69   *Direct infection of unspecified knee in infectious and parasitic diseases classified elsewhere*

✓6ᵗʰ   **M01.x7**   **Direct infection of ankle and foot in infectious and parasitic diseases classified elsewhere**
Direct infection of tarsus, metatarsus and phalanges in infectious and parasitic diseases classified elsewhere

M01.x71   *Direct infection of right ankle and foot in infectious and parasitic diseases classified elsewhere*

M01.x72   *Direct infection of left ankle and foot in infectious and parasitic diseases classified elsewhere*

M01.x79   *Direct infection of unspecified ankle and foot in infectious and parasitic diseases classified elsewhere*

M01.x8   *Direct infection of vertebrae in infectious and parasitic diseases classified elsewhere*

M01.x9   *Direct infection of multiple joints in infectious and parasitic diseases classified elsewhere*

✓4ᵗʰ   **M02**   **Postinfective and reactive arthropathies**
Code first underlying disease, such as:
congenital syphilis [Clutton's joints] (A50.5)
enteritis due to Yersinia enterocolitica (A04.6)
infective endocarditis (I33.0)
viral hepatitis (B15-B19)
EXCLUDES 1   Behçet's disease (M35.2)
direct infections of joint in infectious and parasitic diseases classified elsewhere (M01.-)
postinfectious arthritis (in):
meningococcal (A39.84)
mumps (B26.85)
rheumatic fever (I00)
rubella (B06.82)
syphilis (late) (A52.77)
tabetic arthropathy [Charcôt's] (A52.16)

✓5ᵗʰ   **M02.0**   **Arthropathy following intestinal bypass**
M02.00   **Arthropathy following intestinal bypass, unspecified site**

✓6ᵗʰ   **M02.01**   **Arthropathy following intestinal bypass, shoulder**
M02.011   **Arthropathy following intestinal bypass, right shoulder**
M02.012   **Arthropathy following intestinal bypass, left shoulder**
M02.019   **Arthropathy following intestinal bypass, unspecified shoulder**

✓6ᵗʰ   **M02.02**   **Arthropathy following intestinal bypass, elbow**
M02.021   **Arthropathy following intestinal bypass, right elbow**
M02.022   **Arthropathy following intestinal bypass, left elbow**
M02.029   **Arthropathy following intestinal bypass, unspecified elbow**

✓6ᵗʰ   **M02.03**   **Arthropathy following intestinal bypass, wrist**
Arthropathy following intestinal bypass, carpal bones
M02.031   **Arthropathy following intestinal bypass, right wrist**
M02.032   **Arthropathy following intestinal bypass, left wrist**
M02.039   **Arthropathy following intestinal bypass, unspecified wrist**

✓6ᵗʰ   **M02.04**   **Arthropathy following intestinal bypass, hand**
Arthropathy following intestinal bypass, metacarpals and phalanges
M02.041   **Arthropathy following intestinal bypass, right hand**
M02.042   **Arthropathy following intestinal bypass, left hand**
M02.049   **Arthropathy following intestinal bypass, unspecified hand**

✓6ᵗʰ   **M02.05**   **Arthropathy following intestinal bypass, hip**
M02.051   **Arthropathy following intestinal bypass, right hip**
M02.052   **Arthropathy following intestinal bypass, left hip**
M02.059   **Arthropathy following intestinal bypass, unspecified hip**

✓6ᵗʰ   **M02.06**   **Arthropathy following intestinal bypass, knee**
M02.061   **Arthropathy following intestinal bypass, right knee**
M02.062   **Arthropathy following intestinal bypass, left knee**
M02.069   **Arthropathy following intestinal bypass, unspecified knee**

✓6ᵗʰ   **M02.07**   **Arthropathy following intestinal bypass, ankle and foot**
Arthropathy following intestinal bypass, tarsus, metatarsus and phalanges
M02.071   **Arthropathy following intestinal bypass, right ankle and foot**
M02.072   **Arthropathy following intestinal bypass, left ankle and foot**
M02.079   **Arthropathy following intestinal bypass, unspecified ankle and foot**

M02.08   **Arthropathy following intestinal bypass, vertebrae**

M02.09   **Arthropathy following intestinal bypass, multiple sites**

✓5ᵗʰ   **M02.1**   **Postdysenteric arthropathy**
M02.10   **Postdysenteric arthropathy, unspecified site**

✓6ᵗʰ   **M02.11**   **Postdysenteric arthropathy, shoulder**
M02.111   **Postdysenteric arthropathy, right shoulder**
M02.112   **Postdysenteric arthropathy, left shoulder**
M02.119   **Postdysenteric arthropathy, unspecified shoulder**

✓6ᵗʰ   **M02.12**   **Postdysenteric arthropathy, elbow**
M02.121   **Postdysenteric arthropathy, right elbow**
M02.122   **Postdysenteric arthropathy, left elbow**
M02.129   **Postdysenteric arthropathy, unspecified elbow**

✓6ᵗʰ   **M02.13**   **Postdysenteric arthropathy, wrist**
Postdysenteric arthropathy, carpal bones
M02.131   **Postdysenteric arthropathy, right wrist**
M02.132   **Postdysenteric arthropathy, left wrist**

        M02.139 **Postdysenteric arthropathy, unspecified wrist**

✓6ᵗʰ M02.14 **Postdysenteric arthropathy, hand**
    Postdysenteric arthropathy, metacarpus and phalanges
        M02.141 **Postdysenteric arthropathy, right hand**
        M02.142 **Postdysenteric arthropathy, left hand**
        M02.149 **Postdysenteric arthropathy, unspecified hand**

✓6ᵗʰ M02.15 **Postdysenteric arthropathy, hip**
        M02.151 **Postdysenteric arthropathy, right hip**
        M02.152 **Postdysenteric arthropathy, left hip**
        M02.159 **Postdysenteric arthropathy, unspecified hip**

✓6ᵗʰ M02.16 **Postdysenteric arthropathy, knee**
        M02.161 **Postdysenteric arthropathy, right knee**
        M02.162 **Postdysenteric arthropathy, left knee**
        M02.169 **Postdysenteric arthropathy, unspecified knee**

✓6ᵗʰ M02.17 **Postdysenteric arthropathy, ankle and foot**
    Postdysenteric arthropathy, tarsus, metatarsus and phalanges
        M02.171 **Postdysenteric arthropathy, right ankle and foot**
        M02.172 **Postdysenteric arthropathy, left ankle and foot**
        M02.179 **Postdysenteric arthropathy, unspecified ankle and foot**

        M02.18 **Postdysenteric arthropathy, vertebrae**
        M02.19 **Postdysenteric arthropathy, multiple sites**

✓5ᵗʰ M02.2 **Postimmunization arthropathy**
        M02.20 **Postimmunization arthropathy, unspecified site**

✓6ᵗʰ M02.21 **Postimmunization arthropathy, shoulder**
        M02.211 **Postimmunization arthropathy, right shoulder**
        M02.212 **Postimmunization arthropathy, left shoulder**
        M02.219 **Postimmunization arthropathy, unspecified shoulder**

✓6ᵗʰ M02.22 **Postimmunization arthropathy, elbow**
        M02.221 **Postimmunization arthropathy, right elbow**
        M02.222 **Postimmunization arthropathy, left elbow**
        M02.229 **Postimmunization arthropathy, unspecified elbow**

✓6ᵗʰ M02.23 **Postimmunization arthropathy, wrist**
    Postimmunization arthropathy, carpal bones
        M02.231 **Postimmunization arthropathy, right wrist**
        M02.232 **Postimmunization arthropathy, left wrist**
        M02.239 **Postimmunization arthropathy, unspecified wrist**

✓6ᵗʰ M02.24 **Postimmunization arthropathy, hand**
    Postimmunization arthropathy, metacarpus and phalanges
        M02.241 **Postimmunization arthropathy, right hand**
        M02.242 **Postimmunization arthropathy, left hand**
        M02.249 **Postimmunization arthropathy, unspecified hand**

✓6ᵗʰ M02.25 **Postimmunization arthropathy, hip**
        M02.251 **Postimmunization arthropathy, right hip**
        M02.252 **Postimmunization arthropathy, left hip**
        M02.259 **Postimmunization arthropathy, unspecified hip**

✓6ᵗʰ M02.26 **Postimmunization arthropathy, knee**
        M02.261 **Postimmunization arthropathy, right knee**
        M02.262 **Postimmunization arthropathy, left knee**
        M02.269 **Postimmunization arthropathy, unspecified knee**

✓6ᵗʰ M02.27 **Postimmunization arthropathy, ankle and foot**
    Postimmunization arthropathy, tarsus, metatarsus and phalanges
        M02.271 **Postimmunization arthropathy, right ankle and foot**
        M02.272 **Postimmunization arthropathy, left ankle and foot**
        M02.279 **Postimmunization arthropathy, unspecified ankle and foot**

        M02.28 **Postimmunization arthropathy, vertebrae**
        M02.29 **Postimmunization arthropathy, multiple sites**

✓5ᵗʰ M02.3 **Reiter's disease**
        M02.30 **Reiter's disease, unspecified site**

✓6ᵗʰ M02.31 **Reiter's disease, shoulder**
        M02.311 **Reiter's disease, right shoulder**
        M02.312 **Reiter's disease, left shoulder**
        M02.319 **Reiter's disease, unspecified shoulder**

✓6ᵗʰ M02.32 **Reiter's disease, elbow**
        M02.321 **Reiter's disease, right elbow**
        M02.322 **Reiter's disease, left elbow**
        M02.329 **Reiter's disease, unspecified elbow**

✓6ᵗʰ M02.33 **Reiter's disease, wrist**
    Reiter's disease, carpal bones
        M02.331 **Reiter's disease, right wrist**
        M02.332 **Reiter's disease, left wrist**
        M02.339 **Reiter's disease, unspecified wrist**

✓6ᵗʰ M02.34 **Reiter's disease, hand**
    Reiter's disease, metacarpus and phalanges
        M02.341 **Reiter's disease, right hand**
        M02.342 **Reiter's disease, left hand**
        M02.349 **Reiter's disease, unspecified hand**

✓6ᵗʰ M02.35 **Reiter's disease, hip**
        M02.351 **Reiter's disease, right hip**
        M02.352 **Reiter's disease, left hip**
        M02.359 **Reiter's disease, unspecified hip**

✓6ᵗʰ M02.36 **Reiter's disease, knee**
        M02.361 **Reiter's disease, right knee**
        M02.362 **Reiter's disease, left knee**
        M02.369 **Reiter's disease, unspecified knee**

✓6ᵗʰ M02.37 **Reiter's disease, ankle and foot**
    Reiter's disease, tarsus, metatarsus and phalanges
        M02.371 **Reiter's disease, right ankle and foot**
        M02.372 **Reiter's disease, left ankle and foot**
        M02.379 **Reiter's disease, unspecified ankle and foot**

        M02.38 **Reiter's disease, vertebrae**
        M02.39 **Reiter's disease, multiple sites**

✓5ᵗʰ M02.8 **Other reactive arthropathies**
        M02.80 **Other reactive arthropathies, unspecified site**

✓6ᵗʰ M02.81 **Other reactive arthropathies, shoulder**
        M02.811 **Other reactive arthropathies, right shoulder**
        M02.812 **Other reactive arthropathies, left shoulder**
        M02.819 **Other reactive arthropathies, unspecified shoulder**

✓6ᵗʰ M02.82 **Other reactive arthropathies, elbow**
        M02.821 **Other reactive arthropathies, right elbow**
        M02.822 **Other reactive arthropathies, left elbow**
        M02.829 **Other reactive arthropathies, unspecified elbow**

✓6ᵗʰ M02.83 **Other reactive arthropathies, wrist**
    Other reactive arthropathies, carpal bones
        M02.831 **Other reactive arthropathies, right wrist**
        M02.832 **Other reactive arthropathies, left wrist**
        M02.839 **Other reactive arthropathies, unspecified wrist**

✓6ᵗʰ M02.84 **Other reactive arthropathies, hand**
    Other reactive arthropathies, metacarpus and phalanges
        M02.841 **Other reactive arthropathies, right hand**
        M02.842 **Other reactive arthropathies, left hand**
        M02.849 **Other reactive arthropathies, unspecified hand**

EXCLUDES 1 Not coded here   **EXCLUDES 2** Not included here   ***Manifestation Code***

☑6ᵗʰ **M02.85 Other reactive arthropathies, hip**
    M02.851 Other reactive arthropathies, right hip
    M02.852 Other reactive arthropathies, left hip
    M02.859 Other reactive arthropathies, unspecified hip

☑6ᵗʰ **M02.86 Other reactive arthropathies, knee**
    M02.861 Other reactive arthropathies, right knee
    M02.862 Other reactive arthropathies, left knee
    M02.869 Other reactive arthropathies, unspecified knee

☑6ᵗʰ **M02.87 Other reactive arthropathies, ankle and foot**
    Other reactive arthropathies, tarsus, metatarsus and phalanges
    M02.871 Other reactive arthropathies, right ankle and foot
    M02.872 Other reactive arthropathies, left ankle and foot
    M02.879 Other reactive arthropathies, unspecified ankle and foot
  M02.88 Other reactive arthropathies, vertebrae
  M02.89 Other reactive arthropathies, multiple sites
M02.9 Reactive arthropathy, unspecified

Inflammatory polyarthropathies (M05-M14)

☑4ᵗʰ **M05 Rheumatoid arthritis with rheumatoid factor**
  EXCLUDES 1 *rheumatic fever (I00)*
        juvenile rheumatoid arthritis (M08-)
        rheumatoid arthritis of spine (M45-)

☑5ᵗʰ **M05.0 Felty's syndrome**
    Rheumatoid arthritis with splenoadenomegaly and leukopenia
  M05.00 Felty's syndrome, unspecified site
☑6ᵗʰ **M05.01 Felty's syndrome, shoulder**
    M05.011 Felty's syndrome, right shoulder
    M05.012 Felty's syndrome, left shoulder
    M05.019 Felty's syndrome, unspecified shoulder
☑6ᵗʰ **M05.02 Felty's syndrome, elbow**
    M05.021 Felty's syndrome, right elbow
    M05.022 Felty's syndrome, left elbow
    M05.029 Felty's syndrome, unspecified elbow
☑6ᵗʰ **M05.03 Felty's syndrome, wrist**
    Felty's syndrome, carpal bones
    M05.031 Felty's syndrome, right wrist
    M05.032 Felty's syndrome, left wrist
    M05.039 Felty's syndrome, unspecified wrist
☑6ᵗʰ **M05.04 Felty's syndrome, hand**
    Felty's syndrome, metacarpus and phalanges
    M05.041 Felty's syndrome, right hand
    M05.042 Felty's syndrome, left hand
    M05.049 Felty's syndrome, unspecified hand
☑6ᵗʰ **M05.05 Felty's syndrome, hip**
    M05.051 Felty's syndrome, right hip
    M05.052 Felty's syndrome, left hip
    M05.059 Felty's syndrome, unspecified hip
☑6ᵗʰ **M05.06 Felty's syndrome, knee**
    M05.061 Felty's syndrome, right knee
    M05.062 Felty's syndrome, left knee
    M05.069 Felty's syndrome, unspecified knee
☑6ᵗʰ **M05.07 Felty's syndrome, ankle and foot**
    Felty's syndrome, tarsus, metatarsus and phalanges
    M05.071 Felty's syndrome, right ankle and foot
    M05.072 Felty's syndrome, left ankle and foot
    M05.079 Felty's syndrome, unspecified ankle and foot
  M05.09 Felty's syndrome, multiple sites
☑5ᵗʰ **M05.1 Rheumatoid lung disease with rheumatoid arthritis**
  M05.10 Rheumatoid lung disease with rheumatoid arthritis of unspecified site
☑6ᵗʰ **M05.11 Rheumatoid lung disease with rheumatoid arthritis of shoulder**
    M05.111 Rheumatoid lung disease with rheumatoid arthritis of right shoulder
    M05.112 Rheumatoid lung disease with rheumatoid arthritis of left shoulder

    M05.119 Rheumatoid lung disease with rheumatoid arthritis of unspecified shoulder
☑6ᵗʰ **M05.12 Rheumatoid lung disease with rheumatoid arthritis of elbow**
    M05.121 Rheumatoid lung disease with rheumatoid arthritis of right elbow
    M05.122 Rheumatoid lung disease with rheumatoid arthritis of left elbow
    M05.129 Rheumatoid lung disease with rheumatoid arthritis of unspecified elbow
☑6ᵗʰ **M05.13 Rheumatoid lung disease with rheumatoid arthritis of wrist**
    Rheumatoid lung disease with rheumatoid arthritis, carpal bones
    M05.131 Rheumatoid lung disease with rheumatoid arthritis of right wrist
    M05.132 Rheumatoid lung disease with rheumatoid arthritis of left wrist
    M05.139 Rheumatoid lung disease with rheumatoid arthritis of unspecified wrist
☑6ᵗʰ **M05.14 Rheumatoid lung disease with rheumatoid arthritis of hand**
    Rheumatoid lung disease with rheumatoid arthritis, metacarpus and phalanges
    M05.141 Rheumatoid lung disease with rheumatoid arthritis of right hand
    M05.142 Rheumatoid lung disease with rheumatoid arthritis of left hand
    M05.149 Rheumatoid lung disease with rheumatoid arthritis of unspecified hand
☑6ᵗʰ **M05.15 Rheumatoid lung disease with rheumatoid arthritis of hip**
    M05.151 Rheumatoid lung disease with rheumatoid arthritis of right hip
    M05.152 Rheumatoid lung disease with rheumatoid arthritis of left hip
    M05.159 Rheumatoid lung disease with rheumatoid arthritis of unspecified hip
☑6ᵗʰ **M05.16 Rheumatoid lung disease with rheumatoid arthritis of knee**
    M05.161 Rheumatoid lung disease with rheumatoid arthritis of right knee
    M05.162 Rheumatoid lung disease with rheumatoid arthritis of left knee
    M05.169 Rheumatoid lung disease with rheumatoid arthritis of unspecified knee
☑6ᵗʰ **M05.17 Rheumatoid lung disease with rheumatoid arthritis of ankle and foot**
    Rheumatoid lung disease with rheumatoid arthritis, tarsus, metatarsus and phalanges
    M05.171 Rheumatoid lung disease with rheumatoid arthritis of right ankle and foot
    M05.172 Rheumatoid lung disease with rheumatoid arthritis of left ankle and foot
    M05.179 Rheumatoid lung disease with rheumatoid arthritis of unspecified ankle and foot
  M05.19 Rheumatoid lung disease with rheumatoid arthritis of multiple sites
☑5ᵗʰ **M05.2 Rheumatoid vasculitis with rheumatoid arthritis**
  M05.20 Rheumatoid vasculitis with rheumatoid arthritis of unspecified site
☑6ᵗʰ **M05.21 Rheumatoid vasculitis with rheumatoid arthritis of shoulder**
    M05.211 Rheumatoid vasculitis with rheumatoid arthritis of right shoulder
    M05.212 Rheumatoid vasculitis with rheumatoid arthritis of left shoulder
    M05.219 Rheumatoid vasculitis with rheumatoid arthritis of unspecified shoulder

☑ Appropriate additional character required   ☑7ᵗʰ Requires 7th character, placeholder x must fill empty characters

✓6ᵗʰ **M05.22** **Rheumatoid vasculitis with rheumatoid arthritis of elbow**
　　M05.221 **Rheumatoid vasculitis with rheumatoid arthritis of right elbow**
　　M05.222 **Rheumatoid vasculitis with rheumatoid arthritis of left elbow**
　　M05.229 **Rheumatoid vasculitis with rheumatoid arthritis of unspecified elbow**

✓6ᵗʰ **M05.23** **Rheumatoid vasculitis with rheumatoid arthritis of wrist**
　　Rheumatoid vasculitis with rheumatoid arthritis, carpal bones
　　M05.231 **Rheumatoid vasculitis with rheumatoid arthritis of right wrist**
　　M05.232 **Rheumatoid vasculitis with rheumatoid arthritis of left wrist**
　　M05.239 **Rheumatoid vasculitis with rheumatoid arthritis of unspecified wrist**

✓6ᵗʰ **M05.24** **Rheumatoid vasculitis with rheumatoid arthritis of hand**
　　Rheumatoid vasculitis with rheumatoid arthritis, metacarpus and phalanges
　　M05.241 **Rheumatoid vasculitis with rheumatoid arthritis of right hand**
　　M05.242 **Rheumatoid vasculitis with rheumatoid arthritis of left hand**
　　M05.249 **Rheumatoid vasculitis with rheumatoid arthritis of unspecified hand**

✓6ᵗʰ **M05.25** **Rheumatoid vasculitis with rheumatoid arthritis of hip**
　　M05.251 **Rheumatoid vasculitis with rheumatoid arthritis of right hip**
　　M05.252 **Rheumatoid vasculitis with rheumatoid arthritis of left hip**
　　M05.259 **Rheumatoid vasculitis with rheumatoid arthritis of unspecified hip**

✓6ᵗʰ **M05.26** **Rheumatoid vasculitis with rheumatoid arthritis of knee**
　　M05.261 **Rheumatoid vasculitis with rheumatoid arthritis of right knee**
　　M05.262 **Rheumatoid vasculitis with rheumatoid arthritis of left knee**
　　M05.269 **Rheumatoid vasculitis with rheumatoid arthritis of unspecified knee**

✓6ᵗʰ **M05.27** **Rheumatoid vasculitis with rheumatoid arthritis of ankle and foot**
　　Rheumatoid vasculitis with rheumatoid arthritis, tarsus, metatarsus and phalanges
　　M05.271 **Rheumatoid vasculitis with rheumatoid arthritis of right ankle and foot**
　　M05.272 **Rheumatoid vasculitis with rheumatoid arthritis of left ankle and foot**
　　M05.279 **Rheumatoid vasculitis with rheumatoid arthritis of unspecified ankle and foot**

　M05.29 **Rheumatoid vasculitis with rheumatoid arthritis of multiple sites**

✓5ᵗʰ **M05.3** **Rheumatoid heart disease with rheumatoid arthritis**
　　Rheumatoid carditis
　　Rheumatoid endocarditis
　　Rheumatoid myocarditis
　　Rheumatoid pericarditis
　　M05.30 **Rheumatoid heart disease with rheumatoid arthritis of unspecified site**

✓6ᵗʰ **M05.31** **Rheumatoid heart disease with rheumatoid arthritis of shoulder**
　　M05.311 **Rheumatoid heart disease with rheumatoid arthritis of right shoulder**
　　M05.312 **Rheumatoid heart disease with rheumatoid arthritis of left shoulder**
　　M05.319 **Rheumatoid heart disease with rheumatoid arthritis of unspecified shoulder**

✓6ᵗʰ **M05.32** **Rheumatoid heart disease with rheumatoid arthritis of elbow**
　　M05.321 **Rheumatoid heart disease with rheumatoid arthritis of right elbow**
　　M05.322 **Rheumatoid heart disease with rheumatoid arthritis of left elbow**

　　M05.329 **Rheumatoid heart disease with rheumatoid arthritis of unspecified elbow**

✓6ᵗʰ **M05.33** **Rheumatoid heart disease with rheumatoid arthritis of wrist**
　　Rheumatoid heart disease with rheumatoid arthritis, carpal bones
　　M05.331 **Rheumatoid heart disease with rheumatoid arthritis of right wrist**
　　M05.332 **Rheumatoid heart disease with rheumatoid arthritis of left wrist**
　　M05.339 **Rheumatoid heart disease with rheumatoid arthritis of unspecified wrist**

✓6ᵗʰ **M05.34** **Rheumatoid heart disease with rheumatoid arthritis of hand**
　　Rheumatoid heart disease with rheumatoid arthritis, metacarpus and phalanges
　　M05.341 **Rheumatoid heart disease with rheumatoid arthritis of right hand**
　　M05.342 **Rheumatoid heart disease with rheumatoid arthritis of left hand**
　　M05.349 **Rheumatoid heart disease with rheumatoid arthritis of unspecified hand**

✓6ᵗʰ **M05.35** **Rheumatoid heart disease with rheumatoid arthritis of hip**
　　M05.351 **Rheumatoid heart disease with rheumatoid arthritis of right hip**
　　M05.352 **Rheumatoid heart disease with rheumatoid arthritis of left hip**
　　M05.359 **Rheumatoid heart disease with rheumatoid arthritis of unspecified hip**

✓6ᵗʰ **M05.36** **Rheumatoid heart disease with rheumatoid arthritis of knee**
　　M05.361 **Rheumatoid heart disease with rheumatoid arthritis of right knee**
　　M05.362 **Rheumatoid heart disease with rheumatoid arthritis of left knee**
　　M05.369 **Rheumatoid heart disease with rheumatoid arthritis of unspecified knee**

✓6ᵗʰ **M05.37** **Rheumatoid heart disease with rheumatoid arthritis of ankle and foot**
　　Rheumatoid heart disease with rheumatoid arthritis, tarsus, metatarsus and phalanges
　　M05.371 **Rheumatoid heart disease with rheumatoid arthritis of right ankle and foot**
　　M05.372 **Rheumatoid heart disease with rheumatoid arthritis of left ankle and foot**
　　M05.379 **Rheumatoid heart disease with rheumatoid arthritis of unspecified ankle and foot**

　M05.39 **Rheumatoid heart disease with rheumatoid arthritis of multiple sites**

✓5ᵗʰ **M05.4** **Rheumatoid myopathy with rheumatoid arthritis**
　　M05.40 **Rheumatoid myopathy with rheumatoid arthritis of unspecified site**

✓6ᵗʰ **M05.41** **Rheumatoid myopathy with rheumatoid arthritis of shoulder**
　　M05.411 **Rheumatoid myopathy with rheumatoid arthritis of right shoulder**
　　M05.412 **Rheumatoid myopathy with rheumatoid arthritis of left shoulder**
　　M05.419 **Rheumatoid myopathy with rheumatoid arthritis of unspecified shoulder**

✓6ᵗʰ **M05.42** **Rheumatoid myopathy with rheumatoid arthritis of elbow**
　　M05.421 **Rheumatoid myopathy with rheumatoid arthritis of right elbow**
　　M05.422 **Rheumatoid myopathy with rheumatoid arthritis of left elbow**
　　M05.429 **Rheumatoid myopathy with rheumatoid arthritis of unspecified elbow**

✓6ᵗʰ **M05.43** **Rheumatoid myopathy with rheumatoid arthritis of wrist**
　　Rheumatoid myopathy with rheumatoid arthritis, carpal bones

---

EXCLUDES 1　Not coded here　　　　EXCLUDES 2　Not included here　　　　*Manifestation Code*

MØ5.431 **Rheumatoid myopathy with rheumatoid arthritis of right wrist**

MØ5.432 **Rheumatoid myopathy with rheumatoid arthritis of left wrist**

MØ5.439 **Rheumatoid myopathy with rheumatoid arthritis of unspecified wrist**

✓6ᵗʰ MØ5.44 **Rheumatoid myopathy with rheumatoid arthritis of hand**
Rheumatoid myopathy with rheumatoid arthritis, metacarpus and phalanges

MØ5.441 **Rheumatoid myopathy with rheumatoid arthritis of right hand**

MØ5.442 **Rheumatoid myopathy with rheumatoid arthritis of left hand**

MØ5.449 **Rheumatoid myopathy with rheumatoid arthritis of unspecified hand**

✓6ᵗʰ MØ5.45 **Rheumatoid myopathy with rheumatoid arthritis of hip**

MØ5.451 **Rheumatoid myopathy with rheumatoid arthritis of right hip**

MØ5.452 **Rheumatoid myopathy with rheumatoid arthritis of left hip**

MØ5.459 **Rheumatoid myopathy with rheumatoid arthritis of unspecified hip**

✓6ᵗʰ MØ5.46 **Rheumatoid myopathy with rheumatoid arthritis of knee**

MØ5.461 **Rheumatoid myopathy with rheumatoid arthritis of right knee**

MØ5.462 **Rheumatoid myopathy with rheumatoid arthritis of left knee**

MØ5.469 **Rheumatoid myopathy with rheumatoid arthritis of unspecified knee**

✓6ᵗʰ MØ5.47 **Rheumatoid myopathy with rheumatoid arthritis of ankle and foot**
Rheumatoid myopathy with rheumatoid arthritis, tarsus, metatarsus and phalanges

MØ5.471 **Rheumatoid myopathy with rheumatoid arthritis of right ankle and foot**

MØ5.472 **Rheumatoid myopathy with rheumatoid arthritis of left ankle and foot**

MØ5.479 **Rheumatoid myopathy with rheumatoid arthritis of unspecified ankle and foot**

MØ5.49 **Rheumatoid myopathy with rheumatoid arthritis of multiple sites**

✓5ᵗʰ MØ5.5 **Rheumatoid polyneuropathy with rheumatoid arthritis**

MØ5.5Ø **Rheumatoid polyneuropathy with rheumatoid arthritis of unspecified site**

✓6ᵗʰ MØ5.51 **Rheumatoid polyneuropathy with rheumatoid arthritis of shoulder**

MØ5.511 **Rheumatoid polyneuropathy with rheumatoid arthritis of right shoulder**

MØ5.512 **Rheumatoid polyneuropathy with rheumatoid arthritis of left shoulder**

MØ5.519 **Rheumatoid polyneuropathy with rheumatoid arthritis of unspecified shoulder**

✓6ᵗʰ MØ5.52 **Rheumatoid polyneuropathy with rheumatoid arthritis of elbow**

MØ5.521 **Rheumatoid polyneuropathy with rheumatoid arthritis of right elbow**

MØ5.522 **Rheumatoid polyneuropathy with rheumatoid arthritis of left elbow**

MØ5.529 **Rheumatoid polyneuropathy with rheumatoid arthritis of unspecified elbow**

✓6ᵗʰ MØ5.53 **Rheumatoid polyneuropathy with rheumatoid arthritis of wrist**
Rheumatoid polyneuropathy with rheumatoid arthritis, carpal bones

MØ5.531 **Rheumatoid polyneuropathy with rheumatoid arthritis of right wrist**

MØ5.532 **Rheumatoid polyneuropathy with rheumatoid arthritis of left wrist**

MØ5.539 **Rheumatoid polyneuropathy with rheumatoid arthritis of unspecified wrist**

✓6ᵗʰ MØ5.54 **Rheumatoid polyneuropathy with rheumatoid arthritis of hand**
Rheumatoid polyneuropathy with rheumatoid arthritis, metacarpus and phalanges

MØ5.541 **Rheumatoid polyneuropathy with rheumatoid arthritis of right hand**

MØ5.542 **Rheumatoid polyneuropathy with rheumatoid arthritis of left hand**

MØ5.549 **Rheumatoid polyneuropathy with rheumatoid arthritis of unspecified hand**

✓6ᵗʰ MØ5.55 **Rheumatoid polyneuropathy with rheumatoid arthritis of hip**

MØ5.551 **Rheumatoid polyneuropathy with rheumatoid arthritis of right hip**

MØ5.552 **Rheumatoid polyneuropathy with rheumatoid arthritis of left hip**

MØ5.559 **Rheumatoid polyneuropathy with rheumatoid arthritis of unspecified hip**

✓6ᵗʰ MØ5.56 **Rheumatoid polyneuropathy with rheumatoid arthritis of knee**

MØ5.561 **Rheumatoid polyneuropathy with rheumatoid arthritis of right knee**

MØ5.562 **Rheumatoid polyneuropathy with rheumatoid arthritis of left knee**

MØ5.569 **Rheumatoid polyneuropathy with rheumatoid arthritis of unspecified knee**

✓6ᵗʰ MØ5.57 **Rheumatoid polyneuropathy with rheumatoid arthritis of ankle and foot**
Rheumatoid polyneuropathy with rheumatoid arthritis, tarsus, metatarsus and phalanges

MØ5.571 **Rheumatoid polyneuropathy with rheumatoid arthritis of right ankle and foot**

MØ5.572 **Rheumatoid polyneuropathy with rheumatoid arthritis of left ankle and foot**

MØ5.579 **Rheumatoid polyneuropathy with rheumatoid arthritis of unspecified ankle and foot**

MØ5.59 **Rheumatoid polyneuropathy with rheumatoid arthritis of multiple sites**

✓5ᵗʰ MØ5.6 **Rheumatoid arthritis with involvement of other organs and systems**

MØ5.6Ø **Rheumatoid arthritis of unspecified site with involvement of other organs and systems**

✓6ᵗʰ MØ5.61 **Rheumatoid arthritis of shoulder with involvement of other organs and systems**

MØ5.611 **Rheumatoid arthritis of right shoulder with involvement of other organs and systems**

MØ5.612 **Rheumatoid arthritis of left shoulder with involvement of other organs and systems**

MØ5.619 **Rheumatoid arthritis of unspecified shoulder with involvement of other organs and systems**

✓6ᵗʰ MØ5.62 **Rheumatoid arthritis of elbow with involvement of other organs and systems**

MØ5.621 **Rheumatoid arthritis of right elbow with involvement of other organs and systems**

MØ5.622 **Rheumatoid arthritis of left elbow with involvement of other organs and systems**

MØ5.629 **Rheumatoid arthritis of unspecified elbow with involvement of other organs and systems**

✓6ᵗʰ MØ5.63 **Rheumatoid arthritis of wrist with involvement of other organs and systems**
Rheumatoid arthritis of carpal bones with involvement of other organs and systems

MØ5.631 **Rheumatoid arthritis of right wrist with involvement of other organs and systems**

MØ5.632 **Rheumatoid arthritis of left wrist with involvement of other organs and systems**

✓ **Appropriate additional character required**   ✓ˣ7ᵗʰ **Requires 7th character, placeholder x must fill empty characters**

M05.639 Rheumatoid arthritis of unspecified wrist with involvement of other organs and systems

✓6ᵗʰ **M05.64** Rheumatoid arthritis of hand with involvement of other organs and systems
Rheumatoid arthritis of metacarpus and phalanges with involvement of other organs and systems

M05.641 Rheumatoid arthritis of right hand with involvement of other organs and systems

M05.642 Rheumatoid arthritis of left hand with involvement of other organs and systems

M05.649 Rheumatoid arthritis of unspecified hand with involvement of other organs and systems

✓6ᵗʰ **M05.65** Rheumatoid arthritis of hip with involvement of other organs and systems

M05.651 Rheumatoid arthritis of right hip with involvement of other organs and systems

M05.652 Rheumatoid arthritis of left hip with involvement of other organs and systems

M05.659 Rheumatoid arthritis of unspecified hip with involvement of other organs and systems

✓6ᵗʰ **M05.66** Rheumatoid arthritis of knee with involvement of other organs and systems

M05.661 Rheumatoid arthritis of right knee with involvement of other organs and systems

M05.662 Rheumatoid arthritis of left knee with involvement of other organs and systems

M05.669 Rheumatoid arthritis of unspecified knee with involvement of other organs and systems

✓6ᵗʰ **M05.67** Rheumatoid arthritis of ankle and foot with involvement of other organs and systems
Rheumatoid arthritis of tarsus, metatarsus and phalanges with involvement of other organs and systems

M05.671 Rheumatoid arthritis of right ankle and foot with involvement of other organs and systems

M05.672 Rheumatoid arthritis of left ankle and foot with involvement of other organs and systems

M05.679 Rheumatoid arthritis of unspecified ankle and foot with involvement of other organs and systems

M05.69 Rheumatoid arthritis of multiple sites with involvement of other organs and systems

✓5ᵗʰ **M05.7** Rheumatoid arthritis with rheumatoid factor without organ or systems involvement

M05.70 Rheumatoid arthritis with rheumatoid factor of unspecified site without organ or systems involvement

✓6ᵗʰ **M05.71** Rheumatoid arthritis with rheumatoid factor of shoulder without organ or systems involvement

M05.711 Rheumatoid arthritis with rheumatoid factor of right shoulder without organ or systems involvement

M05.712 Rheumatoid arthritis with rheumatoid factor of left shoulder without organ or systems involvement

M05.719 Rheumatoid arthritis with rheumatoid factor of unspecified shoulder without organ or systems involvement

✓6ᵗʰ **M05.72** Rheumatoid arthritis with rheumatoid factor of elbow without organ or systems involvement

M05.721 Rheumatoid arthritis with rheumatoid factor of right elbow without organ or systems involvement

M05.722 Rheumatoid arthritis with rheumatoid factor of left elbow without organ or systems involvement

M05.729 Rheumatoid arthritis with rheumatoid factor of unspecified elbow without organ or systems involvement

✓6ᵗʰ **M05.73** Rheumatoid arthritis with rheumatoid factor of wrist without organ or systems involvement

M05.731 Rheumatoid arthritis with rheumatoid factor of right wrist without organ or systems involvement

M05.732 Rheumatoid arthritis with rheumatoid factor of left wrist without organ or systems involvement

M05.739 Rheumatoid arthritis with rheumatoid factor of unspecified wrist without organ or systems involvement

✓6ᵗʰ **M05.74** Rheumatoid arthritis with rheumatoid factor of hand without organ or systems involvement

M05.741 Rheumatoid arthritis with rheumatoid factor of right hand without organ or systems involvement

M05.742 Rheumatoid arthritis with rheumatoid factor of left hand without organ or systems involvement

M05.749 Rheumatoid arthritis with rheumatoid factor of unspecified hand without organ or systems involvement

✓6ᵗʰ **M05.75** Rheumatoid arthritis with rheumatoid factor of hip without organ or systems involvement

M05.751 Rheumatoid arthritis with rheumatoid factor of right hip without organ or systems involvement

M05.752 Rheumatoid arthritis with rheumatoid factor of left hip without organ or systems involvement

M05.759 Rheumatoid arthritis with rheumatoid factor of unspecified hip without organ or systems involvement

✓6ᵗʰ **M05.76** Rheumatoid arthritis with rheumatoid factor of knee without organ or systems involvement

M05.761 Rheumatoid arthritis with rheumatoid factor of right knee without organ or systems involvement

M05.762 Rheumatoid arthritis with rheumatoid factor of left knee without organ or systems involvement

M05.769 Rheumatoid arthritis with rheumatoid factor of unspecified knee without organ or systems involvement

✓6ᵗʰ **M05.77** Rheumatoid arthritis with rheumatoid factor of ankle and foot without organ or systems involvement

M05.771 Rheumatoid arthritis with rheumatoid factor of right ankle and foot without organ or systems involvement

M05.772 Rheumatoid arthritis with rheumatoid factor of left ankle and foot without organ or systems involvement

M05.779 Rheumatoid arthritis with rheumatoid factor of unspecified ankle and foot without organ or systems involvement

M05.79 Rheumatoid arthritis with rheumatoid factor of multiple sites without organ or systems involvement

✓5ᵗʰ **M05.8** Other rheumatoid arthritis with rheumatoid factor

M05.80 Other rheumatoid arthritis with rheumatoid factor of unspecified site

✓6ᵗʰ **M05.81** Other rheumatoid arthritis with rheumatoid factor of shoulder

M05.811 Other rheumatoid arthritis with rheumatoid factor of right shoulder

M05.812 Other rheumatoid arthritis with rheumatoid factor of left shoulder

M05.819 Other rheumatoid arthritis with rheumatoid factor of unspecified shoulder

✓6ᵗʰ **M05.82** Other rheumatoid arthritis with rheumatoid factor of elbow

M05.821 Other rheumatoid arthritis with rheumatoid factor of right elbow

M05.822 **Other rheumatoid arthritis with rheumatoid factor of left elbow**

M05.829 **Other rheumatoid arthritis with rheumatoid factor of unspecified elbow**

✓6th M05.83 **Other rheumatoid arthritis with rheumatoid factor of wrist**

M05.831 **Other rheumatoid arthritis with rheumatoid factor of right wrist**

M05.832 **Other rheumatoid arthritis with rheumatoid factor of left wrist**

M05.839 **Other rheumatoid arthritis with rheumatoid factor of unspecified wrist**

✓6th M05.84 **Other rheumatoid arthritis with rheumatoid factor of hand**

M05.841 **Other rheumatoid arthritis with rheumatoid factor of right hand**

M05.842 **Other rheumatoid arthritis with rheumatoid factor of left hand**

M05.849 **Other rheumatoid arthritis with rheumatoid factor of unspecified hand**

✓6th M05.85 **Other rheumatoid arthritis with rheumatoid factor of hip**

M05.851 **Other rheumatoid arthritis with rheumatoid factor of right hip**

M05.852 **Other rheumatoid arthritis with rheumatoid factor of left hip**

M05.859 **Other rheumatoid arthritis with rheumatoid factor of unspecified hip**

✓6th M05.86 **Other rheumatoid arthritis with rheumatoid factor of knee**

M05.861 **Other rheumatoid arthritis with rheumatoid factor of right knee**

M05.862 **Other rheumatoid arthritis with rheumatoid factor of left knee**

M05.869 **Other rheumatoid arthritis with rheumatoid factor of unspecified knee**

✓6th M05.87 **Other rheumatoid arthritis with rheumatoid factor of ankle and foot**

M05.871 **Other rheumatoid arthritis with rheumatoid factor of right ankle and foot**

M05.872 **Other rheumatoid arthritis with rheumatoid factor of left ankle and foot**

M05.879 **Other rheumatoid arthritis with rheumatoid factor of unspecified ankle and foot**

M05.89 **Other rheumatoid arthritis with rheumatoid factor of multiple sites**

M05.9 **Rheumatoid arthritis with rheumatoid factor, unspecified**

✓4th **M06 Other rheumatoid arthritis**

✓5th M06.0 **Rheumatoid arthritis without rheumatoid factor**

M06.00 **Rheumatoid arthritis without rheumatoid factor, unspecified site**

✓6th M06.01 **Rheumatoid arthritis without rheumatoid factor, shoulder**

M06.011 **Rheumatoid arthritis without rheumatoid factor, right shoulder**

M06.012 **Rheumatoid arthritis without rheumatoid factor, left shoulder**

M06.019 **Rheumatoid arthritis without rheumatoid factor, unspecified shoulder**

✓6th M06.02 **Rheumatoid arthritis without rheumatoid factor, elbow**

M06.021 **Rheumatoid arthritis without rheumatoid factor, right elbow**

M06.022 **Rheumatoid arthritis without rheumatoid factor, left elbow**

M06.029 **Rheumatoid arthritis without rheumatoid factor, unspecified elbow**

✓6th M06.03 **Rheumatoid arthritis without rheumatoid factor, wrist**

M06.031 **Rheumatoid arthritis without rheumatoid factor, right wrist**

M06.032 **Rheumatoid arthritis without rheumatoid factor, left wrist**

M06.039 **Rheumatoid arthritis without rheumatoid factor, unspecified wrist**

✓6th M06.04 **Rheumatoid arthritis without rheumatoid factor, hand**

M06.041 **Rheumatoid arthritis without rheumatoid factor, right hand**

M06.042 **Rheumatoid arthritis without rheumatoid factor, left hand**

M06.049 **Rheumatoid arthritis without rheumatoid factor, unspecified hand**

✓6th M06.05 **Rheumatoid arthritis without rheumatoid factor, hip**

M06.051 **Rheumatoid arthritis without rheumatoid factor, right hip**

M06.052 **Rheumatoid arthritis without rheumatoid factor, left hip**

M06.059 **Rheumatoid arthritis without rheumatoid factor, unspecified hip**

✓6th M06.06 **Rheumatoid arthritis without rheumatoid factor, knee**

M06.061 **Rheumatoid arthritis without rheumatoid factor, right knee**

M06.062 **Rheumatoid arthritis without rheumatoid factor, left knee**

M06.069 **Rheumatoid arthritis without rheumatoid factor, unspecified knee**

✓6th M06.07 **Rheumatoid arthritis without rheumatoid factor, ankle and foot**

M06.071 **Rheumatoid arthritis without rheumatoid factor, right ankle and foot**

M06.072 **Rheumatoid arthritis without rheumatoid factor, left ankle and foot**

M06.079 **Rheumatoid arthritis without rheumatoid factor, unspecified ankle and foot**

M06.08 **Rheumatoid arthritis without rheumatoid factor, vertebrae**

M06.09 **Rheumatoid arthritis without rheumatoid factor, multiple sites**

M06.1 **Adult-onset Still's disease**

EXCLUDES 1 *Still's disease NOS (M08.2-)*

✓5th M06.2 **Rheumatoid bursitis**

M06.20 **Rheumatoid bursitis, unspecified site**

✓6th M06.21 **Rheumatoid bursitis, shoulder**

M06.211 **Rheumatoid bursitis, right shoulder**

M06.212 **Rheumatoid bursitis, left shoulder**

M06.219 **Rheumatoid bursitis, unspecified shoulder**

✓6th M06.22 **Rheumatoid bursitis, elbow**

M06.221 **Rheumatoid bursitis, right elbow**

M06.222 **Rheumatoid bursitis, left elbow**

M06.229 **Rheumatoid bursitis, unspecified elbow**

✓6th M06.23 **Rheumatoid bursitis, wrist**

M06.231 **Rheumatoid bursitis, right wrist**

M06.232 **Rheumatoid bursitis, left wrist**

M06.239 **Rheumatoid bursitis, unspecified wrist**

✓6th M06.24 **Rheumatoid bursitis, hand**

M06.241 **Rheumatoid bursitis, right hand**

M06.242 **Rheumatoid bursitis, left hand**

M06.249 **Rheumatoid bursitis, unspecified hand**

✓6th M06.25 **Rheumatoid bursitis, hip**

M06.251 **Rheumatoid bursitis, right hip**

M06.252 **Rheumatoid bursitis, left hip**

M06.259 **Rheumatoid bursitis, unspecified hip**

✓6th M06.26 **Rheumatoid bursitis, knee**

M06.261 **Rheumatoid bursitis, right knee**

M06.262 **Rheumatoid bursitis, left knee**

M06.269 **Rheumatoid bursitis, unspecified knee**

✓6th M06.27 **Rheumatoid bursitis, ankle and foot**

M06.271 **Rheumatoid bursitis, right ankle and foot**

M06.272 **Rheumatoid bursitis, left ankle and foot**

M06.279 **Rheumatoid bursitis, unspecified ankle and foot**

M06.28 **Rheumatoid bursitis, vertebrae**

M06.29 **Rheumatoid bursitis, multiple sites**

✓5th M06.3 **Rheumatoid nodule**

M06.30 **Rheumatoid nodule, unspecified site**

☑ Appropriate additional character required

✓x7th Requires 7th character, placeholder x must fill empty characters

✓6ᵗʰ **M06.31 Rheumatoid nodule, shoulder**
     M06.311 Rheumatoid nodule, right shoulder
     M06.312 Rheumatoid nodule, left shoulder
     M06.319 Rheumatoid nodule, unspecified shoulder

✓6ᵗʰ **M06.32 Rheumatoid nodule, elbow**
     M06.321 Rheumatoid nodule, right elbow
     M06.322 Rheumatoid nodule, left elbow
     M06.329 Rheumatoid nodule, unspecified elbow

✓6ᵗʰ **M06.33 Rheumatoid nodule, wrist**
     M06.331 Rheumatoid nodule, right wrist
     M06.332 Rheumatoid nodule, left wrist
     M06.339 Rheumatoid nodule, unspecified wrist

✓6ᵗʰ **M06.34 Rheumatoid nodule, hand**
     M06.341 Rheumatoid nodule, right hand
     M06.342 Rheumatoid nodule, left hand
     M06.349 Rheumatoid nodule, unspecified hand

✓6ᵗʰ **M06.35 Rheumatoid nodule, hip**
     M06.351 Rheumatoid nodule, right hip
     M06.352 Rheumatoid nodule, left hip
     M06.359 Rheumatoid nodule, unspecified hip

✓6ᵗʰ **M06.36 Rheumatoid nodule, knee**
     M06.361 Rheumatoid nodule, right knee
     M06.362 Rheumatoid nodule, left knee
     M06.369 Rheumatoid nodule, unspecified knee

✓6ᵗʰ **M06.37 Rheumatoid nodule, ankle and foot**
     M06.371 Rheumatoid nodule, right ankle and foot
     M06.372 Rheumatoid nodule, left ankle and foot
     M06.379 Rheumatoid nodule, unspecified ankle and foot

     M06.38 Rheumatoid nodule, vertebrae
     M06.39 Rheumatoid nodule, multiple sites

M06.4 Inflammatory polyarthropathy
     EXCLUDES 1 *polyarthritis NOS (M13.0)*

✓5ᵗʰ **M06.8 Other specified rheumatoid arthritis**
     M06.80 Other specified rheumatoid arthritis, unspecified site

✓6ᵗʰ **M06.81 Other specified rheumatoid arthritis, shoulder**
     M06.811 Other specified rheumatoid arthritis, right shoulder
     M06.812 Other specified rheumatoid arthritis, left shoulder
     M06.819 Other specified rheumatoid arthritis, unspecified shoulder

✓6ᵗʰ **M06.82 Other specified rheumatoid arthritis, elbow**
     M06.821 Other specified rheumatoid arthritis, right elbow
     M06.822 Other specified rheumatoid arthritis, left elbow
     M06.829 Other specified rheumatoid arthritis, unspecified elbow

✓6ᵗʰ **M06.83 Other specified rheumatoid arthritis, wrist**
     M06.831 Other specified rheumatoid arthritis, right wrist
     M06.832 Other specified rheumatoid arthritis, left wrist
     M06.839 Other specified rheumatoid arthritis, unspecified wrist

✓6ᵗʰ **M06.84 Other specified rheumatoid arthritis, hand**
     M06.841 Other specified rheumatoid arthritis, right hand
     M06.842 Other specified rheumatoid arthritis, left hand
     M06.849 Other specified rheumatoid arthritis, unspecified hand

✓6ᵗʰ **M06.85 Other specified rheumatoid arthritis, hip**
     M06.851 Other specified rheumatoid arthritis, right hip
     M06.852 Other specified rheumatoid arthritis, left hip
     M06.859 Other specified rheumatoid arthritis, unspecified hip

✓6ᵗʰ **M06.86 Other specified rheumatoid arthritis, knee**
     M06.861 Other specified rheumatoid arthritis, right knee

     M06.862 Other specified rheumatoid arthritis, left knee
     M06.869 Other specified rheumatoid arthritis, unspecified knee

✓6ᵗʰ **M06.87 Other specified rheumatoid arthritis, ankle and foot**
     M06.871 Other specified rheumatoid arthritis, right ankle and foot
     M06.872 Other specified rheumatoid arthritis, left ankle and foot
     M06.879 Other specified rheumatoid arthritis, unspecified ankle and foot

     M06.88 Other specified rheumatoid arthritis, vertebrae
     M06.89 Other specified rheumatoid arthritis, multiple sites

     M06.9 Rheumatoid arthritis, unspecified

✓4ᵗʰ **M07 Enteropathic arthropathies**
     Code also associated enteropathy, such as:
       regional enteritis [Crohn's disease] (K50-)
       ulcerative colitis (K51-)
     EXCLUDES 1 *psoriatic arthropathies (L40.5-)*

✓5ᵗʰ **M07.6 Enteropathic arthropathies**
     M07.60 Enteropathic arthropathies, unspecified site

✓6ᵗʰ **M07.61 Enteropathic arthropathies, shoulder**
     M07.611 Enteropathic arthropathies, right shoulder
     M07.612 Enteropathic arthropathies, left shoulder
     M07.619 Enteropathic arthropathies, unspecified shoulder

✓6ᵗʰ **M07.62 Enteropathic arthropathies, elbow**
     M07.621 Enteropathic arthropathies, right elbow
     M07.622 Enteropathic arthropathies, left elbow
     M07.629 Enteropathic arthropathies, unspecified elbow

✓6ᵗʰ **M07.63 Enteropathic arthropathies, wrist**
     M07.631 Enteropathic arthropathies, right wrist
     M07.632 Enteropathic arthropathies, left wrist
     M07.639 Enteropathic arthropathies, unspecified wrist

✓6ᵗʰ **M07.64 Enteropathic arthropathies, hand**
     M07.641 Enteropathic arthropathies, right hand
     M07.642 Enteropathic arthropathies, left hand
     M07.649 Enteropathic arthropathies, unspecified hand

✓6ᵗʰ **M07.65 Enteropathic arthropathies, hip**
     M07.651 Enteropathic arthropathies, right hip
     M07.652 Enteropathic arthropathies, left hip
     M07.659 Enteropathic arthropathies, unspecified hip

✓6ᵗʰ **M07.66 Enteropathic arthropathies, knee**
     M07.661 Enteropathic arthropathies, right knee
     M07.662 Enteropathic arthropathies, left knee
     M07.669 Enteropathic arthropathies, unspecified knee

✓6ᵗʰ **M07.67 Enteropathic arthropathies, ankle and foot**
     M07.671 Enteropathic arthropathies, right ankle and foot
     M07.672 Enteropathic arthropathies, left ankle and foot
     M07.679 Enteropathic arthropathies, unspecified ankle and foot

     M07.68 Enteropathic arthropathies, vertebrae
     M07.69 Enteropathic arthropathies, multiple sites

EXCLUDES 1 Not coded here   EXCLUDES 2 Not included here   *Manifestation Code*

✓4th **M08 Juvenile arthritis**

Code also any associated underlying condition, such as:
regional enteritis [Crohn's disease] (K50-)
ulcerative colitis (K51-)

> EXCLUDES 1 *arthropathy in Whipple's disease (M14.8)*
> *Felty's syndrome (M05.0)*
> *juvenile dermatomyositis (M33.0-)*
> *psoriatic juvenile arthropathy (L40.54)*

✓5th **M08.0 Unspecified juvenile rheumatoid arthritis**

Juvenile rheumatoid arthritis with or without rheumatoid factor

M08.00 Unspecified juvenile rheumatoid arthritis of unspecified site

✓6th **M08.01 Unspecified juvenile rheumatoid arthritis, shoulder**

M08.011 Unspecified juvenile rheumatoid arthritis, right shoulder

M08.012 Unspecified juvenile rheumatoid arthritis, left shoulder

M08.019 Unspecified juvenile rheumatoid arthritis, unspecified shoulder

✓6th **M08.02 Unspecified juvenile rheumatoid arthritis of elbow**

M08.021 Unspecified juvenile rheumatoid arthritis, right elbow

M08.022 Unspecified juvenile rheumatoid arthritis, left elbow

M08.029 Unspecified juvenile rheumatoid arthritis, unspecified elbow

✓6th **M08.03 Unspecified juvenile rheumatoid arthritis, wrist**

M08.031 Unspecified juvenile rheumatoid arthritis, right wrist

M08.032 Unspecified juvenile rheumatoid arthritis, left wrist

M08.039 Unspecified juvenile rheumatoid arthritis, unspecified wrist

✓6th **M08.04 Unspecified juvenile rheumatoid arthritis, hand**

M08.041 Unspecified juvenile rheumatoid arthritis, right hand

M08.042 Unspecified juvenile rheumatoid arthritis, left hand

M08.049 Unspecified juvenile rheumatoid arthritis, unspecified hand

✓6th **M08.05 Unspecified juvenile rheumatoid arthritis, hip**

M08.051 Unspecified juvenile rheumatoid arthritis, right hip

M08.052 Unspecified juvenile rheumatoid arthritis, left hip

M08.059 Unspecified juvenile rheumatoid arthritis, unspecified hip

✓6th **M08.06 Unspecified juvenile rheumatoid arthritis, knee**

M08.061 Unspecified juvenile rheumatoid arthritis, right knee

M08.062 Unspecified juvenile rheumatoid arthritis, left knee

M08.069 Unspecified juvenile rheumatoid arthritis, unspecified knee

✓6th **M08.07 Unspecified juvenile rheumatoid arthritis, ankle and foot**

M08.071 Unspecified juvenile rheumatoid arthritis, right ankle and foot

M08.072 Unspecified juvenile rheumatoid arthritis, left ankle and foot

M08.079 Unspecified juvenile rheumatoid arthritis, unspecified ankle and foot

M08.08 Unspecified juvenile rheumatoid arthritis, vertebrae

M08.09 Unspecified juvenile rheumatoid arthritis, multiple sites

M08.1 Juvenile ankylosing spondylitis

> EXCLUDES 1 *ankylosing spondylitis in adults (M45.0-)*

✓5th **M08.2 Juvenile rheumatoid arthritis with systemic onset**

Still's disease NOS

> EXCLUDES 1 *adult-onset Still's disease (M06.1-)*

M08.20 Juvenile rheumatoid arthritis with systemic onset, unspecified site

✓6th **M08.21 Juvenile rheumatoid arthritis with systemic onset, shoulder**

M08.211 Juvenile rheumatoid arthritis with systemic onset, right shoulder

M08.212 Juvenile rheumatoid arthritis with systemic onset, left shoulder

M08.219 Juvenile rheumatoid arthritis with systemic onset, unspecified shoulder

✓6th **M08.22 Juvenile rheumatoid arthritis with systemic onset, elbow**

M08.221 Juvenile rheumatoid arthritis with systemic onset, right elbow

M08.222 Juvenile rheumatoid arthritis with systemic onset, left elbow

M08.229 Juvenile rheumatoid arthritis with systemic onset, unspecified elbow

✓6th **M08.23 Juvenile rheumatoid arthritis with systemic onset, wrist**

M08.231 Juvenile rheumatoid arthritis with systemic onset, right wrist

M08.232 Juvenile rheumatoid arthritis with systemic onset, left wrist

M08.239 Juvenile rheumatoid arthritis with systemic onset, unspecified wrist

✓6th **M08.24 Juvenile rheumatoid arthritis with systemic onset, hand**

M08.241 Juvenile rheumatoid arthritis with systemic onset, right hand

M08.242 Juvenile rheumatoid arthritis with systemic onset, left hand

M08.249 Juvenile rheumatoid arthritis with systemic onset, unspecified hand

✓6th **M08.25 Juvenile rheumatoid arthritis with systemic onset, hip**

M08.251 Juvenile rheumatoid arthritis with systemic onset, right hip

M08.252 Juvenile rheumatoid arthritis with systemic onset, left hip

M08.259 Juvenile rheumatoid arthritis with systemic onset, unspecified hip

✓6th **M08.26 Juvenile rheumatoid arthritis with systemic onset, knee**

M08.261 Juvenile rheumatoid arthritis with systemic onset, right knee

M08.262 Juvenile rheumatoid arthritis with systemic onset, left knee

M08.269 Juvenile rheumatoid arthritis with systemic onset, unspecified knee

✓6th **M08.27 Juvenile rheumatoid arthritis with systemic onset, ankle and foot**

M08.271 Juvenile rheumatoid arthritis with systemic onset, right ankle and foot

M08.272 Juvenile rheumatoid arthritis with systemic onset, left ankle and foot

M08.279 Juvenile rheumatoid arthritis with systemic onset, unspecified ankle and foot

M08.28 Juvenile rheumatoid arthritis with systemic onset, vertebrae

M08.29 Juvenile rheumatoid arthritis with systemic onset, multiple sites

M08.3 Juvenile rheumatoid polyarthritis (seronegative)

✓5th **M08.4 Pauciarticular juvenile rheumatoid arthritis**

M08.40 Pauciarticular juvenile rheumatoid arthritis, unspecified site

✓6th **M08.41 Pauciarticular juvenile rheumatoid arthritis, shoulder**

M08.411 Pauciarticular juvenile rheumatoid arthritis, right shoulder

M08.412 Pauciarticular juvenile rheumatoid arthritis, left shoulder

M08.419 Pauciarticular juvenile rheumatoid arthritis, unspecified shoulder

✓6th **M08.42 Pauciarticular juvenile rheumatoid arthritis, elbow**

M08.421 Pauciarticular juvenile rheumatoid arthritis, right elbow

M08.422 Pauciarticular juvenile rheumatoid arthritis, left elbow

---

✓ Appropriate additional character required   ✓x7th Requires 7th character, placeholder x must fill empty characters

M08.429   Pauciarticular juvenile rheumatoid arthritis, unspecified elbow

✓6ᵗʰ M08.43   Pauciarticular juvenile rheumatoid arthritis, wrist

M08.431   Pauciarticular juvenile rheumatoid arthritis, right wrist

M08.432   Pauciarticular juvenile rheumatoid arthritis, left wrist

M08.439   Pauciarticular juvenile rheumatoid arthritis, unspecified wrist

✓6ᵗʰ M08.44   Pauciarticular juvenile rheumatoid arthritis, hand

M08.441   Pauciarticular juvenile rheumatoid arthritis, right hand

M08.442   Pauciarticular juvenile rheumatoid arthritis, left hand

M08.449   Pauciarticular juvenile rheumatoid arthritis, unspecified hand

✓6ᵗʰ M08.45   Pauciarticular juvenile rheumatoid arthritis, hip

M08.451   Pauciarticular juvenile rheumatoid arthritis, right hip

M08.452   Pauciarticular juvenile rheumatoid arthritis, left hip

M08.459   Pauciarticular juvenile rheumatoid arthritis, unspecified hip

✓6ᵗʰ M08.46   Pauciarticular juvenile rheumatoid arthritis, knee

M08.461   Pauciarticular juvenile rheumatoid arthritis, right knee

M08.462   Pauciarticular juvenile rheumatoid arthritis, left knee

M08.469   Pauciarticular juvenile rheumatoid arthritis, unspecified knee

✓6ᵗʰ M08.47   Pauciarticular juvenile rheumatoid arthritis, ankle and foot

M08.471   Pauciarticular juvenile rheumatoid arthritis, right ankle and foot

M08.472   Pauciarticular juvenile rheumatoid arthritis, left ankle and foot

M08.479   Pauciarticular juvenile rheumatoid arthritis, unspecified ankle and foot

M08.48   Pauciarticular juvenile rheumatoid arthritis, vertebrae

✓5ᵗʰ M08.8   Other juvenile arthritis

M08.80   Other juvenile arthritis, unspecified site

✓6ᵗʰ M08.81   Other juvenile arthritis, shoulder

M08.811   Other juvenile arthritis, right shoulder

M08.812   Other juvenile arthritis, left shoulder

M08.819   Other juvenile arthritis, unspecified shoulder

✓6ᵗʰ M08.82   Other juvenile arthritis, elbow

M08.821   Other juvenile arthritis, right elbow

M08.822   Other juvenile arthritis, left elbow

M08.829   Other juvenile arthritis, unspecified elbow

✓6ᵗʰ M08.83   Other juvenile arthritis, wrist

M08.831   Other juvenile arthritis, right wrist

M08.832   Other juvenile arthritis, left wrist

M08.839   Other juvenile arthritis, unspecified wrist

✓6ᵗʰ M08.84   Other juvenile arthritis, hand

M08.841   Other juvenile arthritis, right hand

M08.842   Other juvenile arthritis, left hand

M08.849   Other juvenile arthritis, unspecified hand

✓6ᵗʰ M08.85   Other juvenile arthritis, hip

M08.851   Other juvenile arthritis, right hip

M08.852   Other juvenile arthritis, left hip

M08.859   Other juvenile arthritis, unspecified hip

✓6ᵗʰ M08.86   Other juvenile arthritis, knee

M08.861   Other juvenile arthritis, right knee

M08.862   Other juvenile arthritis, left knee

M08.869   Other juvenile arthritis, unspecified knee

✓6ᵗʰ M08.87   Other juvenile arthritis, ankle and foot

M08.871   Other juvenile arthritis, right ankle and foot

M08.872   Other juvenile arthritis, left ankle and foot

M08.879   Other juvenile arthritis, unspecified ankle and foot

M08.88   Other juvenile arthritis, vertebrae

M08.89   Other juvenile arthritis, multiple sites

✓5ᵗʰ M08.9   Juvenile arthritis, unspecified

EXCLUDES 1   *juvenile rheumatoid arthritis, unspecified (M08.0-)*

M08.90   Juvenile arthritis, unspecified, unspecified site

✓6ᵗʰ M08.91   Juvenile arthritis, unspecified, shoulder

M08.911   Juvenile arthritis, unspecified, right shoulder

M08.912   Juvenile arthritis, unspecified, left shoulder

M08.919   Juvenile arthritis, unspecified, unspecified shoulder

✓6ᵗʰ M08.92   Juvenile arthritis, unspecified, elbow

M08.921   Juvenile arthritis, unspecified, right elbow

M08.922   Juvenile arthritis, unspecified, left elbow

M08.929   Juvenile arthritis, unspecified, unspecified elbow

✓6ᵗʰ M08.93   Juvenile arthritis, unspecified, wrist

M08.931   Juvenile arthritis, unspecified, right wrist

M08.932   Juvenile arthritis, unspecified, left wrist

M08.939   Juvenile arthritis, unspecified, unspecified wrist

✓6ᵗʰ M08.94   Juvenile arthritis, unspecified, hand

M08.941   Juvenile arthritis, unspecified, right hand

M08.942   Juvenile arthritis, unspecified, left hand

M08.949   Juvenile arthritis, unspecified, unspecified hand

✓6ᵗʰ M08.95   Juvenile arthritis, unspecified, hip

M08.951   Juvenile arthritis, unspecified, right hip

M08.952   Juvenile arthritis, unspecified, left hip

M08.959   Juvenile arthritis, unspecified, unspecified hip

✓6ᵗʰ M08.96   Juvenile arthritis, unspecified, knee

M08.961   Juvenile arthritis, unspecified, right knee

M08.962   Juvenile arthritis, unspecified, left knee

M08.969   Juvenile arthritis, unspecified, unspecified knee

✓6ᵗʰ M08.97   Juvenile arthritis, unspecified, ankle and foot

M08.971   Juvenile arthritis, unspecified, right ankle and foot

M08.972   Juvenile arthritis, unspecified, left ankle and foot

M08.979   Juvenile arthritis, unspecified, unspecified ankle and foot

M08.98   Juvenile arthritis, unspecified, vertebrae

M08.99   Juvenile arthritis, unspecified, multiple sites

✓4ᵗʰ **M1a   Chronic gout**

Use additional code to identify:

autonomic neuropathy in diseases classified elsewhere (G99.0)

calculus of urinary tract in diseases classified elsewhere (N22)

cardiomyopathy in diseases classified elsewhere (I43)

disorders of external ear in diseases classified elsewhere (H61.1-, H62.8-)

disorders of iris and ciliary body in diseases classified elsewhere (H22)

glomerular disorders in diseases classified elsewhere (N08)

The appropriate 7th character is to be added to each code from category M1a.
0   without tophus (tophi)
1   with tophus (tophi)

EXCLUDES 1   *acute gout (M10-)*
     gout NOS (M10-)

✓5ᵗʰ M1a.0   Idiopathic chronic gout

Chronic gouty bursitis
Primary chronic gout

✓x7ᵗʰ M1a.00   Idiopathic chronic gout, unspecified site

✓6ᵗʰ M1a.01   Idiopathic chronic gout, shoulder

✓7ᵗʰ M1a.011   Idiopathic chronic gout, right shoulder

✓7ᵗʰ M1a.012   Idiopathic chronic gout, left shoulder

EXCLUDES 1   Not coded here   EXCLUDES 2   Not included here   *Manifestation Code*

√7ᵗʰ **M1a.019** Idiopathic chronic gout, unspecified shoulder

√6ᵗʰ **M1a.02** Idiopathic chronic gout, elbow
  √7ᵗʰ **M1a.021** Idiopathic chronic gout, right elbow
  √7ᵗʰ **M1a.022** Idiopathic chronic gout, left elbow
  √7ᵗʰ **M1a.029** Idiopathic chronic gout, unspecified elbow

√6ᵗʰ **M1a.03** Idiopathic chronic gout, wrist
  √7ᵗʰ **M1a.031** Idiopathic chronic gout, right wrist
  √7ᵗʰ **M1a.032** Idiopathic chronic gout, left wrist
  √7ᵗʰ **M1a.039** Idiopathic chronic gout, unspecified wrist

√6ᵗʰ **M1a.04** Idiopathic chronic gout, hand
  √7ᵗʰ **M1a.041** Idiopathic chronic gout, right hand
  √7ᵗʰ **M1a.042** Idiopathic chronic gout, left hand
  √7ᵗʰ **M1a.049** Idiopathic chronic gout, unspecified hand

√6ᵗʰ **M1a.05** Idiopathic chronic gout, hip
  √7ᵗʰ **M1a.051** Idiopathic chronic gout, right hip
  √7ᵗʰ **M1a.052** Idiopathic chronic gout, left hip
  √7ᵗʰ **M1a.059** Idiopathic chronic gout, unspecified hip

√6ᵗʰ **M1a.06** Idiopathic chronic gout, knee
  √7ᵗʰ **M1a.061** Idiopathic chronic gout, right knee
  √7ᵗʰ **M1a.062** Idiopathic chronic gout, left knee
  √7ᵗʰ **M1a.069** Idiopathic chronic gout, unspecified knee

√6ᵗʰ **M1a.07** Idiopathic chronic gout, ankle and foot
  √7ᵗʰ **M1a.071** Idiopathic chronic gout, right ankle and foot
  √7ᵗʰ **M1a.072** Idiopathic chronic gout, left ankle and foot
  √7ᵗʰ **M1a.079** Idiopathic chronic gout, unspecified ankle and foot

√x7ᵗʰ **M1a.08** Idiopathic chronic gout, vertebrae
√x7ᵗʰ **M1a.09** Idiopathic chronic gout, multiple sites

√5ᵗʰ **M1a.1** Lead-induced chronic gout
  Code first: toxic effects of lead and its compounds (T56.0-)

√x7ᵗʰ **M1a.10** Lead-induced chronic gout, unspecified site
√6ᵗʰ **M1a.11** Lead-induced chronic gout, shoulder
  √7ᵗʰ **M1a.111** Lead-induced chronic gout, right shoulder
  √7ᵗʰ **M1a.112** Lead-induced chronic gout, left shoulder
  √7ᵗʰ **M1a.119** Lead-induced chronic gout, unspecified shoulder

√6ᵗʰ **M1a.12** Lead-induced chronic gout, elbow
  √7ᵗʰ **M1a.121** Lead-induced chronic gout, right elbow
  √7ᵗʰ **M1a.122** Lead-induced chronic gout, left elbow
  √7ᵗʰ **M1a.129** Lead-induced chronic gout, unspecified elbow

√6ᵗʰ **M1a.13** Lead-induced chronic gout, wrist
  √7ᵗʰ **M1a.131** Lead-induced chronic gout, right wrist
  √7ᵗʰ **M1a.132** Lead-induced chronic gout, left wrist
  √7ᵗʰ **M1a.139** Lead-induced chronic gout, unspecified wrist

√6ᵗʰ **M1a.14** Lead-induced chronic gout, hand
  √7ᵗʰ **M1a.141** Lead-induced chronic gout, right hand
  √7ᵗʰ **M1a.142** Lead-induced chronic gout, left hand
  √7ᵗʰ **M1a.149** Lead-induced chronic gout, unspecified hand

√6ᵗʰ **M1a.15** Lead-induced chronic gout, hip
  √7ᵗʰ **M1a.151** Lead-induced chronic gout, right hip
  √7ᵗʰ **M1a.152** Lead-induced chronic gout, left hip
  √7ᵗʰ **M1a.159** Lead-induced chronic gout, unspecified hip

√6ᵗʰ **M1a.16** Lead-induced chronic gout, knee
  √7ᵗʰ **M1a.161** Lead-induced chronic gout, right knee
  √7ᵗʰ **M1a.162** Lead-induced chronic gout, left knee
  √7ᵗʰ **M1a.169** Lead-induced chronic gout, unspecified knee

√6ᵗʰ **M1a.17** Lead-induced chronic gout, ankle and foot
  √7ᵗʰ **M1a.171** Lead-induced chronic gout, right ankle and foot
  √7ᵗʰ **M1a.172** Lead-induced chronic gout, left ankle and foot

√7ᵗʰ **M1a.179** Lead-induced chronic gout, unspecified ankle and foot

√x7ᵗʰ **M1a.18** Lead-induced chronic gout, vertebrae
√x7ᵗʰ **M1a.19** Lead-induced chronic gout, multiple sites

√5ᵗʰ **M1a.2** Drug-induced chronic gout
  Code first (T36-T50) to identify drug

√x7ᵗʰ **M1a.20** Drug-induced chronic gout, unspecified site
√6ᵗʰ **M1a.21** Drug-induced chronic gout, shoulder
  √7ᵗʰ **M1a.211** Drug-induced chronic gout, right shoulder
  √7ᵗʰ **M1a.212** Drug-induced chronic gout, left shoulder
  √7ᵗʰ **M1a.219** Drug-induced chronic gout, unspecified shoulder

√6ᵗʰ **M1a.22** Drug-induced chronic gout, elbow
  √7ᵗʰ **M1a.221** Drug-induced chronic gout, right elbow
  √7ᵗʰ **M1a.222** Drug-induced chronic gout, left elbow
  √7ᵗʰ **M1a.229** Drug-induced chronic gout, unspecified elbow

√6ᵗʰ **M1a.23** Drug-induced chronic gout, wrist
  √7ᵗʰ **M1a.231** Drug-induced chronic gout, right wrist
  √7ᵗʰ **M1a.232** Drug-induced chronic gout, left wrist
  √7ᵗʰ **M1a.239** Drug-induced chronic gout, unspecified wrist

√6ᵗʰ **M1a.24** Drug-induced chronic gout, hand
  √7ᵗʰ **M1a.241** Drug-induced chronic gout, right hand
  √7ᵗʰ **M1a.242** Drug-induced chronic gout, left hand
  √7ᵗʰ **M1a.249** Drug-induced chronic gout, unspecified hand

√6ᵗʰ **M1a.25** Drug-induced chronic gout, hip
  √7ᵗʰ **M1a.251** Drug-induced chronic gout, right hip
  √7ᵗʰ **M1a.252** Drug-induced chronic gout, left hip
  √7ᵗʰ **M1a.259** Drug-induced chronic gout, unspecified hip

√6ᵗʰ **M1a.26** Drug-induced chronic gout, knee
  √7ᵗʰ **M1a.261** Drug-induced chronic gout, right knee
  √7ᵗʰ **M1a.262** Drug-induced chronic gout, left knee
  √7ᵗʰ **M1a.269** Drug-induced chronic gout, unspecified knee

√6ᵗʰ **M1a.27** Drug-induced chronic gout, ankle and foot
  √7ᵗʰ **M1a.271** Drug-induced chronic gout, right ankle and foot
  √7ᵗʰ **M1a.272** Drug-induced chronic gout, left ankle and foot
  √7ᵗʰ **M1a.279** Drug-induced chronic gout, unspecified ankle and foot

√x7ᵗʰ **M1a.28** Drug-induced chronic gout, vertebrae
√x7ᵗʰ **M1a.29** Drug-induced chronic gout, multiple sites

√5ᵗʰ **M1a.3** Chronic gout due to renal impairment
  Code first associated renal disease

√x7ᵗʰ **M1a.30** Chronic gout due to renal impairment, unspecified site
√6ᵗʰ **M1a.31** Chronic gout due to renal impairment, shoulder
  √7ᵗʰ **M1a.311** Chronic gout due to renal impairment, right shoulder
  √7ᵗʰ **M1a.312** Chronic gout due to renal impairment, left shoulder
  √7ᵗʰ **M1a.319** Chronic gout due to renal impairment, unspecified shoulder

√6ᵗʰ **M1a.32** Chronic gout due to renal impairment, elbow
  √7ᵗʰ **M1a.321** Chronic gout due to renal impairment, right elbow
  √7ᵗʰ **M1a.322** Chronic gout due to renal impairment, left elbow
  √7ᵗʰ **M1a.329** Chronic gout due to renal impairment, unspecified elbow

√6ᵗʰ **M1a.33** Chronic gout due to renal impairment, wrist
  √7ᵗʰ **M1a.331** Chronic gout due to renal impairment, right wrist
  √7ᵗʰ **M1a.332** Chronic gout due to renal impairment, left wrist
  √7ᵗʰ **M1a.339** Chronic gout due to renal impairment, unspecified wrist

---

☑ Appropriate additional character required √x7ᵗʰ Requires 7th character, placeholder x must fill empty characters

√6th **M1a.34 Chronic gout due to renal impairment, hand**

√7th M1a.341 Chronic gout due to renal impairment, right hand

√7th M1a.342 Chronic gout due to renal impairment, left hand

√7th M1a.349 Chronic gout due to renal impairment, unspecified hand

√6th **M1a.35 Chronic gout due to renal impairment, hip**

√7th M1a.351 Chronic gout due to renal impairment, right hip

√7th M1a.352 Chronic gout due to renal impairment, left hip

√7th M1a.359 Chronic gout due to renal impairment, unspecified hip

√6th **M1a.36 Chronic gout due to renal impairment, knee**

√7th M1a.361 Chronic gout due to renal impairment, right knee

√7th M1a.362 Chronic gout due to renal impairment, left knee

√7th M1a.369 Chronic gout due to renal impairment, unspecified knee

√6th **M1a.37 Chronic gout due to renal impairment, ankle and foot**

√7th M1a.371 Chronic gout due to renal impairment, right ankle and foot

√7th M1a.372 Chronic gout due to renal impairment, left ankle and foot

√7th M1a.379 Chronic gout due to renal impairment, unspecified ankle and foot

√x7th M1a.38 Chronic gout due to renal impairment, vertebrae

√x7th M1a.39 Chronic gout due to renal impairment, multiple sites

√5th **M1a.4 Other secondary chronic gout**

Code first associated condition

√x7th M1a.40 Other secondary chronic gout, unspecified site

√6th **M1a.41 Other secondary chronic gout, shoulder**

√7th M1a.411 Other secondary chronic gout, right shoulder

√7th M1a.412 Other secondary chronic gout, left shoulder

√7th M1a.419 Other secondary chronic gout, unspecified shoulder

√6th **M1a.42 Other secondary chronic gout, elbow**

√7th M1a.421 Other secondary chronic gout, right elbow

√7th M1a.422 Other secondary chronic gout, left elbow

√7th M1a.429 Other secondary chronic gout, unspecified elbow

√6th **M1a.43 Other secondary chronic gout, wrist**

√7th M1a.431 Other secondary chronic gout, right wrist

√7th M1a.432 Other secondary chronic gout, left wrist

√7th M1a.439 Other secondary chronic gout, unspecified wrist

√6th **M1a.44 Other secondary chronic gout, hand**

√7th M1a.441 Other secondary chronic gout, right hand

√7th M1a.442 Other secondary chronic gout, left hand

√7th M1a.449 Other secondary chronic gout, unspecified hand

√6th **M1a.45 Other secondary chronic gout, hip**

√7th M1a.451 Other secondary chronic gout, right hip

√7th M1a.452 Other secondary chronic gout, left hip

√7th M1a.459 Other secondary chronic gout, unspecified hip

√6th **M1a.46 Other secondary chronic gout, knee**

√7th M1a.461 Other secondary chronic gout, right knee

√7th M1a.462 Other secondary chronic gout, left knee

√7th M1a.469 Other secondary chronic gout, unspecified knee

√6th **M1a.47 Other secondary chronic gout, ankle and foot**

√7th M1a.471 Other secondary chronic gout, right ankle and foot

√7th M1a.472 Other secondary chronic gout, left ankle and foot

√7th M1a.479 Other secondary chronic gout, unspecified ankle and foot

√x7th M1a.48 Other secondary chronic gout, vertebrae

√x7th M1a.49 Other secondary chronic gout, multiple sites

√x7th **M1a.9 Chronic gout, unspecified**

√4th **M10 Gout**

Acute gout
Gout attack
Gout flare
Gout NOS
Podagra

Use additional code to identify:
autonomic neuropathy in diseases classified elsewhere (G99.0)
calculus of urinary tract in diseases classified elsewhere (N22)
cardiomyopathy in diseases classified elsewhere (I43)
disorders of external ear in diseases classified elsewhere (H61.1-, H62.8-)
disorders of iris and ciliary body in diseases classified elsewhere (H22)
glomerular disorders in diseases classified elsewhere (N08)

EXCLUDES 1   chronic gout (M1a-)

√5th **M10.0 Idiopathic gout**

Gouty bursitis
Primary gout

M10.00 Idiopathic gout, unspecified site

√6th **M10.01 Idiopathic gout, shoulder**

M10.011 Idiopathic gout, right shoulder

M10.012 Idiopathic gout, left shoulder

M10.019 Idiopathic gout, unspecified shoulder

√6th **M10.02 Idiopathic gout, elbow**

M10.021 Idiopathic gout, right elbow

M10.022 Idiopathic gout, left elbow

M10.029 Idiopathic gout, unspecified elbow

√6th **M10.03 Idiopathic gout, wrist**

M10.031 Idiopathic gout, right wrist

M10.032 Idiopathic gout, left wrist

M10.039 Idiopathic gout, unspecified wrist

√6th **M10.04 Idiopathic gout, hand**

M10.041 Idiopathic gout, right hand

M10.042 Idiopathic gout, left hand

M10.049 Idiopathic gout, unspecified hand

√6th **M10.05 Idiopathic gout, hip**

M10.051 Idiopathic gout, right hip

M10.052 Idiopathic gout, left hip

M10.059 Idiopathic gout, unspecified hip

√6th **M10.06 Idiopathic gout, knee**

M10.061 Idiopathic gout, right knee

M10.062 Idiopathic gout, left knee

M10.069 Idiopathic gout, unspecified knee

√6th **M10.07 Idiopathic gout, ankle and foot**

M10.071 Idiopathic gout, right ankle and foot

M10.072 Idiopathic gout, left ankle and foot

M10.079 Idiopathic gout, unspecified ankle and foot

M10.08 Idiopathic gout, vertebrae

M10.09 Idiopathic gout, multiple sites

√5th **M10.1 Lead-induced gout**

Code first: toxic effects of lead and its compounds (T56.0-)

M10.10 Lead-induced gout, unspecified site

√6th **M10.11 Lead-induced gout, shoulder**

M10.111 Lead-induced gout, right shoulder

M10.112 Lead-induced gout, left shoulder

M10.119 Lead-induced gout, unspecified shoulder

√6th **M10.12 Lead-induced gout, elbow**

M10.121 Lead-induced gout, right elbow

M10.122 Lead-induced gout, left elbow

M10.129 Lead-induced gout, unspecified elbow

√6th **M10.13 Lead-induced gout, wrist**

M10.131 Lead-induced gout, right wrist

M10.132 Lead-induced gout, left wrist

M10.139 Lead-induced gout, unspecified wrist

√6th **M10.14 Lead-induced gout, hand**

M10.141 Lead-induced gout, right hand

EXCLUDES 1 Not coded here   EXCLUDES 2 Not included here   *Manifestation Code*

           M10.142   Lead-induced gout, left hand
           M10.149   Lead-induced gout, unspecified hand

✓6th   **M10.15**   **Lead-induced gout, hip**
           M10.151   Lead-induced gout, right hip
           M10.152   Lead-induced gout, left hip
           M10.159   Lead-induced gout, unspecified hip

✓6th   **M10.16**   **Lead-induced gout, knee**
           M10.161   Lead-induced gout, right knee
           M10.162   Lead-induced gout, left knee
           M10.169   Lead-induced gout, unspecified knee

✓6th   **M10.17**   **Lead-induced gout, ankle and foot**
           M10.171   Lead-induced gout, right ankle and foot
           M10.172   Lead-induced gout, left ankle and foot
           M10.179   Lead-induced gout, unspecified ankle and foot

       M10.18   **Lead-induced gout, vertebrae**
       M10.19   **Lead-induced gout, multiple sites**

✓5th   **M10.2**   **Drug-induced gout**
       Code first (T36-T50) to identify drug
       M10.20   **Drug-induced gout, unspecified site**

✓6th   **M10.21**   **Drug-induced gout, shoulder**
           M10.211   Drug-induced gout, right shoulder
           M10.212   Drug-induced gout, left shoulder
           M10.219   Drug-induced gout, unspecified shoulder

✓6th   **M10.22**   **Drug-induced gout, elbow**
           M10.221   Drug-induced gout, right elbow
           M10.222   Drug-induced gout, left elbow
           M10.229   Drug-induced gout, unspecified elbow

✓6th   **M10.23**   **Drug-induced gout, wrist**
           M10.231   Drug-induced gout, right wrist
           M10.232   Drug-induced gout, left wrist
           M10.239   Drug-induced gout, unspecified wrist

✓6th   **M10.24**   **Drug-induced gout, hand**
           M10.241   Drug-induced gout, right hand
           M10.242   Drug-induced gout, left hand
           M10.249   Drug-induced gout, unspecified hand

✓6th   **M10.25**   **Drug-induced gout, hip**
           M10.251   Drug-induced gout, right hip
           M10.252   Drug-induced gout, left hip
           M10.259   Drug-induced gout, unspecified hip

✓6th   **M10.26**   **Drug-induced gout, knee**
           M10.261   Drug-induced gout, right knee
           M10.262   Drug-induced gout, left knee
           M10.269   Drug-induced gout, unspecified knee

✓6th   **M10.27**   **Drug-induced gout, ankle and foot**
           M10.271   Drug-induced gout, right ankle and foot
           M10.272   Drug-induced gout, left ankle and foot
           M10.279   Drug-induced gout, unspecified ankle and foot

       M10.28   **Drug-induced gout, vertebrae**
       M10.29   **Drug-induced gout, multiple sites**

✓5th   **M10.3**   **Gout due to renal impairment**
       Code first associated renal disease
       M10.30   **Gout due to renal impairment, unspecified site**

✓6th   **M10.31**   **Gout due to renal impairment, shoulder**
           M10.311   Gout due to renal impairment, right shoulder
           M10.312   Gout due to renal impairment, left shoulder
           M10.319   Gout due to renal impairment, unspecified shoulder

✓6th   **M10.32**   **Gout due to renal impairment, elbow**
           M10.321   Gout due to renal impairment, right elbow
           M10.322   Gout due to renal impairment, left elbow
           M10.329   Gout due to renal impairment, unspecified elbow

✓6th   **M10.33**   **Gout due to renal impairment, wrist**
           M10.331   Gout due to renal impairment, right wrist
           M10.332   Gout due to renal impairment, left wrist
           M10.339   Gout due to renal impairment, unspecified wrist

✓6th   **M10.34**   **Gout due to renal impairment, hand**
           M10.341   Gout due to renal impairment, right hand
           M10.342   Gout due to renal impairment, left hand
           M10.349   Gout due to renal impairment, unspecified hand

✓6th   **M10.35**   **Gout due to renal impairment, hip**
           M10.351   Gout due to renal impairment, right hip
           M10.352   Gout due to renal impairment, left hip
           M10.359   Gout due to renal impairment, unspecified hip

✓6th   **M10.36**   **Gout due to renal impairment, knee**
           M10.361   Gout due to renal impairment, right knee
           M10.362   Gout due to renal impairment, left knee
           M10.369   Gout due to renal impairment, unspecified knee

✓6th   **M10.37**   **Gout due to renal impairment, ankle and foot**
           M10.371   Gout due to renal impairment, right ankle and foot
           M10.372   Gout due to renal impairment, left ankle and foot
           M10.379   Gout due to renal impairment, unspecified ankle and foot

       M10.38   **Gout due to renal impairment, vertebrae**
       M10.39   **Gout due to renal impairment, multiple sites**

✓5th   **M10.4**   **Other secondary gout**
       Code first associated condition
       M10.40   **Other secondary gout, unspecified site**

✓6th   **M10.41**   **Other secondary gout, shoulder**
           M10.411   Other secondary gout, right shoulder
           M10.412   Other secondary gout, left shoulder
           M10.419   Other secondary gout, unspecified shoulder

✓6th   **M10.42**   **Other secondary gout, elbow**
           M10.421   Other secondary gout, right elbow
           M10.422   Other secondary gout, left elbow
           M10.429   Other secondary gout, unspecified elbow

✓6th   **M10.43**   **Other secondary gout, wrist**
           M10.431   Other secondary gout, right wrist
           M10.432   Other secondary gout, left wrist
           M10.439   Other secondary gout, unspecified wrist

✓6th   **M10.44**   **Other secondary gout, hand**
           M10.441   Other secondary gout, right hand
           M10.442   Other secondary gout, left hand
           M10.449   Other secondary gout, unspecified hand

✓6th   **M10.45**   **Other secondary gout, hip**
           M10.451   Other secondary gout, right hip
           M10.452   Other secondary gout, left hip
           M10.459   Other secondary gout, unspecified hip

✓6th   **M10.46**   **Other secondary gout, knee**
           M10.461   Other secondary gout, right knee
           M10.462   Other secondary gout, left knee
           M10.469   Other secondary gout, unspecified knee

✓6th   **M10.47**   **Other secondary gout, ankle and foot**
           M10.471   Other secondary gout, right ankle and foot
           M10.472   Other secondary gout, left ankle and foot
           M10.479   Other secondary gout, unspecified ankle and foot

       M10.48   **Other secondary gout, vertebrae**
       M10.49   **Other secondary gout, multiple sites**

    M10.9   **Gout, unspecified**
       Gout NOS

✓4th   **M11**   **Other crystal arthropathies**
✓5th   **M11.0**   **Hydroxyapatite deposition disease**
       M11.00   **Hydroxyapatite deposition disease, unspecified site**

✓6th   **M11.01**   **Hydroxyapatite deposition disease, shoulder**
           M11.011   Hydroxyapatite deposition disease, right shoulder
           M11.012   Hydroxyapatite deposition disease, left shoulder

---

✓ Appropriate additional character required   ✓x7th Requires 7th character, placeholder x must fill empty characters

M11.019   Hydroxyapatite deposition disease, unspecified shoulder

✓6ᵗʰ   **M11.02**   Hydroxyapatite deposition disease, elbow

M11.021   Hydroxyapatite deposition disease, right elbow

M11.022   Hydroxyapatite deposition disease, left elbow

M11.029   Hydroxyapatite deposition disease, unspecified elbow

✓6ᵗʰ   **M11.03**   Hydroxyapatite deposition disease, wrist

M11.031   Hydroxyapatite deposition disease, right wrist

M11.032   Hydroxyapatite deposition disease, left wrist

M11.039   Hydroxyapatite deposition disease, unspecified wrist

✓6ᵗʰ   **M11.04**   Hydroxyapatite deposition disease, hand

M11.041   Hydroxyapatite deposition disease, right hand

M11.042   Hydroxyapatite deposition disease, left hand

M11.049   Hydroxyapatite deposition disease, unspecified hand

✓6ᵗʰ   **M11.05**   Hydroxyapatite deposition disease, hip

M11.051   Hydroxyapatite deposition disease, right hip

M11.052   Hydroxyapatite deposition disease, left hip

M11.059   Hydroxyapatite deposition disease, unspecified hip

✓6ᵗʰ   **M11.06**   Hydroxyapatite deposition disease, knee

M11.061   Hydroxyapatite deposition disease, right knee

M11.062   Hydroxyapatite deposition disease, left knee

M11.069   Hydroxyapatite deposition disease, unspecified knee

✓6ᵗʰ   **M11.07**   Hydroxyapatite deposition disease, ankle and foot

M11.071   Hydroxyapatite deposition disease, right ankle and foot

M11.072   Hydroxyapatite deposition disease, left ankle and foot

M11.079   Hydroxyapatite deposition disease, unspecified ankle and foot

M11.08   Hydroxyapatite deposition disease, vertebrae

M11.09   Hydroxyapatite deposition disease, multiple sites

✓5ᵗʰ   **M11.1**   **Familial chondrocalcinosis**

M11.10   Familial chondrocalcinosis, unspecified site

✓6ᵗʰ   **M11.11**   Familial chondrocalcinosis, shoulder

M11.111   Familial chondrocalcinosis, right shoulder

M11.112   Familial chondrocalcinosis, left shoulder

M11.119   Familial chondrocalcinosis, unspecified shoulder

✓6ᵗʰ   **M11.12**   Familial chondrocalcinosis, elbow

M11.121   Familial chondrocalcinosis, right elbow

M11.122   Familial chondrocalcinosis, left elbow

M11.129   Familial chondrocalcinosis, unspecified elbow

✓6ᵗʰ   **M11.13**   Familial chondrocalcinosis, wrist

M11.131   Familial chondrocalcinosis, right wrist

M11.132   Familial chondrocalcinosis, left wrist

M11.139   Familial chondrocalcinosis, unspecified wrist

✓6ᵗʰ   **M11.14**   Familial chondrocalcinosis, hand

M11.141   Familial chondrocalcinosis, right hand

M11.142   Familial chondrocalcinosis, left hand

M11.149   Familial chondrocalcinosis, unspecified hand

✓6ᵗʰ   **M11.15**   Familial chondrocalcinosis, hip

M11.151   Familial chondrocalcinosis, right hip

M11.152   Familial chondrocalcinosis, left hip

M11.159   Familial chondrocalcinosis, unspecified hip

✓6ᵗʰ   **M11.16**   Familial chondrocalcinosis, knee

M11.161   Familial chondrocalcinosis, right knee

M11.162   Familial chondrocalcinosis, left knee

M11.169   Familial chondrocalcinosis, unspecified knee

✓6ᵗʰ   **M11.17**   Familial chondrocalcinosis, ankle and foot

M11.171   Familial chondrocalcinosis, right ankle and foot

M11.172   Familial chondrocalcinosis, left ankle and foot

M11.179   Familial chondrocalcinosis, unspecified ankle and foot

M11.18   Familial chondrocalcinosis, vertebrae

M11.19   Familial chondrocalcinosis, multiple sites

✓5ᵗʰ   **M11.2**   **Other chondrocalcinosis**

Chondrocalcinosis NOS

M11.20   Other chondrocalcinosis, unspecified site

✓6ᵗʰ   **M11.21**   Other chondrocalcinosis, shoulder

M11.211   Other chondrocalcinosis, right shoulder

M11.212   Other chondrocalcinosis, left shoulder

M11.219   Other chondrocalcinosis, unspecified shoulder

✓6ᵗʰ   **M11.22**   Other chondrocalcinosis, elbow

M11.221   Other chondrocalcinosis, right elbow

M11.222   Other chondrocalcinosis, left elbow

M11.229   Other chondrocalcinosis, unspecified elbow

✓6ᵗʰ   **M11.23**   Other chondrocalcinosis, wrist

M11.231   Other chondrocalcinosis, right wrist

M11.232   Other chondrocalcinosis, left wrist

M11.239   Other chondrocalcinosis, unspecified wrist

✓6ᵗʰ   **M11.24**   Other chondrocalcinosis, hand

M11.241   Other chondrocalcinosis, right hand

M11.242   Other chondrocalcinosis, left hand

M11.249   Other chondrocalcinosis, unspecified hand

✓6ᵗʰ   **M11.25**   Other chondrocalcinosis, hip

M11.251   Other chondrocalcinosis, right hip

M11.252   Other chondrocalcinosis, left hip

M11.259   Other chondrocalcinosis, unspecified hip

✓6ᵗʰ   **M11.26**   Other chondrocalcinosis, knee

M11.261   Other chondrocalcinosis, right knee

M11.262   Other chondrocalcinosis, left knee

M11.269   Other chondrocalcinosis, unspecified knee

✓6ᵗʰ   **M11.27**   Other chondrocalcinosis, ankle and foot

M11.271   Other chondrocalcinosis, right ankle and foot

M11.272   Other chondrocalcinosis, left ankle and foot

M11.279   Other chondrocalcinosis, unspecified ankle and foot

M11.28   Other chondrocalcinosis, vertebrae

M11.29   Other chondrocalcinosis, multiple sites

✓5ᵗʰ   **M11.8**   **Other specified crystal arthropathies**

M11.80   Other specified crystal arthropathies, unspecified site

✓6ᵗʰ   **M11.81**   Other specified crystal arthropathies, shoulder

M11.811   Other specified crystal arthropathies, right shoulder

M11.812   Other specified crystal arthropathies, left shoulder

M11.819   Other specified crystal arthropathies, unspecified shoulder

✓6ᵗʰ   **M11.82**   Other specified crystal arthropathies, elbow

M11.821   Other specified crystal arthropathies, right elbow

M11.822   Other specified crystal arthropathies, left elbow

M11.829   Other specified crystal arthropathies, unspecified elbow

✓6ᵗʰ   **M11.83**   Other specified crystal arthropathies, wrist

M11.831   Other specified crystal arthropathies, right wrist

M11.832   Other specified crystal arthropathies, left wrist

M11.839   Other specified crystal arthropathies, unspecified wrist

---

EXCLUDES 1   Not coded here   EXCLUDES 2   Not included here   *Manifestation Code*

✓6th **M11.84 Other specified crystal arthropathies, hand**
    M11.841 Other specified crystal arthropathies, right hand
    M11.842 Other specified crystal arthropathies, left hand
    M11.849 Other specified crystal arthropathies, unspecified hand

✓6th **M11.85 Other specified crystal arthropathies, hip**
    M11.851 Other specified crystal arthropathies, right hip
    M11.852 Other specified crystal arthropathies, left hip
    M11.859 Other specified crystal arthropathies, unspecified hip

✓6th **M11.86 Other specified crystal arthropathies, knee**
    M11.861 Other specified crystal arthropathies, right knee
    M11.862 Other specified crystal arthropathies, left knee
    M11.869 Other specified crystal arthropathies, unspecified knee

✓6th **M11.87 Other specified crystal arthropathies, ankle and foot**
    M11.871 Other specified crystal arthropathies, right ankle and foot
    M11.872 Other specified crystal arthropathies, left ankle and foot
    M11.879 Other specified crystal arthropathies, unspecified ankle and foot

M11.88 Other specified crystal arthropathies, vertebrae
M11.89 Other specified crystal arthropathies, multiple sites

M11.9 Crystal arthropathy, unspecified

✓4th **M12 Other and unspecified arthropathy**
    EXCLUDES 1 *arthrosis (M15-M19)*
              cricoarytenoid arthropathy (J38.7)

✓5th **M12.0 Chronic postrheumatic arthropathy [Jaccoud]**
    M12.00 Chronic postrheumatic arthropathy [Jaccoud], unspecified site

✓6th **M12.01 Chronic postrheumatic arthropathy [Jaccoud], shoulder**
    M12.011 Chronic postrheumatic arthropathy [Jaccoud], right shoulder
    M12.012 Chronic postrheumatic arthropathy [Jaccoud], left shoulder
    M12.019 Chronic postrheumatic arthropathy [Jaccoud], unspecified shoulder

✓6th **M12.02 Chronic postrheumatic arthropathy [Jaccoud], elbow**
    M12.021 Chronic postrheumatic arthropathy [Jaccoud], right elbow
    M12.022 Chronic postrheumatic arthropathy [Jaccoud], left elbow
    M12.029 Chronic postrheumatic arthropathy [Jaccoud], unspecified elbow

✓6th **M12.03 Chronic postrheumatic arthropathy [Jaccoud], wrist**
    M12.031 Chronic postrheumatic arthropathy [Jaccoud], right wrist
    M12.032 Chronic postrheumatic arthropathy [Jaccoud], left wrist
    M12.039 Chronic postrheumatic arthropathy [Jaccoud], unspecified wrist

✓6th **M12.04 Chronic postrheumatic arthropathy [Jaccoud], hand**
    M12.041 Chronic postrheumatic arthropathy [Jaccoud], right hand
    M12.042 Chronic postrheumatic arthropathy [Jaccoud], left hand
    M12.049 Chronic postrheumatic arthropathy [Jaccoud], unspecified hand

✓6th **M12.05 Chronic postrheumatic arthropathy [Jaccoud], hip**
    M12.051 Chronic postrheumatic arthropathy [Jaccoud], right hip
    M12.052 Chronic postrheumatic arthropathy [Jaccoud], left hip
    M12.059 Chronic postrheumatic arthropathy [Jaccoud], unspecified hip

✓6th **M12.06 Chronic postrheumatic arthropathy [Jaccoud], knee**
    M12.061 Chronic postrheumatic arthropathy [Jaccoud], right knee
    M12.062 Chronic postrheumatic arthropathy [Jaccoud], left knee
    M12.069 Chronic postrheumatic arthropathy [Jaccoud], unspecified knee

✓6th **M12.07 Chronic postrheumatic arthropathy [Jaccoud], ankle and foot**
    M12.071 Chronic postrheumatic arthropathy [Jaccoud], right ankle and foot
    M12.072 Chronic postrheumatic arthropathy [Jaccoud], left ankle and foot
    M12.079 Chronic postrheumatic arthropathy [Jaccoud], unspecified ankle and foot

M12.08 Chronic postrheumatic arthropathy [Jaccoud], vertebrae
M12.09 Chronic postrheumatic arthropathy [Jaccoud], multiple sites

✓5th **M12.1 Kaschin-Beck disease**
    Osteochondroarthrosis deformans endemica
    M12.10 Kaschin-Beck disease, unspecified site

✓6th **M12.11 Kaschin-Beck disease, shoulder**
    M12.111 Kaschin-Beck disease, right shoulder
    M12.112 Kaschin-Beck disease, left shoulder
    M12.119 Kaschin-Beck disease, unspecified shoulder

✓6th **M12.12 Kaschin-Beck disease, elbow**
    M12.121 Kaschin-Beck disease, right elbow
    M12.122 Kaschin-Beck disease, left elbow
    M12.129 Kaschin-Beck disease, unspecified elbow

✓6th **M12.13 Kaschin-Beck disease, wrist**
    M12.131 Kaschin-Beck disease, right wrist
    M12.132 Kaschin-Beck disease, left wrist
    M12.139 Kaschin-Beck disease, unspecified wrist

✓6th **M12.14 Kaschin-Beck disease, hand**
    M12.141 Kaschin-Beck disease, right hand
    M12.142 Kaschin-Beck disease, left hand
    M12.149 Kaschin-Beck disease, unspecified hand

✓6th **M12.15 Kaschin-Beck disease, hip**
    M12.151 Kaschin-Beck disease, right hip
    M12.152 Kaschin-Beck disease, left hip
    M12.159 Kaschin-Beck disease, unspecified hip

✓6th **M12.16 Kaschin-Beck disease, knee**
    M12.161 Kaschin-Beck disease, right knee
    M12.162 Kaschin-Beck disease, left knee
    M12.169 Kaschin-Beck disease, unspecified knee

✓6th **M12.17 Kaschin-Beck disease, ankle and foot**
    M12.171 Kaschin-Beck disease, right ankle and foot
    M12.172 Kaschin-Beck disease, left ankle and foot
    M12.179 Kaschin-Beck disease, unspecified ankle and foot

M12.18 Kaschin-Beck disease, vertebrae
M12.19 Kaschin-Beck disease, multiple sites

✓5th **M12.2 Villonodular synovitis (pigmented)**
    M12.20 Villonodular synovitis (pigmented), unspecified site

✓6th **M12.21 Villonodular synovitis (pigmented), shoulder**
    M12.211 Villonodular synovitis (pigmented), right shoulder
    M12.212 Villonodular synovitis (pigmented), left shoulder
    M12.219 Villonodular synovitis (pigmented), unspecified shoulder

✓6th **M12.22 Villonodular synovitis (pigmented), elbow**
    M12.221 Villonodular synovitis (pigmented), right elbow
    M12.222 Villonodular synovitis (pigmented), left elbow
    M12.229 Villonodular synovitis (pigmented), unspecified elbow

√6th **M12.23** Villonodular synovitis (pigmented), wrist
   M12.231 Villonodular synovitis (pigmented), right wrist
   M12.232 Villonodular synovitis (pigmented), left wrist
   M12.239 Villonodular synovitis (pigmented), unspecified wrist

√6th **M12.24** Villonodular synovitis (pigmented), hand
   M12.241 Villonodular synovitis (pigmented), right hand
   M12.242 Villonodular synovitis (pigmented), left hand
   M12.249 Villonodular synovitis (pigmented), unspecified hand

√6th **M12.25** Villonodular synovitis (pigmented), hip
   M12.251 Villonodular synovitis (pigmented), right hip
   M12.252 Villonodular synovitis (pigmented), left hip
   M12.259 Villonodular synovitis (pigmented), unspecified hip

√6th **M12.26** Villonodular synovitis (pigmented), knee
   M12.261 Villonodular synovitis (pigmented), right knee
   M12.262 Villonodular synovitis (pigmented), left knee
   M12.269 Villonodular synovitis (pigmented), unspecified knee

√6th **M12.27** Villonodular synovitis (pigmented), ankle and foot
   M12.271 Villonodular synovitis (pigmented), right ankle and foot
   M12.272 Villonodular synovitis (pigmented), left ankle and foot
   M12.279 Villonodular synovitis (pigmented), unspecified ankle and foot

   M12.28 Villonodular synovitis (pigmented), vertebrae
   M12.29 Villonodular synovitis (pigmented), multiple sites

√5th **M12.3** Palindromic rheumatism
   M12.30 Palindromic rheumatism, unspecified site

√6th **M12.31** Palindromic rheumatism, shoulder
   M12.311 Palindromic rheumatism, right shoulder
   M12.312 Palindromic rheumatism, left shoulder
   M12.319 Palindromic rheumatism, unspecified shoulder

√6th **M12.32** Palindromic rheumatism, elbow
   M12.321 Palindromic rheumatism, right elbow
   M12.322 Palindromic rheumatism, left elbow
   M12.329 Palindromic rheumatism, unspecified elbow

√6th **M12.33** Palindromic rheumatism, wrist
   M12.331 Palindromic rheumatism, right wrist
   M12.332 Palindromic rheumatism, left wrist
   M12.339 Palindromic rheumatism, unspecified wrist

√6th **M12.34** Palindromic rheumatism, hand
   M12.341 Palindromic rheumatism, right hand
   M12.342 Palindromic rheumatism, left hand
   M12.349 Palindromic rheumatism, unspecified hand

√6th **M12.35** Palindromic rheumatism, hip
   M12.351 Palindromic rheumatism, right hip
   M12.352 Palindromic rheumatism, left hip
   M12.359 Palindromic rheumatism, unspecified hip

√6th **M12.36** Palindromic rheumatism, knee
   M12.361 Palindromic rheumatism, right knee
   M12.362 Palindromic rheumatism, left knee
   M12.369 Palindromic rheumatism, unspecified knee

√6th **M12.37** Palindromic rheumatism, ankle and foot
   M12.371 Palindromic rheumatism, right ankle and foot
   M12.372 Palindromic rheumatism, left ankle and foot
   M12.379 Palindromic rheumatism, unspecified ankle and foot

   M12.38 Palindromic rheumatism, vertebrae

   M12.39 Palindromic rheumatism, multiple sites

√5th **M12.4** Intermittent hydrarthrosis
   M12.40 Intermittent hydrarthrosis, unspecified site

√6th **M12.41** Intermittent hydrarthrosis, shoulder
   M12.411 Intermittent hydrarthrosis, right shoulder
   M12.412 Intermittent hydrarthrosis, left shoulder
   M12.419 Intermittent hydrarthrosis, unspecified shoulder

√6th **M12.42** Intermittent hydrarthrosis, elbow
   M12.421 Intermittent hydrarthrosis, right elbow
   M12.422 Intermittent hydrarthrosis, left elbow
   M12.429 Intermittent hydrarthrosis, unspecified elbow

√6th **M12.43** Intermittent hydrarthrosis, wrist
   M12.431 Intermittent hydrarthrosis, right wrist
   M12.432 Intermittent hydrarthrosis, left wrist
   M12.439 Intermittent hydrarthrosis, unspecified wrist

√6th **M12.44** Intermittent hydrarthrosis, hand
   M12.441 Intermittent hydrarthrosis, right hand
   M12.442 Intermittent hydrarthrosis, left hand
   M12.449 Intermittent hydrarthrosis, unspecified hand

√6th **M12.45** Intermittent hydrarthrosis, hip
   M12.451 Intermittent hydrarthrosis, right hip
   M12.452 Intermittent hydrarthrosis, left hip
   M12.459 Intermittent hydrarthrosis, unspecified hip

√6th **M12.46** Intermittent hydrarthrosis, knee
   M12.461 Intermittent hydrarthrosis, right knee
   M12.462 Intermittent hydrarthrosis, left knee
   M12.469 Intermittent hydrarthrosis, unspecified knee

√6th **M12.47** Intermittent hydrarthrosis, ankle and foot
   M12.471 Intermittent hydrarthrosis, right ankle and foot
   M12.472 Intermittent hydrarthrosis, left ankle and foot
   M12.479 Intermittent hydrarthrosis, unspecified ankle and foot

   M12.48 Intermittent hydrarthrosis, other site
   M12.49 Intermittent hydrarthrosis, multiple sites

√5th **M12.5** Traumatic arthropathy
   EXCLUDES 1   current injury–see Alphabetic Index
     post-traumatic osteoarthritis (of):
     NOS (M19.1-)
     first carpometacarpal joint (M18.2-M18.3)
     hip (M16.4-M16.5)
     knee (M17.2-M17.3)
     other single joints (M19.1-)

   M12.50 Traumatic arthropathy, unspecified site

√6th **M12.51** Traumatic arthropathy, shoulder
   M12.511 Traumatic arthropathy, right shoulder
   M12.512 Traumatic arthropathy, left shoulder
   M12.519 Traumatic arthropathy, unspecified shoulder

√6th **M12.52** Traumatic arthropathy, elbow
   M12.521 Traumatic arthropathy, right elbow
   M12.522 Traumatic arthropathy, left elbow
   M12.529 Traumatic arthropathy, unspecified elbow

√6th **M12.53** Traumatic arthropathy, wrist
   M12.531 Traumatic arthropathy, right wrist
   M12.532 Traumatic arthropathy, left wrist
   M12.539 Traumatic arthropathy, unspecified wrist

√6th **M12.54** Traumatic arthropathy, hand
   M12.541 Traumatic arthropathy, right hand
   M12.542 Traumatic arthropathy, left hand
   M12.549 Traumatic arthropathy, unspecified hand

√6th **M12.55** Traumatic arthropathy, hip
   M12.551 Traumatic arthropathy, right hip
   M12.552 Traumatic arthropathy, left hip
   M12.559 Traumatic arthropathy, unspecified hip

EXCLUDES 1 Not coded here   **EXCLUDES 2** Not included here   *Manifestation Code*

✓6th **M12.56 Traumatic arthropathy, knee**
  M12.561 Traumatic arthropathy, right knee
  M12.562 Traumatic arthropathy, left knee
  M12.569 Traumatic arthropathy, unspecified knee

✓6th **M12.57 Traumatic arthropathy, ankle and foot**
  M12.571 Traumatic arthropathy, right ankle and foot
  M12.572 Traumatic arthropathy, left ankle and foot
  M12.579 Traumatic arthropathy, unspecified ankle and foot

M12.58 Traumatic arthropathy, vertebrae
M12.59 Traumatic arthropathy, multiple sites

✓5th **M12.8 Other specific arthropathies, not elsewhere classified**
  Transient arthropathy
  M12.80 Other specific arthropathies, not elsewhere classified, unspecified site
✓6th **M12.81 Other specific arthropathies, not elsewhere classified, shoulder**
  M12.811 Other specific arthropathies, not elsewhere classified, right shoulder
  M12.812 Other specific arthropathies, not elsewhere classified, left shoulder
  M12.819 Other specific arthropathies, not elsewhere classified, unspecified shoulder
✓6th **M12.82 Other specific arthropathies, not elsewhere classified, elbow**
  M12.821 Other specific arthropathies, not elsewhere classified, right elbow
  M12.822 Other specific arthropathies, not elsewhere classified, left elbow
  M12.829 Other specific arthropathies, not elsewhere classified, unspecified elbow
✓6th **M12.83 Other specific arthropathies, not elsewhere classified, wrist**
  M12.831 Other specific arthropathies, not elsewhere classified, right wrist
  M12.832 Other specific arthropathies, not elsewhere classified, left wrist
  M12.839 Other specific arthropathies, not elsewhere classified, unspecified wrist
✓6th **M12.84 Other specific arthropathies, not elsewhere classified, hand**
  M12.841 Other specific arthropathies, not elsewhere classified, right hand
  M12.842 Other specific arthropathies, not elsewhere classified, left hand
  M12.849 Other specific arthropathies, not elsewhere classified, unspecified hand
✓6th **M12.85 Other specific arthropathies, not elsewhere classified, hip**
  M12.851 Other specific arthropathies, not elsewhere classified, right hip
  M12.852 Other specific arthropathies, not elsewhere classified, left hip
  M12.859 Other specific arthropathies, not elsewhere classified, unspecified hip
✓6th **M12.86 Other specific arthropathies, not elsewhere classified, knee**
  M12.861 Other specific arthropathies, not elsewhere classified, right knee
  M12.862 Other specific arthropathies, not elsewhere classified, left knee
  M12.869 Other specific arthropathies, not elsewhere classified, unspecified knee
✓6th **M12.87 Other specific arthropathies, not elsewhere classified, ankle and foot**
  M12.871 Other specific arthropathies, not elsewhere classified, right ankle and foot
  M12.872 Other specific arthropathies, not elsewhere classified, left ankle and foot
  M12.879 Other specific arthropathies, not elsewhere classified, unspecified ankle and foot

M12.88 Other specific arthropathies, not elsewhere classified, vertebrae
M12.89 Other specific arthropathies, not elsewhere classified, multiple sites
M12.9 Arthropathy, unspecified

✓4th **M13 Other arthritis**
  EXCLUDES 1   arthrosis (M15-M19)
        osteoarthritis (M15-M19)
  M13.0 Polyarthritis, unspecified
✓5th **M13.1 Monoarthritis, not elsewhere classified**
  M13.10 Monoarthritis, not elsewhere classified, unspecified site
✓6th **M13.11 Monoarthritis, not elsewhere classified, shoulder**
  M13.111 Monoarthritis, not elsewhere classified, right shoulder
  M13.112 Monoarthritis, not elsewhere classified, left shoulder
  M13.119 Monoarthritis, not elsewhere classified, unspecified shoulder
✓6th **M13.12 Monoarthritis, not elsewhere classified, elbow**
  M13.121 Monoarthritis, not elsewhere classified, right elbow
  M13.122 Monoarthritis, not elsewhere classified, left elbow
  M13.129 Monoarthritis, not elsewhere classified, unspecified elbow
✓6th **M13.13 Monoarthritis, not elsewhere classified, wrist**
  M13.131 Monoarthritis, not elsewhere classified, right wrist
  M13.132 Monoarthritis, not elsewhere classified, left wrist
  M13.139 Monoarthritis, not elsewhere classified, unspecified wrist
✓6th **M13.14 Monoarthritis, not elsewhere classified, hand**
  M13.141 Monoarthritis, not elsewhere classified, right hand
  M13.142 Monoarthritis, not elsewhere classified, left hand
  M13.149 Monoarthritis, not elsewhere classified, unspecified hand
✓6th **M13.15 Monoarthritis, not elsewhere classified, hip**
  M13.151 Monoarthritis, not elsewhere classified, right hip
  M13.152 Monoarthritis, not elsewhere classified, left hip
  M13.159 Monoarthritis, not elsewhere classified, unspecified hip
✓6th **M13.16 Monoarthritis, not elsewhere classified, knee**
  M13.161 Monoarthritis, not elsewhere classified, right knee
  M13.162 Monoarthritis, not elsewhere classified, left knee
  M13.169 Monoarthritis, not elsewhere classified, unspecified knee
✓6th **M13.17 Monoarthritis, not elsewhere classified, ankle and foot**
  M13.171 Monoarthritis, not elsewhere classified, right ankle and foot
  M13.172 Monoarthritis, not elsewhere classified, left ankle and foot
  M13.179 Monoarthritis, not elsewhere classified, unspecified ankle and foot

✓5th **M13.8 Other specified arthritis**
  Allergic arthritis
  EXCLUDES 1   osteoarthritis (M15-M19)
  M13.80 Other specified arthritis, unspecified site
✓6th **M13.81 Other specified arthritis, shoulder**
  M13.811 Other specified arthritis, right shoulder
  M13.812 Other specified arthritis, left shoulder
  M13.819 Other specified arthritis, unspecified shoulder
✓6th **M13.82 Other specified arthritis, elbow**
  M13.821 Other specified arthritis, right elbow
  M13.822 Other specified arthritis, left elbow
  M13.829 Other specified arthritis, unspecified elbow

✓ Appropriate additional character required   ✓x7th Requires 7th character, placeholder x must fill empty characters

✓6th **M13.83 Other specified arthritis, wrist**
     M13.831   Other specified arthritis, right wrist
     M13.832   Other specified arthritis, left wrist
     M13.839   Other specified arthritis, unspecified wrist

✓6th **M13.84 Other specified arthritis, hand**
     M13.841   Other specified arthritis, right hand
     M13.842   Other specified arthritis, left hand
     M13.849   Other specified arthritis, unspecified hand

✓6th **M13.85 Other specified arthritis, hip**
     M13.851   Other specified arthritis, right hip
     M13.852   Other specified arthritis, left hip
     M13.859   Other specified arthritis, unspecified hip

✓6th **M13.86 Other specified arthritis, knee**
     M13.861   Other specified arthritis, right knee
     M13.862   Other specified arthritis, left knee
     M13.869   Other specified arthritis, unspecified knee

✓6th **M13.87 Other specified arthritis, ankle and foot**
     M13.871   Other specified arthritis, right ankle and foot
     M13.872   Other specified arthritis, left ankle and foot
     M13.879   Other specified arthritis, unspecified ankle and foot

M13.88 Other specified arthritis, vertebrae
M13.89 Other specified arthritis, multiple sites

✓4th **M14 Arthropathies in other diseases classified elsewhere**
     EXCLUDES 1   arthropathy in:
          diabetes mellitus (E08-E13 with 4th and 5th characters 61)
          hematological disorders (M36.2-M36.3)
          hypersensitivity reactions (M36.4)
          neoplastic disease (M36.1)
          neurosyphillis (A52.16)
          sarcoidosis (D86.86)
          enteropathic arthropathies (M07.-)
          juvenile psoriatic arthropathy (L40.54)
          lipoid dermatoarthritis (E78.81)

✓5th **M14.6 Charcôt's joint**
     Neuropathic arthropathy
     EXCLUDES 1   Charcôt's joint in diabetes mellitus (E08-E13 with final characters 610)
          Charcôt's joint in tabes dorsalis (A52.16)

     M14.60 Charcôt's joint, unspecified site
✓6th **M14.61 Charcôt's joint, shoulder**
     M14.611   Charcôt's joint, right shoulder
     M14.612   Charcôt's joint, left shoulder
     M14.619   Charcôt's joint, unspecified shoulder

✓6th **M14.62 Charcôt's joint, elbow**
     M14.621   Charcôt's joint, right elbow
     M14.622   Charcôt's joint, left elbow
     M14.629   Charcôt's joint, unspecified elbow

✓6th **M14.63 Charcôt's joint, wrist**
     M14.631   Charcôt's joint, right wrist
     M14.632   Charcôt's joint, left wrist
     M14.639   Charcôt's joint, unspecified wrist

✓6th **M14.64 Charcôt's joint, hand**
     M14.641   Charcôt's joint, right hand
     M14.642   Charcôt's joint, left hand
     M14.649   Charcôt's joint, unspecified hand

✓6th **M14.65 Charcôt's joint, hip**
     M14.651   Charcôt's joint, right hip
     M14.652   Charcôt's joint, left hip
     M14.659   Charcôt's joint, unspecified hip

✓6th **M14.66 Charcôt's joint, knee**
     M14.661   Charcôt's joint, right knee
     M14.662   Charcôt's joint, left knee
     M14.669   Charcôt's joint, unspecified knee

✓6th **M14.67 Charcôt's joint, ankle and foot**
     M14.671   Charcôt's joint, right ankle and foot
     M14.672   Charcôt's joint, left ankle and foot
     M14.679   Charcôt's joint, unspecified ankle and foot

M14.68 Charcôt's joint, vertebrae
M14.69 Charcôt's joint, multiple sites

✓5th **M14.8 Arthropathies in other specified diseases classified elsewhere**
     Code first underlying disease, such as:
          amyloidosis (E85-)
          erythema multiforme (L51-)
          erythema nodosum (L52)
          hemochromatosis (E83.11-)
          hyperparathyroidism (E21-)
          hypothyroidism (E00-E03)
          sickle-cell disorders (D57-)
          thyrotoxicosis [hyperthyroidism] (E05-)
          Whipple's disease (K90.8)

     M14.80   Arthropathies in other specified diseases classified elsewhere, unspecified site
✓6th **M14.81 Arthropathies in other specified diseases classified elsewhere, shoulder**
     M14.811   Arthropathies in other specified diseases classified elsewhere, right shoulder
     M14.812   Arthropathies in other specified diseases classified elsewhere, left shoulder
     M14.819   Arthropathies in other specified diseases classified elsewhere, unspecified shoulder

✓6th **M14.82 Arthropathies in other specified diseases classified elsewhere, elbow**
     M14.821   Arthropathies in other specified diseases classified elsewhere, right elbow
     M14.822   Arthropathies in other specified diseases classified elsewhere, left elbow
     M14.829   Arthropathies in other specified diseases classified elsewhere, unspecified elbow

✓6th **M14.83 Arthropathies in other specified diseases classified elsewhere, wrist**
     M14.831   Arthropathies in other specified diseases classified elsewhere, right wrist
     M14.832   Arthropathies in other specified diseases classified elsewhere, left wrist
     M14.839   Arthropathies in other specified diseases classified elsewhere, unspecified wrist

✓6th **M14.84 Arthropathies in other specified diseases classified elsewhere, hand**
     M14.841   Arthropathies in other specified diseases classified elsewhere, right hand
     M14.842   Arthropathies in other specified diseases classified elsewhere, left hand
     M14.849   Arthropathies in other specified diseases classified elsewhere, unspecified hand

✓6th **M14.85 Arthropathies in other specified diseases classified elsewhere, hip**
     M14.851   Arthropathies in other specified diseases classified elsewhere, right hip
     M14.852   Arthropathies in other specified diseases classified elsewhere, left hip
     M14.859   Arthropathies in other specified diseases classified elsewhere, unspecified hip

✓6th **M14.86 Arthropathies in other specified diseases classified elsewhere, knee**
     M14.861   Arthropathies in other specified diseases classified elsewhere, right knee
     M14.862   Arthropathies in other specified diseases classified elsewhere, left knee
     M14.869   Arthropathies in other specified diseases classified elsewhere, unspecified knee

---

EXCLUDES 1   Not coded here   EXCLUDES 2   Not included here   *Manifestation Code*

✓6th **M14.87** **Arthropathies in other specified diseases classified elsewhere, ankle and foot**

    M14.871 *Arthropathies in other specified diseases classified elsewhere, right ankle and foot*

    M14.872 *Arthropathies in other specified diseases classified elsewhere, left ankle and foot*

    M14.879 *Arthropathies in other specified diseases classified elsewhere, unspecified ankle and foot*

    M14.88 *Arthropathies in other specified diseases classified elsewhere, vertebrae*

    M14.89 *Arthropathies in other specified diseases classified elsewhere, multiple sites*

Osteoarthritis (M15-M19)

EXCLUDES 2   *osteoarthritis of spine (M47-)*

✓4th **M15** **Polyosteoarthritis**

   INCLUDES   arthritis of multiple sites

   EXCLUDES 1   *bilateral involvement of single joint (M16-M19)*

    M15.0 **Primary generalized (osteo)arthritis**

    M15.1 **Heberden's nodes (with arthropathy)**

       Interphalangeal distal osteoarthritis

    M15.2 **Bouchard's nodes (with arthropathy)**

       Juxtaphalangeal distal osteoarthritis

    M15.3 **Secondary multiple arthritis**

       Post-traumatic polyosteoarthritis

    M15.4 **Erosive (osteo)arthritis**

    M15.8 **Other polyosteoarthritis**

    M15.9 **Polyosteoarthritis, unspecified**

       Generalized osteoarthritis NOS

✓4th **M16** **Osteoarthritis of hip**

    M16.0 **Bilateral primary osteoarthritis of hip**

  ✓5th **M16.1** **Unilateral primary osteoarthritis of hip**

       Primary osteoarthritis of hip NOS

     M16.10 **Unilateral primary osteoarthritis, unspecified hip**

     M16.11 **Unilateral primary osteoarthritis, right hip**

     M16.12 **Unilateral primary osteoarthritis, left hip**

    M16.2 **Bilateral osteoarthritis resulting from hip dysplasia**

  ✓5th **M16.3** **Unilateral osteoarthritis resulting from hip dysplasia**

       Dysplastic osteoarthritis of hip NOS

     M16.30 **Unilateral osteoarthritis resulting from hip dysplasia, unspecified hip**

     M16.31 **Unilateral osteoarthritis resulting from hip dysplasia, right hip**

     M16.32 **Unilateral osteoarthritis resulting from hip dysplasia, left hip**

    M16.4 **Bilateral post-traumatic osteoarthritis of hip**

  ✓5th **M16.5** **Unilateral post-traumatic osteoarthritis of hip**

       Post-traumatic osteoarthritis of hip NOS

     M16.50 **Unilateral post-traumatic osteoarthritis, unspecified hip**

     M16.51 **Unilateral post-traumatic osteoarthritis, right hip**

     M16.52 **Unilateral post-traumatic osteoarthritis, left hip**

    M16.6 **Other bilateral secondary osteoarthritis of hip**

    M16.7 **Other unilateral secondary osteoarthritis of hip**

       Secondary osteoarthritis of hip NOS

    M16.9 **Osteoarthritis of hip, unspecified**

✓4th **M17** **Osteoarthritis of knee**

    M17.0 **Bilateral primary osteoarthritis of knee**

  ✓5th **M17.1** **Unilateral primary osteoarthritis of knee**

       Primary osteoarthritis of knee NOS

     M17.10 **Unilateral primary osteoarthritis, unspecified knee**

     M17.11 **Unilateral primary osteoarthritis, right knee**

     M17.12 **Unilateral primary osteoarthritis, left knee**

    M17.2 **Bilateral post-traumatic osteoarthritis of knee**

  ✓5th **M17.3** **Unilateral post-traumatic osteoarthritis of knee**

       Post-traumatic osteoarthritis of knee NOS

     M17.30 **Unilateral post-traumatic osteoarthritis, unspecified knee**

     M17.31 **Unilateral post-traumatic osteoarthritis, right knee**

     M17.32 **Unilateral post-traumatic osteoarthritis, left knee**

    M17.4 **Other bilateral secondary osteoarthritis of knee**

    M17.5 **Other unilateral secondary osteoarthritis of knee**

       Secondary osteoarthritis of knee NOS

    M17.9 **Osteoarthritis of knee, unspecified**

✓4th **M18** **Osteoarthritis of first carpometacarpal joint**

    M18.0 **Bilateral primary osteoarthritis of first carpometacarpal joints**

  ✓5th **M18.1** **Unilateral primary osteoarthritis of first carpometacarpal joint**

       Primary osteoarthritis of first carpometacarpal joint NOS

     M18.10 **Unilateral primary osteoarthritis of first carpometacarpal joint, unspecified hand**

     M18.11 **Unilateral primary osteoarthritis of first carpometacarpal joint, right hand**

     M18.12 **Unilateral primary osteoarthritis of first carpometacarpal joint, left hand**

    M18.2 **Bilateral post-traumatic osteoarthritis of first carpometacarpal joints**

  ✓5th **M18.3** **Unilateral post-traumatic osteoarthritis of first carpometacarpal joint**

       Post-traumatic osteoarthritis of first carpometacarpal joint NOS

     M18.30 **Unilateral post-traumatic osteoarthritis of first carpometacarpal joint, unspecified hand**

     M18.31 **Unilateral post-traumatic osteoarthritis of first carpometacarpal joint, right hand**

     M18.32 **Unilateral post-traumatic osteoarthritis of first carpometacarpal joint, left hand**

    M18.4 **Other bilateral secondary osteoarthritis of first carpometacarpal joints**

  ✓5th **M18.5** **Other unilateral secondary osteoarthritis of first carpometacarpal joint**

       Secondary osteoarthritis of first carpometacarpal joint NOS

     M18.50 **Other unilateral secondary osteoarthritis of first carpometacarpal joint, unspecified hand**

     M18.51 **Other unilateral secondary osteoarthritis of first carpometacarpal joint, right hand**

     M18.52 **Other unilateral secondary osteoarthritis of first carpometacarpal joint, left hand**

    M18.9 **Osteoarthritis of first carpometacarpal joint, unspecified**

✓4th **M19** **Other and unspecified osteoarthritis**

   EXCLUDES 1   *polyarthritis (M15-)*

   EXCLUDES 2   *arthrosis of spine (M47-)*

       hallux rigidus (M20.2)

       osteoarthritis of spine (M47-)

  ✓5th **M19.0** **Primary osteoarthritis of other joints**

   ✓6th **M19.01** **Primary osteoarthritis, shoulder**

      M19.011 **Primary osteoarthritis, right shoulder**

      M19.012 **Primary osteoarthritis, left shoulder**

      M19.019 **Primary osteoarthritis, unspecified shoulder**

   ✓6th **M19.02** **Primary osteoarthritis, elbow**

      M19.021 **Primary osteoarthritis, right elbow**

      M19.022 **Primary osteoarthritis, left elbow**

      M19.029 **Primary osteoarthritis, unspecified elbow**

   ✓6th **M19.03** **Primary osteoarthritis, wrist**

      M19.031 **Primary osteoarthritis, right wrist**

      M19.032 **Primary osteoarthritis, left wrist**

      M19.039 **Primary osteoarthritis, unspecified wrist**

   ✓6th **M19.04** **Primary osteoarthritis, hand**

      EXCLUDES 2   *primary osteoarthritis of first carpometacarpal joint (M18.0-, M18.1-)*

      M19.041 **Primary osteoarthritis, right hand**

      M19.042 **Primary osteoarthritis, left hand**

      M19.049 **Primary osteoarthritis, unspecified hand**

   ✓6th **M19.07** **Primary osteoarthritis ankle and foot**

      M19.071 **Primary osteoarthritis, right ankle and foot**

      M19.072 **Primary osteoarthritis, left ankle and foot**

      M19.079 **Primary osteoarthritis, unspecified ankle and foot**

☑ Appropriate additional character required   ✓x7th Requires 7th character, placeholder x must fill empty characters

Diseases of the Musculoskeletal System and Connective Tissue

M19.1–M20.62

✓5ᵗʰ **M19.1 Post-traumatic osteoarthritis of other joints**

  ✓6ᵗʰ **M19.11 Post-traumatic osteoarthritis, shoulder**

    M19.111 Post-traumatic osteoarthritis, right shoulder

    M19.112 Post-traumatic osteoarthritis, left shoulder

    M19.119 Post-traumatic osteoarthritis, unspecified shoulder

  ✓6ᵗʰ **M19.12 Post-traumatic osteoarthritis, elbow**

    M19.121 Post-traumatic osteoarthritis, right elbow

    M19.122 Post-traumatic osteoarthritis, left elbow

    M19.129 Post-traumatic osteoarthritis, unspecified elbow

  ✓6ᵗʰ **M19.13 Post-traumatic osteoarthritis, wrist**

    M19.131 Post-traumatic osteoarthritis, right wrist

    M19.132 Post-traumatic osteoarthritis, left wrist

    M19.139 Post-traumatic osteoarthritis, unspecified wrist

  ✓6ᵗʰ **M19.14 Post-traumatic osteoarthritis, hand**

    EXCLUDES 2 *post-traumatic osteoarthritis of first carpometacarpal joint (M18.2-, M18.3-)*

    M19.141 Post-traumatic osteoarthritis, right hand

    M19.142 Post-traumatic osteoarthritis, left hand

    M19.149 Post-traumatic osteoarthritis, unspecified hand

  ✓6ᵗʰ **M19.17 Post-traumatic osteoarthritis, ankle and foot**

    M19.171 Post-traumatic osteoarthritis, right ankle and foot

    M19.172 Post-traumatic osteoarthritis, left ankle and foot

    M19.179 Post-traumatic osteoarthritis, unspecified ankle and foot

✓5ᵗʰ **M19.2 Secondary osteoarthritis of other joints**

  ✓6ᵗʰ **M19.21 Secondary osteoarthritis, shoulder**

    M19.211 Secondary osteoarthritis, right shoulder

    M19.212 Secondary osteoarthritis, left shoulder

    M19.219 Secondary osteoarthritis, unspecified shoulder

  ✓6ᵗʰ **M19.22 Secondary osteoarthritis, elbow**

    M19.221 Secondary osteoarthritis, right elbow

    M19.222 Secondary osteoarthritis, left elbow

    M19.229 Secondary osteoarthritis, unspecified elbow

  ✓6ᵗʰ **M19.23 Secondary osteoarthritis, wrist**

    M19.231 Secondary osteoarthritis, right wrist

    M19.232 Secondary osteoarthritis, left wrist

    M19.239 Secondary osteoarthritis, unspecified wrist

  ✓6ᵗʰ **M19.24 Secondary osteoarthritis, hand**

    M19.241 Secondary osteoarthritis, right hand

    M19.242 Secondary osteoarthritis, left hand

    M19.249 Secondary osteoarthritis, unspecified hand

  ✓6ᵗʰ **M19.27 Secondary osteoarthritis, ankle and foot**

    M19.271 Secondary osteoarthritis, right ankle and foot

    M19.272 Secondary osteoarthritis, left ankle and foot

    M19.279 Secondary osteoarthritis, unspecified ankle and foot

✓5ᵗʰ **M19.9 Osteoarthritis, unspecified site**

  M19.90 Unspecified osteoarthritis, unspecified site
    Arthrosis NOS
    Arthritis NOS
    Osteoarthritis NOS

  M19.91 Primary osteoarthritis, unspecified site
    Primary osteoarthritis NOS

  M19.92 Post-traumatic osteoarthritis, unspecified site
    Post-traumatic osteoarthritis NOS

  M19.93 Secondary osteoarthritis, unspecified site
    Secondary osteoarthritis NOS

Other joint disorders (M20-M25)

  EXCLUDES 2 *joints of the spine (M40-M54)*

✓4ᵗʰ **M20 Acquired deformities of fingers and toes**

  EXCLUDES 1 *acquired absence of fingers and toes (Z89-)*
    congenital absence of fingers and toes (Q71.3-, Q72.3-)
    congenital deformities and malformations of fingers and toes (Q66-, Q68-Q70, Q74-)

  ✓5ᵗʰ **M20.0 Deformity of finger(s)**

    EXCLUDES 1 *clubbing of fingers (R68.3)*
     palmar fascial fibromatosis [Dupuytren] (M72.0)
     trigger finger (M65.3)

    ✓6ᵗʰ **M20.00 Unspecified deformity of finger(s)**

      M20.001 Unspecified deformity of right finger(s)

      M20.002 Unspecified deformity of left finger(s)

      M20.009 Unspecified deformity of unspecified finger(s)

    ✓6ᵗʰ **M20.01 Mallet finger**

      M20.011 Mallet finger of right finger(s)

      M20.012 Mallet finger of left finger(s)

      M20.019 Mallet finger of unspecified finger(s)

    ✓6ᵗʰ **M20.02 Boutonnière deformity**

      M20.021 Boutonnière deformity of right finger(s)

      M20.022 Boutonnière deformity of left finger(s)

      M20.029 Boutonnière deformity of unspecified finger(s)

    ✓6ᵗʰ **M20.03 Swan-neck deformity**

      M20.031 Swan-neck deformity of right finger(s)

      M20.032 Swan-neck deformity of left finger(s)

      M20.039 Swan-neck deformity of unspecified finger(s)

    ✓6ᵗʰ **M20.09 Other deformity of finger(s)**

      M20.091 Other deformity of right finger(s)

      M20.092 Other deformity of left finger(s)

      M20.099 Other deformity of finger(s), unspecified finger(s)

  ✓5ᵗʰ **M20.1 Hallux valgus (acquired)**
    Bunion

    M20.10 Hallux valgus (acquired), unspecified foot

    M20.11 Hallux valgus (acquired), right foot

    M20.12 Hallux valgus (acquired), left foot

  ✓5ᵗʰ **M20.2 Hallux rigidus**

    M20.20 Hallux rigidus, unspecified foot

    M20.21 Hallux rigidus, right foot

    M20.22 Hallux rigidus, left foot

  ✓5ᵗʰ **M20.3 Hallux varus (acquired)**

    M20.30 Hallux varus (acquired), unspecified foot

    M20.31 Hallux varus (acquired), right foot

    M20.32 Hallux varus (acquired), left foot

  ✓5ᵗʰ **M20.4 Other hammer toe(s) (acquired)**

    M20.40 Other hammer toe(s) (acquired), unspecified foot

    M20.41 Other hammer toe(s) (acquired), right foot

    M20.42 Other hammer toe(s) (acquired), left foot

  ✓5ᵗʰ **M20.5 Other deformities of toe(s) (acquired)**

    ✓6ᵗʰ **M20.5x Other deformities of toe(s) (acquired)**

      M20.5x1 Other deformities of toe(s) (acquired), right foot

      M20.5x2 Other deformities of toe(s) (acquired), left foot

      M20.5x9 Other deformities of toe(s) (acquired), unspecified foot

  ✓5ᵗʰ **M20.6 Acquired deformities of toe(s), unspecified**

    M20.60 Acquired deformities of toe(s), unspecified, unspecified foot

    M20.61 Acquired deformities of toe(s), unspecified, right foot

    M20.62 Acquired deformities of toe(s), unspecified, left foot

---

EXCLUDES 1 Not coded here   EXCLUDES 2 Not included here   *Manifestation Code*

☑4ᵗʰ **M21 Other acquired deformities of limbs**

EXCLUDES 1 *acquired absence of limb (Z89-)*
congenital absence of limbs (Q71-Q73)
congenital deformities and malformations of limbs (Q65-Q66, Q68-Q74)

EXCLUDES 2 *acquired deformities of fingers or toes (M20-)*
coxa plana (M91.2)

☑5ᵗʰ **M21.0 Valgus deformity, not elsewhere classified**

EXCLUDES 1 *metatarsus valgus (Q66.6)*
talipes calcaneovalgus (Q66.4)

M21.00 Valgus deformity, not elsewhere classified, unspecified site

☑6ᵗʰ **M21.02 Valgus deformity, not elsewhere classified, elbow**
Cubitus valgus

M21.021 Valgus deformity, not elsewhere classified, right elbow

M21.022 Valgus deformity, not elsewhere classified, left elbow

M21.029 Valgus deformity, not elsewhere classified, unspecified elbow

☑6ᵗʰ **M21.06 Valgus deformity, not elsewhere classified, knee**
Genu valgum
Knock knee

M21.061 Valgus deformity, not elsewhere classified, right knee

M21.062 Valgus deformity, not elsewhere classified, left knee

M21.069 Valgus deformity, not elsewhere classified, unspecified knee

☑6ᵗʰ **M21.07 Valgus deformity, not elsewhere classified, ankle**

M21.071 Valgus deformity, not elsewhere classified, right ankle

M21.072 Valgus deformity, not elsewhere classified, left ankle

M21.079 Valgus deformity, not elsewhere classified, unspecified ankle

☑5ᵗʰ **M21.1 Varus deformity, not elsewhere classified**

EXCLUDES 1 *metatarsus varus (Q66.2)*
tibia vara (M92.5)

M21.10 Varus deformity, not elsewhere classified, unspecified site

☑6ᵗʰ **M21.12 Varus deformity, not elsewhere classified, elbow**
Cubitus varus, elbow

M21.121 Varus deformity, not elsewhere classified, right elbow

M21.122 Varus deformity, not elsewhere classified, left elbow

M21.129 Varus deformity, not elsewhere classified, unspecified elbow

☑6ᵗʰ **M21.16 Varus deformity, not elsewhere classified, knee**
Bow leg
Genu varum

M21.161 Varus deformity, not elsewhere classified, right knee

M21.162 Varus deformity, not elsewhere classified, left knee

M21.169 Varus deformity, not elsewhere classified, unspecified knee

☑6ᵗʰ **M21.17 Varus deformity, not elsewhere classified, ankle**

M21.171 Varus deformity, not elsewhere classified, right ankle

M21.172 Varus deformity, not elsewhere classified, left ankle

M21.179 Varus deformity, not elsewhere classified, unspecified ankle

☑5ᵗʰ **M21.2 Flexion deformity**

M21.20 Flexion deformity, unspecified site

☑6ᵗʰ **M21.21 Flexion deformity, shoulder**

M21.211 Flexion deformity, right shoulder

M21.212 Flexion deformity, left shoulder

M21.219 Flexion deformity, unspecified shoulder

☑6ᵗʰ **M21.22 Flexion deformity, elbow**

M21.221 Flexion deformity, right elbow

M21.222 Flexion deformity, left elbow

M21.229 Flexion deformity, unspecified elbow

☑6ᵗʰ **M21.23 Flexion deformity, wrist**

M21.231 Flexion deformity, right wrist

M21.232 Flexion deformity, left wrist

M21.239 Flexion deformity, unspecified wrist

☑6ᵗʰ **M21.24 Flexion deformity, finger joints**

M21.241 Flexion deformity, right finger joints

M21.242 Flexion deformity, left finger joints

M21.249 Flexion deformity, unspecified finger joints

☑6ᵗʰ **M21.25 Flexion deformity, hip**

M21.251 Flexion deformity, right hip

M21.252 Flexion deformity, left hip

M21.259 Flexion deformity, unspecified hip

☑6ᵗʰ **M21.26 Flexion deformity, knee**

M21.261 Flexion deformity, right knee

M21.262 Flexion deformity, left knee

M21.269 Flexion deformity, unspecified knee

☑6ᵗʰ **M21.27 Flexion deformity, ankle and toes**

M21.271 Flexion deformity, right ankle and toes

M21.272 Flexion deformity, left ankle and toes

M21.279 Flexion deformity, unspecified ankle and toes

☑5ᵗʰ **M21.3 Wrist or foot drop (acquired)**

☑6ᵗʰ **M21.33 Wrist drop (acquired)**

M21.331 Wrist drop, right wrist

M21.332 Wrist drop, left wrist

M21.339 Wrist drop, unspecified wrist

☑6ᵗʰ **M21.37 Foot drop (acquired)**

M21.371 Foot drop, right foot

M21.372 Foot drop, left foot

M21.379 Foot drop, unspecified foot

☑5ᵗʰ **M21.4 Flat foot [pes planus] (acquired)**

EXCLUDES 1 *congenital pes planus (Q66.5)*

M21.40 Flat foot [pes planus] (acquired), unspecified foot

M21.41 Flat foot [pes planus] (acquired), right foot

M21.42 Flat foot [pes planus] (acquired), left foot

☑5ᵗʰ **M21.5 Acquired clawhand, clubhand, clawfoot and clubfoot**

EXCLUDES 1 *clubfoot, not specified as acquired (Q66.8)*

☑6ᵗʰ **M21.51 Acquired clawhand**

M21.511 Acquired clawhand, right hand

M21.512 Acquired clawhand, left hand

M21.519 Acquired clawhand, unspecified hand

☑6ᵗʰ **M21.52 Acquired clubhand**

M21.521 Acquired clubhand, right hand

M21.522 Acquired clubhand, left hand

M21.529 Acquired clubhand, unspecified hand

☑6ᵗʰ **M21.53 Acquired clawfoot**

M21.531 Acquired clawfoot, right foot

M21.532 Acquired clawfoot, left foot

M21.539 Acquired clawfoot, unspecified foot

☑6ᵗʰ **M21.54 Acquired clubfoot**

M21.541 Acquired clubfoot, right foot

M21.542 Acquired clubfoot, left foot

M21.549 Acquired clubfoot, unspecified foot

☑5ᵗʰ **M21.6 Other acquired deformities of foot**

EXCLUDES 2 *deformities of toe (acquired) (M20.1-M20.6)*

☑6ᵗʰ **M21.6x Other acquired deformities of foot**

M21.6x1 Other acquired deformities of right foot

M21.6x2 Other acquired deformities of left foot

M21.6x9 Other acquired deformities of unspecified foot

☑5ᵗʰ **M21.7 Unequal limb length (acquired)**

NOTE The site used should correspond to the shorter limb

M21.70 Unequal limb length (acquired), unspecified site

☑6ᵗʰ **M21.72 Unequal limb length (acquired), humerus**

M21.721 Unequal limb length (acquired), right humerus

M21.722 Unequal limb length (acquired), left humerus

M21.729 Unequal limb length (acquired), unspecified humerus

☑6ᵗʰ **M21.73 Unequal limb length (acquired), ulna and radius**

M21.731 Unequal limb length (acquired), right ulna

M21.732 Unequal limb length (acquired), left ulna

☑ Appropriate additional character required   ☑x7ᵗʰ Requires 7th character, placeholder x must fill empty characters

M21.733   Unequal limb length (acquired), right radius

M21.734   Unequal limb length (acquired), left radius

M21.739   Unequal limb length (acquired), unspecified ulna and radius

✓6th   M21.75   Unequal limb length (acquired), femur

M21.751   Unequal limb length (acquired), right femur

M21.752   Unequal limb length (acquired), left femur

M21.759   Unequal limb length (acquired), unspecified femur

✓6th   M21.76   Unequal limb length (acquired), tibia and fibula

M21.761   Unequal limb length (acquired), right tibia

M21.762   Unequal limb length (acquired), left tibia

M21.763   Unequal limb length (acquired), right fibula

M21.764   Unequal limb length (acquired), left fibula

M21.769   Unequal limb length (acquired), unspecified tibia and fibula

✓5th   M21.8   Other specified acquired deformities of limbs

     EXCLUDES 2   coxa plana (M91.2)

M21.80   Other specified acquired deformities of unspecified limb

✓6th   M21.82   Other specified acquired deformities of upper arm

M21.821   Other specified acquired deformities of right upper arm

M21.822   Other specified acquired deformities of left upper arm

M21.829   Other specified acquired deformities of unspecified upper arm

✓6th   M21.83   Other specified acquired deformities of forearm

M21.831   Other specified acquired deformities of right forearm

M21.832   Other specified acquired deformities of left forearm

M21.839   Other specified acquired deformities of unspecified forearm

✓6th   M21.85   Other specified acquired deformities of thigh

M21.851   Other specified acquired deformities of right thigh

M21.852   Other specified acquired deformities of left thigh

M21.859   Other specified acquired deformities of unspecified thigh

✓6th   M21.86   Other specified acquired deformities of lower leg

M21.861   Other specified acquired deformities of right lower leg

M21.862   Other specified acquired deformities of left lower leg

M21.869   Other specified acquired deformities of unspecified lower leg

✓5th   M21.9   Unspecified acquired deformity of limb and hand

M21.90   Unspecified acquired deformity of unspecified limb

✓6th   M21.92   Unspecified acquired deformity of upper arm

M21.921   Unspecified acquired deformity of right upper arm

M21.922   Unspecified acquired deformity of left upper arm

M21.929   Unspecified acquired deformity of unspecified upper arm

✓6th   M21.93   Unspecified acquired deformity of forearm

M21.931   Unspecified acquired deformity of right forearm

M21.932   Unspecified acquired deformity of left forearm

M21.939   Unspecified acquired deformity of unspecified forearm

✓6th   M21.94   Unspecified acquired deformity of hand

M21.941   Unspecified acquired deformity of hand, right hand

M21.942   Unspecified acquired deformity of hand, left hand

M21.949   Unspecified acquired deformity of hand, unspecified hand

✓6th   M21.95   Unspecified acquired deformity of thigh

M21.951   Unspecified acquired deformity of right thigh

M21.952   Unspecified acquired deformity of left thigh

M21.959   Unspecified acquired deformity of unspecified thigh

✓6th   M21.96   Unspecified acquired deformity of lower leg

M21.961   Unspecified acquired deformity of right lower leg

M21.962   Unspecified acquired deformity of left lower leg

M21.969   Unspecified acquired deformity of unspecified lower leg

✓4th   M22   Disorder of patella

     EXCLUDES 1   traumatic dislocation of patella (S83.0-)

✓5th   M22.0   Recurrent dislocation of patella

M22.00   Recurrent dislocation of patella, unspecified knee

M22.01   Recurrent dislocation of patella, right knee

M22.02   Recurrent dislocation of patella, left knee

✓5th   M22.1   Recurrent subluxation of patella

     Incomplete dislocation of patella

M22.10   Recurrent subluxation of patella, unspecified knee

M22.11   Recurrent subluxation of patella, right knee

M22.12   Recurrent subluxation of patella, left knee

✓5th   M22.2   Patellofemoral disorders

✓6th   M22.2x   Patellofemoral disorders

M22.2x1   Patellofemoral disorders, right knee

M22.2x2   Patellofemoral disorders, left knee

M22.2x9   Patellofemoral disorders, unspecified knee

✓5th   M22.3   Other derangements of patella

✓6th   M22.3x   Other derangements of patella

M22.3x1   Other derangements of patella, right knee

M22.3x2   Other derangements of patella, left knee

M22.3x9   Other derangements of patella, unspecified knee

✓5th   M22.4   Chondromalacia patellae

M22.40   Chondromalacia patellae, unspecified knee

M22.41   Chondromalacia patellae, right knee

M22.42   Chondromalacia patellae, left knee

✓5th   M22.8   Other disorders of patella

✓6th   M22.8x   Other disorders of patella

M22.8x1   Other disorders of patella, right knee

M22.8x2   Other disorders of patella, left knee

M22.8x9   Other disorders of patella, unspecified knee

✓5th   M22.9   Unspecified disorder of patella

M22.90   Unspecified disorder of patella, unspecified knee

M22.91   Unspecified disorder of patella, right knee

M22.92   Unspecified disorder of patella, left knee

✓4th   M23   Internal derangement of knee

     EXCLUDES 1   ankylosis (M24.66)

          current injury—see injury of knee and lower leg (S80-S89)

          deformity of knee (M21-)

          osteochondritis dissecans (M93.2)

          recurrent dislocation or subluxation of joints (M24.4)

          recurrent dislocation or subluxation of patella (M22.0-M22.1)

✓5th   M23.0   Cystic meniscus

✓6th   M23.00   Cystic meniscus, unspecified meniscus

     Cystic meniscus, unspecified lateral meniscus

     Cystic meniscus, unspecified medial meniscus

M23.000   Cystic meniscus, unspecified lateral meniscus, right knee

M23.001   Cystic meniscus, unspecified lateral meniscus, left knee

M23.002   Cystic meniscus, unspecified lateral meniscus, unspecified knee

M23.003   Cystic meniscus, unspecified medial meniscus, right knee

M23.004   Cystic meniscus, unspecified medial meniscus, left knee

---

EXCLUDES 1   Not coded here   EXCLUDES 2   Not included here   *Manifestation Code*

M23.005   Cystic meniscus, unspecified medial meniscus, unspecified knee

M23.006   Cystic meniscus, unspecified meniscus, right knee

M23.007   Cystic meniscus, unspecified meniscus, left knee

M23.009   Cystic meniscus, unspecified meniscus, unspecified knee

√6th   **M23.01**   **Cystic meniscus, anterior horn of medial meniscus**

M23.011   Cystic meniscus, anterior horn of medial meniscus, right knee

M23.012   Cystic meniscus, anterior horn of medial meniscus, left knee

M23.019   Cystic meniscus, anterior horn of medial meniscus, unspecified knee

√6th   **M23.02**   **Cystic meniscus, posterior horn of medial meniscus**

M23.021   Cystic meniscus, posterior horn of medial meniscus, right knee

M23.022   Cystic meniscus, posterior horn of medial meniscus, left knee

M23.029   Cystic meniscus, posterior horn of medial meniscus, unspecified knee

√6th   **M23.03**   **Cystic meniscus, other medial meniscus**

M23.031   Cystic meniscus, other medial meniscus, right knee

M23.032   Cystic meniscus, other medial meniscus, left knee

M23.039   Cystic meniscus, other medial meniscus, unspecified knee

√6th   **M23.04**   **Cystic meniscus, anterior horn of lateral meniscus**

M23.041   Cystic meniscus, anterior horn of lateral meniscus, right knee

M23.042   Cystic meniscus, anterior horn of lateral meniscus, left knee

M23.049   Cystic meniscus, anterior horn of lateral meniscus, unspecified knee

√6th   **M23.05**   **Cystic meniscus, posterior horn of lateral meniscus**

M23.051   Cystic meniscus, posterior horn of lateral meniscus, right knee

M23.052   Cystic meniscus, posterior horn of lateral meniscus, left knee

M23.059   Cystic meniscus, posterior horn of lateral meniscus, unspecified knee

√6th   **M23.06**   **Cystic meniscus, other lateral meniscus**

M23.061   **Cystic meniscus, other lateral meniscus, right knee**

M23.062   Cystic meniscus, other lateral meniscus, left knee

M23.069   Cystic meniscus, other lateral meniscus, unspecified knee

√5th   **M23.2**   **Derangement of meniscus due to old tear or injury**
Old bucket-handle tear

√6th   **M23.20**   **Derangement of unspecified meniscus due to old tear or injury**
Derangement of unspecified lateral meniscus due to old tear or injury
Derangement of unspecified medial meniscus due to old tear or injury

M23.200   Derangement of unspecified lateral meniscus due to old tear or injury, right knee

M23.201   Derangement of unspecified lateral meniscus due to old tear or injury, left knee

M23.202   Derangement of unspecified lateral meniscus due to old tear or injury, unspecified knee

M23.203   Derangement of unspecified medial meniscus due to old tear or injury, right knee

M23.204   Derangement of unspecified medial meniscus due to old tear or injury, left knee

M23.205   Derangement of unspecified medial meniscus due to old tear or injury, unspecified knee

M23.206   Derangement of unspecified meniscus due to old tear or injury, right knee

M23.207   Derangement of unspecified meniscus due to old tear or injury, left knee

M23.209   Derangement of unspecified meniscus due to old tear or injury, unspecified knee

√6th   **M23.21**   **Derangement of anterior horn of medial meniscus due to old tear or injury**

M23.211   Derangement of anterior horn of medial meniscus due to old tear or injury, right knee

M23.212   Derangement of anterior horn of medial meniscus due to old tear or injury, left knee

M23.219   Derangement of anterior horn of medial meniscus due to old tear or injury, unspecified knee

√6th   **M23.22**   **Derangement of posterior horn of medial meniscus due to old tear or injury**

M23.221   Derangement of posterior horn of medial meniscus due to old tear or injury, right knee

M23.222   Derangement of posterior horn of medial meniscus due to old tear or injury, left knee

M23.229   Derangement of posterior horn of medial meniscus due to old tear or injury, unspecified knee

√6th   **M23.23**   **Derangement of other medial meniscus due to old tear or injury**

M23.231   Derangement of other medial meniscus due to old tear or injury, right knee

M23.232   Derangement of other medial meniscus due to old tear or injury, left knee

M23.239   Derangement of other medial meniscus due to old tear or injury, unspecified knee

√6th   **M23.24**   **Derangement of anterior horn of lateral meniscus due to old tear or injury**

M23.241   Derangement of anterior horn of lateral meniscus due to old tear or injury, right knee

M23.242   Derangement of anterior horn of lateral meniscus due to old tear or injury, left knee

M23.249   Derangement of anterior horn of lateral meniscus due to old tear or injury, unspecified knee

√6th   **M23.25**   **Derangement of posterior horn of lateral meniscus due to old tear or injury**

M23.251   Derangement of posterior horn of lateral meniscus due to old tear or injury, right knee

M23.252   Derangement of posterior horn of lateral meniscus due to old tear or injury, left knee

M23.259   Derangement of posterior horn of lateral meniscus due to old tear or injury, unspecified knee

√6th   **M23.26**   **Derangement of other lateral meniscus due to old tear or injury**

M23.261   Derangement of other lateral meniscus due to old tear or injury, right knee

M23.262   Derangement of other lateral meniscus due to old tear or injury, left knee

M23.269   Derangement of other lateral meniscus due to old tear or injury, unspecified knee

---

✓ Appropriate additional character required   √x7th Requires 7th character, placeholder x must fill empty characters

☑5ᵗʰ **M23.3 Other meniscus derangements**
Degenerate meniscus
Detached meniscus
Retained meniscus

☑6ᵗʰ **M23.30 Other meniscus derangements, unspecified meniscus**
Other meniscus derangements, unspecified lateral meniscus
Other meniscus derangements, unspecified medial meniscus

M23.300 Other meniscus derangements, unspecified lateral meniscus, right knee

M23.301 Other meniscus derangements, unspecified lateral meniscus, left knee

M23.302 Other meniscus derangements, unspecified lateral meniscus, unspecified knee

M23.303 Other meniscus derangements, unspecified medial meniscus, right knee

M23.304 Other meniscus derangements, unspecified medial meniscus, left knee

M23.305 Other meniscus derangements, unspecified medial meniscus, unspecified knee

M23.306 Other meniscus derangements, unspecified meniscus, right knee

M23.307 Other meniscus derangements, unspecified meniscus, left knee

M23.309 Other meniscus derangements, unspecified meniscus, unspecified knee

☑6ᵗʰ **M23.31 Other meniscus derangements, anterior horn of medial meniscus**

M23.311 Other meniscus derangements, anterior horn of medial meniscus, right knee

M23.312 Other meniscus derangements, anterior horn of medial meniscus, left knee

M23.319 Other meniscus derangements, anterior horn of medial meniscus, unspecified knee

☑6ᵗʰ **M23.32 Other meniscus derangements, posterior horn of medial meniscus**

M23.321 Other meniscus derangements, posterior horn of medial meniscus, right knee

M23.322 Other meniscus derangements, posterior horn of medial meniscus, left knee

M23.329 Other meniscus derangements, posterior horn of medial meniscus, unspecified knee

☑6ᵗʰ **M23.33 Other meniscus derangements, other medial meniscus**

M23.331 Other meniscus derangements, other medial meniscus, right knee

M23.332 Other meniscus derangements, other medial meniscus, left knee

M23.339 Other meniscus derangements, other medial meniscus, unspecified knee

☑6ᵗʰ **M23.34 Other meniscus derangements, anterior horn of lateral meniscus**

M23.341 Other meniscus derangements, anterior horn of lateral meniscus, right knee

M23.342 Other meniscus derangements, anterior horn of lateral meniscus, left knee

M23.349 Other meniscus derangements, anterior horn of lateral meniscus, unspecified knee

☑6ᵗʰ **M23.35 Other meniscus derangements, posterior horn of lateral meniscus**

M23.351 Other meniscus derangements, posterior horn of lateral meniscus, right knee

M23.352 Other meniscus derangements, posterior horn of lateral meniscus, left knee

M23.359 Other meniscus derangements, posterior horn of lateral meniscus, unspecified knee

☑6ᵗʰ **M23.36 Other meniscus derangements, other lateral meniscus**

M23.361 Other meniscus derangements, other lateral meniscus, right knee

M23.362 Other meniscus derangements, other lateral meniscus, left knee

M23.369 Other meniscus derangements, other lateral meniscus, unspecified knee

☑5ᵗʰ **M23.4 Loose body in knee**

M23.40 Loose body in knee, unspecified knee

M23.41 Loose body in knee, right knee

M23.42 Loose body in knee, left knee

☑5ᵗʰ **M23.5 Chronic instability of knee**

M23.50 Chronic instability of knee, unspecified knee

M23.51 Chronic instability of knee, right knee

M23.52 Chronic instability of knee, left knee

☑5ᵗʰ **M23.6 Other spontaneous disruption of ligament(s) of knee**

☑6ᵗʰ **M23.60 Other spontaneous disruption of unspecified ligament of knee**

M23.601 Other spontaneous disruption of unspecified ligament of right knee

M23.602 Other spontaneous disruption of unspecified ligament of left knee

M23.609 Other spontaneous disruption of unspecified ligament of unspecified knee

☑6ᵗʰ **M23.61 Other spontaneous disruption of anterior cruciate ligament of knee**

M23.611 Other spontaneous disruption of anterior cruciate ligament of right knee

M23.612 Other spontaneous disruption of anterior cruciate ligament of left knee

M23.619 Other spontaneous disruption of anterior cruciate ligament of unspecified knee

☑6ᵗʰ **M23.62 Other spontaneous disruption of posterior cruciate ligament of knee**

M23.621 Other spontaneous disruption of posterior cruciate ligament of right knee

M23.622 Other spontaneous disruption of posterior cruciate ligament of left knee

M23.629 Other spontaneous disruption of posterior cruciate ligament of unspecified knee

☑6ᵗʰ **M23.63 Other spontaneous disruption of medial collateral ligament of knee**

M23.631 Other spontaneous disruption of medial collateral ligament of right knee

M23.632 Other spontaneous disruption of medial collateral ligament of left knee

M23.639 Other spontaneous disruption of medial collateral ligament of unspecified knee

☑6ᵗʰ **M23.64 Other spontaneous disruption of lateral collateral ligament of knee**

M23.641 Other spontaneous disruption of lateral collateral ligament of right knee

M23.642 Other spontaneous disruption of lateral collateral ligament of left knee

M23.649 Other spontaneous disruption of lateral collateral ligament of unspecified knee

☑6ᵗʰ **M23.67 Other spontaneous disruption of capsular ligament of knee**

M23.671 Other spontaneous disruption of capsular ligament of right knee

M23.672 Other spontaneous disruption of capsular ligament of left knee

M23.679 Other spontaneous disruption of capsular ligament of unspecified knee

☑5ᵗʰ **M23.8 Other internal derangements of knee**
Laxity of ligament of knee
Snapping knee

☑6ᵗʰ **M23.8x Other internal derangements of knee**

M23.8x1 Other internal derangements of right knee

M23.8x2 Other internal derangements of left knee

M23.8x9 Other internal derangements of unspecified knee

EXCLUDES 1 Not coded here   **EXCLUDES 2** Not included here   *Manifestation Code*

✓5ᵗʰ **M23.9 Unspecified internal derangement of knee**
    M23.90 Unspecified internal derangement of unspecified knee
    M23.91 Unspecified internal derangement of right knee
    M23.92 Unspecified internal derangement of left knee

✓4ᵗʰ **M24 Other specific joint derangements**
    EXCLUDES 1 *current injury—see injury of joint by body region*
    EXCLUDES 2 *ganglion (M67.4)*
    snapping knee (M23.8-)
    temporomandibular joint disorders (M26.6-)

✓5ᵗʰ **M24.0 Loose body in joint**
    EXCLUDES 2 *loose body in knee (M23.4)*
    M24.00 Loose body in unspecified joint
    ✓6ᵗʰ **M24.01 Loose body in shoulder**
        M24.011 Loose body in right shoulder
        M24.012 Loose body in left shoulder
        M24.019 Loose body in unspecified shoulder
    ✓6ᵗʰ **M24.02 Loose body in elbow**
        M24.021 Loose body in right elbow
        M24.022 Loose body in left elbow
        M24.029 Loose body in unspecified elbow
    ✓6ᵗʰ **M24.03 Loose body in wrist**
        M24.031 Loose body in right wrist
        M24.032 Loose body in left wrist
        M24.039 Loose body in unspecified wrist
    ✓6ᵗʰ **M24.04 Loose body in finger joints**
        M24.041 Loose body in right finger joint(s)
        M24.042 Loose body in left finger joint(s)
        M24.049 Loose body in unspecified finger joint(s)
    ✓6ᵗʰ **M24.05 Loose body in hip**
        M24.051 Loose body in right hip
        M24.052 Loose body in left hip
        M24.059 Loose body in unspecified hip
    ✓6ᵗʰ **M24.07 Loose body in ankle and toe joints**
        M24.071 Loose body in right ankle
        M24.072 Loose body in left ankle
        M24.073 Loose body in unspecified ankle
        M24.074 Loose body in right toe joint(s)
        M24.075 Loose body in left toe joint(s)
        M24.076 Loose body in unspecified toe joints
    M24.08 Loose body, other site

✓5ᵗʰ **M24.1 Other articular cartilage disorders**
    EXCLUDES 2 *chondrocalcinosis (M11.1, M11.2-)*
    internal derangement of knee (M23-)
    metastatic calcification (E83.5)
    ochronosis (E70.2)
    M24.10 Other articular cartilage disorders, unspecified site
    ✓6ᵗʰ **M24.11 Other articular cartilage disorders, shoulder**
        M24.111 Other articular cartilage disorders, right shoulder
        M24.112 Other articular cartilage disorders, left shoulder
        M24.119 Other articular cartilage disorders, unspecified shoulder
    ✓6ᵗʰ **M24.12 Other articular cartilage disorders, elbow**
        M24.121 Other articular cartilage disorders, right elbow
        M24.122 Other articular cartilage disorders, left elbow
        M24.129 Other articular cartilage disorders, unspecified elbow
    ✓6ᵗʰ **M24.13 Other articular cartilage disorders, wrist**
        M24.131 Other articular cartilage disorders, right wrist
        M24.132 Other articular cartilage disorders, left wrist
        M24.139 Other articular cartilage disorders, unspecified wrist
    ✓6ᵗʰ **M24.14 Other articular cartilage disorders, hand**
        M24.141 Other articular cartilage disorders, right hand
        M24.142 Other articular cartilage disorders, left hand
        M24.149 Other articular cartilage disorders, unspecified hand

✓6ᵗʰ **M24.15 Other articular cartilage disorders, hip**
    M24.151 Other articular cartilage disorders, right hip
    M24.152 Other articular cartilage disorders, left hip
    M24.159 Other articular cartilage disorders, unspecified hip
✓6ᵗʰ **M24.17 Other articular cartilage disorders, ankle and foot**
    M24.171 Other articular cartilage disorders, right ankle
    M24.172 Other articular cartilage disorders, left ankle
    M24.173 Other articular cartilage disorders, unspecified ankle
    M24.174 Other articular cartilage disorders, right foot
    M24.175 Other articular cartilage disorders, left foot
    M24.176 Other articular cartilage disorders, unspecified foot

✓5ᵗʰ **M24.2 Disorder of ligament**
    Instability secondary to old ligament injury
    Ligamentous laxity NOS
    EXCLUDES 1 *familial ligamentous laxity (M35.7)*
    EXCLUDES 2 *internal derangement of knee (M23.5-M23.89)*
    M24.20 Disorder of ligament, unspecified site
    ✓6ᵗʰ **M24.21 Disorder of ligament, shoulder**
        M24.211 Disorder of ligament, right shoulder
        M24.212 Disorder of ligament, left shoulder
        M24.219 Disorder of ligament, unspecified shoulder
    ✓6ᵗʰ **M24.22 Disorder of ligament, elbow**
        M24.221 Disorder of ligament, right elbow
        M24.222 Disorder of ligament, left elbow
        M24.229 Disorder of ligament, unspecified elbow
    ✓6ᵗʰ **M24.23 Disorder of ligament, wrist**
        M24.231 Disorder of ligament, right wrist
        M24.232 Disorder of ligament, left wrist
        M24.239 Disorder of ligament, unspecified wrist
    ✓6ᵗʰ **M24.24 Disorder of ligament, hand**
        M24.241 Disorder of ligament, right hand
        M24.242 Disorder of ligament, left hand
        M24.249 Disorder of ligament, unspecified hand
    ✓6ᵗʰ **M24.25 Disorder of ligament, hip**
        M24.251 Disorder of ligament, right hip
        M24.252 Disorder of ligament, left hip
        M24.259 Disorder of ligament, unspecified hip
    ✓6ᵗʰ **M24.27 Disorder of ligament, ankle and foot**
        M24.271 Disorder of ligament, right ankle
        M24.272 Disorder of ligament, left ankle
        M24.273 Disorder of ligament, unspecified ankle
        M24.274 Disorder of ligament, right foot
        M24.275 Disorder of ligament, left foot
        M24.276 Disorder of ligament, unspecified foot
    M24.28 Disorder of ligament, vertebrae

✓5ᵗʰ **M24.3 Pathological dislocation of joint, not elsewhere classified**
    EXCLUDES 1 *congenital dislocation or displacement of joint—see congenital malformations and deformations of the musculoskeletal system (Q65-Q79)*
    current injury—see injury of joints and ligaments by body region
    recurrent dislocation of joint (M24.4-)
    M24.30 Pathological dislocation of unspecified joint, not elsewhere classified
    ✓6ᵗʰ **M24.31 Pathological dislocation of shoulder, not elsewhere classified**
        M24.311 Pathological dislocation of right shoulder, not elsewhere classified
        M24.312 Pathological dislocation of left shoulder, not elsewhere classified
        M24.319 Pathological dislocation of unspecified shoulder, not elsewhere classified
    ✓6ᵗʰ **M24.32 Pathological dislocation of elbow, not elsewhere classified**
        M24.321 Pathological dislocation of right elbow, not elsewhere classified

M24.322   Pathological dislocation of left elbow, not elsewhere classified

M24.329   Pathological dislocation of unspecified elbow, not elsewhere classified

√6ᵗʰ   **M24.33**   Pathological dislocation of wrist, not elsewhere classified

M24.331   Pathological dislocation of right wrist, not elsewhere classified

M24.332   Pathological dislocation of left wrist, not elsewhere classified

M24.339   Pathological dislocation of unspecified wrist, not elsewhere classified

√6ᵗʰ   **M24.34**   Pathological dislocation of hand, not elsewhere classified

M24.341   Pathological dislocation of right hand, not elsewhere classified

M24.342   Pathological dislocation of left hand, not elsewhere classified

M24.349   Pathological dislocation of unspecified hand, not elsewhere classified

√6ᵗʰ   **M24.35**   Pathological dislocation of hip, not elsewhere classified

M24.351   Pathological dislocation of right hip, not elsewhere classified

M24.352   Pathological dislocation of left hip, not elsewhere classified

M24.359   Pathological dislocation of unspecified hip, not elsewhere classified

√6ᵗʰ   **M24.36**   Pathological dislocation of knee, not elsewhere classified

M24.361   Pathological dislocation of right knee, not elsewhere classified

M24.362   Pathological dislocation of left knee, not elsewhere classified

M24.369   Pathological dislocation of unspecified knee, not elsewhere classified

√6ᵗʰ   **M24.37**   Pathological dislocation of ankle and foot, not elsewhere classified

M24.371   Pathological dislocation of right ankle, not elsewhere classified

M24.372   Pathological dislocation of left ankle, not elsewhere classified

M24.373   Pathological dislocation of unspecified ankle, not elsewhere classified

M24.374   Pathological dislocation of right foot, not elsewhere classified

M24.375   Pathological dislocation of left foot, not elsewhere classified

M24.376   Pathological dislocation of unspecified foot, not elsewhere classified

√5ᵗʰ   **M24.4**   **Recurrent dislocation of joint**
Recurrent subluxation of joint

EXCLUDES 2   recurrent dislocation of patella (M22.0-M22.1)
recurrent vertebral dislocation (M43.3-, M43.4, M43.5-)

M24.40   Recurrent dislocation, unspecified joint

√6ᵗʰ   **M24.41**   Recurrent dislocation, shoulder

M24.411   Recurrent dislocation, right shoulder

M24.412   Recurrent dislocation, left shoulder

M24.419   Recurrent dislocation, unspecified shoulder

√6ᵗʰ   **M24.42**   Recurrent dislocation, elbow

M24.421   Recurrent dislocation, right elbow

M24.422   Recurrent dislocation, left elbow

M24.429   Recurrent dislocation, unspecified elbow

√6ᵗʰ   **M24.43**   Recurrent dislocation, wrist

M24.431   Recurrent dislocation, right wrist

M24.432   Recurrent dislocation, left wrist

M24.439   Recurrent dislocation, unspecified wrist

√6ᵗʰ   **M24.44**   Recurrent dislocation, hand and finger(s)

M24.441   Recurrent dislocation, right hand

M24.442   Recurrent dislocation, left hand

M24.443   Recurrent dislocation, unspecified hand

M24.444   Recurrent dislocation, right finger

M24.445   Recurrent dislocation, left finger

M24.446   Recurrent dislocation, unspecified finger

√6ᵗʰ   **M24.45**   Recurrent dislocation, hip

M24.451   Recurrent dislocation, right hip

M24.452   Recurrent dislocation, left hip

M24.459   Recurrent dislocation, unspecified hip

√6ᵗʰ   **M24.46**   Recurrent dislocation, knee

M24.461   Recurrent dislocation, right knee

M24.462   Recurrent dislocation, left knee

M24.469   Recurrent dislocation, unspecified knee

√6ᵗʰ   **M24.47**   Recurrent dislocation, ankle, foot and toes

M24.471   Recurrent dislocation, right ankle

M24.472   Recurrent dislocation, left ankle

M24.473   Recurrent dislocation, unspecified ankle

M24.474   Recurrent dislocation, right foot

M24.475   Recurrent dislocation, left foot

M24.476   Recurrent dislocation, unspecified foot

M24.477   Recurrent dislocation, right toe(s)

M24.478   Recurrent dislocation, left toe(s)

M24.479   Recurrent dislocation, unspecified toe(s)

√5ᵗʰ   **M24.5**   **Contracture of joint**

EXCLUDES 1   contracture of muscle without contracture of joint (M62.4-)
contracture of tendon (sheath) without contracture of joint (M62.4-)
Dupuytren's contracture (M72.0)

EXCLUDES 2   acquired deformities of limbs (M20-M21)

M24.50   Contracture, unspecified joint

√6ᵗʰ   **M24.51**   Contracture, shoulder

M24.511   Contracture, right shoulder

M24.512   Contracture, left shoulder

M24.519   Contracture, unspecified shoulder

√6ᵗʰ   **M24.52**   Contracture, elbow

M24.521   Contracture, right elbow

M24.522   Contracture, left elbow

M24.529   Contracture, unspecified elbow

√6ᵗʰ   **M24.53**   Contracture, wrist

M24.531   Contracture, right wrist

M24.532   Contracture, left wrist

M24.539   Contracture, unspecified wrist

√6ᵗʰ   **M24.54**   Contracture, hand

M24.541   Contracture, right hand

M24.542   Contracture, left hand

M24.549   Contracture, unspecified hand

√6ᵗʰ   **M24.55**   Contracture, hip

M24.551   Contracture, right hip

M24.552   Contracture, left hip

M24.559   Contracture, unspecified hip

√6ᵗʰ   **M24.56**   Contracture, knee

M24.561   Contracture, right knee

M24.562   Contracture, left knee

M24.569   Contracture, unspecified knee

√6ᵗʰ   **M24.57**   Contracture, ankle and foot

M24.571   Contracture, right ankle

M24.572   Contracture, left ankle

M24.573   Contracture, unspecified ankle

M24.574   Contracture, right foot

M24.575   Contracture, left foot

M24.576   Contracture, unspecified foot

√5ᵗʰ   **M24.6**   **Ankylosis of joint**

EXCLUDES 1   stiffness of joint without ankylosis (M25.6-)

EXCLUDES 2   spine (M43.2-)

M24.60   Ankylosis, unspecified joint

√6ᵗʰ   **M24.61**   Ankylosis, shoulder

M24.611   Ankylosis, right shoulder

M24.612   Ankylosis, left shoulder

M24.619   Ankylosis, unspecified shoulder

√6ᵗʰ   **M24.62**   Ankylosis, elbow

M24.621   Ankylosis, right elbow

M24.622   Ankylosis, left elbow

M24.629   Ankylosis, unspecified elbow

√6ᵗʰ   **M24.63**   Ankylosis, wrist

M24.631   Ankylosis, right wrist

M24.632   Ankylosis, left wrist

M24.639   Ankylosis, unspecified wrist

EXCLUDES 1   Not coded here   *EXCLUDES 2*   Not included here   **Manifestation Code**

✓6ᵗʰ **M24.64 Ankylosis, hand**
     M24.641 Ankylosis, right hand
     M24.642 Ankylosis, left hand
     M24.649 Ankylosis, unspecified hand

✓6ᵗʰ **M24.65 Ankylosis, hip**
     M24.651 Ankylosis, right hip
     M24.652 Ankylosis, left hip
     M24.659 Ankylosis, unspecified hip

✓6ᵗʰ **M24.66 Ankylosis, knee**
     M24.661 Ankylosis, right knee
     M24.662 Ankylosis, left knee
     M24.669 Ankylosis, unspecified knee

✓6ᵗʰ **M24.67 Ankylosis, ankle and foot**
     M24.671 Ankylosis, right ankle
     M24.672 Ankylosis, left ankle
     M24.673 Ankylosis, unspecified ankle
     M24.674 Ankylosis, right foot
     M24.675 Ankylosis, left foot
     M24.676 Ankylosis, unspecified foot

M24.7 Protrusio acetabuli

✓5ᵗʰ **M24.8 Other specific joint derangements, not elsewhere classified**
     EXCLUDES 2 *iliotibial band syndrome (M76.3)*

     M24.80 Other specific joint derangements of unspecified joint, not elsewhere classified

✓6ᵗʰ   **M24.81 Other specific joint derangements of shoulder, not elsewhere classified**
         M24.811 Other specific joint derangements of right shoulder, not elsewhere classified
         M24.812 Other specific joint derangements of left shoulder, not elsewhere classified
         M24.819 Other specific joint derangements of unspecified shoulder, not elsewhere classified

✓6ᵗʰ   **M24.82 Other specific joint derangements of elbow, not elsewhere classified**
         M24.821 Other specific joint derangements of right elbow, not elsewhere classified
         M24.822 Other specific joint derangements of left elbow, not elsewhere classified
         M24.829 Other specific joint derangements of unspecified elbow, not elsewhere classified

✓6ᵗʰ   **M24.83 Other specific joint derangements of wrist, not elsewhere classified**
         M24.831 Other specific joint derangements of right wrist, not elsewhere classified
         M24.832 Other specific joint derangements of left wrist, not elsewhere classified
         M24.839 Other specific joint derangements of unspecified wrist, not elsewhere classified

✓6ᵗʰ   **M24.84 Other specific joint derangements of hand, not elsewhere classified**
         M24.841 Other specific joint derangements of right hand, not elsewhere classified
         M24.842 Other specific joint derangements of left hand, not elsewhere classified
         M24.849 Other specific joint derangements of unspecified hand, not elsewhere classified

✓6ᵗʰ   **M24.85 Other specific joint derangements of hip, not elsewhere classified**
         Irritable hip
         M24.851 Other specific joint derangements of right hip, not elsewhere classified
         M24.852 Other specific joint derangements of left hip, not elsewhere classified
         M24.859 Other specific joint derangements of unspecified hip, not elsewhere classified

✓6ᵗʰ   **M24.87 Other specific joint derangements of ankle and foot, not elsewhere classified**
         M24.871 Other specific joint derangements of right ankle, not elsewhere classified
         M24.872 Other specific joint derangements of left ankle, not elsewhere classified

     M24.873 Other specific joint derangements of unspecified ankle, not elsewhere classified
     M24.874 Other specific joint derangements of right foot, not elsewhere classified
     M24.875 Other specific joint derangements left foot, not elsewhere classified
     M24.876 Other specific joint derangements of unspecified foot, not elsewhere classified

M24.9 Joint derangement, unspecified

M25 Other joint disorder, not elsewhere classified
     EXCLUDES 2 *abnormality of gait and mobility (R26-)*
         acquired deformities of limb (M20-M21)
         calcification of bursa (M71.4-)
         calcification of shoulder (joint) (M75.3)
         calcification of tendon (M65.2-)
         difficulty in walking (R26.2)
         temporomandibular joint disorder (M26.6-)

✓5ᵗʰ **M25.0 Hemarthrosis**
     EXCLUDES 1 *current injury—see injury of joint by body region*
         hemophilic arthropathy (M36.2)

     M25.00 Hemarthrosis, unspecified joint

✓6ᵗʰ   **M25.01 Hemarthrosis, shoulder**
         M25.011 Hemarthrosis, right shoulder
         M25.012 Hemarthrosis, left shoulder
         M25.019 Hemarthrosis, unspecified shoulder

✓6ᵗʰ   **M25.02 Hemarthrosis, elbow**
         M25.021 Hemarthrosis, right elbow
         M25.022 Hemarthrosis, left elbow
         M25.029 Hemarthrosis, unspecified elbow

✓6ᵗʰ   **M25.03 Hemarthrosis, wrist**
         M25.031 Hemarthrosis, right wrist
         M25.032 Hemarthrosis, left wrist
         M25.039 Hemarthrosis, unspecified wrist

✓6ᵗʰ   **M25.04 Hemarthrosis, hand**
         M25.041 Hemarthrosis, right hand
         M25.042 Hemarthrosis, left hand
         M25.049 Hemarthrosis, unspecified hand

✓6ᵗʰ   **M25.05 Hemarthrosis, hip**
         M25.051 Hemarthrosis, right hip
         M25.052 Hemarthrosis, left hip
         M25.059 Hemarthrosis, unspecified hip

✓6ᵗʰ   **M25.06 Hemarthrosis, knee**
         M25.061 Hemarthrosis, right knee
         M25.062 Hemarthrosis, left knee
         M25.069 Hemarthrosis, unspecified knee

✓6ᵗʰ   **M25.07 Hemarthrosis, ankle and foot**
         M25.071 Hemarthrosis, right ankle
         M25.072 Hemarthrosis, left ankle
         M25.073 Hemarthrosis, unspecified ankle
         M25.074 Hemarthrosis, right foot
         M25.075 Hemarthrosis, left foot
         M25.076 Hemarthrosis, unspecified foot

     M25.08 Hemarthrosis, vertebrae

✓5ᵗʰ **M25.1 Fistula of joint**
     M25.10 Fistula, unspecified joint

✓6ᵗʰ   **M25.11 Fistula, shoulder**
         M25.111 Fistula, right shoulder
         M25.112 Fistula, left shoulder
         M25.119 Fistula, unspecified shoulder

✓6ᵗʰ   **M25.12 Fistula, elbow**
         M25.121 Fistula, right elbow
         M25.122 Fistula, left elbow
         M25.129 Fistula, unspecified elbow

✓6ᵗʰ   **M25.13 Fistula, wrist**
         M25.131 Fistula, right wrist
         M25.132 Fistula, left wrist
         M25.139 Fistula, unspecified wrist

✓6ᵗʰ   **M25.14 Fistula, hand**
         M25.141 Fistula, right hand
         M25.142 Fistula, left hand
         M25.149 Fistula, unspecified hand

✓6ᵗʰ   **M25.15 Fistula, hip**
         M25.151 Fistula, right hip

☑ Appropriate additional character required   ✓x7ᵗʰ Requires 7th character, placeholder x must fill empty characters

        M25.152   Fistula, left hip
        M25.159   Fistula, unspecified hip
   ✓6th   M25.16   Fistula, knee
        M25.161   Fistula, right knee
        M25.162   Fistula, left knee
        M25.169   Fistula, unspecified knee
   ✓6th   M25.17   Fistula, ankle and foot
        M25.171   Fistula, right ankle
        M25.172   Fistula, left ankle
        M25.173   Fistula, unspecified ankle
        M25.174   Fistula, right foot
        M25.175   Fistula, left foot
        M25.176   Fistula, unspecified foot
      M25.18   Fistula, vertebrae
 ✓5th   **M25.2   Flail joint**
      M25.20   Flail joint, unspecified joint
   ✓6th   M25.21   Flail joint, shoulder
        M25.211   Flail joint, right shoulder
        M25.212   Flail joint, left shoulder
        M25.219   Flail joint, unspecified shoulder
   ✓6th   M25.22   Flail joint, elbow
        M25.221   Flail joint, right elbow
        M25.222   Flail joint, left elbow
        M25.229   Flail joint, unspecified elbow
   ✓6th   M25.23   Flail joint, wrist
        M25.231   Flail joint, right wrist
        M25.232   Flail joint, left wrist
        M25.239   Flail joint, unspecified wrist
   ✓6th   M25.24   Flail joint, hand
        M25.241   Flail joint, right hand
        M25.242   Flail joint, left hand
        M25.249   Flail joint, unspecified hand
   ✓6th   M25.25   Flail joint, hip
        M25.251   Flail joint, right hip
        M25.252   Flail joint, left hip
        M25.259   Flail joint, unspecified hip
   ✓6th   M25.26   Flail joint, knee
        M25.261   Flail joint, right knee
        M25.262   Flail joint, left knee
        M25.269   Flail joint, unspecified knee
   ✓6th   M25.27   Flail joint, ankle and foot
        M25.271   Flail joint, right ankle and foot
        M25.272   Flail joint, left ankle and foot
        M25.279   Flail joint, unspecified ankle and foot
      M25.28   Flail joint, other site
 ✓5th   **M25.3   Other instability of joint**
      EXCLUDES 1   *instability of joint secondary to old ligament injury (M24.2-)*
            instability of joint secondary to removal of joint prosthesis (M96.8-)
      EXCLUDES 2   *spinal instabilities (M53.2-)*
      M25.30   Other instability, unspecified joint
   ✓6th   M25.31   Other instability, shoulder
        M25.311   Other instability, right shoulder
        M25.312   Other instability, left shoulder
        M25.319   Other instability, unspecified shoulder
   ✓6th   M25.32   Other instability, elbow
        M25.321   Other instability, right elbow
        M25.322   Other instability, left elbow
        M25.329   Other instability, unspecified elbow
   ✓6th   M25.33   Other instability, wrist
        M25.331   Other instability, right wrist
        M25.332   Other instability, left wrist
        M25.339   Other instability, unspecified wrist
   ✓6th   M25.34   Other instability, hand
        M25.341   Other instability, right hand
        M25.342   Other instability, left hand
        M25.349   Other instability, unspecified hand
   ✓6th   M25.35   Other instability, hip
        M25.351   Other instability, right hip
        M25.352   Other instability, left hip
        M25.359   Other instability, unspecified hip
   ✓6th   M25.36   Other instability, knee
        M25.361   Other instability, right knee

        M25.362   Other instability, left knee
        M25.369   Other instability, unspecified knee
   ✓6th   M25.37   Other instability, ankle and foot
        M25.371   Other instability, right ankle
        M25.372   Other instability, left ankle
        M25.373   Other instability, unspecified ankle
        M25.374   Other instability, right foot
        M25.375   Other instability, left foot
        M25.376   Other instability, unspecified foot
 ✓5th   **M25.4   Effusion of joint**
      EXCLUDES 1   *hydrarthrosis in yaws (A66.6)*
            intermittent hydrarthrosis (M12.4-)
            other infective (teno)synovitis (M65.1-)
      M25.40   Effusion, unspecified joint
   ✓6th   M25.41   Effusion, shoulder
        M25.411   Effusion, right shoulder
        M25.412   Effusion, left shoulder
        M25.419   Effusion, unspecified shoulder
   ✓6th   M25.42   Effusion, elbow
        M25.421   Effusion, right elbow
        M25.422   Effusion, left elbow
        M25.429   Effusion, unspecified elbow
   ✓6th   M25.43   Effusion, wrist
        M25.431   Effusion, right wrist
        M25.432   Effusion, left wrist
        M25.439   Effusion, unspecified wrist
   ✓6th   M25.44   Effusion, hand
        M25.441   Effusion, right hand
        M25.442   Effusion, left hand
        M25.449   Effusion, unspecified hand
   ✓6th   M25.45   Effusion, hip
        M25.451   Effusion, right hip
        M25.452   Effusion, left hip
        M25.459   Effusion, unspecified hip
   ✓6th   M25.46   Effusion, knee
        M25.461   Effusion, right knee
        M25.462   Effusion, left knee
        M25.469   Effusion, unspecified knee
   ✓6th   M25.47   Effusion, ankle and foot
        M25.471   Effusion, right ankle
        M25.472   Effusion, left ankle
        M25.473   Effusion, unspecified ankle
        M25.474   Effusion, right foot
        M25.475   Effusion, left foot
        M25.476   Effusion, unspecified foot
      M25.48   Effusion, other site
 ✓5th   **M25.5   Pain in joint**
      EXCLUDES 2   *pain in hand (M79.64-)*
            pain in fingers (M79.64-)
            pain in foot (M79.67-)
            pain in limb (M79.6-)
            pain in toes (M79.67-)
      M25.50   Pain in unspecified joint
   ✓6th   M25.51   Pain in shoulder
        M25.511   Pain in right shoulder
        M25.512   Pain in left shoulder
        M25.519   Pain in unspecified shoulder
   ✓6th   M25.52   Pain in elbow
        M25.521   Pain in right elbow
        M25.522   Pain in left elbow
        M25.529   Pain in unspecified elbow
   ✓6th   M25.53   Pain in wrist
        M25.531   Pain in right wrist
        M25.532   Pain in left wrist
        M25.539   Pain in unspecified wrist
   ✓6th   M25.55   Pain in hip
        M25.551   Pain in right hip
        M25.552   Pain in left hip
        M25.559   Pain in unspecified hip
   ✓6th   M25.56   Pain in knee
        M25.561   Pain in right knee
        M25.562   Pain in left knee
        M25.569   Pain in unspecified knee
   ✓6th   M25.57   Pain in ankle
        M25.571   Pain in right ankle

EXCLUDES 1   Not coded here   EXCLUDES 2   Not included here   *Manifestation Code*

          M25.572 Pain in left ankle

          M25.579 Pain in unspecified ankle

✓5th **M25.6 Stiffness of joint, not elsewhere classified**

    EXCLUDES1 *ankylosis of joint (M24.6-)*

            contracture of joint (M24.5-)

    M25.60 **Stiffness of unspecified joint, not elsewhere classified**

    ✓6th M25.61 **Stiffness of shoulder, not elsewhere classified**

        M25.611 **Stiffness of right shoulder, not elsewhere classified**

        M25.612 **Stiffness of left shoulder, not elsewhere classified**

        M25.619 **Stiffness of unspecified shoulder, not elsewhere classified**

    ✓6th M25.62 **Stiffness of elbow, not elsewhere classified**

        M25.621 **Stiffness of right elbow, not elsewhere classified**

        M25.622 **Stiffness of left elbow, not elsewhere classified**

        M25.629 **Stiffness of unspecified elbow, not elsewhere classified**

    ✓6th M25.63 **Stiffness of wrist, not elsewhere classified**

        M25.631 **Stiffness of right wrist, not elsewhere classified**

        M25.632 **Stiffness of left wrist, not elsewhere classified**

        M25.639 **Stiffness of unspecified wrist, not elsewhere classified**

    ✓6th M25.64 **Stiffness of hand, not elsewhere classified**

        M25.641 **Stiffness of right hand, not elsewhere classified**

        M25.642 **Stiffness of left hand, not elsewhere classified**

        M25.649 **Stiffness of unspecified hand, not elsewhere classified**

    ✓6th M25.65 **Stiffness of hip, not elsewhere classified**

        M25.651 **Stiffness of right hip, not elsewhere classified**

        M25.652 **Stiffness of left hip, not elsewhere classified**

        M25.659 **Stiffness of unspecified hip, not elsewhere classified**

    ✓6th M25.66 **Stiffness of knee, not elsewhere classified**

        M25.661 **Stiffness of right knee, not elsewhere classified**

        M25.662 **Stiffness of left knee, not elsewhere classified**

        M25.669 **Stiffness of unspecified knee, not elsewhere classified**

    ✓6th M25.67 **Stiffness of ankle and foot, not elsewhere classified**

        M25.671 **Stiffness of right ankle, not elsewhere classified**

        M25.672 **Stiffness of left ankle, not elsewhere classified**

        M25.673 **Stiffness of unspecified ankle, not elsewhere classified**

        M25.674 **Stiffness of right foot, not elsewhere classified**

        M25.675 **Stiffness of left foot, not elsewhere classified**

        M25.676 **Stiffness of unspecified foot, not elsewhere classified**

✓5th **M25.7 Osteophyte**

    M25.70 **Osteophyte, unspecified joint**

    ✓6th M25.71 **Osteophyte, shoulder**

        M25.711 **Osteophyte, right shoulder**

        M25.712 **Osteophyte, left shoulder**

        M25.719 **Osteophyte, unspecified shoulder**

    ✓6th M25.72 **Osteophyte, elbow**

        M25.721 **Osteophyte, right elbow**

        M25.722 **Osteophyte, left elbow**

        M25.729 **Osteophyte, unspecified elbow**

    ✓6th M25.73 **Osteophyte, wrist**

        M25.731 **Osteophyte, right wrist**

        M25.732 **Osteophyte, left wrist**

        M25.739 **Osteophyte, unspecified wrist**

    ✓6th M25.74 **Osteophyte, hand**

        M25.741 **Osteophyte, right hand**

        M25.742 **Osteophyte, left hand**

        M25.749 **Osteophyte, unspecified hand**

    ✓6th M25.75 **Osteophyte, hip**

        M25.751 **Osteophyte, right hip**

        M25.752 **Osteophyte, left hip**

        M25.759 **Osteophyte, unspecified hip**

    ✓6th M25.76 **Osteophyte, knee**

        M25.761 **Osteophyte, right knee**

        M25.762 **Osteophyte, left knee**

        M25.769 **Osteophyte, unspecified knee**

    ✓6th M25.77 **Osteophyte, ankle and foot**

        M25.771 **Osteophyte, right ankle**

        M25.772 **Osteophyte, left ankle**

        M25.773 **Osteophyte, unspecified ankle**

        M25.774 **Osteophyte, right foot**

        M25.775 **Osteophyte, left foot**

        M25.776 **Osteophyte, unspecified foot**

    M25.78 **Osteophyte, vertebrae**

✓5th **M25.8 Other specified joint disorders**

    M25.80 **Other specified joint disorders, unspecified joint**

    ✓6th M25.81 **Other specified joint disorders, shoulder**

        M25.811 **Other specified joint disorders, right shoulder**

        M25.812 **Other specified joint disorders, left shoulder**

        M25.819 **Other specified joint disorders, unspecified shoulder**

    ✓6th M25.82 **Other specified joint disorders, elbow**

        M25.821 **Other specified joint disorders, right elbow**

        M25.822 **Other specified joint disorders, left elbow**

        M25.829 **Other specified joint disorders, unspecified elbow**

    ✓6th M25.83 **Other specified joint disorders, wrist**

        M25.831 **Other specified joint disorders, right wrist**

        M25.832 **Other specified joint disorders, left wrist**

        M25.839 **Other specified joint disorders, unspecified wrist**

    ✓6th M25.84 **Other specified joint disorders, hand**

        M25.841 **Other specified joint disorders, right hand**

        M25.842 **Other specified joint disorders, left hand**

        M25.849 **Other specified joint disorders, unspecified hand**

    ✓6th M25.85 **Other specified joint disorders, hip**

        M25.851 **Other specified joint disorders, right hip**

        M25.852 **Other specified joint disorders, left hip**

        M25.859 **Other specified joint disorders, unspecified hip**

    ✓6th M25.86 **Other specified joint disorders, knee**

        M25.861 **Other specified joint disorders, right knee**

        M25.862 **Other specified joint disorders, left knee**

        M25.869 **Other specified joint disorders, unspecified knee**

    ✓6th M25.87 **Other specified joint disorders, ankle and foot**

        M25.871 **Other specified joint disorders, right ankle and foot**

        M25.872 **Other specified joint disorders, left ankle and foot**

        M25.879 **Other specified joint disorders, unspecified ankle and foot**

M25.9 Joint disorder, unspecified

✓ Appropriate additional character required   ✓x7th Requires 7th character, placeholder x must fill empty characters

Dentofacial anomalies [including malocclusion] and other disorders of jaw (M26-M27)

> **EXCLUDES 1**   hemifacial atrophy or hypertrophy (Q67.4)
> unilateral condylar hyperplasia or hypoplasia (M27.8)

√4th **M26 Dentofacial anomalies [including malocclusion]**

√5th **M26.0 Major anomalies of jaw size**

> **EXCLUDES 1**   acromegaly (E22.0)
> Robin's syndrome (Q87.0)

    M26.00 Unspecified anomaly of jaw size
    M26.01 Maxillary hyperplasia
    M26.02 Maxillary hypoplasia
    M26.03 Mandibular hyperplasia
    M26.04 Mandibular hypoplasia
    M26.05 Macrogenia
    M26.06 Microgenia
    M26.07 Excessive tuberosity of jaw
         Entire maxillary tuberosity
    M26.09 Other specified anomalies of jaw size

√5th **M26.1 Anomalies of jaw-cranial base relationship**

    M26.10 Unspecified anomaly of jaw-cranial base relationship
    M26.11 Maxillary asymmetry
    M26.12 Other jaw asymmetry
    M26.19 Other specified anomalies of jaw-cranial base relationship

√5th **M26.2 Anomalies of dental arch relationship**

    M26.20 Unspecified anomaly of dental arch relationship
    √6th **M26.21 Malocclusion, Angle's class**
        M26.211 Malocclusion, Angle's class I
             Neutro-occlusion
        M26.212 Malocclusion, Angle's class II
             Disto-occlusion Division I
             Disto-occlusion Division II
        M26.213 Malocclusion, Angle's class III
             Mesio-occlusion
        M26.219 Malocclusion, Angle's class, unspecified
    √6th **M26.22 Open occlusal relationship**
        M26.220 Open anterior occlusal relationship
             Anterior openbite
        M26.221 Open posterior occlusal relationship
             Posterior openbite
    M26.23 Excessive horizontal overlap
         Excessive horizontal overjet
    M26.24 Reverse articulation
         Crossbite (anterior) (posterior)
    M26.25 Anomalies of interarch distance
    M26.29 Other anomalies of dental arch relationship
         Midline deviation of dental arch
         Overbite (excessive) deep
         Overbite (excessive) horizontal
         Overbite (excessive) vertical
         Posterior lingual occlusion of mandibular teeth

√5th **M26.3 Anomalies of tooth position of fully erupted tooth or teeth**

> **EXCLUDES 2**   embedded and impacted teeth (K01-)

    M26.30 Unspecified anomaly of tooth position of fully erupted tooth or teeth
         Abnormal spacing of fully erupted tooth or teeth NOS
         Displacement of fully erupted tooth or teeth NOS
         Transposition of fully erupted tooth or teeth NOS
    M26.31 Crowding of fully erupted teeth
    M26.32 Excessive spacing of fully erupted teeth
         Diastema of fully erupted tooth or teeth NOS
    M26.33 Horizontal displacement of fully erupted tooth or teeth
         Tipped tooth or teeth
         Tipping of fully erupted tooth
    M26.34 Vertical displacement of fully erupted tooth or teeth
         Extruded tooth
         Infraeruption of tooth or teeth
         Supraeruption of tooth or teeth
    M26.35 Rotation of fully erupted tooth or teeth
    M26.36 Insufficient interocclusal distance of fully erupted teeth (ridge)
         Lack of adequate intermaxillary vertical dimension of fully erupted teeth

---

    M26.37 Excessive interocclusal distance of fully erupted teeth
         Excessive intermaxillary vertical dimension of fully erupted teeth
         Loss of occlusal vertical dimension of fully erupted teeth
    M26.39 Other anomalies of tooth position of fully erupted tooth or teeth

M26.4 Malocclusion, unspecified

√5th **M26.5 Dentofacial functional abnormalities**

> **EXCLUDES 1**   bruxism (F45.8)
> teeth-grinding NOS (F45.8)

    M26.50 Dentofacial functional abnormalities, unspecified
    M26.51 Abnormal jaw closure
    M26.52 Limited mandibular range of motion
    M26.53 Deviation in opening and closing of the mandible
    M26.54 Insufficient anterior guidance
         Insufficient anterior occlusal guidance
    M26.55 Centric occlusion maximum intercuspation discrepancy

> **EXCLUDES 1**   centric occlusion NOS (M26.59)

    M26.56 Non-working side interference
         Balancing side interference
    M26.57 Lack of posterior occlusal support
    M26.59 Other dentofacial functional abnormalities
         Centric occlusion (of teeth) NOS
         Malocclusion due to abnormal swallowing
         Malocclusion due to mouth breathing
         Malocclusion due to tongue, lip or finger habits

√5th **M26.6 Temporomandibular joint disorders**

> **EXCLUDES 2**   current temporomandibular joint dislocation (S03.0)
> current temporomandibular joint sprain (S03.4)

    M26.60 Temporomandibular joint disorder, unspecified
    M26.61 Adhesions and ankylosis of temporomandibular joint
    M26.62 Arthralgia of temporomandibular joint
    M26.63 Articular disc disorder of temporomandibular joint
    M26.69 Other specified disorders of temporomandibular joint

√5th **M26.7 Dental alveolar anomalies**

    M26.70 Unspecified alveolar anomaly
    M26.71 Alveolar maxillary hyperplasia
    M26.72 Alveolar mandibular hyperplasia
    M26.73 Alveolar maxillary hypoplasia
    M26.74 Alveolar mandibular hypoplasia
    M26.79 Other specified alveolar anomalies

√5th **M26.8 Other dentofacial anomalies**

    M26.81 Anterior soft tissue impingement
         Anterior soft tissue impingement on teeth
    M26.82 Posterior soft tissue impingement
         Posterior soft tissue impingement on teeth
    M26.89 Other dentofacial anomalies

M26.9 Dentofacial anomaly, unspecified

√4th **M27 Other diseases of jaws**

M27.0 Developmental disorders of jaws
     Latent bone cyst of jaw
     Stafne's cyst
     Torus mandibularis
     Torus palatinus

M27.1 Giant cell granuloma, central
     Giant cell granuloma NOS

> **EXCLUDES 1**   peripheral giant cell granuloma (K06.8)

M27.2 Inflammatory conditions of jaws
     Osteitis of jaw(s)
     Osteomyelitis (neonatal) jaw(s)
     Osteoradionecrosis jaw(s)
     Periostitis jaw(s)
     Sequestrum of jaw bone
     Use additional code (W88-W90, X39.0) to identify radiation, if radiation-induced

> **EXCLUDES 2**   osteonecrosis of jaw due to drug (M87.180)

M27.3 Alveolitis of jaws
     Alveolar osteitis
     Dry socket

EXCLUDES 1 Not coded here   **EXCLUDES 2** Not included here   *Manifestation Code*

✓5ᵗʰ M27.4　Other and unspecified cysts of jaw
　　EXCLUDES 1　*cysts of oral region (K09-)*
　　　　　　　　latent bone cyst of jaw (M27.0)
　　　　　　　　Stafne's cyst (M27.0)
　　M27.40　Unspecified cyst of jaw
　　　　　　Cyst of jaw NOS
　　M27.49　Other cysts of jaw
　　　　　　Aneurysmal cyst of jaw
　　　　　　Hemorrhagic cyst of jaw
　　　　　　Traumatic cyst of jaw

✓5ᵗʰ M27.5　Periradicular pathology associated with previous endodontic treatment
　　M27.51　Perforation of root canal space due to endodontic treatment
　　M27.52　Endodontic overfill
　　M27.53　Endodontic underfill
　　M27.59　Other periradicular pathology associated with previous endodontic treatment

✓5ᵗʰ M27.6　Endosseous dental implant failure
　　M27.61　Osseointegration failure of dental implant
　　　　　　Hemorrhagic complications of dental implant placement
　　　　　　Iatrogenic osseointegration failure of dental implant
　　　　　　Osseointegration failure of dental implant due to complications of systemic disease
　　　　　　Osseointegration failure of dental implant due to poor bone quality
　　　　　　Pre-integration failure of dental implant NOS
　　　　　　Pre-osseointegration failure of dental implant
　　M27.62　Post-osseointegration biological failure of dental implant
　　　　　　Failure of dental implant due to lack of attached gingiva
　　　　　　Failure of dental implant due to occlusal trauma (caused by poor prosthetic design)
　　　　　　Failure of dental implant due to parafunctional habits
　　　　　　Failure of dental implant due to periodontal infection (peri-implantitis)
　　　　　　Failure of dental implant due to poor oral hygiene
　　　　　　Iatrogenic post-osseointegration failure of dental implant
　　　　　　Post-osseointegration failure of dental implant due to complications of systemic disease
　　M27.63　Post-osseointegration mechanical failure of dental implant
　　　　　　Failure of dental prosthesis causing loss of dental implant
　　　　　　Fracture of dental implant
　　　　　　EXCLUDES 2　*cracked tooth (K03.81)*
　　　　　　　　　　fractured dental restorative material with loss of material (K08.531)
　　　　　　　　　　fractured dental restorative material without loss of material (K08.530)
　　　　　　　　　　fractured tooth (S02.5)
　　M27.69　Other endosseous dental implant failure
　　　　　　Dental implant failure NOS

M27.8　Other specified diseases of jaws
　　　　Cherubism
　　　　Exostosis
　　　　Fibrous dysplasia
　　　　Unilateral condylar hyperplasia
　　　　Unilateral condylar hypoplasia
　　　　EXCLUDES 1　*jaw pain (R68.84)*

M27.9　Disease of jaws, unspecified

Systemic connective tissue disorders (M30-M36)

INCLUDES　autoimmune disease NOS
　　　　collagen (vascular) disease NOS
　　　　systemic autoimmune disease
　　　　systemic collagen (vascular) disease
EXCLUDES 1　*autoimmune disease, single organ or single cell-type—code to relevant condition category*

✓4ᵗʰ M30　Polyarteritis nodosa and related conditions
　　EXCLUDES 1　*microscopic polyarteritis (M31.7)*
　　M30.0　Polyarteritis nodosa
　　M30.1　Polyarteritis with lung involvement [Churg-Strauss]
　　　　　　Allergic granulomatous angiitis
　　M30.2　Juvenile polyarteritis

M30.3　Mucocutaneous lymph node syndrome [Kawasaki]
M30.8　Other conditions related to polyarteritis nodosa
　　　　Polyangiitis overlap syndrome

✓4ᵗʰ M31　Other necrotizing vasculopathies
　　M31.0　Hypersensitivity angiitis
　　　　　　Goodpasture's syndrome
　　M31.1　Thrombotic microangiopathy
　　　　　　Thrombotic thrombocytopenic purpura
　　M31.2　Lethal midline granuloma
　　✓5ᵗʰ M31.3　Wegener's granulomatosis
　　　　　　Necrotizing respiratory granulomatosis
　　　　M31.30　Wegener's granulomatosis without renal involvement
　　　　　　　　Wegener's granulomatosis NOS
　　　　M31.31　Wegener's granulomatosis with renal involvement
　　M31.4　Aortic arch syndrome [Takayasu]
　　M31.5　Giant cell arteritis with polymyalgia rheumatica
　　M31.6　Other giant cell arteritis
　　M31.7　Microscopic polyangiitis
　　　　　　Microscopic polyarteritis
　　　　　　EXCLUDES 1　*polyarteritis nodosa (M30.0)*
　　M31.8　Other specified necrotizing vasculopathies
　　　　　　Hypocomplementemic vasculitis
　　　　　　Septic vasculitis
　　M31.9　Necrotizing vasculopathy, unspecified

✓4ᵗʰ M32　Systemic lupus erythematosus (SLE)
　　EXCLUDES 1　*lupus erythematosus (discoid) (NOS) (L93.0)*
　　M32.0　Drug-induced systemic lupus erythematosus
　　　　　　Code first (T36-T50) to identify drug
　　✓5ᵗʰ M32.1　Systemic lupus erythematosus with organ or system involvement
　　　　M32.10　Systemic lupus erythematosus, organ or system involvement unspecified
　　　　M32.11　Endocarditis in systemic lupus erythematosus
　　　　　　　　Libman-Sacks disease
　　　　M32.12　Pericarditis in systemic lupus erythematosus
　　　　　　　　Lupus pericarditis
　　　　M32.13　Lung involvement in systemic lupus erythematosus
　　　　　　　　Pleural effusion due to systemic lupus erythematosus
　　　　M32.14　Glomerular disease in systemic lupus erythematosus
　　　　　　　　Lupus renal disease NOS
　　　　M32.15　Tubulo-interstitial nephropathy in systemic lupus erythematosus
　　　　M32.19　Other organ or system involvement in systemic lupus erythematosus
　　M32.8　Other forms of systemic lupus erythematosus
　　M32.9　Systemic lupus erythematosus, unspecified
　　　　　　SLE NOS
　　　　　　Systemic lupus erythematosus NOS
　　　　　　Systemic lupus erythematosus without organ involvement

✓4ᵗʰ M33　Dermatopolymyositis
　　✓5ᵗʰ M33.0　Juvenile dermatopolymyositis
　　　　M33.00　Juvenile dermatopolymyositis, organ involvement unspecified
　　　　M33.01　Juvenile dermatopolymyositis with respiratory involvement
　　　　M33.02　Juvenile dermatopolymyositis with myopathy
　　　　M33.09　Juvenile dermatopolymyositis with other organ involvement
　　✓5ᵗʰ M33.1　Other dermatopolymyositis
　　　　M33.10　Other dermatopolymyositis, organ involvement unspecified
　　　　M33.11　Other dermatopolymyositis with respiratory involvement
　　　　M33.12　Other dermatopolymyositis with myopathy
　　　　M33.19　Other dermatopolymyositis with other organ involvement
　　✓5ᵗʰ M33.2　Polymyositis
　　　　M33.20　Polymyositis, organ involvement unspecified
　　　　M33.21　Polymyositis with respiratory involvement
　　　　M33.22　Polymyositis with myopathy
　　　　M33.29　Polymyositis with other organ involvement

✓5ᵗʰ **M33.9 Dermatopolymyositis, unspecified**

    M33.90 Dermatopolymyositis, unspecified, organ involvement unspecified

    M33.91 Dermatopolymyositis, unspecified with respiratory involvement

    M33.92 Dermatopolymyositis, unspecified with myopathy

    M33.99 Dermatopolymyositis, unspecified with other organ involvement

✓4ᵗʰ **M34 Systemic sclerosis [scleroderma]**

    EXCLUDES 1   *circumscribed scleroderma (L94.0)*
                neonatal scleroderma (P83.8)

    M34.0 Progressive systemic sclerosis

    M34.1 CR(E)ST syndrome

        Combination of calcinosis, Raynaud's phenomenon, esophageal dysfunction, sclerodactyly, telangiectasia

    M34.2 Systemic sclerosis induced by drug and chemical

        Code first (T36-T65) to identify agent

✓5ᵗʰ   **M34.8 Other forms of systemic sclerosis**

    M34.81 Systemic sclerosis with lung involvement

    M34.82 Systemic sclerosis with myopathy

    M34.83 Systemic sclerosis with polyneuropathy

    M34.89 Other systemic sclerosis

    M34.9 Systemic sclerosis, unspecified

✓4ᵗʰ **M35 Other systemic involvement of connective tissue**

    EXCLUDES 1   *reactive perforating collagenosis (L87.1)*

✓5ᵗʰ   **M35.0 Sicca syndrome [Sjögren]**

    M35.00 Sicca syndrome, unspecified

    M35.01 Sicca syndrome with keratoconjunctivitis

    M35.02 Sicca syndrome with lung involvement

    M35.03 Sicca syndrome with myopathy

    M35.04 Sicca syndrome with tubulo-interstitial nephropathy

        Renal tubular acidosis in sicca syndrome

    M35.09 Sicca syndrome with other organ involvement

    M35.1 Other overlap syndromes

        Mixed connective tissue disease

        EXCLUDES 1   *polyangiitis overlap syndrome (M30.8)*

    M35.2 Behçet's disease

    M35.3 Polymyalgia rheumatica

        EXCLUDES 1   *polymyalgia rheumatica with giant cell arteritis (M31.5)*

    M35.4 Diffuse (eosinophilic) fasciitis

    M35.5 Multifocal fibrosclerosis

    M35.6 Relapsing panniculitis [Weber-Christian]

        EXCLUDES 1   *lupus panniculitis (L93.2)*
                 panniculitis NOS (M79.3-)

    M35.7 Hypermobility syndrome

        Familial ligamentous laxity

        EXCLUDES 1   *Ehlers-Danlos syndrome (Q79.6)*
                 ligamentous laxity, NOS (M24.2-)

    M35.8 Other specified systemic involvement of connective tissue

    M35.9 Systemic involvement of connective tissue, unspecified

        Autoimmune disease (systemic) NOS

        Collagen (vascular) disease NOS

✓4ᵗʰ **M36 Systemic disorders of connective tissue in diseases classified elsewhere**

    EXCLUDES 2   *arthropathies in diseases classified elsewhere (M14-)*

    M36.0   *Dermato(poly)myositis in neoplastic disease*

        Code first underlying neoplasm (C00-D49)

    M36.1   *Arthropathy in neoplastic disease*

        Code first underlying neoplasm, such as:
           leukemia (C91-C95)
           malignant histiocytosis (C96.a)
           multiple myeloma (C90.0)

    M36.2   *Hemophilic arthropathy*

        Hemarthrosis in hemophilic arthropathy

        Code first underlying disease, such as:
           factor VIII deficiency (D66)
           with vascular defect (D68.0)
           factor IX deficiency (D67)
           hemophilia (classical) (D66)
           hemophilia B (D67)
           hemophilia C (D68.1)

    M36.3   *Arthropathy in other blood disorders*

    M36.4   *Arthropathy in hypersensitivity reactions classified elsewhere*

        Code first underlying disease, such as:
           Henoch (-Schönlein) purpura (D69.0)

    M36.8   *Systemic disorders of connective tissue in other diseases classified elsewhere*

        Code first underlying disease, such as:
           alkaptonuria (E70.2)
           hypogammaglobulinemia (D80-)
           ochronosis (E70.2)

DORSOPATHIES (M40-M54)

Deforming dorsopathies (M40-M43)

✓4ᵗʰ **M40 Kyphosis and lordosis**

    EXCLUDES 1   *congenital kyphosis and lordosis (Q76.4)*
                 kyphoscoliosis (M41-)
                 postprocedural kyphosis and lordosis (M96-)

✓5ᵗʰ   **M40.0 Postural kyphosis**

        EXCLUDES 1   *osteochondrosis of spine (M42-)*

    M40.00 Postural kyphosis, site unspecified

    M40.03 Postural kyphosis, cervicothoracic region

    M40.04 Postural kyphosis, thoracic region

    M40.05 Postural kyphosis, thoracolumbar region

✓5ᵗʰ   **M40.1 Other secondary kyphosis**

    M40.10 Other secondary kyphosis, site unspecified

    M40.12 Other secondary kyphosis, cervical region

    M40.13 Other secondary kyphosis, cervicothoracic region

    M40.14 Other secondary kyphosis, thoracic region

    M40.15 Other secondary kyphosis, thoracolumbar region

✓5ᵗʰ   **M40.2 Other and unspecified kyphosis**

    ✓6ᵗʰ **M40.20 Unspecified kyphosis**

        M40.202 Unspecified kyphosis, cervical region

        M40.203 Unspecified kyphosis, cervicothoracic region

        M40.204 Unspecified kyphosis, thoracic region

        M40.205 Unspecified kyphosis, thoracolumbar region

        M40.209 Unspecified kyphosis, site unspecified

    ✓6ᵗʰ **M40.29 Other kyphosis**

        M40.292 Other kyphosis, cervical region

        M40.293 Other kyphosis, cervicothoracic region

        M40.294 Other kyphosis, thoracic region

        M40.295 Other kyphosis, thoracolumbar region

        M40.299 Other kyphosis, site unspecified

✓5ᵗʰ   **M40.3 Flatback syndrome**

    M40.30 Flatback syndrome, site unspecified

    M40.35 Flatback syndrome, thoracolumbar region

    M40.36 Flatback syndrome, lumbar region

    M40.37 Flatback syndrome, lumbosacral region

✓5ᵗʰ   **M40.4 Postural lordosis**

        Acquired lordosis

    M40.40 Postural lordosis, site unspecified

    M40.45 Postural lordosis, thoracolumbar region

    M40.46 Postural lordosis, lumbar region

    M40.47 Postural lordosis, lumbosacral region

✓5ᵗʰ   **M40.5 Lordosis, unspecified**

    M40.50 Lordosis, unspecified, site unspecified

    M40.55 Lordosis, unspecified, thoracolumbar region

    M40.56 Lordosis, unspecified, lumbar region

    M40.57 Lordosis, unspecified, lumbosacral region

✓4ᵗʰ **M41 Scoliosis**

    INCLUDES   kyphoscoliosis

    EXCLUDES 1   *congenital scoliosis NOS (Q67.5)*
                 congenital scoliosis due to bony malformation (Q76.3)
                 kyphoscoliotic heart disease (I27.1)
                 postprocedural scoliosis (M96-)
                 postural congenital scoliosis (Q67.5)

✓5ᵗʰ   **M41.0 Infantile idiopathic scoliosis**

        NOTE   Infantile is defined as birth through 4 years of age

    M41.00 Infantile idiopathic scoliosis, site unspecified

    M41.02 Infantile idiopathic scoliosis, cervical region

    M41.03 Infantile idiopathic scoliosis, cervicothoracic region

    M41.04 Infantile idiopathic scoliosis, thoracic region

EXCLUDES 1   Not coded here   EXCLUDES 2   Not included here   *Manifestation Code*

M41.05　Infantile idiopathic scoliosis, thoracolumbar region

M41.06　Infantile idiopathic scoliosis, lumbar region

M41.07　Infantile idiopathic scoliosis, lumbosacral region

M41.08　Infantile idiopathic scoliosis, sacral and sacrococcygeal region

✓5th　M41.1　Juvenile and adolescent idiopathic scoliosis

✓6th　M41.11　Juvenile idiopathic scoliosis

NOTE　Juvenile is defined as 5 through 10 years of age

M41.112　Juvenile idiopathic scoliosis, cervical region

M41.113　Juvenile idiopathic scoliosis, cervicothoracic region

M41.114　Juvenile idiopathic scoliosis, thoracic region

M41.115　Juvenile idiopathic scoliosis, thoracolumbar region

M41.116　Juvenile idiopathic scoliosis, lumbar region

M41.117　Juvenile idiopathic scoliosis, lumbosacral region

M41.119　Juvenile idiopathic scoliosis, site unspecified

✓6th　M41.12　Adolescent scoliosis

NOTE　Adolescent is defined as 11 through 17 years of age

M41.122　Adolescent idiopathic scoliosis, cervical region

M41.123　Adolescent idiopathic scoliosis, cervicothoracic region

M41.124　Adolescent idiopathic scoliosis, thoracic region

M41.125　Adolescent idiopathic scoliosis, thoracolumbar region

M41.126　Adolescent idiopathic scoliosis, lumbar region

M41.127　Adolescent idiopathic scoliosis, lumbosacral region

M41.129　Adolescent idiopathic scoliosis, site unspecified

✓5th　M41.2　Other idiopathic scoliosis

M41.20　Other idiopathic scoliosis, site unspecified

M41.22　Other idiopathic scoliosis, cervical region

M41.23　Other idiopathic scoliosis, cervicothoracic region

M41.24　Other idiopathic scoliosis, thoracic region

M41.25　Other idiopathic scoliosis, thoracolumbar region

M41.26　Other idiopathic scoliosis, lumbar region

M41.27　Other idiopathic scoliosis, lumbosacral region

✓5th　M41.3　Thoracogenic scoliosis

M41.30　Thoracogenic scoliosis, site unspecified

M41.34　Thoracogenic scoliosis, thoracic region

M41.35　Thoracogenic scoliosis, thoracolumbar region

✓5th　M41.4　Neuromuscular scoliosis

Scoliosis secondary to cerebral palsy, Friedreich's ataxia, poliomyelitis and other neuromuscular disorders

Code also underlying condition

M41.40　Neuromuscular scoliosis, site unspecified

M41.41　Neuromuscular scoliosis, occipito-atlanto-axial region

M41.42　Neuromuscular scoliosis, cervical region

M41.43　Neuromuscular scoliosis, cervicothoracic region

M41.44　Neuromuscular scoliosis, thoracic region

M41.45　Neuromuscular scoliosis, thoracolumbar region

M41.46　Neuromuscular scoliosis, lumbar region

M41.47　Neuromuscular scoliosis, lumbosacral region

✓5th　M41.5　Other secondary scoliosis

M41.50　Other secondary scoliosis, site unspecified

M41.52　Other secondary scoliosis, cervical region

M41.53　Other secondary scoliosis, cervicothoracic region

M41.54　Other secondary scoliosis, thoracic region

M41.55　Other secondary scoliosis, thoracolumbar region

M41.56　Other secondary scoliosis, lumbar region

M41.57　Other secondary scoliosis, lumbosacral region

✓5th　M41.8　Other forms of scoliosis

M41.80　Other forms of scoliosis, site unspecified

M41.82　Other forms of scoliosis, cervical region

M41.83　Other forms of scoliosis, cervicothoracic region

M41.84　Other forms of scoliosis, thoracic region

M41.85　Other forms of scoliosis, thoracolumbar region

M41.86　Other forms of scoliosis, lumbar region

M41.87　Other forms of scoliosis, lumbosacral region

M41.9　Scoliosis, unspecified

✓4th　M42　Spinal osteochondrosis

✓5th　M42.0　Juvenile osteochondrosis of spine

Calvé's disease

Scheuermann's disease

EXCLUDES 1　postural kyphosis (M40.0)

M42.00　Juvenile osteochondrosis of spine, site unspecified

M42.01　Juvenile osteochondrosis of spine, occipito-atlanto-axial region

M42.02　Juvenile osteochondrosis of spine, cervical region

M42.03　Juvenile osteochondrosis of spine, cervicothoracic region

M42.04　Juvenile osteochondrosis of spine, thoracic region

M42.05　Juvenile osteochondrosis of spine, thoracolumbar region

M42.06　Juvenile osteochondrosis of spine, lumbar region

M42.07　Juvenile osteochondrosis of spine, lumbosacral region

M42.08　Juvenile osteochondrosis of spine, sacral and sacrococcygeal region

M42.09　Juvenile osteochondrosis of spine, multiple sites in spine

✓5th　M42.1　Adult osteochondrosis of spine

M42.10　Adult osteochondrosis of spine, site unspecified

M42.11　Adult osteochondrosis of spine, occipito-atlanto-axial region

M42.12　Adult osteochondrosis of spine, cervical region

M42.13　Adult osteochondrosis of spine, cervicothoracic region

M42.14　Adult osteochondrosis of spine, thoracic region

M42.15　Adult osteochondrosis of spine, thoracolumbar region

M42.16　Adult osteochondrosis of spine, lumbar region

M42.17　Adult osteochondrosis of spine, lumbosacral region

M42.18　Adult osteochondrosis of spine, sacral and sacrococcygeal region

M42.19　Adult osteochondrosis of spine, multiple sites in spine

M42.9　Spinal osteochondrosis, unspecified

✓4th　M43　Other deforming dorsopathies

EXCLUDES 1　congenital spondylolysis and spondylolisthesis (Q76.2)

hemivertebra (Q76.3-Q76.4)

Klippel-Feil syndrome (Q76.1)

lumbarization and sacralization (Q76.4)

platyspondylisis (Q76.4)

spina bifida occulta (Q76.0)

spinal curvature in osteoporosis (M80-)

spinal curvature in Paget's disease of bone [osteitis deformans] (M88-)

✓5th　M43.0　Spondylolysis

EXCLUDES 1　congenital spondylolysis (Q76.2)

spondylolisthesis (M43.1)

M43.00　Spondylolysis, site unspecified

M43.01　Spondylolysis, occipito-atlanto-axial region

M43.02　Spondylolysis, cervical region

M43.03　Spondylolysis, cervicothoracic region

M43.04　Spondylolysis, thoracic region

M43.05　Spondylolysis, thoracolumbar region

M43.06　Spondylolysis, lumbar region

M43.07　Spondylolysis, lumbosacral region

M43.08　Spondylolysis, sacral and sacrococcygeal region

M43.09　Spondylolysis, multiple sites in spine

✓5th　M43.1　Spondylolisthesis

EXCLUDES 1　acute traumatic of lumbosacral region (S33.1)

acute traumatic of sites other than lumbosacral— code to Fracture, vertebra, by region

congenital spondylolisthesis (Q76.2)

M43.10　Spondylolisthesis, site unspecified

M43.11　Spondylolisthesis, occipito-atlanto-axial region

☑ Appropriate additional character required　　　　√x7th Requires 7th character, placeholder x must fill empty characters

M43.12   Spondylolisthesis, cervical region
M43.13   Spondylolisthesis, cervicothoracic region
M43.14   Spondylolisthesis, thoracic region
M43.15   Spondylolisthesis, thoracolumbar region
M43.16   Spondylolisthesis, lumbar region
M43.17   Spondylolisthesis, lumbosacral region
M43.18   Spondylolisthesis, sacral and sacrococcygeal region
M43.19   Spondylolisthesis, multiple sites in spine

✓5ᵗʰ **M43.2 Fusion of spine**
    Ankylosis of spinal joint
    EXCLUDES 1   *ankylosing spondylitis (M45.0-)*
               congenital fusion of spine (Q76.4)
    EXCLUDES 2   *arthrodesis status (Z98.1)*
               pseudoarthrosis after fusion or arthrodesis (M96.0)

M43.20   Fusion of spine, site unspecified
M43.21   Fusion of spine, occipito-atlanto-axial region
M43.22   Fusion of spine, cervical region
M43.23   Fusion of spine, cervicothoracic region
M43.24   Fusion of spine, thoracic region
M43.25   Fusion of spine, thoracolumbar region
M43.26   Fusion of spine, lumbar region
M43.27   Fusion of spine, lumbosacral region
M43.28   Fusion of spine, sacral and sacrococcygeal region

M43.3   **Recurrent atlantoaxial dislocation with myelopathy**
M43.4   **Other recurrent atlantoaxial dislocation**

✓5ᵗʰ **M43.5 Other recurrent vertebral dislocation**
    EXCLUDES 1   *biomechanical lesions NEC (M99-)*

✓6ᵗʰ **M43.5x Other recurrent vertebral dislocation**
M43.5x2   Other recurrent vertebral dislocation, cervical region
M43.5x3   Other recurrent vertebral dislocation, cervicothoracic region
M43.5x4   Other recurrent vertebral dislocation, thoracic region
M43.5x5   Other recurrent vertebral dislocation, thoracolumbar region
M43.5x6   Other recurrent vertebral dislocation, lumbar region
M43.5x7   Other recurrent vertebral dislocation, lumbosacral region
M43.5x8   Other recurrent vertebral dislocation, sacral and sacrococcygeal region
M43.5x9   Other recurrent vertebral dislocation, site unspecified

M43.6   **Torticollis**
    EXCLUDES 1   *congenital (sternomastoid) torticollis (Q68.0)*
               current injury—see Injury, of spine, by body region
               ocular torticollis (R29.891)
               psychogenic torticollis (F45.8)
               spasmodic torticollis (G24.3)
               torticollis due to birth injury (P15.2)

✓5ᵗʰ **M43.8 Other specified deforming dorsopathies**
    EXCLUDES 2   *kyphosis and lordosis (M40-)*
               scoliosis (M41-)

✓6ᵗʰ **M43.8x Other specified deforming dorsopathies**
M43.8x1   Other specified deforming dorsopathies, occipito-atlanto-axial region
M43.8x2   Other specified deforming dorsopathies, cervical region
M43.8x3   Other specified deforming dorsopathies, cervicothoracic region
M43.8x4   Other specified deforming dorsopathies, thoracic region
M43.8x5   Other specified deforming dorsopathies, thoracolumbar region
M43.8x6   Other specified deforming dorsopathies, lumbar region
M43.8x7   Other specified deforming dorsopathies, lumbosacral region
M43.8x8   Other specified deforming dorsopathies, sacral and sacrococcygeal region
M43.8x9   Other specified deforming dorsopathies, site unspecified

M43.9   **Deforming dorsopathy, unspecified**
    Curvature of spine NOS

Spondylopathies (M45-M49)

✓4ᵗʰ **M45 Ankylosing spondylitis**
    Rheumatoid arthritis of spine
    EXCLUDES 1   *arthropathy in Reiter's disease (M02.3-)*
               juvenile (ankylosing) spondylitis (M08.1)
    EXCLUDES 2   *Behçet's disease (M35.2)*

M45.0   Ankylosing spondylitis of multiple sites in spine
M45.1   Ankylosing spondylitis of occipito-atlanto-axial region
M45.2   Ankylosing spondylitis of cervical region
M45.3   Ankylosing spondylitis of cervicothoracic region
M45.4   Ankylosing spondylitis of thoracic region
M45.5   Ankylosing spondylitis of thoracolumbar region
M45.6   Ankylosing spondylitis lumbar region
M45.7   Ankylosing spondylitis of lumbosacral region
M45.8   Ankylosing spondylitis sacral and sacrococcygeal region
M45.9   Ankylosing spondylitis of unspecified sites in spine

✓4ᵗʰ **M46 Other inflammatory spondylopathies**

✓5ᵗʰ **M46.0 Spinal enthesopathy**
    Disorder of ligamentous or muscular attachments of spine
M46.00   Spinal enthesopathy, site unspecified
M46.01   Spinal enthesopathy, occipito-atlanto-axial region
M46.02   Spinal enthesopathy, cervical region
M46.03   Spinal enthesopathy, cervicothoracic region
M46.04   Spinal enthesopathy, thoracic region
M46.05   Spinal enthesopathy, thoracolumbar region
M46.06   Spinal enthesopathy, lumbar region
M46.07   Spinal enthesopathy, lumbosacral region
M46.08   Spinal enthesopathy, sacral and sacrococcygeal region
M46.09   Spinal enthesopathy, multiple sites in spine

M46.1   **Sacroiliitis, not elsewhere classified**

✓5ᵗʰ **M46.2 Osteomyelitis of vertebra**
M46.20   Osteomyelitis of vertebra, site unspecified
M46.21   Osteomyelitis of vertebra, occipito-atlanto-axial region
M46.22   Osteomyelitis of vertebra, cervical region
M46.23   Osteomyelitis of vertebra, cervicothoracic region
M46.24   Osteomyelitis of vertebra, thoracic region
M46.25   Osteomyelitis of vertebra, thoracolumbar region
M46.26   Osteomyelitis of vertebra, lumbar region
M46.27   Osteomyelitis of vertebra, lumbosacral region
M46.28   Osteomyelitis of vertebra, sacral and sacrococcygeal region

✓5ᵗʰ **M46.3 Infection of intervertebral disc (pyogenic)**
    Use additional code (B95-B97) to identify infectious agent
M46.30   Infection of intervertebral disc (pyogenic), site unspecified
M46.31   Infection of intervertebral disc (pyogenic), occipito-atlanto-axial region
M46.32   Infection of intervertebral disc (pyogenic), cervical region
M46.33   Infection of intervertebral disc (pyogenic), cervicothoracic region
M46.34   Infection of intervertebral disc (pyogenic), thoracic region
M46.35   Infection of intervertebral disc (pyogenic), thoracolumbar region
M46.36   Infection of intervertebral disc (pyogenic), lumbar region
M46.37   Infection of intervertebral disc (pyogenic), lumbosacral region
M46.38   Infection of intervertebral disc (pyogenic), sacral and sacrococcygeal region
M46.39   Infection of intervertebral disc (pyogenic), multiple sites in spine

✓5ᵗʰ **M46.4 Discitis, unspecified**
M46.40   Discitis, unspecified, site unspecified
M46.41   Discitis, unspecified, occipito-atlanto-axial region
M46.42   Discitis, unspecified, cervical region
M46.43   Discitis, unspecified, cervicothoracic region
M46.44   Discitis, unspecified, thoracic region
M46.45   Discitis, unspecified, thoracolumbar region

EXCLUDES 1   Not coded here   EXCLUDES 2   Not included here   *Manifestation Code*

M46.46　Discitis, unspecified, lumbar region
M46.47　Discitis, unspecified, lumbosacral region
M46.48　Discitis, unspecified, sacral and sacrococcygeal region
M46.49　Discitis, unspecified, multiple sites in spine

√5th　M46.5　Other infective spondylopathies
M46.50　Other infective spondylopathies, site unspecified
M46.51　Other infective spondylopathies, occipito-atlanto-axial region
M46.52　Other infective spondylopathies, cervical region
M46.53　Other infective spondylopathies, cervicothoracic region
M46.54　Other infective spondylopathies, thoracic region
M46.55　Other infective spondylopathies, thoracolumbar region
M46.56　Other infective spondylopathies, lumbar region
M46.57　Other infective spondylopathies, lumbosacral region
M46.58　Other infective spondylopathies, sacral and sacrococcygeal region
M46.59　Other infective spondylopathies, multiple sites in spine

√5th　M46.8　Other specified inflammatory spondylopathies
M46.80　Other specified inflammatory spondylopathies, site unspecified
M46.81　Other specified inflammatory spondylopathies, occipito-atlanto-axial region
M46.82　Other specified inflammatory spondylopathies, cervical region
M46.83　Other specified inflammatory spondylopathies, cervicothoracic region
M46.84　Other specified inflammatory spondylopathies, thoracic region
M46.85　Other specified inflammatory spondylopathies, thoracolumbar region
M46.86　Other specified inflammatory spondylopathies, lumbar region
M46.87　Other specified inflammatory spondylopathies, lumbosacral region
M46.88　Other specified inflammatory spondylopathies, sacral and sacrococcygeal region
M46.89　Other specified inflammatory spondylopathies, multiple sites in spine

√5th　M46.9　Unspecified inflammatory spondylopathy
M46.90　Unspecified inflammatory spondylopathy, site unspecified
M46.91　Unspecified inflammatory spondylopathy, occipito-atlanto-axial region
M46.92　Unspecified inflammatory spondylopathy, cervical region
M46.93　Unspecified inflammatory spondylopathy, cervicothoracic region
M46.94　Unspecified inflammatory spondylopathy, thoracic region
M46.95　Unspecified inflammatory spondylopathy, thoracolumbar region
M46.96　Unspecified inflammatory spondylopathy, lumbar region
M46.97　Unspecified inflammatory spondylopathy, lumbosacral region
M46.98　Unspecified inflammatory spondylopathy, sacral and sacrococcygeal region
M46.99　Unspecified inflammatory spondylopathy, multiple sites in spine

√4th　M47　Spondylosis
INCLUDES　arthrosis or osteoarthritis of spine
degeneration of facet joints

√5th　M47.0　Anterior spinal and vertebral artery compression syndromes
√6th　M47.01　Anterior spinal artery compression syndromes
M47.011　Anterior spinal artery compression syndromes, occipito-atlanto-axial region
M47.012　Anterior spinal artery compression syndromes, cervical region
M47.013　Anterior spinal artery compression syndromes, cervicothoracic region

M47.014　Anterior spinal artery compression syndromes, thoracic region
M47.015　Anterior spinal artery compression syndromes, thoracolumbar region
M47.016　Anterior spinal artery compression syndromes, lumbar region
M47.019　Anterior spinal artery compression syndromes, site unspecified
√6th　M47.02　Vertebral artery compression syndromes
M47.021　Vertebral artery compression syndromes, occipito-atlanto-axial region
M47.022　Vertebral artery compression syndromes, cervical region
M47.029　Vertebral artery compression syndromes, site unspecified

√5th　M47.1　Other spondylosis with myelopathy
Spondylogenic compression of spinal cord
EXCLUDES 1　vertebral subluxation (M43.3-M43.5x9)
M47.10　Other spondylosis with myelopathy, site unspecified
M47.11　Other spondylosis with myelopathy, occipito-atlanto-axial region
M47.12　Other spondylosis with myelopathy, cervical region
M47.13　Other spondylosis with myelopathy, cervicothoracic region
M47.14　Other spondylosis with myelopathy, thoracic region
M47.15　Other spondylosis with myelopathy, thoracolumbar region
M47.16　Other spondylosis with myelopathy, lumbar region
M47.17　Other spondylosis with myelopathy, lumbosacral region
M47.18　Other spondylosis with myelopathy, sacral and sacrococcygeal region

√5th　M47.2　Other spondylosis with radiculopathy
M47.20　Other spondylosis with radiculopathy, site unspecified
M47.21　Other spondylosis with radiculopathy, occipito-atlanto-axial region
M47.22　Other spondylosis with radiculopathy, cervical region
M47.23　Other spondylosis with radiculopathy, cervicothoracic region
M47.24　Other spondylosis with radiculopathy, thoracic region
M47.25　Other spondylosis with radiculopathy, thoracolumbar region
M47.26　Other spondylosis with radiculopathy, lumbar region
M47.27　Other spondylosis with radiculopathy, lumbosacral region
M47.28　Other spondylosis with radiculopathy, sacral and sacrococcygeal region

√5th　M47.8　Other spondylosis
√6th　M47.81　Spondylosis without myelopathy or radiculopathy
M47.811　Spondylosis without myelopathy or radiculopathy, occipito-atlanto-axial region
M47.812　Spondylosis without myelopathy or radiculopathy, cervical region
M47.813　Spondylosis without myelopathy or radiculopathy, cervicothoracic region
M47.814　Spondylosis without myelopathy or radiculopathy, thoracic region
M47.815　Spondylosis without myelopathy or radiculopathy, thoracolumbar region
M47.816　Spondylosis without myelopathy or radiculopathy, lumbar region
M47.817　Spondylosis without myelopathy or radiculopathy, lumbosacral region
M47.818　Spondylosis without myelopathy or radiculopathy, sacral and sacrococcygeal region
M47.819　Spondylosis without myelopathy or radiculopathy, site unspecified

✔ Appropriate additional character required　　　√x7th Requires 7th character, placeholder x must fill empty characters

✓6ᵗʰ M47.89 Other spondylosis
   M47.891 Other spondylosis, occipito-atlanto-axial region
   M47.892 Other spondylosis, cervical region
   M47.893 Other spondylosis, cervicothoracic region
   M47.894 Other spondylosis, thoracic region
   M47.895 Other spondylosis, thoracolumbar region
   M47.896 Other spondylosis, lumbar region
   M47.897 Other spondylosis, lumbosacral region
   M47.898 Other spondylosis, sacral and sacrococcygeal region
   M47.899 Other spondylosis, site unspecified
  M47.9 Spondylosis, unspecified

✓4ᵗʰ M48 Other spondylopathies

✓5ᵗʰ M48.0 Spinal stenosis
Caudal stenosis
   M48.00 Spinal stenosis, site unspecified
   M48.01 Spinal stenosis, occipito-atlanto-axial region
   M48.02 Spinal stenosis, cervical region
   M48.03 Spinal stenosis, cervicothoracic region
   M48.04 Spinal stenosis, thoracic region
   M48.05 Spinal stenosis, thoracolumbar region
   M48.06 Spinal stenosis, lumbar region
   M48.07 Spinal stenosis, lumbosacral region
   M48.08 Spinal stenosis, sacral and sacrococcygeal region

✓5ᵗʰ M48.1 Ankylosing hyperostosis [Forestier]
Diffuse idiopathic skeletal hyperostosis [DISH]
   M48.10 Ankylosing hyperostosis [Forestier], site unspecified
   M48.11 Ankylosing hyperostosis [Forestier], occipito-atlanto-axial region
   M48.12 Ankylosing hyperostosis [Forestier], cervical region
   M48.13 Ankylosing hyperostosis [Forestier], cervicothoracic region
   M48.14 Ankylosing hyperostosis [Forestier], thoracic region
   M48.15 Ankylosing hyperostosis [Forestier], thoracolumbar region
   M48.16 Ankylosing hyperostosis [Forestier], lumbar region
   M48.17 Ankylosing hyperostosis [Forestier], lumbosacral region
   M48.18 Ankylosing hyperostosis [Forestier], sacral and sacrococcygeal region
   M48.19 Ankylosing hyperostosis [Forestier], multiple sites in spine

✓5ᵗʰ M48.2 Kissing spine
   M48.20 Kissing spine, site unspecified
   M48.21 Kissing spine, occipito-atlanto-axial region
   M48.22 Kissing spine, cervical region
   M48.23 Kissing spine, cervicothoracic region
   M48.24 Kissing spine, thoracic region
   M48.25 Kissing spine, thoracolumbar region
   M48.26 Kissing spine, lumbar region
   M48.27 Kissing spine, lumbosacral region

✓5ᵗʰ M48.3 Traumatic spondylopathy
   M48.30 Traumatic spondylopathy, site unspecified
   M48.31 Traumatic spondylopathy, occipito-atlanto-axial region
   M48.32 Traumatic spondylopathy, cervical region
   M48.33 Traumatic spondylopathy, cervicothoracic region
   M48.34 Traumatic spondylopathy, thoracic region
   M48.35 Traumatic spondylopathy, thoracolumbar region
   M48.36 Traumatic spondylopathy, lumbar region
   M48.37 Traumatic spondylopathy, lumbosacral region
   M48.38 Traumatic spondylopathy, sacral and sacrococcygeal region

✓5ᵗʰ M48.4 Fatigue fracture of vertebra
Stress fracture of vertebra
EXCLUDES 1   pathological fracture NOS (M84.4-)
    pathological fracture of vertebra due to neoplasm (M84.58)
    pathological fracture of vertebra due to other diagnosis (M84.68)
    pathological fracture of vertebra due to osteoporosis (M80-)
    traumatic fracture of vertebrae (S12.0-S12.3-, S22.0-, S32.0-)

The appropriate 7th character is to be added to each code from subcategory M48.4.
A   initial encounter for fracture
D   subsequent encounter for fracture with routine healing
G   subsequent encounter for fracture with delayed healing
S   sequela of fracture

  ✓x7ᵗʰ M48.40 Fatigue fracture of vertebra, site unspecified
  ✓x7ᵗʰ M48.41 Fatigue fracture of vertebra, occipito-atlanto-axial region
  ✓x7ᵗʰ M48.42 Fatigue fracture of vertebra, cervical region
  ✓x7ᵗʰ M48.43 Fatigue fracture of vertebra, cervicothoracic region
  ✓x7ᵗʰ M48.44 Fatigue fracture of vertebra, thoracic region
  ✓x7ᵗʰ M48.45 Fatigue fracture of vertebra, thoracolumbar region
  ✓x7ᵗʰ M48.46 Fatigue fracture of vertebra, lumbar region
  ✓x7ᵗʰ M48.47 Fatigue fracture of vertebra, lumbosacral region
  ✓x7ᵗʰ M48.48 Fatigue fracture of vertebra, sacral and sacrococcygeal region

✓5ᵗʰ M48.5 Collapsed vertebra, not elsewhere classified
Collapsed vertebra NOS
Wedging of vertebra NOS
EXCLUDES 1   current injury—see Injury of spine, by body region
    fatigue fracture of vertebra (M48.4)
    pathological fracture of vertebra due to neoplasm (M84.58)
    pathological fracture of vertebra due to other diagnosis (M84.68)
    pathological fracture of vertebra due to osteoporosis (M80-)
    pathological fracture NOS (M84.4-)
    stress fracture of vertebra (M48.4-)
    traumatic fracture of vertebra (S12-, S22-, S32-)

The appropriate 7th character is to be added to each code from subcategory M48.5.
A   initial encounter for fracture
D   subsequent encounter for fracture with routine healing
G   subsequent encounter for fracture with delayed healing
S   sequela of fracture

  ✓x7ᵗʰ M48.50 Collapsed vertebra, not elsewhere classified, site unspecified
  ✓x7ᵗʰ M48.51 Collapsed vertebra, not elsewhere classified, occipito-atlanto-axial region
  ✓x7ᵗʰ M48.52 Collapsed vertebra, not elsewhere classified, cervical region
  ✓x7ᵗʰ M48.53 Collapsed vertebra, not elsewhere classified, cervicothoracic region
  ✓x7ᵗʰ M48.54 Collapsed vertebra, not elsewhere classified, thoracic region
  ✓x7ᵗʰ M48.55 Collapsed vertebra, not elsewhere classified, thoracolumbar region
  ✓x7ᵗʰ M48.56 Collapsed vertebra, not elsewhere classified, lumbar region
  ✓x7ᵗʰ M48.57 Collapsed vertebra, not elsewhere classified, lumbosacral region
  ✓x7ᵗʰ M48.58 Collapsed vertebra, not elsewhere classified, sacral and sacrococcygeal region

✓5ᵗʰ M48.8 Other specified spondylopathies
Ossification of posterior longitudinal ligament
  ✓6ᵗʰ M48.8x Other specified spondylopathies
    M48.8x1 Other specified spondylopathies, occipito-atlanto-axial region

EXCLUDES 1 Not coded here   EXCLUDES 2 Not included here   *Manifestation Code*

M48.8x2   **Other specified spondylopathies, cervical region**

M48.8x3   **Other specified spondylopathies, cervicothoracic region**

M48.8x4   **Other specified spondylopathies, thoracic region**

M48.8x5   **Other specified spondylopathies, thoracolumbar region**

M48.8x6   **Other specified spondylopathies, lumbar region**

M48.8x7   **Other specified spondylopathies, lumbosacral region**

M48.8x8   **Other specified spondylopathies, sacral and sacrococcygeal region**

M48.8x9   **Other specified spondylopathies, site unspecified**

M48.9   **Spondylopathy, unspecified**

✓4ᵗʰ M49 Spondylopathies in diseases classified elsewhere

Curvature of spine in diseases classified elsewhere
Deformity of spine in diseases classified elsewhere
Kyphosis in diseases classified elsewhere
Scoliosis in diseases classified elsewhere
Spondylopathy in diseases classified elsewhere

> **EXCLUDES 1**   *curvature of spine in tuberculosis [Pott's] (A18.01)*
> *enteropathic arthropathies (M07-)*
> *neuropathic spondylopathy (in):*
>   *nonsyphilitic NEC (G98.0)*
>   *syringomyelia (G95.0)*
>   *tabes dorsalis (A52.11)*
> *spondylitis (in):*
>   *gonococcal (A54.41)*
>   *syphilis (acquired) (A52.77)*
>   *neuropathic [tabes dorsalis] (A52.11)*
>   *tuberculosis (A18.01)*
>   *typhoid fever (A01.05)*

> *Code first underlying disease, such as:*
>   *brucellosis (A23-)*
>   *Charcôt-Marie-Tooth disease (G60.0)*
>   *enterobacterial infections (A01-A04)*
>   *osteitis fibrosa cystica (E21.0)*

✓5ᵗʰ M49.8 Spondylopathy in diseases classified elsewhere

M49.80   *Spondylopathy in diseases classified elsewhere, site unspecified*

M49.81   *Spondylopathy in diseases classified elsewhere, occipito-atlanto-axial region*

M49.82   *Spondylopathy in diseases classified elsewhere, cervical region*

M49.83   *Spondylopathy in diseases classified elsewhere, cervicothoracic region*

M49.84   *Spondylopathy in diseases classified elsewhere, thoracic region*

M49.85   *Spondylopathy in diseases classified elsewhere, thoracolumbar region*

M49.86   *Spondylopathy in diseases classified elsewhere, lumbar region*

M49.87   *Spondylopathy in diseases classified elsewhere, lumbosacral region*

M49.88   *Spondylopathy in diseases classified elsewhere, sacral and sacrococcygeal region*

M49.89   *Spondylopathy in diseases classified elsewhere, multiple sites in spine*

Other dorsopathies (M50-M54)

> **EXCLUDES 1**   *current injury—see injury of spine by body region*
> *discitis NOS (M46.4-)*

✓4ᵗʰ M50 Cervical disc disorders

> **INCLUDES**   cervicothoracic disc disorders with cervicalgia
> cervicothoracic disc disorders

> **NOTE**   Code to the most superior level of disorder

✓5ᵗʰ M50.0 Cervical disc disorder with myelopathy

M50.00   **Cervical disc disorder with myelopathy, unspecified cervical region**

M50.01   **Cervical disc disorder with myelopathy, occipito-atlanto-axial region**

M50.02   **Cervical disc disorder with myelopathy, mid-cervical region**

M50.03   **Cervical disc disorder with myelopathy, cervicothoracic region**

✓5ᵗʰ M50.1 Cervical disc disorder with radiculopathy

> **EXCLUDES 2**   *brachial radiculitis NOS (M54.13)*

M50.10   **Cervical disc disorder with radiculopathy, unspecified cervical region**

M50.11   **Cervical disc disorder with radiculopathy, occipito-atlanto-axial region**

M50.12   **Cervical disc disorder with radiculopathy, mid-cervical region**

M50.13   **Cervical disc disorder with radiculopathy, cervicothoracic region**

✓5ᵗʰ M50.2 Other cervical disc displacement

M50.20   **Other cervical disc displacement, unspecified cervical region**

M50.21   **Other cervical disc displacement, occipito-atlanto-axial region**

M50.22   **Other cervical disc displacement, mid-cervical region**

M50.23   **Other cervical disc displacement, cervicothoracic region**

✓5ᵗʰ M50.3 Other cervical disc degeneration

M50.30   **Other cervical disc degeneration, unspecified cervical region**

M50.31   **Other cervical disc degeneration, occipito-atlanto-axial region**

M50.32   **Other cervical disc degeneration, mid-cervical region**

M50.33   **Other cervical disc degeneration, cervicothoracic region**

✓5ᵗʰ M50.8 Other cervical disc disorders

M50.80   **Other cervical disc disorders, unspecified cervical region**

M50.81   **Other cervical disc disorders, occipito-atlanto-axial region**

M50.82   **Other cervical disc disorders, mid-cervical region**

M50.83   **Other cervical disc disorders, cervicothoracic region**

✓5ᵗʰ M50.9 Cervical disc disorder, unspecified

M50.90   **Cervical disc disorder, unspecified, unspecified cervical region**

M50.91   **Cervical disc disorder, unspecified, occipito-atlanto-axial region**

M50.92   **Cervical disc disorder, unspecified, mid-cervical region**

M50.93   **Cervical disc disorder, unspecified, cervicothoracic region**

✓4ᵗʰ M51 Thoracic, thoracolumbar, and lumbosacral intervertebral disc disorders

> **EXCLUDES 2**   *cervical and cervicothoracic disc disorders (M50-)*
> *sacral and sacrococcygeal disorders (M53.3)*

✓5ᵗʰ M51.0 Thoracic, thoracolumbar and lumbosacral intervertebral disc disorders with myelopathy

M51.04   **Intervertebral disc disorders with myelopathy, thoracic region**

M51.05   **Intervertebral disc disorders with myelopathy, thoracolumbar region**

M51.06   **Intervertebral disc disorders with myelopathy, lumbar region**

M51.07   **Intervertebral disc disorders with myelopathy, lumbosacral region**

✓5ᵗʰ M51.1 Thoracic, thoracolumbar and lumbosacral intervertebral disc disorders with radiculopathy

Sciatica due to intervertebral disc disorder

> **EXCLUDES 1**   *lumbar radiculitis NOS (M54.16)*
> *sciatica NOS (M54.3)*

M51.14   **Intervertebral disc disorders with radiculopathy, thoracic region**

M51.15   **Intervertebral disc disorders with radiculopathy, thoracolumbar region**

M51.16   **Intervertebral disc disorders with radiculopathy, lumbar region**

M51.17   **Intervertebral disc disorders with radiculopathy, lumbosacral region**

✓5ᵗʰ M51.2 Other thoracic, thoracolumbar and lumbosacral intervertebral disc displacement

Lumbago due to displacement of intervertebral disc

M51.24   **Other intervertebral disc displacement, thoracic region**

☑ Appropriate additional character required   ✓x7ᵗʰ Requires 7th character, placeholder x must fill empty characters

M51.25 Other intervertebral disc displacement, thoracolumbar region

M51.26 Other intervertebral disc displacement, lumbar region

M51.27 Other intervertebral disc displacement, lumbosacral region

√5ᵗʰ **M51.3 Other thoracic, thoracolumbar and lumbosacral intervertebral disc degeneration**

M51.34 Other intervertebral disc degeneration, thoracic region

M51.35 Other intervertebral disc degeneration, thoracolumbar region

M51.36 Other intervertebral disc degeneration, lumbar region

M51.37 Other intervertebral disc degeneration, lumbosacral region

√5ᵗʰ **M51.4 Schmorl's nodes**

M51.44 Schmorl's nodes, thoracic region

M51.45 Schmorl's nodes, thoracolumbar region

M51.46 Schmorl's nodes, lumbar region

M51.47 Schmorl's nodes, lumbosacral region

√5ᵗʰ **M51.8 Other thoracic, thoracolumbar and lumbosacral intervertebral disc disorders**

M51.84 Other intervertebral disc disorders, thoracic region

M51.85 Other intervertebral disc disorders, thoracolumbar region

M51.86 Other intervertebral disc disorders, lumbar region

M51.87 Other intervertebral disc disorders, lumbosacral region

M51.9 Unspecified thoracic, thoracolumbar and lumbosacral intervertebral disc disorder

√4ᵗʰ **M53 Other and unspecified dorsopathies, not elsewhere classified**

M53.0 Cervicocranial syndrome
Posterior cervical sympathetic syndrome

M53.1 Cervicobrachial syndrome
EXCLUDES 2   *cervical disc disorder (M50-)*
thoracic outlet syndrome (G54.0)

√5ᵗʰ **M53.2 Spinal instabilities**
  √6ᵗʰ **M53.2x Spinal instabilities**

M53.2x1 Spinal instabilities, occipito-atlanto-axial region

M53.2x2 Spinal instabilities, cervical region

M53.2x3 Spinal instabilities, cervicothoracic region

M53.2x4 Spinal instabilities, thoracic region

M53.2x5 Spinal instabilities, thoracolumbar region

M53.2x6 Spinal instabilities, lumbar region

M53.2x7 Spinal instabilities, lumbosacral region

M53.2x8 Spinal instabilities, sacral and sacrococcygeal region

M53.2x9 Spinal instabilities, site unspecified

M53.3 Sacrococcygeal disorders, not elsewhere classified
Coccygodynia

√5ᵗʰ **M53.8 Other specified dorsopathies**

M53.80 Other specified dorsopathies, site unspecified

M53.81 Other specified dorsopathies, occipito-atlanto-axial region

M53.82 Other specified dorsopathies, cervical region

M53.83 Other specified dorsopathies, cervicothoracic region

M53.84 Other specified dorsopathies, thoracic region

M53.85 Other specified dorsopathies, thoracolumbar region

M53.86 Other specified dorsopathies, lumbar region

M53.87 Other specified dorsopathies, lumbosacral region

M53.88 Other specified dorsopathies, sacral and sacrococcygeal region

M53.9 Dorsopathy, unspecified

√4ᵗʰ **M54 Dorsalgia**
EXCLUDES 1   *psychogenic dorsalgia (F45.41)*

√5ᵗʰ **M54.0 Panniculitis affecting regions of neck and back**
EXCLUDES 1   *lupus panniculitis (L93.2)*
panniculitis NOS (M79.3)
relapsing [Weber-Christian] panniculitis (M35.6)

M54.00 Panniculitis affecting regions of neck and back, site unspecified

M54.01 Panniculitis affecting regions of neck and back, occipito-atlanto-axial region

M54.02 Panniculitis affecting regions of neck and back, cervical region

M54.03 Panniculitis affecting regions of neck and back, cervicothoracic region

M54.04 Panniculitis affecting regions of neck and back, thoracic region

M54.05 Panniculitis affecting regions of neck and back, thoracolumbar region

M54.06 Panniculitis affecting regions of neck and back, lumbar region

M54.07 Panniculitis affecting regions of neck and back, lumbosacral region

M54.08 Panniculitis affecting regions of neck and back, sacral and sacrococcygeal region

M54.09 Panniculitis affecting regions, neck and back, multiple sites in spine

√5ᵗʰ **M54.1 Radiculopathy**
Brachial neuritis or radiculitis NOS
Lumbar neuritis or radiculitis NOS
Lumbosacral neuritis or radiculitis NOS
Thoracic neuritis or radiculitis NOS
Radiculitis NOS
EXCLUDES 1   *neuralgia and neuritis NOS (M79.2)*
radiculopathy with cervical disc disorder (M50.1)
radiculopathy with lumbar and other intervertebral disc disorder (M51.1-)
radiculopathy with spondylosis (M47.2-)

M54.10 Radiculopathy, site unspecified

M54.11 Radiculopathy, occipito-atlanto-axial region

M54.12 Radiculopathy, cervical region

M54.13 Radiculopathy, cervicothoracic region

M54.14 Radiculopathy, thoracic region

M54.15 Radiculopathy, thoracolumbar region

M54.16 Radiculopathy, lumbar region

M54.17 Radiculopathy, lumbosacral region

M54.18 Radiculopathy, sacral and sacrococcygeal region

M54.2 Cervicalgia
EXCLUDES 1   *cervicalgia due to intervertebral cervical disc disorder (M50-)*

√5ᵗʰ **M54.3 Sciatica**
EXCLUDES 1   *lesion of sciatic nerve (G57.0)*
sciatica due to intervertebral disc disorder (M51.1-)
sciatica with lumbago (M54.4-)

M54.30 Sciatica, unspecified side

M54.31 Sciatica, right side

M54.32 Sciatica, left side

√5ᵗʰ **M54.4 Lumbago with sciatica**
EXCLUDES 1   *lumbago with sciatica due to intervertebral disc disorder (M51.1-)*

M54.40 Lumbago with sciatica, unspecified side

M54.41 Lumbago with sciatica, right side

M54.42 Lumbago with sciatica, left side

M54.5 Low back pain
Loin pain
Lumbago NOS
EXCLUDES 1   *low back strain S39.012*
lumbago due to intervertebral disc displacement (M51.2-)
lumbago with sciatica (M54.4-)

M54.6 Pain in thoracic spine
EXCLUDES 1   *pain in thoracic spine due to intervertebral disc disorder (M51-)*

√5ᵗʰ **M54.8 Other dorsalgia**
EXCLUDES 1   *dorsalgia in thoracic region (M54.6)*
low back pain (M54.5)

M54.81 Occipital neuralgia

M54.89 Other dorsalgia

EXCLUDES 1   Not coded here   EXCLUDES 2   Not included here   *Manifestation Code*

M54.9 **Dorsalgia, unspecified**
Backache NOS
Back pain NOS

SOFT TISSUE DISORDERS (M60-M79)

Disorders of muscles (M60-M63)

EXCLUDES 1   *dermatopolymyositis (M33-)*
muscular dystrophies and myopathies (G71-G72)
myopathy in:
    amyloidosis (E85-)
    polyarteritis nodosa (M30.0)
    rheumatoid arthritis (M05.32)
    scleroderma (M34-)
    Sjögren's syndrome (M35.03)
    systemic lupus erythematosus (M32-)

√4th **M60 Myositis**
     EXCLUDES 2   *inclusion body myositis [IBM] (G72.41)*
√5th   **M60.0 Infective myositis**
     Tropical pyomyositis
     Use additional code (B95-B97) to identify infectious agent
√6th   **M60.00 Infective myositis, unspecified site**
     M60.000 Infective myositis, unspecified right arm
        Infective myositis, right upper limb NOS
     M60.001 Infective myositis, unspecified left arm
        Infective myositis, left upper limb NOS
     M60.002 Infective myositis, unspecified arm
        Infective myositis, upper limb NOS
     M60.003 Infective myositis, unspecified right leg
        Infective myositis, right lower limb NOS
     M60.004 Infective myositis, unspecified left leg
        Infective myositis, left lower limb NOS
     M60.005 Infective myositis, unspecified leg
        Infective myositis, lower limb NOS
     M60.009 Infective myositis, unspecified site
√6th   **M60.01 Infective myositis, shoulder**
     M60.011 Infective myositis, right shoulder
     M60.012 Infective myositis, left shoulder
     M60.019 Infective myositis, unspecified shoulder
√6th   **M60.02 Infective myositis, upper arm**
     M60.021 Infective myositis, right upper arm
     M60.022 Infective myositis, left upper arm
     M60.029 Infective myositis, unspecified upper arm
√6th   **M60.03 Infective myositis, forearm**
     M60.031 Infective myositis, right forearm
     M60.032 Infective myositis, left forearm
     M60.039 Infective myositis, unspecified forearm
√6th   **M60.04 Infective myositis, hand and fingers**
     M60.041 Infective myositis, right hand
     M60.042 Infective myositis, left hand
     M60.043 Infective myositis, unspecified hand
     M60.044 Infective myositis, right finger(s)
     M60.045 Infective myositis, left finger(s)
     M60.046 Infective myositis, unspecified finger(s)
√6th   **M60.05 Infective myositis, thigh**
     M60.051 Infective myositis, right thigh
     M60.052 Infective myositis, left thigh
     M60.059 Infective myositis, unspecified thigh
√6th   **M60.06 Infective myositis, lower leg**
     M60.061 Infective myositis, right lower leg
     M60.062 Infective myositis, left lower leg
     M60.069 Infective myositis, unspecified lower leg
√6th   **M60.07 Infective myositis, ankle, foot and toes**
     M60.070 Infective myositis, right ankle
     M60.071 Infective myositis, left ankle
     M60.072 Infective myositis, unspecified ankle
     M60.073 Infective myositis, right foot
     M60.074 Infective myositis, left foot
     M60.075 Infective myositis, unspecified foot
     M60.076 Infective myositis, right toe(s)
     M60.077 Infective myositis, left toe(s)
     M60.078 Infective myositis, unspecified toe(s)
   M60.08 Infective myositis, other site
   M60.09 Infective myositis, multiple sites

√5th **M60.1 Interstitial myositis**
   M60.10 Interstitial myositis of unspecified site
√6th   **M60.11 Interstitial myositis, shoulder**
     M60.111 Interstitial myositis, right shoulder
     M60.112 Interstitial myositis, left shoulder
     M60.119 Interstitial myositis, unspecified shoulder
√6th   **M60.12 Interstitial myositis, upper arm**
     M60.121 Interstitial myositis, right upper arm
     M60.122 Interstitial myositis, left upper arm
     M60.129 Interstitial myositis, unspecified upper arm
√6th   **M60.13 Interstitial myositis, forearm**
     M60.131 Interstitial myositis, right forearm
     M60.132 Interstitial myositis, left forearm
     M60.139 Interstitial myositis, unspecified forearm
√6th   **M60.14 Interstitial myositis, hand**
     M60.141 Interstitial myositis, right hand
     M60.142 Interstitial myositis, left hand
     M60.149 Interstitial myositis, unspecified hand
√6th   **M60.15 Interstitial myositis, thigh**
     M60.151 Interstitial myositis, right thigh
     M60.152 Interstitial myositis, left thigh
     M60.159 Interstitial myositis, unspecified thigh
√6th   **M60.16 Interstitial myositis, lower leg**
     M60.161 Interstitial myositis, right lower leg
     M60.162 Interstitial myositis, left lower leg
     M60.169 Interstitial myositis, unspecified lower leg
√6th   **M60.17 Interstitial myositis, ankle and foot**
     M60.171 Interstitial myositis, right ankle and foot
     M60.172 Interstitial myositis, left ankle and foot
     M60.179 Interstitial myositis, unspecified ankle and foot
   M60.18 Interstitial myositis, other site
   M60.19 Interstitial myositis, multiple sites
√5th **M60.2 Foreign body granuloma of soft tissue, not elsewhere classified**
     Use additional code to identify the type of retained foreign body (Z18.-)
     EXCLUDES 1   *foreign body granuloma of skin and subcutaneous tissue (L92.3)*
   M60.20 Foreign body granuloma of soft tissue, not elsewhere classified, unspecified site
√6th   **M60.21 Foreign body granuloma of soft tissue, not elsewhere classified, shoulder**
     M60.211 Foreign body granuloma of soft tissue, not elsewhere classified, right shoulder
     M60.212 Foreign body granuloma of soft tissue, not elsewhere classified, left shoulder
     M60.219 Foreign body granuloma of soft tissue, not elsewhere classified, unspecified shoulder
√6th   **M60.22 Foreign body granuloma of soft tissue, not elsewhere classified, upper arm**
     M60.221 Foreign body granuloma of soft tissue, not elsewhere classified, right upper arm
     M60.222 Foreign body granuloma of soft tissue, not elsewhere classified, left upper arm
     M60.229 Foreign body granuloma of soft tissue, not elsewhere classified, unspecified upper arm
√6th   **M60.23 Foreign body granuloma of soft tissue, not elsewhere classified, forearm**
     M60.231 Foreign body granuloma of soft tissue, not elsewhere classified, right forearm
     M60.232 Foreign body granuloma of soft tissue, not elsewhere classified, left forearm
     M60.239 Foreign body granuloma of soft tissue, not elsewhere classified, unspecified forearm
√6th   **M60.24 Foreign body granuloma of soft tissue, not elsewhere classified, hand**
     M60.241 Foreign body granuloma of soft tissue, not elsewhere classified, right hand

M60.242 Foreign body granuloma of soft tissue, not elsewhere classified, left hand	
M60.249 Foreign body granuloma of soft tissue, not elsewhere classified, unspecified hand	
✓6th **M60.25** Foreign body granuloma of soft tissue, not elsewhere classified, thigh	
M60.251 Foreign body granuloma of soft tissue, not elsewhere classified, right thigh	
M60.252 Foreign body granuloma of soft tissue, not elsewhere classified, left thigh	
M60.259 Foreign body granuloma of soft tissue, not elsewhere classified, unspecified thigh	
✓6th **M60.26** Foreign body granuloma of soft tissue, not elsewhere classified, lower leg	
M60.261 Foreign body granuloma of soft tissue, not elsewhere classified, right lower leg	
M60.262 Foreign body granuloma of soft tissue, not elsewhere classified, left lower leg	
M60.269 Foreign body granuloma of soft tissue, not elsewhere classified, unspecified lower leg	
✓6th **M60.27** Foreign body granuloma of soft tissue, not elsewhere classified, ankle and foot	
M60.271 Foreign body granuloma of soft tissue, not elsewhere classified, right ankle and foot	
M60.272 Foreign body granuloma of soft tissue, not elsewhere classified, left ankle and foot	
M60.279 Foreign body granuloma of soft tissue, not elsewhere classified, unspecified ankle and foot	
M60.28 Foreign body granuloma of soft tissue, not elsewhere classified, other site	
✓5th **M60.8** Other myositis	
M60.80 Other myositis, unspecified site	
✓6th **M60.81** Other myositis shoulder	
M60.811 Other myositis, right shoulder	
M60.812 Other myositis, left shoulder	
M60.819 Other myositis, unspecified shoulder	
✓6th **M60.82** Other myositis, upper arm	
M60.821 Other myositis, right upper arm	
M60.822 Other myositis, left upper arm	
M60.829 Other myositis, unspecified upper arm	
✓6th **M60.83** Other myositis, forearm	
M60.831 Other myositis, right forearm	
M60.832 Other myositis, left forearm	
M60.839 Other myositis, unspecified forearm	
✓6th **M60.84** Other myositis, hand	
M60.841 Other myositis, right hand	
M60.842 Other myositis, left hand	
M60.849 Other myositis, unspecified hand	
✓6th **M60.85** Other myositis, thigh	
M60.851 Other myositis, right thigh	
M60.852 Other myositis, left thigh	
M60.859 Other myositis, unspecified thigh	
✓6th **M60.86** Other myositis, lower leg	
M60.861 Other myositis, right lower leg	
M60.862 Other myositis, left lower leg	
M60.869 Other myositis, unspecified lower leg	
✓6th **M60.87** Other myositis, ankle and foot	
M60.871 Other myositis, right ankle and foot	
M60.872 Other myositis, left ankle and foot	
M60.879 Other myositis, unspecified ankle and foot	
M60.88 Other myositis, other site	
M60.89 Other myositis, multiple sites	
M60.9 Myositis, unspecified	
✓4th **M61** **Calcification and ossification of muscle**	
✓5th **M61.0** Myositis ossificans traumatica	
M61.00 Myositis ossificans traumatica, unspecified site	
✓6th **M61.01** Myositis ossificans traumatica, shoulder	
M61.011 Myositis ossificans traumatica, right shoulder	

M61.012 Myositis ossificans traumatica, left shoulder

M61.019 Myositis ossificans traumatica, unspecified shoulder

✓6th **M61.02** Myositis ossificans traumatica, upper arm

M61.021 Myositis ossificans traumatica, right upper arm

M61.022 Myositis ossificans traumatica, left upper arm

M61.029 Myositis ossificans traumatica, unspecified upper arm

✓6th **M61.03** Myositis ossificans traumatica, forearm

M61.031 Myositis ossificans traumatica, right forearm

M61.032 Myositis ossificans traumatica, left forearm

M61.039 Myositis ossificans traumatica, unspecified forearm

✓6th **M61.04** Myositis ossificans traumatica, hand

M61.041 Myositis ossificans traumatica, right hand

M61.042 Myositis ossificans traumatica, left hand

M61.049 Myositis ossificans traumatica, unspecified hand

✓6th **M61.05** Myositis ossificans traumatica, thigh

M61.051 Myositis ossificans traumatica, right thigh

M61.052 Myositis ossificans traumatica, left thigh

M61.059 Myositis ossificans traumatica, unspecified thigh

✓6th **M61.06** Myositis ossificans traumatica, lower leg

M61.061 Myositis ossificans traumatica, right lower leg

M61.062 Myositis ossificans traumatica, left lower leg

M61.069 Myositis ossificans traumatica, unspecified lower leg

✓6th **M61.07** Myositis ossificans traumatica, ankle and foot

M61.071 Myositis ossificans traumatica, right ankle and foot

M61.072 Myositis ossificans traumatica, left ankle and foot

M61.079 Myositis ossificans traumatica, unspecified ankle and foot

M61.08 Myositis ossificans traumatica, other site

M61.09 Myositis ossificans traumatica, multiple sites

✓5th **M61.1** Myositis ossificans progressiva

Fibrodysplasia ossificans progressiva

M61.10 Myositis ossificans progressiva, unspecified site

✓6th **M61.11** Myositis ossificans progressiva, shoulder

M61.111 Myositis ossificans progressiva, right shoulder

M61.112 Myositis ossificans progressiva, left shoulder

M61.119 Myositis ossificans progressiva, unspecified shoulder

✓6th **M61.12** Myositis ossificans progressiva, upper arm

M61.121 Myositis ossificans progressiva, right upper arm

M61.122 Myositis ossificans progressiva, left upper arm

M61.129 Myositis ossificans progressiva, unspecified arm

✓6th **M61.13** Myositis ossificans progressiva, forearm

M61.131 Myositis ossificans progressiva, right forearm

M61.132 Myositis ossificans progressiva, left forearm

M61.139 Myositis ossificans progressiva, unspecified forearm

✓6th **M61.14** Myositis ossificans progressiva, hand and finger(s)

M61.141 Myositis ossificans progressiva, right hand

M61.142 Myositis ossificans progressiva, left hand

M61.143 Myositis ossificans progressiva, unspecified hand

EXCLUDES 1 Not coded here   EXCLUDES 2 Not included here   *Manifestation Code*

M61.144 Myositis ossificans progressiva, right finger(s)

M61.145 Myositis ossificans progressiva, left finger(s)

M61.146 Myositis ossificans progressiva, unspecified finger(s)

√6ᵗʰ M61.15 Myositis ossificans progressiva, thigh

M61.151 Myositis ossificans progressiva, right thigh

M61.152 Myositis ossificans progressiva, left thigh

M61.159 Myositis ossificans progressiva, unspecified thigh

√6ᵗʰ M61.16 Myositis ossificans progressiva, lower leg

M61.161 Myositis ossificans progressiva, right lower leg

M61.162 Myositis ossificans progressiva, left lower leg

M61.169 Myositis ossificans progressiva, unspecified lower leg

√6ᵗʰ M61.17 Myositis ossificans progressiva, ankle, foot and toe(s)

M61.171 Myositis ossificans progressiva, right ankle

M61.172 Myositis ossificans progressiva, left ankle

M61.173 Myositis ossificans progressiva, unspecified ankle

M61.174 Myositis ossificans progressiva, right foot

M61.175 Myositis ossificans progressiva, left foot

M61.176 Myositis ossificans progressiva, unspecified foot

M61.177 Myositis ossificans progressiva, right toe(s)

M61.178 Myositis ossificans progressiva, left toe(s)

M61.179 Myositis ossificans progressiva, unspecified toe(s)

M61.18 Myositis ossificans progressiva, other site

M61.19 Myositis ossificans progressiva, multiple sites

√5ᵗʰ M61.2 Paralytic calcification and ossification of muscle

Myositis ossificans associated with quadriplegia or paraplegia

M61.20 Paralytic calcification and ossification of muscle, unspecified site

√6ᵗʰ M61.21 Paralytic calcification and ossification of muscle, shoulder

M61.211 Paralytic calcification and ossification of muscle, right shoulder

M61.212 Paralytic calcification and ossification of muscle, left shoulder

M61.219 Paralytic calcification and ossification of muscle, unspecified shoulder

√6ᵗʰ M61.22 Paralytic calcification and ossification of muscle, upper arm

M61.221 Paralytic calcification and ossification of muscle, right upper arm

M61.222 Paralytic calcification and ossification of muscle, left upper arm

M61.229 Paralytic calcification and ossification of muscle, unspecified upper arm

√6ᵗʰ M61.23 Paralytic calcification and ossification of muscle, forearm

M61.231 Paralytic calcification and ossification of muscle, right forearm

M61.232 Paralytic calcification and ossification of muscle, left forearm

M61.239 Paralytic calcification and ossification of muscle, unspecified forearm

√6ᵗʰ M61.24 Paralytic calcification and ossification of muscle, hand

M61.241 Paralytic calcification and ossification of muscle, right hand

M61.242 Paralytic calcification and ossification of muscle, left hand

M61.249 Paralytic calcification and ossification of muscle, unspecified hand

√6ᵗʰ M61.25 Paralytic calcification and ossification of muscle, thigh

M61.251 Paralytic calcification and ossification of muscle, right thigh

M61.252 Paralytic calcification and ossification of muscle, left thigh

M61.259 Paralytic calcification and ossification of muscle, unspecified thigh

√6ᵗʰ M61.26 Paralytic calcification and ossification of muscle, lower leg

M61.261 Paralytic calcification and ossification of muscle, right lower leg

M61.262 Paralytic calcification and ossification of muscle, left lower leg

M61.269 Paralytic calcification and ossification of muscle, unspecified lower leg

√6ᵗʰ M61.27 Paralytic calcification and ossification of muscle, ankle and foot

M61.271 Paralytic calcification and ossification of muscle, right ankle and foot

M61.272 Paralytic calcification and ossification of muscle, left ankle and foot

M61.279 Paralytic calcification and ossification of muscle, unspecified ankle and foot

M61.28 Paralytic calcification and ossification of muscle, other site

M61.29 Paralytic calcification and ossification of muscle, multiple sites

√5ᵗʰ M61.3 Calcification and ossification of muscles associated with burns

Myositis ossificans associated with burns

M61.30 Calcification and ossification of muscles associated with burns, unspecified site

√6ᵗʰ M61.31 Calcification and ossification of muscles associated with burns, shoulder

M61.311 Calcification and ossification of muscles associated with burns, right shoulder

M61.312 Calcification and ossification of muscles associated with burns, left shoulder

M61.319 Calcification and ossification of muscles associated with burns, unspecified shoulder

√6ᵗʰ M61.32 Calcification and ossification of muscles associated with burns, upper arm

M61.321 Calcification and ossification of muscles associated with burns, right upper arm

M61.322 Calcification and ossification of muscles associated with burns, left upper arm

M61.329 Calcification and ossification of muscles associated with burns, unspecified upper arm

√6ᵗʰ M61.33 Calcification and ossification of muscles associated with burns, forearm

M61.331 Calcification and ossification of muscles associated with burns, right forearm

M61.332 Calcification and ossification of muscles associated with burns, left forearm

M61.339 Calcification and ossification of muscles associated with burns, unspecified forearm

√6ᵗʰ M61.34 Calcification and ossification of muscles associated with burns, hand

M61.341 Calcification and ossification of muscles associated with burns, right hand

M61.342 Calcification and ossification of muscles associated with burns, left hand

M61.349 Calcification and ossification of muscles associated with burns, unspecified hand

√6ᵗʰ M61.35 Calcification and ossification of muscles associated with burns, thigh

M61.351 Calcification and ossification of muscles associated with burns, right thigh

M61.352 Calcification and ossification of muscles associated with burns, left thigh

M61.359 Calcification and ossification of muscles associated with burns, unspecified thigh

✓6ᵗʰ **M61.36** Calcification and ossification of muscles associated with burns, lower leg

  M61.361 Calcification and ossification of muscles associated with burns, right lower leg

  M61.362 Calcification and ossification of muscles associated with burns, left lower leg

  M61.369 Calcification and ossification of muscles associated with burns, unspecified lower leg

✓6ᵗʰ **M61.37** Calcification and ossification of muscles associated with burns, ankle and foot

  M61.371 Calcification and ossification of muscles associated with burns, right ankle and foot

  M61.372 Calcification and ossification of muscles associated with burns, left ankle and foot

  M61.379 Calcification and ossification of muscles associated with burns, unspecified ankle and foot

  M61.38 Calcification and ossification of muscles associated with burns, other site

  M61.39 Calcification and ossification of muscles associated with burns, multiple sites

✓5ᵗʰ **M61.4** Other calcification of muscle

  EXCLUDES 1   *calcific tendinitis NOS (M65.2-)*
           calcific tendinitis of shoulder (M75.3)

  M61.40 Other calcification of muscle, unspecified site

✓6ᵗʰ **M61.41** Other calcification of muscle, shoulder

  M61.411 Other calcification of muscle, right shoulder

  M61.412 Other calcification of muscle, left shoulder

  M61.419 Other calcification of muscle, unspecified shoulder

✓6ᵗʰ **M61.42** Other calcification of muscle, upper arm

  M61.421 Other calcification of muscle, right upper arm

  M61.422 Other calcification of muscle, left upper arm

  M61.429 Other calcification of muscle, unspecified upper arm

✓6ᵗʰ **M61.43** Other calcification of muscle, forearm

  M61.431 Other calcification of muscle, right forearm

  M61.432 Other calcification of muscle, left forearm

  M61.439 Other calcification of muscle, unspecified forearm

✓6ᵗʰ **M61.44** Other calcification of muscle, hand

  M61.441 Other calcification of muscle, right hand

  M61.442 Other calcification of muscle, left hand

  M61.449 Other calcification of muscle, unspecified hand

✓6ᵗʰ **M61.45** Other calcification of muscle, thigh

  M61.451 Other calcification of muscle, right thigh

  M61.452 Other calcification of muscle, left thigh

  M61.459 Other calcification of muscle, unspecified thigh

✓6ᵗʰ **M61.46** Other calcification of muscle, lower leg

  M61.461 Other calcification of muscle, right lower leg

  M61.462 Other calcification of muscle, left lower leg

  M61.469 Other calcification of muscle, unspecified lower leg

✓6ᵗʰ **M61.47** Other calcification of muscle, ankle and foot

  M61.471 Other calcification of muscle, right ankle and foot

  M61.472 Other calcification of muscle, left ankle and foot

  M61.479 Other calcification of muscle, unspecified ankle and foot

  M61.48 Other calcification of muscle, other site

  M61.49 Other calcification of muscle, multiple sites

✓5ᵗʰ **M61.5** Other ossification of muscle

  M61.50 Other ossification of muscle, unspecified site

✓6ᵗʰ **M61.51** Other ossification of muscle, shoulder

  M61.511 Other ossification of muscle, right shoulder

  M61.512 Other ossification of muscle, left shoulder

  M61.519 Other ossification of muscle, unspecified shoulder

✓6ᵗʰ **M61.52** Other ossification of muscle, upper arm

  M61.521 Other ossification of muscle, right upper arm

  M61.522 Other ossification of muscle, left upper arm

  M61.529 Other ossification of muscle, unspecified upper arm

✓6ᵗʰ **M61.53** Other ossification of muscle, forearm

  M61.531 Other ossification of muscle, right forearm

  M61.532 Other ossification of muscle, left forearm

  M61.539 Other ossification of muscle, unspecified forearm

✓6ᵗʰ **M61.54** Other ossification of muscle, hand

  M61.541 Other ossification of muscle, right hand

  M61.542 Other ossification of muscle, left hand

  M61.549 Other ossification of muscle, unspecified hand

✓6ᵗʰ **M61.55** Other ossification of muscle, thigh

  M61.551 Other ossification of muscle, right thigh

  M61.552 Other ossification of muscle, left thigh

  M61.559 Other ossification of muscle, unspecified thigh

✓6ᵗʰ **M61.56** Other ossification of muscle, lower leg

  M61.561 Other ossification of muscle, right lower leg

  M61.562 Other ossification of muscle, left lower leg

  M61.569 Other ossification of muscle, unspecified lower leg

✓6ᵗʰ **M61.57** Other ossification of muscle, ankle and foot

  M61.571 Other ossification of muscle, right ankle and foot

  M61.572 Other ossification of muscle, left ankle and foot

  M61.579 Other ossification of muscle, unspecified ankle and foot

  M61.58 Other ossification of muscle, other site

  M61.59 Other ossification of muscle, multiple sites

  M61.9 Calcification and ossification of muscle, unspecified

✓4ᵗʰ **M62 Other disorders of muscle**

  EXCLUDES 1   *alcoholic myopathy (G72.1)*
           cramp and spasm (R25.2)
           drug-induced myopathy (G72.0)
           myalgia (M79.1)
           stiff-man syndrome (G25.82)

  EXCLUDES 2   *nontraumatic hematoma of muscle (M79.81)*

✓5ᵗʰ **M62.0** Separation of muscle (nontraumatic)

  Diastasis of muscle

  EXCLUDES 1   *diastasis recti complicating pregnancy, labor and delivery (O71.8)*
           traumatic separation of muscle—see strain of muscle by body region

  M62.00 Separation of muscle (nontraumatic), unspecified site

✓6ᵗʰ **M62.01** Separation of muscle (nontraumatic), shoulder

  M62.011 Separation of muscle (nontraumatic), right shoulder

  M62.012 Separation of muscle (nontraumatic), left shoulder

  M62.019 Separation of muscle (nontraumatic), unspecified shoulder

✓6ᵗʰ **M62.02** Separation of muscle (nontraumatic), upper arm

  M62.021 Separation of muscle (nontraumatic), right upper arm

  M62.022 Separation of muscle (nontraumatic), left upper arm

  M62.029 Separation of muscle (nontraumatic), unspecified upper arm

---

EXCLUDES 1 Not coded here   EXCLUDES 2 Not included here   *Manifestation Code*

☑6ᵗʰ **M62.03 Separation of muscle (nontraumatic), forearm**
      M62.031 Separation of muscle (nontraumatic), right forearm
      M62.032 Separation of muscle (nontraumatic), left forearm
      M62.039 Separation of muscle (nontraumatic), unspecified forearm

☑6ᵗʰ **M62.04 Separation of muscle (nontraumatic), hand**
      M62.041 Separation of muscle (nontraumatic), right hand
      M62.042 Separation of muscle (nontraumatic), left hand
      M62.049 Separation of muscle (nontraumatic), unspecified hand

☑6ᵗʰ **M62.05 Separation of muscle (nontraumatic), thigh**
      M62.051 Separation of muscle (nontraumatic), right thigh
      M62.052 Separation of muscle (nontraumatic), left thigh
      M62.059 Separation of muscle (nontraumatic), unspecified thigh

☑6ᵗʰ **M62.06 Separation of muscle (nontraumatic), lower leg**
      M62.061 Separation of muscle (nontraumatic), right lower leg
      M62.062 Separation of muscle (nontraumatic), left lower leg
      M62.069 Separation of muscle (nontraumatic), unspecified lower leg

☑6ᵗʰ **M62.07 Separation of muscle (nontraumatic), ankle and foot**
      M62.071 Separation of muscle (nontraumatic), right ankle and foot
      M62.072 Separation of muscle (nontraumatic), left ankle and foot
      M62.079 Separation of muscle (nontraumatic), unspecified ankle and foot

    M62.08 Separation of muscle (nontraumatic), other site

☑5ᵗʰ **M62.1 Other rupture of muscle (nontraumatic)**

> **EXCLUDES 1** *traumatic rupture of muscle—see strain of muscle by body region*
> **EXCLUDES 2** *rupture of tendon (M66-)*

    M62.10 Other rupture of muscle (nontraumatic), unspecified site

☑6ᵗʰ **M62.11 Other rupture of muscle (nontraumatic), shoulder**
      M62.111 Other rupture of muscle (nontraumatic), right shoulder
      M62.112 Other rupture of muscle (nontraumatic), left shoulder
      M62.119 Other rupture of muscle (nontraumatic), unspecified shoulder

☑6ᵗʰ **M62.12 Other rupture of muscle (nontraumatic), upper arm**
      M62.121 Other rupture of muscle (nontraumatic), right upper arm
      M62.122 Other rupture of muscle (nontraumatic), left upper arm
      M62.129 Other rupture of muscle (nontraumatic), unspecified upper arm

☑6ᵗʰ **M62.13 Other rupture of muscle (nontraumatic), forearm**
      M62.131 Other rupture of muscle (nontraumatic), right forearm
      M62.132 Other rupture of muscle (nontraumatic), left forearm
      M62.139 Other rupture of muscle (nontraumatic), unspecified forearm

☑6ᵗʰ **M62.14 Other rupture of muscle (nontraumatic), hand**
      M62.141 Other rupture of muscle (nontraumatic), right hand
      M62.142 Other rupture of muscle (nontraumatic), left hand
      M62.149 Other rupture of muscle (nontraumatic), unspecified hand

☑6ᵗʰ **M62.15 Other rupture of muscle (nontraumatic), thigh**
      M62.151 Other rupture of muscle (nontraumatic), right thigh
      M62.152 Other rupture of muscle (nontraumatic), left thigh
      M62.159 Other rupture of muscle (nontraumatic), unspecified thigh

☑6ᵗʰ **M62.16 Other rupture of muscle (nontraumatic), lower leg**
      M62.161 Other rupture of muscle (nontraumatic), right lower leg
      M62.162 Other rupture of muscle (nontraumatic), left lower leg
      M62.169 Other rupture of muscle (nontraumatic), unspecified lower leg

☑6ᵗʰ **M62.17 Other rupture of muscle (nontraumatic), ankle and foot**
      M62.171 Other rupture of muscle (nontraumatic), right ankle and foot
      M62.172 Other rupture of muscle (nontraumatic), left ankle and foot
      M62.179 Other rupture of muscle (nontraumatic), unspecified ankle and foot

    M62.18 Other rupture of muscle (nontraumatic), other site

☑5ᵗʰ **M62.2 Nontraumatic ischemic infarction of muscle**

> **EXCLUDES 1** *compartment syndrome (traumatic) (T79.a-)*
> *nontraumatic compartment syndrome (M79.a-)*
> *rhabdomyolysis (M62.82)*
> *traumatic ischemia of muscle (T79.6)*
> *Volkmann's ischemic contracture (T79.6)*

    M62.20 Nontraumatic ischemic infarction of muscle, unspecified site

☑6ᵗʰ **M62.21 Nontraumatic ischemic infarction of muscle, shoulder**
      M62.211 Nontraumatic ischemic infarction of muscle, right shoulder
      M62.212 Nontraumatic ischemic infarction of muscle, left shoulder
      M62.219 Nontraumatic ischemic infarction of muscle, unspecified shoulder

☑6ᵗʰ **M62.22 Nontraumatic ischemic infarction of muscle, upper arm**
      M62.221 Nontraumatic ischemic infarction of muscle, right upper arm
      M62.222 Nontraumatic ischemic infarction of muscle, left upper arm
      M62.229 Nontraumatic ischemic infarction of muscle, unspecified upper arm

☑6ᵗʰ **M62.23 Nontraumatic ischemic infarction of muscle, forearm**
      M62.231 Nontraumatic ischemic infarction of muscle, right forearm
      M62.232 Nontraumatic ischemic infarction of muscle, left forearm
      M62.239 Nontraumatic ischemic infarction of muscle, unspecified forearm

☑6ᵗʰ **M62.24 Nontraumatic ischemic infarction of muscle, hand**
      M62.241 Nontraumatic ischemic infarction of muscle, right hand
      M62.242 Nontraumatic ischemic infarction of muscle, left hand
      M62.249 Nontraumatic ischemic infarction of muscle, unspecified hand

☑6ᵗʰ **M62.25 Nontraumatic ischemic infarction of muscle, thigh**
      M62.251 Nontraumatic ischemic infarction of muscle, right thigh
      M62.252 Nontraumatic ischemic infarction of muscle, left thigh
      M62.259 Nontraumatic ischemic infarction of muscle, unspecified thigh

☑6ᵗʰ **M62.26 Nontraumatic ischemic infarction of muscle, lower leg**
      M62.261 Nontraumatic ischemic infarction of muscle, right lower leg
      M62.262 Nontraumatic ischemic infarction of muscle, left lower leg
      M62.269 Nontraumatic ischemic infarction of muscle, unspecified lower leg

☑6ᵗʰ **M62.27 Nontraumatic ischemic infarction of muscle, ankle and foot**
      M62.271 Nontraumatic ischemic infarction of muscle, right ankle and foot
      M62.272 Nontraumatic ischemic infarction of muscle, left ankle and foot

---

☑ Appropriate additional character required   ✓x7ᵗʰ Requires 7th character, placeholder x must fill empty characters

M62.279   Nontraumatic ischemic infarction of muscle, unspecified ankle and foot

M62.28   Nontraumatic ischemic infarction of muscle, other site

M62.3   Immobility syndrome (paraplegic)

✓5th M62.4   Contracture of muscle

     Contracture of tendon (sheath)

     EXCLUDES 1   contracture of joint (M24.5-)

M62.40   Contracture of muscle, unspecified site

✓6th M62.41   Contracture of muscle, shoulder

M62.411   Contracture of muscle, right shoulder

M62.412   Contracture of muscle, left shoulder

M62.419   Contracture of muscle, unspecified shoulder

✓6th M62.42   Contracture of muscle, upper arm

M62.421   Contracture of muscle, right upper arm

M62.422   Contracture of muscle, left upper arm

M62.429   Contracture of muscle, unspecified upper arm

✓6th M62.43   Contracture of muscle, forearm

M62.431   Contracture of muscle, right forearm

M62.432   Contracture of muscle, left forearm

M62.439   Contracture of muscle, unspecified forearm

✓6th M62.44   Contracture of muscle, hand

M62.441   Contracture of muscle, right hand

M62.442   Contracture of muscle, left hand

M62.449   Contracture of muscle, unspecified hand

✓6th M62.45   Contracture of muscle, thigh

M62.451   Contracture of muscle, right thigh

M62.452   Contracture of muscle, left thigh

M62.459   Contracture of muscle, unspecified thigh

✓6th M62.46   Contracture of muscle, lower leg

M62.461   Contracture of muscle, right lower leg

M62.462   Contracture of muscle, left lower leg

M62.469   Contracture of muscle, unspecified lower leg

✓6th M62.47   Contracture of muscle, ankle and foot

M62.471   Contracture of muscle, right ankle and foot

M62.472   Contracture of muscle, left ankle and foot

M62.479   Contracture of muscle, unspecified ankle and foot

M62.48   Contracture of muscle, other site

M62.49   Contracture of muscle, multiple sites

✓5th M62.5   Muscle wasting and atrophy, not elsewhere classified

     Disuse atrophy NEC

     EXCLUDES 1   neuralgic amyotrophy (G54.5)

            progressive muscular atrophy (G12.29)

     EXCLUDES 2   pelvic muscle wasting (N81.84)

M62.50   Muscle wasting and atrophy, not elsewhere classified, unspecified site

✓6th M62.51   Muscle wasting and atrophy, not elsewhere classified, shoulder

M62.511   Muscle wasting and atrophy, not elsewhere classified, right shoulder

M62.512   Muscle wasting and atrophy, not elsewhere classified, left shoulder

M62.519   Muscle wasting and atrophy, not elsewhere classified, unspecified shoulder

✓6th M62.52   Muscle wasting and atrophy, not elsewhere classified, upper arm

M62.521   Muscle wasting and atrophy, not elsewhere classified, right upper arm

M62.522   Muscle wasting and atrophy, not elsewhere classified, left upper arm

M62.529   Muscle wasting and atrophy, not elsewhere classified, unspecified upper arm

✓6th M62.53   Muscle wasting and atrophy, not elsewhere classified, forearm

M62.531   Muscle wasting and atrophy, not elsewhere classified, right forearm

M62.532   Muscle wasting and atrophy, not elsewhere classified, left forearm

M62.539   Muscle wasting and atrophy, not elsewhere classified, unspecified forearm

✓6th M62.54   Muscle wasting and atrophy, not elsewhere classified, hand

M62.541   Muscle wasting and atrophy, not elsewhere classified, right hand

M62.542   Muscle wasting and atrophy, not elsewhere classified, left hand

M62.549   Muscle wasting and atrophy, not elsewhere classified, unspecified hand

✓6th M62.55   Muscle wasting and atrophy, not elsewhere classified, thigh

M62.551   Muscle wasting and atrophy, not elsewhere classified, right thigh

M62.552   Muscle wasting and atrophy, not elsewhere classified, left thigh

M62.559   Muscle wasting and atrophy, not elsewhere classified, unspecified thigh

✓6th M62.56   Muscle wasting and atrophy, not elsewhere classified, lower leg

M62.561   Muscle wasting and atrophy, not elsewhere classified, right lower leg

M62.562   Muscle wasting and atrophy, not elsewhere classified, left lower leg

M62.569   Muscle wasting and atrophy, not elsewhere classified, unspecified lower leg

✓6th M62.57   Muscle wasting and atrophy, not elsewhere classified, ankle and foot

M62.571   Muscle wasting and atrophy, not elsewhere classified, right ankle and foot

M62.572   Muscle wasting and atrophy, not elsewhere classified, left ankle and foot

M62.579   Muscle wasting and atrophy, not elsewhere classified, unspecified ankle and foot

M62.58   Muscle wasting and atrophy, not elsewhere classified, other site

M62.59   Muscle wasting and atrophy, not elsewhere classified, multiple sites

✓5th M62.8   Other specified disorders of muscle

     EXCLUDES 2   nontraumatic hematoma of muscle (M79.81)

M62.81   Muscle weakness (generalized)

M62.82   Rhabdomyolysis

     EXCLUDES 1   traumatic rhabdomyolysis (T79.6)

✓6th M62.83   Muscle spasm

M62.830   Muscle spasm of back

M62.831   Muscle spasm of calf

     Charley-horse

M62.838   Other muscle spasm

M62.89   Other specified disorders of muscle

     Muscle (sheath) hernia

M62.9   Disorder of muscle, unspecified

✓4th **M63   Disorders of muscle in diseases classified elsewhere**

     EXCLUDES 1   myopathy in:

            cysticercosis (B69.81)

            endocrine diseases (G73.7)

            metabolic diseases (G73.7)

            sarcoidosis (D86.87)

            syphilis (late) (A52.78)

            secondary (A51.49)

            toxoplasmosis (B58.82)

            tuberculosis (A18.09)

     Code first underlying disease, such as:

         leprosy (A30-)

         neoplasm (C49-, C79.89, D21-, D48.1)

         schistosomiasis (B65-)

         trichinellosis (B75)

✓5th M63.8   Disorders of muscle in diseases classified elsewhere

M63.80   *Disorders of muscle in diseases classified elsewhere, unspecified site*

✓6th **M63.81** Disorders of muscle in diseases classified elsewhere, shoulder

 M63.811 *Disorders of muscle in diseases classified elsewhere, right shoulder*

 M63.812 *Disorders of muscle in diseases classified elsewhere, left shoulder*

 M63.819 *Disorders of muscle in diseases classified elsewhere, unspecified shoulder*

✓6th **M63.82** Disorders of muscle in diseases classified elsewhere, upper arm

 M63.821 *Disorders of muscle in diseases classified elsewhere, right upper arm*

 M63.822 *Disorders of muscle in diseases classified elsewhere, left upper arm*

 M63.829 *Disorders of muscle in diseases classified elsewhere, unspecified upper arm*

✓6th **M63.83** Disorders of muscle in diseases classified elsewhere, forearm

 M63.831 *Disorders of muscle in diseases classified elsewhere, right forearm*

 M63.832 *Disorders of muscle in diseases classified elsewhere, left forearm*

 M63.839 *Disorders of muscle in diseases classified elsewhere, unspecified forearm*

✓6th **M63.84** Disorders of muscle in diseases classified elsewhere, hand

 M63.841 *Disorders of muscle in diseases classified elsewhere, right hand*

 M63.842 *Disorders of muscle in diseases classified elsewhere, left hand*

 M63.849 *Disorders of muscle in diseases classified elsewhere, unspecified hand*

✓6th **M63.85** Disorders of muscle in diseases classified elsewhere, thigh

 M63.851 *Disorders of muscle in diseases classified elsewhere, right thigh*

 M63.852 *Disorders of muscle in diseases classified elsewhere, left thigh*

 M63.859 *Disorders of muscle in diseases classified elsewhere, unspecified thigh*

✓6th **M63.86** Disorders of muscle in diseases classified elsewhere, lower leg

 M63.861 *Disorders of muscle in diseases classified elsewhere, right lower leg*

 M63.862 *Disorders of muscle in diseases classified elsewhere, left lower leg*

 M63.869 *Disorders of muscle in diseases classified elsewhere, unspecified lower leg*

✓6th **M63.87** Disorders of muscle in diseases classified elsewhere, ankle and foot

 M63.871 *Disorders of muscle in diseases classified elsewhere, right ankle and foot*

 M63.872 *Disorders of muscle in diseases classified elsewhere, left ankle and foot*

 M63.879 *Disorders of muscle in diseases classified elsewhere, unspecified ankle and foot*

 M63.88 *Disorders of muscle in diseases classified elsewhere, other site*

 M63.89 *Disorders of muscle in diseases classified elsewhere, multiple sites*

Disorders of synovium and tendon (M65-M67)

✓4th **M65 Synovitis and tenosynovitis**

 EXCLUDES 1 *chronic crepitant synovitis of hand and wrist (M70.0-)*
  current injury—see injury of ligament or tendon by body region
  soft tissue disorders related to use, overuse and pressure (M70-)

✓5th **M65.0** Abscess of tendon sheath

 Use additional code (B95-B96) to identify bacterial agent.

 M65.00 Abscess of tendon sheath, unspecified site

✓6th **M65.01** Abscess of tendon sheath, shoulder

 M65.011 Abscess of tendon sheath, right shoulder

 M65.012 Abscess of tendon sheath, left shoulder

 M65.019 Abscess of tendon sheath, unspecified shoulder

✓6th **M65.02** Abscess of tendon sheath, upper arm

 M65.021 Abscess of tendon sheath, right upper arm

 M65.022 Abscess of tendon sheath, left upper arm

 M65.029 Abscess of tendon sheath, unspecified upper arm

✓6th **M65.03** Abscess of tendon sheath, forearm

 M65.031 Abscess of tendon sheath, right forearm

 M65.032 Abscess of tendon sheath, left forearm

 M65.039 Abscess of tendon sheath, unspecified forearm

✓6th **M65.04** Abscess of tendon sheath, hand

 M65.041 Abscess of tendon sheath, right hand

 M65.042 Abscess of tendon sheath, left hand

 M65.049 Abscess of tendon sheath, unspecified hand

✓6th **M65.05** Abscess of tendon sheath, thigh

 M65.051 Abscess of tendon sheath, right thigh

 M65.052 Abscess of tendon sheath, left thigh

 M65.059 Abscess of tendon sheath, unspecified thigh

✓6th **M65.06** Abscess of tendon sheath, lower leg

 M65.061 Abscess of tendon sheath, right lower leg

 M65.062 Abscess of tendon sheath, left lower leg

 M65.069 Abscess of tendon sheath, unspecified lower leg

✓6th **M65.07** Abscess of tendon sheath, ankle and foot

 M65.071 Abscess of tendon sheath, right ankle and foot

 M65.072 Abscess of tendon sheath, left ankle and foot

 M65.079 Abscess of tendon sheath, unspecified ankle and foot

 M65.08 Abscess of tendon sheath, other site

✓5th **M65.1** Other infective (teno)synovitis

 M65.10 Other infective (teno)synovitis, unspecified site

✓6th **M65.11** Other infective (teno)synovitis, shoulder

 M65.111 Other infective (teno)synovitis, right shoulder

 M65.112 Other infective (teno)synovitis, left shoulder

 M65.119 Other infective (teno)synovitis, unspecified shoulder

✓6th **M65.12** Other infective (teno)synovitis, elbow

 M65.121 Other infective (teno)synovitis, right elbow

 M65.122 Other infective (teno)synovitis, left elbow

 M65.129 Other infective (teno)synovitis, unspecified elbow

✓6th **M65.13** Other infective (teno)synovitis, wrist

 M65.131 Other infective (teno)synovitis, right wrist

 M65.132 Other infective (teno)synovitis, left wrist

 M65.139 Other infective (teno)synovitis, unspecified wrist

✓6th **M65.14** Other infective (teno)synovitis, hand

 M65.141 Other infective (teno)synovitis, right hand

 M65.142 Other infective (teno)synovitis, left hand

 M65.149 Other infective (teno)synovitis, unspecified hand

✓6th **M65.15** Other infective (teno)synovitis, hip

 M65.151 Other infective (teno)synovitis, right hip

 M65.152 Other infective (teno)synovitis, left hip

 M65.159 Other infective (teno)synovitis, unspecified hip

☑ Appropriate additional character required   ✓x7th Requires 7th character, placeholder x must fill empty characters

√6th **M65.16 Other infective (teno)synovitis, knee**
- **M65.161 Other infective (teno)synovitis, right knee**
- **M65.162 Other infective (teno)synovitis, left knee**
- **M65.169 Other infective (teno)synovitis, unspecified knee**

√6th **M65.17 Other infective (teno)synovitis, ankle and foot**
- **M65.171 Other infective (teno)synovitis, right ankle and foot**
- **M65.172 Other infective (teno)synovitis, left ankle and foot**
- **M65.179 Other infective (teno)synovitis, unspecified ankle and foot**

M65.18 Other infective (teno)synovitis, other site

M65.19 Other infective (teno)synovitis, multiple sites

√5th **M65.2 Calcific tendinitis**

> EXCLUDES 1   *tendinitis as classified in M75-M77*
> *calcified tendinitis of shoulder (M75.3)*

M65.20 Calcific tendinitis, unspecified site

√6th **M65.22 Calcific tendinitis, upper arm**
- **M65.221 Calcific tendinitis, right upper arm**
- **M65.222 Calcific tendinitis, left upper arm**
- **M65.229 Calcific tendinitis, unspecified upper arm**

√6th **M65.23 Calcific tendinitis, forearm**
- **M65.231 Calcific tendinitis, right forearm**
- **M65.232 Calcific tendinitis, left forearm**
- **M65.239 Calcific tendinitis, unspecified forearm**

√6th **M65.24 Calcific tendinitis, hand**
- **M65.241 Calcific tendinitis, right hand**
- **M65.242 Calcific tendinitis, left hand**
- **M65.249 Calcific tendinitis, unspecified hand**

√6th **M65.25 Calcific tendinitis, thigh**
- **M65.251 Calcific tendinitis, right thigh**
- **M65.252 Calcific tendinitis, left thigh**
- **M65.259 Calcific tendinitis, unspecified thigh**

√6th **M65.26 Calcific tendinitis, lower leg**
- **M65.261 Calcific tendinitis, right lower leg**
- **M65.262 Calcific tendinitis, left lower leg**
- **M65.269 Calcific tendinitis, unspecified lower leg**

√6th **M65.27 Calcific tendinitis, ankle and foot**
- **M65.271 Calcific tendinitis, right ankle and foot**
- **M65.272 Calcific tendinitis, left ankle and foot**
- **M65.279 Calcific tendinitis, unspecified ankle and foot**

M65.28 Calcific tendinitis, other site

M65.29 Calcific tendinitis, multiple sites

√5th **M65.3 Trigger finger**

> Nodular tendinous disease

M65.30 Trigger finger, unspecified finger

√6th **M65.31 Trigger thumb**
- **M65.311 Trigger thumb, right thumb**
- **M65.312 Trigger thumb, left thumb**
- **M65.319 Trigger thumb, unspecified thumb**

√6th **M65.32 Trigger finger, index finger**
- **M65.321 Trigger finger, right index finger**
- **M65.322 Trigger finger, left index finger**
- **M65.329 Trigger finger, unspecified index finger**

√6th **M65.33 Trigger finger, middle finger**
- **M65.331 Trigger finger, right middle finger**
- **M65.332 Trigger finger, left middle finger**
- **M65.339 Trigger finger, unspecified middle finger**

√6th **M65.34 Trigger finger, ring finger**
- **M65.341 Trigger finger, right ring finger**
- **M65.342 Trigger finger, left ring finger**
- **M65.349 Trigger finger, unspecified ring finger**

√6th **M65.35 Trigger finger, little finger**
- **M65.351 Trigger finger, right little finger**
- **M65.352 Trigger finger, left little finger**
- **M65.359 Trigger finger, unspecified little finger**

M65.4 Radial styloid tenosynovitis [de Quervain]

√5th **M65.8 Other synovitis and tenosynovitis**

M65.80 Other synovitis and tenosynovitis, unspecified site

√6th **M65.81 Other synovitis and tenosynovitis, shoulder**
- **M65.811 Other synovitis and tenosynovitis, right shoulder**
- **M65.812 Other synovitis and tenosynovitis, left shoulder**
- **M65.819 Other synovitis and tenosynovitis, unspecified shoulder**

√6th **M65.82 Other synovitis and tenosynovitis, upper arm**
- **M65.821 Other synovitis and tenosynovitis, right upper arm**
- **M65.822 Other synovitis and tenosynovitis, left upper arm**
- **M65.829 Other synovitis and tenosynovitis, unspecified upper arm**

√6th **M65.83 Other synovitis and tenosynovitis, forearm**
- **M65.831 Other synovitis and tenosynovitis, right forearm**
- **M65.832 Other synovitis and tenosynovitis, left forearm**
- **M65.839 Other synovitis and tenosynovitis, unspecified forearm**

√6th **M65.84 Other synovitis and tenosynovitis, hand**
- **M65.841 Other synovitis and tenosynovitis, right hand**
- **M65.842 Other synovitis and tenosynovitis, left hand**
- **M65.849 Other synovitis and tenosynovitis, unspecified hand**

√6th **M65.85 Other synovitis and tenosynovitis, thigh**
- **M65.851 Other synovitis and tenosynovitis, right thigh**
- **M65.852 Other synovitis and tenosynovitis, left thigh**
- **M65.859 Other synovitis and tenosynovitis, unspecified thigh**

√6th **M65.86 Other synovitis and tenosynovitis, lower leg**
- **M65.861 Other synovitis and tenosynovitis, right lower leg**
- **M65.862 Other synovitis and tenosynovitis, left lower leg**
- **M65.869 Other synovitis and tenosynovitis, unspecified lower leg**

√6th **M65.87 Other synovitis and tenosynovitis, ankle and foot**
- **M65.871 Other synovitis and tenosynovitis, right ankle and foot**
- **M65.872 Other synovitis and tenosynovitis, left ankle and foot**
- **M65.879 Other synovitis and tenosynovitis, unspecified ankle and foot**

M65.88 Other synovitis and tenosynovitis, other site

M65.89 Other synovitis and tenosynovitis, multiple sites

M65.9 Synovitis and tenosynovitis, unspecified

√4th **M66 Spontaneous rupture of synovium and tendon**

> NOTE   A spontaneous rupture is one that occurs when a normal force is applied to tissues that are inferred to have less than normal strength
>
> EXCLUDES 2   *rotator cuff syndrome (M75.1)*
> *rupture where an abnormal force is applied to normal tissue—see injury of tendon by body region*

M66.0 Rupture of popliteal cyst

√5th **M66.1 Rupture of synovium**

> Rupture of synovial cyst
>
> EXCLUDES 2   *rupture of popliteal cyst (M66.0)*

M66.10 Rupture of synovium, unspecified joint

√6th **M66.11 Rupture of synovium, shoulder**
- **M66.111 Rupture of synovium, right shoulder**
- **M66.112 Rupture of synovium, left shoulder**
- **M66.119 Rupture of synovium, unspecified shoulder**

√6th **M66.12 Rupture of synovium, elbow**
- **M66.121 Rupture of synovium, right elbow**
- **M66.122 Rupture of synovium, left elbow**
- **M66.129 Rupture of synovium, unspecified elbow**

√6th **M66.13 Rupture of synovium, wrist**
- **M66.131 Rupture of synovium, right wrist**
- **M66.132 Rupture of synovium, left wrist**
- **M66.139 Rupture of synovium, unspecified wrist**

EXCLUDES 1   Not coded here   EXCLUDES 2   Not included here   *Manifestation Code*

☑6ᵗʰ **M66.14 Rupture of synovium, hand and fingers**
    M66.141 **Rupture of synovium, right hand**
    M66.142 **Rupture of synovium, left hand**
    M66.143 **Rupture of synovium, unspecified hand**
    M66.144 **Rupture of synovium, right finger(s)**
    M66.145 **Rupture of synovium, left finger(s)**
    M66.146 **Rupture of synovium, unspecified finger(s)**

☑6ᵗʰ **M66.15 Rupture of synovium, hip**
    M66.151 **Rupture of synovium, right hip**
    M66.152 **Rupture of synovium, left hip**
    M66.159 **Rupture of synovium, unspecified hip**

☑6ᵗʰ **M66.17 Rupture of synovium, ankle, foot and toes**
    M66.171 **Rupture of synovium, right ankle**
    M66.172 **Rupture of synovium, left ankle**
    M66.173 **Rupture of synovium, unspecified ankle**
    M66.174 **Rupture of synovium, right foot**
    M66.175 **Rupture of synovium, left foot**
    M66.176 **Rupture of synovium, unspecified foot**
    M66.177 **Rupture of synovium, right toe(s)**
    M66.178 **Rupture of synovium, left toe(s)**
    M66.179 **Rupture of synovium, unspecified toe(s)**

  M66.18 Rupture of synovium, other site

☑5ᵗʰ **M66.2 Spontaneous rupture of extensor tendons**
  M66.20 Spontaneous rupture of extensor tendons, unspecified site

☑6ᵗʰ **M66.21 Spontaneous rupture of extensor tendons, shoulder**
    M66.211 **Spontaneous rupture of extensor tendons, right shoulder**
    M66.212 **Spontaneous rupture of extensor tendons, left shoulder**
    M66.219 **Spontaneous rupture of extensor tendons, unspecified shoulder**

☑6ᵗʰ **M66.22 Spontaneous rupture of extensor tendons, upper arm**
    M66.221 **Spontaneous rupture of extensor tendons, right upper arm**
    M66.222 **Spontaneous rupture of extensor tendons, left upper arm**
    M66.229 **Spontaneous rupture of extensor tendons, unspecified upper arm**

☑6ᵗʰ **M66.23 Spontaneous rupture of extensor tendons, forearm**
    M66.231 **Spontaneous rupture of extensor tendons, right forearm**
    M66.232 **Spontaneous rupture of extensor tendons, left forearm**
    M66.239 **Spontaneous rupture of extensor tendons, unspecified forearm**

☑6ᵗʰ **M66.24 Spontaneous rupture of extensor tendons, hand**
    M66.241 **Spontaneous rupture of extensor tendons, right hand**
    M66.242 **Spontaneous rupture of extensor tendons, left hand**
    M66.249 **Spontaneous rupture of extensor tendons, unspecified hand**

☑6ᵗʰ **M66.25 Spontaneous rupture of extensor tendons, thigh**
    M66.251 **Spontaneous rupture of extensor tendons, right thigh**
    M66.252 **Spontaneous rupture of extensor tendons, left thigh**
    M66.259 **Spontaneous rupture of extensor tendons, unspecified thigh**

☑6ᵗʰ **M66.26 Spontaneous rupture of extensor tendons, lower leg**
    M66.261 **Spontaneous rupture of extensor tendons, right lower leg**
    M66.262 **Spontaneous rupture of extensor tendons, left lower leg**
    M66.269 **Spontaneous rupture of extensor tendons, unspecified lower leg**

☑6ᵗʰ **M66.27 Spontaneous rupture of extensor tendons, ankle and foot**
    M66.271 **Spontaneous rupture of extensor tendons, right ankle and foot**

    M66.272 **Spontaneous rupture of extensor tendons, left ankle and foot**
    M66.279 **Spontaneous rupture of extensor tendons, unspecified ankle and foot**

  M66.28 Spontaneous rupture of extensor tendons, other site
  M66.29 Spontaneous rupture of extensor tendons, multiple sites

☑5ᵗʰ **M66.3 Spontaneous rupture of flexor tendons**
  M66.30 Spontaneous rupture of flexor tendons, unspecified site

☑6ᵗʰ **M66.31 Spontaneous rupture of flexor tendons, shoulder**
    M66.311 **Spontaneous rupture of flexor tendons, right shoulder**
    M66.312 **Spontaneous rupture of flexor tendons, left shoulder**
    M66.319 **Spontaneous rupture of flexor tendons, unspecified shoulder**

☑6ᵗʰ **M66.32 Spontaneous rupture of flexor tendons, upper arm**
    M66.321 **Spontaneous rupture of flexor tendons, right upper arm**
    M66.322 **Spontaneous rupture of flexor tendons, left upper arm**
    M66.329 **Spontaneous rupture of flexor tendons, unspecified upper arm**

☑6ᵗʰ **M66.33 Spontaneous rupture of flexor tendons, forearm**
    M66.331 **Spontaneous rupture of flexor tendons, right forearm**
    M66.332 **Spontaneous rupture of flexor tendons, left forearm**
    M66.339 **Spontaneous rupture of flexor tendons, unspecified forearm**

☑6ᵗʰ **M66.34 Spontaneous rupture of flexor tendons, hand**
    M66.341 **Spontaneous rupture of flexor tendons, right hand**
    M66.342 **Spontaneous rupture of flexor tendons, left hand**
    M66.349 **Spontaneous rupture of flexor tendons, unspecified hand**

☑6ᵗʰ **M66.35 Spontaneous rupture of flexor tendons, thigh**
    M66.351 **Spontaneous rupture of flexor tendons, right thigh**
    M66.352 **Spontaneous rupture of flexor tendons, left thigh**
    M66.359 **Spontaneous rupture of flexor tendons, unspecified thigh**

☑6ᵗʰ **M66.36 Spontaneous rupture of flexor tendons, lower leg**
    M66.361 **Spontaneous rupture of flexor tendons, right lower leg**
    M66.362 **Spontaneous rupture of flexor tendons, left lower leg**
    M66.369 **Spontaneous rupture of flexor tendons, unspecified lower leg**

☑6ᵗʰ **M66.37 Spontaneous rupture of flexor tendons, ankle and foot**
    M66.371 **Spontaneous rupture of flexor tendons, right ankle and foot**
    M66.372 **Spontaneous rupture of flexor tendons, left ankle and foot**
    M66.379 **Spontaneous rupture of flexor tendons, unspecified ankle and foot**

  M66.38 Spontaneous rupture of flexor tendons, other site
  M66.39 Spontaneous rupture of flexor tendons, multiple sites

☑5ᵗʰ **M66.8 Spontaneous rupture of other tendons**
  M66.80 Spontaneous rupture of other tendons, unspecified site

☑6ᵗʰ **M66.81 Spontaneous rupture of other tendons, shoulder**
    M66.811 **Spontaneous rupture of other tendons, right shoulder**
    M66.812 **Spontaneous rupture of other tendons, left shoulder**
    M66.819 **Spontaneous rupture of other tendons, unspecified shoulder**

☑6ᵗʰ **M66.82 Spontaneous rupture of other tendons, upper arm**
    M66.821 **Spontaneous rupture of other tendons, right upper arm**

☑ Appropriate additional character required   ☑x7ᵗʰ Requires 7th character, placeholder x must fill empty characters

       M66.822 Spontaneous rupture of other tendons, left upper arm

       M66.829 Spontaneous rupture of other tendons, unspecified upper arm

  ✔6th **M66.83** Spontaneous rupture of other tendons, forearm

       M66.831 Spontaneous rupture of other tendons, right forearm

       M66.832 Spontaneous rupture of other tendons, left forearm

       M66.839 Spontaneous rupture of other tendons, unspecified forearm

  ✔6th **M66.84** Spontaneous rupture of other tendons, hand

       M66.841 Spontaneous rupture of other tendons, right hand

       M66.842 Spontaneous rupture of other tendons, left hand

       M66.849 Spontaneous rupture of other tendons, unspecified hand

  ✔6th **M66.85** Spontaneous rupture of other tendons, thigh

       M66.851 Spontaneous rupture of other tendons, right thigh

       M66.852 Spontaneous rupture of other tendons, left thigh

       M66.859 Spontaneous rupture of other tendons, unspecified thigh

  ✔6th **M66.86** Spontaneous rupture of other tendons, lower leg

       M66.861 Spontaneous rupture of other tendons, right lower leg

       M66.862 Spontaneous rupture of other tendons, left lower leg

       M66.869 Spontaneous rupture of other tendons, unspecified lower leg

  ✔6th **M66.87** Spontaneous rupture of other tendons, ankle and foot

       M66.871 Spontaneous rupture of other tendons, right ankle and foot

       M66.872 Spontaneous rupture of other tendons, left ankle and foot

       M66.879 Spontaneous rupture of other tendons, unspecified ankle and foot

     M66.88 Spontaneous rupture of other tendons, other

     M66.89 Spontaneous rupture of other tendons, multiple sites

  M66.9 Spontaneous rupture of unspecified tendon

     Rupture at musculotendinous junction, nontraumatic

✔4th **M67** **Other disorders of synovium and tendon**

     EXCLUDES 1 *palmar fascial fibromatosis [Dupuytren] (M72.0)*
             tendinitis NOS (M77.9-)
             xanthomatosis localized to tendons (E78.2)

  ✔5th **M67.0** **Short Achilles tendon (acquired)**

     M67.00 Short Achilles tendon (acquired), unspecified ankle

     M67.01 Short Achilles tendon (acquired), right ankle

     M67.02 Short Achilles tendon (acquired), left ankle

  ✔5th **M67.2** **Synovial hypertrophy, not elsewhere classified**

     EXCLUDES 1 *villonodular synovitis (pigmented) (M12.2-)*

     M67.20 Synovial hypertrophy, not elsewhere classified, unspecified site

  ✔6th **M67.21** Synovial hypertrophy, not elsewhere classified, shoulder

       M67.211 Synovial hypertrophy, not elsewhere classified, right shoulder

       M67.212 Synovial hypertrophy, not elsewhere classified, left shoulder

       M67.219 Synovial hypertrophy, not elsewhere classified, unspecified shoulder

  ✔6th **M67.22** Synovial hypertrophy, not elsewhere classified, upper arm

       M67.221 Synovial hypertrophy, not elsewhere classified, right upper arm

       M67.222 Synovial hypertrophy, not elsewhere classified, left upper arm

       M67.229 Synovial hypertrophy, not elsewhere classified, unspecified upper arm

  ✔6th **M67.23** Synovial hypertrophy, not elsewhere classified, forearm

       M67.231 Synovial hypertrophy, not elsewhere classified, right forearm

       M67.232 Synovial hypertrophy, not elsewhere classified, left forearm

       M67.239 Synovial hypertrophy, not elsewhere classified, unspecified forearm

  ✔6th **M67.24** Synovial hypertrophy, not elsewhere classified, hand

       M67.241 Synovial hypertrophy, not elsewhere classified, right hand

       M67.242 Synovial hypertrophy, not elsewhere classified, left hand

       M67.249 Synovial hypertrophy, not elsewhere classified, unspecified hand

  ✔6th **M67.25** Synovial hypertrophy, not elsewhere classified, thigh

       M67.251 Synovial hypertrophy, not elsewhere classified, right thigh

       M67.252 Synovial hypertrophy, not elsewhere classified, left thigh

       M67.259 Synovial hypertrophy, not elsewhere classified, unspecified thigh

  ✔6th **M67.26** Synovial hypertrophy, not elsewhere classified, lower leg

       M67.261 Synovial hypertrophy, not elsewhere classified, right lower leg

       M67.262 Synovial hypertrophy, not elsewhere classified, left lower leg

       M67.269 Synovial hypertrophy, not elsewhere classified, unspecified lower leg

  ✔6th **M67.27** Synovial hypertrophy, not elsewhere classified, ankle and foot

       M67.271 Synovial hypertrophy, not elsewhere classified, right ankle and foot

       M67.272 Synovial hypertrophy, not elsewhere classified, left ankle and foot

       M67.279 Synovial hypertrophy, not elsewhere classified, unspecified ankle and foot

     M67.28 Synovial hypertrophy, not elsewhere classified, other site

     M67.29 Synovial hypertrophy, not elsewhere classified, multiple sites

  ✔5th **M67.3** **Transient synovitis**

     Toxic synovitis

     EXCLUDES 1 *palindromic rheumatism (M12.3-)*

     M67.30 Transient synovitis, unspecified site

  ✔6th **M67.31** Transient synovitis, shoulder

       M67.311 Transient synovitis, right shoulder

       M67.312 Transient synovitis, left shoulder

       M67.319 Transient synovitis, unspecified shoulder

  ✔6th **M67.32** Transient synovitis, elbow

       M67.321 Transient synovitis, right elbow

       M67.322 Transient synovitis, left elbow

       M67.329 Transient synovitis, unspecified elbow

  ✔6th **M67.33** Transient synovitis, wrist

       M67.331 Transient synovitis, right wrist

       M67.332 Transient synovitis, left wrist

       M67.339 Transient synovitis, unspecified wrist

  ✔6th **M67.34** Transient synovitis, hand

       M67.341 Transient synovitis, right hand

       M67.342 Transient synovitis, left hand

       M67.349 Transient synovitis, unspecified hand

  ✔6th **M67.35** Transient synovitis, hip

       M67.351 Transient synovitis, right hip

       M67.352 Transient synovitis, left hip

       M67.359 Transient synovitis, unspecified hip

  ✔6th **M67.36** Transient synovitis, knee

       M67.361 Transient synovitis, right knee

       M67.362 Transient synovitis, left knee

       M67.369 Transient synovitis, unspecified knee

  ✔6th **M67.37** Transient synovitis, ankle and foot

       M67.371 Transient synovitis, right ankle and foot

       M67.372 Transient synovitis, left ankle and foot

EXCLUDES 1 Not coded here   EXCLUDES 2 Not included here   ***Manifestation Code***

M67.379 Transient synovitis, unspecified ankle and foot

M67.38 Transient synovitis, other site

M67.39 Transient synovitis, multiple sites

✓5ᵗʰ M67.4 **Ganglion**
Ganglion of joint or tendon (sheath)
EXCLUDES 1 *ganglion in yaws (A66.6)*
EXCLUDES 2 *cyst of bursa (M71.2-M71.3)*
cyst of synovium (M71.2-M71.3)

M67.40 Ganglion, unspecified site

✓6ᵗʰ M67.41 Ganglion, shoulder
M67.411 Ganglion, right shoulder
M67.412 Ganglion, left shoulder
M67.419 Ganglion, unspecified shoulder

✓6ᵗʰ M67.42 Ganglion, elbow
M67.421 Ganglion, right elbow
M67.422 Ganglion, left elbow
M67.429 Ganglion, unspecified elbow

✓6ᵗʰ M67.43 Ganglion, wrist
M67.431 Ganglion, right wrist
M67.432 Ganglion, left wrist
M67.439 Ganglion, unspecified wrist

✓6ᵗʰ M67.44 Ganglion, hand
M67.441 Ganglion, right hand
M67.442 Ganglion, left hand
M67.449 Ganglion, unspecified hand

✓6ᵗʰ M67.45 Ganglion, hip
M67.451 Ganglion, right hip
M67.452 Ganglion, left hip
M67.459 Ganglion, unspecified hip

✓6ᵗʰ M67.46 Ganglion, knee
M67.461 Ganglion, right knee
M67.462 Ganglion, left knee
M67.469 Ganglion, unspecified knee

✓6ᵗʰ M67.47 Ganglion, ankle and foot
M67.471 Ganglion, right ankle and foot
M67.472 Ganglion, left ankle and foot
M67.479 Ganglion, unspecified ankle and foot

M67.48 Ganglion, other site

M67.49 Ganglion, multiple sites

✓5ᵗʰ M67.5 **Plica syndrome**
Plica knee

M67.50 Plica syndrome, unspecified knee
M67.51 Plica syndrome, right knee
M67.52 Plica syndrome, left knee

✓5ᵗʰ M67.8 **Other specified disorders of synovium and tendon**

M67.80 Other specified disorders of synovium and tendon, unspecified site

✓6ᵗʰ M67.81 Other specified disorders of synovium and tendon, shoulder
M67.811 Other specified disorders of synovium, right shoulder
M67.812 Other specified disorders of synovium, left shoulder
M67.813 Other specified disorders of tendon, right shoulder
M67.814 Other specified disorders of tendon, left shoulder
M67.819 Other specified disorders of synovium and tendon, unspecified shoulder

✓6ᵗʰ M67.82 Other specified disorders of synovium and tendon, elbow
M67.821 Other specified disorders of synovium, right elbow
M67.822 Other specified disorders of synovium, left elbow
M67.823 Other specified disorders of tendon, right elbow
M67.824 Other specified disorders of tendon, left elbow
M67.829 Other specified disorders of synovium and tendon, unspecified elbow

✓6ᵗʰ M67.83 Other specified disorders of synovium and tendon, wrist
M67.831 Other specified disorders of synovium, right wrist

M67.832 Other specified disorders of synovium, left wrist
M67.833 Other specified disorders of tendon, right wrist
M67.834 Other specified disorders of tendon, left wrist
M67.839 Other specified disorders of synovium and tendon, unspecified forearm

✓6ᵗʰ M67.84 Other specified disorders of synovium and tendon, hand
M67.841 Other specified disorders of synovium, right hand
M67.842 Other specified disorders of synovium, left hand
M67.843 Other specified disorders of tendon, right hand
M67.844 Other specified disorders of tendon, left hand
M67.849 Other specified disorders of synovium and tendon, unspecified hand

✓6ᵗʰ M67.85 Other specified disorders of synovium and tendon, hip
M67.851 Other specified disorders of synovium, right hip
M67.852 Other specified disorders of synovium, left hip
M67.853 Other specified disorders of tendon, right hip
M67.854 Other specified disorders of tendon, left hip
M67.859 Other specified disorders of synovium and tendon, unspecified hip

✓6ᵗʰ M67.86 Other specified disorders of synovium and tendon, knee
M67.861 Other specified disorders of synovium, right knee
M67.862 Other specified disorders of synovium, left knee
M67.863 Other specified disorders of tendon, right knee
M67.864 Other specified disorders of tendon, left knee
M67.869 Other specified disorders of synovium and tendon, unspecified knee

✓6ᵗʰ M67.87 Other specified disorders of synovium and tendon, ankle and foot
M67.871 Other specified disorders of synovium, right ankle and foot
M67.872 Other specified disorders of synovium, left ankle and foot
M67.873 Other specified disorders of tendon, right ankle and foot
M67.874 Other specified disorders of tendon, left ankle and foot
M67.879 Other specified disorders of synovium and tendon, unspecified ankle and foot

M67.88 Other specified disorders of synovium and tendon, other site

M67.89 Other specified disorders of synovium and tendon, multiple sites

✓5ᵗʰ M67.9 **Unspecified disorder of synovium and tendon**

M67.90 Unspecified disorder of synovium and tendon, unspecified site

✓6ᵗʰ M67.91 Unspecified disorder of synovium and tendon, shoulder
M67.911 Unspecified disorder of synovium and tendon, right shoulder
M67.912 Unspecified disorder of synovium and tendon, left shoulder
M67.919 Unspecified disorder of synovium and tendon, unspecified shoulder

✓6ᵗʰ M67.92 Unspecified disorder of synovium and tendon, upper arm
M67.921 Unspecified disorder of synovium and tendon, right upper arm
M67.922 Unspecified disorder of synovium and tendon, left upper arm

---

✓ Appropriate additional character required   ✓x7ᵗʰ Requires 7th character, placeholder x must fill empty characters

M67.929 **Unspecified disorder of synovium and tendon, unspecified upper arm**

√6th M67.93 **Unspecified disorder of synovium and tendon, forearm**

M67.931 **Unspecified disorder of synovium and tendon, right forearm**

M67.932 **Unspecified disorder of synovium and tendon, left forearm**

M67.939 **Unspecified disorder of synovium and tendon, unspecified forearm**

√6th M67.94 **Unspecified disorder of synovium and tendon, hand**

M67.941 **Unspecified disorder of synovium and tendon, right hand**

M67.942 **Unspecified disorder of synovium and tendon, left hand**

M67.949 **Unspecified disorder of synovium and tendon, unspecified hand**

√6th M67.95 **Unspecified disorder of synovium and tendon, thigh**

M67.951 **Unspecified disorder of synovium and tendon, right thigh**

M67.952 **Unspecified disorder of synovium and tendon, left thigh**

M67.959 **Unspecified disorder of synovium and tendon, unspecified thigh**

√6th M67.96 **Unspecified disorder of synovium and tendon, lower leg**

M67.961 **Unspecified disorder of synovium and tendon, right lower leg**

M67.962 **Unspecified disorder of synovium and tendon, left lower leg**

M67.969 **Unspecified disorder of synovium and tendon, unspecified lower leg**

√6th M67.97 **Unspecified disorder of synovium and tendon, ankle and foot**

M67.971 **Unspecified disorder of synovium and tendon, right ankle and foot**

M67.972 **Unspecified disorder of synovium and tendon, left ankle and foot**

M67.979 **Unspecified disorder of synovium and tendon, unspecified ankle and foot**

M67.98 **Unspecified disorder of synovium and tendon, other site**

M67.99 **Unspecified disorder of synovium and tendon, multiple sites**

Other soft tissue disorders (M70-M79)

√4th **M70 Soft tissue disorders related to use, overuse and pressure**

INCLUDES soft tissue disorders of occupational origin

EXCLUDES 1 *bursitis NOS (M71.9-)*

EXCLUDES 2 *bursitis of shoulder (M75.5)*
enthesopathies (M76-M77)
pressure ulcer (pressure area) (L89-)

Use additional external cause code to identify activity causing disorder (Y93-)

√5th M70.0 **Crepitant synovitis (acute) (chronic) of hand and wrist**

√6th M70.03 **Crepitant synovitis (acute) (chronic), wrist**

M70.031 **Crepitant synovitis (acute) (chronic), right wrist**

M70.032 **Crepitant synovitis (acute) (chronic), left wrist**

M70.039 **Crepitant synovitis (acute) (chronic), unspecified wrist**

√6th M70.04 **Crepitant synovitis (acute) (chronic), hand**

M70.041 **Crepitant synovitis (acute) (chronic), right hand**

M70.042 **Crepitant synovitis (acute) (chronic), left hand**

M70.049 **Crepitant synovitis (acute) (chronic), unspecified hand**

√5th M70.1 **Bursitis of hand**

M70.10 **Bursitis, unspecified hand**

M70.11 **Bursitis, right hand**

M70.12 **Bursitis, left hand**

√5th M70.2 **Olecranon bursitis**

M70.20 **Olecranon bursitis, unspecified elbow**

M70.21 **Olecranon bursitis, right elbow**

M70.22 **Olecranon bursitis, left elbow**

√5th M70.3 **Other bursitis of elbow**

M70.30 **Other bursitis of elbow, unspecified elbow**

M70.31 **Other bursitis of elbow, right elbow**

M70.32 **Other bursitis of elbow, left elbow**

√5th M70.4 **Prepatellar bursitis**

M70.40 **Prepatellar bursitis, unspecified knee**

M70.41 **Prepatellar bursitis, right knee**

M70.42 **Prepatellar bursitis, left knee**

√5th M70.5 **Other bursitis of knee**

M70.50 **Other bursitis of knee, unspecified knee**

M70.51 **Other bursitis of knee, right knee**

M70.52 **Other bursitis of knee, left knee**

√5th M70.6 **Trochanteric bursitis**

Trochanteric tendinitis

M70.60 **Trochanteric bursitis, unspecified hip**

M70.61 **Trochanteric bursitis, right hip**

M70.62 **Trochanteric bursitis, left hip**

√5th M70.7 **Other bursitis of hip**

Ischial bursitis

M70.70 **Other bursitis of hip, unspecified hip**

M70.71 **Other bursitis of hip, right hip**

M70.72 **Other bursitis of hip, left hip**

√5th M70.8 **Other soft tissue disorders related to use, overuse and pressure**

M70.80 **Other soft tissue disorders related to use, overuse and pressure of unspecified site**

√6th M70.81 **Other soft tissue disorders related to use, overuse and pressure of shoulder**

M70.811 **Other soft tissue disorders related to use, overuse and pressure, right shoulder**

M70.812 **Other soft tissue disorders related to use, overuse and pressure, left shoulder**

M70.819 **Other soft tissue disorders related to use, overuse and pressure, unspecified shoulder**

√6th M70.82 **Other soft tissue disorders related to use, overuse and pressure of upper arm**

M70.821 **Other soft tissue disorders related to use, overuse and pressure, right upper arm**

M70.822 **Other soft tissue disorders related to use, overuse and pressure, left upper arm**

M70.829 **Other soft tissue disorders related to use, overuse and pressure, unspecified upper arms**

√6th M70.83 **Other soft tissue disorders related to use, overuse and pressure of forearm**

M70.831 **Other soft tissue disorders related to use, overuse and pressure, right forearm**

M70.832 **Other soft tissue disorders related to use, overuse and pressure, left forearm**

M70.839 **Other soft tissue disorders related to use, overuse and pressure, unspecified forearm**

√6th M70.84 **Other soft tissue disorders related to use, overuse and pressure of hand**

M70.841 **Other soft tissue disorders related to use, overuse and pressure, right hand**

M70.842 **Other soft tissue disorders related to use, overuse and pressure, left hand**

M70.849 **Other soft tissue disorders related to use, overuse and pressure, unspecified hand**

√6th M70.85 **Other soft tissue disorders related to use, overuse and pressure of thigh**

M70.851 **Other soft tissue disorders related to use, overuse and pressure, right thigh**

M70.852 **Other soft tissue disorders related to use, overuse and pressure, left thigh**

M70.859 **Other soft tissue disorders related to use, overuse and pressure, unspecified thigh**

EXCLUDES 1 Not coded here   EXCLUDES 2 Not included here   *Manifestation Code*

✓6ᵗʰ **M70.86 Other soft tissue disorders related to use, overuse and pressure lower leg**
 M70.861 Other soft tissue disorders related to use, overuse and pressure, right lower leg
 M70.862 Other soft tissue disorders related to use, overuse and pressure, left lower leg
 M70.869 Other soft tissue disorders related to use, overuse and pressure, unspecified leg

✓6ᵗʰ **M70.87 Other soft tissue disorders related to use, overuse and pressure of ankle and foot**
 M70.871 Other soft tissue disorders related to use, overuse and pressure, right ankle and foot
 M70.872 Other soft tissue disorders related to use, overuse and pressure, left ankle and foot
 M70.879 Other soft tissue disorders related to use, overuse and pressure, unspecified ankle and foot

 M70.88 Other soft tissue disorders related to use, overuse and pressure other site

 M70.89 Other soft tissue disorders related to use, overuse and pressure multiple sites

✓5ᵗʰ **M70.9 Unspecified soft tissue disorder related to use, overuse and pressure**
 M70.90 Unspecified soft tissue disorder related to use, overuse and pressure of unspecified site

✓6ᵗʰ **M70.91 Unspecified soft tissue disorder related to use, overuse and pressure of shoulder**
 M70.911 Unspecified soft tissue disorder related to use, overuse and pressure, right shoulder
 M70.912 Unspecified soft tissue disorder related to use, overuse and pressure, left shoulder
 M70.919 Unspecified soft tissue disorder related to use, overuse and pressure, unspecified shoulder

✓6ᵗʰ **M70.92 Unspecified soft tissue disorder related to use, overuse and pressure of upper arm**
 M70.921 Unspecified soft tissue disorder related to use, overuse and pressure, right upper arm
 M70.922 Unspecified soft tissue disorder related to use, overuse and pressure, left upper arm
 M70.929 Unspecified soft tissue disorder related to use, overuse and pressure, unspecified upper arm

✓6ᵗʰ **M70.93 Unspecified soft tissue disorder related to use, overuse and pressure of forearm**
 M70.931 Unspecified soft tissue disorder related to use, overuse and pressure, right forearm
 M70.932 Unspecified soft tissue disorder related to use, overuse and pressure, left forearm
 M70.939 Unspecified soft tissue disorder related to use, overuse and pressure, unspecified forearm

✓6ᵗʰ **M70.94 Unspecified soft tissue disorder related to use, overuse and pressure of hand**
 M70.941 Unspecified soft tissue disorder related to use, overuse and pressure, right hand
 M70.942 Unspecified soft tissue disorder related to use, overuse and pressure, left hand
 M70.949 Unspecified soft tissue disorder related to use, overuse and pressure, unspecified hand

✓6ᵗʰ **M70.95 Unspecified soft tissue disorder related to use, overuse and pressure of thigh**
 M70.951 Unspecified soft tissue disorder related to use, overuse and pressure, right thigh
 M70.952 Unspecified soft tissue disorder related to use, overuse and pressure, left thigh

 M70.959 Unspecified soft tissue disorder related to use, overuse and pressure, unspecified thigh

✓6ᵗʰ **M70.96 Unspecified soft tissue disorder related to use, overuse and pressure lower leg**
 M70.961 Unspecified soft tissue disorder related to use, overuse and pressure, right lower leg
 M70.962 Unspecified soft tissue disorder related to use, overuse and pressure, left lower leg
 M70.969 Unspecified soft tissue disorder related to use, overuse and pressure, unspecified lower leg

✓6ᵗʰ **M70.97 Unspecified soft tissue disorder related to use, overuse and pressure of ankle and foot**
 M70.971 Unspecified soft tissue disorder related to use, overuse and pressure, right ankle and foot
 M70.972 Unspecified soft tissue disorder related to use, overuse and pressure, left ankle and foot
 M70.979 Unspecified soft tissue disorder related to use, overuse and pressure, unspecified ankle and foot

 M70.98 Unspecified soft tissue disorder related to use, overuse and pressure other

 M70.99 Unspecified soft tissue disorder related to use, overuse and pressure multiple sites

✓4ᵗʰ **M71 Other bursopathies**
 EXCLUDES 1 *bunion (M20.1)*
 bursitis related to use, overuse or pressure (M70-)
 enthesopathies (M76-M77)

✓5ᵗʰ **M71.0 Abscess of bursa**
 Use additional code (B95-, B96-) to identify causative organism
 M71.00 Abscess of bursa, unspecified site
✓6ᵗʰ **M71.01 Abscess of bursa, shoulder**
 M71.011 Abscess of bursa, right shoulder
 M71.012 Abscess of bursa, left shoulder
 M71.019 Abscess of bursa, unspecified shoulder
✓6ᵗʰ **M71.02 Abscess of bursa, elbow**
 M71.021 Abscess of bursa, right elbow
 M71.022 Abscess of bursa, left elbow
 M71.029 Abscess of bursa, unspecified elbow
✓6ᵗʰ **M71.03 Abscess of bursa, wrist**
 M71.031 Abscess of bursa, right wrist
 M71.032 Abscess of bursa, left wrist
 M71.039 Abscess of bursa, unspecified wrist
✓6ᵗʰ **M71.04 Abscess of bursa, hand**
 M71.041 Abscess of bursa, right hand
 M71.042 Abscess of bursa, left hand
 M71.049 Abscess of bursa, unspecified hand
✓6ᵗʰ **M71.05 Abscess of bursa, hip**
 M71.051 Abscess of bursa, right hip
 M71.052 Abscess of bursa, left hip
 M71.059 Abscess of bursa, unspecified hip
✓6ᵗʰ **M71.06 Abscess of bursa, knee**
 M71.061 Abscess of bursa, right knee
 M71.062 Abscess of bursa, left knee
 M71.069 Abscess of bursa, unspecified knee
✓6ᵗʰ **M71.07 Abscess of bursa, ankle and foot**
 M71.071 Abscess of bursa, right ankle and foot
 M71.072 Abscess of bursa, left ankle and foot
 M71.079 Abscess of bursa, unspecified ankle and foot
 M71.08 Abscess of bursa, other site
 M71.09 Abscess of bursa, multiple sites

✓5ᵗʰ **M71.1 Other infective bursitis**
 Use additional code (B95-, B96-) to identify causative organism
 M71.10 Other infective bursitis, unspecified site
✓6ᵗʰ **M71.11 Other infective bursitis, shoulder**
 M71.111 Other infective bursitis, right shoulder
 M71.112 Other infective bursitis, left shoulder

    M71.119 Other infective bursitis, unspecified shoulder
✓6th **M71.12** **Other infective bursitis, elbow**
    M71.121 Other infective bursitis, right elbow
    M71.122 Other infective bursitis, left elbow
    M71.129 Other infective bursitis, unspecified elbow
✓6th **M71.13** **Other infective bursitis, wrist**
    M71.131 Other infective bursitis, right wrist
    M71.132 Other infective bursitis, left wrist
    M71.139 Other infective bursitis, unspecified wrist
✓6th **M71.14** **Other infective bursitis, hand**
    M71.141 Other infective bursitis, right hand
    M71.142 Other infective bursitis, left hand
    M71.149 Other infective bursitis, unspecified hand
✓6th **M71.15** **Other infective bursitis, hip**
    M71.151 Other infective bursitis, right hip
    M71.152 Other infective bursitis, left hip
    M71.159 Other infective bursitis, unspecified hip
✓6th **M71.16** **Other infective bursitis, knee**
    M71.161 Other infective bursitis, right knee
    M71.162 Other infective bursitis, left knee
    M71.169 Other infective bursitis, unspecified knee
✓6th **M71.17** **Other infective bursitis, ankle and foot**
    M71.171 Other infective bursitis, right ankle and foot
    M71.172 Other infective bursitis, left ankle and foot
    M71.179 Other infective bursitis, unspecified ankle and foot
    M71.18 Other infective bursitis, other site
    M71.19 Other infective bursitis, multiple sites
✓5th **M71.2** **Synovial cyst of popliteal space [Baker]**
    EXCLUDES 1 *synovial cyst of popliteal space with rupture (M66.0)*
    M71.20 Synovial cyst of popliteal space [Baker], unspecified knee
    M71.21 Synovial cyst of popliteal space [Baker], right knee
    M71.22 Synovial cyst of popliteal space [Baker], left knee
✓5th **M71.3** **Other bursal cyst**
    Synovial cyst NOS
    EXCLUDES 1 *synovial cyst with rupture (M66.1-)*
    M71.30 Other bursal cyst, unspecified site
✓6th **M71.31** **Other bursal cyst, shoulder**
    M71.311 Other bursal cyst, right shoulder
    M71.312 Other bursal cyst, left shoulder
    M71.319 Other bursal cyst, unspecified shoulder
✓6th **M71.32** **Other bursal cyst, elbow**
    M71.321 Other bursal cyst, right elbow
    M71.322 Other bursal cyst, left elbow
    M71.329 Other bursal cyst, unspecified elbow
✓6th **M71.33** **Other bursal cyst, wrist**
    M71.331 Other bursal cyst, right wrist
    M71.332 Other bursal cyst, left wrist
    M71.339 Other bursal cyst, unspecified wrist
✓6th **M71.34** **Other bursal cyst, hand**
    M71.341 Other bursal cyst, right hand
    M71.342 Other bursal cyst, left hand
    M71.349 Other bursal cyst, unspecified hand
✓6th **M71.35** **Other bursal cyst, hip**
    M71.351 Other bursal cyst, right hip
    M71.352 Other bursal cyst, left hip
    M71.359 Other bursal cyst, unspecified hip
✓6th **M71.37** **Other bursal cyst, ankle and foot**
    M71.371 Other bursal cyst, right ankle and foot
    M71.372 Other bursal cyst, left ankle and foot
    M71.379 Other bursal cyst, unspecified ankle and foot
    M71.38 Other bursal cyst, other site
    M71.39 Other bursal cyst, multiple sites
✓5th **M71.4** **Calcium deposit in bursa**
    EXCLUDES 2 *calcium deposit in bursa of shoulder (M75.3)*
    M71.40 Calcium deposit in bursa, unspecified site

✓6th **M71.42** **Calcium deposit in bursa, elbow**
    M71.421 Calcium deposit in bursa, right elbow
    M71.422 Calcium deposit in bursa, left elbow
    M71.429 Calcium deposit in bursa, unspecified elbow
✓6th **M71.43** **Calcium deposit in bursa, wrist**
    M71.431 Calcium deposit in bursa, right wrist
    M71.432 Calcium deposit in bursa, left wrist
    M71.439 Calcium deposit in bursa, unspecified wrist
✓6th **M71.44** **Calcium deposit in bursa, hand**
    M71.441 Calcium deposit in bursa, right hand
    M71.442 Calcium deposit in bursa, left hand
    M71.449 Calcium deposit in bursa, unspecified hand
✓6th **M71.45** **Calcium deposit in bursa, hip**
    M71.451 Calcium deposit in bursa, right hip
    M71.452 Calcium deposit in bursa, left hip
    M71.459 Calcium deposit in bursa, unspecified hip
✓6th **M71.46** **Calcium deposit in bursa, knee**
    M71.461 Calcium deposit in bursa, right knee
    M71.462 Calcium deposit in bursa, left knee
    M71.469 Calcium deposit in bursa, unspecified knee
✓6th **M71.47** **Calcium deposit in bursa, ankle and foot**
    M71.471 Calcium deposit in bursa, right ankle and foot
    M71.472 Calcium deposit in bursa, left ankle and foot
    M71.479 Calcium deposit in bursa, unspecified ankle and foot
    M71.48 Calcium deposit in bursa, other site
    M71.49 Calcium deposit in bursa, multiple sites
✓5th **M71.5** **Other bursitis, not elsewhere classified**
    EXCLUDES 1 *bursitis NOS (M71.9-)*
    EXCLUDES 2 *bursitis of shoulder (M75.5)*
        bursitis of tibial collateral [Pellegrini-Stieda] (M76.4)
    M71.50 Other bursitis, not elsewhere classified, unspecified site
✓6th **M71.52** **Other bursitis, not elsewhere classified, elbow**
    M71.521 Other bursitis, not elsewhere classified, right elbow
    M71.522 Other bursitis, not elsewhere classified, left elbow
    M71.529 Other bursitis, not elsewhere classified, unspecified elbow
✓6th **M71.53** **Other bursitis, not elsewhere classified, wrist**
    M71.531 Other bursitis, not elsewhere classified, right wrist
    M71.532 Other bursitis, not elsewhere classified, left wrist
    M71.539 Other bursitis, not elsewhere classified, unspecified wrist
✓6th **M71.54** **Other bursitis, not elsewhere classified, hand**
    M71.541 Other bursitis, not elsewhere classified, right hand
    M71.542 Other bursitis, not elsewhere classified, left hand
    M71.549 Other bursitis, not elsewhere classified, unspecified hand
✓6th **M71.55** **Other bursitis, not elsewhere classified, hip**
    M71.551 Other bursitis, not elsewhere classified, right hip
    M71.552 Other bursitis, not elsewhere classified, left hip
    M71.559 Other bursitis, not elsewhere classified, unspecified hip
✓6th **M71.56** **Other bursitis, not elsewhere classified, knee**
    M71.561 Other bursitis, not elsewhere classified, right knee
    M71.562 Other bursitis, not elsewhere classified, left knee
    M71.569 Other bursitis, not elsewhere classified, unspecified knee

---

EXCLUDES 1 Not coded here   EXCLUDES 2 Not included here   *Manifestation Code*

☑6ᵗʰ **M71.57** Other bursitis, not elsewhere classified, ankle and foot

    M71.571 Other bursitis, not elsewhere classified, right ankle and foot

    M71.572 Other bursitis, not elsewhere classified, left ankle and foot

    M71.579 Other bursitis, not elsewhere classified, unspecified ankle and foot

  M71.58 Other bursitis, not elsewhere classified, other site

☑5ᵗʰ **M71.8** Other specified bursopathies

  M71.80 Other specified bursopathies, unspecified site

☑6ᵗʰ **M71.81** Other specified bursopathies, shoulder

    M71.811 Other specified bursopathies, right shoulder

    M71.812 Other specified bursopathies, left shoulder

    M71.819 Other specified bursopathies, unspecified shoulder

☑6ᵗʰ **M71.82** Other specified bursopathies, elbow

    M71.821 Other specified bursopathies, right elbow

    M71.822 Other specified bursopathies, left elbow

    M71.829 Other specified bursopathies, unspecified elbow

☑6ᵗʰ **M71.83** Other specified bursopathies, wrist

    M71.831 Other specified bursopathies, right wrist

    M71.832 Other specified bursopathies, left wrist

    M71.839 Other specified bursopathies, unspecified wrist

☑6ᵗʰ **M71.84** Other specified bursopathies, hand

    M71.841 Other specified bursopathies, right hand

    M71.842 Other specified bursopathies, left hand

    M71.849 Other specified bursopathies, unspecified hand

☑6ᵗʰ **M71.85** Other specified bursopathies, hip

    M71.851 Other specified bursopathies, right hip

    M71.852 Other specified bursopathies, left hip

    M71.859 Other specified bursopathies, unspecified hip

☑6ᵗʰ **M71.86** Other specified bursopathies, knee

    M71.861 Other specified bursopathies, right knee

    M71.862 Other specified bursopathies, left knee

    M71.869 Other specified bursopathies, unspecified knee

☑6ᵗʰ **M71.87** Other specified bursopathies, ankle and foot

    M71.871 Other specified bursopathies, right ankle and foot

    M71.872 Other specified bursopathies, left ankle and foot

    M71.879 Other specified bursopathies, unspecified ankle and foot

  M71.88 Other specified bursopathies, other site

  M71.89 Other specified bursopathies, multiple sites

M71.9 Bursopathy, unspecified
  Bursitis NOS

☑4ᵗʰ **M72 Fibroblastic disorders**

  EXCLUDES 2   retroperitoneal fibromatosis (D48.3)

M72.0 Palmar fascial fibromatosis [Dupuytren]

M72.1 Knuckle pads

M72.2 Plantar fascial fibromatosis
  Plantar fasciitis

M72.4 Pseudosarcomatous fibromatosis
  Nodular fasciitis

M72.6 Necrotizing fasciitis
  Use additional code (B95-, B96-) to identify causative organism

M72.8 Other fibroblastic disorders
  Abscess of fascia
  Fasciitis NEC
  Other infective fasciitis
  Use additional code to (B95-, B96-) identify causative organism

  EXCLUDES 1   diffuse (eosinophilic) fasciitis (M35.4)
    necrotizing fasciitis (M72.6)
    nodular fasciitis (M72.4)
    perirenal fasciitis NOS (N13.5)
    perirenal fasciitis with infection (N13.6)
    plantar fasciitis (M72.2)

M72.9 Fibroblastic disorder, unspecified
  Fasciitis NOS
  Fibromatosis NOS

☑4ᵗʰ **M75 Shoulder lesions**

  EXCLUDES 2   shoulder-hand syndrome (M89.0-)

☑5ᵗʰ **M75.0** Adhesive capsulitis of shoulder
  Frozen shoulder
  Periarthritis of shoulder

  M75.00 Adhesive capsulitis of unspecified shoulder

  M75.01 Adhesive capsulitis of right shoulder

  M75.02 Adhesive capsulitis of left shoulder

☑5ᵗʰ **M75.1** Rotator cuff syndrome
  Rotator cuff or supraspinatus tear or rupture (complete) (incomplete), not specified as traumatic
  Supraspinatus syndrome

  M75.10 Rotator cuff syndrome, unspecified shoulder

  M75.11 Rotator cuff syndrome, right shoulder

  M75.12 Rotator cuff syndrome, left shoulder

☑5ᵗʰ **M75.2** Bicipital tendinitis

  M75.20 Bicipital tendinitis, unspecified shoulder

  M75.21 Bicipital tendinitis, right shoulder

  M75.22 Bicipital tendinitis, left shoulder

☑5ᵗʰ **M75.3** Calcific tendinitis of shoulder
  Calcified bursa of shoulder

  M75.30 Calcific tendinitis of unspecified shoulder

  M75.31 Calcific tendinitis of right shoulder

  M75.32 Calcific tendinitis of left shoulder

☑5ᵗʰ **M75.4** Impingement syndrome of shoulder

  M75.40 Impingement syndrome of unspecified shoulder

  M75.41 Impingement syndrome of right shoulder

  M75.42 Impingement syndrome of left shoulder

☑5ᵗʰ **M75.5** Bursitis of shoulder

  M75.50 Bursitis of unspecified shoulder

  M75.51 Bursitis of right shoulder

  M75.52 Bursitis of left shoulder

☑5ᵗʰ **M75.8** Other shoulder lesions

  M75.80 Other shoulder lesions, unspecified shoulder

  M75.81 Other shoulder lesions, right shoulder

  M75.82 Other shoulder lesions, left shoulder

☑5ᵗʰ **M75.9** Shoulder lesion, unspecified

  M75.90 Shoulder lesion, unspecified, unspecified shoulder

  M75.91 Shoulder lesion, unspecified, right shoulder

  M75.92 Shoulder lesion, unspecified, left shoulder

☑4ᵗʰ **M76 Enthesopathies, lower limb, excluding foot**

  EXCLUDES 2   bursitis due to use, overuse and pressure (M70-)
    enthesopathies of ankle and foot (M77.5-)

☑5ᵗʰ **M76.0** Gluteal tendinitis

  M76.00 Gluteal tendinitis, unspecified hip

  M76.01 Gluteal tendinitis, right hip

  M76.02 Gluteal tendinitis, left hip

☑5ᵗʰ **M76.1** Psoas tendinitis

  M76.10 Psoas tendinitis, unspecified hip

  M76.11 Psoas tendinitis, right hip

  M76.12 Psoas tendinitis, left hip

☑5ᵗʰ **M76.2** Iliac crest spur

  M76.20 Iliac crest spur, unspecified hip

  M76.21 Iliac crest spur, right hip

  M76.22 Iliac crest spur, left hip

☑5ᵗʰ **M76.3** Iliotibial band syndrome

  M76.30 Iliotibial band syndrome, unspecified leg

  M76.31 Iliotibial band syndrome, right leg

  M76.32 Iliotibial band syndrome, left leg

✓5th **M76.4 Tibial collateral bursitis [Pellegrini-Stieda]**
     M76.40 Tibial collateral bursitis [Pellegrini-Stieda], unspecified leg
     M76.41 Tibial collateral bursitis [Pellegrini-Stieda], right leg
     M76.42 Tibial collateral bursitis [Pellegrini-Stieda], left leg

✓5th **M76.5 Patellar tendinitis**
     M76.50 Patellar tendinitis, unspecified knee
     M76.51 Patellar tendinitis, right knee
     M76.52 Patellar tendinitis, left knee

✓5th **M76.6 Achilles tendinitis**
     Achilles bursitis
     M76.60 Achilles tendinitis, unspecified leg
     M76.61 Achilles tendinitis, right leg
     M76.62 Achilles tendinitis, left leg

✓5th **M76.7 Peroneal tendinitis**
     M76.70 Peroneal tendinitis, unspecified leg
     M76.71 Peroneal tendinitis, right leg
     M76.72 Peroneal tendinitis, left leg

✓5th **M76.8 Other specified enthesopathies of lower limb, excluding foot**
     ✓6th **M76.81 Anterior tibial syndrome**
         M76.811 Anterior tibial syndrome, right leg
         M76.812 Anterior tibial syndrome, left leg
         M76.819 Anterior tibial syndrome, unspecified leg
     ✓6th **M76.82 Posterior tibial tendinitis**
         M76.821 Posterior tibial tendinitis, right leg
         M76.822 Posterior tibial tendinitis, left leg
         M76.829 Posterior tibial tendinitis, unspecified leg
     ✓6th **M76.89 Other specified enthesopathies of lower limb, excluding foot**
         M76.891 Other specified enthesopathies of right lower limb, excluding foot
         M76.892 Other specified enthesopathies of left lower limb, excluding foot
         M76.899 Other specified enthesopathies of unspecified lower limb, excluding foot

✓5th **M76.9 Unspecified enthesopathy, lower limb, excluding foot**

✓4th **M77 Other enthesopathies**
     EXCLUDES 1   bursitis NOS (M71.9-)
     EXCLUDES 2   bursitis due to use, overuse and pressure (M70-)
         osteophyte (M25.7)
         spinal enthesopathy (M46.0-)

✓5th **M77.0 Medial epicondylitis**
     M77.00 Medial epicondylitis, unspecified elbow
     M77.01 Medial epicondylitis, right elbow
     M77.02 Medial epicondylitis, left elbow

✓5th **M77.1 Lateral epicondylitis**
     Tennis elbow
     M77.10 Lateral epicondylitis, unspecified elbow
     M77.11 Lateral epicondylitis, right elbow
     M77.12 Lateral epicondylitis, left elbow

✓5th **M77.2 Periarthritis of wrist**
     M77.20 Periarthritis, unspecified wrist
     M77.21 Periarthritis, right wrist
     M77.22 Periarthritis, left wrist

✓5th **M77.3 Calcaneal spur**
     M77.30 Calcaneal spur, unspecified foot
     M77.31 Calcaneal spur, right foot
     M77.32 Calcaneal spur, left foot

✓5th **M77.4 Metatarsalgia**
     EXCLUDES 1   Morton's metatarsalgia (G57.6)
     M77.40 Metatarsalgia, unspecified foot
     M77.41 Metatarsalgia, right foot
     M77.42 Metatarsalgia, left foot

✓5th **M77.5 Other enthesopathy of foot**
     M77.50 Other enthesopathy of unspecified foot
     M77.51 Other enthesopathy of right foot
     M77.52 Other enthesopathy of left foot

M77.8 Other enthesopathies, not elsewhere classified

M77.9 Enthesopathy, unspecified
     Bone spur NOS
     Capsulitis NOS
     Periarthritis NOS
     Tendinitis NOS

✓4th **M79 Other and unspecified soft tissue disorders, not elsewhere classified**
     EXCLUDES 1   psychogenic rheumatism (F45.8)
         soft tissue pain, psychogenic (F45.41)

M79.0 Rheumatism, unspecified
     EXCLUDES 1   fibromyalgia (M79.7)
         palindromic rheumatism (M12.3-)

M79.1 Myalgia
     Myofascial pain syndrome
     EXCLUDES 1   fibromyalgia (M79.7)
         myositis (M60-)

M79.2 Neuralgia and neuritis, unspecified
     EXCLUDES 1   brachial radiculitis NOS (M54.1)
         lumbosacral radiculitis NOS (M54.1)
         mononeuropathies (G56-G58)
         radiculitis NOS (M54.1)
         sciatica (M54.3-M54.4)

M79.3 Panniculitis, unspecified
     EXCLUDES 1   lupus panniculitis (L93.2)
         neck and back panniculitis (M54.0-)
         relapsing [Weber-Christian] panniculitis (M35.6)

M79.4 Hypertrophy of (infrapatellar) fat pad

M79.5 Residual foreign body in soft tissue
     EXCLUDES 1   foreign body granuloma of skin and subcutaneous tissue (L92.3)
         foreign body granuloma of soft tissue (M60.2-)

✓5th **M79.6 Pain in limb, hand, foot, fingers and toes**
     EXCLUDES 2   pain in joint (M25.5-)
     ✓6th **M79.60 Pain in limb, unspecified**
         M79.601 Pain in right arm
         Pain in right upper limb NOS
         M79.602 Pain in left arm
         Pain in left upper limb NOS
         M79.603 Pain in arm, unspecified
         Pain in upper limb NOS
         M79.604 Pain in right leg
         Pain in right lower limb NOS
         M79.605 Pain in left leg
         Pain in left lower limb NOS
         M79.606 Pain in leg, unspecified
         Pain in lower limb NOS
         M79.609 Pain in unspecified limb
         Pain in limb NOS
     ✓6th **M79.62 Pain in upper arm**
         Pain in axillary region
         M79.621 Pain in right upper arm
         M79.622 Pain in left upper arm
         M79.629 Pain in unspecified upper arm
     ✓6th **M79.63 Pain in forearm**
         M79.631 Pain in right forearm
         M79.632 Pain in left forearm
         M79.639 Pain in unspecified forearm
     ✓6th **M79.64 Pain in hand and fingers**
         M79.641 Pain in right hand
         M79.642 Pain in left hand
         M79.643 Pain in unspecified hand
         M79.644 Pain in right finger(s)
         M79.645 Pain in left finger(s)
         M79.646 Pain in unspecified finger(s)
     ✓6th **M79.65 Pain in thigh**
         M79.651 Pain in right thigh
         M79.652 Pain in left thigh
         M79.659 Pain in unspecified thigh
     ✓6th **M79.66 Pain in lower leg**
         M79.661 Pain in right lower leg
         M79.662 Pain in left lower leg
         M79.669 Pain in unspecified lower leg
     ✓6th **M79.67 Pain in foot and toes**
         M79.671 Pain in right foot
         M79.672 Pain in left foot
         M79.673 Pain in unspecified foot

EXCLUDES 1   Not coded here   EXCLUDES 2   Not included here   *Manifestation Code*

     © 2011 Ingenix

M79.674 Pain in right toe(s)
M79.675 Pain in left toe(s)
M79.676 Pain in unspecified toe(s)

M79.7 Fibromyalgia
Fibromyositis
Fibrositis
Myofibrositis

✓5ᵗʰ **M79.a Nontraumatic compartment syndrome**
Code first, if applicable, associated postprocedural complication

EXCLUDES 1 compartment syndrome NOS (T79.a-)
fibromyalgia (M79.7)
nontraumatic ischemic infarction of muscle (M62.2-)
traumatic compartment syndrome (T79.a-)

✓6ᵗʰ **M79.a1 Nontraumatic compartment syndrome of upper extremity**
Nontraumatic compartment syndrome of shoulder, arm, forearm, wrist, hand, and fingers

M79.a11 **Nontraumatic compartment syndrome of right upper extremity**

M79.a12 **Nontraumatic compartment syndrome of left upper extremity**

M79.a19 **Nontraumatic compartment syndrome of unspecified upper extremity**

✓6ᵗʰ **M79.a2 Nontraumatic compartment syndrome of lower extremity**
Nontraumatic compartment syndrome of hip, buttock, thigh, leg, foot, and toes

M79.a21 **Nontraumatic compartment syndrome of right lower extremity**

M79.a22 **Nontraumatic compartment syndrome of left lower extremity**

M79.a29 **Nontraumatic compartment syndrome of unspecified lower extremity**

M79.a3 **Nontraumatic compartment syndrome of abdomen**

M79.a9 **Nontraumatic compartment syndrome of other sites**

✓5ᵗʰ **M79.8 Other specified soft tissue disorders**

M79.81 **Nontraumatic hematoma of soft tissue**
Nontraumatic hematoma of muscle
Nontraumatic seroma of muscle and soft tissue

M79.89 **Other specified soft tissue disorders**
Polyalgia

M79.9 Soft tissue disorder, unspecified

OSTEOPATHIES AND CHONDROPATHIES (M80-M94)

Disorders of bone density and structure (M80-M85)

✓4ᵗʰ **M80 Osteoporosis with current pathological fracture**
INCLUDES osteoporosis with current fragility fracture
NOTE Fragility fracture is defined as a fracture sustained with trauma no more than a fall from a standing height or less that occurs under circumstances that would not cause a fracture in a normal healthy bone
Use additional code to identify major osseous defect, if applicable (M89.7-)

EXCLUDES 1 collapsed vertebra NOS (M48.5)
pathological fracture NOS (M84.4)
wedging of vertebra NOS (M48.5)

EXCLUDES 2 personal history of (healed) osteoporosis fracture (Z87.310)

The appropriate 7th character is to be added to each code from category M80.
A   initial encounter for fracture
D   subsequent encounter for fracture with routine healing
G   subsequent encounter for fracture with delayed healing
K   subsequent encounter for fracture with nonunion
P   subsequent encounter for fracture with malunion
S   sequela

✓5ᵗʰ **M80.0 Age-related osteoporosis with current pathological fracture**
Involutional osteoporosis with current pathological fracture
Osteoporosis NOS with current pathological fracture
Postmenopausal osteoporosis with current pathological fracture
Senile osteoporosis with current pathological fracture

✓x7ᵗʰ M80.00 **Age-related osteoporosis with current pathological fracture, unspecified site**

✓6ᵗʰ M80.01 **Age-related osteoporosis with current pathological fracture, shoulder**

✓7ᵗʰ M80.011 **Age-related osteoporosis with current pathological fracture, right shoulder**

✓7ᵗʰ M80.012 **Age-related osteoporosis with current pathological fracture, left shoulder**

✓7ᵗʰ M80.019 **Age-related osteoporosis with current pathological fracture, unspecified shoulder**

✓6ᵗʰ M80.02 **Age-related osteoporosis with current pathological fracture, humerus**

✓7ᵗʰ M80.021 **Age-related osteoporosis with current pathological fracture, right humerus**

✓7ᵗʰ M80.022 **Age-related osteoporosis with current pathological fracture, left humerus**

✓7ᵗʰ M80.029 **Age-related osteoporosis with current pathological fracture, unspecified humerus**

✓6ᵗʰ M80.03 **Age-related osteoporosis with current pathological fracture, forearm**
Age-related osteoporosis with current pathological fracture of wrist

✓7ᵗʰ M80.031 **Age-related osteoporosis with current pathological fracture, right forearm**

✓7ᵗʰ M80.032 **Age-related osteoporosis with current pathological fracture, left forearm**

✓7ᵗʰ M80.039 **Age-related osteoporosis with current pathological fracture, unspecified forearm**

✓6ᵗʰ M80.04 **Age-related osteoporosis with current pathological fracture, hand**

✓7ᵗʰ M80.041 **Age-related osteoporosis with current pathological fracture, right hand**

✓7ᵗʰ M80.042 **Age-related osteoporosis with current pathological fracture, left hand**

✓7ᵗʰ M80.049 **Age-related osteoporosis with current pathological fracture, unspecified hand**

✓6ᵗʰ M80.05 **Age-related osteoporosis with current pathological fracture, femur**
Age-related osteoporosis with current pathological fracture of hip

✓7ᵗʰ M80.051 **Age-related osteoporosis with current pathological fracture, right femur**

✓7ᵗʰ M80.052 **Age-related osteoporosis with current pathological fracture, left femur**

✓7ᵗʰ M80.059 **Age-related osteoporosis with current pathological fracture, unspecified femur**

✓6ᵗʰ M80.06 **Age-related osteoporosis with current pathological fracture, lower leg**

✓7ᵗʰ M80.061 **Age-related osteoporosis with current pathological fracture, right lower leg**

✓7ᵗʰ M80.062 **Age-related osteoporosis with current pathological fracture, left lower leg**

✓7ᵗʰ M80.069 **Age-related osteoporosis with current pathological fracture, unspecified lower leg**

✓6ᵗʰ M80.07 **Age-related osteoporosis with current pathological fracture, ankle and foot**

✓7ᵗʰ M80.071 **Age-related osteoporosis with current pathological fracture, right ankle and foot**

✓7ᵗʰ M80.072 **Age-related osteoporosis with current pathological fracture, left ankle and foot**

✓7ᵗʰ M80.079 **Age-related osteoporosis with current pathological fracture, unspecified ankle and foot**

✓x7ᵗʰ M80.08 **Age-related osteoporosis with current pathological fracture, vertebra(e)**

☑ Appropriate additional character required
✓x7ᵗʰ Requires 7th character, placeholder x must fill empty characters

✓5ᵗʰ M80.8 Other osteoporosis with current pathological fracture
Drug-induced osteoporosis with current pathological fracture
Idiopathic osteoporosis with current pathological fracture
Osteoporosis of disuse with current pathological fracture
Postoophorectomy osteoporosis with current pathological fracture
Postsurgical malabsorption osteoporosis with current pathological fracture
Post-traumatic osteoporosis with current pathological fracture

    ✓x7ᵗʰ M80.80 Other osteoporosis with current pathological fracture, unspecified site
    ✓6ᵗʰ M80.81 Other osteoporosis with pathological fracture, shoulder
       ✓7ᵗʰ M80.811 Other osteoporosis with current pathological fracture, right shoulder
       ✓7ᵗʰ M80.812 Other osteoporosis with current pathological fracture, left shoulder
       ✓7ᵗʰ M80.819 Other osteoporosis with current pathological fracture, unspecified shoulder
    ✓6ᵗʰ M80.82 Other osteoporosis with current pathological fracture, humerus
       ✓7ᵗʰ M80.821 Other osteoporosis with current pathological fracture, right humerus
       ✓7ᵗʰ M80.822 Other osteoporosis with current pathological fracture, left humerus
       ✓7ᵗʰ M80.829 Other osteoporosis with current pathological fracture, unspecified humerus
    ✓6ᵗʰ M80.83 Other osteoporosis with current pathological fracture, forearm
Other osteoporosis with current pathological fracture of wrist
       ✓7ᵗʰ M80.831 Other osteoporosis with current pathological fracture, right forearm
       ✓7ᵗʰ M80.832 Other osteoporosis with current pathological fracture, left forearm
       ✓7ᵗʰ M80.839 Other osteoporosis with current pathological fracture, unspecified forearm
    ✓6ᵗʰ M80.84 Other osteoporosis with current pathological fracture, hand
       ✓7ᵗʰ M80.841 Other osteoporosis with current pathological fracture, right hand
       ✓7ᵗʰ M80.842 Other osteoporosis with current pathological fracture, left hand
       ✓7ᵗʰ M80.849 Other osteoporosis with current pathological fracture, unspecified hand
    ✓6ᵗʰ M80.85 Other osteoporosis with current pathological fracture, femur
Other osteoporosis with current pathological fracture of hip
       ✓7ᵗʰ M80.851 Other osteoporosis with current pathological fracture, right femur
       ✓7ᵗʰ M80.852 Other osteoporosis with current pathological fracture, left femur
       ✓7ᵗʰ M80.859 Other osteoporosis with current pathological fracture, unspecified femur
    ✓6ᵗʰ M80.86 Other osteoporosis with current pathological fracture, lower leg
       ✓7ᵗʰ M80.861 Other osteoporosis with current pathological fracture, right lower leg
       ✓7ᵗʰ M80.862 Other osteoporosis with current pathological fracture, left lower leg
       ✓7ᵗʰ M80.869 Other osteoporosis with current pathological fracture, unspecified lower leg
    ✓6ᵗʰ M80.87 Other osteoporosis with current pathological fracture, ankle and foot
       ✓7ᵗʰ M80.871 Other osteoporosis with current pathological fracture, right ankle and foot
       ✓7ᵗʰ M80.872 Other osteoporosis with current pathological fracture, left ankle and foot
       ✓7ᵗʰ M80.879 Other osteoporosis with current pathological fracture, unspecified ankle and foot

    ✓x7ᵗʰ M80.88 Other osteoporosis with current pathological fracture, vertebra(e)

✓4ᵗʰ M81 Osteoporosis without current pathological fracture
Use additional code to identify:
major osseous defect, if applicable (M89.7-)
personal history of (healed) osteoporosis fracture, if applicable (Z87.310)
> **EXCLUDES 1** *osteoporosis with current pathological fracture (M80-)*
> *Sudeck's atrophy (M89.0)*

M81.0 Age-related osteoporosis without current pathological fracture
Involutional osteoporosis without current pathological fracture
Osteoporosis NOS
Postmenopausal osteoporosis without current pathological fracture
Senile osteoporosis without current pathological fracture

M81.6 Localized osteoporosis [Lequesne]
> **EXCLUDES 1** *Sudeck's atrophy (M89.0)*

M81.8 Other osteoporosis without current pathological fracture
Drug-induced osteoporosis without current pathological fracture
Idiopathic osteoporosis without current pathological fracture
Osteoporosis of disuse without current pathological fracture
Postoophorectomy osteoporosis without current pathological fracture
Postsurgical malabsorption osteoporosis without current pathological fracture
Post-traumatic osteoporosis without current pathological fracture

✓4ᵗʰ M83 Adult osteomalacia
> **EXCLUDES 1** *infantile and juvenile osteomalacia (E55.0)*
> *renal osteodystrophy (N25.0)*
> *rickets (active) (E55.0)*
> *rickets (active) sequelae (E64.3)*
> *vitamin D-resistant osteomalacia (E83.3)*
> *vitamin D-resistant rickets (active) (E83.3)*

M83.0 Puerperal osteomalacia
M83.1 Senile osteomalacia
M83.2 Adult osteomalacia due to malabsorption
Postsurgical malabsorption osteomalacia in adults
M83.3 Adult osteomalacia due to malnutrition
M83.4 Aluminum bone disease
M83.5 Other drug-induced osteomalacia in adults
Code first (T36-T50) to identify drug
M83.8 Other adult osteomalacia
M83.9 Adult osteomalacia, unspecified

✓4ᵗʰ M84 Disorder of continuity of bone
> **EXCLUDES 2** *traumatic fracture of bone-see fracture, by site*

    ✓5ᵗʰ M84.3 Stress fracture
Fatigue fracture
March fracture
Stress fracture NOS
Stress reaction
Use additional external cause code(s) to identify the cause of the stress fracture
> **EXCLUDES 1** *pathological fracture NOS (M84.4-)*
> *pathological fracture due to osteoporosis (M80-)*
> *traumatic fracture (S12-, S22-, S32-, S42-, S52-, S62-, S72-, S82-, S92-)*
> **EXCLUDES 2** *personal history of (healed) stress (fatigue) fracture (Z87.312)*
> *stress fracture of vertebra (M48.4-)*

> The appropriate 7th character is to be added to each code from subcategory M84.3.
> A   initial encounter for fracture
> D   subsequent encounter for fracture with routine healing
> G   subsequent encounter for fracture with delayed healing
> K   subsequent encounter for fracture with nonunion
> P   subsequent encounter for fracture with malunion
> S   sequela

    ✓x7ᵗʰ M84.30 Stress fracture, unspecified site
    ✓6ᵗʰ M84.31 Stress fracture, shoulder
       ✓7ᵗʰ M84.311 Stress fracture, right shoulder
       ✓7ᵗʰ M84.312 Stress fracture, left shoulder

EXCLUDES 1 Not coded here   *EXCLUDES 2* Not included here   ***Manifestation Code***

√7th M84.319 Stress fracture, unspecified shoulder
√6th M84.32 Stress fracture, humerus
  √7th M84.321 Stress fracture, right humerus
  √7th M84.322 Stress fracture, left humerus
  √7th M84.329 Stress fracture, unspecified humerus
√6th M84.33 Stress fracture, ulna and radius
  √7th M84.331 Stress fracture, right ulna
  √7th M84.332 Stress fracture, left ulna
  √7th M84.333 Stress fracture, right radius
  √7th M84.334 Stress fracture, left radius
  √7th M84.339 Stress fracture, unspecified ulna and radius
√6th M84.34 Stress fracture, hand and fingers
  √7th M84.341 Stress fracture, right hand
  √7th M84.342 Stress fracture, left hand
  √7th M84.343 Stress fracture, unspecified hand
  √7th M84.344 Stress fracture, right finger(s)
  √7th M84.345 Stress fracture, left finger(s)
  √7th M84.346 Stress fracture, unspecified finger(s)
√6th M84.35 Stress fracture, pelvis and femur
  Stress fracture, hip
  √7th M84.350 Stress fracture, pelvis
  √7th M84.351 Stress fracture, right femur
  √7th M84.352 Stress fracture, left femur
  √7th M84.353 Stress fracture, unspecified femur
  √7th M84.359 Stress fracture, hip, unspecified
√6th M84.36 Stress fracture, tibia and fibula
  √7th M84.361 Stress fracture, right tibia
  √7th M84.362 Stress fracture, left tibia
  √7th M84.363 Stress fracture, right fibula
  √7th M84.364 Stress fracture, left fibula
  √7th M84.369 Stress fracture, unspecified tibia and fibula
√6th M84.37 Stress fracture, ankle, foot and toes
  √7th M84.371 Stress fracture, right ankle
  √7th M84.372 Stress fracture, left ankle
  √7th M84.373 Stress fracture, unspecified ankle
  √7th M84.374 Stress fracture, right foot
  √7th M84.375 Stress fracture, left foot
  √7th M84.376 Stress fracture, unspecified foot
  √7th M84.377 Stress fracture, right toe(s)
  √7th M84.378 Stress fracture, left toe(s)
  √7th M84.379 Stress fracture, unspecified toe(s)
√x7th M84.38 Stress fracture, other site
  EXCLUDES 2 stress fracture of vertebra (M48.4-)

√5th M84.4 Pathological fracture, not elsewhere classified
  Chronic fracture
  Pathological fracture NOS
  EXCLUDES 1 collapsed vertebra NEC (M48.5)
    pathological fracture in neoplastic disease (M84.5-)
    pathological fracture in osteoporosis (M80-)
    pathological fracture in other disease (M84.6-)
    stress fracture (M84.3-)
    traumatic fracture (S12-, S22-, S32-, S42-, S52-, S62-, S72-, S82-, S92-)
  EXCLUDES 2 personal history of (healed) pathological fracture (Z87.311)

> The appropriate 7th character is to be added to each code from subcategory M84.4.
> A   initial encounter for fracture
> D   subsequent encounter for fracture with routine healing
> G   subsequent encounter for fracture with delayed healing
> K   subsequent encounter for fracture with nonunion
> P   subsequent encounter for fracture with malunion
> S   sequela

√x7th M84.40 Pathological fracture, unspecified site
√6th M84.41 Pathological fracture, shoulder
  √7th M84.411 Pathological fracture, right shoulder
  √7th M84.412 Pathological fracture, left shoulder
  √7th M84.419 Pathological fracture, unspecified shoulder
√6th M84.42 Pathological fracture, humerus

√7th M84.421 Pathological fracture, right humerus
√7th M84.422 Pathological fracture, left humerus
√7th M84.429 Pathological fracture, unspecified humerus
√6th M84.43 Pathological fracture, ulna and radius
  √7th M84.431 Pathological fracture, right ulna
  √7th M84.432 Pathological fracture, left ulna
  √7th M84.433 Pathological fracture, right radius
  √7th M84.434 Pathological fracture, left radius
  √7th M84.439 Pathological fracture, unspecified ulna and radius
√6th M84.44 Pathological fracture, hand and fingers
  √7th M84.441 Pathological fracture, right hand
  √7th M84.442 Pathological fracture, left hand
  √7th M84.443 Pathological fracture, unspecified hand
  √7th M84.444 Pathological fracture, right finger(s)
  √7th M84.445 Pathological fracture, left finger(s)
  √7th M84.446 Pathological fracture, unspecified finger(s)
√6th M84.45 Pathological fracture, femur and pelvis
  √7th M84.451 Pathological fracture, right femur
  √7th M84.452 Pathological fracture, left femur
  √7th M84.453 Pathological fracture, unspecified femur
  √7th M84.454 Pathological fracture, pelvis
  √7th M84.459 Pathological fracture, hip, unspecified
√6th M84.46 Pathological fracture, tibia and fibula
  √7th M84.461 Pathological fracture, right tibia
  √7th M84.462 Pathological fracture, left tibia
  √7th M84.463 Pathological fracture, right fibula
  √7th M84.464 Pathological fracture, left fibula
  √7th M84.469 Pathological fracture, unspecified tibia and fibula
√6th M84.47 Pathological fracture, ankle, foot and toes
  √7th M84.471 Pathological fracture, right ankle
  √7th M84.472 Pathological fracture, left ankle
  √7th M84.473 Pathological fracture, unspecified ankle
  √7th M84.474 Pathological fracture, right foot
  √7th M84.475 Pathological fracture, left foot
  √7th M84.476 Pathological fracture, unspecified foot
  √7th M84.477 Pathological fracture, right toe(s)
  √7th M84.478 Pathological fracture, left toe(s)
  √7th M84.479 Pathological fracture, unspecified toe(s)
√x7th M84.48 Pathological fracture, other site
√6th M84.5 Pathological fracture in neoplastic disease
  Code also underlying neoplasm

> The appropriate 7th character is to be added to each code from subcategory M84.5.
> A   initial encounter for fracture
> D   subsequent encounter for fracture with routine healing
> G   subsequent encounter for fracture with delayed healing
> K   subsequent encounter for fracture with nonunion
> P   subsequent encounter for fracture with malunion
> S   sequela

√x7th M84.50 Pathological fracture in neoplastic disease, unspecified site
√6th M84.51 Pathological fracture in neoplastic disease, shoulder
  √7th M84.511 Pathological fracture in neoplastic disease, right shoulder
  √7th M84.512 Pathological fracture in neoplastic disease, left shoulder
  √7th M84.519 Pathological fracture in neoplastic disease, unspecified shoulder
√6th M84.52 Pathological fracture in neoplastic disease, humerus
  √7th M84.521 Pathological fracture in neoplastic disease, right humerus
  √7th M84.522 Pathological fracture in neoplastic disease, left humerus
  √7th M84.529 Pathological fracture in neoplastic disease, unspecified humerus

---

☑ Appropriate additional character required   √x7th Requires 7th character, placeholder x must fill empty characters

√6th **M84.53 Pathological fracture in neoplastic disease, ulna and radius**
- √7th **M84.531 Pathological fracture in neoplastic disease, right ulna**
- √7th **M84.532 Pathological fracture in neoplastic disease, left ulna**
- √7th **M84.533 Pathological fracture in neoplastic disease, right radius**
- √7th **M84.534 Pathological fracture in neoplastic disease, left radius**
- √7th **M84.539 Pathological fracture in neoplastic disease, unspecified ulna and radius**

√6th **M84.54 Pathological fracture in neoplastic disease, hand**
- √7th **M84.541 Pathological fracture in neoplastic disease, right hand**
- √7th **M84.542 Pathological fracture in neoplastic disease, left hand**
- √7th **M84.549 Pathological fracture in neoplastic disease, unspecified hand**

√6th **M84.55 Pathological fracture in neoplastic disease, pelvis and femur**
- √7th **M84.550 Pathological fracture in neoplastic disease, pelvis**
- √7th **M84.551 Pathological fracture in neoplastic disease, right femur**
- √7th **M84.552 Pathological fracture in neoplastic disease, left femur**
- √7th **M84.553 Pathological fracture in neoplastic disease, unspecified femur**
- √7th **M84.559 Pathological fracture in neoplastic disease, hip, unspecified**

√6th **M84.56 Pathological fracture in neoplastic disease, tibia and fibula**
- √7th **M84.561 Pathological fracture in neoplastic disease, right tibia**
- √7th **M84.562 Pathological fracture in neoplastic disease, left tibia**
- √7th **M84.563 Pathological fracture in neoplastic disease, right fibula**
- √7th **M84.564 Pathological fracture in neoplastic disease, left fibula**
- √7th **M84.569 Pathological fracture in neoplastic disease, unspecified tibia and fibula**

√6th **M84.57 Pathological fracture in neoplastic disease, ankle and foot**
- √7th **M84.571 Pathological fracture in neoplastic disease, right ankle**
- √7th **M84.572 Pathological fracture in neoplastic disease, left ankle**
- √7th **M84.573 Pathological fracture in neoplastic disease, unspecified ankle**
- √7th **M84.574 Pathological fracture in neoplastic disease, right foot**
- √7th **M84.575 Pathological fracture in neoplastic disease, left foot**
- √7th **M84.576 Pathological fracture in neoplastic disease, unspecified foot**

√x7th **M84.58 Pathological fracture in neoplastic disease, vertebrae**

√5th **M84.6 Pathological fracture in other disease**

Code also underlying condition

EXCLUDES 1   *pathological fracture in osteoporosis (M80-)*

The appropriate 7th character is to be added to each code from subcategory M84.6.
- A   initial encounter for fracture
- D   subsequent encounter for fracture with routine healing
- G   subsequent encounter for fracture with delayed healing
- K   subsequent encounter for fracture with nonunion
- P   subsequent encounter for fracture with malunion
- S   sequela

√x7th **M84.60 Pathological fracture in other disease, unspecified site**

√6th **M84.61 Pathological fracture in other disease, shoulder**

- √7th **M84.611 Pathological fracture in other disease, right shoulder**
- √7th **M84.612 Pathological fracture in other disease, left shoulder**
- √7th **M84.619 Pathological fracture in other disease, unspecified shoulder**

√6th **M84.62 Pathological fracture in other disease, humerus**
- √7th **M84.621 Pathological fracture in other disease, right humerus**
- √7th **M84.622 Pathological fracture in other disease, left humerus**
- √7th **M84.629 Pathological fracture in other disease, unspecified humerus**

√6th **M84.63 Pathological fracture in other disease, ulna and radius**
- √7th **M84.631 Pathological fracture in other disease, right ulna**
- √7th **M84.632 Pathological fracture in other disease, left ulna**
- √7th **M84.633 Pathological fracture in other disease, right radius**
- √7th **M84.634 Pathological fracture in other disease, left radius**
- √7th **M84.639 Pathological fracture in other disease, unspecified ulna and radius**

√6th **M84.64 Pathological fracture in other disease, hand**
- √7th **M84.641 Pathological fracture in other disease, right hand**
- √7th **M84.642 Pathological fracture in other disease, left hand**
- √7th **M84.649 Pathological fracture in other disease, unspecified hand**

√6th **M84.65 Pathological fracture in other disease, pelvis and femur**
- √7th **M84.650 Pathological fracture in other disease, pelvis**
- √7th **M84.651 Pathological fracture in other disease, right femur**
- √7th **M84.652 Pathological fracture in other disease, left femur**
- √7th **M84.653 Pathological fracture in other disease, unspecified femur**
- √7th **M84.659 Pathological fracture in other disease, hip, unspecified**

√6th **M84.66 Pathological fracture in other disease, tibia and fibula**
- √7th **M84.661 Pathological fracture in other disease, right tibia**
- √7th **M84.662 Pathological fracture in other disease, left tibia**
- √7th **M84.663 Pathological fracture in other disease, right fibula**
- √7th **M84.664 Pathological fracture in other disease, left fibula**
- √7th **M84.669 Pathological fracture in other disease, unspecified tibia and fibula**

√6th **M84.67 Pathological fracture in other disease, ankle and foot**
- √7th **M84.671 Pathological fracture in other disease, right ankle**
- √7th **M84.672 Pathological fracture in other disease, left ankle**
- √7th **M84.673 Pathological fracture in other disease, unspecified ankle**
- √7th **M84.674 Pathological fracture in other disease, right foot**
- √7th **M84.675 Pathological fracture in other disease, left foot**
- √7th **M84.676 Pathological fracture in other disease, unspecified foot**

√x7th **M84.68 Pathological fracture in other disease, other site**

√5th **M84.8 Other disorders of continuity of bone**

M84.80 Other disorders of continuity of bone, unspecified site

√6th **M84.81 Other disorders of continuity of bone, shoulder**

M84.811 Other disorders of continuity of bone, right shoulder

---

EXCLUDES 1 Not coded here   EXCLUDES 2 Not included here   *Manifestation Code*

M84.812 Other disorders of continuity of bone, left shoulder

M84.819 Other disorders of continuity of bone, unspecified shoulder

✓6th M84.82 Other disorders of continuity of bone, humerus

M84.821 Other disorders of continuity of bone, right humerus

M84.822 Other disorders of continuity of bone, left humerus

M84.829 Other disorders of continuity of bone, unspecified humerus

✓6th M84.83 Other disorders of continuity of bone, ulna and radius

M84.831 Other disorders of continuity of bone, right ulna

M84.832 Other disorders of continuity of bone, left ulna

M84.833 Other disorders of continuity of bone, right radius

M84.834 Other disorders of continuity of bone, left radius

M84.839 Other disorders of continuity of bone, unspecified ulna and radius

✓6th M84.84 Other disorders of continuity of bone, hand

M84.841 Other disorders of continuity of bone, right hand

M84.842 Other disorders of continuity of bone, left hand

M84.849 Other disorders of continuity of bone, unspecified hand

✓6th M84.85 Other disorders of continuity of bone, pelvic region and thigh

M84.851 Other disorders of continuity of bone, right pelvic region and thigh

M84.852 Other disorders of continuity of bone, left pelvic region and thigh

M84.859 Other disorders of continuity of bone, unspecified pelvic region and thigh

✓6th M84.86 Other disorders of continuity of bone, tibia and fibula

M84.861 Other disorders of continuity of bone, right tibia

M84.862 Other disorders of continuity of bone, left tibia

M84.863 Other disorders of continuity of bone, right fibula

M84.864 Other disorders of continuity of bone, left fibula

M84.869 Other disorders of continuity of bone, unspecified tibia and fibula

✓6th M84.87 Other disorders of continuity of bone, ankle and foot

M84.871 Other disorders of continuity of bone, right ankle and foot

M84.872 Other disorders of continuity of bone, left ankle and foot

M84.879 Other disorders of continuity of bone, unspecified ankle and foot

M84.88 Other disorders of continuity of bone, other site

M84.9 Disorder of continuity of bone, unspecified

✓4th M85 Other disorders of bone density and structure

EXCLUDES 1 osteogenesis imperfecta (Q78.0)
osteopetrosis (Q78.2)
osteopoikilosis (Q78.8)
polyostotic fibrous dysplasia (Q78.1)

✓5th M85.0 Fibrous dysplasia (monostotic)

EXCLUDES 2 fibrous dysplasia of jaw (M27.8)

M85.00 Fibrous dysplasia (monostotic), unspecified site

✓6th M85.01 Fibrous dysplasia (monostotic), shoulder

M85.011 Fibrous dysplasia (monostotic), right shoulder

M85.012 Fibrous dysplasia (monostotic), left shoulder

M85.019 Fibrous dysplasia (monostotic), unspecified shoulder

✓6th M85.02 Fibrous dysplasia (monostotic), upper arm

M85.021 Fibrous dysplasia (monostotic), right upper arm

M85.022 Fibrous dysplasia (monostotic), left upper arm

M85.029 Fibrous dysplasia (monostotic), unspecified upper arm

✓6th M85.03 Fibrous dysplasia (monostotic), forearm

M85.031 Fibrous dysplasia (monostotic), right forearm

M85.032 Fibrous dysplasia (monostotic), left forearm

M85.039 Fibrous dysplasia (monostotic), unspecified forearm

✓6th M85.04 Fibrous dysplasia (monostotic), hand

M85.041 Fibrous dysplasia (monostotic), right hand

M85.042 Fibrous dysplasia (monostotic), left hand

M85.049 Fibrous dysplasia (monostotic), unspecified hand

✓6th M85.05 Fibrous dysplasia (monostotic), thigh

M85.051 Fibrous dysplasia (monostotic), right thigh

M85.052 Fibrous dysplasia (monostotic), left thigh

M85.059 Fibrous dysplasia (monostotic), unspecified thigh

✓6th M85.06 Fibrous dysplasia (monostotic), lower leg

M85.061 Fibrous dysplasia (monostotic), right lower leg

M85.062 Fibrous dysplasia (monostotic), left lower leg

M85.069 Fibrous dysplasia (monostotic), unspecified lower leg

✓6th M85.07 Fibrous dysplasia (monostotic), ankle and foot

M85.071 Fibrous dysplasia (monostotic), right ankle and foot

M85.072 Fibrous dysplasia (monostotic), left ankle and foot

M85.079 Fibrous dysplasia (monostotic), unspecified ankle and foot

M85.08 Fibrous dysplasia (monostotic), other site

M85.09 Fibrous dysplasia (monostotic), multiple sites

✓5th M85.1 Skeletal fluorosis

M85.10 Skeletal fluorosis, unspecified site

✓6th M85.11 Skeletal fluorosis, shoulder

M85.111 Skeletal fluorosis, right shoulder

M85.112 Skeletal fluorosis, left shoulder

M85.119 Skeletal fluorosis, unspecified shoulder

✓6th M85.12 Skeletal fluorosis, upper arm

M85.121 Skeletal fluorosis, right upper arm

M85.122 Skeletal fluorosis, left upper arm

M85.129 Skeletal fluorosis, unspecified upper arm

✓6th M85.13 Skeletal fluorosis, forearm

M85.131 Skeletal fluorosis, right forearm

M85.132 Skeletal fluorosis, left forearm

M85.139 Skeletal fluorosis, unspecified forearm

✓6th M85.14 Skeletal fluorosis, hand

M85.141 Skeletal fluorosis, right hand

M85.142 Skeletal fluorosis, left hand

M85.149 Skeletal fluorosis, unspecified hand

✓6th M85.15 Skeletal fluorosis, thigh

M85.151 Skeletal fluorosis, right thigh

M85.152 Skeletal fluorosis, left thigh

M85.159 Skeletal fluorosis, unspecified thigh

✓6th M85.16 Skeletal fluorosis, lower leg

M85.161 Skeletal fluorosis, right lower leg

M85.162 Skeletal fluorosis, left lower leg

M85.169 Skeletal fluorosis, unspecified lower leg

✓6th M85.17 Skeletal fluorosis, ankle and foot

M85.171 Skeletal fluorosis, right ankle and foot

M85.172 Skeletal fluorosis, left ankle and foot

M85.179 Skeletal fluorosis, unspecified ankle and foot

✓ Appropriate additional character required   ✓x7th Requires 7th character, placeholder x must fill empty characters

M85.18 **Skeletal fluorosis, other site**
M85.19 **Skeletal fluorosis, multiple sites**
M85.2 **Hyperostosis of skull**
✓5ᵗʰ M85.3 **Osteitis condensans**
   M85.30 **Osteitis condensans, unspecified site**
  ✓6ᵗʰ M85.31 **Osteitis condensans, shoulder**
    M85.311 **Osteitis condensans, right shoulder**
    M85.312 **Osteitis condensans, left shoulder**
    M85.319 **Osteitis condensans, unspecified shoulder**
  ✓6ᵗʰ M85.32 **Osteitis condensans, upper arm**
    M85.321 **Osteitis condensans, right upper arm**
    M85.322 **Osteitis condensans, left upper arm**
    M85.329 **Osteitis condensans, unspecified upper arm**
  ✓6ᵗʰ M85.33 **Osteitis condensans, forearm**
    M85.331 **Osteitis condensans, right forearm**
    M85.332 **Osteitis condensans, left forearm**
    M85.339 **Osteitis condensans, unspecified forearm**
  ✓6ᵗʰ M85.34 **Osteitis condensans, hand**
    M85.341 **Osteitis condensans, right hand**
    M85.342 **Osteitis condensans, left hand**
    M85.349 **Osteitis condensans, unspecified hand**
  ✓6ᵗʰ M85.35 **Osteitis condensans, thigh**
    M85.351 **Osteitis condensans, right thigh**
    M85.352 **Osteitis condensans, left thigh**
    M85.359 **Osteitis condensans, unspecified thigh**
  ✓6ᵗʰ M85.36 **Osteitis condensans, lower leg**
    M85.361 **Osteitis condensans, right lower leg**
    M85.362 **Osteitis condensans, left lower leg**
    M85.369 **Osteitis condensans, unspecified lower leg**
  ✓6ᵗʰ M85.37 **Osteitis condensans, ankle and foot**
    M85.371 **Osteitis condensans, right ankle and foot**
    M85.372 **Osteitis condensans, left ankle and foot**
    M85.379 **Osteitis condensans, unspecified ankle and foot**
   M85.38 **Osteitis condensans, vertebrae**
   M85.39 **Osteitis condensans, multiple sites**
✓5ᵗʰ M85.4 **Solitary bone cyst**
    EXCLUDES 2 *solitary cyst of jaw (M27.4)*
   M85.40 **Solitary bone cyst, unspecified site**
  ✓6ᵗʰ M85.41 **Solitary bone cyst, shoulder**
    M85.411 **Solitary bone cyst, right shoulder**
    M85.412 **Solitary bone cyst, left shoulder**
    M85.419 **Solitary bone cyst, unspecified shoulder**
  ✓6ᵗʰ M85.42 **Solitary bone cyst, humerus**
    M85.421 **Solitary bone cyst, right humerus**
    M85.422 **Solitary bone cyst, left humerus**
    M85.429 **Solitary bone cyst, unspecified humerus**
  ✓6ᵗʰ M85.43 **Solitary bone cyst, ulna and radius**
    M85.431 **Solitary bone cyst, right ulna and radius**
    M85.432 **Solitary bone cyst, left ulna and radius**
    M85.439 **Solitary bone cyst, unspecified ulna and radius**
  ✓6ᵗʰ M85.44 **Solitary bone cyst, hand**
    M85.441 **Solitary bone cyst, right hand**
    M85.442 **Solitary bone cyst, left hand**
    M85.449 **Solitary bone cyst, unspecified hand**
  ✓6ᵗʰ M85.45 **Solitary bone cyst, pelvis**
    M85.451 **Solitary bone cyst, right pelvis**
    M85.452 **Solitary bone cyst, left pelvis**
    M85.459 **Solitary bone cyst, unspecified pelvis**
  ✓6ᵗʰ M85.46 **Solitary bone cyst, tibia and fibula**
    M85.461 **Solitary bone cyst, right tibia and fibula**
    M85.462 **Solitary bone cyst, left tibia and fibula**
    M85.469 **Solitary bone cyst, unspecified tibia and fibula**
  ✓6ᵗʰ M85.47 **Solitary bone cyst, ankle and foot**
    M85.471 **Solitary bone cyst, right ankle and foot**
    M85.472 **Solitary bone cyst, left ankle and foot**
    M85.479 **Solitary bone cyst, unspecified ankle and foot**

M85.48 **Solitary bone cyst, other site**
✓5ᵗʰ M85.5 **Aneurysmal bone cyst**
    EXCLUDES 2 *aneurysmal cyst of jaw (M27.4)*
   M85.50 **Aneurysmal bone cyst, unspecified site**
  ✓6ᵗʰ M85.51 **Aneurysmal bone cyst, shoulder**
    M85.511 **Aneurysmal bone cyst, right shoulder**
    M85.512 **Aneurysmal bone cyst, left shoulder**
    M85.519 **Aneurysmal bone cyst, unspecified shoulder**
  ✓6ᵗʰ M85.52 **Aneurysmal bone cyst, upper arm**
    M85.521 **Aneurysmal bone cyst, right upper arm**
    M85.522 **Aneurysmal bone cyst, left upper arm**
    M85.529 **Aneurysmal bone cyst, unspecified upper arm**
  ✓6ᵗʰ M85.53 **Aneurysmal bone cyst, forearm**
    M85.531 **Aneurysmal bone cyst, right forearm**
    M85.532 **Aneurysmal bone cyst, left forearm**
    M85.539 **Aneurysmal bone cyst, unspecified forearm**
  ✓6ᵗʰ M85.54 **Aneurysmal bone cyst, hand**
    M85.541 **Aneurysmal bone cyst, right hand**
    M85.542 **Aneurysmal bone cyst, left hand**
    M85.549 **Aneurysmal bone cyst, unspecified hand**
  ✓6ᵗʰ M85.55 **Aneurysmal bone cyst, thigh**
    M85.551 **Aneurysmal bone cyst, right thigh**
    M85.552 **Aneurysmal bone cyst, left thigh**
    M85.559 **Aneurysmal bone cyst, unspecified thigh**
  ✓6ᵗʰ M85.56 **Aneurysmal bone cyst, lower leg**
    M85.561 **Aneurysmal bone cyst, right lower leg**
    M85.562 **Aneurysmal bone cyst, left lower leg**
    M85.569 **Aneurysmal bone cyst, unspecified lower leg**
  ✓6ᵗʰ M85.57 **Aneurysmal bone cyst, ankle and foot**
    M85.571 **Aneurysmal bone cyst, right ankle and foot**
    M85.572 **Aneurysmal bone cyst, left ankle and foot**
    M85.579 **Aneurysmal bone cyst, unspecified ankle and foot**
   M85.58 **Aneurysmal bone cyst, other site**
   M85.59 **Aneurysmal bone cyst, multiple sites**
✓5ᵗʰ M85.6 **Other cyst of bone**
    EXCLUDES 1 *cyst of jaw NEC (M27.4)*
          osteitis fibrosa cystica generalisata [von Recklinghausen's disease of bone] (E21.0)
   M85.60 **Other cyst of bone, unspecified site**
  ✓6ᵗʰ M85.61 **Other cyst of bone, shoulder**
    M85.611 **Other cyst of bone, right shoulder**
    M85.612 **Other cyst of bone, left shoulder**
    M85.619 **Other cyst of bone, unspecified shoulder**
  ✓6ᵗʰ M85.62 **Other cyst of bone, upper arm**
    M85.621 **Other cyst of bone, right upper arm**
    M85.622 **Other cyst of bone, left upper arm**
    M85.629 **Other cyst of bone, unspecified upper arm**
  ✓6ᵗʰ M85.63 **Other cyst of bone, forearm**
    M85.631 **Other cyst of bone, right forearm**
    M85.632 **Other cyst of bone, left forearm**
    M85.639 **Other cyst of bone, unspecified forearm**
  ✓6ᵗʰ M85.64 **Other cyst of bone, hand**
    M85.641 **Other cyst of bone, right hand**
    M85.642 **Other cyst of bone, left hand**
    M85.649 **Other cyst of bone, unspecified hand**
  ✓6ᵗʰ M85.65 **Other cyst of bone, thigh**
    M85.651 **Other cyst of bone, right thigh**
    M85.652 **Other cyst of bone, left thigh**
    M85.659 **Other cyst of bone, unspecified thigh**
  ✓6ᵗʰ M85.66 **Other cyst of bone, lower leg**
    M85.661 **Other cyst of bone, right lower leg**
    M85.662 **Other cyst of bone, left lower leg**
    M85.669 **Other cyst of bone, unspecified lower leg**
  ✓6ᵗʰ M85.67 **Other cyst of bone, ankle and foot**
    M85.671 **Other cyst of bone, right ankle and foot**

EXCLUDES 1 Not coded here   *EXCLUDES 2* Not included here   ***Manifestation Code***

M85.672 Other cyst of bone, left ankle and foot

M85.679 Other cyst of bone, unspecified ankle and foot

M85.68 Other cyst of bone, other site

M85.69 Other cyst of bone, multiple sites

☑5ᵗʰ M85.8 Other specified disorders of bone density and structure

Hyperostosis of bones, except skull

Osteosclerosis, acquired

EXCLUDES 1 *diffuse idiopathic skeletal hyperostosis [DISH] (M48.1)*

osteosclerosis congenita (Q77.4)

osteosclerosis fragilitas (generalista) (Q78.2)

osteosclerosis myelofibrosis (D75.81)

M85.80 Other specified disorders of bone density and structure, unspecified site

☑6ᵗʰ M85.81 Other specified disorders of bone density and structure, shoulder

M85.811 Other specified disorders of bone density and structure, right shoulder

M85.812 Other specified disorders of bone density and structure, left shoulder

M85.819 Other specified disorders of bone density and structure, unspecified shoulder

☑6ᵗʰ M85.82 Other specified disorders of bone density and structure, upper arm

M85.821 Other specified disorders of bone density and structure, right upper arm

M85.822 Other specified disorders of bone density and structure, left upper arm

M85.829 Other specified disorders of bone density and structure, unspecified upper arm

☑6ᵗʰ M85.83 Other specified disorders of bone density and structure, forearm

M85.831 Other specified disorders of bone density and structure, right forearm

M85.832 Other specified disorders of bone density and structure, left forearm

M85.839 Other specified disorders of bone density and structure, unspecified forearm

☑6ᵗʰ M85.84 Other specified disorders of bone density and structure, hand

M85.841 Other specified disorders of bone density and structure, right hand

M85.842 Other specified disorders of bone density and structure, left hand

M85.849 Other specified disorders of bone density and structure, unspecified hand

☑6ᵗʰ M85.85 Other specified disorders of bone density and structure, thigh

M85.851 Other specified disorders of bone density and structure, right thigh

M85.852 Other specified disorders of bone density and structure, left thigh

M85.859 Other specified disorders of bone density and structure, unspecified thigh

☑6ᵗʰ M85.86 Other specified disorders of bone density and structure, lower leg

M85.861 Other specified disorders of bone density and structure, right lower leg

M85.862 Other specified disorders of bone density and structure, left lower leg

M85.869 Other specified disorders of bone density and structure, unspecified lower leg

☑6ᵗʰ M85.87 Other specified disorders of bone density and structure, ankle and foot

M85.871 Other specified disorders of bone density and structure, right ankle and foot

M85.872 Other specified disorders of bone density and structure, left ankle and foot

M85.879 Other specified disorders of bone density and structure, unspecified ankle and foot

M85.88 Other specified disorders of bone density and structure, other site

M85.89 Other specified disorders of bone density and structure, multiple sites

M85.9 Disorder of bone density and structure, unspecified

Other osteopathies (M86-M90)

EXCLUDES 1 *postprocedural osteopathies (M96-)*

☑4ᵗʰ M86 Osteomyelitis

Use additional code (B95-B97) to identify infectious agent

Use additional code to identify major osseous defect, if applicable (M89.7-)

EXCLUDES 1 *osteomyelitis due to:*

echinococcus (B67.2)

gonococcus (A54.43)

salmonella (A02.24)

EXCLUDES 2 *osteomyelitis of:*

orbit (H05.0-)

petrous bone (H70.2-)

vertebra (M46.2-)

☑5ᵗʰ M86.0 Acute hematogenous osteomyelitis

M86.00 Acute hematogenous osteomyelitis, unspecified site

☑6ᵗʰ M86.01 Acute hematogenous osteomyelitis, shoulder

M86.011 Acute hematogenous osteomyelitis, right shoulder

M86.012 Acute hematogenous osteomyelitis, left shoulder

M86.019 Acute hematogenous osteomyelitis, unspecified shoulder

☑6ᵗʰ M86.02 Acute hematogenous osteomyelitis, humerus

M86.021 Acute hematogenous osteomyelitis, right humerus

M86.022 Acute hematogenous osteomyelitis, left humerus

M86.029 Acute hematogenous osteomyelitis, unspecified humerus

☑6ᵗʰ M86.03 Acute hematogenous osteomyelitis, radius and ulna

M86.031 Acute hematogenous osteomyelitis, right radius and ulna

M86.032 Acute hematogenous osteomyelitis, left radius and ulna

M86.039 Acute hematogenous osteomyelitis, unspecified radius and ulna

☑6ᵗʰ M86.04 Acute hematogenous osteomyelitis, hand

M86.041 Acute hematogenous osteomyelitis, right hand

M86.042 Acute hematogenous osteomyelitis, left hand

M86.049 Acute hematogenous osteomyelitis, unspecified hand

☑6ᵗʰ M86.05 Acute hematogenous osteomyelitis, femur

M86.051 Acute hematogenous osteomyelitis, right femur

M86.052 Acute hematogenous osteomyelitis, left femur

M86.059 Acute hematogenous osteomyelitis, unspecified femur

☑6ᵗʰ M86.06 Acute hematogenous osteomyelitis, tibia and fibula

M86.061 Acute hematogenous osteomyelitis, right tibia and fibula

M86.062 Acute hematogenous osteomyelitis, left tibia and fibula

M86.069 Acute hematogenous osteomyelitis, unspecified tibia and fibula

☑6ᵗʰ M86.07 Acute hematogenous osteomyelitis, ankle and foot

M86.071 Acute hematogenous osteomyelitis, right ankle and foot

M86.072 Acute hematogenous osteomyelitis, left ankle and foot

M86.079 Acute hematogenous osteomyelitis, unspecified ankle and foot

M86.08 Acute hematogenous osteomyelitis, other sites

M86.09 Acute hematogenous osteomyelitis, multiple sites

☑ Appropriate additional character required

✓x7ᵗʰ Requires 7th character, placeholder x must fill empty characters

√5th **M86.1 Other acute osteomyelitis**
     M86.10 Other acute osteomyelitis, unspecified site
     √6th M86.11 Other acute osteomyelitis, shoulder
         M86.111 Other acute osteomyelitis, right shoulder
         M86.112 Other acute osteomyelitis, left shoulder
         M86.119 Other acute osteomyelitis, unspecified shoulder
     √6th M86.12 Other acute osteomyelitis, humerus
         M86.121 Other acute osteomyelitis, right humerus
         M86.122 Other acute osteomyelitis, left humerus
         M86.129 Other acute osteomyelitis, unspecified humerus
     √6th M86.13 Other acute osteomyelitis, radius and ulna
         M86.131 Other acute osteomyelitis, right radius and ulna
         M86.132 Other acute osteomyelitis, left radius and ulna
         M86.139 Other acute osteomyelitis, unspecified radius and ulna
     √6th M86.14 Other acute osteomyelitis, hand
         M86.141 Other acute osteomyelitis, right hand
         M86.142 Other acute osteomyelitis, left hand
         M86.149 Other acute osteomyelitis, unspecified hand
     √6th M86.15 Other acute osteomyelitis, femur
         M86.151 Other acute osteomyelitis, right femur
         M86.152 Other acute osteomyelitis, left femur
         M86.159 Other acute osteomyelitis, unspecified femur
     √6th M86.16 Other acute osteomyelitis, tibia and fibula
         M86.161 Other acute osteomyelitis, right tibia and fibula
         M86.162 Other acute osteomyelitis, left tibia and fibula
         M86.169 Other acute osteomyelitis, unspecified tibia and fibula
     √6th M86.17 Other acute osteomyelitis, ankle and foot
         M86.171 Other acute osteomyelitis, right ankle and foot
         M86.172 Other acute osteomyelitis, left ankle and foot
         M86.179 Other acute osteomyelitis, unspecified ankle and foot
     M86.18 Other acute osteomyelitis, other site
     M86.19 Other acute osteomyelitis, multiple sites
√5th **M86.2 Subacute osteomyelitis**
     M86.20 Subacute osteomyelitis, unspecified site
     √6th M86.21 Subacute osteomyelitis, shoulder
         M86.211 Subacute osteomyelitis, right shoulder
         M86.212 Subacute osteomyelitis, left shoulder
         M86.219 Subacute osteomyelitis, unspecified shoulder
     √6th M86.22 Subacute osteomyelitis, humerus
         M86.221 Subacute osteomyelitis, right humerus
         M86.222 Subacute osteomyelitis, left humerus
         M86.229 Subacute osteomyelitis, unspecified humerus
     √6th M86.23 Subacute osteomyelitis, radius and ulna
         M86.231 Subacute osteomyelitis, right radius and ulna
         M86.232 Subacute osteomyelitis, left radius and ulna
         M86.239 Subacute osteomyelitis, unspecified radius and ulna
     √6th M86.24 Subacute osteomyelitis, hand
         M86.241 Subacute osteomyelitis, right hand
         M86.242 Subacute osteomyelitis, left hand
         M86.249 Subacute osteomyelitis, unspecified hand
     √6th M86.25 Subacute osteomyelitis, femur
         M86.251 Subacute osteomyelitis, right femur
         M86.252 Subacute osteomyelitis, left femur
         M86.259 Subacute osteomyelitis, unspecified femur

     √6th M86.26 Subacute osteomyelitis, tibia and fibula
         M86.261 Subacute osteomyelitis, right tibia and fibula
         M86.262 Subacute osteomyelitis, left tibia and fibula
         M86.269 Subacute osteomyelitis, unspecified tibia and fibula
     √6th M86.27 Subacute osteomyelitis, ankle and foot
         M86.271 Subacute osteomyelitis, right ankle and foot
         M86.272 Subacute osteomyelitis, left ankle and foot
         M86.279 Subacute osteomyelitis, unspecified ankle and foot
     M86.28 Subacute osteomyelitis, other site
     M86.29 Subacute osteomyelitis, multiple sites
√5th **M86.3 Chronic multifocal osteomyelitis**
     M86.30 Chronic multifocal osteomyelitis, unspecified site
     √6th M86.31 Chronic multifocal osteomyelitis, shoulder
         M86.311 Chronic multifocal osteomyelitis, right shoulder
         M86.312 Chronic multifocal osteomyelitis, left shoulder
         M86.319 Chronic multifocal osteomyelitis, unspecified shoulder
     √6th M86.32 Chronic multifocal osteomyelitis, humerus
         M86.321 Chronic multifocal osteomyelitis, right humerus
         M86.322 Chronic multifocal osteomyelitis, left humerus
         M86.329 Chronic multifocal osteomyelitis, unspecified humerus
     √6th M86.33 Chronic multifocal osteomyelitis, radius and ulna
         M86.331 Chronic multifocal osteomyelitis, right radius and ulna
         M86.332 Chronic multifocal osteomyelitis, left radius and ulna
         M86.339 Chronic multifocal osteomyelitis, unspecified radius and ulna
     √6th M86.34 Chronic multifocal osteomyelitis, hand
         M86.341 Chronic multifocal osteomyelitis, right hand
         M86.342 Chronic multifocal osteomyelitis, left hand
         M86.349 Chronic multifocal osteomyelitis, unspecified hand
     √6th M86.35 Chronic multifocal osteomyelitis, femur
         M86.351 Chronic multifocal osteomyelitis, right femur
         M86.352 Chronic multifocal osteomyelitis, left femur
         M86.359 Chronic multifocal osteomyelitis, unspecified femur
     √6th M86.36 Chronic multifocal osteomyelitis, tibia and fibula
         M86.361 Chronic multifocal osteomyelitis, right tibia and fibula
         M86.362 Chronic multifocal osteomyelitis, left tibia and fibula
         M86.369 Chronic multifocal osteomyelitis, unspecified tibia and fibula
     √6th M86.37 Chronic multifocal osteomyelitis, ankle and foot
         M86.371 Chronic multifocal osteomyelitis, right ankle and foot
         M86.372 Chronic multifocal osteomyelitis, left ankle and foot
         M86.379 Chronic multifocal osteomyelitis, unspecified ankle and foot
     M86.38 Chronic multifocal osteomyelitis, other site
     M86.39 Chronic multifocal osteomyelitis, multiple sites
√5th **M86.4 Chronic osteomyelitis with draining sinus**
     M86.40 Chronic osteomyelitis with draining sinus, unspecified site
     √6th M86.41 Chronic osteomyelitis with draining sinus, shoulder
         M86.411 Chronic osteomyelitis with draining sinus, right shoulder

---

M86.412 Chronic osteomyelitis with draining sinus, left shoulder

M86.419 Chronic osteomyelitis with draining sinus, unspecified shoulder

☑6ᵗʰ M86.42 Chronic osteomyelitis with draining sinus, humerus

M86.421 Chronic osteomyelitis with draining sinus, right humerus

M86.422 Chronic osteomyelitis with draining sinus, left humerus

M86.429 Chronic osteomyelitis with draining sinus, unspecified humerus

☑6ᵗʰ M86.43 Chronic osteomyelitis with draining sinus, forearm

M86.431 Chronic osteomyelitis with draining sinus, right forearm

M86.432 Chronic osteomyelitis with draining sinus, left forearm

M86.439 Chronic osteomyelitis with draining sinus, unspecified forearm

☑6ᵗʰ M86.44 Chronic osteomyelitis with draining sinus, hand

M86.441 Chronic osteomyelitis with draining sinus, right hand

M86.442 Chronic osteomyelitis with draining sinus, left hand

M86.449 Chronic osteomyelitis with draining sinus, unspecified hand

☑6ᵗʰ M86.45 Chronic osteomyelitis with draining sinus, femur

M86.451 Chronic osteomyelitis with draining sinus, right femur

M86.452 Chronic osteomyelitis with draining sinus, left femur

M86.459 Chronic osteomyelitis with draining sinus, unspecified femur

☑6ᵗʰ M86.46 Chronic osteomyelitis with draining sinus, lower leg

M86.461 Chronic osteomyelitis with draining sinus, right lower leg

M86.462 Chronic osteomyelitis with draining sinus, left lower leg

M86.469 Chronic osteomyelitis with draining sinus, unspecified lower leg

☑6ᵗʰ M86.47 Chronic osteomyelitis with draining sinus, ankle and foot

M86.471 Chronic osteomyelitis with draining sinus, right ankle and foot

M86.472 Chronic osteomyelitis with draining sinus, left ankle and foot

M86.479 Chronic osteomyelitis with draining sinus, unspecified ankle and foot

M86.48 Chronic osteomyelitis with draining sinus, other site

M86.49 Chronic osteomyelitis with draining sinus, multiple sites

☑5ᵗʰ M86.5 Other chronic hematogenous osteomyelitis

M86.50 Other chronic hematogenous osteomyelitis, unspecified site

☑6ᵗʰ M86.51 Other chronic hematogenous osteomyelitis, shoulder

M86.511 Other chronic hematogenous osteomyelitis, right shoulder

M86.512 Other chronic hematogenous osteomyelitis, left shoulder

M86.519 Other chronic hematogenous osteomyelitis, unspecified shoulder

☑6ᵗʰ M86.52 Other chronic hematogenous osteomyelitis, humerus

M86.521 Other chronic hematogenous osteomyelitis, right humerus

M86.522 Other chronic hematogenous osteomyelitis, left humerus

M86.529 Other chronic hematogenous osteomyelitis, unspecified humerus

☑6ᵗʰ M86.53 Other chronic hematogenous osteomyelitis, forearm

M86.531 Other chronic hematogenous osteomyelitis, right forearm

M86.532 Other chronic hematogenous osteomyelitis, left forearm

M86.539 Other chronic hematogenous osteomyelitis, unspecified forearm

☑6ᵗʰ M86.54 Other chronic hematogenous osteomyelitis, hand

M86.541 Other chronic hematogenous osteomyelitis, right hand

M86.542 Other chronic hematogenous osteomyelitis, left hand

M86.549 Other chronic hematogenous osteomyelitis, unspecified hand

☑6ᵗʰ M86.55 Other chronic hematogenous osteomyelitis, femur

M86.551 Other chronic hematogenous osteomyelitis, right femur

M86.552 Other chronic hematogenous osteomyelitis, left femur

M86.559 Other chronic hematogenous osteomyelitis, unspecified femur

☑6ᵗʰ M86.56 Other chronic hematogenous osteomyelitis, lower leg

M86.561 Other chronic hematogenous osteomyelitis, right lower leg

M86.562 Other chronic hematogenous osteomyelitis, left lower leg

M86.569 Other chronic hematogenous osteomyelitis, unspecified lower leg

☑6ᵗʰ M86.57 Other chronic hematogenous osteomyelitis, ankle and foot

M86.571 Other chronic hematogenous osteomyelitis, right ankle and foot

M86.572 Other chronic hematogenous osteomyelitis, left ankle and foot

M86.579 Other chronic hematogenous osteomyelitis, unspecified ankle and foot

M86.58 Other chronic hematogenous osteomyelitis, other site

M86.59 Other chronic hematogenous osteomyelitis, multiple sites

☑5ᵗʰ M86.6 Other chronic osteomyelitis

M86.60 Other chronic osteomyelitis, unspecified site

☑6ᵗʰ M86.61 Other chronic osteomyelitis, shoulder

M86.611 Other chronic osteomyelitis, right shoulder

M86.612 Other chronic osteomyelitis, left shoulder

M86.619 Other chronic osteomyelitis, unspecified shoulder

☑6ᵗʰ M86.62 Other chronic osteomyelitis, upper arm

M86.621 Other chronic osteomyelitis, right upper arm

M86.622 Other chronic osteomyelitis, left upper arm

M86.629 Other chronic osteomyelitis, unspecified upper arm

☑6ᵗʰ M86.63 Other chronic osteomyelitis, forearm

M86.631 Other chronic osteomyelitis, right forearm

M86.632 Other chronic osteomyelitis, left forearm

M86.639 Other chronic osteomyelitis, unspecified forearm

☑6ᵗʰ M86.64 Other chronic osteomyelitis, hand

M86.641 Other chronic osteomyelitis, right hand

M86.642 Other chronic osteomyelitis, left hand

M86.649 Other chronic osteomyelitis, unspecified hand

☑6ᵗʰ M86.65 Other chronic osteomyelitis, thigh

M86.651 Other chronic osteomyelitis, right thigh

M86.652 Other chronic osteomyelitis, left thigh

M86.659 Other chronic osteomyelitis, unspecified thigh

☑6ᵗʰ M86.66 Other chronic osteomyelitis, lower leg

M86.661 Other chronic osteomyelitis, right lower leg

M86.662 Other chronic osteomyelitis, left lower leg

M86.669 Other chronic osteomyelitis, unspecified lower leg

☑ Appropriate additional character required   ☑x7ᵗʰ Requires 7th character, placeholder x must fill empty characters

Diseases of the Musculoskeletal System and Connective Tissue

M86.412–M86.669

Diseases of the Musculoskeletal System and Connective Tissue

M86.67–M87.145

✓6th **M86.67 Other chronic osteomyelitis, ankle and foot**
- **M86.671 Other chronic osteomyelitis, right ankle and foot**
- **M86.672 Other chronic osteomyelitis, left ankle and foot**
- **M86.679 Other chronic osteomyelitis, unspecified ankle and foot**

M86.68 Other chronic osteomyelitis, other site

M86.69 Other chronic osteomyelitis, multiple sites

✓5th **M86.8 Other osteomyelitis**
Brodie's abscess

    ✓6th **M86.8x Other osteomyelitis**
- **M86.8x0 Other osteomyelitis, multiple sites**
- **M86.8x1 Other osteomyelitis, shoulder**
- **M86.8x2 Other osteomyelitis, upper arm**
- **M86.8x3 Other osteomyelitis, forearm**
- **M86.8x4 Other osteomyelitis, hand**
- **M86.8x5 Other osteomyelitis, thigh**
- **M86.8x6 Other osteomyelitis, lower leg**
- **M86.8x7 Other osteomyelitis, ankle and foot**
- **M86.8x8 Other osteomyelitis, other site**
- **M86.8x9 Other osteomyelitis, unspecified sites**

M86.9 Osteomyelitis, unspecified
Infection of bone NOS
Periostitis without osteomyelitis

✓4th **M87 Osteonecrosis**
INCLUDES   avascular necrosis of bone
Use additional code to identify major osseous defect, if applicable (M89.7-)
    EXCLUDES 1   juvenile osteonecrosis (M91-M92)
                  osteochondropathies (M90-M93)

✓5th **M87.0 Idiopathic aseptic necrosis of bone**
M87.00 Idiopathic aseptic necrosis of unspecified bone

    ✓6th **M87.01 Idiopathic aseptic necrosis of shoulder**
Idiopathic aseptic necrosis of clavicle and scapula
- **M87.011 Idiopathic aseptic necrosis of right shoulder**
- **M87.012 Idiopathic aseptic necrosis of left shoulder**
- **M87.019 Idiopathic aseptic necrosis of unspecified shoulder**

    ✓6th **M87.02 Idiopathic aseptic necrosis of humerus**
- **M87.021 Idiopathic aseptic necrosis of right humerus**
- **M87.022 Idiopathic aseptic necrosis of left humerus**
- **M87.029 Idiopathic aseptic necrosis of unspecified humerus**

    ✓6th **M87.03 Idiopathic aseptic necrosis of radius, ulna and carpus**
- **M87.031 Idiopathic aseptic necrosis of right radius**
- **M87.032 Idiopathic aseptic necrosis of left radius**
- **M87.033 Idiopathic aseptic necrosis of unspecified radius**
- **M87.034 Idiopathic aseptic necrosis of right ulna**
- **M87.035 Idiopathic aseptic necrosis of left ulna**
- **M87.036 Idiopathic aseptic necrosis of unspecified ulna**
- **M87.037 Idiopathic aseptic necrosis of right carpus**
- **M87.038 Idiopathic aseptic necrosis of left carpus**
- **M87.039 Idiopathic aseptic necrosis of unspecified carpus**

    ✓6th **M87.04 Idiopathic aseptic necrosis of hand and fingers**
Idiopathic aseptic necrosis of metacarpals and phalanges of hands
- **M87.041 Idiopathic aseptic necrosis of right hand**
- **M87.042 Idiopathic aseptic necrosis of left hand**
- **M87.043 Idiopathic aseptic necrosis of unspecified hand**
- **M87.044 Idiopathic aseptic necrosis of right finger(s)**
- **M87.045 Idiopathic aseptic necrosis of left finger(s)**
- **M87.046 Idiopathic aseptic necrosis of unspecified finger(s)**

✓6th **M87.05 Idiopathic aseptic necrosis of pelvis and femur**
- **M87.050 Idiopathic aseptic necrosis of pelvis**
- **M87.051 Idiopathic aseptic necrosis of right femur**
- **M87.052 Idiopathic aseptic necrosis of left femur**
- **M87.059 Idiopathic aseptic necrosis of unspecified femur**
Idiopathic aseptic necrosis of hip NOS

✓6th **M87.06 Idiopathic aseptic necrosis of tibia and fibula**
- **M87.061 Idiopathic aseptic necrosis of right tibia**
- **M87.062 Idiopathic aseptic necrosis of left tibia**
- **M87.063 Idiopathic aseptic necrosis of unspecified tibia**
- **M87.064 Idiopathic aseptic necrosis of right fibula**
- **M87.065 Idiopathic aseptic necrosis of left fibula**
- **M87.066 Idiopathic aseptic necrosis of unspecified fibula**

✓6th **M87.07 Idiopathic aseptic necrosis of ankle, foot and toes**
Idiopathic aseptic necrosis of metatarsus, tarsus, and phalanges of toes
- **M87.071 Idiopathic aseptic necrosis of right ankle**
- **M87.072 Idiopathic aseptic necrosis of left ankle**
- **M87.073 Idiopathic aseptic necrosis of unspecified ankle**
- **M87.074 Idiopathic aseptic necrosis of right foot**
- **M87.075 Idiopathic aseptic necrosis of left foot**
- **M87.076 Idiopathic aseptic necrosis of unspecified foot**
- **M87.077 Idiopathic aseptic necrosis of right toe(s)**
- **M87.078 Idiopathic aseptic necrosis of left toe(s)**
- **M87.079 Idiopathic aseptic necrosis of unspecified toe(s)**

M87.08 Idiopathic aseptic necrosis of bone, other site

M87.09 Idiopathic aseptic necrosis of bone, multiple sites

✓5th **M87.1 Osteonecrosis due to drugs**
Code first (T36-T50) to identify drug
M87.10 Osteonecrosis due to drugs, unspecified bone

    ✓6th **M87.11 Osteonecrosis due to drugs, shoulder**
- **M87.111 Osteonecrosis due to drugs, right shoulder**
- **M87.112 Osteonecrosis due to drugs, left shoulder**
- **M87.119 Osteonecrosis due to drugs, unspecified shoulder**

    ✓6th **M87.12 Osteonecrosis due to drugs, humerus**
- **M87.121 Osteonecrosis due to drugs, right humerus**
- **M87.122 Osteonecrosis due to drugs, left humerus**
- **M87.129 Osteonecrosis due to drugs, unspecified humerus**

    ✓6th **M87.13 Osteonecrosis due to drugs of radius, ulna and carpus**
- **M87.131 Osteonecrosis due to drugs of right radius**
- **M87.132 Osteonecrosis due to drugs of left radius**
- **M87.133 Osteonecrosis due to drugs of unspecified radius**
- **M87.134 Osteonecrosis due to drugs of right ulna**
- **M87.135 Osteonecrosis due to drugs of left ulna**
- **M87.136 Osteonecrosis due to drugs of unspecified ulna**
- **M87.137 Osteonecrosis due to drugs of right carpus**
- **M87.138 Osteonecrosis due to drugs of left carpus**
- **M87.139 Osteonecrosis due to drugs of unspecified carpus**

    ✓6th **M87.14 Osteonecrosis due to drugs, hand and fingers**
- **M87.141 Osteonecrosis due to drugs, right hand**
- **M87.142 Osteonecrosis due to drugs, left hand**
- **M87.143 Osteonecrosis due to drugs, unspecified hand**
- **M87.144 Osteonecrosis due to drugs, right finger(s)**
- **M87.145 Osteonecrosis due to drugs, left finger(s)**

M87.146 Osteonecrosis due to drugs, unspecified finger(s)

✓6ᵗʰ **M87.15 Osteonecrosis due to drugs, pelvis and femur**
M87.150 Osteonecrosis due to drugs, pelvis
M87.151 Osteonecrosis due to drugs, right femur
M87.152 Osteonecrosis due to drugs, left femur
M87.159 Osteonecrosis due to drugs, unspecified femur

✓6ᵗʰ **M87.16 Osteonecrosis due to drugs, tibia and fibula**
M87.161 Osteonecrosis due to drugs, right tibia
M87.162 Osteonecrosis due to drugs, left tibia
M87.163 Osteonecrosis due to drugs, unspecified tibia
M87.164 Osteonecrosis due to drugs, right fibula
M87.165 Osteonecrosis due to drugs, left fibula
M87.166 Osteonecrosis due to drugs, unspecified fibula

✓6ᵗʰ **M87.17 Osteonecrosis due to drugs, ankle, foot and toes**
M87.171 Osteonecrosis due to drugs, right ankle
M87.172 Osteonecrosis due to drugs, left ankle
M87.173 Osteonecrosis due to drugs, unspecified ankle
M87.174 Osteonecrosis due to drugs, right foot
M87.175 Osteonecrosis due to drugs, left foot
M87.176 Osteonecrosis due to drugs, unspecified foot
M87.177 Osteonecrosis due to drugs, right toe(s)
M87.178 Osteonecrosis due to drugs, left toe(s)
M87.179 Osteonecrosis due to drugs, unspecified toe(s)

✓6ᵗʰ **M87.18 Osteonecrosis due to drugs, other site**
M87.180 Osteonecrosis due to drugs, jaw
M87.188 Osteonecrosis due to drugs, other site
M87.19 Osteonecrosis due to drugs, multiple sites

✓5ᵗʰ **M87.2 Osteonecrosis due to previous trauma**
M87.20 Osteonecrosis due to previous trauma, unspecified bone

✓6ᵗʰ **M87.21 Osteonecrosis due to previous trauma, shoulder**
M87.211 Osteonecrosis due to previous trauma, right shoulder
M87.212 Osteonecrosis due to previous trauma, left shoulder
M87.219 Osteonecrosis due to previous trauma, unspecified shoulder

✓6ᵗʰ **M87.22 Osteonecrosis due to previous trauma, humerus**
M87.221 Osteonecrosis due to previous trauma, right humerus
M87.222 Osteonecrosis due to previous trauma, left humerus
M87.229 Osteonecrosis due to previous trauma, unspecified humerus

✓6ᵗʰ **M87.23 Osteonecrosis due to previous trauma of radius, ulna and carpus**
M87.231 Osteonecrosis due to previous trauma of right radius
M87.232 Osteonecrosis due to previous trauma of left radius
M87.233 Osteonecrosis due to previous trauma of unspecified radius
M87.234 Osteonecrosis due to previous trauma of right ulna
M87.235 Osteonecrosis due to previous trauma of left ulna
M87.236 Osteonecrosis due to previous trauma of unspecified ulna
M87.237 Osteonecrosis due to previous trauma of right carpus
M87.238 Osteonecrosis due to previous trauma of left carpus
M87.239 Osteonecrosis due to previous trauma of unspecified carpus

✓6ᵗʰ **M87.24 Osteonecrosis due to previous trauma, hand and fingers**
M87.241 Osteonecrosis due to previous trauma, right hand
M87.242 Osteonecrosis due to previous trauma, left hand

M87.243 Osteonecrosis due to previous trauma, unspecified hand
M87.244 Osteonecrosis due to previous trauma, right finger(s)
M87.245 Osteonecrosis due to previous trauma, left finger(s)
M87.246 Osteonecrosis due to previous trauma, unspecified finger(s)

✓6ᵗʰ **M87.25 Osteonecrosis due to previous trauma, pelvis and femur**
M87.250 Osteonecrosis due to previous trauma, pelvis
M87.251 Osteonecrosis due to previous trauma, right femur
M87.252 Osteonecrosis due to previous trauma, left femur
M87.256 Osteonecrosis due to previous trauma, unspecified femur

✓6ᵗʰ **M87.26 Osteonecrosis due to previous trauma, tibia and fibula**
M87.261 Osteonecrosis due to previous trauma, right tibia
M87.262 Osteonecrosis due to previous trauma, left tibia
M87.263 Osteonecrosis due to previous trauma, unspecified tibia
M87.264 Osteonecrosis due to previous trauma, right fibula
M87.265 Osteonecrosis due to previous trauma, left fibula
M87.266 Osteonecrosis due to previous trauma, unspecified fibula

✓6ᵗʰ **M87.27 Osteonecrosis due to previous trauma, ankle, foot and toes**
M87.271 Osteonecrosis due to previous trauma, right ankle
M87.272 Osteonecrosis due to previous trauma, left ankle
M87.273 Osteonecrosis due to previous trauma, unspecified ankle
M87.274 Osteonecrosis due to previous trauma, right foot
M87.275 Osteonecrosis due to previous trauma, left foot
M87.276 Osteonecrosis due to previous trauma, unspecified foot
M87.277 Osteonecrosis due to previous trauma, right toe(s)
M87.278 Osteonecrosis due to previous trauma, left toe(s)
M87.279 Osteonecrosis due to previous trauma, unspecified toe(s)
M87.28 Osteonecrosis due to previous trauma, other site
M87.29 Osteonecrosis due to previous trauma, multiple sites

✓5ᵗʰ **M87.3 Other secondary osteonecrosis**
M87.30 Other secondary osteonecrosis, unspecified bone

✓6ᵗʰ **M87.31 Other secondary osteonecrosis, shoulder**
M87.311 Other secondary osteonecrosis, right shoulder
M87.312 Other secondary osteonecrosis, left shoulder
M87.319 Other secondary osteonecrosis, unspecified shoulder

✓6ᵗʰ **M87.32 Other secondary osteonecrosis, humerus**
M87.321 Other secondary osteonecrosis, right humerus
M87.322 Other secondary osteonecrosis, left humerus
M87.329 Other secondary osteonecrosis, unspecified humerus

✓6ᵗʰ **M87.33 Other secondary osteonecrosis of radius, ulna and carpus**
M87.331 Other secondary osteonecrosis of right radius
M87.332 Other secondary osteonecrosis of left radius

M87.333 Other secondary osteonecrosis of unspecified radius

M87.334 Other secondary osteonecrosis of right ulna

M87.335 Other secondary osteonecrosis of left ulna

M87.336 Other secondary osteonecrosis of unspecified ulna

M87.337 Other secondary osteonecrosis of right carpus

M87.338 Other secondary osteonecrosis of left carpus

M87.339 Other secondary osteonecrosis of unspecified carpus

✓6th M87.34 Other secondary osteonecrosis, hand and fingers

M87.341 Other secondary osteonecrosis, right hand

M87.342 Other secondary osteonecrosis, left hand

M87.343 Other secondary osteonecrosis, unspecified hand

M87.344 Other secondary osteonecrosis, right finger(s)

M87.345 Other secondary osteonecrosis, left finger(s)

M87.346 Other secondary osteonecrosis, unspecified finger(s)

✓6th M87.35 Other secondary osteonecrosis, pelvis and femur

M87.350 Other secondary osteonecrosis, pelvis

M87.351 Other secondary osteonecrosis, right femur

M87.352 Other secondary osteonecrosis, left femur

M87.353 Other secondary osteonecrosis, unspecified femur

✓6th M87.36 Other secondary osteonecrosis, tibia and fibula

M87.361 Other secondary osteonecrosis, right tibia

M87.362 Other secondary osteonecrosis, left tibia

M87.363 Other secondary osteonecrosis, unspecified tibia

M87.364 Other secondary osteonecrosis, right fibula

M87.365 Other secondary osteonecrosis, left fibula

M87.366 Other secondary osteonecrosis, unspecified fibula

✓6th M87.37 Other secondary osteonecrosis, ankle and foot

M87.371 Other secondary osteonecrosis, right ankle

M87.372 Other secondary osteonecrosis, left ankle

M87.373 Other secondary osteonecrosis, unspecified ankle

M87.374 Other secondary osteonecrosis, right foot

M87.375 Other secondary osteonecrosis, left foot

M87.376 Other secondary osteonecrosis, unspecified foot

M87.377 Other secondary osteonecrosis, right toe(s)

M87.378 Other secondary osteonecrosis, left toe(s)

M87.379 Other secondary osteonecrosis, unspecified toe(s)

M87.38 Other secondary osteonecrosis, other site

M87.39 Other secondary osteonecrosis, multiple sites

✓5th M87.8 Other osteonecrosis

M87.80 Other osteonecrosis, unspecified bone

✓6th M87.81 Other osteonecrosis, shoulder

M87.811 Other osteonecrosis, right shoulder

M87.812 Other osteonecrosis, left shoulder

M87.819 Other osteonecrosis, unspecified shoulder

✓6th M87.82 Other osteonecrosis, humerus

M87.821 Other osteonecrosis, right humerus

M87.822 Other osteonecrosis, left humerus

M87.829 Other osteonecrosis, unspecified humerus

✓6th M87.83 Other osteonecrosis of radius, ulna and carpus

M87.831 Other osteonecrosis of right radius

M87.832 Other osteonecrosis of left radius

M87.833 Other osteonecrosis of unspecified radius

M87.834 Other osteonecrosis of right ulna

M87.835 Other osteonecrosis of left ulna

M87.836 Other osteonecrosis of unspecified ulna

M87.837 Other osteonecrosis of right carpus

M87.838 Other osteonecrosis of left carpus

M87.839 Other osteonecrosis of unspecified carpus

✓6th M87.84 Other osteonecrosis, hand and fingers

M87.841 Other osteonecrosis, right hand

M87.842 Other osteonecrosis, left hand

M87.843 Other osteonecrosis, unspecified hand

M87.844 Other osteonecrosis, right finger(s)

M87.845 Other osteonecrosis, left finger(s)

M87.849 Other osteonecrosis, unspecified finger(s)

✓6th M87.85 Other osteonecrosis, pelvis and femur

M87.850 Other osteonecrosis, pelvis

M87.851 Other osteonecrosis, right femur

M87.852 Other osteonecrosis, left femur

M87.859 Other osteonecrosis, unspecified femur

✓6th M87.86 Other osteonecrosis, tibia and fibula

M87.861 Other osteonecrosis, right tibia

M87.862 Other osteonecrosis, left tibia

M87.863 Other osteonecrosis, unspecified tibia

M87.864 Other osteonecrosis, right fibula

M87.865 Other osteonecrosis, left fibula

M87.869 Other osteonecrosis, unspecified fibula

✓6th M87.87 Other osteonecrosis, ankle, foot and toes

M87.871 Other osteonecrosis, right ankle

M87.872 Other osteonecrosis, left ankle

M87.873 Other osteonecrosis, unspecified ankle

M87.874 Other osteonecrosis, right foot

M87.875 Other osteonecrosis, left foot

M87.876 Other osteonecrosis, unspecified foot

M87.877 Other osteonecrosis, right toe(s)

M87.878 Other osteonecrosis, left toe(s)

M87.879 Other osteonecrosis, unspecified toe(s)

M87.88 Other osteonecrosis, other site

M87.89 Other osteonecrosis, multiple sites

M87.9 Osteonecrosis, unspecified
Necrosis of bone NOS

✓4th M88 Osteitis deformans [Paget's disease of bone]
EXCLUDES 1 osteitis deformans in neoplastic disease (M90.6)

M88.0 Osteitis deformans of skull

M88.1 Osteitis deformans of vertebrae

✓5th M88.8 Osteitis deformans of other bones

✓6th M88.81 Osteitis deformans of shoulder

M88.811 Osteitis deformans of right shoulder

M88.812 Osteitis deformans of left shoulder

M88.819 Osteitis deformans of unspecified shoulder

✓6th M88.82 Osteitis deformans of upper arm

M88.821 Osteitis deformans of right upper arm

M88.822 Osteitis deformans of left upper arm

M88.829 Osteitis deformans of unspecified upper arm

✓6th M88.83 Osteitis deformans of forearm

M88.831 Osteitis deformans of right forearm

M88.832 Osteitis deformans of left forearm

M88.839 Osteitis deformans of unspecified forearm

✓6th M88.84 Osteitis deformans of hand

M88.841 Osteitis deformans of right hand

M88.842 Osteitis deformans of left hand

M88.849 Osteitis deformans of unspecified hand

✓6th M88.85 Osteitis deformans of thigh

M88.851 Osteitis deformans of right thigh

M88.852 Osteitis deformans of left thigh

EXCLUDES 1 Not coded here   EXCLUDES 2 Not included here   *Manifestation Code*

         M88.859   Osteitis deformans of unspecified thigh

✓6th   **M88.86**   **Osteitis deformans of lower leg**
         M88.861   Osteitis deformans of right lower leg
         M88.862   Osteitis deformans of left lower leg
         M88.869   Osteitis deformans of unspecified lower leg

✓6th   **M88.87**   **Osteitis deformans of ankle and foot**
         M88.871   Osteitis deformans of right ankle and foot
         M88.872   Osteitis deformans of left ankle and foot
         M88.879   Osteitis deformans of unspecified ankle and foot

     M88.88   **Osteitis deformans of other bones**
         EXCLUDES 2   *osteitis deformans of skull (M88.0)*
                  osteitis deformans of vertebrae (M88.1)

     M88.89   **Osteitis deformans of multiple sites**
   M88.9   **Osteitis deformans of unspecified bone**

✓4th   **M89**   **Other disorders of bone**
✓5th   **M89.0**   **Algoneurodystrophy**
         Shoulder-hand syndrome
         Sudeck's atrophy
         EXCLUDES 1   *causalgia, lower limb (G57.7-)*
                  causalgia, upper limb (G56.4-)
                  complex regional pain syndrome II, lower limb (G57.7-)
                  complex regional pain syndrome II, upper limb (G56.4-)
                  reflex sympathetic dystrophy (G90.5-)

     M89.00   **Algoneurodystrophy, unspecified site**
✓6th   **M89.01**   **Algoneurodystrophy, shoulder**
         M89.011   Algoneurodystrophy, right shoulder
         M89.012   Algoneurodystrophy, left shoulder
         M89.019   Algoneurodystrophy, unspecified shoulder

✓6th   **M89.02**   **Algoneurodystrophy, upper arm**
         M89.021   Algoneurodystrophy, right upper arm
         M89.022   Algoneurodystrophy, left upper arm
         M89.029   Algoneurodystrophy, unspecified upper arm

✓6th   **M89.03**   **Algoneurodystrophy, forearm**
         M89.031   Algoneurodystrophy, right forearm
         M89.032   Algoneurodystrophy, left forearm
         M89.039   Algoneurodystrophy, unspecified forearm

✓6th   **M89.04**   **Algoneurodystrophy, hand**
         M89.041   Algoneurodystrophy, right hand
         M89.042   Algoneurodystrophy, left hand
         M89.049   Algoneurodystrophy, unspecified hand

✓6th   **M89.05**   **Algoneurodystrophy, thigh**
         M89.051   Algoneurodystrophy, right thigh
         M89.052   Algoneurodystrophy, left thigh
         M89.059   Algoneurodystrophy, unspecified thigh

✓6th   **M89.06**   **Algoneurodystrophy, lower leg**
         M89.061   Algoneurodystrophy, right lower leg
         M89.062   Algoneurodystrophy, left lower leg
         M89.069   Algoneurodystrophy, unspecified lower leg

✓6th   **M89.07**   **Algoneurodystrophy, ankle and foot**
         M89.071   Algoneurodystrophy, right ankle and foot
         M89.072   Algoneurodystrophy, left ankle and foot
         M89.079   Algoneurodystrophy, unspecified ankle and foot

     M89.08   **Algoneurodystrophy, other site**
     M89.09   **Algoneurodystrophy, multiple sites**

✓5th   **M89.1**   **Physeal arrest**
         Arrest of growth plate
         Epiphyseal arrest
         Growth plate arrest

✓6th   **M89.12**   **Physeal arrest, humerus**
         M89.121   Complete physeal arrest, right proximal humerus
         M89.122   Complete physeal arrest, left proximal humerus
         M89.123   Partial physeal arrest, right proximal humerus

         M89.124   Partial physeal arrest, left proximal humerus
         M89.125   Complete physeal arrest, right distal humerus
         M89.126   Complete physeal arrest, left distal humerus
         M89.127   Partial physeal arrest, right distal humerus
         M89.128   Partial physeal arrest, left distal humerus
         M89.129   Physeal arrest, humerus, unspecified

✓6th   **M89.13**   **Physeal arrest, forearm**
         M89.131   Complete physeal arrest, right distal radius
         M89.132   Complete physeal arrest, left distal radius
         M89.133   Partial physeal arrest, right distal radius
         M89.134   Partial physeal arrest, left distal radius
         M89.138   Other physeal arrest of forearm
         M89.139   Physeal arrest, forearm, unspecified

✓6th   **M89.15**   **Physeal arrest, femur**
         M89.151   Complete physeal arrest, right proximal femur
         M89.152   Complete physeal arrest, left proximal femur
         M89.153   Partial physeal arrest, right proximal femur
         M89.154   Partial physeal arrest, left proximal femur
         M89.155   Complete physeal arrest, right distal femur
         M89.156   Complete physeal arrest, left distal femur
         M89.157   Partial physeal arrest, right distal femur
         M89.158   Partial physeal arrest, left distal femur
         M89.159   Physeal arrest, femur, unspecified

✓6th   **M89.16**   **Physeal arrest, lower leg**
         M89.160   Complete physeal arrest, right proximal tibia
         M89.161   Complete physeal arrest, left proximal tibia
         M89.162   Partial physeal arrest, right proximal tibia
         M89.163   Partial physeal arrest, left proximal tibia
         M89.164   Complete physeal arrest, right distal tibia
         M89.165   Complete physeal arrest, left distal tibia
         M89.166   Partial physeal arrest, right distal tibia
         M89.167   Partial physeal arrest, left distal tibia
         M89.168   Other physeal arrest of lower leg
         M89.169   Physeal arrest, lower leg, unspecified

     M89.18   **Physeal arrest, other site**

✓5th   **M89.2**   **Other disorders of bone development and growth**
     M89.20   **Other disorders of bone development and growth, unspecified site**

✓6th   **M89.21**   **Other disorders of bone development and growth, shoulder**
         M89.211   Other disorders of bone development and growth, right shoulder
         M89.212   Other disorders of bone development and growth, left shoulder
         M89.219   Other disorders of bone development and growth, unspecified shoulder

✓6th   **M89.22**   **Other disorders of bone development and growth, humerus**
         M89.221   Other disorders of bone development and growth, right humerus
         M89.222   Other disorders of bone development and growth, left humerus
         M89.229   Other disorders of bone development and growth, unspecified humerus

✓6th   **M89.23**   **Other disorders of bone development and growth, ulna and radius**
         M89.231   Other disorders of bone development and growth, right ulna
         M89.232   Other disorders of bone development and growth, left ulna

      M89.233 **Other disorders of bone development and growth, right radius**

      M89.234 **Other disorders of bone development and growth, left radius**

      M89.239 **Other disorders of bone development and growth, unspecified ulna and radius**

✓6th   M89.24 **Other disorders of bone development and growth, hand**

      M89.241 **Other disorders of bone development and growth, right hand**

      M89.242 **Other disorders of bone development and growth, left hand**

      M89.249 **Other disorders of bone development and growth, unspecified hand**

✓6th   M89.25 **Other disorders of bone development and growth, femur**

      M89.251 **Other disorders of bone development and growth, right femur**

      M89.252 **Other disorders of bone development and growth, left femur**

      M89.259 **Other disorders of bone development and growth, unspecified femur**

✓6th   M89.26 **Other disorders of bone development and growth, tibia and fibula**

      M89.261 **Other disorders of bone development and growth, right tibia**

      M89.262 **Other disorders of bone development and growth, left tibia**

      M89.263 **Other disorders of bone development and growth, right fibula**

      M89.264 **Other disorders of bone development and growth, left fibula**

      M89.269 **Other disorders of bone development and growth, unspecified lower leg**

✓6th   M89.27 **Other disorders of bone development and growth, ankle and foot**

      M89.271 **Other disorders of bone development and growth, right ankle and foot**

      M89.272 **Other disorders of bone development and growth, left ankle and foot**

      M89.279 **Other disorders of bone development and growth, unspecified ankle and foot**

    M89.28 **Other disorders of bone development and growth, other site**

    M89.29 **Other disorders of bone development and growth, multiple sites**

✓5th   M89.3 **Hypertrophy of bone**

    M89.30 **Hypertrophy of bone, unspecified site**

✓6th   M89.31 **Hypertrophy of bone, shoulder**

      M89.311 **Hypertrophy of bone, right shoulder**

      M89.312 **Hypertrophy of bone, left shoulder**

      M89.319 **Hypertrophy of bone, unspecified shoulder**

✓6th   M89.32 **Hypertrophy of bone, humerus**

      M89.321 **Hypertrophy of bone, right humerus**

      M89.322 **Hypertrophy of bone, left humerus**

      M89.329 **Hypertrophy of bone, unspecified humerus**

✓6th   M89.33 **Hypertrophy of bone, ulna and radius**

      M89.331 **Hypertrophy of bone, right ulna**

      M89.332 **Hypertrophy of bone, left ulna**

      M89.333 **Hypertrophy of bone, right radius**

      M89.334 **Hypertrophy of bone, left radius**

      M89.339 **Hypertrophy of bone, unspecified ulna and radius**

✓6th   M89.34 **Hypertrophy of bone, hand**

      M89.341 **Hypertrophy of bone, right hand**

      M89.342 **Hypertrophy of bone, left hand**

      M89.349 **Hypertrophy of bone, unspecified hand**

✓6th   M89.35 **Hypertrophy of bone, femur**

      M89.351 **Hypertrophy of bone, right femur**

      M89.352 **Hypertrophy of bone, left femur**

      M89.359 **Hypertrophy of bone, unspecified femur**

✓6th   M89.36 **Hypertrophy of bone, tibia and fibula**

      M89.361 **Hypertrophy of bone, right tibia**

      M89.362 **Hypertrophy of bone, left tibia**

      M89.363 **Hypertrophy of bone, right fibula**

      M89.364 **Hypertrophy of bone, left fibula**

      M89.369 **Hypertrophy of bone, unspecified tibia and fibula**

✓6th   M89.37 **Hypertrophy of bone, ankle and foot**

      M89.371 **Hypertrophy of bone, right ankle and foot**

      M89.372 **Hypertrophy of bone, left ankle and foot**

      M89.379 **Hypertrophy of bone, unspecified ankle and foot**

    M89.38 **Hypertrophy of bone, other site**

    M89.39 **Hypertrophy of bone, multiple sites**

✓5th   M89.4 **Other hypertrophic osteoarthropathy**

    Marie-Bamberger disease

    Pachydermoperiostosis

    M89.40 **Other hypertrophic osteoarthropathy, unspecified site**

✓6th   M89.41 **Other hypertrophic osteoarthropathy, shoulder**

      M89.411 **Other hypertrophic osteoarthropathy, right shoulder**

      M89.412 **Other hypertrophic osteoarthropathy, left shoulder**

      M89.419 **Other hypertrophic osteoarthropathy, unspecified shoulder**

✓6th   M89.42 **Other hypertrophic osteoarthropathy, upper arm**

      M89.421 **Other hypertrophic osteoarthropathy, right upper arm**

      M89.422 **Other hypertrophic osteoarthropathy, left upper arm**

      M89.429 **Other hypertrophic osteoarthropathy, unspecified upper arm**

✓6th   M89.43 **Other hypertrophic osteoarthropathy, forearm**

      M89.431 **Other hypertrophic osteoarthropathy, right forearm**

      M89.432 **Other hypertrophic osteoarthropathy, left forearm**

      M89.439 **Other hypertrophic osteoarthropathy, unspecified forearm**

✓6th   M89.44 **Other hypertrophic osteoarthropathy, hand**

      M89.441 **Other hypertrophic osteoarthropathy, right hand**

      M89.442 **Other hypertrophic osteoarthropathy, left hand**

      M89.449 **Other hypertrophic osteoarthropathy, unspecified hand**

✓6th   M89.45 **Other hypertrophic osteoarthropathy, thigh**

      M89.451 **Other hypertrophic osteoarthropathy, right thigh**

      M89.452 **Other hypertrophic osteoarthropathy, left thigh**

      M89.459 **Other hypertrophic osteoarthropathy, unspecified thigh**

✓6th   M89.46 **Other hypertrophic osteoarthropathy, lower leg**

      M89.461 **Other hypertrophic osteoarthropathy, right lower leg**

      M89.462 **Other hypertrophic osteoarthropathy, left lower leg**

      M89.469 **Other hypertrophic osteoarthropathy, unspecified lower leg**

✓6th   M89.47 **Other hypertrophic osteoarthropathy, ankle and foot**

      M89.471 **Other hypertrophic osteoarthropathy, right ankle and foot**

      M89.472 **Other hypertrophic osteoarthropathy, left ankle and foot**

      M89.479 **Other hypertrophic osteoarthropathy, unspecified ankle and foot**

    M89.48 **Other hypertrophic osteoarthropathy, other site**

    M89.49 **Other hypertrophic osteoarthropathy, multiple sites**

✓5th   M89.5 **Osteolysis**

    Use additional code to identify major osseous defect, if applicable (M89.7-)

    EXCLUDES 2   *periprosthetic osteolysis of internal prosthetic joint (T84.05-)*

    M89.50 **Osteolysis, unspecified site**

✓6th   M89.51 **Osteolysis, shoulder**

      M89.511 **Osteolysis, right shoulder**

EXCLUDES 1 Not coded here   **EXCLUDES 2** Not included here   *Manifestation Code*

M89.512 Osteolysis, left shoulder
M89.519 Osteolysis, unspecified shoulder
√6ᵗʰ M89.52 Osteolysis, upper arm
M89.521 Osteolysis, right upper arm
M89.522 Osteolysis, left upper arm
M89.529 Osteolysis, unspecified upper arm
√6ᵗʰ M89.53 Osteolysis, forearm
M89.531 Osteolysis, right forearm
M89.532 Osteolysis, left forearm
M89.539 Osteolysis, unspecified forearm
√6ᵗʰ M89.54 Osteolysis, hand
M89.541 Osteolysis, right hand
M89.542 Osteolysis, left hand
M89.549 Osteolysis, unspecified hand
√6ᵗʰ M89.55 Osteolysis, thigh
M89.551 Osteolysis, right thigh
M89.552 Osteolysis, left thigh
M89.559 Osteolysis, unspecified thigh
√6ᵗʰ M89.56 Osteolysis, lower leg
M89.561 Osteolysis, right lower leg
M89.562 Osteolysis, left lower leg
M89.569 Osteolysis, unspecified lower leg
√6ᵗʰ M89.57 Osteolysis, ankle and foot
M89.571 Osteolysis, right ankle and foot
M89.572 Osteolysis, left ankle and foot
M89.579 Osteolysis, unspecified ankle and foot
M89.58 Osteolysis, other site
M89.59 Osteolysis, multiple sites
√5ᵗʰ M89.6 Osteopathy after poliomyelitis
Use additional code (B91) to identify previous poliomyelitis
EXCLUDES 1 *postpolio syndrome (G14)*
M89.60 Osteopathy after poliomyelitis, unspecified site
√6ᵗʰ M89.61 Osteopathy after poliomyelitis, shoulder
M89.611 Osteopathy after poliomyelitis, right shoulder
M89.612 Osteopathy after poliomyelitis, left shoulder
M89.619 Osteopathy after poliomyelitis, unspecified shoulder
√6ᵗʰ M89.62 Osteopathy after poliomyelitis, upper arm
M89.621 Osteopathy after poliomyelitis, right upper arm
M89.622 Osteopathy after poliomyelitis, left upper arm
M89.629 Osteopathy after poliomyelitis, unspecified upper arm
√6ᵗʰ M89.63 Osteopathy after poliomyelitis, forearm
M89.631 Osteopathy after poliomyelitis, right forearm
M89.632 Osteopathy after poliomyelitis, left forearm
M89.639 Osteopathy after poliomyelitis, unspecified forearm
√6ᵗʰ M89.64 Osteopathy after poliomyelitis, hand
M89.641 Osteopathy after poliomyelitis, right hand
M89.642 Osteopathy after poliomyelitis, left hand
M89.649 Osteopathy after poliomyelitis, unspecified hand
√6ᵗʰ M89.65 Osteopathy after poliomyelitis, thigh
M89.651 Osteopathy after poliomyelitis, right thigh
M89.652 Osteopathy after poliomyelitis, left thigh
M89.659 Osteopathy after poliomyelitis, unspecified thigh
√6ᵗʰ M89.66 Osteopathy after poliomyelitis, lower leg
M89.661 Osteopathy after poliomyelitis, right lower leg
M89.662 Osteopathy after poliomyelitis, left lower leg
M89.669 Osteopathy after poliomyelitis, unspecified lower leg

√6ᵗʰ M89.67 Osteopathy after poliomyelitis, ankle and foot
M89.671 Osteopathy after poliomyelitis, right ankle and foot
M89.672 Osteopathy after poliomyelitis, left ankle and foot
M89.679 Osteopathy after poliomyelitis, unspecified ankle and foot
M89.68 Osteopathy after poliomyelitis, other site
M89.69 Osteopathy after poliomyelitis, multiple sites
√5ᵗʰ M89.7 Major osseous defect
Code first underlying disease, if known, such as:
aseptic necrosis of bone (M87-)
malignant neoplasm of bone (C40-)
osteolysis (M89.5)
osteomyelitis (M86-)
osteonecrosis (M87-)
osteoporosis (M80-, M81-)
periprosthetic osteolysis (T84.05-)
M89.70 Major osseous defect, unspecified site
√6ᵗʰ M89.71 Major osseous defect, shoulder region
Major osseous defect clavicle or scapula
M89.711 Major osseous defect, right shoulder region
M89.712 Major osseous defect, left shoulder region
M89.719 Major osseous defect, unspecified shoulder region
√6ᵗʰ M89.72 Major osseous defect, humerus
M89.721 Major osseous defect, right humerus
M89.722 Major osseous defect, left humerus
M89.729 Major osseous defect, unspecified humerus
√6ᵗʰ M89.73 Major osseous defect, forearm
Major osseous defect of radius and ulna
M89.731 Major osseous defect, right forearm
M89.732 Major osseous defect, left forearm
M89.739 Major osseous defect, unspecified forearm
√6ᵗʰ M89.74 Major osseous defect, hand
Major osseous defect of carpus, fingers, metacarpus
M89.741 Major osseous defect, right hand
M89.742 Major osseous defect, left hand
M89.749 Major osseous defect, unspecified hand
√6ᵗʰ M89.75 Major osseous defect, pelvic region and thigh
Major osseous defect of femur and pelvis
M89.751 Major osseous defect, right pelvic region and thigh
M89.752 Major osseous defect, left pelvic region and thigh
M89.759 Major osseous defect, unspecified pelvic region and thigh
√6ᵗʰ M89.76 Major osseous defect, lower leg
Major osseous defect of fibula and tibia
M89.761 Major osseous defect, right lower leg
M89.762 Major osseous defect, left lower leg
M89.769 Major osseous defect, unspecified lower leg
√6ᵗʰ M89.77 Major osseous defect, ankle and foot
Major osseous defect of metatarsus, tarsus, toes
M89.771 Major osseous defect, right ankle and foot
M89.772 Major osseous defect, left ankle and foot
M89.779 Major osseous defect, unspecified ankle and foot
M89.78 Major osseous defect, other site
M89.79 Major osseous defect, multiple sites
√5ᵗʰ M89.8 Other specified disorders of bone
Infantile cortical hyperostoses
Post-traumatic subperiosteal ossification
√6ᵗʰ M89.8x Other specified disorders of bone
M89.8x0 Other specified disorders of bone, multiple sites
M89.8x1 Other specified disorders of bone, shoulder
M89.8x2 Other specified disorders of bone, upper arm

✔ Appropriate additional character required   √x7ᵗʰ Requires 7th character, placeholder x must fill empty characters

         M89.8x3   Other specified disorders of bone, forearm

         M89.8x4   Other specified disorders of bone, hand

         M89.8x5   Other specified disorders of bone, thigh

         M89.8x6   Other specified disorders of bone, lower leg

         M89.8x7   Other specified disorders of bone, ankle and foot

         M89.8x8   Other specified disorders of bone, other site

         M89.8x9   Other specified disorders of bone, unspecified site

     M89.9   Disorder of bone, unspecified

✓4th **M90**   **Osteopathies in diseases classified elsewhere**

     EXCLUDES 1   *osteochondritis, osteomyelitis, and osteopathy (in):*
         cryptococcosis (B45.3)
         diabetes mellitus (E08-E13 with 4th character .61-)
         gonococcal (A54.43)
         neurogenic syphilis (A52.11)
         renal osteodystrophy (N25.0)
         salmonellosis (A02.24)
         secondary syphilis (A51.46)
         syphilis (late) (A52.77)

✓5th **M90.5**   **Osteonecrosis in diseases classified elsewhere**

     Code first underlying disease, such as:
     caisson disease (T70.3)
     hemoglobinopathy (D50-D64)

     M90.50   *Osteonecrosis in diseases classified elsewhere, unspecified site*

     ✓6th **M90.51**   Osteonecrosis in diseases classified elsewhere, shoulder

         M90.511   *Osteonecrosis in diseases classified elsewhere, right shoulder*

         M90.512   *Osteonecrosis in diseases classified elsewhere, left shoulder*

         M90.519   *Osteonecrosis in diseases classified elsewhere, unspecified shoulder*

     ✓6th **M90.52**   Osteonecrosis in diseases classified elsewhere, upper arm

         M90.521   *Osteonecrosis in diseases classified elsewhere, right upper arm*

         M90.522   *Osteonecrosis in diseases classified elsewhere, left upper arm*

         M90.529   *Osteonecrosis in diseases classified elsewhere, unspecified upper arm*

     ✓6th **M90.53**   Osteonecrosis in diseases classified elsewhere, forearm

         M90.531   *Osteonecrosis in diseases classified elsewhere, right forearm*

         M90.532   *Osteonecrosis in diseases classified elsewhere, left forearm*

         M90.539   *Osteonecrosis in diseases classified elsewhere, unspecified forearm*

     ✓6th **M90.54**   Osteonecrosis in diseases classified elsewhere, hand

         M90.541   *Osteonecrosis in diseases classified elsewhere, right hand*

         M90.542   *Osteonecrosis in diseases classified elsewhere, left hand*

         M90.549   *Osteonecrosis in diseases classified elsewhere, unspecified hand*

     ✓6th **M90.55**   Osteonecrosis in diseases classified elsewhere, thigh

         M90.551   *Osteonecrosis in diseases classified elsewhere, right thigh*

         M90.552   *Osteonecrosis in diseases classified elsewhere, left thigh*

         M90.559   *Osteonecrosis in diseases classified elsewhere, unspecified thigh*

     ✓6th **M90.56**   Osteonecrosis in diseases classified elsewhere, lower leg

         M90.561   *Osteonecrosis in diseases classified elsewhere, right lower leg*

         M90.562   *Osteonecrosis in diseases classified elsewhere, left lower leg*

         M90.569   *Osteonecrosis in diseases classified elsewhere, unspecified lower leg*

     ✓6th **M90.57**   Osteonecrosis in diseases classified elsewhere, ankle and foot

         M90.571   *Osteonecrosis in diseases classified elsewhere, right ankle and foot*

         M90.572   *Osteonecrosis in diseases classified elsewhere, left ankle and foot*

         M90.579   *Osteonecrosis in diseases classified elsewhere, unspecified ankle and foot*

     M90.58   *Osteonecrosis in diseases classified elsewhere, other site*

     M90.59   *Osteonecrosis in diseases classified elsewhere, multiple sites*

✓5th **M90.6**   **Osteitis deformans in neoplastic diseases**

     Osteitis deformans in malignant neoplasm of bone
     Code first the neoplasm (C40-, C41-)
     EXCLUDES 1   *osteitis deformans [Paget's disease of bone] (M88-)*

     M90.60   *Osteitis deformans in neoplastic diseases, unspecified site*

     ✓6th **M90.61**   Osteitis deformans in neoplastic diseases, shoulder

         M90.611   *Osteitis deformans in neoplastic diseases, right shoulder*

         M90.612   *Osteitis deformans in neoplastic diseases, left shoulder*

         M90.619   *Osteitis deformans in neoplastic diseases, unspecified shoulder*

     ✓6th **M90.62**   Osteitis deformans in neoplastic diseases, upper arm

         M90.621   *Osteitis deformans in neoplastic diseases, right upper arm*

         M90.622   *Osteitis deformans in neoplastic diseases, left upper arm*

         M90.629   *Osteitis deformans in neoplastic diseases, unspecified upper arm*

     ✓6th **M90.63**   Osteitis deformans in neoplastic diseases, forearm

         M90.631   *Osteitis deformans in neoplastic diseases, right forearm*

         M90.632   *Osteitis deformans in neoplastic diseases, left forearm*

         M90.639   *Osteitis deformans in neoplastic diseases, unspecified forearm*

     ✓6th **M90.64**   Osteitis deformans in neoplastic diseases, hand

         M90.641   *Osteitis deformans in neoplastic diseases, right hand*

         M90.642   *Osteitis deformans in neoplastic diseases, left hand*

         M90.649   *Osteitis deformans in neoplastic diseases, unspecified hand*

     ✓6th **M90.65**   Osteitis deformans in neoplastic diseases, thigh

         M90.651   *Osteitis deformans in neoplastic diseases, right thigh*

         M90.652   *Osteitis deformans in neoplastic diseases, left thigh*

         M90.659   *Osteitis deformans in neoplastic diseases, unspecified thigh*

     ✓6th **M90.66**   Osteitis deformans in neoplastic diseases, lower leg

         M90.661   *Osteitis deformans in neoplastic diseases, right lower leg*

         M90.662   *Osteitis deformans in neoplastic diseases, left lower leg*

         M90.669   *Osteitis deformans in neoplastic diseases, unspecified lower leg*

     ✓6th **M90.67**   Osteitis deformans in neoplastic diseases, ankle and foot

         M90.671   *Osteitis deformans in neoplastic diseases, right ankle and foot*

         M90.672   *Osteitis deformans in neoplastic diseases, left ankle and foot*

         M90.679   *Osteitis deformans in neoplastic diseases, unspecified ankle and foot*

     M90.68   *Osteitis deformans in neoplastic diseases, other site*

     M90.69   *Osteitis deformans in neoplastic diseases, multiple sites*

√5th **M90.8 Osteopathy in diseases classified elsewhere**
  Code first underlying disease, such as:
    rickets (E55.0)
    vitamin-D-resistant rickets (E83.3)
    M90.80 *Osteopathy in diseases classified elsewhere, unspecified site*
    √6th *M90.81* *Osteopathy in diseases classified elsewhere, shoulder*
      M90.811 *Osteopathy in diseases classified elsewhere, right shoulder*
      M90.812 *Osteopathy in diseases classified elsewhere, left shoulder*
      M90.819 *Osteopathy in diseases classified elsewhere, unspecified shoulder*
    √6th *M90.82* *Osteopathy in diseases classified elsewhere, upper arm*
      M90.821 *Osteopathy in diseases classified elsewhere, right upper arm*
      M90.822 *Osteopathy in diseases classified elsewhere, left upper arm*
      M90.829 *Osteopathy in diseases classified elsewhere, unspecified upper arm*
    √6th *M90.83* *Osteopathy in diseases classified elsewhere, forearm*
      M90.831 *Osteopathy in diseases classified elsewhere, right forearm*
      M90.832 *Osteopathy in diseases classified elsewhere, left forearm*
      M90.839 *Osteopathy in diseases classified elsewhere, unspecified forearm*
    √6th *M90.84* *Osteopathy in diseases classified elsewhere, hand*
      M90.841 *Osteopathy in diseases classified elsewhere, right hand*
      M90.842 *Osteopathy in diseases classified elsewhere, left hand*
      M90.849 *Osteopathy in diseases classified elsewhere, unspecified hand*
    √6th *M90.85* *Osteopathy in diseases classified elsewhere, thigh*
      M90.851 *Osteopathy in diseases classified elsewhere, right thigh*
      M90.852 *Osteopathy in diseases classified elsewhere, left thigh*
      M90.859 *Osteopathy in diseases classified elsewhere, unspecified thigh*
    √6th *M90.86* *Osteopathy in diseases classified elsewhere, lower leg*
      M90.861 *Osteopathy in diseases classified elsewhere, right lower leg*
      M90.862 *Osteopathy in diseases classified elsewhere, left lower leg*
      M90.869 *Osteopathy in diseases classified elsewhere, unspecified lower leg*
    √6th *M90.87* *Osteopathy in diseases classified elsewhere, ankle and foot*
      M90.871 *Osteopathy in diseases classified elsewhere, right ankle and foot*
      M90.872 *Osteopathy in diseases classified elsewhere, left ankle and foot*
      M90.879 *Osteopathy in diseases classified elsewhere, unspecified ankle and foot*
    M90.88 *Osteopathy in diseases classified elsewhere, other site*
    M90.89 *Osteopathy in diseases classified elsewhere, multiple sites*

Chondropathies (M91-M94)

EXCLUDES 1 *postprocedural chondropathies (M96-)*

√4th **M91 Juvenile osteochondrosis of hip and pelvis**
  EXCLUDES 1 *slipped upper femoral epiphysis (nontraumatic) (M93.0)*
  M91.0 Juvenile osteochondrosis of pelvis
    Osteochondrosis (juvenile) of:
      acetabulum
      iliac crest [Buchanan]
      ischiopubic synchondrosis [van Neck]
      symphysis pubis [Pierson]

√5th **M91.1 Juvenile osteochondrosis of head of femur [Legg-Calvé-Perthes]**
  M91.10 Juvenile osteochondrosis of head of femur [Legg-Calvé-Perthes], unspecified leg
  M91.11 Juvenile osteochondrosis of head of femur [Legg-Calvé-Perthes], right leg
  M91.12 Juvenile osteochondrosis of head of femur [Legg-Calvé-Perthes], left leg
√5th **M91.2 Coxa plana**
  Hip deformity due to previous juvenile osteochondrosis
  M91.20 Coxa plana, unspecified hip
  M91.21 Coxa plana, right hip
  M91.22 Coxa plana, left hip
√5th **M91.3 Pseudocoxalgia**
  M91.30 Pseudocoxalgia, unspecified hip
  M91.31 Pseudocoxalgia, right hip
  M91.32 Pseudocoxalgia, left hip
√5th **M91.4 Coxa magna**
  M91.40 Coxa magna, unspecified hip
  M91.41 Coxa magna, right hip
  M91.42 Coxa magna, left hip
√5th **M91.8 Other juvenile osteochondrosis of hip and pelvis**
  Juvenile osteochondrosis after reduction of congenital dislocation of hip
  M91.80 Other juvenile osteochondrosis of hip and pelvis, unspecified leg
  M91.81 Other juvenile osteochondrosis of hip and pelvis, right leg
  M91.82 Other juvenile osteochondrosis of hip and pelvis, left leg
√5th **M91.9 Juvenile osteochondrosis of hip and pelvis, unspecified**
  M91.90 Juvenile osteochondrosis of hip and pelvis, unspecified, unspecified leg
  M91.91 Juvenile osteochondrosis of hip and pelvis, unspecified, right leg
  M91.92 Juvenile osteochondrosis of hip and pelvis, unspecified, left leg

√4th **M92 Other juvenile osteochondrosis**
√5th **M92.0 Juvenile osteochondrosis of humerus**
  Osteochondrosis (juvenile) of capitulum of humerus [Panner]
  Osteochondrosis (juvenile) of head of humerus [Haas]
  M92.00 Juvenile osteochondrosis of humerus, unspecified arm
  M92.01 Juvenile osteochondrosis of humerus, right arm
  M92.02 Juvenile osteochondrosis of humerus, left arm
√5th **M92.1 Juvenile osteochondrosis of radius and ulna**
  Osteochondrosis (juvenile) of lower ulna [Burns]
  Osteochondrosis (juvenile) of radial head [Brailsford]
  M92.10 Juvenile osteochondrosis of radius and ulna, unspecified arm
  M92.11 Juvenile osteochondrosis of radius and ulna, right arm
  M92.12 Juvenile osteochondrosis of radius and ulna, left arm
√5th **M92.2 Juvenile osteochondrosis, hand**
  √6th **M92.20 Unspecified juvenile osteochondrosis, hand**
    M92.201 Unspecified juvenile osteochondrosis, right hand
    M92.202 Unspecified juvenile osteochondrosis, left hand
    M92.209 Unspecified juvenile osteochondrosis, unspecified hand
  √6th **M92.21 Osteochondrosis (juvenile) of carpal lunate [Kienböck]**
    M92.211 Osteochondrosis (juvenile) of carpal lunate [Kienböck], right hand
    M92.212 Osteochondrosis (juvenile) of carpal lunate [Kienböck], left hand
    M92.219 Osteochondrosis (juvenile) of carpal lunate [Kienböck], unspecified hand
  √6th **M92.22 Osteochondrosis (juvenile) of metacarpal heads [Mauclaire]**
    M92.221 Osteochondrosis (juvenile) of metacarpal heads [Mauclaire], right hand
    M92.222 Osteochondrosis (juvenile) of metacarpal heads [Mauclaire], left hand

---

☑ Appropriate additional character required   √x7th Requires 7th character, placeholder x must fill empty characters

    M92.229 Osteochondrosis (juvenile) of metacarpal heads [Mauclaire], unspecified hand

✓6th **M92.29** Other juvenile osteochondrosis, hand

    M92.291 Other juvenile osteochondrosis, right hand

    M92.292 Other juvenile osteochondrosis, left hand

    M92.299 Other juvenile osteochondrosis, unspecified hand

✓5th **M92.3** Other juvenile osteochondrosis, upper limb

    M92.30 Other juvenile osteochondrosis, unspecified upper limb

    M92.31 Other juvenile osteochondrosis, right upper limb

    M92.32 Other juvenile osteochondrosis, left upper limb

✓5th **M92.4** Juvenile osteochondrosis of patella

    Osteochondrosis (juvenile) of primary patellar center [Köhler]

    Osteochondrosis (juvenile) of secondary patellar centre [Sinding Larsen]

    M92.40 Juvenile osteochondrosis of patella, unspecified knee

    M92.41 Juvenile osteochondrosis of patella, right knee

    M92.42 Juvenile osteochondrosis of patella, left knee

✓5th **M92.5** Juvenile osteochondrosis of tibia and fibula

    Osteochondrosis (juvenile) of proximal tibia [Blount]

    Osteochondrosis (juvenile) of tibial tubercle [Osgood-Schlatter]

    Tibia vara

    M92.50 Juvenile osteochondrosis of tibia and fibula, unspecified leg

    M92.51 Juvenile osteochondrosis of tibia and fibula, right leg

    M92.52 Juvenile osteochondrosis of tibia and fibula, left leg

✓5th **M92.6** Juvenile osteochondrosis of tarsus

    Osteochondrosis (juvenile) of calcaneum [Sever]

    Osteochondrosis (juvenile) of os tibiale externum [Haglund]

    Osteochondrosis (juvenile) of talus [Diaz]

    Osteochondrosis (juvenile) of tarsal navicular [Köhler]

    M92.60 Juvenile osteochondrosis of tarsus, unspecified ankle

    M92.61 Juvenile osteochondrosis of tarsus, right ankle

    M92.62 Juvenile osteochondrosis of tarsus, left ankle

✓5th **M92.7** Juvenile osteochondrosis of metatarsus

    Osteochondrosis (juvenile) of fifth metatarsus [Iselin]

    Osteochondrosis (juvenile) of second metatarsus [Freiberg]

    M92.70 Juvenile osteochondrosis of metatarsus, unspecified foot

    M92.71 Juvenile osteochondrosis of metatarsus, right foot

    M92.72 Juvenile osteochondrosis of metatarsus, left foot

M92.8 Other specified juvenile osteochondrosis

    Calcaneal apophysitis

M92.9 Juvenile osteochondrosis, unspecified

    Juvenile apophysitis NOS

    Juvenile epiphysitis NOS

    Juvenile osteochondritis NOS

    Juvenile osteochondrosis NOS

✓4th **M93** Other osteochondropathies

    EXCLUDES 2   osteochondrosis of spine (M42-)

✓5th **M93.0** Slipped upper femoral epiphysis (nontraumatic)

    Use additional code for associated chondrolysis (M94.3)

    ✓6th **M93.00** Unspecified slipped upper femoral epiphysis (nontraumatic)

    M93.001 Unspecified slipped upper femoral epiphysis (nontraumatic), right hip

    M93.002 Unspecified slipped upper femoral epiphysis (nontraumatic), left hip

    M93.003 Unspecified slipped upper femoral epiphysis (nontraumatic), unspecified hip

    ✓6th **M93.01** Acute slipped upper femoral epiphysis (nontraumatic)

    M93.011 Acute slipped upper femoral epiphysis (nontraumatic), right hip

    M93.012 Acute slipped upper femoral epiphysis (nontraumatic), left hip

    M93.013 Acute slipped upper femoral epiphysis (nontraumatic), unspecified hip

    ✓6th **M93.02** Chronic slipped upper femoral epiphysis (nontraumatic)

    M93.021 Chronic slipped upper femoral epiphysis (nontraumatic), right hip

    M93.022 Chronic slipped upper femoral epiphysis (nontraumatic), left hip

    M93.023 Chronic slipped upper femoral epiphysis (nontraumatic), unspecified hip

    ✓6th **M93.03** Acute on chronic slipped upper femoral epiphysis (nontraumatic)

    M93.031 Acute on chronic slipped upper femoral epiphysis (nontraumatic), right hip

    M93.032 Acute on chronic slipped upper femoral epiphysis (nontraumatic), left hip

    M93.033 Acute on chronic slipped upper femoral epiphysis (nontraumatic), unspecified hip

M93.1 Kienböck's disease of adults

    Adult osteochondrosis of carpal lunates

✓5th **M93.2** Osteochondritis dissecans

    M93.20 Osteochondritis dissecans of unspecified site

    ✓6th **M93.21** Osteochondritis dissecans of shoulder

    M93.211 Osteochondritis dissecans, right shoulder

    M93.212 Osteochondritis dissecans, left shoulder

    M93.219 Osteochondritis dissecans, unspecified shoulder

    ✓6th **M93.22** Osteochondritis dissecans of elbow

    M93.221 Osteochondritis dissecans, right elbow

    M93.222 Osteochondritis dissecans, left elbow

    M93.229 Osteochondritis dissecans, unspecified elbow

    ✓6th **M93.23** Osteochondritis dissecans of wrist

    M93.231 Osteochondritis dissecans, right wrist

    M93.232 Osteochondritis dissecans, left wrist

    M93.239 Osteochondritis dissecans, unspecified wrist

    ✓6th **M93.24** Osteochondritis dissecans of joints of hand

    M93.241 Osteochondritis dissecans, joints of right hand

    M93.242 Osteochondritis dissecans, joints of left hand

    M93.249 Osteochondritis dissecans, joints of unspecified hand

    ✓6th **M93.25** Osteochondritis dissecans of hip

    M93.251 Osteochondritis dissecans, right hip

    M93.252 Osteochondritis dissecans, left hip

    M93.259 Osteochondritis dissecans, unspecified hip

    ✓6th **M93.26** Osteochondritis dissecans knee

    M93.261 Osteochondritis dissecans, right knee

    M93.262 Osteochondritis dissecans, left knee

    M93.269 Osteochondritis dissecans, unspecified knee

    ✓6th **M93.27** Osteochondritis dissecans of ankle and joints of foot

    M93.271 Osteochondritis dissecans, right ankle and joints of right foot

    M93.272 Osteochondritis dissecans, left ankle and joints of left foot

    M93.279 Osteochondritis dissecans, unspecified ankle and joints of foot

    M93.28 Osteochondritis dissecans other site

    M93.29 Osteochondritis dissecans multiple sites

✓5th **M93.8** Other specified osteochondropathies

    M93.80 Other specified osteochondropathies of unspecified site

    ✓6th **M93.81** Other specified osteochondropathies of shoulder

    M93.811 Other specified osteochondropathies, right shoulder

    M93.812 Other specified osteochondropathies, left shoulder

    M93.819 Other specified osteochondropathies, unspecified shoulder

    ✓6th **M93.82** Other specified osteochondropathies of upper arm

    M93.821 Other specified osteochondropathies, right upper arm

---

EXCLUDES 1   Not coded here   EXCLUDES 2   Not included here   *Manifestation Code*

          M93.822 Other specified osteochondropathies, left upper arm

          M93.829 Other specified osteochondropathies, unspecified upper arm

✓6th **M93.83** Other specified osteochondropathies of forearm

          M93.831 Other specified osteochondropathies, right forearm

          M93.832 Other specified osteochondropathies, left forearm

          M93.839 Other specified osteochondropathies, unspecified forearm

✓6th **M93.84** Other specified osteochondropathies of hand

          M93.841 Other specified osteochondropathies, right hand

          M93.842 Other specified osteochondropathies, left hand

          M93.849 Other specified osteochondropathies, unspecified hand

✓6th **M93.85** Other specified osteochondropathies of thigh

          M93.851 Other specified osteochondropathies, right thigh

          M93.852 Other specified osteochondropathies, left thigh

          M93.859 Other specified osteochondropathies, unspecified thigh

✓6th **M93.86** Other specified osteochondropathies lower leg

          M93.861 Other specified osteochondropathies, right lower leg

          M93.862 Other specified osteochondropathies, left lower leg

          M93.869 Other specified osteochondropathies, unspecified lower leg

✓6th **M93.87** Other specified osteochondropathies of ankle and foot

          M93.871 Other specified osteochondropathies, right ankle and foot

          M93.872 Other specified osteochondropathies, left ankle and foot

          M93.879 Other specified osteochondropathies, unspecified ankle and foot

    M93.88 Other specified osteochondropathies other

    M93.89 Other specified osteochondropathies multiple sites

✓5th **M93.9** Osteochondropathy, unspecified

Apophysitis NOS

Epiphysitis NOS

Osteochondritis NOS

Osteochondrosis NOS

    M93.90 Osteochondropathy, unspecified of unspecified site

✓6th **M93.91** Osteochondropathy, unspecified of shoulder

          M93.911 Osteochondropathy, unspecified, right shoulder

          M93.912 Osteochondropathy, unspecified, left shoulder

          M93.919 Osteochondropathy, unspecified, unspecified shoulder

✓6th **M93.92** Osteochondropathy, unspecified of upper arm

          M93.921 Osteochondropathy, unspecified, right upper arm

          M93.922 Osteochondropathy, unspecified, left upper arm

          M93.929 Osteochondropathy, unspecified, unspecified upper arm

✓6th **M93.93** Osteochondropathy, unspecified of forearm

          M93.931 Osteochondropathy, unspecified, right forearm

          M93.932 Osteochondropathy, unspecified, left forearm

          M93.939 Osteochondropathy, unspecified, unspecified forearm

✓6th **M93.94** Osteochondropathy, unspecified of hand

          M93.941 Osteochondropathy, unspecified, right hand

          M93.942 Osteochondropathy, unspecified, left hand

          M93.949 Osteochondropathy, unspecified, unspecified hand

✓6th **M93.95** Osteochondropathy, unspecified of thigh

          M93.951 Osteochondropathy, unspecified, right thigh

          M93.952 Osteochondropathy, unspecified, left thigh

          M93.959 Osteochondropathy, unspecified, unspecified thigh

✓6th **M93.96** Osteochondropathy, unspecified lower leg

          M93.961 Osteochondropathy, unspecified, right lower leg

          M93.962 Osteochondropathy, unspecified, left lower leg

          M93.969 Osteochondropathy, unspecified, unspecified lower leg

✓6th **M93.97** Osteochondropathy, unspecified of ankle and foot

          M93.971 Osteochondropathy, unspecified, right ankle and foot

          M93.972 Osteochondropathy, unspecified, left ankle and foot

          M93.979 Osteochondropathy, unspecified, unspecified ankle and foot

    M93.98 Osteochondropathy, unspecified other

    M93.99 Osteochondropathy, unspecified multiple sites

✓4th **M94** Other disorders of cartilage

    M94.0 Chondrocostal junction syndrome [Tietze]

Costochondritis

    M94.1 Relapsing polychondritis

✓5th **M94.2** Chondromalacia

      EXCLUDES 1 chondromalacia patellae (M22.4)

    M94.20 Chondromalacia, unspecified site

✓6th **M94.21** Chondromalacia, shoulder

          M94.211 Chondromalacia, right shoulder

          M94.212 Chondromalacia, left shoulder

          M94.219 Chondromalacia, unspecified shoulder

✓6th **M94.22** Chondromalacia, elbow

          M94.221 Chondromalacia, right elbow

          M94.222 Chondromalacia, left elbow

          M94.229 Chondromalacia, unspecified elbow

✓6th **M94.23** Chondromalacia, wrist

          M94.231 Chondromalacia, right wrist

          M94.232 Chondromalacia, left wrist

          M94.239 Chondromalacia, unspecified wrist

✓6th **M94.24** Chondromalacia, joints of hand

          M94.241 Chondromalacia, joints of right hand

          M94.242 Chondromalacia, joints of left hand

          M94.249 Chondromalacia, joints of unspecified hand

✓6th **M94.25** Chondromalacia, hip

          M94.251 Chondromalacia, right hip

          M94.252 Chondromalacia, left hip

          M94.259 Chondromalacia, unspecified hip

✓6th **M94.26** Chondromalacia, knee

          M94.261 Chondromalacia, right knee

          M94.262 Chondromalacia, left knee

          M94.269 Chondromalacia, unspecified knee

✓6th **M94.27** Chondromalacia, ankle and joints of foot

          M94.271 Chondromalacia, right ankle and joints of right foot

          M94.272 Chondromalacia, left ankle and joints of left foot

          M94.279 Chondromalacia, unspecified ankle and joints of foot

    M94.28 Chondromalacia, other site

    M94.29 Chondromalacia, multiple sites

✓5th **M94.3** Chondrolysis

Code first any associated slipped upper femoral epiphysis (nontraumatic) (M93.0-)

✓6th **M94.35** Chondrolysis, hip

          M94.351 Chondrolysis, right hip

          M94.352 Chondrolysis, left hip

          M94.359 Chondrolysis, unspecified hip

✓5th **M94.8** Other specified disorders of cartilage

✓6th **M94.8x** Other specified disorders of cartilage

          M94.8x0 Other specified disorders of cartilage, multiple sites

---

☑ Appropriate additional character required   √x7th Requires 7th character, placeholder x must fill empty characters

Diseases of the Musculoskeletal System and Connective Tissue

M94.8x1–M96.831

M94.8x1   **Other specified disorders of cartilage, shoulder**

M94.8x2   **Other specified disorders of cartilage, upper arm**

M94.8x3   **Other specified disorders of cartilage, forearm**

M94.8x4   **Other specified disorders of cartilage, hand**

M94.8x5   **Other specified disorders of cartilage, thigh**

M94.8x6   **Other specified disorders of cartilage, lower leg**

M94.8x7   **Other specified disorders of cartilage, ankle and foot**

M94.8x8   **Other specified disorders of cartilage, other site**

M94.8x9   **Other specified disorders of cartilage, unspecified sites**

M94.9   **Disorder of cartilage, unspecified**

Other disorders of the musculoskeletal system and connective tissue (M95)

✓4th **M95   Other acquired deformities of musculoskeletal system and connective tissue**

> EXCLUDES 2   *acquired absence of limbs and organs (Z89-Z90)*
> *acquired deformities of limbs (M20-M21)*
> *congenital malformations and deformations of the musculoskeletal system (Q65-Q79)*
> *deforming dorsopathies (M40-M43)*
> *dentofacial anomalies [including malocclusion] (M26-)*
> *postprocedural musculoskeletal disorders (M96-)*

M95.0   **Acquired deformity of nose**

> EXCLUDES 2   *deviated nasal septum (J34.2)*

✓5th   M95.1   **Cauliflower ear**

> EXCLUDES 2   *other acquired deformities of ear (H61.1)*

M95.10   **Cauliflower ear, unspecified ear**

M95.11   **Cauliflower ear, right ear**

M95.12   **Cauliflower ear, left ear**

M95.2   **Other acquired deformity of head**

M95.3   **Acquired deformity of neck**

M95.4   **Acquired deformity of chest and rib**

M95.5   **Acquired deformity of pelvis**

> EXCLUDES 1   *maternal care for known or suspected disproportion (O33-)*

M95.8   **Other specified acquired deformities of musculoskeletal system**

M95.9   **Acquired deformity of musculoskeletal system, unspecified**

Intraoperative and postprocedural complications and disorders of musculoskeletal system, not elsewhere classified (M96)

✓4th **M96   Intraoperative and postprocedural complications and disorders of musculoskeletal system, not elsewhere classified**

> EXCLUDES 2   *arthropathy following intestinal bypass (M02.0-)*
> *complications of internal orthopedic prosthetic devices, implants and grafts (T84-)*
> *disorders associated with osteoporosis (M80)*
> *presence of functional implants and other devices (Z96-Z97)*

M96.0   **Pseudarthrosis after fusion or arthrodesis**

M96.1   **Postlaminectomy syndrome, not elsewhere classified**

M96.2   **Postradiation kyphosis**

M96.3   **Postlaminectomy kyphosis**

M96.4   **Postsurgical lordosis**

M96.5   **Postradiation scoliosis**

✓5th   M96.6   **Fracture of bone following insertion of orthopedic implant, joint prosthesis, or bone plate**

> Intraoperative fracture of bone during insertion of orthopedic implant, joint prosthesis, or bone plate

> EXCLUDES 2   *complication of internal orthopedic devices, implants or grafts (T84-)*

✓6th   M96.62   **Fracture of humerus following insertion of orthopedic implant, joint prosthesis, or bone plate**

M96.621   **Fracture of humerus following insertion of orthopedic implant, joint prosthesis, or bone plate, right arm**

M96.622   **Fracture of humerus following insertion of orthopedic implant, joint prosthesis, or bone plate, left arm**

M96.629   **Fracture of humerus following insertion of orthopedic implant, joint prosthesis, or bone plate, unspecified arm**

✓6th   M96.63   **Fracture of radius or ulna following insertion of orthopedic implant, joint prosthesis, or bone plate**

M96.631   **Fracture of radius or ulna following insertion of orthopedic implant, joint prosthesis, or bone plate, right arm**

M96.632   **Fracture of radius or ulna following insertion of orthopedic implant, joint prosthesis, or bone plate, left arm**

M96.639   **Fracture of radius or ulna following insertion of orthopedic implant, joint prosthesis, or bone plate, unspecified arm**

M96.65   **Fracture of pelvis following insertion of orthopedic implant, joint prosthesis, or bone plate**

✓6th   M96.66   **Fracture of femur following insertion of orthopedic implant, joint prosthesis, or bone plate**

M96.661   **Fracture of femur following insertion of orthopedic implant, joint prosthesis, or bone plate, right leg**

M96.662   **Fracture of femur following insertion of orthopedic implant, joint prosthesis, or bone plate, left leg**

M96.669   **Fracture of femur following insertion of orthopedic implant, joint prosthesis, or bone plate, unspecified leg**

✓6th   M96.67   **Fracture of tibia or fibula following insertion of orthopedic implant, joint prosthesis, or bone plate**

M96.671   **Fracture of tibia or fibula following insertion of orthopedic implant, joint prosthesis, or bone plate, right leg**

M96.672   **Fracture of tibia or fibula following insertion of orthopedic implant, joint prosthesis, or bone plate, left leg**

M96.679   **Fracture of tibia or fibula following insertion of orthopedic implant, joint prosthesis, or bone plate, unspecified leg**

M96.69   **Fracture of other bone following insertion of orthopedic implant, joint prosthesis, or bone plate**

✓5th   M96.8   **Other intraoperative and postprocedural complications and disorders of musculoskeletal system, not elsewhere classified**

✓6th   M96.81   **Intraoperative hemorrhage and hematoma of a musculoskeletal structure complicating a procedure**

> EXCLUDES 1   *intraoperative hemorrhage and hematoma of a musculoskeletal structure due to accidental puncture and laceration during a procedure (M98.82-)*

M96.810   **Intraoperative hemorrhage and hematoma of a musculoskeletal structure complicating a musculoskeletal system procedure**

M96.811   **Intraoperative hemorrhage and hematoma of a musculoskeletal structure complicating other procedure**

✓6th   M96.82   **Accidental puncture and laceration of a musculoskeletal structure during a procedure**

M96.820   **Accidental puncture and laceration of a musculoskeletal structure during a musculoskeletal system procedure**

M96.821   **Accidental puncture and laceration of a musculoskeletal structure during other procedure**

✓6th   M96.83   **Postprocedural hemorrhage and hematoma of a musculoskeletal structure following a procedure**

M96.830   **Postprocedural hemorrhage and hematoma of a musculoskeletal structure following a musculoskeletal system procedure**

M96.831   **Postprocedural hemorrhage and hematoma of a musculoskeletal structure following other procedure**

EXCLUDES 1   Not coded here   EXCLUDES 2   Not included here   *Manifestation Code*

M96.89 **Other intraoperative and postprocedural complications and disorders of the musculoskeletal system**
    Instability of joint secondary to removal of joint prosthesis
    Use additional code, if applicable, to further specify disorder

Biomechanical lesions, not elsewhere classified (M99)

✓4ᵗʰ **M99 Biomechanical lesions, not elsewhere classified**
    NOTE This category should not be used if the condition can be classified elsewhere.

✓5ᵗʰ **M99.0 Segmental and somatic dysfunction**
    M99.00 **Segmental and somatic dysfunction of head region**
    M99.01 **Segmental and somatic dysfunction of cervical region**
    M99.02 **Segmental and somatic dysfunction of thoracic region**
    M99.03 **Segmental and somatic dysfunction of lumbar region**
    M99.04 **Segmental and somatic dysfunction of sacral region**
    M99.05 **Segmental and somatic dysfunction of pelvic region**
    M99.06 **Segmental and somatic dysfunction of lower extremity**
    M99.07 **Segmental and somatic dysfunction of upper extremity**
    M99.08 **Segmental and somatic dysfunction of rib cage**
    M99.09 **Segmental and somatic dysfunction of abdomen and other regions**

✓5ᵗʰ **M99.1 Subluxation complex (vertebral)**
    M99.10 **Subluxation complex (vertebral) of head region**
    M99.11 **Subluxation complex (vertebral) of cervical region**
    M99.12 **Subluxation complex (vertebral) of thoracic region**
    M99.13 **Subluxation complex (vertebral) of lumbar region**
    M99.14 **Subluxation complex (vertebral) of sacral region**
    M99.15 **Subluxation complex (vertebral) of pelvic region**
    M99.16 **Subluxation complex (vertebral) of lower extremity**
    M99.17 **Subluxation complex (vertebral) of upper extremity**
    M99.18 **Subluxation complex (vertebral) of rib cage**
    M99.19 **Subluxation complex (vertebral) of abdomen and other regions**

✓5ᵗʰ **M99.2 Subluxation stenosis of neural canal**
    M99.20 **Subluxation stenosis of neural canal of head region**
    M99.21 **Subluxation stenosis of neural canal of cervical region**
    M99.22 **Subluxation stenosis of neural canal of thoracic region**
    M99.23 **Subluxation stenosis of neural canal of lumbar region**
    M99.24 **Subluxation stenosis of neural canal of sacral region**
    M99.25 **Subluxation stenosis of neural canal of pelvic region**
    M99.26 **Subluxation stenosis of neural canal of lower extremity**
    M99.27 **Subluxation stenosis of neural canal of upper extremity**
    M99.28 **Subluxation stenosis of neural canal of rib cage**
    M99.29 **Subluxation stenosis of neural canal of abdomen and other regions**

✓5ᵗʰ **M99.3 Osseous stenosis of neural canal**
    M99.30 **Osseous stenosis of neural canal of head region**
    M99.31 **Osseous stenosis of neural canal of cervical region**
    M99.32 **Osseous stenosis of neural canal of thoracic region**
    M99.33 **Osseous stenosis of neural canal of lumbar region**
    M99.34 **Osseous stenosis of neural canal of sacral region**
    M99.35 **Osseous stenosis of neural canal of pelvic region**
    M99.36 **Osseous stenosis of neural canal of lower extremity**
    M99.37 **Osseous stenosis of neural canal of upper extremity**

M99.38 **Osseous stenosis of neural canal of rib cage**
M99.39 **Osseous stenosis of neural canal of abdomen and other regions**

✓5ᵗʰ **M99.4 Connective tissue stenosis of neural canal**
    M99.40 **Connective tissue stenosis of neural canal of head region**
    M99.41 **Connective tissue stenosis of neural canal of cervical region**
    M99.42 **Connective tissue stenosis of neural canal of thoracic region**
    M99.43 **Connective tissue stenosis of neural canal of lumbar region**
    M99.44 **Connective tissue stenosis of neural canal of sacral region**
    M99.45 **Connective tissue stenosis of neural canal of pelvic region**
    M99.46 **Connective tissue stenosis of neural canal of lower extremity**
    M99.47 **Connective tissue stenosis of neural canal of upper extremity**
    M99.48 **Connective tissue stenosis of neural canal of rib cage**
    M99.49 **Connective tissue stenosis of neural canal of abdomen and other regions**

✓5ᵗʰ **M99.5 Intervertebral disc stenosis of neural canal**
    M99.50 **Intervertebral disc stenosis of neural canal of head region**
    M99.51 **Intervertebral disc stenosis of neural canal of cervical region**
    M99.52 **Intervertebral disc stenosis of neural canal of thoracic region**
    M99.53 **Intervertebral disc stenosis of neural canal of lumbar region**
    M99.54 **Intervertebral disc stenosis of neural canal of sacral region**
    M99.55 **Intervertebral disc stenosis of neural canal of pelvic region**
    M99.56 **Intervertebral disc stenosis of neural canal of lower extremity**
    M99.57 **Intervertebral disc stenosis of neural canal of upper extremity**
    M99.58 **Intervertebral disc stenosis of neural canal of rib cage**
    M99.59 **Intervertebral disc stenosis of neural canal of abdomen and other regions**

✓5ᵗʰ **M99.6 Osseous and subluxation stenosis of intervertebral foramina**
    M99.60 **Osseous and subluxation stenosis of intervertebral foramina of head region**
    M99.61 **Osseous and subluxation stenosis of intervertebral foramina of cervical region**
    M99.62 **Osseous and subluxation stenosis of intervertebral foramina of thoracic region**
    M99.63 **Osseous and subluxation stenosis of intervertebral foramina of lumbar region**
    M99.64 **Osseous and subluxation stenosis of intervertebral foramina of sacral region**
    M99.65 **Osseous and subluxation stenosis of intervertebral foramina of pelvic region**
    M99.66 **Osseous and subluxation stenosis of intervertebral foramina of lower extremity**
    M99.67 **Osseous and subluxation stenosis of intervertebral foramina of upper extremity**
    M99.68 **Osseous and subluxation stenosis of intervertebral foramina of rib cage**
    M99.69 **Osseous and subluxation stenosis of intervertebral foramina of abdomen and other regions**

✓5ᵗʰ **M99.7 Connective tissue and disc stenosis of intervertebral foramina**
    M99.70 **Connective tissue and disc stenosis of intervertebral foramina of head region**
    M99.71 **Connective tissue and disc stenosis of intervertebral foramina of cervical region**
    M99.72 **Connective tissue and disc stenosis of intervertebral foramina of thoracic region**
    M99.73 **Connective tissue and disc stenosis of intervertebral foramina of lumbar region**

✓ Appropriate additional character required   ✓x7ᵗʰ Requires 7th character, placeholder x must fill empty characters

    M99.74   **Connective tissue and disc stenosis of intervertebral foramina of sacral region**

    M99.75   **Connective tissue and disc stenosis of intervertebral foramina of pelvic region**

    M99.76   **Connective tissue and disc stenosis of intervertebral foramina of lower extremity**

    M99.77   **Connective tissue and disc stenosis of intervertebral foramina of upper extremity**

    M99.78   **Connective tissue and disc stenosis of intervertebral foramina of rib cage**

    M99.79   **Connective tissue and disc stenosis of intervertebral foramina of abdomen and other regions**

✓5th   M99.8   **Other biomechanical lesions**

    M99.80   **Other biomechanical lesions of head region**

    M99.81   **Other biomechanical lesions of cervical region**

    M99.82   **Other biomechanical lesions of thoracic region**

    M99.83   **Other biomechanical lesions of lumbar region**

    M99.84   **Other biomechanical lesions of sacral region**

    M99.85   **Other biomechanical lesions of pelvic region**

    M99.86   **Other biomechanical lesions of lower extremity**

    M99.87   **Other biomechanical lesions of upper extremity**

    M99.88   **Other biomechanical lesions of rib cage**

    M99.89   **Other biomechanical lesions of abdomen and other regions**

    M99.9   **Biomechanical lesion, unspecified**

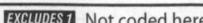

    EXCLUDES 1   Not coded here   EXCLUDES 2   Not included here   *Manifestation Code*

Chapter 14. Diseases of the Genitourinary System (N00-N99)

EXCLUDES 2   certain conditions originating in the perinatal period (P04-P96)
certain infectious and parasitic diseases (A00-B99)
complications of pregnancy, childbirth and the puerperium (O00-O99)
congenital malformations, deformations and chromosomal abnormalities (Q00-Q99)
endocrine, nutritional and metabolic diseases (E00-E88)
injury, poisoning and certain other consequences of external causes (S00-T88)
neoplasms (C00-D49)
symptoms, signs and abnormal clinical and laboratory findings, not elsewhere classified (R00-R94)

This chapter contains the following blocks:
N00-N08   Glomerular diseases
N10-N16   Renal tubulo-interstitial diseases
N17-N19   Acute kidney failure and chronic kidney disease
N20-N23   Urolithiasis
N25-N29   Other disorders of kidney and ureter
N30-N39   Other diseases of the urinary system
N40-N53   Diseases of male genital organs
N60-N65   Disorders of breast
N70-N77   Inflammatory diseases of female pelvic organs
N80-N98   Noninflammatory disorders of female genital tract
N99   Intraoperative and postprocedural complications and disorders of genitourinary system, not elsewhere classified

Glomerular diseases (N00-N08)
Code also any associated kidney failure (N17-N19).
EXCLUDES 1   hypertensive chronic kidney disease (I12-)

☑4ᵗʰ N00   Acute nephritic syndrome
INCLUDES   acute glomerular disease
acute glomerulonephritis
acute nephritis
EXCLUDES 1   acute tubulo-interstitial nephritis (N10)
nephritic syndrome NOS (N05-)

N00.0   Acute nephritic syndrome with minor glomerular abnormality
Acute nephritic syndrome with minimal change lesion

N00.1   Acute nephritic syndrome with focal and segmental glomerular lesions
Acute nephritic syndrome with focal and segmental hyalinosis
Acute nephritic syndrome with focal and segmental sclerosis
Acute nephritic syndrome with focal glomerulonephritis

N00.2   Acute nephritic syndrome with diffuse membranous glomerulonephritis

N00.3   Acute nephritic syndrome with diffuse mesangial proliferative glomerulonephritis

N00.4   Acute nephritic syndrome with diffuse endocapillary proliferative glomerulonephritis

N00.5   Acute nephritic syndrome with diffuse mesangiocapillary glomerulonephritis
Acute nephritic syndrome with membranoproliferative glomerulonephritis, types 1 and 3, or NOS

N00.6   Acute nephritic syndrome with dense deposit disease
Acute nephritic syndrome with membranoproliferative glomerulonephritis, type 2

N00.7   Acute nephritic syndrome with diffuse crescentic glomerulonephritis
Acute nephritic syndrome with extracapillary glomerulonephritis

N00.8   Acute nephritic syndrome with other morphologic changes
Acute nephritic syndrome with proliferative glomerulonephritis NOS

N00.9   Acute nephritic syndrome with unspecified morphologic changes

☑4ᵗʰ N01   Rapidly progressive nephritic syndrome
INCLUDES   rapidly progressive glomerular disease
rapidly progressive glomerulonephritis
rapidly progressive nephritis
EXCLUDES 1   nephritic syndrome NOS (N05-)

N01.0   Rapidly progressive nephritic syndrome with minor glomerular abnormality
Rapidly progressive nephritic syndrome with minimal change lesion

N01.1   Rapidly progressive nephritic syndrome with focal and segmental glomerular lesions
Rapidly progressive nephritic syndrome with focal and segmental hyalinosis
Rapidly progressive nephritic syndrome with focal and segmental sclerosis
Rapidly progressive nephritic syndrome with focal glomerulonephritis

N01.2   Rapidly progressive nephritic syndrome with diffuse membranous glomerulonephritis

N01.3   Rapidly progressive nephritic syndrome with diffuse mesangial proliferative glomerulonephritis

N01.4   Rapidly progressive nephritic syndrome with diffuse endocapillary proliferative glomerulonephritis

N01.5   Rapidly progressive nephritic syndrome with diffuse mesangiocapillary glomerulonephritis
Rapidly progressive nephritic syndrome with membranoproliferative glomerulonephritis, types 1 and 3, or NOS

N01.6   Rapidly progressive nephritic syndrome with dense deposit disease
Rapidly progressive nephritic syndrome with membranoproliferative glomerulonephritis, type 2

N01.7   Rapidly progressive nephritic syndrome with diffuse crescentic glomerulonephritis
Rapidly progressive nephritic syndrome with extracapillary glomerulonephritis

N01.8   Rapidly progressive nephritic syndrome with other morphologic changes
Rapidly progressive nephritic syndrome with proliferative glomerulonephritis NOS

N01.9   Rapidly progressive nephritic syndrome with unspecified morphologic changes

☑4ᵗʰ N02   Recurrent and persistent hematuria
EXCLUDES 1   acute cystitis with hematuria (N30.01)
acute prostatitis with hematuria (N41.01)
chronic prostatitis with hematuria (N41.11)
hematuria NOS (R31.9)
hematuria not associated with specified morphologic lesions (R31-)

N02.0   Recurrent and persistent hematuria with minor glomerular abnormality
Recurrent and persistent hematuria with minimal change lesion

N02.1   Recurrent and persistent hematuria with focal and segmental glomerular lesions
Recurrent and persistent hematuria with focal and segmental hyalinosis
Recurrent and persistent hematuria with focal and segmental sclerosis
Recurrent and persistent hematuria with focal glomerulonephritis

N02.2   Recurrent and persistent hematuria with diffuse membranous glomerulonephritis

N02.3   Recurrent and persistent hematuria with diffuse mesangial proliferative glomerulonephritis

N02.4   Recurrent and persistent hematuria with diffuse endocapillary proliferative glomerulonephritis

N02.5   Recurrent and persistent hematuria with diffuse mesangiocapillary glomerulonephritis
Recurrent and persistent hematuria with membranoproliferative glomerulonephritis, types 1 and 3, or NOS

N02.6   Recurrent and persistent hematuria with dense deposit disease
Recurrent and persistent hematuria with membranoproliferative glomerulonephritis, type 2

N02.7   Recurrent and persistent hematuria with diffuse crescentic glomerulonephritis
Recurrent and persistent hematuria with extracapillary glomerulonephritis

N02.8   Recurrent and persistent hematuria with other morphologic changes
Recurrent and persistent hematuria with proliferative glomerulonephritis NOS

N02.9   Recurrent and persistent hematuria with unspecified morphologic changes

☑4th **N03 Chronic nephritic syndrome**
    INCLUDES   chronic glomerular disease
             chronic glomerulonephritis
             chronic nephritis
    EXCLUDES 1   *chronic tubulo-interstitial nephritis (N11-)*
             diffuse sclerosing glomerulonephritis (N05.8-)
             nephritic syndrome NOS (N05-)

N03.0 Chronic nephritic syndrome with minor glomerular abnormality
Chronic nephritic syndrome with minimal change lesion

N03.1 Chronic nephritic syndrome with focal and segmental glomerular lesions
Chronic nephritic syndrome with focal and segmental hyalinosis
Chronic nephritic syndrome with focal and segmental sclerosis
Chronic nephritic syndrome with focal glomerulonephritis

N03.2 Chronic nephritic syndrome with diffuse membranous glomerulonephritis

N03.3 Chronic nephritic syndrome with diffuse mesangial proliferative glomerulonephritis

N03.4 Chronic nephritic syndrome with diffuse endocapillary proliferative glomerulonephritis

N03.5 Chronic nephritic syndrome with diffuse mesangiocapillary glomerulonephritis
Chronic nephritic syndrome with membranoproliferative glomerulonephritis, types 1 and 3, or NOS

N03.6 Chronic nephritic syndrome with dense deposit disease
Chronic nephritic syndrome with membranoproliferative glomerulonephritis, type 2

N03.7 Chronic nephritic syndrome with diffuse crescentic glomerulonephritis
Chronic nephritic syndrome with extracapillary glomerulonephritis

N03.8 Chronic nephritic syndrome with other morphologic changes
Chronic nephritic syndrome with proliferative glomerulonephritis NOS

N03.9 Chronic nephritic syndrome with unspecified morphologic changes

☑4th **N04 Nephrotic syndrome**
    INCLUDES   congenital nephrotic syndrome
             lipoid nephrosis

N04.0 Nephrotic syndrome with minor glomerular abnormality
Nephrotic syndrome with minimal change lesion

N04.1 Nephrotic syndrome with focal and segmental glomerular lesions
Nephrotic syndrome with focal and segmental hyalinosis
Nephrotic syndrome with focal and segmental sclerosis
Nephrotic syndrome with focal glomerulonephritis

N04.2 Nephrotic syndrome with diffuse membranous glomerulonephritis

N04.3 Nephrotic syndrome with diffuse mesangial proliferative glomerulonephritis

N04.4 Nephrotic syndrome with diffuse endocapillary proliferative glomerulonephritis

N04.5 Nephrotic syndrome with diffuse mesangiocapillary glomerulonephritis
Nephrotic syndrome with membranoproliferative glomerulonephritis, types 1 and 3, or NOS

N04.6 Nephrotic syndrome with dense deposit disease
Nephrotic syndrome with membranoproliferative glomerulonephritis, type 2

N04.7 Nephrotic syndrome with diffuse crescentic glomerulonephritis
Nephrotic syndrome with extracapillary glomerulonephritis

N04.8 Nephrotic syndrome with other morphologic changes
Nephrotic syndrome with proliferative glomerulonephritis NOS

N04.9 Nephrotic syndrome with unspecified morphologic changes

☑4th **N05 Unspecified nephritic syndrome**
    INCLUDES   glomerular disease NOS
             glomerulonephritis NOS
             nephritis NOS
             nephropathy NOS and renal disease NOS with morphological lesion specified in .0-.8
    EXCLUDES 1   *nephropathy NOS with no stated morphological lesion (N28.9)*
             renal disease NOS with no stated morphological lesion (N28.9)
             tubulo-interstitial nephritis NOS (N12)

N05.0 Unspecified nephritic syndrome with minor glomerular abnormality
Unspecified nephritic syndrome with minimal change lesion

N05.1 Unspecified nephritic syndrome with focal and segmental glomerular lesions
Unspecified nephritic syndrome with focal and segmental hyalinosis
Unspecified nephritic syndrome with focal and segmental sclerosis
Unspecified nephritic syndrome with focal glomerulonephritis

N05.2 Unspecified nephritic syndrome with diffuse membranous glomerulonephritis

N05.3 Unspecified nephritic syndrome with diffuse mesangial proliferative glomerulonephritis

N05.4 Unspecified nephritic syndrome with diffuse endocapillary proliferative glomerulonephritis

N05.5 Unspecified nephritic syndrome with diffuse mesangiocapillary glomerulonephritis
Unspecified nephritic syndrome with membranoproliferative glomerulonephritis, types 1 and 3, or NOS

N05.6 Unspecified nephritic syndrome with dense deposit disease
Unspecified nephritic syndrome with membranoproliferative glomerulonephritis, type 2

N05.7 Unspecified nephritic syndrome with diffuse crescentic glomerulonephritis
Unspecified nephritic syndrome with extracapillary glomerulonephritis

N05.8 Unspecified nephritic syndrome with other morphologic changes
Unspecified nephritic syndrome with proliferative glomerulonephritis NOS

N05.9 Unspecified nephritic syndrome with unspecified morphologic changes

☑4th **N06 Isolated proteinuria with specified morphological lesion**
    EXCLUDES 1   *proteinuria not associated with specific morphologic lesions (R80.0)*

N06.0 Isolated proteinuria with minor glomerular abnormality
Isolated proteinuria with minimal change lesion

N06.1 Isolated proteinuria with focal and segmental glomerular lesions
Isolated proteinuria with focal and segmental hyalinosis
Isolated proteinuria with focal and segmental sclerosis
Isolated proteinuria with focal glomerulonephritis

N06.2 Isolated proteinuria with diffuse membranous glomerulonephritis

N06.3 Isolated proteinuria with diffuse mesangial proliferative glomerulonephritis

N06.4 Isolated proteinuria with diffuse endocapillary proliferative glomerulonephritis

N06.5 Isolated proteinuria with diffuse mesangiocapillary glomerulonephritis
Isolated proteinuria with membranoproliferative glomerulonephritis, types 1 and 3, or NOS

N06.6 Isolated proteinuria with dense deposit disease
Isolated proteinuria with membranoproliferative glomerulonephritis, type 2

N06.7 Isolated proteinuria with diffuse crescentic glomerulonephritis
Isolated proteinuria with extracapillary glomerulonephritis

N06.8 Isolated proteinuria with other morphologic lesion
Isolated proteinuria with proliferative glomerulonephritis NOS

N06.9 Isolated proteinuria with unspecified morphologic lesion

✓4ᵗʰ N07 Hereditary nephropathy, not elsewhere classified

EXCLUDES 2   *Alport's syndrome (Q87.81-)*
hereditary amyloid nephropathy (E85-)
nail patella syndrome (Q87.2)
non-neuropathic heredofamilial amyloidosis (E85-)

N07.0 Hereditary nephropathy, not elsewhere classified with minor glomerular abnormality
Hereditary nephropathy, not elsewhere classified with minimal change lesion

N07.1 Hereditary nephropathy, not elsewhere classified with focal and segmental glomerular lesions
Hereditary nephropathy, not elsewhere classified with focal and segmental hyalinosis
Hereditary nephropathy, not elsewhere classified with focal and segmental sclerosis
Hereditary nephropathy, not elsewhere classified with focal glomerulonephritis

N07.2 Hereditary nephropathy, not elsewhere classified with diffuse membranous glomerulonephritis

N07.3 Hereditary nephropathy, not elsewhere classified with diffuse mesangial proliferative glomerulonephritis

N07.4 Hereditary nephropathy, not elsewhere classified with diffuse endocapillary proliferative glomerulonephritis

N07.5 Hereditary nephropathy, not elsewhere classified with diffuse mesangiocapillary glomerulonephritis
Hereditary nephropathy, not elsewhere classified with membranoproliferative glomerulonephritis, types 1 and 3, or NOS

N07.6 Hereditary nephropathy, not elsewhere classified with dense deposit disease
Hereditary nephropathy, not elsewhere classified with membranoproliferative glomerulonephritis, type 2

N07.7 Hereditary nephropathy, not elsewhere classified with diffuse crescentic glomerulonephritis
Hereditary nephropathy, not elsewhere classified with extracapillary glomerulonephritis

N07.8 Hereditary nephropathy, not elsewhere classified with other morphologic lesions
Hereditary nephropathy, not elsewhere classified with proliferative glomerulonephritis NOS

N07.9 Hereditary nephropathy, not elsewhere classified with unspecified morphologic lesions

N08 *Glomerular disorders in diseases classified elsewhere*
Glomerulonephritis
Nephritis
Nephropathy
Code first underlying disease, such as:
amyloidosis (E85-)
congenital syphilis (A50.5)
cryoglobulinemia (D89.1)
disseminated intravascular coagulation (D65)
gout (M1a-, M10-)
microscopic polyangiitis (M31.7)
multiple myeloma (C90.0-)
sepsis (A40.0-A41.9)
sickle-cell disease (D57.0-D57.8)

EXCLUDES 1   *glomerulonephritis, nephritis and nephropathy (in):*
antiglomerular basement membrane disease (M31.0)
diabetes (E08-E13 with .21)
gonococcal (A54.21)
Goodpasture's syndrome (M31.0)
hemolytic-uremic syndrome (D59.3)
lupus (M32.14)
mumps (B26.83)
syphilis (A52.75)
systemic lupus erythematosus (M32.14)
Wegener's granulomatosis (M31.31)
pyelonephritis in diseases classified elsewhere (N16)
renal tubulo-interstitial disorders classified elsewhere (N16)

Renal tubulo-interstitial diseases (N10-N16)

INCLUDES   pyelonephritis
EXCLUDES 1   *pyeloureteritis cystica (N28.85)*

N10 Acute tubulo-interstitial nephritis
Acute infectious interstitial nephritis
Acute pyelitis
Acute pyelonephritis
Acute tubular necrosis
Hemoglobin nephrosis
Myoglobin nephrosis
Use additional code (B95-B97), to identify infectious agent

✓4ᵗʰ N11 Chronic tubulo-interstitial nephritis
INCLUDES   chronic infectious interstitial nephritis
chronic pyelitis
chronic pyelonephritis
Use additional code (B95-B97), to identify infectious agent

N11.0 Nonobstructive reflux-associated chronic pyelonephritis
Pyelonephritis (chronic) associated with (vesicoureteral) reflux
EXCLUDES 1   *vesicoureteral reflux NOS (N13.70)*

N11.1 Chronic obstructive pyelonephritis
Pyelonephritis (chronic) associated with anomaly of pelviureteric junction
Pyelonephritis (chronic) associated with anomaly of pyeloureteric junction
Pyelonephritis (chronic) associated with crossing of vessel
Pyelonephritis (chronic) associated with kinking of ureter
Pyelonephritis (chronic) associated with obstruction of ureter
Pyelonephritis (chronic) associated with stricture of pelviureteric junction
Pyelonephritis (chronic) associated with stricture of ureter
EXCLUDES 1   *calculous pyelonephritis (N20.9)*
obstructive uropathy (N13-)

N11.8 Other chronic tubulo-interstitial nephritis
Nonobstructive chronic pyelonephritis NOS

N11.9 Chronic tubulo-interstitial nephritis, unspecified
Chronic interstitial nephritis NOS
Chronic pyelitis NOS
Chronic pyelonephritis NOS

N12 Tubulo-interstitial nephritis, not specified as acute or chronic
Interstitial nephritis NOS
Pyelitis NOS
Pyelonephritis NOS
EXCLUDES 1   *calculous pyelonephritis (N20.9)*

✓4ᵗʰ N13 Obstructive and reflux uropathy
EXCLUDES 2   *calculus of kidney and ureter without hydronephrosis (N20-)*
congenital obstructive defects of renal pelvis and ureter (Q62.0-Q62.3)
hydronephrosis with ureteropelvic junction obstruction (Q62.1)
obstructive pyelonephritis (N11.1)

N13.1 Hydronephrosis with ureteral stricture, not elsewhere classified
EXCLUDES 1   *hydronephrosis with ureteral stricture with infection (N13.6)*

N13.2 Hydronephrosis with renal and ureteral calculous obstruction
EXCLUDES 1   *hydronephrosis with renal and ureteral calculous obstruction with infection (N13.6)*

✓5ᵗʰ N13.3 Other and unspecified hydronephrosis
EXCLUDES 1   *hydronephrosis with infection (N13.6)*
N13.30 Unspecified hydronephrosis
N13.39 Other hydronephrosis

N13.4 Hydroureter
EXCLUDES 1   *congenital hydroureter (Q62.3)*
hydroureter with infection (N13.6)
vesicoureteral-reflux with hydroureter (N13.73-)

N13.5 Crossing vessel and stricture of ureter without hydronephrosis
Kinking and stricture of ureter without hydronephrosis
EXCLUDES 1   *crossing vessel and stricture of ureter without hydronephrosis with infection (N13.6)*

N13.6 Pyonephrosis
Conditions in N13.0-N13.5 with infection
Obstructive uropathy with infection
Use additional code (B95-B97), to identify infectious agent

Diseases of the Genitourinary System

N13.7–N20

✓5ᵗʰ **N13.7 Vesicoureteral-reflux**

> EXCLUDES 1   *reflux-associated pyelonephritis (N11.0)*

N13.70 Vesicoureteral-reflux, unspecified
Vesicoureteral-reflux NOS

N13.71 Vesicoureteral-reflux without reflux nephropathy

✓6ᵗʰ **N13.72 Vesicoureteral-reflux with reflux nephropathy without hydroureter**

N13.721 Vesicoureteral-reflux with reflux nephropathy without hydroureter, unilateral

N13.722 Vesicoureteral-reflux with reflux nephropathy without hydroureter, bilateral

N13.729 Vesicoureteral-reflux with reflux nephropathy without hydroureter, unspecified

✓6ᵗʰ **N13.73 Vesicoureteral-reflux with reflux nephropathy with hydroureter**

N13.731 Vesicoureteral-reflux with reflux nephropathy with hydroureter, unilateral

N13.732 Vesicoureteral-reflux with reflux nephropathy with hydroureter, bilateral

N13.739 Vesicoureteral-reflux with reflux nephropathy with hydroureter, unspecified

N13.8 Other obstructive and reflux uropathy
Urinary tract obstruction due to specified cause
Code, if applicable, any causal condition first, such as:
enlarged prostate (N40.1)

N13.9 Obstructive and reflux uropathy, unspecified
Urinary tract obstruction NOS

✓4ᵗʰ **N14 Drug- and heavy-metal-induced tubulo-interstitial and tubular conditions**
Code first (T36-T65) to identify drug and toxic agent

N14.0 Analgesic nephropathy

N14.1 Nephropathy induced by other drugs, medicaments and biological substances

N14.2 Nephropathy induced by unspecified drug, medicament or biological substance

N14.3 Nephropathy induced by heavy metals

N14.4 Toxic nephropathy, not elsewhere classified

✓4ᵗʰ **N15 Other renal tubulo-interstitial diseases**

N15.0 Balkan nephropathy
Balkan endemic nephropathy

N15.1 Renal and perinephric abscess

N15.8 Other specified renal tubulo-interstitial diseases

N15.9 Renal tubulo-interstitial disease, unspecified
Infection of kidney NOS

> EXCLUDES 1   *urinary tract infection NOS (N39.0)*

N16 *Renal tubulo-interstitial disorders in diseases classified elsewhere*
Pyelonephritis
Tubulo-interstitial nephritis
Code first underlying disease, such as:
brucellosis (A23.0-A23.9)
cryoglobulinemia (D89.1)
glycogen storage disease (E74.0)
leukemia (C91-C95)
lymphoma (C81.0-C85.9, C96.0-C96.9)
multiple myeloma (C90.0-)
sepsis (A40.0-A41.9)
Wilson's disease (E83.0)

> EXCLUDES 1   *pyelonephritis and tubulo-interstitial nephritis (in):*
> *candidiasis (B37.49)*
> *cystinosis (E72.0)*
> *diphtheritic (A36.84)*
> *salmonella infection (A02.25)*
> *sarcoidosis (D86.84)*
> *sicca syndrome [Sjogren's] (M35.04)*
> *syphilitic (A52.75)*
> *systemic lupus erythematosus (M32.15)*
> *toxoplasmosis (B58.83)*
> *renal tubular degeneration in diabetes (E08-E13 with .22)*

Acute kidney failure and chronic kidney disease (N17-N19)

> EXCLUDES 2   *congenital renal failure (P96.0)*
> *drug- and heavy-metal-induced tubulo-interstitial and tubular conditions (N14-)*
> *extrarenal uremia (R39.2)*
> *hemolytic-uremic syndrome (D59.3)*
> *hepatorenal syndrome (K76.7)*
> *postpartum hepatorenal syndrome (O90.4)*
> *posttraumatic renal failure (T79.5)*
> *prerenal uremia (R39.2)*
> *renal failure:*
> *complicating abortion or ectopic or molar pregnancy (O00-O07, O08.4)*
> *following labor and delivery (O90.4)*
> *postprocedural (N99.0)*

✓4ᵗʰ **N17 Acute kidney failure**
Code also associated underlying condition

> EXCLUDES 1   *posttraumatic renal failure (T79.5)*

N17.0 Acute kidney failure with tubular necrosis
Acute tubular necrosis
Renal tubular necrosis
Tubular necrosis NOS

N17.1 Acute kidney failure with acute cortical necrosis
Acute cortical necrosis
Cortical necrosis NOS
Renal cortical necrosis

N17.2 Acute kidney failure with medullary necrosis
Medullary [papillary] necrosis NOS
Acute medullary [papillary] necrosis
Renal medullary [papillary] necrosis

N17.8 Other acute kidney failure

N17.9 Acute kidney failure, unspecified
Acute kidney injury (nontraumatic)

> EXCLUDES 2   *traumatic kidney injury (S37.0-)*

✓4ᵗʰ **N18 Chronic kidney disease (CKD)**
Code first any associated:
diabetic chronic kidney disease (E08.22, E09.22, E10.22, E11.22, E13.22)
hypertensive chronic kidney disease (I12-, I13-)
Use additional code to identify kidney transplant status, if applicable, (Z94.0)

N18.1 Chronic kidney disease, stage 1

N18.2 Chronic kidney disease, stage 2 (mild)

N18.3 Chronic kidney disease, stage 3 (moderate)

N18.4 Chronic kidney disease, stage 4 (severe)

N18.5 Chronic kidney disease, stage 5

> EXCLUDES 1   *chronic kidney disease, stage 5 requiring chronic dialysis (N18.6)*

N18.6 End stage renal disease
Chronic kidney disease requiring chronic dialysis
Use additional code to identify dialysis status (Z99.2)

N18.9 Chronic kidney disease, unspecified
Chronic renal disease
Chronic renal failure NOS
Chronic renal insufficiency
Chronic uremia
Renal disease NOS

N19 Unspecified kidney failure
Uremia NOS

> EXCLUDES 1   *acute kidney failure (N17-)*
> *chronic kidney disease (N18-)*
> *chronic uremia (N18.9)*
> *extrarenal uremia (R39.2)*
> *prerenal uremia (R39.2)*
> *renal insufficiency (acute) (N28.9)*
> *uremia of newborn (P96.0)*

Urolithiasis (N20-N23)

✓4ᵗʰ **N20 Calculus of kidney and ureter**
Calculous pyelonephritis

> EXCLUDES 1   *nephrocalcinosis (E83.5)*
> *that with hydronephrosis (N13.2)*

EXCLUDES 1   Not coded here   EXCLUDES 2   Not included here   ***Manifestation Code***

N20.0   **Calculus of kidney**
- Nephrolithiasis NOS
- Renal calculus
- Renal stone
- Staghorn calculus
- Stone in kidney

N20.1   **Calculus of ureter**
- Ureteric stone

N20.2   **Calculus of kidney with calculus of ureter**

N20.9   **Urinary calculus, unspecified**

✓4ᵗʰ **N21**   **Calculus of lower urinary tract**
> Calculus of lower urinary tract with cystitis and urethritis

N21.0   **Calculus in bladder**
- Calculus in diverticulum of bladder
- Urinary bladder stone
  > EXCLUDES 2   *staghorn calculus (N20.0)*

N21.1   **Calculus in urethra**
> EXCLUDES 2   *calculus of prostate (N42.0)*

N21.8   **Other lower urinary tract calculus**

N21.9   **Calculus of lower urinary tract, unspecified**
> EXCLUDES 1   *calculus of urinary tract NOS (N20.9)*

N22   *Calculus of urinary tract in diseases classified elsewhere*
> Code first underlying disease, such as:
> gout (M1a-, M10-)
> schistosomiasis (B65.0-B65.9)

N23   **Unspecified renal colic**

Other disorders of kidney and ureter (N25-N29)
> EXCLUDES 2   *disorders of kidney and ureter with urolithiasis (N20-N23)*

✓4ᵗʰ **N25**   **Disorders resulting from impaired renal tubular function**
> EXCLUDES 1   *metabolic disorders classifiable to E70-E88*

N25.0   **Renal osteodystrophy**
- Azotemic osteodystrophy
- Phosphate-losing tubular disorders
- Renal rickets
- Renal short stature

N25.1   **Nephrogenic diabetes insipidus**
> EXCLUDES 1   *diabetes insipidus NOS (E23.2)*

✓5ᵗʰ **N25.8**   **Other disorders resulting from impaired renal tubular function**

     N25.81   **Secondary hyperparathyroidism of renal origin**
> EXCLUDES 1   *secondary hyperparathyroidism, non-renal (E21.1)*

     N25.89   **Other disorders resulting from impaired renal tubular function**
- Hypokalemic nephropathy
- Lightwood-Albright syndrome
- Renal tubular acidosis NOS

N25.9   **Disorder resulting from impaired renal tubular function, unspecified**

✓4ᵗʰ **N26**   **Unspecified contracted kidney**
> EXCLUDES 1   *contracted kidney due to hypertension (I12-)*
> *diffuse sclerosing glomerulonephritis (N05.8-)*
> *hypertensive nephrosclerosis (arteriolar) (arteriosclerotic) (I12-)*
> *small kidney of unknown cause (N27-)*

N26.1   **Atrophy of kidney (terminal)**

N26.2   **Page kidney**

N26.9   **Renal sclerosis, unspecified**

✓4ᵗʰ **N27**   **Small kidney of unknown cause**
> INCLUDES   oligonephronia

N27.0   **Small kidney, unilateral**

N27.1   **Small kidney, bilateral**

N27.9   **Small kidney, unspecified**

✓4ᵗʰ **N28**   **Other disorders of kidney and ureter, not elsewhere classified**

N28.0   **Ischemia and infarction of kidney**
- Renal artery embolism
- Renal artery obstruction
- Renal artery occlusion
- Renal artery thrombosis
- Renal infarct
  > EXCLUDES 1   *atherosclerosis of renal artery (extrarenal part) (I70.1)*
  > *congenital stenosis of renal artery (Q27.1)*
  > *Goldblatt's kidney (I70.1)*

N28.1   **Cyst of kidney, acquired**
- Cyst (multiple)(solitary) of kidney, acquired
  > EXCLUDES 1   *cystic kidney disease (congenital) (Q61-)*

✓5ᵗʰ **N28.8**   **Other specified disorders of kidney and ureter**
> EXCLUDES 1   *hydroureter (N13.4)*
> *ureteric stricture with hydronephrosis (N13.1)*
> *ureteric stricture without hydronephrosis (N13.5)*

     N28.81   **Hypertrophy of kidney**

     N28.82   **Megaloureter**

     N28.83   **Nephroptosis**

     N28.84   **Pyelitis cystica**

     N28.85   **Pyeloureteritis cystica**

     N28.86   **Ureteritis cystica**

     N28.89   **Other specified disorders of kidney and ureter**

N28.9   **Disorder of kidney and ureter, unspecified**
- Nephropathy NOS
- Renal disease (acute) NOS
- Renal insufficiency (acute)
  > EXCLUDES 1   *chronic renal insufficiency (N18.9)*
  > *unspecified nephritic syndrome (N05-)*

N29   *Other disorders of kidney and ureter in diseases classified elsewhere*
> Code first underlying disease, such as:
> amyloidosis (E85-)
> nephrocalcinosis (E83.5)
> schistosomiasis (B65.0-B65.9)
> EXCLUDES 1   *disorders of kidney and ureter in:*
> *cystinosis (E72.0)*
> *gonorrhea (A54.21)*
> *syphilis (A52.75)*
> *tuberculosis (A18.11)*

Other diseases of the urinary system (N30-N39)
> EXCLUDES 1   *urinary infection (complicating):*
> *abortion or ectopic or molar pregnancy (O00-O07, O08.8)*
> *pregnancy, childbirth and the puerperium (O23-, O75.3, O86.2-)*

✓4ᵗʰ **N30**   **Cystitis**
> Use additional code to identify infectious agent (B95-B97)
> EXCLUDES 1   *prostatocystitis (N41.3)*

✓5ᵗʰ **N30.0**   **Acute cystitis**
> EXCLUDES 1   *irradiation cystitis (N30.4-)*
> *trigonitis (N30.3-)*

     N30.00   **Acute cystitis without hematuria**

     N30.01   **Acute cystitis with hematuria**

✓5ᵗʰ **N30.1**   **Interstitial cystitis (chronic)**

     N30.10   **Interstitial cystitis (chronic) without hematuria**

     N30.11   **Interstitial cystitis (chronic) with hematuria**

✓5ᵗʰ **N30.2**   **Other chronic cystitis**

     N30.20   **Other chronic cystitis without hematuria**

     N30.21   **Other chronic cystitis with hematuria**

✓5ᵗʰ **N30.3**   **Trigonitis**
- Urethrotrigonitis

     N30.30   **Trigonitis without hematuria**

     N30.31   **Trigonitis with hematuria**

✓5ᵗʰ **N30.4**   **Irradiation cystitis**

     N30.40   **Irradiation cystitis without hematuria**

     N30.41   **Irradiation cystitis with hematuria**

✓5ᵗʰ **N30.8**   **Other cystitis**
- Abscess of bladder

     N30.80   **Other cystitis without hematuria**

     N30.81   **Other cystitis with hematuria**

✓5ᵗʰ **N30.9**   **Cystitis, unspecified**

     N30.90   **Cystitis, unspecified without hematuria**

     N30.91   **Cystitis, unspecified with hematuria**

✓4ᵗʰ **N31**   **Neuromuscular dysfunction of bladder, not elsewhere classified**
> Use additional code to identify any associated urinary incontinence (N39.3-N39.4-)
> EXCLUDES 1   *cord bladder NOS (G95.8)*
> *neurogenic bladder due to cauda equina syndrome (G83.4)*
> *neuromuscular dysfunction due to spinal cord lesion (G95.8)*

N31.0   **Uninhibited neuropathic bladder, not elsewhere classified**

N31.1   **Reflex neuropathic bladder, not elsewhere classified**

N31.2   **Flaccid neuropathic bladder, not elsewhere classified**
Atonic (motor) (sensory) neuropathic bladder
Autonomous neuropathic bladder
Nonreflex neuropathic bladder

N31.8   **Other neuromuscular dysfunction of bladder**

N31.9   **Neuromuscular dysfunction of bladder, unspecified**
Neurogenic bladder dysfunction NOS

✓4ᵗʰ **N32**   **Other disorders of bladder**
> EXCLUDES 2   *calculus of bladder (N21.0)*
> *cystocele (N81.1-)*
> *hernia or prolapse of bladder, female (N81.1-)*

N32.0   **Bladder-neck obstruction**
Bladder-neck stenosis (acquired)
> EXCLUDES 1   *congenital bladder-neck obstruction (Q64.3-)*

N32.1   **Vesicointestinal fistula**
Vesicorectal fistula

N32.2   **Vesical fistula, not elsewhere classified**
> EXCLUDES 1   *fistula between bladder and female genital tract*
> *(N82.0-N82.1)*

N32.3   **Diverticulum of bladder**
> EXCLUDES 1   *congenital diverticulum of bladder (Q64.6)*
> *diverticulitis of bladder (N30.8-)*

✓5ᵗʰ **N32.8**   **Other specified disorders of bladder**

N32.81   **Overactive bladder**
Detrusor muscle hyperactivity
> EXCLUDES 1   *frequent urination due to specified bladder*
> *condition—code to condition*

N32.89   **Other specified disorders of bladder**
Calcified bladder
Contracted bladder

N32.9   **Bladder disorder, unspecified**

N33   *Bladder disorders in diseases classified elsewhere*
Code first underlying disease, such as:
schistosomiasis (B65.0-B65.9)
> EXCLUDES 1   *bladder disorder in:*
> *syphilis (A52.76)*
> *tuberculosis (A18.12)*
> *cystitis (in):*
> *candidal infection (B37.41)*
> *chlamydial (A56.01)*
> *diphtheritic (A36.85)*
> *gonorrhea (A54.01)*
> *syphilitic (A52.76)*
> *trichomonal infection (A59.03)*
> *neurogenic bladder (N31-)*

✓4ᵗʰ **N34**   **Urethritis and urethral syndrome**
Use additional code (B95-B97), to identify infectious agent
> EXCLUDES 2   *Reiter's disease (M02.3-)*
> *urethritis in diseases with a predominantly sexual mode of*
> *transmission (A50-A64)*
> *urethrotrigonitis (N30.3-)*

N34.0   **Urethral abscess**
Abscess (of) Cowper's gland
Abscess (of) Littrés gland
Abscess (of) urethral (gland)
Periurethral abscess
> EXCLUDES 1   *urethral caruncle (N36.2)*

N34.1   **Nonspecific urethritis**
Nongonococcal urethritis
Nonvenereal urethritis

N34.2   **Other urethritis**
Meatitis, urethral
Postmenopausal urethritis
Ulcer of urethra (meatus)
Urethritis NOS

N34.3   **Urethral syndrome, unspecified**

✓4ᵗʰ **N35**   **Urethral stricture**
> EXCLUDES 1   *congenital urethral stricture (Q64.3-)*
> *postprocedural urethral stricture (N99.1-)*

✓5ᵗʰ **N35.0**   **Post-traumatic urethral stricture**
Urethral stricture due to injury
> EXCLUDES 1   *postprocedural urethral stricture (N99.1-)*

✓6ᵗʰ **N35.01**   **Post-traumatic urethral stricture, male**
N35.010   **Post-traumatic urethral stricture, male, meatal**
N35.011   **Post-traumatic bulbous urethral stricture**

N35.012   **Post-traumatic membranous urethral stricture**
N35.013   **Post-traumatic anterior urethral stricture**
N35.014   **Post-traumatic urethral stricture, male, unspecified**

✓6ᵗʰ **N35.02**   **Post-traumatic urethral stricture, female**
N35.021   **Urethral stricture due to childbirth**
N35.028   **Other post-traumatic urethral stricture, female**

✓5ᵗʰ **N35.1**   **Postinfective urethral stricture, not elsewhere classified**
> EXCLUDES 1   *urethral stricture associated with schistosomiasis*
> *(B65-, N29)*
> *gonococcal urethral stricture (A54.01)*
> *syphilitic urethral stricture (A52.76)*

✓6ᵗʰ **N35.11**   **Postinfective urethral stricture, not elsewhere classified, male**
N35.111   **Postinfective urethral stricture, not elsewhere classified, male, meatal**
N35.112   **Postinfective bulbous urethral stricture, not elsewhere classified**
N35.113   **Postinfective membranous urethral stricture, not elsewhere classified**
N35.114   **Postinfective anterior urethral stricture, not elsewhere classified**
N35.119   **Postinfective urethral stricture, not elsewhere classified, male, unspecified**

N35.12   **Postinfective urethral stricture, not elsewhere classified, female**

N35.8   **Other urethral stricture**
> EXCLUDES 1   *postprocedural urethral stricture (N99.1-)*

N35.9   **Urethral stricture, unspecified**

✓4ᵗʰ **N36**   **Other disorders of urethra**
N36.0   **Urethral fistula**
False urethral passage
Urethroperineal fistula
Urethrorectal fistula
Urinary fistula NOS
> EXCLUDES 1   *urethroscrotal fistula (N50.8)*
> *urethrovaginal fistula (N82.1)*
> *urethrovesicovaginal fistula (N82.1)*

N36.1   **Urethral diverticulum**

N36.2   **Urethral caruncle**

✓5ᵗʰ **N36.4**   **Urethral functional and muscular disorders**
Use additional code to identify associated urinary stress
incontinence (N39.3)

N36.41   **Hypermobility of urethra**

N36.42   **Intrinsic sphincter deficiency (ISD)**

N36.43   **Combined hypermobility of urethra and intrinsic sphincter deficiency**

N36.44   **Muscular disorders of urethra**
Bladder sphincter dyssynergy

N36.8   **Other specified disorders of urethra**

N36.9   **Urethral disorder, unspecified**

N37   *Urethral disorders in diseases classified elsewhere*
Code first underlying disease.
> EXCLUDES 1   *urethritis (in):*
> *candidal infection (B37.41)*
> *chlamydial (A56.01)*
> *gonorrhea (A54.01)*
> *syphilis (A52.76)*
> *trichomonal infection (A59.03)*
> *tuberculosis (A18.13)*

✓4ᵗʰ **N39**   **Other disorders of urinary system**
> EXCLUDES 2   *hematuria NOS (R31-)*
> *recurrent or persistent hematuria (N02-)*
> *recurrent or persistent hematuria with specified*
> *morphological lesion (N02-)*
> *proteinuria NOS (R80-)*

N39.0   **Urinary tract infection, site not specified**
Use additional code (B95-B97), to identify infectious agent
> EXCLUDES 1   *candidiasis of urinary tract (B37.4-)*
> *neonatal urinary tract infection (P39.3)*
> *urinary tract infection of specified site, such as:*
> *cystitis (30-)*
> *urethritis (N34-)*

EXCLUDES 1   Not coded here   EXCLUDES 2   Not included here   *Manifestation Code*

N39.3 **Stress incontinence (female) (male)**
Code also any associated overactive bladder (N32.81)
EXCLUDES 1 *mixed incontinence (N39.46)*

✓5th **N39.4** **Other specified urinary incontinence**
Code also any associated overactive bladder (N32.81)
EXCLUDES 1 *enuresis NOS (R32)*
functional urinary incontinence (R39.81)
urinary incontinence associated with cognitive
impairment (R39.81)
urinary incontinence NOS (R32)
urinary incontinence of nonorganic origin (F98.0)

N39.41 **Urge incontinence**
EXCLUDES 1 *mixed incontinence (N39.46)*

N39.42 **Incontinence without sensory awareness**
N39.43 **Post-void dribbling**
N39.44 **Nocturnal enuresis**
N39.45 **Continuous leakage**
N39.46 **Mixed incontinence**
Urge and stress incontinence

✓6th **N39.49** **Other specified urinary incontinence**
N39.490 **Overflow incontinence**
N39.498 **Other specified urinary incontinence**
Reflex incontinence
Total incontinence

N39.8 **Other specified disorders of urinary system**
N39.9 **Disorder of urinary system, unspecified**

Diseases of male genital organs (N40-N53)

✓4th **N40** **Enlarged prostate [EP]**
Adenofibromatous hypertrophy of prostate
Benign hypertrophy of the prostate
Benign prostatic hyperplasia
Benign prostatic hypertrophy (BPH)
Nodular prostate
Polyp of prostate
EXCLUDES 1 *benign neoplasms of prostate (adenoma, benign)*
(fibroadenoma) (fibroma) (myoma) (D29.1)
EXCLUDES 2 *malignant neoplasm of prostate (C61)*

N40.0 **Enlarged prostate without lower urinary tract symptoms [LUTS]**
Enlarged prostate NOS

N40.1 **Enlarged prostate with lower urinary tract symptoms [LUTS]**
Use additional code for associated symptoms, when specified:
incomplete bladder emptying (R39.14)
nocturia (R35.1)
straining on urination (R39.16)
urinary frequency (R35.0)
urinary hesitancy (R39.11)
urinary incontinence (N39.4-)
urinary obstruction (N13.8)
urinary retention (R33.8)
urinary urgency (R39.15)
weak urinary stream (R39.12)

✓4th **N41** **Inflammatory diseases of prostate**
Use additional code (B95-B97), to identify infectious agent

✓5th **N41.0** **Acute prostatitis**
N41.00 **Acute prostatitis without hematuria**
N41.01 **Acute prostatitis with hematuria**

✓5th **N41.1** **Chronic prostatitis**
N41.10 **Chronic prostatitis without hematuria**
N41.11 **Chronic prostatitis with hematuria**

N41.2 **Abscess of prostate**
N41.3 **Prostatocystitis**
N41.4 **Granulomatous prostatitis**
N41.8 **Other inflammatory diseases of prostate**
N41.9 **Inflammatory disease of prostate, unspecified**
Prostatitis NOS

✓4th **N42** **Other and unspecified disorders of prostate**
N42.0 **Calculus of prostate**
Prostatic stone
N42.1 **Congestion and hemorrhage of prostate**
EXCLUDES 1 *enlarged prostate (N40-)*
hematuria (R31-)
hyperplasia of prostate (N40-)
inflammatory diseases of prostate (N41-)

N42.3 **Dysplasia of prostate**
Prostatic intraepithelial neoplasia I (PIN I)
Prostatic intraepithelial neoplasia II (PIN II)
EXCLUDES 1 *prostatic intraepithelial neoplasia III (PIN III) (D07.5)*

✓5th **N42.8** **Other specified disorders of prostate**
N42.81 **Prostatodynia syndrome**
Painful prostate syndrome
N42.82 **Prostatosis syndrome**
N42.89 **Other specified disorders of prostate**
Cyst of prostate

N42.9 **Disorder of prostate, unspecified**

✓4th **N43** **Hydrocele and spermatocele**
INCLUDES hydrocele of spermatic cord, testis or tunica vaginalis
EXCLUDES 1 *congenital hydrocele (P83.5)*

N43.0 **Encysted hydrocele**
N43.1 **Infected hydrocele**
Use additional code (B95-B97), to identify infectious agent
N43.2 **Other hydrocele**
N43.3 **Hydrocele, unspecified**

✓5th **N43.4** **Spermatocele of epididymis**
Spermatic cyst
N43.40 **Spermatocele of epididymis, unspecified**
N43.41 **Spermatocele of epididymis, single**
N43.42 **Spermatocele of epididymis, multiple**

✓4th **N44** **Noninflammatory disorders of testis**
✓5th **N44.0** **Torsion of testis**
N44.00 **Torsion of testis, unspecified**
N44.01 **Extravaginal torsion of spermatic cord**
N44.02 **Intravaginal torsion of spermatic cord**
Torsion of spermatic cord NOS
N44.03 **Torsion of appendix testis**
N44.04 **Torsion of appendix epididymis**

N44.1 **Cyst of tunica albuginea testis**
N44.2 **Benign cyst of testis**
N44.8 **Other noninflammatory disorders of the testis**

✓4th **N45** **Orchitis and epididymitis**
Use additional code (B95-B97), to identify infectious agent
N45.1 **Epididymitis**
N45.2 **Orchitis**
N45.3 **Epididymo-orchitis**
N45.4 **Abscess of epididymis or testis**

✓4th **N46** **Male infertility**
EXCLUDES 1 *vasectomy status (Z98.52)*

✓5th **N46.0** **Azoospermia**
Absolute male infertility
Male infertility due to germinal (cell) aplasia
Male infertility due to spermatogenic arrest (complete)
N46.01 **Organic azoospermia**
Azoospermia NOS

✓6th **N46.02** **Azoospermia due to extratesticular causes**
Code also associated cause
N46.021 **Azoospermia due to drug therapy**
N46.022 **Azoospermia due to infection**
N46.023 **Azoospermia due to obstruction of efferent ducts**
N46.024 **Azoospermia due to radiation**
N46.025 **Azoospermia due to systemic disease**
N46.029 **Azoospermia due to other extratesticular causes**

✓5th **N46.1** **Oligospermia**
Male infertility due to germinal cell desquamation
Male infertility due to hypospermatogenesis
Male infertility due to incomplete spermatogenic arrest
N46.11 **Organic oligospermia**
Oligospermia NOS

✓6th **N46.12** **Oligospermia due to extratesticular causes**
Code also associated cause
N46.121 **Oligospermia due to drug therapy**
N46.122 **Oligospermia due to infection**
N46.123 **Oligospermia due to obstruction of efferent ducts**
N46.124 **Oligospermia due to radiation**
N46.125 **Oligospermia due to systemic disease**
N46.129 **Oligospermia due to other extratesticular causes**

✓ Appropriate additional character required   ✓x7th Requires 7th character, placeholder x must fill empty characters

Diseases of the Genitourinary System

N46.8–N60.09

N46.8   **Other male infertility**

N46.9   **Male infertility, unspecified**

✓4ᵗʰ **N47**   **Disorders of prepuce**

     N47.0   **Adherent prepuce, newborn**

     N47.1   **Phimosis**

     N47.2   **Paraphimosis**

     N47.3   **Deficient foreskin**

     N47.4   **Benign cyst of prepuce**

     N47.5   **Adhesions of prepuce and glans penis**

     N47.6   **Balanoposthitis**

         EXCLUDES 1   *balanitis (N48.1)*

         Use additional code (B95-B97), to identify infectious agent

     N47.7   **Other inflammatory diseases of prepuce**

         Use additional code (B95-B97), to identify infectious agent

     N47.8   **Other disorders of prepuce**

✓4ᵗʰ **N48**   **Other disorders of penis**

     N48.0   **Leukoplakia of penis**

         Balanitis xerotica obliterans

         Kraurosis of penis

         Lichen sclerosus of external male genital organs

         EXCLUDES 1   *carcinoma in situ of penis (D07.4)*

     N48.1   **Balanitis**

         EXCLUDES 1   *amebic balanitis (A06.8)*

                balanitis xerotica obliterans (N48.0)

                candidal balanitis (B37.42)

                gonococcal balanitis (A54.23)

                herpesviral [herpes simplex] balanitis (A60.01)

         Use additional code (B95-B97), to identify infectious agent

✓5ᵗʰ   N48.2   **Other inflammatory disorders of penis**

         Use additional code (B95-B97), to identify infectious agent

         EXCLUDES 1   *balanitis (N48.1)*

                balanitis xerotica obliterans (N48.0)

                balanoposthitis (N47.6)

         N48.21   **Abscess of corpus cavernosum and penis**

         N48.22   **Cellulitis of corpus cavernosum and penis**

         N48.29   **Other inflammatory disorders of penis**

✓5ᵗʰ   N48.3   **Priapism**

         Painful erection

         Code first underlying cause

         N48.30   **Priapism, unspecified**

         N48.31   **Priapism due to trauma**

         N48.32   **Priapism due to disease classified elsewhere**

         N48.33   **Priapism, drug-induced**

         N48.39   **Other priapism**

     N48.5   **Ulcer of penis**

     N48.6   **Induration penis plastica**

         Peyronie's disease

         Plastic induration of penis

✓5ᵗʰ   N48.8   **Other specified disorders of penis**

         N48.81   **Thrombosis of superficial vein of penis**

         N48.89   **Other specified disorders of penis**

     N48.9   **Disorder of penis, unspecified**

✓4ᵗʰ **N49**   **Inflammatory disorders of male genital organs, not elsewhere classified**

         Use additional code (B95-B97), to identify infectious agent

         EXCLUDES 1   *inflammation of penis (N48.1, N48.2-)*

                orchitis and epididymitis (N45-)

     N49.0   **Inflammatory disorders of seminal vesicle**

         Vesiculitis NOS

     N49.1   **Inflammatory disorders of spermatic cord, tunica vaginalis and vas deferens**

         Vasitis

     N49.2   **Inflammatory disorders of scrotum**

     N49.3   **Fournier gangrene**

     N49.8   **Inflammatory disorders of other specified male genital organs**

         Inflammation of multiple sites in male genital organs

     N49.9   **Inflammatory disorder of unspecified male genital organ**

         Abscess of unspecified male genital organ

         Boil of unspecified male genital organ

         Carbuncle of unspecified male genital organ

         Cellulitis of unspecified male genital organ

✓4ᵗʰ **N50**   **Other and unspecified disorders of male genital organs**

         EXCLUDES 2   *torsion of testis (N44.0-)*

     N50.0   **Atrophy of testis**

N50.1   **Vascular disorders of male genital organs**

         Hematocele, NOS, of male genital organs

         Hemorrhage of male genital organs

         Thrombosis of male genital organs

N50.8   **Other specified disorders of male genital organs**

         Atrophy of scrotum, seminal vesicle, spermatic cord, tunica vaginalis and vas deferens

         Chylocele, tunica vaginalis (nonfilarial) NOS

         Edema of scrotum, seminal vesicle, spermatic cord, testis, tunica vaginalis and vas deferens

         Hypertrophy of scrotum, seminal vesicle, spermatic cord, testis, tunica vaginalis and vas deferens

         Stricture of spermatic cord, tunica vaginalis, and vas deferens

         Ulcer of scrotum, seminal vesicle, spermatic cord, testis, tunica vaginalis and vas deferens

         Urethroscrotal fistula

N50.9   **Disorder of male genital organs, unspecified**

N51   *Disorders of male genital organs in diseases classified elsewhere*

         Code first underlying disease, such as:

         filariasis (B74.0-B74.9)

         EXCLUDES 1   *amebic balanitis (A06.8)*

                candidal balanitis (B37.42)

                gonococcal balanitis (A54.23)

                gonococcal prostatitis (A54.22)

                herpesviral [herpes simplex] balanitis (A60.01)

                trichomonal prostatitis (A59.02)

                tuberculous prostatitis (A18.14)

✓4ᵗʰ **N52**   **Male erectile dysfunction**

         EXCLUDES 1   *psychogenic impotence (F52.21)*

✓5ᵗʰ   N52.0   **Vasculogenic erectile dysfunction**

         N52.01   **Erectile dysfunction due to arterial insufficiency**

         N52.02   **Corporo-venous occlusive erectile dysfunction**

         N52.03   **Combined arterial insufficiency and corporo-venous occlusive erectile dysfunction**

N52.1   *Erectile dysfunction due to diseases classified elsewhere*

         Code first underlying disease

N52.2   **Drug-induced erectile dysfunction**

✓5ᵗʰ   N52.3   **Post-surgical erectile dysfunction**

         N52.31   **Erectile dysfunction following radical prostatectomy**

         N52.32   **Erectile dysfunction following radical cystectomy**

         N52.33   **Erectile dysfunction following urethral surgery**

         N52.34   **Erectile dysfunction following simple prostatectomy**

         N52.39   **Other post-surgical erectile dysfunction**

N52.8   **Other male erectile dysfunction**

N52.9   **Male erectile dysfunction, unspecified**

         Impotence NOS

✓4ᵗʰ **N53**   **Other male sexual dysfunction**

         EXCLUDES 1   *psychogenic sexual dysfunction (F52-)*

✓5ᵗʰ   N53.1   **Ejaculatory dysfunction**

         EXCLUDES 1   *premature ejaculation (F52.4)*

         N53.11   **Retarded ejaculation**

         N53.12   **Painful ejaculation**

         N53.13   **Anejaculatory orgasm**

         N53.14   **Retrograde ejaculation**

         N53.19   **Other ejaculatory dysfunction**

                Ejaculatory dysfunction NOS

N53.8   **Other male sexual dysfunction**

N53.9   **Unspecified male sexual dysfunction**

Disorders of breast (N60-N65)

         EXCLUDES 1   *disorders of breast associated with childbirth (O91-O92)*

✓4ᵗʰ **N60**   **Benign mammary dysplasia**

         INCLUDES   fibrocystic mastopathy

✓5ᵗʰ   N60.0   **Solitary cyst of breast**

         Cyst of breast

         N60.01   **Solitary cyst of right breast**

         N60.02   **Solitary cyst of left breast**

         N60.09   **Solitary cyst of unspecified breast**

EXCLUDES 1   Not coded here   EXCLUDES 2   Not included here   *Manifestation Code*

✓5th **N60.1 Diffuse cystic mastopathy**
Cystic breast
Fibrocystic disease of breast
EXCLUDES 1 *diffuse cystic mastopathy with epithelial proliferation (N60.3-)*

N60.11 Diffuse cystic mastopathy of right breast
N60.12 Diffuse cystic mastopathy of left breast
N60.19 Diffuse cystic mastopathy of unspecified breast

✓5th **N60.2 Fibroadenosis of breast**
Adenofibrosis of breast
EXCLUDES 2 *fibroadenoma of breast (D24-)*

N60.21 Fibroadenosis of right breast
N60.22 Fibroadenosis of left breast
N60.29 Fibroadenosis of unspecified breast

✓5th **N60.3 Fibrosclerosis of breast**
Cystic mastopathy with epithelial proliferation

N60.31 Fibrosclerosis of right breast
N60.32 Fibrosclerosis of left breast
N60.39 Fibrosclerosis of unspecified breast

✓5th **N60.4 Mammary duct ectasia**
N60.41 Mammary duct ectasia of right breast
N60.42 Mammary duct ectasia of left breast
N60.49 Mammary duct ectasia of unspecified breast

✓5th **N60.8 Other benign mammary dysplasias**
N60.81 Other benign mammary dysplasias of right breast
N60.82 Other benign mammary dysplasias of left breast
N60.89 Other benign mammary dysplasias of unspecified breast

✓5th **N60.9 Unspecified benign mammary dysplasia**
N60.91 Unspecified benign mammary dysplasia of right breast
N60.92 Unspecified benign mammary dysplasia of left breast
N60.99 Unspecified benign mammary dysplasia of unspecified breast

N61 Inflammatory disorders of breast
Abscess (acute) (chronic) (nonpuerperal) of areola
Abscess (acute) (chronic) (nonpuerperal) of breast
Carbuncle of breast
Infective mastitis (acute) (subacute) (nonpuerperal)
Mastitis (acute) (subacute) (nonpuerperal) NOS
EXCLUDES 1 *inflammatory carcinoma of breast (C50.9)*
inflammatory disorder of breast associated with childbirth (O91-)
neonatal infective mastitis (P39.0)
thrombophlebitis of breast [Mondor's disease] (I80.8)

N62 Hypertrophy of breast
Gynecomastia
Hypertrophy of breast NOS
Massive pubertal hypertrophy of breast
EXCLUDES 1 *breast engorgement of newborn (P83.4)*
disproportion of reconstructed breast (N65.1)

N63 Unspecified lump in breast
Nodule(s) NOS in breast

✓4th **N64 Other disorders of breast**
EXCLUDES 2 *mechanical complication of breast prosthesis and implant (T85.4-)*

N64.0 Fissure and fistula of nipple
N64.1 Fat necrosis of breast
Fat necrosis (segmental) of breast
Code first breast necrosis due to breast graft (T85.89)

N64.2 Atrophy of breast
N64.3 Galactorrhea not associated with childbirth
N64.4 Mastodynia

✓5th **N64.5 Other signs and symptoms in breast**
EXCLUDES 2 *abnormal findings on diagnostic imaging of breast (R92-)*

N64.51 Induration of breast
N64.52 Nipple discharge
EXCLUDES 1 *abnormal findings in nipple discharge (R89-)*

N64.53 Retraction of nipple
N64.59 Other signs and symptoms in breast

✓5th **N64.8 Other specified disorders of breast**
N64.81 Ptosis of breast
EXCLUDES 1 *ptosis of native breast in relation to reconstructed breast (N65.1)*

N64.82 Hypoplasia of breast
Micromastia
EXCLUDES 1 *congenital absence of breast (Q83.0)*
hypoplasia of native breast in relation to reconstructed breast (N65.1)

N64.89 Other specified disorders of breast
Galactocele
Subinvolution of breast (postlactational)

N64.9 Disorder of breast, unspecified

✓4th **N65 Deformity and disproportion of reconstructed breast**
N65.0 Deformity of reconstructed breast
Contour irregularity in reconstructed breast
Excess tissue in reconstructed breast
Misshapen reconstructed breast

N65.1 Disproportion of reconstructed breast
Breast asymmetry between native breast and reconstructed breast
Disproportion between native breast and reconstructed breast

Inflammatory diseases of female pelvic organs (N70-N77)

EXCLUDES 1 *inflammatory diseases of female pelvic organs complicating:*
abortion or ectopic or molar pregnancy (O00-O07, O08.0)
pregnancy, childbirth and the puerperium (O23-, O75.3, O85, O86-)

✓4th **N70 Salpingitis and oophoritis**
INCLUDES abscess (of) fallopian tube
abscess (of) ovary
pyosalpinx
salpingo-oophoritis
tubo-ovarian abscess
tubo-ovarian inflammatory disease
Use additional code (B95-B97), to identify infectious agent
EXCLUDES 1 *gonococcal infection (A54.24)*
tuberculous infection (A18.17)

✓5th **N70.0 Acute salpingitis and oophoritis**
N70.01 Acute salpingitis
N70.02 Acute oophoritis
N70.03 Acute salpingitis and oophoritis

✓5th **N70.1 Chronic salpingitis and oophoritis**
Hydrosalpinx
N70.11 Chronic salpingitis
N70.12 Chronic oophoritis
N70.13 Chronic salpingitis and oophoritis

✓5th **N70.9 Salpingitis and oophoritis, unspecified**
N70.91 Salpingitis, unspecified
N70.92 Oophoritis, unspecified
N70.93 Salpingitis and oophoritis, unspecified

✓4th **N71 Inflammatory disease of uterus, except cervix**
Endo (myo) metritis
Metritis
Myometritis
Pyometra
Uterine abscess
Use additional code (B95-B97), to identify infectious agent
EXCLUDES 1 *hyperplastic endometritis (N85.0-)*
infection of uterus following delivery (O85, O86-)

N71.0 Acute inflammatory disease of uterus
N71.1 Chronic inflammatory disease of uterus
N71.9 Inflammatory disease of uterus, unspecified

N72 Inflammatory disease of cervix uteri
Cervicitis (with or without erosion or ectropion)
Endocervicitis (with or without erosion or ectropion)
Exocervicitis (with or without erosion or ectropion)
Use additional code (B95-B97), to identify infectious agent
EXCLUDES 1 *erosion and ectropion of cervix without cervicitis (N86)*

✓4th **N73 Other female pelvic inflammatory diseases**
Use additional code (B95-B97), to identify infectious agent
N73.0 Acute parametritis and pelvic cellulitis
Abscess of broad ligament
Abscess of parametrium
Pelvic cellulitis, female

N73.1   **Chronic parametritis and pelvic cellulitis**
Any condition in N73.0 specified as chronic
EXCLUDES 1   *tuberculous parametritis and pelvic cellulitis (A18.17)*

N73.2   **Unspecified parametritis and pelvic cellulitis**
Any condition in N73.0 unspecified whether acute or chronic

N73.3   **Female acute pelvic peritonitis**

N73.4   **Female chronic pelvic peritonitis**
EXCLUDES 1   *tuberculous pelvic (female) peritonitis (A18.17)*

N73.5   **Female pelvic peritonitis, unspecified**

N73.6   **Female pelvic peritoneal adhesions (postinfective)**
EXCLUDES 2   *postprocedural pelvic peritoneal adhesions (N99.4)*

N73.8   **Other specified female pelvic inflammatory diseases**

N73.9   **Female pelvic inflammatory disease, unspecified**
Female pelvic infection or inflammation NOS

N74   *Female pelvic inflammatory disorders in diseases classified elsewhere*
Code first underlying disease
EXCLUDES 1   cervicitis:
chlamydial (A56.02)
gonococcal (A54.03)
herpesviral [herpes simplex] (A60.03)
syphilitic (A52.76)
trichomonal (A59.09)
tuberculous (A18.16)
pelvic inflammatory disease:
chlamydial (A56.11)
gonococcal (A54.24)
herpesviral [herpes simplex] (A60.09)
syphilitic (A52.76)
tuberculous (A18.17)

✓4ᵗʰ **N75**   **Diseases of Bartholin's gland**

N75.0   **Cyst of Bartholin's gland**

N75.1   **Abscess of Bartholin's gland**

N75.8   **Other diseases of Bartholin's gland**
Bartholinitis

N75.9   **Disease of Bartholin's gland, unspecified**

✓4ᵗʰ **N76**   **Other inflammation of vagina and vulva**
Use additional code (B95-B97), to identify infectious agent
EXCLUDES 2   *senile (atrophic) vaginitis (N95.2)*
vulvar vestibulitis (N94.810)

N76.0   **Acute vaginitis**
Acute vulvovaginitis
Vaginitis NOS
Vulvovaginitis NOS

N76.1   **Subacute and chronic vaginitis**
Chronic vulvovaginitis
Subacute vulvovaginitis

N76.2   **Acute vulvitis**
Vulvitis NOS

N76.3   **Subacute and chronic vulvitis**

N76.4   **Abscess of vulva**
Furuncle of vulva

N76.5   **Ulceration of vagina**

N76.6   **Ulceration of vulva**

✓5ᵗʰ **N76.8**   **Other specified inflammation of vagina and vulva**

N76.81   **Mucositis (ulcerative) of vagina and vulva**
Code also type of associated therapy, such as:
antineoplastic and immunosuppressive drugs
(T45.1x-)
radiological procedure and radiotherapy (Y84.2)
EXCLUDES 2   *gastrointestinal mucositis (ulcerative)*
(K92.81)
nasal mucositis (ulcerative) (J34.81)
oral mucositis (ulcerative) (K12.3-)

N76.89   **Other specified inflammation of vagina and vulva**

✓4ᵗʰ **N77**   **Vulvovaginal ulceration and inflammation in diseases classified elsewhere**

N77.0   *Ulceration of vulva in diseases classified elsewhere*
Code first underlying disease, such as:
Behçet's disease (M35.2)
EXCLUDES 1   *ulceration of vulva in gonococcal infection (A54.02)*
ulceration of vulva in herpesviral [herpes simplex]
infection (A60.04)
ulceration of vulva in syphilis (A51.0)
ulceration of vulva in tuberculosis (A18.18)

N77.1   *Vaginitis, vulvitis and vulvovaginitis in diseases classified elsewhere*
Code first underlying disease, such as:
pinworm (B80)
EXCLUDES 1   *vaginitis, vulvitis and vulvovaginitis (in):*
candidiasis (B37.3)
chlamydial (A56.02)
gonococcal infection (A54.02)
herpesviral [herpes simplex] infection (A60.04)
syphilitic, early (A51.0)
syphilitic, late (A52.76)
trichomonal (A59.01)
tuberculous (A18.18)

Noninflammatory disorders of female genital tract (N80-N98)

✓4ᵗʰ **N80**   **Endometriosis**

N80.0   **Endometriosis of uterus**
Adenomyosis
EXCLUDES 1   *stromal endometriosis (D39.0)*

N80.1   **Endometriosis of ovary**

N80.2   **Endometriosis of fallopian tube**

N80.3   **Endometriosis of pelvic peritoneum**

N80.4   **Endometriosis of rectovaginal septum and vagina**

N80.5   **Endometriosis of intestine**

N80.6   **Endometriosis in cutaneous scar**

N80.8   **Other endometriosis**

N80.9   **Endometriosis, unspecified**

✓4ᵗʰ **N81**   **Female genital prolapse**
EXCLUDES 1   *genital prolapse complicating pregnancy, labor or delivery*
(O34.5-)
prolapse and hernia of ovary and fallopian tube (N83.4)
prolapse of vaginal vault after hysterectomy (N99.3)

N81.0   **Urethrocele**
EXCLUDES 1   *urethrocele with cystocele (N81.1-)*
urethrocele with prolapse of uterus (N81.2-N81.4)

✓5ᵗʰ **N81.1**   **Cystocele**
Cystocele with urethrocele
Cystourethrocele
EXCLUDES 1   *cystocele with prolapse of uterus (N81.2-N81.4)*

N81.10   **Cystocele, unspecified**
Prolapse of (anterior) vaginal wall NOS

N81.11   **Cystocele, midline**

N81.12   **Cystocele, lateral**
Paravaginal cystocele

N81.2   **Incomplete uterovaginal prolapse**
First degree uterine prolapse
Prolapse of cervix NOS
Second degree uterine prolapse
EXCLUDES 1   *cervical stump prolapse (N81.85)*

N81.3   **Complete uterovaginal prolapse**
Procidentia (uteri) NOS
Third degree uterine prolapse

N81.4   **Uterovaginal prolapse, unspecified**
Prolapse of uterus NOS

N81.5   **Vaginal enterocele**
EXCLUDES 1   *enterocele with prolapse of uterus (N81.2-N81.4)*

N81.6   **Rectocele**
Prolapse of posterior vaginal wall
Use additional code for associated fecal incontinence, if
applicable (R15.-)
EXCLUDES 2   *perineocele N81.81*
rectal prolapse (K62.3)
rectocele with prolapse of uterus (N81.2-N81.4)

✓5ᵗʰ **N81.8**   **Other female genital prolapse**

N81.81   **Perineocele**

N81.82   **Incompetence or weakening of pubocervical tissue**

N81.83   **Incompetence or weakening of rectovaginal tissue**

N81.84   **Pelvic muscle wasting**
Disuse atrophy of pelvic muscles and anal sphincter

N81.85   **Cervical stump prolapse**

N81.89   **Other female genital prolapse**
Deficient perineum
Old laceration of muscles of pelvic floor

N81.9   **Female genital prolapse, unspecified**

EXCLUDES 1   Not coded here   EXCLUDES 2   Not included here   *Manifestation Code*

✓4th N82   Fistulae involving female genital tract
> EXCLUDES 1   *vesicointestinal fistulae (N32.1)*

     N82.0   Vesicovaginal fistula

     N82.1   Other female urinary-genital tract fistulae
         Cervicovesical fistula
         Ureterovaginal fistula
         Urethrovaginal fistula
         Uteroureteric fistula
         Uterovesical fistula

     N82.2   Fistula of vagina to small intestine

     N82.3   Fistula of vagina to large intestine
         Rectovaginal fistula

     N82.4   Other female intestinal-genital tract fistulae
         Intestinouterine fistula

     N82.5   Female genital tract-skin fistulae
         Uterus to abdominal wall fistula
         Vaginoperineal fistula

     N82.8   Other female genital tract fistulae

     N82.9   Female genital tract fistula, unspecified

✓4th N83   Noninflammatory disorders of ovary, fallopian tube and broad ligament
> EXCLUDES 2   *hydrosalpinx (N70.1-)*

     N83.0   Follicular cyst of ovary
         Cyst of graafian follicle
         Hemorrhagic follicular cyst (of ovary)

     N83.1   Corpus luteum cyst
         Hemorrhagic corpus luteum cyst

     ✓5th N83.2   Other and unspecified ovarian cysts
> EXCLUDES 1   *developmental ovarian cyst (Q50.1)*
>   *neoplastic ovarian cyst (D27-)*
>   *polycystic ovarian syndrome (E28.2)*
>   *Stein-Leventhal syndrome (E28.2)*

         N83.20   Unspecified ovarian cysts

         N83.29   Other ovarian cysts
               Retention cyst of ovary
               Simple cyst of ovary

     ✓5th N83.3   Acquired atrophy of ovary and fallopian tube

         N83.31   Acquired atrophy of ovary

         N83.32   Acquired atrophy of fallopian tube

         N83.33   Acquired atrophy of ovary and fallopian tube

     N83.4   Prolapse and hernia of ovary and fallopian tube

     ✓5th N83.5   Torsion of ovary, ovarian pedicle and fallopian tube
         Torsion of accessory tube

         N83.51   Torsion of ovary and ovarian pedicle

         N83.52   Torsion of fallopian tube
               Torsion of hydatid of Morgagni

         N83.53   Torsion of ovary, ovarian pedicle and fallopian tube

     N83.6   Hematosalpinx
> EXCLUDES 1   *hematosalpinx (with) (in):*
>   *hematocolpos (N89.7)*
>   *hematometra (N85.7)*
>   *tubal pregnancy (O00.1)*

     N83.7   Hematoma of broad ligament

     N83.8   Other noninflammatory disorders of ovary, fallopian tube and broad ligament
         Broad ligament laceration syndrome [Allen-Masters]

     N83.9   Noninflammatory disorder of ovary, fallopian tube and broad ligament, unspecified

✓4th N84   Polyp of female genital tract
> EXCLUDES 1   *adenomatous polyp (D28-)*
>   *placental polyp (O90.89)*

     N84.0   Polyp of corpus uteri
         Polyp of endometrium
         Polyp of uterus NOS
> EXCLUDES 1   *polypoid endometrial hyperplasia (N85.0-)*

     N84.1   Polyp of cervix uteri
         Mucous polyp of cervix

     N84.2   Polyp of vagina

     N84.3   Polyp of vulva
         Polyp of labia

     N84.8   Polyp of other parts of female genital tract

     N84.9   Polyp of female genital tract, unspecified

✓4th N85   Other noninflammatory disorders of uterus, except cervix
> EXCLUDES 1   *endometriosis (N80-)*
>   *inflammatory diseases of uterus (N71-)*
>   *noninflammatory disorders of cervix, except malposition (N86-N88)*
>   *polyp of corpus uteri (N84.0)*
>   *uterine prolapse (N81-)*

     ✓5th N85.0   Endometrial hyperplasia

         N85.00   Endometrial hyperplasia, unspecified
               Hyperplasia (adenomatous) (cystic) (glandular) of endometrium
               Hyperplastic endometritis

         N85.01   Benign endometrial hyperplasia
               Endometrial hyperplasia (complex) (simple) without atypia

         N85.02   Endometrial intraepithelial neoplasia [EIN]
               Endometrial hyperplasia with atypia
> EXCLUDES 1   *malignant neoplasm of endometrium (with endometrial intraepithelial neoplasia [EIN]) (C54.1)*

     N85.2   Hypertrophy of uterus
         Bulky or enlarged uterus
> EXCLUDES 1   *puerperal hypertrophy of uterus (O90.89)*

     N85.3   Subinvolution of uterus
> EXCLUDES 1   *puerperal subinvolution of uterus (O90.89)*

     N85.4   Malposition of uterus
         Anteversion of uterus
         Retroflexion of uterus
         Retroversion of uterus
> EXCLUDES 1   *malposition of uterus complicating pregnancy, labor or delivery (O34.5-, O65.5)*

     N85.5   Inversion of uterus
> EXCLUDES 1   *current obstetric trauma (O71.2)*
>   *postpartum inversion of uterus (O71.2)*

     N85.6   Intrauterine synechiae

     N85.7   Hematometra
         Hematosalpinx with hematometra
> EXCLUDES 1   *hematometra with hematocolpos (N89.7)*

     N85.8   Other specified noninflammatory disorders of uterus
         Atrophy of uterus, acquired
         Fibrosis of uterus NOS

     N85.9   Noninflammatory disorder of uterus, unspecified
         Disorder of uterus NOS

N86   Erosion and ectropion of cervix uteri
     Decubitus (trophic) ulcer of cervix
     Eversion of cervix
> EXCLUDES 1   *erosion and ectropion of cervix with cervicitis (N72)*

✓4th N87   Dysplasia of cervix uteri
> EXCLUDES 1   *abnormal results from cervical cytologic examination without histologic confirmation (R87.61-)*
>   *carcinoma in situ of cervix uteri (D06-)*
>   *cervical intraepithelial neoplasia III [CIN III] (D06-)*
>   *HGSIL of cervix (R87.613)*
>   *severe dysplasia of cervix uteri (D06-)*

     N87.0   Mild cervical dysplasia
         Cervical intraepithelial neoplasia I [CIN I]

     N87.1   Moderate cervical dysplasia
         Cervical intraepithelial neoplasia II [CIN II]

     N87.9   Dysplasia of cervix uteri, unspecified
         Anaplasia of cervix
         Cervical atypism
         Cervical dysplasia NOS

✓4th N88   Other noninflammatory disorders of cervix uteri
> EXCLUDES 2   *inflammatory disease of cervix (N72)*
>   *polyp of cervix (N84.1)*

     N88.0   Leukoplakia of cervix uteri

     N88.1   Old laceration of cervix uteri
         Adhesions of cervix
> EXCLUDES 1   *current obstetric trauma (O71.3)*

     N88.2   Stricture and stenosis of cervix uteri
> EXCLUDES 1   *stricture and stenosis of cervix uteri complicating labor (O65.5)*

     N88.3   Incompetence of cervix uteri
         Investigation and management of (suspected) cervical incompetence in a nonpregnant woman
> EXCLUDES 1   *cervical incompetence complicating pregnancy (O34.3-)*

☑ Appropriate additional character required   ✓x7th Requires 7th character, placeholder x must fill empty characters

N88.4   **Hypertrophic elongation of cervix uteri**

N88.8   **Other specified noninflammatory disorders of cervix uteri**
> *EXCLUDES 1*   *current obstetric trauma (O71.3)*

N88.9   **Noninflammatory disorder of cervix uteri, unspecified**

✓4ᵗʰ **N89**   **Other noninflammatory disorders of vagina**
> *EXCLUDES 1*   *abnormal results from vaginal cytologic examination without histologic confirmation (R87.62-)*
> *carcinoma in situ of vagina (D07.2)*
> *HGSIL of vagina (R87.623)*
> *inflammation of vagina (N76-)*
> *senile (atrophic) vaginitis (N95.2)*
> *severe dysplasia of vagina (D07.2)*
> *trichomonal leukorrhea (A59.00)*
> *vaginal intraepithelial neoplasia [VAIN], grade III (D07.2)*

N89.0   **Mild vaginal dysplasia**
Vaginal intraepithelial neoplasia [VAIN], grade I

N89.1   **Moderate vaginal dysplasia**
Vaginal intraepithelial neoplasia [VAIN], grade II

N89.3   **Dysplasia of vagina, unspecified**

N89.4   **Leukoplakia of vagina**

N89.5   **Stricture and atresia of vagina**
Vaginal adhesions
Vaginal stenosis
> *EXCLUDES 1*   *congenital atresia or stricture (Q52.4)*
> *postprocedural adhesions of vagina (N99.2)*

N89.6   **Tight hymenal ring**
Rigid hymen
Tight introitus
> *EXCLUDES 1*   *imperforate hymen (Q52.3)*

N89.7   **Hematocolpos**
Hematocolpos with hematometra or hematosalpinx

N89.8   **Other specified noninflammatory disorders of vagina**
Leukorrhea NOS
Old vaginal laceration
Pessary ulcer of vagina
> *EXCLUDES 1*   *current obstetric trauma (O70-, O71.4, O71.7-O71.8)*
> *old laceration involving muscles of pelvic floor (N81.8)*

N89.9   **Noninflammatory disorder of vagina, unspecified**

✓4ᵗʰ **N90**   **Other noninflammatory disorders of vulva and perineum**
> *EXCLUDES 1*   *anogenital (venereal) warts (A63.0)*
> *carcinoma in situ of vulva (D07.1)*
> *condyloma acuminatum (A63.0)*
> *current obstetric trauma (O70-, O71.7-O71.8)*
> *inflammation of vulva (N76-)*
> *severe dysplasia of vulva (D07.1)*
> *vulvar intraepithelial neoplasm III [VIN III] (D07.1)*

N90.0   **Mild vulvar dysplasia**
Vulvar intraepithelial neoplasia [VIN], grade I

N90.1   **Moderate vulvar dysplasia**
Vulvar intraepithelial neoplasia [VIN], grade II

N90.3   **Dysplasia of vulva, unspecified**

N90.4   **Leukoplakia of vulva**
Dystrophy of vulva
Kraurosis of vulva
Lichen sclerosus of external female genital organs

N90.5   **Atrophy of vulva**
Stenosis of vulva

N90.6   **Hypertrophy of vulva**
Hypertrophy of labia

N90.7   **Vulvar cyst**

✓5ᵗʰ **N90.8**   **Other specified noninflammatory disorders of vulva and perineum**

   ✓6ᵗʰ **N90.81**   **Female genital mutilation status**
Female genital cutting status

     N90.810   **Female genital mutilation status, unspecified**
Female genital cutting status, unspecified
Female genital mutilation status NOS

     N90.811   **Female genital mutilation Type I status**
Clitorectomy status
Female genital cutting Type I status

     N90.812   **Female genital mutilation Type II status**
Clitorectomy with excision of labia minora status
Female genital cutting Type II status

     N90.813   **Female genital mutilation Type III status**
Female genital cutting Type III status
Infibulation status

     N90.818   **Other female genital mutilation status**
Female genital cutting Type IV status
Female genital mutilation Type IV status
Other female genital cutting status

   N90.89   **Other specified noninflammatory disorders of vulva and perineum**
Adhesions of vulva
Hypertrophy of clitoris

N90.9   **Noninflammatory disorder of vulva and perineum, unspecified**

✓4ᵗʰ **N91**   **Absent, scanty and rare menstruation**
> *EXCLUDES 1*   *ovarian dysfunction (E28-)*

N91.0   **Primary amenorrhea**

N91.1   **Secondary amenorrhea**

N91.2   **Amenorrhea, unspecified**

N91.3   **Primary oligomenorrhea**

N91.4   **Secondary oligomenorrhea**

N91.5   **Oligomenorrhea, unspecified**
Hypomenorrhea NOS

✓4ᵗʰ **N92**   **Excessive, frequent and irregular menstruation**
> *EXCLUDES 1*   *postmenopausal bleeding (N95.0)*
> *precocious puberty (menstruation) (E30.1)*

N92.0   **Excessive and frequent menstruation with regular cycle**
Heavy periods NOS
Menorrhagia NOS
Polymenorrhea

N92.1   **Excessive and frequent menstruation with irregular cycle**
Irregular intermenstrual bleeding
Irregular, shortened intervals between menstrual bleeding
Menometrorrhagia
Metrorrhagia

N92.2   **Excessive menstruation at puberty**
Excessive bleeding associated with onset of menstrual periods
Pubertal menorrhagia
Puberty bleeding

N92.3   **Ovulation bleeding**
Regular intermenstrual bleeding

N92.4   **Excessive bleeding in the premenopausal period**
Climacteric menorrhagia or metrorrhagia
Menopausal menorrhagia or metrorrhagia
Preclimacteric menorrhagia or metrorrhagia
Premenopausal menorrhagia or metrorrhagia

N92.5   **Other specified irregular menstruation**

N92.6   **Irregular menstruation, unspecified**
Irregular bleeding NOS
Irregular periods NOS
> *EXCLUDES 1*   *irregular menstruation with:*
> *lengthened intervals or scanty bleeding (N91.3-N91.5)*
> *shortened intervals or excessive bleeding (N92.1)*

✓4ᵗʰ **N93**   **Other abnormal uterine and vaginal bleeding**
> *EXCLUDES 1*   *neonatal vaginal hemorrhage (P54.6)*
> *precocious puberty (menstruation) (E30.1)*
> *pseudomenses (P54.6)*

N93.0   **Postcoital and contact bleeding**

N93.8   **Other specified abnormal uterine and vaginal bleeding**
Dysfunctional or functional uterine or vaginal bleeding NOS

N93.9   **Abnormal uterine and vaginal bleeding, unspecified**

✓4ᵗʰ **N94**   **Pain and other conditions associated with female genital organs and menstrual cycle**

N94.0   **Mittelschmerz**

N94.1   **Dyspareunia**
> *EXCLUDES 1*   *psychogenic dyspareunia (F52.6)*

N94.2   **Vaginismus**
> *EXCLUDES 1*   *psychogenic vaginismus (F52.5)*

N94.3   **Premenstrual tension syndrome**
Premenstrual dysphoric disorder
Code also associated menstrual migraine (G43.d-)

N94.4   **Primary dysmenorrhea**

N94.5   **Secondary dysmenorrhea**

N94.6   **Dysmenorrhea, unspecified**
> *EXCLUDES 1*   *psychogenic dysmenorrhea (F45.8)*

EXCLUDES 1   Not coded here   *EXCLUDES 2*   Not included here   ***Manifestation Code***

✓5th **N94.8** **Other specified conditions associated with female genital organs and menstrual cycle**

    ✓6th **N94.81** **Vulvodynia**

        N94.810 **Vulvar vestibulitis**

        N94.818 **Other vulvodynia**

        N94.819 **Vulvodynia, unspecified**

            Vulvodynia NOS

    N94.89 **Other specified conditions associated with female genital organs and menstrual cycle**

N94.9 **Unspecified condition associated with female genital organs and menstrual cycle**

✓4th **N95** **Menopausal and other perimenopausal disorders**

    Menopausal and other perimenopausal disorders due to naturally occurring (age-related) menopause and perimenopause

    EXCLUDES 1 *excessive bleeding in the premenopausal period (N92.4)*

        menopausal and perimenopausal disorders due to artificial or premature menopause (E89.4-, E28.31-)

        premature menopause (E28.31-)

    EXCLUDES 2 *postmenopausal osteoporosis (M81.0-)*

        postmenopausal osteoporosis with current pathological fracture (M80.0-)

        postmenopausal urethritis (N34.2)

N95.0 **Postmenopausal bleeding**

N95.1 **Menopausal and female climacteric states**

    Symptoms such as flushing, sleeplessness, headache, lack of concentration, associated with natural (age-related) menopause

    Use additional code for associated symptoms

    EXCLUDES 1 *asymptomatic menopausal state (Z78.0)*

        symptoms associated with artificial menopause (E89.41)

        symptoms associated with premature menopause (E28.310)

N95.2 **Postmenopausal atrophic vaginitis**

    Senile (atrophic) vaginitis

N95.8 **Other specified menopausal and perimenopausal disorders**

N95.9 **Unspecified menopausal and perimenopausal disorder**

N96 **Recurrent pregnancy loss**

    Investigation or care in a nonpregnant woman with history of recurrent pregnancy loss

    EXCLUDES 1 *recurrent pregnancy loss with current pregnancy (O26.2-)*

✓4th **N97** **Female infertility**

    INCLUDES inability to achieve a pregnancy

        sterility, female NOS

    EXCLUDES 1 *female infertility associated with:*

        hypopituitarism (E23.0)

        Stein-Leventhal syndrome (E28.2)

    EXCLUDES 2 *incompetence of cervix uteri (N88.3)*

N97.0 **Female infertility associated with anovulation**

N97.1 **Female infertility of tubal origin**

    Female infertility associated with congenital anomaly of tube

    Female infertility due to tubal block

    Female infertility due to tubal occlusion

    Female infertility due to tubal stenosis

N97.2 **Female infertility of uterine origin**

    Female infertility associated with congenital anomaly of uterus

    Female infertility due to nonimplantation of ovum

N97.8 **Female infertility of other origin**

N97.9 **Female infertility, unspecified**

✓4th **N98** **Complications associated with artificial fertilization**

N98.0 **Infection associated with artificial insemination**

N98.1 **Hyperstimulation of ovaries**

    Hyperstimulation of ovaries NOS

    Hyperstimulation of ovaries associated with induced ovulation

N98.2 **Complications of attempted introduction of fertilized ovum following in vitro fertilization**

N98.3 **Complications of attempted introduction of embryo in embryo transfer**

N98.8 **Other complications associated with artificial fertilization**

N98.9 **Complication associated with artificial fertilization, unspecified**

Intraoperative and postprocedural complications and disorders of genitourinary system, not elsewhere classified (N99)

✓4th **N99** **Intraoperative and postprocedural complications and disorders of genitourinary system, not elsewhere classified**

    EXCLUDES 2 *irradiation cystitis (N30.4-)*

        postoophorectomy osteoporosis with current pathological fracture (M80.8-)

        postoophorectomy osteoporosis without current pathological fracture (M81.8)

N99.0 **Postprocedural (acute) (chronic) kidney failure**

    Use additional code to type of kidney disease

✓5th **N99.1** **Postprocedural urethral stricture**

    Postcatheterization urethral stricture

    ✓6th **N99.11** **Postprocedural urethral stricture, male**

        N99.110 **Postprocedural urethral stricture, male, meatal**

        N99.111 **Postprocedural bulbous urethral stricture**

        N99.112 **Postprocedural membranous urethral stricture**

        N99.113 **Postprocedural anterior urethral stricture**

        N99.114 **Postprocedural urethral stricture, male, unspecified**

    N99.12 **Postprocedural urethral stricture, female**

N99.2 **Postprocedural adhesions of vagina**

N99.3 **Prolapse of vaginal vault after hysterectomy**

N99.4 **Postprocedural pelvic peritoneal adhesions**

    EXCLUDES 2 *pelvic peritoneal adhesions NOS (N73.6)*

        postinfective pelvic peritoneal adhesions (N73.6)

✓5th **N99.5** **Complications of stoma of urinary tract**

    EXCLUDES 2 *mechanical complication of urinary (indwelling) catheter (T83.0-)*

    ✓6th **N99.51** **Complication of cystostomy**

        N99.510 **Cystostomy hemorrhage**

        N99.511 **Cystostomy infection**

        N99.512 **Cystostomy malfunction**

        N99.518 **Other cystostomy complication**

    ✓6th **N99.52** **Complication of other external stoma of urinary tract**

        N99.520 **Hemorrhage of other external stoma of urinary tract**

        N99.521 **Infection of other external stoma of urinary tract**

        N99.522 **Malfunction of other external stoma of urinary tract**

        N99.528 **Other complication of other external stoma of urinary tract**

    ✓6th **N99.53** **Complication of other stoma of urinary tract**

        N99.530 **Hemorrhage of other stoma of urinary tract**

        N99.531 **Infection of other stoma of urinary tract**

        N99.532 **Malfunction of other stoma of urinary tract**

        N99.538 **Other complication of other stoma of urinary tract**

✓5th **N99.6** **Intraoperative hemorrhage and hematoma of a genitourinary system organ or structure complicating a procedure**

    EXCLUDES 1 *intraoperative hemorrhage and hematoma of a genitourinary system organ or structure due to accidental puncture or laceration during a procedure (N99.7-)*

    N99.61 **Intraoperative hemorrhage and hematoma of a genitourinary system organ or structure complicating a genitourinary system procedure**

    N99.62 **Intraoperative hemorrhage and hematoma of a genitourinary system organ or structure complicating other procedure**

✓5th **N99.7** **Accidental puncture and laceration of a genitourinary system organ or structure during a procedure**

    N99.71 **Accidental puncture and laceration of a genitourinary system organ or structure during a genitourinary system procedure**

    N99.72 **Accidental puncture and laceration of a genitourinary system organ or structure during other procedure**

☑ Appropriate additional character required   ✓x7th Requires 7th character, placeholder x must fill empty characters

√5ᵗʰ **N99.8** **Other intraoperative and postprocedural complications and disorders of genitourinary system**

    N99.81 **Other intraoperative complications of genitourinary system**

√6ᵗʰ **N99.82** **Postprocedural hemorrhage and hematoma of a genitourinary system organ or structure following a procedure**

      N99.820 **Postprocedural hemorrhage and hematoma of a genitourinary system organ or structure following a genitourinary system procedure**

      N99.821 **Postprocedural hemorrhage and hematoma of a genitourinary system organ or structure following other procedure**

    N99.83 **Residual ovary syndrome**

    N99.89 **Other postprocedural complications and disorders of genitourinary system**

Chapter 15. Pregnancy, Childbirth and the Puerperium (O00-O9a)

NOTE   CODES FROM THIS CHAPTER ARE FOR USE ONLY ON MATERNAL RECORDS, NEVER ON NEWBORN RECORDS.

Codes from this chapter are for use for conditions related to or aggrevated by the pregnancy, childbirth, or by the puerperium (maternal causes or obstetric causes).

NOTE   Trimesters are counted from the first day of the last menstrual period. They are defined as follows:

1st trimester- less than 14 weeks 0 days
2nd trimester- 14 weeks 0 days to less than 28 weeks 0 days
3rd trimester- 28 weeks 0 days until delivery

EXCLUDES 1   *supervision of normal pregnancy (Z34-)*
EXCLUDES 2   *mental and behavioral disorders associated with the puerperium (F53)*
obstetrical tetanus (A34)
postpartum necrosis of pituitary gland (E23.0)
puerperal osteomalacia (M83.0)

This chapter contains the following blocks:

O00-O08	Pregnancy with abortive outcome
O09	Supervision of high risk pregnancy
O10-O16	Edema, proteinuria and hypertensive disorders in pregnancy, childbirth and the puerperium
O20-O29	Other maternal disorders predominantly related to pregnancy
O30-O48	Maternal care related to the fetus and amniotic cavity and possible delivery problems
O60-O77	Complications of labor and delivery
O80, O82	Encounter for delivery
O85-O92	Complications predominantly related to the puerperium
O94-O9a	Other obstetric conditions, not elsewhere classified

Pregnancy with abortive outcome (O00-O08)

EXCLUDES 1   *continuing pregnancy in multiple gestation after abortion of one fetus or more (O31.1-, O31.3-)*

☑4th **O00 Ectopic pregnancy**

INCLUDES   ruptured ectopic pregnancy

Use additional code from category O08 to identify any associated complication

O00.0 Abdominal pregnancy

EXCLUDES 1   *maternal care for viable fetus in abdominal pregnancy (O36.7-)*

O00.1 Tubal pregnancy
Fallopian pregnancy
Rupture of (fallopian) tube due to pregnancy
Tubal abortion

O00.2 Ovarian pregnancy

O00.8 Other ectopic pregnancy
Cervical pregnancy
Cornual pregnancy
Intraligamentous pregnancy
Mural pregnancy

O00.9 Ectopic pregnancy, unspecified

☑4th **O01 Hydatidiform mole**

Use additional code from category O08 to identify any associated complication

EXCLUDES 1   *chorioadenoma (destruens) (D39.2)*
malignant hydatidiform mole (D39.2)

O01.0 Classical hydatidiform mole
Complete hydatidiform mole

O01.1 Incomplete and partial hydatidiform mole

O01.9 Hydatidiform mole, unspecified
Trophoblastic disease NOS
Vesicular mole NOS

☑4th **O02 Other abnormal products of conception**

Use additional code from category O08 to identify any associated complication

EXCLUDES 1   *papyraceous fetus (O31.0-)*

O02.0 Blighted ovum and nonhydatidiform mole
Carneous mole
Fleshy mole
Intrauterine mole NOS
Molar pregnancy NEC
Pathological ovum

O02.1 Missed abortion
Early fetal death, before completion of 20 weeks of gestation, with retention of dead fetus

EXCLUDES 1   *failed induced abortion (O07-)*
fetal death (intrauterine) (late) (O36.4)
missed abortion with blighted ovum (O02.0)
missed abortion with hydatidiform mole (O01-)
missed abortion with nonhydatidiform (O02.0)
missed delivery (O36.4)
stillbirth (P95)

O02.8 Other specified abnormal products of conception

EXCLUDES 1   *abnormal products of conception with blighted ovum (O02.0)*
abnormal products of conception with hydatidiform mole (O01-)
abnormal products of conception with nonhydatidiform mole (O02.0)

O02.9 Abnormal product of conception, unspecified

☑4th **O03 Spontaneous abortion**

NOTE   Incomplete abortion includes retained products of conception following spontaneous abortion

INCLUDES   miscarriage

O03.0 Genital tract and pelvic infection following incomplete spontaneous abortion
Endometritis following incomplete spontaneous abortion
Oophoritis following incomplete spontaneous abortion
Parametritis following incomplete spontaneous abortion
Pelvic peritonitis following incomplete spontaneous abortion
Salpingitis following incomplete spontaneous abortion
Salpingo-oophoritis following incomplete spontaneous abortion

EXCLUDES 1   *sepsis following incomplete spontaneous abortion (O03.37)*
urinary tract infection following incomplete spontaneous abortion (O03.38)

O03.1 Delayed or excessive hemorrhage following incomplete spontaneous abortion
Afibrinogenemia following incomplete spontaneous abortion
Defibrination syndrome following incomplete spontaneous abortion
Hemolysis following incomplete spontaneous abortion
Intravascular coagulation following incomplete spontaneous abortion

O03.2 Embolism following incomplete spontaneous abortion
Air embolism following incomplete spontaneous abortion
Amniotic fluid embolism following incomplete spontaneous abortion
Blood-clot embolism following incomplete spontaneous abortion
Embolism NOS following incomplete spontaneous abortion
Fat embolism following incomplete spontaneous abortion
Pulmonary embolism following incomplete spontaneous abortion
Pyemic embolism following incomplete spontaneous abortion
Septic or septicopyemic embolism following incomplete spontaneous abortion
Soap embolism following incomplete spontaneous abortion

☑5th **O03.3 Other and unspecified complications following incomplete spontaneous abortion**

O03.30 Unspecified complication following incomplete spontaneous abortion

O03.31 Shock following incomplete spontaneous abortion
Circulatory collapse following incomplete spontaneous abortion
Shock (postprocedural) following incomplete spontaneous abortion

EXCLUDES 1   *shock due to infection following incomplete spontaneous abortion (O03.37)*

O03.32 Renal failure following incomplete spontaneous abortion
Kidney failure (acute) following incomplete spontaneous abortion
Oliguria following incomplete spontaneous abortion
Renal shutdown following incomplete spontaneous abortion
Renal tubular necrosis following incomplete spontaneous abortion
Uremia following incomplete spontaneous abortion

O03.33   **Metabolic disorder following incomplete spontaneous abortion**

O03.34   **Damage to pelvic organs following incomplete spontaneous abortion**

     Laceration, perforation, tear or chemical damage of bladder following incomplete spontaneous abortion

     Laceration, perforation, tear or chemical damage of bowel following incomplete spontaneous abortion

     Laceration, perforation, tear or chemical damage of broad ligament following incomplete spontaneous abortion

     Laceration, perforation, tear or chemical damage of cervix following incomplete spontaneous abortion

     Laceration, perforation, tear or chemical damage of periurethral tissue following incomplete spontaneous abortion

     Laceration, perforation, tear or chemical damage of uterus following incomplete spontaneous abortion

     Laceration, perforation, tear or chemical damage of vagina following incomplete spontaneous abortion

O03.35   **Other venous complications following incomplete spontaneous abortion**

O03.36   **Cardiac arrest following incomplete spontaneous abortion**

O03.37   **Sepsis following incomplete spontaneous abortion**

     Use additional code (B95-B97), to identify infectious agent

     Use additional code (R65.2-) to identify severe sepsis, if applicable

     EXCLUDES 1   *septic or septicopyemic embolism following incomplete spontaneous abortion (O03.2)*

O03.38   **Urinary tract infection following incomplete spontaneous abortion**

     Cystitis following incomplete spontaneous abortion

O03.39   **Incomplete spontaneous abortion with other complications**

O03.4   **Incomplete spontaneous abortion without complication**

O03.5   **Genital tract and pelvic infection following complete or unspecified spontaneous abortion**

     Endometritis following complete or unspecified spontaneous abortion

     Oophoritis following complete or unspecified spontaneous abortion

     Parametritis following complete or unspecified spontaneous abortion

     Pelvic peritonitis following complete or unspecified spontaneous abortion

     Salpingitis following complete or unspecified spontaneous abortion

     Salpingo-oophoritis following complete or unspecified spontaneous abortion

     EXCLUDES 1   *sepsis following complete or unspecified spontaneous abortion (O03.87)*
urinary tract infection following complete or unspecified spontaneous abortion (O03.88)

O03.6   **Delayed or excessive hemorrhage following complete or unspecified spontaneous abortion**

     Afibrinogenemia following complete or unspecified spontaneous abortion

     Defibrination syndrome following complete or unspecified spontaneous abortion

     Hemolysis following complete or unspecified spontaneous abortion

     Intravascular coagulation following complete or unspecified spontaneous abortion

O03.7   **Embolism following complete or unspecified spontaneous abortion**

     Air embolism following complete or unspecified spontaneous abortion

     Amniotic fluid embolism following complete or unspecified spontaneous abortion

     Blood-clot embolism following complete or unspecified spontaneous abortion

     Embolism NOS following complete or unspecified spontaneous abortion

     Fat embolism following complete or unspecified spontaneous abortion

     Pulmonary embolism following complete or unspecified spontaneous abortion

     Pyemic embolism following complete or unspecified spontaneous abortion

     Septic or septicopyemic embolism following complete or unspecified spontaneous abortion

     Soap embolism following complete or unspecified spontaneous abortion

√5ᵗʰ   **O03.8**   **Other and unspecified complications following complete or unspecified spontaneous abortion**

O03.80   **Unspecified complication following complete or unspecified spontaneous abortion**

O03.81   **Shock following complete or unspecified spontaneous abortion**

     Circulatory collapse following complete or unspecified spontaneous abortion

     Shock (postprocedural) following complete or unspecified spontaneous abortion

     EXCLUDES 1   *shock due to infection following complete or unspecified spontaneous abortion (O03.87)*

O03.82   **Renal failure following complete or unspecified spontaneous abortion**

     Kidney failure (acute) following complete or unspecified spontaneous abortion

     Oliguria following complete or unspecified spontaneous abortion

     Renal shutdown following complete or unspecified spontaneous abortion

     Renal tubular necrosis following complete or unspecified spontaneous abortion

     Uremia following complete or unspecified spontaneous abortion

O03.83   **Metabolic disorder following complete or unspecified spontaneous abortion**

O03.84   **Damage to pelvic organs following complete or unspecified spontaneous abortion**

     Laceration, perforation, tear or chemical damage of bladder following complete or unspecified spontaneous abortion

     Laceration, perforation, tear or chemical damage of bowel following complete or unspecified spontaneous abortion

     Laceration, perforation, tear or chemical damage of broad ligament following complete or unspecified spontaneous abortion

     Laceration, perforation, tear or chemical damage of cervix following complete or unspecified spontaneous abortion

     Laceration, perforation, tear or chemical damage of periurethral tissue following complete or unspecified spontaneous abortion

     Laceration, perforation, tear or chemical damage of uterus following complete or unspecified spontaneous abortion

     Laceration, perforation, tear or chemical damage of vagina following complete or unspecified spontaneous abortion

O03.85   **Other venous complications following complete or unspecified spontaneous abortion**

O03.86   **Cardiac arrest following complete or unspecified spontaneous abortion**

O03.87 Sepsis following complete or unspecified spontaneous abortion
Use additional code (B95-B97), to identify infectious agent
Use additional code (R65.2-) to identify severe sepsis, if applicable
EXCLUDES 1 septic or septicopyemic embolism following complete or unspecified spontaneous abortion (O03.7)

O03.88 Urinary tract infection following complete or unspecified spontaneous abortion
Cystitis following complete or unspecified spontaneous abortion

O03.89 Complete or unspecified spontaneous abortion with other complications

O03.9 Complete or unspecified spontaneous abortion without complication
Miscarriage NOS
Spontaneous abortion NOS

☑4th **O04 Complications following (induced) termination of pregnancy**
INCLUDES complications following (induced) termination of pregnancy
EXCLUDES 1 encounter for elective termination of pregnancy, uncomplicated (Z33.2)
failed attempted termination of pregnancy (O07-)

O04.5 Genital tract and pelvic infection following (induced) termination of pregnancy
Endometritis following (induced) termination of pregnancy
Oophoritis following (induced) termination of pregnancy
Parametritis following (induced) termination of pregnancy
Pelvic peritonitis following (induced) termination of pregnancy
Salpingitis following (induced) termination of pregnancy
Salpingo-oophoritis following (induced) termination of pregnancy
EXCLUDES 1 sepsis following (induced) termination of pregnancy (O04.87)
urinary tract infection following (induced) termination of pregnancy (O04.88)

O04.6 Delayed or excessive hemorrhage following (induced) termination of pregnancy
Afibrinogenemia following (induced) termination of pregnancy
Defibrination syndrome following (induced) termination of pregnancy
Hemolysis following (induced) termination of pregnancy
Intravascular coagulation following (induced) termination of pregnancy

O04.7 Embolism following (induced) termination of pregnancy
Air embolism following (induced) termination of pregnancy
Amniotic fluid embolism following (induced) termination of pregnancy
Blood-clot embolism following (induced) termination of pregnancy
Embolism NOS following (induced) termination of pregnancy
Fat embolism following (induced) termination of pregnancy
Pulmonary embolism following (induced) termination of pregnancy
Pyemic embolism following (induced) termination of pregnancy
Septic or septicopyemic embolism following (induced) termination of pregnancy
Soap embolism following (induced) termination of pregnancy

☑5th **O04.8 (Induced) termination of pregnancy with other and unspecified complications**

O04.80 (Induced) termination of pregnancy with unspecified complications

O04.81 Shock following (induced) termination of pregnancy
Circulatory collapse following (induced) termination of pregnancy
Shock (postprocedural) following (induced) termination of pregnancy
EXCLUDES 1 shock due to infection following (induced) termination of pregnancy (O04.87)

O04.82 Renal failure following (induced) termination of pregnancy
Kidney failure (acute) following (induced) termination of pregnancy
Oliguria following (induced) termination of pregnancy
Renal shutdown following (induced) termination of pregnancy
Renal tubular necrosis following (induced) termination of pregnancy
Uremia following (induced) termination of pregnancy

O04.83 Metabolic disorder following (induced) termination of pregnancy

O04.84 Damage to pelvic organs following (induced) termination of pregnancy
Laceration, perforation, tear or chemical damage of bladder following (induced) termination of pregnancy
Laceration, perforation, tear or chemical damage of bowel following (induced) termination of pregnancy
Laceration, perforation, tear or chemical damage of broad ligament following (induced) termination of pregnancy
Laceration, perforation, tear or chemical damage of cervix following (induced) termination of pregnancy
Laceration, perforation, tear or chemical damage of periurethral tissue following (induced) termination of pregnancy
Laceration, perforation, tear or chemical damage of uterus following (induced) termination of pregnancy
Laceration, perforation, tear or chemical damage of vagina following (induced) termination of pregnancy

O04.85 Other venous complications following (induced) termination of pregnancy

O04.86 Cardiac arrest following (induced) termination of pregnancy

O04.87 Sepsis following (induced) termination of pregnancy
Use additional code (B95-B97), to identify infectious agent
Use additional code (R65.2-) to identify severe sepsis, if applicable
EXCLUDES 1 septic or septicopyemic embolism following (induced) termination of pregnancy (O04.7)

O04.88 Urinary tract infection following (induced) termination of pregnancy
Cystitis following (induced) termination of pregnancy

O04.89 (Induced) termination of pregnancy with other complications

☑4th **O07 Failed attempted termination of pregnancy**
INCLUDES failure of attempted induction of termination of pregnancy
incomplete elective abortion
EXCLUDES 1 incomplete spontaneous abortion (O03.0-)

O07.0 Genital tract and pelvic infection following failed attempted termination of pregnancy
Endometritis following failed attempted termination of pregnancy
Oophoritis following failed attempted termination of pregnancy
Parametritis following failed attempted termination of pregnancy
Pelvic peritonitis following failed attempted termination of pregnancy
Salpingitis following failed attempted termination of pregnancy
Salpingo-oophoritis following failed attempted termination of pregnancy
EXCLUDES 1 sepsis following failed attempted termination of pregnancy (O07.37)
urinary tract infection following failed attempted termination of pregnancy (O07.38)

O07.1   Delayed or excessive hemorrhage following failed attempted termination of pregnancy

Afibrinogenemia following failed attempted termination of pregnancy

Defibrination syndrome following failed attempted termination of pregnancy

Hemolysis following failed attempted termination of pregnancy

Intravascular coagulation following failed attempted termination of pregnancy

O07.2   Embolism following failed attempted termination of pregnancy

Air embolism following failed attempted termination of pregnancy

Amniotic fluid embolism following failed attempted termination of pregnancy

Blood-clot embolism following failed attempted termination of pregnancy

Embolism NOS following failed attempted termination of pregnancy

Fat embolism following failed attempted termination of pregnancy

Pulmonary embolism following failed attempted termination of pregnancy

Pyemic embolism following failed attempted termination of pregnancy

Septic or septicopyemic embolism following failed attempted termination of pregnancy

Soap embolism following failed attempted termination of pregnancy

☑5ᵗʰ O07.3   Failed attempted termination of pregnancy with other and unspecified complications

O07.30   Failed attempted termination of pregnancy with unspecified complications

O07.31   Shock following failed attempted termination of pregnancy

Circulatory collapse following failed attempted termination of pregnancy

Shock (postprocedural) following failed attempted termination of pregnancy

EXCLUDES 1   shock due to infection following failed attempted termination of pregnancy (O07.37)

O07.32   Renal failure following failed attempted termination of pregnancy

Kidney failure (acute) following failed attempted termination of pregnancy

Oliguria following failed attempted termination of pregnancy

Renal shutdown following failed attempted termination of pregnancy

Renal tubular necrosis following failed attempted termination of pregnancy

Uremia following failed attempted termination of pregnancy

O07.33   Metabolic disorder following failed attempted termination of pregnancy

O07.34   Damage to pelvic organs following failed attempted termination of pregnancy

Laceration, perforation, tear or chemical damage of bladder following failed attempted termination of pregnancy

Laceration, perforation, tear or chemical damage of bowel following failed attempted termination of pregnancy

Laceration, perforation, tear or chemical damage of broad ligament following failed attempted termination of pregnancy

Laceration, perforation, tear or chemical damage of cervix following failed attempted termination of pregnancy

Laceration, perforation, tear or chemical damage of periurethral tissue following failed attempted termination of pregnancy

Laceration, perforation, tear or chemical damage of uterus following failed attempted termination of pregnancy

Laceration, perforation, tear or chemical damage of vagina following failed attempted termination of pregnancy

O07.35   Other venous complications following failed attempted termination of pregnancy

O07.36   Cardiac arrest following failed attempted termination of pregnancy

O07.37   Sepsis following failed attempted termination of pregnancy

Use additional code (B95-B97), to identify infectious agent

Use additional code (R65.2-) to identify severe sepsis, if applicable

EXCLUDES 1   septic or septicopyemic embolism following failed attempted termination of pregnancy (O07.2)

O07.38   Urinary tract infection following failed attempted termination of pregnancy

Cystitis following failed attempted termination of pregnancy

O07.39   Failed attempted termination of pregnancy with other complications

O07.4   Failed attempted termination of pregnancy without complication

☑4ᵗʰ O08   Complications following ectopic and molar pregnancy

This category is for use with categories O00-O02 to identify any associated complications

O08.0   Genital tract and pelvic infection following ectopic and molar pregnancy

Endometritis following ectopic and molar pregnancy

Oophoritis following ectopic and molar pregnancy

Parametritis following ectopic and molar pregnancy

Pelvic peritonitis following ectopic and molar pregnancy

Salpingitis following ectopic and molar pregnancy

Salpingo-oophoritis following ectopic and molar pregnancy

EXCLUDES 1   sepsis following ectopic and molar pregnancy (O08.82)

urinary tract infection (O08.83)

O08.1   Delayed or excessive hemorrhage following ectopic and molar pregnancy

Afibrinogenemia following ectopic and molar pregnancy

Defibrination syndrome following ectopic and molar pregnancy

Hemolysis following ectopic and molar pregnancy

Intravascular coagulation following ectopic and molar pregnancy

EXCLUDES 1   delayed or excessive hemorrhage due to incomplete abortion (O03.1)

O08.2   Embolism following ectopic and molar pregnancy

Air embolism following ectopic and molar pregnancy

Amniotic fluid embolism following ectopic and molar pregnancy

Blood-clot embolism following ectopic and molar pregnancy

Embolism NOS following ectopic and molar pregnancy

Fat embolism following ectopic and molar pregnancy

Pulmonary embolism following ectopic and molar pregnancy

Pyemic embolism following ectopic and molar pregnancy

Septic or septicopyemic embolism following ectopic and molar pregnancy

Soap embolism following ectopic and molar pregnancy

O08.3   Shock following ectopic and molar pregnancy

Circulatory collapse following ectopic and molar pregnancy

Shock (postprocedural) following ectopic and molar pregnancy

EXCLUDES 1   shock due to infection following ectopic and molar pregnancy (O08.82)

O08.4   Renal failure following ectopic and molar pregnancy

Kidney failure (acute) following ectopic and molar pregnancy

Oliguria following ectopic and molar pregnancy

Renal shutdown following ectopic and molar pregnancy

Renal tubular necrosis following ectopic and molar pregnancy

Uremia following ectopic and molar pregnancy

O08.5   Metabolic disorders following an ectopic and molar pregnancy

---

EXCLUDES 1   Not coded here   *EXCLUDES 2*   Not included here   ***Manifestation Code***

O08.6 **Damage to pelvic organs and tissues following an ectopic and molar pregnancy**
Laceration, perforation, tear or chemical damage of bladder following an ectopic and molar pregnancy
Laceration, perforation, tear or chemical damage of bowel following an ectopic and molar pregnancy
Laceration, perforation, tear or chemical damage of broad ligament following an ectopic and molar pregnancy
Laceration, perforation, tear or chemical damage of cervix following an ectopic and molar pregnancy
Laceration, perforation, tear or chemical damage of periurethral tissue following an ectopic and molar pregnancy
Laceration, perforation, tear or chemical damage of uterus following an ectopic and molar pregnancy
Laceration, perforation, tear or chemical damage of vagina following an ectopic and molar pregnancy

O08.7 **Other venous complications following an ectopic and molar pregnancy**

✓5th **O08.8** **Other complications following an ectopic and molar pregnancy**

  O08.81 **Cardiac arrest following an ectopic and molar pregnancy**

  O08.82 **Sepsis following ectopic and molar pregnancy**
Use additional code (B95-B97), to identify infectious agent
Use additional code (R65.2-) to identify severe sepsis, if applicable
EXCLUDES 1 *septic or septicopyemic embolism following ectopic and molar pregnancy (O08.2)*

  O08.83 **Urinary tract infection following an ectopic and molar pregnancy**
Cystitis following an ectopic and molar pregnancy

  O08.89 **Other complications following an ectopic and molar pregnancy**

O08.9 **Unspecified complication following an ectopic and molar pregnancy**

Supervision of high risk pregnancy (O09)

✓4th **O09** **Supervision of high risk pregnancy**

✓5th **O09.0** **Supervision of pregnancy with history of infertility**

  O09.00 **Supervision of pregnancy with history of infertility, unspecified trimester**

  O09.01 **Supervision of pregnancy with history of infertility, first trimester**

  O09.02 **Supervision of pregnancy with history of infertility, second trimester**

  O09.03 **Supervision of pregnancy with history of infertility, third trimester**

✓5th **O09.1** **Supervision of pregnancy with history of ectopic or molar pregnancy**

  O09.10 **Supervision of pregnancy with history of ectopic or molar pregnancy, unspecified trimester**

  O09.11 **Supervision of pregnancy with history of ectopic or molar pregnancy, first trimester**

  O09.12 **Supervision of pregnancy with history of ectopic or molar pregnancy, second trimester**

  O09.13 **Supervision of pregnancy with history of ectopic or molar pregnancy, third trimester**

✓5th **O09.2** **Supervision of pregnancy with other poor reproductive or obstetric history**
EXCLUDES 2 *pregnancy care for patient with history of recurrent pregnancy loss (O26.2-)*

  ✓6th **O09.21** **Supervision of pregnancy with history of pre-term labor**

    O09.211 **Supervision of pregnancy with history of pre-term labor, first trimester**

    O09.212 **Supervision of pregnancy with history of pre-term labor, second trimester**

    O09.213 **Supervision of pregnancy with history of pre-term labor, third trimester**

    O09.219 **Supervision of pregnancy with history of pre-term labor, unspecified trimester**

  ✓6th **O09.29** **Supervision of pregnancy with other poor reproductive or obstetric history**
Supervision of pregnancy with history of neonatal death
Supervision of pregnancy with history of stillbirth

    O09.291 **Supervision of pregnancy with other poor reproductive or obstetric history, first trimester**

    O09.292 **Supervision of pregnancy with other poor reproductive or obstetric history, second trimester**

    O09.293 **Supervision of pregnancy with other poor reproductive or obstetric history, third trimester**

    O09.299 **Supervision of pregnancy with other poor reproductive or obstetric history, unspecified trimester**

✓5th **O09.3** **Supervision of pregnancy with insufficient antenatal care**
Supervision of concealed pregnancy
Supervision of hidden pregnancy

  O09.30 **Supervision of pregnancy with insufficient antenatal care, unspecified trimester**

  O09.31 **Supervision of pregnancy with insufficient antenatal care, first trimester**

  O09.32 **Supervision of pregnancy with insufficient antenatal care, second trimester**

  O09.33 **Supervision of pregnancy with insufficient antenatal care, third trimester**

✓5th **O09.4** **Supervision of pregnancy with grand multiparity**

  O09.40 **Supervision of pregnancy with grand multiparity, unspecified trimester**

  O09.41 **Supervision of pregnancy with grand multiparity, first trimester**

  O09.42 **Supervision of pregnancy with grand multiparity, second trimester**

  O09.43 **Supervision of pregnancy with grand multiparity, third trimester**

✓5th **O09.5** **Supervision of elderly primigravida and multigravida**
Pregnancy for a female 35 years and older at expected date of delivery

  ✓6th **O09.51** **Supervision of elderly primigravida**

    O09.511 **Supervision of elderly primigravida, first trimester**

    O09.512 **Supervision of elderly primigravida, second trimester**

    O09.513 **Supervision of elderly primigravida, third trimester**

    O09.519 **Supervision of elderly primigravida, unspecified trimester**

  ✓6th **O09.52** **Supervision of elderly multigravida**

    O09.521 **Supervision of elderly multigravida, first trimester**

    O09.522 **Supervision of elderly multigravida, second trimester**

    O09.523 **Supervision of elderly multigravida, third trimester**

    O09.529 **Supervision of elderly multigravida, unspecified trimester**

✓5th **O09.6** **Supervision of young primigravida and multigravida**
Supervision of pregnancy for a female less than 16 years old at expected date of delivery

  ✓6th **O09.61** **Supervision of young primigravida**

    O09.611 **Supervision of young primigravida, first trimester**

    O09.612 **Supervision of young primigravida, second trimester**

    O09.613 **Supervision of young primigravida, third trimester**

    O09.619 **Supervision of young primigravida, unspecified trimester**

  ✓6th **O09.62** **Supervision of young multigravida**

    O09.621 **Supervision of young multigravida, first trimester**

    O09.622 **Supervision of young multigravida, second trimester**

    O09.623 **Supervision of young multigravida, third trimester**

    O09.629 **Supervision of young multigravida, unspecified trimester**

✓5th **O09.7** **Supervision of high risk pregnancy due to social problems**

  O09.70 **Supervision of high risk pregnancy due to social problems, unspecified trimester**

☑ Appropriate additional character required   ✓x7th Requires 7th character, placeholder x must fill empty characters

Pregnancy, Childbirth and the Puerperium

O09.71 Supervision of high risk pregnancy due to social problems, first trimester

O09.72 Supervision of high risk pregnancy due to social problems, second trimester

O09.73 Supervision of high risk pregnancy due to social problems, third trimester

✓5th **O09.8** Supervision of other high risk pregnancies

✓6th **O09.81** Supervision of pregnancy resulting from assisted reproductive technology
Supervision of pregnancy resulting from in-vitro fertilization

O09.811 Supervision of pregnancy resulting from assisted reproductive technology, first trimester

O09.812 Supervision of pregnancy resulting from assisted reproductive technology, second trimester

O09.813 Supervision of pregnancy resulting from assisted reproductive technology, third trimester

O09.819 Supervision of pregnancy resulting from assisted reproductive technology, unspecified trimester

✓6th **O09.82** Supervision of pregnancy with history of in utero procedure during previous pregnancy

O09.821 Supervision of pregnancy with history of in utero procedure during previous pregnancy, first trimester

O09.822 Supervision of pregnancy with history of in utero procedure during previous pregnancy, second trimester

O09.823 Supervision of pregnancy with history of in utero procedure during previous pregnancy, third trimester

O09.829 Supervision of pregnancy with history of in utero procedure during previous pregnancy, unspecified trimester

EXCLUDES 1 *supervision of pregnancy affected by in utero procedure during current pregnancy (O35.7)*

✓6th **O09.89** Supervision of other high risk pregnancies

O09.891 Supervision of other high risk pregnancies, first trimester

O09.892 Supervision of other high risk pregnancies, second trimester

O09.893 Supervision of other high risk pregnancies, third trimester

O09.899 Supervision of other high risk pregnancies, unspecified trimester

✓5th **O09.9** Supervision of high risk pregnancy, unspecified

O09.90 Supervision of high risk pregnancy, unspecified, unspecified trimester

O09.91 Supervision of high risk pregnancy, unspecified, first trimester

O09.92 Supervision of high risk pregnancy, unspecified, second trimester

O09.93 Supervision of high risk pregnancy, unspecified, third trimester

Edema, proteinuria and hypertensive disorders in pregnancy, childbirth and the puerperium (O10-O16)

✓4th **O10** Pre-existing hypertension complicating pregnancy, childbirth and the puerperium
Pre-existing hypertension with pre-existing proteinuria complicating pregnancy, childbirth and the puerperium

EXCLUDES 2 *pre-existing hypertension with superimposed pre-eclampsia complicating pregnancy, childbirth and the puerperium (O11.-)*

✓5th **O10.0** Pre-existing essential hypertension complicating pregnancy, childbirth and the puerperium
Any condition in I10 specified as a reason for obstetric care during pregnancy, childbirth or the puerperium

✓6th **O10.01** Pre-existing essential hypertension complicating pregnancy,

O10.011 Pre-existing essential hypertension complicating pregnancy, first trimester

O10.012 Pre-existing essential hypertension complicating pregnancy, second trimester

O10.013 Pre-existing essential hypertension complicating pregnancy, third trimester

O10.019 Pre-existing essential hypertension complicating pregnancy, unspecified trimester

O10.02 Pre-existing essential hypertension complicating childbirth

O10.03 Pre-existing essential hypertension complicating the puerperium

✓5th **O10.1** Pre-existing hypertensive heart disease complicating pregnancy, childbirth and the puerperium
Any condition in I11 specified as a reason for obstetric care during pregnancy, childbirth or the puerperium
Use additional code from I11 to identify the type of hypertensive heart disease

✓6th **O10.11** Pre-existing hypertensive heart disease complicating pregnancy

O10.111 Pre-existing hypertensive heart disease complicating pregnancy, first trimester

O10.112 Pre-existing hypertensive heart disease complicating pregnancy, second trimester

O10.113 Pre-existing hypertensive heart disease complicating pregnancy, third trimester

O10.119 Pre-existing hypertensive heart disease complicating pregnancy, unspecified trimester

O10.12 Pre-existing hypertensive heart disease complicating childbirth

O10.13 Pre-existing hypertensive heart disease complicating the puerperium

✓5th **O10.2** Pre-existing hypertensive chronic kidney disease complicating pregnancy, childbirth and the puerperium
Any condition in I12 specified as a reason for obstetric care during pregnancy, childbirth or the puerperium
Use additional code from I12 to identify the type of hypertensive chronic kidney disease

✓6th **O10.21** Pre-existing hypertensive chronic kidney disease complicating pregnancy

O10.211 Pre-existing hypertensive chronic kidney disease complicating pregnancy, first trimester

O10.212 Pre-existing hypertensive chronic kidney disease complicating pregnancy, second trimester

O10.213 Pre-existing hypertensive chronic kidney disease complicating pregnancy, third trimester

O10.219 Pre-existing hypertensive chronic kidney disease complicating pregnancy, unspecified trimester

O10.22 Pre-existing hypertensive chronic kidney disease complicating childbirth

O10.23 Pre-existing hypertensive chronic kidney disease complicating the puerperium

✓5th **O10.3** Pre-existing hypertensive heart and chronic kidney disease complicating pregnancy, childbirth and the puerperium
Any condition in I13 specified as a reason for obstetric care during pregnancy, childbirth or the puerperium
Use additional code from I13 to identify the type of hypertensive heart and chronic kidney disease

✓6th **O10.31** Pre-existing hypertensive heart and chronic kidney disease complicating pregnancy

O10.311 Pre-existing hypertensive heart and chronic kidney disease complicating pregnancy, first trimester

O10.312 Pre-existing hypertensive heart and chronic kidney disease complicating pregnancy, second trimester

O10.313 Pre-existing hypertensive heart and chronic kidney disease complicating pregnancy, third trimester

O10.319 Pre-existing hypertensive heart and chronic kidney disease complicating pregnancy, unspecified trimester

EXCLUDES 1 Not coded here   EXCLUDES 2 Not included here   *Manifestation Code*

© 2011 Ingenix

O10.32   Pre-existing hypertensive heart and chronic kidney disease complicating childbirth
O10.33   Pre-existing hypertensive heart and chronic kidney disease complicating the puerperium

✓5th O10.4 **Pre-existing secondary hypertension complicating pregnancy, childbirth and the puerperium**
Any condition in I15 specified as a reason for obstetric care during pregnancy, childbirth or the puerperium
Use additional code from I15 to identify the type of secondary hypertension

✓6th O10.41 **Pre-existing secondary hypertension complicating pregnancy**
O10.411   Pre-existing secondary hypertension complicating pregnancy, first trimester
O10.412   Pre-existing secondary hypertension complicating pregnancy, second trimester
O10.413   Pre-existing secondary hypertension complicating pregnancy, third trimester
O10.419   Pre-existing secondary hypertension complicating pregnancy, unspecified trimester

O10.42   Pre-existing secondary hypertension complicating childbirth
O10.43   Pre-existing secondary hypertension complicating the puerperium

✓5th O10.9 **Unspecified pre-existing hypertension complicating pregnancy, childbirth and the puerperium**

✓6th O10.91 **Unspecified pre-existing hypertension complicating pregnancy**
O10.911   Unspecified pre-existing hypertension complicating pregnancy, first trimester
O10.912   Unspecified pre-existing hypertension complicating pregnancy, second trimester
O10.913   Unspecified pre-existing hypertension complicating pregnancy, third trimester
O10.919   Unspecified pre-existing hypertension complicating pregnancy, unspecified trimester

O10.92   Unspecified pre-existing hypertension complicating childbirth
O10.93   Unspecified pre-existing hypertension complicating the puerperium

✓4th O11 **Pre-existing hypertension with pre-eclampsia**
Conditions in O10 complicated by pre-eclampsia
Pre-eclampsia superimposed pre-existing hypertension
Use additional code from O10 to identify the type of hypertension
O11.1   Pre-existing hypertension with pre-eclampsia, first trimester
O11.2   Pre-existing hypertension with pre-eclampsia, second trimester
O11.3   Pre-existing hypertension with pre-eclampsia, third trimester
O11.9   Pre-existing hypertension with pre-eclampsia, unspecified trimester

✓4th O12 **Gestational [pregnancy-induced] edema and proteinuria without hypertension**

✓5th O12.0 **Gestational edema**
O12.00   Gestational edema, unspecified trimester
O12.01   Gestational edema, first trimester
O12.02   Gestational edema, second trimester
O12.03   Gestational edema, third trimester

✓5th O12.1 **Gestational proteinuria**
O12.10   Gestational proteinuria, unspecified trimester
O12.11   Gestational proteinuria, first trimester
O12.12   Gestational proteinuria, second trimester
O12.13   Gestational proteinuria, third trimester

✓5th O12.2 **Gestational edema with proteinuria**
O12.20   Gestational edema with proteinuria, unspecified trimester
O12.21   Gestational edema with proteinuria, first trimester
O12.22   Gestational edema with proteinuria, second trimester
O12.23   Gestational edema with proteinuria, third trimester

✓4th O13 **Gestational [pregnancy-induced] hypertension without significant proteinuria**
INCLUDES   gestational hypertension NOS
O13.1   Gestational [pregnancy-induced] hypertension without significant proteinuria, first trimester
O13.2   Gestational [pregnancy-induced] hypertension without significant proteinuria, second trimester
O13.3   Gestational [pregnancy-induced] hypertension without significant proteinuria, third trimester
O13.9   Gestational [pregnancy-induced] hypertension without significant proteinuria, unspecified trimester

✓4th O14 **Pre-eclampsia**
EXCLUDES 1   pre-existing hypertension with pre-eclampsia (O11)

✓5th O14.0 **Mild to moderate pre-eclampsia**
O14.00   Mild to moderate pre-eclampsia, unspecified trimester
O14.02   Mild to moderate pre-eclampsia, second trimester
O14.03   Mild to moderate pre-eclampsia, third trimester

✓5th O14.1 **Severe pre-eclampsia**
EXCLUDES 1   HELLP syndrome (O14.2-)
O14.10   Severe pre-eclampsia, unspecified trimester
O14.12   Severe pre-eclampsia, second trimester
O14.13   Severe pre-eclampsia, third trimester

✓5th O14.2 **HELLP syndrome (HELLP)**
Severe pre-eclampsia with hemolysis, elevated liver enzymes and low platelet count
O14.20   HELLP syndrome (HELLP), unspecified trimester
O14.22   HELLP syndrome (HELLP), second trimester
O14.23   HELLP syndrome (HELLP), third trimester

✓5th O14.9 **Unspecified pre-eclampsia**
O14.90   Unspecified pre-eclampsia, unspecified trimester
O14.92   Unspecified pre-eclampsia, second trimester
O14.93   Unspecified pre-eclampsia, third trimester

✓4th O15 **Eclampsia**
INCLUDES   convulsions following conditions in O10-O14 and O16

✓5th O15.0 **Eclampsia in pregnancy**
O15.00   Eclampsia in pregnancy, unspecified trimester
O15.02   Eclampsia in pregnancy, second trimester
O15.03   Eclampsia in pregnancy, third trimester

O15.1   Eclampsia in labor
O15.2   Eclampsia in the puerperium
O15.9   Eclampsia, unspecified as to time period
Eclampsia NOS

✓4th O16 **Unspecified maternal hypertension**
O16.1   Unspecified maternal hypertension, first trimester
O16.2   Unspecified maternal hypertension, second trimester
O16.3   Unspecified maternal hypertension, third trimester
O16.9   Unspecified maternal hypertension, unspecified trimester

Other maternal disorders predominantly related to pregnancy (O20-O29)

EXCLUDES 2   maternal care related to the fetus and amniotic cavity and possible delivery problems (O30-O48)
maternal diseases classifiable elsewhere but complicating pregnancy, labor and delivery, and the puerperium (O98-O99)

✓4th O20 **Hemorrhage in early pregnancy**
Hemorrhage before completion of 20 weeks gestation
EXCLUDES 1   pregnancy with abortive outcome (O00-O08)
O20.0   **Threatened abortion**
Hemorrhage specified as due to threatened abortion
O20.8   **Other hemorrhage in early pregnancy**
O20.9   **Hemorrhage in early pregnancy, unspecified**

✓4th O21 **Excessive vomiting in pregnancy**
O21.0   **Mild hyperemesis gravidarum**
Hyperemesis gravidarum, mild or unspecified, starting before the end of the 20th week of gestation

---

☑ Appropriate additional character required   ✓x7th Requires 7th character, placeholder x must fill empty characters

O21.1   **Hyperemesis gravidarum with metabolic disturbance**

Hyperemesis gravidarum, starting before the end of the 20th week of gestation, with metabolic disturbance such as carbohydrate depletion

Hyperemesis gravidarum, starting before the end of the 20th week of gestation, with metabolic disturbance such as dehydration

Hyperemesis gravidarum, starting before the end of the 20th week of gestation, with metabolic disturbance such as electrolyte imbalance

O21.2   **Late vomiting of pregnancy**

Excessive vomiting starting after 20 completed weeks of gestation

O21.8   **Other vomiting complicating pregnancy**

Vomiting due to diseases classified elsewhere, complicating pregnancy

Use additional code, to identify cause

O21.9   **Vomiting of pregnancy, unspecified**

✓4th **O22**   **Venous complications in pregnancy**

> EXCLUDES 1   venous complications of:
> abortion NOS (O03.9)
> ectopic or molar pregnancy (O08.7)
> failed attempted abortion (O07.35)
> induced abortion (O04.85)
> spontaneous abortion (O03.89)

> EXCLUDES 2   obstetric pulmonary embolism (O88-)
> venous complications of childbirth and the puerperium (O87-)

✓5th **O22.0**   **Varicose veins of lower extremity in pregnancy**

Varicose veins NOS in pregnancy

O22.00   **Varicose veins of lower extremity in pregnancy, unspecified trimester**

O22.01   **Varicose veins of lower extremity in pregnancy, first trimester**

O22.02   **Varicose veins of lower extremity in pregnancy, second trimester**

O22.03   **Varicose veins of lower extremity in pregnancy, third trimester**

✓5th **O22.1**   **Genital varices in pregnancy**

Perineal varices in pregnancy
Vaginal varices in pregnancy
Vulval varices in pregnancy

O22.10   **Genital varices in pregnancy, unspecified trimester**

O22.11   **Genital varices in pregnancy, first trimester**

O22.12   **Genital varices in pregnancy, second trimester**

O22.13   **Genital varices in pregnancy, third trimester**

✓5th **O22.2**   **Superficial thrombophlebitis in pregnancy**

Phlebitis in pregnancy NOS
Thrombophlebitis of legs in pregnancy
Thrombosis in pregnancy NOS

Use additional code to identify the superficial thrombophlebitis (I80.0-)

O22.20   **Superficial thrombophlebitis in pregnancy, unspecified trimester**

O22.21   **Superficial thrombophlebitis in pregnancy, first trimester**

O22.22   **Superficial thrombophlebitis in pregnancy, second trimester**

O22.23   **Superficial thrombophlebitis in pregnancy, third trimester**

✓5th **O22.3**   **Deep phlebothrombosis in pregnancy**

Deep vein thrombosis, antepartum

Use additional code to identify the deep vein thrombosis (I82.4-, I82.5-, I82.62-, I82.72-)

Use additional code, if applicable, for associated long-term (current) use of anticoagulants (Z79.01)

O22.30   **Deep phlebothrombosis in pregnancy, unspecified trimester**

O22.31   **Deep phlebothrombosis in pregnancy, first trimester**

O22.32   **Deep phlebothrombosis in pregnancy, second trimester**

O22.33   **Deep phlebothrombosis in pregnancy, third trimester**

✓5th **O22.4**   **Hemorrhoids in pregnancy**

O22.40   **Hemorrhoids in pregnancy, unspecified trimester**

O22.41   **Hemorrhoids in pregnancy, first trimester**

O22.42   **Hemorrhoids in pregnancy, second trimester**

O22.43   **Hemorrhoids in pregnancy, third trimester**

✓5th **O22.5**   **Cerebral venous thrombosis in pregnancy**

Cerebrovenous sinus thrombosis in pregnancy

O22.50   **Cerebral venous thrombosis in pregnancy, unspecified trimester**

O22.51   **Cerebral venous thrombosis in pregnancy, first trimester**

O22.52   **Cerebral venous thrombosis in pregnancy, second trimester**

O22.53   **Cerebral venous thrombosis in pregnancy, third trimester**

✓5th **O22.8**   **Other venous complications in pregnancy**

✓6th **O22.8x**   **Other venous complications in pregnancy**

O22.8x1   **Other venous complications in pregnancy, first trimester**

O22.8x2   **Other venous complications in pregnancy, second trimester**

O22.8x3   **Other venous complications in pregnancy, third trimester**

O22.8x9   **Other venous complications in pregnancy, unspecified trimester**

✓5th **O22.9**   **Venous complication in pregnancy, unspecified**

Gestational phlebitis NOS
Gestational phlebopathy NOS
Gestational thrombosis NOS

O22.90   **Venous complication in pregnancy, unspecified, unspecified trimester**

O22.91   **Venous complication in pregnancy, unspecified, first trimester**

O22.92   **Venous complication in pregnancy, unspecified, second trimester**

O22.93   **Venous complication in pregnancy, unspecified, third trimester**

✓4th **O23**   **Infections of genitourinary tract in pregnancy**

Use additional code to identify organism (B95-, B96-)

✓5th **O23.0**   **Infections of kidney in pregnancy**

Pyelonephritis in pregnancy

O23.00   **Infections of kidney in pregnancy, unspecified trimester**

O23.01   **Infections of kidney in pregnancy, first trimester**

O23.02   **Infections of kidney in pregnancy, second trimester**

O23.03   **Infections of kidney in pregnancy, third trimester**

✓5th **O23.1**   **Infections of bladder in pregnancy**

O23.10   **Infections of bladder in pregnancy, unspecified trimester**

O23.11   **Infections of bladder in pregnancy, first trimester**

O23.12   **Infections of bladder in pregnancy, second trimester**

O23.13   **Infections of bladder in pregnancy, third trimester**

✓5th **O23.2**   **Infections of urethra in pregnancy**

O23.20   **Infections of urethra in pregnancy, unspecified trimester**

O23.21   **Infections of urethra in pregnancy, first trimester**

O23.22   **Infections of urethra in pregnancy, second trimester**

O23.23   **Infections of urethra in pregnancy, third trimester**

✓5th **O23.3**   **Infections of other parts of urinary tract in pregnancy**

O23.30   **Infections of other parts of urinary tract in pregnancy, unspecified trimester**

O23.31   **Infections of other parts of urinary tract in pregnancy, first trimester**

O23.32   **Infections of other parts of urinary tract in pregnancy, second trimester**

O23.33   **Infections of other parts of urinary tract in pregnancy, third trimester**

✓5th **O23.4**   **Unspecified infection of urinary tract in pregnancy**

O23.40   **Unspecified infection of urinary tract in pregnancy, unspecified trimester**

O23.41   **Unspecified infection of urinary tract in pregnancy, first trimester**

O23.42   **Unspecified infection of urinary tract in pregnancy, second trimester**

O23.43   **Unspecified infection of urinary tract in pregnancy, third trimester**

EXCLUDES 1   Not coded here   EXCLUDES 2   Not included here   *Manifestation Code*

☑5ᵗʰ **O23.5 Infections of the genital tract in pregnancy**
  ☑6ᵗʰ **O23.51 Infection of cervix in pregnancy**
        O23.511 Infections of cervix in pregnancy, first trimester
        O23.512 Infections of cervix in pregnancy, second trimester
        O23.513 Infections of cervix in pregnancy, third trimester
        O23.519 Infections of cervix in pregnancy, unspecified trimester
  ☑6ᵗʰ **O23.52 Salpingo-oophoritis in pregnancy**
        Oophoritis in pregnancy
        Salpingitis in pregnancy
        O23.521 Salpingo-oophoritis in pregnancy, first trimester
        O23.522 Salpingo-oophoritis in pregnancy, second trimester
        O23.523 Salpingo-oophoritis in pregnancy, third trimester
        O23.529 Salpingo-oophoritis in pregnancy, unspecified trimester
  ☑6ᵗʰ **O23.59 Infection of other part of genital tract in pregnancy**
        O23.591 Infection of other part of genital tract in pregnancy, first trimester
        O23.592 Infection of other part of genital tract in pregnancy, second trimester
        O23.593 Infection of other part of genital tract in pregnancy, third trimester
        O23.599 Infection of other part of genital tract in pregnancy, unspecified trimester
☑5ᵗʰ **O23.9 Unspecified genitourinary tract infection in pregnancy**
        Genitourinary tract Infection in pregnancy NOS
        O23.90 Unspecified genitourinary tract infection in pregnancy, unspecified trimester
        O23.91 Unspecified genitourinary tract infection in pregnancy, first trimester
        O23.92 Unspecified genitourinary tract infection in pregnancy, second trimester
        O23.93 Unspecified genitourinary tract infection in pregnancy, third trimester

☑4ᵗʰ **O24 Diabetes mellitus in pregnancy, childbirth, and the puerperium**
  ☑5ᵗʰ **O24.0 Pre-existing diabetes mellitus, type 1, in pregnancy, childbirth and the puerperium**
        Juvenile onset diabetes mellitus, in pregnancy, childbirth and the puerperium
        Ketosis-prone diabetes mellitus in pregnancy, childbirth and the puerperium
        Use additional code from category E10 to further identify any manifestations
    ☑6ᵗʰ **O24.01 Pre-existing diabetes mellitus, type 1, in pregnancy**
        O24.011 Pre-existing diabetes mellitus, type 1, in pregnancy, first trimester
        O24.012 Pre-existing diabetes mellitus, type 1, in pregnancy, second trimester
        O24.013 Pre-existing diabetes mellitus, type 1, in pregnancy, third trimester
        O24.019 Pre-existing diabetes mellitus, type 1, in pregnancy, unspecified trimester
    O24.02 Pre-existing diabetes mellitus, type 1, in childbirth
    O24.03 Pre-existing diabetes mellitus, type 1, in the puerperium
  ☑5ᵗʰ **O24.1 Pre-existing diabetes mellitus, type 2, in pregnancy, childbirth and the puerperium**
        Insulin-resistant diabetes mellitus in pregnancy, childbirth and the puerperium
        Use additional code (for):
          from category E11 to further identify any manifestations
          long-term (current) use of insulin (Z79.4)
    ☑6ᵗʰ **O24.11 Pre-existing diabetes mellitus, type 2, in pregnancy**
        O24.111 Pre-existing diabetes mellitus, type 2, in pregnancy, first trimester
        O24.112 Pre-existing diabetes mellitus, type 2, in pregnancy, second trimester
        O24.113 Pre-existing diabetes mellitus, type 2, in pregnancy, third trimester

        O24.119 Pre-existing diabetes mellitus, type 2, in pregnancy, unspecified trimester
    O24.12 Pre-existing diabetes mellitus, type 2, in childbirth
    O24.13 Pre-existing diabetes mellitus, type 2, in the puerperium
  ☑5ᵗʰ **O24.3 Unspecified pre-existing diabetes mellitus in pregnancy, childbirth and the puerperium**
        Use additional code (for):
          from category E11 to further identify any manifestation
          long-term (current) use of insulin (Z79.4)
    ☑6ᵗʰ **O24.31 Unspecified pre-existing diabetes mellitus in pregnancy**
        O24.311 Unspecified pre-existing diabetes mellitus in pregnancy, first trimester
        O24.312 Unspecified pre-existing diabetes mellitus in pregnancy, second trimester
        O24.313 Unspecified pre-existing diabetes mellitus in pregnancy, third trimester
        O24.319 Unspecified pre-existing diabetes mellitus in pregnancy, unspecified trimester
    O24.32 Unspecified pre-existing diabetes mellitus in childbirth
    O24.33 Unspecified pre-existing diabetes mellitus in the puerperium
  ☑5ᵗʰ **O24.4 Gestational diabetes mellitus**
        Diabetes mellitus arising in pregnancy
        Gestational diabetes mellitus NOS
    ☑6ᵗʰ **O24.41 Gestational diabetes mellitus in pregnancy**
        O24.410 Gestational diabetes mellitus in pregnancy, diet controlled
        O24.414 Gestational diabetes mellitus in pregnancy, insulin controlled
        O24.419 Gestational diabetes mellitus in pregnancy, unspecified control
    ☑6ᵗʰ **O24.42 Gestational diabetes mellitus in childbirth**
        O24.420 Gestational diabetes mellitus in childbirth, diet controlled
        O24.424 Gestational diabetes mellitus in childbirth, insulin controlled
        O24.429 Gestational diabetes mellitus in childbirth, unspecified control
    ☑6ᵗʰ **O24.43 Gestational diabetes mellitus in the puerperium**
        O24.430 Gestational diabetes mellitus in the puerperium, diet controlled
        O24.434 Gestational diabetes mellitus in the puerperium, insulin controlled
        O24.439 Gestational diabetes mellitus in the puerperium, unspecified control
  ☑5ᵗʰ **O24.8 Other pre-existing diabetes mellitus in pregnancy, childbirth, and the puerperium**
        Use additional code (for):
          from categories E08, E09 and E13 to further identify any manifestation
          long-term (current) use of insulin (Z79.4)
    ☑6ᵗʰ **O24.81 Other pre-existing diabetes mellitus in pregnancy**
        O24.811 Other pre-existing diabetes mellitus in pregnancy, first trimester
        O24.812 Other pre-existing diabetes mellitus in pregnancy, second trimester
        O24.813 Other pre-existing diabetes mellitus in pregnancy, third trimester
        O24.819 Other pre-existing diabetes mellitus in pregnancy, unspecified trimester
    O24.82 Other pre-existing diabetes mellitus in childbirth
    O24.83 Other pre-existing diabetes mellitus in the puerperium
  ☑5ᵗʰ **O24.9 Unspecified diabetes mellitus in pregnancy, childbirth and the puerperium**
        Use additional code for long-term (current) use of insulin (Z79.4)
    ☑6ᵗʰ **O24.91 Unspecified diabetes mellitus in pregnancy**
        O24.911 Unspecified diabetes mellitus in pregnancy, first trimester
        O24.912 Unspecified diabetes mellitus in pregnancy, second trimester
        O24.913 Unspecified diabetes mellitus in pregnancy, third trimester

---

☑ Appropriate additional character required   ☑x7ᵗʰ Requires 7th character, placeholder x must fill empty characters

Pregnancy, Childbirth and the Puerperium

O24.919–O26.879

O24.919   Unspecified diabetes mellitus in pregnancy, unspecified trimester

O24.92   Unspecified diabetes mellitus in childbirth

O24.93   Unspecified diabetes mellitus in the puerperium

✓4ᵗʰ **O25 Malnutrition in pregnancy, childbirth and the puerperium**

   ✓5ᵗʰ **O25.1 Malnutrition in pregnancy**

     O25.10   Malnutrition in pregnancy, unspecified trimester

     O25.11   Malnutrition in pregnancy, first trimester

     O25.12   Malnutrition in pregnancy, second trimester

     O25.13   Malnutrition in pregnancy, third trimester

   O25.2 Malnutrition in childbirth

   O25.3 Malnutrition in the puerperium

✓4ᵗʰ **O26 Maternal care for other conditions predominantly related to pregnancy**

   ✓5ᵗʰ **O26.0 Excessive weight gain in pregnancy**

     EXCLUDES 2   gestational edema (O12.0, O12.2)

     O26.00   Excessive weight gain in pregnancy, unspecified trimester

     O26.01   Excessive weight gain in pregnancy, first trimester

     O26.02   Excessive weight gain in pregnancy, second trimester

     O26.03   Excessive weight gain in pregnancy, third trimester

   ✓5ᵗʰ **O26.1 Low weight gain in pregnancy**

     O26.10   Low weight gain in pregnancy, unspecified trimester

     O26.11   Low weight gain in pregnancy, first trimester

     O26.12   Low weight gain in pregnancy, second trimester

     O26.13   Low weight gain in pregnancy, third trimester

   ✓5ᵗʰ **O26.2 Pregnancy care for patient with recurrent pregnancy loss**

     O26.20   Pregnancy care for patient with recurrent pregnancy loss, unspecified trimester

     O26.21   Pregnancy care for patient with recurrent pregnancy loss, first trimester

     O26.22   Pregnancy care for patient with recurrent pregnancy loss, second trimester

     O26.23   Pregnancy care for patient with recurrent pregnancy loss, third trimester

   ✓5ᵗʰ **O26.3 Retained intrauterine contraceptive device in pregnancy**

     O26.30   Retained intrauterine contraceptive device in pregnancy, unspecified trimester

     O26.31   Retained intrauterine contraceptive device in pregnancy, first trimester

     O26.32   Retained intrauterine contraceptive device in pregnancy, second trimester

     O26.33   Retained intrauterine contraceptive device in pregnancy, third trimester

   ✓5ᵗʰ **O26.4 Herpes gestationis**

     O26.40   Herpes gestationis, unspecified trimester

     O26.41   Herpes gestationis, first trimester

     O26.42   Herpes gestationis, second trimester

     O26.43   Herpes gestationis, third trimester

   ✓5ᵗʰ **O26.5 Maternal hypotension syndrome**

     Supine hypotensive syndrome

     O26.50   Maternal hypotension syndrome, unspecified trimester

     O26.51   Maternal hypotension syndrome, first trimester

     O26.52   Maternal hypotension syndrome, second trimester

     O26.53   Maternal hypotension syndrome, third trimester

   ✓5ᵗʰ **O26.6 Liver disorders in pregnancy, childbirth and the puerperium**

     Use additional code to identify the specific disorder

     EXCLUDES 2   hepatorenal syndrome following labor and delivery (O90.4)

     ✓6ᵗʰ O26.61   Liver disorders in pregnancy

       O26.611   Liver disorders in pregnancy, first trimester

       O26.612   Liver disorders in pregnancy, second trimester

       O26.613   Liver disorders in pregnancy, third trimester

       O26.619   Liver disorders in pregnancy, unspecified trimester

     O26.62   Liver disorders in childbirth

     O26.63   Liver disorders in the puerperium

   ✓5ᵗʰ **O26.7 Subluxation of symphysis (pubis) in pregnancy, childbirth and the puerperium**

     EXCLUDES 1   traumatic separation of symphysis (pubis) during childbirth (O71.6)

     ✓6ᵗʰ O26.71   Subluxation of symphysis (pubis) in pregnancy

       O26.711   Subluxation of symphysis (pubis) in pregnancy, first trimester

       O26.712   Subluxation of symphysis (pubis) in pregnancy, second trimester

       O26.713   Subluxation of symphysis (pubis) in pregnancy, third trimester

       O26.719   Subluxation of symphysis (pubis) in pregnancy, unspecified trimester

     O26.72   Subluxation of symphysis (pubis) in childbirth

     O26.73   Subluxation of symphysis (pubis) in the puerperium

   ✓5ᵗʰ **O26.8 Other specified pregnancy related conditions**

     ✓6ᵗʰ O26.81   Pregnancy related exhaustion and fatigue

       O26.811   Pregnancy related exhaustion and fatigue, first trimester

       O26.812   Pregnancy related exhaustion and fatigue, second trimester

       O26.813   Pregnancy related exhaustion and fatigue, third trimester

       O26.819   Pregnancy related exhaustion and fatigue, unspecified trimester

     ✓6ᵗʰ O26.82   Pregnancy related peripheral neuritis

       O26.821   Pregnancy related peripheral neuritis, first trimester

       O26.822   Pregnancy related peripheral neuritis, second trimester

       O26.823   Pregnancy related peripheral neuritis, third trimester

       O26.829   Pregnancy related peripheral neuritis, unspecified trimester

     ✓6ᵗʰ O26.83   Pregnancy related renal disease

       Use additional code to identify the specific disorder

       O26.831   Pregnancy related renal disease, first trimester

       O26.832   Pregnancy related renal disease, second trimester

       O26.833   Pregnancy related renal disease, third trimester

       O26.839   Pregnancy related renal disease, unspecified trimester

     ✓6ᵗʰ O26.84   Uterine size-date discrepancy complicating pregnancy

       EXCLUDES 1   encounter for suspected problem with fetal growth ruled out (Z03.74)

       O26.841   Uterine size-date discrepancy, first trimester

       O26.842   Uterine size-date discrepancy, second trimester

       O26.843   Uterine size-date discrepancy, third trimester

       O26.849   Uterine size-date discrepancy, unspecified trimester

     ✓6ᵗʰ O26.85   Spotting complicating pregnancy

       O26.851   Spotting complicating pregnancy, first trimester

       O26.852   Spotting complicating pregnancy, second trimester

       O26.853   Spotting complicating pregnancy, third trimester

       O26.859   Spotting complicating pregnancy, unspecified trimester

     O26.86   Pruritic urticarial papules and plaques of pregnancy (PUPPP)

       Polymorphic eruption of pregnancy

     ✓6ᵗʰ O26.87   Cervical shortening

       EXCLUDES 1   encounter for suspected cervical shortening ruled out (Z03.75)

       O26.872   Cervical shortening, second trimester

       O26.873   Cervical shortening, third trimester

       O26.879   Cervical shortening, unspecified trimester

EXCLUDES 1 Not coded here   *EXCLUDES 2* Not included here   **Manifestation Code**

☑6ᵗʰ **O26.89** Other specified pregnancy related conditions
  O26.891 Other specified pregnancy related conditions, first trimester
  O26.892 Other specified pregnancy related conditions, second trimester
  O26.893 Other specified pregnancy related conditions, third trimester
  O26.899 Other specified pregnancy related conditions, unspecified trimester

☑5ᵗʰ **O26.9** Pregnancy related conditions, unspecified
  O26.90 Pregnancy related conditions, unspecified, unspecified trimester
  O26.91 Pregnancy related conditions, unspecified, first trimester
  O26.92 Pregnancy related conditions, unspecified, second trimester
  O26.93 Pregnancy related conditions, unspecified, third trimester

☑4ᵗʰ **O28 Abnormal findings on antenatal screening of mother**
  EXCLUDES 1 *diagnostic findings classified elsewhere—see Alphabetical Index*
  O28.0 Abnormal hematological finding on antenatal screening of mother
  O28.1 Abnormal biochemical finding on antenatal screening of mother
  O28.2 Abnormal cytological finding on antenatal screening of mother
  O28.3 Abnormal ultrasonic finding on antenatal screening of mother
  O28.4 Abnormal radiological finding on antenatal screening of mother
  O28.5 Abnormal chromosomal and genetic finding on antenatal screening of mother
  O28.8 Other abnormal findings on antenatal screening of mother
  O28.9 Unspecified abnormal findings on antenatal screening of mother

☑4ᵗʰ **O29 Complications of anesthesia during pregnancy**
  INCLUDES maternal complications arising from the administration of a general, regional or local anesthetic, analgesic or other sedation during pregnancy
  Use additional code, if necessary, to identify the complication
  EXCLUDES 2 *complications of anesthesia during labor and delivery (O74-)*
  complications of anesthesia during the puerperium (O89-)

☑5ᵗʰ **O29.0** Pulmonary complications of anesthesia during pregnancy
  ☑6ᵗʰ **O29.01** Aspiration pneumonitis due to anesthesia during pregnancy
    Inhalation of stomach contents or secretions NOS due to anesthesia during pregnancy
    Mendelson's syndrome due to anesthesia during pregnancy
    O29.011 Aspiration pneumonitis due to anesthesia during pregnancy, first trimester
    O29.012 Aspiration pneumonitis due to anesthesia during pregnancy, second trimester
    O29.013 Aspiration pneumonitis due to anesthesia during pregnancy, third trimester
    O29.019 Aspiration pneumonitis due to anesthesia during pregnancy, unspecified trimester
  ☑6ᵗʰ **O29.02** Pressure collapse of lung due to anesthesia during pregnancy
    O29.021 Pressure collapse of lung due to anesthesia during pregnancy, first trimester
    O29.022 Pressure collapse of lung due to anesthesia during pregnancy, second trimester
    O29.023 Pressure collapse of lung due to anesthesia during pregnancy, third trimester
    O29.029 Pressure collapse of lung due to anesthesia during pregnancy, unspecified trimester

☑6ᵗʰ **O29.09** Other pulmonary complications of anesthesia during pregnancy
    O29.091 Other pulmonary complications of anesthesia during pregnancy, first trimester
    O29.092 Other pulmonary complications of anesthesia during pregnancy, second trimester
    O29.093 Other pulmonary complications of anesthesia during pregnancy, third trimester
    O29.099 Other pulmonary complications of anesthesia during pregnancy, unspecified trimester

☑5ᵗʰ **O29.1** Cardiac complications of anesthesia during pregnancy
  ☑6ᵗʰ **O29.11** Cardiac arrest due to anesthesia during pregnancy
    O29.111 Cardiac arrest due to anesthesia during pregnancy, first trimester
    O29.112 Cardiac arrest due to anesthesia during pregnancy, second trimester
    O29.113 Cardiac arrest due to anesthesia during pregnancy, third trimester
    O29.119 Cardiac arrest due to anesthesia during pregnancy, unspecified trimester
  ☑6ᵗʰ **O29.12** Cardiac failure due to anesthesia during pregnancy
    O29.121 Cardiac failure due to anesthesia during pregnancy, first trimester
    O29.122 Cardiac failure due to anesthesia during pregnancy, second trimester
    O29.123 Cardiac failure due to anesthesia during pregnancy, third trimester
    O29.129 Cardiac failure due to anesthesia during pregnancy, unspecified trimester
  ☑6ᵗʰ **O29.19** Other cardiac complications of anesthesia during pregnancy
    O29.191 Other cardiac complications of anesthesia during pregnancy, first trimester
    O29.192 Other cardiac complications of anesthesia during pregnancy, second trimester
    O29.193 Other cardiac complications of anesthesia during pregnancy, third trimester
    O29.199 Other cardiac complications of anesthesia during pregnancy, unspecified trimester

☑5ᵗʰ **O29.2** Central nervous system complications of anesthesia during pregnancy
  ☑6ᵗʰ **O29.21** Cerebral anoxia due to anesthesia during pregnancy
    O29.211 Cerebral anoxia due to anesthesia during pregnancy, first trimester
    O29.212 Cerebral anoxia due to anesthesia during pregnancy, second trimester
    O29.213 Cerebral anoxia due to anesthesia during pregnancy, third trimester
    O29.219 Cerebral anoxia due to anesthesia during pregnancy, unspecified trimester
  ☑6ᵗʰ **O29.29** Other central nervous system complications of anesthesia during pregnancy
    O29.291 Other central nervous system complications of anesthesia during pregnancy, first trimester
    O29.292 Other central nervous system complications of anesthesia during pregnancy, second trimester
    O29.293 Other central nervous system complications of anesthesia during pregnancy, third trimester
    O29.299 Other central nervous system complications of anesthesia during pregnancy, unspecified trimester

☑5ᵗʰ **O29.3** Toxic reaction to local anesthesia during pregnancy
  ☑6ᵗʰ **O29.3x** Toxic reaction to local anesthesia during pregnancy
    O29.3x1 Toxic reaction to local anesthesia during pregnancy, first trimester

☑ Appropriate additional character required   ☑x7ᵗʰ Requires 7th character, placeholder x must fill empty characters

O29.3x2	Toxic reaction to local anesthesia during pregnancy, second trimester
O29.3x3	Toxic reaction to local anesthesia during pregnancy, third trimester
O29.3x9	Toxic reaction to local anesthesia during pregnancy, unspecified trimester

✓5ᵗʰ **O29.4** Spinal and epidural anesthesia induced headache during pregnancy

   O29.40 Spinal and epidural anesthesia induced headache during pregnancy, unspecified trimester

   O29.41 Spinal and epidural anesthesia induced headache during pregnancy, first trimester

   O29.42 Spinal and epidural anesthesia induced headache during pregnancy, second trimester

   O29.43 Spinal and epidural anesthesia induced headache during pregnancy, third trimester

✓5ᵗʰ **O29.5** Other complications of spinal and epidural anesthesia during pregnancy

  ✓6ᵗʰ **O29.5x** Other complications of spinal and epidural anesthesia during pregnancy

   O29.5x1 Other complications of spinal and epidural anesthesia during pregnancy, first trimester

   O29.5x2 Other complications of spinal and epidural anesthesia during pregnancy, second trimester

   O29.5x3 Other complications of spinal and epidural anesthesia during pregnancy, third trimester

   O29.5x9 Other complications of spinal and epidural anesthesia during pregnancy, unspecified trimester

✓5ᵗʰ **O29.6** Failed or difficult intubation for anesthesia during pregnancy

   O29.60 Failed or difficult intubation for anesthesia during pregnancy, unspecified trimester

   O29.61 Failed or difficult intubation for anesthesia during pregnancy, first trimester

   O29.62 Failed or difficult intubation for anesthesia during pregnancy, second trimester

   O29.63 Failed or difficult intubation for anesthesia during pregnancy, third trimester

✓5ᵗʰ **O29.8** Other complications of anesthesia during pregnancy

  ✓6ᵗʰ **O29.8x** Other complications of anesthesia during pregnancy

   O29.8x1 Other complications of anesthesia during pregnancy, first trimester

   O29.8x2 Other complications of anesthesia during pregnancy, second trimester

   O29.8x3 Other complications of anesthesia during pregnancy, third trimester

   O29.8x9 Other complications of anesthesia during pregnancy, unspecified trimester

✓5ᵗʰ **O29.9** Unspecified complication of anesthesia during pregnancy

   O29.90 Unspecified complication of anesthesia during pregnancy, unspecified trimester

   O29.91 Unspecified complication of anesthesia during pregnancy, first trimester

   O29.92 Unspecified complication of anesthesia during pregnancy, second trimester

   O29.93 Unspecified complication of anesthesia during pregnancy, third trimester

Maternal care related to the fetus and amniotic cavity and possible delivery problems (O30-O48)

✓4ᵗʰ **O30** **Multiple gestation**

Code also any complications specific to multiple gestation

✓5ᵗʰ **O30.0** Twin pregnancy

  ✓6ᵗʰ **O30.00** Twin pregnancy, unspecified number of placenta and unspecified number of amniotic sacs

   O30.001 Twin pregnancy, unspecified number of placenta and unspecified number of amniotic sacs, first trimester

   O30.002 Twin pregnancy, unspecified number of placenta and unspecified number of amniotic sacs, second trimester

   O30.003 Twin pregnancy, unspecified number of placenta and unspecified number of amniotic sacs, third trimester

   O30.009 Twin pregnancy, unspecified number of placenta and unspecified number of amniotic sacs, unspecified trimester

  ✓6ᵗʰ **O30.01** Twin pregnancy, monochorionic/monoamniotic

Twin pregnancy, one placenta, one amniotic sac

EXCLUDES 1   conjoined twins (O30.02-)

   O30.011 Twin pregnancy, monochorionic/monoamniotic, first trimester

   O30.012 Twin pregnancy, monochorionic/monoamniotic, second trimester

   O30.013 Twin pregnancy, monochorionic/monoamniotic, third trimester

   O30.019 Twin pregnancy, monochorionic/monoamniotic, unspecified trimester

  ✓6ᵗʰ **O30.02** Conjoined twins

   O30.021 Conjoined twins, first trimester

   O30.022 Conjoined twins, second trimester

   O30.023 Conjoined twins, third trimester

   O30.029 Conjoined twins, unspecified trimester

  ✓6ᵗʰ **O30.03** Twin pregnancy, monochorionic/diamniotic

Twin pregnancy, one placenta, two amniotic sacs

   O30.031 Twin pregnancy, monochorionic/diamniotic, first trimester

   O30.032 Twin pregnancy, monochorionic/diamniotic, second trimester

   O30.033 Twin pregnancy, monochorionic/diamniotic, third trimester

   O30.039 Twin pregnancy, monochorionic/diamniotic, unspecified trimester

  ✓6ᵗʰ **O30.04** Twin pregnancy, dichorionic/diamniotic

Twin pregnancy, two placentae, two amniotic sacs

   O30.041 Twin pregnancy, dichorionic/diamniotic, first trimester

   O30.042 Twin pregnancy, dichorionic/diamniotic, second trimester

   O30.043 Twin pregnancy, dichorionic/diamniotic, third trimester

   O30.049 Twin pregnancy, dichorionic/diamniotic, unspecified trimester

  ✓6ᵗʰ **O30.09** Twin pregnancy, unable to determine number of placenta and number of anmiotic sacs

   O30.091 Twin pregnancy, unable to determine number of placenta and number of amniotic sacs, first trimester

   O30.092 Twin pregnancy, unable to determine number of placenta and number of amniotic sacs, second trimester

   O30.093 Twin pregnancy, unable to determine number of placenta and number of amniotic sacs, third trimester

   O30.099 Twin pregnancy, unable to determine number of placenta and number of amniotic sacs, unspecified trimester

✓5ᵗʰ **O30.1** Triplet pregnancy, unspecified number of placenta and unspecified number of amniotic sacs

  ✓6ᵗʰ **O30.10** Triplet pregnancy, unspecified number of placenta and unspecified number of amniotic sacs

   O30.101 Triplet pregnancy, unspecified number of placenta and unspecified number of amniotic sacs, first trimester

   O30.102 Triplet pregnancy, unspecified number of placenta and unspecified number of amniotic sacs, second trimester

   O30.103 Triplet pregnancy, unspecified number of placenta and unspecified number of amniotic sacs, third trimester

   O30.109 Triplet pregnancy, unspecified number of placenta and unspecified number of amniotic sacs, unspecified trimester

  ✓6ᵗʰ **O30.11** Triplet pregnancy with two or more monochorionic fetuses

   O30.111 Triplet pregnancy with two or more monochorionic fetuses, first trimester

---

EXCLUDES 1 Not coded here   EXCLUDES 2 Not included here   *Manifestation Code*

O30.112 Triplet pregnancy with two or more monochorionic fetuses, second trimester

O30.113 Triplet pregnancy with two or more monochorionic fetuses, third trimester

O30.119 Triplet pregnancy with two or more monochorionic fetuses, unspecified trimester

✓6th O30.12 **Triplet pregnancy with two or more monoamniotic fetuses**

O30.121 Triplet pregnancy with two or more monoamniotic fetuses, first trimester

O30.122 Triplet pregnancy with two or more monoamniotic fetuses, second trimester

O30.123 Triplet pregnancy with two or more monoamniotic fetuses, third trimester

O30.129 Triplet pregnancy with two or more monoamniotic fetuses, unspecified trimester

✓6th O30.19 **Triplet pregnancy, unable to determine number of placenta and number of amniotic sacs**

O30.191 Triplet pregnancy, unable to determine number of placenta and number of amnioticsacs, first trimester

O30.192 Triplet pregnancy, unable to determine number of placenta and number of amnioticsacs, second trimester

O30.193 Triplet pregnancy, unable to determine number of placenta and number of amnioticsacs, third trimester

O30.199 Triplet pregnancy, unable to determine number of placenta and number of amnioticsacs, unspecified trimester

✓6th O30.2 **Quadruplet pregnancy**

✓6th O30.20 **Quadruplet pregnancy, unspecified number of placenta and unspecified number of amniotic sacs**

O30.201 Quadruplet pregnancy, unspecified number of placenta and unspecified number of amniotic sacs, first trimester

O30.202 Quadruplet pregnancy, unspecified number of placenta and unspecified number of amniotic sacs, second trimester

O30.203 Quadruplet pregnancy, unspecified number of placenta and unspecified number of amniotic sacs, third trimester

O30.209 Quadruplet pregnancy, unspecified number of placenta and unspecified number of amniotic sacs, unspecified trimester

✓6th O30.21 **Quadruplet pregnancy with two or more monochorionic fetuses**

O30.211 Quadruplet pregnancy with two or more monochorionic fetuses, first trimester

O30.212 Quadruplet pregnancy with two or more monochorionic fetuses, second trimester

O30.213 Quadruplet pregnancy with two or more monochorionic fetuses, third trimester

O30.219 Quadruplet pregnancy with two or more monochorionic fetuses, unspecified trimester

✓6th O30.22 **Quadruplet pregnancy with two or more monoamniotic fetuses**

O30.221 Quadruplet pregnancy with two or more monoamniotic fetuses, first trimester

O30.222 Quadruplet pregnancy with two or more monoamniotic fetuses, second trimester

O30.223 Quadruplet pregnancy with two or more monoamniotic fetuses, third trimester

O30.229 Quadruplet pregnancy with two or more monoamniotic fetuses, unspecified trimester

✓6th O30.29 **Quadruplet pregnancy, unable to determine number of placenta and number of amniotic sacs**

O30.291 Quadruplet pregnancy, unable to determine number of placenta and number of amniotic sacs, first trimester

O30.292 Quadruplet pregnancy, unable to determine number of placenta and number of amniotic sacs, second trimester

O30.293 Quadruplet pregnancy, unable to determine number of placenta and number of amniotic sacs, third trimester

O30.299 Quadruplet pregnancy, unable to determine number of placenta and number of amniotic sacs, unspecified trimester

✓5th O30.8 **Other specified multiple gestation**
Multiple gestation pregnancy greater than quadruplets

✓6th O30.80 **Other specified multiple gestation, unspecified number of placenta and unspecified number of amniotic sacs**

O30.801 Other specified multiple gestation, unspecified number of placenta and unspecified number of amniotic sacs, first trimester

O30.802 Other specified multiple gestation, unspecified number of placenta and unspecified number of amniotic sacs, second trimester

O30.803 Other specified multiple gestation, unspecified number of placenta and unspecified number of amniotic sacs, third trimester

O30.809 Other specified multiple gestation, unspecified number of placenta and unspecified number of amniotic sacs, unspecified trimester

✓6th O30.81 **Other specified multiple gestation with two or more monochorionic fetuses**

O30.811 Other specified multiple gestation with two or more monochorionic fetuses, first trimester

O30.812 Other specified multiple gestation with two or more monochorionic fetuses, second trimester

O30.813 Other specified multiple gestation with two or more monochorionic fetuses, third trimester

O30.819 Other specified multiple gestation with two or more monochorionic fetuses, unspecified trimester

✓6th O30.82 **Other specified multiple gestation with two or more monoamniotic fetuses**

O30.821 Other specified multiple gestation with two or more monoamniotic fetuses, first trimester

O30.822 Other specified multiple gestation with two or more monoamniotic fetuses, second trimester

O30.823 Other specified multiple gestation with two or more monoamniotic fetuses, third trimester

O30.829 Other specified multiple gestation with two or more monoamniotic fetuses, unspecified trimester

✓6th O30.89 **Other specified multiple gestation, unable to determine number of placenta and number of amniotic sacs**

O30.891 Other specified multiple gestation, unable to determine number of placenta and number of amniotic sacs, first trimester

O30.892 Other specified multiple gestation, unable to determine number of placenta and number of amniotic sacs, second trimester

O30.893 Other specified multiple gestation, unable to determine number of placenta and number of amniotic sacs, third trimester

O30.899 Other specified multiple gestation, unable to determine number of placenta and number of amniotic sacs, unspecified trimester

---

☑ Appropriate additional character required   ✓x7th Requires 7th character, placeholder x must fill empty characters

Pregnancy, Childbirth and the Puerperium

O30.9–O33.3

✓5ᵗʰ **O30.9**   **Multiple gestation, unspecified**
Multiple pregnancy NOS

     O30.90   **Multiple gestation, unspecified, unspecified trimester**

     O30.91   **Multiple gestation, unspecified, first trimester**

     O30.92   **Multiple gestation, unspecified, second trimester**

     O30.93   **Multiple gestation, unspecified, third trimester**

✓4ᵗʰ **O31**   **Complications specific to multiple gestation**

     EXCLUDES 2   *delayed delivery of second twin, triplet, etc. (O63.2)*
malpresentation of one fetus or more (O32.5)
placental transfusion syndromes (O43.0-)

> One of the following 7th characters is to be assigned to each code under category O31. 7th character 0 is for single gestations and multiple gestations where the fetus is unspecified. 7th characters 1 through 9 are for cases of multiple gestations to identify the fetus for which the code applies. The appropriate code from category O30, Multiple gestation, must also be assigned when assigning a code from category O31 that has a 7th character of 1 through 9.
> 0   not applicable or unspecified
> 1   fetus 1
> 2   fetus 2
> 3   fetus 3
> 4   fetus 4
> 5   fetus 5
> 9   other fetus

✓5ᵗʰ **O31.0**   **Papyraceous fetus**
Fetus compressus

   ✓7ᵗʰ **O31.00**   **Papyraceous fetus, unspecified trimester**

   ✓7ᵗʰ **O31.01**   **Papyraceous fetus, first trimester**

   ✓7ᵗʰ **O31.02**   **Papyraceous fetus, second trimester**

   ✓7ᵗʰ **O31.03**   **Papyraceous fetus, third trimester**

✓5ᵗʰ **O31.1**   **Continuing pregnancy after spontaneous abortion of one fetus or more**

   ✓7ᵗʰ **O31.10**   **Continuing pregnancy after spontaneous abortion of one fetus or more, unspecified trimester**

   ✓7ᵗʰ **O31.11**   **Continuing pregnancy after spontaneous abortion of one fetus or more, first trimester**

   ✓7ᵗʰ **O31.12**   **Continuing pregnancy after spontaneous abortion of one fetus or more, second trimester**

   ✓7ᵗʰ **O31.13**   **Continuing pregnancy after spontaneous abortion of one fetus or more, third trimester**

✓5ᵗʰ **O31.2**   **Continuing pregnancy after intrauterine death of one fetus or more**

   ✓7ᵗʰ **O31.20**   **Continuing pregnancy after intrauterine death of one fetus or more, unspecified trimester**

   ✓7ᵗʰ **O31.21**   **Continuing pregnancy after intrauterine death of one fetus or more, first trimester**

   ✓7ᵗʰ **O31.22**   **Continuing pregnancy after intrauterine death of one fetus or more, second trimester**

   ✓7ᵗʰ **O31.23**   **Continuing pregnancy after intrauterine death of one fetus or more, third trimester**

✓5ᵗʰ **O31.3**   **Continuing pregnancy after elective fetal reduction of one fetus or more**
Continuing pregnancy after selective termination of one fetus or more

   ✓7ᵗʰ **O31.30**   **Continuing pregnancy after elective fetal reduction of one fetus or more, unspecified trimester**

   ✓7ᵗʰ **O31.31**   **Continuing pregnancy after elective fetal reduction of one fetus or more, first trimester**

   ✓7ᵗʰ **O31.32**   **Continuing pregnancy after elective fetal reduction of one fetus or more, second trimester**

   ✓7ᵗʰ **O31.33**   **Continuing pregnancy after elective fetal reduction of one fetus or more, third trimester**

✓5ᵗʰ **O31.8**   **Other complications specific to multiple gestation**

   ✓6ᵗʰ **O31.8x**   **Other complications specific to multiple gestation**

     ✓7ᵗʰ **O31.8x1**   **Other complications specific to multiple gestation, first trimester**

     ✓7ᵗʰ **O31.8x2**   **Other complications specific to multiple gestation, second trimester**

     ✓7ᵗʰ **O31.8x3**   **Other complications specific to multiple gestation, third trimester**

     ✓7ᵗʰ **O31.8x9**   **Other complications specific to multiple gestation, unspecified trimester**

✓4ᵗʰ **O32**   **Maternal care for malpresentation of fetus**

   INCLUDES   the listed conditions as a reason for observation, hospitalization or other obstetric care of the mother, or for cesarean delivery before onset of labor

   EXCLUDES 1   *malpresentation of fetus with obstructed labor (O64-)*

> One of the following 7th characters is to be assigned to each code under category O32. 7th character 0 is for single gestations and multiple gestations where the fetus is unspecified. 7th characters 1 through 9 are for cases of multiple gestations to identify the fetus for which the code applies. The appropriate code from category O30, Multiple gestation, must also be assigned when assigning a code from category O32 that has a 7th character of 1 through 9.
> 0   not applicable or unspecified
> 1   fetus 1
> 2   fetus 2
> 3   fetus 3
> 4   fetus 4
> 5   fetus 5
> 9   other fetus

✓x7ᵗʰ **O32.0**   **Maternal care for unstable lie**

✓x7ᵗʰ **O32.1**   **Maternal care for breech presentation**
Maternal care for buttocks presentation
Maternal care for complete breech
Maternal care for frank breech

     EXCLUDES 1   *footling presentation (O32.8)*
incomplete breech (O32.8)

✓x7ᵗʰ **O32.2**   **Maternal care for transverse and oblique lie**
Maternal care for oblique presentation
Maternal care for transverse presentation

✓x7ᵗʰ **O32.3**   **Maternal care for face, brow and chin presentation**

✓x7ᵗʰ **O32.4**   **Maternal care for high head at term**
Maternal care for failure of head to enter pelvic brim

✓x7ᵗʰ **O32.6**   **Maternal care for compound presentation**

✓x7ᵗʰ **O32.8**   **Maternal care for other malpresentation of fetus**
Maternal care for footling presentation
Maternal care for incomplete breech

✓x7ᵗʰ **O32.9**   **Maternal care for malpresentation of fetus, unspecified**

✓4ᵗʰ **O33**   **Maternal care for disproportion**

   INCLUDES   the listed conditions as a reason for observation, hospitalization or other obstetric care of the mother, or for cesarean delivery before onset of labor

   EXCLUDES 1   *disproportion with obstructed labor (O65- O66)*

     O33.0   **Maternal care for disproportion due to deformity of maternal pelvic bones**
Maternal care for disproportion due to pelvic deformity causing disproportion NOS

     O33.1   **Maternal care for disproportion due to generally contracted pelvis**
Maternal care for disproportion due to contracted pelvis NOS causing disproportion

     O33.2   **Maternal care for disproportion due to inlet contraction of pelvis**
Maternal care for disproportion due to inlet contraction (pelvis) causing disproportion

   ✓x7ᵗʰ **O33.3**   **Maternal care for disproportion due to outlet contraction of pelvis**
Maternal care for disproportion due to mid-cavity contraction (pelvis)
Maternal care for disproportion due to outlet contraction (pelvis)

> One of the following 7th characters is to be assigned to code O33.3. 7th character 0 is for single gestations and multiple gestations where the fetus is unspecified. 7th characters 1 through 9 are for cases of multiple gestations to identify the fetus for which the code applies. The appropriate code from category O30, Multiple gestation, must also be assigned when assigning code O33.3 with a 7th character of 1 through 9.
> 0   not applicable or unspecified
> 1   fetus 1
> 2   fetus 2
> 3   fetus 3
> 4   fetus 4
> 5   fetus 5
> 9   other fetus

EXCLUDES 1 Not coded here   EXCLUDES 2 Not included here   ***Manifestation Code***

√x7ᵗʰ **O33.4 Maternal care for disproportion of mixed maternal and fetal origin**

One of the following 7th characters is to be assigned to code O33.4. 7th character 0 is for single gestations and multiple gestations where the fetus is unspecified. 7th characters 1 through 9 are for cases of multiple gestations to identify the fetus for which the code applies. The appropriate code from category O30, Multiple gestation, must also be assigned when assigning code O33.4 with a 7th character of 1 through 9.
0   not applicable or unspecified
1   fetus 1
2   fetus 2
3   fetus 3
4   fetus 4
5   fetus 5
9   other fetus

√x7ᵗʰ **O33.5 Maternal care for disproportion due to unusually large fetus**
Maternal care for disproportion due to disproportion of fetal origin with normally formed fetus
Maternal care for disproportion due to fetal disproportion NOS

One of the following 7th characters is to be assigned to code O33.5. 7th character 0 is for single gestations and multiple gestations where the fetus is unspecified. 7th characters 1 through 9 are for cases of multiple gestations to identify the fetus for which the code applies. The appropriate code from category O30, Multiple gestation, must also be assigned when assigning code O33.5 with a 7th character of 1 through 9.
0   not applicable or unspecified
1   fetus 1
2   fetus 2
3   fetus 3
4   fetus 4
5   fetus 5
9   other fetus

√x7ᵗʰ **O33.6 Maternal care for disproportion due to hydrocephalic fetus**

One of the following 7th characters is to be assigned to code O33.6. 7th character 0 is for single gestations and multiple gestations where the fetus is unspecified. 7th characters 1 through 9 are for cases of multiple gestations to identify the fetus for which the code applies. The appropriate code from category O30, Multiple gestation, must also be assigned when assigning code O33.6 with a 7th character of 1 through 9.
0   not applicable or unspecified
1   fetus 1
2   fetus 2
3   fetus 3
4   fetus 4
5   fetus 5
9   other fetus

√x7ᵗʰ **O33.7 Maternal care for disproportion due to other fetal deformities**

One of the following 7th characters is to be assigned to code O33.7. 7th character 0 is for single gestations and multiple gestations where the fetus is unspecified. 7th characters 1 through 9 are for cases of multiple gestations to identify the fetus for which the code applies. The appropriate code from category O30, Multiple gestation, must also be assigned when assigning code O33.7 with a 7th character of 1 through 9.
0   not applicable or unspecified
1   fetus 1
2   fetus 2
3   fetus 3
4   fetus 4
5   fetus 5
9   other fetus

Maternal care for disproportion due to fetal ascites
Maternal care for disproportion due to fetal hydrops
Maternal care for disproportion due to fetal meningomyelocele
Maternal care for disproportion due to fetal sacral teratoma
Maternal care for disproportion due to fetal tumor
EXCLUDES 1 *obstructed labor due to other fetal deformities (O66.3)*

O33.8 Maternal care for disproportion of other origin

O33.9 Maternal care for disproportion, unspecified
Maternal care for disproportion due to cephalopelvic disproportion NOS
Maternal care for disproportion due to fetopelvic disproportion NOS

√4ᵗʰ **O34 Maternal care for abnormality of pelvic organs**
INCLUDES the listed conditions as a reason for hospitalization or other obstetric care of the mother, or for cesarean delivery before onset of labor
Code first any associated obstructed labor (O65.5)
Use additional code for specific condition

√5ᵗʰ **O34.0 Maternal care for congenital malformation of uterus**
O34.00 Maternal care for unspecified congenital malformation of uterus, unspecified trimester
O34.01 Maternal care for unspecified congenital malformation of uterus, first trimester
O34.02 Maternal care for unspecified congenital malformation of uterus, second trimester
O34.03 Maternal care for unspecified congenital malformation of uterus, third trimester

√5ᵗʰ **O34.1 Maternal care for benign tumor of corpus uteri**
EXCLUDES 2 *maternal care for benign tumor of cervix (O34.4-)*
maternal care for malignant neoplasm of uterus (O9a.1-)
O34.10 Maternal care for benign tumor of corpus uteri, unspecified trimester
O34.11 Maternal care for benign tumor of corpus uteri, first trimester
O34.12 Maternal care for benign tumor of corpus uteri, second trimester
O34.13 Maternal care for benign tumor of corpus uteri, third trimester

√5ᵗʰ **O34.2 Maternal care due to uterine scar from previous surgery**
O34.21 Maternal care for scar from previous cesarean delivery
O34.29 Maternal care due to uterine scar from other previous surgery

√5ᵗʰ **O34.3 Maternal care for cervical incompetence**
Maternal care for cerclage with or without cervical incompetence
Maternal care for Shirodkar suture with or without cervical incompetence
O34.30 Maternal care for cervical incompetence, unspecified trimester
O34.31 Maternal care for cervical incompetence, first trimester
O34.32 Maternal care for cervical incompetence, second trimester
O34.33 Maternal care for cervical incompetence, third trimester

---

√5ᵗʰ **O34.4** **Maternal care for other abnormalities of cervix**

     O34.40 Maternal care for other abnormalities of cervix, unspecified trimester

     O34.41 Maternal care for other abnormalities of cervix, first trimester

     O34.42 Maternal care for other abnormalities of cervix, second trimester

     O34.43 Maternal care for other abnormalities of cervix, third trimester

√5ᵗʰ **O34.5** **Maternal care for other abnormalities of gravid uterus**

√6ᵗʰ   **O34.51** **Maternal care for incarceration of gravid uterus**

     O34.511 Maternal care for incarceration of gravid uterus, first trimester

     O34.512 Maternal care for incarceration of gravid uterus, second trimester

     O34.513 Maternal care for incarceration of gravid uterus, third trimester

     O34.519 Maternal care for incarceration of gravid uterus, unspecified trimester

√6ᵗʰ   **O34.52** **Maternal care for prolapse of gravid uterus**

     O34.521 Maternal care for prolapse of gravid uterus, first trimester

     O34.522 Maternal care for prolapse of gravid uterus, second trimester

     O34.523 Maternal care for prolapse of gravid uterus, third trimester

     O34.529 Maternal care for prolapse of gravid uterus, unspecified trimester

√6ᵗʰ   **O34.53** **Maternal care for retroversion of gravid uterus**

     O34.531 Maternal care for retroversion of gravid uterus, first trimester

     O34.532 Maternal care for retroversion of gravid uterus, second trimester

     O34.533 Maternal care for retroversion of gravid uterus, third trimester

     O34.539 Maternal care for retroversion of gravid uterus, unspecified trimester

√6ᵗʰ   **O34.59** **Maternal care for other abnormalities of gravid uterus**

     O34.591 Maternal care for other abnormalities of gravid uterus, first trimester

     O34.592 Maternal care for other abnormalities of gravid uterus, second trimester

     O34.593 Maternal care for other abnormalities of gravid uterus, third trimester

     O34.599 Maternal care for other abnormalities of gravid uterus, unspecified trimester

√5ᵗʰ **O34.6** **Maternal care for abnormality of vagina**

     EXCLUDES 2   *maternal care for vaginal varices in pregnancy (O22.1-)*

     O34.60 Maternal care for abnormality of vagina, unspecified trimester

     O34.61 Maternal care for abnormality of vagina, first trimester

     O34.62 Maternal care for abnormality of vagina, second trimester

     O34.63 Maternal care for abnormality of vagina, third trimester

√5ᵗʰ **O34.7** **Maternal care for abnormality of vulva and perineum**

     EXCLUDES 2   *maternal care for perineal and vulval varices in pregnancy (O22.1-)*

     O34.70 Maternal care for abnormality of vulva and perineum, unspecified trimester

     O34.71 Maternal care for abnormality of vulva and perineum, first trimester

     O34.72 Maternal care for abnormality of vulva and perineum, second trimester

     O34.73 Maternal care for abnormality of vulva and perineum, third trimester

√5ᵗʰ **O34.8** **Maternal care for other abnormalities of pelvic organs**

     O34.80 Maternal care for other abnormalities of pelvic organs, unspecified trimester

     O34.81 Maternal care for other abnormalities of pelvic organs, first trimester

     O34.82 Maternal care for other abnormalities of pelvic organs, second trimester

     O34.83 Maternal care for other abnormalities of pelvic organs, third trimester

√5ᵗʰ **O34.9** **Maternal care for abnormality of pelvic organ, unspecified**

     O34.90 Maternal care for abnormality of pelvic organ, unspecified, unspecified trimester

     O34.91 Maternal care for abnormality of pelvic organ, unspecified, first trimester

     O34.92 Maternal care for abnormality of pelvic organ, unspecified, second trimester

     O34.93 Maternal care for abnormality of pelvic organ, unspecified, third trimester

√4ᵗʰ **O35** **Maternal care for known or suspected fetal abnormality and damage**

     INCLUDES   the listed conditions in the fetus as a reason for hospitalization or other obstetric care to the mother, or for termination of pregnancy

     Code also any associated maternal condition

     EXCLUDES 1   *encounter for suspected maternal and fetal conditions ruled out (Z03.7-)*

One of the following 7th characters is to be assigned to each code under category O35. 7th character 0 is for single gestations and multiple gestations where the fetus is unspecified. 7th characters 1 through 9 are for cases of multiple gestations to identify the fetus for which the code applies. The appropriate code from category O30, Multiple gestation, must also be assigned when assigning a code from category O35 that has a 7th character of 1 through 9.

  0   not applicable or unspecified

  1   fetus 1

  2   fetus 2

  3   fetus 3

  4   fetus 4

  5   fetus 5

  9   other fetus

√x7ᵗʰ **O35.0** **Maternal care for (suspected) central nervous system malformation in fetus**

     Maternal care for fetal anencephaly

     Maternal care for fetal hydrocephalus

     Maternal care for fetal spina bifida

     EXCLUDES 2   *chromosomal abnormality in fetus (O35.1)*

√x7ᵗʰ **O35.1** **Maternal care for (suspected) chromosomal abnormality in fetus**

√x7ᵗʰ **O35.2** **Maternal care for (suspected) hereditary disease in fetus**

     EXCLUDES 2   *chromosomal abnormality in fetus (O35.1)*

√x7ᵗʰ **O35.3** **Maternal care for (suspected) damage to fetus from viral disease in mother**

     Maternal care for damage to fetus from maternal cytomegalovirus infection

     Maternal care for damage to fetus from maternal rubella

√x7ᵗʰ **O35.4** **Maternal care for (suspected) damage to fetus from alcohol**

√x7ᵗʰ **O35.5** **Maternal care for (suspected) damage to fetus by drugs**

     Maternal care for damage to fetus from drug addiction

√x7ᵗʰ **O35.6** **Maternal care for (suspected) damage to fetus by radiation**

√x7ᵗʰ **O35.7** **Maternal care for (suspected) damage to fetus by other medical procedures**

     Maternal care for damage to fetus by amniocentesis

     Maternal care for damage to fetus by biopsy procedures

     Maternal care for damage to fetus by hematological investigation

     Maternal care for damage to fetus by intrauterine contraceptive device

     Maternal care for damage to fetus by intrauterine surgery

√x7ᵗʰ **O35.8** **Maternal care for other (suspected) fetal abnormality and damage**

     Maternal care for damage to fetus from maternal listeriosis

     Maternal care for damage to fetus from maternal toxoplasmosis

√x7ᵗʰ **O35.9** **Maternal care for (suspected) fetal abnormality and damage, unspecified**

EXCLUDES 1   Not coded here   EXCLUDES 2   Not included here   *Manifestation Code*

✓4ᵗʰ **O36 Maternal care for other fetal problems**

INCLUDES the listed conditions in the fetus as a reason for hospitalization or other obstetric care of the mother, or for termination of pregnancy

EXCLUDES 1 *encounter for suspected maternal and fetal conditions ruled out (Z03.7-)*
placental transfusion syndromes (O43.0-)

EXCLUDES 2 *labor and delivery complicated by fetal stress (O77-)*

One of the following 7th characters is to be assigned to each code under category O36. 7th character 0 is for single gestations and multiple gestations where the fetus is unspecified. 7th characters 1 through 9 are for cases of multiple gestations to identify the fetus for which the code applies. The appropriate code from category O30, Multiple gestation, must also be assigned when assigning a code from category O36 that has a 7th character of 1 through 9.

0   not applicable or unspecified
1   fetus 1
2   fetus 2
3   fetus 3
4   fetus 4
5   fetus 5
9   other fetus

✓5ᵗʰ **O36.0 Maternal care for rhesus isoimmunization**
Maternal care for Rh incompatibility (with hydrops fetalis)

✓6ᵗʰ **O36.01 Maternal care for anti-D [Rh] antibodies**

✓7ᵗʰ **O36.011 Maternal care for anti-D [Rh] antibodies, first trimester**

✓7ᵗʰ **O36.012 Maternal care for anti-D [Rh] antibodies, second trimester**

✓7ᵗʰ **O36.013 Maternal care for anti-D [Rh] antibodies, third trimester**

✓7ᵗʰ **O36.019 Maternal care for anti-D [Rh] antibodies, unspecified trimester**

✓6ᵗʰ **O36.09 Maternal care for other rhesus isoimmunization**

✓7ᵗʰ **O36.091 Maternal care for other rhesus isoimmunization, first trimester**

✓7ᵗʰ **O36.092 Maternal care for other rhesus isoimmunization, second trimester**

✓7ᵗʰ **O36.093 Maternal care for other rhesus isoimmunization, third trimester**

✓7ᵗʰ **O36.099 Maternal care for other rhesus isoimmunization, unspecified trimester**

✓5ᵗʰ **O36.1 Maternal care for other isoimmunization**
Maternal care for ABO isoimmunization

✓6ᵗʰ **O36.11 Maternal care for Anti-A sensitization**
Maternal care for isoimmunization NOS (with hydrops fetalis)

✓7ᵗʰ **O36.111 Maternal care for Anti-A sensitization, first trimester**

✓7ᵗʰ **O36.112 Maternal care for Anti-A sensitization, second trimester**

✓7ᵗʰ **O36.113 Maternal care for Anti-A sensitization, third trimester**

✓7ᵗʰ **O36.119 Maternal care for Anti-A sensitization, unspecified trimester**

✓6ᵗʰ **O36.19 Maternal care for other isoimmunization**
Maternal care for Anti-B sensitization

✓7ᵗʰ **O36.191 Maternal care for other isoimmunization, first trimester**

✓7ᵗʰ **O36.192 Maternal care for other isoimmunization, second trimester**

✓7ᵗʰ **O36.193 Maternal care for other isoimmunization, third trimester**

✓7ᵗʰ **O36.199 Maternal care for other isoimmunization, unspecified trimester**

✓5ᵗʰ **O36.2 Maternal care for hydrops fetalis**
Maternal care for hydrops fetalis NOS
Maternal care for hydrops fetalis not associated with isoimmunization

EXCLUDES 1 *hydrops fetalis associated with ABO isoimmunization (O36.1-)*
hydrops fetalis associated with rhesus isoimmunization (O36.0-)

✓x7ᵗʰ **O36.20 Maternal care for hydrops fetalis, unspecified trimester**

✓x7ᵗʰ **O36.21 Maternal care for hydrops fetalis, first trimester**

✓x7ᵗʰ **O36.22 Maternal care for hydrops fetalis, second trimester**

✓x7ᵗʰ **O36.23 Maternal care for hydrops fetalis, third trimester**

✓x7ᵗʰ **O36.4 Maternal care for intrauterine death**
Maternal care for intrauterine fetal death NOS
Maternal care for intrauterine fetal death after completion of 20 weeks of gestation
Maternal care for late fetal death
Maternal care for missed delivery

EXCLUDES 1 *missed abortion (O02.1)*
stillbirth (P95)

✓5ᵗʰ **O36.5 Maternal care for known or suspected poor fetal growth**

✓6ᵗʰ **O36.51 Maternal care for known or suspected placental insufficiency**

✓7ᵗʰ **O36.511 Maternal care for known or suspected placental insufficiency, first trimester**

✓7ᵗʰ **O36.512 Maternal care for known or suspected placental insufficiency, second trimester**

✓7ᵗʰ **O36.513 Maternal care for known or suspected placental insufficiency, third trimester**

✓7ᵗʰ **O36.519 Maternal care for known or suspected placental insufficiency, unspecified trimester**

✓6ᵗʰ **O36.59 Maternal care for other known or suspected poor fetal growth**
Maternal care for known or suspected light-for-dates NOS
Maternal care for known or suspected small-for-dates NOS

✓7ᵗʰ **O36.591 Maternal care for other known or suspected poor fetal growth, first trimester**

✓7ᵗʰ **O36.592 Maternal care for other known or suspected poor fetal growth, second trimester**

✓7ᵗʰ **O36.593 Maternal care for other known or suspected poor fetal growth, third trimester**

✓7ᵗʰ **O36.599 Maternal care for other known or suspected poor fetal growth, unspecified trimester**

✓5ᵗʰ **O36.6 Maternal care for excessive fetal growth**
Maternal care for known or suspected large-for-dates

✓x7ᵗʰ **O36.60 Maternal care for excessive fetal growth, unspecified trimester**

✓x7ᵗʰ **O36.61 Maternal care for excessive fetal growth, first trimester**

✓x7ᵗʰ **O36.62 Maternal care for excessive fetal growth, second trimester**

✓x7ᵗʰ **O36.63 Maternal care for excessive fetal growth, third trimester**

✓5ᵗʰ **O36.7 Maternal care for viable fetus in abdominal pregnancy**

✓x7ᵗʰ **O36.70 Maternal care for viable fetus in abdominal pregnancy, unspecified trimester**

✓x7ᵗʰ **O36.71 Maternal care for viable fetus in abdominal pregnancy, first trimester**

✓x7ᵗʰ **O36.72 Maternal care for viable fetus in abdominal pregnancy, second trimester**

✓x7ᵗʰ **O36.73 Maternal care for viable fetus in abdominal pregnancy, third trimester**

✓5ᵗʰ **O36.8 Maternal care for other specified fetal problems**

✓6ᵗʰ **O36.81 Decreased fetal movements**

✓7ᵗʰ **O36.812 Decreased fetal movements, second trimester**

✓7ᵗʰ **O36.813 Decreased fetal movements, third trimester**

✓7ᵗʰ **O36.819 Decreased fetal movements, unspecified trimester**

✓6ᵗʰ **O36.82 Fetal anemia and thrombocytopenia**

✓7ᵗʰ **O36.821 Fetal anemia and thrombocytopenia, first trimester**

✓7ᵗʰ **O36.822 Fetal anemia and thrombocytopenia, second trimester**

✓7ᵗʰ **O36.823 Fetal anemia and thrombocytopenia, third trimester**

✓7ᵗʰ **O36.829 Fetal anemia and thrombocytopenia, unspecified trimester**

✔ Appropriate additional character required   ✓x7ᵗʰ Requires 7th character, placeholder x must fill empty characters

Pregnancy, Childbirth and the Puerperium

O36.89–O42.112

√6ᵗʰ **O36.89** **Maternal care for other specified fetal problems**

    √7ᵗʰ **O36.891** **Maternal care for other specified fetal problems, first trimester**

    √7ᵗʰ **O36.892** **Maternal care for other specified fetal problems, second trimester**

    √7ᵗʰ **O36.893** **Maternal care for other specified fetal problems, third trimester**

    √7ᵗʰ **O36.899** **Maternal care for other specified fetal problems, unspecified trimester**

√5ᵗʰ **O36.9** **Maternal care for fetal problem, unspecified**

    √x7ᵗʰ **O36.90** **Maternal care for fetal problem, unspecified, unspecified trimester**

    √x7ᵗʰ **O36.91** **Maternal care for fetal problem, unspecified, first trimester**

    √x7ᵗʰ **O36.92** **Maternal care for fetal problem, unspecified, second trimester**

    √x7ᵗʰ **O36.93** **Maternal care for fetal problem, unspecified, third trimester**

√4ᵗʰ **O40** **Polyhydramnios**

    Hydramnios

    EXCLUDES 1 *encounter for suspected maternal and fetal conditions ruled out (Z03.7-)*

> One of the following 7th characters is to be assigned to each code under category O40. 7th character 0 is for single gestations and multiple gestations where the fetus is unspecified. 7th characters 1 through 9 are for cases of multiple gestations to identify the fetus for which the code applies. The appropriate code from category O30, Multiple gestation, must also be assigned when assigning a code from category O40 that has a 7th character of 1 through 9.
>
> 0   not applicable or unspecified
> 1   fetus 1
> 2   fetus 2
> 3   fetus 3
> 4   fetus 4
> 5   fetus 5
> 9   other fetus

√x7ᵗʰ **O40.1** **Polyhydramnios, first trimester**
√x7ᵗʰ **O40.2** **Polyhydramnios, second trimester**
√x7ᵗʰ **O40.3** **Polyhydramnios, third trimester**
√x7ᵗʰ **O40.9** **Polyhydramnios, unspecified trimester**

√4ᵗʰ **O41** **Other disorders of amniotic fluid and membranes**

    EXCLUDES 1 *encounter for suspected maternal and fetal conditions ruled out (Z03.7-)*

> One of the following 7th characters is to be assigned to each code under category O41. 7th character 0 is for single gestations and multiple gestations where the fetus is unspecified. 7th characters 1 through 9 are for cases of multiple gestations to identify the fetus for which the code applies. The appropriate code from category O30, Multiple gestation, must also be assigned when assigning a code from category O41 that has a 7th character of 1 through 9.
>
> 0   not applicable or unspecified
> 1   fetus 1
> 2   fetus 2
> 3   fetus 3
> 4   fetus 4
> 5   fetus 5
> 9   other fetus

√5ᵗʰ **O41.0** **Oligohydramnios**

    Oligohydramnios without rupture of membranes

    √x7ᵗʰ **O41.00** **Oligohydramnios, unspecified trimester**
    √x7ᵗʰ **O41.01** **Oligohydramnios, first trimester**
    √x7ᵗʰ **O41.02** **Oligohydramnios, second trimester**
    √x7ᵗʰ **O41.03** **Oligohydramnios, third trimester**

√5ᵗʰ **O41.1** **Infection of amniotic sac and membranes**

    √6ᵗʰ **O41.10** **Infection of amniotic sac and membranes, unspecified**

      √7ᵗʰ **O41.101** **Infection of amniotic sac and membranes, unspecified, first trimester**

      √7ᵗʰ **O41.102** **Infection of amniotic sac and membranes, unspecified, second trimester**

      √7ᵗʰ **O41.103** **Infection of amniotic sac and membranes, unspecified, third trimester**

      √7ᵗʰ **O41.109** **Infection of amniotic sac and membranes, unspecified, unspecified trimester**

    √6ᵗʰ **O41.12** **Chorioamnionitis**

      √7ᵗʰ **O41.121** **Chorioamnionitis, first trimester**
      √7ᵗʰ **O41.122** **Chorioamnionitis, second trimester**
      √7ᵗʰ **O41.123** **Chorioamnionitis, third trimester**
      √7ᵗʰ **O41.129** **Chorioamnionitis, unspecified trimester**

    √6ᵗʰ **O41.14** **Placentitis**

      √7ᵗʰ **O41.141** **Placentitis, first trimester**
      √7ᵗʰ **O41.142** **Placentitis, second trimester**
      √7ᵗʰ **O41.143** **Placentitis, third trimester**
      √7ᵗʰ **O41.149** **Placentitis, unspecified trimester**

√5ᵗʰ **O41.8** **Other specified disorders of amniotic fluid and membranes**

    √6ᵗʰ **O41.8x** **Other specified disorders of amniotic fluid and membranes**

      √7ᵗʰ **O41.8x1** **Other specified disorders of amniotic fluid and membranes, first trimester**

      √7ᵗʰ **O41.8x2** **Other specified disorders of amniotic fluid and membranes, second trimester**

      √7ᵗʰ **O41.8x3** **Other specified disorders of amniotic fluid and membranes, third trimester**

      √7ᵗʰ **O41.8x9** **Other specified disorders of amniotic fluid and membranes, unspecified trimester**

√5ᵗʰ **O41.9** **Disorder of amniotic fluid and membranes, unspecified**

    √x7ᵗʰ **O41.90** **Disorder of amniotic fluid and membranes, unspecified, unspecified trimester**

    √x7ᵗʰ **O41.91** **Disorder of amniotic fluid and membranes, unspecified, first trimester**

    √x7ᵗʰ **O41.92** **Disorder of amniotic fluid and membranes, unspecified, second trimester**

    √x7ᵗʰ **O41.93** **Disorder of amniotic fluid and membranes, unspecified, third trimester**

√4ᵗʰ **O42** **Premature rupture of membranes**

√5ᵗʰ **O42.0** **Premature rupture of membranes, onset of labor within 24 hours of rupture**

    O42.00 **Premature rupture of membranes, onset of labor within 24 hours of rupture, unspecified weeks of gestation**

    √6ᵗʰ **O42.01** **Preterm premature rupture of membranes, onset of labor within 24 hours of rupture**

      Premature rupture of membranes before 37 completed weeks of gestation

      O42.011 **Preterm premature rupture of membranes, onset of labor within 24 hours of rupture, first trimester**

      O42.012 **Preterm premature rupture of membranes, onset of labor within 24 hours of rupture, second trimester**

      O42.013 **Preterm premature rupture of membranes, onset of labor within 24 hours of rupture, third trimester**

      O42.019 **Preterm premature rupture of membranes, onset of labor within 24 hours of rupture, unspecified trimester**

    O42.02 **Full-term premature rupture of membranes, onset of labor within 24 hours of rupture**

      Premature rupture of membranes after 37 completed weeks of gestation

√5ᵗʰ **O42.1** **Premature rupture of membranes, onset of labor more than 24 hours following rupture**

    O42.10 **Premature rupture of membranes, onset of labor more than 24 hours following rupture, unspecified weeks of gestation**

    √6ᵗʰ **O42.11** **Preterm premature rupture of membranes, onset of labor more than 24 hours following rupture**

      Premature rupture of membranes before 37 completed weeks of gestation

      O42.111 **Preterm premature rupture of membranes, onset of labor more than 24 hours following rupture, first trimester**

      O42.112 **Preterm premature rupture of membranes, onset of labor more than 24 hours following rupture, second trimester**

    EXCLUDES 1 Not coded here   **EXCLUDES 2** Not included here   *Manifestation Code*

O42.113 **Preterm premature rupture of membranes, onset of labor more than 24 hours following rupture, third trimester**

O42.119 **Preterm premature rupture of membranes, onset of labor more than 24 hours following rupture, unspecified trimester**

O42.12 **Full-term premature rupture of membranes, onset of labor more than 24 hours following rupture**
Premature rupture of membranes after 37 completed weeks of gestation

✓5th O42.9 **Premature rupture of membranes, unspecified as to length of time between rupture and onset of labor**

O42.90 **Premature rupture of membranes, unspecified as to length of time between rupture and onset of labor, unspecified weeks of gestation**

✓6th O42.91 **Preterm premature rupture of membranes, unspecified as to length of time between rupture and onset of labor**
Premature rupture of membranes before 37 completed weeks of gestation

O42.911 **Preterm premature rupture of membranes, unspecified as to length of time between rupture and onset of labor, first trimester**

O42.912 **Preterm premature rupture of membranes, unspecified as to length of time between rupture and onset of labor, second trimester**

O42.913 **Preterm premature rupture of membranes, unspecified as to length of time between rupture and onset of labor, third trimester**

O42.919 **Preterm premature rupture of membranes, unspecified as to length of time between rupture and onset of labor, unspecified trimester**

O42.92 **Full-term premature rupture of membranes, unspecified as to length of time between rupture and onset of labor**
Premature rupture of membranes after 37 completed weeks of gestation

✓4th O43 **Placental disorders**
EXCLUDES 2 *maternal care for poor fetal growth due to placental insufficiency (O36.5-)*
placenta previa (O44-)
placental polyp (O90.89)
placentitis (O41.14-)
premature separation of placenta [abruptio placentae] (O45-)

✓5th O43.0 **Placental transfusion syndromes**

✓6th O43.01 **Fetomaternal placental transfusion syndrome**
Maternofetal placental transfusion syndrome

O43.011 **Fetomaternal placental transfusion syndrome, first trimester**

O43.012 **Fetomaternal placental transfusion syndrome, second trimester**

O43.013 **Fetomaternal placental transfusion syndrome, third trimester**

O43.019 **Fetomaternal placental transfusion syndrome, unspecified trimester**

✓6th O43.02 **Fetus-to-fetus placental transfusion syndrome**

O43.021 **Fetus-to-fetus placental transfusion syndrome, first trimester**

O43.022 **Fetus-to-fetus placental transfusion syndrome, second trimester**

O43.023 **Fetus-to-fetus placental transfusion syndrome, third trimester**

O43.029 **Fetus-to-fetus placental transfusion syndrome, unspecified trimester**

✓5th O43.1 **Malformation of placenta**

✓6th O43.10 **Malformation of placenta, unspecified**
Abnormal placenta NOS

O43.101 **Malformation of placenta, unspecified, first trimester**

O43.102 **Malformation of placenta, unspecified, second trimester**

O43.103 **Malformation of placenta, unspecified, third trimester**

O43.109 **Malformation of placenta, unspecified, unspecified trimester**

✓6th O43.11 **Circumvallate placenta**

O43.111 **Circumvallate placenta, first trimester**

O43.112 **Circumvallate placenta, second trimester**

O43.113 **Circumvallate placenta, third trimester**

O43.119 **Circumvallate placenta, unspecified trimester**

✓6th O43.12 **Velamentous insertion of umbilical cord**

O43.121 **Velamentous insertion of umbilical cord, first trimester**

O43.122 **Velamentous insertion of umbilical cord, second trimester**

O43.123 **Velamentous insertion of umbilical cord, third trimester**

O43.129 **Velamentous insertion of umbilical cord, unspecified trimester**

✓6th O43.19 **Other malformation of placenta**

O43.191 **Other malformation of placenta, first trimester**

O43.192 **Other malformation of placenta, second trimester**

O43.193 **Other malformation of placenta, third trimester**

O43.199 **Other malformation of placenta, unspecified trimester**

✓5th O43.2 **Morbidly adherent placenta**
Code also associated third stage postpartum hemorrhage, if applicable (O72.0)
EXCLUDES 1 *retained placenta (O73-)*

✓6th O43.21 **Placenta accreta**

O43.211 **Placenta accreta, first trimester**

O43.212 **Placenta accreta, second trimester**

O43.213 **Placenta accreta, third trimester**

O43.219 **Placenta accreta, unspecified trimester**

✓6th O43.22 **Placenta increta**

O43.221 **Placenta increta, first trimester**

O43.222 **Placenta increta, second trimester**

O43.223 **Placenta increta, third trimester**

O43.229 **Placenta increta, unspecified trimester**

✓6th O43.23 **Placenta percreta**

O43.231 **Placenta percreta, first trimester**

O43.232 **Placenta percreta, second trimester**

O43.233 **Placenta percreta, third trimester**

O43.239 **Placenta percreta, unspecified trimester**

✓5th O43.8 **Other placental disorders**

✓6th O43.81 **Placental infarction**

O43.811 **Placental infarction, first trimester**

O43.812 **Placental infarction, second trimester**

O43.813 **Placental infarction, third trimester**

O43.819 **Placental infarction, unspecified trimester**

✓6th O43.89 **Other placental disorders**
Placental dysfunction

O43.891 **Other placental disorders, first trimester**

O43.892 **Other placental disorders, second trimester**

O43.893 **Other placental disorders, third trimester**

O43.899 **Other placental disorders, unspecified trimester**

✓5th O43.9 **Unspecified placental disorder**

O43.90 **Unspecified placental disorder, unspecified trimester**

O43.91 **Unspecified placental disorder, first trimester**

O43.92 **Unspecified placental disorder, second trimester**

O43.93 **Unspecified placental disorder, third trimester**

✓4th O44 **Placenta previa**

✓5th O44.0 **Placenta previa specified as without hemorrhage**
Low implantation of placenta specified as without hemorrhage

O44.00 **Placenta previa specified as without hemorrhage, unspecified trimester**

O44.01 **Placenta previa specified as without hemorrhage, first trimester**

☑ Appropriate additional character required   ✓x7th Requires 7th character, placeholder x must fill empty characters

O44.02 Placenta previa specified as without hemorrhage, second trimester

O44.03 Placenta previa specified as without hemorrhage, third trimester

√5th **O44.1** Placenta previa with hemorrhage
Low implantation of placenta, NOS or with hemorrhage
Marginal placenta previa, NOS or with hemorrhage
Partial placenta previa, NOS or with hemorrhage
Total placenta previa, NOS or with hemorrhage
EXCLUDES 1 labor and delivery complicated by hemorrhage from vasa previa (O69.4)

O44.10 Placenta previa with hemorrhage, unspecified trimester

O44.11 Placenta previa with hemorrhage, first trimester

O44.12 Placenta previa with hemorrhage, second trimester

O44.13 Placenta previa with hemorrhage, third trimester

√4th **O45** Premature separation of placenta [abruptio placentae]

√5th **O45.0** Premature separation of placenta with coagulation defect

√6th **O45.00** Premature separation of placenta with coagulation defect, unspecified

O45.001 Premature separation of placenta with coagulation defect, unspecified, first trimester

O45.002 Premature separation of placenta with coagulation defect, unspecified, second trimester

O45.003 Premature separation of placenta with coagulation defect, unspecified, third trimester

O45.009 Premature separation of placenta with coagulation defect, unspecified, unspecified trimester

√6th **O45.01** Premature separation of placenta with afibrinogenemia
Premature separation of placenta with hypofibrinogenemia

O45.011 Premature separation of placenta with afibrinogenemia, first trimester

O45.012 Premature separation of placenta with afibrinogenemia, second trimester

O45.013 Premature separation of placenta with afibrinogenemia, third trimester

O45.019 Premature separation of placenta with afibrinogenemia, unspecified trimester

√6th **O45.02** Premature separation of placenta with disseminated intravascular coagulation

O45.021 Premature separation of placenta with disseminated intravascular coagulation, first trimester

O45.022 Premature separation of placenta with disseminated intravascular coagulation, second trimester

O45.023 Premature separation of placenta with disseminated intravascular coagulation, third trimester

O45.029 Premature separation of placenta with disseminated intravascular coagulation, unspecified trimester

√6th **O45.09** Premature separation of placenta with other coagulation defect

O45.091 Premature separation of placenta with other coagulation defect, first trimester

O45.092 Premature separation of placenta with other coagulation defect, second trimester

O45.093 Premature separation of placenta with other coagulation defect, third trimester

O45.099 Premature separation of placenta with other coagulation defect, unspecified trimester

√5th **O45.8** Other premature separation of placenta

√6th **O45.8x** Other premature separation of placenta

O45.8x1 Other premature separation of placenta, first trimester

O45.8x2 Other premature separation of placenta, second trimester

O45.8x3 Other premature separation of placenta, third trimester

O45.8x9 Other premature separation of placenta, unspecified trimester

√5th **O45.9** Premature separation of placenta, unspecified
Abruptio placentae NOS

O45.90 Premature separation of placenta, unspecified, unspecified trimester

O45.91 Premature separation of placenta, unspecified, first trimester

O45.92 Premature separation of placenta, unspecified, second trimester

O45.93 Premature separation of placenta, unspecified, third trimester

√4th **O46** Antepartum hemorrhage, not elsewhere classified
EXCLUDES 1 hemorrhage in early pregnancy (O20-)
intrapartum hemorrhage NEC (O67-)
placenta previa (O44-)
premature separation of placenta [abruptio placentae] (O45-)

√5th **O46.0** Antepartum hemorrhage with coagulation defect

√6th **O46.00** Antepartum hemorrhage with coagulation defect, unspecified

O46.001 Antepartum hemorrhage with coagulation defect, unspecified, first trimester

O46.002 Antepartum hemorrhage with coagulation defect, unspecified, second trimester

O46.003 Antepartum hemorrhage with coagulation defect, unspecified, third trimester

O46.009 Antepartum hemorrhage with coagulation defect, unspecified, unspecified trimester

√6th **O46.01** Antepartum hemorrhage with afibrinogenemia
Antepartum hemorrhage with hypofibrinogenemia

O46.011 Antepartum hemorrhage with afibrinogenemia, first trimester

O46.012 Antepartum hemorrhage with afibrinogenemia, second trimester

O46.013 Antepartum hemorrhage with afibrinogenemia, third trimester

O46.019 Antepartum hemorrhage with afibrinogenemia, unspecified trimester

√6th **O46.02** Antepartum hemorrhage with disseminated intravascular coagulation

O46.021 Antepartum hemorrhage with disseminated intravascular coagulation, first trimester

O46.022 Antepartum hemorrhage with disseminated intravascular coagulation, second trimester

O46.023 Antepartum hemorrhage with disseminated intravascular coagulation, third trimester

O46.029 Antepartum hemorrhage with disseminated intravascular coagulation, unspecified trimester

√6th **O46.09** Antepartum hemorrhage with other coagulation defect

O46.091 Antepartum hemorrhage with other coagulation defect, first trimester

O46.092 Antepartum hemorrhage with other coagulation defect, second trimester

O46.093 Antepartum hemorrhage with other coagulation defect, third trimester

O46.099 Antepartum hemorrhage with other coagulation defect, unspecified trimester

√5th **O46.8** Other antepartum hemorrhage

√6th **O46.8x** Other antepartum hemorrhage

O46.8x1 Other antepartum hemorrhage, first trimester

O46.8x2 Other antepartum hemorrhage, second trimester

O46.8x3 Other antepartum hemorrhage, third trimester

EXCLUDES 1 Not coded here   EXCLUDES 2 Not included here   *Manifestation Code*

O46.8x9   Other antepartum hemorrhage, unspecified trimester

☑5ᵗʰ   O46.9   **Antepartum hemorrhage, unspecified**
O46.90   **Antepartum hemorrhage, unspecified, unspecified trimester**
O46.91   **Antepartum hemorrhage, unspecified, first trimester**
O46.92   **Antepartum hemorrhage, unspecified, second trimester**
O46.93   **Antepartum hemorrhage, unspecified, third trimester**

☑4ᵗʰ   O47   **False labor**
Braxton Hicks contractions
Threatened labor
EXCLUDES 1   *preterm labor (O60-)*

☑5ᵗʰ   O47.0   **False labor before 37 completed weeks of gestation**
O47.00   **False labor before 37 completed weeks of gestation, unspecified trimester**
O47.02   **False labor before 37 completed weeks of gestation, second trimester**
O47.03   **False labor before 37 completed weeks of gestation, third trimester**
O47.1   **False labor at or after 37 completed weeks of gestation**
O47.9   **False labor, unspecified**

☑4ᵗʰ   O48   **Late pregnancy**
O48.0   **Post-term pregnancy**
Pregnancy over 40 completed weeks to 42 completed weeks gestation
O48.1   **Prolonged pregnancy**
Pregnancy which has advanced beyond 42 completed weeks gestation

Complications of labor and delivery (O60-O77)

☑4ᵗʰ   O60   **Preterm labor**
INCLUDES   onset (spontaneous) of labor before 37 completed weeks of gestation
EXCLUDES 1   *false labor (O47.0-)*
threatened labor NOS (O47.0-)

☑5ᵗʰ   O60.0   **Preterm labor without delivery**
O60.00   **Preterm labor without delivery, unspecified trimester**
O60.02   **Preterm labor without delivery, second trimester**
O60.03   **Preterm labor without delivery, third trimester**

☑5ᵗʰ   O60.1   **Preterm labor with preterm delivery**

> One of the following 7th characters is to be assigned to each code under subcategory O60.1. 7th character 0 is for single gestations and multiple gestations where the fetus is unspecified. 7th characters 1 through 9 are for cases of multiple gestations to identify the fetus for which the code applies. The appropriate code from category O30, Multiple gestation, must also be assigned when assigning a code from subcategory O60.1 that has a 7th character of 1 through 9.
> 0   not applicable or unspecified
> 1   fetus 1
> 2   fetus 2
> 3   fetus 3
> 4   fetus 4
> 5   fetus 5
> 9   other fetus

☑x7ᵗʰ   O60.10   **Preterm labor with preterm delivery, unspecified trimester**
Preterm labor with delivery NOS
☑x7ᵗʰ   O60.12   **Preterm labor second trimester with preterm delivery second trimester**
☑x7ᵗʰ   O60.13   **Preterm labor second trimester with preterm delivery third trimester**
☑x7ᵗʰ   O60.14   **Preterm labor third trimester with preterm delivery third trimester**

☑5ᵗʰ   O60.2   **Term delivery with preterm labor**

> One of the following 7th characters is to be assigned to each code under subcategory O60.2. 7th character 0 is for single gestations and multiple gestations where the fetus is unspecified. 7th characters 1 through 9 are for cases of multiple gestations to identify the fetus for which the code applies. The appropriate code from category O30, Multiple gestation, must also be assigned when assigning a code from subcategory O60.2 that has a 7th character of 1 through 9.
> 0   not applicable or unspecified
> 1   fetus 1
> 2   fetus 2
> 3   fetus 3
> 4   fetus 4
> 5   fetus 5
> 9   other fetus

☑x7ᵗʰ   O60.20   **Term delivery with preterm labor, unspecified trimester**
☑x7ᵗʰ   O60.22   **Term delivery with preterm labor, second trimester**
☑x7ᵗʰ   O60.23   **Term delivery with preterm labor, third trimester**

☑4ᵗʰ   O61   **Failed induction of labor**
O61.0   **Failed medical induction of labor**
Failed induction (of labor) by oxytocin
Failed induction (of labor) by prostaglandins
O61.1   **Failed instrumental induction of labor**
Failed mechanical induction (of labor)
Failed surgical induction (of labor)
O61.8   **Other failed induction of labor**
O61.9   **Failed induction of labor, unspecified**

☑4ᵗʰ   O62   **Abnormalities of forces of labor**
O62.0   **Primary inadequate contractions**
Failure of cervical dilatation
Primary hypotonic uterine dysfunction
Uterine inertia during latent phase of labor
O62.1   **Secondary uterine inertia**
Arrested active phase of labor
Secondary hypotonic uterine dysfunction
O62.2   **Other uterine inertia**
Atony of uterus without hemorrhage
Atony of uterus NOS
Desultory labor
Hypotonic uterine dysfunction NOS
Irregular labor
Poor contractions
Slow slope active phase of labor
Uterine inertia NOS
EXCLUDES 1   *atony of uterus with hemorrhage (postpartum) (O72.1)*
postpartum atony of uterus without hemorrhage (O75.89)
O62.3   **Precipitate labor**
O62.4   **Hypertonic, incoordinate, and prolonged uterine contractions**
Cervical spasm
Contraction ring dystocia
Dyscoordinate labor
Hour-glass contraction of uterus
Hypertonic uterine dysfunction
Incoordinate uterine action
Tetanic contractions
Uterine dystocia NOS
Uterine spasm
EXCLUDES 1   *dystocia (fetal) (maternal) NOS (O66.9)*
O62.8   **Other abnormalities of forces of labor**
O62.9   **Abnormality of forces of labor, unspecified**

☑4ᵗʰ   O63   **Long labor**
O63.0   **Prolonged first stage (of labor)**
O63.1   **Prolonged second stage (of labor)**
O63.2   **Delayed delivery of second twin, triplet, etc.**
O63.9   **Long labor, unspecified**
Prolonged labor NOS

☑ Appropriate additional character required   ☑x7ᵗʰ Requires 7th character, placeholder x must fill empty characters

Pregnancy, Childbirth and the Puerperium

O64–O69.3

✓4ᵗʰ O64 Obstructed labor due to malposition and malpresentation of fetus

One of the following 7th characters is to be assigned to each code under category O64. 7th character Ø is for single gestations and multiple gestations where the fetus is unspecified. 7th characters 1 through 9 are for cases of multiple gestations to identify the fetus for which the code applies. The appropriate code from category O3Ø, Multiple gestation, must also be assigned when assigning a code from category O64 that has a 7th character of 1 through 9.

Ø   not applicable or unspecified
1   fetus 1
2   fetus 2
3   fetus 3
4   fetus 4
5   fetus 5
9   other fetus

✓x7ᵗʰ O64.Ø   Obstructed labor due to incomplete rotation of fetal head
Deep transverse arrest
Obstructed labor due to persistent occipitoiliac (position)
Obstructed labor due to persistent occipitoposterior (position)
Obstructed labor due to persistent occipitosacral (position)
Obstructed labor due to persistent occipitotransverse (position)

✓x7ᵗʰ O64.1   Obstructed labor due to breech presentation
Obstructed labor due to buttocks presentation
Obstructed labor due to complete breech presentation
Obstructed labor due to frank breech presentation

✓x7ᵗʰ O64.2   Obstructed labor due to face presentation
Obstructed labor due to chin presentation

✓x7ᵗʰ O64.3   Obstructed labor due to brow presentation

✓x7ᵗʰ O64.4   Obstructed labor due to shoulder presentation
Prolapsed arm
EXCLUDES 1   impacted shoulders (O66.Ø)
         shoulder dystocia (O66.Ø)

✓x7ᵗʰ O64.5   Obstructed labor due to compound presentation

✓x7ᵗʰ O64.8   Obstructed labor due to other malposition and malpresentation
Obstructed labor due to footling presentation
Obstructed labor due to incomplete breech presentation

✓x7ᵗʰ O64.9   Obstructed labor due to malposition and malpresentation, unspecified

✓4ᵗʰ O65 Obstructed labor due to maternal pelvic abnormality

O65.Ø   Obstructed labor due to deformed pelvis

O65.1   Obstructed labor due to generally contracted pelvis

O65.2   Obstructed labor due to pelvic inlet contraction

O65.3   Obstructed labor due to pelvic outlet and mid-cavity contraction

O65.4   Obstructed labor due to fetopelvic disproportion, unspecified
EXCLUDES 1   dystocia due to abnormality of fetus (O66.2-O66.3)

O65.5   Obstructed labor due to abnormality of maternal pelvic organs
Obstructed labor due to conditions listed in O34-
Use additional code to identify abnormality of pelvic organs (O34-)

O65.8   Obstructed labor due to other maternal pelvic abnormalities

O65.9   Obstructed labor due to maternal pelvic abnormality, unspecified

✓4ᵗʰ O66 Other obstructed labor

O66.Ø   Obstructed labor due to shoulder dystocia
Impacted shoulders

O66.1   Obstructed labor due to locked twins

O66.2   Obstructed labor due to unusually large fetus

O66.3   Obstructed labor due to other abnormalities of fetus
Dystocia due to fetal ascites
Dystocia due to fetal hydrops
Dystocia due to fetal meningomyelocele
Dystocia due to fetal sacral teratoma
Dystocia due to fetal tumor
Dystocia due to hydrocephalic fetus
Use additional code to identify cause of obstruction

✓5ᵗʰ O66.4   Failed trial of labor

O66.4Ø   Failed trial of labor, unspecified

O66.41   Failed attempted vaginal birth after previous cesarean delivery
Code first rupture of uterus, if applicable (O71.Ø-, O71.1)

O66.5   Attempted application of vacuum extractor and forceps
Attempted application of vacuum or forceps, with subsequent delivery by forceps or cesarean delivery

O66.6   Obstructed labor due to other multiple fetuses

O66.8   Other specified obstructed labor
Use additional code to identify cause of obstruction

O66.9   Obstructed labor, unspecified
Dystocia NOS
Fetal dystocia NOS
Maternal dystocia NOS

✓4ᵗʰ O67 Labor and delivery complicated by intrapartum hemorrhage, not elsewhere classified

EXCLUDES 1   antepartum hemorrhage NEC (O46-)
         placenta previa (O44-)
         premature separation of placenta [abruptio placentae] (O45-)
EXCLUDES 2   postpartum hemorrhage (O72-)

O67.Ø   Intrapartum hemorrhage with coagulation defect
Intrapartum hemorrhage (excessive) associated with afibrinogenemia
Intrapartum hemorrhage (excessive) associated with disseminated intravascular coagulation
Intrapartum hemorrhage (excessive) associated with hyperfibrinolysis
Intrapartum hemorrhage (excessive) associated with hypofibrinogenemia

O67.8   Other intrapartum hemorrhage
Excessive intrapartum hemorrhage

O67.9   Intrapartum hemorrhage, unspecified

✓4ᵗʰ O68 Labor and delivery complicated by abnormality of fetal acid-base balance

Fetal acidemia complicating labor and delivery
Fetal acidosis complicating labor and delivery
Fetal alkalosis complicating labor and delivery
Fetal metabolic acidemia complicating labor and delivery
EXCLUDES 1   fetal stress NOS (O77.9)
         labor and delivery complicated by electrocardiographic evidence of fetal stress (O77.8)
         labor and delivery complicated by ultrasonic evidence of fetal stress (O77.8)
EXCLUDES 2   abnormality in fetal heart rate or rhythm (O76)
         labor and delivery complicated by meconium in amniotic fluid (O77.Ø)

✓4ᵗʰ O69 Labor and delivery complicated by umbilical cord complications

One of the following 7th characters is to be assigned to each code under category O69. 7th character Ø is for single gestations and multiple gestations where the fetus is unspecified. 7th characters 1 through 9 are for cases of multiple gestations to identify the fetus for which the code applies. The appropriate code from category O3Ø, Multiple gestation, must also be assigned when assigning a code from category O69 that has a 7th character of 1 through 9.

Ø   not applicable or unspecified
1   fetus 1
2   fetus 2
3   fetus 3
4   fetus 4
5   fetus 5
9   other fetus

✓x7ᵗʰ O69.Ø   Labor and delivery complicated by prolapse of cord

✓x7ᵗʰ O69.1   Labor and delivery complicated by cord around neck, with compression
EXCLUDES 1   labor and delivery complicated by cord around neck, without compression (O69.81)

✓x7ᵗʰ O69.2   Labor and delivery complicated by other cord entanglement, with compression
Labor and delivery complicated by compression of cord NOS
Labor and delivery complicated by entanglement of cords of twins in monoamniotic sac
Labor and delivery complicated by knot in cord
EXCLUDES 1   labor and delivery complicated by other cord entanglement, without compression (O69.82)

✓x7ᵗʰ O69.3   Labor and delivery complicated by short cord

EXCLUDES 1   Not coded here   *EXCLUDES 2*   Not included here   **Manifestation Code**

Pregnancy, Childbirth and the Puerperium

☑x7ᵗʰ **O69.4 Labor and delivery complicated by vasa previa**
Labor and delivery complicated by hemorrhage from vasa previa

☑x7ᵗʰ **O69.5 Labor and delivery complicated by vascular lesion of cord**
Labor and delivery complicated by cord bruising
Labor and delivery complicated by cord hematoma
Labor and delivery complicated by thrombosis of umbilical vessels

☑5ᵗʰ **O69.8 Labor and delivery complicated by other cord complications**

    ☑x7ᵗʰ **O69.81 Labor and delivery complicated by cord around neck, without compression**

    ☑x7ᵗʰ **O69.82 Labor and delivery complicated by other cord entanglement, without compression**

    ☑x7ᵗʰ **O69.89 Labor and delivery complicated by other cord complications**

☑x7ᵗʰ **O69.9 Labor and delivery complicated by cord complication, unspecified**

☑4ᵗʰ **O70 Perineal laceration during delivery**
Episiotomy extended by laceration
EXCLUDES 1 *obstetric high vaginal laceration alone (O71.4)*

    O70.0 First degree perineal laceration during delivery
Perineal laceration, rupture or tear involving fourchette during delivery
Perineal laceration, rupture or tear involving labia during delivery
Perineal laceration, rupture or tear involving skin during delivery
Perineal laceration, rupture or tear involving vagina during delivery
Perineal laceration, rupture or tear involving vulva during delivery
Slight perineal laceration, rupture or tear during delivery

    O70.1 Second degree perineal laceration during delivery
Perineal laceration, rupture or tear during delivery as in O70.0, also involving pelvic floor
Perineal laceration, rupture or tear during delivery as in O70.0, also involving perineal muscles
Perineal laceration, rupture or tear during delivery as in O70.0, also involving vaginal muscles
EXCLUDES 1 *perineal laceration involving anal sphincter (O70.2)*

    O70.2 Third degree perineal laceration during delivery
Perineal laceration, rupture or tear during delivery as in O70.1, also involving anal sphincter
Perineal laceration, rupture or tear during delivery as in O70.1, also involving rectovaginal septum
Perineal laceration, rupture or tear during delivery as in O70.1, also involving sphincter NOS
EXCLUDES 1 *anal sphincter tear during delivery without third degree perineal laceration (O70.4)*
perineal laceration involving anal or rectal mucosa (O70.3)

    O70.3 Fourth degree perineal laceration during delivery
Perineal laceration, rupture or tear during delivery as in O70.2, also involving anal mucosa
Perineal laceration, rupture or tear during delivery as in O70.2, also involving rectal mucosa

    O70.4 Anal sphincter tear complicating delivery, not associated with third degree laceration
EXCLUDES 1 *anal sphincter tear with third degree perineal laceration (O70.2)*

    O70.9 Perineal laceration during delivery, unspecified

☑4ᵗʰ **O71 Other obstetric trauma**
Obstetric damage from instruments

    ☑5ᵗʰ **O71.0 Rupture of uterus (spontaneous) before onset of labor**
EXCLUDES 1 *disruption of (current) cesarean delivery wound (O90.0)*
laceration of uterus, NEC (O71.81)

        O71.00 Rupture of uterus before onset of labor, unspecified trimester

        O71.02 Rupture of uterus before onset of labor, second trimester

        O71.03 Rupture of uterus before onset of labor, third trimester

    O71.1 Rupture of uterus during labor
Rupture of uterus not stated as occurring before onset of labor
EXCLUDES 1 *disruption of cesarean delivery wound (O90.0)*
laceration of uterus, NEC (O71.81)

    O71.2 Postpartum inversion of uterus

    O71.3 Obstetric laceration of cervix
Annular detachment of cervix

    O71.4 Obstetric high vaginal laceration alone
Laceration of vaginal wall without perineal laceration
EXCLUDES 1 *obstetric high vaginal laceration with perineal laceration (O70-)*

    O71.5 Other obstetric injury to pelvic organs
Obstetric injury to bladder
Obstetric injury to urethra
EXCLUDES 2 *obstetric periurethral trauma (O71.82)*

    O71.6 Obstetric damage to pelvic joints and ligaments
Obstetric avulsion of inner symphyseal cartilage
Obstetric damage to coccyx
Obstetric traumatic separation of symphysis (pubis)

    O71.7 Obstetric hematoma of pelvis
Obstetric hematoma of perineum
Obstetric hematoma of vagina
Obstetric hematoma of vulva

    ☑5ᵗʰ **O71.8 Other specified obstetric trauma**

        O71.81 Laceration of uterus, not elsewhere classified

        O71.82 Other specified trauma to perineum and vulva
Obstetric periurethral trauma

        O71.89 Other specified obstetric trauma

    O71.9 Obstetric trauma, unspecified

☑4ᵗʰ **O72 Postpartum hemorrhage**
INCLUDES hemorrhage after delivery of fetus or infant

    O72.0 Third-stage hemorrhage
Hemorrhage associated with retained, trapped or adherent placenta
Retained placenta NOS
Code also type of adherent placenta (O43.2-)

    O72.1 Other immediate postpartum hemorrhage
Hemorrhage following delivery of placenta
Postpartum hemorrhage (atonic) NOS
Uterine atony with hemorrhage
EXCLUDES 1 *uterine atony NOS (O62.2)*
uterine atony without hemorrhage (O62.2)
postpartum atony of uterus without hemorrhage (O75.89)

    O72.2 Delayed and secondary postpartum hemorrhage
Hemorrhage associated with retained portions of placenta or membranes after the first 24 hours following delivery of placenta
Retained products of conception NOS, following delivery

    O72.3 Postpartum coagulation defects
Postpartum afibrinogenemia
Postpartum fibrinolysis

☑4ᵗʰ **O73 Retained placenta and membranes, without hemorrhage**
EXCLUDES 1 *placenta accreta (O43.21-)*
placenta increta (O43.22-)
placenta percreta (O43.23-)

    O73.0 Retained placenta without hemorrhage
Adherent placenta, without hemorrhage
Trapped placenta without hemorrhage

    O73.1 Retained portions of placenta and membranes, without hemorrhage
Retained products of conception following delivery, without hemorrhage

☑4ᵗʰ **O74 Complications of anesthesia during labor and delivery**
INCLUDES maternal complications arising from the administration of a general, regional or local anesthetic, analgesic or other sedation during labor and delivery
Use additional code, if applicable, to identify specific complication

    O74.0 Aspiration pneumonitis due to anesthesia during labor and delivery
Inhalation of stomach contents or secretions NOS due to anesthesia during labor and delivery
Mendelson's syndrome due to anesthesia during labor and delivery

    O74.1 Other pulmonary complications of anesthesia during labor and delivery

    O74.2 Cardiac complications of anesthesia during labor and delivery

    O74.3 Central nervous system complications of anesthesia during labor and delivery

    O74.4 Toxic reaction to local anesthesia during labor and delivery

    O74.5 Spinal and epidural anesthesia-induced headache during labor and delivery

---

O74.6 **Other complications of spinal and epidural anesthesia during labor and delivery**

O74.7 **Failed or difficult intubation for anesthesia during labor and delivery**

O74.8 **Other complications of anesthesia during labor and delivery**

O74.9 **Complication of anesthesia during labor and delivery, unspecified**

✓4ᵗʰ O75 **Other complications of labor and delivery, not elsewhere classified**

> EXCLUDES 2   puerperal (postpartum) infection (O86-)
> puerperal (postpartum) sepsis (O85)

O75.0 **Maternal distress during labor and delivery**

O75.1 **Shock during or following labor and delivery**
Obstetric shock following labor and delivery

O75.2 **Pyrexia during labor, not elsewhere classified**

O75.3 **Other infection during labor**
Sepsis during labor
Use additional code (B95-B97), to identify infectious agent

O75.4 **Other complications of obstetric surgery and procedures**
Cardiac arrest following obstetric surgery or procedures
Cardiac failure following obstetric surgery or procedures
Cerebral anoxia following obstetric surgery or procedures
Pulmonary edema following obstetric surgery or procedures
Use additional code to identify specific complication

> EXCLUDES 2   complications of anesthesia during labor and
> delivery (O74-)
> disruption of obstetrical (surgical) wound
> (O90.0-O90.1)
> hematoma of obstetrical (surgical) wound (O90.2)
> infection of obstetrical (surgical) wound (O86.0)

O75.5 **Delayed delivery after artificial rupture of membranes**

✓5ᵗʰ O75.8 **Other specified complications of labor and delivery**

O75.81 **Maternal exhaustion complicating labor and delivery**

O75.89 **Other specified complications of labor and delivery**

O75.9 **Complication of labor and delivery, unspecified**

O76 **Abnormality in fetal heart rate and rhythm complicating labor and delivery**
Depressed fetal heart rate tones complicating labor and delivery
Fetal bradycardia complicating labor and delivery
Fetal heart rate decelerations complicating labor and delivery
Fetal heart rate irregularity complicating labor and delivery
Fetal heart rate abnormal variability complicating labor and delivery
Fetal tachycardia complicating labor and delivery
Non-reassuring fetal heart rate or rhythm complicating labor and delivery

> EXCLUDES 1   fetal stress NOS (O77.9)
> labor and delivery complicated by electrocardiographic
> evidence of fetal stress (O77.8)
> labor and delivery complicated by ultrasonic evidence of fetal
> stress (O77.8)

> EXCLUDES 2   fetal metabolic acidemia (O68)
> other fetal stress (O77.0-O77.1)

✓4ᵗʰ O77 **Other fetal stress complicating labor and delivery**

O77.0 **Labor and delivery complicated by meconium in amniotic fluid**

O77.1 **Fetal stress in labor or delivery due to drug administration**

O77.8 **Labor and delivery complicated by other evidence of fetal stress**
Labor and delivery complicated by electrocardiographic evidence of fetal stress
Labor and delivery complicated by ultrasonic evidence of fetal stress

> EXCLUDES 1   abnormality of fetal acid-base balance (O68)
> abnormality in fetal heart rate or rhythm (O76)
> fetal metabolic acidemia (O68)

O77.9 **Labor and delivery complicated by fetal stress, unspecified**

> EXCLUDES 1   abnormality of fetal acid-base balance (O68)
> abnormality in fetal heart rate or rhythm (O76)
> fetal metabolic acidemia (O68)

Encounter for delivery (O80, O82)

O80 **Encounter for full-term uncomplicated delivery**

> NOTE   Delivery requiring minimal or no assistance, with or without episiotomy, without fetal manipulation [e.g., rotation version] or instrumentation [forceps] of a spontaneous, cephalic, vaginal, full-term, single, live-born infant. This code is for use as a single diagnosis code and is not to be used with any other code from chapter 15. This code must be accompanied by a delivery code from the appropriate procedure classification.

Use additional code to indicate outcome of delivery (Z37.0)

O82 **Encounter for cesarean delivery without indication**

> NOTE   This code must be accompanied by a delivery code from the appropriate procedure classification.

Use additional code to indicate outcome of delivery (Z37.0)

Complications predominantly related to the puerperium (O85-O92)

> EXCLUDES 2   mental and behavioral disorders associated with the puerperium
> (F53)
> obstetrical tetanus (A34)
> puerperal osteomalacia (M83.0)

O85 **Puerperal sepsis**
Postpartum sepsis
Puerperal peritonitis
Puerperal pyemia
Use additional code (B95-B97), to identify infectious agent
Use additional code (R65.2-) to identify severe sepsis, if applicable

> EXCLUDES 1   fever of unknown origin following delivery (O86.4)
> genital tract infection following delivery (O86.1-)
> obstetric pyemic and septic embolism (O88.3-)
> puerperal septic thrombophlebitis (O86.81)
> urinary tract infection following delivery (O86.2-)

> EXCLUDES 2   sepsis during labor (O75.3)

✓4ᵗʰ O86 **Other puerperal infections**
Use additional code (B95-B97), to identify infectious agent

> EXCLUDES 2   infection during labor (O75.3)
> obstetrical tetanus (A34)

O86.0 **Infection of obstetric surgical wound**
Infected cesarean delivery wound following delivery
Infected perineal repair following delivery

✓5ᵗʰ O86.1 **Other infection of genital tract following delivery**

O86.11 **Cervicitis following delivery**

O86.12 **Endometritis following delivery**

O86.13 **Vaginitis following delivery**

O86.19 **Other infection of genital tract following delivery**

✓5ᵗʰ O86.2 **Urinary tract infection following delivery**

O86.20 **Urinary tract infection following delivery, unspecified**
Puerperal urinary tract infection NOS

O86.21 **Infection of kidney following delivery**

O86.22 **Infection of bladder following delivery**
Infection of urethra following delivery

O86.29 **Other urinary tract infection following delivery**

O86.4 **Pyrexia of unknown origin following delivery**
Puerperal infection NOS following delivery
Puerperal pyrexia NOS following delivery

> EXCLUDES 2   pyrexia during labor (O75.2)

✓5ᵗʰ O86.8 **Other specified puerperal infections**

O86.81 **Puerperal septic thrombophlebitis**

O86.89 **Other specified puerperal infections**

✓4ᵗʰ O87 **Venous complications in the puerperium**
Venous complications in labor, delivery and the puerperium

> EXCLUDES 2   obstetric embolism (O88-)
> puerperal septic thrombophlebitis (O86.81)
> venous complications in pregnancy (O22-)

O87.0 **Superficial thrombophlebitis in the puerperium**
Puerperal phlebitis NOS
Puerperal thrombosis NOS

O87.1 **Deep phlebothrombosis in the puerperium**
Deep vein thrombosis, postpartum
Pelvic thrombophlebitis, postpartum
Use additional code to identify the deep vein thrombosis
(I82.4-, I82.5-, I82.62-, I82.72-)
Use additional code, if applicable, for associated long-term (current) use of anticoagulants (Z79.01)

EXCLUDES 1 Not coded here   EXCLUDES 2 Not included here   *Manifestation Code*

O87.2   **Hemorrhoids in the puerperium**
O87.3   **Cerebral venous thrombosis in the puerperium**
         Cerebrovenous sinus thrombosis in the puerperium
O87.4   **Varicose veins of lower extremity in the puerperium**
O87.8   **Other venous complications in the puerperium**
         Genital varices in the puerperium
O87.9   **Venous complication in the puerperium, unspecified**
         Puerperal phlebopathy NOS

✓4ᵗʰ **O88 Obstetric embolism**
         EXCLUDES 1 *embolism complicating abortion NOS (O03.2)*
                     embolism complicating ectopic or molar pregnancy (O08.2)
                     embolism complicating failed attempted abortion (O07.2,
                     O07.7)
                     embolism complicating induced abortion (O04.7)
                     embolism complicating spontaneous abortion (O03.2, O03.7)

✓5ᵗʰ O88.0 **Obstetric air embolism**
       ✓6ᵗʰ O88.01 **Obstetric air embolism in pregnancy**
                     O88.011 **Air embolism in pregnancy, first**
                              trimester
                     O88.012 **Air embolism in pregnancy, second**
                              trimester
                     O88.013 **Air embolism in pregnancy, third**
                              trimester
                     O88.019 **Air embolism in pregnancy, unspecified**
                              trimester
             O88.02 **Air embolism in childbirth**
             O88.03 **Air embolism in the puerperium**

✓5ᵗʰ O88.1 **Amniotic fluid embolism**
             Anaphylactoid syndrome in pregnancy
       ✓6ᵗʰ O88.11 **Amniotic fluid embolism in pregnancy**
                     O88.111 **Amniotic fluid embolism in pregnancy,**
                              first trimester
                     O88.112 **Amniotic fluid embolism in pregnancy,**
                              second trimester
                     O88.113 **Amniotic fluid embolism in pregnancy,**
                              third trimester
                     O88.119 **Amniotic fluid embolism in pregnancy,**
                              unspecified trimester
             O88.12 **Amniotic fluid embolism in childbirth**
             O88.13 **Amniotic fluid embolism in the puerperium**

✓5ᵗʰ O88.2 **Obstetric thromboembolism**
       ✓6ᵗʰ O88.21 **Thromboembolism in pregnancy**
                     Obstetric (pulmonary) embolism NOS
                     O88.211 **Thromboembolism in pregnancy, first**
                              trimester
                     O88.212 **Thromboembolism in pregnancy,**
                              second trimester
                     O88.213 **Thromboembolism in pregnancy, third**
                              trimester
                     O88.219 **Thromboembolism in pregnancy,**
                              unspecified trimester
             O88.22 **Thromboembolism in childbirth**
             O88.23 **Thromboembolism in the puerperium**
                     Puerperal (pulmonary) embolism NOS

✓5ᵗʰ O88.3 **Obstetric pyemic and septic embolism**
       ✓6ᵗʰ O88.31 **Pyemic and septic embolism in pregnancy**
                     O88.311 **Pyemic and septic embolism in**
                              pregnancy, first trimester
                     O88.312 **Pyemic and septic embolism in**
                              pregnancy, second trimester
                     O88.313 **Pyemic and septic embolism in**
                              pregnancy, third trimester
                     O88.319 **Pyemic and septic embolism in**
                              pregnancy, unspecified trimester
             O88.32 **Pyemic and septic embolism in childbirth**
             O88.33 **Pyemic and septic embolism in the puerperium**

✓5ᵗʰ O88.8 **Other obstetric embolism**
             Obstetric fat embolism
       ✓6ᵗʰ O88.81 **Other embolism in pregnancy**
                     O88.811 **Other embolism in pregnancy, first**
                              trimester
                     O88.812 **Other embolism in pregnancy, second**
                              trimester
                     O88.813 **Other embolism in pregnancy, third**
                              trimester
                     O88.819 **Other embolism in pregnancy,**
                              unspecified trimester

             O88.82 **Other embolism in childbirth**
             O88.83 **Other embolism in the puerperium**

✓4ᵗʰ **O89 Complications of anesthesia during the puerperium**
         INCLUDES   maternal complications arising from the administration of a
                    general, regional or local anesthetic, analgesic or other
                    sedation during the puerperium
         Use additional code, if applicable, to identify specific complication

✓5ᵗʰ O89.0 **Pulmonary complications of anesthesia during the**
             puerperium
             O89.01 **Aspiration pneumonitis due to anesthesia during**
                     the puerperium
                     Inhalation of stomach contents or secretions NOS
                        due to anesthesia during the puerperium
                     Mendelson's syndrome due to anesthesia during the
                        puerperium
             O89.09 **Other pulmonary complications of anesthesia**
                     during the puerperium
       O89.1 **Cardiac complications of anesthesia during the puerperium**
       O89.2 **Central nervous system complications of anesthesia during**
              the puerperium
       O89.3 **Toxic reaction to local anesthesia during the puerperium**
       O89.4 **Spinal and epidural anesthesia-induced headache during**
              the puerperium
       O89.5 **Other complications of spinal and epidural anesthesia**
              during the puerperium
       O89.6 **Failed or difficult intubation for anesthesia during the**
              puerperium
       O89.8 **Other complications of anesthesia during the puerperium**
       O89.9 **Complication of anesthesia during the puerperium,**
              unspecified

✓4ᵗʰ **O90 Complications of the puerperium, not elsewhere classified**
       O90.0 **Disruption of cesarean delivery wound**
              Dehiscence of cesarean delivery wound
              EXCLUDES 1 *rupture of uterus (spontaneous) before onset of labor*
                          (O71.0-)
                          rupture of uterus during labor (O71.1)
       O90.1 **Disruption of perineal obstetric wound**
              Disruption of wound of episiotomy
              Disruption of wound of perineal laceration
              Secondary perineal tear
       O90.2 **Hematoma of obstetric wound**
       O90.3 **Peripartum cardiomyopathy**
              Conditions in I42- arising during pregnancy and the
                 puerperium
              EXCLUDES 1 *pre-existing heart disease complicating pregnancy*
                          and the puerperium (O99.4-)
       O90.4 **Postpartum acute kidney failure**
              Hepatorenal syndrome following labor and delivery
       O90.5 **Postpartum thyroiditis**
       O90.6 **Postpartum mood disturbance**
              Postpartum blues
              Postpartum dysphoria
              Postpartum sadness
              EXCLUDES 1 *postpartum depression (F53)*
                          puerperal psychosis (F53)

✓5ᵗʰ O90.8 **Other complications of the puerperium, not elsewhere**
             classified
             O90.81 **Anemia of the puerperium**
                     Postpartum anemia NOS
                     EXCLUDES 1 *pre-existing anemia complicating the*
                                 puerperium (O99.0-)
             O90.89 **Other complications of the puerperium, not**
                     elsewhere classified
                     Placental polyp
       O90.9 **Complication of the puerperium, unspecified**

✓4ᵗʰ **O91 Infections of breast associated with pregnancy, the**
       puerperium and lactation
       Use additional code to identify infection
✓5ᵗʰ O91.0 **Infection of nipple associated with pregnancy, the**
             puerperium and lactation
       ✓6ᵗʰ O91.01 **Infection of nipple associated with pregnancy**
                     Gestational abscess of nipple
                     O91.011 **Infection of nipple associated with**
                              pregnancy, first trimester
                     O91.012 **Infection of nipple associated with**
                              pregnancy, second trimester

Pregnancy, Childbirth and the Puerperium

O91.013–O98.112

         O91.013   **Infection of nipple associated with pregnancy, third trimester**
         O91.019   **Infection of nipple associated with pregnancy, unspecified trimester**
      O91.02   **Infection of nipple associated with the puerperium**
         Puerperal abscess of nipple
      O91.03   **Infection of nipple associated with lactation**
         Abscess of nipple associated with lactation

✓5th   **O91.1**   **Abscess of breast associated with pregnancy, the puerperium and lactation**

    ✓6th   **O91.11**   **Abscess of breast associated with pregnancy**
         Gestational mammary abscess
         Gestational purulent mastitis
         Gestational subareolar abscess
         O91.111   **Abscess of breast associated with pregnancy, first trimester**
         O91.112   **Abscess of breast associated with pregnancy, second trimester**
         O91.113   **Abscess of breast associated with pregnancy, third trimester**
         O91.119   **Abscess of breast associated with pregnancy, unspecified trimester**
      O91.12   **Abscess of breast associated with the puerperium**
         Puerperal mammary abscess
         Puerperal purulent mastitis
         Puerperal subareolar abscess
      O91.13   **Abscess of breast associated with lactation**
         Mammary abscess associated with lactation
         Purulent mastitis associated with lactation
         Subareolar abscess associated with lactation

✓5th   **O91.2**   **Nonpurulent mastitis associated with pregnancy, the puerperium and lactation**

    ✓6th   **O91.21**   **Nonpurulent mastitis associated with pregnancy**
         Gestational interstitial mastitis
         Gestational lymphangitis of breast
         Gestational mastitis NOS
         Gestational parenchymatous mastitis
         O91.211   **Nonpurulent mastitis associated with pregnancy, first trimester**
         O91.212   **Nonpurulent mastitis associated with pregnancy, second trimester**
         O91.213   **Nonpurulent mastitis associated with pregnancy, third trimester**
         O91.219   **Nonpurulent mastitis associated with pregnancy, unspecified trimester**
      O91.22   **Nonpurulent mastitis associated with the puerperium**
         Puerperal interstitial mastitis
         Puerperal lymphangitis of breast
         Puerperal mastitis NOS
         Puerperal parenchymatous mastitis
      O91.23   **Nonpurulent mastitis associated with lactation**
         Interstitial mastitis associated with lactation
         Lymphangitis of breast associated with lactation
         Mastitis NOS associated with lactation
         Parenchymatous mastitis associated with lactation

✓4th   **O92**   **Other disorders of breast and disorders of lactation associated with pregnancy and the puerperium**

   ✓5th   **O92.0**   **Retracted nipple associated with pregnancy, the puerperium, and lactation**

    ✓6th   **O92.01**   **Retracted nipple associated with pregnancy**
         O92.011   **Retracted nipple associated with pregnancy, first trimester**
         O92.012   **Retracted nipple associated with pregnancy, second trimester**
         O92.013   **Retracted nipple associated with pregnancy, third trimester**
         O92.019   **Retracted nipple associated with pregnancy, unspecified trimester**
      O92.02   **Retracted nipple associated with the puerperium**
      O92.03   **Retracted nipple associated with lactation**

   ✓5th   **O92.1**   **Cracked nipple associated with pregnancy, the puerperium, and lactation**
         Fissure of nipple, gestational or puerperal

    ✓6th   **O92.11**   **Cracked nipple associated with pregnancy**
         O92.111   **Cracked nipple associated with pregnancy, first trimester**
         O92.112   **Cracked nipple associated with pregnancy, second trimester**

         O92.113   **Cracked nipple associated with pregnancy, third trimester**
         O92.119   **Cracked nipple associated with pregnancy, unspecified trimester**
      O92.12   **Cracked nipple associated with the puerperium**
      O92.13   **Cracked nipple associated with lactation**

   ✓5th   **O92.2**   **Other and unspecified disorders of breast associated with pregnancy and the puerperium**
      O92.20   **Unspecified disorder of breast associated with pregnancy and the puerperium**
      O92.29   **Other disorders of breast associated with pregnancy and the puerperium**

   O92.3   **Agalactia**
       Primary agalactia
       EXCLUDES 1   *elective agalactia (O92.5)*
                secondary agalactia (O92.5)
                therapeutic agalactia (O92.5)

   O92.4   **Hypogalactia**

   O92.5   **Suppressed lactation**
       Elective agalactia
       Secondary agalactia
       Therapeutic agalactia
       EXCLUDES 1   *primary agalactia (O92.3)*

   O92.6   **Galactorrhea**

   ✓5th   **O92.7**   **Other and unspecified disorders of lactation**
      O92.70   **Unspecified disorders of lactation**
      O92.79   **Other disorders of lactation**
         Puerperal galactocele

Other obstetric conditions, not elsewhere classified (O94-O9A)

   O94   **Sequelae of complication of pregnancy, childbirth, and the puerperium**
       NOTE   This category is to be used to indicate conditions in O00-O77-, O85-O94 and O98-O99- as the cause of late effects. The sequelae include conditions specified as such, or as late effects, which may occur at any time after the puerperium
       Code first condition resulting from (sequela) of complication of pregnancy, childbirth, and the puerperium

✓4th   **O98**   **Maternal infectious and parasitic diseases classifiable elsewhere but complicating pregnancy, childbirth and the puerperium**
       INCLUDES   the listed conditions when complicating the pregnant state, when aggravated by the pregnancy, or as a reason for obstetric care
       Use additional code (Chapter 1), to identify specific infectious or parasitic disease
       EXCLUDES 2   *herpes gestationis (O26.4-)*
                infectious carrier state (O99.82-, O99.83-)
                obstetrical tetanus (A34)
                puerperal infection (O86-)
                puerperal sepsis (O85)
                when the reason for maternal care is that the disease is known or suspected to have affected the fetus (O35-O36)

   ✓5th   **O98.0**   **Tuberculosis complicating pregnancy, childbirth and the puerperium**
       Conditions in A15-A19

    ✓6th   **O98.01**   **Tuberculosis complicating pregnancy**
         O98.011   **Tuberculosis complicating pregnancy, first trimester**
         O98.012   **Tuberculosis complicating pregnancy, second trimester**
         O98.013   **Tuberculosis complicating pregnancy, third trimester**
         O98.019   **Tuberculosis complicating pregnancy, unspecified trimester**
      O98.02   **Tuberculosis complicating childbirth**
      O98.03   **Tuberculosis complicating the puerperium**

   ✓5th   **O98.1**   **Syphilis complicating pregnancy, childbirth and the puerperium**
       Conditions in A50-A53

    ✓6th   **O98.11**   **Syphilis complicating pregnancy**
         O98.111   **Syphilis complicating pregnancy, first trimester**
         O98.112   **Syphilis complicating pregnancy, second trimester**

EXCLUDES 1   Not coded here   EXCLUDES 2   Not included here   *Manifestation Code*

O98.113   Syphilis complicating pregnancy, third trimester

O98.119   Syphilis complicating pregnancy, unspecified trimester

O98.12   **Syphilis complicating childbirth**

O98.13   **Syphilis complicating the puerperium**

☑5ᵗʰ O98.2   **Gonorrhea complicating pregnancy, childbirth and the puerperium**
    Conditions in A54-

   ☑6ᵗʰ O98.21   **Gonorrhea complicating pregnancy**

O98.211   Gonorrhea complicating pregnancy, first trimester

O98.212   Gonorrhea complicating pregnancy, second trimester

O98.213   Gonorrhea complicating pregnancy, third trimester

O98.219   Gonorrhea complicating pregnancy, unspecified trimester

O98.22   **Gonorrhea complicating childbirth**

O98.23   **Gonorrhea complicating the puerperium**

☑5ᵗʰ O98.3   **Other infections with a predominantly sexual mode of transmission complicating pregnancy, childbirth and the puerperium**
    Conditions in A55-A64

   ☑6ᵗʰ O98.31   **Other infections with a predominantly sexual mode of transmission complicating pregnancy**

O98.311   Other infections with a predominantly sexual mode of transmission complicating pregnancy, first trimester

O98.312   Other infections with a predominantly sexual mode of transmission complicating pregnancy, second trimester

O98.313   Other infections with a predominantly sexual mode of transmission complicating pregnancy, third trimester

O98.319   Other infections with a predominantly sexual mode of transmission complicating pregnancy, unspecified trimester

O98.32   **Other infections with a predominantly sexual mode of transmission complicating childbirth**

O98.33   **Other infections with a predominantly sexual mode of transmission complicating the puerperium**

☑5ᵗʰ O98.4   **Viral hepatitis complicating pregnancy, childbirth and the puerperium**
    Conditions in B15-B19

   ☑6ᵗʰ O98.41   **Viral hepatitis complicating pregnancy**

O98.411   Viral hepatitis complicating pregnancy, first trimester

O98.412   Viral hepatitis complicating pregnancy, second trimester

O98.413   Viral hepatitis complicating pregnancy, third trimester

O98.419   Viral hepatitis complicating pregnancy, unspecified trimester

O98.42   **Viral hepatitis complicating childbirth**

O98.43   **Viral hepatitis complicating the puerperium**

☑5ᵗʰ O98.5   **Other viral diseases complicating pregnancy, childbirth and the puerperium**
    Conditions in A80-B09, B25-B34, R87.81-, R87.82-
    EXCLUDES 1 *human immunodeficiency [HIV] disease complicating pregnancy, childbirth and the puerperium (O98.7-)*

   ☑6ᵗʰ O98.51   **Other viral diseases complicating pregnancy**

O98.511   Other viral diseases complicating pregnancy, first trimester

O98.512   Other viral diseases complicating pregnancy, second trimester

O98.513   Other viral diseases complicating pregnancy, third trimester

O98.519   Other viral diseases complicating pregnancy, unspecified trimester

O98.52   **Other viral diseases complicating childbirth**

O98.53   **Other viral diseases complicating the puerperium**

☑5ᵗʰ O98.6   **Protozoal diseases complicating pregnancy, childbirth and the puerperium**
    Conditions in B50-B64

   ☑6ᵗʰ O98.61   **Protozoal diseases complicating pregnancy**

O98.611   Protozoal diseases complicating pregnancy, first trimester

O98.612   Protozoal diseases complicating pregnancy, second trimester

O98.613   Protozoal diseases complicating pregnancy, third trimester

O98.619   Protozoal diseases complicating pregnancy, unspecified trimester

O98.62   **Protozoal diseases complicating childbirth**

O98.63   **Protozoal diseases complicating the puerperium**

☑5ᵗʰ O98.7   **Human immunodeficiency [HIV] disease complicating pregnancy, childbirth and the puerperium**
    Use additional code to identify the type of HIV disease:
    acquired immune deficiency syndrome (AIDS) (B20)
    asymptomatic HIV status (Z21)
    HIV positive NOS (Z21)
    symptomatic HIV disease (B20)

   ☑6ᵗʰ O98.71   **Human immunodeficiency [HIV] disease complicating pregnancy**

O98.711   Human immunodeficiency [HIV] disease complicating pregnancy, first trimester

O98.712   Human immunodeficiency [HIV] disease complicating pregnancy, second trimester

O98.713   Human immunodeficiency [HIV] disease complicating pregnancy, third trimester

O98.719   Human immunodeficiency [HIV] disease complicating pregnancy, unspecified trimester

O98.72   **Human immunodeficiency [HIV] disease complicating childbirth**

O98.73   **Human immunodeficiency [HIV] disease complicating the puerperium**

☑5ᵗʰ O98.8   **Other maternal infectious and parasitic diseases complicating pregnancy, childbirth and the puerperium**

   ☑6ᵗʰ O98.81   **Other maternal infectious and parasitic diseases complicating pregnancy**

O98.811   Other maternal infectious and parasitic diseases complicating pregnancy, first trimester

O98.812   Other maternal infectious and parasitic diseases complicating pregnancy, second trimester

O98.813   Other maternal infectious and parasitic diseases complicating pregnancy, third trimester

O98.819   Other maternal infectious and parasitic diseases complicating pregnancy, unspecified trimester

O98.82   **Other maternal infectious and parasitic diseases complicating childbirth**

O98.83   **Other maternal infectious and parasitic diseases complicating the puerperium**

☑5ᵗʰ O98.9   **Unspecified maternal infectious and parasitic disease complicating pregnancy, childbirth and the puerperium**

   ☑6ᵗʰ O98.91   **Unspecified maternal infectious and parasitic disease complicating pregnancy**

O98.911   Unspecified maternal infectious and parasitic disease complicating pregnancy, first trimester

O98.912   Unspecified maternal infectious and parasitic disease complicating pregnancy, second trimester

O98.913   Unspecified maternal infectious and parasitic disease complicating pregnancy, third trimester

O98.919   Unspecified maternal infectious and parasitic disease complicating pregnancy, unspecified trimester

O98.92   **Unspecified maternal infectious and parasitic disease complicating childbirth**

O98.93   **Unspecified maternal infectious and parasitic disease complicating the puerperium**

☑ Appropriate additional character required   ☑x7ᵗʰ Requires 7th character, placeholder x must fill empty characters

☑4ᵗʰ **O99 Other maternal diseases classifiable elsewhere but complicating pregnancy, childbirth and the puerperium**
Conditions which complicate the pregnant state, are aggravated by the pregnancy or are a main reason for obstetric care
Use additional code to identify specific condition
EXCLUDES 2 *when the reason for maternal care is that the condition is known or suspected to have affected the fetus (O35–O36)*

☑5ᵗʰ **O99.0 Anemia complicating pregnancy, childbirth and the puerperium**
Conditions in D50-D64
EXCLUDES 1 *anemia arising in the puerperium (O90.81)*
postpartum anemia NOS (O90.81)

☑6ᵗʰ **O99.01 Anemia complicating pregnancy**

O99.011 Anemia complicating pregnancy, first trimester

O99.012 Anemia complicating pregnancy, second trimester

O99.013 Anemia complicating pregnancy, third trimester

O99.019 Anemia complicating pregnancy, unspecified trimester

O99.02 Anemia complicating childbirth

O99.03 Anemia complicating the puerperium
EXCLUDES 1 *postpartum anemia not pre-existing prior to delivery (O90-.81)*

☑5ᵗʰ **O99.1 Other diseases of the blood and blood-forming organs and certain disorders involving the immune mechanism complicating pregnancy, childbirth and the puerperium**
Conditions in D65-D89
EXCLUDES 2 *hemorrhage with coagulation defects (O45-, O46.0-, O67.0, O72.3)*

☑6ᵗʰ **O99.11 Other diseases of the blood and blood-forming organs and certain disorders involving the immune mechanism complicating pregnancy**

O99.111 Other diseases of the blood and blood-forming organs and certain disorders involving the immune mechanism complicating pregnancy, first trimester

O99.112 Other diseases of the blood and blood-forming organs and certain disorders involving the immune mechanism complicating pregnancy, second trimester

O99.113 Other diseases of the blood and blood-forming organs and certain disorders involving the immune mechanism complicating pregnancy, third trimester

O99.119 Other diseases of the blood and blood-forming organs and certain disorders involving the immune mechanism complicating pregnancy, unspecified trimester

O99.12 Other diseases of the blood and blood-forming organs and certain disorders involving the immune mechanism complicating childbirth

O99.13 Other diseases of the blood and blood-forming organs and certain disorders involving the immune mechanism complicating the puerperium

☑5ᵗʰ **O99.2 Endocrine, nutritional and metabolic diseases complicating pregnancy, childbirth and the puerperium**
Conditions in E00-E88
EXCLUDES 2 *diabetes mellitus (O24-)*
malnutrition (O25-)
postpartum thyroiditis (O90.5)

☑6ᵗʰ **O99.21 Obesity complicating pregnancy, childbirth, and the puerperium**
Use additional code to identify the type of obesity (E66-)

O99.210 Obesity complicating pregnancy, unspecified trimester

O99.211 Obesity complicating pregnancy, first trimester

O99.212 Obesity complicating pregnancy, second trimester

O99.213 Obesity complicating pregnancy, third trimester

O99.214 Obesity complicating childbirth

O99.215 Obesity complicating the puerperium

☑6ᵗʰ **O99.28 Other endocrine, nutritional and metabolic diseases complicating pregnancy, childbirth and the puerperium**

O99.280 Endocrine, nutritional and metabolic diseases complicating pregnancy, unspecified trimester

O99.281 Endocrine, nutritional and metabolic diseases complicating pregnancy, first trimester

O99.282 Endocrine, nutritional and metabolic diseases complicating pregnancy, second trimester

O99.283 Endocrine, nutritional and metabolic diseases complicating pregnancy, third trimester

O99.284 Endocrine, nutritional and metabolic diseases complicating childbirth

O99.285 Endocrine, nutritional and metabolic diseases complicating the puerperium

☑5ᵗʰ **O99.3 Mental disorders and diseases of the nervous system complicating pregnancy, childbirth and the puerperium**

☑6ᵗʰ **O99.31 Alcohol use complicating pregnancy, childbirth, and the puerperium**
Use additional code(s) from F10 to identify manifestations of the alcohol use

O99.310 Alcohol use complicating pregnancy, unspecified trimester

O99.311 Alcohol use complicating pregnancy, first trimester

O99.312 Alcohol use complicating pregnancy, second trimester

O99.313 Alcohol use complicating pregnancy, third trimester

O99.314 Alcohol use complicating childbirth

O99.315 Alcohol use complicating the puerperium

☑6ᵗʰ **O99.32 Drug use complicating pregnancy, childbirth, and the puerperium**
Use additional code(s) from F11-F16 and F18-F19 to identify manifestations of the drug use

O99.320 Drug use complicating pregnancy, unspecified trimester

O99.321 Drug use complicating pregnancy, first trimester

O99.322 Drug use complicating pregnancy, second trimester

O99.323 Drug use complicating pregnancy, third trimester

O99.324 Drug use complicating childbirth

O99.325 Drug use complicating the puerperium

☑6ᵗʰ **O99.33 Smoking (tobacco) complicating pregnancy, childbirth, and the puerperium**
Use additional code from F17 to identify type of tobacco

O99.330 Smoking (tobacco) complicating pregnancy, unspecified trimester

O99.331 Smoking (tobacco) complicating pregnancy, first trimester

O99.332 Smoking (tobacco) complicating pregnancy, second trimester

O99.333 Smoking (tobacco) complicating pregnancy, third trimester

O99.334 Smoking (tobacco) complicating childbirth

O99.335 Smoking (tobacco) complicating the puerperium

☑6ᵗʰ **O99.34 Other mental disorders complicating pregnancy, childbirth, and the puerperium**
Conditions in F01-F09 and F20-F99
EXCLUDES 2 *postpartum mood disturbance (O90.6)*
postnatal psychosis (F53)
puerperal psychosis (F53)

O99.340 Other mental disorders complicating pregnancy, unspecified trimester

O99.341 Other mental disorders complicating pregnancy, first trimester

O99.342 Other mental disorders complicating pregnancy, second trimester

---

EXCLUDES 1 Not coded here   EXCLUDES 2 Not included here   *Manifestation Code*

O99.343 Other mental disorders complicating pregnancy, third trimester

O99.344 Other mental disorders complicating childbirth

O99.345 Other mental disorders complicating the puerperium

✓6th **O99.35** Diseases of the nervous system complicating pregnancy, childbirth, and the puerperium
Conditions in G00-G99
EXCLUDES 2   *pregnancy related peripheral neuritis (O26.8-)*

O99.350 Diseases of the nervous system complicating pregnancy, unspecified trimester

O99.351 Diseases of the nervous system complicating pregnancy, first trimester

O99.352 Diseases of the nervous system complicating pregnancy, second trimester

O99.353 Diseases of the nervous system complicating pregnancy, third trimester

O99.354 Diseases of the nervous system complicating childbirth

O99.355 Diseases of the nervous system complicating the puerperium

✓5th **O99.4** Diseases of the circulatory system complicating pregnancy, childbirth and the puerperium
Conditions in I00-I99
EXCLUDES 1   *peripartum cardiomyopathy (O90.3)*
EXCLUDES 2   *hypertensive disorders (O10-O16)*
obstetric embolism (O88-)
venous complications and cerebrovenous sinus thrombosis in:
labor, childbirth and the puerperium (O87-)
pregnancy (O22-)

✓6th **O99.41** Diseases of the circulatory system complicating pregnancy

O99.411 Diseases of the circulatory system complicating pregnancy, first trimester

O99.412 Diseases of the circulatory system complicating pregnancy, second trimester

O99.413 Diseases of the circulatory system complicating pregnancy, third trimester

O99.419 Diseases of the circulatory system complicating pregnancy, unspecified trimester

O99.42 Diseases of the circulatory system complicating childbirth

O99.43 Diseases of the circulatory system complicating the puerperium

✓5th **O99.5** Diseases of the respiratory system complicating pregnancy, childbirth and the puerperium
Conditions in J00-J99

✓6th **O99.51** Diseases of the respiratory system complicating pregnancy

O99.511 Diseases of the respiratory system complicating pregnancy, first trimester

O99.512 Diseases of the respiratory system complicating pregnancy, second trimester

O99.513 Diseases of the respiratory system complicating pregnancy, third trimester

O99.519 Diseases of the respiratory system complicating pregnancy, unspecified trimester

O99.52 Diseases of the respiratory system complicating childbirth

O99.53 Diseases of the respiratory system complicating the puerperium

✓5th **O99.6** Diseases of the digestive system complicating pregnancy, childbirth and the puerperium
Conditions in K00-K93
EXCLUDES 2   *liver disorders in pregnancy, childbirth and the puerperium (O26.6)*

✓6th **O99.61** Diseases of the digestive system complicating pregnancy

O99.611 Diseases of the digestive system complicating pregnancy, first trimester

O99.612 Diseases of the digestive system complicating pregnancy, second trimester

O99.613 Diseases of the digestive system complicating pregnancy, third trimester

O99.619 Diseases of the digestive system complicating pregnancy, unspecified trimester

O99.62 Diseases of the digestive system complicating childbirth

O99.63 Diseases of the digestive system complicating the puerperium

✓5th **O99.7** Diseases of the skin and subcutaneous tissue complicating pregnancy, childbirth and the puerperium
Conditions in L00-L99
EXCLUDES 2   *herpes gestationis (O26.4)*
pruritic urticarial papules and plaques of pregnancy (PUPPP) (O26.86)

✓6th **O99.71** Diseases of the skin and subcutaneous tissue complicating pregnancy

O99.711 Diseases of the skin and subcutaneous tissue complicating pregnancy, first trimester

O99.712 Diseases of the skin and subcutaneous tissue complicating pregnancy, second trimester

O99.713 Diseases of the skin and subcutaneous tissue complicating pregnancy, third trimester

O99.719 Diseases of the skin and subcutaneous tissue complicating pregnancy, unspecified trimester

O99.72 Diseases of the skin and subcutaneous tissue complicating childbirth

O99.73 Diseases of the skin and subcutaneous tissue complicating the puerperium

✓5th **O99.8** Other specified diseases and conditions complicating pregnancy, childbirth and the puerperium
Conditions in D00-D48, H00-H95, M00-N99, and Q00-Q99
Use additional code to identify condition
EXCLUDES 2   *genitourinary infections in pregnancy (O23.-)*
infection of genitourinary tract following delivery (O86.1-O86.3)
malignant neoplasm complicating pregnancy, childbirth and the puerperium (O9a.1-)
maternal care for known or suspected abnormality of maternal pelvic organs (O34.-)
postpartum acute kidney failure (O90.4)
traumatic injuries in pregnancy (O94)

✓6th **O99.81** Abnormal glucose complicating pregnancy, childbirth and the puerperium
EXCLUDES 1   *gestational diabetes (O24.4-)*

O99.810 Abnormal glucose complicating pregnancy

O99.814 Abnormal glucose complicating childbirth

O99.815 Abnormal glucose complicating the puerperium

✓6th **O99.82** Streptococcus B carrier state complicating pregnancy, childbirth and the puerperium

O99.820 Streptococcus B carrier state complicating pregnancy

O99.824 Streptococcus B carrier state complicating childbirth

O99.825 Streptococcus B carrier state complicating the puerperium

✓6th **O99.83** Other infection carrier state complicating pregnancy, childbirth and the puerperium
Use additional code to identify the carrier state (Z22-)

O99.830 Other infection carrier state complicating pregnancy

O99.834 Other infection carrier state complicating childbirth

O99.835 Other infection carrier state complicating the puerperium

---

☑ Appropriate additional character required   ✓x7th Requires 7th character, placeholder x must fill empty characters

✓6ᵗʰ **O99.84** **Bariatric surgery status complicating pregnancy, childbirth and the puerperium**
> Gastric banding status complicating pregnancy, childbirth and the puerperium
> Gastric bypass status for obesity complicating pregnancy, childbirth and the puerperium
> Obesity surgery status complicating pregnancy, childbirth and the puerperium

O99.840 **Bariatric surgery status complicating pregnancy, unspecified trimester**

O99.841 **Bariatric surgery status complicating pregnancy, first trimester**

O99.842 **Bariatric surgery status complicating pregnancy, second trimester**

O99.843 **Bariatric surgery status complicating pregnancy, third trimester**

O99.844 **Bariatric surgery status complicating childbirth**

O99.845 **Bariatric surgery status complicating the puerperium**

O99.89 **Other specified diseases and conditions complicating pregnancy, childbirth and the puerperium**

✓4ᵗʰ **O9a** **Maternal malignant neoplasms, traumatic injuries and abuse classifiable elsewhere but complicating pregnancy, childbirth and the puerperium**

✓5ᵗʰ **O9a.1** **Malignant neoplasm complicating pregnancy, childbirth and the puerperium**
> Conditions in C00-C97
> Use additional code to identify neoplasm
> > *EXCLUDES 2*   *maternal care for benign tumor of corpus uteri (O34.1-)*
> > *maternal care for benign tumor of cervix (O34.4-)*

✓6ᵗʰ **O9a.11** **Malignant neoplasm complicating pregnancy**

O9a.111 **Malignant neoplasm complicating pregnancy, first trimester**

O9a.112 **Malignant neoplasm complicating pregnancy, second trimester**

O9a.113 **Malignant neoplasm complicating pregnancy, third trimester**

O9a.119 **Malignant neoplasm complicating pregnancy, unspecified trimester**

O9a.12 **Malignant neoplasm complicating childbirth**

O9a.13 **Malignant neoplasm complicating the puerperium**

✓5ᵗʰ **O9a.2** **Injury, poisoning and certain other consequences of external causes complicating pregnancy, childbirth and the puerperium**
> Conditions in S00-T88, except T74 and T76
> Use additional code(s) to identify the injury or poisoning
> > *EXCLUDES 2*   *physical, sexual and psychological abuse complicating pregnancy, childbirth and the puerperium (O94)*

✓6ᵗʰ **O9a.21** **Injury, poisoning and certain other consequences of external causes complicating pregnancy**

O9a.211 **Injury, poisoning and certain other consequences of external causes complicating pregnancy, first trimester**

O9a.212 **Injury, poisoning and certain other consequences of external causes complicating pregnancy, second trimester**

O9a.213 **Injury, poisoning and certain other consequences of external causes complicating pregnancy, third trimester**

O9a.219 **Injury, poisoning and certain other consequences of external causes complicating pregnancy, unspecified trimester**

O9a.22 **Injury, poisoning and certain other consequences of external causes complicating childbirth**

O9a.23 **Injury, poisoning and certain other consequences of external causes complicating the puerperium**

✓5ᵗʰ **O9a.3** **Physical abuse complicating pregnancy, childbirth and the puerperium**
> Conditions in T74.11 or T76.11
> Use additional code (if applicable):
> > to identify any associated current injury due to physical abuse
> > to identify the perpetrator of abuse (Y07-)
> > *EXCLUDES 2*   *sexual abuse complicating pregnancy, childbirth and the puerperium (O94)*

✓6ᵗʰ **O9a.31** **Physical abuse complicating pregnancy**

O9a.311 **Physical abuse complicating pregnancy, first trimester**

O9a.312 **Physical abuse complicating pregnancy, second trimester**

O9a.313 **Physical abuse complicating pregnancy, third trimester**

O9a.319 **Physical abuse complicating pregnancy, unspecified trimester**

O9a.32 **Physical abuse complicating childbirth**

O9a.33 **Physical abuse complicating the puerperium**

✓5ᵗʰ **O9a.4** **Sexual abuse complicating pregnancy, childbirth and the puerperium**
> Conditions in T74.21 or T76.21
> Use additional code (if applicable):
> > to identify any associated current injury due to sexual abuse
> > to identify the perpetrator of abuse (Y07-)

✓6ᵗʰ **O9a.41** **Sexual abuse complicating pregnancy**

O9a.411 **Sexual abuse complicating pregnancy, first trimester**

O9a.412 **Sexual abuse complicating pregnancy, second trimester**

O9a.413 **Sexual abuse complicating pregnancy, third trimester**

O9a.419 **Sexual abuse complicating pregnancy, unspecified trimester**

O9a.42 **Sexual abuse complicating childbirth**

O9a.43 **Sexual abuse complicating the puerperium**

✓5ᵗʰ **O9a.5** **Psychological abuse complicating pregnancy, childbirth and the puerperium**
> Conditions in T74.31 or T76.31
> Use additional code to identify the perpetrator of abuse (Y07-)

✓6ᵗʰ **O9a.51** **Psychological abuse complicating pregnancy**

O9a.511 **Psychological abuse complicating pregnancy, first trimester**

O9a.512 **Psychological abuse complicating pregnancy, second trimester**

O9a.513 **Psychological abuse complicating pregnancy, third trimester**

O9a.519 **Psychological abuse complicating pregnancy, unspecified trimester**

O9a.52 **Psychological abuse complicating childbirth**

O9a.53 **Psychological abuse complicating the puerperium**

EXCLUDES 1   Not coded here   *EXCLUDES 2*   Not included here   *Manifestation Code*

Chapter 16. Certain Conditions Originating in the Perinatal Period (P00-P96)

NOTE   Codes from this chapter are for use on newborn records only, never on maternal records

INCLUDES   conditions that have their origin in the fetal or perinatal period (before birth through the first 28 days after birth) even if morbidity occurs later

EXCLUDES 2   congenital malformations, deformations and chromosomal abnormalities (Q00-Q99)
endocrine, nutritional and metabolic diseases (E00-E88)
injury, poisoning and certain other consequences of external causes (S00-T88)
neoplasms (C00-D49)
tetanus neonatorum (A33)

This chapter contains the following blocks:

P00-P04   Newborn affected by maternal factors and by complications of pregnancy, labor, and delivery
P05-P08   Disorders related to length of gestation and fetal growth
P09   Abnormal findings on neonatal screening
P10-P15   Birth trauma
P19-P29   Respiratory and cardiovascular disorders specific to the perinatal period
P35-P39   Infections specific to the perinatal period
P50-P61   Hemorrhagic and hematological disorders of newborn
P70-P74   Transitory endocrine and metabolic disorders specific to newborn
P76-P78   Digestive system disorders of newborn
P80-P83   Conditions involving the integument and temperature regulation of newborn
P84   Other problems with newborn
P90-P96   Other disorders originating in the perinatal period

Newborn affected by maternal factors and by complications of pregnancy, labor, and delivery (P00-P04)

NOTE   These codes are for use when the listed maternal conditions are specified as the cause of confirmed morbidity or potential morbidity which have their origin in the perinatal period (before birth through the first 28 days after birth). Codes from these categories are also for use for newborns who are suspected of having an abnormal condition resulting from exposure from the mother or the birth process, but without signs or symptoms, and, which after examination and observation, is found not to exist. These codes may be used even if treatment is begun for a suspected condition that is ruled out.

✓4th **P00   Newborn (suspected to be) affected by maternal conditions that may be unrelated to present pregnancy**
Code first any current condition in newborn
EXCLUDES 2   newborn (suspected to be) affected by maternal complications of pregnancy (P01-)
newborn affected by maternal endocrine and metabolic disorders (P70-P74)
newborn affected by noxious substances transmitted via placenta or breast milk (P04-)

P00.0   Newborn (suspected to be) affected by maternal hypertensive disorders
Newborn (suspected to be) affected by maternal conditions classifiable to O10-O11, O13-O16

P00.1   Newborn (suspected to be) affected by maternal renal and urinary tract diseases
Newborn (suspected to be) affected by maternal conditions classifiable to N00-N39

P00.2   Newborn (suspected to be) affected by maternal infectious and parasitic diseases
Newborn (suspected to be) affected by maternal infectious disease classifiable to A00-B99, J09 and J10
EXCLUDES 1   infections specific to the perinatal period (P35-P39)
maternal genital tract or other localized infections (P00.8)

P00.3   Newborn (suspected to be) affected by other maternal circulatory and respiratory diseases
Newborn (suspected to be) affected by maternal conditions classifiable to I00-I99, J00-J99, Q20-Q34 and not included in P00.0, P00.2

P00.4   Newborn (suspected to be) affected by maternal nutritional disorders
Newborn (suspected to be) affected by maternal disorders classifiable to E40-E64
Maternal malnutrition NOS

P00.5   Newborn (suspected to be) affected by maternal injury
Newborn (suspected to be) affected by maternal conditions classifiable to O97.2

P00.6   Newborn (suspected to be) affected by surgical procedure on mother
Newborn (suspected to be) affected by amniocentesis
EXCLUDES 1   Cesarean delivery for present delivery (P03.4)
damage to placenta from amniocentesis, Cesarean delivery or surgical induction (P02.1)
previous surgery to uterus or pelvic organs (P03.89)
EXCLUDES 2   newborn affected by complication of (fetal) intrauterine procedure (P96.5)

P00.7   Newborn (suspected to be) affected by other medical procedures on mother, not elsewhere classified
Newborn (suspected to be) affected by radiation to mother
EXCLUDES 1   damage to placenta from amniocentesis, cesarean delivery or surgical induction (P02.1)
newborn affected by other complications of labor and delivery (P03-)

✓5th **P00.8   Newborn (suspected to be) affected by other maternal conditions**

P00.81   Newborn (suspected to be) affected by periodontal disease in mother

P00.89   Newborn (suspected to be) affected by other maternal conditions
Newborn (suspected to be) affected by conditions classifiable to T80-T88
Newborn (suspected to be) affected by maternal genital tract or other localized infections
Newborn (suspected to be) affected by maternal systemic lupus erythematosus

P00.9   Newborn (suspected to be) affected by unspecified maternal condition

✓4th **P01   Newborn (suspected to be) affected by maternal complications of pregnancy**
Code first any current condition in newborn
P01.0   Newborn (suspected to be) affected by incompetent cervix
P01.1   Newborn (suspected to be) affected by premature rupture of membranes
P01.2   Newborn (suspected to be) affected by oligohydramnios
EXCLUDES 1   oligohydramnios due to premature rupture of membranes (P01.1)
P01.3   Newborn (suspected to be) affected by polyhydramnios
Newborn (suspected to be) affected by hydramnios
P01.4   Newborn (suspected to be) affected by ectopic pregnancy
Newborn (suspected to be) affected by abdominal pregnancy
P01.5   Newborn (suspected to be) affected by multiple pregnancy
Newborn (suspected to be) affected by triplet (pregnancy)
Newborn (suspected to be) affected by twin (pregnancy)
P01.6   Newborn (suspected to be) affected by maternal death
P01.7   Newborn (suspected to be) affected by malpresentation before labor
Newborn (suspected to be) affected by breech presentation before labor
Newborn (suspected to be) affected by external version before labor
Newborn (suspected to be) affected by face presentation before labor
Newborn (suspected to be) affected by transverse lie before labor
Newborn (suspected to be) affected by unstable lie before labor
P01.8   Newborn (suspected to be) affected by other maternal complications of pregnancy
P01.9   Newborn (suspected to be) affected by maternal complication of pregnancy, unspecified

✓4th **P02   Newborn (suspected to be) affected by complications of placenta, cord and membranes**
Code first any current condition in newborn
P02.0   Newborn (suspected to be) affected by placenta previa

✓ Appropriate additional character required

✓x7th Requires 7th character, placeholder x must fill empty characters

P02.1 Newborn (suspected to be) affected by other forms of placental separation and hemorrhage
Newborn (suspected to be) affected by abruptio placenta
Newborn (suspected to be) affected by accidental hemorrhage
Newborn (suspected to be) affected by antepartum hemorrhage
Newborn (suspected to be) affected by damage to placenta from amniocentesis, cesarean delivery or surgical induction
Newborn (suspected to be) affected by maternal blood loss
Newborn (suspected to be) affected by premature separation of placenta

√5th **P02.2 Newborn (suspected to be) affected by other and unspecified morphological and functional abnormalities of placenta**

P02.20 **Newborn (suspected to be) affected by unspecified morphological and functional abnormalities of placenta**

P02.29 **Newborn (suspected to be) affected by other morphological and functional abnormalities of placenta**
Newborn (suspected to be) affected by placental dysfunction
Newborn (suspected to be) affected by placental infarction
Newborn (suspected to be) affected by placental insufficiency

P02.3 Newborn (suspected to be) affected by placental transfusion syndromes
Newborn (suspected to be) affected by placental and cord abnormalities resulting in twin-to-twin or other transplacental transfusion

P02.4 Newborn (suspected to be) affected by prolapsed cord

P02.5 Newborn (suspected to be) affected by other compression of umbilical cord
Newborn (suspected to be) affected by umbilical cord (tightly) around neck
Newborn (suspected to be) affected by entanglement of umbilical cord
Newborn (suspected to be) affected by knot in umbilical cord

√5th **P02.6 Newborn (suspected to be) affected by other and unspecified conditions of umbilical cord**

P02.60 **Newborn (suspected to be) affected by unspecified conditions of umbilical cord**

P02.69 **Newborn (suspected to be) affected by other conditions of umbilical cord**
Newborn (suspected to be) affected by short umbilical cord
Newborn (suspected to be) affected by vasa previa
EXCLUDES 1 *newborn affected by single umbilical artery (Q27.0)*

P02.7 Newborn (suspected to be) affected by chorioamnionitis
Newborn (suspected to be) affected by amnionitis
Newborn (suspected to be) affected by membranitis
Newborn (suspected to be) affected by placentitis

P02.8 Newborn (suspected to be) affected by other abnormalities of membranes

P02.9 Newborn (suspected to be) affected by abnormality of membranes, unspecified

√4th **P03 Newborn (suspected to be) affected by other complications of labor and delivery**
Code first any current condition in newborn

P03.0 **Newborn (suspected to be) affected by breech delivery and extraction**

P03.1 **Newborn (suspected to be) affected by other malpresentation, malposition and disproportion during labor and delivery**
Newborn (suspected to be) affected by contracted pelvis
Newborn (suspected to be) affected by conditions classifiable to O64-O66
Newborn (suspected to be) affected by persistent occipitoposterior
Newborn (suspected to be) affected by transverse lie

P03.2 **Newborn (suspected to be) affected by forceps delivery**

P03.3 **Newborn (suspected to be) affected by delivery by vacuum extractor [ventouse]**

P03.4 **Newborn (suspected to be) affected by Cesarean delivery**

P03.5 **Newborn (suspected to be) affected by precipitate delivery**
Newborn (suspected to be) affected by rapid second stage

P03.6 Newborn (suspected to be) affected by abnormal uterine contractions
Newborn (suspected to be) affected by conditions classifiable to O62-, except O62.3
Newborn (suspected to be) affected by hypertonic labor
Newborn (suspected to be) affected by uterine inertia

√5th **P03.8 Newborn (suspected to be) affected by other specified complications of labor and delivery**

√6th P03.81 **Newborn (suspected to be) affected by abnormality in fetal (intrauterine) heart rate or rhythm**
EXCLUDES 1 *neonatal cardiac dysrhythmia (P29.1)*

P03.810 **Newborn (suspected to be) affected by abnormality in fetal (intrauterine) heart rate or rhythm before the onset of labor**

P03.811 **Newborn (suspected to be) affected by abnormality in fetal (intrauterine) heart rate or rhythm during labor**

P03.819 **Newborn (suspected to be) affected by abnormality in fetal (intrauterine) heart rate or rhythm, unspecified as to time of onset**

P03.82 **Meconium passage during delivery**
EXCLUDES 1 *meconium aspiration (P24.00, P24.01)*
meconium staining (P96.83)

P03.89 **Newborn (suspected to be) affected by other specified complications of labor and delivery**
Newborn (suspected to be) affected by abnormality of maternal soft tissues
Newborn (suspected to be) affected by conditions classifiable to O60-O75 and by procedures used in labor and delivery not included in P02- and P03.0-P03.6
Newborn (suspected to be) affected by induction of labor

P03.9 Newborn (suspected to be) affected by complication of labor and delivery, unspecified

√4th **P04 Newborn (suspected to be) affected by noxious substances transmitted via placenta or breast milk**
INCLUDES nonteratogenic effects of substances transmitted via placenta
EXCLUDES 2 *congenital malformations (Q00-Q99)*
neonatal jaundice from excessive hemolysis due to drugs or toxins transmitted from mother (P58.4)
newborn in contact with and (suspected) exposures hazardous to health not transmitted via placenta or breast milk (Z77-)

P04.0 Newborn (suspected to be) affected by maternal anesthesia and analgesia in pregnancy, labor and delivery
Newborn (suspected to be) affected by reactions and intoxications from maternal opiates and tranquilizers administered during labor and delivery

P04.1 Newborn (suspected to be) affected by other maternal medication
Newborn (suspected to be) affected by cancer chemotherapy
Newborn (suspected to be) affected by cytotoxic drugs
EXCLUDES 1 *dysmorphism due to warfarin (Q86.2)*
fetal hydantoin syndrome (Q86.1)
maternal use of drugs of addiction (P04.4-)

P04.2 Newborn (suspected to be) affected by maternal use of tobacco
Newborn (suspected to be) affected by exposure in utero to tobacco smoke
EXCLUDES 2 *newborn exposure to environmental tobacco smoke (P96.81)*

P04.3 Newborn (suspected to be) affected by maternal use of alcohol
EXCLUDES 1 *fetal alcohol syndrome (Q86.0)*

√5th **P04.4 Newborn (suspected to be) affected by maternal use of drugs of addiction**

P04.41 **Newborn (suspected to be) affected by maternal use of cocaine**
"Crack baby"

P04.49 **Newborn (suspected to be) affected by maternal use of other drugs of addiction**
EXCLUDES 2 *newborn (suspected to be) affected by maternal anesthesia and analgesia (P04.0)*
withdrawal symptoms from maternal use of drugs of addiction (P96.1)

EXCLUDES 1 Not coded here   EXCLUDES 2 Not included here   *Manifestation Code*

P04.5　Newborn (suspected to be) affected by maternal use of nutritional chemical substances

P04.6　Newborn (suspected to be) affected by maternal exposure to environmental chemical substances

P04.8　Newborn (suspected to be) affected by other maternal noxious substances

P04.9　Newborn (suspected to be) affected by maternal noxious substance, unspecified

Disorders of newborn related to length of gestation and fetal growth (P05-P08)

✓4ᵗʰ **P05　Disorders of newborn related to slow fetal growth and fetal malnutrition**

　✓5ᵗʰ **P05.0　Newborn light for gestational age**
　　　Newborn light-for-dates
　　P05.00　Newborn light for gestational age, unspecified weight
　　P05.01　Newborn light for gestational age, less than 500 grams
　　P05.02　Newborn light for gestational age, 500-749 grams
　　P05.03　Newborn light for gestational age, 750-999 grams
　　P05.04　Newborn light for gestational age, 1000-1249 grams
　　P05.05　Newborn light for gestational age, 1250-1499 grams
　　P05.06　Newborn light for gestational age, 1500-1749 grams
　　P05.07　Newborn light for gestational age, 1750-1999 grams
　　P05.08　Newborn light for gestational age, 2000-2499 grams

　✓5ᵗʰ **P05.1　Newborn small for gestational age**
　　　Newborn small-and-light-for-dates
　　　Newborn small-for-dates
　　P05.10　Newborn small for gestational age, unspecified weight
　　P05.11　Newborn small for gestational age, less than 500 grams
　　P05.12　Newborn small for gestational age, 500-749 grams
　　P05.13　Newborn small for gestational age, 750-999 grams
　　P05.14　Newborn small for gestational age, 1000-1249 grams
　　P05.15　Newborn small for gestational age, 1250-1499 grams
　　P05.16　Newborn small for gestational age, 1500-1749 grams
　　P05.17　Newborn small for gestational age, 1750-1999 grams
　　P05.18　Newborn small for gestational age, 2000-2499 grams

　P05.2　Newborn affected by fetal (intrauterine) malnutrition not light or small for gestational age
　　　Infant, not light or small for gestational age, showing signs of fetal malnutrition, such as dry, peeling skin and loss of subcutaneous tissue
　　　EXCLUDES 1　*newborn affected by fetal malnutrition with light for gestational age (P05.0-)*
　　　　　newborn affected by fetal malnutrition with small for gestational age (P05.1-)

　P05.9　Newborn affected by slow intrauterine growth, unspecified
　　　Newborn affected by fetal growth retardation NOS

✓4ᵗʰ **P07　Disorders of newborn related to short gestation and low birth weight, not elsewhere classified**

　NOTE　When both birth weight and gestational age of the newborn are available, both should be coded with birth weight sequenced before gestational age
　The listed conditions, without further specification, as the cause of morbidity or additional care, in newborn
　EXCLUDES 1　*low birth weight due to slow fetal growth and fetal malnutrition (P05-)*

　✓5ᵗʰ **P07.0　Extremely low birth weight newborn**
　　　Newborn birth weight 999 g. or less
　　P07.00　Extremely low birth weight newborn, unspecified weight
　　P07.01　Extremely low birth weight newborn, less than 500 grams
　　P07.02　Extremely low birth weight newborn, 500-749 grams
　　P07.03　Extremely low birth weight newborn, 750-999 grams

　✓5ᵗʰ **P07.1　Other low birth weight newborn**
　　　Newborn birth weight 1000-2499 g.
　　P07.10　Other low birth weight newborn, unspecified weight
　　P07.14　Other low birth weight newborn, 1000-1249 grams
　　P07.15　Other low birth weight newborn, 1250-1499 grams
　　P07.16　Other low birth weight newborn, 1500-1749 grams
　　P07.17　Other low birth weight newborn, 1750-1999 grams
　　P07.18　Other low birth weight newborn, 2000-2499 grams

　✓5ᵗʰ **P07.2　Extreme immaturity of newborn**
　　　Less than 28 completed weeks (less than 196 completed days) of gestation.
　　P07.20　Extreme immaturity of newborn, unspecified weeks
　　P07.21　Extreme immaturity of newborn, less than 24 completed weeks
　　P07.22　Extreme immaturity of newborn, 24-26 completed weeks
　　P07.23　Extreme immaturity of newborn, 27 completed weeks

　✓5ᵗʰ **P07.3　Other preterm newborn**
　　　28 completed weeks or more but less than 37 completed weeks (196 completed days but less than 259 completed days) of gestation
　　　Prematurity NOS
　　P07.30　Other preterm newborn, unspecified weeks
　　P07.31　Other preterm newborn, 28-31 completed weeks
　　P07.32　Other preterm newborn, 32-36 completed weeks

✓4ᵗʰ **P08　Disorders of newborn related to long gestation and high birth weight**

　NOTE　When both birth weight and gestational age of the newborn are available, priority of assignment should be given to birth weight
　INCLUDES　the listed conditions, without further specification, as causes of morbidity or additional care, in newborn

　P08.0　Exceptionally large newborn baby
　　　Usually implies a birth weight of 4500 g. or more
　　　EXCLUDES 1　*syndrome of infant of diabetic mother (P70.1)*
　　　　　syndrome of infant of mother with gestational diabetes (P70.0)

　P08.1　Other heavy for gestational age newborn
　　　Other newborn heavy- or large-for-dates regardless of period of gestation
　　　Usually implies a birth weight of 4000 g. to 4499 g.
　　　EXCLUDES 1　*newborn with a birth weight of 4500 or more (P08.0)*
　　　　　syndrome of infant of diabetic mother (P70.1)
　　　　　syndrome of infant of mother with gestational diabetes (P70.0).

　✓5ᵗʰ **P08.2　Late newborn, not heavy for gestational age**
　　P08.21　Post-term newborn
　　　　Newborn with gestation period over 40 completed weeks to 42 completed weeks

---

P08.22   Prolonged gestation of newborn
Newborn with gestation period over 42 completed weeks (294 days or more), not heavy- or large-for-dates.
Postmaturity NOS

Abnormal findings on neonatal screening (P09)

P09   Abnormal findings on neonatal screening
Use additional code to identify signs, symptoms and conditions associated with the screening
EXCLUDES 2   *nonspecific serologic evidence of human immunodeficiency virus [HIV] (R75)*

Birth trauma (P10-P15)

✓4ᵗʰ **P10   Intracranial laceration and hemorrhage due to birth injury**
EXCLUDES 1   *intracranial hemorrhage of newborn NOS (P52.9)*
intracranial hemorrhage of newborn due to anoxia or hypoxia (P52-)
nontraumatic intracranial hemorrhage of newborn (P52-)

P10.0   Subdural hemorrhage due to birth injury
Subdural hematoma (localized) due to birth injury
EXCLUDES 1   *subdural hemorrhage accompanying tentorial tear (P10.4)*

P10.1   Cerebral hemorrhage due to birth injury
P10.2   Intraventricular hemorrhage due to birth injury
P10.3   Subarachnoid hemorrhage due to birth injury
P10.4   Tentorial tear due to birth injury
P10.8   Other intracranial lacerations and hemorrhages due to birth injury
P10.9   Unspecified intracranial laceration and hemorrhage due to birth injury

✓4ᵗʰ **P11   Other birth injuries to central nervous system**
P11.0   Cerebral edema due to birth injury
P11.1   Other specified brain damage due to birth injury
P11.2   Unspecified brain damage due to birth injury
P11.3   Birth injury to facial nerve
Facial palsy due to birth injury
P11.4   Birth injury to other cranial nerves
P11.5   Birth injury to spine and spinal cord
Fracture of spine due to birth injury
P11.9   Birth injury to central nervous system, unspecified

✓4ᵗʰ **P12   Birth injury to scalp**
P12.0   Cephalhematoma due to birth injury
P12.1   Chignon (from vacuum extraction) due to birth injury
P12.2   Epicranial subaponeurotic hemorrhage due to birth injury
Subgaleal hemorrhage
P12.3   Bruising of scalp due to birth injury
P12.4   Injury of scalp of newborn due to monitoring equipment
Sampling incision of scalp of newborn
Scalp clip (electrode) injury of newborn
✓5ᵗʰ **P12.8   Other birth injuries to scalp**
P12.81   Caput succedaneum
P12.89   Other birth injuries to scalp
P12.9   Birth injury to scalp, unspecified

✓4ᵗʰ **P13   Birth injury to skeleton**
EXCLUDES 2   *birth injury to spine (P11.5)*
P13.0   Fracture of skull due to birth injury
P13.1   Other birth injuries to skull
EXCLUDES 1   *cephalhematoma (P12.0)*
P13.2   Birth injury to femur
P13.3   Birth injury to other long bones
P13.4   Fracture of clavicle due to birth injury
P13.8   Birth injuries to other parts of skeleton
P13.9   Birth injury to skeleton, unspecified

✓4ᵗʰ **P14   Birth injury to peripheral nervous system**
P14.0   Erb's paralysis due to birth injury
P14.1   Klumpke's paralysis due to birth injury
P14.2   Phrenic nerve paralysis due to birth injury
P14.3   Other brachial plexus birth injuries
P14.8   Birth injuries to other parts of peripheral nervous system
P14.9   Birth injury to peripheral nervous system, unspecified

✓4ᵗʰ **P15   Other birth injuries**
P15.0   Birth injury to liver
Rupture of liver due to birth injury
P15.1   Birth injury to spleen
Rupture of spleen due to birth injury
P15.2   Sternomastoid injury due to birth injury
P15.3   Birth injury to eye
Subconjunctival hemorrhage due to birth injury
Traumatic glaucoma due to birth injury
P15.4   Birth injury to face
Facial congestion due to birth injury
P15.5   Birth injury to external genitalia
P15.6   Subcutaneous fat necrosis due to birth injury
P15.8   Other specified birth injuries
P15.9   Birth injury, unspecified

Respiratory and cardiovascular disorders specific to the perinatal period (P19-P29)

✓4ᵗʰ **P19   Metabolic acidemia in newborn**
Metabolic acidemia in newborn
P19.0   Metabolic acidemia in newborn first noted before onset of labor
P19.1   Metabolic acidemia in newborn first noted during labor
P19.2   Metabolic acidemia noted at birth
P19.9   Metabolic acidemia, unspecified

✓4ᵗʰ **P22   Respiratory distress of newborn**
EXCLUDES 1   *respiratory arrest of newborn (P28.81)*
respiratory failure of newborn NOS (P28.5)
P22.0   Respiratory distress syndrome of newborn
Cardiorespiratory distress syndrome of newborn
Hyaline membrane disease
Idiopathic respiratory distress syndrome [IRDS or RDS] of newborn
Pulmonary hypoperfusion syndrome
Respiratory distress syndrome, type I
P22.1   Transient tachypnea of newborn
Idiopathic tachypnea of newborn
Respiratory distress syndrome, type II
Wet lung syndrome
P22.8   Other respiratory distress of newborn
P22.9   Respiratory distress of newborn, unspecified

✓4ᵗʰ **P23   Congenital pneumonia**
INCLUDES   infective pneumonia acquired in utero or during birth
EXCLUDES 1   *neonatal pneumonia resulting from aspiration (P24-)*
P23.0   Congenital pneumonia due to viral agent
EXCLUDES 1   *congenital rubella pneumonitis (P35.0)*
P23.1   Congenital pneumonia due to Chlamydia
P23.2   Congenital pneumonia due to staphylococcus
P23.3   Congenital pneumonia due to streptococcus, group B
P23.4   Congenital pneumonia due to Escherichia coli
P23.5   Congenital pneumonia due to Pseudomonas
P23.6   Congenital pneumonia due to other bacterial agents
Congenital pneumonia due to Hemophilus influenzae
Congenital pneumonia due to Klebsiella pneumoniae
Congenital pneumonia due to Mycoplasma
Congenital pneumonia due to Streptococcus, except group B
Use additional code (B95-B96) to identify organism
P23.8   Congenital pneumonia due to other organisms
Use additional code (B97) to identify organism
P23.9   Congenital pneumonia, unspecified

✓4ᵗʰ **P24   Neonatal aspiration**
INCLUDES   aspiration in utero and during delivery
✓5ᵗʰ **P24.0   Meconium aspiration**
EXCLUDES 1   *meconium passage (without aspiration) during delivery (P03.82)*
meconium staining (P96.83)
P24.00   Meconium aspiration without respiratory symptoms
Meconium aspiration NOS
P24.01   Meconium aspiration with respiratory symptoms
Meconium aspiration pneumonia
Meconium aspiration pneumonitis
Meconium aspiration syndrome NOS
Use additional code to identify any secondary pulmonary hypertension (I27.81), if applicable

---

EXCLUDES 1   Not coded here   EXCLUDES 2   Not included here   *Manifestation Code*

✓5th **P24.1** **Neonatal aspiration of (clear) amniotic fluid and mucus**
Neonatal aspiration of liquor (amnii)

P24.10 **Neonatal aspiration of (clear) amniotic fluid and mucus without respiratory symptoms**
Neonatal aspiration of amniotic fluid and mucus NOS

P24.11 **Neonatal aspiration of (clear) amniotic fluid and mucus with respiratory symptoms**
Neonatal aspiration of amniotic fluid and mucus with pneumonia
Neonatal aspiration of amniotic fluid and mucus with pneumonitis
Use additional code to identify any secondary pulmonary hypertension (I27.81), if applicable

✓5th **P24.2** **Neonatal aspiration of blood**

P24.20 **Neonatal aspiration of blood without respiratory symptoms**
Neonatal aspiration of blood NOS

P24.21 **Neonatal aspiration of blood with respiratory symptoms**
Neonatal aspiration of blood with pneumonia
Neonatal aspiration of blood with pneumonitis
Use additional code to identify any secondary pulmonary hypertension (I27.81), if applicable

✓5th **P24.3** **Neonatal aspiration of milk and regurgitated food**
Neonatal aspiration of stomach contents

P24.30 **Neonatal aspiration of milk and regurgitated food without respiratory symptoms**
Neonatal aspiration of milk and regurgitated food NOS

P24.31 **Neonatal aspiration of milk and regurgitated food with respiratory symptoms**
Neonatal aspiration of milk and regurgitated food with pneumonia
Neonatal aspiration of milk and regurgitated food with pneumonitis
Use additional code to identify any secondary pulmonary hypertension (I27.81), if applicable

✓5th **P24.8** **Other neonatal aspiration**

P24.80 **Other neonatal aspiration without respiratory symptoms**
Neonatal aspiration NEC

P24.81 **Other neonatal aspiration with respiratory symptoms**
Neonatal aspiration pneumonia NEC
Neonatal aspiration with pneumonitis NEC
Neonatal aspiration with pneumonia NOS
Neonatal aspiration with pneumonitis NOS
Use additional code to identify any secondary pulmonary hypertension (I27.81), if applicable

P24.9 **Neonatal aspiration, unspecified**

✓4th **P25** **Interstitial emphysema and related conditions originating in the perinatal period**

P25.0 **Interstitial emphysema originating in the perinatal period**

P25.1 **Pneumothorax originating in the perinatal period**

P25.2 **Pneumomediastinum originating in the perinatal period**

P25.3 **Pneumopericardium originating in the perinatal period**

P25.8 **Other conditions related to interstitial emphysema originating in the perinatal period**

✓4th **P26** **Pulmonary hemorrhage originating in the perinatal period**
EXCLUDES 1 *acute idiopathic hemorrhage in infants over 28 days old (R04.81)*

P26.0 **Tracheobronchial hemorrhage originating in the perinatal period**

P26.1 **Massive pulmonary hemorrhage originating in the perinatal period**

P26.8 **Other pulmonary hemorrhages originating in the perinatal period**

P26.9 **Unspecified pulmonary hemorrhage originating in the perinatal period**

✓4th **P27** **Chronic respiratory disease originating in the perinatal period**
EXCLUDES 1 *respiratory distress of newborn (P22.0-P22.9)*

P27.0 **Wilson-Mikity syndrome**
Pulmonary dysmaturity

P27.1 **Bronchopulmonary dysplasia originating in the perinatal period**

P27.8 **Other chronic respiratory diseases originating in the perinatal period**
Congenital pulmonary fibrosis
Ventilator lung in newborn

P27.9 **Unspecified chronic respiratory disease originating in the perinatal period**

✓4th **P28** **Other respiratory conditions originating in the perinatal period**
EXCLUDES 1 *congenital malformations of the respiratory system (Q30-Q34)*

P28.0 **Primary atelectasis of newborn**
Primary failure to expand terminal respiratory units
Pulmonary hypoplasia associated with short gestation
Pulmonary immaturity NOS

✓5th **P28.1** **Other and unspecified atelectasis of newborn**

P28.10 **Unspecified atelectasis of newborn**
Atelectasis of newborn NOS

P28.11 **Resorption atelectasis without respiratory distress syndrome**
EXCLUDES 1 *resorption atelectasis with respiratory distress syndrome (P22.0)*

P28.19 **Other atelectasis of newborn**
Partial atelectasis of newborn
Secondary atelectasis of newborn

P28.2 **Cyanotic attacks of newborn**
EXCLUDES 1 *apnea of newborn (P28.3-P28.4)*

P28.3 **Primary sleep apnea of newborn**
Central sleep apnea of newborn
Obstructive sleep apnea of newborn
Sleep apnea of newborn NOS

P28.4 **Other apnea of newborn**
Apnea of prematurity
Obstructive apnea of newborn
EXCLUDES 1 *obstructive sleep apnea of newborn (P28.3)*

P28.5 **Respiratory failure of newborn**
EXCLUDES 1 *respiratory arrest of newborn (P28.81)*
respiratory distress of newborn (P22.0-)

✓5th **P28.8** **Other specified respiratory conditions of newborn**

P28.81 **Respiratory arrest of newborn**

P28.89 **Other specified respiratory conditions of newborn**
Congenital laryngeal stridor
Sniffles in newborn
Snuffles in newborn
EXCLUDES 1 *early congenital syphilitic rhinitis (A50.0)*

P28.9 **Respiratory condition of newborn, unspecified**
Respiratory depression in newborn

✓4th **P29** **Cardiovascular disorders originating in the perinatal period**
EXCLUDES 1 *congenital malformations of the circulatory system (Q20-Q28)*

P29.0 **Neonatal cardiac failure**

✓5th **P29.1** **Neonatal cardiac dysrhythmia**

P29.11 **Neonatal tachycardia**

P29.12 **Neonatal bradycardia**

P29.2 **Neonatal hypertension**

P29.3 **Persistent fetal circulation**
Delayed closure of ductus arteriosus
(Persistent) pulmonary hypertension of newborn

P29.4 **Transient myocardial ischemia in newborn**

✓5th **P29.8** **Other cardiovascular disorders originating in the perinatal period**

P29.81 **Cardiac arrest of newborn**

P29.89 **Other cardiovascular disorders originating in the perinatal period**

P29.9 **Cardiovascular disorder originating in the perinatal period, unspecified**

✓ Appropriate additional character required   ✓x7th Requires 7th character, placeholder x must fill empty characters

Infections specific to the perinatal period (P35-P39)

Infections acquired in utero, during birth via the umbilicus, or during the first 28 days after birth

> EXCLUDES 2   asymptomatic human immunodeficiency virus [HIV] infection status (Z21)
> congenital gonococcal infection (A54-)
> congenital pneumonia (P23-)
> congenital syphilis (A50-)
> human immunodeficiency virus [HIV] disease (B20)
> infant botulism (A48.51)
> infectious diseases not specific to the perinatal period (A00-B99, J09, J10-)
> intestinal infectious disease (A00-A09)
> laboratory evidence of human immunodeficiency virus [HIV] (R75)
> tetanus neonatorum (A33)

✓4ᵗʰ **P35 Congenital viral diseases**

   INCLUDES   infections acquired in utero or during birth

P35.0 Congenital rubella syndrome
Congenital rubella pneumonitis

P35.1 Congenital cytomegalovirus infection

P35.2 Congenital herpesviral [herpes simplex] infection

P35.3 Congenital viral hepatitis

P35.8 Other congenital viral diseases
Congenital varicella [chickenpox]

P35.9 Congenital viral disease, unspecified

✓4ᵗʰ **P36 Bacterial sepsis of newborn**

   INCLUDES   congenital sepsis

Use additional code(s), if applicable, to identify severe sepsis (R65.2-) and associated acute organ dysfunction(s)

P36.0 Sepsis of newborn due to streptococcus, group B

✓5ᵗʰ **P36.1 Sepsis of newborn due to other and unspecified streptococci**

    P36.10 Sepsis of newborn due to unspecified streptococci

    P36.19 Sepsis of newborn due to other streptococci

P36.2 Sepsis of newborn due to Staphylococcus aureus

✓5ᵗʰ **P36.3 Sepsis of newborn due to other and unspecified staphylococci**

    P36.30 Sepsis of newborn due to unspecified staphylococci

    P36.39 Sepsis of newborn due to other staphylococci

P36.4 Sepsis of newborn due to Escherichia coli

P36.5 Sepsis of newborn due to anaerobes

P36.8 Other bacterial sepsis of newborn
Use additional code from category B96 to identify organism

P36.9 Bacterial sepsis of newborn, unspecified

✓4ᵗʰ **P37 Other congenital infectious and parasitic diseases**

> EXCLUDES 2   congenital syphilis (A50-)
> infectious neonatal diarrhea (A00-A09)
> necrotizing enterocolitis in newborn (P77-)
> noninfectious neonatal diarrhea (P78.3)
> ophthalmia neonatorum due to gonococcus (A54.31)
> tetanus neonatorum (A33)

P37.0 Congenital tuberculosis

P37.1 Congenital toxoplasmosis
Hydrocephalus due to congenital toxoplasmosis

P37.2 Neonatal (disseminated) listeriosis

P37.3 Congenital falciparum malaria

P37.4 Other congenital malaria

P37.5 Neonatal candidiasis

P37.8 Other specified congenital infectious and parasitic diseases

P37.9 Congenital infectious or parasitic disease, unspecified

✓4ᵗʰ **P38 Omphalitis of newborn**

> EXCLUDES 1   omphalitis not of newborn (L08.82)
> tetanus omphalitis (A33)
> umbilical hemorrhage of newborn (P51-)

P38.1 Omphalitis with mild hemorrhage

P38.9 Omphalitis without hemorrhage
Omphalitis of newborn NOS

✓4ᵗʰ **P39 Other infections specific to the perinatal period**

Use additional code to identify organism or specific infection

P39.0 Neonatal infective mastitis

> EXCLUDES 1   breast engorgement of newborn (P83.4)
> noninfective mastitis of newborn (P83.4)

P39.1 Neonatal conjunctivitis and dacryocystitis
Neonatal chlamydial conjunctivitis
Ophthalmia neonatorum NOS

> EXCLUDES 1   gonococcal conjunctivitis (A54.31)

P39.2 Intra-amniotic infection affecting newborn, not elsewhere classified

P39.3 Neonatal urinary tract infection

P39.4 Neonatal skin infection
Neonatal pyoderma

> EXCLUDES 1   pemphigus neonatorum (L00)
> staphylococcal scalded skin syndrome (L00)

P39.8 Other specified infections specific to the perinatal period

P39.9 Infection specific to the perinatal period, unspecified

Hemorrhagic and hematological disorders of newborn (P50-P61)

> EXCLUDES 1   congenital stenosis and stricture of bile ducts (Q44.3)
> Crigler-Najjar syndrome (E80.5)
> Dubin-Johnson syndrome (E80.6)
> Gilbert syndrome (E80.4)
> hereditary hemolytic anemias (D55-D58)

✓4ᵗʰ **P50 Newborn affected by intrauterine (fetal) blood loss**

> EXCLUDES 1   congenital anemia from intrauterine (fetal) blood loss (P61.3)

P50.0 Newborn affected by intrauterine (fetal) blood loss from vasa previa

P50.1 Newborn affected by intrauterine (fetal) blood loss from ruptured cord

P50.2 Newborn affected by intrauterine (fetal) blood loss from placenta

P50.3 Newborn affected by hemorrhage into co-twin

P50.4 Newborn affected by hemorrhage into maternal circulation

P50.5 Newborn affected by intrauterine (fetal) blood loss from cut end of co-twin's cord

P50.8 Newborn affected by other intrauterine (fetal) blood loss

P50.9 Newborn affected by intrauterine (fetal) blood loss, unspecified
Newborn affected by fetal hemorrhage NOS

✓4ᵗʰ **P51 Umbilical hemorrhage of newborn**

> EXCLUDES 1   omphalitis with mild hemorrhage (P38.1)
> umbilical hemorrhage from cut end of co-twins cord (P50.5)

P51.0 Massive umbilical hemorrhage of newborn

P51.8 Other umbilical hemorrhages of newborn
Slipped umbilical ligature NOS

P51.9 Umbilical hemorrhage of newborn, unspecified

✓4ᵗʰ **P52 Intracranial nontraumatic hemorrhage of newborn**
Intracranial hemorrhage due to anoxia or hypoxia

> EXCLUDES 1   intracranial hemorrhage due to birth injury (P10-)
> intracranial hemorrhage due to other injury (S06-)

P52.0 Intraventricular (nontraumatic) hemorrhage, grade 1, of newborn
Subependymal hemorrhage (without intraventricular extension)
Bleeding into germinal matrix

P52.1 Intraventricular (nontraumatic) hemorrhage, grade 2, of newborn
Subependymal hemorrhage with intraventricular extension
Bleeding into ventricle

✓5ᵗʰ **P52.2 Intraventricular (nontraumatic) hemorrhage, grade 3 and grade 4, of newborn**

    P52.21 Intraventricular (nontraumatic) hemorrhage, grade 3, of newborn
Subependymal hemorrhage with intraventricular extension with enlargement of ventricle

    P52.22 Intraventricular (nontraumatic) hemorrhage, grade 4, of newborn
Bleeding into cerebral cortex
Subependymal hemorrhage with intracerebral extension

P52.3 Unspecified intraventricular (nontraumatic) hemorrhage of newborn

P52.4 Intracerebral (nontraumatic) hemorrhage of newborn

P52.5 Subarachnoid (nontraumatic) hemorrhage of newborn

P52.6 Cerebellar (nontraumatic) and posterior fossa hemorrhage of newborn

P52.8 Other intracranial (nontraumatic) hemorrhages of newborn

P52.9 Intracranial (nontraumatic) hemorrhage of newborn, unspecified

---

EXCLUDES 1   Not coded here   EXCLUDES 2   Not included here   *Manifestation Code*

P53 Hemorrhagic disease of newborn
  Vitamin K deficiency of newborn

☑️4th **P54 Other neonatal hemorrhages**
  EXCLUDES 1 *newborn affected by (intrauterine) blood loss (P50-)*
      pulmonary hemorrhage originating in the perinatal period
      (P26-)

  P54.0 **Neonatal hematemesis**
      EXCLUDES 1 *neonatal hematemesis due to swallowed maternal*
          blood (P78.2)

  P54.1 **Neonatal melena**
      EXCLUDES 1 *neonatal melena due to swallowed maternal blood*
          (P78.2)

  P54.2 **Neonatal rectal hemorrhage**
  P54.3 **Other neonatal gastrointestinal hemorrhage**
  P54.4 **Neonatal adrenal hemorrhage**
  P54.5 **Neonatal cutaneous hemorrhage**
      Neonatal bruising
      Neonatal ecchymoses
      Neonatal petechiae
      Neonatal superficial hematomata
      EXCLUDES 2 *bruising of scalp due to birth injury (P12.3)*
          cephalhematoma due to birth injury (P12.0)

  P54.6 **Neonatal vaginal hemorrhage**
      Neonatal pseudomenses
  P54.8 **Other specified neonatal hemorrhages**
  P54.9 **Neonatal hemorrhage, unspecified**

☑️4th **P55 Hemolytic disease of newborn**
  P55.0 **Rh isoimmunization of newborn**
  P55.1 **ABO isoimmunization of newborn**
  P55.8 **Other hemolytic diseases of newborn**
  P55.9 **Hemolytic disease of newborn, unspecified**

☑️4th **P56 Hydrops fetalis due to hemolytic disease**
  EXCLUDES 1 *hydrops fetalis NOS (P83.2)*

  P56.0 **Hydrops fetalis due to isoimmunization**
☑️5th P56.9 **Hydrops fetalis due to other and unspecified hemolytic**
      disease
      P56.90 **Hydrops fetalis due to unspecified hemolytic**
          disease
      P56.99 **Hydrops fetalis due to other hemolytic disease**

☑️4th **P57 Kernicterus**
  P57.0 **Kernicterus due to isoimmunization**
  P57.8 **Other specified kernicterus**
      EXCLUDES 1 *Crigler-Najjar syndrome (E80.5)*

  P57.9 **Kernicterus, unspecified**

☑️4th **P58 Neonatal jaundice due to other excessive hemolysis**
  EXCLUDES 1 *jaundice due to isoimmunization (P55-P57)*

  P58.0 **Neonatal jaundice due to bruising**
  P58.1 **Neonatal jaundice due to bleeding**
  P58.2 **Neonatal jaundice due to infection**
  P58.3 **Neonatal jaundice due to polycythemia**
☑️5th P58.4 **Neonatal jaundice due to drugs or toxins transmitted from**
      mother or given to newborn
      Code first (T36-T65) to identify drug or toxin
      P58.41 **Neonatal jaundice due to drugs or toxins**
          transmitted from mother
      P58.42 **Neonatal jaundice due to drugs or toxins given to**
          newborn
  P58.5 **Neonatal jaundice due to swallowed maternal blood**
  P58.8 **Neonatal jaundice due to other specified excessive**
      hemolysis
  P58.9 **Neonatal jaundice due to excessive hemolysis, unspecified**

☑️4th **P59 Neonatal jaundice from other and unspecified causes**
  EXCLUDES 1 *jaundice due to inborn errors of metabolism (E70-E88)*
      kernicterus (P57-)

  P59.0 **Neonatal jaundice associated with preterm delivery**
      Hyperbilirubinemia of prematurity
      Jaundice due to delayed conjugation associated with preterm
          delivery
  P59.1 **Inspissated bile syndrome**
☑️5th P59.2 **Neonatal jaundice from other and unspecified**
      hepatocellular damage
      EXCLUDES 1 *congenital viral hepatitis (P35.3)*
      P59.20 **Neonatal jaundice from unspecified**
          hepatocellular damage

  P59.29 **Neonatal jaundice from other hepatocellular**
      damage
      Giant cell hepatitis
      Neonatal (idiopathic) hepatitis
  P59.3 **Neonatal jaundice from breast milk inhibitor**
  P59.8 **Neonatal jaundice from other specified causes**
  P59.9 **Neonatal jaundice, unspecified**
      Neonatal physiological jaundice (intense)(prolonged) NOS

P60 Disseminated intravascular coagulation of newborn
  Defibrination syndrome of newborn

☑️4th **P61 Other perinatal hematological disorders**
  EXCLUDES 1 *transient hypogammaglobulinemia of infancy (D80.7)*

  P61.0 **Transient neonatal thrombocytopenia**
      Neonatal thrombocytopenia due to exchange transfusion
      Neonatal thrombocytopenia due to idiopathic maternal
          thrombocytopenia
      Neonatal thrombocytopenia due to isoimmunization
  P61.1 **Polycythemia neonatorum**
  P61.2 **Anemia of prematurity**
  P61.3 **Congenital anemia from fetal blood loss**
  P61.4 **Other congenital anemias, not elsewhere classified**
      Congenital anemia NOS
  P61.5 **Transient neonatal neutropenia**
      EXCLUDES 1 *congenital neutropenia (nontransient) (D70.0)*
  P61.6 **Other transient neonatal disorders of coagulation**
  P61.8 **Other specified perinatal hematological disorders**
  P61.9 **Perinatal hematological disorder, unspecified**

Transitory endocrine and metabolic disorders specific to newborn (P70-P74)

  INCLUDES transitory endocrine and metabolic disturbances caused by the
      infant's response to maternal endocrine and metabolic
      factors, or its adjustment to extrauterine environment

☑️4th **P70 Transitory disorders of carbohydrate metabolism specific to**
      newborn
  P70.0 **Syndrome of infant of mother with gestational diabetes**
      Newborn (with hypoglycemia) affected by maternal
          gestational diabetes
      EXCLUDES 1 *newborn (with hypoglycemia) affected by maternal*
          (pre-existing) diabetes mellitus (P70.1)
          syndrome of infant of a diabetic mother (P70.1)
  P70.1 **Syndrome of infant of a diabetic mother**
      Newborn (with hypoglycemia) affected by maternal
          (pre-existing) diabetes mellitus
      EXCLUDES 1 *newborn (with hypoglycemia) affected by maternal*
          gestational diabetes (P70.0)
          syndrome of infant of mother with gestational
          diabetes (P70.0)
  P70.2 **Neonatal diabetes mellitus**
  P70.3 **Iatrogenic neonatal hypoglycemia**
  P70.4 **Other neonatal hypoglycemia**
      Transitory neonatal hypoglycemia
  P70.8 **Other transitory disorders of carbohydrate metabolism of**
      newborn
  P70.9 **Transitory disorder of carbohydrate metabolism of**
      newborn, unspecified

☑️4th **P71 Transitory neonatal disorders of calcium and magnesium**
      metabolism
  P71.0 **Cow's milk hypocalcemia in newborn**
  P71.1 **Other neonatal hypocalcemia**
      EXCLUDES 1 *neonatal hypoparathyroidism (P71.4)*
  P71.2 **Neonatal hypomagnesemia**
  P71.3 **Neonatal tetany without calcium or magnesium deficiency**
      Neonatal tetany NOS
  P71.4 **Transitory neonatal hypoparathyroidism**
  P71.8 **Other transitory neonatal disorders of calcium and**
      magnesium metabolism
  P71.9 **Transitory neonatal disorder of calcium and magnesium**
      metabolism, unspecified

☑️ Appropriate additional character required   ☑️x7th Requires 7th character, placeholder x must fill empty characters

Certain Conditions Originating in the Perinatal Period

P72–P91.61

☑4ᵗʰ **P72** **Other transitory neonatal endocrine disorders**
      EXCLUDES 1 *congenital hypothyroidism with or without goiter (E03.0–E03.1)*
          dyshormogenetic goiter (E07.1)
          Pendred's syndrome (E07.1)

     P72.0 **Neonatal goiter, not elsewhere classified**
           Transitory congenital goiter with normal functioning

     P72.1 **Transitory neonatal hyperthyroidism**
           Neonatal thyrotoxicosis

     P72.2 **Other transitory neonatal disorders of thyroid function, not elsewhere classified**
           Transitory neonatal hypothyroidism

     P72.8 **Other specified transitory neonatal endocrine disorders**

     P72.9 **Transitory neonatal endocrine disorder, unspecified**

☑4ᵗʰ **P74** **Other transitory neonatal electrolyte and metabolic disturbances**
     P74.0 **Late metabolic acidosis of newborn**
          EXCLUDES 1 *(fetal) metabolic acidosis of newborn (P19)*

     P74.1 **Dehydration of newborn**
     P74.2 **Disturbances of sodium balance of newborn**
     P74.3 **Disturbances of potassium balance of newborn**
     P74.4 **Other transitory electrolyte disturbances of newborn**
     P74.5 **Transitory tyrosinemia of newborn**
     P74.6 **Transitory hyperammonemia of newborn**
     P74.8 **Other transitory metabolic disturbances of newborn**
           Amino-acid metabolic disorders described as transitory
     P74.9 **Transitory metabolic disturbance of newborn, unspecified**

Digestive system disorders of newborn (P76-P78)

☑4ᵗʰ **P76** **Other intestinal obstruction of newborn**
     P76.0 **Meconium plug syndrome**
           Meconium ileus NOS
          EXCLUDES 1 *meconium ileus in cystic fibrosis (E84.11)*

     P76.1 **Transitory ileus of newborn**
          EXCLUDES 1 *Hirschsprung's disease (Q43.1)*

     P76.2 **Intestinal obstruction due to inspissated milk**

     P76.8 **Other specified intestinal obstruction of newborn**
          EXCLUDES 1 *intestinal obstruction classifiable to K56-*

     P76.9 **Intestinal obstruction of newborn, unspecified**

☑4ᵗʰ **P77** **Necrotizing enterocolitis of newborn**
     P77.1 **Stage 1 necrotizing enterocolitis in newborn**
           Necrotizing enterocolitis without pneumatosis, without perforation

     P77.2 **Stage 2 necrotizing enterocolitis in newborn**
           Necrotizing enterocolitis with pneumatosis, without perforation

     P77.3 **Stage 3 necrotizing enterocolitis in newborn**
           Necrotizing enterocolitis with perforation
           Necrotizing enterocolitis with pneumatosis and perforation

     P77.9 **Necrotizing enterocolitis in newborn, unspecified**
           Necrotizing enterocolitis in newborn, NOS

☑4ᵗʰ **P78** **Other perinatal digestive system disorders**
      EXCLUDES 1 *cystic fibrosis (E84.0–E84.9)*
          neonatal gastrointestinal hemorrhages (P54.0–P54.3)

     P78.0 **Perinatal intestinal perforation**
           Meconium peritonitis

     P78.1 **Other neonatal peritonitis**
           Neonatal peritonitis NOS

     P78.2 **Neonatal hematemesis and melena due to swallowed maternal blood**

     P78.3 **Noninfective neonatal diarrhea**
           Neonatal diarrhea NOS

    ☑5ᵗʰ **P78.8** **Other specified perinatal digestive system disorders**
         P78.81 **Congenital cirrhosis (of liver)**
         P78.82 **Peptic ulcer of newborn**
         P78.83 **Newborn esophageal reflux**
             Neonatal esophageal reflux
         P78.89 **Other specified perinatal digestive system disorders**

     P78.9 **Perinatal digestive system disorder, unspecified**

Conditions involving the integument and temperature regulation of newborn (P80-P83)

☑4ᵗʰ **P80** **Hypothermia of newborn**
     P80.0 **Cold injury syndrome**
           Severe and usually chronic hypothermia associated with a pink flushed appearance, edema and neurological and biochemical abnormalities.
          EXCLUDES 1 *mild hypothermia of newborn (P80.8)*

     P80.8 **Other hypothermia of newborn**
           Mild hypothermia of newborn

     P80.9 **Hypothermia of newborn, unspecified**

☑4ᵗʰ **P81** **Other disturbances of temperature regulation of newborn**
     P81.0 **Environmental hyperthermia of newborn**
     P81.8 **Other specified disturbances of temperature regulation of newborn**
     P81.9 **Disturbance of temperature regulation of newborn, unspecified**
           Fever of newborn NOS

☑4ᵗʰ **P83** **Other conditions of integument specific to newborn**
      EXCLUDES 1 *congenital malformations of skin and integument (Q80–Q84)*
          hydrops fetalis due to hemolytic disease (P56-)
          neonatal skin infection (P39.4)
          staphylococcal scalded skin syndrome (L00)
      EXCLUDES 2 *cradle cap (L21.0)*
          diaper [napkin] dermatitis (L22)

     P83.0 **Sclerema neonatorum**
     P83.1 **Neonatal erythema toxicum**
     P83.2 **Hydrops fetalis not due to hemolytic disease**
           Hydrops fetalis NOS

    ☑5ᵗʰ **P83.3** **Other and unspecified edema specific to newborn**
         P83.30 **Unspecified edema specific to newborn**
         P83.39 **Other edema specific to newborn**

     P83.4 **Breast engorgement of newborn**
           Noninfective mastitis of newborn

     P83.5 **Congenital hydrocele**
     P83.6 **Umbilical polyp of newborn**
     P83.8 **Other specified conditions of integument specific to newborn**
           Bronze baby syndrome
           Neonatal scleroderma
           Urticaria neonatorum

     P83.9 **Condition of the integument specific to newborn, unspecified**

Other problems with newborn (P84)

P84 **Other problems with newborn**
         Acidemia of newborn
         Acidosis of newborn
         Anoxia of newborn NOS
         Asphyxia of newborn NOS
         Hypercapnia of newborn
         Hypoxemia of newborn
         Hypoxia of newborn NOS
         Mixed metabolic and respiratory acidosis of newborn
      EXCLUDES 1 *intracranial hemorrhage due to anoxia or hypoxia (P52-)*
          hypoxic ischemic encephalopathy [HIE] (P91.6-)
          late metabolic acidosis of newborn (P74.0)

Other disorders originating in the perinatal period (P90-P96)

P90 **Convulsions of newborn**
      EXCLUDES 1 *benign myoclonic epilepsy in infancy (G40.3-)*
          benign neonatal convulsions (familial) (G40.3-)

☑4ᵗʰ **P91** **Other disturbances of cerebral status of newborn**
     P91.0 **Neonatal cerebral ischemia**
     P91.1 **Acquired periventricular cysts of newborn**
     P91.2 **Neonatal cerebral leukomalacia**
           Periventricular leukomalacia
     P91.3 **Neonatal cerebral irritability**
     P91.4 **Neonatal cerebral depression**
     P91.5 **Neonatal coma**
    ☑5ᵗʰ **P91.6** **Hypoxic ischemic encephalopathy [HIE]**
         P91.60 **Hypoxic ischemic encephalopathy [HIE], unspecified**
         P91.61 **Mild hypoxic ischemic encephalopathy [HIE]**

EXCLUDES 1 Not coded here   **EXCLUDES 2** Not included here   *Manifestation Code*

P91.62　Moderate hypoxic ischemic encephalopathy [HIE]
P91.63　Severe hypoxic ischemic encephalopathy [HIE]
P91.8　Other specified disturbances of cerebral status of newborn
P91.9　Disturbance of cerebral status of newborn, unspecified

✓4ᵗʰ **P92　Feeding problems of newborn**
　　EXCLUDES 1　*feeding problems in child over 28 days old (R63.3)*
　✓5ᵗʰ **P92.0　Vomiting of newborn**
　　　EXCLUDES 1　*vomiting of child over 28 days old (R11-)*
　　　P92.01　Bilious vomiting of newborn
　　　　　EXCLUDES 1　*bilious vomiting in child over 28 days old (R11.4)*
　　　P92.09　Other vomiting of newborn
　　　　　EXCLUDES 1　*regurgitation of food in newborn (P92.1)*
　　P92.1　Regurgitation and rumination of newborn
　　P92.2　Slow feeding of newborn
　　P92.3　Underfeeding of newborn
　　P92.4　Overfeeding of newborn
　　P92.5　Neonatal difficulty in feeding at breast
　　P92.6　Failure to thrive in newborn
　　　　EXCLUDES 1　*failure to thrive in child over 28 days old (R62.51)*
　　P92.8　Other feeding problems of newborn
　　P92.9　Feeding problem of newborn, unspecified

✓4ᵗʰ **P93　Reactions and intoxications due to drugs administered to newborn**
　　INCLUDES　reactions and intoxications due to drugs administered to fetus affecting newborn
　　EXCLUDES 1　*jaundice due to drugs or toxins transmitted from mother or given to newborn (P58.4-)*
　　　　reactions and intoxications from maternal opiates, tranquilizers and other medication (P04.0-P04.1, P04.4)
　　　　withdrawal symptoms from maternal use of drugs of addiction (P96.1)
　　　　withdrawal symptoms from therapeutic use of drugs in newborn (P96.2)
　　P93.0　Grey baby syndrome
　　　　Grey syndrome from chloramphenicol administration in newborn
　　P93.8　Other reactions and intoxications due to drugs administered to newborn
　　　　Code first (T36-T50) to identify drug

✓4ᵗʰ **P94　Disorders of muscle tone of newborn**
　　P94.0　Transient neonatal myasthenia gravis
　　　　EXCLUDES 1　*myasthenia gravis (G70.0)*
　　P94.1　Congenital hypertonia
　　P94.2　Congenital hypotonia
　　　　Floppy baby syndrome, unspecified
　　P94.8　Other disorders of muscle tone of newborn
　　P94.9　Disorder of muscle tone of newborn, unspecified

P95　Stillbirth
　　Deadborn fetus NOS
　　Fetal death of unspecified cause
　　Stillbirth NOS
　　EXCLUDES 1　*maternal care for intrauterine death (O36.4)*
　　　　missed abortion (O02.1)
　　　　outcome of delivery, stillbirth (Z37.1, Z37.3, Z37.4, Z37.7)

✓4ᵗʰ **P96　Other conditions originating in the perinatal period**
　　P96.0　Congenital renal failure
　　　　Uremia of newborn
　　P96.1　Neonatal withdrawal symptoms from maternal use of drugs of addiction
　　　　Drug withdrawal syndrome in infant of dependent mother
　　　　Neonatal abstinence syndrome
　　　　EXCLUDES 1　*reactions and intoxications from maternal opiates and tranquilizers administered during labor and delivery (P04.0)*
　　P96.2　Withdrawal symptoms from therapeutic use of drugs in newborn
　　P96.3　Wide cranial sutures of newborn
　　　　Neonatal craniotabes
　　P96.5　Complication to newborn due to (fetal) intrauterine procedure
　　　　EXCLUDES 2　*newborn (suspected to be) affected by amniocentesis (P00.6)*

✓5ᵗʰ **P96.8　Other specified conditions originating in the perinatal period**
　　P96.81　Exposure to (parental) (environmental) tobacco smoke in the perinatal period
　　　　EXCLUDES 2　*newborn affected by in utero exposure to tobacco (P04.2)*
　　　　exposure to environmental tobacco smoke after the perinatal period (Z77.22)
　　P96.82　Delayed separation of umbilical cord
　　P96.83　Meconium staining
　　　　EXCLUDES 1　*meconium aspiration (P24.00, P24.01)*
　　　　meconium passage during delivery (P03.82)
　　P96.89　Other specified conditions originating in the perinatal period
　　　　Use additional code to specify condition
　P96.9　Condition originating in the perinatal period, unspecified
　　　　Congenital debility NOS

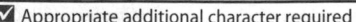 ✓ Appropriate additional character required　　　✓x7ᵗʰ Requires 7th character, placeholder x must fill empty characters

Chapter 17. Congenital Malformations, Deformations and Chromosomal Abnormalities (Q00-Q99)

NOTE   Codes from this chapter are not for use on maternal or fetal records

EXCLUDES 1   *inborn errors of metabolism (E70-E88)*

This chapter contains the following blocks:

Q00-Q07   Congenital malformations of the nervous system
Q10-Q18   Congenital malformations of eye, ear, face and neck
Q20-Q28   Congenital malformations of the circulatory system
Q30-Q34   Congenital malformations of the respiratory system
Q35-Q37   Cleft lip and cleft palate
Q38-Q45   Other congenital malformations of the digestive system
Q50-Q56   Congenital malformations of genital organs
Q60-Q64   Congenital malformations of the urinary system
Q65-Q79   Congenital malformations and deformations of the musculoskeletal system
Q80-Q89   Other congenital malformations
Q90-Q99   Chromosomal abnormalities, not elsewhere classified

Congenital malformations of the nervous system (Q00-Q07)

✓4ᵗʰ Q00 Anencephaly and similar malformations

     Q00.0 Anencephaly
         Acephaly
         Acrania
         Amyelencephaly
         Hemianencephaly
         Hemicephaly

     Q00.1 Craniorachischisis

     Q00.2 Iniencephaly

✓4ᵗʰ Q01 Encephalocele

     INCLUDES   Arnold-Chiari syndrome, type III
         encephalocystocele
         encephalomyelocele
         hydroencephalocele
         hydromeningocele, cranial
         meningocele, cerebral
         meningoencephalocele

     EXCLUDES 1   *Meckel-Gruber syndrome (Q61.9)*

     Q01.0 Frontal encephalocele

     Q01.1 Nasofrontal encephalocele

     Q01.2 Occipital encephalocele

     Q01.8 Encephalocele of other sites

     Q01.9 Encephalocele, unspecified

Q02 Microcephaly

     INCLUDES   hydromicrocephaly
         micrencephalon

     EXCLUDES 1   *Meckel-Gruber syndrome (Q61.9)*

✓4ᵗʰ Q03 Congenital hydrocephalus

     INCLUDES   hydrocephalus in newborn

     EXCLUDES 1   *Arnold-Chiari syndrome, type II (Q07.0-)*
         acquired hydrocephalus (G91-)
         hydrocephalus due to congenital toxoplasmosis (P37.1)
         hydrocephalus with spina bifida (Q05.0-Q05.4)

     Q03.0 Malformations of aqueduct of Sylvius
         Anomaly of aqueduct of Sylvius
         Obstruction of aqueduct of Sylvius, congenital
         Stenosis of aqueduct of Sylvius

     Q03.1 Atresia of foramina of Magendie and Luschka
         Dandy-Walker syndrome

     Q03.8 Other congenital hydrocephalus

     Q03.9 Congenital hydrocephalus, unspecified

✓4ᵗʰ Q04 Other congenital malformations of brain

     EXCLUDES 1   *cyclopia (Q87.0)*
         macrocephaly (Q75.3)

     Q04.0 Congenital malformations of corpus callosum
         Agenesis of corpus callosum

     Q04.1 Arhinencephaly

     Q04.2 Holoprosencephaly

     Q04.3 Other reduction deformities of brain
         Absence of part of brain
         Agenesis of part of brain
         Agyria
         Aplasia of part of brain
         Hydranencephaly
         Hypoplasia of part of brain
         Lissencephaly
         Microgyria
         Pachygyria

     EXCLUDES 1   *congenital malformations of corpus callosum (Q04.0)*

     Q04.4 Septo-optic dysplasia of brain

     Q04.5 Megalencephaly

     Q04.6 Congenital cerebral cysts
         Porencephaly
         Schizencephaly

     EXCLUDES 1   *acquired porencephalic cyst (G93.0)*

     Q04.8 Other specified congenital malformations of brain
         Arnold-Chiari syndrome, type IV
         Macrogyria

     Q04.9 Congenital malformation of brain, unspecified
         Congenital anomaly NOS of brain
         Congenital deformity NOS of brain
         Congenital disease or lesion NOS of brain
         Multiple anomalies NOS of brain, congenital

✓4ᵗʰ Q05 Spina bifida

     Hydromeningocele (spinal)
     Meningocele (spinal)
     Meningomyelocele
     Myelocele
     Myelomeningocele
     Rachischisis
     Spina bifida (aperta)(cystica)
     Syringomyelocele
     Use additional code for any associated paraplegia (paraparesis) (G82.2-)

     EXCLUDES 1   *Arnold-Chiari syndrome, type II (Q07.0-)*
         spina bifida occulta (Q76.0)

     Q05.0 Cervical spina bifida with hydrocephalus

     Q05.1 Thoracic spina bifida with hydrocephalus
         Dorsal spina bifida with hydrocephalus
         Thoracolumbar spina bifida with hydrocephalus

     Q05.2 Lumbar spina bifida with hydrocephalus
         Lumbosacral spina bifida with hydrocephalus

     Q05.3 Sacral spina bifida with hydrocephalus

     Q05.4 Unspecified spina bifida with hydrocephalus

     Q05.5 Cervical spina bifida without hydrocephalus

     Q05.6 Thoracic spina bifida without hydrocephalus
         Dorsal spina bifida NOS
         Thoracolumbar spina bifida NOS

     Q05.7 Lumbar spina bifida without hydrocephalus
         Lumbosacral spina bifida NOS

     Q05.8 Sacral spina bifida without hydrocephalus

     Q05.9 Spina bifida, unspecified

✓4ᵗʰ Q06 Other congenital malformations of spinal cord

     Q06.0 Amyelia

     Q06.1 Hypoplasia and dysplasia of spinal cord
         Atelomyelia
         Myelatelia
         Myelodysplasia of spinal cord

     Q06.2 Diastematomyelia

     Q06.3 Other congenital cauda equina malformations

     Q06.4 Hydromyelia
         Hydrorachis

     Q06.8 Other specified congenital malformations of spinal cord

     Q06.9 Congenital malformation of spinal cord, unspecified
         Congenital anomaly NOS of spinal cord
         Congenital deformity NOS of spinal cord
         Congenital disease or lesion NOS of spinal cord

EXCLUDES 1 Not coded here   **EXCLUDES 2** Not included here   *Manifestation Code*

✓4th **Q07 Other congenital malformations of nervous system**

> EXCLUDES 2   *congenital central alveolar hypoventilation syndrome (G47.35)*
> *familial dysautonomia [Riley-Day] (G90.1)*
> *neurofibromatosis (nonmalignant) (Q85.0-)*

✓5th **Q07.0 Arnold-Chiari syndrome**
Arnold-Chiari syndrome, type II

> EXCLUDES 1 *Arnold-Chiari syndrome, type III (Q01-)*
> *Arnold-Chiari syndrome, type IV (Q04.8)*

    Q07.00 Arnold-Chiari syndrome without spina bifida or hydrocephalus
    Q07.01 Arnold-Chiari syndrome with spina bifida
    Q07.02 Arnold-Chiari syndrome with hydrocephalus
    Q07.03 Arnold-Chiari syndrome with spina bifida and hydrocephalus

  Q07.8 Other specified congenital malformations of nervous system
Agenesis of nerve
Displacement of brachial plexus
Jaw-winking syndrome
Marcus Gunn's syndrome

  Q07.9 Congenital malformation of nervous system, unspecified
Congenital anomaly NOS of nervous system
Congenital deformity NOS of nervous system
Congenital disease or lesion NOS of nervous system

Congenital malformations of eye, ear, face and neck (Q10-Q18)

> EXCLUDES 2 *cleft lip and cleft palate (Q35-Q37)*
> *congenital malformation of:*
>   *cervical spine (Q05.0, Q05.5, Q67.5, Q76.0-Q76.4)*
>   *larynx (Q31-)*
>   *lip NEC (Q38.0)*
>   *nose (Q30-)*
>   *parathyroid gland (Q89.2)*
>   *thyroid gland (Q89.2)*

✓4th **Q10 Congenital malformations of eyelid, lacrimal apparatus and orbit**

> EXCLUDES 1 *cryptophthalmos NOS (Q11.2)*
> *cryptophthalmos syndrome (Q87.0)*

  Q10.0 Congenital ptosis
  Q10.1 Congenital ectropion
  Q10.2 Congenital entropion
  Q10.3 Other congenital malformations of eyelid
Ablepharon
Blepharophimosis, congenital
Coloboma of eyelid
Congenital absence or agenesis of cilia
Congenital absence or agenesis of eyelid
Congenital accessory eyelid
Congenital accessory eye muscle
Congenital malformation of eyelid NOS

  Q10.4 Absence and agenesis of lacrimal apparatus
Congenital absence of punctum lacrimale

  Q10.5 Congenital stenosis and stricture of lacrimal duct
  Q10.6 Other congenital malformations of lacrimal apparatus
Congenital malformation of lacrimal apparatus NOS

  Q10.7 Congenital malformation of orbit

✓4th **Q11 Anophthalmos, microphthalmos and macrophthalmos**

  Q11.0 Cystic eyeball
  Q11.1 Other anophthalmos
Anophthalmos NOS
Agenesis of eye
Aplasia of eye

  Q11.2 Microphthalmos
Cryptophthalmos NOS
Dysplasia of eye
Hypoplasia of eye
Rudimentary eye

> EXCLUDES 1 *cryptophthalmos syndrome (Q87.0)*

  Q11.3 Macrophthalmos

> EXCLUDES 1 *macrophthalmos in congenital glaucoma (Q15.0)*

✓4th **Q12 Congenital lens malformations**

  Q12.0 Congenital cataract
  Q12.1 Congenital displaced lens
  Q12.2 Coloboma of lens
  Q12.3 Congenital aphakia
  Q12.4 Spherophakia

  Q12.8 Other congenital lens malformations
Microphakia

  Q12.9 Congenital lens malformation, unspecified

✓4th **Q13 Congenital malformations of anterior segment of eye**

  Q13.0 Coloboma of iris
Coloboma NOS

  Q13.1 Absence of iris
Aniridia
Use additional code for associated glaucoma (H42)

  Q13.2 Other congenital malformations of iris
Anisocoria, congenital
Atresia of pupil
Congenital malformation of iris NOS
Corectopia

  Q13.3 Congenital corneal opacity
  Q13.4 Other congenital corneal malformations
Congenital malformation of cornea NOS
Microcornea
Peter's anomaly

  Q13.5 Blue sclera

✓5th **Q13.8 Other congenital malformations of anterior segment of eye**
    Q13.81 Rieger's anomaly
Use additional code for associated glaucoma (H42)
    Q13.89 Other congenital malformations of anterior segment of eye

  Q13.9 Congenital malformation of anterior segment of eye, unspecified

✓4th **Q14 Congenital malformations of posterior segment of eye**

> EXCLUDES 2 *optic nerve hypoplasia (H47.03-)*

  Q14.0 Congenital malformation of vitreous humor
Congenital vitreous opacity

  Q14.1 Congenital malformation of retina
Congenital retinal aneurysm

  Q14.2 Congenital malformation of optic disc
Coloboma of optic disc

  Q14.3 Congenital malformation of choroid
  Q14.8 Other congenital malformations of posterior segment of eye
Coloboma of the fundus

  Q14.9 Congenital malformation of posterior segment of eye, unspecified

✓4th **Q15 Other congenital malformations of eye**

> EXCLUDES 1 *congenital nystagmus (H55.01)*
> *ocular albinism (E70.31-)*
> *optic nerve hypoplasia (H47.03-)*
> *retinitis pigmentosa (H35.52)*

  Q15.0 Congenital glaucoma
Axenfeld's anomaly
Buphthalmos
Glaucoma of childhood
Glaucoma of newborn
Hydrophthalmos
Keratoglobus, congenital, with glaucoma
Macrocornea with glaucoma
Macrophthalmos in congenital glaucoma
Megalocornea with glaucoma

  Q15.8 Other specified congenital malformations of eye
  Q15.9 Congenital malformation of eye, unspecified
Congenital anomaly of eye
Congenital deformity of eye

✓4th **Q16 Congenital malformations of ear causing impairment of hearing**

> EXCLUDES 1 *congenital deafness (H90-)*

  Q16.0 Congenital absence of (ear) auricle
  Q16.1 Congenital absence, atresia and stricture of auditory canal (external)
Congenital atresia or stricture of osseous meatus

  Q16.2 Absence of eustachian tube
  Q16.3 Congenital malformation of ear ossicles
Congenital fusion of ear ossicles

  Q16.4 Other congenital malformations of middle ear
Congenital malformation of middle ear NOS

  Q16.5 Congenital malformation of inner ear
Congenital anomaly of membranous labyrinth
Congenital anomaly of organ of Corti

☑ Appropriate additional character required   ✓x7th Requires 7th character, placeholder x must fill empty characters

Q16.9 Congenital malformation of ear causing impairment of hearing, unspecified
Congenital absence of ear NOS

☑4ᵗʰ Q17 Other congenital malformations of ear
> EXCLUDES 1   congenital malformations of ear with impairment of hearing (Q16.0- Q16.9)
> preauricular sinus (Q18.1)

Q17.0 Accessory auricle
Accessory tragus
Polyotia
Preauricular appendage or tag
Supernumerary ear
Supernumerary lobule

Q17.1 Macrotia

Q17.2 Microtia

Q17.3 Other misshapen ear
Pointed ear

Q17.4 Misplaced ear
Low-set ears
> EXCLUDES 1   cervical auricle (Q18.2)

Q17.5 Prominent ear
Bat ear

Q17.8 Other specified congenital malformations of ear
Congenital absence of lobe of ear

Q17.9 Congenital malformation of ear, unspecified
Congenital anomaly of ear NOS

☑4ᵗʰ Q18 Other congenital malformations of face and neck
> EXCLUDES 1   cleft lip and cleft palate (Q35-Q37)
> conditions classified to Q67.0-Q67.4
> congenital malformations of skull and face bones (Q75-)
> cyclopia (Q87.0)
> dentofacial anomalies [including malocclusion] (M26-)
> malformation syndromes affecting facial appearance (Q87.0)
> persistent thyroglossal duct (Q89.2)

Q18.0 Sinus, fistula and cyst of branchial cleft
Branchial vestige

Q18.1 Preauricular sinus and cyst
Fistula of auricle, congenital
Cervicoaural fistula

Q18.2 Other branchial cleft malformations
Branchial cleft malformation NOS
Cervical auricle
Otocephaly

Q18.3 Webbing of neck
Pterygium colli

Q18.4 Macrostomia

Q18.5 Microstomia

Q18.6 Macrocheilia
Hypertrophy of lip, congenital

Q18.7 Microcheilia

Q18.8 Other specified congenital malformations of face and neck
Medial cyst of face and neck
Medial fistula of face and neck
Medial sinus of face and neck

Q18.9 Congenital malformation of face and neck, unspecified
Congenital anomaly NOS of face and neck

Congenital malformations of the circulatory system (Q20-Q28)

☑4ᵗʰ Q20 Congenital malformations of cardiac chambers and connections
> EXCLUDES 1   dextrocardia with situs inversus (Q89.3)
> mirror-image atrial arrangement with situs inversus (Q89.3)

Q20.0 Common arterial trunk
Persistent truncus arteriosus
> EXCLUDES 1   aortic septal defect (Q21.4)

Q20.1 Double outlet right ventricle
Taussig-Bing syndrome

Q20.2 Double outlet left ventricle

Q20.3 Discordant ventriculoarterial connection
Dextrotransposition of aorta
Transposition of great vessels (complete)

Q20.4 Double inlet ventricle
Common ventricle
Cor triloculare biatriatum
Single ventricle

Q20.5 Discordant atrioventricular connection
Corrected transposition
Levotransposition
Ventricular inversion

Q20.6 Isomerism of atrial appendages
Isomerism of atrial appendages with asplenia or polysplenia

Q20.8 Other congenital malformations of cardiac chambers and connections
Cor binoculare

Q20.9 Congenital malformation of cardiac chambers and connections, unspecified

☑4ᵗʰ Q21 Congenital malformations of cardiac septa
> EXCLUDES 1   acquired cardiac septal defect (I51.0)

Q21.0 Ventricular septal defect
Roger's disease

Q21.1 Atrial septal defect
Coronary sinus defect
Patent or persistent foramen ovale
Patent or persistent ostium secundum defect (type II)
Patent or persistent sinus venosus defect

Q21.2 Atrioventricular septal defect
Common atrioventricular canal
Endocardial cushion defect
Ostium primum atrial septal defect (type I)

Q21.3 Tetralogy of Fallot
Ventricular septal defect with pulmonary stenosis or atresia, dextroposition of aorta and hypertrophy of right ventricle.

Q21.4 Aortopulmonary septal defect
Aortic septal defect
Aortopulmonary window

Q21.8 Other congenital malformations of cardiac septa
Eisenmenger's defect
Pentalogy of Fallot
> EXCLUDES 1   Eisenmenger's complex (I27.8)
> Eisenmenger's syndrome (I27.8)

Q21.9 Congenital malformation of cardiac septum, unspecified
Septal (heart) defect NOS

☑4ᵗʰ Q22 Congenital malformations of pulmonary and tricuspid valves

Q22.0 Pulmonary valve atresia

Q22.1 Congenital pulmonary valve stenosis

Q22.2 Congenital pulmonary valve insufficiency
Congenital pulmonary valve regurgitation

Q22.3 Other congenital malformations of pulmonary valve
Congenital malformation of pulmonary valve NOS
Supernumerary cusps of pulmonary valve

Q22.4 Congenital tricuspid stenosis
Congenital tricuspid atresia

Q22.5 Ebstein's anomaly

Q22.6 Hypoplastic right heart syndrome

Q22.8 Other congenital malformations of tricuspid valve

Q22.9 Congenital malformation of tricuspid valve, unspecified

☑4ᵗʰ Q23 Congenital malformations of aortic and mitral valves

Q23.0 Congenital stenosis of aortic valve
Congenital aortic atresia
Congenital aortic stenosis NOS
> EXCLUDES 1   congenital stenosis of aortic valve in hypoplastic left heart syndrome (Q23.4)
> congenital subaortic stenosis (Q24.4)
> supravalvular aortic stenosis (congenital) (Q25.3)

Q23.1 Congenital insufficiency of aortic valve
Bicuspid aortic valve
Congenital aortic insufficiency

Q23.2 Congenital mitral stenosis
Congenital mitral atresia

Q23.3 Congenital mitral insufficiency

Q23.4 Hypoplastic left heart syndrome

Q23.8 Other congenital malformations of aortic and mitral valves

Q23.9 Congenital malformation of aortic and mitral valves, unspecified

---

EXCLUDES 1   Not coded here   EXCLUDES 2   Not included here   *Manifestation Code*

✓4th **Q24 Other congenital malformations of heart**
EXCLUDES 1 *endocardial fibroelastosis (I42.4)*

  Q24.0 Dextrocardia
    EXCLUDES 1 *dextrocardia with situs inversus (Q89.3)*
      isomerism of atrial appendages (with asplenia or polysplenia) (Q20.6)
      mirror-image atrial arrangement with situs inversus (Q89.3)

  Q24.1 Levocardia
  Q24.2 Cor triatriatum
  Q24.3 Pulmonary infundibular stenosis
    Subvalvular pulmonic stenosis
  Q24.4 Congenital subaortic stenosis
  Q24.5 Malformation of coronary vessels
    Congenital coronary (artery) aneurysm
  Q24.6 Congenital heart block
  Q24.8 Other specified congenital malformations of heart
    Congenital diverticulum of left ventricle
    Congenital malformation of myocardium
    Congenital malformation of pericardium
    Malposition of heart
    Uhl's disease
  Q24.9 Congenital malformation of heart, unspecified
    Congenital anomaly of heart
    Congenital disease of heart

✓4th **Q25 Congenital malformations of great arteries**
  Q25.0 Patent ductus arteriosus
    Patent ductus Botallo
    Persistent ductus arteriosus
  Q25.1 Coarctation of aorta
    Coarctation of aorta (preductal) (postductal)
  Q25.2 Atresia of aorta
  Q25.3 Supravalvular aortic stenosis
    EXCLUDES 1 *congenital aortic stenosis NOS (Q23.0)*
      congenital aortic valve stenosis (Q23.0)
  Q25.4 Other congenital malformations of aorta
    Absence of aorta
    Aneurysm of sinus of Valsalva (ruptured)
    Aplasia of aorta
    Congenital aneurysm of aorta
    Congenital malformations of aorta
    Congenital dilatation of aorta
    Double aortic arch [vascular ring of aorta]
    Hypoplasia of aorta
    Persistent convolutions of aortic arch
    Persistent right aortic arch
    EXCLUDES 1 *hypoplasia of aorta in hypoplastic left heart syndrome (Q23.4)*
  Q25.5 Atresia of pulmonary artery
  Q25.6 Stenosis of pulmonary artery
    Supravalvular pulmonary stenosis
  Q25.7 Other congenital malformations of pulmonary artery
    Aberrant pulmonary artery
    Agenesis of pulmonary artery
    Congenital aneurysm of pulmonary artery
    Congenital anomaly of pulmonary artery
    Congenital pulmonary arteriovenous aneurysm
    Hypoplasia of pulmonary artery
  Q25.8 Other congenital malformations of other great arteries
  Q25.9 Congenital malformation of great arteries, unspecified

✓4th **Q26 Congenital malformations of great veins**
  Q26.0 Congenital stenosis of vena cava
    Congenital stenosis of vena cava (inferior)(superior)
  Q26.1 Persistent left superior vena cava
  Q26.2 Total anomalous pulmonary venous connection
    Total anomalous pulmonary venous return [TAPVR], subdiaphragmatic
    Total anomalous pulmonary venous return [TAPVR], supradiaphragmatic
  Q26.3 Partial anomalous pulmonary venous connection
    Partial anomalous pulmonary venous return
  Q26.4 Anomalous pulmonary venous connection, unspecified
  Q26.5 Anomalous portal venous connection
  Q26.6 Portal vein-hepatic artery fistula

  Q26.8 Other congenital malformations of great veins
    Absence of vena cava (inferior) (superior)
    Azygos continuation of inferior vena cava
    Persistent left posterior cardinal vein
    Scimitar syndrome
  Q26.9 Congenital malformation of great vein, unspecified
    Congenital anomaly of vena cava (inferior) (superior) NOS

✓4th **Q27 Other congenital malformations of peripheral vascular system**
  EXCLUDES 2 *anomalies of cerebral and precerebral vessels (Q28.0-Q28.3)*
    anomalies of coronary vessels (Q24.5)
    anomalies of pulmonary artery (Q25.5-Q25.7)
    congenital retinal aneurysm (Q14.1)
    hemangioma and lymphangioma (D18-)

  Q27.0 Congenital absence and hypoplasia of umbilical artery
    Single umbilical artery
  Q27.1 Congenital renal artery stenosis
  Q27.2 Other congenital malformations of renal artery
    Congenital malformation of renal artery NOS
    Multiple renal arteries

✓5th **Q27.3 Arteriovenous malformation (peripheral)**
    Arteriovenous aneurysm
    EXCLUDES 1 *acquired arteriovenous aneurysm (I77.0)*
    EXCLUDES 2 *arteriovenous malformation of cerebral vessels (Q28.2)*
      arteriovenous malformation of precerebral vessels (Q28.0)

    Q27.30 Arteriovenous malformation, site unspecified
    Q27.31 Arteriovenous malformation of vessel of upper limb
    Q27.32 Arteriovenous malformation of vessel of lower limb
    Q27.33 Arteriovenous malformation of digestive system vessel
    Q27.34 Arteriovenous malformation of renal vessel
    Q27.39 Arteriovenous malformation, other site

  Q27.4 Congenital phlebectasia
  Q27.8 Other specified congenital malformations of peripheral vascular system
    Absence of peripheral vascular system
    Atresia of peripheral vascular system
    Congenital aneurysm (peripheral)
    Congenital stricture, artery
    Congenital varix
    EXCLUDES 1 *arteriovenous malformation (Q27.3-)*
  Q27.9 Congenital malformation of peripheral vascular system, unspecified
    Anomaly of artery or vein NOS

✓4th **Q28 Other congenital malformations of circulatory system**
  EXCLUDES 1 *congenital aneurysm NOS (Q27.8)*
    congenital coronary aneurysm (Q24.5)
    ruptured cerebral arteriovenous malformation (I60.8)
    ruptured malformation of precerebral vessels (I72.0)
  EXCLUDES 2 *congenital peripheral aneurysm (Q27.8)*
    congenital pulmonary aneurysm (Q25.7)
    congenital retinal aneurysm (Q14.1)

  Q28.0 Arteriovenous malformation of precerebral vessels
    Congenital arteriovenous precerebral aneurysm (nonruptured)
  Q28.1 Other malformations of precerebral vessels
    Congenital malformation of precerebral vessels NOS
    Congenital precerebral aneurysm (nonruptured)
  Q28.2 Arteriovenous malformation of cerebral vessels
    Arteriovenous malformation of brain NOS
    Congenital arteriovenous cerebral aneurysm (nonruptured)
  Q28.3 Other malformations of cerebral vessels
    Congenital cerebral aneurysm (nonruptured)
    Congenital malformation of cerebral vessels NOS
  Q28.8 Other specified congenital malformations of circulatory system
    Congenital aneurysm, specified site NEC
    Spinal vessel anomaly
  Q28.9 Congenital malformation of circulatory system, unspecified

---

☑ Appropriate additional character required   ✓x7th Requires 7th character, placeholder x must fill empty characters

Congenital malformations of the respiratory system (Q30-Q34)

✓4ᵗʰ Q30   Congenital malformations of nose
     EXCLUDES 1   *congenital deviation of nasal septum (Q67.4)*

   Q30.0   Choanal atresia
      Atresia of nares (anterior) (posterior)
      Congenital stenosis of nares (anterior) (posterior)

   Q30.1   Agenesis and underdevelopment of nose
      Congenital absent of nose

   Q30.2   Fissured, notched and cleft nose

   Q30.3   Congenital perforated nasal septum

   Q30.8   Other congenital malformations of nose
      Accessory nose
      Congenital anomaly of nasal sinus wall

   Q30.9   Congenital malformation of nose, unspecified

✓4ᵗʰ Q31   Congenital malformations of larynx
     EXCLUDES 1   *congenital laryngeal stridor NOS (P28.89)*

   Q31.0   Web of larynx
      Glottic web of larynx
      Subglottic web of larynx
      Web of larynx NOS

   Q31.1   Congenital subglottic stenosis

   Q31.2   Laryngeal hypoplasia

   Q31.3   Laryngocele

   Q31.5   Congenital laryngomalacia

   Q31.8   Other congenital malformations of larynx
      Absence of larynx
      Agenesis of larynx
      Atresia of larynx
      Congenital cleft thyroid cartilage
      Congenital fissure of epiglottis
      Congenital stenosis of larynx NEC
      Posterior cleft of cricoid cartilage

   Q31.9   Congenital malformation of larynx, unspecified

✓4ᵗʰ Q32   Congenital malformations of trachea and bronchus
     EXCLUDES 1   *congenital bronchiectasis (Q33.4)*

   Q32.0   Congenital tracheomalacia

   Q32.1   Other congenital malformations of trachea
      Atresia of trachea
      Congenital anomaly of tracheal cartilage
      Congenital dilatation of trachea
      Congenital malformation of trachea
      Congenital stenosis of trachea
      Congenital tracheocele

   Q32.2   Congenital bronchomalacia

   Q32.3   Congenital stenosis of bronchus

   Q32.4   Other congenital malformations of bronchus
      Absence of bronchus
      Agenesis of bronchus
      Atresia of bronchus
      Congenital diverticulum of bronchus
      Congenital malformation of bronchus NOS

✓4ᵗʰ Q33   Congenital malformations of lung

   Q33.0   Congenital cystic lung
      Congenital cystic lung disease
      Congenital honeycomb lung
      Congenital polycystic lung disease
     EXCLUDES 1   *cystic fibrosis (E84.0)*
            cystic lung disease, acquired or unspecified (J98.4)

   Q33.1   Accessory lobe of lung
      Azygos lobe (fissured), lung

   Q33.2   Sequestration of lung

   Q33.3   Agenesis of lung
      Congenital absence of lung (lobe)

   Q33.4   Congenital bronchiectasis

   Q33.5   Ectopic tissue in lung

   Q33.6   Congenital hypoplasia and dysplasia of lung
     EXCLUDES 1   *pulmonary hypoplasia associated with short gestation (P28.0)*

   Q33.8   Other congenital malformations of lung

   Q33.9   Congenital malformation of lung, unspecified

✓4ᵗʰ Q34   Other congenital malformations of respiratory system
     EXCLUDES 2   *congenital central alveolar hypoventilation syndrome (G47.35)*

   Q34.0   Anomaly of pleura

   Q34.1   Congenital cyst of mediastinum

   Q34.8   Other specified congenital malformations of respiratory system
      Atresia of nasopharynx

   Q34.9   Congenital malformation of respiratory system, unspecified
      Congenital absence of respiratory system
      Congenital anomaly of respiratory system NOS

Cleft lip and cleft palate (Q35-Q37)

Use additional code to identify associated malformation of the nose (Q30.2)
     EXCLUDES 1   *Robin syndrome (Q87.0)*

✓4ᵗʰ Q35   Cleft palate
      Fissure of palate
      Palatoschisis
     EXCLUDES 1   *cleft palate with cleft lip (Q37-)*

   Q35.1   Cleft hard palate

   Q35.3   Cleft soft palate

   Q35.5   Cleft hard palate with cleft soft palate

   Q35.7   Cleft uvula

   Q35.9   Cleft palate, unspecified
      Cleft palate NOS

✓4ᵗʰ Q36   Cleft lip
      Cheiloschisis
      Congenital fissure of lip
      Harelip
      Labium leporinum
     EXCLUDES 1   *cleft lip with cleft palate (Q37-)*

   Q36.0   Cleft lip, bilateral

   Q36.1   Cleft lip, median

   Q36.9   Cleft lip, unilateral
      Cleft lip NOS

✓4ᵗʰ Q37   Cleft palate with cleft lip
      Cheilopalatoschisis

   Q37.0   Cleft hard palate with bilateral cleft lip

   Q37.1   Cleft hard palate with unilateral cleft lip
      Cleft hard palate with cleft lip NOS

   Q37.2   Cleft soft palate with bilateral cleft lip

   Q37.3   Cleft soft palate with unilateral cleft lip
      Cleft soft palate with cleft lip NOS

   Q37.4   Cleft hard and soft palate with bilateral cleft lip

   Q37.5   Cleft hard and soft palate with unilateral cleft lip
      Cleft hard and soft palate with cleft lip NOS

   Q37.8   Unspecified cleft palate with bilateral cleft lip

   Q37.9   Unspecified cleft palate with unilateral cleft lip
      Cleft palate with cleft lip NOS

Other congenital malformations of the digestive system (Q38-Q45)

✓4ᵗʰ Q38   Other congenital malformations of tongue, mouth and pharynx
     EXCLUDES 1   *dentofacial anomalies (M26-)*
            macrostomia (Q18.4)
            microstomia (Q18.5)

   Q38.0   Congenital malformations of lips, not elsewhere classified
      Congenital fistula of lip
      Congenital malformation of lip NOS
      Van der Woude's syndrome
     EXCLUDES 1   *cleft lip (Q36-)*
            cleft lip with cleft palate (Q37-)
            macrocheilia (Q18.6)
            microcheilia (Q18.7)

   Q38.1   Ankyloglossia
      Tongue tie

   Q38.2   Macroglossia
      Congenital hypertrophy of tongue

   Q38.3   Other congenital malformations of tongue
      Aglossia
      Bifid tongue
      Congenital adhesion of tongue
      Congenital fissure of tongue
      Congenital malformation of tongue NOS
      Double tongue
      Hypoglossia
      Hypoplasia of tongue
      Microglossia

Q38.4 **Congenital malformations of salivary glands and ducts**
Atresia of salivary glands and ducts
Congenital absence of salivary glands and ducts
Congenital accessory salivary glands and ducts
Congenital fistula of salivary gland

Q38.5 **Congenital malformations of palate, not elsewhere classified**
Congenital absence of uvula
Congenital malformation of palate NOS
Congenital high arched palate
EXCLUDES 1 *cleft palate (Q35-)*
cleft palate with cleft lip (Q37-)

Q38.6 **Other congenital malformations of mouth**
Congenital malformation of mouth NOS

Q38.7 **Congenital pharyngeal pouch**
Congenital diverticulum of pharynx
EXCLUDES 1 *pharyngeal pouch syndrome (D82.1)*

Q38.8 **Other congenital malformations of pharynx**
Congenital malformation of pharynx NOS
Imperforate pharynx

✓4ᵗʰ **Q39** **Congenital malformations of esophagus**
Q39.0 **Atresia of esophagus without fistula**
Atresia of esophagus NOS

Q39.1 **Atresia of esophagus with tracheo-esophageal fistula**
Atresia of esophagus with broncho-esophageal fistula

Q39.2 **Congenital tracheo-esophageal fistula without atresia**
Congenital tracheo-esophageal fistula NOS

Q39.3 **Congenital stenosis and stricture of esophagus**

Q39.4 **Esophageal web**

Q39.5 **Congenital dilatation of esophagus**
Congenital cardiospasm

Q39.6 **Congenital diverticulum of esophagus**
Congenital esophageal pouch

Q39.8 **Other congenital malformations of esophagus**
Congenital absence of esophagus
Congenital displacement of esophagus
Congenital duplication of esophagus

Q39.9 **Congenital malformation of esophagus, unspecified**

✓4ᵗʰ **Q40** **Other congenital malformations of upper alimentary tract**
Q40.0 **Congenital hypertrophic pyloric stenosis**
Congenital or infantile constriction
Congenital or infantile hypertrophy
Congenital or infantile spasm
Congenital or infantile stenosis
Congenital or infantile stricture

Q40.1 **Congenital hiatus hernia**
Congenital displacement of cardia through esophageal hiatus
EXCLUDES 1 *congenital diaphragmatic hernia (Q79.0)*

Q40.2 **Other specified congenital malformations of stomach**
Congenital displacement of stomach
Congenital diverticulum of stomach
Congenital hourglass stomach
Congenital duplication of stomach
Megalogastria
Microgastria

Q40.3 **Congenital malformation of stomach, unspecified**

Q40.8 **Other specified congenital malformations of upper alimentary tract**

Q40.9 **Congenital malformation of upper alimentary tract, unspecified**
Congenital anomaly of upper alimentary tract
Congenital deformity of upper alimentary tract

✓4ᵗʰ **Q41** **Congenital absence, atresia and stenosis of small intestine**
Congenital obstruction, occlusion or stricture of small intestine or intestine NOS
EXCLUDES 1 *cystic fibrosis with intestinal manifestation (E84.11)*
meconium ileus NOS (without cystic fibrosis) (P76.0)

Q41.0 **Congenital absence, atresia and stenosis of duodenum**

Q41.1 **Congenital absence, atresia and stenosis of jejunum**
Apple peel syndrome
Imperforate jejunum

Q41.2 **Congenital absence, atresia and stenosis of ileum**

Q41.8 **Congenital absence, atresia and stenosis of other specified parts of small intestine**

Q41.9 **Congenital absence, atresia and stenosis of small intestine, part unspecified**
Congenital absence, atresia and stenosis of intestine NOS

✓4ᵗʰ **Q42** **Congenital absence, atresia and stenosis of large intestine**
Congenital obstruction, occlusion and stricture of large intestine

Q42.0 **Congenital absence, atresia and stenosis of rectum with fistula**

Q42.1 **Congenital absence, atresia and stenosis of rectum without fistula**
Imperforate rectum

Q42.2 **Congenital absence, atresia and stenosis of anus with fistula**

Q42.3 **Congenital absence, atresia and stenosis of anus without fistula**
Imperforate anus

Q42.8 **Congenital absence, atresia and stenosis of other parts of large intestine**

Q42.9 **Congenital absence, atresia and stenosis of large intestine, part unspecified**

✓4ᵗʰ **Q43** **Other congenital malformations of intestine**
Q43.0 **Meckel's diverticulum (displaced) (hypertrophic)**
Persistent omphalomesenteric duct
Persistent vitelline duct

Q43.1 **Hirschsprung's disease**
Aganglionosis
Congenital (aganglionic) megacolon

Q43.2 **Other congenital functional disorders of colon**
Congenital dilatation of colon

Q43.3 **Congenital malformations of intestinal fixation**
Congenital omental, anomalous adhesions [bands]
Congenital peritoneal adhesions [bands]
Incomplete rotation of cecum and colon
Insufficient rotation of cecum and colon
Jackson's membrane
Malrotation of colon
Rotation failure of cecum and colon
Universal mesentery

Q43.4 **Duplication of intestine**

Q43.5 **Ectopic anus**

Q43.6 **Congenital fistula of rectum and anus**
EXCLUDES 1 *congenital fistula of anus with absence, atresia and stenosis (Q42.2)*
congenital fistula of rectum with absence, atresia and stenosis (Q42.0)
congenital rectovaginal fistula (Q52.2)
congenital urethrorectal fistula (Q64.7)
pilonidal fistula or sinus (L05-)

Q43.7 **Persistent cloaca**
Cloaca NOS

Q43.8 **Other specified congenital malformations of intestine**
Congenital blind loop syndrome
Congenital diverticulitis, colon
Congenital diverticulum, intestine
Dolichocolon
Megaloappendix
Megaloduodenum
Microcolon
Transposition of appendix
Transposition of colon
Transposition of intestine

Q43.9 **Congenital malformation of intestine, unspecified**

✓4ᵗʰ **Q44** **Congenital malformations of gallbladder, bile ducts and liver**
Q44.0 **Agenesis, aplasia and hypoplasia of gallbladder**
Congenital absence of gallbladder

Q44.1 **Other congenital malformations of gallbladder**
Congenital malformation of gallbladder NOS
Intrahepatic gallbladder

Q44.2 **Atresia of bile ducts**

Q44.3 **Congenital stenosis and stricture of bile ducts**

Q44.4 **Choledochal cyst**

Q44.5 **Other congenital malformations of bile ducts**
Accessory hepatic duct
Biliary duct duplication
Congenital malformation of bile duct NOS
Cystic duct duplication

Q44.6 **Cystic disease of liver**
Fibrocystic disease of liver

☑ Appropriate additional character required   ✓×7ᵗʰ Requires 7th character, placeholder x must fill empty characters

Q44.7 Other congenital malformations of liver
Accessory liver
Alagille's syndrome
Congenital absence of liver
Congenital hepatomegaly
Congenital malformation of liver NOS

✓4th **Q45 Other congenital malformations of digestive system**
     EXCLUDES 2   *congenital diaphragmatic hernia (Q79.0)*
              congenital hiatus hernia (Q40.1)

Q45.0 Agenesis, aplasia and hypoplasia of pancreas
Congenital absence of pancreas

Q45.1 Annular pancreas

Q45.2 Congenital pancreatic cyst

Q45.3 Other congenital malformations of pancreas and pancreatic duct
Accessory pancreas
Congenital malformation of pancreas or pancreatic duct NOS
     EXCLUDES 1   *congenital diabetes mellitus (E10-)*
              cystic fibrosis (E84.0-E84.9)
              fibrocystic disease of pancreas (E84-)
              neonatal diabetes mellitus (P70.2)

Q45.8 Other specified congenital malformations of digestive system
Absence (complete) (partial) of alimentary tract NOS
Duplication of digestive system
Malposition, congenital of digestive system

Q45.9 Congenital malformation of digestive system, unspecified
Congenital anomaly of digestive system
Congenital deformity of digestive system

Congenital malformations of genital organs (Q50-Q56)

     EXCLUDES 1   *androgen insensitivity syndrome (E34.5-)*
              syndromes associated with anomalies in the number and form of chromosomes (Q90-Q99)

✓4th **Q50 Congenital malformations of ovaries, fallopian tubes and broad ligaments**
  ✓5th **Q50.0 Congenital absence of ovary**
      EXCLUDES 1   *Turner's syndrome (Q96-)*
       Q50.01 Congenital absence of ovary, unilateral
       Q50.02 Congenital absence of ovary, bilateral
     Q50.1 Developmental ovarian cyst
     Q50.2 Congenital torsion of ovary
  ✓5th **Q50.3 Other congenital malformations of ovary**
       Q50.31 Accessory ovary
       Q50.32 Ovarian streak
            46, XX with streak gonads
       Q50.39 Other congenital malformation of ovary
            Congenital malformation of ovary NOS
     Q50.4 Embryonic cyst of fallopian tube
       Fimbrial cyst
     Q50.5 Embryonic cyst of broad ligament
       Epoophoron cyst
       Parovarian cyst
     Q50.6 Other congenital malformations of fallopian tube and broad ligament
       Absence of fallopian tube and broad ligament
       Accessory fallopian tube and broad ligament
       Atresia of fallopian tube and broad ligament
       Congenital malformation of fallopian tube or broad ligament NOS

✓4th **Q51 Congenital malformations of uterus and cervix**
     Q51.0 Agenesis and aplasia of uterus
       Congenital absence of uterus
  ✓5th **Q51.1 Doubling of uterus with doubling of cervix and vagina**
       Q51.10 Doubling of uterus with doubling of cervix and vagina without obstruction
            Doubling of uterus with doubling of cervix and vagina NOS
       Q51.11 Doubling of uterus with doubling of cervix and vagina with obstruction
     Q51.2 Other doubling of uterus
       Doubling of uterus NOS
       Septate uterus, complete or partial
     Q51.3 Bicornate uterus
       Bicornate uterus, complete or partial

Q51.4 Unicornate uterus
Unicornate uterus with or without a separate uterine horn
Uterus with only one functioning horn

Q51.5 Agenesis and aplasia of cervix
Congenital absence of cervix

Q51.6 Embryonic cyst of cervix

Q51.7 Congenital fistulae between uterus and digestive and urinary tracts

✓5th **Q51.8 Other congenital malformations of uterus and cervix**
  ✓6th **Q51.81 Other congenital malformations of uterus**
       Q51.810 Arcuate uterus
          Arcuatus uterus
       Q51.811 Hypoplasia of uterus
       Q51.818 Other congenital malformations of uterus
          Müllerian anomaly of uterus NEC
  ✓6th **Q51.82 Other congenital malformations of cervix**
       Q51.820 Cervical duplication
       Q51.821 Hypoplasia of cervix
       Q51.828 Other congenital malformations of cervix

Q51.9 Congenital malformation of uterus and cervix, unspecified

✓4th **Q52 Other congenital malformations of female genitalia**
     Q52.0 Congenital absence of vagina
       Vaginal agenesis, total or partial
  ✓5th **Q52.1 Doubling of vagina**
      EXCLUDES 1   *doubling of vagina with doubling of uterus and cervix (Q51.1-)*
       Q52.10 Doubling of vagina, unspecified
          Septate vagina NOS
       Q52.11 Transverse vaginal septum
       Q52.12 Longitudinal vaginal septum
          Longitudinal vaginal septum with or without obstruction
     Q52.2 Congenital rectovaginal fistula
      EXCLUDES 1   *cloaca (Q43.7)*
     Q52.3 Imperforate hymen
     Q52.4 Other congenital malformations of vagina
       Canal of Nuck cyst, congenital
       Congenital malformation of vagina NOS
       Embryonic vaginal cyst
       Gartner's duct cyst
     Q52.5 Fusion of labia
     Q52.6 Congenital malformation of clitoris
  ✓5th **Q52.7 Other and unspecified congenital malformations of vulva**
       Q52.70 Unspecified congenital malformations of vulva
          Congenital malformation of vulva NOS
       Q52.71 Congenital absence of vulva
       Q52.79 Other congenital malformations of vulva
          Congenital cyst of vulva
     Q52.8 Other specified congenital malformations of female genitalia
     Q52.9 Congenital malformation of female genitalia, unspecified

✓4th **Q53 Undescended and ectopic testicle**
  ✓5th **Q53.0 Ectopic testis**
       Q53.00 Ectopic testis, unspecified
       Q53.01 Ectopic testis, unilateral
       Q53.02 Ectopic testes, bilateral
  ✓5th **Q53.1 Undescended testicle, unilateral**
       Q53.10 Unspecified undescended testicle, unilateral
       Q53.11 Abdominal testis, unilateral
       Q53.12 Ectopic perineal testis, unilateral
  ✓5th **Q53.2 Undescended testicle, bilateral**
       Q53.20 Undescended testicle, unspecified, bilateral
       Q53.21 Abdominal testis, bilateral
       Q53.22 Ectopic perineal testis, bilateral
     Q53.9 Undescended testicle, unspecified
       Cryptorchism NOS

✓4th **Q54 Hypospadias**
     EXCLUDES 1   *epispadias (Q64.0)*
     Q54.0 Hypospadias, balanic
       Hypospadias, coronal
       Hypospadias, glandular
     Q54.1 Hypospadias, penile
     Q54.2 Hypospadias, penoscrotal
     Q54.3 Hypospadias, perineal

EXCLUDES 1   Not coded here   EXCLUDES 2   Not included here   *Manifestation Code*

Q54.4   **Congenital chordee**
Chordee without hypospadias

Q54.8   **Other hypospadias**
Hypospadias with intersex state

Q54.9   **Hypospadias, unspecified**

☑4th **Q55**   **Other congenital malformations of male genital organs**
> EXCLUDES 1   *congenital hydrocele (P83.5)*
> *hypospadias (Q54-)*

Q55.0   **Absence and aplasia of testis**
Monorchism

Q55.1   **Hypoplasia of testis and scrotum**
Fusion of testes

☑5th **Q55.2**   **Other and unspecified congenital malformations of testis and scrotum**

   Q55.20   **Unspecified congenital malformations of testis and scrotum**
     Congenital malformation of testis or scrotum NOS

   Q55.21   **Polyorchism**

   Q55.22   **Retractile testis**

   Q55.23   **Scrotal transposition**

   Q55.29   **Other congenital malformations of testis and scrotum**

Q55.3   **Atresia of vas deferens**
Code first any associated cystic fibrosis (E84-)

Q55.4   **Other congenital malformations of vas deferens, epididymis, seminal vesicles and prostate**
Absence or aplasia of prostate
Absence or aplasia of spermatic cord
Congenital malformation of vas deferens, epididymis, seminal vesicles or prostate NOS

Q55.5   **Congenital absence and aplasia of penis**

☑5th **Q55.6**   **Other congenital malformations of penis**

   Q55.61   **Curvature of penis (lateral)**

   Q55.62   **Hypoplasia of penis**
     Micropenis

   Q55.69   **Other congenital malformation of penis**
     Congenital malformation of penis NOS

Q55.7   **Congenital vasocutaneous fistula**

Q55.8   **Other specified congenital malformations of male genital organs**

Q55.9   **Congenital malformation of male genital organ, unspecified**
Congenital anomaly of male genital organ
Congenital deformity of male genital organ

☑4th **Q56**   **Indeterminate sex and pseudohermaphroditism**
> EXCLUDES 1   *46, XX true hermaphrodite (Q99.1)*
> *androgen insensitivity syndrome (E34.5-)*
> *chimera 46, XX/46, XY true hermaphrodite (Q99.0)*
> *female pseudohermaphroditism with adrenocortical disorder (E25-)*
> *pseudohermaphroditism with specified chromosomal anomaly (Q96-Q99)*
> *pure gonadal dysgenesis (Q99.1)*

Q56.0   **Hermaphroditism, not elsewhere classified**
Ovotestis

Q56.1   **Male pseudohermaphroditism, not elsewhere classified**
46, XY with streak gonads
Male pseudohermaphroditism NOS

Q56.2   **Female pseudohermaphroditism, not elsewhere classified**
Female pseudohermaphroditism NOS

Q56.3   **Pseudohermaphroditism, unspecified**

Q56.4   **Indeterminate sex, unspecified**
Ambiguous genitalia

Congenital malformations of the urinary system (Q60-Q64)

☑4th **Q60**   **Renal agenesis and other reduction defects of kidney**
Congenital absence of kidney
Congenital atrophy of kidney
Infantile atrophy of kidney

Q60.0   **Renal agenesis, unilateral**

Q60.1   **Renal agenesis, bilateral**

Q60.2   **Renal agenesis, unspecified**

Q60.3   **Renal hypoplasia, unilateral**

Q60.4   **Renal hypoplasia, bilateral**

Q60.5   **Renal hypoplasia, unspecified**

Q60.6   **Potter's syndrome**

☑4th **Q61**   **Cystic kidney disease**
> EXCLUDES 1   *acquired cyst of kidney (N28.1)*
> *Potter's syndrome (Q60.6)*

☑5th **Q61.0**   **Congenital renal cyst**

   Q61.00   **Congenital renal cyst, unspecified**
     Cyst of kidney NOS (congenital)

   Q61.01   **Congenital single renal cyst**

   Q61.02   **Congenital multiple renal cysts**

☑5th **Q61.1**   **Polycystic kidney, infantile type**
Polycystic kidney, autosomal recessive

   Q61.11   **Cystic dilatation of collecting ducts**

   Q61.19   **Other polycystic kidney, infantile type**

Q61.2   **Polycystic kidney, adult type**
Polycystic kidney, autosomal dominant

Q61.3   **Polycystic kidney, unspecified**

Q61.4   **Renal dysplasia**
Multicystic dysplastic kidney
Multicystic kidney (development)
Multicystic kidney disease
Multicystic renal dysplasia
> EXCLUDES 1   *polycystic kidney disease (Q61.11-Q61.3)*

Q61.5   **Medullary cystic kidney**
Nephronopthisis
Sponge kidney NOS

Q61.8   **Other cystic kidney diseases**
Fibrocystic kidney
Fibrocystic renal degeneration or disease

Q61.9   **Cystic kidney disease, unspecified**
Meckel-Gruber syndrome

☑4th **Q62**   **Congenital obstructive defects of renal pelvis and congenital malformations of ureter**

Q62.0   **Congenital hydronephrosis**

☑5th **Q62.1**   **Congenital occlusion of ureter**
Atresia and stenosis of ureter

   Q62.10   **Congenital occlusion of ureter, unspecified**

   Q62.11   **Congenital occlusion of ureteropelvic junction**

   Q62.12   **Congenital occlusion of ureterovesical orifice**

Q62.2   **Congenital megaureter**
Congenital dilatation of ureter

☑5th **Q62.3**   **Other obstructive defects of renal pelvis and ureter**

   Q62.31   **Congenital ureterocele, orthotopic**

   Q62.32   **Cecoureterocele**
     Ectopic ureterocele

   Q62.39   **Other obstructive defects of renal pelvis and ureter**
     Ureteropelvic junction obstruction NOS

Q62.4   **Agenesis of ureter**
Congenital absence ureter

Q62.5   **Duplication of ureter**
Accessory ureter
Double ureter

☑5th **Q62.6**   **Malposition of ureter**

   Q62.60   **Malposition of ureter, unspecified**

   Q62.61   **Deviation of ureter**

   Q62.62   **Displacement of ureter**

   Q62.63   **Anomalous implantation of ureter**
     Ectopia of ureter
     Ectopic ureter

   Q62.69   **Other malposition of ureter**

Q62.7   **Congenital vesico-uretero-renal reflux**

Q62.8   **Other congenital malformations of ureter**
Anomaly of ureter NOS

☑4th **Q63**   **Other congenital malformations of kidney**
> EXCLUDES 1   *congenital nephrotic syndrome (N04-)*

Q63.0   **Accessory kidney**

Q63.1   **Lobulated, fused and horseshoe kidney**

Q63.2   **Ectopic kidney**
Congenital displaced kidney
Malrotation of kidney

Q63.3   **Hyperplastic and giant kidney**
Compensatory hypertrophy of kidney

Q63.8   **Other specified congenital malformations of kidney**
Congenital renal calculi

Q63.9   **Congenital malformation of kidney, unspecified**

☑ Appropriate additional character required   ☑x7th Requires 7th character, placeholder x must fill empty characters

✓4th Q64 Other congenital malformations of urinary system

Q64.0 Epispadias
> EXCLUDES 1   *hypospadias (Q54-)*

✓5th Q64.1 Exstrophy of urinary bladder

Q64.10 Exstrophy of urinary bladder, unspecified
Ectopia vesicae

Q64.11 Supravesical fissure of urinary bladder

Q64.12 Cloacal extrophy of urinary bladder

Q64.19 Other exstrophy of urinary bladder
Extroversion of bladder

Q64.2 Congenital posterior urethral valves

✓5th Q64.3 Other atresia and stenosis of urethra and bladder neck

Q64.31 Congenital bladder neck obstruction
Congenital obstruction of vesicourethral orifice

Q64.32 Congenital stricture of urethra

Q64.33 Congenital stricture of urinary meatus

Q64.39 Other atresia and stenosis of urethra and bladder neck
Atresia and stenosis of urethra and bladder neck NOS

Q64.4 Malformation of urachus
Cyst of urachus
Patent urachus
Prolapse of urachus

Q64.5 Congenital absence of bladder and urethra

Q64.6 Congenital diverticulum of bladder

✓5th Q64.7 Other and unspecified congenital malformations of bladder and urethra
> EXCLUDES 1   *congenital prolapse of bladder (mucosa) (Q79.4)*

Q64.70 Unspecified congenital malformation of bladder and urethra
Malformation of bladder or urethra NOS

Q64.71 Congenital prolapse of urethra

Q64.72 Congenital prolapse of urinary meatus

Q64.73 Congenital urethrorectal fistula

Q64.74 Double urethra

Q64.75 Double urinary meatus

Q64.79 Other congenital malformations of bladder and urethra

Q64.8 Other specified congenital malformations of urinary system

Q64.9 Congenital malformation of urinary system, unspecified
Congenital anomaly NOS of urinary system
Congenital deformity NOS of urinary system

Congenital malformations and deformations of the musculoskeletal system (Q65-Q79)

✓4th Q65 Congenital deformities of hip
> EXCLUDES 1   *clicking hip (R29.4)*

✓5th Q65.0 Congenital dislocation of hip, unilateral

Q65.00 Congenital dislocation of unspecified hip, unilateral

Q65.01 Congenital dislocation of right hip, unilateral

Q65.02 Congenital dislocation of left hip, unilateral

Q65.1 Congenital dislocation of hip, bilateral

Q65.2 Congenital dislocation of hip, unspecified

✓5th Q65.3 Congenital partial dislocation of hip, unilateral

Q65.30 Congenital partial dislocation of unspecified hip, unilateral

Q65.31 Congenital partial dislocation of right hip, unilateral

Q65.32 Congenital partial dislocation of left hip, unilateral

Q65.4 Congenital partial dislocation of hip, bilateral

Q65.5 Congenital partial dislocation of hip, unspecified

Q65.6 Congenital unstable hip
Congenital dislocatable hip

Q65.8 Other congenital deformities of hip
Anteversion of femoral neck
Congenital acetabular dysplasia
Congenital coxa valga
Congenital coxa vara

Q65.9 Congenital deformity of hip, unspecified

✓4th Q66 Congenital deformities of feet
> EXCLUDES 1   *reduction defects of feet (Q72-)*
> *valgus deformities (acquired) (M21.0)*
> *varus deformities (acquired) (M21.1)*

Q66.0 Congenital talipes equinovarus

Q66.1 Congenital talipes calcaneovarus

Q66.2 Congenital metatarsus (primus) varus

Q66.3 Other congenital varus deformities of feet
Hallux varus, congenital

Q66.4 Congenital talipes calcaneovalgus

Q66.5 Congenital pes planus
Congenital flat foot
Congenital rigid flat foot
Congenital spastic (everted) flat foot
> EXCLUDES 1   *pes planus, acquired (M21.4)*

Q66.6 Other congenital valgus deformities of feet
Congenital metatarsus valgus

Q66.7 Congenital pes cavus

Q66.8 Other congenital deformities of feet
Congenital asymmetric talipes
Congenital clubfoot NOS
Congenital talipes NOS
Congenital tarsal coalition
Congenital vertical talus
Hammer toe, congenital

Q66.9 Congenital deformity of feet, unspecified

✓4th Q67 Congenital musculoskeletal deformities of head, face, spine and chest
> EXCLUDES 1   *congenital malformation syndromes classified to Q87-*
> *Potter's syndrome (Q60.6)*

Q67.0 Congenital facial asymmetry

Q67.1 Congenital compression facies

Q67.2 Dolichocephaly

Q67.3 Plagiocephaly

Q67.4 Other congenital deformities of skull, face and jaw
Congenital depressions in skull
Congenital hemifacial atrophy or hypertrophy
Deviation of nasal septum, congenital
Squashed or bent nose, congenital
> EXCLUDES 1   *dentofacial anomalies [including malocclusion] (M26-)*
> *syphilitic saddle nose (A50.5)*

Q67.5 Congenital deformity of spine
Congenital postural scoliosis
Congenital scoliosis NOS
> EXCLUDES 1   *infantile idiopathic scoliosis (M41.0)*
> *scoliosis due to congenital bony malformation (Q76.3)*

Q67.6 Pectus excavatum
Congenital funnel chest

Q67.7 Pectus carinatum
Congenital pigeon chest

Q67.8 Other congenital deformities of chest
Congenital deformity of chest wall NOS

✓4th Q68 Other congenital musculoskeletal deformities
> EXCLUDES 1   *reduction defects of limb(s) (Q71-Q73)*
> EXCLUDES 2   *congenital myotonic chondrodystrophy (G71.13)*

Q68.0 Congenital deformity of sternocleidomastoid muscle
Congenital contracture of sternocleidomastoid (muscle)
Congenital (sternomastoid) torticollis
Sternomastoid tumor (congenital)

Q68.1 Congenital deformity of finger(s) and hand
Congenital clubfinger
Spade-like hand (congenital)

Q68.2 Congenital deformity of knee
Congenital dislocation of knee
Congenital genu recurvatum

Q68.3 Congenital bowing of femur
> EXCLUDES 1   *anteversion of femur (neck) (Q65.8)*

Q68.4 Congenital bowing of tibia and fibula

Q68.5 Congenital bowing of long bones of leg, unspecified

Q68.6 Discoid meniscus

EXCLUDES 1   Not coded here   EXCLUDES 2   Not included here   *Manifestation Code*

Q68.8 Other specified congenital musculoskeletal deformities
Congenital deformity of clavicle
Congenital deformity of elbow
Congenital deformity of forearm
Congenital deformity of scapula
Congenital deformity of wrist
Congenital dislocation of elbow
Congenital dislocation of shoulder
Congenital dislocation of wrist

✓4th **Q69 Polydactyly**
Q69.0 Accessory finger(s)
Q69.1 Accessory thumb(s)
Q69.2 Accessory toe(s)
Accessory hallux
Q69.9 Polydactyly, unspecified
Supernumerary digit(s) NOS

✓4th **Q70 Syndactyly**
✓5th **Q70.0 Fused fingers**
Complex syndactly of fingers with synostosis
Q70.00 Fused fingers, unspecified hand
Q70.01 Fused fingers, right hand
Q70.02 Fused fingers, left hand
Q70.03 Fused fingers, bilateral
✓5th **Q70.1 Webbed fingers**
Simple syndactly of fingers without synostosis
Q70.10 Webbed fingers, unspecified hand
Q70.11 Webbed fingers, right hand
Q70.12 Webbed fingers, left hand
Q70.13 Webbed fingers, bilateral
✓5th **Q70.2 Fused toes**
Complex syndactly of toes with synostosis
Q70.20 Fused toes, unspecified foot
Q70.21 Fused toes, right foot
Q70.22 Fused toes, left foot
Q70.23 Fused toes, bilateral
✓5th **Q70.3 Webbed toes**
Simple syndactly of toes without synostosis
Q70.30 Webbed toes, unspecified foot
Q70.31 Webbed toes, right foot
Q70.32 Webbed toes, left foot
Q70.33 Webbed toes, bilateral
Q70.4 Polysyndactyly, unspecified
EXCLUDES 1 *specified syndactyly of hand and feet - code to specified conditions (Q70.0- - Q70.3-)*
Q70.9 Syndactyly, unspecified
Symphalangy NOS

✓4th **Q71 Reduction defects of upper limb**
✓5th **Q71.0 Congenital complete absence of upper limb**
Q71.00 Congenital complete absence of unspecified upper limb
Q71.01 Congenital complete absence of right upper limb
Q71.02 Congenital complete absence of left upper limb
Q71.03 Congenital complete absence of upper limb, bilateral
✓5th **Q71.1 Congenital absence of upper arm and forearm with hand present**
Q71.10 Congenital absence of unspecified upper arm and forearm with hand present
Q71.11 Congenital absence of right upper arm and forearm with hand present
Q71.12 Congenital absence of left upper arm and forearm with hand present
Q71.13 Congenital absence of upper arm and forearm with hand present, bilateral
✓5th **Q71.2 Congenital absence of both forearm and hand**
Q71.20 Congenital absence of both forearm and hand, unspecified upper limb
Q71.21 Congenital absence of both forearm and hand, right upper limb
Q71.22 Congenital absence of both forearm and hand, left upper limb
Q71.23 Congenital absence of both forearm and hand, bilateral
✓5th **Q71.3 Congenital absence of hand and finger**
Q71.30 Congenital absence of unspecified hand and finger
Q71.31 Congenital absence of right hand and finger

Q71.32 Congenital absence of left hand and finger
Q71.33 Congenital absence of hand and finger, bilateral
✓5th **Q71.4 Longitudinal reduction defect of radius**
Clubhand (congenital)
Radial clubhand
Q71.40 Longitudinal reduction defect of unspecified radius
Q71.41 Longitudinal reduction defect of right radius
Q71.42 Longitudinal reduction defect of left radius
Q71.43 Longitudinal reduction defect of radius, bilateral
✓5th **Q71.5 Longitudinal reduction defect of ulna**
Q71.50 Longitudinal reduction defect of unspecified ulna
Q71.51 Longitudinal reduction defect of right ulna
Q71.52 Longitudinal reduction defect of left ulna
Q71.53 Longitudinal reduction defect of ulna, bilateral
✓5th **Q71.6 Lobster-claw hand**
Q71.60 Lobster-claw hand, unspecified hand
Q71.61 Lobster-claw right hand
Q71.62 Lobster-claw left hand
Q71.63 Lobster-claw hand, bilateral
✓5th **Q71.8 Other reduction defects of upper limb**
✓6th **Q71.81 Congenital shortening of upper limb**
Q71.811 Congenital shortening of right upper limb
Q71.812 Congenital shortening of left upper limb
Q71.813 Congenital shortening of upper limb, bilateral
Q71.819 Congenital shortening of unspecified upper limb
✓6th **Q71.89 Other reduction defects of upper limb**
Q71.891 Other reduction defects of right upper limb
Q71.892 Other reduction defects of left upper limb
Q71.893 Other reduction defects of upper limb, bilateral
Q71.899 Other reduction defects of unspecified upper limb
✓5th **Q71.9 Unspecified reduction defect of upper limb**
Q71.90 Unspecified reduction defect of upper limb
Q71.91 Unspecified reduction defect of right upper limb
Q71.92 Unspecified reduction defect of left upper limb
Q71.93 Unspecified reduction defect of upper limb, bilateral

✓4th **Q72 Reduction defects of lower limb**
✓5th **Q72.0 Congenital complete absence of lower limb**
Q72.00 Congenital complete absence of unspecified lower limb
Q72.01 Congenital complete absence of right lower limb
Q72.02 Congenital complete absence of left lower limb
Q72.03 Congenital complete absence of lower limb, bilateral
✓5th **Q72.1 Congenital absence of thigh and lower leg with foot present**
Q72.10 Congenital absence of unspecified thigh and lower leg with foot present
Q72.11 Congenital absence of right thigh and lower leg with foot present
Q72.12 Congenital absence of left thigh and lower leg with foot present
Q72.13 Congenital absence of thigh and lower leg with foot present, bilateral
✓5th **Q72.2 Congenital absence of both lower leg and foot**
Q72.20 Congenital absence of both lower leg and foot, unspecified lower limb
Q72.21 Congenital absence of both lower leg and foot, right lower limb
Q72.22 Congenital absence of both lower leg and foot, left lower limb
Q72.23 Congenital absence of both lower leg and foot, bilateral
✓5th **Q72.3 Congenital absence of foot and toe(s)**
Q72.30 Congenital absence of unspecified foot and toe(s)
Q72.31 Congenital absence of right foot and toe(s)
Q72.32 Congenital absence of left foot and toe(s)
Q72.33 Congenital absence of foot and toe(s), bilateral

☑ Appropriate additional character required   ✓x7th Requires 7th character, placeholder x must fill empty characters

✓5th **Q72.4** **Longitudinal reduction defect of femur**
Proximal femoral focal deficiency
     Q72.40 **Longitudinal reduction defect of unspecified femur**
     Q72.41 **Longitudinal reduction defect of right femur**
     Q72.42 **Longitudinal reduction defect of left femur**
     Q72.43 **Longitudinal reduction defect of femur, bilateral**

✓5th **Q72.5** **Longitudinal reduction defect of tibia**
     Q72.50 **Longitudinal reduction defect of unspecified tibia**
     Q72.51 **Longitudinal reduction defect of right tibia**
     Q72.52 **Longitudinal reduction defect of left tibia**
     Q72.53 **Longitudinal reduction defect of tibia, bilateral**

✓5th **Q72.6** **Longitudinal reduction defect of fibula**
     Q72.60 **Longitudinal reduction defect of unspecified fibula**
     Q72.61 **Longitudinal reduction defect of right fibula**
     Q72.62 **Longitudinal reduction defect of left fibula**
     Q72.63 **Longitudinal reduction defect of fibula, bilateral**

✓5th **Q72.7** **Split foot**
     Q72.70 **Split foot, unspecified lower limb**
     Q72.71 **Split foot, right lower limb**
     Q72.72 **Split foot, left lower limb**
     Q72.73 **Split foot, bilateral**

✓5th **Q72.8** **Other reduction defects of lower limb**
     ✓6th **Q72.81** **Congenital shortening of lower limb**
         Q72.811 **Congenital shortening of right lower limb**
         Q72.812 **Congenital shortening of left lower limb**
         Q72.813 **Congenital shortening of lower limb, bilateral**
         Q72.819 **Congenital shortening of unspecified lower limb**
     ✓6th **Q72.89** **Other reduction defects of lower limb**
         Q72.891 **Other reduction defects of right lower limb**
         Q72.892 **Other reduction defects of left lower limb**
         Q72.893 **Other reduction defects of lower limb, bilateral**
         Q72.899 **Other reduction defects of unspecified lower limb**

✓5th **Q72.9** **Unspecified reduction defect of lower limb**
     Q72.90 **Unspecified reduction defect of unspecified lower limb**
     Q72.91 **Unspecified reduction defect of right lower limb**
     Q72.92 **Unspecified reduction defect of left lower limb**
     Q72.93 **Unspecified reduction defect of lower limb, bilateral**

✓4th **Q73** **Reduction defects of unspecified limb**
     Q73.0 **Congenital absence of unspecified limb(s)**
Amelia NOS
     Q73.1 **Phocomelia, unspecified limb(s)**
Phocomelia NOS
     Q73.8 **Other reduction defects of unspecified limb(s)**
Longitudinal reduction deformity of unspecified limb(s)
Ectromelia of limb NOS
Hemimelia of limb NOS
Reduction defect of limb NOS

✓4th **Q74** **Other congenital malformations of limb(s)**
     EXCLUDES 1   *polydactyly (Q69-)*
               reduction defect of limb (Q71-Q73)
               syndactyly (Q70-)
     Q74.0 **Other congenital malformations of upper limb(s), including shoulder girdle**
Accessory carpal bones
Cleidocranial dysostosis
Congenital pseudarthrosis of clavicle
Macrodactylia (fingers)
Madelung's deformity
Radioulnar synostosis
Sprengel's deformity
Triphalangeal thumb

Q74.1 **Congenital malformation of knee**
Congenital absence of patella
Congenital dislocation of patella
Congenital genu valgum
Congenital genu varum
Rudimentary patella
     EXCLUDES 1   *congenital dislocation of knee (Q68.2)*
               congenital genu recurvatum (Q68.2)
               nail patella syndrome (Q87.2)

Q74.2 **Other congenital malformations of lower limb(s), including pelvic girdle**
Congenital fusion of sacroiliac joint
Congenital malformation of ankle joint
Congenital malformation of sacroiliac joint
     EXCLUDES 1   *anteversion of femur (neck) (Q65.8)*

Q74.3 **Arthrogryposis multiplex congenita**

Q74.8 **Other specified congenital malformations of limb(s)**

Q74.9 **Unspecified congenital malformation of limb(s)**
Congenital anomaly of limb(s) NOS

✓4th **Q75** **Other congenital malformations of skull and face bones**
     EXCLUDES 1   *congenital malformation of face NOS (Q18-)*
               congenital malformation syndromes classified to Q87-
               dentofacial anomalies [including malocclusion] (M26-)
               musculoskeletal deformities of head and face (Q67.0-Q67.4)
               skull defects associated with congenital anomalies of brain
                   such as:
                   anencephaly (Q00.0)
                   encephalocele (Q01-)
                   hydrocephalus (Q03-)
                   microcephaly (Q02)

Q75.0 **Craniosynostosis**
Acrocephaly
Imperfect fusion of skull
Oxycephaly
Trigonocephaly

Q75.1 **Craniofacial dysostosis**
Crouzon's disease

Q75.2 **Hypertelorism**

Q75.3 **Macrocephaly**

Q75.4 **Mandibulofacial dysostosis**
Franceschetti syndrome
Treacher Collins syndrome

Q75.5 **Oculomandibular dysostosis**

Q75.8 **Other specified congenital malformations of skull and face bones**
Absence of skull bone, congenital
Congenital deformity of forehead
Platybasia

Q75.9 **Congenital malformation of skull and face bones, unspecified**
Congenital anomaly of face bones NOS
Congenital anomaly of skull NOS

✓4th **Q76** **Congenital malformations of spine and bony thorax**
     EXCLUDES 1   *congenital musculoskeletal deformities of spine and chest (Q67.5-Q67.8)*
     Q76.0 **Spina bifida occulta**
         EXCLUDES 1   *meningocele (spinal) (Q05-)*
                 spina bifida (aperta) (cystica) (Q05-)
     Q76.1 **Klippel-Feil syndrome**
Cervical fusion syndrome
     Q76.2 **Congenital spondylolisthesis**
Congenital spondylolysis
         EXCLUDES 1   *spondylolisthesis (acquired) (M43.1-)*
                 spondylolysis (acquired) (M43.0-)
     Q76.3 **Congenital scoliosis due to congenital bony malformation**
Hemivertebra fusion or failure of segmentation with scoliosis
     ✓5th **Q76.4** **Other congenital malformations of spine, not associated with scoliosis**
         ✓6th **Q76.41** **Congenital kyphosis**
             Q76.411 **Congenital kyphosis, occipito-atlanto-axial region**
             Q76.412 **Congenital kyphosis, cervical region**
             Q76.413 **Congenital kyphosis, cervicothoracic region**
             Q76.414 **Congenital kyphosis, thoracic region**
             Q76.415 **Congenital kyphosis, thoracolumbar region**
             Q76.419 **Congenital kyphosis, unspecified region**

EXCLUDES 1   Not coded here   EXCLUDES 2   Not included here   *Manifestation Code*

✓6ᵗʰ **Q76.42 Congenital lordosis**
    Q76.425 Congenital lordosis, thoracolumbar region
    Q76.426 Congenital lordosis, lumbar region
    Q76.427 Congenital lordosis, lumbosacral region
    Q76.428 Congenital lordosis, sacral and sacrococcygeal region
    Q76.429 Congenital lordosis, unspecified region
Q76.49 Other congenital malformations of spine, not associated with scoliosis
    Congenital absence of vertebra NOS
    Congenital fusion of spine NOS
    Congenital malformation of lumbosacral (joint) (region) NOS
    Congenital malformation of spine NOS
    Hemivertebra NOS
    Malformation of spine NOS
    Platyspondylisis NOS
    Supernumerary vertebra NOS

Q76.5 Cervical rib
    Supernumerary rib in cervical region

Q76.6 Other congenital malformations of ribs
    Accessory rib
    Congenital absence of rib
    Congenital fusion of ribs
    Congenital malformation of ribs NOS
    EXCLUDES 1 *short rib syndrome (Q77.2)*

Q76.7 Congenital malformation of sternum
    Congenital absence of sternum
    Sternum bifidum

Q76.8 Other congenital malformations of bony thorax

Q76.9 Congenital malformation of bony thorax, unspecified

✓4ᵗʰ **Q77 Osteochondrodysplasia with defects of growth of tubular bones and spine**
    EXCLUDES 1 *mucopolysaccharidosis (E76.0-E76.3)*
    EXCLUDES 2 *congenital myotonic chondrodystrophy (G71.13)*

Q77.0 Achondrogenesis
    Hypochondrogenesis

Q77.1 Thanatophoric short stature

Q77.2 Short rib syndrome
    Asphyxiating thoracic dysplasia [Jeune]

Q77.3 Chondrodysplasia punctata
    EXCLUDES 1 *Rhizomelic chondrodysplasia punctata (E71.43)*

Q77.4 Achondroplasia
    Hypochondroplasia
    Osteosclerosis congenita

Q77.5 Diastrophic dysplasia

Q77.6 Chondroectodermal dysplasia
    Ellis-van Creveld syndrome

Q77.7 Spondyloepiphyseal dysplasia

Q77.8 Other osteochondrodysplasia with defects of growth of tubular bones and spine

Q77.9 Osteochondrodysplasia with defects of growth of tubular bones and spine, unspecified

✓4ᵗʰ **Q78 Other osteochondrodysplasias**
    EXCLUDES 2 *congenital myotonic chondrodystrophy (G71.13)*

Q78.0 Osteogenesis imperfecta
    Fragilitas ossium
    Osteopsathyrosis

Q78.1 Polyostotic fibrous dysplasia
    Albright(-McCune)(-Sternberg) syndrome

Q78.2 Osteopetrosis
    Albers-Schönberg syndrome
    Osteosclerosis NOS

Q78.3 Progressive diaphyseal dysplasia
    Camurati-Engelmann syndrome

Q78.4 Enchondromatosis
    Maffucci's syndrome
    Ollier's disease

Q78.5 Metaphyseal dysplasia
    Pyle's syndrome

Q78.6 Multiple congenital exostoses
    Diaphyseal aclasis

Q78.8 Other specified osteochondrodysplasias
    Osteopoikilosis

Q78.9 Osteochondrodysplasia, unspecified
    Chondrodystrophy NOS
    Osteodystrophy NOS

✓4ᵗʰ **Q79 Congenital malformations of musculoskeletal system, not elsewhere classified**
    EXCLUDES 2 *congenital (sternomastoid) torticollis (Q68.0)*

Q79.0 Congenital diaphragmatic hernia
    EXCLUDES 1 *congenital hiatus hernia (Q40.1)*

Q79.1 Other congenital malformations of diaphragm
    Absence of diaphragm
    Congenital malformation of diaphragm NOS
    Eventration of diaphragm

Q79.2 Exomphalos
    Omphalocele
    EXCLUDES 1 *umbilical hernia (K42-)*

Q79.3 Gastroschisis

Q79.4 Prune belly syndrome
    Congenital prolapse of bladder mucosa
    Eagle-Barrett syndrome

✓5ᵗʰ **Q79.5 Other congenital malformations of abdominal wall**
    EXCLUDES 1 *umbilical hernia (K42-)*
    Q79.51 Congenital hernia of bladder
    Q79.59 Other congenital malformations of abdominal wall

Q79.6 Ehlers-Danlos syndrome

Q79.8 Other congenital malformations of musculoskeletal system
    Absence of muscle
    Absence of tendon
    Accessory muscle
    Amyotrophia congenita
    Congenital constricting bands
    Congenital shortening of tendon
    Poland syndrome

Q79.9 Congenital malformation of musculoskeletal system, unspecified
    Congenital anomaly of musculoskeletal system NOS
    Congenital deformity of musculoskeletal system NOS

Other congenital malformations (Q80-Q89)

✓4ᵗʰ **Q80 Congenital ichthyosis**
    EXCLUDES 1 *Refsum's disease (G60.1)*

Q80.0 Ichthyosis vulgaris

Q80.1 X-linked ichthyosis

Q80.2 Lamellar ichthyosis
    Collodion baby

Q80.3 Congenital bullous ichthyosiform erythroderma

Q80.4 Harlequin fetus

Q80.8 Other congenital ichthyosis

Q80.9 Congenital ichthyosis, unspecified

✓4ᵗʰ **Q81 Epidermolysis bullosa**

Q81.0 Epidermolysis bullosa simplex
    EXCLUDES 1 *Cockayne's syndrome (Q87.1)*

Q81.1 Epidermolysis bullosa letalis
    Herlitz' syndrome

Q81.2 Epidermolysis bullosa dystrophica

Q81.8 Other epidermolysis bullosa

Q81.9 Epidermolysis bullosa, unspecified

✓4ᵗʰ **Q82 Other congenital malformations of skin**
    EXCLUDES 1 *acrodermatitis enteropathica (E83.2)*
    congenital erythropoietic porphyria (E80.0)
    pilonidal cyst or sinus (L05-)
    Sturge-Weber (-Dimitri) syndrome (Q85.8)

Q82.0 Hereditary lymphedema

Q82.1 Xeroderma pigmentosum

Q82.2 Mastocytosis
    Urticaria pigmentosa
    EXCLUDES 1 *malignant mastocytosis (C96.2)*

Q82.3 Incontinentia pigmenti

Q82.4 Ectodermal dysplasia (anhidrotic)
    EXCLUDES 1 *Ellis-van Creveld syndrome (Q77.6)*

Q82.5 **Congenital non-neoplastic nevus**
Birthmark NOS
Flammeus Nevus
Portwine Nevus
Sanguineous Nevus
Strawberry Nevus
Vascular Nevus NOS
Verrucous Nevus
　EXCLUDES 2　*araneus nevus (I78.1)*
　　café au lait spots (L81.3)
　　lentigo (L81.4)
　　melanocytic nevus (D22-)
　　nevus NOS (D22-)
　　pigmented nevus (D22-)
　　spider nevus (I78.1)
　　stellar nevus (I78.1)

Q82.8 **Other specified congenital malformations of skin**
Abnormal palmar creases
Accessory skin tags
Benign familial pemphigus [Hailey-Hailey]
Congenital poikiloderma
Cutis laxa (hyperelastica)
Dermatoglyphic anomalies
Inherited keratosis palmaris et plantaris
Keratosis follicularis [Darier-White]
　EXCLUDES 1　*Ehlers-Danlos syndrome (Q79.6)*

Q82.9 **Congenital malformation of skin, unspecified**

✓4th **Q83** **Congenital malformations of breast**
　EXCLUDES 2　*absence of pectoral muscle (Q79.8)*
　　hypoplasia of breast (N64.82)
　　micromastia (N64.82)

Q83.0 **Congenital absence of breast with absent nipple**

Q83.1 **Accessory breast**
Supernumerary breast

Q83.2 **Absent nipple**

Q83.3 **Accessory nipple**
Supernumerary nipple

Q83.8 **Other congenital malformations of breast**

Q83.9 **Congenital malformation of breast, unspecified**

✓4th **Q84** **Other congenital malformations of integument**

Q84.0 **Congenital alopecia**
Congenital atrichosis

Q84.1 **Congenital morphological disturbances of hair, not elsewhere classified**
Beaded hair
Monilethrix
Pili annulati
　EXCLUDES 1　*Menkes' kinky hair syndrome (E83.0)*

Q84.2 **Other congenital malformations of hair**
Congenital hypertrichosis
Congenital malformation of hair NOS
Persistent lanugo

Q84.3 **Anonychia**
　EXCLUDES 1　*nail patella syndrome (Q87.2)*

Q84.4 **Congenital leukonychia**

Q84.5 **Enlarged and hypertrophic nails**
Congenital onychauxis
Pachyonychia

Q84.6 **Other congenital malformations of nails**
Congenital clubnail
Congenital koilonychia
Congenital malformation of nail NOS

Q84.8 **Other specified congenital malformations of integument**
Aplasia cutis congenita

Q84.9 **Congenital malformation of integument, unspecified**
Congenital anomaly of integument NOS
Congenital deformity of integument NOS

✓4th **Q85** **Phakomatoses, not elsewhere classified**
　EXCLUDES 1　*ataxia telangiectasia [Louis-Bar] (G11.3)*
　　familial dysautonomia [Riley-Day] (G90.1)

✓5th **Q85.0** **Neurofibromatosis (nonmalignant)**

Q85.00 **Neurofibromatosis, unspecified**

Q85.01 **Neurofibromatosis, type 1**
Von Recklinghausen disease

Q85.02 **Neurofibromatosis, type 2**
Acoustic neurofibromatosis

Q85.03 **Schwannomatosis**

Q85.09 **Other neurofibromatosis**

Q85.1 **Tuberous sclerosis**
Bourneville's disease
Epiloia

Q85.8 **Other phakomatoses, not elsewhere classified**
Peutz-Jeghers Syndrome
Sturge-Weber(-Dimitri) syndrome
von Hippel-Lindau syndrome
　EXCLUDES 1　*Meckel-Gruber syndrome (Q61.9)*

Q85.9 **Phakomatosis, unspecified**
Hamartosis NOS

✓4th **Q86** **Congenital malformation syndromes due to known exogenous causes, not elsewhere classified**
　EXCLUDES 2　*iodine-deficiency-related hypothyroidism (E00-E02)*
　　nonteratogenic effects of substances transmitted via placenta or breast milk (P04-)

Q86.0 **Fetal alcohol syndrome (dysmorphic)**

Q86.1 **Fetal hydantoin syndrome**
Meadow's syndrome

Q86.2 **Dysmorphism due to warfarin**

Q86.8 **Other congenital malformation syndromes due to known exogenous causes**

✓4th **Q87** **Other specified congenital malformation syndromes affecting multiple systems**
Use additional code(s) to identify all associated manifestations

Q87.0 **Congenital malformation syndromes predominantly affecting facial appearance**
Acrocephalopolysyndactyly
Acrocephalosyndactyly [Apert]
Cryptophthalmos syndrome
Cyclopia
Goldenhar syndrome
Moebius syndrome
Oro-facial-digital syndrome
Robin syndrome
Whistling face

Q87.1 **Congenital malformation syndromes predominantly associated with short stature**
Aarskog syndrome
Cockayne syndrome
De Lange syndrome
Dubowitz syndrome
Noonan syndrome
Prader-Willi syndrome
Robinow-Silverman-Smith syndrome
Russell-Silver syndrome
Seckel syndrome
Smith-Lemli-Opitz syndrome
　EXCLUDES 1　*Ellis-van Creveld syndrome (Q77.6)*

Q87.2 **Congenital malformation syndromes predominantly involving limbs**
Holt-Oram syndrome
Klippel-Trenaunay-Weber syndrome
Nail patella syndrome
Rubinstein-Taybi syndrome
Sirenomelia syndrome
Thrombocytopenia with absent radius [TAR] syndrome
VATER syndrome

Q87.3 **Congenital malformation syndromes involving early overgrowth**
Beckwith-Wiedemann syndrome
Sotos syndrome
Weaver syndrome

✓5th **Q87.4** **Marfan's syndrome**

Q87.40 **Marfan's syndrome, unspecified**

✓6th **Q87.41** **Marfan's syndrome with cardiovascular manifestations**

Q87.410 **Marfan's syndrome with aortic dilation**

Q87.418 **Marfan's syndrome with other cardiovascular manifestations**

Q87.42 **Marfan's syndrome with ocular manifestations**

Q87.43 **Marfan's syndrome with skeletal manifestation**

Q87.5 **Other congenital malformation syndromes with other skeletal changes**

✓5th **Q87.8** **Other specified congenital malformation syndromes, not elsewhere classified**
　EXCLUDES 1　*Zellweger syndrome (E71.510)*

Q87.81 **Alport syndrome**
Use additional code to identify stage of chronic kidney disease (N18.1-N18.6)

EXCLUDES 1　Not coded here　　　　EXCLUDES 2　Not included here　　　　*Manifestation Code*

Q87.89 Other specified congenital malformation syndromes, not elsewhere classified
    Laurence-Moon (-Bardet)-Biedl syndrome

✓4th **Q89 Other congenital malformations, not elsewhere classified**

  ✓5th **Q89.0 Congenital absence and malformations of spleen**
    EXCLUDES 1 *isomerism of atrial appendages (with asplenia or polysplenia) (Q20.6)*

    Q89.01 Asplenia (congenital)

    Q89.09 Congenital malformations of spleen
      Congenital splenomegaly

  Q89.1 Congenital malformations of adrenal gland
    EXCLUDES 1 *adrenogenital disorders (E25-)*
      congenital adrenal hyperplasia (E25.0)

  Q89.2 Congenital malformations of other endocrine glands
    Congenital malformation of parathyroid or thyroid gland
    Persistent thyroglossal duct
    Thyroglossal cyst
    EXCLUDES 1 *congenital goiter (E03.0)*
      congenital hypothyroidism (E03.1)

  Q89.3 Situs inversus
    Dextrocardia with situs inversus
    Mirror-image atrial arrangement with situs inversus
    Situs inversus or transversus abdominalis
    Situs inversus or transversus thoracis
    Transposition of abdominal viscera
    Transposition of thoracic viscera
    EXCLUDES 1 *dextrocardia NOS (Q24.0)*

  Q89.4 Conjoined twins
    Craniopagus
    Dicephaly
    Pygopagus
    Thoracopagus

  Q89.7 Multiple congenital malformations, not elsewhere classified
    Multiple congenital anomalies NOS
    Multiple congenital deformities NOS
    EXCLUDES 1 *congenital malformation syndromes affecting multiple systems (Q87-)*

  Q89.8 Other specified congenital malformations
    Use additional code(s) to identify all associated manifestations

  Q89.9 Congenital malformation, unspecified
    Congenital anomaly NOS
    Congenital deformity NOS

Chromosomal abnormalities, not elsewhere classified (Q90-Q99)

EXCLUDES 2 *mitochondrial metabolic disorders (E88.3-)*

✓4th **Q90 Down syndrome**
  Use additional code(s) to identify any associated physical conditions and degree of mental retardation (F70-F79)

  Q90.0 Trisomy 21, nonmosaicism (meiotic nondisjunction)
  Q90.1 Trisomy 21, mosaicism (mitotic nondisjunction)
  Q90.2 Trisomy 21, translocation
  Q90.9 Down syndrome, unspecified
    Trisomy 21 NOS

✓4th **Q91 Trisomy 18 and Trisomy 13**
  Q91.0 Trisomy 18, nonmosaicism (meiotic nondisjunction)
  Q91.1 Trisomy 18, mosaicism (mitotic nondisjunction)
  Q91.2 Trisomy 18, translocation
  Q91.3 Trisomy 18, unspecified
  Q91.4 Trisomy 13, nonmosaicism (meiotic nondisjunction)
  Q91.5 Trisomy 13, mosaicism (mitotic nondisjunction)
  Q91.6 Trisomy 13, translocation
  Q91.7 Trisomy 13, unspecified

✓4th **Q92 Other trisomies and partial trisomies of the autosomes, not elsewhere classified**
  INCLUDES unbalanced translocations and insertions
  EXCLUDES 1 *trisomies of chromosomes 13, 18, 21 (Q90-Q91)*

  Q92.0 Whole chromosome trisomy, nonmosaicism (meiotic nondisjunction)
  Q92.1 Whole chromosome trisomy, mosaicism (mitotic nondisjunction)
  Q92.2 Partial trisomy
    Less than whole arm duplicated
    Whole arm or more duplicated
    EXCLUDES 1 *partial trisomy due to unbalanced translocation (Q92.5)*

  Q92.5 Duplications with other complex rearrangements
    Partial trisomy due to unbalanced translocations
    Code also any associated deletions due to unbalanced translocations, inversions and insertions (Q93.7)

  ✓5th **Q92.6 Marker chromosomes**
    Trisomies due to dicentrics
    Trisomies due to extra rings
    Trisomies due to isochromosomes
    Individual with marker heterochromatin

    Q92.61 Marker chromosomes in normal individual
    Q92.62 Marker chromosomes in abnormal individual

  Q92.7 Triploidy and polyploidy

  Q92.8 Other specified trisomies and partial trisomies of autosomes
    Duplications identified by fluorescence in situ hybridization (FISH)
    Duplications identified by in situ hybridization (ISH)
    Duplications seen only at prometaphase

  Q92.9 Trisomy and partial trisomy of autosomes, unspecified

✓4th **Q93 Monosomies and deletions from the autosomes, not elsewhere classified**

  Q93.0 Whole chromosome monosomy, nonmosaicism (meiotic nondisjunction)
  Q93.1 Whole chromosome monosomy, mosaicism (mitotic nondisjunction)
  Q93.2 Chromosome replaced with ring, dicentric or isochromosome
  Q93.3 Deletion of short arm of chromosome 4
    Wolff-Hirschorn syndrome
  Q93.4 Deletion of short arm of chromosome 5
    Cri-du-chat syndrome
  Q93.5 Other deletions of part of a chromosome
    Angelman syndrome
  Q93.7 Deletions with other complex rearrangements
    Deletions due to unbalanced translocations, inversions and insertions
    Code also any associated duplications due to unbalanced translocations, inversions and insertions (Q92.5)

  ✓5th **Q93.8 Other deletions from the autosomes**
    Q93.81 Velo-cardio-facial syndrome
      Deletion 22q11.2
    Q93.88 Other microdeletions
      Miller-Dieker syndrome
      Smith-Magenis syndrome
    Q93.89 Other deletions from the autosomes
      Deletions identified by fluorescence in situ hybridization (FISH)
      Deletions identified by in situ hybridization (ISH)
      Deletions seen only at prometaphase

  Q93.9 Deletion from autosomes, unspecified

✓4th **Q95 Balanced rearrangements and structural markers, not elsewhere classified**
  INCLUDES Robertsonian and balanced reciprocal translocations and insertions

  Q95.0 Balanced translocation and insertion in normal individual
  Q95.1 Chromosome inversion in normal individual
  Q95.2 Balanced autosomal rearrangement in abnormal individual
  Q95.3 Balanced sex/autosomal rearrangement in abnormal individual
  Q95.5 Individual with autosomal fragile site
  Q95.8 Other balanced rearrangements and structural markers
  Q95.9 Balanced rearrangement and structural marker, unspecified

✓4th **Q96 Turner's syndrome**
  EXCLUDES 1 *Noonan syndrome (Q87.1)*

  Q96.0 Karyotype 45, X
  Q96.1 Karyotype 46, X iso (Xq)
    Karyotype 46, isochromosome Xq
  Q96.2 Karyotype 46, X with abnormal sex chromosome, except iso (Xq)
    Karyotype 46, X with abnormal sex chromosome, except isochromosome Xq
  Q96.3 Mosaicism, 45, X/46, XX or XY
  Q96.4 Mosaicism, 45, X/other cell line(s) with abnormal sex chromosome
  Q96.8 Other variants of Turner's syndrome
  Q96.9 Turner's syndrome, unspecified

✓ Appropriate additional character required   ✓x7th Requires 7th character, placeholder x must fill empty characters

✓4ᵗʰ **Q97** **Other sex chromosome abnormalities, female phenotype, not elsewhere classified**

     EXCLUDES 1   *Turner's syndrome (Q96-)*

     Q97.0 **Karyotype 47, XXX**

     Q97.1 **Female with more than three X chromosomes**

     Q97.2 **Mosaicism, lines with various numbers of X chromosomes**

     Q97.3 **Female with 46, XY karyotype**

     Q97.8 **Other specified sex chromosome abnormalities, female phenotype**

     Q97.9 **Sex chromosome abnormality, female phenotype, unspecified**

✓4ᵗʰ **Q98** **Other sex chromosome abnormalities, male phenotype, not elsewhere classified**

     Q98.0 **Klinefelter syndrome karyotype 47, XXY**

     Q98.1 **Klinefelter syndrome, male with more than two X chromosomes**

     Q98.3 **Other male with 46, XX karyotype**

     Q98.4 **Klinefelter syndrome, unspecified**

     Q98.5 **Karyotype 47, XYY**

     Q98.6 **Male with structurally abnormal sex chromosome**

     Q98.7 **Male with sex chromosome mosaicism**

     Q98.8 **Other specified sex chromosome abnormalities, male phenotype**

     Q98.9 **Sex chromosome abnormality, male phenotype, unspecified**

✓4ᵗʰ **Q99** **Other chromosome abnormalities, not elsewhere classified**

     Q99.0 **Chimera 46, XX/46, XY**

         Chimera 46, XX/46, XY true hermaphrodite

     Q99.1 **46, XX true hermaphrodite**

         46, XX with streak gonads

         46, XY with streak gonads

         Pure gonadal dysgenesis

     Q99.2 **Fragile X chromosome**

         Fragile X syndrome

     Q99.8 **Other specified chromosome abnormalities**

     Q99.9 **Chromosomal abnormality, unspecified**

Chapter 18. Symptoms, Signs and Abnormal Clinical and Laboratory Findings, Not Elsewhere Classified (R00-R99)

This chapter includes symptoms, signs, abnormal results of clinical or other investigative procedures, and ill-defined conditions regarding which no diagnosis classifiable elsewhere is recorded.

Signs and symptoms that point rather definitely to a given diagnosis have been assigned to a category in other chapters of the classification. In general, categories in this chapter include the less well-defined conditions and symptoms that, without the necessary study of the case to establish a final diagnosis, point perhaps equally to two or more diseases or to two or more systems of the body. Practically all categories in the chapter could be designated "not otherwise specified", "unknown etiology" or "transient". The Alphabetical Index should be consulted to determine which symptoms and signs are to be allocated here and which to other chapters. The residual subcategories, numbered .8, are generally provided for other relevant symptoms that cannot be allocated elsewhere in the classification.

The conditions and signs or symptoms included in categories R00-R94 consist of: (a) cases for which no more specific diagnosis can be made even after all the facts bearing on the case have been investigated; (b) signs or symptoms existing at the time of initial encounter that proved to be transient and whose causes could not be determined; (c) provisional diagnosis in a patient who failed to return for further investigation or care;(d) cases referred elsewhere for investigation or treatment before the diagnosis was made; (e) cases in which a more precise diagnosis was not available for any other reason; (f) certain symptoms, for which supplementary information is provided, that represent important problems in medical care in their own right.

EXCLUDES 2　abnormal findings on antenatal screening of mother (O28-)
certain conditions originating in the perinatal period (P04-P96)
signs and symptoms classified in the body system chapters
signs and symptoms of breast (N63, N64.5)

This chapter contains the following blocks:

R00-R09	Symptoms and signs involving the circulatory and respiratory systems
R10-R19	Symptoms and signs involving the digestive system and abdomen
R20-R23	Symptoms and signs involving the skin and subcutaneous tissue
R25-R29	Symptoms and signs involving the nervous and musculoskeletal systems
R30-R39	Symptoms and signs involving the urinary system
R40-R46	Symptoms and signs involving cognition, perception, emotional state and behavior
R47-R49	Symptoms and signs involving speech and voice
R50-R69	General symptoms and signs
R70-R79	Abnormal findings on examination of blood, without diagnosis
R80-R82	Abnormal findings on examination of urine, without diagnosis
R83-R89	Abnormal findings on examination of other body fluids, substances and tissues, without diagnosis
R90-R94	Abnormal findings on diagnostic imaging and in function studies, without diagnosis
R97	Abnormal tumor markers
R99	Ill-defined and unknown cause of mortality

Symptoms and signs involving the circulatory and respiratory systems (R00-R09)

✓4ᵗʰ R00　Abnormalities of heart beat
EXCLUDES 1　abnormalities originating in the perinatal period (P29.1)
specified arrhythmias (I47-I49)

R00.0　Tachycardia, unspecified
Rapid heart beat
Sinoauricular tachycardia NOS
Sinus [sinusal] tachycardia NOS
EXCLUDES 1　neonatal tachycardia (P29.11)
paroxysmal tachycardia (I47-)

R00.1　Bradycardia, unspecified
Sinoatrial bradycardia
Sinus bradycardia
Slow heart beat
Vagal bradycardia
EXCLUDES 1　neonatal bradycardia (P29.12)

R00.2　Palpitations
Awareness of heart beat

R00.8　Other abnormalities of heart beat

R00.9　Unspecified abnormalities of heart beat

✓4ᵗʰ R01　Cardiac murmurs and other cardiac sounds
EXCLUDES 1　cardiac murmurs and sounds originating in the perinatal period (P29.8)

R01.0　Benign and innocent cardiac murmurs
Functional cardiac murmur

R01.1　Cardiac murmur, unspecified
Cardiac bruit NOS
Heart murmur NOS

R01.2　Other cardiac sounds
Cardiac dullness, increased or decreased
Precordial friction

✓4ᵗʰ R03　Abnormal blood-pressure reading, without diagnosis

R03.0　Elevated blood-pressure reading, without diagnosis of hypertension
NOTE　This category is to be used to record an episode of elevated blood pressure in a patient in whom no formal diagnosis of hypertension has been made, or as an isolated incidental finding.

R03.1　Nonspecific low blood-pressure reading
EXCLUDES 1　hypotension (I95-)
maternal hypotension syndrome (O26.5-)
neurogenic orthostatic hypotension (G90.3)

✓4ᵗʰ R04　Hemorrhage from respiratory passages

R04.0　Epistaxis
Hemorrhage from nose
Nosebleed

R04.1　Hemorrhage from throat
EXCLUDES 2　hemoptysis (R04.2)

R04.2　Hemoptysis
Blood-stained sputum
Cough with hemorrhage

✓5ᵗʰ R04.8　Hemorrhage from other sites in respiratory passages

R04.81　Acute idiopathic pulmonary hemorrhage in infants
AIPHI
Acute idiopathic hemorrhage in infants over 28 days old
EXCLUDES 1　perinatal pulmonary hemorrhage (P26.-)
von Willebrand's disease (D68.0)

R04.89　Hemorrhage from other sites in respiratory passages
Pulmonary hemorrhage NOS

R04.9　Hemorrhage from respiratory passages, unspecified

R05　Cough
EXCLUDES 1　cough with hemorrhage (R04.2)
smoker's cough (J41.0)

✓4ᵗʰ R06　Abnormalities of breathing
EXCLUDES 1　acute respiratory distress syndrome (J80)
respiratory arrest (R09.2)
respiratory arrest of newborn (P28.81)
respiratory distress syndrome of newborn (P22-)
respiratory failure (J96-)
respiratory failure of newborn (P28.5)

✓5ᵗʰ R06.0　Dyspnea
EXCLUDES 1　tachypnea NOS (R06.82)
transient tachypnea of newborn (P22.1)

R06.00　Dyspnea, unspecified

R06.01　Orthopnea

R06.02　Shortness of breath

R06.09　Other forms of dyspnea

R06.1　Stridor
EXCLUDES 1　congenital laryngeal stridor (P28.89)
laryngismus (stridulus) (J38.5)

R06.2　Wheezing
EXCLUDES 1　asthma (J45-)

R06.3　Periodic breathing
Cheyne-Stokes breathing

R06.4　Hyperventilation
EXCLUDES 1　psychogenic hyperventilation (F45.8)

R06.5　Mouth breathing
EXCLUDES 2　dry mouth NOS (R68.2)

R06.6　Hiccough
EXCLUDES 1　psychogenic hiccough (F45.8)

R06.7　Sneezing

✓ Appropriate additional character required　　　✓x7ᵗʰ Requires 7th character, placeholder x must fill empty characters

✓5ᵗʰ **R06.8**   **Other abnormalities of breathing**

     R06.81   **Apnea, not elsewhere classified**
         Apnea NOS
         EXCLUDES 1   *apnea (of) newborn (P28.4)*
                 sleep apnea (G47.3-)
                 sleep apnea of newborn (primary) (P28.3)

     R06.82   **Tachypnea, not elsewhere classified**
         Tachypnea NOS
         EXCLUDES 1   *transitory tachypnea of newborn (P22.1)*

     R06.83   **Snoring**

     R06.89   **Other abnormalities of breathing**
         Breath-holding (spells)
         Sighing

   R06.9   **Unspecified abnormalities of breathing**

✓4ᵗʰ **R07**   **Pain in throat and chest**
     EXCLUDES 1   *epidemic myalgia (B33.0)*
     EXCLUDES 2   *jaw pain (R68.84)*
                 pain in breast (N64.4)

   R07.0   **Pain in throat**
     EXCLUDES 1   *chronic sore throat (J31.2)*
                 sore throat (acute) NOS (J02.9)
     EXCLUDES 2   *dysphagia (R13.1-)*
                 pain in neck (M54.2)

   R07.1   **Chest pain on breathing**
         Painful respiration

   R07.2   **Precordial pain**

✓5ᵗʰ **R07.8**   **Other chest pain**

     R07.81   **Pleurodynia**
         Pleurodynia NOS
         EXCLUDES 1   *epidemic pleurodynia (B33.0)*

     R07.82   **Intercostal pain**

     R07.89   **Other chest pain**
         Anterior chest-wall pain NOS

   R07.9   **Chest pain, unspecified**

✓4ᵗʰ **R09**   **Other symptoms and signs involving the circulatory and respiratory system**
     EXCLUDES 1   *acute respiratory distress syndrome (J80)*
                 respiratory arrest of newborn (P28.81)
                 respiratory distress syndrome of newborn (P22.0)
                 respiratory failure (J96-)
                 respiratory failure of newborn (P28.5)

✓5ᵗʰ **R09.0**   **Asphyxia and hypoxemia**
     EXCLUDES 1   *asphyxia due to carbon monoxide (T58-)*
                 asphyxia due to foreign body in respiratory tract (T17-)
                 birth (intrauterine) asphyxia (P84)
                 hypercapnia (R06.4)
                 hyperventilation (R06.4)
                 traumatic asphyxia (T71-)

     R09.01   **Asphyxia**

     R09.02   **Hypoxemia**

   R09.1   **Pleurisy**
     EXCLUDES 1   *pleurisy with effusion (J90)*

   R09.2   **Respiratory arrest**
         Cardiorespiratory failure
     EXCLUDES 1   *cardiac arrest (I46-)*
                 respiratory arrest of newborn (P28.81)
                 respiratory distress of newborn (P22.0)
                 respiratory failure (J96-)
                 respiratory failure of newborn (P28.5)
                 respiratory insufficiency (R06.89)
                 respiratory insufficiency of newborn (P28.5)

   R09.3   **Abnormal sputum**
         Abnormal amount of sputum
         Abnormal color of sputum
         Abnormal odor of sputum
         Excessive sputum
     EXCLUDES 1   *blood-stained sputum (R04.2)*

✓5ᵗʰ **R09.8**   **Other specified symptoms and signs involving the circulatory and respiratory systems**

     R09.81   **Nasal congestion**

     R09.82   **Postnasal drip**

     R09.89   **Other specified symptoms and signs involving the circulatory and respiratory systems**
         Abnormal chest percussion
         Bruit (arterial)
         Chest tympany
         Choking sensation
         Feeling of foreign body in throat
         Friction sounds in chest
         Rales
         Weak pulse
     EXCLUDES 2   *foreign body in throat (T17.2-)*
                 wheezing (R06.2)

Symptoms and signs involving the digestive system and abdomen (R10-R19)

   EXCLUDES 1   *congenital or infantile pylorospasm (Q40.0)*
                 gastrointestinal hemorrhage (K92.0-K92.2)
                 intestinal obstruction (K56-)
                 newborn gastrointestinal hemorrhage (P54.0-P54.3)
                 newborn intestinal obstruction (P76-)
                 pylorospasm (K31.3)
                 signs and symptoms involving the urinary system (R30-R39)
                 symptoms referable to female genital organs (N94-)
                 symptoms referable to male genital organs male (N48-N50)

✓4ᵗʰ **R10**   **Abdominal and pelvic pain**
     EXCLUDES 1   *renal colic (N23)*
     EXCLUDES 2   *dorsalgia (M54-)*
                 flatulence and related conditions (R14-)

   R10.0   **Acute abdomen**
         Severe abdominal pain (generalized) (with abdominal rigidity)
     EXCLUDES 1   *abdominal rigidity NOS (R19.3)*
                 generalized abdominal pain NOS (R10.84)
                 localized abdominal pain (R10.1-R10.3-)

✓5ᵗʰ **R10.1**   **Pain localized to upper abdomen**

     R10.10   **Upper abdominal pain, unspecified**

     R10.11   **Right upper quadrant pain**

     R10.12   **Left upper quadrant pain**

     R10.13   **Epigastric pain**
         Dyspepsia
         EXCLUDES 1   *functional dyspepsia (K30)*

   R10.2   **Pelvic and perineal pain**
     EXCLUDES 1   *vulvodynia (N94.81)*

✓5ᵗʰ **R10.3**   **Pain localized to other parts of lower abdomen**

     R10.30   **Lower abdominal pain, unspecified**

     R10.31   **Right lower quadrant pain**

     R10.32   **Left lower quadrant pain**

     R10.33   **Periumbilical pain**

✓5ᵗʰ **R10.8**   **Other abdominal pain**

✓6ᵗʰ **R10.81**   **Abdominal tenderness**
         Abdominal tenderness NOS

         R10.811   **Right upper quadrant abdominal tenderness**

         R10.812   **Left upper quadrant abdominal tenderness**

         R10.813   **Right lower quadrant abdominal tenderness**

         R10.814   **Left lower quadrant abdominal tenderness**

         R10.815   **Periumbilic abdominal tenderness**

         R10.816   **Epigastric abdominal tenderness**

         R10.817   **Generalized abdominal tenderness**

         R10.819   **Abdominal tenderness, unspecified site**

✓6ᵗʰ **R10.82**   **Rebound abdominal tenderness**

         R10.821   **Right upper quadrant rebound abdominal tenderness**

         R10.822   **Left upper quadrant rebound abdominal tenderness**

         R10.823   **Right lower quadrant rebound abdominal tenderness**

         R10.824   **Left lower quadrant rebound abdominal tenderness**

         R10.825   **Periumbilic rebound abdominal tenderness**

         R10.826   **Epigastric rebound abdominal tenderness**

         R10.827   **Generalized rebound abdominal tenderness**

EXCLUDES 1   Not coded here   EXCLUDES 2   Not included here   *Manifestation Code*

R10.829 **Rebound abdominal tenderness, unspecified site**

R10.83 **Colic**
Colic NOS
Infantile colic
EXCLUDES 1   *colic in adult and child over 12 months old (R10.84)*

R10.84 **Generalized abdominal pain**
EXCLUDES 1   *generalized abdominal pain associated with acute abdomen (R10.0)*

R10.9 **Unspecified abdominal pain**

✓4th **R11** **Nausea and vomiting**
EXCLUDES 1   *cyclical vomiting associated with migraine (G43.a-)*
excessive vomiting in pregnancy (O21-)
hematemesis (K92.0)
neonatal hematemesis (P54.0)
newborn vomiting (P92.0-)
psychogenic vomiting (F50.8)
vomiting associated with bulimia nervosa (F50.2)
vomiting following gastrointestinal surgery (K91.0)

R11.0 **Nausea**
Nausea NOS
Nausea without vomiting

✓5th R11.1 **Vomiting**
R11.10 **Vomiting, unspecified**
Vomiting NOS
R11.11 **Vomiting without nausea**
R11.12 **Projectile vomiting**
R11.13 **Vomiting of fecal matter**
R11.14 **Bilious vomiting**
Bilious emesis

R11.2 **Nausea with vomiting, unspecified**
Persistent nausea with vomiting NOS

R12 **Heartburn**
EXCLUDES 1   *dyspepsia NOS (R10.13)*
functional dyspepsia (K30)

✓4th **R13** **Aphagia and dysphagia**
R13.0 **Aphagia**
Inability to swallow
EXCLUDES 1   *psychogenic aphagia (F50.9)*

✓5th R13.1 **Dysphagia**
Code first, if applicable, dysphagia following cerebrovascular disease (I69. with final characters -91)
EXCLUDES 1   *psychogenic dysphagia (F45.8)*
R13.10 **Dysphagia, unspecified**
Difficulty in swallowing NOS
R13.11 **Dysphagia, oral phase**
R13.12 **Dysphagia, oropharyngeal phase**
R13.13 **Dysphagia, pharyngeal phase**
R13.14 **Dysphagia, pharyngoesophageal phase**
R13.19 **Other dysphagia**
Cervical dysphagia
Neurogenic dysphagia

✓4th **R14** **Flatulence and related conditions**
EXCLUDES 1   *psychogenic aerophagy (F45.8)*
R14.0 **Abdominal distension (gaseous)**
Bloating
Tympanites (abdominal) (intestinal)
R14.1 **Gas pain**
R14.2 **Eructation**
R14.3 **Flatulence**

✓4th **R15** **Fecal incontinence**
Encopresis NOS
EXCLUDES 1   *fecal incontinence of nonorganic origin (F98.1)*
R15.0 **Incomplete defecation**
EXCLUDES 1   *constipation (K59.0-)*
fecal impaction (K56.41)
R15.1 **Fecal smearing**
Fecal soiling
R15.2 **Fecal urgency**
R15.9 **Full incontinence of feces**
Fecal incontinence NOS

✓4th **R16** **Hepatomegaly and splenomegaly, not elsewhere classified**
R16.0 **Hepatomegaly, not elsewhere classified**
Hepatomegaly NOS

R16.1 **Splenomegaly, not elsewhere classified**
Splenomegaly NOS

R16.2 **Hepatomegaly with splenomegaly, not elsewhere classified**
Hepatosplenomegaly NOS

R17 **Unspecified jaundice**
EXCLUDES 1   *neonatal jaundice (P55, P57-P59)*

✓4th **R18** **Ascites**
INCLUDES   fluid in peritoneal cavity
EXCLUDES 1   *ascites in alcoholic cirrhosis (K70.31)*
ascites in alcoholic hepatitis (K70.11)
ascites in toxic liver disease with chronic active hepatitis (K71.51)

R18.0 **Malignant ascites**
Code first malignancy, such as:
malignant neoplasm of ovary (C56-)
secondary malignant neoplasm of retroperitoneum and peritoneum (C78.6)

R18.8 **Other ascites**
Ascites NOS
Peritoneal effusion (chronic)

✓4th **R19** **Other symptoms and signs involving the digestive system and abdomen**
EXCLUDES 1   *acute abdomen (R10.0)*

✓5th R19.0 **Intra-abdominal and pelvic swelling, mass and lump**
EXCLUDES 1   *abdominal distension (gaseous) (R14-)*
ascites (R18-)
R19.00 **Intra-abdominal and pelvic swelling, mass and lump, unspecified site**
R19.01 **Right upper quadrant abdominal swelling, mass and lump**
R19.02 **Left upper quadrant abdominal swelling, mass and lump**
R19.03 **Right lower quadrant abdominal swelling, mass and lump**
R19.04 **Left lower quadrant abdominal swelling, mass and lump**
R19.05 **Periumbilic swelling, mass or lump**
Diffuse or generalized umbilical swelling or mass
R19.06 **Epigastric swelling, mass or lump**
R19.07 **Generalized intra-abdominal and pelvic swelling, mass and lump**
Diffuse or generalized intra-abdominal swelling or mass NOS
Diffuse or generalized pelvic swelling or mass NOS
R19.09 **Other intra-abdominal and pelvic swelling, mass and lump**

✓5th R19.1 **Abnormal bowel sounds**
R19.11 **Absent bowel sounds**
R19.12 **Hyperactive bowel sounds**
R19.15 **Other abnormal bowel sounds**
Abnormal bowel sounds NOS

R19.2 **Visible peristalsis**
Hyperperistalsis

✓5th R19.3 **Abdominal rigidity**
EXCLUDES 1   *abdominal rigidity with severe abdominal pain (R10.0)*
R19.30 **Abdominal rigidity, unspecified site**
R19.31 **Right upper quadrant abdominal rigidity**
R19.32 **Left upper quadrant abdominal rigidity**
R19.33 **Right lower quadrant abdominal rigidity**
R19.34 **Left lower quadrant abdominal rigidity**
R19.35 **Periumbilic abdominal rigidity**
R19.36 **Epigastric abdominal rigidity**
R19.37 **Generalized abdominal rigidity**

R19.4 **Change in bowel habit**
EXCLUDES 1   *constipation (K59.0-)*
functional diarrhea (K59.1)

R19.5 **Other fecal abnormalities**
Abnormal stool color
Bulky stools
Mucus in stools
Occult blood in feces
Occult blood in stools
EXCLUDES 1   *melena (K92.1)*
neonatal melena (P54.1)

R19.6 **Halitosis**

☑ Appropriate additional character required   ✓x7th Requires 7th character, placeholder x must fill empty characters

R19.7   **Diarrhea, unspecified**
Diarrhea NOS
EXCLUDES 1   *functional diarrhea (K59.1)*
neonatal diarrhea (P78.3)
psychogenic diarrhea (F45.8)

R19.8   **Other specified symptoms and signs involving the digestive system and abdomen**

Symptoms and signs involving the skin and subcutaneous tissue (R20-R23)

EXCLUDES 2   *symptoms relating to breast (N64.4-N64.5)*

✓4th **R20**   **Disturbances of skin sensation**
EXCLUDES 1   *dissociative anesthesia and sensory loss (F44.6)*
psychogenic disturbances (F45.8)

R20.0   **Anesthesia of skin**

R20.1   **Hypoesthesia of skin**

R20.2   **Paresthesia of skin**
Formication
Pins and needles
Tingling skin
EXCLUDES 1   *acroparesthesia (I73.8)*

R20.3   **Hyperesthesia**

R20.8   **Other disturbances of skin sensation**

R20.9   **Unspecified disturbances of skin sensation**

R21   **Rash and other nonspecific skin eruption**
Rash NOS
EXCLUDES 1   *specified type of rash—code to condition*
vesicular eruption (R23.8)

✓4th **R22**   **Localized swelling, mass and lump of skin and subcutaneous tissue**
Subcutaneous nodules (localized)(superficial)
EXCLUDES 1   *abnormal findings on diagnostic imaging (R90-R93)*
edema (R60-)
enlarged lymph nodes (R59-)
localized adiposity (E65)
swelling of joint (M25.4-)

R22.0   **Localized swelling, mass and lump, head**

R22.1   **Localized swelling, mass and lump, neck**

R22.2   **Localized swelling, mass and lump, trunk**
EXCLUDES 1   *intra-abdominal or pelvic mass and lump (R19.0-)*
intra-abdominal or pelvic swelling (R19.0-)
EXCLUDES 2   *breast mass and lump (N63)*

✓5th **R22.3**   **Localized swelling, mass and lump, upper limb**

R22.30   **Localized swelling, mass and lump, unspecified upper limb**

R22.31   **Localized swelling, mass and lump, right upper limb**

R22.32   **Localized swelling, mass and lump, left upper limb**

R22.33   **Localized swelling, mass and lump, upper limb, bilateral**

✓5th **R22.4**   **Localized swelling, mass and lump, lower limb**

R22.40   **Localized swelling, mass and lump, unspecified lower limb**

R22.41   **Localized swelling, mass and lump, right lower limb**

R22.42   **Localized swelling, mass and lump, left lower limb**

R22.43   **Localized swelling, mass and lump, lower limb, bilateral**

R22.9   **Localized swelling, mass and lump, unspecified**

✓4th **R23**   **Other skin changes**

R23.0   **Cyanosis**
EXCLUDES 1   *acrocyanosis (I73.8)*
cyanotic attacks of newborn (P28.2)

R23.1   **Pallor**
Clammy skin

R23.2   **Flushing**
Excessive blushing
Code first, if applicable, menopausal and female climacteric states (N95.1)

R23.3   **Spontaneous ecchymoses**
Petechiae
EXCLUDES 1   *ecchymoses of newborn (P54.5)*
purpura (D69-)

R23.4   **Changes in skin texture**
Desquamation of skin
Induration of skin
Scaling of skin
EXCLUDES 1   *epidermal thickening NOS (L85.9)*

R23.8   **Other skin changes**

R23.9   **Unspecified skin changes**

Symptoms and signs involving the nervous and musculoskeletal systems (R25-R29)

✓4th **R25**   **Abnormal involuntary movements**
EXCLUDES 1   *specific movement disorders (G20-G26)*
stereotyped movement disorders (F98.4)
tic disorders (F95-)

R25.0   **Abnormal head movements**

R25.1   **Tremor, unspecified**
EXCLUDES 1   *chorea NOS (G25.5)*
essential tremor (G25.0)
hysterical tremor (F44.4)
intention tremor (G25.2)

R25.2   **Cramp and spasm**
EXCLUDES 2   *carpopedal spasm (R29.0)*
charley-horse (M62.831)
infantile spasms (G40.4-)
muscle spasm of back (M62.830)
muscle spasm of calf (M62.831)

R25.3   **Fasciculation**
Twitching NOS

R25.8   **Other abnormal involuntary movements**

R25.9   **Unspecified abnormal involuntary movements**

✓4th **R26**   **Abnormalities of gait and mobility**
EXCLUDES 1   *ataxia NOS (R27.0)*
hereditary ataxia (G11-)
locomotor (syphilitic) ataxia (A52.11)
immobility syndrome (paraplegic) (M62.3)

R26.0   **Ataxic gait**
Staggering gait

R26.1   **Paralytic gait**
Spastic gait

R26.2   **Difficulty in walking, not elsewhere classified**
EXCLUDES 1   *falling (R29.6)*
unsteadiness on feet (R26.81)

✓5th **R26.8**   **Other abnormalities of gait and mobility**

R26.81   **Unsteadiness on feet**

R26.89   **Other abnormalities of gait and mobility**

R26.9   **Unspecified abnormalities of gait and mobility**

✓4th **R27**   **Other lack of coordination**
EXCLUDES 1   *ataxic gait (R26.0)*
hereditary ataxia (G11-)
vertigo NOS (R42)

R27.0   **Ataxia, unspecified**
EXCLUDES 1   *ataxia following cerebrovascular disease (I69. with final characters -93)*

R27.8   **Other lack of coordination**

R27.9   **Unspecified lack of coordination**

✓4th **R29**   **Other symptoms and signs involving the nervous and musculoskeletal systems**

R29.0   **Tetany**
Carpopedal spasm
EXCLUDES 1   *hysterical tetany (F44.5)*
neonatal tetany (P71.3)
parathyroid tetany (E20.9)
post-thyroidectomy tetany (E89.2)

R29.1   **Meningismus**

R29.2   **Abnormal reflex**
EXCLUDES 2   *abnormal pupillary reflex (H57.0)*
hyperactive gag reflex (J39.2)
vasovagal reaction or syncope (R55)

R29.3   **Abnormal posture**

R29.4   **Clicking hip**
EXCLUDES 1   *congenital deformities of hip (Q65-)*

R29.5   **Transient paralysis**
Code first any associated spinal cord injury (S14.0, S14.1-, S24.0, S24.1-, S34.0-, S34.1-)
EXCLUDES 1   *transient ischemic attack (G45.9)*

EXCLUDES 1   Not coded here   EXCLUDES 2   Not included here   *Manifestation Code*

R29.6   Repeated falls
Falling
Tendency to fall
EXCLUDES 2   at risk for falling (Z91.81)
history of falling (Z91.81)

✓5ᵗʰ **R29.8   Other symptoms and signs involving the nervous and musculoskeletal systems**

✓6ᵗʰ **R29.81   Other symptoms and signs involving the nervous system**

R29.810   Facial weakness
Facial droop
EXCLUDES 1   Bell's palsy (G51.0)
facial weakness following cerebrovascular disease (I69. with final characters -92)

R29.818   Other symptoms and signs involving the nervous system

✓6ᵗʰ **R29.89   Other symptoms and signs involving the musculoskeletal system**
EXCLUDES 2   pain in limb (M79.6-)

R29.890   Loss of height
EXCLUDES 1   osteoporosis (M80-M82)

R29.891   Ocular torticollis
EXCLUDES 1   congenital (sternomastoid) torticollis Q68.0
psychogenic torticollis (F45.8)
spasmodic torticollis (G24.3)
torticollis due to birth injury (P15.8)
torticollis NOS M43.6

R29.898   Other symptoms and signs involving the musculoskeletal system

✓5ᵗʰ **R29.9   Unspecified symptoms and signs involving the nervous and musculoskeletal systems**

R29.90   Unspecified symptoms and signs involving the nervous system

R29.91   Unspecified symptoms and signs involving the musculoskeletal system

Symptoms and signs involving the genitourinary system (R30-R39)

✓4ᵗʰ **R30   Pain associated with micturition**
EXCLUDES 1   psychogenic pain associated with micturition (F45.8)

R30.0   Dysuria
Strangury

R30.1   Vesical tenesmus

R30.9   Painful micturition, unspecified
Painful urination NOS

✓4ᵗʰ **R31   Hematuria**
EXCLUDES 1   hematuria included with underlying conditions, such as:
acute cystitis with hematuria (N30.01)
acute prostatitis with hematuria (N41.01)
recurrent and persistent hematuria in glomerular diseases (N02-)

R31.0   Gross hematuria

R31.1   Benign essential microscopic hematuria

R31.2   Other microscopic hematuria

R31.9   Hematuria, unspecified

R32   Unspecified urinary incontinence
Enuresis NOS
EXCLUDES 1   functional urinary incontinence (R39.81)
nonorganic enuresis (F98.0)
stress incontinence and other specified urinary incontinence (N39.3-N39.4-)
urinary incontinence associated with cognitive impairment (R39.81)

✓4ᵗʰ **R33   Retention of urine**
EXCLUDES 1   psychogenic retention of urine (F45.8)

R33.0   Drug induced retention of urine
Code first (T36-T50) to identify the drug

R33.8   Other retention of urine
Code, if applicable, any causal condition first, such as:
enlarged prostate (N40.1)

R33.9   Retention of urine, unspecified

R34   Anuria and oliguria
EXCLUDES 1   anuria and oliguria complicating abortion or ectopic or molar pregnancy (O00-O07, O08.4)
anuria and oliguria complicating pregnancy (O26.83-)
anuria and oliguria complicating the puerperium (O90.4)

✓4ᵗʰ **R35   Polyuria**
Code, if applicable, any causal condition first, such as:
enlarged prostate (N40.1)
EXCLUDES 1   psychogenic polyuria (F45.8)

R35.0   Frequency of micturition

R35.1   Nocturia

R35.8   Other polyuria
Polyuria NOS

✓4ᵗʰ **R36   Urethral discharge**

R36.0   Urethral discharge without blood

R36.1   Hematospermia

R36.9   Urethral discharge, unspecified
Penile discharge NOS
Urethrorrhea

R37   Sexual dysfunction, unspecified

✓4ᵗʰ **R39   Other and unspecified symptoms and signs involving the genitourinary system**

R39.0   Extravasation of urine

✓5ᵗʰ **R39.1   Other difficulties with micturition**
Code, if applicable, any causal condition first, such as:
enlarged prostate (N40.1)

R39.11   Hesitancy of micturition

R39.12   Poor urinary stream
Weak urinary steam

R39.13   Splitting of urinary stream

R39.14   Feeling of incomplete bladder emptying

R39.15   Urgency of urination
EXCLUDES 1   urge incontinence (N39.41, N39.46)

R39.16   Straining to void

R39.19   Other difficulties with micturition

R39.2   Extrarenal uremia
Prerenal uremia
EXCLUDES 1   uremia NOS (N19)

✓5ᵗʰ **R39.8   Other symptoms and signs involving the genitourinary system**

R39.81   Functional urinary incontinence
Urinary incontinence due to cognitive impairment, or severe physical disability or immobility
EXCLUDES 1   stress incontinence and other specified urinary incontinence (N39.3-N39.4-)
urinary incontinence NOS (R32)

R39.89   Other symptoms and signs involving the genitourinary system

R39.9   Unspecified symptoms and signs involving the genitourinary system

Symptoms and signs involving cognition, perception, emotional state and behavior (R40-R46)

EXCLUDES 1   symptoms and signs constituting part of a pattern of mental disorder (F01-F99)

✓4ᵗʰ **R40   Somnolence, stupor and coma**
EXCLUDES 1   neonatal coma (P91.5)
somnolence, stupor and coma in diabetes (E08-E13)
somnolence, stupor and coma in hepatic failure (K72-)
somnolence, stupor and coma in hypoglycemia (nondiabetic) (E15)

R40.0   Somnolence
Drowsiness
EXCLUDES 1   coma (R40.2-)

R40.1   Stupor
Catatonic stupor
Semicoma
EXCLUDES 1   catatonic schizophrenia (F20.2)
coma (R40.2-)
depressive stupor (F31-F33)
dissociative stupor (F44.2)
manic stupor (F30.2)

✓ Appropriate additional character required   ✓x7ᵗʰ Requires 7th character, placeholder x must fill empty characters

Symptoms, Signs and Abnormal Clinical and Laboratory Findings

R40.2–R45.84

✓5ᵗʰ **R40.2 Coma**
Coma NOS
Unconsciousness NOS
Codes first any associated:
coma in fracture of skull (S02-)
coma in intracranial injury (S06-)

> The appropriate 7th character is to be added to each code from subcategory R40.21-, R40.22-, R40.23-.
> Ø   unspecified time
> 1   in the field [EMT or ambulance]
> 2   at arrival to emergency department
> 3   at hospital admission
> 4   24 hours or more after hospital admission

A code from each subcategory is required to complete the coma scale

NOTE   These codes are intended primarily for trauma registry and research use but may be utilized by all users of the classification who wish to collect this information

     R40.20 Unspecified coma
✓6ᵗʰ   **R40.21 Coma scale, eyes open**
       ✓7ᵗʰ   **R40.211 Coma scale, eyes open, never**
       ✓7ᵗʰ   **R40.212 Coma scale, eyes open, to pain**
       ✓7ᵗʰ   **R40.213 Coma scale, eyes open, to sound**
       ✓7ᵗʰ   **R40.214 Coma scale, eyes open, spontaneous**
✓6ᵗʰ   **R40.22 Coma scale, best verbal response**
       ✓7ᵗʰ   **R40.221 Coma scale, best verbal response, none**
       ✓7ᵗʰ   **R40.222 Coma scale, best verbal response, incomprehensible words**
       ✓7ᵗʰ   **R40.223 Coma scale, best verbal response, inappropriate words**
       ✓7ᵗʰ   **R40.224 Coma scale, best verbal response, confused conversation**
       ✓7ᵗʰ   **R40.225 Coma scale, best verbal response, oriented**
✓6ᵗʰ   **R40.23 Coma scale, best motor response**
       ✓7ᵗʰ   **R40.231 Coma scale, best motor response, none**
       ✓7ᵗʰ   **R40.232 Coma scale, best motor response, extension**
       ✓7ᵗʰ   **R40.233 Coma scale, best motor response, abnormal**
       ✓7ᵗʰ   **R40.234 Coma scale, best motor response, flexion withdrawal**
       ✓7ᵗʰ   **R40.235 Coma scale, best motor response, localizes pain**
       ✓7ᵗʰ   **R40.236 Coma scale, best motor response, obeys commands**

     R40.3 Persistent vegetative state
     R40.4 Transient alteration of awareness

✓4ᵗʰ **R41 Other symptoms and signs involving cognitive functions and awareness**
   EXCLUDES 1   *dissociative [conversion] disorders (F44-)*
             mild cognitive impairment, so stated (G31.84)

     R41.0 Disorientation, unspecified
Confusion NOS
Delirium NOS
     R41.1 Anterograde amnesia
     R41.2 Retrograde amnesia
     R41.3 Other amnesia
Amnesia NOS
Memory loss NOS
   EXCLUDES 1   *amnestic disorder due to known physiologic condition (F04)*
             amnestic syndrome due to psychoactive substance use (F10-F19 with 5th character .6)
             transient global amnesia (G45.4)
     R41.4 Neurologic neglect syndrome
Asomatognosia
Hemi-akinesia
Hemi-inattention
Hemispatial neglect
Left-sided neglect
Sensory neglect
Visuospatial neglect
   EXCLUDES 1   *visuospatial deficit (R41.842)*

✓5ᵗʰ **R41.8 Other symptoms and signs involving cognitive functions and awareness**
     R41.81 Age-related cognitive decline
Senility NOS
     R41.82 Altered mental status, unspecified
Change in mental status NOS
   EXCLUDES 1   *altered level of consciousness (R40-)*
             altered mental status due to known condition—code to condition
             delirium NOS (R41.0)
     R41.83 Borderline intellectual functioning
IQ level 71 to 84
   EXCLUDES 1   *mental retardation (F70-F79)*
✓6ᵗʰ   **R41.84 Other specified cognitive deficit**
       R41.840 Attention and concentration deficit
         EXCLUDES 1   *attention-deficit hyperactivity disorders (F90.-)*
       R41.841 Cognitive communication deficit
       R41.842 Visuospatial deficit
       R41.843 Psychomotor deficit
       R41.844 Frontal lobe and executive function deficit
     R41.89 Other symptoms and signs involving cognitive functions and awareness
Anosognosia
     R41.9 Unspecified symptoms and signs involving cognitive functions and awareness

R42 Dizziness and giddiness
Light-headedness
Vertigo NOS
   EXCLUDES 1   *vertiginous syndromes (H81-)*
             vertigo from infrasound (T75.23)

✓4ᵗʰ **R43 Disturbances of smell and taste**
     R43.0 Anosmia
     R43.1 Parosmia
     R43.2 Parageusia
     R43.8 Other disturbances of smell and taste
Mixed disturbance of smell and taste
     R43.9 Unspecified disturbances of smell and taste

✓4ᵗʰ **R44 Other symptoms and signs involving general sensations and perceptions**
   EXCLUDES 1   *alcoholic hallucinations (F1.5)*
             hallucinations in drug psychosis (F11-F19 with .5)
             hallucinations in mood disorders with psychotic symptoms (F30.2, F31.5, F32.3, F33.3)
             hallucinations in schizophrenia, schizotypal and delusional disorders (F20-F29)
   EXCLUDES 2   *disturbances of skin sensation (R20-)*
     R44.0 Auditory hallucinations
     R44.1 Visual hallucinations
     R44.2 Other hallucinations
     R44.3 Hallucinations, unspecified
     R44.8 Other symptoms and signs involving general sensations and perceptions
     R44.9 Unspecified symptoms and signs involving general sensations and perceptions

✓4ᵗʰ **R45 Symptoms and signs involving emotional state**
     R45.0 Nervousness
Nervous tension
     R45.1 Restlessness and agitation
     R45.2 Unhappiness
     R45.3 Demoralization and apathy
   EXCLUDES 1   *anhedonia (R45.84)*
     R45.4 Irritability and anger
     R45.5 Hostility
     R45.6 Violent behavior
     R45.7 State of emotional shock and stress, unspecified
✓5ᵗʰ   **R45.8 Other symptoms and signs involving emotional state**
       R45.81 Low self-esteem
       R45.82 Worries
       R45.83 Excessive crying of child, adolescent or adult
         EXCLUDES 1   *excessive crying of infant (baby) R68.11*
       R45.84 Anhedonia

EXCLUDES 1   Not coded here   EXCLUDES 2   Not included here   ***Manifestation Code***

✓6th R45.85 Homicidal and suicidal ideations
EXCLUDES 1 *suicide attempt (T14.91)*
R45.850 Homicidal ideations
R45.851 Suicidal ideations
R45.86 Emotional lability
R45.87 Impulsiveness
R45.89 Other symptoms and signs involving emotional state

✓4th R46 Symptoms and signs involving appearance and behavior
EXCLUDES 1 *appearance and behavior in schizophrenia, schizotypal and delusional disorders (F20-F29)*
mental and behavioral disorders (F01-F99)
R46.0 Very low level of personal hygiene
R46.1 Bizarre personal appearance
R46.2 Strange and inexplicable behavior
R46.3 Overactivity
R46.4 Slowness and poor responsiveness
EXCLUDES 1 *stupor (R40.1)*
R46.5 Suspiciousness and marked evasiveness
R46.6 Undue concern and preoccupation with stressful events
R46.7 Verbosity and circumstantial detail obscuring reason for contact
✓5th R46.8 Other symptoms and signs involving appearance and behavior
R46.81 Obsessive-compulsive behavior
EXCLUDES 1 *obsessive-compulsive disorder (F42)*
R46.89 Other symptoms and signs involving appearance and behavior

Symptoms and signs involving speech and voice (R47-R49)

✓4th R47 Speech disturbances, not elsewhere classified
EXCLUDES 1 *autism (F84.0)*
cluttering (F80.81)
specific developmental disorders of speech and language (F80-)
stuttering (F80.81)
✓5th R47.0 Dysphasia and aphasia
R47.01 Aphasia
EXCLUDES 1 *aphasia following cerebrovascular disease (I69. with final characters -20)*
progressive isolated aphasia (G31.01)
R47.02 Dysphasia
EXCLUDES 1 *dysphasia following cerebrovascular disease (I69. with final characters -21)*
R47.1 Dysarthria and anarthria
EXCLUDES 1 *dysarthria following cerebrovascular disease (I69. with final characters -22)*
✓5th R47.8 Other speech disturbances
EXCLUDES 1 *dysarthria following cerebrovascular disease (I69. with final characters -28)*
R47.81 Slurred speech
R47.82 Fluency disorder in conditions classified elsewhere
Stuttering in conditions classified elsewhere
Code first underlying disease or condition, such as:
Parkinson's disease (G20)
EXCLUDES 1 *adult onset fluency disorder (F98.5)*
childhood onset fluency disorder (F80.81)
fluency disorder (stuttering) following cerebrovascular disease (I69. with final characters-23)
R47.89 Other speech disturbances
R47.9 Unspecified speech disturbances

✓4th R48 Dyslexia and other symbolic dysfunctions, not elsewhere classified
EXCLUDES 1 *specific developmental disorders of scholastic skills (F81-)*
R48.0 Dyslexia and alexia
R48.1 Agnosia
Astereognosia (astereognosis)
Autotopagnosia
EXCLUDES 1 *visual object agnosia H53.16*
R48.2 Apraxia
EXCLUDES 1 *apraxia following cerebrovascular disease (I69. with final characters -90)*

R48.8 Other symbolic dysfunctions
Acalculia
Agraphia
R48.9 Unspecified symbolic dysfunctions

✓4th R49 Voice and resonance disorders
EXCLUDES 1 *psychogenic voice and resonance disorders (F44.4)*
R49.0 Dysphonia
Hoarseness
R49.1 Aphonia
Loss of voice
✓5th R49.2 Hypernasality and hyponasality
R49.21 Hypernasality
R49.22 Hyponasality
R49.8 Other voice and resonance disorders
R49.9 Unspecified voice and resonance disorder
Change in voice NOS
Resonance disorder NOS

General symptoms and signs (R50-R69)

✓4th R50 Fever of other and unknown origin
EXCLUDES 1 *chills without fever (R68.83)*
febrile convulsions (R56.0-)
fever of unknown origin during labor (O75.2)
fever of unknown origin in newborn (P81.9)
hypothermia due to illness (R68.0)
malignant hyperthermia due to anesthesia (T88.3)
puerperal pyrexia NOS (O86.4)
R50.2 Drug induced fever
Code first (T36-T50) to identify drug
EXCLUDES 1 *postvaccination (postimmunization) fever (R50.83)*
✓5th R50.8 Other specified fever
R50.81 Fever presenting with conditions classified elsewhere
Code first underlying condition when associated fever is present, such as with:
leukemia (C91-C95)
neutropenia (D70-)
sickle cell disease (D57-)
R50.82 Postprocedural fever
EXCLUDES 1 *postprocedural infection (T81.4)*
posttransfusion fever (R50.84)
postvaccination (postimmunization) fever (R50.83)
R50.83 Postvaccination fever
Postimmunization fever
R50.84 Febrile nonhemolytic transfusion reaction
FNHTR
Posttransfusion fever
R50.9 Fever, unspecified
Fever NOS
Fever of unknown origin [FUO]
Fever with chills
Fever with rigors
Hyperpyrexia NOS
Persistent fever
Pyrexia NOS

R51 Headache
Facial pain NOS
EXCLUDES 1 *atypical face pain (G50.1)*
migraine and other headache syndromes (G43-G44)
trigeminal neuralgia (G50.0)

☑ Appropriate additional character required   ✓x7th Requires 7th character, placeholder x must fill empty characters

R52 Pain, unspecified
  Acute pain NOS
  Chronic pain NOS
  Generalized pain NOS
  Pain NOS
  EXCLUDES 1 *acute and chronic pain, not elsewhere classified (G89-)*
        localized pain, unspecified type—code to pain by site, such as:
          abdomen pain (R10-)
          back pain (M54.9)
          breast pain (N64.4)
          chest pain (R07.1-R07.9)
          ear pain (H92.0-)
          eye pain (H57.1)
          headache (R51)
          joint pain (M25.5-)
          limb pain (M79.6-)
          lumbar region pain (M54.5)
          pelvic and perineal pain (R10.2)
          shoulder pain (M25.51-)
          spine pain (M54-)
          throat pain (R07.0)
          tongue pain (K14.6)
          tooth pain (K08.8)
          renal colic (N23)
        pain disorders exclusively related to psychological factors
            (F45.41)

☑4ᵗʰ **R53 Malaise and fatigue**
  R53.0 Neoplastic (malignant) related fatigue
        Code first associated neoplasm
  R53.1 Weakness
        Asthenia NOS
        EXCLUDES 1 *age-related weakness (R54)*
              muscle weakness (M62.8-)
              senile asthenia (R54)

  R53.2 Functional quadriplegia
        Complete immobility due to severe physical disability or frailty
        EXCLUDES 1 *frailty NOS (R54)*
              hysterical paralysis (F44.4)
              immobility syndrome (M62.3)
              neurologic quadriplegia (G82.5-)
              quadriplegia (G82.50)

☑5ᵗʰ **R53.8 Other malaise and fatigue**
        EXCLUDES 1 *combat exhaustion and fatigue (F43.0)*
              congenital debility (P96.9)
              exhaustion and fatigue due to:
              depressive episode (F32-)
              excessive exertion (T73.3)
              exposure (T73.2)
              heat (T67-)
              pregnancy (O26.8-)
              recurrent depressive episode (F33)
              senile debility (R54)
    R53.81 Other malaise
          Chronic debility
          Debility NOS
          General physical deterioration
          Malaise NOS
          Nervous debility
          EXCLUDES 1 *age-related physical debility (R54)*
    R53.82 Chronic fatigue, unspecified
          Chronic fatigue syndrome NOS
          EXCLUDES 1 *postviral fatigue syndrome (G93.3)*
    R53.83 Other fatigue
          Fatigue NOS
          Lack of energy
          Lethargy
          Tiredness

R54 Age-related physical debility
  Frailty
  Old age
  Senescence
  Senile asthenia
  Senile debility
  EXCLUDES 1 *age-related cognitive decline (R41.81)*
        senile psychosis (F03)
        senility NOS (R41.81)

R55 Syncope and collapse
  Blackout
  Fainting
  Vasovagal attack
  EXCLUDES 1 *cardiogenic shock (R57.0)*
        carotid sinus syncope (G90.01)
        heat syncope (T67.1)
        neurocirculatory asthenia (F45.8)
        neurogenic orthostatic hypotension (G90.3)
        orthostatic hypotension (I95.1)
        postprocedural shock (T81.1)
        psychogenic syncope (F48.8)
        shock NOS (R57.9)
        shock complicating or following abortion or ectopic or molar
            pregnancy (O00-O07, O08.3)
        shock complicating or following labor and delivery (O75.1)
        Stokes-Adams attack (I45.9)
        unconsciousness NOS (R40.2-)

☑4ᵗʰ **R56 Convulsions, not elsewhere classified**
  EXCLUDES 1 *dissociative convulsions and seizures (F44.5)*
        epileptic convulsions and seizures (G40-)
        newborn convulsions and seizures (P90)
  ☑5ᵗʰ **R56.0 Febrile convulsions**
    R56.00 Simple febrile convulsions
          Febrile convulsion NOS
          Febrile seizure NOS
    R56.01 Complex febrile convulsions
          Atypical febrile seizure
          Complex febrile seizure
          Complicated febrile seizure
          EXCLUDES 1 *status epilepticus (G40.901)*
  R56.1 Post traumatic seizures
        EXCLUDES 1 *post traumatic epilepsy (G40.-)*
  R56.9 Unspecified convulsions
        Convulsion disorder
        Fit NOS
        Recurrent convulsions
        Seizure(s) (convulsive) NOS

☑4ᵗʰ **R57 Shock, not elsewhere classified**
  EXCLUDES 1 *anaphylactic shock NOS (T78.2)*
        anaphylactic shock (reaction) due to adverse food reaction
            (T78.0-)
        anaphylactic shock due to serum (T80.5)
        anesthetic shock (T88.3)
        electric shock (T75.4)
        obstetric shock (O75.1)
        postprocedural shock (T81.1)
        psychic shock (F43.0)
        septic shock (R65.21)
        shock complicating or following ectopic or molar pregnancy
            (O00-O07, O08.3)
        shock due to lightning (T75.01)
        traumatic shock (T79.4)
        toxic shock syndrome (A48.3)
  R57.0 Cardiogenic shock
  R57.1 Hypovolemic shock
  R57.8 Other shock
  R57.9 Shock, unspecified
        Failure of peripheral circulation NOS

R58 Hemorrhage, not elsewhere classified
  Hemorrhage NOS
  EXCLUDES 1 *hemorrhage included with underlying conditions, such as:*
        acute duodenal ulcer with hemorrhage (K26.0)
        acute gastritis with bleeding (K29.01)
        ulcerative enterocolitis with rectal bleeding (K51.01)

☑4ᵗʰ **R59 Enlarged lymph nodes**
  INCLUDES swollen glands
  EXCLUDES 1 *acute lymphadenitis (L04-)*
        chronic lymphadenitis (I88.1)
        lymphadenitis NOS (I88.9)
        mesenteric (acute) (chronic) lymphadenitis (I88.0)
  R59.0 Localized enlarged lymph nodes
  R59.1 Generalized enlarged lymph nodes
        Lymphadenopathy NOS
  R59.9 Enlarged lymph nodes, unspecified

EXCLUDES 1 Not coded here   EXCLUDES 2 Not included here   *Manifestation Code*

✓4th **R60   Edema, not elsewhere classified**
   EXCLUDES 1   *angioneurotic edema (T78.3)*
               ascites (R18-)
               cerebral edema (G93.6)
               cerebral edema due to birth injury (P11.0)
               edema of larynx (J38.4)
               edema of nasopharynx (J39.2)
               edema of pharynx (J39.2)
               gestational edema (O12.0-)
               hereditary edema (Q82.0)
               hydrops fetalis NOS (P83.2)
               hydrothorax (J94.8)
               nutritional edema (E40-E46)
               hydrops fetalis NOS (P83.2)
               newborn edema (P83.3)
               pulmonary edema (J81-)

   R60.0   Localized edema
   R60.1   Generalized edema
   R60.9   Edema, unspecified
               Fluid retention NOS

R61   Generalized hyperhidrosis
         Excessive sweating
         Night sweats
         Secondary hyperhidrosis
         Code first, if applicable, menopausal and female climacteric states
            (N95.1)
   EXCLUDES 1   *focal (primary) (secondary) hyperhidrosis (L74.5-)*
               Frey's syndrome (L74.52)
               localized (primary) (secondary) hyperhidrosis (L74.5-)

✓4th **R62   Lack of expected normal physiological development in
         childhood and adults**
   EXCLUDES 1   *delayed puberty (E30.0)*
               gonadal dysgenesis (Q99.1)
               hypopituitarism (E23.0)

   R62.0   Delayed milestone in childhood
               Delayed attainment of expected physiological developmental
                  stage
               Late talker
               Late walker

   ✓5th **R62.5   Other and unspecified lack of expected normal
               physiological development in childhood**
      EXCLUDES 1   *HIV disease resulting in failure to thrive (B20)*
                  physical retardation due to malnutrition (E45)

      **R62.50   Unspecified lack of expected normal physiological
                  development in childhood**
                  Infantilism NOS
      R62.51   Failure to thrive (child)
                  Failure to gain weight
         EXCLUDES 1   *failure to thrive in child under 28 days old
                     (P92.6)*
      R62.52   Short stature (child)
                  Lack of growth
                  Physical retardation
                  Short stature NOS
         EXCLUDES 1   *short stature due to endocrine disorder
                     (E34.3)*
      **R62.59   Other lack of expected normal physiological
                  development in childhood**

   R62.7   Adult failure to thrive

✓4th **R63   Symptoms and signs concerning food and fluid intake**
   EXCLUDES 1   *bulimia NOS (F50.2)*
               eating disorders of nonorganic origin (F50-)
               malnutrition (E40-E46)

   R63.0   Anorexia
               Loss of appetite
      EXCLUDES 1   *anorexia nervosa (F50.0-)*
                  loss of appetite of nonorganic origin (F50.8)
   R63.1   Polydipsia
               Excessive thirst
   R63.2   Polyphagia
               Excessive eating
               Hyperalimentation NOS
   R63.3   Feeding difficulties
               Feeding problem (elderly) (infant) NOS
      EXCLUDES 1   *feeding problems of newborn (P92-)*
                  infant feeding disorder of nonorganic origin (F98.2-)
   R63.4   Abnormal weight loss

   R63.5   Abnormal weight gain
      EXCLUDES 1   *excessive weight gain in pregnancy (O26.0-)*
                  obesity (E66-)
   R63.6   Underweight
               Use additional code to identify body mass index (BMI), if
                  known (Z68-)
      EXCLUDES 1   *abnormal weight loss (R63.4)*
                  anorexia nervosa (F50.0-)
                  malnutrition (E40-E46)
   R63.8   Other symptoms and signs concerning food and fluid intake

R64   Cachexia
         Wasting syndrome
         Code first underlying condition, if known
   EXCLUDES 1   *abnormal weight loss (R63.4)*
               nutritional marasmus (E41)

✓4th **R65   Symptoms and signs specifically associated with systemic
         inflammation and infection**
   ✓5th **R65.1   Systemic inflammatory response syndrome [SIRS] of
               non-infectious origin**
               Code first underlying condition, such as:
                  heatstroke (T67.0)
                  injury and trauma (S00-T88)
      EXCLUDES 1   *sepsis—code to infection*
                  severe sepsis (R65.2)

      **R65.10   Systemic inflammatory response syndrome [SIRS]
                  of non-infectious origin without acute organ
                  dysfunction**
                  Systemic inflammatory response syndrome (SIRS)
                     NOS
      **R65.11   Systemic inflammatory response syndrome [SIRS]
                  of non-infectious origin with acute organ
                  dysfunction**
                  Use additional code to identify specific acute organ
                     dysfunction, such as:
                     acute kidney failure (N17-)
                     acute respiratory failure (J96.0-)
                     critical illness myopathy (G72.81)
                     critical illness polyneuropathy (G62.81)
                     disseminated intravascular coagulopathy [DIC]
                        (D65)
                     encephalopathy (metabolic) (septic) (G93.41)
                     hepatic failure (K72.0-)

   R65.2   Severe sepsis
               Infection with associated acute organ dysfunction
               Sepsis with acute organ dysfunction
               Sepsis with multiple organ dysfunction
               Systemic inflammatory response syndrome due to infectious
                  process with acute organ dysfunction
               Code first underlying infection, such as:
                  infection following a procedure (T81.4)
                  infections following infusion, transfusion and therapeutic
                     injection (T80.2)
                  puerperal sepsis (O85)
                  sepsis following complete or unspecified spontaneous
                     abortion (O03.87)
                  sepsis following ectopic and molar pregnancy (O08.82)
                  sepsis following incomplete spontaneous abortion (O03.37)
                  sepsis following (induced) termination of pregnancy
                     (O04.87)
                  sepsis NOS A41.9
               Use additional code to identify specific acute organ
                  dysfunction, such as:
                  acute kidney failure (N17-)
                  acute respiratory failure (J96.0-)
                  critical illness myopathy (G72.81)
                  critical illness polyneuropathy (G62.81)
                  disseminated intravascular coagulopathy [DIC] (D65)
                  encephalopathy (metabolic) (septic) (G93.41)
                  hepatic failure (K72.0-)
      R65.20   Severe sepsis without septic shock
                  Severe sepsis NOS
      R65.21   Severe sepsis with septic shock

☑ Appropriate additional character required   ✓x7th Requires 7th character, placeholder x must fill empty characters

✓4th **R68** **Other general symptoms and signs**

  R68.0 **Hypothermia, not associated with low environmental temperature**

    EXCLUDES 1   *hypothermia NOS (accidental) (T68)*
         hypothermia due to anesthesia (T88.51)
         hypothermia due to low environmental temperature (T68)
         newborn hypothermia (P80-)

✓5th   **R68.1** **Nonspecific symptoms peculiar to infancy**

    EXCLUDES 1   *colic, infantile (R10.83)*
         neonatal cerebral irritability (P91.3)
         teething syndrome (K00.7)

    R68.11 **Excessive crying of infant (baby)**

      EXCLUDES 1   *excessive crying of child, adolescent, or adult (R45.83)*

    R68.12 **Fussy infant (baby)**
         Irritable infant

    R68.13 **Apparent life threatening event in infant [ALTE]**
         Apparent life threatening event in newborn
         Code first confirmed diagnosis, if known
         Use additional code(s) for associated signs and symptoms if no confirmed diagnosis established, or if signs and symptoms are not associated routinely with confirmed diagnosis, or provide additional information for cause of ALTE

    R68.19 **Other nonspecific symptoms peculiar to infancy**

  R68.2 **Dry mouth, unspecified**

    EXCLUDES 1   *dry mouth due to dehydration (E86.0)*
         dry mouth due to sicca syndrome [Sjögren] (M35.0-)
         salivary gland hyposecretion (K11.7)

  R68.3 **Clubbing of fingers**
     Clubbing of nails

    EXCLUDES 1   *congenital clubfinger (Q68.1)*

✓5th   **R68.8** **Other general symptoms and signs**

    R68.81 **Early satiety**

    R68.82 **Decreased libido**
         Decreased sexual desire

    R68.83 **Chills (without fever)**
         Chills NOS

      EXCLUDES 1   *chills with fever (R50.9)*

    R68.84 **Jaw pain**
         Mandibular pain
         Maxilla pain

      EXCLUDES 1   *temporomandibular joint arthralgia (M26.62)*

    R68.89 **Other general symptoms and signs**

 R69 **Illness, unspecified**
     Unknown and unspecified cases of morbidity

Abnormal findings on examination of blood, without diagnosis (R70-R79)

  EXCLUDES 1   *abnormalities (of)(on):*
       abnormal findings on antenatal screening of mother (O28-)
       coagulation hemorrhagic disorders (D65-D68)
       lipids (E78-)
       platelets and thrombocytes (D69-)
       white blood cells classified elsewhere (D70-D72)
     diagnostic abnormal findings classified elsewhere—see Alphabetical Index
     hemorrhagic and hematological disorders of newborn (P50-P61)

✓4th **R70** **Elevated erythrocyte sedimentation rate and abnormality of plasma viscosity**

  R70.0 **Elevated erythrocyte sedimentation rate**

  R70.1 **Abnormal plasma viscosity**

✓4th **R71** **Abnormality of red blood cells**

  EXCLUDES 1   *anemias (D50-D64)*
     anemia of premature infant (P61.2)
     benign (familial) polycythemia (D75.0)
     congenital anemias (P61.2-P61.4)
     newborn anemia due to isoimmunization (P55-)
     polycythemia neonatorum (P61.1)
     polycythemia NOS (D75.1)
     polycythemia vera (D45)
     secondary polycythemia (D75.1)

  R71.0 **Precipitous drop in hematocrit**
     Drop (precipitous) in hemoglobin
     Drop in hematocrit

  R71.8 **Other abnormality of red blood cells**
     Abnormal red-cell morphology NOS
     Abnormal red-cell volume NOS
     Anisocytosis
     Poikilocytosis

✓4th **R73** **Elevated blood glucose level**

  EXCLUDES 1   *diabetes mellitus (E08-E13)*
     diabetes mellitus in pregnancy, childbirth and the puerperium (O24-)
     neonatal disorders (P70.0-P70.2)
     postsurgical hypoinsulinemia (E89.1)

✓5th   **R73.0** **Abnormal glucose**

    EXCLUDES 1   *abnormal glucose in pregnancy (O99.81-)*
       diabetes mellitus (E08-E13)
       dysmetabolic syndrome X (E88.81)
       gestational diabetes (O24.4-)
       glycosuria (R81)
       hypoglycemia (E16.2)

    R73.01 **Impaired fasting glucose**
         Elevated fasting glucose

    R73.02 **Impaired glucose tolerance (oral)**
         Elevated glucose tolerance

    R73.09 **Other abnormal glucose**
         Abnormal glucose NOS
         Abnormal non-fasting glucose tolerance
         Latent diabetes
         Prediabetes

  R73.9 **Hyperglycemia, unspecified**

✓4th **R74** **Abnormal serum enzyme levels**

  R74.0 **Nonspecific elevation of levels of transaminase and lactic acid dehydrogenase [LDH]**

  R74.8 **Abnormal levels of other serum enzymes**
     Abnormal level of acid phosphatase
     Abnormal level of alkaline phosphatase
     Abnormal level of amylase
     Abnormal level of lipase [triacylglycerol lipase]

  R74.9 **Abnormal serum enzyme level, unspecified**

 R75 **Inconclusive laboratory evidence of human immunodeficiency virus [HIV]**
     Nonconclusive HIV-test finding in infants

  EXCLUDES 1   *asymptomatic human immunodeficiency virus [HIV] infection status (Z21)*
     human immunodeficiency virus [HIV] disease (B20)

✓4th **R76** **Other abnormal immunological findings in serum**

  R76.0 **Raised antibody titer**

    EXCLUDES 1   *isoimmunization in pregnancy (O36.0-O36.1)*
       isoimmunization affecting newborn (P55-)

  R76.1 **Abnormal reaction to tuberculin test**
     Abnormal result of Mantoux test

  R76.8 **Other specified abnormal immunological findings in serum**
     Raised level of immunoglobulins NOS

  R76.9 **Abnormal immunological finding in serum, unspecified**

✓4th **R77** **Other abnormalities of plasma proteins**

  EXCLUDES 1   *disorders of plasma-protein metabolism (E88.0)*

  R77.0 **Abnormality of albumin**

  R77.1 **Abnormality of globulin**
     Hyperglobulinemia NOS

  R77.2 **Abnormality of alphafetoprotein**

  R77.8 **Other specified abnormalities of plasma proteins**

  R77.9 **Abnormality of plasma protein, unspecified**

✓4th **R78** **Findings of drugs and other substances, not normally found in blood**

     Use additional code to identify any retained foreign body, if applicable (Z18.-)

  EXCLUDES 1   *mental or behavioral disorders due to psychoactive substance use (F10-F19)*

  R78.0 **Finding of alcohol in blood**
     Use additional external cause code (Y90-), for detail regarding alcohol level

  R78.1 **Finding of opiate drug in blood**

  R78.2 **Finding of cocaine in blood**

  R78.3 **Finding of hallucinogen in blood**

  R78.4 **Finding of other drugs of addictive potential in blood**

R78.5   **Finding of other psychotropic drug in blood**
R78.6   **Finding of steroid agent in blood**
✓5ᵗʰ   R78.7   **Finding of abnormal level of heavy metals in blood**
    R78.71   **Abnormal lead level in blood**
        EXCLUDES 1   *lead poisoning (T56.0-)*
    R78.79   **Finding of abnormal level of heavy metals in blood**
✓5ᵗʰ   R78.8   **Finding of other specified substances, not normally found in blood**
    R78.81   **Bacteremia**
        EXCLUDES 1   *sepsis—code to specified infection (A00-B99)*
    R78.89   **Finding of other specified substances, not normally found in blood**
        Finding of abnormal level of lithium in blood
R78.9   **Finding of unspecified substance, not normally found in blood**

✓4ᵗʰ   R79   **Other abnormal findings of blood chemistry**
    Use additional code to identify any retained foreign body, if applicable (Z18.-)
    EXCLUDES 1   *abnormality of fluid, electrolyte or acid-base balance (E86-E87)*
        asymptomatic hyperuricemia (E79.0)
        hyperglycemia NOS (R73.9)
        hypoglycemia NOS (E16.2)
        neonatal hypoglycemia (P70.3-P70.4)
        specific findings indicating disorder of:
        amino-acid metabolism (E70-E72)
        carbohydrate metabolism (E73-E74)
        lipid metabolism (E75-)
    R79.0   **Abnormal level of blood mineral**
        Abnormal blood level of cobalt
        Abnormal blood level of copper
        Abnormal blood level of iron
        Abnormal blood level of magnesium
        Abnormal blood level of mineral NEC
        Abnormal blood level of zinc
        EXCLUDES 1   *abnormal level of lithium (R78.89)*
            disorders of mineral metabolism (E83-)
            neonatal hypomagnesemia (P71.2)
            nutritional mineral deficiency (E58-E61)
    R79.1   **Abnormal coagulation profile**
        Abnormal or prolonged bleeding time
        Abnormal or prolonged coagulation time
        Abnormal or prolonged partial thromboplastin time [PTT]
        Abnormal or prolonged prothrombin time [PT]
        EXCLUDES 1   *coagulation defects (D68-)*
✓5ᵗʰ   R79.8   **Other specified abnormal findings of blood chemistry**
    R79.81   **Abnormal blood-gas level**
    R79.82   **Elevated C-reactive protein [CRP]**
    R79.89   **Other specified abnormal findings of blood chemistry**
    R79.9   **Abnormal finding of blood chemistry, unspecified**

Abnormal findings on examination of urine, without diagnosis (R80-R82)

    EXCLUDES 1   *abnormal findings on antenatal screening of mother (O28-)*
        diagnostic abnormal findings classified elsewhere—see Alphabetical Index
        specific findings indicating disorder of:
        amino-acid metabolism (E70-E72)
        carbohydrate metabolism (E73-E74)

✓4ᵗʰ   R80   **Proteinuria**
    EXCLUDES 1   *gestational proteinuria (O12.1-)*
    R80.0   **Isolated proteinuria**
        Idiopathic proteinuria
        EXCLUDES 1   *isolated proteinuria with specific morphological lesion (N06-)*
    R80.1   **Persistent proteinuria, unspecified**
    R80.2   **Orthostatic proteinuria, unspecified**
        Postural proteinuria
    R80.3   **Bence Jones proteinuria**
    R80.8   **Other proteinuria**
    R80.9   **Proteinuria, unspecified**
        Albuminuria NOS

R81   **Glycosuria**
    EXCLUDES 1   *renal glycosuria (E74.8)*

✓4ᵗʰ   R82   **Other and unspecified abnormal findings in urine**
    Chromoabnormalities in urine
    Use additional code to identify any retained foreign body, if applicable (Z18.-)
    EXCLUDES 2   *hematuria (R31-)*
    R82.0   **Chyluria**
        EXCLUDES 1   *filarial chyluria (B74-)*
    R82.1   **Myoglobinuria**
    R82.2   **Biliuria**
    R82.3   **Hemoglobinuria**
        EXCLUDES 1   *hemoglobinuria due to hemolysis from external causes NEC (D59.6)*
            hemoglobinuria due to paroxysmal nocturnal [Marchiafava-Micheli] (D59.5)
    R82.4   **Acetonuria**
        Ketonuria
    R82.5   **Elevated urine levels of drugs, medicaments and biological substances**
        Elevated urine levels of catecholamines
        Elevated urine levels of indoleacetic acid
        Elevated urine levels of 17-ketosteroids
        Elevated urine levels of steroids
    R82.6   **Abnormal urine levels of substances chiefly nonmedicinal as to source**
        Abnormal urine level of heavy metals
    R82.7   **Abnormal findings on microbiological examination of urine**
        Positive culture findings of urine
        EXCLUDES 1   *colonization status (Z22-)*
    R82.8   **Abnormal findings on cytological and histological examination of urine**
✓5ᵗʰ   R82.9   **Other and unspecified abnormal findings in urine**
    R82.90   **Unspecified abnormal findings in urine**
    R82.91   **Other chromoabnormalities of urine**
        Chromoconversion (dipstick)
        Idiopathic dipstick converts positive for blood with no cellular forms in sediment
        EXCLUDES 1   *hemoglobinuria (R82.3)*
            myoglobinuria (R82.1)
    R82.99   **Other abnormal findings in urine**
        Cells and casts in urine
        Crystalluria
        Melanuria

Abnormal findings on examination of other body fluids, substances and tissues, without diagnosis (R83-R89)

    EXCLUDES 1   *abnormal findings on antenatal screening of mother (O28-)*
        diagnostic abnormal findings classified elsewhere—see Alphabetical Index
    EXCLUDES 2   *abnormal findings on examination of blood, without diagnosis (R70-R79)*
        abnormal findings on examination of urine, without diagnosis (R80-R82)
        abnormal tumor markers (R97-)

✓4ᵗʰ   R83   **Abnormal findings in cerebrospinal fluid**
    R83.0   **Abnormal level of enzymes in cerebrospinal fluid**
    R83.1   **Abnormal level of hormones in cerebrospinal fluid**
    R83.2   **Abnormal level of other drugs, medicaments and biological substances in cerebrospinal fluid**
    R83.3   **Abnormal level of substances chiefly nonmedicinal as to source in cerebrospinal fluid**
    R83.4   **Abnormal immunological findings in cerebrospinal fluid**
    R83.5   **Abnormal microbiological findings in cerebrospinal fluid**
        Positive culture findings in cerebrospinal fluid
        EXCLUDES 1   *colonization status (Z22-)*
    R83.6   **Abnormal cytological findings in cerebrospinal fluid**
    R83.8   **Other abnormal findings in cerebrospinal fluid**
        Abnormal chromosomal findings in cerebrospinal fluid
    R83.9   **Unspecified abnormal finding in cerebrospinal fluid**

✓4th **R84** **Abnormal findings in specimens from respiratory organs and thorax**
Abnormal findings in bronchial washings
Abnormal findings in nasal secretions
Abnormal findings in pleural fluid
Abnormal findings in sputum
Abnormal findings in throat scrapings
EXCLUDES1 blood-stained sputum (R04.2)

R84.0 **Abnormal level of enzymes in specimens from respiratory organs and thorax**

R84.1 **Abnormal level of hormones in specimens from respiratory organs and thorax**

R84.2 **Abnormal level of other drugs, medicaments and biological substances in specimens from respiratory organs and thorax**

R84.3 **Abnormal level of substances chiefly nonmedicinal as to source in specimens from respiratory organs and thorax**

R84.4 **Abnormal immunological findings in specimens from respiratory organs and thorax**

R84.5 **Abnormal microbiological findings in specimens from respiratory organs and thorax**
Positive culture findings in specimens from respiratory organs and thorax
EXCLUDES1 colonization status (Z22-)

R84.6 **Abnormal cytological findings in specimens from respiratory organs and thorax**

R84.7 **Abnormal histological findings in specimens from respiratory organs and thorax**

R84.8 **Other abnormal findings in specimens from respiratory organs and thorax**
Abnormal chromosomal findings in specimens from respiratory organs and thorax

R84.9 **Unspecified abnormal finding in specimens from respiratory organs and thorax**

✓4th **R85** **Abnormal findings in specimens from digestive organs and abdominal cavity**
INCLUDES abnormal findings in peritoneal fluid
abnormal findings in saliva
EXCLUDES1 cloudy peritoneal dialysis effluent (R88.0)
fecal abnormalities (R19.5)

R85.0 **Abnormal level of enzymes in specimens from digestive organs and abdominal cavity**

R85.1 **Abnormal level of hormones in specimens from digestive organs and abdominal cavity**

R85.2 **Abnormal level of other drugs, medicaments and biological substances in specimens from digestive organs and abdominal cavity**

R85.3 **Abnormal level of substances chiefly nonmedicinal as to source in specimens from digestive organs and abdominal cavity**

R85.4 **Abnormal immunological findings in specimens from digestive organs and abdominal cavity**

R85.5 **Abnormal microbiological findings in specimens from digestive organs and abdominal cavity**
Positive culture findings in specimens from digestive organs and abdominal cavity
EXCLUDES1 colonization status (Z22-)

✓5th **R85.6** **Abnormal cytological findings in specimens from digestive organs and abdominal cavity**

✓6th **R85.61** **Abnormal cytologic smear of anus**
EXCLUDES1 abnormal cytological findings in specimens from other digestive organs and abdominal cavity (R85.69)
carcinoma in situ of anus (histologically confirmed) (D01.3)
anal intraepithelial neoplasia I [AIN I] (K62.82)
anal intraepithelial neoplasia II [AIN II] (K62.82)
anal intraepithelial neoplasia III [AIN III] (D01.3)
dysplasia (mild) (moderate) of anus (histologically confirmed) (K62.82)
severe dysplasia of anus (histologically confirmed) (D01.3)
EXCLUDES2 anal high risk human papillomavirus (HPV) DNA test positive (R85.81)
anal low risk human papillomavirus (HPV) DNA test positive (R85.82)

R85.610 **Atypical squamous cells of undetermined significance on cytologic smear of anus [ASC-US]**

R85.611 **Atypical squamous cells cannot exclude high grade squamous intraepithelial lesion on cytologic smear of anus [ASC-H]**

R85.612 **Low grade squamous intraepithelial lesion on cytologic smear of anus [LGSIL]**

R85.613 **High grade squamous intraepithelial lesion on cytologic smear of anus [HGSIL]**

R85.614 **Cytologic evidence of malignancy on smear of anus**

R85.615 **Unsatisfactory cytologic smear of anus**
Inadequate sample of cytologic smear of anus

R85.616 **Satisfactory anal smear but lacking transformation zone**

R85.618 **Other abnormal cytological findings on specimens from anus**

R85.619 **Unspecified abnormal cytological findings in specimens from anus**
Abnormal anal cytology NOS
Atypical glandular cells of anus NOS

R85.69 **Abnormal cytological findings in specimens from other digestive organs and abdominal cavity**

R85.7 **Abnormal histological findings in specimens from digestive organs and abdominal cavity**

✓5th **R85.8** **Other abnormal findings in specimens from digestive organs and abdominal cavity**

R85.81 **Anal high risk human papillomavirus [HPV] DNA test positive**
EXCLUDES1 anogenital warts due to human papillomavirus (HPV) (A63.0)
condyloma acuminatum (A63.0)

R85.82 **Anal low risk human papillomavirus [HPV] DNA test positive**
Use additional code for associated human papillomavirus (B97.7)

R85.89 **Other abnormal findings in specimens from digestive organs and abdominal cavity**
Abnormal chromosomal findings in specimens from digestive organs and abdominal cavity

R85.9 **Unspecified abnormal finding in specimens from digestive organs and abdominal cavity**

✓4th **R86** **Abnormal findings in specimens from male genital organs**
INCLUDES abnormal findings in prostatic secretions
abnormal findings in semen, seminal fluid
abnormal spermatozoa
EXCLUDES1 azoospermia (N46.0-)
oligospermia (N46.1-)

R86.0 **Abnormal level of enzymes in specimens from male genital organs**

R86.1 **Abnormal level of hormones in specimens from male genital organs**

EXCLUDES1 Not coded here   EXCLUDES2 Not included here   *Manifestation Code*

R86.2　Abnormal level of other drugs, medicaments and biological substances in specimens from male genital organs

R86.3　Abnormal level of substances chiefly nonmedicinal as to source in specimens from male genital organs

R86.4　Abnormal immunological findings in specimens from male genital organs

R86.5　Abnormal microbiological findings in specimens from male genital organs

　　　Positive culture findings in specimens from male genital organs

　　　EXCLUDES 1　colonization status (Z22-)

R86.6　Abnormal cytological findings in specimens from male genital organs

R86.7　Abnormal histological findings in specimens from male genital organs

R86.8　Other abnormal findings in specimens from male genital organs

　　　Abnormal chromosomal findings in specimens from male genital organs

R86.9　Unspecified abnormal finding in specimens from male genital organs

✓4ᵗʰ **R87**　**Abnormal findings in specimens from female genital organs**

　　　Abnormal findings in secretion and smears from cervix uteri
　　　Abnormal findings in secretion and smears from vagina
　　　Abnormal findings in secretion and smears from vulva

R87.0　Abnormal level of enzymes in specimens from female genital organs

R87.1　Abnormal level of hormones in specimens from female genital organs

R87.2　Abnormal level of other drugs, medicaments and biological substances in specimens from female genital organs

R87.3　Abnormal level of substances chiefly nonmedicinal as to source in specimens from female genital organs

R87.4　Abnormal immunological findings in specimens from female genital organs

R87.5　Abnormal microbiological findings in specimens from female genital organs

　　　Positive culture findings in specimens from female genital organs

　　　EXCLUDES 1　colonization status (Z22-)

✓5ᵗʰ **R87.6**　Abnormal cytological findings in specimens from female genital organs

✓6ᵗʰ　**R87.61**　Abnormal cytological findings in specimens from cervix uteri

　　　　EXCLUDES 1　abnormal cytological findings in specimens from other female genital organs (R87.69)
　　　　　abnormal cytological findings in specimens from vagina (R87.62-)
　　　　　carcinoma in situ of cervix uteri (histologically confirmed) (D06-)
　　　　　cervical intraepithelial neoplasia I [CIN I] (N87.0)
　　　　　cervical intraepithelial neoplasia II [CIN II] (N87.1)
　　　　　cervical intraepithelial neoplasia III [CIN III] (D06-)
　　　　　dysplasia (mild) (moderate) of cervix uteri (histologically confirmed) (N87-)
　　　　　severe dysplasia of cervix uteri (histologically confirmed) (D06-)

　　　　EXCLUDES 2　cervical high risk human papillomavirus (HPV) DNA test positive (R87.810)
　　　　　cervical low risk human papillomavirus (HPV) DNA test positive (R87.820)

　　　　R87.610　Atypical squamous cells of undetermined significance on cytologic smear of cervix [ASC-US]

　　　　R87.611　Atypical squamous cells cannot exclude high grade squamous intraepithelial lesion on cytologic smear of cervix [ASC-H]

　　　　R87.612　Low grade squamous intraepithelial lesion on cytologic smear of cervix [LGSIL]

　　　　R87.613　High grade squamous intraepithelial lesion on cytologic smear of cervix [HGSIL]

　　　　R87.614　Cytologic evidence of malignancy on smear of cervix

　　　　R87.615　Unsatisfactory cytologic smear of cervix
　　　　　Inadequate sample of cytologic smear of cervix

　　　　R87.616　Satisfactory cervical smear but lacking transformation zone

　　　　R87.618　Other abnormal cytological findings on specimens from cervix uteri

　　　　R87.619　Unspecified abnormal cytological findings in specimens from cervix uteri
　　　　　Abnormal cervical cytology NOS
　　　　　Abnormal Papanicolaou smear of cervix NOS
　　　　　Abnormal thin preparation smear of cervix NOS
　　　　　Atypical endocervial cells of cervix NOS
　　　　　Atypical endometrial cells of cervix NOS
　　　　　Atypical glandular cells of cervix NOS

✓6ᵗʰ　**R87.62**　Abnormal cytological findings in specimens from vagina

　　　　Use additional code to identify acquired absence of uterus and cervix, if applicable (Z90.71-)

　　　　EXCLUDES 1　abnormal cytological findings in specimens from cervix uteri (R87.61-)
　　　　　abnormal cytological findings in specimens from other female genital organs (R87.69)
　　　　　carcinoma in situ of vagina (histologically confirmed) (D07.2)
　　　　　dysplasia (mild) (moderate) of vagina (histologically confirmed) (N89-)
　　　　　severe dysplasia of vagina (histologically confirmed) (D07.2)
　　　　　vaginal intraepithelial neoplasia I [VAIN I] (N89.0)
　　　　　vaginal intraepithelial neoplasia II [VAIN II] (N89.1)
　　　　　vaginal intraepithelial neoplasia III [VAIN III] (D07.2)

　　　　EXCLUDES 2　vaginal high risk human papillomavirus (HPV) DNA test positive (R87.811)
　　　　　vaginal low risk human papillomavirus (HPV) DNA test positive (R87.821)

　　　　R87.620　Atypical squamous cells of undetermined significance on cytologic smear of vagina [ASC-US]

　　　　R87.621　Atypical squamous cells cannot exclude high grade squamous intraepithelial lesion on cytologic smear of vagina [ASC-H]

　　　　R87.622　Low grade squamous intraepithelial lesion on cytologic smear of vagina [LGSIL]

　　　　R87.623　High grade squamous intraepithelial lesion on cytologic smear of vagina [HGSIL]

　　　　R87.624　Cytologic evidence of malignancy on smear of vagina

　　　　R87.625　Unsatisfactory cytologic smear of vagina
　　　　　Inadequate sample of cytologic smear of vagina

　　　　R87.628　Other abnormal cytological findings on specimens from vagina

　　　　R87.629　Unspecified abnormal cytological findings in specimens from vagina
　　　　　Abnormal Papanicolaou smear of vagina NOS
　　　　　Abnormal thin preparation smear of vagina NOS
　　　　　Abnormal vaginal cytology NOS
　　　　　Atypical endocervical cells of vagina NOS
　　　　　Atypical endometrial cells of vagina NOS
　　　　　Atypical glandular cells of vagina NOS

　　R87.69　Abnormal cytological findings in specimens from other female genital organs
　　　　Abnormal cytological findings in specimens from female genital organs NOS

　　　　EXCLUDES 1　dysplasia of vulva (histologically confirmed) (N90.0-N90.3)

Symptoms, Signs and Abnormal Clinical and Laboratory Findings

R87.7–R93.7

R87.7 Abnormal histological findings in specimens from female genital organs

EXCLUDES 1   *carcinoma in situ (histologically confirmed) of female genital organs (D06-D07.3)*
cervical intraepithelial neoplasia I [CIN I] (N87.0)
cervical intraepithelial neoplasia II [CIN II] (N87.1)
cervical intraepithelial neoplasia III [CIN III] (D06-)
dysplasia (mild) (moderate) of cervix uteri (histologically confirmed) (N87-)
dysplasia (mild) (moderate) of vagina (histologically confirmed) (N89-)
severe dysplasia of cervix uteri (histologically confirmed) (D06-)
severe dysplasia of vagina (histologically confirmed) (D07.2)
vaginal intraepithelial neoplasia I [VAIN I] (N89.0)
vaginal intraepithelial neoplasia II [VAIN II] (N89.1)
vaginal intraepithelial neoplasia III [VAIN III] (D07.2)

✓5ᵗʰ **R87.8 Other abnormal findings in specimens from female genital organs**

✓6ᵗʰ **R87.81 High risk human papillomavirus [HPV] DNA test positive from female genital organs**

EXCLUDES 1   *anogenital warts due to human papillomavirus (HPV) (A63.0)*
condyloma acuminatum (A63.0)

R87.810 Cervical high risk human papillomavirus [HPV] DNA test positive

R87.811 Vaginal high risk human papillomavirus [HPV] DNA test positive

✓6ᵗʰ **R87.82 Low risk human papillomavirus [HPV] DNA test positive from female genital organs**

Use additional code for associated human papillomavirus (B97.7)

R87.820 Cervical low risk human papillomavirus [HPV] DNA test positive

R87.821 Vaginal low risk human papillomavirus [HPV] DNA test positive

R87.89 Other abnormal findings in specimens from female genital organs

Abnormal chromosomal findings in specimens from female genital organs

R87.9 Unspecified abnormal finding in specimens from female genital organs

✓4ᵗʰ **R88 Abnormal findings in other body fluids and substances**

R88.0 Cloudy (hemodialysis) (peritoneal) dialysis effluent

R88.8 Abnormal findings in other body fluids and substances

✓4ᵗʰ **R89 Abnormal findings in specimens from other organs, systems and tissues**

INCLUDES   abnormal findings in nipple discharge
abnormal findings in synovial fluid
abnormal findings in wound secretions

R89.0 Abnormal level of enzymes in specimens from other organs, systems and tissues

R89.1 Abnormal level of hormones in specimens from other organs, systems and tissues

R89.2 Abnormal level of other drugs, medicaments and biological substances in specimens from other organs, systems and tissues

R89.3 Abnormal level of substances chiefly nonmedicinal as to source in specimens from other organs, systems and tissues

R89.4 Abnormal immunological findings in specimens from other organs, systems and tissues

R89.5 Abnormal microbiological findings in specimens from other organs, systems and tissues

Positive culture findings in specimens from other organs, systems and tissues

EXCLUDES 1   *colonization status (Z22-)*

R89.6 Abnormal cytological findings in specimens from other organs, systems and tissues

R89.7 Abnormal histological findings in specimens from other organs, systems and tissues

R89.8 Other abnormal findings in specimens from other organs, systems and tissues

Abnormal chromosomal findings in specimens from other organs, systems and tissues

R89.9 Unspecified abnormal finding in specimens from other organs, systems and tissues

Abnormal findings on diagnostic imaging and in function studies, without diagnosis (R90-R94)

INCLUDES   nonspecific abnormal findings on diagnostic imaging by computerized axial tomography [CAT scan]
nonspecific abnormal findings on diagnostic imaging by magnetic resonance imaging [MRI][NMR]
nonspecific abnormal findings on diagnostic imaging by positron emission tomography [PET scan]
nonspecific abnormal findings on diagnostic imaging by thermography
nonspecific abnormal findings on diagnostic imaging by ultrasound [echogram]
nonspecific abnormal findings on diagnostic imaging by X-ray examination

EXCLUDES 1   *abnormal findings on antenatal screening of mother (O28-)*
diagnostic abnormal findings classified elsewhere—see Alphabetical Index

✓4ᵗʰ **R90 Abnormal findings on diagnostic imaging of central nervous system**

R90.0 Intracranial space-occupying lesion found on diagnostic imaging of central nervous system

✓5ᵗʰ **R90.8 Other abnormal findings on diagnostic imaging of central nervous system**

R90.81 Abnormal echoencephalogram

R90.82 White matter disease, unspecified

R90.89 Other abnormal findings on diagnostic imaging of central nervous system

Other cerebrovascular abnormality found on diagnostic imaging of central nervous system

R91 Abnormal findings on diagnostic imaging of lung

Coin lesion NOS found on diagnostic imaging of lung
Lung mass NOS found on diagnostic imaging of lung

✓4ᵗʰ **R92 Abnormal and inconclusive findings on diagnostic imaging of breast**

R92.0 Mammographic microcalcification found on diagnostic imaging of breast

EXCLUDES 2   *mammographic calcification (calculus) found on diagnostic imaging of breast (R92.1)*

R92.1 Mammographic calcification found on diagnostic imaging of breast

Mammographic calculus found on diagnostic imaging of breast

R92.2 Inconclusive mammogram

Dense breasts NOS
Inconclusive mammogram NEC
Inconclusive mammography due to dense breasts
Inconclusive mammography NEC

R92.8 Other abnormal and inconclusive findings on diagnostic imaging of breast

✓4ᵗʰ **R93 Abnormal findings on diagnostic imaging of other body structures**

R93.0 Abnormal findings on diagnostic imaging of skull and head, not elsewhere classified

EXCLUDES 1   *intracranial space-occupying lesion found on diagnostic imaging (R90.0)*

R93.1 Abnormal findings on diagnostic imaging of heart and coronary circulation

Abnormal echocardiogram NOS
Abnormal heart shadow

R93.2 Abnormal findings on diagnostic imaging of liver and biliary tract

Nonvisualization of gallbladder

R93.3 Abnormal findings on diagnostic imaging of other parts of digestive tract

R93.4 Abnormal findings on diagnostic imaging of urinary organs

Filling defect of bladder found on diagnostic imaging
Filling defect of kidney found on diagnostic imaging
Filling defect of ureter found on diagnostic imaging

EXCLUDES 1   *hypertrophy of kidney (N28.81)*

R93.5 Abnormal findings on diagnostic imaging of other abdominal regions, including retroperitoneum

R93.6 Abnormal findings on diagnostic imaging of limbs

EXCLUDES 2   *abnormal finding in skin and subcutaneous tissue (R93.8)*

R93.7 Abnormal findings on diagnostic imaging of other parts of musculoskeletal system

EXCLUDES 2   *abnormal findings on diagnostic imaging of skull (R93.0)*

EXCLUDES 1   Not coded here   EXCLUDES 2   Not included here   *Manifestation Code*

R93.8   Abnormal findings on diagnostic imaging of other specified body structures
Abnormal finding by radioisotope localization of placenta
Abnormal radiological finding in skin and subcutaneous tissue
Mediastinal shift

R93.9   Diagnostic imaging inconclusive due to excess body fat of patient

☑4ᵗʰ **R94   Abnormal results of function studies**
INCLUDES   abnormal results of radionuclide [radioisotope] uptake studies
abnormal results of scintigraphy

☑5ᵗʰ **R94.0   Abnormal results of function studies of central nervous system**

R94.01   Abnormal electroencephalogram [EEG]
R94.02   Abnormal brain scan
R94.09   Abnormal results of other function studies of central nervous system

☑5ᵗʰ **R94.1   Abnormal results of function studies of peripheral nervous system and special senses**

☑6ᵗʰ **R94.11   Abnormal results of function studies of eye**
R94.110   Abnormal electro-oculogram [EOG]
R94.111   Abnormal electroretinogram [ERG]
Abnormal retinal function study
R94.112   Abnormal visually evoked potential [VEP]
R94.113   Abnormal oculomotor study
R94.118   Abnormal results of other function studies of eye

☑6ᵗʰ **R94.12   Abnormal results of function studies of ear and other special senses**
R94.120   Abnormal auditory function study
R94.121   Abnormal vestibular function study
R94.128   Abnormal results of other function studies of ear and other special senses

☑6ᵗʰ **R94.13   Abnormal results of function studies of peripheral nervous system**
R94.130   Abnormal response to nerve stimulation, unspecified
R94.131   Abnormal electromyogram [EMG]
EXCLUDES 1   *electromyogram of eye (R94.113)*
R94.138   Abnormal results of other function studies of peripheral nervous system

R94.2   Abnormal results of pulmonary function studies
Reduced ventilatory capacity
Reduced vital capacity

☑5ᵗʰ **R94.3   Abnormal results of cardiovascular function studies**
R94.30   Abnormal result of cardiovascular function study, unspecified
R94.31   Abnormal electrocardiogram [ECG] [EKG]
EXCLUDES 1   *long QT syndrome (I45.81)*
R94.39   Abnormal result of other cardiovascular function study
Abnormal electrophysiological intracardiac studies
Abnormal phonocardiogram
Abnormal vectorcardiogram

R94.4   Abnormal results of kidney function studies
Abnormal renal function test

R94.5   Abnormal results of liver function studies

R94.6   Abnormal results of thyroid function studies

R94.7   Abnormal results of other endocrine function studies
EXCLUDES 2   *abnormal glucose (R73.0-)*

R94.8   Abnormal results of function studies of other organs and systems
Abnormal basal metabolic rate [BMR]
Abnormal bladder function test
Abnormal splenic function test

Abnormal tumor markers (R97)

☑4ᵗʰ **R97   Abnormal tumor markers**
Elevated tumor associated antigens [TAA]
Elevated tumor specific antigens [TSA]
R97.0   Elevated carcinoembryonic antigen [CEA]
R97.1   Elevated cancer antigen 125 [CA 125]
R97.2   Elevated prostate specific antigen [PSA]
R97.8   Other abnormal tumor markers

Ill-defined and unknown cause of mortality (R99)

R99   Ill-defined and unknown cause of mortality
Death (unexplained) NOS
Unspecified cause of mortality

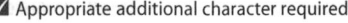 Appropriate additional character required   ☑x7ᵗʰ Requires 7th character, placeholder x must fill empty characters

Chapter 19. Injury, Poisoning and Certain Other Consequences of External Causes (S00-T88)

NOTE   Use secondary code(s) from Chapter 20, External causes of morbidity, to indicate cause of injury. Codes within the T section that include the external cause do not require an additional external cause code

Use additional code to identify any retained foreign body, if applicable (Z18.-)

EXCLUDES 1   birth trauma (P10-P15)
obstetric trauma (O70-O71)

This chapter contains the following blocks:

S00-S09	Injuries to the head
S10-S19	Injuries to the neck
S20-S29	Injuries to the thorax
S30-S39	Injuries to the abdomen, lower back, lumbar spine, pelvis and external genitals
S40-S49	Injuries to the shoulder and upper arm
S50-S59	Injuries to the elbow and forearm
S60-S69	Injuries to the wrist and hand
S70-S79	Injuries to the hip and thigh
S80-S89	Injuries to the knee and lower leg
S90-S99	Injuries to the ankle and foot
T07	Unspecified multiple injuries
T14	Injury of unspecified body region
T15-T19	Effects of foreign body entering through natural orifice
T20-T32	Burns and corrosions
T33-T34	Frostbite
T36-T50	Poisoning by, adverse effect of and underdosing of drugs, medicaments and biological substances
T51-T65	Toxic effects of substances chiefly nonmedicinal as to source
T66-T78	Other and unspecified effects of external causes
T79	Certain early complications of trauma
T80-T88	Complications of surgical and medical care, not elsewhere classified

The chapter uses the S-section for coding different types of injuries related to single body regions and the T-section to cover injuries to unspecified body regions as well as poisoning and certain other consequences of external causes.

Injuries to the head (S00-S09)

INCLUDES   injuries of ear
injuries of eye
injuries of face [any part]
injuries of gum
injuries of jaw
injuries of oral cavity
injuries of palate
injuries of periocular area
injuries of scalp
injuries of temporomandibular joint area
injuries of tongue
injuries of tooth

Code also for any associated infection

EXCLUDES 2   burns and corrosions (T20-T32)
effects of foreign body in ear (T16)
effects of foreign body in larynx (T17.3)
effects of foreign body in mouth NOS (T18.0)
effects of foreign body in nose (T17.0-T17.1)
effects of foreign body in pharynx (T17.2)
effects of foreign body on external eye (T15-)
frostbite (T33-T34)
insect bite or sting, venomous (T63.4)

✓4ᵗʰ **S00**   **Superficial injury of head**

EXCLUDES 1   diffuse cerebral contusion (S06.2-)
focal cerebral contusion (S06.3-)
injury of eye and orbit (S05-)
open wound of head (S01-)

The appropriate 7th character is to be added to each code from category S00.
A   initial encounter
D   subsequent encounter
S   sequela

✓5ᵗʰ   **S00.0**   **Superficial injury of scalp**
   ✓x7ᵗʰ   **S00.00**   **Unspecified superficial injury of scalp**
   ✓x7ᵗʰ   **S00.01**   **Abrasion of scalp**
   ✓x7ᵗʰ   **S00.02**   **Blister (nonthermal) of scalp**

✓x7ᵗʰ   **S00.03**   **Contusion of scalp**
   Bruise of scalp
   Hematoma of scalp
✓x7ᵗʰ   **S00.04**   **External constriction of part of scalp**
✓x7ᵗʰ   **S00.05**   **Superficial foreign body of scalp**
   Splinter in the scalp
✓x7ᵗʰ   **S00.06**   **Insect bite (nonvenomous) of scalp**
✓x7ᵗʰ   **S00.07**   **Other superficial bite of scalp**
   EXCLUDES 1   open bite of scalp (S01.05)

✓5ᵗʰ   **S00.1**   **Contusion of eyelid and periocular area**
   Black eye
   EXCLUDES 2   contusion of eyeball and orbital tissues (S05.1)
   ✓x7ᵗʰ   **S00.10**   **Contusion of unspecified eyelid and periocular area**
   ✓x7ᵗʰ   **S00.11**   **Contusion of right eyelid and periocular area**
   ✓x7ᵗʰ   **S00.12**   **Contusion of left eyelid and periocular area**

✓5ᵗʰ   **S00.2**   **Other and unspecified superficial injuries of eyelid and periocular area**
   EXCLUDES 2   superficial injury of conjunctiva and cornea (S05.0-)
   ✓6ᵗʰ   **S00.20**   **Unspecified superficial injury of eyelid and periocular area**
     ✓7ᵗʰ   **S00.201**   **Unspecified superficial injury of right eyelid and periocular area**
     ✓7ᵗʰ   **S00.202**   **Unspecified superficial injury of left eyelid and periocular area**
     ✓7ᵗʰ   **S00.209**   **Unspecified superficial injury of unspecified eyelid and periocular area**
   ✓6ᵗʰ   **S00.21**   **Abrasion of eyelid and periocular area**
     ✓7ᵗʰ   **S00.211**   **Abrasion of right eyelid and periocular area**
     ✓7ᵗʰ   **S00.212**   **Abrasion of left eyelid and periocular area**
     ✓7ᵗʰ   **S00.219**   **Abrasion of unspecified eyelid and periocular area**
   ✓6ᵗʰ   **S00.22**   **Blister (nonthermal) of eyelid and periocular area**
     ✓7ᵗʰ   **S00.221**   **Blister (nonthermal) of right eyelid and periocular area**
     ✓7ᵗʰ   **S00.222**   **Blister (nonthermal) of left eyelid and periocular area**
     ✓7ᵗʰ   **S00.229**   **Blister (nonthermal) of unspecified eyelid and periocular area**
   ✓6ᵗʰ   **S00.24**   **External constriction of eyelid and periocular area**
     ✓7ᵗʰ   **S00.241**   **External constriction of right eyelid and periocular area**
     ✓7ᵗʰ   **S00.242**   **External constriction of left eyelid and periocular area**
     ✓7ᵗʰ   **S00.249**   **External constriction of unspecified eyelid and periocular area**
   ✓6ᵗʰ   **S00.25**   **Superficial foreign body of eyelid and periocular area**
     Splinter of eyelid and periocular area
     EXCLUDES 2   retained foreign body in eyelid (H02.81-)
     ✓7ᵗʰ   **S00.251**   **Superficial foreign body of right eyelid and periocular area**
     ✓7ᵗʰ   **S00.252**   **Superficial foreign body of left eyelid and periocular area**
     ✓7ᵗʰ   **S00.259**   **Superficial foreign body of unspecified eyelid and periocular area**
   ✓6ᵗʰ   **S00.26**   **Insect bite (nonvenomous) of eyelid and periocular area**
     ✓7ᵗʰ   **S00.261**   **Insect bite (nonvenomous) of right eyelid and periocular area**
     ✓7ᵗʰ   **S00.262**   **Insect bite (nonvenomous) of left eyelid and periocular area**
     ✓7ᵗʰ   **S00.269**   **Insect bite (nonvenomous) of unspecified eyelid and periocular area**
   ✓6ᵗʰ   **S00.27**   **Other superficial bite of eyelid and periocular area**
     EXCLUDES 1   open bite of eyelid and periocular area (S01.15)
     ✓7ᵗʰ   **S00.271**   **Other superficial bite of right eyelid and periocular area**
     ✓7ᵗʰ   **S00.272**   **Other superficial bite of left eyelid and periocular area**
     ✓7ᵗʰ   **S00.279**   **Other superficial bite of unspecified eyelid and periocular area**

✓5ᵗʰ   **S00.3**   **Superficial injury of nose**
   ✓x7ᵗʰ   **S00.30**   **Unspecified superficial injury of nose**

EXCLUDES 1   Not coded here   **EXCLUDES 2**   Not included here   *Manifestation Code*

✓x7ᵗʰ **S00.31** **Abrasion of nose**

✓x7ᵗʰ **S00.32** **Blister (nonthermal) of nose**

✓x7ᵗʰ **S00.33** **Contusion of nose**
　　　Bruise of nose
　　　Hematoma of nose

✓x7ᵗʰ **S00.34** **External constriction of nose**

✓x7ᵗʰ **S00.35** **Superficial foreign body of nose**
　　　Splinter in the nose

✓x7ᵗʰ **S00.36** **Insect bite (nonvenomous) of nose**

✓x7ᵗʰ **S00.37** **Other superficial bite of nose**
　　　EXCLUDES 1　*open bite of nose (S01.25)*

✓5ᵗʰ **S00.4** **Superficial injury of ear**

　✓6ᵗʰ **S00.40** **Unspecified superficial injury of ear**

　　✓7ᵗʰ **S00.401** **Unspecified superficial injury of right ear**

　　✓7ᵗʰ **S00.402** **Unspecified superficial injury of left ear**

　　✓7ᵗʰ **S00.409** **Unspecified superficial injury of unspecified ear**

　✓6ᵗʰ **S00.41** **Abrasion of ear**

　　✓7ᵗʰ **S00.411** **Abrasion of right ear**

　　✓7ᵗʰ **S00.412** **Abrasion of left ear**

　　✓7ᵗʰ **S00.419** **Abrasion of unspecified ear**

　✓6ᵗʰ **S00.42** **Blister (nonthermal) of ear**

　　✓7ᵗʰ **S00.421** **Blister (nonthermal) of right ear**

　　✓7ᵗʰ **S00.422** **Blister (nonthermal) of left ear**

　　✓7ᵗʰ **S00.429** **Blister (nonthermal) of unspecified ear**

　✓6ᵗʰ **S00.43** **Contusion of ear**
　　　Bruise of ear
　　　Hematoma of ear

　　✓7ᵗʰ **S00.431** **Contusion of right ear**

　　✓7ᵗʰ **S00.432** **Contusion of left ear**

　　✓7ᵗʰ **S00.439** **Contusion of unspecified ear**

　✓6ᵗʰ **S00.44** **External constriction of ear**

　　✓7ᵗʰ **S00.441** **External constriction of right ear**

　　✓7ᵗʰ **S00.442** **External constriction of left ear**

　　✓7ᵗʰ **S00.449** **External constriction of unspecified ear**

　✓6ᵗʰ **S00.45** **Superficial foreign body of ear**
　　　Splinter in the ear

　　✓7ᵗʰ **S00.451** **Superficial foreign body of right ear**

　　✓7ᵗʰ **S00.452** **Superficial foreign body of left ear**

　　✓7ᵗʰ **S00.459** **Superficial foreign body of unspecified ear**

　✓6ᵗʰ **S00.46** **Insect bite (nonvenomous) of ear**

　　✓7ᵗʰ **S00.461** **Insect bite (nonvenomous) of right ear**

　　✓7ᵗʰ **S00.462** **Insect bite (nonvenomous) of left ear**

　　✓7ᵗʰ **S00.469** **Insect bite (nonvenomous) of unspecified ear**

　✓6ᵗʰ **S00.47** **Other superficial bite of ear**
　　　EXCLUDES 1　*open bite of ear (S01.35)*

　　✓7ᵗʰ **S00.471** **Other superficial bite of right ear**

　　✓7ᵗʰ **S00.472** **Other superficial bite of left ear**

　　✓7ᵗʰ **S00.479** **Other superficial bite of unspecified ear**

✓5ᵗʰ **S00.5** **Superficial injury of lip and oral cavity**

　✓6ᵗʰ **S00.50** **Unspecified superficial injury of lip and oral cavity**

　　✓7ᵗʰ **S00.501** **Unspecified superficial injury of lip**

　　✓7ᵗʰ **S00.502** **Unspecified superficial injury of oral cavity**

　✓6ᵗʰ **S00.51** **Abrasion of lip and oral cavity**

　　✓7ᵗʰ **S00.511** **Abrasion of lip**

　　✓7ᵗʰ **S00.512** **Abrasion of oral cavity**

　✓6ᵗʰ **S00.52** **Blister (nonthermal) of lip and oral cavity**

　　✓7ᵗʰ **S00.521** **Blister (nonthermal) of lip**

　　✓7ᵗʰ **S00.522** **Blister (nonthermal) of oral cavity**

　✓6ᵗʰ **S00.53** **Contusion of lip and oral cavity**

　　✓7ᵗʰ **S00.531** **Contusion of lip**
　　　　Bruise of lip
　　　　Hematoma of oral cavity

　　✓7ᵗʰ **S00.532** **Contusion of oral cavity**
　　　　Bruise of lip
　　　　Hematoma of oral cavity

　✓6ᵗʰ **S00.54** **External constriction of lip and oral cavity**

　　✓7ᵗʰ **S00.541** **External constriction of lip**

　　✓7ᵗʰ **S00.542** **External constriction of oral cavity**

　✓6ᵗʰ **S00.55** **Superficial foreign body of lip and oral cavity**

　　✓7ᵗʰ **S00.551** **Superficial foreign body of lip**
　　　　Splinter of lip and oral cavity

　　✓7ᵗʰ **S00.552** **Superficial foreign body of oral cavity**
　　　　Splinter of lip and oral cavity

　✓6ᵗʰ **S00.56** **Insect bite (nonvenomous) of lip and oral cavity**

　　✓7ᵗʰ **S00.561** **Insect bite (nonvenomous) of lip**

　　✓7ᵗʰ **S00.562** **Insect bite (nonvenomous) of oral cavity**

　✓6ᵗʰ **S00.57** **Other superficial bite of lip and oral cavity**

　　✓7ᵗʰ **S00.571** **Other superficial bite of lip**
　　　　EXCLUDES 1　*open bite of lip (S01.551)*

　　✓7ᵗʰ **S00.572** **Other superficial bite of oral cavity**
　　　　EXCLUDES 1　*open bite of oral cavity (S01.552)*

✓5ᵗʰ **S00.8** **Superficial injury of other parts of head**

　✓x7ᵗʰ **S00.80** **Unspecified superficial injury of other part of head**

　✓x7ᵗʰ **S00.81** **Abrasion of other part of head**

　✓x7ᵗʰ **S00.82** **Blister (nonthermal) of other part of head**

　✓x7ᵗʰ **S00.83** **Contusion of other part of head**
　　　Bruise of other part of head
　　　Hematoma of other part of head

　✓x7ᵗʰ **S00.84** **External constriction of other part of head**

　✓x7ᵗʰ **S00.85** **Superficial foreign body of other part of head**
　　　Splinter in other part of head

　✓x7ᵗʰ **S00.86** **Insect bite (nonvenomous) of other part of head**

　✓x7ᵗʰ **S00.87** **Other superficial bite of other part of head**
　　　EXCLUDES 1　*open bite of other part of head (S01.85)*

✓5ᵗʰ **S00.9** **Superficial injury of unspecified part of head**

　✓x7ᵗʰ **S00.90** **Unspecified superficial injury of unspecified part of head**

　✓x7ᵗʰ **S00.91** **Abrasion of unspecified part of head**

　✓x7ᵗʰ **S00.92** **Blister (nonthermal) of unspecified part of head**

　✓x7ᵗʰ **S00.93** **Contusion of unspecified part of head**
　　　Bruise of head
　　　Hematoma of head

　✓x7ᵗʰ **S00.94** **External constriction of unspecified part of head**

　✓x7ᵗʰ **S00.95** **Superficial foreign body of unspecified part of head**
　　　Splinter of head

　✓x7ᵗʰ **S00.96** **Insect bite (nonvenomous) of unspecified part of head**

　✓x7ᵗʰ **S00.97** **Other superficial bite of unspecified part of head**
　　　EXCLUDES 1　*open bite of head (S01.95)*

✓4ᵗʰ **S01** **Open wound of head**
　　Code also any associated:
　　　injury of cranial nerve (S04-)
　　　injury of muscle and tendon of head (S09.1-)
　　　intracranial injury (S06-)
　　　wound infection
　　EXCLUDES 1　*open skull fracture (S02- with 7th character B)*
　　EXCLUDES 2　*injury of eye and orbit (S05-)*
　　　　　　　　traumatic amputation of part of head (S08-)

> The appropriate 7th character is to be added to each code from category S01.
> A　initial encounter
> D　subsequent encounter
> S　sequela

✓5ᵗʰ **S01.0** **Open wound of scalp**
　　EXCLUDES 1　*avulsion of scalp (S08.0)*

　✓x7ᵗʰ **S01.00** **Unspecified open wound of scalp**

　✓x7ᵗʰ **S01.01** **Laceration without foreign body of scalp**

　✓x7ᵗʰ **S01.02** **Laceration with foreign body of scalp**

　✓x7ᵗʰ **S01.03** **Puncture wound without foreign body of scalp**

　✓x7ᵗʰ **S01.04** **Puncture wound with foreign body of scalp**

　✓x7ᵗʰ **S01.05** **Open bite of scalp**
　　　Bite of scalp NOS
　　　EXCLUDES 1　*superficial bite of scalp (S00.06, S00.07-)*

✓5ᵗʰ **S01.1** **Open wound of eyelid and periocular area**
　　Open wound of eyelid and periocular area with or without involvement of lacrimal passages

　✓6ᵗʰ **S01.10** **Unspecified open wound of eyelid and periocular area**

　　✓7ᵗʰ **S01.101** **Unspecified open wound of right eyelid and periocular area**

✓ Appropriate additional character required　　　　✓x7ᵗʰ Requires 7th character, placeholder x must fill empty characters

✓7th   **S01.102**   **Unspecified open wound of left eyelid and periocular area**

✓7th   **S01.109**   **Unspecified open wound of unspecified eyelid and periocular area**

✓6th   **S01.11**   **Laceration without foreign body of eyelid and periocular area**

✓7th   **S01.111**   **Laceration without foreign body of right eyelid and periocular area**

✓7th   **S01.112**   **Laceration without foreign body of left eyelid and periocular area**

✓7th   **S01.119**   **Laceration without foreign body of unspecified eyelid and periocular area**

✓6th   **S01.12**   **Laceration with foreign body of eyelid and periocular area**

✓7th   **S01.121**   **Laceration with foreign body of right eyelid and periocular area**

✓7th   **S01.122**   **Laceration with foreign body of left eyelid and periocular area**

✓7th   **S01.129**   **Laceration with foreign body of unspecified eyelid and periocular area**

✓6th   **S01.13**   **Puncture wound without foreign body of eyelid and periocular area**

✓7th   **S01.131**   **Puncture wound without foreign body of right eyelid and periocular area**

✓7th   **S01.132**   **Puncture wound without foreign body of left eyelid and periocular area**

✓7th   **S01.139**   **Puncture wound without foreign body of unspecified eyelid and periocular area**

✓6th   **S01.14**   **Puncture wound with foreign body of eyelid and periocular area**

✓7th   **S01.141**   **Puncture wound with foreign body of right eyelid and periocular area**

✓7th   **S01.142**   **Puncture wound with foreign body of left eyelid and periocular area**

✓7th   **S01.149**   **Puncture wound with foreign body of unspecified eyelid and periocular area**

✓6th   **S01.15**   **Open bite of eyelid and periocular area**

Bite of eyelid and periocular area NOS

EXCLUDES 1   *superficial bite of eyelid and periocular area (S00.26, S00.27)*

✓7th   **S01.151**   **Open bite of right eyelid and periocular area**

✓7th   **S01.152**   **Open bite of left eyelid and periocular area**

✓7th   **S01.159**   **Open bite of unspecified eyelid and periocular area**

✓5th   **S01.2**   **Open wound of nose**

✓x 7th   **S01.20**   **Unspecified open wound of nose**

✓x 7th   **S01.21**   **Laceration without foreign body of nose**

✓x 7th   **S01.22**   **Laceration with foreign body of nose**

✓x 7th   **S01.23**   **Puncture wound without foreign body of nose**

✓x 7th   **S01.24**   **Puncture wound with foreign body of nose**

✓x 7th   **S01.25**   **Open bite of nose**

Bite of nose NOS

EXCLUDES 1   *superficial bite of nose (S00.36, S00.37)*

✓5th   **S01.3**   **Open wound of ear**

✓6th   **S01.30**   **Unspecified open wound of ear**

✓7th   **S01.301**   **Unspecified open wound of right ear**

✓7th   **S01.302**   **Unspecified open wound of left ear**

✓7th   **S01.309**   **Unspecified open wound of unspecified ear**

✓6th   **S01.31**   **Laceration without foreign body of ear**

✓7th   **S01.311**   **Laceration without foreign body of right ear**

✓7th   **S01.312**   **Laceration without foreign body of left ear**

✓7th   **S01.319**   **Laceration without foreign body of unspecified ear**

✓6th   **S01.32**   **Laceration with foreign body of ear**

✓7th   **S01.321**   **Laceration with foreign body of right ear**

✓7th   **S01.322**   **Laceration with foreign body of left ear**

✓7th   **S01.329**   **Laceration with foreign body of unspecified ear**

✓6th   **S01.33**   **Puncture wound without foreign body of ear**

✓7th   **S01.331**   **Puncture wound without foreign body of right ear**

✓7th   **S01.332**   **Puncture wound without foreign body of left ear**

✓7th   **S01.339**   **Puncture wound without foreign body of unspecified ear**

✓6th   **S01.34**   **Puncture wound with foreign body of ear**

✓7th   **S01.341**   **Puncture wound with foreign body of right ear**

✓7th   **S01.342**   **Puncture wound with foreign body of left ear**

✓7th   **S01.349**   **Puncture wound with foreign body of unspecified ear**

✓6th   **S01.35**   **Open bite of ear**

Bite of ear NOS

EXCLUDES 1   *superficial bite of ear (S00.46, S00.47)*

✓7th   **S01.351**   **Open bite of right ear**

✓7th   **S01.352**   **Open bite of left ear**

✓7th   **S01.359**   **Open bite of unspecified ear**

✓5th   **S01.4**   **Open wound of cheek and temporomandibular area**

✓6th   **S01.40**   **Unspecified open wound of cheek and temporomandibular area**

✓7th   **S01.401**   **Unspecified open wound of right cheek and temporomandibular area**

✓7th   **S01.402**   **Unspecified open wound of left cheek and temporomandibular area**

✓7th   **S01.409**   **Unspecified open wound of unspecified cheek and temporomandibular area**

✓6th   **S01.41**   **Laceration without foreign body of cheek and temporomandibular area**

✓7th   **S01.411**   **Laceration without foreign body of right cheek and temporomandibular area**

✓7th   **S01.412**   **Laceration without foreign body of left cheek and temporomandibular area**

✓7th   **S01.419**   **Laceration without foreign body of unspecified cheek and temporomandibular area**

✓6th   **S01.42**   **Laceration with foreign body of cheek and temporomandibular area**

✓7th   **S01.421**   **Laceration with foreign body of right cheek and temporomandibular area**

✓7th   **S01.422**   **Laceration with foreign body of left cheek and temporomandibular area**

✓7th   **S01.429**   **Laceration with foreign body of unspecified cheek and temporomandibular area**

✓6th   **S01.43**   **Puncture wound without foreign body of cheek and temporomandibular area**

✓7th   **S01.431**   **Puncture wound without foreign body of right cheek and temporomandibular area**

✓7th   **S01.432**   **Puncture wound without foreign body of left cheek and temporomandibular area**

✓7th   **S01.439**   **Puncture wound without foreign body of unspecified cheek and temporomandibular area**

✓6th   **S01.44**   **Puncture wound with foreign body of cheek and temporomandibular area**

✓7th   **S01.441**   **Puncture wound with foreign body of right cheek and temporomandibular area**

✓7th   **S01.442**   **Puncture wound with foreign body of left cheek and temporomandibular area**

✓7th   **S01.449**   **Puncture wound with foreign body of unspecified cheek and temporomandibular area**

✓6th   **S01.45**   **Open bite of cheek and temporomandibular area**

Bite of cheek and temporomandibular area NOS

EXCLUDES 2   *superficial bite of cheek and temporomandibular area (S00.86, S00.87)*

✓7th   **S01.451**   **Open bite of right cheek and temporomandibular area**

✓7th   **S01.452**   **Open bite of left cheek and temporomandibular area**

EXCLUDES 1   Not coded here   **EXCLUDES 2**   Not included here   *Manifestation Code*

✓7ᵗʰ **S01.459** Open bite of unspecified cheek and temporomandibular area

✓5ᵗʰ **S01.5** **Open wound of lip and oral cavity**
> *EXCLUDES 2* *tooth dislocation (S03.2)*
> *tooth fracture (S02.5)*

✓6ᵗʰ **S01.50** Unspecified open wound of lip and oral cavity
✓7ᵗʰ **S01.501** Unspecified open wound of lip
✓7ᵗʰ **S01.502** Unspecified open wound of oral cavity

✓6ᵗʰ **S01.51** Laceration of lip and oral cavity without foreign body
✓7ᵗʰ **S01.511** Laceration without foreign body of lip
✓7ᵗʰ **S01.512** Laceration without foreign body of oral cavity

✓6ᵗʰ **S01.52** Laceration of lip and oral cavity with foreign body
✓7ᵗʰ **S01.521** Laceration with foreign body of lip
✓7ᵗʰ **S01.522** Laceration with foreign body of oral cavity

✓6ᵗʰ **S01.53** Puncture wound of lip and oral cavity without foreign body
✓7ᵗʰ **S01.531** Puncture wound without foreign body of lip
✓7ᵗʰ **S01.532** Puncture wound without foreign body of oral cavity

✓6ᵗʰ **S01.54** Puncture wound of lip and oral cavity with foreign body
✓7ᵗʰ **S01.541** Puncture wound with foreign body of lip
✓7ᵗʰ **S01.542** Puncture wound with foreign body of oral cavity

✓6ᵗʰ **S01.55** Open bite of lip and oral cavity
✓7ᵗʰ **S01.551** Open bite of lip
> Bite of lip NOS
> *EXCLUDES 1* *superficial bite of lip (S00.571)*

✓7ᵗʰ **S01.552** Open bite of oral cavity
> Bite of oral cavity NOS
> *EXCLUDES 1* *superficial bite of oral cavity (S00.572)*

✓5ᵗʰ **S01.8** **Open wound of other parts of head**
✓x7ᵗʰ **S01.80** Unspecified open wound of other part of head
✓x7ᵗʰ **S01.81** Laceration without foreign body of other part of head
✓x7ᵗʰ **S01.82** Laceration with foreign body of other part of head
✓x7ᵗʰ **S01.83** Puncture wound without foreign body of other part of head
✓x7ᵗʰ **S01.84** Puncture wound with foreign body of other part of head
✓x7ᵗʰ **S01.85** Open bite of other part of head
> Bite of other part of head NOS
> *EXCLUDES 1* *superficial bite of other part of head (S00.85)*

✓5ᵗʰ **S01.9** **Open wound of unspecified part of head**
✓x7ᵗʰ **S01.90** Unspecified open wound of unspecified part of head
✓x7ᵗʰ **S01.91** Laceration without foreign body of unspecified part of head
✓x7ᵗʰ **S01.92** Laceration with foreign body of unspecified part of head
✓x7ᵗʰ **S01.93** Puncture wound without foreign body of unspecified part of head
✓x7ᵗʰ **S01.94** Puncture wound with foreign body of unspecified part of head
✓x7ᵗʰ **S01.95** Open bite of unspecified part of head
> Bite of head NOS
> *EXCLUDES 1* *superficial bite of head NOS (S00.97)*

✓4ᵗʰ **S02** **Fracture of skull and facial bones**
> **NOTE** A fracture not indicated as open or closed should be coded to closed
> Code also any associated intracranial injury (S06-).

> The appropriate 7th character is to be added to each code from category S02.
> A   initial encounter for closed fracture
> B   initial encounter for open fracture
> D   subsequent encounter for fracture with routine healing
> G   subsequent encounter for fracture with delayed healing
> K   subsequent encounter for fracture with nonunion
> S   sequela

✓x7ᵗʰ **S02.0** **Fracture of vault of skull**
> Fracture of frontal bone
> Fracture of parietal bone

✓5ᵗʰ **S02.1** **Fracture of base of skull**
> *EXCLUDES 1* *orbit NOS (S02.89)*
> *EXCLUDES 2* *orbital floor (S02.3-)*

✓x7ᵗʰ **S02.10** Unspecified fracture of base of skull
✓6ᵗʰ **S02.11** Fracture of occiput
✓7ᵗʰ **S02.110** Type I occipital condyle fracture
✓7ᵗʰ **S02.111** Type II occipital condyle fracture
✓7ᵗʰ **S02.112** Type III occipital condyle fracture
✓7ᵗʰ **S02.113** Unspecified occipital condyle fracture
✓7ᵗʰ **S02.118** Other fracture of occiput
✓7ᵗʰ **S02.119** Unspecified fracture of occiput

✓x7ᵗʰ **S02.19** Other fracture of base of skull
> Fracture of anterior fossa of base of skull
> Fracture of ethmoid sinus
> Fracture of frontal sinus
> Fracture of middle fossa of base of skull
> Fracture of orbital roof
> Fracture of posterior fossa of base of skull
> Fracture of sphenoid
> Fracture of temporal bone

✓x7ᵗʰ **S02.2** **Fracture of nasal bones**
✓x7ᵗʰ **S02.3** **Fracture of orbital floor**
> *EXCLUDES 1* *orbit NOS (S02.89)*
> *EXCLUDES 2* *orbital roof (S02.1-)*

✓5ᵗʰ **S02.4** **Fracture of malar, maxillary and zygoma bones**
> Fracture of superior maxilla
> Fracture of upper jaw (bone)
> Fracture of zygomatic process of temporal bone

✓6ᵗʰ **S02.40** Fracture of malar, maxillary and zygoma bones, unspecified
✓7ᵗʰ **S02.400** Malar fracture unspecified
✓7ᵗʰ **S02.401** Maxillary fracture, unspecified
✓7ᵗʰ **S02.402** Zygomatic fracture, unspecified

✓6ᵗʰ **S02.41** LeFort fracture
✓7ᵗʰ **S02.411** LeFort I fracture
✓7ᵗʰ **S02.412** LeFort II fracture
✓7ᵗʰ **S02.413** LeFort III fracture
✓x7ᵗʰ **S02.42** Fracture of alveolus of maxilla

✓x7ᵗʰ **S02.5** **Fracture of tooth (traumatic)**
> Broken tooth
> *EXCLUDES 1* *cracked tooth (nontraumatic) (K03.81)*

✓5ᵗʰ **S02.6** **Fracture of mandible**
> Fracture of lower jaw (bone)

✓6ᵗʰ **S02.60** Fracture of mandible, unspecified
✓7ᵗʰ **S02.600** Fracture of unspecified part of body of mandible
✓7ᵗʰ **S02.609** Fracture of mandible, unspecified

✓x7ᵗʰ **S02.61** Fracture of condylar process of mandible
✓x7ᵗʰ **S02.62** Fracture of subcondylar process of mandible
✓x7ᵗʰ **S02.63** Fracture of coronoid process of mandible
✓x7ᵗʰ **S02.64** Fracture of ramus of mandible
✓x7ᵗʰ **S02.65** Fracture of angle of mandible
✓x7ᵗʰ **S02.66** Fracture of symphysis of mandible
✓x7ᵗʰ **S02.67** Fracture of alveolus of mandible
✓x7ᵗʰ **S02.69** Fracture of mandible of other specified site

---

☑ Appropriate additional character required   ✓x7ᵗʰ Requires 7th character, placeholder x must fill empty characters

√x7ᵗʰ **S02.8** **Fractures of other specified skull and facial bones**
Fracture of orbit NOS
Fracture of palate
EXCLUDES 1 *fracture of orbital floor (S02.3-)*
fracture of orbital roof (S02.1-)

√5ᵗʰ **S02.9** **Fracture of unspecified skull and facial bones**
√x7ᵗʰ **S02.91** **Unspecified fracture of skull**
√x7ᵗʰ **S02.92** **Unspecified fracture of facial bones**

√4ᵗʰ **S03** **Dislocation and sprain of joints and ligaments of head**
INCLUDES   avulsion of joint (capsule) or ligament of head
laceration of cartilage, joint (capsule) or ligament of head
sprain of cartilage, joint (capsule) or ligament of head
traumatic hemarthrosis of joint or ligament of head
traumatic rupture of joint or ligament of head
traumatic subluxation of joint or ligament of head
traumatic tear of joint or ligament of head
Code also any associated open wound
EXCLUDES 2 *strain of muscle or tendon of head (S09.1)*

The appropriate 7th character is to be added to each code from
category S03.
A   initial encounter
D   subsequent encounter
S   sequela

√x7ᵗʰ **S03.0** **Dislocation of jaw**
Dislocation of jaw (cartilage) (meniscus)
Dislocation of mandible
Dislocation of temporomandibular (joint)
√x7ᵗʰ **S03.1** **Dislocation of septal cartilage of nose**
√x7ᵗʰ **S03.2** **Dislocation of tooth**
√x7ᵗʰ **S03.4** **Sprain of jaw**
Sprain of temporomandibular (joint) (ligament)
√x7ᵗʰ **S03.8** **Sprain of joints and ligaments of other parts of head**
√x7ᵗʰ **S03.9** **Sprain of joints and ligaments of unspecified parts of head**

√4ᵗʰ **S04** **Injury of cranial nerve**
The selection of side should be based on the side of the body being
affected
Codes first any associated intracranial injury (S06-)
Code also any associated:
open wound of head (S01-)
skull fracture (S02-)

The appropriate 7th character is to be added to each code from
category S04.
A   initial encounter
D   subsequent encounter
S   sequela

√5ᵗʰ **S04.0** **Injury of optic nerve and pathways**
Use additional code to identify any visual field defect or
blindness (H53.4-, H54)
√6ᵗʰ **S04.01** **Injury of optic nerve**
Injury of 2nd cranial nerve
√7ᵗʰ **S04.011** **Injury of optic nerve, right eye**
√7ᵗʰ **S04.012** **Injury of optic nerve, left eye**
√7ᵗʰ **S04.019** **Injury of optic nerve, unspecified eye**
Injury of optic nerve NOS
√x7ᵗʰ **S04.02** **Injury of optic chiasm**
√6ᵗʰ **S04.03** **Injury of optic tract and pathways**
Injury of optic radiation
√7ᵗʰ **S04.031** **Injury of optic tract and pathways, right eye**
√7ᵗʰ **S04.032** **Injury of optic tract and pathways, left eye**
√7ᵗʰ **S04.039** **Injury of optic tract and pathways, unspecified eye**
Injury of optic tract and pathways NOS
√6ᵗʰ **S04.04** **Injury of visual cortex**
√7ᵗʰ **S04.041** **Injury of visual cortex, right eye**
√7ᵗʰ **S04.042** **Injury of visual cortex, left eye**
√7ᵗʰ **S04.049** **Injury of visual cortex, unspecified eye**
Injury of visual cortex NOS
√5ᵗʰ **S04.1** **Injury of oculomotor nerve**
Injury of 3rd cranial nerve
√x7ᵗʰ **S04.10** **Injury of oculomotor nerve, unspecified side**
√x7ᵗʰ **S04.11** **Injury of oculomotor nerve, right side**
√x7ᵗʰ **S04.12** **Injury of oculomotor nerve, left side**

√5ᵗʰ **S04.2** **Injury of trochlear nerve**
Injury of 4th cranial nerve
√x7ᵗʰ **S04.20** **Injury of trochlear nerve, unspecified side**
√x7ᵗʰ **S04.21** **Injury of trochlear nerve, right side**
√x7ᵗʰ **S04.22** **Injury of trochlear nerve, left side**
√5ᵗʰ **S04.3** **Injury of trigeminal nerve**
Injury of 5th cranial nerve
√x7ᵗʰ **S04.30** **Injury of trigeminal nerve, unspecified side**
√x7ᵗʰ **S04.31** **Injury of trigeminal nerve, right side**
√x7ᵗʰ **S04.32** **Injury of trigeminal nerve, left side**
√5ᵗʰ **S04.4** **Injury of abducent nerve**
Injury of 6th cranial nerve
√x7ᵗʰ **S04.40** **Injury of abducent nerve, unspecified side**
√x7ᵗʰ **S04.41** **Injury of abducent nerve, right side**
√x7ᵗʰ **S04.42** **Injury of abducent nerve, left side**
√5ᵗʰ **S04.5** **Injury of facial nerve**
Injury of 7th cranial nerve
√x7ᵗʰ **S04.50** **Injury of facial nerve, unspecified side**
√x7ᵗʰ **S04.51** **Injury of facial nerve, right side**
√x7ᵗʰ **S04.52** **Injury of facial nerve, left side**
√5ᵗʰ **S04.6** **Injury of acoustic nerve**
Injury of auditory nerve
Injury of 8th cranial nerve
√x7ᵗʰ **S04.60** **Injury of acoustic nerve, unspecified side**
√x7ᵗʰ **S04.61** **Injury of acoustic nerve, right side**
√x7ᵗʰ **S04.62** **Injury of acoustic nerve, left side**
√5ᵗʰ **S04.7** **Injury of accessory nerve**
Injury of 11th cranial nerve
√x7ᵗʰ **S04.70** **Injury of accessory nerve, unspecified side**
√x7ᵗʰ **S04.71** **Injury of accessory nerve, right side**
√x7ᵗʰ **S04.72** **Injury of accessory nerve, left side**
√5ᵗʰ **S04.8** **Injury of other cranial nerves**
√6ᵗʰ **S04.81** **Injury of olfactory [1st] nerve**
√7ᵗʰ **S04.811** **Injury of olfactory [1st] nerve, right side**
√7ᵗʰ **S04.812** **Injury of olfactory [1st] nerve, left side**
√7ᵗʰ **S04.819** **Injury of olfactory [1st] nerve, unspecified side**
√6ᵗʰ **S04.89** **Injury of other cranial nerves**
Injury of vagus [10th] nerve
√7ᵗʰ **S04.891** **Injury of other cranial nerves, right side**
√7ᵗʰ **S04.892** **Injury of other cranial nerves, left side**
√7ᵗʰ **S04.899** **Injury of other cranial nerves, unspecified side**
S04.9 **Injury of unspecified cranial nerve**

√4ᵗʰ **S05** **Injury of eye and orbit**
Open wound of eye and orbit
EXCLUDES 2 *2nd cranial [optic] nerve injury (S04.0-)*
3rd cranial [oculomotor] nerve injury (S04.1-)
open wound of eyelid and periocular area (S01.1-)
orbital bone fracture (S02.1-, S02.3-, S02.8-)
superficial injury of eyelid (S00.1-S00.2)

The appropriate 7th character is to be added to each code from
category S05.
A   initial encounter
D   subsequent encounter
S   sequela

√5ᵗʰ **S05.0** **Injury of conjunctiva and corneal abrasion without foreign body**
EXCLUDES 1 *foreign body in conjunctival sac (T15.1)*
foreign body in cornea (T15.0)
√x7ᵗʰ **S05.00** **Injury of conjunctiva and corneal abrasion without foreign body, unspecified eye**
√x7ᵗʰ **S05.01** **Injury of conjunctiva and corneal abrasion without foreign body, right eye**
√x7ᵗʰ **S05.02** **Injury of conjunctiva and corneal abrasion without foreign body, left eye**
√5ᵗʰ **S05.1** **Contusion of eyeball and orbital tissues**
Traumatic hyphema
EXCLUDES 2 *black eye NOS (S00.1)*
contusion of eyelid and periocular area (S00.1)
√x7ᵗʰ **S05.10** **Contusion of eyeball and orbital tissues, unspecified eye**
√x7ᵗʰ **S05.11** **Contusion of eyeball and orbital tissues, right eye**
√x7ᵗʰ **S05.12** **Contusion of eyeball and orbital tissues, left eye**

EXCLUDES 1 Not coded here   EXCLUDES 2 Not included here   *Manifestation Code*

✓5th **S05.2** **Ocular laceration and rupture with prolapse or loss of intraocular tissue**
    ✓x7th **S05.20** **Ocular laceration and rupture with prolapse or loss of intraocular tissue, unspecified eye**
    ✓x7th **S05.21** **Ocular laceration and rupture with prolapse or loss of intraocular tissue, right eye**
    ✓x7th **S05.22** **Ocular laceration and rupture with prolapse or loss of intraocular tissue, left eye**

✓5th **S05.3** **Ocular laceration without prolapse or loss of intraocular tissue**
    Laceration of eye NOS
    ✓x7th **S05.30** **Ocular laceration without prolapse or loss of intraocular tissue, unspecified eye**
    ✓x7th **S05.31** **Ocular laceration without prolapse or loss of intraocular tissue, right eye**
    ✓x7th **S05.32** **Ocular laceration without prolapse or loss of intraocular tissue, left eye**

✓5th **S05.4** **Penetrating wound of orbit with or without foreign body**
    EXCLUDES 2 *retained (old) foreign body following penetrating wound in orbit (H05.5-)*
    ✓x7th **S05.40** **Penetrating wound of orbit with or without foreign body, unspecified eye**
    ✓x7th **S05.41** **Penetrating wound of orbit with or without foreign body, right eye**
    ✓x7th **S05.42** **Penetrating wound of orbit with or without foreign body, left eye**

✓5th **S05.5** **Penetrating wound with foreign body of eyeball**
    EXCLUDES 2 *retained (old) intraocular foreign body (H44.6-, H44.7)*
    ✓x7th **S05.50** **Penetrating wound with foreign body of unspecified eyeball**
    ✓x7th **S05.51** **Penetrating wound with foreign body of right eyeball**
    ✓x7th **S05.52** **Penetrating wound with foreign body of left eyeball**

✓5th **S05.6** **Penetrating wound without foreign body of eyeball**
    Ocular penetration NOS
    ✓x7th **S05.60** **Penetrating wound without foreign body of unspecified eyeball**
    ✓x7th **S05.61** **Penetrating wound without foreign body of right eyeball**
    ✓x7th **S05.62** **Penetrating wound without foreign body of left eyeball**

✓5th **S05.7** **Avulsion of eye**
    Traumatic enucleation
    ✓x7th **S05.70** **Avulsion of unspecified eye**
    ✓x7th **S05.71** **Avulsion of right eye**
    ✓x7th **S05.72** **Avulsion of left eye**

✓5th **S05.8** **Other injuries of eye and orbit**
    Lacrimal duct injury
    ✓6th **S05.8x** **Other injuries of eye and orbit**
      ✓7th **S05.8x1** **Other injuries of right eye and orbit**
      ✓7th **S05.8x2** **Other injuries of left eye and orbit**
      ✓7th **S05.8x9** **Other injuries of unspecified eye and orbit**

✓5th **S05.9** **Unspecified injury of eye and orbit**
    Injury of eye NOS
    ✓x7th **S05.90** **Unspecified injury of unspecified eye and orbit**
    ✓x7th **S05.91** **Unspecified injury of right eye and orbit**
    ✓x7th **S05.92** **Unspecified injury of left eye and orbit**

✓4th **S06** **Intracranial injury**
    Traumatic brain injury
    Code also any associated:
      open wound of head (S01-)
      skull fracture (S02-)
    EXCLUDES 1 *head injury NOS (S09.90)*

> The appropriate 7th character is to be added to each code from category S06.
> A   initial encounter
> D   subsequent encounter
> S   sequela

✓5th **S06.0** **Concussion**
    Commotio cerebri
    EXCLUDES 1 *concussion with other intracranial injuries classified in category S06—code to specified intracranial injury*

✓6th **S06.0x** **Concussion**
    ✓7th **S06.0x0** **Concussion without loss of consciousness**
    ✓7th **S06.0x1** **Concussion with loss of consciousness of 30 minutes or less**
    ✓7th **S06.0x2** **Concussion with loss of consciousness of 31 minutes to 59 minutes**
    ✓7th **S06.0x3** **Concussion with loss of consciousness of 1 hour to 5 hours 59 minutes**
    ✓7th **S06.0x4** **Concussion with loss of consciousness of 6 hours to 24 hours**
    ✓7th **S06.0x5** **Concussion with loss of consciousness greater than 24 hours with return to pre-existing conscious level**
    ✓7th **S06.0x6** **Concussion with loss of consciousness greater than 24 hours without return to pre-existing conscious level with patient surviving**
    ✓7th **S06.0x7** **Concussion with loss of consciousness of any duration with death due to brain injury prior to regaining consciousness**
    ✓7th **S06.0x8** **Concussion with loss of consciousness of any duration with death due to other cause prior to regaining consciousness**
    ✓7th **S06.0x9** **Concussion with loss of consciousness of unspecified duration**
      Concussion NOS

✓5th **S06.1** **Traumatic cerebral edema**
    Diffuse traumatic cerebral edema
    Focal traumatic cerebral edema
    ✓6th **S06.1x** **Traumatic cerebral edema**
      ✓7th **S06.1x0** **Traumatic cerebral edema without loss of consciousness**
      ✓7th **S06.1x1** **Traumatic cerebral edema with loss of consciousness of 30 minutes or less**
      ✓7th **S06.1x2** **Traumatic cerebral edema with loss of consciousness of 31 minutes to 59 minutes**
      ✓7th **S06.1x3** **Traumatic cerebral edema with loss of consciousness of 1 hour to 5 hours 59 minutes**
      ✓7th **S06.1x4** **Traumatic cerebral edema with loss of consciousness of 6 hours to 24 hours**
      ✓7th **S06.1x5** **Traumatic cerebral edema with loss of consciousness greater than 24 hours with return to pre-existing conscious level**
      ✓7th **S06.1x6** **Traumatic cerebral edema with loss of consciousness greater than 24 hours without return to pre-existing conscious level with patient surviving**
      ✓7th **S06.1x7** **Traumatic cerebral edema with loss of consciousness of any duration with death due to brain injury prior to regaining consciousness**
      ✓7th **S06.1x8** **Traumatic cerebral edema with loss of consciousness of any duration with death due to other cause prior to regaining consciousness**
      ✓7th **S06.1x9** **Traumatic cerebral edema with loss of consciousness of unspecified duration**
        Traumatic cerebral edema NOS

✓5th **S06.2** **Diffuse traumatic brain injury**
    Diffuse axonal brain injury
    EXCLUDES 1 *traumatic diffuse cerebral edema (S06.1x)*
    ✓6th **S06.2x** **Diffuse traumatic brain injury**
      ✓7th **S06.2x0** **Diffuse traumatic brain injury without loss of consciousness**
      ✓7th **S06.2x1** **Diffuse traumatic brain injury with loss of consciousness of 30 minutes or less**
      ✓7th **S06.2x2** **Diffuse traumatic brain injury with loss of consciousness of 31 minutes to 59 minutes**
      ✓7th **S06.2x3** **Diffuse traumatic brain injury with loss of consciousness of 1 hour to 5 hours 59 minutes**

√7ᵗʰ **S06.2x4** **Diffuse traumatic brain injury with loss of consciousness of 6 hours to 24 hours**

√7ᵗʰ **S06.2x5** **Diffuse traumatic brain injury with loss of consciousness greater than 24 hours with return to pre-existing conscious levels**

√7ᵗʰ **S06.2x6** **Diffuse traumatic brain injury with loss of consciousness greater than 24 hours without return to pre-existing conscious level with patient surviving**

√7ᵗʰ **S06.2x7** **Diffuse traumatic brain injury with loss of consciousness of any duration with death due to brain injury prior to regaining consciousness**

√7ᵗʰ **S06.2x8** **Diffuse traumatic brain injury with loss of consciousness of any duration with death due to other cause prior to regaining consciousness**

√7ᵗʰ **S06.2x9** **Diffuse traumatic brain injury with loss of consciousness of unspecified duration**
Diffuse traumatic brain injury NOS

√5ᵗʰ **S06.3** **Focal traumatic brain injury**
EXCLUDES 1   *any condition classifiable to S06.4-S06.6*
focal cerebral edema (S06.1)

√6ᵗʰ **S06.30** **Unspecified focal traumatic brain injury**

√7ᵗʰ **S06.300** **Unspecified focal traumatic brain injury without loss of consciousness**

√7ᵗʰ **S06.301** **Unspecified focal traumatic brain injury with loss of consciousness of 30 minutes or less**

√7ᵗʰ **S06.302** **Unspecified focal traumatic brain injury with loss of consciousness of 31 minutes to 59 minutes**

√7ᵗʰ **S06.303** **Unspecified focal traumatic brain injury with loss of consciousness of 1 hour to 5 hours 59 minutes**

√7ᵗʰ **S06.304** **Unspecified focal traumatic brain injury with loss of consciousness of 6 hours to 24 hours**

√7ᵗʰ **S06.305** **Unspecified focal traumatic brain injury with loss of consciousness greater than 24 hours with return to pre-existing conscious level**

√7ᵗʰ **S06.306** **Unspecified focal traumatic brain injury with loss of consciousness greater than 24 hours without return to pre-existing conscious level with patient surviving**

√7ᵗʰ **S06.307** **Unspecified focal traumatic brain injury with loss of consciousness of any duration with death due to brain injury prior to regaining consciousness**

√7ᵗʰ **S06.308** **Unspecified focal traumatic brain injury with loss of consciousness of any duration with death due to other cause prior to regaining consciousness**

√7ᵗʰ **S06.309** **Unspecified focal traumatic brain injury with loss of consciousness of unspecified duration**
Unspecified focal traumatic brain injury NOS

√6ᵗʰ **S06.31** **Contusion and laceration of right cerebrum**

√7ᵗʰ **S06.310** **Contusion and laceration of right cerebrum without loss of consciousness**

√7ᵗʰ **S06.311** **Contusion and laceration of right cerebrum with loss of consciousness of 30 minutes or less**

√7ᵗʰ **S06.312** **Contusion and laceration of right cerebrum with loss of consciousness of 31 minutes to 59 minutes**

√7ᵗʰ **S06.313** **Contusion and laceration of right cerebrum with loss of consciousness of 1 hour to 5 hours 59 minutes**

√7ᵗʰ **S06.314** **Contusion and laceration of right cerebrum with loss of consciousness of 6 hours to 24 hours**

√7ᵗʰ **S06.315** **Contusion and laceration of right cerebrum with loss of consciousness greater than 24 hours with return to pre-existing conscious level**

√7ᵗʰ **S06.316** **Contusion and laceration of right cerebrum with loss of consciousness greater than 24 hours without return to pre-existing conscious level with patient surviving**

√7ᵗʰ **S06.317** **Contusion and laceration of right cerebrum with loss of consciousness of any duration with death due to brain injury prior to regaining consciousness**

√7ᵗʰ **S06.318** **Contusion and laceration of right cerebrum with loss of consciousness of any duration with death due to other cause prior to regaining consciousness**

√7ᵗʰ **S06.319** **Contusion and laceration of right cerebrum with loss of consciousness of unspecified duration**
Contusion and laceration of right cerebrum NOS

√6ᵗʰ **S06.32** **Contusion and laceration of left cerebrum**

√7ᵗʰ **S06.320** **Contusion and laceration of left cerebrum without loss of consciousness**

√7ᵗʰ **S06.321** **Contusion and laceration of left cerebrum with loss of consciousness of 30 minutes or less**

√7ᵗʰ **S06.322** **Contusion and laceration of left cerebrum with loss of consciousness of 31 minutes to 59 minutes**

√7ᵗʰ **S06.323** **Contusion and laceration of left cerebrum with loss of consciousness of 1 hour to 5 hours 59 minutes**

√7ᵗʰ **S06.324** **Contusion and laceration of left cerebrum with loss of consciousness of 6 hours to 24 hours**

√7ᵗʰ **S06.325** **Contusion and laceration of left cerebrum with loss of consciousness greater than 24 hours with return to pre-existing conscious level**

√7ᵗʰ **S06.326** **Contusion and laceration of left cerebrum with loss of consciousness greater than 24 hours without return to pre-existing conscious level with patient surviving**

√7ᵗʰ **S06.327** **Contusion and laceration of left cerebrum with loss of consciousness of any duration with death due to brain injury prior to regaining consciousness**

√7ᵗʰ **S06.328** **Contusion and laceration of left cerebrum with loss of consciousness of any duration with death due to other cause prior to regaining consciousness**

√7ᵗʰ **S06.329** **Contusion and laceration of left cerebrum with loss of consciousness of unspecified duration**
Contusion and laceration of left cerebrum NOS

√6ᵗʰ **S06.33** **Contusion and laceration of cerebrum, unspecified**

√7ᵗʰ **S06.330** **Contusion and laceration of cerebrum, unspecified, without loss of consciousness**

√7ᵗʰ **S06.331** **Contusion and laceration of cerebrum, unspecified, with loss of consciousness of 30 minutes or less**

√7ᵗʰ **S06.332** **Contusion and laceration of cerebrum, unspecified, with loss of consciousness of 31 minutes to 59 minutes**

√7ᵗʰ **S06.333** **Contusion and laceration of cerebrum, unspecified, with loss of consciousness of 1 hour to 5 hours 59 minutes**

√7ᵗʰ **S06.334** **Contusion and laceration of cerebrum, unspecified, with loss of consciousness of 6 hours to 24 hours**

√7ᵗʰ **S06.335** **Contusion and laceration of cerebrum, unspecified, with loss of consciousness greater than 24 hours with return to pre-existing conscious level**

EXCLUDES 1   Not coded here   EXCLUDES 2   Not included here   *Manifestation Code*

✓7th **S06.336** **Contusion and laceration of cerebrum, unspecified, with loss of consciousness greater than 24 hours without return to pre-existing conscious level with patient surviving**

✓7th **S06.337** **Contusion and laceration of cerebrum, unspecified, with loss of consciousness of any duration with death due to brain injury prior to regaining consciousness**

✓7th **S06.338** **Contusion and laceration of cerebrum, unspecified, with loss of consciousness of any duration with death due to other cause prior to regaining consciousness**

✓7th **S06.339** **Contusion and laceration of cerebrum, unspecified, with loss of consciousness of unspecified duration**
Contusion and laceration of cerebrum NOS

✓6th **S06.34** **Traumatic hemorrhage of right cerebrum**
Traumatic intracerebral hemorrhage and hematoma of right cerebrum

✓7th **S06.340** **Traumatic hemorrhage of right cerebrum without loss of consciousness**

✓7th **S06.341** **Traumatic hemorrhage of right cerebrum with loss of consciousness of 30 minutes or less**

✓7th **S06.342** **Traumatic hemorrhage of right cerebrum with loss of consciousness of 31 minutes to 59 minutes**

✓7th **S06.343** **Traumatic hemorrhage of right cerebrum with loss of consciousness of 1 hours to 5 hours 59 minutes**

✓7th **S06.344** **Traumatic hemorrhage of right cerebrum with loss of consciousness of 6 hours to 24 hours**

✓7th **S06.345** **Traumatic hemorrhage of right cerebrum with loss of consciousness greater than 24 hours with return to pre-existing conscious level**

✓7th **S06.346** **Traumatic hemorrhage of right cerebrum with loss of consciousness greater than 24 hours without return to pre-existing conscious level with patient surviving**

✓7th **S06.347** **Traumatic hemorrhage of right cerebrum with loss of consciousness of any duration with death due to brain injury prior to regaining consciousness**

✓7th **S06.348** **Traumatic hemorrhage of right cerebrum with loss of consciousness of any duration with death due to other cause prior to regaining consciousness**

✓7th **S06.349** **Traumatic hemorrhage of right cerebrum with loss of consciousness of unspecified duration**
Traumatic hemorrhage of right cerebrum NOS

✓6th **S06.35** **Traumatic hemorrhage of left cerebrum**
Traumatic intracerebral hemorrhage and hematoma of left cerebrum

✓7th **S06.350** **Traumatic hemorrhage of left cerebrum without loss of consciousness**

✓7th **S06.351** **Traumatic hemorrhage of left cerebrum with loss of consciousness of 30 minutes or less**

✓7th **S06.352** **Traumatic hemorrhage of left cerebrum with loss of consciousness of 31 minutes to 59 minutes**

✓7th **S06.353** **Traumatic hemorrhage of left cerebrum with loss of consciousness of 1 hours to 5 hours 59 minutes**

✓7th **S06.354** **Traumatic hemorrhage of left cerebrum with loss of consciousness of 6 hours to 24 hours**

✓7th **S06.355** **Traumatic hemorrhage of left cerebrum with loss of consciousness greater than 24 hours with return to pre-existing conscious level**

✓7th **S06.356** **Traumatic hemorrhage of left cerebrum with loss of consciousness greater than 24 hours without return to pre-existing conscious level with patient surviving**

✓7th **S06.357** **Traumatic hemorrhage of left cerebrum with loss of consciousness of any duration with death due to brain injury prior to regaining consciousness**

✓7th **S06.358** **Traumatic hemorrhage of left cerebrum with loss of consciousness of any duration with death due to other cause prior to regaining consciousness**

✓7th **S06.359** **Traumatic hemorrhage of left cerebrum with loss of consciousness of unspecified duration**
Traumatic hemorrhage of left cerebrum NOS

✓6th **S06.36** **Traumatic hemorrhage of cerebrum, unspecified**
Traumatic intracerebral hemorrhage and hematoma, unspecified

✓7th **S06.360** **Traumatic hemorrhage of cerebrum, unspecified, without loss of consciousness**

✓7th **S06.361** **Traumatic hemorrhage of cerebrum, unspecified, with loss of consciousness of 30 minutes or less**

✓7th **S06.362** **Traumatic hemorrhage of cerebrum, unspecified, with loss of consciousness of 31 minutes to 59 minutes**

✓7th **S06.363** **Traumatic hemorrhage of cerebrum, unspecified, with loss of consciousness of 1 hours to 5 hours 59 minutes**

✓7th **S06.364** **Traumatic hemorrhage of cerebrum, unspecified, with loss of consciousness of 6 hours to 24 hours**

✓7th **S06.365** **Traumatic hemorrhage of cerebrum, unspecified, with loss of consciousness greater than 24 hours with return to pre-existing conscious level**

✓7th **S06.366** **Traumatic hemorrhage of cerebrum, unspecified, with loss of consciousness greater than 24 hours without return to pre-existing conscious level with patient surviving**

✓7th **S06.367** **Traumatic hemorrhage of cerebrum, unspecified, with loss of consciousness of any duration with death due to brain injury prior to regaining consciousness**

✓7th **S06.368** **Traumatic hemorrhage of cerebrum, unspecified, with loss of consciousness of any duration with death due to other cause prior to regaining consciousness**

✓7th **S06.369** **Traumatic hemorrhage of cerebrum, unspecified, with loss of consciousness of unspecified duration**
Traumatic hemorrhage of cerebrum NOS

✓6th **S06.37** **Contusion, laceration, and hemorrhage of cerebellum**

✓7th **S06.370** **Contusion, laceration, and hemorrhage of cerebellum without loss of consciousness**

✓7th **S06.371** **Contusion, laceration, and hemorrhage of cerebellum with loss of consciousness of 30 minutes or less**

✓7th **S06.372** **Contusion, laceration, and hemorrhage of cerebellum with loss of consciousness of 31 minutes to 59 minutes**

✓7th **S06.373** **Contusion, laceration, and hemorrhage of cerebellum with loss of consciousness of 1 hour to 5 hours 59 minutes**

✓7th **S06.374** **Contusion, laceration, and hemorrhage of cerebellum with loss of consciousness of 6 hours to 24 hours**

✓7th **S06.375** **Contusion, laceration, and hemorrhage of cerebellum with loss of consciousness greater than 24 hours with return to pre-existing conscious level**

☑ Appropriate additional character required　　✓x7th Requires 7th character, placeholder x must fill empty characters

✓7ᵗʰ **S06.376** **Contusion, laceration, and hemorrhage of cerebellum with loss of consciousness greater than 24 hours without return to pre-existing conscious level with patient surviving**

✓7ᵗʰ **S06.377** **Contusion, laceration, and hemorrhage of cerebellum with loss of consciousness of any duration with death due to brain injury prior to regaining consciousness**

✓7ᵗʰ **S06.378** **Contusion, laceration, and hemorrhage of cerebellum with loss of consciousness of any duration with death due to other cause prior to regaining consciousness**

✓7ᵗʰ **S06.379** **Contusion, laceration, and hemorrhage of cerebellum with loss of consciousness of unspecified duration**
Contusion, laceration, and hemorrhage of cerebellum NOS

✓6ᵗʰ **S06.38** **Contusion, laceration, and hemorrhage of brainstem**

✓7ᵗʰ **S06.380** **Contusion, laceration, and hemorrhage of brainstem without loss of consciousness**

✓7ᵗʰ **S06.381** **Contusion, laceration, and hemorrhage of brainstem with loss of consciousness of 30 minutes or less**

✓7ᵗʰ **S06.382** **Contusion, laceration, and hemorrhage of brainstem with loss of consciousness of 31 minutes to 59 minutes**

✓7ᵗʰ **S06.383** **Contusion, laceration, and hemorrhage of brainstem with loss of consciousness of 1 hour to 5 hours 59 minutes**

✓7ᵗʰ **S06.384** **Contusion, laceration, and hemorrhage of brainstem with loss of consciousness of 6 hours to 24 hours**

✓7ᵗʰ **S06.385** **Contusion, laceration, and hemorrhage of brainstem with loss of consciousness greater than 24 hours with return to pre-existing conscious level**

✓7ᵗʰ **S06.386** **Contusion, laceration, and hemorrhage of brainstem with loss of consciousness greater than 24 hours without return to pre-existing conscious level with patient surviving**

✓7ᵗʰ **S06.387** **Contusion, laceration, and hemorrhage of brainstem with loss of consciousness of any duration with death due to brain injury prior to regaining consciousness**

✓7ᵗʰ **S06.388** **Contusion, laceration, and hemorrhage of brainstem with loss of consciousness of any duration with death due to other cause prior to regaining consciousness**

✓7ᵗʰ **S06.389** **Contusion, laceration, and hemorrhage of brainstem with loss of consciousness of unspecified duration**
Contusion, laceration, and hemorrhage of brainstem NOS

✓5ᵗʰ **S06.4** **Epidural hemorrhage**
Extradural hemorrhage NOS
Extradural hemorrhage (traumatic)

✓6ᵗʰ **S06.4x** **Epidural hemorrhage**

✓7ᵗʰ **S06.4x0** **Epidural hemorrhage without loss of consciousness**

✓7ᵗʰ **S06.4x1** **Epidural hemorrhage with loss of consciousness of 30 minutes or less**

✓7ᵗʰ **S06.4x2** **Epidural hemorrhage with loss of consciousness of 31 minutes to 59 minutes**

✓7ᵗʰ **S06.4x3** **Epidural hemorrhage with loss of consciousness of 1 hour to 5 hours 59 minutes**

✓7ᵗʰ **S06.4x4** **Epidural hemorrhage with loss of consciousness of 6 hours to 24 hours**

✓7ᵗʰ **S06.4x5** **Epidural hemorrhage with loss of consciousness greater than 24 hours with return to pre-existing conscious level**

✓7ᵗʰ **S06.4x6** **Epidural hemorrhage with loss of consciousness greater than 24 hours without return to pre-existing conscious level with patient surviving**

✓7ᵗʰ **S06.4x7** **Epidural hemorrhage with loss of consciousness of any duration with death due to brain injury prior to regaining consciousness**

✓7ᵗʰ **S06.4x8** **Epidural hemorrhage with loss of consciousness of any duration with death due to other causes prior to regaining consciousness**

✓7ᵗʰ **S06.4x9** **Epidural hemorrhage with loss of consciousness of unspecified duration**
Epidural hemorrhage NOS

✓5ᵗʰ **S06.5** **Traumatic subdural hemorrhage**

✓6ᵗʰ **S06.5x** **Traumatic subdural hemorrhage**

✓7ᵗʰ **S06.5x0** **Traumatic subdural hemorrhage without loss of consciousness**

✓7ᵗʰ **S06.5x1** **Traumatic subdural hemorrhage with loss of consciousness of 30 minutes or less**

✓7ᵗʰ **S06.5x2** **Traumatic subdural hemorrhage with loss of consciousness of 31 minutes to 59 minutes**

✓7ᵗʰ **S06.5x3** **Traumatic subdural hemorrhage with loss of consciousness of 1 hour to 5 hours 59 minutes**

✓7ᵗʰ **S06.5x4** **Traumatic subdural hemorrhage with loss of consciousness of 6 hours to 24 hours**

✓7ᵗʰ **S06.5x5** **Traumatic subdural hemorrhage with loss of consciousness greater than 24 hours with return to pre-existing conscious level**

✓7ᵗʰ **S06.5x6** **Traumatic subdural hemorrhage with loss of consciousness greater than 24 hours without return to pre-existing conscious level with patient surviving**

✓7ᵗʰ **S06.5x7** **Traumatic subdural hemorrhage with loss of consciousness of any duration with death due to brain injury before regaining consciousness**

✓7ᵗʰ **S06.5x8** **Traumatic subdural hemorrhage with loss of consciousness of any duration with death due to other cause before regaining consciousness**

✓7ᵗʰ **S06.5x9** **Traumatic subdural hemorrhage with loss of consciousness of unspecified duration**
Traumatic subdural hemorrhage NOS

✓5ᵗʰ **S06.6** **Traumatic subarachnoid hemorrhage**

✓6ᵗʰ **S06.6x** **Traumatic subarachnoid hemorrhage**

✓7ᵗʰ **S06.6x0** **Traumatic subarachnoid hemorrhage without loss of consciousness**

✓7ᵗʰ **S06.6x1** **Traumatic subarachnoid hemorrhage with loss of consciousness of 30 minutes or less**

✓7ᵗʰ **S06.6x2** **Traumatic subarachnoid hemorrhage with loss of consciousness of 31 minutes to 59 minutes**

✓7ᵗʰ **S06.6x3** **Traumatic subarachnoid hemorrhage with loss of consciousness of 1 hour to 5 hours 59 minutes**

✓7ᵗʰ **S06.6x4** **Traumatic subarachnoid hemorrhage with loss of consciousness of 6 hours to 24 hours**

✓7ᵗʰ **S06.6x5** **Traumatic subarachnoid hemorrhage with loss of consciousness greater than 24 hours with return to pre-existing conscious level**

✓7ᵗʰ **S06.6x6** **Traumatic subarachnoid hemorrhage with loss of consciousness greater than 24 hours without return to pre-existing conscious level with patient surviving**

✓7ᵗʰ **S06.6x7** **Traumatic subarachnoid hemorrhage with loss of consciousness of any duration with death due to brain injury prior to regaining consciousness**

EXCLUDES 1 Not coded here   **EXCLUDES 2** Not included here   *Manifestation Code*

✓7ᵗʰ **S06.6x8** **Traumatic subarachnoid hemorrhage with loss of consciousness of any duration with death due to other cause prior to regaining consciousness**

✓7ᵗʰ **S06.6x9** **Traumatic subarachnoid hemorrhage with loss of consciousness of unspecified duration**

Traumatic subarachnoid hemorrhage NOS

✓5ᵗʰ **S06.8** **Other specified intracranial injuries**

✓6ᵗʰ **S06.81** **Injury of right internal carotid artery, intracranial portion, not elsewhere classified**

✓7ᵗʰ **S06.810** **Injury of right internal carotid artery, intracranial portion, not elsewhere classified without loss of consciousness**

✓7ᵗʰ **S06.811** **Injury of right internal carotid artery, intracranial portion, not elsewhere classified with loss of consciousness of 30 minutes or less**

✓7ᵗʰ **S06.812** **Injury of right internal carotid artery, intracranial portion, not elsewhere classified with loss of consciousness of 31 minutes to 59 minutes**

✓7ᵗʰ **S06.813** **Injury of right internal carotid artery, intracranial portion, not elsewhere classified with loss of consciousness of 1 hour to 5 hours 59 minutes**

✓7ᵗʰ **S06.814** **Injury of right internal carotid artery, intracranial portion, not elsewhere classified with loss of consciousness of 6 hours to 24 hours**

✓7ᵗʰ **S06.815** **Injury of right internal carotid artery, intracranial portion, not elsewhere classified with loss of consciousness greater than 24 hours with return to pre-existing conscious level**

✓7ᵗʰ **S06.816** **Injury of right internal carotid artery, intracranial portion, not elsewhere classified with loss of consciousness greater than 24 hours without return to pre-existing conscious level with patient surviving**

✓7ᵗʰ **S06.817** **Injury of right internal carotid artery, intracranial portion, not elsewhere classified with loss of consciousness of any duration with death due to brain injury prior to regaining consciousness**

✓7ᵗʰ **S06.818** **Injury of right internal carotid artery, intracranial portion, not elsewhere classified with loss of consciousness of any duration with death due to other cause prior to regaining consciousness**

✓7ᵗʰ **S06.819** **Injury of right internal carotid artery, intracranial portion, not elsewhere classified with loss of consciousness of unspecified duration**

Injury of right internal carotid artery, intracranial portion, not elsewhere classified NOS

✓6ᵗʰ **S06.82** **Injury of left internal carotid artery, intracranial portion, not elsewhere classified**

✓7ᵗʰ **S06.820** **Injury of left internal carotid artery, intracranial portion, not elsewhere classified without loss of consciousness**

✓7ᵗʰ **S06.821** **Injury of left internal carotid artery, intracranial portion, not elsewhere classified with loss of consciousness of 30 minutes or less**

✓7ᵗʰ **S06.822** **Injury of left internal carotid artery, intracranial portion, not elsewhere classified with loss of consciousness of 31 minutes to 59 minutes**

✓7ᵗʰ **S06.823** **Injury of left internal carotid artery, intracranial portion, not elsewhere classified with loss of consciousness of 1 hour to 5 hours 59 minutes**

✓7ᵗʰ **S06.824** **Injury of left internal carotid artery, intracranial portion, not elsewhere classified with loss of consciousness of 6 hours to 24 hours**

✓7ᵗʰ **S06.825** **Injury of left internal carotid artery, intracranial portion, not elsewhere classified with loss of consciousness greater than 24 hours with return to pre-existing conscious level**

✓7ᵗʰ **S06.826** **Injury of left internal carotid artery, intracranial portion, not elsewhere classified with loss of consciousness greater than 24 hours without return to pre-existing conscious level with patient surviving**

✓7ᵗʰ **S06.827** **Injury of left internal carotid artery, intracranial portion, not elsewhere classified with loss of consciousness of any duration with death due to brain injury prior to regaining consciousness**

✓7ᵗʰ **S06.828** **Injury of left internal carotid artery, intracranial portion, not elsewhere classified with loss of consciousness of any duration with death due to other cause prior to regaining consciousness**

✓7ᵗʰ **S06.829** **Injury of left internal carotid artery, intracranial portion, not elsewhere classified with loss of consciousness of unspecified duration**

Injury of left internal carotid artery, intracranial portion, not elsewhere classified NOS

✓6ᵗʰ **S06.89** **Other specified intracranial injury**

✓7ᵗʰ **S06.890** **Other specified intracranial injury without loss of consciousness**

✓7ᵗʰ **S06.891** **Other specified intracranial injury with loss of consciousness of 30 minutes or less**

✓7ᵗʰ **S06.892** **Other specified intracranial injury with loss of consciousness of 31 minutes to 59 minutes**

✓7ᵗʰ **S06.893** **Other specified intracranial injury with loss of consciousness of 1 hour to 5 hours 59 minutes**

✓7ᵗʰ **S06.894** **Other specified intracranial injury with loss of consciousness of 6 hours to 24 hours**

✓7ᵗʰ **S06.895** **Other specified intracranial injury with loss of consciousness greater than 24 hours with return to pre-existing conscious level**

✓7ᵗʰ **S06.896** **Other specified intracranial injury with loss of consciousness greater than 24 hours without return to pre-existing conscious level with patient surviving**

✓7ᵗʰ **S06.897** **Other specified intracranial injury with loss of consciousness of any duration with death due to brain injury prior to regaining consciousness**

✓7ᵗʰ **S06.898** **Other specified intracranial injury with loss of consciousness of any duration with death due to other cause prior to regaining consciousness**

✓7ᵗʰ **S06.899** **Other specified intracranial injury with loss of consciousness of unspecified duration**

✓5ᵗʰ **S06.9** **Unspecified intracranial injury**

Brain injury NOS

Head injury NOS with loss of consciousness

EXCLUDES 1 *head injury NOS (S09.90)*

✓6ᵗʰ **S06.9x** **Unspecified intracranial injury**

✓7ᵗʰ **S06.9x0** **Unspecified intracranial injury without loss of consciousness**

✓7ᵗʰ **S06.9x1** **Unspecified intracranial injury with loss of consciousness of 30 minutes or less**

✓7ᵗʰ **S06.9x2** **Unspecified intracranial injury with loss of consciousness of 31 minutes to 59 minutes**

☑ Appropriate additional character required   ✓x7ᵗʰ Requires 7th character, placeholder x must fill empty characters

☑7th **S06.9x3** **Unspecified intracranial injury with loss of consciousness of 1 hour to 5 hours 59 minutes**

☑7th **S06.9x4** **Unspecified intracranial injury with loss of consciousness of 6 hours to 24 hours**

☑7th **S06.9x5** **Unspecified intracranial injury with loss of consciousness greater than 24 hours with return to pre-existing conscious level**

☑7th **S06.9x6** **Unspecified intracranial injury with loss of consciousness greater than 24 hours without return to pre-existing conscious level with patient surviving**

☑7th **S06.9x7** **Unspecified intracranial injury with loss of consciousness of any duration with death due to brain injury prior to regaining consciousness**

☑7th **S06.9x8** **Unspecified intracranial injury with loss of consciousness of any duration with death due to other cause prior to regaining consciousness**

☑7th **S06.9x9** **Unspecified intracranial injury with loss of consciousness of unspecified duration**

☑4th **S07 Crushing injury of head**

Use additional code for all associated injuries, such as:
     intracranial injuries (S06-)
        skull fractures (S02-)

The appropriate 7th character is to be added to each code from category S07.
   A   initial encounter
   D   subsequent encounter
   S   sequela

☑×7th **S07.0 Crushing injury of face**

☑×7th **S07.1 Crushing injury of skull**

☑×7th **S07.8 Crushing injury of other parts of head**

☑×7th **S07.9 Crushing injury of head, part unspecified**

☑4th **S08 Avulsion and traumatic amputation of part of head**

NOTE   An amputation not identified as partial or complete should be coded to complete

The appropriate 7th character is to be added to each code from category S08.
   A   initial encounter
   D   subsequent encounter
   S   sequela

☑×7th **S08.0 Avulsion of scalp**

☑5th **S08.1 Traumatic amputation of ear**

☑6th **S08.11 Complete traumatic amputation of ear**

☑7th **S08.111 Complete traumatic amputation of right ear**

☑7th **S08.112 Complete traumatic amputation of left ear**

☑7th **S08.119 Complete traumatic amputation of unspecified ear**

☑6th **S08.12 Partial traumatic amputation of ear**

☑7th **S08.121 Partial traumatic amputation of right ear**

☑7th **S08.122 Partial traumatic amputation of left ear**

☑7th **S08.129 Partial traumatic amputation of unspecified ear**

☑5th **S08.8 Traumatic amputation of other parts of head**

☑6th **S08.81 Traumatic amputation of nose**

☑7th **S08.811 Complete traumatic amputation of nose**

☑7th **S08.812 Partial traumatic amputation of nose**

☑×7th **S08.89 Traumatic amputation of other parts of head**

☑4th **S09 Other and unspecified injuries of head**

The appropriate 7th character is to be added to each code from category S09.
   A   initial encounter
   D   subsequent encounter
   S   sequela

☑×7th **S09.0 Injury of blood vessels of head, not elsewhere classified**

    EXCLUDES 1   *injury of cerebral blood vessels (S06-)*
                   injury of precerebral blood vessels (S15-)

☑5th **S09.1 Injury of muscle and tendon of head**

Code also any associated open wound (S01-)

    EXCLUDES 2   *sprain to joints and ligament of head (S03.9)*

☑×7th **S09.10 Unspecified injury of muscle and tendon of head**

Injury of muscle and tendon of head NOS

☑×7th **S09.11 Strain of muscle and tendon of head**

☑×7th **S09.12 Laceration of muscle and tendon of head**

☑×7th **S09.19 Other specified injury of muscle and tendon of head**

☑5th **S09.2 Traumatic rupture of ear drum**

    EXCLUDES 1   *traumatic rupture of ear drum due to blast injury (S09.31-)*

☑×7th **S09.20 Traumatic rupture of unspecified ear drum**

☑×7th **S09.21 Traumatic rupture of right ear drum**

☑×7th **S09.22 Traumatic rupture of left ear drum**

☑5th **S09.3 Other specified and unspecified injury of middle and inner ear**

    EXCLUDES 1   *injury to ear NOS (S09.91-)*

    EXCLUDES 2   *injury to external ear (S00.4-, S01.3-, S08.1-)*

☑6th **S09.30 Unspecified injury of middle and inner ear**

☑7th **S09.301 Unspecified injury of right middle and inner ear**

☑7th **S09.302 Unspecified injury of left middle and inner ear**

☑7th **S09.309 Unspecified injury of unspecified middle and inner ear**

☑6th **S09.31 Primary blast injury of ear**

Blast injury of ear NOS

☑7th **S09.311 Primary blast injury of right ear**

☑7th **S09.312 Primary blast injury of left ear**

☑7th **S09.313 Primary blast injury of ear, bilateral**

☑7th **S09.319 Primary blast injury of unspecified ear**

☑6th **S09.39 Other specified injury of middle and inner ear**

Secondary blast injury to ear

☑7th **S09.391 Other specified injury of right middle and inner ear**

☑7th **S09.392 Other specified injury of left middle and inner ear**

☑7th **S09.399 Other specified injury of unspecified middle and inner ear**

☑×7th **S09.8 Other specified injuries of head**

☑5th **S09.9 Unspecified injury of face and head**

☑×7th **S09.90 Unspecified injury of head**

Head injury NOS

    EXCLUDES 1   *brain injury NOS (S06.9-)*
                   head injury NOS with loss of consciousness (S06.9-)
                   intracranial injury NOS (S06.9-)

☑×7th **S09.91 Unspecified injury of ear**

Injury of ear NOS

☑×7th **S09.92 Unspecified injury of nose**

Injury of nose NOS

☑×7th **S09.93 Unspecified injury of face**

Injury of face NOS

EXCLUDES 1 Not coded here   EXCLUDES 2 Not included here   *Manifestation Code*

Injuries to the neck (S10-S19)

INCLUDES   injuries of nape
               injuries of supraclavicular region
               injuries of throat

EXCLUDES 2   burns and corrosions (T20-T32)
               effects of foreign body in esophagus (T18.1)
               effects of foreign body in larynx (T17.3)
               effects of foreign body in pharynx (T17.2)
               effects of foreign body in trachea (T17.4)
               frostbite (T33-T34)
               insect bite or sting, venomous (T63.4)

√4th **S10**   **Superficial injury of neck**

> The appropriate 7th character is to be added to each code from category S10.
> A   initial encounter
> D   subsequent encounter
> S   sequela

  √x7th **S10.0**   **Contusion of throat**
        Contusion of cervical esophagus
        Contusion of larynx
        Contusion of pharynx
        Contusion of trachea

  √5th **S10.1**   **Other and unspecified superficial injuries of throat**
    √x7th **S10.10**   **Unspecified superficial injuries of throat**
    √x7th **S10.11**   **Abrasion of throat**
    √x7th **S10.12**   **Blister (nonthermal) of throat**
    √x7th **S10.14**   **External constriction of part of throat**
    √x7th **S10.15**   **Superficial foreign body of throat**
          Splinter in the throat
    √x7th **S10.16**   **Insect bite (nonvenomous) of throat**
    √x7th **S10.17**   **Other superficial bite of throat**
          EXCLUDES 1   open bite of throat (S11.85)

  √5th **S10.8**   **Superficial injury of other specified parts of neck**
    √x7th **S10.80**   **Unspecified superficial injury of other specified part of neck**
    √x7th **S10.81**   **Abrasion of other specified part of neck**
    √x7th **S10.82**   **Blister (nonthermal) of other specified part of neck**
    √x7th **S10.83**   **Contusion of other specified part of neck**
    √x7th **S10.84**   **External constriction of other specified part of neck**
    √x7th **S10.85**   **Superficial foreign body of other specified part of neck**
          Splinter in other specified part of neck
    √x7th **S10.86**   **Insect bite of other specified part of neck**
    √x7th **S10.87**   **Other superficial bite of other specified part of neck**
          EXCLUDES 1   open bite of other specified parts of neck (S11.85)

  √5th **S10.9**   **Superficial injury of unspecified part of neck**
    √x7th **S10.90**   **Unspecified superficial injury of unspecified part of neck**
    √x7th **S10.91**   **Abrasion of unspecified part of neck**
    √x7th **S10.92**   **Blister (nonthermal) of unspecified part of neck**
    √x7th **S10.93**   **Contusion of unspecified part of neck**
    √x7th **S10.94**   **External constriction of unspecified part of neck**
    √x7th **S10.95**   **Superficial foreign body of unspecified part of neck**
    √x7th **S10.96**   **Insect bite of unspecified part of neck**
    √x7th **S10.97**   **Other superficial bite of unspecified part of neck**

√4th **S11**   **Open wound of neck**
    Code also any associated:
      spinal cord injury (S14.0, S14.1-)
      wound infection
    EXCLUDES 2   open fracture of vertebra (S12- with 7th character B)

> The appropriate 7th character is to be added to each code from category S11.
> A   initial encounter
> D   subsequent encounter
> S   sequela

  √5th **S11.0**   **Open wound of larynx and trachea**
    √6th **S11.01**   **Open wound of larynx**
          EXCLUDES 2   open wound of vocal cord (S11.03)
      √7th **S11.011**   **Laceration without foreign body of larynx**
      √7th **S11.012**   **Laceration with foreign body of larynx**

      √7th **S11.013**   **Puncture wound without foreign body of larynx**
      √7th **S11.014**   **Puncture wound with foreign body of larynx**
      √7th **S11.015**   **Open bite of larynx**
          Bite of larynx NOS
      √7th **S11.019**   **Unspecified open wound of larynx**
    √6th **S11.02**   **Open wound of trachea**
        Open wound of cervical trachea
        Open wound of trachea NOS
        EXCLUDES 2   open wound of thoracic trachea (S27.5-)
      √7th **S11.021**   **Laceration without foreign body of trachea**
      √7th **S11.022**   **Laceration with foreign body of trachea**
      √7th **S11.023**   **Puncture wound without foreign body of trachea**
      √7th **S11.024**   **Puncture wound with foreign body of trachea**
      √7th **S11.025**   **Open bite of trachea**
          Bite of trachea NOS
      √7th **S11.029**   **Unspecified open wound of trachea**
    √6th **S11.03**   **Open wound of vocal cord**
      √7th **S11.031**   **Laceration without foreign body of vocal cord**
      √7th **S11.032**   **Laceration with foreign body of vocal cord**
      √7th **S11.033**   **Puncture wound without foreign body of vocal cord**
      √7th **S11.034**   **Puncture wound with foreign body of vocal cord**
      √7th **S11.035**   **Open bite of vocal cord**
          Bite of vocal cord NOS
      √7th **S11.039**   **Unspecified open wound of vocal cord**

  √5th **S11.1**   **Open wound of thyroid gland**
    √x7th **S11.10**   **Unspecified open wound of thyroid gland**
    √x7th **S11.11**   **Laceration without foreign body of thyroid gland**
    √x7th **S11.12**   **Laceration with foreign body of thyroid gland**
    √x7th **S11.13**   **Puncture wound without foreign body of thyroid gland**
    √x7th **S11.14**   **Puncture wound with foreign body of thyroid gland**
    √x7th **S11.15**   **Open bite of thyroid gland**
          Bite of thyroid gland NOS

  √5th **S11.2**   **Open wound of pharynx and cervical esophagus**
      EXCLUDES 1   open wound of esophagus NOS (S27.8-)
    √x7th **S11.20**   **Unspecified open wound of pharynx and cervical esophagus**
    √x7th **S11.21**   **Laceration without foreign body of pharynx and cervical esophagus**
    √x7th **S11.22**   **Laceration with foreign body of pharynx and cervical esophagus**
    √x7th **S11.23**   **Puncture wound without foreign body of pharynx and cervical esophagus**
    √x7th **S11.24**   **Puncture wound with foreign body of pharynx and cervical esophagus**
    √x7th **S11.25**   **Open bite of pharynx and cervical esophagus**
          Bite of pharynx and cervical esophagus NOS

  √5th **S11.8**   **Open wound of other specified parts of neck**
    √x7th **S11.80**   **Unspecified open wound of other specified part of neck**
    √x7th **S11.81**   **Laceration without foreign body of other specified part of neck**
    √x7th **S11.82**   **Laceration with foreign body of other specified part of neck**
    √x7th **S11.83**   **Puncture wound without foreign body of other specified part of neck**
    √x7th **S11.84**   **Puncture wound with foreign body of other specified part of neck**
    √x7th **S11.85**   **Open bite of other specified part of neck**
          Bite of other specified part of neck NOS
          EXCLUDES 1   superficial bite of other specified part of neck (S10.87)
    √x7th **S11.89**   **Other open wound of other specified part of neck**

  √5th **S11.9**   **Open wound of unspecified part of neck**
    √x7th **S11.90**   **Unspecified open wound of unspecified part of neck**

☑ Appropriate additional character required   √x7th Requires 7th character, placeholder x must fill empty characters

√x7ᵗʰ **S11.91** Laceration without foreign body of unspecified part of neck

√x7ᵗʰ **S11.92** Laceration with foreign body of unspecified part of neck

√x7ᵗʰ **S11.93** Puncture wound without foreign body of unspecified part of neck

√x7ᵗʰ **S11.94** Puncture wound with foreign body of unspecified part of neck

√x7ᵗʰ **S11.95** Open bite of unspecified part of neck
Bite of neck NOS
EXCLUDES 1   superficial bite of neck (S10.97)

√4ᵗʰ **S12** **Fracture of cervical vertebra and other parts of neck**
NOTE   A fracture not indicated as nondisplaced or displaced should be classified to displaced
A fracture not indicated as open or closed should be coded to closed.
INCLUDES   fracture of cervical neural arch
fracture of cervical spine
fracture of cervical spinous process
fracture of cervical transverse process
fracture of cervical vertebral arch
fracture of neck
Code also any associated cervical spinal cord injury (S14.0, S14.1-)

> The appropriate 7th character is to be added to all codes from subcategories S12.0-S12.6.
> A   initial encounter for closed fracture
> B   initial encounter for open fracture
> D   subsequent encounter for fracture with routine healing
> G   subsequent encounter for fracture with delayed healing
> K   subsequent encounter for fracture with nonunion
> S   sequela

√5ᵗʰ **S12.0** **Fracture of first cervical vertebra**
Atlas
√6ᵗʰ **S12.00** Unspecified fracture of first cervical vertebra
√7ᵗʰ **S12.000** Unspecified displaced fracture of first cervical vertebra
√7ᵗʰ **S12.001** Unspecified nondisplaced fracture of first cervical vertebra
√x7ᵗʰ **S12.01** Stable burst fracture of first cervical vertebra
√x7ᵗʰ **S12.02** Unstable burst fracture of first cervical vertebra
√6ᵗʰ **S12.03** Posterior arch fracture of first cervical vertebra
√7ᵗʰ **S12.030** Displaced posterior arch fracture of first cervical vertebra
√7ᵗʰ **S12.031** Nondisplaced posterior arch fracture of first cervical vertebra
√6ᵗʰ **S12.04** Lateral mass fracture of first cervical vertebra
√7ᵗʰ **S12.040** Displaced lateral mass fracture of first cervical vertebra
√7ᵗʰ **S12.041** Nondisplaced lateral mass fracture of first cervical vertebra
√x7ᵗʰ **S12.09** Other fracture of first cervical vertebra
√7ᵗʰ **S12.090** Other displaced fracture of first cervical vertebra
√7ᵗʰ **S12.091** Other nondisplaced fracture of first cervical vertebra

√5ᵗʰ **S12.1** **Fracture of second cervical vertebra**
Axis
√6ᵗʰ **S12.10** Unspecified fracture of second cervical vertebra
√7ᵗʰ **S12.100** Unspecified displaced fracture of second cervical vertebra
√7ᵗʰ **S12.101** Unspecified nondisplaced fracture of second cervical vertebra
√6ᵗʰ **S12.11** Type II dens fracture
√7ᵗʰ **S12.110** Anterior displaced Type II dens fracture
√7ᵗʰ **S12.111** Posterior displaced Type II dens fracture
√7ᵗʰ **S12.112** Nondisplaced Type II dens fracture
√6ᵗʰ **S12.12** Other dens fracture
√7ᵗʰ **S12.120** Other displaced dens fracture
√7ᵗʰ **S12.121** Other nondisplaced dens fracture
√6ᵗʰ **S12.13** Unspecified traumatic spondylolisthesis of second cervical vertebra
√7ᵗʰ **S12.130** Unspecified traumatic displaced spondylolisthesis of second cervical vertebra

√7ᵗʰ **S12.131** Unspecified traumatic nondisplaced spondylolisthesis of second cervical vertebra
√x7ᵗʰ **S12.14** Type III traumatic spondylolisthesis of second cervical vertebra
√6ᵗʰ **S12.15** Other traumatic spondylolisthesis of second cervical vertebra
√7ᵗʰ **S12.150** Other traumatic displaced spondylolisthesis of second cervical vertebra
√7ᵗʰ **S12.151** Other traumatic nondisplaced spondylolisthesis of second cervical vertebra
√6ᵗʰ **S12.19** Other fracture of second cervical vertebra
√7ᵗʰ **S12.190** Other displaced fracture of second cervical vertebra
√7ᵗʰ **S12.191** Other nondisplaced fracture of second cervical vertebra

√5ᵗʰ **S12.2** **Fracture of third cervical vertebra**
√6ᵗʰ **S12.20** Unspecified fracture of third cervical vertebra
√7ᵗʰ **S12.200** Unspecified displaced fracture of third cervical vertebra
√7ᵗʰ **S12.201** Unspecified nondisplaced fracture of third cervical vertebra
√6ᵗʰ **S12.23** Unspecified traumatic spondylolisthesis of third cervical vertebra
√7ᵗʰ **S12.230** Unspecified traumatic displaced spondylolisthesis of third cervical vertebra
√7ᵗʰ **S12.231** Unspecified traumatic nondisplaced spondylolisthesis of third cervical vertebra
√x7ᵗʰ **S12.24** Type III traumatic spondylolisthesis of third cervical vertebra
√6ᵗʰ **S12.25** Other traumatic spondylolisthesis of third cervical vertebra
√7ᵗʰ **S12.250** Other traumatic displaced spondylolisthesis of third cervical vertebra
√7ᵗʰ **S12.251** Other traumatic nondisplaced spondylolisthesis of third cervical vertebra
√6ᵗʰ **S12.29** Other fracture of third cervical vertebra
√7ᵗʰ **S12.290** Other displaced fracture of third cervical vertebra
√7ᵗʰ **S12.291** Other nondisplaced fracture of third cervical vertebra

√5ᵗʰ **S12.3** **Fracture of fourth cervical vertebra**
√6ᵗʰ **S12.30** Unspecified fracture of fourth cervical vertebra
√7ᵗʰ **S12.300** Unspecified displaced fracture of fourth cervical vertebra
√7ᵗʰ **S12.301** Unspecified nondisplaced fracture of fourth cervical vertebra
√6ᵗʰ **S12.33** Unspecified traumatic spondylolisthesis of fourth cervical vertebra
√7ᵗʰ **S12.330** Unspecified traumatic displaced spondylolisthesis of fourth cervical vertebra
√7ᵗʰ **S12.331** Unspecified traumatic nondisplaced spondylolisthesis of fourth cervical vertebra
√x7ᵗʰ **S12.34** Type III traumatic spondylolisthesis of fourth cervical vertebra
√6ᵗʰ **S12.35** Other traumatic spondylolisthesis of fourth cervical vertebra
√7ᵗʰ **S12.350** Other traumatic displaced spondylolisthesis of fourth cervical vertebra
√7ᵗʰ **S12.351** Other traumatic nondisplaced spondylolisthesis of fourth cervical vertebra
√6ᵗʰ **S12.39** Other fracture of fourth cervical vertebra
√7ᵗʰ **S12.390** Other displaced fracture of fourth cervical vertebra
√7ᵗʰ **S12.391** Other nondisplaced fracture of fourth cervical vertebra

EXCLUDES 1   Not coded here   EXCLUDES 2   Not included here   *Manifestation Code*

✓5th **S12.4** **Fracture of fifth cervical vertebra**
 ✓6th **S12.40** **Unspecified fracture of fifth cervical vertebra**
  ✓7th **S12.400** **Unspecified displaced fracture of fifth cervical vertebra**
  ✓7th **S12.401** **Unspecified nondisplaced fracture of fifth cervical vertebra**
 ✓6th **S12.43** **Unspecified traumatic spondylolisthesis of fifth cervical vertebra**
  ✓7th **S12.430** **Unspecified traumatic displaced spondylolisthesis of fifth cervical vertebra**
  ✓7th **S12.431** **Unspecified traumatic nondisplaced spondylolisthesis of fifth cervical vertebra**
 ✓x7th **S12.44** **Type III traumatic spondylolisthesis of fifth cervical vertebra**
 ✓6th **S12.45** **Other traumatic spondylolisthesis of fifth cervical vertebra**
  ✓7th **S12.450** **Other traumatic displaced spondylolisthesis of fifth cervical vertebra**
  ✓7th **S12.451** **Other traumatic nondisplaced spondylolisthesis of fifth cervical vertebra**
 ✓6th **S12.49** **Other fracture of fifth cervical vertebra**
  ✓7th **S12.490** **Other displaced fracture of fifth cervical vertebra**
  ✓7th **S12.491** **Other nondisplaced fracture of fifth cervical vertebra**

✓5th **S12.5** **Fracture of sixth cervical vertebra**
 ✓6th **S12.50** **Unspecified fracture of sixth cervical vertebra**
  ✓7th **S12.500** **Unspecified displaced fracture of sixth cervical vertebra**
  ✓7th **S12.501** **Unspecified nondisplaced fracture of sixth cervical vertebra**
 ✓6th **S12.53** **Unspecified traumatic spondylolisthesis of sixth cervical vertebra**
  ✓7th **S12.530** **Unspecified traumatic displaced spondylolisthesis of sixth cervical vertebra**
  ✓7th **S12.531** **Unspecified traumatic nondisplaced spondylolisthesis of sixth cervical vertebra**
 ✓x7th **S12.54** **Type III traumatic spondylolisthesis of sixth cervical vertebra**
 ✓6th **S12.55** **Other traumatic spondylolisthesis of sixth cervical vertebra**
  ✓7th **S12.550** **Other traumatic displaced spondylolisthesis of sixth cervical vertebra**
  ✓7th **S12.551** **Other traumatic nondisplaced spondylolisthesis of sixth cervical vertebra**
 ✓6th **S12.59** **Other fracture of sixth cervical vertebra**
  ✓7th **S12.590** **Other displaced fracture of sixth cervical vertebra**
  ✓7th **S12.591** **Other nondisplaced fracture of sixth cervical vertebra**

✓5th **S12.6** **Fracture of seventh cervical vertebra**
 ✓6th **S12.60** **Unspecified fracture of seventh cervical vertebra**
  ✓7th **S12.600** **Unspecified displaced fracture of seventh cervical vertebra**
  ✓7th **S12.601** **Unspecified nondisplaced fracture of seventh cervical vertebra**
 ✓6th **S12.63** **Unspecified traumatic spondylolisthesis of seventh cervical vertebra**
  ✓7th **S12.630** **Unspecified traumatic displaced spondylolisthesis of seventh cervical vertebra**
  ✓7th **S12.631** **Unspecified traumatic nondisplaced spondylolisthesis of seventh cervical vertebra**
 ✓x7th **S12.64** **Type III traumatic spondylolisthesis of seventh cervical vertebra**
 ✓6th **S12.65** **Other traumatic spondylolisthesis of seventh cervical vertebra**
  ✓7th **S12.650** **Other traumatic displaced spondylolisthesis of seventh cervical vertebra**
  ✓7th **S12.651** **Other traumatic nondisplaced spondylolisthesis of seventh cervical vertebra**
 ✓6th **S12.69** **Other fracture of seventh cervical vertebra**
  ✓7th **S12.690** **Other displaced fracture of seventh cervical vertebra**
  ✓7th **S12.691** **Other nondisplaced fracture of seventh cervical vertebra**

✓x7th **S12.8** **Fracture of other parts of neck**
 Hyoid bone
 Larynx
 Thyroid cartilage
 Trachea

> The appropriate 7th character is to be added to code S12.8.
> A initial encounter
> D subsequent encounter
> S sequela

✓x7th **S12.9** **Fracture of neck, unspecified**
 Fracture of neck NOS
 Fracture of cervical spine NOS
 Fracture of cervical vertebra NOS

> The appropriate 7th character is to be added to code S12.9.
> A initial encounter
> D subsequent encounter
> S sequela

✓4th **S13** **Dislocation and sprain of joints and ligaments at neck level**
 INCLUDES avulsion of joint or ligament at neck level
  laceration of cartilage, joint or ligament at neck level
  sprain of cartilage, joint or ligament at neck level
  traumatic hemarthrosis of joint or ligament at neck level
  traumatic rupture of joint or ligament at neck level
  traumatic subluxation of joint or ligament at neck level
  traumatic tear of joint or ligament at neck level
 Code also: any associated open wound
 EXCLUDES 2 *strain of muscle or tendon at neck level (S16.1)*

> The appropriate 7th character is to be added to each code from category S13.
> A initial encounter
> D subsequent encounter
> S sequela

✓x7th **S13.0** **Traumatic rupture of cervical intervertebral disc**
 EXCLUDES 1 *rupture or displacement (nontraumatic) of cervical intervertebral disc NOS (M50-)*

✓5th **S13.1** **Subluxation and dislocation of cervical vertebrae**
 Code also any associated:
  open wound of neck (S11-)
  spinal cord injury (S14.1-)
 EXCLUDES 2 *fracture of cervical vertebrae (S12.0--S12.3-)*
 ✓6th **S13.10** **Subluxation and dislocation of unspecified cervical vertebrae**
  ✓7th **S13.100** **Subluxation of unspecified cervical vertebrae**
  ✓7th **S13.101** **Dislocation of unspecified cervical vertebrae**
 ✓6th **S13.11** **Subluxation and dislocation of C0/C1 cervical vertebrae**
  Subluxation and dislocation of atlantooccipital joint
  Subluxation and dislocation of atloidooccipital joint
  Subluxation and dislocation of occipitoatloid joint
  ✓7th **S13.110** **Subluxation of C0/C1 cervical vertebrae**
  ✓7th **S13.111** **Dislocation of C0/C1 cervical vertebrae**
 ✓6th **S13.12** **Subluxation and dislocation of C1/C2 cervical vertebrae**
  Subluxation and dislocation of atlantoaxial joint
  ✓7th **S13.120** **Subluxation of C1/C2 cervical vertebrae**
  ✓7th **S13.121** **Dislocation of C1/C2 cervical vertebrae**
 ✓6th **S13.13** **Subluxation and dislocation of C2/C3 cervical vertebrae**
  ✓7th **S13.130** **Subluxation of C2/C3 cervical vertebrae**
  ✓7th **S13.131** **Dislocation of C2/C3 cervical vertebrae**

√6th **S13.14　Subluxation and dislocation of C3/C4 cervical vertebrae**
　　　√7th **S13.140　Subluxation of C3/C4 cervical vertebrae**
　　　√7th **S13.141　Dislocation of C3/C4 cervical vertebrae**
√6th **S13.15　Subluxation and dislocation of C4/C5 cervical vertebrae**
　　　√7th **S13.150　Subluxation of C4/C5 cervical vertebrae**
　　　√7th **S13.151　Dislocation of C4/C5 cervical vertebrae**
√6th **S13.16　Subluxation and dislocation of C5/C6 cervical vertebrae**
　　　√7th **S13.160　Subluxation of C5/C6 cervical vertebrae**
　　　√7th **S13.161　Dislocation of C5/C6 cervical vertebrae**
√6th **S13.17　Subluxation and dislocation of C6/C7 cervical vertebrae**
　　　√7th **S13.170　Subluxation of C6/C7 cervical vertebrae**
　　　√7th **S13.171　Dislocation of C6/C7 cervical vertebrae**
√6th **S13.18　Subluxation and dislocation of C7/T1 cervical vertebrae**
　　　√7th **S13.180　Subluxation of C7/T1 cervical vertebrae**
　　　√7th **S13.181　Dislocation of C7/T1 cervical vertebrae**
√5th **S13.2　Dislocation of other and unspecified parts of neck**
　　S13.20　Dislocation of unspecified parts of neck
　　S13.29　Dislocation of other parts of neck
√x7th **S13.4　Sprain of ligaments of cervical spine**
　　Sprain of anterior longitudinal (ligament), cervical
　　Sprain of atlanto-axial (joints)
　　Sprain of atlanto-occipital (joints)
　　Whiplash injury of cervical spine
√x7th **S13.5　Sprain of thyroid region**
　　Sprain of cricoarytenoid (joint) (ligament)
　　Sprain of cricothyroid (joint) (ligament)
　　Sprain of thyroid cartilage
√x7th **S13.8　Sprain of joints and ligaments of other parts of neck**
√x7th **S13.9　Sprain of joints and ligaments of unspecified parts of neck**
√4th **S14　Injury of nerves and spinal cord at neck level**
　　Code to highest level of cervical cord injury
　　Code also any associated:
　　　fracture of cervical vertebra (S12.0--S12.6-)
　　　open wound of neck (S11-)
　　　transient paralysis (R29.5)

> The appropriate 7th character is to be added to each code from category S14.
> A　initial encounter
> D　subsequent encounter
> S　sequela

√x7th **S14.0　Concussion and edema of cervical spinal cord**
√5th **S14.1　Other and unspecified injuries of cervical spinal cord**
　√6th **S14.10　Unspecified injury of cervical spinal cord**
　　√7th **S14.101　Unspecified injury at C1 level of cervical spinal cord**
　　√7th **S14.102　Unspecified injury at C2 level of cervical spinal cord**
　　√7th **S14.103　Unspecified injury at C3 level of cervical spinal cord**
　　√7th **S14.104　Unspecified injury at C4 level of cervical spinal cord**
　　√7th **S14.105　Unspecified injury at C5 level of cervical spinal cord**
　　√7th **S14.106　Unspecified injury at C6 level of cervical spinal cord**
　　√7th **S14.107　Unspecified injury at C7 level of cervical spinal cord**
　　√7th **S14.108　Unspecified injury at C8 level of cervical spinal cord**
　　√7th **S14.109　Unspecified injury at unspecified level of cervical spinal cord**
　　　　Injury of cervical spinal cord NOS
　√6th **S14.11　Complete lesion of cervical spinal cord**
　　√7th **S14.111　Complete lesion at C1 level of cervical spinal cord**
　　√7th **S14.112　Complete lesion at C2 level of cervical spinal cord**
　　√7th **S14.113　Complete lesion at C3 level of cervical spinal cord**

　　√7th **S14.114　Complete lesion at C4 level of cervical spinal cord**
　　√7th **S14.115　Complete lesion at C5 level of cervical spinal cord**
　　√7th **S14.116　Complete lesion at C6 level of cervical spinal cord**
　　√7th **S14.117　Complete lesion at C7 level of cervical spinal cord**
　　√7th **S14.118　Complete lesion at C8 level of cervical spinal cord**
　　√7th **S14.119　Complete lesion at unspecified level of cervical spinal cord**
　√6th **S14.12　Central cord syndrome of cervical spinal cord**
　　√7th **S14.121　Central cord syndrome at C1 level of cervical spinal cord**
　　√7th **S14.122　Central cord syndrome at C2 level of cervical spinal cord**
　　√7th **S14.123　Central cord syndrome at C3 level of cervical spinal cord**
　　√7th **S14.124　Central cord syndrome at C4 level of cervical spinal cord**
　　√7th **S14.125　Central cord syndrome at C5 level of cervical spinal cord**
　　√7th **S14.126　Central cord syndrome at C6 level of cervical spinal cord**
　　√7th **S14.127　Central cord syndrome at C7 level of cervical spinal cord**
　　√7th **S14.128　Central cord syndrome at C8 level of cervical spinal cord**
　　√7th **S14.129　Central cord syndrome at unspecified level of cervical spinal cord**
　√6th **S14.13　Anterior cord syndrome of cervical spinal cord**
　　√7th **S14.131　Anterior cord syndrome at C1 level of cervical spinal cord**
　　√7th **S14.132　Anterior cord syndrome at C2 level of cervical spinal cord**
　　√7th **S14.133　Anterior cord syndrome at C3 level of cervical spinal cord**
　　√7th **S14.134　Anterior cord syndrome at C4 level of cervical spinal cord**
　　√7th **S14.135　Anterior cord syndrome at C5 level of cervical spinal cord**
　　√7th **S14.136　Anterior cord syndrome at C6 level of cervical spinal cord**
　　√7th **S14.137　Anterior cord syndrome at C7 level of cervical spinal cord**
　　√7th **S14.138　Anterior cord syndrome at C8 level of cervical spinal cord**
　　√7th **S14.139　Anterior cord syndrome at unspecified level of cervical spinal cord**
　√6th **S14.14　Brown-Séquard syndrome of cervical spinal cord**
　　√7th **S14.141　Brown-Séquard syndrome at C1 level of cervical spinal cord**
　　√7th **S14.142　Brown-Séquard syndrome at C2 level of cervical spinal cord**
　　√7th **S14.143　Brown-Séquard syndrome at C3 level of cervical spinal cord**
　　√7th **S14.144　Brown-Séquard syndrome at C4 level of cervical spinal cord**
　　√7th **S14.145　Brown-Séquard syndrome at C5 level of cervical spinal cord**
　　√7th **S14.146　Brown-Séquard syndrome at C6 level of cervical spinal cord**
　　√7th **S14.147　Brown-Séquard syndrome at C7 level of cervical spinal cord**
　　√7th **S14.148　Brown-Séquard syndrome at C8 level of cervical spinal cord**
　　√7th **S14.149　Brown-Séquard syndrome at unspecified level of cervical spinal cord**
　√6th **S14.15　Other incomplete lesions of cervical spinal cord**
　　　Incomplete lesion of cervical spinal cord NOS
　　　Posterior cord syndrome of cervical spinal cord
　　√7th **S14.151　Other incomplete lesion at C1 level of cervical spinal cord**
　　√7th **S14.152　Other incomplete lesion at C2 level of cervical spinal cord**

EXCLUDES 1　Not coded here　　　　EXCLUDES 2　Not included here　　　　*Manifestation Code*

✓7ᵗʰ **S14.153** **Other incomplete lesion at C3 level of cervical spinal cord**

✓7ᵗʰ **S14.154** **Other incomplete lesion at C4 level of cervical spinal cord**

✓7ᵗʰ **S14.155** **Other incomplete lesion at C5 level of cervical spinal cord**

✓7ᵗʰ **S14.156** **Other incomplete lesion at C6 level of cervical spinal cord**

✓7ᵗʰ **S14.157** **Other incomplete lesion at C7 level of cervical spinal cord**

✓7ᵗʰ **S14.158** **Other incomplete lesion at C8 level of cervical spinal cord**

✓7ᵗʰ **S14.159** **Other incomplete lesion at unspecified level of cervical spinal cord**

✓x7ᵗʰ **S14.2** **Injury of nerve root of cervical spine**

✓x7ᵗʰ **S14.3** **Injury of brachial plexus**

✓x7ᵗʰ **S14.4** **Injury of peripheral nerves of neck**

✓x7ᵗʰ **S14.5** **Injury of cervical sympathetic nerves**

✓x7ᵗʰ **S14.8** **Injury of other specified nerves of neck**

✓x7ᵗʰ **S14.9** **Injury of unspecified nerves of neck**

✓4ᵗʰ **S15** **Injury of blood vessels at neck level**
　Code also any associated open wound (S11-)

> The appropriate 7th character is to be added to each code from category S15.
> A　initial encounter
> D　subsequent encounter
> S　sequela

✓5ᵗʰ **S15.0** **Injury of carotid artery of neck**
　Injury of carotid artery (common) (external) (internal, extracranial portion)
　Injury of carotid artery NOS
　　EXCLUDES 1　*injury of internal carotid artery, intracranial portion (S06.8)*

✓6ᵗʰ **S15.00** **Unspecified injury of carotid artery**

✓7ᵗʰ **S15.001** **Unspecified injury of right carotid artery**

✓7ᵗʰ **S15.002** **Unspecified injury of left carotid artery**

✓7ᵗʰ **S15.009** **Unspecified injury of unspecified carotid artery**

✓6ᵗʰ **S15.01** **Minor laceration of carotid artery**
　Incomplete transection of carotid artery
　Laceration of carotid artery NOS
　Superficial laceration of carotid artery

✓7ᵗʰ **S15.011** **Minor laceration of right carotid artery**

✓7ᵗʰ **S15.012** **Minor laceration of left carotid artery**

✓7ᵗʰ **S15.019** **Minor laceration of unspecified carotid artery**

✓6ᵗʰ **S15.02** **Major laceration of carotid artery**
　Complete transection of carotid artery
　Traumatic rupture of carotid artery

✓7ᵗʰ **S15.021** **Major laceration of right carotid artery**

✓7ᵗʰ **S15.022** **Major laceration of left carotid artery**

✓7ᵗʰ **S15.029** **Major laceration of unspecified carotid artery**

✓6ᵗʰ **S15.09** **Other specified injury of carotid artery**

✓7ᵗʰ **S15.091** **Other specified injury of right carotid artery**

✓7ᵗʰ **S15.092** **Other specified injury of left carotid artery**

✓7ᵗʰ **S15.099** **Other specified injury of unspecified carotid artery**

✓5ᵗʰ **S15.1** **Injury of vertebral artery**

✓6ᵗʰ **S15.10** **Unspecified injury of vertebral artery**

✓7ᵗʰ **S15.101** **Unspecified injury of right vertebral artery**

✓7ᵗʰ **S15.102** **Unspecified injury of left vertebral artery**

✓7ᵗʰ **S15.109** **Unspecified injury of unspecified vertebral artery**

✓6ᵗʰ **S15.11** **Minor laceration of vertebral artery**
　Incomplete transection of vertebral artery
　Laceration of vertebral artery NOS
　Superficial laceration of vertebral artery

✓7ᵗʰ **S15.111** **Minor laceration of right vertebral artery**

✓7ᵗʰ **S15.112** **Minor laceration of left vertebral artery**

✓7ᵗʰ **S15.119** **Minor laceration of unspecified vertebral artery**

✓6ᵗʰ **S15.12** **Major laceration of vertebral artery**
　Complete transection of vertebral artery
　Traumatic rupture of vertebral artery

✓7ᵗʰ **S15.121** **Major laceration of right vertebral artery**

✓7ᵗʰ **S15.122** **Major laceration of left vertebral artery**

✓7ᵗʰ **S15.129** **Major laceration of unspecified vertebral artery**

✓6ᵗʰ **S15.19** **Other specified injury of vertebral artery**

✓7ᵗʰ **S15.191** **Other specified injury of right vertebral artery**

✓7ᵗʰ **S15.192** **Other specified injury of left vertebral artery**

✓7ᵗʰ **S15.199** **Other specified injury of unspecified vertebral artery**

✓5ᵗʰ **S15.2** **Injury of external jugular vein**

✓6ᵗʰ **S15.20** **Unspecified injury of external jugular vein**

✓7ᵗʰ **S15.201** **Unspecified injury of right external jugular vein**

✓7ᵗʰ **S15.202** **Unspecified injury of left external jugular vein**

✓7ᵗʰ **S15.209** **Unspecified injury of unspecified external jugular vein**

✓6ᵗʰ **S15.21** **Minor laceration of external jugular vein**
　Incomplete transection of external jugular vein
　Laceration of external jugular vein NOS
　Superficial laceration of external jugular vein

✓7ᵗʰ **S15.211** **Minor laceration of right external jugular vein**

✓7ᵗʰ **S15.212** **Minor laceration of left external jugular vein**

✓7ᵗʰ **S15.219** **Minor laceration of unspecified external jugular vein**

✓6ᵗʰ **S15.22** **Major laceration of external jugular vein**
　Complete transection of external jugular vein
　Traumatic rupture of external jugular vein

✓7ᵗʰ **S15.221** **Major laceration of right external jugular vein**

✓7ᵗʰ **S15.222** **Major laceration of left external jugular vein**

✓7ᵗʰ **S15.229** **Major laceration of unspecified external jugular vein**

✓6ᵗʰ **S15.29** **Other specified injury of external jugular vein**

✓7ᵗʰ **S15.291** **Other specified injury of right external jugular vein**

✓7ᵗʰ **S15.292** **Other specified injury of left external jugular vein**

✓7ᵗʰ **S15.299** **Other specified injury of unspecified external jugular vein**

✓5ᵗʰ **S15.3** **Injury of internal jugular vein**

✓6ᵗʰ **S15.30** **Unspecified injury of internal jugular vein**

✓7ᵗʰ **S15.301** **Unspecified injury of right internal jugular vein**

✓7ᵗʰ **S15.302** **Unspecified injury of left internal jugular vein**

✓7ᵗʰ **S15.309** **Unspecified injury of unspecified internal jugular vein**

✓6ᵗʰ **S15.31** **Minor laceration of internal jugular vein**
　Incomplete transection of internal jugular vein
　Laceration of internal jugular vein NOS
　Superficial laceration of internal jugular vein

✓7ᵗʰ **S15.311** **Minor laceration of right internal jugular vein**

✓7ᵗʰ **S15.312** **Minor laceration of left internal jugular vein**

✓7ᵗʰ **S15.319** **Minor laceration of unspecified internal jugular vein**

✓6ᵗʰ **S15.32** **Major laceration of internal jugular vein**
　Complete transection of internal jugular vein
　Traumatic rupture of internal jugular vein

✓7ᵗʰ **S15.321** **Major laceration of right internal jugular vein**

✓7ᵗʰ **S15.322** **Major laceration of left internal jugular vein**

✓ Appropriate additional character required　　✓x7ᵗʰ Requires 7th character, placeholder x must fill empty characters

√7ᵗʰ   **S15.329**   **Major laceration of unspecified internal jugular vein**

√6ᵗʰ   **S15.39**   **Other specified injury of internal jugular vein**

√7ᵗʰ   **S15.391**   **Other specified injury of right internal jugular vein**

√7ᵗʰ   **S15.392**   **Other specified injury of left internal jugular vein**

√7ᵗʰ   **S15.399**   **Other specified injury of unspecified internal jugular vein**

√x7ᵗʰ   **S15.8**   **Injury of other specified blood vessels at neck level**

√x7ᵗʰ   **S15.9**   **Injury of unspecified blood vessel at neck level**

√4ᵗʰ   **S16**   **Injury of muscle, fascia and tendon at neck level**

Code also any associated open wound (S11-)

EXCLUDES 2   *sprain of joint or ligament at neck level (S13.9)*

The appropriate 7th character is to be added to each code from category S16.
A   initial encounter
D   subsequent encounter
S   sequela

√x7ᵗʰ   **S16.1**   **Strain of muscle, fascia and tendon at neck level**

√x7ᵗʰ   **S16.2**   **Laceration of muscle, fascia and tendon at neck level**

√x7ᵗʰ   **S16.8**   **Other specified injury of muscle, fascia and tendon at neck level**

√x7ᵗʰ   **S16.9**   **Unspecified injury of muscle, fascia and tendon at neck level**

√4ᵗʰ   **S17**   **Crushing injury of neck**

Use additional code for all associated injuries, such as:
injury of blood vessels (S15-)
open wound of neck (S11-)
spinal cord injury (S14.0, S14.1-)
vertebral fracture (S12.0--S12.3-)

The appropriate 7th character is to be added to each code from category S17.
A   initial encounter
D   subsequent encounter
S   sequela

√x7ᵗʰ   **S17.0**   **Crushing injury of larynx and trachea**

√x7ᵗʰ   **S17.8**   **Crushing injury of other specified parts of neck**

√x7ᵗʰ   **S17.9**   **Crushing injury of neck, part unspecified**

√4ᵗʰ   **S19**   **Other specified and unspecified injuries of neck**

The appropriate 7th character is to be added to each code from category S19.
A   initial encounter
D   subsequent encounter
S   sequela

√5ᵗʰ   **S19.8**   **Other specified injuries of neck**

√x7ᵗʰ   **S19.80**   **Other specified injuries of unspecified part of neck**

√x7ᵗʰ   **S19.81**   **Other specified injuries of larynx**

√x7ᵗʰ   **S19.82**   **Other specified injuries of cervical trachea**

EXCLUDES 2   *other specified injury of thoracic trachea (S27.5-)*

√x7ᵗʰ   **S19.83**   **Other specified injuries of vocal cord**

√x7ᵗʰ   **S19.84**   **Other specified injuries of thyroid gland**

√x7ᵗʰ   **S19.85**   **Other specified injuries of pharynx and cervical esophagus**

√x7ᵗʰ   **S19.89**   **Other specified injuries of other specified part of neck**

√x7ᵗʰ   **S19.9**   **Unspecified injury of neck**

Injuries to the thorax (S20-S29)

INCLUDES   injuries of breast
injuries of chest (wall)
injuries of interscapular area

EXCLUDES 2   *burns and corrosions (T20-T32)*
effects of foreign body in bronchus (T17.5)
effects of foreign body in esophagus (T18.1)
effects of foreign body in lung (T17.8)
effects of foreign body in trachea (T17.4)
frostbite (T33-T34)
injuries of axilla
injuries of clavicle
injuries of scapular region
injuries of shoulder
insect bite or sting, venomous (T63.4)

√4ᵗʰ   **S20**   **Superficial injury of thorax**

The appropriate 7th character is to be added to each code from category S20.
A   initial encounter
D   subsequent encounter
S   sequela

√5ᵗʰ   **S20.0**   **Contusion of breast**

√x7ᵗʰ   **S20.00**   **Contusion of breast, unspecified breast**

√x7ᵗʰ   **S20.01**   **Contusion of right breast**

√x7ᵗʰ   **S20.02**   **Contusion of left breast**

√5ᵗʰ   **S20.1**   **Other and unspecified superficial injuries of breast**

√6ᵗʰ   **S20.10**   **Unspecified superficial injuries of breast**

√7ᵗʰ   **S20.101**   **Unspecified superficial injuries of breast, right breast**

√7ᵗʰ   **S20.102**   **Unspecified superficial injuries of breast, left breast**

√7ᵗʰ   **S20.109**   **Unspecified superficial injuries of breast, unspecified breast**

√6ᵗʰ   **S20.11**   **Abrasion of breast**

√7ᵗʰ   **S20.111**   **Abrasion of breast, right breast**

√7ᵗʰ   **S20.112**   **Abrasion of breast, left breast**

√7ᵗʰ   **S20.119**   **Abrasion of breast, unspecified breast**

√6ᵗʰ   **S20.12**   **Blister (nonthermal) of breast**

√7ᵗʰ   **S20.121**   **Blister (nonthermal) of breast, right breast**

√7ᵗʰ   **S20.122**   **Blister (nonthermal) of breast, left breast**

√7ᵗʰ   **S20.129**   **Blister (nonthermal) of breast, unspecified breast**

√6ᵗʰ   **S20.14**   **External constriction of part of breast**

√7ᵗʰ   **S20.141**   **External constriction of part of breast, right breast**

√7ᵗʰ   **S20.142**   **External constriction of part of breast, left breast**

√7ᵗʰ   **S20.149**   **External constriction of part of breast, unspecified breast**

√6ᵗʰ   **S20.15**   **Superficial foreign body of breast**
Splinter in the breast

√7ᵗʰ   **S20.151**   **Superficial foreign body of breast, right breast**

√7ᵗʰ   **S20.152**   **Superficial foreign body of breast, left breast**

√7ᵗʰ   **S20.159**   **Superficial foreign body of breast, unspecified breast**

√6ᵗʰ   **S20.16**   **Insect bite (nonvenomous) of breast**

√7ᵗʰ   **S20.161**   **Insect bite (nonvenomous) of breast, right breast**

√7ᵗʰ   **S20.162**   **Insect bite (nonvenomous) of breast, left breast**

√7ᵗʰ   **S20.169**   **Insect bite (nonvenomous) of breast, unspecified breast**

√6ᵗʰ   **S20.17**   **Other superficial bite of breast**

EXCLUDES 1   *open bite of breast (S21.05-)*

√7ᵗʰ   **S20.171**   **Other superficial bite of breast, right breast**

√7ᵗʰ   **S20.172**   **Other superficial bite of breast, left breast**

√7ᵗʰ   **S20.179**   **Other superficial bite of breast, unspecified breast**

√5ᵗʰ   **S20.2**   **Contusion of thorax**

√x7ᵗʰ   **S20.20**   **Contusion of thorax, unspecified**

EXCLUDES 1   Not coded here   EXCLUDES 2   Not included here   *Manifestation Code*

✓6th **S20.21 Contusion of front wall of thorax**
- ✓7th **S20.211 Contusion of right front wall of thorax**
- ✓7th **S20.212 Contusion of left front wall of thorax**
- ✓7th **S20.219 Contusion of unspecified front wall of thorax**

✓6th **S20.22 Contusion of back wall of thorax**
- ✓7th **S20.221 Contusion of right back wall of thorax**
- ✓7th **S20.222 Contusion of left back wall of thorax**
- ✓7th **S20.229 Contusion of unspecified back wall of thorax**

✓5th **S20.3 Other and unspecified superficial injuries of front wall of thorax**

✓6th **S20.30 Unspecified superficial injuries of front wall of thorax**
- ✓7th **S20.301 Unspecified superficial injuries of right front wall of thorax**
- ✓7th **S20.302 Unspecified superficial injuries of left front wall of thorax**
- ✓7th **S20.309 Unspecified superficial injuries of unspecified front wall of thorax**

✓6th **S20.31 Abrasion of front wall of thorax**
- ✓7th **S20.311 Abrasion of right front wall of thorax**
- ✓7th **S20.312 Abrasion of left front wall of thorax**
- ✓7th **S20.319 Abrasion of unspecified front wall of thorax**

✓6th **S20.32 Blister (nonthermal) of front wall of thorax**
- ✓7th **S20.321 Blister (nonthermal) of right front wall of thorax**
- ✓7th **S20.322 Blister (nonthermal) of left front wall of thorax**
- ✓7th **S20.329 Blister (nonthermal) of unspecified front wall of thorax**

✓6th **S20.34 External constriction of front wall of thorax**
- ✓7th **S20.341 External constriction of right front wall of thorax**
- ✓7th **S20.342 External constriction of left front wall of thorax**
- ✓7th **S20.349 External constriction of unspecified front wall of thorax**

✓6th **S20.35 Superficial foreign body of front wall of thorax**
Splinter in front wall of thorax
- ✓7th **S20.351 Superficial foreign body of right front wall of thorax**
- ✓7th **S20.352 Superficial foreign body of left front wall of thorax**
- ✓7th **S20.359 Superficial foreign body of unspecified front wall of thorax**

✓6th **S20.36 Insect bite (nonvenomous) of front wall of thorax**
- ✓7th **S20.361 Insect bite (nonvenomous) of right front wall of thorax**
- ✓7th **S20.362 Insect bite (nonvenomous) of left front wall of thorax**
- ✓7th **S20.369 Insect bite (nonvenomous) of unspecified front wall of thorax**

✓6th **S20.37 Other superficial bite of front wall of thorax**
EXCLUDES 1 *open bite of front wall of thorax (S21.15)*
- ✓7th **S20.371 Other superficial bite of right front wall of thorax**
- ✓7th **S20.372 Other superficial bite of left front wall of thorax**
- ✓7th **S20.379 Other superficial bite of unspecified front wall of thorax**

✓5th **S20.4 Other and unspecified superficial injuries of back wall of thorax**

✓6th **S20.40 Unspecified superficial injuries of back wall of thorax**
- ✓7th **S20.401 Unspecified superficial injuries of right back wall of thorax**
- ✓7th **S20.402 Unspecified superficial injuries of left back wall of thorax**
- ✓7th **S20.409 Unspecified superficial injuries of unspecified back wall of thorax**

✓6th **S20.41 Abrasion of back wall of thorax**
- ✓7th **S20.411 Abrasion of right back wall of thorax**
- ✓7th **S20.412 Abrasion of left back wall of thorax**
- ✓7th **S20.419 Abrasion of unspecified back wall of thorax**

✓6th **S20.42 Blister (nonthermal) of back wall of thorax**
- ✓7th **S20.421 Blister (nonthermal) of right back wall of thorax**
- ✓7th **S20.422 Biister (nonthermal) of left back wall of thorax**
- ✓7th **S20.429 Blister (nonthermal) of unspecified back wall of thorax**

✓6th **S20.44 External constriction of back wall of thorax**
- ✓7th **SS20.441 External constriction of right back wall of thorax**
- ✓7th **S20.442 External constriction of left back wall of thorax**
- ✓7th **S20.449 External constriction of unspecified back wall of thorax**

✓6th **S20.45 Superficial foreign body of back wall of thorax**
Splinter of back wall of thorax
- ✓7th **S20.451 Superficial foreign body of right back wall of thorax**
- ✓7th **S20.452 Superficial foreign body of left back wall of thorax**
- ✓7th **S20.459 Superficial foreign body of unspecified back wall of thorax**

✓6th **S20.46 Insect bite (nonvenomous) of back wall of thorax**
- ✓7th **S20.461 Insect bite (nonvenomous) of right back wall of thorax**
- ✓7th **S20.462 Insect bite (nonvenomous) of left back wall of thorax**
- ✓7th **S20.469 Insect bite (nonvenomous) of unspecified back wall of thorax**

✓6th **S20.47 Other superficial bite of back wall of thorax**
EXCLUDES 1 *open bite of back wall of thorax (S21.25)*
- ✓7th **S20.471 Other superficial bite of right back wall of thorax**
- ✓7th **S20.472 Other superficial bite of left back wall of thorax**
- ✓7th **S20.479 Other superficial bite of unspecified back wall of thorax**

✓5th **S20.9 Superficial injury of unspecified parts of thorax**
EXCLUDES 1 *contusion of thorax NOS (S20.20)*

✓x7th **S20.90 Unspecified superficial injury of unspecified parts of thorax**
Superficial injury of thoracic wall NOS

✓x7th **S20.91 Abrasion of unspecified parts of thorax**
✓x7th **S20.92 Blister (nonthermal) of unspecified parts of thorax**
✓x7th **S20.94 External constriction of unspecified parts of thorax**
✓x7th **S20.95 Superficial foreign body of unspecified parts of thorax**
Splinter in thorax NOS

✓x7th **S20.96 Insect bite (nonvenomous) of unspecified parts of thorax**
✓x7th **S20.97 Other superficial bite of unspecified parts of thorax**
EXCLUDES 1 *open bite of thorax NOS (S21.95)*

✓4th **S21 Open wound of thorax**
Code also any associated injury (to) (such as) :
heart (S26-)
intrathoracic organs (S27-)
rib fracture (S22.3-, S22.4-)
spinal cord injury (S24.0-, S24.1-)
traumatic hemothorax (S27.1)
traumatic hemopneumothorax (S27.3)
traumatic pneumothorax (S27.0)
wound infection
EXCLUDES 1 *traumatic amputation (partial) of thorax (S28.1)*

The appropriate 7th character is to be added to each code from category S21.
A   initial encounter
D   subsequent encounter
S   sequela

✓5th **S21.0 Open wound of breast**
✓6th **S21.00 Unspecified open wound of breast**
- ✓7th **S21.001 Unspecified open wound of right breast**
- ✓7th **S21.002 Unspecified open wound of left breast**

☑ Appropriate additional character required   ✓x7th Requires 7th character, placeholder x must fill empty characters

√7ᵗʰ **S21.009** **Unspecified open wound of unspecified breast**

√6ᵗʰ **S21.01** **Laceration without foreign body of breast**

√7ᵗʰ **S21.011** **Laceration without foreign body of right breast**

√7ᵗʰ **S21.012** **Laceration without foreign body of left breast**

√7ᵗʰ **S21.019** **Laceration without foreign body of unspecified breast**

√6ᵗʰ **S21.02** **Laceration with foreign body of breast**

√7ᵗʰ **S21.021** **Laceration with foreign body of right breast**

√7ᵗʰ **S21.022** **Laceration with foreign body of left breast**

√7ᵗʰ **S21.029** **Laceration with foreign body of unspecified breast**

√6ᵗʰ **S21.03** **Puncture wound without foreign body of breast**

√7ᵗʰ **S21.031** **Puncture wound without foreign body of right breast**

√7ᵗʰ **S21.032** **Puncture wound without foreign body of left breast**

√7ᵗʰ **S21.039** **Puncture wound without foreign body of unspecified breast**

√6ᵗʰ **S21.04** **Puncture wound with foreign body of breast**

√7ᵗʰ **S21.041** **Puncture wound with foreign body of right breast**

√7ᵗʰ **S21.042** **Puncture wound with foreign body of left breast**

√7ᵗʰ **S21.049** **Puncture wound with foreign body of unspecified breast**

√6ᵗʰ **S21.05** **Open bite of breast**

Bite of breast NOS

EXCLUDES 1   *superficial bite of breast (S20.17)*

√7ᵗʰ **S21.051** **Open bite of right breast**

√7ᵗʰ **S21.052** **Open bite of left breast**

√7ᵗʰ **S21.059** **Open bite of unspecified breast**

√5ᵗʰ **S21.1** **Open wound of front wall of thorax without penetration into thoracic cavity**

Open wound of chest without penetration into thoracic cavity

√6ᵗʰ **S21.10** **Unspecified open wound of front wall of thorax without penetration into thoracic cavity**

√7ᵗʰ **S21.101** **Unspecified open wound of right front wall of thorax without penetration into thoracic cavity**

√7ᵗʰ **S21.102** **Unspecified open wound of left front wall of thorax without penetration into thoracic cavity**

√7ᵗʰ **S21.109** **Unspecified open wound of unspecified front wall of thorax without penetration into thoracic cavity**

√6ᵗʰ **S21.11** **Laceration without foreign body of front wall of thorax without penetration into thoracic cavity**

√7ᵗʰ **S21.111** **Laceration without foreign body of right front wall of thorax without penetration into thoracic cavity**

√7ᵗʰ **S21.112** **Laceration without foreign body of left front wall of thorax without penetration into thoracic cavity**

√7ᵗʰ **S21.119** **Laceration without foreign body of unspecified front wall of thorax without penetration into thoracic cavity**

√6ᵗʰ **S21.12** **Laceration with foreign body of front wall of thorax without penetration into thoracic cavity**

√7ᵗʰ **S21.121** **Laceration with foreign body of right front wall of thorax without penetration into thoracic cavity**

√7ᵗʰ **S21.122** **Laceration with foreign body of left front wall of thorax without penetration into thoracic cavity**

√7ᵗʰ **S21.129** **Laceration with foreign body of unspecified front wall of thorax without penetration into thoracic cavity**

√6ᵗʰ **S21.13** **Puncture wound without foreign body of front wall of thorax without penetration into thoracic cavity**

√7ᵗʰ **S21.131** **Puncture wound without foreign body of right front wall of thorax without penetration into thoracic cavity**

√7ᵗʰ **S21.132** **Puncture wound without foreign body of left front wall of thorax without penetration into thoracic cavity**

√7ᵗʰ **S21.139** **Puncture wound without foreign body of unspecified front wall of thorax without penetration into thoracic cavity**

√6ᵗʰ **S21.14** **Puncture wound with foreign body of front wall of thorax without penetration into thoracic cavity**

√7ᵗʰ **S21.141** **Puncture wound with foreign body of right front wall of thorax without penetration into thoracic cavity**

√7ᵗʰ **S21.142** **Puncture wound with foreign body of left front wall of thorax without penetration into thoracic cavity**

√7ᵗʰ **S21.149** **Puncture wound with foreign body of unspecified front wall of thorax without penetration into thoracic cavity**

√6ᵗʰ **S21.15** **Open bite of front wall of thorax without penetration into thoracic cavity**

Bite of front wall of thorax NOS

EXCLUDES 1   *superficial bite of front wall of thorax (S20.37)*

√7ᵗʰ **S21.151** **Open bite of right front wall of thorax without penetration into thoracic cavity**

√7ᵗʰ **S21.152** **Open bite of left front wall of thorax without penetration into thoracic cavity**

√7ᵗʰ **S21.159** **Open bite of unspecified front wall of thorax without penetration into thoracic cavity**

√5ᵗʰ **S21.2** **Open wound of back wall of thorax without penetration into thoracic cavity**

√6ᵗʰ **S21.20** **Unspecified open wound of back wall of thorax without penetration into thoracic cavity**

√7ᵗʰ **S21.201** **Unspecified open wound of right back wall of thorax without penetration into thoracic cavity**

√7ᵗʰ **S21.202** **Unspecified open wound of left back wall of thorax without penetration into thoracic cavity**

√7ᵗʰ **S21.209** **Unspecified open wound of unspecified back wall of thorax without penetration into thoracic cavity**

√6ᵗʰ **S21.21** **Laceration without foreign body of back wall of thorax without penetration into thoracic cavity**

√7ᵗʰ **S21.211** **Laceration without foreign body of right back wall of thorax without penetration into thoracic cavity**

√7ᵗʰ **S21.212** **Laceration without foreign body of left back wall of thorax without penetration into thoracic cavity**

√7ᵗʰ **S21.219** **Laceration without foreign body of unspecified back wall of thorax without penetration into thoracic cavity**

√6ᵗʰ **S21.22** **Laceration with foreign body of back wall of thorax without penetration into thoracic cavity**

√7ᵗʰ **S21.221** **Laceration with foreign body of right back wall of thorax without penetration into thoracic cavity**

√7ᵗʰ **S21.222** **Laceration with foreign body of left back wall of thorax without penetration into thoracic cavity**

√7ᵗʰ **S21.229** **Laceration with foreign body of unspecified back wall of thorax without penetration into thoracic cavity**

√6ᵗʰ **S21.23** **Puncture wound without foreign body of back wall of thorax without penetration into thoracic cavity**

√7ᵗʰ **S21.231** **Puncture wound without foreign body of right back wall of thorax without penetration into thoracic cavity**

√7ᵗʰ **S21.232** **Puncture wound without foreign body of left back wall of thorax without penetration into thoracic cavity**

EXCLUDES 1   Not coded here   EXCLUDES 2   Not included here   *Manifestation Code*

☑7ᵗʰ **S21.239** **Puncture wound without foreign body of unspecified back wall of thorax without penetration into thoracic cavity**

☑6ᵗʰ **S21.24** **Puncture wound with foreign body of back wall of thorax without penetration into thoracic cavity**

☑7ᵗʰ **S21.241** **Puncture wound with foreign body of right back wall of thorax without penetration into thoracic cavity**

☑7ᵗʰ **S21.242** **Puncture wound with foreign body of left back wall of thorax without penetration into thoracic cavity**

☑7ᵗʰ **S21.249** **Puncture wound with foreign body of unspecified back wall of thorax without penetration into thoracic cavity**

☑6ᵗʰ **S21.25** **Open bite of back wall of thorax without penetration into thoracic cavity**
Bite of back wall of thorax NOS
EXCLUDES 1 *superficial bite of back wall of thorax (S20.47)*

☑7ᵗʰ **S21.251** **Open bite of right back wall of thorax without penetration into thoracic cavity**

☑7ᵗʰ **S21.252** **Open bite of left back wall of thorax without penetration into thoracic cavity**

☑7ᵗʰ **S21.259** **Open bite of unspecified back wall of thorax without penetration into thoracic cavity**

☑5ᵗʰ **S21.3** **Open wound of front wall of thorax with penetration into thoracic cavity**
Open wound of chest with penetration into thoracic cavity

☑6ᵗʰ **S21.30** **Unspecified open wound of front wall of thorax with penetration into thoracic cavity**

☑7ᵗʰ **S21.301** **Unspecified open wound of right front wall of thorax with penetration into thoracic cavity**

☑7ᵗʰ **S21.302** **Unspecified open wound of left front wall of thorax with penetration into thoracic cavity**

☑7ᵗʰ **S21.309** **Unspecified open wound of unspecified front wall of thorax with penetration into thoracic cavity**

☑6ᵗʰ **S21.31** **Laceration without foreign body of front wall of thorax with penetration into thoracic cavity**

☑7ᵗʰ **S21.311** **Laceration without foreign body of right front wall of thorax with penetration into thoracic cavity**

☑7ᵗʰ **S21.312** **Laceration without foreign body of left front wall of thorax with penetration into thoracic cavity**

☑7ᵗʰ **S21.319** **Laceration without foreign body of unspecified front wall of thorax with penetration into thoracic cavity**

☑6ᵗʰ **S21.32** **Laceration with foreign body of front wall of thorax with penetration into thoracic cavity**

☑7ᵗʰ **S21.321** **Laceration with foreign body of right front wall of thorax with penetration into thoracic cavity**

☑7ᵗʰ **S21.322** **Laceration with foreign body of left front wall of thorax with penetration into thoracic cavity**

☑7ᵗʰ **S21.329** **Laceration with foreign body of unspecified front wall of thorax with penetration into thoracic cavity**

☑6ᵗʰ **S21.33** **Puncture wound without foreign body of front wall of thorax with penetration into thoracic cavity**

☑7ᵗʰ **S21.331** **Puncture wound without foreign body of right front wall of thorax with penetration into thoracic cavity**

☑7ᵗʰ **S21.332** **Puncture wound without foreign body of left front wall of thorax with penetration into thoracic cavity**

☑7ᵗʰ **S21.339** **Puncture wound without foreign body of unspecified front wall of thorax with penetration into thoracic cavity**

☑6ᵗʰ **S21.34** **Puncture wound with foreign body of front wall of thorax with penetration into thoracic cavity**

☑7ᵗʰ **S21.341** **Puncture wound with foreign body of right front wall of thorax with penetration into thoracic cavity**

☑7ᵗʰ **S21.342** **Puncture wound with foreign body of left front wall of thorax with penetration into thoracic cavity**

☑7ᵗʰ **S21.349** **Puncture wound with foreign body of unspecified front wall of thorax with penetration into thoracic cavity**

☑6ᵗʰ **S21.35** **Open bite of front wall of thorax with penetration into thoracic cavity**
EXCLUDES 1 *superficial bite of front wall of thorax (S20.37)*

☑7ᵗʰ **S21.351** **Open bite of right front wall of thorax with penetration into thoracic cavity**

☑7ᵗʰ **S21.352** **Open bite of left front wall of thorax with penetration into thoracic cavity**

☑7ᵗʰ **S21.359** **Open bite of unspecified front wall of thorax with penetration into thoracic cavity**

☑5ᵗʰ **S21.4** **Open wound of back wall of thorax with penetration into thoracic cavity**

☑6ᵗʰ **S21.40** **Unspecified open wound of back wall of thorax with penetration into thoracic cavity**

☑7ᵗʰ **S21.401** **Unspecified open wound of right back wall of thorax with penetration into thoracic cavity**

☑7ᵗʰ **S21.402** **Unspecified open wound of left back wall of thorax with penetration into thoracic cavity**

☑7ᵗʰ **S21.409** **Unspecified open wound of unspecified back wall of thorax with penetration into thoracic cavity**

☑6ᵗʰ **S21.41** **Laceration without foreign body of back wall of thorax with penetration into thoracic cavity**

☑7ᵗʰ **S21.411** **Laceration without foreign body of right back wall of thorax with penetration into thoracic cavity**

☑7ᵗʰ **S21.412** **Laceration without foreign body of left back wall of thorax with penetration into thoracic cavity**

☑7ᵗʰ **S21.419** **Laceration without foreign body of unspecified back wall of thorax with penetration into thoracic cavity**

☑6ᵗʰ **S21.42** **Laceration with foreign body of back wall of thorax with penetration into thoracic cavity**

☑7ᵗʰ **S21.421** **Laceration with foreign body of right back wall of thorax with penetration into thoracic cavity**

☑7ᵗʰ **S21.422** **Laceration with foreign body of left back wall of thorax with penetration into thoracic cavity**

☑7ᵗʰ **S21.429** **Laceration with foreign body of unspecified back wall of thorax with penetration into thoracic cavity**

☑6ᵗʰ **S21.43** **Puncture wound without foreign body of back wall of thorax with penetration into thoracic cavity**

☑7ᵗʰ **S21.431** **Puncture wound without foreign body of right back wall of thorax with penetration into thoracic cavity**

☑7ᵗʰ **S21.432** **Puncture wound without foreign body of left back wall of thorax with penetration into thoracic cavity**

☑7ᵗʰ **S21.439** **Puncture wound without foreign body of unspecified back wall of thorax with penetration into thoracic cavity**

☑6ᵗʰ **S21.44** **Puncture wound with foreign body of back wall of thorax with penetration into thoracic cavity**

☑7ᵗʰ **S21.441** **Puncture wound with foreign body of right back wall of thorax with penetration into thoracic cavity**

☑7ᵗʰ **S21.442** **Puncture wound with foreign body of left back wall of thorax with penetration into thoracic cavity**

☑7ᵗʰ **S21.449** **Puncture wound with foreign body of unspecified back wall of thorax with penetration into thoracic cavity**

☑ Appropriate additional character required   ☑x7ᵗʰ Requires 7th character, placeholder x must fill empty characters

Injury, Poisoning and Certain Other Consequences of External Causes *(left margin)*

S21.45–S22.42 *(left margin)*

- **6th** S21.45 **Open bite of back wall of thorax with penetration into thoracic cavity**
  - Bite of back wall of thorax NOS
  - EXCLUDES 1 *superficial bite of back wall of thorax (S20.47)*
  - **7th** S21.451 **Open bite of right back wall of thorax with penetration into thoracic cavity**
  - **7th** S21.452 **Open bite of left back wall of thorax with penetration into thoracic cavity**
  - **7th** S21.459 **Open bite of unspecified back wall of thorax with penetration into thoracic cavity**
- **5th** S21.9 **Open wound of unspecified part of thorax**
  - Open wound of thoracic wall NOS
  - **x 7th** S21.90 **Unspecified open wound of unspecified part of thorax**
  - **x 7th** S21.91 **Laceration without foreign body of unspecified part of thorax**
  - **x 7th** S21.92 **Laceration with foreign body of unspecified part of thorax**
  - **x 7th** S21.93 **Puncture wound without foreign body of unspecified part of thorax**
  - **x 7th** S21.94 **Puncture wound with foreign body of unspecified part of thorax**
  - **x 7th** S21.95 **Open bite of unspecified part of thorax**
    - EXCLUDES 1 *superficial bite of thorax (S20.97)*

- **4th** **S22 Fracture of rib(s), sternum and thoracic spine**
  - NOTE   A fracture not indicated as nondisplaced or displaced should be classified to displaced
  -          A fracture not indicated as open or closed should be coded to closed
  - Fracture of thoracic neural arch
  - Fracture of thoracic spinous process
  - Fracture of thoracic transverse process
  - Fracture of thoracic vertebra
  - Fracture of thoracic vertebral arch
  - Codes first any associated:
    - injury of intrathoracic organ (S27-)
    - spinal cord injury (S24.0-, S24.1-)
  - EXCLUDES 1 *transection of thorax (S28.1)*
  - EXCLUDES 2 *fracture of clavicle (S42.0-)*
  - *fracture of scapula (S42.1-)*

  > The appropriate 7th character is to be added to each code from category S22.
  > A   initial encounter for closed fracture
  > B   initial encounter for open fracture
  > D   subsequent encounter for fracture with routine healing
  > G   subsequent encounter for fracture with delayed healing
  > K   subsequent encounter for fracture with nonunion
  > S   sequela

  - **5th** S22.0 **Fracture of thoracic vertebra**
    - **6th** S22.00 **Fracture of unspecified thoracic vertebra**
      - **7th** S22.000 **Wedge compression fracture of unspecified thoracic vertebra**
      - **7th** S22.001 **Stable burst fracture of unspecified thoracic vertebra**
      - **7th** S22.002 **Unstable burst fracture of unspecified thoracic vertebra**
      - **7th** S22.008 **Other fracture of unspecified thoracic vertebra**
      - **7th** S22.009 **Unspecified fracture of unspecified thoracic vertebra**
    - **6th** S22.01 **Fracture of first thoracic vertebra**
      - **7th** S22.010 **Wedge compression fracture of first thoracic vertebra**
      - **7th** S22.011 **Stable burst fracture of first thoracic vertebra**
      - **7th** S22.012 **Unstable burst fracture of first thoracic vertebra**
      - **7th** S22.018 **Other fracture of first thoracic vertebra**
      - **7th** S22.019 **Unspecified fracture of first thoracic vertebra**
    - **6th** S22.02 **Fracture of second thoracic vertebra**
      - **7th** S22.020 **Wedge compression fracture of second thoracic vertebra**
      - **7th** S22.021 **Stable burst fracture of second thoracic vertebra**

- **7th** S22.022 **Unstable burst fracture of second thoracic vertebra**
- **7th** S22.028 **Other fracture of second thoracic vertebra**
- **7th** S22.029 **Unspecified fracture of second thoracic vertebra**
- **6th** S22.03 **Fracture of third thoracic vertebra**
  - **7th** S22.030 **Wedge compression fracture of third thoracic vertebra**
  - **7th** S22.031 **Stable burst fracture of third thoracic vertebra**
  - **7th** S22.032 **Unstable burst fracture of third thoracic vertebra**
  - **7th** S22.038 **Other fracture of third thoracic vertebra**
  - **7th** S22.039 **Unspecified fracture of third thoracic vertebra**
- **6th** S22.04 **Fracture of fourth thoracic vertebra**
  - **7th** S22.040 **Wedge compression fracture of fourth thoracic vertebra**
  - **7th** S22.041 **Stable burst fracture of fourth thoracic vertebra**
  - **7th** S22.042 **Unstable burst fracture of fourth thoracic vertebra**
  - **7th** S22.048 **Other fracture of fourth thoracic vertebra**
  - **7th** S22.049 **Unspecified fracture of fourth thoracic vertebra**
- **6th** S22.05 **Fracture of T5-T6 vertebra**
  - **7th** S22.050 **Wedge compression fracture of T5-T6 vertebra**
  - **7th** S22.051 **Stable burst fracture of T5-T6 vertebra**
  - **7th** S22.052 **Unstable burst fracture of T5-T6 vertebra**
  - **7th** S22.058 **Other fracture of T5-T6 vertebra**
  - **7th** S22.059 **Unspecified fracture of T5-T6 vertebra**
- **6th** S22.06 **Fracture of T7-T8 vertebra**
  - **7th** S22.060 **Wedge compression fracture of T7-T8 vertebra**
  - **7th** S22.061 **Stable burst fracture of T7-T8 vertebra**
  - **7th** S22.062 **Unstable burst fracture of T7-T8 vertebra**
  - **7th** S22.068 **Other fracture of T7-T8 thoracic vertebra**
  - **7th** S22.069 **Unspecified fracture of T7-T8 vertebra**
- **6th** S22.07 **Fracture of T9-T10 vertebra**
  - **7th** S22.070 **Wedge compression fracture of T9-T10 vertebra**
  - **7th** S22.071 **Stable burst fracture of T9-T10 vertebra**
  - **7th** S22.072 **Unstable burst fracture of T9-T10 vertebra**
  - **7th** S22.078 **Other fracture of T9-T10 vertebra**
  - **7th** S22.079 **Unspecified fracture of T9-T10 vertebra**
- **6th** S22.08 **Fracture of T11-T12 vertebra**
  - **7th** S22.080 **Wedge compression fracture of T11-T12 vertebra**
  - **7th** S22.081 **Stable burst fracture of T11-T12 vertebra**
  - **7th** S22.082 **Unstable burst fracture of T11-T12 vertebra**
  - **7th** S22.088 **Other fracture of T11-T12 vertebra**
  - **7th** S22.089 **Unspecified fracture of T11-T12 vertebra**
- **5th** S22.2 **Fracture of sternum**
  - **x 7th** S22.20 **Unspecified fracture of sternum**
  - **x 7th** S22.21 **Fracture of manubrium**
  - **x 7th** S22.22 **Fracture of body of sternum**
  - **x 7th** S22.23 **Sternal manubrial dissociation**
  - **x 7th** S22.24 **Fracture of xiphoid process**
- **5th** S22.3 **Fracture of one rib**
  - **x 7th** S22.31 **Fracture of one rib, right side**
  - **x 7th** S22.32 **Fracture of one rib, left side**
  - **x 7th** S22.39 **Fracture of one rib, unspecified side**
- **5th** S22.4 **Multiple fractures of ribs**
  - Fractures of two or more ribs
  - EXCLUDES 1 *flail chest (S22.5-)*
  - **x 7th** S22.41 **Multiple fractures of ribs, right side**
  - **x 7th** S22.42 **Multiple fractures of ribs, left side**

EXCLUDES 1 Not coded here   EXCLUDES 2 Not included here   *Manifestation Code*

✓x7ᵗʰ **S22.43**　**Multiple fractures of ribs, bilateral**
✓x7ᵗʰ **S22.49**　**Multiple fractures of ribs, unspecified side**
✓x7ᵗʰ **S22.5**　**Flail chest**
✓x7ᵗʰ **S22.9**　**Fracture of bony thorax, part unspecified**

✓4ᵗʰ **S23**　**Dislocation and sprain of joints and ligaments of thorax**
　　INCLUDES　avulsion of joint or ligament of thorax
　　　　　laceration of cartilage, joint or ligament of thorax
　　　　　sprain of cartilage, joint or ligament of thorax
　　　　　traumatic hemarthrosis of joint or ligament of thorax
　　　　　traumatic rupture of joint or ligament of thorax
　　　　　traumatic subluxation of joint or ligament of thorax
　　　　　traumatic tear of joint or ligament of thorax
　　Code also any associated open wound
　　EXCLUDES 2　*dislocation, sprain of sternoclavicular joint (S43.2, S43.6)*
　　　　　strain of muscle or tendon of thorax (S29.01-)

The appropriate 7th character is to be added to each code from category S23.
　A　initial encounter
　D　subsequent encounter
　S　sequela

✓x7ᵗʰ **S23.0**　**Traumatic rupture of thoracic intervertebral disc**
　　EXCLUDES 1　*rupture or displacement (nontraumatic) of thoracic intervertebral disc NOS (M51- with fifth character 4)*
✓5ᵗʰ **S23.1**　**Subluxation and dislocation of thoracic vertebra**
　　Code also any associated
　　　open wound of thorax (S21-)
　　　spinal cord injury (S24.0-, S24.1-)
　　EXCLUDES 2　*fracture of thoracic vertebrae (S22.0-)*
　✓6ᵗʰ **S23.10**　**Subluxation and dislocation of unspecified thoracic vertebra**
　　✓7ᵗʰ **S23.100**　**Subluxation of unspecified thoracic vertebra**
　　✓7ᵗʰ **S23.101**　**Dislocation of unspecified thoracic vertebra**
　✓6ᵗʰ **S23.11**　**Subluxation and dislocation of T1/T2 thoracic vertebra**
　　✓7ᵗʰ **S23.110**　**Subluxation of T1/T2 thoracic vertebra**
　　✓7ᵗʰ **S23.111**　**Dislocation of T1/T2 thoracic vertebra**
　✓6ᵗʰ **S23.12**　**Subluxation and dislocation of T2/T3-T3/T4 thoracic vertebra**
　　✓7ᵗʰ **S23.120**　**Subluxation of T2/T3 thoracic vertebra**
　　✓7ᵗʰ **S23.121**　**Dislocation of T2/T3 thoracic vertebra**
　　✓7ᵗʰ **S23.122**　**Subluxation of T3/T4 thoracic vertebra**
　　✓7ᵗʰ **S23.123**　**Dislocation of T3/T4 thoracic vertebra**
　✓6ᵗʰ **S23.13**　**Subluxation and dislocation of T4/T5-T5/T6 thoracic vertebra**
　　✓7ᵗʰ **S23.130**　**Subluxation of T4/T5 thoracic vertebra**
　　✓7ᵗʰ **S23.131**　**Dislocation of T4/T5 thoracic vertebra**
　　✓7ᵗʰ **S23.132**　**Subluxation of T5/T6 thoracic vertebra**
　　✓7ᵗʰ **S23.133**　**Dislocation of T5/T6 thoracic vertebra**
　✓6ᵗʰ **S23.14**　**Subluxation and dislocation of T6/T7-T7/T8 thoracic vertebra**
　　✓7ᵗʰ **S23.140**　**Subluxation of T6/T7 thoracic vertebra**
　　✓7ᵗʰ **S23.141**　**Dislocation of T6/T7 thoracic vertebra**
　　✓7ᵗʰ **S23.142**　**Subluxation of T7/T8 thoracic vertebra**
　　✓7ᵗʰ **S23.143**　**Dislocation of T7/T8 thoracic vertebra**
　✓6ᵗʰ **S23.15**　**Subluxation and dislocation of T8/T9-T9/T10 thoracic vertebra**
　　✓7ᵗʰ **S23.150**　**Subluxation of T8/T9 thoracic vertebra**
　　✓7ᵗʰ **S23.151**　**Dislocation of T8/T9 thoracic vertebra**
　　✓7ᵗʰ **S23.152**　**Subluxation of T9/T10 thoracic vertebra**
　　✓7ᵗʰ **S23.153**　**Dislocation of T9/T10 thoracic vertebra**
　✓6ᵗʰ **S23.16**　**Subluxation and dislocation of T10/T11-T11/T12 thoracic vertebra**
　　✓7ᵗʰ **S23.160**　**Subluxation of T10/T11 thoracic vertebra**
　　✓7ᵗʰ **S23.161**　**Dislocation of T10/T11 thoracic vertebra**
　　✓7ᵗʰ **S23.162**　**Subluxation of T11/T12 thoracic vertebra**
　　✓7ᵗʰ **S23.163**　**Dislocation of T11/T12 thoracic vertebra**
　✓6ᵗʰ **S23.17**　**Subluxation and dislocation of T12/L1 thoracic vertebra**
　　✓7ᵗʰ **S23.170**　**Subluxation of T12/L1 thoracic vertebra**

　　✓7ᵗʰ **S23.171**　**Dislocation of T12/L1 thoracic vertebra**
✓5ᵗʰ **S23.2**　**Dislocation of other and unspecified parts of thorax**
　✓x7ᵗʰ **S23.20**　**Dislocation of unspecified part of thorax**
　✓x7ᵗʰ **S23.29**　**Dislocation of other parts of thorax**
✓x7ᵗʰ **S23.3**　**Sprain of ligaments of thoracic spine**
✓5ᵗʰ **S23.4**　**Sprain of ribs and sternum**
　✓x7ᵗʰ **S23.41**　**Sprain of ribs**
　✓6ᵗʰ **S23.42**　**Sprain of sternum**
　　✓7ᵗʰ **S23.420**　**Sprain of sternoclavicular (joint) (ligament)**
　　✓7ᵗʰ **S23.421**　**Sprain of chondrosternal joint**
　　✓7ᵗʰ **S23.428**　**Other sprain of sternum**
　　✓7ᵗʰ **S23.429**　**Unspecified sprain of sternum**
✓x7ᵗʰ **S23.8**　**Sprain of other specified parts of thorax**
✓x7ᵗʰ **S23.9**　**Sprain of unspecified parts of thorax**

✓4ᵗʰ **S24**　**Injury of nerves and spinal cord at thorax level**
　　NOTE　　Code to highest level of thoracic spinal cord injury
　　Code also any associated:
　　　fracture of thoracic vertebra (S22.0-)
　　　open wound of thorax (S21-)
　　　transient paralysis (R29.5)
　　EXCLUDES 2　*injury of brachial plexus (S14.3)*

The appropriate 7th character is to be added to each code from category S24.
　A　initial encounter
　D　subsequent encounter
　S　sequela

✓x7ᵗʰ **S24.0**　**Concussion and edema of thoracic spinal cord**
✓5ᵗʰ **S24.1**　**Other and unspecified injuries of thoracic spinal cord**
　✓6ᵗʰ **S24.10**　**Unspecified injury of thoracic spinal cord**
　　✓7ᵗʰ **S24.101**　**Unspecified injury at T1 level of thoracic spinal cord**
　　✓7ᵗʰ **S24.102**　**Unspecified injury at T2-T6 level of thoracic spinal cord**
　　✓7ᵗʰ **S24.103**　**Unspecified injury at T7-T10 level of thoracic spinal cord**
　　✓7ᵗʰ **S24.104**　**Unspecified injury at T11-T12 level of thoracic spinal cord**
　　✓7ᵗʰ **S24.109**　**Unspecified injury at unspecified level of thoracic spinal cord**
　　　　　Injury of thoracic spinal cord NOS
　✓6ᵗʰ **S24.11**　**Complete lesion of thoracic spinal cord**
　　✓7ᵗʰ **S24.111**　**Complete lesion at T1 level of thoracic spinal cord**
　　✓7ᵗʰ **S24.112**　**Complete lesion at T2-T6 level of thoracic spinal cord**
　　✓7ᵗʰ **S24.113**　**Complete lesion at T7-T10 level of thoracic spinal cord**
　　✓7ᵗʰ **S24.114**　**Complete lesion at T11-T12 level of thoracic spinal cord**
　　✓7ᵗʰ **S24.119**　**Complete lesion at unspecified level of thoracic spinal cord**
　✓6ᵗʰ **S24.13**　**Anterior cord syndrome of thoracic spinal cord**
　　✓7ᵗʰ **S24.131**　**Anterior cord syndrome at T1 level of thoracic spinal cord**
　　✓7ᵗʰ **S24.132**　**Anterior cord syndrome at T2-T6 level of thoracic spinal cord**
　　✓7ᵗʰ **S24.133**　**Anterior cord syndrome at T7-T10 level of thoracic spinal cord**
　　✓7ᵗʰ **S24.134**　**Anterior cord syndrome at T11-T12 level of thoracic spinal cord**
　　✓7ᵗʰ **S24.139**　**Anterior cord syndrome at unspecified level of thoracic spinal cord**
　✓6ᵗʰ **S24.14**　**Brown-Séquard syndrome of thoracic spinal cord**
　　✓7ᵗʰ **S24.141**　**Brown-Séquard syndrome at T1 level of thoracic spinal cord**
　　✓7ᵗʰ **S24.142**　**Brown-Séquard syndrome at T2-T6 level of thoracic spinal cord**
　　✓7ᵗʰ **S24.143**　**Brown-Séquard syndrome at T7-T10 level of thoracic spinal cord**
　　✓7ᵗʰ **S24.144**　**Brown-Séquard syndrome at T11-T12 level of thoracic spinal cord**
　　✓7ᵗʰ **S24.149**　**Brown-Séquard syndrome at unspecified level of thoracic spinal cord**

√6th **S24.15 Other incomplete lesions of thoracic spinal cord**
Incomplete lesion of thoracic spinal cord NOS
Posterior cord syndrome of thoracic spinal cord

√7th   **S24.151 Other incomplete lesion at T1 level of thoracic spinal cord**

√7th   **S24.152 Other incomplete lesion at T2-T6 level of thoracic spinal cord**

√7th   **S24.153 Other incomplete lesion at T7-T10 level of thoracic spinal cord**

√7th   **S24.154 Other incomplete lesion at T11-T12 level of thoracic spinal cord**

√7th   **S24.159 Other incomplete lesion at unspecified level of thoracic spinal cord**

√x7th **S24.2 Injury of nerve root of thoracic spine**

√x7th **S24.3 Injury of peripheral nerves of thorax**

√x7th **S24.4 Injury of thoracic sympathetic nervous system**
Injury of cardiac plexus
Injury of esophageal plexus
Injury of pulmonary plexus
Injury of stellate ganglion
Injury of thoracic sympathetic ganglion

√x7th **S24.8 Injury of other specified nerves of thorax**

√x7th **S24.9 Injury of unspecified nerve of thorax**

√4th **S25 Injury of blood vessels of thorax**
Code also any associated open wound (S21-)

> The appropriate 7th character is to be added to each code from category S25.
> A   initial encounter
> D   subsequent encounter
> S   sequela

√5th **S25.0 Injury of thoracic aorta**
Injury of aorta NOS

√x7th **S25.00 Unspecified injury of thoracic aorta**

√x7th **S25.01 Minor laceration of thoracic aorta**
Incomplete transection of thoracic aorta
Laceration of thoracic aorta NOS
Superficial laceration of thoracic aorta

√x7th **S25.02 Major laceration of thoracic aorta**
Complete transection of thoracic aorta
Traumatic rupture of thoracic aorta

√x7th **S25.09 Other specified injury of thoracic aorta**

√5th **S25.1 Injury of innominate or subclavian artery**

√6th **S25.10 Unspecified injury of innominate or subclavian artery**

√7th   **S25.101 Unspecified injury of right innominate or subclavian artery**

√7th   **S25.102 Unspecified injury of left innominate or subclavian artery**

√7th   **S25.109 Unspecified injury of unspecified innominate or subclavian artery**

√6th **S25.11 Minor laceration of innominate or subclavian artery**
Incomplete transection of innominate or subclavian artery
Laceration of innominate or subclavian artery NOS
Superficial laceration of innominate or subclavian artery

√7th   **S25.111 Minor laceration of right innominate or subclavian artery**

√7th   **S25.112 Minor laceration of left innominate or subclavian artery**

√7th   **S25.119 Minor laceration of unspecified innominate or subclavian artery**

√6th **S25.12 Major laceration of innominate or subclavian artery**
Complete transection of innominate or subclavian artery
Traumatic rupture of innominate or subclavian artery

√7th   **S25.121 Major laceration of right innominate or subclavian artery**

√7th   **S25.122 Major laceration of left innominate or subclavian artery**

√7th   **S25.129 Major laceration of unspecified innominate or subclavian artery**

√6th **S25.19 Other specified injury of innominate or subclavian artery**

√7th   **S25.191 Other specified injury of right innominate or subclavian artery**

√7th   **S25.192 Other specified injury of left innominate or subclavian artery**

√7th   **S25.199 Other specified injury of unspecified innominate or subclavian artery**

√5th **S25.2 Injury of superior vena cava**
Injury of vena cava NOS

√x7th **S25.20 Unspecified injury of superior vena cava**

√x7th **S25.21 Minor laceration of superior vena cava**
Incomplete transection of superior vena cava
Laceration of superior vena cava NOS
Superficial laceration of superior vena cava

√x7th **S25.22 Major laceration of superior vena cava**
Complete transection of superior vena cava
Traumatic rupture of superior vena cava

√x7th **S25.29 Other specified injury of superior vena cava**

√5th **S25.3 Injury of innominate or subclavian vein**

√6th **S25.30 Unspecified injury of innominate or subclavian vein**

√7th   **S25.301 Unspecified injury of right innominate or subclavian vein**

√7th   **S25.302 Unspecified injury of left innominate or subclavian vein**

√7th   **S25.309 Unspecified injury of unspecified innominate or subclavian vein**

√6th **S25.31 Minor laceration of innominate or subclavian vein**
Incomplete transection of innominate or subclavian vein
Laceration of innominate or subclavian vein NOS
Superficial laceration of innominate or subclavian vein

√7th   **S25.311 Minor laceration of right innominate or subclavian vein**

√7th   **S25.312 Minor laceration of left innominate or subclavian vein**

√7th   **S25.319 Minor laceration of unspecified innominate or subclavian vein**

√6th **S25.32 Major laceration of innominate or subclavian vein**
Complete transection of innominate or subclavian vein
Traumatic rupture of innominate or subclavian vein

√7th   **S25.321 Major laceration of right innominate or subclavian vein**

√7th   **S25.322 Major laceration of left innominate or subclavian vein**

√7th   **S25.329 Major laceration of unspecified innominate or subclavian vein**

√6th **S25.39 Other specified injury of innominate or subclavian vein**

√7th   **S25.391 Other specified injury of right innominate or subclavian vein**

√7th   **S25.392 Other specified injury of left innominate or subclavian vein**

√7th   **S25.399 Other specified injury of unspecified innominate or subclavian vein**

√5th **S25.4 Injury of pulmonary blood vessels**

√6th **S25.40 Unspecified injury of pulmonary blood vessels**

√7th   **S25.401 Unspecified injury of right pulmonary blood vessels**

√7th   **S25.402 Unspecified injury of left pulmonary blood vessels**

√7th   **S25.409 Unspecified injury of unspecified pulmonary blood vessels**

√6th **S25.41 Minor laceration of pulmonary blood vessels**
Incomplete transection of pulmonary blood vessels
Laceration of pulmonary blood vessels NOS
Superficial laceration of pulmonary blood vessels

√7th   **S25.411 Minor laceration of right pulmonary blood vessels**

√7th   **S25.412 Minor laceration of left pulmonary blood vessels**

√7th   **S25.419 Minor laceration of unspecified pulmonary blood vessels**

EXCLUDES 1 Not coded here   **EXCLUDES 2** Not included here   *Manifestation Code*

√6ᵗʰ **S25.42 Major laceration of pulmonary blood vessels**
  Complete transection of pulmonary blood vessels
  Traumatic rupture of pulmonary blood vessels
  √7ᵗʰ **S25.421 Major laceration of right pulmonary blood vessels**
  √7ᵗʰ **S25.422 Major laceration of left pulmonary blood vessels**
  √7ᵗʰ **S25.429 Major laceration of unspecified pulmonary blood vessels**

√6ᵗʰ **S25.49 Other specified injury of pulmonary blood vessels**
  √7ᵗʰ **S25.491 Other specified injury of right pulmonary blood vessels**
  √7ᵗʰ **S25.492 Other specified injury of left pulmonary blood vessels**
  √7ᵗʰ **S25.499 Other specified injury of unspecified pulmonary blood vessels**

√5ᵗʰ **S25.5 Injury of intercostal blood vessels**
  √6ᵗʰ **S25.50 Unspecified injury of intercostal blood vessels**
    √7ᵗʰ **S25.501 Unspecified injury of intercostal blood vessels, right side**
    √7ᵗʰ **S25.502 Unspecified injury of intercostal blood vessels, left side**
    √7ᵗʰ **S25.509 Unspecified injury of intercostal blood vessels, unspecified side**
  √6ᵗʰ **S25.51 Laceration of intercostal blood vessels**
    √7ᵗʰ **S25.511 Laceration of intercostal blood vessels, right side**
    √7ᵗʰ **S25.512 Laceration of intercostal blood vessels, left side**
    √7ᵗʰ **S25.519 Laceration of intercostal blood vessels, unspecified side**
  √6ᵗʰ **S25.59 Other specified injury of intercostal blood vessels**
    √7ᵗʰ **S25.591 Other specified injury of intercostal blood vessels, right side**
    √7ᵗʰ **S25.592 Other specified injury of intercostal blood vessels, left side**
    √7ᵗʰ **S25.599 Other specified injury of intercostal blood vessels, unspecified side**

√5ᵗʰ **S25.8 Injury of other blood vessels of thorax**
  Injury of azygos vein
  Injury of mammary artery or vein
  √6ᵗʰ **S25.80 Unspecified injury of other blood vessels of thorax**
    √7ᵗʰ **S25.801 Unspecified injury of other blood vessels of thorax, right side**
    √7ᵗʰ **S25.802 Unspecified injury of other blood vessels of thorax, left side**
    √7ᵗʰ **S25.809 Unspecified injury of other blood vessels of thorax, unspecified side**
  √6ᵗʰ **S25.81 Laceration of other blood vessels of thorax**
    √7ᵗʰ **S25.811 Laceration of other blood vessels of thorax, right side**
    √7ᵗʰ **S25.812 Laceration of other blood vessels of thorax, left side**
    √7ᵗʰ **S25.819 Laceration of other blood vessels of thorax, unspecified side**
  √6ᵗʰ **S25.89 Other specified injury of other blood vessels of thorax**
    √7ᵗʰ **S25.891 Other specified injury of other blood vessels of thorax, right side**
    √7ᵗʰ **S25.892 Other specified injury of other blood vessels of thorax, left side**
    √7ᵗʰ **S25.899 Other specified injury of other blood vessels of thorax, unspecified side**

√5ᵗʰ **S25.9 Injury of unspecified blood vessel of thorax**
  √x7ᵗʰ **S25.90 Unspecified injury of unspecified blood vessel of thorax**
  √x7ᵗʰ **S25.91 Laceration of unspecified blood vessel of thorax**
  √x7ᵗʰ **S25.99 Other specified injury of unspecified blood vessel of thorax**

√4ᵗʰ **S26 Injury of heart**
  Code also any associated:
    open wound of thorax (S21-)
    traumatic hemopneumothorax (S27.2)
    traumatic hemothorax (S27.1)
    traumatic pneumothorax (S27.0)

  The appropriate 7th character is to be added to each code from category S26.
  A   initial encounter
  D   subsequent encounter
  S   sequela

  √5ᵗʰ **S26.0 Injury of heart with hemopericardium**
    √x7ᵗʰ **S26.00 Unspecified injury of heart with hemopericardium**
    √x7ᵗʰ **S26.01 Contusion of heart with hemopericardium**
    √6ᵗʰ **S26.02 Laceration of heart with hemopericardium**
      √7ᵗʰ **S26.020 Mild laceration of heart with hemopericardium**
        Laceration of heart without penetration of heart chamber
      √7ᵗʰ **S26.021 Moderate laceration of heart with hemopericardium**
        Laceration of heart with penetration of heart chamber
      √7ᵗʰ **S26.022 Major laceration of heart with hemopericardium**
        Laceration of heart with penetration of multiple heart chambers
    √x7ᵗʰ **S26.09 Other injury of heart with hemopericardium**
  √5ᵗʰ **S26.1 Injury of heart without hemopericardium**
    √x7ᵗʰ **S26.10 Unspecified injury of heart without hemopericardium**
    √x7ᵗʰ **S26.11 Contusion of heart without hemopericardium**
    √x7ᵗʰ **S26.12 Laceration of heart without hemopericardium**
    √x7ᵗʰ **S26.19 Other injury of heart without hemopericardium**
  √5ᵗʰ **S26.9 Injury of heart, unspecified with or without hemopericardium**
    √x7ᵗʰ **S26.90 Unspecified injury of heart, unspecified with or without hemopericardium**
    √x7ᵗʰ **S26.91 Contusion of heart, unspecified with or without hemopericardium**
    √x7ᵗʰ **S26.92 Laceration of heart, unspecified with or without hemopericardium**
      Laceration of heart NOS
    √x7ᵗʰ **S26.99 Other injury of heart, unspecified with or without hemopericardium**

√4ᵗʰ **S27 Injury of other and unspecified intrathoracic organs**
  Code also any associated open wound of thorax (S21-)
  EXCLUDES 2   injury of cervical esophagus (S10-S19)
        injury of trachea (cervical) (S10-S19)

  The appropriate 7th character is to be added to each code from category S27.
  A   initial encounter
  D   subsequent encounter
  S   sequela

  √x7ᵗʰ **S27.0 Traumatic pneumothorax**
    EXCLUDES 1 spontaneous pneumothorax (J93-)
  √x7ᵗʰ **S27.1 Traumatic hemothorax**
  √x7ᵗʰ **S27.2 Traumatic hemopneumothorax**
  √5ᵗʰ **S27.3 Other and unspecified injuries of lung**
    √6ᵗʰ **S27.30 Unspecified injury of lung**
      √7ᵗʰ **S27.301 Unspecified injury of lung, unilateral**
      √7ᵗʰ **S27.302 Unspecified injury of lung, bilateral**
      √7ᵗʰ **S27.309 Unspecified injury of lung, unspecified**
    √6ᵗʰ **S27.31 Primary blast injury of lung**
      Blast injury of lung NOS
      √7ᵗʰ **S27.311 Primary blast injury of lung, unilateral**
      √7ᵗʰ **S27.312 Primary blast injury of lung, bilateral**
      √7ᵗʰ **S27.319 Primary blast injury of lung, unspecified**
    √6ᵗʰ **S27.32 Contusion of lung**
      √7ᵗʰ **S27.321 Contusion of lung, unilateral**
      √7ᵗʰ **S27.322 Contusion of lung, bilateral**
      √7ᵗʰ **S27.329 Contusion of lung, unspecified**

☑ Appropriate additional character required   √x7ᵗʰ Requires 7th character, placeholder x must fill empty characters

✓6th **S27.33** **Laceration of lung**
- ✓7th S27.331 Laceration of lung, unilateral
- ✓7th S27.332 Laceration of lung, bilateral
- ✓7th S27.339 Laceration of lung, unspecified

✓6th **S27.39** **Other injuries of lung**
Secondary blast injury of lung
- ✓7th S27.391 Other injuries of lung, unilateral
- ✓7th S27.392 Other injuries of lung, bilateral
- ✓7th S27.399 Other injuries of lung, unspecified

✓5th **S27.4** **Injury of bronchus**

✓6th **S27.40** **Unspecified injury of bronchus**
- ✓7th S27.401 Unspecified injury of bronchus, unilateral
- ✓7th S27.402 Unspecified injury of bronchus, bilateral
- ✓7th S27.409 Unspecified injury of bronchus, unspecified

✓6th **S27.41** **Primary blast injury of bronchus**
Blast injury of bronchus NOS
- ✓7th S27.411 Primary blast injury of bronchus, unilateral
- ✓7th S27.412 Primary blast injury of bronchus, bilateral
- ✓7th S27.419 Primary blast injury of bronchus, unspecified

✓6th **S27.42** **Contusion of bronchus**
- ✓7th S27.421 Contusion of bronchus, unilateral
- ✓7th S27.422 Contusion of bronchus, bilateral
- ✓7th S27.429 Contusion of bronchus, unspecified

✓6th **S27.43** **Laceration of bronchus**
- ✓7th S27.431 Laceration of bronchus, unilateral
- ✓7th S27.432 Laceration of bronchus, bilateral
- ✓7th S27.439 Laceration of bronchus, unspecified

✓6th **S27.49** **Other injury of bronchus**
Secondary blast injury of bronchus
- ✓7th S27.491 Other injury of bronchus, unilateral
- ✓7th S27.492 Other injury of bronchus, bilateral
- ✓7th S27.499 Other injury of bronchus, unspecified

✓5th **S27.5** **Injury of thoracic trachea**
- ✓x7th **S27.50** **Unspecified injury of thoracic trachea**
- ✓x7th **S27.51** **Primary blast injury of thoracic trachea**
Blast injury of thoracic trachea NOS
- ✓x7th **S27.52** **Contusion of thoracic trachea**
- ✓x7th **S27.53** **Laceration of thoracic trachea**
- ✓x7th **S27.59** **Other injury of thoracic trachea**
Secondary blast injury of thoracic trachea

✓5th **S27.6** **Injury of pleura**
- ✓x7th **S27.60** **Unspecified injury of pleura**
- ✓x7th **S27.63** **Laceration of pleura**
- ✓x7th **S27.69** **Other injury of pleura**

✓5th **S27.8** **Injury of other specified intrathoracic organs**

✓6th **S27.80** **Injury of diaphragm**
- ✓7th S27.802 Contusion of diaphragm
- ✓7th S27.803 Laceration of diaphragm
- ✓7th S27.808 Other injury of diaphragm
- ✓7th S27.809 Unspecified injury of diaphragm

✓6th **S27.81** **Injury of esophagus (thoracic part)**
- ✓7th S27.812 Contusion of esophagus (thoracic part)
- ✓7th S27.813 Laceration of esophagus (thoracic part)
- ✓7th S27.818 Other injury of esophagus (thoracic part)
- ✓7th S27.819 Unspecified injury of esophagus (thoracic part)

✓6th **S27.89** **Injury of other specified intrathoracic organs**
Injury of lymphatic thoracic duct
Injury of thymus gland
- ✓7th S27.892 Contusion of other specified intrathoracic organs
- ✓7th S27.893 Laceration of other specified intrathoracic organs
- ✓7th S27.898 Other injury of other specified intrathoracic organs
- ✓7th S27.899 Unspecified injury of other specified intrathoracic organs

✓x7th **S27.9** **Injury of unspecified intrathoracic organ**

✓4th **S28** **Crushing injury of thorax, and traumatic amputation of part of thorax**

The appropriate 7th character is to be added to each code from category S28.
A   initial encounter
D   subsequent encounter
S   sequela

✓x7th **S28.0** **Crushed chest**
Use additional code for all associated injuries
EXCLUDES 1   *flail chest (S22.5)*

✓x7th **S28.1** **Traumatic amputation (partial) of part of thorax, except breast**

✓5th **S28.2** **Traumatic amputation of breast**

✓6th **S28.21** **Complete traumatic amputation of breast**
Traumatic amputation of breast NOS
- ✓7th S28.211 Complete traumatic amputation of right breast
- ✓7th S28.212 Complete traumatic amputation of left breast
- ✓7th S28.219 Complete traumatic amputation of unspecified breast

✓6th **S28.22** **Partial traumatic amputation of breast**
- ✓7th S28.221 Partial traumatic amputation of right breast
- ✓7th S28.222 Partial traumatic amputation of left breast
- ✓7th S28.229 Partial traumatic amputation of unspecified breast

✓4th **S29** **Other and unspecified injuries of thorax**
Code also any associated open wound (S21-)

The appropriate 7th character is to be added to each code from category S29.
A   initial encounter
D   subsequent encounter
S   sequela

✓5th **S29.0** **Injury of muscle and tendon at thorax level**

✓6th **S29.00** **Unspecified injury of muscle and tendon of thorax**
- ✓7th S29.001 Unspecified injury of muscle and tendon of front wall of thorax
- ✓7th S29.002 Unspecified injury of muscle and tendon of back wall of thorax
- ✓7th S29.009 Unspecified injury of muscle and tendon of unspecified wall of thorax

✓6th **S29.01** **Strain of muscle and tendon of thorax**
- ✓7th S29.011 Strain of muscle and tendon of front wall of thorax
- ✓7th S29.012 Strain of muscle and tendon of back wall of thorax
- ✓7th S29.019 Strain of muscle and tendon of unspecified wall of thorax

✓6th **S29.02** **Laceration of muscle and tendon of thorax**
- ✓7th S29.021 Laceration of muscle and tendon of front wall of thorax
- ✓7th S29.022 Laceration of muscle and tendon of back wall of thorax
- ✓7th S29.029 Laceration of muscle and tendon of unspecified wall of thorax

✓6th **S29.09** **Other injury of muscle and tendon of thorax**
- ✓7th S29.091 Other injury of muscle and tendon of front wall of thorax
- ✓7th S29.092 Other injury of muscle and tendon of back wall of thorax
- ✓7th S29.099 Other injury of muscle and tendon of unspecified wall of thorax

✓x7th **S29.8** **Other specified injuries of thorax**
✓x7th **S29.9** **Unspecified injury of thorax**

EXCLUDES 1   Not coded here   EXCLUDES 2   Not included here   *Manifestation Code*

Injuries to the abdomen, lower back, lumbar spine, pelvis and external genitals (S30-S39)

INCLUDES injuries to the abdominal wall
injuries to the anus
injuries to the buttock
injuries to the external genitalia
injuries to the flank
injuries to the groin

EXCLUDES 2 burns and corrosions (T20-T32)
effects of foreign body in anus and rectum (T18.5)
effects of foreign body in genitourinary tract (T19-)
effects of foreign body in stomach, small intestine and colon (T18.2-T18.4)
frostbite (T33-T34)
insect bite or sting, venomous (T63.4)

√4th **S30 Superficial injury of abdomen, lower back, pelvis and external genitals**

EXCLUDES 2 *superficial injury of hip (S70-)*

The appropriate 7th character is to be added to each code from category S30.
A   initial encounter
D   subsequent encounter
S   sequela

√x7th **S30.0 Contusion of lower back and pelvis**
Contusion of buttock

√x7th **S30.1 Contusion of abdominal wall**
Contusion of flank
Contusion of groin

√5th **S30.2 Contusion of external genital organs**
√6th **S30.20 Contusion of unspecified external genital organ**
√7th **S30.201 Contusion of unspecified external genital organ, male**
√7th **S30.202 Contusion of unspecified external genital organ, female**
√x7th **S30.21 Contusion of penis**
√x7th **S30.22 Contusion of scrotum and testes**
√x7th **S30.23 Contusion of vagina and vulva**

√x7th **S30.3 Contusion of anus**

√5th **S30.8 Other superficial injuries of abdomen, lower back, pelvis and external genitals**
√6th **S30.81 Abrasion of abdomen, lower back, pelvis and external genitals**
√7th **S30.810 Abrasion of lower back and pelvis**
√7th **S30.811 Abrasion of abdominal wall**
√7th **S30.812 Abrasion of penis**
√7th **S30.813 Abrasion of scrotum and testes**
√7th **S30.814 Abrasion of vagina and vulva**
√7th **S30.815 Abrasion of unspecified external genital organs, male**
√7th **S30.816 Abrasion of unspecified external genital organs, female**
√7th **S30.817 Abrasion of anus**
√6th **S30.82 Blister (nonthermal) of abdomen, lower back, pelvis and external genitals**
√7th **S30.820 Blister (nonthermal) of lower back and pelvis**
√7th **S30.821 Blister (nonthermal) of abdominal wall**
√7th **S30.822 Blister (nonthermal) of penis**
√7th **S30.823 Blister (nonthermal) of scrotum and testes**
√7th **S30.824 Blister (nonthermal) of vagina and vulva**
√7th **S30.825 Blister (nonthermal) of unspecified external genital organs, male**
√7th **S30.826 Blister (nonthermal) of unspecified external genital organs, female**
√7th **S30.827 Blister (nonthermal) of anus**
√6th **S30.84 External constriction of abdomen, lower back, pelvis and external genitals**
√7th **S30.840 External constriction of lower back and pelvis**
√7th **S30.841 External constriction of abdominal wall**
√7th **S30.842 External constriction of penis**
Hair tourniquet syndrome of penis
Use additional cause code to identify the constricting item (W49.0-)

√7th **S30.843 External constriction of scrotum and testes**
√7th **S30.844 External constriction of vagina and vulva**
√7th **S30.845 External constriction of unspecified external genital organs, male**
√7th **S30.846 External constriction of unspecified external genital organs, female**
√6th **S30.85 Superficial foreign body of abdomen, lower back, pelvis and external genitals**
Splinter in the abdomen, lower back, pelvis and external genitals
√7th **S30.850 Superficial foreign body of lower back and pelvis**
√7th **S30.851 Superficial foreign body of abdominal wall**
√7th **S30.852 Superficial foreign body of penis**
√7th **S30.853 Superficial foreign body of scrotum and testes**
√7th **S30.854 Superficial foreign body of vagina and vulva**
√7th **S30.855 Superficial foreign body of unspecified external genital organs, male**
√7th **S30.856 Superficial foreign body of unspecified external genital organs, female**
√7th **S30.857 Superficial foreign body of anus**
√6th **S30.86 Insect bite (nonvenomous) of abdomen, lower back, pelvis and external genitals**
√7th **S30.860 Insect bite (nonvenomous) of lower back and pelvis**
√7th **S30.861 Insect bite (nonvenomous) of abdominal wall**
√7th **S30.862 Insect bite (nonvenomous) of penis**
√7th **S30.863 Insect bite (nonvenomous) of scrotum and testes**
√7th **S30.864 Insect bite (nonvenomous) of vagina and vulva**
√7th **S30.865 Insect bite (nonvenomous) of unspecified external genital organs, male**
√7th **S30.866 Insect bite (nonvenomous) of unspecified external genital organs, female**
√7th **S30.867 Insect bite (nonvenomous) of anus**
√6th **S30.87 Other superficial bite of abdomen, lower back, pelvis and external genitals**
EXCLUDES 1 *open bite of abdomen, lower back, pelvis and external genitals (S31.05, S31.15, S31.25, S31.35, S31.45, S31.55)*
√7th **S30.870 Other superficial bite of lower back and pelvis**
√7th **S30.871 Other superficial bite of abdominal wall**
√7th **S30.872 Other superficial bite of penis**
√7th **S30.873 Other superficial bite of scrotum and testes**
√7th **S30.874 Other superficial bite of vagina and vulva**
√7th **S30.875 Other superficial bite of unspecified external genital organs, male**
√7th **S30.876 Other superficial bite of unspecified external genital organs, female**
√7th **S30.877 Other superficial bite of anus**

√5th **S30.9 Unspecified superficial injury of abdomen, lower back, pelvis and external genitals**
√x7th **S30.91 Unspecified superficial injury of lower back and pelvis**
√x7th **S30.92 Unspecified superficial injury of abdominal wall**
√x7th **S30.93 Unspecified superficial injury of penis**
√x7th **S30.94 Unspecified superficial injury of scrotum and testes**
√x7th **S30.95 Unspecified superficial injury of vagina and vulva**
√x7th **S30.96 Unspecified superficial injury of unspecified external genital organs, male**
√x7th **S30.97 Unspecified superficial injury of unspecified external genital organs, female**
√x7th **S30.98 Unspecified superficial injury of anus**

☑ Appropriate additional character required   √x7th Requires 7th character, placeholder x must fill empty characters

☑4ᵗʰ S31   Open wound of abdomen, lower back, pelvis and external genitals

Code also any associated:
spinal cord injury (S24.0, S24.1-, S34.0-, S34.1-)
wound infection

> **EXCLUDES 1**   *traumatic amputation of part of abdomen, lower back and pelvis (S38.2-, S38.3)*

> **EXCLUDES 2**   *open wound of hip (S71.00-S71.02)*
> *open fracture of pelvis (S32.1--S32.9 with 7th character B)*

> The appropriate 7th character is to be added to each code from category S31.
> A   initial encounter
> D   subsequent encounter
> S   sequela

☑5ᵗʰ S31.0   Open wound of lower back and pelvis

☑6ᵗʰ S31.00   Unspecified open wound of lower back and pelvis

- ☑7ᵗʰ **S31.000**   **Unspecified open wound of lower back and pelvis without penetration into retroperitoneum**
  Unspecified open wound of lower back and pelvis NOS

- ☑7ᵗʰ **S31.001**   **Unspecified open wound of lower back and pelvis with penetration into retroperitoneum**

☑6ᵗʰ S31.01   Laceration without foreign body of lower back and pelvis

- ☑7ᵗʰ **S31.010**   **Laceration without foreign body of lower back and pelvis without penetration into retroperitoneum**
  Laceration without foreign body of lower back and pelvis NOS

- ☑7ᵗʰ **S31.011**   **Laceration without foreign body of lower back and pelvis with penetration into retroperitoneum**

☑6ᵗʰ S31.02   Laceration with foreign body of lower back and pelvis

- ☑7ᵗʰ **S31.020**   **Laceration with foreign body of lower back and pelvis without penetration into retroperitoneum**
  Laceration with foreign body of lower back and pelvis NOS

- ☑7ᵗʰ **S31.021**   **Laceration with foreign body of lower back and pelvis with penetration into retroperitoneum**

☑6ᵗʰ S31.03   Puncture wound without foreign body of lower back and pelvis

- ☑7ᵗʰ **S31.030**   **Puncture wound without foreign body of lower back and pelvis without penetration into retroperitoneum**
  Puncture wound without foreign body of lower back and pelvis NOS

- ☑7ᵗʰ **S31.031**   **Puncture wound without foreign body of lower back and pelvis with penetration into retroperitoneum**

☑6ᵗʰ S31.04   Puncture wound with foreign body of lower back and pelvis

- ☑7ᵗʰ **S31.040**   **Puncture wound with foreign body of lower back and pelvis without penetration into retroperitoneum**
  Puncture wound with foreign body of lower back and pelvis NOS

- ☑7ᵗʰ **S31.041**   **Puncture wound with foreign body of lower back and pelvis with penetration into retroperitoneum**

☑6ᵗʰ S31.05   Open bite of lower back and pelvis

Bite of lower back and pelvis NOS

> **EXCLUDES 1**   *superficial bite of lower back and pelvis (S30.860, S30.870)*

- ☑7ᵗʰ **S31.050**   **Open bite of lower back and pelvis without penetration into retroperitoneum**
  Open bite of lower back and pelvis NOS

- ☑7ᵗʰ **S31.051**   **Open bite of lower back and pelvis with penetration into retroperitoneum**

☑5ᵗʰ S31.1   Open wound of abdominal wall without penetration into peritoneal cavity

Open wound of abdominal wall NOS

> **EXCLUDES 2**   *open wound of abdominal wall with penetration into peritoneal cavity (S31.6-)*

☑6ᵗʰ S31.10   Unspecified open wound of abdominal wall without penetration into peritoneal cavity

- ☑7ᵗʰ **S31.100**   **Unspecified open wound of abdominal wall, right upper quadrant without penetration into peritoneal cavity**

- ☑7ᵗʰ **S31.101**   **Unspecified open wound of abdominal wall, left upper quadrant without penetration into peritoneal cavity**

- ☑7ᵗʰ **S31.102**   **Unspecified open wound of abdominal wall, epigastric region without penetration into peritoneal cavity**

- ☑7ᵗʰ **S31.103**   **Unspecified open wound of abdominal wall, right lower quadrant without penetration into peritoneal cavity**

- ☑7ᵗʰ **S31.104**   **Unspecified open wound of abdominal wall, left lower quadrant without penetration into peritoneal cavity**

- ☑7ᵗʰ **S31.105**   **Unspecified open wound of abdominal wall, periumbilic region without penetration into peritoneal cavity**

- ☑7ᵗʰ **S31.109**   **Unspecified open wound of abdominal wall, unspecified quadrant without penetration into peritoneal cavity**
  Unspecified open wound of abdominal wall NOS

☑6ᵗʰ S31.11   Laceration without foreign body of abdominal wall without penetration into peritoneal cavity

- ☑7ᵗʰ **S31.110**   **Laceration without foreign body of abdominal wall, right upper quadrant without penetration into peritoneal cavity**

- ☑7ᵗʰ **S31.111**   **Laceration without foreign body of abdominal wall, left upper quadrant without penetration into peritoneal cavity**

- ☑7ᵗʰ **S31.112**   **Laceration without foreign body of abdominal wall, epigastric region without penetration into peritoneal cavity**

- ☑7ᵗʰ **S31.113**   **Laceration without foreign body of abdominal wall, right lower quadrant without penetration into peritoneal cavity**

- ☑7ᵗʰ **S31.114**   **Laceration without foreign body of abdominal wall, left lower quadrant without penetration into peritoneal cavity**

- ☑7ᵗʰ **S31.115**   **Laceration without foreign body of abdominal wall, periumbilic region without penetration into peritoneal cavity**

- ☑7ᵗʰ **S31.119**   **Laceration without foreign body of abdominal wall, unspecified quadrant without penetration into peritoneal cavity**

☑6ᵗʰ S31.12   Laceration with foreign body of abdominal wall without penetration into peritoneal cavity

- ☑7ᵗʰ **S31.120**   **Laceration of abdominal wall with foreign body, right upper quadrant without penetration into peritoneal cavity**

- ☑7ᵗʰ **S31.121**   **Laceration of abdominal wall with foreign body, left upper quadrant without penetration into peritoneal cavity**

- ☑7ᵗʰ **S31.122**   **Laceration of abdominal wall with foreign body, epigastric region without penetration into peritoneal cavity**

- ☑7ᵗʰ **S31.123**   **Laceration of abdominal wall with foreign body, right lower quadrant without penetration into peritoneal cavity**

√7th S31.124 Laceration of abdominal wall with foreign body, left lower quadrant without penetration into peritoneal cavity

√7th S31.125 Laceration of abdominal wall with foreign body, periumbilic region without penetration into peritoneal cavity

√7th S31.129 Laceration of abdominal wall with foreign body, unspecified quadrant without penetration into peritoneal cavity

√6th S31.13 Puncture wound of abdominal wall without foreign body without penetration into peritoneal cavity

√7th S31.130 Puncture wound of abdominal wall without foreign body, right upper quadrant without penetration into peritoneal cavity

√7th S31.131 Puncture wound of abdominal wall without foreign body, left upper quadrant without penetration into peritoneal cavity

√7th S31.132 Puncture wound of abdominal wall without foreign body, epigastric region without penetration into peritoneal cavity

√7th S31.133 Puncture wound of abdominal wall without foreign body, right lower quadrant without penetration into peritoneal cavity

√7th S31.134 Puncture wound of abdominal wall without foreign body, left lower quadrant without penetration into peritoneal cavity

√7th S31.135 Puncture wound of abdominal wall without foreign body, periumbilic region without penetration into peritoneal cavity

√7th S31.139 Puncture wound of abdominal wall without foreign body, unspecified quadrant without penetration into peritoneal cavity

√6th S31.14 Puncture wound of abdominal wall with foreign body without penetration into peritoneal cavity

√7th S31.140 Puncture wound of abdominal wall with foreign body, right upper quadrant without penetration into peritoneal cavity

√7th S31.141 Puncture wound of abdominal wall with foreign body, left upper quadrant without penetration into peritoneal cavity

√7th S31.142 Puncture wound of abdominal wall with foreign body, epigastric region without penetration into peritoneal cavity

√7th S31.143 Puncture wound of abdominal wall with foreign body, right lower quadrant without penetration into peritoneal cavity

√7th S31.144 Puncture wound of abdominal wall with foreign body, left lower quadrant without penetration into peritoneal cavity

√7th S31.145 Puncture wound of abdominal wall with foreign body, periumbilic region without penetration into peritoneal cavity

√7th S31.149 Puncture wound of abdominal wall with foreign body, unspecified quadrant without penetration into peritoneal cavity

√6th S31.15 Open bite of abdominal wall without penetration into peritoneal cavity

Bite of abdominal wall NOS

EXCLUDES 1 superficial bite of abdominal wall (S30.871)

√7th S31.150 Open bite of abdominal wall, right upper quadrant without penetration into peritoneal cavity

√7th S31.151 Open bite of abdominal wall, left upper quadrant without penetration into peritoneal cavity

√7th S31.152 Open bite of abdominal wall, epigastric region without penetration into peritoneal cavity

√7th S31.153 Open bite of abdominal wall, right lower quadrant without penetration into peritoneal cavity

√7th S31.154 Open bite of abdominal wall, left lower quadrant without penetration into peritoneal cavity

√7th S31.155 Open bite of abdominal wall, periumbilic region without penetration into peritoneal cavity

√7th S31.159 Open bite of abdominal wall, unspecified quadrant without penetration into peritoneal cavity

√5th S31.2 Open wound of penis

√x7th S31.20 Unspecified open wound of penis
√x7th S31.21 Laceration without foreign body of penis
√x7th S31.22 Laceration with foreign body of penis
√x7th S31.23 Puncture wound without foreign body of penis
√x7th S31.24 Puncture wound with foreign body of penis
√x7th S31.25 Open bite of penis

Bite of penis NOS

EXCLUDES 1 superficial bite of penis (S30.862, S30.872)

√5th S31.3 Open wound of scrotum and testes

√x7th S31.30 Unspecified open wound of scrotum and testes
√x7th S31.31 Laceration without foreign body of scrotum and testes
√x7th S31.32 Laceration with foreign body of scrotum and testes
√x7th S31.33 Puncture wound without foreign body of scrotum and testes
√x7th S31.34 Puncture wound with foreign body of scrotum and testes
√x7th S31.35 Open bite of scrotum and testes

Bite of scrotum and testes NOS

EXCLUDES 1 superficial bite of scrotum and testes (S30.863, S30.873)

√5th S31.4 Open wound of vagina and vulva

EXCLUDES 1 injury to vagina and vulva during delivery (O70-, O71.4)

√x7th S31.40 Unspecified open wound of vagina and vulva
√x7th S31.41 Laceration without foreign body of vagina and vulva
√x7th S31.42 Laceration with foreign body of vagina and vulva
√x7th S31.43 Puncture wound without foreign body of vagina and vulva
√x7th S31.44 Puncture wound with foreign body of vagina and vulva
√x7th S31.45 Open bite of vagina and vulva

Bite of vagina and vulva NOS

EXCLUDES 1 superficial bite of vagina and vulva (S30.864, S30.874)

√5th S31.5 Open wound of unspecified external genital organs

EXCLUDES 1 traumatic amputation of external genital organs (S38.21, S38.22)

√6th S31.50 Unspecified open wound of unspecified external genital organs

√7th S31.501 Unspecified open wound of unspecified external genital organs, male

√7th S31.502 Unspecified open wound of unspecified external genital organs, female

√6th S31.51 Laceration without foreign body of unspecified external genital organs

√7th S31.511 Laceration without foreign body of unspecified external genital organs, male

---

☑ Appropriate additional character required   √x7th Requires 7th character, placeholder x must fill empty characters

√7th **S31.512** **Laceration without foreign body of unspecified external genital organs, female**

√6th **S31.52** **Laceration with foreign body of unspecified external genital organs**

√7th **S31.521** **Laceration with foreign body of unspecified external genital organs, male**

√7th **S31.522** **Laceration with foreign body of unspecified external genital organs, female**

√6th **S31.53** **Puncture wound without foreign body of unspecified external genital organs**

√7th **S31.531** **Puncture wound without foreign body of unspecified external genital organs, male**

√7th **S31.532** **Puncture wound without foreign body of unspecified external genital organs, female**

√6th **S31.54** **Puncture wound with foreign body of unspecified external genital organs**

√7th **S31.541** **Puncture wound with foreign body of unspecified external genital organs, male**

√7th **S31.542** **Puncture wound with foreign body of unspecified external genital organs, female**

√6th **S31.55** **Open bite of unspecified external genital organs**
Bite of unspecified external genital organs NOS
EXCLUDES 1 *superficial bite of unspecified external genital organs (S30.865, S30.866, S30.875, S30.876)*

√7th **S31.551** **Open bite of unspecified external genital organs, male**

√7th **S31.552** **Open bite of unspecified external genital organs, female**

√5th **S31.6** **Open wound of abdominal wall with penetration into peritoneal cavity**

√6th **S31.60** **Unspecified open wound of abdominal wall with penetration into peritoneal cavity**

√7th **S31.600** **Unspecified open wound of abdominal wall, right upper quadrant with penetration into peritoneal cavity**

√7th **S31.601** **Unspecified open wound of abdominal wall, left upper quadrant with penetration into peritoneal cavity**

√7th **S31.602** **Unspecified open wound of abdominal wall, epigastric region with penetration into peritoneal cavity**

√7th **S31.603** **Unspecified open wound of abdominal wall, right lower quadrant with penetration into peritoneal cavity**

√7th **S31.604** **Unspecified open wound of abdominal wall, left lower quadrant with penetration into peritoneal cavity**

√7th **S31.605** **Unspecified open wound of abdominal wall, periumbilic region with penetration into peritoneal cavity**

√7th **S31.609** **Unspecified open wound of abdominal wall, unspecified quadrant with penetration into peritoneal cavity**

√6th **S31.61** **Laceration without foreign body of abdominal wall with penetration into peritoneal cavity**

√7th **S31.610** **Laceration without foreign body of abdominal wall, right upper quadrant with penetration into peritoneal cavity**

√7th **S31.611** **Laceration without foreign body of abdominal wall, left upper quadrant with penetration into peritoneal cavity**

√7th **S31.612** **Laceration without foreign body of abdominal wall, epigastric region with penetration into peritoneal cavity**

√7th **S31.613** **Laceration without foreign body of abdominal wall, right lower quadrant with penetration into peritoneal cavity**

√7th **S31.614** **Laceration without foreign body of abdominal wall, left lower quadrant with penetration into peritoneal cavity**

√7th **S31.615** **Laceration without foreign body of abdominal wall, periumbilic region with penetration into peritoneal cavity**

√7th **S31.619** **Laceration without foreign body of abdominal wall, unspecified quadrant with penetration into peritoneal cavity**

√6th **S31.62** **Laceration with foreign body of abdominal wall with penetration into peritoneal cavity**

√7th **S31.620** **Laceration with foreign body of abdominal wall, right upper quadrant with penetration into peritoneal cavity**

√7th **S31.621** **Laceration with foreign body of abdominal wall, left upper quadrant with penetration into peritoneal cavity**

√7th **S31.622** **Laceration with foreign body of abdominal wall, epigastric region with penetration into peritoneal cavity**

√7th **S31.623** **Laceration with foreign body of abdominal wall, right lower quadrant with penetration into peritoneal cavity**

√7th **S31.624** **Laceration with foreign body of abdominal wall, left lower quadrant with penetration into peritoneal cavity**

√7th **S31.625** **Laceration with foreign body of abdominal wall, periumbilic region with penetration into peritoneal cavity**

√7th **S31.629** **Laceration with foreign body of abdominal wall, unspecified quadrant with penetration into peritoneal cavity**

√6th **S31.63** **Puncture wound without foreign body of abdominal wall with penetration into peritoneal cavity**

√7th **S31.630** **Puncture wound without foreign body of abdominal wall, right upper quadrant with penetration into peritoneal cavity**

√7th **S31.631** **Puncture wound without foreign body of abdominal wall, left upper quadrant with penetration into peritoneal cavity**

√7th **S31.632** **Puncture wound without foreign body of abdominal wall, epigastric region with penetration into peritoneal cavity**

√7th **S31.633** **Puncture wound without foreign body of abdominal wall, right lower quadrant with penetration into peritoneal cavity**

√7th **S31.634** **Puncture wound without foreign body of abdominal wall, left lower quadrant with penetration into peritoneal cavity**

√7th **S31.635** **Puncture wound without foreign body of abdominal wall, periumbilic region with penetration into peritoneal cavity**

√7th **S31.639** **Puncture wound without foreign body of abdominal wall, unspecified quadrant with penetration into peritoneal cavity**

√6th **S31.64** **Puncture wound with foreign body of abdominal wall with penetration into peritoneal cavity**

√7th **S31.640** **Puncture wound with foreign body of abdominal wall, right upper quadrant with penetration into peritoneal cavity**

√7th **S31.641** **Puncture wound with foreign body of abdominal wall, left upper quadrant with penetration into peritoneal cavity**

√7th **S31.642** **Puncture wound with foreign body of abdominal wall, epigastric region with penetration into peritoneal cavity**

√7th **S31.643** **Puncture wound with foreign body of abdominal wall, right lower quadrant with penetration into peritoneal cavity**

√7th **S31.644** **Puncture wound with foreign body of abdominal wall, left lower quadrant with penetration into peritoneal cavity**

√7th **S31.645** **Puncture wound with foreign body of abdominal wall, periumbilic region with penetration into peritoneal cavity**

√7th **S31.649** **Puncture wound with foreign body of abdominal wall, unspecified quadrant with penetration into peritoneal cavity**

✓6th **S31.65 Open bite of abdominal wall with penetration into peritoneal cavity**
> EXCLUDES 1 *superficial bite of abdominal wall (S30.861, S30.871)*

✓7th **S31.650 Open bite of abdominal wall, right upper quadrant with penetration into peritoneal cavity**

✓7th **S31.651 Open bite of abdominal wall, left upper quadrant with penetration into peritoneal cavity**

✓7th **S31.652 Open bite of abdominal wall, epigastric region with penetration into peritoneal cavity**

✓7th **S31.653 Open bite of abdominal wall, right lower quadrant with penetration into peritoneal cavity**

✓7th **S31.654 Open bite of abdominal wall, left lower quadrant with penetration into peritoneal cavity**

✓7th **S31.655 Open bite of abdominal wall, periumbilic region with penetration into peritoneal cavity**

✓7th **S31.659 Open bite of abdominal wall, unspecified quadrant with penetration into peritoneal cavity**

✓5th **S31.8 Open wound of other parts of abdomen, lower back and pelvis**

✓6th **S31.80 Open wound of unspecified buttock**

✓7th **S31.801 Laceration without foreign body of unspecified buttock**

✓7th **S31.802 Laceration with foreign body of unspecified buttock**

✓7th **S31.803 Puncture wound without foreign body of unspecified buttock**

✓7th **S31.804 Puncture wound with foreign body of unspecified buttock**

✓7th **S31.805 Open bite of unspecified buttock**
> Bite of buttock NOS
> EXCLUDES 1 *superficial bite of buttock (S30.870)*

✓7th **S31.809 Unspecified open wound of unspecified buttock**

✓6th **S31.81 Open wound of right buttock**

✓7th **S31.811 Laceration without foreign body of right buttock**

✓7th **S31.812 Laceration with foreign body of right buttock**

✓7th **S31.813 Puncture wound without foreign body of right buttock**

✓7th **S31.814 Puncture wound with foreign body of right buttock**

✓7th **S31.815 Open bite of right buttock**
> Bite of right buttock NOS
> EXCLUDES 1 *superficial bite of buttock (S30.870)*

✓7th **S31.819 Unspecified open wound of right buttock**

✓6th **S31.82 Open wound of left buttock**

✓7th **S31.821 Laceration without foreign body of left buttock**

✓7th **S31.822 Laceration with foreign body of left buttock**

✓7th **S31.823 Puncture wound without foreign body of left buttock**

✓7th **S31.824 Puncture wound with foreign body of left buttock**

✓7th **S31.825 Open bite of left buttock**
> Bite of left buttock NOS
> EXCLUDES 1 *superficial bite of buttock (S30.870)*

✓7th **S31.829 Unspecified open wound of left buttock**

✓6th **S31.83 Open wound of anus**

✓7th **S31.831 Laceration without foreign body of anus**

✓7th **S31.832 Laceration with foreign body of anus**

✓7th **S31.833 Puncture wound without foreign body of anus**

✓7th **S31.834 Puncture wound with foreign body of anus**

✓7th **S31.835 Open bite of anus**
> Bite of anus NOS
> EXCLUDES 1 *superficial bite of anus (S30.877)*

✓7th **S31.839 Unspecified open wound of anus**

✓4th **S32 Fracture of lumbar spine and pelvis**

> NOTE   A fracture not indicated as displaced or nondisplaced should be coded to displaced
> A fracture not indicated as opened or closed should be coded to closed

> INCLUDES   fracture of lumbosacral neural arch
> fracture of lumbosacral spinous process
> fracture of lumbosacral transverse process
> fracture of lumbosacral vertebra
> fracture of lumbosacral vertebral arch

Codes first any associated spinal cord and spinal nerve injury (S34-)

> EXCLUDES 1 *transection of abdomen (S38.3)*
> EXCLUDES 2 *fracture of hip NOS (S72.0-)*

The appropriate 7th character is to be added to each code from category S32.
A   initial encounter for closed fracture
B   initial encounter for open fracture
D   subsequent encounter for fracture with routine healing
G   subsequent encounter for fracture with delayed healing
K   subsequent encounter for fracture with nonunion
S   sequela

✓5th **S32.0 Fracture of lumbar vertebra**
> Fracture of lumbar spine NOS

✓6th **S32.00 Fracture of unspecified lumbar vertebra**

✓7th **S32.000 Wedge compression fracture of unspecified lumbar vertebra**

✓7th **S32.001 Stable burst fracture of unspecified lumbar vertebra**

✓7th **S32.002 Unstable burst fracture of unspecified lumbar vertebra**

✓7th **S32.008 Other fracture of unspecified lumbar vertebra**

✓7th **S32.009 Unspecified fracture of unspecified lumbar vertebra**

✓6th **S32.01 Fracture of first lumbar vertebra**

✓7th **S32.010 Wedge compression fracture of first lumbar vertebra**

✓7th **S32.011 Stable burst fracture of first lumbar vertebra**

✓7th **S32.012 Unstable burst fracture of first lumbar vertebra**

✓7th **S32.018 Other fracture of first lumbar vertebra**

✓7th **S32.019 Unspecified fracture of first lumbar vertebra**

✓6th **S32.02 Fracture of second lumbar vertebra**

✓7th **S32.020 Wedge compression fracture of second lumbar vertebra**

✓7th **S32.021 Stable burst fracture of second lumbar vertebra**

✓7th **S32.022 Unstable burst fracture of second lumbar vertebra**

✓7th **S32.028 Other fracture of second lumbar vertebra**

✓7th **S32.029 Unspecified fracture of second lumbar vertebra**

✓6th **S32.03 Fracture of third lumbar vertebra**

✓7th **S32.030 Wedge compression fracture of third lumbar vertebra**

✓7th **S32.031 Stable burst fracture of third lumbar vertebra**

✓7th **S32.032 Unstable burst fracture of third lumbar vertebra**

✓7th **S32.038 Other fracture of third lumbar vertebra**

✓7th **S32.039 Unspecified fracture of third lumbar vertebra**

✓ Appropriate additional character required   ✓x7th Requires 7th character, placeholder x must fill empty characters

✓6ᵗʰ **S32.04 Fracture of fourth lumbar vertebra**

    ✓7ᵗʰ **S32.040 Wedge compression fracture of fourth lumbar vertebra**

    ✓7ᵗʰ **S32.041 Stable burst fracture of fourth lumbar vertebra**

    ✓7ᵗʰ **S32.042 Unstable burst fracture of fourth lumbar vertebra**

    ✓7ᵗʰ **S32.048 Other fracture of fourth lumbar vertebra**

    ✓7ᵗʰ **S32.049 Unspecified fracture of fourth lumbar vertebra**

✓6ᵗʰ **S32.05 Fracture of fifth lumbar vertebra**

    ✓7ᵗʰ **S32.050 Wedge compression fracture of fifth lumbar vertebra**

    ✓7ᵗʰ **S32.051 Stable burst fracture of fifth lumbar vertebra**

    ✓7ᵗʰ **S32.052 Unstable burst fracture of fifth lumbar vertebra**

    ✓7ᵗʰ **S32.058 Other fracture of fifth lumbar vertebra**

    ✓7ᵗʰ **S32.059 Unspecified fracture of fifth lumbar vertebra**

✓5ᵗʰ **S32.1 Fracture of sacrum**

    NOTE For vertical fractures, code to most medial fracture extension
        Use two codes if both a vertical and transverse fracture are present

    Code also any associated fracture of pelvic ring (S32.8-)

    ✓x7ᵗʰ **S32.10 Unspecified fracture of sacrum**

    ✓6ᵗʰ **S32.11 Zone I fracture of sacrum**
        Vertical sacral ala fracture of sacrum

        ✓7ᵗʰ **S32.110 Nondisplaced Zone I fracture of sacrum**

        ✓7ᵗʰ **S32.111 Minimally displaced Zone I fracture of sacrum**

        ✓7ᵗʰ **S32.112 Severely displaced Zone I fracture of sacrum**

        ✓7ᵗʰ **S32.119 Unspecified Zone I fracture of sacrum**

    ✓6ᵗʰ **S32.12 Zone II fracture of sacrum**
        Vertical foraminal region fracture of sacrum

        ✓7ᵗʰ **S32.120 Nondisplaced Zone II fracture of sacrum**

        ✓7ᵗʰ **S32.121 Minimally displaced Zone II fracture of sacrum**

        ✓7ᵗʰ **S32.122 Severely displaced Zone II fracture of sacrum**

        ✓7ᵗʰ **S32.129 Unspecified Zone II fracture of sacrum**

    ✓6ᵗʰ **S32.13 Zone III fracture of sacrum**
        Vertical fracture into spinal canal region of sacrum

        ✓7ᵗʰ **S32.130 Nondisplaced Zone III fracture of sacrum**

        ✓7ᵗʰ **S32.131 Minimally displaced Zone III fracture of sacrum**

        ✓7ᵗʰ **S32.132 Severely displaced Zone III fracture of sacrum**

        ✓7ᵗʰ **S32.139 Unspecified Zone III fracture of sacrum**

    ✓x7ᵗʰ **S32.14 Type 1 fracture of sacrum**
        Transverse flexion fracture of sacrum without displacement

    ✓x7ᵗʰ **S32.15 Type 2 fracture of sacrum**
        Transverse flexion fracture of sacrum with posterior displacement

    ✓x7ᵗʰ **S32.16 Type 3 fracture of sacrum**
        Transverse extension fracture of sacrum with anterior displacement

    ✓x7ᵗʰ **S32.17 Type 4 fracture of sacrum**
        Transverse segmental comminution of upper sacrum

    ✓x7ᵗʰ **S32.19 Other fracture of sacrum**

✓x7ᵗʰ **S32.2 Fracture of coccyx**

✓5ᵗʰ **S32.3 Fracture of ilium**

    EXCLUDES 1 fracture of ilium with associated disruption of pelvic ring (S32.8-)

    ✓6ᵗʰ **S32.30 Unspecified fracture of ilium**

        ✓7ᵗʰ **S32.301 Unspecified fracture of right ilium**

        ✓7ᵗʰ **S32.302 Unspecified fracture of left ilium**

        ✓7ᵗʰ **S32.309 Unspecified fracture of unspecified ilium**

    ✓6ᵗʰ **S32.31 Avulsion fracture of ilium**

        ✓7ᵗʰ **S32.311 Displaced avulsion fracture of right ilium**

        ✓7ᵗʰ **S32.312 Displaced avulsion fracture of left ilium**

        ✓7ᵗʰ **S32.313 Displaced avulsion fracture of unspecified ilium**

        ✓7ᵗʰ **S32.314 Nondisplaced avulsion fracture of right ilium**

        ✓7ᵗʰ **S32.315 Nondisplaced avulsion fracture of left ilium**

        ✓7ᵗʰ **S32.316 Nondisplaced avulsion fracture of unspecified ilium**

    ✓6ᵗʰ **S32.39 Other fracture of ilium**

        ✓7ᵗʰ **S32.391 Other fracture of right ilium**

        ✓7ᵗʰ **S32.392 Other fracture of left ilium**

        ✓7ᵗʰ **S32.399 Other fracture of unspecified ilium**

✓5ᵗʰ **S32.4 Fracture of acetabulum**

    Code also any associated fracture of pelvic ring (S32.8-)

    ✓6ᵗʰ **S32.40 Unspecified fracture of acetabulum**

        ✓7ᵗʰ **S32.401 Unspecified fracture of right acetabulum**

        ✓7ᵗʰ **S32.402 Unspecified fracture of left acetabulum**

        ✓7ᵗʰ **S32.409 Unspecified fracture of unspecified acetabulum**

    ✓6ᵗʰ **S32.41 Fracture of anterior wall of acetabulum**

        ✓7ᵗʰ **S32.411 Displaced fracture of anterior wall of right acetabulum**

        ✓7ᵗʰ **S32.412 Displaced fracture of anterior wall of left acetabulum**

        ✓7ᵗʰ **S32.413 Displaced fracture of anterior wall of unspecified acetabulum**

        ✓7ᵗʰ **S32.414 Nondisplaced fracture of anterior wall of right acetabulum**

        ✓7ᵗʰ **S32.415 Nondisplaced fracture of anterior wall of left acetabulum**

        ✓7ᵗʰ **S32.416 Nondisplaced fracture of anterior wall of unspecified acetabulum**

    ✓6ᵗʰ **S32.42 Fracture of posterior wall of acetabulum**

        ✓7ᵗʰ **S32.421 Displaced fracture of posterior wall of right acetabulum**

        ✓7ᵗʰ **S32.422 Displaced fracture of posterior wall of left acetabulum**

        ✓7ᵗʰ **S32.423 Displaced fracture of posterior wall of unspecified acetabulum**

        ✓7ᵗʰ **S32.424 Nondisplaced fracture of posterior wall of right acetabulum**

        ✓7ᵗʰ **S32.425 Nondisplaced fracture of posterior wall of left acetabulum**

        ✓7ᵗʰ **S32.426 Nondisplaced fracture of posterior wall of unspecified acetabulum**

    ✓6ᵗʰ **S32.43 Fracture of anterior column [iliopubic] of acetabulum**

        ✓7ᵗʰ **S32.431 Displaced fracture of anterior column [iliopubic] of right acetabulum**

        ✓7ᵗʰ **S32.432 Displaced fracture of anterior column [iliopubic] of left acetabulum**

        ✓7ᵗʰ **S32.433 Displaced fracture of anterior column [iliopubic] of unspecified acetabulum**

        ✓7ᵗʰ **S32.434 Nondisplaced fracture of anterior column [iliopubic] of right acetabulum**

        ✓7ᵗʰ **S32.435 Nondisplaced fracture of anterior column [iliopubic] of left acetabulum**

        ✓7ᵗʰ **S32.436 Nondisplaced fracture of anterior column [iliopubic] of unspecified acetabulum**

    ✓6ᵗʰ **S32.44 Fracture of posterior column [ilioischial] of acetabulum**

        ✓7ᵗʰ **S32.441 Displaced fracture of posterior column [ilioischial] of right acetabulum**

        ✓7ᵗʰ **S32.442 Displaced fracture of posterior column [ilioischial] of left acetabulum**

        ✓7ᵗʰ **S32.443 Displaced fracture of posterior column [ilioischial] of unspecified acetabulum**

        ✓7ᵗʰ **S32.444 Nondisplaced fracture of posterior column [ilioischial] of right acetabulum**

        ✓7ᵗʰ **S32.445 Nondisplaced fracture of posterior column [ilioischial] of left acetabulum**

EXCLUDES 1 Not coded here   **EXCLUDES 2** Not included here   *Manifestation Code*

✓7ᵗʰ **S32.446** **Nondisplaced fracture of posterior column [ilioischial] of unspecified acetabulum**

✓6ᵗʰ **S32.45** **Transverse fracture of acetabulum**

✓7ᵗʰ **S32.451** **Displaced transverse fracture of right acetabulum**

✓7ᵗʰ **S32.452** **Displaced transverse fracture of left acetabulum**

✓7ᵗʰ **S32.453** **Displaced transverse fracture of unspecified acetabulum**

✓7ᵗʰ **S32.454** **Nondisplaced transverse fracture of right acetabulum**

✓7ᵗʰ **S32.455** **Nondisplaced transverse fracture of left acetabulum**

✓7ᵗʰ **S32.456** **Nondisplaced transverse fracture of unspecified acetabulum**

✓6ᵗʰ **S32.46** **Associated transverse-posterior fracture of acetabulum**

✓7ᵗʰ **S32.461** **Displaced associated transverse-posterior fracture of right acetabulum**

✓7ᵗʰ **S32.462** **Displaced associated transverse-posterior fracture of left acetabulum**

✓7ᵗʰ **S32.463** **Displaced associated transverse-posterior fracture of unspecified acetabulum**

✓7ᵗʰ **S32.464** **Nondisplaced associated transverse-posterior fracture of right acetabulum**

✓7ᵗʰ **S32.465** **Nondisplaced associated transverse-posterior fracture of left acetabulum**

✓7ᵗʰ **S32.466** **Nondisplaced associated transverse-posterior fracture of unspecified acetabulum**

✓6ᵗʰ **S32.47** **Fracture of medial wall of acetabulum**

✓7ᵗʰ **S32.471** **Displaced fracture of medial wall of right acetabulum**

✓7ᵗʰ **S32.472** **Displaced fracture of medial wall of left acetabulum**

✓7ᵗʰ **S32.473** **Displaced fracture of medial wall of unspecified acetabulum**

✓7ᵗʰ **S32.474** **Nondisplaced fracture of medial wall of right acetabulum**

✓7ᵗʰ **S32.475** **Nondisplaced fracture of medial wall of left acetabulum**

✓7ᵗʰ **S32.476** **Nondisplaced fracture of medial wall of unspecified acetabulum**

✓6ᵗʰ **S32.48** **Dome fracture of acetabulum**

✓7ᵗʰ **S32.481** **Displaced dome fracture of right acetabulum**

✓7ᵗʰ **S32.482** **Displaced dome fracture of left acetabulum**

✓7ᵗʰ **S32.483** **Displaced dome fracture of unspecified acetabulum**

✓7ᵗʰ **S32.484** **Nondisplaced dome fracture of right acetabulum**

✓7ᵗʰ **S32.485** **Nondisplaced dome fracture of left acetabulum**

✓7ᵗʰ **S32.486** **Nondisplaced dome fracture of unspecified acetabulum**

✓6ᵗʰ **S32.49** **Other specified fracture of acetabulum**

✓7ᵗʰ **S32.491** **Other specified fracture of right acetabulum**

✓7ᵗʰ **S32.492** **Other specified fracture of left acetabulum**

✓7ᵗʰ **S32.499** **Other specified fracture of unspecified acetabulum**

✓5ᵗʰ **S32.5** **Fracture of pubis**

> **EXCLUDES 1** *fracture of pubis with associated disruption of pelvic ring (S32.8-)*

✓6ᵗʰ **S32.50** **Unspecified fracture of pubis**

✓7ᵗʰ **S32.501** **Unspecified fracture of right pubis**

✓7ᵗʰ **S32.502** **Unspecified fracture of left pubis**

✓7ᵗʰ **S32.509** **Unspecified fracture of unspecified pubis**

✓6ᵗʰ **S32.51** **Fracture of superior rim of pubis**

✓7ᵗʰ **S32.511** **Fracture of superior rim of right pubis**

✓7ᵗʰ **S32.512** **Fracture of superior rim of left pubis**

✓7ᵗʰ **S32.519** **Fracture of superior rim of unspecified pubis**

✓6ᵗʰ **S32.59** **Other specified fracture of pubis**

✓7ᵗʰ **S32.591** **Other specified fracture of right pubis**

✓7ᵗʰ **S32.592** **Other specified fracture of left pubis**

✓7ᵗʰ **S32.599** **Other specified fracture of unspecified pubis**

✓5ᵗʰ **S32.6** **Fracture of ischium**

> **EXCLUDES 1** *fracture of ischium with associated disruption of pelvic ring (S32.8-)*

✓6ᵗʰ **S32.60** **Unspecified fracture of ischium**

✓7ᵗʰ **S32.601** **Unspecified fracture of right ischium**

✓7ᵗʰ **S32.602** **Unspecified fracture of left ischium**

✓7ᵗʰ **S32.609** **Unspecified fracture of unspecified ischium**

✓6ᵗʰ **S32.61** **Avulsion fracture of ischium**

✓7ᵗʰ **S32.611** **Displaced avulsion fracture of right ischium**

✓7ᵗʰ **S32.612** **Displaced avulsion fracture of left ischium**

✓7ᵗʰ **S32.613** **Displaced avulsion fracture of unspecified ischium**

✓7ᵗʰ **S32.614** **Nondisplaced avulsion fracture of right ischium**

✓7ᵗʰ **S32.615** **Nondisplaced avulsion fracture of left ischium**

✓7ᵗʰ **S32.616** **Nondisplaced avulsion fracture of unspecified ischium**

✓6ᵗʰ **S32.69** **Other specified fracture of ischium**

✓7ᵗʰ **S32.691** **Other specified fracture of right ischium**

✓7ᵗʰ **S32.692** **Other specified fracture of left ischium**

✓7ᵗʰ **S32.699** **Other specified fracture of unspecified ischium**

✓5ᵗʰ **S32.8** **Fracture of other parts of pelvis**

Code also any associated:
    fracture of acetabulum (S32.4-)
    sacral fracture (S32.1-)

✓6ᵗʰ **S32.81** **Multiple fractures of pelvis with disruption of pelvic ring**

✓7ᵗʰ **S32.810** **Multiple fractures of pelvis with stable disruption of pelvic ring**

✓7ᵗʰ **S32.811** **Multiple fractures of pelvis with unstable disruption of pelvic ring**

✓x7ᵗʰ **S32.89** **Fracture of other parts of pelvis**

✓x7ᵗʰ **S32.9** **Fracture of unspecified parts of lumbosacral spine and pelvis**

Fracture of lumbosacral spine NOS
Fracture of pelvis NOS

✓ Appropriate additional character required   ✓x7ᵗʰ Requires 7th character, placeholder x must fill empty characters

✓4ᵗʰ S33 Dislocation and sprain of joints and ligaments of lumbar spine and pelvis

> **INCLUDES**   avulsion of joint or ligament of lumbar spine and pelvis
> laceration of cartilage, joint or ligament of lumbar spine and pelvis
> sprain of cartilage, joint or ligament of lumbar spine and pelvis
> traumatic hemarthrosis of joint or ligament of lumbar spine and pelvis
> traumatic rupture of joint or ligament of lumbar spine and pelvis
> traumatic subluxation of joint or ligament of lumbar spine and pelvis
> traumatic tear of joint or ligament of lumbar spine and pelvis

> Code also any associated open wound
> **EXCLUDES 1**   *nontraumatic rupture or displacement of lumbar intervertebral disc NOS (M51-)*
> *obstetric damage to pelvic joints and ligaments (O71.6)*
> **EXCLUDES 2**   *dislocation and sprain of joints and ligaments of hip (S73-)*
> *strain of muscle of lower back and pelvis (S39.01-)*

> The appropriate 7th character is to be added to each code from category S33.
> A   initial encounter
> D   subsequent encounter
> S   sequela

✓x7ᵗʰ S33.0 Traumatic rupture of lumbar intervertebral disc
> **EXCLUDES 1**   *rupture or displacement (nontraumatic) of lumbar intervertebral disc NOS (M51- with fifth character 6)*

✓5ᵗʰ S33.1 Subluxation and dislocation of lumbar vertebra
> Code also any associated:
> open wound of abdomen, lower back and pelvis (S31)
> spinal cord injury (S24.0, S24.1-, S34.0-, S34.1-)
> **EXCLUDES 2**   *fracture of lumbar vertebrae (S32.0-)*

   ✓6ᵗʰ S33.10 Subluxation and dislocation of unspecified lumbar vertebra
     ✓7ᵗʰ S33.100 Subluxation of unspecified lumbar vertebra
     ✓7ᵗʰ S33.101 Dislocation of unspecified lumbar vertebra
   ✓6ᵗʰ S33.11 Subluxation and dislocation of L1/L2 lumbar vertebra
     ✓7ᵗʰ S33.110 Subluxation of L1/L2 lumbar vertebra
     ✓7ᵗʰ S33.111 Dislocation of L1/L2 lumbar vertebra
   ✓6ᵗʰ S33.12 Subluxation and dislocation of L2/L3 lumbar vertebra
     ✓7ᵗʰ S33.120 Subluxation of L2/L3 lumbar vertebra
     ✓7ᵗʰ S33.121 Dislocation of L2/L3 lumbar vertebra
   ✓6ᵗʰ S33.13 Subluxation and dislocation of L3/L4 lumbar vertebra
     ✓7ᵗʰ S33.130 Subluxation of L3/L4 lumbar vertebra
     ✓7ᵗʰ S33.131 Dislocation of L3/L4 lumbar vertebra
   ✓6ᵗʰ S33.14 Subluxation and dislocation of L4/L5 lumbar vertebra
     ✓7ᵗʰ S33.140 Subluxation of L4/L5 lumbar vertebra
     ✓7ᵗʰ S33.141 Dislocation of L4/L5 lumbar vertebra

✓x7ᵗʰ S33.2 Dislocation of sacroiliac and sacrococcygeal joint
✓5ᵗʰ S33.3 Dislocation of other and unspecified parts of lumbar spine and pelvis
   ✓x7ᵗʰ S33.30 Dislocation of unspecified parts of lumbar spine and pelvis
   ✓x7ᵗʰ S33.39 Dislocation of other parts of lumbar spine and pelvis
✓x7ᵗʰ S33.4 Traumatic rupture of symphysis pubis
✓x7ᵗʰ S33.5 Sprain of ligaments of lumbar spine
✓x7ᵗʰ S33.6 Sprain of sacroiliac joint
✓x7ᵗʰ S33.8 Sprain of other parts of lumbar spine and pelvis
✓x7ᵗʰ S33.9 Sprain of unspecified parts of lumbar spine and pelvis

✓4ᵗʰ S34 Injury of lumbar and sacral spinal cord and nerves at abdomen, lower back and pelvis level

> **NOTE**   Code to highest level of lumbar cord injury
> Code also any associated:
> fracture of vertebra (S22.0-, S32.0-)
> open wound of abdomen, lower back and pelvis (S31-)
> transient paralysis (R29.5)

> The appropriate 7th character is to be added to each code from category S34.
> A   initial encounter
> D   subsequent encounter
> S   sequela

✓5ᵗʰ S34.0 Concussion and edema of lumbar and sacral spinal cord
   ✓x7ᵗʰ S34.01 Concussion and edema of lumbar spinal cord
   ✓x7ᵗʰ S34.02 Concussion and edema of sacral spinal cord
     Concussion and edema of conus medullaris
✓5ᵗʰ S34.1 Other and unspecified injury of lumbar and sacral spinal cord
   ✓6ᵗʰ S34.10 Unspecified injury to lumbar spinal cord
     ✓7ᵗʰ S34.101 Unspecified injury to L1 level of lumbar spinal cord
     ✓7ᵗʰ S34.102 Unspecified injury to L2 level of lumbar spinal cord
     ✓7ᵗʰ S34.103 Unspecified injury to L3 level of lumbar spinal cord
     ✓7ᵗʰ S34.104 Unspecified injury to L4 level of lumbar spinal cord
     ✓7ᵗʰ S34.105 Unspecified injury to L5 level of lumbar spinal cord
     ✓7ᵗʰ S34.109 Unspecified injury to unspecified level of lumbar spinal cord
   ✓6ᵗʰ S34.11 Complete lesion of lumbar spinal cord
     ✓7ᵗʰ S34.111 Complete lesion of L1 level of lumbar spinal cord
     ✓7ᵗʰ S34.112 Complete lesion of L2 level of lumbar spinal cord
     ✓7ᵗʰ S34.113 Complete lesion of L3 level of lumbar spinal cord
     ✓7ᵗʰ S34.114 Complete lesion of L4 level of lumbar spinal cord
     ✓7ᵗʰ S34.115 Complete lesion of L5 level of lumbar spinal cord
     ✓7ᵗʰ S34.119 Complete lesion of unspecified level of lumbar spinal cord
   ✓6ᵗʰ S34.12 Incomplete lesion of lumbar spinal cord
     ✓7ᵗʰ S34.121 Incomplete lesion of L1 level of lumbar spinal cord
     ✓7ᵗʰ S34.122 Incomplete lesion of L2 level of lumbar spinal cord
     ✓7ᵗʰ S34.123 Incomplete lesion of L3 level of lumbar spinal cord
     ✓7ᵗʰ S34.124 Incomplete lesion of L4 level of lumbar spinal cord
     ✓7ᵗʰ S34.125 Incomplete lesion of L5 level of lumbar spinal cord
     ✓7ᵗʰ S34.129 Incomplete lesion of unspecified level of lumbar spinal cord
   ✓6ᵗʰ S34.13 Other and unspecified injury to sacral spinal cord
     Other injury to conus medullaris
     ✓7ᵗʰ S34.131 Complete lesion of sacral spinal cord
      Complete lesion of conus medullaris
     ✓7ᵗʰ S34.132 Incomplete lesion of sacral spinal cord
      Incomplete lesion of conus medullaris
     ✓7ᵗʰ S34.139 Unspecified injury to sacral spinal cord
      Unspecified injury of conus medullaris
✓5ᵗʰ S34.2 Injury of nerve root of lumbar and sacral spine
   ✓x7ᵗʰ S34.21 Injury of nerve root of lumbar spine
   ✓x7ᵗʰ S34.22 Injury of nerve root of sacral spine
✓x7ᵗʰ S34.3 Injury of cauda equina
✓x7ᵗʰ S34.4 Injury of lumbosacral plexus
✓x7ᵗʰ S34.5 Injury of lumbar, sacral and pelvic sympathetic nerves
   Injury of celiac ganglion or plexus
   Injury of hypogastric plexus
   Injury of mesenteric plexus (inferior) (superior)
   Injury of splanchnic nerve

EXCLUDES 1 Not coded here   **EXCLUDES 2** Not included here   *Manifestation Code*

√x7ᵗʰ **S34.6** **Injury of peripheral nerve(s) at abdomen, lower back and pelvis level**

√x7ᵗʰ **S34.8** **Injury of other nerves at abdomen, lower back and pelvis level**

√x7ᵗʰ **S34.9** **Injury of unspecified nerves at abdomen, lower back and pelvis level**

√4ᵗʰ **S35** **Injury of blood vessels at abdomen, lower back and pelvis level**
Code also any associated open wound (S31-)

> The appropriate 7th character is to be added to each code from category S35.
> A   initial encounter
> D   subsequent encounter
> S   sequela

√5ᵗʰ **S35.0** **Injury of abdominal aorta**
> EXCLUDES 1   *injury of aorta NOS (S25.0)*

√x7ᵗʰ **S35.00** **Unspecified injury of abdominal aorta**

√x7ᵗʰ **S35.01** **Minor laceration of abdominal aorta**
Incomplete transection of abdominal aorta
Laceration of abdominal aorta NOS
Superficial laceration of abdominal aorta

√x7ᵗʰ **S35.02** **Major laceration of abdominal aorta**
Complete transection of abdominal aorta
Traumatic rupture of abdominal aorta

√x7ᵗʰ **S35.09** **Other injury of abdominal aorta**

√5ᵗʰ **S35.1** **Injury of inferior vena cava**
Injury of hepatic vein
> EXCLUDES 1   *injury of vena cava NOS (S25.2)*

√x7ᵗʰ **S35.10** **Unspecified injury of inferior vena cava**

√x7ᵗʰ **S35.11** **Minor laceration of inferior vena cava**
Incomplete transection of inferior vena cava
Laceration of inferior vena cava NOS
Superficial laceration of inferior vena cava

√x7ᵗʰ **S35.12** **Major laceration of inferior vena cava**
Complete transection of inferior vena cava
Traumatic rupture of inferior vena cava

√x7ᵗʰ **S35.19** **Other injury of inferior vena cava**

√5ᵗʰ **S35.2** **Injury of celiac or mesenteric artery and branches**

√6ᵗʰ **S35.21** **Injury of celiac artery**

√7ᵗʰ **S35.211** **Minor laceration of celiac artery**
Incomplete transection of celiac artery
Laceration of celiac artery NOS
Superficial laceration of celiac artery

√7ᵗʰ **S35.212** **Major laceration of celiac artery**
Complete transection of celiac artery
Traumatic rupture of celiac artery

√7ᵗʰ **S35.218** **Other injury of celiac artery**

√7ᵗʰ **S35.219** **Unspecified injury of celiac artery**

√6ᵗʰ **S35.22** **Injury of superior mesenteric artery**

√7ᵗʰ **S35.221** **Minor laceration of superior mesenteric artery**
Incomplete transection of superior mesenteric artery
Laceration of superior mesenteric artery NOS
Superficial laceration of superior mesenteric artery

√7ᵗʰ **S35.222** **Major laceration of superior mesenteric artery**
Complete transection of superior mesenteric artery
Traumatic rupture of superior mesenteric artery

√7ᵗʰ **S35.228** **Other injury of superior mesenteric artery**

√7ᵗʰ **S35.229** **Unspecified injury of superior mesenteric artery**

√6ᵗʰ **S35.23** **Injury of inferior mesenteric artery**

√7ᵗʰ **S35.231** **Minor laceration of inferior mesenteric artery**
Incomplete transection of inferior mesenteric artery
Laceration of inferior mesenteric artery NOS
Superficial laceration of inferior mesenteric artery

√7ᵗʰ **S35.232** **Major laceration of inferior mesenteric artery**
Complete transection of inferior mesenteric artery
Traumatic rupture of inferior mesenteric artery

√7ᵗʰ **S35.238** **Other injury of inferior mesenteric artery**

√7ᵗʰ **S35.239** **Unspecified injury of inferior mesenteric artery**

√6ᵗʰ **S35.29** **Injury of branches of celiac and mesenteric artery**
Injury of gastric artery
Injury of gastroduodenal artery
Injury of hepatic artery
Injury of splenic artery

√7ᵗʰ **S35.291** **Minor laceration of branches of celiac and mesenteric artery**
Incomplete transection of branches of celiac and mesenteric artery
Laceration of branches of celiac and mesenteric artery NOS
Superficial laceration of branches of celiac and mesenteric artery

√7ᵗʰ **S35.292** **Major laceration of branches of celiac and mesenteric artery**
Complete transection of branches of celiac and mesenteric artery
Traumatic rupture of branches of celiac and mesenteric artery

√7ᵗʰ **S35.298** **Other injury of branches of celiac and mesenteric artery**

√7ᵗʰ **S35.299** **Unspecified injury of branches of celiac and mesenteric artery**

√5ᵗʰ **S35.3** **Injury of portal or splenic vein and branches**

√6ᵗʰ **S35.31** **Injury of portal vein**

√7ᵗʰ **S35.311** **Laceration of portal vein**

√7ᵗʰ **S35.318** **Other specified injury of portal vein**

√7ᵗʰ **S35.319** **Unspecified injury of portal vein**

√6ᵗʰ **S35.32** **Injury of splenic vein**

√7ᵗʰ **S35.321** **Laceration of splenic vein**

√7ᵗʰ **S35.328** **Other specified injury of splenic vein**

√7ᵗʰ **S35.329** **Unspecified injury of splenic vein**

√6ᵗʰ **S35.33** **Injury of superior mesenteric vein**

√7ᵗʰ **S35.331** **Laceration of superior mesenteric vein**

√7ᵗʰ **S35.338** **Other specified injury of superior mesenteric vein**

√7ᵗʰ **S35.339** **Unspecified injury of superior mesenteric vein**

√6ᵗʰ **S35.34** **Injury of inferior mesenteric vein**

√7ᵗʰ **S35.341** **Laceration of inferior mesenteric vein**

√7ᵗʰ **S35.348** **Other specified injury of inferior mesenteric vein**

√7ᵗʰ **S35.349** **Unspecified injury of inferior mesenteric vein**

√5ᵗʰ **S35.4** **Injury of renal blood vessels**

√6ᵗʰ **S35.40** **Unspecified injury of renal blood vessel**

√7ᵗʰ **S35.401** **Unspecified injury of right renal artery**

√7ᵗʰ **S35.402** **Unspecified injury of left renal artery**

√7ᵗʰ **S35.403** **Unspecified injury of unspecified renal artery**

√7ᵗʰ **S35.404** **Unspecified injury of right renal vein**

√7ᵗʰ **S35.405** **Unspecified injury of left renal vein**

√7ᵗʰ **S35.406** **Unspecified injury of unspecified renal vein**

√6ᵗʰ **S35.41** **Laceration of renal blood vessel**

√7ᵗʰ **S35.411** **Laceration of right renal artery**

√7ᵗʰ **S35.412** **Laceration of left renal artery**

√7ᵗʰ **S35.413** **Laceration of unspecified renal artery**

√7ᵗʰ **S35.414** **Laceration of right renal vein**

√7ᵗʰ **S35.415** **Laceration of left renal vein**

√7ᵗʰ **S35.416** **Laceration of unspecified renal vein**

√6ᵗʰ **S35.49** **Other specified injury of renal blood vessel**

√7ᵗʰ **S35.491** **Other specified injury of right renal artery**

√7ᵗʰ **S35.492** **Other specified injury of left renal artery**

√7ᵗʰ   **S35.493**   **Other specified injury of unspecified renal artery**

√7ᵗʰ   **S35.494**   **Other specified injury of right renal vein**

√7ᵗʰ   **S35.495**   **Other specified injury of left renal vein**

√7ᵗʰ   **S35.496**   **Other specified injury of unspecified renal vein**

√5ᵗʰ   **S35.5**   **Injury of iliac blood vessels**

  √x7ᵗʰ   **S35.50**   **Injury of unspecified iliac blood vessel(s)**

  √6ᵗʰ   **S35.51**   **Injury of iliac artery or vein**

         Injury of hypogastric artery or vein

    √7ᵗʰ   **S35.511**   **Injury of right iliac artery**

    √7ᵗʰ   **S35.512**   **Injury of left iliac artery**

    √7ᵗʰ   **S35.513**   **Injury of unspecified iliac artery**

    √7ᵗʰ   **S35.514**   **Injury of right iliac vein**

    √7ᵗʰ   **S35.515**   **Injury of left iliac vein**

    √7ᵗʰ   **S35.516**   **Injury of unspecified iliac vein**

  √6ᵗʰ   **S35.53**   **Injury of uterine artery or vein**

    √7ᵗʰ   **S35.531**   **Injury of right uterine artery**

    √7ᵗʰ   **S35.532**   **Injury of left uterine artery**

    √7ᵗʰ   **S35.533**   **Injury of unspecified uterine artery**

    √7ᵗʰ   **S35.534**   **Injury of right uterine vein**

    √7ᵗʰ   **S35.535**   **Injury of left uterine vein**

    √7ᵗʰ   **S35.536**   **Injury of unspecified uterine vein**

  √x7ᵗʰ   **S35.59**   **Injury of other iliac blood vessels**

√5ᵗʰ   **S35.8**   **Injury of other blood vessels at abdomen, lower back and pelvis level**

        Injury of ovarian artery or vein

  √6ᵗʰ   **S35.8x**   **Injury of other blood vessels at abdomen, lower back and pelvis level**

    √7ᵗʰ   **S35.8x1**   **Laceration of other blood vessels at abdomen, lower back and pelvis level**

    √7ᵗʰ   **S35.8x8**   **Other specified injury of other blood vessels at abdomen, lower back and pelvis level**

    √7ᵗʰ   **S35.8x9**   **Unspecified injury of other blood vessels at abdomen, lower back and pelvis level**

√5ᵗʰ   **S35.9**   **Injury of unspecified blood vessel at abdomen, lower back and pelvis level**

  √x7ᵗʰ   **S35.90**   **Unspecified injury of unspecified blood vessel at abdomen, lower back and pelvis level**

  √x7ᵗʰ   **S35.91**   **Laceration of unspecified blood vessel at abdomen, lower back and pelvis level**

  √x7ᵗʰ   **S35.99**   **Other specified injury of unspecified blood vessel at abdomen, lower back and pelvis level**

√4ᵗʰ   **S36**   **Injury of intra-abdominal organs**

     Code also any associated open wound (S31-)

> The appropriate 7th character is to be added to each code from category S36.
> A   initial encounter
> D   subsequent encounter
> S   sequela

√5ᵗʰ   **S36.0**   **Injury of spleen**

  √x7ᵗʰ   **S36.00**   **Unspecified injury of spleen**

  √6ᵗʰ   **S36.02**   **Contusion of spleen**

    √7ᵗʰ   **S36.020**   **Minor contusion of spleen**

         Contusion of spleen less than 2 cm

    √7ᵗʰ   **S36.021**   **Major contusion of spleen**

         Contusion of spleen greater than 2 cm

    √7ᵗʰ   **S36.029**   **Unspecified contusion of spleen**

  √6ᵗʰ   **S36.03**   **Laceration of spleen**

    √7ᵗʰ   **S36.030**   **Superficial (capsular) laceration of spleen**

         Laceration of spleen less than 1 cm

         Minor laceration of spleen

    √7ᵗʰ   **S36.031**   **Moderate laceration of spleen**

         Laceration of spleen 1 to 3 cm

    √7ᵗʰ   **S36.032**   **Major laceration of spleen**

         Avulsion of spleen

         Laceration of spleen greater than 3 cm

         Massive laceration of spleen

         Multiple moderate lacerations of spleen

         Stellate laceration of spleen

    √7ᵗʰ   **S36.039**   **Unspecified laceration of spleen**

  √x7ᵗʰ   **S36.09**   **Other injury of spleen**

√5ᵗʰ   **S36.1**   **Injury of liver and gallbladder and bile duct**

  √6ᵗʰ   **S36.11**   **Injury of liver**

    √7ᵗʰ   **S36.112**   **Contusion of liver**

    √7ᵗʰ   **S36.113**   **Laceration of liver, unspecified degree**

    √7ᵗʰ   **S36.114**   **Minor laceration of liver**

         Laceration involving capsule only, or, without significant involvement of hepatic parenchyma [i.e., less than 1 cm deep]

    √7ᵗʰ   **S36.115**   **Moderate laceration of liver**

         Laceration involving parenchyma but without major disruption of parenchyma [i.e., less than 10 cm long and less than 3 cm deep]

    √7ᵗʰ   **S36.116**   **Major laceration of liver**

         Laceration with significant disruption of hepatic parenchyma [i.e., greater than 10 cm long and 3 cm deep]

         Multiple moderate lacerations, with or without hematoma

         Stellate laceration of liver

    √7ᵗʰ   **S36.118**   **Other injury of liver**

    √7ᵗʰ   **S36.119**   **Unspecified injury of liver**

  √6ᵗʰ   **S36.12**   **Injury of gallbladder**

    √7ᵗʰ   **S36.122**   **Contusion of gallbladder**

    √7ᵗʰ   **S36.123**   **Laceration of gallbladder**

    √7ᵗʰ   **S36.128**   **Other injury of gallbladder**

    √7ᵗʰ   **S36.129**   **Unspecified injury of gallbladder**

  √x7ᵗʰ   **S36.13**   **Injury of bile duct**

√5ᵗʰ   **S36.2**   **Injury of pancreas**

  √6ᵗʰ   **S36.20**   **Unspecified injury of pancreas**

    √7ᵗʰ   **S36.200**   **Unspecified injury of head of pancreas**

    √7ᵗʰ   **S36.201**   **Unspecified injury of body of pancreas**

    √7ᵗʰ   **S36.202**   **Unspecified injury of tail of pancreas**

    √7ᵗʰ   **S36.209**   **Unspecified injury of unspecified part of pancreas**

  √6ᵗʰ   **S36.22**   **Contusion of pancreas**

    √7ᵗʰ   **S36.220**   **Contusion of head of pancreas**

    √7ᵗʰ   **S36.221**   **Contusion of body of pancreas**

    √7ᵗʰ   **S36.222**   **Contusion of tail of pancreas**

    √7ᵗʰ   **S36.229**   **Contusion of unspecified part of pancreas**

  √6ᵗʰ   **S36.23**   **Laceration of pancreas, unspecified degree**

    √7ᵗʰ   **S36.230**   **Laceration of head of pancreas, unspecified degree**

    √7ᵗʰ   **S36.231**   **Laceration of body of pancreas, unspecified degree**

    √7ᵗʰ   **S36.232**   **Laceration of tail of pancreas, unspecified degree**

    √7ᵗʰ   **S36.239**   **Laceration of unspecified part of pancreas, unspecified degree**

  √6ᵗʰ   **S36.24**   **Minor laceration of pancreas**

    √7ᵗʰ   **S36.240**   **Minor laceration of head of pancreas**

    √7ᵗʰ   **S36.241**   **Minor laceration of body of pancreas**

    √7ᵗʰ   **S36.242**   **Minor laceration of tail of pancreas**

    √7ᵗʰ   **S36.249**   **Minor laceration of unspecified part of pancreas**

  √6ᵗʰ   **S36.25**   **Moderate laceration of pancreas**

    √7ᵗʰ   **S36.250**   **Moderate laceration of head of pancreas**

    √7ᵗʰ   **S36.251**   **Moderate laceration of body of pancreas**

    √7ᵗʰ   **S36.252**   **Moderate laceration of tail of pancreas**

    √7ᵗʰ   **S36.259**   **Moderate laceration of unspecified part of pancreas**

  √6ᵗʰ   **S36.26**   **Major laceration of pancreas**

    √7ᵗʰ   **S36.260**   **Major laceration of head of pancreas**

    √7ᵗʰ   **S36.261**   **Major laceration of body of pancreas**

    √7ᵗʰ   **S36.262**   **Major laceration of tail of pancreas**

    √7ᵗʰ   **S36.269**   **Major laceration of unspecified part of pancreas**

  √6ᵗʰ   **S36.29**   **Other injury of pancreas**

    √7ᵗʰ   **S36.290**   **Other injury of head of pancreas**

    √7ᵗʰ   **S36.291**   **Other injury of body of pancreas**

    √7ᵗʰ   **S36.292**   **Other injury of tail of pancreas**

    √7ᵗʰ   **S36.299**   **Other injury of unspecified part of pancreas**

EXCLUDES 1 Not coded here   **EXCLUDES 2** Not included here   *Manifestation Code*

√5ᵗʰ **S36.3 Injury of stomach**
  √x7ᵗʰ **S36.30 Unspecified injury of stomach**
  √x7ᵗʰ **S36.32 Contusion of stomach**
  √x7ᵗʰ **S36.33 Laceration of stomach**
  √x7ᵗʰ **S36.39 Other injury of stomach**
√5ᵗʰ **S36.4 Injury of small intestine**
  √6ᵗʰ **S36.40 Unspecified injury of small intestine**
    √7ᵗʰ **S36.400 Unspecified injury of duodenum**
    √7ᵗʰ **S36.408 Unspecified injury of other part of small intestine**
    √7ᵗʰ **S36.409 Unspecified injury of unspecified part of small intestine**
  √6ᵗʰ **S36.41 Primary blast injury of small intestine**
    Blast injury of small intestine NOS
    √7ᵗʰ **S36.410 Primary blast injury of duodenum**
    √7ᵗʰ **S36.418 Primary blast injury of other part of small intestine**
    √7ᵗʰ **S36.419 Primary blast injury of unspecified part of small intestine**
  √6ᵗʰ **S36.42 Contusion of small intestine**
    √7ᵗʰ **S36.420 Contusion of duodenum**
    √7ᵗʰ **S36.428 Contusion of other part of small intestine**
    √7ᵗʰ **S36.429 Contusion of unspecified part of small intestine**
  √6ᵗʰ **S36.43 Laceration of small intestine**
    √7ᵗʰ **S36.430 Laceration of duodenum**
    √7ᵗʰ **S36.438 Laceration of other part of small intestine**
    √7ᵗʰ **S36.439 Laceration of unspecified part of small intestine**
  √6ᵗʰ **S36.49 Other injury of small intestine**
    √7ᵗʰ **S36.490 Other injury of duodenum**
    √7ᵗʰ **S36.498 Other injury of other part of small intestine**
    √7ᵗʰ **S36.499 Other injury of unspecified part of small intestine**
√5ᵗʰ **S36.5 Injury of colon**
  EXCLUDES 2   injury of rectum (S36.6-)
  √6ᵗʰ **S36.50 Unspecified injury of colon**
    √7ᵗʰ **S36.500 Unspecified injury of ascending [right] colon**
    √7ᵗʰ **S36.501 Unspecified injury of transverse colon**
    √7ᵗʰ **S36.502 Unspecified injury of descending [left] colon**
    √7ᵗʰ **S36.503 Unspecified injury of sigmoid colon**
    √7ᵗʰ **S36.508 Unspecified injury of other part of colon**
    √7ᵗʰ **S36.509 Unspecified injury of unspecified part of colon**
  √6ᵗʰ **S36.51 Primary blast injury of colon**
    Blast injury of colon NOS
    √7ᵗʰ **S36.510 Primary blast injury of ascending [right] colon**
    √7ᵗʰ **S36.511 Primary blast injury of transverse colon**
    √7ᵗʰ **S36.512 Primary blast injury of descending [left] colon**
    √7ᵗʰ **S36.513 Primary blast injury of sigmoid colon**
    √7ᵗʰ **S36.518 Primary blast injury of other part of colon**
    √7ᵗʰ **S36.519 Primary blast injury of unspecified part of colon**
  √6ᵗʰ **S36.52 Contusion of colon**
    √7ᵗʰ **S36.520 Contusion of ascending [right] colon**
    √7ᵗʰ **S36.521 Contusion of transverse colon**
    √7ᵗʰ **S36.522 Contusion of descending [left] colon**
    √7ᵗʰ **S36.523 Contusion of sigmoid colon**
    √7ᵗʰ **S36.528 Contusion of other part of colon**
    √7ᵗʰ **S36.529 Contusion of unspecified part of colon**
  √6ᵗʰ **S36.53 Laceration of colon**
    √7ᵗʰ **S36.530 Laceration of ascending [right] colon**
    √7ᵗʰ **S36.531 Laceration of transverse colon**
    √7ᵗʰ **S36.532 Laceration of descending [left] colon**
    √7ᵗʰ **S36.533 Laceration of sigmoid colon**
    √7ᵗʰ **S36.538 Laceration of other part of colon**
    √7ᵗʰ **S36.539 Laceration of unspecified part of colon**

  √6ᵗʰ **S36.59 Other injury of colon**
    Secondary blast injury of colon
    √7ᵗʰ **S36.590 Other injury of ascending [right] colon**
    √7ᵗʰ **S36.591 Other injury of transverse colon**
    √7ᵗʰ **S36.592 Other injury of descending [left] colon**
    √7ᵗʰ **S36.593 Other injury of sigmoid colon**
    √7ᵗʰ **S36.598 Other injury of other part of colon**
    √7ᵗʰ **S36.599 Other injury of unspecified part of colon**
√5ᵗʰ **S36.6 Injury of rectum**
  √x7ᵗʰ **S36.60 Unspecified injury of rectum**
  √x7ᵗʰ **S36.61 Primary blast injury of rectum**
    Blast injury of rectum NOS
  √x7ᵗʰ **S36.62 Contusion of rectum**
  √x7ᵗʰ **S36.63 Laceration of rectum**
  √x7ᵗʰ **S36.69 Other injury of rectum**
    Secondary blast injury of rectum
√5ᵗʰ **S36.8 Injury of other intra-abdominal organs**
  √x7ᵗʰ **S36.81 Injury of peritoneum**
  √6ᵗʰ **S36.89 Injury of other intra-abdominal organs**
    Injury of retroperitoneum
    √7ᵗʰ **S36.892 Contusion of other intra-abdominal organs**
    √7ᵗʰ **S36.893 Laceration of other intra-abdominal organs**
    √7ᵗʰ **S36.898 Other injury of other intra-abdominal organs**
    √7ᵗʰ **S36.899 Unspecified injury of other intra-abdominal organs**
√5ᵗʰ **S36.9 Injury of unspecified intra-abdominal organ**
  √x7ᵗʰ **S36.90 Unspecified injury of unspecified intra-abdominal organ**
  √x7ᵗʰ **S36.92 Contusion of unspecified intra-abdominal organ**
  √x7ᵗʰ **S36.93 Laceration of unspecified intra-abdominal organ**
  √x7ᵗʰ **S36.99 Other injury of unspecified intra-abdominal organ**
√4ᵗʰ **S37 Injury of urinary and pelvic organs**
  Code also any associated open wound (S31-)
  EXCLUDES 1   obstetric trauma to pelvic organs (O71-)
  EXCLUDES 2   injury of peritoneum (S36.81)
              injury of retroperitoneum (S36.89-)

The appropriate 7th character is to be added to each code from category S37.
A   initial encounter
D   subsequent encounter
S   sequela

√5ᵗʰ **S37.0 Injury of kidney**
  EXCLUDES 2   acute kidney injury (nontraumatic) (N17.9)
  √6ᵗʰ **S37.00 Unspecified injury of kidney**
    √7ᵗʰ **S37.001 Unspecified injury of right kidney**
    √7ᵗʰ **S37.002 Unspecified injury of left kidney**
    √7ᵗʰ **S37.009 Unspecified injury of unspecified kidney**
  √6ᵗʰ **S37.01 Minor contusion of kidney**
    Contusion of kidney less than 2 cm
    Contusion of kidney NOS
    √7ᵗʰ **S37.011 Minor contusion of right kidney**
    √7ᵗʰ **S37.012 Minor contusion of left kidney**
    √7ᵗʰ **S37.019 Minor contusion of unspecified kidney**
  √6ᵗʰ **S37.02 Major contusion of kidney**
    Contusion of kidney greater than 2 cm
    √7ᵗʰ **S37.021 Major contusion of right kidney**
    √7ᵗʰ **S37.022 Major contusion of left kidney**
    √7ᵗʰ **S37.029 Major contusion of unspecified kidney**
  √6ᵗʰ **S37.03 Laceration of kidney, unspecified degree**
    √7ᵗʰ **S37.031 Laceration of right kidney, unspecified degree**
    √7ᵗʰ **S37.032 Laceration of left kidney, unspecified degree**
    √7ᵗʰ **S37.039 Laceration of unspecified kidney, unspecified degree**
  √6ᵗʰ **S37.04 Minor laceration of kidney**
    Laceration of kidney less than 1 cm
    √7ᵗʰ **S37.041 Minor laceration of right kidney**
    √7ᵗʰ **S37.042 Minor laceration of left kidney**
    √7ᵗʰ **S37.049 Minor laceration of unspecified kidney**

☑ Appropriate additional character required   √x7ᵗʰ Requires 7th character, placeholder x must fill empty characters

√6th **S37.05 Moderate laceration of kidney**
Laceration of kidney 1 to 3 cm
    √7th **S37.051 Moderate laceration of right kidney**
    √7th **S37.052 Moderate laceration of left kidney**
    √7th **S37.059 Moderate laceration of unspecified kidney**
√6th **S37.06 Major laceration of kidney**
Avulsion of kidney
Laceration of kidney greater than 3 cm
Massive laceration of kidney
Multiple moderate lacerations of kidney
Stellate laceration of kidney
    √7th **S37.061 Major laceration of right kidney**
    √7th **S37.062 Major laceration of left kidney**
    √7th **S37.069 Major laceration of unspecified kidney**
√6th **S37.09 Other injury of kidney**
    √7th **S37.091 Other injury of right kidney**
    √7th **S37.092 Other injury of left kidney**
    √7th **S37.099 Other injury of unspecified kidney**

√5th **S37.1 Injury of ureter**
 √x7th **S37.10 Unspecified injury of ureter**
 √x7th **S37.12 Contusion of ureter**
 √x7th **S37.13 Laceration of ureter**
 √x7th **S37.19 Other injury of ureter**

√5th **S37.2 Injury of bladder**
 √x7th **S37.20 Unspecified injury of bladder**
 √x7th **S37.22 Contusion of bladder**
 √x7th **S37.23 Laceration of bladder**
 √x7th **S37.29 Other injury of bladder**

√5th **S37.3 Injury of urethra**
 √x7th **S37.30 Unspecified injury of urethra**
 √x7th **S37.32 Contusion of urethra**
 √x7th **S37.33 Laceration of urethra**
 √x7th **S37.39 Other injury of urethra**

√5th **S37.4 Injury of ovary**
√6th **S37.40 Unspecified injury of ovary**
    √7th **S37.401 Unspecified injury of ovary, unilateral**
    √7th **S37.402 Unspecified injury of ovary, bilateral**
    √7th **S37.409 Unspecified injury of ovary, unspecified**
√6th **S37.42 Contusion of ovary**
    √7th **S37.421 Contusion of ovary, unilateral**
    √7th **S37.422 Contusion of ovary, bilateral**
    √7th **S37.429 Contusion of ovary, unspecified**
√6th **S37.43 Laceration of ovary**
    √7th **S37.431 Laceration of ovary, unilateral**
    √7th **S37.432 Laceration of ovary, bilateral**
    √7th **S37.439 Laceration of ovary, unspecified**
√6th **S37.49 Other injury of ovary**
    √7th **S37.491 Other injury of ovary, unilateral**
    √7th **S37.492 Other injury of ovary, bilateral**
    √7th **S37.499 Other injury of ovary, unspecified**

√5th **S37.5 Injury of fallopian tube**
√6th **S37.50 Unspecified injury of fallopian tube**
    √7th **S37.501 Unspecified injury of fallopian tube, unilateral**
    √7th **S37.502 Unspecified injury of fallopian tube, bilateral**
    √7th **S37.509 Unspecified injury of fallopian tube, unspecified**
√6th **S37.51 Primary blast injury of fallopian tube**
Blast injury of fallopian tube NOS
    √7th **S37.511 Primary blast injury of fallopian tube, unilateral**
    √7th **S37.512 Primary blast injury of fallopian tube, bilateral**
    √7th **S37.519 Primary blast injury of fallopian tube, unspecified**
√6th **S37.52 Contusion of fallopian tube**
    √7th **S37.521 Contusion of fallopian tube, unilateral**
    √7th **S37.522 Contusion of fallopian tube, bilateral**
    √7th **S37.529 Contusion of fallopian tube, unspecified**
√6th **S37.53 Laceration of fallopian tube**
    √7th **S37.531 Laceration of fallopian tube, unilateral**
    √7th **S37.532 Laceration of fallopian tube, bilateral**

    √7th **S37.539 Laceration of fallopian tube, unspecified**
√6th **S37.59 Other injury of fallopian tube**
Secondary blast injury of fallopian tube
    √7th **S37.591 Other injury of fallopian tube, unilateral**
    √7th **S37.592 Other injury of fallopian tube, bilateral**
    √7th **S37.599 Other injury of fallopian tube, unspecified**

√5th **S37.6 Injury of uterus**
   EXCLUDES 1   *injury to gravid uterus (O9A.2-)*
           injury to uterus during delivery (O71-)
 √x7th **S37.60 Unspecified injury of uterus**
 √x7th **S37.62 Contusion of uterus**
 √x7th **S37.63 Laceration of uterus**
 √x7th **S37.69 Other injury of uterus**

√5th **S37.8 Injury of other urinary and pelvic organs**
√6th **S37.81 Injury of adrenal gland**
    √7th **S37.812 Contusion of adrenal gland**
    √7th **S37.813 Laceration of adrenal gland**
    √7th **S37.818 Other injury of adrenal gland**
    √7th **S37.819 Unspecified injury of adrenal gland**
√6th **S37.82 Injury of prostate**
    √7th **S37.822 Contusion of prostate**
    √7th **S37.823 Laceration of prostate**
    √7th **S37.828 Other injury of prostate**
    √7th **S37.829 Unspecified injury of prostate**
√6th **S37.89 Injury of other urinary and pelvic organ**
    √7th **S37.892 Contusion of other urinary and pelvic organ**
    √7th **S37.893 Laceration of other urinary and pelvic organ**
    √7th **S37.898 Other injury of other urinary and pelvic organ**
    √7th **S37.899 Unspecified injury of other urinary and pelvic organ**

√5th **S37.9 Injury of unspecified urinary and pelvic organ**
 √x7th **S37.90 Unspecified injury of unspecified urinary and pelvic organ**
 √x7th **S37.92 Contusion of unspecified urinary and pelvic organ**
 √x7th **S37.93 Laceration of unspecified urinary and pelvic organ**
 √x7th **S37.99 Other injury of unspecified urinary and pelvic organ**

√4th **S38 Crushing injury and traumatic amputation of abdomen, lower back, pelvis and external genitals**
   NOTE   An amputation not identified as partial or complete should be coded to complete

The appropriate 7th character is to be added to each code from category S38.
A   initial encounter
D   subsequent encounter
S   sequela

√5th **S38.0 Crushing injury of external genital organs**
Use additional code for any associated injuries
√6th **S38.00 Crushing injury of unspecified external genital organs**
    √7th **S38.001 Crushing injury of unspecified external genital organs, male**
    √7th **S38.002 Crushing injury of unspecified external genital organs, female**
 √x7th **S38.01 Crushing injury of penis**
 √x7th **S38.02 Crushing injury of scrotum and testis**
 √x7th **S38.03 Crushing injury of vulva**
√x7th **S38.1 Crushing injury of abdomen, lower back, and pelvis**
Use additional code for all associated injuries, such as:
    fracture of thoracic or lumbar spine and pelvis (S22.0-, S32-)
    injury to intra-abdominal organs (S36-)
    injury to urinary and pelvic organs (S37-)
    open wound of abdominal wall (S31-)
    spinal cord injury (S34.0, S34.1-)
    EXCLUDES 2   *crushing injury of external genital organs (S38.2-)*
√5th **S38.2 Traumatic amputation of external genital organs**
√6th **S38.21 Traumatic amputation of female external genital organs**
Traumatic amputation of clitoris
Traumatic amputation of labium (majus) (minus)
Traumatic amputation of vulva

EXCLUDES 1   Not coded here   EXCLUDES 2   Not included here   *Manifestation Code*

☑7ᵗʰ **S38.211** Complete traumatic amputation of female external genital organs

☑7ᵗʰ **S38.212** Partial traumatic amputation of female external genital organs

✓6ᵗʰ **S38.22** **Traumatic amputation of penis**

☑7ᵗʰ **S38.221** Complete traumatic amputation of penis

☑7ᵗʰ **S38.222** Partial traumatic amputation of penis

✓6ᵗʰ **S38.23** **Traumatic amputation of scrotum and testis**

☑7ᵗʰ **S38.231** Complete traumatic amputation of scrotum and testis

☑7ᵗʰ **S38.232** Partial traumatic amputation of scrotum and testis

✓x7ᵗʰ **S38.3** **Transection (partial) of abdomen**

✓4ᵗʰ **S39** **Other and unspecified injuries of abdomen, lower back, pelvis and external genitals**

Code also any associated open wound (S31-)

EXCLUDES 2 *sprain of joints and ligaments of lumbar spine and pelvis (S33.-)*

The appropriate 7th character is to be added to each code from category S39.
A   initial encounter
D   subsequent encounter
S   sequela

✓5ᵗʰ **S39.0** **Injury of muscle, fascia and tendon of abdomen, lower back and pelvis**

✓6ᵗʰ **S39.00** Unspecified injury of muscle, fascia and tendon of abdomen, lower back and pelvis

☑7ᵗʰ **S39.001** Unspecified injury of muscle, fascia and tendon of abdomen

☑7ᵗʰ **S39.002** Unspecified injury of muscle, fascia and tendon of lower back

☑7ᵗʰ **S39.003** Unspecified injury of muscle, fascia and tendon of pelvis

✓6ᵗʰ **S39.01** Strain of muscle, fascia and tendon of abdomen, lower back and pelvis

☑7ᵗʰ **S39.011** Strain of muscle, fascia and tendon of abdomen

☑7ᵗʰ **S39.012** Strain of muscle, fascia and tendon of lower back

☑7ᵗʰ **S39.013** Strain of muscle, fascia and tendon of pelvis

✓6ᵗʰ **S39.02** Laceration of muscle, fascia and tendon of abdomen, lower back and pelvis

☑7ᵗʰ **S39.021** Laceration of muscle, fascia and tendon of abdomen

☑7ᵗʰ **S39.022** Laceration of muscle, fascia and tendon of lower back

☑7ᵗʰ **S39.023** Laceration of muscle, fascia and tendon of pelvis

✓6ᵗʰ **S39.09** Other injury of muscle, fascia and tendon of abdomen, lower back and pelvis

☑7ᵗʰ **S39.091** Other injury of muscle, fascia and tendon of abdomen

☑7ᵗʰ **S39.092** Other injury of muscle, fascia and tendon of lower back

☑7ᵗʰ **S39.093** Other injury of muscle, fascia and tendon of pelvis

✓5ᵗʰ **S39.8** **Other specified injuries of abdomen, lower back, pelvis and external genitals**

✓x7ᵗʰ **S39.81** Other specified injuries of abdomen

✓x7ᵗʰ **S39.82** Other specified injuries of lower back

✓x7ᵗʰ **S39.83** Other specified injuries of pelvis

✓6ᵗʰ **S39.84** Other specified injuries of external genitals

☑7ᵗʰ **S39.840** Fracture of corpus cavernosum penis

☑7ᵗʰ **S39.848** Other specified injuries of external genitals

✓5ᵗʰ **S39.9** **Unspecified injury of abdomen, lower back, pelvis and external genitals**

✓x7ᵗʰ **S39.91** Unspecified injury of abdomen

✓x7ᵗʰ **S39.92** Unspecified injury of lower back

✓x7ᵗʰ **S39.93** Unspecified injury of pelvis

✓x7ᵗʰ **S39.94** Unspecified injury of external genitals

Injuries to the shoulder and upper arm (S40-S49)

INCLUDES injuries of axilla
injuries of scapular region

EXCLUDES 2 *burns and corrosions (T20-T32)*
frostbite (T33-T34)
injuries of elbow (S50-S59)
insect bite or sting, venomous (T63.4)

✓4ᵗʰ **S40** **Superficial injury of shoulder and upper arm**

The appropriate 7th character is to be added to each code from category S40.
A   initial encounter
D   subsequent encounter
S   sequela

✓5ᵗʰ **S40.0** **Contusion of shoulder and upper arm**

✓6ᵗʰ **S40.01** **Contusion of shoulder**

☑7ᵗʰ **S40.011** Contusion of right shoulder

☑7ᵗʰ **S40.012** Contusion of left shoulder

☑7ᵗʰ **S40.019** Contusion of unspecified shoulder

✓6ᵗʰ **S40.02** **Contusion of upper arm**

☑7ᵗʰ **S40.021** Contusion of right upper arm

☑7ᵗʰ **S40.022** Contusion of left upper arm

☑7ᵗʰ **S40.029** Contusion of unspecified upper arm

✓5ᵗʰ **S40.2** **Other superficial injuries of shoulder**

✓6ᵗʰ **S40.21** **Abrasion of shoulder**

☑7ᵗʰ **S40.211** Abrasion of right shoulder

☑7ᵗʰ **S40.212** Abrasion of left shoulder

☑7ᵗʰ **S40.219** Abrasion of unspecified shoulder

✓6ᵗʰ **S40.22** **Blister (nonthermal) of shoulder**

☑7ᵗʰ **S40.221** Blister (nonthermal) of right shoulder

☑7ᵗʰ **S40.222** Blister (nonthermal) of left shoulder

☑7ᵗʰ **S40.229** Blister (nonthermal) of unspecified shoulder

✓6ᵗʰ **S40.24** **External constriction of shoulder**

☑7ᵗʰ **S40.241** External constriction of right shoulder

☑7ᵗʰ **S40.242** External constriction of left shoulder

☑7ᵗʰ **S40.249** External constriction of unspecified shoulder

✓6ᵗʰ **S40.25** **Superficial foreign body of shoulder**
Splinter in the shoulder

☑7ᵗʰ **S40.251** Superficial foreign body of right shoulder

☑7ᵗʰ **S40.252** Superficial foreign body of left shoulder

☑7ᵗʰ **S40.259** Superficial foreign body of unspecified shoulder

✓6ᵗʰ **S40.26** **Insect bite (nonvenomous) of shoulder**

☑7ᵗʰ **S40.261** Insect bite (nonvenomous) of right shoulder

☑7ᵗʰ **S40.262** Insect bite (nonvenomous) of left shoulder

☑7ᵗʰ **S40.269** Insect bite (nonvenomous) of unspecified shoulder

✓6ᵗʰ **S40.27** **Other superficial bite of shoulder**

EXCLUDES 1 *open bite of shoulder (S41.05)*

☑7ᵗʰ **S40.271** Other superficial bite of right shoulder

☑7ᵗʰ **S40.272** Other superficial bite of left shoulder

☑7ᵗʰ **S40.279** Other superficial bite of unspecified shoulder

✓5ᵗʰ **S40.8** **Other superficial injuries of upper arm**

✓6ᵗʰ **S40.81** **Abrasion of upper arm**

☑7ᵗʰ **S40.811** Abrasion of right upper arm

☑7ᵗʰ **S40.812** Abrasion of left upper arm

☑7ᵗʰ **S40.819** Abrasion of unspecified upper arm

✓6ᵗʰ **S40.82** **Blister (nonthermal) of upper arm**

☑7ᵗʰ **S40.821** Blister (nonthermal) of right upper arm

☑7ᵗʰ **S40.822** Blister (nonthermal) of left upper arm

☑7ᵗʰ **S40.829** Blister (nonthermal) of unspecified upper arm

✓6ᵗʰ **S40.84** **External constriction of upper arm**

☑7ᵗʰ **S40.841** External constriction of right upper arm

☑7ᵗʰ **S40.842** External constriction of left upper arm

☑7ᵗʰ **S40.849** External constriction of unspecified upper arm

✓6th **S40.85** **Superficial foreign body of upper arm**
Splinter in the upper arm

    ✓7th **S40.851** **Superficial foreign body of right upper arm**

    ✓7th **S40.852** **Superficial foreign body of left upper arm**

    ✓7th **S40.859** **Superficial foreign body of unspecified upper arm**

✓6th **S40.86** **Insect bite (nonvenomous) of upper arm**

    ✓7th **S40.861** **Insect bite (nonvenomous) of right upper arm**

    ✓7th **S40.862** **Insect bite (nonvenomous) of left upper arm**

    ✓7th **S40.869** **Insect bite (nonvenomous) of unspecified upper arm**

✓6th **S40.87** **Other superficial bite of upper arm**
    EXCLUDES 1 *open bite of upper arm (S41.14)*
    EXCLUDES 2 *other superficial bite of shoulder (S40.27-)*

    ✓7th **S40.871** **Other superficial bite of right upper arm**

    ✓7th **S40.872** **Other superficial bite of left upper arm**

    ✓7th **S40.879** **Other superficial bite of unspecified upper arm**

✓5th **S40.9** **Unspecified superficial injury of shoulder and upper arm**

✓6th **S40.91** **Unspecified superficial injury of shoulder**

    ✓7th **S40.911** **Unspecified superficial injury of right shoulder**

    ✓7th **S40.912** **Unspecified superficial injury of left shoulder**

    ✓7th **S40.919** **Unspecified superficial injury of unspecified shoulder**

✓6th **S40.92** **Unspecified superficial injury of upper arm**

    ✓7th **S40.921** **Unspecified superficial injury of right upper arm**

    ✓7th **S40.922** **Unspecified superficial injury of left upper arm**

    ✓7th **S40.929** **Unspecified superficial injury of unspecified upper arm**

✓4th **S41** **Open wound of shoulder and upper arm**
Code also any associated wound infection
    EXCLUDES 1 *traumatic amputation of shoulder and upper arm (S48-)*
    EXCLUDES 2 *open fracture of shoulder and upper arm (S42- with 7th character B)*

The appropriate 7th character is to be added to each code from category S41.
A   initial encounter
D   subsequent encounter
S   sequela

✓5th **S41.0** **Open wound of shoulder**

✓6th **S41.00** **Unspecified open wound of shoulder**

    ✓7th **S41.001** **Unspecified open wound of right shoulder**

    ✓7th **S41.002** **Unspecified open wound of left shoulder**

    ✓7th **S41.009** **Unspecified open wound of unspecified shoulder**

✓6th **S41.01** **Laceration without foreign body of shoulder**

    ✓7th **S41.011** **Laceration without foreign body of right shoulder**

    ✓7th **S41.012** **Laceration without foreign body of left shoulder**

    ✓7th **S41.019** **Laceration without foreign body of unspecified shoulder**

✓6th **S41.02** **Laceration with foreign body of shoulder**

    ✓7th **S41.021** **Laceration with foreign body of right shoulder**

    ✓7th **S41.022** **Laceration with foreign body of left shoulder**

    ✓7th **S41.029** **Laceration with foreign body of unspecified shoulder**

✓6th **S41.03** **Puncture wound without foreign body of shoulder**

    ✓7th **S41.031** **Puncture wound without foreign body of right shoulder**

    ✓7th **S41.032** **Puncture wound without foreign body of left shoulder**

    ✓7th **S41.039** **Puncture wound without foreign body of unspecified shoulder**

✓6th **S41.04** **Puncture wound with foreign body of shoulder**

    ✓7th **S41.041** **Puncture wound with foreign body of right shoulder**

    ✓7th **S41.042** **Puncture wound with foreign body of left shoulder**

    ✓7th **S41.049** **Puncture wound with foreign body of unspecified shoulder**

✓6th **S41.05** **Open bite of shoulder**
Bite of shoulder NOS
    EXCLUDES 1 *superficial bite of shoulder (S40.27)*

    ✓7th **S41.051** **Open bite of right shoulder**

    ✓7th **S41.052** **Open bite of left shoulder**

    ✓7th **S41.059** **Open bite of unspecified shoulder**

✓5th **S41.1** **Open wound of upper arm**

✓6th **S41.10** **Unspecified open wound of upper arm**

    ✓7th **S41.101** **Unspecified open wound of right upper arm**

    ✓7th **S41.102** **Unspecified open wound of left upper arm**

    ✓7th **S41.109** **Unspecified open wound of unspecified upper arm**

✓6th **S41.11** **Laceration without foreign body of upper arm**

    ✓7th **S41.111** **Laceration without foreign body of right upper arm**

    ✓7th **S41.112** **Laceration without foreign body of left upper arm**

    ✓7th **S41.119** **Laceration without foreign body of unspecified upper arm**

✓6th **S41.12** **Laceration with foreign body of upper arm**

    ✓7th **S41.121** **Laceration with foreign body of right upper arm**

    ✓7th **S41.122** **Laceration with foreign body of left upper arm**

    ✓7th **S41.129** **Laceration with foreign body of unspecified upper arm**

✓6th **S41.13** **Puncture wound without foreign body of upper arm**

    ✓7th **S41.131** **Puncture wound without foreign body of right upper arm**

    ✓7th **S41.132** **Puncture wound without foreign body of left upper arm**

    ✓7th **S41.139** **Puncture wound without foreign body of unspecified upper arm**

✓6th **S41.14** **Puncture wound with foreign body of upper arm**

    ✓7th **S41.141** **Puncture wound with foreign body of right upper arm**

    ✓7th **S41.142** **Puncture wound with foreign body of left upper arm**

    ✓7th **S41.149** **Puncture wound with foreign body of unspecified upper arm**

✓6th **S41.15** **Open bite of upper arm**
Bite of upper arm NOS
    EXCLUDES 1 *superficial bite of upper arm (S40.87)*

    ✓7th **S41.151** **Open bite of right upper arm**

    ✓7th **S41.152** **Open bite of left upper arm**

    ✓7th **S41.159** **Open bite of unspecified upper arm**

✓4th **S42** **Fracture of shoulder and upper arm**
    NOTE   A fracture not indicated as displaced or nondisplaced should be coded to displaced
    A fracture not indicated as open or closed should be coded to closed
    EXCLUDES 1 *traumatic amputation of shoulder and upper arm (S48-)*

The appropriate 7th character is to be added to all codes from category S42.
A   initial encounter for closed fracture
B   initial encounter for open fracture
D   subsequent encounter for fracture with routine healing
G   subsequent encounter for fracture with delayed healing
K   subsequent encounter for fracture with nonunion
P   subsequent encounter for fracture with malunion
S   sequela

✓5th **S42.0** **Fracture of clavicle**

✓6th **S42.00** **Fracture of unspecified part of clavicle**

EXCLUDES 1 Not coded here   EXCLUDES 2 Not included here   *Manifestation Code*

✓7ᵗʰ **S42.001 Fracture of unspecified part of right clavicle**

✓7ᵗʰ **S42.002 Fracture of unspecified part of left clavicle**

✓7ᵗʰ **S42.009 Fracture of unspecified part of unspecified clavicle**

✓6ᵗʰ **S42.01 Fracture of sternal end of clavicle**

✓7ᵗʰ **S42.011 Anterior displaced fracture of sternal end of right clavicle**

✓7ᵗʰ **S42.012 Anterior displaced fracture of sternal end of left clavicle**

✓7ᵗʰ **S42.013 Anterior displaced fracture of sternal end of unspecified clavicle**
Displaced fracture of sternal end of clavicle NOS

✓7ᵗʰ **S42.014 Posterior displaced fracture of sternal end of right clavicle**

✓7ᵗʰ **S42.015 Posterior displaced fracture of sternal end of left clavicle**

✓7ᵗʰ **S42.016 Posterior displaced fracture of sternal end of unspecified clavicle**

✓7ᵗʰ **S42.017 Nondisplaced fracture of sternal end of right clavicle**

✓7ᵗʰ **S42.018 Nondisplaced fracture of sternal end of left clavicle**

✓7ᵗʰ **S42.019 Nondisplaced fracture of sternal end of unspecified clavicle**

✓6ᵗʰ **S42.02 Fracture of shaft of clavicle**

✓7ᵗʰ **S42.021 Displaced fracture of shaft of right clavicle**

✓7ᵗʰ **S42.022 Displaced fracture of shaft of left clavicle**

✓7ᵗʰ **S42.023 Displaced fracture of shaft of unspecified clavicle**

✓7ᵗʰ **S42.024 Nondisplaced fracture of shaft of right clavicle**

✓7ᵗʰ **S42.025 Nondisplaced fracture of shaft of left clavicle**

✓7ᵗʰ **S42.026 Nondisplaced fracture of shaft of unspecified clavicle**

✓6ᵗʰ **S42.03 Fracture of lateral end of clavicle**
Fracture of acromial end of clavicle

✓7ᵗʰ **S42.031 Displaced fracture of lateral end of right clavicle**

✓7ᵗʰ **S42.032 Displaced fracture of lateral end of left clavicle**

✓7ᵗʰ **S42.033 Displaced fracture of lateral end of unspecified clavicle**

✓7ᵗʰ **S42.034 Nondisplaced fracture of lateral end of right clavicle**

✓7ᵗʰ **S42.035 Nondisplaced fracture of lateral end of left clavicle**

✓7ᵗʰ **S42.036 Nondisplaced fracture of lateral end of unspecified clavicle**

✓5ᵗʰ **S42.1 Fracture of scapula**

✓6ᵗʰ **S42.10 Fracture of unspecified part of scapula**

✓7ᵗʰ **S42.101 Fracture of unspecified part of scapula, right shoulder**

✓7ᵗʰ **S42.102 Fracture of unspecified part of scapula, left shoulder**

✓7ᵗʰ **S42.109 Fracture of unspecified part of scapula, unspecified shoulder**

✓6ᵗʰ **S42.11 Fracture of body of scapula**

✓7ᵗʰ **S42.111 Displaced fracture of body of scapula, right shoulder**

✓7ᵗʰ **S42.112 Displaced fracture of body of scapula, left shoulder**

✓7ᵗʰ **S42.113 Displaced fracture of body of scapula, unspecified shoulder**

✓7ᵗʰ **S42.114 Nondisplaced fracture of body of scapula, right shoulder**

✓7ᵗʰ **S42.115 Nondisplaced fracture of body of scapula, left shoulder**

✓7ᵗʰ **S42.116 Nondisplaced fracture of body of scapula, unspecified shoulder**

✓6ᵗʰ **S42.12 Fracture of acromial process**

✓7ᵗʰ **S42.121 Displaced fracture of acromial process, right shoulder**

✓7ᵗʰ **S42.122 Displaced fracture of acromial process, left shoulder**

✓7ᵗʰ **S42.123 Displaced fracture of acromial process, unspecified shoulder**

✓7ᵗʰ **S42.124 Nondisplaced fracture of acromial process, right shoulder**

✓7ᵗʰ **S42.125 Nondisplaced fracture of acromial process, left shoulder**

✓7ᵗʰ **S42.126 Nondisplaced fracture of acromial process, unspecified shoulder**

✓6ᵗʰ **S42.13 Fracture of coracoid process**

✓7ᵗʰ **S42.131 Displaced fracture of coracoid process, right shoulder**

✓7ᵗʰ **S42.132 Displaced fracture of coracoid process, left shoulder**

✓7ᵗʰ **S42.133 Displaced fracture of coracoid process, unspecified shoulder**

✓7ᵗʰ **S42.134 Nondisplaced fracture of coracoid process, right shoulder**

✓7ᵗʰ **S42.135 Nondisplaced fracture of coracoid process, left shoulder**

✓7ᵗʰ **S42.136 Nondisplaced fracture of coracoid process, unspecified shoulder**

✓6ᵗʰ **S42.14 Fracture of glenoid cavity of scapula**

✓7ᵗʰ **S42.141 Displaced fracture of glenoid cavity of scapula, right shoulder**

✓7ᵗʰ **S42.142 Displaced fracture of glenoid cavity of scapula, left shoulder**

✓7ᵗʰ **S42.143 Displaced fracture of glenoid cavity of scapula, unspecified shoulder**

✓7ᵗʰ **S42.144 Nondisplaced fracture of glenoid cavity of scapula, right shoulder**

✓7ᵗʰ **S42.145 Nondisplaced fracture of glenoid cavity of scapula, left shoulder**

✓7ᵗʰ **S42.146 Nondisplaced fracture of glenoid cavity of scapula, unspecified shoulder**

✓6ᵗʰ **S42.15 Fracture of neck of scapula**

✓7ᵗʰ **S42.151 Displaced fracture of neck of scapula, right shoulder**

✓7ᵗʰ **S42.152 Displaced fracture of neck of scapula, left shoulder**

✓7ᵗʰ **S42.153 Displaced fracture of neck of scapula, unspecified shoulder**

✓7ᵗʰ **S42.154 Nondisplaced fracture of neck of scapula, right shoulder**

✓7ᵗʰ **S42.155 Nondisplaced fracture of neck of scapula, left shoulder**

✓7ᵗʰ **S42.156 Nondisplaced fracture of neck of scapula, unspecified shoulder**

✓6ᵗʰ **S42.19 Fracture of other part of scapula**

✓7ᵗʰ **S42.191 Fracture of other part of scapula, right shoulder**

✓7ᵗʰ **S42.192 Fracture of other part of scapula, left shoulder**

✓7ᵗʰ **S42.199 Fracture of other part of scapula, unspecified shoulder**

✓5ᵗʰ **S42.2 Fracture of upper end of humerus**
Fracture of proximal end of humerus
EXCLUDES 2 *fracture of shaft of humerus (S42.3-)*
physeal fracture of upper end of humerus (S49.0-)

✓6ᵗʰ **S42.20 Unspecified fracture of upper end of humerus**

✓7ᵗʰ **S42.201 Unspecified fracture of upper end of right humerus**

✓7ᵗʰ **S42.202 Unspecified fracture of upper end of left humerus**

✓7ᵗʰ **S42.209 Unspecified fracture of upper end of unspecified humerus**

✓6ᵗʰ **S42.21 Unspecified fracture of surgical neck of humerus**
Fracture of neck of humerus NOS

✓7ᵗʰ **S42.211 Unspecified displaced fracture of surgical neck of right humerus**

✓7ᵗʰ **S42.212 Unspecified displaced fracture of surgical neck of left humerus**

☑ Appropriate additional character required ✓ₓ7ᵗʰ Requires 7th character, placeholder x must fill empty characters

√7ᵗʰ **S42.213**   **Unspecified displaced fracture of surgical neck of unspecified humerus**

√7ᵗʰ **S42.214**   **Unspecified nondisplaced fracture of surgical neck of right humerus**

√7ᵗʰ **S42.215**   **Unspecified nondisplaced fracture of surgical neck of left humerus**

√7ᵗʰ **S42.216**   **Unspecified nondisplaced fracture of surgical neck of unspecified humerus**

√6ᵗʰ **S42.22**   **2-part fracture of surgical neck of humerus**

√7ᵗʰ **S42.221**   **2-part displaced fracture of surgical neck of right humerus**

√7ᵗʰ **S42.222**   **2-part displaced fracture of surgical neck of left humerus**

√7ᵗʰ **S42.223**   **2-part displaced fracture of surgical neck of unspecified humerus**

√7ᵗʰ **S42.224**   **2-part nondisplaced fracture of surgical neck of right humerus**

√7ᵗʰ **S42.225**   **2-part nondisplaced fracture of surgical neck of left humerus**

√7ᵗʰ **S42.226**   **2-part nondisplaced fracture of surgical neck of unspecified humerus**

√6ᵗʰ **S42.23**   **3-part fracture of surgical neck of humerus**

√7ᵗʰ **S42.231**   **3-part fracture of surgical neck of right humerus**

√7ᵗʰ **S42.232**   **3-part fracture of surgical neck of left humerus**

√7ᵗʰ **S42.239**   **3-part fracture of surgical neck of unspecified humerus**

√6ᵗʰ **S42.24**   **4-part fracture of surgical neck of humerus**

√7ᵗʰ **S42.241**   **4-part fracture of surgical neck of right humerus**

√7ᵗʰ **S42.242**   **4-part fracture of surgical neck of left humerus**

√7ᵗʰ **S42.249**   **4-part fracture of surgical neck of unspecified humerus**

√6ᵗʰ **S42.25**   **Fracture of greater tuberosity of humerus**

√7ᵗʰ **S42.251**   **Displaced fracture of greater tuberosity of right humerus**

√7ᵗʰ **S42.252**   **Displaced fracture of greater tuberosity of left humerus**

√7ᵗʰ **S42.253**   **Displaced fracture of greater tuberosity of unspecified humerus**

√7ᵗʰ **S42.254**   **Nondisplaced fracture of greater tuberosity of right humerus**

√7ᵗʰ **S42.255**   **Nondisplaced fracture of greater tuberosity of left humerus**

√7ᵗʰ **S42.256**   **Nondisplaced fracture of greater tuberosity of unspecified humerus**

√6ᵗʰ **S42.26**   **Fracture of lesser tuberosity of humerus**

√7ᵗʰ **S42.261**   **Displaced fracture of lesser tuberosity of right humerus**

√7ᵗʰ **S42.262**   **Displaced fracture of lesser tuberosity of left humerus**

√7ᵗʰ **S42.263**   **Displaced fracture of lesser tuberosity of unspecified humerus**

√7ᵗʰ **S42.264**   **Nondisplaced fracture of lesser tuberosity of right humerus**

√7ᵗʰ **S42.265**   **Nondisplaced fracture of lesser tuberosity of left humerus**

√7ᵗʰ **S42.266**   **Nondisplaced fracture of lesser tuberosity of unspecified humerus**

√6ᵗʰ **S42.27**   **Torus fracture of upper end of humerus**

    NOTE   7th character B is not applicable to codes under subcategory S42.27

√7ᵗʰ **S42.271**   **Torus fracture of upper end of right humerus**

√7ᵗʰ **S42.272**   **Torus fracture of upper end of left humerus**

√7ᵗʰ **S42.279**   **Torus fracture of upper end of unspecified humerus**

√6ᵗʰ **S42.29**   **Other fracture of upper end of humerus**

    Fracture of anatomical neck of humerus
    Fracture of articular head of humerus

√7ᵗʰ **S42.291**   **Other displaced fracture of upper end of right humerus**

√7ᵗʰ **S42.292**   **Other displaced fracture of upper end of left humerus**

√7ᵗʰ **S42.293**   **Other displaced fracture of upper end of unspecified humerus**

√7ᵗʰ **S42.294**   **Other nondisplaced fracture of upper end of right humerus**

√7ᵗʰ **S42.295**   **Other nondisplaced fracture of upper end of left humerus**

√7ᵗʰ **S42.296**   **Other nondisplaced fracture of upper end of unspecified humerus**

√5ᵗʰ **S42.3**   **Fracture of shaft of humerus**

    Fracture of humerus NOS
    Fracture of upper arm NOS

    EXCLUDES 2   *physeal fractures of upper end of humerus (S49.0-)*
       physeal fractures of lower end of humerus (S49.1-)

√6ᵗʰ **S42.30**   **Unspecified fracture of shaft of humerus**

√7ᵗʰ **S42.301**   **Unspecified fracture of shaft of humerus, right arm**

√7ᵗʰ **S42.302**   **Unspecified fracture of shaft of humerus, left arm**

√7ᵗʰ **S42.309**   **Unspecified fracture of shaft of humerus, unspecified arm**

√6ᵗʰ **S42.31**   **Greenstick fracture of shaft of humerus**

    NOTE   7th character B is not applicable to codes under subcategory S42.31

√7ᵗʰ **S42.311**   **Greenstick fracture of shaft of humerus, right arm**

√7ᵗʰ **S42.312**   **Greenstick fracture of shaft of humerus, left arm**

√7ᵗʰ **S42.319**   **Greenstick fracture of shaft of humerus, unspecified arm**

√6ᵗʰ **S42.32**   **Transverse fracture of shaft of humerus**

√7ᵗʰ **S42.321**   **Displaced transverse fracture of shaft of humerus, right arm**

√7ᵗʰ **S42.322**   **Displaced transverse fracture of shaft of humerus, left arm**

√7ᵗʰ **S42.323**   **Displaced transverse fracture of shaft of humerus, unspecified arm**

√7ᵗʰ **S42.324**   **Nondisplaced transverse fracture of shaft of humerus, right arm**

√7ᵗʰ **S42.325**   **Nondisplaced transverse fracture of shaft of humerus, left arm**

√7ᵗʰ **S42.326**   **Nondisplaced transverse fracture of shaft of humerus, unspecified arm**

√6ᵗʰ **S42.33**   **Oblique fracture of shaft of humerus**

√7ᵗʰ **S42.331**   **Displaced oblique fracture of shaft of humerus, right arm**

√7ᵗʰ **S42.332**   **Displaced oblique fracture of shaft of humerus, left arm**

√7ᵗʰ **S42.333**   **Displaced oblique fracture of shaft of humerus, unspecified arm**

√7ᵗʰ **S42.334**   **Nondisplaced oblique fracture of shaft of humerus, right arm**

√7ᵗʰ **S42.335**   **Nondisplaced oblique fracture of shaft of humerus, left arm**

√7ᵗʰ **S42.336**   **Nondisplaced oblique fracture of shaft of humerus, unspecified arm**

√6ᵗʰ **S42.34**   **Spiral fracture of shaft of humerus**

√7ᵗʰ **S42.341**   **Displaced spiral fracture of shaft of humerus, right arm**

√7ᵗʰ **S42.342**   **Displaced spiral fracture of shaft of humerus, left arm**

√7ᵗʰ **S42.343**   **Displaced spiral fracture of shaft of humerus, unspecified arm**

√7ᵗʰ **S42.344**   **Nondisplaced spiral fracture of shaft of humerus, right arm**

√7ᵗʰ **S42.345**   **Nondisplaced spiral fracture of shaft of humerus, left arm**

√7ᵗʰ **S42.346**   **Nondisplaced spiral fracture of shaft of humerus, unspecified arm**

√6ᵗʰ **S42.35**   **Comminuted fracture of shaft of humerus**

√7ᵗʰ **S42.351**   **Displaced comminuted fracture of shaft of humerus, right arm**

√7ᵗʰ **S42.352**   **Displaced comminuted fracture of shaft of humerus, left arm**

√7ᵗʰ **S42.353**   **Displaced comminuted fracture of shaft of humerus, unspecified arm**

√7ᵗʰ **S42.354**   **Nondisplaced comminuted fracture of shaft of humerus, right arm**

EXCLUDES 1 Not coded here   **EXCLUDES 2** Not included here   *Manifestation Code*

✓7th **S42.355 Nondisplaced comminuted fracture of shaft of humerus, left arm**

✓7th **S42.356 Nondisplaced comminuted fracture of shaft of humerus, unspecified arm**

✓6th **S42.36 Segmental fracture of shaft of humerus**

✓7th **S42.361 Displaced segmental fracture of shaft of humerus, right arm**

✓7th **S42.362 Displaced segmental fracture of shaft of humerus, left arm**

✓7th **S42.363 Displaced segmental fracture of shaft of humerus, unspecified arm**

✓7th **S42.364 Nondisplaced segmental fracture of shaft of humerus, right arm**

✓7th **S42.365 Nondisplaced segmental fracture of shaft of humerus, left arm**

✓7th **S42.366 Nondisplaced segmental fracture of shaft of humerus, unspecified arm**

✓6th **S42.39 Other fracture of shaft of humerus**

✓7th **S42.391 Other fracture of shaft of right humerus**

✓7th **S42.392 Other fracture of shaft of left humerus**

✓7th **S42.399 Other fracture of shaft of unspecified humerus**

✓5th **S42.4 Fracture of lower end of humerus**
Fracture of distal end of humerus

EXCLUDES 2 *fracture of shaft of humerus (S42.3-)*
physeal fracture of lower end of humerus (S49.1-)

✓6th **S42.40 Unspecified fracture of lower end of humerus**
Fracture of elbow NOS

✓7th **S42.401 Unspecified fracture of lower end of right humerus**

✓7th **S42.402 Unspecified fracture of lower end of left humerus**

✓7th **S42.409 Unspecified fracture of lower end of unspecified humerus**

✓6th **S42.41 Simple supracondylar fracture without intercondylar fracture of humerus**

✓7th **S42.411 Displaced simple supracondylar fracture without intercondylar fracture of right humerus**

✓7th **S42.412 Displaced simple supracondylar fracture without intercondylar fracture of left humerus**

✓7th **S42.413 Displaced simple supracondylar fracture without intercondylar fracture of unspecified humerus**

✓7th **S42.414 Nondisplaced simple supracondylar fracture without intercondylar fracture of right humerus**

✓7th **S42.415 Nondisplaced simple supracondylar fracture without intercondylar fracture of left humerus**

✓7th **S42.416 Nondisplaced simple supracondylar fracture without intercondylar fracture of unspecified humerus**

✓6th **S42.42 Comminuted supracondylar fracture without intercondylar fracture of humerus**

✓7th **S42.421 Displaced comminuted supracondylar fracture without intercondylar fracture of right humerus**

✓7th **S42.422 Displaced comminuted supracondylar fracture without intercondylar fracture of left humerus**

✓7th **S42.423 Displaced comminuted supracondylar fracture without intercondylar fracture of unspecified humerus**

✓7th **S42.424 Nondisplaced comminuted supracondylar fracture without intercondylar fracture of right humerus**

✓7th **S42.425 Nondisplaced comminuted supracondylar fracture without intercondylar fracture of left humerus**

✓7th **S42.426 Nondisplaced comminuted supracondylar fracture without intercondylar fracture of unspecified humerus**

✓6th **S42.43 Fracture (avulsion) of lateral epicondyle of humerus**

✓7th **S42.431 Displaced fracture (avulsion) of lateral epicondyle of right humerus**

✓7th **S42.432 Displaced fracture (avulsion) of lateral epicondyle of left humerus**

✓7th **S42.433 Displaced fracture (avulsion) of lateral epicondyle of unspecified humerus**

✓7th **S42.434 Nondisplaced fracture (avulsion) of lateral epicondyle of right humerus**

✓7th **S42.435 Nondisplaced fracture (avulsion) of lateral epicondyle of left humerus**

✓7th **S42.436 Nondisplaced fracture (avulsion) of lateral epicondyle of unspecified humerus**

✓6th **S42.44 Fracture (avulsion) of medial epicondyle of humerus**

S42.441 Displaced fracture (avulsion) of medial epicondyle of right humerus

✓7th **S42.442 Displaced fracture (avulsion) of medial epicondyle of left humerus**

✓7th **S42.443 Displaced fracture (avulsion) of medial epicondyle of unspecified humerus**

✓7th **S42.444 Nondisplaced fracture (avulsion) of medial epicondyle of right humerus**

✓7th **S42.445 Nondisplaced fracture (avulsion) of medial epicondyle of left humerus**

✓7th **S42.446 Nondisplaced fracture (avulsion) of medial epicondyle of unspecified humerus**

✓7th **S42.447 Incarcerated fracture (avulsion) of medial epicondyle of right humerus**

✓7th **S42.448 Incarcerated fracture (avulsion) of medial epicondyle of left humerus**

✓7th **S42.449 Incarcerated fracture (avulsion) of medial epicondyle of unspecified humerus**

✓6th **S42.45 Fracture of lateral condyle of humerus**
Fracture of capitellum of humerus

✓7th **S42.451 Displaced fracture of lateral condyle of right humerus**

✓7th **S42.452 Displaced fracture of lateral condyle of left humerus**

✓7th **S42.453 Displaced fracture of lateral condyle of unspecified humerus**

✓7th **S42.454 Nondisplaced fracture of lateral condyle of right humerus**

✓7th **S42.455 Nondisplaced fracture of lateral condyle of left humerus**

✓7th **S42.456 Nondisplaced fracture of lateral condyle of unspecified humerus**

✓6th **S42.46 Fracture of medial condyle of humerus**
Trochlea fracture of humerus

✓7th **S42.461 Displaced fracture of medial condyle of right humerus**

✓7th **S42.462 Displaced fracture of medial condyle of left humerus**

✓7th **S42.463 Displaced fracture of medial condyle of unspecified humerus**

✓7th **S42.464 Nondisplaced fracture of medial condyle of right humerus**

✓7th **S42.465 Nondisplaced fracture of medial condyle of left humerus**

✓7th **S42.466 Nondisplaced fracture of medial condyle of unspecified humerus**

✓6th **S42.47 Transcondylar fracture of humerus**

✓7th **S42.471 Displaced transcondylar fracture of right humerus**

✓7th **S42.472 Displaced transcondylar fracture of left humerus**

✓7th **S42.473 Displaced transcondylar fracture of unspecified humerus**

✓7th **S42.474 Nondisplaced transcondylar fracture of right humerus**

✓7th **S42.475 Nondisplaced transcondylar fracture of left humerus**

☑ Appropriate additional character required   ✓x7th Requires 7th character, placeholder x must fill empty characters

✓7th **S42.476** **Nondisplaced transcondylar fracture of unspecified humerus**

✓6th **S42.48** **Torus fracture of lower end of humerus**

> NOTE   7th character B is not applicable to codes under subcategory S42.48

   ✓7th **S42.481** **Torus fracture of lower end of right humerus**

   ✓7th **S42.482** **Torus fracture of lower end of left humerus**

   ✓7th **S42.489** **Torus fracture of lower end of unspecified humerus**

✓6th **S42.49** **Other fracture of lower end of humerus**

   ✓7th **S42.491** **Other displaced fracture of lower end of right humerus**

   ✓7th **S42.492** **Other displaced fracture of lower end of left humerus**

   ✓7th **S42.493** **Other displaced fracture of lower end of unspecified humerus**

   ✓7th **S42.494** **Other nondisplaced fracture of lower end of right humerus**

   ✓7th **S42.495** **Other nondisplaced fracture of lower end of left humerus**

   ✓7th **S42.496** **Other nondisplaced fracture of lower end of unspecified humerus**

✓5th **S42.9** **Fracture of shoulder girdle, part unspecified**

   Fracture of shoulder NOS

   ✓x7th **S42.90** **Fracture of unspecified shoulder girdle, part unspecified**

   ✓x7th **S42.91** **Fracture of right shoulder girdle, part unspecified**

   ✓x7th **S42.92** **Fracture of left shoulder girdle, part unspecified**

✓4th **S43** **Dislocation and sprain of joints and ligaments of shoulder girdle**

> INCLUDES   avulsion of joint or ligament of shoulder girdle
> laceration of cartilage, joint or ligament of shoulder girdle
> sprain of cartilage, joint or ligament of shoulder girdle
> traumatic hemarthrosis of joint or ligament of shoulder girdle
> traumatic rupture of joint or ligament of shoulder girdle
> traumatic subluxation of joint or ligament of shoulder girdle
> traumatic tear of joint or ligament of shoulder girdle

Code also any associated open wound

> EXCLUDES 2   strain of muscle, fascia and tendon of shoulder and upper arm (S46-)

The appropriate 7th character is to be added to each code from category S43.
A   initial encounter
D   subsequent encounter
S   sequela

✓5th **S43.0** **Subluxation and dislocation of shoulder joint**

   Dislocation of glenohumeral joint
   Subluxation of glenohumeral joint

✓6th **S43.00** **Unspecified subluxation and dislocation of shoulder joint**

   Dislocation of humerus NOS
   Subluxation of humerus NOS

   ✓7th **S43.001** **Unspecified subluxation of right shoulder joint**

   ✓7th **S43.002** **Unspecified subluxation of left shoulder joint**

   ✓7th **S43.003** **Unspecified subluxation of unspecified shoulder joint**

   ✓7th **S43.004** **Unspecified dislocation of right shoulder joint**

   ✓7th **S43.005** **Unspecified dislocation of left shoulder joint**

   ✓7th **S43.006** **Unspecified dislocation of unspecified shoulder joint**

✓6th **S43.01** **Anterior subluxation and dislocation of humerus**

   ✓7th **S43.011** **Anterior subluxation of right humerus**

   ✓7th **S43.012** **Anterior subluxation of left humerus**

   ✓7th **S43.013** **Anterior subluxation of unspecified humerus**

   ✓7th **S43.014** **Anterior dislocation of right humerus**

   ✓7th **S43.015** **Anterior dislocation of left humerus**

   ✓7th **S43.016** **Anterior dislocation of unspecified humerus**

✓6th **S43.02** **Posterior subluxation and dislocation of humerus**

   ✓7th **S43.021** **Posterior subluxation of right humerus**

   ✓7th **S43.022** **Posterior subluxation of left humerus**

   ✓7th **S43.023** **Posterior subluxation of unspecified humerus**

   ✓7th **S43.024** **Posterior dislocation of right humerus**

   ✓7th **S43.025** **Posterior dislocation of left humerus**

   ✓7th **S43.026** **Posterior dislocation of unspecified humerus**

✓6th **S43.03** **Inferior subluxation and dislocation of humerus**

   ✓7th **S43.031** **Inferior subluxation of right humerus**

   ✓7th **S43.032** **Inferior subluxation of left humerus**

   ✓7th **S43.033** **Inferior subluxation of unspecified humerus**

   ✓7th **S43.034** **Inferior dislocation of right humerus**

   ✓7th **S43.035** **Inferior dislocation of left humerus**

   ✓7th **S43.036** **Inferior dislocation of unspecified humerus**

✓6th **S43.08** **Other subluxation and dislocation of shoulder joint**

   ✓7th **S43.081** **Other subluxation of right shoulder joint**

   ✓7th **S43.082** **Other subluxation of left shoulder joint**

   ✓7th **S43.083** **Other subluxation of unspecified shoulder joint**

   ✓7th **S43.084** **Other dislocation of right shoulder joint**

   ✓7th **S43.085** **Other dislocation of left shoulder joint**

   ✓7th **S43.086** **Other dislocation of unspecified shoulder joint**

✓5th **S43.1** **Subluxation and dislocation of acromioclavicular joint**

✓6th **S43.10** **Unspecified dislocation of acromioclavicular joint**

   ✓7th **S43.101** **Unspecified dislocation of right acromioclavicular joint**

   ✓7th **S43.102** **Unspecified dislocation of left acromioclavicular joint**

   ✓7th **S43.109** **Unspecified dislocation of unspecified acromioclavicular joint**

✓6th **S43.11** **Subluxation of acromioclavicular joint**

   ✓7th **S43.111** **Subluxation of right acromioclavicular joint**

   ✓7th **S43.112** **Subluxation of left acromioclavicular joint**

   ✓7th **S43.119** **Subluxation of unspecified acromioclavicular joint**

✓6th **S43.12** **Dislocation of acromioclavicular joint, 100%-200% displacement**

   ✓7th **S43.121** **Dislocation of right acromioclavicular joint, 100%-200% displacement**

   ✓7th **S43.122** **Dislocation of left acromioclavicular joint, 100%-200% displacement**

   ✓7th **S43.129** **Dislocation of unspecified acromioclavicular joint, 100%-200% displacement**

✓6th **S43.13** **Dislocation of acromioclavicular joint, greater than 200% displacement**

   ✓7th **S43.131** **Dislocation of right acromioclavicular joint, greater than 200% displacement**

   ✓7th **S43.132** **Dislocation of left acromioclavicular joint, greater than 200% displacement**

   ✓7th **S43.139** **Dislocation of unspecified acromioclavicular joint, greater than 200% displacement**

✓6th **S43.14** **Inferior dislocation of acromioclavicular joint**

   ✓7th **S43.141** **Inferior dislocation of right acromioclavicular joint**

   ✓7th **S43.142** **Inferior dislocation of left acromioclavicular joint**

   ✓7th **S43.149** **Inferior dislocation of unspecified acromioclavicular joint**

✓6th **S43.15** **Posterior dislocation of acromioclavicular joint**

   ✓7th **S43.151** **Posterior dislocation of right acromioclavicular joint**

   ✓7th **S43.152** **Posterior dislocation of left acromioclavicular joint**

EXCLUDES 1   Not coded here   EXCLUDES 2   Not included here   *Manifestation Code*

✓7th **S43.159 Posterior dislocation of unspecified acromioclavicular joint**

✓5th **S43.2 Subluxation and dislocation of sternoclavicular joint**

✓6th **S43.20 Unspecified subluxation and dislocation of sternoclavicular joint**

✓7th **S43.201 Unspecified subluxation of right sternoclavicular joint**

✓7th **S43.202 Unspecified subluxation of left sternoclavicular joint**

✓7th **S43.203 Unspecified subluxation of unspecified sternoclavicular joint**

✓7th **S43.204 Unspecified dislocation of right sternoclavicular joint**

✓7th **S43.205 Unspecified dislocation of left sternoclavicular joint**

✓7th **S43.206 Unspecified dislocation of unspecified sternoclavicular joint**

✓6th **S43.21 Anterior subluxation and dislocation of sternoclavicular joint**

✓7th **S43.211 Anterior subluxation of right sternoclavicular joint**

✓7th **S43.212 Anterior subluxation of left sternoclavicular joint**

✓7th **S43.213 Anterior subluxation of unspecified sternoclavicular joint**

✓7th **S43.214 Anterior dislocation of right sternoclavicular joint**

✓7th **S43.215 Anterior dislocation of left sternoclavicular joint**

✓7th **S43.216 Anterior dislocation of unspecified sternoclavicular joint**

✓6th **S43.22 Posterior subluxation and dislocation of sternoclavicular joint**

✓7th **S43.221 Posterior subluxation of right sternoclavicular joint**

✓7th **S43.222 Posterior subluxation of left sternoclavicular joint**

✓7th **S43.223 Posterior subluxation of unspecified sternoclavicular joint**

✓7th **S43.224 Posterior dislocation of right sternoclavicular joint**

✓7th **S43.225 Posterior dislocation of left sternoclavicular joint**

✓7th **S43.226 Posterior dislocation of unspecified sternoclavicular joint**

✓5th **S43.3 Subluxation and dislocation of other and unspecified parts of shoulder girdle**

✓6th **S43.30 Subluxation and dislocation of unspecified parts of shoulder girdle**
Dislocation of shoulder girdle NOS
Subluxation of shoulder girdle NOS

✓7th **S43.301 Subluxation of unspecified parts of right shoulder girdle**

✓7th **S43.302 Subluxation of unspecified parts of left shoulder girdle**

✓7th **S43.303 Subluxation of unspecified parts of unspecified shoulder girdle**

✓7th **S43.304 Dislocation of unspecified parts of right shoulder girdle**

✓7th **S43.305 Dislocation of unspecified parts of left shoulder girdle**

✓7th **S43.306 Dislocation of unspecified parts of unspecified shoulder girdle**

✓6th **S43.31 Subluxation and dislocation of scapula**

✓7th **S43.311 Subluxation of right scapula**

✓7th **S43.312 Subluxation of left scapula**

✓7th **S43.313 Subluxation of unspecified scapula**

✓7th **S43.314 Dislocation of right scapula**

✓7th **S43.315 Dislocation of left scapula**

✓7th **S43.316 Dislocation of unspecified scapula**

✓6th **S43.39 Subluxation and dislocation of other parts of shoulder girdle**

✓7th **S43.391 Subluxation of other parts of right shoulder girdle**

✓7th **S43.392 Subluxation of other parts of left shoulder girdle**

✓7th **S43.393 Subluxation of other parts of unspecified shoulder girdle**

✓7th **S43.394 Dislocation of other parts of right shoulder girdle**

✓7th **S43.395 Dislocation of other parts of left shoulder girdle**

✓7th **S43.396 Dislocation of other parts of unspecified shoulder girdle**

✓5th **S43.4 Sprain of shoulder joint**

✓6th **S43.40 Unspecified sprain of shoulder joint**

✓7th **S43.401 Unspecified sprain of right shoulder joint**

✓7th **S43.402 Unspecified sprain of left shoulder joint**

✓7th **S43.409 Unspecified sprain of unspecified shoulder joint**

✓6th **S43.41 Sprain of coracohumeral (ligament)**

✓7th **S43.411 Sprain of right coracohumeral (ligament)**

✓7th **S43.412 Sprain of left coracohumeral (ligament)**

✓7th **S43.419 Sprain of unspecified coracohumeral (ligament)**

✓6th **S43.42 Sprain of rotator cuff capsule**
EXCLUDES 1 rotator cuff syndrome (complete) (incomplete), not specified as traumatic (M75.1-)
EXCLUDES 2 injury of tendon of rotator cuff (S46.0-)

✓7th **S43.421 Sprain of right rotator cuff capsule**

✓7th **S43.422 Sprain of left rotator cuff capsule**

✓7th **S43.429 Sprain of unspecified rotator cuff capsule**

✓6th **S43.43 Superior glenoid labrum lesion**
SLAP lesion

✓7th **S43.431 Superior glenoid labrum lesion of right shoulder**

✓7th **S43.432 Superior glenoid labrum lesion of left shoulder**

✓7th **S43.439 Superior glenoid labrum lesion of unspecified shoulder**

✓6th **S43.49 Other sprain of shoulder joint**

✓7th **S43.491 Other sprain of right shoulder joint**

✓7th **S43.492 Other sprain of left shoulder joint**

✓7th **S43.499 Other sprain of unspecified shoulder joint**

✓5th **S43.5 Sprain of acromioclavicular joint**
Sprain of acromioclavicular ligament

✓x7th **S43.50 Sprain of unspecified acromioclavicular joint**

✓x7th **S43.51 Sprain of right acromioclavicular joint**

✓x7th **S43.52 Sprain of left acromioclavicular joint**

✓5th **S43.6 Sprain of sternoclavicular joint**

✓x7th **S43.60 Sprain of unspecified sternoclavicular joint**

✓x7th **S43.61 Sprain of right sternoclavicular joint**

✓x7th **S43.62 Sprain of left sternoclavicular joint**

✓5th **S43.8 Sprain of other specified parts of shoulder girdle**

✓x7th **S43.80 Sprain of other specified parts of unspecified shoulder girdle**

✓x7th **S43.81 Sprain of other specified parts of right shoulder girdle**

✓x7th **S43.82 Sprain of other specified parts of left shoulder girdle**

✓5th **S43.9 Sprain of unspecified parts of shoulder girdle**

✓x7th **S43.90 Sprain of unspecified parts of unspecified shoulder girdle**
Sprain of shoulder girdle NOS

✓x7th **S43.91 Sprain of unspecified parts of right shoulder girdle**

✓x7th **S43.92 Sprain of unspecified parts of left shoulder girdle**

✓4th **S44 Injury of nerves at shoulder and upper arm level**
Code also any associated open wound (S41-)
EXCLUDES 2 injury of brachial plexus (S14.3-)

The appropriate 7th character is to be added to each code from category S44.
A   initial encounter
D   subsequent encounter
S   sequela

✓5th **S44.0 Injury of ulnar nerve at upper arm level**
EXCLUDES 1 ulnar nerve NOS (S54.0)

☑ Appropriate additional character required

✓x7th Requires 7th character, placeholder x must fill empty characters

√x7th **S44.00** Injury of ulnar nerve at upper arm level, unspecified arm

√x7th **S44.01** Injury of ulnar nerve at upper arm level, right arm

√x7th **S44.02** Injury of ulnar nerve at upper arm level, left arm

√5th **S44.1** Injury of median nerve at upper arm level

> EXCLUDES 1   *median nerve NOS (S54.1)*

√x7th **S44.10** Injury of median nerve at upper arm level, unspecified arm

√x7th **S44.11** Injury of median nerve at upper arm level, right arm

√x7th **S44.12** Injury of median nerve at upper arm level, left arm

√5th **S44.2** Injury of radial nerve at upper arm level

> EXCLUDES 1   *radial nerve NOS (S54.2)*

√x7th **S44.20** Injury of radial nerve at upper arm level, unspecified arm

√x7th **S44.21** Injury of radial nerve at upper arm level, right arm

√x7th **S44.22** Injury of radial nerve at upper arm level, left arm

√5th **S44.3** Injury of axillary nerve

S44.30 Injury of axillary nerve, unspecified arm

√x7th **S44.31** Injury of axillary nerve, right arm

√x7th **S44.32** Injury of axillary nerve, left arm

√5th **S44.4** Injury of musculocutaneous nerve

√x7th **S44.40** Injury of musculocutaneous nerve, unspecified arm

√x7th **S44.41** Injury of musculocutaneous nerve, right arm

√x7th **S44.42** Injury of musculocutaneous nerve, left arm

√5th **S44.5** Injury of cutaneous sensory nerve at shoulder and upper arm level

√x7th **S44.50** Injury of cutaneous sensory nerve at shoulder and upper arm level, unspecified arm

√x7th **S44.51** Injury of cutaneous sensory nerve at shoulder and upper arm level, right arm

√x7th **S44.52** Injury of cutaneous sensory nerve at shoulder and upper arm level, left arm

√5th **S44.8** Injury of other nerves at shoulder and upper arm level

√6th **S44.8x** Injury of other nerves at shoulder and upper arm level

√7th **S44.8x1** Injury of other nerves at shoulder and upper arm level, right arm

√7th **S44.8x2** Injury of other nerves at shoulder and upper arm level, left arm

√7th **S44.8x9** Injury of other nerves at shoulder and upper arm level, unspecified arm

√5th **S44.9** Injury of unspecified nerve at shoulder and upper arm level

√x7th **S44.90** Injury of unspecified nerve at shoulder and upper arm level, unspecified arm

√x7th **S44.91** Injury of unspecified nerve at shoulder and upper arm level, right arm

√x7th **S44.92** Injury of unspecified nerve at shoulder and upper arm level, left arm

√4th **S45** **Injury of blood vessels at shoulder and upper arm level**

Code also any associated open wound (S41-)

> EXCLUDES 2   *injury of subclavian artery (S25.1)*
> *injury of subclavian vein (S25.3)*

> The appropriate 7th character is to be added to each code from category S45.
> A   initial encounter
> D   subsequent encounter
> S   sequela

√5th **S45.0** Injury of axillary artery

√6th **S45.00** Unspecified injury of axillary artery

√7th **S45.001** Unspecified injury of axillary artery, right side

√7th **S45.002** Unspecified injury of axillary artery, left side

√7th **S45.009** Unspecified injury of axillary artery, unspecified side

√6th **S45.01** Laceration of axillary artery

√7th **S45.011** Laceration of axillary artery, right side

√7th **S45.012** Laceration of axillary artery, left side

√7th **S45.019** Laceration of axillary artery, unspecified side

√6th **S45.09** Other specified injury of axillary artery

√7th **S45.091** Other specified injury of axillary artery, right side

√7th **S45.092** Other specified injury of axillary artery, left side

√7th **S45.099** Other specified injury of axillary artery, unspecified side

√5th **S45.1** Injury of brachial artery

√6th **S45.10** Unspecified injury of brachial artery

√7th **S45.101** Unspecified injury of brachial artery, right side

√7th **S45.102** Unspecified injury of brachial artery, left side

√7th **S45.109** Unspecified injury of brachial artery, unspecified side

√6th **S45.11** Laceration of brachial artery

√7th **S45.111** Laceration of brachial artery, right side

√7th **S45.112** Laceration of brachial artery, left side

√7th **S45.119** Laceration of brachial artery, unspecified side

√6th **S45.19** Other specified injury of brachial artery

√7th **S45.191** Other specified injury of brachial artery, right side

√7th **S45.192** Other specified injury of brachial artery, left side

√7th **S45.199** Other specified injury of brachial artery, unspecified side

√5th **S45.2** Injury of axillary or brachial vein

√6th **S45.20** Unspecified injury of axillary or brachial vein

√7th **S45.201** Unspecified injury of axillary or brachial vein, right side

√7th **S45.202** Unspecified injury of axillary or brachial vein, left side

√7th **S45.209** Unspecified injury of axillary or brachial vein, unspecified side

√6th **S45.21** Laceration of axillary or brachial vein

√7th **S45.211** Laceration of axillary or brachial vein, right side

√7th **S45.212** Laceration of axillary or brachial vein, left side

√7th **S45.219** Laceration of axillary or brachial vein, unspecified side

√6th **S45.29** Other specified injury of axillary or brachial vein

√7th **S45.291** Other specified injury of axillary or brachial vein, right side

√7th **S45.292** Other specified injury of axillary or brachial vein, left side

√7th **S45.299** Other specified injury of axillary or brachial vein, unspecified side

√5th **S45.3** Injury of superficial vein at shoulder and upper arm level

√6th **S45.30** Unspecified injury of superficial vein at shoulder and upper arm level

√7th **S45.301** Unspecified injury of superficial vein at shoulder and upper arm level, right arm

√7th **S45.302** Unspecified injury of superficial vein at shoulder and upper arm level, left arm

√7th **S45.309** Unspecified injury of superficial vein at shoulder and upper arm level, unspecified arm

√6th **S45.31** Laceration of superficial vein at shoulder and upper arm level

√7th **S45.311** Laceration of superficial vein at shoulder and upper arm level, right arm

√7th **S45.312** Laceration of superficial vein at shoulder and upper arm level, left arm

√7th **S45.319** Laceration of superficial vein at shoulder and upper arm level, unspecified arm

√6th **S45.39** Other specified injury of superficial vein at shoulder and upper arm level

√7th **S45.391** Other specified injury of superficial vein at shoulder and upper arm level, right arm

√7th **S45.392** Other specified injury of superficial vein at shoulder and upper arm level, left arm

√7th **S45.399** Other specified injury of superficial vein at shoulder and upper arm level, unspecified arm

---

EXCLUDES 1   Not coded here   EXCLUDES 2   Not included here   *Manifestation Code*

☑5ᵗʰ **S45.8** **Injury of other specified blood vessels at shoulder and upper arm level**

  ☑6ᵗʰ **S45.80** **Unspecified injury of other specified blood vessels at shoulder and upper arm level**

    ☑7ᵗʰ **S45.801** **Unspecified injury of other specified blood vessels at shoulder and upper arm level, right arm**

    ☑7ᵗʰ **S45.802** **Unspecified injury of other specified blood vessels at shoulder and upper arm level, left arm**

    ☑7ᵗʰ **S45.809** **Unspecified injury of other specified blood vessels at shoulder and upper arm level, unspecified arm**

  ☑6ᵗʰ **S45.81** **Laceration of other specified blood vessels at shoulder and upper arm level**

    ☑7ᵗʰ **S45.811** **Laceration of other specified blood vessels at shoulder and upper arm level, right arm**

    ☑7ᵗʰ **S45.812** **Laceration of other specified blood vessels at shoulder and upper arm level, left arm**

    ☑7ᵗʰ **S45.819** **Laceration of other specified blood vessels at shoulder and upper arm level, unspecified arm**

  ☑6ᵗʰ **S45.89** **Other specified injury of other specified blood vessels at shoulder and upper arm level**

    ☑7ᵗʰ **S45.891** **Other specified injury of other specified blood vessels at shoulder and upper arm level, right arm**

    ☑7ᵗʰ **S45.892** **Other specified injury of other specified blood vessels at shoulder and upper arm level, left arm**

    ☑7ᵗʰ **S45.899** **Other specified injury of other specified blood vessels at shoulder and upper arm level, unspecified arm**

☑5ᵗʰ **S45.9** **Injury of unspecified blood vessel at shoulder and upper arm level**

  ☑6ᵗʰ **S45.90** **Unspecified injury of unspecified blood vessel at shoulder and upper arm level**

    ☑7ᵗʰ **S45.901** **Unspecified injury of unspecified blood vessel at shoulder and upper arm level, right arm**

    ☑7ᵗʰ **S45.902** **Unspecified injury of unspecified blood vessel at shoulder and upper arm level, left arm**

    ☑7ᵗʰ **S45.909** **Unspecified injury of unspecified blood vessel at shoulder and upper arm level, unspecified arm**

  ☑6ᵗʰ **S45.91** **Laceration of unspecified blood vessel at shoulder and upper arm level**

    ☑7ᵗʰ **S45.911** **Laceration of unspecified blood vessel at shoulder and upper arm level, right arm**

    ☑7ᵗʰ **S45.912** **Laceration of unspecified blood vessel at shoulder and upper arm level, left arm**

    ☑7ᵗʰ **S45.919** **Laceration of unspecified blood vessel at shoulder and upper arm level, unspecified arm**

  ☑6ᵗʰ **S45.99** **Other specified injury of unspecified blood vessel at shoulder and upper arm level**

    ☑7ᵗʰ **S45.991** **Other specified injury of unspecified blood vessel at shoulder and upper arm level, right arm**

    ☑7ᵗʰ **S45.992** **Other specified injury of unspecified blood vessel at shoulder and upper arm level, left arm**

    ☑7ᵗʰ **S45.999** **Other specified injury of unspecified blood vessel at shoulder and upper arm level, unspecified arm**

☑4ᵗʰ **S46** **Injury of muscle, fascia and tendon at shoulder and upper arm level**

  Code also any associated open wound (S41-)

  EXCLUDES 2 *injury of muscle, fascia and tendon at elbow (S56-)*
    sprain of joints and ligaments of shoulder girdle (S43.9)

  The appropriate 7th character is to be added to each code from category S46.
  A   initial encounter
  D   subsequent encounter
  S   sequela

☑5ᵗʰ **S46.0** **Injury of muscle(s) and tendon(s) of the rotator cuff of shoulder**

  ☑6ᵗʰ **S46.00** **Unspecified injury of muscle(s) and tendon(s) of the rotator cuff of shoulder**

    ☑7ᵗʰ **S46.001** **Unspecified injury of muscle(s) and tendon(s) of the rotator cuff of right shoulder**

    ☑7ᵗʰ **S46.002** **Unspecified injury of muscle(s) and tendon(s) of the rotator cuff of left shoulder**

    ☑7ᵗʰ **S46.009** **Unspecified injury of muscle(s) and tendon(s) of the rotator cuff of unspecified shoulder**

  ☑6ᵗʰ **S46.01** **Strain of muscle(s) and tendon(s) of the rotator cuff of shoulder**

    ☑7ᵗʰ **S46.011** **Strain of muscle(s) and tendon(s) of the rotator cuff of right shoulder**

    ☑7ᵗʰ **S46.012** **Strain of muscle(s) and tendon(s) of the rotator cuff of left shoulder**

    ☑7ᵗʰ **S46.019** **Strain of muscle(s) and tendon(s) of the rotator cuff of unspecified shoulder**

  ☑6ᵗʰ **S46.02** **Laceration of muscle(s) and tendon(s) of the rotator cuff of shoulder**

    ☑7ᵗʰ **S46.021** **Laceration of muscle(s) and tendon(s) of the rotator cuff of right shoulder**

    ☑7ᵗʰ **S46.022** **Laceration of muscle(s) and tendon(s) of the rotator cuff of left shoulder**

    ☑7ᵗʰ **S46.029** **Laceration of muscle(s) and tendon(s) of the rotator cuff of unspecified shoulder**

  ☑6ᵗʰ **S46.09** **Other injury of muscle(s) and tendon(s) of the rotator cuff of shoulder**

    ☑7ᵗʰ **S46.091** **Other injury of muscle(s) and tendon(s) of the rotator cuff of right shoulder**

    ☑7ᵗʰ **S46.092** **Other injury of muscle(s) and tendon(s) of the rotator cuff of left shoulder**

    ☑7ᵗʰ **S46.099** **Other injury of muscle(s) and tendon(s) of the rotator cuff of unspecified shoulder**

☑5ᵗʰ **S46.1** **Injury of muscle, fascia and tendon of long head of biceps**

  ☑6ᵗʰ **S46.10** **Unspecified injury of muscle, fascia and tendon of long head of biceps**

    ☑7ᵗʰ **S46.101** **Unspecified injury of muscle, fascia and tendon of long head of biceps, right arm**

    ☑7ᵗʰ **S46.102** **Unspecified injury of muscle, fascia and tendon of long head of biceps, left arm**

    ☑7ᵗʰ **S46.109** **Unspecified injury of muscle, fascia and tendon of long head of biceps, unspecified arm**

  ☑6ᵗʰ **S46.11** **Strain of muscle, fascia and tendon of long head of biceps**

    ☑7ᵗʰ **S46.111** **Strain of muscle, fascia and tendon of long head of biceps, right arm**

    ☑7ᵗʰ **S46.112** **Strain of muscle, fascia and tendon of long head of biceps, left arm**

    ☑7ᵗʰ **S46.119** **Strain of muscle, fascia and tendon of long head of biceps, unspecified arm**

  ☑6ᵗʰ **S46.12** **Laceration of muscle, fascia and tendon of long head of biceps**

    ☑7ᵗʰ **S46.121** **Laceration of muscle, fascia and tendon of long head of biceps, right arm**

    ☑7ᵗʰ **S46.122** **Laceration of muscle, fascia and tendon of long head of biceps, left arm**

    ☑7ᵗʰ **S46.129** **Laceration of muscle, fascia and tendon of long head of biceps, unspecified arm**

√6th **S46.19** Other injury of muscle, fascia and tendon of long head of biceps
- √7th **S46.191** Other injury of muscle, fascia and tendon of long head of biceps, right arm
- √7th **S46.192** Other injury of muscle, fascia and tendon of long head of biceps, left arm
- √7th **S46.199** Other injury of muscle, fascia and tendon of long head of biceps, unspecified arm

√5th **S46.2** Injury of muscle, fascia and tendon of other parts of biceps
- √6th **S46.20** Unspecified injury of muscle, fascia and tendon of other parts of biceps
  - √7th **S46.201** Unspecified injury of muscle, fascia and tendon of other parts of biceps, right arm
  - √7th **S46.202** Unspecified injury of muscle, fascia and tendon of other parts of biceps, left arm
  - √7th **S46.209** Unspecified injury of muscle, fascia and tendon of other parts of biceps, unspecified arm
- √6th **S46.21** Strain of muscle, fascia and tendon of other parts of biceps
  - √7th **S46.211** Strain of muscle, fascia and tendon of other parts of biceps, right arm
  - √7th **S46.212** Strain of muscle, fascia and tendon of other parts of biceps, left arm
  - √7th **S46.219** Strain of muscle, fascia and tendon of other parts of biceps, unspecified arm
- √6th **S46.22** Laceration of muscle, fascia and tendon of other parts of biceps
  - √7th **S46.221** Laceration of muscle, fascia and tendon of other parts of biceps, right arm
  - √7th **S46.222** Laceration of muscle, fascia and tendon of other parts of biceps, left arm
  - √7th **S46.229** Laceration of muscle, fascia and tendon of other parts of biceps, unspecified arm
- √6th **S46.29** Other injury of muscle, fascia and tendon of other parts of biceps
  - √7th **S46.291** Other injury of muscle, fascia and tendon of other parts of biceps, right arm
  - √7th **S46.292** Other injury of muscle, fascia and tendon of other parts of biceps, left arm
  - √7th **S46.299** Other injury of muscle, fascia and tendon of other parts of biceps, unspecified arm

√5th **S46.3** Injury of muscle, fascia and tendon of triceps
- √6th **S46.30** Unspecified injury of muscle, fascia and tendon of triceps
  - √7th **S46.301** Unspecified injury of muscle, fascia and tendon of triceps, right arm
  - √7th **S46.302** Unspecified injury of muscle, fascia and tendon of triceps, left arm
  - √7th **S46.309** Unspecified injury of muscle, fascia and tendon of triceps, unspecified arm
- √6th **S46.31** Strain of muscle, fascia and tendon of triceps
  - √7th **S46.311** Strain of muscle, fascia and tendon of triceps, right arm
  - √7th **S46.312** Strain of muscle, fascia and tendon of triceps, left arm
  - √7th **S46.319** Strain of muscle, fascia and tendon of triceps, unspecified arm
- √6th **S46.32** Laceration of muscle, fascia and tendon of triceps
  - √7th **S46.321** Laceration of muscle, fascia and tendon of triceps, right arm
  - √7th **S46.322** Laceration of muscle, fascia and tendon of triceps, left arm
  - √7th **S46.329** Laceration of muscle, fascia and tendon of triceps, unspecified arm
- √6th **S46.39** Other injury of muscle, fascia and tendon of triceps
  - √7th **S46.391** Other injury of muscle, fascia and tendon of triceps, right arm
  - √7th **S46.392** Other injury of muscle, fascia and tendon of triceps, left arm
  - √7th **S46.399** Other injury of muscle, fascia and tendon of triceps, unspecified arm

√5th **S46.8** Injury of other muscles, fascia and tendons at shoulder and upper arm level
- √6th **S46.80** Unspecified injury of other muscles, fascia and tendons at shoulder and upper arm level
  - √7th **S46.801** Unspecified injury of other muscles, fascia and tendons at shoulder and upper arm level, right arm
  - √7th **S46.802** Unspecified injury of other muscles, fascia and tendons at shoulder and upper arm level, left arm
  - √7th **S46.809** Unspecified injury of other muscles, fascia and tendons at shoulder and upper arm level, unspecified arm
- √6th **S46.81** Strain of other muscles, fascia and tendons at shoulder and upper arm level
  - √7th **S46.811** Strain of other muscles, fascia and tendons at shoulder and upper arm level, right arm
  - √7th **S46.812** Strain of other muscles, fascia and tendons at shoulder and upper arm level, left arm
  - √7th **S46.819** Strain of other muscles, fascia and tendons at shoulder and upper arm level, unspecified arm
- √6th **S46.82** Laceration of other muscles, fascia and tendons at shoulder and upper arm level
  - √7th **S46.821** Laceration of other muscles, fascia and tendons at shoulder and upper arm level, right arm
  - √7th **S46.822** Laceration of other muscles, fascia and tendons at shoulder and upper arm level, left arm
  - √7th **S46.829** Laceration of other muscles, fascia and tendons at shoulder and upper arm level, unspecified arm
- √6th **S46.89** Other injury of other muscles, fascia and tendons at shoulder and upper arm level
  - √7th **S46.891** Other injury of other muscles, fascia and tendons at shoulder and upper arm level, right arm
  - √7th **S46.892** Other injury of other muscles, fascia and tendons at shoulder and upper arm level, left arm
  - √7th **S46.899** Other injury of other muscles, fascia and tendons at shoulder and upper arm level, unspecified arm

√5th **S46.9** Injury of unspecified muscle, fascia and tendon at shoulder and upper arm level
- √6th **S46.90** Unspecified injury of unspecified muscle, fascia and tendon at shoulder and upper arm level
  - √7th **S46.901** Unspecified injury of unspecified muscle, fascia and tendon at shoulder and upper arm level, right arm
  - √7th **S46.902** Unspecified injury of unspecified muscle, fascia and tendon at shoulder and upper arm level, left arm
  - √7th **S46.909** Unspecified injury of unspecified muscle, fascia and tendon at shoulder and upper arm level, unspecified arm
- √6th **S46.91** Strain of unspecified muscle, fascia and tendon at shoulder and upper arm level
  - √7th **S46.911** Strain of unspecified muscle, fascia and tendon at shoulder and upper arm level, right arm
  - √7th **S46.912** Strain of unspecified muscle, fascia and tendon at shoulder and upper arm level, left arm
  - √7th **S46.919** Strain of unspecified muscle, fascia and tendon at shoulder and upper arm level, unspecified arm
- √6th **S46.92** Laceration of unspecified muscle, fascia and tendon at shoulder and upper arm level
  - √7th **S46.921** Laceration of unspecified muscle, fascia and tendon at shoulder and upper arm level, right arm
  - √7th **S46.922** Laceration of unspecified muscle, fascia and tendon at shoulder and upper arm level, left arm

---

EXCLUDES 1 Not coded here   EXCLUDES 2 Not included here   *Manifestation Code*

☑7ᵗʰ **S46.929** Laceration of unspecified muscle, fascia and tendon at shoulder and upper arm level, unspecified arm

☑6ᵗʰ **S46.99** Other injury of unspecified muscle, fascia and tendon at shoulder and upper arm level

☑7ᵗʰ **S46.991** Other injury of unspecified muscle, fascia and tendon at shoulder and upper arm level, right arm

☑7ᵗʰ **S46.992** Other injury of unspecified muscle, fascia and tendon at shoulder and upper arm level, left arm

☑7ᵗʰ **S46.999** Other injury of unspecified muscle, fascia and tendon at shoulder and upper arm level, unspecified arm

☑4ᵗʰ **S47** **Crushing injury of shoulder and upper arm**

Use additional code for all associated injuries

EXCLUDES 2 *crushing injury of elbow (S57.0-)*

The appropriate 7th character is to be added to each code from category S47.
A   initial encounter
D   subsequent encounter
S   sequela

√x7ᵗʰ **S47.1** Crushing injury of right shoulder and upper arm
√x7ᵗʰ **S47.2** Crushing injury of left shoulder and upper arm
√x7ᵗʰ **S47.9** Crushing injury of shoulder and upper arm, unspecified arm

☑4ᵗʰ **S48** **Traumatic amputation of shoulder and upper arm**

NOTE   An amputation not identified as partial or complete should be coded to complete

EXCLUDES 1 *traumatic amputation at elbow level (S58.0)*

The appropriate 7th character is to be added to each code from category S48.
A   initial encounter
D   subsequent encounter
S   sequela

☑5ᵗʰ **S48.0** Traumatic amputation at shoulder joint

☑6ᵗʰ **S48.01** Complete traumatic amputation at shoulder joint

☑7ᵗʰ **S48.011** Complete traumatic amputation at right shoulder joint

☑7ᵗʰ **S48.012** Complete traumatic amputation at left shoulder joint

☑7ᵗʰ **S48.019** Complete traumatic amputation at unspecified shoulder joint

☑6ᵗʰ **S48.02** Partial traumatic amputation at shoulder joint

☑7ᵗʰ **S48.021** Partial traumatic amputation at right shoulder joint

☑7ᵗʰ **S48.022** Partial traumatic amputation at left shoulder joint

☑7ᵗʰ **S48.029** Partial traumatic amputation at unspecified shoulder joint

☑5ᵗʰ **S48.1** Traumatic amputation at level between shoulder and elbow

☑6ᵗʰ **S48.11** Complete traumatic amputation at level between shoulder and elbow

☑7ᵗʰ **S48.111** Complete traumatic amputation at level between right shoulder and elbow

☑7ᵗʰ **S48.112** Complete traumatic amputation at level between left shoulder and elbow

☑7ᵗʰ **S48.119** Complete traumatic amputation at level between unspecified shoulder and elbow

☑6ᵗʰ **S48.12** Partial traumatic amputation at level between shoulder and elbow

☑7ᵗʰ **S48.121** Partial traumatic amputation at level between right shoulder and elbow

☑7ᵗʰ **S48.122** Partial traumatic amputation at level between left shoulder and elbow

☑7ᵗʰ **S48.129** Partial traumatic amputation at level between unspecified shoulder and elbow

☑5ᵗʰ **S48.9** Traumatic amputation of shoulder and upper arm, level unspecified

☑6ᵗʰ **S48.91** Complete traumatic amputation of shoulder and upper arm, level unspecified

☑7ᵗʰ **S48.911** Complete traumatic amputation of right shoulder and upper arm, level unspecified

☑7ᵗʰ **S48.912** Complete traumatic amputation of left shoulder and upper arm, level unspecified

☑7ᵗʰ **S48.919** Complete traumatic amputation of unspecified shoulder and upper arm, level unspecified

☑6ᵗʰ **S48.92** Partial traumatic amputation of shoulder and upper arm, level unspecified

☑7ᵗʰ **S48.921** Partial traumatic amputation of right shoulder and upper arm, level unspecified

☑7ᵗʰ **S48.922** Partial traumatic amputation of left shoulder and upper arm, level unspecified

☑7ᵗʰ **S48.929** Partial traumatic amputation of unspecified shoulder and upper arm, level unspecified

☑4ᵗʰ **S49** **Other and unspecified injuries of shoulder and upper arm**

The appropriate 7th character is to be added to each code from subcategories S49.0 and S49.1.
A   initial encounter for closed fracture
D   subsequent encounter for fracture with routine healing
G   subsequent encounter for fracture with delayed healing
K   subsequent encounter for fracture with nonunion
P   subsequent encounter for fracture with malunion
S   sequela

☑5ᵗʰ **S49.0** Physeal fracture of upper end of humerus

☑6ᵗʰ **S49.00** Unspecified physeal fracture of upper end of humerus

☑7ᵗʰ **S49.001** Unspecified physeal fracture of upper end of humerus, right arm

☑7ᵗʰ **S49.002** Unspecified physeal fracture of upper end of humerus, left arm

☑7ᵗʰ **S49.009** Unspecified physeal fracture of upper end of humerus, unspecified arm

☑6ᵗʰ **S49.01** Salter-Harris Type I physeal fracture of upper end of humerus

☑7ᵗʰ **S49.011** Salter-Harris Type I physeal fracture of upper end of humerus, right arm

☑7ᵗʰ **S49.012** Salter-Harris Type I physeal fracture of upper end of humerus, left arm

☑7ᵗʰ **S49.019** Salter-Harris Type I physeal fracture of upper end of humerus, unspecified arm

☑6ᵗʰ **S49.02** Salter-Harris Type II physeal fracture of upper end of humerus

☑7ᵗʰ **S49.021** Salter-Harris Type II physeal fracture of upper end of humerus, right arm

☑7ᵗʰ **S49.022** Salter-Harris Type II physeal fracture of upper end of humerus, left arm

☑7ᵗʰ **S49.029** Salter-Harris Type II physeal fracture of upper end of humerus, unspecified arm

☑6ᵗʰ **S49.03** Salter-Harris Type III physeal fracture of upper end of humerus

☑7ᵗʰ **S49.031** Salter Harris Type III physeal fracture of upper end of humerus, right arm

☑7ᵗʰ **S49.032** Salter Harris Type III physeal fracture of upper end of humerus, left arm

☑7ᵗʰ **S49.039** Salter Harris Type III physeal fracture of upper end of humerus, unspecified arm

☑6ᵗʰ **S49.04** Salter-Harris Type IV physeal fracture of upper end of humerus

☑7ᵗʰ **S49.041** Salter-Harris Type IV physeal fracture of upper end of humerus, right arm

☑7ᵗʰ **S49.042** Salter-Harris Type IV physeal fracture of upper end of humerus, left arm

☑7ᵗʰ **S49.049** Salter-Harris Type IV physeal fracture of upper end of humerus, unspecified arm

☑6ᵗʰ **S49.09** Other physeal fracture of upper end of humerus

☑7ᵗʰ **S49.091** Other physeal fracture of upper end of humerus, right arm

☑7ᵗʰ **S49.092** Other physeal fracture of upper end of humerus, left arm

---

☑ Appropriate additional character required   √x7ᵗʰ Requires 7th character, placeholder x must fill empty characters

☑7ᵗʰ **S49.099 Other physeal fracture of upper end of humerus, unspecified arm**

☑5ᵗʰ **S49.1 Physeal fracture of lower end of humerus**

 ☑6ᵗʰ **S49.10 Unspecified physeal fracture of lower end of humerus**

  ☑7ᵗʰ **S49.101 Unspecified physeal fracture of lower end of humerus, right arm**

  ☑7ᵗʰ **S49.102 Unspecified physeal fracture of lower end of humerus, left arm**

  ☑7ᵗʰ **S49.109 Unspecified physeal fracture of lower end of humerus, unspecified arm**

 ☑6ᵗʰ **S49.11 Salter-Harris Type I physeal fracture of lower end of humerus**

  ☑7ᵗʰ **S49.111 Salter-Harris Type I physeal fracture of lower end of humerus, right arm**

  ☑7ᵗʰ **S49.112 Salter-Harris Type I physeal fracture of lower end of humerus, left arm**

  ☑7ᵗʰ **S49.119 Salter-Harris Type I physeal fracture of lower end of humerus, unspecified arm**

 ☑6ᵗʰ **S49.12 Salter-Harris Type II physeal fracture of lower end of humerus**

  ☑7ᵗʰ **S49.121 Salter-Harris Type II physeal fracture of lower end of humerus, right arm**

  ☑7ᵗʰ **S49.122 Salter-Harris Type II physeal fracture of lower end of humerus, left arm**

  ☑7ᵗʰ **S49.129 Salter-Harris Type II physeal fracture of lower end of humerus, unspecified arm**

 ☑6ᵗʰ **S49.13 Salter Harris Type III physeal fracture of lower end of humerus**

  ☑7ᵗʰ **S49.131 Salter Harris Type III physeal fracture of lower end of humerus, right arm**

  ☑7ᵗʰ **S49.132 Salter Harris Type III physeal fracture of lower end of humerus, left arm**

  ☑7ᵗʰ **S49.139 Salter Harris Type III physeal fracture of lower end of humerus, unspecified arm**

 ☑6ᵗʰ **S49.14 Salter-Harris Type IV physeal fracture of lower end of humerus**

  ☑7ᵗʰ **S49.141 Salter-Harris Type IV physeal fracture of lower end of humerus, right arm**

  ☑7ᵗʰ **S49.142 Salter-Harris Type IV physeal fracture of lower end of humerus, left arm**

  ☑7ᵗʰ **S49.149 Salter-Harris Type IV physeal fracture of lower end of humerus, unspecified arm**

 ☑6ᵗʰ **S49.19 Other physeal fracture of lower end of humerus**

  ☑7ᵗʰ **S49.191 Other physeal fracture of lower end of humerus, right arm**

  ☑7ᵗʰ **S49.192 Other physeal fracture of lower end of humerus, left arm**

  ☑7ᵗʰ **S49.199 Other physeal fracture of lower end of humerus, unspecified arm**

☑5ᵗʰ **S49.8 Other specified injuries of shoulder and upper arm**

The appropriate 7th character is to be added to each code from subcategories S49.8.
A   initial encounter
D   subsequent encounter
S   sequela

 ☑x7ᵗʰ **S49.80 Other specified injuries of shoulder and upper arm, unspecified arm**

 ☑x7ᵗʰ **S49.81 Other specified injuries of right shoulder and upper arm**

 ☑x7ᵗʰ **S49.82 Other specified injuries of left shoulder and upper arm**

☑5ᵗʰ **S49.9 Unspecified injury of shoulder and upper arm**

The appropriate 7th character is to be added to each code from subcategories S49.9.
A   initial encounter
D   subsequent encounter
S   sequela

 ☑x7ᵗʰ **S49.90 Unspecified injury of shoulder and upper arm, unspecified arm**

 ☑x7ᵗʰ **S49.91 Unspecified injury of right shoulder and upper arm**

 ☑x7ᵗʰ **S49.92 Unspecified injury of left shoulder and upper arm**

Injuries to the elbow and forearm (S50-S59)

EXCLUDES 2 *burns and corrosions (T20-T32)*
frostbite (T33-T34)
injuries of wrist and hand (S60-S69)
insect bite or sting, venomous (T63.4)

☑4ᵗʰ **S50 Superficial injury of elbow and forearm**

EXCLUDES 2 *superficial injury of wrist and hand (S60-)*

The appropriate 7th character is to be added to each code from category S50.
A   initial encounter
D   subsequent encounter
S   sequela

☑5ᵗʰ **S50.0 Contusion of elbow**

 ☑x7ᵗʰ **S50.00 Contusion of unspecified elbow**

 ☑x7ᵗʰ **S50.01 Contusion of right elbow**

 ☑x7ᵗʰ **S50.02 Contusion of left elbow**

☑5ᵗʰ **S50.1 Contusion of forearm**

 ☑x7ᵗʰ **S50.10 Contusion of unspecified forearm**

 ☑x7ᵗʰ **S50.11 Contusion of right forearm**

 ☑x7ᵗʰ **S50.12 Contusion of left forearm**

☑5ᵗʰ **S50.3 Other superficial injuries of elbow**

 ☑6ᵗʰ **S50.31 Abrasion of elbow**

  ☑7ᵗʰ **S50.311 Abrasion of right elbow**

  ☑7ᵗʰ **S50.312 Abrasion of left elbow**

  ☑7ᵗʰ **S50.319 Abrasion of unspecified elbow**

 ☑6ᵗʰ **S50.32 Blister (nonthermal) of elbow**

  ☑7ᵗʰ **S50.321 Blister (nonthermal) of right elbow**

  ☑7ᵗʰ **S50.322 Blister (nonthermal) of left elbow**

  ☑7ᵗʰ **S50.329 Blister (nonthermal) of unspecified elbow**

 ☑6ᵗʰ **S50.34 External constriction of elbow**

  ☑7ᵗʰ **S50.341 External constriction of right elbow**

  ☑7ᵗʰ **S50.342 External constriction of left elbow**

  ☑7ᵗʰ **S50.349 External constriction of unspecified elbow**

 ☑6ᵗʰ **S50.35 Superficial foreign body of elbow**
   Splinter in the elbow

  ☑7ᵗʰ **S50.351 Superficial foreign body of right elbow**

  ☑7ᵗʰ **S50.352 Superficial foreign body of left elbow**

  ☑7ᵗʰ **S50.359 Superficial foreign body of unspecified elbow**

 ☑6ᵗʰ **S50.36 Insect bite (nonvenomous) of elbow**

  ☑7ᵗʰ **S50.361 Insect bite (nonvenomous) of right elbow**

  ☑7ᵗʰ **S50.362 Insect bite (nonvenomous) of left elbow**

  ☑7ᵗʰ **S50.369 Insect bite (nonvenomous) of unspecified elbow**

 ☑6ᵗʰ **S50.37 Other superficial bite of elbow**

EXCLUDES 1 *open bite of elbow (S51.05)*

  ☑7ᵗʰ **S50.371 Other superficial bite of right elbow**

  ☑7ᵗʰ **S50.372 Other superficial bite of left elbow**

  ☑7ᵗʰ **S50.379 Other superficial bite of unspecified elbow**

☑5ᵗʰ **S50.8 Other superficial injuries of forearm**

 ☑6ᵗʰ **S50.81 Abrasion of forearm**

  ☑7ᵗʰ **S50.811 Abrasion of right forearm**

  ☑7ᵗʰ **S50.812 Abrasion of left forearm**

  ☑7ᵗʰ **S50.819 Abrasion of unspecified forearm**

 ☑6ᵗʰ **S50.82 Blister (nonthermal) of forearm**

  ☑7ᵗʰ **S50.821 Blister (nonthermal) of right forearm**

  ☑7ᵗʰ **S50.822 Blister (nonthermal) of left forearm**

  ☑7ᵗʰ **S50.829 Blister (nonthermal) of unspecified forearm**

 ☑6ᵗʰ **S50.84 External constriction of forearm**

  ☑7ᵗʰ **S50.841 External constriction of right forearm**

  ☑7ᵗʰ **S50.842 External constriction of left forearm**

  ☑7ᵗʰ **S50.849 External constriction of unspecified forearm**

 ☑6ᵗʰ **S50.85 Superficial foreign body of forearm**
   Splinter in the forearm

  ☑7ᵗʰ **S50.851 Superficial foreign body of right forearm**

  ☑7ᵗʰ **S50.852 Superficial foreign body of left forearm**

EXCLUDES 1 Not coded here   EXCLUDES 2 Not included here   *Manifestation Code*

✓7th **S50.859** Superficial foreign body of unspecified forearm

✓6th **S50.86** **Insect bite (nonvenomous) of forearm**
  ✓7th **S50.861** Insect bite (nonvenomous) of right forearm
  ✓7th **S50.862** Insect bite (nonvenomous) of left forearm
  ✓7th **S50.869** Insect bite (nonvenomous) of unspecified forearm

✓6th **S50.87** **Other superficial bite of forearm**
  EXCLUDES 1 *open bite of forearm (S51.85)*
  ✓7th **S50.871** Other superficial bite of right forearm
  ✓7th **S50.872** Other superficial bite of left forearm
  ✓7th **S50.879** Other superficial bite of unspecified forearm

✓5th **S50.9** **Unspecified superficial injury of elbow and forearm**
  ✓6th **S50.90** **Unspecified superficial injury of elbow**
    ✓7th **S50.901** Unspecified superficial injury of right elbow
    ✓7th **S50.902** Unspecified superficial injury of left elbow
    ✓7th **S50.909** Unspecified superficial injury of unspecified elbow
  ✓6th **S50.91** **Unspecified superficial injury of forearm**
    ✓7th **S50.911** Unspecified superficial injury of right forearm
    ✓7th **S50.912** Unspecified superficial injury of left forearm
    ✓7th **S50.919** Unspecified superficial injury of unspecified forearm

✓4th **S51** **Open wound of elbow and forearm**
  Code also any associated wound infection
  EXCLUDES 1 *open fracture of elbow and forearm (S52- with open fracture 7th character)*
  traumatic amputation of elbow and forearm (S58-)
  EXCLUDES 2 *open wound of wrist and hand (S61-)*

  The appropriate 7th character is to be added to each code from category S51.
  A   initial encounter
  D   subsequent encounter
  S   sequela

✓5th **S51.0** **Open wound of elbow**
  ✓6th **S51.00** **Unspecified open wound of elbow**
    ✓7th **S51.001** Unspecified open wound of right elbow
    ✓7th **S51.002** Unspecified open wound of left elbow
    ✓7th **S51.009** Unspecified open wound of unspecified elbow
      Open wound of elbow NOS
  ✓6th **S51.01** **Laceration without foreign body of elbow**
    ✓7th **S51.011** Laceration without foreign body of right elbow
    ✓7th **S51.012** Laceration without foreign body of left elbow
    ✓7th **S51.019** Laceration without foreign body of unspecified elbow
  ✓6th **S51.02** **Laceration with foreign body of elbow**
    ✓7th **S51.021** Laceration with foreign body of right elbow
    ✓7th **S51.022** Laceration with foreign body of left elbow
    ✓7th **S51.029** Laceration with foreign body of unspecified elbow
  ✓6th **S51.03** **Puncture wound without foreign body of elbow**
    ✓7th **S51.031** Puncture wound without foreign body of right elbow
    ✓7th **S51.032** Puncture wound without foreign body of left elbow
    ✓7th **S51.039** Puncture wound without foreign body of unspecified elbow
  ✓6th **S51.04** **Puncture wound with foreign body of elbow**
    ✓7th **S51.041** Puncture wound with foreign body of right elbow
    ✓7th **S51.042** Puncture wound with foreign body of left elbow

✓7th **S51.049** Puncture wound with foreign body of unspecified elbow
✓6th **S51.05** **Open bite of elbow**
  Bite of elbow NOS
  EXCLUDES 1 *superficial bite of elbow (S50.36, S50.37)*
  ✓7th **S51.051** Open bite, right elbow
  ✓7th **S51.052** Open bite, left elbow
  ✓7th **S51.059** Open bite, unspecified elbow

✓5th **S51.8** **Open wound of forearm**
  EXCLUDES 2 *open wound of elbow (S51.0-)*
  ✓6th **S51.80** **Unspecified open wound of forearm**
    ✓7th **S51.801** Unspecified open wound of right forearm
    ✓7th **S51.802** Unspecified open wound of left forearm
    ✓7th **S51.809** Unspecified open wound of unspecified forearm
      Open wound of forearm NOS
  ✓6th **S51.81** **Laceration without foreign body of forearm**
    ✓7th **S51.811** Laceration without foreign body of right forearm
    ✓7th **S51.812** Laceration without foreign body of left forearm
    ✓7th **S51.819** Laceration without foreign body of unspecified forearm
  ✓6th **S51.82** **Laceration with foreign body of forearm**
    ✓7th **S51.821** Laceration with foreign body of right forearm
    ✓7th **S51.822** Laceration with foreign body of left forearm
    ✓7th **S51.829** Laceration with foreign body of unspecified forearm
  ✓6th **S51.83** **Puncture wound without foreign body of forearm**
    ✓7th **S51.831** Puncture wound without foreign body of right forearm
    ✓7th **S51.832** Puncture wound without foreign body of left forearm
    ✓7th **S51.839** Puncture wound without foreign body of unspecified forearm
  ✓6th **S51.84** **Puncture wound with foreign body of forearm**
    ✓7th **S51.841** Puncture wound with foreign body of right forearm
    ✓7th **S51.842** Puncture wound with foreign body of left forearm
    ✓7th **S51.849** Puncture wound with foreign body of unspecified forearm
  ✓6th **S51.85** **Open bite of forearm**
    Bite of forearm NOS
    EXCLUDES 1 *superficial bite of forearm (S50.86, S50.87)*
    ✓7th **S51.851** Open bite of right forearm
    ✓7th **S51.852** Open bite of left forearm
    ✓7th **S51.859** Open bite of unspecified forearm

✓ Appropriate additional character required   ✓x7th Requires 7th character, placeholder x must fill empty characters

✓4ᵗʰ S52 Fracture of forearm

NOTE A fracture not indicated as displaced or nondisplaced should be coded to displaced

A fracture not indicated as open or closed should be coded to closed.

The open fracture designations are based on the Gustilo open fracture classification.

EXCLUDES 1 traumatic amputation of forearm (S58-)

EXCLUDES 2 fracture at wrist and hand level (S62-)

The appropriate 7th character is to be added to each code from category S52.

A   initial encounter for closed fracture
B   initial encounter for open fracture type I or II initial encounter for open fracture NOS
C   initial encounter for open fracture type IIIA, IIIB, or IIIC
D   subsequent encounter for closed fracture with routine healing
E   subsequent encounter for open fracture type I or II with routine healing
F   subsequent encounter for open fracture type IIIA, IIIB, or IIIC with routine healing
G   subsequent encounter for closed fracture with delayed healing
H   subsequent encounter for open fracture type I or II with delayed healing
J   subsequent encounter for open fracture type IIIA, IIIB, or IIIC with delayed healing
K   subsequent encounter for closed fracture with nonunion
M   subsequent encounter for open fracture type I or II with nonunion
N   subsequent encounter for open fracture type IIIA, IIIB, or IIIC with nonunion
P   subsequent encounter for closed fracture with malunion
Q   subsequent encounter for open fracture type I or II with malunion
R   subsequent encounter for open fracture type IIIA, IIIB, or IIIC with malunion
S   sequela

✓5ᵗʰ S52.0 Fracture of upper end of ulna
Fracture of proximal end of ulna

EXCLUDES 2 fracture of elbow NOS (S42.40-)
fractures of shaft of ulna (S52.2-)

✓6ᵗʰ S52.00 Unspecified fracture of upper end of ulna
- ✓7ᵗʰ S52.001 Unspecified fracture of upper end of right ulna
- ✓7ᵗʰ S52.002 Unspecified fracture of upper end of left ulna
- ✓7ᵗʰ S52.009 Unspecified fracture of upper end of unspecified ulna

✓6ᵗʰ S52.01 Torus fracture of upper end of ulna
NOTE Open fracture 7th characters do not apply to codes under subcategory S52.01
- ✓7ᵗʰ S52.011 Torus fracture of upper end of right ulna
- ✓7ᵗʰ S52.012 Torus fracture of upper end of left ulna
- ✓7ᵗʰ S52.019 Torus fracture of upper end of unspecified ulna

✓6ᵗʰ S52.02 Fracture of olecranon process without intraarticular extension of ulna
- ✓7ᵗʰ S52.021 Displaced fracture of olecranon process without intraarticular extension of right ulna
- ✓7ᵗʰ S52.022 Displaced fracture of olecranon process without intraarticular extension of left ulna
- ✓7ᵗʰ S52.023 Displaced fracture of olecranon process without intraarticular extension of unspecified ulna
- ✓7ᵗʰ S52.024 Nondisplaced fracture of olecranon process without intraarticular extension of right ulna
- ✓7ᵗʰ S52.025 Nondisplaced fracture of olecranon process without intraarticular extension of left ulna
- ✓7ᵗʰ S52.026 Nondisplaced fracture of olecranon process without intraarticular extension of unspecified ulna

✓6ᵗʰ S52.03 Fracture of olecranon process with intraarticular extension of ulna
- ✓7ᵗʰ S52.031 Displaced fracture of olecranon process with intraarticular extension of right ulna
- ✓7ᵗʰ S52.032 Displaced fracture of olecranon process with intraarticular extension of left ulna
- ✓7ᵗʰ S52.033 Displaced fracture of olecranon process with intraarticular extension of unspecified ulna
- ✓7ᵗʰ S52.034 Nondisplaced fracture of olecranon process with intraarticular extension of right ulna
- ✓7ᵗʰ S52.035 Nondisplaced fracture of olecranon process with intraarticular extension of left ulna
- ✓7ᵗʰ S52.036 Nondisplaced fracture of olecranon process with intraarticular extension of unspecified ulna

✓6ᵗʰ S52.04 Fracture of coronoid process of ulna
- ✓7ᵗʰ S52.041 Displaced fracture of coronoid process of right ulna
- ✓7ᵗʰ S52.042 Displaced fracture of coronoid process of left ulna
- ✓7ᵗʰ S52.043 Displaced fracture of coronoid process of unspecified ulna
- ✓7ᵗʰ S52.044 Nondisplaced fracture of coronoid process of right ulna
- ✓7ᵗʰ S52.045 Nondisplaced fracture of coronoid process of left ulna
- ✓7ᵗʰ S52.046 Nondisplaced fracture of coronoid process of unspecified ulna

✓6ᵗʰ S52.09 Other fracture of upper end of ulna
- ✓7ᵗʰ S52.091 Other fracture of upper end of right ulna
- ✓7ᵗʰ S52.092 Other fracture of upper end of left ulna
- ✓7ᵗʰ S52.099 Other fracture of upper end of unspecified ulna

✓5ᵗʰ S52.1 Fracture of upper end of radius
Fracture of proximal end of radius

EXCLUDES 2 physeal fractures of upper end of radius (S59.2-)
fracture of shaft of radius (S52.3-)

✓6ᵗʰ S52.10 Unspecified fracture of upper end of radius
- ✓7ᵗʰ S52.101 Unspecified fracture of upper end of right radius
- ✓7ᵗʰ S52.102 Unspecified fracture of upper end of left radius
- ✓7ᵗʰ S52.109 Unspecified fracture of upper end of unspecified radius

✓6ᵗʰ S52.11 Torus fracture of upper end of radius
NOTE Open fracture 7th characters do not apply to codes under subcategory S52.11
- ✓7ᵗʰ S52.111 Torus fracture of upper end of right radius
- ✓7ᵗʰ S52.112 Torus fracture of upper end of left radius
- ✓7ᵗʰ S52.119 Torus fracture of upper end of unspecified radius

✓6ᵗʰ S52.12 Fracture of head of radius
- ✓7ᵗʰ S52.121 Displaced fracture of head of right radius
- ✓7ᵗʰ S52.122 Displaced fracture of head of left radius
- ✓7ᵗʰ S52.123 Displaced fracture of head of unspecified radius
- ✓7ᵗʰ S52.124 Nondisplaced fracture of head of right radius
- ✓7ᵗʰ S52.125 Nondisplaced fracture of head of left radius
- ✓7ᵗʰ S52.126 Nondisplaced fracture of head of unspecified radius

✓6ᵗʰ S52.13 Fracture of neck of radius
- ✓7ᵗʰ S52.131 Displaced fracture of neck of right radius
- ✓7ᵗʰ S52.132 Displaced fracture of neck of left radius
- ✓7ᵗʰ S52.133 Displaced fracture of neck of unspecified radius
- ✓7ᵗʰ S52.134 Nondisplaced fracture of neck of right radius
- ✓7ᵗʰ S52.135 Nondisplaced fracture of neck of left radius

EXCLUDES 1 Not coded here   **EXCLUDES 2** Not included here   *Manifestation Code*

☑7th **S52.136** Nondisplaced fracture of neck of unspecified radius

☑6th **S52.18** **Other fracture of upper end of radius**

 ☑7th **S52.181** Other fracture of upper end of right radius

 ☑7th **S52.182** Other fracture of upper end of left radius

 ☑7th **S52.189** Other fracture of upper end of unspecified radius

☑5th **S52.2** **Fracture of shaft of ulna**

 ☑6th **S52.20** **Unspecified fracture of shaft of ulna**
  Fracture of ulna NOS

  ☑7th **S52.201** Unspecified fracture of shaft of right ulna

  ☑7th **S52.202** Unspecified fracture of shaft of left ulna

  ☑7th **S52.209** Unspecified fracture of shaft of unspecified ulna

 ☑6th **S52.21** **Greenstick fracture of shaft of ulna**

  ☑7th **S52.211** Greenstick fracture of shaft of right ulna

  ☑7th **S52.212** Greenstick fracture of shaft of left ulna

  ☑7th **S52.219** Greenstick fracture of shaft of unspecified ulna

 ☑6th **S52.22** **Transverse fracture of shaft of ulna**

  ☑7th **S52.221** Displaced transverse fracture of shaft of right ulna

  ☑7th **S52.222** Displaced transverse fracture of shaft of left ulna

  ☑7th **S52.223** Displaced transverse fracture of shaft of unspecified ulna

  ☑7th **S52.224** Nondisplaced transverse fracture of shaft of right ulna

  ☑7th **S52.225** Nondisplaced transverse fracture of shaft of left ulna

  ☑7th **S52.226** Nondisplaced transverse fracture of shaft of unspecified ulna

 ☑6th **S52.23** **Oblique fracture of shaft of ulna**

  ☑7th **S52.231** Displaced oblique fracture of shaft of right ulna

  ☑7th **S52.232** Displaced oblique fracture of shaft of left ulna

  ☑7th **S52.233** Displaced oblique fracture of shaft of unspecified ulna

  ☑7th **S52.234** Nondisplaced oblique fracture of shaft of right ulna

  ☑7th **S52.235** Nondisplaced oblique fracture of shaft of left ulna

  ☑7th **S52.236** Nondisplaced oblique fracture of shaft of unspecified ulna

 ☑6th **S52.24** **Spiral fracture of shaft of ulna**

  ☑7th **S52.241** Displaced spiral fracture of shaft of ulna, right arm

  ☑7th **S52.242** Displaced spiral fracture of shaft of ulna, left arm

  ☑7th **S52.243** Displaced spiral fracture of shaft of ulna, unspecified arm

  ☑7th **S52.244** Nondisplaced spiral fracture of shaft of ulna, right arm

  ☑7th **S52.245** Nondisplaced spiral fracture of shaft of ulna, left arm

  ☑7th **S52.246** Nondisplaced spiral fracture of shaft of ulna, unspecified arm

 ☑6th **S52.25** **Comminuted fracture of shaft of ulna**

  ☑7th **S52.251** Displaced comminuted fracture of shaft of ulna, right arm

  ☑7th **S52.252** Displaced comminuted fracture of shaft of ulna, left arm

  ☑7th **S52.253** Displaced comminuted fracture of shaft of ulna, unspecified arm

  ☑7th **S52.254** Nondisplaced comminuted fracture of shaft of ulna, right arm

  ☑7th **S52.255** Nondisplaced comminuted fracture of shaft of ulna, left arm

  ☑7th **S52.256** Nondisplaced comminuted fracture of shaft of ulna, unspecified arm

☑6th **S52.26** **Segmental fracture of shaft of ulna**

 ☑7th **S52.261** Displaced segmental fracture of shaft of ulna, right arm

 ☑7th **S52.262** Displaced segmental fracture of shaft of ulna, left arm

 ☑7th **S52.263** Displaced segmental fracture of shaft of ulna, unspecified arm

 ☑7th **S52.264** Nondisplaced segmental fracture of shaft of ulna, right arm

 ☑7th **S52.265** Nondisplaced segmental fracture of shaft of ulna, left arm

 ☑7th **S52.266** Nondisplaced segmental fracture of shaft of ulna, unspecified arm

☑6th **S52.27** **Monteggia's fracture of ulna**
 Fracture of upper shaft of ulna with dislocation of radial head

 ☑7th **S52.271** Monteggia's fracture of right ulna

 ☑7th **S52.272** Monteggia's fracture of left ulna

 ☑7th **S52.279** Monteggia's fracture of unspecified ulna

☑6th **S52.28** **Bent bone of ulna**

 ☑7th **S52.281** Bent bone of right ulna

 ☑7th **S52.282** Bent bone of left ulna

 ☑7th **S52.283** Bent bone of unspecified ulna

☑6th **S52.29** **Other fracture of shaft of ulna**

 ☑7th **S52.291** Other fracture of shaft of right ulna

 ☑7th **S52.292** Other fracture of shaft of left ulna

 ☑7th **S52.299** Other fracture of shaft of unspecified ulna

☑5th **S52.3** **Fracture of shaft of radius**

 ☑6th **S52.30** **Unspecified fracture of shaft of radius**

  ☑7th **S52.301** Unspecified fracture of shaft of right radius

  ☑7th **S52.302** Unspecified fracture of shaft of left radius

  ☑7th **S52.309** Unspecified fracture of shaft of unspecified radius

 ☑6th **S52.31** **Greenstick fracture of shaft of radius**

  ☑7th **S52.311** Greenstick fracture of shaft of radius, right arm

  ☑7th **S52.312** Greenstick fracture of shaft of radius, left arm

  ☑7th **S52.319** Greenstick fracture of shaft of radius, unspecified arm

 ☑6th **S52.32** **Transverse fracture of shaft of radius**

  ☑7th **S52.321** Displaced transverse fracture of shaft of right radius

  ☑7th **S52.322** Displaced transverse fracture of shaft of left radius

  ☑7th **S52.323** Displaced transverse fracture of shaft of unspecified radius

  ☑7th **S52.324** Nondisplaced transverse fracture of shaft of right radius

  ☑7th **S52.325** Nondisplaced transverse fracture of shaft of left radius

  ☑7th **S52.326** Nondisplaced transverse fracture of shaft of unspecified radius

 ☑6th **S52.33** **Oblique fracture of shaft of radius**

  ☑7th **S52.331** Displaced oblique fracture of shaft of right radius

  ☑7th **S52.332** Displaced oblique fracture of shaft of left radius

  ☑7th **S52.333** Displaced oblique fracture of shaft of unspecified radius

  ☑7th **S52.334** Nondisplaced oblique fracture of shaft of right radius

  ☑7th **S52.335** Nondisplaced oblique fracture of shaft of left radius

  ☑7th **S52.336** Nondisplaced oblique fracture of shaft of unspecified radius

 ☑6th **S52.34** **Spiral fracture of shaft of radius**

  ☑7th **S52.341** Displaced spiral fracture of shaft of radius, right arm

  ☑7th **S52.342** Displaced spiral fracture of shaft of radius, left arm

  ☑7th **S52.343** Displaced spiral fracture of shaft of radius, unspecified arm

---

☑ Appropriate additional character required ☑x7th Requires 7th character, placeholder x must fill empty characters

    ☑7ᵗʰ **S52.344** **Nondisplaced spiral fracture of shaft of radius, right arm**

    ☑7ᵗʰ **S52.345** **Nondisplaced spiral fracture of shaft of radius, left arm**

    ☑7ᵗʰ **S52.346** **Nondisplaced spiral fracture of shaft of radius, unspecified arm**

☑6ᵗʰ **S52.35** **Comminuted fracture of shaft of radius**

    ☑7ᵗʰ **S52.351** **Displaced comminuted fracture of shaft of radius, right arm**

    ☑7ᵗʰ **S52.352** **Displaced comminuted fracture of shaft of radius, left arm**

    ☑7ᵗʰ **S52.353** **Displaced comminuted fracture of shaft of radius, unspecified arm**

    ☑7ᵗʰ **S52.354** **Nondisplaced comminuted fracture of shaft of radius, right arm**

    ☑7ᵗʰ **S52.355** **Nondisplaced comminuted fracture of shaft of radius, left arm**

    ☑7ᵗʰ **S52.356** **Nondisplaced comminuted fracture of shaft of radius, unspecified arm**

☑6ᵗʰ **S52.36** **Segmental fracture of shaft of radius**

    ☑7ᵗʰ **S52.361** **Displaced segmental fracture of shaft of radius, right arm**

    ☑7ᵗʰ **S52.362** **Displaced segmental fracture of shaft of radius, left arm**

    ☑7ᵗʰ **S52.363** **Displaced segmental fracture of shaft of radius, unspecified arm**

    ☑7ᵗʰ **S52.364** **Nondisplaced segmental fracture of shaft of radius, right arm**

    ☑7ᵗʰ **S52.365** **Nondisplaced segmental fracture of shaft of radius, left arm**

    ☑7ᵗʰ **S52.366** **Nondisplaced segmental fracture of shaft of radius, unspecified arm**

☑6ᵗʰ **S52.37** **Galeazzi's fracture**
       Fracture of lower shaft of radius with radioulnar joint dislocation

    ☑7ᵗʰ **S52.371** **Galeazzi's fracture of right radius**

    ☑7ᵗʰ **S52.372** **Galeazzi's fracture of left radius**

    ☑7ᵗʰ **S52.379** **Galeazzi's fracture of unspecified radius**

☑6ᵗʰ **S52.38** **Bent bone of radius**

    ☑7ᵗʰ **S52.381** **Bent bone of right radius**

    ☑7ᵗʰ **S52.382** **Bent bone of left radius**

    ☑7ᵗʰ **S52.389** **Bent bone of unspecified radius**

☑6ᵗʰ **S52.39** **Other fracture of shaft of radius**

    ☑7ᵗʰ **S52.391** **Other fracture of shaft of radius, right arm**

    ☑7ᵗʰ **S52.392** **Other fracture of shaft of radius, left arm**

    ☑7ᵗʰ **S52.399** **Other fracture of shaft of radius, unspecified arm**

☑5ᵗʰ **S52.5** **Fracture of lower end of radius**
       Fracture of distal end of radius
       EXCLUDES 2 *physeal fractures of lower end of radius (S59.2-)*

☑6ᵗʰ **S52.50** **Unspecified fracture of the lower end of radius**

    ☑7ᵗʰ **S52.501** **Unspecified fracture of the lower end of right radius**

    ☑7ᵗʰ **S52.502** **Unspecified fracture of the lower end of left radius**

    ☑7ᵗʰ **S52.509** **Unspecified fracture of the lower end of unspecified radius**

☑6ᵗʰ **S52.51** **Fracture of radial styloid process**

    ☑7ᵗʰ **S52.511** **Displaced fracture of right radial styloid process**

    ☑7ᵗʰ **S52.512** **Displaced fracture of left radial styloid process**

    ☑7ᵗʰ **S52.513** **Displaced fracture of unspecified radial styloid process**

    ☑7ᵗʰ **S52.514** **Nondisplaced fracture of right radial styloid process**

    ☑7ᵗʰ **S52.515** **Nondisplaced fracture of left radial styloid process**

    ☑7ᵗʰ **S52.516** **Nondisplaced fracture of unspecified radial styloid process**

☑6ᵗʰ **S52.52** **Torus fracture of lower end of radius**

    ☑7ᵗʰ **S52.521** **Torus fracture of lower end of right radius**

    ☑7ᵗʰ **S52.522** **Torus fracture of lower end of left radius**

    ☑7ᵗʰ **S52.529** **Torus fracture of lower end of unspecified radius**

☑6ᵗʰ **S52.53** **Colles' fracture**

    ☑7ᵗʰ **S52.531** **Colles' fracture of right radius**

    ☑7ᵗʰ **S52.532** **Colles' fracture of left radius**

    ☑7ᵗʰ **S52.539** **Colles' fracture of unspecified radius**

☑6ᵗʰ **S52.54** **Smith's fracture**

    ☑7ᵗʰ **S52.541** **Smith's fracture of right radius**

    ☑7ᵗʰ **S52.542** **Smith's fracture of left radius**

    ☑7ᵗʰ **S52.549** **Smith's fracture of unspecified radius**

☑6ᵗʰ **S52.55** **Other extraarticular fracture of lower end of radius**

    ☑7ᵗʰ **S52.551** **Other extraarticular fracture of lower end of right radius**

    ☑7ᵗʰ **S52.552** **Other extraarticular fracture of lower end of left radius**

    ☑7ᵗʰ **S52.559** **Other extraarticular fracture of lower end of unspecified radius**

☑6ᵗʰ **S52.56** **Barton's fracture**

    ☑7ᵗʰ **S52.561** **Barton's fracture of right radius**

    ☑7ᵗʰ **S52.562** **Barton's fracture of left radius**

    ☑7ᵗʰ **S52.569** **Barton's fracture of unspecified radius**

☑6ᵗʰ **S52.57** **Other intraarticular fracture of lower end of radius**

    ☑7ᵗʰ **S52.571** **Other intraarticular fracture of lower end of right radius**

    ☑7ᵗʰ **S52.572** **Other intraarticular fracture of lower end of left radius**

    ☑7ᵗʰ **S52.579** **Other intraarticular fracture of lower end of unspecified radius**

☑6ᵗʰ **S52.59** **Other fractures of lower end of radius**

    ☑7ᵗʰ **S52.591** **Other fractures of lower end of right radius**

    ☑7ᵗʰ **S52.592** **Other fractures of lower end of left radius**

    ☑7ᵗʰ **S52.599** **Other fractures of lower end of unspecified radius**

☑5ᵗʰ **S52.6** **Fracture of lower end of ulna**

☑6ᵗʰ **S52.60** **Unspecified fracture of lower end of ulna**

    ☑7ᵗʰ **S52.601** **Unspecified fracture of lower end of right ulna**

    ☑7ᵗʰ **S52.602** **Unspecified fracture of lower end of left ulna**

    ☑7ᵗʰ **S52.609** **Unspecified fracture of lower end of unspecified ulna**

☑6ᵗʰ **S52.61** **Fracture of ulna styloid process**

    ☑7ᵗʰ **S52.611** **Displaced fracture of right ulna styloid process**

    ☑7ᵗʰ **S52.612** **Displaced fracture of left ulna styloid process**

    ☑7ᵗʰ **S52.613** **Displaced fracture of unspecified ulna styloid process**

    ☑7ᵗʰ **S52.614** **Nondisplaced fracture of right ulna styloid process**

    ☑7ᵗʰ **S52.615** **Nondisplaced fracture of left ulna styloid process**

    ☑7ᵗʰ **S52.616** **Nondisplaced fracture of unspecified ulna styloid process**

☑6ᵗʰ **S52.62** **Torus fracture of lower end of ulna**

    ☑7ᵗʰ **S52.621** **Torus fracture of lower end of right ulna**

    ☑7ᵗʰ **S52.622** **Torus fracture of lower end of left ulna**

    ☑7ᵗʰ **S52.629** **Torus fracture of lower end of unspecified ulna**

☑6ᵗʰ **S52.69** **Other fracture of lower end of ulna**

    ☑7ᵗʰ **S52.691** **Other fracture of lower end of right ulna**

    ☑7ᵗʰ **S52.692** **Other fracture of lower end of left ulna**

    ☑7ᵗʰ **S52.699** **Other fracture of lower end of unspecified ulna**

☑5ᵗʰ **S52.9** **Unspecified fracture of forearm**

    ☑x 7ᵗʰ **S52.90** **Unspecified fracture of unspecified forearm**

    ☑x 7ᵗʰ **S52.91** **Unspecified fracture of right forearm**

    ☑x 7ᵗʰ **S52.92** **Unspecified fracture of left forearm**

EXCLUDES 1 Not coded here   **EXCLUDES 2** Not included here   *Manifestation Code*

☑4ᵗʰ **S53   Dislocation and sprain of joints and ligaments of elbow**

INCLUDES   avulsion of joint or ligament of elbow
laceration of cartilage, joint or ligament of elbow
sprain of cartilage, joint or ligament of elbow
traumatic hemarthrosis of joint or ligament of elbow
traumatic rupture of joint or ligament of elbow
traumatic subluxation of joint or ligament of elbow
traumatic tear of joint or ligament of elbow

Code also any associated open wound

EXCLUDES 2   *strain of muscle, fascia and tendon at forearm level (S56-)*

> The appropriate 7th character is to be added to each code from category S53.
> A   initial encounter
> D   subsequent encounter
> S   sequela

☑5ᵗʰ **S53.0   Subluxation and dislocation of radial head**
Dislocation of radiohumeral joint
Subluxation of radiohumeral joint

EXCLUDES 1   *Monteggia's fracture-dislocation (S52.27-)*

☑6ᵗʰ **S53.00   Unspecified subluxation and dislocation of radial head**

☑7ᵗʰ **S53.001   Unspecified subluxation of right radial head**
☑7ᵗʰ **S53.002   Unspecified subluxation of left radial head**
☑7ᵗʰ **S53.003   Unspecified subluxation of unspecified radial head**
☑7ᵗʰ **S53.004   Unspecified dislocation of right radial head**
☑7ᵗʰ **S53.005   Unspecified dislocation of left radial head**
☑7ᵗʰ **S53.006   Unspecified dislocation of unspecified radial head**

☑6ᵗʰ **S53.01   Anterior subluxation and dislocation of radial head**
Anteriomedial subluxation and dislocation of radial head

☑7ᵗʰ **S53.011   Anterior subluxation of right radial head**
☑7ᵗʰ **S53.012   Anterior subluxation of left radial head**
☑7ᵗʰ **S53.013   Anterior subluxation of unspecified radial head**
☑7ᵗʰ **S53.014   Anterior dislocation of right radial head**
☑7ᵗʰ **S53.015   Anterior dislocation of left radial head**
☑7ᵗʰ **S53.016   Anterior dislocation of unspecified radial head**

☑6ᵗʰ **S53.02   Posterior subluxation and dislocation of radial head**
Posteriolateral subluxation and dislocation of radial head

☑7ᵗʰ **S53.021   Posterior subluxation of right radial head**
☑7ᵗʰ **S53.022   Posterior subluxation of left radial head**
☑7ᵗʰ **S53.023   Posterior subluxation of unspecified radial head**
☑7ᵗʰ **S53.024   Posterior dislocation of right radial head**
☑7ᵗʰ **S53.025   Posterior dislocation of left radial head**
☑7ᵗʰ **S53.026   Posterior dislocation of unspecified radial head**

☑6ᵗʰ **S53.03   Nursemaid's elbow**
☑7ᵗʰ **S53.031   Nursemaid's elbow, right elbow**
☑7ᵗʰ **S53.032   Nursemaid's elbow, left elbow**
☑7ᵗʰ **S53.033   Nursemaid's elbow, unspecified elbow**

☑6ᵗʰ **S53.09   Other subluxation and dislocation of radial head**
☑7ᵗʰ **S53.091   Other subluxation of right radial head**
☑7ᵗʰ **S53.092   Other subluxation of left radial head**
☑7ᵗʰ **S53.093   Other subluxation of unspecified radial head**
☑7ᵗʰ **S53.094   Other dislocation of right radial head**
☑7ᵗʰ **S53.095   Other dislocation of left radial head**
☑7ᵗʰ **S53.096   Other dislocation of unspecified radial head**

☑5ᵗʰ **S53.1   Subluxation and dislocation of ulnohumeral joint**
Subluxation and dislocation of elbow NOS

EXCLUDES 1   *dislocation of radial head alone (S53.0-)*

☑6ᵗʰ **S53.10   Unspecified subluxation and dislocation of ulnohumeral joint**

☑7ᵗʰ **S53.101   Unspecified subluxation of right ulnohumeral joint**
☑7ᵗʰ **S53.102   Unspecified subluxation of left ulnohumeral joint**
☑7ᵗʰ **S53.103   Unspecified subluxation of unspecified ulnohumeral joint**
☑7ᵗʰ **S53.104   Unspecified dislocation of right ulnohumeral joint**
☑7ᵗʰ **S53.105   Unspecified dislocation of left ulnohumeral joint**
☑7ᵗʰ **S53.106   Unspecified dislocation of unspecified ulnohumeral joint**

☑6ᵗʰ **S53.11   Anterior subluxation and dislocation of ulnohumeral joint**

☑7ᵗʰ **S53.111   Anterior subluxation of right ulnohumeral joint**
☑7ᵗʰ **S53.112   Anterior subluxation of left ulnohumeral joint**
☑7ᵗʰ **S53.113   Anterior subluxation of unspecified ulnohumeral joint**
☑7ᵗʰ **S53.114   Anterior dislocation of right ulnohumeral joint**
☑7ᵗʰ **S53.115   Anterior dislocation of left ulnohumeral joint**
☑7ᵗʰ **S53.116   Anterior dislocation of unspecified ulnohumeral joint**

☑6ᵗʰ **S53.12   Posterior subluxation and dislocation of ulnohumeral joint**

☑7ᵗʰ **S53.121   Posterior subluxation of right ulnohumeral joint**
☑7ᵗʰ **S53.122   Posterior subluxation of left ulnohumeral joint**
☑7ᵗʰ **S53.123   Posterior subluxation of unspecified ulnohumeral joint**
☑7ᵗʰ **S53.124   Posterior dislocation of right ulnohumeral joint**
☑7ᵗʰ **S53.125   Posterior dislocation of left ulnohumeral joint**
☑7ᵗʰ **S53.126   Posterior dislocation of unspecified ulnohumeral joint**

☑6ᵗʰ **S53.13   Medial subluxation and dislocation of ulnohumeral joint**

☑7ᵗʰ **S53.131   Medial subluxation of right ulnohumeral joint**
☑7ᵗʰ **S53.132   Medial subluxation of left ulnohumeral joint**
☑7ᵗʰ **S53.133   Medial subluxation of unspecified ulnohumeral joint**
☑7ᵗʰ **S53.134   Medial dislocation of right ulnohumeral joint**
☑7ᵗʰ **S53.135   Medial dislocation of left ulnohumeral joint**
☑7ᵗʰ **S53.136   Medial dislocation of unspecified ulnohumeral joint**

☑6ᵗʰ **S53.14   Lateral subluxation and dislocation of ulnohumeral joint**

☑7ᵗʰ **S53.141   Lateral subluxation of right ulnohumeral joint**
☑7ᵗʰ **S53.142   Lateral subluxation of left ulnohumeral joint**
☑7ᵗʰ **S53.143   Lateral subluxation of unspecified ulnohumeral joint**
☑7ᵗʰ **S53.144   Lateral dislocation of right ulnohumeral joint**
☑7ᵗʰ **S53.145   Lateral dislocation of left ulnohumeral joint**
☑7ᵗʰ **S53.146   Lateral dislocation of unspecified ulnohumeral joint**

☑6ᵗʰ **S53.19   Other subluxation and dislocation of ulnohumeral joint**

☑7ᵗʰ **S53.191   Other subluxation of right ulnohumeral joint**

☑ Appropriate additional character required   ☑x7ᵗʰ Requires 7th character, placeholder x must fill empty characters

✓7th **S53.192 Other subluxation of left ulnohumeral joint**

✓7th **S53.193 Other subluxation of unspecified ulnohumeral joint**

✓7th **S53.194 Other dislocation of right ulnohumeral joint**

✓7th **S53.195 Other dislocation of left ulnohumeral joint**

✓7th **S53.196 Other dislocation of unspecified ulnohumeral joint**

✓5th **S53.2 Traumatic rupture of radial collateral ligament**

> EXCLUDES 1 *sprain of radial collateral ligament NOS (S53.43-)*

✓x7th **S53.20 Traumatic rupture of unspecified radial collateral ligament**

✓x7th **S53.21 Traumatic rupture of right radial collateral ligament**

✓x7th **S53.22 Traumatic rupture of left radial collateral ligament**

✓5th **S53.3 Traumatic rupture of ulnar collateral ligament**

> EXCLUDES 1 *sprain of ulnar collateral ligament (S53.44-)*

✓x7th **S53.30 Traumatic rupture of unspecified ulnar collateral ligament**

✓x7th **S53.31 Traumatic rupture of right ulnar collateral ligament**

✓x7th **S53.32 Traumatic rupture of left ulnar collateral ligament**

✓5th **S53.4 Sprain of elbow**

> EXCLUDES 2 *traumatic rupture of radial collateral ligament (S53.2-)*
>
> *traumatic rupture of ulnar collateral ligament (S53.3-)*

✓6th **S53.40 Unspecified sprain of elbow**

✓7th **S53.401 Unspecified sprain of right elbow**

✓7th **S53.402 Unspecified sprain of left elbow**

✓7th **S53.409 Unspecified sprain of unspecified elbow**
Sprain of elbow NOS

✓6th **S53.41 Radiohumeral (joint) sprain**

✓7th **S53.411 Radiohumeral (joint) sprain of right elbow**

✓7th **S53.412 Radiohumeral (joint) sprain of left elbow**

✓7th **S53.419 Radiohumeral (joint) sprain of unspecified elbow**

✓6th **S53.42 Ulnohumeral (joint) sprain**

✓7th **S53.421 Ulnohumeral (joint) sprain of right elbow**

✓7th **S53.422 Ulnohumeral (joint) sprain of left elbow**

✓7th **S53.429 Ulnohumeral (joint) sprain of unspecified elbow**

✓6th **S53.43 Radial collateral ligament sprain**

✓7th **S53.431 Radial collateral ligament sprain of right elbow**

✓7th **S53.432 Radial collateral ligament sprain of left elbow**

✓7th **S53.439 Radial collateral ligament sprain of unspecified elbow**

✓6th **S53.44 Ulnar collateral ligament sprain**

✓7th **S53.441 Ulnar collateral ligament sprain of right elbow**

✓7th **S53.442 Ulnar collateral ligament sprain of left elbow**

✓7th **S53.449 Ulnar collateral ligament sprain of unspecified elbow**

✓6th **S53.49 Other sprain of elbow**

✓7th **S53.491 Other sprain of right elbow**

✓7th **S53.492 Other sprain of left elbow**

✓7th **S53.499 Other sprain of unspecified elbow**

✓4th **S54 Injury of nerves at forearm level**

Code also any associated open wound (S51-)

> EXCLUDES 2 *injury of nerves at wrist and hand level (S64-)*

> The appropriate 7th character is to be added to each code from category S54.
> A initial encounter
> D subsequent encounter
> S sequela

✓5th **S54.0 Injury of ulnar nerve at forearm level**
Injury of ulnar nerve NOS

✓x7th **S54.00 Injury of ulnar nerve at forearm level, unspecified arm**

✓x7th **S54.01 Injury of ulnar nerve at forearm level, right arm**

✓x7th **S54.02 Injury of ulnar nerve at forearm level, left arm**

✓5th **S54.1 Injury of median nerve at forearm level**
Injury of median nerve NOS

✓x7th **S54.10 Injury of median nerve at forearm level, unspecified arm**

✓x7th **S54.11 Injury of median nerve at forearm level, right arm**

✓x7th **S54.12 Injury of median nerve at forearm level, left arm**

✓5th **S54.2 Injury of radial nerve at forearm level**
Injury of radial nerve NOS

✓x7th **S54.20 Injury of radial nerve at forearm level, unspecified arm**

✓x7th **S54.21 Injury of radial nerve at forearm level, right arm**

✓x7th **S54.22 Injury of radial nerve at forearm level, left arm**

✓5th **S54.3 Injury of cutaneous sensory nerve at forearm level**

✓x7th **S54.30 Injury of cutaneous sensory nerve at forearm level, unspecified arm**

✓x7th **S54.31 Injury of cutaneous sensory nerve at forearm level, right arm**

✓x7th **S54.32 Injury of cutaneous sensory nerve at forearm level, left arm**

✓5th **S54.8 Injury of other nerves at forearm level**

✓6th **S54.8x Injury of other nerves at forearm level**

✓7th **S54.8x1 Unspecified injury of other nerves at forearm level, right ar**

✓7th **S54.8x2 Unspecified injury of other nerves at forearm level, left arm**

✓7th **S54.8x9 Unspecified injury of other nerves at forearm level, unspecified arm**

✓5th **S54.9 Injury of unspecified nerve at forearm level**

✓x7th **S54.90 Injury of unspecified nerve at forearm level, unspecified arm**

✓x7th **S54.91 Injury of unspecified nerve at forearm level, right arm**

✓x7th **S54.92 Injury of unspecified nerve at forearm level, left arm**

✓4th **S55 Injury of blood vessels at forearm level**

Code also any associated open wound (S51-)

> EXCLUDES 2 *injury of blood vessels at wrist and hand level (S65-)*
> *injury of brachial vessels (S45.1-S45.2)*

> The appropriate 7th character is to be added to each code from category S55.
> A initial encounter
> D subsequent encounter
> S sequela

✓5th **S55.0 Injury of ulnar artery at forearm level**

✓6th **S55.00 Unspecified injury of ulnar artery at forearm level**

✓7th **S55.001 Unspecified injury of ulnar artery at forearm level, right arm**

✓7th **S55.002 Unspecified injury of ulnar artery at forearm level, left arm**

✓7th **S55.009 Unspecified injury of ulnar artery at forearm level, unspecified arm**

✓6th **S55.01 Laceration of ulnar artery at forearm level**

✓7th **S55.011 Laceration of ulnar artery at forearm level, right arm**

✓7th **S55.012 Laceration of ulnar artery at forearm level, left arm**

✓7th **S55.019 Laceration of ulnar artery at forearm level, unspecified arm**

EXCLUDES 1 Not coded here   EXCLUDES 2 Not included here   *Manifestation Code*

☑6ᵗʰ **S55.09** **Other specified injury of ulnar artery at forearm level**
  ☑7ᵗʰ S55.091 Other specified injury of ulnar artery at forearm level, right arm
  ☑7ᵗʰ S55.092 Other specified injury of ulnar artery at forearm level, left arm
  ☑7ᵗʰ S55.099 Other specified injury of ulnar artery at forearm level, unspecified arm
☑5ᵗʰ **S55.1** **Injury of radial artery at forearm level**
  ☑6ᵗʰ **S55.10** **Unspecified injury of radial artery at forearm level**
    ☑7ᵗʰ S55.101 Unspecified injury of radial artery at forearm level, right arm
    ☑7ᵗʰ S55.102 Unspecified injury of radial artery at forearm level, left arm
    ☑7ᵗʰ S55.109 Unspecified injury of radial artery at forearm level, unspecified arm
  ☑6ᵗʰ **S55.11** **Laceration of radial artery at forearm level**
    ☑7ᵗʰ S55.111 Laceration of radial artery at forearm level, right arm
    ☑7ᵗʰ S55.112 Laceration of radial artery at forearm level, left arm
    ☑7ᵗʰ S55.119 Laceration of radial artery at forearm level, unspecified arm
  ☑6ᵗʰ **S55.19** **Other specified injury of radial artery at forearm level**
    ☑7ᵗʰ S55.191 Other specified injury of radial artery at forearm level, right arm
    ☑7ᵗʰ S55.192 Other specified injury of radial artery at forearm level, left arm
    ☑7ᵗʰ S55.199 Other specified injury of radial artery at forearm level, unspecified arm
☑5ᵗʰ **S55.2** **Injury of vein at forearm level**
  ☑6ᵗʰ **S55.20** **Unspecified injury of vein at forearm level**
    ☑7ᵗʰ S55.201 Unspecified injury of vein at forearm level, right arm
    ☑7ᵗʰ S55.202 Unspecified injury of vein at forearm level, left arm
    ☑7ᵗʰ S55.209 Unspecified injury of vein at forearm level, unspecified arm
  ☑6ᵗʰ **S55.21** **Laceration of vein at forearm level**
    ☑7ᵗʰ S55.211 Laceration of vein at forearm level, right arm
    ☑7ᵗʰ S55.212 Laceration of vein at forearm level, left arm
    ☑7ᵗʰ S55.219 Laceration of vein at forearm level, unspecified arm
  ☑6ᵗʰ **S55.29** **Other specified injury of vein at forearm level**
    ☑7ᵗʰ S55.291 Other specified injury of vein at forearm level, right arm
    ☑7ᵗʰ S55.292 Other specified injury of vein at forearm level, left arm
    ☑7ᵗʰ S55.299 Other specified injury of vein at forearm level, unspecified arm
☑5ᵗʰ **S55.8** **Injury of other blood vessels at forearm level**
  ☑6ᵗʰ **S55.80** **Unspecified injury of other blood vessels at forearm level**
    ☑7ᵗʰ S55.801 Unspecified injury of other blood vessels at forearm level, right arm
    ☑7ᵗʰ S55.802 Unspecified injury of other blood vessels at forearm level, left arm
    ☑7ᵗʰ S55.809 Unspecified injury of other blood vessels at forearm level, unspecified arm
  ☑6ᵗʰ **S55.81** **Laceration of other blood vessels at forearm level**
    ☑7ᵗʰ S55.811 Laceration of other blood vessels at forearm level, right arm
    ☑7ᵗʰ S55.812 Laceration of other blood vessels at forearm level, left arm
    ☑7ᵗʰ S55.819 Laceration of other blood vessels at forearm level, unspecified arm
  ☑6ᵗʰ **S55.89** **Other specified injury of other blood vessels at forearm level**
    ☑7ᵗʰ S55.891 Other specified injury of other blood vessels at forearm level, right arm
    ☑7ᵗʰ S55.892 Other specified injury of other blood vessels at forearm level, left arm

    ☑7ᵗʰ S55.899 Other specified injury of other blood vessels at forearm level, unspecified arm
☑5ᵗʰ **S55.9** **Injury of unspecified blood vessel at forearm level**
  ☑6ᵗʰ **S55.90** **Unspecified injury of unspecified blood vessel at forearm level**
    ☑7ᵗʰ S55.901 Unspecified injury of unspecified blood vessel at forearm level, right arm
    ☑7ᵗʰ S55.902 Unspecified injury of unspecified blood vessel at forearm level, left arm
    ☑7ᵗʰ S55.909 Unspecified injury of unspecified blood vessel at forearm level, unspecified arm
  ☑6ᵗʰ **S55.91** **Laceration of unspecified blood vessel at forearm level**
    ☑7ᵗʰ S55.911 Laceration of unspecified blood vessel at forearm level, right arm
    ☑7ᵗʰ S55.912 Laceration of unspecified blood vessel at forearm level, left arm
    ☑7ᵗʰ S55.919 Laceration of unspecified blood vessel at forearm level, unspecified arm
  ☑6ᵗʰ **S55.99** **Other specified injury of unspecified blood vessel at forearm level**
    ☑7ᵗʰ S55.991 Other specified injury of unspecified blood vessel at forearm level, right arm
    ☑7ᵗʰ S55.992 Other specified injury of unspecified blood vessel at forearm level, left arm
    ☑7ᵗʰ S55.999 Other specified injury of unspecified blood vessel at forearm level, unspecified arm

☑4ᵗʰ **S56** **Injury of muscle, fascia and tendon at forearm level**
Code also any associated open wound (S51-)
EXCLUDES 2 *injury of muscle, fascia and tendon at or below wrist (S66-)*
sprain of joints and ligaments of elbow (S53.4-)

> The appropriate 7th character is to be added to each code from category S56.
> A initial encounter
> D subsequent encounter
> S sequela

☑5ᵗʰ **S56.0** **Injury of flexor muscle, fascia and tendon of thumb at forearm level**
  ☑6ᵗʰ **S56.00** **Unspecified injury of flexor muscle, fascia and tendon of thumb at forearm level**
    ☑7ᵗʰ S56.001 Unspecified injury of flexor muscle, fascia and tendon of right thumb at forearm level
    ☑7ᵗʰ S56.002 Unspecified injury of flexor muscle, fascia and tendon of left thumb at forearm level
    ☑7ᵗʰ S56.009 Unspecified injury of flexor muscle, fascia and tendon of unspecified thumb at forearm level
  ☑6ᵗʰ **S56.01** **Strain of flexor muscle, fascia and tendon of thumb at forearm level**
    ☑7ᵗʰ S56.011 Strain of flexor muscle, fascia and tendon of right thumb at forearm level
    ☑7ᵗʰ S56.012 Strain of flexor muscle, fascia and tendon of left thumb at forearm level
    ☑7ᵗʰ S56.019 Strain of flexor muscle, fascia and tendon of unspecified thumb at forearm level
  ☑6ᵗʰ **S56.02** **Laceration of flexor muscle, fascia and tendon of thumb at forearm level**
    ☑7ᵗʰ S56.021 Laceration of flexor muscle, fascia and tendon of right thumb at forearm level
    ☑7ᵗʰ S56.022 Laceration of flexor muscle, fascia and tendon of left thumb at forearm level
    ☑7ᵗʰ S56.029 Laceration of flexor muscle, fascia and tendon of unspecified thumb at forearm level
  ☑6ᵗʰ **S56.09** **Other injury of flexor muscle, fascia and tendon of thumb at forearm level**
    ☑7ᵗʰ S56.091 Other injury of flexor muscle, fascia and tendon of right thumb at forearm level
    ☑7ᵗʰ S56.092 Other injury of flexor muscle, fascia and tendon of left thumb at forearm level

---

☑ Appropriate additional character required   ☑x7ᵗʰ Requires 7th character, placeholder x must fill empty characters

✓7th **S56.099** Other injury of flexor muscle, fascia and tendon of unspecified thumb at forearm level

✓5th **S56.1** Injury of flexor muscle, fascia and tendon of other and unspecified finger at forearm level

✓6th **S56.10** Unspecified injury of flexor muscle, fascia and tendon of other and unspecified finger at forearm level

✓7th **S56.101** Unspecified injury of flexor muscle, fascia and tendon of right index finger at forearm level

✓7th **S56.102** Unspecified injury of flexor muscle, fascia and tendon of left index finger at forearm level

✓7th **S56.103** Unspecified injury of flexor muscle, fascia and tendon of right middle finger at forearm level

✓7th **S56.104** Unspecified injury of flexor muscle, fascia and tendon of left middle finger at forearm level

✓7th **S56.105** Unspecified injury of flexor muscle, fascia and tendon of right ring finger at forearm level

✓7th **S56.106** Unspecified injury of flexor muscle, fascia and tendon of left ring finger at forearm level

✓7th **S56.107** Unspecified injury of flexor muscle, fascia and tendon of right little finger at forearm level

✓7th **S56.108** Unspecified injury of flexor muscle, fascia and tendon of left little finger at forearm level

✓7th **S56.109** Unspecified injury of flexor muscle, fascia and tendon of unspecified finger at forearm level

✓6th **S56.11** Strain of flexor muscle, fascia and tendon of other and unspecified finger at forearm level

✓7th **S56.111** Strain of flexor muscle, fascia and tendon of right index finger at forearm level

✓7th **S56.112** Strain of flexor muscle, fascia and tendon of left index finger at forearm level

✓7th **S56.113** Strain of flexor muscle, fascia and tendon of right middle finger at forearm level

✓7th **S56.114** Strain of flexor muscle, fascia and tendon of left middle finger at forearm level

✓7th **S56.115** Strain of flexor muscle, fascia and tendon of right ring finger at forearm level

✓7th **S56.116** Strain of flexor muscle, fascia and tendon of left ring finger at forearm level

✓7th **S56.117** Strain of flexor muscle, fascia and tendon of right little finger at forearm level

✓7th **S56.118** Strain of flexor muscle, fascia and tendon of left little finger at forearm level

✓7th **S56.119** Strain of flexor muscle, fascia and tendon of finger of unspecified finger at forearm level

✓6th **S56.12** Laceration of flexor muscle, fascia and tendon of other and unspecified finger at forearm level

✓7th **S56.121** Laceration of flexor muscle, fascia and tendon of right index finger at forearm level

✓7th **S56.122** Laceration of flexor muscle, fascia and tendon of left index finger at forearm level

✓7th **S56.123** Laceration of flexor muscle, fascia and tendon of right middle finger at forearm level

✓7th **S56.124** Laceration of flexor muscle, fascia and tendon of left middle finger at forearm level

✓7th **S56.125** Laceration of flexor muscle, fascia and tendon of right ring finger at forearm level

✓7th **S56.126** Laceration of flexor muscle, fascia and tendon of left ring finger at forearm level

✓7th **S56.127** Laceration of flexor muscle, fascia and tendon of right little finger at forearm level

✓7th **S56.128** Laceration of flexor muscle, fascia and tendon of left little finger at forearm level

✓7th **S56.129** Laceration of flexor muscle, fascia and tendon of unspecified finger at forearm level

✓6th **S56.19** Other injury of flexor muscle, fascia and tendon of other and unspecified finger at forearm level

✓7th **S56.191** Other injury of flexor muscle, fascia and tendon of right index finger at forearm level

✓7th **S56.192** Other injury of flexor muscle, fascia and tendon of left index finger at forearm level

✓7th **S56.193** Other injury of flexor muscle, fascia and tendon of right middle finger at forearm level

✓7th **S56.194** Other injury of flexor muscle, fascia and tendon of left middle finger at forearm level

✓7th **S56.195** Other injury of flexor muscle, fascia and tendon of right ring finger at forearm level

✓7th **S56.196** Other injury of flexor muscle, fascia and tendon of left ring finger at forearm level

✓7th **S56.197** Other injury of flexor muscle, fascia and tendon of right little finger at forearm level

✓7th **S56.198** Other injury of flexor muscle, fascia and tendon of left little finger at forearm level

✓7th **S56.199** Other injury of flexor muscle, fascia and tendon of unspecified finger at forearm level

✓5th **S56.2** Injury of other flexor muscle, fascia and tendon at forearm level

✓6th **S56.20** Unspecified injury of other flexor muscle, fascia and tendon at forearm level

✓7th **S56.201** Unspecified injury of other flexor muscle, fascia and tendon at forearm level, right arm

✓7th **S56.202** Unspecified injury of other flexor muscle, fascia and tendon at forearm level, left arm

✓7th **S56.209** Unspecified injury of other flexor muscle, fascia and tendon at forearm level, unspecified arm

✓6th **S56.21** Strain of other flexor muscle, fascia and tendon at forearm level

✓7th **S56.211** Strain of other flexor muscle, fascia and tendon at forearm level, right arm

✓7th **S56.212** Strain of other flexor muscle, fascia and tendon at forearm level, left arm

✓7th **S56.219** Strain of other flexor muscle, fascia and tendon at forearm level, unspecified arm

✓6th **S56.22** Laceration of other flexor muscle, fascia and tendon at forearm level

✓7th **S56.221** Laceration of other flexor muscle, fascia and tendon at forearm level, right arm

✓7th **S56.222** Laceration of other flexor muscle, fascia and tendon at forearm level, left arm

✓7th **S56.229** Laceration of other flexor muscle, fascia and tendon at forearm level, unspecified arm

---

EXCLUDES 1   Not coded here   EXCLUDES 2   Not included here   *Manifestation Code*

✓6th **S56.29**   **Other injury of other flexor muscle, fascia and tendon at forearm level**
- ✓7th **S56.291**   Other injury of other flexor muscle, fascia and tendon at forearm level, right arm
- ✓7th **S56.292**   Other injury of other flexor muscle, fascia and tendon at forearm level, left arm
- ✓7th **S56.299**   Other injury of other flexor muscle, fascia and tendon at forearm level, unspecified arm

✓5th **S56.3**   **Injury of extensor or abductor muscles, fascia and tendons of thumb at forearm level**

✓6th **S56.30**   **Unspecified injury of extensor or abductor muscles, fascia and tendons of thumb at forearm level**
- ✓7th **S56.301**   Unspecified injury of extensor or abductor muscles, fascia and tendons of right thumb at forearm level
- ✓7th **S56.302**   Unspecified injury of extensor or abductor muscles, fascia and tendons of left thumb at forearm level
- ✓7th **S56.309**   Unspecified injury of extensor or abductor muscles, fascia and tendons of unspecified thumb at forearm level

✓6th **S56.31**   **Strain of extensor or abductor muscles, fascia and tendons of thumb at forearm level**
- ✓7th **S56.311**   Strain of extensor or abductor muscles, fascia and tendons of right thumb at forearm level
- ✓7th **S56.312**   Strain of extensor or abductor muscles, fascia and tendons of left thumb at forearm level
- ✓7th **S56.319**   Strain of extensor or abductor muscles, fascia and tendons of unspecified thumb at forearm level

✓6th **S56.32**   **Laceration of extensor or abductor muscles, fascia and tendons of thumb at forearm level**
- ✓7th **S56.321**   Laceration of extensor or abductor muscles, fascia and tendons of right thumb at forearm level
- ✓7th **S56.322**   Laceration of extensor or abductor muscles, fascia and tendons of left thumb at forearm level
- ✓7th **S56.329**   Laceration of extensor or abductor muscles, fascia and tendons of unspecified thumb at forearm level

✓6th **S56.39**   **Other injury of extensor or abductor muscles, fascia and tendons of thumb at forearm level**
- ✓7th **S56.391**   Other injury of extensor or abductor muscles, fascia and tendons of right thumb at forearm level
- ✓7th **S56.392**   Other injury of extensor or abductor muscles, fascia and tendons of left thumb at forearm level
- ✓7th **S56.399**   Other injury of extensor or abductor muscles, fascia and tendons of unspecified thumb at forearm level

✓5th **S56.4**   **Injury of extensor muscle, fascia and tendon of other and unspecified finger at forearm level**

✓6th **S56.40**   **Unspecified injury of extensor muscle, fascia and tendon of other and unspecified finger at forearm level**
- ✓7th **S56.401**   Unspecified injury of extensor muscle, fascia and tendon of right index finger at forearm level
- ✓7th **S56.402**   Unspecified injury of extensor muscle, fascia and tendon of left index finger at forearm level
- ✓7th **S56.403**   Unspecified injury of extensor muscle, fascia and tendon of right middle finger at forearm level
- ✓7th **S56.404**   Unspecified injury of extensor muscle, fascia and tendon of left middle finger at forearm level
- ✓7th **S56.405**   Unspecified Injury of extensor muscle, fascia and tendon of right ring finger at forearm level

- ✓7th **S56.406**   Unspecified injury of extensor muscle, fascia and tendon of left ring finger at forearm level
- ✓7th **S56.407**   Unspecified injury of extensor muscle, fascia and tendon of right little finger at forearm level
- ✓7th **S56.408**   Unspecified injury of extensor muscle, fascia and tendon of left little finger at forearm level
- ✓7th **S56.409**   Unspecified injury of extensor muscle, fascia and tendon of unspecified finger at forearm level

✓6th **S56.41**   **Strain of extensor muscle, fascia and tendon of other and unspecified finger at forearm level**
- **S56.411**   Strain of extensor muscle, fascia and tendon of right index finger at forearm level
- ✓7th **S56.412**   Strain of extensor muscle, fascia and tendon of left index finger at forearm level
- ✓7th **S56.413**   Strain of extensor muscle, fascia and tendon of right middle finger at forearm level
- ✓7th **S56.414**   Strain of extensor muscle, fascia and tendon of left middle finger at forearm level
- ✓7th **S56.415**   Strain of extensor muscle, fascia and tendon of right ring finger at forearm level
- ✓7th **S56.416**   Strain of extensor muscle, fascia and tendon of left ring finger at forearm level
- ✓7th **S56.417**   Strain of extensor muscle, fascia and tendon of right little finger at forearm level
- ✓7th **S56.418**   Strain of extensor muscle, fascia and tendon of left little finger at forearm level
- ✓7th **S56.419**   Strain of extensor muscle, fascia and tendon of finger, unspecified finger at forearm level

✓6th **S56.42**   **Laceration of extensor muscle, fascia and tendon of other and unspecified finger at forearm level**
- **S56.421**   Laceration of extensor muscle, fascia and tendon of right index finger at forearm level
- ✓7th **S56.422**   Laceration of extensor muscle, fascia and tendon of left index finger at forearm level
- ✓7th **S56.423**   Laceration of extensor muscle, fascia and tendon of right middle finger at forearm level
- ✓7th **S56.424**   Laceration of extensor muscle, fascia and tendon of left middle finger at forearm level
- ✓7th **S56.425**   Laceration of extensor muscle, fascia and tendon of right ring finger at forearm level
- ✓7th **S56.426**   Laceration of extensor muscle, fascia and tendon of left ring finger at forearm level
- ✓7th **S56.427**   Laceration of extensor muscle, fascia and tendon of right little finger at forearm level
- ✓7th **S56.428**   Laceration of extensor muscle, fascia and tendon of left little finger at forearm level
- ✓7th **S56.429**   Laceration of extensor muscle, fascia and tendon of unspecified finger at forearm level

✓6th **S56.49**   **Other injury of extensor muscle, fascia and tendon of other and unspecified finger at forearm level**
- ✓7th **S56.491**   Other injury of extensor muscle, fascia and tendon of right index finger at forearm level
- ✓7th **S56.492**   Other injury of extensor muscle, fascia and tendon of left index finger at forearm level

---

✓ Appropriate additional character required   ✓x7th Requires 7th character, placeholder x must fill empty characters

✓7th **S56.493** Other injury of extensor muscle, fascia and tendon of right middle finger at forearm level

✓7th **S56.494** Other injury of extensor muscle, fascia and tendon of left middle finger at forearm level

✓7th **S56.495** Other injury of extensor muscle, fascia and tendon of right ring finger at forearm level

✓7th **S56.496** Other injury of extensor muscle, fascia and tendon of left ring finger at forearm level

✓7th **S56.497** Other injury of extensor muscle, fascia and tendon of right little finger at forearm level

✓7th **S56.498** Other injury of extensor muscle, fascia and tendon of left little finger at forearm level

✓7th **S56.499** Other injury of extensor muscle, fascia and tendon of unspecified finger at forearm level

✓5th **S56.5** Injury of other extensor muscle, fascia and tendon at forearm level

    ✓6th **S56.50** Unspecified injury of other extensor muscle, fascia and tendon at forearm level

      ✓7th **S56.501** Unspecified injury of other extensor muscle, fascia and tendon at forearm level, right arm

      ✓7th **S56.502** Unspecified injury of other extensor muscle, fascia and tendon at forearm level, left arm

      ✓7th **S56.509** Unspecified injury of other extensor muscle, fascia and tendon at forearm level, unspecified arm

    ✓6th **S56.51** Strain of other extensor muscle, fascia and tendon at forearm level

      ✓7th **S56.511** Strain of other extensor muscle, fascia and tendon at forearm level, right arm

      ✓7th **S56.512** Strain of other extensor muscle, fascia and tendon at forearm level, left arm

      ✓7th **S56.519** Strain of other extensor muscle, fascia and tendon at forearm level, unspecified arm

    ✓6th **S56.52** Laceration of other extensor muscle, fascia and tendon at forearm level

      ✓7th **S56.521** Laceration of other extensor muscle, fascia and tendon at forearm level, right arm

      ✓7th **S56.522** Laceration of other extensor muscle, fascia and tendon at forearm level, left arm

      ✓7th **S56.529** Laceration of other extensor muscle, fascia and tendon at forearm level, unspecified arm

    ✓6th **S56.59** Other injury of other extensor muscle, fascia and tendon at forearm level

      ✓7th **S56.591** Other injury of other extensor muscle, fascia and tendon at forearm level, right arm

      ✓7th **S56.592** Other injury of other extensor muscle, fascia and tendon at forearm level, left arm

      ✓7th **S56.599** Other injury of other extensor muscle, fascia and tendon at forearm level, unspecified arm

✓5th **S56.8** Injury of other muscles, fascia and tendons at forearm level

    ✓6th **S56.80** Unspecified injury of other muscles, fascia and tendons at forearm level

      ✓7th **S56.801** Unspecified injury of other muscles, fascia and tendons at forearm level, right arm

      ✓7th **S56.802** Unspecified injury of other muscles, fascia and tendons at forearm level, left arm

      ✓7th **S56.809** Unspecified injury of other muscles, fascia and tendons at forearm level, unspecified arm

✓6th **S56.81** Strain of other muscles, fascia and tendons at forearm level

    ✓7th **S56.811** Strain of other muscles, fascia and tendons at forearm level, right arm

    ✓7th **S56.812** Strain of other muscles, fascia and tendons at forearm level, left arm

    ✓7th **S56.819** Strain of other muscles, fascia and tendons at forearm level, unspecified arm

✓6th **S56.82** Laceration of other muscles, fascia and tendons at forearm level

    ✓7th **S56.821** Laceration of other muscles, fascia and tendons at forearm level, right arm

    ✓7th **S56.822** Laceration of other muscles, fascia and tendons at forearm level, left arm

    ✓7th **S56.829** Laceration of other muscles, fascia and tendons at forearm level, unspecified arm

✓6th **S56.89** Other injury of other muscles, fascia and tendons at forearm level

    ✓7th **S56.891** Other injury of other muscles, fascia and tendons at forearm level, right arm

    ✓7th **S56.892** Other injury of other muscles, fascia and tendons at forearm level, left arm

    ✓7th **S56.899** Other injury of other muscles, fascia and tendons at forearm level, unspecified arm

✓5th **S56.9** Injury of unspecified muscles, fascia and tendons at forearm level

    ✓6th **S56.90** Unspecified injury of unspecified muscles, fascia and tendons at forearm level

      ✓7th **S56.901** Unspecified injury of unspecified muscles, fascia and tendons at forearm level, right arm

      ✓7th **S56.902** Unspecified injury of unspecified muscles, fascia and tendons at forearm level, left arm

      ✓7th **S56.909** Unspecified injury of unspecified muscles, fascia and tendons at forearm level, unspecified arm

    ✓6th **S56.91** Strain of unspecified muscles, fascia and tendons at forearm level

      ✓7th **S56.911** Strain of unspecified muscles, fascia and tendons at forearm level, right arm

      ✓7th **S56.912** Strain of unspecified muscles, fascia and tendons at forearm level, left arm

      ✓7th **S56.919** Strain of unspecified muscles, fascia and tendons at forearm level, unspecified arm

    ✓6th **S56.92** Laceration of unspecified muscles, fascia and tendons at forearm level

      ✓7th **S56.921** Laceration of unspecified muscles, fascia and tendons at forearm level, right arm

      ✓7th **S56.922** Laceration of unspecified muscles, fascia and tendons at forearm level, left arm

      ✓7th **S56.929** Laceration of unspecified muscles, fascia and tendons at forearm level, unspecified arm

    ✓6th **S56.99** Other injury of unspecified muscles, fascia and tendons at forearm level

      ✓7th **S56.991** Other injury of unspecified muscles, fascia and tendons at forearm level, right arm

      ✓7th **S56.992** Other injury of unspecified muscles, fascia and tendons at forearm level, left arm

      ✓7th **S56.999** Other injury of unspecified muscles, fascia and tendons at forearm level, unspecified arm

---

EXCLUDES 1 Not coded here   **EXCLUDES 2** Not included here   *Manifestation Code*

✓4th **S57   Crushing injury of elbow and forearm**
Use additional code(s) for all associated injuries
EXCLUDES 2   crushing injury of wrist and hand (S67-)

The appropriate 7th character is to be added to each code from category S57.
A   initial encounter
D   subsequent encounter
S   sequela

✓5th   **S57.0   Crushing injury of elbow**
✓x7th   **S57.00   Crushing injury of unspecified elbow**
✓x7th   **S57.01   Crushing injury of right elbow**
✓x7th   **S57.02   Crushing injury of left elbow**
✓5th   **S57.8   Crushing injury of forearm**
✓x7th   **S57.80   Crushing injury of unspecified forearm**
✓x7th   **S57.81   Crushing injury of right forearm**
✓x7th   **S57.82   Crushing injury of left forearm**

✓4th **S58   Traumatic amputation of elbow and forearm**
NOTE   An amputation not identified as partial or complete should be coded to complete
EXCLUDES 1   traumatic amputation of wrist and hand (S68-)

The appropriate 7th character is to be added to each code from category S58.
A   initial encounter
D   subsequent encounter
S   sequela

✓5th   **S58.0   Traumatic amputation at elbow level**
✓6th   **S58.01   Complete traumatic amputation at elbow level**
✓7th   **S58.011   Complete traumatic amputation at elbow level, right arm**
✓7th   **S58.012   Complete traumatic amputation at elbow level, left arm**
✓7th   **S58.019   Complete traumatic amputation at elbow level, unspecified arm**
✓6th   **S58.02   Partial traumatic amputation at elbow level**
✓7th   **S58.021   Partial traumatic amputation at elbow level, right arm**
✓7th   **S58.022   Partial traumatic amputation at elbow level, left arm**
✓7th   **S58.029   Partial traumatic amputation at elbow level, unspecified arm**
✓5th   **S58.1   Traumatic amputation at level between elbow and wrist**
✓6th   **S58.11   Complete traumatic amputation at level between elbow and wrist**
✓7th   **S58.111   Complete traumatic amputation at level between elbow and wrist, right arm**
✓7th   **S58.112   Complete traumatic amputation at level between elbow and wrist, left arm**
✓7th   **S58.119   Complete traumatic amputation at level between elbow and wrist, unspecified arm**
✓6th   **S58.12   Partial traumatic amputation at level between elbow and wrist**
✓7th   **S58.121   Partial traumatic amputation at level between elbow and wrist, right arm**
✓7th   **S58.122   Partial traumatic amputation at level between elbow and wrist, left arm**
✓7th   **S58.129   Partial traumatic amputation at level between elbow and wrist, unspecified arm**
✓5th   **S58.9   Traumatic amputation of forearm, level unspecified**
EXCLUDES 1   traumatic amputation of wrist (S68-)
✓6th   **S58.91   Complete traumatic amputation of forearm, level unspecified**
✓7th   **S58.911   Complete traumatic amputation of right forearm, level unspecified**
✓7th   **S58.912   Complete traumatic amputation of left forearm, level unspecified**
✓7th   **S58.919   Complete traumatic amputation of unspecified forearm, level unspecified**
✓6th   **S58.92   Partial traumatic amputation of forearm, level unspecified**
✓7th   **S58.921   Partial traumatic amputation of right forearm, level unspecified**

✓7th   **S58.922   Partial traumatic amputation of left forearm, level unspecified**
✓7th   **S58.929   Partial traumatic amputation of unspecified forearm, level unspecified**

✓4th **S59   Other and unspecified injuries of elbow and forearm**
EXCLUDES 2   other and unspecified injuries of wrist and hand (S69-)

The appropriate 7th character is to be added to each code from subcategories S59.0, S59.1, and S59.2.
A   initial encounter for closed fracture
D   subsequent encounter for fracture with routine healing
G   subsequent encounter for fracture with delayed healing
K   subsequent encounter for fracture with nonunion
P   subsequent encounter for fracture with malunion
S   sequela

✓5th   **S59.0   Physeal fracture of lower end of ulna**
✓6th   **S59.00   Unspecified physeal fracture of lower end of ulna**
✓7th   **S59.001   Unspecified physeal fracture of lower end of ulna, right arm**
✓7th   **S59.002   Unspecified physeal fracture of lower end of ulna, left arm**
✓7th   **S59.009   Unspecified physeal fracture of lower end of ulna, unspecified arm**
✓6th   **S59.01   Salter-Harris Type I physeal fracture of lower end of ulna**
✓7th   **S59.011   Salter-Harris Type I physeal fracture of lower end of ulna, right arm**
✓7th   **S59.012   Salter-Harris Type I physeal fracture of lower end of ulna, left arm**
✓7th   **S59.019   Salter-Harris Type I physeal fracture of lower end of ulna, unspecified arm**
✓6th   **S59.02   Salter-Harris Type II physeal fracture of lower end of ulna**
✓7th   **S59.021   Salter-Harris Type II physeal fracture of lower end of ulna, right arm**
✓7th   **S59.022   Salter-Harris Type II physeal fracture of lower end of ulna, left arm**
✓7th   **S59.029   Salter-Harris Type II physeal fracture of lower end of ulna, unspecified arm**
✓6th   **S59.03   Salter-Harris Type III physeal fracture of lower end of ulna**
✓7th   **S59.031   Salter-Harris Type III physeal fracture of lower end of ulna, right arm**
✓7th   **S59.032   Salter-Harris Type III physeal fracture of lower end of ulna, left arm**
✓7th   **S59.039   Salter-Harris Type III physeal fracture of lower end of ulna, unspecified arm**
✓6th   **S59.04   Salter-Harris Type IV physeal fracture of lower end of ulna**
✓7th   **S59.041   Salter-Harris Type IV physeal fracture of lower end of ulna, right arm**
✓7th   **S59.042   Salter-Harris Type IV physeal fracture of lower end of ulna, left arm**
✓7th   **S59.049   Salter-Harris Type IV physeal fracture of lower end of ulna, unspecified arm**
✓6th   **S59.09   Other physeal fracture of lower end of ulna**
✓7th   **S59.091   Other physeal fracture of lower end of ulna, right arm**
✓7th   **S59.092   Other physeal fracture of lower end of ulna, left arm**
✓7th   **S59.099   Other physeal fracture of lower end of ulna, unspecified arm**
✓5th   **S59.1   Physeal fracture of upper end of radius**
✓6th   **S59.10   Unspecified physeal fracture of upper end of radius**
✓7th   **S59.101   Unspecified physeal fracture of upper end of radius, right arm**
✓7th   **S59.102   Unspecified physeal fracture of upper end of radius, left arm**
✓7th   **S59.109   Unspecified physeal fracture of upper end of radius, unspecified arm**
✓6th   **S59.11   Salter-Harris Type I physeal fracture of upper end of radius**
✓7th   **S59.111   Salter-Harris Type I physeal fracture of upper end of radius, right arm**
✓7th   **S59.112   Salter-Harris Type I physeal fracture of upper end of radius, left arm**

☑ Appropriate additional character required   ✓x7th Requires 7th character, placeholder x must fill empty characters

Injury, Poisoning and Certain Other Consequences of External Causes

S59.119–S60.032

✓7th **S59.119** Salter-Harris Type I physeal fracture of upper end of radius, unspecified arm

✓6th **S59.12** Salter-Harris Type II physeal fracture of upper end of radius

   ✓7th **S59.121** Salter-Harris Type II physeal fracture of upper end of radius, right arm

   ✓7th **S59.122** Salter-Harris Type II physeal fracture of upper end of radius, left arm

   ✓7th **S59.129** Salter-Harris Type II physeal fracture of upper end of radius, unspecified arm

✓6th **S59.13** Salter-Harris Type III physeal fracture of upper end of radius

   ✓7th **S59.131** Salter-Harris Type III physeal fracture of upper end of radius, right arm

   ✓7th **S59.132** Salter-Harris Type III physeal fracture of upper end of radius, left arm

   ✓7th **S59.139** Salter-Harris Type III physeal fracture of upper end of radius, unspecified arm

✓6th **S59.14** Salter-Harris Type IV physeal fracture of upper end of radius

   ✓7th **S59.141** Salter-Harris Type IV physeal fracture of upper end of radius, right arm

   ✓7th **S59.142** Salter-Harris Type IV physeal fracture of upper end of radius, left arm

   ✓7th **S59.149** Salter-Harris Type IV physeal fracture of upper end of radius, unspecified arm

✓6th **S59.19** Other physeal fracture of upper end of radius

   ✓7th **S59.191** Other physeal fracture of upper end of radius, right arm

   ✓7th **S59.192** Other physeal fracture of upper end of radius, left arm

   ✓7th **S59.199** Other physeal fracture of upper end of radius, unspecified arm

✓5th **S59.2** Physeal fracture of lower end of radius

✓6th **S59.20** Unspecified physeal fracture of lower end of radius

   ✓7th **S59.201** Unspecified physeal fracture of lower end of radius, right arm

   ✓7th **S59.202** Unspecified physeal fracture of lower end of radius, left arm

   ✓7th **S59.209** Unspecified physeal fracture of lower end of radius, unspecified arm

✓6th **S59.21** Salter-Harris Type I physeal fracture of lower end of radius

   ✓7th **S59.211** Salter-Harris Type I physeal fracture of lower end of radius, right arm

   ✓7th **S59.212** Salter-Harris Type I physeal fracture of lower end of radius, left arm

   ✓7th **S59.219** Salter-Harris Type I physeal fracture of lower end of radius, unspecified arm

✓6th **S59.22** Salter-Harris Type II physeal fracture of lower end of radius

   ✓7th **S59.221** Salter-Harris Type II physeal fracture of lower end of radius, right arm

   ✓7th **S59.222** Salter-Harris Type II physeal fracture of lower end of radius, left arm

   ✓7th **S59.229** Salter-Harris Type II physeal fracture of lower end of radius, unspecified arm

✓6th **S59.23** Salter-Harris Type III physeal fracture of lower end of radius

   ✓7th **S59.231** Salter-Harris Type III physeal fracture of lower end of radius, right arm

   ✓7th **S59.232** Salter-Harris Type III physeal fracture of lower end of radius, left arm

   ✓7th **S59.239** Salter-Harris Type III physeal fracture of lower end of radius, unspecified arm

✓6th **S59.24** Salter-Harris Type IV physeal fracture of lower end of radius

   ✓7th **S59.241** Salter-Harris Type IV physeal fracture of lower end of radius, right arm

   ✓7th **S59.242** Salter-Harris Type IV physeal fracture of lower end of radius, left arm

   ✓7th **S59.249** Salter-Harris Type IV physeal fracture of lower end of radius, unspecified arm

✓6th **S59.29** Other physeal fracture of lower end of radius

---

   ✓7th **S59.291** Other physeal fracture of lower end of radius, right arm

   ✓7th **S59.292** Other physeal fracture of lower end of radius, left arm

   ✓7th **S59.299** Other physeal fracture of lower end of radius, unspecified arm

✓5th **S59.8** Other specified injuries of elbow and forearm

> The appropriate 7th character is to be added to each code from subcategory S59.8.
> A   initial encounter
> D   subsequent encounter
> S   sequela

✓6th **S59.80** Other specified injuries of elbow

   ✓7th **S59.801** Other specified injuries of right elbow

   ✓7th **S59.802** Other specified injuries of left elbow

   ✓7th **S59.809** Other specified injuries of unspecified elbow

✓6th **S59.81** Other specified injuries of forearm

   ✓7th **S59.811** Other specified injuries right forearm

   ✓7th **S59.812** Other specified injuries left forearm

   ✓7th **S59.819** Other specified injuries unspecified forearm

✓5th **S59.9** Unspecified injury of elbow and forearm

> The appropriate 7th character is to be added to each code from subcategory S59.9.
> A   initial encounter
> D   subsequent encounter
> S   sequela

✓6th **S59.90** Unspecified injury of elbow

   ✓7th **S59.901** Unspecified injury of right elbow

   ✓7th **S59.902** Unspecified injury of left elbow

   ✓7th **S59.909** Unspecified injury of unspecified elbow

✓6th **S59.91** Unspecified injury of forearm

   ✓7th **S59.911** Unspecified injury of right forearm

   ✓7th **S59.912** Unspecified injury of left forearm

   ✓7th **S59.919** Unspecified injury of unspecified forearm

Injuries to the wrist, hand and fingers (S60-S69)

EXCLUDES2   burns and corrosions (T20-T32)
frostbite (T33-T34)
insect bite or sting, venomous (T63.4)

✓4th **S60** Superficial injury of wrist, hand and fingers

> The appropriate 7th character is to be added to each code from category S60.
> A   initial encounter
> D   subsequent encounter
> S   sequela

✓5th **S60.0** Contusion of finger without damage to nail

   EXCLUDES1   contusion involving nail (matrix) (S60.1)

✓x7th **S60.00** Contusion of unspecified finger without damage to nail

   Contusion of finger(s) NOS

✓6th **S60.01** Contusion of thumb without damage to nail

   ✓7th **S60.011** Contusion of right thumb without damage to nail

   ✓7th **S60.012** Contusion of left thumb without damage to nail

   ✓7th **S60.019** Contusion of unspecified thumb without damage to nail

✓6th **S60.02** Contusion of index finger without damage to nail

   ✓7th **S60.021** Contusion of right index finger without damage to nail

   ✓7th **S60.022** Contusion of left index finger without damage to nail

   ✓7th **S60.029** Contusion of unspecified index finger without damage to nail

✓6th **S60.03** Contusion of middle finger without damage to nail

   ✓7th **S60.031** Contusion of right middle finger without damage to nail

   ✓7th **S60.032** Contusion of left middle finger without damage to nail

---

EXCLUDES1 Not coded here   EXCLUDES2 Not included here   *Manifestation Code*

√7ᵗʰ **S60.039** **Contusion of unspecified middle finger without damage to nail**

√6ᵗʰ **S60.04** **Contusion of ring finger without damage to nail**

√7ᵗʰ **S60.041** **Contusion of right ring finger without damage to nail**

√7ᵗʰ **S60.042** **Contusion of left ring finger without damage to nail**

√7ᵗʰ **S60.049** **Contusion of unspecified ring finger without damage to nail**

√6ᵗʰ **S60.05** **Contusion of little finger without damage to nail**

√7ᵗʰ **S60.051** **Contusion of right little finger without damage to nail**

√7ᵗʰ **S60.052** **Contusion of left little finger without damage to nail**

√7ᵗʰ **S60.059** **Contusion of unspecified little finger without damage to nail**

√5ᵗʰ **S60.1** **Contusion of finger with damage to nail**

√x7ᵗʰ **S60.10** **Contusion of unspecified finger with damage to nail**

√6ᵗʰ **S60.11** **Contusion of thumb with damage to nail**

√7ᵗʰ **S60.111** **Contusion of right thumb with damage to nail**

√7ᵗʰ **S60.112** **Contusion of left thumb with damage to nail**

√7ᵗʰ **S60.119** **Contusion of unspecified thumb with damage to nail**

√6ᵗʰ **S60.12** **Contusion of index finger with damage to nail**

√7ᵗʰ **S60.121** **Contusion of right index finger with damage to nail**

√7ᵗʰ **S60.122** **Contusion of left index finger with damage to nail**

√7ᵗʰ **S60.129** **Contusion of unspecified index finger with damage to nail**

√6ᵗʰ **S60.13** **Contusion of middle finger with damage to nail**

√7ᵗʰ **S60.131** **Contusion of right middle finger with damage to nail**

√7ᵗʰ **S60.132** **Contusion of left middle finger with damage to nail**

√7ᵗʰ **S60.139** **Contusion of unspecified middle finger with damage to nail**

√6ᵗʰ **S60.14** **Contusion of ring finger with damage to nail**

√7ᵗʰ **S60.141** **Contusion of right ring finger with damage to nail**

√7ᵗʰ **S60.142** **Contusion of left ring finger with damage to nail**

√7ᵗʰ **S60.149** **Contusion of unspecified ring finger with damage to nail**

√6ᵗʰ **S60.15** **Contusion of little finger with damage to nail**

√7ᵗʰ **S60.151** **Contusion of right little finger with damage to nail**

√7ᵗʰ **S60.152** **Contusion of left little finger with damage to nail**

√7ᵗʰ **S60.159** **Contusion of unspecified little finger with damage to nail**

√5ᵗʰ **S60.2** **Contusion of wrist and hand**

EXCLUDES 2   *contusion of fingers (S60.0-, S60.1-)*

√6ᵗʰ **S60.21** **Contusion of wrist**

√7ᵗʰ **S60.211** **Contusion of right wrist**

√7ᵗʰ **S60.212** **Contusion of left wrist**

√7ᵗʰ **S60.219** **Contusion of unspecified wrist**

√6ᵗʰ **S60.22** **Contusion of hand**

√7ᵗʰ **S60.221** **Contusion of right hand**

√7ᵗʰ **S60.222** **Contusion of left hand**

√7ᵗʰ **S60.229** **Contusion of unspecified hand**

√5ᵗʰ **S60.3** **Other superficial injuries of thumb**

√6ᵗʰ **S60.31** **Abrasion of thumb**

√7ᵗʰ **S60.311** **Abrasion of right thumb**

√7ᵗʰ **S60.312** **Abrasion of left thumb**

√7ᵗʰ **S60.319** **Abrasion of unspecified thumb**

√6ᵗʰ **S60.32** **Blister (nonthermal) of thumb**

√7ᵗʰ **S60.321** **Blister (nonthermal) of right thumb**

√7ᵗʰ **S60.322** **Blister (nonthermal) of left thumb**

√7ᵗʰ **S60.329** **Blister (nonthermal) of unspecified thumb**

√6ᵗʰ **S60.34** **External constriction of thumb**

Hair tourniquet syndrome of thumb

Use additional cause code to identify the constricting item (W49.0-)

√7ᵗʰ **S60.341** **External constriction of right thumb**

√7ᵗʰ **S60.342** **External constriction of left thumb**

√7ᵗʰ **S60.349** **External constriction of unspecified thumb**

√6ᵗʰ **S60.35** **Superficial foreign body of thumb**

Splinter in the thumb

√7ᵗʰ **S60.351** **Superficial foreign body of right thumb**

√7ᵗʰ **S60.352** **Superficial foreign body of left thumb**

√7ᵗʰ **S60.359** **Superficial foreign body of unspecified thumb**

√6ᵗʰ **S60.36** **Insect bite (nonvenomous) of thumb**

√7ᵗʰ **S60.361** **Insect bite (nonvenomous) of right thumb**

√7ᵗʰ **S60.362** **Insect bite (nonvenomous) of left thumb**

√7ᵗʰ **S60.369** **Insect bite (nonvenomous) of unspecified thumb**

√6ᵗʰ **S60.37** **Other superficial bite of thumb**

EXCLUDES 1   *open bite of thumb (S61.05-, S61.15-)*

√7ᵗʰ **S60.371** **Other superficial bite of right thumb**

√7ᵗʰ **S60.372** **Other superficial bite of left thumb**

√7ᵗʰ **S60.379** **Other superficial bite of unspecified thumb**

√6ᵗʰ **S60.39** **Other superficial injuries of thumb**

√7ᵗʰ **S60.391** **Other superficial injuries of right thumb**

√7ᵗʰ **S60.392** **Other superficial injuries of left thumb**

√7ᵗʰ **S60.399** **Other superficial injuries of unspecified thumb**

√5ᵗʰ **S60.4** **Other superficial injuries of other fingers**

√6ᵗʰ **S60.41** **Abrasion of fingers**

√7ᵗʰ **S60.410** **Abrasion of right index finger**

√7ᵗʰ **S60.411** **Abrasion of left index finger**

√7ᵗʰ **S60.412** **Abrasion of right middle finger**

√7ᵗʰ **S60.413** **Abrasion of left middle finger**

√7ᵗʰ **S60.414** **Abrasion of right ring finger**

√7ᵗʰ **S60.415** **Abrasion of left ring finger**

√7ᵗʰ **S60.416** **Abrasion of right little finger**

√7ᵗʰ **S60.417** **Abrasion of left little finger**

√7ᵗʰ **S60.418** **Abrasion of other finger**

Abrasion of specified finger with unspecified laterality

√7ᵗʰ **S60.419** **Abrasion of unspecified finger**

√6ᵗʰ **S60.42** **Blister (nonthermal) of fingers**

√7ᵗʰ **S60.420** **Blister (nonthermal) of right index finger**

√7ᵗʰ **S60.421** **Blister (nonthermal) of left index finger**

√7ᵗʰ **S60.422** **Blister (nonthermal) of right middle finger**

√7ᵗʰ **S60.423** **Blister (nonthermal) of left middle finger**

√7ᵗʰ **S60.424** **Blister (nonthermal) of right ring finger**

√7ᵗʰ **S60.425** **Blister (nonthermal) of left ring finger**

√7ᵗʰ **S60.426** **Blister (nonthermal) of right little finger**

√7ᵗʰ **S60.427** **Blister (nonthermal) of left little finger**

√7ᵗʰ **S60.428** **Blister (nonthermal) of other finger**

Blister (nonthermal) of specified finger with unspecified laterality

√7ᵗʰ **S60.429** **Blister (nonthermal) of unspecified finger**

√6ᵗʰ **S60.44** **External constriction of fingers**

Hair tourniquet syndrome of finger

Use additional cause code to identify the constricting item (W49.0-)

√7ᵗʰ **S60.440** **External constriction of right index finger**

√7ᵗʰ **S60.441** **External constriction of left index finger**

√7ᵗʰ **S60.442** **External constriction of right middle finger**

√7ᵗʰ **S60.443** **External constriction of left middle finger**

√7ᵗʰ **S60.444** **External constriction of right ring finger**

√7ᵗʰ **S60.445** **External constriction of left ring finger**

√7th **S60.446** **External constriction of right little finger**

√7th **S60.447** **External constriction of left little finger**

√7th **S60.448** **External constriction of other finger**
External constriction of specified finger with unspecified laterality

√7th **S60.449** **External constriction of unspecified finger**

√6th **S60.45** **Superficial foreign body of fingers**
Splinter in the finger(s)

√7th **S60.450** **Superficial foreign body of right index finger**

√7th **S60.451** **Superficial foreign body of left index finger**

√7th **S60.452** **Superficial foreign body of right middle finger**

√7th **S60.453** **Superficial foreign body of left middle finger**

√7th **S60.454** **Superficial foreign body of right ring finger**

√7th **S60.455** **Superficial foreign body of left ring finger**

√7th **S60.456** **Superficial foreign body of right little finger**

√7th **S60.457** **Superficial foreign body of left little finger**

√7th **S60.458** **Superficial foreign body of other finger**
Superficial foreign body of specified finger with unspecified laterality

√7th **S60.459** **Superficial foreign body of unspecified finger**

√6th **S60.46** **Insect bite (nonvenomous) of fingers**

√7th **S60.460** **Insect bite (nonvenomous) of right index finger**

√7th **S60.461** **Insect bite (nonvenomous) of left index finger**

√7th **S60.462** **Insect bite (nonvenomous) of right middle finger**

√7th **S60.463** **Insect bite (nonvenomous) of left middle finger**

√7th **S60.464** **Insect bite (nonvenomous) of right ring finger**

√7th **S60.465** **Insect bite (nonvenomous) of left ring finger**

√7th **S60.466** **Insect bite (nonvenomous) of right little finger**

√7th **S60.467** **Insect bite (nonvenomous) of left little finger**

√7th **S60.468** **Insect bite (nonvenomous) of other finger**
Insect bite (nonvenomous) of specified finger with unspecified laterality

√7th **S60.469** **Insect bite (nonvenomous) of unspecified finger**

√6th **S60.47** **Other superficial bite of fingers**
EXCLUDES 1   *open bite of fingers (S61.25-, S61.35-)*

√7th **S60.470** **Other superficial bite of right index finger**

√7th **S60.471** **Other superficial bite of left index finger**

√7th **S60.472** **Other superficial bite of right middle finger**

√7th **S60.473** **Other superficial bite of left middle finger**

√7th **S60.474** **Other superficial bite of right ring finger**

√7th **S60.475** **Other superficial bite of left ring finger**

√7th **S60.476** **Other superficial bite of right little finger**

√7th **S60.477** **Other superficial bite of left little finger**

√7th **S60.478** **Other superficial bite of other finger**
Other superficial bite of specified finger with unspecified laterality

√7th **S60.479** **Other superficial bite of unspecified finger**

√5th **S60.5** **Other superficial injuries of hand**
EXCLUDES 2   *superficial injuries of fingers (S60.3-, S60.4-)*

√6th **S60.51** **Abrasion of hand**

√7th **S60.511** **Abrasion of right hand**

√7th **S60.512** **Abrasion of left hand**

√7th **S60.519** **Abrasion of unspecified hand**

√6th **S60.52** **Blister (nonthermal) of hand**

√7th **S60.521** **Blister (nonthermal) of right hand**

√7th **S60.522** **Blister (nonthermal) of left hand**

√7th **S60.529** **Blister (nonthermal) of unspecified hand**

√6th **S60.54** **External constriction of hand**

√7th **S60.541** **External constriction of right hand**

√7th **S60.542** **External constriction of left hand**

√7th **S60.549** **External constriction of unspecified hand**

√6th **S60.55** **Superficial foreign body of hand**
Splinter in the hand

√7th **S60.551** **Superficial foreign body of right hand**

√7th **S60.552** **Superficial foreign body of left hand**

√7th **S60.559** **Superficial foreign body of unspecified hand**

√6th **S60.56** **Insect bite (nonvenomous) of hand**

√7th **S60.561** **Insect bite (nonvenomous) of right hand**

√7th **S60.562** **Insect bite (nonvenomous) of left hand**

√7th **S60.569** **Insect bite (nonvenomous) of unspecified hand**

√6th **S60.57** **Other superficial bite of hand**
EXCLUDES 1   *open bite of hand (S61.45-)*

√7th **S60.571** **Other superficial bite of hand of right hand**

√7th **S60.572** **Other superficial bite of hand of left hand**

√7th **S60.579** **Other superficial bite of hand of unspecified hand**

√5th **S60.8** **Other superficial injuries of wrist**

√6th **S60.81** **Abrasion of wrist**

√7th **S60.811** **Abrasion of right wrist**

√7th **S60.812** **Abrasion of left wrist**

√7th **S60.819** **Abrasion of unspecified wrist**

√6th **S60.82** **Blister (nonthermal) of wrist**

√7th **S60.821** **Blister (nonthermal) of right wrist**

√7th **S60.822** **Blister (nonthermal) of left wrist**

√7th **S60.829** **Blister (nonthermal) of unspecified wrist**

√6th **S60.84** **External constriction of wrist**

√7th **S60.841** **External constriction of right wrist**

√7th **S60.842** **External constriction of left wrist**

√7th **S60.849** **External constriction of unspecified wrist**

√6th **S60.85** **Superficial foreign body of wrist**
Splinter in the wrist

√7th **S60.851** **Superficial foreign body of right wrist**

√7th **S60.852** **Superficial foreign body of left wrist**

√7th **S60.859** **Superficial foreign body of unspecified wrist**

√6th **S60.86** **Insect bite (nonvenomous) of wrist**

√7th **S60.861** **Insect bite (nonvenomous) of right wrist**

√7th **S60.862** **Insect bite (nonvenomous) of left wrist**

√7th **S60.869** **Insect bite (nonvenomous) of unspecified wrist**

√6th **S60.87** **Other superficial bite of wrist**
EXCLUDES 1   *open bite of wrist (S61.55)*

√7th **S60.871** **Other superficial bite of right wrist**

√7th **S60.872** **Other superficial bite of left wrist**

√7th **S60.879** **Other superficial bite of unspecified wrist**

√5th **S60.9** **Unspecified superficial injury of wrist, hand and fingers**

√6th **S60.91** **Unspecified superficial injury of wrist**

√7th **S60.911** **Unspecified superficial injury of right wrist**

√7th **S60.912** **Unspecified superficial injury of left wrist**

√7th **S60.919** **Unspecified superficial injury of unspecified wrist**

√6th **S60.92** **Unspecified superficial injury of hand**

√7th **S60.921** **Unspecified superficial injury of right hand**

EXCLUDES 1 Not coded here   EXCLUDES 2 Not included here   *Manifestation Code*

√7ᵗʰ **S60.922** **Unspecified superficial injury of left hand**

√7ᵗʰ **S60.929** **Unspecified superficial injury of unspecified hand**

√6ᵗʰ **S60.93** **Unspecified superficial injury of thumb**

√7ᵗʰ **S60.931** **Unspecified superficial injury of right thumb**

√7ᵗʰ **S60.932** **Unspecified superficial injury of left thumb**

√7ᵗʰ **S60.939** **Unspecified superficial injury of unspecified thumb**

√6ᵗʰ **S60.94** **Unspecified superficial injury of other fingers**

√7ᵗʰ **S60.940** **Unspecified superficial injury of right index finger**

√7ᵗʰ **S60.941** **Unspecified superficial injury of left index finger**

√7ᵗʰ **S60.942** **Unspecified superficial injury of right middle finger**

√7ᵗʰ **S60.943** **Unspecified superficial injury of left middle finger**

√7ᵗʰ **S60.944** **Unspecified superficial injury of right ring finger**

√7ᵗʰ **S60.945** **Unspecified superficial injury of left ring finger**

√7ᵗʰ **S60.946** **Unspecified superficial injury of right little finger**

√7ᵗʰ **S60.947** **Unspecified superficial injury of left little finger**

√7ᵗʰ **S60.948** **Unspecified superficial injury of other finger**
Unspecified superficial injury of specified finger with unspecified laterality

√7ᵗʰ **S60.949** **Unspecified superficial injury of unspecified finger**

√4ᵗʰ **S61** **Open wound of wrist, hand and fingers**
Code also any associated wound infection
EXCLUDES 1   *open fracture of wrist, hand and finger (S62- with 7th character B)*
traumatic amputation of wrist and hand (S68-)

The appropriate 7th character is to be added to each code from category S61.
A   initial encounter
D   subsequent encounter
S   sequela

√5ᵗʰ **S61.0** **Open wound of thumb without damage to nail**
EXCLUDES 1   *open wound of thumb with damage to nail (S61.1-)*

√6ᵗʰ **S61.00** **Unspecified open wound of thumb without damage to nail**

√7ᵗʰ **S61.001** **Unspecified open wound of right thumb without damage to nail**

√7ᵗʰ **S61.002** **Unspecified open wound of left thumb without damage to nail**

√7ᵗʰ **S61.009** **Unspecified open wound of unspecified thumb without damage to nail**

√6ᵗʰ **S61.01** **Laceration without foreign body of thumb without damage to nail**

√7ᵗʰ **S61.011** **Laceration without foreign body of right thumb without damage to nail**

√7ᵗʰ **S61.012** **Laceration without foreign body of left thumb without damage to nail**

√7ᵗʰ **S61.019** **Laceration without foreign body of unspecified thumb without damage to nail**

√6ᵗʰ **S61.02** **Laceration with foreign body of thumb without damage to nail**

√7ᵗʰ **S61.021** **Laceration with foreign body of right thumb without damage to nail**

√7ᵗʰ **S61.022** **Laceration with foreign body of left thumb without damage to nail**

√7ᵗʰ **S61.029** **Laceration with foreign body of unspecified thumb without damage to nail**

√6ᵗʰ **S61.03** **Puncture wound without foreign body of thumb without damage to nail**

√7ᵗʰ **S61.031** **Puncture wound without foreign body of right thumb without damage to nail**

√7ᵗʰ **S61.032** **Puncture wound without foreign body of left thumb without damage to nail**

√7ᵗʰ **S61.039** **Puncture wound without foreign body of thumb without damage to nail**

√6ᵗʰ **S61.04** **Puncture wound with foreign body of thumb without damage to nail**

√7ᵗʰ **S61.041** **Puncture wound with foreign body of right thumb without damage to nail**

√7ᵗʰ **S61.042** **Puncture wound with foreign body of left thumb without damage to nail**

√7ᵗʰ **S61.049** **Puncture wound with foreign body of unspecified thumb without damage to nail**

√6ᵗʰ **S61.05** **Open bite of thumb without damage to nail**
Bite of thumb NOS
EXCLUDES 1   *superficial bite of thumb (S60.36-, S60.37-)*

√7ᵗʰ **S61.051** **Open bite of right thumb without damage to nail**

√7ᵗʰ **S61.052** **Open bite of left thumb without damage to nail**

√7ᵗʰ **S61.059** **Open bite of unspecified thumb without damage to nail**

√5ᵗʰ **S61.1** **Open wound of thumb with damage to nail**

√6ᵗʰ **S61.10** **Unspecified open wound of thumb with damage to nail**

√7ᵗʰ **S61.101** **Unspecified open wound of right thumb with damage to nail**

√7ᵗʰ **S61.102** **Unspecified open wound of left thumb with damage to nail**

√7ᵗʰ **S61.109** **Unspecified open wound of unspecified thumb with damage to nail**

√6ᵗʰ **S61.11** **Laceration without foreign body of thumb with damage to nail**

√7ᵗʰ **S61.111** **Laceration without foreign body of right thumb with damage to nail**

√7ᵗʰ **S61.112** **Laceration without foreign body of left thumb with damage to nail**

√7ᵗʰ **S61.119** **Laceration without foreign body of unspecified thumb with damage to nail**

√6ᵗʰ **S61.12** **Laceration with foreign body of thumb with damage to nail**

√7ᵗʰ **S61.121** **Laceration with foreign body of right thumb with damage to nail**

√7ᵗʰ **S61.122** **Laceration with foreign body of left thumb with damage to nail**

√7ᵗʰ **S61.129** **Laceration with foreign body of unspecified thumb with damage to nail**

√6ᵗʰ **S61.13** **Puncture wound without foreign body of thumb with damage to nail**

√7ᵗʰ **S61.131** **Puncture wound without foreign body of right thumb with damage to nail**

√7ᵗʰ **S61.132** **Puncture wound without foreign body of left thumb with damage to nail**

√7ᵗʰ **S61.139** **Puncture wound without foreign body of unspecified thumb with damage to nail**

√6ᵗʰ **S61.14** **Puncture wound with foreign body of thumb with damage to nail**

√7ᵗʰ **S61.141** **Puncture wound with foreign body of right thumb with damage to nail**

√7ᵗʰ **S61.142** **Puncture wound with foreign body of left thumb with damage to nail**

√7ᵗʰ **S61.149** **Puncture wound with foreign body of unspecified thumb with damage to nail**

√6ᵗʰ **S61.15** **Open bite of thumb with damage to nail**
Bite of thumb with damage to nail NOS
EXCLUDES 1   *superficial bite of thumb (S60.36-, S60.37-)*

√7ᵗʰ **S61.151** **Open bite of right thumb with damage to nail**

√7ᵗʰ **S61.152** **Open bite of left thumb with damage to nail**

√7ᵗʰ **S61.159** **Open bite of unspecified thumb with damage to nail**

☑ Appropriate additional character required   √x7ᵗʰ Requires 7th character, placeholder x must fill empty characters

✓5th **S61.2 Open wound of other finger without damage to nail**
> EXCLUDES 1 *open wound of finger involving nail (matrix) (S61.3-)*
> EXCLUDES 2 *open wound of thumb without damage to nail (S61.0-)*

✓6th **S61.20 Unspecified open wound of other finger without damage to nail**

✓7th **S61.200 Unspecified open wound of right index finger without damage to nail**

✓7th **S61.201 Unspecified open wound of left index finger without damage to nail**

✓7th **S61.202 Unspecified open wound of right middle finger without damage to nail**

✓7th **S61.203 Unspecified open wound of left middle finger without damage to nail**

✓7th **S61.204 Unspecified open wound of right ring finger without damage to nail**

✓7th **S61.205 Unspecified open wound of left ring finger without damage to nail**

✓7th **S61.206 Unspecified open wound of right little finger without damage to nail**

✓7th **S61.207 Unspecified open wound of left little finger without damage to nail**

✓7th **S61.208 Unspecified open wound of other finger without damage to nail**
> Unspecified open wound of specified finger with unspecified laterality without damage to nail

✓7th **S61.209 Unspecified open wound of unspecified finger without damage to nail**

✓6th **S61.21 Laceration without foreign body of finger without damage to nail**

✓7th **S61.210 Laceration without foreign body of right index finger without damage to nail**

✓7th **S61.211 Laceration without foreign body of left index finger without damage to nail**

✓7th **S61.212 Laceration without foreign body of right middle finger without damage to nail**

✓7th **S61.213 Laceration without foreign body of left middle finger without damage to nail**

✓7th **S61.214 Laceration without foreign body of right ring finger without damage to nail**

✓7th **S61.215 Laceration without foreign body of left ring finger without damage to nail**

✓7th **S61.216 Laceration without foreign body of right little finger without damage to nail**

✓7th **S61.217 Laceration without foreign body of left little finger without damage to nail**

✓7th **S61.218 Laceration without foreign body of other finger without damage to nail**
> Laceration without foreign body of specified finger with unspecified laterality without damage to nail

✓7th **S61.219 Laceration without foreign body of unspecified finger without damage to nail**

✓6th **S61.22 Laceration with foreign body of finger without damage to nail**

✓7th **S61.220 Laceration with foreign body of right index finger without damage to nail**

✓7th **S61.221 Laceration with foreign body of left index finger without damage to nail**

✓7th **S61.222 Laceration with foreign body of right middle finger without damage to nail**

✓7th **S61.223 Laceration with foreign body of left middle finger without damage to nail**

✓7th **S61.224 Laceration with foreign body of right ring finger without damage to nail**

✓7th **S61.225 Laceration with foreign body of left ring finger without damage to nail**

✓7th **S61.226 Laceration with foreign body of right little finger without damage to nail**

✓7th **S61.227 Laceration with foreign body of left little finger without damage to nail**

✓7th **S61.228 Laceration with foreign body of other finger without damage to nail**
> Laceration with foreign body of specified finger with unspecified laterality without damage to nail

✓7th **S61.229 Laceration with foreign body of unspecified finger without damage to nail**

✓6th **S61.23 Puncture wound without foreign body of finger without damage to nail**

✓7th **S61.230 Puncture wound without foreign body of right index finger without damage to nail**

✓7th **S61.231 Puncture wound without foreign body of left index finger without damage to nail**

✓7th **S61.232 Puncture wound without foreign body of right middle finger without damage to nail**

✓7th **S61.233 Puncture wound without foreign body of left middle finger without damage to nail**

✓7th **S61.234 Puncture wound without foreign body of right ring finger without damage to nail**

✓7th **S61.235 Puncture wound without foreign body of left ring finger without damage to nail**

✓7th **S61.236 Puncture wound without foreign body of right little finger without damage to nail**

✓7th **S61.237 Puncture wound without foreign body of left little finger without damage to nail**

✓7th **S61.238 Puncture wound without foreign body of other finger without damage to nail**
> Puncture wound without foreign body of specified finger with unspecified laterality without damage to nail

✓7th **S61.239 Puncture wound without foreign body of unspecified finger without damage to nail**

✓6th **S61.24 Puncture wound with foreign body of finger without damage to nail**

✓7th **S61.240 Puncture wound with foreign body of right index finger without damage to nail**

✓7th **S61.241 Puncture wound with foreign body of left index finger without damage to nail**

✓7th **S61.242 Puncture wound with foreign body of right middle finger without damage to nail**

✓7th **S61.243 Puncture wound with foreign body of left middle finger without damage to nail**

✓7th **S61.244 Puncture wound with foreign body of right ring finger without damage to nail**

✓7th **S61.245 Puncture wound with foreign body of left ring finger without damage to nail**

✓7th **S61.246 Puncture wound with foreign body of right little finger without damage to nail**

✓7th **S61.247 Puncture wound with foreign body of left little finger without damage to nail**

✓7th **S61.248 Puncture wound with foreign body of other finger without damage to nail**
> Puncture wound with foreign body of specified finger with unspecified laterality without damage to nail

✓7th **S61.249 Puncture wound with foreign body of unspecified finger without damage to nail**

✓6th **S61.25 Open bite of finger without damage to nail**
> Bite of finger without damage to nail NOS
> EXCLUDES 1 *superficial bite of finger (S60.46-, S60.47-)*

✓7th **S61.250 Open bite of right index finger without damage to nail**

✓7th **S61.251 Open bite of left index finger without damage to nail**

EXCLUDES 1 Not coded here   EXCLUDES 2 Not included here   *Manifestation Code*

✓7ᵗʰ **S61.252** **Open bite of right middle finger without damage to nail**

✓7ᵗʰ **S61.253** **Open bite of left middle finger without damage to nail**

✓7ᵗʰ **S61.254** **Open bite of right ring finger without damage to nail**

✓7ᵗʰ **S61.255** **Open bite of left ring finger without damage to nail**

✓7ᵗʰ **S61.256** **Open bite of right little finger without damage to nail**

✓7ᵗʰ **S61.257** **Open bite of left little finger without damage to nail**

✓7ᵗʰ **S61.258** **Open bite of other finger without damage to nail**
Open bite of specified finger with unspecified laterality without damage to nail

✓7ᵗʰ **S61.259** **Open bite of unspecified finger without damage to nail**

✓5ᵗʰ **S61.3** **Open wound of other finger with damage to nail**

✓6ᵗʰ **S61.30** **Unspecified open wound of finger with damage to nail**

✓7ᵗʰ **S61.300** **Unspecified open wound of right index finger with damage to nail**

✓7ᵗʰ **S61.301** **Unspecified open wound of left index finger with damage to nail**

✓7ᵗʰ **S61.302** **Unspecified open wound of right middle finger with damage to nail**

✓7ᵗʰ **S61.303** **Unspecified open wound of left middle finger with damage to nail**

✓7ᵗʰ **S61.304** **Unspecified open wound of right ring finger with damage to nail**

✓7ᵗʰ **S61.305** **Unspecified open wound of left ring finger with damage to nail**

✓7ᵗʰ **S61.306** **Unspecified open wound of right little finger with damage to nail**

✓7ᵗʰ **S61.307** **Unspecified open wound of left little finger with damage to nail**

✓7ᵗʰ **S61.308** **Unspecified open wound of other finger with damage to nail**
Unspecified open wound of specified finger with unspecified laterality with damage to nail

✓7ᵗʰ **S61.309** **Unspecified open wound of unspecified finger with damage to nail**

✓6ᵗʰ **S61.31** **Laceration without foreign body of finger with damage to nail**

✓7ᵗʰ **S61.310** **Laceration without foreign body of right index finger with damage to nail**

✓7ᵗʰ **S61.311** **Laceration without foreign body of left index finger with damage to nail**

✓7ᵗʰ **S61.312** **Laceration without foreign body of right middle finger with damage to nail**

✓7ᵗʰ **S61.313** **Laceration without foreign body of left middle finger with damage to nail**

✓7ᵗʰ **S61.314** **Laceration without foreign body of right ring finger with damage to nail**

✓7ᵗʰ **S61.315** **Laceration without foreign body of left ring finger with damage to nail**

✓7ᵗʰ **S61.316** **Laceration without foreign body of right little finger with damage to nail**

✓7ᵗʰ **S61.317** **Laceration without foreign body of left little finger with damage to nail**

✓7ᵗʰ **S61.318** **Laceration without foreign body of other finger with damage to nail**
Laceration without foreign body of specified finger with unspecified laterality with damage to nail

✓7ᵗʰ **S61.319** **Laceration without foreign body of unspecified finger with damage to nail**

✓6ᵗʰ **S61.32** **Laceration with foreign body of finger with damage to nail**

✓7ᵗʰ **S61.320** **Laceration with foreign body of right index finger with damage to nail**

✓7ᵗʰ **S61.321** **Laceration with foreign body of left index finger with damage to nail**

✓7ᵗʰ **S61.322** **Laceration with foreign body of right middle finger with damage to nail**

✓7ᵗʰ **S61.323** **Laceration with foreign body of left middle finger with damage to nail**

✓7ᵗʰ **S61.324** **Laceration with foreign body of right ring finger with damage to nail**

✓7ᵗʰ **S61.325** **Laceration with foreign body of left ring finger with damage to nail**

✓7ᵗʰ **S61.326** **Laceration with foreign body of right little finger with damage to nail**

✓7ᵗʰ **S61.327** **Laceration with foreign body of left little finger with damage to nail**

✓7ᵗʰ **S61.328** **Laceration with foreign body of other finger with damage to nail**
Laceration with foreign body of specified finger with unspecified laterality with damage to nail

✓7ᵗʰ **S61.329** **Laceration with foreign body of unspecified finger with damage to nail**

✓6ᵗʰ **S61.33** **Puncture wound without foreign body of finger with damage to nail**

✓7ᵗʰ **S61.330** **Puncture wound without foreign body of right index finger with damage to nail**

✓7ᵗʰ **S61.331** **Puncture wound without foreign body of left index finger with damage to nail**

✓7ᵗʰ **S61.332** **Puncture wound without foreign body of right middle finger with damage to nail**

✓7ᵗʰ **S61.333** **Puncture wound without foreign body of left middle finger with damage to nail**

✓7ᵗʰ **S61.334** **Puncture wound without foreign body of right ring finger with damage to nail**

✓7ᵗʰ **S61.335** **Puncture wound without foreign body of left ring finger with damage to nail**

✓7ᵗʰ **S61.336** **Puncture wound without foreign body of right little finger with damage to nail**

✓7ᵗʰ **S61.337** **Puncture wound without foreign body of left little finger with damage to nail**

✓7ᵗʰ **S61.338** **Puncture wound without foreign body of other finger with damage to nail**
Puncture wound without foreign body of specified finger with unspecified laterality with damage to nail

✓7ᵗʰ **S61.339** **Puncture wound without foreign body of unspecified finger with damage to nail**

✓6ᵗʰ **S61.34** **Puncture wound with foreign body of finger with damage to nail**

✓7ᵗʰ **S61.340** **Puncture wound with foreign body of right index finger with damage to nail**

✓7ᵗʰ **S61.341** **Puncture wound with foreign body of left index finger with damage to nail**

✓7ᵗʰ **S61.342** **Puncture wound with foreign body of right middle finger with damage to nail**

✓7ᵗʰ **S61.343** **Puncture wound with foreign body of left middle finger with damage to nail**

✓7ᵗʰ **S61.344** **Puncture wound with foreign body of right ring finger with damage to nail**

✓7ᵗʰ **S61.345** **Puncture wound with foreign body of left ring finger with damage to nail**

✓7ᵗʰ **S61.346** **Puncture wound with foreign body of right little finger with damage to nail**

✓7ᵗʰ **S61.347** **Puncture wound with foreign body of left little finger with damage to nail**

✓7ᵗʰ **S61.348** **Puncture wound with foreign body of other finger with damage to nail**
Puncture wound with foreign body of specified finger with unspecified laterality with damage to nail

✓7ᵗʰ **S61.349** **Puncture wound with foreign body of unspecified finger with damage to nail**

✓6ᵗʰ **S61.35** **Open bite of finger with damage to nail**
Bite of finger with damage to nail NOS
EXCLUDES 1 superficial bite of finger (S60.46-, S60.47-)

✓7ᵗʰ **S61.350** **Open bite of right index finger with damage to nail**

√7th **S61.351 Open bite of left index finger with damage to nail**

√7th **S61.352 Open bite of right middle finger with damage to nail**

√7th **S61.353 Open bite of left middle finger with damage to nail**

√7th **S61.354 Open bite of right ring finger with damage to nail**

√7th **S61.355 Open bite of left ring finger with damage to nail**

√7th **S61.356 Open bite of right little finger with damage to nail**

√7th **S61.357 Open bite of left little finger with damage to nail**

√7th **S61.358 Open bite of other finger with damage to nail**
Open bite of specified finger with unspecified laterality with damage to nail

√7th **S61.359 Open bite of unspecified finger with damage to nail**

√5th **S61.4 Open wound of hand**

√6th **S61.40 Unspecified open wound of hand**

√7th **S61.401 Unspecified open wound of right hand**

√7th **S61.402 Unspecified open wound of left hand**

√7th **S61.409 Unspecified open wound of unspecified hand**

√6th **S61.41 Laceration without foreign body of hand**

√7th **S61.411 Laceration without foreign body of right hand**

√7th **S61.412 Laceration without foreign body of left hand**

√7th **S61.419 Laceration without foreign body of unspecified hand**

√6th **S61.42 Laceration with foreign body of hand**

√7th **S61.421 Laceration with foreign body of right hand**

√7th **S61.422 Laceration with foreign body of left hand**

√7th **S61.429 Laceration with foreign body of unspecified hand**

√6th **S61.43 Puncture wound without foreign body of hand**

√7th **S61.431 Puncture wound without foreign body of right hand**

√7th **S61.432 Puncture wound without foreign body of left hand**

√7th **S61.439 Puncture wound without foreign body of unspecified hand**

√6th **S61.44 Puncture wound with foreign body of hand**

√7th **S61.441 Puncture wound with foreign body of right hand**

√7th **S61.442 Puncture wound with foreign body of left hand**

√7th **S61.449 Puncture wound with foreign body of unspecified hand**

√6th **S61.45 Open bite of hand**
Bite of hand NOS
EXCLUDES 1   superficial bite of hand (S60.56-, S60.57-)

√7th **S61.451 Open bite of right hand**

√7th **S61.452 Open bite of left hand**

√7th **S61.459 Open bite of unspecified hand**

√5th **S61.5 Open wound of wrist**

√6th **S61.50 Unspecified open wound of wrist**

√7th **S61.501 Unspecified open wound of right wrist**

√7th **S61.502 Unspecified open wound of left wrist**

√7th **S61.509 Unspecified open wound of unspecified wrist**

√6th **S61.51 Laceration without foreign body of wrist**

√7th **S61.511 Laceration without foreign body of right wrist**

√7th **S61.512 Laceration without foreign body of left wrist**

√7th **S61.519 Laceration without foreign body of unspecified wrist**

√6th **S61.52 Laceration with foreign body of wrist**

√7th **S61.521 Laceration with foreign body of right wrist**

√7th **S61.522 Laceration with foreign body of left wrist**

√7th **S61.529 Laceration with foreign body of unspecified wrist**

√6th **S61.53 Puncture wound without foreign body of wrist**

√7th **S61.531 Puncture wound without foreign body of right wrist**

√7th **S61.532 Puncture wound without foreign body of left wrist**

√7th **S61.539 Puncture wound without foreign body of unspecified wrist**

√6th **S61.54 Puncture wound with foreign body of wrist**

√7th **S61.541 Puncture wound with foreign body of right wrist**

√7th **S61.542 Puncture wound with foreign body of left wrist**

√7th **S61.549 Puncture wound with foreign body of unspecified wrist**

√6th **S61.55 Open bite of wrist**
Bite of wrist NOS
EXCLUDES 1   superficial bite of wrist (S60.86-, S60.87-)

√7th **S61.551 Open bite of right wrist**

√7th **S61.552 Open bite of left wrist**

√7th **S61.559 Open bite of unspecified wrist**

√4th **S62 Fracture at wrist and hand level**
NOTE   A fracture not indicated as displaced or nondisplaced should be coded to displaced
A fracture not indicated as open or closed should be coded to closed.
EXCLUDES 1   traumatic amputation of wrist and hand (S68-)
EXCLUDES 2   fracture of distal parts of ulna and radius (S52-)

The appropriate 7th character is to be added to each code from category S62.
A   initial encounter for closed fracture
B   initial encounter for open fracture
D   subsequent encounter for fracture with routine healing
G   subsequent encounter for fracture with delayed healing
K   subsequent encounter for fracture with nonunion
P   subsequent encounter for fracture with malunion
S   sequela

√5th **S62.0 Fracture of navicular [scaphoid] bone of wrist**

√6th **S62.00 Unspecified fracture of navicular [scaphoid] bone of wrist**

√7th **S62.001 Unspecified fracture of navicular [scaphoid] bone of right wrist**

√7th **S62.002 Unspecified fracture of navicular [scaphoid] bone of left wrist**

√7th **S62.009 Unspecified fracture of navicular [scaphoid] bone of unspecified wrist**

√6th **S62.01 Fracture of distal pole of navicular [scaphoid] bone of wrist**
Fracture of volar tuberosity of navicular [scaphoid] bone of wrist

√7th **S62.011 Displaced fracture of distal pole of navicular [scaphoid] bone of right wrist**

√7th **S62.012 Displaced fracture of distal pole of navicular [scaphoid] bone of left wrist**

√7th **S62.013 Displaced fracture of distal pole of navicular [scaphoid] bone of unspecified wrist**

√7th **S62.014 Nondisplaced fracture of distal pole of navicular [scaphoid] bone of right wrist**

√7th **S62.015 Nondisplaced fracture of distal pole of navicular [scaphoid] bone of left wrist**

√7th **S62.016 Nondisplaced fracture of distal pole of navicular [scaphoid] bone of unspecified wrist**

√6th **S62.02 Fracture of middle third of navicular [scaphoid] bone of wrist**

√7th **S62.021 Displaced fracture of middle third of navicular [scaphoid] bone of right wrist**

√7th **S62.022 Displaced fracture of middle third of navicular [scaphoid] bone of left wrist**

√7th **S62.023** Displaced fracture of middle third of navicular [scaphoid] bone of unspecified wrist

√7th **S62.024** Nondisplaced fracture of middle third of navicular [scaphoid] bone of right wrist

√7th **S62.025** Nondisplaced fracture of middle third of navicular [scaphoid] bone of left wrist

√7th **S62.026** Nondisplaced fracture of middle third of navicular [scaphoid] bone of unspecified wrist

√6th **S62.03** Fracture of proximal third of navicular [scaphoid] bone of wrist

√7th **S62.031** Displaced fracture of proximal third of navicular [scaphoid] bone of right wrist

√7th **S62.032** Displaced fracture of proximal third of navicular [scaphoid] bone of left wrist

√7th **S62.033** Displaced fracture of proximal third of navicular [scaphoid] bone of unspecified wrist

√7th **S62.034** Nondisplaced fracture of proximal third of navicular [scaphoid] bone of right wrist

√7th **S62.035** Nondisplaced fracture of proximal third of navicular [scaphoid] bone of left wrist

√7th **S62.036** Nondisplaced fracture of proximal third of navicular [scaphoid] bone of unspecified wrist

√5th **S62.1** Fracture of other and unspecified carpal bone(s)

EXCLUDES 2 *fracture of scaphoid of wrist (S62.0-)*

√6th **S62.10** Fracture of unspecified carpal bone

Fracture of wrist NOS

√7th **S62.101** Fracture of unspecified carpal bone, right wrist

√7th **S62.102** Fracture of unspecified carpal bone, left wrist

√7th **S62.109** Fracture of unspecified carpal bone, unspecified wrist

√6th **S62.11** Fracture of triquetrum [cuneiform] bone of wrist

√7th **S62.111** Displaced fracture of triquetrum [cuneiform] bone, right wrist

√7th **S62.112** Displaced fracture of triquetrum [cuneiform] bone, left wrist

√7th **S62.113** Displaced fracture of triquetrum [cuneiform] bone, unspecified wrist

√7th **S62.114** Nondisplaced fracture of triquetrum [cuneiform] bone, right wrist

√7th **S62.115** Nondisplaced fracture of triquetrum [cuneiform] bone, left wrist

√7th **S62.116** Nondisplaced fracture of triquetrum [cuneiform] bone, unspecified wrist

√6th **S62.12** Fracture of lunate [semilunar]

√7th **S62.121** Displaced fracture of lunate [semilunar], right wrist

√7th **S62.122** Displaced fracture of lunate [semilunar], left wrist

√7th **S62.123** Displaced fracture of lunate [semilunar], unspecified wrist

√7th **S62.124** Nondisplaced fracture of lunate [semilunar], right wrist

√7th **S62.125** Nondisplaced fracture of lunate [semilunar], left wrist

√7th **S62.126** Nondisplaced fracture of lunate [semilunar], unspecified wrist

√6th **S62.13** Fracture of capitate [os magnum]

√7th **S62.131** Displaced fracture of capitate [os magnum] bone, right wrist

√7th **S62.132** Displaced fracture of capitate [os magnum] bone, left wrist

√7th **S62.133** Displaced fracture of capitate [os magnum] bone, unspecified wrist

√7th **S62.134** Nondisplaced fracture of capitate [os magnum] bone, right wrist

√7th **S62.135** Nondisplaced fracture of capitate [os magnum] bone, left wrist

√7th **S62.136** Nondisplaced fracture of capitate [os magnum] bone, unspecified wrist

√6th **S62.14** Fracture of body of hamate [unciform] bone

Fracture of hamate [unciform] bone NOS

√7th **S62.141** Displaced fracture of body of hamate [unciform] bone, right wrist

√7th **S62.142** Displaced fracture of body of hamate [unciform] bone, left wrist

√7th **S62.143** Displaced fracture of body of hamate [unciform] bone, unspecified wrist

√7th **S62.144** Nondisplaced fracture of body of hamate [unciform] bone, right wrist

√7th **S62.145** Nondisplaced fracture of body of hamate [unciform] bone, left wrist

√7th **S62.146** Nondisplaced fracture of body of hamate [unciform] bone, unspecified wrist

√6th **S62.15** Fracture of hook process of hamate [unciform] bone

Fracture of unciform process of hamate [unciform] bone

√7th **S62.151** Displaced fracture of hook process of hamate [unciform] bone, right wrist

√7th **S62.152** Displaced fracture of hook process of hamate [unciform] bone, left wrist

√7th **S62.153** Displaced fracture of hook process of hamate [unciform] bone, unspecified wrist

√7th **S62.154** Nondisplaced fracture of hook process of hamate [unciform] bone, right wrist

√7th **S62.155** Nondisplaced fracture of hook process of hamate [unciform] bone, left wrist

√7th **S62.156** Nondisplaced fracture of hook process of hamate [unciform] bone, unspecified wrist

√6th **S62.16** Fracture of pisiform

√7th **S62.161** Displaced fracture of pisiform, right wrist

√7th **S62.162** Displaced fracture of pisiform, left wrist

√7th **S62.163** Displaced fracture of pisiform, unspecified wrist

√7th **S62.164** Nondisplaced fracture of pisiform, right wrist

√7th **S62.165** Nondisplaced fracture of pisiform, left wrist

√7th **S62.166** Nondisplaced fracture of pisiform, unspecified wrist

√6th **S62.17** Fracture of trapezium [larger multangular]

√7th **S62.171** Displaced fracture of trapezium [larger multangular], right wrist

√7th **S62.172** Displaced fracture of trapezium [larger multangular], left wrist

√7th **S62.173** Displaced fracture of trapezium [larger multangular], unspecified wrist

√7th **S62.174** Nondisplaced fracture of trapezium [larger multangular], right wrist

√7th **S62.175** Nondisplaced fracture of trapezium [larger multangular], left wrist

√7th **S62.176** Nondisplaced fracture of trapezium [larger multangular], unspecified wrist

√6th **S62.18** Fracture of trapezoid [smaller multangular]

√7th **S62.181** Displaced fracture of trapezoid [smaller multangular], right wrist

√7th **S62.182** Displaced fracture of trapezoid [smaller multangular], left wrist

√7th **S62.183** Displaced fracture of trapezoid [smaller multangular], unspecified wrist

√7th **S62.184** Nondisplaced fracture of trapezoid [smaller multangular], right wrist

√7th **S62.185** Nondisplaced fracture of trapezoid [smaller multangular], left wrist

√7th **S62.186** Nondisplaced fracture of trapezoid [smaller multangular], unspecified wrist

√5th **S62.2** Fracture of first metacarpal bone

√6th **S62.20** Unspecified fracture of first metacarpal bone

√7th **S62.201** Unspecified fracture of first metacarpal bone, right hand

√7th **S62.202** Unspecified fracture of first metacarpal bone, left hand

---

✔ Appropriate additional character required   √x7th Requires 7th character, placeholder x must fill empty characters

Injury, Poisoning and Certain Other Consequences of External Causes

S62.209–S62.335

√7th **S62.209** Unspecified fracture of first metacarpal bone, unspecified hand

√6th **S62.21** Bennett's fracture

√7th **S62.211** Bennett's fracture, right hand

√7th **S62.212** Bennett's fracture, left hand

√7th **S62.213** Bennett's fracture, unspecified hand

√6th **S62.22** Rolando's fracture

√7th **S62.221** Displaced Rolando's fracture, right hand

√7th **S62.222** Displaced Rolando's fracture, left hand

√7th **S62.223** Displaced Rolando's fracture, unspecified hand

√7th **S62.224** Nondisplaced Rolando's fracture, right hand

√7th **S62.225** Nondisplaced Rolando's fracture, left hand

√7th **S62.226** Nondisplaced Rolando's fracture, unspecified hand

√6th **S62.23** Other fracture of base of first metacarpal bone

√7th **S62.231** Other displaced fracture of base of first metacarpal bone, right hand

√7th **S62.232** Other displaced fracture of base of first metacarpal bone, left hand

√7th **S62.233** Other displaced fracture of base of first metacarpal bone, unspecified hand

√7th **S62.234** Other nondisplaced fracture of base of first metacarpal bone, right hand

√7th **S62.235** Other nondisplaced fracture of base of first metacarpal bone, left hand

√7th **S62.236** Other nondisplaced fracture of base of first metacarpal bone, unspecified hand

√6th **S62.24** Fracture of shaft of first metacarpal bone

√7th **S62.241** Displaced fracture of shaft of first metacarpal bone, right hand

√7th **S62.242** Displaced fracture of shaft of first metacarpal bone, left hand

√7th **S62.243** Displaced fracture of shaft of first metacarpal bone, unspecified hand

√7th **S62.244** Nondisplaced fracture of shaft of first metacarpal bone, right hand

√7th **S62.245** Nondisplaced fracture of shaft of first metacarpal bone, left hand

√7th **S62.246** Nondisplaced fracture of shaft of first metacarpal bone, unspecified hand

√6th **S62.25** Fracture of neck of first metacarpal bone

√7th **S62.251** Displaced fracture of neck of first metacarpal bone, right hand

√7th **S62.252** Displaced fracture of neck of first metacarpal bone, left hand

√7th **S62.253** Displaced fracture of neck of first metacarpal bone, unspecified hand

√7th **S62.254** Nondisplaced fracture of neck of first metacarpal bone, right hand

√7th **S62.255** Nondisplaced fracture of neck of first metacarpal bone, left hand

√7th **S62.256** Nondisplaced fracture of neck of first metacarpal bone, unspecified hand

√6th **S62.29** Other fracture of first metacarpal bone

√7th **S62.291** Other fracture of first metacarpal bone, right hand

√7th **S62.292** Other fracture of first metacarpal bone, left hand

√7th **S62.299** Other fracture of first metacarpal bone, unspecified hand

√5th **S62.3** Fracture of other and unspecified metacarpal bone

EXCLUDES 2   fracture of first metacarpal bone (S62.2-)

√6th **S62.30** Unspecified fracture of other metacarpal bone

√7th **S62.300** Unspecified fracture of second metacarpal bone, right hand

√7th **S62.301** Unspecified fracture of second metacarpal bone, left hand

√7th **S62.302** Unspecified fracture of third metacarpal bone, right hand

√7th **S62.303** Unspecified fracture of third metacarpal bone, left hand

√7th **S62.304** Unspecified fracture of fourth metacarpal bone, right hand

√7th **S62.305** Unspecified fracture of fourth metacarpal bone, left hand

√7th **S62.306** Unspecified fracture of fifth metacarpal bone, right hand

√7th **S62.307** Unspecified fracture of fifth metacarpal bone, left hand

√7th **S62.308** Unspecified fracture of other metacarpal bone

Unspecified fracture of specified metacarpal bone with unspecified laterality

√7th **S62.309** Unspecified fracture of unspecified metacarpal bone

√6th **S62.31** Displaced fracture of base of other metacarpal bone

√7th **S62.310** Displaced fracture of base of second metacarpal bone, right hand

√7th **S62.311** Displaced fracture of base of second metacarpal bone. left hand

√7th **S62.312** Displaced fracture of base of third metacarpal bone, right hand

√7th **S62.313** Displaced fracture of base of third metacarpal bone, left hand

√7th **S62.314** Displaced fracture of base of fourth metacarpal bone, right hand

√7th **S62.315** Displaced fracture of base of fourth metacarpal bone, left hand

√7th **S62.316** Displaced fracture of base of fifth metacarpal bone, right hand

√7th **S62.317** Displaced fracture of base of fifth metacarpal bone. left hand

√7th **S62.318** Displaced fracture of base of other metacarpal bone

Displaced fracture of base of specified metacarpal bone with unspecified laterality

√7th **S62.319** Displaced fracture of base of unspecified metacarpal bone

√6th **S62.32** Displaced fracture of shaft of other metacarpal bone

√7th **S62.320** Displaced fracture of shaft of second metacarpal bone, right hand

√7th **S62.321** Displaced fracture of shaft of second metacarpal bone, left hand

√7th **S62.322** Displaced fracture of shaft of third metacarpal bone, right hand

√7th **S62.323** Displaced fracture of shaft of third metacarpal bone, left hand

√7th **S62.324** Displaced fracture of shaft of fourth metacarpal bone, right hand

√7th **S62.325** Displaced fracture of shaft of fourth metacarpal bone, left hand

√7th **S62.326** Displaced fracture of shaft of fifth metacarpal bone, right hand

√7th **S62.327** Displaced fracture of shaft of fifth metacarpal bone, left hand

√7th **S62.328** Displaced fracture of shaft of other metacarpal bone

Displaced fracture of shaft of specified metacarpal bone with unspecified laterality

√7th **S62.329** Displaced fracture of shaft of unspecified metacarpal bone

√6th **S62.33** Displaced fracture of neck of other metacarpal bone

√7th **S62.330** Displaced fracture of neck of second metacarpal bone, right hand

√7th **S62.331** Displaced fracture of neck of second metacarpal bone, left hand

√7th **S62.332** Displaced fracture of neck of third metacarpal bone, right hand

√7th **S62.333** Displaced fracture of neck of third metacarpal bone, left hand

√7th **S62.334** Displaced fracture of neck of fourth metacarpal bone, right hand

√7th **S62.335** Displaced fracture of neck of fourth metacarpal bone, left hand

---

EXCLUDES 1   Not coded here   EXCLUDES 2   Not included here   *Manifestation Code*

✓7ᵗʰ **S62.336** **Displaced fracture of neck of fifth metacarpal bone, right hand**

✓7ᵗʰ **S62.337** **Displaced fracture of neck of fifth metacarpal bone, left hand**

✓7ᵗʰ **S62.338** **Displaced fracture of neck of other metacarpal bone**
Displaced fracture of neck of specified metacarpal bone with unspecified laterality

✓7ᵗʰ **S62.339** **Displaced fracture of neck of unspecified metacarpal bone**

✓6ᵗʰ **S62.34** **Nondisplaced fracture of base of other metacarpal bone**

S62.340 **Nondisplaced fracture of base of second metacarpal bone, right hand**

✓7ᵗʰ **S62.341** **Nondisplaced fracture of base of second metacarpal bone. left hand**

✓7ᵗʰ **S62.342** **Nondisplaced fracture of base of third metacarpal bone, right hand**

✓7ᵗʰ **S62.343** **Nondisplaced fracture of base of third metacarpal bone, left hand**

✓7ᵗʰ **S62.344** **Nondisplaced fracture of base of fourth metacarpal bone, right hand**

✓7ᵗʰ **S62.345** **Nondisplaced fracture of base of fourth metacarpal bone, left hand**

✓7ᵗʰ **S62.346** **Nondisplaced fracture of base of fifth metacarpal bone, right hand**

✓7ᵗʰ **S62.347** **Nondisplaced fracture of base of fifth metacarpal bone. left hand**

✓7ᵗʰ **S62.348** **Nondisplaced fracture of base of other metacarpal bone**
Nondisplaced fracture of base of specified metacarpal bone with unspecified laterality

✓7ᵗʰ **S62.349** **Nondisplaced fracture of base of unspecified metacarpal bone**

✓6ᵗʰ **S62.35** **Nondisplaced fracture of shaft of other metacarpal bone**

✓7ᵗʰ **S62.350** **Nondisplaced fracture of shaft of second metacarpal bone, right hand**

✓7ᵗʰ **S62.351** **Nondisplaced fracture of shaft of second metacarpal bone, left hand**

✓7ᵗʰ **S62.352** **Nondisplaced fracture of shaft of third metacarpal bone, right hand**

✓7ᵗʰ **S62.353** **Nondisplaced fracture of shaft of third metacarpal bone, left hand**

✓7ᵗʰ **S62.354** **Nondisplaced fracture of shaft of fourth metacarpal bone, right hand**

✓7ᵗʰ **S62.355** **Nondisplaced fracture of shaft of fourth metacarpal bone, left hand**

✓7ᵗʰ **S62.356** **Nondisplaced fracture of shaft of fifth metacarpal bone, right hand**

✓7ᵗʰ **S62.357** **Nondisplaced fracture of shaft of fifth metacarpal bone, left hand**

✓7ᵗʰ **S62.358** **Nondisplaced fracture of shaft of other metacarpal bone**
Nondisplaced fracture of shaft of specified metacarpal bone with unspecified laterality

✓7ᵗʰ **S62.359** **Nondisplaced fracture of shaft of unspecified metacarpal bone**

✓6ᵗʰ **S62.36** **Nondisplaced fracture of neck of other metacarpal bone**

✓7ᵗʰ **S62.360** **Nondisplaced fracture of neck of second metacarpal bone, right hand**

✓7ᵗʰ **S62.361** **Nondisplaced fracture of neck of second metacarpal bone, left hand**

✓7ᵗʰ **S62.362** **Nondisplaced fracture of neck of third metacarpal bone, right hand**

✓7ᵗʰ **S62.363** **Nondisplaced fracture of neck of third metacarpal bone, left hand**

✓7ᵗʰ **S62.364** **Nondisplaced fracture of neck of fourth metacarpal bone, right hand**

✓7ᵗʰ **S62.365** **Nondisplaced fracture of neck of fourth metacarpal bone, left hand**

✓7ᵗʰ **S62.366** **Nondisplaced fracture of neck of fifth metacarpal bone, right hand**

✓7ᵗʰ **S62.367** **Nondisplaced fracture of neck of fifth metacarpal bone, left hand**

✓7ᵗʰ **S62.368** **Nondisplaced fracture of neck of other metacarpal bone**
Nondisplaced fracture of neck of specified metacarpal bone with unspecified laterality

✓7ᵗʰ **S62.369** **Nondisplaced fracture of neck of unspecified metacarpal bone**

✓6ᵗʰ **S62.39** **Other fracture of other metacarpal bone**

✓7ᵗʰ **S62.390** **Other fracture of second metacarpal bone, right hand**

✓7ᵗʰ **S62.391** **Other fracture of second metacarpal bone, left hand**

✓7ᵗʰ **S62.392** **Other fracture of third metacarpal bone, right hand**

✓7ᵗʰ **S62.393** **Other fracture of third metacarpal bone, left hand**

✓7ᵗʰ **S62.394** **Other fracture of fourth metacarpal bone, right hand**

✓7ᵗʰ **S62.395** **Other fracture of fourth metacarpal bone, left hand**

✓7ᵗʰ **S62.396** **Other fracture of fifth metacarpal bone, right hand**

✓7ᵗʰ **S62.397** **Other fracture of fifth metacarpal bone, left hand**

✓7ᵗʰ **S62.398** **Other fracture of other metacarpal bone**
Other fracture of specified metacarpal bone with unspecified laterality

✓7ᵗʰ **S62.399** **Other fracture of unspecified metacarpal bone**

✓5ᵗʰ **S62.5** **Fracture of thumb**

✓6ᵗʰ **S62.50** **Fracture of unspecified phalanx of thumb**

✓7ᵗʰ **S62.501** **Fracture of unspecified phalanx of right thumb**

✓7ᵗʰ **S62.502** **Fracture of unspecified phalanx of left thumb**

✓7ᵗʰ **S62.509** **Fracture of unspecified phalanx of unspecified thumb**

✓6ᵗʰ **S62.51** **Fracture of proximal phalanx of thumb**

✓7ᵗʰ **S62.511** **Displaced fracture of proximal phalanx of right thumb**

✓7ᵗʰ **S62.512** **Displaced fracture of proximal phalanx of left thumb**

✓7ᵗʰ **S62.513** **Displaced fracture of proximal phalanx of unspecified thumb**

✓7ᵗʰ **S62.514** **Nondisplaced fracture of proximal phalanx of right thumb**

✓7ᵗʰ **S62.515** **Nondisplaced fracture of proximal phalanx of left thumb**

✓7ᵗʰ **S62.516** **Nondisplaced fracture of proximal phalanx of unspecified thumb**

✓6ᵗʰ **S62.52** **Fracture of distal phalanx of thumb**

✓7ᵗʰ **S62.521** **Displaced fracture of distal phalanx of right thumb**

✓7ᵗʰ **S62.522** **Displaced fracture of distal phalanx of left thumb**

✓7ᵗʰ **S62.523** **Displaced fracture of distal phalanx of unspecified thumb**

✓7ᵗʰ **S62.524** **Nondisplaced fracture of distal phalanx of right thumb**

✓7ᵗʰ **S62.525** **Nondisplaced fracture of distal phalanx of left thumb**

✓7ᵗʰ **S62.526** **Nondisplaced fracture of distal phalanx of unspecified thumb**

✓5ᵗʰ **S62.6** **Fracture of other and unspecified finger(s)**
EXCLUDES 2 *fracture of thumb (S62.5-)*

✓6ᵗʰ **S62.60** **Fracture of unspecified phalanx of finger**

✓7ᵗʰ **S62.600** **Fracture of unspecified phalanx of right index finger**

✓7ᵗʰ **S62.601** **Fracture of unspecified phalanx of left index finger**

✓7ᵗʰ **S62.602** **Fracture of unspecified phalanx of right middle finger**

✓7ᵗʰ **S62.603** **Fracture of unspecified phalanx of left middle finger**

✓ Appropriate additional character required   ✓x7ᵗʰ Requires 7th character, placeholder x must fill empty characters

√7th **S62.604** **Fracture of unspecified phalanx of right ring finger**

√7th **S62.605** **Fracture of unspecified phalanx of left ring finger**

√7th **S62.606** **Fracture of unspecified phalanx of right little finger**

√7th **S62.607** **Fracture of unspecified phalanx of left little finger**

√7th **S62.608** **Fracture of unspecified phalanx of other finger**

Fracture of unspecified phalanx of specified finger with unspecified laterality

√7th **S62.609** **Fracture of unspecified phalanx of unspecified finger**

√6th **S62.61** **Displaced fracture of proximal phalanx of finger**

√7th **S62.610** **Displaced fracture of proximal phalanx of right index finger**

√7th **S62.611** **Displaced fracture of proximal phalanx of left index finger**

√7th **S62.612** **Displaced fracture of proximal phalanx of right middle finger**

√7th **S62.613** **Displaced fracture of proximal phalanx of left middle finger**

√7th **S62.614** **Displaced fracture of proximal phalanx of right ring finger**

√7th **S62.615** **Displaced fracture of proximal phalanx of left ring finger**

√7th **S62.616** **Displaced fracture of proximal phalanx of right little finger**

√7th **S62.617** **Displaced fracture of proximal phalanx of left little finger**

√7th **S62.618** **Displaced fracture of proximal phalanx of other finger**

Displaced fracture of proximal phalanx of specified finger with unspecified laterality

√7th **S62.619** **Displaced fracture of proximal phalanx of unspecified finger**

√6th **S62.62** **Displaced fracture of middle phalanx of finger**

√7th **S62.620** **Displaced fracture of middle phalanx of right index finger**

√7th **S62.621** **Displaced fracture of middle phalanx of left index finger**

√7th **S62.622** **Displaced fracture of middle phalanx of right middle finger**

√7th **S62.623** **Displaced fracture of middle phalanx of left middle finger**

√7th **S62.624** **Displaced fracture of middle phalanx of right ring finger**

√7th **S62.625** **Displaced fracture of middle phalanx of left ring finger**

√7th **S62.626** **Displaced fracture of middle phalanx of right little finger**

√7th **S62.627** **Displaced fracture of middle phalanx of left little finger**

√7th **S62.628** **Displaced fracture of middle phalanx of other finger**

Displaced fracture of middle phalanx of specified finger with unspecified laterality

√7th **S62.629** **Displaced fracture of middle phalanx of unspecified finger**

√6th **S62.63** **Displaced fracture of distal phalanx of finger**

√7th **S62.630** **Displaced fracture of distal phalanx of right index finger**

√7th **S62.631** **Displaced fracture of distal phalanx of left index finger**

√7th **S62.632** **Displaced fracture of distal phalanx of right middle finger**

√7th **S62.633** **Displaced fracture of distal phalanx of left middle finger**

√7th **S62.634** **Displaced fracture of distal phalanx of right ring finger**

√7th **S62.635** **Displaced fracture of distal phalanx of left ring finger**

√7th **S62.636** **Displaced fracture of distal phalanx of right little finger**

√7th **S62.637** **Displaced fracture of distal phalanx of left little finger**

√7th **S62.638** **Displaced fracture of distal phalanx of other finger**

Displaced fracture of distal phalanx of specified finger with unspecified laterality

√7th **S62.639** **Displaced fracture of distal phalanx of unspecified finger**

√6th **S62.64** **Nondisplaced fracture of proximal phalanx of finger**

√7th **S62.640** **Nondisplaced fracture of proximal phalanx of right index finger**

√7th **S62.641** **Nondisplaced fracture of proximal phalanx of left index finger**

√7th **S62.642** **Nondisplaced fracture of proximal phalanx of right middle finger**

√7th **S62.643** **Nondisplaced fracture of proximal phalanx of left middle finger**

√7th **S62.644** **Nondisplaced fracture of proximal phalanx of right ring finger**

√7th **S62.645** **Nondisplaced fracture of proximal phalanx of left ring finger**

√7th **S62.646** **Nondisplaced fracture of proximal phalanx of right little finger**

√7th **S62.647** **Nondisplaced fracture of proximal phalanx of left little finger**

√7th **S62.648** **Nondisplaced fracture of proximal phalanx of other finger**

Nondisplaced fracture of proximal phalanx of specified finger with unspecified laterality

√7th **S62.649** **Nondisplaced fracture of proximal phalanx of unspecified finger**

√6th **S62.65** **Nondisplaced fracture of middle phalanx of finger**

√7th **S62.650** **Nondisplaced fracture of middle phalanx of right index finger**

√7th **S62.651** **Nondisplaced fracture of middle phalanx of left index finger**

√7th **S62.652** **Nondisplaced fracture of middle phalanx of right middle finger**

√7th **S62.653** **Nondisplaced fracture of middle phalanx of left middle finger**

√7th **S62.654** **Nondisplaced fracture of middle phalanx of right ring finger**

√7th **S62.655** **Nondisplaced fracture of middle phalanx of left ring finger**

√7th **S62.656** **Nondisplaced fracture of middle phalanx of right little finger**

√7th **S62.657** **Nondisplaced fracture of middle phalanx of left little finger**

√7th **S62.658** **Nondisplaced fracture of middle phalanx of other finger**

Nondisplaced fracture of middle phalanx of specified finger with unspecified laterality

√7th **S62.659** **Nondisplaced fracture of middle phalanx of unspecified finger**

√6th **S62.66** **Nondisplaced fracture of distal phalanx of finger**

√7th **S62.660** **Nondisplaced fracture of distal phalanx of right index finger**

√7th **S62.661** **Nondisplaced fracture of distal phalanx of left index finger**

√7th **S62.662** **Nondisplaced fracture of distal phalanx of right middle finger**

√7th **S62.663** **Nondisplaced fracture of distal phalanx of left middle finger**

√7th **S62.664** **Nondisplaced fracture of distal phalanx of right ring finger**

√7th **S62.665** **Nondisplaced fracture of distal phalanx of left ring finger**

√7th **S62.666** **Nondisplaced fracture of distal phalanx of right little finger**

√7th **S62.667** **Nondisplaced fracture of distal phalanx of left little finger**

EXCLUDES 1 Not coded here   **EXCLUDES 2** Not included here   *Manifestation Code*

✓7th **S62.668 Nondisplaced fracture of distal phalanx of other finger**
   Nondisplaced fracture of distal phalanx of specified finger with unspecified laterality

✓7th **S62.669 Nondisplaced fracture of distal phalanx of unspecified finger**

✓5th **S62.9 Unspecified fracture of wrist and hand**

✓x7th **S62.90 Unspecified fracture of unspecified wrist and hand**

✓x7th **S62.91 Unspecified fracture of right wrist and hand**

✓x7th **S62.92 Unspecified fracture of left wrist and hand**

✓4th **S63 Dislocation and sprain of joints and ligaments at wrist and hand level**

INCLUDES avulsion of joint or ligament at wrist and hand level
   laceration of cartilage, joint or ligament at wrist and hand level
   sprain of cartilage, joint or ligament at wrist and hand level
   traumatic hemarthrosis of joint or ligament at wrist and hand level
   traumatic rupture of joint or ligament at wrist and hand level
   traumatic subluxation of joint or ligament at wrist and hand level
   traumatic tear of joint or ligament at wrist and hand level

Code also any associated open wound

EXCLUDES 2 strain of muscle, fascia and tendon of wrist and hand (S66-)

The appropriate 7th character is to be added to each code from category S63.
   A   initial encounter
   D   subsequent encounter
   S   sequela

✓5th **S63.0 Subluxation and dislocation of wrist and hand joints**

✓6th **S63.00 Unspecified subluxation and dislocation of wrist and hand**
   Dislocation of carpal bone NOS
   Dislocation of distal end of radius NOS
   Subluxation of carpal bone NOS
   Subluxation of distal end of radius NOS

✓7th **S63.001 Unspecified subluxation of right wrist and hand**

✓7th **S63.002 Unspecified subluxation of left wrist and hand**

✓7th **S63.003 Unspecified subluxation of unspecified wrist and hand**

✓7th **S63.004 Unspecified dislocation of right wrist and hand**

✓7th **S63.005 Unspecified dislocation of left wrist and hand**

✓7th **S63.006 Unspecified dislocation of unspecified wrist and hand**

✓6th **S63.01 Subluxation and dislocation of distal radioulnar joint**

✓7th **S63.011 Subluxation of distal radioulnar joint of right wrist**

✓7th **S63.012 Subluxation of distal radioulnar joint of left wrist**

✓7th **S63.013 Subluxation of distal radioulnar joint of unspecified wrist**

✓7th **S63.014 Dislocation of distal radioulnar joint of right wrist**

✓7th **S63.015 Dislocation of distal radioulnar joint of left wrist**

✓7th **S63.016 Dislocation of distal radioulnar joint of unspecified wrist**

✓6th **S63.02 Subluxation and dislocation of radiocarpal joint**

✓7th **S63.021 Subluxation of radiocarpal joint of right wrist**

✓7th **S63.022 Subluxation of radiocarpal joint of left wrist**

✓7th **S63.023 Subluxation of radiocarpal joint of unspecified wrist**

✓7th **S63.024 Dislocation of radiocarpal joint of right wrist**

✓7th **S63.025 Dislocation of radiocarpal joint of left wrist**

✓7th **S63.026 Dislocation of radiocarpal joint of unspecified wrist**

✓6th **S63.03 Subluxation and dislocation of midcarpal joint**

✓7th **S63.031 Subluxation of midcarpal joint of right wrist**

✓7th **S63.032 Subluxation of midcarpal joint of left wrist**

✓7th **S63.033 Subluxation of midcarpal joint of unspecified wrist**

✓7th **S63.034 Dislocation of midcarpal joint of right wrist**

✓7th **S63.035 Dislocation of midcarpal joint of left wrist**

✓7th **S63.036 Dislocation of midcarpal joint of unspecified wrist**

✓6th **S63.04 Subluxation and dislocation of carpometacarpal joint of thumb**

EXCLUDES 2 interphalangeal subluxation and dislocation of thumb (S63.1-)

✓7th **S63.041 Subluxation of carpometacarpal joint of right thumb**

✓7th **S63.042 Subluxation of carpometacarpal joint of left thumb**

✓7th **S63.043 Subluxation of carpometacarpal joint of unspecified thumb**

✓7th **S63.044 Dislocation of carpometacarpal joint of right thumb**

✓7th **S63.045 Dislocation of carpometacarpal joint of left thumb**

✓7th **S63.046 Dislocation of carpometacarpal joint of unspecified thumb**

✓6th **S63.05 Subluxation and dislocation of other carpometacarpal joint**

EXCLUDES 2 subluxation and dislocation of carpometacarpal joint of thumb (S63.04-)

✓7th **S63.051 Subluxation of other carpometacarpal joint of right hand**

✓7th **S63.052 Subluxation of other carpometacarpal joint of left hand**

✓7th **S63.053 Subluxation of other carpometacarpal joint of unspecified hand**

✓7th **S63.054 Dislocation of other carpometacarpal joint of right hand**

✓7th **S63.055 Dislocation of other carpometacarpal joint of left hand**

✓7th **S63.056 Dislocation of other carpometacarpal joint of unspecified hand**

✓6th **S63.06 Subluxation and dislocation of metacarpal (bone), proximal end**

✓7th **S63.061 Subluxation of metacarpal (bone), proximal end of right hand**

✓7th **S63.062 Subluxation of metacarpal (bone), proximal end of left hand**

✓7th **S63.063 Subluxation of metacarpal (bone), proximal end of unspecified hand**

✓7th **S63.064 Dislocation of metacarpal (bone), proximal end of right hand**

✓7th **S63.065 Dislocation of metacarpal (bone), proximal end of left hand**

✓7th **S63.066 Dislocation of metacarpal (bone), proximal end of unspecified hand**

✓6th **S63.07 Subluxation and dislocation of distal end of ulna**

✓7th **S63.071 Subluxation of distal end of right ulna**

✓7th **S63.072 Subluxation of distal end of left ulna**

✓7th **S63.073 Subluxation of distal end of unspecified ulna**

✓7th **S63.074 Dislocation of distal end of right ulna**

✓7th **S63.075 Dislocation of distal end of left ulna**

✓7th **S63.076 Dislocation of distal end of unspecified ulna**

✓6th **S63.09 Other subluxation and dislocation of wrist and hand**

✓7th **S63.091 Other subluxation of right wrist and hand**

✓7th **S63.092 Other subluxation of left wrist and hand**

✓7th **S63.093 Other subluxation of unspecified wrist and hand**

✓7th **S63.094 Other dislocation of right wrist and hand**

(left margin, rotated) **Injury, Poisoning and Certain Other Consequences of External Causes**   **S63.095–S63.229**

✓7ᵗʰ **S63.095** Other dislocation of left wrist and hand

✓7ᵗʰ **S63.096** Other dislocation of unspecified wrist and hand

✓5ᵗʰ **S63.1** **Subluxation and dislocation of thumb**

✓6ᵗʰ **S63.10** **Unspecified subluxation and dislocation of thumb**

✓7ᵗʰ **S63.101** Unspecified subluxation of right thumb

✓7ᵗʰ **S63.102** Unspecified subluxation of left thumb

✓7ᵗʰ **S63.103** Unspecified subluxation of unspecified thumb

✓7ᵗʰ **S63.104** Unspecified dislocation of right thumb

✓7ᵗʰ **S63.105** Unspecified dislocation of left thumb

✓7ᵗʰ **S63.106** Unspecified dislocation of unspecified thumb

✓6ᵗʰ **S63.11** **Subluxation and dislocation of metacarpophalangeal joint of thumb**

✓7ᵗʰ **S63.111** Subluxation of metacarpophalangeal joint of right thumb

✓7ᵗʰ **S63.112** Subluxation of metacarpophalangeal joint of left thumb

✓7ᵗʰ **S63.113** Subluxation of metacarpophalangeal joint of unspecified thumb

✓7ᵗʰ **S63.114** Dislocation of metacarpophalangeal joint of right thumb

✓7ᵗʰ **S63.115** Dislocation of metacarpophalangeal joint of left thumb

✓7ᵗʰ **S63.116** Dislocation of metacarpophalangeal joint of unspecified thumb

✓6ᵗʰ **S63.12** **Subluxation and dislocation of unspecified interphalangeal joint of thumb**

✓7ᵗʰ **S63.121** Subluxation of unspecified interphalangeal joint of right thumb

✓7ᵗʰ **S63.122** Subluxation of unspecified interphalangeal joint of left thumb

✓7ᵗʰ **S63.123** Subluxation of unspecified interphalangeal joint of unspecified thumb

✓7ᵗʰ **S63.124** Dislocation of unspecified interphalangeal joint of right thumb

✓7ᵗʰ **S63.125** Dislocation of unspecified interphalangeal joint of left thumb

✓7ᵗʰ **S63.126** Dislocation of unspecified interphalangeal joint of unspecified thumb

✓6ᵗʰ **S63.13** **Subluxation and dislocation of proximal interphalangeal joint of thumb**

✓7ᵗʰ **S63.131** Subluxation of proximal interphalangeal joint of right thumb

✓7ᵗʰ **S63.132** Subluxation of proximal interphalangeal joint of left thumb

✓7ᵗʰ **S63.133** Subluxation of proximal interphalangeal joint of unspecified thumb

✓7ᵗʰ **S63.134** Dislocation of proximal interphalangeal joint of right thumb

✓7ᵗʰ **S63.135** Dislocation of proximal interphalangeal joint of left thumb

✓7ᵗʰ **S63.136** Dislocation of proximal interphalangeal joint of unspecified thumb

✓6ᵗʰ **S63.14** **Subluxation and dislocation of distal interphalangeal joint of thumb**

✓7ᵗʰ **S63.141** Subluxation of distal interphalangeal joint of right thumb

✓7ᵗʰ **S63.142** Subluxation of distal interphalangeal joint of left thumb

✓7ᵗʰ **S63.143** Subluxation of distal interphalangeal joint of unspecified thumb

✓7ᵗʰ **S63.144** Dislocation of distal interphalangeal joint of right thumb

✓7ᵗʰ **S63.145** Dislocation of distal interphalangeal joint of left thumb

✓7ᵗʰ **S63.146** Dislocation of distal interphalangeal joint of unspecified thumb

✓5ᵗʰ **S63.2** **Subluxation and dislocation of other finger(s)**

EXCLUDES 2 *subluxation and dislocation of thumb (S63.1-)*

✓6ᵗʰ **S63.20** **Unspecified subluxation of other finger**

✓7ᵗʰ **S63.200** Unspecified subluxation of right index finger

✓7ᵗʰ **S63.201** Unspecified subluxation of left index finger

✓7ᵗʰ **S63.202** Unspecified subluxation of right middle finger

✓7ᵗʰ **S63.203** Unspecified subluxation of left middle finger

✓7ᵗʰ **S63.204** Unspecified subluxation of right ring finger

✓7ᵗʰ **S63.205** Unspecified subluxation of left ring finger

✓7ᵗʰ **S63.206** Unspecified subluxation of right little finger

✓7ᵗʰ **S63.207** Unspecified subluxation of left little finger

✓7ᵗʰ **S63.208** Unspecified subluxation of other finger

Unspecified subluxation of specified finger with unspecified laterality

✓7ᵗʰ **S63.209** Unspecified subluxation of unspecified finger

✓6ᵗʰ **S63.21** **Subluxation of metacarpophalangeal joint of finger**

✓7ᵗʰ **S63.210** Subluxation of metacarpophalangeal joint of right index finger

✓7ᵗʰ **S63.211** Subluxation of metacarpophalangeal joint of left index finger

✓7ᵗʰ **S63.212** Subluxation of metacarpophalangeal joint of right middle finger

✓7ᵗʰ **S63.213** Subluxation of metacarpophalangeal joint of left middle finger

✓7ᵗʰ **S63.214** Subluxation of metacarpophalangeal joint of right ring finger

✓7ᵗʰ **S63.215** Subluxation of metacarpophalangeal joint of left ring finger

✓7ᵗʰ **S63.216** Subluxation of metacarpophalangeal joint of right little finger

✓7ᵗʰ **S63.217** Subluxation of metacarpophalangeal joint of left little finger

✓7ᵗʰ **S63.218** Subluxation of metacarpophalangeal joint of other finger

Subluxation of metacarpophalangeal joint of specified finger with unspecified laterality

✓7ᵗʰ **S63.219** Subluxation of metacarpophalangeal joint of unspecified finger

✓6ᵗʰ **S63.22** **Subluxation of unspecified interphalangeal joint of finger**

✓7ᵗʰ **S63.220** Subluxation of unspecified interphalangeal joint of right index finger

✓7ᵗʰ **S63.221** Subluxation of unspecified interphalangeal joint of left index finger

✓7ᵗʰ **S63.222** Subluxation of unspecified interphalangeal joint of right middle finger

✓7ᵗʰ **S63.223** Subluxation of unspecified interphalangeal joint of left middle finger

✓7ᵗʰ **S63.224** Subluxation of unspecified interphalangeal joint of right ring finger

✓7ᵗʰ **S63.225** Subluxation of unspecified interphalangeal joint of left ring finger

✓7ᵗʰ **S63.226** Subluxation of unspecified interphalangeal joint of right little finger

✓7ᵗʰ **S63.227** Subluxation of unspecified interphalangeal joint of left little finger

✓7ᵗʰ **S63.228** Subluxation of unspecified interphalangeal joint of other finger

Subluxation of unspecified interphalangeal joint of specified finger with unspecified laterality

✓7ᵗʰ **S63.229** Subluxation of unspecified interphalangeal joint of unspecified finger

---

EXCLUDES 1 Not coded here   EXCLUDES 2 Not included here   *Manifestation Code*

☑6ᵗʰ **S63.23 Subluxation of proximal interphalangeal joint of finger**

☑7ᵗʰ **S63.230 Subluxation of proximal interphalangeal joint of right index finger**

☑7ᵗʰ **S63.231 Subluxation of proximal interphalangeal joint of left index finger**

☑7ᵗʰ **S63.232 Subluxation of proximal interphalangeal joint of right middle finger**

☑7ᵗʰ **S63.233 Subluxation of proximal interphalangeal joint of left middle finger**

☑7ᵗʰ **S63.234 Subluxation of proximal interphalangeal joint of right ring finger**

☑7ᵗʰ **S63.235 Subluxation of proximal interphalangeal joint of left ring finger**

☑7ᵗʰ **S63.236 Subluxation of proximal interphalangeal joint of right little finger**

☑7ᵗʰ **S63.237 Subluxation of proximal interphalangeal joint of left little finger**

☑7ᵗʰ **S63.238 Subluxation of proximal interphalangeal joint of other finger**
Subluxation of proximal interphalangeal joint of specified finger with unspecified laterality

☑7ᵗʰ **S63.239 Subluxation of proximal interphalangeal joint of unspecified finger**

☑6ᵗʰ **S63.24 Subluxation of distal interphalangeal joint of finger**

☑7ᵗʰ **S63.240 Subluxation of distal interphalangeal joint of right index finger**

☑7ᵗʰ **S63.241 Subluxation of distal interphalangeal joint of left index finger**

☑7ᵗʰ **S63.242 Subluxation of distal interphalangeal joint of right middle finger**

☑7ᵗʰ **S63.243 Subluxation of distal interphalangeal joint of left middle finger**

☑7ᵗʰ **S63.244 Subluxation of distal interphalangeal joint of right ring finger**

☑7ᵗʰ **S63.245 Subluxation of distal interphalangeal joint of left ring finger**

☑7ᵗʰ **S63.246 Subluxation of distal interphalangeal joint of right little finger**

☑7ᵗʰ **S63.247 Subluxation of distal interphalangeal joint of left little finger**

☑7ᵗʰ **S63.248 Subluxation of distal interphalangeal joint of other finger**
Subluxation of distal interphalangeal joint of specified finger with unspecified laterality

☑7ᵗʰ **S63.249 Subluxation of distal interphalangeal joint of unspecified finger**

☑6ᵗʰ **S63.25 Unspecified dislocation of other finger**

☑7ᵗʰ **S63.250 Unspecified dislocation of right index finger**

☑7ᵗʰ **S63.251 Unspecified dislocation of left index finger**

☑7ᵗʰ **S63.252 Unspecified dislocation of right middle finger**

☑7ᵗʰ **S63.253 Unspecified dislocation of left middle finger**

☑7ᵗʰ **S63.254 Unspecified dislocation of right ring finger**

☑7ᵗʰ **S63.255 Unspecified dislocation of left ring finger**

☑7ᵗʰ **S63.256 Unspecified dislocation of right little finger**

☑7ᵗʰ **S63.257 Unspecified dislocation of left little finger**

☑7ᵗʰ **S63.258 Unspecified dislocation of other finger**
Unspecified dislocation of specified finger with unspecified laterality

☑7ᵗʰ **S63.259 Unspecified dislocation of unspecified finger**
Unspecified dislocation of specified finger with unspecified laterality

☑6ᵗʰ **S63.26 Dislocation of metacarpophalangeal joint of finger**

☑7ᵗʰ **S63.260 Dislocation of metacarpophalangeal joint of right index finger**

☑7ᵗʰ **S63.261 Dislocation of metacarpophalangeal joint of left index finger**

☑7ᵗʰ **S63.262 Dislocation of metacarpophalangeal joint of right middle finger**

☑7ᵗʰ **S63.263 Dislocation of metacarpophalangeal joint of left middle finger**

☑7ᵗʰ **S63.264 Dislocation of metacarpophalangeal joint of right ring finger**

☑7ᵗʰ **S63.265 Dislocation of metacarpophalangeal joint of left ring finger**

☑7ᵗʰ **S63.266 Dislocation of metacarpophalangeal joint of right little finger**

☑7ᵗʰ **S63.267 Dislocation of metacarpophalangeal joint of left little finger**

☑7ᵗʰ **S63.268 Dislocation of metacarpophalangeal joint of other finger**
Dislocation of metacarpophalangeal joint of specified finger with unspecified laterality

☑7ᵗʰ **S63.269 Dislocation of metacarpophalangeal joint of unspecified finger**

☑6ᵗʰ **S63.27 Dislocation of unspecified interphalangeal joint of finger**

☑7ᵗʰ **S63.270 Dislocation of unspecified interphalangeal joint of right index finger**

☑7ᵗʰ **S63.271 Dislocation of unspecified interphalangeal joint of left index finger**

☑7ᵗʰ **S63.272 Dislocation of unspecified interphalangeal joint of right middle finger**

☑7ᵗʰ **S63.273 Dislocation of unspecified interphalangeal joint of left middle finger**

☑7ᵗʰ **S63.274 Dislocation of unspecified interphalangeal joint of right ring finger**

☑7ᵗʰ **S63.275 Dislocation of unspecified interphalangeal joint of left ring finger**

☑7ᵗʰ **S63.276 Dislocation of unspecified interphalangeal joint of right little finger**

☑7ᵗʰ **S63.277 Dislocation of unspecified interphalangeal joint of left little finger**

☑7ᵗʰ **S63.278 Dislocation of unspecified interphalangeal joint of other finger**
Dislocation of unspecified interphalangeal joint of specified finger with unspecified laterality

☑7ᵗʰ **S63.279 Dislocation of unspecified interphalangeal joint of unspecified finger**
Dislocation of unspecified interphalangeal joint of specified finger without specified laterality

☑6ᵗʰ **S63.28 Dislocation of proximal interphalangeal joint of finger**

☑7ᵗʰ **S63.280 Dislocation of proximal interphalangeal joint of right index finger**

☑7ᵗʰ **S63.281 Dislocation of proximal interphalangeal joint of left index finger**

☑7ᵗʰ **S63.282 Dislocation of proximal interphalangeal joint of right middle finger**

☑7ᵗʰ **S63.283 Dislocation of proximal interphalangeal joint of left middle finger**

☑7ᵗʰ **S63.284 Dislocation of proximal interphalangeal joint of right ring finger**

☑7ᵗʰ **S63.285 Dislocation of proximal interphalangeal joint of left ring finger**

☑7ᵗʰ **S63.286 Dislocation of proximal interphalangeal joint of right little finger**

☑ Appropriate additional character required   ☑ₓ7ᵗʰ Requires 7th character, placeholder x must fill empty characters

✓7ᵗʰ **S63.287** **Dislocation of proximal interphalangeal joint of left little finger**

✓7ᵗʰ **S63.288** **Dislocation of proximal interphalangeal joint of other finger**

Dislocation of proximal interphalangeal joint of specified finger with unspecified laterality

✓7ᵗʰ **S63.289** **Dislocation of proximal interphalangeal joint of unspecified finger**

✓6ᵗʰ **S63.29** **Dislocation of distal interphalangeal joint of finger**

✓7ᵗʰ **S63.290** **Dislocation of distal interphalangeal joint of right index finger**

✓7ᵗʰ **S63.291** **Dislocation of distal interphalangeal joint of left index finger**

✓7ᵗʰ **S63.292** **Dislocation of distal interphalangeal joint of right middle finger**

✓7ᵗʰ **S63.293** **Dislocation of distal interphalangeal joint of left middle finger**

✓7ᵗʰ **S63.294** **Dislocation of distal interphalangeal joint of right ring finger**

✓7ᵗʰ **S63.295** **Dislocation of distal interphalangeal joint of left ring finger**

✓7ᵗʰ **S63.296** **Dislocation of distal interphalangeal joint of right little finger**

✓7ᵗʰ **S63.297** **Dislocation of distal interphalangeal joint of left little finger**

✓7ᵗʰ **S63.298** **Dislocation of distal interphalangeal joint of other finger**

Dislocation of distal interphalangeal joint of specified finger with unspecified laterality

✓7ᵗʰ **S63.299** **Dislocation of distal interphalangeal joint of unspecified finger**

✓5ᵗʰ **S63.3** **Traumatic rupture of ligament of wrist**

✓6ᵗʰ **S63.30** **Traumatic rupture of unspecified ligament of wrist**

✓7ᵗʰ **S63.301** **Traumatic rupture of unspecified ligament of right wrist**

✓7ᵗʰ **S63.302** **Traumatic rupture of unspecified ligament of left wrist**

✓7ᵗʰ **S63.309** **Traumatic rupture of unspecified ligament of unspecified wrist**

✓6ᵗʰ **S63.31** **Traumatic rupture of collateral ligament of wrist**

✓7ᵗʰ **S63.311** **Traumatic rupture of collateral ligament of right wrist**

✓7ᵗʰ **S63.312** **Traumatic rupture of collateral ligament of left wrist**

✓7ᵗʰ **S63.319** **Traumatic rupture of collateral ligament of unspecified wrist**

✓6ᵗʰ **S63.32** **Traumatic rupture of radiocarpal ligament**

✓7ᵗʰ **S63.321** **Traumatic rupture of right radiocarpal ligament**

✓7ᵗʰ **S63.322** **Traumatic rupture of left radiocarpal ligament**

✓7ᵗʰ **S63.329** **Traumatic rupture of unspecified radiocarpal ligament**

✓6ᵗʰ **S63.33** **Traumatic rupture of ulnocarpal (palmar) ligament**

✓7ᵗʰ **S63.331** **Traumatic rupture of right ulnocarpal (palmar) ligament**

✓7ᵗʰ **S63.332** **Traumatic rupture of left ulnocarpal (palmar) ligament**

✓7ᵗʰ **S63.339** **Traumatic rupture of unspecified ulnocarpal (palmar) ligament**

✓6ᵗʰ **S63.39** **Traumatic rupture of other ligament of wrist**

✓7ᵗʰ **S63.391** **Traumatic rupture of other ligament of right wrist**

✓7ᵗʰ **S63.392** **Traumatic rupture of other ligament of left wrist**

✓7ᵗʰ **S63.399** **Traumatic rupture of other ligament of unspecified wrist**

✓5ᵗʰ **S63.4** **Traumatic rupture of ligament of finger at metacarpophalangeal and interphalangeal joint(s)**

✓6ᵗʰ **S63.40** **Traumatic rupture of unspecified ligament of finger at metacarpophalangeal and interphalangeal joint**

✓7ᵗʰ **S63.400** **Traumatic rupture of unspecified ligament of right index finger at metacarpophalangeal and interphalangeal joint**

✓7ᵗʰ **S63.401** **Traumatic rupture of unspecified ligament of left index finger at metacarpophalangeal and interphalangeal joint**

✓7ᵗʰ **S63.402** **Traumatic rupture of unspecified ligament of right middle finger at metacarpophalangeal and interphalangeal joint**

✓7ᵗʰ **S63.403** **Traumatic rupture of unspecified ligament of left middle finger at metacarpophalangeal and interphalangeal joint**

✓7ᵗʰ **S63.404** **Traumatic rupture of unspecified ligament of right ring finger at metacarpophalangeal and interphalangeal joint**

✓7ᵗʰ **S63.405** **Traumatic rupture of unspecified ligament of left ring finger at metacarpophalangeal and interphalangeal joint**

✓7ᵗʰ **S63.406** **Traumatic rupture of unspecified ligament of right little finger at metacarpophalangeal and interphalangeal joint**

✓7ᵗʰ **S63.407** **Traumatic rupture of unspecified ligament of left little finger at metacarpophalangeal and interphalangeal joint**

✓7ᵗʰ **S63.408** **Traumatic rupture of unspecified ligament of other finger at metacarpophalangeal and interphalangeal joint**

Traumatic rupture of unspecified ligament of specified finger with unspecified laterality at metacarpophalangeal and interphalangeal joint

✓7ᵗʰ **S63.409** **Traumatic rupture of unspecified ligament of unspecified finger at metacarpophalangeal and interphalangeal joint**

✓6ᵗʰ **S63.41** **Traumatic rupture of collateral ligament of finger at metacarpophalangeal and interphalangeal joint**

✓7ᵗʰ **S63.410** **Traumatic rupture of collateral ligament of right index finger at metacarpophalangeal and interphalangeal joint**

✓7ᵗʰ **S63.411** **Traumatic rupture of collateral ligament of left index finger at metacarpophalangeal and interphalangeal joint**

✓7ᵗʰ **S63.412** **Traumatic rupture of collateral ligament of right middle finger at metacarpophalangeal and interphalangeal joint**

✓7ᵗʰ **S63.413** **Traumatic rupture of collateral ligament of left middle finger at metacarpophalangeal and interphalangeal joint**

✓7ᵗʰ **S63.414** **Traumatic rupture of collateral ligament of right ring finger at metacarpophalangeal and interphalangeal joint**

✓7ᵗʰ **S63.415** **Traumatic rupture of collateral ligament of left ring finger at metacarpophalangeal and interphalangeal joint**

✓7ᵗʰ **S63.416** **Traumatic rupture of collateral ligament of right little finger at metacarpophalangeal and interphalangeal joint**

✓7ᵗʰ **S63.417** **Traumatic rupture of collateral ligament of left little finger at metacarpophalangeal and interphalangeal joint**

EXCLUDES 1 Not coded here   EXCLUDES 2 Not included here   *Manifestation Code*

√7ᵗʰ **S63.418 Traumatic rupture of collateral ligament of other finger at metacarpophalangeal and interphalangeal joint**
Traumatic rupture of collateral ligament of specified finger with unspecified laterality at metacarpophalangeal and interphalangeal joint

√7ᵗʰ **S63.419 Traumatic rupture of collateral ligament of unspecified finger at metacarpophalangeal and interphalangeal joint**

√6ᵗʰ **S63.42 Traumatic rupture of palmar ligament of finger at metacarpophalangeal and interphalangeal joint**

√7ᵗʰ **S63.420 Traumatic rupture of palmar ligament of right index finger at metacarpophalangeal and interphalangeal joint**

√7ᵗʰ **S63.421 Traumatic rupture of palmar ligament of left index finger at metacarpophalangeal and interphalangeal joint**

√7ᵗʰ **S63.422 Traumatic rupture of palmar ligament of right middle finger at metacarpophalangeal and interphalangeal joint**

√7ᵗʰ **S63.423 Traumatic rupture of palmar ligament of left middle finger at metacarpophalangeal and interphalangeal joint**

√7ᵗʰ **S63.424 Traumatic rupture of palmar ligament of right ring finger at metacarpophalangeal and interphalangeal joint**

√7ᵗʰ **S63.425 Traumatic rupture of palmar ligament of left ring finger at metacarpophalangeal and interphalangeal joint**

√7ᵗʰ **S63.426 Traumatic rupture of palmar ligament of right little finger at metacarpophalangeal and interphalangeal joint**

√7ᵗʰ **S63.427 Traumatic rupture of palmar ligament of left little finger at metacarpophalangeal and interphalangeal joint**

√7ᵗʰ **S63.428 Traumatic rupture of palmar ligament of other finger at metacarpophalangeal and interphalangeal joint**
Traumatic rupture of palmar ligament of specified finger with unspecified laterality at metacarpophalangeal and interphalangeal joint

√7ᵗʰ **S63.429 Traumatic rupture of palmar ligament of unspecified finger at metacarpophalangeal and interphalangeal joint**

√6ᵗʰ **S63.43 Traumatic rupture of volar plate of finger at metacarpophalangeal and interphalangeal joint**

√7ᵗʰ **S63.430 Traumatic rupture of volar plate of right index finger at metacarpophalangeal and interphalangeal joint**

√7ᵗʰ **S63.431 Traumatic rupture of volar plate of left index finger at metacarpophalangeal and interphalangeal joint**

√7ᵗʰ **S63.432 Traumatic rupture of volar plate of right middle finger at metacarpophalangeal and interphalangeal joint**

√7ᵗʰ **S63.433 Traumatic rupture of volar plate of left middle finger at metacarpophalangeal and interphalangeal joint**

√7ᵗʰ **S63.434 Traumatic rupture of volar plate of right ring finger at metacarpophalangeal and interphalangeal joint**

√7ᵗʰ **S63.435 Traumatic rupture of volar plate of left ring finger at metacarpophalangeal and interphalangeal joint**

√7ᵗʰ **S63.436 Traumatic rupture of volar plate of right little finger at metacarpophalangeal and interphalangeal joint**

√7ᵗʰ **S63.437 Traumatic rupture of volar plate of left little finger at metacarpophalangeal and interphalangeal joint**

√7ᵗʰ **S63.438 Traumatic rupture of volar plate of other finger at metacarpophalangeal and interphalangeal joint**
Traumatic rupture of volar plate of specified finger with unspecified laterality at metacarpophalangeal and interphalangeal joint

√7ᵗʰ **S63.439 Traumatic rupture of volar plate of unspecified finger at metacarpophalangeal and interphalangeal joint**

√6ᵗʰ **S63.49 Traumatic rupture of other ligament of finger at metacarpophalangeal and interphalangeal joint**

√7ᵗʰ **S63.490 Traumatic rupture of other ligament of right index finger at metacarpophalangeal and interphalangeal joint**

√7ᵗʰ **S63.491 Traumatic rupture of other ligament of left index finger at metacarpophalangeal and interphalangeal joint**

√7ᵗʰ **S63.492 Traumatic rupture of other ligament of right middle finger at metacarpophalangeal and interphalangeal joint**

√7ᵗʰ **S63.493 Traumatic rupture of other ligament of left middle finger at metacarpophalangeal and interphalangeal joint**

√7ᵗʰ **S63.494 Traumatic rupture of other ligament of right ring finger at metacarpophalangeal and interphalangeal joint**

√7ᵗʰ **S63.495 Traumatic rupture of other ligament of left ring finger at metacarpophalangeal and interphalangeal joint**

√7ᵗʰ **S63.496 Traumatic rupture of other ligament of right little finger at metacarpophalangeal and interphalangeal joint**

√7ᵗʰ **S63.497 Traumatic rupture of other ligament of left little finger at metacarpophalangeal and interphalangeal joint**

√7ᵗʰ **S63.498 Traumatic rupture of other ligament of other finger at metacarpophalangeal and interphalangeal joint**
Traumatic rupture of ligament of specified finger with unspecified laterality at metacarpophalangeal and interphalangeal joint

√7ᵗʰ **S63.499 Traumatic rupture of other ligament of unspecified finger at metacarpophalangeal and interphalangeal joint**

√5ᵗʰ **S63.5 Other and unspecified sprain of wrist**

√6ᵗʰ **S63.50 Unspecified sprain of wrist**

√7ᵗʰ **S63.501 Unspecified sprain of right wrist**

√7ᵗʰ **S63.502 Unspecified sprain of left wrist**

√7ᵗʰ **S63.509 Unspecified sprain of unspecified wrist**

√6ᵗʰ **S63.51 Sprain of carpal (joint)**

√7ᵗʰ **S63.511 Sprain of carpal joint of right wrist**

√7ᵗʰ **S63.512 Sprain of carpal joint of left wrist**

√7ᵗʰ **S63.519 Sprain of carpal joint of unspecified wrist**

√6ᵗʰ **S63.52 Sprain of radiocarpal joint**
EXCLUDES 1 *traumatic rupture of radiocarpal ligament (S63.32-)*

√7ᵗʰ **S63.521 Sprain of radiocarpal joint of right wrist**

√7ᵗʰ **S63.522 Sprain of radiocarpal joint of left wrist**

√7ᵗʰ **S63.529 Sprain of radiocarpal joint of unspecified wrist**

√6ᵗʰ **S63.59 Other specified sprain of wrist**

√7ᵗʰ **S63.591 Other specified sprain of right wrist**

√7ᵗʰ **S63.592 Other specified sprain of left wrist**

√7ᵗʰ **S63.599** **Other specified sprain of unspecified wrist**

√5ᵗʰ **S63.6** **Other and unspecified sprain of finger(s)**

> EXCLUDES 1   *traumatic rupture of ligament of finger at metacarpophalangeal and interphalangeal joint(s) (S63.4-)*

√6ᵗʰ **S63.60** **Unspecified sprain of thumb**

√7ᵗʰ **S63.601** **Unspecified sprain of right thumb**

√7ᵗʰ **S63.602** **Unspecified sprain of left thumb**

√7ᵗʰ **S63.609** **Unspecified sprain of unspecified thumb**

√6ᵗʰ **S63.61** **Unspecified sprain of other and unspecified finger(s)**

√7ᵗʰ **S63.610** **Unspecified sprain of right index finger**

√7ᵗʰ **S63.611** **Unspecified sprain of left index finger**

√7ᵗʰ **S63.612** **Unspecified sprain of right middle finger**

√7ᵗʰ **S63.613** **Unspecified sprain of left middle finger**

√7ᵗʰ **S63.614** **Unspecified sprain of right ring finger**

√7ᵗʰ **S63.615** **Unspecified sprain of left ring finger**

√7ᵗʰ **S63.616** **Unspecified sprain of right little finger**

√7ᵗʰ **S63.617** **Unspecified sprain of left little finger**

√7ᵗʰ **S63.618** **Unspecified sprain of other finger**

> Unspecified sprain of specified finger with unspecified laterality

√7ᵗʰ **S63.619** **Unspecified sprain of unspecified finger**

√6ᵗʰ **S63.62** **Sprain of interphalangeal joint of thumb**

√7ᵗʰ **S63.621** **Sprain of interphalangeal joint of right thumb**

√7ᵗʰ **S63.622** **Sprain of interphalangeal joint of left thumb**

√7ᵗʰ **S63.629** **Sprain of interphalangeal joint of unspecified thumb**

√6ᵗʰ **S63.63** **Sprain of interphalangeal joint of other and unspecified finger(s)**

√7ᵗʰ **S63.630** **Sprain of interphalangeal joint of right index finger**

√7ᵗʰ **S63.631** **Sprain of interphalangeal joint of left index finger**

√7ᵗʰ **S63.632** **Sprain of interphalangeal joint of right middle finger**

√7ᵗʰ **S63.633** **Sprain of interphalangeal joint of left middle finger**

√7ᵗʰ **S63.634** **Sprain of interphalangeal joint of right ring finger**

√7ᵗʰ **S63.635** **Sprain of interphalangeal joint of left ring finger**

√7ᵗʰ **S63.636** **Sprain of interphalangeal joint of right little finger**

√7ᵗʰ **S63.637** **Sprain of interphalangeal joint of left little finger**

√7ᵗʰ **S63.638** **Sprain of interphalangeal joint of other finger**

√7ᵗʰ **S63.639** **Sprain of interphalangeal joint of unspecified finger**

√6ᵗʰ **S63.64** **Sprain of metacarpophalangeal joint of thumb**

√7ᵗʰ **S63.641** **Sprain of metacarpophalangeal joint of right thumb**

√7ᵗʰ **S63.642** **Sprain of metacarpophalangeal joint of left thumb**

√7ᵗʰ **S63.649** **Sprain of metacarpophalangeal joint of unspecified thumb**

√6ᵗʰ **S63.65** **Sprain of metacarpophalangeal joint of other and unspecified finger(s)**

√7ᵗʰ **S63.650** **Sprain of metacarpophalangeal joint of right index finger**

√7ᵗʰ **S63.651** **Sprain of metacarpophalangeal joint of left index finger**

√7ᵗʰ **S63.652** **Sprain of metacarpophalangeal joint of right middle finger**

√7ᵗʰ **S63.653** **Sprain of metacarpophalangeal joint of left middle finger**

√7ᵗʰ **S63.654** **Sprain of metacarpophalangeal joint of right ring finger**

√7ᵗʰ **S63.655** **Sprain of metacarpophalangeal joint of left ring finger**

√7ᵗʰ **S63.656** **Sprain of metacarpophalangeal joint of right little finger**

√7ᵗʰ **S63.657** **Sprain of metacarpophalangeal joint of left little finger**

√7ᵗʰ **S63.658** **Sprain of metacarpophalangeal joint of other finger**

> Sprain of metacarpophalangeal joint of specified finger with unspecified laterality

√7ᵗʰ **S63.659** **Sprain of metacarpophalangeal joint of unspecified finger**

√6ᵗʰ **S63.68** **Other sprain of thumb**

√7ᵗʰ **S63.681** **Other sprain of right thumb**

√7ᵗʰ **S63.682** **Other sprain of left thumb**

√7ᵗʰ **S63.689** **Other sprain of unspecified thumb**

√6ᵗʰ **S63.69** **Other sprain of other and unspecified finger(s)**

√7ᵗʰ **S63.690** **Other sprain of right index finger**

√7ᵗʰ **S63.691** **Other sprain of left index finger**

√7ᵗʰ **S63.692** **Other sprain of right middle finger**

√7ᵗʰ **S63.693** **Other sprain of left middle finger**

√7ᵗʰ **S63.694** **Other sprain of right ring finger**

√7ᵗʰ **S63.695** **Other sprain of left ring finger**

√7ᵗʰ **S63.696** **Other sprain of right little finger**

√7ᵗʰ **S63.697** **Other sprain of left little finger**

√7ᵗʰ **S63.698** **Other sprain of other finger**

> Other sprain of specified finger with unspecified laterality

√7ᵗʰ **S63.699** **Other sprain of unspecified finger**

√5ᵗʰ **S63.8** **Sprain of other part of wrist and hand**

√6ᵗʰ **S63.8x** **Sprain of other part of wrist and hand**

√7ᵗʰ **S63.8x1** **Sprain of other part of right wrist and hand**

√7ᵗʰ **S63.8x2** **Sprain of other part of left wrist and hand**

√7ᵗʰ **S63.8x9** **Sprain of other part of unspecified wrist and hand**

√5ᵗʰ **S63.9** **Sprain of unspecified part of wrist and hand**

√x7ᵗʰ **S63.90** **Sprain of unspecified part of unspecified wrist and hand**

√x7ᵗʰ **S63.91** **Sprain of unspecified part of right wrist and hand**

√x7ᵗʰ **S63.92** **Sprain of unspecified part of left wrist and hand**

√4ᵗʰ **S64** **Injury of nerves at wrist and hand level**

Code also any associated open wound (S61-)

> The appropriate 7th character is to be added to each code from category S64.
> A   initial encounter
> D   subsequent encounter
> S   sequela

√5ᵗʰ **S64.0** **Injury of ulnar nerve at wrist and hand level**

√x7ᵗʰ **S64.00** **Injury of ulnar nerve at wrist and hand level of unspecified arm**

√x7ᵗʰ **S64.01** **Injury of ulnar nerve at wrist and hand level of right arm**

√x7ᵗʰ **S64.02** **Injury of ulnar nerve at wrist and hand level of left arm**

√5ᵗʰ **S64.1** **Injury of median nerve at wrist and hand level**

√x7ᵗʰ **S64.10** **Injury of median nerve at wrist and hand level of unspecified arm**

√x7ᵗʰ **S64.11** **Injury of median nerve at wrist and hand level of right arm**

√x7ᵗʰ **S64.12** **Injury of median nerve at wrist and hand level of left arm**

√5ᵗʰ **S64.2** **Injury of radial nerve at wrist and hand level**

√x7ᵗʰ **S64.20** **Injury of radial nerve at wrist and hand level of unspecified arm**

√x7ᵗʰ **S64.21** **Injury of radial nerve at wrist and hand level of right arm**

√x7ᵗʰ **S64.22** **Injury of radial nerve at wrist and hand level of left arm**

√5ᵗʰ **S64.3** **Injury of digital nerve of thumb**

√x7ᵗʰ **S64.30** **Injury of digital nerve of unspecified thumb**

√x7ᵗʰ **S64.31** **Injury of digital nerve of right thumb**

√x7ᵗʰ **S64.32** **Injury of digital nerve of left thumb**

√5ᵗʰ **S64.4** **Injury of digital nerve of other and unspecified finger**

√x7ᵗʰ **S64.40** **Injury of digital nerve of unspecified finger**

EXCLUDES 1   Not coded here   EXCLUDES 2   Not included here   *Manifestation Code*

√6th **S64.49** Injury of digital nerve of other finger
- √7th **S64.490** Injury of digital nerve of right index finger
- √7th **S64.491** Injury of digital nerve of left index finger
- √7th **S64.492** Injury of digital nerve of right middle finger
- √7th **S64.493** Injury of digital nerve of left middle finger
- √7th **S64.494** Injury of digital nerve of right ring finger
- √7th **S64.495** Injury of digital nerve of left ring finger
- √7th **S64.496** Injury of digital nerve of right little finger
- √7th **S64.497** Injury of digital nerve of left little finger
- √7th **S64.498** Injury of digital nerve of other finger
  Injury of digital nerve of specified finger with unspecified laterality

√5th **S64.8** Injury of other nerves at wrist and hand level
- √6th **S64.8x** Injury of other nerves at wrist and hand level
  - √7th **S64.8x1** Injury of other nerves at wrist and hand level of right arm
  - √7th **S64.8x2** Injury of other nerves at wrist and hand level of left arm
  - √7th **S64.8x9** Injury of other nerves at wrist and hand level of unspecified arm

√5th **S64.9** Injury of unspecified nerve at wrist and hand level
- √x7th **S64.90** Injury of unspecified nerve at wrist and hand level of unspecified arm
- √x7th **S64.91** Injury of unspecified nerve at wrist and hand level of right arm
- √x7th **S64.92** Injury of unspecified nerve at wrist and hand level of left arm

√4th **S65** **Injury of blood vessels at wrist and hand level**
Code also any associated open wound (S61-)

The appropriate 7th character is to be added to each code from category S65.
A   initial encounter
D   subsequent encounter
S   sequela

√5th **S65.0** Injury of ulnar artery at wrist and hand level
- √6th **S65.00** Unspecified injury of ulnar artery at wrist and hand level
  - √7th **S65.001** Unspecified injury of ulnar artery at wrist and hand level of right arm
  - √7th **S65.002** Unspecified injury of ulnar artery at wrist and hand level of left arm
  - √7th **S65.009** Unspecified injury of ulnar artery at wrist and hand level of unspecified arm
- √6th **S65.01** Laceration of ulnar artery at wrist and hand level
  - √7th **S65.011** Laceration of ulnar artery at wrist and hand level of right arm
  - √7th **S65.012** Laceration of ulnar artery at wrist and hand level of left arm
  - √7th **S65.019** Laceration of ulnar artery at wrist and hand level of unspecified arm
- √6th **S65.09** Other specified injury of ulnar artery at wrist and hand level
  - √7th **S65.091** Other specified injury of ulnar artery at wrist and hand level of right arm
  - √7th **S65.092** Other specified injury of ulnar artery at wrist and hand level of left arm
  - √7th **S65.099** Other specified injury of ulnar artery at wrist and hand level of unspecified arm

√5th **S65.1** Injury of radial artery at wrist and hand level
- √6th **S65.10** Unspecified injury of radial artery at wrist and hand level
  - √7th **S65.101** Unspecified injury of radial artery at wrist and hand level of right arm
  - √7th **S65.102** Unspecified injury of radial artery at wrist and hand level of left arm
  - √7th **S65.109** Unspecified injury of radial artery at wrist and hand level of unspecified arm

√6th **S65.11** Laceration of radial artery at wrist and hand level
- √7th **S65.111** Laceration of radial artery at wrist and hand level of right arm
- √7th **S65.112** Laceration of radial artery at wrist and hand level of left arm
- √7th **S65.119** Laceration of radial artery at wrist and hand level of unspecified arm

√6th **S65.19** Other specified injury of radial artery at wrist and hand level
- √7th **S65.191** Other specified injury of radial artery at wrist and hand level of right arm
- √7th **S65.192** Other specified injury of radial artery at wrist and hand level of left arm
- √7th **S65.199** Other specified injury of radial artery at wrist and hand level of unspecified arm

√5th **S65.2** Injury of superficial palmar arch
- √6th **S65.20** Unspecified injury of superficial palmar arch
  - √7th **S65.201** Unspecified injury of superficial palmar arch of right hand
  - √7th **S65.202** Unspecified injury of superficial palmar arch of left hand
  - √7th **S65.209** Unspecified injury of superficial palmar arch of unspecified hand
- √6th **S65.21** Laceration of superficial palmar arch
  - √7th **S65.211** Laceration of superficial palmar arch of right hand
  - √7th **S65.212** Laceration of superficial palmar arch of left hand
  - √7th **S65.219** Laceration of superficial palmar arch of unspecified hand
- √6th **S65.29** Other specified injury of superficial palmar arch
  - √7th **S65.291** Other specified injury of superficial palmar arch of right hand
  - √7th **S65.292** Other specified injury of superficial palmar arch of left hand
  - √7th **S65.299** Other specified injury of superficial palmar arch of unspecified hand

√5th **S65.3** Injury of deep palmar arch
- √6th **S65.30** Unspecified injury of deep palmar arch
  - √7th **S65.301** Unspecified injury of deep palmar arch of right hand
  - √7th **S65.302** Unspecified injury of deep palmar arch of left hand
  - √7th **S65.309** Unspecified injury of deep palmar arch of unspecified hand
- √6th **S65.31** Laceration of deep palmar arch
  - √7th **S65.311** Laceration of deep palmar arch of right hand
  - √7th **S65.312** Laceration of deep palmar arch of left hand
  - √7th **S65.319** Laceration of deep palmar arch of unspecified hand
- √6th **S65.39** Other specified injury of deep palmar arch
  - √7th **S65.391** Other specified injury of deep palmar arch of right hand
  - √7th **S65.392** Other specified injury of deep palmar arch of left hand
  - √7th **S65.399** Other specified injury of deep palmar arch of unspecified hand

√5th **S65.4** Injury of blood vessel of thumb
- √6th **S65.40** Unspecified injury of blood vessel of thumb
  - √7th **S65.401** Unspecified injury of blood vessel of right thumb
  - √7th **S65.402** Unspecified injury of blood vessel of left thumb
  - √7th **S65.409** Unspecified injury of blood vessel of unspecified thumb
- √6th **S65.41** Laceration of blood vessel of thumb
  - √7th **S65.411** Laceration of blood vessel of right thumb
  - √7th **S65.412** Laceration of blood vessel of left thumb
  - √7th **S65.419** Laceration of blood vessel of unspecified thumb
- √6th **S65.49** Other specified injury of blood vessel of thumb
  - √7th **S65.491** Other specified injury of blood vessel of right thumb

---

☑ Appropriate additional character required   √x7th Requires 7th character, placeholder x must fill empty characters

√7th **S65.492** Other specified injury of blood vessel of left thumb

√7th **S65.499** Other specified injury of blood vessel of unspecified thumb

√5th **S65.5** Injury of blood vessel of other and unspecified finger

√6th **S65.50** Unspecified injury of blood vessel of other and unspecified finger

√7th **S65.500** Unspecified injury of blood vessel of right index finger

√7th **S65.501** Unspecified injury of blood vessel of left index finger

√7th **S65.502** Unspecified injury of blood vessel of right middle finger

√7th **S65.503** Unspecified injury of blood vessel of left middle finger

√7th **S65.504** Unspecified injury of blood vessel of right ring finger

√7th **S65.505** Unspecified injury of blood vessel of left ring finger

√7th **S65.506** Unspecified injury of blood vessel of right little finger

√7th **S65.507** Unspecified injury of blood vessel of left little finger

√7th **S65.508** Unspecified injury of blood vessel of other finger

     Unspecified injury of blood vessel of specified finger with unspecified laterality

√7th **S65.509** Unspecified injury of blood vessel of unspecified finger

√6th **S65.51** Laceration of blood vessel of other and unspecified finger

√7th **S65.510** Laceration of blood vessel of right index finger

√7th **S65.511** Laceration of blood vessel of left index finger

√7th **S65.512** Laceration of blood vessel of right middle finger

√7th **S65.513** Laceration of blood vessel of left middle finger

√7th **S65.514** Laceration of blood vessel of right ring finger

√7th **S65.515** Laceration of blood vessel of left ring finger

√7th **S65.516** Laceration of blood vessel of right little finger

√7th **S65.517** Laceration of blood vessel of left little finger

√7th **S65.518** Laceration of blood vessel of other finger

     Laceration of blood vessel of specified finger with unspecified laterality

√7th **S65.519** Laceration of blood vessel of unspecified finger

√6th **S65.59** Other specified injury of blood vessel of other and unspecified finger

√7th **S65.590** Other specified injury of blood vessel of right index finger

√7th **S65.591** Other specified injury of blood vessel of left index finger

√7th **S65.592** Other specified injury of blood vessel of right middle finger

√7th **S65.593** Other specified injury of blood vessel of left middle finger

√7th **S65.594** Other specified injury of blood vessel of right ring finger

√7th **S65.595** Other specified injury of blood vessel of left ring finger

√7th **S65.596** Other specified injury of blood vessel of right little finger

√7th **S65.597** Other specified injury of blood vessel of left little finger

√7th **S65.598** Other specified injury of blood vessel of other finger

     Other specified injury of blood vessel of specified finger with unspecified laterality

√7th **S65.599** Other specified injury of blood vessel of unspecified finger

√5th **S65.8** Injury of other blood vessels at wrist and hand level

√6th **S65.80** Unspecified injury of other blood vessels at wrist and hand level

√7th **S65.801** Unspecified injury of other blood vessels at wrist and hand level of right arm

√7th **S65.802** Unspecified injury of other blood vessels at wrist and hand level of left arm

√7th **S65.809** Unspecified injury of other blood vessels at wrist and hand level of unspecified arm

√6th **S65.81** Laceration of other blood vessels at wrist and hand level

√7th **S65.811** Laceration of other blood vessels at wrist and hand level of right arm

√7th **S65.812** Laceration of other blood vessels at wrist and hand level of left arm

√7th **S65.819** Laceration of other blood vessels at wrist and hand level of unspecified arm

√6th **S65.89** Other specified injury of other blood vessels at wrist and hand level

√7th **S65.891** Other specified injury of other blood vessels at wrist and hand level of right arm

√7th **S65.892** Other specified injury of other blood vessels at wrist and hand level of left arm

√7th **S65.899** Other specified injury of other blood vessels at wrist and hand level of unspecified arm

√5th **S65.9** Injury of unspecified blood vessel at wrist and hand level

√6th **S65.90** Unspecified injury of unspecified blood vessel at wrist and hand level

√7th **S65.901** Unspecified injury of unspecified blood vessel at wrist and hand level of right arm

√7th **S65.902** Unspecified injury of unspecified blood vessel at wrist and hand level of left arm

√7th **S65.909** Unspecified injury of unspecified blood vessel at wrist and hand level of unspecified arm

√6th **S65.91** Laceration of unspecified blood vessel at wrist and hand level

√7th **S65.911** Laceration of unspecified blood vessel at wrist and hand level of right arm

√7th **S65.912** Laceration of unspecified blood vessel at wrist and hand level of left arm

√7th **S65.919** Laceration of unspecified blood vessel at wrist and hand level of unspecified arm

√6th **S65.99** Other specified injury of unspecified blood vessel at wrist and hand level

√7th **S65.991** Other specified injury of unspecified blood vessel at wrist and hand of right arm

√7th **S65.992** Other specified injury of unspecified blood vessel at wrist and hand of left arm

√7th **S65.999** Other specified injury of unspecified blood vessel at wrist and hand of unspecified arm

√4th **S66** **Injury of muscle, fascia and tendon at wrist and hand level**

     Code also any associated open wound (S61-)

     EXCLUDES 2   sprain of joints and ligaments of wrist and hand (S63-)

> The appropriate 7th character is to be added to each code from category S66.
> A   initial encounter
> D   subsequent encounter
> S   sequela

√5th **S66.0** Injury of long flexor muscle, fascia and tendon of thumb at wrist and hand level

√6th **S66.00** Unspecified injury of long flexor muscle, fascia and tendon of thumb at wrist and hand level

☑7ᵗʰ **S66.001** Unspecified injury of long flexor muscle, fascia and tendon of right thumb at wrist and hand level

☑7ᵗʰ **S66.002** Unspecified injury of long flexor muscle, fascia and tendon of left thumb at wrist and hand level

☑7ᵗʰ **S66.009** Unspecified injury of long flexor muscle, fascia and tendon of unspecified thumb at wrist and hand level

☑6ᵗʰ **S66.01** Strain of long flexor muscle, fascia and tendon of thumb at wrist and hand level

☑7ᵗʰ **S66.011** Strain of long flexor muscle, fascia and tendon of right thumb at wrist and hand level

☑7ᵗʰ **S66.012** Strain of long flexor muscle, fascia and tendon of left thumb at wrist and hand level

☑7ᵗʰ **S66.019** Strain of long flexor muscle, fascia and tendon of unspecified thumb at wrist and hand level

☑6ᵗʰ **S66.02** Laceration of long flexor muscle, fascia and tendon of thumb at wrist and hand level

☑7ᵗʰ **S66.021** Laceration of long flexor muscle, fascia and tendon of right thumb at wrist and hand level

☑7ᵗʰ **S66.022** Laceration of long flexor muscle, fascia and tendon of left thumb at wrist and hand level

☑7ᵗʰ **S66.029** Laceration of long flexor muscle, fascia and tendon of unspecified thumb at wrist and hand level

☑6ᵗʰ **S66.09** Other specified injury of long flexor muscle, fascia and tendon of thumb at wrist and hand level

☑7ᵗʰ **S66.091** Other specified injury of long flexor muscle, fascia and tendon of right thumb at wrist and hand level

☑7ᵗʰ **S66.092** Other specified injury of long flexor muscle, fascia and tendon of left thumb at wrist and hand level

☑7ᵗʰ **S66.099** Other specified injury of long flexor muscle, fascia and tendon of unspecified thumb at wrist and hand level

☑5ᵗʰ **S66.1** Injury of flexor muscle, fascia and tendon of other and unspecified finger at wrist and hand level

EXCLUDES 2   *Injury of long flexor muscle, fascia and tendon of thumb at wrist and hand level (S66.0-)*

☑6ᵗʰ **S66.10** Unspecified injury of flexor muscle, fascia and tendon of other and unspecified finger at wrist and hand level

☑7ᵗʰ **S66.100** Unspecified injury of flexor muscle, fascia and tendon of right index finger at wrist and hand level

☑7ᵗʰ **S66.101** Unspecified injury of flexor muscle, fascia and tendon of left index finger at wrist and hand level

☑7ᵗʰ **S66.102** Unspecified injury of flexor muscle, fascia and tendon of right middle finger at wrist and hand level

☑7ᵗʰ **S66.103** Unspecified injury of flexor muscle, fascia and tendon of left middle finger at wrist and hand level

☑7ᵗʰ **S66.104** Unspecified injury of flexor muscle, fascia and tendon of right ring finger at wrist and hand level

☑7ᵗʰ **S66.105** Unspecified injury of flexor muscle, fascia and tendon of left ring finger at wrist and hand level

☑7ᵗʰ **S66.106** Unspecified injury of flexor muscle, fascia and tendon of right little finger at wrist and hand level

☑7ᵗʰ **S66.107** Unspecified injury of flexor muscle, fascia and tendon of left little finger at wrist and hand level

☑7ᵗʰ **S66.108** Unspecified injury of flexor muscle, fascia and tendon of other finger at wrist and hand level

Unspecified injury of flexor muscle, fascia and tendon of specified finger with unspecified laterality at wrist and hand level

☑7ᵗʰ **S66.109** Unspecified injury of flexor muscle, fascia and tendon of unspecified finger at wrist and hand level

☑6ᵗʰ **S66.11** Strain of flexor muscle, fascia and tendon of other and unspecified finger at wrist and hand level

☑7ᵗʰ **S66.110** Strain of flexor muscle, fascia and tendon of right index finger at wrist and hand level

☑7ᵗʰ **S66.111** Strain of flexor muscle, fascia and tendon of left index finger at wrist and hand level

☑7ᵗʰ **S66.112** Strain of flexor muscle, fascia and tendon of right middle finger at wrist and hand level

☑7ᵗʰ **S66.113** Strain of flexor muscle, fascia and tendon of left middle finger at wrist and hand level

☑7ᵗʰ **S66.114** Strain of flexor muscle, fascia and tendon of right ring finger at wrist and hand level

☑7ᵗʰ **S66.115** Strain of flexor muscle, fascia and tendon of left ring finger at wrist and hand level

☑7ᵗʰ **S66.116** Strain of flexor muscle, fascia and tendon of right little finger at wrist and hand level

☑7ᵗʰ **S66.117** Strain of flexor muscle, fascia and tendon of left little finger at wrist and hand level

☑7ᵗʰ **S66.118** Strain of flexor muscle, fascia and tendon of other finger at wrist and hand level

Strain of flexor muscle, fascia and tendon of specified finger with unspecified laterality at wrist and hand level

☑7ᵗʰ **S66.119** Strain of flexor muscle, fascia and tendon of unspecified finger at wrist and hand level

☑6ᵗʰ **S66.12** Laceration of flexor muscle, fascia and tendon of other and unspecified finger at wrist and hand level

☑7ᵗʰ **S66.120** Laceration of flexor muscle, fascia and tendon of right index finger at wrist and hand level

☑7ᵗʰ **S66.121** Laceration of flexor muscle, fascia and tendon of left index finger at wrist and hand level

☑7ᵗʰ **S66.122** Laceration of flexor muscle, fascia and tendon of right middle finger at wrist and hand level

☑7ᵗʰ **S66.123** Laceration of flexor muscle, fascia and tendon of left middle finger at wrist and hand level

☑7ᵗʰ **S66.124** Laceration of flexor muscle, fascia and tendon of right ring finger at wrist and hand level

☑7ᵗʰ **S66.125** Laceration of flexor muscle, fascia and tendon of left ring finger at wrist and hand level

☑7ᵗʰ **S66.126** Laceration of flexor muscle, fascia and tendon of right little finger at wrist and hand level

☑7ᵗʰ **S66.127** Laceration of flexor muscle, fascia and tendon of left little finger at wrist and hand level

☑7ᵗʰ **S66.128** Laceration of flexor muscle, fascia and tendon of other finger at wrist and hand level

Laceration of flexor muscle, fascia and tendon of specified finger with unspecified laterality at wrist and hand level

---

☑ Appropriate additional character required   ☑x7ᵗʰ Requires 7th character, placeholder x must fill empty characters

√7th **S66.129** Laceration of flexor muscle, fascia and tendon of unspecified finger at wrist and hand level

√6th **S66.19** Other injury of flexor muscle, fascia and tendon of other and unspecified finger at wrist and hand level

    √7th **S66.190** Other injury of flexor muscle, fascia and tendon of right index finger at wrist and hand level

    √7th **S66.191** Other injury of flexor muscle, fascia and tendon of left index finger at wrist and hand level

    √7th **S66.192** Other injury of flexor muscle, fascia and tendon of right middle finger at wrist and hand level

    √7th **S66.193** Other injury of flexor muscle, fascia and tendon of left middle finger at wrist and hand level

    √7th **S66.194** Other injury of flexor muscle, fascia and tendon of right ring finger at wrist and hand level

    √7th **S66.195** Other injury of flexor muscle, fascia and tendon of left ring finger at wrist and hand level

    √7th **S66.196** Other injury of flexor muscle, fascia and tendon of right little finger at wrist and hand level

    √7th **S66.197** Other injury of flexor muscle, fascia and tendon of left little finger at wrist and hand level

    √7th **S66.198** Other injury of flexor muscle, fascia and tendon of other finger at wrist and hand level

      Other injury of flexor muscle, fascia and tendon of specified finger with unspecified laterality at wrist and hand level

    √7th **S66.199** Other injury of flexor muscle, fascia and tendon of unspecified finger at wrist and hand level

√5th **S66.2** Injury of extensor muscle, fascia and tendon of thumb at wrist and hand level

√6th **S66.20** Unspecified injury of extensor muscle, fascia and tendon of thumb at wrist and hand level

    √7th **S66.201** Unspecified injury of extensor muscle, fascia and tendon of right thumb at wrist and hand level

    √7th **S66.202** Unspecified injury of extensor muscle, fascia and tendon of left thumb at wrist and hand level

    √7th **S66.209** Unspecified injury of extensor muscle, fascia and tendon of unspecified thumb at wrist and hand level

√6th **S66.21** Strain of extensor muscle, fascia and tendon of thumb at wrist and hand level

    √7th **S66.211** Strain of extensor muscle, fascia and tendon of right thumb at wrist and hand level

    √7th **S66.212** Strain of extensor muscle, fascia and tendon of left thumb at wrist and hand level

    √7th **S66.219** Strain of extensor muscle, fascia and tendon of unspecified thumb at wrist and hand level

√6th **S66.22** Laceration of extensor muscle, fascia and tendon of thumb at wrist and hand level

    √7th **S66.221** Laceration of extensor muscle, fascia and tendon of right thumb at wrist and hand level

    √7th **S66.222** Laceration of extensor muscle, fascia and tendon of left thumb at wrist and hand level

    √7th **S66.229** Laceration of extensor muscle, fascia and tendon of unspecified thumb at wrist and hand level

√6th **S66.29** Other specified injury of extensor muscle, fascia and tendon of thumb at wrist and hand level

    √7th **S66.291** Other specified injury of extensor muscle, fascia and tendon of right thumb at wrist and hand level

    √7th **S66.292** Other specified injury of extensor muscle, fascia and tendon of left thumb at wrist and hand level

    √7th **S66.299** Other specified injury of extensor muscle, fascia and tendon of unspecified thumb at wrist and hand level

√5th **S66.3** Injury of extensor muscle, fascia and tendon of other and unspecified finger at wrist and hand level

    EXCLUDES 2   *Injury of extensor muscle, fascia and tendon of thumb at wrist and hand level (S66.2-)*

√6th **S66.30** Unspecified injury of extensor muscle, fascia and tendon of other and unspecified finger at wrist and hand level

    √7th **S66.300** Unspecified injury of extensor muscle, fascia and tendon of right index finger at wrist and hand level

    √7th **S66.301** Unspecified injury of extensor muscle, fascia and tendon of left index finger at wrist and hand level

    √7th **S66.302** Unspecified injury of extensor muscle, fascia and tendon of right middle finger at wrist and hand level

    √7th **S66.303** Unspecified injury of extensor muscle, fascia and tendon of left middle finger at wrist and hand level

    √7th **S66.304** Unspecified injury of extensor muscle, fascia and tendon of right ring finger at wrist and hand level

    √7th **S66.305** Unspecified injury of extensor muscle, fascia and tendon of left ring finger at wrist and hand level

    √7th **S66.306** Unspecified injury of extensor muscle, fascia and tendon of right little finger at wrist and hand level

    √7th **S66.307** Unspecified injury of extensor muscle, fascia and tendon of left little finger at wrist and hand level

    √7th **S66.308** Unspecified injury of extensor muscle, fascia and tendon of other finger at wrist and hand level

      Unspecified injury of extensor muscle, fascia and tendon of specified finger with unspecified laterality at wrist and hand level

    √7th **S66.309** Unspecified injury of extensor muscle, fascia and tendon of unspecified finger at wrist and hand level

√6th **S66.31** Strain of extensor muscle, fascia and tendon of other and unspecified finger at wrist and hand level

    √7th **S66.310** Strain of extensor muscle, fascia and tendon of right index finger at wrist and hand level

    √7th **S66.311** Strain of extensor muscle, fascia and tendon of left index finger at wrist and hand level

    √7th **S66.312** Strain of extensor muscle, fascia and tendon of right middle finger at wrist and hand level

    √7th **S66.313** Strain of extensor muscle, fascia and tendon of left middle finger at wrist and hand level

    √7th **S66.314** Strain of extensor muscle, fascia and tendon of right ring finger at wrist and hand level

    √7th **S66.315** Strain of extensor muscle, fascia and tendon of left ring finger at wrist and hand level

    √7th **S66.316** Strain of extensor muscle, fascia and tendon of right little finger at wrist and hand level

    √7th **S66.317** Strain of extensor muscle, fascia and tendon of left little finger at wrist and hand level

---

EXCLUDES 1   Not coded here   EXCLUDES 2   Not included here   *Manifestation Code*

✓7th **S66.318** **Strain of extensor muscle, fascia and tendon of other finger at wrist and hand level**

Strain of extensor muscle, fascia and tendon of specified finger with unspecified laterality at wrist and hand level

✓7th **S66.319** **Strain of extensor muscle, fascia and tendon of unspecified finger at wrist and hand level**

✓6th **S66.32** **Laceration of extensor muscle, fascia and tendon of other and unspecified finger at wrist and hand level**

✓7th **S66.320** **Laceration of extensor muscle, fascia and tendon of right index finger at wrist and hand level**

✓7th **S66.321** **Laceration of extensor muscle, fascia and tendon of left index finger at wrist and hand level**

✓7th **S66.322** **Laceration of extensor muscle, fascia and tendon of right middle finger at wrist and hand level**

✓7th **S66.323** **Laceration of extensor muscle, fascia and tendon of left middle finger at wrist and hand level**

✓7th **S66.324** **Laceration of extensor muscle, fascia and tendon of right ring finger at wrist and hand level**

✓7th **S66.325** **Laceration of extensor muscle, fascia and tendon of left ring finger at wrist and hand level**

✓7th **S66.326** **Laceration of extensor muscle, fascia and tendon of right little finger at wrist and hand level**

✓7th **S66.327** **Laceration of extensor muscle, fascia and tendon of left little finger at wrist and hand level**

✓7th **S66.328** **Laceration of extensor muscle, fascia and tendon of other finger at wrist and hand level**

Laceration of extensor muscle, fascia and tendon of specified finger with unspecified laterality at wrist and hand level

✓7th **S66.329** **Laceration of extensor muscle, fascia and tendon of unspecified finger at wrist and hand level**

✓6th **S66.39** **Other injury of extensor muscle, fascia and tendon of other and unspecified finger at wrist and hand level**

✓7th **S66.390** **Other injury of extensor muscle, fascia and tendon of right index finger at wrist and hand level**

✓7th **S66.391** **Other injury of extensor muscle, fascia and tendon of left index finger at wrist and hand level**

✓7th **S66.392** **Other injury of extensor muscle, fascia and tendon of right middle finger at wrist and hand level**

✓7th **S66.393** **Other injury of extensor muscle, fascia and tendon of left middle finger at wrist and hand level**

✓7th **S66.394** **Other injury of extensor muscle, fascia and tendon of right ring finger at wrist and hand level**

✓7th **S66.395** **Other injury of extensor muscle, fascia and tendon of left ring finger at wrist and hand level**

✓7th **S66.396** **Other injury of extensor muscle, fascia and tendon of right little finger at wrist and hand level**

✓7th **S66.397** **Other injury of extensor muscle, fascia and tendon of left little finger at wrist and hand level**

✓7th **S66.398** **Other injury of extensor muscle, fascia and tendon of other finger at wrist and hand level**

Other injury of extensor muscle, fascia and tendon of specified finger with unspecified laterality at wrist and hand level

✓7th **S66.399** **Other injury of extensor muscle, fascia and tendon of unspecified finger at wrist and hand level**

✓5th **S66.4** **Injury of intrinsic muscle, fascia and tendon of thumb at wrist and hand level**

✓6th **S66.40** **Unspecified injury of intrinsic muscle, fascia and tendon of thumb at wrist and hand level**

✓7th **S66.401** **Unspecified injury of intrinsic muscle, fascia and tendon of right thumb at wrist and hand level**

✓7th **S66.402** **Unspecified injury of intrinsic muscle, fascia and tendon of left thumb at wrist and hand level**

✓7th **S66.409** **Unspecified injury of intrinsic muscle, fascia and tendon of unspecified thumb at wrist and hand level**

✓6th **S66.41** **Strain of intrinsic muscle, fascia and tendon of thumb at wrist and hand level**

✓7th **S66.411** **Strain of intrinsic muscle, fascia and tendon of right thumb at wrist and hand level**

✓7th **S66.412** **Strain of intrinsic muscle, fascia and tendon of left thumb at wrist and hand level**

✓7th **S66.419** **Strain of intrinsic muscle, fascia and tendon of unspecified thumb at wrist and hand level**

✓6th **S66.42** **Laceration of intrinsic muscle, fascia and tendon of thumb at wrist and hand level**

✓7th **S66.421** **Laceration of intrinsic muscle, fascia and tendon of right thumb at wrist and hand level**

✓7th **S66.422** **Laceration of intrinsic muscle, fascia and tendon of left thumb at wrist and hand**

✓7th **S66.429** **Laceration of intrinsic muscle, fascia and tendon of unspecified thumb at wrist and hand level of side**

✓6th **S66.49** **Other specified injury of intrinsic muscle, fascia and tendon of thumb at wrist and hand level**

✓7th **S66.491** **Other specified injury of intrinsic muscle, fascia and tendon of right thumb at wrist and hand level**

✓7th **S66.492** **Other specified injury of intrinsic muscle, fascia and tendon of left thumb at wrist and hand level**

✓7th **S66.499** **Other specified injury of intrinsic muscle, fascia and tendon of unspecified thumb at wrist and hand level**

✓5th **S66.5** **Injury of intrinsic muscle, fascia and tendon of other and unspecified finger at wrist and hand level**

EXCLUDES 2 *injury of intrinsic muscle, fascia and tendon of thumb at wrist and hand level (S66.4-)*

✓6th **S66.50** **Unspecified injury of intrinsic muscle, fascia and tendon of other and unspecified finger at wrist and hand level**

✓7th **S66.500** **Unspecified injury of intrinsic muscle, fascia and tendon of right index finger at wrist and hand level**

✓7th **S66.501** **Unspecified injury of intrinsic muscle, fascia and tendon of left index finger at wrist and hand level**

✓7th **S66.502** **Unspecified injury of intrinsic muscle, fascia and tendon of right middle finger at wrist and hand level**

✓7th **S66.503** **Unspecified injury of intrinsic muscle, fascia and tendon of left middle finger at wrist and hand level**

✓7th **S66.504** **Unspecified injury of intrinsic muscle, fascia and tendon of right ring finger at wrist and hand level**

✓ Appropriate additional character required   ✓x7th Requires 7th character, placeholder x must fill empty characters

√7th **S66.505** **Unspecified injury of intrinsic muscle, fascia and tendon of left ring finger at wrist and hand level**

√7th **S66.506** **Unspecified injury of intrinsic muscle, fascia and tendon of right little finger at wrist and hand level**

√7th **S66.507** **Unspecified injury of intrinsic muscle, fascia and tendon of left little finger at wrist and hand level**

√7th **S66.508** **Unspecified injury of intrinsic muscle, fascia and tendon of other finger at wrist and hand level**

Unspecified injury of intrinsic muscle, fascia and tendon of specified finger with unspecified laterality at wrist and hand level

√7th **S66.509** **Unspecified injury of intrinsic muscle, fascia and tendon of unspecified finger at wrist and hand level**

√6th **S66.51** **Strain of intrinsic muscle, fascia and tendon of other and unspecified finger at wrist and hand level**

√7th **S66.510** **Strain of intrinsic muscle, fascia and tendon of right index finger at wrist and hand level**

√7th **S66.511** **Strain of intrinsic muscle, fascia and tendon of left index finger at wrist and hand level**

√7th **S66.512** **Strain of intrinsic muscle, fascia and tendon of right middle finger at wrist and hand level**

√7th **S66.513** **Strain of intrinsic muscle, fascia and tendon of left middle finger at wrist and hand level**

√7th **S66.514** **Strain of intrinsic muscle, fascia and tendon of right ring finger at wrist and hand level**

√7th **S66.515** **Strain of intrinsic muscle, fascia and tendon of left ring finger at wrist and hand level**

√7th **S66.516** **Strain of intrinsic muscle, fascia and tendon of right little finger at wrist and hand level**

√7th **S66.517** **Strain of intrinsic muscle, fascia and tendon of left little finger at wrist and hand level**

√7th **S66.518** **Strain of intrinsic muscle, fascia and tendon of other finger at wrist and hand level**

Strain of intrinsic muscle, fascia and tendon of specified finger with unspecified laterality at wrist and hand level

√7th **S66.519** **Strain of intrinsic muscle, fascia and tendon of unspecified finger at wrist and hand level**

√6th **S66.52** **Laceration of intrinsic muscle, fascia and tendon of other and unspecified finger at wrist and hand level**

√7th **S66.520** **Laceration of intrinsic muscle, fascia and tendon of right index finger at wrist and hand level**

√7th **S66.521** **Laceration of intrinsic muscle, fascia and tendon of left index finger at wrist and hand level**

√7th **S66.522** **Laceration of intrinsic muscle, fascia and tendon of right middle finger at wrist and hand level**

√7th **S66.523** **Laceration of intrinsic muscle, fascia and tendon of left middle finger at wrist and hand level**

√7th **S66.524** **Laceration of intrinsic muscle, fascia and tendon of right ring finger at wrist and hand level**

√7th **S66.525** **Laceration of intrinsic muscle, fascia and tendon of left ring finger at wrist and hand level**

√7th **S66.526** **Laceration of intrinsic muscle, fascia and tendon of right little finger at wrist and hand level**

√7th **S66.527** **Laceration of intrinsic muscle, fascia and tendon of left little finger at wrist and hand level**

√7th **S66.528** **Laceration of intrinsic muscle, fascia and tendon of other finger at wrist and hand level**

Laceration of intrinsic muscle, fascia and tendon of specified finger with unspecified laterality at wrist and hand level

√7th **S66.529** **Laceration of intrinsic muscle, fascia and tendon of unspecified finger at wrist and hand level**

√6th **S66.59** **Other injury of intrinsic muscle, fascia and tendon of other and unspecified finger at wrist and hand level**

√7th **S66.590** **Other injury of intrinsic muscle, fascia and tendon of right index finger at wrist and hand level**

√7th **S66.591** **Other injury of intrinsic muscle, fascia and tendon of left index finger at wrist and hand level**

√7th **S66.592** **Other injury of intrinsic muscle, fascia and tendon of right middle finger at wrist and hand level**

√7th **S66.593** **Other injury of intrinsic muscle, fascia and tendon of left middle finger at wrist and hand level**

√7th **S66.594** **Other injury of intrinsic muscle, fascia and tendon of right ring finger at wrist and hand level**

√7th **S66.595** **Other injury of intrinsic muscle, fascia and tendon of left ring finger at wrist and hand level**

√7th **S66.596** **Other injury of intrinsic muscle, fascia and tendon of right little finger at wrist and hand level**

√7th **S66.597** **Other injury of intrinsic muscle, fascia and tendon of left little finger at wrist and hand level**

√7th **S66.598** **Other injury of intrinsic muscle, fascia and tendon of other finger at wrist and hand level**

Other injury of intrinsic muscle, fascia and tendon of specified finger with unspecified laterality at wrist and hand level

√7th **S66.599** **Other injury of intrinsic muscle, fascia and tendon of unspecified finger at wrist and hand level**

√5th **S66.8** **Injury of other specified muscles, fascia and tendons at wrist and hand level**

√6th **S66.80** **Unspecified injury of other specified muscles, fascia and tendons at wrist and hand level**

√7th **S66.801** **Unspecified injury of other specified muscles, fascia and tendons at wrist and hand level, right hand**

√7th **S66.802** **Unspecified injury of other specified muscles, fascia and tendons at wrist and hand level, left hand**

√7th **S66.809** **Unspecified injury of other specified muscles, fascia and tendons at wrist and hand level, unspecified hand**

√6th **S66.81** **Strain of other specified muscles, fascia and tendons at wrist and hand level**

√7th **S66.811** **Strain of other specified muscles, fascia and tendons at wrist and hand level, right hand**

√7th **S66.812** **Strain of other specified muscles, fascia and tendons at wrist and hand level, left hand**

√7th **S66.819** **Strain of other specified muscles, fascia and tendons at wrist and hand level, unspecified hand**

EXCLUDES 1   Not coded here   EXCLUDES 2   Not included here   *Manifestation Code*

√6ᵗʰ **S66.82 Laceration of other specified muscles, fascia and tendons at wrist and hand level**

√7ᵗʰ **S66.821 Laceration of other specfed muscles, fascia and tendons at wrist and hand level, right hand**

√7ᵗʰ **S66.822 Laceration of other specified muscles, fascia and tendons at wrist and hand level, left hand**

√7ᵗʰ **S66.829 Laceration of other specified muscles, fascia and tendons at wrist and hand level, unspecified hand**

√6ᵗʰ **S66.89 Other injury of other specified muscles, fascia and tendons at wrist and hand level**

√7ᵗʰ **S66.891 Other injury of other specified muscles, fascia and tendons at wrist and hand level, right hand**

√7ᵗʰ **S66.892 Other injury of other specified muscles, fascia and tendons at wrist and hand level, left hand**

√7ᵗʰ **S66.899 Other injury of other specified muscles, fascia and tendons at wrist and hand level, unspecified hand**

√5ᵗʰ **S66.9 Injury of unspecified muscle, fascia and tendon at wrist and hand level**

√6ᵗʰ **S66.90 Unspecified injury of unspecified muscle, fascia and tendon at wrist and hand level**

√7ᵗʰ **S66.901 Unspecified injury of unspecified muscle, fascia and tendon at wrist and hand level, right hand**

√7ᵗʰ **S66.902 Unspecified injury of unspecified muscle, fascia and tendon at wrist and hand level, left hand**

√7ᵗʰ **S66.909 Unspecified injury of unspecified muscle, fascia and tendon at wrist and hand level, unspecified hand**

√6ᵗʰ **S66.91 Strain of unspecified muscle, fascia and tendon at wrist and hand level**

√7ᵗʰ **S66.911 Strain of unspecified muscle, fascia and tendon at wrist and hand level, right hand**

√7ᵗʰ **S66.912 Strain of unspecified muscle, fascia and tendon at wrist and hand level, left hand**

√7ᵗʰ **S66.919 Strain of unspecified muscle, fascia and tendon at wrist and hand level of unspecified hand**

√6ᵗʰ **S66.92 Laceration of unspecified muscle, fascia and tendon at wrist and hand level**

√7ᵗʰ **S66.921 Laceration of unspecified muscle, fascia and tendon at wrist and hand level, right hand**

√7ᵗʰ **S66.922 Laceration of unspecified muscle, fascia and tendon at wrist and hand level, left hand**

√7ᵗʰ **S66.929 Laceration of unspecified muscle, fascia and tendon at wrist and hand level of unspecified hand**

√6ᵗʰ **S66.99 Other injury of unspecified muscle, fascia and tendon at wrist and hand level**

√7ᵗʰ **S66.991 Other injury of unspecified muscle, fascia and tendon at wrist and hand level, right hand**

√7ᵗʰ **S66.992 Other injury of unspecified muscle, fascia and tendon at wrist and hand level, left hand**

√7ᵗʰ **S66.999 Other injury of unspecified muscle, fascia and tendon at wrist and hand level of unspecified hand**

√4ᵗʰ **S67 Crushing injury of wrist, hand and fingers**

Use additional code for all associated injuries, such as:
fracture of wrist and hand (S62-)
open wound of wrist and hand (S61-)

The appropriate 7th character is to be added to each code from category S67.
A   initial encounter
D   subsequent encounter
S   sequela

√5ᵗʰ **S67.0 Crushing injury of thumb**

√x7ᵗʰ **S67.00 Crushing injury of unspecified thumb**

√x7ᵗʰ **S67.01 Crushing injury of right thumb**

√x7ᵗʰ **S67.02 Crushing injury of left thumb**

√5ᵗʰ **S67.1 Crushing injury of other and unspecified finger(s)**

EXCLUDES 2   *crushing injury of thumb (S67.0-)*

√x7ᵗʰ **S67.10 Crushing injury of unspecified finger(s)**

√6ᵗʰ **S67.19 Crushing injury of other finger(s)**

√7ᵗʰ **S67.190 Crushing injury of right index finger**

√7ᵗʰ **S67.191 Crushing injury of left index finger**

√7ᵗʰ **S67.192 Crushing injury of right middle finger**

√7ᵗʰ **S67.193 Crushing injury of left middle finger**

√7ᵗʰ **S67.194 Crushing injury of right ring finger**

√7ᵗʰ **S67.195 Crushing injury of left ring finger**

√7ᵗʰ **S67.196 Crushing injury of right little finger**

√7ᵗʰ **S67.197 Crushing injury of left little finger**

√7ᵗʰ **S67.198 Crushing injury of other finger**
Crushing injury of specified finger with unspecified laterality

√5ᵗʰ **S67.2 Crushing injury of hand**

EXCLUDES 2   *crushing injury of fingers (S67.1-)*
crushing injury of thumb (S67.0-)

√x7ᵗʰ **S67.20 Crushing injury of unspecified hand**

√x7ᵗʰ **S67.21 Crushing injury of right hand**

√x7ᵗʰ **S67.22 Crushing injury of left hand**

√5ᵗʰ **S67.3 Crushing injury of wrist**

√x7ᵗʰ **S67.30 Crushing injury of unspecified wrist**

√x7ᵗʰ **S67.31 Crushing injury of right wrist**

√x7ᵗʰ **S67.32 Crushing injury of left wrist**

√5ᵗʰ **S67.4 Crushing injury of wrist and hand**

EXCLUDES 1   *crushing injury of hand alone (S67.2-)*
crushing injury of wrist alone (S67.3-)

EXCLUDES 2   *crushing injury of fingers (S67.1-)*
crushing injury of thumb (S67.0-)

√x7ᵗʰ **S67.40 Crushing injury of unspecified wrist and hand**

√x7ᵗʰ **S67.41 Crushing injury of right wrist and hand**

√x7ᵗʰ **S67.42 Crushing injury of left wrist and hand**

√5ᵗʰ **S67.9 Crushing injury of unspecified part(s) of wrist, hand and fingers**

√x7ᵗʰ **S67.90 Crushing injury of unspecified part(s) of unspecified wrist, hand and fingers**

√x7ᵗʰ **S67.91 Crushing injury of unspecified part(s) of right wrist, hand and fingers**

√x7ᵗʰ **S67.92 Crushing injury of unspecified part(s) of left wrist, hand and fingers**

√4ᵗʰ **S68 Traumatic amputation of wrist, hand and fingers**

NOTE   An amputation not identified as partial or complete should be coded to complete

The appropriate 7th character is to be added to each code from category S68.
A   initial encounter
D   subsequent encounter
S   sequela

√5ᵗʰ **S68.0 Traumatic metacarpophalangeal amputation of thumb**
Traumatic amputation of thumb NOS

√6ᵗʰ **S68.01 Complete traumatic metacarpophalangeal amputation of thumb**

√7ᵗʰ **S68.011 Complete traumatic metacarpophalangeal amputation of right thumb**

√7ᵗʰ **S68.012 Complete traumatic metacarpophalangeal amputation of left thumb**

√7ᵗʰ **S68.019 Complete traumatic metacarpophalangeal amputation of unspecified thumb**

√6ᵗʰ **S68.02 Partial traumatic metacarpophalangeal amputation of thumb**

√7ᵗʰ **S68.021 Partial traumatic metacarpophalangeal amputation of right thumb**

√7ᵗʰ **S68.022 Partial traumatic metacarpophalangeal amputation of left thumb**

√7ᵗʰ **S68.029 Partial traumatic metacarpophalangeal amputation of unspecified thumb**

√5ᵗʰ **S68.1   Traumatic metacarpophalangeal amputation of other and unspecified finger**
Traumatic amputation of finger NOS
EXCLUDES 2   *traumatic metacarpophalangeal amputation of thumb (S68.0-)*

   √6ᵗʰ **S68.11   Complete traumatic metacarpophalangeal amputation of other and unspecified finger**

      √7ᵗʰ **S68.110   Complete traumatic metacarpophalangeal amputation of right index finger**

      √7ᵗʰ **S68.111   Complete traumatic metacarpophalangeal amputation of left index finger**

      √7ᵗʰ **S68.112   Complete traumatic metacarpophalangeal amputation of right middle finger**

      √7ᵗʰ **S68.113   Complete traumatic metacarpophalangeal amputation of left middle finger**

      √7ᵗʰ **S68.114   Complete traumatic metacarpophalangeal amputation of right ring finger**

      √7ᵗʰ **S68.115   Complete traumatic metacarpophalangeal amputation of left ring finger**

      √7ᵗʰ **S68.116   Complete traumatic metacarpophalangeal amputation of right little finger**

      √7ᵗʰ **S68.117   Complete traumatic metacarpophalangeal amputation of left little finger**

      √7ᵗʰ **S68.118   Complete traumatic metacarpophalangeal amputation of other finger**
Complete traumatic metacarpophalangeal amputation of specified finger with unspecified laterality

      √7ᵗʰ **S68.119   Complete traumatic metacarpophalangeal amputation of unspecified finger**

   √6ᵗʰ **S68.12   Partial traumatic metacarpophalangeal amputation of other and unspecified finger**

      √7ᵗʰ **S68.120   Partial traumatic metacarpophalangeal amputation of right index finger**

      √7ᵗʰ **S68.121   Partial traumatic metacarpophalangeal amputation of left index finger**

      √7ᵗʰ **S68.122   Partial traumatic metacarpophalangeal amputation of right middle finger**

      √7ᵗʰ **S68.123   Partial traumatic metacarpophalangeal amputation of left middle finger**

      √7ᵗʰ **S68.124   Partial traumatic metacarpophalangeal amputation of right ring finger**

      √7ᵗʰ **S68.125   Partial traumatic metacarpophalangeal amputation of left ring finger**

      √7ᵗʰ **S68.126   Partial traumatic metacarpophalangeal amputation of right little finger**

      √7ᵗʰ **S68.127   Partial traumatic metacarpophalangeal amputation of left little finger**

      √7ᵗʰ **S68.128   Partial traumatic metacarpophalangeal amputation of other finger**
Partial traumatic metacarpophalangeal amputation of specified finger with unspecified laterality

      √7ᵗʰ **S68.129   Partial traumatic metacarpophalangeal amputation of unspecified finger**

√5ᵗʰ **S68.4   Traumatic amputation of hand at wrist level**
Traumatic amputation of hand NOS
Traumatic amputation of wrist

   √6ᵗʰ **S68.41   Complete traumatic amputation of hand at wrist level**

      √7ᵗʰ **S68.411   Complete traumatic amputation of right hand at wrist level**

      √7ᵗʰ **S68.412   Complete traumatic amputation of left hand at wrist level**

      √7ᵗʰ **S68.419   Complete traumatic amputation of unspecified hand at wrist level**

   √6ᵗʰ **S68.42   Partial traumatic amputation of hand at wrist level**

      √7ᵗʰ **S68.421   Partial traumatic amputation of right hand at wrist level**

      √7ᵗʰ **S68.422   Partial traumatic amputation of left hand at wrist level**

      √7ᵗʰ **S68.429   Partial traumatic amputation of unspecified hand at wrist level**

S68.5   Traumatic transphalangeal amputation of thumb
Traumatic interphalangeal joint amputation of thumb

   √6ᵗʰ **S68.51   Complete traumatic transphalangeal amputation of thumb**

      √7ᵗʰ **S68.511   Complete traumatic transphalangeal amputation of right thumb**

      √7ᵗʰ **S68.512   Complete traumatic transphalangeal amputation of left thumb**

      √7ᵗʰ **S68.519   Complete traumatic transphalangeal amputation of unspecified thumb**

   √6ᵗʰ **S68.52   Partial traumatic transphalangeal amputation of thumb**

      √7ᵗʰ **S68.521   Partial traumatic transphalangeal amputation of right thumb**

      √7ᵗʰ **S68.522   Partial traumatic transphalangeal amputation of left thumb**

      √7ᵗʰ **S68.529   Partial traumatic transphalangeal amputation of unspecified thumb**

√5ᵗʰ **S68.6   Traumatic transphalangeal amputation of other and unspecified finger**

   √6ᵗʰ **S68.61   Complete traumatic transphalangeal amputation of other and unspecified finger(s)**

      √7ᵗʰ **S68.610   Complete traumatic transphalangeal amputation of right index finger**

      √7ᵗʰ **S68.611   Complete traumatic transphalangeal amputation of left index finger**

      √7ᵗʰ **S68.612   Complete traumatic transphalangeal amputation of right middle finger**

      √7ᵗʰ **S68.613   Complete traumatic transphalangeal amputation of left middle finger**

      √7ᵗʰ **S68.614   Complete traumatic transphalangeal amputation of right ring finger**

      √7ᵗʰ **S68.615   Complete traumatic transphalangeal amputation of left ring finger**

      √7ᵗʰ **S68.616   Complete traumatic transphalangeal amputation of right little finger**

      √7ᵗʰ **S68.617   Complete traumatic transphalangeal amputation of left little finger**

      √7ᵗʰ **S68.618   Complete traumatic transphalangeal amputation of other finger**
Complete traumatic transphalangeal amputation of specified finger with unspecified laterality

      √7ᵗʰ **S68.619   Complete traumatic transphalangeal amputation of unspecified finger**

   √6ᵗʰ **S68.62   Partial traumatic transphalangeal amputation of other and unspecified finger**

      √7ᵗʰ **S68.620   Partial traumatic transphalangeal amputation of right index finger**

      √7ᵗʰ **S68.621   Partial traumatic transphalangeal amputation of left index finger**

      √7ᵗʰ **S68.622   Partial traumatic transphalangeal amputation of right middle finger**

      √7ᵗʰ **S68.623   Partial traumatic transphalangeal amputation of left middle finger**

      √7ᵗʰ **S68.624   Partial traumatic transphalangeal amputation of right ring finger**

      √7ᵗʰ **S68.625   Partial traumatic transphalangeal amputation of left ring finger**

      √7ᵗʰ **S68.626   Partial traumatic transphalangeal amputation of right little finger**

      √7ᵗʰ **S68.627   Partial traumatic transphalangeal amputation of left little finger**

      √7ᵗʰ **S68.628   Partial traumatic transphalangeal amputation of other finger**
Partial traumatic transphalangeal amputation of specified finger with unspecified laterality

      √7ᵗʰ **S68.629   Partial traumatic transphalangeal amputation of unspecified finger**

☑5th **S68.7   Traumatic transmetacarpal amputation of hand**
  ☑6th **S68.71   Complete traumatic transmetacarpal amputation of hand**
    ☑7th **S68.711   Complete traumatic transmetacarpal amputation of right hand**
    ☑7th **S68.712   Complete traumatic transmetacarpal amputation of left hand**
    ☑7th **S68.719   Complete traumatic transmetacarpal amputation of unspecified hand**
  ☑6th **S68.72   Partial traumatic transmetacarpal amputation of hand**
    ☑7th **S68.721   Partial traumatic transmetacarpal amputation of right hand**
    ☑7th **S68.722   Partial traumatic transmetacarpal amputation of left hand**
    ☑7th **S68.729   Partial traumatic transmetacarpal amputation of unspecified hand**

☑4th **S69   Other and unspecified injuries of wrist, hand and finger(s)**

> The appropriate 7th character is to be added to each code from category S69.
> A   initial encounter
> D   subsequent encounter
> S   sequela

☑5th **S69.8   Other specified injuries of wrist, hand and finger(s)**
  ☑x7th **S69.80   Other specified injuries of unspecified wrist, hand and finger(s)**
  ☑x7th **S69.81   Other specified injuries of right wrist, hand and finger(s)**
  ☑x7th **S69.82   Other specified injuries of left wrist, hand and finger(s)**
☑5th **S69.9   Unspecified injury of wrist, hand and finger(s)**
  ☑x7th **S69.90   Unspecified injury of unspecified wrist, hand and finger(s)**
  ☑x7th **S69.91   Unspecified injury of right wrist, hand and finger(s)**
  ☑x7th **S69.92   Unspecified injury of left wrist, hand and finger(s)**

Injuries to the hip and thigh (S70-S79)

EXCLUDES 2   *burns and corrosions (T20-T32)*
              frostbite (T33-T34)
              snake bite (T63.0-)
              venomous insect bite or sting (T63.4-)

☑4th **S70   Superficial injury of hip and thigh**

> The appropriate 7th character is to be added to each code from category S70.
> A   initial encounter
> D   subsequent encounter
> S   sequela

☑5th **S70.0   Contusion of hip**
  ☑x7th **S70.00   Contusion of unspecified hip**
  ☑x7th **S70.01   Contusion of right hip**
  ☑x7th **S70.02   Contusion of left hip**
☑5th **S70.1   Contusion of thigh**
  ☑x7th **S70.10   Contusion of unspecified thigh**
  ☑x7th **S70.11   Contusion of right thigh**
  ☑x7th **S70.12   Contusion of left thigh**
☑5th **S70.2   Other superficial injuries of hip**
  ☑6th **S70.21   Abrasion of hip**
    ☑7th **S70.211   Abrasion, right hip**
    ☑7th **S70.212   Abrasion, left hip**
    ☑7th **S70.219   Abrasion, unspecified hip**
  ☑6th **S70.22   Blister (nonthermal) of hip**
    ☑7th **S70.221   Blister (nonthermal), right hip**
    ☑7th **S70.222   Blister (nonthermal), left hip**
    ☑7th **S70.229   Blister (nonthermal), unspecified hip**
  ☑6th **S70.24   External constriction of hip**
    ☑7th **S70.241   External constriction, right hip**
    ☑7th **S70.242   External constriction, left hip**
    ☑7th **S70.249   External constriction, unspecified hip**
  ☑6th **S70.25   Superficial foreign body of hip**
      Splinter in the hip
    ☑7th **S70.251   Superficial foreign body, right hip**
    ☑7th **S70.252   Superficial foreign body, left hip**

  ☑7th **S70.259   Superficial foreign body, unspecified hip**
  ☑6th **S70.26   Insect bite (nonvenomous) of hip**
    ☑7th **S70.261   Insect bite (nonvenomous), right hip**
    ☑7th **S70.262   Insect bite (nonvenomous), left hip**
    ☑7th **S70.269   Insect bite (nonvenomous), unspecified hip**
  ☑6th **S70.27   Other superficial bite of hip**
      EXCLUDES 1   *open bite of hip (S71.05-)*
    ☑7th **S70.271   Other superficial bite of hip, right hip**
    ☑7th **S70.272   Other superficial bite of hip, left hip**
    ☑7th **S70.279   Other superficial bite of hip, unspecified hip**
☑5th **S70.3   Other superficial injuries of thigh**
  ☑6th **S70.31   Abrasion of thigh**
    ☑7th **S70.311   Abrasion, right thigh**
    ☑7th **S70.312   Abrasion, left thigh**
    ☑7th **S70.319   Abrasion, unspecified thigh**
  ☑6th **S70.32   Blister (nonthermal) of thigh**
    ☑7th **S70.321   Blister (nonthermal), right thigh**
    ☑7th **S70.322   Blister (nonthermal), left thigh**
    ☑7th **S70.329   Blister (nonthermal), unspecified thigh**
  ☑6th **S70.34   External constriction of thigh**
    ☑7th **S70.341   External constriction, right thigh**
    ☑7th **S70.342   External constriction, left thigh**
    ☑7th **S70.349   External constriction, unspecified thigh**
  ☑6th **S70.35   Superficial foreign body of thigh**
      Splinter in the thigh
    ☑7th **S70.351   Superficial foreign body, right thigh**
    ☑7th **S70.352   Superficial foreign body, left thigh**
    ☑7th **S70.359   Superficial foreign body, unspecified thigh**
  ☑6th **S70.36   Insect bite (nonvenomous) of thigh**
    ☑7th **S70.361   Insect bite (nonvenomous), right thigh**
    ☑7th **S70.362   Insect bite (nonvenomous), left thigh**
    ☑7th **S70.369   Insect bite (nonvenomous), unspecified thigh**
  ☑6th **S70.37   Other superficial bite of thigh**
      EXCLUDES 1   *open bite of thigh (S71.15)*
    ☑7th **S70.371   Other superficial bite of right thigh**
    ☑7th **S70.372   Other superficial bite of left thigh**
    ☑7th **S70.379   Other superficial bite of unspecified thigh**
☑5th **S70.9   Unspecified superficial injury of hip and thigh**
  ☑6th **S70.91   Unspecified superficial injury of hip**
    ☑7th **S70.911   Unspecified superficial injury of right hip**
    ☑7th **S70.912   Unspecified superficial injury of left hip**
    ☑7th **S70.919   Unspecified superficial injury of unspecified hip**
  ☑6th **S70.92   Unspecified superficial injury of thigh**
    ☑7th **S70.921   Unspecified superficial injury of right thigh**
    ☑7th **S70.922   Unspecified superficial injury of left thigh**
    ☑7th **S70.929   Unspecified superficial injury of unspecified thigh**

☑4th **S71   Open wound of hip and thigh**
    Code also any associated wound infection
    EXCLUDES 1   *open fracture of hip and thigh (S72-)*
                  traumatic amputation of hip and thigh (S78-)
    EXCLUDES 2   *bite of venomous animal (T63-)*
                  open wound of ankle, foot and toes (S91-)
                  open wound of knee and lower leg (S81-)

> The appropriate 7th character is to be added to each code from category S71.
> A   initial encounter
> D   subsequent encounter
> S   sequela

☑5th **S71.0   Open wound of hip**
  ☑6th **S71.00   Unspecified open wound of hip**
    ☑7th **S71.001   Unspecified open wound, right hip**
    ☑7th **S71.002   Unspecified open wound, left hip**

☑ Appropriate additional character required   ☑x7th Requires 7th character, placeholder x must fill empty characters

✓7th **S71.009** **Unspecified open wound, unspecified hip**

✓6th **S71.01** **Laceration without foreign body of hip**

    ✓7th **S71.011** **Laceration without foreign body, right hip**

    ✓7th **S71.012** **Laceration without foreign body, left hip**

    ✓7th **S71.019** **Laceration without foreign body, unspecified hip**

✓6th **S71.02** **Laceration with foreign body of hip**

    ✓7th **S71.021** **Laceration with foreign body, right hip**

    ✓7th **S71.022** **Laceration with foreign body, left hip**

    ✓7th **S71.029** **Laceration with foreign body, unspecified hip**

✓6th **S71.03** **Puncture wound without foreign body of hip**

    ✓7th **S71.031** **Puncture wound without foreign body, right hip**

    ✓7th **S71.032** **Puncture wound without foreign body, left hip**

    ✓7th **S71.039** **Puncture wound without foreign body, unspecified hip**

✓6th **S71.04** **Puncture wound with foreign body of hip**

    ✓7th **S71.041** **Puncture wound with foreign body, right hip**

    ✓7th **S71.042** **Puncture wound with foreign body, left hip**

    ✓7th **S71.049** **Puncture wound with foreign body, unspecified hip**

✓6th **S71.05** **Open bite of hip**
    Bite of hip NOS
    EXCLUDES 1   *superficial bite of hip (S70.26, S70.27)*

    ✓7th **S71.051** **Open bite, right hip**

    ✓7th **S71.052** **Open bite, left hip**

    ✓7th **S71.059** **Open bite, unspecified hip**

✓5th **S71.1** **Open wound of thigh**

✓6th **S71.10** **Unspecified open wound of thigh**

    ✓7th **S71.101** **Unspecified open wound, right thigh**

    ✓7th **S71.102** **Unspecified open wound, left thigh**

    ✓7th **S71.109** **Unspecified open wound, unspecified thigh**

✓6th **S71.11** **Laceration without foreign body of thigh**

    ✓7th **S71.111** **Laceration without foreign body, right thigh**

    ✓7th **S71.112** **Laceration without foreign body, left thigh**

    ✓7th **S71.119** **Laceration without foreign body, unspecified thigh**

✓6th **S71.12** **Laceration with foreign body of thigh**

    ✓7th **S71.121** **Laceration with foreign body, right thigh**

    ✓7th **S71.122** **Laceration with foreign body, left thigh**

    ✓7th **S71.129** **Laceration with foreign body, unspecified thigh**

✓6th **S71.13** **Puncture wound without foreign body of thigh**

    ✓7th **S71.131** **Puncture wound without foreign body, right thigh**

    ✓7th **S71.132** **Puncture wound without foreign body, left thigh**

    ✓7th **S71.139** **Puncture wound without foreign body, unspecified thigh**

✓6th **S71.14** **Puncture wound with foreign body of thigh**

    ✓7th **S71.141** **Puncture wound with foreign body, right thigh**

    ✓7th **S71.142** **Puncture wound with foreign body, left thigh**

    ✓7th **S71.149** **Puncture wound with foreign body, unspecified thigh**

✓6th **S71.15** **Open bite of thigh**
    Bite of thigh NOS
    EXCLUDES 1   *superficial bite of thigh (S70.37-)*

    ✓7th **S71.151** **Open bite, right thigh**

    ✓7th **S71.152** **Open bite, left thigh**

    ✓7th **S71.159** **Open bite, unspecified thigh**

✓4th **S72** **Fracture of femur**
    NOTE   A fracture not indicated as displaced or nondisplaced should be coded to displaced

    The open fracture designations are based on the Gustilo open fracture classification A fracture not indicated as open or closed should be coded to closed

    EXCLUDES 1   *traumatic amputation of hip and thigh (S78-)*

    EXCLUDES 2   *fracture of lower leg and ankle (S82-)*
                  fracture of foot (S92-)
                   periprosthetic fracture of prosthetic implant of hip (T84.040, T84.041)

The appropriate 7th character is to be added to each code from category S72.

A	initial encounter for closed fracture
B	initial encounter for open fracture type I or II
	initial encounter for open fracture NOS
C	initial encounter for open fracture type IIIA, IIIB, or IIIC
D	subsequent encounter for closed fracture with routine healing
E	subsequent encounter for open fracture type I or II with routine healing
F	subsequent encounter for open fracture type IIIA, IIIB, or IIIC with routine healing
G	subsequent encounter for closed fracture with delayed healing
H	subsequent encounter for open fracture type I or II with delayed healing
J	subsequent encounter for open fracture type IIIA, IIIB, or IIIC with delayed healing
K	subsequent encounter for closed fracture with nonunion
M	subsequent encounter for open fracture type I or I with nonunion
N	subsequent encounter for open fracture type IIIA, IIIB, or IIIC with nonunion
P	subsequent encounter for closed fracture with malunion
Q	subsequent encounter for open fracture type I or II with malunion
R	subsequent encounter for open fracture type IIIA, IIIB, or IIIC with malunion
S	sequela

✓5th **S72.0** **Fracture of head and neck of femur**
    EXCLUDES 2   *physeal fracture of upper end of femur (S79.0-)*

✓6th **S72.00** **Fracture of unspecified part of neck of femur**
    Fracture of hip NOS
    Fracture of neck of femur NOS

    ✓7th **S72.001** **Fracture of unspecified part of neck of right femur**

    ✓7th **S72.002** **Fracture of unspecified part of neck of left femur**

    ✓7th **S72.009** **Fracture of unspecified part of neck of unspecified femur**

✓6th **S72.01** **Unspecified intracapsular fracture of femur**
    Subcapital fracture of femur

    ✓7th **S72.011** **Unspecified intracapsular fracture of right femur**

    ✓7th **S72.012** **Unspecified intracapsular fracture of left femur**

    ✓7th **S72.019** **Unspecified intracapsular fracture of unspecified femur**

✓6th **S72.02** **Fracture of epiphysis (separation) (upper) of femur**
    Transepiphyseal fracture of femur
    EXCLUDES 1   *capital femoral epiphyseal fracture (pediatric) of femur (S79.01-)*
                   Salter-Harris Type I physeal fracture of upper end of femur (S79.01-)

    ✓7th **S72.021** **Displaced fracture of epiphysis (separation) (upper) of right femur**

    ✓7th **S72.022** **Displaced fracture of epiphysis (separation) (upper) of left femur**

    ✓7th **S72.023** **Displaced fracture of epiphysis (separation) (upper) of unspecified femur**

    ✓7th **S72.024** **Nondisplaced fracture of epiphysis (separation) (upper) of right femur**

    ✓7th **S72.025** **Nondisplaced fracture of epiphysis (separation) (upper) of left femur**

✓7ᵗʰ **S72.026** **Nondisplaced fracture of epiphysis (separation) (upper) of unspecified femur**

✓6ᵗʰ **S72.03** **Midcervical fracture of femur**
Transcervical fracture of femur NOS

✓7ᵗʰ **S72.031** **Displaced midcervical fracture of right femur**

✓7ᵗʰ **S72.032** **Displaced midcervical fracture of left femur**

✓7ᵗʰ **S72.033** **Displaced midcervical fracture of unspecified femur**

✓7ᵗʰ **S72.034** **Nondisplaced midcervical fracture of right femur**

✓7ᵗʰ **S72.035** **Nondisplaced midcervical fracture of left femur**

✓7ᵗʰ **S72.036** **Nondisplaced midcervical fracture of unspecified femur**

✓6ᵗʰ **S72.04** **Fracture of base of neck of femur**
Cervicotrochanteric fracture of femur

✓7ᵗʰ **S72.041** **Displaced fracture of base of neck of right femur**

✓7ᵗʰ **S72.042** **Displaced fracture of base of neck of left femur**

✓7ᵗʰ **S72.043** **Displaced fracture of base of neck of unspecified femur**

✓7ᵗʰ **S72.044** **Nondisplaced fracture of base of neck of right femur**

✓7ᵗʰ **S72.045** **Nondisplaced fracture of base of neck of left femur**

✓7ᵗʰ **S72.046** **Nondisplaced fracture of base of neck of unspecified femur**

✓6ᵗʰ **S72.05** **Unspecified fracture of head of femur**
Fracture of head of femur NOS

✓7ᵗʰ **S72.051** **Unspecified fracture of head of right femur**

✓7ᵗʰ **S72.052** **Unspecified fracture of head of left femur**

✓7ᵗʰ **S72.059** **Unspecified fracture of head of unspecified femur**

✓6ᵗʰ **S72.06** **Articular fracture of head of femur**

✓7ᵗʰ **S72.061** **Displaced articular fracture of head of right femur**

✓7ᵗʰ **S72.062** **Displaced articular fracture of head of left femur**

✓7ᵗʰ **S72.063** **Displaced articular fracture of head of unspecified femur**

✓7ᵗʰ **S72.064** **Nondisplaced articular fracture of head of right femur**

✓7ᵗʰ **S72.065** **Nondisplaced articular fracture of head of left femur**

✓7ᵗʰ **S72.066** **Nondisplaced articular fracture of head of unspecified femur**

✓6ᵗʰ **S72.09** **Other fracture of head and neck of femur**

✓7ᵗʰ **S72.091** **Other fracture of head and neck of right femur**

✓7ᵗʰ **S72.092** **Other fracture of head and neck of left femur**

✓7ᵗʰ **S72.099** **Other fracture of head and neck of unspecified femur**

✓5ᵗʰ **S72.1** **Pertrochanteric fracture**

✓6ᵗʰ **S72.10** **Unspecified trochanteric fracture of femur**
Fracture of trochanter NOS

✓7ᵗʰ **S72.101** **Unspecified trochanteric fracture of right femur**

✓7ᵗʰ **S72.102** **Unspecified trochanteric fracture of left femur**

✓7ᵗʰ **S72.109** **Unspecified trochanteric fracture of unspecified femur**

✓6ᵗʰ **S72.11** **Fracture of greater trochanter of femur**

✓7ᵗʰ **S72.111** **Displaced fracture of greater trochanter of right femur**

✓7ᵗʰ **S72.112** **Displaced fracture of greater trochanter of left femur**

✓7ᵗʰ **S72.113** **Displaced fracture of greater trochanter of unspecified femur**

✓7ᵗʰ **S72.114** **Nondisplaced fracture of greater trochanter of right femur**

✓7ᵗʰ **S72.115** **Nondisplaced fracture of greater trochanter of left femur**

✓7ᵗʰ **S72.116** **Nondisplaced fracture of greater trochanter of unspecified femur**

✓6ᵗʰ **S72.12** **Fracture of lesser trochanter of femur**

✓7ᵗʰ **S72.121** **Displaced fracture of lesser trochanter of right femur**

✓7ᵗʰ **S72.122** **Displaced fracture of lesser trochanter of left femur**

✓7ᵗʰ **S72.123** **Displaced fracture of lesser trochanter of unspecified femur**

✓7ᵗʰ **S72.124** **Nondisplaced fracture of lesser trochanter of right femur**

✓7ᵗʰ **S72.125** **Nondisplaced fracture of lesser trochanter of left femur**

✓7ᵗʰ **S72.126** **Nondisplaced fracture of lesser trochanter of unspecified femur**

✓6ᵗʰ **S72.13** **Apophyseal fracture of femur**
EXCLUDES 1   *chronic (nontraumatic) slipped upper femoral epiphysis (M93.0-)*

✓7ᵗʰ **S72.131** **Displaced apophyseal fracture of right femur**

✓7ᵗʰ **S72.132** **Displaced apophyseal fracture of left femur**

✓7ᵗʰ **S72.133** **Displaced apophyseal fracture of unspecified femur**

✓7ᵗʰ **S72.134** **Nondisplaced apophyseal fracture of right femur**

✓7ᵗʰ **S72.135** **Nondisplaced apophyseal fracture of left femur**

✓7ᵗʰ **S72.136** **Nondisplaced apophyseal fracture of unspecified femur**

✓6ᵗʰ **S72.14** **Intertrochanteric fracture of femur**

✓7ᵗʰ **S72.141** **Displaced intertrochanteric fracture of right femur**

✓7ᵗʰ **S72.142** **Displaced intertrochanteric fracture of left femur**

✓7ᵗʰ **S72.143** **Displaced intertrochanteric fracture of unspecified femur**

✓7ᵗʰ **S72.144** **Nondisplaced intertrochanteric fracture of right femur**

✓7ᵗʰ **S72.145** **Nondisplaced intertrochanteric fracture of left femur**

✓7ᵗʰ **S72.146** **Nondisplaced intertrochanteric fracture of unspecified femur**

✓5ᵗʰ **S72.2** **Subtrochanteric fracture of femur**

✓x7ᵗʰ **S72.21** **Displaced subtrochanteric fracture of right femur**

✓x7ᵗʰ **S72.22** **Displaced subtrochanteric fracture of left femur**

✓x7ᵗʰ **S72.23** **Displaced subtrochanteric fracture of unspecified femur**

✓x7ᵗʰ **S72.24** **Nondisplaced subtrochanteric fracture of right femur**

✓x7ᵗʰ **S72.25** **Nondisplaced subtrochanteric fracture of left femur**

✓x7ᵗʰ **S72.26** **Nondisplaced subtrochanteric fracture of unspecified femur**

✓5ᵗʰ **S72.3** **Fracture of shaft of femur**

✓6ᵗʰ **S72.30** **Unspecified fracture of shaft of femur**

✓7ᵗʰ **S72.301** **Unspecified fracture of shaft of right femur**

✓7ᵗʰ **S72.302** **Unspecified fracture of shaft of left femur**

✓7ᵗʰ **S72.309** **Unspecified fracture of shaft of unspecified femur**

✓6ᵗʰ **S72.32** **Transverse fracture of shaft of femur**

✓7ᵗʰ **S72.321** **Displaced transverse fracture of shaft of right femur**

✓7ᵗʰ **S72.322** **Displaced transverse fracture of shaft of left femur**

✓7ᵗʰ **S72.323** **Displaced transverse fracture of shaft of unspecified femur**

✓7ᵗʰ **S72.324** **Nondisplaced transverse fracture of shaft of right femur**

✓7ᵗʰ **S72.325** **Nondisplaced transverse fracture of shaft of left femur**

✓7ᵗʰ **S72.326** **Nondisplaced transverse fracture of shaft of unspecified femur**

☑ Appropriate additional character required   ✓x7ᵗʰ Requires 7th character, placeholder x must fill empty characters

√6ᵗʰ **S72.33 Oblique fracture of shaft of femur**

√7ᵗʰ **S72.331** Displaced oblique fracture of shaft of right femur

√7ᵗʰ **S72.332** Displaced oblique fracture of shaft of left femur

√7ᵗʰ **S72.333** Displaced oblique fracture of shaft of unspecified femur

√7ᵗʰ **S72.334** Nondisplaced oblique fracture of shaft of right femur

√7ᵗʰ **S72.335** Nondisplaced oblique fracture of shaft of left femur

√7ᵗʰ **S72.336** Nondisplaced oblique fracture of shaft of unspecified femur

√6ᵗʰ **S72.34 Spiral fracture of shaft of femur**

√7ᵗʰ **S72.341** Displaced spiral fracture of shaft of right femur

√7ᵗʰ **S72.342** Displaced spiral fracture of shaft of left femur

√7ᵗʰ **S72.343** Displaced spiral fracture of shaft of unspecified femur

√7ᵗʰ **S72.344** Nondisplaced spiral fracture of shaft of right femur

√7ᵗʰ **S72.345** Nondisplaced spiral fracture of shaft of left femur

√7ᵗʰ **S72.346** Nondisplaced spiral fracture of shaft of unspecified femur

√6ᵗʰ **S72.35 Comminuted fracture of shaft of femur**

√7ᵗʰ **S72.351** Displaced comminuted fracture of shaft of right femur

√7ᵗʰ **S72.352** Displaced comminuted fracture of shaft of left femur

√7ᵗʰ **S72.353** Displaced comminuted fracture of shaft of unspecified femur

√7ᵗʰ **S72.354** Nondisplaced comminuted fracture of shaft of right femur

√7ᵗʰ **S72.355** Nondisplaced comminuted fracture of shaft of left femur

√7ᵗʰ **S72.356** Nondisplaced comminuted fracture of shaft of unspecified femur

√6ᵗʰ **S72.36 Segmental fracture of shaft of femur**

√7ᵗʰ **S72.361** Displaced segmental fracture of shaft of right femur

√7ᵗʰ **S72.362** Displaced segmental fracture of shaft of left femur

√7ᵗʰ **S72.363** Displaced segmental fracture of shaft of unspecified femur

√7ᵗʰ **S72.364** Nondisplaced segmental fracture of shaft of right femur

√7ᵗʰ **S72.365** Nondisplaced segmental fracture of shaft of left femur

√7ᵗʰ **S72.366** Nondisplaced segmental fracture of shaft of unspecified femur

√6ᵗʰ **S72.39 Other fracture of shaft of femur**

√7ᵗʰ **S72.391** Other fracture of shaft of right femur

√7ᵗʰ **S72.392** Other fracture of shaft of left femur

√7ᵗʰ **S72.399** Other fracture of shaft of unspecified femur

√5ᵗʰ **S72.4 Fracture of lower end of femur**

Fracture of distal end of femur

EXCLUDES 2   fracture of shaft of femur (S72.3-)

    physeal fracture of lower end of femur (S79.1-)

√6ᵗʰ **S72.40 Unspecified fracture of lower end of femur**

√7ᵗʰ **S72.401** Unspecified fracture of lower end of right femur

√7ᵗʰ **S72.402** Unspecified fracture of lower end of left femur

√7ᵗʰ **S72.409** Unspecified fracture of lower end of unspecified femur

√6ᵗʰ **S72.41 Unspecified condyle fracture of lower end of femur**

Condyle fracture of femur NOS

√7ᵗʰ **S72.411** Displaced unspecified condyle fracture of lower end of right femur

√7ᵗʰ **S72.412** Displaced unspecified condyle fracture of lower end of left femur

√7ᵗʰ **S72.413** Displaced unspecified condyle fracture of lower end of unspecified femur

√7ᵗʰ **S72.414** Nondisplaced unspecified condyle fracture of lower end of right femur

√7ᵗʰ **S72.415** Nondisplaced unspecified condyle fracture of lower end of left femur

√7ᵗʰ **S72.416** Nondisplaced unspecified condyle fracture of lower end of unspecified femur

√6ᵗʰ **S72.42 Fracture of lateral condyle of femur**

√7ᵗʰ **S72.421** Displaced fracture of lateral condyle of right femur

√7ᵗʰ **S72.422** Displaced fracture of lateral condyle of left femur

√7ᵗʰ **S72.423** Displaced fracture of lateral condyle of unspecified femur

√7ᵗʰ **S72.424** Nondisplaced fracture of lateral condyle of right femur

√7ᵗʰ **S72.425** Nondisplaced fracture of lateral condyle of left femur

√7ᵗʰ **S72.426** Nondisplaced fracture of lateral condyle of unspecified femur

√6ᵗʰ **S72.43 Fracture of medial condyle of femur**

√7ᵗʰ **S72.431** Displaced fracture of medial condyle of right femur

√7ᵗʰ **S72.432** Displaced fracture of medial condyle of left femur

√7ᵗʰ **S72.433** Displaced fracture of medial condyle of unspecified femur

√7ᵗʰ **S72.434** Nondisplaced fracture of medial condyle of right femur

√7ᵗʰ **S72.435** Nondisplaced fracture of medial condyle of left femur

√7ᵗʰ **S72.436** Nondisplaced fracture of medial condyle of unspecified femur

√6ᵗʰ **S72.44 Fracture of lower epiphysis (separation) of femur**

EXCLUDES 1   Salter-Harris Type I physeal fracture of lower end of femur (S79.11-)

√7ᵗʰ **S72.441** Displaced fracture of lower epiphysis (separation) of right femur

√7ᵗʰ **S72.442** Displaced fracture of lower epiphysis (separation) of left femur

√7ᵗʰ **S72.443** Displaced fracture of lower epiphysis (separation) of unspecified femur

√7ᵗʰ **S72.444** Nondisplaced fracture of lower epiphysis (separation) of right femur

√7ᵗʰ **S72.445** Nondisplaced fracture of lower epiphysis (separation) of left femur

√7ᵗʰ **S72.446** Nondisplaced fracture of lower epiphysis (separation) of unspecified femur

√6ᵗʰ **S72.45 Supracondylar fracture without intracondylar extension of lower end of femur**

Supracondylar fracture of lower end of femur NOS

EXCLUDES 1   supracondylar fracture with intracondylar extension of lower end of femur (S72.46-)

√7ᵗʰ **S72.451** Displaced supracondylar fracture without intracondylar extension of lower end of right femur

√7ᵗʰ **S72.452** Displaced supracondylar fracture without intracondylar extension of lower end of left femur

√7ᵗʰ **S72.453** Displaced supracondylar fracture without intracondylar extension of lower end of unspecified femur

√7ᵗʰ **S72.454** Nondisplaced supracondylar fracture without intracondylar extension of lower end of right femur

√7ᵗʰ **S72.455** Nondisplaced supracondylar fracture without intracondylar extension of lower end of left femur

√7ᵗʰ **S72.456** Nondisplaced supracondylar fracture without intracondylar extension of lower end of unspecified femur

√6ᵗʰ **S72.46 Supracondylar fracture with intracondylar extension of lower end of femur**

EXCLUDES 1   supracondylar fracture without intracondylar extension of lower end of femur (S72.45-)

EXCLUDES 1 Not coded here   *EXCLUDES 2* Not included here   *Manifestation Code*

✓7th **S72.461** **Displaced supracondylar fracture with intracondylar extension of lower end of right femur**

✓7th **S72.462** **Displaced supracondylar fracture with intracondylar extension of lower end of left femur**

✓7th **S72.463** **Displaced supracondylar fracture with intracondylar extension of lower end of unspecified femur**

✓7th **S72.464** **Nondisplaced supracondylar fracture with intracondylar extension of lower end of right femur**

✓7th **S72.465** **Nondisplaced supracondylar fracture with intracondylar extension of lower end of left femur**

✓7th **S72.466** **Nondisplaced supracondylar fracture with intracondylar extension of lower end of unspecified femur**

✓6th **S72.47** **Torus fracture of lower end of femur**
　　　NOTE　Open fracture 7th characters do not apply to codes under subcategory S72.47

✓7th **S72.471** **Torus fracture of lower end of right femur**

✓7th **S72.472** **Torus fracture of lower end of left femur**

✓7th **S72.479** **Torus fracture of lower end of unspecified femur**

✓6th **S72.49** **Other fracture of lower end of femur**

✓7th **S72.491** **Other fracture of lower end of right femur**

✓7th **S72.492** **Other fracture of lower end of left femur**

✓7th **S72.499** **Other fracture of lower end of unspecified femur**

✓5th **S72.8** **Other fracture of femur**

✓6th **S72.8x** **Other fracture of femur**

✓7th **S72.8x1** **Other fracture of right femur**

✓7th **S72.8x2** **Other fracture of left femur**

✓7th **S72.8x9** **Other fracture of unspecified femur**

✓5th **S72.9** **Unspecified fracture of femur**
　　Fracture of thigh NOS
　　Fracture of upper leg NOS
　　EXCLUDES1　*fracture of hip NOS (S72.00-, S72.01-)*

✓x7th **S72.90** **Unspecified fracture of unspecified femur**

✓x7th **S72.91** **Unspecified fracture of right femur**

✓x7th **S72.92** **Unspecified fracture of left femur**

✓4th **S73** **Dislocation and sprain of joint and ligaments of hip**
　　INCLUDES　avulsion of joint or ligament of hip
　　　　laceration of cartilage, joint or ligament of hip
　　　　sprain of cartilage, joint or ligament of hip
　　　　traumatic hemarthrosis of joint or ligament of hip
　　　　traumatic rupture of joint or ligament of hip
　　　　traumatic subluxation of joint or ligament of hip
　　　　traumatic tear of joint or ligament of hip
　　Code also any associated open wound
　　EXCLUDES2　*strain of muscle, fascia and tendon of hip and thigh (S76-)*

> The appropriate 7th character is to be added to each code from category S73.
> A　initial encounter
> D　subsequent encounter
> S　sequela

✓5th **S73.0** **Subluxation and dislocation of hip**
　　EXCLUDES2　*dislocation and subluxation of hip prosthesis (T84.020, T84.021)*

✓6th **S73.00** **Unspecified subluxation and dislocation of hip**
　　Dislocation of hip NOS
　　Subluxation of hip NOS

✓7th **S73.001** **Unspecified subluxation of right hip**

✓7th **S73.002** **Unspecified subluxation of left hip**

✓7th **S73.003** **Unspecified subluxation of unspecified hip**

✓7th **S73.004** **Unspecified dislocation of right hip**

✓7th **S73.005** **Unspecified dislocation of left hip**

✓7th **S73.006** **Unspecified dislocation of unspecified hip**

✓6th **S73.01** **Posterior subluxation and dislocation of hip**

✓7th **S73.011** **Posterior subluxation of right hip**

✓7th **S73.012** **Posterior subluxation of left hip**

✓7th **S73.013** **Posterior subluxation of unspecified hip**

✓7th **S73.014** **Posterior dislocation of right hip**

✓7th **S73.015** **Posterior dislocation of left hip**

✓7th **S73.016** **Posterior dislocation of unspecified hip**

✓6th **S73.02** **Obturator subluxation and dislocation of hip**

✓7th **S73.021** **Obturator subluxation of right hip**

✓7th **S73.022** **Obturator subluxation of left hip**

✓7th **S73.023** **Obturator subluxation of unspecified hip**

✓7th **S73.024** **Obturator dislocation of right hip**

✓7th **S73.025** **Obturator dislocation of left hip**

✓7th **S73.026** **Obturator dislocation of unspecified hip**

✓6th **S73.03** **Other anterior dislocation of hip**

✓7th **S73.031** **Other anterior subluxation of right hip**

✓7th **S73.032** **Other anterior subluxation of left hip**

✓7th **S73.033** **Other anterior subluxation of unspecified hip**

✓7th **S73.034** **Other anterior dislocation of right hip**

✓7th **S73.035** **Other anterior dislocation of left hip**

✓7th **S73.036** **Other anterior dislocation of unspecified hip**

✓6th **S73.04** **Central dislocation of hip**

✓7th **S73.041** **Central subluxation of right hip**

✓7th **S73.042** **Central subluxation of left hip**

✓7th **S73.043** **Central subluxation of unspecified hip**

✓7th **S73.044** **Central dislocation of right hip**

✓7th **S73.045** **Central dislocation of left hip**

✓7th **S73.046** **Central dislocation of unspecified hip**

✓5th **S73.1** **Sprain of hip**

✓6th **S73.10** **Unspecified sprain of hip**

✓7th **S73.101** **Unspecified sprain of right hip**

✓7th **S73.102** **Unspecified sprain of left hip**

✓7th **S73.109** **Unspecified sprain of unspecified hip**

✓6th **S73.11** **Iliofemoral ligament sprain of hip**

✓7th **S73.111** **Iliofemoral ligament sprain of right hip**

✓7th **S73.112** **Iliofemoral ligament sprain of left hip**

✓7th **S73.119** **Iliofemoral ligament sprain of unspecified hip**

✓6th **S73.12** **Ischiocapsular (ligament) sprain of hip**

✓7th **S73.121** **Ischiocapsular ligament sprain of right hip**

✓7th **S73.122** **Ischiocapsular ligament sprain of left hip**

✓7th **S73.129** **Ischiocapsular ligament sprain of unspecified hip**

✓6th **S73.19** **Other sprain of hip**

✓7th **S73.191** **Other sprain of right hip**

✓7th **S73.192** **Other sprain of left hip**

✓7th **S73.199** **Other sprain of unspecified hip**

✓4th **S74** **Injury of nerves at hip and thigh level**
　　Code also any associated open wound (S71-)
　　EXCLUDES2　*injury of nerves at ankle and foot level (S94-)*
　　　　injury of nerves at lower leg level (S84-)

> The appropriate 7th character is to be added to each code from category S74.
> A　initial encounter
> D　subsequent encounter
> S　sequela

✓5th **S74.0** **Injury of sciatic nerve at hip and thigh level**

✓x7th **S74.00** **Injury of sciatic nerve at hip and thigh level, unspecified leg**

✓x7th **S74.01** **Injury of sciatic nerve at hip and thigh level, right leg**

✓x7th **S74.02** **Injury of sciatic nerve at hip and thigh level, left leg**

✓5th **S74.1** **Injury of femoral nerve at hip and thigh level**

✓x7th **S74.10** **Injury of femoral nerve at hip and thigh level, unspecified leg**

✓x7th **S74.11** **Injury of femoral nerve at hip and thigh level, right leg**

✓x7th **S74.12** **Injury of femoral nerve at hip and thigh level, left leg**

✔ Appropriate additional character required　　　✓x7th Requires 7th character, placeholder x must fill empty characters

Injury, Poisoning and Certain Other Consequences of External Causes

S74.2–S75.291

√5th   **S74.2**   **Injury of cutaneous sensory nerve at hip and thigh level**
- √x7th   **S74.20**   **Injury of cutaneous sensory nerve at hip and thigh level, unspecified leg**
- √x7th   **S74.21**   **Injury of cutaneous sensory nerve at hip and high level, right leg**
- √x7th   **S74.22**   **Injury of cutaneous sensory nerve at hip and thigh level, left leg**

√5th   **S74.8**   **Injury of other nerves at hip and thigh level**
- √6th   **S74.8x**   **Injury of other nerves at hip and thigh level**
  - √7th   **S74.8x1**   **Injury of other nerves at hip and thigh level, right leg**
  - √7th   **S74.8x2**   **Injury of other nerves at hip and thigh level, left leg**
  - √7th   **S74.8x9**   **Injury of other nerves at hip and thigh level, unspecified leg**

√5th   **S74.9**   **Injury of unspecified nerve at hip and thigh level**
- √x7th   **S74.90**   **Injury of unspecified nerve at hip and thigh level, unspecified leg**
- √x7th   **S74.91**   **Injury of unspecified nerve at hip and thigh level, right leg**
- √x7th   **S74.92**   **Injury of unspecified nerve at hip and thigh level, left leg**

√4th   **S75**   **Injury of blood vessels at hip and thigh level**

Code also any associated open wound (S71-)

EXCLUDES 2   *injury of blood vessels at lower leg level (S85-)*
                injury of popliteal artery (S85.0)

> The appropriate 7th character is to be added to each code from category S75.
> A   initial encounter
> D   subsequent encounter
> S   sequela

√5th   **S75.0**   **Injury of femoral artery**
- √6th   **S75.00**   **Unspecified injury of femoral artery**
  - √7th   **S75.001**   **Unspecified injury of femoral artery, right leg**
  - √7th   **S75.002**   **Unspecified injury of femoral artery, left leg**
  - √7th   **S75.009**   **Unspecified injury of femoral artery, unspecified leg**
- √6th   **S75.01**   **Minor laceration of femoral artery**
  Incomplete transection of femoral artery
  Laceration of femoral artery NOS
  Superficial laceration of femoral artery
  - √7th   **S75.011**   **Minor laceration of femoral artery, right leg**
  - √7th   **S75.012**   **Minor laceration of femoral artery, left leg**
  - √7th   **S75.019**   **Minor laceration of femoral artery, unspecified leg**
- √6th   **S75.02**   **Major laceration of femoral artery**
  Complete transection of femoral artery
  Traumatic rupture of femoral artery
  - √7th   **S75.021**   **Major laceration of femoral artery, right leg**
  - √7th   **S75.022**   **Major laceration of femoral artery, left leg**
  - √7th   **S75.029**   **Major laceration of femoral artery, unspecified leg**
- √6th   **S75.09**   **Other specified injury of femoral artery**
  - √7th   **S75.091**   **Other specified injury of femoral artery, right leg**
  - √7th   **S75.092**   **Other specified injury of femoral artery, left leg**
  - √7th   **S75.099**   **Other specified injury of femoral artery, unspecified leg**

√5th   **S75.1**   **Injury of femoral vein at hip and thigh level**
- √6th   **S75.10**   **Unspecified injury of femoral vein at hip and thigh level**
  - √7th   **S75.101**   **Unspecified injury of femoral vein at hip and thigh level, right leg**
  - √7th   **S75.102**   **Unspecified injury of femoral vein at hip and thigh level, left leg**
  - √7th   **S75.109**   **Unspecified injury of femoral vein at hip and thigh level, unspecified leg**

- √6th   **S75.11**   **Minor laceration of femoral vein at hip and thigh level**
  Incomplete transection of femoral vein at hip and thigh level
  Laceration of femoral vein at hip and thigh level NOS
  Superficial laceration of femoral vein at hip and thigh level
  - √7th   **S75.111**   **Minor laceration of femoral vein at hip and thigh level, right leg**
  - √7th   **S75.112**   **Minor laceration of femoral vein at hip and thigh level, left leg**
  - √7th   **S75.119**   **Minor laceration of femoral vein at hip and thigh level, unspecified leg**
- √6th   **S75.12**   **Major laceration of femoral vein at hip and thigh level**
  Complete transection of femoral vein at hip and thigh level
  Traumatic rupture of femoral vein at hip and thigh level
  - √7th   **S75.121**   **Major laceration of femoral vein at hip and thigh level, right leg**
  - √7th   **S75.122**   **Major laceration of femoral vein at hip and thigh level, left leg**
  - √7th   **S75.129**   **Major laceration of femoral vein at hip and thigh level, unspecified leg**
- √6th   **S75.19**   **Other specified injury of femoral vein at hip and thigh level**
  - √7th   **S75.191**   **Other specified injury of femoral vein at hip and thigh level, right leg**
  - √7th   **S75.192**   **Other specified injury of femoral vein at hip and thigh level, left leg**
  - √7th   **S75.199**   **Other specified injury of femoral vein at hip and thigh level, unspecified leg**

√5th   **S75.2**   **Injury of greater saphenous vein at hip and thigh level**

EXCLUDES 1   *greater saphenous vein NOS (S85.3)*

- √6th   **S75.20**   **Unspecified injury of greater saphenous vein at hip and thigh level**
  - √7th   **S75.201**   **Unspecified injury of greater saphenous vein at hip and thigh level, right leg**
  - √7th   **S75.202**   **Unspecified injury of greater saphenous vein at hip and thigh level, left leg**
  - √7th   **S75.209**   **Unspecified injury of greater saphenous vein at hip and thigh level, unspecified leg**
- √6th   **S75.21**   **Minor laceration of greater saphenous vein at hip and thigh level**
  Incomplete transection of greater saphenous vein at hip and thigh level
  Laceration of greater saphenous vein at hip and thigh level NOS
  Superficial laceration of greater saphenous vein at hip and thigh level
  - √7th   **S75.211**   **Minor laceration of greater saphenous vein at hip and thigh level, right leg**
  - √7th   **S75.212**   **Minor laceration of greater saphenous vein at hip and thigh level, left leg**
  - √7th   **S75.219**   **Minor laceration of greater saphenous vein at hip and thigh level, unspecified leg**
- √6th   **S75.22**   **Major laceration of greater saphenous vein at hip and thigh level**
  Complete transection of greater saphenous vein at hip and thigh level
  Traumatic rupture of greater saphenous vein at hip and thigh level
  - √7th   **S75.221**   **Major laceration of greater saphenous vein at hip and thigh level, right leg**
  - √7th   **S75.222**   **Major laceration of greater saphenous vein at hip and thigh level, left leg**
  - √7th   **S75.229**   **Major laceration of greater saphenous vein at hip and thigh level, unspecified leg**
- √6th   **S75.29**   **Other specified injury of greater saphenous vein at hip and thigh level**
  - √7th   **S75.291**   **Other specified injury of greater saphenous vein at hip and thigh level, right leg**

EXCLUDES 1   Not coded here   EXCLUDES 2   Not included here   *Manifestation Code*

☑7th **S75.292** Other specified injury of greater saphenous vein at hip and thigh level, left leg

☑7th **S75.299** Other specified injury of greater saphenous vein at hip and thigh level, unspecified leg

☑5th **S75.8** Injury of other blood vessels at hip and thigh level

  ☑6th **S75.80** Unspecified injury of other blood vessels at hip and thigh level

    ☑7th **S75.801** Unspecified injury of other blood vessels at hip and thigh level, right leg

    ☑7th **S75.802** Unspecified injury of other blood vessels at hip and thigh level, left leg

    ☑7th **S75.809** Unspecified injury of other blood vessels at hip and thigh level, unspecified leg

  ☑6th **S75.81** Laceration of other blood vessels at hip and thigh level

    ☑7th **S75.811** Laceration of other blood vessels at hip and thigh level, right leg

    ☑7th **S75.812** Laceration of other blood vessels at hip and thigh level, left leg

    ☑7th **S75.819** Laceration of other blood vessels at hip and thigh level, unspecified leg

  ☑6th **S75.89** Other specified injury of other blood vessels at hip and thigh level

    ☑7th **S75.891** Other specified injury of other blood vessels at hip and thigh level, right leg

    ☑7th **S75.892** Other specified injury of other blood vessels at hip and thigh level, left leg

    ☑7th **S75.899** Other specified injury of other blood vessels at hip and thigh level, unspecified leg

☑5th **S75.9** Injury of unspecified blood vessel at hip and thigh level

  ☑6th **S75.90** Unspecified injury of unspecified blood vessel at hip and thigh level

    ☑7th **S75.901** Unspecified injury of unspecified blood vessel at hip and thigh level, right leg

    ☑7th **S75.902** Unspecified injury of unspecified blood vessel at hip and thigh level, left leg

    ☑7th **S75.909** Unspecified injury of unspecified blood vessel at hip and thigh level, unspecified leg

  ☑6th **S75.91** Laceration of unspecified blood vessel at hip and thigh level

    ☑7th **S75.911** Laceration of unspecified blood vessel at hip and thigh level, right leg

    ☑7th **S75.912** Laceration of unspecified blood vessel at hip and thigh level, left leg

    ☑7th **S75.919** Laceration of unspecified blood vessel at hip and thigh level, unspecified leg

  ☑6th **S75.99** Other specified injury of unspecified blood vessel at hip and thigh level

    ☑7th **S75.991** Other specified injury of unspecified blood vessel at hip and thigh level, right leg

    ☑7th **S75.992** Other specified injury of unspecified blood vessel at hip and thigh level, left leg

    ☑7th **S75.999** Other specified injury of unspecified blood vessel at hip and thigh level, unspecified leg

☑4th **S76** **Injury of muscle, fascia and tendon at hip and thigh level**

Code also any associated open wound (S71-)

> EXCLUDES 2 injury of muscle, fascia and tendon at lower leg level (S86)
> sprain of joint and ligament of hip (S73.1)

> The appropriate 7th character is to be added to each code from category S76.
> A   initial encounter
> D   subsequent encounter
> S   sequela

☑5th **S76.0** Injury of muscle, fascia and tendon of hip

  ☑6th **S76.00** Unspecified injury of muscle, fascia and tendon of hip

    ☑7th **S76.001** Unspecified injury of muscle, fascia and tendon of right hip

    ☑7th **S76.002** Unspecified injury of muscle, fascia and tendon of left hip

    ☑7th **S76.009** Unspecified injury of muscle, fascia and tendon of unspecified hip

  ☑6th **S76.01** Strain of muscle, fascia and tendon of hip

    ☑7th **S76.011** Strain of muscle, fascia and tendon of right hip

    ☑7th **S76.012** Strain of muscle, fascia and tendon of left hip

    ☑7th **S76.019** Strain of muscle, fascia and tendon of unspecified hip

  ☑6th **S76.02** Laceration of muscle, fascia and tendon of hip

    ☑7th **S76.021** Laceration of muscle, fascia and tendon of right hip

    ☑7th **S76.022** Laceration of muscle, fascia and tendon of left hip

    ☑7th **S76.029** Laceration of muscle, fascia and tendon of unspecified hip

  ☑6th **S76.09** Other specified injury of muscle, fascia and tendon of hip

    ☑7th **S76.091** Other specified injury of muscle, fascia and tendon of right hip

    ☑7th **S76.092** Other specified injury of muscle, fascia and tendon of left hip

    ☑7th **S76.099** Other specified injury of muscle, fascia and tendon of unspecified hip

☑5th **S76.1** Injury of quadriceps muscle, fascia and tendon

Injury of patellar ligament (tendon)

  ☑6th **S76.10** Unspecified injury of quadriceps muscle, fascia and tendon

    ☑7th **S76.101** Unspecified injury of right quadriceps muscle, fascia and tendon

    ☑7th **S76.102** Unspecified injury of left quadriceps muscle, fascia and tendon

    ☑7th **S76.109** Unspecified injury of unspecified quadriceps muscle, fascia and tendon

  ☑6th **S76.11** Strain of quadriceps muscle, fascia and tendon

    ☑7th **S76.111** Strain of right quadriceps muscle, fascia and tendon

    ☑7th **S76.112** Strain of left quadriceps muscle, fascia and tendon

    ☑7th **S76.119** Strain of unspecified quadriceps muscle, fascia and tendon

  ☑6th **S76.12** Laceration of quadriceps muscle, fascia and tendon

    ☑7th **S76.121** Laceration of right quadriceps muscle, fascia and tendon

    ☑7th **S76.122** Laceration of left quadriceps muscle, fascia and tendon

    ☑7th **S76.129** Laceration of unspecified quadriceps muscle, fascia and tendon

  ☑6th **S76.19** Other specified injury of quadriceps muscle, fascia and tendon

    ☑7th **S76.191** Other specified injury of right quadriceps muscle, fascia and tendon

    ☑7th **S76.192** Other specified injury of left quadriceps muscle, fascia and tendon

    ☑7th **S76.199** Other specified injury of unspecified quadriceps muscle, fascia and tendon

☑5th **S76.2** Injury of adductor muscle, fascia and tendon of thigh

  ☑6th **S76.20** Unspecified injury of adductor muscle, fascia and tendon of thigh

    ☑7th **S76.201** Unspecified injury of adductor muscle, fascia and tendon of right thigh

    ☑7th **S76.202** Unspecified injury of adductor muscle, fascia and tendon of left thigh

    ☑7th **S76.209** Unspecified injury of adductor muscle, fascia and tendon of unspecified thigh

  ☑6th **S76.21** Strain of adductor muscle, fascia and tendon of thigh

    ☑7th **S76.211** Strain of adductor muscle, fascia and tendon of right thigh

    ☑7th **S76.212** Strain of adductor muscle, fascia and tendon of left thigh

    ☑7th **S76.219** Strain of adductor muscle, fascia and tendon of unspecified thigh

---

☑ Appropriate additional character required   ☑x7th Requires 7th character, placeholder x must fill empty characters

√6th **S76.22 Laceration of adductor muscle, fascia and tendon of thigh**

√7th S76.221 Laceration of adductor muscle, fascia and tendon of right thigh

√7th S76.222 Laceration of adductor muscle, fascia and tendon of left thigh

√7th S76.229 Laceration of adductor muscle, fascia and tendon of unspecified thigh

√6th **S76.29 Other injury of adductor muscle, fascia and tendon of thigh**

√7th S76.291 Other injury of adductor muscle, fascia and tendon of right thigh

√7th S76.292 Other injury of adductor muscle, fascia and tendon of left thigh

√7th S76.299 Other injury of adductor muscle, fascia and tendon of unspecified thigh

√5th **S76.3 Injury of muscle, fascia and tendon of the posterior muscle group at thigh level**

√6th **S76.30 Unspecified injury of muscle, fascia and tendon of the posterior muscle group at thigh level**

√7th S76.301 Unspecified injury of muscle, fascia and tendon of the posterior muscle group at thigh level, right thigh

√7th S76.302 Unspecified injury of muscle, fascia and tendon of the posterior muscle group at thigh level, left thigh

√7th S76.309 Unspecified injury of muscle, fascia and tendon of the posterior muscle group at thigh level, unspecified thigh

√6th **S76.31 Strain of muscle, fascia and tendon of the posterior muscle group at thigh level**

√7th S76.311 Strain of muscle, fascia and tendon of the posterior muscle group at thigh level, right thigh

√7th S76.312 Strain of muscle, fascia and tendon of the posterior muscle group at thigh level, left thigh

√7th S76.319 Strain of muscle, fascia and tendon of the posterior muscle group at thigh level, unspecified thigh

√6th **S76.32 Laceration of muscle, fascia and tendon of the posterior muscle group at thigh level**

√7th S76.321 Laceration of muscle, fascia and tendon of the posterior muscle group at thigh level, right thigh

√7th S76.322 Laceration of muscle, fascia and tendon of the posterior muscle group at thigh level, left thigh

√7th S76.329 Laceration of muscle, fascia and tendon of the posterior muscle group at thigh level, unspecified thigh

√6th **S76.39 Other specified injury of muscle, fascia and tendon of the posterior muscle group at thigh level**

√7th S76.391 Other specified injury of muscle, fascia and tendon of the posterior muscle group at thigh level, right thigh

√7th S76.392 Other secified injury of muscle, fascia and tendon of the posterior muscle group at thigh level, left thigh

√7th S76.399 Other specified injury of muscle, fascia and tendon of the posterior muscle group at thigh level, unspecified thigh

√5th **S76.8 Injury of other specified muscles, fascia and tendons at thigh level**

√6th **S76.80 Unspecified injury of other specified muscles, fascia and tendons at thigh level**

√7th S76.801 Unspecified injury of other specified muscles, fascia and tendons at thigh level, right thigh

√7th S76.802 Unspecified injury of other specified muscles, fascia and tendons at thigh level, left thigh

√7th S76.809 Unspecified injury of other specified muscles, fascia and tendons at thigh level, unspecified thigh

√6th **S76.81 Strain of other specified muscles, fascia and tendons at thigh level**

√7th S76.811 Strain of other specified muscles, fascia and tendons at thigh level, right thigh

√7th S76.812 Strain of other specified muscles, fascia and tendons at thigh level, left thigh

√7th S76.819 Strain of other specified muscles, fascia and tendons at thigh level, unspecified thigh

√6th **S76.82 Laceration of other specified muscles, fascia and tendons at thigh level**

√7th S76.821 Laceration of other specified muscles, fascia and tendons at thigh level, right thigh

√7th S76.822 Laceration of other specified muscles, fascia and tendons at thigh level, left thigh

√7th S76.829 Laceration of other specified muscles, fascia and tendons at thigh level, unspecified thigh

√6th **S76.89 Other injury of other specified muscles, fascia and tendons at thigh level**

√7th S76.891 Other injury of other specified muscles, fascia and tendons at thigh level, right thigh

√7th S76.892 Other injury of other specified muscles, fascia and tendons at thigh level, left thigh

√7th S76.899 Other injury of other specified muscles, fascia and tendons at thigh level, unspecified thigh

√5th **S76.9 Injury of unspecified muscles, fascia and tendons at thigh level**

√6th **S76.90 Unspecified injury of unspecified muscles, fascia and tendons at thigh level**

√7th S76.901 Unspecified injury of unspecified muscles, fascia and tendons at thigh level, right thigh

√7th S76.902 Unspecified injury of unspecified muscles, fascia and tendons at thigh level, left thigh

√7th S76.909 Unspecified injury of unspecified muscles, fascia and tendons at thigh level, unspecified thigh

√6th **S76.91 Strain of unspecified muscles, fascia and tendons at thigh level**

√7th S76.911 Strain of unspecified muscles, fascia and tendons at thigh level, right thigh

√7th S76.912 Strain of unspecified muscles, fascia and tendons at thigh level, left thigh

√7th S76.919 Strain of unspecified muscles, fascia and tendons at thigh level, unspecified thigh

√6th **S76.92 Laceration of unspecified muscles, fascia and tendons at thigh level**

√7th S76.921 Laceration of unspecified muscles, fascia and tendons at thigh level, right thigh

√7th S76.922 Laceration of unspecified muscles, fascia and tendons at thigh level, left thigh

√7th S76.929 Laceration of unspecified muscles, fascia and tendons at thigh level, unspecified thigh

√6th **S76.99 Other specified injury of unspecified muscles, fascia and tendons at thigh level**

√7th S76.991 Other specified injury of unspecified muscles, fascia and tendons at thigh level, right thigh

√7th S76.992 Other specified injury of unspecified muscles, fascia and tendons at thigh level, left thigh

√7th S76.999 Other specified injury of unspecified muscles, fascia and tendons at thigh level, unspecified thigh

---

EXCLUDES 1 Not coded here   EXCLUDES 2 Not included here   *Manifestation Code*

☑4ᵗʰ **S77 Crushing injury of hip and thigh**
Use additional code(s) for all associated injuries
EXCLUDES 2 *crushing injury of ankle and foot (S97-)*
crushing injury of lower leg (S87-)

The appropriate 7th character is to be added to each code from category S77.
A   initial encounter
D   subsequent encounter
S   sequela

☑5ᵗʰ **S77.0 Crushing injury of hip**
✓x7ᵗʰ   **S77.00 Crushing injury of unspecified hip**
✓x7ᵗʰ   **S77.01 Crushing injury of right hip**
✓x7ᵗʰ   **S77.02 Crushing injury of left hip**

☑5ᵗʰ **S77.1 Crushing injury of thigh**
✓x7ᵗʰ   **S77.10 Crushing injury of unspecified thigh**
✓x7ᵗʰ   **S77.11 Crushing injury of right thigh**
✓x7ᵗʰ   **S77.12 Crushing injury of left thigh**

☑5ᵗʰ **S77.2 Crushing injury of hip with thigh**
✓x7ᵗʰ   **S77.20 Crushing injury of unspecified hip with thigh**
✓x7ᵗʰ   **S77.21 Crushing injury of right hip with thigh**
✓x7ᵗʰ   **S77.22 Crushing injury of left hip with thigh**

☑4ᵗʰ **S78 Traumatic amputation of hip and thigh**
NOTE   An amputation not identified and partial or complete should be coded to complete.
EXCLUDES 1 *traumatic amputation of knee (S88.0-)*

The appropriate 7th character is to be added to each code from category S78.
A   initial encounter
D   subsequent encounter
S   sequela

☑5ᵗʰ **S78.0 Traumatic amputation at hip joint**
☑6ᵗʰ   **S78.01 Complete traumatic amputation at hip joint**
✓7ᵗʰ   **S78.011 Complete traumatic amputation at right hip joint**
✓7ᵗʰ   **S78.012 Complete traumatic amputation at left hip joint**
✓7ᵗʰ   **S78.019 Complete traumatic amputation at unspecified hip joint**
☑6ᵗʰ   **S78.02 Partial traumatic amputation at hip joint**
✓7ᵗʰ   **S78.021 Partial traumatic amputation at right hip joint**
✓7ᵗʰ   **S78.022 Partial traumatic amputation at left hip joint**
✓7ᵗʰ   **S78.029 Partial traumatic amputation at unspecified hip joint**

☑5ᵗʰ **S78.1 Traumatic amputation at level between hip and knee**
EXCLUDES 1 *traumatic amputation of knee (S88.0-)*
☑6ᵗʰ   **S78.11 Complete traumatic amputation at level between hip and knee**
✓7ᵗʰ   **S78.111 Complete traumatic amputation at level between right hip and knee**
✓7ᵗʰ   **S78.112 Complete traumatic amputation at level between left hip and knee**
✓7ᵗʰ   **S78.119 Complete traumatic amputation at level between unspecified hip and knee**
☑6ᵗʰ   **S78.12 Partial traumatic amputation at level between hip and knee**
✓7ᵗʰ   **S78.121 Partial traumatic amputation at level between right hip and knee**
✓7ᵗʰ   **S78.122 Partial traumatic amputation at level between left hip and knee**
✓7ᵗʰ   **S78.129 Partial traumatic amputation at level between unspecified hip and knee**

☑5ᵗʰ **S78.9 Traumatic amputation of hip and thigh, level unspecified**
☑6ᵗʰ   **S78.91 Complete traumatic amputation of hip and thigh, level unspecified**
✓7ᵗʰ   **S78.911 Complete traumatic amputation of right hip and thigh, level unspecified**
✓7ᵗʰ   **S78.912 Complete traumatic amputation of left hip and thigh, level unspecified**
✓7ᵗʰ   **S78.919 Complete traumatic amputation of unspecified hip and thigh, level unspecified**

☑6ᵗʰ   **S78.92 Partial traumatic amputation of hip and thigh, level unspecified**
✓7ᵗʰ   **S78.921 Partial traumatic amputation of right hip and thigh, level unspecified**
✓7ᵗʰ   **S78.922 Partial traumatic amputation of left hip and thigh, level unspecified**
✓7ᵗʰ   **S78.929 Partial traumatic amputation of unspecified hip and thigh, level unspecified**

☑4ᵗʰ **S79 Other and unspecified injuries of hip and thigh**
☑5ᵗʰ **S79.0 Physeal fracture of upper end of femur**
NOTE   A fracture not indicated as open or closed should be coded to closed.
EXCLUDES 1 *apophyseal fracture of upper end of femur (S72.13-)*
nontraumatic slipped upper femoral epiphysis (M93.0-)

The appropriate 7th character is to be added to each code from subcategory S79.0.
A   initial encounter for closed fracture
D   subsequent encounter for fracture with routine healing
G   subsequent encounter for fracture with delayed healing
K   subsequent encounter for fracture with nonunion
P   subsequent encounter for fracture with malunion
S   sequela

☑6ᵗʰ   **S79.00 Unspecified physeal fracture of upper end of femur**
✓7ᵗʰ   **S79.001 Unspecified physeal fracture of upper end of right femur**
✓7ᵗʰ   **S79.002 Unspecified physeal fracture of upper end of left femur**
✓7ᵗʰ   **S79.009 Unspecified physeal fracture of upper end of unspecified femur**

☑6ᵗʰ   **S79.01 Salter-Harris Type I physeal fracture of upper end of femur**
Acute on chronic slipped capital femoral epiphysis (traumatic)
Acute slipped capital femoral epiphysis (traumatic)
Capital femoral epiphyseal fracture
EXCLUDES 1 *chronic slipped upper femoral epiphysis (nontraumatic) (M93.02-)*
✓7ᵗʰ   **S79.011 Salter-Harris Type I physeal fracture of upper end of right femur**
✓7ᵗʰ   **S79.012 Salter-Harris Type I physeal fracture of upper end of left femur**
✓7ᵗʰ   **S79.019 Salter-Harris Type I physeal fracture of upper end of unspecified femur**

☑6ᵗʰ   **S79.09 Other physeal fracture of upper end of femur**
✓7ᵗʰ   **S79.091 Other physeal fracture of upper end of right femur**
✓7ᵗʰ   **S79.092 Other physeal fracture of upper end of left femur**
✓7ᵗʰ   **S79.099 Other physeal fracture of upper end of unspecified femur**

☑5ᵗʰ **S79.1 Physeal fracture of lower end of femur**
NOTE   A fracture not indicated as open or closed should be coded to closed.

The appropriate 7th character is to be added to each code from subcategory S79.1.
A   initial encounter for closed fracture
D   subsequent encounter for fracture with routine healing
G   subsequent encounter for fracture with delayed healing
K   subsequent encounter for fracture with nonunion
P   subsequent encounter for fracture with malunion
S   sequela

☑6ᵗʰ   **S79.10 Unspecified physeal fracture of lower end of femur**
✓7ᵗʰ   **S79.101 Unspecified physeal fracture of lower end of right femur**
✓7ᵗʰ   **S79.102 Unspecified physeal fracture of lower end of left femur**
✓7ᵗʰ   **S79.109 Unspecified physeal fracture of lower end of unspecified femur**

√6ᵗʰ **S79.11** Salter-Harris Type I physeal fracture of lower end of femur

  √7ᵗʰ **S79.111** Salter-Harris Type I physeal fracture of lower end of right femur

  √7ᵗʰ **S79.112** Salter-Harris Type I physeal fracture of lower end of left femur

  √7ᵗʰ **S79.119** Salter-Harris Type I physeal fracture of lower end of unspecified femur

√6ᵗʰ **S79.12** Salter-Harris Type II physeal fracture of lower end of femur

  √7ᵗʰ **S79.121** Salter-Harris Type II physeal fracture of lower end of right femur

  √7ᵗʰ **S79.122** Salter-Harris Type II physeal fracture of lower end of left femur

  √7ᵗʰ **S79.129** Salter-Harris Type II physeal fracture of lower end of unspecified femur

√6ᵗʰ **S79.13** Salter-Harris Type III physeal fracture of lower end of femur

  √7ᵗʰ **S79.131** Salter-Harris Type III physeal fracture of lower end of right femur

  √7ᵗʰ **S79.132** Salter-Harris Type III physeal fracture of lower end of left femur

  √7ᵗʰ **S79.139** Salter-Harris Type III physeal fracture of lower end of unspecified femur

√6ᵗʰ **S79.14** Salter-Harris Type IV physeal fracture of lower end of femur

  √7ᵗʰ **S79.141** Salter-Harris Type IV physeal fracture of lower end of right femur

  √7ᵗʰ **S79.142** Salter-Harris Type IV physeal fracture of lower end of left femur

  √7ᵗʰ **S79.149** Salter-Harris Type IV physeal fracture of lower end of unspecified femur

√6ᵗʰ **S79.19** Other physeal fracture of lower end of femur

  √7ᵗʰ **S79.191** Other physeal fracture of lower end of right femur

  √7ᵗʰ **S79.192** Other physeal fracture of lower end of left femur

  √7ᵗʰ **S79.199** Other physeal fracture of lower end of unspecified femur

√5ᵗʰ **S79.8** Other specified injuries of hip and thigh

> The appropriate 7th character is to be added to each code for subcategory S79.8.
> A   initial encounter
> D   subsequent encounter
> S   sequela

√6ᵗʰ **S79.81** Other specified injuries of hip

  √7ᵗʰ **S79.811** Other specified injuries of right hip

  √7ᵗʰ **S79.812** Other specified injuries of left hip

  √7ᵗʰ **S79.819** Other specified injuries of unspecified hip

√6ᵗʰ **S79.82** Other specified injuries of thigh

  √7ᵗʰ **S79.821** Other specified injuries of right thigh

  √7ᵗʰ **S79.822** Other specified injuries of left thigh

  √7ᵗʰ **S79.829** Other specified injuries of unspecified thigh

√5ᵗʰ **S79.9** Unspecified injury of hip and thigh

> The appropriate 7th character is to be added to each code for subcategory S79.9.
> A   initial encounter
> D   subsequent encounter
> S   sequela

√6ᵗʰ **S79.91** Unspecified injury of hip

  √7ᵗʰ **S79.911** Unspecified injury of right hip

  √7ᵗʰ **S79.912** Unspecified injury of left hip

  √7ᵗʰ **S79.919** Unspecified injury of unspecified hip

√6ᵗʰ **S79.92** Unspecified injury of thigh

  √7ᵗʰ **S79.921** Unspecified injury of right thigh

  √7ᵗʰ **S79.922** Unspecified injury of left thigh

  √7ᵗʰ **S79.929** Unspecified injury of unspecified thigh

Injuries to the knee and lower leg (S80-S89)

EXCLUDES 2   burns and corrosions (T20-T32)
frostbite (T33-T34)
injuries of ankle and foot, except fracture of ankle and malleolus (S90-S99)
insect bite or sting, venomous (T63.4)

√4ᵗʰ **S80** Superficial injury of knee and lower leg

EXCLUDES 2   superficial injury of ankle and foot (S90-)

> The appropriate 7th character is to be added to each code from category S80.
> A   initial encounter
> D   subsequent encounter
> S   sequela

√5ᵗʰ **S80.0** Contusion of knee

  √x7ᵗʰ **S80.00** Contusion of unspecified knee

  √x7ᵗʰ **S80.01** Contusion of right knee

  √x7ᵗʰ **S80.02** Contusion of left knee

√5ᵗʰ **S80.1** Contusion of lower leg

  √x7ᵗʰ **S80.10** Contusion of unspecified lower leg

  √x7ᵗʰ **S80.11** Contusion of right lower leg

  √x7ᵗʰ **S80.12** Contusion of left lower leg

√5ᵗʰ **S80.2** Other superficial injuries of knee

√6ᵗʰ **S80.21** Abrasion of knee

  √7ᵗʰ **S80.211** Abrasion, right knee

  √7ᵗʰ **S80.212** Abrasion, left knee

  √7ᵗʰ **S80.219** Abrasion, unspecified knee

√6ᵗʰ **S80.22** Blister (nonthermal) of knee

  √7ᵗʰ **S80.221** Blister (nonthermal), right knee

  √7ᵗʰ **S80.222** Blister (nonthermal), left knee

  √7ᵗʰ **S80.229** Blister (nonthermal), unspecified knee

√6ᵗʰ **S80.24** External constriction of knee

  √7ᵗʰ **S80.241** External constriction, right knee

  √7ᵗʰ **S80.242** External constriction, left knee

  √7ᵗʰ **S80.249** External constriction, unspecified knee

√6ᵗʰ **S80.25** Superficial foreign body of knee
Splinter in the knee

  √7ᵗʰ **S80.251** Superficial foreign body, right knee

  √7ᵗʰ **S80.252** Superficial foreign body, left knee

  √7ᵗʰ **S80.259** Superficial foreign body, unspecified knee

√6ᵗʰ **S80.26** Insect bite (nonvenomous) of knee

  √7ᵗʰ **S80.261** Insect bite (nonvenomous), right knee

  √7ᵗʰ **S80.262** Insect bite (nonvenomous), left knee

  √7ᵗʰ **S80.269** Insect bite (nonvenomous), unspecified knee

√6ᵗʰ **S80.27** Other superficial bite of knee

  EXCLUDES 1   open bite of knee (S81.05-)

  √7ᵗʰ **S80.271** Other superficial bite of right knee

  √7ᵗʰ **S80.272** Other superficial bite of left knee

  √7ᵗʰ **S80.279** Other superficial bite of unspecified knee

√5ᵗʰ **S80.8** Other superficial injuries of lower leg

√6ᵗʰ **S80.81** Abrasion of lower leg

  √7ᵗʰ **S80.811** Abrasion, right lower leg

  √7ᵗʰ **S80.812** Abrasion, left lower leg

  √7ᵗʰ **S80.819** Abrasion, unspecified lower leg

√6ᵗʰ **S80.82** Blister (nonthermal) of lower leg

  √7ᵗʰ **S80.821** Blister (nonthermal), right lower leg

  √7ᵗʰ **S80.822** Blister (nonthermal), left lower leg

  √7ᵗʰ **S80.829** Blister (nonthermal), unspecified lower leg

√6ᵗʰ **S80.84** External constriction of lower leg

  √7ᵗʰ **S80.841** External constriction, right lower leg

  √7ᵗʰ **S80.842** External constriction, left lower leg

  √7ᵗʰ **S80.849** External constriction, unspecified lower leg

√6ᵗʰ **S80.85** Superficial foreign body of lower leg
Splinter in the lower leg

  √7ᵗʰ **S80.851** Superficial foreign body, right lower leg

  √7ᵗʰ **S80.852** Superficial foreign body, left lower leg

  √7ᵗʰ **S80.859** Superficial foreign body, unspecified lower leg

---

EXCLUDES 1 Not coded here   **EXCLUDES 2** Not included here   **Manifestation Code**

✓6ᵗʰ **S80.86** **Insect bite (nonvenomous) of lower leg**

  ✓7ᵗʰ **S80.861** **Insect bite (nonvenomous), right lower leg**

  ✓7ᵗʰ **S80.862** **Insect bite (nonvenomous), left lower leg**

  ✓7ᵗʰ **S80.869** **Insect bite (nonvenomous), unspecified lower leg**

✓6ᵗʰ **S80.87** **Other superficial bite of lower leg**

  EXCLUDES 1 *open bite of lower leg (S81.85-)*

  ✓7ᵗʰ **S80.871** **Other superficial bite, right lower leg**

  ✓7ᵗʰ **S80.872** **Other superficial bite, left lower leg**

  ✓7ᵗʰ **S80.879** **Other superficial bite, unspecified lower leg**

✓5ᵗʰ **S80.9** **Unspecified superficial injury of knee and lower leg**

✓6ᵗʰ **S80.91** **Unspecified superficial injury of knee**

  ✓7ᵗʰ **S80.911** **Unspecified superficial injury of right knee**

  ✓7ᵗʰ **S80.912** **Unspecified superficial injury of left knee**

  ✓7ᵗʰ **S80.919** **Unspecified superficial injury of unspecified knee**

✓6ᵗʰ **S80.92** **Unspecified superficial injury of lower leg**

  ✓7ᵗʰ **S80.921** **Unspecified superficial injury of right lower leg**

  ✓7ᵗʰ **S80.922** **Unspecified superficial injury of left lower leg**

  ✓7ᵗʰ **S80.929** **Unspecified superficial injury of unspecified lower leg**

✓4ᵗʰ **S81** **Open wound of knee and lower leg**

Code also any associated wound infection

EXCLUDES 1 *open fracture of knee and lower leg (S82-)*
       traumatic amputation of lower leg (S88-)

EXCLUDES 2 *open wound of ankle and foot (S91-)*

The appropriate 7th character is to be added to each code from category S81.
A   initial encounter
D   subsequent encounter
S   sequela

✓5ᵗʰ **S81.0** **Open wound of knee**

✓6ᵗʰ **S81.00** **Unspecified open wound of knee**

  ✓7ᵗʰ **S81.001** **Unspecified open wound, right knee**

  ✓7ᵗʰ **S81.002** **Unspecified open wound, left knee**

  ✓7ᵗʰ **S81.009** **Unspecified open wound, unspecified knee**

✓6ᵗʰ **S81.01** **Laceration without foreign body of knee**

  ✓7ᵗʰ **S81.011** **Laceration without foreign body, right knee**

  ✓7ᵗʰ **S81.012** **Laceration without foreign body, left knee**

  ✓7ᵗʰ **S81.019** **Laceration without foreign body, unspecified knee**

✓6ᵗʰ **S81.02** **Laceration with foreign body of knee**

  ✓7ᵗʰ **S81.021** **Laceration with foreign body, right knee**

  ✓7ᵗʰ **S81.022** **Laceration with foreign body, left knee**

  ✓7ᵗʰ **S81.029** **Laceration with foreign body, unspecified knee**

✓6ᵗʰ **S81.03** **Puncture wound without foreign body of knee**

  ✓7ᵗʰ **S81.031** **Puncture wound without foreign body, right knee**

  ✓7ᵗʰ **S81.032** **Puncture wound without foreign body, left knee**

  ✓7ᵗʰ **S81.039** **Puncture wound without foreign body, unspecified knee**

✓6ᵗʰ **S81.04** **Puncture wound with foreign body of knee**

  ✓7ᵗʰ **S81.041** **Puncture wound with foreign body, right knee**

  ✓7ᵗʰ **S81.042** **Puncture wound with foreign body, left knee**

  ✓7ᵗʰ **S81.049** **Puncture wound with foreign body, unspecified knee**

✓6ᵗʰ **S81.05** **Open bite of knee**

Bite of knee NOS

  EXCLUDES 1 *superficial bite of knee (S80.27-)*

  ✓7ᵗʰ **S81.051** **Open bite, right knee**

  ✓7ᵗʰ **S81.052** **Open bite, left knee**

  ✓7ᵗʰ **S81.059** **Open bite, unspecified knee**

✓5ᵗʰ **S81.8** **Open wound of lower leg**

✓6ᵗʰ **S81.80** **Unspecified open wound of lower leg**

  ✓7ᵗʰ **S81.801** **Unspecified open wound, right lower leg**

  ✓7ᵗʰ **S81.802** **Unspecified open wound, left lower leg**

  ✓7ᵗʰ **S81.809** **Unspecified open wound, unspecified lower leg**

✓6ᵗʰ **S81.81** **Laceration without foreign body of lower leg**

  ✓7ᵗʰ **S81.811** **Laceration without foreign body, right lower leg**

  ✓7ᵗʰ **S81.812** **Laceration without foreign body, left lower leg**

  ✓7ᵗʰ **S81.819** **Laceration without foreign body, unspecified lower leg**

✓6ᵗʰ **S81.82** **Laceration with foreign body of lower leg**

  ✓7ᵗʰ **S81.821** **Laceration with foreign body, right lower leg**

  ✓7ᵗʰ **S81.822** **Laceration with foreign body, left lower leg**

  ✓7ᵗʰ **S81.829** **Laceration with foreign body, unspecified lower leg**

✓6ᵗʰ **S81.83** **Puncture wound without foreign body of lower leg**

  ✓7ᵗʰ **S81.831** **Puncture wound without foreign body, right lower leg**

  ✓7ᵗʰ **S81.832** **Puncture wound without foreign body, left lower leg**

  ✓7ᵗʰ **S81.839** **Puncture wound without foreign body, unspecified lower leg**

✓6ᵗʰ **S81.84** **Puncture wound with foreign body of lower leg**

  ✓7ᵗʰ **S81.841** **Puncture wound with foreign body, right lower leg**

  ✓7ᵗʰ **S81.842** **Puncture wound with foreign body, left lower leg**

  ✓7ᵗʰ **S81.849** **Puncture wound with foreign body, unspecified lower leg**

✓6ᵗʰ **S81.85** **Open bite of lower leg**

Bite of lower leg NOS

  EXCLUDES 1 *superficial bite of lower leg (S80.86-, S80.87-)*

  ✓7ᵗʰ **S81.851** **Open bite, right lower leg**

  ✓7ᵗʰ **S81.852** **Open bite, left lower leg**

  ✓7ᵗʰ **S81.859** **Open bite, unspecified lower leg**

☑ Appropriate additional character required   ✓x7ᵗʰ Requires 7th character, placeholder x must fill empty characters

✓4ᵗʰ S82   Fracture of lower leg, including ankle

> **NOTE**   A fracture not indicated as displaced or nondisplaced should be coded to displaced.
> A fracture not designated as open or closed should be coded to closed.
> The open fracture designations are based on the Gustilo open fracture classification.

> **INCLUDES**   fracture of malleolus
> **EXCLUDES 1**   traumatic amputation of lower leg (S88-)
> **EXCLUDES 2**   fracture of foot, except ankle (S92-)
> periprosthetic fracture of prosthetic implant of knee (T84.042, T84.043)

> The appropriate 7th character is to be added to each code from category S82.
> A   initial encounter for closed fracture
> B   initial encounter for open fracture type I or II
>   initial encounter for open fracture NOS
> C   initial encounter for open fracture type IIIA, IIIB, or IIIC
> D   subsequent encounter for closed fracture with routine healing
> E   subsequent encounter for open fracture type I or II with routine healing
> F   subsequent encounter for open fracture type IIIA, IIIB, or IIIC with routine healing
> G   subsequent encounter for closed fracture with delayed healing
> H   subsequent encounter for open fracture type I or II with delayed healing
> J   subsequent encounter for open fracture type IIIA, IIIB or IIIC with delayed healing
> K   subsequent encounter for closed fracture with nonunion
> M   subsequent encounter for open fracture type I or II with nonunion
> N   subsequent encounter for open fracture type IIIA, IIIB or IIIC with nonunion
> P   subsequent encounter for closed fracture with malunion
> Q   subsequent encounter for open fracture type I or II with malunion
> R   subsequent encounter for open fracture type IIIA, IIIB or IIIC with malunion
> S   sequela

✓5ᵗʰ S82.0   Fracture of patella
Knee cap
> **NOTE**   7th characters C, F, J, N, or R do not apply to codes under subcategory S82.0

   ✓6ᵗʰ S82.00   Unspecified fracture of patella
     ✓7ᵗʰ **S82.001   Unspecified fracture of right patella**
     ✓7ᵗʰ **S82.002   Unspecified fracture of left patella**
     ✓7ᵗʰ **S82.009   Unspecified fracture of unspecified patella**

   ✓6ᵗʰ S82.01   Osteochondral fracture of patella
     ✓7ᵗʰ **S82.011   Displaced osteochondral fracture of right patella**
     ✓7ᵗʰ **S82.012   Displaced osteochondral fracture of left patella**
     ✓7ᵗʰ **S82.013   Displaced osteochondral fracture of unspecified patella**
     ✓7ᵗʰ **S82.014   Nondisplaced osteochondral fracture of right patella**
     ✓7ᵗʰ **S82.015   Nondisplaced osteochondral fracture of left patella**
     ✓7ᵗʰ **S82.016   Nondisplaced osteochondral fracture of unspecified patella**

   ✓6ᵗʰ S82.02   Longitudinal fracture of patella
     ✓7ᵗʰ **S82.021   Displaced longitudinal fracture of right patella**
     ✓7ᵗʰ **S82.022   Displaced longitudinal fracture of left patella**
     ✓7ᵗʰ **S82.023   Displaced longitudinal fracture of unspecified patella**
     ✓7ᵗʰ **S82.024   Nondisplaced longitudinal fracture of right patella**
     ✓7ᵗʰ **S82.025   Nondisplaced longitudinal fracture of left patella**
     ✓7ᵗʰ **S82.026   Nondisplaced longitudinal fracture of unspecified patella**

   ✓6ᵗʰ S82.03   Transverse fracture of patella
     ✓7ᵗʰ **S82.031   Displaced transverse fracture of right patella**
     ✓7ᵗʰ **S82.032   Displaced transverse fracture of left patella**
     ✓7ᵗʰ **S82.033   Displaced transverse fracture of unspecified patella**
     ✓7ᵗʰ **S82.034   Nondisplaced transverse fracture of right patella**
     ✓7ᵗʰ **S82.035   Nondisplaced transverse fracture of left patella**
     ✓7ᵗʰ **S82.036   Nondisplaced transverse fracture of unspecified patella**

   ✓6ᵗʰ S82.04   Comminuted fracture of patella
     ✓7ᵗʰ **S82.041   Displaced comminuted fracture of right patella**
     ✓7ᵗʰ **S82.042   Displaced comminuted fracture of left patella**
     ✓7ᵗʰ **S82.043   Displaced comminuted fracture of unspecified patella**
     ✓7ᵗʰ **S82.044   Nondisplaced comminuted fracture of right patella**
     ✓7ᵗʰ **S82.045   Nondisplaced comminuted fracture of left patella**
     ✓7ᵗʰ **S82.046   Nondisplaced comminuted fracture of unspecified patella**

   ✓6ᵗʰ S82.09   Other fracture of patella
     ✓7ᵗʰ **S82.091   Other fracture of right patella**
     ✓7ᵗʰ **S82.092   Other fracture of left patella**
     ✓7ᵗʰ **S82.099   Other fracture of unspecified patella**

✓5ᵗʰ S82.1   Fracture of upper end of tibia
Fracture of proximal end of tibia
> **EXCLUDES 2**   fracture of shaft of tibia (S82.2-)
> physeal fracture of upper end of tibia (S89.0-)

   ✓6ᵗʰ S82.10   Unspecified fracture of upper end of tibia
     ✓7ᵗʰ **S82.101   Unspecified fracture of upper end of right tibia**
     ✓7ᵗʰ **S82.102   Unspecified fracture of upper end of left tibia**
     ✓7ᵗʰ **S82.109   Unspecified fracture of upper end of unspecified tibia**

   ✓6ᵗʰ S82.11   Fracture of tibial spine
     ✓7ᵗʰ **S82.111   Displaced fracture of right tibial spine**
     ✓7ᵗʰ **S82.112   Displaced fracture of left tibial spine**
     ✓7ᵗʰ **S82.113   Displaced fracture of unspecified tibial spine**
     ✓7ᵗʰ **S82.114   Nondisplaced fracture of right tibial spine**
     ✓7ᵗʰ **S82.115   Nondisplaced fracture of left tibial spine**
     ✓7ᵗʰ **S82.116   Nondisplaced fracture of unspecified tibial spine**

   ✓6ᵗʰ S82.12   Fracture of lateral condyle of tibia
     ✓7ᵗʰ **S82.121   Displaced fracture of lateral condyle of right tibia**
     ✓7ᵗʰ **S82.122   Displaced fracture of lateral condyle of left tibia**
     ✓7ᵗʰ **S82.123   Displaced fracture of lateral condyle of unspecified tibia**
     ✓7ᵗʰ **S82.124   Nondisplaced fracture of lateral condyle of right tibia**
     ✓7ᵗʰ **S82.125   Nondisplaced fracture of lateral condyle of left tibia**
     ✓7ᵗʰ **S82.126   Nondisplaced fracture of lateral condyle of unspecified tibia**

   ✓6ᵗʰ S82.13   Fracture of medial condyle of tibia
     ✓7ᵗʰ **S82.131   Displaced fracture of medial condyle of right tibia**
     ✓7ᵗʰ **S82.132   Displaced fracture of medial condyle of left tibia**
     ✓7ᵗʰ **S82.133   Displaced fracture of medial condyle of unspecified tibia**
     ✓7ᵗʰ **S82.134   Nondisplaced fracture of medial condyle of right tibia**
     ✓7ᵗʰ **S82.135   Nondisplaced fracture of medial condyle of left tibia**

EXCLUDES 1 Not coded here   **EXCLUDES 2** Not included here   *Manifestation Code*

☑7ᵗʰ **S82.136** **Nondisplaced fracture of medial condyle of unspecified tibia**

☑6ᵗʰ **S82.14** **Bicondylar fracture of tibia**
Fracture of tibial plateau NOS

☑7ᵗʰ **S82.141** **Displaced bicondylar fracture of right tibia**

☑7ᵗʰ **S82.142** **Displaced bicondylar fracture of left tibia**

☑7ᵗʰ **S82.143** **Displaced bicondylar fracture of unspecified tibia**

☑7ᵗʰ **S82.144** **Nondisplaced bicondylar fracture of right tibia**

☑7ᵗʰ **S82.145** **Nondisplaced bicondylar fracture of left tibia**

☑7ᵗʰ **S82.146** **Nondisplaced bicondylar fracture of unspecified tibia**

☑6ᵗʰ **S82.15** **Fracture of tibial tuberosity**

☑7ᵗʰ **S82.151** **Displaced fracture of right tibial tuberosity**

☑7ᵗʰ **S82.152** **Displaced fracture of left tibial tuberosity**

☑7ᵗʰ **S82.153** **Displaced fracture of unspecified tibial tuberosity**

☑7ᵗʰ **S82.154** **Nondisplaced fracture of right tibial tuberosity**

☑7ᵗʰ **S82.155** **Nondisplaced fracture of left tibial tuberosity**

☑7ᵗʰ **S82.156** **Nondisplaced fracture of unspecified tibial tuberosity**

☑6ᵗʰ **S82.16** **Torus fracture of upper end of tibia)**

> The appropriate 7th character is to be added to all codes from category S82.16
> A   initial encounter for fracture
> D   subsequent encounter for fracture with routine healing
> G   subsequent encounter for fracture with delayed healing
> K   subsequent encounter for fracture with nonunion
> P   subsequent encounter for fracture with malunion
> S   sequela

☑7ᵗʰ **S82.161** **Torus fracture of upper end of right tibia**

☑7ᵗʰ **S82.162** **Torus fracture of upper end of left tibia**

☑7ᵗʰ **S82.169** **Torus fracture of upper end of unspecified tibia**

☑6ᵗʰ **S82.19** **Other fracture of upper end of tibia**

☑7ᵗʰ **S82.191** **Other fracture of upper end of right tibia**

☑7ᵗʰ **S82.192** **Other fracture of upper end of left tibia**

☑7ᵗʰ **S82.199** **Other fracture of upper end of unspecified tibia**

☑5ᵗʰ **S82.2** **Fracture of shaft of tibia**

☑6ᵗʰ **S82.20** **Unspecified fracture of shaft of tibia**
Fracture of tibia NOS

☑7ᵗʰ **S82.201** **Unspecified fracture of shaft of right tibia**

☑7ᵗʰ **S82.202** **Unspecified fracture of shaft of left tibia**

☑7ᵗʰ **S82.209** **Unspecified fracture of shaft of unspecified tibia**

☑6ᵗʰ **S82.22** **Transverse fracture of shaft of tibia**

☑7ᵗʰ **S82.221** **Displaced transverse fracture of shaft of right tibia**

☑7ᵗʰ **S82.222** **Displaced transverse fracture of shaft of left tibia**

☑7ᵗʰ **S82.223** **Displaced transverse fracture of shaft of unspecified tibia**

☑7ᵗʰ **S82.224** **Nondisplaced transverse fracture of shaft of right tibia**

☑7ᵗʰ **S82.225** **Nondisplaced transverse fracture of shaft of left tibia**

☑7ᵗʰ **S82.226** **Nondisplaced transverse fracture of shaft of unspecified tibia**

☑6ᵗʰ **S82.23** **Oblique fracture of shaft of tibia**

☑7ᵗʰ **S82.231** **Displaced oblique fracture of shaft of right tibia**

☑7ᵗʰ **S82.232** **Displaced oblique fracture of shaft of left tibia**

☑7ᵗʰ **S82.233** **Displaced oblique fracture of shaft of unspecified tibia**

☑7ᵗʰ **S82.234** **Nondisplaced oblique fracture of shaft of right tibia**

☑7ᵗʰ **S82.235** **Nondisplaced oblique fracture of shaft of left tibia**

☑7ᵗʰ **S82.236** **Nondisplaced oblique fracture of shaft of unspecified tibia**

☑6ᵗʰ **S82.24** **Spiral fracture of shaft of tibia**
Toddler fracture

☑7ᵗʰ **S82.241** **Displaced spiral fracture of shaft of right tibia**

☑7ᵗʰ **S82.242** **Displaced spiral fracture of shaft of left tibia**

☑7ᵗʰ **S82.243** **Displaced spiral fracture of shaft of unspecified tibia**

☑7ᵗʰ **S82.244** **Nondisplaced spiral fracture of shaft of right tibia**

☑7ᵗʰ **S82.245** **Nondisplaced spiral fracture of shaft of left tibia**

☑7ᵗʰ **S82.246** **Nondisplaced spiral fracture of shaft of unspecified tibia**

☑6ᵗʰ **S82.25** **Comminuted fracture of shaft of tibia**

☑7ᵗʰ **S82.251** **Displaced comminuted fracture of shaft of right tibia**

☑7ᵗʰ **S82.252** **Displaced comminuted fracture of shaft of left tibia**

☑7ᵗʰ **S82.253** **Displaced comminuted fracture of shaft of unspecified tibia**

☑7ᵗʰ **S82.254** **Nondisplaced comminuted fracture of shaft of right tibia**

☑7ᵗʰ **S82.255** **Nondisplaced comminuted fracture of shaft of left tibia**

☑7ᵗʰ **S82.256** **Nondisplaced comminuted fracture of shaft of unspecified tibia**

☑6ᵗʰ **S82.26** **Segmental fracture of shaft of tibia**

☑7ᵗʰ **S82.261** **Displaced segmental fracture of shaft of right tibia**

☑7ᵗʰ **S82.262** **Displaced segmental fracture of shaft of left tibia**

☑7ᵗʰ **S82.263** **Displaced segmental fracture of shaft of unspecified tibia**

☑7ᵗʰ **S82.264** **Nondisplaced segmental fracture of shaft of right tibia**

☑7ᵗʰ **S82.265** **Nondisplaced segmental fracture of shaft of left tibia**

☑7ᵗʰ **S82.266** **Nondisplaced segmental fracture of shaft of unspecified tibia**

☑6ᵗʰ **S82.29** **Other fracture of shaft of tibia**

☑7ᵗʰ **S82.291** **Other fracture of shaft of right tibia**

☑7ᵗʰ **S82.292** **Other fracture of shaft of left tibia**

☑7ᵗʰ **S82.299** **Other fracture of shaft of unspecified tibia**

☑5ᵗʰ **S82.3** **Fracture of lower end of tibia**

EXCLUDES 1   *bimalleolar fracture of lower leg (S82.84-)*
fracture of medial malleolus alone (S82.5-)
Maisonneuve's fracture (S82.86-)
pilon fracture of distal tibia (S82.87-)
trimalleolar fractures of lower leg (S82.85-)

☑6ᵗʰ **S82.30** **Unspecified fracture of lower end of tibia**

☑7ᵗʰ **S82.301** **Unspecified fracture of lower end of right tibia**

☑7ᵗʰ **S82.302** **Unspecified fracture of lower end of left tibia**

☑7ᵗʰ **S82.309** **Unspecified fracture of lower end of unspecified tibia**

☑ Appropriate additional character required   ☑x7ᵗʰ Requires 7th character, placeholder x must fill empty characters

Injury, Poisoning and Certain Other Consequences of External Causes

S82.31–S82.819

√6ᵗʰ **S82.31** Torus fracture of lower end of tibia)

> The appropriate 7th character is to be added to all codes from category S82.31
> A   initial encounter for fracture
> D   subsequent encounter for fracture with routine healing
> G   subsequent encounter for fracture with delayed healing
> K   subsequent encounter for fracture with nonunion
> P   subsequent encounter for fracture with malunion
> S   sequela

     √7ᵗʰ **S82.311** Torus fracture of lower end of right tibia
     √7ᵗʰ **S82.312** Torus fracture of lower end of left tibia
     √7ᵗʰ **S82.319** Torus fracture of lower end of unspecified tibia

√6ᵗʰ **S82.39** Other fracture of lower end of tibia
     √7ᵗʰ **S82.391** Other fracture of lower end of right tibia
     √7ᵗʰ **S82.392** Other fracture of lower end of left tibia
     √7ᵗʰ **S82.399** Other fracture of lower end of unspecified tibia

√5ᵗʰ **S82.4** Fracture of shaft of fibula
     EXCLUDES 2 *fracture of lateral malleolus alone (S82.6-)*

√6ᵗʰ **S82.40** Unspecified fracture of shaft of fibula
     √7ᵗʰ **S82.401** Unspecified fracture of shaft of right fibula
     √7ᵗʰ **S82.402** Unspecified fracture of shaft of left fibula
     √7ᵗʰ **S82.409** Unspecified fracture of shaft of unspecified fibula

√6ᵗʰ **S82.42** Transverse fracture of shaft of fibula
     √7ᵗʰ **S82.421** Displaced transverse fracture of shaft of right fibula
     √7ᵗʰ **S82.422** Displaced transverse fracture of shaft of left fibula
     √7ᵗʰ **S82.423** Displaced transverse fracture of shaft of unspecified fibula
     √7ᵗʰ **S82.424** Nondisplaced transverse fracture of shaft of right fibula
     √7ᵗʰ **S82.425** Nondisplaced transverse fracture of shaft of left fibula
     √7ᵗʰ **S82.426** Nondisplaced transverse fracture of shaft of unspecified fibula

√6ᵗʰ **S82.43** Oblique fracture of shaft of fibula
     √7ᵗʰ **S82.431** Displaced oblique fracture of shaft of right fibula
     √7ᵗʰ **S82.432** Displaced oblique fracture of shaft of left fibula
     √7ᵗʰ **S82.433** Displaced oblique fracture of shaft of unspecified fibula
     √7ᵗʰ **S82.434** Nondisplaced oblique fracture of shaft of right fibula
     √7ᵗʰ **S82.435** Nondisplaced oblique fracture of shaft of left fibula
     √7ᵗʰ **S82.436** Nondisplaced oblique fracture of shaft of unspecified fibula

√6ᵗʰ **S82.44** Spiral fracture of shaft of fibula
     √7ᵗʰ **S82.441** Displaced spiral fracture of shaft of right fibula
     √7ᵗʰ **S82.442** Displaced spiral fracture of shaft of left fibula
     √7ᵗʰ **S82.443** Displaced spiral fracture of shaft of unspecified fibula
     √7ᵗʰ **S82.444** Nondisplaced spiral fracture of shaft of right fibula
     √7ᵗʰ **S82.445** Nondisplaced spiral fracture of shaft of left fibula
     √7ᵗʰ **S82.446** Nondisplaced spiral fracture of shaft of unspecified fibula

√6ᵗʰ **S82.45** Comminuted fracture of shaft of fibula
     √7ᵗʰ **S82.451** Displaced comminuted fracture of shaft of right fibula
     √7ᵗʰ **S82.452** Displaced comminuted fracture of shaft of left fibula

√7ᵗʰ **S82.453** Displaced comminuted fracture of shaft of unspecified fibula
√7ᵗʰ **S82.454** Nondisplaced comminuted fracture of shaft of right fibula
√7ᵗʰ **S82.455** Nondisplaced comminuted fracture of shaft of left fibula
√7ᵗʰ **S82.456** Nondisplaced comminuted fracture of shaft of unspecified fibula

√6ᵗʰ **S82.46** Segmental fracture of shaft of fibula
     √7ᵗʰ **S82.461** Displaced segmental fracture of shaft of right fibula
     √7ᵗʰ **S82.462** Displaced segmental fracture of shaft of left fibula
     √7ᵗʰ **S82.463** Displaced segmental fracture of shaft of unspecified fibula
     √7ᵗʰ **S82.464** Nondisplaced segmental fracture of shaft of right fibula
     √7ᵗʰ **S82.465** Nondisplaced segmental fracture of shaft of left fibula
     √7ᵗʰ **S82.466** Nondisplaced segmental fracture of shaft of unspecified fibula

√6ᵗʰ **S82.49** Other fracture of shaft of fibula
     √7ᵗʰ **S82.491** Other fracture of shaft of right fibula
     √7ᵗʰ **S82.492** Other fracture of shaft of left fibula
     √7ᵗʰ **S82.499** Other fracture of shaft of unspecified fibula

√5ᵗʰ **S82.5** Fracture of medial malleolus
     EXCLUDES 1 *pilon fracture of distal tibia (S82.84-)*
                   Salter-Harris type III of lower end of tibia (S89.13-)
                   Salter-Harris type IV of lower end of tibia (S89.14-)
     √x7ᵗʰ **S82.51** Displaced fracture of medial malleolus of right tibia
     √x7ᵗʰ **S82.52** Displaced fracture of medial malleolus of left tibia
     √x7ᵗʰ **S82.53** Displaced fracture of medial malleolus of unspecified tibia
     √x7ᵗʰ **S82.54** Nondisplaced fracture of medial malleolus of right tibia
     √x7ᵗʰ **S82.55** Nondisplaced fracture of medial malleolus of left tibia
     √x7ᵗʰ **S82.56** Nondisplaced fracture of medial malleolus of unspecified tibia

√5ᵗʰ **S82.6** Fracture of lateral malleolus
     EXCLUDES 1 *pilon fracture of distal tibia (S82.84-)*
     √x7ᵗʰ **S82.61** Displaced fracture of lateral malleolus of right fibula
     √x7ᵗʰ **S82.62** Displaced fracture of lateral malleolus of left fibula
     √x7ᵗʰ **S82.63** Displaced fracture of lateral malleolus of unspecified fibula
     √x7ᵗʰ **S82.64** Nondisplaced fracture of lateral malleolus of right fibula
     √x7ᵗʰ **S82.65** Nondisplaced fracture of lateral malleolus of left fibula
     √x7ᵗʰ **S82.66** Nondisplaced fracture of lateral malleolus of unspecified fibula

√5ᵗʰ **S82.8** Other fractures of lower leg
√6ᵗʰ **S82.81** Torus fracture of upper end of fibula

> The appropriate 7th character is to be added to all codes from category S82.81
> A   initial encounter for fracture
> D   subsequent encounter for fracture with routine healing
> G   subsequent encounter for fracture with delayed healing
> K   subsequent encounter for fracture with nonunion
> P   subsequent encounter for fracture with malunion
> S   sequela

     √7ᵗʰ **S82.811** Torus fracture of upper end of right fibula
     √7ᵗʰ **S82.812** Torus fracture of upper end of left fibula
     √7ᵗʰ **S82.819** Torus fracture of upper end of unspecified fibula

---

EXCLUDES 1 Not coded here   **EXCLUDES 2** Not included here   *Manifestation Code*

✓6th **S82.82   Torus fracture of lower end of fibula**

> The appropriate 7th character is to be added to all codes from category S82.82
> A initial encounter for fracture
> D subsequent encounter for fracture with routine healing
> G subsequent encounter for fracture with delayed healing
> K subsequent encounter for fracture with nonunion
> P subsequent encounter for fracture with malunion
> S sequela

   ✓7th **S82.821   Torus fracture of lower end of right fibula**
   ✓7th **S82.822   Torus fracture of lower end of left fibula**
   ✓7th **S82.829   Torus fracture of lower end of unspecified fibula**

✓6th **S82.83   Other fracture of upper and lower end of fibula**
   ✓7th **S82.831   Other fracture of upper and lower end of right fibula**
   ✓7th **S82.832   Other fracture of upper and lower end of left fibula**
   ✓7th **S82.839   Other fracture of upper and lower end of unspecified fibula**

✓6th **S82.84   Bimalleolar fracture of lower leg**
   ✓7th **S82.841   Displaced bimalleolar fracture of right lower leg**
   ✓7th **S82.842   Displaced bimalleolar fracture of left lower leg**
   ✓7th **S82.843   Displaced bimalleolar fracture of unspecified lower leg**
   ✓7th **S82.844   Nondisplaced bimalleolar fracture of right lower leg**
   ✓7th **S82.845   Nondisplaced bimalleolar fracture of left lower leg**
   ✓7th **S82.846   Nondisplaced bimalleolar fracture of unspecified lower leg**

✓6th **S82.85   Trimalleolar fracture of lower leg**
   ✓7th **S82.851   Displaced trimalleolar fracture of right lower leg**
   ✓7th **S82.852   Displaced trimalleolar fracture of left lower leg**
   ✓7th **S82.853   Displaced trimalleolar fracture of unspecified lower leg**
   ✓7th **S82.854   Nondisplaced trimalleolar fracture of right lower leg**
   ✓7th **S82.855   Nondisplaced trimalleolar fracture of left lower leg**
   ✓7th **S82.856   Nondisplaced trimalleolar fracture of unspecified lower leg**

✓6th **S82.86   Maisonneuve's fracture**
   ✓7th **S82.861   Displaced Maisonneuve's fracture of right leg**
   ✓7th **S82.862   Displaced Maisonneuve's fracture of left leg**
   ✓7th **S82.863   Displaced Maisonneuve's fracture of unspecified leg**
   ✓7th **S82.864   Nondisplaced Maisonneuve's fracture of right leg**
   ✓7th **S82.865   Nondisplaced Maisonneuve's fracture of left leg**
   ✓7th **S82.866   Nondisplaced Maisonneuve's fracture of unspecified leg**

✓6th **S82.87   Pilon fracture of tibia**
   ✓7th **S82.871   Displaced pilon fracture of right tibia**
   ✓7th **S82.872   Displaced pilon fracture of left tibia**
   ✓7th **S82.873   Displaced pilon fracture of unspecified tibia**
   ✓7th **S82.874   Nondisplaced pilon fracture of right tibia**
   ✓7th **S82.875   Nondisplaced pilon fracture of left tibia**
   ✓7th **S82.876   Nondisplaced pilon fracture of unspecified tibia**

✓6th **S82.89   Other fractures of lower leg**
   Fracture of ankle NOS
   ✓7th **S82.891   Other fracture of right lower leg**
   ✓7th **S82.892   Other fracture of left lower leg**
   ✓7th **S82.899   Other fracture of unspecified lower leg**

✓5th **S82.9   Unspecified fracture of lower leg**
   ✓7th **S82.90   Unspecified fracture of unspecified lower leg**
   ✓x7th **S82.91   Unspecified fracture of right lower leg**
   ✓x7th **S82.92   Unspecified fracture of left lower leg**

✓4th **S83   Dislocation and sprain of joints and ligaments of knee**
   INCLUDES   avulsion of joint or ligament of knee
       laceration of cartilage, joint or ligament of knee
       sprain of cartilage, joint or ligament of knee
       traumatic hemarthrosis of joint or ligament of knee
       traumatic rupture of joint or ligament of knee
       traumatic subluxation of joint or ligament of knee
       traumatic tear of joint or ligament of knee
   Code also any associated open wound
   EXCLUDES 1   derangement of patella (M22.0-M22.3)
       injury of patellar ligament (tendon) (S76.1-)
       internal derangement of knee (M23-)
       old dislocation of knee (M23.8x-)
       pathological dislocation of knee (M24.36)
       recurrent dislocation of knee (M22.0)
   EXCLUDES 2   strain of muscle, fascia and tendon of lower leg (S86-)

> The appropriate 7th character is to be added to each code from category S83.
> A initial encounter
> D subsequent encounter
> S sequela

✓5th **S83.0   Subluxation and dislocation of patella**
   ✓6th **S83.00   Unspecified subluxation and dislocation of patella**
     ✓7th **S83.001   Unspecified subluxation of right patella**
     ✓7th **S83.002   Unspecified subluxation of left patella**
     ✓7th **S83.003   Unspecified subluxation of unspecified patella**
     ✓7th **S83.004   Unspecified dislocation of right patella**
     ✓7th **S83.005   Unspecified dislocation of left patella**
     ✓7th **S83.006   Unspecified dislocation of unspecified patella**

   ✓6th **S83.01   Lateral subluxation and dislocation of patella**
     ✓7th **S83.011   Lateral subluxation of right patella**
     ✓7th **S83.012   Lateral subluxation of left patella**
     ✓7th **S83.013   Lateral subluxation of unspecified patella**
     ✓7th **S83.014   Lateral dislocation of right patella**
     ✓7th **S83.015   Lateral dislocation of left patella**
     ✓7th **S83.016   Lateral dislocation of unspecified patella**

   ✓6th **S83.09   Other subluxation and dislocation of patella**
     ✓7th **S83.091   Other subluxation of right patella**
     ✓7th **S83.092   Other subluxation of left patella**
     ✓7th **S83.093   Other subluxation of unspecified patella**
     ✓7th **S83.094   Other dislocation of right patella**
     ✓7th **S83.095   Other dislocation of left patella**
     ✓7th **S83.096   Other dislocation of unspecified patella**

✓5th **S83.1   Subluxation and dislocation of knee**
   EXCLUDES 2   dislocation and subluxation of knee prosthesis (T84.022, T84.023)
   ✓6th **S83.10   Unspecified subluxation and dislocation of knee**
     ✓7th **S83.101   Unspecified subluxation of right knee**
     ✓7th **S83.102   Unspecified subluxation of left knee**
     ✓7th **S83.103   Unspecified subluxation of unspecified knee**
     ✓7th **S83.104   Unspecified dislocation of right knee**
     ✓7th **S83.105   Unspecified dislocation of left knee**
     ✓7th **S83.106   Unspecified dislocation of unspecified knee**

   ✓6th **S83.11   Anterior subluxation and dislocation of proximal end of tibia**
     Posterior subluxation and dislocation of distal end of femur
     ✓7th **S83.111   Anterior subluxation of proximal end of tibia, right knee**

☑ Appropriate additional character required
✓x7th Requires 7th character, placeholder x must fill empty characters

√7th **S83.112** Anterior subluxation of proximal end of tibia, left knee

√7th **S83.113** Anterior subluxation of proximal end of tibia, unspecified knee

√7th **S83.114** Anterior dislocation of proximal end of tibia, right knee

√7th **S83.115** Anterior dislocation of proximal end of tibia, left knee

√7th **S83.116** Anterior dislocation of proximal end of tibia, unspecified knee

√6th **S83.12** Posterior subluxation and dislocation of proximal end of tibia
  Anterior dislocation of distal end of femur

√7th **S83.121** Posterior subluxation of proximal end of tibia, right knee

√7th **S83.122** Posterior subluxation of proximal end of tibia, left knee

√7th **S83.123** Posterior subluxation of proximal end of tibia, unspecified knee

√7th **S83.124** Posterior dislocation of proximal end of tibia, right knee

√7th **S83.125** Posterior dislocation of proximal end of tibia, left knee

√7th **S83.126** Posterior dislocation of proximal end of tibia, unspecified knee

√6th **S83.13** Medial subluxation and dislocation of proximal end of tibia

√7th **S83.131** Medial subluxation of proximal end of tibia, right knee

√7th **S83.132** Medial subluxation of proximal end of tibia, left knee

√7th **S83.133** Medial subluxation of proximal end of tibia, unspecified knee

√7th **S83.134** Medial dislocation of proximal end of tibia, right knee

√7th **S83.135** Medial dislocation of proximal end of tibia, left knee

√7th **S83.136** Medial dislocation of proximal end of tibia, unspecified knee

√6th **S83.14** Lateral subluxation and dislocation of proximal end of tibia

√7th **S83.141** Lateral subluxation of proximal end of tibia, right knee

√7th **S83.142** Lateral subluxation of proximal end of tibia, left knee

√7th **S83.143** Lateral subluxation of proximal end of tibia, unspecified knee

√7th **S83.144** Lateral dislocation of proximal end of tibia, right knee

√7th **S83.145** Lateral dislocation of proximal end of tibia, left knee

√7th **S83.146** Lateral dislocation of proximal end of tibia, unspecified knee

√6th **S83.19** Other subluxation and dislocation of knee

√7th **S83.191** Other subluxation of right knee

√7th **S83.192** Other subluxation of left knee

√7th **S83.193** Other subluxation of unspecified knee

√7th **S83.194** Other dislocation of right knee

√7th **S83.195** Other dislocation of left knee

√7th **S83.196** Other dislocation of unspecified knee

√5th **S83.2** Tear of meniscus, current injury
  EXCLUDES 1 old bucket-handle tear (M23.2)

√6th **S83.20** Tear of unspecified meniscus, current injury
  Tear of meniscus of knee NOS

√7th **S83.200** Bucket-handle tear of unspecified meniscus, current injury, right knee

√7th **S83.201** Bucket-handle tear of unspecified meniscus, current injury, left knee

√7th **S83.202** Bucket-handle tear of unspecified meniscus, current injury, unspecified knee

√7th **S83.203** Other tear of unspecified meniscus, current injury, right knee

√7th **S83.204** Other tear of unspecified meniscus, current injury, left knee

√7th **S83.205** Other tear of unspecified meniscus, current injury, unspecified knee

√7th **S83.206** Unspecified tear of unspecified meniscus, current injury, right knee

√7th **S83.207** Unspecified tear of unspecified meniscus, current injury, left knee

√7th **S83.209** Unspecified tear of unspecified meniscus, current injury, unspecified knee

√6th **S83.21** Bucket-handle tear of medial meniscus, current injury

√7th **S83.211** Bucket-handle tear of medial meniscus, current injury, right knee

√7th **S83.212** Bucket-handle tear of medial meniscus, current injury, left knee

√7th **S83.219** Bucket-handle tear of medial meniscus, current injury, unspecified knee

√6th **S83.22** Peripheral tear of medial meniscus, current injury

√7th **S83.221** Peripheral tear of medial meniscus, current injury, right knee

√7th **S83.222** Peripheral tear of medial meniscus, current injury, left knee

√7th **S83.229** Peripheral tear of medial meniscus, current injury, unspecified knee

√6th **S83.23** Complex tear of medial meniscus, current injury

√7th **S83.231** Complex tear of medial meniscus, current injury, right knee

√7th **S83.232** Complex tear of medial meniscus, current injury, left knee

√7th **S83.239** Complex tear of medial meniscus, current injury, unspecified knee

√6th **S83.24** Other tear of medial meniscus, current injury

√7th **S83.241** Other tear of medial meniscus, current injury, right knee

√7th **S83.242** Other tear of medial meniscus, current injury, left knee

√7th **S83.249** Other tear of medial meniscus, current injury, unspecified knee

√6th **S83.25** Bucket-handle tear of lateral meniscus, current injury

√7th **S83.251** Bucket-handle tear of lateral meniscus, current injury, right knee

√7th **S83.252** Bucket-handle tear of lateral meniscus, current injury, left knee

√7th **S83.259** Bucket-handle tear of lateral meniscus, current injury, unspecified knee

√6th **S83.26** Peripheral tear of lateral meniscus, current injury

√7th **S83.261** Peripheral tear of lateral meniscus, current injury, right knee

√7th **S83.262** Peripheral tear of lateral meniscus, current injury, left knee

√7th **S83.269** Peripheral tear of lateral meniscus, current injury, unspecified knee

√6th **S83.27** Complex tear of lateral meniscus, current injury

√7th **S83.271** Complex tear of lateral meniscus, current injury, right knee

√7th **S83.272** Complex tear of lateral meniscus, current injury, left knee

√7th **S83.279** Complex tear of lateral meniscus, current injury, unspecified knee

√6th **S83.28** Other tear of lateral meniscus, current injury

√7th **S83.281** Other tear of lateral meniscus, current injury, right knee

√7th **S83.282** Other tear of lateral meniscus, current injury, left knee

√7th **S83.289** Other tear of lateral meniscus, current injury, unspecified knee

√5th **S83.3** Tear of articular cartilage of knee, current

√x7th **S83.30** Tear of articular cartilage of unspecified knee, current

√x7th **S83.31** Tear of articular cartilage of right knee, current

√x7th **S83.32** Tear of articular cartilage of left knee, current

√5th **S83.4** Sprain of collateral ligament of knee

√6th **S83.40** Sprain of unspecified collateral ligament of knee

√7th **S83.401** Sprain of unspecified collateral ligament of right knee

---

EXCLUDES 1 Not coded here   **EXCLUDES 2** Not included here   *Manifestation Code*

✓7ᵗʰ **S83.402** Sprain of unspecified collateral ligament of left knee

✓7ᵗʰ **S83.409** Sprain of unspecified collateral ligament of unspecified knee

✓6ᵗʰ **S83.41** Sprain of medial collateral ligament of knee
Sprain of tibial collateral ligament

✓7ᵗʰ **S83.411** Sprain of medial collateral ligament of right knee

✓7ᵗʰ **S83.412** Sprain of medial collateral ligament of left knee

✓7ᵗʰ **S83.419** Sprain of medial collateral ligament of unspecified knee

✓6ᵗʰ **S83.42** Sprain of lateral collateral ligament of knee
Sprain of fibular collateral ligament

✓7ᵗʰ **S83.421** Sprain of lateral collateral ligament of right knee

✓7ᵗʰ **S83.422** Sprain of lateral collateral ligament of left knee

✓7ᵗʰ **S83.429** Sprain of lateral collateral ligament of unspecified knee

✓5ᵗʰ **S83.5** Sprain of cruciate ligament of knee

✓6ᵗʰ **S83.50** Sprain of unspecified cruciate ligament of knee

✓7ᵗʰ **S83.501** Sprain of unspecified cruciate ligament of right knee

✓7ᵗʰ **S83.502** Sprain of unspecified cruciate ligament of left knee

✓7ᵗʰ **S83.509** Sprain of unspecified cruciate ligament of unspecified knee

✓6ᵗʰ **S83.51** Sprain of anterior cruciate ligament of knee

✓7ᵗʰ **S83.511** Sprain of anterior cruciate ligament of right knee

✓7ᵗʰ **S83.512** Sprain of anterior cruciate ligament of left knee

✓7ᵗʰ **S83.519** Sprain of anterior cruciate ligament of unspecified knee

✓6ᵗʰ **S83.52** Sprain of posterior cruciate ligament of knee

✓7ᵗʰ **S83.521** Sprain of posterior cruciate ligament of right knee

✓7ᵗʰ **S83.522** Sprain of posterior cruciate ligament of left knee

✓7ᵗʰ **S83.529** Sprain of posterior cruciate ligament of unspecified knee

✓5ᵗʰ **S83.6** Sprain of the superior tibiofibular joint and ligament

✓ˣ7ᵗʰ **S83.60** Sprain of the superior tibiofibular joint and ligament, unspecified knee

✓ˣ7ᵗʰ **S83.61** Sprain of the superior tibiofibular joint and ligament, right knee

✓ˣ7ᵗʰ **S83.62** Sprain of the superior tibiofibular joint and ligament, left knee

✓5ᵗʰ **S83.8** Sprain of other specified parts of knee

✓6ᵗʰ **S83.8x** Sprain of other specified parts of knee

✓7ᵗʰ **S83.8x1** Sprain of other specified parts of right knee

✓7ᵗʰ **S83.8x2** Sprain of other specified parts of left knee

✓7ᵗʰ **S83.8x9** Sprain of other specified parts of unspecified knee

✓5ᵗʰ **S83.9** Sprain of unspecified site of knee

✓ˣ7ᵗʰ **S83.90** Sprain of unspecified site of unspecified knee

✓ˣ7ᵗʰ **S83.91** Sprain of unspecified site of right knee

✓ˣ7ᵗʰ **S83.92** Sprain of unspecified site of left knee

✓4ᵗʰ **S84** **Injury of nerves at lower leg level**
Code also any associated open wound (S81-)
EXCLUDES 2 *injury of nerves at ankle and foot level (S94-)*

The appropriate 7th character is to be added to each code from category S84.
A   initial encounter
D   subsequent encounter
S   sequela

✓5ᵗʰ **S84.0** Injury of tibial nerve at lower leg level

✓ˣ7ᵗʰ **S84.00** Injury of tibial nerve at lower leg level, unspecified leg

✓ˣ7ᵗʰ **S84.01** Injury of tibial nerve at lower leg level, right leg

✓ˣ7ᵗʰ **S84.02** Injury of tibial nerve at lower leg level, left leg

✓5ᵗʰ **S84.1** Injury of peroneal nerve at lower leg level

✓ˣ7ᵗʰ **S84.10** Injury of peroneal nerve at lower leg level, unspecified leg

✓ˣ7ᵗʰ **S84.11** Injury of peroneal nerve at lower leg level, right leg

✓ˣ7ᵗʰ **S84.12** Injury of peroneal nerve at lower leg level, left leg

✓5ᵗʰ **S84.2** Injury of cutaneous sensory nerve at lower leg level

✓ˣ7ᵗʰ **S84.20** Injury of cutaneous sensory nerve at lower leg level, unspecified leg

✓ˣ7ᵗʰ **S84.21** Injury of cutaneous sensory nerve at lower leg level, right leg

✓ˣ7ᵗʰ **S84.22** Injury of cutaneous sensory nerve at lower leg level, left leg

✓5ᵗʰ **S84.8** Injury of other nerves at lower leg level

✓6ᵗʰ **S84.80** Injury of other nerves at lower leg level

✓7ᵗʰ **S84.801** Injury of other nerves at lower leg level, right leg

✓7ᵗʰ **S84.802** Injury of other nerves at lower leg level, left leg

✓7ᵗʰ **S84.809** Injury of other nerves at lower leg level, unspecified leg

✓5ᵗʰ **S84.9** Injury of unspecified nerve at lower leg level

✓ˣ7ᵗʰ **S84.90** Injury of unspecified nerve at lower leg level, unspecified leg

✓ˣ7ᵗʰ **S84.91** Injury of unspecified nerve at lower leg level, right leg

✓ˣ7ᵗʰ **S84.92** Injury of unspecified nerve at lower leg level, left leg

✓4ᵗʰ **S85** **Injury of blood vessels at lower leg level**
Code also any associated open wound (S81-)
EXCLUDES 2 *injury of blood vessels at ankle and foot level (S95-)*

The appropriate 7th character is to be added to each code from category S85.
A   initial encounter
D   subsequent encounter
S   sequela

✓5ᵗʰ **S85.0** Injury of popliteal artery

✓6ᵗʰ **S85.00** Unspecified injury of popliteal artery

✓7ᵗʰ **S85.001** Unspecified injury of popliteal artery, right leg

✓7ᵗʰ **S85.002** Unspecified injury of popliteal artery, left leg

✓7ᵗʰ **S85.009** Unspecified injury of popliteal artery, unspecified leg

✓6ᵗʰ **S85.01** Laceration of popliteal artery

✓7ᵗʰ **S85.011** Laceration of popliteal artery, right leg

✓7ᵗʰ **S85.012** Laceration of popliteal artery, left leg

✓7ᵗʰ **S85.019** Laceration of popliteal artery, unspecified leg

✓6ᵗʰ **S85.09** Other specified injury of popliteal artery

✓7ᵗʰ **S85.091** Other specified injury of popliteal artery, right leg

✓7ᵗʰ **S85.092** Other specified injury of popliteal artery, left leg

✓7ᵗʰ **S85.099** Other specified injury of popliteal artery, unspecified leg

✓5ᵗʰ **S85.1** Injury of tibial artery

✓6ᵗʰ **S85.10** Unspecified injury of unspecified tibial artery
Injury of tibial artery NOS

✓7ᵗʰ **S85.101** Unspecified injury of unspecified tibial artery, right leg

✓7ᵗʰ **S85.102** Unspecified injury of unspecified tibial artery, left leg

✓7ᵗʰ **S85.109** Unspecified injury of unspecified tibial artery, unspecified leg

✓6ᵗʰ **S85.11** Laceration of unspecified tibial artery

✓7ᵗʰ **S85.111** Laceration of unspecified tibial artery, right leg

✓7ᵗʰ **S85.112** Laceration of unspecified tibial artery, left leg

✓7ᵗʰ **S85.119** Laceration of unspecified tibial artery, unspecified leg

✓6ᵗʰ **S85.12** Other specified injury of unspecified tibial artery

---

✓ Appropriate additional character required   ✓ˣ7ᵗʰ Requires 7th character, placeholder x must fill empty characters

√7th **S85.121** Other specified injury of unspecified tibial artery, right leg

√7th **S85.122** Other specified injury of unspecified tibial artery, left leg

√7th **S85.129** Other specified injury of unspecified tibial artery, unspecified leg

√6th **S85.13** Unspecified injury of anterior tibial artery

√7th **S85.131** Unspecified injury of anterior tibial artery, right leg

√7th **S85.132** Unspecified injury of anterior tibial artery, left leg

√7th **S85.139** Unspecified injury of anterior tibial artery, unspecified leg

√6th **S85.14** Laceration of anterior tibial artery

√7th **S85.141** Laceration of anterior tibial artery, right leg

√7th **S85.142** Laceration of anterior tibial artery, left leg

√7th **S85.149** Laceration of anterior tibial artery, unspecified leg

√6th **S85.15** Other specified injury of anterior tibial artery

√7th **S85.151** Other specified injury of anterior tibial artery, right leg

√7th **S85.152** Other specified injury of anterior tibial artery, left leg

√7th **S85.159** Other specified injury of anterior tibial artery, unspecified leg

√6th **S85.16** Unspecified injury of posterior tibial artery

√7th **S85.161** Unspecified injury of posterior tibial artery, right leg

√7th **S85.162** Unspecified injury of posterior tibial artery, left leg

√7th **S85.169** Unspecified injury of posterior tibial artery, unspecified leg

√6th **S85.17** Laceration of posterior tibial artery

√7th **S85.171** Laceration of posterior tibial artery, right leg

√7th **S85.172** Laceration of posterior tibial artery, left leg

√7th **S85.179** Laceration of posterior tibial artery, unspecified leg

√6th **S85.18** Other specified injury of posterior tibial artery

√7th **S85.181** Other specified injury of posterior tibial artery, right leg

√7th **S85.182** Other specified injury of posterior tibial artery, left leg

√7th **S85.189** Other specified injury of posterior tibial artery, unspecified leg

√5th **S85.2** Injury of peroneal artery

√6th **S85.20** Unspecified injury of peroneal artery

√7th **S85.201** Unspecified injury of peroneal artery, right leg

√7th **S85.202** Unspecified injury of peroneal artery, left leg

√7th **S85.209** Unspecified injury of peroneal artery, unspecified leg

√6th **S85.21** Laceration of peroneal artery

√7th **S85.211** Laceration of peroneal artery, right leg

√7th **S85.212** Laceration of peroneal artery, left leg

√7th **S85.219** Laceration of peroneal artery, unspecified leg

√6th **S85.29** Other specified injury of peroneal artery

√7th **S85.291** Other specified injury of peroneal artery, right leg

√7th **S85.292** Other specified injury of peroneal artery, left leg

√7th **S85.299** Other specified injury of peroneal artery, unspecified leg

√5th **S85.3** Injury of greater saphenous vein at lower leg level
Injury of greater saphenous vein NOS
Injury of saphenous vein NOS

√6th **S85.30** Unspecified injury of greater saphenous vein at lower leg level

√7th **S85.301** Unspecified injury of greater saphenous vein at lower leg level, right leg

√7th **S85.302** Unspecified injury of greater saphenous vein at lower leg level, left leg

√7th **S85.309** Unspecified injury of greater saphenous vein at lower leg level, unspecified leg

√6th **S85.31** Laceration of greater saphenous vein at lower leg level

√7th **S85.311** Laceration of greater saphenous vein at lower leg level, right leg

√7th **S85.312** Laceration of greater saphenous vein at lower leg level, left leg

√7th **S85.319** Laceration of greater saphenous vein at lower leg level, unspecified leg

√6th **S85.39** Other specified injury of greater saphenous vein at lower leg level

√7th **S85.391** Other specified injury of greater saphenous vein at lower leg level, right leg

√7th **S85.392** Other specified injury of greater saphenous vein at lower leg level, left leg

√7th **S85.399** Other specified injury of greater saphenous vein at lower leg level, unspecified leg

√5th **S85.4** Injury of lesser saphenous vein at lower leg level

√6th **S85.40** Unspecified injury of lesser saphenous vein at lower leg level

√7th **S85.401** Unspecified injury of lesser saphenous vein at lower leg level, right leg

√7th **S85.402** Unspecified injury of lesser saphenous vein at lower leg level, left leg

√7th **S85.409** Unspecified injury of lesser saphenous vein at lower leg level, unspecified leg

√6th **S85.41** Laceration of lesser saphenous vein at lower leg level

√7th **S85.411** Laceration of lesser saphenous vein at lower leg level, right leg

√7th **S85.412** Laceration of lesser saphenous vein at lower leg level, left leg

√7th **S85.419** Laceration of lesser saphenous vein at lower leg level, unspecified leg

√6th **S85.49** Other specified injury of lesser saphenous vein at lower leg level

√7th **S85.491** Other specified injury of lesser saphenous vein at lower leg level, right leg

√7th **S85.492** Other specified injury of lesser saphenous vein at lower leg level, left leg

√7th **S85.499** Other specified injury of lesser saphenous vein at lower leg level, unspecified leg

√5th **S85.5** Injury of popliteal vein

√6th **S85.50** Unspecified injury of popliteal vein

√7th **S85.501** Unspecified injury of popliteal vein, right leg

√7th **S85.502** Unspecified injury of popliteal vein, left leg

√7th **S85.509** Unspecified injury of popliteal vein, unspecified leg

√6th **S85.51** Laceration of popliteal vein

√7th **S85.511** Laceration of popliteal vein, right leg

√7th **S85.512** Laceration of popliteal vein, left leg

√7th **S85.519** Laceration of popliteal vein, unspecified leg

√6th **S85.59** Other specified injury of popliteal vein

√7th **S85.591** Other specified injury of popliteal vein, right leg

√7th **S85.592** Other specified injury of popliteal vein, left leg

√7th **S85.599** Other specified injury of popliteal vein, unspecified leg

√5th **S85.8** Injury of other blood vessels at lower leg level

√6th **S85.80** Unspecified injury of other blood vessels at lower leg level

√7th **S85.801** Unspecified injury of other blood vessels at lower leg level, right leg

---

EXCLUDES 1 Not coded here   EXCLUDES 2 Not included here   *Manifestation Code*

☑7ᵗʰ **S85.802** Unspecified injury of other blood vessels at lower leg level, left leg

☑7ᵗʰ **S85.809** Unspecified injury of other blood vessels at lower leg level, unspecified leg

☑6ᵗʰ **S85.81** Laceration of other blood vessels at lower leg level

☑7ᵗʰ **S85.811** Laceration of other blood vessels at lower leg level, right leg

☑7ᵗʰ **S85.812** Laceration of other blood vessels at lower leg level, left leg

☑7ᵗʰ **S85.819** Laceration of other blood vessels at lower leg level, unspecified leg

☑6ᵗʰ **S85.89** Other specified injury of other blood vessels at lower leg level

☑7ᵗʰ **S85.891** Other specified injury of other blood vessels at lower leg level, right leg

☑7ᵗʰ **S85.892** Other specified injury of other blood vessels at lower leg level, left leg

☑7ᵗʰ **S85.899** Other specified injury of other blood vessels at lower leg level, unspecified leg

☑5ᵗʰ **S85.9** Injury of unspecified blood vessel at lower leg level

☑6ᵗʰ **S85.90** Unspecified injury of unspecified blood vessel at lower leg level

☑7ᵗʰ **S85.901** Unspecified injury of unspecified blood vessel at lower leg level, right leg

☑7ᵗʰ **S85.902** Unspecified injury of unspecified blood vessel at lower leg level, left leg

☑7ᵗʰ **S85.909** Unspecified injury of unspecified blood vessel at lower leg level, unspecified leg

☑6ᵗʰ **S85.91** Laceration of unspecified blood vessel at lower leg level

☑7ᵗʰ **S85.911** Laceration of unspecified blood vessel at lower leg level, right leg

☑7ᵗʰ **S85.912** Laceration of unspecified blood vessel at lower leg level, left leg

☑7ᵗʰ **S85.919** Laceration of unspecified blood vessel at lower leg level, unspecified leg

☑6ᵗʰ **S85.99** Other specified injury of unspecified blood vessel at lower leg level

☑7ᵗʰ **S85.991** Other specified injury of unspecified blood vessel at lower leg level, right leg

☑7ᵗʰ **S85.992** Other specified injury of unspecified blood vessel at lower leg level, left leg

☑7ᵗʰ **S85.999** Other specified injury of unspecified blood vessel at lower leg level, unspecified leg

☑4ᵗʰ **S86** **Injury of muscle, fascia and tendon at lower leg level**

Code also any associated open wound (S81-)

EXCLUDES 2 *injury of muscle, fascia and tendon at ankle (S96-)*
injury of patellar ligament (tendon) (S76.1-)
sprain of joints and ligaments of knee (S83-)

The appropriate 7th character is to be added to each code from category S86.
A   initial encounter
D   subsequent encounter
S   sequela

☑5ᵗʰ **S86.0** **Injury of Achilles tendon**

☑6ᵗʰ **S86.00** Unspecified injury of Achilles tendon

☑7ᵗʰ **S86.001** Unspecified injury of right Achilles tendon

☑7ᵗʰ **S86.002** Unspecified injury of left Achilles tendon

☑7ᵗʰ **S86.009** Unspecified injury of unspecified Achilles tendon

☑6ᵗʰ **S86.01** Strain of Achilles tendon

☑7ᵗʰ **S86.011** Strain of right Achilles tendon

☑7ᵗʰ **S86.012** Strain of left Achilles tendon

☑7ᵗʰ **S86.019** Strain of unspecified Achilles tendon

☑6ᵗʰ **S86.02** Laceration of Achilles tendon

☑7ᵗʰ **S86.021** Laceration of right Achilles tendon

☑7ᵗʰ **S86.022** Laceration of left Achilles tendon

☑7ᵗʰ **S86.029** Laceration of unspecified Achilles tendon

☑6ᵗʰ **S86.09** Other specified injury of Achilles tendon

☑7ᵗʰ **S86.091** Other specified injury of right Achilles tendon

☑7ᵗʰ **S86.092** Other specified injury of left Achilles tendon

☑7ᵗʰ **S86.099** Other specified injury of unspecified Achilles tendon

☑5ᵗʰ **S86.1** Injury of other muscle(s) and tendon(s) of posterior muscle group at lower leg level

☑6ᵗʰ **S86.10** Unspecified injury of other muscle(s) and tendon(s) of posterior muscle group at lower leg level

☑7ᵗʰ **S86.101** Unspecified injury of other muscle(s) and tendon(s) of posterior muscle group at lower leg level, right leg

☑7ᵗʰ **S86.102** Unspecified injury of other muscle(s) and tendon(s) of posterior muscle group at lower leg level, left leg

☑7ᵗʰ **S86.109** Unspecified injury of other muscle(s) and tendon(s) of posterior muscle group at lower leg level, unspecified leg

☑6ᵗʰ **S86.11** Strain of other muscle(s) and tendon(s) of posterior muscle group at lower leg level

☑7ᵗʰ **S86.111** Strain of other muscle(s) and tendon(s) of posterior muscle group at lower leg level, right leg

☑7ᵗʰ **S86.112** Strain of other muscle(s) and tendon(s) of posterior muscle group at lower leg level, left leg

☑7ᵗʰ **S86.119** Strain of other muscle(s) and tendon(s) of posterior muscle group at lower leg level, unspecified leg

☑6ᵗʰ **S86.12** Laceration of other muscle(s) and tendon(s) of posterior muscle group at lower leg level

☑7ᵗʰ **S86.121** Laceration of other muscle(s) and tendon(s) of posterior muscle group at lower leg level, right leg

☑7ᵗʰ **S86.122** Laceration of other muscle(s) and tendon(s) of posterior muscle group at lower leg level, left leg

☑7ᵗʰ **S86.129** Laceration of other muscle(s) and tendon(s) of posterior muscle group at lower leg level, unspecified leg

☑6ᵗʰ **S86.19** Other injury of other muscle(s) and tendon(s) of posterior muscle group at lower leg level

☑7ᵗʰ **S86.191** Other injury of other muscle(s) and tendon(s) of posterior muscle group at lower leg level, right leg

☑7ᵗʰ **S86.192** Other injury of other muscle(s) and tendon(s) of posterior muscle group at lower leg level, left leg

☑7ᵗʰ **S86.199** Other injury of other muscle(s) and tendon(s) of posterior muscle group at lower leg level, unspecified leg

☑5ᵗʰ **S86.2** Injury of muscle(s) and tendon(s) of anterior muscle group at lower leg level

☑6ᵗʰ **S86.20** Unspecified injury of muscle(s) and tendon(s) of anterior muscle group at lower leg level

☑7ᵗʰ **S86.201** Unspecified injury of muscle(s) and tendon(s) of anterior muscle group at lower leg level, right leg

☑7ᵗʰ **S86.202** Unspecified injury of muscle(s) and tendon(s) of anterior muscle group at lower leg level, left leg

☑7ᵗʰ **S86.209** Unspecified injury of muscle(s) and tendon(s) of anterior muscle group at lower leg level, unspecified leg

☑6ᵗʰ **S86.21** Strain of muscle(s) and tendon(s) of anterior muscle group at lower leg level

☑7ᵗʰ **S86.211** Strain of muscle(s) and tendon(s) of anterior muscle group at lower leg level, right leg

☑7ᵗʰ **S86.212** Strain of muscle(s) and tendon(s) of anterior muscle group at lower leg level, left leg

☑7ᵗʰ **S86.219** Strain of muscle(s) and tendon(s) of anterior muscle group at lower leg level, unspecified leg

☑ Appropriate additional character required   ☑x7ᵗʰ Requires 7th character, placeholder x must fill empty characters

√6ᵗʰ **S86.22** **Laceration of muscle(s) and tendon(s) of anterior muscle group at lower leg level**

√7ᵗʰ **S86.221** Laceration of muscle(s) and tendon(s) of anterior muscle group at lower leg level, right leg

√7ᵗʰ **S86.222** Laceration of muscle(s) and tendon(s) of anterior muscle group at lower leg level, left leg

√7ᵗʰ **S86.229** Laceration of muscle(s) and tendon(s) of anterior muscle group at lower leg level, unspecified leg

√6ᵗʰ **S86.29** **Other injury of muscle(s) and tendon(s) of anterior muscle group at lower leg level**

√7ᵗʰ **S86.291** Other injury of muscle(s) and tendon(s) of anterior muscle group at lower leg level, right leg

√7ᵗʰ **S86.292** Other injury of muscle(s) and tendon(s) of anterior muscle group at lower leg level, left leg

√7ᵗʰ **S86.299** Other injury of muscle(s) and tendon(s) of anterior muscle group at lower leg level, unspecified leg

√5ᵗʰ **S86.3** **Injury of muscle(s) and tendon(s) of peroneal muscle group at lower leg level**

√6ᵗʰ **S86.30** **Unspecified injury of muscle(s) and tendon(s) of peroneal muscle group at lower leg level**

√7ᵗʰ **S86.301** Unspecified injury of muscle(s) and tendon(s) of peroneal muscle group at lower leg level, right leg

√7ᵗʰ **S86.302** Unspecified injury of muscle(s) and tendon(s) of peroneal muscle group at lower leg level, left leg

√7ᵗʰ **S86.309** Unspecified injury of muscle(s) and tendon(s) of peroneal muscle group at lower leg level, unspecified leg

√6ᵗʰ **S86.31** **Strain of muscle(s) and tendon(s) of peroneal muscle group at lower leg level**

√7ᵗʰ **S86.311** Strain of muscle(s) and tendon(s) of peroneal muscle group at lower leg level, right leg

√7ᵗʰ **S86.312** Strain of muscle(s) and tendon(s) of peroneal muscle group at lower leg level, left leg

√7ᵗʰ **S86.319** Strain of muscle(s) and tendon(s) of peroneal muscle group at lower leg level, unspecified leg

√6ᵗʰ **S86.32** **Laceration of muscle(s) and tendon(s) of peroneal muscle group at lower leg level**

√7ᵗʰ **S86.321** Laceration of muscle(s) and tendon(s) of peroneal muscle group at lower leg level, right leg

√7ᵗʰ **S86.322** Laceration of muscle(s) and tendon(s) of peroneal muscle group at lower leg level, left leg

√7ᵗʰ **S86.329** Laceration of muscle(s) and tendon(s) of peroneal muscle group at lower leg level, unspecified leg

√6ᵗʰ **S86.39** **Other injury of muscle(s) and tendon(s) of peroneal muscle group at lower leg level**

√7ᵗʰ **S86.391** Other injury of muscle(s) and tendon(s) of peroneal muscle group at lower leg level, right leg

√7ᵗʰ **S86.392** Other injury of muscle(s) and tendon(s) of peroneal muscle group at lower leg level, left leg

√7ᵗʰ **S86.399** Other injury of muscle(s) and tendon(s) of peroneal muscle group at lower leg level, unspecified leg

√5ᵗʰ **S86.8** **Injury of other muscles and tendons at lower leg level**

√6ᵗʰ **S86.80** **Unspecified injury of other muscles and tendons at lower leg level**

√7ᵗʰ **S86.801** Unspecified injury of other muscle(s) and tendon(s) at lower leg level, right leg

√7ᵗʰ **S86.802** Unspecified injury of other muscle(s) and tendon(s) at lower leg level, left leg

√7ᵗʰ **S86.809** Unspecified injury of other muscle(s) and tendon(s) at lower leg level, unspecified leg

√6ᵗʰ **S86.81** **Strain of other muscles and tendons at lower leg level**

√7ᵗʰ **S86.811** Strain of other muscle(s) and tendon(s) at lower leg level, right leg

√7ᵗʰ **S86.812** Strain of other muscle(s) and tendon(s) at lower leg level, left leg

√7ᵗʰ **S86.819** Strain of other muscle(s) and tendon(s) at lower leg level, unspecified leg

√6ᵗʰ **S86.82** **Laceration of other muscles and tendons at lower leg level**

√7ᵗʰ **S86.821** Laceration of other muscle(s) and tendon(s) at lower leg level, right leg

√7ᵗʰ **S86.822** Laceration of other muscle(s) and tendon(s) at lower leg level, left leg

√7ᵗʰ **S86.829** Laceration of other muscle(s) and tendon(s) at lower leg level, unspecified leg

√6ᵗʰ **S86.89** **Other injury of other muscles and tendons at lower leg level**

√7ᵗʰ **S86.891** Other injury of other muscle(s) and tendon(s) at lower leg level, right leg

√7ᵗʰ **S86.892** Other injury of other muscle(s) and tendon(s) at lower leg level, left leg

√7ᵗʰ **S86.899** Other injury of other muscle(s) and tendon(s) at lower leg level, unspecified leg

√5ᵗʰ **S86.9** **Injury of unspecified muscle and tendon at lower leg level**

√6ᵗʰ **S86.90** **Unspecified injury of unspecified muscle and tendon at lower leg level**

√7ᵗʰ **S86.901** Unspecified injury of unspecified muscle(s) and tendon(s) at lower leg level, right leg

√7ᵗʰ **S86.902** Unspecified injury of unspecified muscle(s) and tendon(s) at lower leg level, left leg

√7ᵗʰ **S86.909** Unspecified injury of unspecified muscle(s) and tendon(s) at lower leg level, unspecified leg

√6ᵗʰ **S86.91** **Strain of unspecified muscle and tendon at lower leg level**

√7ᵗʰ **S86.911** Strain of unspecified muscle(s) and tendon(s) at lower leg level, right leg

√7ᵗʰ **S86.912** Strain of unspecified muscle(s) and tendon(s) at lower leg level, left leg

√7ᵗʰ **S86.919** Strain of unspecified muscle(s) and tendon(s) at lower leg level, unspecified leg

√6ᵗʰ **S86.92** **Laceration of unspecified muscle and tendon at lower leg level**

√7ᵗʰ **S86.921** Laceration of unspecified muscle(s) and tendon(s) at lower leg level, right leg

√7ᵗʰ **S86.922** Laceration of unspecified muscle(s) and tendon(s) at lower leg level, left leg

√7ᵗʰ **S86.929** Laceration of unspecified muscle(s) and tendon(s) at lower leg level, unspecified leg

√6ᵗʰ **S86.99** **Other injury of unspecified muscle and tendon at lower leg level**

√7ᵗʰ **S86.991** Other injury of unspecified muscle(s) and tendon(s) at lower leg level, right leg

√7ᵗʰ **S86.992** Other injury of unspecified muscle(s) and tendon(s) at lower leg level, left leg

√7ᵗʰ **S86.999** Other injury of unspecified muscle(s) and tendon(s) at lower leg level, unspecified leg

---

EXCLUDES 1 Not coded here   **EXCLUDES 2** Not included here   *Manifestation Code*

☑4th **S87 Crushing injury of lower leg**
Use additional code(s) for all associated injuries
EXCLUDES 2 *crushing injury of ankle and foot (S97-)*

> The appropriate 7th character is to be added to each code from category S87.
> A   initial encounter
> D   subsequent encounter
> S   sequela

☑5th **S87.0 Crushing injury of knee**
  ☑x7th **S87.00 Crushing injury of unspecified knee**
  ☑x7th **S87.01 Crushing injury of right knee**
  ☑x7th **S87.02 Crushing injury of left knee**

☑5th **S87.8 Crushing injury of lower leg**
  ☑x7th **S87.80 Crushing injury of unspecified lower leg**
  ☑x7th **S87.81 Crushing injury of right lower leg**
  ☑x7th **S87.82 Crushing injury of left lower leg**

☑4th **S88 Traumatic amputation of lower leg**
  NOTE   An amputation not identified and partial or complete should be coded to complete
  EXCLUDES 1 *traumatic amputation of ankle and foot (S98-)*

> The appropriate 7th character is to be added to each code from category S88.
> A   initial encounter
> D   subsequent encounter
> S   sequela

☑5th **S88.0 Traumatic amputation at knee level**
  ☑6th **S88.01 Complete traumatic amputation at knee level**
    ☑7th **S88.011 Complete traumatic amputation at knee level, right lower leg**
    ☑7th **S88.012 Complete traumatic amputation at knee level, left lower leg**
    ☑7th **S88.019 Complete traumatic amputation at knee level, unspecified lower leg**
  ☑6th **S88.02 Partial traumatic amputation at knee level**
    ☑7th **S88.021 Partial traumatic amputation at knee level, right lower leg**
    ☑7th **S88.022 Partial traumatic amputation at knee level, left lower leg**
    ☑7th **S88.029 Partial traumatic amputation at knee level, unspecified lower leg**

☑5th **S88.1 Traumatic amputation at level between knee and ankle**
  ☑6th **S88.11 Complete traumatic amputation at level between knee and ankle**
    ☑7th **S88.111 Complete traumatic amputation at level between knee and ankle, right lower leg**
    ☑7th **S88.112 Complete traumatic amputation at level between knee and ankle, left lower leg**
    ☑7th **S88.119 Complete traumatic amputation at level between knee and ankle, unspecified lower leg**
  ☑6th **S88.12 Partial traumatic amputation at level between knee and ankle**
    ☑7th **S88.121 Partial traumatic amputation at level between knee and ankle, right lower leg**
    ☑7th **S88.122 Partial traumatic amputation at level between knee and ankle, left lower leg**
    ☑7th **S88.129 Partial traumatic amputation at level between knee and ankle, unspecified lower leg**

☑5th **S88.9 Traumatic amputation of lower leg, level unspecified**
  ☑6th **S88.91 Complete traumatic amputation of lower leg, level unspecified**
    ☑7th **S88.911 Complete traumatic amputation of right lower leg, level unspecified**
    ☑7th **S88.912 Complete traumatic amputation of left lower leg, level unspecified**
    ☑7th **S88.919 Complete traumatic amputation of unspecified lower leg, level unspecified**
  ☑6th **S88.92 Partial traumatic amputation of lower leg, level unspecified**
    ☑7th **S88.921 Partial traumatic amputation of right lower leg, level unspecified**
    ☑7th **S88.922 Partial traumatic amputation of left lower leg, level unspecified**

    ☑7th **S88.929 Partial traumatic amputation of unspecified lower leg, level unspecified**

☑4th **S89 Other and unspecified injuries of lower leg**
  NOTE   A fracture not indicated as open or closed should be coded to closed.
  EXCLUDES 2 *other and unspecified injuries of ankle and foot (S99-)*

> The appropriate 7th character is to be added to each code from subcategories S89.0, S89.1, S89.2, and S89.3.
> A   initial encounter for closed fracture
> D   subsequent encounter for fracture with routine healing
> G   subsequent encounter for fracture with delayed healing
> K   subsequent encounter for fracture with nonunion
> P   subsequent encounter for fracture with malunion
> S   sequela

☑5th **S89.0 Physeal fracture of upper end of tibia**
  ☑6th **S89.00 Unspecified physeal fracture of upper end of tibia**
    ☑7th **S89.001 Unspecified physeal fracture of upper end of right tibia**
    ☑7th **S89.002 Unspecified physeal fracture of upper end of left tibia**
    ☑7th **S89.009 Unspecified physeal fracture of upper end of unspecified tibia**
  ☑6th **S89.01 Salter-Harris Type I physeal fracture of upper end of tibia**
    ☑7th **S89.011 Salter-Harris Type I physeal fracture of upper end of right tibia**
    ☑7th **S89.012 Salter-Harris Type I physeal fracture of upper end of left tibia**
    ☑7th **S89.019 Salter-Harris Type I physeal fracture of upper end of unspecified tibia**
  ☑6th **S89.02 Salter-Harris Type II physeal fracture of upper end of tibia**
    ☑7th **S89.021 Salter-Harris Type II physeal fracture of upper end of right tibia**
    ☑7th **S89.022 Salter-Harris Type II physeal fracture of upper end of left tibia**
    ☑7th **S89.029 Salter-Harris Type II physeal fracture of upper end of unspecified tibia**
  ☑6th **S89.03 Salter-Harris Type III physeal fracture of upper end of tibia**
    ☑7th **S89.031 Salter-Harris Type III physeal fracture of upper end of right tibia**
    ☑7th **S89.032 Salter-Harris Type III physeal fracture of upper end of left tibia**
    ☑7th **S89.039 Salter-Harris Type III physeal fracture of upper end of unspecified tibia**
  ☑6th **S89.04 Salter-Harris Type IV physeal fracture of upper end of tibia**
    ☑7th **S89.041 Salter-Harris Type IV physeal fracture of upper end of right tibia**
    ☑7th **S89.042 Salter-Harris Type IV physeal fracture of upper end of left tibia**
    ☑7th **S89.049 Salter-Harris Type IV physeal fracture of upper end of unspecified tibia**
  ☑6th **S89.09 Other physeal fracture of upper end of tibia**
    ☑7th **S89.091 Other physeal fracture of upper end of right tibia**
    ☑7th **S89.092 Other physeal fracture of upper end of left tibia**
    ☑7th **S89.099 Other physeal fracture of upper end of unspecified tibia**

☑5th **S89.1 Physeal fracture of lower end of tibia**
  ☑6th **S89.10 Unspecified physeal fracture of lower end of tibia**
    ☑7th **S89.101 Unspecified physeal fracture of lower end of right tibia**
    ☑7th **S89.102 Unspecified physeal fracture of lower end of left tibia**
    ☑7th **S89.109 Unspecified physeal fracture of lower end of unspecified tibia**
  ☑6th **S89.11 Salter-Harris Type I physeal fracture of ower end of tibia**
    ☑7th **S89.111 Salter-Harris Type I physeal fracture of lower end of right tibia**
    ☑7th **S89.112 Salter-Harris Type I physeal fracture of lower end of left tibia**

☑ Appropriate additional character required   ☑x7th Requires 7th character, placeholder x must fill empty characters

    ✓7ᵗʰ **S89.119** Salter-Harris Type I physeal fracture of lower end of unspecified tibia

   ✓6ᵗʰ **S89.12** Salter-Harris Type II physeal fracture of lower end of tibia

    ✓7ᵗʰ **S89.121** Salter-Harris Type II physeal fracture of lower end of right tibia

    ✓7ᵗʰ **S89.122** Salter-Harris Type II physeal fracture of lower end of left tibia

    ✓7ᵗʰ **S89.129** Salter-Harris Type II physeal fracture of lower end of unspecified tibia

   ✓6ᵗʰ **S89.13** Salter-Harris Type III physeal fracture of lower end of tibia

      EXCLUDES 1   *fracture of medial malleolus (adult) (S82.5-)*

    ✓7ᵗʰ **S89.131** Salter-Harris Type III physeal fracture of lower end of right tibia

    ✓7ᵗʰ **S89.132** Salter-Harris Type III physeal fracture of lower end of left tibia

    ✓7ᵗʰ **S89.139** Salter-Harris Type III physeal fracture of lower end of unspecified tibia

   ✓6ᵗʰ **S89.14** Salter-Harris Type IV physeal fracture of lower end of tibia

      EXCLUDES 1   *fracture of medial malleolus (adult) (S82.5-)*

    ✓7ᵗʰ **S89.141** Salter-Harris Type IV physeal fracture of lower end of right tibia

    ✓7ᵗʰ **S89.142** Salter-Harris Type IV physeal fracture of lower end of left tibia

    ✓7ᵗʰ **S89.149** Salter-Harris Type IV physeal fracture of lower end of unspecified tibia

   ✓6ᵗʰ **S89.19** Other physeal fracture of lower end of tibia

    ✓7ᵗʰ **S89.191** Other physeal fracture of lower end of right tibia

    ✓7ᵗʰ **S89.192** Other physeal fracture of lower end of left tibia

    ✓7ᵗʰ **S89.199** Other physeal fracture of lower end of unspecified tibia

  ✓5ᵗʰ **S89.2** Physeal fracture of upper end of fibula

   ✓6ᵗʰ **S89.20** Unspecified physeal fracture of upper end of fibula

    ✓7ᵗʰ **S89.201** Unspecified physeal fracture of upper end of right fibula

    ✓7ᵗʰ **S89.202** Unspecified physeal fracture of upper end of left fibula

    ✓7ᵗʰ **S89.209** Unspecified physeal fracture of upper end of unspecified fibula

   ✓6ᵗʰ **S89.21** Salter-Harris Type I physeal fracture of upper end of fibula

    ✓7ᵗʰ **S89.211** Salter-Harris Type I physeal fracture of upper end of right fibula

    ✓7ᵗʰ **S89.212** Salter-Harris Type I physeal fracture of upper end of left fibula

    ✓7ᵗʰ **S89.219** Salter-Harris Type I physeal fracture of upper end of unspecified fibula

   ✓6ᵗʰ **S89.22** Salter-Harris Type II physeal fracture of upper end of fibula

    ✓7ᵗʰ **S89.221** Salter-Harris Type II physeal fracture of upper end of right fibula

    ✓7ᵗʰ **S89.222** Salter-Harris Type II physeal fracture of upper end of left fibula

    ✓7ᵗʰ **S89.229** Salter-Harris Type II physeal fracture of upper end of unspecified fibula

   ✓6ᵗʰ **S89.29** Other physeal fracture of upper end of fibula

    ✓7ᵗʰ **S89.291** Other physeal fracture of upper end of right fibula

    ✓7ᵗʰ **S89.292** Other physeal fracture of upper end of left fibula

    ✓7ᵗʰ **S89.299** Other physeal fracture of upper end of unspecified fibula

  ✓5ᵗʰ **S89.3** Physeal fracture of lower end of fibula

   ✓6ᵗʰ **S89.30** Unspecified physeal fracture of lower end of fibula

    ✓7ᵗʰ **S89.301** Unspecified physeal fracture of lower end of right fibula

    ✓7ᵗʰ **S89.302** Unspecified physeal fracture of lower end of left fibula

    ✓7ᵗʰ **S89.309** Unspecified physeal fracture of lower end of unspecified fibula

   ✓6ᵗʰ **S89.31** Salter-Harris Type I physeal fracture of lower end of fibula

    ✓7ᵗʰ **S89.311** Salter-Harris Type I physeal fracture of lower end of right fibula

    ✓7ᵗʰ **S89.312** Salter-Harris Type I physeal fracture of lower end of left fibula

    ✓7ᵗʰ **S89.319** Salter-Harris Type I physeal fracture of lower end of unspecified fibula

   ✓6ᵗʰ **S89.32** Salter-Harris Type II physeal fracture of lower end of fibula

    ✓7ᵗʰ **S89.321** Salter-Harris Type II physeal fracture of lower end of right fibula

    ✓7ᵗʰ **S89.322** Salter-Harris Type II physeal fracture of lower end of left fibula

    ✓7ᵗʰ **S89.329** Salter-Harris Type II physeal fracture of lower end of unspecified fibula

   ✓6ᵗʰ **S89.39** Other physeal fracture of lower end of fibula

    ✓7ᵗʰ **S89.391** Other physeal fracture of lower end of right fibula

    ✓7ᵗʰ **S89.392** Other physeal fracture of lower end of left fibula

    ✓7ᵗʰ **S89.399** Other physeal fracture of lower end of unspecified fibula

  ✓5ᵗʰ **S89.8** Other specified injuries of lower leg

> The appropriate 7th character is to be added to each code from subcategory S89.8.
> A   initial encounter
> D   subsequent encounter
> S   sequela

   ✓x7ᵗʰ **S89.80** Other specified injuries of unspecified lower leg

   ✓x7ᵗʰ **S89.81** Other specified injuries of right lower leg

   ✓x7ᵗʰ **S89.82** Other specified injuries of left lower leg

  ✓5ᵗʰ **S89.9** Unspecified injury of lower leg

> The appropriate 7th character is to be added to each code from subcategory S89.9.
> A   initial encounter
> D   subsequent encounter
> S   sequela

   ✓x7ᵗʰ **S89.90** Unspecified injury of unspecified lower leg

   ✓x7ᵗʰ **S89.91** Unspecified injury of right lower leg

   ✓x7ᵗʰ **S89.92** Unspecified injury of left lower leg

Injuries to the ankle and foot (S90-S99)

EXCLUDES 2   *burns and corrosions (T20-T32)*
fracture of ankle and malleolus (S82-)
frostbite (T33-T34)
insect bite or sting, venomous (T63.4)

✓4ᵗʰ **S90 Superficial injury of ankle, foot and toes**

> The appropriate 7th character is to be added to each code from category S90.
> A   initial encounter
> D   subsequent encounter
> S   sequela

  ✓5ᵗʰ **S90.0** Contusion of ankle

   ✓x7ᵗʰ **S90.00** Contusion of unspecified ankle

   ✓x7ᵗʰ **S90.01** Contusion of right ankle

   ✓x7ᵗʰ **S90.02** Contusion of left ankle

  ✓5ᵗʰ **S90.1** Contusion of toe without damage to nail

   ✓6ᵗʰ **S90.11** Contusion of great toe without damage to nail

    ✓7ᵗʰ **S90.111** Contusion of right great toe without damage to nail

    ✓7ᵗʰ **S90.112** Contusion of left great toe without damage to nail

    ✓7ᵗʰ **S90.119** Contusion of unspecified great toe without damage to nail

   ✓6ᵗʰ **S90.12** Contusion of lesser toe without damage to nail

    ✓7ᵗʰ **S90.121** Contusion of right lesser toe(s) without damage to nail

    ✓7ᵗʰ **S90.122** Contusion of left lesser toe(s) without damage to nail

    ✓7ᵗʰ **S90.129** Contusion of unspecified lesser toe(s) without damage to nail
       Contusion of toe NOS

EXCLUDES 1   Not coded here   EXCLUDES 2   Not included here   *Manifestation Code*

☑5ᵗʰ S90.2 Contusion of toe with damage to nail

    ☑6ᵗʰ S90.21 Contusion of great toe with damage to nail

        √7ᵗʰ S90.211 Contusion of right great toe with damage to nail

        √7ᵗʰ S90.212 Contusion of left great toe with damage to nail

        √7ᵗʰ S90.219 Contusion of unspecified great toe with damage to nail

    ☑6ᵗʰ S90.22 Contusion of lesser toe with damage to nail

        √7ᵗʰ S90.221 Contusion of right lesser toe(s) with damage to nail

        √7ᵗʰ S90.222 Contusion of left lesser toe(s) with damage to nail

        √7ᵗʰ S90.229 Contusion of unspecified lesser toe(s) with damage to nail

☑5ᵗʰ S90.3 Contusion of foot

    EXCLUDES 2 contusion of toes (S90.1-, S90.2-)

    ☑x7ᵗʰ S90.30 Contusion of unspecified foot

        Contusion of foot NOS

    ☑x7ᵗʰ S90.31 Contusion of right foot

    ☑x7ᵗʰ S90.32 Contusion of left foot

☑5ᵗʰ S90.4 Other superficial injuries of toe

    ☑6ᵗʰ S90.41 Abrasion of toe

        √7ᵗʰ S90.411 Abrasion, right great toe

        √7ᵗʰ S90.412 Abrasion, left great toe

        √7ᵗʰ S90.413 Abrasion, unspecified great toe

        √7ᵗʰ S90.414 Abrasion, right lesser toe(s)

        √7ᵗʰ S90.415 Abrasion, left lesser toe(s)

        √7ᵗʰ S90.416 Abrasion, unspecified lesser toe(s)

    ☑6ᵗʰ S90.42 Blister (nonthermal) of toe

        √7ᵗʰ S90.421 Blister (nonthermal), right great toe

        √7ᵗʰ S90.422 Blister (nonthermal), left great toe

        √7ᵗʰ S90.423 Blister (nonthermal), unspecified great toe

        √7ᵗʰ S90.424 Blister (nonthermal), right lesser toe(s)

        √7ᵗʰ S90.425 Blister (nonthermal), left lesser toe(s)

        √7ᵗʰ S90.426 Blister (nonthermal), unspecified lesser toe(s)

    ☑6ᵗʰ S90.44 External constriction of toe

        Hair tourniquet syndrome of toe

        √7ᵗʰ S90.441 External constriction, right great toe

        √7ᵗʰ S90.442 External constriction, left great toe

        √7ᵗʰ S90.443 External constriction, unspecified great toe

        √7ᵗʰ S90.444 External constriction, right lesser toe(s)

        √7ᵗʰ S90.445 External constriction, left lesser toe(s)

        √7ᵗʰ S90.446 External constriction, unspecified lesser toe(s)

    ☑6ᵗʰ S90.45 Superficial foreign body of toe

        Splinter in the toe

        √7ᵗʰ S90.451 Superficial foreign body, right great toe

        √7ᵗʰ S90.452 Superficial foreign body, left great toe

        √7ᵗʰ S90.453 Superficial foreign body, unspecified great toe

        √7ᵗʰ S90.454 Superficial foreign body, right lesser toe(s)

        √7ᵗʰ S90.455 Superficial foreign body, left lesser toe(s)

        √7ᵗʰ S90.456 Superficial foreign body, unspecified lesser toe(s)

    ☑6ᵗʰ S90.46 Insect bite (nonvenomous) of toe

        √7ᵗʰ S90.461 Insect bite (nonvenomous), right great toe

        √7ᵗʰ S90.462 Insect bite (nonvenomous), left great toe

        √7ᵗʰ S90.463 Insect bite (nonvenomous), unspecified great toe

        √7ᵗʰ S90.464 Insect bite (nonvenomous), right lesser toe(s)

        √7ᵗʰ S90.465 Insect bite (nonvenomous), left lesser toe(s)

        √7ᵗʰ S90.466 Insect bite (nonvenomous), unspecified lesser toe(s)

☑6ᵗʰ S90.47 Other superficial bite of toe

    EXCLUDES 1 open bite of toe (S91.15-, S91.25-)

    √7ᵗʰ S90.471 Other superficial bite of right great toe

    √7ᵗʰ S90.472 Other superficial bite of left great toe

    √7ᵗʰ S90.473 Other superficial bite of unspecified great toe

    √7ᵗʰ S90.474 Other superficial bite of right lesser toe(s)

    √7ᵗʰ S90.475 Other superficial bite of left lesser toe(s)

    √7ᵗʰ S90.476 Other superficial bite of unspecified lesser toe(s)

☑5ᵗʰ S90.5 Other superficial injuries of ankle

    ☑6ᵗʰ S90.51 Abrasion of ankle

        √7ᵗʰ S90.511 Abrasion, right ankle

        √7ᵗʰ S90.512 Abrasion, left ankle

        √7ᵗʰ S90.519 Abrasion, unspecified ankle

    ☑6ᵗʰ S90.52 Blister (nonthermal) of ankle

        √7ᵗʰ S90.521 Blister (nonthermal), right ankle

        √7ᵗʰ S90.522 Blister (nonthermal), left ankle

        √7ᵗʰ S90.529 Blister (nonthermal), unspecified ankle

    ☑6ᵗʰ S90.54 External constriction of ankle

        √7ᵗʰ S90.541 External constriction, right ankle

        √7ᵗʰ S90.542 External constriction, left ankle

        √7ᵗʰ S90.549 External constriction, unspecified ankle

    ☑6ᵗʰ S90.55 Superficial foreign body of ankle

        Splinter in the ankle

        √7ᵗʰ S90.551 Superficial foreign body, right ankle

        √7ᵗʰ S90.552 Superficial foreign body, left ankle

        √7ᵗʰ S90.559 Superficial foreign body, unspecified ankle

    ☑6ᵗʰ S90.56 Insect bite (nonvenomous) of ankle

        √7ᵗʰ S90.561 Insect bite (nonvenomous), right ankle

        √7ᵗʰ S90.562 Insect bite (nonvenomous), left ankle

        √7ᵗʰ S90.569 Insect bite (nonvenomous), unspecified ankle

    ☑6ᵗʰ S90.57 Other superficial bite of ankle

        EXCLUDES 1 open bite of ankle (S91.05-)

        √7ᵗʰ S90.571 Other superficial bite of ankle, right ankle

        √7ᵗʰ S90.572 Other superficial bite of ankle, left ankle

        √7ᵗʰ S90.579 Other superficial bite of ankle, unspecified ankle

☑5ᵗʰ S90.8 Other superficial injuries of foot

    ☑6ᵗʰ S90.81 Abrasion of foot

        √7ᵗʰ S90.811 Abrasion, right foot

        √7ᵗʰ S90.812 Abrasion, left foot

        √7ᵗʰ S90.819 Abrasion, unspecified foot

    ☑6ᵗʰ S90.82 Blister (nonthermal) of foot

        √7ᵗʰ S90.821 Blister (nonthermal), right foot

        √7ᵗʰ S90.822 Blister (nonthermal), left foot

        √7ᵗʰ S90.829 Blister (nonthermal), unspecified foot

    ☑6ᵗʰ S90.84 External constriction of foot

        √7ᵗʰ S90.841 External constriction, right foot

        √7ᵗʰ S90.842 External constriction, left foot

        √7ᵗʰ S90.849 External constriction, unspecified foot

    ☑6ᵗʰ S90.85 Superficial foreign body of foot

        Splinter in the foot

        √7ᵗʰ S90.851 Superficial foreign body, right foot

        √7ᵗʰ S90.852 Superficial foreign body, left foot

        √7ᵗʰ S90.859 Superficial foreign body, unspecified foot

    ☑6ᵗʰ S90.86 Insect bite (nonvenomous) of foot

        √7ᵗʰ S90.861 Insect bite (nonvenomous), right foot

        √7ᵗʰ S90.862 Insect bite (nonvenomous), left foot

        √7ᵗʰ S90.869 Insect bite (nonvenomous), unspecified foot

    ☑6ᵗʰ S90.87 Other superficial bite of foot

        EXCLUDES 1 open bite of foot (S91.35-)

        √7ᵗʰ S90.871 Other superficial bite of right foot

        √7ᵗʰ S90.872 Other superficial bite of left foot

        √7ᵗʰ S90.879 Other superficial bite of unspecified foot

---

☑ Appropriate additional character required   √x7ᵗʰ Requires 7th character, placeholder x must fill empty characters

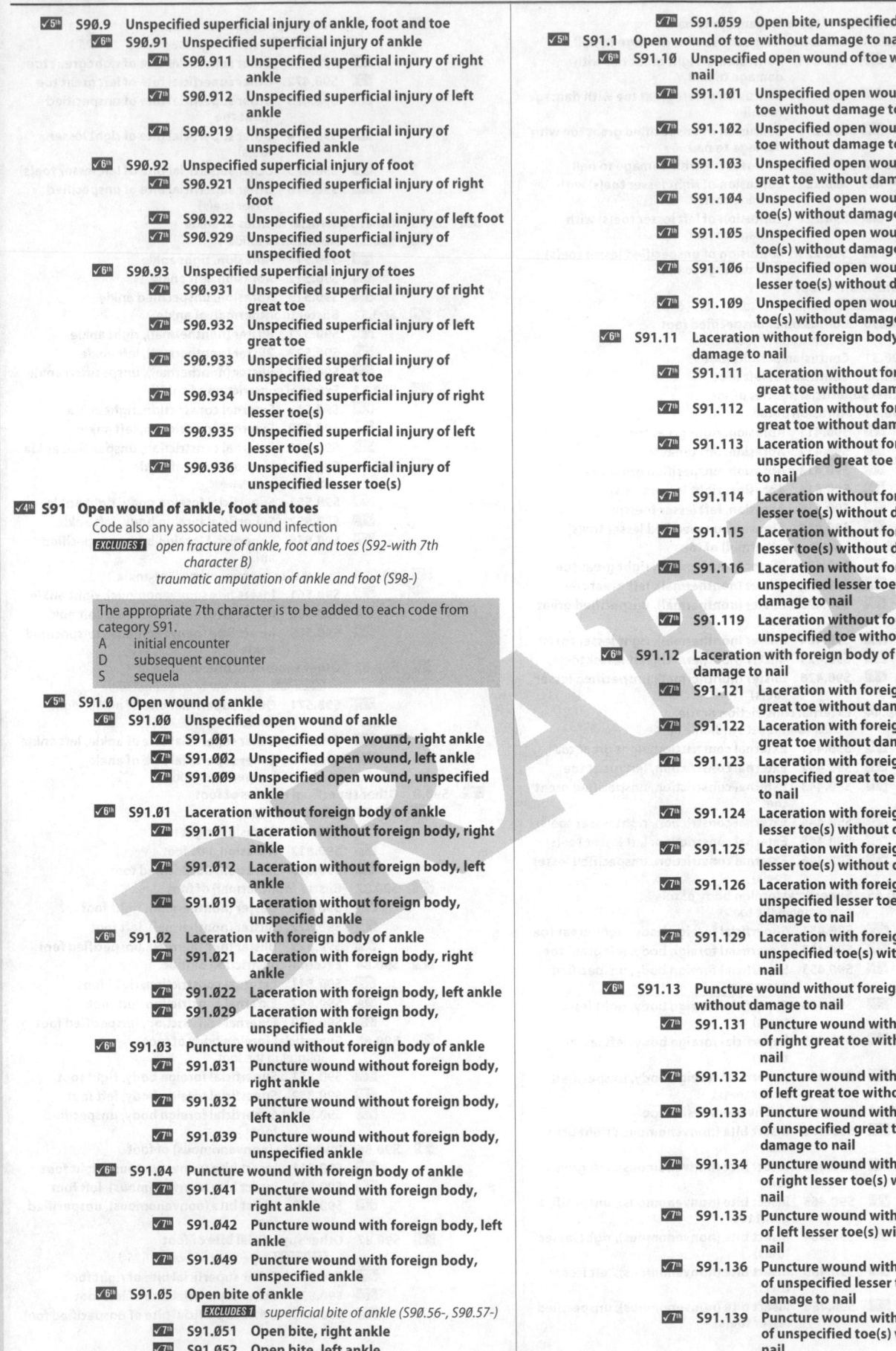

✓5ᵗʰ **S90.9 Unspecified superficial injury of ankle, foot and toe**
- ✓6ᵗʰ **S90.91 Unspecified superficial injury of ankle**
  - ✓7ᵗʰ **S90.911 Unspecified superficial injury of right ankle**
  - ✓7ᵗʰ **S90.912 Unspecified superficial injury of left ankle**
  - ✓7ᵗʰ **S90.919 Unspecified superficial injury of unspecified ankle**
- ✓6ᵗʰ **S90.92 Unspecified superficial injury of foot**
  - ✓7ᵗʰ **S90.921 Unspecified superficial injury of right foot**
  - ✓7ᵗʰ **S90.922 Unspecified superficial injury of left foot**
  - ✓7ᵗʰ **S90.929 Unspecified superficial injury of unspecified foot**
- ✓6ᵗʰ **S90.93 Unspecified superficial injury of toes**
  - ✓7ᵗʰ **S90.931 Unspecified superficial injury of right great toe**
  - ✓7ᵗʰ **S90.932 Unspecified superficial injury of left great toe**
  - ✓7ᵗʰ **S90.933 Unspecified superficial injury of unspecified great toe**
  - ✓7ᵗʰ **S90.934 Unspecified superficial injury of right lesser toe(s)**
  - ✓7ᵗʰ **S90.935 Unspecified superficial injury of left lesser toe(s)**
  - ✓7ᵗʰ **S90.936 Unspecified superficial injury of unspecified lesser toe(s)**

✓4ᵗʰ **S91 Open wound of ankle, foot and toes**
    Code also any associated wound infection
    EXCLUDES 1 *open fracture of ankle, foot and toes (S92-with 7th character B)*
                traumatic amputation of ankle and foot (S98-)

> The appropriate 7th character is to be added to each code from category S91.
> A   initial encounter
> D   subsequent encounter
> S   sequela

- ✓5ᵗʰ **S91.0 Open wound of ankle**
  - ✓6ᵗʰ **S91.00 Unspecified open wound of ankle**
    - ✓7ᵗʰ **S91.001 Unspecified open wound, right ankle**
    - ✓7ᵗʰ **S91.002 Unspecified open wound, left ankle**
    - ✓7ᵗʰ **S91.009 Unspecified open wound, unspecified ankle**
  - ✓6ᵗʰ **S91.01 Laceration without foreign body of ankle**
    - ✓7ᵗʰ **S91.011 Laceration without foreign body, right ankle**
    - ✓7ᵗʰ **S91.012 Laceration without foreign body, left ankle**
    - ✓7ᵗʰ **S91.019 Laceration without foreign body, unspecified ankle**
  - ✓6ᵗʰ **S91.02 Laceration with foreign body of ankle**
    - ✓7ᵗʰ **S91.021 Laceration with foreign body, right ankle**
    - ✓7ᵗʰ **S91.022 Laceration with foreign body, left ankle**
    - ✓7ᵗʰ **S91.029 Laceration with foreign body, unspecified ankle**
  - ✓6ᵗʰ **S91.03 Puncture wound without foreign body of ankle**
    - ✓7ᵗʰ **S91.031 Puncture wound without foreign body, right ankle**
    - ✓7ᵗʰ **S91.032 Puncture wound without foreign body, left ankle**
    - ✓7ᵗʰ **S91.039 Puncture wound without foreign body, unspecified ankle**
  - ✓6ᵗʰ **S91.04 Puncture wound with foreign body of ankle**
    - ✓7ᵗʰ **S91.041 Puncture wound with foreign body, right ankle**
    - ✓7ᵗʰ **S91.042 Puncture wound with foreign body, left ankle**
    - ✓7ᵗʰ **S91.049 Puncture wound with foreign body, unspecified ankle**
  - ✓6ᵗʰ **S91.05 Open bite of ankle**
    - **EXCLUDES 1** *superficial bite of ankle (S90.56-, S90.57-)*
    - ✓7ᵗʰ **S91.051 Open bite, right ankle**
    - ✓7ᵗʰ **S91.052 Open bite, left ankle**
    - ✓7ᵗʰ **S91.059 Open bite, unspecified ankle**

- ✓5ᵗʰ **S91.1 Open wound of toe without damage to nail**
  - ✓6ᵗʰ **S91.10 Unspecified open wound of toe without damage to nail**
    - ✓7ᵗʰ **S91.101 Unspecified open wound of right great toe without damage to nail**
    - ✓7ᵗʰ **S91.102 Unspecified open wound of left great toe without damage to nail**
    - ✓7ᵗʰ **S91.103 Unspecified open wound of unspecified great toe without damage to nail**
    - ✓7ᵗʰ **S91.104 Unspecified open wound of right lesser toe(s) without damage to nail**
    - ✓7ᵗʰ **S91.105 Unspecified open wound of left lesser toe(s) without damage to nail**
    - ✓7ᵗʰ **S91.106 Unspecified open wound of unspecified lesser toe(s) without damage to nail**
    - ✓7ᵗʰ **S91.109 Unspecified open wound of unspecified toe(s) without damage to nail**
  - ✓6ᵗʰ **S91.11 Laceration without foreign body of toe without damage to nail**
    - ✓7ᵗʰ **S91.111 Laceration without foreign body of right great toe without damage to nail**
    - ✓7ᵗʰ **S91.112 Laceration without foreign body of left great toe without damage to nail**
    - ✓7ᵗʰ **S91.113 Laceration without foreign body of unspecified great toe without damage to nail**
    - ✓7ᵗʰ **S91.114 Laceration without foreign body of right lesser toe(s) without damage to nail**
    - ✓7ᵗʰ **S91.115 Laceration without foreign body of left lesser toe(s) without damage to nail**
    - ✓7ᵗʰ **S91.116 Laceration without foreign body of unspecified lesser toe(s) without damage to nail**
    - ✓7ᵗʰ **S91.119 Laceration without foreign body of unspecified toe without damage to nail**
  - ✓6ᵗʰ **S91.12 Laceration with foreign body of toe without damage to nail**
    - ✓7ᵗʰ **S91.121 Laceration with foreign body of right great toe without damage to nail**
    - ✓7ᵗʰ **S91.122 Laceration with foreign body of left great toe without damage to nail**
    - ✓7ᵗʰ **S91.123 Laceration with foreign body of unspecified great toe without damage to nail**
    - ✓7ᵗʰ **S91.124 Laceration with foreign body of right lesser toe(s) without damage to nail**
    - ✓7ᵗʰ **S91.125 Laceration with foreign body of left lesser toe(s) without damage to nail**
    - ✓7ᵗʰ **S91.126 Laceration with foreign body of unspecified lesser toe(s) without damage to nail**
    - ✓7ᵗʰ **S91.129 Laceration with foreign body of unspecified toe(s) without damage to nail**
  - ✓6ᵗʰ **S91.13 Puncture wound without foreign body of toe without damage to nail**
    - ✓7ᵗʰ **S91.131 Puncture wound without foreign body of right great toe without damage to nail**
    - ✓7ᵗʰ **S91.132 Puncture wound without foreign body of left great toe without damage to nail**
    - ✓7ᵗʰ **S91.133 Puncture wound without foreign body of unspecified great toe without damage to nail**
    - ✓7ᵗʰ **S91.134 Puncture wound without foreign body of right lesser toe(s) without damage to nail**
    - ✓7ᵗʰ **S91.135 Puncture wound without foreign body of left lesser toe(s) without damage to nail**
    - ✓7ᵗʰ **S91.136 Puncture wound without foreign body of unspecified lesser toe(s) without damage to nail**
    - ✓7ᵗʰ **S91.139 Puncture wound without foreign body of unspecified toe(s) without damage to nail**

✓6ᵗʰ **S91.14** **Puncture wound with foreign body of toe without damage to nail**

✓7ᵗʰ **S91.141** Puncture wound with foreign body of right great toe without damage to nail

✓7ᵗʰ **S91.142** Puncture wound with foreign body of left great toe without damage to nail

✓7ᵗʰ **S91.143** Puncture wound with foreign body of unspecified great toe without damage to nail

✓7ᵗʰ **S91.144** Puncture wound with foreign body of right lesser toe(s) without damage to nail

✓7ᵗʰ **S91.145** Puncture wound with foreign body of left lesser toe(s) without damage to nail

✓7ᵗʰ **S91.146** Puncture wound with foreign body of unspecified lesser toe(s) without damage to nail

✓7ᵗʰ **S91.149** Puncture wound with foreign body of unspecified toe(s) without damage to nail

✓6ᵗʰ **S91.15** **Open bite of toe without damage to nail**
Bite of toe NOS
EXCLUDES 1 *superficial bite of toe (S90.46-, S90.47-)*

✓7ᵗʰ **S91.151** Open bite of right great toe without damage to nail

✓7ᵗʰ **S91.152** Open bite of left great toe without damage to nail

✓7ᵗʰ **S91.153** Open bite of unspecified great toe without damage to nail

✓7ᵗʰ **S91.154** Open bite of right lesser toe(s) without damage to nail

✓7ᵗʰ **S91.155** Open bite of left lesser toe(s) without damage to nail

✓7ᵗʰ **S91.156** Open bite of unspecified lesser toe(s) without damage to nail

✓7ᵗʰ **S91.159** Open bite of unspecified toe(s) without damage to nail

✓5ᵗʰ **S91.2** **Open wound of toe with damage to nail**

✓6ᵗʰ **S91.20** **Unspecified open wound of toe with damage to nail**

✓7ᵗʰ **S91.201** Unspecified open wound of right great toe with damage to nail

✓7ᵗʰ **S91.202** Unspecified open wound of left great toe with damage to nail

✓7ᵗʰ **S91.203** Unspecified open wound of unspecified great toe with damage to nail

✓7ᵗʰ **S91.204** Unspecified open wound of right lesser toe(s) with damage to nail

✓7ᵗʰ **S91.205** Unspecified open wound of left lesser toe(s) with damage to nail

✓7ᵗʰ **S91.206** Unspecified open wound of unspecified lesser toe(s) with damage to nail

✓7ᵗʰ **S91.209** Unspecified open wound of unspecified toe(s) with damage to nail

✓6ᵗʰ **S91.21** **Laceration without foreign body of toe with damage to nail**

✓7ᵗʰ **S91.211** Laceration without foreign body of right great toe with damage to nail

✓7ᵗʰ **S91.212** Laceration without foreign body of left great toe with damage to nail

✓7ᵗʰ **S91.213** Laceration without foreign body of unspecified great toe with damage to nail

✓7ᵗʰ **S91.214** Laceration without foreign body of right lesser toe(s) with damage to nail

✓7ᵗʰ **S91.215** Laceration without foreign body of left lesser toe(s) with damage to nail

✓7ᵗʰ **S91.216** Laceration without foreign body of unspecified lesser toe(s) with damage to nail

✓7ᵗʰ **S91.219** Laceration without foreign body of unspecified toe(s) with damage to nail

✓6ᵗʰ **S91.22** **Laceration with foreign body of toe with damage to nail**

✓7ᵗʰ **S91.221** Laceration with foreign body of right great toe with damage to nail

✓7ᵗʰ **S91.222** Laceration with foreign body of left great toe with damage to nail

✓7ᵗʰ **S91.223** Laceration with foreign body of unspecified great toe with damage to nail

✓7ᵗʰ **S91.224** Laceration with foreign body of right lesser toe(s) with damage to nail

✓7ᵗʰ **S91.225** Laceration with foreign body of left lesser toe(s) with damage to nail

✓7ᵗʰ **S91.226** Laceration with foreign body of unspecified lesser toe(s) with damage to nail

✓7ᵗʰ **S91.229** Laceration with foreign body of unspecified toe(s) with damage to nail

✓6ᵗʰ **S91.23** **Puncture wound without foreign body of toe with damage to nail**

✓7ᵗʰ **S91.231** Puncture wound without foreign body of right great toe with damage to nail

✓7ᵗʰ **S91.232** Puncture wound without foreign body of left great toe with damage to nail

✓7ᵗʰ **S91.233** Puncture wound without foreign body of unspecified great toe with damage to nail

✓7ᵗʰ **S91.234** Puncture wound without foreign body of right lesser toe(s) with damage to nail

✓7ᵗʰ **S91.235** Puncture wound without foreign body of left lesser toe(s) with damage to nail

✓7ᵗʰ **S91.236** Puncture wound without foreign body of unspecified lesser toe(s) with damage to nail

✓7ᵗʰ **S91.239** Puncture wound without foreign body of unspecified toe(s) with damage to nail

✓6ᵗʰ **S91.24** **Puncture wound with foreign body of toe with damage to nail**

✓7ᵗʰ **S91.241** Puncture wound with foreign body of right great toe with damage to nail

✓7ᵗʰ **S91.242** Puncture wound with foreign body of left great toe with damage to nail

✓7ᵗʰ **S91.243** Puncture wound with foreign body of unspecified great toe with damage to nail

✓7ᵗʰ **S91.244** Puncture wound with foreign body of right lesser toe(s) with damage to nail

✓7ᵗʰ **S91.245** Puncture wound with foreign body of left lesser toe(s) with damage to nail

✓7ᵗʰ **S91.246** Puncture wound with foreign body of unspecified lesser toe(s) with damage to nail

✓7ᵗʰ **S91.249** Puncture wound with foreign body of unspecified toe(s) with damage to nail

✓6ᵗʰ **S91.25** **Open bite of toe with damage to nail**
Bite of toe with damage to nail NOS
EXCLUDES 1 *superficial bite of toe (S90.46-, S90.47-)*

✓7ᵗʰ **S91.251** Open bite of right great toe with damage to nail

✓7ᵗʰ **S91.252** Open bite of left great toe with damage to nail

✓7ᵗʰ **S91.253** Open bite of unspecified great toe with damage to nail

✓7ᵗʰ **S91.254** Open bite of right lesser toe(s) with damage to nail

✓7ᵗʰ **S91.255** Open bite of left lesser toe(s) with damage to nail

✓7ᵗʰ **S91.256** Open bite of unspecified lesser toe(s) with damage to nail

✓7ᵗʰ **S91.259** Open bite of unspecified toe(s) with damage to nail

✓5ᵗʰ **S91.3** **Open wound of foot**

✓6ᵗʰ **S91.30** **Unspecified open wound of foot**

✓7ᵗʰ **S91.301** Unspecified open wound, right foot

✓7ᵗʰ **S91.302** Unspecified open wound, left foot

✓7ᵗʰ **S91.309** Unspecified open wound, unspecified foot

✓6ᵗʰ **S91.31** **Laceration without foreign body of foot**

✓7ᵗʰ **S91.311** Laceration without foreign body, right foot

☑ Appropriate additional character required   ✓x7ᵗʰ Requires 7th character, placeholder x must fill empty characters

√7ᵗʰ **S91.312** Laceration without foreign body, left foot

√7ᵗʰ **S91.319** Laceration without foreign body, unspecified foot

√6ᵗʰ **S91.32** Laceration with foreign body of foot

√7ᵗʰ **S91.321** Laceration with foreign body, right foot

√7ᵗʰ **S91.322** Laceration with foreign body, left foot

√7ᵗʰ **S91.329** Laceration with foreign body, unspecified foot

√6ᵗʰ **S91.33** Puncture wound without foreign body of foot

√7ᵗʰ **S91.331** Puncture wound without foreign body, right foot

√7ᵗʰ **S91.332** Puncture wound without foreign body, left foot

√7ᵗʰ **S91.339** Puncture wound without foreign body, unspecified foot

√6ᵗʰ **S91.34** Puncture wound with foreign body of foot

√7ᵗʰ **S91.341** Puncture wound with foreign body, right foot

√7ᵗʰ **S91.342** Puncture wound with foreign body, left foot

√7ᵗʰ **S91.349** Puncture wound with foreign body, unspecified foot

√6ᵗʰ **S91.35** Open bite of foot

    EXCLUDES 1   *superficial bite of foot (S90.86-, S90.87-)*

√7ᵗʰ **S91.351** Open bite, right foot

√7ᵗʰ **S91.352** Open bite, left foot

√7ᵗʰ **S91.359** Open bite, unspecified foot

√4ᵗʰ **S92** **Fracture of foot and toe, except ankle**

    NOTE   A fracture not indicated as displaced or nondisplaced should be coded to displaced

       A fracture not indicated as open or closed should be coded to closed.

    EXCLUDES 1   *traumatic amputation of ankle and foot (S98-)*

    EXCLUDES 2   *fracture of ankle (S82-)*

           fracture of malleolus (S82-)

The appropriate 7th character is to be added to each code from category S92.

A   initial encounter for closed fracture

B   initial encounter for open fracture

D   subsequent encounter for fracture with routine healing

G   subsequent encounter for fracture with delayed healing

K   subsequent encounter for fracture with nonunion

P   subsequent encounter for fracture with malunion

S   sequela

√5ᵗʰ **S92.0** **Fracture of calcaneus**

    Heel bone

    Os calcis

√6ᵗʰ **S92.00** Unspecified fracture of calcaneus

√7ᵗʰ **S92.001** Unspecified fracture of right calcaneus

√7ᵗʰ **S92.002** Unspecified fracture of left calcaneus

√7ᵗʰ **S92.009** Unspecified fracture of unspecified calcaneus

√6ᵗʰ **S92.01** Fracture of body of calcaneus

√7ᵗʰ **S92.011** Displaced fracture of body of right calcaneus

√7ᵗʰ **S92.012** Displaced fracture of body of left calcaneus

√7ᵗʰ **S92.013** Displaced fracture of body of unspecified calcaneus

√7ᵗʰ **S92.014** Nondisplaced fracture of body of right calcaneus

√7ᵗʰ **S92.015** Nondisplaced fracture of body of left calcaneus

√7ᵗʰ **S92.016** Nondisplaced fracture of body of unspecified calcaneus

√6ᵗʰ **S92.02** Fracture of anterior process of calcaneus

√7ᵗʰ **S92.021** Displaced fracture of anterior process of right calcaneus

√7ᵗʰ **S92.022** Displaced fracture of anterior process of left calcaneus

√7ᵗʰ **S92.023** Displaced fracture of anterior process of unspecified calcaneus

√7ᵗʰ **S92.024** Nondisplaced fracture of anterior process of right calcaneus

√7ᵗʰ **S92.025** Nondisplaced fracture of anterior process of left calcaneus

√7ᵗʰ **S92.026** Nondisplaced fracture of anterior process of unspecified calcaneus

√6ᵗʰ **S92.03** Avulsion fracture of tuberosity of calcaneus

√7ᵗʰ **S92.031** Displaced avulsion fracture of tuberosity of right calcaneus

√7ᵗʰ **S92.032** Displaced avulsion fracture of tuberosity of left calcaneus

√7ᵗʰ **S92.033** Displaced avulsion fracture of tuberosity of unspecified calcaneus

√7ᵗʰ **S92.034** Nondisplaced avulsion fracture of tuberosity of right calcaneus

√7ᵗʰ **S92.035** Nondisplaced avulsion fracture of tuberosity of left calcaneus

√7ᵗʰ **S92.036** Nondisplaced avulsion fracture of tuberosity of unspecified calcaneus

√6ᵗʰ **S92.04** Other fracture of tuberosity of calcaneus

√7ᵗʰ **S92.041** Displaced other fracture of tuberosity of right calcaneus

√7ᵗʰ **S92.042** Displaced other fracture of tuberosity of left calcaneus

√7ᵗʰ **S92.043** Displaced other fracture of tuberosity of unspecified calcaneus

√7ᵗʰ **S92.044** Nondisplaced other fracture of tuberosity of right calcaneus

√7ᵗʰ **S92.045** Nondisplaced other fracture of tuberosity of left calcaneus

√7ᵗʰ **S92.046** Nondisplaced other fracture of tuberosity of unspecified calcaneus

√6ᵗʰ **S92.05** Other extraarticular fracture of calcaneus

√7ᵗʰ **S92.051** Displaced other extraarticular fracture of right calcaneus

√7ᵗʰ **S92.052** Displaced other extraarticular fracture of left calcaneus

√7ᵗʰ **S92.053** Displaced other extraarticular fracture of unspecified calcaneus

√7ᵗʰ **S92.054** Nondisplaced other extraarticular fracture of right calcaneus

√7ᵗʰ **S92.055** Nondisplaced other extraarticular fracture of left calcaneus

√7ᵗʰ **S92.056** Nondisplaced other extraarticular fracture of unspecified calcaneus

√6ᵗʰ **S92.06** Intraarticular fracture of calcaneus

√7ᵗʰ **S92.061** Displaced intraarticular fracture of right calcaneus

√7ᵗʰ **S92.062** Displaced intraarticular fracture of left calcaneus

√7ᵗʰ **S92.063** Displaced intraarticular fracture of unspecified calcaneus

√7ᵗʰ **S92.064** Nondisplaced intraarticular fracture of right calcaneus

√7ᵗʰ **S92.065** Nondisplaced intraarticular fracture of left calcaneus

√7ᵗʰ **S92.066** Nondisplaced intraarticular fracture of unspecified calcaneus

√5ᵗʰ **S92.1** **Fracture of talus**

    Astragalus

√6ᵗʰ **S92.10** Unspecified fracture of talus

√7ᵗʰ **S92.101** Unspecified fracture of right talus

√7ᵗʰ **S92.102** Unspecified fracture of left talus

√7ᵗʰ **S92.109** Unspecified fracture of unspecified talus

√6ᵗʰ **S92.11** Fracture of neck of talus

√7ᵗʰ **S92.111** Displaced fracture of neck of right talus

√7ᵗʰ **S92.112** Displaced fracture of neck of left talus

√7ᵗʰ **S92.113** Displaced fracture of neck of unspecified talus

√7ᵗʰ **S92.114** Nondisplaced fracture of neck of right talus

√7ᵗʰ **S92.115** Nondisplaced fracture of neck of left talus

√7ᵗʰ **S92.116** Nondisplaced fracture of neck of unspecified talus

√6ᵗʰ **S92.12** Fracture of body of talus

√7ᵗʰ **S92.121** Displaced fracture of body of right talus

√7ᵗʰ **S92.122** Displaced fracture of body of left talus

√7ᵗʰ **S92.123** Displaced fracture of body of unspecified talus

√7ᵗʰ **S92.124** Nondisplaced fracture of body of right talus

√7ᵗʰ **S92.125** Nondisplaced fracture of body of left talus

√7ᵗʰ **S92.126** Nondisplaced fracture of body of unspecified talus

√6ᵗʰ **S92.13** Fracture of posterior process of talus

√7ᵗʰ **S92.131** Displaced fracture of posterior process of right talus

√7ᵗʰ **S92.132** Displaced fracture of posterior process of left talus

√7ᵗʰ **S92.133** Displaced fracture of posterior process of unspecified talus

√7ᵗʰ **S92.134** Nondisplaced fracture of posterior process of right talus

√7ᵗʰ **S92.135** Nondisplaced fracture of posterior process of left talus

√7ᵗʰ **S92.136** Nondisplaced fracture of posterior process of unspecified talus

√6ᵗʰ **S92.14** Dome fracture of talus

> EXCLUDES 1 *osteochondritis dissecans (M93.2)*

√7ᵗʰ **S92.141** Displaced dome fracture of right talus

√7ᵗʰ **S92.142** Displaced dome fracture of left talus

√7ᵗʰ **S92.143** Displaced dome fracture of unspecified talus

√7ᵗʰ **S92.144** Nondisplaced dome fracture of right talus

√7ᵗʰ **S92.145** Nondisplaced dome fracture of left talus

√7ᵗʰ **S92.146** Nondisplaced dome fracture of unspecified talus

√6ᵗʰ **S92.15** Avulsion fracture (chip fracture) of talus

√7ᵗʰ **S92.151** Displaced avulsion fracture (chip fracture) of right talus

√7ᵗʰ **S92.152** Displaced avulsion fracture (chip fracture) of left talus

√7ᵗʰ **S92.153** Displaced avulsion fracture (chip fracture) of unspecified talus

√7ᵗʰ **S92.154** Nondisplaced avulsion fracture (chip fracture) of right talus

√7ᵗʰ **S92.155** Nondisplaced avulsion fracture (chip fracture) of left talus

√7ᵗʰ **S92.156** Nondisplaced avulsion fracture (chip fracture) of unspecified talus

√6ᵗʰ **S92.19** Other fracture of talus

√7ᵗʰ **S92.191** Other fracture of right talus

√7ᵗʰ **S92.192** Other fracture of left talus

√7ᵗʰ **S92.199** Other fracture of unspecified talus

√5ᵗʰ **S92.2** Fracture of other and unspecified tarsal bone(s)

√6ᵗʰ **S92.20** Fracture of unspecified tarsal bone(s)

√7ᵗʰ **S92.201** Fracture of unspecified tarsal bone(s) of right foot

√7ᵗʰ **S92.202** Fracture of unspecified tarsal bone(s) of left foot

√7ᵗʰ **S92.209** Fracture of unspecified tarsal bone(s) of unspecified foot

√6ᵗʰ **S92.21** Fracture of cuboid bone

√7ᵗʰ **S92.211** Displaced fracture of cuboid bone of right foot

√7ᵗʰ **S92.212** Displaced fracture of cuboid bone of left foot

√7ᵗʰ **S92.213** Displaced fracture of cuboid bone of unspecified foot

√7ᵗʰ **S92.214** Nondisplaced fracture of cuboid bone of right foot

√7ᵗʰ **S92.215** Nondisplaced fracture of cuboid bone of left foot

√7ᵗʰ **S92.216** Nondisplaced fracture of cuboid bone of unspecified foot

√6ᵗʰ **S92.22** Fracture of lateral cuneiform

√7ᵗʰ **S92.221** Displaced fracture of lateral cuneiform of right foot

√7ᵗʰ **S92.222** Displaced fracture of lateral cuneiform of left foot

√7ᵗʰ **S92.223** Displaced fracture of lateral cuneiform of unspecified foot

√7ᵗʰ **S92.224** Nondisplaced fracture of lateral cuneiform of right foot

√7ᵗʰ **S92.225** Nondisplaced fracture of lateral cuneiform of left foot

√7ᵗʰ **S92.226** Nondisplaced fracture of lateral cuneiform of unspecified foot

√6ᵗʰ **S92.23** Fracture of intermediate cuneiform

√7ᵗʰ **S92.231** Displaced fracture of intermediate cuneiform of right foot

√7ᵗʰ **S92.232** Displaced fracture of intermediate cuneiform of left foot

√7ᵗʰ **S92.233** Displaced fracture of intermediate cuneiform of unspecified foot

√7ᵗʰ **S92.234** Nondisplaced fracture of intermediate cuneiform of right foot

√7ᵗʰ **S92.235** Nondisplaced fracture of intermediate cuneiform of left foot

√7ᵗʰ **S92.236** Nondisplaced fracture of intermediate cuneiform of unspecified foot

√6ᵗʰ **S92.24** Fracture of medial cuneiform

√7ᵗʰ **S92.241** Displaced fracture of medial cuneiform of right foot

√7ᵗʰ **S92.242** Displaced fracture of medial cuneiform of left foot

√7ᵗʰ **S92.243** Displaced fracture of medial cuneiform of unspecified foot

√7ᵗʰ **S92.244** Nondisplaced fracture of medial cuneiform of right foot

√7ᵗʰ **S92.245** Nondisplaced fracture of medial cuneiform of left foot

√7ᵗʰ **S92.246** Nondisplaced fracture of medial cuneiform of unspecified foot

√6ᵗʰ **S92.25** Fracture of navicular [scaphoid] of foot

√7ᵗʰ **S92.251** Displaced fracture of navicular [scaphoid] of right foot

√7ᵗʰ **S92.252** Displaced fracture of navicular [scaphoid] of left foot

√7ᵗʰ **S92.253** Displaced fracture of navicular [scaphoid] of unspecified foot

√7ᵗʰ **S92.254** Nondisplaced fracture of navicular [scaphoid] of right foot

√7ᵗʰ **S92.255** Nondisplaced fracture of navicular [scaphoid] of left foot

√7ᵗʰ **S92.256** Nondisplaced fracture of navicular [scaphoid] of unspecified foot

√5ᵗʰ **S92.3** Fracture of metatarsal bone(s)

√6ᵗʰ **S92.30** Fracture of unspecified metatarsal bone(s)

√7ᵗʰ **S92.301** Fracture of unspecified metatarsal bone(s), right foot

√7ᵗʰ **S92.302** Fracture of unspecified metatarsal bone(s), left foot

√7ᵗʰ **S92.309** Fracture of unspecified metatarsal bone(s), unspecified foot

√6ᵗʰ **S92.31** Fracture of first metatarsal bone

√7ᵗʰ **S92.311** Displaced fracture of first metatarsal bone, right foot

√7ᵗʰ **S92.312** Displaced fracture of first metatarsal bone, left foot

√7ᵗʰ **S92.313** Displaced fracture of first metatarsal bone, unspecified foot

√7ᵗʰ **S92.314** Nondisplaced fracture of first metatarsal bone, right foot

√7ᵗʰ **S92.315** Nondisplaced fracture of first metatarsal bone, left foot

√7ᵗʰ **S92.316** Nondisplaced fracture of first metatarsal bone, unspecified foot

√6ᵗʰ **S92.32** Fracture of second metatarsal bone

√7ᵗʰ **S92.321** Displaced fracture of second metatarsal bone, right foot

√7ᵗʰ **S92.322** Displaced fracture of second metatarsal bone, left foot

√7ᵗʰ **S92.323** Displaced fracture of second metatarsal bone, unspecified foot

√7th **S92.324** Nondisplaced fracture of second metatarsal bone, right foot

√7th **S92.325** Nondisplaced fracture of second metatarsal bone, left foot

√7th **S92.326** Nondisplaced fracture of second metatarsal bone, unspecified foot

√6th **S92.33** Fracture of third metatarsal bone

√7th **S92.331** Displaced fracture of third metatarsal bone, right foot

√7th **S92.332** Displaced fracture of third metatarsal bone, left foot

√7th **S92.333** Displaced fracture of third metatarsal bone, unspecified foot

√7th **S92.334** Nondisplaced fracture of third metatarsal bone, right foot

√7th **S92.335** Nondisplaced fracture of third metatarsal bone, left foot

√7th **S92.336** Nondisplaced fracture of third metatarsal bone, unspecified foot

√6th **S92.34** Fracture of fourth metatarsal bone

√7th **S92.341** Displaced fracture of fourth metatarsal bone, right foot

√7th **S92.342** Displaced fracture of fourth metatarsal bone, left foot

√7th **S92.343** Displaced fracture of fourth metatarsal bone, unspecified foot

√7th **S92.344** Nondisplaced fracture of fourth metatarsal bone, right foot

√7th **S92.345** Nondisplaced fracture of fourth metatarsal bone, left foot

√7th **S92.346** Nondisplaced fracture of fourth metatarsal bone, unspecified foot

√6th **S92.35** Fracture of fifth metatarsal bone

√7th **S92.351** Displaced fracture of fifth metatarsal bone, right foot

√7th **S92.352** Displaced fracture of fifth metatarsal bone, left foot

√7th **S92.353** Displaced fracture of fifth metatarsal bone, unspecified foot

√7th **S92.354** Nondisplaced fracture of fifth metatarsal bone, right foot

√7th **S92.355** Nondisplaced fracture of fifth metatarsal bone, left foot

√7th **S92.356** Nondisplaced fracture of fifth metatarsal bone, unspecified foot

√5th **S92.4** Fracture of great toe

√6th **S92.40** Unspecified fracture of great toe

√7th **S92.401** Displaced unspecified fracture of right great toe

√7th **S92.402** Displaced unspecified fracture of left great toe

√7th **S92.403** Displaced unspecified fracture of unspecified great toe

√7th **S92.404** Nondisplaced unspecified fracture of right great toe

√7th **S92.405** Nondisplaced unspecified fracture of left great toe

√7th **S92.406** Nondisplaced unspecified fracture of unspecified great toe

√6th **S92.41** Fracture of proximal phalanx of great toe

√7th **S92.411** Displaced fracture of proximal phalanx of right great toe

√7th **S92.412** Displaced fracture of proximal phalanx of left great toe

√7th **S92.413** Displaced fracture of proximal phalanx of unspecified great toe

√7th **S92.414** Nondisplaced fracture of proximal phalanx of right great toe

√7th **S92.415** Nondisplaced fracture of proximal phalanx of left great toe

√7th **S92.416** Nondisplaced fracture of proximal phalanx of unspecified great toe

√6th **S92.42** Fracture of distal phalanx of great toe

√7th **S92.421** Displaced fracture of distal phalanx of right great toe

√7th **S92.422** Displaced fracture of distal phalanx of left great toe

√7th **S92.423** Displaced fracture of distal phalanx of unspecified great toe

√7th **S92.424** Nondisplaced fracture of distal phalanx of right great toe

√7th **S92.425** Nondisplaced fracture of distal phalanx of left great toe

√7th **S92.426** Nondisplaced fracture of distal phalanx of unspecified great toe

√6th **S92.49** Other fracture of great toe

√7th **S92.491** Other fracture of right great toe

√7th **S92.492** Other fracture of left great toe

√7th **S92.499** Other fracture of unspecified great toe

√5th **S92.5** Fracture of lesser toe(s)

√6th **S92.50** Unspecified fracture of lesser toe(s)

√7th **S92.501** Displaced unspecified fracture of right lesser toe(s)

√7th **S92.502** Displaced unspecified fracture of left lesser toe(s)

√7th **S92.503** Displaced unspecified fracture of unspecified lesser toe(s)

√7th **S92.504** Nondisplaced unspecified fracture of right lesser toe(s)

√7th **S92.505** Nondisplaced unspecified fracture of left lesser toe(s)

√7th **S92.506** Nondisplaced unspecified fracture of unspecified lesser toe(s)

√6th **S92.51** Fracture of proximal phalanx of lesser toe(s)

√7th **S92.511** Displaced fracture of proximal phalanx of right lesser toe(s)

√7th **S92.512** Displaced fracture of proximal phalanx of left lesser toe(s)

√7th **S92.513** Displaced fracture of proximal phalanx of unspecified lesser toe(s)

√7th **S92.514** Nondisplaced fracture of proximal phalanx of right lesser toe(s)

√7th **S92.515** Nondisplaced fracture of proximal phalanx of left lesser toe(s)

√7th **S92.516** Nondisplaced fracture of proximal phalanx of unspecified lesser toe(s)

√6th **S92.52** Fracture of medial phalanx of lesser toe(s)

√7th **S92.521** Displaced fracture of medial phalanx of right lesser toe(s)

√7th **S92.522** Displaced fracture of medial phalanx of left lesser toe(s)

√7th **S92.523** Displaced fracture of medial phalanx of unspecified lesser toe(s)

√7th **S92.524** Nondisplaced fracture of medial phalanx of right lesser toe(s)

√7th **S92.525** Nondisplaced fracture of medial phalanx of left lesser toe(s)

√7th **S92.526** Nondisplaced fracture of medial phalanx of unspecified lesser toe(s)

√6th **S92.53** Fracture of distal phalanx of lesser toe(s)

√7th **S92.531** Displaced fracture of distal phalanx of right lesser toe(s)

√7th **S92.532** Displaced fracture of distal phalanx of left lesser toe(s)

√7th **S92.533** Displaced fracture of distal phalanx of unspecified lesser toe(s)

√7th **S92.534** Nondisplaced fracture of distal phalanx of right lesser toe(s)

√7th **S92.535** Nondisplaced fracture of distal phalanx of left lesser toe(s)

√7th **S92.536** Nondisplaced fracture of distal phalanx of unspecified lesser toe(s)

√6th **S92.59** Other fracture of lesser toe(s)

√7th **S92.591** Other fracture of right lesser toe(s)

√7th **S92.592** Other fracture of left lesser toe(s)

√7th **S92.599** Other fracture of unspecified lesser toe(s)

√5th **S92.9** Unspecified fracture of foot and toe

√6th **S92.90** Unspecified fracture of foot

√7th **S92.901** Unspecified fracture of right foot

√7th **S92.902** Unspecified fracture of left foot

EXCLUDES 1 Not coded here   **EXCLUDES 2** Not included here   *Manifestation Code*

　✓7ᵗʰ　**S92.909**　Unspecified fracture of unspecified foot

✓6ᵗʰ　**S92.91**　**Unspecified fracture of toe**

　✓7ᵗʰ　**S92.911**　Unspecified fracture of right toe(s)

　✓7ᵗʰ　**S92.912**　Unspecified fracture of left toe(s)

　✓7ᵗʰ　**S92.919**　Unspecified fracture of unspecified toe(s)

✓4ᵗʰ　**S93**　**Dislocation and sprain of joints and ligaments at ankle, foot and toe level**

　　INCLUDES　avulsion of joint or ligament of ankle, foot and toe
　　laceration of cartilage, joint or ligament of ankle, foot and toe
　　sprain of cartilage, joint or ligament of ankle, foot and toe
　　traumatic hemarthrosis of joint or ligament of ankle, foot and toe
　　traumatic rupture of joint or ligament of ankle, foot and toe
　　traumatic subluxation of joint or ligament of ankle, foot and toe
　　traumatic tear of joint or ligament of ankle, foot and toe

　　Code also any associated open wound

　　EXCLUDES 2　*strain of muscle and tendon of ankle and foot (S96-)*

　　The appropriate 7th character is to be added to each code from category S93.
　　A　initial encounter
　　D　subsequent encounter
　　S　sequela

✓5ᵗʰ　**S93.0**　**Subluxation and dislocation of ankle joint**
　　Subluxation and dislocation of astragalus
　　Subluxation and dislocation of fibula, lower end
　　Subluxation and dislocation of talus
　　Subluxation and dislocation of tibia, lower end

　✓x7ᵗʰ　**S93.01**　Subluxation of right ankle joint

　✓x7ᵗʰ　**S93.02**　Subluxation of left ankle joint

　✓x7ᵗʰ　**S93.03**　Subluxation of unspecified ankle joint

　✓x7ᵗʰ　**S93.04**　Dislocation of right ankle joint

　✓x7ᵗʰ　**S93.05**　Dislocation of left ankle joint

　✓x7ᵗʰ　**S93.06**　Dislocation of unspecified ankle joint

✓5ᵗʰ　**S93.1**　**Subluxation and dislocation of toe**

　✓6ᵗʰ　**S93.10**　**Unspecified subluxation and dislocation of toe**
　　　Dislocation of toe NOS
　　　Subluxation of toe NOS

　　✓7ᵗʰ　**S93.101**　Unspecified subluxation of right toe(s)

　　✓7ᵗʰ　**S93.102**　Unspecified subluxation of left toe(s)

　　✓7ᵗʰ　**S93.103**　Unspecified subluxation of unspecified toe(s)

　　✓7ᵗʰ　**S93.104**　Unspecified dislocation of right toe(s)

　　✓7ᵗʰ　**S93.105**　Unspecified dislocation of left toe(s)

　　✓7ᵗʰ　**S93.106**　Unspecified dislocation of unspecified toe(s)

　✓6ᵗʰ　**S93.11**　**Dislocation of interphalangeal joint**

　　✓7ᵗʰ　**S93.111**　Dislocation of interphalangeal joint of right great toe

　　✓7ᵗʰ　**S93.112**　Dislocation of interphalangeal joint of left great toe

　　✓7ᵗʰ　**S93.113**　Dislocation of interphalangeal joint of unspecified great toe

　　✓7ᵗʰ　**S93.114**　Dislocation of interphalangeal joint of right lesser toe(s)

　　✓7ᵗʰ　**S93.115**　Dislocation of interphalangeal joint of left lesser toe(s)

　　✓7ᵗʰ　**S93.116**　Dislocation of interphalangeal joint of unspecified lesser toe(s)

　　✓7ᵗʰ　**S93.119**　Dislocation of interphalangeal joint of unspecified toe(s)

　✓6ᵗʰ　**S93.12**　**Dislocation of metatarsophalangeal joint**

　　✓7ᵗʰ　**S93.121**　Dislocation of metatarsophalangeal joint of right great toe

　　✓7ᵗʰ　**S93.122**　Dislocation of metatarsophalangeal joint of left great toe

　　✓7ᵗʰ　**S93.123**　Dislocation of metatarsophalangeal joint of unspecified great toe

　　✓7ᵗʰ　**S93.124**　Dislocation of metatarsophalangeal joint of right lesser toe(s)

　　✓7ᵗʰ　**S93.125**　Dislocation of metatarsophalangeal joint of left lesser toe(s)

　　✓7ᵗʰ　**S93.126**　Dislocation of metatarsophalangeal joint of unspecified lesser toe(s)

　✓7ᵗʰ　**S93.129**　Dislocation of metatarsophalangeal joint of unspecified toe(s)

　✓6ᵗʰ　**S93.13**　**Subluxation of interphalangeal joint**

　　✓7ᵗʰ　**S93.131**　Subluxation of interphalangeal joint of right great toe

　　✓7ᵗʰ　**S93.132**　Subluxation of interphalangeal joint of left great toe

　　✓7ᵗʰ　**S93.133**　Subluxation of interphalangeal joint of unspecified great toe

　　✓7ᵗʰ　**S93.134**　Subluxation of interphalangeal joint of right lesser toe(s)

　　✓7ᵗʰ　**S93.135**　Subluxation of interphalangeal joint of left lesser toe(s)

　　✓7ᵗʰ　**S93.136**　Subluxation of interphalangeal joint of unspecified lesser toe(s)

　　✓7ᵗʰ　**S93.139**　Subluxation of interphalangeal joint of unspecified toe(s)

　✓6ᵗʰ　**S93.14**　**Subluxation of metatarsophalangeal joint**

　　✓7ᵗʰ　**S93.141**　Subluxation of metatarsophalangeal joint of right great toe

　　✓7ᵗʰ　**S93.142**　Subluxation of metatarsophalangeal joint of left great toe

　　✓7ᵗʰ　**S93.143**　Subluxation of metatarsophalangeal joint of unspecified great toe

　　✓7ᵗʰ　**S93.144**　Subluxation of metatarsophalangeal joint of right lesser toe(s)

　　✓7ᵗʰ　**S93.145**　Subluxation of metatarsophalangeal joint of left lesser toe(s)

　　✓7ᵗʰ　**S93.146**　Subluxation of metatarsophalangeal joint of unspecified lesser toe(s)

　　✓7ᵗʰ　**S93.149**　Subluxation of metatarsophalangeal joint of unspecified toe(s)

✓5ᵗʰ　**S93.3**　**Subluxation and dislocation of foot**
　　EXCLUDES 2　*dislocation of toe (S93.1-)*

　✓6ᵗʰ　**S93.30**　**Unspecified subluxation and dislocation of foot**
　　　Dislocation of foot NOS
　　　Subluxation of foot NOS

　　✓7ᵗʰ　**S93.301**　Unspecified subluxation of right foot

　　✓7ᵗʰ　**S93.302**　Unspecified subluxation of left foot

　　✓7ᵗʰ　**S93.303**　Unspecified subluxation of unspecified foot

　　✓7ᵗʰ　**S93.304**　Unspecified dislocation of right foot

　　✓7ᵗʰ　**S93.305**　Unspecified dislocation of left foot

　　✓7ᵗʰ　**S93.306**　Unspecified dislocation of unspecified foot

　✓6ᵗʰ　**S93.31**　**Subluxation and dislocation of tarsal joint**

　　✓7ᵗʰ　**S93.311**　Subluxation of tarsal joint of right foot

　　✓7ᵗʰ　**S93.312**　Subluxation of tarsal joint of left foot

　　✓7ᵗʰ　**S93.313**　Subluxation of tarsal joint of unspecified foot

　　✓7ᵗʰ　**S93.314**　Dislocation of tarsal joint of right foot

　　✓7ᵗʰ　**S93.315**　Dislocation of tarsal joint of left foot

　　✓7ᵗʰ　**S93.316**　Dislocation of tarsal joint of unspecified foot

　✓6ᵗʰ　**S93.32**　**Subluxation and dislocation of tarsometatarsal joint**

　　✓7ᵗʰ　**S93.321**　Subluxation of tarsometatarsal joint of right foot

　　✓7ᵗʰ　**S93.322**　Subluxation of tarsometatarsal joint of left foot

　　✓7ᵗʰ　**S93.323**　Subluxation of tarsometatarsal joint of unspecified foot

　　✓7ᵗʰ　**S93.324**　Dislocation of tarsometatarsal joint of right foot

　　✓7ᵗʰ　**S93.325**　Dislocation of tarsometatarsal joint of left foot

　　✓7ᵗʰ　**S93.326**　Dislocation of tarsometatarsal joint of unspecified foot

　✓6ᵗʰ　**S93.33**　**Other subluxation and dislocation of foot**

　　✓7ᵗʰ　**S93.331**　Other subluxation of right foot

　　✓7ᵗʰ　**S93.332**　Other subluxation of left foot

　　✓7ᵗʰ　**S93.333**　Other subluxation of unspecified foot

　　✓7ᵗʰ　**S93.334**　Other dislocation of right foot

　　✓7ᵗʰ　**S93.335**　Other dislocation of left foot

　　✓7ᵗʰ　**S93.336**　Other dislocation of unspecified foot

√5ᵗʰ **S93.4 Sprain of ankle**
     EXCLUDES 2   *injury of Achilles tendon (S86.0-)*

     √6ᵗʰ **S93.40 Sprain of unspecified ligament of ankle**
         Sprain of ankle NOS
         Sprained ankle NOS

         √7ᵗʰ **S93.401 Sprain of unspecified ligament of right ankle**

         √7ᵗʰ **S93.402 Sprain of unspecified ligament of left ankle**

         √7ᵗʰ **S93.409 Sprain of unspecified ligament of unspecified ankle**

     √6ᵗʰ **S93.41 Sprain of calcaneofibular ligament**

         √7ᵗʰ **S93.411 Sprain of calcaneofibular ligament of right ankle**

         √7ᵗʰ **S93.412 Sprain of calcaneofibular ligament of left ankle**

         √7ᵗʰ **S93.419 Sprain of calcaneofibular ligament of unspecified ankle**

     √6ᵗʰ **S93.42 Sprain of deltoid ligament**

         √7ᵗʰ **S93.421 Sprain of deltoid ligament of right ankle**

         √7ᵗʰ **S93.422 Sprain of deltoid ligament of left ankle**

         √7ᵗʰ **S93.429 Sprain of deltoid ligament of unspecified ankle**

     √6ᵗʰ **S93.43 Sprain of tibiofibular ligament**

         √7ᵗʰ **S93.431 Sprain of tibiofibular ligament of right ankle**

         √7ᵗʰ **S93.432 Sprain of tibiofibular ligament of left ankle**

         √7ᵗʰ **S93.439 Sprain of tibiofibular ligament of unspecified ankle**

     √6ᵗʰ **S93.49 Sprain of other ligament of ankle**
         Sprain of internal collateral ligament
         Sprain of talofibular ligament

         √7ᵗʰ **S93.491 Sprain of other ligament of right ankle**

         √7ᵗʰ **S93.492 Sprain of other ligament of left ankle**

         √7ᵗʰ **S93.499 Sprain of other ligament of unspecified ankle**

√5ᵗʰ **S93.5 Sprain of toe**

     √6ᵗʰ **S93.50 Unspecified sprain of toe**

         √7ᵗʰ **S93.501 Unspecified sprain of right great toe**

         √7ᵗʰ **S93.502 Unspecified sprain of left great toe**

         √7ᵗʰ **S93.503 Unspecified sprain of unspecified great toe**

         √7ᵗʰ **S93.504 Unspecified sprain of right lesser toe(s)**

         √7ᵗʰ **S93.505 Unspecified sprain of left lesser toe(s)**

         √7ᵗʰ **S93.506 Unspecified sprain of unspecified lesser toe(s)**

         √7ᵗʰ **S93.509 Unspecified sprain of unspecified toe(s)**

     √6ᵗʰ **S93.51 Sprain of interphalangeal joint of toe**

         √7ᵗʰ **S93.511 Sprain of interphalangeal joint of right great toe**

         √7ᵗʰ **S93.512 Sprain of interphalangeal joint of left great toe**

         √7ᵗʰ **S93.513 Sprain of interphalangeal joint of unspecified great toe**

         √7ᵗʰ **S93.514 Sprain of interphalangeal joint of right lesser toe(s)**

         √7ᵗʰ **S93.515 Sprain of interphalangeal joint of left lesser toe(s)**

         √7ᵗʰ **S93.516 Sprain of interphalangeal joint of unspecified lesser toe(s)**

         √7ᵗʰ **S93.519 Sprain of interphalangeal joint of unspecified toe(s)**

     √6ᵗʰ **S93.52 Sprain of metatarsophalangeal joint of toe**

         √7ᵗʰ **S93.521 Sprain of metatarsophalangeal joint of right great toe**

         √7ᵗʰ **S93.522 Sprain of metatarsophalangeal joint of left great toe**

         √7ᵗʰ **S93.523 Sprain of metatarsophalangeal joint of unspecified great toe**

         √7ᵗʰ **S93.524 Sprain of metatarsophalangeal joint of right lesser toe(s)**

         √7ᵗʰ **S93.525 Sprain of metatarsophalangeal joint of left lesser toe(s)**

         √7ᵗʰ **S93.526 Sprain of metatarsophalangeal joint of unspecified lesser toe(s)**

         √7ᵗʰ **S93.529 Sprain of metatarsophalangeal joint of unspecified toe(s)**

√5ᵗʰ **S93.6 Sprain of foot**
     EXCLUDES 2   *sprain of metatarsophalangeal joint of toe (S93.52-)*
                 sprain of toe (S93.5-)

     √6ᵗʰ **S93.60 Unspecified sprain of foot**

         √7ᵗʰ **S93.601 Unspecified sprain of right foot**

         √7ᵗʰ **S93.602 Unspecified sprain of left foot**

         √7ᵗʰ **S93.609 Unspecified sprain of unspecified foot**

     √6ᵗʰ **S93.61 Sprain of tarsal ligament of foot**

         √7ᵗʰ **S93.611 Sprain of tarsal ligament of right foot**

         √7ᵗʰ **S93.612 Sprain of tarsal ligament of left foot**

         √7ᵗʰ **S93.619 Sprain of tarsal ligament of unspecified foot**

     √6ᵗʰ **S93.62 Sprain of tarsometatarsal ligament of foot**

         √7ᵗʰ **S93.621 Sprain of tarsometatarsal ligament of right foot**

         √7ᵗʰ **S93.622 Sprain of tarsometatarsal ligament of left foot**

         √7ᵗʰ **S93.629 Sprain of tarsometatarsal ligament of unspecified foot**

     √6ᵗʰ **S93.69 Other sprain of foot**

         √7ᵗʰ **S93.691 Other sprain of right foot**

         √7ᵗʰ **S93.692 Other sprain of left foot**

         √7ᵗʰ **S93.699 Other sprain of unspecified foot**

√4ᵗʰ **S94 Injury of nerves at ankle and foot level**
     Code also any associated open wound (S91-)

     The appropriate 7th character is to be added to each code from category S94.
     A   initial encounter
     D   subsequent encounter
     S   sequela

     √5ᵗʰ **S94.0 Injury of lateral plantar nerve**

         √x7ᵗʰ **S94.00 Injury of lateral plantar nerve, unspecified leg**

         √x7ᵗʰ **S94.01 Injury of lateral plantar nerve, right leg**

         √x7ᵗʰ **S94.02 Injury of lateral plantar nerve, left leg**

     √5ᵗʰ **S94.1 Injury of medial plantar nerve**

         √x7ᵗʰ **S94.10 Injury of medial plantar nerve, unspecified leg**

         √x7ᵗʰ **S94.11 Injury of medial plantar nerve, right leg**

         √x7ᵗʰ **S94.12 Injury of medial plantar nerve, left leg**

     √5ᵗʰ **S94.2 Injury of deep peroneal nerve at ankle and foot level**
         Injury of terminal, lateral branch of deep peroneal nerve

         √x7ᵗʰ **S94.20 Injury of deep peroneal nerve at ankle and foot level, unspecified leg**

         √x7ᵗʰ **S94.21 Injury of deep peroneal nerve at ankle and foot level, right leg**

         √x7ᵗʰ **S94.22 Injury of deep peroneal nerve at ankle and foot level, left leg**

     √5ᵗʰ **S94.3 Injury of cutaneous sensory nerve at ankle and foot level**

         √x7ᵗʰ **S94.30 Injury of cutaneous sensory nerve at ankle and foot level, unspecified leg**

         √x7ᵗʰ **S94.31 Injury of cutaneous sensory nerve at ankle and foot level, right leg**

         √x7ᵗʰ **S94.32 Injury of cutaneous sensory nerve at ankle and foot level, left leg**

     √5ᵗʰ **S94.8 Injury of other nerves at ankle and foot level**

         √6ᵗʰ **S94.8x Injury of other nerves at ankle and foot level**

             √7ᵗʰ **S94.8x1 Injury of other nerves at ankle and foot level, right leg**

             √7ᵗʰ **S94.8x2 Injury of other nerves at ankle and foot level, left leg**

             √7ᵗʰ **S94.8x9 Injury of other nerves at ankle and foot level, unspecified leg**

     √5ᵗʰ **S94.9 Injury of unspecified nerve at ankle and foot level**

         √x7ᵗʰ **S94.90 Injury of unspecified nerve at ankle and foot level, unspecified leg**

         √x7ᵗʰ **S94.91 Injury of unspecified nerve at ankle and foot level, right leg**

         √x7ᵗʰ **S94.92 Injury of unspecified nerve at ankle and foot level, left leg**

EXCLUDES 1   Not coded here   EXCLUDES 2   Not included here   *Manifestation Code*

✓4th **S95   Injury of blood vessels at ankle and foot level**
　　　Code also any associated open wound (S91-)
　　　EXCLUDES 2 *injury of posterior tibial artery and vein (S85.1-, S85.8-)*

> The appropriate 7th character is to be added to each code from category S95.
> A   initial encounter
> D   subsequent encounter
> S   sequela

✓5th　**S95.0   Injury of dorsal artery of foot**
✓6th　　**S95.00   Unspecified injury of dorsal artery of foot**
✓7th　　　**S95.001   Unspecified injury of dorsal artery of right foot**
✓7th　　　**S95.002   Unspecified injury of dorsal artery of left foot**
✓7th　　　**S95.009   Unspecified injury of dorsal artery of unspecified foot**
✓6th　　**S95.01   Laceration of dorsal artery of foot**
✓7th　　　**S95.011   Laceration of dorsal artery of right foot**
✓7th　　　**S95.012   Laceration of dorsal artery of left foot**
✓7th　　　**S95.019   Laceration of dorsal artery of unspecified foot**
✓6th　　**S95.09   Other specified injury of dorsal artery of foot**
✓7th　　　**S95.091   Other specified injury of dorsal artery of right foot**
✓7th　　　**S95.092   Other specified injury of dorsal artery of left foot**
✓7th　　　**S95.099   Other specified injury of dorsal artery of unspecified foot**

✓5th　**S95.1   Injury of plantar artery of foot**
✓6th　　**S95.10   Unspecified injury of plantar artery of foot**
✓7th　　　**S95.101   Unspecified injury of plantar artery of right foot**
✓7th　　　**S95.102   Unspecified injury of plantar artery of left foot**
✓7th　　　**S95.109   Unspecified injury of plantar artery of unspecified foot**
✓6th　　**S95.11   Laceration of plantar artery of foot**
✓7th　　　**S95.111   Laceration of plantar artery of right foot**
✓7th　　　**S95.112   Laceration of plantar artery of left foot**
✓7th　　　**S95.119   Laceration of plantar artery of unspecified foot**
✓6th　　**S95.19   Other specified injury of plantar artery of foot**
✓7th　　　**S95.191   Other specified injury of plantar artery of right foot**
✓7th　　　**S95.192   Other specified injury of plantar artery of left foot**
✓7th　　　**S95.199   Other specified injury of plantar artery of unspecified foot**

✓5th　**S95.2   Injury of dorsal vein of foot**
✓6th　　**S95.20   Unspecified injury of dorsal vein of foot**
✓7th　　　**S95.201   Unspecified injury of dorsal vein of right foot**
✓7th　　　**S95.202   Unspecified injury of dorsal vein of left foot**
✓7th　　　**S95.209   Unspecified injury of dorsal vein of unspecified foot**
✓6th　　**S95.21   Laceration of dorsal vein of foot**
✓7th　　　**S95.211   Laceration of dorsal vein of right foot**
✓7th　　　**S95.212   Laceration of dorsal vein of left foot**
✓7th　　　**S95.219   Laceration of dorsal vein of unspecified foot**
✓6th　　**S95.29   Other specified injury of dorsal vein of foot**
✓7th　　　**S95.291   Other specified injury of dorsal vein of right foot**
✓7th　　　**S95.292   Other specified injury of dorsal vein of left foot**
✓7th　　　**S95.299   Other specified injury of dorsal vein of unspecified foot**

✓5th　**S95.8   Injury of other blood vessels at ankle and foot level**
✓6th　　**S95.80   Unspecified injury of other blood vessels at ankle and foot level**
✓7th　　　**S95.801   Unspecified injury of other blood vessels at ankle and foot level, right leg**
✓7th　　　**S95.802   Unspecified injury of other blood vessels at ankle and foot level, left leg**

✓7th　　　**S95.809   Unspecified injury of other blood vessels at ankle and foot level, unspecified leg**
✓6th　　**S95.81   Laceration of other blood vessels at ankle and foot level**
✓7th　　　**S95.811   Laceration of other blood vessels at ankle and foot level, right leg**
✓7th　　　**S95.812   Laceration of other blood vessels at ankle and foot level, left leg**
✓7th　　　**S95.819   Laceration of other blood vessels at ankle and foot level, unspecified leg**
✓6th　　**S95.89   Other specified injury of other blood vessels at ankle and foot level**
✓7th　　　**S95.891   Other specified injury of other blood vessels at ankle and foot level, right leg**
✓7th　　　**S95.892   Other specified injury of other blood vessels at ankle and foot level, left leg**
✓7th　　　**S95.899   Other specified injury of other blood vessels at ankle and foot level, unspecified leg**

✓5th　**S95.9   Injury of unspecified blood vessel at ankle and foot level**
✓6th　　**S95.90   Unspecified injury of unspecified blood vessel at ankle and foot level**
✓7th　　　**S95.901   Unspecified injury of unspecified blood vessel at ankle and foot level, right leg**
✓7th　　　**S95.902   Unspecified injury of unspecified blood vessel at ankle and foot level, left leg**
✓7th　　　**S95.909   Unspecified injury of unspecified blood vessel at ankle and foot level, unspecified leg**
✓6th　　**S95.91   Laceration of unspecified blood vessel at ankle and foot level**
✓7th　　　**S95.911   Laceration of unspecified blood vessel at ankle and foot level, right leg**
✓7th　　　**S95.912   Laceration of unspecified blood vessel at ankle and foot level, left leg**
✓7th　　　**S95.919   Laceration of unspecified blood vessel at ankle and foot level, unspecified leg**
✓6th　　**S95.99   Other specified injury of unspecified blood vessel at ankle and foot level**
✓7th　　　**S95.991   Other specified injury of unspecified blood vessel at ankle and foot level, right leg**
✓7th　　　**S95.992   Other specified injury of unspecified blood vessel at ankle and foot level, left leg**
✓7th　　　**S95.999   Other specified injury of unspecified blood vessel at ankle and foot level, unspecified leg**

✓4th **S96   Injury of muscle and tendon at ankle and foot level**
　　　Code also any associated open wound (S91-)
　　　EXCLUDES 2 *injury of Achilles tendon (S86.0-)*
　　　　　　　　sprain of joints and ligaments of ankle and foot (S93-)

> The appropriate 7th character is to be added to each code from category S96.
> A   initial encounter
> D   subsequent encounter
> S   sequela

✓5th　**S96.0   Injury of muscle and tendon of long flexor muscle of toe at ankle and foot level**
✓6th　　**S96.00   Unspecified injury of muscle and tendon of long flexor muscle of toe at ankle and foot level**
✓7th　　　**S96.001   Unspecified injury of muscle and tendon of long flexor muscle of toe at ankle and foot level, right foot**
✓7th　　　**S96.002   Unspecified injury of muscle and tendon of long flexor muscle of toe at ankle and foot level, left foot**
✓7th　　　**S96.009   Unspecified injury of muscle and tendon of long flexor muscle of toe at ankle and foot level, unspecified foot**
✓6th　　**S96.01   Strain of muscle and tendon of long flexor muscle of toe at ankle and foot level**
✓7th　　　**S96.011   Strain of muscle and tendon of long flexor muscle of toe at ankle and foot level, right foot**

✓ Appropriate additional character required　　　　　✓x7th Requires 7th character, placeholder x must fill empty characters

√7th **S96.012** Strain of muscle and tendon of long flexor muscle of toe at ankle and foot level, left foot

√7th **S96.019** Strain of muscle and tendon of long flexor muscle of toe at ankle and foot level, unspecified foot

√6th **S96.02** Laceration of muscle and tendon of long flexor muscle of toe at ankle and foot level

√7th **S96.021** Laceration of muscle and tendon of long flexor muscle of toe at ankle and foot level, right foot

√7th **S96.022** Laceration of muscle and tendon of long flexor muscle of toe at ankle and foot level, left foot

√7th **S96.029** Laceration of muscle and tendon of long flexor muscle of toe at ankle and foot level, unspecified foot

√6th **S96.09** Other injury of muscle and tendon of long flexor muscle of toe at ankle and foot level

√7th **S96.091** Other injury of muscle and tendon of long flexor muscle of toe at ankle and foot level, right foot

√7th **S96.092** Other injury of muscle and tendon of long flexor muscle of toe at ankle and foot level, left foot

√7th **S96.099** Other injury of muscle and tendon of long flexor muscle of toe at ankle and foot level, unspecified foot

√5th **S96.1** Injury of muscle and tendon of long extensor muscle of toe at ankle and foot level

√6th **S96.10** Unspecified injury of muscle and tendon of long extensor muscle of toe at ankle and foot level

√7th **S96.101** Unspecified injury of muscle and tendon of long extensor muscle of toe at ankle and foot level, right foot

√7th **S96.102** Unspecified injury of muscle and tendon of long extensor muscle of toe at ankle and foot level, left foot

√7th **S96.109** Unspecified injury of muscle and tendon of long extensor muscle of toe at ankle and foot level, unspecified foot

√6th **S96.11** Strain of muscle and tendon of long extensor muscle of toe at ankle and foot level

√7th **S96.111** Strain of muscle and tendon of long extensor muscle of toe at ankle and foot level, right foot

√7th **S96.112** Strain of muscle and tendon of long extensor muscle of toe at ankle and foot level, left foot

√7th **S96.119** Strain of muscle and tendon of long extensor muscle of toe at ankle and foot level, unspecified foot

√6th **S96.12** Laceration of muscle and tendon of long extensor muscle of toe at ankle and foot level

√7th **S96.121** Laceration of muscle and tendon of long extensor muscle of toe at ankle and foot level, right foot

√7th **S96.122** Laceration of muscle and tendon of long extensor muscle of toe at ankle and foot level, left foot

√7th **S96.129** Laceration of muscle and tendon of long extensor muscle of toe at ankle and foot level, unspecified foot

√6th **S96.19** Other specified injury of muscle and tendon of long extensor muscle of toe at ankle and foot level

√7th **S96.191** Other specified injury of muscle and tendon of long extensor muscle of toe at ankle and foot level, right foot

√7th **S96.192** Other specified injury of muscle and tendon of long extensor muscle of toe at ankle and foot level, left foot

√7th **S96.199** Other specified injury of muscle and tendon of long extensor muscle of toe at ankle and foot level, unspecified foot

√5th **S96.2** Injury of intrinsic muscle and tendon at ankle and foot level

√6th **S96.20** Unspecified injury of intrinsic muscle and tendon at ankle and foot level

√7th **S96.201** Unspecified injury of intrinsic muscle and tendon at ankle and foot level, right foot

√7th **S96.202** Unspecified injury of intrinsic muscle and tendon at ankle and foot level, left foot

√7th **S96.209** Unspecified injury of intrinsic muscle and tendon at ankle and foot level, unspecified foot

√6th **S96.21** Strain of intrinsic muscle and tendon at ankle and foot level

√7th **S96.211** Strain of intrinsic muscle and tendon at ankle and foot level, right foot

√7th **S96.212** Strain of intrinsic muscle and tendon at ankle and foot level, left foot

√7th **S96.219** Strain of intrinsic muscle and tendon at ankle and foot level, unspecified foot

√6th **S96.22** Laceration of intrinsic muscle and tendon at ankle and foot level

√7th **S96.221** Laceration of intrinsic muscle and tendon at ankle and foot level, right foot

√7th **S96.222** Laceration of intrinsic muscle and tendon at ankle and foot level, left foot

√7th **S96.229** Laceration of intrinsic muscle and tendon at ankle and foot level, unspecified foot

√6th **S96.29** Other specified injury of intrinsic muscle and tendon at ankle and foot level

√7th **S96.291** Other specified injury of intrinsic muscle and tendon at ankle and foot level, right foot

√7th **S96.292** Other specified injury of intrinsic muscle and tendon at ankle and foot level, left foot

√7th **S96.299** Other specified injury of intrinsic muscle and tendon at ankle and foot level, unspecified foot

√5th **S96.8** Injury of other specified muscles and tendons at ankle and foot level

√6th **S96.80** Unspecified injury of other specified muscles and tendons at ankle and foot level

√7th **S96.801** Unspecified injury of other specified muscles and tendons at ankle and foot level, right foot

√7th **S96.802** Unspecified injury of other specified muscles and tendons at ankle and foot level, left foot

√7th **S96.809** Unspecified injury of other specified muscles and tendons at ankle and foot level, unspecified foot

√6th **S96.81** Strain of other specified muscles and tendons at ankle and foot level

√7th **S96.811** Strain of other specified muscles and tendons at ankle and foot level, right foot

√7th **S96.812** Strain of other specified muscles and tendons at ankle and foot level, left foot

√7th **S96.819** Strain of other specified muscles and tendons at ankle and foot level, unspecified foot

√6th **S96.82** Laceration of other specified muscles and tendons at ankle and foot level

√7th **S96.821** Laceration of other specified muscles and tendons at ankle and foot level, right foot

√7th **S96.822** Laceration of other specified muscles and tendons at ankle and foot level, left foot

√7th **S96.829** Laceration of other specified muscles and tendons at ankle and foot level, unspecified foot

√6th **S96.89** Other specified injury of other specified muscles and tendons at ankle and foot level

√7th **S96.891** Other specified injury of other specified muscles and tendons at ankle and foot level, right foot

---

EXCLUDES 1 Not coded here   EXCLUDES 2 Not included here   *Manifestation Code*

☑7th **S96.892** Other specified injury of other specified muscles and tendons at ankle and foot level, left foot

☑7th **S96.899** Other specified injury of other specified muscles and tendons at ankle and foot level, unspecified foot

☑5th **S96.9** Injury of unspecified muscle and tendon at ankle and foot level

  ☑6th **S96.90** Unspecified injury of unspecified muscle and tendon at ankle and foot level

    ☑7th **S96.901** Unspecified injury of unspecified muscle and tendon at ankle and foot level, right foot

    ☑7th **S96.902** Unspecified injury of unspecified muscle and tendon at ankle and foot level, left foot

    ☑7th **S96.909** Unspecified injury of unspecified muscle and tendon at ankle and foot level, unspecified foot

  ☑6th **S96.91** Strain of unspecified muscle and tendon at ankle and foot level

    ☑7th **S96.911** Strain of unspecified muscle and tendon at ankle and foot level, right foot

    ☑7th **S96.912** Strain of unspecified muscle and tendon at ankle and foot level, left foot

    ☑7th **S96.919** Strain of unspecified muscle and tendon at ankle and foot level, unspecified foot

  ☑6th **S96.92** Laceration of unspecified muscle and tendon at ankle and foot level

    ☑7th **S96.921** Laceration of unspecified muscle and tendon at ankle and foot level, right foot

    ☑7th **S96.922** Laceration of unspecified muscle and tendon at ankle and foot level, left foot

    ☑7th **S96.929** Laceration of unspecified muscle and tendon at ankle and foot level, unspecified foot

  ☑6th **S96.99** Other specified injury of unspecified muscle and tendon at ankle and foot level

    ☑7th **S96.991** Other specified injury of unspecified muscle and tendon at ankle and foot level, right foot

    ☑7th **S96.992** Other specified injury of unspecified muscle and tendon at ankle and foot level, left foot

    ☑7th **S96.999** Other specified injury of unspecified muscle and tendon at ankle and foot level, unspecified foot

☑4th **S97 Crushing injury of ankle and foot**
Use additional code(s) for all associated injuries

> The appropriate 7th character is to be added to each code from category S97.
> A   initial encounter
> D   subsequent encounter
> S   sequela

☑5th **S97.0** Crushing injury of ankle

  ☑x7th **S97.00** Crushing injury of unspecified ankle

  ☑x7th **S97.01** Crushing injury of right ankle

  ☑x7th **S97.02** Crushing injury of left ankle

☑5th **S97.1** Crushing injury of toe

  ☑6th **S97.10** Crushing injury of unspecified toe(s)

    ☑7th **S97.101** Crushing injury of unspecified right toe(s)

    ☑7th **S97.102** Crushing injury of unspecified left toe(s)

    ☑7th **S97.109** Crushing injury of unspecified toe(s)
Crushing injury of toe NOS

  ☑6th **S97.11** Crushing injury of great toe

    ☑7th **S97.111** Crushing injury of right great toe

    ☑7th **S97.112** Crushing injury of left great toe

    ☑7th **S97.119** Crushing injury of unspecified great toe

  ☑6th **S97.12** Crushing injury of lesser toe(s)

    ☑7th **S97.121** Crushing injury of right lesser toe(s)

    ☑7th **S97.122** Crushing injury of left lesser toe(s)

    ☑7th **S97.129** Crushing injury of unspecified lesser toe(s)

☑5th **S97.8** Crushing injury of foot

  ☑x7th **S97.80** Crushing injury of unspecified foot
Crushing injury of foot NOS

  ☑x7th **S97.81** Crushing injury of right foot

  ☑x7th **S97.82** Crushing injury of left foot

☑4th **S98 Traumatic amputation of ankle and foot**
An amputation not identified as partial or complete should be coded to complete

> The appropriate 7th character is to be added to each code from category S98.
> A   initial encounter
> D   subsequent encounter
> S   sequela

☑5th **S98.0** Traumatic amputation of foot at ankle level

  ☑6th **S98.01** Complete traumatic amputation of foot at ankle level

    ☑7th **S98.011** Complete traumatic amputation of right foot at ankle level

    ☑7th **S98.012** Complete traumatic amputation of left foot at ankle level

    ☑7th **S98.019** Complete traumatic amputation of unspecified foot at ankle level

  ☑6th **S98.02** Partial traumatic amputation of foot at ankle level

    ☑7th **S98.021** Partial traumatic amputation of right foot at ankle level

    ☑7th **S98.022** Partial traumatic amputation of left foot at ankle level

    ☑7th **S98.029** Partial traumatic amputation of unspecified foot at ankle level

☑5th **S98.1** Traumatic amputation of one toe

  ☑6th **S98.11** Complete traumatic amputation of great toe

    ☑7th **S98.111** Complete traumatic amputation of right great toe

    ☑7th **S98.112** Complete traumatic amputation of left great toe

    ☑7th **S98.119** Complete traumatic amputation of unspecified great toe

  ☑6th **S98.12** Partial traumatic amputation of great toe

    ☑7th **S98.121** Partial traumatic amputation of right great toe

    ☑7th **S98.122** Partial traumatic amputation of left great toe

    ☑7th **S98.129** Partial traumatic amputation of unspecified great toe

  ☑6th **S98.13** Complete traumatic amputation of one lesser toe
Traumatic amputation of toe NOS

    ☑7th **S98.131** Complete traumatic amputation of one right lesser toe

    ☑7th **S98.132** Complete traumatic amputation of one left lesser toe

    ☑7th **S98.139** Complete traumatic amputation of one unspecified lesser toe

  ☑6th **S98.14** Partial traumatic amputation of one lesser toe

    ☑7th **S98.141** Partial traumatic amputation of one right lesser toe

    ☑7th **S98.142** Partial traumatic amputation of one left lesser toe

    ☑7th **S98.149** Partial traumatic amputation of one unspecified lesser toe

☑5th **S98.2** Traumatic amputation of two or more lesser toes

  ☑6th **S98.21** Complete traumatic amputation of two or more lesser toes

    ☑7th **S98.211** Complete traumatic amputation of two or more right lesser toes

    ☑7th **S98.212** Complete traumatic amputation of two or more left lesser toes

    ☑7th **S98.219** Complete traumatic amputation of two or more unspecified lesser toes

  ☑6th **S98.22** Partial traumatic amputation of two or more lesser toes

    ☑7th **S98.221** Partial traumatic amputation of two or more right lesser toes

    ☑7th **S98.222** Partial traumatic amputation of two or more left lesser toes

☑ Appropriate additional character required   ☑x7th Requires 7th character, placeholder x must fill empty characters

Injury, Poisoning and Certain Other Consequences of External Causes

     ✓7ᵗʰ   **S98.229**   **Partial traumatic amputation of two or more unspecified lesser toes**

✓5ᵗʰ   **S98.3**   **Traumatic amputation of midfoot**
     ✓6ᵗʰ   **S98.31**   **Complete traumatic amputation of midfoot**
         ✓7ᵗʰ   **S98.311**   **Complete traumatic amputation of right midfoot**
         ✓7ᵗʰ   **S98.312**   **Complete traumatic amputation of left midfoot**
         ✓7ᵗʰ   **S98.319**   **Complete traumatic amputation of unspecified midfoot**
     ✓6ᵗʰ   **S98.32**   **Partial traumatic amputation of midfoot**
         ✓7ᵗʰ   **S98.321**   **Partial traumatic amputation of right midfoot**
         ✓7ᵗʰ   **S98.322**   **Partial traumatic amputation of left midfoot**
         ✓7ᵗʰ   **S98.329**   **Partial traumatic amputation of unspecified midfoot**

✓5ᵗʰ   **S98.9**   **Traumatic amputation of foot, level unspecified**
     ✓6ᵗʰ   **S98.91**   **Complete traumatic amputation of foot, level unspecified**
         ✓7ᵗʰ   **S98.911**   **Complete traumatic amputation of right foot, level unspecified**
         ✓7ᵗʰ   **S98.912**   **Complete traumatic amputation of left foot, level unspecified**
         ✓7ᵗʰ   **S98.919**   **Complete traumatic amputation of unspecified foot, level unspecified**
     ✓6ᵗʰ   **S98.92**   **Partial traumatic amputation of foot, level unspecified**
         ✓7ᵗʰ   **S98.921**   **Partial traumatic amputation of right foot, level unspecified**
         ✓7ᵗʰ   **S98.922**   **Partial traumatic amputation of left foot, level unspecified**
         ✓7ᵗʰ   **S98.929**   **Partial traumatic amputation of unspecified foot, level unspecified**

✓4ᵗʰ   **S99**   **Other and unspecified injuries of ankle and foot**

> The appropriate 7th character is to be added to each code from category S99.
> A   initial encounter
> D   subsequent encounter
> S   sequela

     ✓5ᵗʰ   **S99.8**   **Other specified injuries of ankle and foot**
         ✓6ᵗʰ   **S99.81**   **Other specified injuries of ankle**
             ✓7ᵗʰ   **S99.811**   **Other specified injuries of right ankle**
             ✓7ᵗʰ   **S99.812**   **Other specified injuries of left ankle**
             ✓7ᵗʰ   **S99.819**   **Other specified injuries of unspecified ankle**
         ✓6ᵗʰ   **S99.82**   **Other specified injuries of foot**
             ✓7ᵗʰ   **S99.821**   **Other specified injuries of right foot**
             ✓7ᵗʰ   **S99.822**   **Other specified injuries of left foot**
             ✓7ᵗʰ   **S99.829**   **Other specified injuries of unspecified foot**
     ✓5ᵗʰ   **S99.9**   **Unspecified injury of ankle and foot**
         ✓6ᵗʰ   **S99.91**   **Unspecified injury of ankle**
             ✓7ᵗʰ   **S99.911**   **Unspecified injury of right ankle**
             ✓7ᵗʰ   **S99.912**   **Unspecified injury of left ankle**
             ✓7ᵗʰ   **S99.919**   **Unspecified injury of unspecified ankle**
         ✓6ᵗʰ   **S99.92**   **Unspecified injury of foot**
             ✓7ᵗʰ   **S99.921**   **Unspecified injury of right foot**
             ✓7ᵗʰ   **S99.922**   **Unspecified injury of left foot**
             ✓7ᵗʰ   **S99.929**   **Unspecified injury of unspecified foot**

Injury, Poisoning And Certain Other Consequences Of External Causes (T07-T88)

T00-T06   **Deactivated**
     Code to individual injuries.

Injuries involving multiple body regions (T07)

EXCLUDES 1   *burns and corrosions (T20-T32)*
     frostbite (T33-T34)
     insect bite or sting, venomous (T63.4)
     sunburn (L55-)

T07   **Unspecified multiple injuries**
     NOTE   This code is for use only when no documentation is available identifying the specific injuries. This code is not for use in the inpatient setting
     EXCLUDES 1   *injury NOS (T14)*

T08-T13   **Deactivated**

Injury of unspecified body region (T14)

✓4ᵗʰ   **T14**   **Injury of unspecified body region**
     EXCLUDES 1   *multiple unspecified injuries (T07)*
     T14.8   **Other injury of unspecified body region**
         Contusion NOS
         Crush injury NOS
         Fracture NOS
         Skin injury NOS
         Vascular injury NOS
     ✓5ᵗʰ   **T14.9**   **Unspecified injury**
         T14.90   **Injury, unspecified**
             NOTE   This code is for use only when no documentation is available identifying the specific injury. This code is not for use in the inpatient setting.
             Injury NOS
         T14.91   **Suicide attempt**
             Attempted suicide NOS

Effects of foreign body entering through natural orifice (T15-T19)

NOTE   Codes within this section that include the external cause do not need an additional external cause code
EXCLUDES 2   *foreign body accidentally left in operation wound (T81.5-)*
     foreign body in penetrating wound—See open wound by body region
     residual foreign body in soft tissue (M79.5)
     splinter, without open wound—See superficial injury by body region

✓4ᵗʰ   **T15**   **Foreign body on external eye**
     EXCLUDES 2   *foreign body in penetrating wound of orbit and eye ball (S05.4-, S05.5-)*
     open wound of eyelid and periocular area (S01.1-)
     retained foreign body in eyelid (H02.8-)
     retained (old) foreign body in penetrating wound of orbit and eye ball (H05.5-, H44.6-, H44.7-)
     superficial foreign body of eyelid and periocular area (S00.25-)

> The appropriate 7th character is to be added to each code from category T15.
> A   initial encounter
> D   subsequent encounter
> S   sequela

     ✓5ᵗʰ   **T15.0**   **Foreign body in cornea**
         ✓x7ᵗʰ   **T15.00**   **Foreign body in cornea, unspecified eye**
         ✓x7ᵗʰ   **T15.01**   **Foreign body in cornea, right eye**
         ✓x7ᵗʰ   **T15.02**   **Foreign body in cornea, left eye**
     ✓5ᵗʰ   **T15.1**   **Foreign body in conjunctival sac**
         ✓x7ᵗʰ   **T15.10**   **Foreign body in conjunctival sac, unspecified eye**
         ✓x7ᵗʰ   **T15.11**   **Foreign body in conjunctival sac, right eye**
         ✓x7ᵗʰ   **T15.12**   **Foreign body in conjunctival sac, left eye**
     ✓5ᵗʰ   **T15.8**   **Foreign body in other and multiple parts of external eye**
         Foreign body in lacrimal punctum
         ✓x7ᵗʰ   **T15.80**   **Foreign body in other and multiple parts of external eye, unspecified eye**
         ✓x7ᵗʰ   **T15.81**   **Foreign body in other and multiple parts of external eye, right eye**
         ✓x7ᵗʰ   **T15.82**   **Foreign body in other and multiple parts of external eye, left eye**

EXCLUDES 1   Not coded here   EXCLUDES 2   Not included here   *Manifestation Code*

√5th **T15.9 Foreign body on external eye, part unspecified**
- √x7th **T15.90** Foreign body on external eye, part unspecified, unspecified eye
- √x7th **T15.91** Foreign body on external eye, part unspecified, right eye
- √x7th **T15.92** Foreign body on external eye, part unspecified, left eye

√4th **T16 Foreign body in ear**
Foreign body in auditory canal

> The appropriate 7th character is to be added to each code from category T16.
> A   initial encounter
> D   subsequent encounter
> S   sequela

- √x7th **T16.1** Foreign body in right ear
- √x7th **T16.2** Foreign body in left ear
- √x7th **T16.9** Foreign body in ear, unspecified ear

√4th **T17 Foreign body in respiratory tract**

> The appropriate 7th character is to be added to each code from category T17.
> A   initial encounter
> D   subsequent encounter
> S   sequela

- √x7th **T17.0** Foreign body in nasal sinus
- √x7th **T17.1** Foreign body in nostril
  Foreign body in nose NOS
- √5th **T17.2 Foreign body in pharynx**
  Foreign body in nasopharynx
  Foreign body in throat NOS
  - √6th **T17.20** Unspecified foreign body in pharynx
    - √7th **T17.200** Unspecified foreign body in pharynx causing asphyxiation
    - √7th **T17.208** Unspecified foreign body in pharynx causing other injury
  - √6th **T17.21** Gastric contents in pharynx
    Aspiration of gastric contents into pharynx
    Vomitus in pharynx
    - √7th **T17.210** Gastric contents in pharynx causing asphyxiation
    - √7th **T17.218** Gastric contents in pharynx causing other injury
  - √6th **T17.22** Food in pharynx
    Bones in pharynx
    Seeds in pharynx
    - √7th **T17.220** Food in pharynx causing asphyxiation
    - √7th **T17.228** Food in pharynx causing other injury
  - √6th **T17.29** Other foreign object in pharynx
    - √7th **T17.290** Other foreign object in pharynx causing asphyxiation
    - √7th **T17.298** Other foreign object in pharynx causing other injury
- √5th **T17.3 Foreign body in larynx**
  - √6th **T17.30** Unspecified foreign body in larynx
    - √7th **T17.300** Unspecified foreign body in larynx causing asphyxiation
    - √7th **T17.308** Unspecified foreign body in larynx causing other injury
  - √6th **T17.31** Gastric contents in larynx
    Aspiration of gastric contents into larynx
    Vomitus in larynx
    - √7th **T17.310** Gastric contents in larynx causing asphyxiation
    - √7th **T17.318** Gastric contents in larynx causing other injury
  - √6th **T17.32** Food in larynx
    Bones in larynx
    Seeds in larynx
    - √7th **T17.320** Food in larynx causing asphyxiation
    - √7th **T17.328** Food in larynx causing other injury
  - √6th **T17.39** Other foreign object in larynx
    - √7th **T17.390** Other foreign object in larynx causing asphyxiation
    - √7th **T17.398** Other foreign object in larynx causing other injury

√5th **T17.4 Foreign body in trachea**
- √6th **T17.40** Unspecified foreign body in trachea
  - √7th **T17.400** Unspecified foreign body in trachea causing asphyxiation
  - √7th **T17.408** Unspecified foreign body in trachea causing other injury
- √6th **T17.41** Gastric contents in trachea
  Aspiration of gastric contents into trachea
  Vomitus in trachea
  - √7th **T17.410** Gastric contents in trachea causing asphyxiation
  - √7th **T17.418** Gastric contents in trachea causing other injury
- √6th **T17.42** Food in trachea
  Bones in trachea
  Seeds in trachea
  - √7th **T17.420** Food in trachea causing asphyxiation
  - √7th **T17.428** Food in trachea causing other injury
- √6th **T17.49** Other foreign object in trachea
  - √7th **T17.490** Other foreign object in trachea causing asphyxiation
  - √7th **T17.498** Other foreign object in trachea causing other injury

√5th **T17.5 Foreign body in bronchus**
- √6th **T17.50** Unspecified foreign body in bronchus
  - √7th **T17.500** Unspecified foreign body in bronchus causing asphyxiation
  - √7th **T17.508** Unspecified foreign body in bronchus causing other injury
- √6th **T17.51** Gastric contents in bronchus
  Aspiration of gastric contents into bronchus
  Vomitus in bronchus
  - √7th **T17.510** Gastric contents in bronchus causing asphyxiation
  - √7th **T17.518** Gastric contents in bronchus causing other injury
- √6th **T17.52** Food in bronchus
  Bones in bronchus
  Seeds in bronchus
  - √7th **T17.520** Food in bronchus causing asphyxiation
  - √7th **T17.528** Food in bronchus causing other injury
- √6th **T17.59** Other foreign object in bronchus
  - √7th **T17.590** Other foreign object in bronchus causing asphyxiation
  - √7th **T17.598** Other foreign object in bronchus causing other injury

√5th **T17.8 Foreign body in other parts of respiratory tract**
Foreign body in bronchioles
Foreign body in lung
- √6th **T17.80** Unspecified foreign body in other parts of respiratory tract
  - √7th **T17.800** Unspecified foreign body in other parts of respiratory tract causing asphyxiation
  - √7th **T17.808** Unspecified foreign body in other parts of respiratory tract causing other injury
- √6th **T17.81** Gastric contents in other parts of respiratory tract
  Aspiration of gastric contents into other parts of respiratory tract
  Vomitus in other parts of respiratory tract
  - √7th **T17.810** Gastric contents in other parts of respiratory tract causing asphyxiation
  - √7th **T17.818** Gastric contents in other parts of respiratory tract causing other injury
- √6th **T17.82** Food in other parts of respiratory tract
  Bones in other parts of respiratory tract
  Seeds in other parts of respiratory tract
  - √7th **T17.820** Food in other parts of respiratory tract causing asphyxiation
  - √7th **T17.828** Food in other parts of respiratory tract causing other injury
- √6th **T17.89** Other foreign object in other parts of respiratory tract
  - √7th **T17.890** Other foreign object in other parts of respiratory tract causing asphyxiation
  - √7th **T17.898** Other foreign object in other parts of respiratory tract causing other injury

Injury, Poisoning and Certain Other Consequences of External Causes

T17.9–T20.05

√5ᵗʰ **T17.9 Foreign body in respiratory tract, part unspecified**

√6ᵗʰ **T17.90 Unspecified foreign body in respiratory tract, part unspecified**

√7ᵗʰ **T17.900 Unspecified foreign body in respiratory tract, part unspecified causing asphyxiation**

√7ᵗʰ **T17.908 Unspecified foreign body in respiratory tract, part unspecified causing other injury**

√6ᵗʰ **T17.91 Gastric contents in respiratory tract, part unspecified**

Aspiration of gastric contents into respiratory tract, part unspecified

Vomitus in trachea respiratory tract, part unspecified

√7ᵗʰ **T17.910 Gastric contents in respiratory tract, part unspecified causing asphyxiation**

√7ᵗʰ **T17.918 Gastric contents in respiratory tract, part unspecified causing other injury**

√6ᵗʰ **T17.92 Food in respiratory tract, part unspecified**

Bones in respiratory tract, part unspecified

Seeds in respiratory tract, part unspecified

√7ᵗʰ **T17.920 Food in respiratory tract, part unspecified causing asphyxiation**

√7ᵗʰ **T17.928 Food in respiratory tract, part unspecified causing other injury**

√6ᵗʰ **T17.99 Other foreign object in respiratory tract, part unspecified**

√7ᵗʰ **T17.990 Other foreign object in respiratory tract, part unspecified in causing asphyxiation**

√7ᵗʰ **T17.998 Other foreign object in respiratory tract, part unspecified causing other injury**

√4ᵗʰ **T18 Foreign body in alimentary tract**

EXCLUDES 2   *foreign body in pharynx (T17.2-)*

The appropriate 7th character is to be added to each code from category T18.
A   initial encounter
D   subsequent encounter
S   sequela

√x7ᵗʰ **T18.0 Foreign body in mouth**

√5ᵗʰ **T18.1 Foreign body in esophagus**

EXCLUDES 2   *foreign body in respiratory tract (T17-)*

√6ᵗʰ **T18.10 Unspecified foreign body in esophagus**

√7ᵗʰ **T18.100 Unspecified foreign body in esophagus causing compression of trachea**

Unspecified foreign body in esophagus causing obstruction of respiration

√7ᵗʰ **T18.108 Unspecified foreign body in esophagus causing other injury**

√6ᵗʰ **T18.11 Gastric contents in esophagus**

Vomitus in esophagus

√7ᵗʰ **T18.110 Gastric contents in esophagus causing compression of trachea**

Gastric contents in esophagus causing obstruction of respiration

√7ᵗʰ **T18.118 Gastric contents in esophagus causing other injury**

√6ᵗʰ **T18.12 Food in esophagus**

Bones in esophagus

Seeds in esophagus

√7ᵗʰ **T18.120 Food in esophagus causing compression of trachea**

Food in esophagus causing obstruction of respiration

√7ᵗʰ **T18.128 Food in esophagus causing other injury**

√6ᵗʰ **T18.19 Other foreign object in esophagus**

√7ᵗʰ **T18.190 Other foreign object in esophagus causing compression of trachea**

Other foreign body in esophagus causing obstruction of respiration

√7ᵗʰ **T18.198 Other foreign object in esophagus causing other injury**

√x7ᵗʰ **T18.2 Foreign body in stomach**

√x7ᵗʰ **T18.3 Foreign body in small intestine**

√x7ᵗʰ **T18.4 Foreign body in colon**

√x7ᵗʰ **T18.5 Foreign body in anus and rectum**

Foreign body in rectosigmoid (junction)

√x7ᵗʰ **T18.8 Foreign body in other parts of alimentary tract**

√x7ᵗʰ **T18.9 Foreign body of alimentary tract, part unspecified**

Foreign body in digestive system NOS

Swallowed foreign body NOS

√4ᵗʰ **T19 Foreign body in genitourinary tract**

EXCLUDES 2   *mechanical complications of contraceptive device (intrauterine) (vaginal) (T83.3-)*

presence of contraceptive device (intrauterine) (vaginal) (Z97.5)

The appropriate 7th character is to be added to each code from category T19.
A   initial encounter
D   subsequent encounter
S   sequela

√x7ᵗʰ **T19.0 Foreign body in urethra**

√x7ᵗʰ **T19.1 Foreign body in bladder**

√x7ᵗʰ **T19.2 Foreign body in vulva and vagina**

√x7ᵗʰ **T19.3 Foreign body in uterus**

√x7ᵗʰ **T19.4 Foreign body in penis**

√x7ᵗʰ **T19.8 Foreign body in other parts of genitourinary tract**

√x7ᵗʰ **T19.9 Foreign body in genitourinary tract, part unspecified**

Burns and corrosions (T20-T32)

INCLUDES   burns (thermal) from electrical heating appliances
burns (thermal) from electricity
burns (thermal) from flame
burns (thermal) from friction
burns (thermal) from hot air and hot gases
burns (thermal) from hot objects
burns (thermal) from lightning
burns (thermal) from radiation
chemical burn [corrosion] (external) (internal)
scalds

EXCLUDES 2   *erythema [dermatitis] ab igne (L59.0)*
radiation-related disorders of the skin and subcutaneous tissue (L55-L59)
sunburn (L55-)

Burns and corrosions of external body surface, specified by site (T20-T25)

INCLUDES   burns and corrosions of first degree [erythema]
burns and corrosions of second degree [blisters][epidermal loss]
burns and corrosions of third degree [deep necrosis of underlying tissue] [full-thickness skin loss]

Use additional code from category T31 or T32 to identify extent of body surface involved

√4ᵗʰ **T20 Burn and corrosion of head, face, and neck**

EXCLUDES 2   *burn and corrosion of ear drum (T28.41, T28.91)*
burn and corrosion of eye and adnexa (T26-)
burn and corrosion of mouth and pharynx (T28.0)

The appropriate 7th character is to be added to each code from category T20.
A   initial encounter
D   subsequent encounter
S   sequela

√5ᵗʰ **T20.0 Burn of unspecified degree of head, face, and neck**

Use additional external cause code to identify the source, place and intent of the burn (X00-X19, X75-X77, X96-X98, Y92)

√x7ᵗʰ **T20.00 Burn of unspecified degree of head, face, and neck, unspecified site**

√6ᵗʰ **T20.01 Burn of unspecified degree of ear [any part, except ear drum]**

EXCLUDES 2   *burn of ear drum (T28.41-)*

√7ᵗʰ **T20.011 Burn of unspecified degree of right ear [any part, except ear drum]**

√7ᵗʰ **T20.012 Burn of unspecified degree of left ear [any part, except ear drum]**

√7ᵗʰ **T20.019 Burn of unspecified degree of unspecified ear [any part, except ear drum]**

√x7ᵗʰ **T20.02 Burn of unspecified degree of lip(s)**

√x7ᵗʰ **T20.03 Burn of unspecified degree of chin**

√x7ᵗʰ **T20.04 Burn of unspecified degree of nose (septum)**

√x7ᵗʰ **T20.05 Burn of unspecified degree of scalp [any part]**

√x7ᵗʰ **T20.06** **Burn of unspecified degree of forehead and cheek**

√x7ᵗʰ **T20.07** **Burn of unspecified degree of neck**

√x7ᵗʰ **T20.09** **Burn of unspecified degree of multiple sites of head, face, and neck**

√5ᵗʰ **T20.1** **Burn of first degree of head, face, and neck**
Use additional external cause code to identify the source, place and intent of the burn (X00-X19, X75-X77, X96-X98, Y92)

√x7ᵗʰ **T20.10** **Burn of first degree of head, face, and neck, unspecified site**

√6ᵗʰ **T20.11** **Burn of first degree of ear [any part, except ear drum]**
EXCLUDES 2 *burn of ear drum (T28.41-)*

√7ᵗʰ **T20.111** **Burn of first degree of right ear [any part, except ear drum]**

√7ᵗʰ **T20.112** **Burn of first degree of left ear [any part, except ear drum]**

√7ᵗʰ **T20.119** **Burn of first degree of unspecified ear [any part, except ear drum]**

√x7ᵗʰ **T20.12** **Burn of first degree of lip(s)**

√x7ᵗʰ **T20.13** **Burn of first degree of chin**

√x7ᵗʰ **T20.14** **Burn of first degree of nose (septum)**

√x7ᵗʰ **T20.15** **Burn of first degree of scalp [any part]**

√x7ᵗʰ **T20.16** **Burn of first degree of forehead and cheek**

√x7ᵗʰ **T20.17** **Burn of first degree of neck**

√x7ᵗʰ **T20.19** **Burn of first degree of multiple sites of head, face, and neck**

√5ᵗʰ **T20.2** **Burn of second degree of head, face, and neck**
Use additional external cause code to identify the source, place and intent of the burn (X00-X19, X75-X77, X96-X98, Y92)

√x7ᵗʰ **T20.20** **Burn of second degree of head, face, and neck, unspecified site**

√6ᵗʰ **T20.21** **Burn of second degree of ear [any part, except ear drum]**
EXCLUDES 2 *burn of ear drum (T28.41-)*

√7ᵗʰ **T20.211** **Burn of second degree of right ear [any part, except ear drum]**

√7ᵗʰ **T20.212** **Burn of second degree of left ear [any part, except ear drum]**

√7ᵗʰ **T20.219** **Burn of second degree of unspecified ear [any part, except ear drum]**

√x7ᵗʰ **T20.22** **Burn of second degree of lip(s)**

√x7ᵗʰ **T20.23** **Burn of second degree of chin**

√x7ᵗʰ **T20.24** **Burn of second degree of nose (septum)**

√x7ᵗʰ **T20.25** **Burn of second degree of scalp [any part]**

√x7ᵗʰ **T20.26** **Burn of second degree of forehead and cheek**

√x7ᵗʰ **T20.27** **Burn of second degree of neck**

√x7ᵗʰ **T20.29** **Burn of second degree of multiple sites of head, face, and neck**

√5ᵗʰ **T20.3** **Burn of third degree of head, face, and neck**
Use additional external cause code to identify the source, place and intent of the burn (X00-X19, X75-X77, X96-X98, Y92)

√x7ᵗʰ **T20.30** **Burn of third degree of head, face, and neck, unspecified site**

√6ᵗʰ **T20.31** **Burn of third degree of ear [any part, except ear drum]**
EXCLUDES 2 *burn of ear drum (T28.41-)*

√7ᵗʰ **T20.311** **Burn of third degree of right ear [any part, except ear drum]**

√7ᵗʰ **T20.312** **Burn of third degree of left ear [any part, except ear drum]**

√7ᵗʰ **T20.319** **Burn of third degree of unspecified ear [any part, except ear drum]**

√x7ᵗʰ **T20.32** **Burn of third degree of lip(s)**

√x7ᵗʰ **T20.33** **Burn of third degree of chin**

√x7ᵗʰ **T20.34** **Burn of third degree of nose (septum)**

√x7ᵗʰ **T20.35** **Burn of third degree of scalp [any part]**

√x7ᵗʰ **T20.36** **Burn of third degree of forehead and cheek**

√x7ᵗʰ **T20.37** **Burn of third degree of neck**

√x7ᵗʰ **T20.39** **Burn of third degree of multiple sites of head, face, and neck**

√5ᵗʰ **T20.4** **Corrosion of unspecified degree of head, face, and neck**
Code first (T51-T65) to identify chemical and intent
Use additional external cause code to identify place (Y92)

√x6ᵗʰ **T20.40** **Corrosion of unspecified degree of head, face, and neck, unspecified site**

√6ᵗʰ **T20.41** **Corrosion of unspecified degree of ear [any part, except ear drum]**
EXCLUDES 2 *corrosion of ear drum (T28.91-)*

√7ᵗʰ **T20.411** **Corrosion of unspecified degree of right ear [any part, except ear drum]**

√7ᵗʰ **T20.412** **Corrosion of unspecified degree of left ear [any part, except ear drum]**

√7ᵗʰ **T20.419** **Corrosion of unspecified degree of unspecified ear [any part, except ear drum]**

√x7ᵗʰ **T20.42** **Corrosion of unspecified degree of lip(s)**

√x7ᵗʰ **T20.43** **Corrosion of unspecified degree of chin**

√x7ᵗʰ **T20.44** **Corrosion of unspecified degree of nose (septum)**

√x7ᵗʰ **T20.45** **Corrosion of unspecified degree of scalp [any part]**

√x7ᵗʰ **T20.46** **Corrosion of unspecified degree of forehead and cheek**

√x7ᵗʰ **T20.47** **Corrosion of unspecified degree of neck**

√x7ᵗʰ **T20.49** **Corrosion of unspecified degree of multiple sites of head, face, and neck**

√5ᵗʰ **T20.5** **Corrosion of first degree of head, face, and neck**
Code first (T51-T65) to identify chemical and intent
Use additional external cause code to identify place (Y92)

√x7ᵗʰ **T20.50** **Corrosion of first degree of head, face, and neck, unspecified site**

√6ᵗʰ **T20.51** **Corrosion of first degree of ear [any part, except ear drum]**
EXCLUDES 2 *corrosion of ear drum (T28.91-)*

√7ᵗʰ **T20.511** **Corrosion of first degree of right ear [any part, except ear drum]**

√7ᵗʰ **T20.512** **Corrosion of first degree of left ear [any part, except ear drum]**

√7ᵗʰ **T20.519** **Corrosion of first degree of unspecified ear [any part, except ear drum]**

√x7ᵗʰ **T20.52** **Corrosion of first degree of lip(s)**

√x7ᵗʰ **T20.53** **Corrosion of first degree of chin**

√x7ᵗʰ **T20.54** **Corrosion of first degree of nose (septum)**

√x7ᵗʰ **T20.55** **Corrosion of first degree of scalp [any part]**

√x7ᵗʰ **T20.56** **Corrosion of first degree of cheek**

√x7ᵗʰ **T20.57** **Corrosion of first degree of neck**

√x7ᵗʰ **T20.59** **Corrosion of first degree of multiple sites of head, face, and neck**

√5ᵗʰ **T20.6** **Corrosion of second degree of head, face, and neck**
Code first (T51-T65) to identify chemical and intent
Use additional external cause code to identify place (Y92)

√x7ᵗʰ **T20.60** **Corrosion of second degree of head, face, and neck, unspecified site**

√6ᵗʰ **T20.61** **Corrosion of second degree of ear [any part, except ear drum]**
EXCLUDES 2 *corrosion of ear drum (T28.91-)*

√7ᵗʰ **T20.611** **Corrosion of second degree of right ear [any part, except ear drum]**

√7ᵗʰ **T20.612** **Corrosion of second degree of left ear [any part, except ear drum]**

√7ᵗʰ **T20.619** **Corrosion of second degree of unspecified ear [any part, except ear drum]**

√x7ᵗʰ **T20.62** **Corrosion of second degree of lip(s)**

√x7ᵗʰ **T20.63** **Corrosion of second degree of chin**

√x7ᵗʰ **T20.64** **Corrosion of second degree of nose (septum)**

√x7ᵗʰ **T20.65** **Corrosion of second degree of scalp [any part]**

√x7ᵗʰ **T20.66** **Corrosion of second degree of forehead and cheek**

√x7ᵗʰ **T20.67** **Corrosion of second degree of neck**

√x7ᵗʰ **T20.69** **Corrosion of second degree of multiple sites of head, face, and neck**

√5ᵗʰ **T20.7** **Corrosion of third degree of head, face, and neck**
Code first (T51-T65) to identify chemical and intent
Use additional external cause code to identify place (Y92)

√x7ᵗʰ **T20.70** **Corrosion of third degree of head, face, and neck, unspecified site**

√6ᵗʰ **T20.71** **Corrosion of third degree of ear [any part, except ear drum]**
EXCLUDES 2 *corrosion of ear drum (T28.91-)*

√7ᵗʰ **T20.711** **Corrosion of third degree of right ear [any part, except ear drum]**

☑ Appropriate additional character required   √x7ᵗʰ Requires 7th character, placeholder x must fill empty characters

Injury, Poisoning and Certain Other Consequences of External Causes

T20.712–T21.47

✓7th T20.712 Corrosion of third degree of left ear [any part, except ear drum]

✓7th T20.719 Corrosion of third degree of unspecified ear [any part, except ear drum]

✓x7th T20.72 Corrosion of third degree of lip(s)

✓x7th T20.73 Corrosion of third degree of chin

✓x7th T20.74 Corrosion of third degree of nose (septum)

✓x7th T20.75 Corrosion of third degree of scalp [any part]

✓x7th T20.76 Corrosion of third degree of forehead and cheek

✓x7th T20.77 Corrosion of third degree of neck

✓x7th T20.79 Corrosion of third degree of multiple sites of head, face, and neck

✓4th T21 Burn and corrosion of trunk

Burns and corrosion of hip region

EXCLUDES 2   *burns and corrosion of:*
axilla (T22- with fifth character 4)
scapular region (T22- with fifth character 6)
shoulder (T22. with fifth character 5)

> The appropriate 7th character is to be added to each code from category T21.
> A   initial encounter
> D   subsequent encounter
> S   sequela

✓5th T21.0 Burn of unspecified degree of trunk

Use additional external cause code to identify the source, place and intent of the burn (X00-X19, X75-X77, X96-X98, Y92)

✓x7th T21.00 Burn of unspecified degree of trunk, unspecified site

✓x7th T21.01 Burn of unspecified degree of chest wall
Burn of of unspecified degree of breast

✓x7th T21.02 Burn of unspecified degree of abdominal wall
Burn of unspecified degree of flank
Burn of unspecified degree of groin

✓x7th T21.03 Burn of unspecified degree of upper back
Burn of unspecified degree of interscapular region

✓x7th T21.04 Burn of unspecified degree of lower back

✓x7th T21.05 Burn of unspecified degree of buttock
Burn of unspecified degree of anus

✓x7th T21.06 Burn of unspecified degree of male genital region
Burn of unspecified degree of penis
Burn of unspecified degree of scrotum
Burn of unspecified degree of testis

✓x7th T21.07 Burn of unspecified degree of female genital region
Burn of unspecified degree of labium (majus) (minus)
Burn of unspecified degree of perineum
Burn of unspecified degree of vulva
EXCLUDES 2   *burn of vagina (T28.3)*

✓x7th T21.09 Burn of unspecified degree of other site of trunk

✓5th T21.1 Burn of first degree of trunk

Use additional external cause code to identify the source, place and intent of the burn (X00-X19, X75-X77, X96-X98, Y92)

✓x7th T21.10 Burn of first degree of trunk, unspecified site

✓x7th T21.11 Burn of first degree of chest wall
Burn of first degree of breast

✓x7th T21.12 Burn of first degree of abdominal wall
Burn of first degree of flank
Burn of first degree of groin

✓x7th T21.13 Burn of first degree of upper back
Burn of first degree of interscapular region

✓x7th T21.14 Burn of first degree of lower back

✓x7th T21.15 Burn of first degree of buttock
Burn of first degree of anus

✓x7th T21.16 Burn of first degree of male genital region
Burn of first degree of penis
Burn of first degree of scrotum
Burn of first degree of testis

✓x7th T21.17 Burn of first degree of female genital region
Burn of first degree of labium (majus) (minus)
Burn of first degree of perineum
Burn of first degree of vulva
EXCLUDES 2   *burn of vagina (T28.3)*

✓x7th T21.19 Burn of first degree of other site of trunk

✓5th T21.2 Burn of second degree of trunk

Use additional external cause code to identify the source, place and intent of the burn (X00-X19, X75-X77, X96-X98, Y92)

✓x7th T21.20 Burn of second degree of trunk, unspecified site

✓x7th T21.21 Burn of second degree of chest wall
Burn of second degree of breast

✓x7th T21.22 Burn of second degree of abdominal wall
Burn of second degree of flank
Burn of second degree of groin

✓x7th T21.23 Burn of second degree of upper back
Burn of second degree of interscapular region

✓x7th T21.24 Burn of second degree of lower back

✓x7th T21.25 Burn of second degree of buttock
Burn of second degree of anus

✓x7th T21.26 Burn of second degree of male genital region
Burn of second degree of penis
Burn of second degree of scrotum
Burn of second degree of testis

✓x7th T21.27 Burn of second degree of female genital region
Burn of second degree of labium (majus) (minus)
Burn of second degree of perineum
Burn of second degree of vulva
EXCLUDES 2   *burn of vagina (T28.3)*

✓x7th T21.29 Burn of second degree of other site of trunk

✓5th T21.3 Burn of third degree of trunk

Use additional external cause code to identify the source, place and intent of the burn (X00-X19, X75-X77, X96-X98, Y92)

✓x7th T21.30 Burn of third degree of trunk, unspecified site

✓x7th T21.31 Burn of third degree of chest wall
Burn of third degree of breast

✓x7th T21.32 Burn of third degree of abdominal wall
Burn of third degree of flank
Burn of third degree of groin

✓x7th T21.33 Burn of third degree of upper back
Burn of third degree of interscapular region

✓x7th T21.34 Burn of third degree of lower back

✓x7th T21.35 Burn of third degree of buttock
Burn of third degree of anus

✓x7th T21.36 Burn of third degree of male genital region
Burn of third degree of penis
Burn of third degree of scrotum
Burn of third degree of testis

✓x7th T21.37 Burn of third degree of female genital region
Burn of third degree of labium (majus) (minus)
Burn of third degree of perineum
Burn of third degree of vulva
EXCLUDES 2   *burn of vagina (T28.3)*

✓x7th T21.39 Burn of third degree of other site of trunk

✓5th T21.4 Corrosion of unspecified degree of trunk

Code first (T51-T65) to identify chemical and intent
Use additional external cause code to identify place (Y92)

✓x7th T21.40 Corrosion of unspecified degree of trunk, unspecified site

✓x7th T21.41 Corrosion of unspecified degree of chest wall
Corrosion of unspecified degree of breast

✓x7th T21.42 Corrosion of unspecified degree of abdominal wall
Corrosion of unspecified degree of flank
Corrosion of unspecified degree of groin

✓x7th T21.43 Corrosion of unspecified degree of upper back
Corrosion of unspecified degree of interscapular region

✓x7th T21.44 Corrosion of unspecified degree of lower back

✓x7th T21.45 Corrosion of unspecified degree of buttock
Corrosion of unspecified degree of anus

✓x7th T21.46 Corrosion of unspecified degree of male genital region
Corrosion of unspecified degree of penis
Corrosion of unspecified degree of scrotum
Corrosion of unspecified degree of testis

✓x7th T21.47 Corrosion of unspecified degree of female genital region
Corrosion of unspecified degree of labium (majus) (minus)
Corrosion of unspecified degree of perineum
Corrosion of unspecified degree of vulva
EXCLUDES 2   *corrosion of vagina (T28.8)*

EXCLUDES 1 Not coded here   *EXCLUDES 2* Not included here   *Manifestation Code*

√x7ᵗʰ **T21.49 Corrosion of unspecified degree of other site of trunk**

√5ᵗʰ **T21.5 Corrosion of first degree of trunk**
Code first (T51-T65) to identify chemical and intent
Use additional external cause code to identify place (Y92)

√x7ᵗʰ **T21.50 Corrosion of first degree of trunk, unspecified site**

√x7ᵗʰ **T21.51 Corrosion of first degree of chest wall**
Corrosion of first degree of breast

√x7ᵗʰ **T21.52 Corrosion of first degree of abdominal wall**
Corrosion of first degree of flank
Corrosion of first degree of groin

√x7ᵗʰ **T21.53 Corrosion of first degree of upper back**
Corrosion of first degree of interscapular region

√x7ᵗʰ **T21.54 Corrosion of first degree of lower back**

√x7ᵗʰ **T21.55 Corrosion of first degree of buttock**
Corrosion of first degree of anus

√x7ᵗʰ **T21.56 Corrosion of first degree of male genital region**
Corrosion of first degree of penis
Corrosion of first degree of scrotum
Corrosion of first degree of testis

√x7ᵗʰ **T21.57 Corrosion of first degree of female genital region**
Corrosion of first degree of labium (majus) (minus)
Corrosion of first degree of perineum
Corrosion of first degree of vulva
EXCLUDES 2 corrosion of vagina (T28.8)

√x7ᵗʰ **T21.59 Corrosion of first degree of other site of trunk**

√5ᵗʰ **T21.6 Corrosion of second degree of trunk**
Code first (T51-T65) to identify chemical and intent
Use additional external cause code to identify place (Y92)

√x7ᵗʰ **T21.60 Corrosion of second degree of trunk, unspecified site**

√x7ᵗʰ **T21.61 Corrosion of second degree of chest wall**
Corrosion of second degree of breast

√x7ᵗʰ **T21.62 Corrosion of second degree of abdominal wall**
Corrosion of second degree of flank
Corrosion of second degree of groin

√x7ᵗʰ **T21.63 Corrosion of second degree of upper back**
Corrosion of second degree of interscapular region

√x7ᵗʰ **T21.64 Corrosion of second degree of lower back**

√x7ᵗʰ **T21.65 Corrosion of second degree of buttock**
Corrosion of second degree of anus

√x7ᵗʰ **T21.66 Corrosion of second degree of male genital region**
Corrosion of second degree of penis
Corrosion of second degree of scrotum
Corrosion of second degree of testis

√x7ᵗʰ **T21.67 Corrosion of second degree of female genital region**
Corrosion of second degree of labium (majus) (minus)
Corrosion of second degree of perineum
Corrosion of second degree of vulva
EXCLUDES 2 corrosion of vagina (T28.8)

√x7ᵗʰ **T21.69 Corrosion of second degree of other site of trunk**

√5ᵗʰ **T21.7 Corrosion of third degree of trunk**
Code first (T51-T65) to identify chemical and intent
Use additional external cause code to identify place (Y92)

√x7ᵗʰ **T21.70 Corrosion of third degree of trunk, unspecified site**

√x7ᵗʰ **T21.71 Corrosion of third degree of chest wall**
Corrosion of third degree of breast

√x7ᵗʰ **T21.72 Corrosion of third degree of abdominal wall**
Corrosion of third degree of flank
Corrosion of third degree of groin

√x7ᵗʰ **T21.73 Corrosion of third degree of upper back**
Corrosion of third degree of interscapular region

√x7ᵗʰ **T21.74 Corrosion of third degree of lower back**

√x7ᵗʰ **T21.75 Corrosion of third degree of buttock**
Corrosion of third degree of anus

√x7ᵗʰ **T21.76 Corrosion of third degree of male genital region**
Corrosion of third degree of penis
Corrosion of third degree of scrotum
Corrosion of third degree of testis

√x7ᵗʰ **T21.77 Corrosion of third degree of female genital region**
Corrosion of third degree of labium (majus) (minus)
Corrosion of third degree of perineum
Corrosion of third degree of vulva
EXCLUDES 2 corrosion of vagina (T28.8)

√x7ᵗʰ **T21.79 Corrosion of third degree of other site of trunk**

√4ᵗʰ **T22 Burn and corrosion of shoulder and upper limb, except wrist and hand**
EXCLUDES 2 burn and corrosion of interscapular region (T21-)
burn and corrosion of wrist and hand (T23-)

The appropriate 7th character is to be added to each code from category T22.
A initial encounter
D subsequent encounter
S sequela

√5ᵗʰ **T22.0 Burn of unspecified degree of shoulder and upper limb, except wrist and hand**
Use additional external cause code to identify the source, place and intent of the burn (X00-X19, X75-X77, X96-X98, Y92)

√x7ᵗʰ **T22.00 Burn of unspecified degree of shoulder and upper limb, except wrist and hand, unspecified site**

√6ᵗʰ **T22.01 Burn of unspecified degree of forearm**
√7ᵗʰ **T22.011 Burn of unspecified degree of right forearm**
√7ᵗʰ **T22.012 Burn of unspecified degree of left forearm**
√7ᵗʰ **T22.019 Burn of unspecified degree of unspecified forearm**

√6ᵗʰ **T22.02 Burn of unspecified degree of elbow**
√7ᵗʰ **T22.021 Burn of unspecified degree of right elbow**
√7ᵗʰ **T22.022 Burn of unspecified degree of left elbow**
√7ᵗʰ **T22.029 Burn of unspecified degree of unspecified elbow**

√6ᵗʰ **T22.03 Burn of unspecified degree of upper arm**
√7ᵗʰ **T22.031 Burn of unspecified degree of right upper arm**
√7ᵗʰ **T22.032 Burn of unspecified degree of left upper arm**
√7ᵗʰ **T22.039 Burn of unspecified degree of unspecified upper arm**

√6ᵗʰ **T22.04 Burn of unspecified degree of axilla**
√7ᵗʰ **T22.041 Burn of unspecified degree of right axilla**
√7ᵗʰ **T22.042 Burn of unspecified degree of left axilla**
√7ᵗʰ **T22.049 Burn of unspecified degree of unspecified axilla**

√6ᵗʰ **T22.05 Burn of unspecified degree of shoulder**
√7ᵗʰ **T22.051 Burn of unspecified degree of right shoulder**
√7ᵗʰ **T22.052 Burn of unspecified degree of left shoulder**
√7ᵗʰ **T22.059 Burn of unspecified degree of unspecified shoulder**

√6ᵗʰ **T22.06 Burn of unspecified degree of scapular region**
√7ᵗʰ **T22.061 Burn of unspecified degree of right scapular region**
√7ᵗʰ **T22.062 Burn of unspecified degree of left scapular region**
√7ᵗʰ **T22.069 Burn of unspecified degree of unspecified scapular region**

√6ᵗʰ **T22.09 Burn of unspecified degree of multiple sites of shoulder and upper limb, except wrist and hand**
√7ᵗʰ **T22.091 Burn of unspecified degree of multiple sites of right shoulder and upper limb, except wrist and hand**
√7ᵗʰ **T22.092 Burn of unspecified degree of multiple sites of left shoulder and upper limb, except wrist and hand**
√7ᵗʰ **T22.099 Burn of unspecified degree of multiple sites of unspecified shoulder and upper limb, except wrist and hand**

√5ᵗʰ **T22.1 Burn of first degree of shoulder and upper limb, except wrist and hand**
Use additional external cause code to identify the source, place and intent of the burn (X00-X19, X75-X77, X96-X98, Y92)

√x7ᵗʰ **T22.10 Burn of first degree of shoulder and upper limb, except wrist and hand, unspecified site**

√6ᵗʰ **T22.11 Burn of first degree of forearm**
√7ᵗʰ **T22.111 Burn of first degree of right forearm**

☑ Appropriate additional character required   √x7ᵗʰ Requires 7th character, placeholder x must fill empty characters

√7ᵗʰ **T22.112** Burn of first degree of left forearm
√7ᵗʰ **T22.119** Burn of first degree of unspecified forearm
√6ᵗʰ **T22.12** Burn of first degree of elbow
√7ᵗʰ **T22.121** Burn of first degree of right elbow
√7ᵗʰ **T22.122** Burn of first degree of left elbow
√7ᵗʰ **T22.129** Burn of first degree of unspecified elbow
√6ᵗʰ **T22.13** Burn of first degree of upper arm
√7ᵗʰ **T22.131** Burn of first degree of right upper arm
√7ᵗʰ **T22.132** Burn of first degree of left upper arm
√7ᵗʰ **T22.139** Burn of first degree of unspecified upper arm
√6ᵗʰ **T22.14** Burn of first degree of axilla
√7ᵗʰ **T22.141** Burn of first degree of right axilla
√7ᵗʰ **T22.142** Burn of first degree of left axilla
√7ᵗʰ **T22.149** Burn of first degree of unspecified axilla
√6ᵗʰ **T22.15** Burn of first degree of shoulder
√7ᵗʰ **T22.151** Burn of first degree of right shoulder
√7ᵗʰ **T22.152** Burn of first degree of left shoulder
√7ᵗʰ **T22.159** Burn of first degree of unspecified shoulder
√6ᵗʰ **T22.16** Burn of first degree of scapular region
√7ᵗʰ **T22.161** Burn of first degree of right scapular region
√7ᵗʰ **T22.162** Burn of first degree of left scapular region
√7ᵗʰ **T22.169** Burn of first degree of unspecified scapular region
√6ᵗʰ **T22.19** Burn of first degree of multiple sites of shoulder and upper limb, except wrist and hand
√7ᵗʰ **T22.191** Burn of first degree of multiple sites of right shoulder and upper limb, except wrist and hand
√7ᵗʰ **T22.192** Burn of first degree of multiple sites of left shoulder and upper limb, except wrist and hand
√7ᵗʰ **T22.199** Burn of first degree of multiple sites of unspecified shoulder and upper limb, except wrist and hand
√5ᵗʰ **T22.2** Burn of second degree of shoulder and upper limb, except wrist and hand
Use additional external cause code to identify the source, place and intent of the burn (X00-X19, X75-X77, X96-X98, Y92)
√x7ᵗʰ **T22.20** Burn of second degree of shoulder and upper limb, except wrist and hand, unspecified site
√6ᵗʰ **T22.21** Burn of second degree of forearm
√7ᵗʰ **T22.211** Burn of second degree of right forearm
√7ᵗʰ **T22.212** Burn of second degree of left forearm
√7ᵗʰ **T22.219** Burn of second degree of unspecified forearm
√6ᵗʰ **T22.22** Burn of second degree of elbow
√7ᵗʰ **T22.221** Burn of second degree of right elbow
√7ᵗʰ **T22.222** Burn of second degree of left elbow
√7ᵗʰ **T22.229** Burn of second degree of unspecified elbow
√6ᵗʰ **T22.23** Burn of second degree of upper arm
√7ᵗʰ **T22.231** Burn of second degree of right upper arm
√7ᵗʰ **T22.232** Burn of second degree of left upper arm
√7ᵗʰ **T22.239** Burn of second degree of unspecified upper arm
√6ᵗʰ **T22.24** Burn of second degree of axilla
√7ᵗʰ **T22.241** Burn of second degree of right axilla
√7ᵗʰ **T22.242** Burn of second degree of left axilla
√7ᵗʰ **T22.249** Burn of second degree of unspecified axilla
√6ᵗʰ **T22.25** Burn of second degree of shoulder
√7ᵗʰ **T22.251** Burn of second degree of right shoulder
√7ᵗʰ **T22.252** Burn of second degree of left shoulder
√7ᵗʰ **T22.259** Burn of second degree of unspecified shoulder

√6ᵗʰ **T22.26** Burn of second degree of scapular region
√7ᵗʰ **T22.261** Burn of second degree of right scapular region
√7ᵗʰ **T22.262** Burn of second degree of left scapular region
√7ᵗʰ **T22.269** Burn of second degree of unspecified scapular region
√6ᵗʰ **T22.29** Burn of second degree of multiple sites of shoulder and upper limb, except wrist and hand
√7ᵗʰ **T22.291** Burn of second degree of multiple sites of right shoulder and upper limb, except wrist and hand
√7ᵗʰ **T22.292** Burn of second degree of multiple sites of left shoulder and upper limb, except wrist and hand
√7ᵗʰ **T22.299** Burn of second degree of multiple sites of unspecified shoulder and upper limb, except wrist and hand
√5ᵗʰ **T22.3** Burn of third degree of shoulder and upper limb, except wrist and hand
Use additional external cause code to identify the source, place and intent of the burn (X00-X19, X75-X77, X96-X98, Y92)
√x7ᵗʰ **T22.30** Burn of third degree of shoulder and upper limb, except wrist and hand, unspecified site
√6ᵗʰ **T22.31** Burn of third degree of forearm
√7ᵗʰ **T22.311** Burn of third degree of right forearm
√7ᵗʰ **T22.312** Burn of third degree of left forearm
√7ᵗʰ **T22.319** Burn of third degree of unspecified forearm
√6ᵗʰ **T22.32** Burn of third degree of elbow
√7ᵗʰ **T22.321** Burn of third degree of right elbow
√7ᵗʰ **T22.322** Burn of third degree of left elbow
√7ᵗʰ **T22.329** Burn of third degree of unspecified elbow
√6ᵗʰ **T22.33** Burn of third degree of upper arm
√7ᵗʰ **T22.331** Burn of third degree of right upper arm
√7ᵗʰ **T22.332** Burn of third degree of left upper arm
√7ᵗʰ **T22.339** Burn of third degree of unspecified upper arm
√6ᵗʰ **T22.34** Burn of third degree of axilla
√7ᵗʰ **T22.341** Burn of third degree of right axilla
√7ᵗʰ **T22.342** Burn of third degree of left axilla
√7ᵗʰ **T22.349** Burn of third degree of unspecified axilla
√6ᵗʰ **T22.35** Burn of third degree of shoulder
√7ᵗʰ **T22.351** Burn of third degree of right shoulder
√7ᵗʰ **T22.352** Burn of third degree of left shoulder
√7ᵗʰ **T22.359** Burn of third degree of unspecified shoulder
√6ᵗʰ **T22.36** Burn of third degree of scapular region
√7ᵗʰ **T22.361** Burn of third degree of right scapular region
√7ᵗʰ **T22.362** Burn of third degree of left scapular region
√7ᵗʰ **T22.369** Burn of third degree of unspecified scapular region
√6ᵗʰ **T22.39** Burn of third degree of multiple sites of shoulder and upper limb, except wrist and hand
√7ᵗʰ **T22.391** Burn of third degree of multiple sites of right shoulder and upper limb, except wrist and hand
√7ᵗʰ **T22.392** Burn of third degree of multiple sites of left shoulder and upper limb, except wrist and hand
√7ᵗʰ **T22.399** Burn of third degree of multiple sites of unspecified shoulder and upper limb, except wrist and hand
√5ᵗʰ **T22.4** Corrosion of unspecified degree of shoulder and upper limb, except wrist and hand
Code first (T51-T65) to identify chemical and intent
Use additional external cause code to identify place (Y92)
√x7ᵗʰ **T22.40** Corrosion of unspecified degree of shoulder and upper limb, except wrist and hand, unspecified site

---

EXCLUDES 1 Not coded here   **EXCLUDES 2** Not included here   *Manifestation Code*

√6ᵗʰ **T22.41 Corrosion of unspecified degree of forearm**
  √7ᵗʰ **T22.411** Corrosion of unspecified degree of right forearm
  √7ᵗʰ **T22.412** Corrosion of unspecified degree of left forearm
  √7ᵗʰ **T22.419** Corrosion of unspecified degree of unspecified forearm

√6ᵗʰ **T22.42 Corrosion of unspecified degree of elbow**
  √7ᵗʰ **T22.421** Corrosion of unspecified degree of right elbow
  √7ᵗʰ **T22.422** Corrosion of unspecified degree of left elbow
  √7ᵗʰ **T22.429** Corrosion of unspecified degree of unspecified elbow

√6ᵗʰ **T22.43 Corrosion of unspecified degree of upper arm**
  √7ᵗʰ **T22.431** Corrosion of unspecified degree of right upper arm
  √7ᵗʰ **T22.432** Corrosion of unspecified degree of left upper arm
  √7ᵗʰ **T22.439** Corrosion of unspecified degree of unspecified upper arm

√6ᵗʰ **T22.44 Corrosion of unspecified degree of axilla**
  √7ᵗʰ **T22.441** Corrosion of unspecified degree of right axilla
  √7ᵗʰ **T22.442** Corrosion of unspecified degree of left axilla
  √7ᵗʰ **T22.449** Corrosion of unspecified degree of unspecified axilla

√6ᵗʰ **T22.45 Corrosion of unspecified degree of shoulder**
  √7ᵗʰ **T22.451** Corrosion of unspecified degree of right shoulder
  √7ᵗʰ **T22.452** Corrosion of unspecified degree of left shoulder
  √7ᵗʰ **T22.459** Corrosion of unspecified degree of unspecified shoulder

√6ᵗʰ **T22.46 Corrosion of unspecified degree of scapular region**
  √7ᵗʰ **T22.461** Corrosion of unspecified degree of right scapular region
  √7ᵗʰ **T22.462** Corrosion of unspecified degree of left scapular region
  √7ᵗʰ **T22.469** Corrosion of unspecified degree of unspecified scapular region

√6ᵗʰ **T22.49 Corrosion of unspecified degree of multiple sites of shoulder and upper limb, except wrist and hand**
  √7ᵗʰ **T22.491** Corrosion of unspecified degree of multiple sites of right shoulder and upper limb, except wrist and hand
  √7ᵗʰ **T22.492** Corrosion of unspecified degree of multiple sites of left shoulder and upper limb, except wrist and hand
  √7ᵗʰ **T22.499** Corrosion of unspecified degree of multiple sites of unspecified shoulder and upper limb, except wrist and hand

√5ᵗʰ **T22.5 Corrosion of first degree of shoulder and upper limb, except wrist and hand**
  Code first (T51-T65) to identify chemical and intent
  Use additional external cause code to identify place (Y92)

√x7ᵗʰ **T22.50 Corrosion of first degree of shoulder and upper limb, except wrist and hand unspecified site**

√6ᵗʰ **T22.51 Corrosion of first degree of forearm**
  √7ᵗʰ **T22.511** Corrosion of first degree of right forearm
  √7ᵗʰ **T22.512** Corrosion of first degree of left forearm
  √7ᵗʰ **T22.519** Corrosion of first degree of unspecified forearm

√6ᵗʰ **T22.52 Corrosion of first degree of elbow**
  √7ᵗʰ **T22.521** Corrosion of first degree of right elbow
  √7ᵗʰ **T22.522** Corrosion of first degree of left elbow
  √7ᵗʰ **T22.529** Corrosion of first degree of unspecified elbow

√6ᵗʰ **T22.53 Corrosion of first degree of upper arm**
  √7ᵗʰ **T22.531** Corrosion of first degree of right upper arm
  √7ᵗʰ **T22.532** Corrosion of first degree of left upper arm

√7ᵗʰ **T22.539** Corrosion of first degree of unspecified upper arm

√6ᵗʰ **T22.54 Corrosion of first degree of axilla**
  √7ᵗʰ **T22.541** Corrosion of first degree of right axilla
  √7ᵗʰ **T22.542** Corrosion of first degree of left axilla
  √7ᵗʰ **T22.549** Corrosion of first degree of unspecified axilla

√6ᵗʰ **T22.55 Corrosion of first degree of shoulder**
  √7ᵗʰ **T22.551** Corrosion of first degree of right shoulder
  √7ᵗʰ **T22.552** Corrosion of first degree of left shoulder
  √7ᵗʰ **T22.559** Corrosion of first degree of unspecified shoulder

√6ᵗʰ **T22.56 Corrosion of first degree of scapular region**
  √7ᵗʰ **T22.561** Corrosion of first degree of right scapular region
  √7ᵗʰ **T22.562** Corrosion of first degree of left scapular region
  √7ᵗʰ **T22.569** Corrosion of first degree of unspecified scapular region

√6ᵗʰ **T22.59 Corrosion of first degree of multiple sites of shoulder and upper limb, except wrist and hand**
  √7ᵗʰ **T22.591** Corrosion of first degree of multiple sites of right shoulder and upper limb, except wrist and hand
  √7ᵗʰ **T22.592** Corrosion of first degree of multiple sites of left shoulder and upper limb, except wrist and hand
  √7ᵗʰ **T22.599** Corrosion of first degree of multiple sites of unspecified shoulder and upper limb, except wrist and hand

√5ᵗʰ **T22.6 Corrosion of second degree of shoulder and upper limb, except wrist and hand**
  Code first (T51-T65) to identify chemical and intent
  Use additional external cause code to identify place (Y92)

√x7ᵗʰ **T22.60 Corrosion of second degree of shoulder and upper limb, except wrist and hand, unspecified site**

√6ᵗʰ **T22.61 Corrosion of second degree of forearm**
  √7ᵗʰ **T22.611** Corrosion of second degree of right forearm
  √7ᵗʰ **T22.612** Corrosion of second degree of left forearm
  √7ᵗʰ **T22.619** Corrosion of second degree of unspecified forearm

√6ᵗʰ **T22.62 Corrosion of second degree of elbow**
  √7ᵗʰ **T22.621** Corrosion of second degree of right elbow
  √7ᵗʰ **T22.622** Corrosion of second degree of left elbow
  √7ᵗʰ **T22.629** Corrosion of second degree of unspecified elbow

√6ᵗʰ **T22.63 Corrosion of second degree of upper arm**
  √7ᵗʰ **T22.631** Corrosion of second degree of right upper arm
  √7ᵗʰ **T22.632** Corrosion of second degree of left upper arm
  √7ᵗʰ **T22.639** Corrosion of second degree of unspecified upper arm

√6ᵗʰ **T22.64 Corrosion of second degree of axilla**
  √7ᵗʰ **T22.641** Corrosion of second degree of right axilla
  √7ᵗʰ **T22.642** Corrosion of second degree of left axilla
  √7ᵗʰ **T22.649** Corrosion of second degree of unspecified axilla

√6ᵗʰ **T22.65 Corrosion of second degree of shoulder**
  √7ᵗʰ **T22.651** Corrosion of second degree of right shoulder
  √7ᵗʰ **T22.652** Corrosion of second degree of left shoulder
  √7ᵗʰ **T22.659** Corrosion of second degree of unspecified shoulder

√6ᵗʰ **T22.66 Corrosion of second degree of scapular region**
  √7ᵗʰ **T22.661** Corrosion of second degree of right scapular region
  √7ᵗʰ **T22.662** Corrosion of second degree of left scapular region

---

☑ Appropriate additional character required   √x7ᵗʰ Requires 7th character, placeholder x must fill empty characters

✓7th T22.669 **Corrosion of second degree of unspecified scapular region**

✓6th T22.69 **Corrosion of second degree of multiple sites of shoulder and upper limb, except wrist and hand**

✓7th T22.691 **Corrosion of second degree of multiple sites of right shoulder and upper limb, except wrist and hand**

✓7th T22.692 **Corrosion of second degree of multiple sites of left shoulder and upper limb, except wrist and hand**

✓7th T22.699 **Corrosion of second degree of multiple sites of unspecified shoulder and upper limb, except wrist and hand**

✓5th T22.7 **Corrosion of third degree of shoulder and upper limb, except wrist and hand**

Code first (T51-T65) to identify chemical and intent

Use additional external cause code to identify place (Y92)

✓x7th T22.70 **Corrosion of third degree of shoulder and upper limb, except wrist and hand, unspecified site**

✓6th T22.71 **Corrosion of third degree of forearm**

✓7th T22.711 **Corrosion of third degree of right forearm**

✓7th T22.712 **Corrosion of third degree of left forearm**

✓7th T22.719 **Corrosion of third degree of unspecified forearm**

✓6th T22.72 **Corrosion of third degree of elbow**

✓7th T22.721 **Corrosion of third degree of right elbow**

✓7th T22.722 **Corrosion of third degree of left elbow**

✓7th T22.729 **Corrosion of third degree of unspecified elbow**

✓6th T22.73 **Corrosion of third degree of upper arm**

✓7th T22.731 **Corrosion of third degree of right upper arm**

✓7th T22.732 **Corrosion of third degree of left upper arm**

✓7th T22.739 **Corrosion of third degree of unspecified upper arm**

✓6th T22.74 **Corrosion of third degree of axilla**

✓7th T22.741 **Corrosion of third degree of right axilla**

✓7th T22.742 **Corrosion of third degree of left axilla**

✓7th T22.749 **Corrosion of third degree of unspecified axilla**

✓6th T22.75 **Corrosion of third degree of shoulder**

✓7th T22.751 **Corrosion of third degree of right shoulder**

✓7th T22.752 **Corrosion of third degree of left shoulder**

✓7th T22.759 **Corrosion of third degree of unspecified shoulder**

✓6th T22.76 **Corrosion of third degree of scapular region**

✓7th T22.761 **Corrosion of third degree of right scapular region**

✓7th T22.762 **Corrosion of third degree of left scapular region**

✓7th T22.769 **Corrosion of third degree of unspecified scapular region**

✓6th T22.79 **Corrosion of third degree of multiple sites of shoulder and upper limb, except wrist and hand**

✓7th T22.791 **Corrosion of third degree of multiple sites of right shoulder and upper limb, except wrist and hand**

✓7th T22.792 **Corrosion of third degree of multiple sites of left shoulder and upper limb, except wrist and hand**

✓7th T22.799 **Corrosion of third degree of multiple sites of unspecified shoulder and upper limb, except wrist and hand**

✓4th **T23 Burn and corrosion of wrist and hand**

The appropriate 7th character is to be added to each code from category T23.
A   initial encounter
D   subsequent encounter
S   sequela

✓5th T23.0 **Burn of unspecified degree of wrist and hand**

Use additional external cause code to identify the source, place and intent of the burn (X00-X19, X75-X77, X96-X98, Y92)

✓6th T23.00 **Burn of unspecified degree of hand, unspecified site**

✓7th T23.001 **Burn of unspecified degree of right hand, unspecified site**

✓7th T23.002 **Burn of unspecified degree of left hand, unspecified site**

✓7th T23.009 **Burn of unspecified degree of unspecified hand, unspecified site**

✓6th T23.01 **Burn of unspecified degree of thumb (nail)**

✓7th T23.011 **Burn of unspecified degree of right thumb (nail)**

✓7th T23.012 **Burn of unspecified degree of left thumb (nail)**

✓7th T23.019 **Burn of unspecified degree of unspecified thumb (nail)**

✓6th T23.02 **Burn of unspecified degree of single finger (nail) except thumb**

✓7th T23.021 **Burn of unspecified degree of single right finger (nail) except thumb**

✓7th T23.022 **Burn of unspecified degree of single left finger (nail) except thumb**

✓7th T23.029 **Burn of unspecified degree of unspecified single finger (nail) except thumb**

✓6th T23.03 **Burn of unspecified degree of multiple fingers (nail), not including thumb**

✓7th T23.031 **Burn of unspecified degree of multiple right fingers (nail), not including thumb**

✓7th T23.032 **Burn of unspecified degree of multiple left fingers (nail), not including thumb**

✓7th T23.039 **Burn of unspecified degree of unspecified multiple fingers (nail), not including thumb**

✓6th T23.04 **Burn of unspecified degree of multiple fingers (nail), including thumb**

✓7th T23.041 **Burn of unspecified degree of multiple right fingers (nail), including thumb**

✓7th T23.042 **Burn of unspecified degree of multiple left fingers (nail), including thumb**

✓7th T23.049 **Burn of unspecified degree of unspecified multiple fingers (nail), including thumb**

✓6th T23.05 **Burn of unspecified degree of palm**

✓7th T23.051 **Burn of unspecified degree of right palm**

✓7th T23.052 **Burn of unspecified degree of left palm**

✓7th T23.059 **Burn of unspecified degree of unspecified palm**

✓6th T23.06 **Burn of unspecified degree of back of hand**

✓7th T23.061 **Burn of unspecified degree of back of right hand**

✓7th T23.062 **Burn of unspecified degree of back of left hand**

✓7th T23.069 **Burn of unspecified degree of back of unspecified hand**

✓6th T23.07 **Burn of unspecified degree of wrist**

✓7th T23.071 **Burn of unspecified degree of right wrist**

✓7th T23.072 **Burn of unspecified degree of left wrist**

✓7th T23.079 **Burn of unspecified degree of unspecified wrist**

✓6th T23.09 **Burn of unspecified degree of multiple sites of wrist and hand**

✓7th T23.091 **Burn of unspecified degree of multiple sites of right wrist and hand**

✓7th T23.092 **Burn of unspecified degree of multiple sites of left wrist and hand**

EXCLUDES 1 Not coded here   **EXCLUDES 2** Not included here   *Manifestation Code*

☑7th **T23.099** Burn of unspecified degree of multiple sites of unspecified wrist and hand

☑5th **T23.1 Burn of first degree of wrist and hand**

Use additional external cause code to identify the source, place and intent of the burn (X00-X19, X75-X77, X96-X98, Y92)

☑6th **T23.10** Burn of first degree of hand, unspecified site

  ☑7th **T23.101** Burn of first degree of right hand, unspecified site

  ☑7th **T23.102** Burn of first degree of left hand, unspecified site

  ☑7th **T23.109** Burn of first degree of unspecified hand, unspecified site

☑6th **T23.11** Burn of first degree of thumb (nail)

  ☑7th **T23.111** Burn of first degree of right thumb (nail)

  ☑7th **T23.112** Burn of first degree of left thumb (nail)

  ☑7th **T23.119** Burn of first degree of unspecified thumb (nail)

☑6th **T23.12** Burn of first degree of single finger (nail) except thumb

  ☑7th **T23.121** Burn of first degree of single right finger (nail) except thumb

  ☑7th **T23.122** Burn of first degree of single left finger (nail) except thumb

  ☑7th **T23.129** Burn of first degree of unspecified single finger (nail) except thumb

☑6th **T23.13** Burn of first degree of multiple fingers (nail), not including thumb

  ☑7th **T23.131** Burn of first degree of multiple right fingers (nail), not including thumb

  ☑7th **T23.132** Burn of first degree of multiple left fingers (nail), not including thumb

  ☑7th **T23.139** Burn of first degree of unspecified multiple fingers (nail), not including thumb

☑6th **T23.14** Burn of first degree of multiple fingers (nail), including thumb

  ☑7th **T23.141** Burn of first degree of multiple right fingers (nail), including thumb

  ☑7th **T23.142** Burn of first degree of multiple left fingers (nail), including thumb

  ☑7th **T23.149** Burn of first degree of unspecified multiple fingers (nail), including thumb

☑6th **T23.15** Burn of first degree of palm

  ☑7th **T23.151** Burn of first degree of right palm

  ☑7th **T23.152** Burn of first degree of left palm

  ☑7th **T23.159** Burn of first degree of unspecified palm

☑6th **T23.16** Burn of first degree of back of hand

  ☑7th **T23.161** Burn of first degree of back of right hand

  ☑7th **T23.162** Burn of first degree of back of left hand

  ☑7th **T23.169** Burn of first degree of back of unspecified hand

☑6th **T23.17** Burn of first degree of wrist

  ☑7th **T23.171** Burn of first degree of right wrist

  ☑7th **T23.172** Burn of first degree of left wrist

  ☑7th **T23.179** Burn of first degree of unspecified wrist

☑6th **T23.19** Burn of first degree of multiple sites of wrist and hand

  ☑7th **T23.191** Burn of first degree of multiple sites of right wrist and hand

  ☑7th **T23.192** Burn of first degree of multiple sites of left wrist and hand

  ☑7th **T23.199** Burn of first degree of multiple sites of unspecified wrist and hand

☑5th **T23.2 Burn of second degree of wrist and hand**

Use additional external cause code to identify the source, place and intent of the burn (X00-X19, X75-X77, X96-X98, Y92)

☑6th **T23.20** Burn of second degree of hand, unspecified site

  ☑7th **T23.201** Burn of second degree of right hand, unspecified site

  ☑7th **T23.202** Burn of second degree of left hand, unspecified site

  ☑7th **T23.209** Burn of second degree of unspecified hand, unspecified site

☑6th **T23.21** Burn of second degree of thumb (nail)

  ☑7th **T23.211** Burn of second degree of right thumb (nail)

  ☑7th **T23.212** Burn of second degree of left thumb (nail)

  ☑7th **T23.219** Burn of second degree of unspecified thumb (nail)

☑6th **T23.22** Burn of second degree of single finger (nail) except thumb

  ☑7th **T23.221** Burn of second degree of single right finger (nail) except thumb

  ☑7th **T23.222** Burn of second degree of single left finger (nail) except thumb

  ☑7th **T23.229** Burn of second degree of unspecified single finger (nail) except thumb

☑6th **T23.23** Burn of second degree of multiple fingers (nail), not including thumb

  ☑7th **T23.231** Burn of second degree of multiple right fingers (nail), not including thumb

  ☑7th **T23.232** Burn of second degree of multiple left fingers (nail), not including thumb

  ☑7th **T23.239** Burn of second degree of unspecified multiple fingers (nail), not including thumb

☑6th **T23.24** Burn of second degree of multiple fingers (nail), including thumb

  ☑7th **T23.241** Burn of second degree of multiple right fingers (nail), including thumb

  ☑7th **T23.242** Burn of second degree of multiple left fingers (nail), including thumb

  ☑7th **T23.249** Burn of second degree of unspecified multiple fingers (nail), including thumb

☑6th **T23.25** Burn of second degree of palm

  ☑7th **T23.251** Burn of second degree of right palm

  ☑7th **T23.252** Burn of second degree of left palm

  ☑7th **T23.259** Burn of second degree of unspecified palm

☑6th **T23.26** Burn of second degree of back of hand

  ☑7th **T23.261** Burn of second degree of back of right hand

  ☑7th **T23.262** Burn of second degree of back of left hand

  ☑7th **T23.269** Burn of second degree of back of unspecified hand

☑6th **T23.27** Burn of second degree of wrist

  ☑7th **T23.271** Burn of second degree of right wrist

  ☑7th **T23.272** Burn of second degree of left wrist

  ☑7th **T23.279** Burn of second degree of unspecified wrist

☑6th **T23.29** Burn of second degree of multiple sites of wrist and hand

  ☑7th **T23.291** Burn of second degree of multiple sites of right wrist and hand

  ☑7th **T23.292** Burn of second degree of multiple sites of left wrist and hand

  ☑7th **T23.299** Burn of second degree of multiple sites of unspecified wrist and hand

☑5th **T23.3 Burn of third degree of wrist and hand**

Use additional external cause code to identify the source, place and intent of the burn (X00-X19, X75-X77, X96-X98, Y92)

☑6th **T23.30** Burn of third degree of hand, unspecified site

  ☑7th **T23.301** Burn of third degree of right hand, unspecified site

  ☑7th **T23.302** Burn of third degree of left hand, unspecified site

  ☑7th **T23.309** Burn of third degree of unspecified hand, unspecified site

☑6th **T23.31** Burn of third degree of thumb (nail)

  ☑7th **T23.311** Burn of third degree of right thumb (nail)

  ☑7th **T23.312** Burn of third degree of left thumb (nail)

  ☑7th **T23.319** Burn of third degree of unspecified thumb (nail)

☑ Appropriate additional character required   ☑x7th Requires 7th character, placeholder x must fill empty characters

✓6th **T23.32** Burn of third degree of single finger (nail) except thumb

    ✓7th **T23.321** Burn of third degree of single right finger (nail) except thumb

    ✓7th **T23.322** Burn of third degree of single left finger (nail) except thumb

    ✓7th **T23.329** Burn of third degree of unspecified single finger (nail) except thumb

✓6th **T23.33** Burn of third degree of multiple fingers (nail), not including thumb

    ✓7th **T23.331** Burn of third degree of multiple right fingers (nail), not including thumb

    ✓7th **T23.332** Burn of third degree of multiple left fingers (nail), not including thumb

    ✓7th **T23.339** Burn of third degree of unspecified multiple fingers (nail), not including thumb

✓6th **T23.34** Burn of third degree of multiple fingers (nail), including thumb

    ✓7th **T23.341** Burn of third degree of multiple right fingers (nail), including thumb

    ✓7th **T23.342** Burn of third degree of multiple left fingers (nail), including thumb

    ✓7th **T23.349** Burn of third degree of unspecified multiple fingers (nail), including thumb

✓6th **T23.35** Burn of third degree of palm

    ✓7th **T23.351** Burn of third degree of right palm

    ✓7th **T23.352** Burn of third degree of left palm

    ✓7th **T23.359** Burn of third degree of unspecified palm

✓6th **T23.36** Burn of third degree of back of hand

    ✓7th **T23.361** Burn of third degree of back of right hand

    ✓7th **T23.362** Burn of third degree of back of left hand

    ✓7th **T23.369** Burn of third degree of back of unspecified hand

✓6th **T23.37** Burn of third degree of wrist

    ✓7th **T23.371** Burn of third degree of right wrist

    ✓7th **T23.372** Burn of third degree of left wrist

    ✓7th **T23.379** Burn of third degree of unspecified wrist

✓6th **T23.39** Burn of third degree of multiple sites of wrist and hand

    ✓7th **T23.391** Burn of third degree of multiple sites of right wrist and hand

    ✓7th **T23.392** Burn of third degree of multiple sites of left wrist and hand

    ✓7th **T23.399** Burn of third degree of multiple sites of unspecified wrist and hand

✓5th **T23.4** Corrosion of unspecified degree of wrist and hand

    Code first (T51-T65) to identify chemical and intent

    Use additional external cause code to identify place (Y92)

✓6th **T23.40** Corrosion of unspecified degree of hand, unspecified site

    ✓7th **T23.401** Corrosion of unspecified degree of right hand, unspecified site

    ✓7th **T23.402** Corrosion of unspecified degree of left hand, unspecified site

    ✓7th **T23.409** Corrosion of unspecified degree of unspecified hand, unspecified site

✓6th **T23.41** Corrosion of unspecified degree of thumb (nail)

    ✓7th **T23.411** Corrosion of unspecified degree of right thumb (nail)

    ✓7th **T23.412** Corrosion of unspecified degree of left thumb (nail)

    ✓7th **T23.419** Corrosion of unspecified degree of unspecified thumb (nail)

✓6th **T23.42** Corrosion of unspecified degree of single finger (nail) except thumb

    ✓7th **T23.421** Corrosion of unspecified degree of single right finger (nail) except thumb

    ✓7th **T23.422** Corrosion of unspecified degree of single left finger (nail) except thumb

    ✓7th **T23.429** Corrosion of unspecified degree of unspecified single finger (nail) except thumb

✓6th **T23.43** Corrosion of unspecified degree of multiple fingers (nail), not including thumb

    ✓7th **T23.431** Corrosion of unspecified degree of multiple right fingers (nail), not including thumb

    ✓7th **T23.432** Corrosion of unspecified degree of multiple left fingers (nail), not including thumb

    ✓7th **T23.439** Corrosion of unspecified degree of unspecified multiple fingers (nail), not including thumb

✓6th **T23.44** Corrosion of unspecified degree of multiple fingers (nail), including thumb

    ✓7th **T23.441** Corrosion of unspecified degree of multiple right fingers (nail), including thumb

    ✓7th **T23.442** Corrosion of unspecified degree of multiple left fingers (nail), including thumb

    ✓7th **T23.449** Corrosion of unspecified degree of unspecified multiple fingers (nail), including thumb

✓6th **T23.45** Corrosion of unspecified degree of palm

    ✓7th **T23.451** Corrosion of unspecified degree of right palm

    ✓7th **T23.452** Corrosion of unspecified degree of left palm

    ✓7th **T23.459** Corrosion of unspecified degree of unspecified palm

✓6th **T23.46** Corrosion of unspecified degree of back of hand

    ✓7th **T23.461** Corrosion of unspecified degree of back of right hand

    ✓7th **T23.462** Corrosion of unspecified degree of back of left hand

    ✓7th **T23.469** Corrosion of unspecified degree of back of unspecified hand

✓6th **T23.47** Corrosion of unspecified degree of wrist

    ✓7th **T23.471** Corrosion of unspecified degree of right wrist

    ✓7th **T23.472** Corrosion of unspecified degree of left wrist

    ✓7th **T23.479** Corrosion of unspecified degree of unspecified wrist

✓6th **T23.49** Corrosion of unspecified degree of multiple sites of wrist and hand

    ✓7th **T23.491** Corrosion of unspecified degree of multiple sites of right wrist and hand

    ✓7th **T23.492** Corrosion of unspecified degree of multiple sites of left wrist and hand

    ✓7th **T23.499** Corrosion of unspecified degree of multiple sites of unspecified wrist and hand

✓5th **T23.5** Corrosion of first degree of wrist and hand

    Code first (T51-T65) to identify chemical and intent

    Use additional external cause code to identify place (Y92)

✓6th **T23.50** Corrosion of first degree of hand, unspecified site

    ✓7th **T23.501** Corrosion of first degree of right hand, unspecified site

    ✓7th **T23.502** Corrosion of first degree of left hand, unspecified site

    ✓7th **T23.509** Corrosion of first degree of unspecified hand, unspecified site

✓6th **T23.51** Corrosion of first degree of thumb (nail)

    ✓7th **T23.511** Corrosion of first degree of right thumb (nail)

    ✓7th **T23.512** Corrosion of first degree of left thumb (nail)

    ✓7th **T23.519** Corrosion of first degree of unspecified thumb (nail)

✓6th **T23.52** Corrosion of first degree of single finger (nail) except thumb

    ✓7th **T23.521** Corrosion of first degree of single right finger (nail) except thumb

    ✓7th **T23.522** Corrosion of first degree of single left finger (nail) except thumb

    ✓7th **T23.529** Corrosion of first degree of unspecified single finger (nail) except thumb

---

EXCLUDES 1 Not coded here   **EXCLUDES 2** Not included here   *Manifestation Code*

✓6th **T23.53** **Corrosion of first degree of multiple fingers (nail), not including thumb**

✓7th **T23.531** **Corrosion of first degree of multiple right fingers (nail), not including thumb**

✓7th **T23.532** **Corrosion of first degree of multiple left fingers (nail), not including thumb**

✓7th **T23.539** **Corrosion of first degree of unspecified multiple fingers (nail), not including thumb**

✓6th **T23.54** **Corrosion of first degree of multiple fingers (nail), including thumb**

✓7th **T23.541** **Corrosion of first degree of multiple right fingers (nail), including thumb**

✓7th **T23.542** **Corrosion of first degree of multiple left fingers (nail), including thumb**

✓7th **T23.549** **Corrosion of first degree of unspecified multiple fingers (nail), including thumb**

✓6th **T23.55** **Corrosion of first degree of palm**

✓7th **T23.551** **Corrosion of first degree of right palm**

✓7th **T23.552** **Corrosion of first degree of left palm**

✓7th **T23.559** **Corrosion of first degree of unspecified palm**

✓6th **T23.56** **Corrosion of first degree of back of hand**

✓7th **T23.561** **Corrosion of first degree of back of right hand**

✓7th **T23.562** **Corrosion of first degree of back of left hand**

✓7th **T23.569** **Corrosion of first degree of back of unspecified hand**

✓6th **T23.57** **Corrosion of first degree of wrist**

✓7th **T23.571** **Corrosion of first degree of right wrist**

✓7th **T23.572** **Corrosion of first degree of left wrist**

✓7th **T23.579** **Corrosion of first degree of unspecified wrist**

✓6th **T23.59** **Corrosion of first degree of multiple sites of wrist and hand**

✓7th **T23.591** **Corrosion of first degree of multiple sites of right wrist and hand**

✓7th **T23.592** **Corrosion of first degree of multiple sites of left wrist and hand**

✓7th **T23.599** **Corrosion of first degree of multiple sites of unspecified wrist and hand**

✓5th **T23.6** **Corrosion of second degree of wrist and hand**

Code first (T51-T65) to identify chemical and intent

Use additional external cause code to identify place (Y92)

✓6th **T23.60** **Corrosion of second degree of hand, unspecified site**

✓7th **T23.601** **Corrosion of second degree of right hand, unspecified site**

✓7th **T23.602** **Corrosion of second degree of left hand, unspecified site**

✓7th **T23.609** **Corrosion of second degree of unspecified hand, unspecified site**

✓6th **T23.61** **Corrosion of second degree of thumb (nail)**

✓7th **T23.611** **Corrosion of second degree of right thumb (nail)**

✓7th **T23.612** **Corrosion of second degree of left thumb (nail)**

✓7th **T23.619** **Corrosion of second degree of unspecified thumb (nail)**

✓6th **T23.62** **Corrosion of second degree of single finger (nail) except thumb**

✓7th **T23.621** **Corrosion of second degree of single right finger (nail) except thumb**

✓7th **T23.622** **Corrosion of second degree of single left finger (nail) except thumb**

✓7th **T23.629** **Corrosion of second degree of unspecified single finger (nail) except thumb**

✓6th **T23.63** **Corrosion of second degree of multiple fingers (nail), not including thumb**

✓7th **T23.631** **Corrosion of second degree of multiple right fingers (nail), not including thumb**

✓7th **T23.632** **Corrosion of second degree of multiple left fingers (nail), not including thumb**

✓7th **T23.639** **Corrosion of second degree of unspecified multiple fingers (nail), not including thumb**

✓6th **T23.64** **Corrosion of second degree of multiple fingers (nail), including thumb**

✓7th **T23.641** **Corrosion of second degree of multiple right fingers (nail), including thumb**

✓7th **T23.642** **Corrosion of second degree of multiple left fingers (nail), including thumb**

✓7th **T23.649** **Corrosion of second degree of unspecified multiple fingers (nail), including thumb**

✓6th **T23.65** **Corrosion of second degree of palm**

✓7th **T23.651** **Corrosion of second degree of right palm**

✓7th **T23.652** **Corrosion of second degree of left palm**

✓7th **T23.659** **Corrosion of second degree of unspecified palm**

✓6th **T23.66** **Corrosion of second degree of back of hand**

✓7th **T23.661** **Corrosion of second degree back of right hand**

✓7th **T23.662** **Corrosion of second degree back of left hand**

✓7th **T23.669** **Corrosion of second degree back of unspecified hand**

✓6th **T23.67** **Corrosion of second degree of wrist**

✓7th **T23.671** **Corrosion of second degree of right wrist**

✓7th **T23.672** **Corrosion of second degree of left wrist**

✓7th **T23.679** **Corrosion of second degree of unspecified wrist**

✓6th **T23.69** **Corrosion of second degree of multiple sites of wrist and hand**

✓7th **T23.691** **Corrosion of second degree of multiple sites of right wrist and hand**

✓7th **T23.692** **Corrosion of second degree of multiple sites of left wrist and hand**

✓7th **T23.699** **Corrosion of second degree of multiple sites of unspecified wrist and hand**

✓5th **T23.7** **Corrosion of third degree of wrist and hand**

Code first (T51-T65) to identify chemical and intent

Use additional external cause code to identify place (Y92)

✓6th **T23.70** **Corrosion of third degree of hand, unspecified site**

✓7th **T23.701** **Corrosion of third degree of right hand, unspecified site**

✓7th **T23.702** **Corrosion of third degree of left hand, unspecified site**

✓7th **T23.709** **Corrosion of third degree of unspecified hand, unspecified site**

✓6th **T23.71** **Corrosion of third degree of thumb (nail)**

✓7th **T23.711** **Corrosion of third degree of right thumb (nail)**

✓7th **T23.712** **Corrosion of third degree of left thumb (nail)**

✓7th **T23.719** **Corrosion of third degree of unspecified thumb (nail)**

✓6th **T23.72** **Corrosion of third degree of single finger (nail) except thumb**

✓7th **T23.721** **Corrosion of third degree of single right finger (nail) except thumb**

✓7th **T23.722** **Corrosion of third degree of single left finger (nail) except thumb**

✓7th **T23.729** **Corrosion of third degree of unspecified single finger (nail) except thumb**

✓6th **T23.73** **Corrosion of third degree of multiple fingers (nail), not including thumb**

✓7th **T23.731** **Corrosion of third degree of multiple right fingers (nail), not including thumb**

✓7th **T23.732** **Corrosion of third degree of multiple left fingers (nail), not including thumb**

✓7th **T23.739** **Corrosion of third degree of unspecified multiple fingers (nail), not including thumb**

✓6th **T23.74** **Corrosion of third degree of multiple fingers (nail), including thumb**

✓7th **T23.741** **Corrosion of third degree of multiple right fingers (nail), including thumb**

☑ Appropriate additional character required   ✓x7th Requires 7th character, placeholder x must fill empty characters

✓7th **T23.742** Corrosion of third degree of multiple left fingers (nail), including thumb

✓7th **T23.749** Corrosion of third degree of unspecified multiple fingers (nail), including thumb

✓6th **T23.75** Corrosion of third degree of palm

✓7th **T23.751** Corrosion of third degree of right palm

✓7th **T23.752** Corrosion of third degree of left palm

✓7th **T23.759** Corrosion of third degree of unspecified palm

✓6th **T23.76** Corrosion of third degree of back of hand

✓7th **T23.761** Corrosion of third degree of back of right hand

✓7th **T23.762** Corrosion of third degree of back of left hand

✓7th **T23.769** Corrosion of third degree back of unspecified hand

✓6th **T23.77** Corrosion of third degree of wrist

✓7th **T23.771** Corrosion of third degree of right wrist

✓7th **T23.772** Corrosion of third degree of left wrist

✓7th **T23.779** Corrosion of third degree of unspecified wrist

✓6th **T23.79** Corrosion of third degree of multiple sites of wrist and hand

✓7th **T23.791** Corrosion of third degree of multiple sites of right wrist and hand

✓7th **T23.792** Corrosion of third degree of multiple sites of left wrist and hand

✓7th **T23.799** Corrosion of third degree of multiple sites of unspecified wrist and hand

✓4th **T24** **Burn and corrosion of lower limb, except ankle and foot**

EXCLUDES 2   *burn and corrosion of ankle and foot (T25-)*
burn and corrosion of hip region (T21-)

> The appropriate 7th character is to be added to each code from category T24.
> A   initial encounter
> D   subsequent encounter
> S   sequela

✓5th **T24.0** **Burn of unspecified degree of lower limb, except ankle and foot**

Use additional external cause code to identify the source, place and intent of the burn (X00-X19, X75-X77, X96-X98, Y92)

✓6th **T24.00** Burn of unspecified degree of unspecified site of lower limb, except ankle and foot

✓7th **T24.001** Burn of unspecified degree of unspecified site of right lower limb, except ankle and foot

✓7th **T24.002** Burn of unspecified degree of unspecified site of left lower limb, except ankle and foot

✓7th **T24.009** Burn of unspecified degree of unspecified site of unspecified lower limb, except ankle and foot

✓6th **T24.01** Burn of unspecified degree of thigh

✓7th **T24.011** Burn of unspecified degree of right thigh

✓7th **T24.012** Burn of unspecified degree of left thigh

✓7th **T24.019** Burn of unspecified degree of unspecified thigh

✓6th **T24.02** Burn of unspecified degree of knee

✓7th **T24.021** Burn of unspecified degree of right knee

✓7th **T24.022** Burn of unspecified degree of left knee

✓7th **T24.029** Burn of unspecified degree of unspecified knee

✓6th **T24.03** Burn of unspecified degree of lower leg

✓7th **T24.031** Burn of unspecified degree of right lower leg

✓7th **T24.032** Burn of unspecified degree of left lower leg

✓7th **T24.039** Burn of unspecified degree of unspecified lower leg

✓6th **T24.09** Burn of unspecified degree of multiple sites of lower limb, except ankle and foot

✓7th **T24.091** Burn of unspecified degree of multiple sites of right lower limb, except ankle and foot

✓7th **T24.092** Burn of unspecified degree of multiple sites of left lower limb, except ankle and foot

✓7th **T24.099** Burn of unspecified degree of multiple sites of unspecified lower limb, except ankle and foot

✓5th **T24.1** **Burn of first degree of lower limb, except ankle and foot**

Use additional external cause code to identify the source, place and intent of the burn (X00-X19, X75-X77, X96-X98, Y92)

✓6th **T24.10** Burn of first degree of unspecified site of lower limb, except ankle and foot

✓7th **T24.101** Burn of first degree of unspecified site of right lower limb, except ankle and foot

✓7th **T24.102** Burn of first degree of unspecified site of left lower limb, except ankle and foot

✓7th **T24.109** Burn of first degree of unspecified site of unspecified lower limb, except ankle and foot

✓6th **T24.11** Burn of first degree of thigh

✓7th **T24.111** Burn of first degree of right thigh

✓7th **T24.112** Burn of first degree of left thigh

✓7th **T24.119** Burn of first degree of unspecified thigh

✓6th **T24.12** Burn of first degree of knee

✓7th **T24.121** Burn of first degree of right knee

✓7th **T24.122** Burn of first degree of left knee

✓7th **T24.129** Burn of first degree of unspecified knee

✓6th **T24.13** Burn of first degree of lower leg

✓7th **T24.131** Burn of first degree of right lower leg

✓7th **T24.132** Burn of first degree of left lower leg

✓7th **T24.139** Burn of first degree of unspecified lower leg

✓6th **T24.19** Burn of first degree of multiple sites of lower limb, except ankle and foot

✓7th **T24.191** Burn of first degree of multiple sites of right lower limb, except ankle and foot

✓7th **T24.192** Burn of first degree of multiple sites of left lower limb, except ankle and foot

✓7th **T24.199** Burn of first degree of multiple sites of unspecified lower limb, except ankle and foot

✓5th **T24.2** **Burn of second degree of lower limb, except ankle and foot**

Use additional external cause code to identify the source, place and intent of the burn (X00-X19, X75-X77, X96-X98, Y92)

✓6th **T24.20** Burn of second degree of unspecified site of lower limb, except ankle and foot

✓7th **T24.201** Burn of second degree of unspecified site of right lower limb, except ankle and foot

✓7th **T24.202** Burn of second degree of unspecified site of left lower limb, except ankle and foot

✓7th **T24.209** Burn of second degree of unspecified site of unspecified lower limb, except ankle and foot

✓6th **T24.21** Burn of second degree of thigh

✓7th **T24.211** Burn of second degree of right thigh

✓7th **T24.212** Burn of second degree of left thigh

✓7th **T24.219** Burn of second degree of unspecified thigh

✓6th **T24.22** Burn of second degree of knee

✓7th **T24.221** Burn of second degree of right knee

✓7th **T24.222** Burn of second degree of left knee

✓7th **T24.229** Burn of second degree of unspecified knee

✓6th **T24.23** Burn of second degree of lower leg

✓7th **T24.231** Burn of second degree of right lower leg

✓7th **T24.232** Burn of second degree of left lower leg

✓7th **T24.239** Burn of second degree of unspecified lower leg

---

√6th **T24.29** **Burn of second degree of multiple sites of lower limb, except ankle and foot**

     √7th **T24.291** **Burn of second degree of multiple sites of right lower limb, except ankle and foot**

     √7th **T24.292** **Burn of second degree of multiple sites of left lower limb, except ankle and foot**

     √7th **T24.299** **Burn of second degree of multiple sites of unspecified lower limb, except ankle and foot**

√5th **T24.3** **Burn of third degree of lower limb, except ankle and foot**

Use additional external cause code to identify the source, place and intent of the burn (X00-X19, X75-X77, X96-X98, Y92)

     √6th **T24.30** **Burn of third degree of unspecified site of lower limb, except ankle and foot**

       √7th **T24.301** **Burn of third degree of unspecified site of right lower limb, except ankle and foot**

       √7th **T24.302** **Burn of third degree of unspecified site of left lower limb, except ankle and foot**

       √7th **T24.309** **Burn of third degree of unspecified site of unspecified lower limb, except ankle and foot**

     √6th **T24.31** **Burn of third degree of thigh**

       √7th **T24.311** **Burn of third degree of right thigh**

       √7th **T24.312** **Burn of third degree of left thigh**

       √7th **T24.319** **Burn of third degree of unspecified thigh**

     √6th **T24.32** **Burn of third degree of knee**

       √7th **T24.321** **Burn of third degree of right knee**

       √7th **T24.322** **Burn of third degree of left knee**

       √7th **T24.329** **Burn of third degree of unspecified knee**

     √6th **T24.33** **Burn of third degree of lower leg**

       √7th **T24.331** **Burn of third degree of right lower leg**

       √7th **T24.332** **Burn of third degree of left lower leg**

       √7th **T24.339** **Burn of third degree of unspecified lower leg**

     √6th **T24.39** **Burn of third degree of multiple sites of lower limb, except ankle and foot**

       √7th **T24.391** **Burn of third degree of multiple sites of right lower limb, except ankle and foot**

       √7th **T24.392** **Burn of third degree of multiple sites of left lower limb, except ankle and foot**

       √7th **T24.399** **Burn of third degree of multiple sites of unspecified lower limb, except ankle and foot**

√5th **T24.4** **Corrosion of unspecified degree of lower limb, except ankle and foot**

Code first (T51-T65) to identify chemical and intent

Use additional external cause code to identify place (Y92)

     √6th **T24.40** **Corrosion of unspecified degree of unspecified site of lower limb, except ankle and foot**

       √7th **T24.401** **Corrosion of unspecified degree of unspecified site of right lower limb, except ankle and foot**

       √7th **T24.402** **Corrosion of unspecified degree of unspecified site of left lower limb, except ankle and foot**

       √7th **T24.409** **Corrosion of unspecified degree of unspecified site of unspecified lower limb, except ankle and foot**

     √6th **T24.41** **Corrosion of unspecified degree of thigh**

       √7th **T24.411** **Corrosion of unspecified degree of right thigh**

       √7th **T24.412** **Corrosion of unspecified degree of left thigh**

       √7th **T24.419** **Corrosion of unspecified degree of unspecified thigh**

     √6th **T24.42** **Corrosion of unspecified degree of knee**

       √7th **T24.421** **Corrosion of unspecified degree of right knee**

       √7th **T24.422** **Corrosion of unspecified degree of left knee**

       √7th **T24.429** **Corrosion of unspecified degree of unspecified knee**

√6th **T24.43** **Corrosion of unspecified degree of lower leg**

     √7th **T24.431** **Corrosion of unspecified degree of right lower leg**

     √7th **T24.432** **Corrosion of unspecified degree of left lower leg**

     √7th **T24.439** **Corrosion of unspecified degree of unspecified lower leg**

√6th **T24.49** **Corrosion of unspecified degree of multiple sites of lower limb, except ankle and foot**

     √7th **T24.491** **Corrosion of unspecified degree of multiple sites of right lower limb, except ankle and foot**

     √7th **T24.492** **Corrosion of unspecified degree of multiple sites of left lower limb, except ankle and foot**

     √7th **T24.499** **Corrosion of unspecified degree of multiple sites of unspecified lower limb, except ankle and foot**

√5th **T24.5** **Corrosion of first degree of lower limb, except ankle and foot**

Code first (T51-T65) to identify chemical and intent

Use additional external cause code to identify place (Y92)

     √6th **T24.50** **Corrosion of first degree of unspecified site of lower limb, except ankle and foot**

       √7th **T24.501** **Corrosion of first degree of unspecified site of right lower limb, except ankle and foot**

       √7th **T24.502** **Corrosion of first degree of unspecified site of left lower limb, except ankle and foot**

       √7th **T24.509** **Corrosion of first degree of unspecified site of unspecified lower limb, except ankle and foot**

     √6th **T24.51** **Corrosion of first degree of thigh**

       √7th **T24.511** **Corrosion of first degree of right thigh**

       √7th **T24.512** **Corrosion of first degree of left thigh**

       √7th **T24.519** **Corrosion of first degree of unspecified thigh**

     √6th **T24.52** **Corrosion of first degree of knee**

       √7th **T24.521** **Corrosion of first degree of right knee**

       √7th **T24.522** **Corrosion of first degree of left knee**

       √7th **T24.529** **Corrosion of first degree of unspecified knee**

     √6th **T24.53** **Corrosion of first degree of lower leg**

       √7th **T24.531** **Corrosion of first degree of right lower leg**

       √7th **T24.532** **Corrosion of first degree of left lower leg**

       √7th **T24.539** **Corrosion of first degree of unspecified lower leg**

     √6th **T24.59** **Corrosion of first degree of multiple sites of lower limb, except ankle and foot**

       √7th **T24.591** **Corrosion of first degree of multiple sites of right lower limb, except ankle and foot**

       √7th **T24.592** **Corrosion of first degree of multiple sites of left lower limb, except ankle and foot**

       √7th **T24.599** **Corrosion of first degree of multiple sites of unspecified lower limb, except ankle and foot**

√5th **T24.6** **Corrosion of second degree of lower limb, except ankle and foot**

Code first (T51-T65) to identify chemical and intent

Use additional external cause code to identify place (Y92)

     √6th **T24.60** **Corrosion of second degree of unspecified site of lower limb, except ankle and foot**

       √7th **T24.601** **Corrosion of second degree of unspecified site of right lower limb, except ankle and foot**

       √7th **T24.602** **Corrosion of second degree of unspecified site of left lower limb, except ankle and foot**

       √7th **T24.609** **Corrosion of second degree of unspecified site of unspecified lower limb, except ankle and foot**

    ☑ Appropriate additional character required   √x7th Requires 7th character, placeholder x must fill empty characters

√6ᵗʰ **T24.61 Corrosion of second degree of thigh**
- √7ᵗʰ **T24.611** Corrosion of second degree of right thigh
- √7ᵗʰ **T24.612** Corrosion of second degree of left thigh
- √7ᵗʰ **T24.619** Corrosion of second degree of unspecified thigh

√6ᵗʰ **T24.62 Corrosion of second degree of knee**
- √7ᵗʰ **T24.621** Corrosion of second degree of right knee
- √7ᵗʰ **T24.622** Corrosion of second degree of left knee
- √7ᵗʰ **T24.629** Corrosion of second degree of unspecified knee

√6ᵗʰ **T24.63 Corrosion of second degree of lower leg**
- √7ᵗʰ **T24.631** Corrosion of second degree of right lower leg
- √7ᵗʰ **T24.632** Corrosion of second degree of left lower leg
- √7ᵗʰ **T24.639** Corrosion of second degree of unspecified lower leg

√6ᵗʰ **T24.69 Corrosion of second degree of multiple sites of lower limb, except ankle and foot**
- √7ᵗʰ **T24.691** Corrosion of second degree of multiple sites of right lower limb, except ankle and foot
- √7ᵗʰ **T24.692** Corrosion of second degree of multiple sites of left lower limb, except ankle and foot
- √7ᵗʰ **T24.699** Corrosion of second degree of multiple sites of unspecified lower limb, except ankle and foot

√5ᵗʰ **T24.7 Corrosion of third degree of lower limb, except ankle and foot**

Code first (T51-T65) to identify chemical and intent
Use additional external cause code to identify place (Y92)

√6ᵗʰ **T24.70 Corrosion of third degree of unspecified site of lower limb, except ankle and foot**
- √7ᵗʰ **T24.701** Corrosion of third degree of unspecified site of right lower limb, except ankle and foot
- √7ᵗʰ **T24.702** Corrosion of third degree of unspecified site of left lower limb, except ankle and foot
- √7ᵗʰ **T24.709** Corrosion of third degree of unspecified site of unspecified lower limb, except ankle and foot

√6ᵗʰ **T24.71 Corrosion of third degree of thigh**
- √7ᵗʰ **T24.711** Corrosion of third degree of right thigh
- √7ᵗʰ **T24.712** Corrosion of third degree of left thigh
- √7ᵗʰ **T24.719** Corrosion of third degree of unspecified thigh

√6ᵗʰ **T24.72 Corrosion of third degree of knee**
- √7ᵗʰ **T24.721** Corrosion of third degree of right knee
- √7ᵗʰ **T24.722** Corrosion of third degree of left knee
- √7ᵗʰ **T24.729** Corrosion of third degree of unspecified knee

√6ᵗʰ **T24.73 Corrosion of third degree of lower leg**
- √7ᵗʰ **T24.731** Corrosion of third degree of right lower leg
- √7ᵗʰ **T24.732** Corrosion of third degree of left lower leg
- √7ᵗʰ **T24.739** Corrosion of third degree of unspecified lower leg

√6ᵗʰ **T24.79 Corrosion of third degree of multiple sites of lower limb, except ankle and foot**
- √7ᵗʰ **T24.791** Corrosion of third degree of multiple sites of right lower limb, except ankle and foot
- √7ᵗʰ **T24.792** Corrosion of third degree of multiple sites of left lower limb, except ankle and foot
- √7ᵗʰ **T24.799** Corrosion of third degree of multiple sites of unspecified lower limb, except ankle and foot

√4ᵗʰ **T25 Burn and corrosion of ankle and foot**

The appropriate 7th character is to be added to each code from category T25.
A   initial encounter
D   subsequent encounter
S   sequela

√5ᵗʰ **T25.0 Burn of unspecified degree of ankle and foot**
Use additional external cause code to identify the source, place and intent of the burn (X00-X19, X75-X77, X96-X98, Y92)

√6ᵗʰ **T25.01 Burn of unspecified degree of ankle**
- √7ᵗʰ **T25.011** Burn of unspecified degree of right ankle
- √7ᵗʰ **T25.012** Burn of unspecified degree of left ankle
- √7ᵗʰ **T25.019** Burn of unspecified degree of unspecified ankle

√6ᵗʰ **T25.02 Burn of unspecified degree of foot**
- EXCLUDES 2   burn of unspecified degree of toe(s) (nail) (T25.03-)
- √7ᵗʰ **T25.021** Burn of unspecified degree of right foot
- √7ᵗʰ **T25.022** Burn of unspecified degree of left foot
- √7ᵗʰ **T25.029** Burn of unspecified degree of unspecified foot

√6ᵗʰ **T25.03 Burn of unspecified degree of toe(s) (nail)**
- √7ᵗʰ **T25.031** Burn of unspecified degree of right toe(s) (nail)
- √7ᵗʰ **T25.032** Burn of unspecified degree of left toe(s) (nail)
- √7ᵗʰ **T25.039** Burn of unspecified degree of unspecified toe(s) (nail)

√6ᵗʰ **T25.09 Burn of unspecified degree of multiple sites of ankle and foot**
- √7ᵗʰ **T25.091** Burn of unspecified degree of multiple sites of right ankle and foot
- √7ᵗʰ **T25.092** Burn of unspecified degree of multiple sites of left ankle and foot
- √7ᵗʰ **T25.099** Burn of unspecified degree of multiple sites of unspecified ankle and foot

√5ᵗʰ **T25.1 Burn of first degree of ankle and foot**
Use additional external cause code to identify the source, place and intent of the burn (X00-X19, X75-X77, X96-X98, Y92)

√6ᵗʰ **T25.11 Burn of first degree of ankle**
- √7ᵗʰ **T25.111** Burn of first degree of right ankle
- √7ᵗʰ **T25.112** Burn of first degree of left ankle
- √7ᵗʰ **T25.119** Burn of first degree of unspecified ankle

√6ᵗʰ **T25.12 Burn of first degree of foot**
- EXCLUDES 2   burn of first degree of toe(s) (nail) (T25.13-)
- √7ᵗʰ **T25.121** Burn of first degree of right foot
- √7ᵗʰ **T25.122** Burn of first degree of left foot
- √7ᵗʰ **T25.129** Burn of first degree of unspecified foot

√6ᵗʰ **T25.13 Burn of first degree of toe(s) (nail)**
- √7ᵗʰ **T25.131** Burn of first degree of right toe(s) (nail)
- √7ᵗʰ **T25.132** Burn of first degree of left toe(s) (nail)
- √7ᵗʰ **T25.139** Burn of first degree of unspecified toe(s) (nail)

√6ᵗʰ **T25.19 Burn of first degree of multiple sites of ankle and foot**
- √7ᵗʰ **T25.191** Burn of first degree of multiple sites of right ankle and foot
- √7ᵗʰ **T25.192** Burn of first degree of multiple sites of left ankle and foot
- √7ᵗʰ **T25.199** Burn of first degree of multiple sites of unspecified ankle and foot

√5ᵗʰ **T25.2 Burn of second degree of ankle and foot**
Use additional external cause code to identify the source, place and intent of the burn (X00-X19, X75-X77, X96-X98, Y92)

√6ᵗʰ **T25.21 Burn of second degree of ankle**
- √7ᵗʰ **T25.211** Burn of second degree of right ankle
- √7ᵗʰ **T25.212** Burn of second degree of left ankle
- √7ᵗʰ **T25.219** Burn of second degree of unspecified ankle

---

EXCLUDES 1   Not coded here   EXCLUDES 2   Not included here   *Manifestation Code*

✓6ᵗʰ **T25.22** **Burn of second degree of foot**
> EXCLUDES 2   *burn of second degree of toe(s) (nail) (T25.23-)*

   ✓7ᵗʰ **T25.221** **Burn of second degree of right foot**
   ✓7ᵗʰ **T25.222** **Burn of second degree of left foot**
   ✓7ᵗʰ **T25.229** **Burn of second degree of unspecified foot**

✓6ᵗʰ **T25.23** **Burn of second degree of toe(s) (nail)**
   ✓7ᵗʰ **T25.231** **Burn of second degree of right toe(s) (nail)**
   ✓7ᵗʰ **T25.232** **Burn of second degree of left toe(s) (nail)**
   ✓7ᵗʰ **T25.239** **Burn of second degree of unspecified toe(s) (nail)**

✓6ᵗʰ **T25.29** **Burn of second degree of multiple sites of ankle and foot**
   ✓7ᵗʰ **T25.291** **Burn of second degree of multiple sites of right ankle and foot**
   ✓7ᵗʰ **T25.292** **Burn of second degree of multiple sites of left ankle and foot**
   ✓7ᵗʰ **T25.299** **Burn of second degree of multiple sites of unspecified ankle and foot**

✓5ᵗʰ **T25.3** **Burn of third degree of ankle and foot**
> Use additional external cause code to identify the source, place and intent of the burn (X00-X19, X75-X77, X96-X98, Y92)

   ✓6ᵗʰ **T25.31** **Burn of third degree of ankle**
      ✓7ᵗʰ **T25.311** **Burn of third degree of right ankle**
      ✓7ᵗʰ **T25.312** **Burn of third degree of left ankle**
      ✓7ᵗʰ **T25.319** **Burn of third degree of unspecified ankle**

   ✓6ᵗʰ **T25.32** **Burn of third degree of foot**
   > EXCLUDES 2   *burn of third degree of toe(s) (nail) (T25.33-)*

      ✓7ᵗʰ **T25.321** **Burn of third degree of right foot**
      ✓7ᵗʰ **T25.322** **Burn of third degree of left foot**
      ✓7ᵗʰ **T25.329** **Burn of third degree of unspecified foot**

   ✓6ᵗʰ **T25.33** **Burn of third degree of toe(s) (nail)**
      ✓7ᵗʰ **T25.331** **Burn of third degree of right toe(s) (nail)**
      ✓7ᵗʰ **T25.332** **Burn of third degree of left toe(s) (nail)**
      ✓7ᵗʰ **T25.339** **Burn of third degree of unspecified toe(s) (nail)**

   ✓6ᵗʰ **T25.39** **Burn of third degree of multiple sites of ankle and foot**
      ✓7ᵗʰ **T25.391** **Burn of third degree of multiple sites of right ankle and foot**
      ✓7ᵗʰ **T25.392** **Burn of third degree of multiple sites of left ankle and foot**
      ✓7ᵗʰ **T25.399** **Burn of third degree of multiple sites of unspecified ankle and foot**

✓5ᵗʰ **T25.4** **Corrosion of unspecified degree of ankle and foot**
> Code first (T51-T65) to identify chemical and intent
> Use additional external cause code to identify place (Y92)

   ✓6ᵗʰ **T25.41** **Corrosion of unspecified degree of ankle**
      ✓7ᵗʰ **T25.411** **Corrosion of unspecified degree of right ankle**
      ✓7ᵗʰ **T25.412** **Corrosion of unspecified degree of left ankle**
      ✓7ᵗʰ **T25.419** **Corrosion of unspecified degree of unspecified ankle**

   ✓6ᵗʰ **T25.42** **Corrosion of unspecified degree of foot**
   > EXCLUDES 2   *corrosion of unspecified degree of toe(s) (nail) (T25.43-)*

      ✓7ᵗʰ **T25.421** **Corrosion of unspecified degree of right foot**
      ✓7ᵗʰ **T25.422** **Corrosion of unspecified degree of left foot**
      ✓7ᵗʰ **T25.429** **Corrosion of unspecified degree of unspecified foot**

   ✓6ᵗʰ **T25.43** **Corrosion of unspecified degree of toe(s) (nail)**
      ✓7ᵗʰ **T25.431** **Corrosion of unspecified degree of right toe(s) (nail)**
      ✓7ᵗʰ **T25.432** **Corrosion of unspecified degree of left toe(s) (nail)**
      ✓7ᵗʰ **T25.439** **Corrosion of unspecified degree of unspecified toe(s) (nail)**

✓6ᵗʰ **T25.49** **Corrosion of unspecified degree of multiple sites of ankle and foot**
   ✓7ᵗʰ **T25.491** **Corrosion of unspecified degree of multiple sites of right ankle and foot**
   ✓7ᵗʰ **T25.492** **Corrosion of unspecified degree of multiple sites of left ankle and foot**
   ✓7ᵗʰ **T25.499** **Corrosion of unspecified degree of multiple sites of unspecified ankle and foot**

✓5ᵗʰ **T25.5** **Corrosion of first degree of ankle and foot**
> Code first (T51-T65) to identify chemical and intent
> Use additional external cause code to identify place (Y92)

   ✓6ᵗʰ **T25.51** **Corrosion of first degree of ankle**
      ✓7ᵗʰ **T25.511** **Corrosion of first degree of right ankle**
      ✓7ᵗʰ **T25.512** **Corrosion of first degree of left ankle**
      ✓7ᵗʰ **T25.519** **Corrosion of first degree of unspecified ankle**

   ✓6ᵗʰ **T25.52** **Corrosion of first degree of foot**
   > EXCLUDES 2   *corrosion of first degree of toe(s) (nail) (T25.53-)*

      ✓7ᵗʰ **T25.521** **Corrosion of first degree of right foot**
      ✓7ᵗʰ **T25.522** **Corrosion of first degree of left foot**
      ✓7ᵗʰ **T25.529** **Corrosion of first degree of unspecified foot**

   ✓6ᵗʰ **T25.53** **Corrosion of first degree of toe(s) (nail)**
      ✓7ᵗʰ **T25.531** **Corrosion of first degree of right toe(s) (nail)**
      ✓7ᵗʰ **T25.532** **Corrosion of first degree of left toe(s) (nail)**
      ✓7ᵗʰ **T25.539** **Corrosion of first degree of unspecified toe(s) (nail)**

   ✓6ᵗʰ **T25.59** **Corrosion of first degree of multiple sites of ankle and foot**
      ✓7ᵗʰ **T25.591** **Corrosion of first degree of multiple sites of right ankle and foot**
      ✓7ᵗʰ **T25.592** **Corrosion of first degree of multiple sites of left ankle and foot**
      ✓7ᵗʰ **T25.599** **Corrosion of first degree of multiple sites of unspecified ankle and foot**

✓5ᵗʰ **T25.6** **Corrosion of second degree of ankle and foot**
> Code first (T51-T65) to identify chemical and intent
> Use additional external cause code to identify place (Y92)

   ✓6ᵗʰ **T25.61** **Corrosion of second degree of ankle**
      ✓7ᵗʰ **T25.611** **Corrosion of second degree of right ankle**
      ✓7ᵗʰ **T25.612** **Corrosion of second degree of left ankle**
      ✓7ᵗʰ **T25.619** **Corrosion of second degree of unspecified ankle**

   ✓6ᵗʰ **T25.62** **Corrosion of second degree of foot**
   > EXCLUDES 2   *corrosion of second degree of toe(s) (nail) (T25.63-)*

      ✓7ᵗʰ **T25.621** **Corrosion of second degree of right foot**
      ✓7ᵗʰ **T25.622** **Corrosion of second degree of left foot**
      ✓7ᵗʰ **T25.629** **Corrosion of second degree of unspecified foot**

   ✓6ᵗʰ **T25.63** **Corrosion of second degree of toe(s) (nail)**
      ✓7ᵗʰ **T25.631** **Corrosion of second degree of right toe(s) (nail)**
      ✓7ᵗʰ **T25.632** **Corrosion of second degree of left toe(s) (nail)**
      ✓7ᵗʰ **T25.639** **Corrosion of second degree of unspecified toe(s) (nail)**

   ✓6ᵗʰ **T25.69** **Corrosion of second degree of multiple sites of ankle and foot**
      ✓7ᵗʰ **T25.691** **Corrosion of second degree of right ankle and foot**
      ✓7ᵗʰ **T25.692** **Corrosion of second degree of left ankle and foot**
      ✓7ᵗʰ **T25.699** **Corrosion of second degree of unspecified ankle and foot**

✓5ᵗʰ **T25.7** **Corrosion of third degree of ankle and foot**
> Code first (T51-T65) to identify chemical and intent
> Use additional external cause code to identify place (Y92)

   ✓6ᵗʰ **T25.71** **Corrosion of third degree of ankle**
      ✓7ᵗʰ **T25.711** **Corrosion of third degree of right ankle**
      ✓7ᵗʰ **T25.712** **Corrosion of third degree of left ankle**

☑ Appropriate additional character required   ✓x7ᵗʰ Requires 7th character, placeholder x must fill empty characters

√7ᵗʰ **T25.719** Corrosion of third degree of unspecified ankle

√6ᵗʰ **T25.72** Corrosion of third degree of foot
    EXCLUDES 2 *corrosion of third degree of toe(s) (nail) (T25.73-)*
√7ᵗʰ **T25.721** Corrosion of third degree of right foot
√7ᵗʰ **T25.722** Corrosion of third degree of left foot
√7ᵗʰ **T25.729** Corrosion of third degree of unspecified foot

√6ᵗʰ **T25.73** Corrosion of third degree of toe(s) (nail)
√7ᵗʰ **T25.731** Corrosion of third degree of right toe(s) (nail)
√7ᵗʰ **T25.732** Corrosion of third degree of left toe(s) (nail)
√7ᵗʰ **T25.739** Corrosion of third degree of unspecified toe(s) (nail)

√6ᵗʰ **T25.79** Corrosion of third degree of multiple sites of ankle and foot
√7ᵗʰ **T25.791** Corrosion of third degree of multiple sites of right ankle and foot
√7ᵗʰ **T25.792** Corrosion of third degree of multiple sites of left ankle and foot
√7ᵗʰ **T25.799** Corrosion of third degree of multiple sites of unspecified ankle and foot

Burns and corrosions confined to eye and internal organs (T26-T28)

√4ᵗʰ **T26 Burn and corrosion confined to eye and adnexa**

> The appropriate 7th character is to be added to each code from category T26.
> A   initial encounter
> D   subsequent encounter
> S   sequela

√5ᵗʰ **T26.0 Burn of eyelid and periocular area**
> Use additional external cause code to identify the source, place and intent of the burn (X00-X19, X75-X77, X96-X98, Y92)
√x7ᵗʰ **T26.00** Burn of unspecified eyelid and periocular area
√x7ᵗʰ **T26.01** Burn of right eyelid and periocular area
√x7ᵗʰ **T26.02** Burn of left eyelid and periocular area

√5ᵗʰ **T26.1 Burn of cornea and conjunctival sac**
> Use additional external cause code to identify the source, place and intent of the burn (X00-X19, X75-X77, X96-X98, Y92)
√x7ᵗʰ **T26.10** Burn of cornea and conjunctival sac, unspecified eye
√x7ᵗʰ **T26.11** Burn of cornea and conjunctival sac, right eye
√x7ᵗʰ **T26.12** Burn of cornea and conjunctival sac, left eye

√5ᵗʰ **T26.2 Burn with resulting rupture and destruction of eyeball**
> Use additional external cause code to identify the source, place and intent of the burn (X00-X19, X75-X77, X96-X98, Y92)
√x7ᵗʰ **T26.20** Burn with resulting rupture and destruction of unspecified eyeball
√x7ᵗʰ **T26.21** Burn with resulting rupture and destruction of right eyeball
√x7ᵗʰ **T26.22** Burn with resulting rupture and destruction of left eyeball

√5ᵗʰ **T26.3 Burns of other specified parts of eye and adnexa**
> Use additional external cause code to identify the source, place and intent of the burn (X00-X19, X75-X77, X96-X98, Y92)
√x7ᵗʰ **T26.30** Burns of other specified parts of unspecified eye and adnexa
√x7ᵗʰ **T26.31** Burns of other specified parts of right eye and adnexa
√x7ᵗʰ **T26.32** Burns of other specified parts of left eye and adnexa

√5ᵗʰ **T26.4 Burn of eye and adnexa, part unspecified**
> Use additional external cause code to identify the source, place and intent of the burn (X00-X19, X75-X77, X96-X98, Y92)
√x7ᵗʰ **T26.40** Burn of unspecified eye and adnexa, part unspecified
√x7ᵗʰ **T26.41** Burn of right eye and adnexa, part unspecified

√x7ᵗʰ **T26.42** Burn of left eye and adnexa, part unspecified

√5ᵗʰ **T26.5 Corrosion of eyelid and periocular area**
> Code first (T51-T65) to identify chemical and intent
> Use additional external cause code to identify place (Y92)
√x7ᵗʰ **T26.50** Corrosion of unspecified eyelid and periocular area
√x7ᵗʰ **T26.51** Corrosion of right eyelid and periocular area
√x7ᵗʰ **T26.52** Corrosion of left eyelid and periocular area

√5ᵗʰ **T26.6 Corrosion of cornea and conjunctival sac**
> Code first (T51-T65) to identify chemical and intent
> Use additional external cause code to identify place (Y92)
√x7ᵗʰ **T26.60** Corrosion of cornea and conjunctival sac, unspecified eye
√x7ᵗʰ **T26.61** Corrosion of cornea and conjunctival sac, right eye
√x7ᵗʰ **T26.62** Corrosion of cornea and conjunctival sac, left eye

√5ᵗʰ **T26.7 Corrosion with resulting rupture and destruction of eyeball**
> Code first (T51-T65) to identify chemical and intent
> Use additional external cause code to identify place (Y92)
√x7ᵗʰ **T26.70** Corrosion with resulting rupture and destruction of unspecified eyeball
√x7ᵗʰ **T26.71** Corrosion with resulting rupture and destruction of right eyeball
√x7ᵗʰ **T26.72** Corrosion with resulting rupture and destruction of left eyeball

√5ᵗʰ **T26.8 Corrosions of other specified parts of eye and adnexa**
> Code first (T51-T65) to identify chemical and intent
> Use additional external cause code to identify place (Y92)
√x7ᵗʰ **T26.80** Corrosions of other specified parts of unspecified eye and adnexa
√x7ᵗʰ **T26.81** Corrosions of other specified parts of right eye and adnexa
√x7ᵗʰ **T26.82** Corrosions of other specified parts of left eye and adnexa

√5ᵗʰ **T26.9 Corrosion of eye and adnexa, part unspecified**
> Code first (T51-T65) to identify chemical and intent
> Use additional external cause code to identify place (Y92)
√x7ᵗʰ **T26.90** Corrosion of unspecified eye and adnexa, part unspecified
√x7ᵗʰ **T26.91** Corrosion of right eye and adnexa, part unspecified
√x7ᵗʰ **T26.92** Corrosion of left eye and adnexa, part unspecified

√4ᵗʰ **T27 Burn and corrosion of respiratory tract**
> Use additional external cause code to identify the source and intent of the burn (X00- X19, X75-X77, X96-X98)
> Use additional external cause code to identify place (Y92)

> The appropriate 7th character is to be added to each code from category T27.
> A   initial encounter
> D   subsequent encounter
> S   sequela

√x7ᵗʰ **T27.0** Burn of larynx and trachea
√x7ᵗʰ **T27.1** Burn involving larynx and trachea with lung
√x7ᵗʰ **T27.2** Burn of other parts of respiratory tract
> Burn of thoracic cavity
√x7ᵗʰ **T27.3** Burn of respiratory tract, part unspecified
> Code first (T51-T65) to identify chemical and intent for codes T27.4-T27.7
√x7ᵗʰ **T27.4** Corrosion of larynx and trachea
√x7ᵗʰ **T27.5** Corrosion involving larynx and trachea with lung
√x7ᵗʰ **T27.6** Corrosion of other parts of respiratory tract
√x7ᵗʰ **T27.7** Corrosion of respiratory tract, part unspecified

√4ᵗʰ **T28 Burn and corrosion of other internal organs**
> Use additional external cause code to identify the source and intent of the burn (X00- X19, X75-X77, X96-X98)
> Use additional external cause code to identify place (Y92)

> The appropriate 7th character is to be added to each code from category T28.
> A   initial encounter
> D   subsequent encounter
> S   sequela

√x7ᵗʰ **T28.0** Burn of mouth and pharynx
√x7ᵗʰ **T28.1** Burn of esophagus
√x7ᵗʰ **T28.2** Burn of other parts of alimentary tract
√x7ᵗʰ **T28.3** Burn of internal genitourinary organs

EXCLUDES 1 Not coded here   EXCLUDES 2 Not included here   *Manifestation Code*

√5ᵗʰ **T28.4** **Burns of other and unspecified internal organs**
- √x7ᵗʰ **T28.40** **Burn of unspecified internal organ**
- √6ᵗʰ **T28.41** **Burn of ear drum**
  - √7ᵗʰ **T28.411** **Burn of right ear drum**
  - √7ᵗʰ **T28.412** **Burn of left ear drum**
  - √7ᵗʰ **T28.419** **Burn of unspecified ear drum**
- √x7ᵗʰ **T28.49** **Burn of other internal organ**
  - Code first (T51-T65) to identify chemical and intent for T28.5-T28.9-

√x7ᵗʰ **T28.5** **Corrosion of mouth and pharynx**

√x7ᵗʰ **T28.6** **Corrosion of esophagus**

√x7ᵗʰ **T28.7** **Corrosion of other parts of alimentary tract**

√x7ᵗʰ **T28.8** **Corrosion of internal genitourinary organs**

√x7ᵗʰ **T28.9** **Corrosions of other and unspecified internal organs**
- √x7ᵗʰ **T28.90** **Corrosions of unspecified internal organs**
- √6ᵗʰ **T28.91** **Corrosions of ear drum**
  - √7ᵗʰ **T28.911** **Corrosions of right ear drum**
  - √7ᵗʰ **T28.912** **Corrosions of left ear drum**
  - √7ᵗʰ **T28.919** **Corrosions of unspecified ear drum**
- √x7ᵗʰ **T28.99** **Corrosions of other internal organs**

Burns and corrosions of multiple and unspecified body regions (T30-T32)

√4ᵗʰ **T30** **Burn and corrosion, body region unspecified**

    T30.0 **Burn of unspecified body region, unspecified degree**
> **NOTE**   This code is not for inpatient use. Code to specified site and degree of burns

    Burn NOS
    Multiple burns NOS

    T30.4 **Corrosion of unspecified body region, unspecified degree**
> **NOTE**   This code is not for inpatient use. Code to specified site and degree of corrosion

    Corrosion NOS
    Multiple corrosion NOS

√4ᵗʰ **T31** **Burns classified according to extent of body surface involved**
> **NOTE**   This category is to be used as the primary code only when the site of the burn is unspecified. It should be used as a supplementary code with categories T20-T25 when the site is specified.

    T31.0 **Burns involving less than 10% of body surface**

√5ᵗʰ **T31.1** **Burns involving 10-19% of body surface**
- **T31.10** **Burns involving 10-19% of body surface with 0% to 9% third degree burns**
  - Burns involving 10-19% of body surface NOS
- **T31.11** **Burns involving 10-19% of body surface with 10-19% third degree burns**

√5ᵗʰ **T31.2** **Burns involving 20-29% of body surface**
- **T31.20** **Burns involving 20-29% of body surface with 0% to 9% third degree burns**
  - Burns involving 20-29% of body surface NOS
- **T31.21** **Burns involving 20-29% of body surface with 10-19% third degree burns**
- **T31.22** **Burns involving 20-29% of body surface with 20-29% third degree burns**

√5ᵗʰ **T31.3** **Burns involving 30-39% of body surface**
- **T31.30** **Burns involving 30-39% of body surface with 0% to 9% third degree burns**
  - Burns involving 30-39% of body surface NOS
- **T31.31** **Burns involving 30-39% of body surface with 10-19% third degree burns**
- **T31.32** **Burns involving 30-39% of body surface with 20-29% third degree burns**
- **T31.33** **Burns involving 30-39% of body surface with 30-39% third degree burns**

√5ᵗʰ **T31.4** **Burns involving 40-49% of body surface**
- **T31.40** **Burns involving 40-49% of body surface with 0% to 9% third degree burns**
  - Burns involving 40-49% of body surface NOS
- **T31.41** **Burns involving 40-49% of body surface with 10-19% third degree burns**
- **T31.42** **Burns involving 40-49% of body surface with 20-29% third degree burns**
- **T31.43** **Burns involving 40-49% of body surface with 30-39% third degree burns**
- **T31.44** **Burns involving 40-49% of body surface with 40-49% third degree burns**

√5ᵗʰ **T31.5** **Burns involving 50-59% of body surface**
- **T31.50** **Burns involving 50-59% of body surface with 0% to 9% third degree burns**
  - Burns involving 50-59% of body surface NOS
- **T31.51** **Burns involving 50-59% of body surface with 10-19% third degree burns**
- **T31.52** **Burns involving 50-59% of body surface with 20-29% third degree burns**
- **T31.53** **Burns involving 50-59% of body surface with 30-39% third degree burns**
- **T31.54** **Burns involving 50-59% of body surface with 40-49% third degree burns**
- **T31.55** **Burns involving 50-59% of body surface with 50-59% third degree burns**

√5ᵗʰ **T31.6** **Burns involving 60-69% of body surface**
- **T31.60** **Burns involving 60-69% of body surface with 0% to 9% third degree burns**
  - Burns involving 60-69% of body surface NOS
- **T31.61** **Burns involving 60-69% of body surface with 10-19% third degree burns**
- **T31.62** **Burns involving 60-69% of body surface with 20-29% third degree burns**
- **T31.63** **Burns involving 60-69% of body surface with 30-39% third degree burns**
- **T31.64** **Burns involving 60-69% of body surface with 40-49% third degree burns**
- **T31.65** **Burns involving 60-69% of body surface with 50-59% third degree burns**
- **T31.66** **Burns involving 60-69% of body surface with 60-69% third degree burns**

√5ᵗʰ **T31.7** **Burns involving 70-79% of body surface**
- **T31.70** **Burns involving 70-79% of body surface with 0% to 9% third degree burns**
  - Burns involving 70-79% of body surface NOS
- **T31.71** **Burns involving 70-79% of body surface with 10-19% third degree burns**
- **T31.72** **Burns involving 70-79% of body surface with 20-29% third degree burns**
- **T31.73** **Burns involving 70-79% of body surface with 30-39% third degree burns**
- **T31.74** **Burns involving 70-79% of body surface with 40-49% third degree burns**
- **T31.75** **Burns involving 70-79% of body surface with 50-59% third degree burns**
- **T31.76** **Burns involving 70-79% of body surface with 60-69% third degree burns**
- **T31.77** **Burns involving 70-79% of body surface with 70-79% third degree burns**

√5ᵗʰ **T31.8** **Burns involving 80-89% of body surface**
- **T31.80** **Burns involving 80-89% of body surface with 0% to 9% third degree burns**
  - Burns involving 80-89% of body surface NOS
- **T31.81** **Burns involving 80-89% of body surface with 10-19% third degree burns**
- **T31.82** **Burns involving 80-89% of body surface with 20-29% third degree burns**
- **T31.83** **Burns involving 80-89% of body surface with 30-39% third degree burns**
- **T31.84** **Burns involving 80-89% of body surface with 40-49% third degree burns**
- **T31.85** **Burns involving 80-89% of body surface with 50-59% third degree burns**
- **T31.86** **Burns involving 80-89% of body surface with 60-69% third degree burns**
- **T31.87** **Burns involving 80-89% of body surface with 70-79% third degree burns**
- **T31.88** **Burns involving 80-89% of body surface with 80-89% third degree burns**

√5ᵗʰ **T31.9** **Burns involving 90% or more of body surface**
- **T31.90** **Burns involving 90% or more of body surface with 0% to 9% third degree burns**
  - Burns involving 90% or more of body surface NOS
- **T31.91** **Burns involving 90% or more of body surface with 10-19% third degree burns**
- **T31.92** **Burns involving 90% or more of body surface with 20-29% third degree burns**
- **T31.93** **Burns involving 90% or more of body surface with 30-39% third degree burns**

✔ Appropriate additional character required   √x7ᵗʰ Requires 7th character, placeholder x must fill empty characters

T31.94   Burns involving 90% or more of body surface with 40-49% third degree burns

T31.95   Burns involving 90% or more of body surface with 50-59% third degree burns

T31.96   Burns involving 90% or more of body surface with 60-69% third degree burns

T31.97   Burns involving 90% or more of body surface with 70-79% third degree burns

T31.98   Burns involving 90% or more of body surface with 80-89% third degree burns

T31.99   Burns involving 90% or more of body surface with 90% or more third degree burns

☑4th **T32**   **Corrosions classified according to extent of body surface involved**

> NOTE   This category is to be used as the primary code only when the site of the corrosion is unspecified. It may be used as a supplementary code with categories T20-T25 when the site is specified.

T32.0   Corrosions involving less than 10% of body surface

☑5th **T32.1**   Corrosions involving 10-19% of body surface

T32.10   Corrosions involving 10-19% of body surface with 0% to 9% third degree corrosion
    Corrosions involving 10-19% of body surface NOS

T32.11   Corrosions involving 10-19% of body surface with 10-19% third degree corrosion

☑5th **T32.2**   Corrosions involving 20-29% of body surface

T32.20   Corrosions involving 20-29% of body surface with 0% to 9% third degree corrosion

T32.21   Corrosions involving 20-29% of body surface with 10-19% third degree corrosion

T32.22   Corrosions involving 20-29% of body surface with 20-29% third degree corrosion

☑5th **T32.3**   Corrosions involving 30-39% of body surface

T32.30   Corrosions involving 30-39% of body surface with 0% to 9% third degree corrosion

T32.31   Corrosions involving 30-39% of body surface with 10-19% third degree corrosion

T32.32   Corrosions involving 30-39% of body surface with 20-29% third degree corrosion

T32.33   Corrosions involving 30-39% of body surface with 30-39% third degree corrosion

☑5th **T32.4**   Corrosions involving 40-49% of body surface

T32.40   Corrosions involving 40-49% of body surface with 0% to 9% third degree corrosion

T32.41   Corrosions involving 40-49% of body surface with 10-19% third degree corrosion

T32.42   Corrosions involving 40-49% of body surface with 20-29% third degree corrosion

T32.43   Corrosions involving 40-49% of body surface with 30-39% third degree corrosion

T32.44   Corrosions involving 40-49% of body surface with 40-49% third degree corrosion

☑5th **T32.5**   Corrosions involving 50-59% of body surface

T32.50   Corrosions involving 50-59% of body surface with 0% to 9% third degree corrosion

T32.51   Corrosions involving 50-59% of body surface with 10-19% third degree corrosion

T32.52   Corrosions involving 50-59% of body surface with 20-29% third degree corrosion

T32.53   Corrosions involving 50-59% of body surface with 30-39% third degree corrosion

T32.54   Corrosions involving 50-59% of body surface with 40-49% third degree corrosion

T32.55   Corrosions involving 50-59% of body surface with 50-59% third degree corrosion

☑5th **T32.6**   Corrosions involving 60-69% of body surface

T32.60   Corrosions involving 60-69% of body surface with 0% to 9% third degree corrosion

T32.61   Corrosions involving 60-69% of body surface with 10-19% third degree corrosion

T32.62   Corrosions involving 60-69% of body surface with 20-29% third degree corrosion

T32.63   Corrosions involving 60-69% of body surface with 30-39% third degree corrosion

T32.64   Corrosions involving 60-69% of body surface with 40-49% third degree corrosion

T32.65   Corrosions involving 60-69% of body surface with 50-59% third degree corrosion

T32.66   Corrosions involving 60-69% of body surface with 60-69% third degree corrosion

☑5th **T32.7**   Corrosions involving 70-79% of body surface

T32.70   Corrosions involving 70-79% of body surface with 0% to 9% third degree corrosion

T32.71   Corrosions involving 70-79% of body surface with 10-19% third degree corrosion

T32.72   Corrosions involving 70-79% of body surface with 20-29% third degree corrosion

T32.73   Corrosions involving 70-79% of body surface with 30-39% third degree corrosion

T32.74   Corrosions involving 70-79% of body surface with 40-49% third degree corrosion

T32.75   Corrosions involving 70-79% of body surface with 50-59% third degree corrosion

T32.76   Corrosions involving 70-79% of body surface with 60-69% third degree corrosion

T32.77   Corrosions involving 70-79% of body surface with 70-79% third degree corrosion

☑5th **T32.8**   Corrosions involving 80-89% of body surface

T32.80   Corrosions involving 80-89% of body surface with 0% to 9% third degree corrosion

T32.81   Corrosions involving 80-89% of body surface with 10-19% third degree corrosion

T32.82   Corrosions involving 80-89% of body surface with 20-29% third degree corrosion

T32.83   Corrosions involving 80-89% of body surface with 30-39% third degree corrosion

T32.84   Corrosions involving 80-89% of body surface with 40-49% third degree corrosion

T32.85   Corrosions involving 80-89% of body surface with 50-59% third degree corrosion

T32.86   Corrosions involving 80-89% of body surface with 60-69% third degree corrosion

T32.87   Corrosions involving 80-89% of body surface with 70-79% third degree corrosion

T32.88   Corrosions involving 80-89% of body surface with 80-89% third degree corrosion

☑5th **T32.9**   Corrosions involving 90% or more of body surface

T32.90   Corrosions involving 90% or more of body surface with 0% to 9% third degree corrosion

T32.91   Corrosions involving 90% or more of body surface with 10-19% third degree corrosion

T32.92   Corrosions involving 90% or more of body surface with 20-29% third degree corrosion

T32.93   Corrosions involving 90% or more of body surface with 30-39% third degree corrosion

T32.94   Corrosions involving 90% or more of body surface with 40-49% third degree corrosion

T32.95   Corrosions involving 90% or more of body surface with 50-59% third degree corrosion

T32.96   Corrosions involving 90% or more of body surface with 60-69% third degree corrosion

T32.97   Corrosions involving 90% or more of body surface with 70-79% third degree corrosion

T32.98   Corrosions involving 90% or more of body surface with 80-89% third degree corrosion

T32.99   Corrosions involving 90% or more of body surface with 90% or more third degree corrosion

Frostbite (T33-T34)

EXCLUDES 2   *hypothermia and other effects of reduced temperature (T68, T69-)*

☑4th **T33**   **Superficial frostbite**

> INCLUDES   frostbite with partial thickness skin loss

> The appropriate 7th character is to be added to each code from category T33.
> A   initial encounter
> D   subsequent encounter
> S   sequela

☑5th **T33.0**   Superficial frostbite of head

☑6th   **T33.01**   Superficial frostbite of ear

☑7th   **T33.011**   Superficial frostbite of right ear

☑7th   **T33.012**   Superficial frostbite of left ear

☑7th   **T33.019**   Superficial frostbite of unspecified ear

☑x7th   **T33.02**   Superficial frostbite of nose

☑x7th   **T33.09**   Superficial frostbite of other part of head

---

EXCLUDES 1   Not coded here   EXCLUDES 2   Not included here   *Manifestation Code*

✓x7th T33.1　**Superficial frostbite of neck**
✓x7th T33.2　**Superficial frostbite of thorax**
✓x7th T33.3　**Superficial frostbite of abdominal wall, lower back and pelvis**
✓5th T33.4　**Superficial frostbite of arm**
　　EXCLUDES 2　*superficial frostbite of wrist and hand (T33.5-)*
　　✓x7th T33.40　**Superficial frostbite of unspecified arm**
　　✓x7th T33.41　**Superficial frostbite of right arm**
　　✓x7th T33.42　**Superficial frostbite of left arm**
✓5th T33.5　**Superficial frostbite of wrist, hand, and fingers**
　　✓6th T33.51　**Superficial frostbite of wrist**
　　　　✓7th T33.511　**Superficial frostbite of right wrist**
　　　　✓7th T33.512　**Superficial frostbite of left wrist**
　　　　✓7th T33.519　**Superficial frostbite of unspecified wrist**
　　✓6th T33.52　**Superficial frostbite of hand**
　　　　EXCLUDES 2　*superficial frostbite of fingers (T33.53-)*
　　　　✓7th T33.521　**Superficial frostbite of right hand**
　　　　✓7th T33.522　**Superficial frostbite of left hand**
　　　　✓7th T33.529　**Superficial frostbite of unspecified hand**
　　✓6th T33.53　**Superficial frostbite of finger(s)**
　　　　✓7th T33.531　**Superficial frostbite of right finger(s)**
　　　　✓7th T33.532　**Superficial frostbite of left finger(s)**
　　　　✓7th T33.539　**Superficial frostbite of unspecified finger(s)**
✓5th T33.6　**Superficial frostbite of hip and thigh**
　　✓x7th T33.60　**Superficial frostbite of unspecified hip and thigh**
　　✓x7th T33.61　**Superficial frostbite of right hip and thigh**
　　✓x7th T33.62　**Superficial frostbite of left hip and thigh**
✓5th T33.7　**Superficial frostbite of knee and lower leg**
　　EXCLUDES 2　*superficial frostbite of ankle and foot (T33.8-)*
　　✓x7th T33.70　**Superficial frostbite of unspecified knee and lower leg**
　　✓x7th T33.71　**Superficial frostbite of right knee and lower leg**
　　✓x7th T33.72　**Superficial frostbite of left knee and lower leg**
✓5th T33.8　**Superficial frostbite of ankle, foot, and toe(s)**
　　✓6th T33.81　**Superficial frostbite of ankle**
　　　　✓7th T33.811　**Superficial frostbite of right ankle**
　　　　✓7th T33.812　**Superficial frostbite of left ankle**
　　　　✓7th T33.819　**Superficial frostbite of unspecified ankle**
　　✓6th T33.82　**Superficial frostbite of foot**
　　　　✓7th T33.821　**Superficial frostbite of right foot**
　　　　✓7th T33.822　**Superficial frostbite of left foot**
　　　　✓7th T33.829　**Superficial frostbite of unspecified foot**
　　✓6th T33.83　**Superficial frostbite of toe(s)**
　　　　✓7th T33.831　**Superficial frostbite of right toe(s)**
　　　　✓7th T33.832　**Superficial frostbite of left toe(s)**
　　　　✓7th T33.839　**Superficial frostbite of unspecified toe(s)**
✓5th T33.9　**Superficial frostbite of other and unspecified sites**
　　✓x7th T33.90　**Superficial frostbite of unspecified sites**
　　　　Superficial frostbite NOS
　　✓x7th T33.99　**Superficial frostbite of other sites**
　　　　Superficial frostbite of leg NOS
　　　　Superficial frostbite of trunk NOS

✓4th T34　**Frostbite with tissue necrosis**

> The appropriate 7th character is to be added to each code from category T34.
> A　initial encounter
> D　subsequent encounter
> S　sequela

✓5th T34.0　**Frostbite with tissue necrosis of head**
　　✓6th T34.01　**Frostbite with tissue necrosis of ear**
　　　　✓7th T34.011　**Frostbite with tissue necrosis of right ear**
　　　　✓7th T34.012　**Frostbite with tissue necrosis of left ear**
　　　　✓7th T34.019　**Frostbite with tissue necrosis of unspecified ear**
　　✓x7th T34.02　**Frostbite with tissue necrosis of nose**
　　✓x7th T34.09　**Frostbite with tissue necrosis of other part of head**
✓x7th T34.1　**Frostbite with tissue necrosis of neck**
✓x7th T34.2　**Frostbite with tissue necrosis of thorax**
✓x7th T34.3　**Frostbite with tissue necrosis of abdominal wall, lower back and pelvis**

✓5th T34.4　**Frostbite with tissue necrosis of arm**
　　EXCLUDES 2　*frostbite with tissue necrosis of wrist and hand (T34.5-)*
　　✓x7th T34.40　**Frostbite with tissue necrosis of unspecified arm**
　　✓x7th T34.41　**Frostbite with tissue necrosis of right arm**
　　✓x7th T34.42　**Frostbite with tissue necrosis of left arm**
✓5th T34.5　**Frostbite with tissue necrosis of wrist, hand, and finger(s)**
　　✓6th T34.51　**Frostbite with tissue necrosis of wrist**
　　　　✓7th T34.511　**Frostbite with tissue necrosis of right wrist**
　　　　✓7th T34.512　**Frostbite with tissue necrosis of left wrist**
　　　　✓7th T34.519　**Frostbite with tissue necrosis of unspecified wrist**
　　✓6th T34.52　**Frostbite with tissue necrosis of hand**
　　　　EXCLUDES 2　*frostbite with tissue necrosis of finger(s) (T34.53-)*
　　　　✓7th T34.521　**Frostbite with tissue necrosis of right hand**
　　　　✓7th T34.522　**Frostbite with tissue necrosis of left hand**
　　　　✓7th T34.529　**Frostbite with tissue necrosis of unspecified hand**
　　✓6th T34.53　**Frostbite with tissue necrosis of finger(s)**
　　　　✓7th T34.531　**Frostbite with tissue necrosis of right finger(s)**
　　　　✓7th T34.532　**Frostbite with tissue necrosis of left finger(s)**
　　　　✓7th T34.539　**Frostbite with tissue necrosis of unspecified finger(s)**
✓5th T34.6　**Frostbite with tissue necrosis of hip and thigh**
　　✓x7th T34.60　**Frostbite with tissue necrosis of unspecified hip and thigh**
　　✓x7th T34.61　**Frostbite with tissue necrosis of right hip and thigh**
　　✓x7th T34.62　**Frostbite with tissue necrosis of left hip and thigh**
✓5th T34.7　**Frostbite with tissue necrosis of knee and lower leg**
　　EXCLUDES 2　*frostbite with tissue necrosis of ankle and foot (T34.8-)*
　　✓x7th T34.70　**Frostbite with tissue necrosis of unspecified knee and lower leg**
　　✓x7th T34.71　**Frostbite with tissue necrosis of right knee and lower leg**
　　✓x7th T34.72　**Frostbite with tissue necrosis of left knee and lower leg**
✓5th T34.8　**Frostbite with tissue necrosis of ankle, foot, and toe(s)**
　　✓6th T34.81　**Frostbite with tissue necrosis of ankle**
　　　　✓7th T34.811　**Frostbite with tissue necrosis of right ankle**
　　　　✓7th T34.812　**Frostbite with tissue necrosis of left ankle**
　　　　✓7th T34.819　**Frostbite with tissue necrosis of unspecified ankle**
　　✓6th T34.82　**Frostbite with tissue necrosis of foot**
　　　　✓7th T34.821　**Frostbite with tissue necrosis of right foot**
　　　　✓7th T34.822　**Frostbite with tissue necrosis of left foot**
　　　　✓7th T34.829　**Frostbite with tissue necrosis of unspecified foot**
　　✓6th T34.83　**Frostbite with tissue necrosis of toe(s)**
　　　　✓7th T34.831　**Frostbite with tissue necrosis of right toe(s)**
　　　　✓7th T34.832　**Frostbite with tissue necrosis of left toe(s)**
　　　　✓7th T34.839　**Frostbite with tissue necrosis of unspecified toe(s)**
✓5th T34.9　**Frostbite with tissue necrosis of other and unspecified sites**
　　✓x7th T34.90　**Frostbite with tissue necrosis of unspecified sites**
　　　　Frostbite with tissue necrosis NOS
　　✓x7th T34.99　**Frostbite with tissue necrosis of other sites**
　　　　Frostbite with tissue necrosis of leg NOS
　　　　Frostbite with tissue necrosis of trunk NOS

Poisoning by, adverse effects of and underdosing of drugs, medicaments and biological substances (T36-T50)

INCLUDES   poisoning is defined as:
    overdose of substances
    wrong substance given or taken in error
  adverse effect is defined as:
    "hypersensitivity", "reaction", etc. of correct substance properly administered
  underdosing is defined as:
    taking less of a medication than is prescribed or instructed by the manufacturer, whether inadvertently or deliberately

Use additional code(s) for all manifestations of poisoning and adverse effects
Use additional code for intent of underdosing:
  failure in dosage during medical and surgical care (Y63.61, Y63.8-Y63.9)
  patient's underdosing of medication regime (Z91.12-, Z91.13-)

EXCLUDES 1   toxic reaction to local anesthesia in pregnancy (O29.3-)

EXCLUDES 2   abuse and dependence of psychoactive substances (F10-F19)
  abuse of non-dependence-producing substances (F55-)
  drug reaction and poisoning affecting newborn (P00-P96)
  pathological drug intoxication (inebriation) (F10-F19)

NOTE   When no intent of poisoning is indicated code to accidental. Undetermined intent is only for use when there is specific documentation in the record that the intent of the poisoning cannot be determined.

√4ᵗʰ **T36**   **Poisoning by, adverse effect of and underdosing of systemic antibiotics**

    EXCLUDES 1   antineoplastic antibiotics (T45.1-)
      locally applied antibiotic NEC (T49.0)
      topically used antibiotic for ear, nose and throat (T49.6)
      topically used antibiotic for eye (T49.5)

    The appropriate 7th character is to be added to each code from category T36.
    A   initial encounter
    D   subsequent encounter
    S   sequela

√5ᵗʰ   **T36.0**   **Poisoning by, adverse effect of and underdosing of penicillins**

  √6ᵗʰ   **T36.0x**   **Poisoning by, adverse effect of and underdosing of penicillins**

    √7ᵗʰ   **T36.0x1**   **Poisoning by penicillins, accidental (utentional)**
        Poisoning by penicillins NOS

    √7ᵗʰ   **T36.0x2**   **Poisoning by penicillins, intentional self-harm**

    √7ᵗʰ   **T36.0x3**   **Poisoning by penicillins, assault**

    √7ᵗʰ   **T36.0x4**   **Poisoning by penicillins, undetermined**

    √7ᵗʰ   **T36.0x5**   **Adverse effect of penicillins**

    √7ᵗʰ   **T36.0x6**   **Underdosing of penicillins**

√5ᵗʰ   **T36.1**   **Poisoning by, adverse effect of and underdosing of cephalosporins and other beta-lactam antibiotics**

  √6ᵗʰ   **T36.1x**   **Poisoning by, adverse effect of and underdosing of cephalosporins and other beta-lactam antibiotics**

    √7ᵗʰ   **T36.1x1**   **Poisoning by cephalosporins and other beta-lactam antibiotics, accidental (unintentional)**
        Poisoning by cephalosporins and other beta-lactam antibiotics NOS

    √7ᵗʰ   **T36.1x2**   **Poisoning by cephalosporins and other beta-lactam antibiotics, intentional self-harm**

    √7ᵗʰ   **T36.1x3**   **Poisoning by cephalosporins and other beta-lactam antibiotics, assault**

    √7ᵗʰ   **T36.1x4**   **Poisoning by cephalosporins and other beta-lactam antibiotics, undetermined**

    √7ᵗʰ   **T36.1x5**   **Adverse effect of cephalosporins and other beta-lactam antibiotics**

    √7ᵗʰ   **T36.1x6**   **Underdosing of cephalosporins and other beta-lactam antibiotics**

√5ᵗʰ   **T36.2**   **Poisoning by, adverse effect of and underdosing of chloramphenicol group**

  √6ᵗʰ   **T36.2x**   **Poisoning by, adverse effect of and underdosing of chloramphenicol group**

    √7ᵗʰ   **T36.2x1**   **Poisoning by chloramphenicol group, accidental (unintentional)**
        Poisoning by chloramphenicol group NOS

    √7ᵗʰ   **T36.2x2**   **Poisoning by chloramphenicol group, intentional self-harm**

    √7ᵗʰ   **T36.2x3**   **Poisoning by chloramphenicol group, assault**

    √7ᵗʰ   **T36.2x4**   **Poisoning by chloramphenicol group, undetermined**

    √7ᵗʰ   **T36.2x5**   **Adverse effect of chloramphenicol group**

    √7ᵗʰ   **T36.2x6**   **Underdosing of chloramphenicol group**

√5ᵗʰ   **T36.3**   **Poisoning by, adverse effect of and underdosing of macrolides**

  √6ᵗʰ   **T36.3x**   **Poisoning by, adverse effect of and underdosing of macrolides**

    √7ᵗʰ   **T36.3x1**   **Poisoning by macrolides, accidental (unintentional)**
        Poisoning by macrolides NOS

    √7ᵗʰ   **T36.3x2**   **Poisoning by macrolides, intentional self-harm**

    √7ᵗʰ   **T36.3x3**   **Poisoning by macrolides, assault**

    √7ᵗʰ   **T36.3x4**   **Poisoning by macrolides, undetermined**

    √7ᵗʰ   **T36.3x5**   **Adverse effect of macrolides**

    √7ᵗʰ   **T36.3x6**   **Underdosing of macrolides**

√5ᵗʰ   **T36.4**   **Poisoning by, adverse effect of and underdosing of tetracyclines**

  √6ᵗʰ   **T36.4x**   **Poisoning by, adverse effect of and underdosing of tetracyclines**

    √7ᵗʰ   **T36.4x1**   **Poisoning by tetracyclines, accidental (unintentional)**
        Poisoning by tetracyclines NOS

    √7ᵗʰ   **T36.4x2**   **Poisoning by tetracyclines, intentional self-harm**

    √7ᵗʰ   **T36.4x3**   **Poisoning by tetracyclines, assault**

    √7ᵗʰ   **T36.4x4**   **Poisoning by tetracyclines, undetermined**

    √7ᵗʰ   **T36.4x5**   **Adverse effect of tetracyclines**

    √7ᵗʰ   **T36.4x6**   **Underdosing of tetracyclines**

√5ᵗʰ   **T36.5**   **Poisoning by, adverse effect of and underdosing of aminoglycosides**
    Poisoning by, adverse effect of and underdosing of streptomycin

  √6ᵗʰ   **T36.5x**   **Poisoning by, adverse effect of and underdosing of aminoglycosides**

    √7ᵗʰ   **T36.5x1**   **Poisoning by aminoglycosides, accidental (unintentional)**
        Poisoning by aminoglycosides NOS

    √7ᵗʰ   **T36.5x2**   **Poisoning by aminoglycosides, intentional self-harm**

    √7ᵗʰ   **T36.5x3**   **Poisoning by aminoglycosides, assault**

    √7ᵗʰ   **T36.5x4**   **Poisoning by aminoglycosides, undetermined**

    √7ᵗʰ   **T36.5x5**   **Adverse effect of aminoglycosides**

    √7ᵗʰ   **T36.5x6**   **Underdosing of aminoglycosides**

√5ᵗʰ   **T36.6**   **Poisoning by, adverse effect of and underdosing of rifampicins**

  √6ᵗʰ   **T36.6x**   **Poisoning by, adverse effect of and underdosing of rifampicins**

    √7ᵗʰ   **T36.6x1**   **Poisoning by rifampicins, accidental (unintentional)**
        Poisoning by rifampicins NOS

    √7ᵗʰ   **T36.6x2**   **Poisoning by rifampicins, intentional self-harm**

    √7ᵗʰ   **T36.6x3**   **Poisoning by rifampicins, assault**

    √7ᵗʰ   **T36.6x4**   **Poisoning by rifampicins, undetermined**

    √7ᵗʰ   **T36.6x5**   **Adverse effect of rifampicins**

    √7ᵗʰ   **T36.6x6**   **Underdosing of rifampicins**

√5ᵗʰ   **T36.7**   **Poisoning by, adverse effect of and underdosing of antifungal antibiotics, systemically used**

  √6ᵗʰ   **T36.7x**   **Poisoning by, adverse effect of and underdosing of antifungal antibiotics, systemically used**

    √7ᵗʰ   **T36.7x1**   **Poisoning by antifungal antibiotics, systemically used, accidental (unintentional)**
        Poisoning by antifungal antibiotics, systemically used NOS

    √7ᵗʰ   **T36.7x2**   **Poisoning by antifungal antibiotics, systemically used, intentional self-harm**

EXCLUDES 1   Not coded here   **EXCLUDES 2**   Not included here   *Manifestation Code*

✓7th **T36.7x3** **Poisoning by antifungal antibiotics, systemically used, assault**

✓7th **T36.7x4** **Poisoning by antifungal antibiotics, systemically used, undetermined**

✓7th **T36.7x5** **Adverse effect of antifungal antibiotics, systemically used**

✓7th **T36.7x6** **Underdosing of antifungal antibiotics, systemically used**

✓5th **T36.8** **Poisoning by, adverse effect of and underdosing of other systemic antibiotics**

✓6th **T36.8x** **Poisoning by, adverse effect of and underdosing of other systemic antibiotics**

✓7th **T36.8x1** **Poisoning by other systemic antibiotics, accidental (unintentional)**
Poisoning by other systemic antibiotics NOS

✓7th **T36.8x2** **Poisoning by other systemic antibiotics, intentional self-harm**

✓7th **T36.8x3** **Poisoning by other systemic antibiotics, assault**

✓7th **T36.8x4** **Poisoning by other systemic antibiotics, undetermined**

✓7th **T36.8x5** **Adverse effect of other systemic antibiotics**

✓7th **T36.8x6** **Underdosing of other systemic antibiotics**

✓5th **T36.9** **Poisoning by, adverse effect of and underdosing of unspecified systemic antibiotic**

✓x7th **T36.91** **Poisoning by unspecified systemic antibiotic, accidental (unintentional)**
Poisoning by systemic antibiotic NOS

✓x7th **T36.92** **Poisoning by unspecified systemic antibiotic, intentional self-harm**

✓x7th **T36.93** **Poisoning by unspecified systemic antibiotic, assault**

✓x7th **T36.94** **Poisoning by unspecified systemic antibiotic, undetermined**

✓x7th **T36.95** **Adverse effect of unspecified systemic antibiotic**

✓x7th **T36.96** **Underdosing of unspecified systemic antibiotic**

✓4th **T37** **Poisoning by, adverse effect of and underdosing of other systemic anti- infectives and antiparasitics**

EXCLUDES 1 *anti-infectives topically used for ear, nose and throat (T49.6-)*
anti-infectives topically used for eye (T49.5-)
locally applied anti-infectives NEC (T49.0-)

The appropriate 7th character is to be added to each code from category T37.
A   initial encounter
D   subsequent encounter
S   sequela

✓5th **T37.0** **Poisoning by, adverse effect of and underdosing of sulfonamides**

✓6th **T37.0x** **Poisoning by, adverse effect of and underdosing of sulfonamides**

✓7th **T37.0x1** **Poisoning by sulfonamides, accidental (unintentional)**
Poisoning by sulfonamides NOS

✓7th **T37.0x2** **Poisoning by sulfonamides, intentional self-harm**

✓7th **T37.0x3** **Poisoning by sulfonamides, assault**

✓7th **T37.0x4** **Poisoning by sulfonamides, undetermined**

✓7th **T37.0x5** **Adverse effect of sulfonamides**

✓7th **T37.0x6** **Underdosing of sulfonamides**

✓5th **T37.1** **Poisoning by, adverse effect of and underdosing of antimycobacterial drugs**

EXCLUDES 1 *rifampicins (T36.6-)*
streptomycin (T36.5-)

✓6th **T37.1x** **Poisoning by, adverse effect of and underdosing of antimycobacterial drugs**

✓7th **T37.1x1** **Poisoning by antimycobacterial drugs, accidental (unintentional)**
Poisoning by antimycobacterial drugs NOS

✓7th **T37.1x2** **Poisoning by antimycobacterial drugs, intentional self-harm**

✓7th **T37.1x3** **Poisoning by antimycobacterial drugs, assault**

✓7th **T37.1x4** **Poisoning by antimycobacterial drugs, undetermined**

✓7th **T37.1x5** **Adverse effect of antimycobacterial drugs**

✓7th **T37.1x6** **Underdosing of antimycobacterial drugs**

✓5th **T37.2** **Poisoning by, adverse effect of and underdosing of antimalarials and drugs acting on other blood protozoa**

EXCLUDES 1 *hydroxyquinoline derivatives (T37.8-)*

✓6th **T37.2x** **Poisoning by, adverse effect of and underdosing of antimalarials and drugs acting on other blood protozoa**

✓7th **T37.2x1** **Poisoning by antimalarials and drugs acting on other blood protozoa, accidental (unintentional)**
Poisoning by antimalarials and drugs acting on other blood protozoa NOS

✓7th **T37.2x2** **Poisoning by antimalarials and drugs acting on other blood protozoa, intentional self-harm**

✓7th **T37.2x3** **Poisoning by antimalarials and drugs acting on other blood protozoa, assault**

✓7th **T37.2x4** **Poisoning by antimalarials and drugs acting on other blood protozoa, undetermined**

✓7th **T37.2x5** **Adverse effect of antimalarials and drugs acting on other blood protozoa**

✓7th **T37.2x6** **Underdosing of antimalarials and drugs acting on other blood protozoa**

✓5th **T37.3** **Poisoning by, adverse effect of and underdosing of other antiprotozoal drugs**

✓6th **T37.3x** **Poisoning by, adverse effect of and underdosing of other antiprotozoal drugs**

✓7th **T37.3x1** **Poisoning by other antiprotozoal drugs, accidental (unintentional)**
Poisoning by other antiprotozoal drugs NOS

✓7th **T37.3x2** **Poisoning by other antiprotozoal drugs, intentional self-harm**

✓7th **T37.3x3** **Poisoning by other antiprotozoal drugs, assault**

✓7th **T37.3x4** **Poisoning by other antiprotozoal drugs, undetermined**

✓7th **T37.3x5** **Adverse effect of other antiprotozoal drugs**

✓7th **T37.3x6** **Underdosing of other antiprotozoal drugs**

✓5th **T37.4** **Poisoning by, adverse effect of and underdosing of anthelminthics**

✓6th **T37.4x** **Poisoning by, adverse effect of and underdosing of anthelminthics**

✓7th **T37.4x1** **Poisoning by anthelminthics, accidental (unintentional)**
Poisoning by anthelminthics NOS

✓7th **T37.4x2** **Poisoning by anthelminthics, intentional self-harm**

✓7th **T37.4x3** **Poisoning by anthelminthics, assault**

✓7th **T37.4x4** **Poisoning by anthelminthics, undetermined**

✓7th **T37.4x5** **Adverse effect of anthelminthics**

✓7th **T37.4x6** **Underdosing of anthelminthics**

✓5th **T37.5** **Poisoning by, adverse effect of and underdosing of antiviral drugs**

EXCLUDES 1 *amantadine (T42.8-)*
cytarabine (T45.1-)

✓6th **T37.5x** **Poisoning by, adverse effect of and underdosing of antiviral drugs**

✓7th **T37.5x1** **Poisoning by antiviral drugs, accidental (unintentional)**
Poisoning by antiviral drugs NOS

✓7th **T37.5x2** **Poisoning by antiviral drugs, intentional self-harm**

✓7th **T37.5x3** **Poisoning by antiviral drugs, assault**

✓7th **T37.5x4** **Poisoning by antiviral drugs, undetermined**

✓7th **T37.5x5** **Adverse effect of antiviral drugs**

Injury, Poisoning and Certain Other Consequences of External Causes

T37.5x6–T38.4x6

    ☑7th   **T37.5x6**   **Underdosing of antiviral drugs**

☑5th   **T37.8**   **Poisoning by, adverse effect of and underdosing of other specified systemic anti-infectives and antiparasitics**
Poisoning by, adverse effect of and underdosing of hydroxyquinoline derivatives
    EXCLUDES 1   *antimalarial drugs (T37.2-)*

  ☑6th   **T37.8x**   **Poisoning by, adverse effect of and underdosing of other specified systemic anti-infectives and antiparasitics**

    ☑7th   **T37.8x1**   **Poisoning by other specified systemic anti-infectives and antiparasitics, accidental (unintentional)**
Poisoning by other specified systemic anti-infectives and antiparasitics NOS

    ☑7th   **T37.8x2**   **Poisoning by other specified systemic anti-infectives and antiparasitics, intentional self-harm**

    ☑7th   **T37.8x3**   **Poisoning by other specified systemic anti-infectives and antiparasitics, assault**

    ☑7th   **T37.8x4**   **Poisoning by other specified systemic anti-infectives and antiparasitics, undetermined**

    ☑7th   **T37.8x5**   **Adverse effect of other specified systemic anti-infectives and antiparasitics**

    ☑7th   **T37.8x6**   **Underdosing of other specified systemic anti-infectives and antiparasitics**

☑5th   **T37.9**   **Poisoning by, adverse effect of and underdosing of unspecified systemic anti-infective and antiparasitics**

  ☑x7th   **T37.91**   **Poisoning by unspecified systemic anti-infective and antiparasitics, accidental (unintentional)**
Poisoning by, adverse effect of and underdosing of systemic anti-infective and antiparasitics NOS

  ☑x7th   **T37.92**   **Poisoning by unspecified systemic anti-infective and antiparasitics, intentional self-harm**

  ☑x7th   **T37.93**   **Poisoning by unspecified systemic anti-infective and antiparasitics, assault**

  ☑x7th   **T37.94**   **Poisoning by unspecified systemic anti-infective and antiparasitics, undetermined**

  ☑x7th   **T37.95**   **Adverse effect of unspecified systemic anti-infective and antiparasitic**

  ☑x7th   **T37.96**   **Underdosing of unspecified systemic anti-infectives and antiparasitics**

☑4th   **T38**   **Poisoning by, adverse effect of and underdosing of hormones and their synthetic substitutes and antagonists, not elsewhere classified**
    EXCLUDES 1   *mineralocorticoids and their antagonists (T50.0-)*
oxytocic hormones (T48.0-)
parathyroid hormones and derivatives (T50.9-)

> The appropriate 7th character is to be added to each code from category T38.
> A   initial encounter
> D   subsequent encounter
> S   sequela

☑5th   **T38.0**   **Poisoning by, adverse effect of and underdosing of glucocorticoids and synthetic analogues**
    EXCLUDES 1   *glucocorticoids, topically used (T49-)*

  ☑6th   **T38.0x**   **Poisoning by, adverse effect of and underdosing of glucocorticoids and synthetic analogues**

    ☑7th   **T38.0x1**   **Poisoning by glucocorticoids and synthetic analogues, accidental (unintentional)**
Poisoning by glucocorticoids and synthetic analogues NOS

    ☑7th   **T38.0x2**   **Poisoning by glucocorticoids and synthetic analogues, intentional self-harm**

    ☑7th   **T38.0x3**   **Poisoning by glucocorticoids and synthetic analogues, assault**

    ☑7th   **T38.0x4**   **Poisoning by glucocorticoids and synthetic analogues, undetermined**

    ☑7th   **T38.0x5**   **Adverse effect of glucocorticoids and synthetic analogues**

    ☑7th   **T38.0x6**   **Underdosing of glucocorticoids and synthetic analogues**

☑5th   **T38.1**   **Poisoning by, adverse effect of and underdosing of thyroid hormones and substitutes**

  ☑6th   **T38.1x**   **Poisoning by, adverse effect of and underdosing of thyroid hormones and substitutes**

    ☑7th   **T38.1x1**   **Poisoning by thyroid hormones and substitutes, accidental (unintentional)**
Poisoning by thyroid hormones and substitutes NOS

    ☑7th   **T38.1x2**   **Poisoning by thyroid hormones and substitutes, intentional self-harm**

    ☑7th   **T38.1x3**   **Poisoning by thyroid hormones and substitutes, assault**

    ☑7th   **T38.1x4**   **Poisoning by thyroid hormones and substitutes, undetermined**

    ☑7th   **T38.1x5**   **Adverse effect of thyroid hormones and substitutes**

    ☑7th   **T38.1x6**   **Underdosing of thyroid hormones and substitutes**

☑5th   **T38.2**   **Poisoning by, adverse effect of and underdosing of antithyroid drugs**

  ☑6th   **T38.2x**   **Poisoning by, adverse effect of and underdosing of antithyroid drugs**

    ☑7th   **T38.2x1**   **Poisoning by antithyroid drugs, accidental (unintentional)**
Poisoning by antithyroid drugs NOS

    ☑7th   **T38.2x2**   **Poisoning by antithyroid drugs, intentional self-harm**

    ☑7th   **T38.2x3**   **Poisoning by antithyroid drugs, assault**

    ☑7th   **T38.2x4**   **Poisoning by antithyroid drugs, undetermined**

    ☑7th   **T38.2x5**   **Adverse effect of antithyroid drugs**

    ☑7th   **T38.2x6**   **Underdosing of antithyroid drugs**

☑5th   **T38.3**   **Poisoning by, adverse effect of and underdosing of insulin and oral hypoglycemic [antidiabetic] drugs**

  ☑6th   **T38.3x**   **Poisoning by, adverse effect of and underdosing of insulin and oral hypoglycemic [antidiabetic] drugs**

    ☑7th   **T38.3x1**   **Poisoning by insulin and oral hypoglycemic [antidiabetic] drugs, accidental (unintentional)**
Poisoning by insulin and oral hypoglycemic [antidiabetic] drugs NOS

    ☑7th   **T38.3x2**   **Poisoning by insulin and oral hypoglycemic [antidiabetic] drugs, intentional self-harm**

    ☑7th   **T38.3x3**   **Poisoning by insulin and oral hypoglycemic [antidiabetic] drugs, assault**

    ☑7th   **T38.3x4**   **Poisoning by insulin and oral hypoglycemic [antidiabetic] drugs, undetermined**

    ☑7th   **T38.3x5**   **Adverse effect of insulin and oral hypoglycemic [antidiabetic] drugs**

    ☑7th   **T38.3x6**   **Underdosing of insulin and oral hypoglycemic [antidiabetic] drugs**

☑5th   **T38.4**   **Poisoning by, adverse effect of and underdosing of oral contraceptives**
Poisoning by, adverse effect of and underdosing of multiple- and single-ingredient oral contraceptive preparations

  ☑6th   **T38.4x**   **Poisoning by, adverse effect of and underdosing of oral contraceptives**

    ☑7th   **T38.4x1**   **Poisoning by oral contraceptives, accidental (unintentional)**
Poisoning by oral contraceptives NOS

    ☑7th   **T38.4x2**   **Poisoning by oral contraceptives, intentional self-harm**

    ☑7th   **T38.4x3**   **Poisoning by oral contraceptives, assault**

    ☑7th   **T38.4x4**   **Poisoning by oral contraceptives, undetermined**

    ☑7th   **T38.4x5**   **Adverse effect of oral contraceptives**

    ☑7th   **T38.4x6**   **Underdosing of oral contraceptives**

EXCLUDES 1   Not coded here   EXCLUDES 2   Not included here   ***Manifestation Code***

√5ᵗʰ **T38.5 Poisoning by, adverse effect of and underdosing of other estrogens and progestogens**

Poisoning by, adverse effect of and underdosing of estrogens and progestogens mixtures and substitutes

√6ᵗʰ **T38.5x Poisoning by, adverse effect of and underdosing of other estrogens and progestogens**

√7ᵗʰ **T38.5x1 Poisoning by other estrogens and progestogens, accidental (unintentional)**

Poisoning by other estrogens and progestogens NOS

√7ᵗʰ **T38.5x2 Poisoning by other estrogens and progestogens, intentional self-harm**

√7ᵗʰ **T38.5x3 Poisoning by other estrogens and progestogens, assault**

√7ᵗʰ **T38.5x4 Poisoning by other estrogens and progestogens, undetermined**

√7ᵗʰ **T38.5x5 Adverse effect of other estrogens and progestogens**

√7ᵗʰ **T38.5x6 Underdosing of other estrogens and progestogens**

√5ᵗʰ **T38.6 Poisoning by, adverse effect of and underdosing of antigonadotrophins, antiestrogens, antiandrogens, not elsewhere classified**

Poisoning by, adverse effect of and underdosing of tamoxifen

√6ᵗʰ **T38.6x Poisoning by, adverse effect of and underdosing of antigonadotrophins, antiestrogens, antiandrogens, not elsewhere classified**

√7ᵗʰ **T38.6x1 Poisoning by antigonadotrophins, antiestrogens, antiandrogens, not elsewhere classified, accidental (unintentional)**

Poisoning by antigonadotrophins, antiestrogens, antiandrogens, not elsewhere classified NOS

√7ᵗʰ **T38.6x2 Poisoning by antigonadotrophins, antiestrogens, antiandrogens, not elsewhere classified, intentional self-harm**

√7ᵗʰ **T38.6x3 Poisoning by antigonadotrophins, antiestrogens, antiandrogens, not elsewhere classified, assault**

√7ᵗʰ **T38.6x4 Poisoning by antigonadotrophins, antiestrogens, antiandrogens, not elsewhere classified, undetermined**

√7ᵗʰ **T38.6x5 Adverse effect of antigonadotrophins, antiestrogens, antiandrogens, not elsewhere classified**

√7ᵗʰ **T38.6x6 Underdosing of antigonadotrophins, antiestrogens, antiandrogens, not elsewhere classified**

√5ᵗʰ **T38.7 Poisoning by, adverse effect of and underdosing of androgens and anabolic congeners**

√6ᵗʰ **T38.7x Poisoning by, adverse effect of and underdosing of androgens and anabolic congeners**

√7ᵗʰ **T38.7x1 Poisoning by androgens and anabolic congeners, accidental (unintentional)**

Poisoning by androgens and anabolic congeners NOS

√7ᵗʰ **T38.7x2 Poisoning by androgens and anabolic congeners, intentional self-harm**

√7ᵗʰ **T38.7x3 Poisoning by androgens and anabolic congeners, assault**

√7ᵗʰ **T38.7x4 Poisoning by androgens and anabolic congeners, undetermined**

√7ᵗʰ **T38.7x5 Adverse effect of androgens and anabolic congeners**

√7ᵗʰ **T38.7x6 Underdosing of androgens and anabolic congeners**

√5ᵗʰ **T38.8 Poisoning by, adverse effect of and underdosing of other and unspecified hormones and synthetic substitutes**

√6ᵗʰ **T38.80 Poisoning by, adverse effect of and underdosing of unspecified hormones and synthetic substitutes**

√7ᵗʰ **T38.801 Poisoning by unspecified hormones and synthetic substitutes, accidental (unintentional)**

Poisoning by unspecified hormones and synthetic substitutes NOS

√7ᵗʰ **T38.802 Poisoning by unspecified hormones and synthetic substitutes, intentional self-harm**

√7ᵗʰ **T38.803 Poisoning by unspecified hormones and synthetic substitutes, assault**

√7ᵗʰ **T38.804 Poisoning by unspecified hormones and synthetic substitutes, undetermined**

√7ᵗʰ **T38.805 Adverse effect of unspecified hormones and synthetic substitutes**

√7ᵗʰ **T38.806 Underdosing of unspecified hormones and synthetic substitutes**

√6ᵗʰ **T38.81 Poisoning by, adverse effect of and underdosing of anterior pituitary [adenohypophyseal] hormones**

√7ᵗʰ **T38.811 Poisoning by anterior pituitary [adenohypophyseal] hormones, accidental (unintentional)**

Poisoning by anterior pituitary [adenohypophyseal] hormones NOS

√7ᵗʰ **T38.812 Poisoning by anterior pituitary [adenohypophyseal] hormones, intentional self-harm**

√7ᵗʰ **T38.813 Poisoning by anterior pituitary [adenohypophyseal] hormones, assault**

√7ᵗʰ **T38.814 Poisoning by anterior pituitary [adenohypophyseal] hormones, undetermined**

√7ᵗʰ **T38.815 Adverse effect of anterior pituitary [adenohypophyseal] hormones**

√7ᵗʰ **T38.816 Underdosing of anterior pituitary [adenohypophyseal] hormones**

√6ᵗʰ **T38.89 Poisoning by, adverse effect of and underdosing of other hormones and synthetic substitutes**

√7ᵗʰ **T38.891 Poisoning by other hormones and synthetic substitutes, accidental (unintentional)**

Poisoning by other hormones and synthetic substitutes NOS

√7ᵗʰ **T38.892 Poisoning by other hormones and synthetic substitutes, intentional self-harm**

√7ᵗʰ **T38.893 Poisoning by other hormones and synthetic substitutes, assault**

√7ᵗʰ **T38.894 Poisoning by other hormones and synthetic substitutes, undetermined**

√7ᵗʰ **T38.895 Adverse effect of other hormones and synthetic substitutes**

√7ᵗʰ **T38.896 Underdosing of other hormones and synthetic substitutes**

√5ᵗʰ **T38.9 Poisoning by, adverse effect of and underdosing of other and unspecified hormone antagonists**

√6ᵗʰ **T38.90 Poisoning by, adverse effect of and underdosing of unspecified hormone antagonists**

√7ᵗʰ **T38.901 Poisoning by unspecified hormone antagonists, accidental (unintentional)**

Poisoning by unspecified hormone antagonists NOS

√7ᵗʰ **T38.902 Poisoning by unspecified hormone antagonists, intentional self-harm**

√7ᵗʰ **T38.903 Poisoning by unspecified hormone antagonists, assault**

√7ᵗʰ **T38.904 Poisoning by unspecified hormone antagonists, undetermined**

√7ᵗʰ **T38.905 Adverse effect of unspecified hormone antagonists**

√7ᵗʰ **T38.906 Underdosing of unspecified hormone antagonists**

√6ᵗʰ **T38.99 Poisoning by, adverse effect of and underdosing of other hormone antagonists**

√7ᵗʰ **T38.991 Poisoning by other hormone antagonists, accidental (unintentional)**

Poisoning by other hormone antagonists NOS

√7ᵗʰ **T38.992 Poisoning by other hormone antagonists, intentional self-harm**

√7ᵗʰ **T38.993 Poisoning by other hormone antagonists, assault**

☑ Appropriate additional character required   √x7ᵗʰ Requires 7th character, placeholder x must fill empty characters

✓7ᵗʰ **T38.994** Poisoning by other hormone antagonists, undetermined

✓7ᵗʰ **T38.995** Adverse effect of other hormone antagonists

✓7ᵗʰ **T38.996** Underdosing of other hormone antagonists

✓4ᵗʰ **T39** Poisoning by, adverse effect of and underdosing of nonopioid analgesics, antipyretics and antirheumatics

> The appropriate 7th character is to be added to each code from category T39.
> A   initial encounter
> D   subsequent encounter
> S   sequela

✓5ᵗʰ **T39.0** Poisoning by, adverse effect of and underdosing of salicylates

  ✓6ᵗʰ **T39.01** Poisoning by, adverse effect of and underdosing of aspirin
     Poisoning by, adverse effect of and underdosing of acetylsalicylic acid

    ✓7ᵗʰ **T39.011** Poisoning by aspirin, accidental (unintentional)

    ✓7ᵗʰ **T39.012** Poisoning by aspirin, intentional self-harm

    ✓7ᵗʰ **T39.013** Poisoning by aspirin, assault

    ✓7ᵗʰ **T39.014** Poisoning by aspirin, undetermined

    ✓7ᵗʰ **T39.015** Adverse effect of aspirin

    ✓7ᵗʰ **T39.016** Underdosing of aspirin

  ✓6ᵗʰ **T39.09** Poisoning by, adverse effect of and underdosing of other salicylates

    ✓7ᵗʰ **T39.091** Poisoning by salicylates, accidental (unintentional)
       Poisoning by salicylates NOS

    ✓7ᵗʰ **T39.092** Poisoning by salicylates, intentional self-harm

    ✓7ᵗʰ **T39.093** Poisoning by salicylates, assault

    ✓7ᵗʰ **T39.094** Poisoning by salicylates, undetermined

    ✓7ᵗʰ **T39.095** Adverse effect of salicylates

    ✓7ᵗʰ **T39.096** Underdosing of salicylates

✓5ᵗʰ **T39.1** Poisoning by, adverse effect of and underdosing of 4-Aminophenol derivatives

  ✓6ᵗʰ **T39.1x** Poisoning by, adverse effect of and underdosing of 4-Aminophenol derivatives

    ✓7ᵗʰ **T39.1x1** Poisoning by 4-Aminophenol derivatives, accidental (unintentional)
       Poisoning by 4-Aminophenol derivatives NOS

    ✓7ᵗʰ **T39.1x2** Poisoning by 4-Aminophenol derivatives, intentional self-harm

    ✓7ᵗʰ **T39.1x3** Poisoning by 4-Aminophenol derivatives, assault

    ✓7ᵗʰ **T39.1x4** Poisoning by 4-Aminophenol derivatives, undetermined

    ✓7ᵗʰ **T39.1x5** Adverse effect of 4-Aminophenol derivatives

    ✓7ᵗʰ **T39.1x6** Underdosing of 4-Aminophenol derivatives

✓5ᵗʰ **T39.2** Poisoning by, adverse effect of and underdosing of pyrazolone derivatives

  ✓6ᵗʰ **T39.2x** Poisoning by, adverse effect of and underdosing of pyrazolone derivatives

    ✓7ᵗʰ **T39.2x1** Poisoning by pyrazolone derivatives, accidental (unintentional)
       Poisoning by pyrazolone derivatives NOS

    ✓7ᵗʰ **T39.2x2** Poisoning by pyrazolone derivatives, intentional self-harm

    ✓7ᵗʰ **T39.2x3** Poisoning by pyrazolone derivatives, assault

    ✓7ᵗʰ **T39.2x4** Poisoning by pyrazolone derivatives, undetermined

    ✓7ᵗʰ **T39.2x5** Adverse effect of pyrazolone derivatives

    ✓7ᵗʰ **T39.2x6** Underdosing of pyrazolone derivatives

✓5ᵗʰ **T39.3** Poisoning by, adverse effect of and underdosing of other nonsteroidal anti-inflammatory drugs [NSAID]

  ✓6ᵗʰ **T39.31** Poisoning by, adverse effect of and underdosing of propionic acid derivatives
     Poisoning by, adverse effect of and underdosing of fenoprofen
     Poisoning by, adverse effect of and underdosing of flurbiprofen
     Poisoning by, adverse effect of and underdosing of ibuprofen
     Poisoning by, adverse effect of and underdosing of ketoprofen
     Poisoning by, adverse effect of and underdosing of naproxen
     Poisoning by, adverse effect of and underdosing of oxaprozin

    ✓7ᵗʰ **T39.311** Poisoning by propionic acid derivatives, accidental (unintentional)

    ✓7ᵗʰ **T39.312** Poisoning by propionic acid derivatives, intentional self-harm

    ✓7ᵗʰ **T39.313** Poisoning by propionic acid derivatives, assault

    ✓7ᵗʰ **T39.314** Poisoning by propionic acid derivatives, undetermined

    ✓7ᵗʰ **T39.315** Adverse effect of propionic acid derivatives

    ✓7ᵗʰ **T39.316** Underdosing of propionic acid derivatives

  ✓6ᵗʰ **T39.39** Poisoning by, adverse effect of and underdosing of other nonsteroidal anti-inflammatory drugs [NSAID]

    ✓7ᵗʰ **T39.391** Poisoning by other nonsteroidal anti-inflammatory drugs [NSAID], accidental (unintentional)
       Poisoning by other nonsteroidal anti-inflammatory drugs NOS

    ✓7ᵗʰ **T39.392** Poisoning by other nonsteroidal anti-inflammatory drugs [NSAID], intentional self-harm

    ✓7ᵗʰ **T39.393** Poisoning by other nonsteroidal anti-inflammatory drugs [NSAID], assault

    ✓7ᵗʰ **T39.394** Poisoning by other nonsteroidal anti-inflammatory drugs [NSAID], undetermined

    ✓7ᵗʰ **T39.395** Adverse effect of other nonsteroidal anti-inflammatory drugs [NSAID]

    ✓7ᵗʰ **T39.396** Underdosing of other nonsteroidal anti-inflammatory drugs [NSAID]

✓5ᵗʰ **T39.4** Poisoning by, adverse effect of and underdosing of antirheumatics, not elsewhere classified

    EXCLUDES 1   *poisoning by, adverse effect of and underdosing of glucocorticoids (T38.0-)*
          poisoning by, adverse effect of and underdosing of salicylates (T39.0-)

  ✓6ᵗʰ **T39.4x** Poisoning by, adverse effect of and underdosing of antirheumatics, not elsewhere classified

    ✓7ᵗʰ **T39.4x1** Poisoning by antirheumatics, not elsewhere classified, accidental (unintentional)
       Poisoning by antirheumatics, not elsewhere classified NOS

    ✓7ᵗʰ **T39.4x2** Poisoning by antirheumatics, not elsewhere classified, intentional self-harm

    ✓7ᵗʰ **T39.4x3** Poisoning by antirheumatics, not elsewhere classified, assault

    ✓7ᵗʰ **T39.4x4** Poisoning by antirheumatics, not elsewhere classified, undetermined

    ✓7ᵗʰ **T39.4x5** Adverse effect of antirheumatics, not elsewhere classified

    ✓7ᵗʰ **T39.4x6** Underdosing of antirheumatics, not elsewhere classified

---

EXCLUDES 1 Not coded here   **EXCLUDES 2** Not included here   *Manifestation Code*

✓5th **T39.8** **Poisoning by, adverse effect of and underdosing of other nonopioid analgesics and antipyretics, not elsewhere classified**

✓6th **T39.8x** **Poisoning by, adverse effect of and underdosing of other nonopioid analgesics and antipyretics, not elsewhere classified**

✓7th **T39.8x1** **Poisoning by other nonopioid analgesics and antipyretics, not elsewhere classified, accidental (unintentional)**
Poisoning by other nonopioid analgesics and antipyretics, not elsewhere classified NOS

✓7th **T39.8x2** **Poisoning by other nonopioid analgesics and antipyretics, not elsewhere classified, intentional self-harm**

✓7th **T39.8x3** **Poisoning by other nonopioid analgesics and antipyretics, not elsewhere classified, assault**

✓7th **T39.8x4** **Poisoning by other nonopioid analgesics and antipyretics, not elsewhere classified, undetermined**

✓7th **T39.8x5** **Adverse effect of other nonopioid analgesics and antipyretics, not elsewhere classified**

✓7th **T39.8x6** **Underdosing of other nonopioid analgesics and antipyretics, not elsewhere classified**

✓5th **T39.9** **Poisoning by, adverse effect of and underdosing of unspecified nonopioid analgesic, antipyretic and antirheumatic**

✓x7th **T39.91** **Poisoning by unspecified nonopioid analgesic, antipyretic and antirheumatic, accidental (unintentional)**
Poisoning by nonopioid analgesic, antipyretic and antirheumatic NOS

✓x7th **T39.92** **Poisoning by unspecified nonopioid analgesic, antipyretic and antirheumatic, intentional self-harm**

✓x7th **T39.93** **Poisoning by unspecified nonopioid analgesic, antipyretic and antirheumatic, assault**

✓x7th **T39.94** **Poisoning by unspecified nonopioid analgesic, antipyretic and antirheumatic, undetermined**

✓x7th **T39.95** **Adverse effect of unspecified nonopioid analgesic, antipyretic and antirheumatic**

✓x7th **T39.96** **Underdosing of unspecified nonopioid analgesic, antipyretic and antirheumatic**

✓4th **T40** **Poisoning by, adverse effect of and underdosing of narcotics and psychodysleptics [hallucinogens]**

EXCLUDES 2 *drug dependence and related mental and behavioral disorders due to psychoactive substance use (F10-F19-)*

The appropriate 7th character is to be added to each code from category T40.
A initial encounter
D subsequent encounter
S sequela

✓5th **T40.0** **Poisoning by, adverse effect of and underdosing of opium**

✓6th **T40.0x** **Poisoning by, adverse effect of and underdosing of opium**

✓7th **T40.0x1** **Poisoning by opium, accidental (unintentional)**
Poisoning by opium NOS

✓7th **T40.0x2** **Poisoning by opium, intentional self-harm**

✓7th **T40.0x3** **Poisoning by opium, assault**

✓7th **T40.0x4** **Poisoning by opium, undetermined**

✓7th **T40.0x5** **Adverse effect of opium**

✓7th **T40.0x6** **Underdosing of opium**

✓5th **T40.1** **Poisoning by, adverse effect of and underdosing of heroin**

✓6th **T40.1x** **Poisoning by and adverse effect of heroin**

✓7th **T40.1x1** **Poisoning by heroin, accidental (unintentional)**
Poisoning by heroin NOS

✓7th **T40.1x2** **Poisoning by heroin, intentional self-harm**

✓7th **T40.1x3** **Poisoning by heroin, assault**

✓7th **T40.1x4** **Poisoning by heroin, undetermined**

✓7th **T40.1x5** **Adverse effect of heroin**

✓7th **T40.1x6** **Underdosing of heroin**

✓5th **T40.2** **Poisoning by, adverse effect of and underdosing of other opioids**

✓6th **T40.2x** **Poisoning by, adverse effect of and underdosing of other opioids**

✓7th **T40.2x1** **Poisoning by other opioids, accidental (unintentional)**
Poisoning by other opioids NOS

✓7th **T40.2x2** **Poisoning by other opioids, intentional self-harm**

✓7th **T40.2x3** **Poisoning by other opioids, assault**

✓7th **T40.2x4** **Poisoning by other opioids, undetermined**

✓7th **T40.2x5** **Adverse effect of other opioids**

✓7th **T40.2x6** **Underdosing of other opioids**

✓5th **T40.3** **Poisoning by, adverse effect of and underdosing of methadone**

✓6th **T40.3x** **Poisoning by, adverse effect of and underdosing of methadone**

✓7th **T40.3x1** **Poisoning by methadone, accidental (unintentional)**
Poisoning by methadone NOS

✓7th **T40.3x2** **Poisoning by methadone, intentional self-harm**

✓7th **T40.3x3** **Poisoning by methadone, assault**

✓7th **T40.3x4** **Poisoning by methadone, undetermined**

✓7th **T40.3x5** **Adverse effect of methadone**

✓7th **T40.3x6** **Underdosing of methadone**

✓5th **T40.4** **Poisoning by, adverse effect of and underdosing of other synthetic narcotics**

✓6th **T40.4x** **Poisoning by, adverse effect of and underdosing of other synthetic narcotics**

✓7th **T40.4x1** **Poisoning by other synthetic narcotics, accidental (unintentional)**
Poisoning by other synthetic narcotics NOS

✓7th **T40.4x2** **Poisoning by other synthetic narcotics, intentional self-harm**

✓7th **T40.4x3** **Poisoning by other synthetic narcotics, assault**

✓7th **T40.4x4** **Poisoning by other synthetic narcotics, undetermined**

✓7th **T40.4x5** **Adverse effect of other synthetic narcotics**

✓7th **T40.4x6** **Underdosing of other synthetic narcotics**

✓5th **T40.5** **Poisoning by, adverse effect of and underdosing of cocaine**

✓6th **T40.5x** **Poisoning by, adverse effect of and underdosing of cocaine**

✓7th **T40.5x1** **Poisoning by cocaine, accidental (unintentional)**
Poisoning by cocaine NOS

✓7th **T40.5x2** **Poisoning by cocaine, intentional self-harm**

✓7th **T40.5x3** **Poisoning by cocaine, assault**

✓7th **T40.5x4** **Poisoning by cocaine, undetermined**

✓7th **T40.5x5** **Adverse effect of cocaine**

✓7th **T40.5x6** **Underdosing of cocaine**

✓5th **T40.6** **Poisoning by, adverse effect of and underdosing of other and unspecified narcotics**

✓6th **T40.60** **Poisoning by, adverse effect of and underdosing of unspecified narcotics**

✓7th **T40.601** **Poisoning by unspecified narcotics, accidental (unintentional)**
Poisoning by narcotics NOS

✓7th **T40.602** **Poisoning by unspecified narcotics, intentional self-harm**

✓7th **T40.603** **Poisoning by unspecified narcotics, assault**

✓7th **T40.604** **Poisoning by unspecified narcotics, undetermined**

✓7th **T40.605** **Adverse effect of unspecified narcotics**

✓7th **T40.606** **Underdosing of unspecified narcotics**

√6th **T40.69** **Poisoning by, adverse effect of and underdosing of other narcotics**

     √7th **T40.691** **Poisoning by other narcotics, accidental (unintentional)**
         Poisoning by other narcotics NOS

     √7th **T40.692** **Poisoning by other narcotics, intentional self-harm**

     √7th **T40.693** **Poisoning by other narcotics, assault**

     √7th **T40.694** **Poisoning by other narcotics, undetermined**

     √7th **T40.695** **Adverse effect of other narcotics**

     √7th **T40.696** **Underdosing of other narcotics**

√5th **T40.7** **Poisoning by, adverse effect of and underdosing of cannabis (derivatives)**

     √6th **T40.7x** **Poisoning by, adverse effect of and underdosing of cannabis (derivatives)**

         √7th **T40.7x1** **Poisoning by cannabis (derivatives), accidental (unintentional)**
             Poisoning by cannabis NOS

         √7th **T40.7x2** **Poisoning by cannabis (derivatives), intentional self-harm**

         √7th **T40.7x3** **Poisoning by cannabis (derivatives), assault**

         √7th **T40.7x4** **Poisoning by cannabis (derivatives), undetermined**

         √7th **T40.7x5** **Adverse effect of cannabis (derivatives)**

         √7th **T40.7x6** **Underdosing of cannabis (derivatives)**

√5th **T40.8** **Poisoning by, adverse effect of and underdosing of lysergide [LSD]**

     √6th **T40.8x** **Poisoning by and adverse effect of lysergide [LSD]**

         √7th **T40.8x1** **Poisoning by lysergide [LSD], accidental (unintentional)**
             Poisoning by lysergide [LSD]NOS

         √7th **T40.8x2** **Poisoning by lysergide [LSD], intentional self-harm**

         √7th **T40.8x3** **Poisoning by lysergide [LSD], assault**

         √7th **T40.8x4** **Poisoning by lysergide [LSD], undetermined**

         √7th **T40.8x5** **Adverse effect of lysergide [LSD]**

         √7th **T40.8x6** **Underdosing of lysergide [LSD]**

√5th **T40.9** **Poisoning by, adverse effect of and underdosing of other and unspecified psychodysleptics [hallucinogens]**

     √6th **T40.90** **Poisoning by, adverse effect of and underdosing of unspecified psychodysleptics [hallucinogens]**

         √7th **T40.901** **Poisoning by unspecified psychodysleptics [hallucinogens], accidental (unintentional)**

         √7th **T40.902** **Poisoning by unspecified psychodysleptics [hallucinogens], intentional self-harm**

         √7th **T40.903** **Poisoning by unspecified psychodysleptics [hallucinogens], assault**

         √7th **T40.904** **Poisoning by unspecified psychodysleptics [hallucinogens], undetermined**

         √7th **T40.905** **Adverse effect of unspecified psychodysleptics [hallucinogens]**

         √7th **T40.906** **Underdosing of unspecified psychodysleptics**

     √6th **T40.99** **Poisoning by, adverse effect of and underdosing of other psychodysleptics [hallucinogens]**

         √7th **T40.991** **Poisoning by other psychodysleptics [hallucinogens], accidental (unintentional)**
             Poisoning by other psychodysleptics [hallucinogens] NOS

         √7th **T40.992** **Poisoning by other psychodysleptics [hallucinogens], intentional self-harm**

         √7th **T40.993** **Poisoning by other psychodysleptics [hallucinogens], assault**

         √7th **T40.994** **Poisoning by other psychodysleptics [hallucinogens], undetermined**

         √7th **T40.995** **Adverse effect of other psychodysleptics [hallucinogens]**

         √7th **T40.996** **Underdosing of other psychodysleptics**

√4th **T41** **Poisoning by, adverse effect of and underdosing of anesthetics and therapeutic gases**

     EXCLUDES 1   *benzodiazepines (T42.4-)*
                 cocaine (T40.5-)
                 complications of anesthesia during pregnancy (O29-)
                 complications of anesthesia during labor and delivery (O74-)
                 complications of anesthesia during the puerperium (O89-)
                 opioids (T40.0-T40.2-)

> The appropriate 7th character is to be added to each code from category T41.
> A   initial encounter
> D   subsequent encounter
> S   sequela

√5th **T41.0** **Poisoning by, adverse effect of and underdosing of inhaled anesthetics**

     EXCLUDES 1   *oxygen (T41.5-)*

     √6th **T41.0x** **Poisoning by, adverse effect of and underdosing of inhaled anesthetics**

         √7th **T41.0x1** **Poisoning by inhaled anesthetics, accidental (unintentional)**
             Poisoning by inhaled anesthetics NOS

         √7th **T41.0x2** **Poisoning by inhaled anesthetics, intentional self-harm**

         √7th **T41.0x3** **Poisoning by inhaled anesthetics, assault**

         √7th **T41.0x4** **Poisoning by inhaled anesthetics, undetermined**

         √7th **T41.0x5** **Adverse effect of inhaled anesthetics**

         √7th **T41.0x6** **Underdosing of inhaled anesthetics**

√5th **T41.1** **Poisoning by, adverse effect of and underdosing of intravenous anesthetics**
       Poisoning by, adverse effect of and underdosing of thiobarbiturates

     √6th **T41.1x** **Poisoning by, adverse effect of and underdosing of intravenous anesthetics**

         √7th **T41.1x1** **Poisoning by intravenous anesthetics, accidental (unintentional)**
             Poisoning by intravenous anesthetics NOS

         √7th **T41.1x2** **Poisoning by intravenous anesthetics, intentional self-harm**

         √7th **T41.1x3** **Poisoning by intravenous anesthetics, assault**

         √7th **T41.1x4** **Poisoning by intravenous anesthetics, undetermined**

         √7th **T41.1x5** **Adverse effect of intravenous anesthetics**

         √7th **T41.1x6** **Underdosing of intravenous anesthetics**

√5th **T41.2** **Poisoning by, adverse effect of and underdosing of other and unspecified general anesthetics**

     √6th **T41.20** **Poisoning by, adverse effect of and underdosing of unspecified general anesthetics**

         √7th **T41.201** **Poisoning by unspecified general anesthetics, accidental (unintentional)**
             Poisoning by general anesthetics NOS

         √7th **T41.202** **Poisoning by unspecified general anesthetics, intentional self-harm**

         √7th **T41.203** **Poisoning by unspecified general anesthetics, assault**

         √7th **T41.204** **Poisoning by unspecified general anesthetics, undetermined**

         √7th **T41.205** **Adverse effect of unspecified general anesthetics**

         √7th **T41.206** **Underdosing of unspecified general anesthetics**

     √6th **T41.29** **Poisoning by, adverse effect of and underdosing of other general anesthetics**

         √7th **T41.291** **Poisoning by other general anesthetics, accidental (unintentional)**
             Poisoning by other general anesthetics NOS

         √7th **T41.292** **Poisoning by other general anesthetics, intentional self-harm**

         √7th **T41.293** **Poisoning by other general anesthetics, assault**

         √7th **T41.294** **Poisoning by other general anesthetics, undetermined**

EXCLUDES 1   Not coded here   EXCLUDES 2   Not included here   *Manifestation Code*

✓7th **T41.295 Adverse effect of other general anesthetics**

✓7th **T41.296 Underdosing of other general anesthetics**

✓5th **T41.3 Poisoning by, adverse effect of and underdosing of local anesthetics**

✓6th **T41.3x Poisoning by, adverse effect of and underdosing of local anesthetics**

✓7th **T41.3x1 Poisoning by local anesthetics, accidental (unintentional)**
Poisoning by local anesthetics NOS

✓7th **T41.3x2 Poisoning by local anesthetics, intentional self-harm**

✓7th **T41.3x3 Poisoning by local anesthetics, assault**

✓7th **T41.3x4 Poisoning by local anesthetics, undetermined**

✓7th **T41.3x5 Adverse effect of local anesthetics**

✓7th **T41.3x6 Underdosing of local anesthetics**

✓5th **T41.4 Poisoning by, adverse effect of and underdosing of unspecified anesthetic**

✓x7th **T41.41 Poisoning by unspecified anesthetic, accidental (unintentional)**
Poisoning by anesthetic NOS

✓x7th **T41.42 Poisoning by unspecified anesthetic, intentional self-harm**

✓x7th **T41.43 Poisoning by unspecified anesthetic, assault**

✓x7th **T41.44 Poisoning by unspecified anesthetic, undetermined**

✓x7th **T41.45 Adverse effect of unspecified anesthetic**

✓x7th **T41.46 Underdosing of unspecified anesthetics**

✓5th **T41.5 Poisoning by, adverse effect of and underdosing of therapeutic gases**

✓6th **T41.5x Poisoning by, adverse effect of and underdosing of therapeutic gases**

✓7th **T41.5x1 Poisoning by therapeutic gases, accidental (unintentional)**
Poisoning by therapeutic gases NOS

✓7th **T41.5x2 Poisoning by therapeutic gases, intentional self-harm**

✓7th **T41.5x3 Poisoning by therapeutic gases, assault**

✓7th **T41.5x4 Poisoning by therapeutic gases, undetermined**

✓7th **T41.5x5 Adverse effect of therapeutic gases**

✓7th **T41.5x6 Underdosing of therapeutic gases**

✓4th **T42 Poisoning by, adverse effect of and underdosing of antiepileptic, sedative- hypnotic and antiparkinsonism drugs**

EXCLUDES 2 *drug dependence and related mental and behavioral disorders due to psychoactive substance use (F10--F19-)*

The appropriate 7th character is to be added to each code from category T42.
A   initial encounter
D   subsequent encounter
S   sequela

✓5th **T42.0 Poisoning by, adverse effect of and underdosing of hydantoin derivatives**

✓6th **T42.0x Poisoning by, adverse effect of and underdosing of hydantoin derivatives**

✓7th **T42.0x1 Poisoning by hydantoin derivatives, accidental (unintentional)**
Poisoning by hydantoin derivatives NOS

✓7th **T42.0x2 Poisoning by hydantoin derivatives, intentional self-harm**

✓7th **T42.0x3 Poisoning by hydantoin derivatives, assault**

✓7th **T42.0x4 Poisoning by hydantoin derivatives, undetermined**

✓7th **T42.0x5 Adverse effect of hydantoin derivatives**

✓7th **T42.0x6 Underdosing of hydantoin derivatives**

✓5th **T42.1 Poisoning by, adverse effect of and underdosing of iminostilbenes**
Poisoning by, adverse effect of and underdosing of carbamazepine

✓6th **T42.1x Poisoning by, adverse effect of and underdosing of iminostilbenes**

✓7th **T42.1x1 Poisoning by iminostilbenes, accidental (unintentional)**
Poisoning by iminostilbenes NOS

✓7th **T42.1x2 Poisoning by iminostilbenes, intentional self-harm**

✓7th **T42.1x3 Poisoning by iminostilbenes, assault**

✓7th **T42.1x4 Poisoning by iminostilbenes, undetermined**

✓7th **T42.1x5 Adverse effect of iminostilbenes**

✓7th **T42.1x6 Underdosing of iminostilbenes**

✓5th **T42.2 Poisoning by, adverse effect of and underdosing of succinimides and oxazolidinediones**

✓6th **T42.2x Poisoning by, adverse effect of and underdosing of succinimides and oxazolidinediones**

✓7th **T42.2x1 Poisoning by succinimides and oxazolidinediones, accidental (unintentional)**
Poisoning by succinimides and oxazolidinediones NOS

✓7th **T42.2x2 Poisoning by succinimides and oxazolidinediones, intentional self-harm**

✓7th **T42.2x3 Poisoning by succinimides and oxazolidinediones, assault**

✓7th **T42.2x4 Poisoning by succinimides and oxazolidinediones, undetermined**

✓7th **T42.2x5 Adverse effect of succinimides and oxazolidinediones**

✓7th **T42.2x6 Underdosing of succinimides and oxazolidinediones**

✓5th **T42.3 Poisoning by, adverse effect of and underdosing of barbiturates**

EXCLUDES 1 *poisoning by, adverse effect of and underdosing of thiobarbiturates (T41.1-)*

✓6th **T42.3x Poisoning by, adverse effect of and underdosing of barbiturates**

✓7th **T42.3x1 Poisoning by barbiturates, accidental (unintentional)**
Poisoning by barbiturates NOS

✓7th **T42.3x2 Poisoning by barbiturates, intentional self-harm**

✓7th **T42.3x3 Poisoning by barbiturates, assault**

✓7th **T42.3x4 Poisoning by barbiturates, undetermined**

✓7th **T42.3x5 Adverse effect of barbiturates**

✓7th **T42.3x6 Underdosing of barbiturates**

✓5th **T42.4 Poisoning by, adverse effect of and underdosing of benzodiazepines**

✓6th **T42.4x Poisoning by, adverse effect of and underdosing of benzodiazepines**

✓7th **T42.4x1 Poisoning by benzodiazepines, accidental (unintentional)**
Poisoning by benzodiazepines NOS

✓7th **T42.4x2 Poisoning by benzodiazepines, intentional self-harm**

✓7th **T42.4x3 Poisoning by benzodiazepines, assault**

✓7th **T42.4x4 Poisoning by benzodiazepines, undetermined**

✓7th **T42.4x5 Adverse effect of benzodiazepines**

✓7th **T42.4x6 Underdosing of benzodiazepines**

✓5th **T42.5 Poisoning by, adverse effect of and underdosing of mixed antiepileptics**

✓6th **T42.5x Poisoning by, adverse effect of and underdosing of antiepileptics**

✓7th **T42.5x1 Poisoning by mixed antiepileptics, accidental (unintentional)**
Poisoning by mixed antiepileptics NOS

✓7th **T42.5x2 Poisoning by mixed antiepileptics, intentional self-harm**

✓7th **T42.5x3 Poisoning by mixed antiepileptics, assault**

✓7th **T42.5x4 Poisoning by mixed antiepileptics, undetermined**

✓7th **T42.5x5 Adverse effect of mixed antiepileptics**

✓7th **T42.5x6 Underdosing of mixed antiepileptics**

✓5ᵗʰ **T42.6 Poisoning by, adverse effect of and underdosing of other antiepileptic and sedative-hypnotic drugs**

Poisoning by, adverse effect of and underdosing of methaqualone

Poisoning by, adverse effect of and underdosing of valproic acid

EXCLUDES 1 *poisoning by, adverse effect of and underdosing of carbamazepine (T42.1-)*

✓6ᵗʰ **T42.6x Poisoning by, adverse effect of and underdosing of other antiepileptic and sedative-hypnotic drugs**

✓7ᵗʰ **T42.6x1 Poisoning by other antiepileptic and sedative-hypnotic drugs, accidental (unintentional)**

Poisoning by other antiepileptic and sedative-hypnotic drugs NOS

✓7ᵗʰ **T42.6x2 Poisoning by other antiepileptic and sedative-hypnotic drugs, intentional self-harm**

✓7ᵗʰ **T42.6x3 Poisoning by other antiepileptic and sedative-hypnotic drugs, assault**

✓7ᵗʰ **T42.6x4 Poisoning by other antiepileptic and sedative-hypnotic drugs, undetermined**

✓7ᵗʰ **T42.6x5 Adverse effect of other antiepileptic and sedative-hypnotic drugs**

✓7ᵗʰ **T42.6x6 Underdosing of other antiepileptic and sedative-hypnotic drugs**

✓5ᵗʰ **T42.7 Poisoning by, adverse effect of and underdosing of unspecified antiepileptic and sedative-hypnotic drugs**

✓x7ᵗʰ **T42.71 Poisoning by unspecified antiepileptic and sedative-hypnotic drugs, accidental (unintentional)**

Poisoning by antiepileptic and sedative-hypnotic drugs NOS

✓x7ᵗʰ **T42.72 Poisoning by unspecified antiepileptic and sedative-hypnotic drugs, intentional self-harm**

✓x7ᵗʰ **T42.73 Poisoning by unspecified antiepileptic and sedative-hypnotic drugs, assault**

✓x7ᵗʰ **T42.74 Poisoning by unspecified antiepileptic and sedative-hypnotic drugs, undetermined**

✓x7ᵗʰ **T42.75 Adverse effect of unspecified antiepileptic and sedative-hypnotic drugs**

✓x7ᵗʰ **T42.76 Underdosing of unspecified antiepileptic and sedative-hypnotic drugs**

✓5ᵗʰ **T42.8 Poisoning by, adverse effect of and underdosing of antiparkinsonism drugs and other central muscle-tone depressants**

Poisoning by, adverse effect of and underdosing of amantadine

✓6ᵗʰ **T42.8x Poisoning by, adverse effect of and underdosing of antiparkinsonism drugs and other central muscle-tone depressants**

✓7ᵗʰ **T42.8x1 Poisoning by antiparkinsonism drugs and other central muscle-tone depressants, accidental (unintentional)**

Poisoning by antiparkinsonism drugs and other central muscle-tone depressants NOS

✓7ᵗʰ **T42.8x2 Poisoning by antiparkinsonism drugs and other central muscle-tone depressants, intentional self-harm**

✓7ᵗʰ **T42.8x3 Poisoning by antiparkinsonism drugs and other central muscle-tone depressants, assault**

✓7ᵗʰ **T42.8x4 Poisoning by antiparkinsonism drugs and other central muscle-tone depressants, undetermined**

✓7ᵗʰ **T42.8x5 Adverse effect of antiparkinsonism drugs and other central muscle-tone depressants**

✓7ᵗʰ **T42.8x6 Underdosing of antiparkinsonism drugs and other central muscle-tone depressants**

✓4ᵗʰ **T43 Poisoning by, adverse effect of and underdosing of psychotropic drugs, not elsewhere classified**

EXCLUDES 1 *appetite depressants (T50.5-)*
barbiturates (T42.3-)
benzodiazepines (T42.4-)
methaqualone (T42.6-)
psychodysleptics [hallucinogens] (T40.7-T40.9-)

EXCLUDES 2 *drug dependence and related mental and behavioral disorders due to psychoactive substance use (F10--F19-)*

The appropriate 7th character is to be added to each code from category T43.
A   initial encounter
D   subsequent encounter
S   sequela

✓5ᵗʰ **T43.0 Poisoning by, adverse effect of and underdosing of tricyclic and tetracyclic antidepressants**

✓6ᵗʰ **T43.01 Poisoning by, adverse effect of and underdosing of tricyclic antidepressants**

✓7ᵗʰ **T43.011 Poisoning by tricyclic antidepressants, accidental (unintentional)**

Poisoning by tricyclic antidepressants NOS

✓7ᵗʰ **T43.012 Poisoning by tricyclic antidepressants, intentional self-harm**

✓7ᵗʰ **T43.013 Poisoning by tricyclic antidepressants, assault**

✓7ᵗʰ **T43.014 Poisoning by tricyclic antidepressants, undetermined**

✓7ᵗʰ **T43.015 Adverse effect of tricyclic antidepressants**

✓7ᵗʰ **T43.016 Underdosing of tricyclic antidepressants**

✓6ᵗʰ **T43.02 Poisoning by, adverse effect of and underdosing of tetracyclic antidepressants**

✓7ᵗʰ **T43.021 Poisoning by tetracyclic antidepressants, accidental (unintentional)**

Poisoning by tetracyclic antidepressants NOS

✓7ᵗʰ **T43.022 Poisoning by tetracyclic antidepressants, intentional self-harm**

✓7ᵗʰ **T43.023 Poisoning by tetracyclic antidepressants, assault**

✓7ᵗʰ **T43.024 Poisoning by tetracyclic antidepressants, undetermined**

✓7ᵗʰ **T43.025 Adverse effect of tetracyclic antidepressants**

✓7ᵗʰ **T43.026 Underdosing of tetracyclic antidepressants**

✓5ᵗʰ **T43.1 Poisoning by, adverse effect of and underdosing of monoamine-oxidase-inhibitor antidepressants**

✓6ᵗʰ **T43.1x Poisoning by, adverse effect of and underdosing of monoamine-oxidase-inhibitor antidepressants**

✓7ᵗʰ **T43.1x1 Poisoning by monoamine-oxidase-inhibitor antidepressants, accidental (unintentional)**

Poisoning by monoamine-oxidase-inhibitor antidepressants NOS

✓7ᵗʰ **T43.1x2 Poisoning by monoamine-oxidase-inhibitor antidepressants, intentional self-harm**

✓7ᵗʰ **T43.1x3 Poisoning by monoamine-oxidase-inhibitor antidepressants, assault**

✓7ᵗʰ **T43.1x4 Poisoning by monoamine-oxidase-inhibitor antidepressants, undetermined**

✓7ᵗʰ **T43.1x5 Adverse effect of monoamine-oxidase-inhibitor antidepressants**

✓7ᵗʰ **T43.1x6 Underdosing of monoamine-oxidase-inhibitor antidepressants**

✓5ᵗʰ **T43.2 Poisoning by, adverse effect of and underdosing of other and unspecified antidepressants**

✓6ᵗʰ **T43.20 Poisoning by, adverse effect of and underdosing of unspecified antidepressants**

✓7ᵗʰ **T43.201 Poisoning by unspecified antidepressants, accidental (unintentional)**

Poisoning by antidepressants NOS

EXCLUDES 1 Not coded here   EXCLUDES 2 Not included here   *Manifestation Code*

✓7ᵗʰ **T43.202** **Poisoning by unspecified antidepressants, intentional self-harm**

✓7ᵗʰ **T43.203** **Poisoning by unspecified antidepressants, assault**

✓7ᵗʰ **T43.204** **Poisoning by unspecified antidepressants, undetermined**

✓7ᵗʰ **T43.205** **Adverse effect of unspecified antidepressants**

✓7ᵗʰ **T43.206** **Underdosing of unspecified antidepressants**

✓6ᵗʰ **T43.21** **Poisoning by, adverse effect of and underdosing of selective serotonin and norepinephrine reuptake inhibitors**

Poisoning by, adverse effect of and underdosing of SSNRI antidepressants

✓7ᵗʰ **T43.211** **Poisoning by selective serotonin and norepinephrine reuptake inhibitors, accidental (unintentional)**

✓7ᵗʰ **T43.212** **Poisoning by selective serotonin and norepinephrine reuptake inhibitors, intentional self-harm**

✓7ᵗʰ **T43.213** **Poisoning by selective serotonin and norepinephrine reuptake inhibitors, assault**

✓7ᵗʰ **T43.214** **Poisoning by selective serotonin and norepinephrine reuptake inhibitors, undetermined**

✓7ᵗʰ **T43.215** **Adverse effect of selective serotonin and norepinephrine reuptake inhibitors**

✓7ᵗʰ **T43.216** **Underdosing of selective serotonin and norepinephrine reuptake inhibitors**

✓6ᵗʰ **T43.22** **Poisoning by, adverse effect of and underdosing of selective serotonin reuptake inhibitors**

Poisoning by, adverse effect of and underdosing of SSRI antidepressants

✓7ᵗʰ **T43.221** **Poisoning by selective serotonin reuptake inhibitors, accidental (unintentional)**

✓7ᵗʰ **T43.222** **Poisoning by selective serotonin reuptake inhibitors, intentional self-harm**

✓7ᵗʰ **T43.223** **Poisoning by selective serotonin reuptake inhibitors, assault**

✓7ᵗʰ **T43.224** **Poisoning by selective serotonin reuptake inhibitors, undetermined**

✓7ᵗʰ **T43.225** **Adverse effect of selective serotonin reuptake inhibitors**

✓7ᵗʰ **T43.226** **Underdosing of selective serotonin reuptake inhibitors**

✓6ᵗʰ **T43.29** **Poisoning by, adverse effect of and underdosing of other antidepressants**

✓7ᵗʰ **T43.291** **Poisoning by other antidepressants, accidental (unintentional)**

Poisoning by other antidepressants NOS

✓7ᵗʰ **T43.292** **Poisoning by other antidepressants, intentional self-harm**

✓7ᵗʰ **T43.293** **Poisoning by other antidepressants, assault**

✓7ᵗʰ **T43.294** **Poisoning by other antidepressants, undetermined**

✓7ᵗʰ **T43.295** **Adverse effect of other antidepressants**

✓7ᵗʰ **T43.296** **Underdosing of other antidepressants**

✓5ᵗʰ **T43.3** **Poisoning by, adverse effect of and underdosing of phenothiazine antipsychotics and neuroleptics**

✓6ᵗʰ **T43.3x** **Poisoning by, adverse effect of and underdosing of phenothiazine antipsychotics and neuroleptics**

✓7ᵗʰ **T43.3x1** **Poisoning by phenothiazine antipsychotics and neuroleptics, accidental (unintentional)**

Poisoning by phenothiazine antipsychotics and neuroleptics NOS

✓7ᵗʰ **T43.3x2** **Poisoning by phenothiazine antipsychotics and neuroleptics, intentional self-harm**

✓7ᵗʰ **T43.3x3** **Poisoning by phenothiazine antipsychotics and neuroleptics, assault**

✓7ᵗʰ **T43.3x4** **Poisoning by phenothiazine antipsychotics and neuroleptics, undetermined**

✓7ᵗʰ **T43.3x5** **Adverse effect of phenothiazine antipsychotics and neuroleptics**

✓7ᵗʰ **T43.3x6** **Underdosing of phenothiazine antipsychotics and neuroleptics**

✓5ᵗʰ **T43.4** **Poisoning by, adverse effect of and underdosing of butyrophenone and thiothixene neuroleptics**

✓6ᵗʰ **T43.4x** **Poisoning by, adverse effect of and underdosing of butyrophenone and thiothixene neuroleptics**

✓7ᵗʰ **T43.4x1** **Poisoning by butyrophenone and thiothixene neuroleptics, accidental (unintentional)**

Poisoning by butyrophenone and thiothixene neuroleptics NOS

✓7ᵗʰ **T43.4x2** **Poisoning by butyrophenone and thiothixene neuroleptics, intentional self-harm**

✓7ᵗʰ **T43.4x3** **Poisoning by butyrophenone and thiothixene neuroleptics, assault**

✓7ᵗʰ **T43.4x4** **Poisoning by butyrophenone and thiothixene neuroleptics, undetermined**

✓7ᵗʰ **T43.4x5** **Adverse effect of butyrophenone and thiothixene neuroleptics**

✓7ᵗʰ **T43.4x6** **Underdosing of butyrophenone and thiothixene neuroleptics**

✓5ᵗʰ **T43.5** **Poisoning by, adverse effect of and underdosing of other and unspecified antipsychotics and neuroleptics**

> **EXCLUDES 1** *poisoning by, adverse effect of and underdosing of rauwolfia (T46.5-)*

✓6ᵗʰ **T43.50** **Poisoning by, adverse effect of and underdosing of unspecified antipsychotics and neuroleptics**

✓7ᵗʰ **T43.501** **Poisoning by unspecified antipsychotics and neuroleptics, accidental (unintentional)**

Poisoning by antipsychotics and neuroleptics NOS

✓7ᵗʰ **T43.502** **Poisoning by unspecified antipsychotics and neuroleptics, intentional self-harm**

✓7ᵗʰ **T43.503** **Poisoning by unspecified antipsychotics and neuroleptics, assault**

✓7ᵗʰ **T43.504** **Poisoning by unspecified antipsychotics and neuroleptics, undetermined**

✓7ᵗʰ **T43.505** **Adverse effect of unspecified antipsychotics and neuroleptics**

✓7ᵗʰ **T43.506** **Underdosing of unspecified antipsychotics and neuroleptics**

✓6ᵗʰ **T43.59** **Poisoning by, adverse effect of and underdosing of other antipsychotics and neuroleptics**

✓7ᵗʰ **T43.591** **Poisoning by other antipsychotics and neuroleptics, accidental (unintentional)**

Poisoning by other antipsychotics and neuroleptics NOS

✓7ᵗʰ **T43.592** **Poisoning by other antipsychotics and neuroleptics, intentional self-harm**

✓7ᵗʰ **T43.593** **Poisoning by other antipsychotics and neuroleptics, assault**

✓7ᵗʰ **T43.594** **Poisoning by other antipsychotics and neuroleptics, undetermined**

✓7ᵗʰ **T43.595** **Adverse effect of other antipsychotics and neuroleptics**

✓7ᵗʰ **T43.596** **Underdosing of other antipsychotics and neuroleptics**

✓5ᵗʰ **T43.6** **Poisoning by, adverse effect of and underdosing of psychostimulants**

> **EXCLUDES 1** *poisoning by, adverse effect of and underdosing of cocaine (T40.5-)*

✓6ᵗʰ **T43.60** **Poisoning by, adverse effect of and underdosing of unspecified psychostimulant**

✓7ᵗʰ **T43.601** **Poisoning by unspecified psychostimulants, accidental (unintentional)**

Poisoning by psychostimulants NOS

✓7ᵗʰ **T43.602** **Poisoning by unspecified psychostimulants, intentional self-harm**

✓7ᵗʰ **T43.603** **Poisoning by unspecified psychostimulants, assault**

☑ Appropriate additional character required   ✓x7ᵗʰ Requires 7th character, placeholder x must fill empty characters

√7th **T43.604** **Poisoning by unspecified psychostimulants, undetermined**

√7th **T43.605** **Adverse effect of unspecified psychostimulants**

√7th **T43.606** **Underdosing of unspecified psychostimulants**

√6th **T43.61** **Poisoning by, adverse effect of and underdosing of caffeine**

    √7th **T43.611** **Poisoning by caffeine, accidental (unintentional)**
        Poisoning by caffeine NOS

    √7th **T43.612** **Poisoning by caffeine, intentional self-harm**

    √7th **T43.613** **Poisoning by caffeine, assault**

    √7th **T43.614** **Poisoning by caffeine, undetermined**

    √7th **T43.615** **Adverse effect of caffeine**

    √7th **T43.616** **Underdosing of caffeine**

√6th **T43.62** **Poisoning by, adverse effect of and underdosing of amphetamines**
    Poisoning by, adverse effect of and underdosing of methamphetamines

    √7th **T43.621** **Poisoning by amphetamines, accidental (unintentional)**
        Poisoning by amphetamines NOS

    √7th **T43.622** **Poisoning by amphetamines, intentional self-harm**

    √7th **T43.623** **Poisoning by amphetamines, assault**

    √7th **T43.624** **Poisoning by amphetamines, undetermined**

    √7th **T43.625** **Adverse effect of amphetamines**

    √7th **T43.626** **Underdosing of amphetamines**

√6th **T43.63** **Poisoning by, adverse effect of and underdosing of methylphenidate**

    √7th **T43.631** **Poisoning by methylphenidate, accidental (unintentional)**
        Poisoning by methylphenidate NOS

    √7th **T43.632** **Poisoning by methylphenidate, intentional self-harm**

    √7th **T43.633** **Poisoning by methylphenidate, assault**

    √7th **T43.634** **Poisoning by methylphenidate, undetermined**

    √7th **T43.635** **Adverse effect of methylphenidate**

    √7th **T43.636** **Underdosing of methylphenidate**

√6th **T43.69** **Poisoning by, adverse effect of and underdosing of other psychostimulants**

    √7th **T43.691** **Poisoning by other psychostimulants, accidental (unintentional)**
        Poisoning by other psychostimulants NOS

    √7th **T43.692** **Poisoning by other psychostimulants, intentional self-harm**

    √7th **T43.693** **Poisoning by other psychostimulants, assault**

    √7th **T43.694** **Poisoning by other psychostimulants, undetermined**

    √7th **T43.695** **Adverse effect of other psychostimulants**

    √7th **T43.696** **Underdosing of other psychostimulants**

√5th **T43.8** **Poisoning by, adverse effect of and underdosing of other psychotropic drugs**

√6th **T43.8x** **Poisoning by, adverse effect of and underdosing of other psychotropic drugs**

    √7th **T43.8x1** **Poisoning by other psychotropic drugs, accidental (unintentional)**
        Poisoning by other psychotropic drugs NOS

    √7th **T43.8x2** **Poisoning by other psychotropic drugs, intentional self-harm**

    √7th **T43.8x3** **Poisoning by other psychotropic drugs, assault**

    √7th **T43.8x4** **Poisoning by other psychotropic drugs, undetermined**

    √7th **T43.8x5** **Adverse effect of other psychotropic drugs**

    √7th **T43.8x6** **Underdosing of other psychotropic drugs**

√5th **T43.9** **Poisoning by, adverse effect of and underdosing of unspecified psychotropic drug**

√x7th **T43.91** **Poisoning by unspecified psychotropic drug, accidental (unintentional)**
    Poisoning by psychotropic drug NOS

√x7th **T43.92** **Poisoning by unspecified psychotropic drug, intentional self-harm**

√x7th **T43.93** **Poisoning by unspecified psychotropic drug, assault**

√x7th **T43.94** **Poisoning by unspecified psychotropic drug, undetermined**

√x7th **T43.95** **Adverse effect of unspecified psychotropic drug**

√x7th **T43.96** **Underdosing of unspecified psychotropic drug**

√4th **T44** **Poisoning by, adverse effect of and underdosing of drugs primarily affecting the autonomic nervous system**

> The appropriate 7th character is to be added to each code from category T44.
> A   initial encounter
> D   subsequent encounter
> S   sequela

√5th **T44.0** **Poisoning by, adverse effect of and underdosing of anticholinesterase agents**

√6th **T44.0x** **Poisoning by, adverse effect of and underdosing of anticholinesterase agents**

    √7th **T44.0x1** **Poisoning by anticholinesterase agents, accidental (unintentional)**
        Poisoning by anticholinesterase agents NOS

    √7th **T44.0x2** **Poisoning by anticholinesterase agents, intentional self-harm**

    √7th **T44.0x3** **Poisoning by anticholinesterase agents, assault**

    √7th **T44.0x4** **Poisoning by anticholinesterase agents, undetermined**

    √7th **T44.0x5** **Adverse effect of anticholinesterase agents**

    √7th **T44.0x6** **Underdosing of anticholinesterase agents**

√5th **T44.1** **Poisoning by, adverse effect of and underdosing of other parasympathomimetics [cholinergics]**

√6th **T44.1x** **Poisoning by, adverse effect of and underdosing of other parasympathomimetics [cholinergics]**

    √7th **T44.1x1** **Poisoning by other parasympathomimetics [cholinergics], accidental (unintentional)**
        Poisoning by other parasympathomimetics [cholinergics] NOS

    √7th **T44.1x2** **Poisoning by other parasympathomimetics [cholinergics], intentional self-harm**

    √7th **T44.1x3** **Poisoning by other parasympathomimetics [cholinergics], assault**

    √7th **T44.1x4** **Poisoning by other parasympathomimetics [cholinergics], undetermined**

    √7th **T44.1x5** **Adverse effect of other parasympathomimetics [cholinergics]**

    √7th **T44.1x6** **Underdosing of other parasympathomimetics**

√5th **T44.2** **Poisoning by, adverse effect of and underdosing of ganglionic blocking drugs**

√6th **T44.2x** **Poisoning by, adverse effect of and underdosing of ganglionic blocking drugs**

    √7th **T44.2x1** **Poisoning by ganglionic blocking drugs, accidental (unintentional)**
        Poisoning by ganglionic blocking drugs NOS

    √7th **T44.2x2** **Poisoning by ganglionic blocking drugs, intentional self-harm**

    √7th **T44.2x3** **Poisoning by ganglionic blocking drugs, assault**

    √7th **T44.2x4** **Poisoning by ganglionic blocking drugs, undetermined**

    √7th **T44.2x5** **Adverse effect of ganglionic blocking drugs**

EXCLUDES 1 Not coded here   **EXCLUDES 2** Not included here   *Manifestation Code*

☑7th **T44.2x6** **Underdosing of ganglionic blocking drugs**

☑5th **T44.3** **Poisoning by, adverse effect of and underdosing of other parasympatholytics [anticholinergics and antimuscarinics] and spasmolytics**
Poisoning by, adverse effect of and underdosing of papaverine

☑6th **T44.3x** **Poisoning by, adverse effect of and underdosing of other parasympatholytics [anticholinergics and antimuscarinics] and spasmolytics**

☑7th **T44.3x1** **Poisoning by other parasympatholytics [anticholinergics and antimuscarinics] and spasmolytics, accidental (unintentional)**
Poisoning by other parasympatholytics [anticholinergics and antimuscarinics] and spasmolytics NOS

☑7th **T44.3x2** **Poisoning by other parasympatholytics [anticholinergics and antimuscarinics] and spasmolytics, intentional self-harm**

☑7th **T44.3x3** **Poisoning by other parasympatholytics [anticholinergics and antimuscarinics] and spasmolytics, assault**

☑7th **T44.3x4** **Poisoning by other parasympatholytics [anticholinergics and antimuscarinics] and spasmolytics, undetermined**

☑7th **T44.3x5** **Adverse effect of other parasympatholytics [anticholinergics and antimuscarinics] and spasmolytics**

☑7th **T44.3x6** **Underdosing of other parasympatholytics [anticholinergics and antimuscarinics] and spasmolytics**

☑5th **T44.4** **Poisoning by, adverse effect of and underdosing of predominantly alpha-adrenoreceptor agonists**
Poisoning by, adverse effect of and underdosing of metaraminol

☑6th **T44.4x** **Poisoning by, adverse effect of and underdosing of predominantly alpha-adrenoreceptor agonists**

☑7th **T44.4x1** **Poisoning by predominantly alpha-adrenoreceptor agonists, accidental (unintentional)**
Poisoning by predominantly alpha-adrenoreceptor agonists NOS

☑7th **T44.4x2** **Poisoning by predominantly alpha-adrenoreceptor agonists, intentional self-harm**

☑7th **T44.4x3** **Poisoning by predominantly alpha-adrenoreceptor agonists, assault**

☑7th **T44.4x4** **Poisoning by predominantly alpha-adrenoreceptor agonists, undetermined**

☑7th **T44.4x5** **Adverse effect of predominantly alpha-adrenoreceptor agonists**

☑7th **T44.4x6** **Underdosing of predominantly alpha-adrenoreceptor agonists**

☑5th **T44.5** **Poisoning by, adverse effect of and underdosing of predominantly beta-adrenoreceptor agonists**
EXCLUDES 1 *poisoning by, adverse effect of and underdosing of beta-adrenoreceptor agonists used in asthma therapy (T48.6-)*

☑6th **T44.5x** **Poisoning by, adverse effect of and underdosing of predominantly beta-adrenoreceptor agonists**

☑7th **T44.5x1** **Poisoning by predominantly beta-adrenoreceptor agonists, accidental (unintentional)**
Poisoning by predominantly beta-adrenoreceptor agonists NOS

☑7th **T44.5x2** **Poisoning by predominantly beta-adrenoreceptor agonists, intentional self-harm**

☑7th **T44.5x3** **Poisoning by predominantly beta-adrenoreceptor agonists, assault**

☑7th **T44.5x4** **Poisoning by predominantly beta-adrenoreceptor agonists, undetermined**

☑7th **T44.5x5** **Adverse effect of predominantly beta-adrenoreceptor agonists**

☑7th **T44.5x6** **Underdosing of predominantly beta-adrenoreceptor agonists**

☑5th **T44.6** **Poisoning by, adverse effect of and underdosing of alpha-adrenoreceptor antagonists**
EXCLUDES 1 *poisoning by, adverse effect of and underdosing of ergot alkaloids (T48.0)*

☑6th **T44.6x** **Poisoning by, adverse effect of and underdosing of alpha-adrenoreceptor antagonists**

☑7th **T44.6x1** **Poisoning by alpha-adrenoreceptor antagonists, accidental (unintentional)**
Poisoning by alpha-adrenoreceptor antagonists NOS

☑7th **T44.6x2** **Poisoning by alpha-adrenoreceptor antagonists, intentional self-harm**

☑7th **T44.6x3** **Poisoning by alpha-adrenoreceptor antagonists, assault**

☑7th **T44.6x4** **Poisoning by alpha-adrenoreceptor antagonists, undetermined**

☑7th **T44.6x5** **Adverse effect of alpha-adrenoreceptor antagonists**

☑7th **T44.6x6** **Underdosing of alpha-adrenoreceptor antagonists**

☑5th **T44.7** **Poisoning by, adverse effect of and underdosing of beta-adrenoreceptor antagonists**

☑6th **T44.7x** **Poisoning by, adverse effect of and underdosing of beta-adrenoreceptor antagonists**

☑7th **T44.7x1** **Poisoning by beta-adrenoreceptor antagonists, accidental (unintentional)**
Poisoning by beta-adrenoreceptor antagonists NOS

☑7th **T44.7x2** **Poisoning by beta-adrenoreceptor antagonists, intentional self-harm**

☑7th **T44.7x3** **Poisoning by beta-adrenoreceptor antagonists, assault**

☑7th **T44.7x4** **Poisoning by beta-adrenoreceptor antagonists, undetermined**

☑7th **T44.7x5** **Adverse effect of beta-adrenoreceptor antagonists**

☑7th **T44.7x6** **Underdosing of beta-adrenoreceptor antagonists**

☑5th **T44.8** **Poisoning by, adverse effect of and underdosing of centrally-acting and adrenergic-neuron- blocking agents**
EXCLUDES 1 *poisoning by, adverse effect of and underdosing of clonidine (T46.5)*
poisoning by, adverse effect of and underdosing of guanethidine (T46.5)

☑6th **T44.8x** **Poisoning by, adverse effect of and underdosing of centrally-acting and adrenergic-neuron-blocking agents**

☑7th **T44.8x1** **Poisoning by centrally-acting and adrenergic-neuron-blocking agents, accidental (unintentional)**
Poisoning by centrally-acting and adrenergic-neuron-blocking agents NOS

☑7th **T44.8x2** **Poisoning by centrally-acting and adrenergic-neuron-blocking agents, intentional self-harm**

☑7th **T44.8x3** **Poisoning by centrally-acting and adrenergic-neuron-blocking agents, assault**

☑7th **T44.8x4** **Poisoning by centrally-acting and adrenergic-neuron-blocking agents, undetermined**

☑7th **T44.8x5** **Adverse effect of centrally-acting and adrenergic-neuron-blocking agents**

☑7th **T44.8x6** **Underdosing of centrally-acting and adrenergic-neuron-blocking agents**

☑ Appropriate additional character required   ☑x7th Requires 7th character, placeholder x must fill empty characters

✓5th **T44.9** **Poisoning by, adverse effect of and underdosing of other and unspecified drugs primarily affecting the autonomic nervous system**
> Poisoning by, adverse effect of and underdosing of drug stimulating both alpha and beta-adrenoreceptors

     ✓6th **T44.90** **Poisoning by, adverse effect of and underdosing of unspecified drugs primarily affecting the autonomic nervous system**

         ✓7th **T44.901** **Poisoning by unspecified drugs primarily affecting the autonomic nervous system, accidental (unintentional)**
> Poisoning by unspecified drugs primarily affecting the autonomic nervous system NOS

         ✓7th **T44.902** **Poisoning by unspecified drugs primarily affecting the autonomic nervous system, intentional self-harm**

         ✓7th **T44.903** **Poisoning by unspecified drugs primarily affecting the autonomic nervous system, assault**

         ✓7th **T44.904** **Poisoning by unspecified drugs primarily affecting the autonomic nervous system, undetermined**

         ✓7th **T44.905** **Adverse effect of unspecified drugs primarily affecting the autonomic nervous system**

         ✓7th **T44.906** **Underdosing of unspecified drugs primarily affecting the autonomic nervous system**

     ✓6th **T44.99** **Poisoning by, adverse effect of and underdosing of other drugs primarily affecting the autonomic nervous system**

         ✓7th **T44.991** **Poisoning by other drug primarily affecting the autonomic nervous system, accidental (unintentional)**
> Poisoning by other drugs primarily affecting the autonomic nervous system NOS

         ✓7th **T44.992** **Poisoning by other drug primarily affecting the autonomic nervous system, intentional self-harm**

         ✓7th **T44.993** **Poisoning by other drug primarily affecting the autonomic nervous system, assault**

         ✓7th **T44.994** **Poisoning by other drug primarily affecting the autonomic nervous system, undetermined**

         ✓7th **T44.995** **Adverse effect of other drug primarily affecting the autonomic nervous system**

         ✓7th **T44.996** **Underdosing of other drug primarily affecting the autonomic nervous system**

✓4th **T45** **Poisoning by, adverse effect of and underdosing of primarily systemic and hematological agents, not elsewhere classified**

> The appropriate 7th character is to be added to each code from category T45.
> A   initial encounter
> D   subsequent encounter
> S   sequela

     ✓5th **T45.0** **Poisoning by, adverse effect of and underdosing of antiallergic and antiemetic drugs**
> EXCLUDES 1   *poisoning by, adverse effect of and underdosing of phenothiazine-based neuroleptics (T43.3)*

     ✓6th **T45.0x** **Poisoning by, adverse effect of and underdosing of antiallergic and antiemetic drugs**

         ✓7th **T45.0x1** **Poisoning by antiallergic and antiemetic drugs, accidental (unintentional)**
> Poisoning by antiallergic and antiemetic drugs NOS

         ✓7th **T45.0x2** **Poisoning by antiallergic and antiemetic drugs, intentional self-harm**

         ✓7th **T45.0x3** **Poisoning by antiallergic and antiemetic drugs, assault**

         ✓7th **T45.0x4** **Poisoning by antiallergic and antiemetic drugs, undetermined**

         ✓7th **T45.0x5** **Adverse effect of antiallergic and antiemetic drugs**

         ✓7th **T45.0x6** **Underdosing of antiallergic and antiemetic drugs**

     ✓5th **T45.1** **Poisoning by, adverse effect of and underdosing of antineoplastic and immunosuppressive drugs**
> EXCLUDES 1   *poisoning by, adverse effect of and underdosing of tamoxifen (T38.6)*

     ✓6th **T45.1x** **Poisoning by, adverse effect of and underdosing of antineoplastic and immunosuppressive drugs**

         ✓7th **T45.1x1** **Poisoning by antineoplastic and immunosuppressive drugs, accidental (unintentional)**
> Poisoning by antineoplastic and immunosuppressive drugs NOS

         ✓7th **T45.1x2** **Poisoning by antineoplastic and immunosuppressive drugs, intentional self-harm**

         ✓7th **T45.1x3** **Poisoning by antineoplastic and immunosuppressive drugs, assault**

         ✓7th **T45.1x4** **Poisoning by antineoplastic and immunosuppressive drugs, undetermined**

         ✓7th **T45.1x5** **Adverse effect of antineoplastic and immunosuppressive drugs**

         ✓7th **T45.1x6** **Underdosing of antineoplastic and immunosuppressive drugs**

     ✓5th **T45.2** **Poisoning by, adverse effect of and underdosing of vitamins**
> EXCLUDES 2   *poisoning by, adverse effect of and underdosing of nicotinic acid (derivatives) (T46.7)*
> *poisoning by, adverse effect of and underdosing of iron (T45.4)*
> *poisoning by, adverse effect of and underdosing of vitamin K (T45.7)*

     ✓6th **T45.2x** **Poisoning by, adverse effect of and underdosing of vitamins**

         ✓7th **T45.2x1** **Poisoning by vitamins, accidental (unintentional)**
> Poisoning by vitamins NOS

         ✓7th **T45.2x2** **Poisoning by vitamins, intentional self-harm**

         ✓7th **T45.2x3** **Poisoning by vitamins, assault**

         ✓7th **T45.2x4** **Poisoning by vitamins, undetermined**

         ✓7th **T45.2x5** **Adverse effect of vitamins**

         ✓7th **T45.2x6** **Underdosing of vitamins**
> EXCLUDES 1   *vitamin deficiencies (E50-E56)*

     ✓5th **T45.3** **Poisoning by, adverse effect of and underdosing of enzymes**

     ✓6th **T45.3x** **Poisoning by, adverse effect of and underdosing of enzymes**

         ✓7th **T45.3x1** **Poisoning by enzymes, accidental (unintentional)**
> Poisoning by enzymes NOS

         ✓7th **T45.3x2** **Poisoning by enzymes, intentional self-harm**

         ✓7th **T45.3x3** **Poisoning by enzymes, assault**

         ✓7th **T45.3x4** **Poisoning by enzymes, undetermined**

         ✓7th **T45.3x5** **Adverse effect of enzymes**

         ✓7th **T45.3x6** **Underdosing of enzymes**

     ✓5th **T45.4** **Poisoning by, adverse effect of and underdosing of iron and its compounds**

     ✓6th **T45.4x** **Poisoning by, adverse effect of and underdosing of iron and its compounds**

         T45.4x1 **Poisoning by iron and its compounds, accidental (unintentional)**
> Poisoning by iron and its compounds NOS

         ✓7th **T45.4x2** **Poisoning by iron and its compounds, intentional self-harm**

         ✓7th **T45.4x3** **Poisoning by iron and its compounds, assault**

         ✓7th **T45.4x4** **Poisoning by iron and its compounds, undetermined**

         ✓7th **T45.4x5** **Adverse effect of iron and its compounds**

         ✓7th **T45.4x6** **Underdosing of iron and its compounds**
> EXCLUDES 1   *iron deficiency (E61.1)*

EXCLUDES 1   Not coded here   EXCLUDES 2   Not included here   *Manifestation Code*

✓5ᵗʰ **T45.5** **Poisoning by, adverse effect of and underdosing of anticoagulants and antithrombotic drugs**

✓6ᵗʰ **T45.51** **Poisoning by, adverse effect of and underdosing of anticoagulants**

✓7ᵗʰ **T45.511** **Poisoning by anticoagulants, accidental (unintentional)**
Poisoning by anticoagulants NOS

✓7ᵗʰ **T45.512** **Poisoning by anticoagulants, intentional self-harm**

✓7ᵗʰ **T45.513** **Poisoning by anticoagulants, assault**

✓7ᵗʰ **T45.514** **Poisoning by anticoagulants, undetermined**

✓7ᵗʰ **T45.515** **Adverse effect of anticoagulants**

✓7ᵗʰ **T45.516** **Underdosing of anticoagulants**

✓6ᵗʰ **T45.52** **Poisoning by, adverse effect of and underdosing of antithrombotic drugs**
Poisoning by, adverse effect of and underdosing of antiplatelet drugs

EXCLUDES 2   *poisoning by, adverse effect of and underdosing of aspirin (T39.01-)*
poisoning by, adverse effect of and underdosing of acetylsalicylic acid (T39.01-)

✓7ᵗʰ **T45.521** **Poisoning by antithrombotic drugs, accidental (unintentional)**
Poisoning by antithrombotic drug NOS

✓7ᵗʰ **T45.522** **Poisoning by antithrombotic drugs, intentional self-harm**

✓7ᵗʰ **T45.523** **Poisoning by antithrombotic drugs, assault**

✓7ᵗʰ **T45.524** **Poisoning by antithrombotic drugs, undetermined**

✓7ᵗʰ **T45.525** **Adverse effect of antithrombotic drugs**

✓7ᵗʰ **T45.526** **Underdosing of antithrombotic drugs**

✓5ᵗʰ **T45.6** **Poisoning by, adverse effect of and underdosing of fibrinolysis-affecting drugs**

✓6ᵗʰ **T45.60** **Poisoning by, adverse effect of and underdosing of unspecified fibrinolysis-affecting drugs**

✓7ᵗʰ **T45.601** **Poisoning by unspecified fibrinolysis-affecting drugs, accidental (unintentional)**
Poisoning by fibrinolysis-affecting drug NOS

✓7ᵗʰ **T45.602** **Poisoning by unspecified fibrinolysis-affecting drugs, intentional self-harm**

✓7ᵗʰ **T45.603** **Poisoning by unspecified fibrinolysis-affecting drugs, assault**

✓7ᵗʰ **T45.604** **Poisoning by unspecified fibrinolysis-affecting drugs, undetermined**

✓7ᵗʰ **T45.605** **Adverse effect of unspecified fibrinolysis-affecting drugs**

✓7ᵗʰ **T45.606** **Underdosing of unspecified fibrinolysis-affecting drugs**

✓6ᵗʰ **T45.61** **Poisoning by, adverse effect of and underdosing of thrombolytic drugs**

✓7ᵗʰ **T45.611** **Poisoning by thrombolytic drug, accidental (unintentional)**
Poisoning by thrombolytic drug NOS

✓7ᵗʰ **T45.612** **Poisoning by thrombolytic drug, intentional self-harm**

✓7ᵗʰ **T45.613** **Poisoning by thrombolytic drug, assault**

✓7ᵗʰ **T45.614** **Poisoning by thrombolytic drug, undetermined**

✓7ᵗʰ **T45.615** **Adverse effect of thrombolytic drugs**

✓7ᵗʰ **T45.616** **Underdosing of thrombolytic drugs**

✓6ᵗʰ **T45.62** **Poisoning by, adverse effect of and underdosing of hemostatic drugs**

✓7ᵗʰ **T45.621** **Poisoning by hemostatic drug, accidental (unintentional)**
Poisoning by hemostatic drug NOS

✓7ᵗʰ **T45.622** **Poisoning by hemostatic drug, intentional self-harm**

✓7ᵗʰ **T45.623** **Poisoning by hemostatic drug, assault**

✓7ᵗʰ **T45.624** **Poisoning by hemostatic drug, undetermined**

✓7ᵗʰ **T45.625** **Adverse effect of hemostatic drug**

✓7ᵗʰ **T45.626** **Underdosing of hemostatic drugs**

✓6ᵗʰ **T45.69** **Poisoning by, adverse effect of and underdosing of other fibrinolysis-affecting drugs**

✓7ᵗʰ **T45.691** **Poisoning by other fibrinolysis-affecting drugs, accidental (unintentional)**
Poisoning by other fibrinolysis-affecting drug NOS

✓7ᵗʰ **T45.692** **Poisoning by other fibrinolysis-affecting drugs, intentional self-harm**

✓7ᵗʰ **T45.693** **Poisoning by other fibrinolysis-affecting drugs, assault**

✓7ᵗʰ **T45.694** **Poisoning by other fibrinolysis-affecting drugs, undetermined**

✓7ᵗʰ **T45.695** **Adverse effect of other fibrinolysis-affecting drugs**

✓7ᵗʰ **T45.696** **Underdosing of other fibrinolysis-affecting drugs**

✓5ᵗʰ **T45.7** **Poisoning by, adverse effect of and underdosing of anticoagulant antagonists, vitamin K and other coagulants**

✓6ᵗʰ **T45.7x** **Poisoning by, adverse effect of and underdosing of anticoagulant antagonists, vitamin K and other coagulants**

✓7ᵗʰ **T45.7x1** **Poisoning by anticoagulant antagonists, vitamin K and other coagulants, accidental (unintentional)**
Poisoning by anticoagulant antagonists, vitamin K and other coagulants NOS

✓7ᵗʰ **T45.7x2** **Poisoning by anticoagulant antagonists, vitamin K and other coagulants, intentional self-harm**

✓7ᵗʰ **T45.7x3** **Poisoning by anticoagulant antagonlsts, vitamin K and other coagulants, assault**

✓7ᵗʰ **T45.7x4** **Poisoning by anticoagulant antagonists, vitamin K and other coagulants, undetermined**

✓7ᵗʰ **T45.7x5** **Adverse effect of anticoagulant antagonists, vitamin K and other coagulants**

✓7ᵗʰ **T45.7x6** **Underdosing of anticoagulant antagonist, vitamin K and other coagulants**
EXCLUDES 1   *vitamin K deficiency (E56.1)*

✓5ᵗʰ **T45.8** **Poisoning by, adverse effect of and underdosing of other primarily systemic and hematological agents**
Poisoning by, adverse effect of and underdosing of liver preparations and other antianemic agents
Poisoning by, adverse effect of and underdosing of natural blood and blood products
Poisoning by, adverse effect of and underdosing of plasma substitute
EXCLUDES 2   *poisoning by, adverse effect of and underdosing of immunoglobulin (T50.z1)*
poisoning by, adverse effect of and underdosing of iron (T45.4)

✓6ᵗʰ **T45.8x** **Poisoning by, adverse effect of and underdosing of other primarily systemic and hematological agents**

✓7ᵗʰ **T45.8x1** **Poisoning by other primarily systemic and hematological agents, accidental (unintentional)**
Poisoning by other primarily systemic and hematological agents NOS

✓7ᵗʰ **T45.8x2** **Poisoning by other primarily systemic and hematological agents, intentional self-harm**

✓7ᵗʰ **T45.8x3** **Poisoning by other primarily systemic and hematological agents, assault**

✓7ᵗʰ **T45.8x4** **Poisoning by other primarily systemic and hematological agents, undetermined**

✓7ᵗʰ **T45.8x5** **Adverse effect of other primarily systemic and hematological agents**

✓7ᵗʰ **T45.8x6** **Underdosing of other primarily systemic and hematological agents**

√5ᵗʰ **T45.9** **Poisoning by, adverse effect of and underdosing of unspecified primarily systemic and hematological agent**

√x7ᵗʰ **T45.91** **Poisoning by unspecified primarily systemic and hematological agent, accidental (unintentional)**
Poisoning by primarily systemic and hematological agent NOS

√7ᵗʰ **T45.92** **Poisoning by unspecified primarily systemic and hematological agent, intentional self-harm**

√x7ᵗʰ **T45.93** **Poisoning by unspecified primarily systemic and hematological agent, assault**

√x7ᵗʰ **T45.94** **Poisoning by unspecified primarily systemic and hematological agent, undetermined**

√x7ᵗʰ **T45.95** **Adverse effect of unspecified primarily systemic and hematological agent**

√x7ᵗʰ **T45.96** **Underdosing of unspecified primarily systemic and hematological agent**

√4ᵗʰ **T46** **Poisoning by, adverse effect of and underdosing of agents primarily affecting the cardiovascular system**

> EXCLUDES 1   *poisoning by, adverse effect of and underdosing of metaraminol (T44.4)*

> The appropriate 7th character is to be added to each code from category T46.
> A   initial encounter
> D   subsequent encounter
> S   sequela

√5ᵗʰ **T46.0** **Poisoning by, adverse effect of and underdosing of cardiac-stimulant glycosides and drugs of similar action**

√6ᵗʰ **T46.0x** **Poisoning by, adverse effect of and underdosing of cardiac-stimulant glycosides and drugs of similar action**

√7ᵗʰ **T46.0x1** **Poisoning by cardiac-stimulant glycosides and drugs of similar action, accidental (unintentional)**
Poisoning by cardiac-stimulant glycosides and drugs of similar action NOS

√7ᵗʰ **T46.0x2** **Poisoning by cardiac-stimulant glycosides and drugs of similar action, intentional self-harm**

√7ᵗʰ **T46.0x3** **Poisoning by cardiac-stimulant glycosides and drugs of similar action, assault**

√7ᵗʰ **T46.0x4** **Poisoning by cardiac-stimulant glycosides and drugs of similar action, undetermined**

√7ᵗʰ **T46.0x5** **Adverse effect of cardiac-stimulant glycosides and drugs of similar action**

√7ᵗʰ **T46.0x6** **Underdosing of cardiac-stimulant glycosides and drugs of similar action**

T46.1 **Poisoning by, adverse effect of and underdosing of calcium-channel blockers**

√6ᵗʰ **T46.1x** **Poisoning by, adverse effect of and underdosing of calcium-channel blockers**

√7ᵗʰ **T46.1x1** **Poisoning by calcium-channel blockers, accidental (unintentional)**
Poisoning by calcium-channel blockers NOS

√7ᵗʰ **T46.1x2** **Poisoning by calcium-channel blockers, intentional self-harm**

√7ᵗʰ **T46.1x3** **Poisoning by calcium-channel blockers, assault**

√7ᵗʰ **T46.1x4** **Poisoning by calcium-channel blockers, undetermined**

√7ᵗʰ **T46.1x5** **Adverse effect of calcium-channel blockers**

√7ᵗʰ **T46.1x6** **Underdosing of calcium-channel blockers**

√5ᵗʰ **T46.2** **Poisoning by, adverse effect of and underdosing of other antidysrhythmic drugs, not elsewhere classified**

> EXCLUDES 1   *poisoning by, adverse effect of and underdosing of beta-adrenoreceptor antagonists (T44.7-)*

√6ᵗʰ **T46.2x** **Poisoning by, adverse effect of and underdosing of other antidysrhythmic drugs**

√7ᵗʰ **T46.2x1** **Poisoning by other antidysrhythmic drugs, accidental (unintentional)**
Poisoning by other antidysrhythmic drugs NOS

√7ᵗʰ **T46.2x2** **Poisoning by other antidysrhythmic drugs, intentional self-harm**

√7ᵗʰ **T46.2x3** **Poisoning by other antidysrhythmic drugs, assault**

√7ᵗʰ **T46.2x4** **Poisoning by other antidysrhythmic drugs, undetermined**

√7ᵗʰ **T46.2x5** **Adverse effect of other antidysrhythmic drugs**

√7ᵗʰ **T46.2x6** **Underdosing of other antidysrhythmic drugs**

√5ᵗʰ **T46.3** **Poisoning by, adverse effect of and underdosing of coronary vasodilators**
Poisoning by, adverse effect of and underdosing of dipyridamole

> EXCLUDES 1   *poisoning by, adverse effect of and underdosing of calcium-channel blockers (T46.1)*

√6ᵗʰ **T46.3x** **Poisoning by, adverse effect of and underdosing of coronary vasodilators**

√7ᵗʰ **T46.3x1** **Poisoning by coronary vasodilators, accidental (unintentional)**
Poisoning by coronary vasodilators NOS

√7ᵗʰ **T46.3x2** **Poisoning by coronary vasodilators, intentional self-harm**

√7ᵗʰ **T46.3x3** **Poisoning by coronary vasodilators, assault**

√7ᵗʰ **T46.3x4** **Poisoning by coronary vasodilators, undetermined**

√7ᵗʰ **T46.3x5** **Adverse effect of coronary vasodilators**

√7ᵗʰ **T46.3x6** **Underdosing of coronary vasodilators**

√5ᵗʰ **T46.4** **Poisoning by, adverse effect of and underdosing of angiotensin-converting-enzyme inhibitors**

√6ᵗʰ **T46.4x** **Poisoning by, adverse effect of and underdosing of angiotensin-converting-enzyme inhibitors**

√7ᵗʰ **T46.4x1** **Poisoning by angiotensin-converting-enzyme inhibitors, accidental (unintentional)**
Poisoning by angiotensin-converting-enzyme inhibitors NOS

√7ᵗʰ **T46.4x2** **Poisoning by angiotensin-converting-enzyme inhibitors, intentional self-harm**

√7ᵗʰ **T46.4x3** **Poisoning by angiotensin-converting-enzyme inhibitors, assault**

√7ᵗʰ **T46.4x4** **Poisoning by angiotensin-converting-enzyme inhibitors, undetermined**

√7ᵗʰ **T46.4x5** **Adverse effect of angiotensin-converting- enzyme inhibitors**

√7ᵗʰ **T46.4x6** **Underdosing of angiotensin-converting-enzyme inhibitors**

√5ᵗʰ **T46.5** **Poisoning by, adverse effect of and underdosing of other antihypertensive drugs**

> EXCLUDES 2   *poisoning by, adverse effect of and underdosing of beta-adrenoreceptor antagonists (T44.7)*
> *poisoning by, adverse effect of and underdosing of calcium-channel blockers (T46.1)*
> *poisoning by, adverse effect of and underdosing of diuretics (T50.0-T50.2)*

√6ᵗʰ **T46.5x** **Poisoning by, adverse effect of and underdosing of other antihypertensive drugs**

√7ᵗʰ **T46.5x1** **Poisoning by other antihypertensive drugs, accidental (unintentional)**
Poisoning by other antihypertensive drugs NOS

√7ᵗʰ **T46.5x2** **Poisoning by other antihypertensive drugs, intentional self-harm**

√7ᵗʰ **T46.5x3** **Poisoning by other antihypertensive drugs, assault**

√7ᵗʰ **T46.5x4** **Poisoning by other antihypertensive drugs, undetermined**

√7ᵗʰ **T46.5x5** **Adverse effect of other antihypertensive drugs**

√7ᵗʰ **T46.5x6** **Underdosing of other antihypertensive drugs**

EXCLUDES 1   Not coded here   EXCLUDES 2   Not included here   *Manifestation Code*

√5ᵗʰ **T46.6**   **Poisoning by, adverse effect of and underdosing of antihyperlipidemic and antiarteriosclerotic drugs**

√6ᵗʰ **T46.6x**   **Poisoning by, adverse effect of and underdosing of antihyperlipidemic and antiarteriosclerotic drugs**

√7ᵗʰ **T46.6x1**   **Poisoning by antihyperlipidemic and antiarteriosclerotic drugs, accidental (unintentional)**
Poisoning by antihyperlipidemic and antiarteriosclerotic drugs NOS

√7ᵗʰ **T46.6x2**   **Poisoning by antihyperlipidemic and antiarteriosclerotic drugs, intentional self-harm**

√7ᵗʰ **T46.6x3**   **Poisoning by antihyperlipidemic and antiarteriosclerotic drugs, assault**

√7ᵗʰ **T46.6x4**   **Poisoning by antihyperlipidemic and antiarteriosclerotic drugs, undetermined**

√7ᵗʰ **T46.6x5**   **Adverse effect of antihyperlipidemic and antiarteriosclerotic drugs**

√7ᵗʰ **T46.6x6**   **Underdosing of antihyperlipidemic and antiarteriosclerotic drugs**

√5ᵗʰ **T46.7**   **Poisoning by, adverse effect of and underdosing of peripheral vasodilators**
Poisoning by, adverse effect of and underdosing of nicotinic acid (derivatives)

EXCLUDES 1   *poisoning by, adverse effect of and underdosing of papaverine (T44.3)*

√6ᵗʰ **T46.7x**   **Poisoning by, adverse effect of and underdosing of peripheral vasodilators**

√7ᵗʰ **T46.7x1**   **Poisoning by peripheral vasodilators, accidental (unintentional)**
Poisoning by peripheral vasodilators NOS

√7ᵗʰ **T46.7x2**   **Poisoning by peripheral vasodilators, intentional self-harm**

√7ᵗʰ **T46.7x3**   **Poisoning by peripheral vasodilators, assault**

√7ᵗʰ **T46.7x4**   **Poisoning by peripheral vasodilators, undetermined**

√7ᵗʰ **T46.7x5**   **Adverse effect of peripheral vasodilators**

√7ᵗʰ **T46.7x6**   **Underdosing of peripheral vasodilators**

√5ᵗʰ **T46.8**   **Poisoning by, adverse effect of and underdosing of antivaricose drugs, including sclerosing agents**

√6ᵗʰ **T46.8x**   **Poisoning by, adverse effect of and underdosing of antivaricose drugs, including sclerosing agents**

√7ᵗʰ **T46.8x1**   **Poisoning by antivaricose drugs, including sclerosing agents, accidental (unintentional)**
Poisoning by antivaricose drugs, including sclerosing agents NOS

√7ᵗʰ **T46.8x2**   **Poisoning by antivaricose drugs, including sclerosing agents, intentional self-harm**

√7ᵗʰ **T46.8x3**   **Poisoning by antivaricose drugs, including sclerosing agents, assault**

√7ᵗʰ **T46.8x4**   **Poisoning by antivaricose drugs, including sclerosing agents, undetermined**

√7ᵗʰ **T46.8x5**   **Adverse effect of antivaricose drugs, including sclerosing agents**

√7ᵗʰ **T46.8x6**   **Underdosing of antivaricose drugs, including sclerosing agents**

√5ᵗʰ **T46.9**   **Poisoning by, adverse effect of and underdosing of other and unspecified agents primarily affecting the cardiovascular system**

√6ᵗʰ **T46.90**   **Poisoning by, adverse effect of and underdosing of unspecified agents primarily affecting the cardiovascular system**

√7ᵗʰ **T46.901**   **Poisoning by unspecified agents primarily affecting the cardiovascular system, accidental (unintentional)**

√7ᵗʰ **T46.902**   **Poisoning by unspecified agents primarily affecting the cardiovascular system, intentional self-harm**

√7ᵗʰ **T46.903**   **Poisoning by unspecified agents primarily affecting the cardiovascular system, assault**

√7ᵗʰ **T46.904**   **Poisoning by unspecified agents primarily affecting the cardiovascular system, undetermined**

√7ᵗʰ **T46.905**   **Adverse effect of unspecified agents primarily affecting the cardiovascular system**

√7ᵗʰ **T46.906**   **Underdosing of unspecified agents primarily affecting the cardiovascular system**

√6ᵗʰ **T46.99**   **Poisoning by, adverse effect of and underdosing of other agents primarily affecting the cardiovascular system**

√7ᵗʰ **T46.991**   **Poisoning by other agents primarily affecting the cardiovascular system, accidental (unintentional)**

√7ᵗʰ **T46.992**   **Poisoning by other agents primarily affecting the cardiovascular system, intentional self-harm**

√7ᵗʰ **T46.993**   **Poisoning by other agents primarily affecting the cardiovascular system, assault**

√7ᵗʰ **T46.994**   **Poisoning by other agents primarily affecting the cardiovascular system, undetermined**

√7ᵗʰ **T46.995**   **Adverse effect of other agents primarily affecting the cardiovascular system**

√7ᵗʰ **T46.996**   **Underdosing of other agents primarily affecting the cardiovascular system**

√4ᵗʰ **T47**   **Poisoning by, adverse effect of and underdosing of agents primarily affecting the gastrointestinal system**

The appropriate 7th character is to be added to each code from category T47.
A   initial encounter
D   subsequent encounter
S   sequela

√5ᵗʰ **T47.0**   **Poisoning by, adverse effect of and underdosing of histamine H2-receptor blockers**

√6ᵗʰ **T47.0X**   **Poisoning by, adverse effect of and underdosing of histamine H2-receptor blockers**

√7ᵗʰ **T47.0x1**   **Poisoning by histamine H2-receptor blockers, accidental (unintentional)**
Poisoning by histamine H2-receptor blockers NOS

√7ᵗʰ **T47.0x2**   **Poisoning by histamine H2-receptor blockers, intentional self-harm**

√7ᵗʰ **T47.0x3**   **Poisoning by histamine H2-receptor blockers, assault**

√7ᵗʰ **T47.0x4**   **Poisoning by histamine H2-receptor blockers, undetermined**

√7ᵗʰ **T47.0x5**   **Adverse effect of histamine H2-receptor blockers**

√7ᵗʰ **T47.0x6**   **Underdosing of histamine H2-receptor blockers**

√5ᵗʰ **T47.1**   **Poisoning by, adverse effect of and underdosing of other antacids and anti-gastric-secretion drugs**

√6ᵗʰ **T47.1x**   **Poisoning by, adverse effect of and underdosing of other antacids and anti-gastric-secretion drugs**

√7ᵗʰ **T47.1x1**   **Poisoning by other antacids and anti-gastric-secretion drugs, accidental (unintentional)**
Poisoning by other antacids and anti-gastric-secretion drugs NOS

√7ᵗʰ **T47.1x2**   **Poisoning by other antacids and anti-gastric-secretion drugs, intentional self-harm**

√7ᵗʰ **T47.1x3**   **Poisoning by other antacids and anti-gastric-secretion drugs, assault**

√7ᵗʰ **T47.1x4**   **Poisoning by other antacids and anti-gastric-secretion drugs, undetermined**

√7ᵗʰ **T47.1x5**   **Adverse effect of other antacids and anti-gastric-secretion drugs**

√7ᵗʰ **T47.1x6**   **Underdosing of other antacids and anti-gastric-secretion drugs**

✓5th T47.2 Poisoning by, adverse effect of and underdosing of stimulant laxatives

     ✓6th T47.2x Poisoning by, adverse effect of and underdosing of stimulant laxatives

         ✓7th T47.2x1 Poisoning by stimulant laxatives, accidental (unintentional)
             Poisoning by stimulant laxatives NOS

         ✓7th T47.2x2 Poisoning by stimulant laxatives, intentional self-harm

         ✓7th T47.2x3 Poisoning by stimulant laxatives, assault

         ✓7th T47.2x4 Poisoning by stimulant laxatives, undetermined

         ✓7th T47.2x5 Adverse effect of stimulant laxatives

         ✓7th T47.2x6 Underdosing of stimulant laxatives

✓5th T47.3 Poisoning by, adverse effect of and underdosing of saline and osmotic laxatives

     ✓6th T47.3x Poisoning by and adverse effect of saline and osmotic laxatives

         ✓7th T47.3x1 Poisoning by saline and osmotic laxatives, accidental (unintentional)
             Poisoning by saline and osmotic laxatives NOS

         ✓7th T47.3x2 Poisoning by saline and osmotic laxatives, intentional self-harm

         ✓7th T47.3x3 Poisoning by saline and osmotic laxatives, assault

         ✓7th T47.3x4 Poisoning by saline and osmotic laxatives, undetermined

         ✓7th T47.3x5 Adverse effect of saline and osmotic laxatives

         ✓7th T47.3x6 Underdosing of saline and osmotic laxatives

✓5th T47.4 Poisoning by, adverse effect of and underdosing of other laxatives

     ✓6th T47.4x Poisoning by, adverse effect of and underdosing of other laxatives

         ✓7th T47.4x1 Poisoning by other laxatives, accidental (unintentional)
             Poisoning by other laxatives NOS

         ✓7th T47.4x2 Poisoning by other laxatives, intentional self-harm

         ✓7th T47.4x3 Poisoning by other laxatives, assault

         ✓7th T47.4x4 Poisoning by other laxatives, undetermined

         ✓7th T47.4x5 Adverse effect of other laxatives

         ✓7th T47.4x6 Underdosing of other laxatives

✓5th T47.5 Poisoning by, adverse effect of and underdosing of digestants

     ✓6th T47.5x Poisoning by, adverse effect of and underdosing of digestants

         ✓7th T47.5x1 Poisoning by digestants, accidental (unintentional)
             Poisoning by digestants NOS

         ✓7th T47.5x2 Poisoning by digestants, intentional self-harm

         ✓7th T47.5x3 Poisoning by digestants, assault

         ✓7th T47.5x4 Poisoning by digestants, undetermined

         ✓7th T47.5x5 Adverse effect of digestants

         ✓7th T47.5x6 Underdosing of digestants

✓5th T47.6 Poisoning by, adverse effect of and underdosing of antidiarrheal drugs

     EXCLUDES 2 *poisoning by, adverse effect of and underdosing of systemic antibiotics and other anti-infectives (T36-T37)*

     ✓6th T47.6x Poisoning by, adverse effect of and underdosing of antidiarrheal drugs

         ✓7th T47.6x1 Poisoning by antidiarrheal drugs, accidental (unintentional)
             Poisoning by antidiarrheal drugs NOS

         ✓7th T47.6x2 Poisoning by antidiarrheal drugs, intentional self-harm

         ✓7th T47.6x3 Poisoning by antidiarrheal drugs, assault

         ✓7th T47.6x4 Poisoning by antidiarrheal drugs, undetermined

         ✓7th T47.6x5 Adverse effect of antidiarrheal drugs

         ✓7th T47.6x6 Underdosing of antidiarrheal drugs

✓5th T47.7 Poisoning by, adverse effect of and underdosing of emetics

     ✓6th T47.7x Poisoning by, adverse effect of and underdosing of emetics

         ✓7th T47.7x1 Poisoning by emetics, accidental (unintentional)
             Poisoning by emetics NOS

         ✓7th T47.7x2 Poisoning by emetics, intentional self-harm

         ✓7th T47.7x3 Poisoning by emetics, assault

         ✓7th T47.7x4 Poisoning by emetics, undetermined

         ✓7th T47.7x5 Adverse effect of emetics

         ✓7th T47.7x6 Underdosing of emetics

✓5th T47.8 Poisoning by, adverse effect of and underdosing of other agents primarily affecting gastrointestinal system

     ✓6th T47.8x Poisoning by, adverse effect of and underdosing of other agents primarily affecting gastrointestinal system

         ✓7th T47.8x1 Poisoning by other agents primarily affecting gastrointestinal system, accidental (unintentional)
             Poisoning by other agents primarily affecting gastrointestinal system NOS

         ✓7th T47.8x2 Poisoning by other agents primarily affecting gastrointestinal system, intentional self-harm

         ✓7th T47.8x3 Poisoning by other agents primarily affecting gastrointestinal system, assault

         ✓7th T47.8x4 Poisoning by other agents primarily affecting gastrointestinal system, undetermined

         ✓7th T47.8x5 Adverse effect of other agents primarily affecting gastrointestinal system

         ✓7th T47.8x6 Underdosing of other agents primarily affecting gastrointestinal system

✓5th T47.9 Poisoning by, adverse effect of and underdosing of unspecified agents primarily affecting the gastrointestinal system

     ✓x7th T47.91 Poisoning by unspecified agents primarily affecting the gastrointestinal system, accidental (unintentional)
             Poisoning by agents primarily affecting the gastrointestinal system NOS

     ✓x7th T47.92 Poisoning by unspecified agents primarily affecting the gastrointestinal system, intentional self-harm

     ✓x7th T47.93 Poisoning by unspecified agents primarily affecting the gastrointestinal system, assault

     ✓x7th T47.94 Poisoning by unspecified agents primarily affecting the gastrointestinal system, undetermined

     ✓x7th T47.95 Adverse effect of unspecified agents primarily affecting the gastrointestinal system

     ✓x7th T47.96 Underdosing of unspecified agents primarily affecting the gastrointestinal system

✓4th T48 Poisoning by, adverse effect of and underdosing of agents primarily acting on smooth and skeletal muscles and the respiratory system

> The appropriate 7th character is to be added to each code from category T48.
> A   initial encounter
> D   subsequent encounter
> S   sequela

✓5th T48.0 Poisoning by, adverse effect of and underdosing of oxytocic drugs

     EXCLUDES 1 *poisoning by, adverse effect of and underdosing of estrogens, progestogens and antagonists (T38.4-T38.6)*

     ✓6th T48.0x Poisoning by, adverse effect of and underdosing of oxytocic drugs

         ✓7th T48.0x1 Poisoning by oxytocic drugs, accidental (unintentional)
             Poisoning by oxytocic drugs NOS

         ✓7th T48.0x2 Poisoning by oxytocic drugs, intentional self-harm

---

EXCLUDES 1 Not coded here   **EXCLUDES 2** Not included here   *Manifestation Code*

✓7th **T48.0x3** Poisoning by oxytocic drugs, assault
✓7th **T48.0x4** Poisoning by oxytocic drugs, undetermined
✓7th **T48.0x5** Adverse effect of oxytocic drugs
✓7th **T48.0x6** Underdosing of oxytocic drugs

✓5th **T48.1** Poisoning by, adverse effect of and underdosing of skeletal muscle relaxants [neuromuscular blocking agents]

✓6th **T48.1x** Poisoning by, adverse effect of and underdosing of skeletal muscle relaxants [neuromuscular blocking agents]

✓7th **T48.1x1** Poisoning by skeletal muscle relaxants [neuromuscular blocking agents], accidental (unintentional)
Poisoning by skeletal muscle relaxants [neuromuscular blocking agents] NOS

✓7th **T48.1x2** Poisoning by skeletal muscle relaxants [neuromuscular blocking agents], intentional self-harm

✓7th **T48.1x3** Poisoning by skeletal muscle relaxants [neuromuscular blocking agents], assault

✓7th **T48.1x4** Poisoning by skeletal muscle relaxants [neuromuscular blocking agents], undetermined

✓7th **T48.1x5** Adverse effect of skeletal muscle relaxants [neuromuscular blocking agents]

✓7th **T48.1x6** Underdosing of skeletal muscle relaxants [neuromuscular blocking agents]

✓5th **T48.2** Poisoning by, adverse effect of and underdosing of other and unspecified drugs acting on muscles

✓6th **T48.20** Poisoning by, adverse effect of and underdosing of unspecified drugs acting on muscles

✓7th **T48.201** Poisoning by unspecified drugs acting on muscles, accidental (unintentional)
Poisoning by unspecified drugs acting on muscles NOS

✓7th **T48.202** Poisoning by unspecified drugs acting on muscles, intentional self-harm

✓7th **T48.203** Poisoning by unspecified drugs acting on muscles, assault

✓7th **T48.204** Poisoning by unspecified drugs acting on muscles, undetermined

✓7th **T48.205** Adverse effect of unspecified drugs acting on muscles

✓7th **T48.206** Underdosing of unspecified drugs acting on muscles

✓6th **T48.29** Poisoning by, adverse effect of and underdosing of other drugs acting on muscles

✓7th **T48.291** Poisoning by other drugs acting on muscles, accidental (unintentional)
Poisoning by other drugs acting on muscles NOS

✓7th **T48.292** Poisoning by other drugs acting on muscles, intentional self-harm

✓7th **T48.293** Poisoning by other drugs acting on muscles, assault

✓7th **T48.294** Poisoning by other drugs acting on muscles, undetermined

✓7th **T48.295** Adverse effect of other drugs acting on muscles

✓7th **T48.296** Underdosing of other drugs acting on muscles

✓5th **T48.3** Poisoning by, adverse effect of and underdosing of antitussives

✓6th **T48.3x** Poisoning by, adverse effect of and underdosing of antitussives

✓7th **T48.3x1** Poisoning by antitussives, accidental (unintentional)
Poisoning by antitussives NOS

✓7th **T48.3x2** Poisoning by antitussives, intentional self-harm

✓7th **T48.3x3** Poisoning by antitussives, assault

✓7th **T48.3x4** Poisoning by antitussives, undetermined

✓7th **T48.3x5** Adverse effect of antitussives

✓7th **T48.3x6** Underdosing of antitussives

✓5th **T48.4** Poisoning by, adverse effect of and underdosing of expectorants

✓6th **T48.4x** Poisoning by, adverse effect of and underdosing of expectorants

✓7th **T48.4x1** Poisoning by expectorants, accidental (unintentional)
Poisoning by expectorants NOS

✓7th **T48.4x2** Poisoning by expectorants, intentional self-harm

✓7th **T48.4x3** Poisoning by expectorants, assault

✓7th **T48.4x4** Poisoning by expectorants, undetermined

✓7th **T48.4x5** Adverse effect of expectorants

✓7th **T48.4x6** Underdosing of expectorants

✓5th **T48.5** Poisoning by, adverse effect of and underdosing of other anti-common-cold drugs
Poisoning by, adverse effect of and underdosing of decongestants
EXCLUDES 2 poisoning by, adverse effect of and underdosing of antipyretics, NEC (T39.9-)
poisoning by, adverse effect of and underdosing of non-steroidal antiinflammatory drugs (T39.3-)
poisoning by, adverse effect of and underdosing of salicylates (T39.0-)

✓6th **T48.5x** Poisoning by, adverse effect of and underdosing of other anti-common-cold drugs

✓7th **T48.5x1** Poisoning by other anti-common-cold drugs, accidental (unintentional)
Poisoning by other anti-common-cold drugs NOS

✓7th **T48.5x2** Poisoning by other anti-common-cold drugs, intentional self-harm

✓7th **T48.5x3** Poisoning by other anti-common-cold drugs, assault

✓7th **T48.5x4** Poisoning by other anti-common-cold drugs, undetermined

✓7th **T48.5x5** Adverse effect of other anti-common-cold drugs

✓7th **T48.5x6** Underdosing of other anti-common-cold drugs

✓5th **T48.6** Poisoning by, adverse effect of and underdosing of antiasthmatics, not elsewhere classified
Poisoning by, adverse effect of and underdosing of beta-adrenoreceptor agonists used in asthma therapy
EXCLUDES 1 poisoning by, adverse effect of and underdosing of beta-adrenoreceptor agonists not used in asthma therapy (T44.5)
poisoning by, adverse effect of and underdosing of anterior pituitary [adenohypophyseal] hormones (T38.8)

✓6th **T48.6x** Poisoning by, adverse effect of and underdosing of antiasthmatics

✓7th **T48.6x1** Poisoning by antiasthmatics, accidental (unintentional)
Poisoning by antiasthmatics NOS

✓7th **T48.6x2** Poisoning by antiasthmatics, intentional self-harm

✓7th **T48.6x3** Poisoning by antiasthmatics, assault

✓7th **T48.6x4** Poisoning by antiasthmatics, undetermined

✓7th **T48.6x5** Adverse effect of antiasthmatics

✓7th **T48.6x6** Underdosing of antiasthmatics

✓5th **T48.9** Poisoning by, adverse effect of and underdosing of other and unspecified agents primarily acting on the respiratory system

✓6th **T48.90** Poisoning by, adverse effect of and underdosing of unspecified agents primarily acting on the respiratory system

✓7th **T48.901** Poisoning by unspecified agents primarily acting on the respiratory system, accidental (unintentional)

✓7th **T48.902** Poisoning by unspecified agents primarily acting on the respiratory system, intentional self-harm

✓7th **T48.903** Poisoning by unspecified agents primarily acting on the respiratory system, assault

  ✓7th **T48.904** Poisoning by unspecified agents primarily acting on the respiratory system, undetermined

  ✓7th **T48.905** Adverse effect of unspecified agents primarily acting on the respiratory system

  ✓7th **T48.906** Underdosing of unspecified agents primarily acting on the respiratory system

✓6th **T48.99** Poisoning by, adverse effect of and underdosing of other agents primarily acting on the respiratory system

  ✓7th **T48.991** Poisoning by other agents primarily acting on the respiratory system, accidental (unintentional)

  ✓7th **T48.992** Poisoning by other agents primarily acting on the respiratory system, intentional self-harm

  ✓7th **T48.993** Poisoning by other agents primarily acting on the respiratory system, assault

  ✓7th **T48.994** Poisoning by other agents primarily acting on the respiratory system, undetermined

  ✓7th **T48.995** Adverse effect of other agents primarily acting on the respiratory system

  ✓7th **T48.996** Underdosing of other agents primarily acting on the respiratory system

✓4th **T49** Poisoning by, adverse effect of and underdosing of topical agents primarily affecting skin and mucous membrane and by ophthalmological, otorhinolaryngological and dental drugs

Poisoning by, adverse effect of and underdosing of glucocorticoids, topically used

> The appropriate 7th character is to be added to each code from category T49.
> A   initial encounter
> D   subsequent encounter
> S   sequela

✓5th **T49.0** Poisoning by, adverse effect of and underdosing of local antifungal, anti-infective and anti-inflammatory drugs

✓6th **T49.0x** Poisoning by, adverse effect of and underdosing of local antifungal, anti-infective and anti-inflammatory drugs

  ✓7th **T49.0x1** Poisoning by local antifungal, anti-infective and anti-inflammatory drugs, accidental (unintentional)

Poisoning by local antifungal, anti-infective and anti-inflammatory drugs NOS

  ✓7th **T49.0x2** Poisoning by local antifungal, anti-infective and anti-inflammatory drugs, intentional self-harm

  ✓7th **T49.0x3** Poisoning by local antifungal, anti-infective and anti-inflammatory drugs, assault

  ✓7th **T49.0x4** Poisoning by local antifungal, anti-infective and anti-inflammatory drugs, undetermined

  ✓7th **T49.0x5** Adverse effect of local antifungal, anti-infective and anti-inflammatory drugs

  ✓7th **T49.0x6** Underdosing of local antifungal, anti-infective and anti-inflammatory drugs

✓5th **T49.1** Poisoning by, adverse effect of and underdosing of antipruritics

✓6th **T49.1x** Poisoning by, adverse effect of and underdosing of antipruritics

  ✓7th **T49.1x1** Poisoning by antipruritics, accidental (unintentional)

Poisoning by antipruritics NOS

  ✓7th **T49.1x2** Poisoning by antipruritics, intentional self-harm

  ✓7th **T49.1x3** Poisoning by antipruritics, assault

  ✓7th **T49.1x4** Poisoning by antipruritics, undetermined

  ✓7th **T49.1x5** Adverse effect of antipruritics

  ✓7th **T49.1x6** Underdosing of antipruritics

✓5th **T49.2** Poisoning by, adverse effect of and underdosing of local astringents and local detergents

✓6th **T49.2x** Poisoning by, adverse effect of and underdosing of local astringents and local detergents

  ✓7th **T49.2x1** Poisoning by local astringents and local detergents, accidental (unintentional)

Poisoning by local astringents and local detergents NOS

  ✓7th **T49.2x2** Poisoning by local astringents and local detergents, intentional self-harm

  ✓7th **T49.2x3** Poisoning by local astringents and local detergents, assault

  ✓7th **T49.2x4** Poisoning by local astringents and local detergents, undetermined

  ✓7th **T49.2x5** Adverse effect of local astringents and local detergents

  ✓7th **T49.2x6** Underdosing of local astringents and local detergents

✓5th **T49.3** Poisoning by, adverse effect of and underdosing of emollients, demulcents and protectants

✓6th **T49.3x** Poisoning by, adverse effect of and underdosing of emollients, demulcents and protectants

  ✓7th **T49.3x1** Poisoning by emollients, demulcents and protectants, accidental (unintentional)

Poisoning by emollients, demulcents and protectants NOS

  ✓7th **T49.3x2** Poisoning by emollients, demulcents and protectants, intentional self-harm

  ✓7th **T49.3x3** Poisoning by emollients, demulcents and protectants, assault

  ✓7th **T49.3x4** Poisoning by emollients, demulcents and protectants, undetermined

  ✓7th **T49.3x5** Adverse effect of emollients, demulcents and protectants

  ✓7th **T49.3x6** Underdosing of emollients, demulcents and protectants

✓5th **T49.4** Poisoning by, adverse effect of and underdosing of keratolytics, keratoplastics, and other hair treatment drugs and preparations

✓6th **T49.4x** Poisoning by, adverse effect of and underdosing of keratolytics, keratoplastics, and other hair treatment drugs and preparations

  ✓7th **T49.4x1** Poisoning by keratolytics, keratoplastics, and other hair treatment drugs and preparations, accidental (unintentional)

Poisoning by keratolytics, keratoplastics, and other hair treatment drugs and preparations NOS

  ✓7th **T49.4x2** Poisoning by keratolytics, keratoplastics, and other hair treatment drugs and preparations, intentional self-harm

  ✓7th **T49.4x3** Poisoning by keratolytics, keratoplastics, and other hair treatment drugs and preparations, assault

  ✓7th **T49.4x4** Poisoning by keratolytics, keratoplastics, and other hair treatment drugs and preparations, undetermined

  ✓7th **T49.4x5** Adverse effect of keratolytics, keratoplastics, and other hair treatment drugs and preparations

  ✓7th **T49.4x6** Underdosing of keratolytics, keratoplastics, and other hair treatment drugs and preparations

✓5th **T49.5** Poisoning by, adverse effect of and underdosing of ophthalmological drugs and preparations

✓6th **T49.5x** Poisoning by, adverse effect of and underdosing of ophthalmological drugs and preparations

  ✓7th **T49.5x1** Poisoning by ophthalmological drugs and preparations, accidental (unintentional)

Poisoning by ophthalmological drugs and preparations NOS

  ✓7th **T49.5x2** Poisoning by ophthalmological drugs and preparations, intentional self-harm

  ✓7th **T49.5x3** Poisoning by ophthalmological drugs and preparations, assault

---

EXCLUDES 1 Not coded here   EXCLUDES 2 Not included here   *Manifestation Code*

√7ᵗʰ **T49.5x4 Poisoning by ophthalmological drugs and preparations, undetermined**

√7ᵗʰ **T49.5x5 Adverse effect of ophthalmological drugs and preparations**

√7ᵗʰ **T49.5x6 Underdosing of ophthalmological drugs and preparations**

√5ᵗʰ **T49.6 Poisoning by, adverse effect of and underdosing of otorhinolaryngological drugs and preparations**

√6ᵗʰ **T49.6x Poisoning by, adverse effect of and underdosing of otorhinolaryngological drugs and preparations**

√7ᵗʰ **T49.6x1 Poisoning by otorhinolaryngological drugs and preparations, accidental (unintentional)**
Poisoning by otorhinolaryngological drugs and preparations NOS

√7ᵗʰ **T49.6x2 Poisoning by otorhinolaryngological drugs and preparations, intentional self-harm**

√7ᵗʰ **T49.6x3 Poisoning by otorhinolaryngological drugs and preparations, assault**

√7ᵗʰ **T49.6x4 Poisoning by otorhinolaryngological drugs and preparations, undetermined**

√7ᵗʰ **T49.6x5 Adverse effect of otorhinolaryngological drugs and preparations**

√7ᵗʰ **T49.6x6 Underdosing of otorhinolaryngological drugs and preparations**

√5ᵗʰ **T49.7 Poisoning by, adverse effect of and underdosing of dental drugs, topically applied**

√6ᵗʰ **T49.7x Poisoning by, adverse effect of and underdosing of dental drugs, topically applied**

√7ᵗʰ **T49.7x1 Poisoning by dental drugs, topically applied, accidental (unintentional)**
Poisoning by dental drugs, topically applied NOS

√7ᵗʰ **T49.7x2 Poisoning by dental drugs, topically applied, intentional self-harm**

√7ᵗʰ **T49.7x3 Poisoning by dental drugs, topically applied, assault**

√7ᵗʰ **T49.7x4 Poisoning by dental drugs, topically applied, undetermined**

√7ᵗʰ **T49.7x5 Adverse effect of dental drugs, topically applied**

√7ᵗʰ **T49.7x6 Underdosing of dental drugs, topically applied**

√5ᵗʰ **T49.8 Poisoning by, adverse effect of and underdosing of other topical agents**
Poisoning by, adverse effect of and underdosing of spermicides

√6ᵗʰ **T49.8x Poisoning by, adverse effect of and underdosing of other topical agents**

√7ᵗʰ **T49.8x1 Poisoning by other topical agents, accidental (unintentional)**
Poisoning by other topical agents NOS

√7ᵗʰ **T49.8x2 Poisoning by other topical agents, intentional self-harm**

√7ᵗʰ **T49.8x3 Poisoning by other topical agents, assault**

√7ᵗʰ **T49.8x4 Poisoning by other topical agents, undetermined**

√7ᵗʰ **T49.8x5 Adverse effect of other topical agents**

√7ᵗʰ **T49.8x6 Underdosing of other topical agents**

√5ᵗʰ **T49.9 Poisoning by, adverse effect of and underdosing of unspecified topical agent**

√x7ᵗʰ **T49.91 Poisoning by unspecified topical agent, accidental (unintentional)**

√x7ᵗʰ **T49.92 Poisoning by unspecified topical agent, intentional self-harm**

√x7ᵗʰ **T49.93 Poisoning by unspecified topical agent, assault**

√x7ᵗʰ **T49.94 Poisoning by unspecified topical agent, undetermined**

√x7ᵗʰ **T49.95 Adverse effect of unspecified topical agent**

√x7ᵗʰ **T49.96 Underdosing of unspecified topical agent**

√4ᵗʰ **T50 Poisoning by, adverse effect of and underdosing of diuretics and other and unspecified drugs, medicaments and biological substances**

> The appropriate 7th character is to be added to each code from category T50.
> A   initial encounter
> D   subsequent encounter
> S   sequela

√5ᵗʰ **T50.0 Poisoning by, adverse effect of and underdosing of mineralocorticoids and their antagonists**

√6ᵗʰ **T50.0x Poisoning by, adverse effect of and underdosing of mineralocorticoids and their antagonists**

√7ᵗʰ **T50.0x1 Poisoning by mineralocorticoids and their antagonists, accidental (unintentional)**
Poisoning by mineralocorticoids and their antagonists NOS

√7ᵗʰ **T50.0x2 Poisoning by mineralocorticoids and their antagonists, intentional self-harm**

√7ᵗʰ **T50.0x3 Poisoning by mineralocorticoids and their antagonists, assault**

√7ᵗʰ **T50.0x4 Poisoning by mineralocorticoids and their antagonists, undetermined**

√7ᵗʰ **T50.0x5 Adverse effect of mineralocorticoids and their antagonists**

√7ᵗʰ **T50.0x6 Underdosing of mineralocorticoids and their antagonists**

√5ᵗʰ **T50.1 Poisoning by, adverse effect of and underdosing of loop [high-ceiling] diuretics**

√6ᵗʰ **T50.1x Poisoning by, adverse effect of and underdosing of loop [high-ceiling] diuretics**

√7ᵗʰ **T50.1x1 Poisoning by loop [high-ceiling] diuretics, accidental (unintentional)**
Poisoning by loop [high-ceiling] diuretics NOS

√7ᵗʰ **T50.1x2 Poisoning by loop [high-ceiling] diuretics, intentional self-harm**

√7ᵗʰ **T50.1x3 Poisoning by loop [high-ceiling] diuretics, assault**

√7ᵗʰ **T50.1x4 Poisoning by loop [high-ceiling] diuretics, undetermined**

√7ᵗʰ **T50.1x5 Adverse effect of loop [high-ceiling] diuretics**

√7ᵗʰ **T50.1x6 Underdosing of loop [high-ceiling] diuretics**

√5ᵗʰ **T50.2 Poisoning by, adverse effect of and underdosing of carbonic-anhydrase inhibitors, benzothiadiazides and other diuretics**
Poisoning by, adverse effect of and underdosing of acetazolamide

√6ᵗʰ **T50.2x Poisoning by, adverse effect of and underdosing of carbonic-anhydrase inhibitors, benzothiadiazides and other diuretics**

√7ᵗʰ **T50.2x1 Poisoning by carbonic-anhydrase inhibitors, benzothiadiazides and other diuretics, accidental (unintentional)**
Poisoning by carbonic-anhydrase inhibitors, benzothiadiazides and other diuretics NOS

√7ᵗʰ **T50.2x2 Poisoning by carbonic-anhydrase inhibitors, benzothiadiazides and other diuretics, intentional self-harm**

√7ᵗʰ **T50.2x3 Poisoning by carbonic-anhydrase inhibitors, benzothiadiazides and other diuretics, assault**

√7ᵗʰ **T50.2x4 Poisoning by carbonic-anhydrase inhibitors, benzothiadiazides and other diuretics, undetermined**

√7ᵗʰ **T50.2x5 Adverse effect of carbonic-anhydrase inhibitors, benzothiadiazides and other diuretics**

√7ᵗʰ **T50.2x6 Underdosing of carbonic-anhydrase inhibitors, benzothiadiazides and other diuretics**

☑ Appropriate additional character required   √x7ᵗʰ Requires 7th character, placeholder x must fill empty characters

✓5th **T50.3** **Poisoning by, adverse effect of and underdosing of electrolytic, caloric and water-balance agents**
> Poisoning by, adverse effect of and underdosing of oral rehydration salts

    ✓6th **T50.3x** **Poisoning by, adverse effect of and underdosing of electrolytic, caloric and water-balance agents**

        ✓7th **T50.3x1** **Poisoning by electrolytic, caloric and water-balance agents, accidental (unintentional)**
> Poisoning by electrolytic, caloric and water-balance agents NOS

        ✓7th **T50.3x2** **Poisoning by electrolytic, caloric and water-balance agents, intentional self-harm**

        ✓7th **T50.3x3** **Poisoning by electrolytic, caloric and water-balance agents, assault**

        ✓7th **T50.3x4** **Poisoning by electrolytic, caloric and water-balance agents, undetermined**

        ✓7th **T50.3x5** **Adverse effect of electrolytic, caloric and water-balance agents**

        ✓7th **T50.3x6** **Underdosing of electrolytic, caloric and water-balance agents**

✓5th **T50.4** **Poisoning by, adverse effect of and underdosing of drugs affecting uric acid metabolism**

    ✓6th **T50.4x** **Poisoning by, adverse effect of and underdosing of drugs affecting uric acid metabolism**

        ✓7th **T50.4x1** **Poisoning by drugs affecting uric acid metabolism, accidental (unintentional)**
> Poisoning by drugs affecting uric acid metabolism NOS

        ✓7th **T50.4x2** **Poisoning by drugs affecting uric acid metabolism, intentional self-harm**

        ✓7th **T50.4x3** **Poisoning by drugs affecting uric acid metabolism, assault**

        ✓7th **T50.4x4** **Poisoning by drugs affecting uric acid metabolism, undetermined**

        ✓7th **T50.4x5** **Adverse effect of drugs affecting uric acid metabolism**

        ✓7th **T50.4x6** **Underdosing of drugs affecting uric acid metabolism**

✓5th **T50.5** **Poisoning by, adverse effect of and underdosing of appetite depressants**

    ✓6th **T50.5x** **Poisoning by, adverse effect of and underdosing of appetite depressants**

        ✓7th **T50.5x1** **Poisoning by appetite depressants, accidental (unintentional)**
> Poisoning by appetite depressants NOS

        ✓7th **T50.5x2** **Poisoning by appetite depressants, intentional self-harm**

        ✓7th **T50.5x3** **Poisoning by appetite depressants, assault**

        ✓7th **T50.5x4** **Poisoning by appetite depressants, undetermined**

        ✓7th **T50.5x5** **Adverse effect of appetite depressants**

        ✓7th **T50.5x6** **Underdosing of appetite depressants**

✓5th **T50.6** **Poisoning by, adverse effect of and underdosing of antidotes and chelating agents**
> Poisoning by, adverse effect of and underdosing of alcohol deterrents

    ✓6th **T50.6x** **Poisoning by, adverse effect of and underdosing of antidotes and chelating agents**

        ✓7th **T50.6x1** **Poisoning by antidotes and chelating agents, accidental (unintentional)**
> Poisoning by antidotes and chelating agents NOS

        ✓7th **T50.6x2** **Poisoning by antidotes and chelating agents, intentional self-harm**

        ✓7th **T50.6x3** **Poisoning by antidotes and chelating agents, assault**

        ✓7th **T50.6x4** **Poisoning by antidotes and chelating agents, undetermined**

        ✓7th **T50.6x5** **Adverse effect of antidotes and chelating agents**

        ✓7th **T50.6x6** **Underdosing of antidotes and chelating agents**

✓5th **T50.7** **Poisoning by, adverse effect of and underdosing of analeptics and opioid receptor antagonists**

    ✓6th **T50.7x** **Poisoning by, adverse effect of and underdosing of analeptics and opioid receptor antagonists**

        ✓7th **T50.7x1** **Poisoning by analeptics and opioid receptor antagonists, accidental (unintentional)**
> Poisoning by analeptics and opioid receptor antagonists NOS

        ✓7th **T50.7x2** **Poisoning by analeptics and opioid receptor antagonists, intentional self-harm**

        ✓7th **T50.7x3** **Poisoning by analeptics and opioid receptor antagonists, assault**

        ✓7th **T50.7x4** **Poisoning by analeptics and opioid receptor antagonists, undetermined**

        ✓7th **T50.7x5** **Adverse effect of analeptics and opioid receptor antagonists**

        ✓7th **T50.7x6** **Underdosing of analeptics and opioid receptor antagonists**

✓5th **T50.8** **Poisoning by, adverse effect of and underdosing of diagnostic agents**

    ✓6th **T50.8x** **Poisoning by, adverse effect of and underdosing of diagnostic agents**

        ✓7th **T50.8x1** **Poisoning by diagnostic agents, accidental (unintentional)**
> Poisoning by diagnostic agents NOS

        ✓7th **T50.8x2** **Poisoning by diagnostic agents, intentional self-harm**

        ✓7th **T50.8x3** **Poisoning by diagnostic agents, assault**

        ✓7th **T50.8x4** **Poisoning by diagnostic agents, undetermined**

        ✓7th **T50.8x5** **Adverse effect of diagnostic agents**

        ✓7th **T50.8x6** **Underdosing of diagnostic agents**

✓5th **T50.a** **Poisoning by, adverse effect of and underdosing of bacterial vaccines**

    ✓6th **T50.a1** **Poisoning by, adverse effect of and underdosing of pertussis vaccine, including combinations with a pertussis component**

        ✓7th **T50.a11** **Poisoning by pertussis vaccine, including combinations with a pertussis component, accidental (unintentional)**

        ✓7th **T50.a12** **Poisoning by pertussis vaccine, including combinations with a pertussis component, intentional self-harm**

        ✓7th **T50.a13** **Poisoning by pertussis vaccine, including combinations with a pertussis component, assault**

        ✓7th **T50.a14** **Poisoning by pertussis vaccine, including combinations with a pertussis component, undetermined**

        ✓7th **T50.a15** **Adverse effect of pertussis vaccine, including combinations with a pertussis component**

        ✓7th **T50.a16** **Underdosing of pertussis vaccine, including combinations with a pertussis component**

    ✓6th **T50.a2** **Poisoning by, adverse effect of and underdosing of mixed bacterial vaccines without a pertussis component**

        ✓7th **T50.a21** **Poisoning by mixed bacterial vaccines without a pertussis component, accidental (unintentional)**

        ✓7th **T50.a22** **Poisoning by mixed bacterial vaccines without a pertussis component, intentional self-harm**

        ✓7th **T50.a23** **Poisoning by mixed bacterial vaccines without a pertussis component, assault**

        ✓7th **T50.a24** **Poisoning by mixed bacterial vaccines without a pertussis component, undetermined**

        ✓7th **T50.a25** **Adverse effect of mixed bacterial vaccines without a pertussis component**

        ✓7th **T50.a26** **Underdosing of mixed bacterial vaccines without a pertussis component**

EXCLUDES 1 Not coded here   **EXCLUDES 2** Not included here   *Manifestation Code*

√6th **T50.a9** **Poisoning by, adverse effect of and underdosing of other bacterial vaccines**

√7th T50.a91 Poisoning by other bacterial vaccines, accidental (unintentional)

√7th T50.a92 Poisoning by other bacterial vaccines, intentional self-harm

√7th T50.a93 Poisoning by other bacterial vaccines, assault

√7th T50.a94 Poisoning by other bacterial vaccines, undetermined

√7th T50.a95 Adverse effect of other bacterial vaccines

√7th T50.a96 Underdosing of other bacterial vaccines

√5th **T50.b** **Poisoning by, adverse effect of and underdosing of viral vaccines**

√6th **T50.b1** **Poisoning by, adverse effect of and underdosing of smallpox vaccines**

√7th T50.b11 Poisoning by smallpox vaccines, accidental (unintentional)

√7th T50.b12 Poisoning by smallpox vaccines, intentional self-harm

√7th T50.b13 Poisoning by smallpox vaccines, assault

√7th T50.b14 Poisoning by smallpox vaccines, undetermined

√7th T50.b15 Adverse effect of smallpox vaccines

√7th T50.b16 Underdosing of smallpox vaccines

√6th **T50.b9** **Poisoning by, adverse effect of and underdosing of other viral vaccines**

√7th T50.b91 Poisoning by other viral vaccines, accidental (unintentional)

√7th T50.b92 Poisoning by other viral vaccines, intentional self-harm

√7th T50.b93 Poisoning by other viral vaccines, assault

√7th T50.b94 Poisoning by other viral vaccines, undetermined

√7th T50.b95 Adverse effect of other viral vaccines

√7th T50.b96 Underdosing of other viral vaccines

√5th **T50.z** **Poisoning by, adverse effect of and underdosing of other vaccines and biological substances**

√6th **T50.z1** **Poisoning by, adverse effect of and underdosing of immunoglobulin**

√7th T50.z11 Poisoning by immunoglobulin, accidental (unintentional)

√7th T50.z12 Poisoning by immunoglobulin, intentional self-harm

√7th T50.z13 Poisoning by immunoglobulin, assault

√7th T50.z14 Poisoning by immunoglobulin, undetermined

√7th T50.z15 Adverse effect of immunoglobulin

√7th T50.z16 Underdosing of immunoglobulin

√6th **T50.z9** **Poisoning by, adverse effect of and underdosing of other vaccines and biological substances**

√7th T50.z91 Poisoning by other vaccines and biological substances, accidental (unintentional)

√7th T50.z92 Poisoning by other vaccines and biological substances, intentional self-harm

√7th T50.z93 Poisoning by other vaccines and biological substances, assault

√7th T50.z94 Poisoning by other vaccines and biological substances, undetermined

√7th T50.z95 Adverse effect of other vaccines and biological substances

√7th T50.z96 Underdosing of other vaccines and biological substances

√5th **T50.9** **Poisoning by, adverse effect of and underdosing of other and unspecified drugs, medicaments and biological substances**

√6th **T50.90** **Poisoning by, adverse effect of and underdosing of unspecified drugs, medicaments and biological substances**

√7th T50.901 Poisoning by unspecified drugs, medicaments and biological substances, accidental (unintentional)

√7th T50.902 Poisoning by unspecified drugs, medicaments and biological substances, intentional self-harm

√7th T50.903 Poisoning by unspecified drugs, medicaments and biological substances, assault

√7th T50.904 Poisoning by unspecified drugs, medicaments and biological substances, undetermined

√7th T50.905 Adverse effect of unspecified drugs, medicaments and biological substances

√7th T50.906 Underdosing of unspecified drugs, medicaments and biological substances

√6th **T50.99** **Poisoning by, adverse effect of and underdosing of other drugs, medicaments and biological substances**

√7th T50.991 Poisoning by other drugs, medicaments and biological substances, accidental (unintentional)

√7th T50.992 Poisoning by other drugs, medicaments and biological substances, intentional self-harm

√7th T50.993 Poisoning by other drugs, medicaments and biological substances, assault

√7th T50.994 Poisoning by other drugs, medicaments and biological substances, undetermined

√7th T50.995 Adverse effect of other drugs, medicaments and biological substances

√7th T50.996 Underdosing of other drugs, medicaments and biological substances

Toxic effects of substances chiefly nonmedicinal as to source (T51-T65)

Use additional code(s) for all associated manifestations of toxic effect, such as:
personal history of foreign body fully removed (Z87.821)
respiratory conditions due to external agents (J60-J70)
to identify any retained foreign body, if applicable (Z18.-)

NOTE   When no intent is indicated code to accidental. Undetermined intent is only for use when there is specific documentation in the record that the intent of the toxic effect cannot be determined

EXCLUDES 1 contact with and (suspected) exposure to toxic substances (Z77-)

√4th **T51** **Toxic effect of alcohol**

> The appropriate 7th character is to be added to each code from category T51.
> A   initial encounter
> D   subsequent encounter
> S   sequela

√5th **T51.0** **Toxic effect of ethanol**
Toxic effect of ethyl alcohol
EXCLUDES 2 acute alcohol intoxication or 'hangover' effects (F10.129, F10.229, F10.929)
drunkenness (F10.129, F10.229, F10.929)
pathological alcohol intoxication (F10.129, F10.229, F10.929)

√6th **T51.0x** **Toxic effect of ethanol**

√7th T51.0x1 Toxic effect of ethanol, accidental (unintentional)
Toxic effect of ethanol NOS

√7th T51.0x2 Toxic effect of ethanol, intentional self-harm

√7th T51.0x3 Toxic effect of ethanol, assault

√7th T51.0x4 Toxic effect of ethanol, undetermined

√5th **T51.1** **Toxic effect of methanol**
Toxic effect of methyl alcohol

√6th **T51.1x** **Toxic effect of methanol**

√7th T51.1x1 Toxic effect of methanol, accidental (unintentional)
Toxic effect of methanol NOS

√7th T51.1x2 Toxic effect of methanol, intentional self-harm

√7th T51.1x3 Toxic effect of methanol, assault

√7th T51.1x4 Toxic effect of methanol, undetermined

✓5th **T51.2   Toxic effect of 2-Propanol**
    Toxic effect of isopropyl alcohol

   ✓6th **T51.2x   Toxic effect of 2-Propanol**

     ✓7th **T51.2x1   Toxic effect of 2-Propanol, accidental (unintentional)**
        Toxic effect of 2-Propanol NOS

     ✓7th **T51.2x2   Toxic effect of 2-Propanol, intentional self-harm**

     ✓7th **T51.2x3   Toxic effect of 2-Propanol, assault**

     ✓7th **T51.2x4   Toxic effect of 2-Propanol, undetermined**

✓5th **T51.3   Toxic effect of fusel oil**
    Toxic effect of amyl alcohol
    Toxic effect of butyl [1-butanol] alcohol
    Toxic effect of propyl [1-propanol] alcohol

   ✓6th **T51.3x   Toxic effect of fusel oil**

     ✓7th **T51.3x1   Toxic effect of fusel oil, accidental (unintentional)**
        Toxic effect of fusel oil NOS

     ✓7th **T51.3x2   Toxic effect of fusel oil, intentional self-harm**

     ✓7th **T51.3x3   Toxic effect of fusel oil, assault**

     ✓7th **T51.3x4   Toxic effect of fusel oil, undetermined**

✓5th **T51.8   Toxic effect of other alcohols**

   ✓6th **T51.8x   Toxic effect of other alcohols**

     ✓7th **T51.8x1   Toxic effect of other alcohols, accidental (unintentional)**
        Toxic effect of other alcohols NOS

     ✓7th **T51.8x2   Toxic effect of other alcohols, intentional self-harm**

     ✓7th **T51.8x3   Toxic effect of other alcohols, assault**

     ✓7th **T51.8x4   Toxic effect of other alcohols, undetermined**

✓5th **T51.9   Toxic effect of unspecified alcohol**

   ✓x7th **T51.91   Toxic effect of unspecified alcohol, accidental (unintentional)**

   ✓x7th **T51.92   Toxic effect of unspecified alcohol, intentional self-harm**

   ✓x7th **T51.93   Toxic effect of unspecified alcohol, assault**

   ✓x7th **T51.94   Toxic effect of unspecified alcohol, undetermined**

✓4th **T52   Toxic effect of organic solvents**

   EXCLUDES 1   *halogen derivatives of aliphatic and aromatic hydrocarbons (T53-)*

   The appropriate 7th character is to be added to each code from category T52.
    A   initial encounter
    D   subsequent encounter
    S   sequela

  ✓5th **T52.0   Toxic effects of petroleum products**
    Toxic effects of gasoline [petrol]
    Toxic effects of kerosene [paraffin oil]
    Toxic effects of paraffin wax
    Toxic effects of ether petroleum
    Toxic effects of naphtha petroleum
    Toxic effects of spirit petroleum

   ✓6th **T52.0x   Toxic effects of petroleum products**

     ✓7th **T52.0x1   Toxic effect of petroleum products, accidental (unintentional)**
        Toxic effects of petroleum products NOS

     ✓7th **T52.0x2   Toxic effect of petroleum products, intentional self-harm**

     ✓7th **T52.0x3   Toxic effect of petroleum products, assault**

     ✓7th **T52.0x4   Toxic effect of petroleum products, undetermined**

  ✓5th **T52.1   Toxic effects of benzene**

   EXCLUDES 1   *homologues of benzene (T52.2)*
       nitroderivatives and aminoderivatives of benzene and its homologues (T65.3)

   ✓6th **T52.1x   Toxic effects of benzene**

     ✓7th **T52.1x1   Toxic effect of benzene, accidental (unintentional)**
        Toxic effects of benzene NOS

     ✓7th **T52.1x2   Toxic effect of benzene, intentional self-harm**

     ✓7th **T52.1x3   Toxic effect of benzene, assault**

     ✓7th **T52.1x4   Toxic effect of benzene, undetermined**

✓5th **T52.2   Toxic effects of homologues of benzene**
    Toxic effects of toluene [methylbenzene]
    Toxic effects of xylene [dimethylbenzene]

   ✓6th **T52.2x   Toxic effects of homologues of benzene**

     ✓7th **T52.2x1   Toxic effects of homologues of benzene, accidental (unintentional)**
        Toxic effects of homologues of benzene NOS

     ✓7th **T52.2x2   Toxic effects of homologues of benzene, intentional self-harm**

     ✓7th **T52.2x3   Toxic effect of homologues of benzene, assault**

     ✓7th **T52.2x4   Toxic effect of homologues of benzene, undetermined**

✓5th **T52.3   Toxic effects of glycols**

   ✓6th **T52.3x   Toxic effects of glycols**

     ✓7th **T52.3x1   Toxic effect of glycols, accidental (unintentional)**
        Toxic effects of glycols NOS

     ✓7th **T52.3x2   Toxic effect of glycols, intentional self-harm**

     ✓7th **T52.3x3   Toxic effect of glycols, assault**

     ✓7th **T52.3x4   Toxic effect of glycols, undetermined**

✓5th **T52.4   Toxic effects of ketones**

   ✓6th **T52.4x   Toxic effects of ketones**

     ✓7th **T52.4x1   Toxic effect of ketones, accidental (unintentional)**
        Toxic effects of ketones NOS

     ✓7th **T52.4x2   Toxic effect of ketones, intentional self-harm**

     ✓7th **T52.4x3   Toxic effect of ketones, assault**

     ✓7th **T52.4x4   Toxic effect of ketones, undetermined**

✓5th **T52.8   Toxic effects of other organic solvents**

   ✓6th **T52.8x   Toxic effect of other organic solvents**

     ✓7th **T52.8x1   Toxic effect of other organic solvents, accidental (unintentional)**
        Toxic effects of other organic solvents NOS

     ✓7th **T52.8x2   Toxic effect of other organic solvents, intentional self-harm**

     ✓7th **T52.8x3   Toxic effect of other organic solvents, assault**

     ✓7th **T52.8x4   Toxic effect of other organic solvents, undetermined**

✓5th **T52.9   Toxic effects of unspecified organic solvent**

   ✓x7th **T52.91   Toxic effect of unspecified organic solvent, accidental (unintentional)**

   ✓x7th **T52.92   Toxic effect of unspecified organic solvent, intentional self-harm**

   ✓x7th **T52.93   Toxic effect of unspecified organic solvent, assault**

   ✓x7th **T52.94   Toxic effect of unspecified organic solvent, undetermined**

✓4th **T53   Toxic effect of halogen derivatives of aliphatic and aromatic hydrocarbons**

   The appropriate 7th character is to be added to each code from category T53.
    A   initial encounter
    D   subsequent encounter
    S   sequela

  ✓5th **T53.0   Toxic effects of carbon tetrachloride**
    Toxic effects of tetrachloromethane

   ✓6th **T53.0x   Toxic effects of carbon tetrachloride**

     ✓7th **T53.0x1   Toxic effect of carbon tetrachloride, accidental (unintentional)**
        Toxic effects of carbon tetrachloride NOS

     ✓7th **T53.0x2   Toxic effect of carbon tetrachloride, intentional self-harm**

     ✓7th **T53.0x3   Toxic effect of carbon tetrachloride, assault**

     ✓7th **T53.0x4   Toxic effect of carbon tetrachloride, undetermined**

EXCLUDES 1 Not coded here   EXCLUDES 2 Not included here   *Manifestation Code*

☑5ᵗʰ **T53.1** **Toxic effects of chloroform**
Toxic effects of trichloromethane

     ☑6ᵗʰ **T53.1x** **Toxic effects of chloroform**

         ☑7ᵗʰ **T53.1x1** **Toxic effect of chloroform, accidental (unintentional)**
Toxic effects of chloroform NOS

         ☑7ᵗʰ **T53.1x2** **Toxic effect of chloroform, intentional self-harm**

         ☑7ᵗʰ **T53.1x3** **Toxic effect of chloroform, assault**

         ☑7ᵗʰ **T53.1x4** **Toxic effect of chloroform, undetermined**

☑5ᵗʰ **T53.2** **Toxic effects of trichloroethylene**
Toxic effects of trichloroethene

     ☑6ᵗʰ **T53.2x** **Toxic effects of trichloroethylene**

         ☑7ᵗʰ **T53.2x1** **Toxic effect of trichloroethylene, accidental (unintentional)**
Toxic effects of trichloroethylene NOS

         ☑7ᵗʰ **T53.2x2** **Toxic effect of trichloroethylene, intentional self-harm**

         ☑7ᵗʰ **T53.2x3** **Toxic effect of trichloroethylene, assault**

         ☑7ᵗʰ **T53.2x4** **Toxic effect of trichloroethylene, undetermined**

☑5ᵗʰ **T53.3** **Toxic effects of tetrachloroethylene**
Toxic effects of perchloroethylene
Toxic effect of tetrachloroethene

     ☑6ᵗʰ **T53.3x** **Toxic effects of tetrachloroethylene**

         ☑7ᵗʰ **T53.3x1** **Toxic effect of tetrachloroethylene, accidental (unintentional)**
Toxic effects of tetrachloroethylene NOS

         ☑7ᵗʰ **T53.3x2** **Toxic effect of tetrachloroethylene, intentional self-harm**

         ☑7ᵗʰ **T53.3x3** **Toxic effect of tetrachloroethylene, assault**

         ☑7ᵗʰ **T53.3x4** **Toxic effect of tetrachloroethylene, undetermined**

☑5ᵗʰ **T53.4** **Toxic effects of dichloromethane**
Toxic effects of methylene chloride

     ☑6ᵗʰ **T53.4x** **Toxic effects of dichloromethane**

         ☑7ᵗʰ **T53.4x1** **Toxic effect of dichloromethane, accidental (unintentional)**
Toxic effects of dichloromethane NOS

         ☑7ᵗʰ **T53.4x2** **Toxic effect of dichloromethane, intentional self-harm**

         ☑7ᵗʰ **T53.4x3** **Toxic effect of dichloromethane, assault**

         ☑7ᵗʰ **T53.4x4** **Toxic effect of dichloromethane, undetermined**

☑5ᵗʰ **T53.5** **Toxic effects of chlorofluorocarbons**

     ☑6ᵗʰ **T53.5x** **Toxic effects of chlorofluorocarbons**

         ☑7ᵗʰ **T53.5x1** **Toxic effect of chlorofluorocarbons, accidental (unintentional)**
Toxic effects of chlorofluorocarbons NOS

         ☑7ᵗʰ **T53.5x2** **Toxic effect of chlorofluorocarbons, intentional self-harm**

         ☑7ᵗʰ **T53.5x3** **Toxic effect of chlorofluorocarbons, assault**

         ☑7ᵗʰ **T53.5x4** **Toxic effect of chlorofluorocarbons, undetermined**

☑5ᵗʰ **T53.6** **Toxic effects of other halogen derivatives of aliphatic hydrocarbons**

     ☑6ᵗʰ **T53.6x** **Toxic effects of other halogen derivatives of aliphatic hydrocarbons**

         ☑7ᵗʰ **T53.6x1** **Toxic effect of other halogen derivatives of aliphatic hydrocarbons, accidental (unintentional)**
Toxic effects of other halogen derivatives of aliphatic hydrocarbons NOS

         ☑7ᵗʰ **T53.6x2** **Toxic effect of other halogen derivatives of aliphatic hydrocarbons, intentional self-harm**

         ☑7ᵗʰ **T53.6x3** **Toxic effect of other halogen derivatives of aliphatic hydrocarbons, assault**

         ☑7ᵗʰ **T53.6x4** **Toxic effect of other halogen derivatives of aliphatic hydrocarbons, undetermined**

☑5ᵗʰ **T53.7** **Toxic effects of other halogen derivatives of aromatic hydrocarbons**

     ☑6ᵗʰ **T53.7x** **Toxic effects of other halogen derivatives of aromatic hydrocarbons**

         ☑7ᵗʰ **T53.7x1** **Toxic effect of other halogen derivatives of aromatic hydrocarbons, accidental (unintentional)**
Toxic effects of other halogen derivatives of aromatic hydrocarbons NOS

         ☑7ᵗʰ **T53.7x2** **Toxic effect of other halogen derivatives of aromatic hydrocarbons, intentional self-harm**

         ☑7ᵗʰ **T53.7x3** **Toxic effect of other halogen derivatives of aromatic hydrocarbons, assault**

         ☑7ᵗʰ **T53.7x4** **Toxic effect of other halogen derivatives of aromatic hydrocarbons, undetermined**

☑5ᵗʰ **T53.9** **Toxic effects of unspecified halogen derivatives of aliphatic and aromatic hydrocarbons**

     ☑x7ᵗʰ **T53.91** **Toxic effect of unspecified halogen derivatives of aliphatic and aromatic hydrocarbons, accidental (unintentional)**

     ☑x7ᵗʰ **T53.92** **Toxic effect of unspecified halogen derivatives of aliphatic and aromatic hydrocarbons, intentional self-harm**

     ☑x7ᵗʰ **T53.93** **Toxic effect of unspecified halogen derivatives of aliphatic and aromatic hydrocarbons, assault**

     ☑x7ᵗʰ **T53.94** **Toxic effect of unspecified halogen derivatives of aliphatic and aromatic hydrocarbons, undetermined**

☑4ᵗʰ **T54** **Toxic effect of corrosive substances**

> The appropriate 7th character is to be added to each code from category T54.
> A   initial encounter
> D   subsequent encounter
> S   sequela

☑5ᵗʰ **T54.0** **Toxic effects of phenol and phenol homologues**

     ☑6ᵗʰ **T54.0x** **Toxic effects of phenol and phenol homologues**

         ☑7ᵗʰ **T54.0x1** **Toxic effect of phenol and phenol homologues, accidental (unintentional)**
Toxic effects of phenol and phenol homologues NOS

         ☑7ᵗʰ **T54.0x2** **Toxic effect of phenol and phenol homologues, intentional self-harm**

         ☑7ᵗʰ **T54.0x3** **Toxic effect of phenol and phenol homologues, assault**

         ☑7ᵗʰ **T54.0x4** **Toxic effect of phenol and phenol homologues, undetermined**

☑5ᵗʰ **T54.1** **Toxic effects of other corrosive organic compounds**

     ☑6ᵗʰ **T54.1x** **Toxic effects of other corrosive organic compounds**

         ☑7ᵗʰ **T54.1x1** **Toxic effect of other corrosive organic compounds, accidental (unintentional)**
Toxic effects of other corrosive organic compounds NOS

         ☑7ᵗʰ **T54.1x2** **Toxic effect of other corrosive organic compounds, intentional self-harm**

         ☑7ᵗʰ **T54.1x3** **Toxic effect of other corrosive organic compounds, assault**

         ☑7ᵗʰ **T54.1x4** **Toxic effect of other corrosive organic compounds, undetermined**

☑5ᵗʰ **T54.2** **Toxic effects of corrosive acids and acid-like substances**
Toxic effects of hydrochloric acid
Toxic effects of sulfuric acid

     ☑6ᵗʰ **T54.2x** **Toxic effects of corrosive acids and acid-like substances**

         ☑7ᵗʰ **T54.2x1** **Toxic effect of corrosive acids and acid-like substances, accidental (unintentional)**
Toxic effects of corrosive acids and acid-like substances NOS

         ☑7ᵗʰ **T54.2x2** **Toxic effect of corrosive acids and acid-like substances, intentional self-harm**

         ☑7ᵗʰ **T54.2x3** **Toxic effect of corrosive acids and acid-like substances, assault**

√7th **T54.2x4** Toxic effect of corrosive acids and acid-like substances, undetermined

√5th **T54.3** **Toxic effects of corrosive alkalis and alkali-like substances**
Toxic effects of potassium hydroxide
Toxic effects of sodium hydroxide

√6th **T54.3x** **Toxic effects of corrosive alkalis and alkali-like substances**

√7th **T54.3x1** **Toxic effect of corrosive alkalis and alkali-like substances, accidental (unintentional)**
Toxic effects of corrosive alkalis and alkali-like substances NOS

√7th **T54.3x2** **Toxic effect of corrosive alkalis and alkali-like substances, intentional self-harm**

√7th **T54.3x3** **Toxic effect of corrosive alkalis and alkali-like substances, assault**

√7th **T54.3x4** **Toxic effect of corrosive alkalis and alkali-like substances, undetermined**

√5th **T54.9** **Toxic effects of unspecified corrosive substance**

√x7th **T54.91** **Toxic effect of unspecified corrosive substance, accidental (unintentional)**

√x7th **T54.92** **Toxic effect of unspecified corrosive substance, intentional self-harm**

√x7th **T54.93** **Toxic effect of unspecified corrosive substance, assault**

√x7th **T54.94** **Toxic effect of unspecified corrosive substance, undetermined**

√4th **T55** **Toxic effect of soaps and detergents**

> The appropriate 7th character is to be added to each code from category T55.
> A   initial encounter
> D   subsequent encounter
> S   sequela

√5th **T55.0** **Toxic effect of soaps**

√6th **T55.0x** **Toxic effect of soaps**

√7th **T55.0x1** **Toxic effect of soaps, accidental (unintentional)**
Toxic effect of soaps NOS

√7th **T55.0x2** **Toxic effect of soaps, intentional self-harm**

√7th **T55.0x3** **Toxic effect of soaps, assault**

√7th **T55.0x4** **Toxic effect of soaps, undetermined**

√5th **T55.1** **Toxic effect of detergents**

√6th **T55.1x** **Toxic effect of detergents**

√7th **T55.1x1** **Toxic effect of detergents, accidental (unintentional)**
Toxic effect of detergents NOS

√7th **T55.1x2** **Toxic effect of detergents, intentional self-harm**

√7th **T55.1x3** **Toxic effect of detergents, assault**

√7th **T55.1x4** **Toxic effect of detergents, undetermined**

√4th **T56** **Toxic effect of metals**

INCLUDES   toxic effects of fumes and vapors of metals
toxic effects of metals from all sources, except medicinal substances
Use additional code to identify any retained metal foreign body, if applicable (Z18.0-, T18.1-)

EXCLUDES 1   *arsenic and its compounds (T57.0)*
manganese and its compounds (T57.2)

> The appropriate 7th character is to be added to each code from category T56.
> A   initial encounter
> D   subsequent encounter
> S   sequela

√5th **T56.0** **Toxic effects of lead and its compounds**

√6th **T56.0x** **Toxic effects of lead and its compounds**

√7th **T56.0x1** **Toxic effect of lead and its compounds, accidental (unintentional)**
Toxic effects of lead and its compounds NOS

√7th **T56.0x2** **Toxic effect of lead and its compounds, intentional self-harm**

√7th **T56.0x3** **Toxic effect of lead and its compounds, assault**

√7th **T56.0x4** **Toxic effect of lead and its compounds, undetermined**

√5th **T56.1** **Toxic effects of mercury and its compounds**

√6th **T56.1x** **Toxic effects of mercury and its compounds**

√7th **T56.1x1** **Toxic effect of mercury and its compounds, accidental (unintentional)**
Toxic effects of mercury and its compounds NOS

√7th **T56.1x2** **Toxic effect of mercury and its compounds, intentional self-harm**

√7th **T56.1x3** **Toxic effect of mercury and its compounds, assault**

√7th **T56.1x4** **Toxic effect of mercury and its compounds, undetermined**

√5th **T56.2** **Toxic effects of chromium and its compounds**

√6th **T56.2x** **Toxic effects of chromium and its compounds**

√7th **T56.2x1** **Toxic effect of chromium and its compounds, accidental (unintentional)**
Toxic effects of chromium and its compounds NOS

√7th **T56.2x2** **Toxic effect of chromium and its compounds, intentional self-harm**

√7th **T56.2x3** **Toxic effect of chromium and its compounds, assault**

√7th **T56.2x4** **Toxic effect of chromium and its compounds, undetermined**

√5th **T56.3** **Toxic effects of cadmium and its compounds**

√6th **T56.3x** **Toxic effects of cadmium and its compounds**

√7th **T56.3x1** **Toxic effect of cadmium and its compounds, accidental (unintentional)**
Toxic effects of cadmium and its compounds NOS

√7th **T56.3x2** **Toxic effect of cadmium and its compounds, intentional self-harm**

√7th **T56.3x3** **Toxic effect of cadmium and its compounds, assault**

√7th **T56.3x4** **Toxic effect of cadmium and its compounds, undetermined**

√5th **T56.4** **Toxic effects of copper and its compounds**

√6th **T56.4x** **Toxic effects of copper and its compounds**

√7th **T56.4x1** **Toxic effect of copper and its compounds, accidental (unintentional)**
Toxic effects of copper and its compounds NOS

√7th **T56.4x2** **Toxic effect of copper and its compounds, intentional self-harm**

√7th **T56.4x3** **Toxic effect of copper and its compounds, assault**

√7th **T56.4x4** **Toxic effect of copper and its compounds, undetermined**

√5th **T56.5** **Toxic effects of zinc and its compounds**

√6th **T56.5x** **Toxic effects of zinc and its compounds**

√7th **T56.5x1** **Toxic effect of zinc and its compounds, accidental (unintentional)**
Toxic effects of zinc and its compounds NOS

√7th **T56.5x2** **Toxic effect of zinc and its compounds, intentional self-harm**

√7th **T56.5x3** **Toxic effect of zinc and its compounds, assault**

√7th **T56.5x4** **Toxic effect of zinc and its compounds, undetermined**

√5th **T56.6** **Toxic effects of tin and its compounds**

√6th **T56.6x** **Toxic effects of tin and its compounds**

√7th **T56.6x1** **Toxic effect of tin and its compounds, accidental (unintentional)**
Toxic effects of tin and its compounds NOS

√7th **T56.6x2** **Toxic effect of tin and its compounds, intentional self-harm**

√7th **T56.6x3** **Toxic effect of tin and its compounds, undetermined**

√7th **T56.6x4** **Toxic effect of tin and its compounds, undetermined**

EXCLUDES 1 Not coded here   **EXCLUDES 2** Not included here   *Manifestation Code*

✓5ᵗʰ **T56.7** **Toxic effects of beryllium and its compounds**
   ✓6ᵗʰ **T56.7x** **Toxic effects of beryllium and its compounds**
      ✓7ᵗʰ **T56.7x1** **Toxic effect of beryllium and its compounds, accidental (unintentional)**
         Toxic effects of beryllium and its compounds NOS
      ✓7ᵗʰ **T56.7x2** **Toxic effect of beryllium and its compounds, intentional self-harm**
      ✓7ᵗʰ **T56.7x3** **Toxic effect of beryllium and its compounds, assault**
      ✓7ᵗʰ **T56.7x4** **Toxic effect of beryllium and its compounds, undetermined**

✓5ᵗʰ **T56.8** **Toxic effects of other metals**
   ✓6ᵗʰ **T56.81** **Toxic effect of thallium**
      ✓7ᵗʰ **T56.811** **Toxic effect of thallium, accidental (unintentional)**
         Toxic effect of thallium NOS
      ✓7ᵗʰ **T56.812** **Toxic effect of thallium, intentional self-harm**
      ✓7ᵗʰ **T56.813** **Toxic effect of thallium, assault**
      ✓7ᵗʰ **T56.814** **Toxic effect of thallium, undetermined**
   ✓6ᵗʰ **T56.89** **Toxic effects of other metals**
      ✓7ᵗʰ **T56.891** **Toxic effect of other metals, accidental (unintentional)**
         Toxic effects of other metals NOS
      ✓7ᵗʰ **T56.892** **Toxic effect of other metals, intentional self-harm**
      ✓7ᵗʰ **T56.893** **Toxic effect of other metals, assault**
      ✓7ᵗʰ **T56.894** **Toxic effect of other metals, undetermined**

✓5ᵗʰ **T56.9** **Toxic effects of unspecified metal**
   ✓x7ᵗʰ **T56.91** **Toxic effect of unspecified metal, accidental (unintentional)**
   ✓x7ᵗʰ **T56.92** **Toxic effect of unspecified metal, intentional self-harm**
   ✓x7ᵗʰ **T56.93** **Toxic effect of unspecified metal, assault**
   ✓x7ᵗʰ **T56.94** **Toxic effect of unspecified metal, undetermined**

✓4ᵗʰ **T57** **Toxic effect of other inorganic substances**

> The appropriate 7th character is to be added to each code from category T57.
> A   initial encounter
> D   subsequent encounter
> S   sequela

✓5ᵗʰ **T57.0** **Toxic effect of arsenic and its compounds**
   ✓6ᵗʰ **T57.0x** **Toxic effect of arsenic and its compounds**
      ✓7ᵗʰ **T57.0x1** **Toxic effect of arsenic and its compounds, accidental (unintentional)**
         Toxic effect of arsenic and its compounds NOS
      ✓7ᵗʰ **T57.0x2** **Toxic effect of arsenic and its compounds, intentional self-harm**
      ✓7ᵗʰ **T57.0x3** **Toxic effect of arsenic and its compounds, assault**
      ✓7ᵗʰ **T57.0x4** **Toxic effect of arsenic and its compounds, undetermined**

✓5ᵗʰ **T57.1** **Toxic effect of phosphorus and its compounds**
   EXCLUDES 1 *organophosphate insecticides (T60.0)*
   ✓6ᵗʰ **T57.1x** **Toxic effect of phosphorus and its compounds**
      ✓7ᵗʰ **T57.1x1** **Toxic effect of phosphorus and its compounds, accidental (unintentional)**
         Toxic effect of phosphorus and its compounds NOS
      ✓7ᵗʰ **T57.1x2** **Toxic effect of phosphorus and its compounds, intentional self-harm**
      ✓7ᵗʰ **T57.1x3** **Toxic effect of phosphorus and its compounds, assault**
      ✓7ᵗʰ **T57.1x4** **Toxic effect of phosphorus and its compounds, undetermined**

✓5ᵗʰ **T57.2** **Toxic effect of manganese and its compounds**
   ✓6ᵗʰ **T57.2x** **Toxic effect of manganese and its compounds**
      ✓7ᵗʰ **T57.2x1** **Toxic effect of manganese and its compounds, accidental (unintentional)**
         Toxic effect of manganese and its compounds NOS
      ✓7ᵗʰ **T57.2x2** **Toxic effect of manganese and its compounds, intentional self-harm**
      ✓7ᵗʰ **T57.2x3** **Toxic effect of manganese and its compounds, assault**
      ✓7ᵗʰ **T57.2x4** **Toxic effect of manganese and its compounds, undetermined**

✓5ᵗʰ **T57.3** **Toxic effect of hydrogen cyanide**
   ✓6ᵗʰ **T57.3x** **Toxic effect of hydrogen cyanide**
      ✓7ᵗʰ **T57.3x1** **Toxic effect of hydrogen cyanide, accidental (unintentional)**
         Toxic effect of hydrogen cyanide NOS
      ✓7ᵗʰ **T57.3x2** **Toxic effect of hydrogen cyanide, intentional self-harm**
      ✓7ᵗʰ **T57.3x3** **Toxic effect of hydrogen cyanide, assault**
      ✓7ᵗʰ **T57.3x4** **Toxic effect of hydrogen cyanide, undetermined**

✓5ᵗʰ **T57.8** **Toxic effect of other specified inorganic substances**
   ✓6ᵗʰ **T57.8x** **Toxic effect of other specified inorganic substances**
      ✓7ᵗʰ **T57.8x1** **Toxic effect of other specified inorganic substances, accidental (unintentional)**
         Toxic effect of other specified inorganic substances NOS
      ✓7ᵗʰ **T57.8x2** **Toxic effect of other specified inorganic substances, intentional self-harm**
      ✓7ᵗʰ **T57.8x3** **Toxic effect of other specified inorganic substances, assault**
      ✓7ᵗʰ **T57.8x4** **Toxic effect of other specified inorganic substances, undetermined**

✓5ᵗʰ **T57.9** **Toxic effect of unspecified inorganic substance**
   ✓x7ᵗʰ **T57.91** **Toxic effect of unspecified inorganic substance, accidental (unintentional)**
   ✓x7ᵗʰ **T57.92** **Toxic effect of unspecified inorganic substance, intentional self-harm**
   ✓x7ᵗʰ **T57.93** **Toxic effect of unspecified inorganic substance, assault**
   ✓x7ᵗʰ **T57.94** **Toxic effect of unspecified inorganic substance, undetermined**

✓4ᵗʰ **T58** **Toxic effect of carbon monoxide**
   INCLUDES asphyxiation from carbon monoxide
         toxic effect of carbon monoxide from all sources

> The appropriate 7th character is to be added to each code from category T58.
> A   initial encounter
> D   subsequent encounter
> S   sequela

✓5ᵗʰ **T58.0** **Toxic effect of carbon monoxide from motor vehicle exhaust**
   Toxic effect of exhaust gas from gas engine
   Toxic effect of exhaust gas from motor pump
   ✓x7ᵗʰ **T58.01** **Toxic effect of carbon monoxide from motor vehicle exhaust, accidental (unintentional)**
   ✓x7ᵗʰ **T58.02** **Toxic effect of carbon monoxide from motor vehicle exhaust, intentional self-harm**
   ✓x7ᵗʰ **T58.03** **Toxic effect of carbon monoxide from motor vehicle exhaust, assault**
   ✓x7ᵗʰ **T58.04** **Toxic effect of carbon monoxide from motor vehicle exhaust, undetermined**

✓5ᵗʰ **T58.1** **Toxic effect of carbon monoxide from utility gas**
   Toxic effect of acetylene
   Toxic effect of gas NOS used for lighting, heating, cooking
   Toxic effect of water gas
   ✓x7ᵗʰ **T58.11** **Toxic effect of carbon monoxide from utility gas, accidental (unintentional)**
   ✓x7ᵗʰ **T58.12** **Toxic effect of carbon monoxide from utility gas, intentional self-harm**
   ✓x7ᵗʰ **T58.13** **Toxic effect of carbon monoxide from utility gas, assault**
   ✓x7ᵗʰ **T58.14** **Toxic effect of carbon monoxide from utility gas, undetermined**

√5th **T58.2 Toxic effect of carbon monoxide from incomplete combustion of other domestic fuels**
Toxic effect of carbon monoxide from incomplete combustion of coal, coke, kerosene, wood

√6th **T58.2x Toxic effect of carbon monoxide from incomplete combustion of other domestic fuels**

√7th **T58.2x1 Toxic effect of carbon monoxide from incomplete combustion of other domestic fuels, accidental (unintentional)**

√7th **T58.2x2 Toxic effect of carbon monoxide from incomplete combustion of other domestic fuels, intentional self-harm**

√7th **T58.2x3 Toxic effect of carbon monoxide from incomplete combustion of other domestic fuels, assault**

√7th **T58.2x4 Toxic effect of carbon monoxide from incomplete combustion of other domestic fuels, undetermined**

√5th **T58.8 Toxic effect of carbon monoxide from other source**
Toxic effect of carbon monoxide from blast furnace gas
Toxic effect of carbon monoxide from fuels in industrial use
Toxic effect of carbon monoxide from kiln vapor

√6th **T58.8x Toxic effect of carbon monoxide from other source**

√7th **T58.8x1 Toxic effect of carbon monoxide from other source, accidental (unintentional)**

√7th **T58.8x2 Toxic effect of carbon monoxide from other source, intentional self-harm**

√7th **T58.8x3 Toxic effect of carbon monoxide from other source, assault**

√7th **T58.8x4 Toxic effect of carbon monoxide from other source, undetermined**

√5th **T58.9 Toxic effect of carbon monoxide from unspecified source**

√x7th **T58.91 Toxic effect of carbon monoxide from unspecified source, accidental (unintentional)**

√x7th **T58.92 Toxic effect of carbon monoxide from unspecified source, intentional self-harm**

√x7th **T58.93 Toxic effect of carbon monoxide from unspecified source, assault**

√x7th **T58.94 Toxic effect of carbon monoxide from unspecified source, undetermined**

√4th **T59 Toxic effect of other gases, fumes and vapors**
INCLUDES aerosol propellants
EXCLUDES 1 *chlorofluorocarbons (T53.5)*

The appropriate 7th character is to be added to each code from category T59.
A initial encounter
D subsequent encounter
S sequela

√5th **T59.0 Toxic effect of nitrogen oxides**

√6th **T59.0x Toxic effect of nitrogen oxides**

√7th **T59.0x1 Toxic effect of nitrogen oxides, accidental (unintentional)**
Toxic effect of nitrogen oxides NOS

√7th **T59.0x2 Toxic effect of nitrogen oxides, intentional self-harm**

√7th **T59.0x3 Toxic effect of nitrogen oxides, assault**

√7th **T59.0x4 Toxic effect of nitrogen oxides, undetermined**

√5th **T59.1 Toxic effect of sulfur dioxide**

√6th **T59.1x Toxic effect of sulfur dioxide**

√7th **T59.1x1 Toxic effect of sulfur dioxide, accidental (unintentional)**
Toxic effect of sulfur dioxide NOS

√7th **T59.1x2 Toxic effect of sulfur dioxide, intentional self-harm**

√7th **T59.1x3 Toxic effect of sulfur dioxide, assault**

√7th **T59.1x4 Toxic effect of sulfur dioxide, undetermined**

√5th **T59.2 Toxic effect of formaldehyde**

√6th **T59.2x Toxic effect of formaldehyde**

√7th **T59.2x1 Toxic effect of formaldehyde, accidental (unintentional)**
Toxic effect of formaldehyde NOS

√7th **T59.2x2 Toxic effect of formaldehyde, intentional self-harm**

√7th **T59.2x3 Toxic effect of formaldehyde, assault**

√7th **T59.2x4 Toxic effect of formaldehyde, undetermined**

√5th **T59.3 Toxic effect of lacrimogenic gas**
Toxic effect of tear gas

√6th **T59.3x Toxic effect of lacrimogenic gas**

√7th **T59.3x1 Toxic effect of lacrimogenic gas, accidental (unintentional)**
Toxic effect of lacrimogenic gas NOS

√7th **T59.3x2 Toxic effect of lacrimogenic gas, intentional self-harm**

√7th **T59.3x3 Toxic effect of lacrimogenic gas, assault**

√7th **T59.3x4 Toxic effect of lacrimogenic gas, undetermined**

√5th **T59.4 Toxic effect of chlorine gas**

√6th **T59.4x Toxic effect of chlorine gas**

√7th **T59.4x1 Toxic effect of chlorine gas, accidental (unintentional)**
Toxic effect of chlorine gas NOS

√7th **T59.4x2 Toxic effect of chlorine gas, intentional self-harm**

√7th **T59.4x3 Toxic effect of chlorine gas, assault**

√7th **T59.4x4 Toxic effect of chlorine gas, undetermined**

√5th **T59.5 Toxic effect of fluorine gas and hydrogen fluoride**

√6th **T59.5x Toxic effect of fluorine gas and hydrogen fluoride**

√7th **T59.5x1 Toxic effect of fluorine gas and hydrogen fluoride, accidental (unintentional)**
Toxic effect of fluorine gas and hydrogen fluoride NOS

√7th **T59.5x2 Toxic effect of fluorine gas and hydrogen fluoride, intentional self-harm**

√7th **T59.5x3 Toxic effect of fluorine gas and hydrogen fluoride, assault**

√7th **T59.5x4 Toxic effect of fluorine gas and hydrogen fluoride, undetermined**

√5th **T59.6 Toxic effect of hydrogen sulfide**

√6th **T59.6x Toxic effect of hydrogen sulfide**

√7th **T59.6x1 Toxic effect of hydrogen sulfide, accidental (unintentional)**
Toxic effect of hydrogen sulfide NOS

√7th **T59.6x2 Toxic effect of hydrogen sulfide, intentional self-harm**

√7th **T59.6x3 Toxic effect of hydrogen sulfide, assault**

√7th **T59.6x4 Toxic effect of hydrogen sulfide, undetermined**

√5th **T59.7 Toxic effect of carbon dioxide**

√6th **T59.7x Toxic effect of carbon dioxide**

√7th **T59.7x1 Toxic effect of carbon dioxide, accidental (unintentional)**
Toxic effect of carbon dioxide NOS

√7th **T59.7x2 Toxic effect of carbon dioxide, intentional self-harm**

√7th **T59.7x3 Toxic effect of carbon dioxide, assault**

√7th **T59.7x4 Toxic effect of carbon dioxide, undetermined**

√5th **T59.8 Toxic effect of other specified gases, fumes and vapors**

√6th **T59.81 Toxic effect of smoke**
Smoke inhalation
EXCLUDES 2 *toxic effect of cigarette (tobacco) smoke (T65.22-)*

√7th **T59.811 Toxic effect of smoke, accidental (unintentional)**
Toxic effect of smoke NOS

√7th **T59.812 Toxic effect of smoke, intentional self-harm**

√7th **T59.813 Toxic effect of smoke, assault**

√7th **T59.814 Toxic effect of smoke, undetermined**

√6th **T59.89 Toxic effect of other specified gases, fumes and vapors**

√7th **T59.891 Toxic effect of other specified gases, fumes and vapors, accidental (unintentional)**

√7th **T59.892 Toxic effect of other specified gases, fumes and vapors, intentional self-harm**

EXCLUDES 1 Not coded here   EXCLUDES 2 Not included here   *Manifestation Code*

√7ᵗʰ **T59.893** **Toxic effect of other specified gases, fumes and vapors, assault**

√7ᵗʰ **T59.894** **Toxic effect of other specified gases, fumes and vapors, undetermined**

√5ᵗʰ **T59.9** **Toxic effect of unspecified gases, fumes and vapors**

√x7ᵗʰ **T59.91** **Toxic effect of unspecified gases, fumes and vapors, accidental (unintentional)**

√x7ᵗʰ **T59.92** **Toxic effect of unspecified gases, fumes and vapors, intentional self-harm**

√x7ᵗʰ **T59.93** **Toxic effect of unspecified gases, fumes and vapors, assault**

√x7ᵗʰ **T59.94** **Toxic effect of unspecified gases, fumes and vapors, undetermined**

√4ᵗʰ **T60** **Toxic effect of pesticides**

INCLUDES   toxic effect of wood preservatives

The appropriate 7th character is to be added to each code from category T60.
A   initial encounter
D   subsequent encounter
S   sequela

√5ᵗʰ **T60.0** **Toxic effect of organophosphate and carbamate insecticides**

√6ᵗʰ **T60.0x** **Toxic effect of organophosphate and carbamate insecticides**

√7ᵗʰ **T60.0x1** **Toxic effect of organophosphate and carbamate insecticides, accidental (unintentional)**
Toxic effect of organophosphate and carbamate insecticides NOS

√7ᵗʰ **T60.0x2** **Toxic effect of organophosphate and carbamate insecticides, intentional self-harm**

√7ᵗʰ **T60.0x3** **Toxic effect of organophosphate and carbamate insecticides, assault**

√7ᵗʰ **T60.0x4** **Toxic effect of organophosphate and carbamate insecticides, undetermined**

√5ᵗʰ **T60.1** **Toxic effect of halogenated insecticides**

EXCLUDES 1   chlorinated hydrocarbon (T53-)

√6ᵗʰ **T60.1x** **Toxic effect of halogenated insecticides**

√7ᵗʰ **T60.1x1** **Toxic effect of halogenated insecticides, accidental (unintentional)**
Toxic effect of halogenated insecticides NOS

√7ᵗʰ **T60.1x2** **Toxic effect of halogenated insecticides, intentional self-harm**

√7ᵗʰ **T60.1x3** **Toxic effect of halogenated insecticides, assault**

√7ᵗʰ **T60.1x4** **Toxic effect of halogenated insecticides, undetermined**

√5ᵗʰ **T60.2** **Toxic effect of other insecticides**

√6ᵗʰ **T60.2x** **Toxic effect of other insecticides**

√7ᵗʰ **T60.2x1** **Toxic effect of other insecticides, accidental (unintentional)**
Toxic effect of other insecticides NOS

√7ᵗʰ **T60.2x2** **Toxic effect of other insecticides, intentional self-harm**

√7ᵗʰ **T60.2x3** **Toxic effect of other insecticides, assault**

√7ᵗʰ **T60.2x4** **Toxic effect of other insecticides, undetermined**

√5ᵗʰ **T60.3** **Toxic effect of herbicides and fungicides**

√6ᵗʰ **T60.3x** **Toxic effect of herbicides and fungicides**

√7ᵗʰ **T60.3x1** **Toxic effect of herbicides and fungicides, accidental (unintentional)**
Toxic effect of herbicides and fungicides NOS

√7ᵗʰ **T60.3x2** **Toxic effect of herbicides and fungicides, intentional self-harm**

√7ᵗʰ **T60.3x3** **Toxic effect of herbicides and fungicides, assault**

√7ᵗʰ **T60.3x4** **Toxic effect of herbicides and fungicides, undetermined**

√5ᵗʰ **T60.4** **Toxic effect of rodenticides**

EXCLUDES 1   strychnine and its salts (T65.1)
thallium (T56.81-)

√6ᵗʰ **T60.4x** **Toxic effect of rodenticides**

√7ᵗʰ **T60.4x1** **Toxic effect of rodenticides, accidental (unintentional)**
Toxic effect of rodenticides NOS

√7ᵗʰ **T60.4x2** **Toxic effect of rodenticides, intentional self-harm**

√7ᵗʰ **T60.4x3** **Toxic effect of rodenticides, assault**

√7ᵗʰ **T60.4x4** **Toxic effect of rodenticides, undetermined**

√5ᵗʰ **T60.8** **Toxic effect of other pesticides**

√6ᵗʰ **T60.8x** **Toxic effect of other pesticides**

√7ᵗʰ **T60.8x1** **Toxic effect of other pesticides, accidental (unintentional)**
Toxic effect of other pesticides NOS

√7ᵗʰ **T60.8x2** **Toxic effect of other pesticides, intentional self-harm**

√7ᵗʰ **T60.8x3** **Toxic effect of other pesticides, assault**

√7ᵗʰ **T60.8x4** **Toxic effect of other pesticides, undetermined**

√5ᵗʰ **T60.9** **Toxic effect of unspecified pesticide**

√x7ᵗʰ **T60.91** **Toxic effect of unspecified pesticide, accidental (unintentional)**

√x7ᵗʰ **T60.92** **Toxic effect of unspecified pesticide, intentional self-harm**

√x7ᵗʰ **T60.93** **Toxic effect of unspecified pesticide, assault**

√x7ᵗʰ **T60.94** **Toxic effect of unspecified pesticide, undetermined**

√4ᵗʰ **T61** **Toxic effect of noxious substances eaten as seafood**

EXCLUDES 1   allergic reaction to food, such as:
anaphylactic shock (reaction) due to adverse food reaction (T78.0-)
dermatitis (L23.6, L25.4, L27.2)
gastroenteritis (noninfective) (K52.2)
anaphylactic shock (T78.02, T78.05)
bacterial foodborne intoxications (A05-)
toxic effect of food contaminants, such as:
aflatoxin and other mycotoxins (T64)
cyanides (T65.0-)
harmful algae bloom (T65.82-)
hydrogen cyanide (T57.3-)
mercury (T56.1-)
red tide (T65.82-)

The appropriate 7th character is to be added to each code from category T61.
A   initial encounter
D   subsequent encounter
S   sequela

√5ᵗʰ **T61.0** **Ciguatera fish poisoning**

√x7ᵗʰ **T61.01** **Ciguatera fish poisoning, accidental (unintentional)**

√x7ᵗʰ **T61.02** **Ciguatera fish poisoning, intentional self-harm**

√x7ᵗʰ **T61.03** **Ciguatera fish poisoning, assault**

√x7ᵗʰ **T61.04** **Ciguatera fish poisoning, undetermined**

√5ᵗʰ **T61.1** **Scombroid fish poisoning**
Histamine-like syndrome

√x7ᵗʰ **T61.11** **Scombroid fish poisoning, accidental (unintentional)**

√x7ᵗʰ **T61.12** **Scombroid fish poisoning, intentional self-harm**

√x7ᵗʰ **T61.13** **Scombroid fish poisoning, assault**

√x7ᵗʰ **T61.14** **Scombroid fish poisoning, undetermined**

√5ᵗʰ **T61.7** **Other fish and shellfish poisoning**

√6ᵗʰ **T61.77** **Other fish poisoning**

√7ᵗʰ **T61.771** **Other fish poisoning, accidental (unintentional)**

√7ᵗʰ **T61.772** **Other fish poisoning, intentional self-harm**

√7ᵗʰ **T61.773** **Other fish poisoning, assault**

√7ᵗʰ **T61.774** **Other fish poisoning, undetermined**

√6ᵗʰ **T61.78** **Other shellfish poisoning**

√7ᵗʰ **T61.781** **Other shellfish poisoning, accidental (unintentional)**

√7ᵗʰ **T61.782** **Other shellfish poisoning, intentional self-harm**

√7th **T61.783** Other shellfish poisoning, assault

√7th **T61.784** Other shellfish poisoning, undetermined

√5th **T61.8** **Toxic effect of other seafood**

√6th **T61.8x** Toxic effect of other seafood

√7th **T61.8x1** Toxic effect of other seafood, accidental (unintentional)

√7th **T61.8x2** Toxic effect of other seafood, intentional self-harm

√7th **T61.8x3** Toxic effect of other seafood, assault

√7th **T61.8x4** Toxic effect of other seafood, undetermined

√5th **T61.9** **Toxic effect of unspecified seafood**

√x7th **T61.91** Toxic effect of unspecified seafood, accidental (unintentional)

√x7th **T61.92** Toxic effect of unspecified seafood, intentional self-harm

√x7th **T61.93** Toxic effect of unspecified seafood, assault

√x7th **T61.94** Toxic effect of unspecified seafood, undetermined

√4th **T62** **Toxic effect of other noxious substances eaten as food**

EXCLUDES 1 allergic reaction to food, such as:
anaphylactic shock (reaction) due to adverse food reaction (T78.0-)
dermatitis (L23.6, L25.4, L27.2)
gastroenteritis (noninfective) (K52.2)
bacterial food borne intoxications (A05-)
toxic effect of food contaminants, such as:
aflatoxin and other mycotoxins (T64)
cyanides (T65.0-)
hydrogen cyanide (T57.3-)
mercury (T56.1-)

The appropriate 7th character is to be added to each code from category T62.
A   initial encounter
D   subsequent encounter
S   sequela

√5th **T62.0** **Toxic effect of ingested mushrooms**

√6th **T62.0x** Toxic effect of ingested mushrooms

√7th **T62.0x1** Toxic effect of ingested mushrooms, accidental (unintentional)
Toxic effect of ingested mushrooms NOS

√7th **T62.0x2** Toxic effect of ingested mushrooms, intentional self-harm

√7th **T62.0x3** Toxic effect of ingested mushrooms, assault

√7th **T62.0x4** Toxic effect of ingested mushrooms, undetermined

√5th **T62.1** **Toxic effect of ingested berries**

√6th **T62.1x** Toxic effect of ingested berries

√7th **T62.1x1** Toxic effect of ingested berries, accidental (unintentional)
Toxic effect of ingested berries NOS

√7th **T62.1x2** Toxic effect of ingested berries, intentional self-harm

√7th **T62.1x3** Toxic effect of ingested berries, assault

√7th **T62.1x4** Toxic effect of ingested berries, undetermined

√5th **T62.2** **Toxic effect of other ingested (parts of) plant(s)**

√6th **T62.2x** Toxic effect of other ingested (parts of) plant(s)

√7th **T62.2x1** Toxic effect of other ingested (parts of) plant(s), accidental (unintentional)
Toxic effect of other ingested (parts of) plant(s) NOS

√7th **T62.2x2** Toxic effect of other ingested (parts of) plant(s), intentional self-harm

√7th **T62.2x3** Toxic effect of other ingested (parts of) plant(s), assault

√7th **T62.2x4** Toxic effect of other ingested (parts of) plant(s), undetermined

√5th **T62.8** **Toxic effect of other specified noxious substances eaten as food**

√6th **T62.8x** Toxic effect of other specified noxious substances eaten as food

√7th **T62.8x1** Toxic effect of other specified noxious substances eaten as food, accidental (unintentional)
Toxic effect of other specified noxious substances eaten as food NOS

√7th **T62.8x2** Toxic effect of other specified noxious substances eaten as food, intentional self-harm

√7th **T62.8x3** Toxic effect of other specified noxious substances eaten as food, assault

√7th **T62.8x4** Toxic effect of other specified noxious substances eaten as food, undetermined

√5th **T62.9** **Toxic effect of unspecified noxious substance eaten as food**

√x7th **T62.91** Toxic effect of unspecified noxious substance eaten as food, accidental (unintentional)
Toxic effect of unspecified noxious substance eaten as food NOS

√x7th **T62.92** Toxic effect of unspecified noxious substance eaten as food, intentional self-harm

√x7th **T62.93** Toxic effect of unspecified noxious substance eaten as food, assault

√x7th **T62.94** Toxic effect of unspecified noxious substance eaten as food, undetermined

√4th **T63** **Toxic effect of contact with venomous animals and plants**

INCLUDES bite or touch of venomous animal
pricked or stuck by thorn or leaf

EXCLUDES 2 ingestion of toxic animal or plant (T61-, T62-))

The appropriate 7th character is to be added to each code from category T63.
A   initial encounter
D   subsequent encounter
S   sequela

√5th **T63.0** **Toxic effect of snake venom**

√6th **T63.00** Toxic effect of unspecified snake venom

√7th **T63.001** Toxic effect of unspecified snake venom, accidental (unintentional)
Toxic effect of unspecified snake venom NOS

√7th **T63.002** Toxic effect of unspecified snake venom, intentional self-harm

√7th **T63.003** Toxic effect of unspecified snake venom, assault

√7th **T63.004** Toxic effect of unspecified snake venom, undetermined

√6th **T63.01** Toxic effect of rattlesnake venom

√7th **T63.011** Toxic effect of rattlesnake venom, accidental (unintentional)
Toxic effect of rattlesnake venom NOS

√7th **T63.012** Toxic effect of rattlesnake venom, intentional self-harm

√7th **T63.013** Toxic effect of rattlesnake venom, assault

√7th **T63.014** Toxic effect of rattlesnake venom, undetermined

√6th **T63.02** Toxic effect of coral snake venom

√7th **T63.021** Toxic effect of coral snake venom, accidental (unintentional)
Toxic effect of coral snake venom NOS

√7th **T63.022** Toxic effect of coral snake venom, intentional self-harm

√7th **T63.023** Toxic effect of coral snake venom, assault

√7th **T63.024** Toxic effect of coral snake venom, undetermined

√6th **T63.03** Toxic effect of taipan venom

√7th **T63.031** Toxic effect of taipan venom, accidental (unintentional)
Toxic effect of taipan venom NOS

√7th **T63.032** Toxic effect of taipan venom, intentional self-harm

√7th **T63.033** Toxic effect of taipan venom, assault

EXCLUDES 1 Not coded here   EXCLUDES 2 Not included here   *Manifestation Code*

✓7th **T63.034** Toxic effect of taipan venom, undetermined

✓6th **T63.04** Toxic effect of cobra venom
 ✓7th **T63.041** Toxic effect of cobra venom, accidental (unintentional)
 Toxic effect of cobra venom NOS
 ✓7th **T63.042** Toxic effect of cobra venom, intentional self-harm
 ✓7th **T63.043** Toxic effect of cobra venom, assault
 ✓7th **T63.044** Toxic effect of cobra venom, undetermined

✓6th **T63.06** Toxic effect of venom of other North and South American snake
 ✓7th **T63.061** Toxic effect of venom of other North and South American snake, accidental (unintentional)
 Toxic effect of venom of other North and South American snake NOS
 ✓7th **T63.062** Toxic effect of venom of other North and South American snake, intentional self-harm
 ✓7th **T63.063** Toxic effect of venom of other North and South American snake, assault
 ✓7th **T63.064** Toxic effect of venom of other North and South American snake, undetermined

✓6th **T63.07** Toxic effect of venom of other Australian snake
 ✓7th **T63.071** Toxic effect of venom of other Australian snake, accidental (unintentional)
 Toxic effect of venom of other Australian snake NOS
 ✓7th **T63.072** Toxic effect of venom of other Australian snake, intentional self-harm
 ✓7th **T63.073** Toxic effect of venom of other Australian snake, assault
 ✓7th **T63.074** Toxic effect of venom of other Australian snake, undetermined

✓6th **T63.08** Toxic effect of venom of other African and Asian snake
 ✓7th **T63.081** Toxic effect of venom of other African and Asian snake, accidental (unintentional)
 Toxic effect of venom of other African and Asian snake NOS
 ✓7th **T63.082** Toxic effect of venom of other African and Asian snake, intentional self-harm
 ✓7th **T63.083** Toxic effect of venom of other African and Asian snake, assault
 ✓7th **T63.084** Toxic effect of venom of other African and Asian snake, undetermined

✓6th **T63.09** Toxic effect of venom of other snake
 ✓7th **T63.091** Toxic effect of venom of other snake, accidental (unintentional)
 Toxic effect of venom of other snake NOS
 ✓7th **T63.092** Toxic effect of venom of other snake, intentional self-harm
 ✓7th **T63.093** Toxic effect of venom of other snake, assault
 ✓7th **T63.094** Toxic effect of venom of other snake, undetermined

✓5th **T63.1** Toxic effect of venom of other reptiles
✓6th **T63.11** Toxic effect of venom of gila monster
 ✓7th **T63.111** Toxic effect of venom of gila monster, accidental (unintentional)
 Toxic effect of venom of gila monster NOS
 ✓7th **T63.112** Toxic effect of venom of gila monster, intentional self-harm
 ✓7th **T63.113** Toxic effect of venom of gila monster, assault
 ✓7th **T63.114** Toxic effect of venom of gila monster, undetermined

✓6th **T63.12** Toxic effect of venom of other venomous lizard
 ✓7th **T63.121** Toxic effect of venom of other venomous lizard, accidental (unintentional)
 Toxic effect of venom of other venomous lizard NOS
 ✓7th **T63.122** Toxic effect of venom of other venomous lizard, intentional self-harm
 ✓7th **T63.123** Toxic effect of venom of other venomous lizard, assault
 ✓7th **T63.124** Toxic effect of venom of other venomous lizard, undetermined

✓6th **T63.19** Toxic effect of venom of other reptiles
 ✓7th **T63.191** Toxic effect of venom of other reptiles, accidental (unintentional)
 Toxic effect of venom of other reptiles NOS
 ✓7th **T63.192** Toxic effect of venom of other reptiles, intentional self-harm
 ✓7th **T63.193** Toxic effect of venom of other reptiles, assault
 ✓7th **T63.194** Toxic effect of venom of other reptiles, undetermined

✓5th **T63.2** Toxic effect of venom of scorpion
✓6th **T63.2x** Toxic effect of venom of scorpion
 ✓7th **T63.2x1** Toxic effect of venom of scorpion, accidental (unintentional)
 Toxic effect of venom of scorpion NOS
 ✓7th **T63.2x2** Toxic effect of venom of scorpion, intentional self-harm
 ✓7th **T63.2x3** Toxic effect of venom of scorpion, assault
 ✓7th **T63.2x4** Toxic effect of venom of scorpion, undetermined

✓5th **T63.3** Toxic effect of venom of spider
✓6th **T63.30** Toxic effect of unspecified spider venom
 ✓7th **T63.301** Toxic effect of unspecified spider venom, accidental (unintentional)
 ✓7th **T63.302** Toxic effect of unspecified spider venom, intentional self-harm
 ✓7th **T63.303** Toxic effect of unspecified spider venom, assault
 ✓7th **T63.304** Toxic effect of unspecified spider venom, undetermined

✓6th **T63.31** Toxic effect of venom of black widow spider
 ✓7th **T63.311** Toxic effect of venom of black widow spider, accidental (unintentional)
 ✓7th **T63.312** Toxic effect of venom of black widow spider, intentional self-harm
 ✓7th **T63.313** Toxic effect of venom of black widow spider, assault
 ✓7th **T63.314** Toxic effect of venom of black widow spider, undetermined

✓6th **T63.32** Toxic effect of venom of tarantula
 ✓7th **T63.321** Toxic effect of venom of tarantula, accidental (unintentional)
 ✓7th **T63.322** Toxic effect of venom of tarantula, intentional self-harm
 ✓7th **T63.323** Toxic effect of venom of tarantula, assault
 ✓7th **T63.324** Toxic effect of venom of tarantula, undetermined

✓6th **T63.33** Toxic effect of venom of brown recluse spider
 ✓7th **T63.331** Toxic effect of venom of brown recluse spider, accidental (unintentional)
 ✓7th **T63.332** Toxic effect of venom of brown recluse spider, intentional self-harm
 ✓7th **T63.333** Toxic effect of venom of brown recluse spider, assault
 ✓7th **T63.334** Toxic effect of venom of brown recluse spider, undetermined

✓6th **T63.39** Toxic effect of venom of other spider
 ✓7th **T63.391** Toxic effect of venom of other spider, accidental (unintentional)
 ✓7th **T63.392** Toxic effect of venom of other spider, intentional self-harm
 ✓7th **T63.393** Toxic effect of venom of other spider, assault
 ✓7th **T63.394** Toxic effect of venom of other spider, undetermined

✓5ᵗʰ **T63.4** **Toxic effect of venom of other arthropods**

  ✓6ᵗʰ **T63.41** **Toxic effect of venom of centipedes and venomous millipedes**

    ✓7ᵗʰ **T63.411** **Toxic effect of venom of centipedes and venomous millipedes, accidental (unintentional)**

    ✓7ᵗʰ **T63.412** **Toxic effect of venom of centipedes and venomous millipedes, intentional self-harm**

    ✓7ᵗʰ **T63.413** **Toxic effect of venom of centipedes and venomous millipedes, assault**

    ✓7ᵗʰ **T63.414** **Toxic effect of venom of centipedes and venomous millipedes, undetermined**

  ✓6ᵗʰ **T63.42** **Toxic effect of venom of ants**

    ✓7ᵗʰ **T63.421** **Toxic effect of venom of ants, accidental (unintentional)**

    ✓7ᵗʰ **T63.422** **Toxic effect of venom of ants, intentional self-harm**

    ✓7ᵗʰ **T63.423** **Toxic effect of venom of ants, assault**

    ✓7ᵗʰ **T63.424** **Toxic effect of venom of ants, undetermined**

  ✓6ᵗʰ **T63.43** **Toxic effect of venom of caterpillars**

    ✓7ᵗʰ **T63.431** **Toxic effect of venom of caterpillars, accidental (unintentional)**

    ✓7ᵗʰ **T63.432** **Toxic effect of venom of caterpillars, intentional self-harm**

    ✓7ᵗʰ **T63.433** **Toxic effect of venom of caterpillars, assault**

    ✓7ᵗʰ **T63.434** **Toxic effect of venom of caterpillars, undetermined**

  ✓6ᵗʰ **T63.44** **Toxic effect of venom of bees**

    ✓7ᵗʰ **T63.441** **Toxic effect of venom of bees, accidental (unintentional)**

    ✓7ᵗʰ **T63.442** **Toxic effect of venom of bees, intentional self-harm**

    ✓7ᵗʰ **T63.443** **Toxic effect of venom of bees, assault**

    ✓7ᵗʰ **T63.444** **Toxic effect of venom of bees, undetermined**

  ✓6ᵗʰ **T63.45** **Toxic effect of venom of hornets**

    ✓7ᵗʰ **T63.451** **Toxic effect of venom of hornets, accidental (unintentional)**

    ✓7ᵗʰ **T63.452** **Toxic effect of venom of hornets, intentional self-harm**

    ✓7ᵗʰ **T63.453** **Toxic effect of venom of hornets, assault**

    ✓7ᵗʰ **T63.454** **Toxic effect of venom of hornets, undetermined**

  ✓6ᵗʰ **T63.46** **Toxic effect of venom of wasps**

    Toxic effect of yellow jacket

    ✓7ᵗʰ **T63.461** **Toxic effect of venom of wasps, accidental (unintentional)**

    ✓7ᵗʰ **T63.462** **Toxic effect of venom of wasps, intentional self-harm**

    ✓7ᵗʰ **T63.463** **Toxic effect of venom of wasps, assault**

    ✓7ᵗʰ **T63.464** **Toxic effect of venom of wasps, undetermined**

  ✓6ᵗʰ **T63.48** **Toxic effect of venom of other arthropod**

    ✓7ᵗʰ **T63.481** **Toxic effect of venom of other arthropod, accidental (unintentional)**

    ✓7ᵗʰ **T63.482** **Toxic effect of venom of other arthropod, intentional self-harm**

    ✓7ᵗʰ **T63.483** **Toxic effect of venom of other arthropod, assault**

    ✓7ᵗʰ **T63.484** **Toxic effect of venom of other arthropod, undetermined**

✓5ᵗʰ **T63.5** **Toxic effect of contact with venomous fish**

  EXCLUDES 2 *poisoning by ingestion of fish (T61-)*

  ✓6ᵗʰ **T63.51** **Toxic effect of contact with stingray**

    ✓7ᵗʰ **T63.511** **Toxic effect of contact with stingray, accidental (unintentional)**

    ✓7ᵗʰ **T63.512** **Toxic effect of contact with stingray, intentional self-harm**

    ✓7ᵗʰ **T63.513** **Toxic effect of contact with stingray, assault**

    ✓7ᵗʰ **T63.514** **Toxic effect of contact with stingray, undetermined**

✓6ᵗʰ **T63.59** **Toxic effect of contact with other venomous fish**

    ✓7ᵗʰ **T63.591** **Toxic effect of contact with other venomous fish, accidental (unintentional)**

    ✓7ᵗʰ **T63.592** **Toxic effect of contact with other venomous fish, intentional self-harm**

    ✓7ᵗʰ **T63.593** **Toxic effect of contact with other venomous fish, assault**

    ✓7ᵗʰ **T63.594** **Toxic effect of contact with other venomous fish, undetermined**

✓5ᵗʰ **T63.6** **Toxic effect of contact with other venomous marine animals**

  EXCLUDES 1 *sea-snake venom (T63.09)*

  EXCLUDES 2 *poisoning by ingestion of shellfish (T61.78-)*

  ✓6ᵗʰ **T63.61** **Toxic effect of contact with Portugese Man-o-war**

    Toxic effect of contact with bluebottle

    ✓7ᵗʰ **T63.611** **Toxic effect of contact with Portugese Man-o-war, accidental (unintentional)**

    ✓7ᵗʰ **T63.612** **Toxic effect of contact with Portugese Man-o-war, intentional self-harm**

    ✓7ᵗʰ **T63.613** **Toxic effect of contact with Portugese Man-o-war, assault**

    ✓7ᵗʰ **T63.614** **Toxic effect of contact with Portugese Man-o-war, undetermined**

  ✓6ᵗʰ **T63.62** **Toxic effect of contact with other jellyfish**

    ✓7ᵗʰ **T63.621** **Toxic effect of contact with other jellyfish, accidental (unintentional)**

    ✓7ᵗʰ **T63.622** **Toxic effect of contact with other jellyfish, intentional self-harm**

    ✓7ᵗʰ **T63.623** **Toxic effect of contact with other jellyfish, assault**

    ✓7ᵗʰ **T63.624** **Toxic effect of contact with other jellyfish, undetermined**

  ✓6ᵗʰ **T63.63** **Toxic effect of contact with sea anemone**

    ✓7ᵗʰ **T63.631** **Toxic effect of contact with sea anemone, accidental (unintentional)**

    ✓7ᵗʰ **T63.632** **Toxic effect of contact with sea anemone, intentional self-harm**

    ✓7ᵗʰ **T63.633** **Toxic effect of contact with sea anemone, assault**

    ✓7ᵗʰ **T63.634** **Toxic effect of contact with sea anemone, undetermined**

  ✓6ᵗʰ **T63.69** **Toxic effect of contact with other venomous marine animals**

    ✓7ᵗʰ **T63.691** **Toxic effect of contact with other venomous marine animals, accidental (unintentional)**

    ✓7ᵗʰ **T63.692** **Toxic effect of contact with other venomous marine animals, intentional self-harm**

    ✓7ᵗʰ **T63.693** **Toxic effect of contact with other venomous marine animals, assault**

    ✓7ᵗʰ **T63.694** **Toxic effect of contact with other venomous marine animals, undetermined**

✓5ᵗʰ **T63.7** **Toxic effect of contact with venomous plant**

  ✓6ᵗʰ **T63.71** **Toxic effect of contact with venomous marine plant**

    ✓7ᵗʰ **T63.711** **Toxic effect of contact with venomous marine plant, accidental (unintentional)**

    ✓7ᵗʰ **T63.712** **Toxic effect of contact with venomous marine plant, intentional self-harm**

    ✓7ᵗʰ **T63.713** **Toxic effect of contact with venomous marine plant, assault**

    ✓7ᵗʰ **T63.714** **Toxic effect of contact with venomous marine plant, undetermined**

  ✓6ᵗʰ **T63.79** **Toxic effect of contact with other venomous plant**

    ✓7ᵗʰ **T63.791** **Toxic effect of contact with other venomous plant, accidental (unintentional)**

    ✓7ᵗʰ **T63.792** **Toxic effect of contact with other venomous plant, intentional self-harm**

    ✓7ᵗʰ **T63.793** **Toxic effect of contact with other venomous plant, assault**

    ✓7ᵗʰ **T63.794** **Toxic effect of contact with other venomous plant, undetermined**

EXCLUDES 1 Not coded here   *EXCLUDES 2* Not included here   ***Manifestation Code***

☑5ᵗʰ **T63.8 Toxic effect of contact with other venomous animals**
  ☑6ᵗʰ **T63.81 Toxic effect of contact with venomous frog**
    EXCLUDES 1 *contact with nonvenomous frog (W62.0)*
    ☑7ᵗʰ **T63.811 Toxic effect of contact with venomous frog, accidental (unintentional)**
    ☑7ᵗʰ **T63.812 Toxic effect of contact with venomous frog, intentional self-harm**
    ☑7ᵗʰ **T63.813 Toxic effect of contact with venomous frog, assault**
    ☑7ᵗʰ **T63.814 Toxic effect of contact with venomous frog, undetermined**
  ☑6ᵗʰ **T63.82 Toxic effect of contact with venomous toad**
    EXCLUDES 1 *contact with nonvenomous toad (W62.1)*
    ☑7ᵗʰ **T63.821 Toxic effect of contact with venomous toad, accidental (unintentional)**
    ☑7ᵗʰ **T63.822 Toxic effect of contact with venomous toad, intentional self-harm**
    ☑7ᵗʰ **T63.823 Toxic effect of contact with venomous toad, assault**
    ☑7ᵗʰ **T63.824 Toxic effect of contact with venomous toad, undetermined**
  ☑6ᵗʰ **T63.83 Toxic effect of contact with other venomous amphibian**
    EXCLUDES 1 *contact with nonvenomous amphibian (W62.9)*
    ☑7ᵗʰ **T63.831 Toxic effect of contact with other venomous amphibian, accidental (unintentional)**
    ☑7ᵗʰ **T63.832 Toxic effect of contact with other venomous amphibian, intentional self-harm**
    ☑7ᵗʰ **T63.833 Toxic effect of contact with other venomous amphibian, assault**
    ☑7ᵗʰ **T63.834 Toxic effect of contact with other venomous amphibian, undetermined**
  ☑6ᵗʰ **T63.89 Toxic effect of contact with other venomous animals**
    ☑7ᵗʰ **T63.891 Toxic effect of contact with other venomous animals, accidental (unintentional)**
    ☑7ᵗʰ **T63.892 Toxic effect of contact with other venomous animals, intentional self-harm**
    ☑7ᵗʰ **T63.893 Toxic effect of contact with other venomous animals, assault**
    ☑7ᵗʰ **T63.894 Toxic effect of contact with other venomous animals, undetermined**
☑5ᵗʰ **T63.9 Toxic effect of contact with unspecified venomous animal**
  ☑x7ᵗʰ **T63.91 Toxic effect of contact with unspecified venomous animal, accidental (unintentional)**
  ☑x7ᵗʰ **T63.92 Toxic effect of contact with unspecified venomous animal, intentional self-harm**
  ☑x7ᵗʰ **T63.93 Toxic effect of contact with unspecified venomous animal, assault**
  ☑x7ᵗʰ **T63.94 Toxic effect of contact with unspecified venomous animal, undetermined**

☑4ᵗʰ **T64 Toxic effect of aflatoxin and other mycotoxin food contaminants**

> The appropriate 7th character is to be added to each code from category T64.
> A   initial encounter
> D   subsequent encounter
> S   sequela

☑5ᵗʰ **T64.0 Toxic effect of aflatoxin**
  ☑x7ᵗʰ **T64.01 Toxic effect of aflatoxin, accidental (unintentional)**
  ☑x7ᵗʰ **T64.02 Toxic effect of aflatoxin, intentional self-harm**
  ☑x7ᵗʰ **T64.03 Toxic effect of aflatoxin, assault**
  ☑x7ᵗʰ **T64.04 Toxic effect of aflatoxin, undetermined**
☑5ᵗʰ **T64.8 Toxic effect of other mycotoxin food contaminants**
  ☑x7ᵗʰ **T64.81 Toxic effect of other mycotoxin food contaminants, accidental (unintentional)**
  ☑x7ᵗʰ **T64.82 Toxic effect of other mycotoxin food contaminants, intentional self-harm**
  ☑x7ᵗʰ **T64.83 Toxic effect of other mycotoxin food contaminants, assault**

☑x7ᵗʰ **T64.84 Toxic effect of other mycotoxin food contaminants, undetermined**

☑4ᵗʰ **T65 Toxic effect of other and unspecified substances**

> The appropriate 7th character is to be added to each code from category T65.
> A   initial encounter
> D   subsequent encounter
> S   sequela

☑5ᵗʰ **T65.0 Toxic effect of cyanides**
    EXCLUDES 1 *hydrogen cyanide (T57.3-)*
  ☑6ᵗʰ **T65.0x Toxic effect of cyanides**
    ☑7ᵗʰ **T65.0x1 Toxic effect of cyanides, accidental (unintentional)**
            Toxic effect of cyanides NOS
    ☑7ᵗʰ **T65.0x2 Toxic effect of cyanides, intentional self-harm**
    ☑7ᵗʰ **T65.0x3 Toxic effect of cyanides, assault**
    ☑7ᵗʰ **T65.0x4 Toxic effect of cyanides, undetermined**
☑5ᵗʰ **T65.1 Toxic effect of strychnine and its salts**
  ☑6ᵗʰ **T65.1x Toxic effect of strychnine and its salts**
    ☑7ᵗʰ **T65.1x1 Toxic effect of strychnine and its salts, accidental (unintentional)**
            Toxic effect of strychnine and its salts NOS
    ☑7ᵗʰ **T65.1x2 Toxic effect of strychnine and its salts, intentional self-harm**
    ☑7ᵗʰ **T65.1x3 Toxic effect of strychnine and its salts, assault**
    ☑7ᵗʰ **T65.1x4 Toxic effect of strychnine and its salts, undetermined**
☑5ᵗʰ **T65.2 Toxic effect of tobacco and nicotine**
    EXCLUDES 2 *nicotine dependence (F17-)*
  ☑6ᵗʰ **T65.21 Toxic effect of chewing tobacco**
    ☑7ᵗʰ **T65.211 Toxic effect of chewing tobacco, accidental (unintentional)**
            Toxic effect of chewing tobacco NOS
    ☑7ᵗʰ **T65.212 Toxic effect of chewing tobacco, intentional self-harm**
    ☑7ᵗʰ **T65.213 Toxic effect of chewing tobacco, assault**
    ☑7ᵗʰ **T65.214 Toxic effect of chewing tobacco, undetermined**
  ☑6ᵗʰ **T65.22 Toxic effect of tobacco cigarettes**
            Toxic effect of tobacco smoke
            Use additional code for exposure to second hand tobacco smoke (Z57.31, Z77.22)
    ☑7ᵗʰ **T65.221 Toxic effect of tobacco cigarettes, accidental (unintentional)**
            Toxic effect of tobacco cigarettes NOS
    ☑7ᵗʰ **T65.222 Toxic effect of tobacco cigarettes, intentional self-harm**
    ☑7ᵗʰ **T65.223 Toxic effect of tobacco cigarettes, assault**
    ☑7ᵗʰ **T65.224 Toxic effect of tobacco cigarettes, undetermined**
  ☑6ᵗʰ **T65.29 Toxic effect of other tobacco and nicotine**
    ☑7ᵗʰ **T65.291 Toxic effect of other tobacco and nicotine, accidental (unintentional)**
            Toxic effect of other tobacco and nicotine NOS
    ☑7ᵗʰ **T65.292 Toxic effect of other tobacco and nicotine, intentional self-harm**
    ☑7ᵗʰ **T65.293 Toxic effect of other tobacco and nicotine, assault**
    ☑7ᵗʰ **T65.294 Toxic effect of other tobacco and nicotine, undetermined**

☑ 5ᵗʰ **T65.3 Toxic effect of nitroderivatives and aminoderivatives of benzene and its homologues**
Toxic effect of anilin [benzenamine]
Toxic effect of nitrobenzene
Toxic effect of trinitrotoluene

   ☑ 6ᵗʰ **T65.3x Toxic effect of nitroderivatives and aminoderivatives of benzene and its homologues**

     ☑ 7ᵗʰ **T65.3x1 Toxic effect of nitroderivatives and aminoderivatives of benzene and its homologues, accidental (unintentional)**
Toxic effect of nitroderivatives and aminoderivatives of benzene and its homologues NOS

     ☑ 7ᵗʰ **T65.3x2 Toxic effect of nitroderivatives and aminoderivatives of benzene and its homologues, intentional self-harm**

     ☑ 7ᵗʰ **T65.3x3 Toxic effect of nitroderivatives and aminoderivatives of benzene and its homologues, assault**

     ☑ 7ᵗʰ **T65.3x4 Toxic effect of nitroderivatives and aminoderivatives of benzene and its homologues, undetermined**

☑ 5ᵗʰ **T65.4 Toxic effect of carbon disulfide**

   ☑ 6ᵗʰ **T65.4x Toxic effect of carbon disulfide**

     ☑ 7ᵗʰ **T65.4x1 Toxic effect of carbon disulfide, accidental (unintentional)**
Toxic effect of carbon disulfide NOS

     ☑ 7ᵗʰ **T65.4x2 Toxic effect of carbon disulfide, intentional self-harm**

     ☑ 7ᵗʰ **T65.4x3 Toxic effect of carbon disulfide, assault**

     ☑ 7ᵗʰ **T65.4x4 Toxic effect of carbon disulfide, undetermined**

☑ 5ᵗʰ **T65.5 Toxic effect of nitroglycerin and other nitric acids and esters**
Toxic effect of 1,2,3-Propanetriol trinitrate

   ☑ 6ᵗʰ **T65.5x Toxic effect of nitroglycerin and other nitric acids and esters**

     ☑ 7ᵗʰ **T65.5x1 Toxic effect of nitroglycerin and other nitric acids and esters, accidental (unintentional)**
Toxic effect of nitroglycerin and other nitric acids and esters NOS

     ☑ 7ᵗʰ **T65.5x2 Toxic effect of nitroglycerin and other nitric acids and esters, intentional self-harm**

     ☑ 7ᵗʰ **T65.5x3 Toxic effect of nitroglycerin and other nitric acids and esters, assault**

     ☑ 7ᵗʰ **T65.5x4 Toxic effect of nitroglycerin and other nitric acids and esters, undetermined**

☑ 5ᵗʰ **T65.6 Toxic effect of paints and dyes, not elsewhere classified**

   ☑ 6ᵗʰ **T65.6x Toxic effect of paints and dyes, not elsewhere classified**

     ☑ 7ᵗʰ **T65.6x1 Toxic effect of paints and dyes, not elsewhere classified, accidental (unintentional)**
Toxic effect of paints and dyes NOS

     ☑ 7ᵗʰ **T65.6x2 Toxic effect of paints and dyes, not elsewhere classified, intentional self-harm**

     ☑ 7ᵗʰ **T65.6x3 Toxic effect of paints and dyes, not elsewhere classified, assault**

     ☑ 7ᵗʰ **T65.6x4 Toxic effect of paints and dyes, not elsewhere classified, undetermined**

☑ 5ᵗʰ **T65.8 Toxic effect of other specified substances**

   ☑ 6ᵗʰ **T65.81 Toxic effect of latex**

     ☑ 7ᵗʰ **T65.811 Toxic effect of latex, accidental (unintentional)**
Toxic effect of latex NOS

     ☑ 7ᵗʰ **T65.812 Toxic effect of latex, intentional self-harm**

     ☑ 7ᵗʰ **T65.813 Toxic effect of latex, assault**

     ☑ 7ᵗʰ **T65.814 Toxic effect of latex, undetermined**

   ☑ 6ᵗʰ **T65.82 Toxic effect of harmful algae and algae toxins**
Toxic effect of (harmful) algae bloom NOS
Toxic effect of blue-green algae bloom
Toxic effect of brown tide
Toxic effect of cyanobacteria bloom
Toxic effect of Florida red tide
Toxic effect of pfiesteria piscicida
Toxic effect of red tide

     ☑ 7ᵗʰ **T65.821 Toxic effect of harmful algae and algae toxins, accidental (unintentional)**
Toxic effect of harmful algae and algae toxins NOS

     ☑ 7ᵗʰ **T65.822 Toxic effect of harmful algae and algae toxins, intentional self-harm**

     ☑ 7ᵗʰ **T65.823 Toxic effect of harmful algae and algae toxins, assault**

     ☑ 7ᵗʰ **T65.824 Toxic effect of harmful algae and algae toxins, undetermined**

   ☑ 6ᵗʰ **T65.83 Toxic effect of fiberglass**

     ☑ 7ᵗʰ **T65.831 Toxic effect of fiberglass, accidental (unintentional)**
Toxic effect of fiberglass NOS

     ☑ 7ᵗʰ **T65.832 Toxic effect of fiberglass, intentional self-harm**

     ☑ 7ᵗʰ **T65.833 Toxic effect of fiberglass, assault**

     ☑ 7ᵗʰ **T65.834 Toxic effect of fiberglass, undetermined**

   ☑ 6ᵗʰ **T65.89 Toxic effect of other specified substances**

     ☑ 7ᵗʰ **T65.891 Toxic effect of other specified substances, accidental (unintentional)**
Toxic effect of other specified substances NOS

     ☑ 7ᵗʰ **T65.892 Toxic effect of other specified substances, intentional self-harm**

     ☑ 7ᵗʰ **T65.893 Toxic effect of other specified substances, assault**

     ☑ 7ᵗʰ **T65.894 Toxic effect of other specified substances, undetermined**

☑ 5ᵗʰ **T65.9 Toxic effect of unspecified substance**

   ☑x7ᵗʰ **T65.91 Toxic effect of unspecified substance, accidental (unintentional)**
Poisoning NOS

   ☑x7ᵗʰ **T65.92 Toxic effect of unspecified substance, intentional self-harm**

   ☑x7ᵗʰ **T65.93 Toxic effect of unspecified substance, assault**

   ☑x7ᵗʰ **T65.94 Toxic effect of unspecified substance, undetermined**

Other and unspecified effects of external causes (T66-T78)

☑x7ᵗʰ **T66 Radiation sickness, unspecified**

   EXCLUDES 1 specified adverse effects of radiation, such as:
     burns (T20-T31)
     leukemia (C91-C95)
     radiation:
       gastroenteritis and colitis (K52.0)
       pneumonitis (J70.0)
       related disorders of the skin and subcutaneous tissue (L55-L59)
       sunburn (L55-)

The appropriate 7th character is to be added to code T66.
A   initial encounter
D   subsequent encounter
S   sequela

☑ 4ᵗʰ **T67 Effects of heat and light**

   EXCLUDES 1 erythema [dermatitis] ab igne (L59.0)
     malignant hyperpyrexia due to anesthesia (T88.3)
     radiation-related disorders of the skin and subcutaneous tissue (L55-L59)
   EXCLUDES 2 burns (T20-T31)
     sunburn (L55-)
     sweat disorder due to heat (L74-L75))

The appropriate 7th character is to be added to each code from category T67.
A   initial encounter
D   subsequent encounter
S   sequela

EXCLUDES 1 Not coded here   *EXCLUDES 2* Not included here   *Manifestation Code*

√x7th **T67.0   Heatstroke and sunstroke**
  Heat apoplexy
  Heat pyrexia
  Siriasis
  Thermoplegia
  Use additional code(s) to identify any associated
      complications of heatstroke, such as:
          coma and stupor (R40.-)
          systemic inflammatory response syndrome (R65.1-)

√x7th **T67.1   Heat syncope**
  Heat collapse

√x7th **T67.2   Heat cramp**

√x7th **T67.3   Heat exhaustion, anhydrotic**
  Heat prostration due to water depletion
  EXCLUDES 1 *heat exhaustion due to salt depletion (T67.4)*

√x7th **T67.4   Heat exhaustion due to salt depletion**
  Heat prostration due to salt (and water) depletion

√x7th **T67.5   Heat exhaustion, unspecified**
  Heat prostration NOS

√x7th **T67.6   Heat fatigue, transient**

√x7th **T67.7   Heat edema**

√x7th **T67.8   Other effects of heat and light**

√x7th **T67.9   Effect of heat and light, unspecified**

√x7th **T68   Hypothermia**
  Accidental hypothermia
  Hypothermia NOS
  EXCLUDES 1 *hypothermia following anesthesia (T88.51)*
              hypothermia not associated with low environmental
                  temperature (R68.0)
              hypothermia of newborn (P80-)
  EXCLUDES 2 *frostbite (T33-T34)*
  Use additional code to identify source of exposure:
      exposure to excessive cold of man-made origin (W93)
      exposure to excessive cold of natural origin (X31)

> The appropriate 7th character is to be added to code T68.
>   A   initial encounter
>   D   subsequent encounter
>   S   sequela

√4th **T69   Other effects of reduced temperature**
  EXCLUDES 2 *frostbite (T33-T34)*
  Use additional code to identify source of exposure:
      exposure to excessive cold of man-made origin (W93)
      exposure to excessive cold of natural origin (X31)

> The appropriate 7th character is to be added to each code from
> category T69.
>   A   initial encounter
>   D   subsequent encounter
>   S   sequela

√5th **T69.0   Immersion hand and foot**
  √6th **T69.01   Immersion hand**
    √7th **T69.011   Immersion hand, right hand**
    √7th **T69.012   Immersion hand, left hand**
    √7th **T69.019   Immersion hand, unspecified hand**
  √6th **T69.02   Immersion foot**
      Trench foot
    √7th **T69.021   Immersion foot, right foot**
    √7th **T69.022   Immersion foot, left foot**
    √7th **T69.029   Immersion foot, unspecified foot**

√x7th **T69.1   Chilblains**

√x7th **T69.8   Other specified effects of reduced temperature**

√x7th **T69.9   Effect of reduced temperature, unspecified**

√4th **T70   Effects of air pressure and water pressure**

> The appropriate 7th character is to be added to each code from
> category T70.
>   A   initial encounter
>   D   subsequent encounter
>   S   sequela

√x7th **T70.0   Otitic barotrauma**
  Aero-otitis media
  Effects of change in ambient atmospheric pressure or water
      pressure on ears

√x7th **T70.1   Sinus barotrauma**
  Aerosinusitis
  Effects of change in ambient atmospheric pressure on sinuses

√5th **T70.2   Other and unspecified effects of high altitude**
  EXCLUDES 2 *polycythemia due to high altitude (D75.1)*
  √x7th **T70.20   Unspecified effects of high altitude**
  √x7th **T70.29   Other effects of high altitude**
      Alpine sickness
      Anoxia due to high altitude
      Barotrauma NOS
      Hypobaropathy
      Mountain sickness

√x7th **T70.3   Caisson disease [decompression sickness]**
  Compressed-air disease
  Diver's palsy or paralysis

√x7th **T70.4   Effects of high-pressure fluids**
  Hydraulic jet injection (industrial)
  Pneumatic jet injection (industrial)
  Traumatic jet injection (industrial)

√x7th **T70.8   Other effects of air pressure and water pressure**

√x7th **T70.9   Effect of air pressure and water pressure, unspecified**

√4th **T71   Asphyxiation**
  Mechanical suffocation
  Traumatic suffocation
  EXCLUDES 1 *acute respiratory distress (syndrome) (J80)*
              anoxia due to high altitude (T70.2)
              asphyxia NOS (R09.01)
              asphyxia from carbon monoxide (T58-)
              asphyxia from inhalation of food or foreign body (T17-)
              asphyxia from other gases, fumes and vapors (T59-)
              respiratory distress (syndrome) in newborn (P22-)

> The appropriate 7th character is to be added to each code from
> category T71.
>   A   initial encounter
>   D   subsequent encounter
>   S   sequela

√5th **T71.1   Asphyxiation due to mechanical threat to breathing**
    Suffocation due to mechanical threat to breathing
  √6th **T71.11   Asphyxiation due to smothering under pillow**
    √7th **T71.111   Asphyxiation due to smothering under pillow, accidental**
        Asphyxiation due to smothering under pillow NOS
    √7th **T71.112   Asphyxiation due to smothering under pillow, intentional self-harm**
    √7th **T71.113   Asphyxiation due to smothering under pillow, assault**
    √7th **T71.114   Asphyxiation due to smothering under pillow, undetermined**
  √6th **T71.12   Asphyxiation due to plastic bag**
    √7th **T71.121   Asphyxiation due to plastic bag, accidental**
        Asphyxiation due to plastic bag NOS
    √7th **T71.122   Asphyxiation due to plastic bag, intentional self-harm**
    √7th **T71.123   Asphyxiation due to plastic bag, assault**
    √7th **T71.124   Asphyxiation due to plastic bag, undetermined**
  √6th **T71.13   Asphyxiation due to being trapped in bed linens**
    √7th **T71.131   Asphyxiation due to being trapped in bed linens, accidental**
        Asphyxiation due to being trapped in bed linens NOS
    √7th **T71.132   Asphyxiation due to being trapped in bed linens, intentional self-harm**
    √7th **T71.133   Asphyxiation due to being trapped in bed linens, assault**
    √7th **T71.134   Asphyxiation due to being trapped in bed linens, undetermined**
  √6th **T71.14   Asphyxiation due to smothering under another person's body (in bed)**
    √7th **T71.141   Asphyxiation due to smothering under another person's body (in bed), accidental**
        Asphyxiation due to smothering under another person's body (in bed) NOS
    √7th **T71.143   Asphyxiation due to smothering under another person's body (in bed), assault**

√7th **T71.144 Asphyxiation due to smothering under another person's body (in bed), undetermined**

√6th **T71.15 Asphyxiation due to smothering in furniture**

   √7th **T71.150 Asphyxiation due to smothering in furniture NOS**

   √7th **T71.151 Asphyxiation due to smothering in furniture, accidental**

   √7th **T71.152 Asphyxiation due to smothering in furniture, intentional self-harm**

   √7th **T71.153 Asphyxiation due to smothering in furniture, assault**

   √7th **T71.154 Asphyxiation due to smothering in furniture, undetermined**

√6th **T71.16 Asphyxiation due to hanging**
     Hanging by window shade cord
     Use additional code for any associated injuries, such as:
       crushing injury of neck (S17-)
       fracture of cervical vertebrae (S12.0-S12.2-)
       open wound of neck (S11-)

   √7th **T71.161 Asphyxiation due to hanging, accidental**
       Asphyxiation due to hanging NOS
       Hanging NOS

   √7th **T71.162 Asphyxiation due to hanging, intentional self-harm**

   √7th **T71.163 Asphyxiation due to hanging, assault**

   √7th **T71.164 Asphyxiation due to hanging, undetermined**

√6th **T71.19 Asphyxiation due to mechanical threat to breathing due to other causes**

   √7th **T71.191 Asphyxiation due to mechanical threat to breathing due to other causes, accidental**
       Asphyxiation due to other causes NOS

   √7th **T71.192 Asphyxiation due to mechanical threat to breathing due to other causes, intentional self-harm**

   √7th **T71.193 Asphyxiation due to mechanical threat to breathing due to other causes, assault**

   √7th **T71.194 Asphyxiation due to mechanical threat to breathing due to other causes, undetermined**

√5th **T71.2 Asphyxiation due to systemic oxygen deficiency due to low oxygen content in ambient air**
     Suffocation due to systemic oxygen deficiency due to low oxygen content in ambient air

  √x7th **T71.20 Asphyxiation due to systemic oxygen deficiency due to low oxygen content in ambient air due to unspecified cause**

  √x7th **T71.21 Asphyxiation due to cave-in or falling earth**
       Use additional code for any associated cataclysm (X34-X38)

√6th **T71.22 Asphyxiation due to being trapped in a car trunk**

   √7th **T71.221 Asphyxiation due to being trapped in a car trunk, accidental**

   √7th **T71.222 Asphyxiation due to being trapped in a car trunk, intentional self-harm**

   √7th **T71.223 Asphyxiation due to being trapped in a car trunk, assault**

   √7th **T71.224 Asphyxiation due to being trapped in a car trunk, undetermined**

√6th **T71.23 Asphyxiation due to being trapped in a (discarded) refrigerator**

   √7th **T71.231 Asphyxiation due to being trapped in a (discarded) refrigerator, accidental**

   √7th **T71.232 Asphyxiation due to being trapped in a (discarded) refrigerator, intentional self-harm**

   √7th **T71.233 Asphyxiation due to being trapped in a (discarded) refrigerator, assault**

   √7th **T71.234 Asphyxiation due to being trapped in a (discarded) refrigerator, undetermined**

  √x7th **T71.29 Asphyxiation due to being trapped in other low oxygen environment**

  √x7th **T71.9 Asphyxiation due to unspecified cause**
     Suffocation (by strangulation) due to unspecified cause
     Suffocation NOS
     Systemic oxygen deficiency due to low oxygen content in ambient air due to unspecified cause
     Systemic oxygen deficiency due to mechanical threat to breathing due to unspecified cause
     Traumatic asphyxia NOS

√4th **T73 Effects of other deprivation**

> The appropriate 7th character is to be added to each code from category T73.
> A   initial encounter
> D   subsequent encounter
> S   sequela

√x7th **T73.0 Starvation**
     Deprivation of food

√x7th **T73.1 Deprivation of water**

√x7th **T73.2 Exhaustion due to exposure**

√x7th **T73.3 Exhaustion due to excessive exertion**
     Exhaustion due to overexertion

√x7th **T73.8 Other effects of deprivation**

√x7th **T73.9 Effect of deprivation, unspecified**

√4th **T74 Adult and child abuse, neglect and other maltreatment, confirmed**

> EXCLUDES 1   *abuse and maltreatment in pregnancy (O94)*
>   *adult and child maltreatment, suspected (T76-)*

> Use additional code, if applicable, to identify any associated current injury
> Use additional external cause code to identify perpetrator, if known (Y07-)

> The appropriate 7th character is to be added to each code from category T74.
> A   initial encounter
> D   subsequent encounter
> S   sequela

√5th **T74.0 Neglect or abandonment, confirmed**

  √x7th **T74.01 Adult neglect or abandonment, confirmed**

  √x7th **T74.02 Child neglect or abandonment, confirmed**

√5th **T74.1 Physical abuse, confirmed**

> EXCLUDES 2   *sexual abuse (T74.2-)*

  √x7th **T74.11 Adult physical abuse, confirmed**

  √x7th **T74.12 Child physical abuse, confirmed**
>   EXCLUDES 2   *shaken infant syndrome (T74.4)*

√5th **T74.2 Sexual abuse, confirmed**
     Rape, confirmed
     Sexual assault, confirmed

  √x7th **T74.21 Adult sexual abuse, confirmed**

  √x7th **T74.22 Child sexual abuse, confirmed**

√5th **T74.3 Psychological abuse, confirmed**

  √x7th **T74.31 Adult psychological abuse, confirmed**

  √x7th **T74.32 Child psychological abuse, confirmed**

√x7th **T74.4 Shaken infant syndrome**

√5th **T74.9 Unspecified maltreatment, confirmed**

  √x7th **T74.91 Unspecified adult maltreatment, confirmed**

  √x7th **T74.92 Unspecified child maltreatment, confirmed**

√4th **T75 Other and unspecified effects of other external causes**

> EXCLUDES 1   *adverse effects NEC (T78-)*
> EXCLUDES 2   *burns (electric) (T20-T31)*

> The appropriate 7th character is to be added to each code from category T75.
> A   initial encounter
> D   subsequent encounter
> S   sequela

√5th **T75.0 Effects of lightning**
     Struck by lightning

  √x7th **T75.00 Unspecified effects of lightning**
       Struck by lightning NOS

  √x7th **T75.01 Shock due to being struck by lightning**

  √x7th **T75.09 Other effects of lightning**
       Use additional code for other effects of lightning

√x7th **T75.1 Unspecified effects of drowning and nonfatal submersion**
     Immersion

> EXCLUDES 1   *specified effects of drowning—code to effects*

EXCLUDES 1   Not coded here   EXCLUDES 2   Not included here   *Manifestation Code*

√5ᵗʰ **T75.2 Effects of vibration**
- √x7ᵗʰ **T75.20 Unspecified effects of vibration**
- √x7ᵗʰ **T75.21 Pneumatic hammer syndrome**
- √x7ᵗʰ **T75.22 Traumatic vasospastic syndrome**
- √x7ᵗʰ **T75.23 Vertigo from infrasound**
  - *EXCLUDES 1*   *vertigo NOS (R42)*
- **T75.29 Other effects of vibration**

√x7ᵗʰ **T75.3 Motion sickness**
Airsickness
Seasickness
Travel sickness
Use additional external cause code to identify vehicle or type of motion (Y92.81-, Y93.5-)

√x7ᵗʰ **T75.4 Electrocution**
Shock from electric current
Shock from electroshock gun (taser)

√5ᵗʰ **T75.8 Other specified effects of external causes**
- √x7ᵗʰ **T75.81 Effects of abnormal gravitation [G] forces**
- √x7ᵗʰ **T75.82 Effects of weightlessness**
- √x7ᵗʰ **T75.89 Other specified effects of external causes**

√4ᵗʰ **T76 Adult and child abuse, neglect and other maltreatment, suspected**
- *EXCLUDES 1*   *adult and child maltreatment, confirmed (T74-)*
  suspected abuse and maltreatment in pregnancy (O94)
  suspected adult physical and sexual abuse, ruled out (Z04.71)
  suspected child physical and sexual abuse, ruled out (Z04.72)

Use additional code, if applicable, to identify any associated current injury

> The appropriate 7th character is to be added to each code from category T76.
> A   initial encounter
> D   subsequent encounter
> S   sequela

√5ᵗʰ **T76.0 Neglect or abandonment, suspected**
- √x7ᵗʰ **T76.01 Adult neglect or abandonment, suspected**
- √x7ᵗʰ **T76.02 Child neglect or abandonment, suspected**

√5ᵗʰ **T76.1 Physical abuse, suspected**
- √x7ᵗʰ **T76.11 Adult physical abuse, suspected**
- √x7ᵗʰ **T76.12 Child physical abuse, suspected**

√5ᵗʰ **T76.2 Sexual abuse, suspected**
Rape, suspected
Sexual abuse, suspected
- *EXCLUDES 1*   *alleged abuse, ruled out (Z04.7)*
- √x7ᵗʰ **T76.21 Adult sexual abuse, suspected**
- √x7ᵗʰ **T76.22 Child sexual abuse, suspected**

√5ᵗʰ **T76.3 Psychological abuse, suspected**
- √x7ᵗʰ **T76.31 Adult psychological abuse, suspected**
- √x7ᵗʰ **T76.32 Child psychological abuse, suspected**

√5ᵗʰ **T76.9 Unspecified maltreatment, suspected**
- √x7ᵗʰ **T76.91 Unspecified adult maltreatment, suspected**
- √x7ᵗʰ **T76.92 Unspecified child maltreatment, suspected**

√4ᵗʰ **T78 Adverse effects, not elsewhere classified**
- *EXCLUDES 2*   *complications of surgical and medical care NEC (T80-T88)*

> The appropriate 7th character is to be added to each code from category T78.
> A   initial encounter
> D   subsequent encounter
> S   sequela

√5ᵗʰ **T78.0 Anaphylactic shock due to adverse food reaction**
Anaphylactic reaction due to food
- √x7ᵗʰ **T78.00 Anaphylactic shock due to unspecified food**
- √x7ᵗʰ **T78.01 Anaphylactic shock due to peanuts**
- √x7ᵗʰ **T78.02 Anaphylactic shock due to shellfish (crustaceans)**
- √x7ᵗʰ **T78.03 Anaphylactic shock due to other fish**
- √x7ᵗʰ **T78.04 Anaphylactic shock due to fruits and vegetables**
- √x7ᵗʰ **T78.05 Anaphylactic shock due to tree nuts and seeds**
  - *EXCLUDES 1*   *anaphylactic shock due to peanuts (T78.01)*
- √x7ᵗʰ **T78.06 Anaphylactic shock due to food additives**
- √x7ᵗʰ **T78.07 Anaphylactic shock due to milk and dairy products**
- √x7ᵗʰ **T78.08 Anaphylactic shock due to eggs**
- √x7ᵗʰ **T78.09 Anaphylactic shock due to other food products**

√x7ᵗʰ **T78.1 Other adverse food reactions, not elsewhere classified**
Use additional code to identify the type of reaction
- *EXCLUDES 1*   *anaphylactic shock due to adverse food reaction (T78.0)*
  anaphylactic reaction due to food (T78.0)
  bacterial food borne intoxications (A05-)
- *EXCLUDES 2*   *allergic and dietetic gastroenteritis and colitis (K52.2)*
  allergic rhinitis due to food (J30.5)
  dermatitis due to food in contact with skin (L23.6, L24.6, L25.4)
  dermatitis due to ingested food (L27.2)

√x7ᵗʰ **T78.2 Anaphylactic shock, unspecified**
Allergic shock
Anaphylactic reaction
Anaphylaxis
- *EXCLUDES 1*   *anaphylactic shock due to:*
  adverse effect of correct medicinal substance properly administered (T88.6)
  adverse food reaction (T78.0-)
  serum (T80.5)

√x7ᵗʰ **T78.3 Angioneurotic edema**
Giant urticaria
Quincke's edema
- *EXCLUDES 1*   *urticaria (L50-)*
  serum (T80.6)

√5ᵗʰ **T78.4 Other and unspecified allergy**
- *EXCLUDES 1*   *specified types of allergic reaction such as:*
  allergic diarrhea (K52.2)
  allergic gastroenteritis and colitis (K52.2)
  dermatitis (L23-L25, L27-)
  hay fever (J30.1)
- √x7ᵗʰ **T78.40 Allergy, unspecified**
  Allergic reaction NOS
  Hypersensitivity NOS
- √x7ᵗʰ **T78.41 Arthus phenomenon**
  Arthus reaction
- √x7ᵗʰ **T78.49 Other allergy**

√x7ᵗʰ **T78.8 Other adverse effects, not elsewhere classified**

Certain early complications of trauma (T79)

√4ᵗʰ **T79 Certain early complications of trauma, not elsewhere classified**
- *EXCLUDES 2*   *acute respiratory distress syndrome (J80)*
  complications occurring during or following medical procedures (T80-T88)
  complications of surgical and medical care NEC (T80-T88)
  newborn respiratory distress syndrome (P22.0)

> The appropriate 7th character is to be added to each code from category T79.
> A   initial encounter
> D   subsequent encounter
> S   sequela

√x7ᵗʰ **T79.0 Air embolism (traumatic)**
- *EXCLUDES 1*   *air embolism complicating:*
  abortion or ectopic or molar pregnancy (O00-O07, O08.2)
  pregnancy, childbirth and the puerperium (O88.0)
  air embolism following:
  infusion, transfusion, and therapeutic injection (T80.0)
  procedure NEC (I81.7-)

√x7ᵗʰ **T79.1 Fat embolism (traumatic)**
- *EXCLUDES 1*   *fat embolism complicating:*
  abortion or ectopic or molar pregnancy (O00-O07, O08.2)
  pregnancy, childbirth and the puerperium (O88.8)

√x7ᵗʰ **T79.2 Traumatic secondary and recurrent hemorrhage and seroma**

Injury, Poisoning and Certain Other Consequences of External Causes

T79.4–T80.29

✓x7ᵗʰ **T79.4** **Traumatic shock**

Shock (immediate) (delayed) following injury

> EXCLUDES 1   anaphylactic shock due to adverse food reaction (T78.0-)
> anaphylactic shock due to correct medicinal substance properly administered (T88.6)
> anaphylactic shock due to serum (T80.5)
> anaphylactic shock NOS (T78.2)
> anesthetic shock (T88.2)
> electric shock (T75.4)
> nontraumatic shock NEC (R57-)
> obstetric shock (O75.1)
> postprocedural shock (T81.1)
> septic shock (R65.21)
> shock complicating abortion or ectopic or molar pregnancy (O00-O07, O08.3)
> shock due to lightning (T75.01)
> shock NOS (R57.9)

✓x7ᵗʰ **T79.5** **Traumatic anuria**

Crush syndrome

Renal failure following crushing

✓x7ᵗʰ **T79.6** **Traumatic ischemia of muscle**

Traumatic rhabdomyolysis

Volkmann's ischemic contracture

> EXCLUDES 2   anterior tibial syndrome (M76.8)
> compartment syndrome (traumatic) (T79.a-)
> nontraumatic ischemia of muscle (M62.2-)

✓x7ᵗʰ **T79.7** **Traumatic subcutaneous emphysema**

> EXCLUDES 1   emphysema NOS (J43)
> emphysema (subcutaneous) resulting from a procedure (T81.82)

✓5ᵗʰ **T79.a** **Traumatic compartment syndrome**

> EXCLUDES 1   fibromyalgia (M79.7)
> nontraumatic compartment syndrome (M79.a-)
> traumatic ischemic infarction of muscle (T79.6)

    ✓x7ᵗʰ **T79.a0** **Compartment syndrome, unspecified**

Compartment syndrome NOS

    ✓6ᵗʰ **T79.a1** **Traumatic compartment syndrome of upper extremity**

Traumatic compartment syndrome of shoulder, arm, forearm, wrist, hand, and fingers

      ✓7ᵗʰ **T79.a11** **Traumatic compartment syndrome of right upper extremity**

      ✓7ᵗʰ **T79.a12** **Traumatic compartment syndrome of left upper extremity**

      ✓7ᵗʰ **T79.a19** **Traumatic compartment syndrome of unspecified upper extremity**

    ✓6ᵗʰ **T79.a2** **Traumatic compartment syndrome of lower extremity**

Traumatic compartment syndrome of hip, buttock, thigh, leg, foot, and toes

      ✓7ᵗʰ **T79.a21** **Traumatic compartment syndrome of right lower extremity**

      ✓7ᵗʰ **T79.a22** **Traumatic compartment syndrome of left lower extremity**

      ✓7ᵗʰ **T79.a29** **Traumatic compartment syndrome of unspecified lower extremity**

    ✓x7ᵗʰ **T79.a3** **Traumatic compartment syndrome of abdomen**

    ✓x7ᵗʰ **T79.a9** **Traumatic compartment syndrome of other sites**

✓x7ᵗʰ **T79.8** **Other early complications of trauma**

✓x7ᵗʰ **T79.9** **Unspecified early complication of trauma**

Complications of surgical and medical care, not elsewhere classified (T80-T88)

Use additional code(s) to identify the specified condition resulting from the complication

Use additional code (Y62-Y82) to identify devices involved and details of circumstances

> EXCLUDES 2   adverse effects of drugs and medicaments (T36-T50 with fifth or sixth character 5)
> any encounters with medical care for postprocedural conditions in which no complications are present, such as:
>   artificial opening status (Z93-)
>   closure of external stoma (Z43-)
>   fitting and adjustment of external prosthetic device (Z44-)
> burns and corrosions from local applications and irradiation (T20-T32)
> complications of surgical procedures during pregnancy, childbirth and the puerperium (O00-O99)
> mechanical complication of respirator [ventilator] (J95.850)
> poisoning and toxic effects of drugs and chemicals (T36-T65 with final characters 1-4)
> postprocedural fever (R50.82)
> specified complications classified elsewhere, such as:
>   cerebrospinal fluid leak from spinal puncture (G97.0)
>   colostomy malfunction (K94.0-)
>   disorders of fluid and electrolyte imbalance (E86- E87)
>   functional disturbances following cardiac surgery (I97.0-I97.1)
>   intraoperative and postprocedural complications of specified body systems (D78-, E36-, E89-, G97.3-, G97.4, H59.3-, H59-, H95.2-, H95.3, I97.4-, I97.5, J95.6-, J95.7, K91.6-, L76-, M96-, N99-)
>   ostomy complications (J95.0-, K94-, N99.5-)
>   postgastric surgery syndromes (K91.1)
>   postlaminectomy syndrome NEC (M96.1)
>   postmastectomy lymphedema syndrome (I97.2)
>   postsurgical blind-loop syndrome (K91.2)
>   ventilator associated pneumonia (J95.851)

✓4ᵗʰ **T80** **Complications following infusion, transfusion and therapeutic injection**

> INCLUDES   complications following perfusion
> EXCLUDES 2   bone marrow transplant rejection (T86.01)
> febrile nonhemolytic transfusion reaction (R50.84)
> fluid overload due to transfusion (E87.71)
> posttransfusion purpura (D69.51)
> transfusion associated circulatory overload (TACO) (E87.71)
> transfusion (red blood cell) associated hemochromatosis (E83.111)
> transfusion related acute lung injury (TRALI) (J95.84)

> The appropriate 7th character is to be added to each code from category T80.
> A   initial encounter
> D   subsequent encounter
> S   sequela

✓x7ᵗʰ **T80.0** **Air embolism following infusion, transfusion and therapeutic injection**

✓x7ᵗʰ **T80.1** **Vascular complications following infusion, transfusion and therapeutic injection**

Use additional code to identify the vascular complication

> EXCLUDES 2   extravasation of vesicant agent (T80.81-)
> infiltration of vesicant agent (T80.81-)
> vascular complications specified as due to prosthetic devices, implants and grafts (T82.8-, T83.8, T84.8-, T85.8)
> postprocedural vascular complications (T81.7-)

✓5ᵗʰ **T80.2** **Infections following infusion, transfusion and therapeutic injection**

Use additional code to identify the specific infection, such as: sepsis (A41.9)

Use additional code (R65.2-) to identify severe sepsis, if applicable

> EXCLUDES 2   infections specified as due to prosthetic devices, implants and grafts (T82.6-T82.7, T83.5-T83.6, T84.5-T84.7, T85.7)
> postprocedural infections (T81.4)

    ✓x7ᵗʰ **T80.21** **Infection due to central venous catheter**

Catheter-related bloodstream infection (CRBSI) NOS

Infection due to portacath (port-a-cath)

Infection due to umbilical venous catheter

    ✓x7ᵗʰ **T80.29** **Infection following other infusion, transfusion and therapeutic injection**

✓5ᵗʰ **T80.3   ABO incompatibility reaction due to transfusion of blood or blood products**

EXCLUDES 1 *minor blood group antigens reactions (Duffy) (E) (K(ell)) (Kidd) (Lewis) (M) (N) (P) (S) (T80.a)*

✓x7ᵗʰ **T80.30   ABO incompatibility reaction due to transfusion of blood or blood products, unspecified**
ABO incompatibility blood transfusion NOS
Reaction to ABO incompatibility from transfusion NOS

✓6ᵗʰ **T80.31   ABO incompatibility with hemolytic transfusion reaction**

✓7ᵗʰ **T80.310   ABO incompatibility with acute hemolytic transfusion reaction**
ABO incompatibility with hemolytic transfusion reaction less than 24 hours after transfusion
Acute hemolytic transfusion reaction (AHTR) due to ABO incompatibility

✓7ᵗʰ **T80.311   ABO incompatibility with delayed hemolytic transfusion reaction**
ABO incompatibility with hemolytic transfusion reaction 24 hours or more after transfusion
Delayed hemolytic transfusion reaction (DHTR) due to ABO incompatibility

✓7ᵗʰ **T80.319   ABO incompatibility with hemolytic transfusion reaction, unspecified**
ABO incompatibility with hemolytic transfusion reaction at unspecified time after transfusion
Hemolytic transfusion reaction (HTR) due to ABO incompatibility NOS

✓x7ᵗʰ **T80.39   Other ABO incompatibility reaction due to transfusion of blood or blood products**
Delayed serologic transfusion reaction (DSTR) from ABO incompatibility
Other ABO incompatible blood transfusion
Other reaction to ABO incompatible blood transfusion

✓x7ᵗʰ **T80.4   Rh incompatibility reaction due to transfusion of blood or blood products**
Reaction due to incompatibility of Rh antigens (C) (c) (D) (E) (e)

✓x7ᵗʰ **T80.40   Rh incompatibility reaction due to transfusion of blood or blood products, unspecified**
Reaction due to Rh factor in transfusion NOS
Rh incompatible blood transfusion NOS

✓6ᵗʰ **T80.41   Rh incompatibility with hemolytic transfusion reaction**

✓7ᵗʰ **T80.410   Rh incompatibility with acute hemolytic transfusion reaction**
Acute hemolytic transfusion reaction (AHTR) due to Rh incompatibility
Rh incompatibility with hemolytic transfusion reaction less than 24 hours after transfusion

✓7ᵗʰ **T80.411   Rh incompatibility with delayed hemolytic transfusion reaction**
Delayed hemolytic transfusion reaction (DHTR) due to Rh incompatibility
Rh incompatibility with hemolytic transfusion reaction 24 hours or more after transfusion

✓7ᵗʰ **T80.419   Rh incompatibility with hemolytic transfusion reaction, unspecified**
Hemolytic transfusion reaction (HTR) due to Rh incompatibility NOS
Rh incompatibility with hemolytic transfusion reaction at unspecified time after transfusion

✓x7ᵗʰ **T80.49   Other Rh incompatibility reaction due to transfusion of blood or blood products**
Delayed serologic transfusion reaction (DSTR) from Rh incompatibility
Other reaction to Rh incompatible blood transfusion

✓5ᵗʰ **T80.a   Non-ABO incompatibility reaction due to transfusion of blood or blood products**
Reaction due to incompatibility of minor antigens (Duffy) (Kell) (Kidd) (Lewis) (M) (N) (P) (S)

✓x7ᵗʰ **T80.a0   Non-ABO incompatibility reaction due to transfusion of blood or blood products, unspecified**
Non-ABO antigen incompatibility reaction from transfusion NOS

✓6ᵗʰ **T80.a1   Non-ABO incompatibility with hemolytic transfusion reaction**

✓7ᵗʰ **T80.a10   Non-ABO incompatibility with acute hemolytic transfusion reaction**
Acute hemolytic transfusion reaction (AHTR) due to non-ABO incompatibility
Non-ABO incompatibility with hemolytic transfusion reaction less than 24 hours after transfusion

✓7ᵗʰ **T80.a11   Non-ABO incompatibility with delayed hemolytic transfusion reaction**
Delayed hemolytic transfusion reaction (DHTR) due to non-ABO incompatibility
Non-ABO incompatibility with hemolytic transfusion reaction 24 or more hours after transfusion

✓7ᵗʰ **T80.a19   Non-ABO incompatibility with hemolytic transfusion reaction, unspecified**
Hemolytic transfusion reaction (HTR) due to non-ABO incompatibility NOS
Non-ABO incompatibility with hemolytic transfusion reaction at unspecified time after transfusion

✓x7ᵗʰ **T80.a9   Other non-ABO incompatibility reaction due to transfusion of blood or blood products**
Delayed serologic transfusion reaction (DSTR) from non-ABO incompatibility
Other reaction to non-ABO incompatible blood transfusion

✓x7ᵗʰ **T80.5   Anaphylactic shock due to serum**
Anaphylactic reaction due to serum

EXCLUDES 1 *allergic shock NOS (T78.2)*
anaphylactic shock NOS (T78.2)
anaphylactic shock due to adverse effect of correct medicinal substance properly administered (T88.6)

✓x7ᵗʰ **T80.6   Other serum reactions**
Intoxication by serum
Protein sickness
Serum rash
Serum sickness
Serum urticaria

EXCLUDES 2 *serum hepatitis (B16-)*

✓5ᵗʰ **T80.8   Other complications following infusion, transfusion and therapeutic injection**

✓6ᵗʰ **T80.81   Extravasation of vesicant agent**
Infiltration of vesicant agent

✓7ᵗʰ **T80.810   Extravasation of vesicant antineoplastic chemotherapy**
Infiltration of vesicant antineoplastic chemotherapy

✓7ᵗʰ **T80.818   Extravasation of other vesicant agent**
Infiltration of other vesicant agent

✓x7ᵗʰ **T80.89   Other complications following infusion, transfusion and therapeutic injection**
Delayed serologic transfusion reaction (DSTR), unspecified incompatibility
Use additional code to identify graft-versus-host reaction, if applicable, (D89.81-)

✓ Appropriate additional character required   ✓x7ᵗʰ Requires 7th character, placeholder x must fill empty characters

√5ᵗʰ **T80.9 Unspecified complication following infusion, transfusion and therapeutic injection**

√7ᵗʰ **T80.90 Unspecified complication following infusion and therapeutic injection**

√6ᵗʰ **T80.91 Hemolytic transfusion reaction, unspecified incompatibility**

> EXCLUDES 1   *ABO incompatibility with hemolytic transfusion reaction (T80.31-)*
> *Non-ABO incompatibility with hemolytic transfusion reaction (T80.a1-)*
> *Rh incompatibility with hemolytic transfusion reaction (T80.41-)*

√7ᵗʰ **T80.910 Acute hemolytic transfusion reaction, unspecified incompatibility**

√7ᵗʰ **T80.911 Delayed hemolytic transfusion reaction, unspecified incompatibility**

√7ᵗʰ **T80.919 Hemolytic transfusion reaction, unspecified incompatibility, unspecified as acute or delayed**
> Hemolytic transfusion reaction NOS

√x7ᵗʰ **T80.92 Unspecified transfusion reaction**
> Transfusion reaction NOS

√4ᵗʰ **T81 Complications of procedures, not elsewhere classified**

> EXCLUDES 2   *complications following immunization (T88.0-T88.1)*
> *complications following infusion, transfusion and therapeutic injection (T80-)*
> *complications of transplanted organs and tissue (T86-)*
> *specified complications classified elsewhere, such as:*
>   *adverse effect, poisoning and toxic effects of drugs and chemicals (T36-T65)*
>   *complication of prosthetic devices, implants and grafts (T82-T85)*
>   *dermatitis due to drugs and medicaments (L23.3, L24.4, L25.1, L27.0-L27.1)*
>   *endosseous dental implant failure (M27.6-)*
>   *floppy iris syndrome (IFIS) (intraoperative) H21.81*
>   *intraoperative and postprocedural complications of specific body system (D78-, E36-, E89-, G97.3-, G97.4, H59.3-, H59-, H95.2-, H95.3, I97.4-, I97.5, J95, K91-, L76-, M96-, N99-)*
>   *ostomy complications (J95.0-, K94-, N99.5-)*
>   *plateau iris syndrome (post-iridectomy) (postprocedural) H21.82*

> The appropriate 7th character is to be added to each code from category T81.
> A   initial encounter
> D   subsequent encounter
> S   sequela

√x7ᵗʰ **T81.1 Shock during or resulting from a procedure, not elsewhere classified**
> Collapse NOS during or resulting from a procedure, not elsewhere classified
> Shock (hypovolemic) during or resulting from a procedure, not elsewhere classified
> Postprocedural shock NOS during or resulting from a procedure, not elsewhere classified

> EXCLUDES 1   *anaphylactic shock NOS (T78.2)*
> *anaphylactic shock due to correct substance properly administered (T88.6)*
> *anaphylactic shock due to serum (T80.5)*
> *anesthetic shock (T88.2)*
> *electric shock (T75.4)*
> *obstetric shock (O75.1)*
> *septic shock (R65.21)*
> *shock following abortion or ectopic or molar pregnancy (O00-O07, O08.3)*
> *traumatic shock (T79.4)*

√5ᵗʰ **T81.3 Disruption of wound, not elsewhere classified**
> Disruption of any suture materials or other closure methods

> EXCLUDES 1   *breakdown (mechanical) of permanent sutures (T85.612)*
> *displacement of permanent sutures (T86.622)*
> *disruption of cesarean delivery wound (O90.0)*
> *disruption of perineal obstetric wound (O90.1)*
> *mechanical complication of permanent sutures NEC (T85.692)*

√x7ᵗʰ **T81.30 Disruption of wound, unspecified**
> Disruption of wound NOS

√x7ᵗʰ **T81.31 Disruption of external operation (surgical) wound, not elsewhere classified**
> Dehiscence of operation wound NOS
> Disruption of operation wound NOS
> Disruption or dehiscence of closure of cornea
> Disruption or dehiscence of closure of mucosa
> Disruption or dehiscence of closure of skin and subcutaneous tissue
> Full-thickness skin disruption or dehiscence
> Superficial disruption or dehiscence of operation wound

√x7ᵗʰ **T81.32 Disruption of internal operation (surgical) wound, not elsewhere classified**
> Deep disruption or dehiscence of operation wound NOS
> Disruption or dehiscence of closure of internal organ or other internal tissue
> Disruption or dehiscence of closure of muscle or muscle flap
> Disruption or dehiscence of closure of ribs or rib cage
> Disruption or dehiscence of closure of skull or craniotomy
> Disruption or dehiscence of closure of sternum or sternotomy
> Disruption or dehiscence of closure of tendon or ligament
> Disruption or dehiscence of closure of superficial or muscular fascia

√x7ᵗʰ **T81.33 Disruption of traumatic injury wound repair**
> Disruption or dehiscence of closure of traumatic laceration (external) (internal)

√x7ᵗʰ **T81.4 Infection following a procedure**
> Intra-abdominal abscess following a procedure
> Postprocedural infection, not elsewhere classified
> Sepsis following a procedure
> Stitch abscess following a procedure
> Subphrenic abscess following a procedure
> Wound abscess following a procedure
> Use additional code to identify infection
> Use additional code (R65.2-) to identify severe sepsis, if applicable

> EXCLUDES 1   *obstetric surgical wound infection (O86.0)*
> *postprocedural fever NOS (R50.82)*
> *postprocedural retroperitoneal abscess (K68.11)*

> EXCLUDES 2   *bleb associated endophthalmitis (H59.4-)*
> *infection due to infusion, transfusion and therapeutic injection (T80.2-)*
> *infection due to prosthetic devices, implants and grafts (T82.6-T82.7, T83.5-T83.6, T84.5-T84.7, T85.7)*

√5ᵗʰ **T81.5 Complications of foreign body accidentally left in body following procedure**

√6ᵗʰ **T81.50 Unspecified complication of foreign body accidentally left in body following procedure**

√7ᵗʰ **T81.500 Unspecified complication of foreign body accidentally left in body following surgical operation**

√7ᵗʰ **T81.501 Unspecified complication of foreign body accidentally left in body following infusion or transfusion**

√7ᵗʰ **T81.502 Unspecified complication of foreign body accidentally left in body following kidney dialysis**

√7ᵗʰ **T81.503 Unspecified complication of foreign body accidentally left in body following injection or immunization**

√7ᵗʰ **T81.504 Unspecified complication of foreign body accidentally left in body following endoscopic examination**

√7ᵗʰ **T81.505 Unspecified complication of foreign body accidentally left in body following heart catheterization**

√7ᵗʰ **T81.506 Unspecified complication of foreign body accidentally left in body following aspiration, puncture or other catheterization**

√7ᵗʰ **T81.507 Unspecified complication of foreign body accidentally left in body following removal of catheter or packing**

√7ᵗʰ **T81.508** **Unspecified complication of foreign body accidentally left in body following other procedure**

√7ᵗʰ **T81.509** **Unspecified complication of foreign body accidentally left in body following unspecified procedure**

√6ᵗʰ **T81.51** **Adhesions due to foreign body accidentally left in body following procedure**

√7ᵗʰ **T81.510** **Adhesions due to foreign body accidentally left in body following surgical operation**

√7ᵗʰ **T81.511** **Adhesions due to foreign body accidentally left in body following infusion or transfusion**

√7ᵗʰ **T81.512** **Adhesions due to foreign body accidentally left in body following kidney dialysis**

√7ᵗʰ **T81.513** **Adhesions due to foreign body accidentally left in body following injection or immunization**

√7ᵗʰ **T81.514** **Adhesions due to foreign body accidentally left in body following endoscopic examination**

√7ᵗʰ **T81.515** **Adhesions due to foreign body accidentally left in body following heart catheterization**

√7ᵗʰ **T81.516** **Adhesions due to foreign body accidentally left in body following aspiration, puncture or other catheterization**

√7ᵗʰ **T81.517** **Adhesions due to foreign body accidentally left in body following removal of catheter or packing**

√7ᵗʰ **T81.518** **Adhesions due to foreign body accidentally left in body following other procedure**

√7ᵗʰ **T81.519** **Adhesions due to foreign body accidentally left in body following unspecified procedure**

√6ᵗʰ **T81.52** **Obstruction due to foreign body accidentally left in body following procedure**

√7ᵗʰ **T81.520** **Obstruction due to foreign body accidentally left in body following surgical operation**

√7ᵗʰ **T81.521** **Obstruction due to foreign body accidentally left in body following infusion or transfusion**

√7ᵗʰ **T81.522** **Obstruction due to foreign body accidentally left in body following kidney dialysis**

√7ᵗʰ **T81.523** **Obstruction due to foreign body accidentally left in body following injection or immunization**

√7ᵗʰ **T81.524** **Obstruction due to foreign body accidentally left in body following endoscopic examination**

√7ᵗʰ **T81.525** **Obstruction due to foreign body accidentally left in body following heart catheterization**

√7ᵗʰ **T81.526** **Obstruction due to foreign body accidentally left in body following aspiration, puncture or other catheterization**

√7ᵗʰ **T81.527** **Obstruction due to foreign body accidentally left in body following removal of catheter or packing**

√7ᵗʰ **T81.528** **Obstruction due to foreign body accidentally left in body following other procedure**

√7ᵗʰ **T81.529** **Obstruction due to foreign body accidentally left in body following unspecified procedure**

√6ᵗʰ **T81.53** **Perforation due to foreign body accidentally left in body following procedure**

√7ᵗʰ **T81.530** **Perforation due to foreign body accidentally left in body following surgical operation**

√7ᵗʰ **T81.531** **Perforation due to foreign body accidentally left in body following infusion or transfusion**

√7ᵗʰ **T81.532** **Perforation due to foreign body accidentally left in body following kidney dialysis**

√7ᵗʰ **T81.533** **Perforation due to foreign body accidentally left in body following injection or immunization**

√7ᵗʰ **T81.534** **Perforation due to foreign body accidentally left in body following endoscopic examination**

√7ᵗʰ **T81.535** **Perforation due to foreign body accidentally left in body following heart catheterization**

√7ᵗʰ **T81.536** **Perforation due to foreign body accidentally left in body following aspiration, puncture or other catheterization**

√7ᵗʰ **T81.537** **Perforation due to foreign body accidentally left in body following removal of catheter or packing**

√7ᵗʰ **T81.538** **Perforation due to foreign body accidentally left in body following other procedure**

√7ᵗʰ **T81.539** **Perforation due to foreign body accidentally left in body following unspecified procedure**

√6ᵗʰ **T81.59** **Other complications of foreign body accidentally left in body following procedure**

> *EXCLUDES 2*   *obstruction or perforation due to prosthetic devices and implants intentionally left in body (T82.0-T82.5, T83.0-T83.4, T84.0-T84.4, T85.0-T85.6)*

√7ᵗʰ **T81.590** **Other complications of foreign body accidentally left in body following surgical operation**

√7ᵗʰ **T81.591** **Other complications of foreign body accidentally left in body following infusion or transfusion**

√7ᵗʰ **T81.592** **Other complications of foreign body accidentally left in body following kidney dialysis**

√7ᵗʰ **T81.593** **Other complications of foreign body accidentally left in body following injection or immunization**

√7ᵗʰ **T81.594** **Other complications of foreign body accidentally left in body following endoscopic examination**

√7ᵗʰ **T81.595** **Other complications of foreign body accidentally left in body following heart catheterization**

√7ᵗʰ **T81.596** **Other complications of foreign body accidentally left in body following aspiration, puncture or other catheterization**

√7ᵗʰ **T81.597** **Other complications of foreign body accidentally left in body following removal of catheter or packing**

√7ᵗʰ **T81.598** **Other complications of foreign body accidentally left in body following other procedure**

√7ᵗʰ **T81.599** **Other complications of foreign body accidentally left in body following unspecified procedure**

√5ᵗʰ **T81.6** **Acute reaction to foreign substance accidentally left during a procedure**

> *EXCLUDES 2*   *complications of foreign body accidentally left in body cavity or operation wound following procedure (T81.5-)*

√x7ᵗʰ **T81.60** **Unspecified acute reaction to foreign substance accidentally left during a procedure**

√x7ᵗʰ **T81.61** **Aseptic peritonitis due to foreign substance accidentally left during a procedure**
Chemical peritonitis

√x7ᵗʰ **T81.69** **Other acute reaction to foreign substance accidentally left during a procedure**

√5ᵗʰ **T81.7** **Vascular complications following a procedure, not elsewhere classified**
Air embolism following procedure NEC
Phlebitis or thrombophlebitis resulting from a procedure
EXCLUDES 1   *embolism complicating abortion or ectopic or molar pregnancy (O00–O07, O08.2)*
embolism complicating pregnancy, childbirth and the puerperium (O88-)
traumatic embolism (T79.0)
EXCLUDES 2   *embolism due to prosthetic devices, implants and grafts (T82.8-, T83.8, T84.8-, T85.8)*
embolism following infusion, transfusion and therapeutic injection (T80.0)

    √6ᵗʰ **T81.71** **Complication of artery following a procedure, not elsewhere classified**

       √7ᵗʰ **T81.710** **Complication of mesenteric artery following a procedure, not elsewhere classified**

       √7ᵗʰ **T81.711** **Complication of renal artery following a procedure, not elsewhere classified**

       √7ᵗʰ **T81.718** **Complication of other artery following a procedure, not elsewhere classified**

       √7ᵗʰ **T81.719** **Complication of unspecified artery following a procedure, not elsewhere classified**

    √x7ᵗʰ **T81.72** **Complication of vein following a procedure, not elsewhere classified**

√5ᵗʰ **T81.8** **Other complications of procedures, not elsewhere classified**
EXCLUDES 2   *hypothermia following anesthesia (T88.51)*
malignant hyperpyrexia due to anesthesia (T88.3)

    √x7ᵗʰ **T81.81** **Complication of inhalation therapy**
    √x7ᵗʰ **T81.82** **Emphysema (subcutaneous) resulting from a procedure**
    √x7ᵗʰ **T81.83** **Persistent postprocedural fistula**
    √x7ᵗʰ **T81.89** **Other complications of procedures, not elsewhere classified**
Use additional code to specify complication, such as: postprocedural delirium (F05)

    √x7ᵗʰ **T81.9** **Unspecified complication of procedure**

√4ᵗʰ **T82** **Complications of cardiac and vascular prosthetic devices, implants and grafts**
EXCLUDES 2   *failure and rejection of transplanted organs and tissue (T86-)*

The appropriate 7th character is to be added to each code from category T82.
A   initial encounter
D   subsequent encounter
S   sequela

√5ᵗʰ **T82.0** **Mechanical complication of heart valve prosthesis**
Mechanical complication of artificial heart valve
EXCLUDES 1   *mechanical complication of biological heart valve graft (T82.22-)*

    √x7ᵗʰ **T82.01** **Breakdown (mechanical) of heart valve prosthesis**
    √x7ᵗʰ **T82.02** **Displacement of heart valve prosthesis**
Malposition of heart valve prosthesis
    √x7ᵗʰ **T82.03** **Leakage of heart valve prosthesis**
    √x7ᵗʰ **T82.09** **Other mechanical complication of heart valve prosthesis**
Obstruction (mechanical) of heart valve prosthesis
Perforation of heart valve prosthesis
Protrusion of heart valve prosthesis

√5ᵗʰ **T82.1** **Mechanical complication of cardiac electronic device**
    √6ᵗʰ **T82.11** **Breakdown (mechanical) of cardiac electronic device**

       √7ᵗʰ **T82.110** **Breakdown (mechanical) of cardiac electrode**

       √7ᵗʰ **T82.111** **Breakdown (mechanical) of cardiac pulse generator (battery)**

       √7ᵗʰ **T82.118** **Breakdown (mechanical) of other cardiac electronic device**

       √7ᵗʰ **T82.119** **Breakdown (mechanical) of unspecified cardiac electronic device**

    √6ᵗʰ **T82.12** **Displacement of cardiac electronic device**
Malposition of cardiac electronic device

       √7ᵗʰ **T82.120** **Displacement of cardiac electrode**

       √7ᵗʰ **T82.121** **Displacement of cardiac pulse generator (battery)**

       √7ᵗʰ **T82.128** **Displacement of other cardiac electronic device**

       √7ᵗʰ **T82.129** **Displacement of unspecified cardiac electronic device**

    √6ᵗʰ **T82.19** **Other mechanical complication of cardiac electronic device**
Leakage of cardiac electronic device
Obstruction of cardiac electronic device
Perforation of cardiac electronic device
Protrusion of cardiac electronic device

       √7ᵗʰ **T82.190** **Other mechanical complication of cardiac electrode**

       √7ᵗʰ **T82.191** **Other mechanical complication of cardiac pulse generator (battery)**

       √7ᵗʰ **T82.198** **Other mechanical complication of other cardiac electronic device**

       √7ᵗʰ **T82.199** **Other mechanical complication of unspecified cardiac device**

√5ᵗʰ **T82.2** **Mechanical complication of coronary artery bypass graft and biological heart valve graft**
EXCLUDES 1   *mechanical complication of artificial heart valve prosthesis (T82.0-)*

    √6ᵗʰ **T82.21** **Mechanical complication of coronary artery bypass graft**

       √7ᵗʰ **T82.211** **Breakdown (mechanical) of coronary artery bypass graft**

       √7ᵗʰ **T82.212** **Displacement of coronary artery bypass graft**
Malposition of coronary artery bypass graft

       √7ᵗʰ **T82.213** **Leakage of coronary artery bypass graft**

       √7ᵗʰ **T82.218** **Other mechanical complication of coronary artery bypass graft**
Obstruction, mechanical of coronary artery bypass graft
Perforation of coronary artery bypass graft
Protrusion of coronary artery bypass graft

    √6ᵗʰ **T82.22** **Mechanical complication of biological heart valve graft**

       √7ᵗʰ **T82.221** **Breakdown (mechanical) of biological heart valve graft**

       √7ᵗʰ **T82.222** **Displacement of biological heart valve graft**
Malposition of biological heart valve graft

       √7ᵗʰ **T82.223** **Leakage of biological heart valve graft**

       √7ᵗʰ **T82.228** **Other mechanical complication of biological heart valve graft**
Obstruction of biological heart valve graft
Perforation of biological heart valve graft
Protrusion of biological heart valve graft

√5ᵗʰ **T82.3** **Mechanical complication of other vascular grafts**
    √6ᵗʰ **T82.31** **Breakdown (mechanical) of other vascular grafts**

       √7ᵗʰ **T82.310** **Breakdown (mechanical) of aortic (bifurcation) graft (replacement)**

       √7ᵗʰ **T82.311** **Breakdown (mechanical) of carotid arterial graft (bypass)**

       √7ᵗʰ **T82.312** **Breakdown (mechanical) of femoral arterial graft (bypass)**

       √7ᵗʰ **T82.318** **Breakdown (mechanical) of other vascular grafts**

       √7ᵗʰ **T82.319** **Breakdown (mechanical) of unspecified vascular grafts**

    √6ᵗʰ **T82.32** **Displacement of other vascular grafts**
Malposition of other vascular grafts

       √7ᵗʰ **T82.320** **Displacement of aortic (bifurcation) graft (replacement)**

       √7ᵗʰ **T82.321** **Displacement of carotid arterial graft (bypass)**

       √7ᵗʰ **T82.322** **Displacement of femoral arterial graft (bypass)**

       √7ᵗʰ **T82.328** **Displacement of other vascular grafts**

       √7ᵗʰ **T82.329** **Displacement of unspecified vascular grafts**

EXCLUDES 1 Not coded here   *EXCLUDES 2* Not included here   *Manifestation Code*

✓6th T82.33 Leakage of other vascular grafts
- **✓7th T82.330 Leakage of aortic (bifurcation) graft (replacement)**
- **✓7th T82.331 Leakage of carotid arterial graft (bypass)**
- **✓7th T82.332 Leakage of femoral arterial graft (bypass)**
- **✓7th T82.338 Leakage of other vascular grafts**
- **✓7th T82.339 Leakage of unspecified vascular graft**

✓6th T82.39 Other mechanical complication of other vascular grafts
- Obstruction (mechanical) of other vascular grafts
- Perforation of other vascular grafts
- Protrusion of other vascular grafts
- **✓7th T82.390 Other mechanical complication of aortic (bifurcation) graft (replacement)**
- **✓7th T82.391 Other mechanical complication of carotid arterial graft (bypass)**
- **✓7th T82.392 Other mechanical complication of femoral arterial graft (bypass)**
- **✓7th T82.398 Other mechanical complication of other vascular grafts**
- **✓7th T82.399 Other mechanical complication of unspecified vascular grafts**

✓5th T82.4 Mechanical complication of vascular dialysis catheter
- Mechanical complication of hemodialysis catheter
- *EXCLUDES 1* *mechanical complication of intraperitoneal dialysis catheter (T85.62)*

✓x7th T82.41 Breakdown (mechanical) of vascular dialysis catheter

✓x7th T82.42 Displacement of vascular dialysis catheter
- Malposition of vascular dialysis catheter

✓x7th T82.43 Leakage of vascular dialysis catheter

✓x7th T82.49 Other complication of vascular dialysis catheter
- Obstruction (mechanical) of vascular dialysis catheter
- Perforation of vascular dialysis catheter
- Protrusion of vascular dialysis catheter

✓5th T82.5 Mechanical complication of other cardiac and vascular devices and implants
- *EXCLUDES 2* *mechanical complication of epidural and subdural infusion catheter (T85.61)*

✓6th T82.51 Breakdown (mechanical) of other cardiac and vascular devices and implants
- **✓7th T82.510 Breakdown (mechanical) of surgically created arteriovenous fistula**
- **✓7th T82.511 Breakdown (mechanical) of surgically created arteriovenous shunt**
- **✓7th T82.512 Breakdown (mechanical) of artificial heart**
- **✓7th T82.513 Breakdown (mechanical) of balloon (counterpulsation) device**
- **✓7th T82.514 Breakdown (mechanical) of infusion catheter**
- **✓7th T82.515 Breakdown (mechanical) of umbrella device**
- **✓7th T82.518 Breakdown (mechanical) of other cardiac and vascular devices and implants**
- **✓7th T82.519 Breakdown (mechanical) of unspecified cardiac and vascular devices and implants**

✓6th T82.52 Displacement of other cardiac and vascular devices and implants
- Malposition of other cardiac and vascular devices and implants
- **✓7th T82.520 Displacement of surgically created arteriovenous fistula**
- **✓7th T82.521 Displacement of surgically created arteriovenous shunt**
- **✓7th T82.522 Displacement of artificial heart**
- **✓7th T82.523 Displacement of balloon (counterpulsation) device**
- **✓7th T82.524 Displacement of infusion catheter**
- **✓7th T82.525 Displacement of umbrella device**
- **✓7th T82.528 Displacement of other cardiac and vascular devices and implants**
- **✓7th T82.529 Displacement of unspecified cardiac and vascular devices and implants**

✓6th T82.53 Leakage of other cardiac and vascular devices and implants
- **✓7th T82.530 Leakage of surgically created arteriovenous fistula**
- **✓7th T82.531 Leakage of surgically created arteriovenous shunt**
- **✓7th T82.532 Leakage of artificial heart**
- **✓7th T82.533 Leakage of balloon (counterpulsation) device**
- **✓7th T82.534 Leakage of infusion catheter**
- **✓7th T82.535 Leakage of umbrella device**
- **✓7th T82.538 Leakage of other cardiac and vascular devices and implants**
- **✓7th T82.539 Leakage of unspecified cardiac and vascular devices and implants**

✓6th T82.59 Other mechanical complication of other cardiac and vascular devices and implants
- Obstruction (mechanical) of other cardiac and vascular devices and implants
- Perforation of other cardiac and vascular devices and implants
- Protrusion of other cardiac and vascular devices and implants
- **✓7th T82.590 Other mechanical complication of surgically created arteriovenous fistula**
- **✓7th T82.591 Other mechanical complication of surgically created arteriovenous shunt**
- **✓7th T82.592 Other mechanical complication of artificial heart**
- **✓7th T82.593 Other mechanical complication of balloon (counterpulsation) device**
- **✓7th T82.594 Other mechanical complication of infusion catheter**
- **✓7th T82.595 Other mechanical complication of umbrella device**
- **✓7th T82.598 Other mechanical complication of other cardiac and vascular devices and implants**
- **✓7th T82.599 Other mechanical complication of unspecified cardiac and vascular devices and implants**

✓x7th T82.6 Infection and inflammatory reaction due to cardiac valve prosthesis
- Use additional code to identify infection

✓x7th T82.7 Infection and inflammatory reaction due to other cardiac and vascular devices, implants and grafts
- Use additional code to identify infection

✓5th T82.8 Other specified complications of cardiac and vascular prosthetic devices, implants and grafts

✓6th T82.81 Embolism of cardiac and vascular prosthetic devices, implants and grafts
- **✓7th T82.817 Embolism of cardiac prosthetic devices, implants and grafts**
- **✓7th T82.818 Embolism of vascular prosthetic devices, implants and grafts**

✓6th T82.82 Fibrosis of cardiac and vascular prosthetic devices, implants and grafts
- **✓7th T82.827 Fibrosis of cardiac prosthetic devices, implants and grafts**
- **✓7th T82.828 Fibrosis of vascular prosthetic devices, implants and grafts**

✓6th T82.83 Hemorrhage of cardiac and vascular prosthetic devices, implants and grafts
- **✓7th T82.837 Hemorrhage of cardiac prosthetic devices, implants and grafts**
- **✓7th T82.838 Hemorrhage of vascular prosthetic devices, implants and grafts**

✓6th T82.84 Pain from cardiac and vascular prosthetic devices, implants and grafts
- **✓7th T82.847 Pain from cardiac prosthetic devices, implants and grafts**
- **✓7th T82.848 Pain from vascular prosthetic devices, implants and grafts**

✔ Appropriate additional character required   ✓x7th Requires 7th character, placeholder x must fill empty characters

√6ᵗʰ **T82.85** **Stenosis of cardiac and vascular prosthetic devices, implants and grafts**

     √7ᵗʰ **T82.857** **Stenosis of cardiac prosthetic devices, implants and grafts**

     √7ᵗʰ **T82.858** **Stenosis of vascular prosthetic devices, implants and grafts**

√6ᵗʰ **T82.86** **Thrombosis of cardiac and vascular prosthetic devices, implants and grafts**

     √7ᵗʰ **T82.867** **Thrombosis of cardiac prosthetic devices, implants and grafts**

     √7ᵗʰ **T82.868** **Thrombosis of vascular prosthetic devices, implants and grafts**

√6ᵗʰ **T82.89** **Other specified complication of cardiac and vascular prosthetic devices, implants and grafts**

     √7ᵗʰ **T82.897** **Other specified complication of cardiac prosthetic devices, implants and grafts**

     √7ᵗʰ **T82.898** **Other specified complication of vascular prosthetic devices, implants and grafts**

√x7ᵗʰ **T82.9** **Unspecified complication of cardiac and vascular prosthetic device, implant and graft**

√4ᵗʰ **T83** **Complications of genitourinary prosthetic devices, implants and grafts**

> **EXCLUDES 2** *failure and rejection of transplanted organs and tissue (T86-)*

> The appropriate 7th character is to be added to each code from category T83.
> A   initial encounter
> D   subsequent encounter
> S   sequela

√5ᵗʰ **T83.0** **Mechanical complication of urinary (indwelling) catheter**

    EXCLUDES 2 *complications of stoma of urinary tract (N99.5-)*

   √6ᵗʰ **T83.01** **Breakdown (mechanical) of urinary (indwelling) catheter**

     √7ᵗʰ **T83.010** **Breakdown (mechanical) of cystostomy catheter**

     √7ᵗʰ **T83.018** **Breakdown (mechanical) of other indwelling urethral catheter**

   √6ᵗʰ **T83.02** **Displacement of urinary (indwelling) catheter**

     Malposition of urinary (indwelling) catheter

     √7ᵗʰ **T83.020** **Displacement of cystostomy catheter**

     √7ᵗʰ **T83.028** **Displacement of other indwelling urethral catheter**

   √6ᵗʰ **T83.03** **Leakage of urinary (indwelling) catheter**

     √7ᵗʰ **T83.030** **Leakage of cystostomy catheter**

     √7ᵗʰ **T83.038** **Leakage of other indwelling urethral catheter**

   √6ᵗʰ **T83.09** **Other mechanical complication of urinary (indwelling) catheter**

     Obstruction (mechanical) of urinary (indwelling) catheter
     Perforation of urinary (indwelling) catheter
     Protrusion of urinary (indwelling) catheter

     √7ᵗʰ **T83.090** **Other mechanical complication of cystostomy catheter**

     √7ᵗʰ **T83.098** **Other mechanical complication of other indwelling urethral catheter**

√5ᵗʰ **T83.1** **Mechanical complication of other urinary devices and implants**

   √6ᵗʰ **T83.11** **Breakdown (mechanical) of other urinary devices and implants**

     √7ᵗʰ **T83.110** **Breakdown (mechanical) of urinary electronic stimulator device**

     √7ᵗʰ **T83.111** **Breakdown (mechanical) of urinary sphincter implant**

     √7ᵗʰ **T83.112** **Breakdown (mechanical) of urinary stent**

     √7ᵗʰ **T83.118** **Breakdown (mechanical) of other urinary devices and implants**

   √6ᵗʰ **T83.12** **Displacement of other urinary devices and implants**

     Malposition of other urinary devices and implants

     √7ᵗʰ **T83.120** **Displacement of urinary electronic stimulator device**

     √7ᵗʰ **T83.121** **Displacement of urinary sphincter implant**

     √7ᵗʰ **T83.122** **Displacement of urinary stent**

     √7ᵗʰ **T83.128** **Displacement of other urinary devices and implants**

   √6ᵗʰ **T83.19** **Other mechanical complication of other urinary devices and implants**

     Leakage of other urinary devices and implants
     Obstruction (mechanical) of other urinary devices and implants
     Perforation of other urinary devices and implants
     Protrusion of other urinary devices and implants

     √7ᵗʰ **T83.190** **Other mechanical complication of urinary electronic stimulator device**

     √7ᵗʰ **T83.191** **Other mechanical complication of urinary sphincter implant**

     √7ᵗʰ **T83.192** **Other mechanical complication of urinary stent**

     √7ᵗʰ **T83.198** **Other mechanical complication of other urinary devices and implants**

√5ᵗʰ **T83.2** **Mechanical complication of graft of urinary organ**

   √x7ᵗʰ **T83.21** **Breakdown (mechanical) of graft of urinary organ**

   √x7ᵗʰ **T83.22** **Displacement of graft of urinary organ**

     Malposition of graft of urinary organ

   √x7ᵗʰ **T83.23** **Leakage of graft of urinary organ**

   √x7ᵗʰ **T83.29** **Other mechanical complication of graft of urinary organ**

     Obstruction (mechanical) of graft of urinary organ
     Perforation of graft of urinary organ
     Protrusion of graft of urinary organ

√5ᵗʰ **T83.3** **Mechanical complication of intrauterine contraceptive device**

   √x7ᵗʰ **T83.31** **Breakdown (mechanical) of intrauterine contraceptive device**

   √x7ᵗʰ **T83.32** **Displacement of intrauterine contraceptive device**

     Malposition of intrauterine contraceptive device

   √x7ᵗʰ **T83.39** **Other mechanical complication of intrauterine contraceptive device**

     Leakage of intrauterine contraceptive device
     Obstruction (mechanical) of intrauterine contraceptive device
     Perforation of intrauterine contraceptive device
     Protrusion of intrauterine contraceptive device

√5ᵗʰ **T83.4** **Mechanical complication of other prosthetic devices, implants and grafts of genital tract**

   √6ᵗʰ **T83.41** **Breakdown (mechanical) of other prosthetic devices, implants and grafts of genital tract**

     √7ᵗʰ **T83.410** **Breakdown (mechanical) of penile (implanted) prosthesis**

     √7ᵗʰ **T83.418** **Breakdown (mechanical) of other prosthetic devices, implants and grafts of genital tract**

   √6ᵗʰ **T83.42** **Displacement of other prosthetic devices, implants and grafts of genital tract**

     Malposition of other prosthetic devices, implants and grafts of genital tract

     √7ᵗʰ **T83.420** **Displacement of penile (implanted) prosthesis**

     √7ᵗʰ **T83.428** **Displacement of other prosthetic devices, implants and grafts of genital tract**

   √6ᵗʰ **T83.49** **Other mechanical complication of other prosthetic devices, implants and grafts of genital tract**

     Leakage of other prosthetic devices, implants and grafts of genital tract
     Obstruction, mechanical of other prosthetic devices, implants and grafts of genital tract
     Perforation of other prosthetic devices, implants and grafts of genital tract
     Protrusion of other prosthetic devices, implants and grafts of genital tract

     √7ᵗʰ **T83.490** **Other mechanical complication of penile (implanted) prosthesis**

     √7ᵗʰ **T83.498** **Other mechanical complication of other prosthetic devices, implants and grafts of genital tract**

√5ᵗʰ **T83.5** **Infection and inflammatory reaction due to prosthetic device, implant and graft in urinary system**

     Use additional code to identify infection

   √x7ᵗʰ **T83.51** **Infection and inflammatory reaction due to indwelling urinary catheter**

✓x7ᵗʰ **T83.59** **Infection and inflammatory reaction due to prosthetic device, implant and graft in urinary system**

✓x7ᵗʰ **T83.6** **Infection and inflammatory reaction due to prosthetic device, implant and graft in genital tract**
　　　Use additional code to identify infection

✓5ᵗʰ **T83.8** **Other specified complications of genitourinary prosthetic devices, implants and grafts**

　　✓x7ᵗʰ **T83.81** **Embolism of genitourinary prosthetic devices, implants and grafts**

　　✓x7ᵗʰ **T83.82** **Fibrosis of genitourinary prosthetic devices, implants and grafts**

　　✓x7ᵗʰ **T83.83** **Hemorrhage of genitourinary prosthetic devices, implants and grafts**

　　✓x7ᵗʰ **T83.84** **Pain from genitourinary prosthetic devices, implants and grafts**

　　✓x7ᵗʰ **T83.85** **Stenosis of genitourinary prosthetic devices, implants and grafts**

　　✓x7ᵗʰ **T83.86** **Thrombosis of genitourinary prosthetic devices, implants and grafts**

　　✓x7ᵗʰ **T83.89** **Other specified complication of genitourinary prosthetic devices, implants and grafts**

✓x7ᵗʰ **T83.9** **Unspecified complication of genitourinary prosthetic device, implant and graft**

✓4ᵗʰ **T84** **Complications of internal orthopedic prosthetic devices, implants and grafts**
　　EXCLUDES 2　*failure and rejection of transplanted organs and tissues (T86-)*
　　　　fracture of bone following insertion of orthopedic implant, joint prosthesis or bone plate (M96.6)

> The appropriate 7th character is to be added to each code from category T84.
> A　initial encounter
> D　subsequent encounter
> S　sequela

✓5ᵗʰ **T84.0** **Mechanical complication of internal joint prosthesis**

　　✓6ᵗʰ **T84.01** **Broken internal joint prosthesis**
　　　　Breakage (fracture) of prosthetic joint
　　　　Broken prosthetic joint implant
　　　　EXCLUDES 1　*periprosthetic joint implant fracture (T84.04)*

　　　　✓7ᵗʰ **T84.010** **Broken internal right hip prosthesis**
　　　　✓7ᵗʰ **T84.011** **Broken internal left hip prosthesis**
　　　　✓7ᵗʰ **T84.012** **Broken internal right knee prosthesis**
　　　　✓7ᵗʰ **T84.013** **Broken internal left knee prosthesis**
　　　　✓7ᵗʰ **T84.018** **Broken internal joint prosthesis, other site**
　　　　　　Use additional code to identify the joint (Z96.6-)
　　　　✓7ᵗʰ **T84.019** **Broken internal joint prosthesis, unspecified site**

　　✓6ᵗʰ **T84.02** **Dislocation of internal joint prosthesis**
　　　　Instability of internal joint prosthesis
　　　　Subluxation of internal joint prosthesis

　　　　✓7ᵗʰ **T84.020** **Dislocation of internal right hip prosthesis**
　　　　✓7ᵗʰ **T84.021** **Dislocation of internal left hip prosthesis**
　　　　✓7ᵗʰ **T84.022** **Dislocation of internal right knee prosthesis**
　　　　✓7ᵗʰ **T84.023** **Dislocation of internal left knee prosthesis**
　　　　✓7ᵗʰ **T84.028** **Dislocation of other internal joint prosthesis**
　　　　　　Use additional code to identify the joint (Z96.6-)
　　　　✓7ᵗʰ **T84.029** **Dislocation of unspecified internal joint prosthesis**

　　✓6ᵗʰ **T84.03** **Mechanical loosening of internal prosthetic joint**
　　　　Aseptic loosening of prosthetic joint

　　　　✓7ᵗʰ **T84.030** **Mechanical loosening of internal right hip prosthetic joint**
　　　　✓7ᵗʰ **T84.031** **Mechanical loosening of internal left hip prosthetic joint**
　　　　✓7ᵗʰ **T84.032** **Mechanical loosening of internal right knee prosthetic joint**

　　　　✓7ᵗʰ **T84.033** **Mechanical loosening of internal left knee prosthetic joint**
　　　　✓7ᵗʰ **T84.038** **Mechanical loosening of other internal prosthetic joint**
　　　　　　Use additional code to identify the joint (Z96.6-)
　　　　✓7ᵗʰ **T84.039** **Mechanical loosening of unspecified internal prosthetic joint**

　　✓6ᵗʰ **T84.04** **Periprosthetic fracture around internal prosthetic joint**
　　　　EXCLUDES 2　*breakage (fracture) of prosthetic joint (T84.01)*

　　　　✓7ᵗʰ **T84.040** **Periprosthetic fracture around internal prosthetic right hip joint**
　　　　✓7ᵗʰ **T84.041** **Periprosthetic fracture around internal prosthetic left hip joint**
　　　　✓7ᵗʰ **T84.042** **Periprosthetic fracture around internal prosthetic right knee joint**
　　　　✓7ᵗʰ **T84.043** **Periprosthetic fracture around internal prosthetic left knee joint**
　　　　✓7ᵗʰ **T84.048** **Periprosthetic fracture around other internal prosthetic joint**
　　　　　　Use additional code to identify the joint (Z96.6-)
　　　　✓7ᵗʰ **T84.049** **Periprosthetic fracture around unspecified internal prosthetic joint**

　　✓6ᵗʰ **T84.05** **Periprosthetic osteolysis of internal prosthetic joint**
　　　　Use additional code to identify major osseous defect, if applicable (M89.7-)

　　　　✓7ᵗʰ **T84.050** **Periprosthetic osteolysis of internal prosthetic right hip joint**
　　　　✓7ᵗʰ **T84.051** **Periprosthetic osteolysis of internal prosthetic left hip joint**
　　　　✓7ᵗʰ **T84.052** **Periprosthetic osteolysis of internal prosthetic right knee joint**
　　　　✓7ᵗʰ **T84.053** **Periprosthetic osteolysis of internal prosthetic left knee joint**
　　　　✓7ᵗʰ **T84.058** **Periprosthetic osteolysis of other internal prosthetic joint**
　　　　　　Use additional code to identify the joint (Z96.6-)
　　　　✓7ᵗʰ **T84.059** **Periprosthetic osteolysis of unspecified internal prosthetic joint**

　　✓6ᵗʰ **T84.06** **Wear of articular bearing surface of internal prosthetic joint**

　　　　✓7ᵗʰ **T84.060** **Wear of articular bearing surface of internal prosthetic right hip joint**
　　　　✓7ᵗʰ **T84.061** **Wear of articular bearing surface of internal prosthetic left hip joint**
　　　　✓7ᵗʰ **T84.062** **Wear of articular bearing surface of internal prosthetic right knee joint**
　　　　✓7ᵗʰ **T84.063** **Wear of articular bearing surface of internal prosthetic left knee joint**
　　　　✓7ᵗʰ **T84.068** **Wear of articular bearing surface of other internal prosthetic joint**
　　　　　　Use additional code to identify the joint (Z96.6-)
　　　　✓7ᵗʰ **T84.069** **Wear of articular bearing surface of unspecified internal prosthetic joint**

　　✓6ᵗʰ **T84.09** **Other mechanical complication of internal joint prosthesis**
　　　　Prosthetic joint implant failure NOS

　　　　✓7ᵗʰ **T84.090** **Other mechanical complication of internal right hip prosthesis**
　　　　✓7ᵗʰ **T84.091** **Other mechanical complication of internal left hip prosthesis**
　　　　✓7ᵗʰ **T84.092** **Other mechanical complication of internal right knee prosthesis**
　　　　✓7ᵗʰ **T84.093** **Other mechanical complication of internal left knee prosthesis**
　　　　✓7ᵗʰ **T84.098** **Other mechanical complication of other internal joint prosthesis**
　　　　　　Use additional code to identify the joint (Z96.6-)
　　　　✓7ᵗʰ **T84.099** **Other mechanical complication of unspecified internal joint prosthesis**

Injury, Poisoning and Certain Other Consequences of External Causes   **T84.1–T84.398**

√5ᵗʰ **T84.1** **Mechanical complication of internal fixation device of bones of limb**

> EXCLUDES 2   *mechanical complication of internal fixation device of bones of feet (T84.2-)*
> *mechanical complication of internal fixation device of bones of fingers (T84.2-)*
> *mechanical complication of internal fixation device of bones of hands (T84.2-)*
> *mechanical complication of internal fixation device of bones of toes (T84.2-)*

√6ᵗʰ **T84.11** **Breakdown (mechanical) of internal fixation device of bones of limb**

√7ᵗʰ **T84.110** **Breakdown (mechanical) of internal fixation device of right humerus**

√7ᵗʰ **T84.111** **Breakdown (mechanical) of internal fixation device of left humerus**

√7ᵗʰ **T84.112** **Breakdown (mechanical) of internal fixation device of bone of right forearm**

√7ᵗʰ **T84.113** **Breakdown (mechanical) of internal fixation device of bone of left forearm**

√7ᵗʰ **T84.114** **Breakdown (mechanical) of internal fixation device of right femur**

√7ᵗʰ **T84.115** **Breakdown (mechanical) of internal fixation device of left femur**

√7ᵗʰ **T84.116** **Breakdown (mechanical) of internal fixation device of bone of right lower leg**

√7ᵗʰ **T84.117** **Breakdown (mechanical) of internal fixation device of bone of left lower leg**

√7ᵗʰ **T84.119** **Breakdown (mechanical) of internal fixation device of unspecified bone of limb**

√6ᵗʰ **T84.12** **Displacement of internal fixation device of bones of limb**

> Malposition of internal fixation device of bones of limb

√7ᵗʰ **T84.120** **Displacement of internal fixation device of right humerus**

√7ᵗʰ **T84.121** **Displacement of internal fixation device of left humerus**

√7ᵗʰ **T84.122** **Displacement of internal fixation device of bone of right forearm**

√7ᵗʰ **T84.123** **Displacement of internal fixation device of bone of left forearm**

√7ᵗʰ **T84.124** **Displacement of internal fixation device of right femur**

√7ᵗʰ **T84.125** **Displacement of internal fixation device of left femur**

√7ᵗʰ **T84.126** **Displacement of internal fixation device of bone of right lower leg**

√7ᵗʰ **T84.127** **Displacement of internal fixation device of bone of left lower leg**

√7ᵗʰ **T84.129** **Displacement of internal fixation device of unspecified bone of limb**

√6ᵗʰ **T84.19** **Other mechanical complication of internal fixation device of bones of limb**

> Obstruction (mechanical) of internal fixation device of bones of limb
> Perforation of internal fixation device of bones of limb
> Protrusion of internal fixation device of bones of limb

√7ᵗʰ **T84.190** **Other mechanical complication of internal fixation device of right humerus**

√7ᵗʰ **T84.191** **Other mechanical complication of internal fixation device of left humerus**

√7ᵗʰ **T84.192** **Other mechanical complication of internal fixation device of bone of right forearm**

√7ᵗʰ **T84.193** **Other mechanical complication of internal fixation device of bone of left forearm**

√7ᵗʰ **T84.194** **Other mechanical complication of internal fixation device of right femur**

√7ᵗʰ **T84.195** **Other mechanical complication of internal fixation device of left femur**

√7ᵗʰ **T84.196** **Other mechanical complication of internal fixation device of bone of right lower leg**

√7ᵗʰ **T84.197** **Other mechanical complication of internal fixation device of bone of left lower leg**

√7ᵗʰ **T84.199** **Other mechanical complication of internal fixation device of unspecified bone of limb**

√5ᵗʰ **T84.2** **Mechanical complication of internal fixation device of other bones**

√6ᵗʰ **T84.21** **Breakdown (mechanical) of internal fixation device of other bones**

√7ᵗʰ **T84.210** **Breakdown (mechanical) of internal fixation device of bones of hand and fingers**

√7ᵗʰ **T84.213** **Breakdown (mechanical) of internal fixation device of bones of foot and toes**

√7ᵗʰ **T84.216** **Breakdown (mechanical) of internal fixation device of vertebrae**

√7ᵗʰ **T84.218** **Breakdown (mechanical) of internal fixation device of other bones**

√6ᵗʰ **T84.22** **Displacement of internal fixation device of other bones**

> Malposition of internal fixation device of other bones

√7ᵗʰ **T84.220** **Displacement of internal fixation device of bones of hand and fingers**

√7ᵗʰ **T84.223** **Displacement of internal fixation device of bones of foot and toes**

√7ᵗʰ **T84.226** **Displacement of internal fixation device of vertebrae**

√7ᵗʰ **T84.228** **Displacement of internal fixation device of other bones**

√6ᵗʰ **T84.29** **Other mechanical complication of internal fixation device of other bones**

> Obstruction (mechanical) of internal fixation device of other bones
> Perforation of internal fixation device of other bones
> Protrusion of internal fixation device of other bones

√7ᵗʰ **T84.290** **Other mechanical complication of internal fixation device of bones of hand and fingers**

√7ᵗʰ **T84.293** **Other mechanical complication of internal fixation device of bones of foot and toes**

√7ᵗʰ **T84.296** **Other mechanical complication of internal fixation device of vertebrae**

√7ᵗʰ **T84.298** **Other mechanical complication of internal fixation device of other bones**

√5ᵗʰ **T84.3** **Mechanical complication of other bone devices, implants and grafts**

> EXCLUDES 2   *other complications of bone graft (T86.83-)*

√6ᵗʰ **T84.31** **Breakdown (mechanical) of other bone devices, implants and grafts**

√7ᵗʰ **T84.310** **Breakdown (mechanical) of electronic bone stimulator**

√7ᵗʰ **T84.318** **Breakdown (mechanical) of other bone devices, implants and grafts**

√6ᵗʰ **T84.32** **Displacement of other bone devices, implants and grafts**

> Malposition of other bone devices, implants and grafts

√7ᵗʰ **T84.320** **Displacement of electronic bone stimulator**

√7ᵗʰ **T84.328** **Displacement of other bone devices, implants and grafts**

√6ᵗʰ **T84.39** **Other mechanical complication of other bone devices, implants and grafts**

> Obstruction (mechanical) of other bone devices, implants and grafts
> Perforation of other bone devices, implants and grafts
> Protrusion of other bone devices, implants and grafts

√7ᵗʰ **T84.390** **Other mechanical complication of electronic bone stimulator**

√7ᵗʰ **T84.398** **Other mechanical complication of other bone devices, implants and grafts**

EXCLUDES 1   Not coded here   EXCLUDES 2   Not included here   *Manifestation Code*

✓5ᵗʰ **T84.4 Mechanical complication of other internal orthopedic devices, implants and grafts**

  ✓6ᵗʰ **T84.41 Breakdown (mechanical) of other internal orthopedic devices, implants and grafts**

    ✓7ᵗʰ **T84.41Ø Breakdown (mechanical) of muscle and tendon graft**

    ✓7ᵗʰ **T84.418 Breakdown (mechanical) of other internal orthopedic devices, implants and grafts**

  ✓6ᵗʰ **T84.42 Displacement of other internal orthopedic devices, implants and grafts**

    Malposition of other internal orthopedic devices, implants and grafts

    ✓7ᵗʰ **T84.42Ø Displacement of muscle and tendon graft**

    ✓7ᵗʰ **T84.428 Displacement of other internal orthopedic devices, implants and grafts**

  ✓6ᵗʰ **T84.49 Other mechanical complication of other internal orthopedic devices, implants and grafts**

    Mechanical complication of other internal orthopedic devices, implants and grafts NOS

    Obstruction (mechanical) of other internal orthopedic devices, implants and grafts

    Perforation of other internal orthopedic devices, implants and grafts

    Protrusion of other internal orthopedic devices, implants and grafts

    ✓7ᵗʰ **T84.49Ø Other mechanical complication of muscle and tendon graft**

    ✓7ᵗʰ **T84.498 Other mechanical complication of other internal orthopedic devices, implants and grafts**

✓5ᵗʰ **T84.5 Infection and inflammatory reaction due to internal joint prosthesis**

  Use additional code to identify infection

  ✓x7ᵗʰ **T84.5Ø Infection and inflammatory reaction due to unspecified internal joint prosthesis**

  ✓x7ᵗʰ **T84.51 Infection and inflammatory reaction due to internal right hip prosthesis**

  ✓x7ᵗʰ **T84.52 Infection and inflammatory reaction due to internal left hip prosthesis**

  ✓x7ᵗʰ **T84.53 Infection and inflammatory reaction due to internal right knee prosthesis**

  ✓x7ᵗʰ **T84.54 Infection and inflammatory reaction due to internal left knee prosthesis**

  ✓x7ᵗʰ **T84.59 Infection and inflammatory reaction due to other internal joint prosthesis**

✓5ᵗʰ **T84.6 Infection and inflammatory reaction due to internal fixation device**

  Use additional code to identify infection

  ✓x7ᵗʰ **T84.6Ø Infection and inflammatory reaction due to internal fixation device of unspecified site**

  ✓6ᵗʰ **T84.61 Infection and inflammatory reaction due to internal fixation device of arm**

    ✓7ᵗʰ **T84.61Ø Infection and inflammatory reaction due to internal fixation device of right humerus**

    ✓7ᵗʰ **T84.611 Infection and inflammatory reaction due to internal fixation device of left humerus**

    ✓7ᵗʰ **T84.612 Infection and inflammatory reaction due to internal fixation device of right radius**

    ✓7ᵗʰ **T84.613 Infection and inflammatory reaction due to internal fixation device of left radius**

    ✓7ᵗʰ **T84.614 Infection and inflammatory reaction due to internal fixation device of right ulna**

    ✓7ᵗʰ **T84.615 Infection and inflammatory reaction due to internal fixation device of left ulna**

    ✓7ᵗʰ **T84.619 Infection and inflammatory reaction due to internal fixation device of unspecified bone of arm**

  ✓6ᵗʰ **T84.62 Infection and inflammatory reaction due to internal fixation device of leg**

    ✓7ᵗʰ **T84.62Ø Infection and inflammatory reaction due to internal fixation device of right femur**

    ✓7ᵗʰ **T84.621 Infection and inflammatory reaction due to internal fixation device of left femur**

    ✓7ᵗʰ **T84.622 Infection and inflammatory reaction due to internal fixation device of right tibia**

    ✓7ᵗʰ **T84.623 Infection and inflammatory reaction due to internal fixation device of left tibia**

    ✓7ᵗʰ **T84.624 Infection and inflammatory reaction due to internal fixation device of right fibula**

    ✓7ᵗʰ **T84.625 Infection and inflammatory reaction due to internal fixation device of left fibula**

    ✓7ᵗʰ **T84.629 Infection and inflammatory reaction due to internal fixation device of unspecified bone of leg**

  ✓x7ᵗʰ **T84.63 Infection and inflammatory reaction due to internal fixation device of spine**

  ✓x7ᵗʰ **T84.69 Infection and inflammatory reaction due to internal fixation device of other site**

✓x7ᵗʰ **T84.7 Infection and inflammatory reaction due to other internal orthopedic prosthetic devices, implants and grafts**

  Use additional code to identify infection

✓5ᵗʰ **T84.8 Other specified complications of internal orthopedic prosthetic devices, implants and grafts**

  ✓x7ᵗʰ **T84.81 Embolism due to internal orthopedic prosthetic devices, implants and grafts**

  ✓x7ᵗʰ **T84.82 Fibrosis due to internal orthopedic prosthetic devices, implants and grafts**

  ✓x7ᵗʰ **T84.83 Hemorrhage due to internal orthopedic prosthetic devices, implants and grafts**

  ✓x7ᵗʰ **T84.84 Pain due to internal orthopedic prosthetic devices, implants and grafts**

  ✓x7ᵗʰ **T84.85 Stenosis due to internal orthopedic prosthetic devices, implants and grafts**

  ✓x7ᵗʰ **T84.86 Thrombosis due to internal orthopedic prosthetic devices, implants and grafts**

  ✓x7ᵗʰ **T84.89 Other specified complication of internal orthopedic prosthetic devices, implants and grafts**

✓x7ᵗʰ **T84.9 Unspecified complication of internal orthopedic prosthetic device, implant and graft**

✓4ᵗʰ **T85 Complications of other internal prosthetic devices, implants and grafts**

  EXCLUDES 2 *failure and rejection of transplanted organs and tissue (T86-)*

The appropriate 7th character is to be added to each code from category T85.
A   initial encounter
D   subsequent encounter
S   sequela

✓5ᵗʰ **T85.Ø Mechanical complication of ventricular intracranial (communicating) shunt**

  ✓x7ᵗʰ **T85.Ø1 Breakdown (mechanical) of ventricular intracranial (communicating) shunt**

  ✓x7ᵗʰ **T85.Ø2 Displacement of ventricular intracranial (communicating) shunt**

    Malposition of ventricular intracranial (communicating) shunt

  ✓x7ᵗʰ **T85.Ø3 Leakage of ventricular intracranial (communicating) shunt**

  ✓x7ᵗʰ **T85.Ø9 Other mechanical complication of ventricular intracranial (communicating) shunt**

    Obstruction (mechanical) of ventricular intracranial (communicating) shunt

    Perforation of ventricular intracranial (communicating) shunt

    Protrusion of ventricular intracranial (communicating) shunt

✓5ᵗʰ **T85.1** **Mechanical complication of implanted electronic stimulator of nervous system**

     ✓6ᵗʰ **T85.11** **Breakdown (mechanical) of implanted electronic stimulator of nervous system**

        ✓7ᵗʰ **T85.110** **Breakdown (mechanical) of implanted electronic neurostimulator (electrode) of brain**

        ✓7ᵗʰ **T85.111** **Breakdown (mechanical) of implanted electronic neurostimulator (electrode) of peripheral nerve**

        ✓7ᵗʰ **T85.112** **Breakdown (mechanical) of implanted electronic neurostimulator (electrode) of spinal cord**

        ✓7ᵗʰ **T85.118** **Breakdown (mechanical) of other implanted electronic stimulator of nervous system**

     ✓6ᵗʰ **T85.12** **Displacement of implanted electronic stimulator of nervous system**

        Malposition of implanted electronic stimulator of nervous system

        ✓7ᵗʰ **T85.120** **Displacement of implanted electronic neurostimulator (electrode) of brain**

        ✓7ᵗʰ **T85.121** **Displacement of implanted electronic neurostimulator (electrode) of peripheral nerve**

        ✓7ᵗʰ **T85.122** **Displacement of implanted electronic neurostimulator (electrode) of spinal cord**

        ✓7ᵗʰ **T85.128** **Displacement of other implanted electronic stimulator of nervous system**

     ✓6ᵗʰ **T85.19** **Other mechanical complication of implanted electronic stimulator of nervous system**

        Leakage of implanted electronic stimulator of nervous system

        Obstruction (mechanical) of implanted electronic stimulator of nervous system

        Perforation of implanted electronic stimulator of nervous system

        Protrusion of implanted electronic stimulator of nervous system

        ✓7ᵗʰ **T85.190** **Other mechanical complication of implanted electronic neurostimulator (electrode) of brain**

        ✓7ᵗʰ **T85.191** **Other mechanical complication of implanted electronic neurostimulator (electrode) of peripheral nerve**

        ✓7ᵗʰ **T85.192** **Other mechanical complication of implanted electronic neurostimulator (electrode) of spinal cord**

        ✓7ᵗʰ **T85.199** **Other mechanical complication of other implanted electronic stimulator of nervous system**

✓5ᵗʰ **T85.2** **Mechanical complication of intraocular lens**

     ✓x7ᵗʰ **T85.21** **Breakdown (mechanical) of intraocular lens**

     ✓x7ᵗʰ **T85.22** **Displacement of intraocular lens**

        Malposition of intraocular lens

     ✓x7ᵗʰ **T85.29** **Other mechanical complication of intraocular lens**

        Obstruction (mechanical) of intraocular lens

        Perforation of intraocular lens

        Protrusion of intraocular lens

✓5ᵗʰ **T85.3** **Mechanical complication of other ocular prosthetic devices, implants and grafts**

        EXCLUDES 2   *other complications of corneal graft (T86.84-)*

     ✓6ᵗʰ **T85.31** **Breakdown (mechanical) of other ocular prosthetic devices, implants and grafts**

        ✓7ᵗʰ **T85.310** **Breakdown (mechanical) of prosthetic orbit of right eye**

        ✓7ᵗʰ **T85.311** **Breakdown (mechanical) of prosthetic orbit of left eye**

        ✓7ᵗʰ **T85.318** **Breakdown (mechanical) of other ocular prosthetic devices, implants and grafts**

     ✓6ᵗʰ **T85.32** **Displacement of other ocular prosthetic devices, implants and grafts**

        Malposition of other ocular prosthetic devices, implants and grafts

        ✓7ᵗʰ **T85.320** **Displacement of prosthetic orbit of right eye**

        ✓7ᵗʰ **T85.321** **Displacement of prosthetic orbit of left eye**

        ✓7ᵗʰ **T85.328** **Displacement of other ocular prosthetic devices, implants and grafts**

     ✓6ᵗʰ **T85.39** **Other mechanical complication of other ocular prosthetic devices, implants and grafts**

        Obstruction (mechanical) of other ocular prosthetic devices, implants and grafts

        Perforation of other ocular prosthetic devices, implants and grafts

        Protrusion of other ocular prosthetic devices, implants and grafts

        ✓7ᵗʰ **T85.390** **Other mechanical complication of prosthetic orbit of right eye**

        ✓7ᵗʰ **T85.391** **Other mechanical complication of prosthetic orbit of left eye**

        ✓7ᵗʰ **T85.398** **Other mechanical complication of other ocular prosthetic devices, implants and grafts**

✓5ᵗʰ **T85.4** **Mechanical complication of breast prosthesis and implant**

     ✓x7ᵗʰ **T85.41** **Breakdown (mechanical) of breast prosthesis and implant**

     ✓x7ᵗʰ **T85.42** **Displacement of breast prosthesis and implant**

        Malposition of breast prosthesis and implant

     ✓x7ᵗʰ **T85.43** **Leakage of breast prosthesis and implant**

     ✓x7ᵗʰ **T85.44** **Capsular contracture of breast implant**

     ✓x7ᵗʰ **T85.49** **Other mechanical complication of breast prosthesis and implant**

        Obstruction (mechanical) of breast prosthesis and implant

        Perforation of breast prosthesis and implant

        Protrusion of breast prosthesis and implant

✓5ᵗʰ **T85.5** **Mechanical complication of gastrointestinal prosthetic devices, implants and grafts**

     ✓6ᵗʰ **T85.51** **Breakdown (mechanical) of gastrointestinal prosthetic devices, implants and grafts**

        ✓7ᵗʰ **T85.510** **Breakdown (mechanical) of bile duct prosthesis**

        ✓7ᵗʰ **T85.511** **Breakdown (mechanical) of esophageal anti-reflux device**

        ✓7ᵗʰ **T85.518** **Breakdown (mechanical) of other gastrointestinal prosthetic devices, implants and grafts**

     ✓6ᵗʰ **T85.52** **Displacement of gastrointestinal prosthetic devices, implants and grafts**

        Malposition of gastrointestinal prosthetic devices, implants and grafts

        ✓7ᵗʰ **T85.520** **Displacement of bile duct prosthesis**

        ✓7ᵗʰ **T85.521** **Displacement of esophageal anti-reflux device**

        ✓7ᵗʰ **T85.528** **Displacement of other gastrointestinal prosthetic devices, implants and grafts**

     ✓6ᵗʰ **T85.59** **Other mechanical complication of gastrointestinal prosthetic devices, implants and**

        Obstruction, mechanical of gastrointestinal prosthetic devices, implants and grafts

        Perforation of gastrointestinal prosthetic devices, implants and grafts

        Protrusion of gastrointestinal prosthetic devices, implants and grafts

        ✓7ᵗʰ **T85.590** **Other mechanical complication of bile duct prosthesis**

        ✓7ᵗʰ **T85.591** **Other mechanical complication of esophageal anti-reflux device**

        ✓7ᵗʰ **T85.598** **Other mechanical complication of other gastrointestinal prosthetic devices, implants and grafts**

✓5ᵗʰ **T85.6** **Mechanical complication of other specified internal and external prosthetic devices, implants and grafts**

     ✓6ᵗʰ **T85.61** **Breakdown (mechanical) of other specified internal prosthetic devices, implants and grafts**

        ✓7ᵗʰ **T85.610** **Breakdown (mechanical) of epidural and subdural infusion catheter**

        ✓7ᵗʰ **T85.611** **Breakdown (mechanical) of intraperitoneal dialysis catheter**

           EXCLUDES 1   *mechanical complication of vascular dialysis catheter (T82.4-)*

EXCLUDES 1   Not coded here   EXCLUDES 2   Not included here   ***Manifestation Code***

✓7th **T85.612 Breakdown (mechanical) of permanent sutures**
EXCLUDES 1 *mechanical complication of permanent (wire) suture used in bone repair (T84.1-T84.2)*

✓7th **T85.613 Breakdown (mechanical) of artificial skin graft and decellularized allodermis**
Failure of artificial skin graft and decellularized allodermis
Non-adherence of artificial skin graft and decellularized allodermis
Poor incorporation of artificial skin graft and decellularized allodermis
Shearing of artificial skin graft and decellularized allodermis

✓7th **T85.614 Breakdown (mechanical) of insulin pump**

✓7th **T85.618 Breakdown (mechanical) of other specified internal prosthetic devices, implants and grafts**

✓6th **T85.62 Displacement of other specified internal prosthetic devices, implants and grafts**
Malposition of other specified internal prosthetic devices, implants and grafts

✓7th **T85.620 Displacement of epidural and subdural infusion catheter**

✓7th **T85.621 Displacement of intraperitoneal dialysis catheter**
EXCLUDES 1 *mechanical complication of vascular dialysis catheter (T82.4-)*

✓7th **T85.622 Displacement of permanent sutures**
EXCLUDES 1 *mechanical complication of permanent (wire) suture used in bone repair (T84.1-T84.2)*

✓7th **T85.623 Displacement of artificial skin graft and decellularized allodermis**
Dislodgement of artificial skin graft and decellularized allodermis
Displacement of artificial skin graft and decellularized allodermis

✓7th **T85.624 Displacement of insulin pump**

✓7th **T85.628 Displacement of other specified internal prosthetic devices, implants and grafts**

✓6th **T85.63 Leakage of other specified internal prosthetic devices, implants and grafts**

✓7th **T85.630 Leakage of epidural and subdural infusion catheter**

✓7th **T85.631 Leakage of intraperitoneal dialysis catheter**
EXCLUDES 1 *mechanical complication of vascular dialysis catheter (T82.4)*

✓7th **T85.633 Leakage of insulin pump**

✓7th **T85.638 Leakage of other specified internal prosthetic devices, implants and grafts**

✓6th **T85.69 Other mechanical complication of other specified internal prosthetic devices, implants and grafts**
Obstruction, mechanical of other specified internal prosthetic devices, implants and grafts
Perforation of other specified internal prosthetic devices, implants and grafts
Protrusion of other specified internal prosthetic devices, implants and grafts

✓7th **T85.690 Other mechanical complication of epidural and subdural infusion catheter**

✓7th **T85.691 Other mechanical complication of intraperitoneal dialysis catheter**
EXCLUDES 1 *mechanical complication of vascular dialysis catheter (T82.4)*

✓7th **T85.692 Other mechanical complication of permanent sutures**
EXCLUDES 1 *mechanical complication of permanent (wire) suture used in bone repair (T84.1-T84.2)*

✓7th **T85.693 Other mechanical complication of artificial skin graft and decellularized allodermis**

✓7th **T85.694 Other mechanical complication of insulin pump**

✓7th **T85.698 Other mechanical complication of other specified internal prosthetic devices, implants and grafts**
Mechanical complication of nonabsorbable surgical material NOS

✓5th **T85.7 Infection and inflammatory reaction due to other internal prosthetic devices, implants and grafts**
Use additional code to identify infection

✓x7th **T85.71 Infection and inflammatory reaction due to peritoneal dialysis catheter**

✓x7th **T85.72 Infection and inflammatory reaction due to insulin pump**

✓x7th **T85.79 Infection and inflammatory reaction due to other internal prosthetic devices, implants and grafts**

✓5th **T85.8 Other specified complications of internal prosthetic devices, implants and grafts, not elsewhere classified**

✓x7th **T85.81 Embolism due to internal prosthetic devices, implants and grafts, not elsewhere classified**

✓x7th **T85.82 Fibrosis due to internal prosthetic devices, implants and grafts, not elsewhere classified**

✓x7th **T85.83 Hemorrhage due to internal prosthetic devices, implants and grafts, not elsewhere classified**

✓x7th **T85.84 Pain due to internal prosthetic devices, implants and grafts, not elsewhere classified**

✓x7th **T85.85 Stenosis due to internal prosthetic devices, implants and grafts, not elsewhere classified**

✓x7th **T85.86 Thrombosis due to internal prosthetic devices, implants and grafts, not elsewhere classified**

✓x7th **T85.89 Other specified complication of internal prosthetic devices, implants and grafts, not elsewhere classified**

✓x7th **T85.9 Unspecified complication of internal prosthetic device, implant and graft**
Complication of internal prosthetic device, implant and graft NOS

✓4th **T86 Complications of transplanted organs and tissue**
Use additional code to identify other transplant complications, such as:
graft-versus-host disease (D89.81-)
malignancy associated with organ transplant (C80.2)
post-transplant lymphoproliferative disorders (PTLD) (D47.z1)

✓5th **T86.0 Complications of bone marrow transplant**

T86.00 Unspecified complication of bone marrow transplant

T86.01 Bone marrow transplant rejection

T86.02 Bone marrow transplant failure

T86.03 Bone marrow transplant infection

T86.09 Other complications of bone marrow transplant

✓5th **T86.1 Complications of kidney transplant**

T86.10 Unspecified complication of kidney transplant

T86.11 Kidney transplant rejection

T86.12 Kidney transplant failure

T86.13 Kidney transplant infection
Use additional code to specify infection

T86.19 Other complication of kidney transplant

✓5th **T86.2 Complications of heart transplant**
EXCLUDES 1 *complication of:*
artificial heart device (T82.5)
heart-lung transplant (T86.3)

T86.20 Unspecified complication of heart transplant

T86.21 Heart transplant rejection

T86.22 Heart transplant failure

T86.23 Heart transplant infection
Use additional code to specify infection

✓6th **T86.29 Other complications of heart transplant**

T86.290 Cardiac allograft vasculopathy
EXCLUDES 1 *atherosclerosis of coronary arteries (I25.75-, I25.76-, I25.81-)*

T86.298 Other complications of heart transplant

✓5th **T86.3 Complications of heart-lung transplant**

T86.30 Unspecified complication of heart-lung transplant

T86.31 Heart-lung transplant rejection

T86.32 Heart-lung transplant failure

T86.33 Heart-lung transplant infection
Use additional code to specify infection

T86.39 Other complications of heart-lung transplant

✓5th **T86.4** Complications of liver transplant

T86.40 Unspecified complication of liver transplant

T86.41 Liver transplant rejection

T86.42 Liver transplant failure

T86.43 Liver transplant infection
Use additional code to identify infection, such as:
cytomegalovirus (CMV) infection (B25-)

T86.49 Other complications of liver transplant

✓5th **T86.8** Complications of other transplanted organs and tissues

✓6th **T86.81** Complications of lung transplant
EXCLUDES 1 complication of heart-lung transplant (T86.3-)

T86.810 Lung transplant rejection

T86.811 Lung transplant failure

T86.812 Lung transplant infection
Use additional code to specify infection

T86.818 Other complications of lung transplant

T86.819 Unspecified complication of lung transplant

✓6th **T86.82** Complications of skin graft (allograft) (autograft)
EXCLUDES 2 complication of artificial skin graft (T85.64)

T86.820 Skin graft (allograft) rejection

T86.821 Skin graft (allograft) (autograft) failure

T86.822 Skin graft (allograft) (autograft) infection
Use additional code to specify infection

T86.828 Other complications of skin graft (allograft) (autograft)

T86.829 Unspecified complication of skin graft (allograft) (autograft)

✓6th **T86.83** Complications of bone graft
EXCLUDES 2 mechanical complications of bone graft (T84.3-)

T86.830 Bone graft rejection

T86.831 Bone graft failure

T86.832 Bone graft infection
Use additional code to specify infection

T86.838 Other complications of bone graft

T86.839 Unspecified complication of bone graft

✓6th **T86.84** Complications of corneal transplant
EXCLUDES 2 mechanical complications of corneal graft (T85.3-)

T86.840 Corneal transplant rejection

T86.841 Corneal transplant failure

T86.842 Corneal transplant infection
Use additional code to specify infection

T86.848 Other complications of corneal transplant

T86.849 Unspecified complication of corneal transplant

✓6th **T86.85** Complication of intestine transplant

T86.850 Intestine transplant rejection

T86.851 Intestine transplant failure

T86.852 Intestine transplant infection
Use additional code to specify infection

T86.858 Other complications of intestine transplant

T86.859 Unspecified complication of intestine transplant

✓6th **T86.89** Complications of other transplanted tissue
Transplant failure or rejection of pancreas

T86.890 Other transplanted tissue rejection

T86.891 Other transplanted tissue failure

T86.892 Other transplanted tissue infection
Use additional code to specify infection

T86.898 Other complications of other transplanted tissue

T86.899 Unspecified complication of other transplanted tissue

✓5th **T86.9** Complication of unspecified transplanted organ and tissue

T86.90 Unspecified complication of unspecified transplanted organ and tissue

T86.91 Unspecified transplanted organ and tissue rejection

T86.92 Unspecified transplanted organ and tissue failure

T86.93 Unspecified transplanted organ and tissue infection
Use additional code to specify infection

T86.99 Other complications of unspecified transplanted organ and tissue

✓4th **T87** Complications peculiar to reattachment and amputation

✓5th **T87.0** Complications of reattached (part of) upper extremity

✓6th **T87.0x** Complications of reattached (part of) upper extremity

T87.0x1 Complications of reattached (part of) right upper extremity

T87.0x2 Complications of reattached (part of) left upper extremity

T87.0x9 Complications of reattached (part of) unspecified upper extremity

✓5th **T87.1** Complications of reattached (part of) lower extremity

✓6th **T87.1x** Complications of reattached (part of) lower extremity

T87.1x1 Complications of reattached (part of) right lower extremity

T87.1x2 Complications of reattached (part of) left lower extremity

T87.1x9 Complications of reattached (part of) unspecified lower extremity

T87.2 Complications of other reattached body part

✓5th **T87.3** Neuroma of amputation stump

T87.30 Neuroma of amputation stump, unspecified extremity

T87.31 Neuroma of amputation stump, right upper extremity

T87.32 Neuroma of amputation stump, left upper extremity

T87.33 Neuroma of amputation stump, right lower extremity

T87.34 Neuroma of amputation stump, left lower extremity

✓5th **T87.4** Infection of amputation stump

T87.40 Infection of amputation stump, unspecified extremity

T87.41 Infection of amputation stump, right upper extremity

T87.42 Infection of amputation stump, left upper extremity

T87.43 Infection of amputation stump, right lower extremity

T87.44 Infection of amputation stump, left lower extremity

✓5th **T87.5** Necrosis of amputation stump

T87.50 Necrosis of amputation stump, unspecified extremity

T87.51 Necrosis of amputation stump, right upper extremity

T87.52 Necrosis of amputation stump, left upper extremity

T87.53 Necrosis of amputation stump, right lower extremity

T87.54 Necrosis of amputation stump, left lower extremity

T87.8 Other complications of amputation stump
Amputation stump contracture
Amputation stump contracture of next proximal joint
Amputation stump flexion
Amputation stump edema
Amputation stump hematoma
EXCLUDES 2 phantom limb syndrome (G54.6-G54.7)

T87.9 Unspecified complications of amputation stump

EXCLUDES 1 Not coded here   EXCLUDES 2 Not included here   *Manifestation Code*

© 2011 Ingenix

☑4ᵗʰ **T88 Other complications of surgical and medical care, not elsewhere classified**

> EXCLUDES 2   complication following infusion, transfusion and therapeutic injection (T80.-)
> complication following procedure NEC (T81.-)
> complications of anesthesia in labor and delivery (O74.-)
> complications of anesthesia in pregnancy (O29.-)
> complications of anesthesia in puerperium (O89.-)
> complications of devices, implants and grafts (T82-T85)
> complications of obstetric surgery and procedure (O75.4)
> dermatitis due to drugs and medicaments (L23.3, L24.4, L25.1, L27.0-L27.1)
> poisoning and toxic effects of drugs and chemicals (T36-T65)
> specified complications classified elsewhere

> The appropriate 7th character is to be added to each code from category T88.
> A   initial encounter
> D   subsequent encounter
> S   sequela

√x7ᵗʰ **T88.0 Infection following immunization**
Sepsis following immunization

√x7ᵗʰ **T88.1 Other complications following immunization, not elsewhere classified**
Generalized vaccinia
Rash following immunization
> EXCLUDES 1   vaccinia not from vaccine (B08.011)
> EXCLUDES 2   anaphylactic shock due to serum (T80.5)
> other serum reactions (T80.6)
> postimmunization:
>   arthropathy (M02.2)
>   encephalitis (G04.0-)
>   fever (R50.83)

√x7ᵗʰ **T88.2 Shock due to anesthesia**
Code first appropriate code from category T41
> EXCLUDES 1   complications of anesthesia (in):
> labor and delivery (O74-)
> pregnancy (O29-)
> puerperium (O89-)
> postprocedural shock NOS (T81.1)

√x7ᵗʰ **T88.3 Malignant hyperthermia due to anesthesia**
Code first appropriate code from category T41

√x7ᵗʰ **T88.4 Failed or difficult intubation**

√5ᵗʰ **T88.5 Other complications of anesthesia**
Code first appropriate code from category T41

   √x7ᵗʰ **T88.51 Hypothermia following anesthesia**

   √x7ᵗʰ **T88.52 Failed moderate sedation during procedure**
Failed conscious sedation during procedure
> EXCLUDES 2   personal history of failed moderate sedation (Z92.83)

   √x7ᵗʰ **T88.59 Other complications of anesthesia**

√x7ᵗʰ **T88.6 Anaphylactic shock due to adverse effect of correct drug or medicament properly administered**
Code first (T36-T50 with fifth or sixth character 5) to identify drug
> EXCLUDES 1   anaphylactic shock due to serum (T80.5)

√x7ᵗʰ **T88.7 Unspecified adverse effect of drug or medicament**
Code first (T36-T50 with fifth or sixth character 5) to identify drug
Drug hypersensitivity NOS
Drug reaction NOS
> EXCLUDES 1   specified adverse effects of drugs and medicaments (A00-R94 and T80-T88.6, T88.8)

√x7ᵗʰ **T88.8 Other specified complications of surgical and medical care, not elsewhere classified**
Use additional code to identify the complication

√x7ᵗʰ **T88.9 Complication of surgical and medical care, unspecified**

T90-T98 Deactivated
Replaced with 7th character S for categories S00-T88

Chapter 20. External Causes of Morbidity (V00-Y99)

NOTE   This chapter permits the classification of environmental events and circumstances as the cause of injury, and other adverse effects. Where a code from this section is applicable, it is intended that it shall be used secondary to a code from another chapter of the Classification indicating the nature of the condition. Most often, the condition will be classifiable to Chapter 19, Injury, poisoning and certain other consequences of external causes (S00-T88). Other conditions that may be stated to be due to external causes are classified in Chapters I to XVIII. For these conditions, codes from Chapter 20 should be used to provide additional information as to the cause of the condition.

This chapter contains the following blocks:

V00-X58	Accidents
V00-V99	Transport accidents
V00-V09	Pedestrian injured in transport accident
V10-V19	Pedal cyclist injured in transport accident
V20-V29	Motorcycle rider injured in transport accident
V30-V39	Occupant of three-wheeled motor vehicle injured in transport accident
V40-V49	Car occupant injured in transport accident
V50-V59	Occupant of pick-up truck or van injured in transport accident
V60-V69	Occupant of heavy transport vehicle injured in transport accident
V70-V79	Bus occupant injured in transport accident
V80-V89	Other land transport accidents
V90-V94	Water transport accidents
V95-V97	Air and space transport accidents
V98-V99	Other and unspecified transport accidents
W00-X58	Other external causes of accidental injury
W00-W19	Slipping, tripping, stumbling and falls
W20-W49	Exposure to inanimate mechanical forces
W50-W64	Exposure to animate mechanical forces
W65-W74	Accidental drowning and submersion
W85-W99	Exposure to electric current, radiation and extreme ambient air temperature and pressure
X00-X08	Exposure to smoke, fire and flames
X10-X19	Contact with heat and hot substances
X30-X39	Exposure to forces of nature
X52, X58	Accidental exposure to other specified factors
X71-X83	Intentional self-harm
X92-Y08	Assault
Y21-Y33	Event of undetermined intent
Y35-Y38	Legal intervention, operations of war, military operations, and terrorism
Y62-Y84	Complications of medical and surgical care
Y62-Y69	Misadventures to patients during surgical and medical care
Y70-Y82	Medical devices associated with adverse incidents in diagnostic and therapeutic use
Y83-Y84	Surgical and other medical procedures as the cause of abnormal reaction of the patient, or of later complication, without mention of misadventure at the time of the procedure
Y90-Y99	Supplementary factors related to causes of morbidity classified elsewhere

Transport accidents (V00-V99)

This section is structured in 12 groups. Those relating to land transport accidents (V01- V89) reflect the victim's mode of transport and are subdivided to identify the victim's "counterpart" or the type of event. The vehicle of which the injured person is an occupant is identified in the first two characters since it is seen as the most important factor to identify for prevention purposes. A transport accident is one in which the vehicle involved must be moving or running or in use for transport purposes at the time of the accident.

Use additional code to identify:
  airbag injury (w22.1)
  type of street or road (y92.4-)
  use of cellular telephone and other electronic equipment at the time of the transport accident (Y93.c-)

EXCLUDES 1   *agricultural vehicles in stationary use or maintenance (W31-)*
  assault by crashing of motor vehicle (Y03-)
  automobile or motor cycle in stationary use or maintenance—code to type of accident
  crashing of motor vehicle, undetermined intent (Y32)
  intentional self-harm by crashing of motor vehicle (X82)

EXCLUDES 2   *transport accidents due to cataclysm (X34-X38)*

Definitions of transport vehicles:

A **transport accident** is any accident involving a device designed primarily for, or used at the time primarily for, conveying persons or good from one place to another.

A **public highway** [trafficway] or street is the entire width between property lines (or other boundary lines) of land open to the public as a matter of right or custom for purposes of moving persons or property from one place to another. A roadway is that part of the public highway designed, improved and customarily used for vehicular traffic.

A **traffic accident** is any vehicle accident occurring on the public highway [i.e. originating on, terminating on, or involving a vehicle partially on the highway]. A vehicle accident is assumed to have occurred on the public highway unless another place is specified, except in the case of accidents involving only off-road motor vehicles, which are classified as nontraffic accidents unless the contrary is stated.

A **nontraffic accident** is any vehicle accident that occurs entirely in any place other than a public highway.

A **pedestrian** is any person involved in an accident who was not at the time of the accident riding in or on a motor vehicle, railway train, streetcar or animal-drawn or other vehicle, or on a pedal cycle or animal. This includes, a person changing a tire or working on a parked car. It also includes the use of a pedestrian conveyance such as a baby carriage, ice-skates, roller skates, a skateboard, nonmotorized or motorized wheelchair, motorized mobility scooter, or nonmotorized scooter.

A **driver** is an occupant of a transport vehicle who is operating or intending to operate it.

A **passenger** is any occupant of a transport vehicle other than the driver, except a person traveling on the outside of the vehicle.

A **person** on the outside of a vehicle is any person being transported by a vehicle but not occupying the space normally reserved for the driver or passengers, or the space intended for the transport of property. This includes the body, bumper, fender, roof, running board or step of a vehicle.

A **pedal cycle** is any land transport vehicle operated solely by nonmotorized pedals including a bicycle or tricycle.

A **pedal cyclist** is any person riding a pedal cycle or in a sidecar or trailer attached to a pedal cycle.

A **motorcycle** is a two-wheeled motor vehicle with one or two riding saddles and sometimes with a third wheel for the support of a sidecar. The sidecar is considered part of the motorcycle.

A **motorcycle rider** is any person riding a motorcycle or in a sidecar or trailer attached to the motorcycle.

A **three-wheeled motor vehicle** is a motorized tricycle designed primarily for on-road use. This includes a motor-driven tricycle, a motorized rickshaw, or a three-wheeled motor car.

A **car [automobile]** is a four-wheeled motor vehicle designed primarily for carrying up to 7 persons. A trailer being towed by the car is considered part of the car.

A **pick-up truck or van** is a four or six-wheeled motor vehicle designed for carrying passengers as well as property or cargo weighing less than the local limit for classification as a heavy goods vehicle, and not requiring a special driver's license. This includes a minivan and a sport-utility vehicle (SUV).

A **heavy transport vehicle** is a motor vehicle designed primarily for carrying property, meeting local criteria for classification as a heavy goods vehicle in terms of weight and requiring a special driver's license.

A **bus (coach)** is a motor vehicle designed or adapted primarily for carrying more than 10 passengers, and requiring a special driver's license.

A **railway train or railway vehicle** is any device, with or without freight or passenger cars couple to it, designed for traffic on a railway track. This includes subterranean (subways) or elevated trains.

A **streetcar**, is a device designed and used primarily for transporting passengers within a municipality, running on rails, usually subject to normal traffic control signals, and operated principally on a right-of-way that forms part of the roadway. This includes a tram or trolley that runs on rails. A trailer being towed by a streetcar is considered part of the streetcar.

A **special vehicle mainly used on industrial premises** is a motor vehicle designed primarily for use within the buildings and premises of industrial or commercial establishments. This includes battery-powered trucks, forklifts, coal-cars in a coal mine, logging cars and trucks used in mines or quarries.

A **special vehicle mainly used in agriculture** is a motor vehicle designed specifically for use in farming and agriculture (horticulture), to work the land, tend and harvest crops and transport materials on the farm. This includes harvesters, farm machinery and tractor and trailers.

A **special construction vehicle** is a motor vehicle designed specifically for use on construction and demolition sites. This includes bulldozers, diggers, earth levellers, dump trucks. backhoes, front-end loaders, pavers, and mechanical shovels.

A **special all-terrain vehicle** is a motor vehicle of special design to enable it to negotiate over rough or soft terrain , snow or sand. This includes snow mobiles, All-terrain vehicles (ATV), and dune buggies. It does not include passenger vehicle designated as Sport Utility Vehicles. (SUV)

A **watercraft** is any device designed for transporting passengers or goods on water. This includes motor or sail boats, ships, and hovercraft.

An **aircraft** is any device for transporting passengers or goods in the air. This includes hot-air balloons, gliders, helicopters and airplanes.

A **military vehicle** is any motorized vehicle operating on a public roadway owned by the military and being operated by a member of the military.

Pedestrian injured in transport accident (V00-V09)

INCLUDES   person changing tire on transport vehicle
person examining engine of vehicle broken down in (on side of) road

EXCLUDES 1   *fall due to non-transport collision with other person (W03)*
pedestrian on foot falling (slipping) on ice and snow (W00-)
struck or bumped by another person (W51)

✓4th **V00 Pedestrian conveyance accident**

Use additional place of occurrence and activity external cause codes, if known (Y92-, Y93-)

EXCLUDES 1   *collision with another person without fall (W51)*
fall due to person on foot colliding with another person on foot (W03)
fall from non-moving wheelchair, nonmotorized scooter and motorized mobility scooter without collision (W05.-)
pedestrian (conveyance) collision with other land transport vehicle (V01-V09)
pedestrian on foot falling (slipping) on ice and snow (W00-)

> The appropriate 7th character is to be added to each code from category V00.
> A   initial encounter
> D   subsequent encounter
> S   sequela

✓5th **V00.0 Pedestrian on foot injured in collision with pedestrian conveyance**

✓x7th **V00.01 Pedestrian on foot injured in collision with roller-skater**

✓x7th **V00.02 Pedestrian on foot injured in collision with skateboarder**

✓x7th **V00.09 Pedestrian on foot injured in collision with other pedestrian conveyance**

✓5th **V00.1 Rolling-type pedestrian conveyance accident**

EXCLUDES 1   *accident with babystroller (V00.82-)*
accident with motorized mobility scooter (V00.83-)
accident with wheelchair (powered) (V00.81-)

✓6th **V00.11 In-line roller-skate accident**

✓7th **V00.111 Fall from in-line roller-skates**

✓7th **V00.112 In-line roller-skater colliding with stationary object**

✓7th **V00.118 Other in-line roller-skate accident**
     EXCLUDES 1   *roller-skater collision with other land transport vehicle (V01-V09 with 5th character 1)*

✓6th **V00.12 Non-in- line roller-skate accident**

✓7th **V00.121 Fall from non-in-line roller-skates**

✓7th **V00.122 Non-in-line roller-skater colliding with stationary object**

✓7th **V00.128 Other non-in-line roller-skating accident**
     EXCLUDES 1   *roller-skater collision with other land transport vehicle (V01-V09 with 5th character 1)*

✓6th **V00.13 Skateboard accident**

✓7th **V00.131 Fall from skateboard**

✓7th **V00.132 Skateboarder colliding with stationary object**

✓7th **V00.138 Other skateboard accident**
     EXCLUDES 1   *skateboarder collision with other land transport vehicle (V01-V09 with 5th character 2)*

✓6th **V00.14 Scooter (nonmotorized) accident**
     EXCLUDES 1   *motorscooter accident (V20-V29)*

✓7th **V00.141 Fall from scooter (nonmotorized)**

✓7th **V00.142 Scooter (nonmotorized) colliding with stationary object**

✓7th **V00.148 Other scooter (nonmotorized) accident**
     EXCLUDES 1   *scooter (nonmotorized) collision with other land transport vehicle (V01-V09 with fifth character 9)*

✓6th **V00.15 Heelies accident**
Rolling shoe
Wheeled shoe
Wheelies accident

✓7th **V00.151 Fall from heelies**

✓7th **V00.152 Heelies colliding with stationary object**

✓7th **V00.158 Other heelies accident**

✓6th **V00.18 Accident on other rolling-type pedestrian conveyance**

✓7th **V00.181 Fall from other rolling-type pedestrian conveyance**

✓7th **V00.182 Pedestrian on other rolling-type pedestrian conveyance colliding with stationary object**

✓7th **V00.188 Other accident on other rolling-type pedestrian conveyance**

✓5th **V00.2 Gliding-type pedestrian conveyance accident**

✓6th **V00.21 Ice-skates accident**

✓7th **V00.211 Fall from ice-skates**

✓7th **V00.212 Ice-skater colliding with stationary object**

✓7th **V00.218 Other ice-skates accident**
     EXCLUDES 1   *ice-skater collision with other land transport vehicle (V01-V09 with 5th digit 9)*

✓6th **V00.22 Sled accident**

✓7th **V00.221 Fall from sled**

✓7th **V00.222 Sledder colliding with stationary object**

✓7th **V00.228 Other sled accident**
     EXCLUDES 1   *sled collision with other land transport vehicle (V01-V09 with 5th digit 9)*

✓6th **V00.28 Other gliding-type pedestrian conveyance accident**

✓7th **V00.281 Fall from other gliding-type pedestrian conveyance**

✓7th **V00.282 Pedestrian on other gliding-type pedestrian conveyance colliding with stationary object**

✓7th **V00.288 Other accident on other gliding-type pedestrian conveyance**
     EXCLUDES 1   *gliding-type pedestrian conveyance collision with other land transport vehicle (V01-V09 with 5th digit 9)*

✓5th **V00.3 Flat-bottomed pedestrian conveyance accident**

✓6th **V00.31 Snowboard accident**

✓7th **V00.311 Fall from snowboard**

✓7th **V00.312 Snowboarder colliding with stationary object**

✓7th **V00.318 Other snowboard accident**
     EXCLUDES 1   *snowboarder collision with other land transport vehicle (V01-V09 with 5th digit 9)*

✓6th **V00.32 Snow-ski accident**

✓7th **V00.321 Fall from snow-skis**

✓7th **V00.322 Snow-skier colliding with stationary object**

✓7th **V00.328 Other snow-ski accident**
     EXCLUDES 1   *snow-skier collision with other land transport vehicle (V01-V09 with 5th digit 9)*

✓6th **V00.38 Other flat-bottomed pedestrian conveyance accident**

✓7th **V00.381 Fall from other flat-bottomed pedestrian conveyance**

✓7th **V00.382 Pedestrian on other flat-bottomed pedestrian conveyance colliding with stationary object**

✓7th **V00.388 Other accident on other flat-bottomed pedestrian conveyance**

✓5th **V00.8 Accident on other pedestrian conveyance**

✓ Appropriate additional character required   ✓x7th Requires 7th character, placeholder x must fill empty characters

√6th **V00.81 Accident with wheelchair (powered)**
√7th **V00.811 Fall from moving wheelchair (powered)**
EXCLUDES 1 *fall from non-moving wheelchair (W05.0)*
√7th **V00.812 Wheelchair (powered) colliding with stationary object**
√7th **V00.818 Other accident with wheelchair (powered)**
√6th **V00.82 Accident with babystroller**
√7th **V00.821 Fall from babystroller**
√7th **V00.822 Babystroller colliding with stationary object**
√7th **V00.828 Other accident with babystroller**
√6th **V00.83 Accident with motorized mobility scooter**
√7th **V00.831 Fall from motorized mobility scooter**
EXCLUDES 1 *fall from non-moving motorized mobility scooter (W05.2)*
√7th **V00.832 Motorized mobility scooter colliding with stationary object**
√7th **V00.838 Other accident with motorized mobility scooter**
√6th **V00.89 Accident on other pedestrian conveyance**
√7th **V00.891 Fall from other pedestrian conveyance**
√7th **V00.892 Pedestrian on other pedestrian conveyance colliding with stationary object**
√7th **V00.898 Other accident on other pedestrian conveyance**
EXCLUDES 1 *other pedestrian (conveyance) collision with other land transport vehicle (V01-V09 with 5th digit 9)*

√4th **V01 Pedestrian injured in collision with pedal cycle**

The appropriate 7th character is to be added to each code from category V01.
A   initial encounter
D   subsequent encounter
S   sequela

√5th **V01.0 Pedestrian injured in collision with pedal cycle in nontraffic accident**
√x7th **V01.00 Pedestrian on foot injured in collision with pedal cycle in nontraffic accident**
Pedestrian NOS injured in collision with pedal cycle in nontraffic accident
√x7th **V01.01 Pedestrian on roller-skates injured in collision with pedal cycle in nontraffic accident**
√x7th **V01.02 Pedestrian on skateboard injured in collision with pedal cycle in nontraffic accident**
√x7th **V01.09 Pedestrian with other conveyance injured in collision with pedal cycle in nontraffic accident**
Pedestrian with babystroller injured in collision with pedal cycle in nontraffic accident
Pedestrian on ice-skates injured in collision with pedal cycle in nontraffic accident
Pedestrian on nonmotorized scooter injured in collision with pedal cycle in nontraffic accident
Pedestrian on sled injured in collision with pedal cycle in nontraffic accident
Pedestrian on snowboard injured in collision with pedal cycle in nontraffic accident
Pedestrian on snow-skis injured in collision with pedal cycle in nontraffic accident
Pedestrian in wheelchair (powered) injured in collision with pedal cycle in nontraffic accident
Pedestrian in motorized mobility scooter injured in collision with pedal cycle in nontraffic accident
√5th **V01.1 Pedestrian injured in collision with pedal cycle in traffic accident**
√x7th **V01.10 Pedestrian on foot injured in collision with pedal cycle in traffic accident**
Pedestrian NOS injured in collision with pedal cycle in traffic accident
√x7th **V01.11 Pedestrian on roller-skates injured in collision with pedal cycle in traffic accident**
√x7th **V01.12 Pedestrian on skateboard injured in collision with pedal cycle in traffic accident**

√x7th **V01.19 Pedestrian with other conveyance injured in collision with pedal cycle in traffic accident**
Pedestrian with babystroller injured in collision with pedal cycle in traffic accident
Pedestrian on ice-skates injured in collision with pedal cycle in traffic accident
Pedestrian on nonmotorized scooter injured in collision with pedal cycle in traffic accident
Pedestrian on sled injured in collision with pedal cycle in traffic accident
Pedestrian on snowboard injured in collision with pedal cycle in traffic accident
Pedestrian on snow-skis injured in collision with pedal cycle in traffic accident
Pedestrian in wheelchair (powered) injured in collision with pedal cycle in traffic accident
Pedestrian in motorized mobility scooter injured in collision with pedal cycle in traffic accident
√5th **V01.9 Pedestrian injured in collision with pedal cycle, unspecified whether traffic or nontraffic accident**
√x7th **V01.90 Pedestrian on foot injured in collision with pedal cycle, unspecified whether traffic or nontraffic accident**
Pedestrian NOS injured in collision with pedal cycle, unspecified whether traffic or nontraffic accident
√x7th **V01.91 Pedestrian on roller-skates injured in collision with pedal cycle, unspecified whether traffic or nontraffic accident**
√x7th **V01.92 Pedestrian on skateboard injured in collision with pedal cycle, unspecified whether traffic or nontraffic accident**
√x7th **V01.99 Pedestrian with other conveyance injured in collision with pedal cycle, unspecified whether traffic or nontraffic accident**
Pedestrian with babystroller injured in collision with pedal cycle, unspecified whether traffic or nontraffic accident
Pedestrian on ice-skates injured in collision with pedal cycle unspecified, whether traffic or nontraffic accident
Pedestrian on nonmotorized scooter injured in collision with pedal cycle, unspecified whether traffic or nontraffic accident
Pedestrian on sled injured in collision with pedal cycle unspecified, whether traffic or nontraffic accident
Pedestrian on snowboard injured in collision with pedal cycle, unspecified whether traffic or nontraffic accident
Pedestrian on snow-skis injured in collision with pedal cycle, unspecified whether traffic or nontraffic accident
Pedestrian in wheelchair (powered) injured in collision with pedal cycle, unspecified whether traffic or nontraffic accident
Pedestrian in motorized mobility scooter injured in collision with pedal cycle, unspecified whether traffic or nontraffic accident

√4th **V02 Pedestrian injured in collision with two- or three-wheeled motor vehicle**

The appropriate 7th character is to be added to each code from category V02.
A   initial encounter
D   subsequent encounter
S   sequela

√5th **V02.0 Pedestrian injured in collision with two- or three-wheeled motor vehicle in nontraffic accident**
√x7th **V02.00 Pedestrian on foot injured in collision with two- or three-wheeled motor vehicle in nontraffic accident**
Pedestrian NOS injured in collision with two- or three-wheeled motor vehicle in nontraffic accident
√x7th **V02.01 Pedestrian on roller-skates injured in collision with two- or three-wheeled motor vehicle in nontraffic accident**
√x7th **V02.02 Pedestrian on skateboard injured in collision with two- or three-wheeled motor vehicle in nontraffic accident**

EXCLUDES 1 Not coded here   EXCLUDES 2 Not included here   *Manifestation Code*

✓x7ᵗʰ **V02.09 Pedestrian with other conveyance injured in collision with two- or three-wheeled motor vehicle in nontraffic accident**

Pedestrian with babystroller injured in collision with two- or three-wheeled motor vehicle in nontraffic accident

Pedestrian on ice-skates injured in collision with two- or three-wheeled motor vehicle in nontraffic accident

Pedestrian on nonmotorized scooter injured in collision with two- or three-wheeled motor vehicle in nontraffic accident

Pedestrian on sled injured in collision with two- or three-wheeled motor vehicle in nontraffic accident

Pedestrian on snowboard injured in collision with two- or three-wheeled motor vehicle in nontraffic accident

Pedestrian on snow-skis injured in collision with two- or three-wheeled motor vehicle in nontraffic accident

Pedestrian in wheelchair (powered) injured in collision with two- or three-wheeled motor vehicle in nontraffic accident

Pedestrian in motorized mobility scooter injured in collision with two- or three-wheeled motor vehicle in nontraffic accident

✓5ᵗʰ **V02.1 Pedestrian injured in collision with two- or three-wheeled motor vehicle in traffic accident**

✓x7ᵗʰ **V02.10 Pedestrian on foot injured in collision with two- or three-wheeled motor vehicle in traffic accident**

Pedestrian NOS injured in collision with two- or three-wheeled motor vehicle in traffic accident

✓x7ᵗʰ **V02.11 Pedestrian on roller-skates injured in collision with two- or three-wheeled motor vehicle in traffic accident**

✓x7ᵗʰ **V02.12 Pedestrian on skateboard injured in collision with two- or three-wheeled motor vehicle in traffic accident**

✓x7ᵗʰ **V02.19 Pedestrian with other conveyance injured in collision with two- or three-wheeled motor vehicle in traffic accident**

Pedestrian with babystroller injured in collision with two- or three-wheeled motor vehicle in traffic accident

Pedestrian on ice-skates injured in collision with two- or three-wheeled motor vehicle in traffic accident

Pedestrian on nonmotorized scooter injured in collision with two- or three-wheeled motor vehicle in traffic accident

Pedestrian on sled injured in collision with two- or three-wheeled motor vehicle in traffic accident

Pedestrian on snowboard injured in collision with two- or three-wheeled motor vehicle in traffic accident

Pedestrian on snow-skis injured in collision with two- or three-wheeled motor vehicle in traffic accident

Pedestrian in wheelchair (powered) injured in collision with two- or three-wheeled motor vehicle in traffic accident

Pedestrian in motorized mobility scooter injured in collision with two- or three-wheeled motor vehicle in traffic accident

✓5ᵗʰ **V02.9 Pedestrian injured in collision with two- or three-wheeled motor vehicle, unspecified whether traffic or nontraffic accident**

✓x7ᵗʰ **V02.90 Pedestrian on foot injured in collision with two- or three-wheeled motor vehicle, unspecified whether traffic or nontraffic accident**

Pedestrian NOS injured in collision with two- or three-wheeled motor vehicle, unspecified whether traffic or nontraffic accident

✓x7ᵗʰ **V02.91 Pedestrian on roller-skates injured in collision with two- or three-wheeled motor vehicle, unspecified whether traffic or nontraffic accident**

✓x7ᵗʰ **V02.92 Pedestrian on skateboard injured in collision with two- or three-wheeled motor vehicle, unspecified whether traffic or nontraffic accident**

✓x7ᵗʰ **V02.99 Pedestrian with other conveyance injured in collision with two- or three-wheeled motor vehicle, unspecified whether traffic or nontraffic accident**

Pedestrian with babystroller injured in collision with two- or three-wheeled motor vehicle, unspecified whether traffic or nontraffic accident

Pedestrian on ice-skates injured in collision with two- or three-wheeled motor vehicle, unspecified whether traffic or nontraffic accident

Pedestrian on nonmotorized scooter injured in collision with two- or three-wheeled motor vehicle, unspecified whether traffic or nontraffic accident

Pedestrian on sled injured in collision with two- or three-wheeled motor vehicle, unspecified whether traffic or nontraffic accident

Pedestrian on snowboard injured in collision with two- or three-wheeled motor vehicle, unspecified whether traffic or nontraffic accident

Pedestrian on snow-skis injured in collision with two- or three-wheeled motor vehicle, unspecified whether traffic or nontraffic accident

Pedestrian in wheelchair (powered) injured in collision with two- or three-wheeled motor vehicle, unspecified whether traffic or nontraffic accident

Pedestrian in motorized mobility scooter injured in collision with two- or three-wheeled motor vehicle, unspecified whether traffic or nontraffic accident

✓4ᵗʰ **V03 Pedestrian injured in collision with car, pick-up truck or van**

> The appropriate 7th character is to be added to each code from category V03.
> A   initial encounter
> D   subsequent encounter
> S   sequela

✓5ᵗʰ **V03.0 Pedestrian injured in collision with car, pick-up truck or van in nontraffic accident**

✓x7ᵗʰ **V03.00 Pedestrian on foot injured in collision with car, pick-up truck or van in nontraffic accident**

Pedestrian NOS injured in collision with car, pick-up truck or van in nontraffic accident

✓x7ᵗʰ **V03.01 Pedestrian on roller-skates injured in collision with car, pick-up truck or van in nontraffic accident**

✓x7ᵗʰ **V03.02 Pedestrian on skateboard injured in collision with car, pick-up truck or van in nontraffic accident**

✓x7ᵗʰ **V03.09 Pedestrian with other conveyance injured in collision with car, pick-up truck or van in nontraffic accident**

Pedestrian with babystroller injured in collision with car, pick-up truck or van in nontraffic accident

Pedestrian on ice-skates injured in collision with car, pick-up truck or van in nontraffic accident

Pedestrian on nonmotorized scooter injured in collision with car, pick-up truck or van in nontraffic accident

Pedestrian on sled Injured in collision with car, pick-up truck or van in nontraffic accident

Pedestrian on snowboard injured in collision with car, pick-up truck or van in nontraffic accident

Pedestrian on snow-skis injured in collision with car, pick-up truck or van in nontraffic accident

Pedestrian in wheelchair (powered) injured in collision with car, pick-up truck or van in nontraffic accident

Pedestrian in motorized mobility scooter injured in collision with car, pick-up truck or van in nontraffic accident

✓5ᵗʰ **V03.1 Pedestrian injured in collision with car, pick-up truck or van in traffic accident**

✓x7ᵗʰ **V03.10 Pedestrian on foot injured in collision with car, pick-up truck or van in traffic accident**

Pedestrian NOS injured in collision with car, pick-up truck or van in traffic accident

---

☑ Appropriate additional character required

✓x7ᵗʰ Requires 7th character, placeholder x must fill empty characters

√x7th **V03.11** **Pedestrian on roller-skates injured in collision with car, pick-up truck or van in traffic accident**

√x7th **V03.12** **Pedestrian on skateboard injured in collision with car, pick-up truck or van in traffic accident**

√x7th **V03.19** **Pedestrian with other conveyance injured in collision with car, pick-up truck or van in traffic accident**

    Pedestrian with babystroller injured in collision with car, pick-up truck or van in traffic accident

    Pedestrian on ice-skates injured in collision with car, pick-up truck or van in traffic accident

    Pedestrian on nonmotorized scooter injured in collision with car, pick-up truck or van in traffic accident

    Pedestrian on sled injured in collision with car, pick-up truck or van in traffic accident

    Pedestrian on snowboard injured in collision with car, pick-up truck or van in traffic accident

    Pedestrian on snow-skis injured in collision with car, pick-up truck or van in traffic accident

    Pedestrian in wheelchair (powered) injured in collision with car, pick-up truck or van in traffic accident

    Pedestrian in motorized mobility scooter injured in collision with car, pick-up truck or van in traffic accident

√5th **V03.9** **Pedestrian injured in collision with car, pick-up truck or van, unspecified whether traffic or nontraffic accident**

√x7th **V03.90** **Pedestrian on foot injured in collision with car, pick-up truck or van, unspecified whether traffic or nontraffic accident**

    Pedestrian NOS injured in collision with car, pick-up truck or van, unspecified whether traffic or nontraffic accident

√x7th **V03.91** **Pedestrian on roller-skates injured in collision with car, pick-up truck or van, unspecified whether traffic or nontraffic accident**

√x7th **V03.92** **Pedestrian on skateboard injured in collision with car, pick-up truck or van, unspecified whether traffic or nontraffic accident**

√x7th **V03.99** **Pedestrian with other conveyance injured in collision with car, pick-up truck or van, unspecified whether traffic or nontraffic accident**

    Pedestrian with babystroller injured in collision with car, pick-up truck or van, unspecified whether traffic or nontraffic accident

    Pedestrian on ice-skates injured in collision with car, pick-up truck or van, unspecified whether traffic or nontraffic accident

    Pedestrian on nonmotorized scooter injured in collision with car, pick-up truck or van, unspecified whether traffic or nontraffic accident

    Pedestrian on sled injured in collision with car, pick-up truck or van in nontraffic accident

    Pedestrian on snowboard injured in collision with car, pick-up truck or van, unspecified whether traffic or nontraffic accident

    Pedestrian on snow-skis injured in collision with car, pick-up truck or van, unspecified whether traffic or nontraffic accident

    Pedestrian in wheelchair (powered) injured in collision with car, pick-up truck or van, unspecified whether traffic or nontraffic accident

    Pedestrian in motorized mobility scooter injured in collision with car, pick-up truck or van, unspecified whether traffic or nontraffic accident

√4th **V04** **Pedestrian injured in collision with heavy transport vehicle or bus**

> *EXCLUDES 1*   *pedestrian injured in collision with military vehicle (V09.01, V09.21)*

The appropriate 7th character is to be added to each code from category V04.
- A   initial encounter
- D   subsequent encounter
- S   sequela

√5th **V04.0** **Pedestrian injured in collision with heavy transport vehicle or bus in nontraffic accident**

√x7th **V04.00** **Pedestrian on foot injured in collision with heavy transport vehicle or bus in nontraffic accident**

    Pedestrian NOS injured in collision with heavy transport vehicle or bus in nontraffic accident

√x7th **V04.01** **Pedestrian on roller-skates injured in collision with heavy transport vehicle or bus in nontraffic accident**

√x7th **V04.02** **Pedestrian on skateboard injured in collision with heavy transport vehicle or bus in nontraffic accident**

√x7th **V04.09** **Pedestrian with other conveyance injured in collision with heavy transport vehicle or bus in nontraffic accident**

    Pedestrian with babystroller injured in collision with heavy transport vehicle or bus in nontraffic accident

    Pedestrian on ice-skates injured in collision with heavy transport vehicle or bus in nontraffic accident

    Pedestrian on nonmotorized scooter injured in collision with heavy transport vehicle or bus in nontraffic accident

    Pedestrian on sled injured in collision with heavy transport vehicle or bus in nontraffic accident

    Pedestrian on snowboard injured in collision with heavy transport vehicle or bus in nontraffic accident

    Pedestrian on snow-skis injured in collision with heavy transport vehicle or bus in nontraffic accident

    Pedestrian in wheelchair (powered) injured in collision with heavy transport vehicle or bus in nontraffic accident

    Pedestrian in motorized mobility scooter injured in collision with heavy transport vehicle or bus in nontraffic accident

√5th **V04.1** **Pedestrian injured in collision with heavy transport vehicle or bus in traffic accident**

√x7th **V04.10** **Pedestrian on foot injured in collision with heavy transport vehicle or bus in traffic accident**

    Pedestrian NOS injured in collision with heavy transport vehicle or bus in traffic accident

√x7th **V04.11** **Pedestrian on roller-skates injured in collision with heavy transport vehicle or bus in traffic accident**

√x7th **V04.12** **Pedestrian on skateboard injured in collision with heavy transport vehicle or bus in traffic accident**

√x7th **V04.19** **Pedestrian with other conveyance injured in collision with heavy transport vehicle or bus in traffic accident**

    Pedestrian with babystroller injured in collision with heavy transport vehicle or bus in traffic accident

    Pedestrian on ice-skates injured in collision with heavy transport vehicle or bus in traffic accident

    Pedestrian on nonmotorized scooter injured in collision with heavy transport vehicle or bus in traffic accident

    Pedestrian on sled injured in collision with heavy transport vehicle or bus in traffic accident

    Pedestrian on snowboard injured in collision with heavy transport vehicle or bus in traffic accident

    Pedestrian on snow-skis injured in collision with heavy transport vehicle or bus in traffic accident

    Pedestrian in wheelchair (powered) injured in collision with heavy transport vehicle or bus in traffic accident

    Pedestrian in motorized mobility scooter injured in collision with heavy transport vehicle or bus in traffic accident

√5th **V04.9** **Pedestrian injured in collision with heavy transport vehicle or bus, unspecified whether traffic or nontraffic accident**

√x7th **V04.90** **Pedestrian on foot injured in collision with heavy transport vehicle or bus, unspecified whether traffic or nontraffic accident**

    Pedestrian NOS injured in collision with heavy transport vehicle or bus, unspecified whether traffic or nontraffic accident

---

EXCLUDES 1 Not coded here   *EXCLUDES 2* Not included here   *Manifestation Code*

√x7th **V04.91** **Pedestrian on roller-skates injured in collision with heavy transport vehicle or bus, unspecified whether traffic or nontraffic accident**

√x7th **V04.92** **Pedestrian on skateboard injured in collision with heavy transport vehicle or bus, unspecified whether traffic or nontraffic accident**

√x7th **V04.99** **Pedestrian with other conveyance injured in collision with heavy transport vehicle or bus, unspecified whether traffic or nontraffic accident**

Pedestrian with babystroller injured in collision with heavy transport vehicle or bus, unspecified whether traffic or nontraffic accident

Pedestrian on ice-skates injured in collision with heavy transport vehicle or bus, unspecified whether traffic or nontraffic accident

Pedestrian on nonmotorized scooter injured in collision with heavy transport vehicle or bus, unspecified whether traffic or nontraffic accident

Pedestrian on sled injured in collision with heavy transport vehicle or bus, unspecified whether traffic or nontraffic accident

Pedestrian on snowboard injured in collision with heavy transport vehicle or bus, unspecified whether traffic or nontraffic accident

Pedestrian on snow-skis injured in collision with heavy transport vehicle or bus, unspecified whether traffic or nontraffic accident

Pedestrian in wheelchair (powered) injured in collision with heavy transport vehicle or bus, unspecified whether traffic or nontraffic accident

Pedestrian in motorized mobility scooter injured in collision with heavy transport vehicle or bus, unspecified whether traffic or nontraffic accident

√4th **V05** **Pedestrian injured in collision with railway train or railway vehicle**

> The appropriate 7th character is to be added to each code from category V05.
> A   initial encounter
> D   subsequent encounter
> S   sequela

√5th **V05.0** **Pedestrian injured in collision with railway train or railway vehicle in nontraffic accident**

√x7th **V05.00** **Pedestrian on foot injured in collision with railway train or railway vehicle in nontraffic accident**

Pedestrian NOS injured in collision with railway train or railway vehicle in nontraffic accident

√x7th **V05.01** **Pedestrian on roller-skates injured in collision with railway train or railway vehicle in nontraffic accident**

√x7th **V05.02** **Pedestrian on skateboard injured in collision with railway train or railway vehicle in nontraffic accident**

√x7th **V05.09** **Pedestrian with other conveyance injured in collision with railway train or railway vehicle in nontraffic accident**

Pedestrian with babystroller injured in collision with railway train or railway vehicle in nontraffic accident

Pedestrian on ice-skates injured in collision with railway train or railway vehicle in nontraffic accident

Pedestrian on nonmotorized scooter injured in collision with railway train or railway vehicle in nontraffic accident

Pedestrian on sled injured in collision with railway train or railway vehicle in nontraffic accident

Pedestrian on snowboard injured in collision with railway train or railway vehicle in nontraffic accident

Pedestrian on snow-skis injured in collision with railway train or railway vehicle in nontraffic accident

Pedestrian in wheelchair (powered) injured in collision with railway train or railway vehicle in nontraffic accident

Pedestrian in motorized mobility scooter injured in collision with railway train or railway vehicle in nontraffic accident

√5th **V05.1** **Pedestrian injured in collision with railway train or railway vehicle in traffic accident**

√x7th **V05.10** **Pedestrian on foot injured in collision with railway train or railway vehicle in traffic accident**

Pedestrian NOS injured in collision with railway train or railway vehicle in traffic accident

√x7th **V05.11** **Pedestrian on roller-skates injured in collision with railway train or railway vehicle in traffic accident**

√x7th **V05.12** **Pedestrian on skateboard injured in collision with railway train or railway vehicle in traffic accident**

√x7th **V05.19** **Pedestrian with other conveyance injured in collision with railway train or railway vehicle in traffic accident**

Pedestrian with babystroller injured in collision with railway train or railway vehicle in traffic accident

Pedestrian on ice-skates injured in collision with railway train or railway vehicle in traffic accident

Pedestrian on nonmotorized scooter injured in collision with railway train or railway vehicle in traffic accident

Pedestrian on sled injured in collision with railway train or railway vehicle in traffic accident

Pedestrian on snowboard injured in collision with railway train or railway vehicle in traffic accident

Pedestrian on snow-skis injured in collision with railway train or railway vehicle in traffic accident

Pedestrian in wheelchair (powered) injured in collision with railway train or railway vehicle in traffic accident

Pedestrian in motorized mobility scooter injured in collision with railway train or railway vehicle in traffic accident

√5th **V05.9** **Pedestrian injured in collision with railway train or railway vehicle, unspecified whether traffic or nontraffic accident**

√x7th **V05.90** **Pedestrian on foot injured in collision with railway train or railway vehicle, unspecified whether traffic or nontraffic accident**

Pedestrian NOS injured in collision with railway train or railway vehicle, unspecified whether traffic or nontraffic accident

√x7th **V05.91** **Pedestrian on roller-skates injured in collision with railway train or railway vehicle, unspecified whether traffic or nontraffic accident**

√x7th **V05.92** **Pedestrian on skateboard injured in collision with railway train or railway vehicle, unspecified whether traffic or nontraffic accident**

√x7ᵗʰ **V05.99** **Pedestrian with other conveyance injured in collision with railway train or railway vehicle, unspecified whether traffic or nontraffic accident**

Pedestrian with babystroller injured in collision with railway train or railway vehicle, unspecified whether traffic or nontraffic

Pedestrian on ice-skates injured in collision with railway train or railway vehicle, unspecified whether traffic or nontraffic

Pedestrian on nonmotorized scooter injured in collision with railway train or railway vehicle, unspecified whether traffic or nontraffic

Pedestrian on sled injured in collision with railway train or railway vehicle, unspecified whether traffic or nontraffic

Pedestrian on snowboard injured in collision with railway train or railway vehicle, unspecified whether traffic or nontraffic

Pedestrian on snow-skis injured in collision with railway train or railway vehicle, unspecified whether traffic or nontraffic

Pedestrian in wheelchair (powered) injured in collision with railway train or railway vehicle, unspecified whether traffic or nontraffic

Pedestrian in motorized mobility scooter injured in collision with railway train or railway vehicle, unspecified whether traffic or nontraffic

√4ᵗʰ **V06** **Pedestrian injured in collision with other nonmotor vehicle**

> **INCLUDES** collision with animal-drawn vehicle, animal being ridden, nonpowered streetcar
>
> **EXCLUDES 1** *pedestrian injured in collision with pedestrian conveyance (V00.0-)*

> The appropriate 7th character is to be added to each code from category V06.
> A   initial encounter
> D   subsequent encounter
> S   sequela

√5ᵗʰ **V06.0** **Pedestrian injured in collision with other nonmotor vehicle in nontraffic accident**

√x7ᵗʰ **V06.00** **Pedestrian on foot injured in collision with other nonmotor vehicle in nontraffic accident**

Pedestrian NOS injured in collision with other nonmotor vehicle in nontraffic accident

√x7ᵗʰ **V06.01** **Pedestrian on roller-skates injured in collision with other nonmotor vehicle in nontraffic accident**

√x7ᵗʰ **V06.02** **Pedestrian on skateboard injured in collision with other nonmotor vehicle in nontraffic accident**

√x7ᵗʰ **V06.09** **Pedestrian with other conveyance injured in collision with other nonmotor vehicle in nontraffic accident**

Pedestrian with babystroller injured in collision with other nonmotor vehicle in nontraffic accident

Pedestrian on ice-skates injured in collision with other nonmotor vehicle in nontraffic accident

Pedestrian on nonmotorized scooter injured in collision with other nonmotor vehicle in nontraffic accident

Pedestrian on sled injured in collision with other nonmotor vehicle in nontraffic accident

Pedestrian on snowboard injured in collision with other nonmotor vehicle in nontraffic accident

Pedestrian on snow-skis injured in collision with other nonmotor vehicle in nontraffic accident

Pedestrian in wheelchair (powered) injured in collision with other nonmotor vehicle in nontraffic accident

Pedestrian in motorized mobility scooter injured in collision with other nonmotor vehicle in nontraffic accident

√5ᵗʰ **V06.1** **Pedestrian injured in collision with other nonmotor vehicle in traffic accident**

√x7ᵗʰ **V06.10** **Pedestrian on foot injured in collision with other nonmotor vehicle in traffic accident**

Pedestrian NOS injured in collision with other nonmotor vehicle in traffic accident

√x7ᵗʰ **V06.11** **Pedestrian on roller-skates injured in collision with other nonmotor vehicle in traffic accident**

√x7ᵗʰ **V06.12** **Pedestrian on skateboard injured in collision with other nonmotor vehicle in traffic accident**

√x7ᵗʰ **V06.19** **Pedestrian with other conveyance injured in collision with other nonmotor vehicle in traffic accident**

Pedestrian with babystroller injured in collision with other nonmotor vehicle in nontraffic accident

Pedestrian on ice-skates injured in collision with other nonmotor vehicle in traffic accident

Pedestrian on nonmotorized scooter injured in collision with other nonmotor vehicle in traffic accident

Pedestrian on sled injured in collision with other nonmotor vehicle in traffic accident

Pedestrian on snowboard injured in collision with other nonmotor vehicle in traffic accident

Pedestrian on snow-skis injured in collision with other nonmotor vehicle in traffic accident

Pedestrian in wheelchair (powered) injured in collision with other nonmotor vehicle in traffic accident

Pedestrian in motorized mobility scooter injured in collision with other nonmotor vehicle in traffic accident

√5ᵗʰ **V06.9** **Pedestrian injured in collision with other nonmotor vehicle, unspecified whether traffic or nontraffic accident**

√x7ᵗʰ **V06.90** **Pedestrian on foot injured in collision with other nonmotor vehicle, unspecified whether traffic or nontraffic accident**

Pedestrian NOS injured in collision with other nonmotor vehicle, unspecified whether traffic or nontraffic accident

√x7ᵗʰ **V06.91** **Pedestrian on roller-skates injured in collision with other nonmotor vehicle, unspecified whether traffic or nontraffic accident**

√x7ᵗʰ **V06.92** **Pedestrian on skateboard injured in collision with other nonmotor vehicle, unspecified whether traffic or nontraffic accident**

√x7ᵗʰ **V06.99** **Pedestrian with other conveyance injured in collision with other nonmotor vehicle, unspecified whether traffic or nontraffic accident**

Pedestrian with babystroller injured in collision with other nonmotor vehicle, unspecified whether traffic or nontraffic accident

Pedestrian on ice-skates injured in collision with other nonmotor vehicle, unspecified whether traffic or nontraffic accident

Pedestrian on nonmotorized scooter injured in collision with other nonmotor vehicle, unspecified whether traffic or nontraffic accident

Pedestrian on sled injured in collision with other nonmotor vehicle, unspecified whether traffic or nontraffic accident

Pedestrian on snowboard injured in collision with other nonmotor vehicle, unspecified whether traffic or nontraffic accident

Pedestrian on snow-skis injured in collision with other nonmotor vehicle, unspecified whether traffic or nontraffic accident

Pedestrian in wheelchair (powered) injured in collision with other nonmotor vehicle, unspecified whether traffic or nontraffic accident

Pedestrian in motorized mobility scooter injured in collision with other nonmotor vehicle, unspecified whether traffic or nontraffic accident

√4ᵗʰ **V09** **Pedestrian injured in other and unspecified transport accidents**

> The appropriate 7th character is to be added to each code from category V09.
> A   initial encounter
> D   subsequent encounter
> S   sequela

√5ᵗʰ **V09.0** **Pedestrian injured in nontraffic accident involving other and unspecified motor vehicles**

√x7ᵗʰ **V09.00** **Pedestrian injured in nontraffic accident involving unspecified motor vehicles**

√x7ᵗʰ **V09.01** **Pedestrian injured in nontraffic accident involving military vehicle**

EXCLUDES 1 Not coded here   **EXCLUDES 2** Not included here   *Manifestation Code*

√x7ᵗʰ **V09.09** **Pedestrian injured in nontraffic accident involving other motor vehicles**
　　　Pedestrian injured in nontraffic accident by special vehicle

√x7ᵗʰ **V09.1** **Pedestrian injured in unspecified nontraffic accident**

√5ᵗʰ **V09.2** **Pedestrian injured in traffic accident involving other and unspecified motor vehicles**

√x7ᵗʰ **V09.20** **Pedestrian injured in traffic accident involving unspecified motor vehicles**

√x7ᵗʰ **V09.21** **Pedestrian injured in traffic accident involving military vehicle**

√x7ᵗʰ **V09.29** **Pedestrian injured in traffic accident involving other motor vehicles**

√x7ᵗʰ **V09.3** **Pedestrian injured in unspecified traffic accident**

√x7ᵗʰ **V09.9** **Pedestrian injured in unspecified transport accident**

Pedal cycle rider injured in transport accident (V10-V19)

INCLUDES　any non-motorized vehicle, excluding an animal-drawn vehicle, or a sidecar or trailer attached to the pedal cycle
EXCLUDES 2　rupture of pedal cycle tire (W37.0)

√4ᵗʰ **V10** **Pedal cycle rider injured in collision with pedestrian or animal**
　　EXCLUDES 1　pedal cycle rider collision with animal-drawn vehicle or animal being ridden (V16-)

The appropriate 7th character is to be added to each code from category V10.
　A　initial encounter
　D　subsequent encounter
　S　sequela

√x7ᵗʰ **V10.0** **Pedal cycle driver injured in collision with pedestrian or animal in nontraffic accident**

√x7ᵗʰ **V10.1** **Pedal cycle passenger injured in collision with pedestrian or animal in nontraffic accident**

√x7ᵗʰ **V10.2** **Unspecified pedal cyclist injured in collision with pedestrian or animal in nontraffic accident**

√x7ᵗʰ **V10.3** **Person boarding or alighting a pedal cycle injured in collision with pedestrian or animal**

√x7ᵗʰ **V10.4** **Pedal cycle driver injured in collision with pedestrian or animal in traffic accident**

√x7ᵗʰ **V10.5** **Pedal cycle passenger injured in collision with pedestrian or animal in traffic accident**

√x7ᵗʰ **V10.9** **Unspecified pedal cyclist injured in collision with pedestrian or animal in traffic accident**

√4ᵗʰ **V11** **Pedal cycle rider injured in collision with other pedal cycle**

The appropriate 7th character is to be added to each code from category V11.
　A　initial encounter
　D　subsequent encounter
　S　sequela

√x7ᵗʰ **V11.0** **Pedal cycle driver injured in collision with other pedal cycle in nontraffic accident**

√x7ᵗʰ **V11.1** **Pedal cycle passenger injured in collision with other pedal cycle in nontraffic accident**

√x7ᵗʰ **V11.2** **Unspecified pedal cyclist injured in collision with other pedal cycle in nontraffic accident**

√x7ᵗʰ **V11.3** **Person boarding or alighting a pedal cycle injured in collision with other pedal cycle**

√x7ᵗʰ **V11.4** **Pedal cycle driver injured in collision with other pedal cycle in traffic accident**

√x7ᵗʰ **V11.5** **Pedal cycle passenger injured in collision with other pedal cycle in traffic accident**

√x7ᵗʰ **V11.9** **Unspecified pedal cyclist injured in collision with other pedal cycle in traffic accident**

√4ᵗʰ **V12** **Pedal cycle rider injured in collision with two- or three-wheeled motor vehicle**

The appropriate 7th character is to be added to each code from category V12.
　A　initial encounter
　D　subsequent encounter
　S　sequela

√x7ᵗʰ **V12.0** **Pedal cycle driver injured in collision with two- or three-wheeled motor vehicle in nontraffic accident**

√x7ᵗʰ **V12.1** **Pedal cycle passenger injured in collision with two- or three-wheeled motor vehicle in nontraffic accident**

√x7ᵗʰ **V12.2** **Unspecified pedal cyclist injured in collision with two- or three-wheeled motor vehicle in nontraffic accident**

√x7ᵗʰ **V12.3** **Person boarding or alighting a pedal cycle injured in collision with two- or three-wheeled motor vehicle**

√x7ᵗʰ **V12.4** **Pedal cycle driver injured in collision with two- or three-wheeled motor vehicle in traffic accident**

√x7ᵗʰ **V12.5** **Pedal cycle passenger injured in collision with two- or three-wheeled motor vehicle in traffic accident**

√x7ᵗʰ **V12.9** **Unspecified pedal cyclist injured in collision with two- or three-wheeled motor vehicle in traffic accident**

√4ᵗʰ **V13** **Pedal cycle rider injured in collision with car, pick-up truck or van**

The appropriate 7th character is to be added to each code from category V13.
　A　initial encounter
　D　subsequent encounter
　S　sequela

√x7ᵗʰ **V13.0** **Pedal cycle driver injured in collision with car, pick-up truck or van in nontraffic accident**

√x7ᵗʰ **V13.1** **Pedal cycle passenger injured in collision with car, pick-up truck or van in nontraffic accident**

√x7ᵗʰ **V13.2** **Unspecified pedal cyclist injured in collision with car, pick-up truck or van in nontraffic accident**

√x7ᵗʰ **V13.3** **Person boarding or alighting a pedal cycle injured in collision with car, pick-up truck or van**

√x7ᵗʰ **V13.4** **Pedal cycle driver injured in collision with car, pick-up truck or van in traffic accident**

√x7ᵗʰ **V13.5** **Pedal cycle passenger injured in collision with car, pick-up truck or van in traffic accident**

√x7ᵗʰ **V13.9** **Unspecified pedal cyclist injured in collision with car, pick-up truck or van in traffic accident**

√4ᵗʰ **V14** **Pedal cycle rider injured in collision with heavy transport vehicle or bus**
　　EXCLUDES 1　pedal cycle rider injured in collision with military vehicle (V19.81)

The appropriate 7th character is to be added to each code from category V14.
　A　initial encounter
　D　subsequent encounter
　S　sequela

√x7ᵗʰ **V14.0** **Pedal cycle driver injured in collision with heavy transport vehicle or bus in nontraffic accident**

√x7ᵗʰ **V14.1** **Pedal cycle passenger injured in collision with heavy transport vehicle or bus in nontraffic accident**

√x7ᵗʰ **V14.2** **Unspecified pedal cyclist injured in collision with heavy transport vehicle or bus in nontraffic accident**

√x7ᵗʰ **V14.3** **Person boarding or alighting a pedal cycle injured in collision with heavy transport vehicle or bus**

√x7ᵗʰ **V14.4** **Pedal cycle driver injured in collision with heavy transport vehicle or bus in traffic accident**

√x7ᵗʰ **V14.5** **Pedal cycle passenger injured in collision with heavy transport vehicle or bus in traffic accident**

√x7ᵗʰ **V14.9** **Unspecified pedal cyclist injured in collision with heavy transport vehicle or bus in traffic accident**

√4ᵗʰ **V15** **Pedal cycle rider injured in collision with railway train or railway vehicle**

The appropriate 7th character is to be added to each code from category V15.
　A　initial encounter
　D　subsequent encounter
　S　sequela

√x7ᵗʰ **V15.0** **Pedal cycle driver injured in collision with railway train or railway vehicle in nontraffic accident**

√x7ᵗʰ **V15.1** **Pedal cycle passenger injured in collision with railway train or railway vehicle in nontraffic accident**

√x7ᵗʰ **V15.2** **Unspecified pedal cyclist injured in collision with railway train or railway vehicle in nontraffic accident**

√x7ᵗʰ **V15.3** **Person boarding or alighting a pedal cycle injured in collision with railway train or railway vehicle**

√x7ᵗʰ **V15.4** **Pedal cycle driver injured in collision with railway train or railway vehicle in traffic accident**

√x7ᵗʰ **V15.5** **Pedal cycle passenger injured in collision with railway train or railway vehicle in traffic accident**

☑ Appropriate additional character required　　　　√x7ᵗʰ Requires 7th character, placeholder x must fill empty characters

√x7ᵗʰ **V15.9** Unspecified pedal cyclist injured in collision with railway train or railway vehicle in traffic accident

√4ᵗʰ **V16 Pedal cycle rider injured in collision with other nonmotor vehicle**

INCLUDES collision with animal-drawn vehicle, animal being ridden, streetcar

The appropriate 7th character is to be added to each code from category V16.
A   initial encounter
D   subsequent encounter
S   sequela

√x7ᵗʰ **V16.0** Pedal cycle driver injured in collision with other nonmotor vehicle in nontraffic accident

√x7ᵗʰ **V16.1** Pedal cycle passenger injured in collision with other nonmotor vehicle in nontraffic accident

√x7ᵗʰ **V16.2** Unspecified pedal cyclist injured in collision with other nonmotor vehicle in nontraffic accident

√x7ᵗʰ **V16.3** Person boarding or alighting a pedal cycle injured in collision with other nonmotor vehicle in nontraffic accident

√x7ᵗʰ **V16.4** Pedal cycle driver injured in collision with other nonmotor vehicle in traffic accident

√x7ᵗʰ **V16.5** Pedal cycle passenger injured in collision with other nonmotor vehicle in traffic accident

√x7ᵗʰ **V16.9** Unspecified pedal cyclist injured in collision with other nonmotor vehicle in traffic accident

√4ᵗʰ **V17 Pedal cycle rider injured in collision with fixed or stationary object**

The appropriate 7th character is to be added to each code from category V17.
A   initial encounter
D   subsequent encounter
S   sequela

√x7ᵗʰ **V17.0** Pedal cycle driver injured in collision with fixed or stationary object in nontraffic accident

√x7ᵗʰ **V17.1** Pedal cycle passenger injured in collision with fixed or stationary object in nontraffic accident

√x7ᵗʰ **V17.2** Unspecified pedal cyclist injured in collision with fixed or stationary object in nontraffic accident

√x7ᵗʰ **V17.3** Person boarding or alighting a pedal cycle injured in collision with fixed or stationary object

√x7ᵗʰ **V17.4** Pedal cycle driver injured in collision with fixed or stationary object in traffic accident

√x7ᵗʰ **V17.5** Pedal cycle passenger injured in collision with fixed or stationary object in traffic accident

√x7ᵗʰ **V17.9** Unspecified pedal cyclist injured in collision with fixed or stationary object in traffic accident

√4ᵗʰ **V18 Pedal cycle rider injured in noncollision transport accident**

INCLUDES fall or thrown from pedal cycle (without antecedent collision)
overturning pedal cycle NOS
overturning pedal cycle without collision

The appropriate 7th character is to be added to each code from category V18.
A   initial encounter
D   subsequent encounter
S   sequela

√x7ᵗʰ **V18.0** Pedal cycle driver injured in noncollision transport accident in nontraffic accident

√x7ᵗʰ **V18.1** Pedal cycle passenger injured in noncollision transport accident in nontraffic accident

√x7ᵗʰ **V18.2** Unspecified pedal cyclist injured in noncollision transport accident in nontraffic accident

√x7ᵗʰ **V18.3** Person boarding or alighting a pedal cycle injured in noncollision transport accident

√x7ᵗʰ **V18.4** Pedal cycle driver injured in noncollision transport accident in traffic accident

√x7ᵗʰ **V18.5** Pedal cycle passenger injured in noncollision transport accident in traffic accident

√x7ᵗʰ **V18.9** Unspecified pedal cyclist injured in noncollision transport accident in traffic accident

√4ᵗʰ **V19 Pedal cycle rider injured in other and unspecified transport accidents**

The appropriate 7th character is to be added to each code from category V19.
A   initial encounter
D   subsequent encounter
S   sequela

√5ᵗʰ **V19.0** Pedal cycle driver injured in collision with other and unspecified motor vehicles in nontraffic accident

√x7ᵗʰ **V19.00** Pedal cycle driver injured in collision with unspecified motor vehicles in nontraffic accident

√x7ᵗʰ **V19.09** Pedal cycle driver injured in collision with other motor vehicles in nontraffic accident

√5ᵗʰ **V19.1** Pedal cycle passenger injured in collision with other and unspecified motor vehicles in nontraffic accident

√x7ᵗʰ **V19.10** Pedal cycle passenger injured in collision with unspecified motor vehicles in nontraffic accident

√x7ᵗʰ **V19.19** Pedal cycle passenger injured in collision with other motor vehicles in nontraffic accident

√5ᵗʰ **V19.2** Unspecified pedal cyclist injured in collision with other and unspecified motor vehicles in nontraffic accident

√x7ᵗʰ **V19.20** Unspecified pedal cyclist injured in collision with unspecified motor vehicles in nontraffic accident
Pedal cycle collision NOS, nontraffic

√x7ᵗʰ **V19.29** Unspecified pedal cyclist injured in collision with other motor vehicles in nontraffic accident

√5ᵗʰ **V19.3** Pedal cyclist (driver) (passenger) injured in unspecified nontraffic accident
Pedal cycle accident NOS, nontraffic
Pedal cyclist injured in nontraffic accident NOS

√5ᵗʰ **V19.4** Pedal cycle driver injured in collision with other and unspecified motor vehicles in traffic accident

√x7ᵗʰ **V19.40** Pedal cycle driver injured in collision with unspecified motor vehicles in traffic accident

√x7ᵗʰ **V19.49** Pedal cycle driver injured in collision with other motor vehicles in traffic accident

√5ᵗʰ **V19.5** Pedal cycle passenger injured in collision with other and unspecified motor vehicles in traffic accident

√x7ᵗʰ **V19.50** Pedal cycle passenger injured in collision with unspecified motor vehicles in traffic accident

√x7ᵗʰ **V19.59** Pedal cycle passenger injured in collision with other motor vehicles in traffic accident

√5ᵗʰ **V19.6** Unspecified pedal cyclist injured in collision with other and unspecified motor vehicles in traffic accident

√x7ᵗʰ **V19.60** Unspecified pedal cyclist injured in collision with unspecified motor vehicles in traffic accident
Pedal cycle collision NOS (traffic)

√x7ᵗʰ **V19.69** Unspecified pedal cyclist injured in collision with other motor vehicles in traffic accident

√5ᵗʰ **V19.8** Pedal cyclist (driver) (passenger) injured in other specified transport accidents

√x7ᵗʰ **V19.81** Pedal cyclist (driver) (passenger) injured in transport accident with military vehicle

√x7ᵗʰ **V19.88** Pedal cyclist (driver) (passenger) injured in other specified transport accidents

√x7ᵗʰ **V19.9** Pedal cyclist (driver) (passenger) injured in unspecified traffic accident
Pedal cycle accident NOS

Motorcycle rider injured in transport accident (V20-V29)

INCLUDES moped
motorcycle with sidecar
motorized bicycle
motor scooter
EXCLUDES 1 three-wheeled motor vehicle (V30-V39)

√4ᵗʰ **V20 Motorcycle rider injured in collision with pedestrian or animal**

EXCLUDES 1 motorcycle rider collision with animal-drawn vehicle or animal being ridden (V26-)

The appropriate 7th character is to be added to each code from category V20.
A   initial encounter
D   subsequent encounter
S   sequela

√x7ᵗʰ **V20.0** Motorcycle driver injured in collision with pedestrian or animal in nontraffic accident

---

EXCLUDES 1 Not coded here   EXCLUDES 2 Not included here   *Manifestation Code*

✓x7ᵗʰ **V20.1** Motorcycle passenger injured in collision with pedestrian or animal in nontraffic accident

✓x7ᵗʰ **V20.2** Unspecified motorcycle rider injured in collision with pedestrian or animal in nontraffic accident

✓x7ᵗʰ **V20.3** Person boarding or alighting a motorcycle injured in collision with pedestrian or animal

✓x7ᵗʰ **V20.4** Motorcycle driver injured in collision with pedestrian or animal in traffic accident

✓x7ᵗʰ **V20.5** Motorcycle passenger injured in collision with pedestrian or animal in traffic accident

✓x7ᵗʰ **V20.9** Unspecified motorcycle rider injured in collision with pedestrian or animal in traffic accident

✓4ᵗʰ **V21** **Motorcycle rider injured in collision with pedal cycle**

The appropriate 7th character is to be added to each code from category V21.
A　initial encounter
D　subsequent encounter
S　sequela

✓x7ᵗʰ **V21.0** Motorcycle driver injured in collision with pedal cycle in nontraffic accident

✓x7ᵗʰ **V21.1** Motorcycle passenger injured in collision with pedal cycle in nontraffic accident

✓x7ᵗʰ **V21.2** Unspecified motorcycle rider injured in collision with pedal cycle in nontraffic accident

✓x7ᵗʰ **V21.3** Person boarding or alighting a motorcycle injured in collision with pedal cycle

✓x7ᵗʰ **V21.4** Motorcycle driver injured in collision with pedal cycle in traffic accident

✓x7ᵗʰ **V21.5** Motorcycle passenger injured in collision with pedal cycle in traffic accident

✓x7ᵗʰ **V21.9** Unspecified motorcycle rider injured in collision with pedal cycle in traffic accident

✓4ᵗʰ **V22** **Motorcycle rider injured in collision with two- or three-wheeled motor vehicle**

The appropriate 7th character is to be added to each code from category V22.
A　initial encounter
D　subsequent encounter
S　sequela

✓x7ᵗʰ **V22.0** Motorcycle driver injured in collision with two- or three-wheeled motor vehicle in nontraffic accident

✓x7ᵗʰ **V22.1** Motorcycle passenger injured in collision with two- or three-wheeled motor vehicle in nontraffic accident

✓x7ᵗʰ **V22.2** Unspecified motorcycle rider injured in collision with two- or three-wheeled motor vehicle in nontraffic accident

✓x7ᵗʰ **V22.3** Person boarding or alighting a motorcycle injured in collision with two- or three-wheeled motor vehicle

✓x7ᵗʰ **V22.4** Motorcycle driver injured in collision with two- or three-wheeled motor vehicle in traffic accident

✓x7ᵗʰ **V22.5** Motorcycle passenger injured in collision with two- or three-wheeled motor vehicle in traffic accident

✓x7ᵗʰ **V22.9** Unspecified motorcycle rider injured in collision with two- or three-wheeled motor vehicle in traffic accident

✓4ᵗʰ **V23** **Motorcycle rider injured in collision with car, pick-up truck or van**

The appropriate 7th character is to be added to each code from category V23.
A　initial encounter
D　subsequent encounter
S　sequela

✓x7ᵗʰ **V23.0** Motorcycle driver injured in collision with car, pick-up truck or van in nontraffic accident

✓x7ᵗʰ **V23.1** Motorcycle passenger injured in collision with car, pick-up truck or van in nontraffic accident

✓x7ᵗʰ **V23.2** Unspecified motorcycle rider injured in collision with car, pick-up truck or van in nontraffic accident

✓x7ᵗʰ **V23.3** Person boarding or alighting a motorcycle injured in collision with car, pick-up truck or van

✓x7ᵗʰ **V23.4** Motorcycle driver injured in collision with car, pick-up truck or van in traffic accident

✓x7ᵗʰ **V23.5** Motorcycle passenger injured in collision with car, pick-up truck or van in traffic accident

✓x7ᵗʰ **V23.9** Unspecified motorcycle rider injured in collision with car, pick-up truck or van in traffic accident

✓4ᵗʰ **V24** **Motorcycle rider injured in collision with heavy transport vehicle or bus**

EXCLUDES 1　motorcycle rider injured in collision with military vehicle (V29.81)

The appropriate 7th character is to be added to each code from category V24.
A　initial encounter
D　subsequent encounter
S　sequela

✓x7ᵗʰ **V24.0** Motorcycle driver injured in collision with heavy transport vehicle or bus in nontraffic accident

✓x7ᵗʰ **V24.1** Motorcycle passenger injured in collision with heavy transport vehicle or bus in nontraffic accident

✓x7ᵗʰ **V24.2** Unspecified motorcycle rider injured in collision with heavy transport vehicle or bus in nontraffic accident

✓x7ᵗʰ **V24.3** Person boarding or alighting a motorcycle injured in collision with heavy transport vehicle or bus

✓x7ᵗʰ **V24.4** Motorcycle driver injured in collision with heavy transport vehicle or bus in traffic accident

✓x7ᵗʰ **V24.5** Motorcycle passenger injured in collision with heavy transport vehicle or bus in traffic accident

✓x7ᵗʰ **V24.9** Unspecified motorcycle rider injured in collision with heavy transport vehicle or bus in traffic accident

✓4ᵗʰ **V25** **Motorcycle rider injured in collision with railway train or railway vehicle**

The appropriate 7th character is to be added to each code from category V25.
A　initial encounter
D　subsequent encounter
S　sequela

✓x7ᵗʰ **V25.0** Motorcycle driver injured in collision with railway train or railway vehicle in nontraffic accident

✓x7ᵗʰ **V25.1** Motorcycle passenger injured in collision with railway train or railway vehicle in nontraffic accident

✓x7ᵗʰ **V25.2** Unspecified motorcycle rider injured in collision with railway train or railway vehicle in nontraffic accident

✓x7ᵗʰ **V25.3** Person boarding or alighting a motorcycle injured in collision with railway train or railway vehicle

✓x7ᵗʰ **V25.4** Motorcycle driver injured in collision with railway train or railway vehicle in traffic accident

✓x7ᵗʰ **V25.5** Motorcycle passenger injured in collision with railway train or railway vehicle in traffic accident

✓x7ᵗʰ **V25.9** Unspecified motorcycle rider injured in collision with railway train or railway vehicle in traffic accident

✓4ᵗʰ **V26** **Motorcycle rider injured in collision with other nonmotor vehicle**

INCLUDES　collision with animal-drawn vehicle, animal being ridden, streetcar

The appropriate 7th character is to be added to each code from category V26.
A　initial encounter
D　subsequent encounter
S　sequela

✓x7ᵗʰ **V26.0** Motorcycle driver injured in collision with other nonmotor vehicle in nontraffic accident

✓x7ᵗʰ **V26.1** Motorcycle passenger injured in collision with other nonmotor vehicle in nontraffic accident

✓x7ᵗʰ **V26.2** Unspecified motorcycle rider injured in collision with other nonmotor vehicle in nontraffic accident

✓x7ᵗʰ **V26.3** Person boarding or alighting a motorcycle injured in collision with other nonmotor vehicle

✓x7ᵗʰ **V26.4** Motorcycle driver injured in collision with other nonmotor vehicle in traffic accident

✓x7ᵗʰ **V26.5** Motorcycle passenger injured in collision with other nonmotor vehicle in traffic accident

✓x7ᵗʰ **V26.9** Unspecified motorcycle rider injured in collision with other nonmotor vehicle in traffic accident

---

✔ Appropriate additional character required　　　　✓x7ᵗʰ Requires 7th character, placeholder x must fill empty characters

√4th **V27 Motorcycle rider injured in collision with fixed or stationary object**

> The appropriate 7th character is to be added to each code from category V27.
> A   initial encounter
> D   subsequent encounter
> S   sequela

√x7th **V27.0 Motorcycle driver injured in collision with fixed or stationary object in nontraffic accident**

√x7th **V27.1 Motorcycle passenger injured in collision with fixed or stationary object in nontraffic accident**

√x7th **V27.2 Unspecified motorcycle rider injured in collision with fixed or stationary object in nontraffic accident**

√x7th **V27.3 Person boarding or alighting a motorcycle injured in collision with fixed or stationary object**

√x7th **V27.4 Motorcycle driver injured in collision with fixed or stationary object in traffic accident**

√x7th **V27.5 Motorcycle passenger injured in collision with fixed or stationary object in traffic accident**

√x7th **V27.9 Unspecified motorcycle rider injured in collision with fixed or stationary object in traffic accident**

√4th **V28 Motorcycle rider injured in noncollision transport accident**
> INCLUDES   fall or thrown from motorcycle (without antecedent collision)
> overturning motorcycle NOS
> overturning motorcycle without collision

> The appropriate 7th character is to be added to each code from category V28.
> A   initial encounter
> D   subsequent encounter
> S   sequela

√x7th **V28.0 Motorcycle driver injured in noncollision transport accident in nontraffic accident**

√x7th **V28.1 Motorcycle passenger injured in noncollision transport accident in nontraffic accident**

√x7th **V28.2 Unspecified motorcycle rider injured in noncollision transport accident in nontraffic accident**

√x7th **V28.3 Person boarding or alighting a motorcycle injured in noncollision transport accident**

√x7th **V28.4 Motorcycle driver injured in noncollision transport accident in traffic accident**

√x7th **V28.5 Motorcycle passenger injured in noncollision transport accident in traffic accident**

√x7th **V28.9 Unspecified motorcycle rider injured in noncollision transport accident in traffic accident**

√4th **V29 Motorcycle rider injured in other and unspecified transport accidents**

> The appropriate 7th character is to be added to each code from category V29.
> A   initial encounter
> D   subsequent encounter
> S   sequela

√5th **V29.0 Motorcycle driver injured in collision with other and unspecified motor vehicles in nontraffic accident**

√x7th **V29.00 Motorcycle driver injured in collision with unspecified motor vehicles in nontraffic accident**

√x7th **V29.09 Motorcycle driver injured in collision with other motor vehicles in nontraffic accident**

√5th **V29.1 Motorcycle passenger injured in collision with other and unspecified motor vehicles in nontraffic accident**

√x7th **V29.10 Motorcycle passenger injured in collision with unspecified motor vehicles in nontraffic accident**

√x7th **V29.19 Motorcycle passenger injured in collision with other motor vehicles in nontraffic accident**

√5th **V29.2 Unspecified motorcycle rider injured in collision with other and unspecified motor vehicles in nontraffic accident**

√x7th **V29.20 Unspecified motorcycle rider injured in collision with unspecified motor vehicles in nontraffic accident**
> Motorcycle collision NOS, nontraffic

√x7th **V29.29 Unspecified motorcycle rider injured in collision with other motor vehicles in nontraffic accident**

√x7th **V29.3 Motorcycle rider (driver) (passenger) injured in unspecified nontraffic accident**
> Motorcycle accident NOS, nontraffic
> Motorcycle rider injured in nontraffic accident NOS

√5th **V29.4 Motorcycle driver injured in collision with other and unspecified motor vehicles in traffic accident**

√x7th **V29.40 Motorcycle driver injured in collision with unspecified motor vehicles in traffic accident**

√x7th **V29.49 Motorcycle driver injured in collision with other motor vehicles in traffic accident**

√5th **V29.5 Motorcycle passenger injured in collision with other and unspecified motor vehicles in traffic accident**

√x7th **V29.50 Motorcycle passenger injured in collision with unspecified motor vehicles in traffic accident**

√x7th **V29.59 Motorcycle passenger injured in collision with other motor vehicles in traffic accident**

√5th **V29.6 Unspecified motorcycle rider injured in collision with other and unspecified motor vehicles in traffic accident**

√x7th **V29.60 Unspecified motorcycle rider injured in collision with unspecified motor vehicles in traffic accident**
> Motorcycle collision NOS (traffic)

√x7th **V29.69 Unspecified motorcycle rider injured in collision with other motor vehicles in traffic accident**

√5th **V29.8 Motorcycle rider (driver) (passenger) injured in other specified transport accidents**

√x7th **V29.81 Motorcycle rider (driver) (passenger) injured in transport accident with military vehicle**

√x7th **V29.88 Motorcycle rider (driver) (passenger) injured in other specified transport accidents**

√x7th **V29.9 Motorcycle rider (driver) (passenger) injured in unspecified traffic accident**
> Motorcycle accident NOS

Occupant of three-wheeled motor vehicle injured in transport accident (V30-V39)

> INCLUDES   motorized tricycle
> motorized rickshaw
> three-wheeled motor car
> EXCLUDES 1   *all-terrain vehicles (V86-)*
> *motorcycle with sidecar (V20-V29)*
> *vehicle designed primarily for off-road use (V86-)*

√4th **V30 Occupant of three-wheeled motor vehicle injured in collision with pedestrian or animal**
> EXCLUDES 1   *three-wheeled motor vehicle collision with animal-drawn vehicle or animal being ridden (V36-)*

> The appropriate 7th character is to be added to each code from category V30.
> A   initial encounter
> D   subsequent encounter
> S   sequela

√x7th **V30.0 Driver of three-wheeled motor vehicle injured in collision with pedestrian or animal in nontraffic accident**

√x7th **V30.1 Passenger in three-wheeled motor vehicle injured in collision with pedestrian or animal in nontraffic accident**

√x7th **V30.2 Person on outside of three-wheeled motor vehicle injured in collision with pedestrian or animal in nontraffic accident**

√x7th **V30.3 Unspecified occupant of three-wheeled motor vehicle injured in collision with pedestrian or animal in nontraffic accident**

√x7th **V30.4 Person boarding or alighting a three-wheeled motor vehicle injured in collision with pedestrian or animal**

√x7th **V30.5 Driver of three-wheeled motor vehicle injured in collision with pedestrian or animal in traffic accident**

√x7th **V30.6 Passenger in three-wheeled motor vehicle injured in collision with pedestrian or animal in traffic accident**

√x7th **V30.7 Person on outside of three-wheeled motor vehicle injured in collision with pedestrian or animal in traffic accident**

√x7th **V30.9 Unspecified occupant of three-wheeled motor vehicle injured in collision with pedestrian or animal in traffic accident**

EXCLUDES 1   Not coded here   EXCLUDES 2   Not included here   *Manifestation Code*

☑4ᵗʰ **V31** **Occupant of three-wheeled motor vehicle injured in collision with pedal cycle**

> The appropriate 7th character is to be added to each code from category V31.
> A   initial encounter
> D   subsequent encounter
> S   sequela

√x7ᵗʰ **V31.0** Driver of three-wheeled motor vehicle injured in collision with pedal cycle in nontraffic accident

√x7ᵗʰ **V31.1** Passenger in three-wheeled motor vehicle injured in collision with pedal cycle in nontraffic accident

√x7ᵗʰ **V31.2** Person on outside of three-wheeled motor vehicle injured in collision with pedal cycle in nontraffic accident

√x7ᵗʰ **V31.3** Unspecified occupant of three-wheeled motor vehicle injured in collision with pedal cycle in nontraffic accident

√x7ᵗʰ **V31.4** Person boarding or alighting a three-wheeled motor vehicle injured in collision with pedal cycle

√x7ᵗʰ **V31.5** Driver of three-wheeled motor vehicle injured in collision with pedal cycle in traffic accident

√x7ᵗʰ **V31.6** Passenger in three-wheeled motor vehicle injured in collision with pedal cycle in traffic accident

√x7ᵗʰ **V31.7** Person on outside of three-wheeled motor vehicle injured in collision with pedal cycle in traffic accident

√x7ᵗʰ **V31.9** Unspecified occupant of three-wheeled motor vehicle injured in collision with pedal cycle in traffic accident

☑4ᵗʰ **V32** **Occupant of three-wheeled motor vehicle injured in collision with two- or three-wheeled motor vehicle**

> The appropriate 7th character is to be added to each code from category V32.
> A   initial encounter
> D   subsequent encounter
> S   sequela

√x7ᵗʰ **V32.0** Driver of three-wheeled motor vehicle injured in collision with two- or three-wheeled motor vehicle in nontraffic accident

√x7ᵗʰ **V32.1** Passenger in three-wheeled motor vehicle injured in collision with two- or three-wheeled motor vehicle in nontraffic accident

√x7ᵗʰ **V32.2** Person on outside of three-wheeled motor vehicle injured in collision with two- or three-wheeled motor vehicle in nontraffic accident

√x7ᵗʰ **V32.3** Unspecified occupant of three-wheeled motor vehicle injured in collision with two- or three-wheeled motor vehicle in nontraffic accident

√x7ᵗʰ **V32.4** Person boarding or alighting a three-wheeled motor vehicle injured in collision with two- or three-wheeled motor vehicle

√x7ᵗʰ **V32.5** Driver of three-wheeled motor vehicle injured in collision with two- or three-wheeled motor vehicle in traffic accident

√x7ᵗʰ **V32.6** Passenger in three-wheeled motor vehicle injured in collision with two- or three-wheeled motor vehicle in traffic accident

√x7ᵗʰ **V32.7** Person on outside of three-wheeled motor vehicle injured in collision with two- or three-wheeled motor vehicle in traffic accident

√x7ᵗʰ **V32.9** Unspecified occupant of three-wheeled motor vehicle injured in collision with two- or three-wheeled motor vehicle in traffic accident

☑4ᵗʰ **V33** **Occupant of three-wheeled motor vehicle injured in collision with car, pick-up truck or van**

> The appropriate 7th character is to be added to each code from category V33.
> A   initial encounter
> D   subsequent encounter
> S   sequela

√x7ᵗʰ **V33.0** Driver of three-wheeled motor vehicle injured in collision with car, pick-up truck or van in nontraffic accident

√x7ᵗʰ **V33.1** Passenger in three-wheeled motor vehicle injured in collision with car, pick-up truck or van in nontraffic accident

√x7ᵗʰ **V33.2** Person on outside of three-wheeled motor vehicle injured in collision with car, pick-up truck or van in nontraffic accident

√x7ᵗʰ **V33.3** Unspecified occupant of three-wheeled motor vehicle injured in collision with car, pick-up truck or van in nontraffic accident

√x7ᵗʰ **V33.4** Person boarding or alighting a three-wheeled motor vehicle injured in collision with car, pick-up truck or van

√x7ᵗʰ **V33.5** Driver of three-wheeled motor vehicle injured in collision with car, pick-up truck or van in traffic accident

√x7ᵗʰ **V33.6** Passenger in three-wheeled motor vehicle injured in collision with car, pick-up truck or van in traffic accident

√x7ᵗʰ **V33.7** Person on outside of three-wheeled motor vehicle injured in collision with car, pick-up truck or van in traffic accident

√x7ᵗʰ **V33.9** Unspecified occupant of three-wheeled motor vehicle injured in collision with car, pick-up truck or van in traffic accident

☑4ᵗʰ **V34** **Occupant of three-wheeled motor vehicle injured in collision with heavy transport vehicle or bus**

> **EXCLUDES 1**   occupant of three-wheeled motor vehicle injured in collision with military vehicle (V39.81)

> The appropriate 7th character is to be added to each code from category V34.
> A   initial encounter
> D   subsequent encounter
> S   sequela

√x7ᵗʰ **V34.0** Driver of three-wheeled motor vehicle injured in collision with heavy transport vehicle or bus in nontraffic accident

√x7ᵗʰ **V34.1** Passenger in three-wheeled motor vehicle injured in collision with heavy transport vehicle or bus in nontraffic accident

√x7ᵗʰ **V34.2** Person on outside of three-wheeled motor vehicle injured in collision with heavy transport vehicle or bus in nontraffic accident

√x7ᵗʰ **V34.3** Unspecified occupant of three-wheeled motor vehicle injured in collision with heavy transport vehicle or bus in nontraffic accident

√x7ᵗʰ **V34.4** Person boarding or alighting a three-wheeled motor vehicle injured in collision with heavy transport vehicle or bus

√x7ᵗʰ **V34.5** Driver of three-wheeled motor vehicle injured in collision with heavy transport vehicle or bus in traffic accident

√x7ᵗʰ **V34.6** Passenger in three-wheeled motor vehicle injured in collision with heavy transport vehicle or bus in traffic accident

√x7ᵗʰ **V34.7** Person on outside of three-wheeled motor vehicle injured in collision with heavy transport vehicle or bus in traffic accident

√x7ᵗʰ **V34.9** Unspecified occupant of three-wheeled motor vehicle injured in collision with heavy transport vehicle or bus in traffic accident

☑4ᵗʰ **V35** **Occupant of three-wheeled motor vehicle injured in collision with railway train or railway vehicle**

> The appropriate 7th character is to be added to each code from category V35.
> A   initial encounter
> D   subsequent encounter
> S   sequela

√x7ᵗʰ **V35.0** Driver of three-wheeled motor vehicle injured in collision with railway train or railway vehicle in nontraffic accident

√x7ᵗʰ **V35.1** Passenger in three-wheeled motor vehicle injured in collision with railway train or railway vehicle in nontraffic accident

√x7ᵗʰ **V35.2** Person on outside of three-wheeled motor vehicle injured in collision with railway train or railway vehicle in nontraffic accident

√x7ᵗʰ **V35.3** Unspecified occupant of three-wheeled motor vehicle injured in collision with railway train or railway vehicle in nontraffic accident

√x7ᵗʰ **V35.4** Person boarding or alighting a three-wheeled motor vehicle injured in collision with railway train or railway vehicle

√x7ᵗʰ **V35.5** Driver of three-wheeled motor vehicle injured in collision with railway train or railway vehicle in traffic accident

√x7ᵗʰ **V35.6** Passenger in three-wheeled motor vehicle injured in collision with railway train or railway vehicle in traffic accident

√x7ᵗʰ **V35.7** Person on outside of three-wheeled motor vehicle injured in collision with railway train or railway vehicle in traffic accident

---

☑ Appropriate additional character required   √x7ᵗʰ Requires 7th character, placeholder x must fill empty characters

External Causes of Morbidity

V35.9–V39.59

√x7ᵗʰ **V35.9** Unspecified occupant of three-wheeled motor vehicle injured in collision with railway train or railway vehicle in traffic accident

√4ᵗʰ **V36** **Occupant of three-wheeled motor vehicle injured in collision with other nonmotor vehicle**

INCLUDES collision with animal-drawn vehicle, animal being ridden, streetcar

The appropriate 7th character is to be added to each code from category V36.
A   initial encounter
D   subsequent encounter
S   sequela

√x7ᵗʰ **V36.0** Driver of three-wheeled motor vehicle injured in collision with other nonmotor vehicle in nontraffic accident

√x7ᵗʰ **V36.1** Passenger in three-wheeled motor vehicle injured in collision with other nonmotor vehicle in nontraffic accident

√x7ᵗʰ **V36.2** Person on outside of three-wheeled motor vehicle injured in collision with other nonmotor vehicle in nontraffic accident

√x7ᵗʰ **V36.3** Unspecified occupant of three-wheeled motor vehicle injured in collision with other nonmotor vehicle in nontraffic accident

√x7ᵗʰ **V36.4** Person boarding or alighting a three-wheeled motor vehicle injured in collision with other nonmotor vehicle

√x7ᵗʰ **V36.5** Driver of three-wheeled motor vehicle injured in collision with other nonmotor vehicle in traffic accident

√x7ᵗʰ **V36.6** Passenger in three-wheeled motor vehicle injured in collision with other nonmotor vehicle in traffic accident

√x7ᵗʰ **V36.7** Person on outside of three-wheeled motor vehicle injured in collision with other nonmotor vehicle in traffic accident

√x7ᵗʰ **V36.9** Unspecified occupant of three-wheeled motor vehicle injured in collision with other nonmotor vehicle in traffic accident

√4ᵗʰ **V37** **Occupant of three-wheeled motor vehicle injured in collision with fixed or stationary object**

The appropriate 7th character is to be added to each code from category V37.
A   initial encounter
D   subsequent encounter
S   sequela

√x7ᵗʰ **V37.0** Driver of three-wheeled motor vehicle injured in collision with fixed or stationary object in nontraffic accident

√x7ᵗʰ **V37.1** Passenger in three-wheeled motor vehicle injured in collision with fixed or stationary object in nontraffic accident

√x7ᵗʰ **V37.2** Person on outside of three-wheeled motor vehicle injured in collision with fixed or stationary object in nontraffic accident

√x7ᵗʰ **V37.3** Unspecified occupant of three-wheeled motor vehicle injured in collision with fixed or stationary object in nontraffic accident

√x7ᵗʰ **V37.4** Person boarding or alighting a three-wheeled motor vehicle injured in collision with fixed or stationary object

√x7ᵗʰ **V37.5** Driver of three-wheeled motor vehicle injured in collision with fixed or stationary object in traffic accident

√x7ᵗʰ **V37.6** Passenger in three-wheeled motor vehicle injured in collision with fixed or stationary object in traffic accident

√x7ᵗʰ **V37.7** Person on outside of three-wheeled motor vehicle injured in collision with fixed or stationary object in traffic accident

√x7ᵗʰ **V37.9** Unspecified occupant of three-wheeled motor vehicle injured in collision with fixed or stationary object in traffic accident

V38 **Occupant of three-wheeled motor vehicle injured in noncollision transport accident**

INCLUDES fall or thrown from three-wheeled motor vehicle
overturning of three-wheeled motor vehicle NOS
overturning of three-wheeled motor vehicle without collision

The appropriate 7th character is to be added to each code from category V38.
A   initial encounter
D   subsequent encounter
S   sequela

√x7ᵗʰ **V38.0** Driver of three-wheeled motor vehicle injured in noncollision transport accident in nontraffic accident

√x7ᵗʰ **V38.1** Passenger in three-wheeled motor vehicle injured in noncollision transport accident in nontraffic accident

√x7ᵗʰ **V38.2** Person on outside of three-wheeled motor vehicle injured in noncollision transport accident in nontraffic accident

√x7ᵗʰ **V38.3** Unspecified occupant of three-wheeled motor vehicle injured in noncollision transport accident in nontraffic accident

√x7ᵗʰ **V38.4** Person boarding or alighting a three-wheeled motor vehicle injured in noncollision transport accident

√x7ᵗʰ **V38.5** Driver of three-wheeled motor vehicle injured in noncollision transport accident in traffic accident

√x7ᵗʰ **V38.6** Passenger in three-wheeled motor vehicle injured in noncollision transport accident in traffic accident

√x7ᵗʰ **V38.7** Person on outside of three-wheeled motor vehicle injured in noncollision transport accident in traffic accident

√x7ᵗʰ **V38.9** Unspecified occupant of three-wheeled motor vehicle injured in noncollision transport accident in traffic accident

√4ᵗʰ **V39** **Occupant of three-wheeled motor vehicle injured in other and unspecified transport accidents**

The appropriate 7th character is to be added to each code from category V39.
A   initial encounter
D   subsequent encounter
S   sequela

√5ᵗʰ **V39.0** Driver of three-wheeled motor vehicle injured in collision with other and unspecified motor vehicles in nontraffic accident

√x7ᵗʰ **V39.00** Driver of three-wheeled motor vehicle injured in collision with unspecified motor vehicles in nontraffic accident

√x7ᵗʰ **V39.09** Driver of three-wheeled motor vehicle injured in collision with other motor vehicles in nontraffic accident

√5ᵗʰ **V39.1** Passenger in three-wheeled motor vehicle injured in collision with other and unspecified motor vehicles in nontraffic accident

√x7ᵗʰ **V39.10** Passenger in three-wheeled motor vehicle injured in collision with unspecified motor vehicles in nontraffic accident

√x7ᵗʰ **V39.19** Passenger in three-wheeled motor vehicle injured in collision with other motor vehicles in nontraffic accident

√5ᵗʰ **V39.2** Unspecified occupant of three-wheeled motor vehicle injured in collision with other and unspecified motor vehicles in nontraffic accident

√x7ᵗʰ **V39.20** Unspecified occupant of three-wheeled motor vehicle injured in collision with unspecified motor vehicles in nontraffic accident
Collision NOS involving three-wheeled motor vehicle, nontraffic

√x7ᵗʰ **V39.29** Unspecified occupant of three-wheeled motor vehicle injured in collision with other motor vehicles in nontraffic accident

√x7ᵗʰ **V39.3** Occupant (driver) (passenger) of three-wheeled motor vehicle injured in unspecified nontraffic accident
Accident NOS involving three-wheeled motor vehicle, nontraffic
Occupant of three-wheeled motor vehicle injured in nontraffic accident NOS

√5ᵗʰ **V39.4** Driver of three-wheeled motor vehicle injured in collision with other and unspecified motor vehicles in traffic accident

√x7ᵗʰ **V39.40** Driver of three-wheeled motor vehicle injured in collision with unspecified motor vehicles in traffic accident

√x7ᵗʰ **V39.49** Driver of three-wheeled motor vehicle injured in collision with other motor vehicles in traffic accident

√5ᵗʰ **V39.5** Passenger in three-wheeled motor vehicle injured in collision with other and unspecified motor vehicles in traffic accident

√x7ᵗʰ **V39.50** Passenger in three-wheeled motor vehicle injured in collision with unspecified motor vehicles in traffic accident

√x7ᵗʰ **V39.59** Passenger in three-wheeled motor vehicle injured in collision with other motor vehicles in traffic accident

EXCLUDES 1 Not coded here   EXCLUDES 2 Not included here   *Manifestation Code*

√5th **V39.6 Unspecified occupant of three-wheeled motor vehicle injured in collision with other and unspecified motor vehicles in traffic accident**

    √x7th **V39.60 Unspecified occupant of three-wheeled motor vehicle injured in collision with unspecified motor vehicles in traffic accident**

         Collision NOS involving three-wheeled motor vehicle (traffic)

    √x7th **V39.69 Unspecified occupant of three-wheeled motor vehicle injured in collision with other motor vehicles in traffic accident**

√5th **V39.8 Occupant (driver) (passenger) of three-wheeled motor vehicle injured in other specified transport accidents**

    √x7th **V39.81 Occupant (driver) (passenger) of three-wheeled motor vehicle injured in transport accident with military vehicle**

    √x7th **V39.89 Occupant (driver) (passenger) of three-wheeled motor vehicle injured in other specified transport accidents**

√x7th **V39.9 Occupant (driver) (passenger) of three-wheeled motor vehicle injured in unspecified traffic accident**

     Accident NOS involving three-wheeled motor vehicle

Car occupant injured in transport accident (V40-V49)

INCLUDES   a four-wheeled motor vehicle designed primarily for carrying passengers

         automobile (pulling a trailer or camper)

EXCLUDES 1   bus (V50-V59)

         minibus (V50-V59)

         minivan (V50-V59)

         motorcoach (V70-V79)

         pick-up truck (V50-V59)

         sport utility vehicle (SUV) (V50-V59)

√4th **V40 Car occupant injured in collision with pedestrian or animal**

     EXCLUDES 1   car collision with animal-drawn vehicle or animal being ridden (V46-)

     The appropriate 7th character is to be added to each code from category V40.
     A   initial encounter
     D   subsequent encounter
     S   sequela

√x7th **V40.0 Car driver injured in collision with pedestrian or animal in nontraffic accident**

√x7th **V40.1 Car passenger injured in collision with pedestrian or animal in nontraffic accident**

√x7th **V40.2 Person on outside of car injured in collision with pedestrian or animal in nontraffic accident**

√x7th **V40.3 Unspecified car occupant injured in collision with pedestrian or animal in nontraffic accident**

√x7th **V40.4 Person boarding or alighting a car injured in collision with pedestrian or animal**

√x7th **V40.5 Car driver injured in collision with pedestrian or animal in traffic accident**

√x7th **V40.6 Car passenger injured in collision with pedestrian or animal in traffic accident**

√x7th **V40.7 Person on outside of car injured in collision with pedestrian or animal in traffic accident**

√x7th **V40.9 Unspecified car occupant injured in collision with pedestrian or animal in traffic accident**

√4th **V41 Car occupant injured in collision with pedal cycle**

     The appropriate 7th character is to be added to each code from category V41.
     A   initial encounter
     D   subsequent encounter
     S   sequela

√x7th **V41.0 Car driver injured in collision with pedal cycle in nontraffic accident**

√x7th **V41.1 Car passenger injured in collision with pedal cycle in nontraffic accident**

√x7th **V41.2 Person on outside of car injured in collision with pedal cycle in nontraffic accident**

√x7th **V41.3 Unspecified car occupant injured in collision with pedal cycle in nontraffic accident**

√x7th **V41.4 Person boarding or alighting a car injured in collision with pedal cycle**

√x7th **V41.5 Car driver injured in collision with pedal cycle in traffic accident**

√x7th **V41.6 Car passenger injured in collision with pedal cycle in traffic accident**

√x7th **V41.7 Person on outside of car injured in collision with pedal cycle in traffic accident**

√x7th **V41.9 Unspecified car occupant injured in collision with pedal cycle in traffic accident**

√4th **V42 Car occupant injured in collision with two- or three-wheeled motor vehicle**

     The appropriate 7th character is to be added to each code from category V42.
     A   initial encounter
     D   subsequent encounter
     S   sequela

√x7th **V42.0 Car driver injured in collision with two- or three-wheeled motor vehicle in nontraffic accident**

√x7th **V42.1 Car passenger injured in collision with two- or three-wheeled motor vehicle in nontraffic accident**

√x7th **V42.2 Person on outside of car injured in collision with two- or three-wheeled motor vehicle in nontraffic accident**

√x7th **V42.3 Unspecified car occupant injured in collision with two- or three-wheeled motor vehicle in nontraffic accident**

√x7th **V42.4 Person boarding or alighting a car injured in collision with two- or three-wheeled motor vehicle**

√x7th **V42.5 Car driver injured in collision with two- or three-wheeled motor vehicle in traffic accident**

√x7th **V42.6 Car passenger injured in collision with two- or three-wheeled motor vehicle in traffic accident**

√x7th **V42.7 Person on outside of car injured in collision with two- or three-wheeled motor vehicle in traffic accident**

√x7th **V42.9 Unspecified car occupant injured in collision with two- or three-wheeled motor vehicle in traffic accident**

√4th **V43 Car occupant injured in collision with car, pick-up truck or van**

     The appropriate 7th character is to be added to each code from category V43.
     A   initial encounter
     D   subsequent encounter
     S   sequela

√5th **V43.0 Car driver injured in collision with car, pick-up truck or van in nontraffic accident**

    √x7th **V43.01 Car driver injured in collision with sport utility vehicle in nontraffic accident**

    √x7th **V43.02 Car driver injured in collision with other type car in nontraffic accident**

    √x7th **V43.03 Car driver injured in collision with pick-up truck in nontraffic accident**

    √x7th **V43.04 Car driver injured in collision with van in nontraffic accident**

√5th **V43.1 Car passenger injured in collision with car, pick-up truck or van in nontraffic accident**

    √x7th **V43.11 Car passenger injured in collision with sport utility vehicle in nontraffic accident**

    √x7th **V43.12 Car passenger injured in collision with other type car in nontraffic accident**

    √x7th **V43.13 Car passenger injured in collision with pick-up in nontraffic accident**

    √x7th **V43.14 Car passenger injured in collision with van in nontraffic accident**

√5th **V43.2 Person on outside of car injured in collision with car, pick-up truck or van in nontraffic accident**

    √x7th **V43.21 Person on outside of car injured in collision with sport utility vehicle in nontraffic accident**

    √x7th **V43.22 Person on outside of car injured in collision with other type car in nontraffic accident**

    √x7th **V43.23 Person on outside of car injured in collision with pick-up truck in nontraffic accident**

    √x7th **V43.24 Person on outside of car injured in collision with van in nontraffic accident**

√5th **V43.3 Unspecified car occupant injured in collision with car, pick-up truck or van in nontraffic accident**

    √x7th **V43.31 Unspecified car occupant injured in collision with sport utility vehicle in nontraffic accident**

    √x7th **V43.32 Unspecified car occupant injured in collision with other type car in nontraffic accident**

√x7ᵗʰ **V43.33** Unspecified car occupant injured in collision with pick-up truck in nontraffic accident

√x7ᵗʰ **V43.34** Unspecified car occupant injured in collision with van in nontraffic accident

√5ᵗʰ **V43.4** Person boarding or alighting a car injured in collision with car, pick-up truck or van

√x7ᵗʰ **V43.41** Person boarding or alighting a car injured in collision with sport utility vehicle

√x7ᵗʰ **V43.42** Person boarding or alighting a car injured in collision with other type car

√x7ᵗʰ **V43.43** Person boarding or alighting a car injured in collision with pick-up truck

√x7ᵗʰ **V43.44** Person boarding or alighting a car injured in collision with van

√5ᵗʰ **V43.5** Car driver injured in collision with car, pick-up truck or van in traffic accident

√x7ᵗʰ **V43.51** Car driver injured in collision with sport utility vehicle in traffic accident

√x7ᵗʰ **V43.52** Car driver injured in collision with other type car in traffic accident

√x7ᵗʰ **V43.53** Car driver injured in collision with pick-up truck in traffic accident

√x7ᵗʰ **V43.54** Car driver injured in collision with van in traffic accident

√5ᵗʰ **V43.6** Car passenger injured in collision with car, pick-up truck or van in traffic accident

√x7ᵗʰ **V43.61** Car passenger injured in collision with sport utility vehicle in traffic accident

√x7ᵗʰ **V43.62** Car passenger injured in collision with other type car in traffic accident

√x7ᵗʰ **V43.63** Car passenger injured in collision with pick-up truck in traffic accident

√x7ᵗʰ **V43.64** Car passenger injured in collision with van in traffic accident

√5ᵗʰ **V43.7** Person on outside of car injured in collision with car, pick-up truck or van in traffic accident

√x7ᵗʰ **V43.71** Person on outside of car injured in collision with sport utility vehicle in traffic accident

√x7ᵗʰ **V43.72** Person on outside of car injured in collision with other type car in traffic accident

√x7ᵗʰ **V43.73** Person on outside of car injured in collision with pick-up truck in traffic accident

√x7ᵗʰ **V43.74** Person on outside of car injured in collision with van in traffic accident

√5ᵗʰ **V43.9** Unspecified car occupant injured in collision with car, pick-up truck or van in traffic accident

√x7ᵗʰ **V43.91** Unspecified car occupant injured in collision with sport utility vehicle in traffic accident

√x7ᵗʰ **V43.92** Unspecified car occupant injured in collision with other type car in traffic accident

√x7ᵗʰ **V43.93** Unspecified car occupant injured in collision with pick-up truck in traffic accident

√x7ᵗʰ **V43.94** Unspecified car occupant injured in collision with van in traffic accident

√4ᵗʰ **V44** **Car occupant injured in collision with heavy transport vehicle or bus**

EXCLUDES 1   *car occupant injured in collision with military vehicle (V49.81)*

The appropriate 7th character is to be added to each code from category V44.
A   initial encounter
D   subsequent encounter
S   sequela

√x7ᵗʰ **V44.0** Car driver injured in collision with heavy transport vehicle or bus in nontraffic accident

√x7ᵗʰ **V44.1** Car passenger injured in collision with heavy transport vehicle or bus in nontraffic accident

√x7ᵗʰ **V44.2** Person on outside of car injured in collision with heavy transport vehicle or bus in nontraffic accident

√x7ᵗʰ **V44.3** Unspecified car occupant injured in collision with heavy transport vehicle or bus in nontraffic accident

√x7ᵗʰ **V44.4** Person boarding or alighting a car injured in collision with heavy transport vehicle or bus

√x7ᵗʰ **V44.5** Car driver injured in collision with heavy transport vehicle or bus in traffic accident

√x7ᵗʰ **V44.6** Car passenger injured in collision with heavy transport vehicle or bus in traffic accident

√x7ᵗʰ **V44.7** Person on outside of car injured in collision with heavy transport vehicle or bus in traffic accident

√x7ᵗʰ **V44.9** Unspecified car occupant injured in collision with heavy transport vehicle or bus in traffic accident

√4ᵗʰ **V45** **Car occupant injured in collision with railway train or railway vehicle**

The appropriate 7th character is to be added to each code from category V45.
A   initial encounter
D   subsequent encounter
S   sequela

√x7ᵗʰ **V45.0** Car driver injured in collision with railway train or railway vehicle in nontraffic accident

√x7ᵗʰ **V45.1** Car passenger injured in collision with railway train or railway vehicle in nontraffic accident

√x7ᵗʰ **V45.2** Person on outside of car injured in collision with railway train or railway vehicle in nontraffic accident

√x7ᵗʰ **V45.3** Unspecified car occupant injured in collision with railway train or railway vehicle in nontraffic accident

√x7ᵗʰ **V45.4** Person boarding or alighting a car injured in collision with railway train or railway vehicle

√x7ᵗʰ **V45.5** Car driver injured in collision with railway train or railway vehicle in traffic accident

√x7ᵗʰ **V45.6** Car passenger injured in collision with railway train or railway vehicle in traffic accident

√x7ᵗʰ **V45.7** Person on outside of car injured in collision with railway train or railway vehicle in traffic accident

√x7ᵗʰ **V45.9** Unspecified car occupant injured in collision with railway train or railway vehicle in traffic accident

√4ᵗʰ **V46** **Car occupant injured in collision with other nonmotor vehicle**

INCLUDES   collision with animal-drawn vehicle, animal being ridden, streetcar

The appropriate 7th character is to be added to each code from category V46.
A   initial encounter
D   subsequent encounter
S   sequela

√x7ᵗʰ **V46.0** Car driver injured in collision with other nonmotor vehicle in nontraffic accident

√x7ᵗʰ **V46.1** Car passenger injured in collision with other nonmotor vehicle in nontraffic accident

√x7ᵗʰ **V46.2** Person on outside of car injured in collision with other nonmotor vehicle in nontraffic accident

√x7ᵗʰ **V46.3** Unspecified car occupant injured in collision with other nonmotor vehicle in nontraffic accident

√x7ᵗʰ **V46.4** Person boarding or alighting a car injured in collision with other nonmotor vehicle

√x7ᵗʰ **V46.5** Car driver injured in collision with other nonmotor vehicle in traffic accident

√x7ᵗʰ **V46.6** Car passenger injured in collision with other nonmotor vehicle in traffic accident

√x7ᵗʰ **V46.7** Person on outside of car injured in collision with other nonmotor vehicle in traffic accident

√x7ᵗʰ **V46.9** Unspecified car occupant injured in collision with other nonmotor vehicle in traffic accident

√4ᵗʰ **V47** **Car occupant injured in collision with fixed or stationary object**

The appropriate 7th character is to be added to each code from category V47.
A   initial encounter
D   subsequent encounter
S   sequela

√5ᵗʰ **V47.0** Car driver injured in collision with fixed or stationary object in nontraffic accident

√x7ᵗʰ **V47.01** Driver of sport utility vehicle injured in collision with fixed or stationary object in nontraffic accident

√x7ᵗʰ **V47.02** Driver of other type car injured in collision with fixed or stationary object in nontraffic accident

√5ᵗʰ **V47.1** Car passenger injured in collision with fixed or stationary object in nontraffic accident

√x7ᵗʰ **V47.11** Passenger of sport utility vehicle injured in collision with fixed or stationary object in nontraffic accident

---

EXCLUDES 1   Not coded here   EXCLUDES 2   Not included here   *Manifestation Code*

√x7ᵗʰ   **V47.12**   Passenger of other type car injured in collision with fixed or stationary object in nontraffic accident

√x7ᵗʰ   **V47.2**   Person on outside of car injured in collision with fixed or stationary object in nontraffic accident

√5ᵗʰ   **V47.3**   Unspecified car occupant injured in collision with fixed or stationary object in nontraffic accident

√x7ᵗʰ   **V47.31**   Unspecified occupant of sport utility vehicle injured in collision with fixed or stationary object in nontraffic accident

√x7ᵗʰ   **V47.32**   Unspecified occupant of other type car injured in collision with fixed or stationary object in nontraffic accident

√x7ᵗʰ   **V47.4**   Person boarding or alighting a car injured in collision with fixed or stationary object

√5ᵗʰ   **V47.5**   Car driver injured in collision with fixed or stationary object in traffic accident

√x7ᵗʰ   **V47.51**   Driver of sport utility vehicle injured in collision with fixed or stationary object in traffic accident

√x7ᵗʰ   **V47.52**   Driver of other type car injured in collision with fixed or stationary object in traffic accident

√5ᵗʰ   **V47.6**   Car passenger injured in collision with fixed or stationary object in traffic accident

√x7ᵗʰ   **V47.61**   Passenger of sport utility vehicle injured in collision with fixed or stationary object in traffic accident

√x7ᵗʰ   **V47.62**   Passenger of other type car injured in collision with fixed or stationary object in traffic accident

√x7ᵗʰ   **V47.7**   Person on outside of car injured in collision with fixed or stationary object in traffic accident

√5ᵗʰ   **V47.9**   Unspecified car occupant injured in collision with fixed or stationary object in traffic accident

√x7ᵗʰ   **V47.91**   Unspecified occupant of sport utility vehicle injured in collision with fixed or stationary object in traffic accident

√x7ᵗʰ   **V47.92**   Unspecified occupant of other type car injured in collision with fixed or stationary object in traffic accident

✓4ᵗʰ   **V48**   **Car occupant injured in noncollision transport accident**
Overturning car NOS
Overturning car without collision

> The appropriate 7th character is to be added to each code from category V48.
> A   initial encounter
> D   subsequent encounter
> S   sequela

√x7ᵗʰ   **V48.0**   Car driver injured in noncollision transport accident in nontraffic accident

√x7ᵗʰ   **V48.1**   Car passenger injured in noncollision transport accident in nontraffic accident

√x7ᵗʰ   **V48.2**   Person on outside of car injured in noncollision transport accident in nontraffic accident

√x7ᵗʰ   **V48.3**   Unspecified car occupant injured in noncollision transport accident in nontraffic accident

√x7ᵗʰ   **V48.4**   Person boarding or alighting a car injured in noncollision transport accident

√x7ᵗʰ   **V48.5**   Car driver injured in noncollision transport accident in traffic accident

√x7ᵗʰ   **V48.6**   Car passenger injured in noncollision transport accident in traffic accident

√x7ᵗʰ   **V48.7**   Person on outside of car injured in noncollision transport accident in traffic accident

√x7ᵗʰ   **V48.9**   Unspecified car occupant injured in noncollision transport accident in traffic accident

✓4ᵗʰ   **V49**   **Car occupant injured in other and unspecified transport accidents**

> The appropriate 7th character is to be added to each code from category V49.
> A   initial encounter
> D   subsequent encounter
> S   sequela

√5ᵗʰ   **V49.0**   Driver injured in collision with other and unspecified motor vehicles in nontraffic accident

√x7ᵗʰ   **V49.00**   Driver injured in collision with unspecified motor vehicles in nontraffic accident

√x7ᵗʰ   **V49.09**   Driver injured in collision with other motor vehicles in nontraffic accident

√5ᵗʰ   **V49.1**   Passenger injured in collision with other and unspecified motor vehicles in nontraffic accident

√x7ᵗʰ   **V49.10**   Passenger injured in collision with unspecified motor vehicles in nontraffic accident

√x7ᵗʰ   **V49.19**   Passenger injured in collision with other motor vehicles in nontraffic accident

√5ᵗʰ   **V49.2**   Unspecified car occupant injured in collision with other and unspecified motor vehicles in nontraffic accident

√x7ᵗʰ   **V49.20**   Unspecified car occupant injured in collision with unspecified motor vehicles in nontraffic accident
Car collision NOS, nontraffic

√x7ᵗʰ   **V49.29**   Unspecified car occupant injured in collision with other motor vehicles in nontraffic accident

√x7ᵗʰ   **V49.3**   Car occupant (driver) (passenger) injured in unspecified nontraffic accident
Car accident NOS, nontraffic
Car occupant injured in nontraffic accident NOS

√5ᵗʰ   **V49.4**   Driver injured in collision with other and unspecified motor vehicles in traffic accident

√x7ᵗʰ   **V49.40**   Driver injured in collision with unspecified motor vehicles in traffic accident

√x7ᵗʰ   **V49.49**   Driver injured in collision with other motor vehicles in traffic accident

√5ᵗʰ   **V49.5**   Passenger injured in collision with other and unspecified motor vehicles in traffic accident

√x7ᵗʰ   **V49.50**   Passenger injured in collision with unspecified motor vehicles in traffic accident

√x7ᵗʰ   **V49.59**   Passenger injured in collision with other motor vehicles in traffic accident

√5ᵗʰ   **V49.6**   Unspecified car occupant injured in collision with other and unspecified motor vehicles in traffic accident

√x7ᵗʰ   **V49.60**   Unspecified car occupant injured in collision with unspecified motor vehicles in traffic accident
Car collision NOS (traffic)

√x7ᵗʰ   **V49.69**   Unspecified car occupant injured in collision with other motor vehicles in traffic accident

√5ᵗʰ   **V49.8**   Car occupant (driver) (passenger) injured in other specified transport accidents

√x7ᵗʰ   **V49.81**   Car occupant (driver) (passenger) injured in transport accident with military vehicle

√x7ᵗʰ   **V49.88**   Car occupant (driver) (passenger) injured in other specified transport accidents

√x7ᵗʰ   **V49.9**   Car occupant (driver) (passenger) injured in unspecified traffic accident
Car accident NOS

Occupant of pick-up truck or van injured in transport accident (V50-V59)

INCLUDES   a four or six wheel motor vehicle designed primarily for carrying passengers and property but weighing less than the local limit for classification as a heavy goods vehicle
minibus
minivan
sport utility vehicle (SUV)
truck
van

EXCLUDES 1   heavy transport vehicle (V60-V69)

✓4ᵗʰ   **V50**   **Occupant of pick-up truck or van injured in collision with pedestrian or animal**

EXCLUDES 1   pick-up truck or van collision with animal-drawn vehicle or animal being ridden (V56-)

> The appropriate 7th character is to be added to each code from category V50.
> A   initial encounter
> D   subsequent encounter
> S   sequela

√x7ᵗʰ   **V50.0**   Driver of pick-up truck or van injured in collision with pedestrian or animal in nontraffic accident

√x7ᵗʰ   **V50.1**   Passenger in pick-up truck or van injured in collision with pedestrian or animal in nontraffic accident

√x7ᵗʰ   **V50.2**   Person on outside of pick-up truck or van injured in collision with pedestrian or animal in nontraffic accident

√x7ᵗʰ   **V50.3**   Unspecified occupant of pick-up truck or van injured in collision with pedestrian or animal in nontraffic accident

---

✓ Appropriate additional character required   √x7ᵗʰ Requires 7th character, placeholder x must fill empty characters

External Causes of Morbidity

V50.4–V55.9

√x7ᵗʰ **V50.4** Person boarding or alighting a pick-up truck or van injured in collision with pedestrian or animal

√x7ᵗʰ **V50.5** Driver of pick-up truck or van injured in collision with pedestrian or animal in traffic accident

√x7ᵗʰ **V50.6** Passenger in pick-up truck or van injured in collision with pedestrian or animal in traffic accident

√x7ᵗʰ **V50.7** Person on outside of pick-up truck or van injured in collision with pedestrian or animal in traffic accident

√x7ᵗʰ **V50.9** Unspecified occupant of pick-up truck or van injured in collision with pedestrian or animal in traffic accident

√4ᵗʰ **V51 Occupant of pick-up truck or van injured in collision with pedal cycle**

> The appropriate 7th character is to be added to each code from category V51.
> A   initial encounter
> D   subsequent encounter
> S   sequela

√x7ᵗʰ **V51.0** Driver of pick-up truck or van injured in collision with pedal cycle in nontraffic accident

√x7ᵗʰ **V51.1** Passenger in pick-up truck or van injured in collision with pedal cycle in nontraffic accident

√x7ᵗʰ **V51.2** Person on outside of pick-up truck or van injured in collision with pedal cycle in nontraffic accident

√x7ᵗʰ **V51.3** Unspecified occupant of pick-up truck or van injured in collision with pedal cycle in nontraffic accident

√x7ᵗʰ **V51.4** Person boarding or alighting a pick-up truck or van injured in collision with pedal cycle

√x7ᵗʰ **V51.5** Driver of pick-up truck or van injured in collision with pedal cycle in traffic accident

√x7ᵗʰ **V51.6** Passenger in pick-up truck or van injured in collision with pedal cycle in traffic accident

√x7ᵗʰ **V51.7** Person on outside of pick-up truck or van injured in collision with pedal cycle in traffic accident

√x7ᵗʰ **V51.9** Unspecified occupant of pick-up truck or van injured in collision with pedal cycle in traffic accident

√4ᵗʰ **V52 Occupant of pick-up truck or van injured in collision with two- or three-wheeled motor vehicle**

> The appropriate 7th character is to be added to each code from category V52.
> A   initial encounter
> D   subsequent encounter
> S   sequela

√x7ᵗʰ **V52.0** Driver of pick-up truck or van injured in collision with two- or three-wheeled motor vehicle in nontraffic accident

√x7ᵗʰ **V52.1** Passenger in pick-up truck or van injured in collision with two- or three-wheeled motor vehicle in nontraffic accident

√x7ᵗʰ **V52.2** Person on outside of pick-up truck or van injured in collision with two- or three-wheeled motor vehicle in nontraffic accident

√x7ᵗʰ **V52.3** Unspecified occupant of pick-up truck or van injured in collision with two- or three-wheeled motor vehicle in nontraffic accident

√x7ᵗʰ **V52.4** Person boarding or alighting a pick-up truck or van injured in collision with two- or three-wheeled motor vehicle

√x7ᵗʰ **V52.5** Driver of pick-up truck or van injured in collision with two- or three-wheeled motor vehicle in traffic accident

√x7ᵗʰ **V52.6** Passenger in pick-up truck or van injured in collision with two- or three-wheeled motor vehicle in traffic accident

√x7ᵗʰ **V52.7** Person on outside of pick-up truck or van injured in collision with two- or three-wheeled motor vehicle in traffic accident

√x7ᵗʰ **V52.9** Unspecified occupant of pick-up truck or van injured in collision with two- or three-wheeled motor vehicle in traffic accident

√4ᵗʰ **V53 Occupant of pick-up truck or van injured in collision with car, pick-up truck or van**

> The appropriate 7th character is to be added to each code from category V53.
> A   initial encounter
> D   subsequent encounter
> S   sequela

√x7ᵗʰ **V53.0** Driver of pick-up truck or van injured in collision with car, pick-up truck or van in nontraffic accident

√x7ᵗʰ **V53.1** Passenger in pick-up truck or van injured in collision with car, pick-up truck or van in nontraffic accident

√x7ᵗʰ **V53.2** Person on outside of pick-up truck or van injured in collision with car, pick-up truck or van in nontraffic accident

√x7ᵗʰ **V53.3** Unspecified occupant of pick-up truck or van injured in collision with car, pick-up truck or van in nontraffic accident

√x7ᵗʰ **V53.4** Person boarding or alighting a pick-up truck or van injured in collision with car, pick-up truck or van

√x7ᵗʰ **V53.5** Driver of pick-up truck or van injured in collision with car, pick-up truck or van in traffic accident

√x7ᵗʰ **V53.6** Passenger in pick-up truck or van injured in collision with car, pick-up truck or van in traffic accident

√x7ᵗʰ **V53.7** Person on outside of pick-up truck or van injured in collision with car, pick-up truck or van in traffic accident

√x7ᵗʰ **V53.9** Unspecified occupant of pick-up truck or van injured in collision with car, pick-up truck or van in traffic accident

√4ᵗʰ **V54 Occupant of pick-up truck or van injured in collision with heavy transport vehicle or bus**

> EXCLUDES 1   *occupant of pick-up truck or van injured in collision with military vehicle (V59.81)*

> The appropriate 7th character is to be added to each code from category V54.
> A   initial encounter
> D   subsequent encounter
> S   sequela

√x7ᵗʰ **V54.0** Driver of pick-up truck or van injured in collision with heavy transport vehicle or bus in nontraffic accident

√x7ᵗʰ **V54.1** Passenger in pick-up truck or van injured in collision with heavy transport vehicle or bus in nontraffic accident

√x7ᵗʰ **V54.2** Person on outside of pick-up truck or van injured in collision with heavy transport vehicle or bus in nontraffic accident

√x7ᵗʰ **V54.3** Unspecified occupant of pick-up truck or van injured in collision with heavy transport vehicle or bus in nontraffic accident

√x7ᵗʰ **V54.4** Person boarding or alighting a pick-up truck or van injured in collision with heavy transport vehicle or bus

√x7ᵗʰ **V54.5** Driver of pick-up truck or van injured in collision with heavy transport vehicle or bus in traffic accident

√x7ᵗʰ **V54.6** Passenger in pick-up truck or van injured in collision with heavy transport vehicle or bus in traffic accident

√x7ᵗʰ **V54.7** Person on outside of pick-up truck or van injured in collision with heavy transport vehicle or bus in traffic accident

√x7ᵗʰ **V54.9** Unspecified occupant of pick-up truck or van injured in collision with heavy transport vehicle or bus in traffic accident

√4ᵗʰ **V55 Occupant of pick-up truck or van injured in collision with railway train or railway vehicle**

> The appropriate 7th character is to be added to each code from category V55.
> A   initial encounter
> D   subsequent encounter
> S   sequela

√x7ᵗʰ **V55.0** Driver of pick-up truck or van injured in collision with railway train or railway vehicle in nontraffic accident

√x7ᵗʰ **V55.1** Passenger in pick-up truck or van injured in collision with railway train or railway vehicle in nontraffic accident

√x7ᵗʰ **V55.2** Person on outside of pick-up truck or van injured in collision with railway train or railway vehicle in nontraffic accident

√x7ᵗʰ **V55.3** Unspecified occupant of pick-up truck or van injured in collision with railway train or railway vehicle in nontraffic accident

√x7ᵗʰ **V55.4** Person boarding or alighting a pick-up truck or van injured in collision with railway train or railway vehicle

√x7ᵗʰ **V55.5** Driver of pick-up truck or van injured in collision with railway train or railway vehicle in traffic accident

√x7ᵗʰ **V55.6** Passenger in pick-up truck or van injured in collision with railway train or railway vehicle in traffic accident

√x7ᵗʰ **V55.7** Person on outside of pick-up truck or van injured in collision with railway train or railway vehicle in traffic accident

√x7ᵗʰ **V55.9** Unspecified occupant of pick-up truck or van injured in collision with railway train or railway vehicle in traffic accident

---

EXCLUDES 1   Not coded here   EXCLUDES 2   Not included here   *Manifestation Code*

☑4ᵗʰ **V56 Occupant of pick-up truck or van injured in collision with other nonmotor vehicle**

> INCLUDES collision with animal-drawn vehicle, animal being ridden, streetcar

> The appropriate 7th character is to be added to each code from category V56.
> A initial encounter
> D subsequent encounter
> S sequela

✓x7ᵗʰ **V56.0** Driver of pick-up truck or van injured in collision with other nonmotor vehicle in nontraffic accident

✓x7ᵗʰ **V56.1** Passenger in pick-up truck or van injured in collision with other nonmotor vehicle in nontraffic accident

✓x7ᵗʰ **V56.2** Person on outside of pick-up truck or van injured in collision with other nonmotor vehicle in nontraffic accident

✓x7ᵗʰ **V56.3** Unspecified occupant of pick-up truck or van injured in collision with other nonmotor vehicle in nontraffic accident

✓x7ᵗʰ **V56.4** Person boarding or alighting a pick-up truck or van injured in collision with other nonmotor vehicle

✓x7ᵗʰ **V56.5** Driver of pick-up truck or van injured in collision with other nonmotor vehicle in traffic accident

✓x7ᵗʰ **V56.6** Passenger in pick-up truck or van injured in collision with other nonmotor vehicle in traffic accident

✓x7ᵗʰ **V56.7** Person on outside of pick-up truck or van injured in collision with other nonmotor vehicle in traffic accident

✓x7ᵗʰ **V56.9** Unspecified occupant of pick-up truck or van injured in collision with other nonmotor vehicle in traffic accident

☑4ᵗʰ **V57 Occupant of pick-up truck or van injured in collision with fixed or stationary object**

> The appropriate 7th character is to be added to each code from category V57.
> A initial encounter
> D subsequent encounter
> S sequela

✓x7ᵗʰ **V57.0** Driver of pick-up truck or van injured in collision with fixed or stationary object in nontraffic accident

✓x7ᵗʰ **V57.1** Passenger in pick-up truck or van injured in collision with fixed or stationary object in nontraffic accident

✓x7ᵗʰ **V57.2** Person on outside of pick-up truck or van injured in collision with fixed or stationary object in nontraffic accident

✓x7ᵗʰ **V57.3** Unspecified occupant of pick-up truck or van injured in collision with fixed or stationary object in nontraffic accident

✓x7ᵗʰ **V57.4** Person boarding or alighting a pick-up truck or van injured in collision with fixed or stationary object

✓x7ᵗʰ **V57.5** Driver of pick-up truck or van injured in collision with fixed or stationary object in traffic accident

✓x7ᵗʰ **V57.6** Passenger in pick-up truck or van injured in collision with fixed or stationary object in traffic accident

✓x7ᵗʰ **V57.7** Person on outside of pick-up truck or van injured in collision with fixed or stationary object in traffic accident

✓x7ᵗʰ **V57.9** Unspecified occupant of pick-up truck or van injured in collision with fixed or stationary object in traffic accident

☑4ᵗʰ **V58 Occupant of pick-up truck or van injured in noncollision transport accident**

> INCLUDES overturning pick-up truck or van NOS
> overturning pick-up truck or van without collision

> The appropriate 7th character is to be added to each code from category V58.
> A initial encounter
> D subsequent encounter
> S sequela

✓x7ᵗʰ **V58.0** Driver of pick-up truck or van injured in noncollision transport accident in nontraffic accident

✓x7ᵗʰ **V58.1** Passenger in pick-up truck or van injured in noncollision transport accident in nontraffic accident

✓x7ᵗʰ **V58.2** Person on outside of pick-up truck or van injured in noncollision transport accident in nontraffic accident

✓x7ᵗʰ **V58.3** Unspecified occupant of pick-up truck or van injured in noncollision transport accident in nontraffic accident

✓x7ᵗʰ **V58.4** Person boarding or alighting a pick-up truck or van injured in noncollision transport accident

✓x7ᵗʰ **V58.5** Driver of pick-up truck or van injured in noncollision transport accident in traffic accident

✓x7ᵗʰ **V58.6** Passenger in pick-up truck or van injured in noncollision transport accident in traffic accident

✓x7ᵗʰ **V58.7** Person on outside of pick-up truck or van injured in noncollision transport accident in traffic accident

✓x7ᵗʰ **V58.9** Unspecified occupant of pick-up truck or van injured in noncollision transport accident in traffic accident

☑4ᵗʰ **V59 Occupant of pick-up truck or van injured in other and unspecified transport accidents**

> The appropriate 7th character is to be added to each code from category V59.
> A initial encounter
> D subsequent encounter
> S sequela

✓5ᵗʰ **V59.0** Driver of pick-up truck or van injured in collision with other and unspecified motor vehicles in nontraffic accident

✓x7ᵗʰ **V59.00** Driver of pick-up truck or van injured in collision with unspecified motor vehicles in nontraffic accident

✓x7ᵗʰ **V59.09** Driver of pick-up truck or van injured in collision with other motor vehicles in nontraffic accident

✓5ᵗʰ **V59.1** Passenger in pick-up truck or van injured in collision with other and unspecified motor vehicles in nontraffic accident

✓x7ᵗʰ **V59.10** Passenger in pick-up truck or van injured in collision with unspecified motor vehicles in nontraffic accident

✓x7ᵗʰ **V59.19** Passenger in pick-up truck or van injured in collision with other motor vehicles in nontraffic accident

✓5ᵗʰ **V59.2** Unspecified occupant of pick-up truck or van injured in collision with other and unspecified motor vehicles in nontraffic accident

✓x7ᵗʰ **V59.20** Unspecified occupant of pick-up truck or van injured in collision with unspecified motor vehicles in nontraffic accident

> Collision NOS involving pick-up truck or van, nontraffic

✓x7ᵗʰ **V59.29** Unspecified occupant of pick-up truck or van injured in collision with other motor vehicles in nontraffic accident

✓x7ᵗʰ **V59.3** Occupant (driver) (passenger) of pick-up truck or van injured in unspecified nontraffic accident

> Accident NOS involving pick-up truck or van, nontraffic
> Occupant of pick-up truck or van injured in nontraffic accident NOS

✓5ᵗʰ **V59.4** Driver of pick-up truck or van injured in collision with other and unspecified motor vehicles in traffic accident

✓x7ᵗʰ **V59.40** Driver of pick-up truck or van injured in collision with unspecified motor vehicles in traffic accident

✓x7ᵗʰ **V59.49** Driver of pick-up truck or van injured in collision with other motor vehicles in traffic accident

✓5ᵗʰ **V59.5** Passenger in pick-up truck or van injured in collision with other and unspecified motor vehicles in traffic accident

✓x7ᵗʰ **V59.50** Passenger in pick-up truck or van injured in collision with unspecified motor vehicles in traffic accident

✓x7ᵗʰ **V59.59** Passenger in pick-up truck or van injured in collision with other motor vehicles in traffic accident

✓5ᵗʰ **V59.6** Unspecified occupant of pick-up truck or van injured in collision with other and unspecified motor vehicles in traffic accident

✓x7ᵗʰ **V59.60** Unspecified occupant of pick-up truck or van injured in collision with unspecified motor vehicles in traffic accident

> Collision NOS involving pick-up truck or van (traffic)

✓x7ᵗʰ **V59.69** Unspecified occupant of pick-up truck or van injured in collision with other motor vehicles in traffic accident

✓5ᵗʰ **V59.8** Occupant (driver) (passenger) of pick-up truck or van injured in other specified transport accidents

✓x7ᵗʰ **V59.81** Occupant (driver) (passenger) of pick-up truck or van injured in transport accident with military vehicle

✓x7ᵗʰ **V59.88** Occupant (driver) (passenger) of pick-up truck or van injured in other specified transport accidents

✓x7ᵗʰ **V59.9** Occupant (driver) (passenger) of pick-up truck or van injured in unspecified traffic accident

> Accident NOS involving pick-up truck or van

☑ Appropriate additional character required   ✓x7ᵗʰ Requires 7th character, placeholder x must fill empty characters

Occupant of heavy transport vehicle injured in transport accident (V60-V69)

18 wheeler
Armored car
Panel truck

EXCLUDES 1   *bus*
                motorcoach

✓4th V60   Occupant of heavy transport vehicle injured in collision with pedestrian or animal

     EXCLUDES 1   *heavy transport vehicle collision with animal-drawn vehicle or animal being ridden (V66-)*

     The appropriate 7th character is to be added to each code from category V60.
       A   initial encounter
       D   subsequent encounter
       S   sequela

✓7th **V60.0**   Driver of heavy transport vehicle injured in collision with pedestrian or animal in nontraffic accident

✓7th **V60.1**   Passenger in heavy transport vehicle injured in collision with pedestrian or animal in nontraffic accident

✓7th **V60.2**   Person on outside of heavy transport vehicle injured in collision with pedestrian or animal in nontraffic accident

✓7th **V60.3**   Unspecified occupant of heavy transport vehicle injured in collision with pedestrian or animal in nontraffic accident

✓7th **V60.4**   Person boarding or alighting a heavy transport vehicle injured in collision with pedestrian or animal

✓7th **V60.5**   Driver of heavy transport vehicle injured in collision with pedestrian or animal in traffic accident

✓7th **V60.6**   Passenger in heavy transport vehicle injured in collision with pedestrian or animal in traffic accident

✓7th **V60.7**   Person on outside of heavy transport vehicle injured in collision with pedestrian or animal in traffic accident

✓7th **V60.9**   Unspecified occupant of heavy transport vehicle injured in collision with pedestrian or animal in traffic accident

✓4th V61   Occupant of heavy transport vehicle injured in collision with pedal cycle

     The appropriate 7th character is to be added to each code from category V61.
       A   initial encounter
       D   subsequent encounter
       S   sequela

✓7th **V61.0**   Driver of heavy transport vehicle injured in collision with pedal cycle in nontraffic accident

✓7th **V61.1**   Passenger in heavy transport vehicle injured in collision with pedal cycle in nontraffic accident

✓7th **V61.2**   Person on outside of heavy transport vehicle injured in collision with pedal cycle in nontraffic accident

✓7th **V61.3**   Unspecified occupant of heavy transport vehicle injured in collision with pedal cycle in nontraffic accident

✓7th **V61.4**   Person boarding or alighting a heavy transport vehicle injured in collision with pedal cycle while boarding or alighting

✓7th **V61.5**   Driver of heavy transport vehicle injured in collision with pedal cycle in traffic accident

✓7th **V61.6**   Passenger in heavy transport vehicle injured in collision with pedal cycle in traffic accident

✓7th **V61.7**   Person on outside of heavy transport vehicle injured in collision with pedal cycle in traffic accident

✓7th **V61.9**   Unspecified occupant of heavy transport vehicle injured in collision with pedal cycle in traffic accident

✓4th V62   Occupant of heavy transport vehicle injured in collision with two- or three-wheeled motor vehicle

     The appropriate 7th character is to be added to each code from category V62.
       A   initial encounter
       D   subsequent encounter
       S   sequela

✓7th **V62.0**   Driver of heavy transport vehicle injured in collision with two- or three-wheeled motor vehicle in nontraffic accident

✓7th **V62.1**   Passenger in heavy transport vehicle injured in collision with two- or three-wheeled motor vehicle in nontraffic accident

✓7th **V62.2**   Person on outside of heavy transport vehicle injured in collision with two- or three-wheeled motor vehicle in nontraffic accident

✓7th **V62.3**   Unspecified occupant of heavy transport vehicle injured in collision with two- or three-wheeled motor vehicle in nontraffic accident

✓7th **V62.4**   Person boarding or alighting a heavy transport vehicle injured in collision with two- or three-wheeled motor vehicle

✓7th **V62.5**   Driver of heavy transport vehicle injured in collision with two- or three-wheeled motor vehicle in traffic accident

✓7th **V62.6**   Passenger in heavy transport vehicle injured in collision with two- or three-wheeled motor vehicle in traffic accident

✓7th **V62.7**   Person on outside of heavy transport vehicle injured in collision with two- or three-wheeled motor vehicle in traffic accident

✓7th **V62.9**   Unspecified occupant of heavy transport vehicle injured in collision with two- or three-wheeled motor vehicle in traffic accident

✓4th V63   Occupant of heavy transport vehicle injured in collision with car, pick-up truck or van

     The appropriate 7th character is to be added to each code from category V63.
       A   initial encounter
       D   subsequent encounter
       S   sequela

✓7th **V63.0**   Driver of heavy transport vehicle injured in collision with car, pick-up truck or van in nontraffic accident

✓7th **V63.1**   Passenger in heavy transport vehicle injured in collision with car, pick-up truck or van in nontraffic accident

✓7th **V63.2**   Person on outside of heavy transport vehicle injured in collision with car, pick-up truck or van in nontraffic accident

✓7th **V63.3**   Unspecified occupant of heavy transport vehicle injured in collision with car, pick-up truck or van in nontraffic accident

✓7th **V63.4**   Person boarding or alighting a heavy transport vehicle injured in collision with car, pick-up truck or van

✓7th **V63.5**   Driver of heavy transport vehicle injured in collision with car, pick-up truck or van in traffic accident

✓7th **V63.6**   Passenger in heavy transport vehicle injured in collision with car, pick-up truck or van in traffic accident

✓7th **V63.7**   Person on outside of heavy transport vehicle injured in collision with car, pick-up truck or van in traffic accident

✓7th **V63.9**   Unspecified occupant of heavy transport vehicle injured in collision with car, pick-up truck or van in traffic accident

✓4th V64   Occupant of heavy transport vehicle injured in collision with heavy transport vehicle or bus

     EXCLUDES 1   *occupant of heavy transport vehicle injured in collision with military vehicle (V69.81)*

     The appropriate 7th character is to be added to each code from category V64.
       A   initial encounter
       D   subsequent encounter
       S   sequela

✓7th **V64.0**   Driver of heavy transport vehicle injured in collision with heavy transport vehicle or bus in nontraffic accident

✓7th **V64.1**   Passenger in heavy transport vehicle injured in collision with heavy transport vehicle or bus in nontraffic accident

✓7th **V64.2**   Person on outside of heavy transport vehicle injured in collision with heavy transport vehicle or bus in nontraffic accident

✓7th **V64.3**   Unspecified occupant of heavy transport vehicle injured in collision with heavy transport vehicle or bus in nontraffic accident

✓7th **V64.4**   Person boarding or alighting a heavy transport vehicle injured in collision with heavy transport vehicle or bus while boarding or alighting

✓7th **V64.5**   Driver of heavy transport vehicle injured in collision with heavy transport vehicle or bus in traffic accident

✓7th **V64.6**   Passenger in heavy transport vehicle injured in collision with heavy transport vehicle or bus in traffic accident

✓7th **V64.7**   Person on outside of heavy transport vehicle injured in collision with heavy transport vehicle or bus in traffic accident

✓7th **V64.9**   Unspecified occupant of heavy transport vehicle injured in collision with heavy transport vehicle or bus in traffic accident

---

EXCLUDES 1 Not coded here   **EXCLUDES 2** Not included here   *Manifestation Code*

✓4th **V65 Occupant of heavy transport vehicle injured in collision with railway train or railway vehicle**

> The appropriate 7th character is to be added to each code from category V65.
> A   initial encounter
> D   subsequent encounter
> S   sequela

✓x7th **V65.0 Driver of heavy transport vehicle injured in collision with railway train or railway vehicle in nontraffic accident**

✓x7th **V65.1 Passenger in heavy transport vehicle injured in collision with railway train or railway vehicle in nontraffic accident**

✓x7th **V65.2 Person on outside of heavy transport vehicle injured in collision with railway train or railway vehicle in nontraffic accident**

✓x7th **V65.3 Unspecified occupant of heavy transport vehicle injured in collision with railway train or railway vehicle in nontraffic accident**

✓x7th **V65.4 Person boarding or alighting a heavy transport vehicle injured in collision with railway train or railway vehicle**

✓x7th **V65.5 Driver of heavy transport vehicle injured in collision with railway train or railway vehicle in traffic accident**

✓x7th **V65.6 Passenger in heavy transport vehicle injured in collision with railway train or railway vehicle in traffic accident**

✓x7th **V65.7 Person on outside of heavy transport vehicle injured in collision with railway train or railway vehicle in traffic accident**

✓x7th **V65.9 Unspecified occupant of heavy transport vehicle injured in collision with railway train or railway vehicle in traffic accident**

✓4th **V66 Occupant of heavy transport vehicle injured in collision with other nonmotor vehicle**
> INCLUDES   collision with animal-drawn vehicle, animal being ridden, streetcar

> The appropriate 7th character is to be added to each code from category V66.
> A   initial encounter
> D   subsequent encounter
> S   sequela

✓x7th **V66.0 Driver of heavy transport vehicle injured in collision with other nonmotor vehicle in nontraffic accident**

✓x7th **V66.1 Passenger in heavy transport vehicle injured in collision with other nonmotor vehicle in nontraffic accident**

✓x7th **V66.2 Person on outside of heavy transport vehicle injured in collision with other nonmotor vehicle in nontraffic accident**

✓x7th **V66.3 Unspecified occupant of heavy transport vehicle injured in collision with other nonmotor vehicle in nontraffic accident**

✓x7th **V66.4 Person boarding or alighting a heavy transport vehicle injured in collision with other nonmotor vehicle**

✓x7th **V66.5 Driver of heavy transport vehicle injured in collision with other nonmotor vehicle in traffic accident**

✓x7th **V66.6 Passenger in heavy transport vehicle injured in collision with other nonmotor vehicle in traffic accident**

✓x7th **V66.7 Person on outside of heavy transport vehicle injured in collision with other nonmotor vehicle in traffic accident**

✓x7th **V66.9 Unspecified occupant of heavy transport vehicle injured in collision with other nonmotor vehicle in traffic accident**

✓4th **V67 Occupant of heavy transport vehicle injured in collision with fixed or stationary object**

> The appropriate 7th character is to be added to each code from category V67.
> A   initial encounter
> D   subsequent encounter
> S   sequela

✓x7th **V67.0 Driver of heavy transport vehicle injured in collision with fixed or stationary object in nontraffic accident**

✓x7th **V67.1 Passenger in heavy transport vehicle injured in collision with fixed or stationary object in nontraffic accident**

✓x7th **V67.2 Person on outside of heavy transport vehicle injured in collision with fixed or stationary object in nontraffic accident**

✓x7th **V67.3 Unspecified occupant of heavy transport vehicle injured in collision with fixed or stationary object in nontraffic accident**

✓x7th **V67.4 Person boarding or alighting a heavy transport vehicle injured in collision with fixed or stationary object**

✓x7th **V67.5 Driver of heavy transport vehicle injured in collision with fixed or stationary object in traffic accident**

✓x7th **V67.6 Passenger in heavy transport vehicle injured in collision with fixed or stationary object in traffic accident**

✓x7th **V67.7 Person on outside of heavy transport vehicle injured in collision with fixed or stationary object in traffic accident**

✓x7th **V67.9 Unspecified occupant of heavy transport vehicle injured in collision with fixed or stationary object in traffic accident**

✓4th **V68 Occupant of heavy transport vehicle injured in noncollision transport accident**
> INCLUDES   overturning heavy transport vehicle NOS
> overturning heavy transport vehicle without collision

> The appropriate 7th character is to be added to each code from category V68.
> A   initial encounter
> D   subsequent encounter
> S   sequela

✓x7th **V68.0 Driver of heavy transport vehicle injured in noncollision transport accident in nontraffic accident**

✓x7th **V68.1 Passenger in heavy transport vehicle injured in noncollision transport accident in nontraffic accident**

✓x7th **V68.2 Person on outside of heavy transport vehicle injured in noncollision transport accident in nontraffic accident**

✓x7th **V68.3 Unspecified occupant of heavy transport vehicle injured in noncollision transport accident in nontraffic accident**

✓x7th **V68.4 Person boarding or alighting a heavy transport vehicle injured in noncollision transport accident**

✓x7th **V68.5 Driver of heavy transport vehicle injured in noncollision transport accident in traffic accident**

✓x7th **V68.6 Passenger in heavy transport vehicle injured in noncollision transport accident in traffic accident**

✓x7th **V68.7 Person on outside of heavy transport vehicle injured in noncollision transport accident in traffic accident**

✓x7th **V68.9 Unspecified occupant of heavy transport vehicle injured in noncollision transport accident in traffic accident**

✓4th **V69 Occupant of heavy transport vehicle injured in other and unspecified transport accidents**

> The appropriate 7th character is to be added to each code from category V69.
> A   initial encounter
> D   subsequent encounter
> S   sequela

✓5th **V69.0 Driver of heavy transport vehicle injured in collision with other and unspecified motor vehicles in nontraffic accident**

    ✓x7th **V69.00 Driver of heavy transport vehicle injured in collision with unspecified motor vehicles in nontraffic accident**

    ✓x7th **V69.09 Driver of heavy transport vehicle injured in collision with other motor vehicles in nontraffic accident**

✓5th **V69.1 Passenger in heavy transport vehicle injured in collision with other and unspecified motor vehicles in nontraffic accident**

    ✓x7th **V69.10 Passenger in heavy transport vehicle injured in collision with unspecified motor vehicles in nontraffic accident**

    ✓x7th **V69.19 Passenger in heavy transport vehicle injured in collision with other motor vehicles in nontraffic accident**

✓5th **V69.2 Unspecified occupant of heavy transport vehicle injured in collision with other and unspecified motor vehicles in nontraffic accident**

    ✓x7th **V69.20 Unspecified occupant of heavy transport vehicle injured in collision with unspecified motor vehicles in nontraffic accident**
> Collision NOS involving heavy transport vehicle, nontraffic

    ✓x7th **V69.29 Unspecified occupant of heavy transport vehicle injured in collision with other motor vehicles in nontraffic accident**

✓x7th **V69.3 Occupant (driver) (passenger) of heavy transport vehicle injured in unspecified nontraffic accident**
> Accident NOS involving heavy transport vehicle, nontraffic
> Occupant of heavy transport vehicle injured in nontraffic accident NOS

✓5ᵗʰ **V69.4** Driver of heavy transport vehicle injured in collision with other and unspecified motor vehicles in traffic accident

    ✓x7ᵗʰ **V69.40** Driver of heavy transport vehicle injured in collision with unspecified motor vehicles in traffic accident

    ✓x7ᵗʰ **V69.49** Driver of heavy transport vehicle injured in collision with other motor vehicles in traffic accident

✓5ᵗʰ **V69.5** Passenger in heavy transport vehicle injured in collision with other and unspecified motor vehicles in traffic accident

    ✓x7ᵗʰ **V69.50** Passenger in heavy transport vehicle injured in collision with unspecified motor vehicles in traffic accident

    ✓x7ᵗʰ **V69.59** Passenger in heavy transport vehicle injured in collision with other motor vehicles in traffic accident

✓5ᵗʰ **V69.6** Unspecified occupant of heavy transport vehicle injured in collision with other and unspecified motor vehicles in traffic accident

    ✓x7ᵗʰ **V69.60** Unspecified occupant of heavy transport vehicle injured in collision with unspecified motor vehicles in traffic accident

        Collision NOS involving heavy transport vehicle (traffic)

    ✓x7ᵗʰ **V69.69** Unspecified occupant of heavy transport vehicle injured in collision with other motor vehicles in traffic accident

✓5ᵗʰ **V69.8** Occupant (driver) (passenger) of heavy transport vehicle injured in other specified transport accidents

    ✓x7ᵗʰ **V69.81** Occupant (driver) (passenger) of heavy transport vehicle injured in transport accidents with military vehicle

    ✓x7ᵗʰ **V69.88** Occupant (driver) (passenger) of heavy transport vehicle injured in other specified transport accidents

✓x7ᵗʰ **V69.9** Occupant (driver) (passenger) of heavy transport vehicle injured in unspecified traffic accident

    Accident NOS involving heavy transport vehicle

Bus occupant injured in transport accident (V70-V79)

INCLUDES   motorcoach

EXCLUDES 1   minibus (V50-V59)

✓4ᵗʰ **V70** Bus occupant injured in collision with pedestrian or animal

> The appropriate 7th character is to be added to each code from category V70.
> A   initial encounter
> D   subsequent encounter
> S   sequela

    EXCLUDES 1   bus collision with animal-drawn vehicle or animal being ridden (V76-)

✓x7ᵗʰ **V70.0** Driver of bus injured in collision with pedestrian or animal in nontraffic accident

✓x7ᵗʰ **V70.1** Passenger on bus injured in collision with pedestrian or animal in nontraffic accident

✓x7ᵗʰ **V70.2** Person on outside of bus injured in collision with pedestrian or animal in nontraffic accident

✓x7ᵗʰ **V70.3** Unspecified occupant of bus injured in collision with pedestrian or animal in nontraffic accident

✓x7ᵗʰ **V70.4** Person boarding or alighting from bus injured in collision with pedestrian or animal

✓x7ᵗʰ **V70.5** Driver of bus injured in collision with pedestrian or animal in traffic accident

✓x7ᵗʰ **V70.6** Passenger on bus injured in collision with pedestrian or animal in traffic accident

✓x7ᵗʰ **V70.7** Person on outside of bus injured in collision with pedestrian or animal in traffic accident

✓x7ᵗʰ **V70.9** Unspecified occupant of bus injured in collision with pedestrian or animal in traffic accident

✓4ᵗʰ **V71** Bus occupant injured in collision with pedal cycle

> The appropriate 7th character is to be added to each code from category V71.
> A   initial encounter
> D   subsequent encounter
> S   sequela

✓x7ᵗʰ **V71.0** Driver of bus injured in collision with pedal cycle in nontraffic accident

✓x7ᵗʰ **V71.1** Passenger on bus injured in collision with pedal cycle in nontraffic accident

✓x7ᵗʰ **V71.2** Person on outside of bus injured in collision with pedal cycle in nontraffic accident

✓x7ᵗʰ **V71.3** Unspecified occupant of bus injured in collision with pedal cycle in nontraffic accident

✓x7ᵗʰ **V71.4** Person boarding or alighting from bus injured in collision with pedal cycle

✓x7ᵗʰ **V71.5** Driver of bus injured in collision with pedal cycle in traffic accident

✓x7ᵗʰ **V71.6** Passenger on bus injured in collision with pedal cycle in traffic accident

✓x7ᵗʰ **V71.7** Person on outside of bus injured in collision with pedal cycle in traffic accident

✓x7ᵗʰ **V71.9** Unspecified occupant of bus injured in collision with pedal cycle in traffic accident

✓4ᵗʰ **V72** Bus occupant injured in collision with two- or three-wheeled motor vehicle

> The appropriate 7th character is to be added to each code from category V72.
> A   initial encounter
> D   subsequent encounter
> S   sequela

✓x7ᵗʰ **V72.0** Driver of bus injured in collision with two- or three-wheeled motor vehicle in nontraffic accident

✓x7ᵗʰ **V72.1** Passenger on bus injured in collision with two- or three-wheeled motor vehicle in nontraffic accident

✓x7ᵗʰ **V72.2** Person on outside of bus injured in collision with two- or three-wheeled motor vehicle in nontraffic accident

✓x7ᵗʰ **V72.3** Unspecified occupant of bus injured in collision with two- or three-wheeled motor vehicle in nontraffic accident

✓x7ᵗʰ **V72.4** Person boarding or alighting from bus injured in collision with two- or three-wheeled motor vehicle

✓x7ᵗʰ **V72.5** Driver of bus injured in collision with two- or three-wheeled motor vehicle in traffic accident

✓x7ᵗʰ **V72.6** Passenger on bus injured in collision with two- or three-wheeled motor vehicle in traffic accident

✓x7ᵗʰ **V72.7** Person on outside of bus injured in collision with two- or three-wheeled motor vehicle in traffic accident

✓x7ᵗʰ **V72.9** Unspecified occupant of bus injured in collision with two- or three-wheeled motor vehicle in traffic accident

✓4ᵗʰ **V73** Bus occupant injured in collision with car, pick-up truck or van

> The appropriate 7th character is to be added to each code from category V73.
> A   initial encounter
> D   subsequent encounter
> S   sequela

✓x7ᵗʰ **V73.0** Driver of bus injured in collision with car, pick-up truck or van in nontraffic accident

✓x7ᵗʰ **V73.1** Passenger on bus injured in collision with car, pick-up truck or van in nontraffic accident

✓x7ᵗʰ **V73.2** Person on outside of bus injured in collision with car, pick-up truck or van in nontraffic accident

✓x7ᵗʰ **V73.3** Unspecified occupant of bus injured in collision with car, pick-up truck or van in nontraffic accident

✓x7ᵗʰ **V73.4** Person boarding or alighting from bus injured in collision with car, pick-up truck or van

✓x7ᵗʰ **V73.5** Driver of bus injured in collision with car, pick-up truck or van in traffic accident

✓x7ᵗʰ **V73.6** Passenger on bus injured in collision with car, pick-up truck or van in traffic accident

✓x7ᵗʰ **V73.7** Person on outside of bus injured in collision with car, pick-up truck or van in traffic accident

✓x7ᵗʰ **V73.9** Unspecified occupant of bus injured in collision with car, pick-up truck or van in traffic accident

---

EXCLUDES 1   Not coded here   EXCLUDES 2   Not included here   *Manifestation Code*

☑4th V74 Bus occupant injured in collision with heavy transport vehicle or bus

> EXCLUDES 1 *bus occupant injured in collision with military vehicle (V79.81)*

> The appropriate 7th character is to be added to each code from category V74.
> A   initial encounter
> D   subsequent encounter
> S   sequela

- ✓x7th **V74.0** Driver of bus injured in collision with heavy transport vehicle or bus in nontraffic accident
- ✓x7th **V74.1** Passenger on bus injured in collision with heavy transport vehicle or bus in nontraffic accident
- ✓x7th **V74.2** Person on outside of bus injured in collision with heavy transport vehicle or bus in nontraffic accident
- ✓x7th **V74.3** Unspecified occupant of bus injured in collision with heavy transport vehicle or bus in nontraffic accident
- ✓x7th **V74.4** Person boarding or alighting from bus injured in collision with heavy transport vehicle or bus
- ✓x7th **V74.5** Driver of bus injured in collision with heavy transport vehicle or bus in traffic accident
- ✓x7th **V74.6** Passenger on bus injured in collision with heavy transport vehicle or bus in traffic accident
- ✓x7th **V74.7** Person on outside of bus injured in collision with heavy transport vehicle or bus in traffic accident
- ✓x7th **V74.9** Unspecified occupant of bus injured in collision with heavy transport vehicle or bus in traffic accident

☑4th V75 Bus occupant injured in collision with railway train or railway vehicle

> The appropriate 7th character is to be added to each code from category V75.
> A   initial encounter
> D   subsequent encounter
> S   sequela

- ✓x7th **V75.0** Driver of bus injured in collision with railway train or railway vehicle in nontraffic accident
- ✓x7th **V75.1** Passenger on bus injured in collision with railway train or railway vehicle in nontraffic accident
- ✓x7th **V75.2** Person on outside of bus injured in collision with railway train or railway vehicle in nontraffic accident
- ✓x7th **V75.3** Unspecified occupant of bus injured in collision with railway train or railway vehicle in nontraffic accident
- ✓x7th **V75.4** Person boarding or alighting from bus injured in collision with railway train or railway vehicle
- ✓x7th **V75.5** Driver of bus injured in collision with railway train or railway vehicle in traffic accident
- ✓x7th **V75.6** Passenger on bus injured in collision with railway train or railway vehicle in traffic accident
- ✓x7th **V75.7** Person on outside of bus injured in collision with railway train or railway vehicle in traffic accident
- ✓x7th **V75.9** Unspecified occupant of bus injured in collision with railway train or railway vehicle in traffic accident

☑4th V76 Bus occupant injured in collision with other nonmotor vehicle

> INCLUDES collision with animal-drawn vehicle, animal being ridden, streetcar

> The appropriate 7th character is to be added to each code from category V76.
> A   initial encounter
> D   subsequent encounter
> S   sequela

- ✓x7th **V76.0** Driver of bus injured in collision with other nonmotor vehicle in nontraffic accident
- ✓x7th **V76.1** Passenger on bus injured in collision with other nonmotor vehicle in nontraffic accident
- ✓x7th **V76.2** Person on outside of bus injured in collision with other nonmotor vehicle in nontraffic accident
- ✓x7th **V76.3** Unspecified occupant of bus injured in collision with other nonmotor vehicle in nontraffic accident
- ✓x7th **V76.4** Person boarding or alighting from bus injured in collision with other nonmotor vehicle
- ✓x7th **V76.5** Driver of bus injured in collision with other nonmotor vehicle in traffic accident
- ✓x7th **V76.6** Passenger on bus injured in collision with other nonmotor vehicle in traffic accident
- ✓x7th **V76.7** Person on outside of bus injured in collision with other nonmotor vehicle in traffic accident

- ✓x7th **V76.9** Unspecified occupant of bus injured in collision with other nonmotor vehicle in traffic accident

☑4th V77 Bus occupant injured in collision with fixed or stationary object

> The appropriate 7th character is to be added to each code from category V77.
> A   initial encounter
> D   subsequent encounter
> S   sequela

- ✓x7th **V77.0** Driver of bus injured in collision with fixed or stationary object in nontraffic accident
- ✓x7th **V77.1** Passenger on bus injured in collision with fixed or stationary object in nontraffic accident
- ✓x7th **V77.2** Person on outside of bus injured in collision with fixed or stationary object in nontraffic accident
- ✓x7th **V77.3** Unspecified occupant of bus injured in collision with fixed or stationary object in nontraffic accident
- ✓x7th **V77.4** Person boarding or alighting from bus injured in collision with fixed or stationary object
- ✓x7th **V77.5** Driver of bus injured in collision with fixed or stationary object in traffic accident
- ✓x7th **V77.6** Passenger on bus injured in collision with fixed or stationary object in traffic accident
- ✓x7th **V77.7** Person on outside of bus injured in collision with fixed or stationary object in traffic accident
- ✓x7th **V77.9** Unspecified occupant of bus injured in collision with fixed or stationary object in traffic accident

☑4th V78 Bus occupant injured in noncollision transport accident

> INCLUDES overturning bus NOS
> overturning bus without collision

> The appropriate 7th character is to be added to each code from category V78.
> A   initial encounter
> D   subsequent encounter
> S   sequela

- ✓x7th **V78.0** Driver of bus injured in noncollision transport accident in nontraffic accident
- ✓x7th **V78.1** Passenger on bus injured in noncollision transport accident in nontraffic accident
- ✓x7th **V78.2** Person on outside of bus injured in noncollision transport accident in nontraffic accident
- ✓x7th **V78.3** Unspecified occupant of bus injured in noncollision transport accident in nontraffic accident
- ✓x7th **V78.4** Person boarding or alighting from bus injured in noncollision transport accident
- ✓x7th **V78.5** Driver of bus injured in noncollision transport accident in traffic accident
- ✓x7th **V78.6** Passenger on bus injured in noncollision transport accident in traffic accident
- ✓x7th **V78.7** Person on outside of bus injured in noncollision transport accident in traffic accident
- ✓x7th **V78.9** Unspecified occupant of bus injured in noncollision transport accident in traffic accident

☑4th V79 Bus occupant injured in other and unspecified transport accidents

> The appropriate 7th character is to be added to each code from category V79.
> A   initial encounter
> D   subsequent encounter
> S   sequela

- ✓5th **V79.0** Driver of bus injured in collision with other and unspecified motor vehicles in nontraffic accident
  - ✓x7th **V79.00** Driver of bus injured in collision with unspecified motor vehicles in nontraffic accident
  - ✓x7th **V79.09** Driver of bus injured in collision with other motor vehicles in nontraffic accident
- ✓5th **V79.1** Passenger on bus injured in collision with other and unspecified motor vehicles in nontraffic accident
  - ✓x7th **V79.10** Passenger on bus injured in collision with unspecified motor vehicles in nontraffic accident
  - ✓x7th **V79.19** Passenger on bus injured in collision with other motor vehicles in nontraffic accident
- ✓5th **V79.2** Unspecified bus occupant injured in collision with other and unspecified motor vehicles in nontraffic accident

---

☑ Appropriate additional character required   ✓x7th Requires 7th character, placeholder x must fill empty characters

√x7ᵗʰ **V79.20 Unspecified bus occupant injured in collision with unspecified motor vehicles in nontraffic accident**
Bus collision NOS, nontraffic

√x7ᵗʰ **V79.29 Unspecified bus occupant injured in collision with other motor vehicles in nontraffic accident**

√x7ᵗʰ **V79.3 Bus occupant (driver) (passenger) injured in unspecified nontraffic accident**
Bus accident NOS, nontraffic
Bus occupant injured in nontraffic accident NOS

√5ᵗʰ **V79.4 Driver of bus injured in collision with other and unspecified motor vehicles in traffic accident**

√x7ᵗʰ **V79.40 Driver of bus injured in collision with unspecified motor vehicles in traffic accident**

√x7ᵗʰ **V79.49 Driver of bus injured in collision with other motor vehicles in traffic accident**

√5ᵗʰ **V79.5 Passenger on bus injured in collision with other and unspecified motor vehicles in traffic accident**

√x7ᵗʰ **V79.50 Passenger on bus injured in collision with unspecified motor vehicles in traffic accident**

√x7ᵗʰ **V79.59 Passenger on bus injured in collision with other motor vehicles in traffic accident**

√5ᵗʰ **V79.6 Unspecified bus occupant injured in collision with other and unspecified motor vehicles in traffic accident**

√x7ᵗʰ **V79.60 Unspecified bus occupant injured in collision with unspecified motor vehicles in traffic accident**
Bus collision NOS (traffic)

√x7ᵗʰ **V79.69 Unspecified bus occupant injured in collision with other motor vehicles in traffic accident**

√5ᵗʰ **V79.8 Bus occupant (driver) (passenger) injured in other specified transport accidents**

√x7ᵗʰ **V79.81 Bus occupant (driver) (passenger) injured in transport accidents with military vehicle**

√x7ᵗʰ **V79.88 Bus occupant (driver) (passenger) injured in other specified transport accidents**

√x7ᵗʰ **V79.9 Bus occupant (driver) (passenger) injured in unspecified traffic accident**
Bus accident NOS

Other land transport accidents (V80-V89)

√4ᵗʰ **V80 Animal-rider or occupant of animal-drawn vehicle injured in transport accident**

> The appropriate 7th character is to be added to each code from category V80.
> A   initial encounter
> D   subsequent encounter
> S   sequela

√5ᵗʰ **V80.0 Animal-rider or occupant of animal drawn vehicle injured by fall from or being thrown from animal or animal-drawn vehicle in noncollision accident**

√6ᵗʰ **V80.01 Animal-rider injured by fall from or being thrown from animal in noncollision accident**

√7ᵗʰ **V80.010 Animal-rider injured by fall from or being thrown from horse in noncollision accident**

√7ᵗʰ **V80.018 Animal-rider injured by fall from or being thrown from other animal in noncollision accident**

√x7ᵗʰ **V80.02 Occupant of animal-drawn vehicle injured by fall from or being thrown from animal-drawn vehicle in noncollision accident**
Overturning animal-drawn vehicle NOS
Overturning animal-drawn vehicle without collision

√5ᵗʰ **V80.1 Animal-rider or occupant of animal-drawn vehicle injured in collision with pedestrian or animal**
EXCLUDES 1 *animal-rider or animal-drawn vehicle collision with animal-drawn vehicle or animal being ridden (V80.7)*

√x7ᵗʰ **V80.11 Animal-rider injured in collision with pedestrian or animal**

√x7ᵗʰ **V80.12 Occupant of animal-drawn vehicle injured in collision with pedestrian or animal**

√5ᵗʰ **V80.2 Animal-rider or occupant of animal-drawn vehicle injured in collision with pedal cycle**

√x7ᵗʰ **V80.21 Animal-rider injured in collision with pedal cycle**

√x7ᵗʰ **V80.22 Occupant of animal-drawn vehicle injured in collision with pedal cycle**

√5ᵗʰ **V80.3 Animal-rider or occupant of animal-drawn vehicle injured in collision with two- or three-wheeled motor vehicle**

√x7ᵗʰ **V80.31 Animal-rider injured in collision with two- or three-wheeled motor vehicle**

√x7ᵗʰ **V80.32 Occupant of animal-drawn vehicle injured in collision with two- or three-wheeled motor vehicle**

√5ᵗʰ **V80.4 Animal-rider or occupant of animal-drawn vehicle injured in collision with car, pick-up truck, van, heavy transport vehicle or bus**
EXCLUDES 1 *animal-rider injured in collision with military vehicle (V80.910)*
occupant of animal-drawn vehicle injured in collision with military vehicle (V80.920)

√x7ᵗʰ **V80.41 Animal-rider injured in collision with car, pick-up truck, van, heavy transport vehicle or bus**

√x7ᵗʰ **V80.42 Occupant of animal-drawn vehicle injured in collision with car, pick-up truck, van, heavy transport vehicle or bus**

√5ᵗʰ **V80.5 Animal-rider or occupant of animal-drawn vehicle injured in collision with other specified motor vehicle**

√x7ᵗʰ **V80.51 Animal-rider injured in collision with other specified motor vehicle**

√x7ᵗʰ **V80.52 Occupant of animal-drawn vehicle injured in collision with other specified motor vehicle**

√5ᵗʰ **V80.6 Animal-rider or occupant of animal-drawn vehicle injured in collision with railway train or railway vehicle**

√x7ᵗʰ **V80.61 Animal-rider injured in collision with railway train or railway vehicle**

√x7ᵗʰ **V80.62 Occupant of animal-drawn vehicle injured in collision with railway train or railway vehicle**

√5ᵗʰ **V80.7 Animal-rider or occupant of animal-drawn vehicle injured in collision with other nonmotor vehicles**

√6ᵗʰ **V80.71 Animal-rider or occupant of animal-drawn vehicle injured in collision with animal being ridden**

√7ᵗʰ **V80.710 Animal-rider injured in collision with other animal being ridden**

√7ᵗʰ **V80.711 Occupant of animal-drawn vehicle injured in collision with animal being ridden**

√6ᵗʰ **V80.72 Animal-rider or occupant of animal-drawn vehicle injured in collision with other animal-drawn vehicle**

√7ᵗʰ **V80.720 Animal-rider injured in collision with animal-drawn vehicle**

√7ᵗʰ **V80.721 Occupant of animal-drawn vehicle injured in collision with other animal-drawn vehicle**

√6ᵗʰ **V80.73 Animal-rider or occupant of animal-drawn vehicle injured in collision with streetcar**

√7ᵗʰ **V80.730 Animal-rider injured in collision with streetcar**

√7ᵗʰ **V80.731 Occupant of animal-drawn vehicle injured in collision with streetcar**

√6ᵗʰ **V80.79 Animal-rider or occupant of animal-drawn vehicle injured in collision with other nonmotor vehicles**

√7ᵗʰ **V80.790 Animal-rider injured in collision with other nonmotor vehicles**

√7ᵗʰ **V80.791 Occupant of animal-drawn vehicle injured in collision with other nonmotor vehicles**

√5ᵗʰ **V80.8 Animal-rider or occupant of animal-drawn vehicle injured in collision with fixed or stationary object**

√x7ᵗʰ **V80.81 Animal-rider injured in collision with fixed or stationary object**

√x7ᵗʰ **V80.82 Occupant of animal-drawn vehicle injured in collision with fixed or stationary object**

√5ᵗʰ **V80.9 Animal-rider or occupant of animal-drawn vehicle injured in other and unspecified transport accidents**

√6ᵗʰ **V80.91 Animal-rider injured in other and unspecified transport accidents**

√7ᵗʰ **V80.910 Animal-rider injured in transport accident with military vehicle**

√7ᵗʰ **V80.918 Animal-rider injured in other transport accident**

√7ᵗʰ **V80.919 Animal-rider injured in unspecified transport accident**
Animal rider accident NOS

EXCLUDES 1 Not coded here   EXCLUDES 2 Not included here   *Manifestation Code*

✓6th **V80.92** **Occupant of animal-drawn vehicle injured in other and unspecified transport accidents**

 ✓7th **V80.920** **Occupant of animal-drawn vehicle injured in transport accident with military vehicle**

 ✓7th **V80.928** **Occupant of animal-drawn vehicle injured in other transport accident**

 ✓7th **V80.929** **Occupant of animal-drawn vehicle injured in unspecified transport accident**
   Animal-drawn vehicle accident NOS

✓4th **V81** **Occupant of railway train or railway vehicle injured in transport accident**
 INCLUDES derailment of railway train or railway vehicle
   person on outside of train
 EXCLUDES 1 *streetcar (V82-)*

> The appropriate 7th character is to be added to each code from category V81.
> A initial encounter
> D subsequent encounter
> S sequela

✓x7th **V81.0** **Occupant of railway train or railway vehicle injured in collision with motor vehicle in nontraffic accident**
 EXCLUDES 1 *occupant of railway train or railway vehicle injured due to collision with military vehicle (V81.83)*

✓x7th **V81.1** **Occupant of railway train or railway vehicle injured in collision with motor vehicle in traffic accident**
 EXCLUDES 1 *occupant of railway train or railway vehicle injured due to collision with military vehicle (V81.83)*

✓x7th **V81.2** **Occupant of railway train or railway vehicle injured in collision with or hit by rolling stock**

✓x7th **V81.3** **Occupant of railway train or railway vehicle injured in collision with other object**
  Railway collision NOS

✓x7th **V81.4** **Person injured while boarding or alighting from railway train or railway vehicle**

✓x7th **V81.5** **Occupant of railway train or railway vehicle injured by fall in railway train or railway vehicle**

✓x7th **V81.6** **Occupant of railway train or railway vehicle injured by fall from railway train or railway vehicle**

✓x7th **V81.7** **Occupant of railway train or railway vehicle injured in derailment without antecedent collision**

✓5th **V81.8** **Occupant of railway train or railway vehicle injured in other specified railway accidents**

 ✓x7th **V81.81** **Occupant of railway train or railway vehicle injured due to explosion or fire on train**

 ✓x7th **V81.82** **Occupant of railway train or railway vehicle injured due to object falling onto train**
   Occupant of railway train or railway vehicle injured due to falling earth onto train
   Occupant of railway train or railway vehicle injured due to falling rocks onto train
   Occupant of railway train or railway vehicle injured due to falling snow onto train
   Occupant of railway train or railway vehicle injured due to falling trees onto train

 ✓x7th **V81.83** **Occupant of railway train or railway vehicle injured due to collision with military vehicle**

 ✓x7th **V81.89** **Occupant of railway train or railway vehicle injured due to other specified railway accident**

✓x7th **V81.9** **Occupant of railway train or railway vehicle injured in unspecified railway accident**
  Railway accident NOS

✓4th **V82** **Occupant of powered streetcar injured in transport accident**
 INCLUDES interurban electric car
   person on outside of streetcar
   tram (car)
   trolley (car)
 EXCLUDES 1 *bus (V70-V79)*
   motorcoach (V70-V79)
   nonpowered streetcar (V76-)
   train (V81-)

> The appropriate 7th character is to be added to each code from category V82.
> A initial encounter
> D subsequent encounter
> S sequela

✓x7th **V82.0** **Occupant of streetcar injured in collision with motor vehicle in nontraffic accident**

✓x7th **V82.1** **Occupant of streetcar injured in collision with motor vehicle in traffic accident**

✓x7th **V82.2** **Occupant of streetcar injured in collision with or hit by rolling stock**

✓x7th **V82.3** **Occupant of streetcar injured in collision with other object**
 EXCLUDES 1 *collision with animal-drawn vehicle or animal being ridden (V82.8)*

✓x7th **V82.4** **Person injured while boarding or alighting from streetcar**

✓x7th **V82.5** **Occupant of streetcar injured by fall in streetcar**
 EXCLUDES 1 *fall in streetcar:*
   while boarding or alighting (V82.4)
   with antecedent collision (V82.0-V82.3)

✓x7th **V82.6** **Occupant of streetcar injured by fall from streetcar**
 EXCLUDES 1 *fall from streetcar:*
   while boarding or alighting (V82.4)
   with antecedent collision (V82.0-V82.3)

✓x7th **V82.7** **Occupant of streetcar injured in derailment without antecedent collision**
 EXCLUDES 1 *occupant of streetcar injured in derailment with antecedent collision (V82.0-V82.3)*

✓x7th **V82.8** **Occupant of streetcar injured in other specified transport accidents**
  Streetcar collision with military vehicle
  Streetcar collision with train or nonmotor vehicles

✓x7th **V82.9** **Occupant of streetcar injured in unspecified traffic accident**
  Streetcar accident NOS

✓4th **V83** **Occupant of special vehicle mainly used on industrial premises injured in transport accident**
 INCLUDES battery-powered airport passenger vehicle
   battery-powered truck (baggage) (mail)
   coal-car in mine
   forklift (truck)
   logging car
   self-propelled industrial truck
   station baggage truck (powered)
   tram, truck, or tub (powered) in mine or quarry
 EXCLUDES 1 *special construction vehicles (V85-)*
   special industrial vehicle in stationary use or maintenance (W31-)

> The appropriate 7th character is to be added to each code from category V83.
> A initial encounter
> D subsequent encounter
> S sequela

✓x7th **V83.0** **Driver of special industrial vehicle injured in traffic accident**

✓x7th **V83.1** **Passenger of special industrial vehicle injured in traffic accident**

✓x7th **V83.2** **Person on outside of special industrial vehicle injured in traffic accident**

✓x7th **V83.3** **Unspecified occupant of special industrial vehicle injured in traffic accident**

✓x7th **V83.4** **Person injured while boarding or alighting from special industrial vehicle**

✓x7th **V83.5** **Driver of special industrial vehicle injured in nontraffic accident**

✓x7th **V83.6** **Passenger of special industrial vehicle injured in nontraffic accident**

✓x7th **V83.7** **Person on outside of special industrial vehicle injured in nontraffic accident**

√x7th V83.9   Unspecified occupant of special industrial vehicle injured in nontraffic accident
     Special-industrial-vehicle accident NOS

√4th V84   Occupant of special vehicle mainly used in agriculture injured in transport accident

    INCLUDES   self-propelled farm machinery
                 tractor (and trailer)
    EXCLUDES 1   animal-powered farm machinery accident (W30.8-)
                 contact with combine harvester (W30.0)
                 special agricultural vehicle in stationary use or maintenance (W30-)

> The appropriate 7th character is to be added to each code from category V84.
> A   initial encounter
> D   subsequent encounter
> S   sequela

√x7th V84.0   Driver of special agricultural vehicle injured in traffic accident

√x7th V84.1   Passenger of special agricultural vehicle injured in traffic accident

√x7th V84.2   Person on outside of special agricultural vehicle injured in traffic accident

√x7th V84.3   Unspecified occupant of special agricultural vehicle injured in traffic accident

√x7th V84.4   Person injured while boarding or alighting from special agricultural vehicle

√x7th V84.5   Driver of special agricultural vehicle injured in nontraffic accident

√x7th V84.6   Passenger of special agricultural vehicle injured in nontraffic accident

√x7th V84.7   Person on outside of special agricultural vehicle injured in nontraffic accident

√x7th V84.9   Unspecified occupant of special agricultural vehicle injured in nontraffic accident
     Special-agricultural vehicle accident NOS

√4th V85   Occupant of special construction vehicle injured in transport accident

    INCLUDES   bulldozer
                 digger
                 dump truck
                 earth-leveller
                 mechanical shovel
                 road-roller
    EXCLUDES 1   special industrial vehicle (V83-)
                 special construction vehicle in stationary use or maintenance (W31-)

> The appropriate 7th character is to be added to each code from category V85.
> A   initial encounter
> D   subsequent encounter
> S   sequela

√x7th V85.0   Driver of special construction vehicle injured in traffic accident

√x7th V85.1   Passenger of special construction vehicle injured in traffic accident

√x7th V85.2   Person on outside of special construction vehicle injured in traffic accident

√x7th V85.3   Unspecified occupant of special construction vehicle injured in traffic accident

√x7th V85.4   Person injured while boarding or alighting from special construction vehicle

√x7th V85.5   Driver of special construction vehicle injured in nontraffic accident

√x7th V85.6   Passenger of special construction vehicle injured in nontraffic accident

√x7th V85.7   Person on outside of special construction vehicle injured in nontraffic accident

√x7th V85.9   Unspecified occupant of special construction vehicle injured in nontraffic accident
     Special-construction-vehicle accident NOS

√4th V86   Occupant of special all-terrain or other off-road motor vehicle, injured in transport accident

    EXCLUDES 1   special all-terrain vehicle in stationary use or maintenance (W31-)
                 sport-utility vehicle (V50-V59)
                 three-wheeled motor vehicle designed for on-road use (V30-V39)

> The appropriate 7th character is to be added to each code from category V86.
> A   initial encounter
> D   subsequent encounter
> S   sequela

√5th V86.0   Driver of special all-terrain or other off-road motor vehicle injured in traffic accident

    √x7th V86.01   Driver of ambulance or fire engine injured in traffic accident

    √x7th V86.02   Driver of snowmobile injured in traffic accident

    √x7th V86.03   Driver of dune buggy injured in traffic accident

    √x7th V86.04   Driver of military vehicle injured in traffic accident

    √x7th V86.09   Driver of other special all-terrain or other off-road motor vehicle injured in traffic accident
       Driver of dirt bike injured in traffic accident
       Driver of go cart injured in traffic accident
       Driver of golf cart injured in traffic accident

√5th V86.1   Passenger of special all-terrain or other off-road motor vehicle injured in traffic accident

    √x7th V86.11   Passenger of ambulance or fire engine injured in traffic accident

    √x7th V86.12   Passenger of snowmobile injured in traffic accident

    √x7th V86.13   Passenger of dune buggy injured in traffic accident

    √x7th V86.14   Passenger of military vehicle injured in traffic accident

    √x7th V86.19   Passenger of other special all-terrain or other off-road motor vehicle injured in traffic accident
       Passenger of dirt bike injured in traffic accident
       Passenger of go cart injured in traffic accident
       Passenger of golf cart injured in traffic accident

√5th V86.2   Person on outside of special all-terrain or other off-road motor vehicle injured in traffic accident

    √x7th V86.21   Person on outside of ambulance or fire engine injured in traffic accident

    √x7th V86.22   Person on outside of snowmobile injured in traffic accident

    √x7th V86.23   Person on outside of dune buggy injured in traffic accident

    √x7th V86.24   Person on outside of military vehicle injured in traffic accident

    √x7th V86.29   Person on outside of other special all-terrain or other off-road motor vehicle injured in traffic accident
       Person on outside of dirt bike injured in traffic accident
       Person on outside of go cart in traffic accident
       Person on outside of golf cart injured in traffic accident

√5th V86.3   Unspecified occupant of special all-terrain or other off-road motor vehicle injured in traffic accident

    √x7th V86.31   Unspecified occupant of ambulance or fire engine injured in traffic accident

    √x7th V86.32   Unspecified occupant of snowmobile injured in traffic accident

    √x7th V86.33   Unspecified occupant of dune buggy injured in traffic accident

    √x7th V86.34   Unspecified occupant of military vehicle injured in traffic accident

    √x7th V86.39   Unspecified occupant of other special all-terrain or other off-road motor vehicle injured in traffic accident
       Unspecified occupant of dirt bike injured in traffic accident
       Unspecified occupant of go cart injured in traffic accident
       Unspecified occupant of golf cart injured in traffic accident

---

EXCLUDES 1   Not coded here   EXCLUDES 2   Not included here   *Manifestation Code*

√5th V86.4 Person injured while boarding or alighting from special all-terrain or other off-road motor vehicle

- **√x7th V86.41 Person injured while boarding or alighting from ambulance or fire engine**
- **√x7th V86.42 Person injured while boarding or alighting from snowmobile**
- **√x7th V86.43 Person injured while boarding or alighting from dune buggy**
- **√x7th V86.44 Person injured while boarding or alighting from military vehicle**
- **√x7th V86.49 Person injured while boarding or alighting from other special all-terrain or other off-road motor vehicle**

  Person injured while boarding or alighting from dirt bike

  Person injured while boarding or alighting from go cart

  Person injured while boarding or alighting from golf cart

√5th V86.5 Driver of special all-terrain or other off-road motor vehicle injured in nontraffic accident

- **√x7th V86.51 Driver of ambulance or fire engine injured in nontraffic accident**
- **√x7th V86.52 Driver of snowmobile injured in nontraffic accident**
- **√x7th V86.53 Driver of dune buggy injured in nontraffic accident**
- **√x7th V86.54 Driver of military vehicle injured in nontraffic accident**
- **√x7th V86.59 Driver of other special all-terrain or other off-road motor vehicle injured in nontraffic accident**

  Driver of dirt bike injured in nontraffic accident

  Driver of go cart injured in nontraffic accident

  Driver of golf cart injured in nontraffic accident

√5th V86.6 Passenger of special all-terrain or other off-road motor vehicle injured in nontraffic accident

- **√x7th V86.61 Passenger of ambulance or fire engine injured in nontraffic accident**
- **√x7th V86.62 Passenger of snowmobile injured in nontraffic accident**
- **√x7th V86.63 Passenger of dune buggy injured in nontraffic accident**
- **√x7th V86.64 Passenger of military vehicle injured in nontraffic accident**
- **√x7th V86.69 Passenger of other special all-terrain or other off-road motor vehicle injured in nontraffic accident**

  Passenger of dirt bike injured in nontraffic accident

  Passenger of go cart injured in nontraffic accident

  Passenger of golf cart injured in nontraffic accident

√5th V86.7 Person on outside of special all-terrain or other off-road motor vehicle injured in nontraffic accident

- **√x7th V86.71 Person on outside of ambulance or fire engine injured in nontraffic accident**
- **√x7th V86.72 Person on outside of snowmobile injured in nontraffic accident**
- **√x7th V86.73 Person on outside of dune buggy injured in nontraffic accident**
- **√x7th V86.74 Person on outside of military vehicle injured in nontraffic accident**
- **√x7th V86.79 Person on outside of other special all-terrain or other off-road motor vehicles injured in nontraffic accident**

  Person on outside of dirt bike injured in nontraffic accident

  Person on outside of go cart injured in nontraffic accident

  Person on outside of golf cart injured in nontraffic accident

√5th V86.9 Unspecified occupant of special all-terrain or other off-road motor vehicle injured in nontraffic accident

- **√x7th V86.91 Unspecified occupant of ambulance or fire engine injured in nontraffic accident**
- **√x7th V86.92 Unspecified occupant of snowmobile injured in nontraffic accident**
- **√x7th V86.93 Unspecified occupant of dune buggy injured in nontraffic accident**
- **√x7th V86.94 Unspecified occupant of military vehicle injured in nontraffic accident**

- **√x7th V86.99 Unspecified occupant of other special all-terrain or other off-road motor vehicle injured in nontraffic accident**

  All-terrain motor-vehicle accident NOS

  Off-road motor-vehicle accident NOS

  Other motor-vehicle accident NOS

  Unspecified occupant of dirt bike injured in nontraffic accident

  Unspecified occupant of go cart injured in nontraffic accident

  Unspecified occupant of golf cart injured in nontraffic accident

√4th V87 Traffic accident of specified type but victim's mode of transport unknown

> **EXCLUDES 1** collision involving:
> pedal cycle (V10-V19)
> pedestrian (V01-V09)

> The appropriate 7th character is to be added to each code from category V87.
> A initial encounter
> D subsequent encounter
> S sequela

- **√x7th V87.0 Person injured in collision between car and two- or three-wheeled powered vehicle (traffic)**
- **√x7th V87.1 Person injured in collision between other motor vehicle and two- or three-wheeled motor vehicle (traffic)**
- **√x7th V87.2 Person injured in collision between car and pick-up truck or van (traffic)**
- **√x7th V87.3 Person injured in collision between car and bus (traffic)**
- **√x7th V87.4 Person injured in collision between car and heavy transport vehicle (traffic)**
- **√x7th V87.5 Person injured in collision between heavy transport vehicle and bus (traffic)**
- **√x7th V87.6 Person injured in collision between railway train or railway vehicle and car (traffic)**
- **√x7th V87.7 Person injured in collision between other specified motor vehicles (traffic)**
- **√x7th V87.8 Person injured in other specified noncollision transport accidents involving motor vehicle (traffic)**
- **√x7th V87.9 Person injured in other specified (collision)(noncollision) transport accidents involving nonmotor vehicle (traffic)**

√4th V88 Nontraffic accident of specified type but victim's mode of transport unknown

> **EXCLUDES 1** collision involving:
> pedal cycle (V10-V19)
> pedestrian (V01-V09)

> The appropriate 7th character is to be added to each code from category V88.
> A initial encounter
> D subsequent encounter
> S sequela

- **√x7th V88.0 Person injured in collision between car and two- or three-wheeled motor vehicle, nontraffic**
- **√x7th V88.1 Person injured in collision between other motor vehicle and two- or three-wheeled motor vehicle, nontraffic**
- **√x7th V88.2 Person injured in collision between car and pick-up truck or van, nontraffic**
- **√x7th V88.3 Person injured in collision between car and bus, nontraffic**
- **√x7th V88.4 Person injured in collision between car and heavy transport vehicle, nontraffic**
- **√x7th V88.5 Person injured in collision between heavy transport vehicle and bus, nontraffic**
- **√x7th V88.6 Person injured in collision between railway train or railway vehicle and car, nontraffic**
- **√x7th V88.7 Person injured in collision between other specified motor vehicle, nontraffic**
- **√x7th V88.8 Person injured in other specified noncollision transport accidents involving motor vehicle, nontraffic**
- **√x7th V88.9 Person injured in other specified (collision)(noncollision) transport accidents involving nonmotor vehicle, nontraffic**

☑ Appropriate additional character required

√x7th Requires 7th character, placeholder x must fill empty characters

✓4ᵗʰ **V89 Motor- or nonmotor-vehicle accident, type of vehicle unspecified**

> The appropriate 7th character is to be added to each code from category V89.
> A   initial encounter
> D   subsequent encounter
> S   sequela

✓x7ᵗʰ **V89.0 Person injured in unspecified motor-vehicle accident, nontraffic**
Motor-vehicle accident NOS, nontraffic

✓x7ᵗʰ **V89.1 Person injured in unspecified nonmotor-vehicle accident, nontraffic**
Nonmotor-vehicle accident NOS (nontraffic)

✓x7ᵗʰ **V89.2 Person injured in unspecified motor-vehicle accident, traffic**
Motor-vehicle accident [MVA] NOS
Road (traffic) accident [RTA] NOS

✓x7ᵗʰ **V89.3 Person injured in unspecified nonmotor-vehicle accident, traffic**
Nonmotor-vehicle traffic accident NOS

✓x7ᵗʰ **V89.9 Person injured in unspecified vehicle accident**
Collision NOS

Water transport accidents (V90-V94)

✓4ᵗʰ **V90 Drowning and submersion due to accident to watercraft**
> EXCLUDES 1   civilian water transport accident involving military watercraft (V94.81-)
> fall into water not from watercraft (W16-)
> military watercraft accident in military or war operations (Y36.0-, Y37.0-)
> water-transport-related drowning or submersion without accident to watercraft (V92-)

> The appropriate 7th character is to be added to each code from category V90.
> A   initial encounter
> D   subsequent encounter
> S   sequela

✓5ᵗʰ **V90.0 Drowning and submersion due to watercraft overturning**
 ✓x7ᵗʰ **V90.00 Drowning and submersion due to merchant ship overturning**
 ✓x7ᵗʰ **V90.01 Drowning and submersion due to passenger ship overturning**
 Drowning and submersion due to Ferry-boat overturning
 Drowning and submersion due to Liner overturning
 ✓x7ᵗʰ **V90.02 Drowning and submersion due to fishing boat overturning**
 ✓x7ᵗʰ **V90.03 Drowning and submersion due to other powered watercraft overturning**
 Drowning and submersion due to Hovercraft (on open water) overturning
 Drowning and submersion due to Jet ski overturning
 ✓x7ᵗʰ **V90.04 Drowning and submersion due to sailboat overturning**
 ✓x7ᵗʰ **V90.05 Drowning and submersion due to canoe or kayak overturning**
 ✓x7ᵗʰ **V90.06 Drowning and submersion due to (nonpowered) inflatable craft overturning**
 ✓x7ᵗʰ **V90.08 Drowning and submersion due to other unpowered watercraft overturning**
 Drowning and submersion due to windsurfer overturning
 ✓x7ᵗʰ **V90.09 Drowning and submersion due to unspecified watercraft overturning**
 Drowning and submersion due to boat NOS overturning
 Drowning and submersion due to ship NOS overturning
 Drowning and submersion due to watercraft NOS overturning

✓5ᵗʰ **V90.1 Drowning and submersion due to watercraft sinking**
 ✓x7ᵗʰ **V90.10 Drowning and submersion due to merchant ship sinking**
 ✓x7ᵗʰ **V90.11 Drowning and submersion due to passenger ship sinking**
 Drowning and submersion due to Ferry-boat sinking
 Drowning and submersion due to Liner sinking
 ✓x7ᵗʰ **V90.12 Drowning and submersion due to fishing boat sinking**
 ✓x7ᵗʰ **V90.13 Drowning and submersion due to other powered watercraft sinking**
 Drowning and submersion due to Hovercraft (on open water) sinking
 Drowning and submersion due to Jet ski sinking
 ✓x7ᵗʰ **V90.14 Drowning and submersion due to sailboat sinking**
 ✓x7ᵗʰ **V90.15 Drowning and submersion due to canoe or kayak sinking**
 ✓x7ᵗʰ **V90.16 Drowning and submersion due to (nonpowered) inflatable craft sinking**
 ✓x7ᵗʰ **V90.18 Drowning and submersion due to other unpowered watercraft sinking**
 ✓x7ᵗʰ **V90.19 Drowning and submersion due to unspecified watercraft sinking**
 Drowning and submersion due to boat NOS sinking
 Drowning and submersion due to ship NOS sinking
 Drowning and submersion due to watercraft NOS sinking

✓5ᵗʰ **V90.2 Drowning and submersion due to falling or jumping from burning watercraft**
 ✓x7ᵗʰ **V90.20 Drowning and submersion due to falling or jumping from burning merchant ship**
 ✓x7ᵗʰ **V90.21 Drowning and submersion due to falling or jumping from burning passenger ship**
 Drowning and submersion due to falling or jumping from burning Ferry-boat
 Drowning and submersion due to falling or jumping from burning Liner
 ✓x7ᵗʰ **V90.22 Drowning and submersion due to falling or jumping from burning fishing boat**
 ✓x7ᵗʰ **V90.23 Drowning and submersion due to falling or jumping from other burning powered watercraft**
 Drowning and submersion due to falling and jumping from burning Hovercraft (on open water)
 Drowning and submersion due to falling and jumping from burning Jet ski
 ✓x7ᵗʰ **V90.24 Drowning and submersion due to falling or jumping from burning sailboat**
 ✓x7ᵗʰ **V90.25 Drowning and submersion due to falling or jumping from burning canoe or kayak**
 ✓x7ᵗʰ **V90.26 Drowning and submersion due to falling or jumping from burning (nonpowered) inflatable craft**
 ✓x7ᵗʰ **V90.27 Drowning and submersion due to falling or jumping from burning water-skis**
 ✓x7ᵗʰ **V90.28 Drowning and submersion due to falling or jumping from other burning unpowered watercraft**
 Drowning and submersion due to falling and jumping from burning surf-board
 Drowning and submersion due to falling and jumping from burning windsurfer
 ✓x7ᵗʰ **V90.29 Drowning and submersion due to falling or jumping from unspecified burning watercraft**
 Drowning and submersion due to falling or jumping from burning boat NOS
 Drowning and submersion due to falling or jumping from burning ship NOS
 Drowning and submersion due to falling or jumping from burning watercraft NOS

✓5ᵗʰ **V90.3 Drowning and submersion due to falling or jumping from crushed watercraft**
 ✓x7ᵗʰ **V90.30 Drowning and submersion due to falling or jumping from crushed merchant ship**
 ✓x7ᵗʰ **V90.31 Drowning and submersion due to falling or jumping from crushed passenger ship**
 Drowning and submersion due to falling and jumping from crushed Ferry boat
 Drowning and submersion due to falling and jumping from crushed Liner
 ✓x7ᵗʰ **V90.32 Drowning and submersion due to falling or jumping from crushed fishing boat**

√x7ᵗʰ **V90.33 Drowning and submersion due to falling or jumping from other crushed powered watercraft**
Drowning and submersion due to falling and jumping from crushed Hovercraft
Drowning and submersion due to falling and jumping from crushed Jet ski

√x7ᵗʰ **V90.34 Drowning and submersion due to falling or jumping from crushed sailboat**

√x7ᵗʰ **V90.35 Drowning and submersion due to falling or jumping from crushed canoe or kayak**

√x7ᵗʰ **V90.36 Drowning and submersion due to falling or jumping from crushed (nonpowered) inflatable craft**

√x7ᵗʰ **V90.37 Drowning and submersion due to falling or jumping from crushed water-skis**

√x7ᵗʰ **V90.38 Drowning and submersion due to falling or jumping from other crushed unpowered watercraft**
Drowning and submersion due to falling and jumping from crushed surf-board
Drowning and submersion due to falling and jumping from crushed windsurfer

√x7ᵗʰ **V90.39 Drowning and submersion due to falling or jumping from crushed unspecified watercraft**
Drowning and submersion due to falling and jumping from crushed boat NOS
Drowning and submersion due to falling and jumping from crushed ship NOS
Drowning and submersion due to falling and jumping from crushed watercraft NOS

√5ᵗʰ **V90.8 Drowning and submersion due to other accident to watercraft**

√x7ᵗʰ **V90.80 Drowning and submersion due to other accident to merchant ship**

√x7ᵗʰ **V90.81 Drowning and submersion due to other accident to passenger ship**
Drowning and submersion due to other accident to Ferry-boat
Drowning and submersion due to other accident to Liner

√x7ᵗʰ **V90.82 Drowning and submersion due to other accident to fishing boat**

√x7ᵗʰ **V90.83 Drowning and submersion due to other accident to other powered watercraft**
Drowning and submersion due to other accident to Hovercraft (on open water)
Drowning and submersion due to other accident to Jet ski

√x7ᵗʰ **V90.84 Drowning and submersion due to other accident to sailboat**

√x7ᵗʰ **V90.85 Drowning and submersion due to other accident to canoe or kayak**

√x7ᵗʰ **V90.86 Drowning and submersion due to other accident to (nonpowered) inflatable craft**

√x7ᵗʰ **V90.87 Drowning and submersion due to other accident to water-skis**

√x7ᵗʰ **V90.88 Drowning and submersion due to other accident to other unpowered watercraft**
Drowning and submersion due to other accident to surf-board
Drowning and submersion due to other accident to windsurfer

√x7ᵗʰ **V90.89 Drowning and submersion due to other accident to unspecified watercraft**
Drowning and submersion due to other accident to boat NOS
Drowning and submersion due to other accident to ship NOS
Drowning and submersion due to other accident to watercraft NOS

√4ᵗʰ **V91 Other injury due to accident to watercraft**
INCLUDES any injury except drowning and submersion as a result of an accident to watercraft
EXCLUDES 1 civilian water transport accident involving military watercraft (V94.81-)
military watercraft accident in military or war operations (Y36, Y37-)
EXCLUDES 2 drowning and submersion due to accident to watercraft (V90-)

The appropriate 7th character is to be added to each code from category V91.
A initial encounter
D subsequent encounter
S sequela

√5ᵗʰ **V91.0 Burn due to watercraft on fire**
EXCLUDES 1 burn from localized fire or explosion on board ship without accident to watercraft (V93-)

√x7ᵗʰ **V91.00 Burn due to merchant ship on fire**

√x7ᵗʰ **V91.01 Burn due to passenger ship on fire**
Burn due to Ferry-boat on fire
Burn due to Liner on fire

√x7ᵗʰ **V91.02 Burn due to fishing boat on fire**

√x7ᵗʰ **V91.03 Burn due to other powered watercraft on fire**
Burn due to Hovercraft (on open water) on fire
Burn due to Jet ski on fire

√x7ᵗʰ **V91.04 Burn due to sailboat on fire**

√x7ᵗʰ **V91.05 Burn due to canoe or kayak on fire**

√x7ᵗʰ **V91.06 Burn due to (nonpowered) inflatable craft on fire**

√x7ᵗʰ **V91.07 Burn due to water-skis on fire**

√x7ᵗʰ **V91.08 Burn due to other unpowered watercraft on fire**

√x7ᵗʰ **V91.09 Burn due to unspecified watercraft on fire**
Burn due to boat NOS on fire
Burn due to ship NOS on fire
Burn due to watercraft NOS on fire

√5ᵗʰ **V91.1 Crushed between watercraft and other watercraft or other object due to collision**
Crushed by lifeboat after abandoning ship in a collision
NOTE select the specified type of watercraft that the victim was on at the time of the collision

√x7ᵗʰ **V91.10 Crushed between merchant ship and other watercraft or other object due to collision**

√x7ᵗʰ **V91.11 Crushed between passenger ship and other watercraft or other object due to collision**
Crushed between Ferry-boat and other watercraft or other object due to collision
Crushed between Liner and other watercraft or other object due to collision

√x7ᵗʰ **V91.12 Crushed between fishing boat and other watercraft or other object due to collision**

√x7ᵗʰ **V91.13 Crushed between other powered watercraft and other watercraft or other object due to collision**
Crushed between Hovercraft (on open water) and other watercraft or other object due to collision
Crushed between Jet ski and other watercraft or other object due to collision

√x7ᵗʰ **V91.14 Crushed between sailboat and other watercraft or other object due to collision**

√x7ᵗʰ **V91.15 Crushed between canoe or kayak and other watercraft or other object due to collision**

√x7ᵗʰ **V91.16 Crushed between (nonpowered) inflatable craft and other watercraft or other object due to collision**

√x7ᵗʰ **V91.18 Crushed between other unpowered watercraft and other watercraft or other object due to collision**
Crushed between surfboard and other watercraft or other object due to collision
Crushed between windsurfer and other watercraft or other object due to collision

√x7ᵗʰ **V91.19 Crushed between unspecified watercraft and other watercraft or other object due to collision**
Crushed between boat NOS and other watercraft or other object due to collision
Crushed between ship NOS and other watercraft or other object due to collision
Crushed between watercraft NOS and other watercraft or other object due to collision

☑5ᵗʰ **V91.2**   **Fall due to collision between watercraft and other watercraft or other object**
Fall while remaining on watercraft after collision
NOTE   Select the specified type of watercraft that the victim was on at the time of the collision
EXCLUDES 1   *crushed between watercraft and other watercraft and other object due to collision (V91.1-)*
drowning and submersion due to falling from crushed watercraft (V90.3-)

☑x7ᵗʰ **V91.20**   **Fall due to collision between merchant ship and other watercraft or other object**

☑x7ᵗʰ **V91.21**   **Fall due to collision between passenger ship and other watercraft or other object**
Fall due to collision between Ferry-boat and other watercraft or other object
Fall due to collision between Liner and other watercraft or other object

☑x7ᵗʰ **V91.22**   **Fall due to collision between fishing boat and other watercraft or other object**

☑x7ᵗʰ **V91.23**   **Fall due to collision between other powered watercraft and other watercraft or other object**
Fall due to collision between Hovercraft (on open water) and other watercraft or other object
Fall due to collision between Jet ski and other watercraft or other object

☑x7ᵗʰ **V91.24**   **Fall due to collision between sailboat and other watercraft or other object**

☑x7ᵗʰ **V91.25**   **Fall due to collision between canoe or kayak and other watercraft or other object**

☑x7ᵗʰ **V91.26**   **Fall due to collision between (nonpowered) inflatable craft and other watercraft or other object**

☑x7ᵗʰ **V91.29**   **Fall due to collision between unspecified watercraft and other watercraft or other object**
Fall due to collision between boat NOS and other watercraft or other object
Fall due to collision between ship NOS and other watercraft or other object
Fall due to collision between watercraft NOS and other watercraft or other object

☑5ᵗʰ **V91.3**   **Hit or struck by falling object due to accident to watercraft**
Hit or struck by falling object (part of damaged watercraft or other object) after falling or jumping from damaged watercraft
EXCLUDES 2   *drowning or submersion due to fall or jumping from damaged watercraft (V90.2-, V90.3-)*

☑x7ᵗʰ **V91.30**   **Hit or struck by falling object due to accident to merchant ship**

☑x7ᵗʰ **V91.31**   **Hit or struck by falling object due to accident to passenger ship**
Hit or struck by falling object due to accident to Ferry-boat
Hit or struck by falling object due to accident to Liner

☑x7ᵗʰ **V91.32**   **Hit or struck by falling object due to accident to fishing boat**

☑x7ᵗʰ **V91.33**   **Hit or struck by falling object due to accident to other powered watercraft**
Hit or struck by falling object due to accident to Hovercraft (on open water)
Hit or struck by falling object due to accident to Jet ski

☑x7ᵗʰ **V91.34**   **Hit or struck by falling object due to accident to sailboat**

☑x7ᵗʰ **V91.35**   **Hit or struck by falling object due to accident to canoe or kayak**

☑x7ᵗʰ **V91.36**   **Hit or struck by falling object due to accident to (nonpowered) inflatable craft**

☑x7ᵗʰ **V91.37**   **Hit or struck by falling object due to accident to water-skis**
Hit by water-skis after jumping off of waterskis

☑x7ᵗʰ **V91.38**   **Hit or struck by falling object due to accident to other unpowered watercraft**
Hit or struck by surf-board after falling off damaged surf-board
Hit or struck by object after falling off damaged windsurfer

☑x7ᵗʰ **V91.39**   **Hit or struck by falling object due to accident to unspecified watercraft**
Hit or struck by falling object due to accident to boat NOS
Hit or struck by falling object due to accident to ship NOS
Hit or struck by falling object due to accident to watercraft NOS

☑5ᵗʰ **V91.8**   **Other injury due to other accident to watercraft**

☑x7ᵗʰ **V91.80**   **Other injury due to other accident to merchant ship**

☑x7ᵗʰ **V91.81**   **Other injury due to other accident to passenger ship**
Other injury due to other accident to Ferry-boat
Other injury due to other accident to Liner

☑x7ᵗʰ **V91.82**   **Other injury due to other accident to fishing boat**

☑x7ᵗʰ **V91.83**   **Other injury due to other accident to other powered watercraft**
Other injury due to other accident to Hovercraft (on open water)
Other injury due to other accident to Jet ski

☑x7ᵗʰ **V91.84**   **Other injury due to other accident to sailboat**

☑x7ᵗʰ **V91.85**   **Other injury due to other accident to canoe or kayak**

☑x7ᵗʰ **V91.86**   **Other injury due to other accident to (nonpowered) inflatable craft**

☑x7ᵗʰ **V91.87**   **Other injury due to other accident to water-skis**

☑x7ᵗʰ **V91.88**   **Other injury due to other accident to other unpowered watercraft**
Other injury due to other accident to surf-board
Other injury due to other accident to windsurfer

☑x7ᵗʰ **V91.89**   **Other injury due to other accident to unspecified watercraft**
Other injury due to other accident to boat NOS
Other injury due to other accident to ship NOS
Other injury due to other accident to watercraft NOS

☑4ᵗʰ **V92**   **Drowning and submersion due to accident on board watercraft, without accident to watercraft**
EXCLUDES 1   *civilian water transport accident involving military watercraft (V94.81-)*
drowning or submersion due to accident to watercraft (V90-V91)
drowning or submersion of diver who voluntarily jumps from boat not involved in an accident (W16.711, W16.721)
fall into water without watercraft (W16-)
military watercraft accident in military or war operations (Y36, Y37)

The appropriate 7th character is to be added to each code from category V92.
A   initial encounter
D   subsequent encounter
S   sequela

☑5ᵗʰ **V92.0**   **Drowning and submersion due to fall off watercraft**
Drowning and submersion due to fall from gangplank of watercraft
Drowning and submersion due to fall overboard watercraft
EXCLUDES 2   *hitting head on object or bottom of body of water due to fall from watercraft (V94.0-)*

☑x7ᵗʰ **V92.00**   **Drowning and submersion due to fall off merchant ship**

☑x7ᵗʰ **V92.01**   **Drowning and submersion due to fall off passenger ship**
Drowning and submersion due to fall off Ferry-boat
Drowning and submersion due to fall off Liner

☑x7ᵗʰ **V92.02**   **Drowning and submersion due to fall off fishing boat**

☑x7ᵗʰ **V92.03**   **Drowning and submersion due to fall off other powered watercraft**
Drowning and submersion due to fall off Hovercraft (on open water)
Drowning and submersion due to fall off Jet ski

☑x7ᵗʰ **V92.04**   **Drowning and submersion due to fall off sailboat**

☑x7ᵗʰ **V92.05**   **Drowning and submersion due to fall off canoe or kayak**

☑x7ᵗʰ **V92.06**   **Drowning and submersion due to fall off (nonpowered) inflatable craft**

EXCLUDES 1   Not coded here   **EXCLUDES 2**   Not included here   *Manifestation Code*

✓x7ᵗʰ **V92.07 Drowning and submersion due to fall off water-skis**

> EXCLUDES 1   *drowning and submersion due to falling off burning water-skis (V90.27)*
> *drowning and submersion due to falling off crushed water-skis (V90.37)*
> *hit by boat while water-skiing NOS (V94.x)*

✓x7ᵗʰ **V92.08 Drowning and submersion due to fall off other unpowered watercraft**

Drowning and submersion due to fall off surf-board
Drowning and submersion due to fall off windsurfer

> EXCLUDES 1   *drowning and submersion due to fall off burning unpowered watercraft (V90.28)*
> *drowning and submersion due to fall off crushed unpowered watercraft (V90.38)*
> *drowning and submersion due to fall off damaged unpowered watercraft (V90.88)*
> *drowning and submersion due to rider of nonpowered watercraft being hit by other watercraft (V94.21)*
> *other injury due to rider of nonpowered watercraft being hit by other watercraft (V94.22)*

✓x7ᵗʰ **V92.09 Drowning and submersion due to fall off unspecified watercraft**

Drowning and submersion due to fall off boat NOS
Drowning and submersion due to fall off ship
Drowning and submersion due to fall off watercraft NOS

✓5ᵗʰ **V92.1 Drowning and submersion due to being thrown overboard by motion of watercraft**

> EXCLUDES 1   *drowning and submersion due to fall off surf-board (V92.08)*
> *drowning and submersion due to fall off water-skis (V92.07)*
> *drowning and submersion due to fall off windsurfer (V92.08)*

✓x7ᵗʰ **V92.10 Drowning and submersion due to being thrown overboard by motion of merchant ship**

✓x7ᵗʰ **V92.11 Drowning and submersion due to being thrown overboard by motion of passenger ship**

Drowning and submersion due to being thrown overboard by motion of Ferry-boat
Drowning and submersion due to being thrown overboard by motion of Liner

✓x7ᵗʰ **V92.12 Drowning and submersion due to being thrown overboard by motion of fishing boat**

✓x7ᵗʰ **V92.13 Drowning and submersion due to being thrown overboard by motion of other powered watercraft**

Drowning and submersion due to being thrown overboard by motion of Hovercraft

✓x7ᵗʰ **V92.14 Drowning and submersion due to being thrown overboard by motion of sailboat**

✓x7ᵗʰ **V92.15 Drowning and submersion due to being thrown overboard by motion of canoe or kayak**

✓x7ᵗʰ **V92.16 Drowning and submersion due to being thrown overboard by motion of (nonpowered) inflatable craft**

✓x7ᵗʰ **V92.19 Drowning and submersion due to being thrown overboard by motion of unspecified watercraft**

Drowning and submersion due to being thrown overboard by motion of boat NOS
Drowning and submersion due to being thrown overboard by motion of ship NOS
Drowning and submersion due to being thrown overboard by motion of watercraft NOS

✓5ᵗʰ **V92.2 Drowning and submersion due to being washed overboard from watercraft**

Code first any associated cataclysm (X37.0-)

✓x7ᵗʰ **V92.20 Drowning and submersion due to being washed overboard from merchant ship**

✓x7ᵗʰ **V92.21 Drowning and submersion due to being washed overboard from passenger ship**

Drowning and submersion due to being washed overboard from Ferry-boat
Drowning and submersion due to being washed overboard from Liner

✓x7ᵗʰ **V92.22 Drowning and submersion due to being washed overboard from fishing boat**

✓x7ᵗʰ **V92.23 Drowning and submersion due to being washed overboard from other powered watercraft**

Drowning and submersion due to being washed overboard from Hovercraft (on open water)
Drowning and submersion due to being washed overboard from Jet ski

✓x7ᵗʰ **V92.24 Drowning and submersion due to being washed overboard from sailboat**

✓x7ᵗʰ **V92.25 Drowning and submersion due to being washed overboard from canoe or kayak**

✓x7ᵗʰ **V92.26 Drowning and submersion due to being washed overboard from (nonpowered) inflatable craft**

✓x7ᵗʰ **V92.27 Drowning and submersion due to being washed overboard from water-skis**

> EXCLUDES 1   *drowning and submersion due to fall off water-skis (V92.07)*

✓x7ᵗʰ **V92.28 Drowning and submersion due to being washed overboard from other unpowered watercraft**

Drowning and submersion due to being washed overboard from surf-board
Drowning and submersion due to being washed overboard from windsurfer

✓x7ᵗʰ **V92.29 Drowning and submersion due to being washed overboard from unspecified watercraft**

Drowning and submersion due to being washed overboard from boat NOS
Drowning and submersion due to being washed overboard from ship NOS
Drowning and submersion due to being washed overboard from watercraft NOS

✓4ᵗʰ **V93 Other injury due to accident on board watercraft, without accident to watercraft**

> EXCLUDES 1   *civilian water transport accident involving military watercraft (V94.81-)*
> *other injury due to accident to watercraft (V91-)*
> *military watercraft accident in military or war operations (Y36, Y37-)*
>
> EXCLUDES 2   *drowning and submersion due to accident on board watercraft, without accident to watercraft (V92-)*

The appropriate 7th character is to be added to each code from category V93.
A   initial encounter
D   subsequent encounter
S   sequela

✓5ᵗʰ **V93.0 Burn due to localized fire on board watercraft**

> EXCLUDES 1   *burn due to watercraft on fire (V91.0-)*

✓x7ᵗʰ **V93.00 Burn due to localized fire on board merchant vessel**

✓x7ᵗʰ **V93.01 Burn due to localized fire on board passenger vessel**

Burn due to localized fire on board Ferry-boat
Burn due to localized fire on board Liner

✓x7ᵗʰ **V93.02 Burn due to localized fire on board fishing boat**

✓x7ᵗʰ **V93.03 Burn due to localized fire on board other powered watercraft**

Burn due to localized fire on board Hovercraft
Burn due to localized fire on board Jet ski

✓x7ᵗʰ **V93.04 Burn due to localized fire on board sailboat**

✓x7ᵗʰ **V93.09 Burn due to localized fire on board unspecified watercraft**

Burn due to localized fire on board boat NOS
Burn due to localized fire on board ship NOS
Burn due to localized fire on board watercraft NOS

✓5ᵗʰ **V93.1 Other burn on board watercraft**

Burn due to source other than fire on board watercraft

> EXCLUDES 1   *burn due to watercraft on fire (V91.0-)*

✓x7ᵗʰ **V93.10 Other burn on board merchant vessel**

✓x7ᵗʰ **V93.11 Other burn on board passenger vessel**

Other burn on board Ferry-boat
Other burn on board Liner

✓x7ᵗʰ **V93.12 Other burn on board fishing boat**

✓x7ᵗʰ **V93.13 Other burn on board other powered watercraft**

Other burn on board Hovercraft
Other burn on board Jet ski

✓x7ᵗʰ **V93.14 Other burn on board sailboat**

√x7ᵗʰ **V93.19 Other burn on board unspecified watercraft**
Other burn on board boat NOS
Other burn on board ship NOS
Other burn on board watercraft NOS

√5ᵗʰ **V93.2 Heat exposure on board watercraft**
    EXCLUDES 1   *exposure to man-made heat not aboard watercraft (W92)*
                    exposure to natural heat while on board watercraft (X30)
                    exposure to sunlight while on board watercraft (X32)
    EXCLUDES 2   *burn due to fire on board watercraft (V93.0-)*

√x7ᵗʰ **V93.20 Heat exposure on board merchant ship**
√x7ᵗʰ **V93.21 Heat exposure on board passenger ship**
Heat exposure on board Ferry-boat
Heat exposure on board Liner
√x7ᵗʰ **V93.22 Heat exposure on board fishing boat**
√x7ᵗʰ **V93.23 Heat exposure on board other powered watercraft**
Heat exposure on board hovercraft
√x7ᵗʰ **V93.24 Heat exposure on board sailboat**
√x7ᵗʰ **V93.29 Heat exposure on board unspecified watercraft**
Heat exposure on board boat NOS
Heat exposure on board ship NOS
Heat exposure on board watercraft NOS

√5ᵗʰ **V93.3 Fall on board watercraft**
    EXCLUDES 1   *fall due to collision of watercraft (V91.2-)*

√x7ᵗʰ **V93.30 Fall on board merchant ship**
√x7ᵗʰ **V93.31 Fall on board passenger ship**
Fall on board Ferry-boat
Fall on board Liner
√x7ᵗʰ **V93.32 Fall on board fishing boat**
√x7ᵗʰ **V93.33 Fall on board other powered watercraft**
Fall on board Hovercraft (on open water)
Fall on board Jet ski
√x7ᵗʰ **V93.34 Fall on board sailboat**
√x7ᵗʰ **V93.35 Fall on board canoe or kayak**
√x7ᵗʰ **V93.36 Fall on board (nonpowered) inflatable craft**
√x7ᵗʰ **V93.38 Fall on board other unpowered watercraft**
√x7ᵗʰ **V93.39 Fall on board unspecified watercraft**
Fall on board boat NOS
Fall on board ship NOS
Fall on board watercraft NOS

√5ᵗʰ **V93.4 Struck by falling object on board watercraft**
Hit by falling object on board watercraft
    EXCLUDES 1   *struck by falling object due to accident to watercraft (V91.3)*

√x7ᵗʰ **V93.40 Struck by falling object on merchant ship**
√x7ᵗʰ **V93.41 Struck by falling object on passenger ship**
Struck by falling object on Ferry-boat
Struck by falling object on Liner
√x7ᵗʰ **V93.42 Struck by falling object on fishing boat**
√x7ᵗʰ **V93.43 Struck by falling object on other powered watercraft**
Struck by falling object on Hovercraft
√x7ᵗʰ **V93.44 Struck by falling object on sailboat**
√x7ᵗʰ **V93.48 Struck by falling object on other unpowered watercraft**
√x7ᵗʰ **V93.49 Struck by falling object on unspecified watercraft**

√5ᵗʰ **V93.5 Explosion on board watercraft**
Boiler explosion on steamship
    EXCLUDES 2   *fire on board watercraft (V93.0-)*

√x7ᵗʰ **V93.50 Explosion on board merchant ship**
√x7ᵗʰ **V93.51 Explosion on board passenger ship**
Explosion on board Ferry-boat
Explosion on board Liner
√x7ᵗʰ **V93.52 Explosion on board fishing boat**
√x7ᵗʰ **V93.53 Explosion on board other powered watercraft**
Explosion on board Hovercraft
Explosion on board Jet ski
√x7ᵗʰ **V93.54 Explosion on board sailboat**
√x7ᵗʰ **V93.59 Explosion on board unspecified watercraft**
Explosion on board boat NOS
Explosion on board ship NOS
Explosion on board watercraft NOS

√5ᵗʰ **V93.6 Machinery accident on board watercraft**
    EXCLUDES 1   *machinery explosion on board watercraft (V93.4-)*
                    machinery fire on board watercraft (V93.0-)

√x7ᵗʰ **V93.60 Machinery accident on board merchant ship**

√x7ᵗʰ **V93.61 Machinery accident on board passenger ship**
Machinery accident on board Ferry-boat
Machinery accident on board Liner
√x7ᵗʰ **V93.62 Machinery accident on board fishing boat**
√x7ᵗʰ **V93.63 Machinery accident on board other powered watercraft**
Machinery accident on board Hovercraft
√x7ᵗʰ **V93.64 Machinery accident on board sailboat**
√x7ᵗʰ **V93.69 Machinery accident on board unspecified watercraft**
Machinery accident on board boat NOS
Machinery accident on board ship NOS
Machinery accident on board watercraft NOS

√5ᵗʰ **V93.8 Other injury due to other accident on board watercraft**
Accidental poisoning by gases or fumes on watercraft

√x7ᵗʰ **V93.80 Other injury due to other accident on board merchant ship**
√x7ᵗʰ **V93.81 Other injury due to other accident on board passenger ship**
Other injury due to other accident on board Ferry-boat
Other injury due to other accident on board Liner
√x7ᵗʰ **V93.82 Other injury due to other accident on board fishing boat**
√x7ᵗʰ **V93.83 Other injury due to other accident on board other powered watercraft**
Other injury due to other accident on board Hovercraft
Other injury due to other accident on board Jet ski
√x7ᵗʰ **V93.84 Other injury due to other accident on board sailboat**
√x7ᵗʰ **V93.85 Other injury due to other accident on board canoe or kayak**
√x7ᵗʰ **V93.86 Other injury due to other accident on board (nonpowered) inflatable craft**
√x7ᵗʰ **V93.87 Other injury due to other accident on board water-skis**
Hit or struck by object while waterskiing
√x7ᵗʰ **V93.88 Other injury due to other accident on board other unpowered watercraft**
Hit or struck by object while surfing
Hit or struck by object while on board windsurfer
√x7ᵗʰ **V93.89 Other injury due to other accident on board unspecified watercraft**
Other injury due to other accident on board boat NOS
Other injury due to other accident on board ship NOS
Other injury due to other accident on board watercraft NOS

√4ᵗʰ **V94 Other and unspecified water transport accidents**
    EXCLUDES 1   *military watercraft accidents in military or war operations (Y36, Y37)*

> The appropriate 7th character is to be added to each code from category V94.
> A   initial encounter
> D   subsequent encounter
> S   sequela

√x7ᵗʰ **V94.0 Hitting object or bottom of body of water due to fall from watercraft**
    EXCLUDES 2   *drowning and submersion due to fall from watercraft (V92.0-)*

√5ᵗʰ **V94.1 Bather struck by watercraft**
Swimmer hit by watercraft
√x7ᵗʰ **V94.11 Bather struck by powered watercraft**
√x7ᵗʰ **V94.12 Bather struck by nonpowered watercraft**

√5ᵗʰ **V94.2 Rider of nonpowered watercraft struck by other watercraft**
√x7ᵗʰ **V94.21 Rider of nonpowered watercraft struck by other nonpowered watercraft**
Canoer hit by other nonpowered watercraft
Surfer hit by other nonpowered watercraft
Windsurfer hit by other nonpowered watercraft
√x7ᵗʰ **V94.22 Rider of nonpowered watercraft struck by powered watercraft**
Canoer hit by motorboat
Surfer hit by motorboat
Windsurfer hit by motorboat

✓5ᵗʰ **V94.3** **Injury to rider of (inflatable) watercraft being pulled behind other watercraft**

    ✓x7ᵗʰ **V94.31** **Injury to rider of (inflatable) recreational watercraft being pulled behind other watercraft**
         Injury to rider of inner-tube pulled behind motor boat

    ✓x7ᵗʰ **V94.32** **Injury to rider of non-recreational watercraft being pulled behind other watercraft**
         Injury to occupant of dingy being pulled behind boat or ship
         Injury to occupant of life-raft being pulled behind boat or ship

✓x7ᵗʰ **V94.4** **Injury to barefoot water-skier**
     Injury to person being pulled behind boat or ship

✓5ᵗʰ **V94.8** **Other water transport accident**

    ✓6ᵗʰ **V94.81** **Water transport accident involving military watercraft**

        ✓7ᵗʰ **V94.810** **Civilian watercraft involved in water transport accident with military watercraft**
             Passenger on civilian watercraft injured due to accident with military watercraft

        ✓7ᵗʰ **V94.811** **Civilian in water injured by military watercraft**

        ✓7ᵗʰ **V94.818** **Other water transport accident involving military watercraft**

    ✓x7ᵗʰ **V94.89** **Other water transport accident**

✓x7ᵗʰ **V94.9** **Unspecified water transport accident**
     Water transport accident NOS

Air and space transport accidents (V95-V97)

EXCLUDES 1   *military aircraft accidents in military or war operations (Y36, Y37)*

✓4ᵗʰ **V95** **Accident to powered aircraft causing injury to occupant**

> The appropriate 7th character is to be added to each code from category V95.
> A   initial encounter
> D   subsequent encounter
> S   sequela

✓5ᵗʰ **V95.0** **Helicopter accident injuring occupant**
    ✓x7ᵗʰ **V95.00** **Unspecified helicopter accident injuring occupant**
    ✓x7ᵗʰ **V95.01** **Helicopter crash injuring occupant**
    ✓x7ᵗʰ **V95.02** **Forced landing of helicopter injuring occupant**
    ✓x7ᵗʰ **V95.03** **Helicopter collision injuring occupant**
         Helicopter collision with any object, fixed, movable or moving
    ✓x7ᵗʰ **V95.04** **Helicopter fire injuring occupant**
    ✓x7ᵗʰ **V95.05** **Helicopter explosion injuring occupant**
    ✓x7ᵗʰ **V95.09** **Other helicopter accident injuring occupant**

✓5ᵗʰ **V95.1** **Ultralight, microlight or powered-glider accident injuring occupant**
    ✓x7ᵗʰ **V95.10** **Unspecified ultralight, microlight or powered-glider accident injuring occupant**
    ✓x7ᵗʰ **V95.11** **Ultralight, microlight or powered-glider crash injuring occupant**
    ✓x7ᵗʰ **V95.12** **Forced landing of ultralight, microlight or powered-glider injuring occupant**
    ✓x7ᵗʰ **V95.13** **Ultralight, microlight or powered-glider collision injuring occupant**
         Ultralight, microlight or powered-glider collision with any object, fixed, movable or moving
    ✓x7ᵗʰ **V95.14** **Ultralight, microlight or powered-glider fire injuring occupant**
    ✓x7ᵗʰ **V95.15** **Ultralight, microlight or powered-glider explosion injuring occupant**
    ✓x7ᵗʰ **V95.19** **Other ultralight, microlight or powered-glider accident injuring occupant**

✓5ᵗʰ **V95.2** **Other private fixed-wing aircraft accident injuring occupant**
    ✓x7ᵗʰ **V95.20** **Unspecified accident to other private fixed-wing aircraft, injuring occupant**
    ✓x7ᵗʰ **V95.21** **Other private fixed-wing aircraft crash injuring occupant**
    ✓x7ᵗʰ **V95.22** **Forced landing of other private fixed-wing aircraft injuring occupant**

    ✓x7ᵗʰ **V95.23** **Other private fixed-wing aircraft collision injuring occupant**
         Other private fixed-wing aircraft collision with any object, fixed, movable or moving
    ✓x7ᵗʰ **V95.24** **Other private fixed-wing aircraft fire injuring occupant**
    ✓x7ᵗʰ **V95.25** **Other private fixed-wing aircraft explosion injuring occupant**
    ✓x7ᵗʰ **V95.29** **Other accident to other private fixed-wing aircraft injuring occupant**

✓5ᵗʰ **V95.3** **Commercial fixed-wing aircraft accident injuring occupant**
    ✓x7ᵗʰ **V95.30** **Unspecified accident to commercial fixed-wing aircraft injuring occupant**
    ✓x7ᵗʰ **V95.31** **Commercial fixed-wing aircraft crash injuring occupant**
    ✓x7ᵗʰ **V95.32** **Forced landing of commercial fixed-wing aircraft injuring occupant**
    ✓x7ᵗʰ **V95.33** **Commercial fixed-wing aircraft collision injuring occupant**
         Commercial fixed-wing aircraft collision with any object, fixed, movable or moving
    ✓x7ᵗʰ **V95.34** **Commercial fixed-wing aircraft fire injuring occupant**
    ✓x7ᵗʰ **V95.35** **Commercial fixed-wing aircraft explosion injuring occupant**
    ✓x7ᵗʰ **V95.39** **Other accident to commercial fixed-wing aircraft injuring occupant**

✓5ᵗʰ **V95.4** **Spacecraft accident injuring occupant**
    ✓x7ᵗʰ **V95.40** **Unspecified spacecraft accident injuring occupant**
    ✓x7ᵗʰ **V95.41** **Spacecraft crash injuring occupant**
    ✓x7ᵗʰ **V95.42** **Forced landing of spacecraft injuring occupant**
    ✓x7ᵗʰ **V95.43** **Spacecraft collision injuring occupant**
         Spacecraft collision with any object, fixed, moveable or moving
    ✓x7ᵗʰ **V95.44** **Spacecraft fire injuring occupant**
    ✓x7ᵗʰ **V95.45** **Spacecraft explosion injuring occupant**
    ✓x7ᵗʰ **V95.49** **Other spacecraft accident injuring occupant**

✓x7ᵗʰ **V95.8** **Other powered aircraft accidents injuring occupant**
✓x7ᵗʰ **V95.9** **Unspecified aircraft accident injuring occupant**
     Aircraft accident NOS
     Air transport accident NOS

✓4ᵗʰ **V96** **Accident to nonpowered aircraft causing injury to occupant**

> The appropriate 7th character is to be added to each code from category V96.
> A   initial encounter
> D   subsequent encounter
> S   sequela

✓5ᵗʰ **V96.0** **Balloon accident injuring occupant**
    ✓x7ᵗʰ **V96.00** **Unspecified balloon accident injuring occupant**
    ✓x7ᵗʰ **V96.01** **Balloon crash injuring occupant**
    ✓x7ᵗʰ **V96.02** **Forced landing of balloon injuring occupant**
    ✓x7ᵗʰ **V96.03** **Balloon collision injuring occupant**
         Balloon collision with any object, fixed, moveable or moving
    ✓x7ᵗʰ **V96.04** **Balloon fire injuring occupant**
    ✓x7ᵗʰ **V96.05** **Balloon explosion injuring occupant**
    ✓x7ᵗʰ **V96.09** **Other balloon accident injuring occupant**

✓5ᵗʰ **V96.1** **Hang-glider accident injuring occupant**
    ✓x7ᵗʰ **V96.10** **Unspecified hang-glider accident injuring occupant**
    ✓x7ᵗʰ **V96.11** **Hang-glider crash injuring occupant**
    ✓x7ᵗʰ **V96.12** **Forced landing of hang-glider injuring occupant**
    ✓x7ᵗʰ **V96.13** **Hang-glider collision injuring occupant**
         Hang-glider collision with any object, fixed, moveable or moving
    ✓x7ᵗʰ **V96.14** **Hang-glider fire injuring occupant**
    ✓x7ᵗʰ **V96.15** **Hang-glider explosion injuring occupant**
    ✓x7ᵗʰ **V96.19** **Other hang-glider accident injuring occupant**

✓5ᵗʰ **V96.2** **Glider (nonpowered) accident injuring occupant**
    ✓x7ᵗʰ **V96.20** **Unspecified glider (nonpowered) accident injuring occupant**
    ✓x7ᵗʰ **V96.21** **Glider (nonpowered) crash injuring occupant**
    ✓x7ᵗʰ **V96.22** **Forced landing of glider (nonpowered) injuring occupant**

☑ Appropriate additional character required   ✓x7ᵗʰ Requires 7th character, placeholder x must fill empty characters

External Causes of Morbidity

V96.23–W01.19

☑x7ᵗʰ **V96.23 Glider (nonpowered) collision injuring occupant**
Glider (nonpowered) collision with any object, fixed, moveable or moving

☑x7ᵗʰ **V96.24 Glider (nonpowered) fire injuring occupant**

☑x7ᵗʰ **V96.25 Glider (nonpowered) explosion injuring occupant**

☑x7ᵗʰ **V96.29 Other glider (nonpowered) accident injuring occupant**

☑x7ᵗʰ **V96.8 Other nonpowered-aircraft accidents injuring occupant**
Kite carrying a person accident injuring occupant

☑x7ᵗʰ **V96.9 Unspecified nonpowered-aircraft accident injuring occupant**
Nonpowered-aircraft accident NOS

☑4ᵗʰ **V97 Other specified air transport accidents**

> The appropriate 7th character is to be added to each code from category V97.
> A   initial encounter
> D   subsequent encounter
> S   sequela

☑x7ᵗʰ **V97.0 Occupant of aircraft injured in other specified air transport accidents**
Fall in, on or from aircraft in air transport accident
EXCLUDES 1   accident while boarding or alighting aircraft (V97.1)

☑x7ᵗʰ **V97.1 Person injured while boarding or alighting from aircraft**

☑5ᵗʰ **V97.2 Parachutist accident**

☑x7ᵗʰ **V97.21 Parachutist entangled in object**
Parachutist landing in tree

☑x7ᵗʰ **V97.22 Parachutist injured on landing**

☑x7ᵗʰ **V97.29 Other parachutist accident**

☑5ᵗʰ **V97.3 Person on ground injured in air transport accident**

☑x7ᵗʰ **V97.31 Hit by object falling from aircraft**
Hit by crashing aircraft
Injured by aircraft hitting house
Injured by aircraft hitting car

☑x7ᵗʰ **V97.32 Injured by rotating propeller**

☑x7ᵗʰ **V97.33 Sucked into jet engine**

☑x7ᵗʰ **V97.39 Other injury to person on ground due to air transport accident**

☑5ᵗʰ **V97.8 Other air transport accidents, not elsewhere classified**
EXCLUDES 1   aircraft accident NOS (V95.9)
exposure to changes in air pressure during ascent or descent (W94-)

☑6ᵗʰ **V97.81 Air transport accident involving military aircraft**

☑7ᵗʰ **V97.810 Civilian aircraft involved in air transport accident with military aircraft**
Passenger in civilian aircraft injured due to accident with military aircraft

☑7ᵗʰ **V97.811 Civilian injured by military aircraft**

☑7ᵗʰ **V97.818 Other air transport accident involving military aircraft**

☑x7ᵗʰ **V97.89 Other air transport accidents, not elsewhere classified**
Injury from machinery on aircraft

Other and unspecified transport accidents (V98-V99)

EXCLUDES 1   vehicle accident, type of vehicle unspecified (V89-)

☑4ᵗʰ **V98 Other specified transport accidents**

> The appropriate 7th character is to be added to each code from category V98.
> A   initial encounter
> D   subsequent encounter
> S   sequela

☑x7ᵗʰ **V98.0 Accident to, on or involving cable-car, not on rails**
Caught or dragged by cable-car, not on rails
Fall or jump from cable-car, not on rails
Object thrown from or in cable-car, not on rails

☑x7ᵗʰ **V98.1 Accident to, on or involving land-yacht**

☑x7ᵗʰ **V98.2 Accident to, on or involving ice yacht**

☑x7ᵗʰ **V98.3 Accident to, on or involving ski lift**
Accident to, on or involving ski chair-lift
Accident to, on or involving ski-lift with gondola

☑x7ᵗʰ **V98.8 Other specified transport accidents**

☑x7ᵗʰ **V99 Unspecified transport accident**

> The appropriate 7th character is to be added to code V99.
> A   initial encounter
> D   subsequent encounter
> S   sequela

OTHER EXTERNAL CAUSES OF ACCIDENTAL INJURY (W00-X58)

Slipping, tripping, stumbling and falls (W00-W19)

EXCLUDES 1   assault involving a fall (Y01-Y02)
fall (in) (from):
   animal (V80-)
   machinery (in operation) (W28-W31)
   transport vehicle (V01-V99)
intentional self-harm involving a fall (X80-X81)
EXCLUDES 2   at risk for fall (history of fall) Z91.81
fall (in) (from):
   burning building (X00-)
   into fire (X00-X04, X08-X09)

☑4ᵗʰ **W00 Fall due to ice and snow**
INCLUDES   pedestrian on foot falling (slipping) on ice and snow
EXCLUDES 1   fall on (from) ice and snow involving pedestrian conveyance (V00-)
fall from stairs and steps not due to ice and snow (W10-)

> The appropriate 7th character is to be added to each code from category W00.
> A   initial encounter
> D   subsequent encounter
> S   sequela

☑x7ᵗʰ **W00.0 Fall on same level due to ice and snow**

☑x7ᵗʰ **W00.1 Fall from stairs and steps due to ice and snow**

☑x7ᵗʰ **W00.2 Other fall from one level to another due to ice and snow**

☑x7ᵗʰ **W00.9 Unspecified fall due to ice and snow**

☑4ᵗʰ **W01 Fall on same level from slipping, tripping and stumbling**
INCLUDES   fall on moving sidewalk
EXCLUDES 1   fall due to bumping (striking) against object (W18.0-)
fall in shower or bathtub (W18.2-)
fall on same level NOS (W18.30)
fall on same level from slipping, tripping and stumbling due to ice or snow (W00.0)
fall off or from toilet (W18.1-)
slipping, tripping and stumbling NOS (W18.40)
slipping, tripping and stumbling without falling (W18.4-)

> The appropriate 7th character is to be added to each code from category W01.
> A   initial encounter
> D   subsequent encounter
> S   sequela

☑x7ᵗʰ **W01.0 Fall on same level from slipping, tripping and stumbling without subsequent striking against object**
Falling over animal

☑5ᵗʰ **W01.1 Fall on same level from slipping, tripping and stumbling with subsequent striking against object**

☑x7ᵗʰ **W01.10 Fall on same level from slipping, tripping and stumbling with subsequent striking against unspecified object**

☑6ᵗʰ **W01.11 Fall on same level from slipping, tripping and stumbling with subsequent striking against sharp object**

☑7ᵗʰ **W01.110 Fall on same level from slipping, tripping and stumbling with subsequent striking against sharp glass**

☑7ᵗʰ **W01.111 Fall on same level from slipping, tripping and stumbling with subsequent striking against power tool or machine**

☑7ᵗʰ **W01.118 Fall on same level from slipping, tripping and stumbling with subsequent striking against other sharp object**

☑7ᵗʰ **W01.119 Fall on same level from slipping, tripping and stumbling with subsequent striking against unspecified sharp object**

☑6ᵗʰ **W01.19 Fall on same level from slipping, tripping and stumbling with subsequent striking against other object**

EXCLUDES 1   Not coded here   EXCLUDES 2   Not included here   **Manifestation Code**

☑7th **W01.190** **Fall on same level from slipping, tripping and stumbling with subsequent striking against furniture**

☑7th **W01.198** **Fall on same level from slipping, tripping and stumbling with subsequent striking against other object**

W02 Deactivated
See category V00

✓☑7th **W03 Other fall on same level due to collision with another person**
Fall due to non-transport collision with other person

EXCLUDES 1 *collision with another person without fall (W51)*
crushed or pushed by a crowd or human stampede (W52)
fall involving pedestrian conveyance (V00-V09)
fall due to ice or snow (W00)
fall on same level NOS (W18.30)

The appropriate 7th character is to be added to code W03.
A　initial encounter
D　subsequent encounter
S　sequela

✓☑7th **W04 Fall while being carried or supported by other persons**
Accidentally dropped while being carried

The appropriate 7th character is to be added to code W04.
A　initial encounter
D　subsequent encounter
S　sequela

☑4th **W05 Fall from non-moving wheelchair, nonmotorized scooter and motorized mobility scooter**

EXCLUDES 1 *fall from moving wheelchair (powered) (V00.811)*
fall from moving motorized mobility scooter (V08.831)
fall from nonmotorized scooter (V08.841)

The appropriate 7th character is to be added to each code from category W05.
A　initial encounter
D　subsequent encounter
S　sequela

✓x7th **W05.0 Fall from non-moving wheelchair**
✓x7th **W05.1 Fall from non-moving nonmotorized scooter**
✓x7th **W05.2 Fall from non-moving motorized mobility scooter**

✓x7th **W06 Fall from bed**

The appropriate 7th character is to be added to code W06.
A　initial encounter
D　subsequent encounter
S　sequela

✓x7th **W07 Fall from chair**

The appropriate 7th character is to be added to code W07.
A　initial encounter
D　subsequent encounter
S　sequela

✓x7th **W08 Fall from other furniture**

The appropriate 7th character is to be added to code W08.
A　initial encounter
D　subsequent encounter
S　sequela

☑4th **W09 Fall on and from playground equipment**

EXCLUDES 1 *fall involving recreational machinery (W31)*

The appropriate 7th character is to be added to each code from category W09.
A　initial encounter
D　subsequent encounter
S　sequela

✓x7th **W09.0 Fall on or from playground slide**
✓x7th **W09.1 Fall from playground swing**
✓x7th **W09.2 Fall on or from jungle gym**
✓x7th **W09.8 Fall on or from other playground equipment**

☑4th **W10 Fall on and from stairs and steps**

EXCLUDES 1 *Fall from stairs and steps due to ice and snow (W00.1)*

The appropriate 7th character is to be added to each code from category W10.
A　initial encounter
D　subsequent encounter
S　sequela

✓x7th **W10.0 Fall (on)(from) escalator**
✓x7th **W10.1 Fall (on)(from) sidewalk curb**
✓x7th **W10.2 Fall (on)(from) incline**
Fall (on) (from) ramp
✓x7th **W10.8 Fall (on) (from) other stairs and steps**
✓x7th **W10.9 Fall (on) (from) unspecified stairs and steps**

✓x7th **W11 Fall on and from ladder**

The appropriate 7th character is to be added code W11.
A　initial encounter
D　subsequent encounter
S　sequela

✓x7th **W12 Fall on and from scaffolding**

The appropriate 7th character is to be added to code W12.
A　initial encounter
D　subsequent encounter
S　sequela

☑4th **W13 Fall from, out of or through building or structure**

The appropriate 7th character is to be added to each code from category W13.
A　initial encounter
D　subsequent encounter
S　sequela

✓x7th **W13.0 Fall from, out of or through balcony**
Fall from, out of or through railing
✓x7th **W13.1 Fall from, out of or through bridge**
✓x7th **W13.2 Fall from, out of or through roof**
✓x7th **W13.3 Fall through floor**
✓x7th **W13.4 Fall from, out of or through window**
EXCLUDES 2 *fall with subsequent striking against sharp glass (W01.110)*
✓x7th **W13.8 Fall from, out of or through other building or structure**
Fall from, out of or through viaduct
Fall from, out of or through wall
Fall from, out of or through flag-pole
✓x7th **W13.9 Fall from, out of or through building, not otherwise specified**
EXCLUDES 1 *collapse of a building or structure (W20-)*
fall or jump from burning building or structure (X00-)

✓x7th **W14 Fall from tree**

The appropriate 7th character is to be added to code W14.
A　initial encounter
D　subsequent encounter
S　sequela

✓x7th **W15 Fall from cliff**

The appropriate 7th character is to be added to code W15.
A　initial encounter
D　subsequent encounter
S　sequela

☑4th **W16 Fall, jump or diving into water**

EXCLUDES 1 *accidental non-watercraft drowning and submersion not involving fall (W65-W74)*
effects of air pressure from diving (W94-)
fall into water from watercraft (V90-V94)
hitting an object or against bottom when falling from watercraft (V94.0)
EXCLUDES 2 *striking or hitting diving board (W21.3)*

The appropriate 7th character is to be added to each code from category W16.
A　initial encounter
D　subsequent encounter
S　sequela

☑ Appropriate additional character required　　✓x7th Requires 7th character, placeholder x must fill empty characters

✓5th **W16.0** **Fall into swimming pool**
Fall into swimming pool NOS
EXCLUDES 1   *fall into empty swimming pool (W17.3)*

  ✓6th **W16.01** **Fall into swimming pool striking water surface**

    ✓7th **W16.011** **Fall into swimming pool striking water surface causing drowning and submersion**
EXCLUDES 1   *drowning and submersion while in swimming pool without fall (W67)*

    ✓7th **W16.012** **Fall into swimming pool striking water surface causing other injury**

  ✓6th **W16.02** **Fall into swimming pool striking bottom**

    ✓7th **W16.021** **Fall into swimming pool striking bottom causing drowning and submersion**
EXCLUDES 1   *drowning and submersion while in swimming pool without fall (W67)*

    ✓7th **W16.022** **Fall into swimming pool striking bottom causing other injury**

  ✓6th **W16.03** **Fall into swimming pool striking wall**

    ✓7th **W16.031** **Fall into swimming pool striking wall causing drowning and submersion**
EXCLUDES 1   *drowning and submersion while in swimming pool without fall (W67)*

    ✓7th **W16.032** **Fall into swimming pool striking wall causing other injury**

✓5th **W16.1** **Fall into natural body of water**
Fall into lake
Fall into open sea
Fall into river
Fall into stream

  ✓6th **W16.11** **Fall into natural body of water striking water surface**

    ✓7th **W16.111** **Fall into natural body of water striking water surface causing drowning and submersion**
EXCLUDES 1   *drowning and submersion while in natural body of water without fall (W69)*

    ✓7th **W16.112** **Fall into natural body of water striking water surface causing other injury**

  ✓6th **W16.12** **Fall into natural body of water striking bottom**

    ✓7th **W16.121** **Fall into natural body of water striking bottom causing drowning and submersion**
EXCLUDES 1   *drowning and submersion while in natural body of water without fall (W69)*

    ✓7th **W16.122** **Fall into natural body of water striking bottom causing other injury**

  ✓6th **W16.13** **Fall into natural body of water striking side**

    ✓7th **W16.131** **Fall into natural body of water striking side causing drowning and submersion**
EXCLUDES 1   *drowning and submersion while in natural body of water without fall (W69)*

    ✓7th **W16.132** **Fall into natural body of water striking side causing other injury**

✓5th **W16.2** **Fall in (into) filled bathtub or bucket of water**

  ✓6th **W16.21** **Fall in (into) filled bathtub**
EXCLUDES 1   *fall into empty bathtub (W18.2)*

    ✓7th **W16.211** **Fall in (into) filled bathtub causing drowning and submersion**
EXCLUDES 1   *drowning and submersion while in filled bathtub without fall (W65)*

    ✓7th **W16.212** **Fall in (into) filled bathtub causing other injury**

  ✓6th **W16.22** **Fall in (into) bucket of water**

    ✓7th **W16.221** **Fall in (into) bucket of water causing drowning and submersion**

    ✓7th **W16.222** **Fall in (into) bucket of water causing other injury**

✓5th **W16.3** **Fall into other water**
Fall into fountain
Fall into reservoir

  ✓6th **W16.31** **Fall into other water striking water surface**

    ✓7th **W16.311** **Fall into other water striking water surface causing drowning and submersion**
EXCLUDES 1   *drowning and submersion while in other water without fall (W73)*

    ✓7th **W16.312** **Fall into other water striking water surface causing other injury**

  ✓6th **W16.32** **Fall into other water striking bottom**

    ✓7th **W16.321** **Fall into other water striking bottom causing drowning and submersion**
EXCLUDES 1   *drowning and submersion while in other water without fall (W73)*

    ✓7th **W16.322** **Fall into other water striking bottom causing other injury**

  ✓6th **W16.33** **Fall into other water striking wall**

    ✓7th **W16.331** **Fall into other water striking wall causing drowning and submersion**
EXCLUDES 1   *drowning and submersion while in other water without fall (W73)*

    ✓7th **W16.332** **Fall into other water striking wall causing other injury**

✓5th **W16.4** **Fall into unspecified water**

  ✓x7th **W16.41** **Fall into unspecified water causing drowning and submersion**

  ✓x7th **W16.42** **Fall into unspecified water causing other injury**

✓5th **W16.5** **Jumping or diving into swimming pool**

  ✓6th **W16.51** **Jumping or diving into swimming pool striking water surface**

    ✓7th **W16.511** **Jumping or diving into swimming pool striking water surface causing drowning and submersion**
EXCLUDES 1   *drowning and submersion while in swimming pool without jumping or diving (W67)*

    ✓7th **W16.512** **Jumping or diving into swimming pool striking water surface causing other injury**

  ✓6th **W16.52** **Jumping or diving into swimming pool striking bottom**

    ✓7th **W16.521** **Jumping or diving into swimming pool striking bottom causing drowning and submersion**
EXCLUDES 1   *drowning and submersion while in swimming pool without jumping or diving (W67)*

    ✓7th **W16.522** **Jumping or diving into swimming pool striking bottom causing other injury**

  ✓6th **W16.53** **Jumping or diving into swimming pool striking wall**

    ✓7th **W16.531** **Jumping or diving into swimming pool striking wall causing drowning and submersion**
EXCLUDES 1   *drowning and submersion while in swimming pool without jumping or diving (W67)*

    ✓7th **W16.532** **Jumping or diving into swimming pool striking wall causing other injury**

✓5th **W16.6** **Jumping or diving into natural body of water**
Jumping or diving into lake
Jumping or diving into open sea
Jumping or diving into river
Jumping or diving into stream

  ✓6th **W16.61** **Jumping or diving into natural body of water striking water surface**

    ✓7th **W16.611** **Jumping or diving into natural body of water striking water surface causing drowning and submersion**
EXCLUDES 1   *drowning and submersion while in natural body of water without jumping or diving (W69)*

EXCLUDES 1   Not coded here   EXCLUDES 2   Not included here   *Manifestation Code*

√7ᵗʰ **W16.612** Jumping or diving into natural body of water striking water surface causing other injury

√6ᵗʰ **W16.62** Jumping or diving into natural body of water striking bottom

√7ᵗʰ **W16.621** Jumping or diving into natural body of water striking bottom causing drowning and submersion

> EXCLUDES 1 *drowning and submersion while in natural body of water without jumping or diving (W69)*

√7ᵗʰ **W16.622** Jumping or diving into natural body of water striking bottom causing other injury

√5ᵗʰ **W16.7** Jumping or diving from boat

> EXCLUDES 1 *Fall from boat into water—see watercraft accident (V90-V94)*

√6ᵗʰ **W16.71** Jumping or diving from boat striking water surface

√7ᵗʰ **W16.711** Jumping or diving from boat striking water surface causing drowning and submersion

√7ᵗʰ **W16.712** Jumping or diving from boat striking water surface causing other injury

√6ᵗʰ **W16.72** Jumping or diving from boat striking bottom

√7ᵗʰ **W16.721** Jumping or diving from boat striking bottom causing drowning and submersion

√7ᵗʰ **W16.722** Jumping or diving from boat striking bottom causing other injury

√5ᵗʰ **W16.8** Jumping or diving into other water

Jumping or diving into fountain
Jumping or diving into reservoir

√6ᵗʰ **W16.81** Jumping or diving into other water striking water surface

√7ᵗʰ **W16.811** Jumping or diving into other water striking water surface causing drowning and submersion

> EXCLUDES 1 *drowning and submersion while in other water without jumping or diving (W73)*

√7ᵗʰ **W16.812** Jumping or diving into other water striking water surface causing other injury

√6ᵗʰ **W16.82** Jumping or diving into other water striking bottom

√7ᵗʰ **W16.821** Jumping or diving into other water striking bottom causing drowning and submersion

> EXCLUDES 1 *drowning and submersion while in other water without jumping or diving (W73)*

√7ᵗʰ **W16.822** Jumping or diving into other water striking bottom causing other injury

√6ᵗʰ **W16.83** Jumping or diving into other water striking wall

√7ᵗʰ **W16.831** Jumping or diving into other water striking wall causing drowning and submersion

> EXCLUDES 1 *drowning and submersion while in other water without jumping or diving (W73)*

√7ᵗʰ **W16.832** Jumping or diving into other water striking wall causing other injury

√5ᵗʰ **W16.9** Jumping or diving into unspecified water

√x7ᵗʰ **W16.91** Jumping or diving into unspecified water causing drowning and submersion

√x7ᵗʰ **W16.92** Jumping or diving into unspecified water causing other injury

√4ᵗʰ **W17** Other fall from one level to another

> The appropriate 7th character is to be added to each code from category W17.
> A   initial encounter
> D   subsequent encounter
> S   sequela

√x7ᵗʰ **W17.0** Fall into well

√x7ᵗʰ **W17.1** Fall into storm drain or manhole

√x7ᵗʰ **W17.2** Fall into hole

Fall into pit

√x7ᵗʰ **W17.3** Fall into empty swimming pool

> EXCLUDES 1 *fall into filled swimming pool (W16.0-)*

√x7ᵗʰ **W17.4** Fall from dock

√5ᵗʰ **W17.8** Other fall from one level to another

√x7ᵗʰ **W17.81** Fall down embankment (hill)

√x7ᵗʰ **W17.82** Fall from (out of) grocery cart

Fall due to grocery cart tipping over

√x7ᵗʰ **W17.89** Other fall from one level to another

√4ᵗʰ **W18** Other slipping, tripping and stumbling and falls

> The appropriate 7th character is to be added to each code from category W18.
> A   initial encounter
> D   subsequent encounter
> S   sequela

√5ᵗʰ **W18.0** Fall due to bumping against object

Striking against object with subsequent fall

> EXCLUDES 1 *fall on same level due to slipping, tripping, or stumbling with subsequent striking against object (W01.1-)*

√x7ᵗʰ **W18.00** Striking against unspecified object with subsequent fall

√x7ᵗʰ **W18.01** Striking against sports equipment with subsequent fall

√x7ᵗʰ **W18.02** Striking against glass with subsequent fall

√x7ᵗʰ **W18.09** Striking against other object with subsequent fall

√5ᵗʰ **W18.1** Fall from or off toilet

√x7ᵗʰ **W18.11** Fall from or off toilet without subsequent striking against object

Fall from (off) toilet NOS

√x7ᵗʰ **W18.12** Fall from or off toilet with subsequent striking against object

√x7ᵗʰ **W18.2** Fall in (into) shower or empty bathtub

> EXCLUDES 1 *fall in full bathtub causing drowning or submersion (W16.21-)*

√5ᵗʰ **W18.3** Other and unspecified fall on same level

√x7ᵗʰ **W18.30** Fall on same level, unspecified

√x7ᵗʰ **W18.31** Fall on same level due to stepping on an object

Fall on same level due to stepping on an animal

> EXCLUDES 1 *slipping, tripping and stumbling without fall due to stepping on animal (W18.41)*

√x7ᵗʰ **W18.39** Other fall on same level

√5ᵗʰ **W18.4** Slipping, tripping and stumbling without falling

> EXCLUDES 1 *collision with another person without fall (W51)*

√x7ᵗʰ **W18.40** Slipping, tripping and stumbling without falling, unspecified

√x7ᵗʰ **W18.41** Slipping, tripping and stumbling without falling due to stepping on object

Slipping, tripping and stumbling without falling due to stepping on animal

> EXCLUDES 1 *slipping, tripping and stumbling with fall due to stepping on animal (W18.31)*

√x7ᵗʰ **W18.42** Slipping, tripping and stumbling without falling due to stepping into hole or opening

√x7ᵗʰ **W18.43** Slipping, tripping and stumbling without falling due to stepping from one level to another

√x7ᵗʰ **W18.49** Other slipping, tripping and stumbling without falling

√x7ᵗʰ **W19** Unspecified fall

Accidental fall NOS

> The appropriate 7th character is to be added to code W19.
> A   initial encounter
> D   subsequent encounter
> S   sequela

☑ Appropriate additional character required

√x7ᵗʰ Requires 7th character, placeholder x must fill empty characters

Exposure to inanimate mechanical forces (W20-W49)

EXCLUDES 1   assault (X91-Y08)
      contact or collision with animals or persons (W50-W64)
      exposure to inanimate mechanical forces involving military or war
         operations (Y36-, Y37-)
      intentional self-harm (X70-X83)

W20   Struck by thrown, projected or falling object
   Code first any associated:
     cataclysm (X34-X39)
     lightning strike (T75.00)
   EXCLUDES 1   falling object in:
         machinery accident (W24, W28-W31)
         transport accident (V01-V99)
       object set in motion by:
         explosion (W35-W40)
         firearm (W32-W34)
         struck by thrown sports equipment (W21-)

> The appropriate 7th character is to be added to each code from category W20.
> A   initial encounter
> D   subsequent encounter
> S   sequela

W20.0   Struck by falling object in cave-in
    EXCLUDES 2   asphyxiation due to cave-in (T71.21)

W20.1   Struck by object due to collapse of building
    EXCLUDES 1   struck by object due to collapse of burning building
            (X00.2, X02.2)

W20.8   Other cause of strike by thrown, projected or falling object
    EXCLUDES 1   struck by thrown sports equipment (W21-)

W21   Striking against or struck by sports equipment
   EXCLUDES 1   assault with sports equipment (Y08.0-)
         striking against or struck by sports equipment with
           subsequent fall (W18.01)

> The appropriate 7th character is to be added to each code from category W21.
> A   initial encounter
> D   subsequent encounter
> S   sequela

W21.0   Struck by hit or thrown ball
    W21.00   Struck by hit or thrown ball, unspecified type
    W21.01   Struck by football
    W21.02   Struck by soccer ball
    W21.03   Struck by baseball
    W21.04   Struck by golf ball
    W21.05   Struck by basketball
    W21.06   Struck by volleyball
    W21.07   Struck by softball
    W21.09   Struck by other hit or thrown ball

W21.1   Struck by bat, racquet or club
    W21.11   Struck by baseball bat
    W21.12   Struck by tennis racquet
    W21.13   Struck by golf club
    W21.19   Struck by other bat, racquet or club

W21.2   Struck by hockey stick or puck
    W21.21   Struck by hockey stick
      W21.210   Struck by ice hockey stick
      W21.211   Struck by field hockey stick
    W21.22   Struck by hockey puck
      W21.220   Struck by ice hockey puck
      W21.221   Struck by field hockey puck

W21.3   Struck by sports foot wear
    W21.31   Struck by shoe cleats
       Stepped on by shoe cleats
    W21.32   Struck by skate blades
       Skated over by skate blades
    W21.39   Struck by other sports foot wear

W21.4   Striking against diving board
     Use additional code for subsequent falling into water, if
     applicable (W16-)

W21.8   Striking against or struck by other sports equipment
    W21.81   Striking against or struck by football helmet
    **W21.89   Striking against or struck by other sports
          equipment**

W21.9   Striking against or struck by unspecified sports equipment

W22   Striking against or struck by other objects
   EXCLUDES 1   striking against or struck by object with subsequent fall
         (W18.09)

> The appropriate 7th character is to be added to each code from category W22.
> A   initial encounter
> D   subsequent encounter
> S   sequela

W22.0   Striking against stationary object
    EXCLUDES 1   striking against stationary sports equipment (W21.8)
    W22.01   Walked into wall
    W22.02   Walked into lamppost
    W22.03   Walked into furniture
    W22.04   Striking against wall of swimming pool
      **W22.041   Striking against wall of swimming pool
            causing drowning and submersion**
         EXCLUDES 1   drowning and submersion
               while swimming without
               striking against wall (W67)
      **W22.042   Striking against wall of swimming pool
            causing other injury**
    W22.09   Striking against other stationary object

W22.1   Striking against or struck by automobile airbag
    **W22.10   Striking against or struck by unspecified
          automobile airbag**
    **W22.11   Striking against or struck by driver side
          automobile airbag**
    **W22.12   Striking against or struck by front passenger side
          automobile airbag**
    **W22.19   Striking against or struck by other automobile
          airbag**

W22.8   Striking against or struck by other objects
    Striking against or struck by object NOS
    EXCLUDES 1   struck by thrown, projected or falling object (W20-)

W23   Caught, crushed, jammed or pinched in or between objects
   EXCLUDES 1   injury caused by cutting or piercing instruments (W25-W27)
         injury caused by firearms malfunction (W32.1, W33.1-,
           W34.1-)
         injury caused by lifting and transmission devices (W24-)
         injury caused by machinery (W28-W31)
         injury caused by nonpowered hand tools (W27-)
         injury caused by transport vehicle being used as a means of
          transportation (V01-V99)
         injury caused by struck by thrown, projected or falling object
          (W20-)

> The appropriate 7th character is to be added to each code from category W23.
> A   initial encounter
> D   subsequent encounter
> S   sequela

**W23.0   Caught, crushed, jammed, or pinched between moving
       objects**

**W23.1   Caught, crushed, jammed, or pinched between stationary
       objects**

**W24   Contact with lifting and transmission devices, not elsewhere
     classified**
   EXCLUDES 1   transport accidents (V01-V99)

> The appropriate 7th character is to be added to each code from category W24.
> A   initial encounter
> D   subsequent encounter
> S   sequela

W24.0   Contact with lifting devices, not elsewhere classified
     Contact with chain hoist
     Contact with drive belt
     Contact with pulley (block)

W24.1   Contact with transmission devices, not elsewhere classified
     Contact with transmission belt or cable

☑×7ᵗʰ W25 Contact with sharp glass
Code first any associated:
injury due to flying glass from explosion or firearm discharge (W32-W40)
transport accident (V00-V99)
EXCLUDES 1 *fall on same level due to slipping, tripping and stumbling with subsequent striking against sharp glass (W01.10)*
striking against sharp glass with subsequent fall (W18.02)

The appropriate 7th character is to be added to code W25.
A   initial encounter
D   subsequent encounter
S   sequela

☑4ᵗʰ W26 Contact with knife, sword or dagger

The appropriate 7th character is to be added to each code from category W26.
A   initial encounter
D   subsequent encounter
S   sequela

☑×7ᵗʰ W26.0 Contact with knife
EXCLUDES 1 *contact with electric knife (W29.1)*

☑×7ᵗʰ W26.1 Contact with sword or dagger

☑4ᵗʰ W27 Contact with nonpowered hand tool

The appropriate 7th character is to be added to each code from category W27.
A   initial encounter
D   subsequent encounter
S   sequela

☑×7ᵗʰ W27.0 Contact with workbench tool
Contact with auger
Contact with axe
Contact with chisel
Contact with handsaw
Contact with screwdriver

☑×7ᵗʰ W27.1 Contact with garden tool
Contact with hoe
Contact with nonpowered lawn mower
Contact with pitchfork
Contact with rake

☑×7ᵗʰ W27.2 Contact with scissors

☑×7ᵗʰ W27.3 Contact with needle (sewing)
EXCLUDES 1 *contact with hypodermic needle (W46-)*

☑×7ᵗʰ W27.4 Contact with kitchen utensil
Contact with fork
Contact with ice-pick
Contact with can-opener NOS

☑×7ᵗʰ W27.5 Contact with paper-cutter

☑×7ᵗʰ W27.8 Contact with other nonpowered hand tool
Contact with nonpowered sewing machine
Contact with shovel

☑×7ᵗʰ W28 Contact with powered lawn mower
Powered lawn mower (commercial) (residential)
EXCLUDES 1 *contact with nonpowered lawn mower (W27.1)*
EXCLUDES 2 *exposure to electric current (W86-)*

The appropriate 7th character is to be added to code W28.
A   initial encounter
D   subsequent encounter
S   sequela

☑4ᵗʰ W29 Contact with other powered hand tools and household machinery
EXCLUDES 1 *contact with commercial machinery (W31.82)*
contact with hot household appliance (X15)
contact with nonpowered hand tool (W27-)
exposure to electric current (W86)

The appropriate 7th character is to be added to each code from category W29.
A   initial encounter
D   subsequent encounter
S   sequela

☑×7ᵗʰ W29.0 Contact with powered kitchen appliance
Contact with blender
Contact with can-opener
Contact with garbage disposal
Contact with mixer

☑×7ᵗʰ W29.1 Contact with electric knife

☑×7ᵗʰ W29.2 Contact with other powered household machinery
Contact with electric fan
Contact with powered dryer (clothes) (powered) (spin)
Contact with washing-machine
Contact with sewing machine

☑×7ᵗʰ W29.3 Contact with powered garden and outdoor hand tools and machinery
Contact with chainsaw
Contact with edger
Contact with garden cultivator (tiller)
Contact with hedge trimmer
Contact with other powered garden tool
EXCLUDES 1 *contact with powered lawn mower (W28)*

☑×7ᵗʰ W29.4 Contact with nail gun

☑×7ᵗʰ W29.8 Contact with other powered powered hand tools and household machinery
Contact with do-it-yourself tool NOS

☑4ᵗʰ W30 Contact with agricultural machinery
INCLUDES animal-powered farm machine
EXCLUDES 1 *agricultural transport vehicle accident (V01-V99)*
explosion of grain store (W40.8)
exposure to electric current (W86-)

The appropriate 7th character is to be added to each code from category W30.
A   initial encounter
D   subsequent encounter
S   sequela

☑×7ᵗʰ W30.0 Contact with combine harvester
Contact with reaper
Contact with thresher

☑×7ᵗʰ W30.1 Contact with power take-off devices (PTO)

☑×7ᵗʰ W30.2 Contact with hay derrick

☑×7ᵗʰ W30.3 Contact with grain storage elevator
EXCLUDES 1 *explosion of grain store (W40.8)*

☑5ᵗʰ W30.8 Contact with other specified agricultural machinery

☑×7ᵗʰ W30.81 Contact with agricultural transport vehicle in stationary use
Contact with agricultural transport vehicle under repair, not on public roadway
EXCLUDES 1 *agricultural transport vehicle accident (V01-V99)*

☑×7ᵗʰ W30.89 Contact with other specified agricultural machinery

☑×7ᵗʰ W30.9 Contact with unspecified agricultural machinery
Contact with farm machinery NOS

☑4ᵗʰ W31 Contact with other and unspecified machinery
EXCLUDES 1 *contact with agricultural machinery (W30-)*
contact with machinery in transport under own power or being towed by a vehicle (V01-V99)
exposure to electric current (W86)

The appropriate 7th character is to be added to each code from category W31.
A   initial encounter
D   subsequent encounter
S   sequela

☑×7ᵗʰ W31.0 Contact with mining and earth-drilling machinery
Contact with bore or drill (land) (seabed)
Contact with shaft hoist
Contact with shaft lift
Contact with undercutter

☑×7ᵗʰ W31.1 Contact with metalworking machines
Contact with abrasive wheel
Contact with forging machine
Contact with lathe
Contact with mechanical shears
Contact with metal drilling machine
Contact with milling machine
Contact with power press
Contact with rolling-mill
Contact with metal sawing machine

☑ Appropriate additional character required   ☑×7ᵗʰ Requires 7th character, placeholder x must fill empty characters

√x7th **W31.2 Contact with powered woodworking and forming machines**
Contact with band saw
Contact with bench saw
Contact with circular saw
Contact with molding machine
Contact with overhead plane
Contact with powered saw
Contact with radial saw
Contact with sander
EXCLUDES 1 *nonpowered woodworking tools (W27.0)*

√x7th **W31.3 Contact with prime movers**
Contact with gas turbine
Contact with internal combustion engine
Contact with steam engine
Contact with water driven turbine

√5th **W31.8 Contact with other specified machinery**

√x7th **W31.81 Contact with recreational machinery**
Contact with roller coaster

√x7th **W31.82 Contact with other commercial machinery**
Contact with commercial electric fan
Contact with commercial kitchen appliances
Contact with commercial powered dryer (clothes) (powered) (spin)
Contact with commercial washing-machine
Contact with commercial sewing machine
EXCLUDES 1 *contact with household machinery (W29-)*
contact with powered lawn mower (W28)

√x7th **W31.83 Contact with special construction vehicle in stationary use**
Contact with special construction vehicle under repair, not on public roadway
EXCLUDES 1 *special construction vehicle accident (V01-V99)*

√x7th **W31.89 Contact with other specified machinery**

√x7th **W31.9 Contact with unspecified machinery**
Contact with machinery NOS

√4th **W32 Accidental handgun discharge and malfunction**
INCLUDES Accidental discharge and malfunction of gun for single hand use
Accidental discharge and malfunction of pistol
Accidental discharge and malfunction of revolver
Handgun discharge and malfunction NOS
EXCLUDES 1 *accidental airgun discharge and malfunction (W34.010, W34.110)*
accidental BB gun discharge and malfunction (W34.010, W34.110)
accidental pellet gun discharge and malfunction (W34.010, W34.110)
accidental shotgun discharge and malfunction (W33.01, W33.11)
assault by handgun discharge (X93)
handgun discharge involving legal intervention (Y35.0-)
handgun discharge involving military or war operations (Y36.4-)
intentional self-harm by handgun discharge (X72)
Very pistol discharge and malfunction (W34.09, W34.19)

The appropriate 7th character is to be added to each code from category W32.
A   initial encounter
D   subsequent encounter
S   sequela

√x7th **W32.0 Accidental handgun discharge**
√x7th **W32.1 Accidental handgun malfunction**
Injury due to explosion of handgun (parts)
Injury due to malfunction of mechanism or component of handgun
Injury due to recoil of handgun
Powder burn from handgun

√4th **W33 Accidental rifle, shotgun and larger firearm discharge and malfunction**
INCLUDES rifle, shotgun and larger firearm discharge and malfunction NOS
EXCLUDES 1 *accidental airgun discharge and malfunction (W34.010, W34.110)*
accidental BB gun discharge and malfunction (W34.010, W34.110)
accidental handgun discharge and malfunction (W32-)
accidental pellet gun discharge and malfunction (W34.010, W34.110)
assault by rifle, shotgun and larger firearm discharge (X94)
firearm discharge involving legal intervention (Y35.0-)
firearm discharge involving military or war operations (Y36.4-)
intentional self-harm by rifle, shotgun and larger firearm discharge (X73)

The appropriate 7th character is to be added to each code from category W33.
A   initial encounter
D   subsequent encounter
S   sequela

√5th **W33.0 Accidental rifle, shotgun and larger firearm discharge**
√x7th **W33.00 Accidental discharge of unspecified larger firearm**
Discharge of unspecified larger firearm NOS
√x7th **W33.01 Accidental discharge of shotgun**
Discharge of shotgun NOS
√x7th **W33.02 Accidental discharge of hunting rifle**
Discharge of hunting rifle NOS
√x7th **W33.03 Accidental discharge of machine gun**
Discharge of machine gun NOS
√x7th **W33.09 Accidental discharge of other larger firearm**
Discharge of other larger firearm NOS

√5th **W33.1 Accidental rifle, shotgun and larger firearm malfunction**
Injury due to explosion of rifle, shotgun and larger firearm (parts)
Injury due to malfunction of mechanism or component of rifle, shotgun and larger firearm
Injury due to piercing, cutting, crushing or pinching due to (by) slide trigger mechanism, scope or other gun part
Injury due to recoil of rifle, shotgun and larger firearm
Powder burn from rifle, shotgun and larger firearm
√x7th **W33.10 Accidental malfunction of unspecified larger firearm**
Malfunction of unspecified larger firearm NOS
√x7th **W33.11 Accidental malfunction of shotgun**
Malfunction of shotgun NOS
√x7th **W33.12 Accidental malfunction of hunting rifle**
Malfunction of hunting rifle NOS
√x7th **W33.13 Accidental malfunction of machine gun**
Malfunction of machine gun NOS
√x7th **W33.19 Accidental malfunction of other larger firearm**
Malfunction of other larger firearm NOS

√4th **W34 Accidental discharge and malfunction from other and unspecified firearms and guns**

The appropriate 7th character is to be added to each code from category W34.
A   initial encounter
D   subsequent encounter
S   sequela

√5th **W34.0 Accidental discharge from other and unspecified firearms and guns**
√x7th **W34.00 Accidental discharge from unspecified firearms or gun**
Discharge from firearm NOS
Gunshot wound NOS
Shot NOS
√6th **W34.01 Accidental discharge of gas, air or spring-operated guns**
√7th **W34.010 Accidental discharge of airgun**
Accidental discharge of BB gun
Accidental discharge of pellet gun
√7th **W34.011 Accidental discharge of paintball gun**
Accidental injury due to paintball discharge
√7th **W34.018 Accidental discharge of other gas, air or spring-operated gun**

√x7th **W34.09** **Accidental discharge from other specified firearms**
Accidental discharge from Very pistol [flare]

√5th **W34.1** **Accidental malfunction from other and unspecified firearms and guns**

√x7th **W34.10** **Accidental malfunction from unspecified firearms or gun**
Firearm malfunction NOS

√6th **W34.11** **Accidental malfunction of gas, air or spring-operated guns**

√7th **W34.110** **Accidental malfunction of airgun**
Accidental malfunction of BB gun
Accidental malfunction of pellet gun

√7th **W34.111** **Accidental malfunction of paintball gun**
Accidental injury due to paintball gun malfunction

√7th **W34.118** **Accidental malfunction of other gas, air or spring-operated gun**

√x7th **W34.19** **Accidental malfunction from other specified firearms**
Accidental malfunction from Very pistol [flare]

√x7th **W35 Explosion and rupture of boiler**
EXCLUDES 1 *explosion and rupture of boiler on watercraft (V93.4)*

The appropriate 7th character is to be added to code W35.
A   initial encounter
D   subsequent encounter
S   sequela

√4th **W36 Explosion and rupture of gas cylinder**

The appropriate 7th character is to be added to each code from category W36.
A   initial encounter
D   subsequent encounter
S   sequela

√x7th **W36.1** **Explosion and rupture of aerosol can**
√x7th **W36.2** **Explosion and rupture of air tank**
√x7th **W36.3** **Explosion and rupture of pressurized-gas tank**
√x7th **W36.8** **Explosion and rupture of other gas cylinder**
√x7th **W36.9** **Explosion and rupture of unspecified gas cylinder**

√4th **W37 Explosion and rupture of pressurized tire, pipe or hose**

The appropriate 7th character is to be added to each code from category W37.
A   initial encounter
D   subsequent encounter
S   sequela

√x7th **W37.0** **Explosion of bicycle tire**
√x7th **W37.8** **Explosion and rupture of other pressurized tire, pipe or hose**

√x7th **W38 Explosion and rupture of other specified pressurized devices**

The appropriate 7th character is to be added to code W38.
A   initial encounter
D   subsequent encounter
S   sequela

√x7th **W39 Discharge of firework**

The appropriate 7th character is to be added to code W39.
A   initial encounter
D   subsequent encounter
S   sequela

√4th **W40 Explosion of other materials**
EXCLUDES 1 *assault by explosive material (X96)*
explosion involving legal intervention (Y35.1-)
explosion involving military or war operations (Y36.0-, Y36.2-)
intentional self-harm by explosive material (X75)

The appropriate 7th character is to be added to each code from category W40.
A   initial encounter
D   subsequent encounter
S   sequela

√x7th **W40.0** **Explosion of blasting material**
Explosion of blasting cap
Explosion of detonator
Explosion of dynamite
Explosion of explosive (any) used in blasting operations

√x7th **W40.1** **Explosion of explosive gases**
Explosion of acetylene
Explosion of butane
Explosion of coal gas
Explosion in mine NOS
Explosion of explosive gas
Explosion of fire damp
Explosion of gasoline fumes
Explosion of methane
Explosion of propane

√x7th **W40.8** **Explosion of other specified explosive materials**
Explosion in dump NOS
Explosion in factory NOS
Explosion in grain store
Explosion in munitions
EXCLUDES 1 *explosion involving legal intervention (Y35.1-)*
explosion involving military or war operations (Y36.0-, Y36.2-)

√x7th **W40.9** **Explosion of unspecified explosive materials**
Explosion NOS

W41 Deactivated
See subcategory T70.4

√4th **W42 Exposure to noise**

The appropriate 7th character is to be added to each code from category W42.
A   initial encounter
D   subsequent encounter
S   sequela

√x7th **W42.0** **Exposure to supersonic waves**
√x7th **W42.9** **Exposure to other noise**
Exposure to sound waves NOS

W43 Deactivated
See subcategory T75.2

W44 Deactivated
See categories T15-T19

√4th **W45 Foreign body or object entering through skin**
EXCLUDES 2 *contact with hand tools (nonpowered) (powered) (W27-W29)*
contact with knife, sword or dagger (W26-)
contact with sharp glass (W25-)
struck by objects (W20-W22)

The appropriate 7th character is to be added to each code from category W45.
A   initial encounter
D   subsequent encounter
S   sequela

√x7th **W45.0** **Nail entering through skin**
√x7th **W45.1** **Paper entering through skin**
Paper cut
√x7th **W45.2** **Lid of can entering through skin**
√x7th **W45.8** **Other foreign body or object entering through skin**
Splinter in skin NOS

√4th **W46 Contact with hypodermic needle**

The appropriate 7th character is to be added to each code from category W46.
A   initial encounter
D   subsequent encounter
S   sequela

√x7th **W46.0** **Contact with hypodermic needle**
Hypodermic needle stick NOS
√x7th **W46.1** **Contact with contaminated hypodermic needle**

☑ Appropriate additional character required   √x7th Requires 7th character, placeholder x must fill empty characters

External Causes of Morbidity

W49–W56.11

✓4ᵗʰ **W49 Exposure to other inanimate mechanical forces**
> INCLUDES exposure to abnormal gravitational [G] forces
> exposure to inanimate mechanical forces NEC
>
> EXCLUDES 1 exposure to inanimate mechanical forces involving military or war operations (Y36-, Y37-)

> The appropriate 7th character is to be added to each code from category W49.
> A   initial encounter
> D   subsequent encounter
> S   sequela

✓5ᵗʰ **W49.0 Item causing external constriction**
   ✓x7ᵗʰ **W49.01 Hair causing external constriction**
   ✓x7ᵗʰ **W49.02 String or thread causing external constriction**
   ✓x7ᵗʰ **W49.03 Rubber band causing external constriction**
   ✓x7ᵗʰ **W49.04 Ring or other jewelry causing external constriction**
   ✓x7ᵗʰ **W49.09 Other specified item causing external constriction**
✓x7ᵗʰ **W49.9 Exposure to other inanimate mechanical forces**

Exposure to animate mechanical forces (W50-W64)
> EXCLUDES 1 Toxic effect of contact with venomous animals and plants (T63-)

✓4ᵗʰ **W50 Accidental hit, strike, kick, twist, bite or scratch by another person**
> Hit, strike, kick, twist, bite, or scratch by another person NOS
>
> EXCLUDES 1 assault by bodily force (Y04)
> struck by objects (W20-W22)

> The appropriate 7th character is to be added to each code from category W50.
> A   initial encounter
> D   subsequent encounter
> S   sequela

✓x7ᵗʰ **W50.0 Accidental hit or strike by another person**
> Hit or strike by another person NOS
✓x7ᵗʰ **W50.1 Accidental kick by another person**
> Kick by another person NOS
✓x7ᵗʰ **W50.2 Accidental twist by another person**
> Twist by another person NOS
✓x7ᵗʰ **W50.3 Accidental bite by another person**
> Human bite
> Bite by another person NOS
✓x7ᵗʰ **W50.4 Accidental scratch by another person**
> Scratch by another person NOS

✓x7ᵗʰ **W51 Accidental striking against or bumped into by another person**
> EXCLUDES 1 assault by striking against or bumping into by another person (Y04.2)
> fall due to collision with another person (W03)

> The appropriate 7th character is to be added to code W51.
> A   initial encounter
> D   subsequent encounter
> S   sequela

✓x7ᵗʰ **W52 Crushed, pushed or stepped on by crowd or human stampede**
> Crushed, pushed or stepped on by crowd or human stampede with or without fall

> The appropriate 7th character is to be added to code W52.
> A   initial encounter
> D   subsequent encounter
> S   sequela

✓4ᵗʰ **W53 Contact with rodent**
> Contact with saliva, feces or urine of rodent

> The appropriate 7th character is to be added to each code from category W53.
> A   initial encounter
> D   subsequent encounter
> S   sequela

✓5ᵗʰ **W53.0 Contact with mouse**
   ✓x7ᵗʰ **W53.01 Bitten by mouse**
   ✓x7ᵗʰ **W53.09 Other contact with mouse**
✓5ᵗʰ **W53.1 Contact with rat**
   ✓x7ᵗʰ **W53.11 Bitten by rat**
   ✓x7ᵗʰ **W53.19 Other contact with rat**
✓5ᵗʰ **W53.2 Contact with squirrel**
   ✓x7ᵗʰ **W53.21 Bitten by squirrel**
   ✓x7ᵗʰ **W53.29 Other contact with squirrel**
✓5ᵗʰ **W53.8 Contact with other rodent**
   ✓x7ᵗʰ **W53.81 Bitten by other rodent**
   ✓x7ᵗʰ **W53.89 Other contact with other rodent**

✓4ᵗʰ **W54 Contact with dog**
> Contact with saliva, feces or urine of dog

> The appropriate 7th character is to be added to each code from category W54.
> A   initial encounter
> D   subsequent encounter
> S   sequela

✓x7ᵗʰ **W54.0 Bitten by dog**
✓x7ᵗʰ **W54.1 Struck by dog**
> Knocked over by dog
✓x7ᵗʰ **W54.8 Other contact with dog**

✓4ᵗʰ **W55 Contact with other mammals**
> Contact with saliva, feces or urine of mammal
>
> EXCLUDES 1 animal being ridden—see transport accidents
> bitten or struck by dog (W54)
> bitten or struck by rodent (W53-)
> contact with marine mammals (W56.x-)

> The appropriate 7th character is to be added to each code from category W55.
> A   initial encounter
> D   subsequent encounter
> S   sequela

✓5ᵗʰ **W55.0 Contact with cat**
   ✓x7ᵗʰ **W55.01 Bitten by cat**
   ✓x7ᵗʰ **W55.03 Scratched by cat**
   ✓x7ᵗʰ **W55.09 Other contact with cat**
✓5ᵗʰ **W55.1 Contact with horse**
   ✓x7ᵗʰ **W55.11 Bitten by horse**
   ✓x7ᵗʰ **W55.12 Struck by horse**
   ✓x7ᵗʰ **W55.19 Other contact with horse**
✓5ᵗʰ **W55.2 Contact with cow**
> Contact with bull
   ✓x7ᵗʰ **W55.21 Bitten by cow**
   ✓x7ᵗʰ **W55.22 Struck by cow**
> Gored by bull
   ✓x7ᵗʰ **W55.29 Other contact with cow**
✓5ᵗʰ **W55.3 Contact with other hoof stock**
> Contact with goats
> Contact with sheep
   ✓x7ᵗʰ **W55.31 Bitten by other hoof stock**
   ✓x7ᵗʰ **W55.32 Struck by other hoof stock**
> Gored by goat
> Gored by ram
   ✓x7ᵗʰ **W55.39 Other contact with other hoof stock**
✓5ᵗʰ **W55.4 Contact with pig**
   ✓x7ᵗʰ **W55.41 Bitten by pig**
   ✓x7ᵗʰ **W55.42 Struck by pig**
   ✓x7ᵗʰ **W55.49 Other contact with pig**
✓5ᵗʰ **W55.5 Contact with raccoon**
   ✓x7ᵗʰ **W55.51 Bitten by raccoon**
   ✓x7ᵗʰ **W55.52 Struck by raccoon**
   ✓x7ᵗʰ **W55.59 Other contact with raccoon**
✓5ᵗʰ **W55.8 Contact with other mammals**
   ✓x7ᵗʰ **W55.81 Bitten by other mammals**
   ✓x7ᵗʰ **W55.82 Struck by other mammals**
   ✓x7ᵗʰ **W55.89 Other contact with other mammals**

✓4ᵗʰ **W56 Contact with nonvenomous marine animal**
> EXCLUDES 1 contact with venomous marine animal (T63-)

> The appropriate 7th character is to be added to each code from category W56.
> A   initial encounter
> D   subsequent encounter
> S   sequela

✓5ᵗʰ **W56.0 Contact with dolphin**
   ✓x7ᵗʰ **W56.01 Bitten by dolphin**
   ✓x7ᵗʰ **W56.02 Struck by dolphin**
   ✓x7ᵗʰ **W56.09 Other contact with dolphin**
✓5ᵗʰ **W56.1 Contact with sea lion**
   ✓x7ᵗʰ **W56.11 Bitten by sea lion**

EXCLUDES 1 Not coded here   EXCLUDES 2 Not included here   *Manifestation Code*

√x7ᵗʰ **W56.12 Struck by sea lion**
W56.19 Other contact with sea lion
√5ᵗʰ **W56.2 Contact with orca**
Contact with killer whale
√x7ᵗʰ **W56.21 Bitten by orca**
√x7ᵗʰ **W56.22 Struck by orca**
√x7ᵗʰ **W56.29 Other contact with orca**
√5ᵗʰ **W56.3 Contact with other marine mammals**
√x7ᵗʰ **W56.31 Bitten by other marine mammals**
√x7ᵗʰ **W56.32 Struck by other marine mammals**
√x7ᵗʰ **W56.39 Other contact with other marine mammals**
√5ᵗʰ **W56.4 Contact with shark**
√x7ᵗʰ **W56.41 Bitten by shark**
√x7ᵗʰ **W56.42 Struck by shark**
√x7ᵗʰ **W56.49 Other contact with shark**
√5ᵗʰ **W56.5 Contact with other fish**
√x7ᵗʰ **W56.51 Bitten by other fish**
√x7ᵗʰ **W56.52 Struck by other fish**
√x7ᵗʰ **W56.59 Other contact with other fish**
√5ᵗʰ **W56.8 Contact with other nonvenomous marine animals**
√x7ᵗʰ **W56.81 Bitten by other nonvenomous marine animals**
√x7ᵗʰ **W56.82 Struck by other nonvenomous marine animals**
√x7ᵗʰ **W56.89 Other contact with other nonvenomous marine animals**

√x7ᵗʰ **W57 Bitten or stung by nonvenomous insect and other nonvenomous arthropods**
EXCLUDES 1   *contact with venomous insects and arthropods (T63.2-, T63.3-, T63.4-)*

The appropriate 7th character is to be added to code W57.
A   initial encounter
D   subsequent encounter
S   sequela

☑4ᵗʰ **W58 Contact with crocodile or alligator**

The appropriate 7th character is to be added to each code from category W58.
A   initial encounter
D   subsequent encounter
S   sequela

√5ᵗʰ **W58.0 Contact with alligator**
√x7ᵗʰ **W58.01 Bitten by alligator**
√x7ᵗʰ **W58.02 Struck by alligator**
√x7ᵗʰ **W58.03 Crushed by alligator**
√x7ᵗʰ **W58.09 Other contact with alligator**
√5ᵗʰ **W58.1 Contact with crocodile**
√x7ᵗʰ **W58.11 Bitten by crocodile**
√x7ᵗʰ **W58.12 Struck by crocodile**
√x7ᵗʰ **W58.13 Crushed by crocodile**
√x7ᵗʰ **W58.19 Other contact with crocodile**

☑4ᵗʰ **W59 Contact with other nonvenomous reptiles**
EXCLUDES 1   *contact with venomous reptile (T63.0-, T63.1-)*

The appropriate 7th character is to be added to each code from category W59.
A   initial encounter
D   subsequent encounter
S   sequela

√5ᵗʰ **W59.0 Contact with nonvenomous lizards**
√x7ᵗʰ **W59.01 Bitten by nonvenomous lizards**
√x7ᵗʰ **W59.02 Struck by nonvenomous lizards**
√x7ᵗʰ **W59.09 Other contact with nonvenomous lizards**
Exposure to nonvenomous lizards
√5ᵗʰ **W59.1 Contact with nonvenomous snakes**
√x7ᵗʰ **W59.11 Bitten by nonvenomous snake**
√x7ᵗʰ **W59.12 Struck by nonvenomous snake**
√x7ᵗʰ **W59.13 Crushed by nonvenomous snake**
√x7ᵗʰ **W59.19 Other contact with nonvenomous snake**
√5ᵗʰ **W59.2 Contact with turtles**
EXCLUDES 1   *contact with tortoises (W59.8-)*
√x7ᵗʰ **W59.21 Bitten by turtle**
√x7ᵗʰ **W59.22 Struck by turtle**
√x7ᵗʰ **W59.29 Other contact with turtle**
Exposure to turtles
√5ᵗʰ **W59.8 Contact with other nonvenomous reptiles**

√x7ᵗʰ **W59.81 Bitten by other nonvenomous reptiles**
√x7ᵗʰ **W59.82 Struck by other nonvenomous reptiles**
√x7ᵗʰ **W59.83 Crushed by other nonvenomous reptiles**
√x7ᵗʰ **W59.89 Other contact with other nonvenomous reptiles**

√x7ᵗʰ **W60 Contact with nonvenomous plant thorns and spines and sharp leaves**
EXCLUDES 1   *contact with venomous plants (T63.x-)*

The appropriate 7th character is to be added to code W56.
A   initial encounter
D   subsequent encounter
S   sequela

☑4ᵗʰ **W61 Contact with birds (domestic) (wild)**
Contact with excreta of birds

The appropriate 7th character is to be added to each code from category W61.
A   initial encounter
D   subsequent encounter
S   sequela

√5ᵗʰ **W61.0 Contact with parrot**
√x7ᵗʰ **W61.01 Bitten by parrot**
√x7ᵗʰ **W61.02 Struck by parrot**
√x7ᵗʰ **W61.09 Other contact with parrot**
Exposure to parrots
√5ᵗʰ **W61.1 Contact with macaw**
√x7ᵗʰ **W61.11 Bitten by macaw**
√x7ᵗʰ **W61.12 Struck by macaw**
√x7ᵗʰ **W61.19 Other contact with macaw**
Exposure to macaws
√5ᵗʰ **W61.2 Contact with other psittacines**
√x7ᵗʰ **W61.21 Bitten by other psittacines**
√x7ᵗʰ **W61.22 Struck by other psittacines**
√x7ᵗʰ **W61.29 Other contact with other psittacines**
Exposure to other psittacines
√5ᵗʰ **W61.3 Contact with chicken**
√x7ᵗʰ **W61.32 Struck by chicken**
√x7ᵗʰ **W61.33 Pecked by chicken**
√x7ᵗʰ **W61.39 Other contact with chicken**
Exposure to chickens
√5ᵗʰ **W61.4 Contact with turkey**
√x7ᵗʰ **W61.42 Struck by turkey**
√x7ᵗʰ **W61.43 Pecked by turkey**
√x7ᵗʰ **W61.49 Other contact with turkey**
√5ᵗʰ **W61.5 Contact with goose**
√x7ᵗʰ **W61.51 Bitten by goose**
√x7ᵗʰ **W61.52 Struck by goose**
√x7ᵗʰ **W61.59 Other contact with goose**
√5ᵗʰ **W61.6 Contact with duck**
√x7ᵗʰ **W61.61 Bitten by duck**
√x7ᵗʰ **W61.62 Struck by duck**
√x7ᵗʰ **W61.69 Other contact with duck**
√5ᵗʰ **W61.9 Contact with other birds**
√x7ᵗʰ **W61.91 Bitten by other birds**
√x7ᵗʰ **W61.92 Struck by other birds**
√x7ᵗʰ **W61.99 Other contact with other birds**
Contact with bird NOS

☑4ᵗʰ **W62 Contact with nonvenomous amphibians**
EXCLUDES 1   *contact with venomous amphibians (T63.81-R63.83)*

The appropriate 7th character is to be added to each code from category W62.
A   initial encounter
D   subsequent encounter
S   sequela

√x7ᵗʰ **W62.0 Contact with nonvenomous frogs**
√x7ᵗʰ **W62.1 Contact with nonvenomous toads**
√x7ᵗʰ **W62.9 Contact with other nonvenomous amphibians**

☑ Appropriate additional character required   √x7ᵗʰ Requires 7th character, placeholder x must fill empty characters

W64 Exposure to other animate mechanical forces
Exposure to nonvenomous animal NOS
EXCLUDES 1   contact with venomous animal (T63-)

The appropriate 7th character is to be added to code W64.
A   initial encounter
D   subsequent encounter
S   sequela

Accidental non-transport drowning and submersion (W65-W74)
EXCLUDES 1   accidental drowning and submersion due to fall into water (W16-)
accidental drowning and submersion due to water transport accident (V90-, V92-)
EXCLUDES 2   accidental drowning and submersion due to cataclysm (X34-X39)

W65 Accidental drowning and submersion while in bath-tub
EXCLUDES 1   accidental drowning and submersion due to fall in (into) bathtub (W16.211)

The appropriate 7th character is to be added to code W65.
A   initial encounter
D   subsequent encounter
S   sequela

W66 Deactivated
See category W16

W67 Accidental drowning and submersion while in swimming-pool
EXCLUDES 1   accidental drowning and submersion due to fall into swimming pool (W16.011, W16.021, W16.031)
accidental drowning and submersion due to striking into wall of swimming pool (W22.041)

The appropriate 7th character is to be added to code W67.
A   initial encounter
D   subsequent encounter
S   sequela

W68 Deactivated
See category W16

W69 Accidental drowning and submersion while in natural water
Accidental drowning and submersion while in lake
Accidental drowning and submersion while in open sea
Accidental drowning and submersion while in river
Accidental drowning and submersion while in stream
EXCLUDES 1   accidental drowning and submersion due to fall into natural body of water (W16.111, W16.121, W16.131)

The appropriate 7th character is to be added to code W69.
A   initial encounter
D   subsequent encounter
S   sequela

W70 Deactivated
See category W16

W73 Other specified cause of accidental non-transport drowning and submersion
Accidental drowning and submersion while in quenching tank
Accidental drowning and submersion while in reservoir
EXCLUDES 1   accidental drowning and submersion due to fall into other water (W16.311, W16.321, W16.331)

The appropriate 7th character is to be added to code W73.
A   initial encounter
D   subsequent encounter
S   sequela

W74 Unspecified cause of accidental drowning and submersion
Drowning NOS

The appropriate 7th character is to be added to code W74.
A   initial encounter
D   subsequent encounter
S   sequela

W75-W77 Deactivated
See category T71

W78 Deactivated
See subcategory T17.81

W79-W80 Deactivated
See categories T17 and T18

W81 Deactivated
See subcategory T71.2

W83 Deactivated
See category T71

W84 Deactivated
See subcategory T71.9

Exposure to electric current, radiation and extreme ambient air temperature and pressure (W85-W99)
EXCLUDES 1   exposure to:
failure in dosage of radiation or temperature during surgical and medical care (Y63.2-Y63.5)
lightning (T75.0-)
natural cold (X31)
natural heat (X30)
natural radiation NOS (X39)
radiological procedure and radiotherapy (Y84.2)
sunlight (X32)

W85 Exposure to electric transmission lines
Broken power line

The appropriate 7th character is to be added to code W85.
A   initial encounter
D   subsequent encounter
S   sequela

W86 Exposure to other specified electric current

The appropriate 7th character is to be added to each code from category W86.
A   initial encounter
D   subsequent encounter
S   sequela

W86.0   Exposure to domestic wiring and appliances
W86.1   Exposure to industrial wiring, appliances and electrical machinery
Exposure to conductors
Exposure to control apparatus
Exposure to electrical equipment and machinery
Exposure to transformers
W86.8   Exposure to other electric current
Exposure to wiring and appliances in or on farm (not farmhouse)
Exposure to wiring and appliances outdoors
Exposure to wiring and appliances in or on public building
Exposure to wiring and appliances in or on residential institutions
Exposure to wiring and appliances in or on schools

W87 Deactivated
See category W86

W88 Exposure to ionizing radiation
EXCLUDES 1   exposure to sunlight (X32)

The appropriate 7th character is to be added to each code from category W88.
A   initial encounter
D   subsequent encounter
S   sequela

W88.0   Exposure to X-rays
W88.1   Exposure to radioactive isotopes
W88.8   Exposure to other ionizing radiation

W89 Exposure to man-made visible and ultraviolet light
Exposure to welding light (arc)
EXCLUDES 2   exposure to sunlight (X32)

The appropriate 7th character is to be added to each code from category W89.
A   initial encounter
D   subsequent encounter
S   sequela

W89.0   Exposure to welding light (arc)
W89.1   Exposure to tanning bed
W89.8   Exposure to other man-made visible and ultraviolet light
W89.9   Exposure to unspecified man-made visible and ultraviolet light

EXCLUDES 1   Not coded here   EXCLUDES 2   Not included here   *Manifestation Code*

√4th **W90 Exposure to other nonionizing radiation**
  EXCLUDES 1 exposure to sunlight (X32)

> The appropriate 7th character is to be added to each code from category W90.
> A   initial encounter
> D   subsequent encounter
> S   sequela

√x7th **W90.0 Exposure to radiofrequency**
√x7th **W90.1 Exposure to infrared radiation**
√x7th **W90.2 Exposure to laser radiation**
√x7th **W90.8 Exposure to other nonionizing radiation**

W91 Deactivated
  See category W90

√x7th **W92 Exposure to excessive heat of man-made origin**

> The appropriate 7th character is to be added to code W92.
> A   initial encounter
> D   subsequent encounter
> S   sequela

√4th **W93 Exposure to excessive cold of man-made origin**

> The appropriate 7th character is to be added to each code from category W93.
> A   initial encounter
> D   subsequent encounter
> S   sequela

√5th **W93.0 Contact with or inhalation of dry ice**
  √x7th **W93.01 Contact with dry ice**
  √x7th **W93.02 Inhalation of dry ice**
√5th **W93.1 Contact with or inhalation of liquid air**
  √x7th **W93.11 Contact with liquid air**
      Contact with liquid hydrogen
      Contact with liquid nitrogen
  √x7th **W93.12 Inhalation of liquid air**
      Inhalation of liquid hydrogen
      Inhalation of liquid nitrogen
√x7th **W93.2 Prolonged exposure in deep freeze unit or refrigerator**
√x7th **W93.8 Exposure to other excessive cold of man-made origin**

√4th **W94 Exposure to high and low air pressure and changes in air pressure**

> The appropriate 7th character is to be added to each code from category W94.
> A   initial encounter
> D   subsequent encounter
> S   sequela

√x7th **W94.0 Exposure to prolonged high air pressure**
√5th **W94.1 Exposure to prolonged low air pressure**
  √x7th **W94.11 Exposure to residence or prolonged visit at high altitude**
  √x7th **W94.12 Exposure to other prolonged low air pressure**
√5th **W94.2 Exposure to rapid changes in air pressure during ascent**
  √x7th **W94.21 Exposure to reduction in atmospheric pressure while surfacing from deep-water diving**
  √x7th **W94.22 Exposure to reduction in atmospheric pressure while surfacing from underground**
  √x7th **W94.23 Exposure to sudden change in air pressure in aircraft during ascent**
  √x7th **W94.29 Exposure to other rapid changes in air pressure during ascent**
√5th **W94.3 Exposure to rapid changes in air pressure during descent**
  √x7th **W94.31 Exposure to sudden change in air pressure in aircraft during ascent or descent**
  √x7th **W94.32 Exposure to high air pressure from rapid descent in water**
  √x7th **W94.39 Exposure to other rapid changes in air pressure during descent**

√x7th **W99 Exposure to other man-made environmental factors**

> The appropriate 7th character is to be added to code W99.
> A   initial encounter
> D   subsequent encounter
> S   sequela

Exposure to smoke, fire and flames (X00-X08)

EXCLUDES 1 arson (X97)
EXCLUDES 2 explosions (W35-W40)
    lightning (T75.0-)
    transport accident (V01-V99)

√4th **X00 Exposure to uncontrolled fire in building or structure**
  Conflagration in building or structure
  Code first any associated cataclysm
  EXCLUDES 2 exposure to ignition or melting of nightwear (X05)
      exposure to ignition or melting of other clothing and apparel (X06-)
      exposure to other specified smoke, fire and flames (X08-)

> The appropriate 7th character is to be added to each code from category X00.
> A   initial encounter
> D   subsequent encounter
> S   sequela

√x7th **X00.0 Exposure to flames in uncontrolled fire in building or structure**
√x7th **X00.1 Exposure to smoke in uncontrolled fire in building or structure**
√x7th **X00.2 Injury due to collapse of burning building or structure in uncontrolled fire**
    EXCLUDES 1 injury due to collapse of building not on fire (W20.1)
√x7th **X00.3 Fall from burning building or structure in uncontrolled fire**
√x7th **X00.4 Hit by object from burning building or structure in uncontrolled fire**
√x7th **X00.5 Jump from burning building or structure in uncontrolled fire**
√x7th **X00.8 Other exposure to uncontrolled fire in building or structure**

√4th **X01 Exposure to uncontrolled fire, not in building or structure**
  Exposure to forest fire

> The appropriate 7th character is to be added to each code from category X01.
> A   initial encounter
> D   subsequent encounter
> S   sequela

√x7th **X01.0 Exposure to flames in uncontrolled fire, not in building or structure**
√x7th **X01.1 Exposure to smoke in uncontrolled fire, not in building or structure**
√x7th **X01.3 Fall due to uncontrolled fire, not in building or structure**
√x7th **X01.4 Hit by object due to uncontrolled fire, not in building or structure**
√x7th **X01.8 Other exposure to uncontrolled fire, not in building or structure**

√4th **X02 Exposure to controlled fire in building or structure**
  Exposure to fire in fireplace
  Exposure to fire in stove

> The appropriate 7th character is to be added to each code from category X02.
> A   initial encounter
> D   subsequent encounter
> S   sequela

√x7th **X02.0 Exposure to flames in controlled fire in building or structure**
√x7th **X02.1 Exposure to smoke in controlled fire in building or structure**
√x7th **X02.2 Injury due to collapse of burning building or structure in controlled fire**
    EXCLUDES 1 injury due to collapse of building not on fire (W20.1)
√x7th **X02.3 Fall from burning building or structure in controlled fire**
√x7th **X02.4 Hit by object from burning building or structure in controlled fire**
√x7th **X02.5 Jump from burning building or structure in controlled fire**
√x7th **X02.8 Other exposure to controlled fire in building or structure**

☑ Appropriate additional character required

√x7th Requires 7th character, placeholder x must fill empty characters

External Causes of Morbidity

X03–X14.1

√4ᵗʰ **X03 Exposure to controlled fire, not in building or structure**
Exposure to bon fire
Exposure to camp-fire
Exposure to trash fire

> The appropriate 7th character is to be added to each code from category X03.
> A   initial encounter
> D   subsequent encounter
> S   sequela

√x7ᵗʰ **X03.0 Exposure to flames in controlled fire, not in building or structure**
√x7ᵗʰ **X03.1 Exposure to smoke in controlled fire, not in building or structure**
√x7ᵗʰ **X03.3 Fall due to controlled fire, not in building or structure**
√x7ᵗʰ **X03.4 Hit by object due to controlled fire, not in building or structure**
√x7ᵗʰ **X03.8 Other exposure to controlled fire, not in building or structure**

√x7ᵗʰ **X04 Exposure to ignition of highly flammable material**
Exposure to ignition of gasoline
Exposure to ignition of kerosene
Exposure to ignition of petrol
EXCLUDES 2   *exposure to ignition or melting of nightwear (X05)*
     exposure to ignition or melting of other clothing and apparel (X06)

> The appropriate 7th character is to be added to code X04.
> A   initial encounter
> D   subsequent encounter
> S   sequela

√x7ᵗʰ **X05 Exposure to ignition or melting of nightwear**
EXCLUDES 2   *exposure to uncontrolled fire in building or structure (X00-)*
     exposure to uncontrolled fire, not in building or structure (X01-)
     exposure to controlled fire in building or structure (X02-)
     exposure to controlled fire, not in building or structure (X03-)
     exposure to ignition of highly flammable materials (X04-)

> The appropriate 7th character is to be added to code X05.
> A   initial encounter
> D   subsequent encounter
> S   sequela

√4ᵗʰ **X06 Exposure to ignition or melting of other clothing and apparel**
EXCLUDES 2   *exposure to uncontrolled fire in building or structure (X00-)*
     exposure to uncontrolled fire, not in building or structure (X01-)
     exposure to controlled fire in building or structure (X02-)
     exposure to controlled fire, not in building or structure (X03-)
     exposure to ignition of highly flammable materials (X04-)

> The appropriate 7th character is to be added to each code from category X06.
> A   initial encounter
> D   subsequent encounter
> S   sequela

√x7ᵗʰ **X06.0 Exposure to ignition of plastic jewelry**
√x7ᵗʰ **X06.1 Exposure to melting of plastic jewelry**
√x7ᵗʰ **X06.2 Exposure to ignition of other clothing and apparel**
√x7ᵗʰ **X06.3 Exposure to melting of other clothing and apparel**

√4ᵗʰ **X08 Exposure to other specified smoke, fire and flames**

> The appropriate 7th character is to be added to each code from category X08.
> A   initial encounter
> D   subsequent encounter
> S   sequela

√5ᵗʰ **X08.0 Exposure to bed fire**
Exposure to mattress fire
√x7ᵗʰ **X08.00 Exposure to bed fire due to unspecified burning material**
√x7ᵗʰ **X08.01 Exposure to bed fire due to burning cigarette**
√x7ᵗʰ **X08.09 Exposure to bed fire due to other burning material**
√5ᵗʰ **X08.1 Exposure to sofa fire**
√x7ᵗʰ **X08.10 Exposure to sofa fire due to unspecified burning material**
√x7ᵗʰ **X08.11 Exposure to sofa fire due to burning cigarette**

√x7ᵗʰ **X08.19 Exposure to sofa fire due to other burning material**
√5ᵗʰ **X08.2 Exposure to other furniture fire**
√x7ᵗʰ **X08.20 Exposure to other furniture fire due to unspecified burning material**
√x7ᵗʰ **X08.21 Exposure to other furniture fire due to burning cigarette**
√x7ᵗʰ **X08.29 Exposure to other furniture fire due to other burning material**
√x7ᵗʰ **X08.8 Exposure to other specified smoke, fire and flames**

X09 Deactivated
See category X08

Contact with heat and hot substances (X10-X19)

EXCLUDES 1   *exposure to excessive natural heat (X30)*
     exposure to fire and flames (X00-X09)

√4ᵗʰ **X10 Contact with hot drinks, food, fats and cooking oils**

> The appropriate 7th character is to be added to each code from category X10.
> A   initial encounter
> D   subsequent encounter
> S   sequela

√x7ᵗʰ **X10.0 Contact with hot drinks**
√x7ᵗʰ **X10.1 Contact with hot food**
√x7ᵗʰ **X10.2 Contact with fats and cooking oils**

√4ᵗʰ **X11 Contact with hot tap-water**
Contact with boiling tap-water
Contact with boiling water NOS
EXCLUDES 1   *contact with water heated on stove (X12)*

> The appropriate 7th character is to be added to each code from category X11.
> A   initial encounter
> D   subsequent encounter
> S   sequela

√x7ᵗʰ **X11.0 Contact with hot water in bath or tub**
EXCLUDES 1   *contact with running hot water in bath or tub (X11.1)*
√x7ᵗʰ **X11.1 Contact with running hot water**
Contact with hot water running out of hose
Contact with hot water running out of tap
√x7ᵗʰ **X11.8 Contact with other hot tap-water**
Contact with hot water in bucket
Contact with hot tap-water NOS

√x7ᵗʰ **X12 Contact with other hot fluids**
Contact with water heated on stove
EXCLUDES 1   *hot (liquid) metals (X18)*

> The appropriate 7th character is to be added to code X12.
> A   initial encounter
> D   subsequent encounter
> S   sequela

√4ᵗʰ **X13 Contact with steam and other hot vapors**

> The appropriate 7th character is to be added to each code from category X13.
> A   initial encounter
> D   subsequent encounter
> S   sequela

√x7ᵗʰ **X13.0 Inhalation of steam and other hot vapors**
√x7ᵗʰ **X13.1 Other contact with steam and other hot vapors**

√4ᵗʰ **X14 Contact with hot air and other hot gases**

> The appropriate 7th character is to be added to each code from category X14.
> A   initial encounter
> D   subsequent encounter
> S   sequela

√x7ᵗʰ **X14.0 Inhalation of hot air and gases**
√x7ᵗʰ **X14.1 Other contact with hot air and other hot gases**

EXCLUDES 1 Not coded here   *EXCLUDES 2* Not included here   **Manifestation Code**

✓4ᵗʰ **X15　Contact with hot household appliances**
　　EXCLUDES 1　*contact with heating appliances (X16)*
　　　　　　contact with powered household appliances (W29-)
　　　　　　exposure to controlled fire in building or structure due to
　　　　　　　　household appliance (X02.8)
　　　　　　exposure to household appliances electrical current (W86.0)

The appropriate 7th character is to be added to each code from category X15.
A　　initial encounter
D　　subsequent encounter
S　　sequela

✓x7ᵗʰ **X15.0　Contact with hot stove (kitchen)**
✓x7ᵗʰ **X15.1　Contact with hot toaster**
✓x7ᵗʰ **X15.2　Contact with hotplate**
✓x7ᵗʰ **X15.3　Contact with hot saucepan or skillet**
✓x7ᵗʰ **X15.8　Contact with other hot household appliances**
　　　　Contact with cooker
　　　　Contact with kettle
　　　　Contact with light bulbs

✓x7ᵗʰ **X16　Contact with hot heating appliances, radiators and pipes**
　　EXCLUDES 1　*contact with powered appliances (W29-)*
　　　　　　exposure to controlled fire in building or structure due to
　　　　　　　　appliance (X02.8)
　　　　　　exposure to industrial appliances electrical current (W86.1)

The appropriate 7th character is to be added to code X16.
A　　initial encounter
D　　subsequent encounter
S　　sequela

✓x7ᵗʰ **X17　Contact with hot engines, machinery and tools**
　　EXCLUDES 1　*contact with hot heating appliances, radiators and pipes (X16)*
　　　　　　contact with hot household appliances (X15)

The appropriate 7th character is to be added to code X17.
A　　initial encounter
D　　subsequent encounter
S　　sequela

✓x7ᵗʰ **X18　Contact with other hot metals**
　　Contact with liquid metal

The appropriate 7th character is to be added to code X18.
A　　initial encounter
D　　subsequent encounter
S　　sequela

✓x7ᵗʰ **X19　Contact with other heat and hot substances**
　　EXCLUDES 1　*objects that are not normally hot, e.g., an object made hot by a*
　　　　　　house fire (X00-X09)

The appropriate 7th character is to be added to code X19.
A　　initial encounter
D　　subsequent encounter
S　　sequela

X20-X29　Deactivated
　　　　See category T63

Exposure to forces of nature (X30-X39)

✓x7ᵗʰ **X30　Exposure to excessive natural heat**
　　Exposure to excessive heat as the cause of sunstroke
　　Exposure to heat NOS
　　EXCLUDES 1　*excessive heat of man-made origin (W92)*
　　　　　　exposure to man-made radiation (W89)
　　　　　　exposure to sunlight (X32)
　　　　　　exposure to tanning bed (W89)

The appropriate 7th character is to be added to code X30.
A　　initial encounter
D　　subsequent encounter
S　　sequela

✓x7ᵗʰ **X31　Exposure to excessive natural cold**
　　Excessive cold as the cause of chilblains NOS
　　Excessive cold as the cause of immersion foot or hand
　　Exposure to cold NOS
　　Exposure to weather conditions
　　EXCLUDES 1　*cold of man-made origin (W93-)*
　　　　　　contact with or inhalation of:
　　　　　　dry ice (W93-)
　　　　　　liquefied gas (W93-)

The appropriate 7th character is to be added to code X31.
A　　initial encounter
D　　subsequent encounter
S　　sequela

✓x7ᵗʰ **X32　Exposure to sunlight**
　　EXCLUDES 1　*radiation-related disorders of the skin and subcutaneous*
　　　　　　tissue (L55-L59)
　　　　　　man-made radiation (tanning bed) (W89)

The appropriate 7th character is to be added to code X32.
A　　initial encounter
D　　subsequent encounter
S　　sequela

✓x7ᵗʰ **X34　Earthquake**
　　EXCLUDES 2　*tidal wave (tsunami) due to earthquake (X37.41)*

The appropriate 7th character is to be added to code X34.
A　　initial encounter
D　　subsequent encounter
S　　sequela

✓x7ᵗʰ **X35　Volcanic eruption**
　　EXCLUDES 2　*tidal wave (tsunami) due to volcanic eruption (X37.41)*

The appropriate 7th character is to be added to code X35.
A　　initial encounter
D　　subsequent encounter
S　　sequela

✓4ᵗʰ **X36　Avalanche, landslide and other earth movements**
　　INCLUDES　victim of mudslide of cataclysmic nature
　　EXCLUDES 1　*earthquake (X34)*
　　EXCLUDES 2　*transport accident involving collision with avalanche or*
　　　　　　landslide not in motion (V01-V99)

The appropriate 7th character is to be added to each code from category X36.
A　　initial encounter
D　　subsequent encounter
S　　sequela

✓x7ᵗʰ **X36.0　Collapse of dam or man-made structure causing earth movement**
✓x7ᵗʰ **X36.1　Avalanche, landslide, or mudslide**

✓4ᵗʰ **X37　Cataclysmic storm**

The appropriate 7th character is to be added to each code from category X37.
A　　initial encounter
D　　subsequent encounter
S　　sequela

✓x7ᵗʰ **X37.0　Hurricane**
　　　　Storm surge
　　　　Typhoon
✓x7ᵗʰ **X37.1　Tornado**
　　　　Cyclone
　　　　Twister
✓x7ᵗʰ **X37.2　Blizzard (snow)(ice)**
✓x7ᵗʰ **X37.3　Dust storm**
✓5ᵗʰ **X37.4　Tidalwave**
　　✓x7ᵗʰ **X37.41　Tidal wave due to earthquake or volcanic eruption**
　　　　　Tidal wave NOS
　　　　　Tsunami
　　✓x7ᵗʰ **X37.42　Tidal wave due to storm**
　　✓x7ᵗʰ **X37.43　Tidal wave due to landslide**
✓x7ᵗʰ **X37.8　Other cataclysmic storms**
　　　　Cloudburst
　　　　Torrential rain
　　　　EXCLUDES 2　*flood (X38)*

√x7ᵗʰ **X37.9** **Unspecified cataclysmic storm**
Storm NOS
EXCLUDES 1 *collapse of dam or man-made structure causing earth movement (X36.0)*

√x7ᵗʰ **X38** **Flood**
Flood arising from remote storm
Flood of cataclysmic nature arising from melting snow
Flood resulting directly from storm
EXCLUDES 1 *collapse of dam or man-made structure causing earth movement (X36.0)*
tidal wave NOS (X37.41)
tidal wave caused by storm (X37.42)

The appropriate 7th character is to be added to code X38.
A   initial encounter
D   subsequent encounter
S   sequela

√4ᵗʰ **X39** **Exposure to other forces of nature**

The appropriate 7th character is to be added to each code from category X39.
A   initial encounter
D   subsequent encounter
S   sequela

√5ᵗʰ **X39.0** **Exposure to natural radiation**
EXCLUDES 1 *contact with and (suspected) exposure to radon and other naturally occuring radiation (Z77.123)*
exposure to man-made radiation (W88-W90)
exposure to sunlight (X32)

√x7ᵗʰ **X39.01** **Exposure to radon**
√x7ᵗʰ **X39.08** **Exposure to other natural radiation**
√x7ᵗʰ **X39.8** **Other exposure to forces of nature**

X40-X49 **Deactivated**
See categories T36-T65 with fifth or sixth character 1

X50-X51 **Deactivated**
See category Y93

Accidental exposure to other specified factors (X52, X58)

√x7ᵗʰ **X52** **Prolonged stay in weightless environment**
Weightlessness in spacecraft (simulator)

The appropriate 7th character is to be added to code X52.
A   initial encounter
D   subsequent encounter
S   sequela

X53 **Deactivated**
See subcategory T73.0

X54 **Deactivated**
See subcategory T73.1

X57 **Deactivated**
See subcategory T73.9

√x7ᵗʰ **X58** **Exposure to other specified factors**
Accident NOS
Exposure NOS

The appropriate 7th character is to be added to code X58.
A   initial encounter
D   subsequent encounter
S   sequela

Intentional self-harm (X71-X83)

Purposely self-inflicted injury
Suicide (attempted)

X60-X69 **Deactivated**
See categories T36-T65 with fifth or sixth character 2

X70 **Deactivated**
See category T71

√4ᵗʰ **X71** **Intentional self-harm by drowning and submersion**

The appropriate 7th character is to be added to each code from category X71.
A   initial encounter
D   subsequent encounter
S   sequela

√x7ᵗʰ **X71.0** **Intentional self-harm by drowning and submersion while in bathtub**
√x7ᵗʰ **X71.1** **Intentional self-harm by drowning and submersion while in swimming pool**
√x7ᵗʰ **X71.2** **Intentional self-harm by drowning and submersion after jump into swimming pool**
√x7ᵗʰ **X71.3** **Intentional self-harm by drowning and submersion in natural water**
√x7ᵗʰ **X71.8** **Other intentional self-harm by drowning and submersion**
√x7ᵗʰ **X71.9** **Intentional self-harm by drowning and submersion, unspecified**

√x7ᵗʰ **X72** **Intentional self-harm by handgun discharge**
Intentional self-harm by gun for single hand use
Intentional self-harm by pistol
Intentional self-harm by revolver
EXCLUDES 1 *Very pistol (X74.8)*

The appropriate 7th character is to be added to code X72.
A   initial encounter
D   subsequent encounter
S   sequela

√4ᵗʰ **X73** **Intentional self-harm by rifle, shotgun and larger firearm discharge**
EXCLUDES 1 *airgun (X74.01)*

The appropriate 7th character is to be added to each code from category X73.
A   initial encounter
D   subsequent encounter
S   sequela

√x7ᵗʰ **X73.0** **Intentional self-harm by shotgun discharge**
√x7ᵗʰ **X73.1** **Intentional self-harm by hunting rifle discharge**
√x7ᵗʰ **X73.2** **Intentional self-harm by machine gun discharge**
√x7ᵗʰ **X73.8** **Intentional self-harm by other larger firearm discharge**
√x7ᵗʰ **X73.9** **Intentional self-harm by unspecified larger firearm discharge**

√4ᵗʰ **X74** **Intentional self-harm by other and unspecified firearm and gun discharge**

The appropriate 7th character is to be added to each code from category X74.
A   initial encounter
D   subsequent encounter
S   sequela

√5ᵗʰ **X74.0** **Intentional self-harm by gas, air or spring-operated guns**
√x7ᵗʰ **X74.01** **Intentional self-harm by airgun**
Intentional self-harm by BB gun discharge
Intentional self-harm by pellet gun discharge
√x7ᵗʰ **X74.02** **Intentional self-harm by paintball gun**
√x7ᵗʰ **X74.09** **Intentional self-harm by other gas, air or spring-operated gun**
√x7ᵗʰ **X74.8** **Intentional self-harm by other firearm discharge**
Intentional self-harm by Very pistol [flare] discharge
√x7ᵗʰ **X74.9** **Intentional self-harm by unspecified firearm discharge**

EXCLUDES 1 Not coded here   EXCLUDES 2 Not included here   *Manifestation Code*

✓x7ᵗʰ **X75　Intentional self-harm by explosive material**

> The appropriate 7th character is to be added to code X75.
> A　initial encounter
> D　subsequent encounter
> S　sequela

✓x7ᵗʰ **X76　Intentional self-harm by smoke, fire and flames**

> The appropriate 7th character is to be added to code X76.
> A　initial encounter
> D　subsequent encounter
> S　sequela

✓4ᵗʰ **X77　Intentional self-harm by steam, hot vapors and hot objects**

> The appropriate 7th character is to be added to each code from category X77.
> A　initial encounter
> D　subsequent encounter
> S　sequela

✓x7ᵗʰ **X77.0　Intentional self-harm by steam or hot vapors**
✓x7ᵗʰ **X77.1　Intentional self-harm by hot tap water**
✓x7ᵗʰ **X77.2　Intentional self-harm by other hot fluids**
✓x7ᵗʰ **X77.3　Intentional self-harm by hot household appliances**
✓x7ᵗʰ **X77.8　Intentional self-harm by other hot objects**
✓x7ᵗʰ **X77.9　Intentional self-harm by unspecified hot objects**

✓4ᵗʰ **X78　Intentional self-harm by sharp object**

> The appropriate 7th character is to be added to each code from category X78.
> A　initial encounter
> D　subsequent encounter
> S　sequela

✓x7ᵗʰ **X78.0　Intentional self-harm by sharp glass**
✓x7ᵗʰ **X78.1　Intentional self-harm by knife**
✓x7ᵗʰ **X78.2　Intentional self-harm by sword or dagger**
✓x7ᵗʰ **X78.8　Intentional self-harm by other sharp object**
✓x7ᵗʰ **X78.9　Intentional self-harm by unspecified sharp object**

✓x7ᵗʰ **X79　Intentional self-harm by blunt object**

> The appropriate 7th character is to be added to code X79.
> A　initial encounter
> D　subsequent encounter
> S　sequela

✓x7ᵗʰ **X80　Intentional self-harm by jumping from a high place**
　　Intentional fall from one level to another

> The appropriate 7th character is to be added to code X80.
> A　initial encounter
> D　subsequent encounter
> S　sequela

✓4ᵗʰ **X81　Intentional self-harm by jumping or lying in front of moving object**

> The appropriate 7th character is to be added to each code from category X81.
> A　initial encounter
> D　subsequent encounter
> S　sequela

✓x7ᵗʰ **X81.0　Intentional self-harm by jumping or lying in front of motor vehicle**
✓x7ᵗʰ **X81.1　Intentional self-harm by jumping or lying in front of (subway) train**
✓x7ᵗʰ **X81.8　Intentional self-harm by jumping or lying in front of other moving object**

✓4ᵗʰ **X82　Intentional self-harm by crashing of motor vehicle**

> The appropriate 7th character is to be added to each code from category X82.
> A　initial encounter
> D　subsequent encounter
> S　sequela

✓x7ᵗʰ **X82.0　Intentional collision of motor vehicle with other motor vehicle**
✓x7ᵗʰ **X82.1　Intentional collision of motor vehicle with train**
✓x7ᵗʰ **X82.2　Intentional collision of motor vehicle with tree**
✓x7ᵗʰ **X82.8　Other intentional self-harm by crashing of motor vehicle**

✓4ᵗʰ **X83　Intentional self-harm by other specified means**

> **EXCLUDES 1**　intentional self-harm by poisoning or contact with toxic substance—see Table of Drugs and Chemicals

> The appropriate 7th character is to be added to each code from category X83.
> A　initial encounter
> D　subsequent encounter
> S　sequela

✓x7ᵗʰ **X83.0　Intentional self-harm by crashing of aircraft**
✓x7ᵗʰ **X83.1　Intentional self-harm by electrocution**
✓x7ᵗʰ **X83.2　Intentional self-harm by exposure to extremes of cold**
✓x7ᵗʰ **X83.8　Intentional self-harm by other specified means**

X84　　Deactivated
　　　　See category T14

Assault (X92-Y08)

INCLUDES　homicide
　　　　injuries inflicted by another person with intent to injure or kill, by any means

EXCLUDES 1　injuries due to legal intervention (Y35-)
　　　　injuries due to operations of war (Y36-)
　　　　injuries due to terrorism (Y38-)

X85-X90　Deactivated
　　　　See categories T36-T65 with fifth or sixth character 3

X91　　Deactivated
　　　　See category T71

✓4ᵗʰ **X92　Assault by drowning and submersion**

> The appropriate 7th character is to be added to each code from category X92.
> A　initial encounter
> D　subsequent encounter
> S　sequela

✓x7ᵗʰ **X92.0　Assault by drowning and submersion while in bathtub**
✓x7ᵗʰ **X92.1　Assault by drowning and submersion while in swimming pool**
✓x7ᵗʰ **X92.2　Assault by drowning and submersion after push into swimming pool**
✓x7ᵗʰ **X92.3　Assault by drowning and submersion in natural water**
✓x7ᵗʰ **X92.8　Other assault by drowning and submersion**
✓x7ᵗʰ **X92.9　Assault by drowning and submersion, unspecified**

✓x7ᵗʰ **X93　Assault by handgun discharge**
　　Assault by discharge of gun for single hand use
　　Assault by discharge of pistol
　　Assault by discharge of revolver
　　EXCLUDES 1　Very pistol (X95.8)

> The appropriate 7th character is to be added to code X93.
> A　initial encounter
> D　subsequent encounter
> S　sequela

✓4ᵗʰ **X94　Assault by rifle, shotgun and larger firearm discharge**
　　EXCLUDES 1　airgun (X95.01)

> The appropriate 7th character is to be added to each code from category X94.
> A　initial encounter
> D　subsequent encounter
> S　sequela

✓x7ᵗʰ **X94.0　Assault by shotgun**
✓x7ᵗʰ **X94.1　Assault by hunting rifle**
✓x7ᵗʰ **X94.2　Assault by machine gun**
✓x7ᵗʰ **X94.8　Assault by other larger firearm discharge**
✓x7ᵗʰ **X94.9　Assault by unspecified larger firearm discharge**

✓4ᵗʰ **X95　Assault by other and unspecified firearm and gun discharge**

> The appropriate 7th character is to be added to each code from category X95.
> A　initial encounter
> D　subsequent encounter
> S　sequela

✓5ᵗʰ **X95.0　Assault by gas, air or spring-operated guns**

✓ Appropriate additional character required

✓x7ᵗʰ Requires 7th character, placeholder x must fill empty characters

√x7ᵗʰ   **X95.Ø1**   **Assault by airgun discharge**
      Assault by BB gun discharge
      Assault by pellet gun discharge
√x7ᵗʰ   **X95.Ø2**   **Assault by paintball gun discharge**
√x7ᵗʰ   **X95.Ø9**   **Assault by other gas, air or spring-operated gun**
√x7ᵗʰ   **X95.8**   **Assault by other firearm discharge**
      Assault by Very pistol [flare] discharge
√x7ᵗʰ   **X95.9**   **Assault by unspecified firearm discharge**

√4ᵗʰ **X96**   **Assault by explosive material**
    EXCLUDES 1   *incendiary device (X97)*
                  terrorism involving explosive material (Y38.2-)

    The appropriate 7th character is to be added to each code from category X96.
      A   initial encounter
      D   subsequent encounter
      S   sequela

√x7ᵗʰ   **X96.Ø**   **Assault by antipersonnel bomb**
        EXCLUDES 1   *antipersonnel bomb use in military or war (Y36.2-)*
√x7ᵗʰ   **X96.1**   **Assault by gasoline bomb**
√x7ᵗʰ   **X96.2**   **Assault by letter bomb**
√x7ᵗʰ   **X96.3**   **Assault by fertilizer bomb**
√x7ᵗʰ   **X96.4**   **Assault by pipe bomb**
√x7ᵗʰ   **X96.8**   **Assault by other specified explosive**
√x7ᵗʰ   **X96.9**   **Assault by unspecified explosive**

√x7ᵗʰ **X97**   **Assault by smoke, fire and flames**
      Assault by arson
      Assault by cigarettes
      Assault by incendiary device

    The appropriate 7th character is to be added to code X97.
      A   initial encounter
      D   subsequent encounter
      S   sequela

√4ᵗʰ **X98**   **Assault by steam, hot vapors and hot objects**

    The appropriate 7th character is to be added to each code from category X98.
      A   initial encounter
      D   subsequent encounter
      S   sequela

√x7ᵗʰ   **X98.Ø**   **Assault by steam or hot vapors**
√x7ᵗʰ   **X98.1**   **Assault by hot tap water**
√x7ᵗʰ   **X98.2**   **Assault by hot fluids**
√x7ᵗʰ   **X98.3**   **Assault by hot household appliances**
√x7ᵗʰ   **X98.8**   **Assault by other hot objects**
√x7ᵗʰ   **X98.9**   **Assault by unspecified hot objects**

√4ᵗʰ **X99**   **Assault by sharp object**
    EXCLUDES 1   *assault by strike by sports equipment (YØ8.Ø-)*

    The appropriate 7th character is to be added to each code from category X99.
      A   initial encounter
      D   subsequent encounter
      S   sequela

√x7ᵗʰ   **X99.Ø**   **Assault by sharp glass**
√x7ᵗʰ   **X99.1**   **Assault by knife**
√x7ᵗʰ   **X99.2**   **Assault by sword or dagger**
√x7ᵗʰ   **X99.8**   **Assault by other sharp object**
√x7ᵗʰ   **X99.9**   **Assault by unspecified sharp object**
      Assault by stabbing NOS

√x7ᵗʰ **YØØ**   **Assault by blunt object**
    EXCLUDES 1   *assault by strike by sports equipment (YØ8.Ø-)*

    The appropriate 7th character is to be added to code YØØ.
      A   initial encounter
      D   subsequent encounter
      S   sequela

√x7ᵗʰ **YØ1**   **Assault by pushing from high place**

    The appropriate 7th character is to be added to code YØ1.
      A   initial encounter
      D   subsequent encounter
      S   sequela

√4ᵗʰ **YØ2**   **Assault by pushing or placing victim in front of moving object**

    The appropriate 7th character is to be added to each code from category YØ2.
      A   initial encounter
      D   subsequent encounter
      S   sequela

√x7ᵗʰ   **YØ2.Ø**   **Assault by pushing or placing victim in front of motor vehicle**
√x7ᵗʰ   **YØ2.1**   **Assault by pushing or placing victim in front of (subway) train**
√x7ᵗʰ   **YØ2.8**   **Assault by pushing or placing victim in front of other moving object**

√4ᵗʰ **YØ3**   **Assault by crashing of motor vehicle**

    The appropriate 7th character is to be added to each code from category YØ3.
      A   initial encounter
      D   subsequent encounter
      S   sequela

√x7ᵗʰ   **YØ3.Ø**   **Assault by being hit or run over by motor vehicle**
√x7ᵗʰ   **YØ3.8**   **Other assault by crashing of motor vehicle**

√4ᵗʰ **YØ4**   **Assault by bodily force**
    EXCLUDES 1   *assault by:*
                submersion (X92-)
                use of weapon (X93-X95, X99, YØØ)

    The appropriate 7th character is to be added to each code from category YØ4.
      A   initial encounter
      D   subsequent encounter
      S   sequela

√x7ᵗʰ   **YØ4.Ø**   **Assault by unarmed brawl or fight**
√x7ᵗʰ   **YØ4.1**   **Assault by human bite**
√x7ᵗʰ   **YØ4.2**   **Assault by strike against or bumped into by another person**
√x7ᵗʰ   **YØ4.8**   **Assault by other bodily force**
      Assault by bodily force NOS

YØ5   **Deactivated**
    See subcategories T74.Ø, T76.Ø

YØ6   **Deactivated**
    See subcategories T74.Ø, T76.Ø

√4ᵗʰ **YØ7**   **Perpetrator of assault, maltreatment and neglect**
    NOTE   Codes from this category are for use only in cases of confirmed abuse (T74-)
          Selection of the correct perpetrator code is based on the relationship between the perpetrator and the victim
    INCLUDES   perpetrator of abandonment
          perpetrator of emotional neglect
          perpetrator of mental cruelty
          perpetrator of physical abuse
          perpetrator of physical neglect
          perpetrator of sexual abuse
          perpetrator of torture

√5ᵗʰ   **YØ7.Ø**   **Spouse or partner, perpetrator of maltreatment and neglect**
        NOTE   Spouse or partner, perpetrator of maltreatment and neglect against spouse or partner
        YØ7.Ø1   **Husband, perpetrator of maltreatment and neglect**
        YØ7.Ø2   **Wife, perpetrator of maltreatment and neglect**
        YØ7.Ø3   **Male partner, perpetrator of maltreatment and neglect**
        YØ7.Ø4   **Female partner, perpetrator of maltreatment and neglect**

√5ᵗʰ   **YØ7.1**   **Parent (adoptive) (biological), perpetrator of maltreatment and neglect**
        YØ7.11   **Biological father, perpetrator of maltreatment and neglect**
        YØ7.12   **Biological mother, perpetrator of maltreatment and neglect**

    EXCLUDES 1   Not coded here   EXCLUDES 2   Not included here   *Manifestation Code*

      Y07.13   **Adoptive father, perpetrator of maltreatment and neglect**

      Y07.14   **Adoptive mother, perpetrator of maltreatment and neglect**

✓5th Y07.4 **Other family member, perpetrator of maltreatment and neglect**

    ✓6th Y07.41 **Sibling, perpetrator of maltreatment and neglect**

          EXCLUDES 1 *stepsibling, perpetrator of maltreatment and neglect (Y07.435, Y07.436)*

        Y07.410 **Brother, perpetrator of maltreatment and neglect**

        Y07.411 **Sister, perpetrator of maltreatment and neglect**

    ✓6th Y07.42 **Foster parent, perpetrator of maltreatment and neglect**

        Y07.420 **Foster father, perpetrator of maltreatment and neglect**

        Y07.421 **Foster mother, perpetrator of maltreatment and neglect**

    ✓6th Y07.43 **Stepparent or stepsibling, perpetrator of maltreatment and neglect**

        Y07.430 **Stepfather, perpetrator of maltreatment and neglect**

        Y07.432 **Male friend of parent (co-residing in household), perpetrator of maltreatment and neglect**

        Y07.433 **Stepmother, perpetrator of maltreatment and neglect**

        Y07.434 **Female friend of parent (co-residing in household), perpetrator of maltreatment and neglect**

        Y07.435 **Stepbrother, perpetrator or maltreatment and neglect**

        Y07.436 **Stepsister, perpetrator of maltreatment and neglect**

    ✓6th Y07.49 **Other family member, perpetrator of maltreatment and neglect**

        Y07.490 **Male cousin, perpetrator of maltreatment and neglect**

        Y07.491 **Female cousin, perpetrator of maltreatment and neglect**

        Y07.499 **Other family member, perpetrator of maltreatment and neglect**

✓5th Y07.5 **Non-family member, perpetrator of maltreatment and neglect**

      Y07.50 **Unspecified non-family member, perpetrator of maltreatment and neglect**

    ✓6th Y07.51 **Daycare provider, perpetrator of maltreatment and neglect**

        Y07.510 **At-home childcare provider, perpetrator of maltreatment and neglect**

        Y07.511 **Daycare center childcare provider, perpetrator of maltreatment and neglect**

        Y07.512 **At-home adultcare provider, perpetrator of maltreatment and neglect**

        Y07.513 **Adultcare center provider, perpetrator of maltreatment and neglect**

        Y07.519 **Unspecified daycare provider, perpetrator of maltreatment and neglect**

    ✓6th Y07.52 **Healthcare provider, perpetrator of maltreatment and neglect**

        Y07.521 **Mental health provider, perpetrator of maltreatment and neglect**

        Y07.528 **Other therapist or healthcare provider, perpetrator of maltreatment and neglect**

          Nurse, perpetrator of maltreatment and neglect

          Occupational therapist, perpetrator of maltreatment and neglect

          Physical therapist, perpetrator of maltreatment and neglect

          Speech therapist, perpetrator of maltreatment and neglect

        Y07.529 **Unspecified healthcare provider, perpetrator of maltreatment and neglect**

      Y07.53 **Teacher or instructor, perpetrator of maltreatment and neglect**

          Coach, perpetrator of maltreatment and neglect

      Y07.59 **Other non-family member, perpetrator of maltreatment and neglect**

  Y07.9 **Unspecified perpetrator of maltreatment and neglect**

✓4th **Y08** **Assault by other specified means**

> The appropriate 7th character is to be added to each code from category Y08.
> A   initial encounter
> D   subsequent encounter
> S   sequela

  ✓5th **Y08.0** **Assault by strike by sport equipment**

    ✓x7th **Y08.01** **Assault by strike by hockey stick**

    ✓x7th **Y08.02** **Assault by strike by baseball bat**

    ✓x7th **Y08.09** **Assault by strike by other specified type of sport equipment**

  ✓5th **Y08.8** **Assault by other specified means**

    ✓x7th **Y08.81** **Assault by crashing of aircraft**

    ✓x7th **Y08.89** **Assault by other specified means**

  Y09 **Assault by unspecified means**

    Assassination (attempted) NOS

    Homicide (attempted) NOS

    Manslaughter (attempted) NOS

    Murder (attempted) NOS

Event of undetermined intent (Y21-Y33)

Undetermined intent is only for use when there is specific documentation in the record that the intent of the injury cannot be determined. If no such documentation is present, code to accidental (unintentional)

Y10-Y19 **Deactivated**

      See codes T36-T65 with fifth or sixth character 4

Y20 **Deactivated**

      See category T71

✓4th **Y21** **Drowning and submersion, undetermined intent**

> The appropriate 7th character is to be added to each code from category Y21.
> A   initial encounter
> D   subsequent encounter
> S   sequela

  ✓x7th **Y21.0** **Drowning and submersion while in bathtub, undetermined intent**

  ✓x7th **Y21.1** **Drowning and submersion after fall into bathtub, undetermined intent**

  ✓x7th **Y21.2** **Drowning and submersion while in swimming pool, undetermined intent**

  ✓x7th **Y21.3** **Drowning and submersion after fall into swimming pool, undetermined intent**

  ✓x7th **Y21.4** **Drowning and submersion in natural water, undetermined intent**

  ✓x7th **Y21.8** **Other drowning and submersion, undetermined intent**

  ✓x7th **Y21.9** **Unspecified drowning and submersion, undetermined intent**

✓x7th **Y22** **Handgun discharge, undetermined intent**

    Discharge of gun for single hand use, undetermined intent

    Discharge of pistol, undetermined intent

    Discharge of revolver, undetermined intent

    EXCLUDES 2 *Very pistol (Y24.8)*

> The appropriate 7th character is to be added to code Y22.
> A   initial encounter
> D   subsequent encounter
> S   sequela

✓ Appropriate additional character required   ✓x7th Requires 7th character, placeholder x must fill empty characters

√4ᵗʰ **Y23 Rifle, shotgun and larger firearm discharge, undetermined intent**

EXCLUDES 2 *airgun (Y24.0)*

The appropriate 7th character is to be added to each code from category Y23.
A   initial encounter
D   subsequent encounter
S   sequela

√x7ᵗʰ **Y23.0 Shotgun discharge, undetermined intent**
√x7ᵗʰ **Y23.1 Hunting rifle discharge, undetermined intent**
√x7ᵗʰ **Y23.2 Military firearm discharge, undetermined intent**
√x7ᵗʰ **Y23.3 Machine gun discharge, undetermined intent**
√x7ᵗʰ **Y23.8 Other larger firearm discharge, undetermined intent**
√x7ᵗʰ **Y23.9 Unspecified larger firearm discharge, undetermined intent**

√4ᵗʰ **Y24 Other and unspecified firearm discharge, undetermined intent**

The appropriate 7th character is to be added to each code from category Y24.
A   initial encounter
D   subsequent encounter
S   sequela

√x7ᵗʰ **Y24.0 Airgun discharge, undetermined intent**
BB gun discharge, undetermined intent
Pellet gun discharge, undetermined intent
√x7ᵗʰ **Y24.8 Other firearm discharge, undetermined intent**
Paintball gun discharge, undetermined intent
Very pistol [flare] discharge, undetermined intent
√x7ᵗʰ **Y24.9 Unspecified firearm discharge, undetermined intent**

√x7ᵗʰ **Y25 Contact with explosive material, undetermined intent**

The appropriate 7th character is to be added to code Y25.
A   initial encounter
D   subsequent encounter
S   sequela

√x7ᵗʰ **Y26 Exposure to smoke, fire and flames, undetermined intent**

The appropriate 7th character is to be added to code Y26.
A   initial encounter
D   subsequent encounter
S   sequela

√4ᵗʰ **Y27 Contact with steam, hot vapors and hot objects, undetermined intent**

The appropriate 7th character is to be added to each code from category Y27.
A   initial encounter
D   subsequent encounter
S   sequela

√x7ᵗʰ **Y27.0 Contact with steam and hot vapors, undetermined intent**
√x7ᵗʰ **Y27.1 Contact with hot tap water, undetermined intent**
√x7ᵗʰ **Y27.2 Contact with hot fluids, undetermined intent**
√x7ᵗʰ **Y27.3 Contact with hot household appliance, undetermined intent**
√x7ᵗʰ **Y27.8 Contact with other hot objects, undetermined intent**
√x7ᵗʰ **Y27.9 Contact with unspecified hot objects, undetermined intent**

√4ᵗʰ **Y28 Contact with sharp object, undetermined intent**

The appropriate 7th character is to be added to each code from category Y28.
A   initial encounter
D   subsequent encounter
S   sequela

√x7ᵗʰ **Y28.0 Contact with sharp glass, undetermined intent**
√x7ᵗʰ **Y28.1 Contact with knife, undetermined intent**
√x7ᵗʰ **Y28.2 Contact with sword or dagger, undetermined intent**
√x7ᵗʰ **Y28.8 Contact with other sharp object, undetermined intent**
√x7ᵗʰ **Y28.9 Contact with unspecified sharp object, undetermined intent**

√x7ᵗʰ **Y29 Contact with blunt object, undetermined intent**

The appropriate 7th character is to be added to code Y29.
A   initial encounter
D   subsequent encounter
S   sequela

√x7ᵗʰ **Y30 Falling, jumping or pushed from a high place, undetermined intent**
Victim falling from one level to another, undetermined intent

The appropriate 7th character is to be added to code Y30.
A   initial encounter
D   subsequent encounter
S   sequela

√x7ᵗʰ **Y31 Falling, lying or running before or into moving object, undetermined intent**

The appropriate 7th character is to be added to code Y31.
A   initial encounter
D   subsequent encounter
S   sequela

√x7ᵗʰ **Y32 Crashing of motor vehicle, undetermined intent**

The appropriate 7th character is to be added to code Y32.
A   initial encounter
D   subsequent encounter
S   sequela

√x7ᵗʰ **Y33 Other specified events, undetermined intent**

The appropriate 7th character is to be added to code Y33.
A   initial encounter
D   subsequent encounter
S   sequela

Legal intervention, operations of war, military operations, and terrorism (Y35-Y38)

√4ᵗʰ **Y35 Legal intervention**
INCLUDES   any injury sustained as a result of an encounter with any law enforcement official, serving in any capacity at the time of the encounter, whether on-duty or off-duty. Includes injury to law enforcement official, suspect and bystander

The appropriate 7th character is to be added to each code from category Y35.
A   initial encounter
D   subsequent encounter
S   sequela

√5ᵗʰ **Y35.0 Legal intervention involving firearm discharge**
√6ᵗʰ **Y35.00 Legal intervention involving unspecified firearm discharge**
Legal intervention involving gunshot wound
Legal intervention involving shot NOS
√7ᵗʰ **Y35.001 Legal intervention involving unspecified firearm discharge, law enforcement official injured**
√7ᵗʰ **Y35.002 Legal intervention involving unspecified firearm discharge, bystander injured**
√7ᵗʰ **Y35.003 Legal intervention involving unspecified firearm discharge, suspect injured**
√6ᵗʰ **Y35.01 Legal intervention involving injury by machine gun**
√7ᵗʰ **Y35.011 Legal intervention involving injury by machine gun, law enforcement official injured**
√7ᵗʰ **Y35.012 Legal intervention involving injury by machine gun, bystander injured**
√7ᵗʰ **Y35.013 Legal intervention involving injury by machine gun, suspect injured**
√6ᵗʰ **Y35.02 Legal intervention involving injury by handgun**
√7ᵗʰ **Y35.021 Legal intervention involving injury by handgun, law enforcement official injured**
√7ᵗʰ **Y35.022 Legal intervention involving injury by handgun, bystander injured**

EXCLUDES 1 Not coded here   EXCLUDES 2 Not included here   *Manifestation Code*

✓7th **Y35.023** Legal intervention involving injury by handgun, suspect injured

✓6th **Y35.03** **Legal intervention involving injury by rifle pellet**

✓7th **Y35.031** **Legal intervention involving injury by rifle pellet, law enforcement official injured**

✓7th **Y35.032** **Legal intervention involving injury by rifle pellet, bystander injured**

✓7th **Y35.033** **Legal intervention involving injury by rifle pellet, suspect injured**

✓6th **Y35.04** **Legal intervention involving injury by rubber bullet**

✓7th **Y35.041** **Legal intervention involving injury by rubber bullet, law enforcement official injured**

✓7th **Y35.042** **Legal intervention involving injury by rubber bullet, bystander injured**

✓7th **Y35.043** **Legal intervention involving injury by rubber bullet, suspect injured**

✓6th **Y35.09** **Legal intervention involving other firearm discharge**

✓7th **Y35.091** **Legal intervention involving other firearm discharge, law enforcement official injured**

✓7th **Y35.092** **Legal intervention involving other firearm discharge, bystander injured**

✓7th **Y35.093** **Legal intervention involving other firearm discharge, suspect injured**

✓5th **Y35.1** **Legal intervention involving explosives**

✓6th **Y35.10** **Legal intervention involving unspecified explosives**

✓7th **Y35.101** **Legal intervention involving unspecified explosives, law enforcement official injured**

✓7th **Y35.102** **Legal intervention involving unspecified explosives, bystander injured**

✓7th **Y35.103** **Legal intervention involving unspecified explosives, suspect injured**

✓6th **Y35.11** **Legal intervention involving injury by dynamite**

✓7th **Y35.111** **Legal intervention involving injury by dynamite, law enforcement official injured**

✓7th **Y35.112** **Legal intervention involving injury by dynamite, bystander injured**

✓7th **Y35.113** **Legal intervention involving injury by dynamite, suspect injured**

✓6th **Y35.12** **Legal intervention involving injury by explosive shell**

✓7th **Y35.121** **Legal intervention involving injury by explosive shell, law enforcement official injured**

✓7th **Y35.122** **Legal intervention involving injury by explosive shell, bystander injured**

✓7th **Y35.123** **Legal intervention involving injury by explosive shell, suspect injured**

✓6th **Y35.19** **Legal intervention involving other explosives**

Legal intervention involving injury by grenade

Legal intervention involving injury by mortar bomb

✓7th **Y35.191** **Legal intervention involving other explosives, law enforcement official injured**

✓7th **Y35.192** **Legal intervention involving other explosives, bystander injured**

✓7th **Y35.193** **Legal intervention involving other explosives, suspect injured**

✓5th **Y35.2** **Legal intervention involving gas**

Legal intervention involving asphyxiation by gas

Legal intervention involving poisoning by gas

✓6th **Y35.20** **Legal intervention involving unspecified gas**

✓7th **Y35.201** **Legal intervention involving unspecified gas, law enforcement official injured**

✓7th **Y35.202** **Legal intervention involving unspecified gas, bystander injured**

✓7th **Y35.203** **Legal intervention involving unspecified gas, suspect injured**

✓6th **Y35.21** **Legal intervention involving injury by tear gas**

✓7th **Y35.211** **Legal intervention involving injury by tear gas, law enforcement official injured**

✓7th **Y35.212** **Legal intervention involving injury by tear gas, bystander injured**

✓7th **Y35.213** **Legal intervention involving injury by tear gas, suspect injured**

✓6th **Y35.29** **Legal intervention involving other gas**

✓7th **Y35.291** **Legal intervention involving other gas, law enforcement official injured**

✓7th **Y35.292** **Legal intervention involving other gas, bystander injured**

✓7th **Y35.293** **Legal intervention involving other gas, suspect injured**

✓5th **Y35.3** **Legal intervention involving blunt objects**

Legal intervention involving being hit or struck by blunt object

✓6th **Y35.30** **Legal intervention involving unspecified blunt objects**

✓7th **Y35.301** **Legal intervention involving unspecified blunt objects, law enforcement official injured**

✓7th **Y35.302** **Legal intervention involving unspecified blunt objects, bystander injured**

✓7th **Y35.303** **Legal intervention involving unspecified blunt objects, suspect injured**

✓6th **Y35.31** **Legal intervention involving baton**

✓7th **Y35.311** **Legal intervention involving baton, law enforcement official injured**

✓7th **Y35.312** **Legal intervention involving baton, bystander injured**

✓7th **Y35.313** **Legal intervention involving baton, suspect injured**

✓6th **Y35.39** **Legal intervention involving other blunt objects**

✓7th **Y35.391** **Legal intervention involving other blunt objects, law enforcement official injured**

✓7th **Y35.392** **Legal intervention involving other blunt objects, bystander injured**

✓7th **Y35.393** **Legal intervention involving other blunt objects, suspect injured**

✓5th **Y35.4** **Legal intervention involving sharp objects**

Legal intervention involving being cut by sharp objects

Legal intervention involving being stabbed by sharp objects

✓6th **Y35.40** **Legal intervention involving unspecified sharp objects**

✓7th **Y35.401** **Legal intervention involving unspecified sharp objects, law enforcement official injured**

✓7th **Y35.402** **Legal intervention involving unspecified sharp objects, bystander injured**

✓7th **Y35.403** **Legal intervention involving unspecified sharp objects, suspect injured**

✓6th **Y35.41** **Legal intervention involving bayonet**

✓7th **Y35.411** **Legal intervention involving bayonet, law enforcement official injured**

✓7th **Y35.412** **Legal intervention involving bayonet, bystander injured**

✓7th **Y35.413** **Legal intervention involving bayonet, suspect injured**

✓6th **Y35.49** **Legal intervention involving other sharp objects**

✓7th **Y35.491** **Legal intervention involving other sharp objects, law enforcement official injured**

✓7th **Y35.492** **Legal intervention involving other sharp objects, bystander injured**

✓7th **Y35.493** **Legal intervention involving other sharp objects, suspect injured**

✓5th **Y35.8** **Legal intervention involving other specified means**

✓6th **Y35.81** **Legal intervention involving manhandling**

✓7th **Y35.811** **Legal intervention involving manhandling, law enforcement official injured**

✓ Appropriate additional character required　　　　✓x7th Requires 7th character, placeholder x must fill empty characters

✓7th **Y35.812 Legal intervention involving manhandling, bystander injured**

✓7th **Y35.813 Legal intervention involving manhandling, suspect injured**

✓6th **Y35.89 Legal intervention involving other specified means**

✓7th **Y35.891 Legal intervention involving other specified means, law enforcement official injured**

✓7th **Y35.892 Legal intervention involving other specified means, bystander injured**

✓7th **Y35.893 Legal intervention involving other specified means, suspect injured**

✓5th **Y35.9 Legal intervention, means unspecified**

✓x7th **Y35.91 Legal intervention, means unspecified, law enforcement official injured**

✓x7th **Y35.92 Legal intervention, means unspecified, bystander injured**

✓x7th **Y35.93 Legal intervention, means unspecified, suspect injured**

✓4th **Y36 Operations of war**

INCLUDES   injuries to military personnel and civilians caused by war, civil insurrection, and peacekeeping missions

EXCLUDES 1   *injury to military personnel occurring during peacetime military operations (Y37-)*

military vehicles involved in transport accidents with non-military vehicle during peacetime (V09.01, V09.21, V19.81, V29.81, V39.81, V49.81, V59.81, V69.81, V79.81)

> The appropriate 7th character is to be added to each code from category Y36.
> A   initial encounter
> D   subsequent encounter
> S   sequela

✓5th **Y36.0 War operations involving explosion of marine weapons**

✓6th **Y36.00 War operations involving explosion of unspecified marine weapon**

War operations involving underwater blast NOS

✓7th **Y36.000 War operations involving explosion of unspecified marine weapon, military personnel**

✓7th **Y36.001 War operations involving explosion of unspecified marine weapon, civilian**

✓6th **Y36.01 War operations involving explosion of depth-charge**

✓7th **Y36.010 War operations involving explosion of depth-charge, military personnel**

✓7th **Y36.011 War operations involving explosion of depth-charge, civilian**

✓6th **Y36.02 War operations involving explosion of marine mine**

War operations involving explosion of marine mine, at sea or in harbor

✓7th **Y36.020 War operations involving explosion of marine mine, military personnel**

✓7th **Y36.021 War operations involving explosion of marine mine, civilian**

✓6th **Y36.03 War operations involving explosion of sea-based artillery shell**

✓7th **Y36.030 War operations involving explosion of sea-based artillery shell, military personnel**

✓7th **Y36.031 War operations involving explosion of sea-based artillery shell, civilian**

✓6th **Y36.04 War operations involving explosion of torpedo**

✓7th **Y36.040 War operations involving explosion of torpedo, military personnel**

✓7th **Y36.041 War operations involving explosion of torpedo, civilian**

✓6th **Y36.05 War operations involving accidental detonation of onboard marine weapons**

✓7th **Y36.050 War operations involving accidental detonation of onboard marine weapons, military personnel**

✓7th **Y36.051 War operations involving accidental detonation of onboard marine weapons, civilian**

✓6th **Y36.09 War operations involving explosion of other marine weapons**

✓7th **Y36.090 War operations involving explosion of other marine weapons, military personnel**

✓7th **Y36.091 War operations involving explosion of other marine weapons, civilian**

✓5th **Y36.1 War operations involving destruction of aircraft**

✓6th **Y36.10 War operations involving unspecified destruction of aircraft**

✓7th **Y36.100 War operations involving unspecified destruction of aircraft, military personnel**

✓7th **Y36.101 War operations involving unspecified destruction of aircraft, civilian**

✓6th **Y36.11 War operations involving destruction of aircraft due to enemy fire or explosives**

War operations involving destruction of aircraft due to air to air missile

War operations involving destruction of aircraft due to explosive placed on aircraft

War operations involving destruction of aircraft due to rocket propelled grenade [RPG]

War operations involving destruction of aircraft due to small arms fire

War operations involving destruction of aircraft due to surface to air missile

✓7th **Y36.110 War operations involving destruction of aircraft due to enemy fire or explosives, military personnel**

✓7th **Y36.111 War operations involving destruction of aircraft due to enemy fire or explosives, civilian**

✓6th **Y36.12 War operations involving destruction of aircraft due to collision with other aircraft**

✓7th **Y36.120 War operations involving destruction of aircraft due to collision with other aircraft, military personnel**

✓7th **Y36.121 War operations involving destruction of aircraft due to collision with other aircraft, civilian**

✓6th **Y36.13 War operations involving destruction of aircraft due to onboard fire**

✓7th **Y36.130 War operations involving destruction of aircraft due to onboard fire, military personnel**

✓7th **Y36.131 War operations involving destruction of aircraft due to onboard fire, civilian**

✓6th **Y36.14 War operations involving destruction of aircraft due to accidental detonation of onboard munitions and explosives**

✓7th **Y36.140 War operations involving destruction of aircraft due to accidental detonation of onboard munitions and explosives, military personnel**

✓7th **Y36.141 War operations involving destruction of aircraft due to accidental detonation of onboard munitions and explosives, civilian**

✓6th **Y36.19 War operations involving other destruction of aircraft**

✓7th **Y36.190 War operations involving other destruction of aircraft, military personnel**

✓7th **Y36.191 War operations involving other destruction of aircraft, civilian**

✓5th **Y36.2 War operations involving other explosions and fragments**

EXCLUDES 1   *war operations involving explosion of aircraft (Y36.1-)*

war operations involving explosion of marine weapons (Y36.0-)

war operations involving explosion of nuclear weapons (Y36.5-)

war operations involving explosion occurring after cessation of hostilities (Y36.8-)

EXCLUDES 1 Not coded here   EXCLUDES 2 Not included here   *Manifestation Code*

√6th **Y36.20 War operations involving unspecified explosion and fragments**
War operations involving air blast NOS
War operations involving blast NOS
War operations involving blast fragments NOS
War operations involving blast wave NOS
War operations involving blast wind NOS
War operations involving explosion NOS
War operations involving explosion of bomb NOS

√7th **Y36.200 War operations involving unspecified explosion and fragments, military personnel**

√7th **Y36.201 War operations involving unspecified explosion and fragments, civilian**

√6th **Y36.21 War operations involving explosion of aerial bomb**

√7th **Y36.210 War operations involving explosion of aerial bomb, military personnel**

√7th **Y36.211 War operations involving explosion of aerial bomb, civilian**

√6th **Y36.22 War operations involving explosion of guided missile**

√7th **Y36.220 War operations involving explosion of guided missile, military personnel**

√7th **Y36.221 War operations involving explosion of guided missile, civilian**

√6th **Y36.23 War operations involving explosion of improvised explosive device [IED]**
War operations involving explosion of person-borne improvised explosive device [IED]
War operations involving explosion of vehicle-borne improvised explosive device [IED]
War operations involving explosion of roadside improvised explosive device [IED]

√7th **Y36.230 War operations involving explosion of improvised explosive device [IED], military personnel**

√7th **Y36.231 War operations involving explosion of improvised explosive device [IED], civilian**

√6th **Y36.24 War operations involving explosion due to accidental detonation and discharge of own munitions or munitions launch device**

√7th **Y36.240 War operations involving explosion due to accidental detonation and discharge of own munitions or munitions launch device, military personnel**

√7th **Y36.241 War operations involving explosion due to accidental detonation and discharge of own munitions or munitions launch device, civilian**

√6th **Y36.25 War operations involving fragments from munitions**

√7th **Y36.250 War operations involving fragments from munitions, military personnel**

√7th **Y36.251 War operations involving fragments from munitions, civilian**

√6th **Y36.26 War operations involving fragments of improvised explosive device [IED]**
War operations involving fragments of person-borne improvised explosive device [IED]
War operations involving fragments of vehicle-borne improvised explosive device [IED]
War operations involving fragments of roadside improvised explosive device [IED]

√7th **Y36.260 War operations involving fragments of improvised explosive device [IED], military personnel**

√7th **Y36.261 War operations involving fragments of improvised explosive device [IED], civilian**

√6th **Y36.27 War operations involving fragments from weapons**

√7th **Y36.270 War operations involving fragments from weapons, military personnel**

√7th **Y36.271 War operations involving fragments from weapons, civilian**

√6th **Y36.29 War operations involving other explosions and fragments**
War operations involving explosion of grenade
War operations involving explosions of land mine
War operations involving shrapnel NOS

√7th **Y36.290 War operations involving other explosions and fragments, military personnel**

√7th **Y36.291 War operations involving other explosions and fragments, civilian**

√5th **Y36.3 War operations involving fires, conflagrations and hot substances**
War operations involving smoke, fumes, and heat from fires, conflagrations and hot substances

EXCLUDES 1 *war operations involving fires and conflagrations aboard military aircraft (Y36.1-)*
war operations involving fires and conflagrations aboard military watercraft (Y36.0-)
war operations involving fires and conflagrations caused indirectly by conventional weapons (Y36.2-)
war operations involving fires and thermal effects of nuclear weapons (Y36.53-)

√6th **Y36.30 War operations involving unspecified fire, conflagration and hot substance**

√7th **Y36.300 War operations involving unspecified fire, conflagration and hot substance, military personnel**

√7th **Y36.301 War operations involving unspecified fire, conflagration and hot substance, civilian**

√6th **Y36.31 War operations involving gasoline bomb**
War operations involving incendiary bomb
War operations involving petrol bomb

√7th **Y36.310 War operations involving gasoline bomb, military personnel**

√7th **Y36.311 War operations involving gasoline bomb, civilian**

√6th **Y36.32 War operations involving incendiary bullet**

√7th **Y36.320 War operations involving incendiary bullet, military personnel**

√7th **Y36.321 War operations involving incendiary bullet, civilian**

√6th **Y36.33 War operations involving flamethrower**

√7th **Y36.330 War operations involving flamethrower, military personnel**

√7th **Y36.331 War operations involving flamethrower, civilian**

√6th **Y36.39 War operations involving other fires, conflagrations and hot substances**

√7th **Y36.390 War operations involving other fires, conflagrations and hot substances, military personnel**

√7th **Y36.391 War operations involving other fires, conflagrations and hot substances, civilian**

√5th **Y36.4 War operations involving firearm discharge and other forms of conventional warfare**

√6th **Y36.41 War operations involving rubber bullets**

√7th **Y36.410 War operations involving rubber bullets, military personnel**

√7th **Y36.411 War operations involving rubber bullets, civilian**

√6th **Y36.42 War operations involving firearms pellets**

√7th **Y36.420 War operations involving firearms pellets, military personnel**

√7th **Y36.421 War operations involving firearms pellets, civilian**

√6th **Y36.43 War operations involving other firearms discharge**
War operations involving bullets NOS

EXCLUDES 1 *war operations involving munitions fragments (Y36.25-)*
war operations involving incendiary bullets (Y36.32-)

√7th **Y36.430 War operations involving other firearms discharge, military personnel**

√7th **Y36.431 War operations involving other firearms discharge, civilian**

☑ Appropriate additional character required   √x7th Requires 7th character, placeholder x must fill empty characters

√6th **Y36.44 War operations involving unarmed hand to hand combat**

> EXCLUDES 1   *war operations involving combat using blunt or piercing object (Y36.45-)*
> *war operations involving intentional restriction of air and airway (Y36.46-)*
> *war operations involving unintentional restriction of air and airway (Y36.47-)*

√7th   **Y36.440 War operations involving unarmed hand to hand combat, military personnel**

√7th   **Y36.441 War operations involving unarmed hand to hand combat, civilian**

√6th **Y36.45 War operations involving combat using blunt or piercing object**

√7th   **Y36.450 War operations involving combat using blunt or piercing object, military personnel**

√7th   **Y36.451 War operations involving combat using blunt or piercing object, civilian**

√6th **Y36.46 War operations involving intentional restriction of air and airway**

√7th   **Y36.460 War operations involving intentional restriction of air and airway, military personnel**

√7th   **Y36.461 War operations involving intentional restriction of air and airway, civilian**

√6th **Y36.47 War operations involving unintentional restriction of air and airway**

√7th   **Y36.470 War operations involving unintentional restriction of air and airway, military personnel**

√7th   **Y36.471 War operations involving unintentional restriction of air and airway, civilian**

√6th **Y36.49 War operations involving other forms of conventional warfare**

√7th   **Y36.490 War operations involving other forms of conventional warfare, military personnel**

√7th   **Y36.491 War operations involving other forms of conventional warfare, civilian**

√5th **Y36.5 War operations involving nuclear weapons**
War operations involving dirty bomb NOS

√6th **Y36.50 War operations involving unspecified effect of nuclear weapon**

√7th   **Y36.500 War operations involving unspecified effect of nuclear weapon, military personnel**

√7th   **Y36.501 War operations involving unspecified effect of nuclear weapon, civilian**

√6th **Y36.51 War operations involving direct blast effect of nuclear weapon**
War operations involving blast pressure of nuclear weapon

√7th   **Y36.510 War operations involving direct blast effect of nuclear weapon, military personnel**

√7th   **Y36.511 War operations involving direct blast effect of nuclear weapon, civilian**

√6th **Y36.52 War operations involving indirect blast effect of nuclear weapon**
War operations involving being thrown by blast of nuclear weapon
War operations involving being struck or crushed by blast debris of nuclear weapon

√7th   **Y36.520 War operations involving indirect blast effect of nuclear weapon, military personnel**

√7th   **Y36.521 War operations involving indirect blast effect of nuclear weapon, civilian**

√6th **Y36.53 War operations involving thermal radiation effect of nuclear weapon**
War operations involving direct heat from nuclear weapon
War operation involving fireball effects from nuclear weapon

√7th   **Y36.530 War operations involving thermal radiation effect of nuclear weapon, military personnel**

√7th   **Y36.531 War operations involving thermal radiation effect of nuclear weapon, civilian**

√6th **Y36.54 War operation involving nuclear radiation effects of nuclear weapon**
War operation involving acute radiation exposure from nuclear weapon
War operation involving exposure to immediate ionizing radiation from nuclear weapon
War operation involving fallout exposure from nuclear weapon
War operation involving secondary effects of nuclear weapons

√7th   **Y36.540 War operation involving nuclear radiation effects of nuclear weapon, military personnel**

√7th   **Y36.541 War operation involving nuclear radiation effects of nuclear weapon, civilian**

√6th **Y36.59 War operation involving other effects of nuclear weapons**

√7th   **Y36.590 War operation involving other effects of nuclear weapons, military personnel**

√7th   **Y36.591 War operation involving other effects of nuclear weapons, civilian**

√5th **Y36.6 War operations involving biological weapons**

√6th **Y36.6x War operations involving biological weapons**

√7th   **Y36.6x0 War operations involving biological weapons, military personnel**

√7th   **Y36.6x1 War operations involving biological weapons, civilian**

√5th **Y36.7 War operations involving chemical weapons and other forms of unconventional warfare**

> EXCLUDES 1   *war operations involving incendiary devices (Y36.3-, Y36.5-)*

√6th **Y36.7x War operations involving chemical weapons and other forms of unconventional warfare**

√7th   **Y36.7x0 War operations involving chemical weapons and other forms of unconventional warfare, military personnel**

√7th   **Y36.7x1 War operations involving chemical weapons and other forms of unconventional warfare, civilian**

√5th **Y36.8 War operations occurring after cessation of hostilities**
War operations classifiable to categories Y36.0-Y36.8 but occurring after cessation of hostilities

√6th **Y36.81 Explosion of mine placed during war operations but exploding after cessation of hostilities**

√7th   **Y36.810 Explosion of mine placed during war operations but exploding after cessation of hostilities, military personnel**

√7th   **Y36.811 Explosion of mine placed during war operations but exploding after cessation of hostilities, civilian**

√6th **Y36.82 Explosion of bomb placed during war operations but exploding after cessation of hostilities**

√7th   **Y36.820 Explosion of bomb placed during war operations but exploding after cessation of hostilities, military personnel**

√7th   **Y36.821 Explosion of bomb placed during war operations but exploding after cessation of hostilities, civilian**

√6th **Y36.88 Other war operations occurring after cessation of hostilities**

√7th   **Y36.880 Other war operations occurring after cessation of hostilities, military personnel**

√7th   **Y36.881 Other war operations occurring after cessation of hostilities, civilian**

√6th **Y36.89 Unspecified war operations occurring after cessation of hostilities**

√7th   **Y36.890 Unspecified war operations occurring after cessation of hostilities, military personnel**

√7th   **Y36.891 Unspecified war operations occurring after cessation of hostilities, civilian**

EXCLUDES 1   Not coded here   EXCLUDES 2   Not included here   *Manifestation Code*

☑5ᵗʰ Y36.9 Other and unspecified war operations
- **☑x7ᵗʰ Y36.90 War operations, unspecified**
- **☑x7ᵗʰ Y36.91 War operations involving unspecified weapon of mass destruction [WMD]**
- **☑x7ᵗʰ Y36.92 War operations involving friendly fire**

☑4ᵗʰ Y37 Military operations
> INCLUDES injuries to military personnel and civilians occurring during peacetime on military property and during routine military exercises and operations
> EXCLUDES 1 military aircraft involved in aircraft accident with civilian aircraft (V97.81-)
> military vehicles involved in transport accident with civilian vehicle (V09.01, V09.21, V19.81, V29.81, V39.81, V49.81, V59.81, V69.81, V79.81)
> military watercraft involved in water transport accident with civilian watercraft (V94.81-)
> war operations (Y36-)

> The appropriate 7th character is to be added to each code from category Y37.
> A initial encounter
> D subsequent encounter
> S sequela

☑5ᵗʰ Y37.0 Military operations involving explosion of marine weapons
- **☑6ᵗʰ Y37.00 Military operations involving explosion of unspecified marine weapon**
  Military operations involving underwater blast NOS
  - **☑7ᵗʰ Y37.000 Military operations involving explosion of unspecified marine weapon, military personnel**
  - **☑7ᵗʰ Y37.001 Military operations involving explosion of unspecified marine weapon, civilian**
- **☑6ᵗʰ Y37.01 Military operations involving explosion of depth-charge**
  - **☑7ᵗʰ Y37.010 Military operations involving explosion of depth-charge, military personnel**
  - **☑7ᵗʰ Y37.011 Military operations involving explosion of depth-charge, civilian**
- **☑6ᵗʰ Y37.02 Military operations involving explosion of marine mine**
  Military operations involving explosion of marine mine, at sea or in harbor
  - **☑7ᵗʰ Y37.020 Military operations involving explosion of marine mine, military personnel**
  - **☑7ᵗʰ Y37.021 Military operations involving explosion of marine mine, civilian**
- **☑6ᵗʰ Y37.03 Military operations involving explosion of sea-based artillery shell**
  - **☑7ᵗʰ Y37.030 Military operations involving explosion of sea-based artillery shell, military personnel**
  - **☑7ᵗʰ Y37.031 Military operations involving explosion of sea-based artillery shell, civilian**
- **☑6ᵗʰ Y37.04 Military operations involving explosion of torpedo**
  - **☑7ᵗʰ Y37.040 Military operations involving explosion of torpedo, military personnel**
  - **☑7ᵗʰ Y37.041 Military operations involving explosion of torpedo, civilian**
- **☑6ᵗʰ Y37.05 Military operations involving accidental detonation of onboard marine weapons**
  - **☑7ᵗʰ Y37.050 Military operations involving accidental detonation of onboard marine weapons, military personnel**
  - **☑7ᵗʰ Y37.051 Military operations involving accidental detonation of onboard marine weapons, civilian**
- **☑6ᵗʰ Y37.09 Military operations involving explosion of other marine weapons**
  - **☑7ᵗʰ Y37.090 Military operations involving explosion of other marine weapons, military personnel**
  - **☑7ᵗʰ Y37.091 Military operations involving explosion of other marine weapons, civilian**

☑5ᵗʰ Y37.1 Military operations involving destruction of aircraft
- **☑6ᵗʰ Y37.10 Military operations involving unspecified destruction of aircraft**
  - **☑7ᵗʰ Y37.100 Military operations involving unspecified destruction of aircraft, military personnel**
  - **☑7ᵗʰ Y37.101 Military operations involving unspecified destruction of aircraft, civilian**
- **☑6ᵗʰ Y37.11 Military operations involving destruction of aircraft due to enemy fire or explosives**
  Military operations involving destruction of aircraft due to air to air missile
  Military operations involving destruction of aircraft due to explosive placed on aircraft
  Military operations involving destruction of aircraft due to rocket propelled grenade [RPG]
  Military operations involving destruction of aircraft due to small arms fire
  Military operations involving destruction of aircraft due to surface to air missile
  - **☑7ᵗʰ Y37.110 Military operations involving destruction of aircraft due to enemy fire or explosives, military personnel**
  - **☑7ᵗʰ Y37.111 Military operations involving destruction of aircraft due to enemy fire or explosives, civilian**
- **☑6ᵗʰ Y37.12 Military operations involving destruction of aircraft due to collision with other aircraft**
  - **☑7ᵗʰ Y37.120 Military operations involving destruction of aircraft due to collision with other aircraft, military personnel**
  - **☑7ᵗʰ Y37.121 Military operations involving destruction of aircraft due to collision with other aircraft, civilian**
- **☑6ᵗʰ Y37.13 Military operations involving destruction of aircraft due to onboard fire**
  - **☑7ᵗʰ Y37.130 Military operations involving destruction of aircraft due to onboard fire, military personnel**
  - **☑7ᵗʰ Y37.131 Military operations involving destruction of aircraft due to onboard fire, civilian**
- **☑6ᵗʰ Y37.14 Military operations involving destruction of aircraft due to accidental detonation of onboard munitions and explosives**
  - **☑7ᵗʰ Y37.140 Military operations involving destruction of aircraft due to accidental detonation of onboard munitions and explosives, military personnel**
  - **☑7ᵗʰ Y37.141 Military operations involving destruction of aircraft due to accidental detonation of onboard munitions and explosives, civilian**
- **☑6ᵗʰ Y37.19 Military operations involving other destruction of aircraft**
  - **☑7ᵗʰ Y37.190 Military operations involving other destruction of aircraft, military personnel**
  - **☑7ᵗʰ Y37.191 Military operations involving other destruction of aircraft, civilian**

☑5ᵗʰ Y37.2 Military operations involving other explosions and fragments
> EXCLUDES 1 military operations involving explosion of aircraft (Y37.1-)
> military operations involving explosion of marine weapons (Y37.0-)
> military operations involving explosion of nuclear weapons (Y37.5-)
- **☑6ᵗʰ Y37.20 Military operations involving unspecified explosion and fragments**
  Military operations involving air blast NOS
  Military operations involving blast NOS
  Military operations involving blast fragments NOS
  Military operations involving blast wave NOS
  Military operations involving blast wind NOS
  Military operations involving explosion NOS
  Military operations involving explosion of bomb NOS
  - **☑7ᵗʰ Y37.200 Military operations involving unspecified explosion and fragments, military personnel**

✓7th   **Y37.201 Military operations involving unspecified explosion and fragments, civilian**

✓6th   **Y37.21 Military operations involving explosion of aerial bomb**

✓7th   **Y37.210 Military operations involving explosion of aerial bomb, military personnel**

✓7th   **Y37.211 Military operations involving explosion of aerial bomb, civilian**

✓6th   **Y37.22 Military operations involving explosion of guided missile**

✓7th   **Y37.220 Military operations involving explosion of guided missile, military personnel**

✓7th   **Y37.221 Military operations involving explosion of guided missile, civilian**

✓6th   **Y37.23 Military operations involving explosion of improvised explosive device [IED]**

Military operations involving explosion of person-borne improvised explosive device [IED]

Military operations involving explosion of vehicle-borne improvised explosive device [IED]

Military operations involving explosion of roadside improvised explosive device [IED]

✓7th   **Y37.230 Military operations involving explosion of improvised explosive device [IED], military personnel**

✓7th   **Y37.231 Military operations involving explosion of improvised explosive device [IED], civilian**

✓6th   **Y37.24 Military operations involving explosion due to accidental detonation and discharge of own munitions or munitions launch device**

✓7th   **Y37.240 Military operations involving explosion due to accidental detonation and discharge of own munitions or munitions launch device, military personnel**

✓7th   **Y37.241 Military operations involving explosion due to accidental detonation and discharge of own munitions or munitions launch device, civilian**

✓6th   **Y37.25 Military operations involving fragments from munitions**

✓7th   **Y37.250 Military operations involving fragments from munitions, military personnel**

✓7th   **Y37.251 Military operations involving fragments from munitions, civilian**

✓6th   **Y37.26 Military operations involving fragments of improvised explosive device [IED]**

Military operations involving fragments of person-borne improvised explosive device [IED]

Military operations involving fragments of vehicle-borne improvised explosive device [IED]

Military operations involving fragments of roadside improvised explosive device [IED]

✓7th   **Y37.260 Military operations involving fragments of improvised explosive device [IED], military personnel**

✓7th   **Y37.261 Military operations involving fragments of improvised explosive device [IED], civilian**

✓6th   **Y37.27 Military operations involving fragments from weapons**

✓7th   **Y37.270 Military operations involving fragments from weapons, military personnel**

✓7th   **Y37.271 Military operations involving fragments from weapons, civilian**

✓6th   **Y37.29 Military operations involving other explosions and fragments**

Military operations involving explosion of grenade

Military operations involving explosions of land mine

Military operations involving shrapnel NOS

✓7th   **Y37.290 Military operations involving other explosions and fragments, military personnel**

✓7th   **Y37.291 Military operations involving other explosions and fragments, civilian**

✓5th   **Y37.3 Military operations involving fires, conflagrations and hot substances**

Military operations involving smoke, fumes, and heat from fires, conflagrations and hot substances

> EXCLUDES 1   *military operations involving fires and conflagrations aboard military aircraft (Y37.1-)*
>
> *military operations involving fires and conflagrations aboard military watercraft (Y37.0-)*
>
> *military operations involving fires and conflagrations caused indirectly by conventional weapons (Y37.2-)*
>
> *military operations involving fires and thermal effects of nuclear weapons (Y36.53-)*

✓6th   **Y37.30 Military operations involving unspecified fire, conflagration and hot substance**

✓7th   **Y37.300 Military operations involving unspecified fire, conflagration and hot substance, military personnel**

✓7th   **Y37.301 Military operations involving unspecified fire, conflagration and hot substance, civilian**

✓6th   **Y37.31 Military operations involving gasoline bomb**

Military operations involving incendiary bomb

Military operations involving petrol bomb

✓7th   **Y37.310 Military operations involving gasoline bomb, military personnel**

✓7th   **Y37.311 Military operations involving gasoline bomb, civilian**

✓6th   **Y37.32 Military operations involving incendiary bullet**

✓7th   **Y37.320 Military operations involving incendiary bullet, military personnel**

✓7th   **Y37.321 Military operations involving incendiary bullet, civilian**

✓6th   **Y37.33 Military operations involving flamethrower**

✓7th   **Y37.330 Military operations involving flamethrower, military personnel**

✓7th   **Y37.331 Military operations involving flamethrower, civilian**

✓6th   **Y37.39 Military operations involving other fires, conflagrations and hot substances**

✓7th   **Y37.390 Military operations involving other fires, conflagrations and hot substances, military personnel**

✓7th   **Y37.391 Military operations involving other fires, conflagrations and hot substances, civilian**

✓5th   **Y37.4 Military operations involving firearm discharge and other forms of conventional warfare**

✓6th   **Y37.41 Military operations involving rubber bullets**

✓7th   **Y37.410 Military operations involving rubber bullets, military personnel**

✓7th   **Y37.411 Military operations involving rubber bullets, civilian**

✓6th   **Y37.42 Military operations involving firearms pellets**

✓7th   **Y37.420 Military operations involving firearms pellets, military personnel**

✓7th   **Y37.421 Military operations involving firearms pellets, civilian**

✓6th   **Y37.43 Military operations involving other firearms discharge**

Military operations involving bullets NOS

> EXCLUDES 1   *military operations involving munitions fragments (Y37.25-)*
>
> *military operations involving incendiary bullets (Y37.32-)*

✓7th   **Y37.430 Military operations involving other firearms discharge, military personnel**

✓7th   **Y37.431 Military operations involving other firearms discharge, civilian**

EXCLUDES 1 Not coded here   **EXCLUDES 2** Not included here   *Manifestation Code*

☑6ᵗʰ **Y37.44** **Military operations involving unarmed hand to hand combat**

> EXCLUDES 1 *military operations involving combat using blunt or piercing object (Y37.45-)*
> *military operations involving intentional restriction of air and airway (Y37.46-)*
> *military operations involving unintentional restriction of air and airway (Y37.47-)*

    ☑7ᵗʰ **Y37.440** **Military operations involving unarmed hand to hand combat, military personnel**

    ☑7ᵗʰ **Y37.441** **Military operations involving unarmed hand to hand combat, civilian**

☑6ᵗʰ **Y37.45** **Military operations involving combat using blunt or piercing object**

    ☑7ᵗʰ **Y37.450** **Military operations involving combat using blunt or piercing object, military personnel**

    ☑7ᵗʰ **Y37.451** **Military operations involving combat using blunt or piercing object, civilian**

☑6ᵗʰ **Y37.46** **Military operations involving intentional restriction of air and airway**

    ☑7ᵗʰ **Y37.460** **Military operations involving intentional restriction of air and airway, military personnel**

    ☑7ᵗʰ **Y37.461** **Military operations involving intentional restriction of air and airway, civilian**

☑6ᵗʰ **Y37.47** **Military operations involving unintentional restriction of air and airway**

    ☑7ᵗʰ **Y37.470** **Military operations involving unintentional restriction of air and airway, military personnel**

    ☑7ᵗʰ **Y37.471** **Military operations involving unintentional restriction of air and airway, civilian**

☑6ᵗʰ **Y37.49** **Military operations involving other forms of conventional warfare**

    ☑7ᵗʰ **Y37.490** **Military operations involving other forms of conventional warfare, military personnel**

    ☑7ᵗʰ **Y37.491** **Military operations involving other forms of conventional warfare, civilian**

☑5ᵗʰ **Y37.5** **Military operations involving nuclear weapons**

Military operation involving dirty bomb NOS

☑6ᵗʰ **Y37.50** **Military operations involving unspecified effect of nuclear weapon**

    ☑7ᵗʰ **Y37.500** **Military operations involving unspecified effect of nuclear weapon, military personnel**

    ☑7ᵗʰ **Y37.501** **Military operations involving unspecified effect of nuclear weapon, civilian**

☑6ᵗʰ **Y37.51** **Military operations involving direct blast effect of nuclear weapon**

Military operations involving blast pressure of nuclear weapon

    ☑7ᵗʰ **Y37.510** **Military operations involving direct blast effect of nuclear weapon, military personnel**

    ☑7ᵗʰ **Y37.511** **Military operations involving direct blast effect of nuclear weapon, civilian**

☑6ᵗʰ **Y37.52** **Military operations involving indirect blast effect of nuclear weapon**

Military operations involving being thrown by blast of nuclear weapon

Military operations involving being struck or crushed by blast debris of nuclear weapon

    ☑7ᵗʰ **Y37.520** **Military operations involving indirect blast effect of nuclear weapon, military personnel**

    ☑7ᵗʰ **Y37.521** **Military operations involving indirect blast effect of nuclear weapon, civilian**

☑6ᵗʰ **Y37.53** **Military operations involving thermal radiation effect of nuclear weapon**

Military operations involving direct heat from nuclear weapon

Military operation involving fireball effects from nuclear weapon

    ☑7ᵗʰ **Y37.530** **Military operations involving thermal radiation effect of nuclear weapon, military personnel**

    ☑7ᵗʰ **Y37.531** **Military operations involving thermal radiation effect of nuclear weapon, civilian**

☑6ᵗʰ **Y37.54** **Military operation involving nuclear radiation effects of nuclear weapon**

Military operation involving acute radiation exposure from nuclear weapon

Military operation involving exposure to immediate ionizing radiation from nuclear weapon

Military operation involving fallout exposure from nuclear weapon

Military operation involving secondary effects of nuclear weapons

    ☑7ᵗʰ **Y37.540** **Military operation involving nuclear radiation effects of nuclear weapon, military personnel**

    ☑7ᵗʰ **Y37.541** **Military operation involving nuclear radiation effects of nuclear weapon, civilian**

☑6ᵗʰ **Y37.59** **Military operation involving other effects of nuclear weapons**

    ☑7ᵗʰ **Y37.590** **Military operation involving other effects of nuclear weapons, military personnel**

    ☑7ᵗʰ **Y37.591** **Military operation involving other effects of nuclear weapons, civilian**

☑5ᵗʰ **Y37.6** **Military operations involving biological weapons**

☑6ᵗʰ **Y37.6x** **Military operations involving biological weapons**

    ☑7ᵗʰ **Y37.6x0** **Military operations involving biological weapons, military personnel**

    ☑7ᵗʰ **Y37.6x1** **Military operations involving biological weapons, civilian**

☑5ᵗʰ **Y37.7** **Military operations involving chemical weapons and other forms of unconventional warfare**

> EXCLUDES 1 *military operations involving incendiary devices (Y36.3-, Y36.5-)*

☑6ᵗʰ **Y37.7x** **Military operations involving chemical weapons and other forms of unconventional warfare**

    ☑7ᵗʰ **Y37.7x0** **Military operations involving chemical weapons and other forms of unconventional warfare, military personnel**

    ☑7ᵗʰ **Y37.7x1** **Military operations involving chemical weapons and other forms of unconventional warfare, civilian**

☑5ᵗʰ **Y37.9** **Other and unspecified military operations**

    ☑x7ᵗʰ **Y37.90** **Military operations, unspecified**

    ☑x7ᵗʰ **Y37.91** **Military operations involving unspecified weapon of mass destruction [WMD]**

    ☑x7ᵗʰ **Y37.92** **Military operations involving friendly fire**

☑4ᵗʰ **Y38** **Terrorism**

> NOTE These codes are for use to identify injuries resulting from the unlawful use of force or violence against persons or property to intimidate or coerce a Government, the civilian population, or any segment thereof, in furtherance of political or social objective

Use additional code for place of occurrence (Y92-)

> The appropriate 7th character is to be added to each code from category Y38.
> A   initial encounter
> D   subsequent encounter
> S   sequela

☑5ᵗʰ **Y38.0** **Terrorism involving explosion of marine weapons**

Terrorism involving depth-charge

Terrorism involving marine mine

Terrorism involving mine NOS, at sea or in harbor

Terrorism involving sea-based artillery shell

Terrorism involving torpedo

Terrorism involving underwater blast

☑6ᵗʰ **Y38.0x** **Terrorism involving explosion of marine weapons**

    ☑7ᵗʰ **Y38.0x1** **Terrorism involving explosion of marine weapons, public safety official injured**

    ☑7ᵗʰ **Y38.0x2** **Terrorism involving explosion of marine weapons, civilian injured**

☑ Appropriate additional character required   ☑x7ᵗʰ Requires 7th character, placeholder x must fill empty characters

External Causes of Morbidity

Y38.0x3–Y60

√7ᵗʰ **Y38.0x3** **Terrorism involving explosion of marine weapons, terrorist injured**

√5ᵗʰ **Y38.1** **Terrorism involving destruction of aircraft**
Terrorism involving aircraft burned
Terrorism involving aircraft exploded
Terrorism involving aircraft being shot down
Terrorism involving aircraft used as a weapon

√6ᵗʰ **Y38.1x** **Terrorism involving destruction of aircraft**

√7ᵗʰ **Y38.1x1** **Terrorism involving destruction of aircraft, public safety official injured**

√7ᵗʰ **Y38.1x2** **Terrorism involving destruction of aircraft, civilian injured**

√7ᵗʰ **Y38.1x3** **Terrorism involving destruction of aircraft, terrorist injured**

√5ᵗʰ **Y38.2** **Terrorism involving other explosions and fragments**
Terrorism involving antipersonnel (fragments) bomb
Terrorism involving blast NOS
Terrorism involving explosion NOS
Terrorism involving explosion of breech block
Terrorism involving explosion of cannon block
Terrorism involving explosion (fragments) of artillery shell
Terrorism involving explosion (fragments) of bomb
Terrorism involving explosion (fragments) of grenade
Terrorism involving explosion (fragments) of guided missile
Terrorism involving explosion (fragments) of land mine
Terrorism involving explosion of mortar bomb
Terrorism involving explosion of munitions
Terrorism involving explosion (fragments) of rocket
Terrorism involving explosion (fragments) of shell
Terrorism involving shrapnel
Terrorism involving mine NOS, on land
     EXCLUDES 1   *terrorism involving explosion of nuclear weapon (Y38.5)*
                terrorism involving suicide bomber (Y38.81)

√6ᵗʰ **Y38.2x** **Terrorism involving other explosions and fragments**

√7ᵗʰ **Y38.2x1** **Terrorism involving other explosions and fragments, public safety official injured**

√7ᵗʰ **Y38.2x2** **Terrorism involving other explosions and fragments, civilian injured**

√7ᵗʰ **Y38.2x3** **Terrorism involving other explosions and fragments, terrorist injured**

√5ᵗʰ **Y38.3** **Terrorism involving fires, conflagration and hot substances**
Terrorism involving conflagration NOS
Terrorism involving fire NOS
Terrorism involving petrol bomb
     EXCLUDES 1   *terrorism involving fire or heat of nuclear weapon (Y38.5)*

√6ᵗʰ **Y38.3x** **Terrorism involving fires, conflagration and hot substances**

√7ᵗʰ **Y38.3x1** **Terrorism involving fires, conflagration and hot substances, public safety official injured**

√7ᵗʰ **Y38.3x2** **Terrorism involving fires, conflagration and hot substances, civilian injured**

√7ᵗʰ **Y38.3x3** **Terrorism involving fires, conflagration and hot substances, terrorist injured**

√5ᵗʰ **Y38.4** **Terrorism involving firearms**
Terrorism involving carbine bullet
Terrorism involving machine gun bullet
Terrorism involving pellets (shotgun)
Terrorism involving pistol bullet
Terrorism involving rifle bullet
Terrorism involving rubber (rifle) bullet

√6ᵗʰ **Y38.4x** **Terrorism involving firearms**

√7ᵗʰ **Y38.4x1** **Terrorism involving firearms, public safety official injured**

√7ᵗʰ **Y38.4x2** **Terrorism involving firearms, civilian injured**

√7ᵗʰ **Y38.4x3** **Terrorism involving firearms, terrorist injured**

√5ᵗʰ **Y38.5** **Terrorism involving nuclear weapons**
Terrorism involving blast effects of nuclear weapon
Terrorism involving exposure to ionizing radiation from nuclear weapon
Terrorism involving fireball effect of nuclear weapon
Terrorism involving heat from nuclear weapon

√6ᵗʰ **Y38.5x** **Terrorism involving nuclear weapons**

√7ᵗʰ **Y38.5x1** **Terrorism involving nuclear weapons, public safety official injured**

√7ᵗʰ **Y38.5x2** **Terrorism involving nuclear weapons, civilian injured**

√7ᵗʰ **Y38.5x3** **Terrorism involving nuclear weapons, terrorist injured**

√5ᵗʰ **Y38.6** **Terrorism involving biological weapons**
Terrorism involving anthrax
Terrorism involving cholera
Terrorism involving smallpox

√6ᵗʰ **Y38.6x** **Terrorism involving biological weapons**

√7ᵗʰ **Y38.6x1** **Terrorism involving biological weapons, public safety official injured**

√7ᵗʰ **Y38.6x2** **Terrorism involving biological weapons, civilian injured**

√7ᵗʰ **Y38.6x3** **Terrorism involving biological weapons, terrorist injured**

√5ᵗʰ **Y38.7** **Terrorism involving chemical weapons**
Terrorism involving gases, fumes, chemicals
Terrorism involving hydrogen cyanide
Terrorism involving phosgene
Terrorism involving sarin

√6ᵗʰ **Y38.7x** **Terrorism involving chemical weapons**

√7ᵗʰ **Y38.7x1** **Terrorism involving chemical weapons, public safety official injured**

√7ᵗʰ **Y38.7x2** **Terrorism involving chemical weapons, civilian injured**

√7ᵗʰ **Y38.7x3** **Terrorism involving chemical weapons, terrorist injured**

√5ᵗʰ **Y38.8** **Terrorism involving other and unspecified means**

Y38.80 **Terrorism involving unspecified means**
Terrorism NOS

√6ᵗʰ **Y38.81** **Terrorism involving suicide bomber**

√7ᵗʰ **Y38.811** **Terrorism involving suicide bomber, public safety official injured**

√7ᵗʰ **Y38.812** **Terrorism involving suicide bomber, civilian injured**

√6ᵗʰ **Y38.89** **Terrorism involving other means**
Terrorism involving drowning and submersion
Terrorism involving lasers
Terrorism involving piercing or stabbing instruments

√7ᵗʰ **Y38.891** **Terrorism involving other means, public safety official injured**

√7ᵗʰ **Y38.892** **Terrorism involving other means, civilian injured**

√7ᵗʰ **Y38.893** **Terrorism involving other means, terrorist injured**

√5ᵗʰ **Y38.9** **Terrorism, secondary effects**
     NOTE   This code is for use to identify injuries occurring subsequent to a terrorist attack, not due to the initial attack itself.

√6ᵗʰ **Y38.9x** **Terrorism, secondary effects**

√7ᵗʰ **Y38.9x1** **Terrorism, secondary effects, public safety official injured**

√7ᵗʰ **Y38.9x2** **Terrorism, secondary effects, civilian injured**

Y40-Y59 **Deactivated**
See T36-T50 with fifth or sixth character 5

Complications of medical and surgical care (Y62-Y84)

   INCLUDES   complications of medical devices
surgical and medical procedures as the cause of abnormal reaction of the patient, or of later complication, without mention of misadventure at the time of the procedure

Misadventures to patients during surgical and medical care (Y62-Y69)

   EXCLUDES 2   *breakdown or malfunctioning of medical device (during procedure) (after implantation) (ongoing use) (Y70-Y82)*
surgical and medical procedures as the cause of abnormal reaction of the patient, without mention of misadventure at the time of the procedure (Y83-Y84)

Y60 **Deactivated**
See complications within body system chapters

   EXCLUDES 1   Not coded here   EXCLUDES 2   Not included here   *Manifestation Code*

Y61 Deactivated
     See subcategory T81.5

✓4th **Y62 Failure of sterile precautions during surgical and medical care**
  Y62.0 Failure of sterile precautions during surgical operation
  Y62.1 Failure of sterile precautions during infusion or transfusion
  Y62.2 Failure of sterile precautions during kidney dialysis and other perfusion
  Y62.3 Failure of sterile precautions during injection or immunization
  Y62.4 Failure of sterile precautions during endoscopic examination
  Y62.5 Failure of sterile precautions during heart catheterization
  Y62.6 Failure of sterile precautions during aspiration, puncture and other catheterization
  Y62.8 Failure of sterile precautions during other surgical and medical care
  Y62.9 Failure of sterile precautions during unspecified surgical and medical care

✓4th **Y63 Failure in dosage during surgical and medical care**
    EXCLUDES 2 *accidental overdose of drug or wrong drug given in error (T36-T50)*
  Y63.0 Excessive amount of blood or other fluid given during transfusion or infusion
  Y63.1 Incorrect dilution of fluid used during infusion
  Y63.2 Overdose of radiation given during therapy
  Y63.3 Inadvertent exposure of patient to radiation during medical care
  Y63.4 Failure in dosage in electroshock or insulin-shock therapy
  Y63.5 Inappropriate temperature in local application and packing
  ✓5th **Y63.6** Underdosing and nonadministration of necessary drug, medicament or biological substance
    Y63.61 Underdosing of necessary drug, medicament or biological substance
    Y63.62 Nonadministration of necessary drug, medicament or biological substance
  Y63.8 Failure in dosage during other surgical and medical care
  Y63.9 Failure in dosage during unspecified surgical and medical care

✓4th **Y64 Contaminated medical or biological substances**
  Y64.0 Contaminated medical or biological substance, transfused or infused
  Y64.1 Contaminated medical or biological substance, injected or used for immunization
  Y64.8 Contaminated medical or biological substance administered by other means
  Y64.9 Contaminated medical or biological substance administered by unspecified means
    Administered contaminated medical or biological substance NOS

✓4th **Y65 Other misadventures during surgical and medical care**
  Y65.0 Mismatched blood in transfusion
  Y65.1 Wrong fluid used in infusion
  Y65.2 Failure in suture or ligature during surgical operation
  Y65.3 Endotracheal tube wrongly placed during anesthetic procedure
  Y65.4 Failure to introduce or to remove other tube or instrument
  ✓5th **Y65.5** Performance of wrong procedure (operation)
    Y65.51 Performance of wrong procedure (operation) on correct patient
      Wrong device implanted into correct surgical site
      EXCLUDES 1 *performance of correct procedure (operation) on wrong side or body part (Y65.53)*
    Y65.52 Performance of procedure (operation) on patient not scheduled for surgery
      Performance of procedure (operation) intended for another patient
      Performance of procedure (operation) on wrong patient
    Y65.53 Performance of correct procedure (operation) on wrong side or body part
      Performance of correct procedure (operation) on wrong side
      Performance of correct procedure (operation) on wrong site

  Y65.8 Other specified misadventures during surgical and medical care

Y66 Nonadministration of surgical and medical care
  Premature cessation of surgical and medical care
  EXCLUDES 1 *DNR status (Z66)*
    palliative care (Z51.5)

Y69 Unspecified misadventure during surgical and medical care

Medical devices associated with adverse incidents in diagnostic and therapeutic use (Y70-Y82)

  INCLUDES breakdown or malfunction of medical devices (during use) (after implantation) (ongoing use)
  EXCLUDES 1 *misadventure to patients during surgical and medical care, classifiable to (Y62-Y69)*
    later complications following use of medical devices without breakdown or malfunctioning of device (Y83-Y84)

✓4th **Y70 Anesthesiology devices associated with adverse incidents**
  Y70.0 Diagnostic and monitoring anesthesiology devices associated with adverse incidents
  Y70.1 Therapeutic (nonsurgical) and rehabilitative anesthesiology devices associated with adverse incidents
  Y70.2 Prosthetic and other implants, materials and accessory anesthesiology devices associated with adverse incidents
  Y70.3 Surgical instruments, materials and anesthesiology devices (including sutures) associated with adverse incidents
  Y70.8 Miscellaneous anesthesiology devices associated with adverse incidents, not elsewhere classified

✓4th **Y71 Cardiovascular devices associated with adverse incidents**
  Y71.0 Diagnostic and monitoring cardiovascular devices associated with adverse incidents
  Y71.1 Therapeutic (nonsurgical) and rehabilitative cardiovascular devices associated with adverse incidents
  Y71.2 Prosthetic and other implants, materials and accessory cardiovascular devices associated with adverse incidents
  Y71.3 Surgical instruments, materials and cardiovascular devices (including sutures) associated with adverse incidents
  Y71.8 Miscellaneous cardiovascular devices associated with adverse incidents, not elsewhere classified

✓4th **Y72 Otorhinolaryngological devices associated with adverse incidents**
  Y72.0 Diagnostic and monitoring otorhinolaryngological devices associated with adverse incidents
  Y72.1 Therapeutic (nonsurgical) and rehabilitative otorhinolaryngological devices associated with adverse incidents
  Y72.2 Prosthetic and other implants, materials and accessory otorhinolaryngological devices associated with adverse incidents
  Y72.3 Surgical instruments, materials and otorhinolaryngological devices (including sutures) associated with adverse incidents
  Y72.8 Miscellaneous otorhinolaryngological devices associated with adverse incidents, not elsewhere classified

✓4th **Y73 Gastroenterology and urology devices associated with adverse incidents**
  Y73.0 Diagnostic and monitoring gastroenterology and urology devices associated with adverse incidents
  Y73.1 Therapeutic (nonsurgical) and rehabilitative gastroenterology and urology devices associated with adverse incidents
  Y73.2 Prosthetic and other implants, materials and accessory gastroenterology and urology devices associated with adverse incidents
  Y73.3 Surgical instruments, materials and gastroenterology and urology devices (including sutures) associated with adverse incidents
  Y73.8 Miscellaneous gastroenterology and urology devices associated with adverse incidents, not elsewhere classified

✓4th **Y74 General hospital and personal-use devices associated with adverse incidents**
  Y74.0 Diagnostic and monitoring general hospital and personal-use devices associated with adverse incidents
  Y74.1 Therapeutic (nonsurgical) and rehabilitative general hospital and personal-use devices associated with adverse incidents

---

✓ Appropriate additional character required   ✓x7th Requires 7th character, placeholder x must fill empty characters

Y74.2 Prosthetic and other implants, materials and accessory general hospital and personal-use devices associated with adverse incidents

Y74.3 Surgical instruments, materials and general hospital and personal-use devices (including sutures) associated with adverse incidents

Y74.8 Miscellaneous general hospital and personal-use devices associated with adverse incidents, not elsewhere classified

✓4ᵗʰ Y75 Neurological devices associated with adverse incidents

Y75.0 Diagnostic and monitoring neurological devices associated with adverse incidents

Y75.1 Therapeutic (nonsurgical) and rehabilitative neurological devices associated with adverse incidents

Y75.2 Prosthetic and other implants, materials and neurological devices associated with adverse incidents

Y75.3 Surgical instruments, materials and neurological devices (including sutures) associated with adverse incidents

Y75.8 Miscellaneous neurological devices associated with adverse incidents, not elsewhere classified

✓4ᵗʰ Y76 Obstetric and gynecological devices associated with adverse incidents

Y76.0 Diagnostic and monitoring obstetric and gynecological devices associated with adverse incidents

Y76.1 Therapeutic (nonsurgical) and rehabilitative obstetric and gynecological devices associated with adverse incidents

Y76.2 Prosthetic and other implants, materials and accessory obstetric and gynecological devices associated with adverse incidents

Y76.3 Surgical instruments, materials and obstetric and gynecological devices (including sutures) associated with adverse incidents

Y76.8 Miscellaneous obstetric and gynecological devices associated with adverse incidents, not elsewhere classified

✓4ᵗʰ Y77 Ophthalmic devices associated with adverse incidents

Y77.0 Diagnostic and monitoring ophthalmic devices associated with adverse incidents

Y77.1 Therapeutic (nonsurgical) and rehabilitative ophthalmic devices associated with adverse incidents

Y77.2 Prosthetic and other implants, materials and accessory ophthalmic devices associated with adverse incidents

Y77.3 Surgical instruments, materials and ophthalmic devices (including sutures) associated with adverse incidents

Y77.8 Miscellaneous ophthalmic devices associated with adverse incidents, not elsewhere classified

✓4ᵗʰ Y78 Radiological devices associated with adverse incidents

Y78.0 Diagnostic and monitoring radiological devices associated with adverse incidents

Y78.1 Therapeutic (nonsurgical) and rehabilitative radiological devices associated with adverse incidents

Y78.2 Prosthetic and other implants, materials and accessory radiological devices associated with adverse incidents

Y78.3 Surgical instruments, materials and radiological devices (including sutures) associated with adverse incidents

Y78.8 Miscellaneous radiological devices associated with adverse incidents, not elsewhere classified

✓4ᵗʰ Y79 Orthopedic devices associated with adverse incidents

Y79.0 Diagnostic and monitoring orthopedic devices associated with adverse incidents

Y79.1 Therapeutic (nonsurgical) and rehabilitative orthopedic devices associated with adverse incidents

Y79.2 Prosthetic and other implants, materials and accessory orthopedic devices associated with adverse incidents

Y79.3 Surgical instruments, materials and orthopedic devices (including sutures) associated with adverse incidents

Y79.8 Miscellaneous orthopedic devices associated with adverse incidents, not elsewhere classified

✓4ᵗʰ Y80 Physical medicine devices associated with adverse incidents

Y80.0 Diagnostic and monitoring physical medicine devices associated with adverse incidents

Y80.1 Therapeutic (nonsurgical) and rehabilitative physical medicine devices associated with adverse incidents

Y80.2 Prosthetic and other implants, materials and accessory physical medicine devices associated with adverse incidents

Y80.3 Surgical instruments, materials and physical medicine devices (including sutures) associated with adverse incidents

Y80.8 Miscellaneous physical medicine devices associated with adverse incidents, not elsewhere classified

✓4ᵗʰ Y81 General- and plastic-surgery devices associated with adverse incidents

Y81.0 Diagnostic and monitoring general- and plastic-surgery devices associated with adverse incidents

Y81.1 Therapeutic (nonsurgical) and rehabilitative general- and plastic-surgery devices associated with adverse incidents

Y81.2 Prosthetic and other implants, materials and accessory general- and plastic-surgery devices associated with adverse incidents

Y81.3 Surgical instruments, materials and general- and plastic-surgery devices (including sutures) associated with adverse incidents

Y81.8 Miscellaneous general- and plastic-surgery devices associated with adverse incidents, not elsewhere classified

✓4ᵗʰ Y82 Other and unspecified medical devices associated with adverse incidents

Y82.8 Other medical devices associated with adverse incidents

Y82.9 Unspecified medical devices associated with adverse incidents

Surgical and other medical procedures as the cause of abnormal reaction of the patient, or of later complication, without mention of misadventure at the time of the procedure (Y83-Y84)

EXCLUDES 1   misadventures to patients during surgical and medical care, classifiable to (Y62-Y69)

✓4ᵗʰ Y83 Surgical operation and other surgical procedures as the cause of abnormal reaction of the patient, or of later complication, without mention of misadventure at the time of the procedure

Y83.0 Surgical operation with transplant of whole organ as the cause of abnormal reaction of the patient, or of later complication, without mention of misadventure at the time of the procedure

Y83.1 Surgical operation with implant of artificial internal device as the cause of abnormal reaction of the patient, or of later complication, without mention of misadventure at the time of the procedure

Y83.2 Surgical operation with anastomosis, bypass or graft as the cause of abnormal reaction of the patient, or of later complication, without mention of misadventure at the time of the procedure

Y83.3 Surgical operation with formation of external stoma as the cause of abnormal reaction of the patient, or of later complication, without mention of misadventure at the time of the procedure

Y83.4 Other reconstructive surgery as the cause of abnormal reaction of the patient, or of later complication, without mention of misadventure at the time of the procedure

Y83.5 Amputation of limb(s) as the cause of abnormal reaction of the patient, or of later complication, without mention of misadventure at the time of the procedure

Y83.6 Removal of other organ (partial) (total) as the cause of abnormal reaction of the patient, or of later complication, without mention of misadventure at the time of the procedure

Y83.8 Other surgical procedures as the cause of abnormal reaction of the patient, or of later complication, without mention of misadventure at the time of the procedure

Y83.9 Surgical procedure, unspecified as the cause of abnormal reaction of the patient, or of later complication, without mention of misadventure at the time of the procedure

✓4ᵗʰ Y84 Other medical procedures as the cause of abnormal reaction of the patient, or of later complication, without mention of misadventure at the time of the procedure

Y84.0 Cardiac catheterization as the cause of abnormal reaction of the patient, or of later complication, without mention of misadventure at the time of the procedure

Y84.1 Kidney dialysis as the cause of abnormal reaction of the patient, or of later complication, without mention of misadventure at the time of the procedure

EXCLUDES 1 Not coded here   EXCLUDES 2 Not included here   *Manifestation Code*

Y84.2　Radiological procedure and radiotherapy as the cause of abnormal reaction of the patient, or of later complication, without mention of misadventure at the time of the procedure

Y84.3　Shock therapy as the cause of abnormal reaction of the patient, or of later complication, without mention of misadventure at the time of the procedure

Y84.4　Aspiration of fluid as the cause of abnormal reaction of the patient, or of later complication, without mention of misadventure at the time of the procedure

Y84.5　Insertion of gastric or duodenal sound as the cause of abnormal reaction of the patient, or of later complication, without mention of misadventure at the time of the procedure

Y84.6　Urinary catheterization as the cause of abnormal reaction of the patient, or of later complication, without mention of misadventure at the time of the procedure

Y84.7　Blood-sampling as the cause of abnormal reaction of the patient, or of later complication, without mention of misadventure at the time of the procedure

Y84.8　Other medical procedures as the cause of abnormal reaction, or of later complication, without mention of misadventure at the time of the procedure

Y84.9　Medical procedure, unspecified as the cause of abnormal reaction of the patient, or of later complication, without mention of misadventure at the time of the procedure

Y85-Y89　Deactivated
Replaced with 7th character S for categories V00-Y38

Supplementary factors related to causes of morbidity classified elsewhere (Y90-Y99)

NOTE　These categories may be used to provide supplementary information concerning causes of morbidity. They are not to be used for single-condition coding.

✓4th **Y90　Evidence of alcohol involvement determined by blood alcohol level**
　　Code first any associated alcohol related disorders (F10)

Y90.0　Blood alcohol level of less than 20 mg/100 ml

Y90.1　Blood alcohol level of 20-39 mg/100 ml

Y90.2　Blood alcohol level of 40-59 mg/100 ml

Y90.3　Blood alcohol level of 60-79 mg/100 ml

Y90.4　Blood alcohol level of 80-99 mg/100 ml

Y90.5　Blood alcohol level of 100-119 mg/100 ml

Y90.6　Blood alcohol level of 120-199 mg/100 ml

Y90.7　Blood alcohol level of 200-239 mg/100 ml

Y90.8　Blood alcohol level of 240 mg/100 ml or more

Y90.9　Presence of alcohol in blood, level not specified

Y91　Deactivated
See category F10

✓4th **Y92　Place of occurrence of the external cause**
　　The following category is for use, when relevant, to identify the place of occurrence of the external cause. Use in conjunction with an activity code.
　　Place of occurrence should be recorded only at the initial encounter for treatment

✓5th **Y92.0　Non-institutional (private) residence as the place of occurrence of the external cause**
　　　EXCLUDES 1　*abandoned or derelict house (Y92.89)*
　　　　home under construction but not yet occupied (Y92.6-)
　　　　institutional place of residence (Y92.1-)

Y92.00　Unspecified non-institutional (private) residence as the place of occurrence of the external cause

✓6th Y92.01　Single-family non-institutional (private) house as the place of occurrence of the external cause
　　　Farmhouse as the place of occurrence of the external cause
　　　EXCLUDES 1　*barn (Y92.71)*
　　　　chicken coop or hen house (Y92.72)
　　　　farm field (Y92.73)
　　　　orchard (Y92.74)
　　　　single family mobile home or trailer (Y92.02-)
　　　　slaughter house (Y92.86)

Y92.010　Kitchen of single-family (private) house as the place of occurrence of the external cause

Y92.011　Dining room of single-family (private) house as the place of occurrence of the external cause

Y92.012　Bathroom of single-family (private) house as the place of occurrence of the external cause

Y92.013　Bedroom of single-family (private) house as the place of occurrence of the external cause

Y92.014　Private driveway to single-family (private) house as the place of occurrence of the external cause

Y92.015　Private garage of single-family (private) house as the place of occurrence of the external cause

Y92.016　Swimming-pool in single-family (private) house or garden as the place of occurrence of the external cause

Y92.017　Garden or yard in single-family (private) house as the place of occurrence of the external cause

Y92.018　Other place in single-family (private) house as the place of occurrence of the external cause

Y92.019　Unspecified place in single-family (private) house as the place of occurrence of the external cause

✓6th Y92.02　Mobile home as the place of occurrence of the external cause

Y92.020　Kitchen in mobile home as the place of occurrence of the external cause

Y92.021　Dining room in mobile home as the place of occurrence of the external cause

Y92.022　Bathroom in mobile home as the place of occurrence of the external cause

Y92.023　Bedroom in mobile home as the place of occurrence of the external cause

Y92.024　Driveway of mobile home as the place of occurrence of the external cause

Y92.025　Garage of mobile home as the place of occurrence of the external cause

Y92.026　Swimming-pool of mobile home as the place of occurrence of the external cause

Y92.027　Garden or yard of mobile home as the place of occurrence of the external cause

Y92.028　Other place in mobile home as the place of occurrence of the external cause

Y92.029　Unspecified place in mobile home as the place of occurrence of the external cause

✓6th Y92.03　Apartment as the place of occurrence of the external cause
　　　Condominium as the place of occurrence of the external cause
　　　Co-op apartment as the place of occurrence of the external cause

Y92.030　Kitchen in apartment as the place of occurrence of the external cause

Y92.031　Bathroom in apartment as the place of occurrence of the external cause

Y92.032　Bedroom in apartment as the place of occurrence of the external cause

Y92.038　Other place in apartment as the place of occurrence of the external cause

Y92.039　Unspecified place in apartment as the place of occurrence of the external cause

✓6th Y92.04　Boarding-house as the place of occurrence of the external cause

Y92.040　Kitchen in boarding-house as the place of occurrence of the external cause

Y92.041　Bathroom in boarding-house as the place of occurrence of the external cause

Y92.042　Bedroom in boarding-house as the place of occurrence of the external cause

Y92.043　Driveway of boarding-house as the place of occurrence of the external cause

Y92.044　Garage of boarding-house as the place of occurrence of the external cause

---

☑ Appropriate additional character required　　　　✓x7th Requires 7th character, placeholder x must fill empty characters

Y92.045   Swimming-pool of boarding-house as the place of occurrence of the external cause

Y92.046   Garden or yard of boarding-house as the place of occurrence of the external cause

Y92.048   Other place in boarding-house as the place of occurrence of the external cause

Y92.049   Unspecified place in boarding-house as the place of occurrence of the external cause

✓6th   Y92.09   Other non-institutional residence as the place of occurrence of the external cause

Y92.090   Kitchen in other non-institutional residence as the place of occurrence of the external cause

Y92.091   Bathroom in other non-institutional residence as the place of occurrence of the external cause

Y92.092   Bedroom in other non-institutional residence as the place of occurrence of the external cause

Y92.093   Driveway of other non-institutional residence as the place of occurrence of the external cause

Y92.094   Garage of other non-institutional residence as the place of occurrence of the external cause

Y92.095   Swimming-pool of other non-institutional residence as the place of occurrence of the external cause

Y92.096   Garden or yard of other non-institutional residence as the place of occurrence of the external cause

Y92.098   Other place in other non-institutional residence as the place of occurrence of the external cause

Y92.099   Unspecified place in other non-institutional residence as the place of occurrence of the external cause

✓5th   Y92.1   Institutional (nonprivate) residence as the place of occurrence of the external cause

Y92.10   Unspecified residential institution as the place of occurrence of the external cause

✓6th   Y92.11   Children's home and orphanage as the place of occurrence of the external cause

Y92.110   Kitchen in children's home and orphanage as the place of occurrence of the external cause

Y92.111   Bathroom in children's home and orphanage as the place of occurrence of the external cause

Y92.112   Bedroom in children's home and orphanage as the place of occurrence of the external cause

Y92.113   Driveway of children's home and orphanage as the place of occurrence of the external cause

Y92.114   Garage of children's home and orphanage as the place of occurrence of the external cause

Y92.115   Swimming-pool of children's home and orphanage as the place of occurrence of the external cause

Y92.116   Garden or yard of children's home and orphanage as the place of occurrence of the external cause

Y92.118   Other place in children's home and orphanage as the place of occurrence of the external cause

Y92.119   Unspecified place in children's home and orphanage as the place of occurrence of the external cause

✓6th   Y92.12   Nursing home as the place of occurrence of the external cause

Home for the sick as the place of occurrence of the external cause

Hospice as the place of occurrence of the external cause

Y92.120   Kitchen in nursing home as the place of occurrence of the external cause

Y92.121   Bathroom in nursing home as the place of occurrence of the external cause

Y92.122   Bedroom in nursing home as the place of occurrence of the external cause

Y92.123   Driveway of nursing home as the place of occurrence of the external cause

Y92.124   Garage of nursing home as the place of occurrence of the external cause

Y92.125   Swimming-pool of nursing home as the place of occurrence of the external cause

Y92.126   Garden or yard of nursing home as the place of occurrence of the external cause

Y92.128   Other place in nursing home as the place of occurrence of the external cause

Y92.129   Unspecified place in nursing home as the place of occurrence of the external cause

✓6th   Y92.13   Military base as the place of occurrence of the external cause

EXCLUDES 1   *military training grounds (Y92.84)*

Y92.130   Kitchen on military base as the place of occurrence of the external cause

Y92.131   Mess hall on military base as the place of occurrence of the external cause

Y92.133   Barracks on military base as the place of occurrence of the external cause

Y92.135   Garage on military base as the place of occurrence of the external cause

Y92.136   Swimming-pool on military base as the place of occurrence of the external cause

Y92.137   Garden or yard on military base as the place of occurrence of the external cause

Y92.138   Other place on military base as the place of occurrence of the external cause

Y92.139   Unspecified place military base as the place of occurrence of the external cause

✓6th   Y92.14   Prison as the place of occurrence of the external cause

Y92.140   Kitchen in prison as the place of occurrence of the external cause

Y92.141   Dining room in prison as the place of occurrence of the external cause

Y92.142   Bathroom in prison as the place of occurrence of the external cause

Y92.143   Cell of prison as the place of occurrence of the external cause

Y92.146   Swimming-pool of prison as the place of occurrence of the external cause

Y92.147   Courtyard of prison as the place of occurrence of the external cause

Y92.148   Other place in prison as the place of occurrence of the external cause

Y92.149   Unspecified place in prison as the place of occurrence of the external cause

✓6th   Y92.15   Reform school as the place of occurrence of the external cause

Y92.150   Kitchen in reform school as the place of occurrence of the external cause

Y92.151   Dining room in reform school as the place of occurrence of the external cause

Y92.152   Bathroom in reform school as the place of occurrence of the external cause

Y92.153   Bedroom in reform school as the place of occurrence of the external cause

Y92.154   Driveway of reform school as the place of occurrence of the external cause

Y92.155   Garage of reform school as the place of occurrence of the external cause

Y92.156   Swimming-pool of reform school as the place of occurrence of the external cause

Y92.157   Garden or yard of reform school as the place of occurrence of the external cause

Y92.158   Other place in reform school as the place of occurrence of the external cause

Y92.159   Unspecified place in reform school as the place of occurrence of the external cause

---

EXCLUDES 1   Not coded here   EXCLUDES 2   Not included here   *Manifestation Code*

☑6ᵗʰ **Y92.16** **School dormitory as the place of occurrence of the external cause**

> EXCLUDES 1 *reform school as the place of occurrence of the external cause (Y92.15-)*
> *school buildings and grounds as the place of occurrence of the external cause (Y92.21-)*
> *school sports and athletic areas as the place of occurrence of the external cause (Y92.3-)*

    Y92.160 **Kitchen in school dormitory as the place of occurrence of the external cause**

    Y92.161 **Dining room in school dormitory as the place of occurrence of the external cause**

    Y92.162 **Bathroom in school dormitory as the place of occurrence of the external cause**

    Y92.163 **Bedroom in school dormitory as the place of occurrence of the external cause**

    Y92.168 **Other place in school dormitory as the place of occurrence of the external cause**

    Y92.169 **Unspecified place in school dormitory as the place of occurrence of the external cause**

☑6ᵗʰ **Y92.19** **Other specified residential institution as the place of occurrence of the external cause**

    Y92.190 **Kitchen in other specified residential institution as the place of occurrence of the external cause**

    Y92.191 **Dining room in other specified residential institution as the place of occurrence of the external cause**

    Y92.192 **Bathroom in other specified residential institution as the place of occurrence of the external cause**

    Y92.193 **Bedroom in other specified residential institution as the place of occurrence of the external cause**

    Y92.194 **Driveway of other specified residential institution as the place of occurrence of the external cause**

    Y92.195 **Garage of other specified residential institution as the place of occurrence of the external cause**

    Y92.196 **Pool of other specified residential institution as the place of occurrence of the external cause**

    Y92.197 **Garden or yard of other specified residential institution as the place of occurrence of the external cause**

    Y92.198 **Other place in other specified residential institution as the place of occurrence of the external cause**

    Y92.199 **Unspecified place in other specified residential institution as the place of occurrence of the external cause**

☑5ᵗʰ **Y92.2** **School, other institution and public administrative area as the place of occurrence of the external cause**

Building and adjacent grounds used by the general public or by a particular group of the public

> EXCLUDES 1 *building under construction as the place of occurrence of the external cause (Y92.6)*
> *residential institution as the place of occurrence of the external cause (Y92.1)*
> *school dormitory as the place of occurrence of the external cause (Y92.16-)*
> *sports and athletics area of schools as the place of occurrence of the external cause (Y92.3-)*

☑6ᵗʰ **Y92.21** **School (private) (public) (state) as the place of occurrence of the external cause**

    Y92.210 **Daycare center as the place of occurrence of the external cause**

    Y92.211 **Elementary school as the place of occurrence of the external cause**

        Kindergarten as the place of occurrence of the external cause

    Y92.212 **Middle school as the place of occurrence of the external cause**

    Y92.213 **High school as the place of occurrence of the external cause**

    Y92.214 **College as the place of occurrence of the external cause**

        University as the place of occurrence of the external cause

    Y92.215 **Trade school as the place of occurrence of the external cause**

    Y92.218 **Other school as the place of occurrence of the external cause**

    Y92.219 **Unspecified school as the place of occurrence of the external cause**

Y92.22 **Religious institution as the place of occurrence of the external cause**

Church as the place of occurrence of the external cause

Mosque as the place of occurrence of the external cause

Synagogue as the place of occurrence of the external cause

☑6ᵗʰ **Y92.23** **Hospital as the place of occurrence of the external cause**

> EXCLUDES 1 *ambulatory (outpatient) health services establishments (Y92.53-)*
> *home for the sick as the place of occurrence of the external cause (Y92.12-)*
> *hospice as the place of occurrence of the external cause (Y92.12-)*
> *nursing home as the place of occurrence of the external cause (Y92.12-)*

    Y92.230 **Patient room in hospital as the place of occurrence of the external cause**

    Y92.231 **Patient bathroom in hospital as the place of occurrence of the external cause**

    Y92.232 **Corridor of hospital as the place of occurrence of the external cause**

    Y92.233 **Cafeteria of hospital as the place of occurrence of the external cause**

    Y92.234 **Operating room of hospital as the place of occurrence of the external cause**

    Y92.238 **Other place in hospital as the place of occurrence of the external cause**

    Y92.239 **Unspecified place in hospital as the place of occurrence of the external cause**

☑6ᵗʰ **Y92.24** **Public administrative building as the place of occurrence of the external cause**

    Y92.240 **Courthouse as the place of occurrence of the external cause**

    Y92.241 **Library as the place of occurrence of the external cause**

    Y92.242 **Post office as the place of occurrence of the external cause**

    Y92.243 **City hall as the place of occurrence of the external cause**

    Y92.248 **Other public administrative building as the place of occurrence of the external cause**

☑6ᵗʰ **Y92.25** **Cultural building as the place of occurrence of the external cause**

    Y92.250 **Art Gallery as the place of occurrence of the external cause**

    Y92.251 **Museum as the place of occurrence of the external cause**

    Y92.252 **Music hall as the place of occurrence of the external cause**

    Y92.253 **Opera house as the place of occurrence of the external cause**

    Y92.254 **Theater (live) as the place of occurrence of the external cause**

    Y92.258 **Other cultural public building as the place of occurrence of the external cause**

Y92.26 **Movie house or cinema as the place of occurrence of the external cause**

Y92.29 **Other specified public building as the place of occurrence of the external cause**

Assembly hall as the place of occurrence of the external cause

Clubhouse as the place of occurrence of the external cause

    ☑ Appropriate additional character required   ☑x7ᵗʰ Requires 7th character, placeholder x must fill empty characters

✓5ᵗʰ **Y92.3** **Sports and athletics area as the place of occurrence of the external cause**

✓6ᵗʰ **Y92.31** **Athletic court as the place of occurrence of the external cause**

EXCLUDES 1 tennis court in private home or garden (Y92.09)

Y92.310 **Basketball court as the place of occurrence of the external cause**

Y92.311 **Squash court as the place of occurrence of the external cause**

Y92.312 **Tennis court as the place of occurrence of the external cause**

Y92.318 **Other athletic court as the place of occurrence of the external cause**

✓6ᵗʰ **Y92.32** **Athletic field as the place of occurrence of the external cause**

Y92.320 **Baseball field as the place of occurrence of the external cause**

Y92.321 **Football field as the place of occurrence of the external cause**

Y92.322 **Soccer field as the place of occurrence of the external cause**

Y92.328 **Other athletic field as the place of occurrence of the external cause**

Cricket field as the place of occurrence of the external cause

Hockey field as the place of occurrence of the external cause

✓6ᵗʰ **Y92.33** **Skating rink as the place of occurrence of the external cause**

Y92.330 **Ice skating rink (indoor) (outdoor) as the place of occurrence of the external cause**

Y92.331 **Roller skating rink as the place of occurrence of the external cause**

Y92.34 **Swimming pool (public) as the place of occurrence of the external cause**

EXCLUDES 1 swimming pool in private home or garden (Y92.016)

Y92.39 **Other specified sports and athletic area as the place of occurrence of the external cause**

Golf-course as the place of occurrence of the external cause

Gymnasium as the place of occurrence of the external cause

Riding-school as the place of occurrence of the external cause

Stadium as the place of occurrence of the external cause

✓5ᵗʰ **Y92.4** **Street , highway and other paved roadways as the place of occurrence of the external cause**

EXCLUDES 1 private driveway of residence (Y92.014, Y92.024, Y92.043)

✓6ᵗʰ **Y92.41** **Street and highway as the place of occurrence of the external cause**

Y92.410 **Unspecified street and highway as the place of occurrence of the external cause**

Road NOS as the place of occurrence of the external cause

Y92.411 **Interstate highway as the place of occurrence of the external cause**

Freeway as the place of occurrence of the external cause

Motorway as the place of occurrence of the external cause

Y92.412 **Parkway as the place of occurrence of the external cause**

Y92.413 **State road as the place of occurrence of the external cause**

Y92.414 **Local residential or business street as the place of occurrence of the external cause**

Y92.415 **Exit ramp or entrance ramp of street or highway as the place of occurrence of the external cause**

✓6ᵗʰ **Y92.48** **Other paved roadways as the place of occurrence of the external cause**

Y92.480 **Sidewalk as the place of occurrence of the external cause**

Y92.481 **Parking lot as the place of occurrence of the external cause**

Y92.482 **Bike path as the place of occurrence of the external cause**

Y92.488 **Other paved roadways as the place of occurrence of the external cause**

✓5ᵗʰ **Y92.5** **Trade and service area as the place of occurrence of the external cause**

EXCLUDES 1 garage in private home (Y92.015)

schools and other public administration buildings (Y92.2-)

✓6ᵗʰ **Y92.51** **Private commercial establishments as the place of occurrence of the external cause**

Y92.510 **Bank as the place of occurrence of the external cause**

Y92.511 **Restaurant or café as the place of occurrence of the external cause**

Y92.512 **Supermarket, store or market as the place of occurrence of the external cause**

Y92.513 **Shop (commercial) as the place of occurrence of the external cause**

✓6ᵗʰ **Y92.52** **Service areas as the place of occurrence of the external cause**

Y92.520 **Airport as the place of occurrence of the external cause**

Y92.521 **Bus station as the place of occurrence of the external cause**

Y92.522 **Railway station as the place of occurrence of the external cause**

Y92.523 **Highway rest stop as the place of occurrence of the external cause**

Y92.524 **Gas station as the place of occurrence of the external cause**

Petroleum station as the place of occurrence of the external cause

Service station as the place of occurrence of the external cause

✓6ᵗʰ **Y92.53** **Ambulatory health services establishments as the place of occurrence of the external cause**

Y92.530 **Ambulatory surgery center as the place of occurrence of the external cause**

Outpatient surgery center, including that connected with a hospital as the place of occurrence of the external cause

Same day surgery center, including that connected with a hospital as the place of occurrence of the external cause

Y92.531 **Health care provider office as the place of occurrence of the external cause**

Physician office as the place of occurrence of the external cause

Y92.532 **Urgent care center as the place of occurrence of the external cause**

Y92.538 **Other ambulatory health services establishments as the place of occurrence of the external cause**

Y92.59 **Other trade areas as the place of occurrence of the external cause**

Office building as the place of occurrence of the external cause

Casino as the place of occurrence of the external cause

Garage (commercial) as the place of occurrence of the external cause

Hotel as the place of occurrence of the external cause

Radio or television station as the place of occurrence of the external cause

Shopping mall as the place of occurrence of the external cause

Warehouse as the place of occurrence of the external cause

✓5ᵗʰ **Y92.6** **Industrial and construction area as the place of occurrence of the external cause**

Y92.61 **Building [any] under construction as the place of occurrence of the external cause**

EXCLUDES 1 Not coded here   *EXCLUDES 2* Not included here   **Manifestation Code**

Y92.62 Dock or shipyard as the place of occurrence of the external cause

Dockyard as the place of occurrence of the external cause

Dry dock as the place of occurrence of the external cause

Shipyard as the place of occurrence of the external cause

Y92.63 Factory as the place of occurrence of the external cause

Factory building as the place of occurrence of the external cause

Factory premises as the place of occurrence of the external cause

Industrial yard as the place of occurrence of the external cause

Y92.64 Mine or pit as the place of occurrence of the external cause

Mine as the place of occurrence of the external cause

Y92.65 Oil rig as the place of occurrence of the external cause

Pit (coal) (gravel) (sand) as the place of occurrence of the external cause

Y92.69 Other specified industrial and construction area as the place of occurrence of the external cause

Gasworks as the place of occurrence of the external cause

Power-station (coal) (nuclear) (oil) as the place of occurrence of the external cause

Tunnel under construction as the place of occurrence of the external cause

Workshop as the place of occurrence of the external cause

✓5th Y92.7 Farm as the place of occurrence of the external cause

Ranch as the place of occurrence of the external cause

EXCLUDES 1 *farmhouse and home premises of farm (Y92.01-)*

Y92.71 Barn as the place of occurrence of the external cause

Y92.72 Chicken coop as the place of occurrence of the external cause

Hen house as the place of occurrence of the external cause

Y92.73 Farm field as the place of occurrence of the external cause

Y92.74 Orchard as the place of occurrence of the external cause

Y92.79 Other farm location as the place of occurrence of the external cause

✓5th Y92.8 Other places as the place of occurrence of the external cause

✓6th Y92.81 Transport vehicle as the place of occurrence of the external cause

EXCLUDES 1 *transport accidents (V00-V99)*

Y92.810 Car as the place of occurrence of the external cause

Y92.811 Bus as the place of occurrence of the external cause

Y92.812 Truck as the place of occurrence of the external cause

Y92.813 Airplane as the place of occurrence of the external cause

Y92.814 Boat as the place of occurrence of the external cause

Y92.815 Train as the place of occurrence of the external cause

Y92.816 Subway car as the place of occurrence of the external cause

Y92.818 Other transport vehicle as the place of occurrence of the external cause

✓6th Y92.82 Wilderness area

Y92.820 Desert as the place of occurrence of the external cause

Y92.821 Forest as the place of occurrence of the external cause

Y92.828 Other wilderness area as the place of occurrence of the external cause

Swamp as the place of occurrence of the external cause

Mountain as the place of occurrence of the external cause

Marsh as the place of occurrence of the external cause

Prairie as the place of occurrence of the external cause

✓6th Y92.83 Recreation area as the place of occurrence of the external cause

Y92.830 Public park as the place of occurrence of the external cause

Y92.831 Amusement park as the place of occurrence of the external cause

Y92.832 Beach as the place of occurrence of the external cause

Seashore as the place of occurrence of the external cause

Y92.833 Campsite as the place of occurrence of the external cause

Y92.834 Zoological garden (Zoo) as the place of occurrence of the external cause

Y92.838 Other recreation area as the place of occurrence of the external cause

Y92.84 Military training ground as the place of occurrence of the external cause

Y92.85 Railroad track as the place of occurrence of the external cause

Y92.86 Slaughter house as the place of occurrence of the external cause

Y92.89 Other specified places as the place of occurrence of the external cause

Derelict house as the place of occurrence of the external cause

Y92.9 Unspecified place or not applicable

☑ Appropriate additional character required   ✓x7th Requires 7th character, placeholder x must fill empty characters

✓4th Y93   Activity codes

NOTE   Category Y93 is provided for use to indicate the activity of the person seeking healthcare for an injury or health condition, such as a heart attack while shoveling snow, which resulted from, or was contributed to, by the activity. These codes are appropriate for use for both acute injuries, such as those from chapter 19, and conditions that are due to the long-term, cumulative effects of an activity, such as those from chapter 13. They are also appropriate for use with external cause codes for cause and intent if identifying the activity provides additional information on the event. These codes should be used in conjunction with codes for external cause status (Y99) and place of occurrence (Y92). This section contains the following broad activity categories:

Y93.0   Activities involving walking and running
Y93.1   Activities involving water and water craft
Y93.2   Activities involving ice and snow
Y93.3   Activities involving climbing, rappelling, and jumping off
Y93.4   Activities involving dancing and other rhythmic movement
Y93.5   Activities involving other sports and athletics played individually
Y93.6   Activities involving other sports and athletics played as a team or group
Y93.7   Activities involving other specified sports and athletics
Y93.a   Activities involving other cardiorespiratory exercise
Y93.b   Activities involving other muscle strengthening exercises
Y93.c   Activities involving computer technology and electronic devices
Y93.d   Activities involving arts and handcrafts
Y93.e   Activities involving personal hygiene and interior property and clothing maintenance
Y93.f   Activities involving caregiving
Y93.g   Activities involving food preparation, cooking and grilling
Y93.h   Activities involving exterior property and land maintenance, building and construction
Y93.i   Activities involving roller coasters and other types of external motion
Y93.j   Activities involving playing musical instrument
Y93.k   Activities involving animal care
Y93.8   Activities, other specified
Y93.9   Activity, unspecified

✓5th Y93.0   Activities involving walking and running

EXCLUDES 1   activity, walking an animal (Y93.k1)
activity. walking or running on a treadmill (Y93.a1)

Y93.01   **Activity, walking, marching and hiking**
Activity, walking, marching and hiking on level or elevated terrain
EXCLUDES 1   activity, mountain climbing (Y93.31)

Y93.02   **Activity, running**

✓5th Y93.1   Activities involving water and water craft

EXCLUDES 1   activities involving ice (Y93.2-)

Y93.11   **Activity, swimming**
Y93.12   **Activity, springboard and platform diving**
Y93.13   **Activity, water polo**
Y93.14   **Activity, water aerobics and water exercise**
Y93.15   **Activity, underwater diving and snorkeling**
Activity, SCUBA diving
Y93.16   **Activity, rowing, canoeing, kayaking, rafting and tubing**
Activity, canoeing, kayaking, rafting and tubing in calm and turbulent water
Y93.17   **Activity, water skiing and wake boarding**
Y93.18   **Activity, surfing, windsurfing and boogie boarding**
Activity, water sliding
Y93.19   **Activity, other activity involving water and watercraft**
Activity involving water NOS
Activity, parasailing
Activity, water survival training and testing

✓5th Y93.2   Activities involving ice and snow

EXCLUDES 1   activity, shoveling ice and snow (Y93.h1)

Y93.21   **Activity, ice skating**
Activity, figure skating (singles) (pairs)
Activity, ice dancing
EXCLUDES 1   activity, ice hockey (Y93.22)

Y93.22   **Activity, ice hockey**
Y93.23   **Activity, snow (alpine) (downhill) skiing, snow boarding, sledding, tobogganing and snow tubing**
EXCLUDES 1   activity, cross country skiing (Y93.24)

Y93.24   **Activity, cross country skiing**
Activity, nordic skiing
Y93.29   **Activity, other involving ice and snow**
Activity involving ice and snow NOS

✓5th Y93.3   Activities involving climbing, rappelling and jumping off

EXCLUDES 1   activity, hiking on level or elevated terrain (Y93.01)
activity, jumping rope (Y93.56)
activity, trampoline jumping (Y93.44)

Y93.31   **Activity, mountain climbing, rock climbing and wall climbing**
Y93.32   **Activity, rappelling**
Y93.33   **Activity, BASE jumping**
Activity, Building, Antenna, Span, Earth jumping
Y93.34   **Activity, bungee jumping**
Y93.35   **Activity, hang gliding**
Y93.39   **Activity, other involving climbing, rappelling and jumping off**

✓5th Y93.4   Activities involving dancing and other rhythmic movement

EXCLUDES 1   activity, martial arts (Y93.75)

Y93.41   **Activity, dancing**
Y93.42   **Activity, yoga**
Y93.43   **Activity, gymnastics**
Activity, rhythmic gymnastics
EXCLUDES 1   activity, trampolining (Y93.44)

Y93.44   **Activity, trampolining**
Y93.45   **Activity, cheerleading**
Y93.49   **Activity, other involving dancing and other rhythmic movements**

✓5th Y93.5   Activities involving other sports and athletics played individually

EXCLUDES 1   activity, dancing (Y93.41)
activity, gymnastic (Y93.43)
activity, trampolining (Y93.44)
activity, yoga (Y93.42)

Y93.51   **Activity, roller skating (inline) and skateboarding**
Y93.52   **Activity, horseback riding**
Y93.53   **Activity, golf**
Y93.54   **Activity, bowling**
Y93.55   **Activity, bike riding**
Y93.56   **Activity, jumping rope**
Y93.57   **Activity, non-running track and field events**
EXCLUDES 1   activity, running (any form) (Y93.02)

Y93.59   **Activity, other involving other sports and athletics played individually**
EXCLUDES 1   activities involving climbing, rappelling, and jumping (Y93.3-)
activities involving ice and snow (Y93.2-)
activities involving walking and running (Y93.0-)
activities involving water and watercraft (Y93.1-)

✓5th Y93.6   Activities involving other sports and athletics played as a team or group

EXCLUDES 1   activity, ice hockey (Y93.22)
activity, water polo (Y93.13)

Y93.61   **Activity, American tackle football**
Activity, football NOS
Y93.62   **Activity, American flag or touch football**
Y93.63   **Activity, rugby**
Y93.64   **Activity, baseball**
Activity, softball
Y93.65   **Activity, lacrosse and field hockey**
Y93.66   **Activity, soccer**
Y93.67   **Activity, basketball**
Y93.68   **Activity, volleyball (beach) (court)**

EXCLUDES 1   Not coded here   **EXCLUDES 2**   Not included here   *Manifestation Code*

Y93.6a　**Activity, physical games generally associated with school recess, summer camp and children**
　　　　Activity, capture the flag
　　　　Activity, dodge ball
　　　　Activity, four square
　　　　Activity, kickball

Y93.69　**Activity, other involving other sports and athletics played as a team or group**
　　　　Activity, cricket

✓5th Y93.7　**Activities involving other specified sports and athletics**

Y93.71　**Activity, boxing**

Y93.72　**Activity, wrestling**

Y93.73　**Activity, racquet and hand sports**
　　　　Activity, handball
　　　　Activity, racquetball
　　　　Activity, squash
　　　　Activity, tennis

Y93.74　**Activity, frisbee**
　　　　Activity, ultimate frisbee

Y93.75　**Activity, martial arts**
　　　　Activity, combatives

Y93.79　**Activity, other specified sports and athletics**
　　　　EXCLUDES 1 *sports and athletics activities specified in categories Y93.0-Y93.6*

✓5th Y93.a　**Activities involving other cardiorespiratory exercise**
　　　Activities involving physical training

Y93.a1　**Activity, exercise machines primarily for cardiorespiratory conditioning**
　　　　Activity, elliptical and stepper machines
　　　　Activity, stationary bike
　　　　Activity, treadmill

Y93.a2　**Activity, calisthenics**
　　　　Activity, jumping jacks
　　　　Activity, warm up and cool down

Y93.a3　**Activity, aerobic and step exercise**

Y93.a4　**Activity, circuit training**

Y93.a5　**Activity, obstacle course**
　　　　Activity, challenge course
　　　　Activity, confidence course

Y93.a6　**Activity, grass drills**
　　　　Activity, guerilla drills

Y93.a9　**Activity, other involving other cardiorespiratory exercise**
　　　　EXCLUDES 1 *activities involving cardiorespiratory exercise specified in categories Y93.0-Y93.7*

✓5th Y93.b　**Activities involving other muscle strengthening exercises**

Y93.b1　**Activity, exercise machines primarily for muscle strengthening**

Y93.b2　**Activity, push-ups, pull-ups, sit-ups**

Y93.b3　**Activity, free weights**
　　　　Activity, barbells
　　　　Activity, dumbbells

Y93.b4　**Activity, pilates**

Y93.b9　**Activity, other involving other muscle strengthening exercises**
　　　　EXCLUDES 1 *activities involving muscle strengthening specified in categories Y93.0-Y93.a*

✓5th Y93.c　**Activities involving computer technology and electronic devices**
　　　　EXCLUDES 1 *activity, electronic musical keyboard or instruments (Y93.j-)*

Y93.c1　**Activity, computer keyboarding**
　　　　Activity, electronic game playing using keyboard or other stationary device

Y93.c2　**Activity, hand held interactive electronic device**
　　　　Activity, cellular telephone and communication device
　　　　Activity, electronic game playing using interactive device
　　　　EXCLUDES 1 *activity, electronic game playing using keyboard or other stationary device (Y93.c1)*

Y93.c9　**Activity, other involving computer technology and electronic devices**

✓5th Y93.d　**Activities involving arts and handcrafts**
　　　　EXCLUDES 1 *activities involving playing musical instrument (Y93.j-)*

Y93.d1　**Activity, knitting and crocheting**

Y93.d2　**Activity, sewing**

Y93.d3　**Activity, furniture building and finishing**
　　　　Activity, furniture repair

Y93.d9　**Activity, involving other arts and handcrafts**

✓5th Y93.e　**Activities involving personal hygiene and interior property and clothing maintenance**
　　　　EXCLUDES 1 *activities involving cooking and grilling (Y93.g-)*
　　　　　　activities involving exterior property and land maintenance, building and construction (Y93.h-)
　　　　　　activities involving caregiving (Y93.f-)
　　　　　　activity, dishwashing (Y93.g1)
　　　　　　activity, food preparation (Y93.g1)
　　　　　　activity, gardening (Y93.h2)

Y93.e1　**Activity, personal bathing and showering**

Y93.e2　**Activity, laundry**

Y93.e3　**Activity, vacuuming**

Y93.e4　**Activity, ironing**

Y93.e5　**Activity, floor mopping and cleaning**

Y93.e6　**Activity, residential relocation**
　　　　Activity, packing up and unpacking involved in moving to a new residence

Y93.e8　**Activity, other personal hygiene**

Y93.e9　**Activity, other interior property and clothing maintenance**

✓5th Y93.f　**Activities involving caregiving**
　　　Activity involving the provider of caregiving

Y93.f1　**Activity, caregiving, bathing**

Y93.f2　**Activity, caregiving, lifting**

Y93.f9　**Activity, other caregiving**

✓5th Y93.g　**Activities involving food preparation, cooking and grilling**

Y93.g1　**Activity, food preparation and clean up**
　　　　Activity, dishwashing

Y93.g2　**Activity, grilling and smoking food**

Y93.g3　**Activity, cooking and baking**
　　　　Activity, use of stove, oven and microwave oven

Y93.g9　**Activity, other involving cooking and grilling**

✓5th Y93.h　**Activities involving exterior property and land maintenance, building and construction**

Y93.h1　**Activity, digging, shoveling and raking**
　　　　Activity, dirt digging
　　　　Activity, raking leaves
　　　　Activity, snow shoveling

Y93.h2　**Activity, gardening and landscaping**
　　　　Activity, pruning, trimming shrubs, weeding

Y93.h3　**Activity, building and construction**

Y93.h9　**Activity, other involving exterior property and land maintenance, building and construction**

✓5th Y93.i　**Activities involving roller coasters and other types of external motion**

Y93.i1　**Activity, rollercoaster riding**

Y93.i9　**Activity, other involving external motion**

✓5th Y93.j　**Activities involving playing musical instrument**
　　　Activity involving playing electric musical instrument

Y93.j1　**Activity, piano playing**
　　　　Activity, musical keyboard (electronic) playing

Y93.j2　**Activity, drum and other percussion instrument playing**

Y93.j3　**Activity, string instrument playing**

Y93.j4　**Activity, winds and brass instrument playing**

✓5th Y93.k　**Activities involving animal care**
　　　　EXCLUDES 1 *activity, horseback riding (Y93.52)*

Y93.k1　**Activity, walking an animal**

Y93.k2　**Activity, milking an animal**

Y93.k3　**Activity, grooming and shearing an animal**

Y93.k9　**Activity, other involving animal care**

✓5th Y93.8　**Activities, other specified**

Y93.81　**Activity, refereeing a sports activity**

Y93.82　**Activity, spectator at an event**

Y93.83　**Activity, rough housing and horseplay**

Y93.84　**Activity, sleeping**

Y93.89　**Activity, other specified**

Y93.9　**Activity, unspecified**

Y95　**Nosocomial condition**

Y96　**Deactivated**
　　　Use code Y99.0

✓ Appropriate additional character required

✓x7th Requires 7th character, placeholder x must fill empty characters

Y97   **Deactivated**
       See categories Z57, Z77

Y98   **Deactivated**
       See categories Z72, Z73

√4ᵗʰ **Y99**   **External cause status**

> **NOTE**   A single code from category Y99 should be used in conjunction with the external cause code(s) assigned to a record to indicate the status of the person at the time the event occurred.

     Y99.0   **Civilian activity done for income or pay**
         Civilian activity done for financial or other compensation
         EXCLUDES 1   *military activity (Y99.1)*
                           volunteer activity (Y99.2)

     Y99.1   **Military activity**
         EXCLUDES 2   *activity of off duty military personnel (Y99.8)*

     Y99.2   **Volunteer activity**
         EXCLUDES 1   *activity of child or other family member assisting in compensated work of other family member (Y99.8)*

     Y99.8   **Other external cause status**
         Activity NEC
         Activity of child or other family member assisting in compensated work of other family member
         Hobby not done for income
         Leisure activity
         Off-duty activity of military personnel
         Recreation or sport not for income or while a student
         Student activity
         EXCLUDES 1   *civilian activity done for income or compensation (Y99.0)*
                           military activity (Y99.1)

     Y99.9   **Unspecified external cause status**

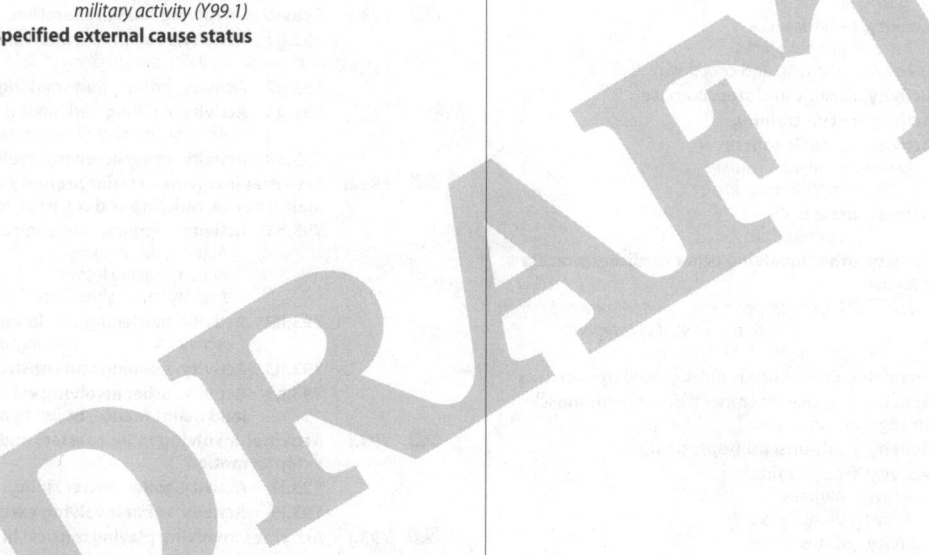

EXCLUDES 1 Not coded here   **EXCLUDES 2** Not included here   *Manifestation Code*

Chapter 21. Factors Influencing Health Status and Contact With Health Services (Z00-Z99)

NOTE Z codes represent reasons for encounters. A corresponding procedure code must accompany a Z code if a procedure is performed. Categories Z00-Z99 are provided for occasions when circumstances other than a disease, injury or external cause classifiable to categories A00-Y89 are recorded as "diagnoses" or "problems". This can arise in two main ways:

(a) When a person who may or may not be sick encounters the health services for some specific purpose, such as to receive limited care or service for a current condition, to donate an organ or tissue, to receive prophylactic vaccination (immunization), or to discuss a problem which is in itself not a disease or injury.

(b) When some circumstance or problem is present which influences the person's health status but is not in itself a current illness or injury.

This chapter contains the following blocks:

Z00-Z13 Persons encountering health services for examination and investigation
Z14-Z15 Genetic carrier and genetic susceptibility to disease
Z16 Infection with drug resistant microorganisms
Z17 Estrogen receptor status
Z18 Retained foreign body fragments
Z20-Z28 Persons with potential health hazards related to communicable diseases
Z30-Z39 Persons encountering health services in circumstances related to reproduction
Z40-Z53 Persons encountering health services for specific procedures and health care
Z55-Z65 Persons with potential health hazards related to socioeconomic and psychosocial circumstances
Z66 Do not resuscitate [DNR] status
Z67 Blood type
Z68 Body mass index (BMI)
Z69-Z76 Persons encountering health services in other circumstances
Z77-Z99 Persons with potential health hazards related to family and personal history and certain conditions influencing health status

Persons encountering health services for examinations (Z00-Z13)

NOTE Nonspecific abnormal findings disclosed at the time of these examinations are classified to categories R70-R94.

EXCLUDES 1 *examinations related to pregnancy and reproduction (Z30-Z36, Z39-)*

☑4th **Z00** **Encounter for general examination without complaint, suspected or reported diagnosis**
    EXCLUDES 1 *encounter for examination for administrative purposes (Z02-)*
    EXCLUDES 2 *encounter for pre-procedural examinations (Z01.81-)*
        special screening examinations (Z11-Z13)

☑5th **Z00.0** **Encounter for general adult medical examination**
        Encounter for adult periodic examination (annual) (physical) and any associated laboratory and radiologic examinations
        EXCLUDES 1 *encounter for examination of sign or symptom—code to sign or symptom*
            general health check-up of infant or child (Z00.12-)

    Z00.00 **Encounter for general adult medical examination without abnormal findings**
        Encounter for adult health check-up NOS

    Z00.01 **Encounter for general adult medical examination with abnormal findings**
        Use additional code to identify abnormal findings

☑5th **Z00.1** **Encounter for newborn, infant and child health examinations**

    ☑6th **Z00.11** **Newborn health examination**
        Health check for child under 29 days old
        Use additional code to identify any abnormal findings
        EXCLUDES 1 *health check for child over 28 days old (Z00.12-)*

        Z00.110 **Health examination for newborn under 8 days old**
            Health check for child under 8 days old

        Z00.111 **Health examination for newborn 8 to 28 days old**
            Health check for newborn 8 to 28 days old
            Newborn weight check

    ☑6th **Z00.12** **Encounter for routine child health examination**
        Encounter for development testing of infant or child
        Health check (routine) for child over 28 days old
        EXCLUDES 1 *health check for child under 29 days old (Z00.11-)*
            health supervision of foundling or other healthy infant or child (Z76.1-Z76.2)
            newborn health examination (Z00.11-)

        Z00.121 **Encounter for routine child health examination with abnormal findings**
            Use additional code to identify abnormal findings

        Z00.129 **Encounter for routine child health examination without abnormal findings**
            Encounter for routine child health examination NOS

    Z00.2 **Encounter for examination for period of rapid growth in childhood**

    Z00.3 **Encounter for examination for adolescent development state**
        Encounter for puberty development state

    Z00.5 **Encounter for examination of potential donor of organ and tissue**

    Z00.6 **Encounter for examination for normal comparison and control in clinical research program**

☑5th **Z00.7** **Encounter for examination for period of delayed growth in childhood**

    Z00.70 **Encounter for examination for period of delayed growth in childhood without abnormal findings**

    Z00.71 **Encounter for examination for period of delayed growth in childhood with abnormal findings**
        Use additional code to identify abnormal findings

    Z00.8 **Encounter for other general examination**
        Encounter for health examination in population surveys

☑4th **Z01** **Encounter for other special examination without complaint, suspected or reported diagnosis**
    INCLUDES routine examination of specific system
    NOTE Codes from category Z01 represent the reason for the encounter. A separate procedure code is required to identify any examinations or procedures performed
    EXCLUDES 1 *encounter for examination for administrative purposes (Z02-)*
        encounter for examination for suspected conditions, proven not to exist (Z03-)
        encounter for laboratory and radiologic examinations as a component of general medical examinations (Z00.0-)
        encounter for laboratory, radiologic and imaging examinations for sign(s) and symptom(s)—code to the sign(s) or symptom(s)
    EXCLUDES 2 *screening examinations (Z11-Z13)*

☑5th **Z01.0** **Encounter for examination of eyes and vision**
    EXCLUDES 1 *examination for driving license (Z02.4)*

    Z01.00 **Encounter for examination of eyes and vision without abnormal findings**
        Encounter for examination of eyes and vision NOS

    Z01.01 **Encounter for examination of eyes and vision with abnormal findings**
        Use additional code to identify abnormal findings

☑5th **Z01.1** **Encounter for examination of ears and hearing**

    Z01.10 **Encounter for examination of ears and hearing without abnormal findings**
        Encounter for examination of ears and hearing NOS

    ☑6th **Z01.11** **Encounter for examination of ears and hearing with abnormal findings**

        Z01.110 **Encounter for hearing examination following failed hearing screening**

        Z01.118 **Encounter for examination of ears and hearing with other abnormal findings**
            Use additional code to identify abnormal findings

    Z01.12 **Encounter for hearing conservation and treatment**

☑5th **Z01.2** **Encounter for dental examination and cleaning**

    Z01.20 **Encounter for dental examination and cleaning without abnormal findings**
        Encounter for dental examination and cleaning NOS

☑ Appropriate additional character required   ☑x7th Requires 7th character, placeholder x must fill empty characters

Z01.21   **Encounter for dental examination and cleaning with abnormal findings**
> Use additional code to identify abnormal findings

√5th   **Z01.3**   **Encounter for examination of blood pressure**

Z01.30   **Encounter for examination of blood pressure without abnormal findings**
> Encounter for examination of blood pressure NOS

Z01.31   **Encounter for examination of blood pressure with abnormal findings**
> Use additional code to identify abnormal findings

√5th   **Z01.4**   **Encounter for gynecological examination**
> *EXCLUDES 2*   *pregnancy examination or test (Z32.0-)*
> *routine examination for contraceptive maintenance (Z30.4)*

√6th   **Z01.41**   **Encounter for routine gynecological examination**
> Encounter for general gynecological examination with or without cervical smear
> Encounter for gynecological examination (general) (routine) NOS
> Encounter for pelvic examination (annual) (periodic)
> Use additional code:
> for screening for human papillomavirus, if applicable, (Z11.51)
> for screening vaginal pap smear, if applicable (Z12.72)
> to identify acquired absence of uterus, if applicable (Z90.71-)
> *EXCLUDES 1*   *gynecologic examination status-post hysterectomy for malignant condition (Z08)*
> *screening cervical pap smear not a part of a routine gynecological examination (Z12.4)*

Z01.411   **Encounter for gynecological examination (general) (routine) with abnormal findings**

Z01.419   **Encounter for gynecological examination (general) (routine) without abnormal findings**
> Use additional code to identify abnormal findings

Z01.42   **Encounter for cervical smear to confirm findings of recent normal smear following initial abnormal smear**

√5th   **Z01.8**   **Encounter for other specified special examinations**

√6th   **Z01.81**   **Encounter for preprocedural examinations**
> Encounter for preoperative examinations
> Encounter for radiological and imaging examinations as part of preprocedural examination

Z01.810   **Encounter for preprocedural cardiovascular examination**

Z01.811   **Encounter for preprocedural respiratory examination**

Z01.812   **Encounter for preprocedural laboratory examination**
> Blood and urine tests prior to treatment or procedure

Z01.818   **Encounter for other preprocedural examination**
> Encounter for preprocedural examination NOS
> Encounter for examinations prior to antineoplastic chemotherapy

Z01.82   **Encounter for allergy testing**
> *EXCLUDES 1*   *encounter for antibody response examination (Z01.84)*

Z01.83   **Encounter for blood typing**
> Encounter for Rh typing

Z01.84   **Encounter for antibody response examination**
> Encounter for immunity status testing
> *EXCLUDES 1*   *encounter for allergy testing (Z01.82)*

Z01.89   **Encounter for other specified special examinations**

√4th   **Z02**   **Encounter for administrative examination**

Z02.0   **Encounter for examination for admission to educational institution**
> Encounter for examination for admission to preschool (education)
> Encounter for examination for re-admission to school following illness or medical treatment

Z02.1   **Encounter for pre-employment examination**

Z02.2   **Encounter for examination for admission to residential institution**
> *EXCLUDES 1*   *examination for admission to prison (Z02.89)*

Z02.3   **Encounter for examination for recruitment to armed forces**

Z02.4   **Encounter for examination for driving license**

Z02.5   **Encounter for examination for participation in sport**
> *EXCLUDES 1*   *blood-alcohol and blood-drug test (Z02.83)*

Z02.6   **Encounter for examination for insurance purposes**

√5th   **Z02.7**   **Encounter for issue of medical certificate**
> *EXCLUDES 1*   *encounter for general medical examination (Z00-Z01, Z02.0-Z02.6, Z02.8-Z02.9,)*

Z02.71   **Encounter for disability determination**
> Encounter for issue of medical certificate of incapacity
> Encounter for issue of medical certificate of invalidity

Z02.79   **Encounter for issue of other medical certificate**

√5th   **Z02.8**   **Encounter for other administrative examinations**

Z02.81   **Encounter for paternity testing**

Z02.82   **Encounter for adoption services**

Z02.83   **Encounter for blood-alcohol and blood-drug test**
> Use additional code for findings of alcohol or drugs in blood (R78-)

Z02.89   **Encounter for other administrative examinations**
> Encounter for examination for admission to prison
> Encounter for examination for admission to summer camp
> Encounter for immigration examination
> Encounter for naturalization examination
> Encounter for premarital examination
> *EXCLUDES 1*   *health supervision of foundling or other healthy infant or child (Z76.1-Z76.2)*

Z02.9   **Encounter for administrative examinations, unspecified**

√4th   **Z03**   **Encounter for medical observation for suspected diseases and conditions ruled out**
> *NOTE*   This category is to be used when a person without a diagnosis is suspected of having an abnormal condition, without signs or symptoms, which requires study, but after examination and observation, is ruled out. This category is also for use for administrative and legal observation status.
> *EXCLUDES 1*   *contact with and (suspected) exposures hazardous to health (Z77-)*
> *newborn observation for suspected condition, ruled out (P00-P04)*
> *person with feared complaint in whom no diagnosis is made (Z71.1)*
> *signs or symptoms under study—code to signs or symptoms*

Z03.6   **Encounter for observation for suspected toxic effect from ingested substance ruled out**
> Encounter for observation for suspected adverse effect from drug
> Encounter for observation for suspected poisoning

√5th   **Z03.7**   **Encounter for suspected maternal and fetal conditions ruled out**
> Encounter for suspected maternal and fetal conditions not found
> *EXCLUDES 1*   *known or suspected fetal anomalies affecting management of mother, not ruled out (O26-, O35-, O36-, O40-, O41-)*

Z03.71   **Encounter for suspected problem with amniotic cavity and membrane ruled out**
> Encounter for suspected oligohydramnios ruled out
> Encounter for suspected polyhydramnios ruled out

Z03.72   **Encounter for suspected placental problem ruled out**

Z03.73   **Encounter for suspected fetal anomaly ruled out**

Z03.74   **Encounter for suspected problem with fetal growth ruled out**

Z03.75   **Encounter for suspected cervical shortening ruled out**

Z03.79   **Encounter for other suspected maternal and fetal conditions ruled out**

√5th   **Z03.8**   **Encounter for observation for other suspected diseases and conditions ruled out**

√6th   **Z03.81**   **Encounter for observation for suspected exposure to biological agents ruled out**

Z03.810   **Encounter for observation for suspected exposure to anthrax ruled out**

EXCLUDES 1   Not coded here   *EXCLUDES 2*   Not included here   *Manifestation Code*

Z03.818 **Encounter for observation for suspected exposure to other biological agents ruled out**

Z03.89 **Encounter for observation for other suspected diseases and conditions ruled out**

✓4ᵗʰ **Z04 Encounter for examination and observation for other reasons**

INCLUDES encounter for examination for medicolegal reasons

NOTE This category is to be used when a person without a diagnosis is suspected of having an abnormal condition, without signs or symptoms, which requires study, but after examination and observation, is ruled-out. This category is also for use for administrative and legal observation status.

Z04.1 **Encounter for examination and observation following transport accident**

EXCLUDES 1 *encounter for examination and observation following work accident (Z04.2)*

Z04.2 **Encounter for examination and observation following work accident**

Z04.3 **Encounter for examination and observation following other accident**

✓5ᵗʰ Z04.4 **Encounter for examination and observation following alleged rape**

Encounter for examination and observation of victim following alleged rape

Encounter for examination and observation of victim following alleged sexual abuse

Z04.41 **Encounter for examination and observation following alleged adult rape**

Suspected adult rape, ruled out

Suspected adult sexual abuse, ruled out

Z04.42 **Encounter for examination and observation following alleged child rape**

Suspected child rape, ruled out

Suspected child sexual abuse, ruled out

Z04.6 **Encounter for general psychiatric examination, requested by authority**

✓5ᵗʰ Z04.7 **Encounter for examination and observation following alleged physical abuse**

Z04.71 **Encounter for examination and observation following alleged adult physical abuse**

Suspected adult physical abuse, ruled out

EXCLUDES 1 *confirmed case of adult physical abuse (T74-)*

encounter for examination and observation following alleged adult sexual abuse (Z04.41)

suspected case of adult physical abuse, not ruled out (T76-)

Z04.72 **Encounter for examination and observation following alleged child physical abuse**

Suspected child physical abuse, ruled out

EXCLUDES 1 *confirmed case of child physical abuse (T74-)*

encounter for examination and observation following alleged child sexual abuse (Z04.42)

suspected case of child physical abuse, not ruled out (T76-)

Z04.8 **Encounter for examination and observation for other specified reasons**

Encounter for examination and observation for request for expert evidence

Z04.9 **Encounter for examination and observation for unspecified reason**

Encounter for observation NOS

Z08 Encounter for follow-up examination after completed treatment for malignant neoplasm

Medical surveillance following completed treatment

Use additional code to identify any acquired absence of organs (Z90-)

Use additional code to identify the personal history of malignant neoplasm (Z85-)

EXCLUDES 1 *aftercare following medical care (Z43-Z49, Z51)*

Z09 Encounter for follow-up examination after completed treatment for conditions other than malignant neoplasm

Medical surveillance following completed treatment

Use additional code to identify any applicable history of disease code (Z86-, Z87-)

EXCLUDES 1 *aftercare following medical care (Z43-Z49, Z51)*

surveillance of contraception (Z30.4-)

surveillance of prosthetic and other medical devices (Z44-Z46)

✓4ᵗʰ **Z11 Encounter for screening for infectious and parasitic diseases**

NOTE Screening is the testing for disease or disease precursors in asymptomatic individuals so that early detection and treatment can be provided for those who test positive for the disease.

EXCLUDES 1 *encounter for diagnostic examination—code to sign or symptom*

Z11.0 **Encounter for screening for intestinal infectious diseases**

Z11.1 **Encounter for screening for respiratory tuberculosis**

Z11.2 **Encounter for screening for other bacterial diseases**

Z11.3 **Encounter for screening for infections with a predominantly sexual mode of transmission**

EXCLUDES 2 *encounter for screening for human immunodeficiency virus [HIV] (Z11.4)*

encounter for screening for human papillomavirus (Z11.51)

Z11.4 **Encounter for screening for human immunodeficiency virus [HIV]**

✓5ᵗʰ Z11.5 **Encounter for screening for other viral diseases**

EXCLUDES 2 *encounter for screening for viral intestinal disease (Z11.0)*

Z11.51 **Encounter for screening for human papillomavirus (HPV)**

Z11.59 **Encounter for screening for other viral diseases**

Z11.6 **Encounter for screening for other protozoal diseases and helminthiases**

EXCLUDES 2 *encounter for screening for protozoal intestinal disease (Z11.0)*

Z11.8 **Encounter for screening for other infectious and parasitic diseases**

Encounter for screening for chlamydia

Encounter for screening for rickettsial

Encounter for screening for spirochetal

Encounter for screening for mycoses

Z11.9 **Encounter for screening for infectious and parasitic diseases, unspecified**

✓4ᵗʰ **Z12 Encounter for screening for malignant neoplasms**

NOTE Screening is the testing for disease or disease precursors in asymptomatic individuals so that early detection and treatment can be provided for those who test positive for the disease.

Use additional code to identify any family history of malignant neoplasm (Z80-)

EXCLUDES 1 *encounter for diagnostic examination—code to sign or symptom*

Z12.0 **Encounter for screening for malignant neoplasm of stomach**

✓5ᵗʰ Z12.1 **Encounter for screening for malignant neoplasm of intestinal tract**

Z12.10 **Encounter for screening for malignant neoplasm of intestinal tract, unspecified**

Z12.11 **Encounter for screening for malignant neoplasm of colon**

Encounter for screening colonoscopy NOS

Z12.12 **Encounter for screening for malignant neoplasm of rectum**

Z12.13 **Encounter for screening for malignant neoplasm of small intestine**

Z12.2 **Encounter for screening for malignant neoplasm of respiratory organs**

✓5ᵗʰ Z12.3 **Encounter for screening for malignant neoplasm of breast**

Z12.31 **Encounter for screening mammogram for malignant neoplasm of breast**

EXCLUDES 1 *inconclusive mammogram (R92.2)*

Z12.39 **Encounter for other screening for malignant neoplasm of breast**

☑ Appropriate additional character required   ✓x7ᵗʰ Requires 7th character, placeholder x must fill empty characters

Z12.4 **Encounter for screening for malignant neoplasm of cervix**
Encounter for screening pap smear for malignant neoplasm of cervix
> EXCLUDES 1   *encounter for screening for human papillomavirus (Z11.51)*
> *when screening is part of general gynecological examination (Z01.4-)*

Z12.5 **Encounter for screening for malignant neoplasm of prostate**

Z12.6 **Encounter for screening for malignant neoplasm of bladder**

✓5th **Z12.7** **Encounter for screening for malignant neoplasm of other genitourinary organs**

   Z12.71 **Encounter for screening for malignant neoplasm of testis**

   Z12.72 **Encounter for screening for malignant neoplasm of vagina**
Vaginal pap smear status-post hysterectomy for non-malignant condition
Use additional code to identify acquired absence of uterus (Z90.71-)
> EXCLUDES 1   *vaginal pap smear status-post hysterectomy for malignant conditions (Z08)*

   Z12.73 **Encounter for screening for malignant neoplasm of ovary**

   Z12.79 **Encounter for screening for malignant neoplasm of other genitourinary organs**

✓5th **Z12.8** **Encounter for screening for malignant neoplasm of other sites**

   Z12.81 **Encounter for screening for malignant neoplasm of oral cavity**

   Z12.82 **Encounter for screening for malignant neoplasm of nervous system**

   Z12.83 **Encounter for screening for malignant neoplasm of skin**

   Z12.89 **Encounter for screening for malignant neoplasm of other sites**

Z12.9 **Encounter for screening for malignant neoplasm, site unspecified**

✓4th **Z13** **Encounter for screening for other diseases and disorders**
> NOTE   Screening is the testing for disease or disease precursors in asymptomatic individuals so that early detection and treatment can be provided for those who test positive for the disease.
> EXCLUDES 1   *encounter for diagnostic examination—code to sign or symptom*

Z13.0 **Encounter for screening for diseases of the blood and blood-forming organs and certain disorders involving the immune mechanism**

Z13.1 **Encounter for screening for diabetes mellitus**

✓5th **Z13.2** **Encounter for screening for nutritional, metabolic and other endocrine disorders**

   Z13.21 **Encounter for screening for nutritional disorder**

✓6th   **Z13.22** **Encounter for screening for metabolic disorder**

     Z13.220 **Encounter for screening for lipoid disorders**
Encounter for screening for cholesterol level
Encounter for screening for hypercholesterolemia
Encounter for screening for hyperlipidemia

     Z13.228 **Encounter for screening for other metabolic disorders**

   Z13.29 **Encounter for screening for other suspected endocrine disorder**
> EXCLUDES 1   *encounter for screening for diabetes mellitus (Z13.1)*

Z13.4 **Encounter for screening for certain developmental disorders in childhood**
Encounter for screening for developmental handicaps in early childhood
> EXCLUDES 1   *routine development testing of infant or child (Z00.1-)*

Z13.5 **Encounter for screening for eye and ear disorders**
> EXCLUDES 2   *encounter for general hearing examination (Z01.1-)*
> *encounter for general vision examination (Z01.0-)*

Z13.6 **Encounter for screening for cardiovascular disorders**

✓5th **Z13.7** **Encounter for screening for genetic and chromosomal anomalies**
> EXCLUDES 1   *genetic testing for procreative management (Z31.4-)*

   Z13.71 **Encounter for nonprocreative screening for genetic disease carrier status**

   Z13.79 **Encounter for other screening for genetic and chromosomal anomalies**

✓5th **Z13.8** **Encounter for screening for other specified diseases and disorders**
> EXCLUDES 2   *screening for malignant neoplasms (Z12-)*

✓6th   **Z13.81** **Encounter for screening for digestive system disorders**

     Z13.810 **Encounter for screening for upper gastrointestinal disorder**

     Z13.811 **Encounter for screening for lower gastrointestinal disorder**
> EXCLUDES 1   *encounter for screening for intestinal infectious disease (Z11.0)*

     Z13.818 **Encounter for screening for other digestive system disorders**

✓6th   **Z13.82** **Encounter for screening for musculoskeletal disorder**

     Z13.820 **Encounter for screening for osteoporosis**

     Z13.828 **Encounter for screening for other musculoskeletal disorder**

   Z13.83 **Encounter for screening for respiratory disorder NEC**
> EXCLUDES 1   *encounter for screening for respiratory tuberculosis (Z11.1)*

   Z13.84 **Encounter for screening for dental disorders**

✓6th   **Z13.85** **Encounter for screening for nervous system disorders**

     Z13.850 **Encounter for screening for traumatic brain injury**

     Z13.858 **Encounter for screening for other nervous system disorders**

   Z13.88 **Encounter for screening for disorder due to exposure to contaminants**
> EXCLUDES 1   *those exposed to contaminants without suspected disorders (Z57-Z77-)*

   Z13.89 **Encounter for screening for other disorder**
Encounter for screening for genitourinary disorders

Z13.9 **Encounter for screening, unspecified**

Genetic carrier and genetic susceptibility to disease (Z14-Z15)

✓4th **Z14** **Genetic carrier**

✓5th **Z14.0** **Hemophilia A carrier**

   Z14.01 **Asymptomatic hemophilia A carrier**

   Z14.02 **Symptomatic hemophilia A carrier**

Z14.1 **Cystic fibrosis carrier**

Z14.8 **Genetic carrier of other disease**

✓4th **Z15** **Genetic susceptibility to disease**
Confirmed abnormal gene
Use additional code, if applicable, for any associated family history of the disease (Z80-Z84)

✓5th **Z15.0** **Genetic susceptibility to malignant neoplasm**
Code first, if applicable, any current malignant neoplasm (C00-C75, C81-C96)
Use additional code, if applicable, for any personal history of malignant neoplasm (Z85-)

   Z15.01 **Genetic susceptibility to malignant neoplasm of breast**

   Z15.02 **Genetic susceptibility to malignant neoplasm of ovary**

   Z15.03 **Genetic susceptibility to malignant neoplasm of prostate**

   Z15.04 **Genetic susceptibility to malignant neoplasm of endometrium**

   Z15.09 **Genetic susceptibility to other malignant neoplasm**

✓5th **Z15.8** **Genetic susceptibility to other disease**

   Z15.81 **Genetic susceptibility to multiple endocrine neoplasia [MEN]**

   Z15.89 **Genetic susceptibility to other disease**

EXCLUDES 1 Not coded here   EXCLUDES 2 Not included here   *Manifestation Code*

Infection with drug resistant microorganisms (Z16)

Z16 Infection with drug resistant microorganisms
> **NOTE**   This category is intended for use as an additional code for infectious conditions classified elsewhere to indicate the presence of drug-resistance of the infectious organism
> Code first the infection

Estrogen receptor status (Z17)

✓4ᵗʰ **Z17 Estrogen receptor status**
> Code first malignant neoplasm of breast (C50-)

Z17.0 Estrogen receptor positive status [ER+]
Z17.1 Estrogen receptor negative status [ER-]

Retained foreign body fragment (Z18)

✓4ᵗʰ **Z18 Retained foreign body fragments**
> Embedded fragment (status)
> Embedded splinter (status)
> Retained foreign body status
> *EXCLUDES 1*   *artificial joint prosthesis status (Z96.6-)*
> *foreign body accidentally left during a procedure (T81.5-)*
> *foreign body entering through orifice (T15-T19)*
> *in situ cardiac device (Z95.-)*
> *organ or tissue replaced by means other than transplant (Z96.-, Z97.-)*
> *organ or tissue replaced by transplant (Z94.-)*
> *personal history of retained foreign body fully removed (Z87.821)*
> *superficial foreign body (non-embedded splinter)—code to superficial foreign body, by site*

✓5ᵗʰ **Z18.0 Retained radioactive fragments**
Z18.01 Retained depleted uranium fragments
Z18.09 Other retained radioactive fragments
> Other retained depleted isotope fragments
> Retained nontherapeutic radioactive fragments

✓5ᵗʰ **Z18.1 Retained metal fragments**
> *EXCLUDES 1*   *retained radioactive metal fragments (Z18.01-Z18.09)*
Z18.10 Retained metal fragments, unspecified
> Retained metal fragment NOS
Z18.11 Retained magnetic metal fragments
Z18.12 Retained nonmagnetic metal fragments
Z18.2 Retained plastic fragments
> Acrylics fragments
> Diethylhexylphthalates fragments
> Isocyanate fragments

✓5ᵗʰ **Z18.3 Retained organic fragments**
Z18.31 Retained animal quills or spines
Z18.32 Retained tooth
Z18.33 Retained wood fragments
Z18.39 Other retained organic fragments

✓5ᵗʰ **Z18.8 Other specified retained foreign body**
Z18.81 Retained glass fragments
Z18.83 Retained stone or crystalline fragments
> Retained concrete or cement fragments
Z18.89 Other specified retained foreign body fragments
Z18.9 Retained foreign body fragments, unspecified material

Persons with potential health hazards related to communicable diseases (Z20-Z28)

✓4ᵗʰ **Z20 Contact with and (suspected) exposure to communicable diseases**
> *EXCLUDES 1*   *carrier of infectious disease (Z22-)*
> *diagnosed current infectious or parasitic disease—see Alphabetic Index*
> *EXCLUDES 2*   *personal history of infectious and parasitic diseases (Z86.1-)*

✓5ᵗʰ **Z20.0 Contact with and (suspected) exposure to intestinal infectious diseases**
Z20.01 Contact with and (suspected) exposure to intestinal infectious diseases due to Escherichia coli (E. coli)
Z20.09 Contact with and (suspected) exposure to other intestinal infectious diseases
Z20.1 Contact with and (suspected) exposure to tuberculosis
Z20.2 Contact with and (suspected) exposure to infections with a predominantly sexual mode of transmission

Z20.3 Contact with and (suspected) exposure to rabies
Z20.4 Contact with and (suspected) exposure to rubella
Z20.5 Contact with and (suspected) exposure to viral hepatitis
Z20.6 Contact with and (suspected) exposure to human immunodeficiency virus [HIV]
> *EXCLUDES 1*   *asymptomatic human immunodeficiency virus [HIV] HIV infection status (Z21)*
Z20.7 Contact with and (suspected) exposure to pediculosis, acariasis and other infestations

✓5ᵗʰ **Z20.8 Contact with and (suspected) exposure to other communicable diseases**
✓6ᵗʰ **Z20.81 Contact with and (suspected) exposure to other bacterial communicable diseases**
Z20.810 Contact with and (suspected) exposure to anthrax
Z20.811 Contact with and (suspected) exposure to meningococcus
Z20.818 Contact with and (suspected) exposure to other bacterial communicable diseases
✓6ᵗʰ **Z20.82 Contact with and (suspected) exposure to other viral communicable diseases**
Z20.820 Contact with and (suspected) exposure to varicella
Z20.828 Contact with and (suspected) exposure to other viral communicable diseases
Z20.89 Contact with and (suspected) exposure to other communicable diseases
Z20.9 Contact with and (suspected) exposure to unspecified communicable disease

Z21 Asymptomatic human immunodeficiency virus [HIV] infection status
> HIV positive NOS
> Code first human immunodeficiency [HIV] disease complicating pregnancy, childbirth and the puerperium, if applicable (O98.7-)
> *EXCLUDES 1*   *acquired immunodeficiency syndrome (B20)*
> *contact with human immunodeficiency virus [HIV] (Z20.6)*
> *exposure to human immunodeficiency virus [HIV] (Z20.6)*
> *human immunodeficiency virus [HIV] disease (B20)*
> *inconclusive laboratory evidence of human immunodeficiency virus [HIV] (R75)*

✓4ᵗʰ **Z22 Carrier of infectious disease**
> Colonization status
> Suspected carrier
Z22.0 Carrier of typhoid
Z22.1 Carrier of other intestinal infectious diseases
Z22.2 Carrier of diphtheria
✓5ᵗʰ **Z22.3 Carrier of other specified bacterial diseases**
Z22.31 Carrier of bacterial disease due to meningococci
Z22.32 Carrier of bacterial disease due to staphylococci
✓6ᵗʰ **Z22.33 Carrier of bacterial disease due to streptococci**
Z22.330 Carrier of Group B streptococcus
Z22.338 Carrier of other streptococcus
Z22.39 Carrier of other specified bacterial diseases
Z22.4 Carrier of infections with a predominantly sexual mode of transmission
✓5ᵗʰ **Z22.5 Carrier of viral hepatitis**
Z22.50 Carrier of unspecified viral hepatitis
Z22.51 Carrier of viral hepatitis B
> Hepatitis B surface antigen [HBsAg] carrier
Z22.52 Carrier of viral hepatitis C
Z22.59 Carrier of other viral hepatitis
Z22.6 Carrier of human T-lymphotropic virus type-1 [HTLV-1] infection
Z22.8 Carrier of other infectious diseases
Z22.9 Carrier of infectious disease, unspecified

Z23 Encounter for immunization
> Code first any routine childhood examination
> **NOTE**   Procedure codes are required to identify the types of immunizations given

✓4ᵗʰ **Z28 Immunization not carried out and underimmunization status**
> Vaccination not carried out
✓5ᵗʰ **Z28.0 Immunization not carried out because of contraindication**
Z28.01 Immunization not carried out because of acute illness of patient

---

✓ Appropriate additional character required   ✓x7ᵗʰ Requires 7th character, placeholder x must fill empty characters

Z28.02   Immunization not carried out because of chronic illness or condition of patient

Z28.03   Immunization not carried out because of immune compromised state of patient

Z28.04   Immunization not carried out because of patient allergy to vaccine or component

Z28.09   Immunization not carried out because of other contraindication

Z28.1   Immunization not carried out because of patient decision for reasons of belief or group pressure

    Immunization not carried out because of religious belief

✓5th **Z28.2**   Immunization not carried out because of patient decision for other and unspecified reason

Z28.20   Immunization not carried out because of patient decision for unspecified reason

Z28.21   Immunization not carried out because of patient refusal

Z28.29   Immunization not carried out because of patient decision for other reason

Z28.3   Underimmunization status

    Delinquent immunization status

    Lapsed immunization schedule status

✓5th **Z28.8**   Immunization not carried out for other reason

Z28.81   Immunization not carried out due to patient having had the disease

Z28.82   Immunization not carried out because of caregiver refusal

    Immunization not carried out because of guardian refusal

    Immunization not carried out because of parent refusal

> EXCLUDES 2   *immunization not carried out because of caregiver refusal because of religious belief (Z28.1)*

Z28.89   Immunization not carried out for other reason

Z28.9   Immunization not carried out for unspecified reason

Persons encountering health services in circumstances related to reproduction (Z30-Z39)

✓4th **Z30**   **Encounter for contraceptive management**

✓5th **Z30.0**   Encounter for general counseling and advice on contraception

✓6th **Z30.01**   Encounter for initial prescription of contraceptives

> EXCLUDES 1   *encounter for surveillance of contraceptives (Z30.4-)*

Z30.011   Encounter for initial prescription of contraceptive pills

Z30.012   Encounter for prescription of emergency contraception

    Encounter for postcoital contraception

Z30.013   Encounter for initial prescription of injectable contraceptive

Z30.014   Encounter for initial prescription of intrauterine contraceptive device

> EXCLUDES 1   *encounter for insertion of intrauterine contraceptive device (Z30.430, Z30.432)*

Z30.018   Encounter for initial prescription of other contraceptives

Z30.019   Encounter for initial prescription of contraceptives, unspecified

Z30.02   Counseling and instruction in natural family planning to avoid pregnancy

Z30.09   Encounter for other general counseling and advice on contraception

    Encounter for family planning advice NOS

Z30.2   Encounter for sterilization

✓5th **Z30.4**   Encounter for surveillance of contraceptives

Z30.40   Encounter for surveillance of contraceptives, unspecified

Z30.41   Encounter for surveillance of contraceptive pills

    Encounter for repeat prescription for contraceptive pill

Z30.42   Encounter for surveillance of injectable contraceptive

---

✓6th **Z30.43**   Encounter for surveillance of intrauterine contraceptive device

Z30.430   Encounter for insertion of intrauterine contraceptive device

Z30.431   Encounter for routine checking of intrauterine contraceptive device

Z30.432   Encounter for removal of intrauterine contraceptive device

Z30.433   Encounter for removal and reinsertion of intrauterine contraceptive device

    Encounter for replacement of intrauterine contraceptive device

Z30.49   Encounter for surveillance of other contraceptives

Z30.8   Encounter for other contraceptive management

    Encounter for postvasectomy sperm count

    Encounter for routine examination for contraceptive maintenance

> EXCLUDES 1   *sperm count following sterilization reversal (Z31.42)*
> *sperm count for fertility testing (Z31.41)*

Z30.9   Encounter for contraceptive management, unspecified

✓4th **Z31**   **Encounter for procreative management**

> EXCLUDES 1   *complications associated with artificial fertilization (N98-)*
> *female infertility (N97-)*
> *male infertility (N46-)*

Z31.0   Encounter for reversal of previous sterilization

✓5th **Z31.4**   Encounter for procreative investigation and testing

> EXCLUDES 1   *postvasectomy sperm count (Z30.8)*

Z31.41   Encounter for fertility testing

    Encounter for fallopian tube patency testing

    Encounter for sperm count for fertility testing

Z31.42   Aftercare following sterilization reversal

    Sperm count following sterilization reversal

✓6th **Z31.43**   Encounter for genetic testing of female for procreative management

    Use additional code for recurrent pregnancy loss, if applicable (N96, O26.2-)

> EXCLUDES 1   *nonprocreative genetic testing (Z13.7-)*

Z31.430   Encounter of female for testing for genetic disease carrier status for procreative management

Z31.438   Encounter for other genetic testing of female for procreative management

✓6th **Z31.44**   Encounter for genetic testing of male for procreative management

> EXCLUDES 1   *nonprocreative genetic testing (Z13.7-)*

Z31.440   Encounter of male for testing for genetic disease carrier status for procreative management

Z31.441   Encounter for testing of male partner of patient with recurrent pregnancy loss

Z31.448   Encounter for other genetic testing of male for procreative management

Z31.49   Encounter for other procreative investigation and testing

Z31.5   Encounter for genetic counseling

✓5th **Z31.6**   Encounter for general counseling and advice on procreation

Z31.61   Procreative counseling and advice using natural family planning

Z31.62   Encounter for fertility preservation counseling

    Encounter for fertility preservation counseling prior to cancer therapy

    Encounter for fertility preservation counseling prior to surgical removal of gonads

Z31.69   Encounter for other general counseling and advice on procreation

✓5th **Z31.8**   Encounter for other procreative management

Z31.81   Encounter for male factor infertility in female patient

Z31.82   Encounter for Rh incompatibility status

Z31.83   Encounter for assisted reproductive fertility procedure cycle

    Patient undergoing in vitro fertilization cycle

    Use additional code to identify the type of infertility

> EXCLUDES 1   *pre-cycle diagnosis and testing—code to reason for encounter*

EXCLUDES 1   Not coded here   EXCLUDES 2   Not included here   *Manifestation Code*

Z31.84 **Encounter for fertility preservation procedure**
Encounter for fertility preservation procedure prior to cancer therapy
Encounter for fertility preservation procedure prior to surgical removal of gonads

Z31.89 **Encounter for other procreative management**

Z31.9 **Encounter for procreative management, unspecified**

✓4th **Z32 Encounter for pregnancy test and childbirth and childcare instruction**

✓5th Z32.0 **Encounter for pregnancy test**

Z32.00 **Encounter for pregnancy test, result unknown**
Encounter for pregnancy test NOS

Z32.01 **Encounter for pregnancy test, result positive**

Z32.02 **Encounter for pregnancy test, result negative**

Z32.2 **Encounter for childbirth instruction**

Z32.3 **Encounter for childcare instruction**
Encounter for prenatal or postpartum childcare instruction

✓4th **Z33 Pregnant state**

Z33.1 **Pregnant state, incidental**
Pregnant state NOS

EXCLUDES 1 *complications of pregnancy (O00-O99)*

Z33.2 **Encounter for elective termination of pregnancy**

EXCLUDES 1 *early fetal death with retention of dead fetus (O02.1)*
late fetal death (O36.4)
spontaneous abortion (O03)

✓4th **Z34 Encounter for supervision of normal pregnancy**

EXCLUDES 1 *any complication of pregnancy (O00-O99)*
encounter for pregnancy test (Z32.0-)
encounter for supervision of high risk pregnancy (O09-)

✓5th Z34.0 **Encounter for supervision of normal first pregnancy**

Z34.00 **Encounter for supervision of normal first pregnancy, unspecified trimester**

Z34.01 **Encounter for supervision of normal first pregnancy, first trimester**

Z34.02 **Encounter for supervision of normal first pregnancy, second trimester**

Z34.03 **Encounter for supervision of normal first pregnancy, third trimester**

✓5th Z34.8 **Encounter for supervision of other normal pregnancy**

Z34.80 **Encounter for supervision of other normal pregnancy, unspecified trimester**

Z34.81 **Encounter for supervision of other normal pregnancy, first trimester**

Z34.82 **Encounter for supervision of other normal pregnancy, second trimester**

Z34.83 **Encounter for supervision of other normal pregnancy, third trimester**

✓5th Z34.9 **Encounter for supervision of normal pregnancy, unspecified**

Z34.90 **Encounter for supervision of normal pregnancy, unspecified, unspecified trimester**

Z34.91 **Encounter for supervision of normal pregnancy, unspecified, first trimester**

Z34.92 **Encounter for supervision of normal pregnancy, unspecified, second trimester**

Z34.93 **Encounter for supervision of normal pregnancy, unspecified, third trimester**

Z36 Encounter for antenatal screening of mother

EXCLUDES 1 *abnormal findings on antenatal screening of mother (O28-)*
diagnostic examination—code to sign or symptom
encounter for suspected maternal and fetal conditions ruled out (Z03.7-)
suspected fetal condition affecting management of pregnancy—code to condition in Chapter 15

EXCLUDES 2 *genetic counseling and testing (Z31.43-, Z31.5)*
routine prenatal care (Z34)

✓4th **Z37 Outcome of delivery**

NOTE This category is intended for use as an additional code to identify the outcome of delivery on the mother's record. It is not for use on the newborn record.

EXCLUDES 1 *stillbirth (P95)*

Z37.0 **Single live birth**

Z37.1 **Single stillbirth**

Z37.2 **Twins, both liveborn**

Z37.3 **Twins, one liveborn and one stillborn**

Z37.4 **Twins, both stillborn**

✓5th Z37.5 **Other multiple births, all liveborn**

Z37.50 **Multiple births, unspecified, all liveborn**

Z37.51 **Triplets, all liveborn**

Z37.52 **Quadruplets, all liveborn**

Z37.53 **Quintuplets, all liveborn**

Z37.54 **Sextuplets, all liveborn**

Z37.59 **Other multiple births, all liveborn**

✓5th Z37.6 **Other multiple births, some liveborn**

Z37.60 **Multiple births, unspecified, some liveborn**

Z37.61 **Triplets, some liveborn**

Z37.62 **Quadruplets, some liveborn**

Z37.63 **Quintuplets, some liveborn**

Z37.64 **Sextuplets, some liveborn**

Z37.69 **Other multiple births, some liveborn**

Z37.7 **Other multiple births, all stillborn**

Z37.9 **Outcome of delivery, unspecified**
Multiple birth NOS
Single birth NOS

✓4th **Z38 Liveborn infants according to place of birth and type of delivery**

NOTE This category is for use as the principal code on the initial record of a newborn baby. It is to be used for the initial birth record only. It is not to be used on the mother's record.

✓5th Z38.0 **Single liveborn infant, born in hospital**
Single liveborn infant, born in birthing center or other health care facility

Z38.00 **Single liveborn infant, delivered vaginally**

Z38.01 **Single liveborn infant, delivered by cesarean**

Z38.1 **Single liveborn infant, born outside hospital**

Z38.2 **Single liveborn infant, unspecified as to place of birth**
Single liveborn infant NOS

✓5th Z38.3 **Twin liveborn infant, born in hospital**

Z38.30 **Twin liveborn infant, delivered vaginally**

Z38.31 **Twin liveborn infant, delivered by cesarean**

Z38.4 **Twin liveborn infant, born outside hospital**

Z38.5 **Twin liveborn infant, unspecified as to place of birth**

✓5th Z38.6 **Other multiple liveborn infant, born in hospital**

Z38.61 **Triplet liveborn infant, delivered vaginally**

Z38.62 **Triplet liveborn infant, delivered by cesarean**

Z38.63 **Quadruplet liveborn infant, delivered vaginally**

Z38.64 **Quadruplet liveborn infant, delivered by cesarean**

Z38.65 **Quintuplet liveborn infant, delivered vaginally**

Z38.66 **Quintuplet liveborn infant, delivered by cesarean**

Z38.68 **Other multiple liveborn infant, delivered vaginally**

Z38.69 **Other multiple liveborn infant, delivered by cesarean**

Z38.7 **Other multiple liveborn infant, born outside hospital**

Z38.8 **Other multiple liveborn infant, unspecified as to place of birth**

✓4th **Z39 Encounter for maternal postpartum care and examination**

Z39.0 **Encounter for care and examination of mother immediately after delivery**
Care and observation in uncomplicated cases when the delivery occurs outside a healthcare facility

EXCLUDES 1 *care for postpartum complication—see Alphabetic index*

Z39.1 **Encounter for care and examination of lactating mother**
Encounter for supervision of lactation

EXCLUDES 1 *disorders of lactation (O92-)*

Z39.2 **Encounter for routine postpartum follow-up**

Encounters for other specific health care (Z40–Z53)

NOTE   Categories Z40-Z53 are intended for use to indicate a reason for care. They may be used for patients who have already been treated for a disease or injury, but who are receiving aftercare or prophylactic care, or care to consolidate the treatment, or to deal with a residual state

EXCLUDES 2   *follow-up examination for medical surveillance after treatment (Z08-Z09)*

✓4ᵗʰ Z40   Encounter for prophylactic surgery

     EXCLUDES 1   *organ donations (Z52-)*
                 therapeutic organ removal—code to condition

   ✓5ᵗʰ Z40.0   Encounter for prophylactic surgery for risk factors related to malignant neoplasms
         Admission for prophylactic organ removal
         Use additional code to identify risk factor

         Z40.00   Encounter for prophylactic removal of unspecified organ

         Z40.01   Encounter for prophylactic removal of breast

         Z40.02   Encounter for prophylactic removal of ovary

         Z40.09   Encounter for prophylactic removal of other organ

   Z40.8   Encounter for other prophylactic surgery

   Z40.9   Encounter for prophylactic surgery, unspecified

✓4ᵗʰ Z41   Encounter for procedures for purposes other than remedying health state

   Z41.1   Encounter for cosmetic surgery
       Encounter for cosmetic breast implant
       Encounter for cosmetic procedure

     EXCLUDES 1   *encounter for breast reduction (N62)*
              encounter for plastic and reconstructive surgery following medical procedure or healed injury (Z42-)
              encounter for post-mastectomy breast implantation (Z42.1)

   Z41.2   Encounter for routine and ritual male circumcision

   Z41.3   Encounter for ear piercing

   Z41.8   Encounter for other procedures for purposes other than remedying health state

   Z41.9   Encounter for procedure for purposes other than remedying health state, unspecified

✓4ᵗʰ Z42   Encounter for plastic and reconstructive surgery following medical procedure or healed injury

     EXCLUDES 1   *encounter for cosmetic plastic surgery (Z41.1)*
              encounter for plastic surgery for treatment of current injury—code to relevent injury

   Z42.1   Encounter for breast reconstruction following mastectomy

     EXCLUDES 1   *deformity and disproportion of reconstructed breast (N65.1-)*

   Z42.8   Encounter for other plastic and reconstructive surgery following medical procedure or healed injury

✓4ᵗʰ Z43   Encounter for attention to artificial openings

     INCLUDES   closure of artificial openings
             passage of sounds or bougies through artificial openings
             reforming artificial openings
             removal of catheter from artificial openings
             toilet or cleansing of artificial openings

     EXCLUDES 1   *artificial opening status only, without need for care (Z93-)*
              complications of external stoma (J95.0-, K94.-, N99.5-)

     EXCLUDES 2   *fitting and adjustment of prosthetic and other devices (Z44-Z46)*

   Z43.0   Encounter for attention to tracheostomy

   Z43.1   Encounter for attention to gastrostomy

   Z43.2   Encounter for attention to ileostomy

   Z43.3   Encounter for attention to colostomy

   Z43.4   Encounter for attention to other artificial openings of digestive tract

   Z43.5   Encounter for attention to cystostomy

   Z43.6   Encounter for attention to other artificial openings of urinary tract
       Encounter for attention to nephrostomy
       Encounter for attention to ureterostomy
       Encounter for attention to urethrostomy

   Z43.7   Encounter for attention to artificial vagina

   Z43.8   Encounter for attention to other artificial openings

   Z43.9   Encounter for attention to unspecified artificial opening

✓4ᵗʰ Z44   Encounter for fitting and adjustment of external prosthetic device

     INCLUDES   removal or replacement of external prosthetic device

     EXCLUDES 1   *malfunction or other complications of device—see Alphabetical Index*
              presence of prosthetic device (Z97-)

   ✓5ᵗʰ Z44.0   Encounter for fitting and adjustment of artificial arm

     ✓6ᵗʰ Z44.00   Encounter for fitting and adjustment of unspecified artificial arm

         Z44.001   Encounter for fitting and adjustment of unspecified right artificial arm

         Z44.002   Encounter for fitting and adjustment of unspecified left artificial arm

         Z44.009   Encounter for fitting and adjustment of unspecified artificial arm, unspecified arm

     ✓6ᵗʰ Z44.01   Encounter for fitting and adjustment of complete artificial arm

         Z44.011   Encounter for fitting and adjustment of complete right artificial arm

         Z44.012   Encounter for fitting and adjustment of complete left artificial arm

         Z44.019   Encounter for fitting and adjustment of complete artificial arm, unspecified arm

     ✓6ᵗʰ Z44.02   Encounter for fitting and adjustment of partial artificial arm

         Z44.021   Encounter for fitting and adjustment of partial artificial right arm

         Z44.022   Encounter for fitting and adjustment of partial artificial left arm

         Z44.029   Encounter for fitting and adjustment of partial artificial arm, unspecified arm

   ✓5ᵗʰ Z44.1   Encounter for fitting and adjustment of artificial leg

     ✓6ᵗʰ Z44.10   Encounter for fitting and adjustment of unspecified artificial leg

         Z44.101   Encounter for fitting and adjustment of unspecified right artificial leg

         Z44.102   Encounter for fitting and adjustment of unspecified left artificial leg

         Z44.109   Encounter for fitting and adjustment of unspecified artificial leg, unspecified leg

     ✓6ᵗʰ Z44.11   Encounter for fitting and adjustment of complete artificial leg

         Z44.111   Encounter for fitting and adjustment of complete right artificial leg

         Z44.112   Encounter for fitting and adjustment of complete left artificial leg

         Z44.119   Encounter for fitting and adjustment of complete artificial leg, unspecified leg

     ✓6ᵗʰ Z44.12   Encounter for fitting and adjustment of partial artificial leg

         Z44.121   Encounter for fitting and adjustment of partial artificial right leg

         Z44.122   Encounter for fitting and adjustment of partial artificial left leg

         Z44.129   Encounter for fitting and adjustment of partial artificial leg, unspecified leg

   ✓5ᵗʰ Z44.2   Encounter for fitting and adjustment of artificial eye

     EXCLUDES 1   *mechanical complication of ocular prosthesis (T85.3)*

     Z44.20   Encounter for fitting and adjustment of artificial eye, unspecified

     Z44.21   Encounter for fitting and adjustment of artificial right eye

     Z44.22   Encounter for fitting and adjustment of artificial left eye

   ✓5ᵗʰ Z44.3   Encounter for fitting and adjustment of external breast prosthesis

     EXCLUDES 1   *complications of breast implant (T85.4-)*
              encounter for adjustment or removal of breast implant (Z45.81-)
              encounter for initial breast implant insertion for cosmetic breast augmentation (Z41.1)
              encounter for breast reconstruction following mastectomy (Z42.1)

     Z44.30   Encounter for fitting and adjustment of external breast prosthesis, unspecified breast

     Z44.31   Encounter for fitting and adjustment of external right breast prosthesis

---

EXCLUDES 1 Not coded here   **EXCLUDES 2** Not included here   *Manifestation Code*

Z44.32 Encounter for fitting and adjustment of external left breast prosthesis

Z44.8 Encounter for fitting and adjustment of other external prosthetic devices

Z44.9 Encounter for fitting and adjustment of unspecified external prosthetic device

✓4ᵗʰ **Z45 Encounter for adjustment and management of implanted device**

INCLUDES removal or replacement of implanted device

EXCLUDES 1 *malfunction or other complications of device—see Alphabetical Index*

presence of prosthetic and other devices (Z95-Z97)

EXCLUDES 2 *encounter for fitting and adjustment of non-implanted device (Z46-)*

✓5ᵗʰ **Z45.0 Encounter for adjustment and management of cardiac device**

✓6ᵗʰ **Z45.01 Encounter for adjustment and management of cardiac pacemaker**

EXCLUDES 1 *encounter for adjustment and management of automatic implantable cardiac defibrillator with synchronous cardiac pacemaker (Z45.02)*

Z45.010 Encounter for checking and testing of cardiac pacemaker pulse generator [battery]

Encounter for replacing cardiac pacemaker pulse generator [battery]

Z45.018 Encounter for adjustment and management of other part of cardiac pacemaker

Z45.02 Encounter for adjustment and management of automatic implantable cardiac defibrillator

Encounter for adjustment and management of automatic implantable cardiac defibrillator with synchronous cardiac pacemaker

Z45.09 Encounter for adjustment and management of other cardiac device

Z45.1 Encounter for adjustment and management of infusion pump

Z45.2 Encounter for adjustment and management of vascular access device

Encounter for adjustment and management of vascular catheters

EXCLUDES 1 *encounter for adjustment and management of renal dialysis catheter (Z49.01)*

✓5ᵗʰ **Z45.3 Encounter for adjustment and management of implanted devices of the special senses**

Z45.31 Encounter for adjustment and management of implanted visual substitution device

✓6ᵗʰ **Z45.32 Encounter for adjustment and management of implanted hearing device**

EXCLUDES 1 *Encounter for fitting and adjustment of hearing aide (Z46.1)*

Z45.320 Encounter for adjustment and management of bone conduction device

Z45.321 Encounter for adjustment and management of cochlear device

Z45.328 Encounter for adjustment and management of other implanted hearing device

✓5ᵗʰ **Z45.4 Encounter for adjustment and management of implanted nervous system device**

Z45.41 Encounter for adjustment and management of cerebrospinal fluid drainage device

Encounter for adjustment and management of cerebral ventricular (communicating) shunt

Z45.42 Encounter for adjustment and management of neuropacemaker (brain) (peripheral nerve) (spinal cord)

Z45.49 Encounter for adjustment and management of other implanted nervous system device

✓5ᵗʰ **Z45.8 Encounter for adjustment and management of other implanted devices**

✓6ᵗʰ **Z45.81 Encounter for adjustment or removal of breast implant**

Encounter for elective implant exchange (different material) (different size)

Encounter removal of tissue expander without synchronous insertion of permanent implant

EXCLUDES 1 *complications of breast implant (T85.4-)*

encounter for initial breast implant insertion for cosmetic breast augmentation (Z41.1)

encounter for breast reconstruction following mastectomy (Z42.1)

Z45.811 Encounter for adjustment or removal of right breast implant

Z45.812 Encounter for adjustment or removal of left breast implant

Z45.819 Encounter for adjustment or removal of unspecified breast implant

Z45.82 Encounter for adjustment or removal of myringotomy device (stent) (tube)

Z45.89 Encounter for adjustment and management of other implanted devices

Z45.9 Encounter for adjustment and management of unspecified implanted device

✓4ᵗʰ **Z46 Encounter for fitting and adjustment of other devices**

INCLUDES removal or replacement of other device

EXCLUDES 1 *malfunction or other complications of device—see Alphabetical Index*

EXCLUDES 2 *encounter for fitting and management of implanted devices (Z45-)*

issue of repeat prescription only (Z76.0)

presence of prosthetic and other devices (Z95-Z97)

Z46.0 Encounter for fitting and adjustment of spectacles and contact lenses

Z46.1 Encounter for fitting and adjustment of hearing aid

EXCLUDES 1 *encounter for adjustment and management of implanted hearing device (Z45.32-)*

Z46.2 Encounter for fitting and adjustment of other devices related to nervous system and special senses

EXCLUDES 2 *encounter for adjustment and management of implanted nervous system device (Z45.4-)*

encounter for adjustment and management of implanted visual substitution device (Z45.31)

Z46.3 Encounter for fitting and adjustment of dental prosthetic device

Encounter for fitting and adjustment of dentures

Z46.4 Encounter for fitting and adjustment of orthodontic device

✓5ᵗʰ **Z46.5 Encounter for fitting and adjustment of other gastrointestinal appliance and device**

EXCLUDES 1 *encounter for attention to artificial openings of digestive tract (Z43.1-Z43.4)*

Z46.51 Encounter for fitting and adjustment of gastric lap band

Z46.59 Encounter for fitting and adjustment of other gastrointestinal appliance and device

Z46.6 Encounter for fitting and adjustment of urinary device

EXCLUDES 2 *attention to artificial openings of urinary tract (Z43.5, Z43.6)*

✓5ᵗʰ **Z46.8 Encounter for fitting and adjustment of other specified devices**

Z46.81 Encounter for fitting and adjustment of insulin pump

Encounter for insulin pump titration

Encounter for insulin pump instruction and training

Z46.82 Encounter for fitting and adjustment of non-vascular catheter

Z46.89 Encounter for fitting and adjustment of other specified devices

Encounter for fitting and adjustment of wheelchair

Z46.9 Encounter for fitting and adjustment of unspecified device

✓4ᵗʰ **Z47 Orthopedic aftercare**

EXCLUDES 1 *aftercare for healing fracture—code to fracture with 7th character D*

Z47.1 Aftercare following joint replacement surgery

Use additional code to identify the joint (Z96.6-)

☑ Appropriate additional character required   ✓x5ᵗʰ Requires 7th character, placeholder x must fill empty characters

Z47.2 Encounter for removal of internal fixation device

EXCLUDES 1   *encounter for adjustment of internal fixation device for fracture treatment—code to fracture with appropriate 7th character*
encounter for removal of external fixation device—code to fracture with 7th character D
infection or inflammatory reaction to internal fixation device (T84.6-)
mechanical complication of internal fixation device (T84.1-)

✓5th **Z47.8 Encounter for other orthopedic aftercare**

Z47.81 Encounter for orthopedic aftercare following surgical amputation
Use additional code to identify the limb amputated (Z89-)

Z47.82 Encounter for orthopedic aftercare following scoliosis surgery

Z47.89 Encounter for other orthopedic aftercare

✓4th **Z48 Encounter for other postprocedural aftercare**

EXCLUDES 1   *encounter for follow-up examination after completed treatment (Z08-Z09)*

EXCLUDES 2   *encounter for attention to artificial openings (Z43-)*
encounter for fitting and adjustment of prosthetic and other devices (Z44-Z46)

✓5th **Z48.0 Encounter for attention to dressings, sutures and drains**

EXCLUDES 1   *encounter for planned postprocedural wound closure (Z48.1)*

Z48.00 Encounter for change or removal of nonsurgical wound dressing
Encounter for change or removal of wound dressing NOS

Z48.01 Encounter for change or removal of surgical wound dressing

Z48.02 Encounter for removal of sutures
Encounter for removal of staples

Z48.03 Encounter for change or removal of drains

Z48.1 Encounter for planned postprocedural wound closure

EXCLUDES 1   *encounter for attention to dressings and sutures (Z48.0-)*

✓5th **Z48.2 Encounter for aftercare following organ transplant**

Z48.21 Encounter for aftercare following heart transplant

Z48.22 Encounter for aftercare following kidney transplant

Z48.23 Encounter for aftercare following liver transplant

Z48.24 Encounter for aftercare following lung transplant

✓6th **Z48.28 Encounter for aftercare following multiple organ transplant**

Z48.280 Encounter for aftercare following heart-lung transplant

Z48.288 Encounter for aftercare following multiple organ transplant

✓6th **Z48.29 Encounter for aftercare following other organ transplant**

Z48.290 Encounter for aftercare following bone marrow transplant

Z48.298 Encounter for aftercare following other organ transplant

Z48.3 Aftercare following surgery for neoplasm
Use additional code to identify the neoplasm

✓5th **Z48.8 Encounter for other specified postprocedural aftercare**

✓6th **Z48.81 Encounter for surgical aftercare following surgery on specified body systems**

NOTE   These codes identify the body system requiring aftercare. They are for use in conjunction with other aftercare codes to fully explain the aftercare encounter. The condition treated should also be coded if still present.

EXCLUDES 1   *aftercare for injury—code the injury with 7th character D*
aftercare following surgery for neoplasm (Z48.3)

EXCLUDES 2   *aftercare following organ transplant (Z48.2-)*
orthopedic aftercare (Z47-)

Z48.810 Encounter for surgical aftercare following surgery on the sense organs

Z48.811 Encounter for surgical aftercare following surgery on the nervous system

EXCLUDES 2   *encounter for surgical aftercare following surgery on the sense organs (Z48.810)*

Z48.812 Encounter for surgical aftercare following surgery on the circulatory system

Z48.813 Encounter for surgical aftercare following surgery on the respiratory system

Z48.814 Encounter for surgical aftercare following surgery on the teeth or oral cavity

Z48.815 Encounter for surgical aftercare following surgery on the digestive system

Z48.816 Encounter for surgical aftercare following surgery on the genitourinary system

EXCLUDES 1   *encounter for aftercare following sterilization reversal (Z31.42)*

Z48.817 Encounter for surgical aftercare following surgery on the skin and subcutaneous tissue

Z48.89 Encounter for other specified surgical aftercare

✓4th **Z49 Encounter for care involving renal dialysis**
Code also associated end stage renal disease (N18.6)

✓5th **Z49.0 Preparatory care for renal dialysis**
Encounter for dialysis instruction and training

Z49.01 Encounter for fitting and adjustment of extracorporeal dialysis catheter
Removal or replacement of renal dialysis catheter
Toilet or cleansing of renal dialysis catheter

Z49.02 Encounter for fitting and adjustment of peritoneal dialysis catheter

✓5th **Z49.3 Encounter for adequacy testing for dialysis**

Z49.31 Encounter for adequacy testing for hemodialysis

Z49.32 Encounter for adequacy testing for peritoneal dialysis
Encounter for peritoneal equilibration test

✓4th **Z51 Encounter for other aftercare**
Code also condition requiring care

EXCLUDES 1   *follow-up examination after treatment (Z08-Z09)*

Z51.0 Encounter for antineoplastic radiation therapy

✓5th **Z51.1 Encounter for antineoplastic chemotherapy and immunotherapy**

EXCLUDES 2   *encounter for chemotherapy and immunotherapy for nonneoplastic condition—code to condition*

Z51.11 Encounter for antineoplastic chemotherapy

Z51.12 Encounter for antineoplastic immunotherapy

Z51.5 Encounter for palliative care

✓5th **Z51.8 Encounter for other specified aftercare**

EXCLUDES 1   *holiday relief care (Z75.5)*

Z51.81 Encounter for therapeutic drug level monitoring
Code also any long-term (current) drug therapy (Z79-)

EXCLUDES 1   *encounter for blood-drug test for administrative or medicolegal reasons (Z02.83)*

Z51.89 Encounter for other specified aftercare

✓4th **Z52 Donors of organs and tissues**

INCLUDES   autologous and other living donors

EXCLUDES 1   *cadaveric donor—omit code*
examination of potential donor (Z00.5)

✓5th **Z52.0 Blood donor**

✓6th **Z52.00 Unspecified blood donor**

Z52.000 Unspecified donor, whole blood

Z52.001 Unspecified donor, stem cells

Z52.008 Unspecified donor, other blood

✓6th **Z52.01 Autologous blood donor**

Z52.010 Autologous donor, whole blood

Z52.011 Autologous donor, stem cells

Z52.018 Autologous donor, other blood

EXCLUDES 1   Not coded here   EXCLUDES 2   Not included here   *Manifestation Code*

✓6ᵗʰ **Z52.09   Other blood donor**
Volunteer donor

Z52.090   Other blood donor, whole blood

Z52.091   Other blood donor, stem cells

Z52.098   Other blood donor, other blood

✓5ᵗʰ **Z52.1   Skin donor**

Z52.10   Skin donor, unspecified

Z52.11   Skin donor, autologous

Z52.19   Skin donor, other

✓5ᵗʰ **Z52.2   Bone donor**

Z52.20   Bone donor, unspecified

Z52.21   Bone donor, autologous

Z52.29   Bone donor, other

Z52.3   Bone marrow donor

Z52.4   Kidney donor

Z52.5   Cornea donor

Z52.6   Liver donor

✓5ᵗʰ **Z52.8   Donor of other specified organs or tissues**

✓6ᵗʰ **Z52.81   Egg (Oocyte) donor**

Z52.810   Egg (Oocyte) donor under age 35, anonymous recipient
Egg donor under age 35 NOS

Z52.811   Egg (Oocyte) donor under age 35, designated recipient

Z52.812   Egg (Oocyte) donor age 35 and over, anonymous recipient
Egg donor age 35 and over NOS

Z52.813   Egg (Oocyte) donor age 35 and over, designated recipient

Z52.819   Egg (Oocyte) donor, unspecified

Z52.89   Donor of other specified organs or tissues

Z52.9   Donor of unspecified organ or tissue
Donor NOS

✓4ᵗʰ **Z53   Persons encountering health services for specific procedures and treatment, not carried out**

✓5ᵗʰ **Z53.0   Procedure and treatment not carried out because of contraindication**

Z53.01   Procedure and treatment not carried out due to patient smoking

Z53.09   Procedure and treatment not carried out because of other contraindication

Z53.1   Procedure and treatment not carried out because of patient's decision for reasons of belief and group pressure

✓5ᵗʰ **Z53.2   Procedure and treatment not carried out because of patient's decision for other and unspecified reasons**

Z53.20   Procedure and treatment not carried out because of patient's decision for unspecified reasons

Z53.21   Procedure and treatment not carried out due to patient leaving prior to being seen by health care provider

Z53.29   Procedure and treatment not carried out because of patient's decision for other reasons

Z53.8   Procedure and treatment not carried out for other reasons

Z53.9   Procedure and treatment not carried out, unspecified reason

Persons with potential health hazards related to socioeconomic and psychosocial circumstances (Z55-Z65)

✓4ᵗʰ **Z55   Problems related to education and literacy**
EXCLUDES 1 *disorders of psychological development (F80-F89)*

Z55.0   Illiteracy and low-level literacy

Z55.1   Schooling unavailable and unattainable

Z55.2   Failed school examinations

Z55.3   Underachievement in school

Z55.4   Educational maladjustment and discord with teachers and classmates

Z55.8   Other problems related to education and literacy
Problems related to inadequate teaching

Z55.9   Problems related to education and literacy, unspecified
Academic problems NOS

✓4ᵗʰ **Z56   Problems related to employment and unemployment**
EXCLUDES 2 *occupational exposure to risk factors (Z57-)*
problems related to housing and economic circumstances (Z59-)

Z56.0   Unemployment, unspecified

Z56.1   Change of job

Z56.2   Threat of job loss

Z56.3   Stressful work schedule

Z56.4   Discord with boss and workmates

Z56.5   Uncongenial work environment
Difficult conditions at work

Z56.6   Other physical and mental strain related to work

✓5ᵗʰ **Z56.8   Other problems related to employment**

Z56.81   Sexual harassment on the job

Z56.82   Military deployment status
Individual (civilian or military) currently deployed in theater or in support of military war, peacekeeping and humanitarian operations

Z56.89   Other problems related to employment

Z56.9   Unspecified problems related to employment
Occupational problems NOS

✓4ᵗʰ **Z57   Occupational exposure to risk factors**

Z57.0   Occupational exposure to noise

Z57.1   Occupational exposure to radiation

Z57.2   Occupational exposure to dust

✓5ᵗʰ **Z57.3   Occupational exposure to other air contaminants**

Z57.31   Occupational exposure to environmental tobacco smoke
EXCLUDES 2 *exposure to environmental tobacco smoke (Z77.22)*

Z57.39   Occupational exposure to other air contaminants

Z57.4   Occupational exposure to toxic agents in agriculture
Occupational exposure to solids, liquids, gases or vapors in agriculture

Z57.5   Occupational exposure to toxic agents in other industries
Occupational exposure to solids, liquids, gases or vapors in other industries

Z57.6   Occupational exposure to extreme temperature

Z57.7   Occupational exposure to vibration

Z57.8   Occupational exposure to other risk factors

Z57.9   Occupational exposure to unspecified risk factor

✓4ᵗʰ **Z59   Problems related to housing and economic circumstances**
EXCLUDES 2 *problems related to upbringing (Z62-)*

Z59.0   Homelessness

Z59.1   Inadequate housing
Lack of heating
Restriction of space
Technical defects in home preventing adequate care
Unsatisfactory surroundings
EXCLUDES 1 *problems related to the natural and physical environment (Z77.1-)*

Z59.2   Discord with neighbors, lodgers and landlord

Z59.3   Problems related to living in residential institution
Boarding-school resident
EXCLUDES 1 *institutional upbringing (Z62.2)*

Z59.4   Lack of adequate food and safe drinking water
Inadequate drinking water supply
EXCLUDES 1 *effects of hunger (T73.0)*
inappropriate diet or eating habits (Z72.4)
malnutrition (E40-E46)

Z59.5   Extreme poverty

Z59.6   Low income

Z59.7   Insufficient social insurance and welfare support

Z59.8   Other problems related to housing and economic circumstances
Foreclosure on loan
Isolated dwelling
Problems with creditors

Z59.9   Problem related to housing and economic circumstances, unspecified

✓4ᵗʰ **Z60   Problems related to social environment**

Z60.0   Problems of adjustment to life-cycle transitions
Empty nest syndrome
Phase of life problem
Problem with adjustment to retirement [pension]

Z60.2   Problems related to living alone

Z60.3   Acculturation difficulty
Problem with migration
Problem with social transplantation

✓ Appropriate additional character required   ✓x7ᵗʰ Requires 7th character, placeholder x must fill empty characters

Z60.4 Social exclusion and rejection
Exclusion and rejection on the basis of personal characteristics, such as unusual physical appearance, illness or behavior.
EXCLUDES 1 *target of adverse discrimination such as for racial or religious reasons (Z60.5)*

Z60.5 Target of (perceived) adverse discrimination and persecution
EXCLUDES 1 *social exclusion and rejection (Z60.4)*

Z60.8 Other problems related to social environment

Z60.9 Problem related to social environment, unspecified

√4th **Z62 Problems related to upbringing**
Current and past negative life events in childhood
Current and past problems of a child related to upbringing
EXCLUDES 2 *maltreatment syndrome (T74-)*
problems related to housing and economic circumstances (Z59-)

Z62.0 Inadequate parental supervision and control

Z62.1 Parental overprotection

√5th **Z62.2 Upbringing away from parents**
EXCLUDES 1 *problems with boarding school (Z59.3)*
Z62.21 Child in welfare custody
Child in care of non-parental family member
Child in foster care
EXCLUDES 2 *problem for parent due to child in welfare custody (Z63.5)*
Z62.22 Institutional upbringing
Child living in orphanage or group home
Z62.29 Other upbringing away from parents

Z62.3 Hostility towards and scapegoating of child

Z62.6 Inappropriate (excessive) parental pressure

√5th **Z62.8 Other specified problems related to upbringing**
√6th **Z62.81 Personal history of abuse in childhood**
Z62.810 Personal history of physical and sexual abuse in childhood
EXCLUDES 1 *current child physical abuse (T74.12, T76.12)*
current child sexual abuse (T74.22, T76.22)
Z62.811 Personal history of psychological abuse in childhood
EXCLUDES 1 *current child psychological abuse (T74.32, T76.32)*
Z62.812 Personal history of neglect in childhood
EXCLUDES 1 *current child neglect (T74.02, T76.02)*
Z62.819 Personal history of unspecified abuse in childhood
EXCLUDES 1 *current child abuse NOS (T74.92, T76.92)*
√6th **Z62.82 Parent-child conflict**
Z62.820 Parent-biological child conflict
Parent-child problem NOS
Z62.821 Parent-adopted child conflict
Z62.822 Parent-foster child conflict
√6th **Z62.89 Other specified problems related to upbringing**
Z62.890 Parent-child estrangement NEC
Z62.891 Sibling rivalry
Z62.898 Other specified problems related to upbringing

Z62.9 Problem related to upbringing, unspecified

√4th **Z63 Other problems related to primary support group, including family circumstances**
EXCLUDES 2 *maltreatment syndrome (T74-, T76)*
parent-child problems (Z62-)
problems related to negative life events in childhood (Z62-)
problems related to upbringing (Z62-)

Z63.0 Problems in relationship with spouse or partner
EXCLUDES 1 *counseling for spousal or partner abuse problems (Z69.1)*
counseling related to sexual attitude, behavior, and orientation (Z70-)

Z63.1 Problems in relationship with in-laws

√5th **Z63.3 Absence of family member**
EXCLUDES 1 *absence of family member due to disappearance and death (Z63.4)*
absence of family member due to separation and divorce (Z63.5)
Z63.31 Absence of family member due to military deployment
Individual or family affected by other family member being on military deployment
EXCLUDES 1 *family disruption due to return of family member from military deployment (Z63.71)*
Z63.32 Other absence of family member

Z63.4 Disappearance and death of family member
Assumed death of family member
Bereavement

Z63.5 Disruption of family by separation and divorce
Marital estrangement

Z63.6 Dependent relative needing care at home

√5th **Z63.7 Other stressful life events affecting family and household**
Z63.71 Stress on family due to return of family member from military deployment
Individual or family affected by family member having returned from military deployment (current or past conflict)
Z63.72 Alcoholism and drug addiction in family
Z63.79 Other stressful life events affecting family and household
Anxiety (normal) about sick person in family
Health problems within family
Ill or disturbed family member
Isolated family

Z63.8 Other specified problems related to primary support group
Family discord NOS
Family estrangement NOS
High expressed emotional level within family
Inadequate family support NOS
Inadequate or distorted communication within family

Z63.9 Problem related to primary support group, unspecified
Relationship disorder NOS

√4th **Z64 Problems related to certain psychosocial circumstances**
Z64.0 Problems related to unwanted pregnancy
Z64.1 Problems related to multiparity
Z64.4 Discord with counselors
Discord with probation officer
Discord with social worker

√4th **Z65 Problems related to other psychosocial circumstances**
Z65.0 Conviction in civil and criminal proceedings without imprisonment
Z65.1 Imprisonment and other incarceration
Z65.2 Problems related to release from prison
Z65.3 Problems related to other legal circumstances
Arrest
Child custody or support proceedings
Litigation
Prosecution
Z65.4 Victim of crime and terrorism
Victim of torture
Z65.5 Exposure to disaster, war and other hostilities
EXCLUDES 1 *target of perceived discrimination or persecution (Z60.5)*
Z65.8 Other specified problems related to psychosocial circumstances
Z65.9 Problem related to unspecified psychosocial circumstances

Do not resuscitate status (Z66)

Z66 Do not resuscitate
DNR status

Blood type (Z67)

√4th **Z67 Blood type**
√5th **Z67.1 Type A blood**
Z67.10 Type A blood, Rh positive
Z67.11 Type A blood, Rh negative
√5th **Z67.2 Type B blood**
Z67.20 Type B blood, Rh positive

EXCLUDES 1 Not coded here   EXCLUDES 2 Not included here   *Manifestation Code*

Z67.21　Type B blood, Rh negative

✓5ᵗʰ Z67.3　Type AB blood
　　　Z67.3Ø　Type AB blood, Rh positive
　　　Z67.31　Type AB blood, Rh negative

✓5ᵗʰ Z67.4　Type O blood
　　　Z67.4Ø　Type O blood, Rh positive
　　　Z67.41　Type O blood, Rh negative

✓5ᵗʰ Z67.9　Unspecified blood type
　　　Z67.9Ø　Unspecified blood type, Rh positive
　　　Z67.91　Unspecified blood type, Rh negative

Body mass index (BMI) (Z68)

✓4ᵗʰ **Z68　Body mass index (BMI)**
　　Kilograms per meters squared
　　NOTE　BMI adult codes are for use for persons 21 years of age or older
　　　　　BMI pediatric codes are for use for persons 2-2Ø years of age. These percentiles are based on the growth charts published by the Centers for Disease Control and Prevention (CDC)

Z68.1　Body mass index (BMI) 19 or less, adult

✓5ᵗʰ Z68.2　Body mass index (BMI) 2Ø-29, adult
　　　Z68.2Ø　Body mass index (BMI) 2Ø.Ø-2Ø.9, adult
　　　Z68.21　Body mass index (BMI) 21.Ø-21.9, adult
　　　Z68.22　Body mass index (BMI) 22.Ø-22.9, adult
　　　Z68.23　Body mass index (BMI) 23.Ø-23.9, adult
　　　Z68.24　Body mass index (BMI) 24.Ø-24.9, adult
　　　Z68.25　Body mass index (BMI) 25.Ø-25.9, adult
　　　Z68.26　Body mass index (BMI) 26.Ø-26.9, adult
　　　Z68.27　Body mass index (BMI) 27.Ø-27.9, adult
　　　Z68.28　Body mass index (BMI) 28.Ø-28.9, adult
　　　Z68.29　Body mass index (BMI) 29.Ø-29.9, adult

✓5ᵗʰ Z68.3　Body mass index (BMI) 3Ø-39, adult
　　　Z68.3Ø　Body mass index (BMI) 3Ø.Ø-3Ø.9, adult
　　　Z68.31　Body mass index (BMI) 31.Ø-31.9, adult
　　　Z68.32　Body mass index (BMI) 32.Ø-32.9, adult
　　　Z68.33　Body mass index (BMI) 33.Ø-33.9, adult
　　　Z68.34　Body mass index (BMI) 34.Ø-34.9, adult
　　　Z68.35　Body mass index (BMI) 35.Ø-35.9, adult
　　　Z68.36　Body mass index (BMI) 36.Ø-36.9, adult
　　　Z68.37　Body mass index (BMI) 37.Ø-37.9, adult
　　　Z68.38　Body mass index (BMI) 38.Ø-38.9, adult
　　　Z68.39　Body mass index (BMI) 39.Ø-39.9, adult

✓5ᵗʰ Z68.4　Body mass index (BMI) 4Ø or greater, adult
　　　Z68.41　Body mass index (BMI) 4Ø.Ø-44.9, adult
　　　Z68.42　Body mass index (BMI) 45.Ø-49.9, adult
　　　Z68.43　Body mass index (BMI) 5Ø-59.9 , adult
　　　Z68.44　Body mass index (BMI) 6Ø.Ø-69.9, adult
　　　Z68.45　Body mass index (BMI) 7Ø or greater, adult

✓5ᵗʰ Z68.5　Body mass index (BMI) pediatric
　　　Z68.51　Body mass index (BMI) pediatric, less than 5th percentile for age
　　　Z68.52　Body mass index (BMI) pediatric, 5th percentile to less than 85th percentile for age
　　　Z68.53　Body mass index (BMI) pediatric, 85th percentile to less than 95th percentile for age
　　　Z68.54　Body mass index (BMI) pediatric, greater than or equal to 95th percentile for age

Persons encountering health services in other circumstances (Z69-Z76)

✓4ᵗʰ **Z69　Encounter for mental health services for victim and perpetrator of abuse**
　　Counseling for victims and perpetrators of abuse

✓5ᵗʰ Z69.Ø　Encounter for mental health services for child abuse problems

✓6ᵗʰ Z69.Ø1　Encounter for mental health services for parental child abuse
　　　Z69.Ø1Ø　Encounter for mental health services for victim of parental child abuse
　　　Z69.Ø11　Encounter for mental health services for perpetrator of parental child abuse
　　　　　EXCLUDES 1　*encounter for mental health services for non-parental child abuse (Z69.Ø2-)*

✓6ᵗʰ Z69.Ø2　Encounter for mental health services for non-parental child abuse
　　　Z69.Ø2Ø　Encounter for mental health services for victim of non-parental child abuse
　　　Z69.Ø21　Encounter for mental health services for perpetrator of non-parental child abuse

✓5ᵗʰ Z69.1　Encounter for mental health services for spousal or partner abuse problems
　　　Z69.11　Encounter for mental health services for victim of spousal or partner abuse
　　　Z69.12　Encounter for mental health services for perpetrator of spousal or partner abuse

✓5ᵗʰ Z69.8　Encounter for mental health services for victim or perpetrator of other abuse
　　　Z69.81　Encounter for mental health services for victim of other abuse
　　　　　Encounter for rape victim counseling
　　　Z69.82　Encounter for mental health services for perpetrator of other abuse

✓4ᵗʰ **Z70　Counseling related to sexual attitude, behavior and orientation**
　　Encounter for mental health services for sexual attitude, behavior and orientation
　　EXCLUDES 2　*contraceptive or procreative counseling (Z3Ø-Z31)*

Z70.Ø　Counseling related to sexual attitude

Z70.1　Counseling related to patient's sexual behavior and orientation
　　Patient concerned regarding impotence
　　Patient concerned regarding non-responsiveness
　　Patient concerned regarding promiscuity
　　Patient concerned regarding sexual orientation

Z70.2　Counseling related to sexual behavior and orientation of third party
　　Advice sought regarding sexual behavior and orientation of child
　　Advice sought regarding sexual behavior and orientation of partner
　　Advice sought regarding sexual behavior and orientation of spouse

Z70.3　Counseling related to combined concerns regarding sexual attitude, behavior and orientation

Z70.8　Other sex counseling
　　Encounter for sex education

Z70.9　Sex counseling, unspecified

✓4ᵗʰ **Z71　Persons encountering health services for other counseling and medical advice, not elsewhere classified**
　　EXCLUDES 2　*contraceptive or procreation counseling (Z3Ø-Z31)*
　　　　　　　sex counseling (Z7Ø-)

Z71.Ø　Person encountering health services to consult on behalf of another person
　　Person encountering health services to seek advice or treatment for non-attending third party
　　EXCLUDES 2　*anxiety (normal) about sick person in family (Z63.7)*
　　　　　　　expectant (adoptive) parent(s) pre-birth pediatrician visit (Z76.81)

Z71.1　Person with feared health complaint in whom no diagnosis is made
　　Person encountering health services with feared condition which was not demonstrated
　　Person encountering health services in which problem was normal state
　　"Worried well"
　　EXCLUDES 1　*medical observation for suspected diseases and conditions proven not to exist (ZØ3-)*

Z71.2　Person consulting for explanation of examination or test findings

Z71.3　Dietary counseling and surveillance
　　Use additional code for any associated underlying medical condition
　　Use additional code to identify body mass index (BMI), if known (Z68-)

✓5ᵗʰ Z71.4　Alcohol abuse counseling and surveillance
　　Use additional code for alcohol abuse or dependence (F1Ø-)
　　　Z71.41　Alcohol abuse counseling and surveillance of alcoholic
　　　Z71.42　Counseling for family member of alcoholic
　　　　　Counseling for significant other, partner, or friend of alcoholic

---

✓ Appropriate additional character required　　　　✓x7ᵗʰ Requires 7th character, placeholder x must fill empty characters

✓5th **Z71.5 Drug abuse counseling and surveillance**
> Use additional code for drug abuse or dependence (F11-F16, F18-F19)

Z71.51 Drug abuse counseling and surveillance of drug abuser

Z71.52 Counseling for family member of drug abuser
> Counseling for significant other, partner, or friend of drug abuser

Z71.6 Tobacco abuse counseling
> Use additional code for nicotine dependence (F17-)

Z71.7 Human immunodeficiency virus [HIV] counseling

✓5th **Z71.8 Other specified counseling**
> EXCLUDES 2   counseling for contraception (Z30.0-)
> counseling for genetics (Z31.5)
> counseling for procreative management (Z31.6-)

Z71.81 Spiritual or religious counseling

Z71.89 Other specified counseling

Z71.9 Counseling, unspecified
> Encounter for medical advice NOS

✓4th **Z72 Problems related to lifestyle**
> EXCLUDES 2   problems related to life-management difficulty (Z73-)
> problems related to socioeconomic and psychosocial circumstances (Z55-Z65)

Z72.0 Tobacco use
> Tobacco use NOS
> EXCLUDES 1   history of tobacco dependence (Z87.891)
> nicotine dependence (F17.2-)
> tobacco dependence (F17.2-)
> tobacco use during pregnancy (O99.33-)

Z72.3 Lack of physical exercise

Z72.4 Inappropriate diet and eating habits
> EXCLUDES 1   behavioral eating disorders of infancy or childhood (F98.2- F98.3)
> eating disorders (F50-)
> lack of adequate food (Z59.4)
> malnutrition and other nutritional deficiencies (E40-E64)

✓5th **Z72.5 High risk sexual behavior**
> Promiscuity
> EXCLUDES 1   paraphilias (F65)

Z72.51 High risk heterosexual behavior

Z72.52 High risk homosexual behavior

Z72.53 High risk bisexual behavior

Z72.6 Gambling and betting
> EXCLUDES 1   compulsive or pathological gambling (F63.0)

Z72.8 Other problems related to lifestyle

✓6th **Z72.81 Antisocial behavior**
> EXCLUDES 1   conduct disorders (F91-)

Z72.810 Child and adolescent antisocial behavior
> Antisocial behavior (child) (adolescent) without manifest psychiatric disorder
> Delinquency NOS
> Group delinquency
> Offenses in the context of gang membership
> Stealing in company with others
> Truancy from school

Z72.811 Adult antisocial behavior
> Adult antisocial behavior without manifest psychiatric disorder

✓6th **Z72.82 Problems related to sleep**

Z72.820 Sleep deprivation
> Lack of adequate sleep
> EXCLUDES 1   insomnia (G47.0-)

Z72.821 Inadequate sleep hygiene
> Bad sleep habits
> Irregular sleep habits
> Unhealthy sleep wake schedule
> EXCLUDES 1   insomnia (F51.0-, G47.0-)

Z72.89 Other problems related to lifestyle
> Self-damaging behavior

Z72.9 Problem related to lifestyle, unspecified

✓4th **Z73 Problems related to life management difficulty**
> EXCLUDES 2   problems related to socioeconomic and psychosocial circumstances (Z55-Z65)

Z73.0 Burn-out

Z73.1 Type A behavior pattern

Z73.2 Lack of relaxation and leisure

Z73.3 Stress, not elsewhere classified
> Physical and mental strain NOS
> EXCLUDES 1   stress related to employment or unemployment (Z56-)

Z73.4 Inadequate social skills, not elsewhere classified

Z73.5 Social role conflict, not elsewhere classified

Z73.6 Limitation of activities due to disability
> EXCLUDES 1   care-provider dependency (Z74-)

✓5th **Z73.8 Other problems related to life management difficulty**

✓6th **Z73.81 Behavioral insomnia of childhood**

Z73.810 Behavioral insomnia of childhood, sleep-onset association type

Z73.811 Behavioral insomnia of childhood, limit setting type

Z73.812 Behavioral insomnia of childhood, combined type

Z73.819 Behavioral insomnia of childhood, unspecified type

Z73.82 Dual sensory impairment

Z73.89 Other problems related to life management difficulty

Z73.9 Problem related to life management difficulty, unspecified

✓4th **Z74 Problems related to care provider dependency**
> EXCLUDES 2   dependence on enabling machines or devices NEC (Z99-)

✓5th **Z74.0 Reduced mobility**

Z74.01 Bed confinement status
> Bedridden

Z74.09 Other reduced mobility
> Chair ridden
> Reduced mobility NOS
> EXCLUDES 2   wheelchair dependence (Z99.3)

Z74.1 Need for assistance with personal care

Z74.2 Need for assistance at home and no other household member able to render care

Z74.3 Need for continuous supervision

Z74.8 Other problems related to care provider dependency

Z74.9 Problem related to care provider dependency, unspecified

✓4th **Z75 Problems related to medical facilities and other health care**

Z75.0 Medical services not available in home
> EXCLUDES 1   no other household member able to render care (Z74.2)

Z75.1 Person awaiting admission to adequate facility elsewhere

Z75.2 Other waiting period for investigation and treatment

Z75.3 Unavailability and inaccessibility of health-care facilities
> EXCLUDES 1   bed unavailable (Z75.1)

Z75.4 Unavailability and inaccessibility of other helping agencies

Z75.5 Holiday relief care

Z75.8 Other problems related to medical facilities and other health care

Z75.9 Unspecified problem related to medical facilities and other health care

✓4th **Z76 Persons encountering health services in other circumstances**

Z76.0 Encounter for issue of repeat prescription
> Encounter for issue of repeat prescription for appliance
> Encounter for issue of repeat prescription for medicaments
> Encounter for issue of repeat prescription for spectacles
> EXCLUDES 2   issue of medical certificate (Z02.7)
> repeat prescription for contraceptive (Z30.4-)

Z76.1 Encounter for health supervision and care of foundling

Z76.2 Encounter for health supervision and care of other healthy infant and child
> Encounter for medical or nursing care or supervision of healthy infant under circumstances such as adverse socioeconomic conditions at home
> Encounter for medical or nursing care or supervision of healthy infant under circumstances such as awaiting foster or adoptive placement
> Encounter for medical or nursing care or supervision of healthy infant under circumstances such as maternal illness
> Encounter for medical or nursing care or supervision of healthy infant under circumstances such as number of children at home preventing or interfering with normal care

Z76.3 Healthy person accompanying sick person

EXCLUDES 1   Not coded here   EXCLUDES 2   Not included here   *Manifestation Code*

Z76.4   **Other boarder to healthcare facility**
> EXCLUDES 1   *homelessness (Z59.0)*

Z76.5   **Malingerer [conscious simulation]**
Person feigning illness (with obvious motivation)
> EXCLUDES 1   *factitious disorder (F68.1-)*
> *peregrinating patient (F68.1-)*

✓5ᵗʰ   Z76.8   **Persons encountering health services in other specified circumstances**

Z76.81   **Expectant parent(s) prebirth pediatrician visit**
Pre-adoption pediatrician visit for adoptive parent(s)

Z76.82   **Awaiting organ transplant status**
Patient waiting for organ availability

Z76.89   **Persons encountering health services in other specified circumstances**
Persons encountering health services NOS

Persons with potential health hazards related to family and personal history and certain conditions influencing health status (Z77-Z99)

Code also any follow-up examination (Z08-Z09)

✓4ᵗʰ   **Z77   Other contact with and (suspected) exposures hazardous to health**
> INCLUDES   contact with and (suspected) exposures to potential hazards to health
> EXCLUDES 2   *contact with and (suspected) exposure to communicable diseases (Z20.-)*
> *exposure to (parental) (environmental) tobacco smoke in the perinatal period (P96.81)*
> *newborn (suspected to be) affected by noxious substances transmitted via placenta or breast milk (P04.-)*
> *occupational exposure to risk factors (Z57.-)*
> *retained foreign body (Z18.-)*
> *retained foreign body fully removed (Z87.821)*
> *toxic effects of substances chiefly nonmedicinal as to source (T51-T65)*

✓5ᵗʰ   Z77.0   **Contact with and (suspected) exposure to hazardous, chiefly nonmedicinal, chemicals**

✓6ᵗʰ   Z77.01   **Contact with and (suspected) exposure to hazardous metals**

Z77.010   **Contact with and (suspected) exposure to arsenic**

Z77.011   **Contact with and (suspected) exposure to lead**

Z77.018   **Contact with and (suspected) exposure to other hazardous metals**
Contact with and (suspected) exposure to chromium compounds
Contact with and (suspected) exposure to nickel dust

✓6ᵗʰ   Z77.02   **Contact with and (suspected) exposure to hazardous aromatic compounds**

Z77.020   **Contact with and (suspected) exposure to aromatic amines**

Z77.021   **Contact with and (suspected) exposure to benzene**

Z77.028   **Contact with and (suspected) exposure to other hazardous aromatic compounds**
Aromatic dyes NOS
Polycyclic aromatic hydrocarbons

✓6ᵗʰ   Z77.09   **Contact with and (suspected) exposure to other hazardous, chiefly nonmedicinal, chemicals**

Z77.090   **Contact with and (suspected) exposure to asbestos**

Z77.098   **Contact with and (suspected) exposure to other hazardous, chiefly nonmedicinal, chemicals**
Dyes NOS

✓5ᵗʰ   Z77.1   **Contact with and (suspected) exposure to environmental pollution and hazards in the physical environment**

✓6ᵗʰ   Z77.11   **Contact with and (suspected) exposure to environmental pollution**

Z77.110   **Contact with and (suspected) exposure to air pollution**

Z77.111   **Contact with and (suspected) exposure to water pollution**

Z77.112   **Contact with and (suspected) exposure to soil pollution**

Z77.118   **Contact with and (suspected) exposure to other environmental pollution**

✓6ᵗʰ   Z77.12   **Contact with and (suspected) exposure to hazards in the physical environment**

Z77.120   **Contact with and (suspected) exposure to mold (toxic)**

Z77.121   **Contact with and (suspected) exposure to harmful algae and algae toxins**
Contact with and (suspected) exposure to (harmful) algae bloom NOS
Contact with and (suspected) exposure to blue-green algae bloom
Contact with and (suspected) exposure to brown tide
Contact with and (suspected) exposure to cyanobacteria bloom
Contact with and (suspected) exposure to Florida red tide
Contact with and (suspected) exposure to pfiesteria piscicida
Contact with and (suspected) exposure to red tide

Z77.122   **Contact with and (suspected) exposure to noise**

Z77.123   **Contact with and (suspected) exposure to radon and other naturally occuring radiation**
> EXCLUDES 2   *radiation exposure as the cause of a confirmed condition (W88-W90, X39.0-)*
> *radiation sickness NOS (T66)*

Z77.128   **Contact with and (suspected) exposure to other hazards in the physical environment**

✓5ᵗʰ   Z77.2   **Contact with and (suspected) exposure to other hazardous substances**

Z77.21   **Contact with and (suspected) exposure to potentially hazardous body fluids**

Z77.22   **Contact with and (suspected) exposure to environmental tobacco smoke (acute) (chronic)**
Exposure to second hand tobacco smoke (acute) (chronic)
Passive smoking (acute) (chronic)
> EXCLUDES 1   *nicotine dependence (F17-)*
> *tobacco use (Z72.0)*
> EXCLUDES 2   *occupational exposure to environmental tobacco smoke (Z57.31)*

Z77.29   **Contact with and (suspected) exposure to other hazardous substances**

Z77.9   **Other contact with and (suspected) exposures hazardous to health**

✓4ᵗʰ   **Z78   Other specified health status**
> EXCLUDES 2   *asymptomatic human immunodeficiency virus [HIV] infection status (Z21)*
> *postprocedural status (Z93- Z99)*
> *sex reassignment status (Z87.890)*

Z78.0   **Asymptomatic menopausal state**
Menopausal state NOS
Postmenopausal status NOS
> EXCLUDES 2   *symptomatic menopausal state (N95.1)*

Z78.1   **Physical restraint status**
> EXCLUDES 1   *physical restraint due to a procedure - omit code*

Z78.9   **Other specified health status**

✓4ᵗʰ   **Z79   Long term (current) drug therapy**
> INCLUDES   long term (current) drug use for prophylactic purposes
Code also any therapeutic drug level monitoring (Z51.81)
> EXCLUDES 2   *drug abuse and dependence (F11-F19)*
> *drug use complicating pregnancy, childbirth, and the puerperium (O99.32-)*

✓5ᵗʰ   Z79.0   **Long term (current) use of anticoagulants and antithrombotics/antiplatelets**
> EXCLUDES 2   *long term (current) use of aspirin (Z79.82)*

Z79.01   **Long term (current) use of anticoagulants**

Z79.02   **Long term (current) use of antithrombotics/antiplatelets**

☑ Appropriate additional character required   ✓x7ᵗʰ Requires 7th character, placeholder x must fill empty characters

Z79.1   **Long term (current) use of non-steroidal anti-inflammatories (NSAID)**
> EXCLUDES 2   *long term (current) use of aspirin (Z79.82)*

Z79.2   **Long term (current) use of antibiotics**

Z79.3   **Long term (current) use of hormonal contraceptives**
> Long term (current) use of birth control pill or patch

Z79.4   **Long term (current) use of insulin**

√5th **Z79.5**   **Long term (current) use of steroids**

     Z79.51   Long term (current) use of inhaled steroids

     Z79.52   Long term (current) use of systemic steroids

√5th **Z79.8**   **Other long term (current) drug therapy**

√6th   **Z79.81**   **Long term (current) use of agents affecting estrogen receptors and estrogen levels**
> Code first, if applicable:
> malignant neoplasm of breast (C50-)
> malignant neoplasm of prostate (C61)
> Use additional code, if applicable, to identify:
> estrogen receptor positive status (Z17.0)
> family history of breast cancer (Z80.3)
> genetic susceptibility to malignant neoplasm (cancer) (Z15.0-)
> personal history of breast cancer (Z85.3)
> personal history of prostate cancer (Z85.46)
> postmenopausal status (Z78.0)
> EXCLUDES 1   *hormone replacement therapy (postmenopausal) (Z79.890)*

       Z79.810   **Long term (current) use of selective estrogen receptor modulators (SERMs)**
> Long term (current) use of raloxifene (Evista)
> Long term (current) use of tamoxifen (Nolvadex)
> Long term (current) use of toremifene (Fareston)

       Z79.811   **Long term (current) use of aromatase inhibitors**
> Long term (current) use of anastrozole (Arimidex)
> Long term (current) use of exemestane (Aromasin)
> Long term (current) use of letrozole (Femara)

       Z79.818   **Long term (current) use of other agents affecting estrogen receptors and estrogen levels**
> Long term (current) use of estrogen receptor downregulators
> Long term (current) use of fulvestrant (Faslodex)
> Long term (current) use of gonadotropin-releasing hormone (GnRH) agonist
> Long term (current) use of goserelin acetate (Zoladex)
> Long term (current) use of leuprolide acetate (leuprorelin) (Lupron)
> Long term (current) use of megestrol acetate (Megace)

   Z79.82   **Long term (current) use of aspirin**

√6th   **Z79.89**   **Other long term (current) drug therapy**

       Z79.890   **Hormone replacement therapy (postmenopausal)**

       Z79.891   **Long term (current) use of opiate analgesic**
> Long term (current) use of methadone for pain management
> EXCLUDES 1   *methadone use NOS (F11.2-)*
> *use of methadone for treatment of heroin addiction (F11.2-)*

       Z79.899   **Other long term (current) drug therapy**

√4th **Z80**   **Family history of primary malignant neoplasm**

   Z80.0   **Family history of malignant neoplasm of digestive organs**
> Conditions classifiable to C15-C26

   Z80.1   **Family history of malignant neoplasm of trachea, bronchus and lung**
> Conditions classifiable to C33-C34

   Z80.2   **Family history of malignant neoplasm of other respiratory and intrathoracic organs**
> Conditions classifiable to C30-C32, C37-C39

Z80.3   **Family history of malignant neoplasm of breast**
> Conditions classifiable to C50-

√5th **Z80.4**   **Family history of malignant neoplasm of genital organs**
> Conditions classifiable to C51-C63

     Z80.41   Family history of malignant neoplasm of ovary

     Z80.42   Family history of malignant neoplasm of prostate

     Z80.43   Family history of malignant neoplasm of testis

     Z80.49   Family history of malignant neoplasm of other genital organs

√5th **Z80.5**   **Family history of malignant neoplasm of urinary tract**
> Conditions classifiable to C64-C68

     Z80.51   Family history of malignant neoplasm of kidney

     Z80.52   Family history of malignant neoplasm of bladder

     Z80.59   Family history of malignant neoplasm of other urinary tract organ

Z80.6   **Family history of leukemia**
> Conditions classifiable to C91-C95

Z80.7   **Family history of other malignant neoplasms of lymphoid, hematopoietic and related tissues**
> Conditions classifiable to C81-C90, C96-

Z80.8   **Family history of malignant neoplasm of other organs or systems**
> Conditions classifiable to C00-C14, C40-C49, C69-C79

Z80.9   **Family history of malignant neoplasm, unspecified**
> Conditions classifiable to C80.1

√4th **Z81**   **Family history of mental and behavioral disorders**

   Z81.0   **Family history of mental retardation**
> Conditions classifiable to F70-F79

   Z81.1   **Family history of alcohol abuse and dependence**
> Conditions classifiable to F10-

   Z81.2   **Family history of tobacco abuse and dependence**
> Conditions classifiable to F17-

   Z81.3   **Family history of other psychoactive substance abuse and dependence**
> Conditions classifiable to F11-F16, F18-F19

   Z81.4   **Family history of other substance abuse and dependence**
> Conditions classifiable to F55

   Z81.8   **Family history of other mental and behavioral disorders**
> Conditions classifiable elsewhere in F01-F99

√4th **Z82**   **Family history of certain disabilities and chronic diseases (leading to disablement)**

   Z82.0   **Family history of epilepsy and other diseases of the nervous system**
> Conditions classifiable to G00-G99

   Z82.1   **Family history of blindness and visual loss**
> Conditions classifiable to H54-

   Z82.2   **Family history of deafness and hearing loss**
> Conditions classifiable to H90-H91

   Z82.3   **Family history of stroke**
> Conditions classifiable to I60-I64

√5th **Z82.4**   **Family history of ischemic heart disease and other diseases of the circulatory system**
> Conditions classifiable to I00-I52, I65-I99

     Z82.41   Family history of sudden cardiac death

     Z82.49   Family history of ischemic heart disease and other diseases of the circulatory system

   Z82.5   **Family history of asthma and other chronic lower respiratory diseases**
> Conditions classifiable to J40-J47
> EXCLUDES 2   *family history of other diseases of the respiratory system (Z83.6)*

√5th **Z82.6**   **Family history of arthritis and other diseases of the musculoskeletal system and connective tissue**
> Conditions classifiable to M00-M99

     Z82.61   Family history of arthritis

     Z82.62   Family history of osteoporosis

     Z82.69   Family history of other diseases of the musculoskeletal system and connective tissue

√5th **Z82.7**   **Family history of congenital malformations, deformations and chromosomal abnormalities**
> Conditions classifiable to Q00-Q99

     Z82.71   Family history of polycystic kidney

     Z82.79   Family history of other congenital malformations, deformations and chromosomal abnormalities

   Z82.8   **Family history of other disabilities and chronic diseases leading to disablement, not elsewhere classified**

EXCLUDES 1   Not coded here   EXCLUDES 2   Not included here   *Manifestation Code*

☑4th Z83　Family history of other specific disorders

EXCLUDES 2　contact with and (suspected) exposure to communicable disease in the family (Z20-)

Z83.0　Family history of human immunodeficiency virus [HIV] disease
Conditions classifiable to B20

Z83.1　Family history of other infectious and parasitic diseases
Conditions classifiable to A00-B19, B25-B94, B99

Z83.2　Family history of diseases of the blood and blood-forming organs and certain disorders involving the immune mechanism
Conditions classifiable to D50-D89

Z83.3　Family history of diabetes mellitus
Conditions classifiable to E08-E13

☑5th **Z83.4　Family history of other endocrine, nutritional and metabolic diseases**
Conditions classifiable to E00-E07, E15-E88

　Z83.41　Family history of multiple endocrine neoplasia [MEN] syndrome

　Z83.49　Family history of other endocrine, nutritional and metabolic diseases

Z83.5　Family history of eye and ear disorders
Conditions classifiable to H00-H53, H55-H83, H92-H95
EXCLUDES 2　family history of blindness and visual loss (Z82.1)
family history of deafness and hearing loss (Z82.2)

Z83.6　Family history of other diseases of the respiratory system
Conditions classifiable to J00-J39, J60-J99
EXCLUDES 2　family history of asthma and other chronic lower respiratory diseases (Z82.5)

☑5th **Z83.7　Family history of diseases of the digestive system**
Conditions classifiable to K00-K93

　Z83.71　Family history of colonic polyps
EXCLUDES 1　family history of malignant neoplasm of digestive organs (Z80.0)

　Z83.79　Family history of other diseases of the digestive system

☑4th Z84　Family history of other conditions

Z84.0　Family history of diseases of the skin and subcutaneous tissue
Conditions classifiable to L00-L99

Z84.1　Family history of disorders of kidney and ureter
Conditions classifiable to N00-N29

Z84.2　Family history of other diseases of the genitourinary system
Conditions classifiable to N30-N99

Z84.3　Family history of consanguinity

☑5th **Z84.8　Family history of other specified conditions**

　Z84.81　Family history of carrier of genetic disease

　Z84.89　Family history of other specified conditions

☑4th Z85　Personal history of malignant neoplasm

Code first any follow-up examination after treatment of malignant neoplasm (Z08)
Use additional code to identify:
alcohol use and dependence (F10-)
exposure to environmental tobacco smoke (Z77.22)
history of tobacco use (Z87.891)
occupational exposure to environmental tobacco smoke (Z57.31)
tobacco dependence (F17-)
tobacco use (Z72.0)
EXCLUDES 2　personal history of benign neoplasm (Z86.01-)
personal history of carcinoma-in-situ (Z86.00-)

☑5th **Z85.0　Personal history of malignant neoplasm of digestive organs**

　Z85.00　Personal history of malignant neoplasm of unspecified digestive organ

　Z85.01　Personal history of malignant neoplasm of esophagus
Conditions classifiable to C15

☑6th　**Z85.02　Personal history of malignant neoplasm of stomach**

　　Z85.020　Personal history of malignant carcinoid tumor of stomach
Conditions classifiable to C7a.092

　　Z85.028　Personal history of other malignant neoplasm of stomach
Conditions classifiable to C16

☑6th **Z85.03　Personal history of malignant neoplasm of large intestine**

　　Z85.030　Personal history of malignant carcinoid tumor of large intestine
Conditions classifiable to C7a.022-C7a.025, C7a.029

　　Z85.038　Personal history of other malignant neoplasm of large intestine
Conditions classifiable to C18

☑6th **Z85.04　Personal history of malignant neoplasm of rectum, rectosigmoid junction, and anus**

　　Z85.040　Personal history of malignant carcinoid tumor of rectum
Conditions classifiable to C7a.026

　　Z85.048　Personal history of other malignant neoplasm of rectum, rectosigmoid junction, and anus
Conditions classifiable to C19-C21

Z85.05　Personal history of malignant neoplasm of liver
Conditions classifiable to C22

☑6th **Z85.06　Personal history of malignant neoplasm of small intestine**

　　Z85.060　Personal history of malignant carcinoid tumor of small intestine
Conditions classifiable to C7a.01-

　　Z85.068　Personal history of other malignant neoplasm of small intestine
Conditions classifiable to C17

Z85.07　Personal history of malignant neoplasm of pancreas
Conditions classifiable to C25

Z85.09　Personal history of malignant neoplasm of other digestive organs

☑5th **Z85.1　Personal history of malignant neoplasm of trachea, bronchus and lung**

☑6th　**Z85.11　Personal history of malignant neoplasm of bronchus and lung**

　　Z85.110　Personal history of malignant carcinoid tumor of bronchus and lung
Conditions classifiable to C7a.090

　　Z85.118　Personal history of other malignant neoplasm of bronchus and lung
Conditions classifiable to C34

　Z85.12　Personal history of malignant neoplasm of trachea
Conditions classifiable to C33

☑5th **Z85.2　Personal history of malignant neoplasm of other respiratory and intrathoracic organs**

　Z85.20　Personal history of malignant neoplasm of unspecified respiratory organ

　Z85.21　Personal history of malignant neoplasm of larynx
Conditions classifiable to C32

　Z85.22　Personal history of malignant neoplasm of nasal cavities, middle ear, and accessory sinuses
Conditions classifiable to C30-C31

☑6th　**Z85.23　Personal history of malignant neoplasm of thymus**

　　Z85.230　Personal history of malignant carcinoid tumor of thymus
Conditions classifiable to C7a.091

　　Z85.238　Personal history of other malignant neoplasm of thymus
Conditions classifiable to C37

　Z85.29　Personal history of malignant neoplasm of other respiratory and intrathoracic organs

Z85.3　Personal history of malignant neoplasm of breast
Conditions classifiable to C50-

☑5th **Z85.4　Personal history of malignant neoplasm of genital organs**
Conditions classifiable to C51-C63

　Z85.40　Personal history of malignant neoplasm of unspecified female genital organ

　Z85.41　Personal history of malignant neoplasm of cervix uteri

　Z85.42　Personal history of malignant neoplasm of other parts of uterus

　Z85.43　Personal history of malignant neoplasm of ovary

　Z85.44　Personal history of malignant neoplasm of other female genital organs

　Z85.45　Personal history of malignant neoplasm of unspecified male genital organ

---

☑　Appropriate additional character required　　　　☑x7th　Requires 7th character, placeholder x must fill empty characters

Z85.46 **Personal history of malignant neoplasm of prostate**

Z85.47 **Personal history of malignant neoplasm of testis**

Z85.48 **Personal history of malignant neoplasm of epididymis**

Z85.49 **Personal history of malignant neoplasm of other male genital organs**

√5th Z85.5 **Personal history of malignant neoplasm of urinary tract**
Conditions classifiable to C64-C68

Z85.50 **Personal history of malignant neoplasm of unspecified urinary tract organ**

Z85.51 **Personal history of malignant neoplasm of bladder**

√6th Z85.52 **Personal history of malignant neoplasm of kidney**
> EXCLUDES 1   *personal history of malignant neoplasm of renal pelvis (Z85.53)*

Z85.520 **Personal history of malignant carcinoid tumor of kidney**
Conditions classifiable to C7a.093

Z85.528 **Personal history of other malignant neoplasm of kidney**
Conditions classifiable to C64

Z85.53 **Personal history of malignant neoplasm of renal pelvis**

Z85.59 **Personal history of malignant neoplasm of other urinary tract organ**

Z85.6 **Personal history of leukemia**
Conditions classifiable to C91-C95
> EXCLUDES 1   *leukemia in remission C91.0-C95.9 with 5th character 1*

√5th Z85.7 **Personal history of other malignant neoplasms of lymphoid, hematopoietic and related tissues**

Z85.71 **Personal history of Hodgkin lymphoma**
Conditions classifiable to C81

Z85.72 **Personal history of non-Hodgkin lymphomas**
Conditions classifiable to C82-C85

Z85.79 **Personal history of other malignant neoplasms of lymphoid, hematopoietic and related tissues**
Conditions classifiable to C88-C90, C96
> EXCLUDES 1   *multiple myeloma in remission (C90.01)*
> *plasma cell leukemia in remission (C90.11)*
> *plasmacytoma in remission (C90.21)*

√5th Z85.8 **Personal history of malignant neoplasms of other organs and systems**
Conditions classifiable to C00-C14, C40-C49, C69-C79, C7a.098

√6th Z85.81 **Personal history of malignant neoplasm of lip, oral cavity, and pharynx**

Z85.810 **Personal history of malignant neoplasm of tongue**

Z85.818 **Personal history of malignant neoplasm of other sites of lip, oral cavity, and pharynx**

Z85.819 **Personal history of malignant neoplasm of unspecified site of lip, oral cavity, and pharynx**

√6th Z85.82 **Personal history of malignant neoplasm of skin**

Z85.820 **Personal history of malignant melanoma of skin**
Conditions classifiable to C43

Z85.821 **Personal history of Merkel cell carcinoma**
Conditions classifiable to C4a

Z85.828 **Personal history of other malignant neoplasm of skin**
Conditions classifiable to C44

√6th Z85.83 **Personal history of malignant neoplasm of bone and soft tissue**

Z85.830 **Personal history of malignant neoplasm of bone**

Z85.831 **Personal history of malignant neoplasm of soft tissue**
> EXCLUDES 2   *personal history of malignant neoplasm of skin (Z85.82-)*

√6th Z85.84 **Personal history of malignant neoplasm of eye and nervous tissue**

Z85.840 **Personal history of malignant neoplasm of eye**

Z85.841 **Personal history of malignant neoplasm of brain**

Z85.848 **Personal history of malignant neoplasm of other parts of nervous tissue**

√6th Z85.85 **Personal history of malignant neoplasm of endocrine glands**

Z85.850 **Personal history of malignant neoplasm of thyroid**

Z85.858 **Personal history of malignant neoplasm of other endocrine glands**

Z85.89 **Personal history of malignant neoplasm of other organs and systems**

Z85.9 **Personal history of malignant neoplasm, unspecified**
Conditions classifiable to C7a.00, C80.1

√4th **Z86 Personal history of certain other diseases**
Code first any follow-up examination after treatment (Z09)

√5th Z86.0 **Personal history of in-situ and benign neoplasms and neoplasms of uncertain behavior**
> EXCLUDES 2   *personal history of malignant neoplasms (Z85-)*

√6th Z86.00 **Personal history of in-situ neoplasm**

Z86.000 **Personal history of in-situ neoplasm of breast**

Z86.001 **Personal history of in-situ neoplasm of cervix uteri**

Z86.008 **Personal history of in-situ neoplasm of other site**

√6th Z86.01 **Personal history of benign neoplasm**

Z86.010 **Personal history of colonic polyps**

Z86.011 **Personal history of benign neoplasm of the brain**

Z86.012 **Personal history of benign carcinoid tumor**

Z86.018 **Personal history of other benign neoplasm**

Z86.03 **Personal history of neoplasm of uncertain behavior**

√5th Z86.1 **Personal history of infectious and parasitic diseases**
Conditions classifiable to A00-B89, B99
> EXCLUDES 1   *personal history of infectious diseases specific to a body system*
> *sequelae of infectious and parasitic diseases (B90-B94)*

Z86.11 **Personal history of tuberculosis**

Z86.12 **Personal history of poliomyelitis**

Z86.13 **Personal history of malaria**

Z86.19 **Personal history of other infectious and parasitic diseases**

Z86.2 **Personal history of diseases of the blood and blood-forming organs and certain disorders involving the immune mechanism**
Conditions classifiable to D50-D89

√5th Z86.3 **Personal history of endocrine, nutritional and metabolic diseases**
Conditions classifiable to E00-E88

Z86.31 **Personal history of diabetic foot ulcer**
> EXCLUDES 2   *current diabetic foot ulcer (E08.621, E09.621, E10.621, E11.621, E13.621)*

Z86.39 **Personal history of other endocrine, nutritional and metabolic disease**

√5th Z86.5 **Personal history of mental and behavioral disorders**
Conditions classifiable to F40-F59
> EXCLUDES 2   *substance abuse and dependence (F10-F19 with final character 1, in remission)*

Z86.51 **Personal history of combat and operational stress reaction**

Z86.59 **Personal history of other mental and behavioral disorders**

√5th Z86.6 **Personal history of diseases of the nervous system and sense organs**
Conditions classifiable to G00-G99, H00-H95

Z86.61 **Personal history of infections of the central nervous system**
Personal history of encephalitis
Personal history of meningitis

Z86.69 **Personal history of other diseases of the nervous system and sense organs**

EXCLUDES 1   Not coded here   EXCLUDES 2   Not included here   *Manifestation Code*

✓5th **Z86.7** **Personal history of diseases of the circulatory system**
Conditions classifiable to I00-I99
EXCLUDES 2 *old myocardial infarction (I25.2)*
postmyocardial infarction syndrome (I24.1)

Z86.71 **Personal history of venous thrombosis and embolism**

Z86.72 **Personal history of thrombophlebitis**

Z86.73 **Personal history of transient ischemic attack (TIA), and cerebral infarction without residual deficits**
Personal history of prolonged reversible ischemic neurological deficit (PRIND)
Personal history of stroke NOS without residual deficits
EXCLUDES 1 *personal history of traumatic brain injury (Z87.820)*
sequelae of cerebrovascular disease (I69-)

Z86.74 **Personal history of sudden cardiac arrest**
Personal history of sudden cardiac death successfully resuscitated

Z86.79 **Personal history of other diseases of the circulatory system**

✓4th **Z87** **Personal history of other diseases and conditions**
Code first any follow-up examination after treatment (Z09)

✓5th **Z87.0** **Personal history of diseases of the respiratory system**
Conditions classifiable to J00-J99

Z87.01 **Personal history of pneumonia (recurrent)**

Z87.09 **Personal history of other diseases of the respiratory system**

✓5th **Z87.1** **Personal history of diseases of the digestive system**
Conditions classifiable to K00-K93

Z87.11 **Personal history of peptic ulcer disease**

Z87.19 **Personal history of other diseases of the digestive system**

Z87.2 **Personal history of diseases of the skin and subcutaneous tissue**
Conditions classifiable to L00-L99
EXCLUDES 2 *personal history of diabetic foot ulcer (Z86.31)*

✓5th **Z87.3** **Personal history of diseases of the musculoskeletal system and connective tissue**
Conditions classifiable to M00-M99
EXCLUDES 2 *personal history of (healed) traumatic fracture (Z87.81)*

✓6th **Z87.31** **Personal history of (healed) nontraumatic fracture**

Z87.310 **Personal history of (healed) osteoporosis fracture**
Personal history of (healed) fragility fracture
Personal history of (healed) collapsed vertebra due to osteoporosis

Z87.311 **Personal history of (healed) other pathological fracture**
Personal history of (healed) collapsed vertebra NOS
EXCLUDES 2 *personal history of osteoporosis fracture (Z87.310)*

Z87.312 **Personal history of (healed) stress fracture**
Personal history of (healed) fatigue fracture

Z87.39 **Personal history of other diseases of the musculoskeletal system and connective tissue**

✓5th **Z87.4** **Personal history of diseases of the genitourinary system**
Conditions classifiable to N00-N99

✓6th **Z87.41** **Personal history of dysplasia of the female genital tract**
EXCLUDES 1 *personal history of malignant neoplasm of female genital tract (Z85.40-Z85.44)*

Z87.410 **Personal history of cervical dysplasia**

Z87.411 **Personal history of vaginal dysplasia**

Z87.412 **Personal history of vulvar dysplasia**

Z87.42 **Personal history of other diseases of the female genital tract**

✓6th **Z87.43** **Personal history of diseases of the male genital organs**

Z87.430 **Personal history of prostatic dysplasia**
EXCLUDES 1 *personal history of malignant neoplasm of prostate (Z85.46)*

Z87.438 **Personal history of other diseases of male genital organs**

✓6th **Z87.44** **Personal history of diseases of the urinary system**
EXCLUDES 1 *personal history of malignant neoplasm of cervix uteri (Z85.41)*

Z87.440 **Personal history of urinary (tract) infections**

Z87.441 **Personal history of nephrotic syndrome**

Z87.442 **Personal history of urinary calculi**
Personal history of kidney stones

Z87.448 **Personal history of other diseases of urinary system**

✓5th **Z87.5** **Personal history of complications of pregnancy, childbirth and the puerperium**
Conditions classifiable to O00-O99
EXCLUDES 2 *recurrent pregnancy loss (N96)*

Z87.51 **Personal history of pre-term labor**
EXCLUDES 1 *current pregnancy with history of pre-term labor (O09.21-)*

Z87.59 **Personal history of other complications of pregnancy, childbirth and the puerperium**
Personal history of trophoblastic disease

✓5th **Z87.7** **Personal history of (corrected) congenital malformations**
Conditions classifiable to Q00-Q89 that have been repaired or corrected
EXCLUDES 1 *congenital malformations that have been partially corrected or repaired but which still require medical treatment—code to condition*
EXCLUDES 2 *other postprocedural states (Z98.-)*
personal history of medical treatment (Z92.-)
presence of cardiac and vascular implants and grafts (Z95.-)
presence of other devices (Z97.-)
presence of other functional implants (Z96.-)
transplanted organ and tissue status (Z94.-)

✓6th **Z87.71** **Personal history of (corrected) congenital malformations of genitourinary system**

Z87.710 **Personal history of (corrected) hypospadias**

Z87.718 **Personal history of other specified (corrected) congenital malformations of genitourinary system**

✓6th **Z87.72** **Personal history of (corrected) congenital malformations of nervous system and sense organs**

Z87.720 **Personal history of (corrected) congenital malformations of eye**

Z87.721 **Personal history of (corrected) congenital malformations of ear**

Z87.728 **Personal history of other specified (corrected) congenital malformations of nervous system and sense organs**

✓6th **Z87.73** **Personal history of (corrected) congenital malformations of digestive system**

Z87.730 **Personal history of (corrected) cleft lip and palate**

Z87.738 **Personal history of other specified (corrected) congenital malformations of digestive system**

Z87.74 **Personal history of (corrected) congenital malformations of heart and circulatory system**

Z87.75 **Personal history of (corrected) congenital malformations of respiratory system**

Z87.76 **Personal history of (corrected) congenital malformations of integument, limbs and musculoskeletal system**

✓6th **Z87.79** **Personal history of other (corrected) congenital malformations**

Z87.790 **Personal history of (corrected) congenital malformations of face and neck**

Z87.798 **Personal history of other (corrected) congenital malformations**

✓5th **Z87.8** **Personal history of other specified conditions**
EXCLUDES 2 *personal history of self harm (Z91.5)*

Z87.81 **Personal history of (healed) traumatic fracture**
EXCLUDES 2 *personal history of (healed) nontraumatic fracture (Z87.31-)*

✔ Appropriate additional character required   ✓x7th Requires 7th character, placeholder x must fill empty characters

Factors Influencing Health Status and Contact With Health Services

Z87.82–Z90.3

√6ᵗʰ **Z87.82 Personal history of other (healed) physical injury and trauma**
Conditions classifiable to S00-T88, except traumatic fractures

     Z87.820 Personal history of traumatic brain injury
         EXCLUDES 1   *personal history of transient ischemic attack (TIA), and cerebral infarction without residual deficits (Z86.73)*

     Z87.821 Personal history of retained foreign body fully removed

     Z87.828 Personal history of other (healed) physical injury and trauma

√6ᵗʰ **Z87.89 Personal history of other specified conditions**
     Z87.890 Personal history of sex reassignment
     Z87.891 Personal history of nicotine dependence
         EXCLUDES 1   *current nicotine dependence (F17.2-)*

     Z87.898 Personal history of other specified conditions

√4ᵗʰ **Z88 Allergy status to drugs, medicaments and biological substances**
     EXCLUDES 2   *allergy status, other than to drugs and biological substances (Z91.0-)*

Z88.0 Allergy status to penicillin
Z88.1 Allergy status to other antibiotic agents status
Z88.2 Allergy status to sulfonamides status
Z88.3 Allergy status to other anti-infective agents status
Z88.4 Allergy status to anesthetic agent status
Z88.5 Allergy status to narcotic agent status
Z88.6 Allergy status to analgesic agent status
Z88.7 Allergy status to serum and vaccine status
Z88.8 Allergy status to other drugs, medicaments and biological substances status
Z88.9 Allergy status to unspecified drugs, medicaments and biological substances status

√4ᵗʰ **Z89 Acquired absence of limb**
     INCLUDES   amputation status
         postprocedural loss of limb
         post-traumatic loss of limb
     EXCLUDES 1   *acquired deformities of limbs (M20-M21)*
         congenital absence of limbs (Q71-Q73)

√5ᵗʰ **Z89.0 Acquired absence of thumb and other finger(s)**
√6ᵗʰ **Z89.01 Acquired absence of thumb**
     Z89.011 Acquired absence of right thumb
     Z89.012 Acquired absence of left thumb
     Z89.019 Acquired absence of unspecified thumb
√6ᵗʰ **Z89.02 Acquired absence of other finger(s)**
     EXCLUDES 2   *acquired absence of thumb (Z89.01-)*
     Z89.021 Acquired absence of right finger(s)
     Z89.022 Acquired absence of left finger(s)
     Z89.029 Acquired absence of unspecified finger(s)

√5ᵗʰ **Z89.1 Acquired absence of hand and wrist**
√6ᵗʰ **Z89.11 Acquired absence of hand**
     Z89.111 Acquired absence of right hand
     Z89.112 Acquired absence of left hand
     Z89.119 Acquired absence of unspecified hand
√6ᵗʰ **Z89.12 Acquired absence of wrist**
     Disarticulation at wrist
     Z89.121 Acquired absence of right wrist
     Z89.122 Acquired absence of left wrist
     Z89.129 Acquired absence of unspecified wrist

√5ᵗʰ **Z89.2 Acquired absence of upper limb above wrist**
√6ᵗʰ **Z89.20 Acquired absence of upper limb, unspecified level**
     Z89.201 Acquired absence of right upper limb, unspecified level
     Z89.202 Acquired absence of left upper limb, unspecified level
     Z89.209 Acquired absence of unspecified upper limb, unspecified level
         Acquired absence of arm NOS

√6ᵗʰ **Z89.21 Acquired absence of upper limb below elbow**

     Z89.211 Acquired absence of right upper limb below elbow
     Z89.212 Acquired absence of left upper limb below elbow
     Z89.219 Acquired absence of unspecified upper limb below elbow
√6ᵗʰ **Z89.22 Acquired absence of upper limb above elbow**
     Disarticulation at elbow
     Z89.221 Acquired absence of right upper limb above elbow
     Z89.222 Acquired absence of left upper limb above elbow
     Z89.229 Acquired absence of unspecified upper limb above elbow
√6ᵗʰ **Z89.23 Acquired absence of shoulder**
     Z89.231 Acquired absence of right shoulder
     Z89.232 Acquired absence of left shoulder
     Z89.239 Acquired absence of unspecified shoulder

√5ᵗʰ **Z89.4 Acquired absence of toe(s), foot, and ankle**
√6ᵗʰ **Z89.41 Acquired absence of great toe**
     Z89.411 Acquired absence of right great toe
     Z89.412 Acquired absence of left great toe
     Z89.419 Acquired absence of unspecified great toe
√6ᵗʰ **Z89.42 Acquired absence of other toe(s)**
     EXCLUDES 2   *acquired absence of great toe (Z89.41-)*
     Z89.421 Acquired absence of other right toe(s)
     Z89.422 Acquired absence of other left toe(s)
     Z89.429 Acquired absence of other toe(s), unspecified side
√6ᵗʰ **Z89.43 Acquired absence of foot**
     Z89.431 Acquired absence of right foot
     Z89.432 Acquired absence of left foot
     Z89.439 Acquired absence of unspecified foot
√6ᵗʰ **Z89.44 Acquired absence of ankle**
     Disarticulation of ankle
     Z89.441 Acquired absence of right ankle
     Z89.442 Acquired absence of left ankle
     Z89.449 Acquired absence of unspecified ankle

√5ᵗʰ **Z89.5 Acquired absence of leg below knee**
     Z89.50 Acquired absence of unspecified leg below knee
     Z89.51 Acquired absence of right leg below knee
     Z89.52 Acquired absence of left leg below knee

√5ᵗʰ **Z89.6 Acquired absence of leg above knee**
√6ᵗʰ **Z89.61 Acquired absence of leg above knee**
     Acquired absence of leg NOS
     Disarticulation at knee
     Z89.611 Acquired absence of right leg above knee
     Z89.612 Acquired absence of left leg above knee
     Z89.619 Acquired absence of unspecified leg above knee
√6ᵗʰ **Z89.62 Acquired absence of hip**
     Disarticulation at hip
     Z89.621 Acquired absence of right hip
     Z89.622 Acquired absence of left hip
     Z89.629 Acquired absence of unspecified hip

Z89.9 Acquired absence of limb, unspecified

√4ᵗʰ **Z90 Acquired absence of organs, not elsewhere classified**
     INCLUDES   postprocedural or post-traumatic loss of body part NEC
     EXCLUDES 1   *congenital absence—see Alphabetical Index*
     EXCLUDES 2   *postprocedural absence of endocrine glands (E89-)*

√5ᵗʰ **Z90.0 Acquired absence of part of head and neck**
     Z90.01 Acquired absence of eye
     Z90.02 Acquired absence of larynx
     Z90.09 Acquired absence of other part of head and neck
         Acquired absence of nose
         EXCLUDES 2   *teeth (K08.1)*

√5ᵗʰ **Z90.1 Acquired absence of breast and nipple**
     Z90.10 Acquired absence of unspecified breast and nipple
     Z90.11 Acquired absence of right breast and nipple
     Z90.12 Acquired absence of left breast and nipple
     Z90.13 Acquired absence of bilateral breasts and nipples

Z90.2 Acquired absence of lung [part of]
Z90.3 Acquired absence of stomach [part of]

EXCLUDES 1   Not coded here   EXCLUDES 2   Not included here   *Manifestation Code*

✓5ᵗʰ **Z90.4** **Acquired absence of other specified parts of digestive tract**

 ✓6ᵗʰ **Z90.41** **Acquired absence of pancreas**
  Use additional code to identify any associated:
   insulin use (Z79.4)
   diabetes mellitus, postpancreatectomy (E13.-)

  Z90.410 **Acquired total absence of pancreas**
   Acquired absence of pancreas NOS

  Z90.411 **Acquired partial absence of pancreas**

 Z90.49 **Acquired absence of other specified parts of digestive tract**

Z90.5 **Acquired absence of kidney**

Z90.6 **Acquired absence of other parts of urinary tract**
 Acquired absence of bladder

✓5ᵗʰ **Z90.7** **Acquired absence of genital organ(s)**
 EXCLUDES 1 *personal history of sex reassignment (Z87.890)*
 EXCLUDES 2 *female genital mutilation status (N90.81-)*

 ✓6ᵗʰ **Z90.71** **Acquired absence of cervix and uterus**
  Z90.710 **Acquired absence of both cervix and uterus**
   Acquired absence of uterus NOS
   Status post total hysterectomy

  Z90.711 **Acquired absence of uterus with remaining cervical stump**
   Status post partial hysterectomy with remaining cervical stump

  Z90.712 **Acquired absence of cervix with remaining uterus**

 ✓6ᵗʰ **Z90.72** **Acquired absence of ovaries**
  Z90.721 **Acquired absence of ovaries, unilateral**
  Z90.722 **Acquired absence of ovaries, bilateral**

 Z90.79 **Acquired absence of other genital organ(s)**

✓5ᵗʰ **Z90.8** **Acquired absence of other organs**
 Z90.81 **Acquired absence of spleen**
 Z90.89 **Acquired absence of other organs**

✓4ᵗʰ **Z91** **Personal risk factors, not elsewhere classified**
 EXCLUDES 2 *contact with and (suspected) exposures hazardous to health (Z77-)*
  exposure to pollution and other problems related to physical environment (Z77.1-)
  personal history of physical injury and trauma (Z87.81, Z87.82-)
  occupational exposure to risk factors (Z57-)

✓5ᵗʰ **Z91.0** **Allergy status, other than to drugs and biological substances**
 EXCLUDES 2 *allergy status to drugs, medicaments, and biological substances (Z88-)*

 ✓6ᵗʰ **Z91.01** **Food allergy status**
  EXCLUDES 2 *food additives allergy status (Z91.02)*

  Z91.010 **Allergy to peanuts**
  Z91.011 **Allergy to milk products**
   EXCLUDES 1 *lactose intolerance (E73-)*
  Z91.012 **Allergy to eggs**
  Z91.013 **Allergy to seafood**
   Allergy to shellfish
   Allergy to octopus or squid ink
  Z91.018 **Allergy to other foods**
   Allergy to nuts other than peanuts

 Z91.02 **Food additives allergy status**

 ✓6ᵗʰ **Z91.03** **Insect allergy status**
  Z91.030 **Bee allergy status**
  Z91.038 **Other insect allergy status**

 ✓6ᵗʰ **Z91.04** **Nonmedicinal substance allergy status**
  Z91.040 **Latex allergy status**
   Latex sensitivity status
  Z91.041 **Radiographic dye allergy status**
   Allergy status to contrast media used for diagnostic x-ray procedure
  Z91.048 **Other nonmedicinal substance allergy status**

 Z91.09 **Other allergy status, other than to drugs and biological substances**

✓5ᵗʰ **Z91.1** **Patient's noncompliance with medical treatment and regimen**
 Z91.11 **Patient's noncompliance with dietary regimen**

 ✓6ᵗʰ **Z91.12** **Patient's intentional underdosing of medication regimen**
  Code first underdosing of medication (T36-T50) with fifth or sixth character 6
  EXCLUDES 1 *adverse effect of prescribed drug taken as directed—code to adverse effect*
   poisoning (overdose)—code to poisoning

  Z91.120 **Patient's intentional underdosing of medication regimen due to financial hardship**

  Z91.128 **Patient's intentional underdosing of medication regimen for other reason**

 ✓6ᵗʰ **Z91.13** **Patient's unintentional underdosing of medication regimen**
  Code first underdosing of medication (T36-T50) with fifth or sixth character 6
  EXCLUDES 1 *adverse effect of prescribed drug taken as directed—code to adverse effect*
   poisoning (overdose)—code to poisoning

  Z91.130 **Patient's unintentional underdosing of medication regimen due to age-related debility**

  Z91.138 **Patient's unintentional underdosing of medication regimen for other reason**

 Z91.14 **Patient's other noncompliance with medication regimen**
  Patient's underdosing of medication NOS

 Z91.15 **Patient's noncompliance with renal dialysis**

 Z91.19 **Patient's noncompliance with other medical treatment and regimen**

✓5ᵗʰ **Z91.4** **Personal history of psychological trauma, not elsewhere classified**

 ✓6ᵗʰ **Z91.41** **Personal history of adult abuse**
  EXCLUDES 2 *personal history of abuse in childhood (Z62.81-)*

  Z91.410 **Personal history of adult physical and sexual abuse**
   EXCLUDES 1 *current adult physical abuse (T74.11, T76.11)*
   current adult sexual abuse (T74. 21, T76.21)

  Z91.411 **Personal history of adult psychological abuse**

  Z91.412 **Personal history of adult neglect**
   EXCLUDES 1 *current adult neglect (T74.01, T76.01)*

  Z91.419 **Personal history of unspecified adult abuse**

 Z91.49 **Other personal history of psychological trauma, not elsewhere classified**

Z91.5 **Personal history of self-harm**
 Personal history of parasuicide
 Personal history of self-poisoning
 Personal history of suicide attempt

✓6ᵗʰ **Z91.8** **Other specified personal risk factors, not elsewhere classified**
 Z91.81 **History of falling**
  At risk for falling

 Z91.82 **Personal history of military deployment**
  Individual (civilian or military) with past history of military war, peacekeeping and humanitarian deployment (current or past conflict)
  Returned from military deployment

 Z91.89 **Other specified personal risk factors, not elsewhere classified**

✓4ᵗʰ **Z92** **Personal history of medical treatment**
 EXCLUDES 2 *postprocedural states (Z98-)*

 Z92.0 **Personal history of contraception**
  EXCLUDES 1 *counseling or management of current contraceptive practices (Z30-)*
   long term (current) use of contraception (Z79.3)
   presence of (intrauterine) contraceptive device (Z97.5)

✓5ᵗʰ **Z92.2** **Personal history of drug therapy**
 EXCLUDES 2 *long term (current) drug therapy (Z79-)*

 Z92.21 **Personal history of antineoplastic chemotherapy**
 Z92.22 **Personal history of monoclonal drug therapy**
 Z92.23 **Personal history of estrogen therapy**

√6th **Z92.24**   **Personal history of steroid therapy**

    Z92.240   **Personal history of inhaled steroid therapy**

    Z92.241   **Personal history of systemic steroid therapy**
       Personal history of steroid therapy NOS

    Z92.25   **Personal history of immunosupression therapy**
     EXCLUDES 2   *personal history of steroid therapy (Z92.24)*

    Z92.29   **Personal history of other drug therapy**

Z92.3   **Personal history of irradiation**
    Personal history of exposure to therapeutic radiation
    EXCLUDES 1   *exposure to radiation in the physical environment (Z77.12)*
       occupational exposure to radiation (Z57.1)

√5th **Z92.8**   **Personal history of other medical treatment**

    Z92.81   **Personal history of extracorporeal membrane oxygenation (ECMO)**

    Z92.82   **Status post administration of tPA (rtPA) in a different facility within the last 24 hours prior to admission to current facility**
     Code first condition requiring tPA administration, such as:
       acute cerebral infarction (I63-)
       acute myocardial infarction (I21-, I22-)

    Z92.83   **Personal history of failed moderate sedation**
     Personal history of failed conscious sedation
     EXCLUDES 2   *failed moderate sedation during procedure (T88.52)*

    Z92.89   **Personal history of other medical treatment**

√4th **Z93**   **Artificial opening status**
    EXCLUDES 1   *artificial openings requiring attention or management (Z43-)*
       complications of external stoma (J95.0-, K94.-, N99.5-)

Z93.0   **Tracheostomy status**

Z93.1   **Gastrostomy status**

Z93.2   **Ileostomy status**

Z93.3   **Colostomy status**

Z93.4   **Other artificial openings of gastrointestinal tract status**

√5th **Z93.5**   **Cystostomy status**

    Z93.50   **Unspecified cystostomy status**

    Z93.51   **Cutaneous-vesicostomy status**

    Z93.52   **Appendico-vesicostomy status**

    Z93.59   **Other cystostomy status**

Z93.6   **Other artificial openings of urinary tract status**
    Nephrostomy status
    Ureterostomy status
    Urethrostomy status

Z93.8   **Other artificial opening status**

Z93.9   **Artificial opening status, unspecified**

√4th **Z94**   **Transplanted organ and tissue status**
    INCLUDES   organ or tissue replaced by heterogenous or homogenous transplant
    EXCLUDES 1   *complications of transplanted organ or tissue—see Alphabetical Index*
    EXCLUDES 2   *presence of vascular grafts (Z95-)*

Z94.0   **Kidney transplant status**

Z94.1   **Heart transplant status**
    EXCLUDES 1   *artificial heart status (Z95.811)*
       heart-valve replacement status (Z95.2-Z95.4)

Z94.2   **Lung transplant status**

Z94.3   **Heart and lungs transplant status**

Z94.4   **Liver transplant status**

Z94.5   **Skin transplant status**
    Autogenous skin transplant status

Z94.6   **Bone transplant status**

Z94.7   **Corneal transplant status**

√5th **Z94.8**   **Other transplanted organ and tissue status**

    Z94.81   **Bone marrow transplant status**

    Z94.82   **Intestine transplant status**

    Z94.83   **Pancreas transplant status**

    Z94.84   **Stem cells transplant status**

    Z94.89   **Other transplanted organ and tissue status**

Z94.9   **Transplanted organ and tissue status, unspecified**

√4th **Z95**   **Presence of cardiac and vascular implants and grafts**
    EXCLUDES 1   *complications of cardiac and vascular devices, implants and grafts (T82-)*

Z95.0   **Presence of cardiac pacemaker**
    EXCLUDES 1   *adjustment or management of cardiac pacemaker (Z45.0)*
       presence of automatic (implantable) cardiac defibrillator with synchronous cardiac pacemaker (Z95.810)

Z95.1   **Presence of aortocoronary bypass graft**

Z95.2   **Presence of prosthetic heart valve**
    Presence of heart valve NOS

Z95.3   **Presence of xenogenic heart valve**

Z95.4   **Presence of other heart-valve replacement**

Z95.5   **Presence of coronary angioplasty implant and graft**
    EXCLUDES 1   *coronary angioplasty status without implant and graft (Z98.61)*

√5th **Z95.8**   **Presence of other cardiac and vascular implants and grafts**

    √6th **Z95.81**   **Presence of other cardiac implants and grafts**

       Z95.810   **Presence of automatic (implantable) cardiac defibrillator**
         Presence of automatic (implantable) cardiac defibrillator with synchronous cardiac pacemaker

       Z95.811   **Presence of heart assist device**

       Z95.812   **Presence of fully implantable artificial heart**

       Z95.818   **Presence of other cardiac implants and grafts**

    √6th **Z95.82**   **Presence of other vascular implants and grafts**

       Z95.820   **Peripheral vascular angioplasty status with implants and grafts**
         EXCLUDES 1   *peripheral vascular angioplasty without implant and graft (Z98.62)*

       Z95.828   **Presence of other vascular implants and grafts**
         Presence of intravascular prosthesis NEC

Z95.9   **Presence of cardiac and vascular implant and graft, unspecified**

√4th **Z96**   **Presence of other functional implants**
    EXCLUDES 1   *complications of internal prosthetic devices, implants and grafts (T82-T85)*
       fitting and adjustment of prosthetic and other devices (Z44-Z46)

Z96.0   **Presence of urogenital implants**

Z96.1   **Presence of intraocular lens**
    Presence of pseudophakia

√5th **Z96.2**   **Presence of otological and audiological implants**

    Z96.20   **Presence of otological and audiological implant, unspecified**

    Z96.21   **Cochlear implant status**

    Z96.22   **Myringotomy tube(s) status**

    Z96.29   **Presence of other otological and audiological implants**
     Presence of bone-conduction hearing device
     Presence of eustachian tube stent
     Stapes replacement

Z96.3   **Presence of artificial larynx**

√5th **Z96.4**   **Presence of endocrine implants**

    Z96.41   **Presence of insulin pump (external) (internal)**

    Z96.49   **Presence of other endocrine implants**

Z96.5   **Presence of tooth-root and mandibular implants**

√5th **Z96.6**   **Presence of orthopedic joint implants**

    Z96.60   **Presence of unspecified orthopedic joint implant**

    √6th **Z96.61**   **Presence of artificial shoulder joint**

       Z96.611   **Presence of right artificial shoulder joint**

       Z96.612   **Presence of left artificial shoulder joint**

       Z96.619   **Presence of unspecified artificial shoulder joint**

    √6th **Z96.62**   **Presence of artificial elbow joint**

       Z96.621   **Presence of right artificial elbow joint**

       Z96.622   **Presence of left artificial elbow joint**

       Z96.629   **Presence of unspecified artificial elbow joint**

    √6th **Z96.63**   **Presence of artificial wrist joint**

       Z96.631   **Presence of right artificial wrist joint**

EXCLUDES 1   Not coded here   EXCLUDES 2   Not included here   *Manifestation Code*

Z96.632   Presence of left artificial wrist joint
Z96.639   Presence of unspecified artificial wrist joint

√6ᵗʰ **Z96.64** **Presence of artificial hip joint**
Hip-joint replacement (partial) (total)
Z96.641   Presence of right artificial hip joint
Z96.642   Presence of left artificial hip joint
Z96.643   Presence of artificial hip joint, bilateral
Z96.649   Presence of unspecified artificial hip joint

√6ᵗʰ **Z96.65** **Presence of artificial knee joint**
Z96.651   Presence of right artificial knee joint
Z96.652   Presence of left artificial knee joint
Z96.653   Presence of artificial knee joint, bilateral
Z96.659   Presence of unspecified artificial knee joint

√6ᵗʰ **Z96.66** **Presence of artificial ankle joint**
Z96.661   Presence of right artificial ankle joint
Z96.662   Presence of left artificial ankle joint
Z96.669   Presence of unspecified artificial ankle joint

√6ᵗʰ **Z96.69** **Presence of other orthopedic joint implants**
Z96.691   Finger-joint replacement of right hand
Z96.692   Finger-joint replacement of left hand
Z96.693   Finger-joint replacement, bilateral
Z96.698   Presence of other orthopedic joint implants

Z96.7 **Presence of other bone and tendon implants**
Presence of skull plate

√5ᵗʰ Z96.8 **Presence of other specified functional implants**
Z96.81 **Presence of artificial skin**
Z96.89 **Presence of other specified functional implants**

Z96.9 **Presence of functional implant, unspecified**

√4ᵗʰ **Z97** **Presence of other devices**
EXCLUDES 1 *complications of internal prosthetic devices, implants and grafts (T82-T85)*
fitting and adjustment of prosthetic and other devices (Z44-Z46)
EXCLUDES 2 *presence of cerebrospinal fluid drainage device (Z98.2)*

Z97.0 **Presence of artificial eye**

√5ᵗʰ Z97.1 **Presence of artificial limb (complete) (partial)**
Z97.10 **Presence of artificial limb (complete) (partial), unspecified**
Z97.11 **Presence of artificial right arm (complete) (partial)**
Z97.12 **Presence of artificial left arm (complete) (partial)**
Z97.13 **Presence of artificial right leg (complete) (partial)**
Z97.14 **Presence of artificial left leg (complete) (partial)**
Z97.15 **Presence of artificial arms, bilateral (complete) (partial)**
Z97.16 **Presence of artificial legs, bilateral (complete) (partial)**

Z97.2 **Presence of dental prosthetic device (complete) (partial)**
Presence of dentures (complete) (partial)

Z97.3 **Presence of spectacles and contact lenses**

Z97.4 **Presence of external hearing-aid**

Z97.5 **Presence of (intrauterine) contraceptive device**
EXCLUDES 1 *checking, reinsertion or removal of contraceptive device (Z30.43)*

Z97.8 **Presence of other specified devices**

√4ᵗʰ **Z98** **Other postprocedural states**
EXCLUDES 2 *aftercare (Z43-Z49, Z51)*
follow-up medical care (Z08- Z09)
postprocedural complication—see Alphabetical Index

Z98.0 **Intestinal bypass and anastomosis status**
EXCLUDES 2 *bariatric surgery status (Z98.84)*
gastric bypass status (Z98.84)
obesity surgery status (Z98.84)

Z98.1 **Arthrodesis status**

Z98.2 **Presence of cerebrospinal fluid drainage device**
Presence of CSF shunt

Z98.3 **Post therapeutic collapse of lung status**
Code first underlying disease

√5ᵗʰ **Z98.4** **Cataract extraction status**
Use additional code to identify intraocular lens implant status (Z96.1)
EXCLUDES 1 *aphakia (H27.0)*
Z98.41 **Cataract extraction status, right eye**
Z98.42 **Cataract extraction status, left eye**
Z98.49 **Cataract extraction status, unspecified eye**

√5ᵗʰ **Z98.5** **Sterilization status**
EXCLUDES 1 *female infertility (N97-)*
male infertility (N46-)
Z98.51 **Tubal ligation status**
Z98.52 **Vasectomy status**

√5ᵗʰ **Z98.6** **Angioplasty status**
Z98.61 **Coronary angioplasty status**
EXCLUDES 1 *coronary angioplasty status with implant and graft (Z95.5)*
Z98.62 **Peripheral vascular angioplasty status**
EXCLUDES 1 *peripheral vascular angioplasty status with implant and graft (Z95.820)*

√5ᵗʰ **Z98.8** **Other specified postprocedural states**
√6ᵗʰ **Z98.81** **Dental procedure status**
Z98.810 **Dental sealant status**
Z98.811 **Dental restoration status**
Dental crown status
Dental fillings status
Z98.818 **Other dental procedure status**

Z98.82 **Breast implant status**
EXCLUDES 1 *breast implant removal status (Z98.86)*

Z98.83 **Filtering (vitreous) bleb after glaucoma surgery status**
EXCLUDES 1 *inflammation (infection) of postprocedural bleb (H59.4-)*

Z98.84 **Bariatric surgery status**
Gastric banding status
Gastric bypass status for obesity
Obesity surgery status
EXCLUDES 1 *bariatric surgery status complicating pregnancy, childbirth, or the puerperium (O99.84)*
EXCLUDES 2 *intestinal bypass and anastomosis status (Z98.0)*

Z98.85 **Transplanted organ removal status**
Transplanted organ previously removed due to complication, failure, rejection or infection
EXCLUDES 1 *encounter for removal of transplanted organ—code to complication of transplanted organ (T86-)*

Z98.86 **Personal history of breast implant removal**

√6ᵗʰ **Z98.87** **Personal history of in utero procedure**
Z98.870 **Personal history of in utero procedure during pregnancy**
EXCLUDES 2 *complications from in utero procedure for current pregnancy (O35.7)*
supervision of current pregnancy with history of in utero procedure during previous pregnancy (O09.82-)
Z98.871 **Personal history of in utero procedure while a fetus**

Z98.89 **Other specified postprocedural states**
Personal history of surgery, not elsewhere classified

√4ᵗʰ **Z99** **Dependence on enabling machines and devices, not elsewhere classified**
EXCLUDES 1 *cardiac pacemaker status (Z95.0)*

Z99.0 **Dependence on aspirator**

√5ᵗʰ Z99.1 **Dependence on respirator**
Dependence on ventilator
Z99.11 **Dependence on respirator [ventilator] status**
Z99.12 **Encounter for respirator [ventilator] dependence during power failure**
EXCLUDES 1 *mechanical complication of respirator [ventilator] (J95.850)*

☑ Appropriate additional character required   √x7ᵗʰ Requires 7th character, placeholder x must fill empty characters

Z99.2   **Dependence on renal dialysis**
Hemodialysis status
Peritoneal dialysis status
Presence of arteriovenous shunt for dialysis
Renal dialysis status NOS

     EXCLUDES 1   *encounter for fitting and adjustment of dialysis*
catheter (Z49.0-)
noncompliance with renal dialysis (Z91.15)

Z99.3   **Dependence on wheelchair**
Wheelchair confinement status

Code first cause of dependence, such as:
muscular dystrophy (G71.0)
obesity (E66-)

✓5ᵗʰ   **Z99.8**   **Dependence on other enabling machines and devices**

     Z99.81   **Dependence on supplemental oxygen**
Dependence on long-term oxygen

     Z99.89   **Dependence on other enabling machines and devices**
Dependence on machine or device NOS

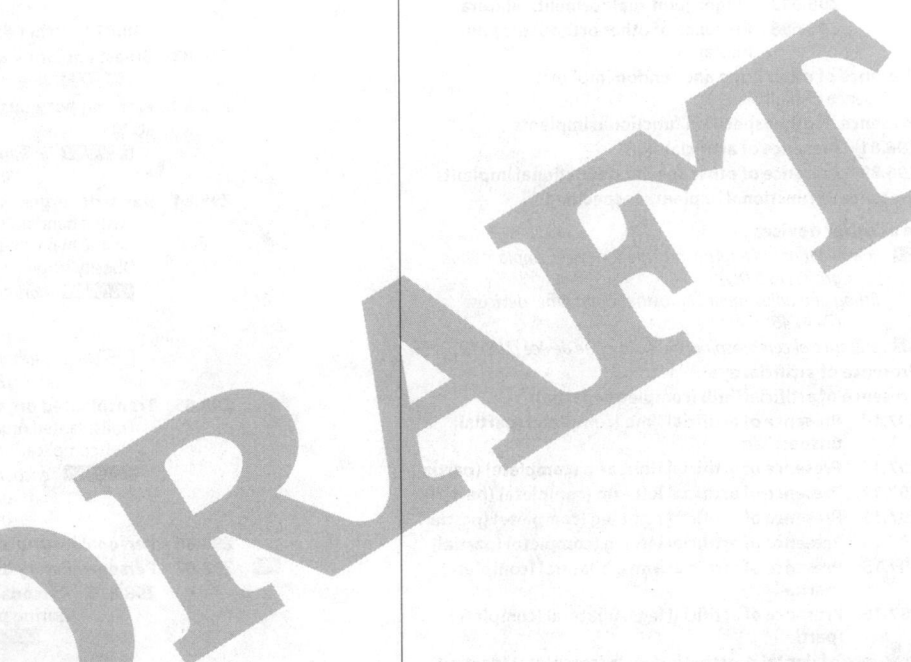